ELSEVIER

evolve

To access your Student Resources, visit the web address below:

http://evolve.elsevier.com/Iggy/

- **Integrated Management of Care Questions for the NCLEX Examination**
  Multiple-choice self-test questions are divided by chapter and focus on delegation and supervision, assignment, and prioritization/decision making. The Integrated Management of Care Questions for the NCLEX Examination help you understand and apply the material covered in the text and integrate it with material you have learned elsewhere in the curriculum—fostering the skills needed to master the NCLEX Examination.

- **Pharmacology Review Questions**
  Safe medication administration is a major theme of the NCLEX Examination. The Pharmacology Review Questions will make you more comfortable with the application of clinical drug therapy and promote readiness for safe drug administration. These questions are keyed to the text—just look for the "Evolve Pharm Review" icons.

- **Answer Guidelines—Critical Thinking Challenges and Study Guide Case Studies**
  Suggested Answer Guidelines are provided for the Critical Thinking Challenges interspersed throughout the text and for the Case Studies within the Critical Thinking Study Guide. These exercises provide a safe and effective means of practicing the on-the-spot decision making that you will face in the fast-paced world of medical-surgical nursing. The Answer Guidelines allow you to gauge your mastery of the text and readiness for your examinations.

- **WebLinks**
  An exciting resource links you to hundreds of carefully chosen websites that supplement the content of the textbook. These WebLinks are regularly updated, and new links are added as they develop.

- **Additional Resources**
  Audio Glossary, "Building" Concept Maps, Concept Map Creator, Fluid and Electrolyte Tutorial, Content Updates, Audio Clips, Video Clips, Animations, Bonus Health Assessment Images.

Medical-Surgical Nursing

CRITICAL THINKING FOR COLLABORATIVE CARE

ELSEVIER
SAUNDERS

5

FIFTH EDITION

Medical-Surgical Nursing

CRITICAL THINKING FOR COLLABORATIVE CARE

Donna D. Ignatavicius, MS, RN, C
Presenter and Consultant for Nursing Programs
President, DI Associates, Inc.
Placitas, New Mexico

M. Linda Workman, PhD, RN, FAAN
Gertrude Perkins Oliva Professor of Oncology
Frances Payne Bolton School of Nursing
Case Western Reserve University
Cleveland, Ohio

ELSEVIER
SAUNDERS

ELSEVIER
SAUNDERS

11830 Westline Industrial Drive
St. Louis, Missouri 63146

MEDICAL-SURGICAL NURSING: CRITICAL THINKING FOR COLLABORATIVE CARE
Single Volume 0-7216-0446-3
2-Volume Set 0-7216-0671-7

NOTICE

Nursing is an ever-changing field. Standard safety precautions must be followed, but as new research and clinical experience broaden our knowledge, changes in treatment and drug therapy may become necessary or appropriate. Readers are advised to check the most current product information provided by the manufacturer of each drug to be administered to verify the recommended dose, the method and duration of administration, and contraindications. It is the responsibility of the licensed health care provider, relying on experience and knowledge of the patient, to determine dosages and the best treatment for each individual patient. Neither the publisher nor the editor assumes any liability for any injury and/or damage to persons or property arising from this publication.

International Standard Book Number 0-7216-0446-3 (Single Volume)
0-7216-0671-7 (2-Volume Set)

Executive Publisher: Barbara Nelson Cullen
Editor: Lee Henderson
Developmental Editor: Laura Sieh Chu, Robin Richman
Publishing Services Manager: Deborah L. Vogel
Senior Project Manager: Jodi M. Willard
Book Designer: Teresa McBryan

Printed in United States of America

Last digit is the print number: 9 8 7 6 5 4 3 2 1

DEDICATION

To Charles and Stephanie
Thanks for your unending support, love, and understanding during every edition; I could not do this without you!

Donna

To my mother, Eunice Workman, from whom I inherited the creativity and persistence to pursue my dream of being an author.

Linda

About the Authors

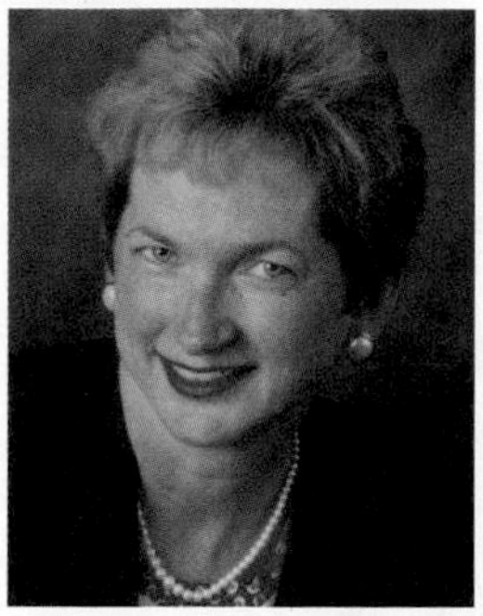

Donna D. Ignatavicius received her diploma in nursing from the Peninsula General School of Nursing in Salisbury, Maryland. After working as a staff and charge nurse in medical-surgical nursing, she became an instructor in Staff Development at the University of Maryland Medical Center. She then received her BSN from the University of Maryland School of Nursing. For 5 years she taught in several schools of nursing while working toward her MS in Nursing, which she received in 1981. Ms. Ignatavicius then taught in the BSN program at the University of Maryland for 6 years, after which she continued to pursue her interest in gerontology and accepted the position of Director of Nursing of a major skilled-nursing facility in her home state of Maryland. She has been a certified gerontologic nurse since 1989 and was certified in nursing case management by the American Nurses Credentialing Center in 1998. Recently she has taught in both diploma and associate degree nursing programs. Through her consulting and seminar business, Ms. Ignatavicius has gained national recognition in nursing education and critical thinking. She is currently the President of DI Associates, Inc. (http://www.diassociates.com/), a company dedicated to improving health care through education and consultation for both faculty and clinicians.

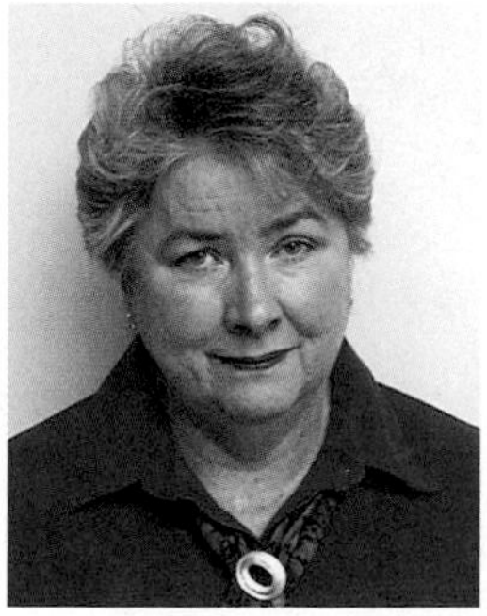

M. Linda Workman received her BSN from the University of Cincinnati College of Nursing and Health. After serving in the U.S. Army Nurse Corps and working as an Assistant Head Nurse and Head Nurse in civilian hospitals, Dr. Workman, a native of Canada, earned her MSN from the University of Cincinnati College of Nursing and Health and a PhD in Developmental Biology from the University of Cincinnati College of Arts and Sciences. Dr. Workman's 25 years of academic experience include teaching at the diploma, associate degree, baccalaureate, and master's levels. Her areas of teaching expertise include medical-surgical nursing, physiology, pathophysiology, genetics, oncology, and immunology. Dr. Workman has been recognized nationally for her teaching expertise and was inducted into the American Academy of Nursing in 1992. She received the Excellence in Teaching award at the University of Cincinnati in 2001 and at Case Western Reserve University in 2004. She is a former American Cancer Society Professor of Oncology Nursing and currently is senior faculty at the Frances Payne Bolton School of Nursing, Case Western Reserve University, where she occupies an endowed chair in oncology.

Consultants

ELAINE BISHOP KENNEDY, EdD, RN
Professor, Department of Nursing
Wor-Wic Community College
Salisbury, Maryland
Concept Maps
Plans of Care

MICHELLE M. BYRNE, PhD, RN, CNOR
Associate Professor
Department of Nursing
North Georgia College and State University
Dahlonega, Georgia
Culture consultant

RICHARD LINTNER, RT(R), (CV), (MR), (CT), ARRT
Program Director
School of Interventional Radiology;
Manager
Interventional Radiology
Kansas University Medical Center
Kansas City, Kansas
Consultant for interventional radiology

Contributors

RICHARD B. ARBOUR, MSN, RN, CCRN, CNRN
Guest Lecturer, Graduate Program
LaSalle University School of Nursing;
Staff Nurse/Clinical Researcher
Albert Einstein Healthcare Network
Philadelphia, Pennsylvania

DEANNE A. BLACH, MSN, RN
Coordinator, CE Programs and Senior Health & Education
University of Arkansas for Medical Sciences
AHEC-NW at Harrison
Harrison, Arkansas

MARCIA M. BOEHMKE, DNS, RN, ANPc
Research Assistant Professor, School of Nursing
University of Buffalo, The State University of New York
Buffalo, New York

MICHELLE M. BYRNE, PhD, RN, CNOR
Associate Professor
Department of Nursing
North Georgia College and State University
Dahlonega, Georgia

LINDA J. CAPUTI, EdD, MSN, RN
Professor, Department of Nursing
College of DuPage
Glen Ellyn, Illinois

JOHN M. CLOCHESY, PhD, RN, FAAN, FCCM
Independence Foundation Professor of Nursing Education
Case Western Reserve University
Cleveland, Ohio

TAMMY L. COFFEE, MSN, ACNP
Acute Care Nurse Practitioner
Metro Health Medical Center
Cleveland, Ohio

JANICE CUZZELL, RN, MA, CWS
Certified Wound Specialist
Savannah, Georgia

KARRIE K. DIETZEN, MSN, RN, CGRN
Assistant Professor, Associate's of Science in Nursing Program
Ivy Tech State College, East Central Region
Muncie, Indiana;
PRN: Staff RN Medical/Surgical Unit & Endoscopy Lab
Community Hospital-Anderson
Anderson, Indiana

MARY R. HERON EVANS, MS, RN, ONC
Assistant Professor, School of Nursing
Gulf Coast Community College;
Staff, Gulf Coast Medical Center
Panama City, Florida

CHRISTINE A. GATES, BS, CRT
Certified Respiratory Therapist
Cincinnati, Ohio

JACQUELYN R. GIBBS, MSN, RN
Assistant Professor, Department of Nursing
Raymond Walters College, University of Cincinnati
Cincinnati, Ohio

GAYLE K. GILMORE, RN, MA, MIS, CIC
Consultant, Infection Control Education and Consultation
Duluth, Minnesota

LYNN C. HADAWAY, MEd, RNC, CRNI
President, Lynn Hadaway Associates, Inc.
Milner, Georgia

WADE HAGAN, MSN, RN, PHN, CCRN
Instructor, Nursing Department
Mt. San Jacinto Community College District
Menifee, California;
Faculty Associate
California State University
Dominguez Hills, California

KATHY A. HAUSMAN, PhD, RN, C
Assistant Professor, School of Nursing
University of Maryland
Baltimore, Maryland

MARY K. KAZANOWSKI, PhD, ARNP, CHPN, BC
Professor, Department of Nursing
Saint Anselm College;
Level III RN
VNA Hospice
Manchester, New Hampshire

ELAINE BISHOP KENNEDY, EdD, RN
Professor, Department of Nursing
Wor-Wic Community College
Salisbury, Maryland

LINDA A. LaCHARITY, PhD, RN
Assistant Professor, College of Nursing
University of Cincinnati
Cincinnati, Ohio

LINDA LASKOWSKI-JONES, RN, MS, APRN, BC, CCRN, CEN
Director, Trauma, Emergency & Aeromedical Services
Christiana Care Health System—Christiana Hospital
Newark, Delaware

RUTH LINDQUIST, PhD, RN, APRN, BC
Professor, School of Nursing;
Senior Associate Dean for Academic Affairs and Administration
University of Minnesota
Minneapolis, Minnesota

DEITRA LEONARD LOWDERMILK, PhD, BSN, RNC, MEd
Clinical Professor, Women's Health, School of Nursing
University of North Carolina at Chapel Hill
Chapel Hill, North Carolina

JUDY MALKIEWICZ, PhD, RN
Professor, School of Nursing
University of Northern Colorado
Greeley, Colorado

JANICE HOOT MARTIN, PhD, RN, GNP
Professor Emeritus, School of Nursing
University of Northern Colorado
Greeley, Colorado

CYNTHIA KINDLER MATZKO, MSN, RN, APRN, BC
Master's Prepared Advanced Practice Nurse;
Rheumatology Clinical Nursing Specialist
Geisinger Medical Center
Danville, Pennsylvania

LORA McGUIRE, RN, MS
Professor, Department of Nursing
Joliet Junior College
Joliet, Illinois

M. ELAINE McLEOD, MSN, APRN, BC-ADM, APRN-BC, CDE
Clinical Nurse Specialist, Diabetes
Tennessee Valley Healthcare System
Nashville, Tennessee

MADELINE B. MURPHY, MSN, NP-C
Coordinator, Adult NP Program
Breen School of Nursing
Ursuline College;
Clinical Faculty, Department of Medicine
University Hospitals of Cleveland
Cleveland, Ohio

CATHY A. MURRAY, MSN, RN, CNS, ONC
Assistant Professor, Department of Nursing
Ivy Tech State College—Community College of Indiana;
PRN Staff Nurse Orthopedics
Ball Memorial Hospital
Muncie, Indiana

FRANK EDWARDS MYERS III, MA, CIC, CPHQ
Manager of Clinical Epidemiology and Safety Systems
Scripps Mercy Hospital/Scripps Health
San Diego, California

KAREN NOVAK, MSN, RN, OCN, ACNP
Nurse Practitioner
Northwestern Medical Faculty Foundation
Chicago, Illinois

REBECCA M. PATTON, MSN, RN, CNOR
Director of Perioperative Services
EMH Regional Healthcare System
Elyria, Ohio

TOMMIE WRIGHT PNIEWSKI, MSN, RN, CNAA
Associate Professor, Department of Nursing
Hopkinsville Community College;
Education Coordinator of Special Projects
Christian Health Center/Christian Church Homes of Kentucky
Hopkinsville, Kentucky

SUZANNE K. POWELL, BSN, RN, MBA, CCM, CPHQ
Editor-in-Chief
Lippincott's Case Management: The Journal for Professional Practice
Lippincott, Williams & Wilkins
Philadelphia, Pennsylvania;
Director, Acute Care Quality Improvement Program
Health Services Advisory Group
Phoenix, Arizona

ANGELA SAMMARCO, PhD, RN
Assistant Professor, Department of Nursing
College of Staten Island, City University of New York
Staten Island, New York

JAMES G. SAMPSON, ND, MSN, ANP-C
Assistant Professor, Adjunct
University of Colorado School of Nursing;
Adult Nurse Practitioner
Denver Health Medical Center
Denver, Colorado

MARIAH SNYDER, PhD, FAAN
Professor Emeritus, School of Nursing
University of Minnesota
Minneapolis, Minnesota

KAREN L. TOULSON, BSN, RN, CEN
Nurse Manager, Emergency Department
Christiana Care Health Systems
Newark, Delaware

SHIRLEY E. VAN ZANDT, MS, MPH, CRNP
Instructor, School of Nursing
Johns Hopkins University
Baltimore, Maryland

CONSTANCE VISOVSKY, PhD, RN, ACNP
Assistant Professor, Frances Payne Bolton School of Nursing
Case Western Reserve University;
Nurse Practitioner, Ireland Cancer Center
University Hospitals of Cleveland
Cleveland, Ohio

CHRIS WINKELMAN, PhD, RN, CNP, CCRN
Assistant Professor, Frances Payne Bolton School of Nursing
Case Western Reserve University;
Staff Nurse, Trauma and Critical Care
MetroHealth Medical Center
Cleveland, Ohio

PAMELA C. ZICKAFOOSE, EdD, MSN, RN, CAN, BC
Instructor, Department of Nursing
Delaware Technical & Community College;
Educator
Bayhealth Medical Center
Dover, Delaware

Reviewers

JOAN P. ANDERSON, MA, RN, MALS
Suffolk County Community College
Selden, New York

MICHELE AUGUST-BRADY, DNSC, RN
Moravian College
Bethlehem, Pennsylvania

GAYLE A. BERO, MSN, RN, FNP, NCC
St. Joseph's Hospital Health Center
St. Joseph's College of Nursing
Syracuse, New York

SANDRA BRANNAN, MSN, RN
Lamar University
Beaumont, Texas

MICHELE BUNNING, MSN, RN
Good Samaritan College of Nursing and Health Science
Cincinnati, Ohio

PAMELA R. CANGELOSI, PhD, RN
George Mason University
College of Nursing and Health Science
Fairfax, Virginia

BARBARA CELIA, EdD, RN
Drexel University
College of Nursing and Health Professions
Philadelphia, Pennsylvania

CATHERINE M. CONCERT, MS, RN, APRN, BC, FNP, CGRN
Wyckoff Heights Medical Center;
Long Island University
Brooklyn, New York

PATSY ELAINE CRIHFIELD, MSN, RN, CCRN, APRN, BC, NP-C
Dyersburg State Community College
Dyersburg, Tennessee

DORIS DENISON, MSN, RN, NP, ACNP
Wayne State University
College of Nursing
Detroit, Michigan

CLAIRE P. DONAGHY, PhD, RN, APN C, CCRN, ACNP
County College of Morris
Randolph, New Jersey;
St. Clare's Health Services;
Morris Anesthesia Group
Denville, New Jersey

SHEILA A. DUNN, MSN, RN, C-ANP
St. Louis VA Medical Center
Belleville, Illinois;
St. Louis University
St. Louis, Missouri

JAYNE EDMAN, MSN, RN
Brookdale Community College
Lincroft, New Jersey

ANN E. FRONCZEK, MSN, RN, NP
Binghamton University
Decker School of Nursing
Binghamton, New York

DAVID GOEDE, MS, RN, APRN, BC
Monroe Community College;
University of Rochester
Strong Memorial Hospital
Rochester, New York

SHARRON E. GUILLETT, PhD, RN
Marymount University
Arlington, VA

ANNETTE GUNDERMAN, EdD, MSN, RN
Bloomsburg University
Bloomsburg, Pennsylvania

SUZY HARRINGTON, MS, RN, CHES
Central Colorado Area Health Education Center
Denver, Colorado

CONNIE S. HEFLIN, MSN, RN
West Kentucky Community and Technical College
Paducah, Kentucky

SARAH M. HOWELL, MSN, RN
Mississippi University for Women
Columbus, Mississippi

SUSAN J. LAMANNA, MA, MSN, RN, ANP
Onondaga Community College
Syracuse, New York

SUSAN B. LEIGHT, EdD, RNCO, CRNP
West Virginia Wesleyan College
Buckhannon, West Virginia

CAROL T. LEMAY, RN
University of Massachusetts, Amherst
Amherst, Massachusetts

JANIE LIPPS, MSN, APRN C, CDE
Vanderbilt University Medical Center
Nashville, Tennessee

JAYNE HANSCHE LOBERT, MS, RN, CS, NP
Oakland Community College
Waterford, Michigan

MARGARET A. LYNCH, MSN, FNP
The Cambridge Hospital
Cambridge, Massachusetts

CYNTHIA GLAWE MAILLOUX, PhD, RN
Pennsylvania State University, Worthington Scranton
Dunmore, Pennsylvania

DOROTHY MATHERS, MSN, RN
Pennsylvania College of Technology
Williamsport, Pennsylvania

ELIZABETH J. MILLER, MSN, MPH, APRN-BC, ABD
John Dingell Detroit VA Medical Center
Detroit, Michigan

IRIS L. MULLINS, PhD, RN
Radford University
School of Nursing
Radford, Virginia

MARIO R. ORTIZ, PhD, RN, FNP
University of Portland
School of Nursing
Portland, Oregon

AMY B. SHARRON, MS, RN, CS, GNP
United Health Care
Evercare
Auburndale, Massachusetts

MARY VIRGINIA SHINDLE, MSN, RNBC, HNC
Shepherd University
Shepherdstown, West Virginia

DARRELL R. SPURLOCK JR., MSN, RN, CCRN, CEN
Mount Carmel College of Nursing
Columbus, Ohio

PATRICIA SWEENEY, MS, APRN, BC
Pennsylvania State University, Worthington Scranton
Dunmore, Pennsylvania;
Emergency Services PC
Scranton, Pennsylvania

SUZANNE E. TATRO, MS, BSN, RN
York Technical College
Rock Hill, South Carolina

JOYCE B. VAZZANO, MSN, RN, CMSRN
John Hopkins University
School of Nursing
Baltimore, Maryland

SHARON HENRY WALICEK, MEd, MSN, RN, CCRN, CCNS, ANP-BC
Elgin Community College;
Elgin Cardiology Associates
Elgin, Illinois

COLEEN WEIL, MSN, RN, C
Wor-Wic Community College
Salisbury, Maryland

JOAN DOMIGAN WENTZ, MSN, RN
Assistant Professor
Jewish Hospital College of Nursing and Allied Health
St. Louis, Missouri

DIANE M. WHEELER, RNCS, ANP
Upper Care Internal Medicine
Falmouth, Massachusetts

CHERYLE I. WHITNEY, MSN, RN, BC
Tomball College
Tomball, Texas

CECILIA ELAINE WILSON, MS, RN, CPN
Texas Woman's University
College of Nursing
Dallas, Texas

RITA E. M. WISE, MSN, RN
Reading Hospital
School of Nursing
West Reading, Pennsylvania

Preface

The first edition of this text, entitled *Medical-Surgical Nursing: A Nursing Process Approach,* received widespread acclaim in the 1990s. The following three editions built on that achievement and further solidified the book's position as a major trendsetter for the practice of adult health nursing. Now in its fifth edition, "Iggy" charts an essential course for the future of adult nursing–a course reflected in its current title: *Medical-Surgical Nursing: Critical Thinking for Collaborative Care.*

This title was carefully chosen to emphasize the importance of developing and enhancing critical thinking skills to help today's nursing students function in interdisciplinary teams in a variety of health care settings, including both acute care and community-based settings.

KEY THEMES FOR THE 5TH EDITION

As in the extraordinarily successful fourth edition, a key theme of this edition–reflected in the book's subtitle–is critical thinking. To help achieve that emphasis on critical thinking, case-based Critical Thinking Challenges are interspersed throughout the text. These exercises provide a safe and effective means of practicing the on-the-spot decision making that students will face in the fast-paced world of medical-surgical nursing. Suggested answer guidelines for these Critical Thinking Challenges are provided on the text's Evolve website.

In addition to this key theme of critical thinking, the fifth edition also emphasizes "readiness"–readiness for the NCLEX® Examination, readiness for major emergencies such as we saw in the aftermath of the events of 9/11, readiness for safe drug administration, and readiness for the new world of genetics that is unfolding before us.

As the nursing shortage becomes more acute, it is more critical than ever that students be ready to pass the licensure exam on the first try. To help both students and faculty in reaching that goal, the fifth edition includes an innovative end-of-chapter feature called "Get Ready for the NCLEX Examination!" These unique learning aids consist of a list of Key Points *organized by NCLEX Client Needs Category* as found in the NCLEX test plan. Also included in these "Get Ready for the NCLEX Examination!" sections are highlighted reminders to go to the Student CD-ROM for "Review Questions for the NCLEX Examination" and to the Evolve website for "Integrated Management of Care Questions for the NCLEX Examination." The Review Questions for the NCLEX Examination (found on the Student CD-ROM) are keyed to the Learning Outcomes at the start of each chapter–one question per Learning Outcome. The "Integrated Management of Care Questions for the NCLEX Examination" (on the Evolve website) focus on delegation and supervision, assignment, and prioritization/decision making. These questions are aimed at stimulating and validating critical thinking to help students understand and apply the material covered in the text and integrate it with material they have learned elsewhere in the curriculum.

To help prepare students for both common medical-surgical emergencies and mass-casualty events such as the terrorist acts and natural disasters that seem to be increasingly in the news, this edition features an entirely new unit–Unit 3 (Concepts of Emergency Nursing)–which consists of two emergency care chapters. Chapter 12 (Emergency and Mass Casualty Nursing) provides an introduction to emergency and mass casualty nursing. At the end of this chapter, the reader is "walked through" a case scenario related to bioterrorism and the response of the emergency health care team. Chapter 13 (Interventions for Clients with Common Environmental Emergencies) describes selected environmental emergencies, such as heatstroke, spider bites, and near-drowning. The first-response/emergency interventions and continuing care are discussed for each emergency.

To promote readiness for safe drug administration, the fifth edition provides Pharmacology Review Questions on the Evolve website. These questions, which are keyed to the text with distinctive "Evolve Pharm Review" icons, give students practice in concepts of safe medication administration–a major theme of the NCLEX Examination.

To promote readiness for the emerging genetic basis of many diseases and disorders, we provide a new chapter, Genetic Concepts for Medical-Surgical Nursing (Chapter 11), as well as Genetic Considerations boxes and "Etiology and Genetic Risk" headings wherever appropriate.

Additional themes carried over from the previous edition are an emphasis on women's health issues, cultural considerations, complementary and alternative therapies, and the special needs of older adults. In addition, concepts of case management and community-based care are interwoven throughout to help the reader understand these growing roles and trends.

CLINICAL CURRENCY AND ACCURACY

To ensure this text's currency and accuracy, we listened to the readers of the previous editions–their impressions of and experiences with the text. Based on this input, we formulated our revision plan. We assembled a team of clinical experts to revise, rewrite and, in some cases, draft entirely new chapters.

We also commissioned in-depth reviews of selected chapters by clinicians and instructors from across the United States and Canada and used their reviews to guide us in revising the chapters into their final form. A nursing expert in sues reviewed the entire fourth edition and made endations for how to best present illustrations, re- findings, and incidence/prevalence data. For this edi- we also enlisted the assistance of an interventional ra- logist to ensure the accuracy of selected diagnostic esting procedures and associated client care.

The results are reflected in the fifth edition's strong, consistent focus on critical thinking, collaborative care, pathophysiology, drug therapy, and community-based care; its foundation of relevant research; and its emphasis on the critical "need to know" information that nurses must master in order to provide safe, effective care based on solid scientific evidence. This base of scientific evidence is emphasized throughout the text and is highlighted in our Best Practice charts. In addition, our Evidence-Based Practice for Nursing boxes now designate the *level of evidence* reflected in the reported research as based on a national standard described in Chapter 1.

OUTSTANDING READABILITY

The fifth edition has been carefully revised from cover to cover for improved readability. Today's students need to be able to read information once and understand it; they do not have time to repeatedly re-read the same information. To achieve this level of readability, we took two steps: (1) We revised the text into a direct-address style, wherever appropriate, that speaks directly to the reader; and (2) we kept sentences as short as possible consistent with the complexity of the content.

Reading level is highly influenced by the length of sentences and the length of words. Thus, while we can control the length of the sentences, medical terms are often 4 to 5 syllables long and will tend to skew a chapter's reading level. Nevertheless, the result of our efforts for the fifth edition is a med-surg text of consistently outstanding readability. The average reading level is 10th-11th grade, with a few chapters above and below that threshold.

It is important to note that reducing the reading level of this edition did not reduce the quality or depth of content that students need to know. Instead, the content is clear and focused.

EASE OF ACCESS

To make the text as easy to use as possible, we have maintained the fourth edition's approach of smaller chapters of more uniform length. The fifth edition has 80 chapters.

We also have maintained the fourth edition's unit structure, with vital body systems (cardiovascular, respiratory, and neurologic) appearing earlier in the book. In these three units, we have continued to provide critical care content in separate chapters that discuss managing critically ill clients with coronary artery disease, respiratory problems, and neurologic problems.

To help break up long blocks of text and also to highlight key information, we have included numerous headings, bulleted lists, tables, charts, and in-text highlights. We end each chapter with a Selected Bibliography (with classic sources before 2000 noted with an asterisk [*]). Key Terms are in boldface type and are defined in the text to foster the learning of need-to-know vocabulary.

A COLLABORATIVE APPROACH

As in the previous four editions, we take a collaborative approach to client care. We believe that in the real world of health care, nurses, clients, and other health care providers (including physicians, advanced-practice nurses, and physician's assistants) *share* responsibility for the management of client problems. Thus we present client care in a collaborative management framework. In this framework we make no artificial distinctions between medical treatment and nursing care. Instead, under each Collaborative Management heading we cover the entire range of approaches taken by health care practitioners of all disciplines when dealing with client problems.

New to this edition are 7 additional Concept Maps (for a total of 15) that underscore this collaborative approach. Also known as *clinical correlation maps,* these Concept Maps now begin with a case scenario. They then demonstrate visually how a complex health problem is addressed. Each Concept Map spells out the steps of the nursing process and related concepts to illustrate the relationships among disease processes, medical treatments, nursing interventions, and more. Identifying these relationships not only underscores the collaborative nature of health care but also stimulates critical thinking and fosters learning.

Although our approach is collaborative, the text is first and foremost a *nursing* text. We therefore use a nursing process approach to organize discussions of client health problems and their management. Discussions of key health problems follow a full nursing process format, with the following structure:

- [Health problem]
  - Pathophysiology
    - Etiology and Genetic Risk
    - Incidence/Prevalence
  - Collaborative Management
    - Assessment
    - Analysis
      - Common Nursing Diagnoses and Collaborative Problems
      - Additional Nursing Diagnoses and Collaborative Problems
    - Planning and Implementation
      - Nursing Diagnosis/Collaborative Problem
        - Planning: Expected Outcomes
        - Interventions
    - Community-Based Care
      - Health Teaching
      - Home Care Management
      - Health Care Resources
    - Evaluation: Outcomes

The nursing diagnoses used in this edition are the 2003-2004 NANDA-approved diagnoses–the most recently approved diagnoses at the time of this revision.

Discussions of less common or less complex disorders, although not given this complete subhead structure, nonetheless follow the same basic format: a discussion of the problem itself (including pertinent information on pathophysiology) followed by a section on collaborative care of clients with the disorder. Common nursing diagnoses/collaborative problems are often identified as well.

appropriate), and nursing interventions with rationales. In addition, "Med Error Alerts" have been added for this edition where common mistakes could be made in medication administration. Medication errors are a major health problem in health care today, and our goal with this new feature is to help students administer drugs safely.

- Key Features charts highlight the clinical manifestations of important health problems.
- Evidence-Based Practice for Nursing boxes, provided in nearly every chapter, give synopses of recent nursing research articles and other scientific articles applicable to nursing. Each box provides a summary of the article, a brief critique, the level of evidence (new to this edition), and a summary of implications for nursing practice. The goal of this feature is to help students identify the strengths and weaknesses of the research and see how research can help guide nursing practice.
- Nursing care plans remain significant tools with which the nursing student must be familiar. The fifth edition therefore includes selected examples of these care-planning tools. It has been retitled "Plan of Care" and incorporates NIC and NOC language. Nursing Plans of Care continue to include a distinctive icon (D) to designate interventions that can be delegated to assistive nursing personnel.
- New to this edition, Home Care Assessment charts serve as a convenient summary of essential assessment points for clients who need follow-up home health nursing care.
- Assessment Using Gordon's Functional Health Patterns charts provide a convenient one-stop list of relevant questions to ask clients regarding the impact of health conditions on everyday function.
- Meeting *Healthy People 2010* Objectives boxes suggest specific activities that nurses can undertake to promote achievement of the specific numbered objectives of the *Healthy People 2010* program.
- Resource Management boxes (formerly "Cost of Care" boxes) provide an important financial/resource context for medical-surgical nurses when managing resources for client care. Nurses must increasingly understand cost and other resource factors in order to help clients work toward wellness.
- Legal/Ethical Issues boxes introduce students to some of the dilemmas they will face in the increasingly high-tech world of medical-surgical nursing.

AN INTEGRATED MULTIMEDIA RESOURCE BASED ON PROVEN LEARNING STRATEGIES

Medical-Surgical Nursing: Critical Thinking for Collaborative Care, 5th edition, is the hub of a comprehensive package of electronic and print publications that break new ground in the application of proven learning strategies and evidence-based educational practice. This integrated multimedia resource actively engages the student in problem solving and critical thinking. Every effort has been made to correlate content among the text and its companion publications. Unlike many textbook authors, we have personally been involved in the development of most of the companion publications to ensure consistency and cohesion between the textbook and the companion publications.

RESOURCES FOR INSTRUCTORS

Resources for instructors include a printed Instructor's Resource Manual, an Instructor's Electronic Resource CD-ROM/DVD, and Evolve Learning Resources for faculty.

The printed Instructor's Resource Manual, written by Susan Behmke and Sharon Souter, along with contributions from four expert authors, continues to serve as a touchstone for new and seasoned faculty alike. The IRM for the 5th edition features a simplified new format as well as four new introductory chapters. The introductory chapters cover evaluation of critical thinking, test construction, incorporation of technology into the classroom, and teaching strategies for students with a variety of learning styles. IRM chapters now correspond directly to textbook chapters and feature Concept Map Case Studies that correspond to the 15 Concept Maps in the text.

The Instructor's Electronic Resource CD-ROM/DVD consists of a Test Bank, Image Collection, Lecture Slides, ready-to-use narrated PowerPoint Lectures, and a Faculty Development Video.

- The Test Bank is a robust 2500-item bank that includes both traditional and NCLEX Examination "alternate" item types, and each question is coded for correct answer, rationale, cognitive type, nursing process step, and NCLEX Client Needs Category. The Test Bank is provided in ExamView, Blackboard, and ParTest formats.
- The expanded Image Collection now consists of 700 images from the text and are delivered in a format that makes incorporation into lectures and presentations easier than ever.
- The Lecture Slides (formerly "LectureView") are a collection of 1200 text slides developed to correspond to each chapter in the text.
- The new, ready-to-use PowerPoint Lectures are narrated lectures by co-author Linda Workman on topics that faculty find particularly challenging.
- The new Faculty Development Video, delivered on DVD-ROM as part of the Instructor's Electronic Resource, is a 60-minute video by Donna Ignatavicius that addresses the implications of changes in the NCLEX Examination for faculty. Excerpted from one of Donna Ignatavicius's popular seminars, this DVD is a unique resource for faculty.

For the convenience of faculty, all of these resources except the Faculty Development Video are also available online on a secure instructor area of the Evolve website entitled Evolve Learning Resources.

RESOURCES FOR STUDENTS

Resources for students include a free Student CD-ROM, a thoroughly revised and updated Critical Thinking Study Guide, a Clinical Companion, a Virtual Clinical Excursions workbook/CD-ROM, and Evolve Learning Resources.

The new Student CD-ROM features Review Questions for the NCLEX Examination–one for each Learning Outcome at the beginning of the chapter. Also included on the

Integral to this collaborative management approach is a clear delineation of just who is responsible for what. When a responsibility is primarily the nurse's, the text says so. When a decision must be made jointly by the client, nurse, physician, and physical therapist, for example, this is clearly stated. When different health care practitioners in different care settings might be involved in the client's care, this is stated.

To further emphasize the nurse's role, we have integrated pertinent components of the Nursing Interventions Classification (NIC) system and the Nursing Outcomes Classification (NOC) system. These systems were developed by the Center for Nursing Classification to standardize nursing interventions and outcomes and the terminology used to describe them. Where appropriate for health problems that receive full nursing process coverage, NIC interventions are clearly identified with a NIC symbol **NIC**. Selected activities associated with each identified intervention are listed in NIC Intervention Activities charts.

The expected outcomes for client care in this edition are consistent with the NOC system. However, NOC continues to be developed and refined to ensure that outcomes are evidence-based. We have therefore included NOC outcomes and specified indicators when appropriate, as well as other outcome statements validated empirically by clinical practice. Those statements that are particularly consistent with NOC language are identified with a NOC symbol ***NOC***.

ORGANIZATION

The 80 chapters of *Medical-Surgical Nursing: Critical Thinking for Collaborative Care* are grouped into 17 units. Unit 1, Health Promotion and Illness, lays the foundation for the health care concepts incorporated throughout the text. Unit 2 covers important biopsychosocial concepts related to health care, including pain and rehabilitation. Chapter 11 is a new chapter in this unit and introduces the major concepts of genetics and related nursing implications for client care. A new unit, Unit 3, consists of two emergency care chapters as previously described.

Unit 4 consists of six chapters on the management of clients with fluid, electrolyte, and acid-base imbalances. This unit includes an expanded chapter on infusion therapy (Chapter 17) and is supplemented with an online fluid and electrolyte tutorial on the companion Evolve website.

Unit 5 presents the perioperative nursing content that medical-surgical nurses need to know. This content provides a solid foundation to help the student better understand the specific surgeries covered throughout the remainder of the text.

Unit 6 provides core content on health problems related to immune system function. This content includes normal inflammation and the immune response, altered cell growth and cancer development, and interventions for clients with connective tissue disease, HIV infection, and other immunologic disorders, cancers, and infections.

The remaining 11 units cover medical-surgical content by body system. Each of these units begins with an Assessment chapter and continues with one or more Interventions chapters for clients with specific health problems in that body system.

MULTINATIONAL, MULTICULTURAL, MULTIGENERATIONAL FOCUS

To reflect the increasing diversity of our society, *Medical-Surgical Nursing: Critical Thinking for Collaborative Care* takes a multinational, multicultural, and multigenerational focus. Addressing the needs of both U.S. and Canadian readers, we have included examples of trade names of drugs available in the United States and those available in Canada. Drugs that are available only in Canada are designated with a ✷ symbol.

To help nurses provide quality care for clients whose cultural background may differ from their own, numerous Cultural Considerations boxes highlight important aspects of culturally competent care throughout the text. A revised cultural health chapter (Chapter 6) is also included in this edition. Located inside the back cover is an innovative Communication Quick Reference for Spanish-Speaking Clients. This Quick Reference helps ensure clear communication between native English speakers and the rapidly growing population who speak Spanish as a first language.

Increases in life expectancy and the "graying" of the baby-boom generation add up to a steadily increasing older adult population. To help equip nurses for this challenge, the fifth edition continues to feature expanded coverage of the care of older adults. It includes a greater number of Nursing Focus on the Older Adult charts and highlights laboratory values and drug dosages typical for older clients. Charts specifying normal physiologic changes to expect in the older population are included in each Assessment chapter. In addition, Considerations for Older Adults boxes are included throughout the text to emphasize key points to keep in mind when caring for these clients.

Also appearing throughout the text is an increased number of Women's Health Considerations boxes, which address topics of concern to women and their health care providers. These in-text highlights alert the reader to gender-related differences in assessment parameters and in the incidence, severity, and treatment of common health problems.

ADDITIONAL LEARNING RESOURCES

As in previous editions, the fifth edition continues to include a rich array of "andragogic" learning aids–learning aids geared toward adult learners–to help students quickly identify and understand key information and to serve as study aids. Several of these features are new to this edition.

- Written in "client-friendly" language, Client Education Guide charts provide the types of instructions that nurses must learn to provide to clients and their families to help them cope with life changes caused by illness.
- Laboratory Profile charts summarize important information on laboratory tests commonly ordered to evaluate health problems. Information typically includes normal ranges of laboratory values (including differences for older adults, when appropriate) and the possible significance of abnormal findings.
- Drug Therapy charts summarize important information about commonly used drugs. These charts include both U.S. and Canadian trade names for typically used drugs, usual dosages (including dosages for older clients, as

Student CD-ROM are animations and video clips (each keyed to the text by a distinctive "clapboard" icon, as well as a new Audio Glossary. The Audio Glossary includes the definitions of all Key Terms from the text, along with audio files for difficult pronunciations. The Student CD-ROM also includes Audio Clips that allow students to hear key sounds in health assessment.

The *Critical Thinking Study Guide* has been carefully revised and updated under the authorship of Julie S. Snyder for an increased emphasis on critical thinking and rigorous accuracy. The Study Guide features a simplified format and a greater variety of question types. Multiple-choice questions are now written in NCLEX format and emphasize the NCLEX priorities of delegation, management of care, and pharmacology. The use of Case Studies is expanded in this edition, and a new chapter on study tips is included.

The pocket-sized *Clinical Companion,* authored by Kathy A. Hausman, retains the alphabetical organization and streamlined format that made it so popular in previous editions. The new edition is printed in color and in a smaller page size for easier portability, and it includes a quick reference to nursing care after incidents of chemical terrorism and bioterrorism. The *Clinical Companion* is a pocket-sized "Iggy" for students going into clinicals and is written by an author who actively supervises clinicals and who knows firsthand what students in clinicals are being asked to know about their clients.

The *Virtual Clinical Excursions* workbook/CD-ROM package, featuring an updated and easy-to-navigate "virtual" clinical setting, will once again be available for the fifth edition. This unique learning tool guides the student through a virtual clinical environment and helps the student apply textbook content in a "safe" context. The clinical simulations and workbook represent the next generation of research-based learning tools to promote critical thinking and meaningful learning.

Also available for students in a dynamic collection of Evolve Learning Resources, available at http://evolve.elsevier.com/Iggy/. Evolve resources include the following:

- Pharmacology Review Questions (keyed to icons in the textbook)
- Integrated Management of Care Questions for the NCLEX Examination
- Answer Guidelines for Critical Thinking Challenges
- Answer Guidelines for Study Guide Case Studies
- "Building" Concept Maps ("building" versions of the 15 Concept Maps from the text)
- Concept Map Creator (a handy tool for creating customized Concept Maps)
- Fluid & Electrolyte Tutorial (a complete self-paced tutorial on this perennially difficult content)
- WebLinks (a dynamic library of Internet links, updated regularly for currency)
- Content Updates
- Health Assessment Image Collection (supplemental images of common assessment findings)
- The Audio Glossary, Audio Clips, Animations, and Video Clips from the Student CD-ROM.

For more information on any of these innovative companion publications, contact your Elsevier sales representative, visit http://www.us.elsevierhealth.com/, or contact Elsevier Faculty Support at 1-800-222-9570 or sales.inquiry@elsevier.com.

• • •

In summary, *Medical-Surgical Nursing: Critical Thinking for Collaborative Care,* 5th edition, together with its fully integrated multimedia ancillary package, provides the tools you will need to meet the challenge of nursing in the first decade of the 21st century and beyond. The only elements that remain to be added to this package are those that you alone can provide–your diligence, your commitment, your innovation, *your nursing care.*

Donna D. Ignatavicius
M. Linda Workman

Acknowledgments

Publishing a textbook and ancillary package of this depth and breadth would not be possible without the combined efforts of many people. Our contributing authors once again provided consistently excellent manuscripts in a timely fashion. Special thanks to Elaine Kennedy, who developed all of our new case-study-based Concept Maps. Our reviewers–expert clinicians and instructors from around the United States and Canada–provided invaluable suggestions and encouragement throughout the book's development.

The staff of W.B. Saunders/Elsevier once again provided us with crucial guidance and support throughout the planning, writing, revision, and production of the fifth edition. In particular, Executive Publisher Barbara Nelson Cullen and Editor Lee Henderson worked closely with us from the early stages of this edition to help us hone and focus our revision plan, and Lee oversaw the project from start to finish. Developmental Editor Laura Sieh Chu and Managing Editor Robin Richman then worked with us step-by-step to bring the fifth edition from vision to publication. Maureen Iannuzzi held the reins of our complex ancillary package and worked with a gifted group of writers and content experts to provide an outstanding library of resources to complement and enhance the text. Special thanks to Senior Editor's Assistant Marie Thomas, who handled the countless administrative details associated with a project of this size. She is without peer among editorial assistants.

Senior Project Manager Jodi Willard was once again a joy to work with. If, as is said, the mark of a good copy editor is that her work is invisible to the reader, then Jodi is the consummate copy editor. Her unwavering attention to detail, flexibility, and conscientiousness not only helped to make this edition the most consistently readable ever, but also made the entire production process incredibly smooth and headache-free.

Special thanks also to Publishing Services Manager Debbie Vogel. For two editions now, Debbie has worked quietly behind the scenes to help bring the book to publication precisely on schedule and with a very high level of quality.

Designer Teresa McBryan is responsible for the beautiful cover and interior design of the fifth edition. The praise of a book designer's work is often unsung, but Teresa's work on this edition has cast important features in exactly the right light, with neither too much nor too little emphasis, making this edition not only practical and easy to read, but beautiful.

Our acknowledgments would not be complete without recognizing Karen McKie, Bob Boehringer, Jo Beth Griffin, our dedicated team of sales representatives, and other key members of the Sales and Marketing staff who helped to put this book into your hands.

Finally, we wish to thank Executive Vice President, Nursing and Health Professions, Sally Schrefer. Sally's personal leadership style continues to create a unique publishing environment in which authors and editors have the freedom to interact creatively to produce the best books in the field.

Donna D. Ignatavicius
M. Linda Workman

Contents

UNIT ONE

HEALTH PROMOTION and ILLNESS

UNIT FOUR

MANAGEMENT of CLIENTS with FLUID, ELECTROLYTE, and ACID-BASE IMBALANCES

UNIT SEVEN

PROBLEMS of OXYGENATION

Management of Clients with Problems of the Respiratory Tract

UNIT EIGHT

PROBLEMS of CARDIAC OUTPUT and TISSUE PERFUSION

Management of Clients with Problems of the Cardiovascular System

UNIT **NINE**

PROBLEMS of TISSUE PERFUSION

Management of Clients with Problems of the Hematologic System

UNIT **TEN**

PROBLEMS of MOBILITY, SENSATION, and COGNITION

Management of Clients with Problems of the Nervous System

UNIT THIRTEEN

PROBLEMS of DIGESTION, NUTRITION, and ELIMINATION

Management of Clients with Problems of the Gastrointestinal System

UNIT SIXTEEN

PROBLEMS of EXCRETION

Management of Clients with Problems of the Renal/Urinary System

UNIT SEVENTEEN

PROBLEMS of REPRODUCTION

Management of Clients with Problems of the Reproductive System

Guide to Special Features

ASSESSMENT USING GORDON'S FUNCTIONAL HEALTH PATTERNS

BEST PRACTICE

BEST PRACTICE for EMERGENCY CARE

CLIENT EDUCATION GUIDE

CONCEPT MAPS

DRUG THERAPY

EVIDENCE-BASED PRACTICE for Nursing

FOCUSED ASSESSMENT

HOME CARE ASSESSMENT

KEY FEATURES

LABORATORY PROFILE

LEGAL/ETHICAL ISSUES

Meeting HEALTHY PEOPLE 2010 Objectives

NIC INTERVENTION ACTIVITIES

NURSING FOCUS on the OLDER ADULT

PLAN of CARE

RESOURCE MANAGEMENT

Reference Guide for Student CD-ROM

The Student CD-ROM provided with this text contains the following features:

- **Review Questions for the NCLEX Examination**
- **Health Assessment Audio Clips**
- **Health Assessment Images**
- **Audio Glossary**
- **Health Assessment Video Clips**
- **Animations**

Look for this multimedia icon in the margins of the text. This icon highlights related animations and health assessment video clips on your Student CD-ROM.

HEALTH ASSESSMENT AUDIO CLIPS

UNIT SIX MANAGEMENT OF CLIENTS WITH PROBLEMS OF THE IMMUNE RESPONSE

CHAPTER 26

Stridor

UNIT SEVEN MANAGEMENT OF CLIENTS WITH PROBLEMS OF THE RESPIRATORY TRACT

CHAPTER 30

Bronchial breath sounds
Bronchovesicular breath sounds
Vesicular breath sounds
High-pitched crackles
Low-pitched crackles
High-pitched wheeze
Low-pitched wheeze
Pleural friction rub

UNIT EIGHT MANAGEMENT OF CLIENTS WITH PROBLEMS OF THE CARDIOVASCULAR SYSTEM

CHAPTER 36

Single S1
S1 at various locations
Single S2
S2 at various locations
The fourth heart sound (S4)
The third heart sound (S3)
Murmurs: High, medium, and low
Murmurs: Blowing, harsh or rough, and rumble
Systolic murmur
Diastolic murmur
Pericardial friction rub

HEALTH ASSESSMENT VIDEO CLIPS

UNIT SEVEN MANAGEMENT OF CLIENTS WITH PROBLEMS OF THE RESPIRATORY TRACT

CHAPTER 30

Inspection: Nose (adult female)
Inspection and palpation: Breathing and respiratory excursion, anterior chest (adult male)
Inspection and palpation: Respirations, respiratory excursion, and tactile fremitus, posterior chest (adult male)
Palpation: Tactile fremitus, posterior chest (adult female)
Inspection and percussion: Diaphragmatic excursion (adult male)
Percussion: Anterior thorax (adult male)

UNIT EIGHT MANAGEMENT OF CLIENTS WITH PROBLEMS OF THE CARDIOVASCULAR SYSTEM

CHAPTER 36

Inspection and palpation: Cardiac, anterior chest (adult female)
Inspection and palpation: Cardiac, auscultatory landmarks (adult male)
Auscultation: Cardiac, with diaphragm (adult male)
Auscultation: Cardiac, with bell (adult male)
Auscultation: Cardiac, with diaphragm and bell (adult female)
Auscultation: Carotid artery (adult male)
Inspection and palpation: Pulses, lower extremities (adult female)

UNIT TEN MANAGEMENT OF CLIENTS WITH PROBLEMS OF THE NERVOUS SYSTEM

CHAPTER 44

Evaluation: Smell, cranial nerve I—olfactory nerve (adult male)
Evaluation: Central vision and visual acuity, cranial nerve II—optic nerve (adult male)
Evaluation: Pupil responses, direct and accommodation, cranial nerves III, IV, and VI—oculomotor, trochlear, and abducens nerves (adult male)
Evaluation: Sensory, light touch; face, upper, and lower extremities, cranial nerve V—trigeminal nerve (older adult female)
Inspection: Fine motor coordination, upper extremities (older adult male)
Inspection: Fine motor coordination, lower extremities (older adult female)
Evaluation: Sensory, face, and upper extremities
Evaluation: Deep tendon reflex, patellar tendon (adult male)

UNIT ELEVEN MANAGEMENT OF CLIENTS WITH PROBLEMS OF THE SENSORY SYSTEM

CHAPTER 49

Inspection and palpation: External eye (adult male)
Evaluation: Central vision and visual acuity (adult male)
Evaluation: Pupil responses, direct and consensual (older adult female)

CHAPTER 51

Inspection and palpation: External ear (older adult male)
Inspection: Ear canal (adult male)

UNIT TWELVE MANAGEMENT OF CLIENTS WITH PROBLEMS OF THE MUSCULOSKELETAL SYSTEM

CHAPTER 53

Inspection: Gait (older adult female)
Inspection: General muscle strength (adult male)
Inspection and palpation: Muscular development (adult male)

UNIT THIRTEEN MANAGEMENT OF CLIENTS WITH PROBLEMS OF THE GASTROINTESTINAL SYSTEM

CHAPTER 56

Auscultation: Abdomen, bowel sounds (adult male)
Auscultation: Percussion: Abdomen (adult male)
Percussion: Liver (adult male)
Percussion: Spleen (adult male)
Palpation: Abdomen, superficial and deep (adult male)

UNIT SEVENTEEN MANAGEMENT OF CLIENTS WITH PROBLEMS OF THE REPRODUCTIVE SYSTEM

CHAPTER 76

Inspection: External genitalia (younger adult female)
Inspection: Speculum examination (younger adult female)
Palpation: Bimanual examination (younger adult female)
Inspection and palpation: Standing position (younger adult male)
Inspection and palpation: Standing position, clip 2 (younger adult male)
Palpation: Inguinal hernia evaluation (younger adult male)

CHAPTER 77

Inspection: Female breasts (sitting position, adult female)
Inspection: Female breasts (supine position, adult female)

HEALTH ASSESSMENT IMAGES

UNIT SEVEN MANAGEMENT OF CLIENTS WITH PROBLEMS OF THE RESPIRATORY TRACT

CHAPTER 30

Anterior lobes of the lung
Posterior lobes of the lung
Chest landmarks
Pleural effusion diagram

CHAPTER 33

Bronchitis diagram
Emphysema diagram

CHAPTER 34

Pneumonia diagram
Atelectasis diagram

CHAPTER 35

Client with pneumothorax

UNIT EIGHT MANAGEMENT OF CLIENTS WITH PROBLEMS OF THE CARDIOVASCULAR SYSTEM

CHAPTER 39

Rubor phase of Raynaud's disease
Cyanotic phase of Raynaud's disease

UNIT NINE MANAGEMENT OF CLIENTS WITH PROBLEMS OF THE HEMATOLOGIC SYSTEM

CHAPTER 42

Pale skin with anemia

UNIT TEN MANAGEMENT OF CLIENTS WITH PROBLEMS OF THE NERVOUS SYSTEM

CHAPTER 44

Sensory pathways of CNS
Major motor pathways of CNS
Reflex arc

CHAPTER 47

Facial presentation of Bell's palsy
Residual slight muscle weakness post-Bell's palsy

UNIT ELEVEN MANAGEMENT OF CLIENTS WITH PROBLEMS OF THE SENSORY SYSTEM

CHAPTER 49

Anatomy of the middle ear
Anatomy of the inner ear
Pathways of hearing

CHAPTER 50

Hordeolum
Chalazion
Acute conjunctivitis

CHAPTER 52

Otitis externa
Causes of conductive hearing loss
Causes of sensorineural hearing loss

UNIT THIRTEEN MANAGEMENT OF CLIENTS WITH PROBLEMS OF THE GASTROINTESTINAL SYSTEM

CHAPTER 56

Abdominal auscultation sites
Abdominal structures that may be palpable
Referred abdominal pain–anterior
Referred abdominal pain–posterior

CHAPTER 57

Lymph nodes–head and neck
Lymph nodes–tongue
Lymph nodes–ear

CHAPTER 60

Inguinal hernia pathway
Femoral hernia pathway

UNIT FOURTEEN MANAGEMENT OF CLIENTS WITH PROBLEMS OF THE ENDOCRINE SYSTEM

CHAPTER 66

Addison's disease

CHAPTER 67

Anterior view of thyroid in Asian female with goiter

UNIT FIFTEEN MANAGEMENT OF CLIENTS WITH PROBLEMS OF THE SKIN, HAIR, AND NAILS

CHAPTER 69

Distribution of eccrine and apocrine sweat glands
Ecchymosis caused by injury from falling on a hard object

CHAPTER 70

Contact dermatitis of hands due to prolonged exposure to bleach
Atopic dermatitis on the cheeks of an infant
Urticaria
Anatomical distribution of psoriasis
Cherry angioma

UNIT SEVENTEEN MANAGEMENT OF CLIENTS WITH PROBLEMS OF THE REPRODUCTIVE SYSTEM

CHAPTER 80

Anatomic distribution of secondary syphilis

ANIMATIONS

UNIT SEVEN MANAGEMENT OF CLIENTS WITH PROBLEMS OF THE RESPIRATORY TRACT

CHAPTER 30

Pulmonary circulation
Anatomic location of sinuses
Percussion tones throughout the chest
Patterns of respiration

UNIT EIGHT MANAGEMENT OF CLIENTS WITH PROBLEMS OF THE CARDIOVASCULAR SYSTEM

CHAPTER 36

Cardiac cycle during systole and diastole
Blood flow: Circulatory system
Pulse variations
Auscultation of heart valves

UNIT TEN MANAGEMENT OF CLIENTS WITH PROBLEMS OF THE NERVOUS SYSTEM

CHAPTER 44

Functional areas of the brain
Reflex arc
Sensory pathways and clinical evaluation of the central nervous system
Motor pathways and clinical evaluation of the central nervous system

UNIT ELEVEN MANAGEMENT OF CLIENTS WITH PROBLEMS OF THE SENSORY SYSTEM

CHAPTER 51

Weber test

UNIT TWELVE MANAGEMENT OF CLIENTS WITH PROBLEMS OF THE MUSCULOSKELETAL SYSTEM

CHAPTER 53

Classification of joints: Hinge joint
Classification of joints: Gliding joint–hand
Classification of joints: Condyloid joint

UNIT SEVENTEEN MANAGEMENT OF CLIENTS WITH PROBLEMS OF THE REPRODUCTIVE SYSTEM

CHAPTER 76

Lymphatic drainage of breast
The menstrual cycle

CHAPTER 79

Rectal examination

CHAPTER 1

Critical Thinking in the Role of the Medical-Surgical Nurse

DONNA D. IGNATAVICIUS

LEARNING OUTCOMES

After studying this chapter, you should be able to:

1. Explain why critical thinking is an essential part of medical-surgical nursing.
2. Compare and contrast common definitions of health.
3. Explain why some populations are more likely to experience health problems than others.
4. Explain the purpose of Healthy People 2010.
5. Differentiate the three levels of illness prevention and provide at least one example of each level.
6. Identify the major roles of the medical-surgical nurse.
7. Explain the relationship between critical thinking and evidence-based practice.
8. Assess factors that may affect the teaching-learning process.
9. Describe best practice interventions for promoting adult learning.
10. Review the key components of the nursing process.
11. Describe the difference between a nursing diagnosis and a medical problem.
12. Identify best practice interventions for clinical documentation.

Go to your Student CD-ROM for Review Questions for the NCLEX Examination keyed to these Learning Outcomes.

The purpose of medical-surgical nursing, sometimes called adult health nursing, is to promote health and prevent illness in individuals from 18 to older than 100 years of age. Nurses who practice medical-surgical nursing are generalists who must have a broad knowledge base to meet the needs of clients in a variety of health care settings. Rapid advances in technology, massive increases in knowledge, and dramatic changes in the health care delivery system require that medical-surgical nurses use expert critical thinking skills to provide complex, holistic health care.

CRITICAL THINKING

Critical thinking, sometimes referred to as clinical reasoning or judgment, is an essential competency that all nurses need to provide quality, cost-effective client care. Alfaro-LeFevre (2003) describes critical thinking as purposeful, outcome-directed thinking that aims to make judgments based on scientific evidence, rather than on tradition or conjecture (guesswork). The best source of evidence is the result of research. Nursing has increased its research findings on which to base its practice.

Evidence-Based Practice

The term **evidence-based practice** is often used to describe the care that nurses provide based on research and identified standards. Throughout this text, Evidence-Based Practice for Nursing boxes summarize and critique some of the most current research for medical-surgical nursing.

However, available nursing research is limited and often does not represent the highest level of evidence. As seen in Table 1-1, the highest level of evidence, or LOE-1, is based on a meta-analysis of multiple well-designed randomized controlled studies. A significant amount of nursing research consists of small pilot studies at LOE-7 or LOE-8. The findings of these studies cannot be generalized, but they provide a basis for future larger and better controlled research. Each study in this text's Evidence-Based Practice for Nursing boxes is rated by level of evidence using the scale in Table

UNIT **ONE**

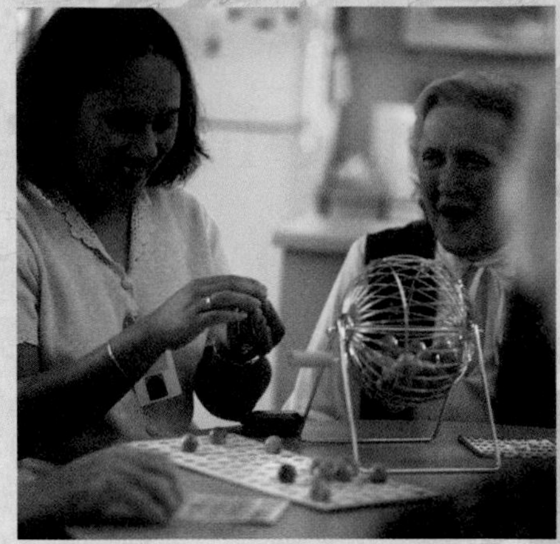

HEALTH PROMOTION and ILLNESS

TABLE 1-1 Level of Evidence (LOE) Rating Scale and Origins of Evidence

LOE	Origin of Evidence
Highest	
LOE-1	Meta-analysis of multiple well-designed randomized controlled trials (RCTs) of adequate quality
LOE-2	At least one properly designed RCT of appropriate size (more than 100 subjects, multiple sites)
LOE-3	Well-designed trial without randomization (e.g., single pretest and post-test, cohort, time series, or meta-analysis of cohort studies)
Moderate	
LOE-4	Well-conducted qualitative systematic review (integrative review on nonexperimental design studies)
LOE-5	Well-conducted case control study
LOE-6	Poorly controlled study (RCT with major flaws) Uncontrolled studies (e.g., correlational descriptive study, case series)
Lowest (Weakest)	
LOE-7	Conflicting evidence with the weight of evidence supporting the recommendation of meta-analysis showing a trend that did not reach statistical significance NIH Consensus Reports Published practice guidelines from professional organizations, health organizations, or federal agencies (e.g., Centers for Disease Control and Prevention)
LOE-8	Qualitative designs with few participants Opinion from expert authorities, agencies, or committees Case studies

Modified from Hadorn, D., et al. (1996). Rating the quality of evidence for clinical practice guidelines. *Journal of Clinical Epidemiology, 49*(7), 749-753; and Rosswurm, M., & Larrabee, J. (1999). A model for change to evidence-based practice. *Image: The Journal of Nursing Scholarship, 31*(4), 317-322.

TABLE 1-2 Examples of Critical Thinking Indicators

Behaviors Demonstrating Critical Thinking Characteristics and Attitudes

Open and fair-minded: Shows tolerance for different viewpoints; questions how own viewpoints are influencing thinking

Creative: Offers alternative solutions and approaches; comes up with useful ideas

Proactive: Anticipates consequences, plans ahead, acts on opportunities

Behaviors Demonstrating Knowledge and Intellectual Skills

Knowledge

- Clarifies reasons behind interventions and diagnostic studies
- Clarifies personal values, beliefs, needs
- Demonstrates focused physical assessment skills (e.g., breath sounds or IV site assessment)

Intellectual Skills/Competencies

- Sets priorities and makes decisions in a timely way; includes key stakeholders in making decisions
- Distinguishes normal from abnormal; identifies risks for abnormal
- Considers multiple explanations and solutions

Data obtained from Alfaro-LeFevre, R. (2003). *Critical thinking in nursing: A practical approach* (3rd ed.). Philadelphia: W.B. Saunders.

1-1. Nursing implications are also discussed to help you consider these findings for daily practice.

Critical Thinking Skills and Behaviors

Alfaro-LeFevre (2004) also developed **Critical Thinking Indicators (CTIs)** that identify the behaviors and skills of a critical thinker. The CTIs are divided into the three aspects of critical thinking: knowledge, affective or emotional behaviors, and cognitive behaviors. Examples of each of these aspects of critical thinking are listed in Table 1-2. Medical-surgical nurses should use all of these behaviors and skills to provide high-quality, excellent care.

Critical Thinking Challenges are threaded throughout this book to help you apply critical thinking for a variety of clinical case scenarios. Additional critical thinking activities may be found at http://www.evolve.elsevier.com/Iggy/.

HEALTH

Beliefs about health and illness are a major feature of every known culture. How one views himself or herself as a person and as a part of the environment affects how health is defined.

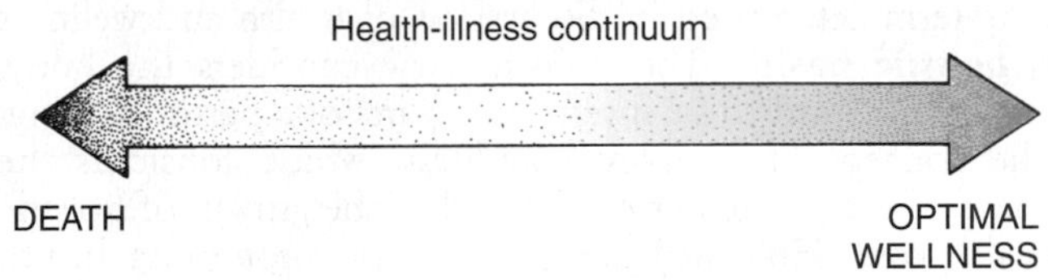

Figure 1-1 ■ Common concept of health as a continuum ranging from optimal wellness at one end to illness culminating in death at the other end.

Health is often viewed as a continuum on which optimal wellness, at one end, is the highest level of function, and illness, at the other end, results in death (Figure 1-1). Every person is somewhere on the continuum. As a person's health state changes, his or her location on the continuum changes.

Although the term *health* is used every day, no universally accepted definition has been established. Over time, the focus and expression of health have varied depending on knowledge, theories, and beliefs. Some individuals view health and disease as a reward or punishment for their actions. Others consider health to be a wholeness of the body; this view is often referred to as holistic health.

Definitions of Health

A typical dictionary may define health in terms of a person's ability to function in society. Some definitions also describe health as a disease-free state or condition. Definitions such as these do not make clear what constitutes health and illness and seem to present an "either/or" situation; that is, a person is either healthy or ill.

WORLD HEALTH ORGANIZATION DEFINITION OF HEALTH

As science has progressed, the definition of **health** has evolved. One of the most commonly quoted definitions is the one presented in 1947 by the World Health Organization (WHO), in which health is defined as "a state of complete physical, mental, and social well-being and not merely the absence of disease or infirmity" (WHO, 1947, p. 1). According to WHO, to be healthy a person must be in a state of physical, mental, and social well-being. Some health care professionals have found this concept problematic because achieving a state of "health" seems to be an unrealistic goal. This definition does not allow for degrees of health or illness, and it fails to reflect the dynamic, ever-changing nature of health.

SOCIOLOGIC DEFINITIONS OF HEALTH

Sociologists view health as a condition that allows for the pursuit and enjoyment of desired cultural values. Researchers who have polled laypersons for their definitions of health concur that health is the absence of symptoms and a feeling of well-being. "Good health" includes the ability to carry out "normal" daily activities, such as going to work and performing household chores.

HOLISTIC HEALTH

One term often used in discussions of health and wellness is **holistic health.** The holistic view considers the body, mind, and spirit to be interrelated parts of a person's being. The concept of high-level wellness, which considers the needs of the whole person, has led to the growth of holistic health care. Holistic health focuses on promoting health and preventing illness, with an emphasis on the person's responsibility to achieve high-level wellness. There is also concern with bringing the person's mind, body, and spirit into harmony with the environment. Various alternative and complementary therapies have been used for many years to promote mind-body-spirit harmony. Chapter 4 describes some commonly used therapies and how they can be incorporated into medical-surgical nursing practice. Additional discussions of these therapies can be found under the text for various disorders throughout the text.

DEFINITION OF HEALTH USED IN THIS TEXT

In this text, health is defined as a person's "level of wellness." This level of wellness is a process in which a person strives to attain his or her full potential. Health reflects a person's biologic, psychological, and sociologic state (Figure 1-2). The *biologic* (physical) state refers to the structure of body tissues and organs as well as to the biochemical interactions and functions within the body. The *psychological* state includes a person's mood, emotions, and personality. The *sociologic* (social) state involves the interaction between a person and the environment.

Spiritual health is sometimes considered to be part of sociologic health but may be described as a separate aspect of the overall health state. Spiritual health often affects both the client's biologic and psychological health state. A study by Narayanasamy & Owens (2001) found that nurses are often confused about the meaning of spirituality and their role related to spiritual health. However, the study sample believed that clients' faith produced a positive effect on clients and families. (See the Evidence-Based Practice for Nursing box above.)

A high level of wellness is achieved when these biopsychosocial needs are met. One of the primary functions of nursing is to assist clients in reaching this high level of wellness. It is therefore essential that you understand the concept of health and wellness. As you assess clients, be aware of factors that affect a person's health state, and select nursing interventions that promote and maintain an optimal level of wellness (Figure 1-3).

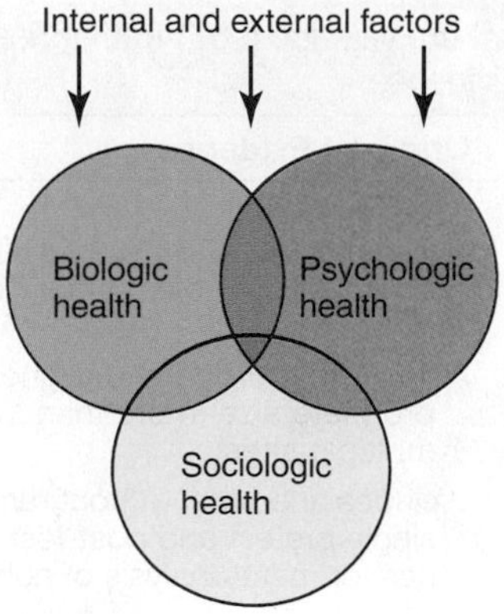

Figure 1-2 ■ Textbook definition of health–a person's biologic, psychological, and sociologic health state. Internal and external factors affect a person's level of wellness.

EVIDENCE-BASED PRACTICE for Nursing

How do nurses intervene to promote spiritual health of clients?

Narayanasamy, A., & Owens, J. (2001). A critical incident study of nurses' responses to the spiritual needs of their patients. *Journal of Advanced Nursing, 33*(4), 446-455.

The purpose of this study was to determine what nurses identify as spiritual needs of clients in an acute care setting and to explore how they responded to those needs. Critical incidents were obtained from 115 volunteer nurses. These data were subjected to content analysis and themes were identified that answered the study questions. The themes were "personal," "procedural," "culturalist," and "evangelical." The findings suggest that nurses are confused about the domain of spiritual health and what it means. They recognized that spirituality plays a positive role in health promotion and the clients' trust in the staff. Nurses did feel that promoting spiritual health was important, but they differed in their approach.

Level of Evidence: 6—Uncontrolled study, but serves as pilot research for nurses' understanding of spiritual health.

Critique. Nurses in acute care often become focused on technical tasks and give less attention and time to meeting other types of needs. This study confirms that nurses believe that spiritual health is an important domain for health promotion, but demonstrates the variety of beliefs and approaches related to spirituality. The data from this convenience sample prevent generalizing these findings, but show the need for further research and education in this area.

Implications for Nursing. Nurses need to recognize the importance of spiritual health in the promotion of overall health. The meaning of spirituality differs from person to person, and nurses need to ask about what it means for each client. Then, a mutual plan for meeting spiritual health needs should be implemented.

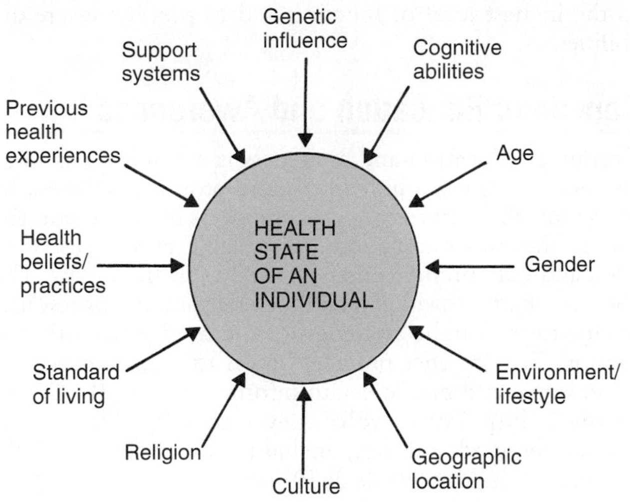

Figure 1-3 ■ Multiple variables influence health and illness.

Quality of Life

Over the past two decades, the concept of **quality of life (QOL)** has emerged as a broad, multidimensional description of a client's health and functional status. Cella (1994) proposed two domains for QOL measurement: subjectivity and multidimensionality. *Subjectivity* refers to clients' perceptions of satisfaction with their functional level, including activities of daily living (e.g., dressing) and independent living skills (e.g., shopping). Older adults typically equate their health status with how well they can function on a daily basis. *Multidimensionality* refers to physical, functional, emotional, and social well-being.

Through her classic nursing research with cancer clients, Ferrell (1996) conceptualized QOL as having four domains: physical, psychological, social, and spiritual well-being. When caring for any client with a major health problem, consider the importance of all domains. Medical-surgical nurses often become focused only on the physical aspects of care, but the other domains are equally important to clients.

A holistic nursing specialty that emphasizes the relationship between spirituality and health is **parish nursing** (Tuck, Wallace, & Pullen, 2001). Parish nurses are generally affiliated with one or more churches, and foster health promotion and education for members of the church, especially those with identified health care needs. Some nurses provide their services on a part-time volunteer basis, whereas others are paid for their services.

Health Promotion and Protection

Health promotion and protection refers to activities that are directed toward developing a person's resources to maintain or enhance well-being as a protection against illness. Reversing the emphasis from curing a disease to promoting health provides a more positive orientation for health care. Illness no longer needs to be the primary focus of health care. In addition, illness care is much more expensive than health promotion.

In 1990, the U.S. Department of Health and Human Services (DHHS) joined the world mission to promote health in its "Healthy People 2000" campaign. The expectation was that individuals would be healthier and would be practicing healthier lifestyles by the year 2000. In particular, the agenda called for health care access for everyone, a longer life expectancy, and equal life expectancy for individuals of all cultures. These goals have not been met. For example, some ethnic groups in the United States–especially Hispanics, black individuals, Asian Americans, and Pacific Islanders–continue to have shorter life expectancies than other groups.

"Healthy People 2010" (DHHS, 2000) has been published to revise these goals and present a more aggressive plan to improve the nation's health by focusing on health promotion practices. This plan has two overall national health goals:

- Increase quality and years of healthy life
- Eliminate health disparities among different demographic groups in the United States

The Healthy People (HP) initiative focuses on 28 areas devoted to an array of diseases, conditions, and public health challenges. Each focus area lists specific health objectives to meet by 2010. These objectives target interventions designed to reduce or eliminate illness, disability, and premature death. This text contains special boxes entitled "Meeting Healthy People 2010 Objectives" that list some of the key objectives from the document and the interventions that nurses can use to help meet those national health objectives.

Several nursing theorists have developed health promotion models for nursing. One of the best known models is that advocated by Pender. In her classic model, Pender (1987) makes a distinction between health promotion and illness prevention: Health promotion is not "health problem specific," but illness prevention (most recently called health protection) is. Pender believes that health promotion is a positive activity, whereas illness prevention is an avoidance activity.

Although this text integrates health promotion and illness prevention (health protection), it recognizes that the two concepts are somewhat different. The goal of both types of activities is to improve or maintain the client's health.

Part of the health promotion movement in nursing is reflected in the use of the term *client* rather than *patient.* The word *patient* is associated with a dependent position in a hospital, whereas the word *client* suggests an active partnership in the process of health care delivery and maintenance in any setting. Therefore *client* is the term used for the health care consumer, or "customer," in this text.

PRACTICES TO PROMOTE HEALTH

Researchers have found that certain health practices have a positive correlation with health promotion in adults. These general health practices include the following:

- Eating well-balanced meals that incorporate foods from the food pyramid, as recommended (see Figure 64-2)
- Eating moderately to maintain ideal weight and prevent obesity
- Exercising moderately on a routine schedule
- Sleeping regularly, about 8 hours each day
- Limiting alcohol consumption to a moderate amount
- Not smoking
- Keeping exposure to the sun to a minimum

These practices have been associated with high-level wellness regardless of gender, age, or economic status. The greater the number of these practices followed in a consistent, routine manner, the better the health state.

PRACTICES TO PREVENT ILLNESS

Illness prevention is related to health protection and maintenance. Prevention is essential for decreasing the occurrence of illness. Preventive health behavior is described as a voluntary action taken by a person or group to decrease the potential or actual threat of illness and its harmful consequences. Ethnic groups vary in the ways that they promote health, especially prevention and early detection. Throughout this text, these cultural considerations are discussed where appropriate.

Individuals must be motivated and educated to make health-related changes. However, each individual must choose whether or not to make these changes. Three levels of illness prevention are summarized in Table 1-3: primary, secondary, and tertiary.

Primary Prevention

Primary prevention is used to avoid or delay the actual occurrence of a specific disease. Strategies for health maintenance raise the general level of health and well-being of a person, family, or community. Attending smoking cessation clinics, receiving immunizations, and using seat belts are examples of primary prevention strategies.

Secondary Prevention

The purpose of **secondary prevention** is early detection of a disease or condition, sometimes before the signs and symptoms are evident. The emphasis is on early diagnosis and treatment as well as on intervention to prevent or limit permanent disability or death. Screening procedures, such as obtaining a Papanicolaou (Pap) smear for detecting cervical cancer, are examples of secondary prevention.

Tertiary Prevention

Tertiary prevention involves rehabilitation and begins when the disease or condition has stabilized and no further healing is expected. An example is cardiac rehabilitation after a myocardial infarction. The goal is to return the person to the highest level of function and to prevent severe disabilities.

TABLE 1-3 Examples of Health Behaviors for the Three Levels of Illness Prevention

Level	Examples of Behaviors
Primary prevention	Wearing seat belts Eating well-balanced meals Not smoking Consuming no or minimal alcohol Being immunized Maintaining ideal body weight
Secondary prevention	Having yearly Papanicolaou (Pap) smear tests Performing a monthly breast or testicular self-examination Having mammograms as recommended Having routine tonometry tests to detect glaucoma
Tertiary prevention	Following a cardiac rehabilitation program Pursuing rehabilitation programs for stroke, head injury, or arthritis

Consumer Education and Awareness

Consumer education and awareness is a major focus in an attempt to influence individuals and promote wellness. Information about nutrition, exercise, stress management, and routine health examinations is available at schools, work sites, and community centers, as well as in the media. This abundance of information and materials is a major resource for increasing public awareness of the need for health promotion. The Internet provides access to a vast amount of professional and public health information. See the Evolve website at http://www.evolve.elsevier.com/Iggy/ for a list of commonly used websites, including the website for the complete "Healthy People 2010" document.

ROLE OF THE MEDICAL-SURGICAL NURSE

Medical-surgical nursing is one of the many specialties in nursing, yet its scope is much broader than other specialties such as cardiovascular or orthopedic nursing. In 1991, the Academy of Medical-Surgical Nurses (AMSN) was formed as the first specialty organization for this group of nurses. AMSN has published standards for medical-surgical nursing and a core curriculum. The official journal of the AMSN is *MEDSURG Nursing: The Journal of Adult Health.*

The focus of **medical-surgical nursing** is on the adult client with acute or chronic illness in any health care setting or on the client who is at risk for illness (Figure 1-4). Nurses who specialize in medical-surgical nursing need to have a broad knowledge of the biologic, psychological, and social sciences because their clients have a range of needs. The overall outcome of care is similar to that for any other specialty—the achievement of an optimal level of wellness and the prevention of illness.

Because the typical client is usually older than 65 years of age, medical-surgical nurses need a strong background in **gerontology,** or the care of older adults. In this text, charts

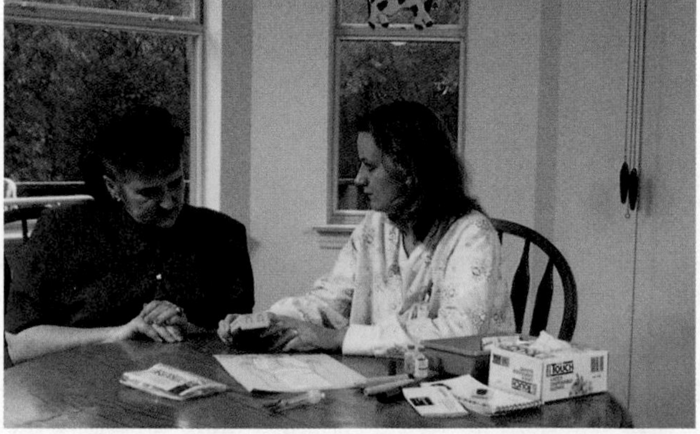

Figure 1-4 ■ Medical-surgical nurses care for adult clients in various settings with such chronic disorders as diabetes mellitus. (From Harkreader, H.C. [2004]. Fundamentals of nursing: Caring and clinical judgment [2nd ed.]. Philadelphia: W.B. Saunders.)

entitled Nursing Focus on the Older Adult highlight the special nursing interventions required for this group of clients. In addition, Considerations for Older Adults are discussed as appropriate throughout this text.

As medical-surgical nursing meets changing health care needs, the expectations for providing client care expand and increase. Medical-surgical nurses assume various roles and functions within a number of health care settings (Figure 1-5). Although each role is associated with specific responsibilities, some aspects are interrelated and are common to all nursing positions and specialties. All roles require the use of critical thinking skills and behaviors.

Coordinator of Care

You cannot provide all of the care that a client needs. As a **care coordinator,** collaborate with the health care team to help the client meet expected outcomes identified as part of the interdisciplinary plan of care. Interdisciplinary clinical rounds and other methods for communication facilitate the process of planning and implementation.

Caregiver

Another role commonly associated with the medical-surgical nurse is that of **caregiver.** In this role, nurses assess clients, analyze collected information to determine clients' needs, develop nursing diagnoses and collaborative problems, plan care and carry out the plan with the health care team, and evaluate the care given. This process, which is referred to as the nursing process (discussion begins on p. 10), is used throughout this text as an organizational and practice framework.

As a caregiver, the nurse provides physical care through skills such as administering medications and performing comprehensive assessments. Some nursing tasks and activities may be delegated to assistive nursing personnel–unlicensed nursing staff members such as patient care technicians (PCTs) or patient care assistants (PCAs). Interventions that you may delegate are indicated throughout this text and in the Client Care Plans. The nurse also implements psychosocial and spiritual interventions, such as encouraging the client to discuss concerns with a clergyperson or offering measures to reduce anxiety.

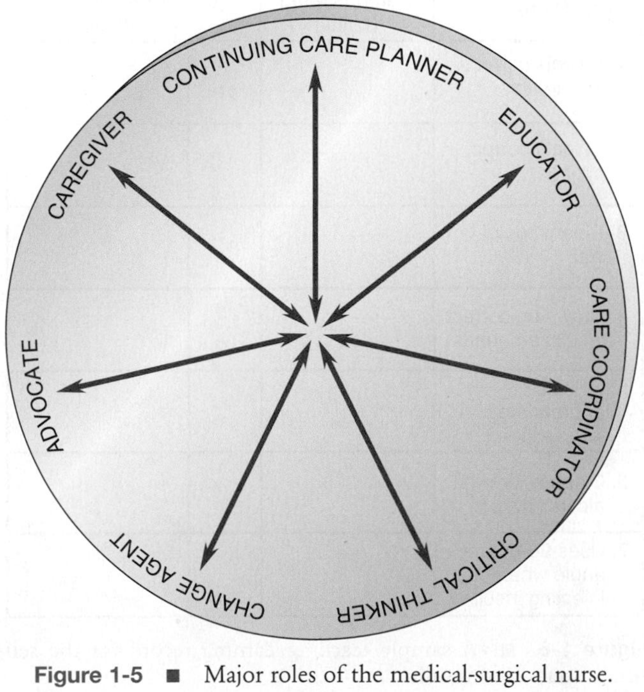

Figure 1-5 ■ Major roles of the medical-surgical nurse.

Activities performed by the nurse caregiver are often categorized as *collaborative* (interdependent) or *independent.* **Collaborative** functions include the following:

- Those that are mutually determined by the nurse and the physician or other health care team member, such as setting activity limitations or providing a special diet
- Those that are directed or prescribed by the health care provider (physician, nurse practitioner, or physician's assistant) but require nursing judgment to perform (e.g., administering medications)

Independent nursing functions are initiated and carried out by the nurse without direction from the health care provider. Examples include the following:

- Weighing a client
- Listening to breath sounds
- Elevating the head of the bed to facilitate breathing

This text discusses both types of functions–collaborative and independent–in an interrelated framework under the heading *Collaborative Management.* Charts entitled Best Practice for Nursing identify the most important nursing care for clients with selected health problems.

Continuing Care Planner

Because health care continues to emphasize early discharge from the hospital, nursing home, and home care, the role of the medical-surgical nurse as a continuing care planner has become increasingly important. This process involves an assessment of the client's health needs across the health care continuum. A large part of this process is health teaching and assessment of the home (or other setting to which the client is discharged) for available resources, support systems, and equipment, if needed.

Continuing care planning may be coordinated by a case manager or by a designated discharge planner employed by the agency in collaboration with the staff nurse. The discharge planner or case manager is usually a nurse or social worker. Chapter 3 describes case management in detail. If the agency does not employ designated discharge planners, you may be responsible for the continuing care planning. Throughout this text, sections entitled Community-Based Care are included to facilitate planning and describe settings in which continuing care may be needed (see also Chapter 2).

Educator

Client education is a major component of medical-surgical nursing care. In collaboration with the interdisciplinary health team, the nurse tries to improve health by facilitating client learning regarding health promotion, disease and illness, and specific treatment. As educators, nurses work with individual clients and family members or other caregivers. The role of education has become increasingly important because clients are discharged "quicker and sicker" from the hospital, subacute unit, or nursing home. Nurses often become frustrated when they feel they do not have the time they need to teach in these fast-paced settings.

THE TEACHING-LEARNING PROCESS

In collaboration with other members of the health care team, assess the client's learning needs and barriers to learning. A client with a disease of 20 years' duration may need as much teaching as one with a newly diagnosed condition. Make no assumptions; instead assess each client individually. Determine the client's goals and willingness to learn. If the client has no interest in learning, wait for another time or setting before beginning client education. Chart 1-1 summarizes the most important teaching-learning principles for adults.

Teaching may occur in a spontaneous, informal manner, or it may follow a more structured, formal approach based on written teaching plans. Most facilities provide written teaching plans and tools for the interdisciplinary team to ensure that every client receives the same accurate information.

The nurse documents on the appropriate record what was taught and what the client learned (Figure 1-6). Some health care agencies use a lay version of the clinical pathway as a learning tool that outlines care in a sequential manner for the client (see Developing the Collaborative Plan of Care, p. 14). In general, a summary of the teaching-learning process for each client becomes a part of the client's medical record. A copy is also given to the client or family member or significant other at discharge. Each Community-Based Care section within this text includes a subsection entitled Health Teaching. Client Education Guides for teaching clients are also included as appropriate throughout the text.

FACTORS AFFECTING THE TEACHING-LEARNING PROCESS

As interdisciplinary team members assess the teaching-learning needs of each client, they evaluate many factors that may enhance or impede learning. Some of the most important factors include the client's educational level, socioeconomic level, support system, age, and culture.

CHART 1-1

BEST PRACTICE for Adult Learning

- Assess the client's goals and willingness to learn.
- Before beginning teaching, assess how the client is feeling (e.g., a client in acute pain is unlikely to learn).
- Include family and significant others in teaching as appropriate.
- Assess factors that may influence the client's ability or motivation to learn, such as educational level, socioeconomic status, and cultural background.
- Provide pictures or other types of visual aids to reinforce learning.
- Break complex information or skills into small parts until the client learns them.
- Provide the client with "hands-on" experience for psychomotor skills, and request a return demonstration by the client (e.g., insulin administration, dressing change, colostomy care).
- Provide the client with a health resource contact for follow-up questions or concerns.

Educational Level

The client's educational level will directly affect your plans for teaching. In the United States it is estimated that more than one third of adults do not have a high school diploma. Consequently, illiteracy in the United States is widespread. Therefore information written for the public should not be above the sixth grade reading level, and it often needs to be lower.

For illiterate clients and for those with limited reading skills, use other types of visual aids (e.g., pictures and videos). When possible, explain and interpret information for clients rather than merely offering them a booklet or instruction sheet.

Socioeconomic Level

Consider the clients' financial resources when teaching them how to care for themselves at home. For example, if a client needs to perform muscle-strengthening exercises using small weights, do not expect the client to purchase expensive commercial weights. Instead, suggest the use of 1- or 2-pound coffee cans or bags, bags of sugar or flour, or similar household items.

Another concern is the cost of required medications, equipment, or supplies. Clients who do not qualify for medical assistance but work for an employer that does not provide group health insurance may not be able to afford the necessary medical items or follow-up care. As part of continuing care planning, attempt to locate resources that can provide the necessary items, such as community health organizations, churches, or lay organizations, such as the Lions Club. Clinics that specialize in providing care for working and uninsured clients are available in some parts of the United States. Some of these clinics are nurse-managed community centers.

Teaching-Learning Record for Insulin Self-Administration			
Client Steps	Taught/ Demonstrated (Initial)	Date	Return Demonstration (Initial)
1. Selects correct insulin type.			
2. Selects correct syringe.			
3. Cleans top of vial.			
4. Draws up correct insulin amount(s).			
5. Selects appropriate site for injection.			
6. Cleans skin with alcohol swipe.			
7. Uses 90-degree angle when injecting insulin.			

Figure 1-6 ■ A sample teaching-learning record for the self-administration of insulin.

Support Systems

Assess the client's support systems, including part or all of these systems in client education. Examples of support systems include families, significant others, churches, and social community clubs and organizations. In general, individuals tend to be more compliant with their health regimen if they have the encouragement of others. Support is particularly important when the client must follow many lifestyle restrictions. For instance, a farmer who is accustomed to eating fried foods and red meat may find it difficult to change to a low-fat, low-sodium diet. If the farmer's wife has always been the cook in the home, the nurse includes her in the teaching process to help ensure compliance with the new dietary restrictions.

Age

Age also affects the teaching-learning process. An older adult may take longer to process information or may have visual or hearing deficits (Chart 1-2). Provide small amounts of information at a time and check with the client before proceeding to make sure that he or she has understood. Too much information is difficult to comprehend and absorb, and this usually results in frustration and noncompliance.

Cultural Considerations

Consider the client's cultural background before teaching. If the client does not clearly understand the primary language, locate resources that can help with the teaching process. For example, many individuals who immigrated to the United States in the 1940s have attempted to retain their language and culture and not become too "Americanized." As a result, when interacting with health care professionals, they may need someone to interpret for them.

Another factor to consider during health teaching is the health practices of various cultures. For example, Mexican Americans, particularly those living near the Mexican border, often use *curandismo* (folk medicine) either because they cannot afford Westernized health care or because they prefer their own medical traditions. These clients may also avoid the health care system because of limitations in speaking, reading, or writing English or Spanish.

The nurse also considers spiritual and religious differences. A client whose spiritual beliefs forbid taking medication is not likely to comply with instructions about drug therapy. This type of information is essential so you can incorporate cultural beliefs and practices into the teaching-learning process.

CHART 1-2

NURSING FOCUS on the OLDER ADULT
Facilitating Learning

- Ensure that the client wears glasses or hearing aids if needed.
- Be sure that the area for teaching has ample lighting and minimal distraction.
- Provide most of the teaching in the morning (after breakfast), before the client becomes too fatigued.
- Speak slowly and provide small amounts of new information at a time.
- Ask the client to repeat the information to make sure that he or she has learned it.
- Provide written information so the client can refer to it later if needed.

Advocate

As a client advocate, the medical-surgical nurse assists the client and family in interpreting information from other health care team members. Offer additional assistance that the client needs in making decisions about health care. Such assistance may include explaining the implications of the client's decisions and ensuring that the client receives appropriate care. For example, a client scheduled for a total knee replacement may not understand that the knee joint will be removed and replaced with a prosthesis. *If the client does not fully understand the operative procedure, notify the surgeon of the need for additional preoperative education.* The information is reinforced even if another health team member has provided it.

Change Agent

The medical-surgical nurse serves as a change agent within the work setting and within the profession. The role of the change agent involves planning and implementing a system to change the client's health-related behaviors. In the work setting, the nurse assesses the health behaviors of the client and family and identifies those that need altering. The most important factor in this process is assessing the client's readiness to change. If the client is not ready, he or she will not comply with the change, and the nurse will be ineffective in this role.

Within the community, medical-surgical nurses serve as role models and assist consumers in bringing about changes to improve the environment, work conditions, or other factors that affect health. Nurses also work together to bring about change through legislation. For example, they provide and support legislative bills that can affect a person's health status, such as those that mandate a client's bill of rights.

THE CONCEPT OF CARING

A critical attribute for medical-surgical nurses is caring. Nurse caring has been broadly described as a process, a set of actions, and an attitude that conveys physical care and emotional concern for others. Nurses have been studying and practicing caring for many years, yet confusion remains about a precise definition of caring. Debate also continues among nursing theorists and researchers regarding the best method for measuring human caring (Beck, 1999).

The results of a classic study by Barr and Bush (1998) found four factors or broad examples of caring in critical care nurses:

- Support from colleagues (nurses they work with)
- Nurses modeling care (and caring)
- Observable client progress and positive client and family interaction
- Economic/bureaucratic factors (negative factors that nurses must overcome)

When providing client care, the nurse subjects in the study stated that listening and caring were key caring techniques. Today's medical-surgical nurses who work in hospitals often feel they do not have time to listen to or show caring toward their clients. The focus of client care is often on technical tasks rather than on outcomes or psychosocial interventions such as caring. However, in keeping with the definition of health and the role of the nurse, clients need to have their biopsychosocial needs met to promote health and prevent illness.

PRACTICE SETTINGS FOR MEDICAL-SURGICAL NURSES

Medical-surgical nurses have opportunities to provide health care in a variety of settings, including hospitals, long-term care facilities, and community-based settings (Figure 1-7). Most acute care hospitals and fewer long-term or community settings are voluntarily accredited by the Joint Commission on Accreditation of Healthcare Organizations (JCAHO). This group sets standards that assure quality health care. The hospital setting is described in this chapter. Chapter 2 discusses community-based settings.

Hospitals, or **acute care facilities**, have historically been the largest employers of nurses, with slightly more than half of all nurses working within hospitals. This percentage is declining as hospitals continue to "rightsize" and as care continues to move into the community. Few hospitals are freestanding today. Most are part of an integrated health care system (IHS) or integrated health care delivery system (IHDS) that typically comprises inpatient and ambulatory facilities, and may include long-term care and home health agencies.

In the United States, most hospital care costs are paid for by third-party payers, either managed care organizations or traditional insurers. Medicare Part A (in-hospital coverage), a federal program, pays for most of the acute care given to individuals who are older than 65 years of age or who have been disabled for at least 2 years. State medical assistance programs, often managed care Medicaid, pay for some of the health care provided to clients of any age who are indigent. Chapter 3 describes managed care and case management.

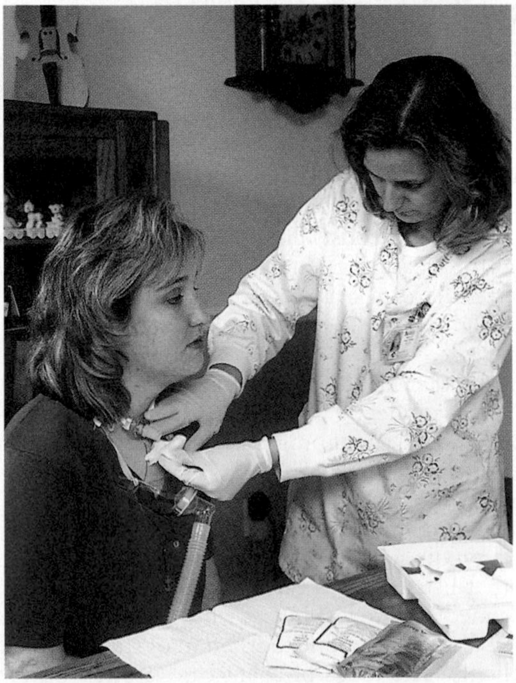

Figure 1-7 ■ Nurses often care for clients in the home. (From Harkreader, H.C. [2004]. Fundamentals of nursing: Caring and clinical judgment [2nd ed.]. Philadelphia: W.B. Saunders.)

In Canada, all individuals are entitled to free comprehensive health care for life. The Canadian government started this system in the 1960s with the belief that health care should be accessible to all Canadian citizens.

There are three general types of inpatient units in most hospital settings:

- Critical care units
- Intermediate or specialty care units
- Long-term care units (including subacute units)

Critical Care Units

Critical care units are areas for the complex, intense care of critically ill clients. Examples are surgical or medical intensive care units, shock trauma and "step-down" units, and neurosurgical intensive care units. Emergency and operating departments are also considered critical care areas because of the acute and intense nature of the care provided in these parts of the hospital. Critical care areas require nurses who thrive in crisis situations and who work effectively under high stress. Nurses in these areas must be highly skilled in making accurate observations of clients' conditions and in interpreting findings quickly and correctly. The nurse-to-client ratio in critical care units is typically 1:2 or 1:3 depending on the acuity of the clients. Critical care nursing is a subspecialty of nursing practice.

Intermediate or Specialty Care Units

Intermediate care units have changed dramatically over the past two decades. The clients in these units are much sicker today than in the past. Examples of specialty intermediate care areas are neuroscience (neurology) units, urology units, and orthopedic units. In hospitals that are too small to separate clients by specialty, intermediate care units provide treatment for a combination of multiple medical and surgical health problems.

Nurses in intermediate care areas must be able to adapt to caring for various types of illness and must be competent in health teaching and discharge planning. As in critical care areas, nurses must also be highly skilled in critical thinking and psychomotor tasks.

Long-Term Care Units

Long-term care (LTC) units may be found within or adjacent to a hospital for clients with chronic illnesses or health problems that require a finite period of medical care or rehabilitation. These units may also be referred to as transitional care units, skilled nursing facilities (SNFs), or subacute units. Most long-term care, though, is provided in freestanding nursing homes. Chapter 2 describes long-term care in more detail.

OVERVIEW OF THE NURSING PROCESS

The nursing process is an organized, systematic approach used by medical-surgical nurses to meet the individualized health care needs of their clients, families, and communities. The term nursing process emerged in the mid-1960s. As nursing became more recognized and respected as a profession, there was a growing need to define more clearly what nurses do.

Comparison of the Nursing Process with the Scientific Method

The **nursing process** is a decision-making approach that requires critical thinking. Many textbooks compare the nursing process with the scientific method of solving problems. The steps in these two approaches are similar–they both proceed from identification of the problem to evaluation of the solution. One difference is that the scientist identifies the problem first and then collects the data, whereas the nurse collects the data first and then determines the problem.

Intuitive Judgment in Nursing Practice

Over the past 20 years, research has shown that nurses sometimes use (and should use) intuitive judgment in clinical practice (Benner & Tanner, 1987). **Intuition** is the ability to understand immediately without using formal analysis; it is based on experience and knowledge, and is therefore used by experts (Alfaro-LeFevre, 2003). Intuition helps the nurse to act quickly if necessary, particularly in critical care settings or emergency situations in which he or she must assess the client and intervene at once.

The authors of this text use the nursing process as the organizing framework for its content. We do not believe that the nursing process is merely a technical skill with rules that apply in all situations but rather that nurses need to use critical thinking based on current evidence and intuition when the situation demands it.

Steps of the Nursing Process

Most literature citations list five steps for the nursing process: assessment, analysis (nursing diagnosis), planning, implementation, and evaluation. The steps are usually followed in sequence, from assessment to evaluation. However, once the nursing process begins, it is continuous or cyclic (Figure 1-8). For example, if the client's outcomes are not met on the basis of the initial evaluation, the nurse may need to reassess the client or implement new actions to help achieve the desired outcomes. To understand the nursing process as a whole, it is first necessary to briefly review each step and its associated activities. A more detailed discussion of the nursing process may be found in basic nursing textbooks.

ASSESSMENT

Assessment, the first step of the nursing process, is a systematic method of collecting data about the client, family, or community for the purpose of identifying actual and potential health problems. The **database** is the organization of assessment data and often refers to the tool or chart form used to record the data.

Admission/First Visit Database

The complete database includes a thorough health history, physical assessment, and psychosocial assessment. In the acute care setting, the admission database is usually completed during the first 8 hours after a client's admission to the hospital. Assessments are updated at least every shift throughout the client's stay. In the home or ambulatory care setting, complete the database during the first visit and update it during subsequent visits.

In the skilled nursing unit or nursing home, the admission nursing assessment is documented within the first 24 hours. The federally mandated and standardized interdisciplinary Minimum Data Set (MDS) requires initial completion within 5 days of admission.

The information collected by the nurse is *not* a repetition of the medical history recorded by the health care provider. A *medical* history is obtained by the health care provider to determine the presence of a pathologic condition and to provide a basis for planning medical care. A **nursing history** is obtained by the nurse and focuses on the meaning of the illness and/or hospitalization to the client and family. It is used as a basis for planning nursing care.

Data may be organized in one of a variety of methods. In clinical practice, data are often collected by body system. In a few health care settings, human response patterns or functional health patterns are used as a framework. Some nursing programs also teach students to organize and collect data by one of these methods.

This text incorporates Gordon's (2002) **Functional Health Patterns** in the Assessment chapters (Table 1-4). In addition, the first page of each unit illustrates the relationship of health patterns, common health concepts, and major health problems discussed in this text.

Episodic, or Problem-Centered, Database

An episodic database is collected for a limited or short-term problem. It focuses on one problem, and the data collected are associated with the problem. For example, an older hospitalized woman falls while trying to get out of bed and

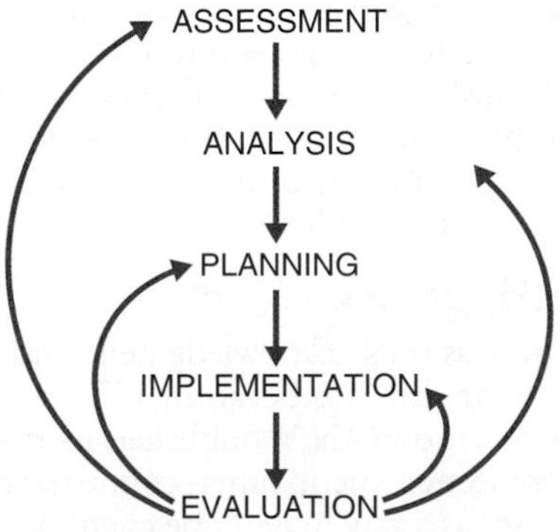

Figure 1-8 ■ The nursing process cycle.

TABLE 1-4 Gordon's Functional Health Patterns

- Health Perception—Health Management Pattern
- Nutritional-Metabolic Pattern
- Elimination Pattern
- Activity-Exercise Pattern
- Sleep-Rest Pattern
- Cognitive-Perceptual Pattern
- Self-Perception—Self-Concept Pattern
- Role-Relationship Pattern
- Sexuality-Reproductive Pattern
- Coping—Stress—Tolerance Pattern
- Value—Belief Pattern

Data from Gordon, M. (2002). *Manual of nursing diagnosis* (10th ed.). St. Louis: Mosby.

complains of hip pain. The nurse's history focuses on how the fall occurred, which parts of the client's body made contact with the floor, and what position she assumed after she fell. The physical assessment is centered on the neurologic and musculoskeletal systems, especially the head, hip, and knee. These data are usually recorded on a variance form, or incident report, according to agency policy.

In other situations, the nurse documents assessment findings on a flow sheet at frequent intervals during the day. For example, the client who is receiving epidural analgesia must be monitored continuously to determine whether the intervention is successful and whether adverse effects occur.

Sources of Data

Obtain and document data from several sources in the client's medical record according to the policies of the health care agency.

CLIENT

The client is the primary source of data. This information is direct and firsthand and is collected during an interview. Interviewing is a communication skill by which you can explore the thoughts, feelings, and perceptions of the client. As in the teaching-learning process, the interview process is affected by many variables, including timing, environment, and demographic factors such as age. Chart 1-3 provides tips for interviewing an older adult.

FAMILY AND SIGNIFICANT OTHERS

The client's family members or significant others are secondary sources of data and can often supplement or verify information provided by the client. They may also be able to offer information about the client before the illness, provide a family history related to health and illness, and describe the client's home environment.

MEDICAL RECORDS

Previous medical histories, laboratory records, vital signs, and diagnostic reports provide pertinent data. These data can validate information identified in the current history and physical examination or can serve as a comparison to indicate changes in the client's health condition. Records from previous hospital admissions supply additional pieces of information. The client's health care provider usually requests the old records from the agency's medical records department or other health care facility where the client has sought health care.

INTERDISCIPLINARY COLLABORATION

A nurse often gathers client information in collaboration with other members of the health care team. The physician or nurse practitioner is a key source of information. A case manager or home care nurse who has worked with the client can also contribute valuable information.

When a client is admitted to the hospital from another health care facility, such as a nursing home, the hospital nurse should contact the nurse who cared for the client in the previous facility for specific client information. Most nursing homes supply a transfer form that accompanies the client to the hospital or other facility. This form describes the client's abilities and limitations, drug therapy, diet therapy, and past and current health state. This information is particularly helpful when the client cannot communicate and when no family is available.

CHART 1-3

NURSING FOCUS on the OLDER ADULT
Interviewing

- Review old records and the medical history, if available, before interviewing the client.
- Provide as much privacy as possible.
- Ask the client whether family or significant others should be present during the interview.
- Refer to the client by his or her last name (e.g., Mrs. Brown) unless he or she prefers another name.
- Make sure that eyeglasses, contact lenses, and hearing aids are available and working properly (if the client wears these devices).
- Conduct the interview when the client is not experiencing pain and after basic comfort needs have been met.
- Before conducting the interview, allow the client to adjust to a new environment.
- Sit at the client's eye level during the interview.
- Speak clearly, slowly, and in a low-pitched voice; do not shout.
- Be aware that the client may not be able to distinguish soft consonant blends such as "sh" or "ch."
- Interview in the morning, after breakfast, or in the early afternoon, after the client has rested.
- Whenever possible, use open-ended questions to gather more information; avoid questions that can be answered "yes" or "no."
- Consider the client's education, culture, and age when phrasing questions, especially about sensitive or controversial issues.
- Observe the client's nonverbal behavior as well as what he or she says.

ANALYSIS

The second step of the nursing process is the analysis of data. In this phase, summarize and analyze the data, and draw conclusions to determine what health problems the client may have or is at risk for. Compare client data with "normal" findings and behaviors for the client's age, education, and cultural background. Review abnormal data to determine patterns of altered functioning. Client health problems are identified and categorized as potential problems requiring prevention or as actual problems being managed or requiring interventions.

In their classic book, Aspinall and Tanner (1981) state that nurses make two types of judgments or conclusions about the health state of a client: (1) those health problems that nurses, "by virtue of their education and experience, are licensed and able to treat" (nursing diagnoses), and (2) those problems that are diagnosed and treated by other members of the health care team but require continued nursing assessment and implementation of therapeutic interventions (collaborative problems) (p. 4). This textbook uses nursing diagnoses and collaborative problems that incorporate both types of client health problems.

Nursing Diagnoses

The nursing profession's acknowledgment and endorsement of the term *nursing diagnosis* began in 1973 when the American Nurses Association (ANA) published its first *Standards of Nursing Practice.* Since then, other countries have adopted nursing diagnoses as a way to describe client health problems.

Although many definitions of nursing diagnosis have been proposed by various nursing leaders, the authors of this text recognize the official definition approved by the North American Nursing Diagnosis Association (NANDA) at its Ninth Conference in 1990: "A nursing diagnosis is a clinical judgment about an individual, family, or community response to actual or potential health problems/life processes which provides the basis for definitive therapy toward achievement of outcomes for which the nurse is accountable" (Carpenito, 1995, p. 65).

Unlike medical diagnoses, which identify illness, nursing diagnoses identify the *responses* to health problems and life processes such as aging or death. A medical diagnosis is the basis for medical interventions; a nursing diagnosis is the basis for nursing interventions. Nursing diagnoses are not diagnostic tests, medical treatments, or problems experienced by the nurse while caring for the client (Table 1-5).

Since 1973, the list of nursing diagnoses has expanded. In 2003, there were 167 NANDA-approved nursing diagnoses (NANDA International, 2003). Even though these diagnoses are heavily emphasized in nursing programs, many health care facilities do not use them as they are stated in practice. JCAHO-accredited health care agencies are mandated to use an interdisciplinary, collaborative approach to client care. Therefore both collaborative problems and nursing diagnoses are discussed in this text.

Collaborative Problems

Collaborative problems, as identified in this text, are potential health problems for which the nurse monitors and helps to prevent. They often require interdisciplinary interventions. Through keen assessment skills, detect the health problem as early as possible if it occurs and notify the health care provider. Then, in collaboration with members of the interdisciplinary care team, carry out interventions to resolve the problem. An example of a collaborative problem is Potential for Hypoglycemia for a client with diabetes.

PLANNING

The planning step follows the analysis step of the nursing process. Throughout the planning process, the nurse performs several important functions: setting priorities and expected outcomes, selecting nursing interventions, and determining resources.

Setting Priorities and Outcomes

After analyzing the needs of the client to identify client health problems, decide on the urgency of these problems. This step is vital because some problems are more critical than others. Problems of higher priority require more immediate intervention than problems of lower priority. Setting priorities helps you to organize and plan care to solve the most urgent problems first.

ESTABLISHING PRIORITIES

In determining the priority of the problems, consider their impact on the client. Priorities may fluctuate as the client's level of wellness changes. Consider both actual and potential problems when establishing priorities. Actual problems are usually more important than potential problems; however, potential problems may at times be more important. For example, in a client who has had a stroke (brain attack), the Risk for Aspiration related to impaired swallowing is potentially more life threatening than the actual problem of Constipation related to immobility. Ensuring that any client has an effective airway is always the most important priority when rendering care. To help you learn and practice priority setting, the critical thinking challenges in this text ask you to establish priorities in specific clinical scenarios.

ESTABLISHING OUTCOMES

If possible, the client and the nurse then try to reach a mutual decision regarding expected outcomes on the basis of identified nursing diagnoses and collaborative problems. Outcomes serve as guides for selecting nursing interventions and for determining criteria for evaluating nursing interventions. The purpose of writing **expected outcomes** is to assist in evaluating the client's progress and in determining the resolution of the client's problem if possible.

Expected outcomes have the following characteristics:

- Client-centered
- Realistic in terms of the client's potential for achievement and the nurse's ability to help the client achieve them
- Specific and measurable to the extent possible, using **indicators**

Moorhead, Johnson, and Maas (2004) updated the Nursing Outcomes Classification (NOC) system, which lists evidence-based expected outcomes with indicators that determine whether outcomes were met. Like the NANDA nursing diagnoses, the outcomes are alphabetized using broad labels. For example, Aspiration Prevention is an NOC outcome that is defined as "personal actions to prevent the passage of fluid and solid particles into the lung (Moorhead, Johnson, & Maas, 2004, p. 153). Two of the indicators for Aspiration Prevention are:

- Positions self upright for eating/drinking
- Selects food according to swallowing ability

For a specific client who is at risk for aspiration, the nurse can rate whether or not the client demonstrated the indicators

TABLE 1-5 Differentiation Between Medical and Nursing Diagnoses

Medical Diagnosis	Nursing Diagnosis
Identifies the pathologic basis for an illness	Identifies a response to illness
Focuses on the physical condition of the client	Focuses on the physical, psychosocial, and spiritual needs of the client
Addresses actual, existing problems	Addresses actual and potential problems
Is not validated with the client	Is validated with the client if possible
Uses standardized goals and treatments	Uses individualized outcomes and interventions
May not be resolvable	Is usually resolvable

using a rating scale of 1 to 5 (5 being the best). If the client received a 4 or 5 for the desired indicators, the outcome of Aspiration Prevention was met. Otherwise, the outcome was not met.

This text incorporates NOC outcomes where appropriate and presents selected indicators to help you determine if the outcomes were met. The rating scales are not included due to space constraints, but you can refer to the NOC text reference listed in this chapter's Selected Bibliography (Moorhead, Johnson, & Maas, 2004) for that information.

Selecting Nursing Interventions

After determining the outcomes, develop strategies to accomplish them. Nursing interventions, also known as nursing actions or measures, are designed to assist the client in achieving the desired outcomes. They are based on the client's health problems and define activities required to promote, maintain, or restore health.

McCloskey and Bulechek (2000) define an **intervention** as "any treatment, based upon clinical judgement and knowledge, that a nurse performs to enhance patient/client outcomes" (p. 3). In 1992 these authors published the results of the first phase of the Iowa Intervention Project. This research produced a Nursing Interventions Classification (NIC) system of 336 standardized nursing interventions. The newest update includes 514 evidence-based interventions that have been supported by a number of nursing specialty organizations (Dochterman & Bulechek, 2004).

As with the development of nursing diagnoses and NOC, NIC is intended to help nurses standardize their terminology and practice.

Using NIC, the primary intervention for a Risk for Aspiration related to impaired swallowing is Aspiration Precautions. This intervention is defined as "prevention or minimization of risk factors in the [client] at risk for aspiration" (Dochterman & Bulechek, 2004, p. 175). A number of specific activities are associated with this intervention, such as the following:

- Maintain an airway.
- Monitor pulmonary status.
- Feed in small amounts.
- Cut food into small pieces.

These actions direct the nurse or other health care team member in providing evidence-based client care.

NIC interventions and activities are included throughout the Interventions chapters of this text as appropriate and space allows. Refer to the NIC text reference listed in the Selected Bibliography (Dochterman & Bulechek, 2004) for more information.

Developing the Collaborative Plan of Care

The Joint Commission on Accreditation of Healthcare Organizations (JCAHO) mandates that its accredited agencies establish a collaborative plan of care for its clients. The **collaborative plan of care (POC)** is an interdisciplinary document that outlines the essential aspects of client care, often across a time sequence. One format that may be used is a clinical pathway, which is also called a critical path, care map, or coordinated POC.

The **clinical pathway (CP)** delineates what care must be provided, who will provide the care, and when the care will be provided. It is a guideline for care that can be individualized if needed. Most pathways also list expected outcomes for the client, which may be hourly, daily, or weekly depending on the nature of the health care setting. CPs are typically used in acute care, subacute care, and rehabilitation settings. This text provides several samples of clinical pathways on the Evolve website.

A number of health care agencies do not use pathways, and instead use interdisciplinary care plans, similar in format to traditional nursing care plans. Various members of the health care team develop the plan of care as appropriate for the client, and all members monitor the client's progress in meeting expected outcomes.

This text includes sample Client Care Plans. Although these plans of care are not interdisciplinary, they are helpful for beginning students to learn the steps of the nursing process and to identify the rationale (scientific evidence) for selected nursing interventions. Interventions that the nurse can delegate to assistive nursing personnel are specified. This format is no longer used in most clinical practice settings because JCAHO does not require the use of columnar care plans. Instead JCAHO requires evidence that nurses plan and implement care on the basis of identified client health problems and in collaboration with the interdisciplinary team.

To save time and duplication, a number of computer programs and books have been developed to create standardized plans of care or clinical pathways that can be individualized as needed. As technology advances, these programs should be more widely available to nurses in all health care settings.

This text also provides examples of visual plans of care known as **concept maps,** sometimes referred to as clinical care maps or clinical correlation maps. These concept maps present assessment data, nursing diagnoses/collaborative problems, and collaborative care for clients with complex health problems. NIC and NOC categories are included as needed. The maps show the relationships among these components, thus enabling you to see the "big picture" regarding the client's interdisciplinary care. Concept maps are not used in the clinical practice setting, but they provide a learning tool for summarizing client care and stimulating critical thinking (Ignatavicius, 2004).

Determining Resources

When planning nursing interventions, determine what resources are necessary for implementation of these interventions. The client is a valuable source of information about health care resources that were successful in the past. For example, the client with an irritated stoma may mention that an enterostomal therapist was helpful with previous problems. Including the client and family in planning care often promotes their cooperation during the implementation phase.

Other nurses and health care team members are valuable resources. An interdisciplinary conference or "walking rounds" during which health care team members identify problems and the resources to solve them may be very helpful, especially in planning community-based care.

When the financial feasibility of the plan is explored, consider the availability of other resources for the client, such as equipment, time, personnel, and money. The client's value system is also considered. For instance, if the client requires dialysis in the home, the type of system implemented depends on the home water supply, electrical capability, space, available money, spiritual beliefs, and personal support system.

IMPLEMENTATION

Implementation involves the actual carrying out of a specific, individualized POC. This step of the nursing process is the action phase, in which the nurse assumes responsibility for implementing the POC based on the nursing diagnosis and collaborative problems. Best practice interventions are based on scientific evidence, identified standards of care and, at times, intuitive judgment. Best Practice for Nursing interventions are summarized in charts throughout this text. Because planning and implementation are closely related, this text discusses them under one heading, Planning and Implementation, with expected outcomes and interventions clearly labeled.

EVALUATION

Evaluation, the fifth step of the nursing process, is a cognitive activity that completes the nursing process by indicating the degree to which the client's expected outcomes have been met.

Although evaluation is given as the final step of the nursing process, it is an ongoing and integral part of each step of the process (see Figure 1-8). Review the data to determine whether sufficient information was collected and whether the appropriate behaviors were identified. Nursing diagnoses and collaborative problems are evaluated for their accuracy and completeness. Examine the expected outcomes, indicators, and interventions to determine whether they were realistic, achievable, and effective.

The result of evaluation may be one or a combination of the following:

- The client responded as expected and the problem is resolved. No additional nursing actions are needed.
- Client behaviors indicate that the client's problem has not been resolved. Re-evaluation will continue.
- Client behaviors are similar to those present initially. Little or no evidence is available to show that the problem has been resolved. Reassessment and replanning are needed.
- Client behaviors indicate a new problem. Assessment, planning, and implementation of an additional plan of action are needed to resolve the problem.

In this text, NOC outcomes are listed under the Planning and Implementation and Evaluation: Outcomes sections.

Documentation

Documentation of each phase of the nursing process is essential and is accomplished by various means. Two general, traditional methods of documentation are still used in many health care settings: (1) source-oriented charting, which usually includes narrative notes that organize varied data and are entered into the medical record by health care professionals (e.g., nurses' notes, physicians' progress notes, dietary notes), and (2) the problem-oriented record (POR), in which a master health problem list is developed. Each problem is numbered, and all chart entries refer to one of the problems identified on the list. This system is used less often.

In the POR system, all health care professionals may record their notes in a SOAP, SOAPIER, or PIE format (or one of its many variations) and on the same progress note form in the chart. The initials represent **S**ubjective data, **Ob**jective data, **A**nalysis, **P**lan of action, **I**nterventions, **E**valuation, and **R**evision of the plan. This technique of documentation is systematic and limits data to only pertinent information related to the identified problem. Although this system assists the nurse in addressing each step of the nursing process, it is very time consuming and promotes duplication of record keeping. Some physicians, social workers, and dietitians still use the SOAP format, but new systems for nursing documentation have been and are being developed.

DOCUMENTATION SYSTEMS

Focus Charting

A useful format in documentation is focus charting. Focus charting is not limited to specific client health problems but instead encourages nurses to document any significant changes in the client's condition, any client concern, or any significant client event. As seen in Figure 1-9, the record has three columns. The actual notes are divided into **D**ata, **Ac**tion, and **R**esponse information. An **E** may be added for documenting client **E**ducation. This technique helps locate desired information but still uses the familiar narrative approach to recording pertinent data.

Charting by Exception

Another system is charting by exception (CBE). CBE was started at St. Luke's Hospital in Milwaukee, Wisconsin, in an attempt to save nursing time. It incorporates three basic components (Burke & Murphy, 1988):

- Comprehensive flow sheets that list normal findings and require the nurse to initial them if they are present. If the findings are not present, the nurse writes an entry into the notes.
- References to preestablished nursing standards. The nurse initials the appropriate space when they are completed.

Date/Time	Focus/Problem	Notes
4/11/05 2:15 P.M.	Fever	D: T = 102.2° (R); face flushed; diaphoretic A: Give Tylenol 2 tab as ordered. Recheck temp. in 1 hr. R. Jones, RN
4/11/05 3:15 P.M.	Fever	R: T = 100.2° (R); face not flushed; not diaphoretic D. Ignas, LPN
4/12/05 3:30 A.M.	Impaired skin	D: 2-cm reddened area over coccyx; blanches A: Positioned on (L) side N. Smith, RNC

Figure 1-9 ■ A sample of focus charting.

- Bedside accessibility of forms. All flow sheets are kept at the bedside, which prevents wasting the nurse's time in looking for a client's chart. Bedside charting also prevents transcription of data from one form to another, which can lead to errors and wasted time. The information is available for any health care professional to read.

Many acute care facilities have a modified form of CBE and use a variety of flowsheets. Many agencies do not have bedside charting due to recent federal laws and regulations that protect the client's privacy.

Computerized Nursing Information Systems (NIS)

One major advantage of documentation systems such as CBE is the ability to transfer the concept to computerization. **Electronic charting**, also known as point-of-care charting and online documentation, is common in hospitals, nursing homes, home care agencies, and ambulatory care settings. The literature suggests that the major advantages of point-of-care documentation are accuracy and time savings. Electronic charting at the bedside also increases the time that the nurse spends in the client's room. The goal of any system should be to streamline or diminish paperwork and save valuable time, giving nurses more time for direct client care. Some health care facilities are adding NANDA diagnoses, NOC, and NIC to their documentation systems.

LEGAL ASPECTS OF DOCUMENTATION

Regardless of the type of documentation system used, remember that the client's chart is a legal document. Chart 1-4 lists basic charting guidelines that all nurses should follow. Further discussion of documentation can be found in basic fundamental nursing texts.

CHART 1-4

BEST PRACTICE for Nursing Documentation

- Write clearly and legibly.
- Do not erase or "white-out" any part of the client's record.
- To correct an error, use one line to cross out the incorrect entry, then initial the change.
- Use only standard and facility-approved abbreviations and symbols.
- Document significant information as close as possible to the time it is collected instead of waiting until the end of a shift.
- Transcribe physicians' orders carefully and correctly.
- If using nurses' notes or progress notes, do not leave blank spaces between entries.
- Time and date each entry on the client's record.
- Use only blue or black ink (it visualizes best for copies or microfilm).
- Document like a reporter: State facts objectively and avoid judgment or criticism.
- Do not state that "an incident report has been completed" or refer to any unusual occurrence or special event as an "incident."
- Follow all facility policies for documentation.
- To add one or two words, use a caret (^) and insert the words, then initial the change; if agency policy does not allow this practice, write a late entry.
- To make a late entry, begin by stating that it is a "Late entry for (date and time);" if the entry is more than a day late, state the reason for the late entry (e.g., "on vacation for 3 days").
- If an order is discontinued on the record as indicated by a highlighter, be sure that the original can still be read, especially on copies.

GET READY for the NCLEX Examination!

KEY POINTS

- Critical Thinking is purposeful, outcome-directed thinking involving judgment based on sound, scientific evidence.
- Evidence-based practice is the care that nurses should provide that is grounded in research and other sources of science.
- Health is a continuum from wellness to death; holistic health considers the interrelationship of the mind, body, and spirit.
- Health promotion and protection (illness prevention) refers to activities that the nurse and other health care professionals implement to maintain or enhance wellness.
- Healthy People 2010 is a set of goals for individuals in the United States to improve health for all.
- Three levels of illness prevention—primary, secondary, and tertiary—are available to help clients stay healthy or achieve optimal wellness (see Table 1-3).
- The medical-surgical nurse functions as a coordinator of care, caregiver, continuing care planner, educator, client advocate, and change agent.
- The teaching-learning process is affected by a person's educational level, age, socioeconomic level, support systems, and culture.
- The information in Chart 1-1 and Chart 1-2 summarizes the important points related to the adult learning process, including special needs of older adults.
- The steps of the nursing process are assessment, analysis (nursing diagnoses), planning Nursing Outcomes Classification), implementation (Nursing Interventions Classification), and evaluation. Gordon's Functional Health Patterns help to organize data collection during the client interview (see Table 1-4).
- Chart 1-4 summarizes important information regarding the legal aspects of clinical documentation.

ADDITIONAL STUDY RESOURCES

Go to your Student CD-ROM for Review Questions for the NCLEX Examination.

evolve Go to http://evolve.elsevier.com/Iggy/ for Integrated Management of Care Questions for the NCLEX Examination.

SELECTED BIBLIOGRAPHY

Asterisk indicates a classic or definitive work on this subject.

Ackley, B.J., & Ladwig, G.B. (2002). *Nursing diagnosis handbook: A guide to planning care.* St. Louis: Mosby.

Alfaro-LeFevre, R. (2002). *Applying the nursing process: Promoting collaborative care.* Philadelphia: J.B. Lippincott.

Alfaro-LeFevre, R. (2003). *Critical thinking in nursing: A practical approach* (3rd ed.). Philadelphia: W.B. Saunders.

Alfaro-LeFevre, R. (2004). Critical thinking indicators: 2004 evidence-based version. www.alfaroteachsmart.com.

*Allen, K.M., & Phillips, J.M. (1997). *Women's health across the life-span: A comprehensive perspective.* Philadelphia: Lippincott-Raven.

*Aspinall, M.J., & Tanner, C. (1981). *Decision-making for patient care.* Norwalk, CT: Appleton & Lange.

*Barr, W.J., & Bush, H.A. (1998). Four factors of nurse caring in the ICU. *Dimensions of Critical Care Nursing, 17*(4), 214-223.

*Beck, C.T. (1999). Quantitative measurement of caring. *Journal of Advanced Nursing, 30*(1), 24-32.

*Benner, P., & Tanner, C. (1987). How expert nurses use intuition. *American Journal of Nursing, 87,* 23-31.

*Bower, F. (1972). The process of planning nursing care. St. Louis: Mosby.

*Burke, L.J., & Murphy, J. (1988). *Charting by exception: A cost-effective, quality approach.* New York: John Wiley & Sons.

*Carpenito, L.J. (1995). *Nursing care plans and documentation: Nursing diagnoses and collaborative problems.* Philadelphia: J.B. Lippincott.

*Cella, D.F. (1994). Quality of life: The concept and definition. *Journal of Pain and Symptom Management, 6,* 186-192.

Coyle, G.A., & Heinen, M. (2002). Scan your way to a comprehensive electronic record. *Nursing Management, 33*(12), 56-60.

*Davis, C.M., & Curley, C.M. (1999). Disparities of health in African Americans. *Nursing Clinics of North America, 34*(2), 345-355.

Dochterman, J.M., & Bulechek, G.M. (2004). *Nursing Interventions Classification (NIC)* (4th ed.). St. Louis: Mosby.

*Dunn, H.L. (1980). *High level wellness.* Thorofare, NJ: Charles B. Slack.

*Eggland, E.T. (1995). Charting smarter: Using new mechanisms to organize your paperwork. *Nursing95, 25*(9), 34-41.

*Facione, N.C., & Facione, P.A. (1996). Externalizing the critical thinking in knowledge development and clinical judgment. *Nursing Outlook, 44*(3), 129-136.

*Ferrell, B.R. (1996). The quality of lives: 1,525 voices of cancer. *Oncology Nursing Forum, 23*(6), 907-916.

*Flaskerud, J.H., & Kim, S. (1999). Health problems of Asian and Latino immigrants. *Nursing Clinics of North America, 34*(2), 359-380.

Gordon, M. (2002). *Manual of nursing diagnosis* (10th ed.). St. Louis: Mosby.

Ignatavicius, D.D. (2001). Six critical thinking skills for at-the-bedside success. *Nursing Management, 32*(1), 37-39.

Ignatavicius, D.D. (2004). From traditional care plans to innovative concept maps. In *Annual Review of Nursing Education.* New York: Springer.

Jarvis, C. (2004). Physical examination and health assessment (4th ed.). Philadelphia: W.B. Saunders.

Lew, P.S., & Latney. C. (2002). Achieve best practices with an evidence-based approach. *Nursing Management, 33*(12), 24-30.

McCloskey, J.C., & Bulechek, G.M. (2000). *Nursing interventions classification (NIC)* (3rd ed.). Philadelphia: W.B. Saunders.

Mohide, E.A., & King, B. (2003). Building a foundation for evidence-based practice: Experiences in a tertiary hospital. *Evidence-Based Nursing, 6*(4), 100-103.

Moorhead, S., Johnson, M., & Maas, M. (2004). *Nursing outcomes classification (NOC)* (3rd ed.). St. Louis: Mosby.

NANDA International (2003). *NANDA nursing diagnoses: Definitions and classification 2003-2004.* Philadelphia: Author.

Narayanasamy, A., & Owens, J. (2001). A critical incident study of nurses' responses to the spiritual needs of their patients. *Journal of Advanced Nursing, 33*(4), 446-455.

Nay, R. (2003). Evidence-based practice: Does it benefit older people and gerontic nursing? *Geriatric Nursing, 24*(6), 338-342.

*Pender, N.J. (1987). *Health promotion in nursing practice* (2nd ed.). Norwalk, CT: Appleton & Lange.

Thurmond, V.A. (2001). The holism in critical thinking. A concept analysis. *Journal of Holistic Nursing, 19*(4), 375-389.

Tuck, I., Wallace, D., & Pullen, L. (2001). Spirituality and spiritual care provided by parish nurses. *Western Journal of Nursing Research, 23*(5), 441-453.

U.S. Department of Health and Human Services, Public Health Service. (2000). *Healthy People 2010: National health promotion and disease prevention objectives.* Washington, DC: U.S. Government Printing Office.

Wilkinson, J.M. (2000). Nursing diagnosis handbook with NIC interventions and NOC outcomes (7th ed.). Upper Saddle River, NJ: Prentice Hall Health.

*World Health Organization. (1947). *Constitution of the World Health Organization: Chronicle of the World Health Organization.* Geneva: Author.

Young, K.M. (2003). Where's the evidence? *American Journal of Nursing, 103*(10), 11.

CHAPTER

2 Community-Based Care

DONNA D. IGNATAVICIUS

LEARNING OUTCOMES

After studying this chapter, you should be able to:

1. Explain the primary purpose of ambulatory care.
2. Identify the unique features of nursing primary care.
3. Discuss the growth of home care in the United States.
4. Describe the role of the nurse in home care.
5. Identify interventions for which Medicare typically pays in home care.
6. State the purpose of OASIS in home care.
7. Compare and contrast the common types of long-term care settings.
8. Differentiate assisted-living from other types of long-term care.
9. Describe the term *transitional care.*

Go to your Student CD-ROM for Review Questions for the NCLEX Examination keyed to these Learning Outcomes.

Care for medical-surgical clients can be provided in a number of settings. Community-based care may be needed after a hospital stay or as an alternative to inpatient hospital care. The current trend is toward care in alternative settings, such as ambulatory care, home care, and long-term care in rehabilitation centers, nursing homes, and chronic care facilities. This chapter provides a brief description of each of these settings, which provide varying opportunities for nursing employment.

This text covers care for clients in numerous settings in which medical-surgical nurses practice. The Community-Based Care sections that follow the discussions of major health problems highlight the most important aspects of care in nonhospital environments.

AMBULATORY CARE

Ambulatory health care is a general term for client care provided in a number of community settings, such as physician offices, hospital or freestanding outpatient clinics, freestanding surgicenters, and health maintenance organizations (a type of managed-care organization) (see Chapter 3). The purpose of ambulatory care is health promotion, health protection (illness prevention), short-term treatment (e.g., surgery), and follow-up for existing health problems.

Client visits to ambulatory care settings are episodic and based on need. For example, clients may visit their health care provider for annual physical examinations (health promotion). In some cases, they seek out providers for acute health care problems, chemotherapy, or selected surgeries, such as cataract removal or laparoscopic cholecystectomy (removal of the gallbladder). Still others are monitored periodically for chronic health conditions such as diabetes mellitus and hypertension.

Clients discharged from the hospital are often followed in one or more ambulatory care settings. Many health care providers in these settings are advanced practice nurses (APNs), such as nurse practitioners and clinical nurse specialists. The cost of ambulatory care is typically far less than that of a long-term or home care agency.

Role of the Nurse in Ambulatory Care

One of the major roles of the nurse working in an ambulatory care setting is performing health promotion activities, including client education, health screening, and comprehensive assessment. In a surgicenter, for example, the nurse provides preoperative teaching to prepare clients for the surgical procedure and postoperative expectations. Their vital signs and general condition are assessed to ensure that they are ready for the surgery.

Many physicians employ nurses to assist in their office practice. These nurses often triage clients by telephone; that is, they decide which clients need priority care and intervene accordingly. In some parts of the country, large physician practices employ nurse case managers who monitor high-risk, high-cost, problem-prone clients throughout the continuum of health care in all settings. Some may also participate in **telephonic case management**. In this case, the nurse provides information to help the client receive care in the appropriate setting. Case management is discussed in Chapter 3.

Nursing Primary Care

Nursing primary care takes place in ambulatory care settings, sometimes called community centers. Health care is provided by nurses, often in underserved areas of the country. Although the organizational structure and services provided vary among centers, most of them are affiliated with large university schools of nursing. The primary health care providers are typically nurse practitioners, nurse midwives, clinical nurse specialists, and students preparing to become one of these advanced practice specialists. The funding for nursing primary care varies. Some funding comes from city, state, and federal governments, whereas other funding comes from grants obtained by university faculty.

HOME CARE

Home care in the United States and other countries is a diverse industry. For many clients the home not only is the preferred health care setting but is also the lowest cost setting. **Home care** is part of a continuum of comprehensive health care in which health services are provided to individuals and families in their place of residence. The goal is to promote, maintain, or restore health or to maximize the level of independence while minimizing the effects of disability and illness, including terminal illness (Marrelli & Krulish, 1999).

Historical Perspective and Trends in Home Care Nursing

Modern home care nursing has its roots in public health and community health nursing models. In the mid-1880s, visiting nurse associations (VNAs) evolved in Philadelphia, Boston, and Buffalo, New York. The traditions of Lillian Wald, who is regarded as the founder of public health nursing, began with the Henry Street Settlement in New York City in 1893. During the early twentieth century, most of the home care in the United States was provided by VNAs and the nursing divisions of governmental health agencies. Public health principles and practices, as well as components of family and community care, were integrated into home health nursing services. Nurses provided health promotion services to individuals, families, and communities while continuing to provide nursing care to the sick.

Many factors have contributed to the acceptance of home care, including the following:

- A continued shift from inpatient-based care to community-based care and home care, including palliative care (care of dying clients)
- Increased acceptance by the medical community and the consumer community that home care is often a viable alternative to institutional care
- Baby boomers who, as they get older, are becoming more educated about health care alternatives and are becoming more involved in the decision-making process
- An aging population that has increased the need for health care for older adults
- Technology such as mobile x-ray machines, apnea monitors, and electrocardiographs, which allow clients to remain safely at home while having their health needs monitored; the introduction of telehealthcare services allows even more ways for clients to be monitored from their home (Kinsella, 2003)
- The generally lower cost of home care (compared to institutional care)
- The increase in managed care, which dictates a lower cost care environment

Although there has been significant growth in home care since the 1960s, the number of Medicare-certified agencies has decreased. The National Association for Home Care (NAHC) believes this recent decline to be the direct result of changes in Medicare home care reimbursement, which is now based on a prospective payment system. The amount of reimbursement using this method has declined to the point that some home care agencies have closed.

Types of Home Care

The term *home care* is used to describe a variety of products and services. There are different specialty areas within the home care industry, and nurses may work in any one of these areas. Some companies may provide all or just one of these home care services. There are generally four types of services provided by the home care industry:

1. *Skilled home care service.* This is the largest type of service, with these agencies employing most of the home care nurses and other health care professionals to provide care as needed. Skilled home care services are provided by home care organizations that are usually Medicare certified and provide two or more of the following services:
   - Nursing (RN and LPN)
   - Physical therapy (LPT, LPTA)
   - Occupational therapy (OTR, COTA)
   - Speech/language pathology
   - Social services (MSW, BSW)
   - Home care aides

   The organization may also provide respiratory therapy and other specialty services (e.g., enterostomal therapy, behavioral health nursing), depending on the specialty programs of the organization. In general, Medicare, Medicaid, and other insurance or managed care programs cover these skilled services when the qualifying criteria of the insurance program are met.
2. *Personal care or private duty service.* This type of service may provide "shifts" of nurses or home care aides to clients in their homes. It may also provide additional services such as homemaker services, transportation, respite for caregivers, meal preparation, and sitter services. Some insurance programs may pay for a limited amount of these services related to health care, but most of them are paid privately by the client or family.
3. *Home medical equipment (HME) service.* This service can also include durable medical equipment (DME). HME companies provide hospital beds, wheelchairs, bath benches, oxygen and related equipment and services, walkers, and other equipment. In general, Medicare and other insurance or managed care programs pay for HME when the qualifying criteria of the insurance program are met.
4. *Home infusion or intravenous service.* Companies providing this type of service have pharmacists that mix the infusion therapies. The company then delivers the infusion, sets it up in the home, trains the client/family on proper administration, and sometimes administers the infusion therapies. Therapies can be enteral or parenteral and can include tube feedings, antibiotics, hyperalimentation, blood and blood products, tocolytic therapy, antineoplastics,

opioid analgesics, and catecholamines. Nursing services for activities such as observation and assessment, therapy administration, site care, and line maintenance may be covered by Medicare and other insurance or managed care programs. The therapies may or may not be covered by the insurance or managed care program depending on the coverage criteria of the specific insurance program.

Role of the Nurse in Home Care

Despite all that is changing in the home care environment, one thing has remained the same: nursing is an essential component. A knowledgeable and experienced nurse is able to draw on existing resources and to "create" resources through the use of family and community support systems. This knowledge and experience, coupled with the fact that nursing is an essential component of home care, makes it possible for nurses to direct and manage home care effectively. Nurses can continue to support client advocacy by promoting nursing's unique contribution to the care of the client and caregivers.

Home care has come to mean a variety of specialized and generalized nursing care provided to clients whose primary site for health care is their home. Adult health (medical-surgical) care, child (pediatric) care, perinatal care, older adult (geriatric) care, behavioral health care, and many other specialties are practiced routinely by home care nurses. Effective home care nursing incorporates the aspects of comprehensive assessment skills with current technology and the "high-touch" care of skilled nurses. Home care *case management* uses the client care plan in conjunction with effective care coordination and ongoing communication to ensure that the client is receiving appropriate care. Collaborative communication among team members and active and ongoing client participation ensures that clients are truly equal partners in their health care. Table 2-1 compares nursing in the home care setting to nursing in the inpatient setting.

Home Visits

Home care provided by private duty or personal care companies is often rendered in "hours" or "shifts" of service delivery. In general, intermittent home care is provided in "visits" by Medicare-certified agencies. The actual visit time is the time spent in the client's home for the provision of the ordered care. The length of the visit depends on the complexity of the care being provided, the type of visit (e.g., the admission visit is typically longer because of the increased amount of data being collected and documented), how well the client tolerates the care, and how efficient the nurse is in providing the care. Although the actual visit time is the time spent in the client's home, several components go into effective visit provision:

- Visit preparation, including phone calls to the physician to clarify orders
- Phone calls to other providers involved in the client's care to coordinate care delivery
- Gathering of required documentation and supplies (wound dressings, catheter, venipuncture)
- Phone calls to insurance companies for visit authorization or care delivery updates
- Travel time to the client's home
- Completion of all necessary documentation
- Further care coordination with the physician and/or other members of the health care team

The number of visits nurses are expected to make per day varies from agency to agency. The average is four to six visits per day. The range depends on the geographic location of the clients, the complexity of the care being rendered, the type of visits, and other factors such as weather. Inclement weather poses another challenge to home care staff. Many staff use four-wheel drive vehicles, boats, and other alternate means of transportation. In areas of extremely heavy snowfall, nurses have even been known to use skis, snowmobiles, or snowshoes to ensure that they can reach their clients. Staff assignments are generally based on the geographic location of the client, the client diagnosis, and/or the service to be delivered (e.g., infusion services, cardiac services, rehabilitative services).

Client Plan of Care

As with other care settings, a physician's order is needed for care interventions and care plan changes. Because home care nursing practice is more autonomous than many inpatient settings, it is imperative that orders be obtained from physicians for care and care changes. Sometimes the physician does not see the client for months and therefore relies on the nurse's assessments and reports to assist with devel-

TABLE 2-1 Major Differences Between Nursing Care in the Home and in Inpatient Settings

Home Setting	Inpatient Setting
Nurse is more autonomous and is many times the "eyes and ears" of the physician.	Nurse relies heavily on physician directives.
Environment is controlled by the client/caregiver. Circumstances are often less than optimal for the provision of skilled care.	Environment is controlled by the facility and its staff.
Nurse must be knowledgeable about the care of all types and ages of clients.	Nurse is typically knowledgeable about the care of specific types of clients, often based on diagnosis.
Nurse must know and understand various reimbursement requirements and document accordingly.	Financial officer and accounting department usually handle reimbursement.
For older adults, only selected skilled and nonskilled services are reimbursed by Medicare.	For older adults, hospital care is largely reimbursed by Medicare.
There is limited direct supervision of assistive staff, such as home care aides.	There is continuous direct supervision of assistive staff. Nurse and staff work as a single unit.

opment and revision of the care plan. Verbal and telephone orders are a large part of the home care practice and communication with physicians. For Medicare clients, agencies generally use the Form 485 from the Centers for Medicare and Medicaid Services as the client plan of care (Figure 2-1). This plan of care is developed with input from the client/caregiver, physician, and other members of the health care team. The plan of care must be signed by the physician before the agency bills for the services rendered under the plan of care.

Medicare usually pays for home care services when the beneficiary meets one or more of certain qualifying conditions:

- The client is confined to the home.
- Services are provided under a plan of care established and approved by a physician.
- The client is under the care of a physician.
- The client needs skilled nursing care on an intermittent basis or needs physical therapy or speech-language pathology services.
- The client has a continued need for occupational therapy services.

Once client eligibility has been established, Medicare usually pays for any or all of the following skilled nursing services:

- Observation and assessment of the client's condition when only the specialized skills of a medical professional can determine a client's status
- Management and evaluation of a client care plan
- Teaching and training activities
- Administration of medications and IV fluids
- Nasopharyngeal and tracheostomy suctioning
- Urinary catheters
- Wound care

Department of Health and Human Services
Health Care Financing Administration

Form Approved
OMB No. 0938-0357

HOME HEALTH CERTIFICATION AND PLAN OF CARE

1. Patient's HI Claim No. | 2. Start Of Care Date | 3. Certification Period From: To: | 4. Medical Record No. | 5. Provider No.

6. Patient's Name and Address | 7. Provider's Name, Address and Telephone Number

8. Date of Birth | 9. Sex ☐ M ☐ F | 10. Medications: Dose/Frequency/Route (N)ew (C)hanged

11. ICD-9-CM | Principal Diagnosis | Date

12. ICD-9-CM | Surgical Procedure | Date

13. ICD-9-CM | Other Pertinent Diagnoses | Date

14. DME and Supplies | 15. Safety Measures:

16. Nutritional Req. | 17. Allergies:

18.A. Functional Limitations
1 ☐ Amputation 5 ☐ Paralysis 9 ☐ Legally Blind
2 ☐ Bowel/Bladder (Incontinence) 6 ☐ Endurance A ☐ Dyspnea With Minimal Exertion
3 ☐ Contracture 7 ☐ Ambulation B ☐ Other (Specify)
4 ☐ Hearing 8 ☐ Speech

18.B. Activities Permitted
1 ☐ Complete Bedrest 6 ☐ Partial Weight Bearing A ☐ Wheelchair
2 ☐ Bedrest BRP 7 ☐ Independent At Home B ☐ Walker
3 ☐ Up As Tolerated 8 ☐ Crutches C ☐ No Restrictions
4 ☐ Transfer Bed/Chair 9 ☐ Cane D ☐ Other (Specify)
5 ☐ Exercises Prescribed

19. Mental Status: 1 ☐ Oriented 3 ☐ Forgetful 5 ☐ Disoriented 7 ☐ Agitated
2 ☐ Comatose 4 ☐ Depressed 6 ☐ Lethargic 8 ☐ Other

20. Prognosis: 1 ☐ Poor 2 ☐ Guarded 3 ☐ Fair 4 ☐ Good 5 ☐ Excellent

21. Orders for Discipline and Treatments (Specify Amount/Frequency/Duration)

22. Goals/Rehabilitation Potential/Discharge Plans

23. Nurse's Signature and Date of Verbal SOC Where Applicable: | 25. Date HHA Received Signed POT

24. Physician's Name and Address | 26. I certify/recertify that this patient is confined to his/her home and needs intermittent skilled nursing care, physical therapy and/or speech therapy or continues to need occupational therapy. The patient is under my care, and I have authorized the services on this plan of care and will periodically review the plan.

27. Attending Physician's Signature and Date Signed | 28. Anyone who misrepresents, falsifies, or conceals essential information required for payment of Federal funds may be subject to fine, imprisonment, or civil penalty under applicable Federal laws.

Figure 2-1 ■ Centers for Medicare and Medicaid Services Form 485.

- Ostomy care
- Rehabilitation nursing
- Psychiatric evaluation, therapy, and teaching

Medicare principles governing reasonable and necessary skilled nursing services include the following (Health Care Financing Administration [HCFA], 1996):

- A skilled nursing service is a service that must be provided by a registered nurse (or a licensed practical [vocational] nurse under the supervision of a registered nurse) to be safe and effective.
- A service is not considered a skilled nursing service merely because it is performed by or under the direct supervision of a licensed nurse. A service is not considered a skilled nursing service if it can be performed safely and effectively by the average nonmedical person (or self-administered) without direct nursing supervision.
- If a service requires the skills of a licensed nurse to be provided safely and effectively, it continues to be a skilled service even if it is taught to the client/caregiver.
- The skilled nursing service must be reasonable and necessary to the diagnosis and treatment of the client's illness or injury within the context of the client's unique medical condition.

Documentation and Home Care

Reimbursement for home care relies heavily on the documentation of care. In many home care and other community-based settings, the research-based **Omaha Problem Classification System** may be used instead of the nursing diagnoses from the North American Nursing Diagnosis Association. The Omaha system delineates four general areas that represent community and home care practice and provide organizational groupings for client problems: environmental, psychosocial, physiologic, and health-related behaviors. More than 40 nursing diagnoses with modifiers such as potential deficit, deficit, and health promotion are then listed within their appropriate domains (Barrera, 2003).

Computerization and Home Care

To facilitate the documentation and communication processes, home care agencies have implemented automation. Most agencies have computerized Form 485 (Plan of Care) from the Centers for Medicare and Medicaid Services, and many agencies have implemented an electronic clinical documentation system for their client care staff. Several software products are on the market and use a variety of hardware products, from the handheld to the personal computer. For agencies that have implemented an electronic clinical documentation system, nurses carry a handheld, laptop, or other computer into the clients' homes to document their assessment findings and care delivery. This information is then transmitted to the main agency server.

One advantage of computerization is immediate access to the information by office personnel or other members of the health care team once the nurse has transmitted it to the agency. Another advantage is that the nurse can readily access client medical record information, day or night, without coming into the office. This allows more flexibility in scheduling the day. Many software programs also reduce the amount of times the information must be entered (or written if documentation is done by hand) because it flows to all appropriate locations within the documentation system. Computer literacy is becoming a requirement for nursing practice in many settings, and home care is no exception.

Telehealth and Home Care

A growing trend in home care is the use of telehealth. **Telehealth** can be defined as the "electronic provision of health care and information services for the direct benefit of individual [clients] and their families" (Russo, 2001, p. 3). This technology includes nurse-client and nurse-provider interactions, as well as education and information for nurses and clients. One of the many benefits to telehealth is increased client participation in his or her care.

Examples of technology devices include interactive video systems, monitoring technology using plain old telephones (POTs), and digital subscriber lines and the Internet. The client can contact an on-call nurse any time and set up a video visit to address the problem. Another use of the technology is nursing case management. Nurses can triage clients and prioritize which clients need attention first. The health status of the client can also be monitored. Photos of wounds, for example, allow the nurse an opportunity to track the progress of wound healing (Russo, 2001).

Outcomes and Home Care

In January 1999, new regulations were put into place that require Medicare-certified home care agencies to track and report client outcomes. The research-based tool for outcome tracking is called the **O**utcome and **AS**sessment **I**nformation **S**et (OASIS). These outcome measures are the crux of Outcome Based Quality Improvement (OBQI), a systematic approach that home care agencies can implement and follow for continuous improvement of quality of care.

Before OASIS, there was no uniform data set that agencies could use to track their own outcomes and, perhaps more important, to compare themselves to similar agencies across the United States. In a sense, the OASIS serves as a "report card" for the performance of the home care agency (Wardell, 2003).

LONG-TERM CARE

In clinical practice, long-term care (LTC) has become synonymous with nursing home care, although many clients do not stay for an extended period of time in a nursing home, and not all LTC clients are in nursing homes. Long-term care for adult clients with medical-surgical problems can occur either in the home or in facilities such as nursing homes, transitional care units, chronic care facilities, or rehabilitation centers. In general, **long-term care** implies that clients receive care for a prolonged period of time, usually weeks or months. A small percentage of clients may remain in a facility indefinitely, perhaps a lifetime. The nursing home is the most common type of LTC setting.

Common Types of Long-Term Care Settings

Long-term care settings can be divided into residential (e.g., assisted-living) facilities, nursing homes, and chronic care/extended care facilities. Some are part of retirement communities, and others have specialty units, such as dementia, ventilator, or transitional care/subacute units.

RESIDENTIAL FACILITIES

The most common type of **residential facilities** include assisted-living facilities and group homes. Some of these facilities are small and much like boarding homes before the advent of Medicare (Ignatavicius, 1998). Others are large communities managed by national corporations. Many of the larger complexes are life care or continuing care retirement centers that offer a continuum of services, from independent living to skilled care. The typical resident in a residential facility is fairly independent and is able to perform most or all self-care activities. Employees in these facilities are usually unlicensed staff, although a licensed nurse may be available during the day.

Assisted-living facilities (ALFs) are nonmedical facilities that have grown rapidly over the past 5 years in response to an expanding older adult population. Assisted-living facilities vary somewhat in their requirements for resident function, depending on available services and resources. Some states regulate these facilities as they do nursing homes because sicker and more dependent residents are being accepted.

NURSING HOMES

Nursing home care can be expensive, with annual costs between $30,000 and $45,000 in the United States. Most facilities are profit-making, proprietary organizations. As the proportion of older adults increases from 13% of the population in 2000 to 20% by 2030, the implication for increasing health care expenditures is profound. Older adults use health care services at a far greater rate than do younger adults.

Nursing homes in the United States provide care for clients with physical and cognitive impairments or chronic illness. Clients admitted to a nursing home are called **residents** because the facility is considered their home. The majority of residents are women older than 65 years of age. However, nursing homes are experiencing an increase in the number of younger residents as individuals live longer with debilitating chronic illnesses such as multiple sclerosis and traumatic brain injury (TBI).

Nursing homes have undergone another major change. Most Medicare-certified facilities are increasingly admitting short-term (less than 1 week to 2 weeks) residents for rehabilitation or recovery from an illness or injury and then discharging them to home or another setting. Clients come from hospitals "quicker and sicker," and they often require complex or continuing care. Examples of common health problems that require short-term care in a nursing home include rehabilitation for total joint replacements, serious fractures, and strokes, and continued postoperative care following major surgeries such as a coronary artery bypass graft (CABG).

Nursing homes may provide intermediate or skilled care, or a combination of these levels. Formerly called intermediate care facilities, **nursing facilities (NFs)** provide a custodial, maintenance level of care. Certified, licensed NFs receive Medicaid funding for the care of residents who cannot perform activities of daily living (ADLs) independently. Each state has specific guidelines for reimbursement.

Skilled nursing facilities (SNFs, pronounced "snifs") provide care that requires licensed health care professionals, such as nurses and therapists. Only a small portion of most nursing home residents are categorized as skilled and are therefore eligible for Medicare reimbursement. Examples of skilled care include new tube feedings, daily rehabilitative care for postoperative fractured hips, and care of stage 3 and stage 4 wounds.

Chronic or extended care facilities provide care for long-term, chronically ill clients, such those with severe head injuries or those who need chronic ventilator support. These facilities are often managed by county or state governments.

Role of the Nurse in Long-Term Care

Before 1965, LTC settings were not carefully monitored by external agencies. Poor sanitation, resident abuse, and inadequate care were common in the nursing home industry. Since 1965, nursing homes and other LTC facilities have been carefully scrutinized and highly regulated by both federal and state agencies. Nurses who work in these facilities must be aware of these laws, which are meant to protect both the residents and the staff.

In general, nurses employed in LTC facilities are more autonomous than nurses working in hospitals. Health care providers are usually not present in the LTC facility on a continuous basis, because residents in these facilities are considered to be more medically "stable" than those in acute care. With early discharge from acute care, however, LTC nurses are caring for sicker residents than in the past and therefore need increased skills and knowledge to manage them.

For the past 15 years, geriatric nursing research has helped validate best practice patterns for nurses who care for older adults in a variety of settings. Most notable is the work led by the John A. Hartford Institute for the Advancement of Geriatric Nursing Practice in New York City. Some of the areas studied include pain management, the use of physical restraints, fall prevention, and medication safety (Mezey, Fulmer, & Abraham, 2003) (Table 2-2).

Most nurses in LTC are placed "in charge" of a unit or shift because there are more unlicensed personnel (certified nursing assistants) than professional nurses. Therefore the LTC nurse needs leadership, management, and clinical competencies to function in this interdisciplinary care environment. There may be only one nurse in charge of 30 to 40 residents and a number of certified nursing assistants.

Documentation in Long-Term Care

Documentation in most LTC settings is highly regulated by both federal and state governments. The Minimum Data Set (MDS), for example, is a federally mandated assessment

TABLE 2-2 Examples of Geriatric Nursing Protocols for Best Practice

- Assessment of Function
- Mealtime Difficulties
- Urinary Incontinence
- Assessment of Cognitive Function
- Delirium
- Preventing Falls
- Depression
- Pain Management
- Physical Restraints
- Advance Directives

Data from Mezey, M.D., Fulmer, T., & Abraham, I. (2003). *Geriatric nursing protocols for best practice,* (2nd ed.). New York: Springer.

form that is completed for all nursing home residents regardless of the level of care or reimbursement system. This document is an interdisciplinary tool completed by each member of the health care team.

The team develops an interdisciplinary care plan for all actual or potential resident problems. Depending on the resident's level of care, this plan is updated every 30 to 60 days, or more often as the resident's condition changes.

TRANSITIONAL CARE

Transitional care units (TCU) or **subacute care units (SAC units)** are designed for clients who are too ill to be discharged from the hospital to a traditional nursing home or the client's own home. These units "fill the gap" between the hospital and the traditional long-term care (LTC) facility. Most units are located in hospital settings and provide a skilled level of care.

Little has been published about the role of the nurse in transitional or subacute care. The ratio of licensed to unlicensed staff is usually better than that in traditional homes. Nurses who work in these settings must be knowledgeable about LTC and have medical-surgical, critical care, or rehabilitation skills depending on the type of unit in which they work. Nurses work closely with rehabilitation therapists to help residents meet functional outcomes. Restorative nursing aides may assist the resident in returning to an optimal level of ADL functioning.

REHABILITATIVE CARE

Rehabilitation is designed for clients who have experienced an acute injury or illness or for those who are coping with chronic conditions. Rehabilitation services may be provided in the home setting, nursing home, or rehabilitation unit or center. Chapter 10 discusses in detail the rehabilitation of individuals with chronic or disabling health problems.

GET READY for the NCLEX Examination!

KEY POINTS

- The purpose of ambulatory care is health promotion, health protection (illness prevention), and short-term treatment or follow-up for selected health problems.
- The primary role of the nurse in ambulatory care is client education and assessment.
- Nursing primary care is provided by advanced practice nurses to promote health and prevent illness, especially in underserved areas of the United States.
- Home care has expanded to care for clients who require skilled health care professional services. Examples of skilled nursing services are administering intravenous therapy and medications, assessing and teaching, and providing selected treatments.
- Telehealth is a growing trend in home health care to more easily monitor and assess clients in the home environment.
- The purpose of OASIS is to track clinical outcomes in home health care.
- Long-term care is a general term that includes care in residential facilities, nursing homes, and chronic/extended care settings.
- Assisted-living facilities are nonmedical settings that have grown rapidly in response to an expanding older adult population. Licensed and/or unlicensed staff may be available as needed.
- Transitional care units are designed to "fill the gap" between acute care and traditional long-term care.

ADDITIONAL STUDY RESOURCES

Go to your Student CD-ROM for Review Questions for the NCLEX Examination.

evolve Go to http://evolve.elsevier.com/Iggy/ for Integrated Management of Care Questions for the NCLEX Examination.

SELECTED BIBLIOGRAPHY

Asterisk indicates a classic or definitive work on this subject.

*Abraham, I., et al. (1999). *Geriatric nursing protocols for best practice.* New York: Springer.

*Anderson, A. (1996). Nursing clinics in urban settings. *Home Healthcare Nurse, 14,* 542-546.

Barrera, C., et al. (2003). Nursing care makes a difference: Application of the Omaha System. *Outcomes Management, 7*(4), 181-185.

*Bohny, B.J. (1997). A time for self-care: Role of the home healthcare nurse. *Home Healthcare Nurse, 15*(4), 281-286.

*Boroughs, D.S. (1999). Documentation in the long-term care setting. *Journal of Nursing Administration, 29*(12), 46-49.

*Catanzaro, J., & Serembus, J.F. (1998). High-tech wound and ostomy care in the home setting. *Critical Care Nursing Clinics of North America, 10*(3), 327-338.

Chetney, R. (2003). Home care's challenge: Move the information…not the patient. *Home Healthcare Nurse, 21*(10), 712.

*Congdon, J.G., & Magilvy, J.K. (1998). Rural nursing homes: A housing option for older adults. *Geriatric Nursing, 19*(3), 157-159.

Fermazin, M., et al. (2003). Nursing home compare: Web site offers critical information to consumers, professionals. *Lippincott's Case Management: Managing the Process of Patient Care, 8*(4), 175-183.

*Hammer, R.M. (1999). The lived experience of being at home: A phenomenological investigation. *Journal of Gerontological Nursing, 25*(11), 10-18.

*Health Care Financing Administration. (1996). *Home health agency manual.* Baltimore: Author.

*Health Care Financing Administration. (1998). *OASIS user's manual.* Baltimore: Author.

*Ignatavicius, D.D. (1998). *Introduction to long term care nursing: Principles and practice.* Philadelphia: F.A. Davis.

*Jones, A.M., & Foster, N. (1997). Transitional care: Bridging the gap. *MEDSURG Nursing, 6*(1), 32-38.

*Kinsella, A. (1998). Home telehealthcare services: Their role on home care today. *Home Care Management, 2*(5), 17-22.

Kinsella, A. (2003). Telehealth opportunities for home care patients. *Home Healthcare Nurse, 21*(10), 661-665.

*Marrelli, T., & Krulish, L. (1999). *Home care therapy: Quality, documentation, and reimbursement.* Boca Grande, FL: Marrelli and Associates.

*Martin, K.S., & Scheet, N.J. (1992). *The Omaha system: Applications for community health nursing.* Philadelphia: W.B. Saunders.

*McNeal, G.J. (1998). Care of the critically ill at home. *Critical Care Nursing Clinics of North America, 10*(3), 267-278.

Mezey, M.D., Fulmer, T., & Abraham, I. (2003). *Geriatric nursing protocols for best practice,* (2nd ed.). New York: Springer.

Milone-Nuzzo, P. (2003). Clinical nurse specialists in home care. *Clinical Nurse Specialist, 17*(5), 234-235.

Mitty, E.L. (2003). Policy perspectives: Assisted living and the role of nursing. *American Journal of Nursing, 103*(8), 32-43.

*National Association for Home Care. (1999). *Basic statistics about home care.* Washington, DC: Author.

Russo, H. (2001). Window of opportunity for home care nurses: Telehealth technologies. *Online Journal of Issues in Nursing, 6*(3), 1-10.

Spillman, B.C., & Lubitz, J. (2000). The effect of longevity on spending for acute and long-term care. *New England Journal of Medicine, 342*(19), 1409-1415.

Tappen, R.M., Hall, R.F., & Folden, S.L. (2001). Impact of comprehensive nurse-managed transitional care. *Clinical Nursing Research, 10*(3), 295-313.

*Vaca, K.J., Vaca, B.L., & Daake, C.J. (1998). Review of nursing home regulations. *MEDSURG Nursing, 7*(3), 165-171.

Wallace, M. (2003). Is there a nurse in the house? The role of nurses in assisted living: Past, present, and future. *Geriatric Nursing, 24*(4), 218-221, 235.

Wardell, R.C. (2003). When OASIS becomes our report card. *Home Healthcare Nurse, 21*(6), 415.

CHAPTER

3 Introduction to Managed Care and Case Management

DONNA D. IGNATAVICIUS • SUZANNE K. POWELL

LEARNING OUTCOMES

After studying this chapter, you should be able to:

1. Explain the primary purpose of managed health care, including factors that drive concerns about cost and quality.
2. Contrast the fee-for-service and capitated reimbursement systems for health care.
3. Compare the health maintenance organization (HMO) with the preferred provider organization (PPO).
4. Delineate the overall goals of case management.
5. Explain the role of case management based on national standards.
6. Identify at least three certifications for case managers.
7. Clarify the differences and similarities between case management and disease management.

Go to your Student CD-ROM for Review Questions for the NCLEX Examination keyed to these Learning Outcomes.

The cost of health care in the United States has dramatically increased over the past 20 years and now accounts for about 15% of the gross national product (GNP). As a result, insurance companies and health care providers have reexamined how health care is paid and how client care is managed. Managed health care has evolved to consider both the quality and the cost of care.

Today managed care has grown to be the largest provider for health care in the United States. **Managed health care** is a system that attempts to control costs by using a select group of providers who have agreed to a set payment *before* delivering care. In this system, client care is outcome driven and is managed by a utilization and/or a case management process. Nurses have many roles in case management and disease management. They work in these roles as they focus on achieving client outcomes while maintaining costs.

There are several factors currently driving concerns about cost and quality in the health care system. These factors include the following (Greenberg, 2003):

- **Aging, chronically ill population:** A large number of Americans are now reaching middle age, bringing chronic illness and higher use of health care services. Availability of new health care technologies and medications, as well as an aging and well-informed population, is driving increased costs in health care.
- **Purchaser pressure to contain costs:** The prices of health care premiums are increasing rapidly. In an effort to manage costs, public and private purchasers are seeking ways to shift the financial burden.
- **Physician and consumer resistance to "tight" management and referral control:** Open access models of health care, such as Preferred Provider Organizations (PPOs), now have the greatest volume of enrollees. Many health care companies no longer rely on utilization management and referral control to manage costs. Financial incentives, personalized care management, and "consumer directed" health care are now used by payers who are attempting to manage care and manage costs.
- **Renewed emphasis on evidence-based practice:** The emergence of disease management reflects a growing trend to align medical practices with evidence-based practice. Health care organizations are seeking to ensure that clients with health care needs are promptly identified and provided with the clinical interventions and resources needed to most effectively manage their illnesses while maintaining health.

MANAGED CARE

The managed care system is very different from the traditional way of paying for health care. Before the managed care movement, hospitals, physicians, and other health care providers were paid by health insurance companies on the basis of what the providers billed for their services. Under this **fee-for-service** arrangement, two physicians could perform identical services but could bill at their own rates. For example, one physician might bill $3000 for a surgical procedure, whereas another might bill $1800 for the same service. Under this fee-for-service system, the financial risk was largely taken by the insurance companies.

Purpose of Managed Care

Managed care organizations (MCOs) standardize and control costs. Under the managed care payment system, health care providers receive a uniform amount of money for each client; this is referred to as a **capitated reimbursement system** (Table 3-1). Unlike the traditional fee-for-service arrangement, the MCO and the providers share the financial risks.

Balancing cost with quality is an important concept for managed care. Health care providers have been concerned that some MCOs may be too focused on saving money rather than on providing high-quality client care (Powell, 2000a). The National Committee for Quality Assurance (NCQA) reviews and accredits MCOs that demonstrate high-quality care.

As discussed in Chapter 1, an important role for the nurse is to advocate for clients to ensure that they receive the necessary and appropriate care. As client advocates, care coordinators, and consumers, nurses need to know about managed care and the need for collaborative management of client care.

Role of Advanced Practice Nurses

Advanced practice nurses, such as nurse practitioners, certified nurse midwives, and clinical nurse specialists, have become more predominant health care providers in the managed care environment because they can deliver more cost-effective health care. In addition, they work from a wellness model, with a focus on empowering clients to stay well and care for themselves. As a result of the increased demand for and success of these advanced practice roles, many schools of nursing are offering new or additional graduate programs.

TABLE 3-1 Glossary of Terms Related to Managed Care and Case Management

authorization The process used by managed health care organizations to grant services for a specified period for reimbursement of specific services

capitation A managed care reimbursement arrangement that prepays the physician or other health care provider a set dollar amount on a per-member, per-month basis for the delivery of services to a specified group of members

deductible The amount of money that an insured person must pay toward health care costs before the insurance company begins reimbursement for health care

disease management A systems-based approach to caring for clients, usually those with high risk or chronic conditions, using standardized treatment strategies that ensure appropriate utilization and high-quality care across the continuum of health care

fee-for-service A reimbursement arrangement in which health care services are paid for as billed by the provider

indemnity An arrangement in which benefits are paid in a predetermined amount in the event of a covered loss

integrated delivery system (IDS) (also know as integrated health care system) A system created to manage or provide health care services ranging from primary to tertiary inpatient care and all other settings for care

risk sharing A mechanism that provides incentives to physicians and other health care providers to deliver cost-effective and efficient services

Types of Managed Care Organizations

Many businesses contract with a variety of MCOs to reduce health benefit costs. Government reimbursement systems have also entered into managed care arrangements to control escalating costs. For example, Medicare, a federal program for older adults and qualified disabled individuals, is expected to become a totally managed care system. Many state Medicaid programs, which pay for health services for the poor, have also entered managed care agreements.

The oldest and most common type of MCO is the **health maintenance organization (HMO)**, which is sometimes referred to as a membership organization. Many models for HMOs are used, but all either employ health care professionals to serve subscribing members (enrollees) in an ambulatory setting, or contract with primary physicians and other providers to treat clients in their private offices. The enrollee usually pays a small copayment, typically $5 or $10, for each visit to the health care provider. A client who wishes to seek services from a specialist typically needs a referral by the primary provider. Hospitalization or other inpatient services are provided by agencies that contract with the HMO.

Another popular type of MCO is the **preferred provider organization (PPO).** PPOs provide contractual arrangements with physicians, hospitals, and other providers who meet their criteria. Clients can seek services from any provider, within or outside of the PPO network, without obtaining a referral from a primary physician. In other words, they can use any of the "preferred" providers who render care to a group of subscribers in the health plan. The co-payment for each office visit to a preferred provider within the PPO network is usually $10 to $20, depending on the PPO.

COLLABORATIVE INTERDISCIPLINARY MANAGEMENT: CASE MANAGEMENT

As the United States moves forward with the managed care system, health care professionals have realized that they must work together as an interdisciplinary team to provide comprehensive, cost-effective care. Although this idea is not new in certain settings (e.g., rehabilitation, home care, and long-term care), health care professionals in hospitals have not always worked in collaborative teams. One of the constraints in acute care is the short-term stay. However, the Joint Commission on Accreditation of Healthcare Organizations (JCAHO) mandates that *all* JCAHO-accredited agencies must provide collaborative, interdisciplinary care for their clients.

This text has advocated collaborative management of care since the publication of its first edition in 1991. This edition continues to discuss client care under Collaborative Management headings. Nurses often take the lead role in the interdisciplinary team because they tend to be with clients for longer periods as they deliver and coordinate comprehensive, holistic care.

Focus on Outcomes

The primary focus of collaborative management is on the outcomes of care. The interdisciplinary team identifies expected outcomes for the client and provides interventions to help the client meet those outcomes. Both clinical and cost outcomes are established. This text identifies common clinical outcomes for clients with a number of diseases and illnesses. When possible, the Nursing Outcome Classification System is used as a guide. However, each client is an individual with unique problems and circumstances that may require modification of the commonly identified expected outcomes.

Resource Management boxes are also found throughout this text to increase awareness of costs and, in some cases, to show how nurses can help manage resources.

Development of Case Management

Although all clients need to have their care managed in a collaborative manner, not all clients need to be case managed. Case management is based on the assumption that certain clients with complex health problems need assistance in using the health care system and its resources effectively.

Case management is not a new concept. Since the turn of the twentieth century, social workers, psychologists, and others have "carried a caseload" of clients in the community for a variety of purposes. For instance, social workers and community health nurses have worked with at-risk older adults to keep them at home rather than admitting them to a nursing home.

In the mid-1980s, Karen Zander and colleagues at the New England Medical Center introduced a nursing case management (NCM) model. In this model, case managers followed up on high-risk, high-cost clients during their hospital stay to coordinate resources and ensure quality outcomes. Physician-nurse collaboration was a primary focus, which increased communication and coordination of care.

The Carondolet integrated health system in Arizona expanded on the NCM model by using case managers across the health care continuum. Sometimes referred to as "beyond the walls" case management, this model incorporated the ethnic values and culture of the community to ensure individualized, holistic care.

Definition and Process of Case Management

Many definitions for case management can be found in the literature. According to the Case Management Society of America (CMSA), "***Case management** is a collaborative process of assessment, planning, facilitation and advocacy for options and services to meet an individual's health needs through communication and available resources to promote quality cost-effective outcomes*" (CMSA, 2002). Sometimes case managers meet the health needs of a population rather than a single individual (e.g., all diabetic clients or all asthmatic school-age children in a given community).

The case management process is reserved for clients who have complex health problems (high risk) and incur a high cost to the health care system. An example of a client who could benefit from case management is an older woman with pulmonary emphysema and congestive heart failure who has had repeated admissions to the hospital for pneumonia and lives alone at home. Where appropriate in this text, the role of the case manager is discussed under Community-Based Care sections.

Part of the definition of case management endorsed by CMSA is similar to the steps of the nursing process (Chart 3-1). Similarly, the American Nurses Association (ANA) states that nursing case management includes five components: assessment, planning, implementation, evaluation, and interaction.

Goals of Case Management

The ANA identifies the goals of case management as follows:

- To provide quality health care along a continuum of care
- To decrease fragmentation (and duplication) of care across many health care settings
- To enhance the client's quality of life
- To increase cost containment (through appropriate use of resources)

The goals of case management as outlined by CMSA (2002) are more specific and include the following:

- To enhance an individual's safety, productivity, satisfaction, and quality of life
- To assure that appropriate services are generated in a timely and cost-effective manner

CHART 3-1

BEST PRACTICE for
The Process of Case Management

Needs Assessment
- Assesses/collects data
- Conducts case screening
- Identifies client's support systems and care providers
- Reviews history and determines current health care needs
- Obtains approvals for contracts

Plan Development
- Identifies services and funding options
- Reviews plan for consensus
- Advocates for client as needed
- Develops plan of care as indicated

Implementation and Coordination
- Communicates regularly with clients and support systems
- Coordinates treatment plan
- Promotes coordinated and efficient care
- Identifies needs for additional services

Outcomes Monitoring and Evaluation
- Assesses benefit value to cost and value to quality of life
- Reviews plan for continuity of care
- Evaluates client satisfaction and compliance with treatment plan

Documentation
- Records services and outcomes
- Submits reports and other documentation as needed

- To assist clients to achieve an enhanced level of health, and to maintain wellness and function by facilitating timely and appropriate health services
- To assist clients to appropriately self-direct care, self-advocate, and make informed health care decisions to the highest degree possible
- To maintain cost effectiveness in the provision of health services
- To facilitate appropriate and timely benefit and treatment decisions
- To maintain ongoing documentation and reporting of goal achievement

Types of Case Managers

In some agencies, the case manager is referred to as the care coordinator or care manager. Most case managers are nurses, but some are social workers or mental health/behavioral health workers. Some case managers have little or no clinical health background.

In general, case managers can be considered as having either an internal or an external role. **Internal case managers** are employed by a health care agency and are usually nurses or social workers. Although these individuals manage resources, their primary focus is clinical care. **External case managers** are either employed by a managed care organization (MCO) or traditional insurance company or are self-employed and contract with the MCO or traditional insurance company. The primary focus of external case managers is the utilization of resources for insurance companies.

In the past decades, there has been a growing number of so-called case managers. This "internal versus external" increase of professionals has caused an emerging challenge: how to integrate the care of clients as they move through the health care system. Case management has the same problem as managed care itself–fragmentation. "Through the continuum" case management is one answer to this dilemma. However, "handing off" clients from one setting to another has been a recurring problem (Powell, 2000a).

Complex, integrated health care systems fuel the problem. To resolve this fragmentation problem, some systems insist that *one case manager be assigned the task of being the central point of contact.* If an integrated system includes managed care case managers, acute care case managers, home health case managers, rehabilitation case mangers, and skilled nursing facility case managers, the model still remains fragmented. However, if the primary managed care case manager is ***accountable*** *for the coordination of the big picture;* the other case managers can manage the crises and details while the client resides in his or her respective level of care (Powell, 2000a).

Standards for Case Management Practice

The Case Management Society of America (CMSA) first published its ***Standards of Practice for Case Management*** in 1995. The 2002 revised standards are recognized nationally by health care organizations, certification and accreditation agencies, and individual case managers as voluntary practice guidelines for the case management profession. The standards are intended to identify and address the foundational knowledge and skill sets of a case manager in today's health care environment. Individual case managers, employers, and organizations may use the guidelines across varying case management practice settings and specialty areas (Moreo & Lamb, 2003).

These standards, both in 1995 and 2002, describe responsibilities, delineate expectations, and define accountabilities. The revised standards have also addressed the following issues (American Health Consultants, 2002; Moreo & Lamb, 2003):

- Client confidentiality issues for case managers
- Cultural competency for case management
- Legal issues of consent for case management
- Emerging trends/evolving practice (e.g., population-based practice; evidence-based practice)
- A shift in focus from resource utilization and cost of care to resource management and care management

As the largest professional case management organization, CMSA published standards that specify the recommended preparation for a case manager. As listed in the criteria, the recommended educational preparation is a baccalaureate degree in a health or human service. Although most case managers today are about 40 years of age and are nurses prepared at the associate degree level, it is likely that new case managers will have at least a baccalaureate degree as the twenty-first century unfolds. An increasing number of nursing programs believe that case management is an advanced practice role and offer masters' preparation in a case manager.

According to CMSA, the criteria for preparation as a case manager also includes working toward obtaining a certified case manager (CCM) credential. Since 1997, this certification process has required that the experienced case manager (with at least 2 years' experience) successfully complete a national standardized examination. The CCM designation is a valued credential in the field of case management for any discipline.

A certification is available for nurses who want credentials by their professional organization as a nursing case manager. In October 1997, the first nursing case management examination was given by the American Nurses Credentialing Center (ANCC). This modular test is available to nurses who are already have credentials in another field by the ANCC. Other certifications may also be acquired by case managers, such as the CRRN certification for case managers in rehabilitation nursing (Table 3-2).

Although models for case management vary, all case managers assume a common set of roles and functions. The CMSA *Standards of Practice* outlines the major roles of the case manager, including assessment, planning, facilitation, and advocacy. For nurses, many of the skills needed to fulfill these roles are learned in basic nursing education programs.

As an assessor, the case manager gathers all relevant data from a variety of sources and evaluates this information to identify barriers, clarify or determine realistic outcomes, and seek potential alternatives. The case manager works with the client and family/significant other to develop a plan that ensures that outcomes will be met and costs will be contained. As a facilitator, the case manager uses expert communication skills with all parties involved, including the care providers, client, family, and managed care payer. The client's best interests are represented by the case manager's advocacy for necessary resources, including funding and the coordination of health care services.

TABLE 3-2 The Most Common Types of Case Manager Certifications

Type of Case Manager	Certification Designation
Case manager (generalist)	Certified Case Manager (CCM)
Disability manager	Certified Disability Management Specialist (CDMS), formerly the Certified Insurance Rehabilitation Specialist (CIRS)
Rehabilitation nurse	Certified Rehabilitation Registered Nurse (CRRN)
Occupational health nurse	Certified Occupational Health Nurse (COHN)
Continuity of care manager	Advanced Certification in Continuity of Care (A-CCC)
Vocational evaluator	Certified Vocational Evaluator (CVE)
Drug and alcohol counselor	Masters Addiction Counselor (MAC)
Life care planner	Certified Life Care Planner (CLCP)

Data taken in part from May, V.R., et al. (2000). The life care planning process and certification: Current trends in health care management. *The Journal of Care Management, 6*(1), 38-40, 45-49.

From Case Management to Disease State Management

Case management models vary depending on the country's health care system or specific health care agency. For example, many case managers in the United States practice disease state management, sometimes called disease management. Put simply, disease state management focuses on the care of clients with chronic disease or illness, such as asthma, diabetes, or heart failure. The purpose of this approach is to keep clients with chronic conditions as healthy as possible in the community. Most chronic disease conditions have been "disease managed" in the past 10 years. The following are some of the more common conditions:

- Asthma
- Coronary artery disease (CAD)
- Chronic obstructive pulmonary disease (COPD)
- Heart failure (HF)
- Diabetes
- High-risk pregnancy
- Human immunodeficiency virus (HIV) infection
- Oncology
- Transplants
- Geriatric issues

There has been much debate as to whether disease management is a part of case management or whether case management is a component of disease management. Furthermore, the process is sometimes referred to as "disease-specific case management." One difference is that case management has been traditionally an individual-based approach in *either* acute *or* post-acute care. Disease management is systems based, integrating the clients through multiple levels of care. The essential idea is that disease management is case management at its finest, and case management *can:*

- Be proactive
- Follow a disease-specific population across the continuum of care
- Allow time to fully utilize the critical educational element to promote wellness
- Generate the improved quality of life case that managers seek for their clients

Powell (2000b) suggests that disease management is a system or program, whereas case management is the *process* used in disease management *programs.*

The Role of Clinical Pathways

As mentioned in Chapter 1, the clinical pathway (CP) is one format used as the client's plan of care. It is an interdisciplinary guideline for care that optimally sequences the interventions and expected outcomes for a client. Other names for the pathway include the collaborative plan of care (POC), multidisciplinary action plan (MAP), critical pathway, and care path.

The CP is developed by clinical experts for diagnoses, treatments, procedures, or symptoms that are costly, complex, and variable. The health care team follows the pathway in managing the client's care. If expected outcomes are not met, the case manager, nurse, or other health professional records these variances, or deviations, on a data collection tool. The variances are then analyzed to identify actual or potential problems. An action plan is implemented and followed up to determine whether the problem was resolved or avoided. This sequence of data collection, problem identification, action plan, and follow-up is part of the continuous quality improvement (CQI) process that every health care agency uses to monitor and improve the care that it provides.

CPs were introduced over two decades ago, yet their popularity has waxed and waned. Some hospitals are only *now* beginning to use them, whereas others have seen them come and go. Some facilities have incorporated the best of clinical pathways into their automated case management tools. Still, clinical pathways have an important focus for health care and case management. The forces that initially demanded them remain today (American Health Consultants, 2003):

- Changes in economics in health care
- Initiatives and regulations for quality improvement and best practice from an expanding body of evidence
- The desire for automation of the health care record
- The search for improved methods to involve clients and families

This text provides several examples of CPs with varying formats on the Evolve website. Traditional client care plans are also included in this text to help students identify the difference between a nursing focused care plan and an interdisciplinary plan of care, such as the clinical pathway.

GET READY for the NCLEX Examination!

KEY POINTS

- The primary purpose of managed health care is to provide quality client care while controlling health care costs.
- One major factor that is driving concerns about cost and quality of health care in the United States is its aging, chronically ill population that requires ongoing, high-cost care.

- Under the traditional fee-for-service reimbursement system, the insurance companies paid on the basis of what providers billed for services; under the capitated reimbursement system, each provider agrees to a set amount of payment before rendering services.
- A health maintenance organization (HMO) is a membership program in which enrollees are treated by providers who contract with the HMO. Referral from a primary physician is required if clients seek services from other providers.
- A preferred provider organization (PPO) allows subscribers to acquire health care services from any "preferred" provider that has contracted with the PPO. Clients do not need a referral from a primary physician.
- Case management is a collaborative process used to meet the client's health needs through communication and available resources to promote quality cost-effective outcomes for the client.
- Case management is reserved for clients with complex, high-risk, and/or chronic health problems.
- The primary goals of case management are to ensure that clients receive high-quality health care throughout the continuum, to decrease fragmentation and duplication of services, to enhance the client's quality of life, and to contain costs.
- The primary roles of the case manager include assessment, planning, facilitation, and advocacy, as published by the Case Management Society of America in its 2002 *Standards of Practice for Case Management*.
- Case managers may be certified as a CCM (certified case manager), as a nursing case manager through the American Nurses' Credentialing Center (ANCC), or in a specialty area, such as rehabilitation or disability.
- Disease management is an across-the-continuum, systems-based approach to care for populations of clients with chronic, complex illnesses, such as asthma, HIV infection, and cancer; it uses case management as the process for providing care.

ADDITIONAL STUDY RESOURCES

Go to your Student CD-ROM for Review Questions for the NCLEX Examination.

evolve Go to http://evolve.elsevier.com/Iggy/ for Integrated Management of Care Questions for the NCLEX Examination.

SELECTED BIBLIOGRAPHY

Asterisk indicates a classic or definitive work on this subject.

Aliotta, S. (2003). Coordination of care: The Council for Case Management accountability's third state of the science paper. *The Case Manager, 14*(2), 49-52.

American Health Consultants (2002). Revised CMSA standards reflect new CM issues. *Hospital Case Management, 10*(12), 192.

American Health Consultants (2003). Old hat or cutting edge? The state of the art of clinical pathways. *Hospital Case Management, 11*(1), 1-3.

Carr, D.D. (2003). Case management as a triad in long-term care: A collaborative approach. *Lippincott's Case Management: Managing the Process of Patient Care, 8*(5), 224-227.

Case Management Society of America (CMSA). (2002). *Standards of Practice for Case Management–Revised 2002.* Little Rock, AK: Author.

Cesta, T., Tahan, H., & Fink, L. (2003). *The case manager's survival guide* (2nd ed.). St. Louis: Mosby.

Creager, L. (2003). Nine steps to effective and efficient hospital case management. *Care Management, 9*(2), 32-34.

*Engen, C. (1998). Critical thinking in case management. *Inside Case Management, 5*(9), 11-12.

Fick, D.M., et al. (2000). Advance practice nursing care management model for elders in a managed care environment. *Journal of Care Management, 6*(1), 28-30, 33-37, 49.

Finkelman, A.W. (2001). *Managed care: A nursing perspective.* Upper Saddle River, NJ: Prentice Hall.

Greenberg, L. (2003). *Leaping the chasm: A discussion of case management's potential to improve safety and quality.* Retrieved on May 25, 2003, from http://www.cmsa.org/Newsletters/CMSAatWorkForYou.

Huston, C.J. (2002). The role of the case manager in a disease management program. *Lippincott's Case Management: Managing the Role of Patient Care, 7*(6), 221-227.

*Ignatavicius, D.D., & Hausman, K. (1995). *Clinical pathways for collaborative practice.* Philadelphia: W.B. Saunders.

Keim, P. (2003). High-risk population: Evolution of disease management. *Continuing Care, 22*(6), 24-26.

Kelly, T.A. (2003). Critical thinking and case management. *The Case Manager, 14*(3), 70-72.

May, V.R., et al. (2000). The life care planning process and certification: Current trends in health care management. *The Journal of Care Management, 6*(1), 38-40, 45-49.

Moreo, K., & Lamb, G. (2003). Providing relevant guidelines for case management practice: Revised CMSA Standards of Practice for Case Management. *Lippincott's Case Management: Managing the Process of Patient Care, 8*(3), 122-124.

*Mullahy, C.M. (1999). *The case manager's handbook.* (2nd ed.). Gaithersburg, MD: Aspen.

*Nash, D. (1997). Disease management: A bumpy road ahead. *The Journal of Outcomes Management, 4*(1), 2.

Powell, S.K. (2000a). *Nursing case management: A practical guide to success in managed care* (2nd ed.). Philadelphia: Lippincott Williams & Wilkins.

Powell, S.K. (2000b). *Advanced case management: Outcomes and beyond.* Philadelphia: Lippincott Williams & Wilkins.

Powell, S.K., & Ignatavicius, D. (2001). *CMSA core curriculum for case management.* Philadelphia: Lippincott Williams & Wilkins.

Upman, C.M.S. (2003). The evolution of case management. *Care Management, 9*(3), 13-17.

*Zander, K. (1996). *Handbook of nursing case management.* Gaithersburg, MD: Aspen.

CHAPTER

4

Introduction to Complementary and Alternative Therapies in Nursing

RUTH LINDQUIST • MARIAH SNYDER

LEARNING OUTCOMES

After studying this chapter, you should be able to:

1. Describe the purposes of the National Center for Complementary and Alternative Medicine (NCCAM).
2. Identify four examples of mind-body therapies.
3. Discuss the scope of complementary and alternative therapies with particular attention to the cultural aspects of their use.
4. Differentiate manipulative and body-based therapies from biologic-based therapies.
5. Provide examples of herbal therapies, their purpose, and their adverse effects.
6. Identify selected complementary and alternative therapies that nurses can use in providing care to a variety of client populations.
7. Explain the purposes of commonly used therapies in nursing practice.
8. Discuss implications for care of clients using complementary and alternative therapies.

Go to your Student CD-ROM for Review Questions for the NCLEX Examination keyed to these Learning Outcomes.

OVERVIEW

Western biomedicine has been the predominant health care system in the United States and other Western countries for the past 100 years. However, during the past 20 years, a growing interest in complementary (additional treatment) and alternative (substitutions for traditional treatment) therapies has evolved. In a national survey in the United States, Eisenberg and colleagues (1998) found that over 40% of Americans used complementary and/or alternative therapies. This number is thought to be a conservative figure in that only English-speaking persons were included and inquiries were only made about the use of 16 therapies. Most persons receiving complementary and alternative therapies pay for them out-of-the pocket, because most third-party payers reimburse for only selected therapies such as chiropractic treatment and acupuncture.

One of the reasons for the increase in nonbiomedical treatments is that individuals wish to be treated in a holistic fashion (Astin, 1998). Biomedicine is based on the Cartesian philosophy in which the body and mind are treated as separate entities. Nurses believe in a holistic, caring philosophy. Therefore complementary and alternative therapies are consistent with nursing and nursing practice.

This chapter describes some of the common therapies used by nurses in a variety of settings. In most cases, no special or advanced training is needed to use these modalities. Some complementary and alternative therapies, such as acupuncture, require specialized education and, in some states, licensure or certification.

NATIONAL CENTER FOR COMPLEMENTARY AND ALTERNATIVE MEDICINE (NCCAM)

Legitimacy was given to complementary and alternative therapies when the National Institutes of Health established the Office of Alternative Medicine in 1992. This office has since been renamed as the National Center for Complementary

and Alternative Medicine (NCCAM). The purposes of the center are to:

- Fund studies examining the effectiveness of various complementary therapies
- Advance the knowledge about complementary therapies of health professionals
- Serve as a clearinghouse for information about these therapies.

NCCAM has defined complementary and alternative medicine in the following manner:

Complementary and alternative medicine covers a broad range of healing philosophies, approaches, and therapies that mainstream Western medicine does not commonly use, accept, study, understand, or make available (National Center for Complementary and Alternative Medicine, 2003). NCCAM has also developed a classification system for the more than 1800 therapies (Kreitzer & Jensen, 2000). Table 4-1 presents the five categories in this system and examples of therapies found in each category.

COMMONLY USED THERAPIES IN NURSING

Systems of Care

As indicated in Table 4-1, numerous systems of care exist. Each of these systems is based on a philosophy that guides the practitioner in the assessments to make and the therapies to use. According to Bodeker (2002), the majority of persons in many countries use therapies other than ones in the traditional biomedical system. With the growing immigrant population in the United States, it is imperative that nurses increase their knowledge about other systems of health care.

Numerous therapies that nurses use come from other systems of care such as yoga from Ayurvedic medicine and Qigong from traditional Chinese medicine (TCM). Understanding the philosophic or theoretic base underlying these therapies helps nurses gain a better perspective about the therapy being used. Nyo-Metzger and colleagues (2003) found that knowledge about non-Western health practices assisted health professionals in avoiding misdiagnoses of illnesses in immigrants.

Acupressure, a traditional Chinese medicine therapy, is used in nursing for a number of conditions, particularly in the treatment of pain, nausea, and vomiting. Gach (1990) defines **acupressure** as "an ancient healing art that used the fingers to press certain points on the body to stimulate the body's self-curative abilities" (p. 3). According to the philosophy of TCM, *qi* or energy flows along 12 major meridians. Illness or pain occurs when the flow of *qi* is blocked or diminished (Weiss, 2002). Acupressure is similar to **acupuncture;** pressure instead of needles is used on one of the 365 to 700 **acupoints** that are located on meridians throughout the body. Although most research has been done on acupuncture, studies on the effectiveness of acupressure are increasing.

One acupoint that is often helpful in reducing or eliminating pain is the *hoku* point. This point is on the back of the hand, and is located halfway between the junction of the first and second metacarpal bones. A valley is formed when the thumb is abducted. Pressure (usually with the thumb of the opposite hand) on this point helps alleviate pain. The *hoku* point has also been found to be helpful in stimulating the immune system, in relieving diarrhea, and helping to cure the common cold. There are a number of precautions to observe when using acupressure. Gach (1990) cautions against brisk rubbing or deep pressure in clients with heart disease, cancer, and high blood pressure to prevent sympathetic system stimulation.

Mind-Body Therapies

A huge number of therapies are classified as being mind-body therapies. Because these therapies are based on a holistic philosophy, they fit with the holistic, caring philosophy of nursing. Nurses have traditionally used a number of mind-body therapies such as journaling, imagery, meditation, and animal-assisted therapy.

JOURNALING

Journaling is one of the reflective therapies (Snyder & Lindquist, 2002); it is a tool for recording the process of one's life. Writing provides a vehicle for a person to express feelings, to gain new perspectives, and to pay attention to what is in the unconscious. A number of techniques for journaling can be used: intensive journaling (Progoff, 1975), focused writing (Pennebaker, 1997), and free-flowing (Bolton, 1999).

Free-flowing journaling is the technique most often used. The person writes whatever comes to mind without censoring any thoughts or feelings or correcting grammar or punctuation. The writing done is for oneself and need not be shared. The expectation to share what is written usually places constraints on what is being recorded. Entries are made in a book dedicated to journaling. This may be a loose-leaf notebook or a special journal entry book.

Although journal writing has been done for centuries, little formal research exists to support its use. Spera, Buhrfeind, and Pennebaker (1994) found that persons who had lost their

TABLE 4-1 CCAM Classification for Complementary Therapies and Examples of Therapies in Each Category: Alternative Systems of Care

Category	Examples
Systems of care	Traditional Chinese medicine, Ayurvedic, Native American/American Indian medicine, homeopathy
Mind-body therapies	Imagery, meditation, music, journaling, humor, biofeedback, yoga, prayer
Biologic-based therapies	Herbs, aromatherapy, special diets (Ornish, Pritikin), nutritional and food supplements
Manipulative and body-based therapies	Chiropractic treatment, massage, rolfing, light and color therapies, hydrotherapy
Energy therapies	Healing touch, Reiki, external Qigong, magnets

jobs and used focused-writing about the event were more likely to obtain employment sooner than persons who did not write or who wrote about superficial events. Bolton (1999) reported improved emotional health and less focus on pain connected with a situation or event in persons who recorded their feelings via journaling.

IMAGERY

Imagery has been used for many years in nursing. While changing dressings or doing other procedures that may produce pain, a nurse may ask a client to think about a pleasant event or a beautiful scene. Post-White and Fitzgerald (2002) define **imagery** as "the formation of a mental representation of an object, place, event, or situation that is perceived through the senses" (p. 44). Visualization is sometimes used interchangeably with imagery, but in reality all senses can be used in imagery.

The scientific base for the use of imagery relates to the reduction of stress, which is mediated through psychoneuroimmune interactions (Post-White & Fitzgerald, 2002). Imagery has been used in a wide variety of conditions, including the following:

- Reducing pain (Broome, Rehwaldt, & Fogg, 1998)
- Reducing nausea and vomiting (Troesch et al., 1993)
- Decreasing anxiety (Thompson & Coppens, 1994)
- Promoting comfort during treatment for cancer

Many techniques can be used to help individuals use their senses to create images. Guided imagery in which the client is provided with images or prompts by a nurse, a family member, or a friend, or via a tape is the technique frequently used by nurses. Before suggestions for imagery are presented, provide the client with instructions that will help produce relaxation. These may include tensing and relaxing muscle groups and focusing attention on one's breathing.

When the individual seems relaxed (slower respirations and relaxed muscles), give specific suggestions for imagery. The client may be asked to choose a place he or she enjoys and to think about the sights, smells, tastes, and feelings associated with the place. Time allowed for imagery varies, but it is usually between 15 and 20 minutes. Opportunities are provided for the person to enjoy being in this place; the client is informed that he or she can return to this "place" at anytime. Some clients like to create their own imagery tape to listen to while others prefer listening to commercial tapes or having the nurse or family member guide them through the session. Use of guided imagery has few risks. However, be attentive to any adverse effects such as heightened anxiety or difficulty in breathing.

MEDITATION

Meditation has been a part of many religions and cultures for thousands of years. Although often thought of in terms of religion, meditation, or focusing on the moment, can be used in a nonreligious context. Kreitzer (2002) defined **meditation** as "a self-directed practice for relaxing the body and calming the mind (p. 101). Everly and Rosenfeld (1981) identified four types of meditation:

- Mental repetition such as using a mantra
- Physical repetition such as focusing on breathing or walking
- Problem contemplation such as solving a riddle or *koan*
- Visual concentration that is similar to imagery

Walking meditation, a commonly used type, contains both active and meditative elements. While walking, the person focuses attention on the sound of the foot hitting the ground, the feelings in the muscles and joints, or the movements of the body. This type of meditation may be appealing to persons who are more active and have difficulty concentrating while sitting. The walking meditation should be done for about 20 minutes.

The labyrinth is an ancient form of walking meditation that has attracted renewed attention. Labyrinths are found in many cultures such as Hindu, Hopi Indians, Crete, and medieval European religions. The labyrinth is not a maze. The person walks the circles meditatively. Persons may ask themselves a question and search for answers while walking, they may pray, or they may just focus on feelings they are experiencing.

Meditation has been used to reduce anxiety, reduce pain, relieve symptoms of psoriasis, lower blood pressure, and promote health (Figure 4-1). In early studies, Benson (1975) explored the effectiveness of transcendental meditation (TM) in reducing hypertension. More recently, Kabat-Zinn and colleagues (1998) found that mindfulness meditation was effective in reducing the symptoms of psoriasis. Research on outcomes of meditation continues.

Animal-Assisted Therapy

It is not unusual to see dogs, birds, or other animals when visiting a hospital or nursing home. Since the 1970s, studies have sought to validate the link between animal companionship and positive health outcomes. Jorgenson (2002) differentiates between animal-assisted therapy (AAT) and pet visitation. In AAT, the animal, often a dog, is an integral part of the treatment plan. For example, a dog may be used to assist a client to improve motor skills or increase ability to concentrate. In contrast, the goal of pet visitation is aimed more at increasing socialization or keeping the person in touch with reality.

Animal-assisted therapy has been used with many different client groups including hospice (Chinner & Dalziel, 1991), behavioral health (Barker & Dawson, 1998), and dementia (Batson et al., 1995). Jorgenson (2002) recommends that any facility planning to implement AAT should first develop

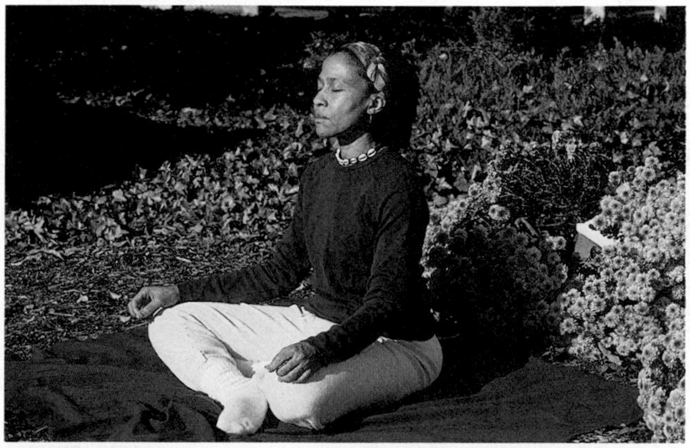

Figure 4-1 ■ Meditation can be used to relax the body and calm the mind. (From Potter, P.A., & Perry, A.G. [2001]. *Fundamentals of nursing* (5th ed.). St. Louis: Mosby.)

guidelines that specify the inclusion and exclusion criteria for clients who might receive AAT, the procedure to be used during the visitation, and the responsibilities of the nursing staff. Some institutions do not allow dogs to be on site for more than 1 hour because the animal becomes exhausted.

Manipulative and Body-Based Therapies

Three large groups of therapies make up the manipulative and body-based NCCAM category: chiropractic, osteopathy, and massage. Movement therapies such as dance and Tai Chi are sometimes also placed in this category. Massage and Tai Chi are common manipulative and body-based therapies that nurses can learn and teach to their clients.

MASSAGE

Massage has a long history within nursing. Until recently, back rubs were a standard nursing procedure administered to all hospitalized clients on a daily basis. **Massage** involves using various strokes and pressure to manipulate soft tissues for therapeutic purposes (Snyder & Lindquist, 2002). Many types of massage exist: Swedish (rather vigorous massage with long, flowing strokes), Esalen (light touch), neuromuscular (deep tissue), Shiatsu (Japanese pressure-point), and reflexology (massage of various points on the foot). Many different strokes are used in massage. Massage can be of the entire body or of selected areas such as foot, hands, shoulder/neck, or back (Figure 4-2).

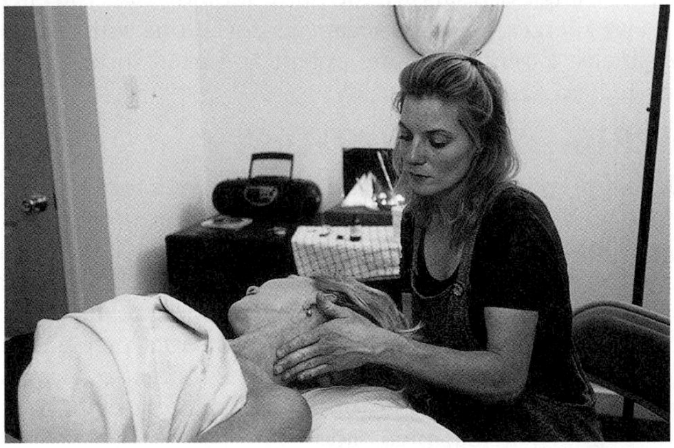

Figure 4-2 ■ Massage therapy can be effectively used to relieve tension. (From Potter, P.A., & Perry, A.G. [2005]. *Fundamentals of nursing* (6th ed.). St. Louis: Mosby.)

Hand massage can be readily used with any client group. Table 4-2 details one technique that can be used. Snyder and colleagues found that hand massage, when used with persons with dementia, produced relaxation and helped to lessen aggressive behaviors (Snyder, Egan, & Burns, 1995).

A growing body of research provides support for massage. As noted in the Evidence-Based Practice for Nursing box on p. 36, back massage produced relaxation in persons undergoing a diagnostic procedure. Massage has been found to reduce pain (Hulme, Waterman, & Hillier, 1999), produce relaxation (Snyder, Egan, & Burns, 1995), and improve sleep (Richards, 1998).

Because of cultural differences related to touch and personal preferences related to touch, the nurse needs to obtain permission of the person before using massage. Massage should not be used over reddened, bruised, or infected areas of skin.

TAI CHI

Tai Chi is a holistic movement therapy that has wide popularity in China, Taiwan, and Japan. **Tai Chi** is a traditional Chinese martial art that has been adapted to be a mind-body exercise. The goal is to integrate body movements, mind concentration, muscle relaxation, and breathing to achieve the desired outcome. Several styles of Tai Chi exist: *chen* (quick and slow large movements), *yang* (slow large movements), *sun* (quick compact), and Tai Chi Chih (simple repetitive movements). The latter is a style that is popular in the United States and originated in the West. Tai Chi is

TABLE 4-2 Directions for Administering Hand Massage

Do not massage the hand if it is injured, reddened, swollen, or infected. Each hand is massaged for about 2½ minutes.

Back of Hand
- Use medium pressure strokes from the wrist to the fingertips.
- Make large half-circle stretching strokes from the center to the side of the hand using moderate pressure.
- Make small circular strokes (like an O) over the entire back of the hand.
- Use light pressure strokes from the wrist to the fingertips.

Palm of Hand
- Make medium pressure strokes from the wrist to the fingertips.
- Use gentle strokes to lift the muscle tissue of the palms.
- Use small circular strokes, applying moderate pressure over the palm.
- Use large stretching strokes from the center of the palm to the sides (like opening up the palm).

Fingers
- Gently squeeze each finger from the base to the tip on both sides using the thumb and index finger.
- Do gentle range of motion.
- Apply gentle pressure on the nail bed.

Completion
- Place the client's hand on yours and cover it with your other hand.
- Gently draw your top hand toward you several times.
- Turn the hand over and gently draw your other hand toward you several times.

Modified from Snyder, M., & Lindquist, R. (Eds.). (2002). *Complementary/alternative therapies in nursing* (4th ed.). New York: Springer.

EVIDENCE-BASED PRACTICE for Nursing

Back massage may reduce stress in clients having cardiac catheterizations

McNamara, M.E., et al. (2003). The effects of back massage before diagnostic cardiac catheterization. *Alternative Therapies in Health and Medicine, 9,* 50-57.

Back massage may be helpful in reducing stress in clients having cardiac catheterizations. The aim of this research was to examine the effects that a 20-minute back massage had on blood pressure, respirations, pain perception, skin temperature, and perceived stress in 46 subjects who were having a diagnostic cardiac catheterization. A repeated measure design was used with a control and an experimental group. Subjects in the control group received the usual care that was provided in the cardiac catheterization laboratory. A 20-minute back massage was administered to the subjects in the experimental group before the test.

Findings showed that subjects receiving the back massage had a 20-mm Hg decline in systolic blood pressure immediately after the massage. The systolic pressure was 7 mm Hg lower than before the catheterization 10 minutes after the completion of the massage. Reductions in pain perception, respirations, and systolic blood pressure and perceived stress occurred in both groups during the waiting period.

Level of Evidence: 5—Well-controlled case study.

Critique. Although this study used a small convenience sample, it was an attempt to examine a nontraditional, yet simple method for minimizing stress in clients having a very stressful procedure. More studies using larger groups of culturally diverse subjects of varying ages need to be done to help generalize findings that can be useful for health care practice.

Implications for Nursing. Back massage could be considered as a possible therapy to use to reduce the stress of clients having cardiac catheterizations and, perhaps, other invasive diagnostic procedures. This intervention requires little time and could be performed by either a nurse or unlicensed nursing personnel before the procedure.

closely tied to the philosophy of traditional Chinese medicine (TCM); the movements promote the flow of *qi* or energy throughout the body.

CONSIDERATIONS FOR OLDER ADULTS

A growing body of research on Tai Chi is evolving. Much of the research on Tai Chi has focused on its use with older adults, particularly in preventing falls (Shih, 1997). Tai Chi has also been shown to promote both physical and mental well-being in older adults (Chen, Snyder, & Kirchbaum, 2001). One notable finding is that many older adults continued to use Tai Chi after the study concluded.

Biologic-Based Therapies

This category of therapies is more similar to the biomedical model. However, the regulations governing herbal preparations and food additives differ from those for pharmaceuticals. This seeming lack of strict regulation has contributed to concerns about these preparations. Use of essential oils in aromatherapy and herbal preparations is becoming more common.

AROMATHERAPY

Aromatherapy is one of the fastest growing areas in complementary therapies. Use of essential oils can be traced back to ancient times. Modern interest in aromatherapy was initiated in France in the 1930s. Clinical **aromatherapy** is defined as "the use of essential oils for their expected outcomes that are measurable" (Buckle, 2002, p. 246). Buckle notes that the term *aromatherapy* conveys that use of the essential oil is via smell. However, essential oils may be applied in compresses, used in baths, or applied topically to the skin. What is common to all of these forms of use is that essential oils, the steam distillate of aromatic plants, are used. Essential oils may be obtained from the flowers, leaves, bark, wood, roots, seeds, or peels of plants.

Numerous essential oils have been identified and used. For example, lavender (*Lavandula officinalis*) and rose (*Rosa damascena)* are two of the oils used to promote relaxation and sleep. Peppermint (*Mentha piperita)* has been used for stimulation and to promote concentration. Sandalwood (*Santalum album)* and lavender (*L. officinalis)* have been used to ease depression. Tea tree has been tested to determine its effectiveness in treating methicillin-resistant *Staphylococcus aureus* (MRSA) infections.

Although only a small body of research on essential oils currently exists, a number of studies are being conducted. Before using essential oils, the nurse should assess the client for any allergies and any negative associations with particular smells. Essential oils are potent and need to be diluted before being applied topically.

HERBAL PREPARATIONS

Herbal preparations are plants that are used for medicinal purposes and have been used by societies for thousands of years. Today they are widely used in the United States where millions of individuals use herbal preparations on a regular basis. In recent years, there has been a dramatic increase in use of herbal remedies by Americans. Herbal preparations have become increasingly popular as a means to promote health, to prevent diseases, or to cure a variety of ailments. For example, herbal preparations are used in an effort to control high blood pressure, relieve abdominal pain, control high serum glucose levels, or manage painful chronic conditions. Several common herbs, their intended purposes, and precautions are listed in Table 4-3.

Herbal preparations are frequently considered an attractive alternative or supplement to conventional health care, and are commonly viewed as "less risky" than conventional drug therapy because they are "natural." However, herbs have pharmacoactive effects that may be serious or deadly as in cases of overuse, inappropriate use, herbal toxicities, and herb-drug and herb-herb interactions. The full range of beneficial and adverse effects of many herbal preparations is not known. Although the effects of some herbs have been studied, others have not. Furthermore, even though herbs have been used for thousands of years, the combination of many of herbs with Western medicine is relatively new (Lu, 2003), and the effects of many herb-drug combinations remain to be determined. Thus with the increased popularity in the use of herbs has come heightened concern about their safety.

There are other drawbacks to herbal therapies. Herbs may be self-administered to treat a serious ailment that could more effectively be treated by conventional medicine, potentially resulting in a delay of diagnosis and treatment by conventional practitioners. In other situations, improper dosages of herbs may be taken when lower dosages or other precautions are indicated due, for example, to a client's

TABLE 4-3 Commonly Used Herbal Preparations

Herb	Intended Effects/Uses	Cautions/Adverse Effects
Gingko biloba	Reduce memory problems, dementia, peripheral vascular disease; has antioxidant and vasodilatory properties.	Use with anticoagulants may cause bleeding; rarely dizziness, headache, GI upset.
Garlic	Lower cholesterol or blood pressure; act as a natural antibiotic; act as an antiplatelet agent.	Bleeding when used with other antiplatelet agents; potentiates antidiabetic drugs; avoid before surgery.
Echinacea	Build immunity; help wound healing.	Not recommended for individuals with immune diseases. May suppress immune function if used for more than 8 weeks.
Ginseng	Promote general well-being; antiaging.	Observe INR with warfarin. Side effects may depend on type of ginseng used.
St. John's wort	Ease mild to moderate depression.	Photosensitivity; avoid use in major depression or with other antidepressants.

INR, International Normalized Ratio; *GI,* gastrointestinal.

poor liver or renal function for detoxification or excretion (Eliopoulos, 1999). In some cases, although herbal intake may contribute to the need for emergency department visits, clients may neglect or choose not to tell their health care providers about their use of herbs.

In the United States, herbal preparations are regulated as food and nutritional supplements by the Food and Drug Administration (FDA). Although regulated by the FDA, regulations are less strict than for drugs. Because herbs are not classified as drugs, they do not receive the same oversight in their preparation and use as drugs. However, even though herbs do not require a prescription, they are the basis of many prescription drugs. It has been observed that of the best selling 150 prescription drugs, 86 contain at least one major active compound from natural sources (Plotnikoff, 2002). Adding to the complexity of herbal therapy, herbal preparations cause a variety of responses depending on the nature of the herb and how it was prepared. There is no guarantee that an herb has been properly prepared, thus there are uncertainties related to product quality. However, herbs that are sold as standardized extracts are viewed as more likely to contain accurate amounts of herbs as reflected on their label and less likely to contain other inactive elements or contamination. Because an herb is natural, it does not mean that it is safe. Because a given herb is considered "safe," it does not mean it is effective. What is on an herbal product's label does not reflect the contents in all cases (Plotnikoff, 2002, p. 263).

Unregulated and unprescribed, herbs may have untoward effects such as liver toxicity; herbs may potentiate other drugs, alter blood pressure, or cause bleeding. Some problems encountered in treating clients who are using herbs with conventional medications and treatments include oversedation, inhibition of coagulation, blood pressure effects (hypertension or hypotension), dysrhythmias, and electrolyte changes.

In any health care setting, it is important to integrate herb usage questions into a client's health history and to interpret findings of physical assessments that are possibly related to the client's herbal use. Ask a client about the intended purpose of herbal use as well as the frequency and dose of the herbs used. If herbal preparations are used, remind the client about the importance of informing future care providers about herbal therapy use. For example, to avoid increased risks of bleeding, one should not use ginkgo, ginseng, and garlic before surgery.

There is increasing need to know the intended effects and side effects of herbal therapies and safety precautions related to their ingestion as the public continues to explore the use of herbs. You can play an important role in the identification of adverse herb effects, herb-herb, and herb-drug interactions, and in the identification and prevention of adverse effects and side effects of herbal therapy. Nurses can inform clients about the use of herbs and discuss dangers of excessive or inappropriate use. You can also explain the importance for clients to monitor their response to herbal preparations over time, so that toxicities and adverse effects may be noted and herbal intake stopped if indicated. Nurses should caution clients about unreliable sources of health information and refer clients to credible resources for herbal remedies. Examples include the National Library of Medicine's PubMed Website: http://www.ncbi.nlm.nih.gov/ PubMed/; the American Botanical Council: http://herbalgram.org; and the Herb Research Foundation: http://www.herbs.org.

Energy Therapies

Energy therapies include both biofield therapies and bioelectromagnetics. Because it is difficult to *see* energy, much skepticism exists about the therapies in this NCCAM category. However, healing touch techniques have a long history of use in nursing. Since the 1970s when Krieger (1976) began her research, nurses have continued to conduct research on the effectiveness of energy therapies in producing positive health outcomes. Umbreit (2002) defined **healing touch** as "a type of complementary therapy that used energy-based techniques to balance and align the human energy field" (p. 165). Healing touch encompasses many techniques. The most well-known energy therapy is therapeutic touch. Therapeutic touch, magnetic unruffling, and magnets are discussed.

THERAPEUTIC TOUCH

According to Quinn (2002), **therapeutic touch** (TT) "is the use of the hands on or near the body with the intention to heal" (p. 183). One of the assumptions upon which TT is based is that illness is an imbalance in the flow of energy or the energy pattern. In TT, the practitioner intervenes in the recipient's energy field to stimulate healing potential.

TT consists of five steps: centering, assessing the energy field, clearing and mobilizing the client's energy field, directing energy for healing, and balancing the energy field. In centering, the practitioner quiets oneself and focuses attention on the client with the intention to heal. The practitioner uses her or his hands to assess the flow of energy in the client; hands are moved from head to foot, noting any blockages in the flow of energy or absences or excesses in energy in a particular spot. In the clearing and mobilizing element, the practitioner holds his or her hands 2 to 4 inches from the client's body and moves the hands with the palms facing the client's, from head to foot in a sweeping motion (Figure 4-3). This process may be repeated. Based on the assessment, the practitioner directs energy so that imbalances are resolved. The practitioner's hands are placed on the client and energy is directed toward the client. Finally, the practitioner seeks to balance the energy in the client by using head-to-toe clearing motions with the intention of smoothing the energy of the client.

TT has been used to achieve numerous health outcomes: reduce anxiety (Quinn & Strelkauskas, 1993), reduce pain (Peck, 1997), improve the immune system (Olson et al., 1997), and improve functional ability (Peck, 1998). Caution should be used in administering TT to the very young and very old.

MAGNETIC UNRUFFLING

Little research has been conducted on **magnetic unruffling.** In this therapy, practitioners move their hands from above the head to past the feet of the client. The practitioner can think of the fingers as magnets collecting excess energy. They may then shake the collected energy from their hands before starting the next sweep. Each sweep takes about 30 seconds. These movements are continued until the body feels like glass (Hover-Kramer, 1999). Magnetic unruffling has been used with clients who have had general anesthesia, have a chemical dependency disorder, are experiencing chronic pain, or have a systemic illness.

MAGNETS

Magnets are another type of energy therapy. One of the prime purposes for using magnets is to relieve chronic pain, particularly back and joint pain. Magnets can be applied via wide belts, orthotics, or in mattresses and pillows. More research is needed about the use of magnets and their effectiveness in managing chronic pain.

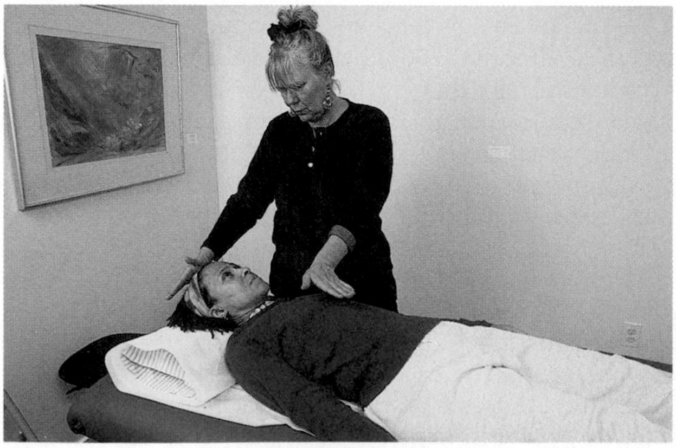

Figure 4-3 ■ In therapeutic touch, the practitioner directs the practitioner's own interpersonal energy to help or heal another. (From Potter, P.A., & Perry, A.G. [2005]. *Fundamentals of nursing.* (6th ed.). St. Louis: Mosby.)

SUMMARY OF IMPLICATIONS FOR NURSING

Complementary and alternative therapies are increasingly being used to promote health, prevent disease, or address illness and symptoms. Increased nursing research is essential to evaluate the usefulness of therapies and their role in medical-surgical nursing practice. Throughout this text, discussions of specific complementary and alternative therapies are included as part of the collaborative management of various diseases and illnesses. These descriptions are labeled with a separate heading to help locate this information.

Nurses have an important role in assessing the clients' use of therapies in order to discuss safety, perceived effectiveness, and satisfaction. Furthermore, the knowledge of clients' use of complementary and alternative therapies is important in the planning of care and in the determination as to how conventional and nonconventional therapies may be safely combined to benefit clients. A better understanding of therapies enhances your ability to educate clients about specific therapies and their effects, to discuss therapies of potential benefit to clients, and to refer clients to appropriate providers for desired therapies.

GET READY for the NCLEX Examination!

KEY POINTS

- Complementary and alternative therapies include a broad range of healing approaches and therapies that are not commonly used as part of Western medicine. Many of these therapies are derived from Eastern medicine, such as traditional Chinese medicine (e.g., acupressure).
- Many individuals living in the United States and other Western countries are using complementary and alternative therapies.
- As part of the National Institutes of Health, the National Center for Complementary and Alternative Medicine is funding research to determine the usefulness of selected therapies.
- Examples of mind-body therapies include journaling, imagery, meditation, and animal-assisted therapy.
- Journaling allows an opportunity for reflection as the individual records thoughts and feelings.
- Imagery is often used for reducing pain, nausea and vomiting, and anxiety.
- Massage is a commonly used manipulative and body-based therapy in nursing, for example, giving a back rub.
- Tai Chi is a popular holistic therapy used in China, Taiwan, and Japan that is gaining interest in the Western sector; it integrates body movements, concentration, and relaxation techniques.
- Aromatherapy and herbal preparations are commonly used biologic therapies; these interventions are used for an assortment of problems (see Table 4-3).
- Therapeutic touch promotes healing by balancing a person's energy field.
- Magnets may be used as an adjunct for chronic pain management, especially for joint and back pain.

ADDITIONAL STUDY RESOURCES

Go to your Student CD-ROM for Review Questions for the NCLEX Examination.

evolve Go to http://evolve.elsevier.com/Iggy/ for Integrated Management of Care Questions for the NCLEX Examination.

SELECTED BIBLIOGRAPHY

Asterisk indicates a classic or definitive work on this subject.

*Astin, J.A. (1998). Why patients use alternative medicine: Results of a national study. *Journal of the American Medical Association, 2799,* 1548-1553.

*Barker, S.B., & Dawson, K.S. (1998). The effects of animal-assisted therapy on anxiety ratings of hospitalizing psychiatric patients. *Psychiatric Service, 49,* 797-801.

*Batson, K., et al. (1995). The effect of a therapy dog on socialization and physiologic indicators of stress in persons diagnosed with Alzheimer's disease. In C.C. Wilson & C.C. Turner (Eds.), *Companion animals in human health* (pp. 203-215). Thousand Oaks, CA: Sage.

*Benson, H. (1975). *The relaxation response.* New York: Avon.

Bodeker, G. (2002). Lessons on integration from the developing world's experience. *British Medical Journal, 322,* 154-167.

*Bolton, G. (1999). *The therapeutic potential of creative writing.* London: Jessica Kingsley Publishers.

*Broome, M.E., Rehwaldt, M., & Fogg, L. (1998). Relationships between cognitive behavioral techniques, temperament, observed distress, and pain reports in children and adolescents during lumbar puncture. *Journal of Pediatric Nursing, 13,* 48-51.

Buckle, J. (2002). Aromatherapy. In M. Snyder & R. Lindquist (Eds.), *Complementary/alternative therapies in nursing* (4th ed., pp. 245-258). New York: Springer.

Chen, K.M., Snyder, M., & Kirchbaum, K. (2001). Clinical use of Tai Chi in elderly populations. *Geriatric Nursing, 22,* 198-200.

*Chinner, T.L., & Dalziel, F.R. (1991). An exploratory study on the viability and efficacy of a pet-facilitated therapy project with a hospice. *Journal of Palliative Care, 7,* 13-20.

*Eisenberg, D.M., et al. (1998). Trends in alternative medicine use in the United States, 1990-1997. *Journal of the American Medical Association, 280,* 1569-1575.

*Eliopoulos, C. (1999). Using complementary and alternative therapies wisely. *Geriatric Nursing, 20,* 139-143.

*Everly, G.S., & Rosenfeld, R. (1981). *The nature and treatment of the stress response.* New York: Plenum.

*Gach, M. (1990). *Acupressure potent points.* New York: Bantam Books.

Hover-Kramer, D. (Ed.). (2001). *Healing touch: A resource for health care professionals.* Albany, NY: Delmar.

*Hulme, J., Waterman, H., & Hillier, V.F. (1999). The effect of foot massage on patients' perception of care following laparoscopic sterilization as day case patients. *Journal of Advanced Nursing, 30,* 460-468.

Jorgenson, J. (2002). Animal-assisted therapy. In M. Snyder & R. Lindquist (Eds.), *Complementary/alternative therapies in nursing* (4th ed., pp. 152-162). New York: Springer.

*Kabat-Zinn, J., et al. (1998). Influence of a mindfulness meditation-based stress reduction intervention on rates of skin clearing in patients with moderate to severe psoriasis undergoing phototherapy (UVB) and photochemotherapy (PUVA). *Psychosomatic Medicine, 60,* 525-632.

Kreitzer, M.J. (2002). Meditation. In M. Snyder & R. Lindquist (Eds.), *Complementary/alternative therapies in nursing* (4th ed., pp. 101-113). New York: Springer.

Kreitzer, M.J., & Jensen, D. (2000). Healing practices: Trends, challenges, and opportunities for nurses in acute and critical care. *AACN Clinical Issues: in Advanced Practice in Acute and Critical Care, 11,* 7-16.

*Krieger, D. (1976). Healing by laying on of hands as facilitators of bioenergetic change: The response of in-vivo hemoglobin. *Psychoenergetic Systems, 1,* 121-129.

Lu, Y. (2003). Herb use in critical care: What to watch for. *Critical Care Nursing Clinics of North America, 15*(3), 313-319.

McNamara, M.E., et al. (2003). The effects of back massage before diagnostic cardiac catheterization. *Alternative Therapies in Health and Medicine, 9,* 50-57.

National Center for Complementary and Alternative Medicine. (2003). Retrieved on June 9, 2003, from www.nccam.gov.

Nyo-Metzger, Q., Massagli, M.P., & Clarridge, B.R. (2003). Linguistic and cultural barriers to care: Perspectives of Chinese and Vietnamese immigrants. *Journal of General Internal Medicine, 18,* 44-52.

*Olson, M., et al. (1997). Stress-induced immunosuppression and therapeutic touch. *Alternative Therapies in Health and Medicine, 3*(2), 68-74.

*Peck, S.D. (1997). The effectiveness of therapeutic touch for decreasing pain in elders with degenerative arthritis. *Journal of Holistic Nursing, 15,* 176-198.

*Peck, S.D. (1998). The efficacy of therapeutic touch for improving functional ability in elders with degenerative arthritis. *Nursing Science Quarterly, 11,* 123-132.

*Pennebaker, J.W. (1997). *Opening up: The healing power of expressing emotions.* New York: Guilford Press.

Plotnikoff, G. (2002). Herbal medicines. In M. Snyder & R. Lindquist (Eds.), *Complementary/alternative therapies in nursing* (4th ed., pp. 259-271). New York: Springer.

Post-White, J., & Fitzgerald, M. (2002). Imagery. In M. Snyder & R. Lindquist (Eds.), *Complementary/alternative therapies in nursing* (4th ed., pp. 43-57). New York: Springer.

*Progoff, I. (1975). *At a journal workshop.* New York: Dialogue House Library.

Quinn, J.F. (2002). Therapeutic touch. In M. Snyder & R. Lindquist (Eds.), *Complementary/alternative therapies in nursing* (4th ed., pp. 183-196). New York: Springer.

*Quinn, J.F., & Strelkauskas, A.J. (1993). Psychoneuroimmunological effects of therapeutic touch on practitioners and recently bereaved recipients: A pilot study. *Advances in Nursing Science, 15*(4), 13-26.

*Richards, K.C. (1998). Effect of a back massage and relaxation intervention on sleep in critically ill patients. *American Journal of Critical Care, 7,* 288-299.

*Shih, J. (1997). Basic Beijing twenty-four forms of Tai Chi exercise and average velocity of sway. *Perceptual and Motor Skills, 84,* 287-290.

Snyder, M., & Lindquist, R. (Eds.). (2002). *Complementary/alternative therapies in nursing* (4th ed.). New York: Springer.

*Snyder, M., Egan, E.C., & Burns, K. (1995). Efficacy of hand massage in decreasing agitation behaviors associated with care activities in persons with dementia. *Geriatric Nursing, 16*(2), 60-63.

Sparber, A. (in press). Complementary therapy in critical care settings. A review of surveys and implication for nurses. *Critical Care Nursing Clinic of North America, 15.*

*Spera, S.P., Buhrfeind, E.D., & Pennebaker, J.W. (1994). Expressive writing and coping with job loss. *Academy of Management Journal, 37,* 722-733.

*Thompson, M.B., & Coppens, N.M. (1994). The effects of guided imagery on anxiety levels and movement of clients undergoing magnetic resonance imaging. *Holistic Nursing Practice, 8*(2), 1179-1185.

*Troesch, L.M., et al. (1993). The influence of guided imagery on chemotherapy-related nausea and vomiting. *Oncology Nursing Forum, 20,* 1179-1185.

Umbreit, A.W. (2002). Healing touch. In M. Snyder & R. Lindquist (Eds.), *Complementary/alternative therapies in nursing* (4th ed., pp. 165-182). New York: Springer.

Weiss, P. (2002). Acupressure. In M. Snyder & R. Lindquist (Eds.), *Complementary/alternative therapies in nursing* (4th ed., pp. 205-220). New York: Springer.

CHAPTER

5 Health Care of Older Adults

DONNA D. IGNATAVICIUS

LEARNING OUTCOMES

After studying this chapter, you should be able to:

1. Identify four subgroups of older adults.
2. Describe nursing interventions for relocation stress syndrome.
3. Discuss common health issues that may concern older adults.
4. Explain why older adults are often at high risk for falls.
5. State common interventions for older clients at high risk for falls.
6. Describe the nursing care required for clients who are restrained.
7. Explain the effects of drugs on the older adult.
8. Compare and contrast delirium and dementia.
9. Interpret the signs and symptoms of elder neglect or abuse.
10. Discuss potential economic issues for older adults.
11. Describe government and community resources that are available for older adults.

Go to your Student CD-ROM for Review Questions
for the NCLEX Examination keyed to these Learning Outcomes.

The percentage of individuals older than age 65 years in the United States is about 13%. Women tend to live longer than men. This number is expected to grow as "baby boomers" approach late adulthood in the next 10 to 15 years. As many as 50% to 80% of hospitalized clients on medical-surgical units are over 65 years of age. Health care professionals need to know about the special needs of older adults as they care for them in a variety of settings.

This chapter describes the major health issues associated with late adulthood. The care of older adults (sometimes referred to as elders) with specific health problems, such as pain, acute and chronic illnesses, and surgical procedures, is discussed in appropriate chapters throughout this text. In addition, Nursing Focus on the Older Adult charts and Considerations for Older Adults headings highlight the most important information.

OVERVIEW

Late adulthood can be divided into four subgroups:

- 65 to 74 years of age: the young old
- 75 to 84 years of age: the middle old
- 85 to 99 years of age: the old old
- 100 years of age or more: the elite old

The fastest growing subgroup is the old old, sometimes referred to as the advanced older adult population. The members of this subgroup are sometimes referred to as the "frail elderly," although a number of 85 to 95 year olds are very healthy. In general, the needs and problems of this subgroup are different from those of adults between 65 and 74 years of age. The incidence of chronic disease increases with advanced age. For example, three fourths of all cancer diagnoses occur after age 75 (Loeb, 2003).

About 80% to 85% of all older adults are relatively healthy and live in the community at home, in assisted-living facilities, or in retirement complexes. Men over 65 years of age are less likely to live in a single-person household than women of that age. Five percent of all older adults reside in long-term care facilities (mostly nursing homes), and another 10% to 15% are ill but are cared for at home. Older adults from any setting usually experience one or more hospitalizations in their lifetime. About half of all older adults are admitted for short-term stays in a nursing home.

Many older adults experience one or more relocations during their "senior" years, such as when selling a house to move into a retirement living center. They usually have more difficulty adjusting to major change when compared to younger and middle-aged adults. Being admitted to a hospital or nursing home is a particularly traumatic experience. Older adults often suffer from relocation stress syndrome, also known as relocation trauma. **Relocation stress syndrome** is defined as a nursing diagnosis by the North American Nursing Diagnosis Association (NANDA). It is described as "physiological and/or psychosocial distress following transfer from one environment to another" (NANDA, 2003, p. 147). Examples of physiologic behaviors include sleep disturbance and in-

CHART 5-1

BEST PRACTICE for
Minimizing the Effects of Relocation Stress in Older Adults

- Provide opportunities for the client to assist in decision making.
- Carefully explain all procedures and routines to the client before they occur.
- Ask the family or significant other to provide familiar or special keepsakes to keep at the client's bedside (e.g., family picture, favorite hairbrush).
- Reorient the client frequently to his or her location.
- Ask the client about his or her expectations during hospitalization or nursing home placement.
- Encourage the client's family and friends to visit often.
- Establish a trusting relationship with the client as early as possible.
- Assess the client's usual lifestyle and daily activities, including food likes and dislikes and preferred time for bathing.
- Avoid unnecessary room changes.
- If possible, have a family member, significant other, staff member, or volunteer accompany the client when leaving the unit for special procedures or therapies.

creased physical symptoms, such as gastrointestinal distress. Examples of psychosocial manifestations are withdrawal, anxiety, anger, and depression. The nurse can be very helpful in assisting clients to adjust to their new environment. Chart 5-1 lists nursing interventions that may help to minimize the effects of relocation.

HEALTH ISSUES FOR OLDER ADULTS

Common health issues and problems that can affect older adults in any setting include the following:

- Health promotion
- Self-management
- Nutritional awareness
- Physical fitness and mobility
- Stress management
- Accidents
- Drug use and misuse
- Mental health/behavioral health problems
- Elder neglect and abuse

Health Promotion

Health is a major concern for most older adults. Health status can affect the ability to perform basic activities of daily living and to participate in social roles. A failure to perform these activities may increase dependence on others and may have a negative effect on morale and life satisfaction. When older adults lose the ability to function independently, they often feel empty and worthless. Loss of autonomy is a painful event related to the physical and mental changes of aging, and it can be the result of physical illness (Davidhizar & Shearer, 2000).

Like younger adults, middle and older adults need to practice health promotion and illness prevention to maintain or achieve a high level of wellness. The risk factors that negatively impact "successful" aging are alcohol abuse, smoking, depression, lack of exercise, and obesity. In addition, being nonwhite and uneducated compounds the risk for health problems (Davidhizar, Eshleman, & Moody, 2002).

CHART 5-2

CLIENT EDUCATION GUIDE
Lifestyles and Practices to Promote Wellness

Health-Protecting Behaviors

- Have yearly influenza vaccinations (after October 1).
- Obtain a pneumococcal vaccination. (A routine revaccination may be necessary.)
- Have a tetanus immunization, and get a booster every 10 years.
- Wear seat belts when you are in an automobile.
- Use alcohol in moderation or not at all.
- Avoid smoking.
- If you smoke at home, do not smoke in bed.
- Install and maintain working smoke detectors.
- Create a hazard-free environment to prevent falls; eliminate hazards such as scatter rugs and waxed floors.
- Use medications according to your physician's prescription.
- Avoid over-the-counter medications unless your physician directs you to use them.
- Take one aspirin every day (any dose between 81 and 325 mg) to decrease the risk of myocardial infarction and colon cancer.

Health-Enhancing Behaviors

- Have a yearly physical examination; see your health care provider more often if health problems occur.
- Reduce dietary fat to not more than 30% of calories; saturated fat should provide less than 10% of your calories.
- Increase your dietary intake of complex carbohydrate and fiber-containing food to five or more servings of fruits and vegetables and six or more servings of grain products daily.
- Increase calcium intake to between 1000 and 1500 mg daily.
- Allow at least 10 to 15 minutes of sun exposure two to three times weekly for vitamin D intake; avoid prolonged sun exposure.
- Exercise regularly three to five times a week for 30 minutes per session.
- Manage stress through coping mechanisms that have been successful in the past.
- Get together with individuals in different settings.
- Reminisce about your life.

Chronic illness is a major problem in older adult population (see Chapter 10). The nurse working with these clients in any setting needs to teach them the importance of promoting wellness and strategies for accomplishing this goal (Chart 5-2).

Self-Management

An older person's ability to maintain a positive self-concept and self-control may be hampered by the loss of resources in the late years of life. Older adults may also experience a number of losses that can affect their sense of control over their lives: the death of a spouse and significant others, the loss of social and work roles, and a decrease in physical mobility. The nurse can support older clients' self-esteem and feelings of independence by encouraging them to maintain as much control as possible over their lives, to participate in decision making, and to perform as many tasks as possible.

Regardless of the situation, it is important that older clients direct their lifestyle in a manner that encourages them to feel capable and valued. Most important, they need to find opportunities to be productive and take care of themselves as well as others.

A number of tools are available to the nurse in the community health or home health setting for assessing the self-care or self-management ability of older adults. (See Chapter 10 for discussion of functional assessment.) When older adults are admitted to a hospital or nursing home, the nurse needs to assess self-management capabilities for discharge planning.

Nutritional Awareness

NUTRITIONAL NEEDS IN THE COMMUNITY

A person's need for adequate nutrition remains constant throughout the life span, yet many older individuals are at risk for undernutrition. Inflation, reduced income, and a lack of transportation are factors that may contribute to inadequate nutrition among older adults. Older adults whose diets consist of inappropriate or unbalanced foods (e.g., an excess of carbohydrates) may also be poorly nourished. Some clients reduce their intake of food to near-starvation levels, even with the availability of assistive programs such as food stamps, free food, and Meals on Wheels. The lack of transportation, the necessity of traveling to obtain such services, and the inability to carry large quantities of groceries prohibit some older adults from taking advantage of food programs. Some older adults are too proud to accept free services.

Poor nutrition may also be related to loneliness. Older adults may respond to loneliness, depression, and boredom by not eating, which can lead to undernutrition. Many clients who live alone lose the incentive to prepare or eat balanced diets. Others respond to stress by overeating, which leads to obesity.

NUTRITIONAL REQUIREMENTS

The minimal nutritional requirements of the human body remain consistent from youth through old age, with a few exceptions. Older adults need an increased dietary intake of calcium, vitamin D, vitamin C, and vitamin A because alterations with age disrupt the ability to store, use, and absorb these substances. A sedentary lifestyle and reduced metabolic rate requires a reduction in total caloric intake to maintain an ideal body weight.

PHYSICAL CHANGES AFFECTING NUTRITION

Other physical aging changes influence nutritional status or the ability to consume needed nutrients. Diminished senses of taste and smell often result in a loss of appeal of food. Older adults experience a greater decline in the ability to taste sweet and salt than in the discrimination of bitter and sour. This physiologic change often results in an overuse of table sugar and salt to compensate. Teach the client to substitute herbs and spices to season food or to vary the textures of food substances to achieve satisfaction from food.

Tooth loss and poorly fitting dentures from inadequate dental care can also cause the older adult to avoid important foodstuffs. Older individuals with dentition problems often resort to eating soft, high-calorie foods such as ice cream and mashed potatoes, which lack roughage and fiber. Unless the person carefully chooses more nutritious soft foods, vitamin deficiencies, constipation, and other disorders can result. The extensive use of prescribed and over-the-counter (OTC) drugs, including herbal supplements, may affect appetite, food tolerances, and food absorption and use.

Older adults sometimes respond to problems associated with mobility, prescribed diuretics, and limited bladder capacity by limiting fluid intake, especially in the evening. Teach older adults that fluid restrictions make them susceptible to dehydration and electrolyte imbalances that can cause serious illness or death.

NUTRITIONAL NEEDS IN THE HOSPITAL AND NURSING HOME

In addition to the nutritional needs described for older adults living in the community, those who are in the hospital or nursing home have special needs related to their illness and general health. For example, an older client with a pressure ulcer needs additional protein, vitamin C, and zinc to heal the open skin lesion. The health care provider, nurse, and dietitian collaborate to determine the best sources of these nutrients. The health care provider may prescribe a multivitamin tablet with zinc to be given every day. The dietitian may recommend that a high-calorie, high-protein supplement such as Ensure Plus be given several times a day. The nurse encourages the client to select and eat high-protein foods to promote healing and prevent undernutrition.

Anorexia and weight loss are the most common nutritional problems in both hospitals and long-term care settings. Common causes of undernutrition include drugs, chewing problems, immobility, infections, and Alzheimer's disease. Another issue may be the lack of foods that are culturally specific. For example, a Mexican man may be used to eating enchiladas, rellenos, and tacos, but is served baked chicken and mashed potatoes. Chapter 64 discusses nutrition in detail, including interdisciplinary interventions for the prevention and management of common problems.

Physical Fitness and Mobility

Exercise and activity are important for older adults as a means of promoting and maintaining health (Figure 5-1). Physical activity can help keep the body in shape and main-

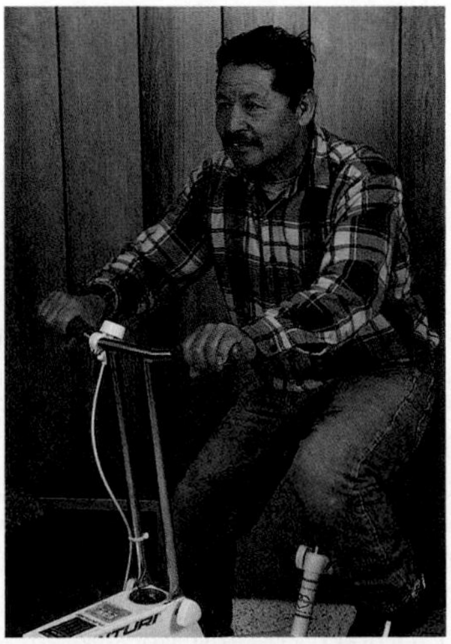

Figure 5-1 ■ Exercise is important to older adults for health promotion and maintenance.

tain an optimal level of functioning. In addition, regular and moderate exercise typically results in feelings of well-being. Numerous studies have shown that exercise has many benefits, including the following (Christmas & Andersen, 2000):

- Decrease falls
- Increase strength
- Reduce arthritis pain
- Reduce depression
- Improve longevity
- Reduce risks for diabetes and coronary artery disease

Nurses and other health care professionals need to teach older adults about the value of physical activity. One of the best exercises for older adults is walking at least 30 minutes, three to five times a week. During the winter, indoor shopping centers and other public places can be used. Swimming is also recommended but does not offer the weight-bearing advantage of walking. Older adults who have been sedentary should start their exercise programs slowly and gradually increase the frequency and duration of activity over time.

A few nursing studies have been conducted to explore exercise habits in the older adult population. One study of Latina older women found that, although the subjects verbalized the benefits of exercise, perceived barriers prevented them from exercising on a regular basis (Juarbe et al., 2002). The common barriers cited were time constraints, spousal and maternal roles, personal health limitations, lack of motivation, and fatigue. External barriers included transportation difficulties and cost. The researchers concluded that health education for this group needed to be culturally relevant, focusing on time and role-constraint barriers.

When any older adult is hospitalized, the opportunity for continuing a program of physical fitness is interrupted, at least temporarily. During severe or prolonged illness, clients are at high risk for complications of decreased physical mobility, such as pneumonia, skin impairment, contractures, muscle atrophy, constipation, and renal calculi. These problems are addressed elsewhere in this text.

Stress Management

FACTORS CONTRIBUTING TO STRESS IN OLDER ADULTS

Stress can speed up the aging process over time, or it can lead to diseases that increase the rate of degeneration. Stress can impair the reserve capacity of older adults and lessen their ability to respond and adapt to changes in their environment.

Although no period of the life cycle is free from stress, the later years can be a time of especially high risk. Frequently observed sources of stress for the older population include rapid environmental changes that require immediate reaction, changes in lifestyle resulting from retirement or physical incapacity, acute or chronic illness, the loss of significant others, financial hardships, and relocation. How individuals react to these stresses depends on their personal coping skills and support networks. The loss of roles experienced by older adults often limits the availability of external support networks. For instance, losses leave many clients without friends to whom they can turn for support and help. As a result, many must rely solely on their personal resources to maintain their mental health/behavioral health. A combination of poor physical health and social problems leaves older adults susceptible to stress overload, which can result in illness and premature death.

COPING WITH STRESS

The ways in which individuals adapt to old age largely depend on the personality traits and coping strategies that have characterized them throughout their lives. Establishing and maintaining relationships with others throughout life is especially important to the older person's happiness. Even more important than having friends is the nature of the friendships. Individuals who have close, intimate, stable relationships with others in whom they confide are more likely to maintain integrity in times of crisis.

A qualitative study by Loeb et al. (2003) found that older adults with at least two chronic illnesses coped by focusing on lifestyle changes to promote health, relying on spirituality and/or religion, and engaging in life. Some older adults sought information about health care, such as asking pharmacists about their medications. A limitation of this study was that all study subjects were white, and coping strategies may be different for various ethnic or racial groups.

ENVIRONMENTAL FACTORS

Most older adults live in and own their own homes. Physical or economic problems may force some to relocate to a retirement center or an assisted-living facility. Family members and facility staff need to be aware that older adults need personal space in their new surroundings. They need to participate in deciding how the space will be arranged and what they can keep in their new home to help offset the feelings of powerlessness. Suggest that the client or family bring in personal items, such as pictures of relatives and friends, favorite clothing, and valued knickknacks to assist in making the new setting seem more familiar and comfortable. This same intervention can be carried out in a hospital setting.

Changes in vision, touch, and motor ability can create difficulties for older adults in any environment. For example, decreased vision in old age, especially the poor perception of distance, may make walking more difficult; the person is less aware of the location of each step. A reduced sense of touch decreases the awareness of body orientation (e.g., whether the foot is squarely on the step). The decreased reaction time that commonly results from age-related changes in the neurologic system may also impair the ability to recognize or move from a dangerous setting.

Accidents

ACCIDENTS IN THE COMMUNITY

Most accidents occur at home. Teach older adults about the need to be aware of safety precautions to prevent accidents, such as falls. Incapacitating accidents are a primary cause of restricted physical fitness and decreased mobility in old age. Some individuals develop **fallophobia** and avoid leaving their homes for fear of falling.

Safeguards such as handrails, slip-proof underpads for rugs, and adequate lighting are essential in the home. Avoiding scatter rugs, slippery floors, and clutter is also important to prevent falls. Remind older adults to avoid going out on days when steps are wet or icy, and to ask for help when ambulating. To minimize sensory overload, advise the older adult to concentrate on one activity at a time. If needed, encourage the use of visual, hearing, or ambulatory assistive devices. High costs and a fear of appearing old sometimes prevent older adults from obtaining or using hearing aids, eyeglasses, walkers, or canes.

ACCIDENTS IN THE HOSPITAL AND NURSING HOME

The most common accident among older clients in a hospital or nursing home setting is falling. A **fall** is an unintentional change in body position that results in the client's body coming to rest on the floor or ground (Resnick, 2003). Some falls result in serious injuries such as fractures and head trauma. Most health care settings require an admission fall risk assessment and a protocol for clients who are at high risk for falls.

Risk Assessment and Interventions for Preventing Falls

Assess the client for risk for falls. Many risk assessment tools have been developed to help the nurse focus on factors that increase an older person's risk of falling (Resnick, 2003). Chart 5-3 lists some of the common risk factors that the nurse should assess and the measures for preventing falls. A history of falling is the single most important predictor for falls.

Once an older client has been identified as being at high risk for falls, choose interventions that help prevent falls and possible serious injury. For clients in the community, Tai Chi exercise is gaining popularity as an important activity to improve balance and functional mobility, as well as to decrease the fear of falling, especially among older women (Taggart, 2002).

Chart 5-3 lists common interventions that should be implemented for all older adults at a high risk for falling. One of the most controversial issues in fall prevention is the use of siderails as a physical restraint, especially in the hospital setting. At this time, hospital staff members are encouraged to evaluate each client as to the need to raise all four rails, two upper rails only, or no rails. In the nursing home, siderails are classified as restraints.

Older clients often have **nocturia** (urination at night) and get out of bed to go to the bathroom. They may forget to ask for assistance and may subsequently fall as a result of disorientation in the darkness in an unfamiliar environment. In some cases, they may crawl over the siderail, which can make the fall more serious. Because of this, siderails are used less often in both hospitals and nursing homes.

Use of Restraints

Similar considerations have been given regarding the use of other physical and chemical restraints. A **restraint** is any device or medication that prevents the client from moving freely. In 1990, the federal government enforced a law that gives nursing home residents the right to be restraint free. Removing physical restraints from nursing home residents has reduced serious injuries, although falls and minor injuries have increased in some cases.

CHART 5-3

BEST PRACTICE for
Assessing Risk Factors and Preventing Falls in Older Adults

Assess for the presence of the following risk factors:
- History of falls
- Advanced age (>80 years)
- Multiple illnesses
- Generalized weakness or decreased mobility
- Disorientation or confusion
- Use of drugs that can cause increased confusion, mobility limitations, or orthostatic hypotension
- Urinary incontinence
- Communication impairments
- Major visual impairments or visual impairment without correction
- Substance abuse
- Location of client's room away from the nurses' station (in the hospital or nursing home)
- Change of shift or mealtime (in the hospital or nursing home)

Implement the following nursing interventions for all clients, regardless of risk:
- Monitor the client's activities and behavior as often as possible, preferably every 30 to 60 minutes.
- Remind the client to call for help before getting out of bed or a chair.
- Help the client to get out of bed or a chair.
- Provide, or remind the client to use, a walker or cane for ambulating.
- Remind the client to wear eyeglasses or a hearing aid if needed.
- Help the incontinent client to toilet every 1 to 2 hours.
- Clean up spills immediately.
- Arrange the furniture in the client's room or hallway to eliminate clutter or obstacles that could contribute to a fall.
- Provide adequate lighting at all times, especially at night.
- Observe for side effects and toxic effects of drug therapy.
- Orient the client to the environment.
- Keep the call light within reach, and ensure that the client can use it.
- Place the bed in the lowest position with the brakes locked.
- Place objects that the client needs within reach.
- Ensure that adequate handrails are present in the client's room, bathroom, and hall.
- Have the physical therapist assess the client for mobility and safety.

For clients at a high risk for falls:
- Implement all interventions listed above.
- Relocate the client for best visibility and supervision.
- Use bed and chair alarms.
- Encourage family members or significant other to stay with the client.

Hospitals have also reduced the use of physical restraints. The Joint Commission on Accreditation of Healthcare Organizations (JCAHO) has specific standards that limit the use of physical restraints in hospitals and nursing homes. Chemical restraints or psychoactive drugs such as haloperidol (Haldol) have sometimes been used in place of physical restraints.

PHYSICAL RESTRAINTS

Experts agree that older adults should not be placed in a physical restraint or sedated just because they are old. Alternatives are used before applying any type of restraint (Chart 5-4). However, if all other interventions (e.g., reminding clients to call for assistance when needed or asking a family member to stay with clients) are ineffective in fall prevention, the nurse may need to use a physical restraint

CHART 5-4

BEST PRACTICE for Restraint Alternatives

- If the client is acutely confused, reorient him or her to reality as often as possible.
- If the client has dementia, use validation to reaffirm his or her feelings and concerns.
- Check the client often, at least every hour.
- If the client pulls tubes and lines, cover them with roller gauze or another protective device.
- Provide activities that keep the client busy, such as an activity pillow or apron, puzzle, or art activity.
- Provide soft, calming music.
- Place the client in an area where he or she can be supervised. (If the client is agitated, do not place him or her in a noisy area.)
- Turn off the television if the client is agitated.
- Ask a family member or friend to stay with the client at night.
- Help the client to toilet every 2 to 3 hours, including during the night.
- Be sure that the client's needs for food, fluids, and comfort are met.
- If agency policy allows, provide the client with a pet visit.
- Provide familiar objects or cherished items that the client can touch.
- Document the use of all alternative interventions.
- If a restraint is applied, use the least restrictive device (e.g., mitts rather than wrist restraints, a roller belt rather than a vest).

for a specified period. Applying a restraint is a serious intervention and should be analyzed for its risk versus its benefit. Check the client in a restraint every 30 to 60 minutes, and release the restraint at least every 2 hours for turning, repositioning, and toileting. Physical restraints such as vests have caused serious injury and even death. If restraint is needed, the least restrictive device should be used.

CHEMICAL RESTRAINTS

Chemical restraints, or psychoactive drugs, are often overused in hospital settings. Clients who are noisy, agitated, abusive, or combative may have an "as needed" order for a psychoactive drug. Such medications include the following:

- Antipsychotic drugs
- Antianxiety drugs
- Antidepressant drugs
- Sedative-hypnotic drugs

These drugs produce serious side effects and toxic effects and therefore should be reserved for clients with a documented mental health or behavioral health problem, such as severe anxiety or psychosis. Clients receiving these medications must be closely monitored for therapeutic and adverse effects.

The most potent group of psychoactive drugs is the antipsychotics. These drugs may be appropriate for the control of certain behavioral symptoms, such as hallucinations, delusions, and violent episodes. However, fewer than half of clients respond to these drugs. If a psychoactive drug is used as a last resort to control behavior, the lowest dose should be given.

Drug Use and Misuse

Drug therapy for the older population in general is another major health issue. Because of the multiple chronic and acute illnesses that occur in this age group, drugs for older adults account for about one third of all prescription drug costs. The term **polypharmacy** has been used to describe the use of multiple drugs by older adults.

Older adults also commonly use nonprescription drugs, such as analgesics, antacids, cold and cough preparations, laxatives, and herbal/vitamin supplements, often without consulting a health care provider. The occurrence of adverse drug reactions is directly related to the number of drugs taken and the frequency with which they are taken. Therefore older adults are at high risk for adverse drug reactions or interactions and are often admitted to the hospital for these problems.

PHYSIOLOGIC CHANGES AFFECTING DRUG USE

Older adults may not tolerate the standard dosage of medications traditionally prescribed for younger adults. The physiologic changes related to aging make drug therapy more complex and challenging. These changes affect the absorption, distribution, metabolism, and excretion of drugs from the body.

Age-related changes that can potentially affect drug absorption from an oral route include an increase in gastric pH, a decrease in gastric blood flow, and a decrease in gastrointestinal motility. Despite these changes, most clients do not have major absorption difficulties because of age-related changes alone.

Age-related changes that affect drug distribution include smaller amounts of total body water, an increased ratio of adipose tissue to lean body mass, a decreased albumin level, and a decreased cardiac output. Increased adipose tissue in proportion to lean body mass can cause increased storage of lipid-soluble drugs. This leads to a decreased concentration of the drug in plasma but an increased concentration in tissue.

Drug metabolism most often occurs in the liver. Age-related changes affecting metabolism include a decrease in liver size, a decrease in liver blood flow, and a decrease in liver enzyme activity. These changes can result in increased plasma concentrations of a drug. Changes in the kidneys can also result in high plasma concentrations of drugs.

The excretion of drugs most often involves the renal system. Age-related changes of the renal system include decreased renal blood flow and reduced glomerular filtration rate. These changes result in a decreased creatinine clearance and thus a slower excretion time for medications. Consequently, serum drug levels can become toxic, and the client can become extremely ill or die.

EFFECTS OF DRUGS ON OLDER ADULTS

Because of age-related physiologic changes, older adults are at a high risk for side effects and toxic effects from drugs. Older adults have less reserve capacity in most organ systems. When chronic disease is added to the physiologic changes of aging, drug reactions have a more dramatic effect and take a longer time to correct. Often a lower dose of medication is necessary to prevent adverse effects. The policy of "start low, go slow" is essential when health care providers prescribe drugs for this group. The physiologic changes of aging are highly individual. Alterations in drug therapy should always be individualized according to the actual physiologic changes present and the occurrence and severity of chronic disease. Common adverse drug reactions are listed in Table 5-1.

Many of these signs and symptoms can be mistakenly attributed to a concurrent illness or assumed to be part of the aging process. Assess all older clients with such symptoms for possible adverse reactions to medications.

SELF-ADMINISTRATION OF MEDICATION

Most individuals older than 65 years of age live at home and are responsible for taking their own medications. Because the risk of drug toxicity is considerably increased in the older population, the nurse should assist clients in assuming this task responsibly. Help prevent problems by educating clients and their caregivers, providing clear and concise directions, and developing ways to assist them in overcoming handicaps or difficulties with self-administration.

Older adults make errors in self-administration for several reasons. First, they may simply forget. In the rush of daily activities, they may not take the drug at all or may take it too often because of an inability to remember when or whether their medications have been taken. It can be helpful for clients to associate pill taking with daily events (e.g., meals) or to keep a simple chart or calendar. Pill boxes have been devised so that a daily, weekly, or monthly supply of medicine can be placed in the appropriate compartments (Figure 5-2). Egg cartons can be very cost-effective pill boxes. Large print on the drug label assists clients who have poor visual acuity. Writing the drug regimen on the top of the bottle with large letters and numbers is also helpful.

A second reason that older adults often commit errors in taking medications is poor communication with health care professionals. These difficulties result from inadequate explanations or explanations that are not understood because of educational limitations or language barriers. Health care professionals often presume that their client has acquired the knowledge if they have told the client about the medications. The nurse or other health care provider needs to help older adults plan their medication schedules.

A third reason for medication errors is attitude and ingrained feelings about taking medicine. Some individuals add to their drug regimen by taking over-the-counter (OTC) drugs, which can interact with prescription drugs and cause serious problems. For example, a client receiving warfarin (Coumadin, Warfilone✱) for anticoagulation may take ibuprofen (Motrin) regularly for arthritis. Because ibuprofen has anticoagulant ability, this combination can cause overt or occult bleeding. When obtaining a medication history, it is important to ask clients about all OTC drugs, including herbal and food supplements.

Other older individuals avoid taking medication whenever they can. The fear of drug dependency or the cost of the drugs may cause many to discontinue their medications too soon. In addition, the actions or side effects of some drugs may not be desirable. For example, diuretics may cause incontinence when clients cannot get to the bathroom quickly enough. Others may think that two pills are twice as effective as one; some older adults take medication that is leftover from a previous illness or take a drug that has been prescribed for someone else.

Health care providers can influence the attitudes of older adults toward their medications and their health problems. One method being tried in some hospitals and nursing homes is supervised drug self-administration, in which clients are allowed to take their own medications under supervision. In this way, the nurse can be sure of a client's understanding and ability to self-administer medications at home or in another health care setting.

TABLE 5-1 Common Adverse Drug Reactions in Older Adults

■ Edema	■ Dizziness
■ Nausea and vomiting	■ Urinary retention
■ Anorexia	■ Diarrhea
■ Dry mouth	■ Constipation
■ Fatigue	■ Confusion
■ Weakness	

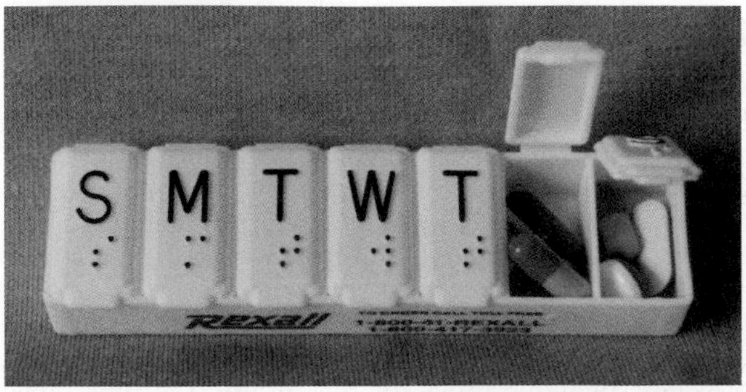

Figure 5-2 ■ A medication system for safe self-administration.

Mental Health/Behavioral Health

Most older adults are mentally sound and competent. A few changes in cognition have been identified as age related and are linked to specific cognitive functions rather than intellectual capacity. These changes include a decreased reaction time to stimuli and an impairment of memory for recent events. However, gross cognitive impairment, depression, hallucinations, and delusions are not part of the normal aging process.

Two forms of competence exist: legal competence and clinical competence. A person is **legally competent** if he or she is:

- 18 years of age or older
- Pregnant or a married minor
- A legally emancipated (free) minor who is self-supporting
- Not declared incompetent by a court of law

If a court determines that a person is not legally competent, a guardian is appointed to make financial and health care decisions.

A person is **clinically competent** if he or she is legally competent and has decisional capacity. Decisional capacity is determined by an individual's ability to identify problems, recognize options, make decisions, and provide the rationale supporting the decisions.

It is not surprising that mental illness does occur among the older population. Losses in income and physical health, a lack of comprehensive health care and social services, a loss of social roles, and the death of significant others may affect a person's emotional stability. Older adults are often unaware of early symptoms of emotional or mental impairments. Their symptoms may go unnoticed by family and friends and thus progress until crisis results. The three most common cognitive problems among older adults are depression, dementia, and delirium.

DEPRESSION

Depression, the most common mental health/behavioral health disorder among older adults, is a response to multiple life stresses, a single situation (situational depression), a primary disorder, or a problem associated with dementia. It can range from mild, transient feelings of sadness to a severe sense of helplessness and hopelessness. Depression is thought to result from a lack of the neurotransmitters norepinephrine and serotonin in the brain. It is often underdiagnosed by physicians and is therefore undertreated (Kurlowicz, 2003).

Families and nurses are often in a position to suspect depression in an older adult. Several screening tools are available to help determine if the client has clinical depression. The Geriatric Depression Scale–Short Form (GDS-SF) is commonly used and completed by the client. A score of 11 or greater is consistent with a diagnosis of clinical depression (Kurlowicz, 2003).

Without diagnosis and subsequent treatment, depression can result in the following:

- Worsening of medical conditions
- Risk of physical illness
- Alcoholism
- Increased pain and disability
- Delayed recovery from illness
- Suicide (especially among older men)

Older adults have the highest suicide rate of any age-group (Uncapher & Arean, 2000). In their study, Uncapher and Arean (2000) sent two case studies of suicidal, depressed clients to primary care physicians to determine if any bias in treatment would be present. The two cases were the same except for age–one client was age 38 years and the other was age 78 years. The 215 physician responses showed that all providers recognized the depression and suicide risk but were less willing to treat the older client. They believed that suicidal ideation was normal for the older client.

CULTURAL CONSIDERATIONS

White men older than 70 years of age, especially those living alone, are at the highest risk for suicide. Older adults contemplating suicide usually do not talk about their plans and choose a method that will ensure death (e.g., a gunshot).

Elders with depression may experience early morning insomnia, excessive daytime sleeping, poor appetite, a lack of energy, and an unwillingness to participate in social and recreational activities. The primary treatment for depression usually includes drug therapy and psychotherapy. In some parts of the country, electroconvulsive therapy (ECT) may be used either as a last resort or when drugs are not effective.

Selective serotonin reuptake inhibitors (SSRIs) are the first choice for drug therapy, but take 2 to 3 weeks to work. They act by increasing the amount of serotonin and norepinephrine at neuronal synapses in the brain. More information about depression is available in mental health/behavioral health nursing textbooks.

DEMENTIA

Dementia is a broad term used for a syndrome that is characterized by a slowly progressive cognitive decline. Formerly called organic brain syndrome (OBS) and chronic brain syndrome (CBS), dementia represents a global impairment of intellectual function and is generally chronic and progressive. There are many types of dementia, the most common being Alzheimer's disease. Multi-infarct dementia, the second most common dementia, is a vascular disorder and accounts for 20% to 25% of all dementias. Chapter 45 discusses dementias in detail, with a focus on Alzheimer's disease.

DELIRIUM

Whereas dementia is a chronic, progressive disorder, **delirium** is an acute state of confusion. Delirium also differs from dementia in that it is usually short-term and reversible within 3 weeks. It is often seen among older adults in a hospital setting or in a setting with which they are unfamiliar. Behavior typically fits into one of two categories: hyperactivity (most common) or hypoactivity (Ignatavicius, 1999). Hyperactive clients may try to climb out of bed or pull out invasive catheters (e.g., urinary catheters or intravenous cannulas), or they may become quite agitated and combative. Hypoactive clients are quiet, apathetic, and withdrawn. Wakefield (2002) found that most nurses in her study did not realize that acutely confused older adults can be quiet.

Multiple factors can cause delirium, including the following:

- Medication (especially anticholinergic drugs)
- Metabolic disturbances
- Infections
- Surgical operations
- Circulatory, renal, and pulmonary disorders
- Nutritional deficiencies
- Major loss

Acutely confused clients who are discharged from the hospital are at an increased risk for functional decline, falls, and incontinence (Wakefield, 2002). Therefore nurses should assess older clients for acute confusion. A number of assessment tools have been developed, including the Confusion Assessment Method (CAM), Delirium Rating Scale (DRS), and NEECHAM Confusion Scale. Although the CAM is easy to use (Table 5-2), Rapp et al. (2000) found that the most useful tool was the nurse-developed NEECHAM Confusion Scale (see the Evidence-Based Practice for Nursing box on p. 48).

TABLE 5-2 The Confusion Assessment Method (CAM)

1. Acute onset and fluctuating course (e.g., Is there evidence of an acute change in mental status from the client's baseline?)
2. Inattention (e.g., Does the client have difficulty focusing attention or keeping track of what is being said?)
3. Disorganized thinking (e.g., Is the client's thinking and conversation disorganized or incoherent?)
4. Altered level of consciousness (e.g., Is the client lethargic, hyperalert, or difficult to arouse?)

The diagnosis of delirium by the CAM is the presence of features 1 *and* 2 and either 3 *or* 4.

To manage delirium, use a calm voice to reorient the client and to divert the client's attention away from devices or tubes. A number of innovative nursing interventions have been used with some success. For example, playing tapes of soothing music in the client's room may have a calming effect. Giving the client a doll or stuffed animal to "fidget" with may prevent the client from removing important medical instrumentation. Some nurses believe that providing dolls and stuffed animals is treating the adult like a child, but this intervention can sometimes be very effective when used for therapeutic purposes. If the client has a favorite item, such as an afghan blanket or a picture, the nurse asks the family or significant others to provide it for the same purpose.

EVIDENCE-BASED PRACTICE for Nursing

Which tool is best for nurses to use when assessing clients who are acutely confused?

Rapp, C.G., et al. (2000). Acute confusion assessment instruments: Clinical versus research usability. *Applied Nursing Research, 13*(1), 37-45.

Acute confusion (AC), also known as delirium, is a common problem seen by nurses in a variety of health care settings. This study examined five AC assessment tools—Confusion Assessment Method (CAM), Delirium Rating Scale (DRS), Delirium Symptom Inventory (DSI), Mini-Mental State Examination (MMSE), and Neelon/Champagne (NEECHAM) Confusion Scale—to determine the most reliable indicator of acute confusion. The researchers also asked evaluators to identify which tool was the easiest to use. The NEECHAM tool was unanimously selected because it specifically assesses for AC and identifies both at-risk clients and those who actually have AC. They also liked the CAM because it was linked to the criteria for delirium as listed in the *Diagnostic and Statistical Manual,* 4th edition (DSM-IV). A protocol that includes both tools was written, and nurses from the authors' health care system have been trained in its use for screening clients.

Level of Evidence: 6—Poorly controlled study, but helps to validate the use of the CAM.

Critique. The authors evaluated tools that had already been tested for reliability and validity and applied them for use in the practice setting. The NEECHAM tool, the only nurse-designed tool, was selected by the raters. Other authors have reported that this tool can be incorporated into daily practice.

Implications for Nursing. This study validated that nurses need to assess for AC using a standardized screening method, especially for older adults. Early identification of delirium alerts the health care team to the need for modifications in the client's plan of care.

Table 5-3 briefly differentiates delirium and dementia and lists the major nursing considerations for each. The most difficult challenge is caring for a client who is experiencing both problems at the same time.

Elder Neglect and Abuse

Another problem sometimes encountered by older adults is neglect and abuse, both verbal and physical. Some older adults are vulnerable to these problems, especially widowed women who may have difficulty being assertive. Older persons who are neglected or abused are often physically dependent. The abuser is often a family member who becomes frustrated or distraught over the burden of caring for the older adult.

Prolonged caregiving by a family member is a new and unexpected role for adult children, most often women. This new role may result in role fatigue and role conflict. Caregiver Role Strain and Risk for Caregiver Role Strain were added to the list of nursing diagnoses approved by the North American Nursing Diagnosis Association (NANDA). From their research, McCloskey and Bulechek (2000) identified Caregiver Support as a major nursing intervention (Chart 5-5).

Gray-Vickery (2000) described four common types of abuse:

- **Neglect** occurs when a caregiver fails to provide for a client's basic needs, such as food, clothing, or assistance with activities of daily living (ADLs). Whether intentional or unintentional, neglect accounts for almost half of all cases of actual elder abuse.
- **Physical abuse** is the use of physical force that results in bodily injury, especially in the "bathing suit" zone (abdomen, buttocks, genital area, upper thighs). Examples of physical abuse include hitting, burning, pushing, and molesting the client. Approximately one fourth of all cases of actual elder abuse involve physical force.
- **Financial abuse** occurs when the client's property or resources are mismanaged or misused; this is more common than physical abuse.
- **Emotional abuse** is the intentional use of threats, humiliation, intimidation, and isolation toward older adults. It occurs in more than one third of all cases of actual elder abuse.

TABLE 5-3 Differences in the Characteristics of Delirium and Dementia

Variable	Dementia	Delirium
Description	A chronic, progressive cognitive decline	An acute confusional state
Onset	Slow	Fast
Duration	Months to years	Hours to less than 1 month
Cause	Unknown, possibly familial, chemical	Multiple, such as surgery, infection, drugs
Reversibility	None	Usually
Management	Treat signs and symptoms	Remove or treat the cause
Nursing interventions	Reorientation not effective in the late stages; use validation therapy (acknowledge the client's feelings and do not argue); provide a safe environment; observe for associated behaviors, such as delusions and hallucinations	Reorient the client to reality; provide a safe environment

Carefully assess the client for signs of abuse, such as bruises in clusters or regular patterns; burns, commonly to the buttocks or the soles of the feet; unusual hair loss; or multiple injuries, especially fractures. If the older adult is too weak or has no other resources or support systems, he or she may not acknowledge that the abuse is occurring. Neglect may be manifested by pressure ulcers, contractures, dehydration or undernutrition, urine burns, excessive body odor, and listlessness (Gray-Vickery, 1999). Dyer et al. (2000) found that depression and dementia were common in community elders who were abused or neglected.

If physical abuse or neglect is suspected, notify the physician and social worker to investigate the situation. All states in the United States and other Western countries have laws requiring health care professionals to report suspected elder abuse.

ECONOMIC ISSUES FOR OLDER ADULTS

Income

Most adults hope to provide for their own needs throughout their life cycle. One of the greatest fears related to aging is becoming dependent on family, friends, or society. In many cases, older adults have not achieved economic self-sufficiency. One fifth of the total population of the United States is poor, and one fifth of the poor are older than age 65 years.

Most individuals expect their financial resources to decline in their retirement years compared with their working years. They also expect their level of expenses to decline, but this may not occur. In the United States, for example, the inflation that began in the 1970s has reduced the value of financial assets. Older adults have been especially hard hit because most rely on Social Security benefits or pension funds for the bulk of their income. Recent declines in the stock market as a result of terrorism and war have added to the reduction in assets. Many older adults are unable to adjust their income to changing economic circumstances and hence are powerless to combat declining real income.

Health care purchases are paid for in large part by private insurance and federal health and social programs. However, the rising cost of these programs contributes substantially to rising government costs and may result in more out-of-pocket costs for the older health care consumer. Health care costs for older adults is a major issue being debated in the United States by Congress and other political bodies. Many elders take multiple medications that are extremely expensive in the United States, but that can be sometimes obtained in other countries such as Canada and Mexico or ordered on the Internet. The quality of these drugs is not guaranteed, but older adults are looking for ways to comply with their treatment plan, while having enough money to meet their basic needs.

Housing

The popular belief that older adults are frail, dependent, senile individuals living out their last years in an institution has no factual basis. Many older adults live in their own homes and have paid off their mortgages. However, living arrangements are a major problem for some individuals as they age. This issue can increase the client's stress level and have an impact on health care planning.

In many countries, the rising costs of energy and housing have joined the high costs of food and health care as factors that contribute to the economic hardship of older adults. In addition to financial difficulties, housing may be a problem because of a lack of environmental supports that would help older adults to continue residing and participating in the community.

Deterioration of property, escalation of property taxes, and maintenance service costs create many problems for older homeowners wishing to keep their homes. In some areas, older renters are extremely vulnerable to high rents, real estate speculation, and the loss of living quarters because of the removal of substandard, low-rent apartment or hotel buildings. Physical impairments and a lack of available and affordable support services (e.g., household help, transportation, home health care, and meal assistance) prevent some older adults from managing adequately in their own homes.

The need for special housing for older adults has long been recognized. Numbers of government and privately funded experiments in alternative housing have been tested. These projects incorporate variables such as personal care services, special health and safety remedies, and recreation and leisure plans. Although most of these projects provide security, improve life satisfaction, and prove to be cost-effective, many areas of the United States have no overall plan for alternative living arrangements for older adults.

RESOURCES FOR OLDER ADULTS

In the United States, Canada, and other countries, a broad range of government benefits and services is available to assist older adults with problems related to income, health in-

CHART 5-5

NIC INTERVENTION ACTIVITIES for Caregiver Support

Caregiver Support: *Provision of the necessary information, advocacy, and support to facilitate primary client care by someone other than a health care professional.*

- Determine caregiver's level of knowledge.
- Determine caregiver's acceptance of role.
- Teach caregiver stress management techniques.
- Monitor for indicators of stress.
- Identify sources of respite care.
- Teach the caregiver health care maintenance strategies to sustain own physical and mental health.
- Encourage caregiver participation in support groups.
- Educate caregiver about the grieving process.
- Teach caregiver strategies to access and maximize health care and community resources.
- Foster caregiver social networking.

surance, housing, and social services. Teach older adults and their families about the types of services available to help them achieve a higher quality of life.

Government Resources

INCOME

In the United States, the major portion of federal funds that support programs for older adults is devoted to the Social Security program. The Social Security Act was passed in 1935, when many individuals were economically impoverished after the Depression. Since that time, there has been a gradual shift from a program intended to provide a minimal supplement to retirees' sources of income to one that is the primary source of retirement income for many individuals. Other provisions of this act that are significant for individuals younger than 65 years of age are the disability and survivors' insurance provisions.

HEALTH INSURANCE

Medicare is a federal health insurance program that was enacted as part of the amendments to the Social Security Act of 1965. This program was created to help older adults, individuals receiving dialysis, and disabled individuals of any age to meet the cost of health care. Despite its deficiencies, Medicare has provided a means for older adults to obtain needed health care in times of escalating costs without decimating their total personal savings.

Medicare provides health insurance to individuals 65 years of age and older and to qualified disabled individuals of any age. **Medicare A** primarily pays for most in-hospital care and is paid for by the federal government. It covers only a very small portion of the care required in long-term care and only minimal home care services. Many clients who are enrolled in Medicare are enrolled in managed care organizations (see Chapter 3). **Medicare B** is an optional insurance and requires payment of a monthly premium. Medicare B pays some of the outpatient costs associated with health care provider visits, medication, and home care services. Some older adults also pay for supplemental private insurance to cover what Medicare does not pay.

Medical assistance (Medicaid) is a program designed to provide payment for medical services for the poor, including older adults who are poor. This program supplements the Medicare insurance program for eligible adults 65 years of age and older. Eligibility is related to determination of poverty level, and each state program determines its own criteria for eligibility. A number of states have completed the transition to managed care for their Medicaid recipients.

HOUSING PROGRAMS

The U.S. Congress has passed a number of legislative acts designed to alleviate housing problems for older citizens. Among these programs is rental assistance for low-income families, older adults, and the disabled. Direct low-interest loans are available to individuals to construct special rental housing facilities. For information related to these housing programs, nurses can contact the local public housing authority or the Housing and Urban Development area office in most communities.

CHART 5-6

NURSING FOCUS on the OLDER ADULT
Social Services Provided by the Older Americans Act of 1965

- Senior centers to meet the need for a central place for older adults to congregate, develop new interests, and socialize
- Nutrition programs to provide nutritious meals in a centralized setting as well as to homebound older adults; recreation, education, and health activities incorporated in many sites as a regular part of the program
- Transportation services to accommodate older adults via special fares on existing public transportation systems and the operation of specially equipped vehicles for frail and handicapped older adults
- Information and referral services to direct older adults to the appropriate agency that provides needed services
- In-home services such as household help, telephone reassurance, chore maintenance, and visitation by home care aides to enable impaired older adults to remain living in the community

SOCIAL SERVICES

The Older Americans Act of 1965 provided social services to older adults. Under this legislation, each state created an office to provide leadership in the coordination and development of services for older adults (Office on Aging). Some of the more significant programs and services carried out under this legislation are described in Chart 5-6.

RESEARCH AGENCIES

The National Institute on Aging was established in 1974. Its purpose is to conduct research on the biologic, population-related, and sociologic aspects of aging at its Gerontology Research Center in Baltimore. It also supports research by others at universities and laboratories across the United States.

One division within the National Institute for Mental Health–the Center for Studies of the Mental Health of the Aging–is devoted exclusively to problems of older adults. Its major role is to stimulate, coordinate, and support research training and to offer technical assistance related to aging and mental health/behavioral health. Although it provides no money for programs of service delivery to older adults, it significantly affects the training of those working with older adults in community mental health/behavioral health centers and other service settings.

Community Resources

Over the years it has become evident that government programs cannot provide all of the services needed by older adults. In many areas, private efforts can supply the same services at lower costs and without the red tape involved with some government programs. Transportation is an area in which the private sector and local, state, and federal governments all have roles.

In many urban areas, governments have established Dial-A-Ride or similar services that provide free transportation. The federal government has subsidized the development and operation of transit systems, but the main focus of this aid has been on high-use systems and routes. For occasional travel, particularly in rural areas, the best solution may be for the older adult to rely on a friend or a neighbor. Churches and community groups often help organize this approach by using sign-up sheets and recruiting volunteers to drive each week.

Education, recreation, and cultural activities help maintain a person's physical condition, mental alertness, and social contact. Education helps older adults keep up with a rapidly changing world. Advances in the Internet and in cable and satellite television systems provide a broad range of new educational experiences at home. Nevertheless, the value of person-to-person discussion and the need to focus some educational activities on local issues means that community discussion groups and other informal education will remain important.

Churches and other religious institutions serve older adults in many ways. In addition to their primary role of providing organized worship, they sponsor many activities that bring individuals together with their peers as well as with younger individuals. Clergypersons and other spiritual leaders are often excellent counselors, and other members of the congregation or religious group are sometimes willing to help older members in time of trouble.

Most libraries have community resource books (e.g., those published by the United Way). Area agencies on aging are excellent referral centers. Some of these agencies publish directories of services that are specifically geared toward the older adult. The nurse can help to inform older clients about the community resources they may need depending on their specific life situation.

THE FUTURE OF GERONTOLOGIC NURSING

Nurses in most adult health care settings encounter the challenges of caring for both healthy and ill older adults. In view of the rapidly increasing older population, especially the over-85 age group, nurses in many settings are specializing in gerontologic nursing or geriatric case management. Nurses can practice these specialties in acute care, long-term care, and community-based settings.

Just as nurses can achieve certification in medical-surgical nursing, they can become certified in gerontologic nursing or case management. The American Nurses Credentialing Center (ANCC) provides three gerontology examinations for the certification of those who qualify: gerontologic nurse, gerontologic clinical specialist, and gerontologic nurse practitioner. The ANCC also offers a nursing case management examination that is broad based and not specific for geriatric case management. Other professional organizations also certify case managers, including geriatric case managers.

GET READY for the NCLEX Examination!

KEY POINTS

- The four subgroups of the older adult population are the young old, middle old, old old, and elite old.
- Relocation stress syndrome is the reaction of an older adult when transferred to a different environment; ways to minimize this problem are listed in Chart 5-1.
- Nutrition and physical fitness are two health problems experienced by older adults.
- The biggest concern regarding accidents among older adults in both the community and inpatient setting is falls.
- Risk factors and common nursing interventions to keep older adults from falling are listed in Chart 5-3.
- Physical and chemical restraints should not be used for older adults until all other alternatives have been tried.
- Physiologic changes of aging predispose older adults to toxic effects of medication; drugs are absorbed, metabolized, and distributed more slowly than in younger individuals. Medications are also excreted more slowly by the kidneys.
- Medication use in older adults is often a problem when they commit errors when self-medicating, avoid needed medications, or have problems understanding their medication regimen.
- Depression is the most common, yet most underdiagnosed and undertreated mental health/behavioral health disorder among older adults.
- Delirium is acute confusion that is short-lived; dementia is chronic confusion that progresses slowly and worsens. Table 5-3 compares these two health problems commonly seen in older adults.
- Elder neglect and abuse are serious problems; family caregivers are most commonly the abusers.
- The nurse and other health care professionals need to assess for signs of elder neglect and abuse; if suspected, it should be reported.
- Many older adults are not prepared for retirement in view of increased expenses and income that is not adequate to meet basic needs, health care treatments, and medications.
- The nurse and other health care professionals need to provide information regarding community resources for older adults to help them meet their basic needs.

ADDITIONAL STUDY RESOURCES

Go to your Student CD-ROM for Review Questions for the NCLEX Examination.

evolve Go to http://evolve.elsevier.com/Iggy/ for Integrated Management of Care Questions for the NCLEX Examination.

SELECTED BIBLIOGRAPHY

Asterisk indicates a classic or definitive work on this subject.

Christmas, C., & Andersen, R.A. (2000). Exercise and older patients: Guidelines for the physician. *Journal of the American Geriatric Society, 48*(3), 318-324.

*Conley, D., Schultz, A.A., & Selvin, R. (1999). The challenge of predicting patients at risk for falling: Development of the Conley Scale. *MEDSURG Nursing: The Journal of Adult Health, 8*(6), 348-354.

Davidhizar, R., & Shearer, R. (2000). Helping elders adjust to losing autonomy. *The Journal of Care Management, 6*(1), 53-54, 69-72.

Davidhizar, R., Eshleman, J., & Moody, M. (2002). Health promotion in aging adults. *Geriatric Nursing, 23*(1), 28-35.

Dochterman, J.M., & Bulechek, G.M. (2004). *Nursing interventions classification (NIC)* (4th ed.). St. Louis: Mosby.

Dyer, C.B., et al. (2000). The high prevalence of depression and dementia in elder abuse or neglect. *Journal of the American Geriatric Society, 48*(2), 205-208.

*Gray-Vickery, P. (1999). Recognizing elder abuse. *Nursing99, 29*(9), 52-63.

Gray-Vickery, P. (2000). Protecting the older adult. *Nursing2000, 30*(7), 34-37.

*Hammond, M., & Levine, J.M. (1999). Bedrails: Choosing the best alternative. *Geriatric Nursing, 20*(6), 297-301.

*Ignatavicius, D.D. (1998). *Introduction to long-term care: Principles and practice.* Philadelphia: F.A. Davis.

*Ignatavicius, D.D. (1999). Resolving the delirium dilemma. *Nursing99, 29*(10), 41-47.

Ignatavicius, D. (2000). Do you help staff rise to the fall-prevention challenge? *Nursing Management, 31*(1), 27-30.

Jacelon, C.S. (2002). Attitudes and behaviors of hospital staff toward elders in an acute care setting, *Applied Nursing Research, 15*(4), 227-234.

Juarbe, T., Turok, X.P., & Perez-Stable, E.J. (2002). Perceived benefits and barriers to physical activity among Latina women. *Western Journal of Nursing Research, 24*(8), 868-886.

Kurlowicz, L.H. (2003). Depression in older adults. In M.D. Mezey, T. Fulmer, & I. Abraham (Eds.), *Geriatric nursing protocols for best practice* (pp. 185-205). New York: Springer.

Loeb, S.J. (2003). The older men's health program and screening inventory: A tool for assessing health practices and beliefs. *Geriatric Nursing, 24*(4), 278-285.

Loeb, S.J., Penrod, J., Falkenstern, S., et al. (2003). Supporting older adults living with multiple chronic conditions. *Western Journal of Nursing Research, 25*(1), 8-29.

McCloskey, J.C., & Bulechek, G.M. (2000). *Nursing interventions classification (NIC)* (3rd ed.). St. Louis: Mosby.

Napierkowski, D. (2002). Using restraints with restraint. *Nursing2002, 32*(1), 58-63.

North American Nursing Diagnosis Association International. (2003). *Nursing diagnoses: Definitions and classification 2003-2004.* Philadelphia: NANDA International.

Rapp, C.G., et al. (2000). Acute confusion assessment instruments: Clinical versus research usability. *Applied Nursing Research, 13*(1), 37-45.

Resnick, B. (2003). Preventing falls in acute care. In M.D. Mezey, T. Fulmer, & I. Abraham (Eds.), *Geriatric nursing protocols for best practice* (pp. 141-164). New York: Springer.

*Schiavento, M. (1997). The Hispanic elderly: Implications for nursing care. *Journal of Gerontological Nursing, 23*(6), 10-15.

Stevens, J.A., & Olson, S. (2000). Reducing falls and resulting hip fractures among older women. *Morbidity and Mortality Weekly Report, 49*(RR02), 1-12.

Taggart, H.M. (2002). Effects of Tai Chi exercise on balance, functional mobility, and fear of falling among older women. *Applied Nursing Research, 15*(4), 235-242.

Theodus, P. (2003). Fall prevention in frail elderly nursing home residents. A challenge to case management: Part I. *Lippincott's Case Management, 8*(6), 246-251.

Uncapher, H., & Arean, P.A. (2000). Physicians are less willing to treat suicidal ideation in older patients. *Journal of the American Geriatric Society, 48*(2), 188-192.

Wakefield, B.J. (2002). Behaviors and outcomes of acute confusion in hospitalized patients. *Applied Nursing Research, 15*(4), 209-216.

Wells, D.L., & Dawson, P. (2000). Description of retained abilities in older persons with dementia. *Research in Nursing and Health Care, 23*(2), 158-166.

UNIT **TWO**

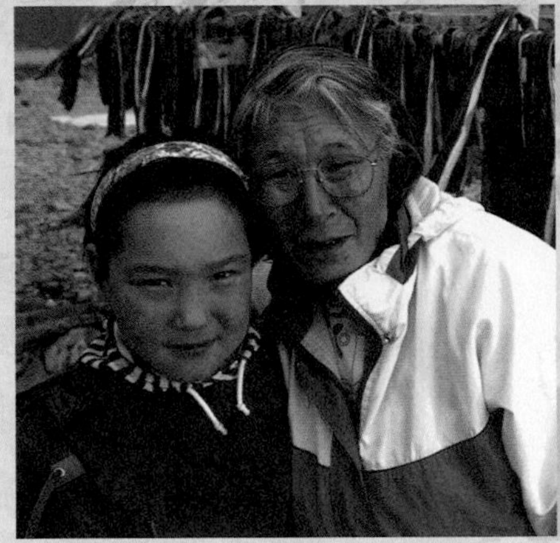

BIOPSYCHOSOCIAL CONCEPTS RELATED to HEALTH CARE

CHAPTER

6 Cultural Aspects of Health

MICHELLE M. BYRNE

LEARNING OUTCOMES

After studying this chapter, you should be able to:

1. Define culture, cultural competence, cultural awareness, and ethnocentrism.
2. Explain the purpose and nursing implications of Healthy People 2010 as related to culture.
3. Identify common factors related to cultural assessment.
4. Describe three methods for cultural assessment.
5. Identify and describe three cultural groups that have often been neglected.
6. Discuss specific cultural practices, such as religion, nutrition, and folk medicine, that the nurse should consider when assessing a client's culture.
7. Describe ways that nurses can communicate sensitively with clients from various cultural groups.

Go to your Student CD-ROM for Review Questions for the NCLEX Examination keyed to these Learning Outcomes.

This century, population diversity is rapidly increasing throughout the world. As a result of the Internet, foreign travel, and global industrialization, there is more interaction between different individuals of the world. A myriad of societies and citizens have their own way of doing things and interacting with others, often with unique beliefs and practices. Although there are cultural similarities among many individuals in specific cultures, there are also diverse groups within each culture. As a nurse, cultural diversity is embedded in the relationships with your clients as well as with your coworkers in the workplace setting (Anderson et al., 2003).

THE NEED FOR CULTURAL CONSIDERATIONS OF HEALTH

Many individuals from differing cultures continue to immigrate to North America in large numbers, bringing new and different ideas with them. These individuals have various cultural needs based on their ethnicity, background, and immigration status. According to the U.S. Census Bureau, the estimated figures for the U.S. population in 2000 showed the following percentages for several large cultural groups:

- European Americans: 71.5%
- African Americans: 12.2%
- Hispanics: 12.6%
- Asian Americans/Pacific Islanders: 3.8%

In 2000, the number of minority populations in the United States accounted for 28% of the total population. It is estimated that minority groups are an emerging majority and will make up 43.8% of the population by 2050. This diversity makes culturally sensitive health care imperative.

The U.S. government has an initiative for health care workers and organizations to become culturally competent. There are many definitions for cultural competence. In 2000, the U.S. Department of Health and Human Services (DHHS) developed a widely recognized definition. **Cultural competence** is the ability of health care providers and organizations to understand and respond effectively to the cultural and linguistic needs that clients bring to the health care setting. Among other standards to achieve cultural competence, the DHHS made several suggestions for health care organizations. First, organizations are to ensure that staff members are trained to work respectfully and effectively with clients in culturally diverse health care environments. Second, organizations are to develop procedures to address cross-cultural ethical and legal conflicts in health care delivery, such as culturally insensitive or discriminatory treatment; difficulty in accessing service; or denial of services. For these reasons, the term **cultural sensitivity** is sometimes used to describe the way that one responds to cultural differences.

HEALTHY PEOPLE 2010

Another program created by the U.S. Department of Health and Human Services (2000) is **Healthy People 2010.** The goal by 2010 is to eliminate the differences in six areas of health status experienced by racial and ethnic minorities while trying to continually improve the overall health of all American individuals. The target areas are the following:

- Infant mortality
- Cancer screening and management
- Cardiovascular disease
- Diabetes mellitus
- Human immunodeficiency virus (HIV) infection/acquired immunodeficiency syndrome (AIDS)
- Immunizations

This goal is to be met through research, preventive programs, and inclusion of members of minority groups.

Currently there are significant differences in health and health care access for ethnic or racial groups as compared to the dominant European American group in the United States. The reasons for these differences include the following (Baldwin, 2003; Freire, 2002):

- Poor socioeconomic status
- Health beliefs and behaviors
- Access to health care
- Environmental factors
- Direct and indirect manifestations of discrimination
- Lack of health insurance
- Insufficient transportation
- Geographic location
- Cost of services
- Language barriers

Oftentimes, complex issues such as racism, "classism," ageism, and sexism are embedded in disparities in health care but ignored due to lack of knowledge or awareness by members of the health care team.

CULTURE AND NURSING

Diverse values, beliefs, and practices impact health, illness, professional health care, and folk health care. Nursing has a long history of addressing the physical and emotional needs of individual clients, and currently there is an increased emphasis on taking care of cultural needs. Therefore nurses and nursing students must learn to integrate cultural considerations as part of holistic client care (Figure 6-1).

Definition of Culture

A dictionary definition of **culture** suggests that it is an integrated pattern of human behavior that includes thought, speech, action, and artifacts. Culture is learned and transmitted to succeeding generations. Culture can include things such as language, art, morals, laws, appearance, customs, rituals, technology, economics, and kinship or family systems.

Many individuals in a culture, especially older individuals, spend years teaching about the importance of keeping the traditions of their culture. Beliefs and rituals often vary within a culture, especially when it is made up of distinct subcultures. An example is the Native American population, which consists of many subcultures, or councils, across the United States. For instance, the Lakota Council is made up of several tribes that have specific customs. These customs differ from those of other groups of Native Americans. According to several treaties between the Lakotas and the U.S. government, the Lakotas are American Indians, not Native Americans. For that reason, many Lakotas and other related subcultures refer to themselves as American Indian because that is their legal designated name (Personal communication, Ogala Lakota College, Pine Ridge, SD, August 6, 2003).

Implications for Nursing Practice

Culture also influences health and nursing care. It influences the way individuals think about health, the ways in which they express pain, what they consider to be symptoms, how they seek and accept help and care, and who they consider to be healers. Madeline Leininger, a nurse anthropologist and theorist, has provided a large body of knowledge integrating nursing care and cultural care.

In the 1950s Leininger combined culture and nursing into a new field called **transcultural nursing.** She developed the theory of Culture Care Diversity and Universality. She specified that transcultural nursing is an area of study and practice that focuses on the care, health, and illness patterns of individuals with similarities and differences in their cultural beliefs, values, and practices. The practice of transcultural nurses

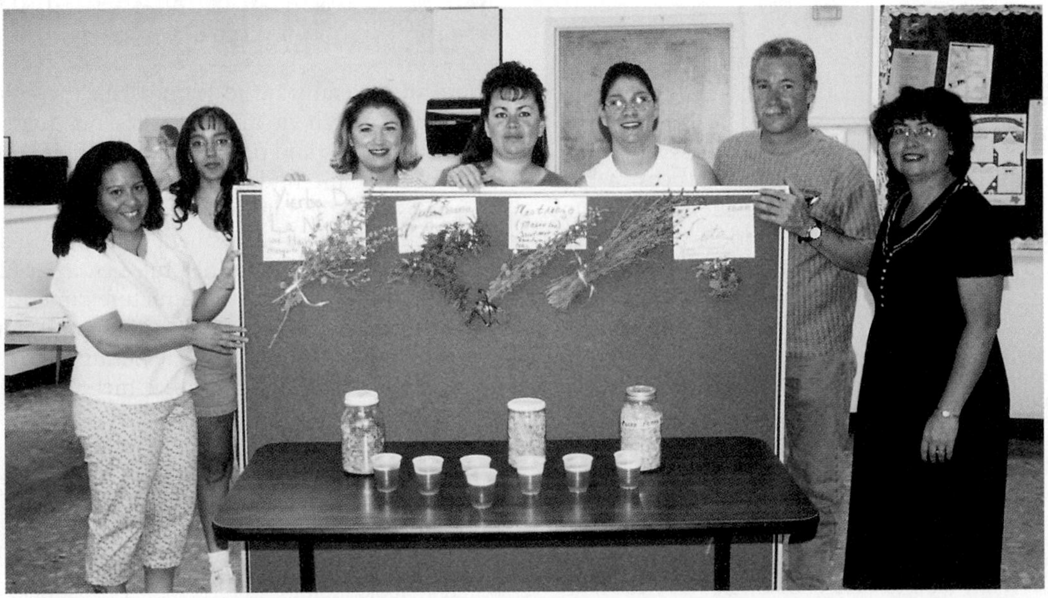

Figure 6-1 ■ Nursing students in an associate degree program learning about the value of herbs for healing in the southwestern part of the United States. (Courtesy Luna Vocational Technical Institute, Las Vegas, NM.)

is to provide care that considers the cultural aspects of the client (Leininger, 2002). Over time, other nurses have become proficient in the field of cultural care, including Andrews, Boyle, Campinha-Bacote, Douglas, Purnell, and Spector.

Cultural considerations should certainly be integrated in the nursing care of all clients. Individuals have diverse needs in health care and may fall into various categories. For example, cultural differences exist between residents of urban and rural areas as well as differing geographic sections of the country. Furthermore, how recently a person has immigrated to the United States can provide insight into cultural variations.

Differences are also found related to age, gender, and sexual orientation. Therefore, it is important that nurses and other health care professionals examine their beliefs and biases about cultural differences (Byrne, 2001, 2002; Byrne et al., 2003). How do you feel about individuals different than yourself? Too often, the term "different" has negative connotations. One of the foundations for becoming culturally competent as a nurse is to examine personal beliefs and biases (Campinha-Bacote, 2001, 2002; Byrne, 2001, 2002; Byrne et al. 2003).

Campinha-Bacote's model of cultural competence includes personal awareness, knowledge, skill, encounters, and desire (Table 6-1). **Cultural awareness** is defined as "the process through which the nurse becomes respectful, appreciative, and sensitive to the values, beliefs, lifeways, practices and problem-solving strategies of a client's culture" (p. 8, 2001). Cultural awareness also includes an examination of one's own prejudice and bias. This awareness is not always easy, in that there is a tendency to be blind to our bias, or ethnocentric in our perspectives. **Ethnocentrism** is the judging of others through the exclusive lens of one's own cultural beliefs. Ethnocentrism has been found to negatively affect client care (Sutherland, 2002). Therefore, explicit examples of bias, stereotypes, and our assumptions may assist health care providers in becoming less ethnocentric in their practice (Byrne, 2001, 2002; Byrne et al., 2003; Sutherland, 2002).

THE CULTURE OF THE HEALTH CARE SYSTEM

Hospitals, nursing homes, and health care offices in both public and private sectors have cultural beliefs, values, and practices, as do nursing programs in schools and universities. Nurses and physicians make up a culture within themselves according to their unique beliefs, values, and practices. If diversity is synonymous with difference, then health care professionals must realize that, if we view a client as different, then a client views us as different as well. Nurses are members of a culture in the health care system. Because each of us has been socialized into the health care team, there are values and belief systems that we hold near and dear to our hearts. We may believe some things so strongly that we do not see our opinions as a value system.

Beliefs can be defined as ideas that a person accepts as true. One belief of health care professionals is a belief of standardization (Spector, 2000). Standardization is implemented through competency statements, policies, procedures, forms, care plans, orders, flow sheets, and critical pathways. Standardization is even embedded in our schooling as we learn via competencies and measurable objectives. However, an emphasis on objectivity and standardization may minimize creativity and individuality.

Another common cultural characteristic found in the health care system is neatness, cleanliness, and timeliness. Disorderliness and disorganization are two attributes that are not highly prized in the health care arena. In addition, perspectives of time among health care workers are future-oriented. Immunizations and prevention measures are directed at minimizing future illnesses. Some cultural groups may blame previous behaviors on present problems or only address health problems that are adversely affecting them at the moment.

Other customs of our health care system is the medicalization of the birthing and dying process. Due to urbanization, reimbursement mandates, and advances in technology, these events usually take place in a hospital setting. Many non-Western cultures do not have the same emphasis on medical intervention during the birth or death of a loved one. It is important to examine the health care culture and determine how our clients may perceive our practices, language, and behaviors as different to bridge cultural differences.

TABLE 6-1 Campinha-Bacote's Asked Model for Cultural Competence

Awareness: Are you aware of your personal biases and prejudices towards cultures different than yours?
Skill: Do you have the skill to conduct a cultural assessment and perform a culturally based physical assessment?
Knowledge: Do you have knowledge of the patient's world view, cultural bound illnesses, and the field of biocultural ecology?
Encounters: How many face-to-face encounters have you had with patients from diverse cultural backgrounds?
Desire: What is your desire to "want to be" culturally competent?

Courtesy of Dr. Josie Campinha-Bacote, expert in cultural nursing.

ASSESSING AND MANAGING THE CULTURAL NEEDS OF CLIENTS

There are several ways to learn about the culture of clients. Cultural research in nursing relies on questioning clients, observing them, and participating in their cultural activities. Each of these methods can also be used in nursing practice.

The aspects of culture that need to be assessed depend on the situation. Several assessment guides created by expert cultural nurses are especially helpful. Leininger (2002) bases her assessment on cultural social structure dimensions (Table 6-2). Purnell developed a model for assessing the cultural aspects of a particular group (Table 6-3). He points out that, although the model is given as a whole for assessment, the situation and culture studied may lead the health care provider to concentrate

TABLE 6-2 Leininger's Factors for Assessing Cultural Groups or Persons

- Worldview of the group
- Technologic factors
- Kinship and social factors
- Economic factors
- Cultural values and lifeways
- Philosophic and religious factors
- Political and legal factors
- Educational factors

on one area before another. In a very religious community, for example, the provider may want to start the assessment with spirituality rather than with another domain.

Many of the same factors are found in various assessment models. Nurses should adapt and integrate assessment models that are most appropriate for their clinical practice arena and types of cultural groups being cared for.

Performing a Cultural Assessment

The three major methods for assessing the culture of a client include observation, interview, and participation. The health care setting often determines the order in which these methods are used.

OBSERVATION

A cultural assessment in the home starts with the observation phase. For example, what are the neighborhood and geographic areas in which the client and family live (Figure 6-2)? Is the street in front of the house a busy one, or is it in a more rural area? Is public transportation available, or do residents have their own cars? Going into the client's house, the nurse observes for Bibles, religious books, and religious symbols on the walls or tables. Evidence of technology, such as air-conditioning, televisions, telephones, kitchen appliances, and computers, is noted. The interactions and communication patterns among family members are also observed.

TABLE 6-3 Purnell's Factors for Assessing Cultural Groups or Persons

▪ Nutrition	▪ Heritage
▪ Communication	▪ Pregnancy and childbirth
▪ Family roles	▪ Death rituals
▪ Work issues	▪ Spirituality
▪ Biocultural ecology	▪ Health care practices
▪ High-risk behaviors	▪ Folk health practices

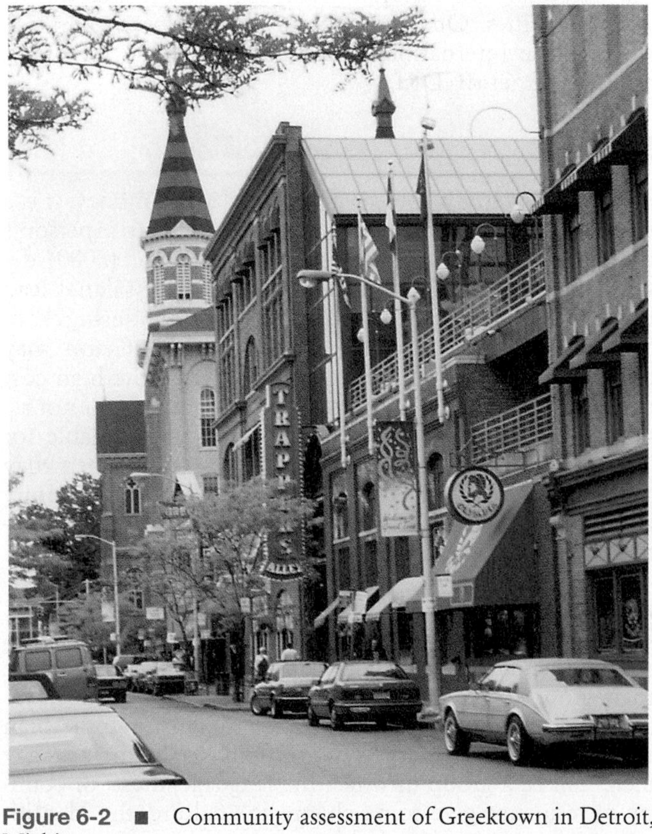

Figure 6-2 ▪ Community assessment of Greektown in Detroit, Michigan.

INTERVIEW

Following observation, you should interview the client and possibly the family. Nurses often obtain health histories from their clients, and cultural interviewing is only slightly different. The best questions for cultural interviews are semistructured and open-ended questions. The nurse usually has an interview guide or an outline for the questions. Spector (2000) has identified nine suggestions for enhancing communication when gathering cultural data:

- Determine the level of fluency in English and arrange for an interpreter if needed.
- Ask how the client prefers to be addressed.
- Allow the client to choose seating for comfortable personal space and eye contact.
- Avoid body language that may be offensive or misunderstood.
- Speak directly to the client, whether an interpreter is present or not.
- Choose a speech rate and style that promotes understanding and demonstrates respect for the client.
- Avoid slang technical jargon and complex sentences.
- Use open-ended questions or questions phrased in several ways to obtain information.
- Determine the client's reading ability before using written materials in the teaching process.

A good interviewer will often deviate from the form if the client shows interest in a particular question. Often more details are learned in such a circumstance. A large amount of information can usually be gleaned from actively listening to a client, whether during an interview or at any other time.

PARTICIPATION

Participation is the third method of collecting data for a cultural assessment. This process is very helpful for understanding a particular cultural population rather than assessing just one client. For example, a nurse may begin working in a community that has had an influx of Hispanic immigrants. To better understand some of the cultural needs of the individual, he or she may begin participating in the community activities.

Trips to local churches can provide insight into the religious life of a culture. Many ethnic communities have festivals with crafts, foods, music, and clothing. Political rallies may also be a good place to interact and learn the beliefs of groups. Similarly, markets held in the community tell a lot about the buying and social habits of a group.

In preparing a cultural assessment, put together the information gathered from the cultural group or from the client about the lifestyles, general beliefs and practices and, specifically, health care beliefs. Cultural data should be integrated in all phases of the nursing process.

Developing the Cultural Care Plan

Use the data gathered about a client or clients from a particular culture to plan, implement, and evaluate culturally competent care. Leininger (2002) has suggested one way of planning cultural care for a client, and this method is used by many nurses. She uses three modes for planning care:

- *Culture care preservation or maintenance* is a way to help "people of a particular culture to retain or preserve relevant care values so they can maintain and/or preserve their well-being, recover from illness, or face handicaps and/or death."
- *Culture care accommodation or negotiation* refers to "professional actions and decisions that help people of a designated culture adapt to or negotiate with others for a beneficial or satisfying health outcome with professional care providers."
- *Culture care repatterning or restructuring* helps clients to "reorder, change or greatly modify their lifeways . . . providing a lifeway more beneficial or healthier than before the changes were co-established with the clients."

Research Applications

It is important for nurses to research the specific health and illness practices for specific cultural groups. One study examined the motivation, health beliefs, and access barriers experienced by older minority women in keeping mammography appointments (Bernstein, Mutschler, & Bernstein, 2000). Minority women have a high mortality rate associated with breast cancer and low rates of routine mammography. The study sample contained mostly African-American women, but also included European American, Hispanic, and Haitian participants. The method used was peer interaction with the participants to educate them about breast health, and offered them a no-cost, next-day appointment for a mammogram. Researchers also assessed their willingness to change behavior. Sixty percent of the study group kept their appointments or had a mammogram within 3 months. According to the authors, the success of the program resulted from the following: (1) the interaction between the women and culturally competent peers who offered education, (2) the use of interpreters for non–English-speaking participants, and (3) the fact that the women in the study group were treated as experts in telling their own experiences and stories related to breast health.

In addition to researching cultural groups, research has explored how nurses respond to the cultural needs of their clients. For example, a sample of 126 United Kingdom registered nurses completed questionnaires that pertained to cultural care (Narayanasamy, 2003). These nurses practiced mostly in adult acute care settings and agreed that their clients presented with cultural needs (80%). However, most nurses focused their cultural assessments and interventions only on religious and dietary practices. The major barriers for culturally focused care identified by this group of nurses was language difficulties, especially the utilization of resources for translation services.

SPECIAL CONSIDERATIONS FOR SELECTED CULTURAL GROUPS

A person's characteristics may be embedded in different cultural groups. For example, there are disabled individuals with Greek-American backgrounds whose cultural care plans would include ethnic and disability characteristics. The same might be true of a lesbian client who is African American. She would need attentive care for her sexual orientation as well as for her ethnicity. Three specific groups in our society–disabled individuals, impoverished persons, and those with diverse sexual orientations–originate from diverse ethnic backgrounds, yet must be assessed from a variety of cultural aspects.

Disability

Disabilities are physical as well as emotional. Some disabilities are visible; others are not. Some disabilities are acquired from various illnesses, conditions, and accidents, whereas others are a result of developmental problems. There are, however, some common themes that describe cultures of individuals with disabilities.

Individuals with disabilities are members of the largest minority group in the United States. Approximately 15% to 20% of U.S. residents have a disabling condition that impacts their life activities (Lipson & Rogers, 2000). Disability activists have argued that health care providers lack knowledge regarding the social nature of disability. Cultural competence must be broadened to include this group (Lipson & Rogers, 2000). Students and nurses should familiarize themselves with the Americans with Disabilities Act, which addresses employment, public services, public accommodations, and telecommunications for these individuals.

It is important for health care professionals to assess their personal attitudes and biases toward clients with disabilities. Nurses can use literature searches to identify specific organizations to assist them in acquiring the knowledge and skills necessary for culturally competent care related to specific disabilities. One such website is http://www.icdri.org, which is the International Center for Disability Resources on the Internet (ICDRI).

Poverty

Although poverty is often defined as a lack of money, it is a much more complex phenomenon that affects a person's health, well-being, and access to care. Spector (2000) describes a cycle of poverty in which insufficient salaries lead to poor nutrition, and densely populated housing contributes to a high incidence of illness. These factors may contribute to a lack of preventive care due to the high cost of health care services. A nurse must be conscious of not assuming that adequate financial resources are available for transportation, prescription, or medical devices when they are not. It is important to be aware of the local community resources for client referral when clients cannot afford nutritious meals, necessary medication, or health care services.

Sexual Orientation

Sexual orientation can influence the delivery of cultural care to a group of individuals. Spinks, Andrews, and Boyle (2000) discuss the provision of cultural care to lesbian clients, but many of their suggestions could include gay men. Unlike a group in which the language, dress, or country of residence give some clue to the culture, the identification of someone in a lesbian or gay community may be more difficult. The nurse may assume incorrectly that a client is heterosexual and thus not provide the unique health care that is needed. A lack of therapeutic communication, along with bias of the health care professional, is often present.

A gay or lesbian client has similar physical health needs in screening and health promotion as most clients but may also have unique issues that need to be addressed. Some examples include whether to have children through adoption, artificial insemination, or intentional heterosexual contact. Substance abuse may be an ineffective coping mechanism because of the inherent stresses in feeling the need to hide one's sexual orientation due societal intolerance. One group in a large city took a proactive role in providing culturally competent care by forming a Feminist Women's Health Center to meet the needs of all women, including lesbian clients (Spinks, Andrews, & Boyle, 2000).

SELECTED CONCEPTS RELATED TO CULTURALLY SENSITIVE NURSING

Specific cultural practices involving spirituality, nutrition, and folk practices should be considered when assessing clients and planning their care.

Religion and Spirituality

The spiritual well-being of clients who practice a religion is an important consideration in nursing in that it has a bearing on many different aspects of health and illness (McEvoy, 2003). Some examples may be the acceptance or nonacceptance of blood products, dietary rules or rituals, the furnishing of religious support for the sick, and beliefs and practices related to birth or death.

In times of crisis, religion often plays a major role in caring for the client. Many individuals are atheists (do not believe in a higher power) or agnostics (question whether there is a God or higher power). It is best to request nonjudgmentally, "Tell me how I can assist you in meeting any religious or spiritual needs you may have." Although Christianity is prevalent in many areas of North America, globalization is bringing together many varied religions that should be considered in planning care. Further discussion of religion and spirituality is found in other fundamental textbooks.

Generic or Folk Medicine

Although many North Americans believe in using the professional medical and nursing system for health care, many more do not seek professional care for many reasons:

- Transportation difficulties
- High cost of care
- Fear and distrust of health care workers
- Poor communication between clients and professionals

Therefore cultural ways of healing might be sought before or while seeking care from the traditional health care system. Although, considered unscientific and strange to many health care workers, it is essential to assess and support clients in their practices when appropriate.

Where do folk health ideas come from? Individuals within certain cultures look at their ideas as ways to preserve both their heritage and their health. Folk health beliefs, practices, and values are learned from experience and observations. They are passed down from generation to generation and have been found to be valuable to cultures and individuals.

Long before there were physicians and nurses, there were systems of caring for and curing individuals. For example, early ancestors found they could prevent or cure disease with plants. Digitalis (which comes from the foxglove plant) and belladonna have been used for many generations to treat heart failure and tuberculosis. Substances other than plants are also used. For example, in the South of the United States (and among Southerners who migrated north), the practice among some black individuals and European Americans from the Appalachian Mountains is to eat clay or dirt to promote maternal wellness. This practice is called **geophagia**. Many southern families have had their own clay banks for years. Some literature suggests that this practice originated in Africa (Spector, 2000). Red clay may be used for anemia, and white clay is preferred for indigestion. White clay consists of kaolin, the same ingredient found in some medications given taken for indigestion today. The cost of these drugs far exceeds that of the natural clay.

There are also numerous hot/cold beliefs related to healing. These beliefs may not necessarily be based on a nurse's definition of temperature. Hot/cold theories of healing are found among Hispanic, Arab, Asian, Southeast Indian, African-American, and Southern Anglo-American cultures. If the nurse provides care to an adult who has some of these beliefs, he or she may find that the client's explanation for the present illness goes back to earlier life. For example, some Hispanic women believe that partaking of "cold" foods and medicines after pregnancy will cause bleeding to stop. They believe this blood is reabsorbed into the body to cause nervousness or insanity later in life. A similar belief is that cold can get into the open vagina after childbirth and stay in the body to cause arthritis in adult life. Health care providers who care for these clients must realize that the client's view of the etiology of the problem may be quite different from the scientific explanation.

The "evil eye" is a prominent belief in some cultures, including Hispanic and Arab cultures. The Spanish term for this belief is *mal de ojo,* and some believe that "the gods" give the evil eye when they become envious or jealous when a person is excessively praised or admired. Another belief is that a person who is angry with another person can "put the evil eye" on him or her. Various amulets are worn to reflect the evil eye back onto the person who caused it (Figure 6-3).

Various methods are used to protect individuals from evil. Garlic or a substance such as asafoetida may be worn around the neck, often in a little red bag. Both of these substances are thought to protect against colds and flu. They both smell so bad that they may indeed work, because other individuals do not want to get close to the wearer.

A very important point to consider with folk medicine is the use of particular phrases to describe health problems. Some African Americans and some Appalachians refer to the blood in various ways that can have several meanings. For example, "high blood" can mean hypertension, or too much blood in the body, or it can mean the movement of

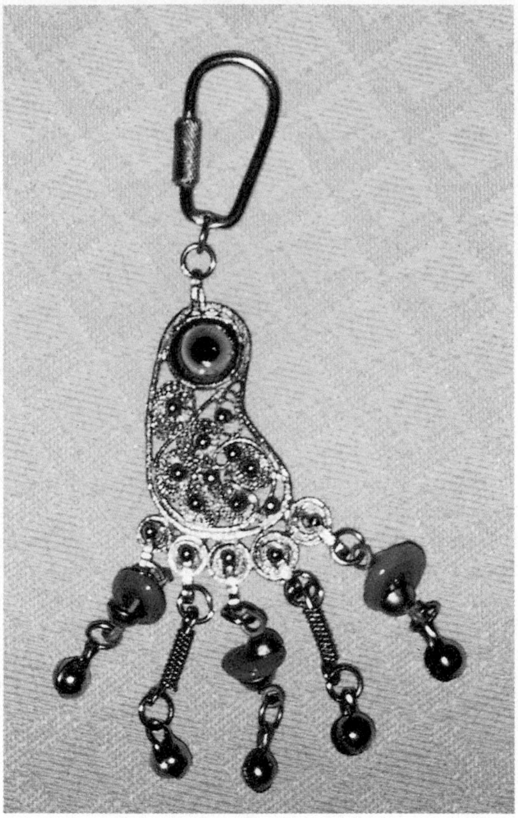

Figure 6-3 ■ "Hand of God" amulet to protect the wearer from the "evil eye."

blood to a higher part of the body such as the brain or head. The movement of blood into the head is commonly believed to cause strokes or nervousness or to make the person "fall out" (faint). A similar situation is "low blood," which can mean low blood pressure or anemia. These different terms can cause communication problems. When taking care of clients, the nurse must sometimes delve deeper into the meaning of certain phrases.

This section has described only a few examples of the generic or folk beliefs that may be found in almost any culture. What must nurses do to help individuals with these beliefs? Most folk practices are not hurtful, but when they are, nurses and physicians must sensitively address them. Belittling of client practices lacks cultural awareness and sensitivity, hence it is imperative for students to learn and appreciate cultural differences.

The subject of folk health is broad; refer to books in the Selected Bibliography for greater detail.

Pain

Pain is universal in all cultures, yet the way in which individuals discuss pain varies greatly among and between cultures. Pain has been labeled the fifth vital sign along with temperature, pulse, respiration, and blood pressure. Nurses routinely assess pain on a Visual Analogue Scale, which is a numerical rating from 0 to 10. Although this technique provides some objectivity among health care providers, it does limit the sensitivity of culturally dependent subjective signs and symptoms of the pain response. Nurses may believe that silent suffering is a valued reaction to pain. Nurses must identify whether they prefer to see self-control in their clients rather than displays of strong feelings related to pain, and how their perceptions impact their nursing interventions addressing pain (Spector, 2000) (see Chapter 7).

The alleviation of pain is also culturally based. Techniques such as acupuncture, long used by the Chinese, have become more widespread in the United States to alleviate pain. Similarly, herbal remedies have been used by many cultures through the ages (see also Chapters 4 and 7). In addition, massage therapy and mind-body techniques of complementary and alternative therapies have also been found to reduce or relieve pain.

Religious practices have a place in pain management and healing. Some Catholics may use their rosaries to guide their prayer. Other denominations in the Christian faith have special healing services either in churches or in the sick room. Jewish clients may ask to speak to a rabbi. Native American/American Indian clients may have shamans who perform religious rituals for healing that involve the client, relatives, and other members of the cultural group. One role of the nurse is to respect and provide privacy for all religious practices.

Nutrition

Culture has a major impact on food and the way in which it is prepared and served. Technology, economics, and religion–all parts of the cultural assessment–influence the food that is eaten by various cultural groups.

Technology affects how food is produced and distributed. High-level technology is involved on large agricultural farms, but very few tools may be necessary to grow a backyard garden. Foods are much less seasonal now than they were before rapid transportation systems could move food from many countries with varying growing seasons.

Economics also affect the production and distribution of food. In some countries, food is produced on small farms. The food that is not needed by the family who produced it is brought to a central market area for sale. Custom also dictates how food is sold. In many European countries, individuals go to specialty stores or markets to buy fresh meat and produce each day. Many economically deprived countries experience famine and starvation.

Religion also dictates what different cultural groups eat and how the food is prepared. Many individuals of the Hindu religion refrain from eating cows; some are lactovegetarians, eating only milk products and vegetables. Some Jewish individuals do not eat pork or shellfish; there are religious rituals for killing the meat to make it kosher. Many Jewish individuals believe that milk and meat should not be eaten at the same meal (Spector, 2000). Religion also influences whether specific things are eaten at different times. Some Christians who are Catholic or Episcopalian "give up" certain foods, commonly meat or desserts, during the Lenten season. Religious holidays may also feature traditional meats, such as the "Christmas turkey" or the "Easter ham."

Beliefs and practices related to the hot/cold theory often involve foods. Illness is often seen as an imbalance between elements, and food or herbs are used to therapeutically restore the body to its natural balance. Therefore curing a "hot" disease such as arthritis may require cold foods or medicines. Beliefs vary about what is hot and what is cold. A similar belief is the Chinese *yin* and *yang* balance of foods for health. When faced with a client who has these beliefs, interview the client and family or refer to books with details about these specific beliefs.

Foods are important in planning care with certain cultural groups. For example, many African and Asian Americans are lactose intolerant and have problems digesting milk and milk products. African Americans also have a tendency to have high blood pressure, which may be diet related. Obesity, overeating, or anorexia nervosa may also have a cultural basis for establishing eating and activity habits.

Communication

One of the stumbling blocks to effective health care is communication. Not only do clients and nurses often speak different languages, there is also miscommunication when nurses use technical language, slang, or jargon. In addition, individuals in every culture have silent ways of expressing themselves through facial expressions, posture, and hand gestures; through the space between individuals; and through touch. Discomfort and a lack of understanding results if efforts are not made to overcome miscommunication or a lack of communication.

When nurses and clients speak an entirely different language, several interventions can be taken to try to effectively communicate with the client and the family. The first step is to assess the population for which care will be provided. If it is primarily a Hispanic group, then learning the language is the ideal answer. Although learning a complete language is often not possible, knowing and using a few words and phrases often goes a long way in making a client comfortable and interested in the care provided.

Interpreters are often used in health care with different cultures. The best situation is to have someone on the health care team act as an interpreter. When this is not possible, arrangements can sometimes be made with individuals in the community. Some health care facilities have found that foreign language professors from nearby schools or colleges can act in this capacity as may the client's friends or family members. An important consideration is the need to maintain confidentiality. With friends and family in the room, the client may be less forthcoming with personal information–information that could be important to diagnosis and treatment.

One helpful resource is the AT&T Language Service ([800] 752-6096). This service offers translation of more than 150 languages. There is a fee for this service, but it can be very helpful.

Another solution is to use pictures identified with both the foreign language word and the English equivalent. For example, Spanish-speaking clients would be shown a picture of a nurse with the words "enfermera" and "nurse" underneath it or a hypodermic syringe and needle with the words "inyección" and "shot" underneath it (Figure 6-4). Many resources are available for nurses to learn Spanish and other languages (Joyce & Villanueva, 2000).

Nonverbal communication can involve space, gestures, posture, and facial expressions, all of which vary with the culture of the person. When someone invades another's personal space, that person can get very uncomfortable and

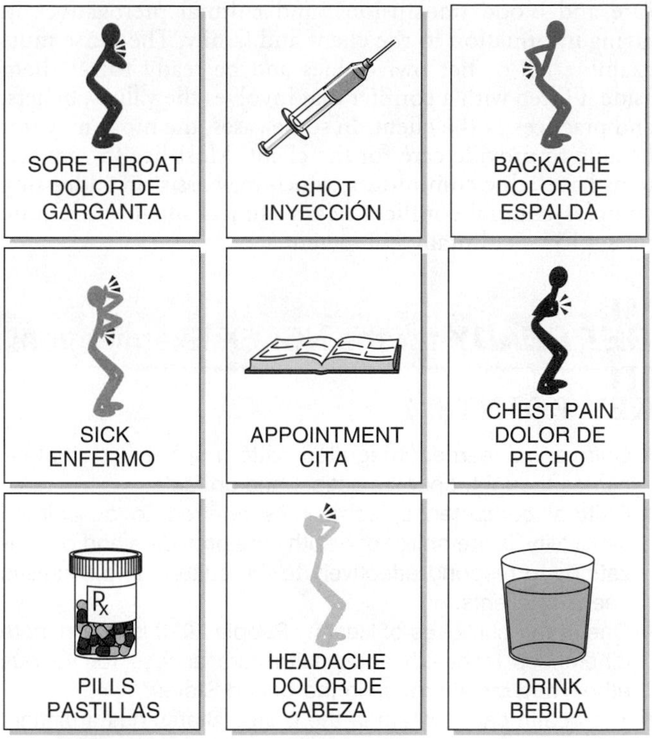

Figure 6-4 ■ English/Spanish pictograph to assist with communication. (Courtesy Anne Grimmer, Xid Design, Tallahassee, FL.)

transmit feelings of discomfort. Understanding that space has culturally embedded relevance can help clients in coping with feelings of being invaded.

Gestures are also culturally embedded ways of communication. They vary between cultures and may be interpreted as unacceptable or threatening depending on the ethnic group. In the European-American culture, the thumb and first finger make a circle and the other fingers are held upright to mean "everything's okay." In some Arab cultures, however, this same hand gesture means a woman's vagina. This example illustrates the concern that the use of certain gestures can cause.

Facial expressions and looking directly at someone can also cause discomfort in certain cultures. Some groups expect their health care providers to be serious and formal, whereas others want a more intimate, personal reaction. European-American nurses value the use of eye-to-eye contact with clients, but some clients may avert their eyes because of cultural differences.

Ethics of Cultural Caring

The ethics of nursing includes, but is not limited to, ensuring client confidentiality, getting informed consent for certain procedures and surgery, and respecting the right of clients to make autonomous decisions about their care. The ethics regarding the cultural care of clients goes further and considers the values of each individual client and his or her cultural beliefs and practices. The nurse must support and advocate for clients to have their unique needs met in the health care system. Some aspects of cultural care involve beliefs related to birth and death, the right to refuse medical care and blood transfusions, and cultural prerogatives in giving information to the client and family. The nurse must examine his or her own values and be ready to set them aside if faced with a conflict that involves the values, beliefs, and practices of the client. In some cases, the nurse may not be able to provide care for the client. Most health care systems have ethic committees, which may assist in addressing complex cultural conflicts. Many clinical situations require nurses to be culturally competent.

GET READY for the NCLEX Examination!

KEY POINTS

- Culture is a learned integrated pattern of behavior that includes thought, speech, action, and artifacts.
- Cultural competence, sometimes referred to as cultural sensitivity, is the ability of health care providers and organizations to respond effectively to the cultural and linguistic needs of clients.
- One of the purposes of Healthy People 2010 is to eliminate differences in health and health care access for various ethnic and racial groups in the United States.
- The health care system in the United States has a distinct culture, including standardization, cleanliness, and medicalization of birthing and dying.
- Factors that are related to cultural assessment are listed in Tables 6-2 and 6-3.
- Three methods of cultural assessment are observation, interview, and participation.
- Special considerations are needed for subcultural groups that may be affiliated with a number of ethnic or racial groups—disabled clients, impoverished persons, and those with diverse sexual orientations.
- Nurses need to be educated in specific cultural practices that affect assessment and planning of client care, including religion, nutrition, and communication.
- Clients may avoid the traditional health care system due to transportation problems, high cost of care, fear and distrust of health care staff, or poor communication between clients and health care providers; generic or folk medicine may be used as an alternative.
- Communication techniques vary among cultural groups and may be misinterpreted; nurses need to learn how groups communicate (verbal and nonverbal) to avoid misperceptions.

ADDITIONAL STUDY RESOURCES

Go to your Student CD-ROM for Review Questions for the NCLEX Examination.

Go to http://evolve.elsevier.com/Iggy/ for Integrated Management of Care Questions for the NCLEX Examination.

SELECTED BIBLIOGRAPHY

Anderson, L., et al., and the Task Force on Community Preventive Services. (2003). Culturally competent healthcare systems: A systematic review. *American Journal of Preventive Medicine, 24*(3S), 68-79.

Baldwin, D. (2003). Disparities in health and health care: Focusing efforts to eliminate unequal burdens. *Online Journal of Issues in Nursing 8*(1), Manuscript 1. Retrieved January 31, 2003, from http://nursingworld.org/ojin/topics20/tpc20_1.htm.

Bernstein, J., Mutschler, P., & Bernstein, E. (2000). Keeping mammography appointments: Motivation, health beliefs, and access barriers experienced by older minority women. *Journal of Midwifery and Women's Health, 45*(4), 308-313.

Byrne, M. (2001) Uncovering racial bias in nursing fundamental textbooks. *Nursing and Health Care Perspectives, 22*(6), 299-303.

Byrne, M. (2002). Instructional bias-awareness and reduction in perioperative education. *AORN Journal, 75*(4), 808-816.

Byrne, M., et al. (2003). The Byrne Guide for Inclusionary Cultural Content. *Journal of Nursing Education, 42*(6), 277-281.

Campinha-Bacote, J. (2001). A model of practice to address cultural competence in rehabilitation nursing. *Rehabilitation Nursing, 26*(1), 8-11.

Campinha-Bacote, J. (2002): *Readings and resources in transcultural health care in mental health* (13th ed.). Cincinnati, OH: Transcultural C.A.R.E. Associates Press.

Freire, G. (2002). Hispanics and the politics of health care. *Journal of Health & Social Policy 14*(4), 21-35.

Joyce, E., & Villanueva, M. (2000): *Say it in Spanish: A guide for health care professionals.* Philadelphia: W.B. Saunders.

Leininger, M. (2002). Culture care theory: A major contribution to advance transcultural nursing knowledge and practices. *Journal of Transcultural Nursing 13*(3), 189-192.

Lipson, J.G., & Rogers, J.G. (2000). Cultural aspects of disability. *Journal of Transcultural Nursing, 11*(3), 212-219.

McEvoy, M. (2003). Culture and spirituality as an integrated concept in pediatric care. *MCN: American Journal of Maternal Child Nursing 28*(1), 39-43.

Narayanasamy, A. (2003). Transcultural nursing: How do nurses respond to cultural needs? *British Journal of Nursing, 12*(3), 185-194.

Purnell, L. (2000). A description of the Purnell model for cultural competence. *Journal of Transcultural Nursing, 11*(1), 40-46.

Spector, R.E. (2000). *Cultural diversity in health and illness* (5th ed.). Upper Saddle River, NJ: Prentice-Hall Health.

Spinks, V.S., Andrews, J., & Boyle, J.S. (2000). Providing health care for lesbian clients. *Journal of Transcultural Nursing, 11*(2), 137-143.

Sutherland, L. (2002). Ethnocentrism in a pluralistic society: A concept analysis. *Journal of Transcultural Nursing, 13*(4), 274-281.

U.S. Department of Health and Human Services, Office of Disease Prevention and Health Promotion. (2000). *Tracking Healthy People 2010* (2nd ed.). Pittsburgh: U.S. Government Printing Office.

CHAPTER 7

Pain: The Fifth Vital Sign

LORA MCGUIRE

LEARNING OUTCOMES

After studying this chapter, you should be able to:

1. Define the concept of pain.
2. Identify three populations at high risk for undertreatment of pain.
3. Discuss the attitudes and knowledge of nurses, physicians, and clients regarding pain assessment and management.
4. Differentiate between addiction, tolerance, and physical dependence.
5. Compare and contrast the characteristics of the major types of pain.
6. Explain the transmission of pain.
7. Describe the components of a comprehensive pain assessment.
8. Describe the use of non-opioid analgesics in pain management.
9. Discuss and compare opioid analgesics, using an equianalgesic chart.
10. Explain the purpose of adjuvant medication in pain management.
11. Differentiate four routes of analgesic administration.
12. Identify special considerations for older adults related to pain assessment and management.
13. Identify physical and cognitive-behavioral therapies for clients experiencing pain.
14. Develop a teaching/learning plan for managing pain as part of community-based care for clients.
15. Describe the role of the nurse as an advocate in pain management.

Go to your Student CD-ROM for Review Questions for the NCLEX Examination keyed to these Learning Outcomes.

Pain is a universal, complex, subjective experience. It is the most common reason for a client to seek medical care, and the number one reason for a person to take medication. It alters or compromises quality of life more than any other single health-related problem. Despite more than 20 years of work by clinicians and professional and lay organizations, unrelieved and undertreated pain remains a major, yet avoidable public health problem in the United States (Berry & Dahl, 2000).

Your primary role in pain management is to advocate for the client by *believing* reports of pain. Because many practitioners may have difficulty with this concept, it must be emphasized repeatedly that there is no diagnostic test for pain. Even though some nurses with many years of experience think that they can identify clients in pain, it is impossible. To assist in advocating for adequate pain relief, the American Pain Foundation has developed a "Pain Care Bill of Rights" (Table 7-1).

OVERVIEW

Everyone experiences pain at some point in life. Because pain is such a private and personal experience, it may be difficult to describe or explain pain to others. The amount of pain and responses to it vary from person to person; therefore interpreting pain solely on actions or behaviors can be misleading.

Pain is generally related to some type of tissue damage and serves as a warning signal (e.g., pain signals a person to immediately remove a hand from a hot stove). Although pain is familiar to everyone, it is so complex that it cannot be easily described, and there is no single, universal treatment.

Definitions of Pain

Although several attempts have been made to define pain in descriptive or measurable terms, the two most accepted definitions have been put forth by the International Association of Pain (1979) and Margo McCaffery (1979). **Pain** is an unpleasant sensory and emotional experience associated with actual or potential tissue damage.

McCaffery offered a more personal explanation of pain when she stated that pain is whatever the experiencing person says it is and exists whenever he or she says it does. This understanding of pain requires that the client be seen as the authority on the pain and as the only one who can define the experience. In other words, *self-report* is always the most reliable indication of pain. Nurses who approach pain from this perspective can help the client achieve effective pain management by advocating for proper control.

TABLE 7-1 Pain Care Bill of Rights

As a person with pain, you have the right to:
- Have your report of pain taken seriously and to be treated with dignity and respect by doctors, nurses, pharmacists, and other health care professionals.
- Have your pain thoroughly assessed and promptly treated.
- Be informed by your health care provider about what may be causing your pain, possible treatments, and the benefits, risks, and costs of each.
- Participate actively in decisions about how to manage your pain.
- Have your pain reassessed regularly and your treatment adjusted if your pain has not been eased.
- Be referred to a pain specialist if your pain persists.
- Get clear and prompt answers to your questions, take time to make decisions, and refuse a particular type of treatment if you choose.

Although not always required by law, these are the rights you should expect for your pain care.

From American Pain Foundation, Baltimore, MD.

TABLE 7-2 Impact of Unrelieved Pain

Physiologic Impact
- Prolongs stress response
- Increases heart rate, blood pressure, and oxygen demand
- Decreases gastrointestinal motility
- Causes immobility
- Decreases immune response
- Delays healing
- Increases risk for chronic pain

Quality of Life Impact
- Interferes with activities of daily living
- Causes anxiety, depression, fear, anger, and sleeplessness
- Impairs family, work, and social relationships

Financial Impact
- Costs Americans $100 billion per year
- Increases hospital lengths of stay
- Leads to lost income and productivity

Modified from McCaffery, M., & Pasero, C. (1999). *Pain: Clinical manual* (2nd ed.) St. Louis: Mosby.

TABLE 7-3 Characteristics of Acute and Chronic Pain

Acute	Chronic*
Has short duration	Lasts more than several months (usually greater than 3)
Usually has a well-defined cause	May or may not have well-defined cause
Decreases with healing	Begins gradually and persists
Is reversible	Is exhausting and useless
Ranges from mild to severe intensity	Ranges from mild to severe intensity
May be accompanied by anxiety and restlessness	May be accompanied by depression and fatigue, as well as decreased functional ability

*Includes chronic cancer pain and chronic noncancer pain.

TABLE 7-4 Examples of Acute and Chronic Pain

Acute Pain
- Postoperative
- Trauma
- Burns
- Procedural
- Obstetric

Chronic Cancer Pain
- Tumor invasion
- Nerve compression
- Bone metastasis
- HIV-related pain
- Treatment-related pain (radiation, surgery, chemotherapy)

Chronic Noncancer Pain
- Arthritis
- Low back pain
- Fibromyalgia
- Neuropathic (diabetic neuropathy, phantom limb, post-herpetic neuralgia)
- Complex regional pain syndrome (CRPS)
- Intermittent causes, such as headaches and sickle cell pain

Scope of the Problem

Pain is a major economic problem and a major cause of disability that hampers the lives of many people. About 9 in 10 Americans regularly suffer pain. Approximately 25 million Americans suffer acute pain related to surgery or injury. Chronic pain is the most common cause of long-term disability, affecting 250 million Americans.

There is overwhelming evidence that pain is undertreated in the United States. In the last decade alone, numerous studies have continued to prove that pain is still not adequately treated in all areas of health care. Populations at the highest risk are older adults, minorities, and addicts. For example, one study of older adults found that 40% to 85% of nursing home residents had undertreated pain. Another study found that Hispanics with pain were half as likely as white clients to receive analgesics (Todd et al., 2000). In clients who are substance abusers, unrelieved pain can contribute to relapses or increased substance use.

Inadequate pain management can lead to many consequences affecting the client and family members. These consequences may affect the client/family physiologically, emotionally, and financially to greatly impair quality of life (Table 7-2).

Types of Pain

There are three main types of pain: acute, chronic cancer pain, and chronic noncancer pain (Tables 7-3 and 7-4). **Acute pain** results from acute injury, disease, or surgery. Chronic pain is divided into two subtypes. **Chronic cancer pain** is pain associated with cancer or another progressive disease such as acquired immunodeficiency syndrome (AIDS). The cause of pain is usually life threatening. **Chronic noncancer pain** is associated with tissue injury that has healed or is not associated with cancer, such as arthritis or chronic back pain. This type of pain is the most common.

ACUTE PAIN

Almost everyone experiences acute pain at some time. Certain characteristics distinguish this type of pain from the more chronic (long-term) pain often associated with chronic illness. A major distinction between acute and chronic pain is the effect on biologic responses. Acute pain serves a biologic purpose. It acts as a warning signal because it can activate the sympathetic nervous system, causing various physiologic responses. These responses are similar to those found in "fight-or-flight" reactions and include the following:

- Increased heart rate
- Increased blood pressure
- Increased respiratory rate
- Dilated pupils
- Sweating

Behavioral signs of acute pain may include restlessness, an inability to concentrate, apprehension, and overall distress.

Acute pain is usually temporary, of sudden onset, and easily localized. The client can often describe the pain, which may subside with or without treatment. Acute pain often results from sudden, accidental trauma (e.g., fractures, burns, and lacerations) or from surgery, ischemia, or acute inflammation. The pain is usually confined to the affected area. As this area heals, the quality of sensation of the pain changes. Although possibly severe, acute pain is limited over time and generally can be managed successfully. Both the caregiver and the client can see an end to the pain, which makes coping somewhat easier.

Pain that accompanies surgery is one of the most common examples of acute pain, but it is not always well managed. Usually this poorly managed postoperative pain is a result of inadequate drug therapy.

The severity of postoperative pain may be a predictor of long-term pain. The use of **preemptive analgesia** is a technique designed to decrease pain in the postoperative period, decrease the requirements for a postoperative analgesic, improve morbidity, and decrease hospital stay. Preemptive analgesia includes administering local anesthetics, opioids, and nonsteroidal anti-inflammatory drugs (NSAIDs) in the preoperative, intraoperative, and/or postoperative period. This intervention may inhibit changes in the spinal cord—changes that can lead to a central sensitization that results in chronic pain.

In general, intrathoracic and upper intra-abdominal surgical approaches are associated with more severe, steady wound pain and with pain on movement in the postoperative period. Many clients who undergo superficial surgery of the head and neck, chest wall, or limbs report minimal postoperative pain. Muscle-splitting procedures are generally far more painful than muscle-stretching procedures.

CHRONIC PAIN

Chronic pain is defined as pain that persists or recurs for indefinite periods, usually for more than 3 months. The onset is gradual, and the character and quality of the pain change over time. Because chronic pain often involves deep body structures, it is usually poorly localized and often difficult to describe. If the underlying cause cannot be treated medically, controlling the long-term effects of chronic pain may be a difficult clinical challenge.

Because chronic pain persists for extended periods, it can interfere with personal relationships and activities of daily living. It can also result in emotional and financial burdens. Thus the efforts of an interdisciplinary health care team are needed to manage the situation effectively. Inadequately managed pain is an overwhelming, frustrating experience for both the sufferer and the caregiver. Over half of clients with chronic pain become clinically depressed. Although many characteristics of chronic pain are similar in different clients, the nurse should be aware that each situation is unique and requires a highly specialized plan of care.

CHRONIC CANCER PAIN. Approximately two thirds of clients with advanced cancer have moderate to severe pain. What is frustrating is that we have known for over 30 years that 90% of cancer pain can be treated simply by giving adequate amounts of oral opioids around-the-clock. Yet clients with terminal cancer are often inadequately treated for their excruciating pain.

Most cancer pain is caused by the disease itself. The sources of pain include nerve compression, invasion of tissue, and/or bone metastasis. Cancer treatments can also cause pain due to surgery, as well as toxicities from chemotherapy and radiation therapy.

Clients with cancer pain generally have pain in two or more areas, but usually only talk about the primary area of pain. Be sure to perform a complete pain assessment to locate all areas of pain.

CHRONIC NONCANCER PAIN. Chronic noncancer pain is a major health problem. In the United States alone it is estimated that 25% of people, many of them older than 65 years of age, are affected with a chronic illness and chronic pain. Unlike acute pain, chronic pain serves no biologic purpose. After the initial warning signal of pain, the body must learn to adapt to the persistent pain impulses by blocking or adjusting to activation of the sympathetic nervous system (which causes the fight-or-flight reaction in acute pain). Because of this adaptation, the symptoms that may be associated with acute pain are *absent* with chronic pain.

Chronic noncancer pain was formerly called chronic nonmalignant pain. However, most pain experts, and certainly clients who suffer with daily pain, believe that all pain is malignant; thus the newer term.

Chronic noncancer pain may be caused by chronic diseases such as rheumatoid arthritis, lupus erythematosus, sickle cell anemia, fibromyalgia, low back pain, chronic headaches, and osteoporosis (see Table 7-4).

Neuropathic pain is one of the most challenging types of chronic noncancer pains; it results from some type of nerve injury. Examples of causes include diabetic neuropathy, postherpetic neuralgia, radiculopathy (spinal nerve damage), and trigeminal neuralgia. Neuropathic pain is described as burning, shooting, stabbing, and feeling "pins and needles."

Theoretical Bases for Pain

GATE CONTROL THEORY

The **gate control theory** was proposed to explain the observed relationship between pain and emotion. Melzack and Wall (1982) first introduced this theory and concluded that pain is not just a physiologic response. Psychological variables such as behavioral and emotional responses also influence the perception of pain.

According to this theory, a gating mechanism occurs in the spinal cord. Nerve fibers (A delta and C fibers) transmit pain impulses from the periphery of the body. These impulses travel to the dorsal horns of the spinal cord, specifically to the *substantia gelatinosa*. The cells of the substantia gelatinosa can inhibit or facilitate the pain impulses transmitted to the trigger cells (T-cells). When T-cell activity is

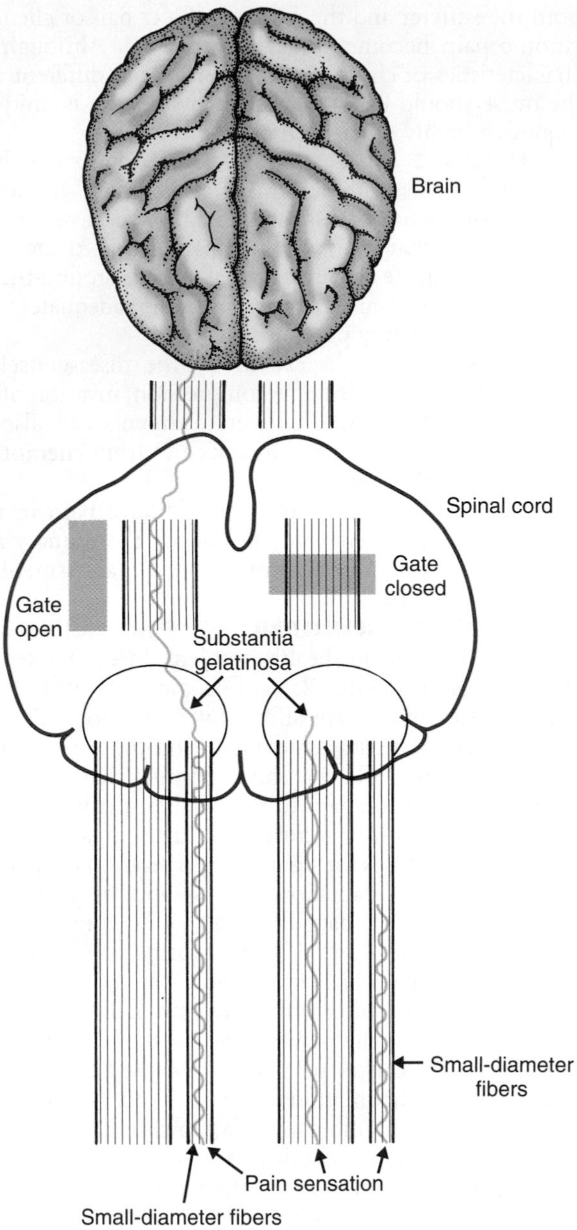

Figure 7-1 ■ The gate control theory of pain.

inhibited, the gate is closed and impulses are less likely to be transmitted to the brain. When the gate is opened, pain impulses ascend to the brain (Figure 7-1).

Similar gating mechanisms exist in the nerve fibers descending from the thalamus and cerebral cortex. These areas of the brain regulate thoughts and emotions, including beliefs and values. When pain occurs, a person's thoughts and emotions can modify perceptual phenomena as they reach the level of conscious awareness.

The gate control theory has helped nurses and other health care professionals to recognize the *holistic* nature of pain. As a result, many cognitive-behavioral therapies (e.g., imagery and distraction (see pp. 84 and 85) are used to help relieve pain.

ANATOMIC AND PHYSIOLOGIC BASES FOR PAIN

PAIN STIMULI. A wide range of sensory input is capable of producing pain. Tissue ischemia and muscle spasm also cause pain. Free nerve endings (receptors capable of responding to painful stimuli) are referred to as nociceptors. Nociceptors are located in various body tissues and are activated by thermal, mechanical, and chemical stimuli. In addition to nociceptors, other receptors in the body respond to almost any type of intense stimulation, which sometimes results in pain.

In most circumstances, painful stimuli cause actual tissue damage, which leads to the release of certain chemical substances called neurotransmitters (e.g., histamine, bradykinin, serotonin, norepinephrine) and certain acids that sensitize nociceptors, including leukotrienes, prostaglandins, and substance P. These chemicals are believed to activate pain receptors.

PAIN FIBERS AND PATHWAYS. Painful stimuli often originate in the periphery (extremities) of the body. To be perceived, the stimuli must be transmitted first to the spinal cord and then to the central areas of the brain, as described by the gate control theory of pain (see Figure 7-1). In the periphery, two specific fibers can transmit stimuli: (1) A delta fibers, which are found primarily in the skin and muscle, and (2) C fibers, which are distributed in muscle, periosteum, and viscera. Both of these nerve fibers are first-order neurons capable of accepting nociceptive stimuli.

A delta fibers are myelinated fibers that carry rapid, sharp, pricking, or piercing sensations. A person feeling these sensations can generally localize them readily to a fairly well-defined area. Because these fibers respond predominately to mechanical rather than chemical or thermal stimuli, they are called mechanical nociceptors.

C fibers are unmyelinated or poorly myelinated fibers that conduct thermal, chemical, and strong mechanical impulses. Pain conduction from C fibers is more diffuse and dull, burning, or achy–quite different from the sensations of A delta fibers. In contrast to the intermittent nature of A delta sensations, C fibers usually produce persistent pain.

Second-order neurons, or pain pathways of the ascending pain tracts, are found in the dorsal horn of the spinal cord and terminate in the thalamus. The spinothalamic tract is divided into two spinal tracts. The lateral, or neospinothalamic, tract is responsible for sensory pain discrimination; it transmits pain stimuli more directly to the sensory cortex, where pain is eventually perceived and interpreted. The paleospinothalamic tract synapses in other parts of the brain, such as the limbic system (emotional center) and the reticular formation (sleep-wake center). The painful stimuli are therefore subjected to emotional and behavioral influences.

CENTRAL NERVOUS SYSTEM PROCESSING. The central processing of pain occurs at three different levels of the brain: the thalamus, midbrain, and cortex. These areas cooperate to raise the awareness of pain, interpret painful stimuli, and produce a response to pain. The thalamus acts as the relay station for sensory input from the spinothalamic tract of the spinal cord. The midbrain signals the cortex to increase awareness of the stimuli. The cortex seems to be involved both in the discrimination of well-localized pain and in the interpretation of the pain experience.

INHIBITORY AND FACILITATORY MECHANISMS. Sensory input to the spinal cord may be influenced by chemical substances known as neuroregulators. Neuroregulators are classified as either neurotransmitters or neuromodulators.

TABLE 7-5 Physiologic Sources of Pain

Physiologic Structure	Characteristics of Pain	Sources of Acute Postoperative Pain	Sources of Chronic Pain Syndromes
Nociceptive Pain			
Somatic Pain			
Cutaneous or superficial: skin and subcutaneous tissues Deep somatic: bone, muscle blood vessels, connective tissues	Sharp, burning Dull, aching, cramping	Incisional pain, pain at insertion sites of tubes and drains, wound complications, orthopaedic procedures, skeletal muscle spasms	Bony metastases, osteoarthritis and rheumatoid arthritis, low back pain, peripheral vascular diseases
Visceral Pain			
Organs and the linings of the body cavities	Poorly localized Diffuse, deep cramping or splitting, sharp, stabbing	Chest tubes, abdominal tubes and drains, bladder distention or spasms, intestinal distention	Pancreatitis, liver metastases, colitis, appendicitis
Neuropathic Pain			
Nerve fibers, spinal cord, and central nervous system	Poorly localized Shooting, burning, fiery, shocklike, sharp, painful numbness	Phantom limb pain, postmastectomy pain, nerve compression	HIV-related pain, diabetic neuropathy, postherpetic neuralgia, chemotherapy-induced neuropathies, cancer-related nerve injury, radiculopathies

Neurotransmitters are the chemicals that exert inhibitory (slowing down) or excitatory (speeding up) activity at postsynaptic nerve cell membranes. Acetylcholine, norepinephrine, epinephrine, dopamine, and serotonin are documented neurotransmitters.

Neuromodulators, also called endogenous opiates, are hormones in the brain. These substances are composed of large amino acid peptides called alpha-**endorphins**, beta-endorphins, and enkephalins. These natural opiate-like substances are responsible for pain relief.

Opioid receptors are binding sites not only for endogenous opiates but also for opioid analgesics taken to relieve pain. There are several types of opioid receptors: mu, kappa, delta, epsilon, and sigma. Mu receptors are found throughout the central nervous system, especially in the brainstem, limbic system, and dorsal horn of the spinal cord. Morphine and morphine agonists bind to mu receptors.

Sources of Pain

There are two major sources of pain—nociceptive and neuropathic. **Somatic pain** (e.g., skin and musculoskeletal structures) and **visceral pain** (body-organ related) are types of **nociceptive pain**. Table 7-5 describes these categories and lists examples of each.

Attitudes and Practices Related to Pain

Negative and mistaken beliefs about pain and its treatment are common in the health care system. Studies have shown that many health care professionals do not have the knowledge and skills to manage pain adequately.

ATTITUDES AND KNOWLEDGE OF NURSES

Nurses' attitudes toward pain influence the way they perceive and interact with clients in pain. Without adequate assessment skills or knowledge of pain and analgesic therapy, nurses may not be able to understand their clients' pain and confidently participate with health care providers and other professionals in its treatment.

Nurses who have little personal experience with pain may not appreciate the magnitude of painful conditions associated with diseases and medical and surgical interventions. They may expect clients with chronic pain to react similarly to those with acute pain. They may assume that reactions to pain fall within a certain norm on the basis of their own cultural values. The more that a client's response varies from these expected norms, the more likely it is that a nurse's attitude toward the client will be positively or negatively biased.

ATTITUDES AND KNOWLEDGE OF HEALTH CARE PROVIDERS

Undertreatment of pain is a serious problem in the United States and elsewhere in the world. Between 50% and 80% of clients with cancer do not receive adequate pain control.

Despite increased education about pain, there are several reasons why many health care providers may underprescribe medication for clients in pain, especially opioids such as morphine. First, cultural and societal attitudes exist regarding opioid use.

Second, fear of regulatory scrutiny may lead to underprescribing of opioids. A physician or other health care provider may be reprimanded by the governing state board for prescribing what the board considers an inappropriate amount or type of pain medication.

Third, there is still a lack of knowledge about the effects of analgesics. Even with knowledge about correct prescribing practices, health care providers may fail to assess and treat the client's pain.

ATTITUDES AND KNOWLEDGE OF CLIENTS

Not only do health care professionals need education about pain management, but the public needs education as well. Nurses can help clients and families maintain successful pain management through education concerning available pain management resources.

Many clients are reluctant to report pain. When they do, they may underestimate its severity (Berry & Dahl, 2000). Clients may not state their pain because they want to be "good" clients or do not want to bother or distract their caregivers from other issues in their care. In clients with a history of cancer, pain can be an unwanted reminder of the disease and its progression.

Clients may also be reluctant to take pain medications, especially opioid analgesics, because they fear becoming addicted to or used to the medication (Berry & Dahl, 2000). These exaggerated fears of addiction must be addressed by the nurse so that the client will comply with the medication regimen.

Pain Perception and Disparities in Care

Many variables affect the perception of and response to pain. Factors such as age, gender, sociocultural background, and even genetics influence the client's ability to process and react to pain. These factors also put clients at risk of undertreatment.

Age can influence how pain is perceived, assessed, and treated. It has been well documented that the incidence of pain in older adults is high, as is risk for undertreatment.

Chart 7-1 addresses key components in assessment and management of pain in older adults.

It is well known that certain painful conditions are more common in either men or women. Seventy-two percent of chronic pain sufferers are women. Women suffer more often from migraine headache, tension headache, rheumatoid arthritis and osteoarthritis, fibromyalgia, and multiple sclerosis. Men suffer more from cluster headache, back pain, gout, peripheral vascular disease, and postherpetic neuralgia.

Women are at a higher risk for undertreatment of pain than men. A classic study by Cleeland et al. (1994) found that female cancer clients were more likely to be undertreated than male clients. It has also been well documented that investigation of chest pain is more extensive in men than women. Researchers are currently exploring gender and cultural differences in response to pain and opioids.

Genetic Considerations

Codeine is a commonly used opioid analgesic used to relieve pain. After ingestion, codeine is converted to morphine in the body's tissues. Thus the morphine is what alters the client's

CHART 7-1

NURSING FOCUS on the OLDER ADULT
Experiencing Pain

Prevalence of Pain
- Recognize that older adults are at great risk for undertreated pain.
- Consider the older adult at risk for the undertreatment of cancer pain because of inappropriate beliefs about pain sensitivity, tolerance, and ability to use opioids.

Beliefs about Pain
- In addition to receiving less analgesia, older adults tend to report pain less often than do younger adults. These findings may be related to beliefs and concerns about pain and the reporting of pain. Many older people hold the following beliefs and concerns about pain:
  - Pain is something that must be lived with.
  - Expressing pain is unacceptable or is a sign of weakness.
  - Complaining of pain will result in being labeled as a "bad" client.
  - Nurses are too busy to listen to complaints of pain.
  - Pain signifies a serious illness or impending death.
- Nurses should be aware of the beliefs of older clients regarding pain management. Nurses and other caregivers often undermedicate these clients and are sometimes reluctant to administer the prescribed analgesics.*

Assessment
- Ask about present pain only.
- Use a standard scale, such as the numerical Faces or Iowa Pain Thermometer rating scales.
- Explain the scale each time it is used.
- Use verbal descriptions other than pain, such as "ache," "sore," and "hurt."
- Use visual representations of pain measures rather than mental images of pain rating scales. Be sure that the client is wearing glasses and hearing aids, if needed and available.
- Alter a written pain scale to include large lettering, adequate space between lines, nonglossy paper, and color for increased visualization.
- Provide adequate lighting and privacy to avoid distracting background noise.

Considerations for Cognitively Impaired Clients
- Assess for nonverbal indicators of pain (facial expressions, grimacing, vocalizations, body movements, behavioral changes).
- Remember to "assume pain is present" (APP) in cognitively impaired clients with diseases and conditions commonly associated with pain.
- Little attention has been given to assessing or managing pain in older adults who are cognitively impaired (confused) and unable to communicate. Feldt (2000) tested a Checklist of Nonverbal Pain Indicators (CNP) to assess cognitively impaired older adults hospitalized for hip fracture. Feldt noted that older adults who were not cognitively impaired received significantly more pain medication in comparison to the impaired group.

Management of Pain
- Use around-the-clock dosing of analgesics.
- Consider an analgesic trial in a cognitively impaired client.
- Beware of adverse effects of acetaminophen (hepatotoxicity and nephrotoxicity) and NSAIDs (GI bleeding nephrotoxicity).
- Start low and go slow with opioid dosing.
- Avoid the use of meperidine, codeine, and propoxyphene (available in combination with acetaminophen, as Darvocet)
- Use methadone and tramadol with caution.
- Older adults and those with renal disease should not take meperidine because of the prolonged half-life of its drug metabolite, normeperidine.
- Use nondrug pain relief measures.

Data is, in part, from The American Geriatrics Society Foundation for Health in Aging. Available at http://www.healthinaging.org; and AGS Panel on Persistent Pain in Older Persons. (2002). The management of persistent pain in older persons. *Journal of the American Geriatrics Society, 50*(6 suppl.), S205-S224.

*Unfounded concerns about overmedication, addiction, and decreases in pain perception may contribute to undermedication (Berry & Dahl, 2000).

pain perception, not the codeine itself. Some clients (as many as 10%) are unable to obtain pain relief from codeine because they have a variation in the gene that codes for the enzyme that converts codeine to morphine (CYP2D6). For these clients, the conversion of codeine is so slow that the drug is excreted before pain is relieved (Burroughs et al., 2002). Therefore when caring for clients who are not obtaining pain relief from codeine, inform the health care provider to determine whether a change to morphine might be appropriate.

CULTURAL CONSIDERATIONS

A person's culture and ethnic background are significant in the meaning of pain and its manifestations. Pain behaviors are learned and influenced by beliefs. Cultural background also influences adherence to treatments.

As mentioned previously, minority clients are at risk for undertreatment of pain. Those at highest risk are clients cared for at centers serving mostly minorities. Different ethnic/racial groups may also experience pain differently. Inadequate and difficult assessment language barriers, attitudes toward pain and opioids, and access to health care may all contribute to undertreatment.

Maintain a nonjudgmental attitude when caring for clients with different cultural backgrounds and avoid stereotyping by ethnic group. Attempt to provide culturally sensitive client-education materials.

It is important to recognize that not all people manifest pain in the same way and that there is no right or wrong way. Accept all clients' expressions of pain, regardless of how different they may be from your own.

Tolerance, Physical Dependence, and Addiction

It is crucial that nurses and other health care professionals not refer to clients as "addict," "clock-watcher," or "drug seeker." These labels have caused biases and impacted the care that these clients have received.

The following descriptions of tolerance, physical dependence, and addiction have come from a consensus document (2001) from the American Academy of Pain Medicine (AAPM), American Pain Society (APS), and American Society of Addiction Medicine (ASAM).

Tolerance is a state of adaptation in which exposure to a drug induces changes that result in a decrease in one or more of the drug's effects over time. **Physical dependence** is the adaptation manifested by a drug-class–specific withdrawal syndrome. It can be produced by abrupt cessation, rapid dose reduction, decreasing blood level of the drug, and/or administration of an antagonist.

Physical dependence occurs in *everyone* who takes opioids over a period of time. It is important to *prevent* physical withdrawal. So-called **withdrawal symptoms** result when a client who is physically dependent on opioids abruptly ceases using them. These symptoms result from autonomic nervous system responses and include nausea and vomiting, abdominal cramping, muscle twitching, profuse perspiration, delirium, and convulsions. When it is necessary to discontinue opioid analgesia for a client who is opioid dependent, a slow tapering (weaning) of the drug dosage lessens or alleviates the physical withdrawal symptoms.

By contrast, **addiction** is a primary, chronic neurobiologic disease with genetic, psychosocial, and environmental factors influencing its development and manifestations. It is characterized by behaviors that include one or more of the following: impaired control over drug use, compulsive use, continued use despite harm, and craving. Addiction occurs over time, not as a result of one hospital stay. The stress of unrelieved pain could cause a relapse in a recovering client or an increase in drug use in the person who is actively using drugs (Nichols, 2003).

Pseudoaddiction is an iatrogenic syndrome created by the undertreatment of pain. It is characterized by client behaviors such as anger and escalating demands for more or different medications, and results in suspicion and avoidance by staff. Pseudoaddiction can be distinguished from true addiction in that the behaviors resolve when pain is effectively treated.

Tolerance, physical dependence, and addiction are separate conditions, but they may coexist. However, it is important to distinguish tolerance and physical dependence from addiction.

The danger of addiction to pain medication is vastly overrated. Although available data on addiction consistently show that it is rarely a result of using opioids for pain relief, health care professionals still have exaggerated fears. Clients and families also have fears related to addiction. Careful explanation of the difference between physical dependence and addiction should be discussed whenever a client starts on opioid therapy.

Clients who are substance abusers often have traumatic injuries and other health problems that cause pain. It is important for the nurse to recognize that substance abusers, typically those abusing opioids, are often tolerant to the pain-relieving effects of opioid analgesics and generally require increased doses. There is always the danger of abrupt physiologic withdrawal when recreational users of opioid agonists are given mixed agonist-antagonists and partial agonists.

Placebos

The clinical use of placebos in non–research-based therapies has not been shown to have a sustained effect on pain relief. McCaffery's definition of a **placebo** is "any medical treatment (medication or procedure, including surgery) or nursing care that produces an effect in a client because of its implicit or explicit or nursing care therapeutic intent and not because of its specific nature (physical or chemical properties)" (1979, p. 160). Placebos are substances or actions that produce an effect regardless of their known intrinsic value. When a client responds favorably to a placebo, it is known as the **placebo effect.** Placebos do not indicate whether or not a client has real pain. Because of the deception involved and the need for informed consent, never administer a placebo to your client.

Health care agencies should develop educational programs to inform professionals about pain management, including the inappropriate use of placebos. Ethics committees should be consulted for assistance in formulating policies and procedures regarding the use of placebos. Because of the Joint Commission's commitment to effective pain control, a policy against the use of placebos is recommended to be in place in all accredited institutions and agencies.

COLLABORATIVE MANAGEMENT

Assessment

HISTORY

Ask the client about the pain experience, including the sequence of events (precipitating and relieving factors); the nature of adjustments, if any, in life or in the family; and beliefs about the cause of the pain and what should be done about it (client's expectations). Personal characteristics (e.g., age and culture) influence attitudes about reporting a pain history. Families and significant others are included in this information-gathering process.

Clients may report pain in the absence of any observable or documented physiologic changes. Respect the client's verbal and nonverbal expressions of pain without making judgments or inferences about the reality of the pain. If clients perceive that health care professionals doubt the existence of their pain, mistrust and other negative feelings can arise and interfere with a therapeutic nurse-client relationship.

Assess the length of time the client has experienced pain. Clients may welcome an opportunity to discuss acute pain with the nurse because it is a relatively short-term experience and is easily described. However, clients with chronic pain can become frustrated when they are unable to adequately describe their vague, diffuse pain experience. Structured interviews using assessment aids (e.g., pain scales and descriptors) often help clients to express their pain.

Information about a client's pain can be helpful in understanding the factors associated with the present pain or previous episodes of pain. If the client is in pain when the nurse is obtaining the history, the session should be kept reasonably short or continued at a later time. Essential data include the following:

- *Precipitating factors.* Does the client associate any activities, food, or other environmental factors with the onset of pain? What does the client think causes the present pain? Was the onset of pain sudden or slow? Has the client done anything or taken anything to relieve the pain? What were the results of the intervention?
- *Aggravating factors.* What factors make the pain worse? What influence has this pain had on the client's activity? What changes of life activity have been affected (e.g., diet, job, sleep)?
- *Localization of pain.* Can the client localize the pain or describe where it travels or radiates?
- *Character and quality of pain.* What words does the client use to describe the pain and its character, quality, or intensity?
- *Duration of pain.* How long has the client experienced this pain?

PHYSICAL ASSESSMENT/CLINICAL MANIFESTATIONS

Although physiologic changes occur in response to acute noxious stimuli, these changes are usually *not* reliable indicators of pain. Acute pain, with its property of warning an individual about harm, *may*, but not always, cause several physiologic manifestations, which are largely a function of sympathetic nervous system stimulation. Clients with acute pain may manifest changes in vital body functions, such as tachycardia and blood pressure changes. Blood pressure is usually increased initially and then decreased. However, not all clients with acute pain have these signs, so *the client's statement of pain is the only reliable indicator.*

Physiologic changes in response to chronic pain are usually adapted to as the body attempts to compensate for and adapt to noxious stimuli. The pain no longer serves as a necessary warning. Chronic pain clients, then, frequently have developed coping skills and may appear to look quite well.

Certain motor or body movements may be associated with either acute or chronic pain. Some may be more exaggerated or obvious than others. Clients in pain may support or shield ("splint"), holding painful body parts while moving, or they may lie listlessly because they are afraid to move. Assess the functional status and degree of impairment in the client with pain.

LOCATION OF PAIN. Assess the pain from two dimensions: the level of pain (deep or superficial) and the position or location of pain. Most clients can usually describe the depth of acute pain or chronic pain. The actual area or location of the pain, however, may not be as easily identified. Ask the client whether the pain is superficial or deep. In general, clients with pain involving superficial or cutaneous (skin) structures describe their pain as superficial and can often localize the pain to a specific area.

Pain may be described as belonging to one of four categories related to its location:

- **Localized pain** is pain confined to the site of origin.
- **Projected pain** is pain along a specific nerve or nerves.
- **Radiating pain** is diffuse pain around the site of origin that is not well localized.
- **Referred pain** is pain perceived in an area distant from the site of painful stimuli.

A client who has difficulty specifying the exact location of pain can be asked to point to the painful areas on his or her own body or on another person. It is sometimes helpful to have the client point to or shade in the painful areas on a diagram on the front and back of the human body (Figure 7-2). Clients who cannot identify the painful areas and state that they just "hurt all over" are encouraged to focus on parts of the body that are *not* painful. Ask the client to concentrate on different body parts, beginning with the hand and fingers of one extremity, and identify the presence or absence of pain. By focusing attention on selected areas of the body, the client is assisted in localizing painful areas. Clients who state that they hurt everywhere often begin to realize that some parts of the body are not painful.

Clients may present with more than one discrete painful site. In fact, about one half of clients with advanced cancer report having pain in more than one location. As painful areas are identified, the nurse helps the client to understand the origin of the pain. This understanding is particularly important for clients with cancer, because every new pain often raises the suspicion of metastasis (spread of disease). The pain may be caused by other reasons, such as immobility or constipation.

OTHER PAIN DATA. After asking the client to locate the pain, ask him or her to describe it. Clients may use one word or a group of words to convey the sensations or feelings of the pain. Avoid suggesting descriptive words for the pain.

Pain is rarely the same at all times. It is perceived differently over time and varies with factors such as physical activity and stress (see the earlier discussion under History).

McGill-Melzack PAIN QUESTIONNAIRE

Patient's name ______________ Age __________

File No. ________________ Date __________

Clinical category (e.g., cardiac, neurologic)

Diagnosis: __________

____

____

Analgesic (if already administered):

1. Type ____________________
2. Dosage ____________________
3. Time given in relation to this test ______

Patient's intelligence: circle number that represents best estimate.

1 (low) 2 3 4 5 (high)

****

This questionnaire has been designed to tell us more about your pain. Four major questions we ask are

1. Where is your pain?
2. What does it feel like?
3. How does it change with time?
4. How strong is it?

It is important that you tell us how your pain feels now. Please follow the instructions at the beginning of each part.

Part 1. Where Is Your Pain?

Please mark, on the drawings below, the areas where you feel pain. Put E if external, or I if internal, near the areas you mark. Put EI if both external and internal.

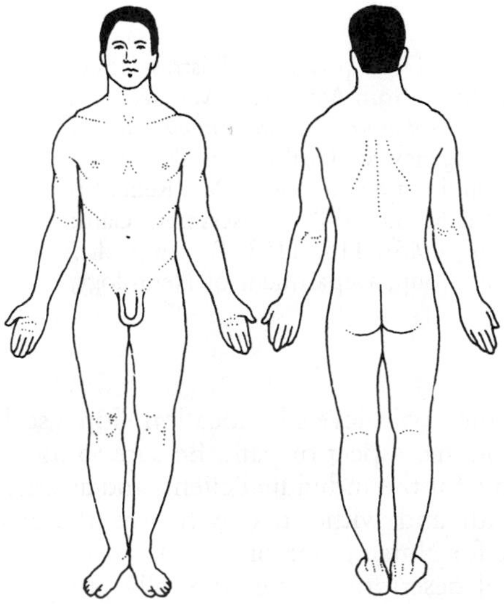

Part 2. What Does Your Pain Feel Like?

Some of the words below describe your *present* pain. Circle *ONLY* those words that best describe it. Leave out any category that is not suitable. Use only a single word in each appropriate category—the one that applies best.

1. Flickering, Quivering, Pulsing, Throbbing, Beating, Pounding
2. Jumping, Flashing, Shooting
3. Pricking, Boring, Drilling, Stabbing, Lancinating
4. Sharp, Cutting, Lacerating
5. Pinching, Pressing, Gnawing, Cramping, Crushing
6. Tugging, Pulling, Wrenching
7. Hot, Burning, Scalding, Searing
8. Tingling, Itchy, Smarting, Stinging
9. Dull, Sore, Hurting, Aching, Heavy
10. Tender, Taut, Rasping, Splitting
11. Tiring, Exhausting
12. Sickening, Suffocat-ing
13. Fearful, Frightful, Terrifying
14. Punishing, Grueling, Cruel, Vicious, Killing
15. Wretched, Blinding
16. Annoying, Troublesome, Miserable, Intense, Unbearable
17. Spreading, Radiating, Penetrating, Piercing
18. Tight, Numb, Drawing, Squeezing, Tearing
19. Cool, Cold, Freezing
20. Nagging, Nauseating, Agonizing, Dreadful, Torturing

Part 3. How Does Your Pain Change With Time?

1. Which word or words would you use to describe the *pattern* of your pain?

1	2	3
Continuous	Rhythmic	Brief
Steady	Periodic	Momentary
Constant	Intermittent	Transient

2. What kind of things *relieve* your pain?
3. What kind of things *increase* your pain?

Part 4. How Strong Is Your Pain?

People agree that the following 5 words represent pain of increasing intensity. They are:

1	2	3	4	5
Mild	Discomforting	Distressing	Horrible	Excruciating

To answer each question below, write the number of the most appropriate word in the space beside the question.

1. Which word describes your pain right now? ____
2. Which word describes it at its worst? ____
3. Which word describes it when it is least? ____
4. Which word describes the worst toothache you ever had? ____
5. Which word describes the worst headache you ever had? ____
6. Which word describes the worst stomachache you ever had? ____

Figure 7-2 ■ The McGill-Melzack Pain Questionnaire. (From Melzack, R. [1975]. The McGill Pain Questionnaire: Major properties and scoring methods. *Pain, 1,* 272-281.)

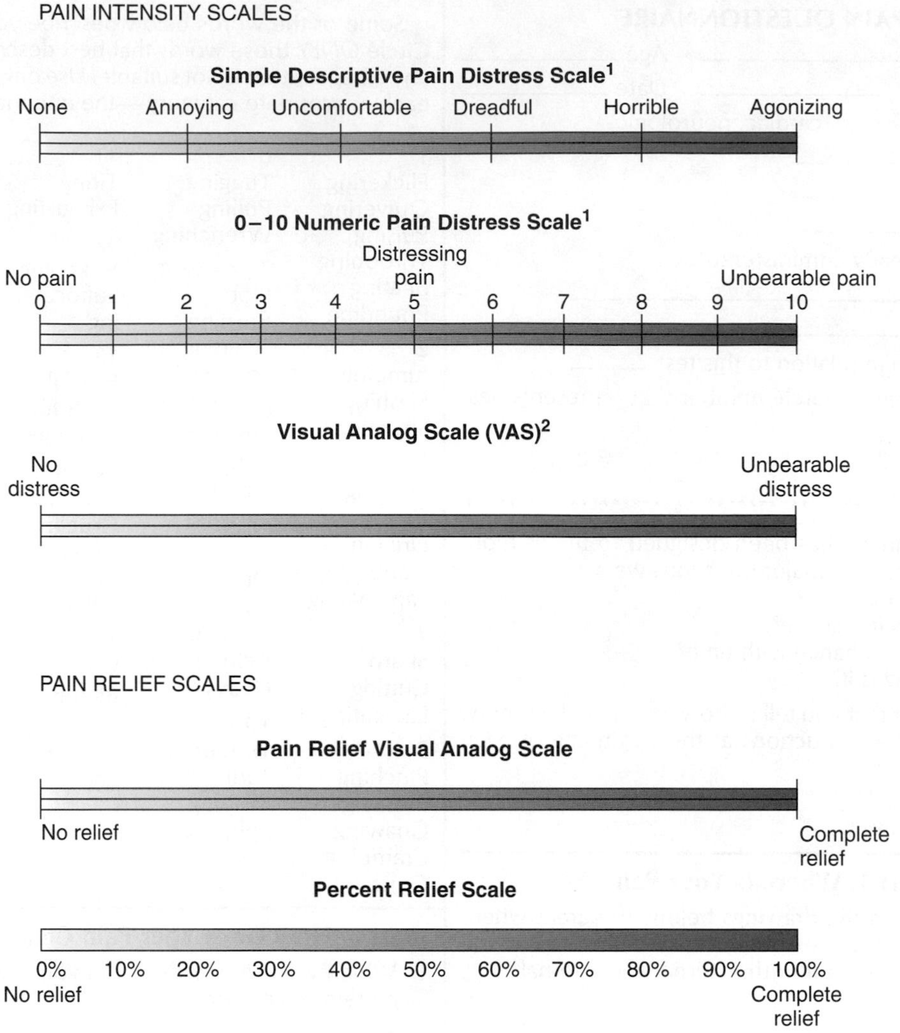

[1]If used as a graphic rating scale, a 10-cm baseline is recommended.

[2]A 10-cm baseline is recommended for VAS scales.

Figure 7-3 ■ Pain rating scales and pain relief scales. (Simple Descriptive Pain Distress Scale, 0-10 Numeric Pain Distress Scale, and Visual Analog Scale redrawn from Acute Pain Management Guideline Panel. [1992]. *Acute pain management: Operative or medical procedures and trauma. Clinical practice guideline.* AHCPR Pub. No. 92-0032. Rockville, MD: Agency for Health Care Policy and Research, Public Health Service, U.S. Department of Health and Human Services; Pain Relief Visual Analog Scale redrawn from Fishman, B., et al. [1987]. The Memorial Pain Assessment Card: A valid instrument for the evaluation of cancer pain. *Cancer, 60*[5], 1151-1158; Percent Relief Scale redrawn from the Brief Pain Inventory. Pain Research Group, Department of Neurology, University of Wisconsin–Madison.)

Subjective measurements of pain intensity by the client are more reliable and accurate than observable qualities of pain. Only the client can determine the amount or severity of pain being experienced. Various visual analog scales (VASs), number rating scales (NRSs), descriptive word scales, and other measures have been designed to help clients communicate the magnitude or severity of pain and to help nurses quantify the pain (Figure 7-3).

Use pain intensity scales to measure pain in the clinical or home setting and to assess and determine the effectiveness of pain relief interventions. The client is presented with a pain scale and asked to rate the amount of painful stimuli. Clients with more than one discrete painful site may wish to specify their pain levels by location. Some scales also assess the emotional aspect of pain. Be sure to use the *same* scale over time for the individual client, and assess pain intensity both with and without activity (see the Evidence-Based Practice for Nursing box on p. 73).

Verbal descriptive scales typically group words such as "none," "moderate," or "severe," and permit an intensity rating of pain. However, the 0 to 10 NRS is most commonly used in clinical practice for adult clients who can communicate in English (see Figure 7-3). For culturally diverse clients with language barriers, the Wong-Baker scale (Faces Pain Rating scale of smile to frown) may be helpful. This scale is also used for children, older adults, and develop-

EVIDENCE-BASED PRACTICE for Nursing

How to assess pain intensity in cognitively impaired African-American older adults

Taylor, L.J. & Jen, K. (2003). Pain intensity assessment: A comparison of selected pain intensity scales for use in cognitively intact and cognitively impaired African American older adults. *Pain Management Nursing, 4*(2), 87-95.

The purpose of this study was to determine the reliability and validity of the Faces Pain Scale, Verbal Description Scale, Numeric Rating Scale, and the Iowa Pain Thermometer for pain assessment in cognitively impaired African-American older adults. Fifty-seven African-American adults participated; 77% had some degree of cognitive impairment, 23% were cognitively intact. All of the participants were able to use all four scales, and both groups preferred the Faces Pain Scale.

Level of Evidence: 6—This study used a small convenience sample. However, it serves as an excellent pilot study to hopefully stimulate further research of larger, randomized groups.

Critique. Very few studies have looked at older African Americans with regard to physical assessment or health care. This study not only used this group as the sample, but also compared cognitively impaired and cognitively intact older adults. In view of growing diversity in the United States, more research of this type is needed to develop best practices for all people of any cultural/ethnic background.

Implications for Nursing. As the population ages, accurate assessment and treatment of pain needs to be a priority. Older and minority clients are each at risk for undertreatment of pain. Use of simple pain scales, such as the Faces Pain Scale, should be a routine part of pain assessment in all clients, both cognitively intact and cognitively impaired.

mentally disabled populations. The book listed in the Selected Bibliography by McCaffery and Pasero (1999) contains 0 to 10 pain rating scales in 25 different languages.

ASSESSING PAIN IN COGNITIVELY IMPAIRED OR CRITICALLY ILL NONVERBAL CLIENTS. Although it seems obvious, nonverbal, intubated, and cognitively impaired clients *do* feel pain! It is important to be proactive and "assume pain is present," or APP (Pasero & McCaffery, 2000).

Clients with painful chronic conditions such as arthritis, osteoporosis, cancer, pressure ulcers, and contractures should receive an analgesic trial of around-the-clock medications. Procedural pain should also be assumed and analgesics given beforehand. Turning, suctioning, drain removal, wound care, and other routine procedures are very painful (Puntillo et al., 2001).

Possible indicators of pain in nonverbal clients include facial expressions, verbalizations, body language, and behavioral changes. There are several behavioral pain indicator checklists or tools available for the nurse to use. In a study of older adults with hip fractures, facial grimaces and restlessness were the two most common pain indicators (Feldt, 2000).

After receiving a 24- to 48-hour analgesic trial, a complete reassessment should be performed. Family members' reports of a client's pain should be incorporated into the plan of care.

PSYCHOSOCIAL ASSESSMENT

ACUTE PAIN. All pain holds significant meaning for the person experiencing it. Clients having acute pain from surgery may interpret their pain as necessary and expected. It may be viewed with relief as a sign that some greater problem has been resolved or alleviated by the surgery. Knowing that the duration of the pain is limited may allow the client to deal with unpleasant sensations without too much difficulty. In contrast, acute chest pain associated with angina may mark the beginning of a life of fear and uncertainty.

CHRONIC PAIN. Various psychosocial factors influence chronic pain. Some factors are similar to those found in the acute pain experience, such as anxiety or fear related to the meaning of the pain. Because chronic pain persists or is perhaps only partially relieved, the client may feel powerless, angry, hostile or desperate. The client is also vulnerable to labels such as "chronic complainer" or "fake."

The status of family and other close relationships, along with the breadth of social resources available to the chronic pain client, must be assessed. The existence of a pain-specific conflict with a spouse or significant other may affect or limit pain coping strategies. Other people may react to chronic pain with depression, social withdrawal, and preoccupation with physical symptoms.

If the chronic pain is associated with a progressive disease such as cancer, rheumatoid arthritis, or peripheral vascular disease, the client may have worries and concerns about the consequences of the illness. Clients with cancer-related pain may fear death or body mutilation. Some may think they are being punished for some wrongdoing in life. Others may attach a religious or spiritual significance to lingering pain.

Ask open-ended questions (e.g., "Tell me how your pain has affected your job or role as a mother") to allow the client to describe personal attitudes about pain and its influence on life. This opportunity can help a client whose life has been changed by pain. However, some clients choose not to share their private information or fears. This decision should be respected. Assess the impact of the pain on their ability to function.

In 2000, the Joint Commission Accreditation of Health Care Organizations (JCAHO) published new pain management standards. The American Pain Society (APS) called pain "the fifth vital sign." Pain documentation as the fifth vital sign is not required by JCAHO or APS, yet most health care agencies use it to ensure all pain is assessed at regular intervals and treated appropriately.

Interventions

Drug Therapy. Medications are the gold-standard form of pain control. However, many nurses and other health professionals have inadequate knowledge regarding the pharmacology of drugs used in pain control. This lack of information, together with the misconceptions and attitudes about pain previously discussed, are the two main reasons why clients have inadequate pain relief.

There are three groups of medications used to manage pain: non-opioids, opioids, and adjuvants. To advocate for your client, a thorough understanding of the medications used to treat pain is necessary (Table 7-6).

Non-Opioid Analgesics. The **non-opioid** (formerly called nonnarcotic) **analgesics** are the first line therapy for mild to moderate pain. The two most common non-opioids are **acetylsalicylic acid** (**aspirin**, Apo-ASA✱) and **acetaminophen** (**Tylenol**, Atasol✱). Studies have shown that their analgesic and antipyretic (fever reduction) effects are the same in equal doses. The single optimal dose of aspirin or acetaminophen is between 650 and 1000 mg.

There is a ceiling to the analgesic effect of these non-opioids. In other words, if the dose of the non-opioid analgesic is greater than 1000 mg, there will be no additional analgesic effect, only more side effects. Aspirin can cause bleeding, and acetaminophen can cause hepatotoxicity (liver toxicity).

TABLE 7-6 Examples of Analgesics by Classification

Non-Opioids	Opioids	Adjuvants
Acetaminophen (Tylenol)	Pure agonists:	Tricyclic antidepressants:
NSAIDs (nonselective):	Morphine	Amitriptyline (Elavil)
Aspirin	Fentanyl (Duragesic, Actiq)	Desipramine (Norpramin)
Ibuprofen (Motrin)	Hydrocodone (Vicoden)	Nortriptyline (Pamelor)
Naproxen (Naprosyn)	Oxycodone (OxyContin, Percodan)	Doxepin (Sinequan)
Etodolac (Lodine)	Hydromorphone (Dilaudid)	Anticonvulsants:
Ketoprofen (Toradol)	Meperidine (Demerol) (outdated drug)	Gabapentin (Neurontin)
Piroxicam (Feldene)	Methadone	Valproic acid (Depakene)
Salsalate (Disalcid)	Codeine	Topiramate (Topamax)
NSAIDs (selective):	Agonist/antagonists (not commonly used):	Clonazepam (Klonopin)
Celecoxib (Celebrex)	Pentazocine (Talwin)	Baclofen (Lioresal)
Valdecoxib (Bextra)	Butorphanol (Stadol)	Alpha-2 adrenergics:
	Nalbuphine (Nubain)	Clonidine (Catapres)
	Buprenorphine (Buprenex)	Tizanidine (Zanaflex)
		Local anesthetics:
		Mexiletine (Mexitil)
		Topical lidocaine (Lidoderm)
		NMDA antagonists:
		Ketamine
		Dextromethorphan

Modified from McCaffery, M., & Pasero, C., (1999). *Pain: Clinical manual* (2nd ed.) St. Louis: Mosby.

Many people underestimate the effectiveness of non-opioid analgesics, also referred to as **peripheral-acting analgesics**. For mild pain, the non-opioids aspirin 650 mg and acetaminophen (Tylenol) 650 mg produce pain relief comparable to that of the opioids codeine 32 mg PO and meperidine (Demerol) 50 mg PO. Most non-opioids (other than acetaminophen) are potent anti-inflammatory agents called **nonsteroidal anti-inflammatory drugs (NSAIDs).**

Nonsteroidal Anti-Inflammatory Drugs. Aspirin and other NSAIDs are very effective for inflammatory type pain, such as rheumatoid arthritis, postoperative pain, dental pain, menstrual pain, migraines, low back pain, sunburn, and bone pain. These agents inhibit the synthesis of prostaglandins, which are fatty-acid substances found throughout the body. The release of prostaglandins in tissues causes pain, edema, and inflammation. By inhibiting the synthesis of prostaglandins, anti-inflammatory drugs decrease inflammation and pain. NSAIDs are particularly useful in the management of acute inflammation such as that which causes postoperative pain. **Ketorolac (Toradol)** is one of the most popular NSAIDs prescribed for short-term use in cases of acute pain because it can be given orally, intramuscularly, or by intravenous (IV) push. A newer COX-2 NSAID, **parecoxib (Dynastat),** should soon be available for either IV or intramuscular injection.

Aspirin and other NSAIDs can cause gastrointestinal (GI) disturbances and can prevent platelet aggregation, which results in a tendency toward bleeding. Therefore observe the client for gastric discomfort or vomiting, and bleeding or bruising. Report these problems to the health care provider immediately.

CONSIDERATIONS FOR OLDER ADULTS

Older adults often take over-the-counter (OTC) NSAIDs for common problems, such as osteoarthritis and back pain. However, while they are usually effective in relieving pain, these drugs can increase or decrease the effects of other drugs that the client is taking. The most serious drug-drug interactions are with anticoagulants, oral hypoglycemics, and antihypertensives, including diuretics (Durrance, 2003). To add to these potential problems, normal physiologic changes of aging affect the protein binding, drug distribution, and renal elimination of NSAIDs. King (2000) reported that almost 17,000 deaths occur among clients with arthritis related to long-term NSAID use. In addition, NSAIDs can cause tinnitus and other peripheral and central nervous system symptoms that can contribute to falls in older adults (King, 2000).

NSAIDs also cause renal toxicity; therefore renal function blood tests should be routinely monitored with long-term therapy, especially in the older adult. In addition, NSAIDs can cause sodium and water retention that may lead to congestive heart failure, more often in an older client.

When taking a client history, ask about the use of NSAIDs, keeping in mind that store brand names may not be considered as NSAIDs. For example, Walprofen is Wal-Mart's brand name for ibuprofen; Walproxen is the name for naproxen. Orudis contains ketoprofen, and Aleve contains naproxen. Ask the client or client's family to provide the name of each drug that the client is taking, as well as the daily dosage. Some clients may unknowingly take several types of NSAIDs at the same time, putting them at a high risk for adverse drug effects.

The side effects of individual NSAIDs differ. For example, ibuprofen (Motrin, Actiprofen✱) and naproxen (Naprosyn, Naxen✱) appear to cause fewer GI problems than ketoprofen (Orudis, Rhodis✱). By adding a GI protective drug such as misoprostol (Cytotec), GI side effects may be reduced.

Because of the high incidence of GI bleeding due to NSAID use, particularly in older adults, the American Pain Society Clinical Practice Guidelines (1999) recommend selective cyclooxygenase-2 (COX-2) inhibitors, such as celecoxib (Celebrex) and valdecoxib (Bextra), for long-term use. This newer class of NSAIDs, COX-2 inhibitors, selectively block the COX-2 enzyme responsible for inflammation and the production of substances associated with pain (e.g., prostaglandins). However, all COX-2 inhibitors have recently been associated with increased cardiovascular disease and may have limited use or be unavailable in the future. Most older NSAIDs block both COX-1 and COX-2 enzymes. The COX-1 enzyme is responsible for the gastric and renal side effects associated with older NSAID use. Studies of clients with dental pain, osteoarthritis, and rheumatoid arthritis treated with COX-2 inhibitors demonstrate effective analgesia without GI side effects. There is no difference in the COX-2 analgesic efficacy or in renal side effects, but the decreased risk of GI bleeding makes these drugs more beneficial.

Acetaminophen. Unlike the rest of the non-opioid analgesics, acetaminophen (Tylenol) has few anti-inflammatory properties. Acetaminophen has some advantages over aspirin in that it is available in a liquid form (which is the best way to take oral analgesics) and it can be taken on an empty stomach. Acetaminophen causes no adverse gastrointestinal (GI) effects. Therefore it is preferred for any client who has a history of ulcer disease. Acetaminophen also has no effect on platelet aggregation as most of the other non-opioids do. This drug is also preferred, then, for clients in whom bleeding is likely, such as preoperative or postoperative clients. Acetaminophen is not without its serious side effects, however. The main adverse effects are hepatotoxicity (liver toxicity) and nephro-toxicity (renal toxicity) with long-term use.

Health care providers commonly prescribe acetaminophen for pain. Acetaminophen exerts its analgesic action by blocking peripheral pain receptors, thus increasing the threshold of these receptors to painful stimuli. Reports of liver toxicity have been associated with higher doses of the drug (1000 mg) taken more frequently than every 4 hours for long-term use. Current recommendations restrict the total daily amount of acetaminophen to no more than 4000 mg (4 g). For long-term use, no more than 3600 mg daily should be taken. Less than 2400 mg daily should be used in older adults. Teach clients to be aware of the amount of acetaminophen in combination products such as Vicodin and Darvocet. The acetaminophen in these products limits their use for chronic pain.

Opioid Analgesics. **Opioid analgesics** are the mainstay in the management of all types of pain. Opioids (formerly called **narcotics**) work centrally by blocking the release of neurotransmitters in the spinal cord. Opioids are classified as full agonists (morphine-like), partial agonists, or mixed agonists/antagonists. There are no advantages to the partial or mixed agonists, and they could precipitate a withdrawal if given to a client taking a full agonist.

Full Agonists. The opioid **full agonists** bind to mu receptors and block the release of substance P, preventing the transmission of pain. The full agonists are the most potent of all analgesics.

Most opioid agonists are similar in pharmacologic effects, so a client does not need more than one. Although the oral route is generally the preferred route, most opioids can be administered in many different routes.

There is no ceiling in the dose of a pure opioid agonist. The use of an equianalgesic chart when changing opioids is necessary, though, because these drugs vary in their oral to parenteral dosages (Table 7-7).

Equianalgesic Chart. Nurses should be familiar with a comparison chart of equivalent opioid dosages. This chart is useful when switching opioids or routes of administration of opioids, and it enables the nurse to learn the dosage of the drugs being administered for pain.

The term **equianalgesic** refers to the dose and route of administration of one drug that produces about the same degree of analgesia as the given dose and route of another drug. Most commonly, 10 mg IM of morphine is the standard dose against which other opioids are measured. Equianalgesic opioid drug guides provide only the comparative analgesic potencies among these drugs. Dose modifications may be necessary according to each client's response and as always, with older adults, the guideline is to "start low and go slow" with drug dosing.

Common Opioids. **Codeine** is a short-acting weak opioid. It is considered a pro-drug, meaning an enzyme is necessary to break it down to be effective. It is estimated that 5% to 10% of the population lack this enzyme, which could account for codeine's ineffectiveness in certain clients. Codeine has limited value for severe pain, and should not be used in older adults due to the possible accumulation of a toxic metabolite, as well as constipation.

Hydrocodone is available as a combination product with acetaminophen (Lortab, Vicodin) and ibuprofen (Vicoprofen). Because of this, the dose cannot be escalated due to the toxicities from the non-opioids. Therefore hydrocodone has limited usefulness for chronic, long-term pain.

Oxycodone is available as a single-agent, both in short- and long-acting preparations (OxyContin). It is also available in combination with aspirin (Percodan, Oxycodone✱) or acetaminophen (Percocet, Tylox, Roxicet, Oxycocet✱). Oxycodone is recommended for acute and chronic pain.

Morphine (Duramorph, Roxanol, Avinza, Kadian, Morphitec✱) is the gold standard opioid for both acute and chronic pain (see the Concept Map on p. 77). It is inexpensive, available in many dosage strengths (both short and long acting), and can be given in virtually any route, including rectally. MS Contin, Avinza, and Kadian are examples of long-acting or slow-release forms of the drug. Ten milligrams of morphine intramuscularly equals 30 mg orally.

Hydromorphone (Dilaudid) is eight times more potent than morphine. It is currently only available in the short-acting form. Like morphine, hydromorphone is useful for all types of moderate to severe pain.

Fentanyl (Sublimaze) is a potent opioid available in two special forms, the 72-hour patch known as **Duragesic,** which is useful for chronic pain, and in the oral transmucosal lozenge (Actiq). **Actiq** lozenges are indicated for breakthrough cancer pain and should not be given to opioid-naive clients. **Breakthrough pain** occurs primarily in clients with severe terminal cancer pain. The client experiences pain between scheduled doses of the drug regimen. Other drugs may also be used for this purpose, but lozenges are less invasive for the client. Actiq is also currently being used "off-label" (not FDA approved) for procedural-type pain.

Methadone (Dolophine) is the only full opioid agonist with a dual mechanism of action. It works on both the mu receptors and the NMDA receptors. Because of its long half-life (24 to 36 hours), always assess for sedation (especially days 2 to 3) and use cautiously in older adults. When managing pain in a client in a methadone maintenance program for substance abuse, be sure to increase the methadone dose for pain relief or add a second opioid.

Tramadol (Ultram) is classified as an atypical opioid. It binds weakly to the mu receptors in the central nervous system and inhibits the reuptake of norepinephrine and serotonin. Tramadol can be used for acute pain and chronic neuropathic pain. It should not be given in doses greater than 400 mg daily because it can cause seizures. It should be

TABLE 7-7 Dose Equivalents for Opioid Analgesics in Opioid-Naive Adults[a]

	Approximate Equianalgesic Dose		Usual Starting Dose for Moderate to Severe Pain	
Drug	**Oral**	**Parenteral**	**Oral**	**Parenteral**
Opioid Agonist[b]				
Morphine[c]	30 mg q3-4h (repeat around-the-clock dosing) 60 mg q3-4h (single dose or intermittent dosing)	10 mg q3-4h	30 mg q3-4h	10 mg q3-4h
Morphine, controlled-release[b,d] (MS Contin, Oramorph)	90-120 mg q12h	N/A	90-120 mg q12h	N/A
Hydromorphone[c] (Dilaudid)	7.5 mg q3-4h	1.5 mg q3-4h	6 mg q3-4h	1.5 mg q3-4h
Levorphanol (Levo-Dromoran)	4 mg q6-8h	2 mg q6-8h	4 mg q6-8h	2 mg q6-8h
Meperidine (Demerol)	300 mg q2-3h	100 mg q3h	N/R	100 mg q3h
Methadone (Dolophine, other)	20 mg q6-8h	10 mg q6-8h	20 mg q6-8h	10 mg q6-8h
Oxymorphone[c] (Numorphan)	N/A	1 mg q3-4h	N/A	1 mg q3-4h
Combination Opioid/NSAID Preparations[e]				
Codeine[f] (with aspirin or acetaminophen)	18-200 mg q3-4h	130 mg q3-4h	60 mg q3-4h	60 mg q2h (IM/SC)
Hydrocodone (in Lorcet, Lortab, Vicodin, others)	30 mg q3-4h	N/A	10 mg q3-4h	N/A
Oxycodone (Roxicodone, also in Percocet, Percodan, Tylox, others)	30 mg q3-4h	N/A	10 mg q3-4h	N/A

From Management of Cancer Pain Guideline Panel. (1994) *Management of cancer pain: Clinical practice guidelines.* AHCPR Pub. No. 94-0592. Rockville, MD: Agency for Health Care Policy and Research, Public Health Service, U.S. Department of Health and Human Services.

N/A, Not available; *N/R,* not recommended; *SC,* subcutaneous.

NOTE: Published tables vary in the suggested doses that are equianalgesic to morphine. Clinical response is the criterion that must be applied for each patient; titration to clinical responses is necessary. Because there is not complete cross tolerance among these drugs, it is usually necessary to use a lower-than-equianalgesic dose when changing drugs and to retitrate to response.

[a]**CAUTION:** Recommended doses do not apply for adult patients with body weight less than 50 kg.

[b]**CAUTION:** Recommended doses do not apply to patients with renal or hepatic insufficiency or other conditions affecting drug metabolism and kinetics.

[c]**CAUTION:** For morphine, hydromorphone, and oxymorphone, rectal administration is an alternate route for patients unable to take oral medications. Equianalgesic doses may differ from oral and parenteral doses because of pharmacokinetic differences.

[d]Transdermal fentanyl (Duragesic) is an alternative option. Transdermal fentanyl dosage is not calculated as equianalgesic to a single morphine dosage. See the package insert for dosing calculations. Doses above 25 mcg/hr should not be used in opioid-naive patients.

[e]**CAUTION:** Doses of aspirin and acetaminophen in combination opioid-NSAID preparations must also be adjusted to the patient's body weight. Aspirin is contraindicated in children in the presence of fever or other viral disease because of its association with Reye's syndrome.

[f]**CAUTION:** Codeine doses above 65 mg often are not appropriate because of diminishing incremental analgesia with increasing doses, as well as a higher incidence of nausea, constipation, and other side effects.

used cautiously in clients who are taking antidepressant medications.

Meperidine (Demerol) used to be routinely prescribed in acute care settings. Most health care agencies now have policies in place restricting its use to less than 48 hours, or no more than 600 mg in 24 hours. Many agencies have discontinued its use altogether for older adults due to the resulting toxicities. Because of the accumulation of the toxic metabolite normeperidine, central nervous system toxicities may occur (Waitman & McCaffery, 2001). Repetitive doses of meperidine, particularly in older adults or in people with decreased renal clearance, may cause numbness, twitching, confusion, and seizures. It is never a good idea to give meperidine orally because of its poor bioavailability–75 mg intramuscularly equals 300 mg orally. *Meperidine use is considered to be outdated pain management.*

Agonists-Antagonists. The **agonist-antagonist drugs** are opioid (agonists) that antagonize the pure agonists (counteract opioid effects). These drugs include mixed agonists (pentazocine [Talwin], nalbuphine [Nubain], butorphanol [Stadol]), and partial agonists (buprenorphine [Buprenex]).

Because of their opioid antagonist properties, administering them after a client has been receiving opioids may cause withdrawal symptoms. If agonist-antagonist anal-

CONCEPT MAP Chronic Cancer Pain

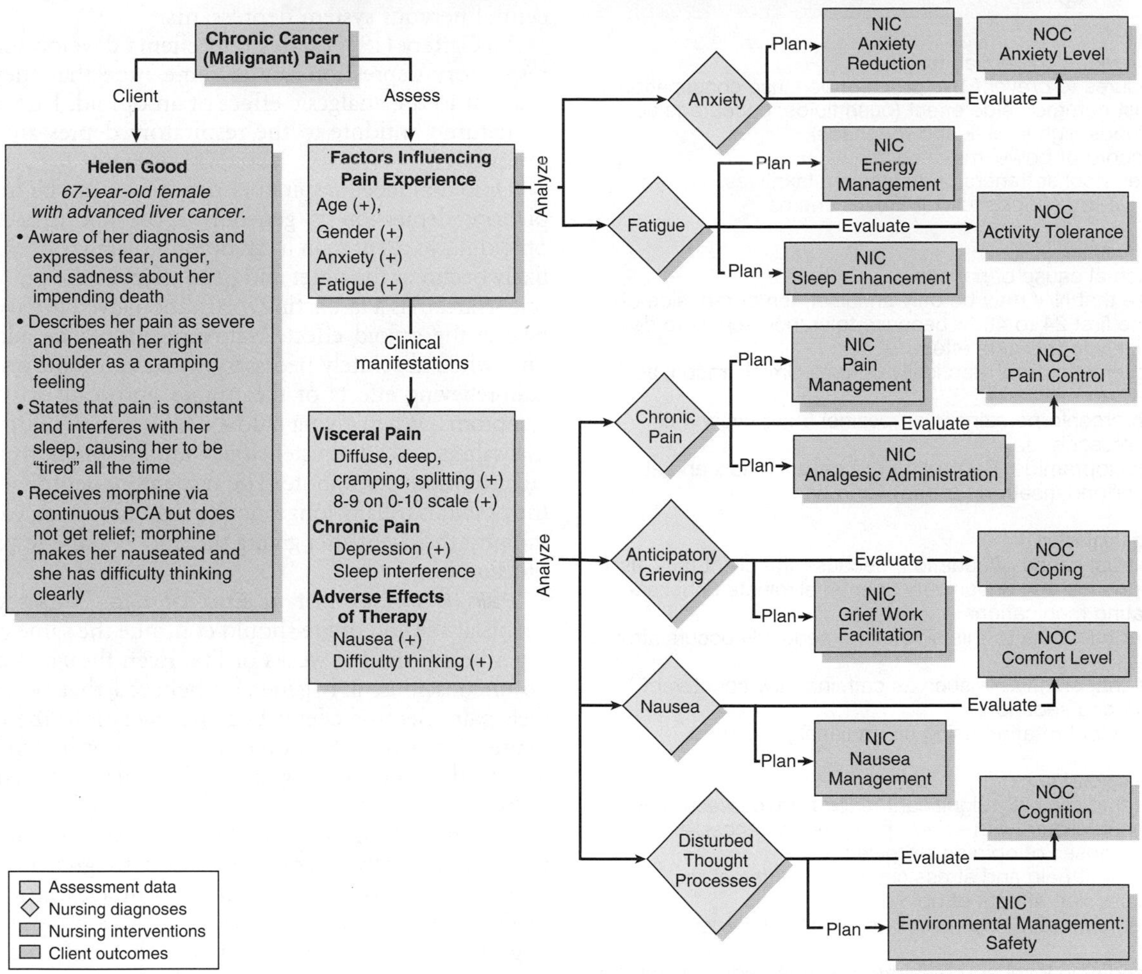

Concept Map by Elaine Bishop Kennedy, EdD, RN

gesics are given together with an opioid, eventually they antagonize opioid analgesia; hence the client has poor pain relief.

The major side effects produced by these drugs are drowsiness, occasional nausea, and psychotomimetic effect such as hallucinations and euphoria. The agonist-antagonist drugs have little place in the management of pain, especially chronic pain. These drugs offer no advantage over morphine-like agonists (American Pain Society, 2003).

Side Effects of Opioids. The most important type of opioid receptor is the mu receptor. **Mu opioids** cause side effects that include constipation, nausea and vomiting, urinary retention, pruritus (itching), sedation, and respiratory depression. These side effects are often mistakenly viewed as allergies, but it is rare to be allergic to morphine-type medications. The side effects (other than constipation) are time limited and easily managed (Table 7-8).

NAUSEA AND VOMITING. Nausea and vomiting often are mistaken for allergic reactions, and clients may be denied opioids. The side effect of nausea or vomiting in clients taking opioids varies from client to client and with opioid to opioid. If a client is nauseated after receiving an opioid, the cause and appropriate treatment must be determined.

Nausea and vomiting may occur initially as a side effect in clients taking opioids for pain relief. Treating the nausea and vomiting with an appropriate antiemetic usually helps. In addition, if client needs to continue the opioid therapy longer than 1 week, the problem usually resolves on its own.

CONSTIPATION. Although constipation may seem like a minor side effect, it is not to the client, especially the older adult. Often the discomfort of constipation is more distressing to the client than the pain itself.

Opioids inhibit peristalsis in the gastrointestinal tract. Clients who take regular doses of opioids almost always become constipated. Also, many clients in pain lack proper exercise and have an inadequate diet, both making the problem of constipation worse.

Whenever a client is started on regular doses of opioids, it is essential that the preventive approach be used. Implement interventions to prevent the problem of constipation (see Table 7-8.)

SEDATION. Because opioids have a depressant effect on the central nervous system, some drowsiness can be anticipated. However, sedation is not always caused by opioids. If the client is still in pain, other causes of sedation should be ruled out before decreasing the opioid dosage or changing medications. For example, other medications, such as hypnotics or tranquilizers (diazepam [Valium], alprazolam [Xanax}, or promethazine [Phenergan], could be causing the

TABLE 7-8 Nursing Interventions to Prevent Side Effects of Opioids

Constipation
- Assess previous bowel habits.
- Use measures to *prevent* this problem because constipation is the most common side effect (push fluids, encourage activity, give foods high in bulk and roughage).
- Keep a record of bowel movements.
- Administer stool softeners and stimulant laxatives.
- If ineffective, try suppository or Fleet's enema.

Nausea and Vomiting (N/V)
- Assess actual cause of nausea.
- Recognize that N/V may be only an initial, temporary side effect for the first 24 to 48 hr because tolerance seems to develop quickly to this side effect.
- Try an antiemetic prophylactically before administration, as prescribed.
- Treat with prochlorperazine (Compazine) 5 mg every 4 hr orally, as prescribed.
- Give metoclopramide (Reglan) 10 mg before meals and at bedtime, or ondansetron (Zofran) 4 mg IV.

Sedation and Confusion
- Assess actual cause of sedation, because the client may also be on hypnotics and antianxiety agents; eliminate unnecessary sedating medications.
- Recall that tolerance to this side effect generally occurs after 2 to 3 days.
- Be aware that stimulants such as caffeine may counteract opioid-induced sedation.
- Consider opioid rotation using an equianalgesic chart.

Respiratory Depression
- Be aware that clinically significant respiratory depression is rarely seen in clients with severe pain due to cancer, even when large doses of opioids are given.
- Recognize that pain and stress seem to counteract the respiratory depression effects of opioids.
- Recall that respiratory depression is usually preceded by sedation.
- Monitor sedation level and respiratory status frequently for the first 24 to 48 hr, especially in opioid-naive clients.
- If increased sedation occurs, decrease opioid dose and attempt to stimulate client.
- Be aware that respiratory rate alone is not indicative of respiratory status.
- If absolutely necessary in an unresponsive client, administer naloxone (Narcan) 0.4 mg diluted in 10 mL of normal saline; push 0.5 mL slowly for 2 min and observe the client.

sedation. Often the elimination of other central nervous system–depressant medications resolves the sedation problem.

Sedation occurs before opioid-induced respiratory depression, so nurse-monitored sedation levels are recommended by use of a sedation scale for opioid-naive clients or clients receiving opioids IV or epidurally. The key to assessing sedation is determining how easily the client is aroused. Assess each client's individual response to the first dose of an opioid. Be sure to assess the client's level of consciousness. Monitor respiratory rate and depth, especially while the client is sleeping.

RESPIRATORY DEPRESSION. A main reason for inadequate pain control is the exaggerated fear of respiratory depression. However, this problem rarely occurs, especially in clients taking opioids for chronic, long-term pain.

The pain, stress, and anxiety experienced by the client are potent respiratory *stimulants* that may override or negate the respiratory depression resulting from the drugs. The nurse also considers that the effect of all opioid analgesics may be greater in a client who is older, has reduced blood volume or renal disease, or has received anesthetic agents or other central nervous system depressants.

McCaffery (1979) states that clients develop tolerance to respiratory depression at the same time that they become tolerant to the analgesic effect of an opioid. Pain appears to be nature's antidote to the respiratory depressant effects of opioids.

Opioid-induced respiratory depression can be treated. Respiratory depression is generally more apt to occur in an opioid-naive client than in an opioid-tolerant one. It also most likely occurs at the onset and peak effect of the opioid. Naloxone (Narcan) is a fast-acting medication given intravenously to reverse the opioid effect. Naloxone should be administered only when absolutely necessary because it removes all of the pain-relieving effects of the opioid and leads to withdrawal symptoms. When giving naloxone, be sure to dilute with normal saline, and administer slowly until respirations increase to eight or more per minute. The respiratory depressant effect of the opioid is usually longer acting than naloxone. Continue to monitor the client after giving the drug because respiratory depression can recur.

Pain Management in End of Life. Nurses caring for clients at the end of life should continue the same opioid regimen before the last weeks of life. Even though a client may be unconscious, it is generally believed that he or she still feels pain. Because clients become tolerant to the respiratory depressant effects of an opioid, it does not hasten death unless the dose was not properly and gradually titrated. Chapter 9 discusses end-of-life issues in further detail.

Routes of Administration. Opioids can be administered in virtually every route used to give medications. Table 7-9 lists the routes with advantages and disadvantages. Effective management of pain requires the knowledge that the oral route is always the preferred route for most types of pain. The IV route is the most efficient route due to its rapid titration. The IM route is no longer acceptable as state-of-the-art pain management, due to its many disadvantages.

PRN Range Orders. Nurses have administered PRN range orders for opioid analgesia for many years. Although this approach is meant to manage the pain of individual clients based on accurate assessments, obvious safety issues are involved.

Patient-Controlled Analgesia. **Patient-controlled analgesia (PCA)** is a common way to combat the problem of inadequate analgesia in the management of acute and chronic pain. This method allows the client to control the dosage of opioid analgesia received. This approach to pain control can improve pain relief and increase client satisfaction. It can also decrease the amount of opioid consumption per day when compared with nurse-administered intermittent dosing methods.

Clients who have ready access to an analgesic are more likely to medicate themselves before the pain becomes severe, and thus they may require a reduced amount. Having such control over drug administration also reduces anxiety, which helps relieve pain.

PCA is achieved through the use of a PCA infusion pump (Figure 7-4). Both stationary pole pumps (for hospital use) and ambulatory pumps (for nursing home or home use) are available. The infusion pump delivers the desired amount of

TABLE 7-9 Routes of Administration

Oral

Advantages

- Preferred route of analgesia
- Allows greater mobility and convenience
- Drug levels peak in 1 to 2 hours
- Greater client satisfaction
- If client is NPO or has a nasogastric or gastrostomy tube, medications can still be given orally
- Cost efficient
- Relatively steady blood levels produced

Disadvantages

- Slow onset
- Long-acting opioids cannot be crushed, broken, or chewed
- Some clients are unable to swallow or are NPO
- Requires functional GI system

Rectal

Advantages

- Good for clients who are NPO, nauseated, or at home
- Easy for clients to self-administer, especially older adults
- Duration of action 4 to 6 hr
- Any opioid can be compounded by a pharmacist for rectal route
- Clinical practice suggests oral and rectal doses of analgesics fairly equal

Disadvantages

- May be more expensive than oral route and difficult to obtain
- Contraindicated in thrombocytopenic clients

Intramuscular

Advantages

- Should be used for acute short-term pain

Disadvantages

- Rapid peak effect but short duration of action and rapid fall-off
- Problems with absorption lead to inconsistent blood levels
- Painful administration
- Not recommended for chronic long-term pain, especially cancer pain
- Client is dependent on others to administer injection
- Not recommended for use with emaciated clients or clients with decreased muscle mass
- Long-term use can cause fibrosis and sterile abscesses

Transdermal

Advantages

- Available as fentanyl (Duragesic)
- Doses of 25, 50, 75, and 100 mcg/hr patches applied every 72 hr
- Noninvasive, easy to use, well accepted by clients

Disadvantages

- Due to gradual increases in plasma concentration, may need to supplement with short-acting analgesics for first 12 to 24 hr after initial application
- Costly
- Difficult to adjust dose
- Febrile clients absorb medication quickly
- Concerns over disposal

OTFC (Oral Transmucosal Fentanyl Citrate)

Advantages

- Good bioavailability, rapid peak effect
- FDA-approved for breakthrough cancer pain
- May be useful off-label for procedural pain

Disadvantages

- Sweetened matrix contains 2 g sugar
- Short-acting, short half-life
- Must be swabbed inside mouth for at least 10 minutes to dissolve completely

Topical

Advantages

- Easy to use
- Little systemic absorption
- Lidoderm patch, EMLA topical cream, capsaicin cream are examples

Disadvantages

- May cause skin reactions
- Capsaicin causes burning initially

Sublingual

Advantages

- Most opioids can be absorbed SL
- Good for clients with no IV access and/or impaired swallowing

Disadvantages

- May not be absorbed or may cause mucosal irritation

Intranasal

Advantages

- Butorphanol (Stadol NS) opioid agonist-antagonist
- Sumatriptan for migraines
- Convenient delivery form
- Good for outpatient use

Disadvantages

- Butorphanol is not to be given to client on pure opioid; can precipitate a withdrawal

Subcutaneous

Advantages

- Available as bolus, continuous infusion, or continuous infusion with PCA
- Avoids need for intravenous access and cheaper than IV
- Readily managed at home
- Recommended for cancer clients who cannot take anything by mouth and in whom IV access is not desirable
- Avoids repetitive injections and is less painful
- Continuous infusion
- Avoids peaks and valleys in bloodstream; maintains steady blood level
- Provides prolonged parenteral administration of opioid
- No delay in drug administration

Disadvantages

- Subcutaneous boluses have slower onset and a lower peak effect than IV boluses
- Requires use of ambulatory infusion pump, which is not always client acceptable

Intravenous

- Available as bolus, continuous infusion, or continuous infusion with PCA IV bolus

Advantages

- Good for acute pain or procedures
- Immediate pain relief
- Provides fastest onset but shortest duration
- Peak in 5 to 15 minutes
- Eliminates anxiety and prevents pain
- Recommended when unable to achieve pain control through oral or rectal routes with high dosages of opioid or unable to use oral/rectal route
- Continuous IV administration provides steady blood level

Disadvantages

- Not recommended for constant pain due to peaks and valleys in bloodstream
- Requires use of infusion pump with an alarm

Continued

TABLE 7-9 Routes of Administration—*cont'd*

Patient-Controlled Analgesia (PCA)	Spinal (Epidural and Intrathecal) Administration
Advantages ▪ Allows client to receive a predetermined intravenous bolus of an opioid by hitting a syringe pump mechanism ▪ Gives client sense of control, less anxiety ▪ Provides quick and consistent pain relief ▪ Maintains a constant level of pain relief ▪ Eliminates the need for repeated injections ▪ Saves time ▪ Especially recommended for acute pain such as postoperative pain	***Advantages*** ▪ Opioid (usually morphine or fentanyl) administered through catheter into epidural or intrathecal space ▪ Preservative-free morphine or fentanyl used ▪ Useful for postoperative pain (abdominal, thoracic, orthopedic) or chronic pain ▪ May be intermittent bolus or by continuous infusion pump
Disadvantages ▪ Requires use of a pump ▪ Requires reinforced client teaching for maximum effectiveness ▪ Requires two nurses to program to prevent errors (in hospitals) ▪ Requires designated person to hit button if client cannot	***Disadvantages*** ▪ Careful client selection is necessary because procedure is expensive and may be risky ▪ Side effects include nausea, vomiting, pruritus, sedation, urinary retention, and respiratory depression ▪ Possible complication of hematoma and infection and/or meningitis

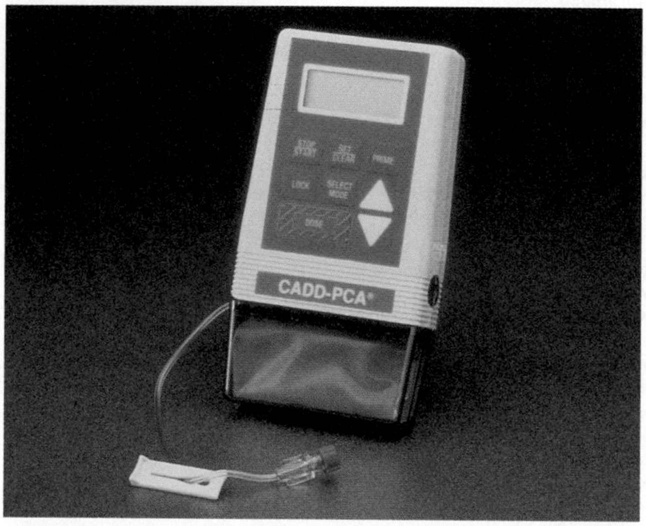

Figure 7-4 ■ An ambulatory patient-controlled analgesia infusion pump. (CADD-PCA is a registered trademark of Pharmacia Deltec, St. Paul, MN.)

medication through a conventional IV route for pain. Morphine is the most commonly used drug for PCA. Meperidine (Demerol) is reserved as a last resort for short-term (usually less than 48 hours) or no more than 600 mg in 24 hours. Its toxic metabolite, normeperidine, may accumulate in the blood and is can induce confusion and seizures. Older adults are particularly at risk. Hydromorphone (Dilaudid) and fentanyl are also used for PCA. Standing or preprinted orders from the health care provider are commonly used for PCA administration.

Drug security to avoid overdosing is achieved through a locked syringe pump system or locked drug reservoir system. The device is programmed to deliver a certain amount of drug (**demand dose**) within a specific interval known as a **lockout interval**. The health care provider specifies the amount of the demand dose. Morphine doses typically range from 1 to 2 mg, hydromorphone from 0.15 to 0.4 mg, and fentanyl from 12.5 to 25 mcg. Doses vary according to the client's degree of pain. The lockout interval is usually 5 to 15 minutes.

To prevent medication errors, it is recommended that two nurses program the dosing parameters into the PCA delivery device. When the client presses the button or pendant (on ambulatory pumps), the appropriate bolus or demand dose is delivered. No drug is administered if the client attempts to access the drug before the designated time interval between doses has elapsed. With this technique, there is little chance that clients will overmedicate themselves.

The PCA regimen may consist of a demand-dosing-only schedule or a continuous infusion or **basal rate** and demand dosing. With demand or self-administered dosing only, the client relies solely on a push of the pendant or bolus feature to seek pain relief. Continuous or basal infusion of the opioid in addition to demand dosing provides more consistent analgesia and allows the client to sleep without fear of missing any pain medication. However, when a continuous infusion is added to the regimen, clients may be at greater risk for opioid-induced side effects (e.g., nausea and vomiting, sedation, respiratory depression), especially if the hourly dose is too much for the client.

Your primary role in caring for clients using PCA is to teach them how to use the device and to report side effects, such as dizziness, nausea and vomiting, and inability to void. As with all opioids, monitor the client's vital signs, particularly respirations, and check sedation level every 2 hours initially.

When a client is cognitively impaired or unable to push the PCA button, another method of administration should be considered. PCA means **patient-controlled**, so having someone else push the button defeats the purpose. More importantly, this practice can cause oversedation and possible serious safety issues. Although controversial, some health care agencies do allow one designee to push the PCA for a client who cannot. If the designee is the nurse, inform the family, visitors, or any health care provider not to push the button. Familiarize yourself with the agency's pain management protocols related to PCA use.

Epidural Analgesia. **Epidural analgesia** (also known as peridural or extradural analgesia) refers to the instillation of a pain-blocking agent, usually an opioid analgesic alone or in combination with a local anesthetic, into the epidural space (the space between the dura mater and the vertebral column). Epidural analgesia is more commonly used for the management acute pain, such as postoperative pain. It has been used since the 1950s but has become more popular as newer and more innovative approaches to acute pain control are explored. Epidural analgesia is used primarily in clients who are predisposed to respiratory complications (including those undergoing thoracic surgery), those with preexisting respiratory disease, and those who are obese.

Intrathecal (subarachnoid) analgesia, in which a pain-blocking agent is introduced into the space between the arachnoid mater and pia mater of the spinal cord (where cerebrospinal fluid is located), may be considered for long-term management of **intractable pain** (chronic pain that cannot be managed using standard therapies). However, it is not used as commonly as epidural analgesia due to increased central nervous system risks.

DESCRIPTION. Morphine (preservative free), hydromorphone (Dilaudid), and fentanyl (Sublimaze) are the most commonly used opioids for epidural administration. Sufentanil (Sufenta), an analogue of fentanyl but more potent, may also be used. A local anesthetic such as bupivacaine (Marcaine), which affects both sensory and motor nerves, may be given alone or in combination with an opioid. *Low* concentrations of local anesthetics are used to prevent significant sensory and motor deficits. The incidence of lower motor weakness is far less common with ropivacaine (Naropin) when compared to bupivacaine because it is more selective for sensory nerves.

Using a combination of opioids, non-opioids, and local anesthetics for postoperative pain (as described above) is sometimes referred to as **multimodal analgesia** or **balanced analgesia**. The advantage of these drug combinations is to provide better pain control at lower doses than any single drug does. Another advantage is that these drugs *decrease* the surgical stress response, which is typically mediated by multiple endocrine and metabolic changes. These changes contribute to increased pain, GI distress, confusion (especially in older adults), and cardiopulmonary complications (Pasero, 2003). Balanced analgesia, then, not only decreases pain, but also helps to decrease other problems that result from the stress of surgery. Balanced analgesia is especially appropriate for clients having complex surgeries, such as those undergoing abdominal or thoracic procedures.

A temporary, externalized epidural catheter is used for acute pain control. This device is not sutured to the skin and is easily dislodged. Be sure to tape the catheter in two places to anchor it properly. Some clinicians do not recommend transparent dressings because the catheter may be dislodged when the dressing is removed. The catheter is generally placed in either the lumbar or the thoracic region. Rarely is the catheter placed above the level of sixth thoracic vertebra, because the diaphragmatic muscle may be affected by the analgesic.

COMPLICATIONS. Complications that occur with epidural analgesia are directly related to catheter placement, catheter maintenance, and the type of analgesic. Infection results from a failure to maintain aseptic technique during catheter placement, direct drug instillation, and infusion solution and tubing changes. Infection also results from a failure to maintain aseptic conditions for indwelling catheters at the site of insertion or at the site of tube junctions. To prevent infections, the nurse ensures that all catheter line connections are secure and that an occlusive sterile dressing is maintained over the catheter site.

Pruritus (itching) and nausea and vomiting are common side effects of epidural opioids. Pruritus is first treated with a small amount of naloxone (Narcan). Because epidural-induced pruritus does not appear to be caused by histamine release, diphenhydramine (Benadryl, Allerdryl✱) may not be effective in relieving itching and may only work via its sedating effects. The health care provider usually prescribes an antiemetic as needed for nausea and vomiting.

Clients who receive epidural opioids are also at risk for respiratory depression resulting from high plasma or cerebrospinal fluid concentrations of the instilled drug. Clients receiving epidural therapy with only a local anesthetic are not at risk for respiratory depression. Because of its potential for greater spread up the spinal cord, morphine is more likely than fentanyl to cause respiratory depression. Morphine is preferred to fentanyl when a larger distribution of analgesia is required (e.g., pain relief from extensive abdominal wounds).

Monitor the client's respirations and sedation level at frequent intervals during and after the administration of epidural opioids and immediately report any concerns to the health care provider. Opioid-induced respiratory depression usually occurs within the first few hours of administering fentanyl, but may not be seen for 12 hours or more when morphine is given. This complication is managed by administering low doses (0.2 mg) of naloxone (Narcan) intravenously.

Urinary retention is another common problem associated with epidural analgesia, but it occurs no more frequently than postoperative urinary retention in clients not receiving epidural analgesia. Although the cause is not clear, this problem usually occurs during the first or second day of analgesia administration and may be treated with bethanechol chloride (Urecholine) or intermittent urinary catheterization. The incidence of this complication is less than 25% and is more likely to occur in men than in woman.

Lower motor weakness is more common when an epidural local anesthetic is used in combination with the opioid. Assist clients who get out of bed for the first time to determine the degree of leg weakness. Do not delegate this activity and assessment to unlicensed assistive personnel.

LONG-TERM USE. Epidural analgesia may also be used for long-term chronic pain relief. Such pain is usually the result of cancer or central sensitization. A permanent epidural catheter may be inserted, and several catheter devices are available for this purpose. The DuPen silastic catheter (Davol) is a commonly used **external catheter**. A portion of the catheter exits the skin. Drugs can be intermittently injected into this portion, or the catheter can be attached to an infusion device for continuous drug administration.

Implantable devices are also used to treat chronic pain. The epidural Port-A-Cath (SIMS Deltec, Inc.) is implanted under the skin, and the catheter portion is inserted into the epidural space. As with the DuPen catheter, this device can be injected with drugs intermittently or can be connected to an infusion device for continuous opioid delivery. Injectable ports have been shown to reduce the incidence of catheter dislodgement and early infection. Systems consisting of either an externalized catheter or a drug delivery device are rarely used for intrathecal drug administration. The SynchroMed pump (Medtronic, Inc.) is a totally implantable system that contains a drug reservoir. The drug reservoir is

A

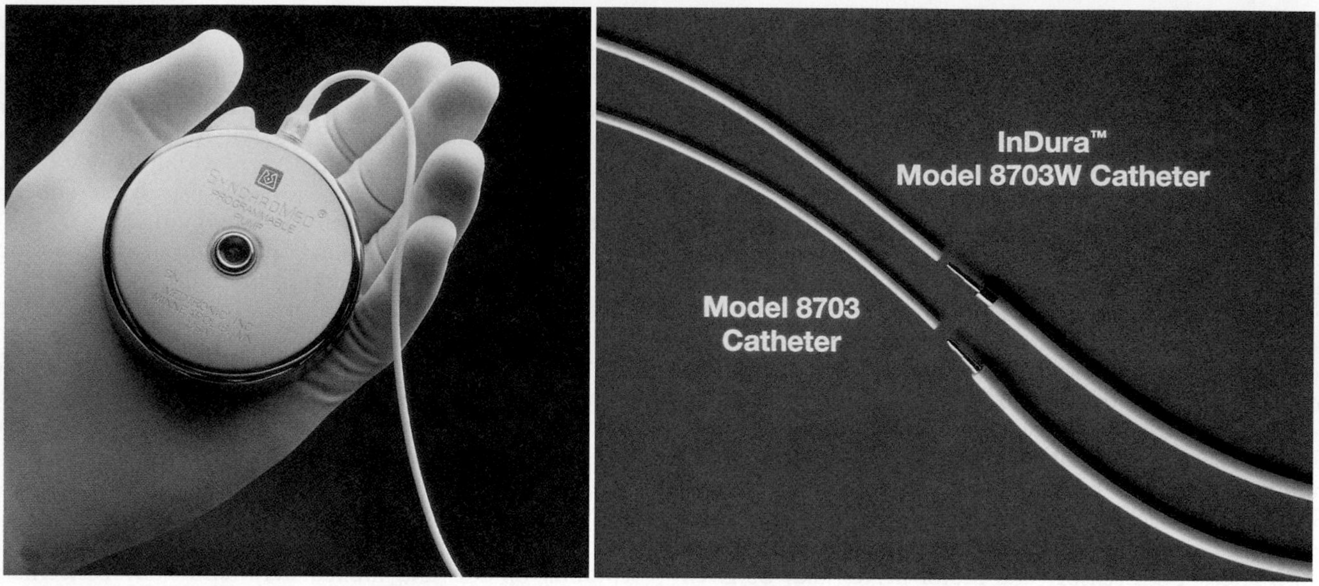

B

Figure 7-5 ■ A SynchroMed implantable pump **(A)** and spinal catheters **(B)** for delivery of a precise volume of long-term intraspinal analgesia each day. (Courtesy of Medtronic, Inc., Columbia Heights, MN.)

filled on a routine basis and is capable of continuously administering a certain volume of drug each day (Figure 7-5).

The side effects of long-term epidural opioids are common in clients who have had little exposure to opioids. Clients who receive this therapy are usually more tolerant of the effects of opioids and may not require the rigorous monitoring needed for postoperative analgesia. Male clients receiving long-term epidural opioids may complain of sexual dysfunction, decreased libido, and difficulty maintaining an erection; female clients may experience amenorrhea. Testosterone injections seem to help improve sexual function in male clients.

Adjuvant Analgesics. Always consider the use of adjuvant analgesics, especially for clients with chronic pain or complex pain syndromes. Adjuvant analgesics can be helpful for many clients in pain. Although not true analgesics, the **adjuvant medications** relieve pain either alone or in combination with analgesics. These drugs can potentiate or enhance the effectiveness of the analgesic.

Some nurses and other health professionals confuse potentiators with additives. **Additives** are drugs that add an effect, either harmful or beneficial. A common example of this is the drug promethazine (Phenergan). Phenergan is a phenothiazine that has been given for years with opioids such as meperidine (Demerol) to enhance the opioid effects. However, it does just the opposite. Phenergan does not have any analgesic or analgesia-potentiating properties. In fact, it is thought to actually have antianalgesic properties.

The use of adjuvant analgesics not only can provide additional pain relief in some cases but also can help control other discomforts associated with pain (anxiety, depression, nausea, insomnia). Table 7-10 gives examples of adjuvant medications.

Some **antiepileptic drugs** (AEDs or anticonvulsants), such as gabapentin (Neurontin), are effective in treating postherpetic neuralgia and the painful neuropathy associated with diabetes mellitus (Rowbotham et al., 1998; Backonja et al., 1998). They have also been useful in many clients with neuropathic pain from back injuries as well. Doses of gabapentin can be escalated up to 3600 mg daily with few side effects compared to other anticonvulsants. Topiramate (Topamax) is a newer AED with promise for neuropathic pain (Jenson et al., 2002). Because most AEDs can cause hyponatremia, monitor electrolyte values carefully, especially in older adults.

The older **tricyclic antidepressants**, such as amitriptyline (Elavil), nortriptyline (Pamelor), and imipramine (Tofranil), may be beneficial in treating chronic neuropathic pain. Both tricyclic antidepressants and other antidepressants such as trazodone (Desyrel), paroxetine (Paxil), and sertraline (Zoloft) help treat the depression that can accompany chronic pain. They also stimulate the activity of endogenous opiates (endorphins and enkephalins) by increasing levels of the neurotransmitter serotonin. Perhaps the greatest advantage of this group of drugs, particularly the tricyclic antidepressants, is the sedative effect. This effect can be helpful in promoting sleep when administered at bedtime. The tricyclics are contraindicated in clients with a history of seizures or cardiac disease. They should also be used with caution in older adults because they have long-half lives and can cause toxicities.

In some cases, antianxiety agents help relax the client and thus help relieve pain. However, many of these drugs cause confusion, drowsiness, and hypotension; the health care provider selects the drugs with the fewest side effects. Examples of antianxiety agents include alprazolam (Xanax), clorazepate (Tranxene, Novo-Clopate✱), Lorazepam (Ativan), and oxazepam (Serax, Zapex✱). Clonazepam (Klonopin), also used for anxiety, has been shown to be particularly helpful for certain types of nerve injury pain.

Oral local anesthetics, such as mexiletine (Mexitil), act by suppressing the electrical activity of both peripheral nerves and neurons in the central nervous system. They are useful for electric shock–like pain and continuous pain. Mexiletine is contraindicated for clients who have cardiac conduction

TABLE 7-10 Examples of Adjuvant Analgesics

Drug Class	Example	Indications
Tricyclic antidepressants	Amitriptyline (Elavil) Nortriptyline (Pamelor) Desipramine (Norpramin)	Multipurpose; any chronic pain; pain associated with depression
Anticonvulsants	Gabapentin (Neurontin) Carbamazepine (Tegretol) Valproic acid (Depakene) Clonazepam (Klonopin)	First-line recommendation for neuropathic pain Any lancinating, burning, neuropathic pain
Stimulants	Methylphenidate (Ritalin) Dextroamphetamine (Dexedrine) Dronabinol (Marinol)	Lethargy: counteract opioid-induced sedation; used for anorexia with associated weight loss in HIV and cancer clients
Steroids	Dexamethasone (Decadron) Prednisone	Severe bone pain; nerve compression; increased intracranial pressure; soft tissue infiltration
Systemic local anesthetics	Lidocaine (Xylocaine) Mexiletine (Mexitil)	Any lancinating, burning pain
Topical anesthetics	EMLA, Numby Capsaicin Lidoderm patch	Procedural, invasive pain Postherpetic neuralgia; diabetic neuropathy; postmastectomy pain
Miscellaneous	Clonidine Baclofen Calcitonin Tizanidine (Zanaflex)	Nonspecific analgesic; may be helpful for select group of chronic pain clients Trigeminal neuralgia; other neuropathic pains Sympathetically maintained pain; phantom limb pain Alpha$_2$-adrenergics useful for spasticity pain

defects or dysrhythmias or are currently taking cardiac antidisrhythmic medications.

Other agents known to have some effect in relieving mild to moderate chronic pain include dextromethorphan (the active ingredient in many cough syrups) and ketamine. Both of these agents are N-methyl-D-aspartate (NMDA) antagonists. NMDA receptors are involved in the development of tolerance to opioids. The administration of NMDA antagonists is thought to potentiate the action of opioids and prevent the development of opioid tolerance.

Topical Medications. Other topical medications can be useful, particularly for localized neuropathic pain. For example, the Lidoderm patch is approved for postherpetic neuralgia. Up to three patches can be applied at once, or they can be cut to the area of pain. The patch should be put on for 12 hours and removed for 12 hours. There is virtually no systemic absorption of lidocaine.

EMLA and ELA-Max creams are combinations of topical lidocaine and prilocaine. These must be applied to intact skin at least 45 minutes before needle sticks. The topical medications for pain relief have rare side effects of local skin reactions.

Local, short-acting gels and creams may provide **cryotherapy** to decrease pain, especially for muscle aches and pains. Bio-Freeze is an example of a commonly used gel that is often used by physical therapists to "cool down" an area after it has been manipulated. Other products can be bought over-the-counter (OTC) (e.g., Ben Gay). The effects of this type of application last about 1 to 2 hours, depending upon the client.

Other Interventions. There are a number of effective interventions for pain that are nonpharmacologic. These modalities may be used alone, for mild to moderate pain, or in combination with drug therapy for more severe pain. These therapies are classified as either physical measures or cognitive-behavioral measures. Some of these measures may be referred to as part of complementary and alternative medicine (CAM), such as imagery, therapeutic touch, and hypnosis. Chapter 4 discusses CAM in more detail.

Physical Measures. Physical measures may be used instead of or in addition to drug therapy to relieve pain. **Cutaneous (skin) stimulation** strategies to relieve pain have been in use for many years. Various types of stimulation to the skin and subcutaneous tissue produce pain relief. Nurses play an important role in educating clients about these techniques. Methods of cutaneous stimulation include techniques such as the following:

- Transcutaneous electrical nerve stimulation (TENS)
- Application of heat, cold, and pressure
- Therapeutic touch
- Massage
- Vibration

Whichever method is used, several characteristics of cutaneous stimulation must be considered:

- The benefits of these techniques are highly unpredictable and may vary from application to application.
- Pain relief is generally sustained only as long as the stimulation continues.
- Multiple trials may be necessary to establish the desired effects.
- Stimulation itself may aggravate pre-existing pain or may produce new pain.

Despite the drawbacks to cutaneous stimulation, it is effective in the management of both acute pain and chronic pain. These techniques have both physiologic and psychological effects on the client. Cutaneous stimulation techniques also give clients an opportunity to participate actively in the management of their pain.

Physical Therapy. Physical therapy is used for clients experiencing pain to increase function, decrease pain, compensate for decreased function, and prevent further deterioration. Exercises and physical modalities such as heat, cold, massage, or TENS units may be used. Measures of client progress include an increase in the range of motion, strength, and function of the affected area as well as impact of pain on quality of life. Collaborate with the physical therapist to evaluate these treatments.

The physical or occupational therapist may also help to decrease pain by making one or more splints to rest severely inflamed joints. These devices are most commonly used short-term for clients with osteoarthritis or rheumatoid arthritis.

Transcutaneous Electrical Nerve Stimulation. **Transcutaneous electrical nerve stimulation (TENS)** (also referred to as **percutaneous electrical nerve stimulation [PENS]**) involves the use of a battery-operated device capable of delivering small electrical currents to the skin and underlying tissues. This technique is not as widely used as when it first was developed. However, for older adults, it may be safer and just as effective as medications (Resnick, 2003). Electrodes connected to a small box are placed over the painful sites. The voltage or current is regulated by adjusting a dial to the point at which the client perceives a prickly, "pins-and-needles" sensation. The current is adjusted on the basis of the client's degree of pain relief and level of comfort.

The health care provider, nurse, or physical therapist (depending on the health care setting) assists the client in applying the electrodes either on the painful area or above or below it (Figure 7-6). A conducting substance (usually a gel) is placed between the electrode and the client's skin.

The advantages of TENS units are that the client can wear the unit and achieve a level of pain relief while participating in activities of daily living. The unit is easy to use and can be worn for several hours. However, the skin may become irritated at the site of the electrode placement. To prevent this, the nurse teaches the client to rotate electrode sites.

In general, clients can use TENS units for the management of both acute pain and chronic pain. This type of therapy is indicated for localized pain, such as postoperative pain or local chronic pain, particularly low back pain.

Other Cutaneous Techniques. Additional cutaneous stimulation techniques, such as touch, pressure, massage, vibration, and heat and cold application, stimulate the skin and somehow interrupt the pain pathway. These interventions are relatively easy for the client to learn and are fairly economical. Cold applications are especially helpful for inflamed areas. Heat is appropriate when an increased blood flow is desired, such as for clients with arthritis. Paraffin dips for the hands are particularly helpful to those clients to increase movement. Warm showers and compresses that can be done at home are also useful in reducing stiffness and promoting movement in clients with arthritis, especially after awakening.

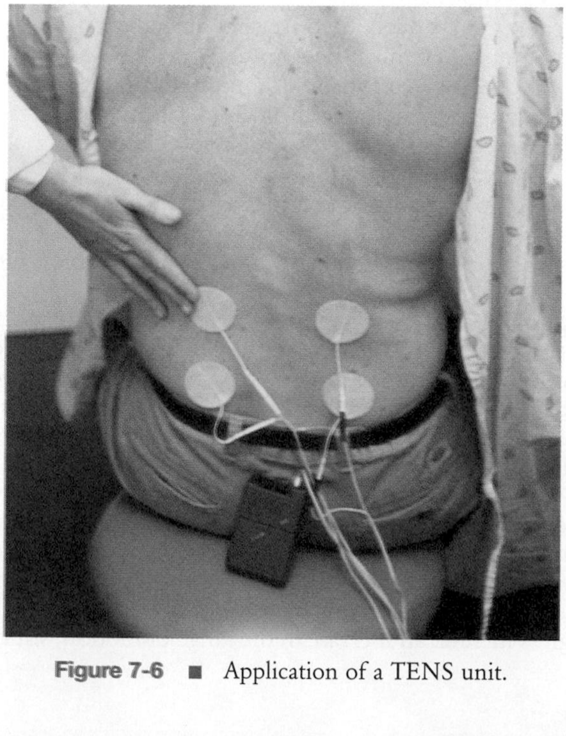

Figure 7-6 ■ Application of a TENS unit.

Cognitive-Behavioral Measures. Cognitive-behavioral strategies to relieve pain (e.g., distraction) have been popular for years, mainly as adjuncts to drug therapy. Theoretic explanations for the effectiveness of these measures reflect the premises of the gate control theory. Examples of cognitive-behavioral measures include distraction, imagery, relaxation, hypnosis, music therapy, aromatherapy, prayer and meditation, and other coping skills (also see Chapter 4).

Distraction. **Distraction** can be an effective method of acute pain relief. Simple measures such as holding a client's hand, taking him or her for a walk, or encouraging deep breathing exercises can divert attention from the pain. Nurses often observe that clients request less pain medication when family members are present and when talking on the phone. After visiting hours are over, many clients request something for pain, because they are no longer distracted.

Instead of viewing distraction as a therapeutic pain relief measure, as they should, some nurses may question the presence or severity of the pain if a client is easily distracted from it. Distraction alters the perception of pain but does not influence the cause or peripheral mechanism of pain. It is a transient method of pain relief and is probably best used with other pain control measures.

You can provide several methods of distraction. For example, visual distractors (e.g., pictures or television) can divert the client's attention to something pleasant or interesting. Auditory distractors, including music or relaxation tapes, can have a calming effect. Changing the environment can remove unpleasant stressors or reminders that may enhance pain. Physical distractions (e.g., deep breathing exercises) help the client concentrate on other physiologic sensations.

Distraction can be particularly useful in the following situations:

- Exacerbations of pain
- Painful procedures (e.g., dressing changes or invasive procedures)
- Interrupting the client's constant perception of pain

Imagery. **Imagery** is a form of distraction in which the client is encouraged to visualize or think about some pleasant or desirable feeling, sensation, or event. Guided imagery occurs when a person, often a nurse, assists the client in sustaining a sequence of thoughts aimed at diverting attention away from the pain. Intense concentration is required to visualize images. Clients who are extremely anxious, agitated, or unable to concentrate may first benefit from mild distraction.

Imagery is particularly useful for chronic pain. Clients who practice this technique can mentally and vividly experience sights, sounds, smells, events, or other sensations. The nurse first assesses the client's level of concentration to determine whether he or she can sustain a particular thought or thoughts for a desired time. The time interval for mental imagery can vary from 5 to 60 minutes. Behaviors that are helpful in assessing a client's capacity for imagery include the following:

- Reading and comprehending the newspaper
- Listening to music or other auditory stimuli
- Having the ability to follow and participate in sustained conversation
- Having an interest in environmental surroundings

When the client has demonstrated some ability to concentrate, assist the client in identifying a pleasant or favorable thought. The client is encouraged to focus on this thought to divert attention away from painful stimuli. Audiotapes may help in forming and maintaining images. The nurse, client, or family may wish to create audiotapes, or commercially available audiotapes may be used. The following is an example of guided imagery instructions: "Imagine yourself on the beach on some deserted island. You can hear the sound of waves rushing onto the shore, the cry of seagulls flying high above, and the rustling of trees as they are brushed gently by the wind. You can feel the warmth of the sun over your body and the cooling breeze."

Imagery works for some clients but not for others. The capacity to become engaged in the reality of the image may be important for the successful use of this therapy.

Relaxation Techniques. Clients may use **relaxation techniques** to reduce anxiety, tension, and emotional stress, all of which may exacerbate pain. Techniques to help clients relax can be both physical and psychological. Physical relaxation techniques include the following:

- Receiving a body massage, back rub, or warm or hot bath
- Modifying the environment to reduce distractions
- Moving into a comfortable position

Psychological relaxation techniques include the following:

- Pleasant conversation
- Music
- Relaxation tapes

Some relaxation tapes assist the client with progressive relaxation of the muscles. Relaxation exercises can be effectively coupled with guided imagery, distraction, and hypnosis.

Hypnosis. **Hypnosis** is defined as an altered state of consciousness in which a person enters a trance and loses an overall sense of reality. Although the person is in a trance, he or she has some sense of awareness and contact with reality and has an understanding of what is actually happening. Hypnosis can be used to treat a variety of pain syndromes, particularly chronic pain. It is used to help clients overcome the emotional consequences of pain and can promote a positive state of mind. Although nurses do not usually teach hypnosis, they are in a key position to help clarify misconceptions, instruct clients about relaxation and distraction, and encourage clients to practice self-hypnosis.

Other Complementary and Alternative Therapies. The data are scarce regarding the usefulness of other pain management techniques, such as magnet therapy, acupuncture, and herbal supplements. Although not supported by research, some clients believe that magnets applied to the skin or worn in shoes can reduce pain. This is a noninvasive therapy, and there is no harm to those who use this modality.

The practice of **acupuncture** originated in China. According to ancient beliefs, the body is divided into sections by lines, or meridians. Specific acupuncture points are located within these meridians. The acupuncturist inserts tiny needles into the skin and subcutaneous tissues at these points, and manual vibration or electrical stimulation is delivered. This technique is used to relieve pain and is thought to cure certain diseases. Several studies have shown that acupuncture can help reduce pain in clients with musculoskeletal problems (Lu, Lu, & Kleinman, 2001; Gilbertson, Wenner, & Russell, 2003).

Acupuncture is still widely acclaimed in China, but is less popular in the West because the physiologic basis for this technique is unclear. Many Western health care professionals are skeptical about its usefulness. Nonetheless, acupuncture is practiced for the treatment of pain and for anesthetic purposes during diagnostic procedures, labor and delivery, and surgery. It is also used to help clients change their behavior (e.g., smoking cessation). Certain parts of the United States (e.g., southwestern states) and other countries are expanding the use of this therapy for various purposes.

Glucosamine is a commonly used supplement for clients who have arthritis. It is believed to restore joint health and thus relieve pain and inflammation. Ask the client about the use of herbal supplements, because some can cause serious interactions with other pharmacologic agents.

Invasive Techniques for Chronic Pain. Invasive techniques are used to interrupt the pain pathways when pain is intractable (not able to be relieved) or severely debilitating. Depending on the technique, some degree of neurologic deficit and nerve destruction is expected. Various invasive techniques are used when chronic or persistent pain can no longer be adequately controlled with drugs or other pain-reducing methods.

Nerve Blocks. **Nerve blocks** can be used for both diagnostic and treatment purposes. These procedures are usually indicated for pain confined to a specific area or nerve distribution. This technique involves localizing a nerve root (or roots) and injecting it with either a local anesthetic for temporary relief or diagnostic evaluations or with a chemical agent (e.g., phenol or alcohol) to achieve permanent **neurolysis** or nerve destruction. Temporary blocks or permanent destruction (neuroablation) might be considered in areas such as the intercostal nerves, celiac plexus, superior hypogastric block, or craniofacial nerves.

The complications associated with nerve block vary. In general, injecting a local anesthetic or chemical agent into a peripheral nerve root leads to decreased sensation in the area; motor function is not affected. Injecting a local anesthetic into the lumbosacral area of the spinal cord area may cause transient motor and bowel and bladder dysfunction. Neurolysis of the lumbosacral nerves can damage motor nerve roots, resulting in lost or impaired bowel, bladder, or sexual function. This procedure is usually reserved for clients with intractable cancer-related pain.

Before permanent neurolysis is considered, a temporary nerve block may be given to determine the degree of relief obtained from disrupting the nerve impulses. Although the intent of neurolysis is to permanently destroy nerve transmission, clients may experience only short-term pain relief because of nerve cell regeneration or the development of alternative pathways capable of transmitting pain. Permanent ablation of nerve roots can be performed with thermal techniques such as **radiofrequency ablation** (uses heat) or **cryoanalgesia** (uses cold).

Because a nerve block is an invasive procedure performed by anesthesiologists, neurosurgeons, surgeons, and neurologists, the health care provider is responsible for informing the client about the procedure and its risks and alternative treatments. The nurse reinforces this information with the client and family.

Spinal Cord Stimulation. Spinal cord stimulator therapy offers a more invasive method of nerve stimulation. This technique involves the use of electrodes implanted under the skin and into the area of the nerve responsible for the pain. At first, a trial of spinal cord stimulation is attempted through the use of temporary externalized electrodes that are implanted and connected to a stimulator device. The amount of electrical current is adjusted to provide pain relief without additional discomfort. If this trial is successful, the client undergoes surgery for placement of a permanent implantable simulator.

Surgical Techniques. The surgical techniques aimed at surgically interrupting the transmission of pain include rhizotomy and cordotomy. These two procedures are not performed as commonly today because of the new, improved pain management measures available (Figure 7-7).

In **rhizotomy,** sensory nerve roots are destroyed where they enter the spinal cord. In a *closed* rhizotomy, a percutaneous catheter is inserted into the area, and the sensory nerve roots are destroyed by chemicals, coagulation, or cryodestruction (extreme cold). A laminectomy is necessary for an *open* rhizotomy. During this surgery, the health care provider isolates and destroys the nerve roots.

In a **cordotomy,** the surgeon cuts the pain pathways at the midline portion of the spinal cord before nerve impulses ascend to the spinothalamic tract. As with the other surgical procedures, clients may experience impaired bowel, bladder, or sexual function. Because of the complexity of the pain experience, the interruption of nerve conduction and pain pathways may not completely interrupt the client's sensation of pain.

After surgical intervention, assess the nature of the neurologic deficits, if any, and teach the client how to adapt to them. If the client has lost sensation in a body area, he or she will need to learn how to protect that area from harm. The nurse also assesses expectations in relation to the surgery and helps the client to express realistic expectations.

Community-Based Care

The pain experience extends beyond hospitalization. Many clients have chronic pain, but are not hospitalized. Others are in nursing homes or assisted-living facilities and have chronic pain, often not well managed. Effective analgesic regimens or pain-relieving strategies should be coordinated before discharge if clients are to leave the hospital still having pain. The nurse ensures that the client, especially one who is on opioids, has enough pain medication to last at least until the first follow-up visit.

HOME CARE MANAGEMENT

Preparation for home care is carried out with the client and family. Together with the client and family, the nurse, discharge planner, or occupational therapist determines whether modifications are necessary for maintaining a reasonably pain-free regimen after discharge. Fatigue heightens the awareness of pain. If physical modifications (e.g., installing a downstairs bathroom) are unrealistic (too expensive or unacceptable to the client or family), suggest schedule changes, role responsibilities, and daily routines to help avoid fatigue.

At home, clients may require a referral for physical therapy, especially to start or continue treatment with cutaneous stimulation, TENS, or heat or cold techniques. Clients may

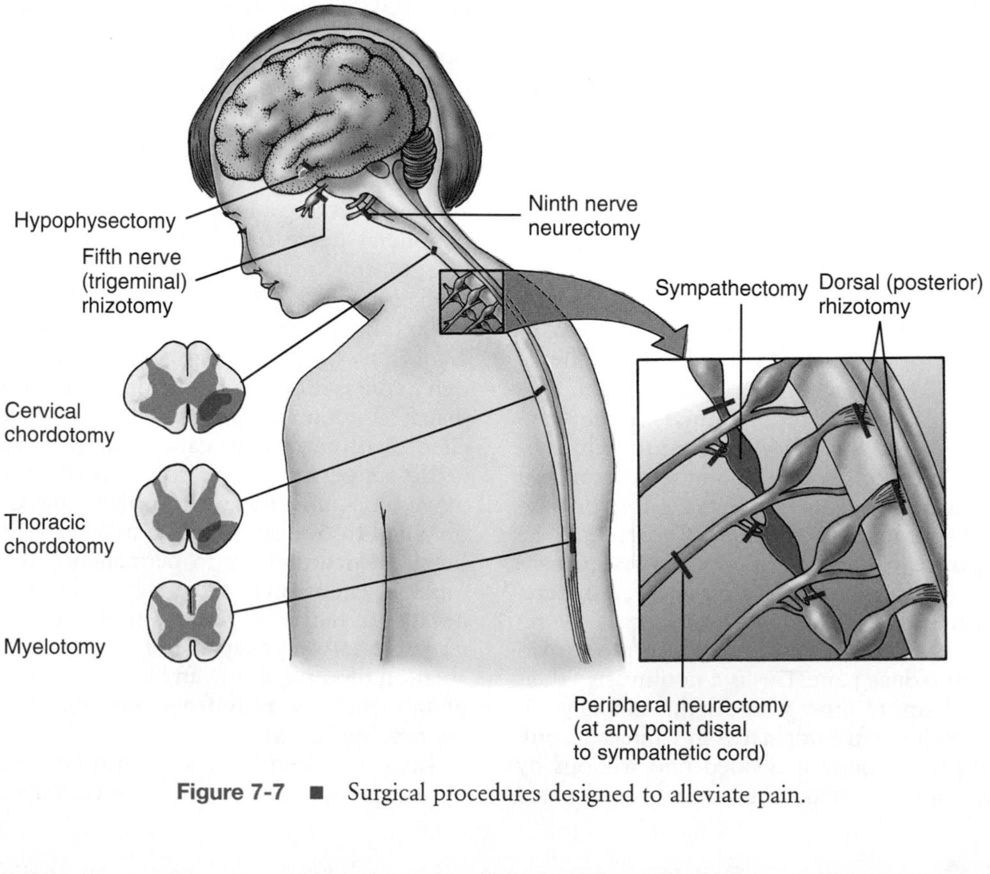

Figure 7-7 ■ Surgical procedures designed to alleviate pain.

need a psychiatric clinical nurse specialist or social worker to assist them in developing coping strategies or maintaining adequate family dynamics. A hospice referral (hospital- or community-based) can help maintain continuity of care in the management of terminally ill clients. Clients with cancer may be at risk for developing uncontrolled pain that results in hospitalization if it cannot be managed at home. It is important that nurses be knowledgeable about palliative care and end-of-life issues so they are better able to manage pain crises (see Chapter 9).

The growing number of home infusion therapy programs provides a wide variety of services to clients who require technology-supported pain care at home. Many of these services depend on approval by the insurance carrier, usually before analgesic options are considered and placement of technology is performed. Well-defined home agency practices and professional support at home are required if clients leave the hospital with infusion therapy for pain management.

HEALTH TEACHING

Direct educational efforts toward involving clients and their families in continuing health care behaviors that relieve pain and improve psychological well-being and overall functional status. Teach the client and family about analgesic regimens, including any technical skills needed to administer or deliver the analgesic, the purpose and action of medications, their side effects or adverse reactions, and the importance of dosage intervals. Also teach the client or family members how to prevent or treat the constipation commonly associated with taking opioid analgesics and other pain medications.

The nurse explains that, ideally, the analgesic regimen should not interfere with the client's sleep, rest, appetite, level of physical mobility, or driving ability. If such interference occurs, encourage the family or significant other to consult with the health care provider or home care nurse.

In clients with pain from advanced cancer, all efforts should be directed toward maximizing pain relief and symptom control at home to eliminate unnecessary readmissions. This may mean that the health care provider prescribes a flexible analgesic schedule that allows the client to adjust analgesics according to the amount of pain. Teach the client and family how to safely increase the medication within the prescribed dosing guidelines.

Evaluate family support systems to assist the client in adhering to and continuing the proposed medical and nursing plans. Family members are informed about and included in activities during and after hospitalization.

To achieve a reasonable level of expectation for the client, suggest ways to continue participation in household, social, sexual, and work-oriented activities after discharge. The nurse can help the client identify important activities and plan them around adequate rest schedules.

The client with chronic pain needs continued support to cope with the anxiety, fear, and powerlessness that often accompany this pain. Help the client and family or significant others to identify coping strategies that have worked in the past. Outside support systems are also identified, such as self-help organizations.

HEALTH CARE RESOURCES

A home care nurse referral is made when it is anticipated that clients will require assistance or supervision with their pain relief regimen at home. This referral should include specific information from the hospital-based staff nurse about the client's overall physical condition, general level of sedation, weakness or fatigue, possible constipation or nutritional problems, sleep patterns, and functional status.

In addition to explaining the client's physical status to the home care nurse, the staff nurse or case manager also describes the client's level of anxiety and general expectations about pain status after discharge. The client's close relationships and available support network are important factors in providing ongoing support for effective pain intervention strategies.

Referral to an advanced practice nurse pain specialist, social worker, or psychologist is an appropriate way to continue providing support to the client and family, reinforce instructions for cognitive-behavioral strategies to deal with pain, and evaluate overall physical and emotional adaptation after discharge. When severe chronic or intractable pain exists, health care professionals should direct the client and family to appropriate resources, such as pain centers or health care providers who specialize in pain management.

Clients with chronic pain often require treatment and support beyond that available in the traditional health care system. For this reason, pain clinics or programs have evolved over the past 25 years. The underlying premise of these resources is to foster independence and self-care behaviors while promoting pain control and maximizing quality of life. These programs use analgesics, adjuvant drug therapy, physical measures, cognitive-behavioral strategies, surgical interventions, and individual and group counseling for clients and family.

GET READY for the NCLEX Examination!

KEY POINTS

- Pain is what the client says it is; self-report is always the most reliable indication of pain.
- Three major types of pain have been identified—acute, chronic cancer, and chronic noncancer.
- Acute pain serves as a warning to the body, causing sympathetic responses, such as increased heart rate, increased blood pressure and pulse, dilated pupils, and sweating.
- Both types of chronic pain do not cause sympathetic reactions; therefore some clients do not appear to be in pain, even when they are (see Table 7-3).
- The gate control theory has helped to explain the mechanism of pain and its management.
- Three populations at risk for undertreatment of pain include older adults, minority clients, and drug addicts.
- Factors that affect pain and its management include age, gender, genetics, and culture.
- Tolerance implies that the client has adapted to a drug and over time its effects decline; physical dependence is manifested by a withdrawal reaction; addiction is a primary, chronic disease that occurs over a long period of time. Behaviors in addiction include craving, compulsive drug use, and continued use despite harm.
- Placebos should never be used on any client; their use in non–research based practice is unethical.
- Assess a client's pain for precipitating factors, aggravating factors, location, character and quality, and duration.

- Standardized pain intensity scales, such as number rating scales and descriptive word scales, are commonly used to quantify the severity of pain.
- Special considerations for older adults experiencing pain are summarized in Chart 7-1.
- Acute and chronic pain can cause anxiety, fear, or depression.
- Non-opioid drugs are the first-line therapy for mild to moderate pain; nonsteroidal anti-inflammatory drugs (NSAIDs) and acetaminophen (Tylenol) are commonly used drugs in this category.
- NSAIDs should be used with caution in older adults due to adverse effects, such as GI disturbances, bleeding, and sodium and water retention.
- Acetaminophen can cause hepatotoxicity with long-term use.
- The opioid full agonists are most effective for both acute and chronic pain management; they bind to mu receptors and block pain transmission.
- Equianalgesic charts are useful when changing from one opioid to another; morphine 10 mg is the standard dose against which other opioids are measured.
- Morphine is the gold standard drug for both acute and chronic pain, and is available in many forms, both short acting and long acting.
- Other commonly used full agonists include codeine, oxycodone, hydromorphone, and fentanyl.
- Meperidine is an outdated drug, but is still sometimes used for acute pain management; its toxic metabolite can cause seizures and confusion.
- Common side effects of opioids include nausea and vomiting, constipation, sedation, and respiratory depression.
- Table 7-9 summarizes the advantages and disadvantages of drug therapy by route of administration.
- Multimodal (balanced) analgesia for epidural pain management is a combination of opioids, non-opioids, and/or local anesthetics to relieve acute pain, usually postoperative pain.
- Sedation is the primary side effect that is assessed for clients receiving PCA or epidural medication.
- Common adjuvant analgesics, as an addition to other drug regimens, are listed in Table 7-10.
- Nonpharmacologic therapies for pain management may be used in place of or in combination with drug therapy; these therapies are classified as physical measures or cognitive-behavioral therapies.
- Examples of physical measures include transcutaneous nerve stimulation (TENS), heat, cold, and massage.
- Distraction, imagery, relaxation techniques, and hypnosis are examples of cognitive-behavioral therapies.
- Acupuncture, magnet therapy, and herbal supplements are examples of other complementary and alternative therapies used for chronic pain management.
- Nerve blocks and surgical techniques are invasive techniques performed by health care specialists to treat chronic pain; rhizotomy and cordotomy are examples of surgeries.
- Pain can be managed in any setting, including the home; some clients require parenteral pain medications at home; therefore health teaching for the client and family is needed.
- Clients whose pain is difficult to manage should be referred to pain specialists and/or pain centers.

ADDITIONAL STUDY RESOURCES

Go to your Student CD-ROM for Review Questions for the NCLEX Examination.

evolve Go to http://evolve.elsevier.com/Iggy/ for Integrated Management of Care Questions for the NCLEX Examination.

SELECTED BIBLIOGRAPHY

Asterisk indicates a classic or definitive work on this subject.

*Acute Pain Management Guideline Panel. (1992). *Acute pain management: Operative or medical procedures and trauma. Clinical Practice Guideline.* AHCPR Pub. No. 92-0032. Rockville, MD: Agency for Health Care Policy and Research, Public Health Service, U.S. Department of Health and Human Services.

AGS, American Geriatric Society. (2002). The management of persistent pain in older persons. *Journal of the American Geriatric Society, 50*(56) 205–224.

*American Pain Society. (1999). *Guideline for the management of pain in osteoarthritis, rheumatoid arthritis, and juvenile chronic arthritis.* Glenview, IL: American Pain Society.

*American Pain Society. (2003). *Principles of analgesic use in the treatment of acute pain and cancer pain* (5th ed.). Glenview, IL: American Pain Society.

American Society of Addiction Medicine. (2001). Definitions related to the use of opioids for the treatment of pain. Consensus document from the American Academy of Pain Medicine, the American Pain Society and the American Society of Addiction Medicine, February 2001. Accessed June 2001 from http://www.asam.org.

Anderson, C. (2000). What's new in pain management. *Home Healthcare Nurse, 18*(10), 649-659.

Ardery, G., et al. Lack of opioid administration in older hip fracture patients. *Geriatric Nursing, 24*(6), 353-359.

*Backonja, M., et al., for the Gabapentin Diabetic Neuropathy Study Group. (1998). Gabapentin for the symptomatic treatment of painful neuropathy in patients with diabetes mellitus. A randomized controlled trial. *Journal of the American Medical Association, 280*(21), 1831-1836.

Berry, P.H., & Dahl, J.L. (2000). The new JCAHO pain standards: Implications for pain management nurses. *Pain Management Nursing, 1*(1), 3-12.

Brookoff, D. (2000). Chronic pain: 1. A new disease. *Hospital Practice, 35,*(7), 306-309.

Burroughs, V.J., et al. (2002). *Cultural and genetic diversity in America: The need for individualized pharmaceutical treatment.* Washington, DC: National Pharmaceutical Council and National Medical Association.

Carter, G., & Galer, B. (2001). Advances in the management of neuropathic pain. *Physical Medicine and Rehabilitation Clinics, 12*(2), 447-459.

Ciccone, D., & Just, N. (2001). Pain expectancy and work disability in patients with acute and chronic pain: A test of the fear avoidance hypothesis. *The Journal of Pain, 2*(3), 181-194.

*Cleeland, C.S., et al. (1994). Pain and its treatment in outpatients with metastatic cancer. *The New England Journal of Medicine, 330*(9), 592-596.

Collins, S., et al. (2000). Antidepressants and anticonvulsants for diabetic neuropathy and postherpetic neuralgia: A quantitative systematic review. *Journal of Pain and Symptom Management, 20*(6), 449-458.

Compton, P., et al. (2000). Pain responses in methadone-maintained opioid abusers. *Journal of Pain and Symptom Management, 20*(4), 237-245.

Coyne, P., & Smith, T. (2002). Nebulized fentanyl citrate improves patients' perception of breathing, respiratory rate, and oxygen

saturation in dyspnea. *Journal of Pain and Symptom Management, 23*(2), 157-160.
Dahl, J., & Gordon, D. (2002). Joint commission pain standards: A progress report. *APS Bulletin, 12*(6), 1, 11-12.
Dallocchio, C., et al. (2000). Gabapentin vs. amitriptyline in painful diabetic neuropathy: An open-label pilot study. *Journal of Pain and Symptom Management, 20*(4), 280-285.
Durrance, S.A. (2003). Older adults and NSAIDs: Avoiding adverse reactions. *Geriatric Nursing, 24*(6), 349-352.
Eastman, P. (2003). Better pain control with pharmacogenetics? *Oncology Times, XXV*(1), 26, 27.
Eksterowica, N. (2003). Meperidine-using evidence-based rationale. *ASPMN Pathways, 12*(1), 4-5.
Ellison, N., McPherson, L., & McGuire, L. (2001). Pain report from the Dannemiller Memorial Educational Foundation. San Antonio: Dannemiller.
Fainsinger, R., Gara, C., & Perez, A. (2000). Amputation and prevention of phantom pain. *Journal of Pain and Symptom Management, 20*(4), 308-312.
Feldt, K.S. (2000). The checklist of nonverbal pain indicators (CNPI). *Pain Management Nursing, 1*(1), 13-21.
Ferrell, B., Stein, W., & Beck, J. (2000). The geriatric pain measure: Validity, reliability and factor analysis. *Journal of the American Geriatrics Society, 48*(12), 1669-1673.
Ferrell, B., et al. (2001). Ethical dilemmas in pain management. *The Journal of Pain, 2*(3), 171-180.
Fine, P. (2000). Pain and aging: Overcoming barriers to treatment and the role of transdermal opioid therapy. *Clinical Geriatrics, 8*(12), 1-6.
Frank-Stromborg, M., & Chistensen, A. (2001). A serious look at the undertreatment of pain: Part 1. *Clinical Journal of Oncology Nursing, 5*(5), 235-236.
Freedman, G. (2002). Clinical management of common causes of geriatric pain. *Geriatrics, 57*(5), 36-42.
Furrow, B. (2001). Pain management and provider liability: No more excuses. *Journal of Law, Medicine & Ethics, 29*, 28-51.
Gerstle, D., All, A., & Wallace, D. (2001). Quality of life and chronic nonmalignant pain. *Pain Management Nursing, 2*(3), 98-109.
Gilbertson, B., Wenner, K., & Russell, L.C. (2003). Acupuncture and arthroscopic acromioplasty. *Journal of Orthopaedic Research, 21*(4), 752-758.
Gordon, D., et al. (2001). A nurse-run inpatient pain consultation service. *Pain Management Nursing, 1*(2), 29-33.
Green, C., Wheeler, J., & LaPorte, F. (2003). Clinical decision making in pain management: Contributions of physician and patient characteristics to variations in practice. *The Journal of Pain, 4*(1): 29-39.
Green, C., et al. (2003). Race and chronic pain: A comparison study of young black and white Americans presenting for management. *The Journal of Pain, 4*(4), 176-183.
Guay, D. (2001). Adjunctive agents in the management of chronic pain. *Pharmacotherapy, 21*(9), 1070-1081.
Hazelett, S., Powell, C., & Androulakakis, V. (2002). Patients' behavior at the time of injury: Effect on nurses' perception of pain level and subsequent treatment. *Pain Management Nursing, 3*(1), 28-35.
Heidrich, D. (2001). Controlled-release oxycodone hydrochloride (OxyContin). *Clinical Nurse Specialist, 15*(5), 207-209.
Hutchison, R. (2004). Pain control: COX-2–selective NSAIDs. *American Journal of Nursing, 104*(3), 52-56.
Jacob, E. (2001). The pain experience of patients with sickle cell anemia. *Pain Management Nursing, 2*(3), 74-83.
*Jacox, A.K., et al. (1994). *Management of cancer pain: Adults. Clinical practice guideline No. 9.* AHCPR Pub. No. 94-0593. Rockville, MD: Agency for Health Care Policy and Research, Public Health Service, U.S. Department of Health and Human Services.
Jenson, M.G., et al. (2002). Topiramate for the treatment of neuropathic and chronic pain syndromes: An open label trial. *American Journal of Pain Management, 12*, 16-23.
Katz, N. (2002). The impact of pain management of quality of life. *Journal of Pain and Symptom Management, 24*(1), S38-S47.
Kedziera, P. (2001). Easing elders' pain. *Holistic Nursing Practice, 15*(2), 4-16.
Kessenich, C. (2001). Cyclo-oxygenase 2 inhibitors: An important new drug classification. *Pain Management Nursing, 2*(1), 13-18.
Kettleman, K. (2000). What's so bad about meperidine? *Nursing 2000, 30*(10), 20.
King, S.A. (2000). The use of NSAIDs for geriatric pain. *Geriatric Times, 1*, 1-6.
Knox, K. (2000). PCA patient education: An essential ingredient for success. *Analgesia, 11*(1), 4-6.
LaDike, S. (2002). Ethical issues in pain management. *Critical Care Nursing Clinics of North America, 14*, 165-170.
Laird, M., & Gidal, B. (2000). Use of gabapentin in the treatment of neuropathic pain. *The Annals of Pharmacotherapy, 34*(6), 802-807.
Lee, K., Ray, J., & Dunn, G. (2001). Chronic pain management and the surgeon: Barriers and opportunities. *Journal of the American College of Surgeons, 193*(6), 689-702.
Lu, D.P., Lu, G.P., & Kleinman, L. (2001). Acupuncture and clinical hypnosis for facial and head and neck pain: A single crossover comparison. *American Journal of Clinical Hypnosis, 44*(2), 141-148.
Lynch, M. (2001). Pain as the fifth vital sign. *Journal of Intravenous Nursing, 24*(2), 85-94.
*McCaffery, M. (1979). *Nursing management of the patient with pain* (2nd ed.). Philadelphia: J.B. Lippincott.
*McCaffery, M., & Pasero, C. (1999). Harmful effects of unrelieved pain. *Pain: Clinical Manual* 15-34.
*McCaffery, M., & Pasero, C. (1999). *Pain: Clinical manual* (2nd ed.). St. Louis: Mosby.
McCaffery, M., & Pasero, C. (2001). Stigmatizing patients as addicts. *American Journal of Nursing, 101*(5), 77-79.
McCaffery, M., & Pasero, C. (2003). Breakthrough pain. *American Journal of Nursing, 103*(4), 83-85.
McCaffery, M., & Robinson, E. (2002). Your patient is in pain: Here is how you respond. *Nursing 2002, 32*(10), 36-47.
McNeil, J., et al. (2001). Pain management outcomes for hospitalized Hispanic patients. *Pain Management Nursing, 2*(1), 25-36.
*Melzack, R., Wall, P.D. (1982). *The challenge of pain.* New York: Basic Books.
Merboth, M., & Barnason, S. (2000). Managing pain: The fifth vital sign. *Nursing Clinics of North America, 35*(2), 375-383.
Miller, K., & Miller, M. (2003). Challenges in end-of-life pain management. *Annals of Long-Term Care, 11*(4), 26-32.
Milligan, K. et al. (2001). Evaluation of long-term efficacy and safety of transdermal fentanyl in the treatment of chronic noncancer pain. *The Journal of Pain, 2*(4), 197-204.
Newshan, G. (2000). Pain management in the addicted patient: Practical considerations. *Nursing Outlook, 48*(2), 81-85.
Nichols, R. (2003). Pain management in patients with addictive disease. *American Journal of Nursing, 103*(3), 87, 89.
Pasero, C. (2002). Subcutaneous opioid infusion. *American Journal of Nursing, 102*(7), 61-62.
Pasero, C. (2003). Epidural analgesia for postoperative pain, Part 2. *American Journal of Nursing, 103*(11), 43-45.
Pasero, C., & McCaffery, M. (2000). When patients can't report pain. *American Journal of Nursing, 100*(9), 22-23.
Pasero, C., & McCaffery, M. (2001). Hydromorphone. *American Journal of Nursing, 101*(2), 22-23.
Pasero, C., & McCaffery, M. (2001). Reversing respiratory depression with naloxone. *American Journal of Nursing, 100*(2), 26.
Pasero, C., & McCaffery, M. (2001). The patient's report of pain. *American Journal of Nursing, 101*(12), 73-74.
Pasero, C., & McCaffery, M. (2001). Undertreatment of pain. *American Journal of Nursing, 101*(11), 62, 64, 66.
Pasero, C., & McCaffery, M. (2002). Monitoring sedation. *American Journal of Nursing, 102*(2), 67-69.

Pasero, C., & McCaffery, M. (2002). Pain in the critically ill. *American Journal of Nursing, 102*(1), 56-60.

Pasero, C., & McCaffery, M. (2003). Lidocaine patch 5%. *American Journal of Nursing, 103*(9), 75-78.

Pasero, C., & McCaffery, M. (2003). Tramadol. *American Journal of Nursing, 103*(2), 71, 73.

Pullen, R. (2002). Pain management for chronic nonmalignant neuropathic pain. *Home Healthcare Nurse, 20*(6), 387-392.

Puntillo, K.A., et al. (2001). Patients' perceptions and responses to procedural pain: Results from Thunder Project II. *Am J Critical Care, 10*(4), 238-251.

Resnick, B. (2003). Managing chronic pain in the older patient. *Geriatric Nursing, 24*(6), 373.

Robinson, M., et al. (2001). Gender role expectations of pain: Relationship to sex differences in pain. *The Journal of Pain, 2*(5), 251-257.

*Rowbotham, M., et al. for the Gabapentin Post-Herpetic Neuralgia Study Group. (1998). Gabapentin for the treatment of postherpetic neuralgia: A randomized controlled trial. *Journal of the American Medical Association, 280*(21), 1837-1842.

Sargent, C. (2002). Naloxone: How well do you know this drug? *Clinical Journal of Oncology Nursing, 6*(1), 17-18.

Schaffer, S.D., & Yucha, C.B. (2004). Relaxation and pain management. *American Journal of Nursing, 104*(8), 75-82.

Slaughter, A., Pasero, C., & Manworren, R. (2002). Unacceptable pain levels. *American Journal of Nursing, 102*(5), 75, 77.

Smith, R., Curci, M., & Silverman, A. (2002). Pain management: The global connection, *Nursing Management, 33*(6), 27-30.

Stegman, M. (2001). Control of pain: Every person's right. *Orthopaedic Nursing, 20*(2), 31-36.

Swenson, C. (2002). Ethical issues in pain management. *Seminars in Oncology Nursing, 18*(2), 135-142.

Todd, K.H., et al. (2000). Ethnicity and analgesic practice. *Annals of Emergency Medicine, 35*, 11-16.

Tucker, K. (2001). Deceptive placebo administration. *American Journal of Nursing, 101*(8), 55-56.

Vallerand, A., & Polomano, R. (2000). The relationship of gender to pain. *Pain Management Nursing, 1*(3), S8-15.

Waitman, J., & McCaffery, M. (2001). Meperidine–A liability. *American Journal of Nursing, 101*(1), 57-58.

Watt-Watson, J., et al. (2000). The impact of nurses' empathic responses on patients' management in acute care. *Nursing Research*, 49(4), 191-200.

Wentz, J. (2001). Assessing pain in the cognitively impaired adult. *Nursing 2001, 31*(7), 26.

Wentz, J. (2003). Understanding neuropathic pain. *Nursing 2003, 33*(1), 22.

Young-McCaughan, S., & Miaskowski, C. (2001). Definition of and mechanism for opioid-induced sedation. *Pain Management Nursing*, *2*(3), 84-97.

Young-McCaughan, S., & Miaskowski, C. (2001). Measurement of opioid-induced sedation. *Pain Management Nursing, 2*(4), 132-149.

CHAPTER 8

Substance Abuse

TOMMIE WRIGHT PNIEWSKI

LEARNING OUTCOMES

After studying this chapter, you should be able to:

1. Discuss substance abuse as a major health issue in the United States.
2. Explain the effects of substance abuse on the mental and physical health of individuals and society.
3. Describe the relationship between stress and substance abuse.
4. Identify assessment findings associated with use of nicotine, alcohol, stimulants, hallucinogens, depressants, opioids, inhalants, and steroids.
5. Prioritize care for clients who exhibit signs or symptoms of substance abuse.
6. Discuss recent biologic and genetic research in the etiology of substance abuse.
7. Identify symptoms that are indicative of emergency situations associated with the use of the following substances: alcohol, nicotine, stimulants, hallucinogens, depressants, opioids, inhalants, and steroids.
8. Identify the responsibilities of the nurse when a peer or other health care worker is suspected of abusing substances.
9. Identify common medication regimens that are used in the emergency treatment of drug withdrawal and adverse reactions to drugs and alcohol.
10. Prioritize nursing care for clients who are in alcohol withdrawal.

Go to your Student CD-ROM for Review Questions for the NCLEX Examination keyed to these Learning Outcomes.

OVERVIEW OF SUBSTANCE ABUSE

Subtance abuse is described as the overindulgence of a chemical substance and the resulting dependence that interferes with life's activities. Each year there are alarming increases in the abuse of mind- and mood-altering substances, such as alcohol, marijuana, cocaine and nontherapeutic use of prescription drugs. The mental and physical health of the individual is affected by substance abuse, which also significantly affects the lives of others. Productivity is drastically reduced, and the costs of abuse to society are enormous. Categories of substances commonly abused include stimulants, hallucinogens, depressants, opioids (narcotics), and other substances that alter the mind. Stimulants are abused by some clients because the need for "faster, better, and longer" exists as a mindset in society. Hallucinogens continue to be popular in various forms but are commonly encountered as mind-altering drugs such as phencyclidine (PCP) and lysergic acid (LSD). Depressants, such as the anxiolytics, are becoming increasingly popular as a maladaptive alternative in responding to the ever-increasing demands of today's busy lifestyles. Opioids and morphine derivatives, although important for therapeutic uses for pain relief, continue to be abused and addictive in the drug community.

Incidence/Prevalence of Substance Abuse

A chronic, long-standing problem, substance abuse continues to be prevalent in the United States. Studies conducted by the National Institute on Drug Abuse (NIDA) (2003) are helpful in assessment of drug abuse. Studies indicate that substance abuse increased from 6.3% of the populations studied in 2000 to 7.1% in 2001. This represents about 15.9 million Americans age 12 years and older being identified as "current users."

Patterns of use among ethnic groups generally remain the same among major racial and ethnic groups. In 2001, the rate among African Americans was 7.4%, white individuals, 7.2%, and Hispanics 6.4%. The highest rates of illicit drug use were among Native Americans/American Indians and Alaskan Natives at 9.9%. The lowest rate of substance use was among Asian Americans at 2.8% (NIDA, 2003).

WOMEN'S HEALTH CONSIDERATIONS

According to the NIDA report, 4 million women in the United States use drugs (Mathias, 2000). Women of all races, ages, educational backgrounds, cultures, and community types are among the drug users in the United States. Drug use

Continued

and abuse data among women are becoming increasingly available as the nursing profession seeks to improve the health of women. Usually women abuse more than one drug. Almost half of all women 15 to 44 years of age have used drugs (including tobacco products and alcohol) at least once in their lifetime. Approximately 2 million women used cocaine and more than 6 million used marijuana in 1999 (Mathias, 2000).

Women are at risk for developing drug dependence as a result of biologic predisposition, stressors in the environment, and availability of quality support services. These factors must be explored during the nursing assessment to be thorough in addressing the specific client's needs.

Cultural Competence Related to Substance Abuse

Culture influences every aspect of the client's life. The nurse needs to demonstrate competence in understanding the cultural influences that are related to drug abuse to plan care that will work for the person with substance abuse problems. In addition, an understanding of the client's culture helps to avoid making assumptions about substance abuse based on the client's body language. Some behaviors (e.g., avoiding eye contact), which are interpreted within the Western culture as negative are considered normal, even reverent, in other cultures (e.g., Asian culture).

Adapt the assessment and subsequent planning of care within the norms of the client's culture. With the stigma associated with substance abuse, be aware of those behaviors and norms that would alienate him or her. Often, substance abuse disorders are a result of interpersonal inadequacies. The user perceives the substance as helpful to reduce stress or assist him or her in coping. Success of drug treatment is often related to the use of external support, forcing the user to rely on other persons rather than the chemical.

Be open to the array of religious preferences to avoid conflicts between treatment modalities and the client's faith. In addition, you need a firm awareness of self to avoid reactive behaviors to the client's beliefs or absence of personal convictions. A posture of judgment is never appropriate and is particularly nontherapeutic when caring for the client with substance abuse. Chapter 6 describes cultural aspects of health in more detail, including how to perform a cultural assessment.

Substance Abuse, Stress, and Addiction

Many clients relate substance abuse to stress relief; however, external situational stress is not the only contributing factor resulting in substance abuse. The role that stress does play in substance abuse occurs more in a biologic response to stress, part of which is a normal response. The introduction of stress in the brain, as perceived by the individual, results in stimulation of the hypothalamus. The hypothalamus, located beneath the thalamus, is the center for emotional responses and houses the limbic system (emotional part of the brain). In addition, the hypothalamus controls the involuntary nervous system and organ functions. Biologic rhythms and internal drives (e.g., sex drive) are directed by the nuclei of the hypothalamus. Perceptions of pleasure, fear, and rage are also found in the hypothalamus. Autonomic nervous system pathways initiate most physical expressions of these emotions, such as a pounding heart, increased blood pressure, pallor, increased perspiration, and a dry mouth.

Responses to external stress (situational or ingested chemicals) or internal stress (disease or withdrawal of drugs) trigger chemical and hormonal responses in the body arising from activity in the hypothalamus. The body reacts to stress by secreting hormones in the blood and neurotransmitters in the brain. Normally, the body secretes stress hormones throughout the day in small amounts. When the body experiences stress, the brain reacts by increasing the level of stress hormones. Corticotropin-releasing factor (CRF) is released into the blood, which carries the CRF to the pituitary gland. This stimulates the release of adrenocorticotropin (ACTH) resulting in stimulation of the release of other hormones, primarily cortisol, from the adrenal glands. Cortisol travels throughout the body, assisting the body to cope with the stress. Cortisol influences the continued response to the stress or reduction depending on the severity of the stressor.

Depending on the source of the stress, the behavioral manifestations frequently have an influence on the quality of the body's response. Stress responses that are frequently triggered can result in a more sensitive response. Continued substance abuse creates a cycle of ever-increasing amounts of the drug to sustain the desired level of response to the drug. As with achieving the desired result, the body also responds with "withdrawal" responses (symptoms of withdrawal) when deprived of the substance. A cyclic ingestion-withdrawal response sets the stage for addiction.

Substance abuse is a documented nursing diagnosis when the following criteria are present:

- The client loses control of use of the drug.
- The client takes the drug even though the drug has caused adverse conditions in the body.
- The client demonstrates cognitive, behavioral, and physiologic disturbances with the abuse of drugs or inhalants.

Dependence is characterized as a condition that causes a habitual, compulsive, and uncontrollable urge to use a substance; and without the substance, the body experiences severe physiologic, psychological, and emotional disturbances. Substance abuse in the presence of medical or surgical problems creates a complicated situation in terms of helping clients to reach their highest level of function.

Genetics of Substance Abuse

Research in the genetic connection between a person's gene makeup and substance abuse has noted associations of genes to cluster and contribute to substance use and/or abuse. A single gene theory has not been substantiated as has the cluster arrangement of groups of genes. A complex interaction between the genetic makeup and the environment has been noted in current research to result in substance abuse and dependence. Even though there have been numerous discoveries by the Human Genome Project, there is still a question as to what mechanisms underlie substance abuse. Drugs that are commonly abused stimulate the reward pathways of the brain.

The exact linkage between genes and their contribution to substance use is not known; however, current projects suggest that there may be activities among genes indicating that one gene influences behavior early in drug use and later another gene may overstimulate the reward center, resulting in "cravings." Current information regarding substance use, abuse, and dependence suggests that common pathways are shared in the reward center of the brain, which perpetuates substance use.

Personality traits are thought to be contributing factors in substance abuse. Genetic factors have been linked to variations in genes among persons with sensation-seeking behavior traits. Persons with the sensation-seeking behaviors have been found to be more susceptible to substance dependence.

Based on clinical research, the strongest risk factor in the assessment of substance use or dependence is the family history. How the individual interprets substance abuse or dependence is important in the planning, intervention, and success of that person. The implication of research linking dependence and drug abuse has profound influence on the perception of the drug user (Hardie, 2002).

Other research findings note that a lack of a specific enzyme (cytochrome P450) may cause more serious reactions to small amounts of "ecstasy" and may be significant in the body's processing of that drug. With further research, there is a potential to predict which persons are at risk for extremely serious reactions to substances such as ecstasy (Tipton, 2003).

Substance abuse, a chronic mental disorder, can be treated effectively, resulting in reduced crime, drug use, and psychological problems associated with drug use. Nursing implications with regard to the genetics of substance use are primarily directed to education in the linkage of substance abuse and genetics.

Substance Abuse and the Hospitalized Client

The client may be hospitalized when he or she can no longer be managed in an ambulatory care setting or when emergencies arise. As part of the comprehensive health assessment, the nurse carefully assesses for any signs, symptoms, or history of substance abuse.

In a comprehensive assessment, alcohol, tobacco, prescription drug, over-the-counter, and illicit drug use must be determined. Obtaining history of herbal treatment is necessary to determine the potential for interactions or symptomatic withdrawal from natural substances. The nurse should be adept in ascertaining substance abuse during the interview process. Failure to include a complete substance use history could have serious adverse effects on the client. The client who habitually uses substances requires closer observation for withdrawal than the occasional user. You need to be knowledgeable of various substances to be alert for signs of complications.

Caring for the client experiencing substance problems includes determining where the client will be going at the time of discharge. If the client has focused on treatment and recovery from the substance, discharge to a residential treatment center may be the environment of choice. If the client's plan includes continuation of the substance use, home may be the choice for discharge. Regardless of the best intentions of health care providers, the client may choose to handle his or her own substance abuse problem. Assist clients in reaching their optimal level of function as determined by both the client and the health care team.

Understanding the influence of abusive substances is an important educational aspect for the hospitalized client. Some chemicals have potentiating effects on therapeutic medications that can lead to serious or life-threatening situations. Room assignment, delegation of personnel, staffing assignments, and other nursing decisions are important with the substance-using client. The course of hospitalization may be altered as a result of substance abuse; treatment, care, and recovery can all be influenced by substance abuse.

Referrals and community-based health resources are important in assisting the client with substance abuse. Emotional support is necessary to help the client cope with the reason for hospitalization, being in the hospital, and dealing with the adverse effects of the substance abuse.

Nurses as Substance Abusers

History has shown a tendency of health care professionals to be susceptible to substance abuse associated with drug availability and job stress. The *ANA Code of Ethics for Nurses* gives a standard of professional behavior that seeks to safeguard and protect the public, as well as preserve integrity within the profession. Nursing practice is governed in each state by a Board of Nursing. In supporting safe and competent nursing, boards of nursing have peer assistance programs to assist in identifying and effectively managing substance abuse in the employment setting. All nurses need to be knowledgeable of their state board of nursing laws and the consequences of unprofessional behavior.

Prescription Drugs and Abuse

Some prescription drugs can easily become addictive because of the nature of their action in the brain. There is a tendency for the client to become comfortable with the effects of the drug long after the therapeutic need is satisfied. Improper use of therapeutic substances can result in addiction; such substances may also be used improperly for pleasure-seeking effects. Examples of therapeutic prescription drugs that can produce addiction or be used for maladaptive purposes are morphine, barbiturates, and benzodiazepines.

Challenges for the health care professional include preparedness to intervene in the risk behaviors created by substance use or abuse. This health problem is not limited to teenagers or to an impoverished population. All age groups and socioeconomic groups are vulnerable to substance abuse. The professional who is knowledgeable about substance abuse will be able to identify and appropriately care for the client experiencing substance use or abuse problems.

CONSIDERATIONS FOR OLDER ADULTS

Substance abuse should not be overlooked in the older adult. The potential for nontherapeutic use or abuse is high because of the number of different types of medications taken. As part the aging process, older adults have more difficulty metabolizing and excreting drugs; therefore toxicity is a common situation. Self-medication is a problem in the older population, increasing the complexity of care. A thorough drug history is necessary for identifying patterns of drug use that are harmful to the client. Misuse of prescription medications can happen quite innocently as memory becomes altered. Regular drug administration times are difficult to remember, resulting in overdosing or underdosing.

Approximately 1 in 4 persons in the United States has a friend or family member with substance abuse problems or a history of drug abuse. Medical-surgical nursing care is affected by substance abuse because of the complications caused by the physical presence or dependence on the substance. Clinical management of client health problems is more complex when the client has an addiction to drugs and/or alcohol.

The following sections describe some of the most common groups of illicit substances and their effects on the body (Table 8-1). Many drugs can cause coma or death. When drug use is suspected, blood and urine testing is done to determine the type of substance ingested. Nursing implications related to assessment and care of clients who abuse drugs and alcohol are also discussed.

STIMULANTS

Stimulants are drugs that excite the cerebral cortex of the brain, producing a variety of behavioral responses (see Table 8-1). Any substance that is introduced into the body that excites or stimulates an increase in body activity is referred to as a stimulant. Examples of stimulants are caffeine, nicotine, amphetamines, and methamphetamines. Although amphetamines and methamphetamines can be used for therapeutic purposes, their use is limited. Agents that are considered to be illicit and abused stimulants are "crack" (a potent form of cocaine), cocaine, and illegally produced methamphetamines. The incidence of stimulant use is varied among age groups and chemicals.

The following are the therapeutic effects of stimulants:

- Increase mental alertness
- Improve one's sense of well-being
- Increase the capacity to work
- Improve the performance of motor skills
- Stimulate general metabolism by increasing respiratory and cardiac function

When a large amount of stimulant is introduced into the body, the effects can cause insomnia, tremor, and restlessness, with resulting loss of motor function. The prolonged and sustained use of a stimulant can result in toxicity; an overdose can cause hallucinations, seizures, and cardiac dysrhythmias.

Amphetamines

OVERVIEW

Amphetamines are stimulants that increase the body's activities. Prescribed therapeutically as psychomotor stimulants, amphetamines and methamphetamines are effective in the treatment of attention deficit hyperactivity disorder (ADHD), obesity, and narcolepsy. When amphetamines are used as for recreation, the desired effect is to achieve a state of euphoria and grandiosity. Names for amphetamines (biphetamine, Dexedrine) in the drug environment include "black beauties," "cross," and "hearts." Knowledge of the "street" names for these drugs assists the nurse in assessment and identification of abusive use of amphetamines. Amphetamines can be ingested by a variety of methods including consumption by mouth, injection, smoking, or sniffing. Amphetamines have a high potential for addiction both physically and psychologically. Use of stimulants results in energy, excitement, relief of fatigue, decreased appetite, insomnia, aggression, and a tendency toward menstrual problems in women.

TABLE 8-1 Commonly Abused Substances

Stimulants
Amphetamines
Methamphetamine
Cocaine
Hallucinogens and Related Compounds
Lysergic Acid (LSD)
Phencyclidine (PCP)
Ketamine
3,4-Methylenedioxymethamphetamine
Marijuana
Depressants
Benzodiazepines
Rohypnol
Gamma hydroxybytyrate (GHB)
Barbiturates
Alcohol
Narcotics: Opioids and Morphine Derivatives
Inhalants
Solvents
Gases
Nitrites
Steroids (Anabolic)

COLLABORATIVE MANAGEMENT

As a result of these effects, assess the client for objective symptoms of stimulant use, overdose, or withdrawal. Table 8-2 lists these clinical manifestations. For both overdose and withdrawal, the priority for care is to maintain a safe environment both physically and psychologically for the client. Close observations are necessary to prevent development of further complications. Supportive communications are necessary to reduce anxiety and fear in the client. A nonjudgmental attitude is essential in establishing a therapeutic rapport. Many times health care providers view substance abuse clients as responsible for their situation and therefore have difficulty maintaining a professional demeanor when providing care.

Methamphetamine

Methamphetamine (Desoxyn) is a powerful substance that is highly addictive. Therapeutically, methamphetamine is available as a Schedule II substance. It is available medically through a prescription for ADHD, narcolepsy, and obesity. Although it is similar to amphetamines, methamphetamine is more powerful and affects the brain more dramatically. High levels of the neurotransmitter dopamine are released as a result of the ingestion of methamphetamine. There is evidence that this drug has neurotoxic effects on the brain, damaging cells that contain other transmitters such as serotonin. Symptoms of parkinsonism can be found in the long-term user. Even small amounts of methamphetamine can result in dramatic results.

Recreational drugs are used to obtain a "rush" or "flash." Commonly known as "chalk," "speed," "crank," "crystal," "glass," and "ice," methamphetamines are manufactured illegally in "meth" labs across the United States. In addition to the results produced by amphetamines, methamphetamine can also produce life-threatening conditions, such as hyperthermia (fever) and convulsions. Irreversible damage to the

TABLE 8-2 Clinical Manifestations and Emergency Care for Clients Who Abuse Stimulants

	Clinical Manifestations	Emergency Care
Stimulant overdose	Respiratory distress Ataxia Fever Convulsions Coma Myocardial infarction Stroke Death	Respiratory support Cooling blanket Anti-epileptic drugs Antipsychotics Ammonium chloride (to acidify urine for excretion of amphetamines [bases])
Stimulant withdrawal	Fatigue Depression Agitation Apathy Anxiety Insomnia Disorientation Craving	Antianxiety medications Antidepressants Dopamine agonists (to reduce tremors)

vessels in the brain can cause strokes. Cardiovascular collapse, resulting in death, can be caused by methamphetamine use.

Assessment findings of methamphetamine use are the same symptoms found in amphetamine use; however, they may be more pronounced or vivid than those for amphetamine use. Nursing care for the client experiencing withdrawal or overdose is the same as that for amphetamine use.

Cocaine

OVERVIEW

Cocaine is a stimulant that is commonly known as "coke," "crack," "flake," "rocks," and "snow." Cocaine, legally used as a Schedule II drug, is valuable as a topical anesthetic or a vasoconstrictor to stop bleeding. The physiologic action of cocaine is interference with the reabsorption process of dopamine. As a chemical messenger related to pleasure and movement, dopamine is released as part of the brain's reward system and is associated with the euphoria achieved with cocaine use. Processing cocaine using ammonia or sodium bicarbonate transforms the cocaine into "crack cocaine," a preparation that can be inhaled. This process is referred to as "freebasing" cocaine. Smoking cocaine is a more direct method of getting the drug to the brain. Physical dependency can occur with psychological dependence being more common. Cocaine use is severely addicting, and withdrawal can be a life-threatening situation. Adverse reactions include all of the reactions listed with stimulant use, including vertigo, nausea, vomiting, abdominal cramps, hypotension or hypertension, chills, fever, tachycardia, and tachypnea, progressing to collapse of the peripheral circulatory system, coma, and death.

COLLABORATIVE MANAGEMENT

Assessment

When caring for the client using cocaine, observe for symptoms that are associated with crack cocaine use. With moderate amounts of this drug, the client may exhibit increased alertness, euphoria, anorexia, high blood pressure, increased heart rate, and dilated pupils. In high doses (overdose), agitation, confusion, hallucinations, panic attacks, paranoia, or convulsions may occur. Withdrawal symptoms include irritability, sluggishness, and prolonged periods of sleep, depression, and nausea. Laboratory results for determining presence in the urine is detectable in the urine 1 to 4 hours after ingestion and may remain in the urine up to 3 days after use. To determine relative time of ingestions, serum levels are necessary.

Interventions

Nursing care of the client with overdose or withdrawal includes astute observation for cardiac symptoms and frequent monitoring of vital signs. Assess for signs of depression and potential suicide gestures during the withdrawal period. Help reduce nausea by ensuring that the environmental temperature is comfortable and that odors are eliminated. Assess nutrition and hydration status due to the tendency of the person to fail to eat or take in fluids during use of the drug.

During the initial and ongoing physical assessment, pay careful attention to the mucous membranes of the nose, because prolonged snorting can deteriorate the membranes and the nasal septum. Nosebleeds are common with snorting the drug and can be a valuable tool in assessment of use. Cardiopulmonary arrest can occur with the first use of cocaine. Generally the medical treatment for cocaine withdrawal or overdose is the same as that for amphetamines.

Nicotine

OVERVIEW

Nicotine is one of the most addictive substances in the United States and is the addictive component of tobacco. Although the U.S. Surgeon General issued a report in 1989 about the health hazards of tobacco and cigarette smoking, tobacco products continue to be used. This report cited nicotine as a major contributing factor to strokes, the third leading cause of death. Today, there is wide use of nicotine products in cigarettes, pipe tobacco, chewing tobacco, and "spit" tobacco (Figure 8-1).

Physiologically, nicotine has both stimulant and sedative properties that affect the central nervous system (CNS). First, nicotine stimulates the discharge of epinephrine from the adrenal cortex, causing a sudden release of glucose. After recovery from the stimulant effects of the nicotine, depressant effects result in feelings of depression and fatigue. Daily

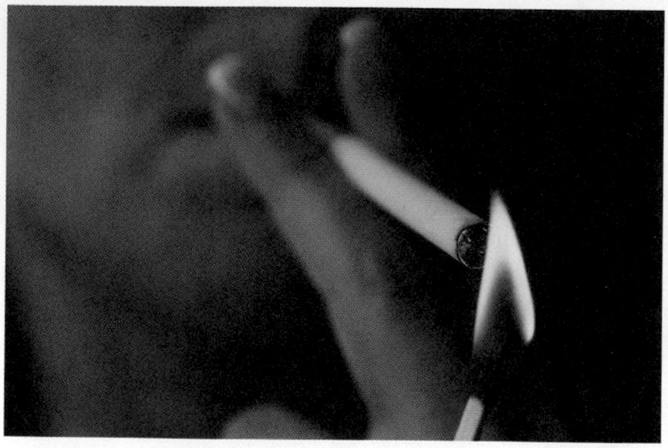

Figure 8-1 ■ The incidence of smoking is increasing among women.

ingestion of nicotine results in accumulation of nicotine in the body, lasting up to 24 hours. Because of the cyclic properties of nicotine, the body begins to require more nicotine usage to maintain the stimulant effects of the drug.

The dependence process begins with the cyclic use of nicotine for continuation of the stimulation experienced by the body. The addictive power of nicotine has been compared to that of cocaine. With the cessation of nicotine use, withdrawal symptoms are observed in the tobacco user. Lack of nicotine use in a 24-hour period can result in aggression, hostility, anger, and inappropriate social interactions. Research into the use of nicotine has resulted in data that show an increased level of dopamine, a neurotransmitter affecting brain pathways that control reward and pleasure. During periods of stress, there is a need for additional nicotine because the stress hormone corticosterone reduces the effects of nicotine. As stress and anxiety increase, the cycle of dependence grows stronger, leading the user to increase consumption of nicotine.

COLLABORATIVE MANAGEMENT

As proponents of good health practices, the nurse may help motivate the client to quit using nicotine by describing the negative effects of smoking, including chronic cardiovascular and respiratory diseases. Secondhand smoke affects other people who are exposed to the smoker. The nurse teaches the importance of smoking cessation. A number of community-based support groups and smoking cessation programs, using behavioral methods, hypnosis, acupressure, or other modalities, are available. Smoking cessation is discussed in the cardiovascular unit of this text.

HALLUCINOGENS AND RELATED COMPOUNDS

Chemical substances that possess mind-altering or mental perception–altering properties are known as **hallucinogens** (see Table 8-1). Examples of hallucinogenic substances are lysergic acid (LSD), phencyclidine (PCP), and marijuana. Of these three, the only therapeutic drug is PCP, which is used as a veterinary anesthetic agent. There are no therapeutic uses acceptable for medical treatment today, although marijuana has been used by some to treat cancer pain.

Hallucinogenic compounds are desirable to the drug user because of their thrill-seeking effects, which are caused by an alteration in perception. These drugs produce changes in the neurotransmitters of the brain. Alterations in mood, sensory distortions, delusions, and depersonalization are some of the resulting behaviors. Physical changes experienced by the user are increased pulse, blood pressure, and respirations, as well as pupillary dilation. A psychological dependence may occur, or the client may experience suicidal or psychotic states. Flashbacks are a common phenomenon when psychedelic drugs are used and can occur at any time. The user is returned to the initial drug experience without warning, which can be very disturbing and can create a threat to safety. Observe for objective signs of use, as well as looking for paranoia and suspicious behavior. Addiction to hallucinogens is psychological in nature rather than physical addiction.

Lysergic Acid

OVERVIEW

Lysergic acid (LSD) is the prototype and major hallucinogenic drug, known as "acid" in the drug community. The drug is odorless and colorless with a slightly bitter taste. Usually taken orally, LSD is often distributed on absorbent, decorative paper, making it very attractive to adolescents and children. The health hazards of LSD are unpredictable and are affected by dose, personality and mood of the user, anticipated outcome, and environment at the time of use. Because the exact mechanism of action is not known, further studies in drug research are being conducted by the National Institute on Drug Abuse (Mathias, 2000). LSD is known to influence neurotransmission in the CNS. The effects of the drug can last up to 12 hours and can result in either pleasant or unpleasant experiences, also known as "good trips" or "bad trips."

Introspective thinking may occur with the person experiencing personal revelations about themselves, the truth of the universe, or other bizarre thoughts. Sensory experiences are powerful in LSD use because of the perception of surroundings. Colors seem more vivid and tangible to the person experiencing the effects of LSD. Thoughts and feelings can be so bizarre that a "trip" can result in suicide. LSD use can also result in severe and chronic mental illness, such as schizophrenia. Because LSD does not result in compulsive drug-seeking behaviors, it is not considered addictive, but a strong tolerance can develop. An increased amount of the drug is needed to attain the same level of stimulation as earlier experiences. LSD stimulates the sympathetic nervous system. Some neuromuscular involvement is noted such as tremors and hyperflexia. Effects of LSD can last from 8 to 12 hours.

COLLABORATIVE MANAGEMENT

Assessment

Observe for intoxication such as:

- Dilated pupils
- Tachycardia
- Palpitations
- Diaphoresis
- Tremors

- Poor coordination
- Elevated temperature
- Increased pulse and respiration

Many psychological symptoms also occur as paranoid ideas, anxiety, depression, and transforming sounds and sights into sensation (hearing colors). Overdose can result in brain damage, psychosis, or death.

Interventions

Treatment options for the person in an LSD crisis include one-to-one observation to keep the client safe and to help the person sort reality as the effects subside. Fears can be comforted and prevent the person from acting on fear or psychotic thoughts. Because there is such a sensory influence on the person, the environment should be calming, at a comfortable temperature with few disturbances. Reducing the stimuli can significantly limit the response to the drug's effects. In an emergency situation, the person is exposed to varied and powerful stimuli that contribute to intense behavioral responses to the powerful stimulus created by LSD. Antianxiety medications (benzodiazepines) or medications to control or eliminate the symptoms of mental illness may be prescribed. Haloperidol (Haldol) has been found to be effective in the treatment of LSD symptoms. Effects created by other hallucinogens such as mescaline and psilocybin (derived from peyote cactus and mushrooms) respond to the same treatment regimen as used with LSD.

Phencyclidine

Phencyclidine, commonly known as PCP, is an animal anesthetic that causes a feeling of detachment in humans. Clients using PCP ("angel dust") are unaware of their surroundings, which causes the detachment. Primarily affecting the CNS, the client exhibits flushing, increased perspiration, aggression, and incoherence. The user may experience feelings of superior strength and physical power. Some users state that their use is related to the numbing effects on the mind. However, the results may progress to a comatose state.

There is no evidence of physical addiction; however, psychological addiction is common. There is evidence to suggest a decrease in the use of PCP, a commonly abused drug in the past. The nurse who suspects PCP abuse assesses for shallow respirations, generalized numbness of the extremities, and psychological effects, including distinct changes in body awareness. High doses of PCP can produce vomiting, loss of balance, visual disturbances, and dizziness. Seizures, coma, and death have resulted from high doses of PCP. Lasting effects of PCP use can include memory loss, speech difficulties, and interference with thinking processes.

Ketamine

Closely associated with PCP, ketamine is a substance classified as a disassociate anesthetic. Because of the short duration, ketamine is sometimes known as "businessman's LSD." Moderate doses produce euphoria, loss of inhibition, confusion, ringing in the ears, a quick burst of energy, and a drunken feeling. Tolerance can occur as well as physical and psychological dependence. Street names for ketamine are "special K," "K", and "kat." Ketamine is also referred to as a "techno" drug because of its attractiveness to the "Rave" culture.

Complications associated with ketamine overdose include the following:

- Tunnel vision
- Shortness of breath
- Loss of balance
- Numbness of the body
- Clinical depression
- No sense of time
- Seizures
- Coma

A calm and stimulus-free environment is important for the client recovering from a ketamine overdose, as well as availability of supportive therapies. Respiratory support is a priority because of the anesthetic effects of the drug.

3,4-Methylenedioxymethamphetamine

OVERVIEW

Amphetamines can be altered to become a hallucinogen, as in the case of **3,4-methylenedioxymethamphetamine (MDMA),** an oral drug that is also called "Adam," "ecstasy," "XTC," "hug," "beans," and the "date rape" drug. Known as the "love drug" in the 1970s and popular in the 1980s in the "Rave" community, MDMA remains an increasingly popular recreational (club drug). MDMA can be ingested orally, smoked, snorted, or injected. The desired effects are development of trust in others, which eases inhibitions between people, and increases in confidence, euphoria, and physical energy. Methylenedioxyamphetamine (MDA) is the parent drug of MDMA, both of which produce psychostimulant and psychedelic effects.

Part of the popularity of the drug includes the relaxation of voluntary muscles and the amnesiac effect for the period in which the drug is most active in the body; hence, the name "date rape" drug. The physiologic effects of MDMA occur at the serotonin receptor sites, which create the inhibition of behaviors. Serotonin plays a vital role in the regulation of aggression, mood, sexual activity, sleep, and pain sensitivity. Action at the serotonin site accounts for the report of heightened sexual experiences and tranquility. Demonstrating a structural relationship to methamphetamine, MDMA also causes a degeneration of neurons containing dopamine, a neurotransmitter, resulting in parkinsonism. MDMA is neurotoxic and can cause brain damage. Interfering with the temperature control mechanism of the body, malignant hyperthermia can also result with the use of MDMA.

COLLABORATIVE MANAGEMENT

Assess the client who has taken MDMA for psychological symptoms, including confusion, depression, sleep disturbances, drug craving, severe anxiety, and paranoia. With moderate doses, other effects are euphoria, nervousness, hyperexcitability, and a rapid heart rate. Physical symptoms of high-dose ingestion are muscle tension, involuntary teeth clenching, nausea, visual disturbances, faintness, and chills or sweating. Abnormal vital signs such as increased heart rate and blood pressure are also observed. Nursing care of the client on MDMA is based on the symptoms that are apparent at the time of assessment.

If acute symptoms are present, the priority for care is safety and symptomatic relief of the psychological manifestations.

Medication regimens are focused on reduction or elimination of the adverse effects of the drug.

Marijuana

OVERVIEW

Marijuana is commonly called "weed," "smoke," "pot," "grass," "Mary Jane," and "herb." Widely used and distributed, this drug is illegal and does not have any accepted legal therapeutic uses. For some clients, it has been used experimentally for chronic pain control. Although there is a considerable and ongoing debate about the uses and need for legalization of marijuana, it remains a contraband substance in the United States. Even though physical dependence for marijuana is seemingly nonexistent, it has a high risk for psychological dependence if it is used over long periods of time. The desired effects of marijuana are sensations of euphoria, sexual arousal, and relaxation. The "high" experience that users feel is a result of the action of tetrahydrocannabinol (THC), the main active substance in marijuana. THC changes the method by which sensory information enters and is processed in the hippocampus. As a component of the brain's limbic system, the hippocampus is necessary for the integration of sensory experiences and emotion, as well as learning and memory. Frequent and long-term use of marijuana can create the same respiratory changes seen in long-term tobacco smokers. Studies of young adults who use marijuana demonstrate that learning and social behavior are affected by heavy marijuana use. Evidence suggests that marijuana use affects critical skills related to attention, memory, and learning. Heavy marijuana users make more mistakes in their work and have more difficulty maintaining attention.

◆ COLLABORATIVE MANAGEMENT

Whether smoked or taken orally, the physical and psychological effects in moderate doses include relaxation, happiness, euphoria, increased heart rate, and impaired short-term memory. High doses produce more pronounced effects such paranoia, restlessness, anxiety attacks, panic attacks, increased appetite, impaired coordination, and altered perceptions. Withdrawal effects include insomnia, decreased appetite, nausea, irritability, and anxiety.

Nursing interventions for the person who is under the influence of marijuana are based on the severity of symptoms presented. A complete physical assessment as well as frequent vital sign assessment is needed to determine stability of the person's physical condition. Communication skills are important to ascertain self-destructive tendencies and the ability to give accurate, relevant data for treatment. Research of marijuana notes that there is no evidence of immediate life-threatening physical complications with use. However, impaired judgment, chromosomal influence on fetuses, and loss of memory are significant long-term effects of marijuana use.

DEPRESSANTS

Drugs that reduce the activity of the central nervous system (CNS) are referred to as **depressants** (see Table 8-1). Benzodiazepines and barbiturates are discussed as depressants because of their activity in the ascending reticular activating system in the CNS. Both classes have valuable therapeutic properties in treating anxiety and emotional disorders. CNS depressants are therapeutically used as adjuncts to sleep and can be used as needed for situational tension. The route of ingestion is either oral or by injection. On the illicit drug market, barbiturates are called "barbs" or "ludes"; depending on the chemical makeup. A commonly abused benzodiazepine, Rohypnol, is referred to as "rophies," "ruffies," "R2s," "Mexican Valium," "rib," "roach," or "Roches." Sometimes Rohypnol (flunitrazepam) is referred to as the "forget me pill" or "forget pill." These are Schedule IV drugs because of their high potential for abuse.

Benzodiazepines

The desired results for the use of prescribed benzodiazepines include relaxation, sleep, seizure control, withdrawal from alcohol, and relief of anxiety. Abuse is present when the client continues to use the drug after the clinical signs have subsided. The street value of benzodiazepines and the drug effects make this drug popular. Physical and psychological dependence on benzodiazepines is prevalent. The user can develop a high tolerance for the drug, causing increasing amounts to be needed to achieve the desired feeling. Benzodiazepines depress the CNS; therefore combination with other CNS substances has a potentiating effect.

ROHYPNOL

Rohypnol (flunitrazepam) is a highly potent benzodiazepine (10 times more potent as diazepam [Valium]) available through a provider prescription. Presently this drug is not available in the United States; however, it is used legally in other countries. Therapeutic use of this drug is for severe sleep disorders and inpatient psychiatric care. Combined with alcohol, this drug is also known to as a date rape drug. It is colorless, tasteless, and is not easily detected in the urine. Rohypnol can be swallowed, inhaled, injected, smoked, or dissolved in a drink. Effects of this drug provide the following:

- Relief from tension
- Anticonvulsant action
- Sedation
- Amnesia
- Muscle relaxation
- Sleep
- Slowing of motor performance, an effect that is greatly increased when combined with alcohol

Young people use this drug to engage in violent or destructive activities without feelings of guilt. Rohypnol has physical and psychological dependence properties. Moderate doses create a loss of inhibition, drunken state, dizziness, tranquility, and slurred speech.

Signs and symptoms associated with withdrawal or overdosing from Rohypnol include the following:

- Headache
- Muscle pain
- Extreme anxiety
- Tension and restlessness
- Confusion and irritability
- Depersonalization
- Hypersensitivity to light, noise, and physical contact
- Delirium

- Convulsions
- Shock
- Respiratory depression
- Cardiovascular collapse

Nursing care should focus on the severity of the symptoms and astute assessment for deterioration in the client's physical condition. Treatment of Rohypnol abuse is aimed at a medical model of detoxification using tapering doses.

GAMMA HYDROXYBUTYRATE

Gamma hydroxybutyrate (GHB) is gaining increased attention as a club drug along with LSD, ecstasy, ketamine, methamphetamine, and Rohypnol. GHB is referred to as "liquid ecstasy." In small amounts, GHB reduces one's social inhibitions and increasing libido. It is produced illegally in the United States and was referred to as the date rape drug of the 1990s. GHB may be inhaled, injected, or swallowed. In small doses, it produces euphoria, anxiety, increased sexual pleasure, impaired judgment, a loss of coordination, and nausea along with the loss of inhibition. Routine urine drug screening does not show GHB, but GHB can be detected if a GHB-specific test is requested.

Results of high doses of GHB range from dizziness to death. Common symptoms of overdose of GHB are respiratory depression, memory loss, bradycardia, muscular fatigue, and coma. The adverse effects of GHB can be devastating. When combined with alcohol, deaths are more prevalent. Anyone presenting at the emergency department in a coma of unknown origin must be evaluated for GHB use.

The nurse needs to be skillful in assessing the client who has taken an overdose of GHB because of the legal ramifications of the drug. Using an open, nonjudgmental approach is necessary to develop a trusting and honest communication. Reactions in the person taking GHB vary with each use and may confuse the client with these different responses.

Barbiturates

Barbiturates are drugs that depress the CNS through action in the cerebral cortex and the reticular formation (helps regulate the sleep-wake cycle). Effects of barbiturates include sedation, drowsiness, and a decrease in motor activity of the body similar to those seen with alcohol use. Therapeutic uses of barbiturates are short-term insomnia, preanesthesia, and anticonvulsant therapy. Because of the aging process, older adults can tolerate only small doses of barbiturates. Dependence on barbiturates can occur in a short time and can lead to withdrawal symptoms if the drug is discontinued abruptly. Initial withdrawal symptoms are anxiety, restlessness, insomnia, irritability, and impaired attention with more severe symptoms if the person has a chronic pattern of use. Physical illness may accompany the withdrawal of barbiturates with nausea, vomiting, abdominal cramping, seizures, and varied behavioral responses. With severe dependence, the effects of withdrawal can be life threatening. Toxic or overdose symptoms include respiratory depression, coma, and pinpoint pupils. Laboratory testing for barbiturates can be done by direct immunoassay from blood, urine, or gastric contents.

Nursing interventions for the client in crisis due to overdose or withdrawal of barbiturates are to ensure safety through frequent vital signs, neurologic checks, and emotional support. Symptomatic treatment such as drug tapering is necessary to avoid the more severe response to drug elimination. Food, fluids, and a calm environment are necessary to achieve the initial outcomes for the client. Because barbiturates are constipating, monitor the client for elimination patterns, being sure to provide high fiber in the diet. Immediate and long-term care of the person with physical addiction requires various members of the health care team to treat and support the planning and implementation of holistic care.

Alcohol

OVERVIEW

Alcohol in various mixed drinks, beer, wine, and liquor provides sedation, relaxation, and release of a person's inhibitions. A substantial number of people in the United States drink alcoholic beverages. For most people, alcohol is used for a pleasure experience. Alcohol acts as a depressant on the CNS and the respiratory system; therefore the signs and symptoms of the effects of alcohol use are primarily neurologic. One of every 13 adults in the United States abuses alcohol (Stewart & Richards, 2003).

Alcoholism (alcohol dependence syndrome) is a disease wherein the person has a strong need or compulsion to consume alcohol, is unable to quit once he or she begins drinking, experiences a physical dependence, and has a need to increase the amount of alcohol to get "high" (high tolerance). Physical dependence occurs when the person experiences withdrawal after alcohol use is stopped after a period of heavy drinking. When drinking alcohol relieves the symptoms of withdrawal, the person has developed a true physical dependence on alcohol, and is considered an alcoholic (Figure 8-2).

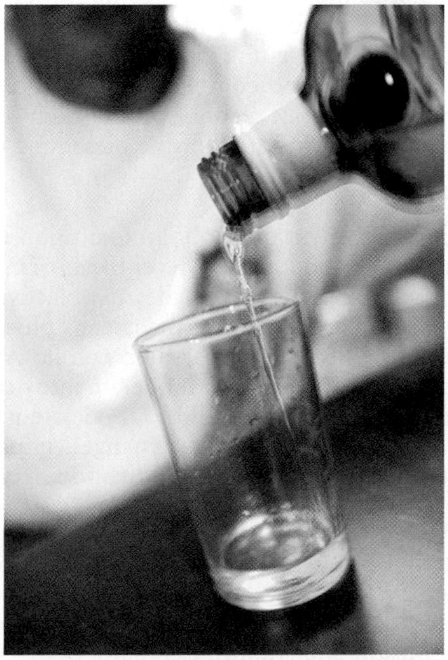

Figure 8-2 ■ Alcohol is commonly used for pleasure and acts as a central nervous system depressant.

Alcohol abuse exists when a person *does not* have a strong craving for alcohol, loss of control, or physical dependence but has problems related to alcohol use. Examples of alcohol abuse are when the person fails to fulfill responsibilities at home, work, or school; when the person drinks in unsafe situations; when the person experiences legal problems that are alcohol related, or when the person continues to drink when problems have been caused or worsened by use of alcohol. When one or more of these events occur within a 12-month period, the person is abusing alcohol.

CONSIDERATIONS FOR OLDER ADULTS

Older adults also face risks for alcohol-related problems. The risk for intoxication and serious drug interactions is increased when alcohol is used in combination with other drugs. Older adults may have experienced a longer history of alcohol use and are at greater risk for severe withdrawal.

Because of the "normal" aging processes, sometimes there is confusion in identification of alcohol withdrawal from expected changes in the aging population. Societal expectations and morés of the older population may make obtaining an accurate substance use history difficult. In treatment of the older person in withdrawal, treatment regimens need to take into consideration the change in function of the aging body. Generally the treatment of the older adult employs adjusted dosages of medications to avoid oversedation and close monitoring for subtle physiologic changes.

COLLABORATIVE MANAGEMENT

Nursing care of the person with alcohol problems or alcoholism is a challenge related to the will of the person and the motivation to reduce or stop alcohol consumption. The person with alcohol problems presents in the emergency department for emergency care when alcohol has been a contributing factor to the situation or a complication to the reason for which the person presents for treatment. The nurse in the medical-surgical setting must be knowledgeable about the signs, symptoms, and complications of alcohol use because of the influence of alcohol on the body and the increase of risk during treatment of the presenting condition.

Assessment

An objective assessment of alcohol intoxication is obtained from obtaining a blood alcohol level (BAL). This measurement is important because it provides an objective reference in which to anticipate severity of the client's physical status.

Toxic levels of alcohol are classified as follows:

- 80 to 200 mg/dL (mild to moderate intoxication). Behaviors consistent with mild to moderate intoxication include mood and behavior changes, impaired judgment, and poor motor coordination. Hypotension may occur in clients with levels greater than 100 mg/dL (Pagana & Pagana, 2002).
- 250 to 400 mg/dL (marked intoxication). Observations noted with this level of intoxication are staggering ataxia and emotional lability. Symptoms may progress to confusion and stupor or coma.
- Greater than 500 mg/dL (severe intoxication). Death is due to respiratory depression.

CHART 8-1

KEY FEATURES of

Disease: Typical Signs and Symptoms of Clients in Alcohol Withdrawal

Objective Symptoms	Subjective Signs
Tremors	No appetite
Jerky movements	Reports "shaking inside"
Vomiting	Nausea
Diaphoresis, tenting skin	Delusional
Undernourished	Hallucinating
Dehydrated	
Increased pulse and blood pressure	
Disoriented to place, time	

The most threatening result of alcohol abuse or alcoholism is withdrawal from the substance. Symptoms of withdrawal range from mild to severe and can progress to death. Alcohol withdrawal can be evaluated by categories according to severity:

- *Minor withdrawal*–restlessness, anxiety, sleeping difficulties, agitation and tremors, tachycardia, low-grade fever, diaphoresis, and elevated blood pressure
- *Major withdrawal*–in addition to the signs and symptoms of mild withdrawal, visual or auditory hallucinations, tremors of the entire body (**delirium tremens,** or **DTs**), heart rate greater than 100 beats/min, diastolic pressure above 100 mm Hg, pronounced diaphoresis, and vomiting
- *Life-threatening withdrawal*–delirium tremens, disorientation times, global confusion, and inability to recognize familiar objects or people

The life-threatening stage of alcohol withdrawal has a 2% to 5% mortality rate, requiring emergency medical interventions. Alcohol seizures may occur 12 to 48 hours after the last drink.

Interventions

When the client is experiencing withdrawal of alcohol–or another depressant–the priority for care is to prevent the client from harming himself or herself or others. Attempt to reorient him or her to reality frequently. The health care provider often prescribes medications to calm or sedate the client according to agency protocol or physician preference. Examples of typical drugs that are used are benzodiazepines, such as chlordiazepoxide (Librium) and diazepam (Valium), to prevent seizures and DTs. Other commonly used drugs include beta-blockers to reduce cravings and decrease pulse and blood pressure, and alpha-adrenergic blockers to decrease withdrawal symptoms. Table 8-2 lists some of the most commonly used medications for alcohol withdrawal. Intravenous fluids and vitamins, such as thiamine, are also prescribed. In collaboration with the dietitian, plan ways to increase protein and calories to address the client's nutritional needs.

Nursing care for the client with alcohol use or abuse includes thorough assessment to identify dependence and frequency of use. Chart 8-1 lists common objective and subjective signs and symptoms of clients in alcohol withdrawal. Chart 8-2 includes nursing activities that you should implement when caring for a client in alcohol withdrawal.

Clients who are alcoholic and their families require extensive rehabilitation and support. Collaborate with the case manager, social worker, or discharge planner to ensure

CHART 8-2

NIC INTERVENTION ACTIVITIES for The Client in Alcohol Withdrawal

Substance Use Treatment: Alcohol Withdrawal: *Care of the client experiencing sudden cessation of alcohol consumption*

- Create a low-stimulation environment.
- Monitor vital signs during withdrawal.
- Monitor for delirium tremens (DTs).
- Administer anticonvulsants or sedatives, as appropriate.
- Medicate to relieve physical discomfort, as needed.
- Address hallucinations in a therapeutic manner.
- Maintain adequate nutrition and fluid intake.
- Administer vitamin therapy as appropriate.
- Provide emotional support to client/family, as appropriate.
- Provide reality orientation, as appropriate.

NIC intervention activities selected from Dochterman, J.M., & Bulechek, G.M. (Eds.) (2004). *Nursing interventions classification (NIC)* (4th ed.). St. Louis: Mosby. No part of this work is to be altered without prior written permission from the Publisher.

that the client and family members are aware of community resources such as Alcoholics Anonymous for clients and Al-Anon for family members and friends. If these programs fail, aversion therapy with disulfiram (Antabuse) may be an option for treatment. Mental health/behavioral health texts discuss psychosocial support and alcohol abuse treatment in more detail.

NARCOTICS: OPIOIDS AND MORPHINE DERIVATIVES

OVERVIEW

Narcotic is a broad term encompassing all drugs that are made from the Asian poppy or produced as a synthetic drug which produces the same effects of the opium plant. A desired (therapeutic) action of narcotics is to reduce the client's perception of pain. Drugs included in this category are codeine, morphine, heroin, methadone, hydromorphone (Dilaudid), meperidine (Demerol), and oxycodone, (OxyContin). These drugs are therapeutically used for relief of severe pain, such as pain experienced in terminal cancer or postoperative pain. Sleep is an added feature of the drug when it is used for pain. Opium and morphine derivatives have become drugs of dependence because of their analgesic and euphoric effects. Common names for heroin and opium in the drug community are "horse" and "smack" for heroin and "Dover's powder" for opium. The sites of action of these drugs are in the brain, binding in the receptor sites of the CNS (causing CNS depression) and in the gastrointestinal system (producing the antidiarrheal effects of opium; Lomotil). Desired effects of substance abuse with these drugs are the escape effect in the mind and analgesia. Aggression and sexual drives are usually minimized with use of the opioids and morphine-like drugs.

A high potential for addiction, tolerance, and dependence occurs with this class of drugs. The withdrawal effects can range from mild withdrawal symptoms to death. According to the National Institute on Drug Abuse, there are four categories of opiate withdrawal (Mathias, 2000):

- Grade 0 is characterized by drug craving, anxiety, and drug-seeking behaviors.
- Grade 1 is characterized by yawning, sweating, lacrimation, and rhinorrhea ("runny nose").
- Grade 2 is characterized by mydriasis (pupillary dilation), gooseflesh, muscle twitching, and anorexia.
- Grade 3, the most dangerous of the grades in opiate withdrawal, is characterized by increased pulse, respiratory rate, and blood pressure; abdominal cramps; diarrhea; vomiting; and weakness.

These drugs may be taken orally, injected, or inhaled. Heroin, a highly addictive drug, is an opiate derivative. Unlike the other opiate drugs noted earlier, heroin has no medical use. The health hazards of heroin are serious and include fatal overdoses and spontaneous abortions. Intravenous use of heroin or other abused substances increases the risk of acquiring infectious diseases such as human immunodeficiency virus infection (HIV) and hepatitis. Short-term effects of heroin are felt immediately and continue for a few hours after a single dose. Heroin users report an immediate feeling of extreme euphoria ("rush"). The person experiences a dry mouth, heavy extremities, and a warm, flushed feeling. Generally, there are alternate sensations of wakefulness and sleep. Common street names for heroin are "horse," "smack," "H," "skag," and "junk." Long-term use of heroin results in many physical problems, such as emaciation, frequent infections, cellulitis, and liver disease. Morphine, heroin, and codeine use can be identified in the urine from 2 hours after ingestion up to 3 days after use.

COLLABORATIVE MANAGEMENT

Care of the client with an opiate or heroin addiction becomes complex because of the physical condition, the addictive behaviors, and the safety concerns both physically and psychologically. The nurse must have an understanding of the withdrawal symptoms to be aware of the severity of the medical condition created by withdrawal from opiates and their derivatives. Implications include the need for current information about addictions and the addictive drug cycle, both physically and mentally.

Assessment

When possible, determine the client's history of drug use, drug of choice, and the last ingestion. A small percentage of clients become addicted to opioids while being treated for severe, chronic pain. For example, clients with sickle cell anemia have episodes of extreme pain during exacerbations of their disease and require large amounts of pain medication.

Three major problems that require emergency intervention may occur when opiates are used: intoxication, overdose, and withdrawal. Assessment findings for each of these conditions are listed in Chart 8-3.

Interventions

Anticonvulsant drugs are commonly prescribed to prevent seizures. Other medications, such as naloxone (Narcan) and naltrexone (ReVia), work as opioid antagonists, competing with opioids at the receptor sites. Midazolam (Versed) may also be given to induce amnesic effects; anxiety-reducing medications (anxiolytics) help to relieve anxiety. In some cases of severe dependence, methadone is prescribed to relieve pain. Other medications may be given to treat symptoms such as diarrhea or nausea.

Provide supportive measures for the client, including nonpharmacologic measures to relieve pain, reduce stimuli, and provide basic comfort measures. Monitor vital signs

CHART 8-3

KEY FEATURES of
Disease: Manifestations of Opiate Use That Require Emergency Interventions

Opiate Intoxication
- Constricted pupils
- Decreased blood pressure
- Decreased respirations
- Drowsiness
- Slurred speech
- Initial euphoria followed by dysphoria (depression)
- Cognitive impairments resulting in judgment and memory losses

Opiate Overdose
- Dilated pupils
- Respiratory depression
- Coma
- Shock
- Convulsions
- Respiratory arrest
- Death

Opiate Withdrawal
- Yawning
- Insomnia
- Irritability
- Rhinorrhea
- Diaphoresis
- Abdominal cramps
- Nausea and vomiting
- Muscle aches
- Chills, cold flashes with goose bumps (referred to as "cold turkey")

frequently and assess for major changes. Pay special attention to alterations in respiratory rate or pattern.

INHALANTS

Breathable chemical vapors that produce psychoactive effects are called **inhalants.** These substances are popular with young people because of their accessibility (in the home) and price. Three categories of inhalants are common household items. **Solvents** produce a "high" when inhaled. Examples of solvents are paint thinners, gasoline, glues, paper correction fluid, felt-tip markers, and electronic contact cleaners. **Gases** are another source of inhalants and include products such as butane lighters, propane tanks, whipping cream aerosols, spray paints, hair or deodorant sprays, chloroform, ether, and nitrous oxide (laughing gas). **Nitrites** are the third source of inhalants and include cyclohexyl nitrite, amyl nitrite, and butyl nitrite. The terms most readily referring to inhalant use are "glue," "kick," "bang," "sniff," "huffing," "poppers," "whippets," and "Texas Shoeshine."

Inhalants produce anesthetic results, consequently slowing body functions. Persons who use inhalants feel intoxicated, less inhibited, and less in control with repeated use. They may inhale to the point of causing unconsciousness. Sniffing highly concentrated chemicals can result in death from cardiac failure. Suffocation can also occur because the inhalant takes the place of oxygen in the lungs and respirations cease. Irreversible effects, including hearing losses, limb spasms, brain damage, and bone marrow suppression, can occur from inhalants. Reversible effects that can occur with inhalants include liver and kidney damage and blood oxygen depletion. Pouring or dispensing the inhalant into a paper bag increases the concentration of the substance, inducing a quicker, more pronounced effect.

Signs of inhalant use follow:
- Slurred speech
- Drunk, dizzy, or dazed appearance
- Chemical smell on the person
- Paint stains on body or face
- Red eyes
- Rhinorrhea

You may come in contact with young adults who have had experience with inhalants. These clients may have been admitted to the hospital for complications of inhalant use or because of medical conditions. Once the client is stabilized, try to determine with the client the reasons for his or her use of inhalants. Management and treatment of chemical ingestions is supportive. There are known antidotes available for inhalant overdose or toxicity.

STEROIDS

Anabolic-androgenic steroids are growing in popularity among young athletes. The term *anabolic* indicates muscle building, and the term *androgenic* refers to increased masculinity. Anabolic steroids are synthetic substances that mimic the actions of testosterone. Steroids are legally available through prescription use for people with hormonal difficulties such as delayed puberty or impotence. Athletes are known to use steroids to increase strength and performance even when it is known to be unhealthy, life threatening, and illegal for use in amateur, professional, and international events. The pressure to become stronger, to achieve, and to succeed many times tempts the person to use steroids to "bulk up" for mastery in selected sports. Misuse of steroids can lead to serious medical problems, some of which are irreversible. Possible effects of steroids include the following:
- For men: shrinking testicles, reduced sperm count, infertility, baldness, development of breasts, and an increased risk for cancer
- For women: growth of facial hair, male pattern baldness, changes or cessation of menses, enlargement of the clitoris, and deepened voice
- For adolescents: premature skeletal maturation and accelerated puberty changes

Aggression is increased by the use of steroids. In addition, there may be a noted increase in mental illness as a result of mood disturbances. Discontinuation of steroids can result in depression.

GET READY for the NCLEX Examination!

KEY POINTS

- Substance abuse interferes with life's activities, which can endanger the client when hospitalized; therefore a complete drug history is essential in identification of substance abuse in the hospitalized client.
- Common drugs of abuse are stimulants, hallucinogens, depressants, opioids, inhalants, and steroids.

- Research findings indicate a link between genetics and substance use. Personality traits are thought to be contributing factors to substance abuse.
- Nursing care of the person using substances must consider the developmental stage, cultural background, and social environment when developing a plan of care for the client.
- Stimulants increase mental alertness, improve a person's sense of well-being, increase the capacity to work, improve performance of motor skills, and increase metabolism through increased respiratory and cardiac function. Examples of stimulants common in the drug culture are amphetamines, methamphetamines, cocaine, and nicotine.
- The following are common slang terms for illicit amphetamine substances:
  - Amphetamines: "crosses," "hearts," "black beauties"
  - Methamphetamines: "crank," "crystal," "ice," "glass," "speed," "chalk"
  - Cocaine: "coke," "snow," "flake," "rocks," "crack"
- Symptoms of stimulant use that require emergency interventions are elevated vital signs (including temperature), dehydration, and neurologic changes, including convulsions or coma.
- Medications common in the treatment of overdose or withdrawal of stimulants include antipsychotics, antiparkinsonism agents, antidepressants, antianxiety medications, and intravenous therapy.
- Hallucinogenic substances, which create an alteration in perception and a subsequent euphoria, include LSD, PCP, ketamine, MDMA (ecstasy), and marijuana. Effects of hallucinogenic substances, such as enhanced sexual arousal, create a safety risk for the person who uses because of the euphoria and false sense of abilities experienced.
- PCP creates a feeling of detachment; referred to as "angel dust," PCP is an animal tranquilizer that creates numbing effects on the mind.
- Depressants, including benzodiazepines, gamma hydroxybutyrate (GHB), barbiturates, alcohol, and narcotics, are among the most popular abused substances.
- Barbiturates are commonly referred to as "barbs" and "ludes"; clients can develop physical withdrawal if they abruptly stop these drugs.
- Alcohol withdrawal is classified as minor, major, and life threatening. Life-threatening symptoms of alcohol withdrawal are delirium tremens (DTs), disorientation, global confusion, and inability to recognize familiar objects or persons.
- Interventions for acute alcohol withdrawal are administration of sedatives, vitamins, magnesium sulfate, anticonvulsants, and folic acid (see Chart 8-2).
- Chart 8-3 summarizes clinical manifestations of alcohol withdrawal that require emergency interventions.
- Minor to moderate symptoms of opiate or narcotic withdrawal are yawning, insomnia, irritability, rhinorrhea, diaphoresis, chills, and "goose bumps."
- The most dangerous grade of opiate withdrawal is characterized by increased pulse and respiratory rates, increased blood pressure, abdominal cramps, diarrhea, vomiting, and weakness. This condition requires emergency intervention to prevent death.
- Interventions for symptoms associated with narcotic withdrawal range from supportive care to use of IV fluids, anticonvulsants, opioid antagonists, methadone substitution, clonidine, and midazolam hydrochloride (Versed).
- Inhalants are used by children and adolescents because of their easy availability; inhalants induce the following effects: slurred speech, drunkenness, dizzy or dazed appearance, red eyes, and rhinorrhea. There may be a chemical odor present or paint smears on the face.
- Inhalants create anesthetic results and slow body functions resulting in feelings of intoxication.
- "Sniffing" can result in unconsciousness and suffocation due to competition for air space in the lungs between the inhalant and oxygen.
- Irreversible effects from inhalant use are limb spasms, brain damage, and hearing loss. Nursing care of the person having used inhalants is symptomatic and supportive.
- Continuous steroid use is found primarily in athletes to build strength and muscle mass. Routine drug screens are helpful in detecting steroids or other drugs that may enhance the athletic ability of a participant.

ADDITIONAL STUDY RESOURCES

Go to your Student CD-ROM for Review Questions for the NCLEX Examination.

evolve Go to http://evolve.elsevier.com/Iggy/ for Integrated Management of Care Questions for the NCLEX Examination.

SELECTED BIBLIOGRAPHY

Asterisk indicates a classic or definitive work on this subject.

Acello, B. (2000). Controlling pain, facing fears about opioid addiction, *Nursing 2000, 30*(5), 72.

American Nurses Association. (2001). *Code for nurses with interpretative statements.* Washington, DC: American Nurses Association.

Club Drugs: Emergency Room Update, (2001) *SAMHSA News* 9(2), 7-8,

Compton, P. (2002) Caring for an alcohol-dependent patient. *Nursing, 32*(12), 58-63.

Elimination of substance abuse in young people. (2002). International Council of Nurses Position Statement. Available at http://www.icn.ch/psabuse.htm.

Gill, M. (2003). MDMA toxicity: The influence of metabolic genotype at CYP2D6. Available at http://www.tcd.ie/Research/projects/drugs/analsci.html.

*Greenblant, J. (1997). Gamma hydroxy butyrate (GHB) abuse in the United States, SAMHSA, OAS Working Paper. Rockville, MD: SAMHSA's Clearinghouse for Alcohol and Drug Abuse.

Hardie, T. (2002). The genetics of substance abuse. *AACN Clinical Issues, 13*(4), 511-522.

Inhalants: Most popular drug for 12-year-olds. (2001). *SAMHSA News*, 23.

Lehne, R. (2001). *Pharmacology for nursing care* (4th ed.). Philadelphia: W.B. Saunders.

Lesher, A. (2000). A club drug alert. *NIDA, 14*(6), 1-4.

Ludwick, R.E., et al. (2000). Alcohol use in elderly women: Nursing considerations in community settings. *Journal of Gerontological Nursing, 26*(2), 44-49.

Malseed, R. (2004). *Nurse's drug guide.* (5th ed.). Philadelphia: Lippincott Williams & Wilkins.

Marijuana abuse. (2002). *National Institute on Drug Abuse: Research Report Series.* National Institutes of Health Publication No. 03-3859, U.S. Department of Health and Human Services. Available at http://drugabuse.gov/PDF/RRmarijuana.pdf.

Martin, K. (2002). Combining medications may be effective treatment for "speedball" abuse. *NIDA Notes, 17*(3), 11.

Mathias, R. (2000). Cocaine, marijuana, and heroin use up, methamphetamine abuse down. Available at http://drugabuse.gov.

McCloskey, J. (2003). *Unifying nursing languages: The harmonization of NANDA, NIC, and NOC.* Washington, DC: American Nurses Association.

Mioto, K., & Roth, B. (2002). GHB: A club drug to watch. *Substance Abuse Treatment Advisory, 2*(1).

Monitoring the Futures Survey Released, *HHS News (*2001).12.19: Media Advisory, 1-5. Available at www.drugabuse.gov/MedAdv/01/NR12-19.html.

National Institute on Drug Abuse, National Institute of Health, U.S. Department of Health and Human Services. (2003). Available at http://www.nida.nih.gov.

National Priorities II: Healing America's drug users national drug control strategy: 2002. Available at http://www.whitehousedrugpolicy.gov/publicatios/policy/03ndcs/2priorities.html.

Pagana, K., Pagana, T. (2002). *Mosby's manual of diagnostic and laboratory tests.* (2nd ed.). St. Louis: Mosby.

*Perkins, S. (1999). *Drug identification: Designer and club drugs quick reference guide.* Knoxville, TN: Alliance Press.

*Position statement: Abuse of prescription drugs. (1997). Washington, DC: American Nurses Association.

Principles of drug addiction treatment. (2000). Washington, DC: National Institute on Drug Abuse.

Sachse, D. (2000). Emergency: Delirium tremens. *American Journal of Nursing, 100*(5), 41-42.

**Standards of addictions: Nursing practice with selected diagnoses and criteria.* (1988). Washington, DC: American Nurses Association.

Stewart, K.B., & Richards, A.B. (2000). Recognizing and managing your patient's alcohol abuse. *Nursing 2000, 30*(2), 56-59.

*Stocker, S. (1999). Studies link stress and drug addiction. *NIDA Notes, 14*(1), 1-4.

Substance abuse increases in New York City in aftermath of September 11th. (2002). *NIDA.* Available at http://www.drugabuse.gov/Newsroom/02/NR5-28.html.

Substance abuse predicting it, preventing it. (2001). *SAMHSA News 9*(2), 1-27.

Substance abuse treatment advisory, GHB: A club drug to watch. (2002). U.S. Department of Health and Human Services. Available at http://www.samhsa.gov.

Teen smoking dropped dramatically in 2002. (2003). *NIDA Notes, 17*(6).

Tips for teens: The truth about inhalants. (2001). Center for Substance Abuse Prevention, Substance Abuse and Mental Health Services Administration. Available at http://www.health.org.

Tipton, D. (2003). Assessment of the neurotoxicity of "ecstasy." Biochemistry/pharmacology. Available at http://www.tcd.ie/Research/projects/drugs/analsci.html.

Use of marijuana, cocaine, pain relievers and tranquilizers increases according to national household survey on drug abuse. (2002). *NHSDA, 9*(5).

Varcarolis, E. (2002). *Foundations of psychiatric mental health nursing: A clinical approach.* (4th ed.). Philadelphia: W.B. Saunders.

*Viera, A. (1999). Toxic ingestion of gamma-hydroxybutyric acid. *Southern Medical Journal, 92*(4), 404-405.

Williams, J. (2002). Prenatal exposure to ecstasy may impair memory and cognition. *NIDA Notes,* 17(3), 8-9.

Youth marijuana admissions by race and ethnicity. (2002). *The DASIS report, 9*(2), 1-4. Available at http://www.samhsa.gov/.

Zerwekh, J., & Claborn, J. (2003). *Nursing today: Transitions and trends.* (4th ed.). St. Louis: W.B. Saunders.

Zickler, P. (2002). Brain imaging studies show long-term damage from amphetamine use. *NIDA Notes, 15*(3).

Zickler, P. (2002). Cannabinoid antagonist reduces marijuana's effects in humans. *NIDA Notes, 17*(3), 1, 10.

Zickler, P.(2002) NIDA initiative targets increasing teen use of anabolic steroids. *NIDA Notes, 15*(3), 1, 6.

Zickler, P. (2002). Study demonstrates that marijuana smokers experience significant withdrawal. *NIDA Notes, 17*(3), 7.

CHAPTER 9

End-of-Life Care

MARY K. KAZANOWSKI

LEARNING OUTCOMES

After studying this chapter, you should be able to:

1. Describe the pathophysiology of death.
2. Explain the purpose for advance directives.
3. Discuss the philosophies of palliative and hospice care.
4. Describe the role of the nurse and the interdisciplinary team in end-of-life care.
5. Interpret the common physical and emotional signs of impending death.
6. Identify common symptoms of distress near death.
7. Prioritize interventions for symptoms experienced by the client near death.
8. Describe common psychosocial issues for clients and their families near death.
9. Develop a plan of care to assist clients and families in coping with the dying process.
10. Explain how variations in culture and religious beliefs can impact the experience of dying and death.
11. Describe care of the client after death.
12. Discuss the ethical and legal obligations of the nurse with regard to end-of-life care.

Go to your Student CD-ROM for Review Questions for the NCLEX Examination keyed to these Learning Outcomes.

OVERVIEW OF DEATH AND DYING

Death occurs when the lungs and heart cease to function. In general, death is caused by an illness or trauma that overwhelms the compensatory mechanisms of the body. Direct causes of death include respiratory failure and shock, which results in lack of blood flow to meet the demands of vital organs such as the kidneys, brain, and heart.

Multiple Organ Dysfunction Syndrome

Inadequate blood flow to body tissues deprives cells of their source of oxygen, which leads to anaerobic metabolism with acidosis, hyperkalemia, and tissue ischemia. Dramatic changes in vital organs lead to release of toxic metabolites and destructive enzymes. This sequence referred to as **multiple organ dysfunction syndrome (MODS).**

MODS occurs first in the liver, heart, brain, and kidney. MODS also occurs in the lungs in clients with septicemia. A lethal dysrhythmia such as ventricular fibrillation, asystole, or pulseless electrical activity can occur at any point during the process of shock and/or hypoxemia, which ultimately leads to the cessation of cardiac output. Shortly after cardiac arrest, respiratory arrest occurs. When respiratory arrest occurs first, cardiac arrest follows within minutes.

Clinical death refers to the short interval after the cessation of heartbeat and breathing when no evidence of brain function is present. If this termination of function occurs suddenly, as in cardiac arrest or massive hemorrhage, a brief time remains before vital organs lose their viability. Initiation of cardiopulmonary resuscitation (CPR) at this time may be successful in a person with healthy organs. However, CPR is likely to be futile in those with terminal disease.

Incidence of Death

Dying is part of the normal life cycle and more than 2.5 million people die in the United States each year. The most common causes of death in the United States are coronary artery disease and cancer.

Almost 80% of people who die are age 65 years or older (Sheehan & Schirm, 2003). Most of these deaths occur after long, progressively debilitating chronic illnesses, such as cancer, cardiac disease, renal disease, and lung disease. Only 25% of all deaths take place at home, with about 50% occurring in hospitals. The remaining 25% occur in nursing homes, but that number is expected to double by 2020 (Sheehan & Schirm, 2003).

Death as a Natural Process

The U.S. health system is based on the acute care model, which is focused on prevention, early detection, and cure of disease. This focus along with advances in health care makes it difficult for many clients and health care providers to accept death as an outcome of disease. Many view death as a failure of treatment.

These views have led to a major deficiency in the care and quality of life for many Americans at the end of life. In 1995, a landmark study highlighted the poor quality of dying that hospitalized clients experienced at the end of their lives. This SUPPORT study showed that more than 50% of a sample of 9105 individuals with a life-threatening disease had moderate to severe pain during the last days of their lives. In addition, they did not have their wishes met, even when they were made known.

As a result of the SUPPORT study, a major initiative was undertaken to improve care at the end of life. The Institute of Medicine was commissioned to study the problem. Core curricula on end-of-life care were developed and implemented to educate medical and nursing students, physicians, and nurses. These courses focus on death as a natural process and provide information on how to ensure quality end-of-life care. In 1998, the American Association of Colleges of Nursing (AACN) published "Peaceful Death," which outlined 15 undergraduate nursing competencies for providing quality end-of-life care (Table 9-1).

The Institute of Medicine's report on Improving Care at the End of Life addresses the deficiencies in our health care system and its care of dying clients. It concluded that each health care facility should be held accountable for identifying its shortcomings and devising strategies to improve the quality and consistency of care at the end of life. One strategy that has been implemented in select hospitals has been the development of a palliative care team or unit, staffed by nurses and physicians with expertise in end-of-life care.

End-of-life care in long-term care settings has not been addressed in most facilities. In general, the assessment tools (e.g., Minimum Data Set) and regulations for nursing homes do not guide care for residents who are dying. Most staff members are not trained in end-of-life care despite the expected increase in terminally ill residents over the next 10 to 15 years (Sheehan & Schirm, 2003).

TABLE 9-1 Peaceful Death AACN Undergraduate Nursing Competencies

1. Recognize dynamic changes in population demographics, health care economics, and service delivery that necessitate improved professional preparation for end-of-life care.
2. Promote the provision of comfort care to the dying as an active, desirable, and important skill, and an integral component of nursing care.
3. Communicate effectively and compassionately with the client, family, and health care team members about end-of-life issues.
4. Recognize one's own attitudes, feelings, values, and expectations about death and the individual, cultural, and spiritual diversity existing in these beliefs and customs.
5. Demonstrate respect for the client's views and wishes during end-of-life care.
6. Collaborate with interdisciplinary team members while implementing the nursing role in end-of-life care.
7. Use scientifically based standardized tools to assess symptoms experienced by clients at the end of life.
8. Use data from symptom assessment to plan and intervene in symptom management using state-of-the-art traditional approaches.
9. Evaluate the impact of traditional, complementary, and technologic therapies on client-centered outcomes.
10. Assess and treat multiple dimensions, including physical, psychological, social, and spiritual needs, to improve quality of care at the end of life.
11. Assist the client, family, colleagues, and one's self to cope with suffering, grief, loss, and bereavement in end-of-life care.
12. Apply legal and ethical principles in the analysis of complex issues in end-of-life care, recognizing the influence of personal values, professional codes, and client preferences.
13. Identify barriers and facilitators to clients' and caregivers' effective use of resources.
14. Demonstrate skill at implementing a plan for improved end-of-life care within a dynamic and complex health care delivery system.
15. Apply knowledge gained from palliative care research to end-of-life education and care.

Palliative Care

Palliative care is a philosophy that provides a compassionate and supportive approach to clients and families who are living with life-threatening illnesses. This holistic approach neither hastens nor postpones death, but provides relief of symptoms experienced by the dying client (Matzo & Sherman, 2001b). Relieving symptoms, while providing emotional and spiritual support improves the quality of care at the end of life.

THE END-OF-LIFE EXPERIENCE

Advance Directives

An **advance directive** is a written document prepared by a competent individual that specifies what, if any, extraordinary actions a person would want when he or she can no longer make decisions about personal health care. Advance directives such as the durable power of attorney (DPOA) for health care and the living will are usually completed long before a medical crisis. A **DPOA for health care** is a legal document in which a person appoints someone else to make his or her health care decisions in the event he or she becomes incapable of making decisions (Figure 9-1). A **living will** is also a legal document that instructs physicians and family members about what life-sustaining treatment one does or does not want at some future time if a person becomes unable to make decisions.

The Patient Self-Determination Act of 1990 requires that all clients admitted to health care agencies be asked if they have drafted advance directives. Clients who have not drafted advance directives should be given information about the process and the implications of having (or not having) these in place, and should be assisted in drafting them. Nurses should document any discussion regarding a person's decision related to end-of-life care.

Advance directives guide physicians in planning care for seriously ill individuals. If the client has advanced or terminal disease and has indicated that he or she does not want cardiopulmonary resuscitation (CPR) performed, then the physician can initiate a "do not resuscitate" (DNR) order. However, most Americans do not have advance directives in place. Many physicians do not discuss a person's wishes for end-of-life care. Nurses are often in the position of initiating discussions with clients about their wishes regarding CPR, especially when their condition declines quickly. Most agencies require that CPR be initiated on clients whose breathing or heartbeat has ceased unless a physician's order of "do not resuscitate" (DNR) is obtained.

DURABLE POWER OF ATTORNEY FOR HEALTH CARE

Power of Attorney made this __________ day of __________, 20____

1. I, the undersigned hereby appoint (insert name and address of agent)

____

as agent to act for me and in my name to make any and all decisions for me concerning my personal care, medical treatment, hospitalization and health care and to require, withhold or withdraw any type of medical treatment or procedure, even though my death may ensue. My agent shall have the same access to my medical records that I have, including the right to disclose the contents to others. My agent shall also have full power to make a disposition of any part or all of my body for medical purposes, authorize an autopsy and direct the disposition of my remains. (Neither the attending physician nor any other health care provider may act as your agent.)

2. The powers granted above shall be subject to the following rules or limitations (if none, leave blank):

____

____

(The subject of life-sustaining treatment is of particular importance. For your convenience in dealing with that subject some general statements concerning the withholding or removal of life-sustaining treatment are set forth below. If you agree with one of these statements, you may initial that statement; but do not initial more than one.)

(I do not want my life to be prolonged nor do I want life-sustaining treatment
(to be provided or continued if my agent believes the burdens of the treatment
(outweigh the expected benefits. I want my agent to consider the relief of
(suffering the expense involved and the quality as well as the possible extension
______(of my life in making decisions concerning life-sustaining treatment.

(I want my life to be prolonged and I want life-sustaining treatment to be
(provided or continued unless I am in a coma which my attending physician
(believes to be irreversible, in accordance with reasonable medical standards at
(the time of reference. If and when I have suffered irreversible coma, I want
______(life-sustaining treatment to be withheld or discontinued.

(I want my life to be prolonged to the greatest extent possible without regard to
______(my condition, the chances I have for recovery or the cost of the procedures.

3. This power of attorney shall become effective on ______________________

____

4. This power of attorney shall terminate on ______________________

____

5. If any agent named by me shall die, become legally disabled, resign, refuse to act or be unavailable, I name the following (each to act alone and successively, in the order named) as successors to such agent:

____

____

6. If a guardian of my person is to be appointed, I nominate the following to serve as such guardian (if same as agent, leave blank):

____

Figure 9-1 ■ An example of a durable power of attorney for health care.

Continued

7. I am fully informed as to all the contents of this form and understand the full import of this grant of power to my agent.

Signed ______________________________
Principal

The principal has had an opportunity to read the above form and has signed the form or acknowledged his or her signature or mark on the form in my presence.

______________________ Residing at ______________________
Witness

(You may, but are not required to, request your agent and successor agents to provide specimen signature below. If you include specimen signature in this Power of Attorney, you must complete the certification opposite the signatures of the agents.)

Specimen signatures of agent (and successors)	**I certify that the signature of my agent (and successors) are correct.**
______________________ **(agent)**	______________________ **(principal)**
______________________ **(successor agent)**	______________________ **(principal)**
______________________ **(successor agent)**	______________________ **(principal)**

Figure 9-1, *cont'd* ■ An example of a durable power of attorney for health care.

It is now believed that CPR causes pain and that it interferes with a person's ability to have a "good death." A good death is one that is free from avoidable distress and suffering for clients, families, and caregivers; one that is in accord with the client's and family's wishes; and one that is reasonably consistent with clinical, cultural, and ethical standards.

Goals for End-of-Life Care

The goals of care for a client near the end of life are as follows:

- Control symptoms
- Identify client needs
- Promote meaningful interactions between the client and significant others
- Facilitate a peaceful death

Interventions that attend to the physical, psychological, social, and spiritual needs of clients require an interdisciplinary approach to care that is accessible and committed to these goals. The interdisciplinary care of hospice is the most successful approach to end-of-life care to date. Although the perception of hospice is that it provides care for the dying, the emphasis of hospice care is on its provision of quality of life for clients.

Hospice Care

The term **hospice**, which shares the same language root as "hospitality," traces back to medieval times, when it referred to a resting place for weary or ill travelers. In the late 1800s, hospice became synonymous with care of the terminally ill with the founding of Our Lady's Hospice in Dublin by Sister May Aikenhead of the Irish Sisters of Charity, a colleague of Florence Nightingale. In the 1960s, Dame Cicely Saunders, M.D., developed the cornerstone of modern hospice care and opened St. Christopher's Hospice in suburban London. In 1963, Cicely Saunders spoke about hospice at Yale University and, in 1974, Connecticut Hospice began to oversee the care of homebound clients. In 1979, Connecticut Hospice opened the first inpatient hospice in the United States. As of 2002, there were about 3100 hospice programs in the United States.

The concept of hospice came about as a grassroots effort in response to the unmet needs of terminally ill people. As both a philosophy and a system of care, **hospice care** seeks to use an interdisciplinary approach to facilitate both quality of life and a "good" death for clients who are nearing the end of their lives. The hospice system of care is provided in a variety of settings. Hospice programs are often affiliated with home care agencies, providing services to clients at home or in an extended care facility. Some communities also have hospice houses, which admit clients in the terminal phase of their lives and provide a comfortable place where they can die.

In 1983, the Medicare Hospice Benefit passed by Congress defined hospice care in the United States. This benefit pays for hospice services for Medicare recipients who have a prognosis of 6 months or less to live and agree to forgo cu-

TABLE 9-2 General Medical Guidelines for Hospice Appropriateness of Noncancer Clients

- Life expectancy less than 6 months
- No definite terminal diagnosis
- Increasing need for medical care
- Dependence in most ADLs
- Weight loss more than 10% over past 6 months
- Failure to maintain adequate nourishment
- Albumin less than 2.5 g/dL
- Cholesterol less than 156 mg/dL
- Resting tachycardia more than 100 beats/min
- No dialysis or renal transplant

rative treatment for their terminal illness. Historically, clients with terminal cancer have most frequently been the recipients of hospice care. However, clients with other life-limiting conditions with life expectancy of 6 months or less are also appropriate for hospice even if they do not have a definitive terminal diagnosis. Guidelines are available to assist health care providers and families in identifying who is entitled to hospice care under the Medicare hospice benefit (Table 9-2). Clients who are hospice appropriate but do not qualify for Medicare also utilize benefits through private insurance or managed care. In some states, Medical Assistance pays for hospice care.

Not all hospices restrict their services to the terminally ill. Some agencies have bridge programs for clients who have a life-limiting disease, but who are not ready to forgo treatment (and hospitalization) for their disease and/or do not have a prognosis of 6 months or less to live. The advantage of bridge programs is that clients, whose condition may decline, have ready access to expert palliative care. Although treatment of symptoms is the focus of palliative care, no specific therapy is excluded from consideration for clients with a palliative plan of care (Hospice and Palliative Nurses Association, 2002).

SYMPTOMS OF DISTRESS AT END OF LIFE

OVERVIEW

As death nears, clients often have physical symptoms of distress that require treatment to control them until death. Pain, dyspnea, agitation, nausea, and vomiting are common problems at the end of life. Other symptoms include, but are not limited to, fatigue, weakness, constipation, anorexia, and delirium. In general, many symptoms require the use of medications. Once these symptoms occur, medications are usually administered around-the-clock until death to prevent recurrence and attain control. With the appropriate knowledge and resources, the management of symptoms near death can usually be achieved with medication. Most studies show that symptoms of distress (e.g., pain near death) can be effectively controlled in more than 90% of cases when clients have access to palliative care providers.

COLLABORATIVE MANAGEMENT

Assessment

Obtain information about the client's diagnosis, past medical history, and recent state of health to identify the risks for symptoms of distress at end of life. For example, clients with lung cancer, cardiac failure, or chronic respiratory disease are at high risk for respiratory distress and dyspnea near death. Clients with a primary brain tumor or metastasis to the brain are at risk for seizure activity. Those with tumors near major arteries, such as with head and neck cancer, are at risk for hemorrhage. Individuals who have been experiencing pain often continue to have pain, and it may increase, decrease, or remain at the same level of intensity.

PHYSICAL ASSESSMENT/CLINICAL MANIFESTATIONS

Near the end of life, the client often grows weak and lethargic and sleeps for longer periods of time. This lethargy and sleep may progress to the point that the client has a decreased level of consciousness and rouses only to touch. In many cases, the ability of the client to communicate verbally diminishes and level of consciousness decreases, making it difficult to assess the client's perception of symptoms. When caring for clients who are unable to communicate their distress or needs, it is essential that health care providers identify alternative ways to assess symptoms of distress. Professional caregivers should teach family caregivers to watch closely for objective signs of discomfort (e.g., restlessness, grimacing, or moaning). They should also identify when these symptoms occur in relation to positioning, movement, medication, or other external stimuli (Chart 9-1). For example, grimacing when turning from side to side in the bed is indicative of pain or discomfort with movement. When the head of the bed is flat, an increase in respiratory rate and effort indicates shortness of breath and is referred to as orthopnea.

Although the client's point of view is the most valid indicator of comfort or distress, the family's perception of symptoms is also important. The family's perceptions of symptoms should be obtained as part of each client's symptom assessment. Family caregivers, health care providers, and clients may differ in their perceptions of symptoms in terms of intensity, significance, and meaning. Whereas health care providers are often more adept at identifying symptoms of distress, families are often more knowledgeable about client habits and preferences. Health care providers need to incorporate all client-related information into the plan for symptom management and work with clients and families toward a common outcome.

When first recognized, a symptom of distress is assessed in terms of intensity, frequency, duration, quality, exacerbating and relieving factors, and effect on the client's sleep and ability to participate in activities of daily living. A method for rating the intensity of that symptom should be used to facilitate ongoing assessments and evaluate treatment response. A rating scale of 0 to 10 is commonly used, with 0 indicating no distress and 10 indicating the worst possible distress. The intensity of the symptom before and after an intervention (e.g., medication) is documented and is referred to daily to evaluate the client's overall comfort. (See Chapter 7 for a complete discussion of pain assessment.)

Constipation and other problems are typical as a result of immobility and drug effects. These problems are discussed elsewhere in Chapter 10.

As death nears, peripheral circulation decreases and the client's skin often becomes cold, mottled, and cyanotic. Blood pressure decreases, becomes inaudible, and often is

CHART 9-1

CLIENT EDUCATION GUIDE
Common Physical Signs and Symptoms of Approaching Death

Coolness of Extremities
Circulation to the extremities is decreased; the skin may become mottled or discolored.
- Cover the person with a blanket.
- Do not use an electric blanket, hot water bottle, electric heating pad, or hair dryer to warm the person.

Increased Sleeping
Metabolism is decreased.
- Spend time sitting quietly with the person.
- Do not force the person to stay awake.
- Talk to the person as you normally would, even if he or she does not respond.

Fluid and Food Decrease
Metabolic needs have decreased.
- Do not force the person to eat or drink.
- Offer ice chips or small sips of liquids at frequent intervals if the person is alert.
- Use glycerin swabs to keep the mouth moist and comfortable.
- Coat the lips with lip balm or petroleum jelly.

Incontinence
The perineal muscles relax.
- Keep the area clean and dry.
- If the person would be more comfortable, use urine catheters.

Congestion and Gurgling
The person is unable to cough up secretions effectively.
- Suctioning can be used to remove secretions, but this may cause discomfort.
- Medications can decrease the production of secretions.

Breathing Pattern Change
Slowed circulation to the brain may cause the breathing pattern to become irregular, with brief periods of no breathing or shallow breathing.
- Elevate the person's head.
- Position the person on his or her side.

Disorientation
Decreased metabolism and slowed circulation to the brain may occur.
- Identify yourself whenever you communicate with the person.
- Speak softly, clearly, and truthfully.

Restlessness
Decreased metabolism and slowed circulation to the brain may occur.
- Play soothing music.
- Do not restrain the person.
- Massage the person's forehead.
- Reduce the number of people in the room.

Modified from the Hospice of North Central Florida, Inc.

only palpable near death. The dying person's pulse may increase in rate, become irregular in rhythm, gradually decrease, and stop. Meanwhile, respirations become shallow until they, too, stop. Death has taken place when respirations and heartbeat cease.

PSYCHOSOCIAL ASSESSMENT

Individuals facing death may have coping difficulties, fear, and anxiety with regard to their decline and/or impending death. Cultural considerations, values, and religious beliefs of the client and family should be assessed for their influence on the dying experience, control of symptoms, and family bereavement. (See Chapter 7 for cultural considerations in pain management.) Families of individuals near death are also likely to manifest fear, anxiety, and knowledge deficits regarding the process of death and their role in caring for the client.

Assess the client and individual family members for their expectations regarding death and for fear and anxiety. Families may have a preconceived notion about the dying process that may or may not be realistic. Chart 9-2 describes the common emotional signs of approaching death that the nurse should explain to the client, family, or significant others.

CHART 9-2

CLIENT EDUCATION GUIDE
Common Emotional Signs of Approaching Death

Withdrawal
The person is preparing to "let go" from surroundings and relationships.

Vision-like Experiences
The person may talk to people you cannot see or hear and see objects and places not visible to you. These are not hallucinations or drug reactions.
- Do not deny or argue with what the person claims.
- Affirm the experience.

Letting Go
The person may become agitated or continue to perform repetitive tasks. Often this indicates that something is unresolved or is preventing the person from letting go. As difficult as it may be to do or say, the dying person takes on a more peaceful demeanor when loved ones are able to say things such as "It's okay to go. We'll be all right."

Saying Goodbye
When the person is ready to die and you are ready to let go, saying "goodbye" is important for both of you. Touching, hugging, crying, and saying "I love you," "Thank you," "I'm sorry," or "I'll miss you so much" are all natural expressions of sadness and loss. Verbalizing these sentiments can bring comfort both to the dying person and to those left behind.

Modified from the Hospice of North Central Florida, Inc.

Interventions

Common symptoms of distress as death nears are fatigue, pain, dyspnea, nausea and vomiting, restlessness, and agitation. Interventions aim to promote comfort and control the symptoms.

FATIGUE MANAGEMENT. Clients near death frequently have profound fatigue, weakness, and a decreased level of consciousness. Therefore anorexia is common and clients often lose their ability to swallow. If the client is not awake, professional and family caregivers should avoid giving food or liquid orally because of the risk of aspiration. Nurses need to reassure the family that anorexia is often normal and that giving fluid or food can actually lead to discomfort. In general, families have great difficulty accepting that their loved ones are not being fed and may request that intravenous (IV) fluids be initiated. With great sensitivity, reinforce that the cessation of food and liquids is a natural process and that hydration can actually increase discomfort in a person with multisystem slowdown. Discomfort from fluid replacement could lead to respiratory secretions (and distress), increased gastrointestinal secretions, nausea, vomiting, edema, and ascites. Applying emollient to the lips and moistening the mouth and lips with applicators and saturated gauze can help prevent and/or relieve the dry mouth that may occur with a decreased oral intake.

Impaired swallowing near death also presents a problem for medication management because clients lose their ability to swallow their oral medications. Although some pills may be crushed, medications such as sustained-release capsules cannot be taken apart. Scheduled medications can often be discontinued, but medications for pain, dyspnea, agitation, nausea, vomiting, and seizures need to be continued to maintain symptom control until death. In collaboration with a physician and pharmacist experienced in palliative care, identify alternative routes and or alternative medications to maintain control of symptoms. The guiding principle for choice of route in clients near death is to choose the least invasive route with the most effective treatment.

PAIN MANAGEMENT. Pain is the symptom that dying clients fear the most. Although it is not universal, it is common and has many possible causes. Diseases such as cancer often cause tumor pain as a result of the infiltration of malignant cells into organs, nerves, and bones. Other causes of pain in dying clients include "disturbance" pain resulting from headaches, osteoarthritis, muscle spasms, and stiff joints caused by immobility.

Clients who have had their pain controlled with long-acting opioids must continue their scheduled doses of opioids to prevent any recurrence of pain. Depending on the brand of long-acting opioid, oral capsules may be given rectally (same dose and same capsule) when clients are no longer able to swallow. Increases in pain require immediate-relief analgesics (e.g., morphine sulfate immediate-release) and possibly an increase in long-acting opioids. Liquid morphine sulfate can be given sublingually, rectally, or via the buccal mucosa, and it is quick acting, effective, and safe to administer, even to comatose clients. Chapter 7 describes in detail the management of chronic malignant and nonmalignant pain, including complementary and alternative therapies.

DYSPNEA MANAGEMENT. Dyspnea is a subjective experience in which the client experiences an uncomfortable awareness of breathing, breathlessness, or severe shortness of breath. This condition can manifest itself as copious secretions, cough, chest pain, fatigue, or air hunger. It is a common symptom of distress near the end of life, occurring in 50% to 70% of dying clients. Many clients, families, and health care providers consider this to be the worst symptom of distress near death.

Dyspnea can be:

- Directly related to the client's primary diagnosis (e.g., lung cancer, breast cancer, or coronary artery disease)
- Secondary to the primary diagnosis (e.g., pleural effusion, metastasis to the lung or pleura)
- Related to treatment of the primary disease (e.g., heart failure caused by chemotherapy, constrictive pericarditis due to radiation therapy, anemia related to chemotherapy)
- Related to an etiology unrelated to the primary disease (e.g., pneumonia)

Depending on the cause, the pathophysiology of dyspnea can involve the following:

- Obstructive, restrictive, or vascular disturbances in the airways with tumor or nodal involvement
- Pulmonary congestion secondary to fluid overload and/or cardiac dysfunction
- Bronchoconstriction and bronchospasm as seen with respiratory infection, chronic obstructive pulmonary disease (COPD), or airway blockage by a tumor
- A decreased hemoglobin-carrying capacity, as with anemia
- Hyperventilation secondary to neuromuscular disease, with limited movement of the diaphragm

The goal for the client with dyspnea near the end of life is to treat the primary cause and relieve the psychological distress and autonomic response that accompany this symptom. Because diagnostic testing to identify the cause of dyspnea at the end of life is usually inappropriate, the cause is determined by physical assessment and knowledge of the underlying condition. If the cause of dyspnea cannot be treated successfully, interventions are aimed at alleviating the distress.

Opioids. Morphine sulfate is the standard treatment for dyspnea near death. Nurses need to understand that individuals who have not been taking daily opioids should initially receive low doses of morphine (e.g., 5 to 10 mg PO), which can be repeated if necessary. Individuals who have been taking opioids for pain will need to have their breakthrough dose of morphine increased by 50% of their usual dose for effective treatment of dyspnea. If IV access is available, health care providers may prescribe 1 to 2 mg of morphine to be given every 5 to 10 minutes until relief is obtained. However, health care providers should not initiate IV access in dying clients unless it is absolutely necessary.

Morphine via a facial nebulizer is another option for dyspnea near the end of life. Although some research suggests that the nebulized route is no more effective than the oral route, anecdotal reports indicate that nebulized morphine is effective, easy to administer, and has few side effects. The suggested dose for nebulized morphine is 4 mg morphine with 3 mL normal saline (Wrede-Seaman, 2002). If not effective, the concentration should be doubled to 8 mg in 3 mL saline. It should be repeated every 4 hours around-the-clock (ATC) and every 1 hour PRN.

Diuretics and Other Drugs. Individuals with signs of fluid volume excess as manifested by dyspnea, crackles on auscultation, peripheral edema, and other signs of heart failure should be given a diuretic such as furosemide (Lasix) to decrease blood volume, reduce vascular congestion, and reduce the workload of the heart. Furosemide can be administered by mouth, intravenously, subcutaneously, or intramuscularly. IV administration, which is effective in the pulmonary system within minutes, may be preferred for treating congestive heart failure and pulmonary edema.

Bronchodilators such as albuterol or ipratropium bromide via a metered dose inhaler (MDI) or nebulizer may be given for symptoms of bronchospasm (wheezes on auscultation of breath sounds). *Corticosteroids* may also be given for bronchospasm and inflammatory problems within and exterior to the lung. Superior vena cava syndrome and lymphangitis carcinomatosis can cause dyspnea and may respond to corticosteroids.

Antibiotics may be indicated in clients with dyspnea secondary to a respiratory infection. A thorough workup for a respiratory infection is not appropriate in clients in whom death is imminent. However, it is safe to assume an upper respiratory infection is present if dyspnea, an elevated temperature, adventitious breath sounds, and a congested cough have developed. A trial of an appropriate antibiotic should be considered if the client is suffering from the infection.

Secretions in the respiratory tract and oral cavity may contribute to a client's dyspnea near death. Loud, wet respirations (referred to as **death rattle**) are disturbing to family and caregivers even when they do not seem to cause dyspnea or respiratory distress. *Anticholinergics* such as oral or sublingual hyoscyamine (Levsin) or transdermal scopolamine are used to reduce the production of secretions.

Sedatives such as benzodiazepines are commonly used when morphine does not fully control the client's dyspnea. Lorazepam (Ativan) 0.5 mg is commonly administered orally or sublingually every 4 hours PRN or around-the-clock to prevent or control dyspnea and anxiety.

Oxygen. Oxygen for dyspnea near death has not been established as a standard of care for all individuals. However, clients who do not respond promptly to morphine or other medications should be given a trial dose of oxygen (2 to 6 L by nasal cannula) to assess its effect. If it provides relief, it should be continued.

Other Nonpharmacologic Interventions. Pharmacologic interventions should be initiated early in the course of dyspnea near death. Nonpharmacologic interventions can be used in conjunction with, but not in place of, medications. Nonpharmacologic interventions include the following:

- Altering the environment to facilitate the circulation of cool air (e.g., via air-conditioner and fan)
- Applying wet cloths on the client's face
- Positioning the client to facilitate chest expansion
- Encouraging imagery and deep breathing
- Intervening to conserve client energy
- Facilitating the client's rest

Positioning the body with the head of the bed elevated and the upper body supported to facilitate diaphragmatic excursion can be accomplished with a hospital bed or pillows or with the client out of bed and in a chair. Insertion of a Foley catheter to avoid the need for exertion with voiding may be considered if the client will benefit.

NAUSEA AND VOMITING MANAGEMENT. Although not as common a problem as pain or dyspnea, nausea and vomiting are thought to occur in about 40% of terminally ill individuals during the last week of life. It is particularly prevalent in individuals with acquired immunodeficiency syndrome (AIDS) or breast, stomach, or gynecologic cancers.

Common causes of nausea and vomiting at the end of life include the following:

- Initiation of upload therapy (nausea usually lasts a few days)
- Uremia
- Hypercalcemia
- Increased intracranial pressure secondary to brain metastasis
- Vagal stimulation secondary to oral candida
- Stretching of the hepatic capsule
- Constipation or impaction
- Bowel obstruction

If constipation is identified as a problem, a biphosphate enema is administered to release stool quickly. If stool in the rectum cannot be evacuated, a mineral oil enema followed by disimpaction may be required to relieve the client's distress.

Nausea and vomiting related to other causes can generally be controlled by one or more antiemetic agents. Combinations of antiemetics as rectal suppositories, gels, or oral troches can be tried and individualized for maximal relief and control (Chart 9-3).

RESTLESSNESS AND AGITATION MANAGEMENT. Agitation at the end of life requires that you assess for pain or urinary retention, constipation, or other reversible cause. If constipation is ruled out as the cause and if analgesia and catheterization do not relieve the restlessness, sedatives should be administered to provide some relief. Consultation with a spiritual and/or bereavement counselor should be considered to assess for unfinished business or spiritual distress as a possible cause of the agitation.

CONSIDERATIONS FOR OLDER ADULTS

In some cases, agitation and anxiety are part of delirium (acute confusional state), particularly in older adults. Chapter 5 discusses delirium in detail.

Benzodiazepines such as lorazepam (Ativan) or alprazolam (Xanax) are often given for anxiety, restlessness, or myoclonus near death. Lorazepam 1 to 2 mg is often crushed and given sublingually with a few drops of water; this is continued at 0.5 to 2 mg every 6 to 8 hours around-the-clock. If paradoxical agitation occurs, another benzodiazepine is substituted for lorazepam. Until recently, long-acting benzodiazepines such as diazepam (Valium) were not recommended for agitation near death. However, long-acting medications such as diazepam (Valium) and

CHART 9-3

BEST PRACTICE for Symptom Relief

- For unrelieved pain: Morphine solution, 0.25 to 0.5 mL (20 mg/1 mL solution) PO/SL q2-3h PRN
- For unrelieved dyspnea: Morphine solution, 0.25 to 0.5 mL (20 mg/1 mL solution) PO/SL q2h PRN
- For nausea or vomiting: Prochlorperazine, 25-mg suppository PR or 25 mg/0.5 mL transdermal gel to inner wrist q8h PRN
- For unrelieved nausea or vomiting, or for agitation/restlessness: ABH* suppository, 1 PR or 25 mg/0.5 mL transdermal gel to inner wrist q8h PRN
- For severe agitation and restlessness:
  - Determine if client is in pain; treat accordingly
  - Determine if client is constipated or experiencing urinary retention; take appropriate action (Foley catheter)
  - If agitation persists and the safety of the client or caregiver is at risk, administer pentobarbital suppository, 1 PR or 60 mg/0.5 mL gel transdermally q4-6h PRN
- For loud, wet respirations or excessive secretions:
  - Hyoscyamine (Levsin) SL tablets, 1 to 2 PO or SL q4-6h PRN
- For unrelieved respiratory fluid accumulation: Furosemide (Lasix), 40 to 80 mg PO, SC, IM, or IV

Printed with permission from VNA Hospice, Visiting Nurse Services, Manchester, NH.
PR, Per rectum; *SC*, subcutaneous; *SL*, sublingual.
*Many hospice and palliative care organizations use pharmacist-compounded medications which combine the therapeutic effects of several drugs to control symptoms of distress. These medications are compounded as suppositories or gels, which can be administered to clients who cannot swallow. For example, ABH contains Ativan (lorazepam) 1 mg, Benadryl (diphenhydramine) 12.5 mg, and Haldol (haloperidol) 1 mg. Reglan (metoclopramide) is often added to treat nausea and vomiting.

clonazepam (Klonopin) are now considered helpful in controlling anxiety near death.

Barbiturates such as phenobarbital or pentobarbital are given when benzodiazepines fail to control anxiety, delirium, or restlessness near death. The neuroleptic haloperidol (Haldol) may be administered when hallucinations or paranoia occur (see Chart 9-3).

MANAGEMENT OF THE REFRACTORY SYMPTOMS OF DISTRESS. Studies show that most clients with access to palliative care achieve control of symptoms such as pain, dyspnea, and agitation near death. However, a small percentage of clients experience symptoms of distress that are refractory or resistant to treatment. They may require such high doses of analgesia that sedation occurs as a side effect, or they may actually need to be sedated to control symptoms of distress. Although sedation is not ideal, its occurrence as a side effect of treatment for symptoms of distress at the end of life may be acceptable if there is no alternative for comfort. It is important that both health care providers and the public understand that adequate symptom management may at times result in sedation. The sedation that occurs is a side effect of treatment–it is not a treatment goal or an effect meant to hasten death.

The administration of medications for symptoms of distress at the end of life is guided by protocols using doses of medications that are considered safe. These guidelines and protocols are used with the intention of alleviating suffering, not hastening death. The occurrence of an untoward effect of a medication is, however, a risk. According to the Guideline Panel for Management of Cancer Pain (1994), the increased risk of earlier death counts little against the benefit of pain relief and painless death in a client who faces imminent death from progression of a primary disease. The ethical duty of the nurse is to assist in relieving pain or other symptoms of distress in a client near death.

PSYCHOSOCIAL MANAGEMENT. The experience of dying for any person can be extremely difficult for any client and family. But unexpected deaths, particularly in young people, tend to be most traumatic. Dying of a chronic, progressively debilitating illness is also traumatic, but this situation generally presents a different set of issues. Knowledge of the expected outcome of a disease in some ways is helpful, in that it allows health care providers the opportunity to assess client preferences and develop plans of care consistent with these needs. Such a goal requires excellent communication among health care providers, clients, and families.

Whereas death is the termination of life, dying is a process. Individuals facing death may demonstrate emotional signs and symptoms of their response to the dying process through behaviors that equate to saying goodbye or through actual withdrawal. Families need to be educated that such behaviors are normal to the process of dying (see Chart 9-2).

Grief is the emotional feeling related to the perception of the loss. **Mourning** is the outward social expression of the loss. Interventions to assist clients and families in grieving and mourning are based on the cultural beliefs, values, and practices of clients and families. Table 9-3 lists basic beliefs regarding death, dying, and afterlife for some of the major subcultures and religions.

Interventions are aimed at providing appropriate emotional support to allow clients and families to verbalize their fears and concerns. Nurses can also assist by keeping families informed of the client's level of comfort, keeping them involved in health care decisions, and reframing the situation to emphasize the goal of keeping the individual comfortable.

Offering Physical and Emotional Support. Intervene with those grieving an impending death by "being with" as opposed to "being there." "Being with" implies that you are physically and psychologically with the grieving client, empathizing to provide emotional support. Listening and somehow acknowledging the legitimacy of the client and/or family's pain are often more therapeutic than speaking; this concept is sometimes referred to as "presence." Nurses facilitate the expression of grief by giving the person who is mourning permission to express herself or himself. Your manner and words show that these expressions of grief are acceptable and expected. Say something such as, "This must be very difficult for you" or "I'm sorry this is happening."

Being Realistic. The pain of loss cannot be, nor should it be, taken away no matter how committed you may be to the client's comfort. Avoid trite assurances such as, "Things will be fine. Don't cry," or "Don't be upset. She wouldn't want it that way," or "In a year you will have forgotten." Such comments can actually be barriers to demonstrating care and concern. Accept whatever the grieving person says about the situation and remain present, ready to listen attentively and guide gently. In this way, you can help the bereaved prepare for the necessary reminiscence and integration of the loss.

Encouraging Reminiscence. Storytelling through reminiscence and life review can be an important activity for clients who are dying. Life review is a structured process of reflecting on one's life and is often facilitated by an interviewer. Reminiscence is the process of randomly reflecting on memories of events in one's life. The benefits of storytelling through either method include catharsis, the ability to attain perspective, and enhancement of meaning. Suggest that the client and family tape autobiographic stories, record memories in a journal, or develop a scrapbook. If the client does not have enough energy for these activities, familiar objects such as photographs and favorite jewelry pieces can be used to spark ideas for stories that the client may want to tell.

Promoting Spirituality. **Spirituality**, a part of every human being, is the connection to self, others, the environment, and a "higher power" (e.g., God, Allah, spirit). **Religion** can be described as the formal expression of one's spirituality. Studies have shown that religious acts (e.g., prayer, meditation, inspirational reading, recitation of mantras) help clients cope with death and the dying process (Cairns, 1999). Perform a spiritual assessment to identify whether God or religion is important to the client and to facilitate open expression of one's beliefs and needs. Offer and arrange for clergy visits to perform sacred rituals or rites if valued by the client.

Clients who have been alienated from their religious or spiritual community and/or have difficulty in finding meaning in their suffering and approaching death may suffer from spiritual distress. Possible causes include guilt, regrets, lack of meaning, poor relationships, and fear of the unknown. Acknowledge the client's spiritual pain, encourage verbalization, and use a family genogram to elicit relationships, fears, hopes, and unfinished business. Explore issues related to forgiveness for possible resolution.

TABLE 9-3 Basic Beliefs Regarding Death, Dying, and Afterlife for Selected Major Cultures and Religions

African American
One cannot make a definitive statement about the dying and mourning process because of the diversity that exists among different communities.
Funerals tend to be highly involved ceremonies with defined rituals; family, friends, and acquaintances of the deceased make an effort to attend.

Asian—encompasses several countries and religions (e.g., Chinese, Filipino, Japanese, Laotian, Cambodian, Korean, Vietnamese)
There is a traditional strong family and extended family with male dominance.
Herbal medicine plays an important role.
Direct eye contact is considered impolite.
For Southeast Asians, discussing dying brings bad luck, and hospitals and treatments are alien. Some Southeast Asians, especially if uneducated, are likely to avoid visiting terminally ill family members for fear of contracting the disease.
The number or character "4" is avoided because it symbolizes death.
Funeral and burial customs vary greatly depending on culture, religion, and generation involved.

Latino/Hispanic
Many subcultures within this population with diverse cultural variations exist (e.g., Mexico, Central America, the Caribbean, South America).
Catholicism is the predominant religion, but many people depend on folk healers for treatment of ailments.
Death is viewed as a direct result of life; one naturally follows the other.
There is an acceptance of death due to poverty, religion, and culture.
Family and family life are important, especially regarding deaths and funerals.
Expression of grief is open, especially among women.

Native Americans/American Indians
Over 350 distinct tribes in the United States exist with variation in cultural practices.
The focus of identity is on the tribe or council, rather than on ancestry; each tribe has its own belief system.
Most tribes have the belief that spirits are attached to living things.
Indian healers (Shamans) are common.
Family is usually a large extended unit, often including as many as a hundred or more.
Family may not want the client to die at home, but to allow a family member to die alone is also not appropriate.
Material possessions often are dispersed before or after death to friends and family members.
Bereavement follow-up may not be appropriate because some tribes have a taboo against speaking of the dead.

Judaism
This religion encompasses Orthodox, Conservative, and Reformed Jews.
There is a strong belief in the sacredness of life and one, indivisible God.
Funerals have two common themes: honor the dead and comfort the mourners.
The body must not be left unattended until burial which should take place as soon as possible (preferably within 24 hours).
Autopsies and cremation are opposed.
The deceased is often dressed in a white shroud and buried in a plain pine box.
A 7-day mourning period, called Shiva, follows the person's death for the immediate next of kin.
Due to acculturation to American society, there may be variations in funeral and mourning traditions.

Modified from Antelope, T., Eighmy, J., & Nahman, E. (2002). Care of the patient and family. In Hospice and Palliative Nurses Association (Eds.), *Core curriculum for the generalist hospice and palliative care nurse.* (pp. 155-180). Dubuque, IA: Kendall/Hunt.

Fostering Hope. Hope involves picturing a reality that is not yet present and imagining what a situation might be like. This image sets the direction for clients and their families to give them purpose in life and to help them find the strength to go forward, even in the darkest times (Wang, 2000). Foster hope for clients and their families by listening and caring.

Avoiding Explanations of the Loss. Do not try to explain the loss in philosophic or religious terms. Statements such as "Everything happens for the best" or "God sends us only as much as we can bear" are not helpful when the bereaved person has yet to express feelings of anguish or anger. Telling someone too soon that they have other children to rely on or that there are other family members who need them does not diminish the intensity of the grief. In fact, doing so can create feelings of anger and resentment toward the nurse because it reflects an insensitivity to client pain. "Being with" remains important as the weeks or months pass and the funeral crisis supports dissipate. The out-of-town relatives return home, and friends and local relatives resume their own lives. Consider contacting family members after the death to allow them the opportunity to voice their perceptions of the experience. In particular, family caregivers who assumed the role of symptom manager in the home often welcome the opportunity to discuss their experience.

Communicating with the Client. Clients near death are often obtunded and/or withdrawn from the external environment. However, their sense of hearing remains intact until death. Conversation in the room and near the client should be conducted as if the client were alert. Caregivers are encouraged to talk softly to the client and to touch and gently stroke the skin. Although the dying person may not respond, these actions foster a sense of communication between the client and the caregiver.

Providing Referrals to Bereavement Specialists. Bereavement includes grief and mourning–the inner feelings and outward reactions of the survivor. Inform the client and family about bereavement counselors who can assist them to cope both before and after the death. Bereavement counselors are extremely knowledgeable about the grieving process and can be accessed through hospice agencies. Any nurse caring for clients who are dying or have died, should know how to access this resource.

Participation in bereavement support groups by individuals who are grieving a person's pending or past death has been shown to facilitate the grieving process. Being a part of a support group (e.g., Alzheimer caregiver support group) can help people to discover that others have suffered through an experience just as devastating as their own. This discovery makes them more likely to share their feelings with others and work toward some resolution of the experience.

Teaching About the Physical Signs of Death. Although emotionally challenging, witnessing the death of a loved one may actually facilitate the family's acceptance of death. Witnessing how ill a person is makes the event real and enhances an understanding of how disease affects bodily function and decline. If death is anticipated, use nontechnical language to give the client and family or significant others information about the signs of death. The physical signs are described in detail–realistic enough to be unmistakable yet not so graphic as to alarm the listeners. Chart 9-1 describes the common signs and symptoms of approaching death. Such charts are often shared with family and friends who are anticipating the death of a loved one.

Ensuring Palliative Care. Family and friends who are anticipating the death of a loved one often fear that the death will be characterized by pain and suffering. Reassure families that clients will be monitored closely for any sign or symptom of distress. Appropriate medications and other measures will be administered as needed until pain or other symptom of distress is controlled. Families are reassured that significant advances have been made in pain and symptom control.

Most people who choose hospice care prefer the home to other environments during the final episodes of illness. Although there are exceptions, being surrounded by familiar people and things, having ready access to friends and relatives, and having the freedom from institutional restriction make the home setting more comfortable and give the client and family more control. If clients are not able to stay at home until death, they should be offered information about the nearest hospice house. Hospice houses are generally staffed by nurses who provide direct care, and families are allowed to remain with clients. Clients whose cases are being followed by either type of hospice have access to nurses, home health aides, social workers, spiritual and/or bereavement counselors, the medical hospice director, and volunteers, each of whom are members of the interdisciplinary team. Interdisciplinary hospice team meetings are scheduled regularly to review client needs and to review the plan of care initiated by the nurse and client.

To ensure that client and family needs are promptly addressed as they arise, hospices provide 24-hour on-call services. It is not always possible to predict the final phase of the terminal process or the development of symptoms of distress. To address this problem, some hospices have arranged for pharmacies to supply clients with "symptom relief kits by prescription." These kits provide a limited amount of commonly used medications that are effective in treating symptoms near death.

CHART 9-4

HOME CARE ASSESSMENT of
The Client with Physical Manifestations of Death

- No breathing
- No heartbeat
- Release of bowel and bladder contents
- No response to name, environmental sounds, touch, or pain
- Eyelids slightly open
- Pupils enlarged and not constricting in response to light
- Eyes fixed on a certain spot
- No blinking in response to air moving over the eyes or to a light touch on the eye
- Jaw relaxed and mouth slightly open

CHART 9-5

BEST PRACTICE for
Postmortem Care

- Ensure that the nurse or physician has completed and signed the death certificate.
- Ask the family or significant others if they wish to wash or help wash the client.
- Remove or cut all tubes and lines according to health care agency policy.
- Close the client's eyes.
- Replace dentures or other dental appliances, if worn.
- Straighten the client and lower the bed to a flat position.
- Place a pillow under the client's head.
- Wash the client as needed; comb and arrange the client's hair.
- Place pads under the client's hips and around the perineum to absorb feces and urine.
- Clean up the client's room or unit.
- Allow the family or significant others to see the client in private and to perform any religious or cultural customs they wish.
- Notify the hospital chaplain or appropriate community religious leader if requested by the family or significant others.
- Prepare the client for transfer to either a morgue or funeral home; wrap the client in a shroud and attach identification tags per agency policy (if the client is to be transferred to the morgue).

POSTMORTEM CARE

Cessation of breathing is usually noticed by nurses and family at the time of death. Chart 9-4 lists other physical manifestations of death.

Depending on the state or county, the nurse or physician pronounces the client as dead in a health care agency. The nurse or the physician then completes a death certificate, which must accompany the body to the funeral home. Before preparing the body for transfer, ask the physician whether an autopsy will be ordered. When the death is expected, an autopsy will likely be deferred. But when the physician or family members do not know the cause of death, an autopsy may be performed. The nurse or unlicensed assistive personnel prepare the body for immediate postmortem viewing by the family as described in Chart 9-5.

After the family or significant others view the body, follow agency procedure for preparing the client for transfer to either the morgue or a funeral home. In the hospital, a postmortem kit is generally used with a shroud and identification tags.

TABLE 9-4 Definitions of Ethical Concepts Related to Issues at End of Life

Passive euthanasia An act of omission (e.g., withholding or withdrawing treatment) that might prolong the life of a person who cannot be cured by the treatment. In this situation, the withdrawal of the intervention does not directly cause the client's death.
Principle of double effect Involves taking an action (e.g., administering an opioid) intended to have a good effect, which also has a known harmful effect. This is not active euthanasia.
Voluntary active euthanasia An act by which the causative agent in the death of a client is administered directly by another.
Involuntary active euthanasia The action to end the client's life is taken without the client's consent.
Physician-assisted suicide Refers to a practice whereby a physician provides a means (e.g., medication) to a client with the knowledge that the client will use the means to commit suicide.

CULTURAL CONSIDERATIONS

Basic beliefs about death, dying, and afterlife vary among groups. Table 9-3 lists some of these common beliefs and practices in selected cultures and religions.

EUTHANASIA

Nurses spend more time with clients and their families than do any other health care professionals. Therefore they are usually in the best and most immediate position to assist clients with dealing with end-of-life care. This includes assisting in the decision-making process related to end-of-life care, whether it be an immediate need or an issue for the future. To do this, nurses must be knowledgeable about terminology and ethical issues related to death and dying (Table 9-4).

There is a great deal of confusion regarding the concepts of euthanasia. It is essential that everyone understand and articulate the distinction between active and passive euthanasia and assisted suicide versus the appropriate treatment of pain and symptoms of distress. **Passive euthanasia** involves the withdrawal or withholding of a treatment that might prolong the life of a person who cannot be cured by the treatment. In this situation the withdrawal of the intervention does not directly cause the client's death. It is the progression of the client's disease or the poor health status of the client that is the cause of death. Professional organizations such as the American Nurses Association, the American Medical Association, and religious communities such as the Catholic Church support the right of clients and their surrogate decision makers to refuse or stop treatment (e.g., mechanical ventilation, tube feedings, antibiotics, and intravenous fluids), which are medically futile and may actually cause discomfort.

Active euthanasia involves a health care provider taking action that purposefully and directly causes the client's death. Active euthanasia is not supported by most professional organizations, including the American Nurses Association. In the state of Oregon, physician-assisted suicide is legal in certain situations.

Nurses should not be involved in active euthanasia or physician-assisted euthanasia. They do, however, play a major role in clients' end-of- life care by advocating for clients' wishes, and ensuring quality symptom management and support at the end of life.

GET READY for the NCLEX Examination!

KEY POINTS

- Death occurs when the lungs and heart no longer function, causing inadequate blood flow to major organs, acidosis, and tissue ischemia (multiple organ dysfunction syndrome [MODS]).
- Clinical death occurs when there is no brain function present.
- Palliative care is a holistic philosophy that provides compassionate and supportive care to clients and families who are living with life-threatening illnesses.
- An advance directive is a written document prepared by a competent person that specifies what, if any, extraordinary actions that person would want if she or he could no longer make decisions about care; examples are living wills and durable powers of attorney for health care.
- Hospice care is an interdisciplinary approach to help clients have a good quality of life and a "good" death, minimizing symptoms of distress.
- Pain, dyspnea, agitation, nausea, and vomiting are common problems at the end of life.
- Chart 9-2 describes the emotional signs of impending death that the nurse should explain to the client and family.
- Common physical signs of approaching death are listed in Chart 9-1.
- Medications are frequently used for unrelieved dyspnea, pain, agitation, and nausea and vomiting (see Chart 9-3).
- Nursing interventions to manage the psychosocial aspects of death and dying include offering physical and emotional support, being realistic, encouraging reminiscence, promoting spirituality, fostering hope, avoiding explanation of loss, and communicating with the client. Bereavement service referral is also important.
- Postmortem care is described in Chart 9-5.
- Passive euthanasia involves withholding treatment that might prolong a client's life; active euthanasia involves giving a client a treatment or agent that causes death.

ADDITIONAL STUDY RESOURCES

Go to your Student CD-ROM for Review Questions for the NCLEX Examination.

evolve Go to http://evolve.elsevier.com/Iggy/ for Integrated Management of Care Questions for the NCLEX Examination.

SELECTED BIBLIOGRAPHY

Asterisk indicates a classic or definitive work on this subject.

Amella, E. (2003). Geriatrics and palliative care: Collaboration for quality of life until death. *Journal of Hospice and Palliative Nursing, 5*(1), 40-48.

*American Association of Colleges of Nursing. (1998). *Peaceful death: Recommended competencies and curricular guidelines for end-of-life nursing care.* Washington, DC: Author.

*American Nurses Association. (1994a). *Position statement on active euthanasia.* Washington, DC: Author.
*American Nurses Association. (1994b). *Position statement on assisted suicide.* Washington, DC: Author.
*Benzein, E., & Saveman, B. (1998). Nurses' perception of hope in patients with cancer: A palliative care perspective. *Cancer Nursing, 21*(1), 10-16.
*Cairns, A.B. (1999). Spirituality and religiosity in palliative care. *Home Healthcare Nurse, 17*(7), 450-455.
Davis, A.J., & Konishi, E. (2000). End-of-life ethical issues in Japan. *Geriatric Nursing, 21*(2), 89-91.
End-of-Life Nursing Education Consortium (ELNEC). (2000). *ELNEC faculty guide.* Washington, DC: American Association of Colleges of Nursing and City of Hope National Medical Center.
*Escalante, C.P., et al. (1996). Dyspnea in cancer patients: Etiology, resource utilization, and survival implications in a managed care world. *Cancer, 78,* 1314-1319.
*Field, M.J., Cassel, C.K., Committee on Care at the End of Life, Institute of Medicine. (1997). *Approaching Death: Improving Care at the End of Life,* Washington, DC: National Academy Press.
Griffie, J., Nelson-Marten, P., & Muchka, S. (2004). Acknowledging the "elephant": Communication in palliative care. *American Journal of Nursing, 104*(1), 48-58.
*Harwood, K.V. (1999). Dyspnea. In C.H. Yarbro, M.H. Frogge, & M. Goodman (Eds.). *Cancer symptom management* (2nd ed., pp. 45-57). Boston: Jones & Bartlett.
*Hospice and Palliative Nurses Association. (1996). *Clinical practice protocol: Dyspnea.* Pittsburgh: Author.
*Hospice and Palliative Nurses Association. (1997). *Clinical practice protocol: Terminal restlessness.* Pittsburgh, PA: Author.
Hospice and Palliative Nurses Association. (2002). *Core curriculum for the generalist hospice and palliative care nurse.* Dubuque, IA: Kendall/Hunt.
Kessler, T.C., et al. (2003). Assessment of dying. *American Journal of Nursing, 103*(11), 52-57.
*Kubler-Ross, E. (1969). *On death and dying.* New York: Macmillan.
*Management of Cancer Pain Guideline Panel. (1994). *Management of cancer pain. Clinical practice guidelines.* AHCPR Publication No. 94-0592. Rockville, MD: Agency for Health Care Policy and Research, Public Health Service, U.S. Department of Health and Human Services.
*March, P.A. (1998). Terminal restlessness. *The American Journal of Hospice and Palliative Care, 15*(1), 51-53.
Matzo, M.L., & Sherman, D.W. (Eds.). (2001a). *Palliative care nursing: Quality care to the end of life.* New York: Springer.
Matzo, M.L. & Sherman, D.W. (2001b). Palliative care: Ensuring competent care at the end of life. *Geriatric Nursing, 22*(6), 288-293.
*McMillan, S.C. (1996). The quality of life of patients with cancer receiving hospice care. *Oncology Nursing Forum, 23,* 1221-1228.
Norton, S.A., & Talerico, K.A. (2000). Facilitating end-of-life decision-making: Strategies for communicating and assessing. *Journal of Gerontological Nursing, 26*(9), 6-13.
Perrin, K.O. (2001). Ethical issues at the end of life. In *Ethics and conflict.* (pp. 127-151). Thorofare, NJ: Slack.
Pitorak, E.F. (2003). Care at the time of death. *American Journal of Nursing, 103*(7), 42-51.
Robinson, C.B., et al. (2000). Development of a protocol to prevent opioid-induced constipation in patients with cancer: A research utilization project. *Clinical Journal of Oncology Nursing, 4,* 79-84.
Sheehan, D.K., & Schirm, V. (2003). End-of-life care of older adults. *American Journal of Nursing, 103*(11), 48-54.
*Support Study Principal Investigators. (1995). A controlled trial to improve care for seriously ill hospitalized patients. *Journal of the American Medical Association, 274,* 1591-1598.
Travis, S.S., et al. (2001). Terminal restlessness in the nursing facility: Assessment, palliation, and symptom management. *Geriatric Nursing, 22*(6), 308-312.
Virani, R., & Sofer, D. (2003). Improving the quality of end-of-life care. *American Journal of Nursing, 103*(5), 52-55.
Wang, C.H. (2000). Knowing and approaching hope as human experience: Implications for the medical-surgical nurse. *MEDSURG Nursing, 9*(4), 189-192.
Wilkie, D.J. (2001). Toolkit for nursing excellence at end-of-life transition for nurse educators (TNEEL-NE). Seattle, WA: University of Washington.
Wrede-Seaman, L. (2002). *Symptom management algorithms: A handbook for palliative care.* Yakima, WA: Intellicard.

CHAPTER

10

Rehabilitation Concepts for Acute and Chronic Problems

DONNA D. IGNATAVICIUS

LEARNING OUTCOMES

After studying this chapter, you should be able to:

1. Differentiate between impairment, disability, and handicap.
2. Identify the roles of each member of the interdisciplinary rehabilitation team.
3. Interpret physical and psychosocial assessment findings for the client in a rehabilitation program.
4. Describe the major components of a functional assessment.
5. Prioritize nursing diagnoses for the client in a rehabilitation program.
6. Develop a teaching plan for the rehabilitation client who has impaired physical mobility.
7. Explain the role of the interdisciplinary team in managing clients with self-care deficits.
8. Analyze risk factors for skin breakdown in clients who are in rehabilitation settings.
9. Differentiate bladder training techniques for a client with spastic versus flaccid bladder.
10. Assess client outcomes of the interdisciplinary rehabilitation program.
11. Explain the primary concerns for clients being discharged to home after rehabilitation.

Go to your Student CD-ROM for Review Questions for the NCLEX Examination keyed to these Learning Outcomes.

A **chronic illness** or condition is one that has existed for at least 3 months. A **disabling condition** is any physical or mental health/behavioral health problem that can cause disability. This text focuses on physical health problems; mental health/behavioral health problems are discussed in textbooks on mental health/behavioral health nursing.

The rate of chronic and disabling illnesses is expected to increase rapidly as baby boomers approach late adulthood. Medical-surgical nurses care for clients with chronic conditions in a variety of health care settings.

Clients with chronic and disabling conditions often participate in rehabilitation programs to prevent disability, maintain functional ability, and restore as much function as possible. The nurse is a vital member of the rehabilitation team.

OVERVIEW

Chronic and disabling illnesses are a major health problem in the United States, with almost half of the population having one or more chronic conditions. Chronic disease accounts for about 70% of all deaths, and associated medical costs account for over 60% of the nation's health care cost (http://www.ncsl.org/programs/health/phchronic.htm).

Some people with chronic and disabling problems are in residential settings, whereas others are managed at home. Disability occurs slightly more often in men than in women and in families with lower incomes (see the Resource Management box on p. 119).

Stroke is the leading cause of disability. Coronary artery disease, cancer, chronic obstructive pulmonary disease (COPD), asthma, and arthritis are other common chronic conditions that may result in varying degrees of disability. Most of these conditions occur in people older than 65 years of age. These health problems are discussed throughout this text.

Chronic and disabling conditions are not always diseases such as heart disease; they may also result from accidents. Accidents are the leading cause of death among young adults and the third leading cause of death in adults 45 to 54 years of age. Increasing numbers of people survive accidents because of advances in medical technology. These survivors are often faced with chronic or disabling conditions, such as traumatic brain injuries (TBIs) and spinal cord injuries (SCIs). Many of them require months to years of follow-up health care after returning to the community. As a result, the need for rehabilitation is on the rise.

RESOURCE MANAGEMENT

CHRONIC AND DISABLING DISEASES IN THE UNITED STATES

Cost of Care

- Direct medical costs for chronic conditions were about $510 billion in 2000.
- Direct costs are expected to increase to almost $2 trillion by 2020 due to the aging baby boomer population.
- The number of Americans with chronic conditions is growing at an explosive rate, with over 125 million having one or more chronic illnesses.
- The most common costly chronic illnesses are diabetes, arthritis, asthma and other chronic lung problems, osteoporosis, mental disorders, Alzheimer's disease, neurologic disorders such as strokes and spinal cord injuries, and hypertension.

Implications for Nursing

Many chronic conditions can be prevented or detected early before they result in life-threatening and costly complications. Health education reduces costs by teaching clients how to care for themselves. Nurses need to be more involved in promoting wellness, even when they are caring for clients who are ill. For example, teach women about ways to minimize risk factors that predispose them to cardiovascular diseases, such as stroke and coronary artery disease. Teach older men about the importance of prostate screening to detect early cancer. Health teaching and promotion interventions are described throughout this textbook.

CONCEPTS RELATED TO REHABILITATION

Rehabilitation is the process of learning to live with chronic and disabling conditions, often those resulting from trauma. The goal of rehabilitation is to return the client to the fullest possible physical, mental, social, vocational, and economic capacity. Rehabilitation is not limited to the return of function in post-traumatic situations. It also includes education and therapy for any chronic illness characterized by a change in a body system function or body structure. Rehabilitation programs related to respiratory, cardiac, and musculoskeletal health problems are common examples that do not involve trauma. Cancer rehabilitation is not as common, but needs to increase as the number of cancer diagnoses and cancer survival rates increase (Beck, 2003).

In any discussion of rehabilitation, it is important to define and distinguish the terms *impairment, disability,* and *handicap.* These terms have been used interchangeably in some settings; for this chapter, the terms are defined according to the classic, but still widely used, *International Classification of Impairments, Disabilities and Handicaps* (World Health Organization, 1980).

Impairment

Impairment is an abnormality of a body structure or structures or an alteration in a body system function resulting from any cause; it represents a disturbance at the organ level. Impairments can be temporary or permanent and may or may not be associated with an active pathologic condition.

Disability

Disability is the consequence of an impairment and is usually described in terms of a client's altered functional ability; it represents a disturbance at the personal level. A variety of diseases or traumas impair mobility and may result in a decreased ability to function.

Handicap

A **handicap** is the disadvantage that a person feels as a result of impairments and disabilities. This disadvantage is based on interactions that the client experiences in society. Although impairments and the disabilities that result from pathologic changes in a body organ are often unpreventable or irreversible, handicaps are both preventable and reversible.

REHABILITATION AS PART OF COMMUNITY-BASED CARE

After the acute condition or injury has been stabilized in a hospital, the client may be discharged to continue the healing process at home, generally under the follow-up care of a nonhospital health care provider (e.g., a family physician). The nurse provides home care preparation, health teaching, psychosocial preparation, and information about various health care resources to help the client resume his or her usual roles in society.

Some health problems require the intermediate step of rehabilitation, which can occur in a number of settings. Rehabilitation starts in the acute care hospital (sometimes called acute rehabilitation) and continues after discharge from the hospital. The nurse's coordination of care from acute care through community-based care is critical to the success of rehabilitation.

Settings for Rehabilitation

For continuing rehabilitation services, the most common settings are freestanding rehabilitation hospitals, rehabilitation units within hospitals, and skilled nursing home units to which the client is typically admitted for 1 to 3 weeks (Figure 10-1). Ambulatory care rehabilitation departments and home rehabilitation programs may be needed for continuing less intensive rehabilitative services.

Some hospitals and nursing homes have converted one or more inpatient units into transitional care units (TCUs). In this way, the client can stay in the same health care system for both acute and continuing rehabilitative care.

After disabled clients become more confident and independent in the inpatient setting, they may choose to live at home or in a group home. Group homes are facilities where clients live independently while together with other disabled adults. Each client or group of clients has a care provider, such as a personal care aide, to assist with the activities of daily living (ADLs) and decisions requiring accurate judgments. The clients may or may not be employed. The goal of these centers is to provide independent living arrangements outside an institution, especially for younger clients with traumatic brain injury (TBI).

The Rehabilitation Team

Successful rehabilitation depends on the coordinated effort of a group of health care professionals, the interdisciplinary rehabilitation team, and the involvement of the client, family, and other support systems in planning and implementing care. The goal of the rehabilitation team is to restore and maintain function.

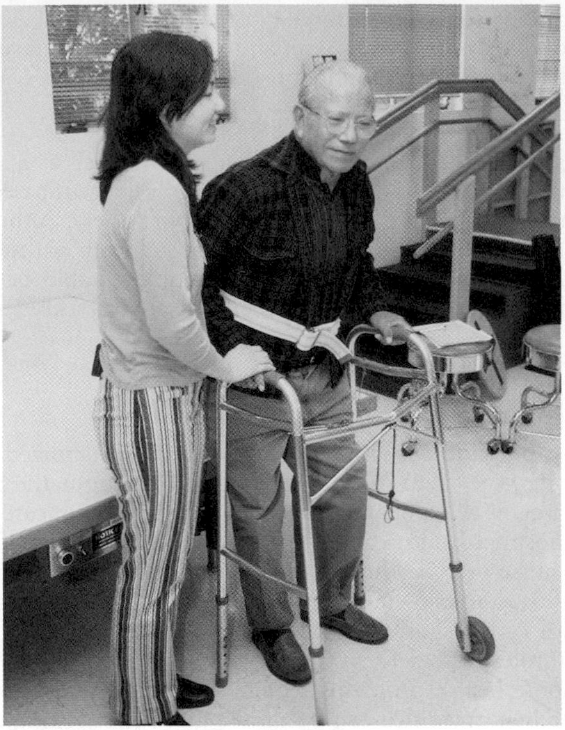

Figure 10-1 ■ A physical therapist helping a client to ambulate.

Members of the interdisciplinary health care team in the rehabilitation setting include physicians, nurses, physical therapists, occupational therapists, speech-language pathologists, recreational or activity therapists, cognitive therapists, aides, social workers, psychologists, vocational counselors, clients, and family members or significant others. Not all settings that offer rehabilitation services have all of these members on their team.

A physician who specializes in rehabilitative medicine is called a **physiatrist.** Except for most freestanding skilled nursing facilities, most inpatient rehabilitation settings employ physiatrists.

The **rehabilitation nurse** in the inpatient setting coordinates the efforts of the team members and therefore may be designated as the client's case manager. Nurses and other health care professionals may be designated as **rehabilitation case managers** in the home or in acute care settings. In clients undergoing rehabilitation, health problems are characterized by an altered functional ability and a diminished quality of life. The goal of rehabilitation nursing is to assist in the restoration and maintenance of optimal health. The rehabilitation nurse must be innovative and patient in helping clients regain independence.

Physical therapists (PTs) intervene to help the client achieve mobility (e.g., by facilitating ambulation and teaching the client to use a walker). They may also teach techniques for performing certain ADLs, such as transferring (e.g., moving into and out of bed), ambulating, and toileting.

Occupational therapists (OTs) work to develop the client's fine motor skills used for ADLs, such as those required for eating, maintaining hygiene, dressing, and driving. OTs may also teach skills related to coordination (e.g., hand movements) and cognitive retraining (Figure 10-2).

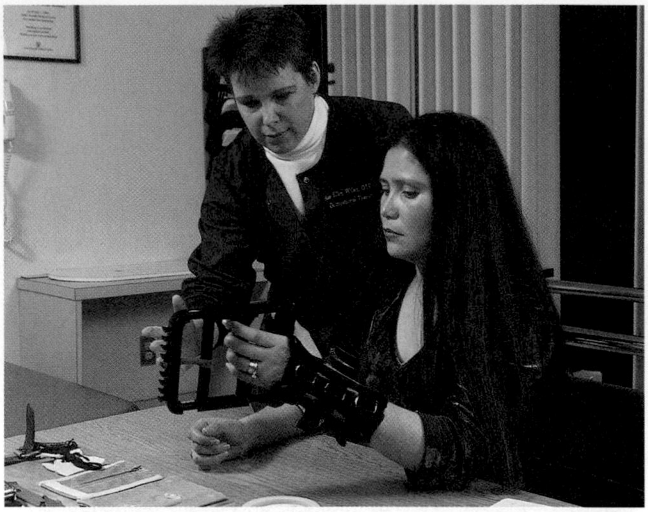

Figure 10-2 ■ An occupational therapist working with a client.

Speech-language pathologists (SLPs) evaluate and retrain clients with speech, language, or swallowing problems. Speech is roughly defined as the ability to say words, and language is the ability to understand and put words together in a meaningful way. Some clients, especially those who have experienced a head injury or stroke, have difficulty with both speech and language. Clients who have experienced a stroke also typically have dysphagia (difficulty with swallowing). SLPs provide screening and testing for dysphagia. If the client has dysphagia, the SLP recommends appropriate foods and feeding techniques.

Recreational or **activity therapists** work to help clients continue or develop hobbies or interests. These therapists often coordinate their efforts with those of the OT.

Cognitive therapists, usually neuropsychologists, work primarily with clients who have experienced head injuries and have cognitive impairments. These therapists often use computers to assist with cognitive retraining.

Nursing or **therapy assistants** work in the nursing or therapy departments to assist in the care of clients. These members of the rehabilitation team are under the direct supervision of the registered nurse or therapist.

Various counselors are helpful in promoting community reintegration of the client and acceptance of the disability or chronic illness. **Social workers** help clients to identify support services and resources, including financial assistance, and they usually coordinate transfers to or discharges from the rehabilitation setting. Psychologists also counsel clients and families on their psychological problems and on strategies to cope with disability.

Vocational counselors assist with job placement, training, or further education. Work-related skills are taught if the client needs to change careers because of the disability. If the client has not yet completed high school, educational tutors may help with completion of the requirements for graduation.

Interdisciplinary team conferences for the exchange of ideas are held on a regular basis with the client, family members and significant others, and health care providers. Chart documentation is shared and read by all team members.

COLLABORATIVE MANAGEMENT

Assessment

HISTORY

Collect the health history, including the history of the client's present condition, any current medications, and any treatment programs in progress. Begin by obtaining general background data about the client and family. These data include financial status, occupations, educational levels, cultural background, and home situation. In collaboration with the occupational therapist, the nurse or case manager addresses the architectural features of the home environment (e.g., the layout of the home). Together they discuss whether the physical layout at home, such as the presence of stairs or the width of doorways, will present a problem to the client. Data are gathered on the client's neighborhood, such as the location of shopping centers and available transportation.

Assess the client's usual daily schedule and habits of everyday living. These include hygiene practices, eating, elimination, sexual activity, and sleep. Ask about the client's preferred method and time of bathing and hygiene activity. In assessing dietary patterns, food likes and dislikes are noted. Information about bowel and bladder function and the normal pattern of elimination is also obtained.

In assessing sexuality patterns, ask about changes in sexual function since the onset of the disability. The client's current and previous sleep habits, patterns, usual number of hours of sleep, and use of hypnotics are also assessed. Question whether the client feels well rested after sleep. Sleep patterns have a significant impact on activity patterns. The assessment of activity patterns focuses on work, exercise, and recreational activities.

TABLE 10-1 Assessment of Clients in Rehabilitation

Body System	Relevant Data
Cardiovascular system	Chest pain Fatigue Fear of cardiac failure
Respiratory system	Shortness of breath or dyspnea Activity tolerance Fear of inability to breathe
Gastrointestinal system and nutrition	Oral intake, eating pattern Anorexia, nausea, and vomiting Dysphagia Laboratory data (e.g., serum prealbumin level) Weight loss or gain Bowel elimination pattern or habits Change in stool Ability to get to toilet
Renal-urinary system	Urinary pattern Fluid intake Urinary incontinence or retention Urine culture or urinalysis
Neurologic system	Motor function Sensation Cognitive abilities
Musculoskeletal system	Functional ability Range of motion Endurance Muscle strength
Integumentary system	Risk of skin breakdown Presence of skin lesions

PHYSICAL ASSESSMENT/CLINICAL MANIFESTATIONS

Collect the physical assessment data systematically according to major body systems on admission for baseline and every day, according to agency policy and type of setting (Table 10-1). The focus of the assessment related to rehabilitation and chronic disease is on the functional abilities of the client.

CARDIOVASCULAR ASSESSMENT. An alteration in cardiac status may affect the client's cardiac output or cause activity intolerance. Assess the manifestations of decreased cardiac output (e.g., chest pain and fatigue). If present, determine when the client experiences these symptoms and what relieves them. The physician may prescribe a change in medications or may prescribe a prophylactic dose of nitroglycerin to be taken before the client resumes activities. Collaborate with the physician and appropriate therapists to determine whether activities need to be modified.

For the client showing fatigue, the nurse and the client plan methods for using limited energy resources. For instance, frequent rest periods can be taken throughout the day, especially before performing activities. Major tasks could be performed in the morning because most people have the most energy at that time.

A great hindrance to rehabilitation for clients with cardiac disorders is fear. These clients may have survived a life-threatening experience (e.g., myocardial infarction) and are now so afraid of recurrence (and death) that they are unable or unwilling to resume any activity. They usually benefit from participation in a structured cardiac rehabilitation program. (See Chapter 38 for a complete description of cardiac rehabilitation.)

RESPIRATORY ASSESSMENT. Ask the client whether he or she is experiencing shortness of breath during or after activity. It is important to determine the level of activity that can be accomplished without experiencing shortness of breath. For example, can the client climb one flight of stairs without shortness of breath, or does shortness of breath occur after climbing only two steps?

The fear associated with any inability to breathe normally can render a person dependent in many aspects of life. Some problems related to disorders of the respiratory system can be resolved or diminished, but some chronic disease, such as emphysema, often continue to worsen.

GASTROINTESTINAL AND NUTRITIONAL ASSESSMENT. Monitor the client's oral intake and pattern of eating. He or she is also assessed for the presence of anorexia, dysphagia (difficulty swallowing), nausea, vomiting, or discomfort that may interfere with oral intake. In collaboration with the physician and the dietitian, review the client's height, weight, hemoglobin and hematocrit levels, and serum prealbumin, and blood glucose concentrations (see Chapter 64 for a complete nutritional assessment). Weight loss or weight gain is particularly significant and may be related to an associated disease or to the illness that caused the disability.

Elimination habits vary from person to person; they are often related to daily job or activity schedules, dietary patterns, and family or cultural background. Elimination habits may be difficult to assess, because many nurses are hesitant to request (and many clients are afraid to volunteer) information pertaining to elimination. When assessing elimination status, the nurse first asks about the client's usual elimination patterns before the injury or the illness.

Note any changes in the client's bowel routine or stool consistency. If the client reports any change in elimination pattern, try to determine whether this alteration is due to a change in diet, activity pattern, or medication use that could cause increased or decreased motility of the gastrointestinal tract. Bowel habits are evaluated on the basis of what is normal for that person.

The nurse also asks whether the client can manage bowel functions independently. Independence in bowel elimination requires cognition, manual dexterity, sensation, muscle control, and mobility. If the client requires help, the nurse determines whether someone is available at home to provide the assistance. The client's (and family's) ability to cope with any dependency in bowel elimination must also be assessed.

RENAL AND URINARY ASSESSMENT. Ask about the client's baseline urinary patterns, including the number of times the client usually voids, and determine whether the client routinely awakens during the night to empty the bladder or has uninterrupted sleep. Fluid intake patterns and volume are recorded, including the type of fluids ingested and the time they were consumed.

The nurse questions whether the client has ever experienced any problems with urinary incontinence or retention. Laboratory reports, especially the results of the urinalysis, are also monitored.

NEUROLOGIC ASSESSMENT. In rehabilitation, the neurologic assessment includes the functional aspects of motor ability, sensation, and cognition. The nurse assesses the client's pre-existing problems, general physical condition, and communication abilities.

The movement of an extremity is compared with the function of the opposite extremity to identify **paresis** (weakness) or **paralysis** (absence of movement). The identification of sensory-perceptual alterations is important in assessing the client's risk for injury. Assess the client's response to light touch, hot or cold temperature, and position change in each extremity and on the trunk. Levels of decreased sensation are identified. For a perceptual assessment, the nurse evaluates the client's ability to receive and understand what is heard and seen and the ability to express appropriate motor and verbal responses. During this portion of the assessment, begin to assess short-term and long-term memory.

The nurse also ascertains the client's cognitive abilities, especially if there is a head injury or stroke. Several tools are available to evaluate cognition. One of the most common is the Mini-Mental State Examination, which is described in detail in Chapter 45.

MUSCULOSKELETAL ASSESSMENT. As with other body systems, the rehabilitation nursing assessment of the musculoskeletal system focuses on function. Assess the client's musculoskeletal status, response to the impairment, and demands of the home, work, or school environment. The client's endurance level is determined, and both active and passive range of motion (ROM) of joints are measured. Review the results of manual muscle testing by physical therapy, which identifies the client's ROM and resistance against gravity. In this procedure, the therapist determines the degree of muscle strength present in each body segment. The grading system usually ranges from 0 (no evidence of muscle contractility) to 5 (normal muscle contractility) (see Chapter 53).

SKIN ASSESSMENT. When assessing a client's skin, the nurse identifies actual or potential interruptions in its integrity.

RISK FOR SKIN BREAKDOWN. To maintain healthy skin, the body must have adequate food, water, and oxygen intake; intact waste removal mechanisms; sensation; and functional mobility. Changes in any of these variables can lead to rapid and extensive skin breakdown. If the client cannot protect or maintain the skin, the nurse must be able to assess and plan for his or her needs. The nurse monitors the client to determine the risk of skin breakdown before it occurs.

Most rehabilitation settings use special skin assessment tools to identify clients at risk for skin breakdown. For example, the classic Braden Scale for Predicting Pressure Sore Risk (see Chapter 70) assesses several areas: sensory perception, skin moisture, activity level, nutritional status, and potential for friction and shear.

Other skin risk assessment tools are available. Some tools also include additional indicators of nutritional status, such as the serum prealbumin. When either of these levels is low, the client is at high risk for pressure ulcers. Some tools include incontinence and altered mental state as risk factors.

ACTUAL SKIN BREAKDOWN. If a pressure ulcer or other change in skin integrity develops, the nurse accurately assesses the problem and its possible causes. If possible, inspect the skin every 2 hours (more often if needed) until the client learns to inspect his or her own skin several times a day. The depth and diameter of the open skin area is measured in centimeters or inches, depending on the policy of the facility. The area around the open lesion must also be assessed to determine the presence of cellulitis or other tissue damage. Chapter 70 includes a widely used classification system for staging skin breakdown. Determine the client's understanding of the cause and treatment of skin breakdown as well as his or her ability to inspect the skin and participate in maintaining skin integrity.

In many health care agencies, a skin assessment and documentation tool ("skin sheet") is used to keep track of each area of skin breakdown. A baseline assessment is conducted on admission to the agency, and the form is updated periodically depending on the agency's policy and the nurse's judgment. In some long-term care, acute care, or rehabilitation settings, and with the client's permission, photographs of the skin are taken on admission and at various intervals to document its condition.

FUNCTIONAL ASSESSMENT

Functional ability refers to the client's ability to perform **activities of daily living (ADLs),** such as bathing, dressing, feeding, and ambulating, as well as independent living skills such as using the telephone, shopping, preparing food, and housekeeping. **Functional assessment** tools are used to assess a client's abilities. Rehabilitation nurses, physiatrists, or therapists complete one or more of these assessment tools on the basis of the client's abilities and the policy of the health care setting. The most commonly used tool is the Functional Independence Measure. Other tools, such as the LORS-II, are referenced in the Selected Bibliography at the end of this chapter.

A uniform data system used for outcome data collection across the United States is the Functional Independence Measure (FIM) developed by Granger and Gresham (1984). As a basic indicator of the severity of a disability, the FIM attempts to quantify what the person actually does, whatever the diagnosis or impairment. It does not measure what a person should do or how the person would perform under a different set of circumstances. To eliminate the bias of a particular discipline, the assessment may be performed by trained clinicians. The entire assessment may be performed by one person, or certain categories may be completed by representatives of various disciplines.

Categories for assessment are self-care, sphincter control, mobility and locomotion, communication, and cognition. Scoring is done with numbers that use predetermined criteria for measurement. The client is evaluated when he or she is admitted to and discharged from a rehabilitation institution and at other specified times to determine client progress. In some settings, it is also being used to help determine staffing levels (Gross, et al., 2001). The FIM assessment system has also been adapted for use in other health care settings, including acute care and home care.

PSYCHOSOCIAL ASSESSMENT

The nurse must understand the theories of body image and self-esteem to assess the client's psychosocial needs adequately. These concepts serve as a basis for understanding psychological responses to chronic illness and the resulting disability. The client's self-esteem and body image are assessed through verbal indicators and descriptions of self-care.

Assess the client's use of defense mechanisms and manifestations of anxiety, such as those noted in facial expressions and communication patterns. To assess the client's response to loss, the nurse asks the client to describe feelings concerning the loss of a body part or function. The presence of any stress-related physical problem is noted. The client may experience symptoms of depression, such as fatigue, a change in appetite, or feelings of powerlessness. See Chapter 9 for a more thorough discussion of loss and grieving.

The nurse assesses the availability of support systems for the client. The major support system is typically the family or significant others. Family interactions and coping patterns are also assessed.

VOCATIONAL ASSESSMENT

The client is assisted in maximizing functional status to allow him or her to resume many usual activities. The nurse should be aware of the appropriate resources for each client in compiling a vocational database. Vocational counselors can help the client find meaningful training, education, or employment after discharge from the rehabilitation setting.

Clients in the United States should be informed about the Americans with Disabilities Act, which was passed by Congress in 1991 to prevent employer discrimination against disabled people. The employer must offer reasonable assistance to a disabled employee to allow him or her to perform the job. For example, if an employee has a severe hearing loss, the employer may need to hire an interpreter for sign language. Workers have a right to ask for special adaptations based on their disabilities.

The rehabilitation team assesses the cognitive and physical demands of the client's job and ascertains whether he or she can return to the former job or whether retraining in another field is necessary. The physical demands of jobs range from light in sedentary occupations (0 to 10 pounds often lifted) to heavy (more than 100 pounds often lifted). The nurse must also consider other aspects of the job, such as strength, mobility, or senses required (e.g., hearing).

Job analysis also involves assessing the work environment of the client's former job. Collaborate with the vocational counselor to determine whether the environment is conducive to the client's return. Union contracts must also be considered, and any job modifications must be noted. If an injured worker requires vocational rehabilitation, refer him or her to vocational rehabilitation personnel to evaluate present skills and learn new skills for employment if needed. In most states, worker's compensation insurance helps to support vocational rehabilitation.

Analysis

COMMON NURSING DIAGNOSES AND COLLABORATIVE PROBLEMS

Regardless of the client's age or specific disability, the following nursing diagnoses are commonly applicable to the client with chronic illness or disability:

1. Impaired Physical Mobility related to neuromuscular impairment, sensory-perceptual impairment, and/or pain
2. Self-Care Deficit (specify deficits) related to neuromuscular impairment and/or perceptual or cognitive impairment
3. Risk for Impaired Skin Integrity related to altered sensation and/or altered nutritional state
4. Impaired Urinary Elimination related to neurologic dysfunction and/or trauma or disease affecting spinal cord nerves
5. Constipation related to neurologic impairment
6. Ineffective Coping related to situational crisis and/or inadequate time to prepare for stressor

ADDITIONAL NURSING DIAGNOSES AND COLLABORATIVE PROBLEMS

Additional nursing diagnoses may apply depending on the client's specific disability. For example, a client with rheumatoid arthritis also experiences Chronic Pain related to chronic physical disability. The client with a spinal cord injury may also have Sexual Dysfunction related to altered body function.

Planning and Implementation

IMPAIRED PHYSICAL MOBILITY

NOC **PLANNING: EXPECTED OUTCOMES.** Most clients with chronic illness or disability are expected to move purposefully in his or her environment with or without assistive device. Not all clients are able to achieve all indicators for this outcome due to physical limitations. Indicators include that the client has noncompromised:

- Balance
- Coordination
- Gait
- Muscle movement
- Body positioning performance
- Transfer performance

INTERVENTIONS. Most problems requiring rehabilitation relate to impaired physical mobility. Clients with neurologic disease or injury, amputations, arthritis, severe burns, and cardiopulmonary disease experience some degree of impaired mobility. Physical and occupational therapists are the key rehabilitation team members in helping clients meet their mobility goals. Depending on the setting, clients often spend several hours every day working in the physical therapy department to regain function and skills.

Transfer Techniques. Clients with decreased mobility may require assistance with transfers, such as from a bed to a chair, commode, or wheelchair. Because the degree of assistance required varies with the client and the specific disability, the nurse carefully assesses mobility status before attempting a transfer. The physical or occupational therapist usually specifies the type of transfer. For example, a quadriplegic client may use a sliding board for transfer, whereas a client with an above-knee amputation may need a wheelchair with removable arms. In any case, the nurse always plans the transfer technique before initiating it. The desired outcome is that the client will eventually be able to transfer independently and safely.

Basic techniques for the nurse to use when assisting in the transfer of the client from a bed to a chair or wheelchair (and vice versa) are identified in Chart 10-1. These techniques are also taught to the family member or other caregiver who will be caring for the client at home. Additional information about transfers can be found in basic nursing textbooks.

Alternative Transfer Techniques. Some clients cannot bear weight. For example, a spinal cord injury resulting in quadriplegia involves using either a **sliding board** (which requires balance skills) or, with the nurse or therapist, a "bear hug" technique. The sitting client places his or her arms around the nurse's neck while being lifted from the bed to the chair or vice versa. Another person assists with the transfer by stabilizing the wheelchair and holding onto the client's waist. Most physical therapists recommend that the client wear pants or a **gait belt** so the assistant can hold onto the belt during the transfer.

Potential Problems with Transfers. Before any transfer, the nurse carefully observes for potential problems. Orthostatic, or postural, hypotension is a common problem in rehabilitation and contributes to falls, which are common in any client with impaired mobility. If the client moves from a lying to a sitting or standing position too quickly, his or her blood pressure drops; as a result, he or she becomes dizzy or faints. This problem is worsened by antihypertensive medications, especially in older adults. To prevent this, help the client change positions slowly, with frequent rest periods to allow the blood pressure to stabilize. The nurse may measure blood pressure with the client in the lying, sitting, and standing positions to examine the differences. Orthostatic hypotension is indicated by a drop of more than 20 mm Hg in systolic pressure or 10 mm Hg in diastolic pressure between positions. Notify the physician about this change.

If the client has problems in maintaining blood pressure while out of bed, the physical therapist usually starts the client on a tilt table to gradually increase tolerance. This is a particularly common problem for clients who are quadriplegic.

Weight gain is another potential problem. Because the client undergoing rehabilitation has impaired mobility, he or she tends to gain weight. Excessive weight hinders transfers both for the nurse or the therapist who is assisting and for the client who is learning to transfer independently. Weight is usually checked every week to monitor gains or losses.

Gait Training. The physical therapist works with clients for gait training if they are able to ambulate. While regaining the ability to ambulate, clients may need to use canes or walkers (Figure 10-3). When working with clients who are using such assistive devices, also known as **ambulatory aids,** the physical therapist ensures that there is a level surface on which to walk. The nurse reinforces the physical therapist's instructions and encourages practice, with the goal being to walk independently with or without an assistive device. Older clients typically use a walker for a broader base of support. Younger or minimally impaired clients often progress to the use of a hemi-cane or straight cane. Chart 10-2 outlines how to use assistive devices for ambulation.

Some clients never regain the ability to walk because of their impairment, such as multiple sclerosis or spinal cord injury. They may become wheelchair dependent and need to learn wheelchair mobility skills. With the help of physical and occupational therapy, most clients can learn to move anywhere in the wheelchair.

Prevention of Complications. During the rehabilitation phase, clients are vulnerable to complications of immobility. Table 10-2 lists the common complications and

CHART 10-1

BEST PRACTICE for
Transfer Techniques

Bed to Wheelchair or Chair

1. Place the chair at an angle to the bed on the client's strong side.
2. Lock the wheelchair brakes or secure the chair position.
3. Assist the client to stand, and move his or her strong hand to the armrest.
4. Keep the client's body weight forward and pivot.
5. When the client's legs touch the chair edge, assist the client in sitting.

Wheelchair or Chair to Bed

1. Place the chair with the client's strong side next to the bed.
2. Lock the wheelchair brakes or secure the chair position.
3. Assist the client to stand, and move his or her strong hand to the armrest.
4. Keep the client's body weight forward and pivot.
5. When the client's legs touch the bed edge, assist the client in sitting and then reclining.

Use of a Sliding Board

1. Place the chair or wheelchair as close to the bed as possible.
2. Remove the armrest from the chair or (if removable) wheelchair.
3. Powder the sliding board.
4. Place the sliding board under the client's buttocks.
5. Instruct the client to reach toward his or her side.
6. Assist the client in sliding gently to the bed.

the major strategies the nurse can use to help prevent each complication. Implementing range-of-motion (ROM) routines, adhering to schedules for turning and repositioning, and maintaining skin care are constant components of rehabilitation nursing care to prevent complications of immobility. The key is to increase mobility.

One way to increase mobility, even with clients who are bedridden, is through ROM exercises. ROM techniques are beneficial for any client with decreased mobility (Table 10-3). Although basic ROM techniques are presented in basic nursing textbooks, a few key principles are pertinent to rehabilitation nursing care:

- The human body contains more joints than simply the knees, hips, elbows, and shoulders. For ROM techniques to be effective in preventing musculoskeletal contractures, the client must exercise all joints, including each joint of the fingers, hands, toes, and so forth.
- In performing ROM activities, the nurse or client completes full-range movement of each joint at least five times and completes the entire process at least three times daily.
- The nurse does not move the joints beyond the point at which the client expresses pain or beyond the point at which the nurse perceives stiffness or difficulty.

Clients with decreased mobility who are able to follow directions are taught by the nurse and the physical therapist to perform active or active-assisted ROM exercises.

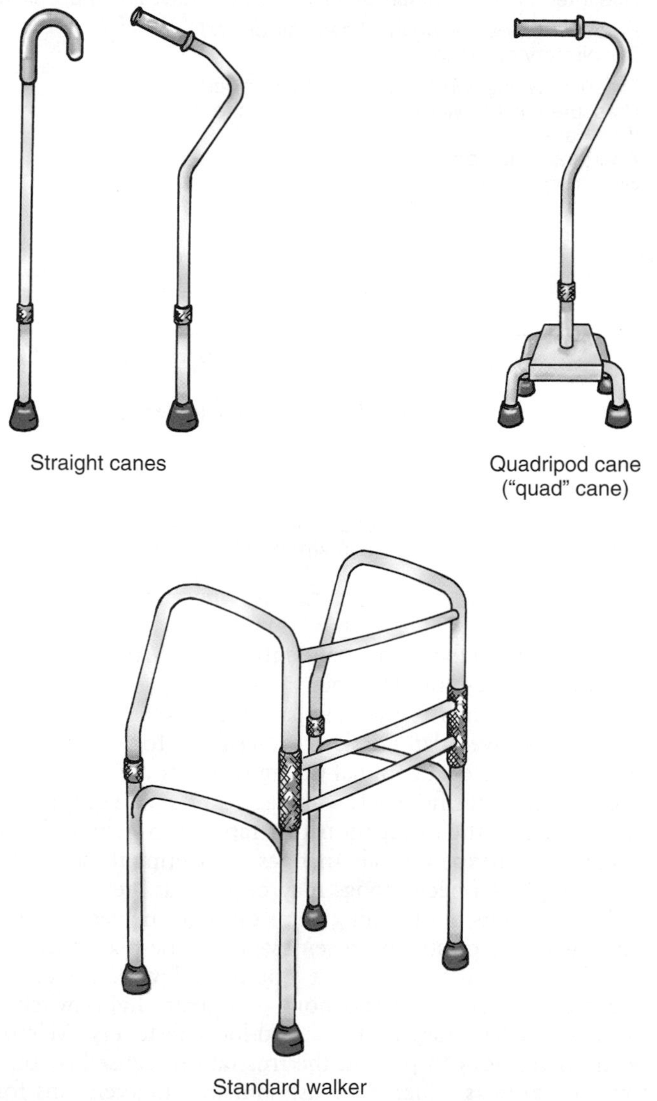

Figure 10-3 ■ Assistive devices for ambulation. Assistive devices vary in the amount of support they provide. A straight cane provides less support than a quadripod cane or walker.

SELF-CARE DEFICIT

NOC **PLANNING: EXPECTED OUTCOMES.** Most clients with chronic illness or disability are expected to perform the most basic physical tasks and personal care activities independently with or without assistive devices. Indicators include that the client demonstrates noncompromised:

- Eating
- Dressing
- Toileting
- Bathing
- Grooming
- Hygiene
- Oral hygiene
- Walking or wheelchair mobility
- Transfer performance
- Positioning of self

INTERVENTIONS. Activities of daily living (ADLs), or self-care activities, include eating, bathing, dressing, grooming, and toileting. Encourage the client to perform as much self-care as possible. The nurse and occupational therapist collaborate to identify ways in which self-care activities can be modified so the client can perform them independently, if possible. For example, the occupational therapist teaches a hemiplegic client to put on a shirt by first placing the affected arm in the sleeve and then putting the unaffected arm in the appropriate sleeve. The nurse reinforces this dressing technique and encourages the client to practice.

CHART 10-2

BEST PRACTICE for
Gait Training

Walker Assisted

1. Apply a gait belt around the client's waist.
2. Assist the client to a standing position.
3. Assist the client in placing both hands on the walker.
4. Ensure that the client is well balanced.
5. Assist the client repeatedly to perform the following sequence:
   a. Lift the walker.
   b. Move the walker 2 feet forward and set it down on all legs.
   c. While resting on the walker, take small steps.
   d. Check balance.

Cane Assisted

1. Apply a gait belt around the client's waist.
2. Assist the client to a standing position.
3. Assist the client in placing his or her strong hand on the cane.
4. Ensure that the client is well balanced.
5. Assist the client to perform the following sequence repeatedly:
   a. Move the cane forward.
   b. Move the weaker leg one step forward.
   c. Move the stronger leg one step forward.
   d. Check balance.

TABLE 10-2 Prevention of the Common Hazards of Immobility

Body System	Complication	Prevention
Musculoskeletal	Contractures	Range-of-motion exercises
	Foot drop	Foot support while in bed, range-of-motion exercises, high-top tennis shoes
	Osteoporosis	Range-of-motion exercises, ambulation if possible (walking)
	Susceptibility to fractures	Weight-bearing exercises
	Muscular atrophy	Passive or active range-of-motion exercises
Gastrointestinal	Constipation	Increased activity level Increased fluid intake, fiber
Cardiovascular	Decreased cardiac output	Range-of-motion exercises
	Increased venous stasis	Exercise, support hose, or antiembolism stockings
	Thrombus formation	Exercise, support hose, or antiembolism stockings
	Embolism	Avoidance of leg massage, low–molecular weight heparin
Neurologic	Disorientation	Sleep-wake schedule in accord with light-dark pattern Reorientation (to person, place, and time) Control of sensory stimulation
	Postural hypotension	Avoidance of sudden position changes, tilt table
Renal/urinary	Calculi	Decreased dietary calcium level Increased fluid intake Maintenance of acidic urine
	Infection	Increase fluids Use intermittent catheterization instead of indwelling if possible
Respiratory	Pneumonia	Frequent repositioning in wheelchair or bed Respiratory exercises
Integumentary	Pressure ulcers	Frequent repositioning in wheelchair or bed Pressure relief devices (bed and wheelchair) Skin care Adequate nutrition Skin monitoring

TABLE 10-3 Types of Range-of-Motion Exercises

Type	Description	Indications
Passive	Exercises are performed by the nurse for the client.	The client is too weak to participate actively.
Active	Exercises are performed by the client.	The client is able to complete range-of-motion movements.
Assisted, or active assisted	Exercises are performed by the client but are guided by the nurse or therapist.	The client is weak and needs assistance.
Resistive	The actions of the client are in opposition to those performed by the nurse or therapist.	The client has full range of motion, and an increase in strength is desired.

In long-term care (LTC) settings (e.g., nursing homes), federal regulations require that residents not lose their functional skills. Therefore most facilities have developed **restorative nursing** programs and have coordinated these programs with rehabilitation therapy and activity therapy. The focus of this coordinated effort includes the following:

- Bed mobility
- Walking
- Transfers
- Dressing
- Grooming
- Active range of motion
- Communication

Nursing assistants in LTC and home health settings are typically involved in restorative programs (Marrelli, 2003).

NIC **Self-Care Assistance.** A variety of **assistive/adaptive devices** are available for clients with chronic illness and disability. An assistive/adaptive device, or self-care support device, is any item that enables the client to perform all or part of an activity independently. Table 10-4 identifies common devices and describes their use.

Many department stores and large pharmacies carry clothing and assistive/adaptive devices designed for clients with disabilities. The occupational therapist works with the client to determine specific needs with regard to such equipment. The nurse and the occupational therapist also help look for creative and inexpensive alternatives to meeting these needs. For example, barbecue tongs may be used as "reachers" for pulling up pants or obtaining items on high shelves. A foam curler with the plastic insert removed may be placed over a pencil or eating utensil to make a built-up device. The client might use an extended shoehorn to operate light switches from wheelchair height. Hook-and-loop fasteners (Velcro) sewn on clothes can prevent the frustrations caused by buttons and zippers. Chart 10-3 lists nursing interventions for clients who need self-care assistance.

Energy Conservation. Fatigue is commonly associated with chronic and disabling conditions. Therefore nurses

TABLE 10-4 Uses of Assistive/Adaptive Devices

Device	Use
Buttonhook	Threaded through the buttonhole to enable clients with weak finger mobility to button shirts Alternative uses include serving as pencil holder or cigarette holder
Extended shoe horn	Assists in the application of shoes for clients with decreased mobility Alternative uses include turning light switches off or on while client is in a wheelchair
Plate guard	Applied to a plate to assist clients with weak hand and arm mobility to feed themselves
Gel pad	Placed under a plate or a glass to prevent dishes from slipping and moving Alternative uses include placement under bathing and grooming items to prevent them from moving
Foam buildups	Applied to eating utensils to assist clients with weak hand grasps to feed themselves Alternative uses include application to pens and pencils to assist with writing or over a buttonhook to assist with grasping the device
Hook and loop fastener (Velcro) straps	Applied to utensils, a buttonhook, or a pencil to slip over the hand and provide a method of stabilizing the device when the client's hand grasp is weak
Long-handled reacher	Assists in obtaining items located on high shelves or at ground level for clients who are unable to change positions easily
Elastic shoelaces or Velcro shoe closure	Prevents the need for tying shoes

CHART 10-3

NIC INTERVENTION ACTIVITIES for The Client in Rehabilitation

Self-Care Assistance: *Assisting another to perform activities of daily living*

- Monitor client's ability for independent self-care.
- Monitor client's need for adaptive devices for personal hygiene, dressing, grooming, toileting, and eating.
- Provide assistance until the client is fully able to assume self-care.
- Use consistent repetition of health routines as a means of establishing them.
- Encourage client to perform normal activities of daily living to level of ability.
- Teach family to encourage independence, to intervene only when the client is unable to perform.
- Establish a routine for self-care activities.

NIC intervention activities selected from Dochterman, J.M., & Bulechek, G.M. (Eds.) (2004). *Nursing interventions classification (NIC).* (4th ed.). St. Louis: Mosby. No part of this work is to be altered without prior written permission from the Publisher.

CHART 10-4

NURSING FOCUS on the OLDER ADULT
Special Considerations in Rehabilitation

- When getting the client out of bed, move him or her (or instruct him or her to move or sit up) slowly to prevent orthostatic hypotension. This problem is most common in older adults who take antihypertensive medications.
- Turn the client more often than every 2 hours, even if it is just a minor position change. Skin becomes thinner and more fragile with age.
- Determine whether the client had any problem with urinary patterns before the illness or rehabilitation. A client with a previous problem may not have a successful bladder training program.
- Be aware that intestinal motility decreases with age, which leads to constipation.
- Assess the client's support system of family and significant others. Many older clients have no spouse or close friends, who would usually serve as a support network.

work with occupational therapists to assess the client's self-care abilities and to determine possible ways of conserving energy. The nurse and the therapist develop strategies for **energy conservation** after evaluating the client's self-care routines. Preparation for ADLs can be helpful in reducing effort and energy expenditure (e.g., gathering all necessary equipment before starting grooming routines). If a client has high energy levels in the morning, he or she can be taught to schedule energy-intensive activities in the morning rather than later in the day or evening. Spacing activities is also helpful for conserving energy. In addition, allowing time to rest before and after eating and toileting decreases the strain on the client's energy level.

RISK FOR IMPAIRED SKIN INTEGRITY

NOC **PLANNING: EXPECTED OUTCOMES.** The client with chronic illness or disability is expected to have structural intactness and physiologic function of the skin as indicated by having none of the following:

- Skin lesions
- Erythema
- Blanching
- Necrosis
- Induration
- Skin flaking

INTERVENTIONS. An enormous variety of topical and mechanical remedies have been used with varying success to prevent and treat pressure ulcers. Pressure reduction is a nursing intervention that may be achieved when the nurse temporarily repositions the client or alters the physical properties of the mattress surface, such as adding a mattress overlay.

Turning and Repositioning. The best intervention to prevent skin impairment is frequent position changes in combination with adequate skin care and sufficient nutritional intake. In general, the nurse turns and repositions the client every 2 hours if the client is unable to perform this activity. This may not be sufficient for people who are frail and have thin skin, especially older adults (Chart 10-4). To determine the best turning schedule, assess the client's skin condition during each turning and repositioning. For example, if the client has been sleeping for 2 hours and the nurse decides to postpone turning for 1 hour, reddened areas over the bony prominences may be present. If such reddened areas do not fade within 30 minutes after pressure relief or do not blanch, they may be classified as preulcer areas, or stage I pressure areas (see Chapter 70).

Clients who sit for prolonged periods in a wheelchair need to be repositioned at least every 1 to 2 hours. Each client is evaluated by the physical or occupational therapist for the best seating pad or cushion that is comfortable yet reduces pressure on bony prominences. Clients who are able are taught to perform "wheelchair push-ups" by using their arms to lift their buttocks off the wheelchair seat for 10 seconds or longer every hour, or more often if needed. The physical therapist helps clients strengthen their arm muscles in preparation for performing wheelchair push-ups.

If the client wears tennis shoes for foot positioning, remove the shoes and assess for pressure areas. Many clients with neurologic problems have decreased or absent sensation and may not be able to feel the discomfort of increased pressure. Also check clients who are sitting in wheelchairs for signs of pressure, especially on the lower legs where the leg of the wheelchair could rub against the skin.

Skin Care. Adequate skin care is an essential component of prevention. The nurse performs or assists clients in completing skin care each time they are turned, repositioned, or bathed. Skin care includes cleaning soiled areas, drying carefully, and applying body lotion. If a client is incontinent, topical barrier creams or ointments can help protect the skin from moisture, which facilitates skin breakdown. Reddened areas are not rubbed because doing so can cause extensive damage to the already fragile capillary system. Instead the nurse carefully observes the areas for further breakdown and relieves pressure on the areas as much as possible. Bed pillows are often good pressure-relieving devices. (See Chapter 70 for a complete discussion of skin care interventions.)

Nutrition. Sufficient nutrition is needed both to repair wounds and to prevent pressure ulcers. The nurse collaborates with the dietitian to assess the client's food selection and ensure that it contains adequate protein and carbohydrates. Both the nurse and the dietitian closely monitor the client's weight and levels of serum prealbumin. If either of these indexes decreases significantly, the client may be given high-protein, high-carbohydrate food supplements (e.g., milkshakes) or commercial preparations (e.g., Ensure Plus) (also see Chapter 64).

Mechanical Devices. Pressure-relieving devices include waterbeds, gel mattresses or pads, air mattresses, low–air loss overlays or beds, and air-fluidized beds. Mattress overlays, such as air and gel types, and replacement mattresses are often effective in reducing pressure. The use of any mechanical device (except air-fluidized beds) does not eliminate the need for turning and repositioning.

Specialty beds are categorized as either "low air loss" or "air fluidized." Air-fluidized therapy (e.g., Clinitron or FluidAir bed) provides the most effective pressure relief; the client is maintained in a nearly pressure-free environment (Figure 10-4). In general, these beds are not used to prevent skin breakdown, because most insurers will not reimburse the agency for the use of the bed. Therefore special beds are usually reserved for severe skin problems that have not healed with the use of a conventional bed or other mechanical device. If optimal nutrition and healing conditions are maintained, skin breakdowns should heal with continued use of air-fluidized therapy. The primary disadvantage of this therapy is its expense, which may exceed several hundred dollars for each day of use. The cost of air-fluidized therapy may be reimbursed by some health insurance providers.

IMPAIRED URINARY ELIMINATION

NOC **PLANNING: EXPECTED OUTCOMES.** Most clients with chronic illness or disability are expected to have a normal collection and discharge of urine. Not all clients are able to meet the following indicators due to physiologic impairment. Indicators include that the client has noncompromised:

- Elimination pattern
- Adequacy of fluid intake
- Emptying of bladder

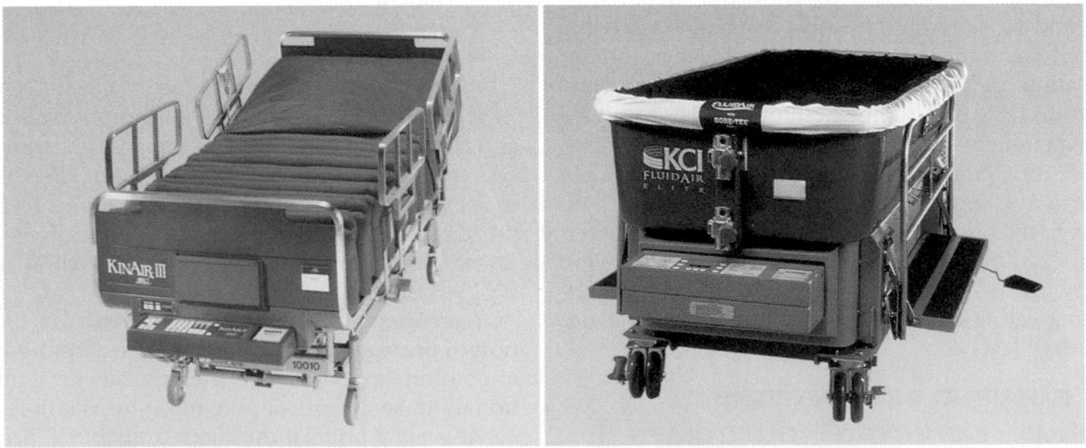

Figure 10-4 ■ Pressure relief devices. *Left,* KinAir III beds provide controlled air suspension to redistribute body weight away from bony prominences. *Right,* FluidAir Elite beds use airflow and bead fluidizations. Both of these beds are covered with Gore-Tex fabric, which resists tearing. This fabric is also waterproof and acts as a barrier against bacteria. (Courtesy Kinetic Concepts, Inc., San Antonio, TX.)

In addition, the client is expected to have none of the following:

- Hesitancy with urination
- Urinary retention
- Urinary incontinence

INTERVENTIONS. Neurologic disabilities may interfere with successful bladder control in a client undergoing rehabilitation. These disabilities result in three basic functional types of neurogenic bladder: reflex (spastic) bladder, flaccid bladder, and uninhibited bladder.

A **reflex** or **spastic** (upper motor neuron) **bladder** causes incontinence that is characterized by sudden, gushing voids. The bladder does not usually empty completely. A reflex bladder is also sometimes referred to as a "spastic" bladder. Neurologic problems affecting the upper motor neuron typically occur with high-level or mid-level spinal cord injuries above the twelfth thoracic vertebra (T12). These injuries result in a failure of impulse transmission from the lower spinal cord areas to the cortex of the brain. When the bladder fills and transmits impulses to the spinal cord, the client is not conscious of the filling sensation. However, because there is no injury to the lower spinal cord and the voiding reflex arc is intact, the efferent (motor) impulse is relayed and the bladder contracts.

A **flaccid** (lower motor neuron) **bladder** results in urinary retention and overflow (dribbling). Injuries that cause damage to the lower motor neuron at the spinal cord level of S2-4 (e.g., multiple sclerosis and spinal cord injury below T12) may directly interfere with the reflex arc or may result in inappropriate interpretation of impulses to the brain. The bladder fills and afferent (sensory) impulses conduct the message via the spinal cord to the cortical region of the brain. Because of the injury, the impulse is not interpreted correctly by the cortical bladder center in the brain, and there is a failure to respond with a message for the bladder to contract.

An **uninhibited bladder** may occur when the client has a neurologic problem that affects the cortical bladder center of the brain (frontal lobe), such as stroke or brain injury. When the bladder needs to empty, the client has little sensorimotor control and cannot wait until he or she is on the commode or bedpan before voiding. The client is incontinent, but the bladder may not completely empty.

Bladder Training. The nurse can teach three techniques to assist the client in "repatterning" voiding (bladder training):

- Facilitating, or triggering, techniques
- Intermittent catheterization
- Consistent scheduling of toileting routines; "timed void"

These techniques may not be as effective in clients with physiologic changes associated with aging.

Facilitating or Triggering Techniques. Facilitating (triggering) techniques are used to stimulate voiding (Table 10-5). If there is an upper motor neuron problem but the reflex arc is intact (reflex bladder pattern), the voiding response can be initiated by any stimulus that sends the message to the spinal cord level S2-4 that the bladder might be full. Such techniques include stroking the medial aspect of the thigh, pinching the area above the groin, pulling pubic hair, massaging the penoscrotal area, pinching the posterior aspect of the glans penis, and providing digital anal stimulation.

When the client has a lower motor neuron problem, the voiding reflex arc is not intact (flaccid bladder pattern), and additional stimulation may be needed to initiate voiding. Two techniques used to facilitate voiding are the Valsalva maneuver and the Credé maneuver. In teaching the Valsalva maneuver, the nurse instructs the client to hold his or her breath and bear down as if trying to defecate. The nurse assists the client in performing the Credé maneuver by placing the client's hand in a cupped position directly over the bladder area and instructing the client to push inward and downward as if massaging the bladder to empty.

Intermittent Catheterization. Intermittent catheterization is often used for disorders that involve a flaccid or spastic bladder. In assisting the client with intermittent catheterization for a flaccid bladder, the nurse initially inserts a urinary catheter every 2 to 3 hours–after the client has attempted voiding and has used the Valsalva and Credé maneuvers. If less than 150 mL of residual urine is obtained, the nurse typically increases the interval between catheterizations. This interval may be up to 3 to 4 hours according to the health care provider's order or health care agency protocol. The interval may be gradually increased to 4 to 6 hours, but the client should not go beyond 8 hours between catheterizations. The exception occurs when the residual urine volume is less than 150 mL each time with an adequate intake of fluids. If the client will be performing intermittent self-catheterization at home after discharge from the rehabilitation facility, the nurse instructs the client about clean (not sterile) technique.

Intermittent catheterizations may also be performed to determine residual urine volumes for the client with a reflex (upper motor neuron) or uninhibited bladder, although this procedure has been largely replaced with the less invasive **bladder ultrasound.** Nurses can perform this test at the bedside to determine postvoiding residuals. The

TABLE 10-5 Management of Impaired Urinary Elimination

Functional Type	Neurologic Disability	Clinical Manifestations	Re-establishing Voiding Patterns
Reflex (spastic)	Upper motor neuron spinal cord injury above T12	Urinary frequency, incontinence	Triggering or facilitating techniques Medications Bedside bladder ultrasound Intermittent catheterization Consistent toileting schedule
Flaccid	Lower motor neuron spinal cord injury below T12 (affects S2-4 reflex arc)	Urinary retention, overflow	Valsalva and Credé maneuvers Medications
Uninhibited	Brain damage from injury or stroke	Frequency, urgency, incontinence, voiding in small amounts	Intermittent catheterization Consistent toileting schedule Regulation of fluid intake

client is catheterized if the bladder volume is greater than 150 mL.

Toileting Schedule. Consistent toileting routines may be the best way to re-establish voiding continence when the client displays an uninhibited bladder pattern (associated with brain damage or head injury). Assess the client's previous voiding pattern and determine his or her daily routine. At a minimum, the nurse assists the client with voiding after awakening in the morning, before and after meals, before and after physical activity, and at bedtime. Most often, the client is toileted every 2 hours during the day and every 4 hours at night.

Consider the client's bladder capacity, which may range from 100 to 500 mL, as well as mobility limitations and restrictive clothing. Bladder capacity is determined by measuring urine output. Ensure that the client is aware of nearby bathrooms at all times or has a call system to contact the nurse or unlicensed assistive personnel for assistance.

Drug Therapy. Medications that may be used for urinary elimination problems include cholinergics (to promote bladder emptying), antispasmodics (to prevent incontinence), and skeletal muscle relaxants (to decrease spasticity, which promotes self-care). Medications are not usually prescribed by the health care provider in the initial management of bladder problems, but may be used to assist with a bladder training program. Report the client's progress in bladder training to the rehabilitation team so that the best decision regarding drug therapy can be made. In general, anticholinergics, antispasmodics, and skeletal muscle relaxants help to promote continence in clients with a reflex (upper motor neuron) bladder. Cholinergics, such as bethanechol chloride (Urecholine), may decrease urinary retention problems resulting from a flaccid bladder. They may also facilitate complete bladder emptying in a client with a large residual volume, which occurs with reflex bladder problems. An uninhibited bladder does not routinely require medications for bladder training programs unless urinary function is affected by additional pathologic changes.

Fluid Intake. Instruct the client to maintain an adequate intake of fluids, at least 2000 to 2500 mL/day. An acidic urine usually minimizes the risk of urinary tract infection and calculus (stone) formation, although this belief is controversial. However, some microorganisms, such as *Escherichia coli,* do grow best in acidic environments. Therefore encourage the client to drink fluids that promote an acidic urine, including large amounts of cranberry juice, prune juice, bouillon, tomato juice, and water. Fluids that promote an alkaline urine are discouraged, including citrus juices, excessive amounts of milk and milk products, and carbonated beverages. Remind the client that drinking water and other liquids helps prevent urinary infection.

In addition, discourage high-calorie fluids for overweight clients. Disabled clients have more difficulty with mobility and self-care if their weight is not controlled.

Prevention of Complications. The client with altered urinary elimination is at risk for skin breakdown from incontinence, urinary tract infection from urinary retention, and urinary calculi from urinary retention and stasis. The nurse keeps the client clean and dry and provides skin care as described under Risk for Impaired Skin Integrity (pp. 127 and 128). (See Chapter 73 for preventive measures for urinary tract infection and calculi.)

CONSTIPATION

NOC **PLANNING: EXPECTED OUTCOMES.** The client with chronic illness or disability is expected to have a normal formation and evacuation of stool. Indicators include that the client has noncompromised:

- Elimination pattern
- Control of bowel movements
- Ease of stool passage
- Comfort of stool passage
- Muscle tone to evacuate stool

INTERVENTIONS. Neurologic problems often affect the client's bowel pattern by causing a reflex (spastic) bowel, a flaccid bowel, or an uninhibited bowel.

Upper motor neuron diseases and injuries, such as a cervical or mid-level spinal cord injury, may result in a reflex (spastic) bowel pattern, with defecation occurring suddenly and without warning. With a reflex pattern, any facilitating or triggering mechanism may lead to defecation if the lower colon contains stool. An example of facilitating or triggering techniques is digital stimulation. For this technique, use a lubricated glove or finger cot and massage the anus in a circular motion for no less than 1 full minute. Digital stimulation should not be used for clients with cardiac disease because of the risk of inducing a vagal response (a rapid decrease in heart rate).

Lower motor neuron diseases and injuries interfere with transmission of the nervous impulse across the reflex arc and may result in a flaccid bowel pattern, with defecation occurring infrequently and in small amounts. The use of facilitating and triggering mechanisms in combination with a toileting schedule, suppository use, and disimpaction yields the best results. Clients may be able to self-administer the suppository or disimpact if necessary.

Neurologic injuries that affect the brain may cause an uninhibited bowel pattern, with frequent defecation, urgency, and complaints of hard stool. Clients may manage uninhibited bowel patterns through a consistent toileting schedule, a high-fiber diet, and the use of stool softeners.

Bowel Training. An overview of management techniques for bowel dysfunction is presented in Table 10-6. In many cases, clients are not able to regain control over their bowel function in the manner previously possible. The rehabilitation team assists in designing a bowel elimination program that accommodates the disability.

The nurse works with clients to schedule bowel elimination as close as possible to their previous routine. For example, a client who had stools at noon every other day before the illness or injury should have the bowel program scheduled in the same way. An exception is the client who prefers another time that best fits into his or her daily routine. If the client is employed during the day, a time-consuming bowel elimination program in the morning may not be reasonable. It may be preferable to change the bowel protocol to the evening, when there is more time.

Drug Therapy. Bowel training programs for clients with neurologic problems are often designed to include a combination of suppository use and a consistent toileting schedule. Although medications should not be a first choice when formulating a bowel training program, consider the need for a suppository if clients do not re-establish defecation habits through a consistent toileting schedule, dietary modification, anal stimulation, and disimpaction.

TABLE 10-6 Management of Bowel Dysfunction

Functional Type	Neurologic Disability	Dysfunction	Re-establishing Defecation Patterns
Reflex (spastic)	Upper motor neuron spinal cord injury above T12	Defecation without warning	Triggering mechanisms Facilitation techniques High-fiber diet Suppository use Consistent toileting schedule
Flaccid	Lower motor neuron spinal cord injury below T12 (affects S2-4 reflex arc)	Infrequent, small stools	Triggering or facilitating techniques High-fiber diet Suppository use Consistent toileting schedule Manual disimpaction
Uninhibited	Brain damage from injury or stroke	Frequency, urgency, and constipation	Consistent toileting schedule High-fiber diet Stool softener use

Bisacodyl (Dulcolax) and glycerin are common agents prescribed by health care providers as suppositories in bowel training programs. Suppositories must be placed against the bowel wall to stimulate the sacral reflex arc and promote rectal emptying. Both agents are equivalent in effect, with results occurring in 15 to 30 minutes. Administer the suppository when the client expects to defecate, for example, after a meal to coincide with the gastrocolic reflex. Administering the suppository every second or third day is usually effective in re-establishing defecation patterns. Depending on each client's need, other medications (e.g., laxatives) may be indicated for bowel training programs.

Nutrition. Bowel elimination is directly related to the type and quality of food and fluid ingested. A high-fiber diet is a mainstay of most bowel training programs and includes whole-grain foods, bran, and fresh and dried fruits. Increasing dietary fiber is effective in facilitating defecation only if the client reduces fat intake. Drinking plenty of fluids also helps with bowel elimination.

Prevention of Complications. Constipation, diarrhea, and flatulence are common complications of any bowel training program. Assess for these complications and modify the bowel training program accordingly in collaboration with the physician and the dietitian.

INEFFECTIVE COPING

NOC **PLANNING: EXPECTED OUTCOMES.** The client with chronic illness or disability is expected to take personal actions to manage stressors that tax the client's resources. Indicators include that the client consistently:

- Identifies ineffective and effective coping patterns
- Verbalizes a sense of control
- Reports decrease in stress
- Seeks information concerning illness and treatment
- Modifies lifestyle as needed
- Adapts to life changes
- Uses available social support

INTERVENTIONS. The client with a disability often has a poor self-concept because of changes in body image from structural or functional changes. The use of an assistive device, such as a wheelchair, also differentiates the client from most other people, and the client may not want to accept the need for the device. Encourage the client to discuss his or her feelings and ask questions to elicit specific information that can help in assessing his or her acceptance of and ability to cope with the disability.

A disability also affects a person's role in society. For instance, a young medical student may fall from a ladder and become a quadriplegic; as a result, plans for a career as a surgeon are altered. A middle-aged farmer may be burned severely when his tractor catches on fire. He can no longer care for his farm, and his wife takes over during his rehabilitation process. An older adult who cares for her grandchildren is crippled with rheumatoid arthritis and can no longer provide child care. Disability requires role changes and always involves losses in the lives of those affected.

In addition to role changes, relationships with people change. Socializing with friends and family may be a strain when a person feels "different." Intimate relationships are affected because sexual dysfunction may result from disability. The nurse should be sensitive to these issues and should not avoid discussing them.

Assess the client's previous coping strategies and support systems so they can be used during rehabilitation if needed. The client is asked what strategies have been used to cope successfully with previous life crises, if any. Spiritual and religious beliefs are important for some people and should not be overlooked when helping to identify sources of support.

Some clients use complementary and alternative medicine (CAM) to cope with chronic disease and disability, especially if chronic pain is a problem. Examples of these therapies include acupuncture, acupressure, imagery, and music. Chapter 4 discusses CAM in detail.

Community-Based Care

Discharge planning begins during the client's admission. If the client is being transferred from a hospital to a rehabilitation unit or facility, orient him or her to the change in routine and emphasize the importance of self-care. When the client is admitted to the rehabilitation unit or facility, the case manager assesses his or her current living situation at home. Together with the client and family members or significant others, the case manager determines the adequacy of the current situation and the potential needs after discharge to home. The client with chronic illness and disability may require home care, assistance with activities of daily living (ADLs), nursing care, or physical or occupational therapy after discharge. The case manager assesses these needs and plans with the client, family or significant other, social worker, physical or vocational therapist, and physician the best ways to meet identified needs.

Other health care professionals may be necessary to meet the unique needs of special populations. For example, clients with brain injury may benefit from life planning, a process that examines and plans to meet lifelong needs. Case managers specializing in life planning may be part of the interdisciplinary rehabilitation team.

HOME CARE MANAGEMENT

Before the client returns home, the nurse assesses his or her readiness for discharge from the rehabilitation facility or hospital. The home may be assessed in multiple ways.

PREDISCHARGE ASSESSMENT. Before discharge, the case manager or occupational therapist may visit the home to assess its layout and accessibility. These professionals may be employed by the health care agency or by a third-party payer, such as a health maintenance organization (see Chapter 3 for a discussion of third-party payers). Because of the stress of hospitalization, a client with a fractured hip who is ambulating well with a walker may neglect to explain to the nurse that the home has three steps at the entrance and that the bathroom is accessible by stairway only. The client may not consider it important to mention that throw rugs, which do not provide a completely level surface on which to use a cane, are scattered throughout the apartment.

During a predischarge visit to the home, the case manager assesses the accessibility of the home in general and of the bathrooms, bedrooms, and kitchen. If the client will be wheelchair dependent after discharge from the facility, ramps are needed to replace steps, and doorways should be checked for adequate width. A doorway width of 36 to 38 inches (slightly less than 1 m) is usually sufficient for a standard-sized wheelchair. Any room that the client needs to use is checked. The bedroom should have sufficient space for the client to maneuver transfers to and from the wheelchair and the bed.

Space requirements depend on the client's need to use a wheelchair, walker, or cane. In the bathroom, grab bars may need to be installed before the client comes home. Bathtub benches can provide support for the client who has difficulty with mobility and, when used in combination with a handheld shower head, can provide easily accessible bathing facilities. Assessment of the kitchen may or may not be critical depending on whether the client has help with cooking and preparing meals. If the client will be responsible for cooking after discharge, the kitchen is assessed for wheelchair or walker accessibility, appliance accessibility, and the need for adaptive equipment.

LEAVE-OF-ABSENCE VISIT. A second method of assessing the client's home is through a brief home visit, also called a leave-of-absence (LOA) visit, by the client before discharge. The nurse explains the need for the trial home visit and assesses the client's comfort level with this idea. The client who has been hospitalized for a lengthy period may feel intense anxiety about returning home. The nurse may allay such anxieties with careful preparation. Before the visit, the rehabilitation nurse meets with the client and family members or significant others to set goals for the visit and to identify specific tasks to be attempted while at home. After the home visit, the client is interviewed to determine the success of the visit and to assess additional education or training needs before final discharge.

Going home may not be an option for everyone. Some clients may not have a support network of family members or significant others. For example, many older adults have no spouse or close friends living nearby. Children may live far away, which can make home care difficult. If no caregiver is available, the family must decide whether care can be provided in the home by an outside resource or whether the client needs to be admitted to a 24-hour supervised health care setting, such as a nursing home. Rehabilitation services are available in most long-term care settings (skilled nursing facilities) at least 5 days a week.

HEALTH TEACHING

Education of the client and the family is the cornerstone of nursing care. Assess every component of care to determine how to teach the client to perform activities of daily living (ADLs) independently. Determine the client's learning potential and cognitive capacity and encourage him or her to perform or direct each skill or technique independently to verify understanding. Written material explaining the steps in the procedure is provided to the client and family members to reinforce learning and to provide support with the technique after discharge. Before distributing written material, the rehabilitation team assesses the reading level of the material and determines whether it is appropriate for the client's reading ability and language skills.

Any chronic illness or disability necessitates changes in lifestyle and body image. The nurse assists in dealing with such changes by encouraging the verbalization of feelings and emotions. A focus on existing capabilities instead of disabilities is emphasized.

The client may fail to relate psychologically to the disability during hospitalization. For example, he or she may display anger or frustration in attempting to perform self-care routines before discharge from the rehabilitation facility. Encourage the client to be open about such feelings and to talk about ways to prevent worries from becoming realities after discharge.

The leave-of-absence home visit assists the client and family members or significant others in psychosocial preparation for discharge. It allows the experience of the home situation while being able to return to the hospital environment after a few hours. Often the client finds that his or her fears were not realized during the home visit but finds new problems in the home that must be addressed before discharge. Review this information with the client in preparation for discharge to the home.

HEALTH CARE RESOURCES

After discharge to the home, various health care resources (e.g., physical therapy, home care nursing, and vocational counseling) are available to the client with chronic illness and disability. Assess the need for additional care and support throughout the hospitalization and collaborate with the case manager and physician in arranging for home services.

Evaluation: Outcomes

The client and rehabilitation team evaluate the effectiveness of interdisciplinary interventions on the basis of the identified nursing diagnoses and collaborative problems. Expected outcomes may include that the client will:

- Move purposefully in his or her environment with or without assistive devices.

- Perform the most basic physical tasks and personal care activities independently with or without assistive devices.
- Have structural intactness and physiologic function of the skin.
- Have normal collection and discharge of urine.
- Have normal formation and evacuation of stool.
- Take personal actions to manage stressors that tax the client's resources.

GET READY for the NCLEX Examination!

KEY POINTS

- Rehabilitation is the process of learning to live with chronic and disabling conditions.
- Clients in a rehabilitation setting are managed by an interdisciplinary team of health care professionals; the client is also a member of the team.
- Assessment of the client in rehabilitation includes the components that are listed in Table 10-1.
- The Functional Independence Measure (FIM) system is used to assess functional ability of the client in rehabilitation.
- The members of the interdisciplinary team teach clients how transfer, bed mobility, and gait training techniques.
- The client is taught how to perform activities of daily living with or without using adaptive devices; the client should be encouraged to be as independent as possible.
- One of the goals of nursing care is to prevent complications of immobility for the client (see Table 10-2).
- Clients in rehabilitation should be assessed for risk factors that make them likely to develop skin breakdown; interventions to prevent skin problems include repositioning and adequate nutrition.
- Clients with bladder and bowel problems are managed by training programs; spastic, flaccid, and uninhibited elimination are managed differently (see Tables 10-5 and 10-6).
- Nurses and other health care team members assist clients to cope with their losses and assess the availability of client support systems.

ADDITIONAL STUDY RESOURCES

Go to your Student CD-ROM for Review Questions for the NCLEX Examination.

evolve Go to http://evolve.elsevier.com/Iggy/ for Integrated Management of Care Questions for the NCLEX Examination.

SELECTED BIBLIOGRAPHY

Asterisk indicates a classic or definitive work on this subject.

Association of Rehabilitation Nurses. (2000a). *Standards and scope of rehabilitation nursing practice.* Glenview, IL: Author.

Association of Rehabilitation Nurses. (2000b). *The specialty practice of rehabilitation nursing: A core curriculum* (4th ed.). Skokie, IL: Author.

Beck, L.A. (2003). Cancer rehabilitation: Does it make a difference? *Rehabilitation Nursing, 28*(2), 42-47.

*Braden, B.J., & Bergstrom, N. (1992). Pressure reduction. In G.M. Bulechek & J.C. McCloskey (Eds.), *Nursing interventions: Essential nursing treatments* (2nd ed., pp. 94-108). Philadelphia: W.B. Saunders.

Bray, J. (2003). Therapeutic relationships: Building blocks for rehabilitation nursing. *Rehabilitation Nursing, 28*(5), 140.

Dochterman, J.M., & Bulechek, G.M. (2004). *Nursing interventions classification (NIC)* (4th ed.). St. Louis: Mosby.

Gallagner, R.M. (2000). How long-term care is changing. *American Journal of Nursing, 100*(2), 65-67.

Gibson, K.L. (2003). Caring for a patient who lives with a spinal cord injury. *Nursing, 33*(7), 36-41.

Glenn, J. (2003). Restorative Nursing Bladder Training Program: Recommending a strategy. *Rehabilitation Nursing, 28*(1), 15-22.

*Granger, C.V., & Gresham, G.E. (1984). *Functional assessment in rehabilitation medicine.* Baltimore: Williams & Wilkins.

*Granger, C.V., et al. (1993). Performance profiles of the Functional Independence Measure. *Journal of Physical Medicine and Rehabilitation, 72,* 84-89.

Gross, J.C., et al. (2001). Determining stroke rehabilitation inpatients' level of nursing care. *Clinical Nursing Research, 10*(1), 40-51.

*Ignatavicius, D.D. (1998). *Introduction to long term care nursing.* Philadelphia: F.A. Davis.

*Institute of Medicine. (1991). *Disability in America.* Washington, DC: National Academy Press.

*Katz, S., et al. (1963). Studies of illness in the aged. The index of ADL: A standardized measure of biological and psychosocial function. *Journal of the American Medical Association, 185,* 914-919.

Lorig, K.R., Ritter, P.L., & Gonzalez, V.M. (2003). Hispanic chronic disease self-management: A randomized community-based outcome trial. *Nursing Research, 52*(6), 361-369.

Maas, M., Buckwalter, M., Hardy, M., et al. (2001). *Nursing care of older adults: Diagnoses, outcomes, and interventions.* St. Louis: Mosby.

Marrelli, T. (2003). Restorative care and home care: New implications for aide and nurse roles? *Geriatric Nursing, 24*(2), 128-129.

Moorhead, S., Johnson, M., & Maas, M. (2004). *Nursing outcomes classification (NOC)* (3rd ed.). St. Louis: Mosby.

*Nazarko, L. (1999). Rehabilitation. *Nursing Management, 6*(5), 24-27.

Nazarko, L. (2003). Rehabilitation and continence promotion following a stroke. *Nursing Times, 99*(44), 52, 55.

*Neal, L.J. (1995). The rehabilitation nurse in the home care setting: Treating chronic wounds as a disability. *Rehabilitation Nursing, 20*(5), 261-264.

Percentage of deaths due to chronic diseases. (2002). Available at http://ncsl.org/programs/health/phchronic.htm.

*Posavec, E.J., & Carey, R.G. (1982). Using a level of function scale (LORS-II) to evaluate the success of inpatient rehabilitation programs. *Rehabilitation Nursing, 7*(6), 17-19.

Pryor, J. (2000). Creating a rehabilitative milieu. *Rehabilitation Nursing, 25*(4), 141-144.

*Sorensen, B., & Luken, K. (1999). Improving functional outcomes with recreational therapy. *The Case Manager, 10*(5), 48-53.

*Wood, C., & Lui, J. (1999). The evolution of disability care and case management: Identifying core competencies. *The Case Manager, 10*(4), 41-46.

*World Health Organization. (1980). *International classification of impairments, disabilities and handicaps.* Geneva: Author.

CHAPTER

11 Genetic Concepts for Medical-Surgical Nursing

M. LINDA WORKMAN

LEARNING OUTCOMES

After studying this chapter, you should be able to:

1. Describe the structure and forms of DNA.
2. List the events and processes involved in DNA replication.
3. Describe the relationship between genes and proteins.
4. Compare the concept of phenotype with that of genotype.
5. Compare the patterns of inheritance for single gene traits.
6. Explain how genetic variations can induce or affect adult health problems.
7. List 10 adult health problems that have a genetic basis.
8. Identify assessment questions that help obtain information for a genetic assessment.
9. Construct a three-generation pedigree.
10. Identify clients at risk for a genetic predisposition for health problems.
11. Explain how genetic testing is different from other laboratory tests.
12. Describe the role of the medical-surgical nurse in genetic counseling.

Go to your Student CD-ROM for Review Questions for the NCLEX Examination keyed to these Learning Outcomes.

Many scientific advances are leading to better health by preventing illness, disease, or disability and by improving interventions to treat health problems that do occur. For example, 50 years ago only about 15% of clients diagnosed with cancer lived 5 years, and even fewer were cured. Today more than 50% of clients diagnosed with cancer in North America are cured of the disease, and many others will live 5 years or longer. Advances in cancer prevention, diagnosis, and treatment have made these improvements possible.

One of the most important areas of advancement is in the understanding of the influence of genetic factors on adult health and adult illness. These advances, marked by completion of the first phase of the Human Genome Project, led to a whole new era, called **genomic medicine.** Genomic medicine, or "genomics," will lead to drug therapies that take into account each client's genetic differences, allowing a drug regimen to be tailored for a specific client. Genomics also will help to identify clients at risk for specific health problems so that prevention and early detection strategies can be better targeted.

Nursing organizations, such as the American Nurses Association and the American Academy of Nursing, support the need for all nurses to have a basic understanding of genetics to provide the best possible care for clients and families (Grady & Collins, 2003; Lea, 2002a). Many common adult health problems (e.g., hypertension, diabetes, heart disease, cancer, arthritis, and many others) have a genetic basis. Changes in genes (mutations or variations) can have serious results. Gene mutations/variations can increase the risk for a disorder and thus are known as "susceptibility" genes or gene differences. Other gene mutations/variations decrease the risk for a disorder and thus are known as "protective" genes or gene differences. The purpose of this chapter is to help you learn more about basic genetics and how this information relates to adult health care. Table 11-1 defines commonly used genetic terms.

GENETIC BIOLOGY

All living things, including people, animals, plants, and microorganisms, have genes. Genes are the instructions for the making of all the different substances any organism makes. Think of all the hormones, enzymes, and other proteins your body makes. It is the specific genes that tell each cell what protein to make, how to make it, when to make it, and how much to make. Think of each gene as a specific "recipe" for making a certain protein.

So where are these genes? The genes are located in the nucleus of most body cells. As shown in Figure 11-1, the cell nucleus contains the DNA in the form of chromosomes. It is interesting that all cells with a nucleus contain all the

TABLE 11-1 Genetic Terms and Concepts

allele One of possible alternate forms of a gene. Can be due to a variation in a gene sequence or to the existence of many slightly different genes (within a species) coding for the same single trait.

base pairs Nucleotides that pair up loosely together when DNA is double-stranded. They are held together with the relatively weak forces of hydrogen bonds. Normally, adenine and thymine form a pair by sharing two hydrogen bonds; cytosine and guanine form a base pair sharing three hydrogen bonds.

complementary bases The nitrogenous bases that normally pair using hydrogen bonds. Adenine and thymine are complementary to each other. Cytosine and guanine are complementary to each other. Because these pairs are complementary (and faithful), if the sequences of bases for one strand of DNA is known, the complementary strand can be predicted.

chromosome A temporary but consistent state of cellular DNA tightly condensed and coiled into dense bodies that take up stain and are visible under a microscope during metaphase of mitosis.

euploid The normal or expected number of chromosomes for the species.

diploid (2N) This is the complete set of chromosome pairs found in all the individual's somatic cells. The normal diploid chromosome number for humans is 46 (23 pairs). The normal diploid chromosome number for mice is 40 (20 pairs).

haploid (1N) A set of chromosomes consisting of half of each pair. The normal haploid number of human chromosomes is 23. Only the sex cells (ova and sperm) have the haploid number so that fertilization results in the normal diploid number.

centromere The "pinched-in" area of a chromosome where the two chromatids are joined.

chromatid The longitudinal half of a metaphase chromosome (split through the centromere). This structure actually is the original and duplicated DNA that has not yet separated during mitosis.

"p" arm The short "arm" of a chromosome above the centromere.

"q" arm The long "arm" of a chromosome below the centromere.

autosomes The 22 pairs of human chromosomes that do not code for the sexual differentiation of the individual.

sex chromosomes The pair of chromosomes that code for the sexual differentiation of the individual. In males the sex chromosomes are usually an X and a Y. In females the sex chromosomes are usually two Xs.

nucleoside A nitrogenous base of adenine, guanine, cytosine, or thymine attached to a five-sided sugar (ribose sugar).

nucleotide A nucleoside (nitrogenous base attached to a five-sided sugar) connected to a phosphate group. It is this structure that assembles into a single strand of DNA.

concordance The frequency with which a specific trait or condition is found in both members of a natural pair. When such a trait/condition is present in both members of a natural pair (as in the case of "identical" twins), the trait/condition is considered genetic in origin.

monozygotic (MZ) siblings These siblings are the product of one fertilized egg that split into two or more equal parts during embryogenesis. The genetic material is identical for all individuals who develop as a result of this split. This is the origin of "identical" twins or triplets.

dizygotic (DZ) siblings Even though these siblings have shared a womb and are born at the same time, they are the result of different fertilized eggs. Their genetic material is not identical and is no more similar than any other siblings. This is the origin of "fraternal" twins, triplets or other multiple births.

codon Think "code"! Each amino acid that makes up a protein has a specific code in the DNA. This is made up of a three-base sequence. For example, the DNA code (codon) for the amino acid methionine is TAC (for thymine, adenine, and cytosine).

anticodon The "anticodon" is actually the complementary code of an amino acid.

RNA RNA, or ribonucleic acid, is a single strand of nitrogenous bases (adenine, guanine, cytosine, and uracil) constructed during transcription from a segment of DNA containing the gene for a specific protein. The RNA is complementary to the "template" DNA. A major difference in RNA is the use of the base "uracil" in place of thymine.

transcription The process of making a new strand of DNA or RNA that is complementary to the original or "template" DNA. When a cell is dividing, both entire strands of DNA are transcribed so that there is sufficient DNA for each of the two new "daughter" cells. When a protein is going to be made, only the segment of DNA that contains the gene for the protein is transcribed into RNA.

translation The using of a messenger RNA molecule as the directions for proper placement of amino acids during protein synthesis.

ribose A five-sided sugar with a hydroxyl group (OH) on the number 2 carbon. This type of sugar forms an attachment with the bases that compose the RNA nucleotides (adenosine, guanosine, cytidine, and uridine).

deoxyribose A five-sided sugar with a hydrogen molecule (and no oxygen) on the number 2 carbon. This type of sugar forms an attachment with the nitrogenous bases that compose DNA nucleotides (adenosine, guanosine, cytidine, and thymidine).

gene expression The activation of a gene leading to the transcription, translation, and synthesis of a specific protein. The result of gene expression is the observable presence of the specific trait or condition coded for by the gene.

genome The complete set of genes for the species.

gene locus The exact location of a gene on a specific chromosome.

genotype The exact allele pair composition for any given single gene trait. When both alleles are identical *(homozygous),* genotype and phenotype are the same. When a gene's alleles are different from each other *(heterozygous),* the actual genotype may be different from what is observed *(phenotype).*

phenotype The observed expression of any given single trait (e.g., blood type, hair color, presence of male secondary sexual characteristics).

homozygous Having identical alleles (two) at a gene chromosome locus for a specific single gene trait.

heterozygous Having two different alleles at a gene chromosome locus for a specific single gene trait.

mutation An alteration in the base sequence of a gene that has deleterious effects on the function of the gene's product.

polymorphism An alteration in the base sequence of a gene that has minimal effects on the function of the gene's product.

genes. At one time, science tried to explain how different cells have different functions by suggesting that the genes of different cells were unique. For example, you make insulin in the beta cells of your pancreas and nowhere else. Wouldn't it make sense that the reason only the beta cells can make insulin is that they are the only cells that have the gene for insulin? Well, even though that theory makes some sense, it is not the case. In fact *all* human cells with a nucleus have the gene for insulin. The only cell type, however, that allows the insulin gene to be active and make insulin is the beta cell of the pancreas. We have the insulin gene in our skin cells, heart cells, brain cells, and other cells, but only in the beta cells is this gene selectively "turned on" **(expressed)** when you need to make insulin.

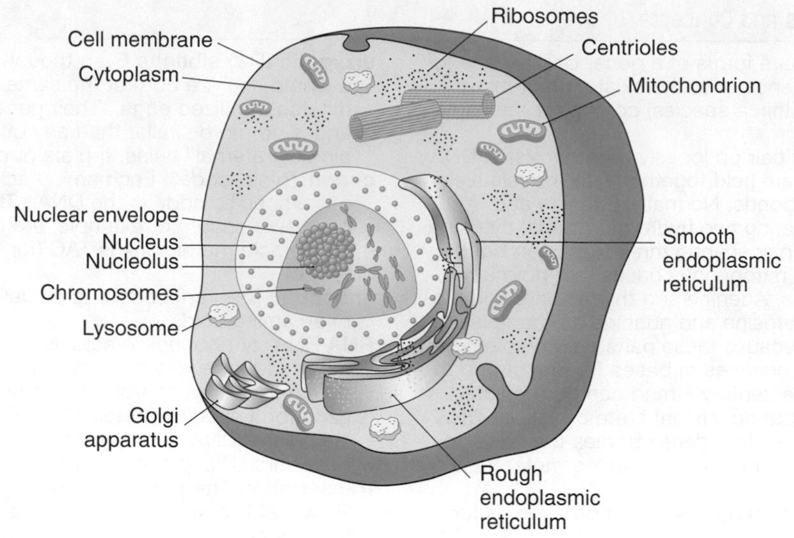

Figure 11-1 ■ Anatomy of a cell.

An important fact to remember is that all human cells with a nucleus each contain the entire set of human genes. This complete set of genes is called the **genome.** The human genome contains about 35,000 individual genes (Collins et al., 2003).

The only exceptions for chromosomes are the mature red blood cells, which have no nucleus, and the sex cells (the eggs and sperm). Sex cells have only one chromosome of each pair (thus 23 chromosomes) so that when an egg is fertilized by a sperm, the chromosomes unite to form a new individual with 46 chromosomes.

One area that is somewhat confusing about genetics is how DNA (deoxyribonucleic acid) is different from the genes and from the chromosomes. DNA, chromosomes, and genes are all the same basic thing; only the structures differ. Figure 11-2 shows that if we pick out any one chromosome in the nucleus, we can "unwind" it and see that the framework of any chromosome is the DNA. Each chromosome has many genes within it. Humans have 23 pairs of chromosomes–46 individual chromosomes. The Y chromosome, a small chromosome, has only 78 genes. Larger chromosomes, such as the number 1 chromosome, contain thousands of genes.

One way to think of it is to consider all the DNA in any cell's nucleus to be a giant "cookbook" containing all the recipes needed to make all the proteins, hormones, enzymes, and other substances your body needs. The chromosome pairs are the different book chapters (so the human genome cookbook has 23 chapters), and the genes are the individual recipes contained within the chapters.

There is a specific chromosome location **(locus)** for every gene. For example, the locus for the gene for blood type is on chromosome 9. The locus for the gene for the beta chain of hemoglobin is on chromosome 11. The first phase of the Human Genome Project determined the exact sequence of DNA and the location of many genes. Figure 11-2 shows that each chromosome is made up of a large chunk of DNA that has been twisted (like a length of rope) until it coils up tightly into a very dense structure. Thus in each cell the DNA is divided into 46 separate chunks.

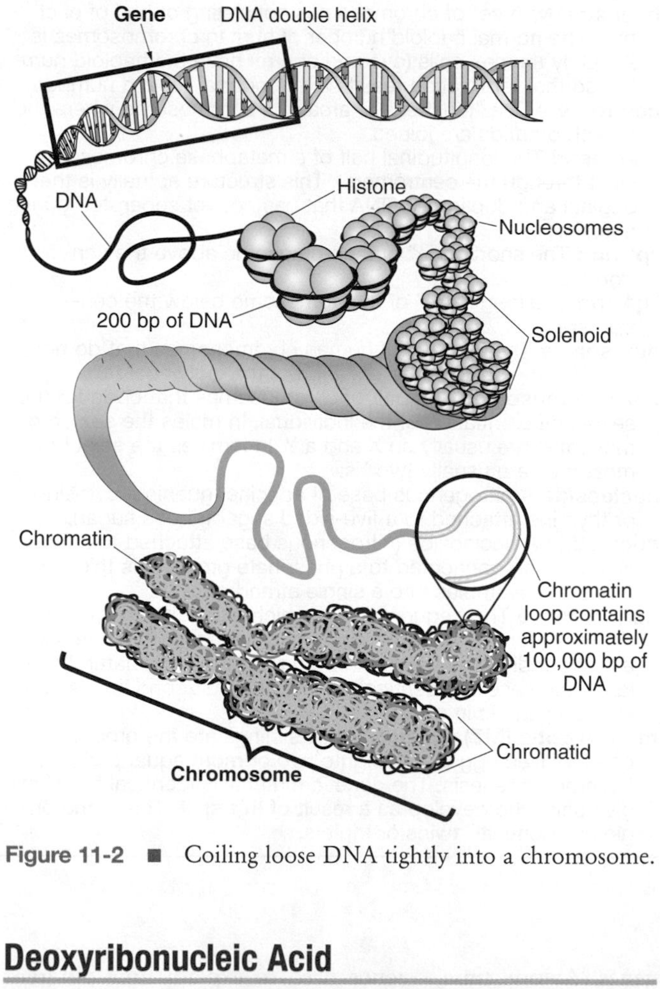

Figure 11-2 ■ Coiling loose DNA tightly into a chromosome.

Deoxyribonucleic Acid

DNA is short for **deoxyribonucleic acid,** which is the basic genetic material in a cell that contains genes. Most DNA (about 99.99%) is in the nucleus. A small amount of DNA is also present in other cell organelles, such as the mitochondria. This chapter focuses on the nuclear DNA.

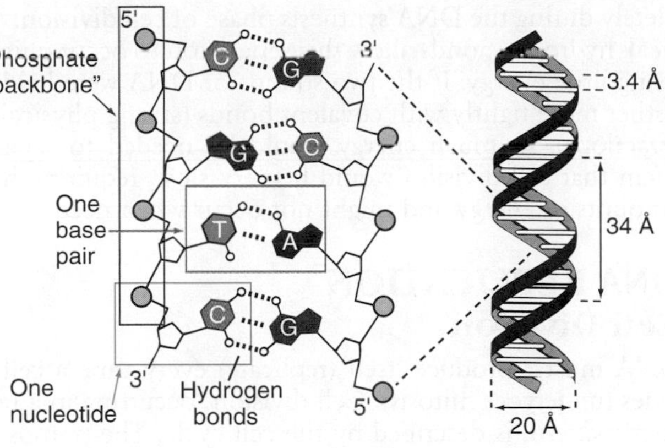

Figure 11-3 ■ The structure of DNA.

DNA STRUCTURE

In humans, DNA is a linear, double-stranded structure composed of multiple units of four different nitrogenous bases, each attached to a sugar molecule. The bases in each strand are connected together by phosphate groups. The two individual strands are held together (loosely) by hydrogen bonds interacting with the base pairs of the two strands.

This double-stranded DNA is arranged like a long set of railroad tracks. The "backbones" of the track are the two long steel rails. For DNA these backbones are the phosphate groups that hold the strand of bases together (like beads on a string with the string being the backbone). The bases are the individual railroad ties (or beads). Think of each tie as having two pieces, one piece attached to the right-handed rail and one piece attached to the left-sided rail.

Figure 11-3 shows a very small piece of double-stranded DNA on the left (containing only four base pairs) taken from the larger piece of DNA on the right. The phosphate groups that hold the nucleotides together as a strand are in the red box. The green box in the lower left-hand section shows a whole nucleotide (a base with the sugar and the phosphate group) in place in the left-hand DNA strand. The blue box in the middle of the two strands shows how the base from the left strand lines up with and pairs to a complementary base in the right strand.

Bases

Many trillions of bases in the double-stranded DNA are found in the nucleus of just one cell. In fact, if you could crack the cell open like an egg, then extract the nucleus (yolk) and open it, the amount of DNA in the nucleus, stretched out, is about 6 feet long. If the DNA in one cell could be made large enough to see and touch (about the width of a tape measure), it would be long enough to stretch out more than 1000 feet! There is much more DNA in each nucleus than is needed for the 35,000 genes. The gene DNA makes up only about 5% of all the DNA in each cell. What is known about all that extra DNA is discussed on p. 139.

The four bases in DNA are adenine (A), guanine (G), cytosine (C), and thymine (T). These four bases are made from vitamins and the nitrogen atoms from amino acids. For example, thymine is made from folic acid and nitrogen. Two of the bases (thymine and cytosine) are called **pyrimidines** because

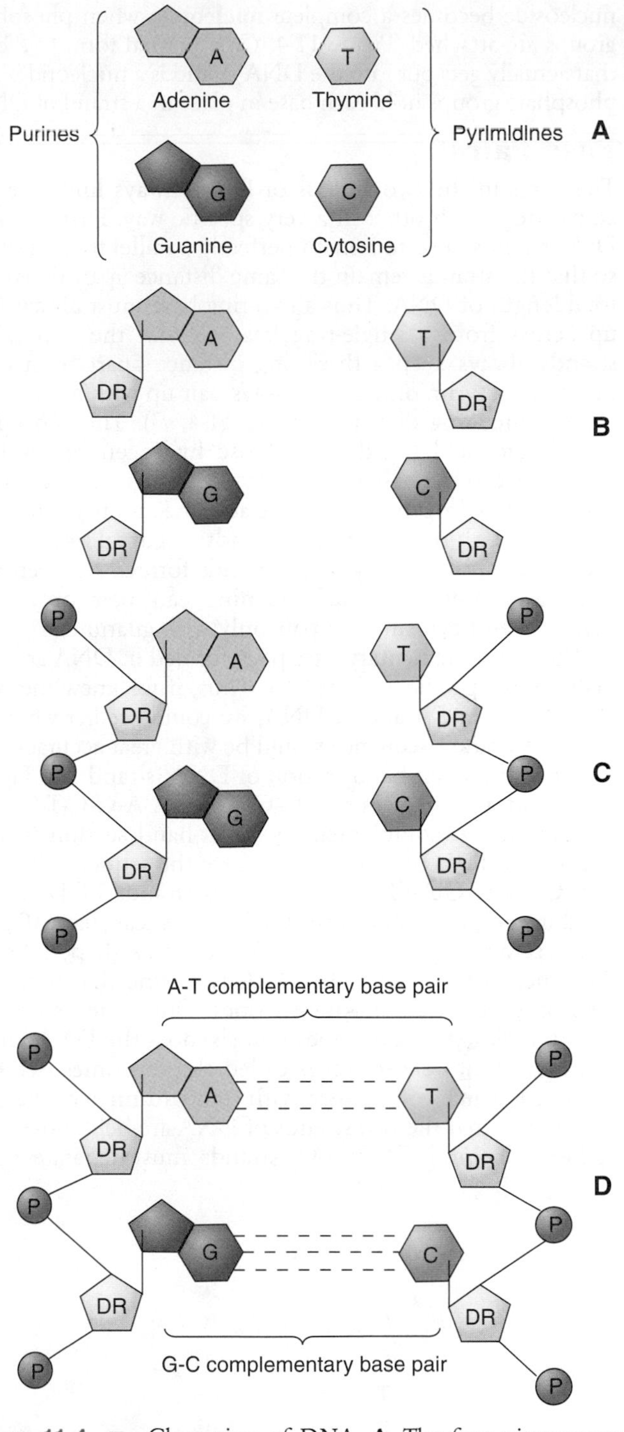

Figure 11-4 ■ Close view of DNA. **A,** The four nitrogenous bases of DNA. **B,** Nitrogenous bases converted into nucleosides by attaching a deoxyribose sugar (DR). **C,** The four nucleosides converted into nucleotides by attaching phosphate groups (P). **D,** Two short strands of DNA held loosely together by hydrogen bonds forming complementary base pairs. ––––, weak hydrogen bonds.

of their single-ringed chemical structures (Figure 11-4, *A*). The other two bases (adenine and guanine) are called **purines** because of their double-ringed chemical structures.

Each base becomes a **nucleoside** when a five-sided sugar (known as a deoxyribose sugar) is attached to it. Figure 11-4, *B* shows how the four bases become four nucleosides. Each nucleoside becomes a complete **nucleotide** when phosphate groups are attached (Figure 11-4, *C*). The final form of a base that actually gets put into the DNA strand is a nucleotide. The phosphate groups hold each base in place in a strand of DNA.

Base Pairs

The bases in the two strands of DNA always link together across from each other in a very specific way. First, the two DNA strands need to remain perfectly parallel to each other so that the strands remain the same distance apart down the total length of DNA. Thus a two-ring base must always line up across from a single-ring base so that the two DNA strands always keep a three-ring distance apart from each other. So a pyrimidine must always pair up with a purine to keep a three-ring distance (Figure 11-4, *D*). The two DNA strands are held together by loose hydrogen bonds that form between the base pairs. Cytosine and guanine connect with three hydrogen bonds while adenine and thymine connect with only two hydrogen bonds (Figure 11-4, *D*). Because the number of hydrogen bonds formed between any two bases must be equal, adenine can pair only with thymine, and cytosine can pair only with guanine.

These complementary base pairs formed in DNA are normally both specific and faithful. Thus, if we knew the base sequence of one strand of DNA, we could predict what the opposite strand's sequence would be with great accuracy. For example, if the left-hand section of DNA (strand 1 in Figure 11-5) had the sequence A-G-G-C-T-C-A-A-C-C-T-G, the corresponding (complementary) right-hand section (strand 2 in Figure 11-5) of DNA would have the sequence T-C-C-G-A-G-T-T-G-G-A-C. When the two strands of DNA are lined up properly, they twist in a loose helical shape (Figure 11-6; see also Figure 11-2). DNA keeps this shape most of the time. In this shape, the DNA is so fine that it can be seen only with electron microscopes. Only when a cell begins to divide (i.e., undergoes mitosis) does the DNA supercoil tightly into dense pieces called chromosomes (see Figure 11-2), which can be seen with standard microscopes.

The fact that the two strands of DNA are held loosely together is helpful. These two strands must separate completely during the DNA synthesis phase of cell division. The weak hydrogen bonds allow this separation to occur quickly, using little energy. If the two strands of DNA were held together more tightly with covalent bonds (strong physical interactions), so much energy would be needed to separate them that cell division would be very slow, requiring huge amounts of energy and might not occur when needed.

DNA REPLICATION

Cell Division

DNA must reproduce itself (replicate) every time a cell divides (undergoes mitosis). Cell division, occurring in a regulated pattern, is described by the cell cycle. The purpose of mitotic cell division is for one cell to reproduce (duplicate) into two new cells. Each of the two new cells is identical to the original cell that started mitosis. In order for each new cell to have exactly the right amount of DNA and genes, the DNA in the dividing cell must exactly replicate. Figure 11-7 shows the phases of the cell cycle.

Living cells that are not actively reproducing are in a reproductive resting state called G_0. During the G_0 period, cells actively carry out their functions but do not divide. Normal cells spend most of their lives in the G_0 state, just as most humans spend the majority of their lives in a nonpregnant state.

Mitotic cell division makes one cell divide into two cells. These two cells are identical to each other and to the origi-

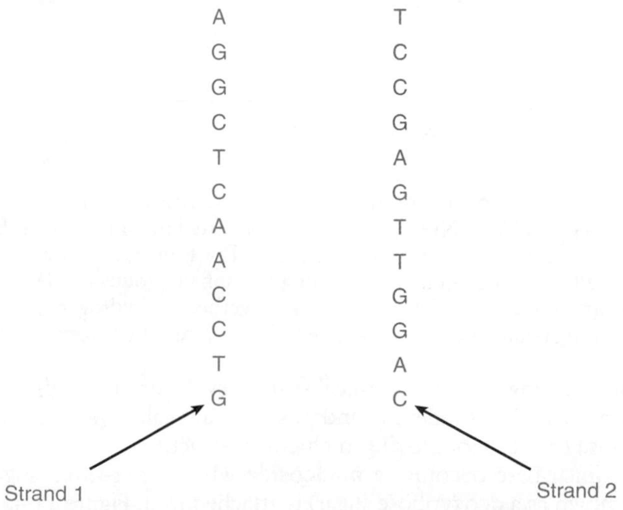

Figure 11-5 ■ Complementary strands of DNA.

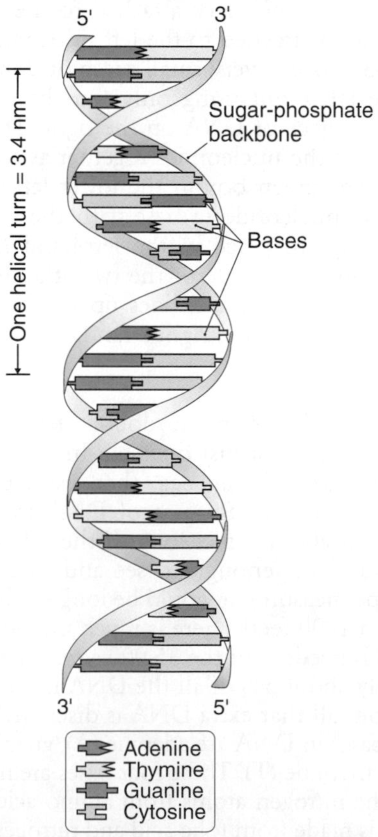

Figure 11-6 ■ Complementary strands of DNA twisted into a loose helical shape.

nal cell that started the mitotic cell division. Cells must go through four phases of the cell cycle to divide:

- *G_1:* The cell is getting ready for division by taking on extra nutrients, making more energy, and growing extra membrane. The amount of cell fluid (cytoplasm) also increases.
- *S:* Because making one cell into two cells requires twice as much of everything, including DNA, the cell must double its DNA content through DNA synthesis. This process occurs in S phase. First the double strands of DNA must separate. Then enzymes read the sequence of one of the original strands and build a new strand complementary to the original strand. The same thing is happening to the other original strand (Figure 11-8). The process of making a new copy of an entire strand of DNA is called **DNA transcription.**

Numerous enzymes are involved in DNA synthesis. Some of the enzymes "relax" and then "unwind" the double-stranded DNA. Other enzymes separate the two strands and keep them separate. Different enzymes "read" the original DNA strands and determine the order of the bases for the new strands. Special enzymes actually build the new strands by placing and linking nucleotides together. Finally, other enzymes actually "spell check" the new strands of DNA to ensure that each base in the new strand is exactly complementary to its base pair on the original strand.

When DNA synthesis is complete, the result is two sets of double-stranded DNA. Each of the two sets has one old strand and one new strand. Notice in Figure 11-7 that the nucleus during S phase is twice as large as it was during G_1 because it now has twice as much DNA.

During M phase of the cell cycle, one set of DNA will move into one of the two new cells made during mitosis and the second set will move into the other new cell. In this way, every new cell ends up with exactly the right amount of DNA with all the genes.

- *G_2:* The cell makes important proteins that will be used in actual cell division and in normal physiologic function after cell division is complete.
- *M:* The single cell splits apart into two cells (actual mitosis). It is in this phase, after the DNA has completely replicated itself, that the 46 separate chunks of DNA twist very tightly, bending around small protein balls called histones, to form very dense bodies that can be seen (when stained) using a standard microscope.

These dense bodies are called "chromosomes" because in this form they can take up stain and have color.

Chromosome Formation

It is during M phase that the fact that there is much more DNA in each cell than just the genes is helpful. The delivery of genes to each new cell during mitosis is critical for the new cells to be able to function. Thus, this DNA delivery must be precise and perfect. Having the DNA pack down into chromosomes makes for precise DNA delivery. This works in much the same way that oral drugs do. For example, think about the size of a single aspirin tablet that contains 325 mg of the drug aspirin. This tablet is not very large, only a little over 1 cm in diameter. This tablet also contains some other material that is not aspirin but helps to form the aspirin tablet. Now think about a drug that contains only 1 mg of drug per tablet. If that tablet contained just the 1 mg of drug, the tablet would be too small to handle (about the size of a grain of sand). Thus more material is added with the 1 mg of drug to make the tablet large enough to handle.

If each cell contained only enough DNA to make up the genes, the process of DNA replication and delivery of DNA to the two new cells would be less precise. So there is at least 20 times more DNA than is needed for the 35,000 genes. This extra DNA allows chromosomes to form, which can then be split exactly in half, allowing very precise delivery of DNA to the new cells.

So, as you can see in Figure 11-2, a chromosome is a specific large chunk of double-stranded DNA, with each chunk containing billions of bases and hundreds (and sometimes thousands) of genes. During M phase, each chromosome forms and moves to the center of the cell that is about to divide. Stringlike fibers form from each side of the cell and attach to each chromosome half (chromatid). This action is shown in Figure 11-9 (using just four chromosomes). Just before the cell splits into two cells *(cytokinesis),* each chro-

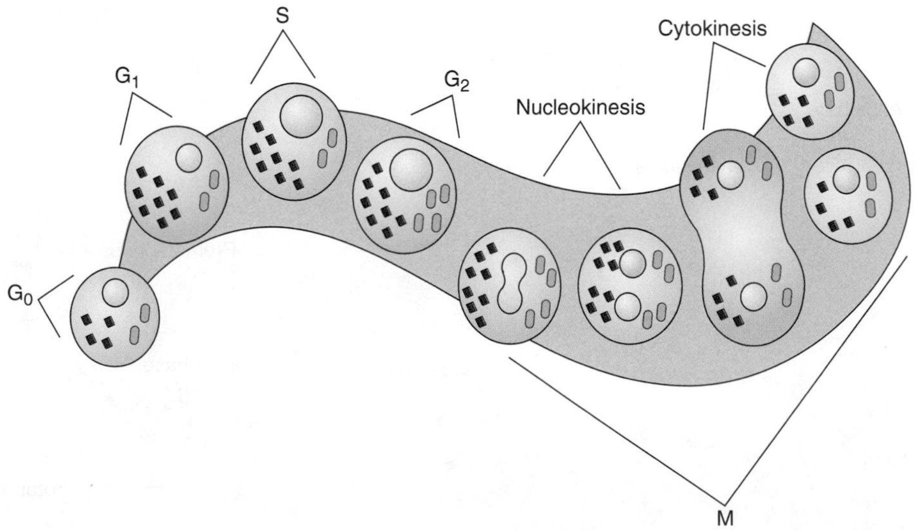

Figure 11-7 ■ The cell cycle.

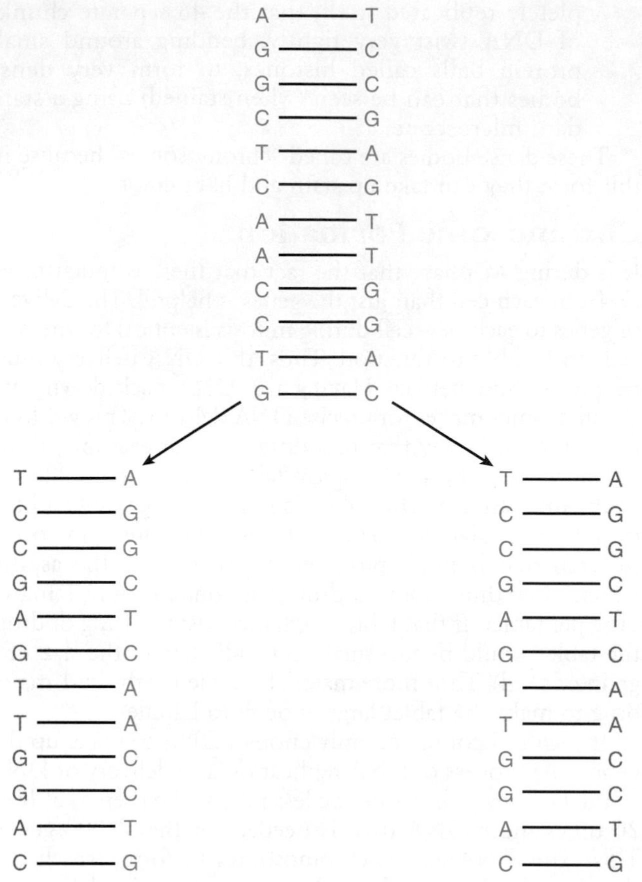

Figure 11-8 ■ DNA replication. *Blue type,* Original DNA; *red type,* newly made (replicated) DNA.

mosome is pulled apart so that half of each chromosome goes into one new cell and the other half goes into the other new cell. The process of pulling the chromosomes apart is called *nucleokinesis.*

Chromosome Function

Chromosomes are temporary structures, but their job is important: precise delivery of DNA to the two new cells. As we have seen, humans have 46 chromosomes divided into 23 pairs. This number is known as the "diploid" number of chromosomes for humans. Remember that each chromosome we view just before cell division actually has twice the DNA in it. This chromosome is going to split down the middle during mitosis, with half of the chromosome going to one new cell and the other half going to the other cell.

Figure 11-10 shows a metaphase chromosome. The "pinched-in" area of the chromosome is the **centromere.** Each longitudinal half of the chromosome is a **chromatid,** shown encircled on the right. The "arms" above the centromere are the short arms, or the "p" arms. The longer arms (not legs) below the centromere are the "q" arms. You may read that a particular gene is located on 9q, meaning that the gene has its location **(locus)** on the long arm of the number 9 chromosome.

The very "tips" of the chromosomes are the **telomeres,** or the telomeric DNA (deep pink area of Figure 11-10 and Figure 11-11). This DNA actually caps each chromosome. Figure 11-11 shows a chromosome lying on its side. The deep pink areas at each end are the telomeres. The inset figure below the chromosome is the enlarged end region and telomere of the chromosome. This region contained many thousands of bases when we were born. With every round of cell

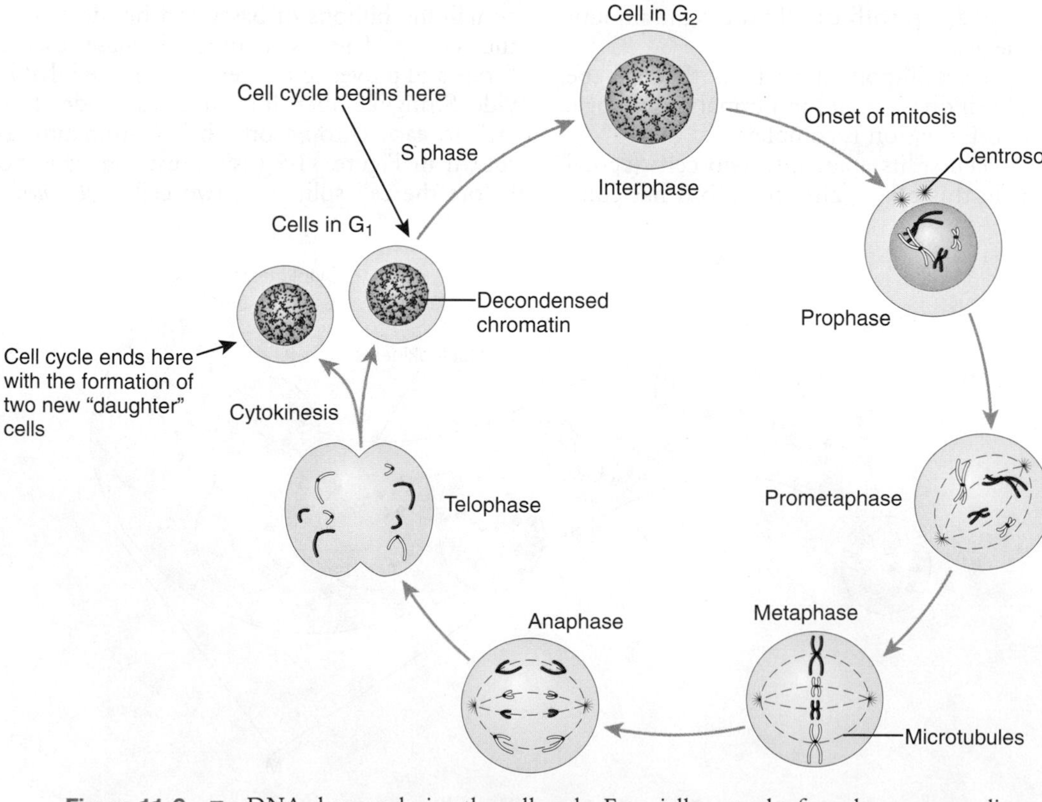

Figure 11-9 ■ DNA changes during the cell cycle. Especially note the four chromosomes lining up during metaphase of mitosis and being pulled apart during anaphase of mitosis.

division, the telomeres of the chromosomes in the cell that just divided are shortened by 50 to 100 bases. Telomeric DNA is not replaced by the cell. As a person ages, the telomeres become shorter. Eventually, the telomere DNA is gone and the chromosomes unravel, which is a signal for the cell to commit "cellular suicide" **(apoptosis)** and die.

Telomeres are related to aging and other important events that happen in the life of the cell. With normal aging, these telomeres shorten until they are gone and the cell then dies. When the cell death rate in any one organ occurs faster than cells can be replaced, the organ cannot function, and death ensues (Novak, 2003). The normal loss of telomeric DNA with each cell division gives all our normal cells a finite life span. The rate at which a person ages is related to the rate of telomere loss. Faster cellular aging occurs with faster rates of telomere loss. Slower cellular aging occurs with slower rates of telomere loss.

Chromosomal Analysis

We can tell some things about a person or their cells by examining chromosomes. It is important to remember that the information that can be obtained by chromosomal analysis is limited because there is a large chunk of DNA in every chromosome. Only very large deletions, additions, or rearrangements of DNA show up at the level of the chromosome. Losses or gains of just a few bases (or even thousands) cannot be detected at the chromosome level. Figure 11-12 shows how the chromosomes of one cell look just before cell division. To analyze chromosomes, they must first be organized into a karyotype.

A **karyotype** is a technique used to make an organized arrangement of all of the chromosomes within one cell during the metaphase section of mitosis (Figure 11-13). A technician first collects the chromosomes into pairs and then lines them up according to size (largest first) and centromere position. This gross organization of DNA can be used to determine missing or extra whole chromosomes and some large structural rearrangements. A missing gene or a mutated gene would not show up at this level of analysis. What we can tell about the person from whom the set of chromosomes in Figure 11-13 was taken is that the person is human, female, and **euploid** (has the correct number of chromosome pairs for the species). We really cannot tell much more than that. This person is chromosomally "normal," although she might have one or more genes that are mutated and "abnormal." If the karyotype is abnormal in any way (had more or less than the normal number or broken chromosomes), the karyotype would be called **aneuploid.**

Autosomes are the 22 pairs of human chromosomes (numbered 1 through 22) that do not code for the sexual differentiation of a person. Autosomal chromosomes contain genes that code for all the structures and regulatory proteins needed for normal function.

Sex chromosomes are the pair of chromosomes that contain the genes for the sexual differentiation of the person. In males the sex chromosomes are an X and a Y. In females the sex chromosomes are two XXs (see Figure 11-13).

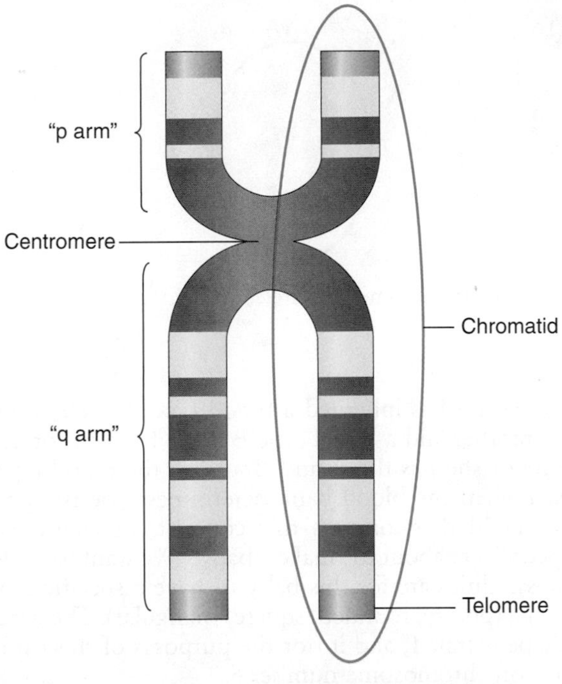

Figure 11-10 ■ A single metaphase chromosome.

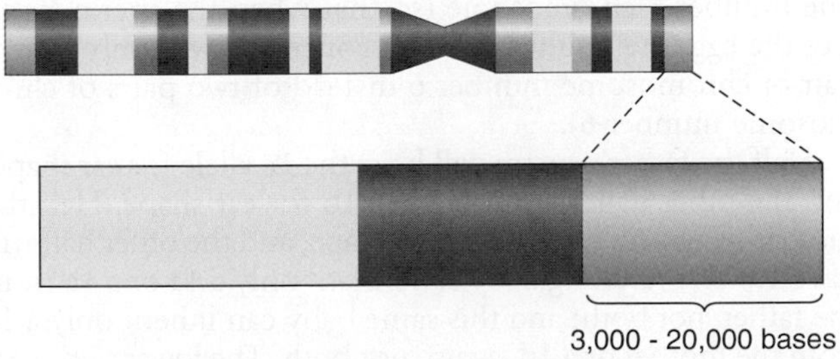

Figure 11-11 ■ Telomeric DNA.

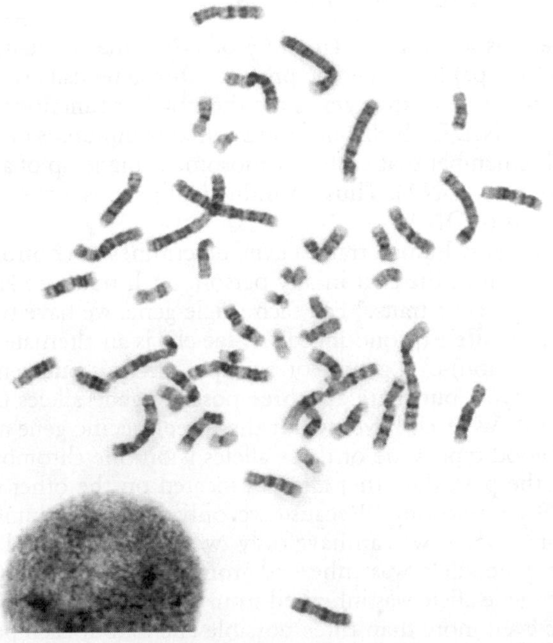

Figure 11-12 ■ A spread of chromosomes from one cell during metaphase of mitosis. (The dark spot in the lower left-hand corner is the nucleus of another cell.)

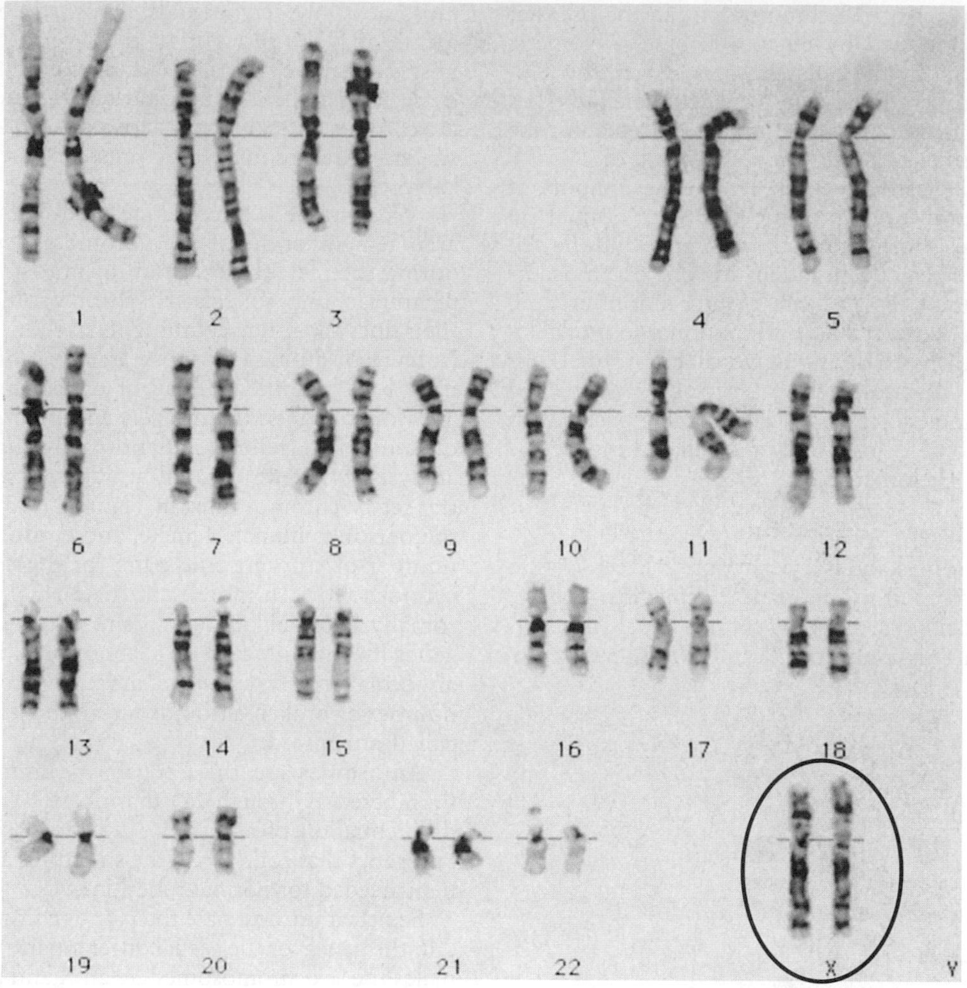

Figure 11-13 ■ A karyotype of a normal female. (The sex chromosomes are circled in red.)

Gene Structure and Function

A **gene** is a specific segment(s) of DNA that contains the code (recipe) for a specific protein. One gene usually codes for one protein; thus genes are the smallest functional unit of the DNA. Each chromosome contains hundreds of genes (and remember that each chromosome is made up of a large segment of DNA). Thus an individual gene is a very small segment of DNA.

For many human traits a gene determines or controls the expression of the trait in any person. Such traits are known as "single gene traits." For each single gene, we have two alleles. An **allele** (pronounced "ah-**lee**-el") is an alternate form (or variation) of a gene. For example, there is one gene for blood type, but there are three possible gene alleles (A, B, and O). We each have two of the three specific gene alleles for blood type. One of these alleles is on one chromosome 9 of the pair; the other allele is located on the other number 9 chromosome. Because we only have two number 9 chromosomes, we can have only two alleles for blood type. One gene allele was inherited from our mothers, and the other gene allele was inherited from our fathers. (Some traits have even more than three possible alleles, but each person only has two.) Which gene alleles we inherit from our parents determines our blood type.

If a person has inherited a blood type A allele from his or her mother and a blood type B allele from his or her father, he or she has the A and B alleles; the blood type expressed when the blood bank determines type is type AB. Figure 11-14 demonstrates this concept. In Figure 11-14, two people are about to "make a baby." We want to see what the possibilities are for this baby to have a specific type of ear shape (pointy, rounded, square, triangular). The gene for ear shape is trait 1, and it (for the purposes of this explanation) is on chromosome number 6.

Each of the father's sperm contains only one number 6 chromosome, and each of the mother's eggs contains only one number 6 chromosome (so that when the sperm fertilizes the egg, the resulting person conceived will only have a pair of chromosome number 6 instead of two pairs of chromosome number 6).

Half the father's sperm will have the 1a allele for ear shape, and the other half will have allele 1b for ear shape. Half the mother's eggs will have 1c for ear shape, and the other half will have 1d. The resulting baby can inherit only a 1a or a 1b from the father, not both; and this same baby can inherit only a 1c from the mother or a 1d, again, not both. The lower potion of Figure 11-14 shows all the combinations possible for each ear shape gene alleles for any child created by these two people.

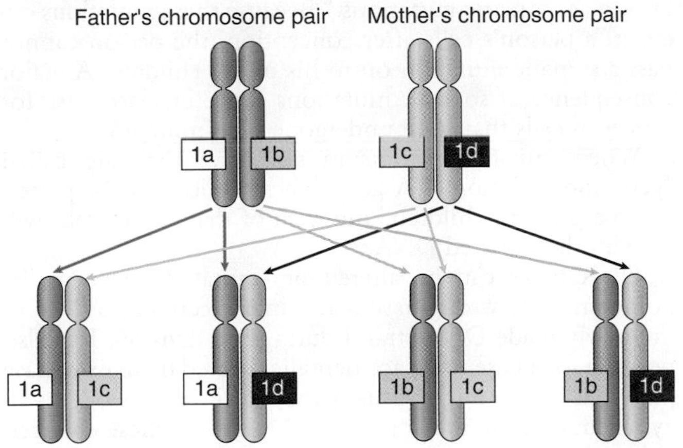

Figure 11-14 ■ Inheritance of four possible alleles for the single gene trait 1. (Any one person can have only two alleles for a single gene trait.)

If a person has two identical alleles for a single gene trait, that person is said to be *homozygous* for that trait. So if a person has an A blood-type gene allele on one number 9 chromosome and an A blood-type gene allele on the other number 9 chromosome, he or she is homozygous for that trait and will express the A blood type.

If a person has two different alleles for a single gene trait, he or she is *heterozygous* for that trait. So if a person has an A blood-type gene allele on one number 9 chromosome and a B blood-type gene allele on the other number 9 chromosome, that person is heterozygous for that trait and will express the AB blood type. Because the A and B alleles are equally dominant *(co-dominant),* they will both be expressed in the actual blood type.

There are differences in expression of the alleles for a trait depending on whether an allele is dominant or is recessive. If a person has an A blood-type gene allele on one number 9 chromosome and an O blood-type gene allele on the other number 9 chromosome, that person is heterozygous for that trait and expresses only the A blood type. Because the A allele is dominant and the O allele is recessive, they will not both be expressed in the actual blood type. Only the dominant allele is expressed, and the recessive allele is "silent." We will learn more about dominant, recessive, and co-dominant expression later under Patterns of Inheritance on p. 146.

PHENOTYPE

The **phenotype** of any gene for a person is what characteristic can actually be observed or, in some cases, determined by a laboratory test. For example, the person who has the AO gene alleles for blood type has the phenotype of type A blood. A person with curly hair has a curly hair phenotype regardless of whether he or she has two alleles for curly hair or one allele for curly hair and one allele for straight hair.

GENOTYPE

The **genotype** for a person's single gene trait is what the actual alleles are for that trait, not just what can be observed. A person with a phenotype of type A blood could have either an AA genotype or an AO genotype. The person who has type O blood would be known to have an OO genotype. When a person has homozygous alleles for a trait, the genotype and phenotype are the same. When a person has heterozygous alleles for a trait, the phenotype and the genotype are not the same. Recessive traits are expressed only when the person is homozygous for the alleles. Thus for recessive traits phenotype and genotype are the same. Dominant traits are expressed when the person is homozygous for the alleles or heterozygous for the alleles. Thus for dominant traits phenotype and genotype can be the same but do not have to be the same.

Gene Expression

The purpose of a gene is to code for the making of a specific protein used by a cell, tissue, or organ within a person. For example, the hormone insulin is a protein. When a person's blood glucose level starts to rise, the beta cells of the pancreas rapidly make insulin to meet the immediate needs of the person for blood glucose homeostasis.

To continue the cookbook analogy, each gene is the recipe needed to make a specific protein. All the "stuff" that our body makes–every hormone, every enzyme, every growth factor, every biologic chemical needed to keep us functioning–is a protein. These proteins are "gene products" because they are produced when the right gene is "turned on" or "expressed." The following are just a few examples of gene products: insulin, hemoglobin, erythropoietin, angiotensin, and estrogen.

Protein Synthesis

Protein synthesis is the process by which we use genes to make proteins that are needed for proper physiologic function. As you may remember from your science classes, proteins are made up of individual amino acids hooked together like beads on a string. There are 22 different amino acids. Every protein has a specific amount of the amino acids and a specific order in which they are put together. If even one amino acid is out of order or completely deleted from the sequence, the protein will be incorrect and unable to do its job in the body.

For example, the hormone insulin is a protein that contains 51 amino acids in a specific sequence. If some of the amino acids are missing or are in the wrong position, the protein made would be different from real insulin and could not reduce blood glucose levels. Therefore the actual order of the amino acids is critical for the final function of any protein.

Within the DNA there is a code for each amino acid (Table 11-2). Each amino acid code is three bases (nucleotides) long. A gene is the recipe for making a specific protein. It contains all the amino acid codes in exactly the right order for that specific protein. For example, the final active form of the protein insulin has 51 amino acids. Thus the minimum number of bases needed in the gene for insulin would be 153 (three bases per amino acid X 51 amino acids). Figure 11-15 shows an example of short protein made up of only seven amino acids.

Figure 11-16 shows the model of using DNA to make proteins. To think of this process in terms of the cookbook, the entire genome in each cell is the giant cookbook in the library. When a specific protein needs to be made, the chapter for that protein is opened (the chromosome), and the right recipe is found (the gene). The recipe is copied (transcribed) onto a note card (messenger ribonucleic acid, or mRNA) and taken to the kitchen (endoplasmic reticulum). In the kitchen, all the ingredients (amino acids) are put together (translated) in the right order with the help of bowls, ovens, pans, potholders, and other kitchen tools (adapter and transfer molecules). Some foods may need to be altered a little before serving, such as carved, frosted, or peeled (removing extra amino acids to activate the protein).

Many of the steps of protein synthesis use the same enzymes and similar processes as in DNA synthesis, although there are a few differences. During DNA synthesis, the entire DNA strand is transcribed into a new DNA strand. For protein synthesis only the area of the DNA that contains the gene for the specific protein needed is transcribed into RNA.

RNA itself is similar to DNA with a few differences. First the sugar attached to the base is a ribose sugar (hence the name "ribo"nucleic acid). In addition, thymine does not exist in RNA. Instead a similar base called uracil is placed in RNA instead of thymine. This means there is a specific three-base RNA code (called a codon) for each amino acid (see Table 11-2). These RNA codes are complementary to the DNA amino acid codes, with uracil in place of thymine. In addition to the amino acid codes, RNA contains some "stop" codes that tell the process when the protein is finished. Last, RNA is single-stranded instead of double-stranded (Figure 11-17).

Mutations

Mutations are DNA changes that are passed from one generation to another and thus are *inherited.* An inherited mutation does not have to mean that the mutation is passed from one human generation to another. It can mean that the mutation is passed from one *cell* generation to another and thus might affect only certain tissues within a person rather than be a problem within a family. These types of mutations occur in general body cells (somatic cells) and are known as "somatic mutations." Because these mutations occur in a person's cells after conception, the person cannot pass a somatic mutation on to his or her children. A major consequence of somatic mutations is the increased risk for cancer in cells that have undergone such mutations.

When mutations occur in sex cells, they are called "germline mutations." A germline mutation can be passed on to a person's children, and each of that child's cells will contain the mutated DNA.

DNA bases can be altered or "mutated" accidentally. Sometimes the wrong base is put into a certain position in the newly made DNA strand during cell division. It is also possible for a base to be accidentally deleted or an extra base placed in to the strand. Usually the "spell check" work of enzymes during the making of DNA prevents these changes, although some changes probably occur daily in any one person. If these changes occur in a gene area of the DNA, the change can alter the expression of that gene, and an incorrect gene product (protein) might result.

The genes for most proteins are generally the same in all people. Sometimes a base in one person's gene for a specific protein is not the same as that in most people. This difference can be either a variation known as a *single nucleotide polymorphism, or SNP* ("snip"), or it can be a mutation. When a base difference allows the protein to be made but there are differences in how well the protein works, the difference is called a variation or a **polymorphism.** When a base difference causes a loss of protein function, it is called a **mutation.**

TABLE 11-2 Examples of DNA Codes and RNA Codons for Selected Amino Acids

Amino Acid	DNA Code(s)	RNA Codons
Alanine	CGA, CGG, CGT, CGC	GCU, GCC, GCA, GCG
Glycine	CCA, CCG, CCT, CCC	GGU, GGC, GGA, GGG
Isoleucine	TAA, TAG, TAT	AUU, AUC, AUA
Lysine	TTT, TTC	AAA, AAG
Tryptophan	ACC	UGG
Tyrosine	ATA, ATG	UAU, UAC
Start		AUG
Stop		UAA, UAG, UGA

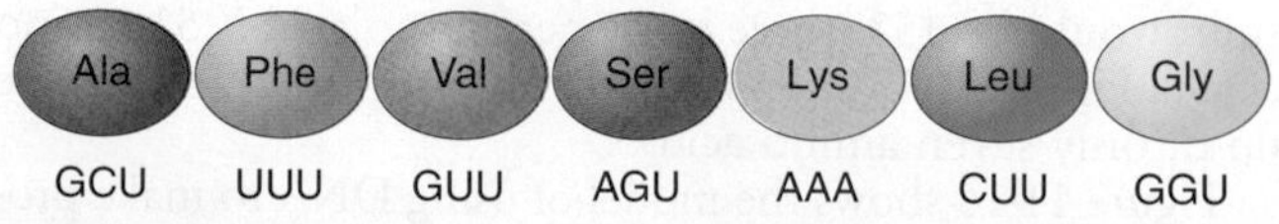

Figure 11-15 ■ A sample protein composed of seven amino acids. The RNA codons for the individual amino acids are listed below each amino acid.

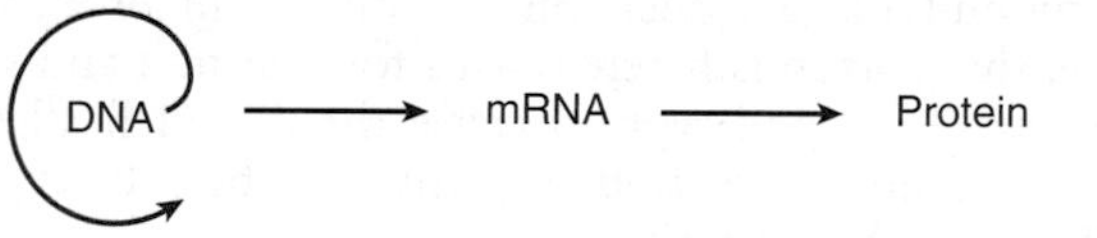

Figure 11-16 ■ The genetic model for protein synthesis.

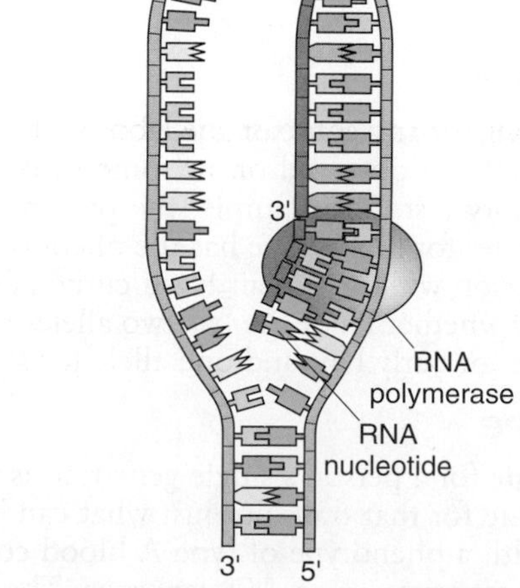

Figure 11-17 ■ RNA transcription for protein synthesis.

POINT MUTATION

The two types of mutations are point mutations and frameshift mutations. **Point mutations** are the substitution of one base for another. A change has been made at a single point of DNA, and the type of change is a base substitution, not a deletion or addition. So the triplets, or three-base codes, remain intact, although one may be incorrect. This change may or may not alter amino acid position or protein synthesis.

Below is an analogy to a point mutation. The top sentence represents the "reading sequence" for a specific gene:

THE BIG DOG ATE THE CAT

THE BIG DOG ATE THE CAP

A point mutation, as seen in the bottom sentence, has changed the *t* in cat to a *p*. The coded message is similar but not exactly the same.

Sometimes a point mutation can change the protein (gene product) a little, but it can still "sort of" work. Sometimes, however, a point mutation changes the protein just enough that it does not work at all. It all depends on how critical the amino acid that changed was to the function of the protein.

For example, the beta chain of hemoglobin in healthy people has the amino acid glutamine in the sixth position (shown in Figure 11-18 in the red box with the DNA code of CTC, the RNA codon of GAG). People who have sickle cell disease have a single base substitution in the gene for the beta chain of hemoglobin, replacing the T with an A (shown in the blue box in Figure 11-18). This results in the DNA code of CAC (instead of CTC), the RNA codon of GUG (instead of GAG), and the placement of valine instead of glutamine in the sixth amino acid position. The altered beta chain will function adequately as part of hemoglobin as long as plenty of oxygen is present. However, when hypoxia occurs in people who have valine rather than glutamine in both of the beta chains of hemoglobin, the chain pulls in on itself and distorts the red blood cell into a sickle shape (see Figure 43-1 in Chapter 43). This shape change causes blood cells to clump and obstruct blood flow to tissues, leading to cell damage and death. So this mutation does not completely disrupt hemoglobin function (which would be incompatible with life) but reduces its efficiency and can have severe consequences.

Sometimes an SNP or base substitution does not change the amino acid sequence. For example, Figure 11-19, *A*, shows the original (and correct) DNA codes in a short gene sequence. In Figure 11-19, *B*, there is a point mutation in which the third G in the third DNA code is substituted with a C. Both GGG and GGC code for the amino acid proline, however, and there is no resulting amino acid change in the final protein. This is an example of a "silent" mutation. The mutation did not affect the amino acid sequence of the protein. In Figure 11-19, *C*, a point mutation in the first DNA code substitutes a C in place of a G. This will cause a different amino acid to be placed in the protein. Usually, a different amino acid at least reduces the effect of the protein and may make it nonfunctional altogether. This type of mutation is a "missense" mutation. Some missense mutations cause mild dysfunction or problems and others cause major dysfunction or problems. A nonsense mutation is one in which a single base change, as in Figure 11-19, *D*, results in a "stop" codon; so translation will stop at this point, and a complete protein is not made.

HbA	1	2	3	4	5	6
DNA	CAC	GTG	GAC	TGA	GGA	CTC
RNA	GUG	CAC	CUG	ACU	CCU	GAG
AAs	val	his	leu	thr	pro	glu

HbS	1	2	3	4	5	6
DNA	CAC	GTG	GAC	TGA	GGA	CAC
RNA	GUG	CAC	CUG	ACU	CCU	GUG
AAs	val	his	leu	thr	pro	val

Figure 11-18 ■ A clinical example of the consequences of a point mutation. *AAs,* Amino acids; *HbA,* adult hemoglobin; *HbS,* sickle cell hemoglobin.

FRAMESHIFT MUTATION

In a **frameshift mutation** a base is added or deleted. This type of mutation always alters amino acid position, disrupts the reading frame, and stops protein synthesis. These changes ruin the reading sequence of the gene from the mutation on down. These changes are very serious because a normal product cannot be made from a gene with such a mutation.

The following is an analogy to a frameshift mutation. The top sentence represents the correct "reading sequence" for a specific gene.

THE BIG DOG ATE THE CAT

THB IGD OGA TET HEC AT

THE PBI GDO GAT ETH ECA T

DNA code	ACG	CTA	GGG	CAC	a. Original DNA codes and amino acids
Amino acid	Cys	Asp	Pro	Val	
DNA code	ACG	CTA	GGC	CAC	b. Silent mutation in which a base substitution does not change the amino acid
Amino acid	Cys	Asp	Pro	Val	
DNA code	ACC	CTA	GGG	CAC	c. Missense mutation in which a base substitution changes the amino acid
Amino acid	Trp	Asp	Pro	Val	
DNA code	ACT	CTA	GGG	CAC	d. Nonsense mutation in which a base substitution causes an early stop signal and an incomplete, nonfunctional protein
Amino acid	Stop	Asp	Pro	Val	

Figure 11-19 ■ Types of point mutations.

A base deletion mutation, as seen in the middle sentence, has removed the *E* in "THE," shifting the rest of the bases to the left (for the three base codes) and disrupting the reading frame. A base addition mutation, as seen in the bottom sentence, has added a *P* to "BIG," shifting the three-base reading codes to the right and disrupting the reading frame. The coded message (recipe) has been lost completely.

Why are we talking about mutations and variations? Changes in genes, even small changes, can have serious results. Some changes would inactivate a protein. Other changes may alter how often or how well a group of cells divides. Gene variations may cause one person to have a greater than normal risk for developing a disease. A different variation in the same gene may cause another person to have a smaller than normal risk for developing the same disease.

PATTERNS OF INHERITANCE

For every single gene trait we each inherit one allele for that gene from our mothers and one allele from our fathers. How these traits are expressed depend on whether one or both alleles are "dominant" or whether one or both alleles are "recessive." Expression also depends on whether the gene for the trait is located on an autosome or on a sex chromosome.

It is possible to determine how the gene for a specific trait is **transmitted** (passed from one human generation to the next). By looking at how that trait is expressed through several generations of a family, patterns emerge that indicate whether that gene is dominant or recessive and whether it is located on an autosomal chromosome or on one of the sex chromosomes. This information can be determined through pedigree analysis. Determining inheritance patterns for a specific trait makes it possible to predict the risk for any one person to have a trait or transmit that trait to his or her children.

Pedigree

A **pedigree** is a graph of a family history for a specific trait or health problem over several generations. Figure 11-20 shows a typical three-generation pedigree. Figure 11-21 shows the accepted symbols used when creating a pedigree. Although the term *pedigree* is the correct genetic term, some clients are offended by this term. You may want to use the term *family tree* in place of pedigree when talking with clients. When analyzing a pedigree, note the answers to the following questions:

- Is any pattern of inheritance present, or does the trait appear sporadic?
- Is the trait expressed equally among males and females or unequally?
- Is the trait present in every generation, or does it skip one or more generations?
- Do only affected individuals have children affected with the trait, or do unaffected individuals also have children who express the trait?

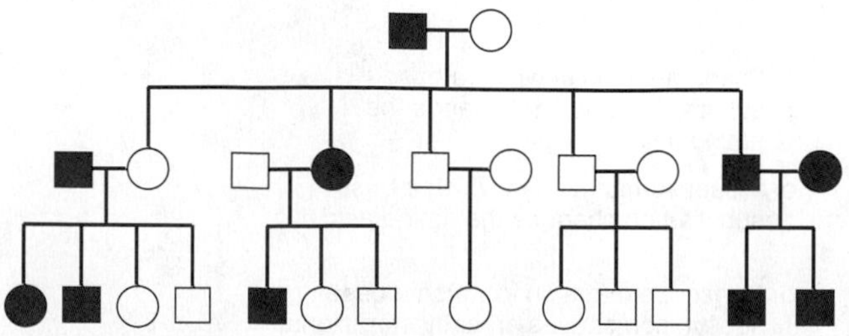

Figure 11-20 ■ A three-generation pedigree showing an autosomal dominant pattern of inheritance.

The four types of inheritance patterns associated with single gene–controlled traits include autosomal dominant, autosomal recessive, sex-linked dominant, and sex-linked recessive. Each inheritance pattern has specific defining criteria. Table 11-3 lists the patterns of inheritance for some disorders that either are identified in adults or may be identified in children who live to adulthood.

Some traits and disorders cluster within a family but do not follow any known pattern of inheritance. Although no specific gene has yet been found for some of these disorders, the clustering suggests a genetic basis. It is thought that for

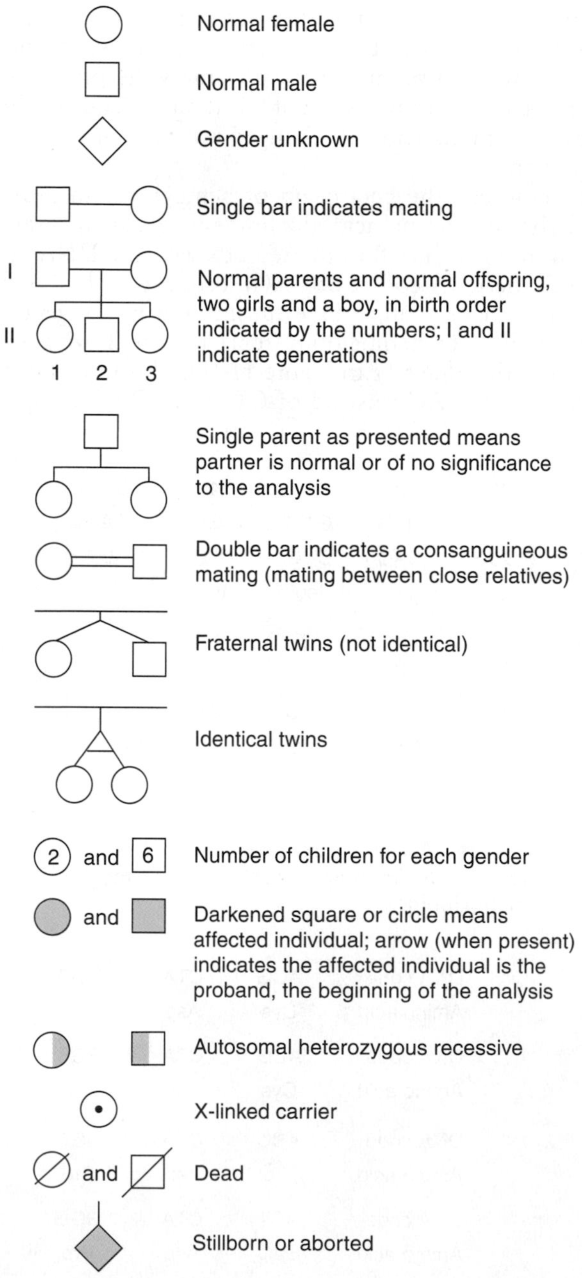

Figure 11-21 ■ Standard pedigree symbols.

some of the disorders that show familial clustering, environmental factors may modify a genetic predisposition. Continued genetic research may solve the familial clustering gene puzzle.

Autosomal Dominant Pattern of Inheritance

Autosomal dominant (AD) single gene traits require that the gene alleles controlling the trait be located on an autosomal chromosome. A dominant gene allele is expressed even when only one allele of the pair is dominant. Other criteria for AD patterns of inheritance include the following:

- The trait appears in every generation with no skipping.
- The risk for an affected person to pass the trait to his or her children is 50% with each pregnancy.
- Unaffected people do not have affected children; therefore their risk is essentially 0%.
- The trait is found equally in males and females.

An example of an AD trait is blood type A. If a person is homozygous for the blood type A allele, he or she will express type A blood (with genotype being identical to the phenotype). If a person is heterozygous for the blood type A allele, with the other allele being type O (which is a recessive trait), he or she will also express type A blood. In this case, however, the phenotype is not identical to the genotype. *When a dominant allele is paired with a recessive allele, only the dominant allele is expressed.* The blood type B allele is also a dominant allele. When a B allele is paired with an O allele, B blood type is expressed. When a person has one blood type A allele and a blood type B allele, however, both alleles are expressed (because they are equally dominant) and the person has type AB blood.

When a person actually has a specific gene allele, he or she is said to "carry" that gene allele. This issue is different from being a "carrier" of a recessive allele. Carrier status is discussed under Autosomal Recessive Patterns of Inheritance on p. 148.

Some health problems are inherited as an autosomal dominant (AD) single gene trait. These problems may not be apparent at birth but develop as the person ages (see Table 11-3). Two factors that affect the expression of some AD single gene traits are penetrance and expressivity.

PENETRANCE

The term **penetrance** describes how often or how well, within a population, a gene is expressed when it is present. Some genes are more penetrant than others. For example, the gene for Huntington disease (HD) is transmitted as an autosomal dominant trait. Therefore, if a person has one HD allele, he or she is at risk for developing HD. This gene is "highly penetrant" (sometimes called "fully penetrant"). This means that if a person has the HD gene allele, his or her risk of expressing the gene and developing the disease is about 99.99%.

Some gene alleles have "reduced" penetrance. This means that even if a person has the gene mutation, his or her risk for this gene being expressed and actually developing the disorder is less than 100%.

Penetrance is calculated by examining a population of people known to have the gene mutation and assessing the percentage that go on to express the gene by developing the disorder. For example, the *BRCA2* gene mutation increases a person's risk for breast cancer. This gene is not fully penetrant, so some women (and men) who have the gene do not develop breast cancer. The penetrance rate for this gene mutation is calculated to be between 60% and 80%, meaning that a person who has the gene mutation has a 60% to 80% risk for developing breast cancer. Although this risk is far higher than among people who do not have this mutant gene, the risk is not 100%. Having the gene mutation does not absolutely predict that the person will develop breast cancer, just that the risk is high.

EXPRESSIVITY

Expressivity is the degree of expression a person has when a specific autosomal dominant gene is present. The gene is always expressed, but some people have more severe results than do other people. For example, the gene mutation for one form of neurofibromatosis (NF1) has an autosomal dominant pattern of inheritance. Some people with this gene have only a few light brown skin tone areas known as café au lait spots. These skin lesions can be so minor that the person may

TABLE 11-3 Patterns of Inheritance for Genetic Disorders Among Adults

Pattern of Inheritance	Disorder
Autosomal dominant	Breast cancer* (mutation of *BRCA1* or *BRCA2* genes) Diabetes mellitus type 2* Familial adenomatous polyposis Familial melanoma Familial hypercholesterolemia Hereditary nonpolyposis colon cancer (HNCC) Huntington disease Long QT syndrome and sudden cardiac death Malignant hyperthermia (MH) Marfan syndrome Myotonic dystrophy Neurofibromatosis (types 1 and 2) Ovarian cancer* (mutation of *BRCA1* genes) Polycystic kidney disease† (types 1 and 2) Retinitis pigmentosa† von Willebrand's disease
Autosomal recessive	Albinism Alpha-1 antitrypsin deficiency Beta thalassemia Bloom syndrome Cystic fibrosis Hereditary hemochromatosis Sickle cell disease Xeroderma pigmentosum
Sex-linked recessive	Glucose-6-phosphate dehydrogenase deficiency Hemophilia Red-green color-blind
Familial clustering	Alzheimer's disease Autoimmune disorders Bipolar disorder Parkinson disease Schizophrenia Hypertension Rheumatoid arthritis

*Some disorders have both a genetic and nongenetic form.
†Some disorders have more than one genetic form and can also be autosomal recessive.

not even be aware that they are present. Other people with the same gene mutation develop hundreds of tumors (neurofibromas) that protrude through the skin. Expressivity accounts for some variation in genetic disease severity.

Autosomal Recessive Pattern of Inheritance

Autosomal recessive (AR) single gene traits require that the gene controlling the trait be located on an autosomal chromosome. The trait can be expressed only when both alleles are present. Table 11-3 lists common adult disorders that have an AR pattern of inheritance. Figure 11-22 shows a typical pedigree for an AR disorder. Criteria for AR patterns of inheritance include the following:

- The trait may not appear in all generations of any one branch of a family.
- The trait or characteristic usually first appears only in siblings rather than in the parents themselves.
- About 25% of a family will be affected and express the trait.
- The children of an affected father and an affected mother will *always* be affected (risk is 100%).
- Unaffected people who are carriers (heterozygous for the trait) and do not express the trait themselves can transmit the trait to their children if their partner is either also a carrier or is affected.
- The trait is found equally in males and females.

An example of an AR trait is type O blood. The blood-type O allele is recessive, and both alleles must be type O (homozygous) for the person to express type O blood. If only one allele is a type O allele and the other allele is either type A or type B, the dominant allele will be expressed and the O allele, although present, is not expressed. For AR single gene traits, phenotype and genotype are always the same.

A person who has one mutated allele for a recessive genetic disorder is a **carrier.** A carrier, even though he or she may have one mutated allele, does not usually have any manifestations of the disorder but can pass this mutated allele on to his or her children. For some autosomal recessive disorders, a carrier may have very mild manifestations. One example is sickle cell trait. A person with two sickle cell alleles has the disease and has many associated health problems. A carrier with one sickle cell allele may be healthy most of the time and have manifestations only under conditions of severe hypoxia.

Sex-Linked Recessive Pattern of Inheritance

Some genes are present only on the sex chromosomes. The Y chromosome has only a few genes that are not also present on the X chromosome. These few genes are important for male sexual development. The X chromosome, however, has many single genes that are not present on the Y or elsewhere in the human genome. Some of these genes are specific for female sexual development, but there are also several hundred other genes on the X chromosome that code for other functions. Thus sex-linked patterns of inheritance issues are really issues of X-linked patterns of inheritance. Few traits or disorders have an X-linked dominant pattern of expression, and they are not discussed in this chapter.

Because the number of X chromosomes in males and females is not the same (1:2), the number of X-linked chromosome genes in the two genders is also unequal. Males have only one X chromosome, a condition called hemizygosity for any gene on the X chromosome. As a result, X-linked recessive genes have a dominant expressive pattern of inheritance in males and a recessive expressive pattern of inheritance females. This difference in expression is because males do not have a second X chromosome to balance the expression of any recessive gene on the first X chromosome.

Sex-linked (X-linked) recessive single gene traits require that the gene allele be present on both of the X chromosomes for the trait to be expressed in females (homozygous) and on only one X chromosome for the trait to be expressed in males (hemizygous). Figure 11-23 shows a typical pedigree for an X-linked recessive disorder. Features of X-linked recessive pattern of inheritance include the following:

- The incidence of the trait is much higher among males in a kinship than among females.
- The trait cannot be transmitted from father to son.
- Transmission of the trait is from father to all daughters (who will be carriers).
- Female carriers have a 50% risk (with each pregnancy) of transmitting the gene to their children.

Familial Clustering

Some disorders appear in families at a rate higher than normal and greater than can be accounted for by chance alone; however, no specific pattern occurs within a family. Although clusters suggest a genetic influence, it is likely that additional factors, such as gender and the environment, also influence disease development or disease severity. Such disorders include Alzheimer's disease, Parkinson disease, type 1 diabetes, and many others. These disorders are often called "multifactorial" because although an increased genetic risk

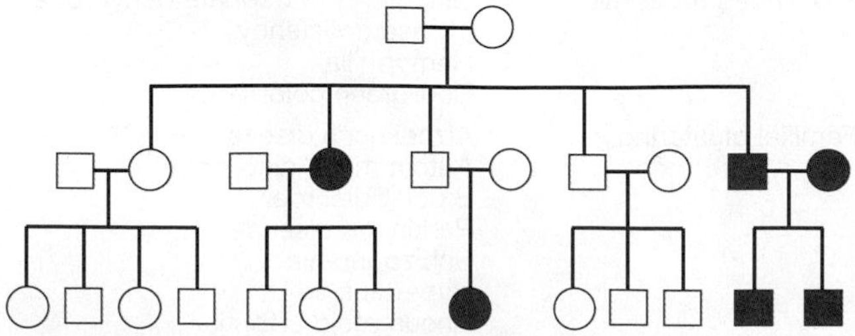

Figure 11-22 ■ A typical pedigree showing an autosomal recessive pattern of inheritance.

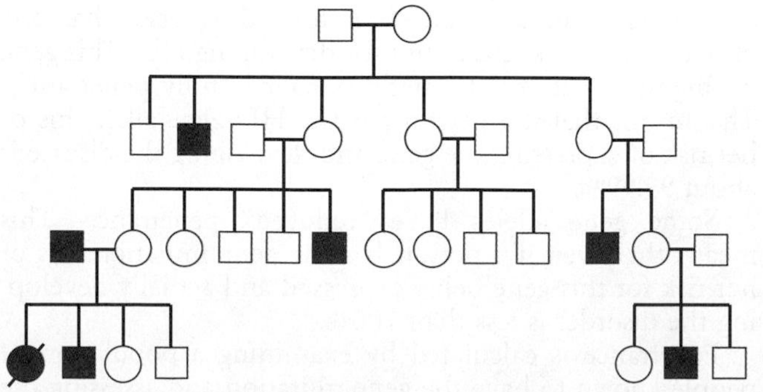

Figure 11-23 ■ A typical pedigree showing a sex-linked (X-linked) recessive pattern of inheritance.

may be present, the risk is changed by diet, lifestyle, exposure to toxins, infectious agents, and other factors.

GENETIC TESTING

PURPOSE OF TESTING

With completion of the first phase of the Human Genome Project, many people are eager to have genetic testing but also are fearful of genetic testing. The lay public often believes that a single genetic test can "tell everything about a person." Although the potential for genetic testing to be all inclusive exists, this is not currently the case. Some people want to identify family members who might have "bad genes." Some people want to identify people with "perfect genes." It is important to remember that no single person is genetically perfect.

Genetic testing can be performed with many different techniques. Some genetic tests are very specific for a disease or disorder. Others may show a gene variation but the significance of the variation may not be known. At times unexpected information is found during genetic testing. Some ordinary tests, such as blood typing and tissue typing, provide genetic information. Laboratory tests that measure the amount of an enzyme or protein a person makes actually provide genetic information.

Actual genetic testing can be performed at many levels. Cellular or biochemical tests provide information about gene products made by a cell, tissue, or organ. Chromosomes can be assessed for missing, extra, or broken chromosomes. Chromosome segments can be analyzed for abnormalities or changes from normal positions. The sequence of an individual gene can be examined to determine variation or mutation. At present not all genes can be analyzed, and the analysis of even one gene is limited by expense and availability. Specific base pairs can be evaluated for mutations. Again, these tests are currently expensive and the results may not be conclusive. Table 11-4 lists purposes of genetic testing for adults.

BENEFITS AND RISKS OF TESTING

Genetic testing is different from any other type of testing for many reasons. *It is important to remember that just because the technology exists does not mean it should be used in all cases.* Informed consent is required before genetic testing is undertaken. At present the person tested is the one who gives consent. Because genetic testing *always* gives information about a family and family members, not just the client, however, there is some debate about who else should give consent.

BENEFITS

Genetic testing can be useful to confirm a diagnosis or to test people who are at risk for a health problem but do not as yet have any symptoms. Presymptomatic testing can help a person, family, and their health care provider develop an appropriate plan of care or screening for early detection. For example, in the case of a strong genetic predisposition of colon cancer, identifying a client before symptoms appear allows interventions to prevent disease development or diagnosis earlier, when cure is more likely.

RISKS

Unlike most tests, genetic testing results do not change. This means that a positive test result cannot be "taken back." Genetic tests pose some unusual risks. The risks of genetic testing may include psychological or social risks as well as a risk for family disruption. Often genetic tests are expensive and may not be covered by insurance. Some genetic tests have limited value for predicting future risk. Testing may identify a client at great risk for the future development of a serious health problem that cannot be prevented. Some disorders, such as Huntington disease (HD), currently have no treatment. Knowing positive test results in these situations can lead to depression, blame, and guilt.

Another risk of genetic testing is that positive results may be used to discriminate against a person or a family. Some protection is in place to prevent health insurance companies from failing to insure a person or dropping the coverage of a person who is at high risk for developing a serious illness (e.g., breast or ovarian cancer). However, there are no protections against rate hikes or exclusions of specific treatments. Clients often fear workplace discrimination and even personal discrimination if positive test results are known.

GENETIC COUNSELING

Genetic testing is not a standard test that any person should have performed without knowing the advantages and disad-

TABLE 11-4 Purposes of Genetic Testing for Adults

Purpose Type	Definition
Carrier testing	Determining whether a client without symptoms has an allele for a recessive disorder that could be transmitted to his or her children. Disorders for which carrier testing is common include sickle cell disease, hemophilia, hereditary hemochromatosis, cystic fibrosis, beta thalassemia, and Tay-Sach's disease.
Diagnostic testing	Determining whether a client has or does not have a mutation that increases the risk for a specific genetic disorder.
Symptomatic	Client has clinical manifestations; test results confirm a diagnosis.
Presymptomatic	Client has no clinical manifestations but is at high risk for inheriting a specific genetic disorder for which there is no known prevention or treatment. A disorder for which presymptomatic testing is commonly performed is Huntington disease.
Predisposition	Family history or genetic testing indicates risk is high for a known genetic disorder. The client does not have any manifestations but wants to know whether he or she has the specific mutation and what the chances are that it will be expressed. Disorders for which predisposition testing is often performed include hereditary breast/ovarian cancer and hereditary colorectal cancers. The advantage of predisposition testing is that the client can then engage in heightened screening activities or medical and surgical interventions that reduce risk.

vantages. Counseling clients before, during, and after testing is critical. Entire families may be a part of the genetic evaluation and follow-up. In fact, it may be difficult to determine just which person is the client. For example, a 45-year-old woman has breast cancer. In her family, her mother, grandmother, brother, and one sister have all had breast cancer. This woman's older daughter wonders whether she has a gene mutation for breast cancer and asks to be tested. This daughter is called the **proband** because she is the person who brought the family's issue to the attention of genetic professionals. When she and her younger sister are tested, the older daughter does not have the mutation but the younger sister does. Thus, although the older sister was considered the client, the younger sister is the one who has a gene mutation.

Genetic counseling is a process, not a single session or a single recommendation. This process should begin when the client or family is first identified as potentially having a genetic problem. The process continues through actual testing, if the decision to test is made, and it continues through interpretation of results and follow-up. Steps in the process are listed in Table 11-5.

Often a client may request genetic testing even when there is no indication of need for the test (evaluation does not indicate an increased risk for a genetic disorder). Genetic counseling and evaluation can help clients understand whether any useful information could be obtained from testing.

Counseling should be performed by a professional or a team that has defined expertise in interpretation of genetic testing results. Such professionals include advanced-practice nurses with specialization in one or more aspects of genetics, certified genetic counselors, clinical geneticists, medical geneticists, and laboratory geneticists. Each of these professionals has a different level of preparation in genetics and thus has different skills and roles in the counseling process (Table 11-6). For example, an advanced-practice nurse may be appropriate to counsel a client about the Huntington disease gene mutation because this test is not ambiguous and the gene is highly penetrant. A person who has a variation or mutation in an unusual gene region or when penetrance is reduced may best be served by counseling from a clinical or medical geneticist.

No matter which professional is involved in genetic counseling, a key feature of this counseling is to be "nondirective." The counselor provides as much information as possible about the risks and benefits but does not in any way influence the client's decision to test or not to test. Once the client has made the decision, the counselor supports the client and the decision. Chart 11-1 lists NIC intervention activities for adult clients considering or having genetic testing.

TABLE 11-5 Steps Involved in the Process of Genetic Testing and Counseling

Pre-testing Assessment and Client Education (may take multiple sessions)
- Determining client understanding and why testing or counseling is being sought
- Determining whether testing is reasonable (considering cost of the test, specificity, probable risk, accuracy of testing)
- Establishing a trusting professional relationship
- Assuring privacy and confidentiality
- Reviewing informed consent procedures
- Assessing the client's ability to communicate accurately (including language issues, cognitive function, and sensory perception)
- Assessing the client's psychosocial status and availability of social support
- Taking a detailed client health history (including drugs, diet, exercise, hormonal history, and lifestyle issues)
- Obtaining physical assessment data relevant to the at-risk disorder
- Taking a detailed family history and constructing a three-generation pedigree (minimum)
- Obtaining and verifying information obtained from the following:
  - Client
  - Family members
  - Medical records
  - Pathology reports
  - Death certificates
- Interpreting the family history
- Discussing the consequences of testing
- Discussing client rights and obligations regarding disclosure of information
- Discussing testing options
- Assessing to determine whether coercion is occurring
- Obtaining material to be tested (usually blood)

Test Result Presentation
- Re-assessing the client's wish to know or not know the test results
- Respecting the client's decision not to know the test results
- Assuring privacy and confidentiality
- Presenting the test results
- Interpreting the test results
- Assessing the client's perception of the test results

Follow-up
- Supporting the client's decision to disclose or not disclose the information to other family members
- Discussing the potential risks for other family members
- Assuring privacy and confidentiality
- Addressing the client's concerns
- Discussing prevention, early detection, and treatment options
- Discussing family concerns
- Addressing psychosocial issues
- Discussing available resources for information, support, further counseling
- Providing summary of results and consultation to the client

ETHICAL ISSUES

THE RIGHT TO KNOW VERSUS THE RIGHT NOT TO KNOW

Many ethical issues must be considered with genetic testing. Individual clients do have a right to know their genetic risk, and they also have a right to choose not to know. Sometimes a client's right to know has an impact on the right of another family member not to know. For example, your maternal grandfather had Huntington disease (HD) and you want to know whether you have that gene, so you are tested. Your mother does not want to know whether she has the gene. If you are tested and found to have the gene, because HD is autosomal dominant, the only way you could have the gene is if your mother also has it. Thus when you find out you are positive and tell your mother your status, your mother will learn that she is also positive, even if she did not want to know.

CONFIDENTIALITY

The results of a genetic test must therefore remain confidential to the client. Currently the results cannot be given to a family member, other health care provider, or insurance

TABLE 11-6 Genetic Professionals

Professional	Educational and Professional Requirements
Certified Genetic Counselor	Master's degree in human genetics or genetic counseling from a program accredited by the American Board of Genetic Counselors. Includes clinical and laboratory training. Successful completion of a certification examination. May specialize in prenatal genetics, cancer genetics, neurogenetic disorders, psychiatric disorders, artificial reproduction, cardiology, or public health.
Clinical Geneticist	Medical doctor (MD) or MD/PhD. Classroom preparation in molecular biology, cytogenetics, biochemical genetics, immunogenetics, and population genetics. Residency in internal medicine, pediatrics, obstetrics, or other area. Completion of an American Board of Medical Genetics fellowship program (usually at least 2 yr). Successful completion of a general certification examination.
Medical Geneticist	PhD; Medical doctor (MD); or MD-PhD. Classroom preparation in molecular biology, cytogenetics, biochemical genetics, immunogenetics, and population genetics. Additional preparation in forensic, pharmaceutical, pathology, and genetic technologies. Completion of an American Board of Medical Genetics genetics fellowship program (usually at least 2 yr). Successful completion of a general certification examination. May also have completed an additional specialty examination.
Advance Practice Nurse with a specialty in genetics	Master's degree in nursing with 16 to 20 semester credits in genetics and counseling. May be eligible to certify through the International Society of Nurses in Genetics (ISONG) after a specified number of clinical practice hours. Current certification is by portfolio.

Data from http://www.kumc.edu/gec/prof/career.html.

CHART 11-1

NIC INTERVENTION ACTIVITIES for The Adult Client with or at Risk for a Genetic Problem

Genetic Counseling: *Use of an interactive helping process focusing on assisting an individual, family, or group, manifesting or at risk for developing or transmitting a birth defect or genetic condition, to cope*

- Provide privacy and ensure confidentiality.
- Establish a therapeutic relationship based on trust and respect.
- Determine the client's purpose, goals, and agenda for the genetic counseling session.
- Determine knowledge base, myths, perceptions, and misperceptions related to a birth defect or genetic condition.
- Determine presence and quality of family support, other support systems, and previous coping skills.
- Provide estimates of client's risk based upon phenotype (client characteristics), family history (pedigree analysis), calculated risk information, or genotype (genetic testing results).
- Provide estimates of occurrence or recurrence risks for client and at-risk family members.
- Provide information on the natural history of the disease or condition, treatment and/or management strategies, and preventions strategies, if known.
- Provide information about the risks, benefits, and limitations of treatment/management options, as well as options for dealing with recurrence risk in a nondirective manner.
- Provide decision-making support as clients consider their options.
- Prioritize areas of risk reduction in collaboration with the individual, family, or group.
- Monitor response when client learns about own genetic risk factors.
- Allow expression of feelings.
- Support client's coping process.
- Institute crisis support measures as needed.
- Provide referral to genetic health care specialists, as necessary.
- Provide referral to community resources, including genetic support groups, as needed.
- Provide client a written summary of genetic counseling session, as indicated.

Coping Enhancement: *Assisting a client to adapt to perceived stressors, changes, or threats that interfere with meeting life demands and roles*

- Appraise the impact of the client's life situation on roles and relationships.
- Appraise the client's understanding of the disease process.
- Appraise and discuss alternative responses to situation.
- Use a calm, reassuring approach.
- Help client to identify the information he/she is most interested in obtaining.
- Provide factual information concerning diagnosis, treatment, and prognosis.
- Evaluate the client's decision-making ability.
- Discourage decision making when the client is under severe stress.
- Acknowledge the client's spiritual/cultural background.
- Confront client's ambivalent (angry or depressed) feelings.
- Arrange situations that encourage client's autonomy.
- Encourage the identification of specific life values.
- Support the use of appropriate defense mechanisms.
- Encourage verbalization of feelings, perceptions, and fears.
- Discuss consequences of not dealing with guilt and shame.
- Appraise the client's needs/desires for social support.
- Determine the risk of the client inflicting self-harm.
- Encourage family involvement, as appropriate.
- Assist the client to clarify misconceptions.

NIC intervention activities selected from Dochterman, J.M., & Bulechek, G.M. (Eds.). (2004). *Nursing interventions classification (NIC)* (4th ed.). St. Louis: Mosby.

carrier without the client's permission. This issue is controversial, as described below under Sharing of Information.

COERCION

The final decision to have genetic testing or to not have rests with the client. Family members or a primary care provider may be urging the client to have the test. However, the client must make the decision without such pressures.

SHARING OF INFORMATION

The client makes the final decision to share the information with family members. Some clients choose not to share this information even when other family members may also be at risk. An area of controversy is one in which the health care provider knows the client has a positive test result for a serious inherited condition, such as hereditary, non-polyposis colon cancer (HNPCC). This condition has an autosomal dominant inheritance pattern, and each child of the client has a 50% risk for having the gene. If the client chooses not to tell his or her grown children, they then do not have the opportunity for increased screening to find the cancer at an early stage when cure is possible. An ethical dilemma arises when the health care provider wants to inform the children of their risk. Different states have different views on whether or not the health care provider has an obligation to inform other family members.

THE ROLE OF THE MEDICAL-SURGICAL NURSE IN GENETIC COUNSELING

Medical-surgical nurses help clients during the assessing, testing, and counseling processes in many areas, although they do not provide in-depth genetic counseling. Clients often feel most comfortable sharing information with nurses and asking nurses to clarify information.

Nurses may be the first health care professionals to identify a client at genetic risk. Some of the following are indicators that a client may have an increased genetic risk for a disease or disorder:

- The disease or disorder occurs at a higher incidence within the family than among the general population.
- The client or close family members have another identified genetic problem.
- The incidence of a specific disease or disorder occurs in the client or in family members at an unusually early age.
- A rare disease is present in two or more family members.
- More than one type of cancer in present in any one person.
- The presence of clinical manifestations is associated with one or more genetic disorders (unusual freckling or skin pigmentation, bicuspid aortic valve, deafness)

A nurse may be the health care professional that verifies information that can bring a genetic problem to light. For example, during an assessment, the client may tell you that her mother died of bone cancer when she was 40 years old. Bone cancer is quite rare among adults; thus you might then ask, "Did your mother ever have any other type of cancer?" Often the client may then tell you that her mother had breast cancer some years before that (and the "bone cancer" was really breast cancer that had spread to the bones). Breast cancer at an early age can indicate a genetic predisposition.

Clients may ask questions that indicate an interest in genetic testing. The following are examples of questions that may be cues that the client has genetic concerns:

- Will my children get this disease?
- Because my sister has this problem, what are the chances I might also develop it?
- Is there a way to test and see whether my chances of getting this disease (or having this problem) are high?

Areas of responsibility for any medical-surgical nurse in working with a client who is considering or having genetic testing include communication, privacy and confidentiality, information accuracy, client advocacy, and support.

COMMUNICATION

As a nurse, you must ensure that communication between the client and whomever is providing the genetic information is clear. First assess the client's ability to receive and process information. Can the client see and hear clearly, or are assistive devices needed? Does the client understand English, or will an interpreter be needed? Is the client's cognition at the time of meeting with the genetic professional adequate, or is it impaired by medication, disease, anxiety, or fear?

If you think the client does not understand terms or jargon during a discussion between the client and a genetic professional, ask the professional to use common terms and examples for the client. Verify with the client that he or she understands.

After any discussion about genetic risk or genetic testing, assess the client's understanding of what was said. Ask the client to explain to you, in his or her own words, what the issue means and what his or her expectations are.

PRIVACY AND CONFIDENTIALITY

All conversations regarding potential diagnoses or genetic testing must occur in a private environment. The client has the right to determine who may be a part of the discussion. The client can decide to exclude his or her primary physician and any family member from the discussion with a genetic professional. It is important that health care professionals who may be present during such discussion do not disclose information, formally or informally, without the client's permission. It is your responsibility to protect this information from improper disclosure to family members, other health care professionals, other clients, insurance providers, or anyone not specifically named by the client.

INFORMATION ACCURACY

As a medical-surgical nurse, you can help correct myths about genetic disorders and teach clients about the nature of genetic testing. In addition, you can help clients to find accurate and helpful resource materials or websites. Medical-surgical nurses are not genetics experts and would not be expected to be the final source of definitive information; however, you can help ensure that the client is referred to the correct level of genetic counseling. If you have been present during the client's discussions with a genetics professional, you can assess whether he or she understands the issues regarding his or her health problem.

CLIENT ADVOCACY

As a client advocate, you must ensure that the client's rights are not neglected or ignored. Ask the client privately what his or her wishes are regarding genetic testing. Ask whether another person or agency is insisting on the testing. Remind the client that he or she does not have to agree to testing. Determine whether the client has signed an informed consent statement for the test.

SUPPORT

Considering or having genetic testing is a stressful experience. The client and family require strong support and may need help to find the best way to cope (see Chart 11-1). Genetic testing should be performed only after genetic counseling has first occurred and should be followed with an opportunity for more counseling.

Clients may feel anger, depression, guilt, or hopelessness. Clients who have positive results from genetic testing may have issues of role changes, risk for early death or disability, and the possibility of having passed the risk for a health problem on to their children. Clients who have an ambiguous test result or one of unknown significance may feel that they have agonized over a decision, spent money, and still have no clear answer or direction. Even clients who have negative genetic test results need counseling and support. Some clients may have an unrealistic view of what a negative result means for their general health. Others may feel guilty that they were "spared" when siblings were not.

Assess the client's response to genetic test results. Ask about how the client may have used coping mechanisms in the past. If the client has disclosed information to family members, assess whether they can help provide client support or need support themselves. Refer the client to appropriate support groups and general counseling services.

GET READY for the NCLEX Examination!

KEY POINTS

- DNA, genes, and chromosomes are different forms of the same substance.
- All human cells with a nucleus contain all the genes.
- Every time a cell divides, it must replicate its DNA.
- The normal human chromosome number is 46.
- The purpose of a gene is to serve as the instructions for making a specific protein.
- Mutations can change the activity of a protein and have adverse effects on health.
- Many common adult diseases or disorders have a genetic basis (hypertension, diabetes, cancer) although some of these diseases also may occur among people with no genetic risk.
- A pedigree with at least three generations is needed when performing a genetic risk assessment.
- Each child of a person who has an autosomal dominant genetic problem has a 50% risk of inheriting the gene for the problem.
- Having a gene for a disorder does not necessarily mean that the disorder will ever develop.
- Genetic testing requires informed consent.
- The results of genetic tests do not change.
- There is no single genetic test that can provide information about all aspects of a client's health risks.
- Genetic testing reveals information about the client and his or her family members.
- Genetic testing is expensive and might not be covered by insurance.
- Genetic testing requires individual genetic risk assessment.
- Just because a genetic test is available does not mean that it is right or necessary that any given client should have the test.
- Clients having genetic testing should have genetic counseling before the testing and follow-up counseling after testing.

ADDITIONAL STUDY RESOURCES

Go to your Student CD-ROM for Review Questions for the NCLEX Examination.

evolve Go to http://evolve.elsevier.com/Iggy/ for Integrated Management of Care Questions for the NCLEX Examination.

SELECTED BIBLIOGRAPHY

American Society of Clinical Oncology. (2003). American Society of Clinical Oncology policy statement update: Genetic testing for cancer susceptibility. *Journal of Clinical Oncology, 21*(12), 2397-2406.

Anionwu, E. (2003). Forum: Genetics is fundamental to quality care. *Nursing Times, 99*(6), 12.

Burke, W. (2002). Genetic testing. *New England Journal of Medicine, 347*(23), 1867-1875.

Burton, H., & Shuttleworth, A. (2003). Genetics education for primary health care nurses. *Primary Health Care, 13*(4), 35-38.

Burton, H., & Stewart, A. (2003). From Mendel to the Human Genome Project: The implications for nurse education. *Nurse Education Today, 23*(5), 380-385.

Calzone, K., Jenkins, J., & Masny, A. (2002). Core competencies in cancer genetics for advanced practice oncology nurses. *Oncology Nursing Forum, 29*(9), 1327-1333.

Cashion, A. (2002). Genetics in transplantation. *MEDSURG Nursing, 11*(2), 91-94.

Cheek, D. (2002). Current issues in genetics. *AACN Clinical Issues: Advanced Practice in Acute and Critical Care, 13*(4), 485.

Cheek, D., & Cesan, A. (2003). Genetic predictors of cardiovascular disease: The use of chip technology. *Journal of Cardiovascular Nursing, 18*(1), 50-56.

Collins, F., et al. (2003). A vision for the future of genomics research. *Nature, 422*(24), 835-847.

Grady, P., & Collins, F. (2003). Genetics and nursing science: Realizing the potential. *Nursing Research, 52*(2), 69.

Greco, K. (2003). Nursing in the genomic era: Nurturing our genetic nature. *MEDSURG Nursing, 12*(5), 307-312.

Guttmacher, A., & Collins, F. (2003). Genomic medicine–A primer. *New England Journal of Medicine, 347*(19), 1512-1520.

Guttmacher, A., Jenkins, J., Uhlmann, W. (2000). Genomic medicine: Who will practice it? A call to open arms. *American Journal of Medical Genetics, 106*(3), 216-222.

Houfek, J., & Atwood, J. (2003). Genetic susceptibility to lung cancer: Implications for smoking cessation. *MEDSURG Nursing, 12*(1), 45-49.

Imperatore, G., et al. (2003). Hereditary hemochromatosis: Perspective of public health, medical genetics, and primary care. *Genetics in Medicine, 5*(1), 1-8.

Jenkins, J. (2002). Genetics competency: New directions for nursing. *AACN Clinical Issues: Advanced Practice in Acute and Critical Care, 13*(4), 486-491.

Jenkins, J. (2000). An historic perspective on genetic care. *Nursing World/Online Journal of Issues in Nursing, 5*(3), 1-17.

Jenkins, J., & Collins, F. (2003). Are you genetically literate? *American Journal of Nursing, 103*(4), 13.

Jenkins, J., & Lea, D. (2005). Nursing care in the genomic era: A case-based approach. Boston: Jones & Bartlett.

Lea, D. (2002a). Position statement: Integrating genetics competencies into baccalaureate and advanced nursing education. *Nursing Outlook, 50*(4), 167-168.

Lea, D. (2002b). What nurses need to know about genetics. *DCCN: Dimensions of Critical Care Nursing, 21*(2), 50-61.

Lea, D., & Williams, J. (2002). Genetic testing and screening: Use them as a part of routine nursing practice. *American Journal of Nursing, 102*(7), 36-43, 49-50.

Lessick, M., et al. (2001). Advances in genetic testing for cancer risk. *MEDSURG Nursing, 10*(3), 123-127.

Loud, J., et al. (2002). Applications of advances in molecular biology and genomics to clinical cancer care. *Cancer Nursing, 25*(2), 110-122.

Middleton, L., et al. (2002). The role of the nurse in cancer genetics. *Cancer Nursing, 25*(3), 196-208.

Nicol, M. (2003). The variation of response to pharmacotherapy: Pharmacogenetics–A new perspective to "the right drug for the right person." *MEDSURG Nursing, 12*(4), 242-249.

Novak, K. (2003). Telomeres and telomerases in cancer. *Medscape General Medicine, 5*(1), 1-5.

Nussbaum, R., McInnes, R., & Willard, H. (2001). *Thompson & Thompson: Genetics in medicine* (6th ed.). Philadelphia: W.B. Saunders.

Olsen, S., et al. (2003). Creating a nursing vision for leadership in genetics. *MEDSURG Nursing, 12*(3), 177-183.

Peska, E. (2003). Genomics offers opportunities for nurses. *Journal of Continuing Education in Nursing, 34*(5), 195-196.

Peters, J., et al. (2001). Cancer genetics fundamentals. *Cancer Nursing, 24*(6), 446-461.

Prows, C., & Prows, D. (2004). Medication selection by genotype. *American Journal of Nursing, 104*(5), 60-70.

Read, C. (2002). Pharmacogenomics: An evolving paradigm for drug therapy. *MEDSURG Nursing, 11*(3), 122-124.

Rieger, P. (2000). The gene genies. *The American Journal of Nursing, 100*(10), 87-90.

Smith, K., (2001). Genetic disease, genetic testing, and the clinician. *Journal of the American Medical Association, 285*(1), 91.

Spahis, J. (2002). Human genetics: Constructing a family pedigree. *The American Journal of Nursing, 102*(7), 44-50.

Varmus H. (2002). Getting ready for gene-based medicine. *New England Journal of Medicine, 347*, 1526-1527.

Williams, J. (2002). Education for genetics and nursing practice. *AACN Clinical Issues: Advanced Practice in Acute and Critical Care, 13*(4), 492-500, 590-595.

Williams, J., & Lessick, M. (2001). Historical evolution of nursing in genetics. *MEDSURG Nursing, 10*(6), 301-307.

Winkelman, C. (2004). What every critical care nurse needs to know about the genetic contribution to critical illness. *Critical Care Nurse, 24*(3), 34-45.

Wung, S. (2002). Genetic advances in coronary disease. *MEDSURG Nursing, 11*(6), 296-300.

UNIT **THREE**

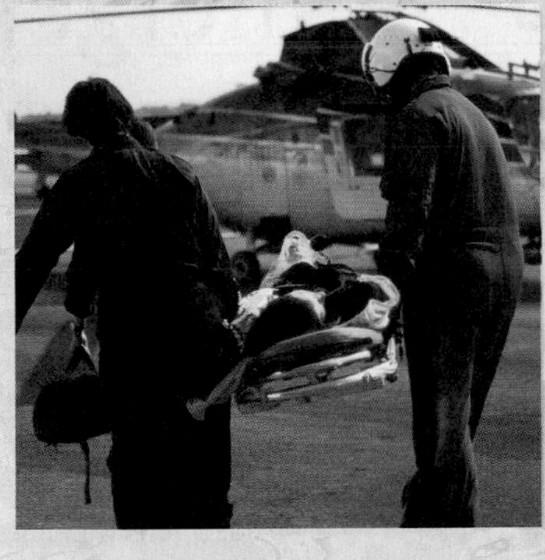

CONCEPTS of EMERGENCY NURSING

CHAPTER

12 Emergency and Mass Casualty Nursing

LINDA LASKOWSKI-JONES • KAREN L. TOULSON

LEARNING OUTCOMES

After studying this chapter, you should be able to:

1. Describe the emergency department (ED) environment, including special populations, cultural considerations, and interdisciplinary team members.
2. Plan and implement best practices to maintain staff and client safety in the ED.
3. Explain the core competencies that nurses need to function in the ED.
4. Identify types of certification that ED nurses can obtain to demonstrate or develop their expertise.
5. Triage clients into emergent, urgent, and nonurgent categories.
6. Prioritize resuscitation interventions based on the primary survey of the ED client.
7. Describe the general process of admission through disposition of a client in the ED.
8. Contrast the triage process under usual conditions with triage in a mass casualty.
9. Identify the components of an Emergency Preparedness and Response Plan.
10. Compare the key personnel roles in an Emergency Preparedness and Response Plan.
11. Differentiate two types of debriefing that occur after a mass casualty incident.
12. Describe the general process that occurs in the ED when a client is suspected of a bioterrorism agent, such as anthrax.

Go to your Student CD-ROM for Review Questions for the NCLEX Examination keyed to these Learning Outcomes.

Emergency department (ED) visits in the United States have increased 14% between 1997 and 2000 (McCaig & Ly, 2002). During this same period of time, the number of EDs has decreased from 4005 to 3934. Thus the remaining EDs are encountering more clients with fewer facilities. To add to this problem, about 41 million people in the United States do not have health insurance and use the ED as their primary health care provider.

The ED is fast paced. Clients seek treatment for many physical, psychological, spiritual, and social reasons. At the height of activity, the ED may appear quite chaotic. In general, nurses are drawn to this environment because they dislike routines and thrive in challenging, stimulating work settings.

THE EMERGENCY DEPARTMENT ENVIRONMENT OF CARE

In the emergency care environment, rapid change is the rule. Although most EDs have treatment areas that are designated for certain populations such as clients with trauma, cardiac, psychiatric, or gynecologic problems, care can actually take place anywhere in this environment. In an overcrowded ED, many clients receive initial treatment outside of the usual treatment rooms, including the waiting room and hallways.

Client care areas are typically alive with activity and noise, although the pace can slow at times. Emergency nurses can expect background sounds that include ringing telephones, monitor alarms, vocal clients, crying children, and radio transmissions between ED staff and incoming ambulance or helicopter personnel. Interruptions are the norm.

Demographic Data

Staff members in the ED provide care for clients across the life span with a broad spectrum of issues, illnesses, and injuries—as well as various cultural and religious values. During a given shift, for example, the emergency nurse may function as a cardiac nurse, a pediatric nurse, a psychiatric nurse, a trauma nurse, and even a maternity nurse. Because of the multispecialty nature of the environment, EDs play a unique role within the U.S. health care system. Between 1992 and 2001, the number of ED visits rose from 89.8 million to 107.5 million visits per year (McCaig & Burt, 2003). The most common reasons that clients seek ED care include chest pain, abdominal pain, headache, and fever. The average age of a person who enters the ED is 35.7 years of age;

clients 75 years of age or older generate the highest ED visit rate (McCaig & Burt, 2003).

Special Populations

The ED serves as an important safety net for clients who are ill or injured but lack access to health care. Especially vulnerable populations include those with Medicare and Medicaid, minorities, and those who are underinsured or uninsured. Because the current health care system is complex, expensive, and difficult to navigate, some clients view the ED as an easy access route to basic health care services. Clients may also use the ED as a temporary bridge to establishing a relationship with a primary care provider or a clinic. A small percentage of clients actively attempt to manipulate the system to their advantage. These clients are commonly referred to as "frequent flyers" by frustrated staff. Some are drug seekers. Others are noncompliant with follow-up instructions that they receive upon discharge. They actively elect not to pursue a relationship with another appropriate health care provider and continue to use the ED for virtually all of their health care needs.

CULTURAL CONSIDERATIONS

The emergency nurse needs to be aware of the various cultural and religious values of clients that may impact emergency department care. Many individuals have distinct beliefs that must be respected in the health care setting. For example, Mexican Americans are typically modest and do not like to have their bodies exposed. They are also family oriented and affectionate toward each other. A religious belief system can affect the delivery of trauma care. For example, Jehovah's Witness clients do not accept blood transfusions. Clients with language barriers also present a challenge for the emergency nurse. The Spanish speaking population in the United States, for instance, is rapidly increasing. When a bilingual staff member is not available to competently interpret, the emergency nurse can employ resources such as telephone language lines and dedicated interpreters contracted by the hospital.

Special Nursing Teams

Many EDs have specialized teams that deal with high-risk populations of clients. One example of this concept is the forensic nurse examiner team. **Forensic nurse examiners** are educated to obtain client histories, collect forensic evidence, and offer counseling and follow-up care for victims of rape, child abuse, and domestic violence. They are trained to recognize evidence of abuse and to intervene on the client's behalf. Interventions may include providing information to the client about developing a safety plan or how to escape a violent relationship. The forensic nurse examiner documents injuries and collects physical and photographic evidence. Nurses from this team may also provide testimony in court as to what was observed during the examination and information about the type of care rendered.

The **psychiatric crisis nurse team** is another example of an ED specialty team. These nurses interact with clients and families in crisis. The sudden illness, serious injury, or death of a loved one may have precipitated the crisis. This team also evaluates individuals with psychiatric complaints or disorders and facilitates the client's follow-up or admission to an appropriate psychiatric facility.

Interdisciplinary Team Members

The **emergency nurse** is one member of the large interdisciplinary team who provides care for clients in the emergency department (ED). A team approach to emergency care is considered a standard of practice. In this setting, the emergency nurse must interact in a professional manner with all levels of health team providers, from prehospital emergency medical services (EMS) personnel to physicians, hospital technicians, and professional and ancillary staff.

PREHOSPITAL CARE PROVIDERS

Prehospital care providers are typically the first caregivers encountered by the client if he or she is transported to the ED by an ambulance or helicopter (Figure 12-1). Local protocols define the skill level of the EMS responders dispatched to render assistance to the client. **Emergency medical technicians (EMTs)** offer basic life support (BLS) interventions such as oxygen, basic wound care, splinting, spinal immobilization, and monitoring of vital signs. Some units carry automatic external defibrillators (AEDs) and may be authorized to administer selected medications such as an EpiPen or nitroglycerin based on established medical control protocols. For clients who require care that exceeds BLS resources, paramedics are usually dispatched. **Paramedics** are advanced life support (ALS) providers who can perform advanced techniques, which may include cardiac monitoring, advanced airway management and intubation, establishing intravenous access, and administering drugs en route to the ED (Figure 12-2).

The prehospital provider is a key source for valuable client data. Emergency nurses rely on these providers to be the eyes and ears of the health team in the prehospital set-

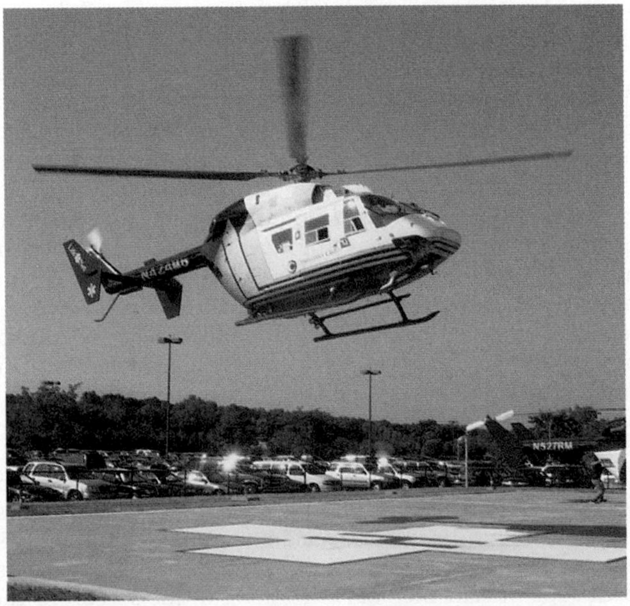

Figure 12-1 ■ Advanced life support helicopter arriving at emergency department landing zone. Helicopters are used to rapidly transport critically ill and injured clients to the hospital for emergent care.

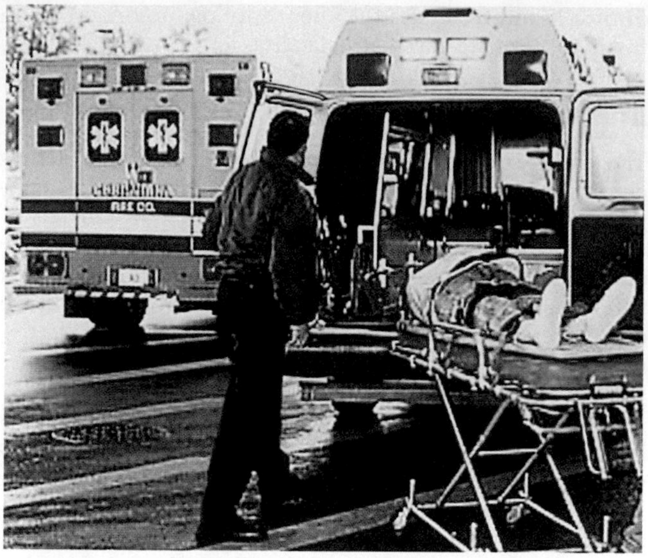

Figure 12-2 ■ Prehospital providers unload a client from the ambulance to be brought into the emergency department.

ting. The emergency nurse must pay close attention to the information that is shared to ensure continuity of care.

PHYSICIANS

Another integral member of the emergency health care team is the **emergency medicine physician**. These doctors receive specialized education and training in emergency client management. In the past, physicians of all types with varying competencies rotated through the ED. As emergency care became increasingly complex and specialized, emergency medicine became a recognized physician specialty practice, complete with board certification requirements. Today, there are emergency medicine residency programs throughout the United States that formally prepare emergency physicians to competently assume responsibility for the emergency client population.

The emergency nurse routinely interacts with a number of staff and community physicians involved in the care of ED clients. On an ongoing basis, however, the emergency nurse works most closely with emergency medicine physicians. Even though other physician specialists may be involved in ED client treatment, the emergency medicine physician typically directs the overall care in the department. Many EDs also employ nurse practitioners and physician's assistants to assume designated roles in client assessment and treatment. These individuals act in collaboration with or under the supervision of the emergency medicine physician to expedite emergency care delivery.

SUPPORT STAFF

The emergency nurse also interacts on a regular basis with professional and ancillary staff who function in support roles. These personnel include x-ray and ultrasound technicians, respiratory therapists, laboratory technicians and social workers. Each support staff member is essential to the success of the emergency health team. It is important for the emergency nurse to gain an understanding of the individual roles and responsibilities of these personnel. The emergency nurse is accountable for communicating pertinent staff considerations, client needs, and restrictions to support staff, such as physical limitations or isolation precautions, to assure that ongoing client and staff safety issues are addressed–and for assuring that clients are properly prepared for diagnostic or therapeutic intervention. Each interaction with a support team member can be viewed as a learning opportunity. These professionals possess unique bodies of knowledge and skill sets that can augment the efforts of the emergency nurse. For example, the respiratory therapist can assist the emergency nurse to trouble shoot mechanical ventilator issues. Laboratory technicians can offer advice regarding specimen collection procedures. During the discharge planning process, social workers can be tremendous client advocates in locating community resources, including temporary housing, durable medical goods, drug and alcohol counseling, health insurance information, prescription services, and health care provider referrals.

INPATIENT UNIT STAFF

The emergency nurse's interactions extend beyond the walls of the ED. Essential to continuity of care is communication with staff nurses from the inpatient units. Providing a concise but comprehensive report of the client's ED experience, including relevant medical history, assessment and diagnostic findings, interventions, and the client's response to those interventions is integral to the transfer process and client safety. Both emergency nurses and nurses on inpatient units should strive to understand the unique aspects of their two practice environments to prevent conflicts. For example, nurses on inpatient units can be critical of the push to move clients out of the ED setting quickly, particularly when the unit activity is high. Similarly, the emergency nurse may be critical of the inpatient unit's lack of understanding or enthusiasm for accepting admissions rapidly. Effective interpersonal communication skills and respectful negotiation can optimize teamwork between the emergency nurse and the inpatient unit nurse. For instance, when ED client volume or acuity is overwhelming, the unit nurse can volunteer to assist the ED nurse by moving a monitored client to the hospital bed. By the same token, the emergency nurse can elect to delay sending admitted clients to inpatient units during change of shift or crisis periods such as a cardiac arrest on the unit whenever possible.

Staff and Client Safety Considerations

In the emergency department (ED) setting, client and staff safety is an ever-present concern for the emergency nurse (Chart 12-1). Some of the most prevalent safety issues involve the following:

- Appropriate client identification
- Fall risk
- Skin breakdown in vulnerable populations
- High risk for medical errors or adverse events due to the emergent nature of care delivery

Staff safety concerns are primarily centered on the potential for transmission of disease and for personal safety when dealing with aggressive, agitated, or violent clients and visitors.

CLIENT IDENTIFICATION

Client identification is a focal point of care in the ED. All clients are issued an identification bracelet at their point of entry of the ED–generally at the triage registration desk or at the bedside if emergent needs exist. For clients with an unknown identity and those with emergent conditions that prevent the proper identification process (e.g., unconscious

CHART 12-1

BEST PRACTICE for
Maintaining Client and Staff Safety in the Emergency Department

Safety Consideration	Interventions to Minimize Risk
Client identification	Provide an ID bracelet for each client. Use two unique identifiers (e.g., name, date of birth). If client identity is unknown, use a special identification system.
Injury prevention for clients	Keep rails up on stretcher. Keep stretcher in lowest position. Remind the client to use call light/bell for assistance. Reorient confused clients frequently. If client is confused, ask a family member or significant other to monitor the client. Implement skin prevention measures for clients at risk for skin breakdown.
Risk for errors and adverse events	Obtain a thorough client and family history. Check the client for a medical alert bracelet or necklace. Search the client's belongings when he or she has altered mental status.
Injury prevention for staff	Use standard precautions at all times. Anticipate hostile, violent client and family behavior. Plan options if violence occurs, including assistance from the security department.

client without identification or emergent trauma client), hospitals commonly use a "Jane/John Doe" or other identification system. Whatever method is used, the emergency nurse is accountable for verifying the client's identity before each intervention and before medication administration. The fast pace of the ED often complicates assuring proper identification. However, the emergency nurse must adhere to client identification standards to optimize client safety and to reduce personal liability risk.

CLIENT SAFETY

The nurse must also ensure that the client is safe in the environment while receiving care. Two primary safety considerations are to protect clients from falls and to prevent skin breakdown.

CONSIDERATIONS FOR OLDER ADULTS

Clients who are on beds or stretchers should have all side rails up and the bed or stretcher in the lowest position. Access to a call light or bell is especially important; the client is instructed to call for the nurse if assistance is needed rather than attempt independent ambulation. Older clients may become confused and need reorientation. In some cases, the nurse should ask a family member, significant other, or sitter to stay with the client to prevent falls.

Some clients spend a lengthy time on stretchers while awaiting inpatient unit bed availability. Protecting skin integrity begins in the ED. Emergency nurses should assess the skin frequently and implement preventive interventions into the ED plan of care, especially when caring for older adults. Interventions that promote clean, dry skin for incontinent clients, mobility techniques that decrease shearing forces when moving the immobile client, and routine turning aid in the prevention of skin breakdown.

RISK FOR ERRORS AND ADVERSE EVENTS

A significant risk for all clients who enter the emergency care environment involves the potential for medical errors or adverse events. Causative factors stem from the episodic and often chaotic nature of emergency management. Clients arrive in the ED with urgent or emergent needs that must be addressed rapidly. They may not know–or even be able to relate–key elements of their medical history such as medical conditions, allergies, or current medications. Gaps in information can lead to prescribing and treatment errors. To reduce the error potential, the emergency nurse makes every attempt to obtain essential medical history information from the client, family, or reliable significant others as necessary. When dealing with clients who arrive with an altered mental status, a quick survey to determine whether the client is wearing a medical alert bracelet or necklace is an important aspect of initial care to gain critical medical information. In addition, a two-person search of client belongings may yield medication containers, the name of a physician, pharmacy, family contact person, or a medication list. In this case, the nurse serves as a detective to find clues, which may not only promote client safety, but which may also help determine the diagnosis and influence the overall emergency treatment plan.

Lastly, emergency nurses need to be aware of their own personal safety while caring for clients. The emergency nurse must use standard precautions at all times when there is a potential for contamination by blood or other body fluids. Clients with tuberculosis can be preferentially placed in a negative pressure room; the nurse can wear a positive air-purifying respirator (PAPR) before engaging in any close interaction.

Hostile behavior also poses a significant injury risk to ED staff members. Recognizing volatile situations or individuals who show evidence of violent tendencies is critical to planning an escape route or attempting de-escalation strategies before harm can occur. Many EDs have at least one security guard in their settings at all times for assistance with these situations.

SCOPE OF EMERGENCY NURSING PRACTICE

The scope of emergency nursing practice encompasses management of clients across the life span–from birth through death–and all health conditions that prompt an individual of any age to seek emergency care. It is the breadth and depth of knowledge as well as the emergency care skills that attract and provide ongoing challenge to nurses who enter into this specialty.

Education

Nurses come to work in the ED in a variety of ways. Traditionally, hospital employers have required nurses to have 6 months to 1 year of experience in an acute care medical-surgical or critical care unit setting before working in the ED.

The rationale for this requirement was that nurses would have developed competencies in basic nursing care and organizational skills before entering ED specialty practice.

The nursing shortage has inspired many emergency nurse leaders to rethink the philosophy of hiring only experienced acute care nurses into the ED when sufficient numbers of them are not available to fulfill staffing needs. Today, many nurses are entering the ED upon graduation from nursing school. Strategies to bridge the knowledge and experience gap include emergency nursing course work and clinical rotations incorporated into senior-level nursing school curricula, extended hospital ED orientation programs, and emergency nursing internship programs (Gurney, 2002).

Core Competencies

Emergency nursing practice requires that nurses be skilled in client assessment, priority setting and critical thinking, multitasking, and communication. A sound knowledge base is essential. Flexibility and adaptability are essential traits of the nurse because situations within the ED, as well as individual clients, can change rapidly.

ASSESSMENT

First and foremost, the foundation of the emergency nurse's skill base is assessment (Twedell, 2000). The emergency nurse not only must rapidly and accurately discern normal from abnormal, but also must categorize assessment findings according to acuity and age. For example, mottling of the extremities may be a normal finding in a newborn, but it may indicate poor peripheral perfusion and a shock state in an older child. The significance of pre-existing disease states, or **comorbidities**, must also be factored into the emergency nurse's assessment in regard to how the condition might adversely affect or complicate a seemingly unrelated health problem. For example, a trauma client who has rib fractures and a past medical history of chronic obstructive pulmonary disease (COPD) may not be able to maintain adequate oxygenation without endotracheal intubation and mechanical ventilatory support in the ED. Another common assessment scenario involves the Type I diabetic client who presents to the ED with an altered mental status after a fall–Is the altered mental status due to hypoglycemia or to intracranial injury? The nurse must quickly act to assess blood glucose in this case, as well as follow trauma protocols for managing a potential head injury.

PRIORITY SETTING/CRITICAL THINKING SKILLS

Another essential skill for the emergency nurse is priority setting, which is inherent in the triage process and is described later in this chapter. Priority setting depends on accurate assessment as well as critical thinking skills. These skills are generally gained through hands-on clinical experience in the ED. However, discussion of case studies and the use of simulation software can help prepare nurses to acquire this skill base in a nonthreatening environment and then apply it in the actual clinical situation.

KNOWLEDGE OF EMERGENCY CARE

The knowledge base for emergency nurses is broad and encompasses not only typical client presentations of common medical and surgical disease entities, but also the less common ones, such as poisonous snake and insect bites, heat stroke, hypothermia, and hazardous materials contamination. These emergency care nursing principles extend to recognition, management, and legal implications of societal problems such as child abuse, domestic violence, elder abuse, and sexual assault.

Although most EDs have physicians available around the clock who are physically located within the ED, the emergency nurse often initiates interdisciplinary protocols to expedite life-saving interventions such as application of cardiac monitoring, oxygen therapy, insertion of intravenous catheters, and infusion of appropriate parenteral solutions. In many EDs, nurses function under medical protocols that allow them to initiate drug therapy for emergent conditions such as anaphylactic shock and cardiac arrest. Emergency care principles extend to knowing what essential laboratory and diagnostic tests may be needed and, when necessary, obtaining them. The Emergency Nurses Association's *Emergency Nursing Core Curriculum* (2000a) is an excellent reference that outlines the fundamental body of knowledge that encompasses the emergency nurse's knowledge and skill base.

TECHNICAL SKILLS

The emergency nurse must also be proficient in performing a variety of technical skills (multitasking), sometimes in a stressful, high-pressure environment such as a cardiac or trauma resuscitation. In addition to basic skills, the emergency nurse may also need to be proficient with equipment most often found in the critical care environment, such as invasive pressure monitoring devices. EDs that are components of a Level I trauma center typically have such critical care equipment in the ED setting.

The emergency nurse assists the physician with a number of procedures. Knowledge and skills related to procedural setup, client preparation, teaching, and post-procedural care are also essential facets of emergency nursing practice. Common ED procedures include the following:

- Simple and complex suturing for wound closure
- Foreign body removal
- Central line insertion
- Endotracheal intubation
- Transvenous pacemaker insertion
- Lumbar puncture
- Pelvic examination
- Chest tube insertion
- Peritoneal lavage
- Fracture management

More than one emergency nurse may be necessary to assist with some procedures. For example, if conscious sedation is used to produce a state of amnesia and relaxation during fracture manipulation, one nurse assists the physician with the actual procedure, while the other nurse is dedicated to monitoring the client before, during, and after the conscious sedation medications are administered.

COMMUNICATION

Finally, an essential aspect of the emergency nurse's skill base is communication. The ED environment is complex–barriers to effective communication exist at virtually all levels of interaction. Overcrowding and insufficient nursing personnel to meet the demand for services create difficulties with communication of pertinent client information and quality of written documentation. The high-stress ED environment also threatens positive, effective interpersonal behaviors, particularly when nurses must deal with hostile, violent, or demanding clientele as well as negative co-workers (Keough, Schlomer & Bollenberg, 2003). Despite the obstacles, the emergency nurse should seek to uphold professional standards of communication to the best of his or her ability when confronted with adversity–and seek administrative support when barriers cannot seem to be overcome. Sometimes practice modifications need to be made based upon overwhelming client volume or acuity, but the nurse should strive to maintain both client safety and dignity and invoke additional resources to manage the burden when possible.

CERTIFICATION

Two general types of certification are referred to in emergency nursing practice: the "certification," which marks successful completion of a particular course of study and emergency nursing specialty certification (Table 12-1). As part of the orientation and employment requirements for staff nurses in most U.S. EDs, successful completion of the Health Care Provider Basic Cardiac Life Support (BCLS) and Advanced Cardiac Life Support (ACLS) provider courses through the American Heart Association (Cummins, 2003) is necessary. These courses provide instruction in fundamental, evidence-based management theory and techniques for cardiopulmonary resuscitation (CPR); course participants include physicians, nurses, and prehospital personnel. BCLS emphasizes hands-on, noninvasive assessment and management skills to restore an effective airway, breathing, and circulation. The participant performs basic airway maneuvers and CPR. The ACLS course builds on the BCLS content to include advanced concepts in cardiac monitoring, invasive airway management skills, pharmacologic and electrical therapies, intravascular access techniques, special resuscitation situations, and postresuscitation management considerations.

Many emergency nurse leaders also require emergency nurses who care for children to successfully complete the Pediatric Advanced Life Support (PALS) course offered jointly by the American Academy of Pediatrics and the American Heart Association (2002). This course teaches the essential concepts of neonatal and pediatric resuscitation to physicians, nurses, and paramedics. Another option for establishing a defined pediatric emergency nursing knowledge base is the Emergency Nurses Association Emergency Nursing Pediatric Course (ENPC) (Eckle, Haley, & Baker, 1998), which offers a broad content area related to nursing management of pediatric conditions, not only resuscitation principles.

For nurses who are employed in EDs that are components of trauma centers, successful completion of the Emergency Nurses Association (2000c) Trauma Nursing Core Course, or a similar program, may be required for employment in addition to BCLS, ACLS, and PALS training. This course includes both lecture and skills stations, and focuses on concepts related to the nursing assessment and management of injuries, particularly during the initial phase of trauma care.

Unlike the "certification" courses, emergency nursing specialty certification through the Emergency Nurses Association's Board Certification for Emergency Nursing (BCEN) program constitutes professional certification in the truest sense of the word. Individuals who both qualify to take the examination and achieve a passing score are authorized to use the initials "CEN"–Certified Emergency Nurse–as part of their professional credentials after their name.

EMERGENCY NURSING PRINCIPLES

Triage

Triage is derived from the French word "trier," which means "to sort" or "to choose" (Gilboy, 2003). The concept of emergency department (ED) **triage** is based upon sorting or classifying clients into priority levels depending on illness or injury severity. The organization of emergency care and even the ED is structured through triage principles. The key concept is that clients who present to the ED with the highest acuity needs receive the quickest evaluation, treatment, and prioritized resource utilization such as x-ray studies, laboratory work, and computed tomography (CT) scans. These clients also have priority for hospital service areas, such as the operating room or cardiac catheterization laboratory. An individual with a lower acuity problem may wait longer in the ED, because the higher acuity client is moved to the "head of the line."

The triage nurse is the gatekeeper in the emergency care system. When clients present to the ED, regulatory standards dictate that a registered nurse (RN), physician, or physician's assistant perform a rapid assessment to determine triage priority (Joint Commission Resources, 2003). The RN is typically the individual assigned to perform the triage function in most hospitals, however. In fact, the Emergency Nurses Association (2001) *Standards of Emergency Nursing Practice* clearly delineate the registered nurse as the health care provider who should triage each ED client. The triage nurse should have appropriate training and experience in both emergency nursing and triage decision-making concepts. Typically, the RN determines the client's triage priority independently. In rare instances, the triage nurse may seek the input of an emergency physician, physician's assistant, or advanced practice nurse to help establish the acuity level if the client's presentation is highly unusual.

TABLE 12-1 Descriptions of Certifications for Emergency Nursing

Certification	Description
Basic Cardiac Life Support (BCLS) (required)	Noninvasive assessment and management skills for airway maintenance and CPR
Advanced Cardiac Life Support (ACLS) (usually required)	Invasive airway management skills, pharmacology, and electrical therapies, special resuscitation
Pediatric Advanced Life Support (PALS) (may be required)	Neonatal and pediatric resuscitation
Certified Emergency Nurse (CEN) (optional)	Validates core emergency nursing knowledge base

Based upon the triage priority, clients may be rushed into a treatment room, directed to a lower acuity area within the ED (e.g., a "**fast track**"), or asked to sit in the waiting room. Variations on this theme include triage nurse–initiated protocols for laboratory work or diagnostic studies that may be performed before the client is actually evaluated by a physician, or even initiation of care on a stretcher in the hallway of an overcrowded ED.

EMERGENT, URGENT, AND NONURGENT CATEGORIES

There are many triage schemes that may be appropriately used by a hospital ED. Whatever scheme is used, it must be applied consistently by all triage nursing staff and endorsed by the emergency medicine physician staff. A basic example of a triage scheme is the commonly used three-tiered model of "emergent, urgent, and nonurgent." In this model, for instance, a client experiencing crushing substernal chest pain, shortness of breath, and diaphoresis would be classified as "emergent" and triaged immediately to a treatment room within the ED. Similarly, a critically injured trauma client or an individual with an active hemorrhage would also be prioritized as "emergent." The **emergent triage** category implies that a condition exists that poses an immediate threat to life or limb.

The **urgent triage** category indicates that the client should be treated quickly, but that an immediate threat to life does not exist at the moment. Reassessment must occur if a physician cannot evaluate the client in a timely manner. In individuals with evidence of clinical deterioration, triage priority may be upgraded from "urgent" to "emergent." Examples of clients who typically fall into the "urgent" category include those with a new onset of pneumonia (as long as respiratory failure does not appear imminent), abdominal pain, renal colic, complex lacerations not associated with major hemorrhage, displaced fractures or dislocations, a history of a seizure before arrival, and temperature greater than 101° F (37° C).

Those categorized as "**nonurgent**" can generally tolerate waiting several hours for health care services without a significant risk of clinical deterioration. Conditions within this classification include clients with sprains and strains, simple fractures, simple lacerations or soft tissue injuries, viral or "cold" symptoms, and skin rashes.

OTHER MULTITIERED MODELS

To further stratify client conditions within an acuity classification or triage priority system, four- and five-tier triage models also exist. Such models are either based on comprehensive lists of conditions that indicate the particular triage priority to which a client should be assigned, or the nature of resources that a client will use in the ED setting. A given client complaint may generate various triage classifications in different hospitals depending upon the triage priority system used at that particular institution. Some schemes may even take into account the presence of pre-existing conditions such as a history of warfarin (Coumadin) use, diabetes, heart disease, and organ transplantation when determining triage priority.

Surprisingly, there is no universally accepted triage system recognized in the United States. Thus there is no standardization of triage acuity data to compare client acuity between hospitals (Travers, 2003). With that said, the Emergency Nurses Association endorses a standardized five-level model known as the **Emergency Severity Index (ESI)** that categorizes both client acuity and resource utilization. "The triage algorithm yields rapid, reproducible, and clinically relevant stratification of clients into five groups, from level 1 (most urgent) to level 5 (least urgent)" (Gilboy et al., 2003). This five-level ESI triage model was found to be safer and provided better discrimination, reliability, sensitivity, and specificity than a three-level triage system in one study involving 15,324 clients at a southeastern tertiary ED (see the Evidence-Based Practice for Nursing box below) (Travers, et al. 2002).

The Primary Survey and Resuscitation Interventions

Perhaps the hallmark public image of emergency nursing is the resuscitation scene as viewed on television where the emergency team acts rapidly and competently to save a human life. This drama is actually played out daily in EDs across the country. Although only a relatively small percentage of clients who seek emergency services actually require this level of care, emergency nurses often define their roles in terms of their resuscitation skills and experience. The opportunity to participate in resuscitation on a regular basis is a primary reason many nurses choose to work in the ED setting. There is much pride in the frequently heard emergency nurse's statement that "we save lives."

Even for the experienced emergency nurse, however, resuscitation can be challenging due to the critical nature of the client's illness or injuries as well as the impact of other issues intrinsic to the emergency environment. There is also

EVIDENCE-BASED PRACTICE for Nursing

Is another triage system better than the traditional three-level triage model?

Travers, D.A., et al. (2002). Five-level triage system more effective than three-level in tertiary emergency department. *Journal of Emergency Nursing, 28*, 395-400.

This retrospective study involved chart reviews at two different times to determine which of two triage systems was the most valid, reliable, and sensitive. At Time I, 305 records were reviewed; at Time II, 303 records were reviewed. Spearman correlations compared the two triage systems. The results showed that the five-level Emergency Severity Index (ESI) was superior to the traditional method—it was more reliable, valid, and stable.

Level of Evidence: 4—Well-conducted qualitative systematic review.

Critique. This study provided evidence that the traditional triage system needs to be revised. The ESI was developed in the United States in the late 1990s. Although this system had strong reliability in other studies, no other study to compare two systems had been published. A retrospective study was the most efficient way to examine large numbers of client records, although all records were from one large medical center. The study should be repeated in other sized hospitals for comparison with this study's results.

Implications for Nursing. Emergency nurses could better depend on the newer system to accurately triage their clients. Emergency departments could start piloting the ESI and collect data on its outcomes, as recommended by the Emergency Nurses Association.

a high risk to the nurse of contamination with blood and body fluids. For this reason, standard precautions attire must be worn in all resuscitation situations and consists an impervious cover gown, gloves, proper eye protection, a face mask, and even a surgical cap and shoe covers if *significant* blood loss is anticipated (e.g., during performance of an ED thoracotomy or when managing a client with gastrointestinal (GI) bleeding).

To remain focused on priorities and keep the situation under control, an organized approach is essential. This approach is applicable for *every* resuscitation situation and promotes rapid identification and intervention techniques to address the most immediate life threats. Although both medical and trauma resuscitation scenes may appear chaotic and complex to the lay person, if performed according to widely accepted protocols and standards, they are actually highly planned events that are based on established priorities of care. These priorities are addressed in order as part of the initial assessment termed the "primary survey." The **primary survey** organizes the approach to the client so that immediate threats to life are rapidly identified and effectively managed. The primary survey is based on a standard "ABC" mnemonic with a "D" and "E" added for trauma clients: airway/cervical spine (**A**), breathing (**B**), circulation (**C**), disability (**D**), and exposure (**E**). Resuscitation efforts occur simultaneously with each element of the primary survey (Cummins, 2003; American College of Surgeons, 1997; Emergency Nurses Association, 2000a). Even though the resuscitation team may encounter multiple clinical problems or injuries, issues identified in the primary survey must be managed before the team engages in interventions of lower priority, such as splinting fractures and dressing wounds.

A: AIRWAY/CERVICAL SPINE

The highest priority intervention in the primary survey is to establish a patent airway. Even minutes without an adequate oxygen supply in humans can lead to cerebral injury that can progress to anoxic brain death. The airway must be cleared of any secretions or debris with either a suction catheter or manually if necessary. The cervical spine must be protected in any trauma client with the potential for spinal injury by manually aligning the neck in a neutral, in-line position and using a jaw thrust maneuver when establishing an airway. Supplemental oxygen is required for all individuals who require resuscitation. In general, a non-rebreather mask is best for the spontaneously breathing client. Bag-valve-mask (BVM) ventilation with the appropriate airway adjunct and a 100% oxygen source is indicated for the individual who needs ventilatory assistance during resuscitation. A client with significantly impaired consciousness, indicated by a Glasgow Coma Score less than or equal to 8, requires a definitive airway such as an endotracheal tube (American College of Surgeons, 1997) (Figure 12-3). After endotracheal intubation, a mechanical ventilator is employed. Initially, oxygen in high concentration (FIO_2 100%) is administered; lower concentrations may be ordered after the client's condition has improved.

B: BREATHING

After the airway is successfully secured, breathing becomes the next priority in the primary survey. This assessment determines whether or not ventilatory efforts are effective–not only whether or not the client is breathing. The focus is on auscultation of breath sounds and evaluation of chest expansion, respiratory effort, and any evidence of chest wall trauma or physical abnormalities. Both apneic clients and those with poor ventilatory effort need bag-valve-mask (BVM) ventilation for support until endotracheal intubation is performed and a mechanical ventilator is used. If cardiopulmonary resuscitation (CPR) becomes necessary, the mechanical ventilator must be disconnected and the client manually ventilated with a BVM device to better sequence ventilations with chest compressions, as well as to assess lung compliance through sensing the degree of difficulty in ventilating the client with the BVM.

Another life-saving intervention that may be performed in this phase is chest decompression, either with a needle or chest tube to vent trapped air. The main indication for chest decompression is clinical evidence of a tension pneumothorax, which can pose a critical threat to both breathing and circulation: decreased to absent breath sounds over the affected side, respiratory distress, hypotension, jugular vein distention, and tracheal deviation. If unrelieved, a tension pneumothorax causes mediastinal shift, cardiovascular collapse, and death. Causes of tension pneumothorax include barotrauma from BVM ventilation or other positive-pressure ventilation, blunt or penetrating chest trauma, and expansion of a simple pneumothorax.

Chest decompression is performed in two ways: needle thoracostomy and tube thoracostomy. **Needle thoracostomy** is a quick, temporary maneuver used in an emergency

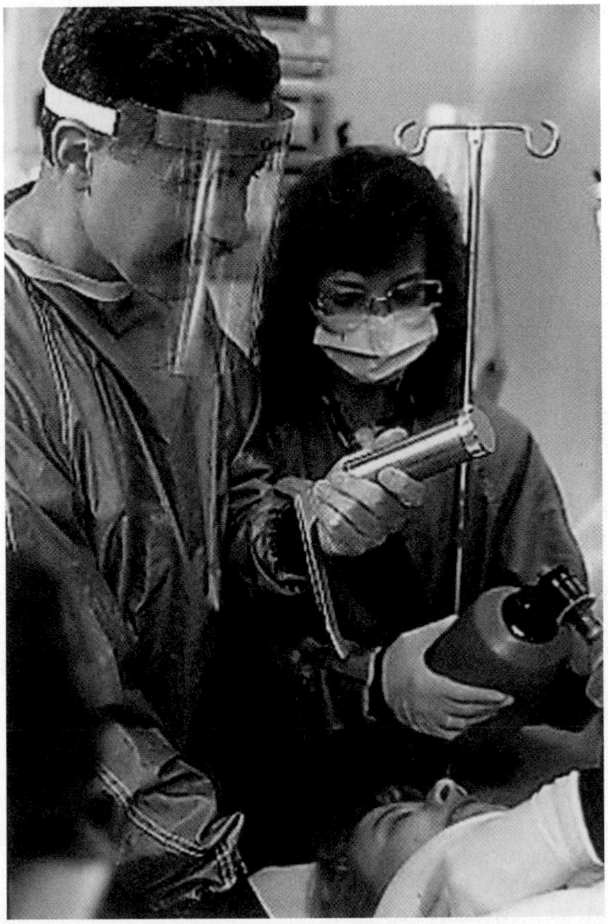

Figure 12-3 ■ Emergency department trauma resuscitation room. Wearing standard precautions attire, trauma team members prepare to intubate the injured client.

to vent trapped air pending chest tube insertion. A large-bore needle (14 or 16 gauge IV catheter, 3 to 6 cm in length) is inserted into the second intercostal space in the midclavicular line; a "rush of air" is expected as the trapped air is expelled from the pleural space under pressure (American College of Surgeons, 1997). Documentation of the air rush out of the catheter confirms the presence of a tension pneumothorax. After needle thoracostomy, a chest tube is inserted **(tube thoracostomy)** in the fifth intercostal space, just anterior to the midaxillary line. Chest tube placement in this anatomic position promotes both air and fluid drainage.

C: CIRCULATION

When effective ventilation is assured, the priority shifts to circulation. The adequacy of heart rate, blood pressure, and overall perfusion become the focus of this element of the primary survey. Common threats to circulation include cardiac arrest, myocardial dysfunction, and hemorrhage leading to a shock state. Interventions are targeted at restoring effective circulation through cardiopulmonary resuscitation, hemorrhage control, intravenous vascular access with fluid and blood administration as necessary, and pharmacologic agents. *External* hemorrhage is best controlled with firm, direct pressure on the bleeding site with thick, dry dressing material. *Internal* hemorrhage is a more covert threat that must be suspected in injured clients or those who present in a shock state.

In a resuscitation situation, blood pressure can be quickly and easily estimated before a manual cuff pressure can be obtained by palpating for the presence or absence of peripheral and central pulses:

- Presence of a radial pulse: BP at least 80 mm Hg systolic
- Presence of a femoral pulse: BP at least 70 mm Hg systolic
- Presence of a carotid pulse: BP at least 60 mm Hg systolic

By the time hypotension occurs, compensatory mechanisms employed by the body in an attempt to maintain vital signs in a shock state have been exhausted. Timely, effective intervention is critical to preserve life and vital organ function.

Intravenous access is best achieved initially with insertion of large-bore peripheral intravenous lines in the antecubital fossae (bend of the elbow). Additional access can be obtained via central veins in the femoral, subclavian, or jugular sites using large-bore ($\geq$8.5 Fr) central venous catheters. Resuscitation solutions of choice are lactated Ringer's and 0.9% normal saline (NS). Fluids and blood products should be warmed before administration to prevent hypothermia. A good rule of thumb is to consider the need for blood product administration in a hemorrhagic shock state when significant hypotension persists after infusion of 2 L of solution.

D: DISABILITY

The disability examination provides a rapid baseline assessment of neurologic status. A simple method to evaluate level of consciousness is the "AVPU" mnemonic:

- A: Alert
- V: Responsive to voice
- P: Responsive to pain
- U: Unresponsive

Another well established means of assessing and documenting level of consciousness that is both objective and widely accepted is the **Glasgow Coma Scale,** which scores eye opening, verbal response, and motor response. The lowest score is 3, which indicates a totally unresponsive client; a normal GCS is 15. Metabolic abnormalities, hypoxia, neurologic injury, and intoxicants can impair level of consciousness. Frequent reassessment is essential to enable rapid intervention in the event of neurologic compromise or deterioration.

E: EXPOSURE

The final component of the primary survey is exposure. All clothing is removed to allow for thorough assessment. In a resuscitation situation, clothing should be cut away to gain rapid access to the body. If evidence preservation is an issue, items should be handled per institutional policy. Evidence may include articles of clothing, impaled objects, weapons, drugs, and bullets. Emergency nurses are often called upon to provide testimony in court regarding their recollections of the presentation and treatment of clients in the ED. Examples of types of cases in which evidence collection is vital include rape, child abuse, domestic violence, homicide, suicide, drug overdose, and assault.

Once clothing is removed, hypothermia (body temperature less than or equal to 36° C) poses a significant risk. In particular, hypothermia complicates management of the injured client by causing vasoconstriction, difficulty with venous access and arterial assessment, impaired oxygenation and ventilation, coagulopathy, increased bleeding, and slowed drug metabolism in the liver (Sedlak, 1995). Interventions to prevent hypothermia are basic: remove wet sheets or clothing, cover the client with blankets, infuse only warm solutions and blood products, set the room temperature at 75° to 80° F, and employ devices such as heat lamps and warming blankets. Table 12-2 highlights the primary survey and associated resuscitation interventions.

The Secondary Survey and Resuscitation Interventions

After the ED resuscitation team addresses the immediate life threats, other activities that the emergency nurse can anticipate include insertion of gastric tubes for decompression of the GI tract to prevent vomiting and aspiration, insertion of a urinary catheter to allow careful measure of urine output, and preparation for diagnostic studies such as bedside ultrasound, 12-lead electrocardiogram (ECG), radiologic studies, and laboratory analysis of blood. The resuscitation team also performs a more comprehensive head-to-toe assessment, known as the **secondary survey,** to identify other injuries or medical issues that need to be managed or that might impact the course of treatment. The client may be transported immediately to the operating room or cardiac catheterization laboratory directly from the ED depending on the nature of the medical problem or injury.

Care of the Emergency Department Client

Most people who come to the ED do not need resuscitation; they come for a variety of reasons. For instance, they are afraid that symptoms they are experiencing may indicate

TABLE 12-2 The Primary Survey and Resuscitation Interventions

Priorities of the Primary Survey	Examples of Specific Interventions
A: Airway/cervical spine	Establish a patent airway by positioning, suctioning, and oxygen, as needed. Protect the cervical spine by maintaining alignment. If the Glasgow Coma Scale (GCS) is ≤8 or the client is at risk for airway compromise, prepare for endotracheal intubation and mechanical ventilation.
B: Breathing	Assess breath sounds and respiratory effort. Observe for chest wall trauma or other physical abnormality. Prepare for chest decompression, if needed.
C: Circulation	Monitor vital signs, especially blood pressure and pulse. Maintain vascular access using a large bore catheter. Use direct pressure for external bleeding.
D: Disability	Evaluate the client's level of consciousness (LOC) using the AVPU system and the GCS. Re-evaluate the client's LOC frequently.
E: Exposure	Remove all clothing for a complete physical assessment. Prevent hypothermia, such as by covering the client with blankets, using heat lamps, and infusing warm solutions.

a very serious condition such as a stroke or heart attack. They have an acute illness, an exacerbation of a chronic illness, or an injury that requires urgent intervention (e.g., asthma, appendicitis, a fracture or laceration). Clients may have nagging problems that they just cannot tolerate until they get an appointment with a primary care physician like a urinary tract infection. Some individuals use the ED as a clinic to meet their episodic health needs in the absence of a primary health care provider.

Because clients have a variety of health care needs in the ED setting, the nursing care needs are highly variable as well. However, certain commonalties for the care of all emergency clients exist. After triage, the emergency nurse assigned to the individual reviews or completes a nursing assessment. Based upon established treatment protocols in some emergency departments (EDs), the nurse may take action when necessary. These interventions may include application of oxygen, cardiac monitoring, intravenous access, and collection of blood or urine specimens, even before the client is seen by a physician.

The client should be undressed to allow for an appropriate examination. Maintaining privacy and dignity, as well as maintaining confidentiality of information, is essential to the ethical provision of nursing care as well as client satisfaction. In a busy ED environment with overcrowding issues, maintaining dignity, privacy, and confidentiality can be challenging, especially when care may sometimes take place on stretchers in the hallway. Keeping voices low when discussing client information, employing alternative areas for clients to undress when no treatment room is available, such as a bathroom or an office with a locking door, and providing two client gowns (one to wear as a robe over the first gown) and a sheet or blanket as a cover are all appropriate strategies. Being creative when confronted with such challenges is a key role expectation of the emergency nurse.

After the physician has evaluated the client, the nurse is responsible for implementing orders. Medication administration, collection of specimens, assistance with bedside procedures such as laceration repair or lumbar puncture, and procuring diagnostic procedures are all in the domain of the emergency nurse. It is the emergency nurse's role to reassess and reprioritize needs whenever necessary, because the client's condition can improve or deteriorate.

Disposition

At the conclusion of the workup, the physician must make a decision regarding client disposition. Should the client be admitted to the hospital or discharged to home with instructions for continued care and follow-up? Usually, the answer is straightforward. A client who has an evolving myocardial infarction, stroke, or acute surgical need will be admitted. Sometimes, though, the ED disposition decision is less clear. Often the emergency nurse and physician discuss this decision collaboratively. The nurse may have a greater sense of how well a client will fare in a home setting depending upon whether or not other family members or friends are available to assist and are reliable. For example, an individual with a minor head injury has suffered a loss of consciousness. Typically, someone is expected to remain with that client for the first 12 to 24 hours after injury to be sure that he does not show any evidence of deterioration. Another common scenario involves the risk to the client in cases of actual or suspected domestic violence or child abuse. If discharge to home is not deemed safe, the client may be admitted to the hospital until resources can be organized to provide for a safe environment. Social workers or case managers are usually consulted to investigate resource needs and to plan accordingly.

Case Management

Some EDs employ registered nurse case managers who can screen ED clients and intervene when necessary to arrange appropriate referral and follow-up. This is a new and evolving role in the ED setting which can be beneficial in the provision of comprehensive care and as a strategy to avoid inappropriate use of resources in an era of profound ED overcrowding.

ED case managers, supported by computer-based information systems, can review the ED census on both a "real-time" as well as on a retrospective basis to determine which clients have visited the ED frequently in a given period of time. The case manager can then determine the reasons why they sought emergency services, such as lack of a primary health care provider, exacerbation of a chronic condition, or lack of health education. Case management interventions include facilitating referrals to primary care providers who are accepting new clients or to subsidized community-based health clinics for individuals or families in need of routine services.

For those with needs related to chronic conditions, the ED case manager can arrange referral into appropriate disease management programs in the community if available (see Chapter 3). Disease management programs are specific to a particular condition such as asthma, COPD, diabetes, hypertension, heart failure, and renal failure. They help clients learn how to properly manage their condition on a day-to-day basis to prevent exacerbations or clinical deterioration. The main goal is to keep the client out of the hospital as long as possible. Health teaching is a key component of these programs. For other health teaching needs, the ED case manager can direct the client to the appropriate educational resources such as a health educator, nutritionist, or organization (e.g., the American Cancer Society, the American Heart Association).

Other functions of the ED case manager might include working with staff to plan disposition for homeless individuals, locating a safe environment for victims of domestic violence or elder abuse, and providing information on community resources for low-cost prescription plans and health insurance.

Client/Family Health Teaching

A key role of the emergency nurse is health teaching. At the most basic level, emergency nurses review discharge instructions with the client and family before signing them out of the department.

CULTURAL CONSIDERATIONS

Most discharge instructions are either preprinted or computer generated, and can be customized to address the individual client's needs. The client's ability to read as well as understand English must be taken into account. Many hospitals have teaching information available in Spanish and other regional languages. However, interpreters may be necessary to assist the health care provider to customize the information appropriately. The emergency nurse may need to demonstrate how to care for a wound, for example, or how to measure the correct dose of a medication. When follow-up is necessary, specific information regarding the timing and type of follow-up must be communicated.

Beyond discharge instructions, the ED environment and community-at-large present many opportunities for health teaching by the nurse. Lassman (2001) asserts that "injury prevention should be an integral part of emergency care" (p. 171) and advocates that emergency nurses are obligated as health care professionals to educate the public about wellness and injury prevention. If the client presented after a motor vehicle crash, for instance, this is an ideal time to reinforce the need to wear seat belts or use child safety seats correctly. ED visits that result from mishaps in the home provide an excellent opportunity to discuss home safety issues, such as the need for smoke detectors and carbon monoxide detectors, and fall prevention tips, such as the need for proper lighting and removal of throw rugs. Safety tips may be based on the developmental stage of children in the home. For example, instructing parents to cover electrical outlets during the toddler years may prevent an electrical injury.

Injury is not the only topic that affords a teaching opportunity. A new onset or an exacerbation of a medical condition also allows for education, such as how to measure blood glucose and ways to control blood pressure or reduce the risk of heart disease.

MASS CASUALTY PRINCIPLES

Mass casualty incidents occur yearly in the United States due to events such as severe weather phenomenon, earthquakes, fire, catastrophic building collapse, and transportation disasters such as plane crashes and train derailments. Emergency preparedness training and drills have been standard functions of EDs and hospitals for many years. The Joint Commission on Accreditation of Health Care Organizations requires that hospitals have an emergency preparedness plan that is tested through drills or actual participation in a real event at least twice yearly, no less than 4 months but no more than 8 months apart. One of these drills or events must involve community-wide resources to assess the efficacy of collaborative efforts and command structures (Joint Commission Resources, 2003).

Even though emergency preparedness is considered a regulatory requirement for hospital accreditation, the degree to which many employees seriously participated in such drills in the past was highly variable. On September 11, 2001, however, the concept of emergency preparedness changed the American way of life and dramatically changed traditional hospital and community disaster planning.

With the catastrophic collapse of the twin towers of the World Trade Center after the terrorist-driven airplanes crashed into them, and the subsequent real and perceived threat of domestic terrorism including anthrax exposure, hospital emergency preparedness concepts became integrated into daily operations of EDs. Suddenly, weapons of mass destruction (WMD) were on the forefront of public health risk to the general population. The term **"NBC"** was coined to refer to nuclear, biologic, and chemical weapons of mass destruction. Hospital ED decontamination facilities and all levels of personal protective gear to protect staff from various types of contaminants are under review and are being upgraded to handle nuclear, chemical, and biologically contaminated clients.

ED physician and nursing staff undergo not only hazardous materials training, but how to recognize patterns of illness in clients who present for treatment that could be indicative of biologic terrorism agents, such as anthrax or smallpox. Protocols for the pharmacologic treatment of infectious disease agents, as well as stockpiles of antibiotics and nerve agent antidotes, are readily available. The most immediate advantage of this intense focus on enhancing emergency preparedness plans is that the ability to competently handle the more typical community mass casualty incident such as a bus crash, tornado, or building collapse has greatly improved in many systems.

Triage

Triage concepts in a mass casualty incident differ from the "civilian triage" covered earlier in this chapter that is practiced during usual ED operations (Table 12-3). In mass casu-

TABLE 12-3 Comparison of Triage Under Usual versus Mass Casualty Operations

Triage Under Usual Conditions	Triage Under Mass Casualty Conditions
Emergent (immediate threat to life)	Emergent or Class I (red tag) (immediate threat to life)
Urgent (major injuries that require immediate treatment)	Urgent or Class II (yellow tag) (major injuries that require immediate treatment)
Nonurgent (minor injuries that do not require immediate treatment)	Nonurgent or Class III (green tag) (minor injuries that do not require immediate treatment)
	Expectant or Class IV (black tag) (expected and allowed to die)

alty or disaster situations, a military form of triage is implemented with the overall goal of doing the greatest good for the greatest number of people (Bracken, 2003). This concept means that clients who are critically ill or injured who might otherwise receive the benefit of an attempted resuscitation during usual operations could be triaged into an "expectant" category and allowed to die. Classic examples of black-tagged clients include those with massive head trauma, extensive full-thickness body burns, and high cervical spinal cord injury requiring mechanical ventilation. The rationale for this seemingly heartless decision is that the limited resources must be dedicated to saving the most lives, rather than expending valuable personnel time, equipment, and supplies to save one life at the possible expense of others.

Triage functions may be performed by emergency medical services (EMS) providers in the field, such as emergency medical technicians (EMTs) and paramedics, nurse and physician field teams who are called from the hospital into a mass casualty scene to assist EMS providers, and nurse and physician hospital teams to assess and reassess incoming clients. Before going to the incident in the field, it is important that nurses and physicians have adequate training to prepare them to recognize risks inherent in an unstable multicasualty environment (e.g., potential for structural collapse; becoming the secondary target of a terrorist attack). They must take measures to protect themselves so that they do not become victims as well.

Mass casualty triage practices can vary in different localities, but some concepts are fairly universal. Most mass casualty teams both in the field and in the hospital setting use a disaster triage tag system that categorizes triage priority by color and number: emergent (class I) clients are identified with a red tag; urgent (class II) clients are marked with a yellow tag; nonurgent (class III) clients are given a green tag; individuals who are expected to die or are dead are issued a black tag (class IV) (Bracken, 2003). In general, red-tagged clients have immediate threats to life such as airway compromise or hemorrhagic shock that require immediate treatment. Yellow-tagged clients have major injuries such as open fractures and large wounds that need treatment within a 30-minute to 2-hour time frame. Green-tagged clients have minor injuries that can be managed in a delayed fashion, generally in more than 2 hours. Examples of minor "green tag" injuries include closed fractures, sprains, strains, contusions, and abrasions.

These green-tagged clients are often referred to as the "walking wounded"; they may actually evacuate themselves from the mass casualty scene and go to the hospital in a private vehicle. Green-tagged clients usually constitute the greatest number in most large-scale multicasualty situations and can overwhelm the system if provisions are not made to handle them as part of the disaster plan. The other issue is that because green-tagged clients may take it upon themselves to come the hospital in their own way, the hospital may not be able to get a sense from the emergency medical providers at the scene just how many actual casualties will arrive at the hospital. A related concern is that green-tagged clients who self-transport may unknowingly carry contaminants from a nuclear, biologic, or chemical incident into the hospital environment with potentially disastrous consequences. ED staff must anticipate these issues and devise emergency response plans accordingly.

A special bracelet with a disaster number is typically applied to each individual in the triage area. Preprinted labels with this specific disaster number can be applied to the client's chart forms and personal belongings; they can even be used as a means to track client movement through the ED (Newberry, 2002). After the client's name has been confirmed, the standard hospital identification bracelet may be used.

Systems Notification/Activation of Emergency Preparedness

A **mass casualty incident** or disaster is commonly defined based on the resource availability of a particular community or hospital facility. When the number of casualties exceeds the resource capabilities, a **disaster** situation is recognized to exist. What may be a routine day in the emergency department (ED) of a large urban trauma center could be defined as a disaster for a small rural community hospital if the same number of clients were to arrive. Each facility, then, must define its own parameters to identify when a disaster situation is present. Flexibility is needed because resources may change by time of day and by day of the week. For instance, hospitals typically have the fewest human resources available after midnight on the weekend. An incident that occurs in this time frame may require activation of the emergency preparedness plan to bring extra resources into the hospital, whereas the same incident during weekday business hours might be handled with on-site personnel alone without activation of the plan.

Notification that a mass casualty situation exists usually occurs by means of radio communication between the ED and EMS providers at the scene. A state or regional emergency management agency may also notify the ED of the event. Each hospital has its own policy that specifies *who* has the authority to activate and *how* to activate the disaster or emergency preparedness plan. Group paging systems, telephone trees, and instant computer-based alert messages constitute the most common means of notifying essential personnel of a mass casualty incident or disaster.

A catastrophic event of great magnitude, such as a devastating earthquake or tornado, or even a terrorist incident involving weapons of mass destruction (WMD) also necessitates volunteer assistance from all levels of health care providers in the region. In this case, the media may be contacted to broadcast messages to the health care community-at-large via television and radio announcements. For such incidents, the National Guard, the American Red Cross, the Public Health Department, various military units, and even a **Disaster Medical Assistance Team (DMAT)** can be activated by state and federal government authorities.

A DMAT is a medical relief team made up of medical, paraprofessional, and support personnel that is deployed to a disaster area with enough medical equipment and supplies to sustain operations for 72 hours (Riley, 2003). DMATs are part of the National Disaster Medical System (NDMS) in the United States and function to provide relief services ranging from primary health care and triage to evacuation and staffing to assist health care facilities that have become overwhelmed with casualties (Riley, 2003). Because licensed health care providers such as nurses act as federal employees when they are deployed, their professional licenses are recognized and valid in all states.

Hospital Emergency Preparedness: Personnel Roles and Responsibilities

The roles and responsibilities of hospital personnel in a mass casualty incident or disaster are defined within the institution's emergency response or preparedness plan (Table 12-4). Each plan can be as individual as the particular hospital's operations. However, virtually all plans identify certain key functions. One of the primary roles to be established at the onset of an incident is the role of a **hospital incident commander** who assumes overall leadership for implementing the institutional plan. This individual is usually either a physician in the ED or a hospital administrator who has the authority to activate resources. The hospital incident commander's role is to take a global view of the entire situation and facilitate client movement through the system as well as bring in both human and supply resources to meet client needs. For example, a hospital incident commander might dictate that all clients due to be discharged from an inpatient unit be moved to a lounge area immediately to free up hospital beds for mass casualty victims. He or she could also direct departments such as physical therapy or a surgical clinic to cancel their usual operations and then convert the space into a minor treatment area to handle numerous "walking wounded" clients. The incident commander assists in the organization of hospital-wide services to rapidly expand hospital capacity, recruit paid or volunteer staff to assume clinical or support assignments, and assure the availability of medical supplies to treat clients.

Another typical role defined in hospital emergency preparedness plans is that of the **medical command physician**. This individual focuses on determining the number, acuity, and medical resource needs of victims arriving from the incident scene to the hospital and organizing the emergency health care team response to the injured or ill clients. Responsibilities include identifying the need for and calling in specialty-trained providers such as the following:

- Trauma surgeons
- Neurosurgeons
- Orthopedic surgeons
- Pulmonologists
- Plastic surgeons
- Burn surgeons
- Infectious disease physicians
- Industrial hygienists
- Radiation safety personnel

In smaller hospitals with limited specialty resources, the medical command physician would also help determine which clients would be transported out of the facility to a higher level of care.

Closely affiliated with the medical command physician is the **triage officer.** Again, this individual is generally a physician in a large hospital who is assisted by triage nurses. When physician resources are limited, a nurse may assume this role. The triage officer rapidly evaluates each individual who presents to the hospital, even those who come in with triage tags in place. Client acuity is re-evaluated for appropriate disposition to the area within the ED or hospital best suited to meet the client's medical needs.

The ED charge nurse, trauma program manager, and other ED nursing leadership personnel act in close collaboration with the medical command physician and triage officer to organize nursing and ancillary services to meet client needs. Telephone trees can be activated to call in off-duty emergency nurses. Nurses from medical-surgical nursing units can be recruited to provide care for stable ED clients, thus freeing up emergency nurses to aid mass casualty victims. Critical care unit nurses can supplement emergency nurses in the resuscitation setting or assist in monitored care and transport to critical care units. Emergency nurse leaders also typically direct the ancillary departments to deliver supplies, instrument trays, medications, food, and personnel to meet service demands.

Many other roles and responsibilities can be defined within the institutional emergency response plan, and may include the supply officer, the communications officer, the infection control officer, and the community relations/public information officer, to name a few. The community

TABLE 12-4 Key Personnel Roles and Functions for Emergency Preparedness and Response Plan

Personnel Role	Personnel Function
Hospital incident commander	Physician or administrator who assumes overall leadership for implementing the emergency plan
Medical command physician	Physician who decides the number, acuity, and resource needs of clients
Triage officer	Physician or nurse who rapidly evaluates each client to determine priorities for treatment
Community relations or public information officer	Person who serves as a liaison between the medical center and media

relations or public information officer is an especially important role to delineate in advance because mass casualty incidents tend to attract a large amount of media attention. This staff member can draw media away from the clinical areas so that essential hospital operations are not hindered. He or she can also serve as the liaison between hospital administration and the media to release only appropriate and accurate information.

Hospital staff of all levels may be required to alter their routine operations to accommodate a high volume of clients. Some plans dictate specific actions by staff members, such as who should be called when the plan is activated, who should report, where to report, what supplies or equipment carts should be brought to a predesignated location, and what type of paperwork or system should be implemented for client identification in a large-scale event. Some staff may even have their roles changed completely, for example, nurses who work in other departments, such as the performance improvement department or case management, may be reassigned to fulfill a clinical responsibility for staffing of a nursing unit. The key concept is that staff members are expected to remain flexible in a mass casualty situation and perform at their highest level to address both the needs of the health care system and those of the clients. The greatest good for the greatest number of people is still the organizing principle when considering roles and responsibilities in mass casualty events, not necessarily individual staff preferences.

Event Resolution

When the last major casualties have been treated and no more are anticipated to arrive in numbers that could overwhelm the health care system, it is time for the incident commander to consider "standing down" or deactivating the emergency response plan. However, although the casualties may have left the ED, other areas in the hospital may still be under great stress and need the support of the supplemental resources brought in by emergency plan activation. Before terminating the response, it is essential to assure that the needs of the other hospital departments have been met and all are in agreement to resume normal operations.

A key consideration in event resolution is staff and supply availability. If nursing staff and other personnel were called in from home during their off hours, or if they worked well beyond their scheduled shifts to meet client and departmental needs, some provision for an adequate rest period should be made. Exhaustion poses a risk not only to client safety but also to the emergency nurse when he or she must drive home. Sleeping quarters at the hospital might be necessary in this case, especially if the disaster event contributed to treacherous travel conditions.

Creativity and flexibility of nursing leaders and emergency nursing staff come together to provide staffing coverage of the ED. A personal emergency preparedness plan for each emergency nurse can help in such situations. It should consist of the preplanned specific arrangements that are to be made for child care, pet care, and elder care if the need arises and the emergency nurse is unable to return home for an extended period of time. Emergency contact names, addresses, and telephone numbers should be included for optimal usefulness in a crisis.

Severe shortages of supplies also pose a threat to normal operations at the conclusion of a mass casualty incident. Taking inventory and restocking the ED are high priority assignments. Close collaboration between the ED and the central supply department are essential to resolving stock availability problems. Instrument trays must be washed, packaged, and resterilized. Critical supplies that have been depleted from hospital stores must be reordered and delivered to the hospital quickly. Contracts with key vendors outlining emergency resupply expectations and arrangements should be a part of the hospital's overall emergency preparedness plan.

Debriefing

CRITICAL INCIDENT STRESS DEBRIEFING

There are two general types of **debriefing** that occur after a mass casualty incident or disaster. The first type of debriefing entails bringing in critical incident stress debriefing (CISD) teams to provide sessions for small groups of staff to promote effective coping strategies. The second type of debriefing involves an administrative review of staff and system performance during the event to determine whether or not opportunities for improvement in the emergency management plan exist.

The concept of CISD began in 1983 as a crisis stress management intervention to decrease the effects of traumatic events and facilitate recovery of high-risk workers such as emergency medical personnel, firefighters, and police officers (Mitchell, Sakraida & Kameg, 2003). CISD is now only one component of a much broader **Critical Incident Stress Management (CISM)** program. CISM programming addresses precrisis through postcrisis interventions for small to large groups, including communities (Everly & Mitchell, 1999). After working through the turmoil and the emotional impact of the incident as well as the aftermath, emergency staff may find it difficult to "get back to normal." Without intervention, staff may develop **post-traumatic stress disorder (PTSD),** which can lead to multiple characteristic psychological and physical effects: flashbacks, avoidance, diminished interest in previously enjoyable events, detachment, and physical manifestations including rapid heart rate, insomnia, and other physiologic effects of anxiety (Mitchell, Kameg & Sakraida, 2003). Individuals suffering from PTSD can have great difficulty relating in their usual way to family and friends. Ultimately, professional "burnout" can stem from the inability to cope with the stress effectively.

A CISD team is comprised of two to three specially trained individuals who come together quickly when called to deal with the emotional needs of health team members after a particularly devastating or disturbing incident. The CISD team leader typically has background in a mental health/behavioral health field; the co-leader is ideally a peer of the group being debriefed (Mitchell, Sakraida & Kameg, 2003). Thus if nurses are to be debriefed, then a nurse member of the CISD team is generally assigned to the session. CISD-trained physicians, police, firefighters, EMTs, and paramedics may also be used depending on the needs of the group. The third member of the team is known as the "doorkeeper" and is responsible for keeping inappropriate individuals out (e.g., media, spectators) and talking with anyone who leaves the session early in an effort to have them return or accept follow-up (Mitchell, Sakraida & Kameg, 2003). Staff involved in the incident need protected time to undergo stress debriefing, which generally lasts from 1 to 3 hours per session.

Typical "ground rules" for stress debriefing include strict confidentiality of information shared during the session and unconditional acceptance of the thoughts and feelings expressed by individuals within the group. The usual arrangement for the most effective group interaction consists of a circular configuration of chairs in a private setting. Food should be available so that hunger is not a distraction. CISD group leaders encourage group discussion through asking a series of questions designed to make everyone involved tell his or her own story about the incident and explain the personal impact. The group leaders enable participants to place the incident into perspective and dispel any feelings of blame or guilt. They also educate participants about self-care concepts and coping strategies to use immediately. Individuals who require more than a CISD session may need referral for mental health/behavioral health counseling. Evidence-based research efforts using meta-analysis techniques have produced mixed results regarding the efficacy of CISD; however, the technique is perceived to be clinically effective (Mitchell, Sakraida & Kameg, 2003).

ADMINISTRATIVE REVIEW

The second type of debriefing is an administrative function directed at analyzing the hospital's response to the event while it is still in the forefront of the minds of everyone who participated in it. The goal of this type of debriefing is to discern what went right and what went wrong during activation and implementation of the emergency preparedness plan so that changes can be made. Typically, representatives from all departments that were involved in the incident come together soon after plan activation has been discontinued. They each are given an opportunity to hear and express both positive and negative comments related to their experiences with the event. Although drills are important, implementing the emergency preparedness plan during an actual mass casualty event is the most effective means of "reality testing" the plan's utility. Information gleaned from participants can be used to modify or revise the plan in preparation for future events. Lessons learned serve as the best catalyst for improvements in the overall system of disaster management.

EMERGENCY DEPARTMENT CASE SCENARIO: POSSIBLE ANTHRAX EXPOSURE

Case Presentation

M.C., a 34-year-old woman, presents to the triage desk of a large suburban emergency department (ED) bearing a box with a dusting of white powder on it. M.C. quickly explains to the triage nurse that she is afraid an employee at her office has contaminated the box with anthrax. She exhibits signs of severe anxiety while she relates that this employee was born in an Arab country and obviously "hates America." Nearly sobbing now, she expresses her fears that she has been deliberately exposed to anthrax by a terrorist and needs treatment.

The triage nurse immediately notifies security and escorts the client outside of the building. The client is confused and angry as to why she cannot be placed in a treatment room. She wants the substance on the box tested to determine if it is indeed anthrax. The emergency nurse instructs M.C. to place the box on the ground in a grassy area outside of the ED. She then asks that the security guard establish a safe perimeter around the box and place calls to both the local law enforcement agency as well as the Department of Public Health. The agency will take possession of the box, investigate the woman's claim, and engage in appropriate testing of the white powder.

In the meantime, the emergency nurse also activates the ED's hazardous materials decontamination plan. Nursing staff don appropriate protective attire which includes an impervious gown, gloves, face mask, and eye protection, and prepare the decontamination facility (Figure 12-4). When ready to begin decontamination, M.C. is directed to enter the decontamination room through the outside door from the parking lot to avoid the potential for contamination of the ED. Staff assist M.C. to remove all of her clothing. She is directed into a shower stall and washed thoroughly with soap and water. When decontamination is complete, she is given a hospital gown, robe, and slippers, and is placed in a wheelchair for transport to an ED treatment room in the "fast track" area for low acuity clients.

Upon arrival to the treatment room, M.C. appears much less anxious. A physician examines her and determines that she has no clinical evidence of infectious disease. For this reason, and because an actual exposure to anthrax has not yet been confirmed by the Public Health Department, the physician elects *not* to prescribe the typical 60-day course of a prophylactic antibiotic for *Bacillus anthracis* such as doxycycline or ciprofloxacin (Cipro). The emergency physician explains that her plan is to discharge the client to home with referral for outpatient follow-up at the Public Health Department. M.C. again becomes tearful and demands that she be given a prescription for an antibiotic because she is afraid she will die. She contends that she will sue the hospital if anything should happen to her.

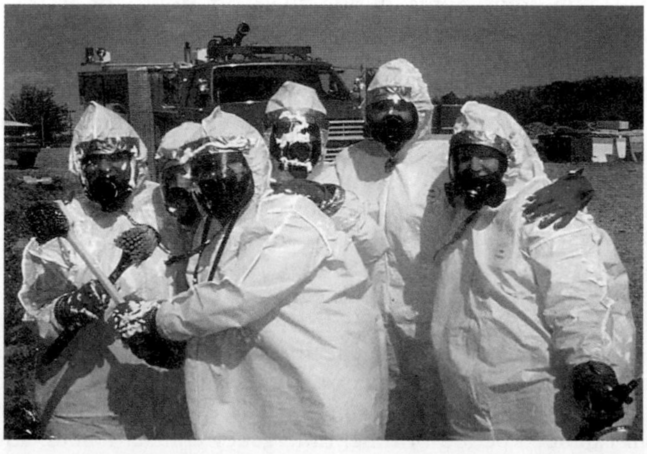

Figure 12-4 ■ Hazardous materials team members wearing protective clothing and respirators prepare to decontaminate individuals exposed to toxic chemicals in an outdoor decontamination area.

The emergency physician and nurse actively engage MC in discharge teaching about anthrax. With compassion and empathy, they explain that taking antibiotics unnecessarily will promote the growth of resistant bacteria and may cause serious drug-related side effects. They tell M.C. that the Department of Public Health will analyze the substance on the box, and if it is found to be *B. anthracis*, she will be notified right away. She will then be re-evaluated by the Public Health Department and started on appropriate postexposure prophylactic antibiotics. M.C. is reassured and offered the services of a community mental health/behavioral health clinic if she desires counseling to address her anxiety about this situation as well as her perceived threat from the Arab employee at her work site. After this teaching episode, M.C. appears to have her anxiety and anger under control. Because M.C.'s own clothing was confiscated and placed in a hazardous materials container for disposal during the decontamination process, the emergency nurse contacts the social worker to request that female apparel be made available from the hospital's supply of donated clothing so that she can get dressed. The client is given written discharge instructions.

Case Discussion

Although it may seem odd that the emergency nurse escorted M.C. outside of the building, this action prevented the potential spread of *B. anthracis* into the ED and potentially the hospital environment. Contamination of innocent bystanders as well as the hospital environment with a hazardous material can force the closure of key areas within the facility and can necessitate evacuation of clients and staff. Because M.C. was a "walk-in" client, she accessed the triage area before undergoing decontamination. Had M.C. been a known potentially contaminated client before arrival (e.g., if she was treated by an ambulance crew), she would have been taken to the decontamination facility upon arrival. Decontamination should precede triage; only the most basic life-sustaining interventions should be performed before or during decontamination (Newberry, 2002). M.C. also brought a potentially contaminated item into the ED. It is important to realize that the ED has no ability to conduct "point of care" testing to determine whether the unknown white powder substance was actually *B. anthracis*, the bacterium responsible for causing anthrax infection. Such testing is the domain of the Public Health Department.

Local, state, and federal law enforcement agencies also must become involved in the overall investigation of an actual or potential bioterrorism event so that the suspected perpetrators can be apprehended, even in the event of a hoax or practical joke. Hoaxes are not taken lightly by law enforcement in this era of heightened terrorist awareness. The practical jokers may find themselves prosecuted as criminals and serving prison time for their actions. More common, however, are the panicked reactions from innocent people like M.C. who come to the ED believing that they have suffered an exposure to a bioterrorism agent.

M.C. was sent into the decontamination room through an outside door. Most ED decontamination facilities have both outside and inside doors. The client enters from the outside, is decontaminated, and is then transported into the ED. Containment tanks to collect wastewater run-off from the decontamination process and separate air handling systems are typical components of new facility designs. Potentially contaminated clothing is removed from the victim and destroyed.

According to Centers for Disease Control and Prevention (2001) guidelines, unless the client exhibits clinical evidence of disease, or the substance under question tests positive for *B. anthracis*, antibiotics are not indicated. Anthrax can manifest disease in three forms: cutaneous, gastrointestinal, and inhalational or pulmonary. Cutaneous anthrax is caused by direct contact with *B. anthracis*. It presents as a pruritic papular lesion that turns into a vesicle, which, in 2 to 6 days, becomes a lesion with depressed black eschar; this form of anthrax is generally nonfatal if treated with antibiotics (CDC, 2001). Gastrointestinal anthrax is caused by ingestion of contaminated food and is characterized by abdominal pain, nausea, vomiting (hematemesis), fever, bloody diarrhea, and sepsis in late stages. There is a high mortality rate, especially after the client exhibits sepsis. Pulmonary or inhalational anthrax stems from inhalation of anthrax spores. This illness begins as a flu-like syndrome with fever and drenching sweats that progresses rapidly to respiratory failure. Classic radiographic evidence consists of a widened mediastinum and pleural effusions on a chest radiograph; these findings may not appear until later in the course of illness (CDC, 2002). Unless treatment is instituted very early in the prodromal stage, mortality rates are exceptionally high.

Once in the fast track setting in this case scenario, attention was directed at reducing the anxiety level of the client and providing effective health teaching. The psychosocial harm that occurs with actual or potential victims of bioterrorism events cannot be underestimated. When large groups of individuals are involved in a potential exposure, there is great potential for hysteria to occur. Effective interventions include calmly providing factual information about the potential threat and offering follow-up with both public health and mental health/behavioral health professionals as needed to address both physical and mental health/behavioral health issues.

GET READY for the NCLEX Examination!

KEY POINTS

- Emergency departments (EDs) are fast-paced and overcrowded environments that process clients across the life span with a variety of health problems.
- The most common reasons that clients seek ED care include chest pain, abdominal pain, headache, and fever.
- The interdisciplinary ED team includes prehospital providers, physicians, nurses, and support (ancillary) staff.
- Use the best practices listed in Chart 12-1 to maintain safety in the ED.
- Core competencies for the ED nurse include assessment, priority setting/critical thinking, knowledge of the ED, technical skills, and communication.
- The most commonly used triage system used under usual conditions is the three-level model: emergent, urgent, and nonurgent.
- Implement the steps of the primary survey and resuscitation interventions outlined in Table 12-2.
- Client education as part of the discharge plan is an important part of ED nursing practice.

- All medical centers must have an emergency preparedness and response team in case of mass casualty.
- The typical triage system for a mass casualty situation includes an additional category for those clients allowed to die (black-tagged).
- Special roles are assigned in a mass casualty incident as identified in Table 12-4.
- In a situation wherein exposure to a biologic agent is suspected, the decontamination team wears special, protective gear and decontaminates the clients who were exposed. Those clients are separated from others in the ED.

ADDITIONAL STUDY RESOURCES

Go to your Student CD-ROM for Review Questions for the NCLEX Examination.

evolve Go to http://evolve.elsevier.com/Iggy/ for Integrated Management of Care Questions for the NCLEX Examination.

SELECTED BIBLIOGRAPHY

Asterisk indicates a classic or definitive work on this subject.

American Academy of Pediatrics & American Heart Association. (2002). *PALS provider manual.* Dallas: American Heart Association.

*American College of Surgeons Committee on Trauma. (1997). *Advanced trauma life support course for physicians student manual* (6th ed.). Chicago: Author.

Bitterman, R. (2000). Overview of hospital and physician responsibilities mandated by EMTALA, In R. Bitterman (Ed.), *Providing emergency care under federal law: EMTALA.* (pp. 15-22). Dallas: American College of Emergency Physicians.

Bracken, J. (2003). Triage. In L. Newberry (Ed.), *Sheehy's emergency nursing principles and practice* (5th ed., pp. 75-83). St. Louis: Mosby.

Case, J., Mowery, M., & Welebob, E. (2002*). The nursing shortage: Can technology help?* Oakland, CA: California Healthcare Foundation.

Centers for Disease Control and Prevention. (2001). Update: Investigation of bioterrorism-related anthrax and interim guidelines for clinical evaluation of persons with possible anthrax. November 02, 2001. *MMWR* 2001, *50*, 941-948. Retrieved September 11, 2003, from http://www.cdc.gov/mmwr/preview/mmwrhtml/mm5043al.htm.

Centers for Disease Control and Prevention. (2002). Clinical issues in the prophylaxis, diagnosis, and treatment of anthrax. *Emerging Infectious Diseases*, *8*(2). Retrieved September 11, 2003, from http://www.cdc.gov/ncidod/EID/vol8no2/01-0521.htm.

*Craig, P.A. (1998). Risk management issues in the emergency department. In B.J. Youngberg (Ed.). *The risk manager's desk reference.* (pp. 1-24). New York: Aspen.

Cummins, R.O. (Ed.). (2003). *ACLS: Principles and practice.* Dallas: American Heart Association.

*Dame, L.A. (1998). The Emergency Medical Treatment and Active Labor Act: The anomalous right to health care. *Health Matrix: Journal of Law Medicine*, *8*, 1.

*Eckle, N., Haley, K., & Baker, P. (Eds.). (1998). *ENPC provider manual* (2nd ed.). Park Ridge, IL: Emergency Nurses Association.

*Emergency Medical Treatment and Active Labor Act, 42 U.S.C.SS 1395dd. (1996).

Emergency Nurses Association. (2000a). *Emergency nursing core curriculum* (5th ed.). Philadelphia: W.B. Saunders.

Emergency Nurses Association. (2000b). *Orientation to emergency nursing: Concepts, competencies & critical thinking* (2nd ed.). Des Plaines, IL: Author.

Emergency Nurses Association. (2000c). *Trauma nursing core course provider manual* (5th ed.). Park Ridge, IL: Author.

Emergency Nurses Association. (2001). *Standards of emergency nursing practice* (4th ed.). Des Plaines, IL: Author.

Emergency Nurses Association. (2002). *Emergency Nurses Association position statements: Stress management strategies.* Retrieved September 23, 2003, from http://www.ena.org/about/position/stressmanagement.asp.

*Everly, G.S., & Mitchell, J.T. (1999). *Critical incident stress management (CISM): A new era and standard of care in crisis intervention.* Ellicott City, MD: Chevron Publishing.

Gilboy, N. (2003). The evolution of triage. In N. Gilboy, et al. (Eds.). *The Emergency Severity Index: Implementation handbook.* (pp. 2-5). Des Plaines, IL: Emergency Nurses Association.

Gilboy, N., et al. (Eds.) (2003). *The Emergency Severity Index: Implementation handbook.* Des Plaines, IL: Emergency Nurses Association.

Gurney, D. (2002). Developing a successful 16-week "Transition ED Nursing" program: One busy community hospital's experience. *Journal of Emergency Nursing, 28*, 505-514.

Heinrich, J. (2001, June 22). EMTALA implementation and enforcement issues. *FDCH Government Account Reports*, Retrieved February 10, 2002, from http://ehostvgw12.epnet.com.

*Hyman, D. (1998). Patient dumping and EMTALA: Past imperfect/future shock. *Health Matrix: Journal of Law Medicine*, *8*, 29-57.

Joint Commission Resources. (2003). *Accreditation issues for emergency departments.* Oakbrook Terrace, IL: Joint Commission on Accreditation of Health Care Organizations.

Kamoie, B. (2000). EMTALA: Reading beyond the emergency room to expand hospital liability. *Journal of Health Law, 33*, 25-55.

Kelly, L.Y. & Joel, L. A. (2001). *The nursing experience: Trends, challenges, and transitions* (4th ed.). New York: McGraw-Hill.

Keough, V.A., Schlomer, R.S., & Bollenberg, B.W. (2003). Serendipitous findings from an Illinois ED nursing educational survey reflect a crisis in emergency nursing. *Journal of Emergency Nursing, 29*, 17-22.

Lassman, J. (2001). Teachable moments: A paradigm shift. *Journal of Emergency Nursing, 27*, 171-175.

Litvak, E., et al. (2001). Emergency department diversion: Causes and solutions. *Academic Emergency Medicine, 8*, 1108-1110.

*Mayer, T.A., & Zimmerman, P.G. (1999). ED customer satisfaction survival skills: One hospital's experience. *Journal of Emergency Nursing, 25*, 187-191.

McCaig, L.F., & Burt, C.W. (2003). National hospital ambulatory medical care survey: 2001 emergency department summary. *Advance Data from Vital Health Statistics, 335,* Hyattsville, MD: National Center for Health Statistics.

McCaig, L. F. & Ly, N. (2002). National hospital ambulatory medical care survey: 2000 emergency department summary. *Advance Data from Vital Health Statistics, 326,* Hyattsville, MD: National Center for Health Statistics.

Mitchell, A.M., Kameg, K., & Sakraida, T.J. (2003). Post-traumatic stress: Clinical implications. *Disaster Management & Response*, *1*(1), 14-18.

Mitchell, A.M., Sakraida, T.J., & Kameg, K. (2003). Critical incident stress debriefing: Implications for best practice. *Disaster Management & Response*, *1*(2), 46-51.

Newberry, L. (2002). Practical suggestions for helping emergency nurses handle mass casualties. *Disaster Management & Response, Premier Issue*, 15-17.

Riley, J.M. (2003). Providing nursing care with federal disaster-relief teams. *Disaster Management & Response*, *1*(3), 76-79.

*Sedlak, S.K. (1995). Hypothermia in trauma: The nurse's role in recognition, prevention, and management. *International Journal of Trauma Nursing*, *1*(1), 19-26.

Travers, D. (2003). Triage acuity systems. In N. Gilboy, et al. (Eds.). *The emergency severity index: Implementation handbook.* (pp. 6-11). Des Plaines, IL: Emergency Nurses Association.

Travers, D.A., et al. (2002). Five-level triage system more effective than three-level in tertiary emergency department. *Journal of Emergency Nursing, 28*, 395-400.

Twedell, D.M. (2000). Nursing process: Assessment and priority setting. In Emergency Nurses Association. *Emergency nursing core curriculum* (5th ed.). Philadelphia: W.B. Saunders.

CHAPTER 13

Interventions for Clients with Common Environmental Emergencies

LINDA LASKOWSKI-JONES

LEARNING OUTCOMES

After studying this chapter, you should be able to:

1. Assess clients for common types of heat-related injuries.
2. Teach clients how to prevent heat-related injuries.
3. Prioritize first aid interventions for clients who have heat-related injuries.
4. Prioritize first aid interventions for clients experiencing snakebites.
5. Differentiate care for clients who have arthropod bites and stings.
6. Develop a plan of care for a client who is allergic to bees and experiences a bee sting.
7. Teach clients how to prevent arthropod bites and stings.
8. Prioritize care for clients who have been struck by lightning.
9. Teach clients how to avoid cold injuries.
10. Explain the rationale for interventions when warming clients who have cold injuries.
11. Describe best practices for clients who are at risk for or experience altitude-related illnesses.
12. Develop a plan of care for a client with near-drowning.

Go to your Student CD-ROM for Review Questions for the NCLEX Examination keyed to these Learning Outcomes.

Recreational pursuits as well as home and work responsibilities summon people of all ages to leave the shelter of their homes for the great outdoors. Seemingly harmless outside activities can have associated environmental risks. Some of these hazards, such as insect bites or stings, reptile bites, and environmental conditions, may also pose threats indoors. This chapter gives an overview of selected environmental emergencies and presents management concepts to address immediate emergency care needs as well as acute care interventions for these hazards. Common sense illness and injury prevention strategies for nurses to incorporate into their own lifestyle and health teaching opportunities are also discussed. The information contained in this chapter is pertinent to everyone who has close encounters with the summer and winter elements, whether driving to work or taking part in an adventure sport.

HEAT-RELATED ILLNESSES

There are several notable predisposing environmental and physical factors associated with heat-related illnesses. High environmental temperature (>95° F) and high humidity (>80%) constitute the most common environmental factors. Physical factors range from extremes of age to a client's current health status. For example, dehydration, fatigue, lack of sleep, obesity, heart disease, fever, strenuous exercise, seizures, and all degrees of burns (even sunburn) cause individuals to become more susceptible to heat stress. In addition, the use of drugs such as anticholinergic agents, beta-adrenergic blockers, angiotensin-converting enzyme (ACE) inhibitors, diuretics, cocaine, and amphetamines also increases the risk of heat-related illness (Auerbach, Donner, & Weiss, 2003). Before participating in any hot weather activity, clients at risk should be taught to consider these risk factors and take the necessary steps to eliminate or minimize them whenever possible.

HEALTH PROMOTION/ILLNESS PREVENTION

Chart 13-1 lists heat-related illness prevention strategies. These strategies are important to incorporate into health teaching opportunities with clients who participate in warm weather activities, as well as those with health risk factors that may predispose them to heat-related illness.

Heat Exhaustion

PATHOPHYSIOLOGY

Heat exhaustion is a syndrome primarily caused by dehydration. It stems from heavy perspiration as well as inadequate fluid and electrolyte consumption during heat exposure over hours to days. Clients complain of feeling quite ill, and their clinical presentation resembles having the flu. Although not considered a true emergency condition, if untreated, heat exhaustion can be a precursor to heat stroke.

COLLABORATIVE MANAGEMENT

In heat exhaustion, clients have a normal mental status in the presence of a flu-like syndrome with headache, weakness, fatigue, anorexia, nausea, and vomiting. The client should be assessed for orthostatic hypotension and tachycardia. It is important to note that the client's body temperature is *not* significantly elevated in this condition. He or she may continue to perspire despite the effects of dehydration.

Treatment consists of immediately terminating physical activity and moving the individual to a cool place. Constrictive clothing should be removed. An oral rehydrating solution such as a sports drink should be provided. Salt tablets should never be given without first crushing and dissolving them in adequate quantities of water–salt tablets alone cause stomach irritation, nausea, and vomiting. Effective cooling measures consist of placing cold packs on the neck, chest, abdomen, and groin; soaking the person in cool water; or fanning the individual while spraying water on the skin (Auerbach, Donner, & Weiss, 2003). If the characteristic signs and symptoms persist, an ambulance should be called to transport the client to the hospital.

CHART 13-1

CLIENT EDUCATION GUIDE
Heat-Related Illness Prevention

- Ensure adequate intake of nutritious foods and fluids such as commercially available sports bars and drinks that contain carbohydrates, sodium, and other essential electrolytes before, during, and after exercise.
- Prevent overexposure to the sun; use a sunscreen with an SPF of at least 30.
- Take time to get used to the heat by gradually increasing time spent working or playing in a hot environment.
- Rest frequently when working in a hot environment. Plan to limit activity at the hottest time of day.
- Wear clothing suited to the environment. Lightweight, light-colored, and loose-fitting clothing is best.
- Pay attention to your personal physical limitations; modify activities accordingly.

In the clinical setting, vital sign assessment and temperature monitoring are necessary. The client is typically rehydrated with intravenous (IV) 0.9% saline solution if nausea or vomiting is present. Blood is drawn for serum electrolyte analysis. Hospital admission is typically indicated for clients with significant comorbid conditions that have been worsened by the heat-related illness or for those with unresolved signs and symptoms after a period of treatment and observation.

Heat Stroke

PATHOPHYSIOLOGY

Heat stroke is a true medical emergency with a mortality rate that can approach 80% for individuals not effectively treated in a timely manner (Auerbach, Donner, & Weiss, 2003). The victim's heat regulatory mechanisms fail and are unable to compensate for a critical elevation in body temperature, which may exceed 105° F (40.5° C). If uncorrected, organ dysfunction and death will ensue.

Two types of heat stroke are (1) exertional and (2) classic. **Exertional heat stroke** has a sudden onset and is typically due to strenuous physical activity in hot, humid conditions. Lack of proper acclimatization to the hot weather and wearing clothing too heavy for the environment are common contributing factors. Conversely, **classic heat stroke** occurs over a period of time as a result of chronic exposure to a hot, humid environment, such as a home without air-conditioning in the high heat of the summer. It generally affects ill and older adults. The body's ability to dissipate heat effectively is significantly impaired in this disorder. All of the risk factors for heat-related illness previously described play an important role in the incidence of heat stroke.

COLLABORATIVE MANAGEMENT

Assessment

Victims of heat stroke have a profoundly elevated body temperature (>105° F or 40.5° C). This disorder is also characterized by mental status changes, which occur as a result of thermal injury to the brain. Typical mental status changes are evidenced by the appearance of anxiety, confusion, bizarre behavior, loss of coordination, hallucinations, agitation, seizures, and coma. Vital sign abnormalities may include hypotension, tachycardia, and tachypnea. Although the client's skin is classically described as hot and dry, the presence of sweating does *not* rule out heat stroke–persons may continue to perspire in this state.

Dematte et al. (1998) studied the sequelae of near-fatal classic heat stroke in 58 clients admitted to a Chicago intensive care unit during a sustained heat wave. They found that multiorgan dysfunction with neurologic impairment developed in 100% of these clients. Approximately one-half had moderate to severe renal insufficiency and disseminated intravascular coagulation (DIC), and 10% experienced acute respiratory distress syndrome. The in-hospital mortality rate was 21% for this group. Related complications that have been widely reported include electrolyte and acid-base disturbances, rhabdomyolysis, cerebral edema, and cerebral hemorrhage.

Interventions

Heat stroke must be recognized and treated immediately and aggressively for optimal client outcome (Chart 13-2).

FIRST AID. In the prehospital setting, rapid cooling is the first priority of care after ensuring a patent airway. According to Auerbach, Donner, and Weiss (2003), the faster the cooling, the lower the morbidity and mortality rates of heat stroke. Methods for rapidly cooling the client include the following:

- Stripping away clothing
- Placing ice packs on the neck, axillae, chest, and groin
- Immersing the victim in cold water
- Wetting the client's body with tepid water and then fanning rapidly to aid in cooling by evaporation.

Immersion in ice is contraindicated because shivering generates additional body heat and increases oxygen consumption. No food or liquid should be given by mouth because vomiting and aspiration are risks in the presence of neurologic impairment. Immediate medical care is essential. An ambulance with advanced life support capabilities should be summoned as soon as possible.

HOSPITAL CARE. Once in a clinical setting, monitor and support the client's airway and circulatory status. Initiation of high concentration oxygen therapy and IV lines with 0.9% saline solution are indicated. Ringer's lactate solution should be avoided because the liver may be unable to metabolize lactate effectively while the client is hyperthermic (Morris, 2003). Aggressive interventions to cool the client must continue until rectal temperature is 102° F or less. Methods include using cooling blankets and applying iced gastric and peritoneal lavage (Morris, 2003). Use a continuous temperature monitoring device, such as a rectal probe or temperature monitoring urinary bladder catheter, to prevent overcorrection of the desired body temperature and hypothermia. If shivering occurs during the cooling process, chlorpromazine (Thorazine) 25 to 50 mg IM or IV may be prescribed.

Seizures pose a serious problem because seizure activity further elevates body temperature. Be sure that a benzodiazepine such as diazepam is immediately available for IV administration. Admission to a critical care unit for continued support and hemodynamic monitoring is usually indicated because complication and mortality rates for heat stroke are high.

CHART 13-2

BEST PRACTICE for
Emergency Care of the Client with Heatstroke

EMERGENCY CARE

At the Scene

- Ensure a patent airway.
- Remove the client from the hot environment (into air-conditioning or into the shade).
- Remove the client's clothing.
- Pour or spray water on the client's body and scalp.
- Fan the client (not only the person providing care, but all surrounding people should fan the client with newspapers or whatever is available).
- If ice is available, place ice in cloth or bags and position the packs on the client's scalp, in the groin area, under the neck, and in the armpits.
- Get the client to the nearest emergency department.

At the Hospital

- Give oxygen by mask or nasal cannula.
- Start at least one IV with a large-bore needle or cannula.
- Administer normal saline (0.9% sodium chloride) as rapidly as possible, using cooled solutions if available.
- Use a cooling blanket.
- **Do not give aspirin or any other antipyretics.**
- Insert a rectal probe to measure core body temperature continuously or use a rectal thermometer and assess temperature every 15 minutes.
- Insert a Foley catheter.
- Monitor vital signs at least every 15 minutes.
- Obtain the following laboratory tests as quickly as possible: serum electrolytes, cardiac enzymes, liver enzymes, and complete blood count (CBC).
- Assess arterial blood gases.
- Administer muscle relaxants (benzodiazepines) if the client begins to shiver.
- Measure urine output and specific gravity to determine fluid needs.
- Slow cooling interventions when core body temperature is reduced to 102° F (38.8° C).

SNAKEBITES

More often than not, people have a fear of snakes. Although most snake species are nonvenomous and harmless, there are one or more species of poisonous snakes found in every U.S. state except Maine, Alaska, and Hawaii. The two families of indigenous poisonous snakes in North America are the Crotalidae and the Elapidae.

The Crotalidae are the "pit vipers," named for the characteristic depression between each eye and nostril that serves as a heat-sensitive organ for locating warm-blooded prey. They include various species of rattlesnakes, copperheads, and water moccasins (also known as "cottonmouths") and account for the vast majority of the poisonous snakebites in the United States (Figures 13-1 and 13-2).

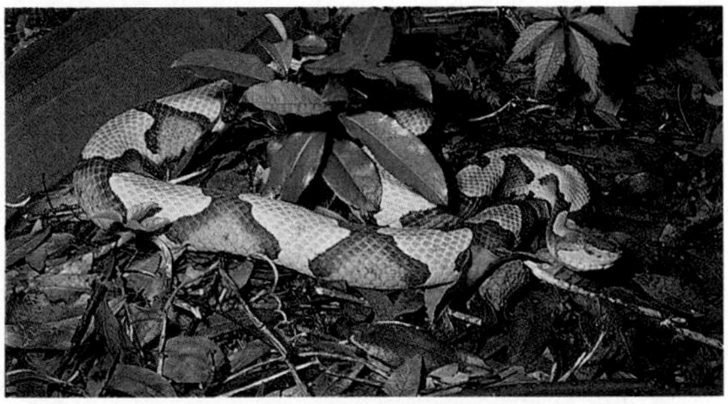

Figure 13-1 ■ Southern copperhead *(Agkistrodon contortrix contortrix)* has markings that make it almost invisible when lying in leaf litter. (From Auerbach, P., Donner, H.J., & Weiss, E.A. [2003]. *Field guide to wilderness medicine* [2nd ed., plate 7]. St. Louis: Mosby.)

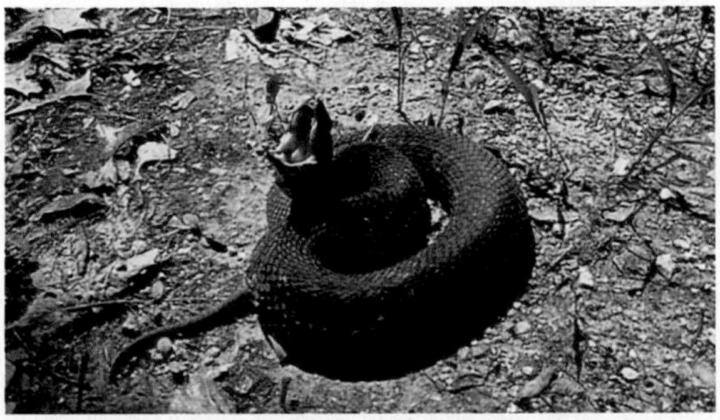

Figure 13-2 ■ Cottonmouth water moccasin *(Agkistrodon piscivoris).* The open-mouthed threat gesture is characteristic of this semiaquatic pit viper. (From Auerbach, P.S., Donner, H.J., & Weiss, E.A. [2003]. *Field guide to wilderness medicine* [2nd ed., plate 6]. St. Louis: Mosby.)

The Elapidae include the coral snakes, which are found from North Carolina to Florida, and in the Gulf states through Texas and Arizona. Coral snakes are accountable for less than 1% of the snakebites in the United States (Lee, 1997). Coral snakes have broad bands of red and black rings, separated by yellow or cream rings. These nonaggressive snakes have short, fixed fangs and inject neurotoxic venom into prey via a chewing motion.

Of the 5000 snakebites that occur each year in the United States, nearly 25% are inflicted by venomous snakes (Holstege et al., 1997). Fatalities are few, but tend to occur in older adults and in individuals who are inadequately treated. Most bites are reported between April and October, with a peak incidence in July and August. This time frame corresponds to an increase in both human and reptile activity in the outdoor environment during the warm weather months. Most snakes fear humans and attempt to avoid contact with them. Sudden, unexpected confrontations at close range are the usual precursors to defensive strikes. Awareness is the key to snakebite prevention.

HEALTH PROMOTION/ILLNESS PREVENTION

Chart 13-3 provides common sense considerations to avoid being bitten by a poisonous snake.

North American Pit Vipers

North American pit vipers can be differentiated from harmless snakes by noting the following key anatomic features:

- The heat-sensing "pit" described on p. 175
- A triangular head that indicates the presence of venom glands
- Two retractable, curved fangs that have canals for venom flow (fangs retract posteriorly when the snake's mouth is closed)
- Up to three sets of developing "replacement" fangs behind the primary fangs

CHART 13-3

CLIENT EDUCATION GUIDE
Snakebite Prevention

- Avoid keeping venomous snakes as pets.
- Be extremely careful in locations that may harbor snakes such as tall grass, rock piles, ledges and crevices, wood piles, brush, swamps, and caves. Snakes are most active on warm nights.
- Don protective attire such as boots, heavy pants, and leather gloves. When walking or hiking, use a walking stick or trekking poles.
- Inspect suspicious areas before placing hands and feet in them.
- Do not harass any snakes you may encounter. Striking distance is at least the length of the snake. Young snakes still pose a threat; they are capable of envenomation from birth.
- Be aware that newly dead or decapitated snakes can inflict a bite for 20 to 60 minutes after death due to persistence of the bite reflex.
- Use extreme caution if attempting to transport the snake with the victim to the medical facility for identification purposes. Ensure that the snake is placed in a sealed container.

Unlike copperheads and water moccasins, rattlesnakes also have interlocking horny rings in their tails that vibrate and serve as a characteristic warning signal to predators. Pit vipers can regulate the amount of venom flow through their fangs depending, in part, on the size of the prey. The quantity of venom injected in defensive bites on humans is highly variable. Approximately 25% of pit viper bites are actually "dry"; that is, there is no envenomation (venom release), yet there are distinctive fang marks on the client (Table 13-1). In contrast, harmless snakes do *not* have venom glands or fangs.

PATHOPHYSIOLOGY

When providing emergency care to a victim of snakebite, the key question is whether or not envenomation has actually occurred. Understanding venom's purpose and function is essential to recognizing the manifestations of envenomation and planning appropriate interventions. The primary functions of venom are to immobilize, kill, and aid in digestion of prey. Venom causes local and systemic toxic effects. The enzymes in venom break down human tissue proteins, alter membrane integrity, and impair blood clotting mechanisms. Not surprisingly, then, the pathophysiologic effects of pit viper envenomation can lead to local tissue necrosis, massive tissue swelling, intravascular fluid shifts and hypovolemic shock, pulmonary edema, renal failure, and hemorrhagic complications from disseminated intravascular coagulation (DIC).

COLLABORATIVE MANAGEMENT

Assessment

The clinical manifestations of envenomation are based on the type and amount of venom injected, the bite location, as well as the age, size, and health status of the victim. Puncture wounds in the skin are a key *local* sign of pit viper envenomation. One or more puncture wounds may be present, depending upon how many fangs the snake has and how many times the snake struck the client. Severe pain, swelling, and redness or ecchymosis (bruising) in the area around the bite are common. Hours later, vesicles or hemorrhagic bullae may form. *Systemic* responses to venom must be distinguished from the psychophysiologic effects of anxiety and panic related to being bitten by a snake. Commonly reported complaints include a minty, rubbery, or metallic taste in the mouth and tingling or paresthesias of the scalp, face, and lips. Other effects include muscle fasciculations and weakness, nausea, vomiting, hypotension, seizures, and coagulopathy (clotting abnormalities) or disseminated intravascular coagulation (DIC). If the bite site

TABLE 13-1 Grades of Pit Viper Envenomation

Envenomation Characteristics

- None. Fang marks, but no local or systemic reactions
- Minimal. Fang marks, local swelling and pain, but no systemic reactions
- Moderate. Fang marks and swelling progressing beyond the site of the bite; systemic signs and symptoms, such as nausea, vomiting, paresthesias, and hypotension
- Severe. Fang marks present with marked swelling of the extremity, subcutaneous ecchymosis, severe symptoms, including manifestations of coagulopathy

From Auerbach, P.S., Donner, H.J., & Weiss, E.A. (2003). Field guide to wilderness medicine (2nd ed.). St. Louis: Mosby.

does not show evidence of local tissue swelling or redness within 8 hours, systemic effects are unlikely to develop.

Interventions

FIRST AID. First aid interventions for snakebite should begin in the field and can improve the victim's outcome. The first priority is to move the person to a safe area away from the snake and encourage rest to decrease venom circulation. Next, jewelry and constricting clothing are removed before swelling becomes significant. Immobilizing the affected extremity in a position of function with a splint is another intervention to limit the spread of the venom. The extremity should be kept below the level of the heart. Keep the individual warm and provide calm reassurance. Do not offer any alcohol or stimulants such as caffeinated beverages because these may speed the absorption of venom (Gold & Wingert, 1994).

HOSPITAL CARE. Acute care in a hospital is warranted as soon as possible. However, if transportation and definitive treatment will be delayed, a 2- to 4-cm constricting band may be applied proximal to an extremity wound to impede venom circulation via lymphatic flow, but it should not be tight enough to impair venous drainage or arterial flow. This band should *not* be used as a tourniquet. Placement of the band may worsen the local tissue necrosis by retaining venom in the tissues–the risk of increased limb damage must be weighed against the consequences of systemic venom effects (Auerbach, Donner, & Weiss, 2003). Assess distal circulation frequently. The band should be loosened if edema renders it too tight. The wound should *not* be incised and sucked, or have ice applied to it. However, a commercially available device called the Sawyer extractor has been found to remove significant amounts of venom if used within 3 minutes of envenomation and left in place for at least 30 minutes (Auerbach, Donner, & Weiss, 2003).

Initial Interventions. Envenomation is a medical emergency. Acute care management in the hospital involves supportive care, which includes supplemental oxygen, two large-bore IV lines, and infusion of crystalloid fluids such as normal saline solution or lactated Ringer's solution. Continuous cardiac and blood pressure monitoring are necessary to quickly detect clinical deterioration. Because envenomation can cause severe pain at the bite site, opioid pain medication is indicated. Snakebite also poses tetanus and wound infection risks. Therefore tetanus prophylaxis, attention to wound care, and broad-spectrum antibiotics must be incorporated into the management plan.

Severe pit viper envenomation causes coagulopathy (clotting abnormalities) and promotes hemorrhage and tissue destruction. Along with typical baseline laboratory studies, a coagulation profile, complete blood count, creatinine kinase, type and crossmatch, and urinalysis should be anticipated. An electrocardiogram (ECG) is necessary to detect evidence of myocardial ischemia or other cardiac abnormalities. Pertinent client history related to the event includes a full account of the snake's appearance, the time the bite was inflicted, prehospital interventions, and any past incidence of snakebite or antivenom use. To accurately assess the development of tissue edema at the bite site, the circumference of the bitten extremity should be measured and recorded every 15 to 30 minutes.

Drug Therapy. Venom potency varies. Not all snake bite victims need antivenom administration. The decision whether or not to give antivenom is based upon the severity of the envenomation. Table 13-1 provides a classification scheme for grading envenomation severity. Conventional pit viper antivenom is most effective within 4 hours of the bite, less effective after 12 hours, but may reverse coagulopathy beyond 24 hours (Gold & Wingert, 1994). Best practice is to contact the regional poison control center so that toxicologists can provide advice in antivenom dosing and medical management.

Until the newest antivenom known as CroFab was introduced in the year 2001, Antivenin Crotalidae Polyvalent was the most commonly used antivenom to treat bites of all North American and South American crotalids (e.g., rattlesnakes, copperheads, and water moccasins). It is considered to be *conventional* antivenom therapy and continues to play a role on a more limited basis in the management of venomous snakebite. The drug is most effective when administered within the first 4 hours of envenomation, but it may reverse coagulopathy even after 24 hours.

The usual dosing regimen is for the drug to be administered over 2 to 4 hours in the following manner:

- Mild envenomation–5 vials
- Moderate envenomation–10 vials
- Severe envenomation–15 to 20 vials

Each vial of powder comes with a bottle of diluent. Do not shake the solution when reconstituting the drug; this action destroys the antivenom proteins and renders the agent ineffective. The vials should be gently rolled to dissolve the powder into the solution, which may take 10 minutes per vial.

The solution from the reconstituted vials is then injected into 250 mL of normal saline. The infusion is begun slowly at a rate of 1 to 5 mL/hr. In general, the rate can be doubled every minute if there is no evidence of an allergic response. The rate of infusion, then, is 10 to 20 minutes per vial. The total infusion time is typically 1 to 2 hours.

Because Antivenin Crotalidae Polyvalent (conventional antivenom) is made from horse serum, there is a high risk of hypersensitivity reactions of varying severity, including life-threatening anaphylactic shock. Administration of this drug requires care in following all dosing guidelines for dilution and infusion. Intradermal skin testing, which was routinely recommended to detect an allergy to horse serum before antivenom administration, is now considered to be inaccurate and not helpful in medical management decisions (Norris & Bush, 2001). Diphenhydramine, epinephrine, and resuscitation equipment must be immediately available to treat anaphylaxis if it occurs. Serum sickness, a type III hypersensitivity reaction, typically follows 7 to 14 days after drug administration and presents as a flu-like syndrome with a skin rash and joint pain. Serum sickness is generally treated with antihistamines and steroids.

Manifestations of an allergic reaction may include anxiety, chills, weakness, wheezing, stridor, vomiting, dyspnea, diaphoresis, throat constriction, sneezing, or red streaking at the IV site. If an allergic reaction is suspected, stop the infusion. Epinephrine may be prescribed if indicated. Other agents to manage the allergic response include IV diphenhydramine (Benadryl) and cimetidine (Tagamet). Both H1 and H2 antagonists are required to treat the reaction effectively. Other measures include further dilution of the antivenom or restarting at a slower rate.

The initial dosage of conventional antivenom is repeated every 2 hours until the progression of local signs ceases and systemic signs resolve. Pregnancy is *not* a contraindication to treatment (Lee, 1997). CroFab or Crotalidae Polyvalent Immune Fab (Ovine) is the newest IV product indicated for the treatment of minimal to moderate crotalid envenomation (First New Management, 2001). CroFab is made from the blood of healthy sheep immunized with North American snake venom. CroFab consists of specific antibody fragments that bind, neutralize and redistribute toxins in crotalid venom so that they may be removed from the client's body ("First New Management," 2001).

CroFab appears to be safer than conventional antivenom therapy. Mild to moderate allergic reactions such as pruritus and urticaria can occur, but anaphylaxis is rare. Skin testing before administration is not necessary. CroFab should be given to clients as soon as possible. The optimal timing is within 6 hours of envenomation ("First New Management," 2001; Hutchinson & Shahan, 2002). Over the first 10 minutes, the infusion should be slow (25 to 50 mL/hr). Monitor the client closely for evidence of an allergic reaction. If symptoms are not effectively controlled with the first dose, including coagulopathy, an additional four to six vials are recommended. Once the client's symptoms are under control, two vials of CroFab are administered every 6 hours for a total of 18 hours of administration (Hutchinson & Shahan, 2002).

If the client has a known hypersensitivity to ovine (sheep) products, CroFab is contraindicated. CroFab is also contraindicated if the client has an allergy to papain or papaya, which is used during the manufacturing process. Give CroFab cautiously to clients who have the following:

- Had an allergic reaction to conventional antivenom therapy in the past
- A hypersensitivity to bromelain (a pineapple-derived enzyme)
- Renal or hepatic impairment
- Pregnancy
- Sensitivity to mercury-containing products (contains ethyl mercury)

At this time, research is limited regarding the efficacy of CroFab with severe envenomation as well as with copperhead envenomation. Finally, if clinical symptoms and coagulopathy recur after the initial infusion, repeat dosing is required.

Coral Snakes

PATHOPHYSIOLOGY

North American coral snakes are found in the southeastern United States and in Texas and Arizona (Figure 13-3). These snakes burrow into the ground and are characteristically nonaggressive. Their ability to inject venom is less efficient than that of the pit vipers. Their maxillary fangs are small and fixed in an upright position. The coral snake must use a chewing motion to inject venom from venom glands through its maxillary fangs. Most bites occur when people attempt to handle the snake. Coral snake venom lacks the complexity of pit viper venom, but can be extremely potent. It has only two primary components: a postsynaptic neurotoxin and a myotoxin. The amount of venom in an adult coral snake is enough to kill a human.

Coral snakes can be recognized by bands of black, red, and yellow coloration that completely encircle the body of the snake. If a black band lies between the red and yellow bands, the snake is most likely nonvenomous. There are several harmless species that closely mimic the appearance of the coral snake. A helpful memory aid for identifying coral snakes is "red on yellow can kill a fellow" and "red and black, venom lack" (Norris & Bush, 2001).

COLLABORATIVE MANAGEMENT

Assessment

Manifestations of coral snake envenomation (venom release) are most closely related to the neurotoxic properties of coral snake venom. The physiologic effect is to block the binding of acetylcholine at the postsynaptic junction (Norris & Bush, 2001). Unlike pit viper envenomation, pain at the bite site may be only mild and transient. Swelling is unlikely. Fang marks may be difficult to visualize due to the coral snake's small teeth. Coagulopathy does not occur as a result of coral snake envenomation. The toxic effects of coral snake venom also may be delayed up to 12 to 13 hours after a bite, but then produce rapid clinical deterioration. Early signs and symptoms consist of nausea, vomiting, headache, pallor, and abdominal pain. Assess for neurologic manifestations, such as paresthesias, numbness, and mental status changes, as well as cranial nerve and peripheral nerve deficits. Total flaccid paralysis may occur later. The client may have difficulty speaking, swallowing, and breathing.

Respiratory insufficiency and cardiovascular collapse can occur in severe cases. Arterial blood gas analysis reveals evidence of respiratory insufficiency. The myotoxic component of the venom can cause an elevation in creatinine kinase (CK) levels due to muscle breakdown and produce myoglobinuria. Despite the pronounced clinical effects, death is rare if the client receives timely management.

Interventions

FIRST AID. Because several varieties of harmless snakes mimic the appearance of the coral snake, the first priority, if possible, is to definitively identify the snake as a coral snake. Identification can be facilitated if the snake is captured and brought to the health care facility with the victim. However, if the snake cannot be caught or positively identified, the vic-

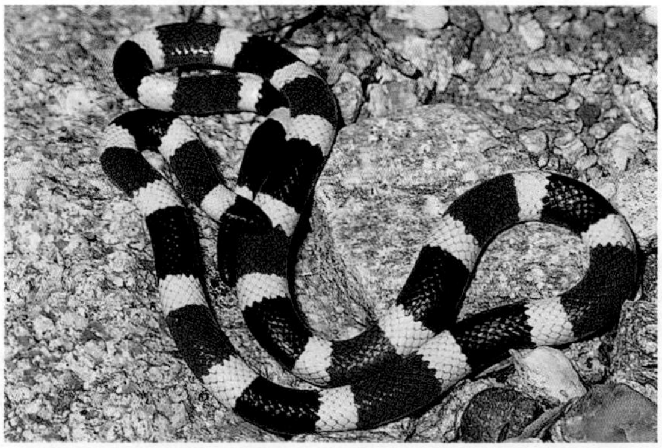

Figure 13-3 ■ Sonoran coral snake *(Micruroides euryxanthus)* is also known as the Arizona coral snake. No documented fatality has followed a bite by this species. (From Auerbach, P.S., Donner, H.J., & Weiss, E.A. [2003]. *Field guide to wilderness medicine* [2nd ed., plate 8]. St. Louis: Mosby.)

tim should be treated as if envenomation has occurred. The field care is the same for that of a pit viper bite without the added concern over tissue necrosis if a constricting band is used, because coral snake venom does not destroy tissue. A field method called the "Australian compression and immobilization technique" in which the extremity is encircled snugly with a roller gauze dressing to impede lymphatic flow and then splinted also may be useful to slow the systemic spread of venom in coral snake bites (Auerbach, Donner, & Weiss, 2003). This compression bandage must not be so tight as to impair arterial flow nor should it be removed until the victim is being managed at an acute care facility.

HOSPITAL CARE. Once in an acute care setting, clients who have had an actual or potential coral snake envenomation should have continuous cardiac, blood pressure, and pulse oximetry monitoring. Prepare to provide aggressive airway management via endotracheal intubation if respiratory insufficiency or severe neurologic impairment occurs. Aspiration of secretions presents a significant risk for this client.

Antivenom administration is recommended even in the absence of clinical evidence of envenomation (Norris & Bush, 2001). The onset of symptoms after coral snake envenomation can be delayed for several hours. However, a delay in antivenom administration can lead to ineffective treatment of neurotoxicity once it develops. The antivenom indicated for the treatment of North American coral snake envenomation is Antivenin *Micrurus fulvius* (Wyeth-Ayerst) made from horse serum. It is effective against the venom of all coral snake species within the United States except the small Sonoran coral snake found in Arizona. No fatalities have been reported as a result of a Sonoran coral snake envenomation; only supportive care is recommended for this type of bite (Norris & Bush, 2001).

The same clinical precautions are applicable when administering coral snake antivenom as with Crotalinae (pit viper) antivenom. The most significant risk to the client is an anaphylactic response to the antivenom. Skin testing is considered inaccurate and not beneficial (Norris & Bush, 2001). Therefore ensure that the client's IV lines are patent and that emergency drugs such as epinephrine as well as resuscitation equipment are immediately available. Premedication with H1- and H2-blocking antihistamines such as diphenhydramine and cimetidine should be anticipated. The adult dose is three to six vials.

Begin the infusion slowly, then increase to enable the entire infusion to be completed within about 2 hours. If an allergic reaction occurs, stop the infusion while the client is treated with epinephrine and/or more antihistamines. The infusion is then restarted at a slower rate. For severe reactions, the physician must determine whether to continue antivenom administration. The initial dose of coral snake antivenom may need to be repeated if neurotoxicity continues to progress. A poison control center should be contacted for assistance with client management and antivenom dosing.

ARTHROPOD BITES AND STINGS

There are several clinically significant insects found in North America that are members of the phylum Arthropoda. These insects include notable species of spiders, scorpions, bees, and wasps. Spiders are carnivorous arthropods that belong to the arachnid class. Unlike snakes, almost all species of spiders are venomous to some degree–most are not harmful to humans either because their mouthparts are too small to pierce human skin, or the quantity of their venom is inadequate to produce significant consequences. However, the venom of some spiders indigenous to the United States does produce significant pathologic effects. Spiders of particular clinical interest are the brown recluse, black widow, and tarantula. Scorpions, bees, and wasps are other venomous arthropods that produce toxic reactions in humans.

Brown Recluse Spider

PATHOPHYSIOLOGY

The brown spiders of the *Loxosceles* genus are known for producing bites that result in ulcerative lesions. In the United States, the brown recluse spider *(L. reclusa)* is the best known culprit of these genera. Brown recluse spiders, also known as "fiddlebacks" or "violin spiders," are medium-sized spiders (body length 8 to 15 mm) that are light brown in color and have a dark brown, fiddle-shaped mark that extends from their eyes down their back (Figure 13-4). Like their name implies, brown recluse spiders are shy and hide in areas that are dark and secluded, such as boxes, closets, basements, sheds, garages, luggage, shoes, clothing, and even bed sheets. Most indoor bites occur when people are sleeping, reaching into boxes or closets, or donning clothing that contains the spider. Few people ever get a look at the spider that bit them. The only evidence may be the characteristic skin lesion and, less often, systemic effects from the injected toxin (commonly referred to as "necrotic arachnidism" or "loxoscelism" in medical literature).

COLLABORATIVE MANAGEMENT

Assessment

Brown recluse spider venom produces cytotoxic effects on tissue. The initial bite has been variously described as painless or stinging to sharp and painful. Some victims are unaware that they were bitten until the telltale lesion with intense local aching and pruritus develops over minutes to hours. The central bite site may appear as a bleb or vesicle surrounded by edema and erythema, which may expand

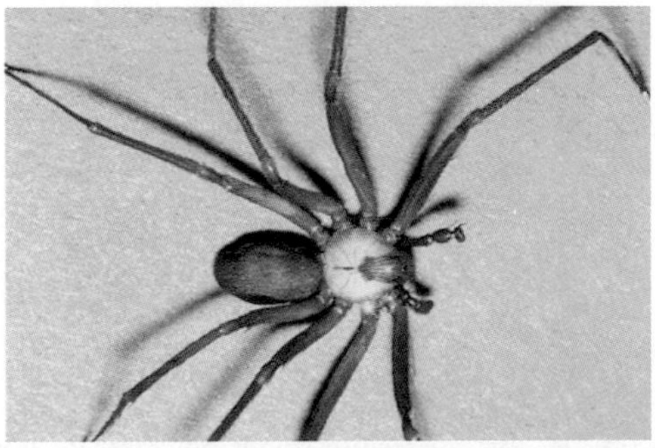

Figure 13-4 ■ Brown recluse spider *(Loxosceles reclusa).* (From Auerbach, P.S., Donner, H.J., & Weiss, E.A. [2003]. *Field guide to wilderness medicine* [2nd ed., plate 12]. St. Louis: Mosby.)

over the course of hours as the toxin spreads to surrounding tissues. Over the next 1 to 3 days, the central lesion typically becomes dark and necrotic (Figure 13-5). Eschar eventually forms. When the eschar sloughs, an open wound or ulcer can remain for weeks to months. Surgical intervention is often necessary to promote wound healing and reduce scarring. Skin grafting may be required for large wounds. In rare cases, some persons may also exhibit manifestations of systemic toxicity to brown recluse spider bites. These can include fever, chills, nausea, vomiting, malaise, joint pain, and petechiae (Morris, 2003). At the extreme end, hemolytic reactions, renal failure, and death have been reported.

Interventions

FIRST AID. The basic first aid for a brown recluse spider bite is to apply cold compresses intermittently during the first 4 days after the bite (Auerbach, Donner, & Weiss, 2003). The cold compress helps decrease the enzymatic activity of the venom and may limit tissue necrosis. Heat should *never* be used because it increases the enzymatic activity and potentially worsens the wound. Rest and elevation of the affected extremity are also recommended (Morris, 2003).

HOSPITAL CARE. For clients with wounds that appear infected, a topical antiseptic and a sterile dressing are necessary; antibiotics are also indicated (Auerbach, Donner, & Weiss, 2003). For severe wounds, therapy with Dapsone may be considered. Dapsone, administered orally in doses of 50 mg twice daily, is a polymorphonuclear leukocyte inhibitor that is effective in treating crater lesions in adults (Morris, 2003). Because there is a risk of blood dyscrasias in persons with glucose-6-phosphate-dehydrogenase G6PD deficiency, G6PD screening and careful monitoring of blood studies are important to detect abnormalities. Methemoglobinemia is another potential adverse effect of Dapsone. An evaluation by a surgeon is usually necessary for clients whose wounds require interventions beyond conservative management. Debridement and skin grafting may be required in order for severe wounds to heal.

Black Widow Spider

PATHOPHYSIOLOGY

Black widow spiders can be found in every state in the United States except Alaska. They have a notorious reputation for inflicting deadly bites. The black widow belongs to the genus *Latrodectus* and prefers a cool, damp environment like outdoor log piles, vegetation, and under rocks. They also commonly inhabit barns, sheds, and garages. The female spider is about 12 to 16 mm in length and is best identified by her shiny black color and the red hourglass pattern on her ventral abdomen. Male spiders are smaller in size and lighter in color with white and gray markings. The hourglass pattern is faint in males. Black widow spiders carry neurotoxic venom. Their usual prey is another arthropod but may include small lizards and snakes. Bites to humans are defensive in nature when the spider is at risk of being crushed.

The initial bite of a black widow spider is variously described as nearly painless to sharply painful. Typically, the client notices a tiny papule or small red punctate mark. The client may experience intense pain, which seems out of proportion to the lesion. In many cases, the symptoms do not progress beyond a local reaction in the area of the bite site. If systemic signs and symptoms do occur, they generally develop within 1 hour and involve the neuromuscular system.

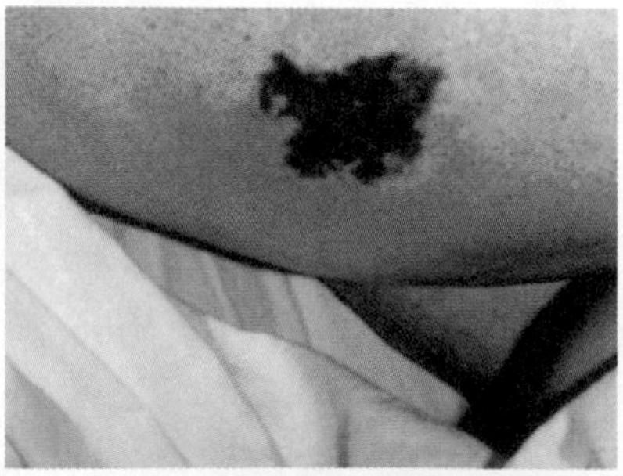

Figure 13-5 ■ Brown recluse spider bite after 24 hours, with central ischemia and rapidly advancing cellulitis. (From Auerbach, P.S., Donner, H.J., & Weiss, E.A. [2003]. *Field guide to wilderness medicine* [2nd ed., plate 13]. St. Louis: Mosby).

COLLABORATIVE MANAGEMENT

Assessment

Envenomation by a black widow spider produces a clinical syndrome known as latrodectism. The neurotoxic venom causes neurotransmitter release from nerve terminals. Severe abdominal pain, muscle rigidity and spasm, hypertension, and nausea and vomiting constitute the classic clinical presentation. In fact, some clinicians erroneously identify the problem as an acute abdomen and consider surgical consultation due to the similar clinical features as peritonitis. The muscle spasms commonly involve the large muscles of the abdomen, back, and limbs. Other noteworthy signs include facial edema (*Latrodectus* facies), ptosis, diaphoresis, weakness, increased salivation, priapism (sustained erection), respiratory difficulty, increased respiratory secretions, fasciculations, and paresthesias. The effects of the bite are self-limited and generally resolve in a few days. However, older adults with significant comorbid conditions such as cardiovascular disease are at much higher risk for a complicated course.

Interventions

FIRST AID. The primary first aid intervention for a black widow spider bite in the prehospital setting is to apply an ice pack. Ice inhibits the action of the neurotoxin. The client should be monitored for evidence of systemic toxicity as described above. If signs or symptoms develop, intervene to support the client's airway, breathing, and circulation. Clients should be transported to a medical facility as soon as possible for advanced life support care.

HOSPITAL CARE. Clients require close monitoring of vital signs, with special attention to blood pressure and respiratory function. Supportive therapy in the hospital includes administration of opioid pain medication and muscle relaxants such as diazepam (Valium). Calcium gluconate (10 mL of a 10% solution) also may be given for muscle spasms, rigidity, and pain. Tetanus prophylaxis is necessary. The client must be observed for the development of seizures related to a rapidly rising blood pressure (Auerbach, Donner,

& Weiss, 2003). Antihypertensive agents may be needed. Although relapses may occur, symptoms usually subside in 48 hours (Morris, 2003). Less often, pulmonary edema, uncontrollable hypertension, and shock ensue. These clients require critical care management. Hospital admission is recommended for all pregnant women and those with a history of hypertension (Boyer, McNally, & Binford, 2001). Antivenom is available for black widow spider bites. However, this agent is rarely used because it carries its own significant risk of anaphylaxis and serum sickness. It is generally administered to treat only severe reactions in which respiratory arrest, seizures, or uncontrolled hypertension occurs. Because pregnant women may have uterine contractions from a black widow spider bite that can cause a premature delivery, antivenom is also indicated for them. The typical dose is one to three ampules. A poison control center can assist in antivenom dosing and client management under these circumstances.

Tarantulas

PATHOPHYSIOLOGY

Tarantulas are members of the Theraphosidae family, the largest sized spiders in the arachnid class. They mainly can be found in the tropical and subtropical areas of the United States and on all continents of the world. However, a number of species are also found in dry, arid states, such as New Mexico and Arizona. Tarantulas can grow to 10 cm in length and live for up to 25 years (Boyer, McNally, & Binford, 2001). These spiders possess venom that paralyzes prey and causes muscle necrosis. However, most bites to humans result in only local effects. A more serious issue is that several genera of tarantulas have *urticating hairs* in their dorsal abdominal area that can be launched into the air as a defensive maneuver and onto a victim. Thousands of these barbed hairs may land on an individual, penetrate skin and eyes, and induce a severe inflammatory reaction.

COLLABORATIVE MANAGEMENT

Assessment

Tarantula bites typically produce pain at the bite site, variously described as mild to moderate to severe. Swelling, redness, numbness, and lymphangitis constitute the usual local effects. Tarantulas found in the United States are not implicated in producing systemic reactions. However, venom from tarantulas in other parts of the world may induce systemic illness. As described earlier, the more troubling aspect of tarantula exposure may be contact with urticating hairs thrown from the spider or rubbed onto a victim's skin during handling. The hairs produce an inflammatory response in skin and mucous membranes consisting of edematous papules that are associated with intense pruritus that can last several weeks. If hairs come into contact with the eyes–sometimes through transfer with hairs on a victim's hands–severe ophthalmic complications can occur (Boyer, McNally, & Binford, 2001).

Interventions

Supportive management is generally all that is required to manage clients who have suffered a venomous bite or exposure to urticating hairs of a tarantula. Pain at the bite site is treated through administration of analgesics appropriate to the level of pain the client is experiencing. The involved extremity can also be immobilized and elevated to decrease pain and swelling. The bite can be expected to heal without sequelae.

Urticating hairs are best removed as soon as possible through repeated use of sticky tape applied to the skin and then removed to pull the hairs from the skin, followed by thorough irrigation (Boyer, McNally, & Binford, 2001). For eye exposure, copious irrigation with saline is required. Oral antihistamines and topical or systemic steroids may be used to treat the intense pruritus associated with urticating hair exposure (Auerbach, Donner, & Weiss, 2003).

Scorpions

PATHOPHYSIOLOGY

Scorpions are found in many states within the United States, although not typically in the Midwest or New England. However, stings are always possible when people keep scorpions as pets or when scorpions are inadvertently transported to nonindigenous areas in baggage and packaging. Unlike spiders that envenom their prey by inflicting a bite, scorpions inject venom through a stinging apparatus on their tail. Most scorpion stings produce a relatively mild reaction characterized by local pain, inflammation, and mild systemic symptoms. These effects are typically self-limiting and best treated by analgesics, supportive management, and basic wound care.

One species of scorpion found in the United States that can inflict a sting associated with a severe, potentially fatal systemic response is the *Centruroides exilicauda,* or the bark scorpion (Figure 13-6). It is often found in trees, wood piles, and around debris. Humans are most often stung when this scorpion gets into clothing, shoes, blankets, and personal items left on the ground. The small bark scorpion is about 5 cm (2 inches) in length and may be solid yellow, brown, or tan in color. There are also some striped varieties, though not as common. While many scorpions have thick claws and thick tails, distinctive features of the bark scorpion

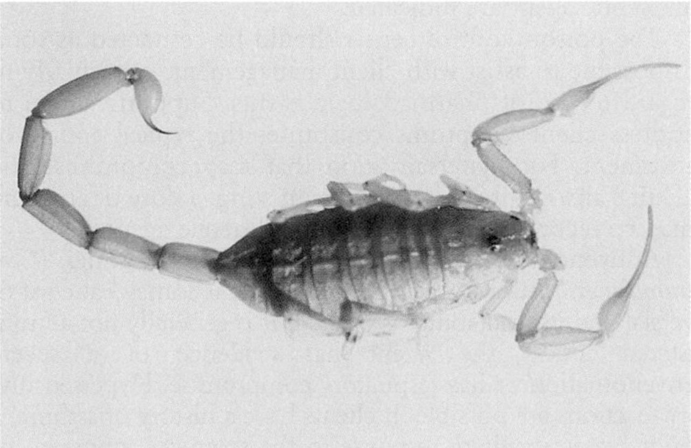

Figure 13-6 ■ *Centruroides exilicauda (C. sculpturatus),* the bark scorpion of Arizona. (From Auerbach, P.S., Donner, H.J., & Weiss, E.A. [2003]. *Field guide to wilderness medicine* [2nd ed., plate 17]. St. Louis: Mosby.)

include thin pincers and a thin tail, as well as the presence of a tubercle, called a subaculeate tooth, at the base of the stinger. This scorpion is found throughout Arizona and in some areas of New Mexico, Texas, Nevada, and California. The venom of the bark scorpion is neurotoxic.

COLLABORATIVE MANAGEMENT

Assessment

Because bark scorpion venom is neurotoxic, manifestations typically involve the cranial nerves and/or the musculoskeletal system. The sting site may or may not show evidence of the envenomation. There may be no redness or other obvious sign of inflammation. Suchard and Connor (2001) advocate the "tap test," that is, a gentle tap at the potential sting site while the client is not looking greatly increases the pain and serves as a confirmatory test for a bark scorpion sting. The severity of the bark scorpion sting is highly variable, from local pain to systemic manifestations, such as respiratory failure, pancreatitis, musculoskeletal dysfunction, and cranial nerve involvement.

Symptoms usually begin immediately after the sting and reach maximum intensity in 5 hours (Suchard & Connor, 2001). Although the symptoms may start to resolve after 9 to 30 hours, the pain and paresthesias can remain for up to 2 weeks.

Interventions

The first priority of client management is vital sign assessment and continuous monitoring for several hours in a hospital emergency department or critical care unit to enable rapid intervention if progression of symptoms occurs. The client may require intubation and mechanical ventilation if signs of respiratory failure occur. Supplemental oxygen and IV fluid replacement should be instituted immediately. Apply an ice pack to the sting site to control pain. Give analgesic and sedative agents with caution in the nonintubated, spontaneously breathing client. Potent opioids, benzodiazepines, and barbiturates can cause loss of airway reflexes and precipitate respiratory failure. Fever is treated with acetaminophen and application of a cooling blanket as needed. Because scorpion stings produce a puncture wound, tetanus prophylaxis and basic wound care with an antiseptic agent are indicated.

The poison control center should be contacted as soon as possible to assist with client management, particularly in regard to use of pharmacologic agents. Supportive care to address client symptoms constitutes the typical course of treatment. For hypersalivation that may compromise the client's airway after a bark scorpion sting, a dose of atropine may be recommended as an anticholinergic agent.

Antivenom is available for bark scorpion stings (*Centruroides exilicauda* Antivenin), but its use is somewhat controversial and its availability is limited. It is generally not administered unless the client has evidence of a severe envenomation or has respiratory compromise. Hypersensitivity reactions are possible. If clients have a history of asthma, a prior hypersensitivity response to the scorpion antivenin, or allergies to goats or goat products, or if the client takes beta blockers or angiotensin-converting (ACE) inhibitors, then antivenom use is contraindicated (Suchard & Connor, 2001). The poison control center should be consulted for preparation and dosing of the antivenom if it is both available and indicated for the client. Be sure that advanced life support equipment is readily available to treat an anaphylactic response to the antivenom if it should occur. Serum sickness may develop after antivenom administration and is generally treated with antihistamines and tapering regimen of corticosteroids.

Bees and Wasps

PATHOPHYSIOLOGY

Bees and wasps are venomous arthropod members of the Hymenoptera order. Stings can produce a wide range of reactions from discomfort at the sting site, to severe pain and life-threatening anaphylaxis in allergic individuals. Bees and wasps are capable of stinging repeatedly when disturbed. Only the honeybee does not have this tendency. "Africanized" or "killer bees" are a very aggressive bee species found in the southwestern states that are known to attack in groups. When an individual sustains multiple stings, reactions are more severe and may be fatal because venom doses have cumulative toxic effects.

HEALTH PROMOTION/ILLNESS PREVENTION

Chart 13-4 lists actions that may help prevent arthropod bites and stings.

COLLABORATIVE MANAGEMENT

Assessment

The client who is stung by a bee or wasp first experiences a local reaction that is characterized by immediate pain and a wheal-and-flare reaction. Swelling can be extensive and involve an entire limb or body area. Systemic effects can then develop based upon the individual's sensitivity to the venom. These effects may include generalized edema, nausea, vomiting, and diarrhea. If the client has an allergy to the

CHART 13-4

CLIENT EDUCATION GUIDE
Arthropod Bite/Sting Prevention

- Wear appropriate protective clothing, including gloves and shoes, when working in areas known to harbor venomous arthropods, such as spiders, scorpions, bees, and wasps.
- Cover garbage cans. Bees and wasps are attracted to uncovered garbage.
- Use screens in windows and doors to prevent flying insects from entering buildings.
- Inspect clothing, shoes, and gear for insects before putting on these items.
- Shake out clothing and gear that has been on the ground to prevent arthropod "stowaways" and inadvertent bites and stings.
- Consult an exterminator to control arthropod populations in and around the home. Eliminating insects that are part of the arthropod's food source may also limit their presence.
- Identify nesting areas such as yard debris and rock piles; remove them whenever possible.
- Do not place unprotected hands where the eyes cannot see.
- Avoid handling insects or keeping them as "pets."
- Carry prescription epinephrine preparations and antihistamines if known to be allergic to bee and wasp stings.

venom, then urticaria, pruritus, and swelling of the lips and tongue may ensue. An allergic response can progress to an anaphylactic reaction rapidly in highly sensitive clients. Anaphylaxis is evidenced by respiratory distress with bronchospasm and laryngeal edema, hypotension, deterioration in mental status, and cardiac dysrhythmias. This type of reaction constitutes a true medical emergency that is imminently life threatening and may lead to cardiac arrest.

Interventions

FIRST AID. Basic emergency care for bee and wasp stings includes quick removal of the stinger and application of an ice pack. Honeybees and yellow jackets are most likely to leave a stinger. Most sources strongly advise against using tweezers to remove a stinger to avoid pinching the venom sac in the stinger and causing additional venom to be injected during removal; the commonly preferred method is to remove the stinger by gently scraping or brushing it off with the edge of a knife blade, credit card, or needle.

HOSPITAL CARE. Advanced emergency care interventions must be prioritized to assure that airway, breathing, and circulation are maintained. First, it is essential to determine whether the client has a history of allergic reactions to bee stings and whether an epinephrine kit has been prescribed. These kits sometimes contain an antihistamine tablet as well. In the presence of a severe allergic reaction characterized by wheezing, facial swelling, and respiratory distress, epinephrine must be administered without delay. Allergic clients typically carry an "EpiPen" (adult). This device enables epinephrine to be administered simply and quickly in an emergency because it delivers the right dose intramuscularly with just a click of a button. Other kits contain a prefilled epinephrine syringe. The standard epinephrine dose for adults is 0.3 to 0.5 mg of a 1:1000 solution given intramuscularly. The IM route is recommended over the subcutaneous route because it has more predictable and rapid absorption (Project Team of the Resuscitation Council [UK], 1999). Usually, directions on the epinephrine delivery device specify that the dose should be repeated in 15 minutes if signs and symptoms persist.

After epinephrine administration, an antihistamine such as diphenhydramine (Benadryl, Allerdryl✱) or chlorpheniramine (Chlor-Trimeton, Novopheniram✱) should also be given immediately. In the field setting, oral liquid diphenhydramine (available over the counter) may be easier for the victim to swallow than the tablet form if there is tongue or pharyngeal edema. For reactions that cause just pruritus and urticaria, only an antihistamine may be indicated initially. It is imperative that the emergency medical system be activated by calling 911 and that the client be transported to a medical facility as soon as possible.

Once in a clinical setting, clients who sustain serious reactions to bee or wasp stings need supplemental oxygen and continuous cardiac and blood pressure monitoring. Establish an IV infusion with normal saline solution to support blood pressure. Advanced life support drugs and equipment should be made immediately available. If epinephrine IM fails to relieve the life-threatening reaction, epinephrine 0.1 mg of a 1:10,000 solution may be ordered as a very slow IV bolus. IV epinephrine administration carries a much greater risk of adverse cardiovascular effects than IM epinephrine. Use the IV form of epinephrine with extreme caution, especially in older adults with cardiovascular disease. Bronchospasm may be treated with albuterol via inhalation or a similar bronchodilating agent.

Parenteral antihistamines and corticosteroids are also commonly prescribed to decrease the immune response. The toxin in the bee and wasp venom may outlast the effects of the initial doses of epinephrine and antihistamines and cause a recurrence of the allergic reaction over time. Corticosteroids prescribed in tapered doses are usually given to manage or prevent delayed allergic effects as well as serum sickness. Anyone who develops an allergic reaction to bee or wasp stings should be strongly encouraged to always carry a prescription epinephrine emergency kit and wear a medical alert tag or bracelet.

LIGHTNING INJURIES

PATHOPHYSIOLOGY

Lightning is a year-round weather problem. It is caused by an electric charge generated within thunderclouds that may propagate downward to become cloud-to-ground lightning, the most dangerous form to people or structures on the ground (Krider & Uman, 1995). Between 1980 and 1995, there were 1318 deaths attributed to lightning in the United States, yielding an average of 82 deaths per year (MMWR, 1998). Males accounted for 85% of the victims of lightning-related death; the majority (68%) were in the 15- to 44-year-old age range (MMWR, 1998). Most lightning-related injuries occur in the summer months due to increased thunderstorm activity and greater numbers of people spending time outdoors. Anyone without adequate shelter, including golfers, hikers, campers, beach goers, and swimmers, are at risk. Lopez and Holle (1995) found that 92% of fatal lightning strikes happened in the months of May through September; of those, 73% occurred in the afternoon and early evening hours.

Lightning has an enormous magnitude of energy and a much shorter duration of contact and a different current flow than a typical high-voltage electric shock. *High-voltage* electricity is considered to exceed 1000 volts. The energy in a single lightning stroke can exceed 1 million volts. The duration of contact, however, is nearly instantaneous, resulting in a flashover phenomenon–an effect that may explain the relatively low overall mortality rate. Because water is a conductor of electricity and current takes the path of least resistance to the ground, any wetness on the body increases the flashover effect of a lightning strike. Lightning flashover can produce an explosive force powerful enough to damage or blow off the victim's clothing and shoes (Cooper, et al., 2001).

Lightning can produce injury by directly striking a victim, by splashing or side flashing off a nearby strike area, and by traveling through the ground–also known as "step voltage" (Cherington, 2003). Although only 30% of victims die, 74% are left with permanent disabilities (MMWR, 1998).

HEALTH PROMOTION/ILLNESS PREVENTION

Perhaps the best remedy for lightning injuries is avoidance. Injuries due to lightning strike are highly preventable. Chart 13-5 lists common sense prevention strategies.

CHART 13-5

CLIENT EDUCATION GUIDE
Lightning Strike Prevention

- Observe weather forecasts when planning to be outside.
- Seek shelter when you hear thunder. Safe areas include the nearest building or an enclosed vehicle. Isolated sheds and the entrances to caves are dangerous, however. Do not stand under an isolated tall tree or structure (e.g., ski lift, flag pole, boat mast, power line) in an open area such as a field, ridge or hilltop; lightning seeks the highest point. A stand of dense trees offers better protection.
- Leave the water immediately (including an indoor shower or bathtub) and move away from any open bodies of water.
- Avoid metal objects: put down tools, fishing rods, garden equipment, golf clubs, and umbrellas; stand clear of fences, exposed pipes, motorcycles, bicycles, tractors, and golf carts.
- If camping in a tent, stay away from the metal tent poles and wet walls.
- Once inside a building, stay away from open doors, windows, fireplaces, metal fixtures, and plumbing.
- Turn off electrical equipment including computers, televisions, and stereos.
- Stay off the telephone. Lightning can enter through the telephone line and produce head and neck trauma, including cataracts and tympanic membrane disruption. Death can result.
- If you are caught out in the open and cannot seek shelter, attempt to move to lower ground such as a ravine or valley; stay away from any tall trees or objects that could result in a lightning strike splashing over to you; place insulating material between you and the ground (e.g., sleeping pad, rain parka, life jacket) and bend down on your knees, bend forward and place your hands on your knees. A lightning strike is imminent if your hair stands on end, you see blue halos around objects, and hear high-pitched or crackling noises. If you cannot move away from the area immediately, crouch on the balls of your feet and tuck your head down to minimize the target size; do not lie down on the ground or have hand contact with the ground.

Data from Auerbach, P.S., Donner, H.J., & Weiss, E.A. [2003]. Field guide to wilderness medicine (2nd ed.). St. Louis: Mosby.

COLLABORATIVE MANAGEMENT

Assessment

Both the cardiopulmonary and the central nervous systems are profoundly affected by lightning injuries. The most lethal initial effect of the massive current discharge on the cardiopulmonary system is either asystole or ventricular fibrillation. It is important to understand that cardiac cells are autorhythmic. An effective cardiac rhythm may return spontaneously. However, prolonged respiratory arrest from impairment of the medullary respiratory center can produce hypoxia and, subsequently, a second cardiac arrest (Cooper, et al., 2001). Therefore the principle of "reverse triage" is the rule when attempting to manage multiple victims of a lightning strike: those who are in cardiopulmonary arrest should be afforded priority resuscitation measures with immediate airway and ventilatory management, chest compressions, and other appropriate life support interventions (Cherington, 2003; Cooper, et al., 2001). Individuals who exhibit signs of life immediately after a lightning strike may be treated in a less emergent fashion because they have the best chance of recovery. Despite survival, victims of lightning strike can suffer serious myocardial injury, which may be manifested by ECG and myocardial perfusion abnormalities. The initial appearance of mottled skin and decreased to absent peripheral pulses usually arises from arterial vasospasm. These findings most often resolve spontaneously in several hours without the need for intervention (Cooper, et al., 2001).

Central nervous system (CNS) injury is a significant result of lightning strike. Typical CNS effects include an immediate but temporary paralysis, known as keraunoparalysis or "muscular stunning," which can persist for minutes to hours, loss of consciousness, amnesia, confusion or disorientation, photophobia, and seizures (Fahmy, et al., 1999). Intracranial hemorrhage, cerebral infarction, encephalopathy, cerebellar dysfunction, and spinal cord injury may also occur (Cherington, 2003). Fatigue and cognitive impairments as well as post-traumatic stress disorder are long-term neuropsychological consequences reported in survivors of lightning injuries (van Zomeren, et al., 1998). Other lightning strike-related effects include ruptured tympanic membranes, blindness, cataracts, and retinal detachment, which may be due to both blast effect and intense heat production (Espaillat, Janigian, & To, 1999).

Lightning strike also causes skin burns. Most burns are superficial and heal without incident. Clients may have punctate full-thickness burns, charring, and contact burns from overlying metal objects. An uncommon but characteristic cutaneous manifestation of lightning is the appearance of branching or ferning marks on the skin called **Lichtenberg figures**, also known as keraunographic markings or erythematous arborization.

Interventions

FIRST AID. Because of lightning's powerful impact to the body, clients are at great risk for the entire spectrum of multisystem trauma. The full extent of injury may not be known until thorough monitoring and diagnostic evaluation can be performed in the hospital. Initial care must include spinal immobilization with attention to stabilization of airway, breathing, and circulation through standard basic and advanced life support measures. As a reminder, reverse triage will potentially do the greatest good for the greatest number of victims in a lightning strike that results in mass casualties. CPR should be performed immediately when a client is in cardiac arrest. In the presence of cardiopulmonary or central nervous system injury, skin burns are an initial priority. However, if time and resources permit, a sterile dressing may be applied to cover the sites. Victims of lightning strike are *not* electrically charged; the rescuer is in no danger from physical contact. Nonetheless, the storm can present a continued threat to everyone in the vicinity who lacks adequate shelter. Contrary to popular belief, lightning can and does strike in the same place more than once.

HOSPITAL CARE. Once in the acute care hospital setting, the client requires advanced life support management, including cardiac monitoring to detect cardiac dysrhythmias. Airway, breathing, and circulatory support are indicated as needed. The client may require a period of mechanical ventilation until spontaneous breathing returns. A thorough physical and diagnostic evaluation to identify both obvious and occult traumatic injuries is important because the client may have suffered a fall or blast effect during the strike. A creatinine kinase (CK) measurement may be ordered to detect skeletal muscle damage resulting from the lightning strike. In severe cases, rhabdomyolysis (muscle destruction) and kidney failure can occur. Burn wounds should be assessed and treated according to standard burn care protocols. Tetanus prophylaxis is necessary. Care of the client is supportive as recovery ensues. Some institutions transfer these clients to a burn center for subsequent management.

COLD INJURIES

Two common cold injuries are hypothermia and frostbite. Both types of injuries can be prevented by implementing protection from the cold. Teach clients at risk ways to prevent these injuries, which can range from mild discomfort to major systemic complications.

HEALTH PROMOTION/ILLNESS PREVENTION

When participating in cold weather activities, clothing choices are critical to the prevention of hypothermia and frostbite. Synthetic clothing is best because it wicks away moisture from the body and dries fast. Cotton clothing, especially as an underlayer, holds moisture, becomes wet, and contributes to the development of hypothermia. Cotton clothing should be strictly avoided in a cold outdoor environment; this rule applies to gloves and socks as well. The mountaineering adage that "cotton kills" is important to remember. Wet socks and gloves promote frostbite in the toes and fingers. Wearing too many pairs of socks can impair circulation and predispose the client to frostbite.

Clothing should be layered so that it can be easily added or removed as the temperature changes. The inner layers should provide warmth (insulation). Polyester fleece is a good choice. The outer layer's purpose is to block the wind and protect the client from moisture. This layer is best made of a windproof, waterproof, breathable fabric such as Gore-Tex. A hat is an essential clothing item that significantly decreases body heat through the head. Face protection with a face mask should be considered on particularly cold days when wind chill poses a risk. Sunscreen (at least SPF 30) and sunglasses are also important to protect skin and eyes from the harmful rays of the sun.

When driving in winter cannot be avoided, water, extra clothing, and food should be kept in the car in case the vehicle becomes stranded. Maintaining personal fitness and conditioning are also important considerations to prevent hypothermia and frostbite. Individuals should not diet or restrict food or fluid intake when participating in winter outdoor activities. Malnutrition and dehydration contribute to cold-related illnesses and injuries. Finally, it is imperative for individuals to know their physical limits and to come in out of the cold when these limits have been met.

Hypothermia

PATHOPHYSIOLOGY

Hypothermia is generally defined as a core body temperature less than 95° F (35° C). An understanding of the etiologies and risk factors involved in the development of hypothermia is key to both recognition and prevention. Predisposing conditions that promote the development of hypothermia include the following:

- Cold water immersion
- Illness
- Injury
- Shock states
- Immobilization
- Weather
- Extremes of age
- Selected medications (e.g., phenothiazines, sedatives, anxiolytics, meperidine, and vasodilating agents)
- Alcohol intoxication
- Malnutrition
- Inadequate clothing or shelter

An important point, however, is that an environmental temperatures less than 82° F can produce hypothermia in any susceptible individual. Therefore clients are actually at risk on a *year-round* basis in most areas of the world. Wind chill is a significant factor: heat loss increases as wind velocity rises. Wet conditions further heat loss through evaporation. Weather is the most notable cause of hypothermia for outdoor sports enthusiasts and for those with inadequate clothing or shelter. The mortality rate for hypothermia exceeds 50% when body temperature falls below 32° C (90° F), and nears 100% in victims who have concurrent illness or injuries (Bowman, et al., 2003).

◆COLLABORATIVE MANAGEMENT

◆Assessment

Hypothermia is divided into the categories of *mild* (32° C to 35° C), *moderate* (28° C to 32° C), and *severe* (<28° C). In the injured client, hypothermia exists when the body temperature is 36° C or below (American College of Surgeons, 1997). Treatment decisions are based on the degree of hypothermia present. *Mild* hypothermia is manifested by shivering, dysarthria, muscular incoordination, and impaired cognitive abilities (i.e., mental slowness) and "cold diuresis." Cold diuresis results from peripheral vasoconstriction and shunting of blood to the core of the body. With core hypervolemia, glomerular filtration rate accelerates causing an increase in urine output. Dehydration occurs and exacerbates the hypothermic condition due to impaired circulation. Shivering and an increased metabolic rate are the body's compensatory mechanisms to stimulate heat production. Early cardiopulmonary manifestations include tachycardia and increased respiratory rate.

Clients with *moderate* (28° C to 32° C) to *severe* hypothermia (<28° C) have obvious motor impairment and weakness. They become uncoordinated and may stumble or fall. Their cognitive abilities and mental processes deteriorate. Confusion and apathy progress to irrationality and incoherence, stupor, and unconsciousness. Shivering stops at this point. Victims may even erroneously perceive warmth and engage in "paradoxical undressing" in which they disrobe, an action that aggravates their already perilous hypothermic condition (Auerbach, Donner, & Weiss, 2003). Vital signs become depressed. Bradycardia and hypotension ensue. Respiratory rate and effort, and cardiac output decline. Prolongation of the P-R, QRS, and Q-Tc intervals occur; J waves or Osborn waves may appear on the ECG (Auerbach, Donner, & Weiss, 2003). A cold heart is an irritable heart; atrial and ventricular dysrhythmias are common. The ventricular fibrillation threshold is decreased. Deterioration to ventricular fibrillation and asystole is easily precipitated by rough handling or jolting of the client's body, as well as by performance of some medical procedures and central line insertion. In severe hypothermia (<28° C), neurologic reflexes and responsiveness to pain are absent. Profound hypotension, acid-base abnormalities, ventricular fibrillation, and asystole are characteristic.

In moderate to severe hypothermia, laboratory values may reveal **coagulopathy**, or blood clotting abnormalities, and platelet dysfunction. Clotting factor function is temperature dependent and is reduced in hypothermia (Watts, 1998). Platelet aggregation is impaired; thrombocytopenia develops due to destruction of platelets in the liver and spleen (Watts, 1998). Prolonged bleeding times result. A very important concept is that hypothermia causes coagulopathy over a range of temperatures–the greater the degree of hypothermia, the more likely the client will hemorrhage from injury or invasive procedures. This concept has especially critical implications for the injured client in a shock state who requires resuscitation: hypothermia must be identified and treated effectively to prevent further blood loss.

Interventions

FIRST AID. Treatment of mild hypothermia is straightforward: the individual needs to be sheltered from the cold environment, have all wet clothing removed, and undergo passive or active external rewarming. Passive methods involve applying warm clothing or blankets. Active methods incorporate heating blankets, warm packs, and convective air heaters or warmers to speed rewarming. If a heating blanket is used, Gentilello (1999) advises that the blanket should be placed on top of the client instead of underneath because greater heat loss occurs from above the body by convection and radiation. In addition, the individual may have a reduced risk of burn injury with this arrangement.

In a camping or wilderness setting, a rescuer can share the same sleeping bag with a hypothermic victim to promote transfer of body heat as a primitive but effective means of active external rewarming. Both the rescuer and the victim should be only minimally clothed to facilitate heat transfer. In the case of mild, uncomplicated hypothermia as the only health problem, having the client drink warm high-carbohydrate liquids that do not contain alcohol or caffeine can aid in rewarming. Alcohol is a peripheral vasodilator; both alcohol and caffeine are diuretics. The effects of these agents can potentially worsen dehydration and hypothermia.

HOSPITAL CARE. Treatment of moderate to severe hypothermia differs from that of mild hypothermia in that active, external rewarming methods are contraindicated. Core temperature "afterdrop" can occur. **Afterdrop** is defined as a continued decrease in core body temperature after the victim is removed from the cold environment due to equilibration of core and peripheral blood temperature and countercurrent cooling of blood perfusing cold tissue (Tisherman, 2002). Applying external heat promotes afterdrop by producing peripheral vasodilation, which stimulates the return of cold blood from the periphery to the warmer core.

Several general management principles apply to both moderate and severe hypothermia. The client should be protected from further heat loss and handled gently to prevent ventricular fibrillation. The client is best kept in a horizontal position to prevent orthostatic changes in blood pressure from cardiovascular instability. Only core rewarming methods are indicated to treat moderate to severe hypothermia. For moderate hypothermia, core rewarming methods include administration of warm IV fluids, heated oxygen or inspired gas to prevent further heat loss via the respiratory tract, and heated peritoneal or pleural lavage (Gentilello, 1999). Even though they are commonly employed, gastric, colonic, and bladder lavage are less effective because of the smaller surface area for heat exchange (Gentilello, 1999). Active rewarming with externally applied heating devices is dangerous in this population because it produces vasodilation in the extremities.

In addition to rewarming interventions, standard resuscitation efforts are indicated with special attention to maintenance of airway, breathing, and circulation. Administer drugs with caution because metabolism is unpredictable in hypothermic conditions. Drugs can accumulate without obvious therapeutic effect while the client is cold, but will become active and potentially lead to drug toxicity as effective rewarming is underway. CPR should be initiated for ventricular fibrillation and asystole. Defibrillation attempts may be ineffective until the core temperature is above 30° C (86° F) (Auerbach, Donner, & Weiss, 2003).

The client who is severely hypothermic is at high risk of cardiac arrest. For these clients, the treatment of choice is to employ extracorporeal rewarming methods such as cardiopulmonary bypass, hemodialysis, or continuous arteriovenous rewarming (CAVR). The advantage of CAVR for the trauma client with hemorrhage is that heparin is not required. A limitation is that the client's systolic blood pressure must be greater than 60 mm Hg for blood to flow through the circuit. Cardiopulmonary bypass is the fastest rewarming technique. It supports the circulation and allows for timely correction of fluid, electrolyte, and metabolic abnormalities. However, this device is not available in all hospitals. It requires specialized personnel and resources to operate it properly. Complications can occur after weaning from cardiopulmonary bypass as well. Common complications include acute respiratory distress syndrome (ARDS), acute renal failure and pneumonia.

A long-standing principle in the treatment of clients with hypothermic cardiac arrest is that "no one is dead until they are warm and dead." There is a factual basis to this statement when considering the number of survivors who have suffered a prolonged hypothermic cardiac arrest. Clinical judgment must always take precedence, however. Prolonged resuscitation efforts may not be reasonable in cases in which survival appears highly unlikely, such as in an anoxic event followed by a hypothermic cardiac arrest. If the arrest victim is rewarmed to a core temperature of 30° to 32° C but continues to have no cardiac activity and dilated nonreactive pupils, consideration should be given to terminating resuscitative efforts (Cummins, 2003).

Frostbite

PATHOPHYSIOLOGY

Another significant cold-related injury that may or may not be associated with hypothermia is frostbite. A principal predisposing factor is inadequate insulation against cold weather, that is, either the skin is exposed to the cold or the individual's clothing offers insufficient protection. Wet clothing, in particular, serves as a poor insulator and facilitates the development of frostbite. Fatigue and poor nutrition are other contributing factors. Clients who smoke, consume alcohol, or have impaired peripheral circulation have a higher incidence of frostbite. These factors aggravate cold injuries. Any previous history of frostbite further increases a client's susceptibility.

COLLABORATIVE MANAGEMENT

Assessment

Frostbite is classified as superficial or mild ("frostnip"), or deep. **Frostnip** may produce initial pain, numbness, and pallor of the affected area, but is easily remedied with application of warmth and does not induce tissue injury. Frostnip typically develops on skin areas such as the face, nose, finger, or toes. The American College of Surgeons (1997) characterizes deep frostbite by the degree of tissue freezing. Like burns, frostbite injuries can be partial or full thickness. First-degree frostbite, the least severe type of deep frostbite, involves hyperemia of the involved area and edema formation. In second-degree frostbite, large fluid-filled blisters develop with a partial thickness skin necrosis (Figure 13-7). Third-degree frostbite appears as small blisters that contain dark fluid and an affected body part that is cool, numb, blue, or red and does not blanch. Full thickness and subcutaneous tissue necrosis occurs and require debridement. In fourth-degree frostbite, there are no blisters or edema; the part is numb, cold, and bloodless. The full thickness necrosis extends into the muscle and bone. At this stage, gangrene develops, which may necessitate amputation of the affected part.

Interventions

FIRST AID. Recognition of frostbite is essential to early, effective intervention and prevention of further tissue damage. Asking a partner to frequently observe for early signs of frostbite such as a white, waxy appearance to exposed skin, especially on the nose, cheeks, and ears, is an effective strategy to identify the problem before it worsens. In this case, the best remedy is to have the individual seek shelter from the wind and cold and to attend to the affected body part. Superficial frostbite is easily managed in the prehospital setting using body heat to warm the affected area. Clients can be taught to place their warm hands over the affected areas on their face or to place cold hands under the arms in the axillary region.

HOSPITAL CARE. Clients with deep frostbite need aggressive management. For all degrees of deep frostbite, rapid rewarming in a water bath at a temperature range of 38° C to 41° C is indicated to thaw the frozen part (Tisherman, 2002). Because clients experience severe pain during the rewarming process, this intervention is best accomplished in a medical facility; however, it may be done in another setting if no other options exist for prompt transport or rescue. Analgesic agents, especially IV opiates, are an essential aspect of this client's care plan as soon as possible. Dry heat should never be applied, nor should the frostbitten areas be rubbed as part of the warming process. These actions produce further tissue injury.

When the rewarming process is complete, elevate the extremity above heart level if possible to decrease tissue edema. Frostbite destroys tissue and produces a deep tetanus-prone wound; the client should be immunized for tetanus prophylaxis (Kanzenbach & Dexter, 1999). Once a client's frozen part has been thawed, do not allow it to refreeze, which worsens the injury. Surgical intervention is ultimately indicated to evaluate tissue viability and provide wound management in cases of deep frostbite. Debridement of necrotic tissue will be necessary. Amputation may be indicated for clients with severe injuries or for those who develop gangrene.

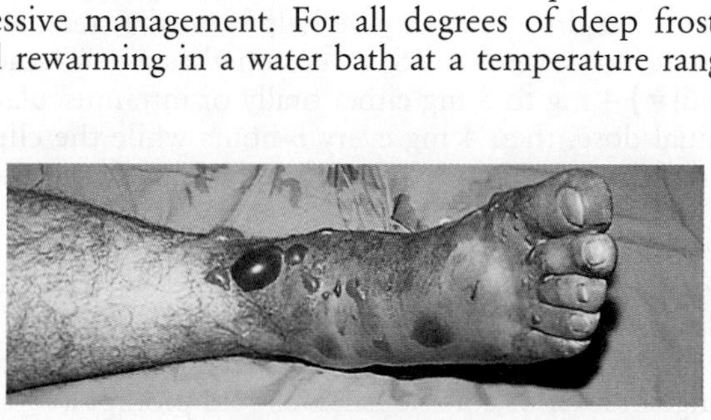

Figure 13-7 ■ Edema and blister formation 24 hours after frostbite injury occurring in an area covered by a tightly fitted boot. (From Auerbach, P.S., Donner, H.J., & Weiss, E.A. [2003]. *Field guide to wilderness medicine* [2nd ed., plate 1]. St. Louis: Mosby.)

ALTITUDE-RELATED ILLNESSES

PATHOPHYSIOLOGY

High altitude, generally defined as elevations above 5000 feet, can produce a range of physiologic consequences in the body. Some of these effects can be quite deleterious to a person's health and, in extreme cases, can be fatal. Because so many people visit mountainous areas for sport and recreation such as skiing and hiking, it is important to have an understanding of altitude physiology and the ability to recognize the most common emergency situations that may be induced by altitude effects on the human body.

As altitude increases, barometric pressure decreases. Oxygen constitutes 21% of the barometric pressure. Therefore as barometric pressure falls, the partial pressure of oxygen decreases, resulting in less available oxygen to humans. The physiologic consequence is hypoxia. Hypoxia becomes more pronounced as elevation increases. High altitude is considered to be about 5000 to 11,500 feet–the same elevation as most Western ski areas in the United States. Very high altitude is defined as altitudes between about 11,500 feet and 18,000 feet. The peaks of some Western ski areas are in the 12,000- to 13,000-foot range. Elevations of greater than 18,000 feet constitute extreme altitude. Supplemental oxygen is necessary at these altitudes to prevent altitude-related illness, including death, from occurring during abrupt ascent.

The process of adapting to high altitude is called **acclimatization**. Acclimatization involves physiologic changes that help the body to compensate for less available oxygen in the atmosphere. As the carotid bodies sense a decline in PaO_2 at about 5000 feet, the respiratory rate increases to improve oxygen delivery. This mechanism is called the hypoxic ventilatory response. Increased respiratory rate causes hypocapnia (decreased carbon dioxide) and respiratory alkalosis, which limits further increases in respiratory rate. At this point, sleep disturbances characterized by periodic respirations are common. REM (rapid eye movement) sleep is impaired. Hypoxia can occur from periods of apnea. Within 24 to 48 hours of being at high altitude, the kidneys excrete the excess bicarbonate and enable the pH to return to normal, and ventilatory rate to again increase as an important compensatory response. Greater sympathetic nervous system activity increases heart rate, blood pressure, and cardiac output. Pulmonary artery pressure rises as an effect of generalized hypoxia-induced pulmonary vasoconstriction. Cerebral blood flow increases to maintain cerebral oxygen delivery. Hypoxia also induces red blood cell production by stimulating the release of erythropoietin. The result is an increase in hemoglobin concentration. Over time, polycythemia can develop in individuals who remain in a high altitude environment.

People who plan to ascend to high altitudes are advised to ascend slowly, over the course of days or even weeks, depending on the degree of elevation. Ascending too rapidly is the primary cause of altitude-related illness, mediated by the effects of hypoxia on the body. Altitude-related illness is more common in individuals who sleep at elevations above 8000 feet.

The three most significant clinical conditions that pose a risk to people at high altitude are acute mountain sickness (AMS), high altitude cerebral edema (HACE), and high altitude pulmonary edema (HAPE). These conditions may overlap in the same individual. The underlying pathophysiology is hypoxia. Although each syndrome has somewhat unique manifestations, the basic assessment and management approach is the same.

◆COLLABORATIVE MANAGEMENT

◆Assessment

Acute mountain sickness (AMS) is often the precursor to high altitude cerebral edema (HACE) and/or high altitude pulmonary edema (HAPE). AMS most often occurs in individuals who make a rapid ascent without acclimatization to altitudes above 8000 feet from altitudes below 5000 feet (Hackett & Roach, 2001). Again, the most important altitude effects occur when an individual who is not acclimated sleeps at elevations over 8000 feet. Assessment of the typical client with AMS reveals complaints of throbbing headache, anorexia, nausea, and vomiting. Feeling chilled, irritable, and apathetic are also symptoms associated with AMS. The syndrome produces effects similar to an alcohol-induced hangover. The client may relate a feeling of extreme illness. Vital signs are variable: the client can be tachycardic or bradycardic, have normal blood pressure, or have postural hypotension. The client may experience dyspnea both on exertion and at rest. Exertional dyspnea is expected as an individual adjusts to high altitude. However, dyspnea at rest is abnormal and may signal the onset of high altitude pulmonary edema.

If AMS progresses to **high altitude cerebral edema (HACE),** which is the extreme form of this disorder, the client will be physically unable to perform activities of daily living and will exhibit extreme apathy. A key sign of HACE is the development of ataxia without focal signs (Hackett & Roach, 2001). Clients have a change in mental status with confusion and impaired judgment. Cranial nerve dysfunction and seizures may occur. If untreated, a further decline in the client's level of consciousness ensues. Stupor, coma, and death can result from brain swelling and the subsequent damage caused by increased intracranial pressure over the course of 1 to 3 days.

High altitude pulmonary edema (HAPE) often appears in conjunction with HACE, but may occur during the progression of AMS within the first 2 to 4 days of a rapid ascent to high altitude, commonly on the second night. It is the most frequent cause of death associated with high altitude (Hackett & Roach, 2001). Clients notice poor exercise tolerance and a prolonged recovery time after exertion. Fatigue and weakness, as well as other signs and symptoms of AMS, are present. Important clinical indicators of HAPE include a persistent dry cough and cyanosis of the lips and nail beds. Tachycardia and tachypnea occur at rest. Rales may be auscultated in one or both lungs. Pink, frothy sputum is a late sign of HAPE. A chest x-ray demonstrates pulmonary infiltrates and pulmonary edema. Arterial blood gas analysis shows respiratory alkalosis and hypoxemia (decreased oxygen). Pneumonia also may be a concurrent finding. If a pulmonary artery catheter is inserted for hemodynamic monitoring, pulmonary artery pressure will be significantly elevated. The client may also have an elevated body temperature.

◆Interventions

FIRST AID. The most important intervention to manage serious altitude-related illnesses is descent to a lower altitude. Clients must be monitored carefully for any evidence of symptom progression. With mild AMS, the client should be allowed to rest and acclimate at the current altitude. The client must be instructed not ascend to a higher altitude, especially for sleep, until symptoms dissipate. If symptoms persist or worsen, the client should be moved to a lower altitude as soon as possible. Even a descent of about 1600 feet to 3300 feet may improve the client's condition and reverse altitude-related pathologic effects. Oxygen should also be administered if available to effectively treat symptoms of AMS.

HOSPITAL CARE. The oral medication acetazolamide (Diamox, Apo-Acetazolamide✱) is used to both prevent and treat AMS. Acetazolamide is a carbonic anhydrase inhibitor. It acts by causing a bicarbonate diuresis, which rids the body of excess fluid, and induces metabolic acidosis. The acidotic state increases respiratory rate and decreases the occurrence of periodic respiration during sleep at night. In this way it helps clients to acclimate faster to a high altitude. For best results, acetazolamide should be taken 24 hours before ascent and be continued for the first 2 days of the trip. Dosing regimens vary. The most common regimens involve taking 125 mg to 250 mg PO twice daily, or one 500 mg sustained-release capsule daily. Acetazolamide is a sulfa drug. It may cause hypersensitivity reactions in allergic individuals.

The other drug that may be helpful in the treatment of moderate to severe AMS is dexamethasone (Decadron, Deronil✱) 4 mg to 8 mg either orally or intramuscularly as an initial dose, then 4 mg every 6 hours while the client is undergoing descent to a lower altitude. This drug's mechanism of action is unclear for AMS treatment. It does not appear to speed acclimatization like acetazolamide, but it does relieve the symptoms of AMS. Symptoms may recur when the drug is stopped.

For the treatment of HACE, early recognition of ataxia or a change in level of consciousness should prompt a rapid descent by rescuers or companions to a lower altitude. While undergoing descent, the client can be given supplemental oxygen and dexamethasone 4 mg to 8 mg initially as an oral, IM, or IV dose, followed by 4 mg every 6 hours if available. If mental status is severely impaired and the client's airway is at risk, all drugs should be given parenterally. Loop diuretics such as furosemide (Lasix) may be prescribed to decrease brain swelling. Ultimately, the client with HACE must be admitted to the hospital. Critical care management may be necessary.

Like HACE, early recognition of HAPE is essential to improve the client's chance for survival. This is a serious condition that requires prompt evacuation to a lower altitude, oxygen administration, and bedrest to save the client's life. If descent must be delayed because of weather conditions or other factors, oxygen administration is essential as soon as possible. Cold stress must be avoided because it can increase pulmonary artery pressure. Keep the client warm at all times. Drugs are not substitutes for descent and oxygen. However, the treatment of HAPE may include administration of diuretics such as furosemide to reduce pulmonary edema, morphine, and vasodilators to decrease pulmonary vascular resistance. Hospital admission is warranted. In uncomplicated cases of HAPE, recovery occurs quickly but effects such as weakness and fatigue may persist for 2 weeks.

Chart 13-6 provides best practice strategies for preventing, recognizing, and treating altitude-related illnesses.

NEAR-DROWNING

PATHOPHYSIOLOGY

Drowning is a leading cause of accidental death in the United States. The victim dies by suffocation from submersion in a liquid medium (usually water). Although suffocation most commonly results from aspiration of fresh or salt water into the lungs, about 10% to 20% of victims experience laryngospasm with subsequent glottic closure followed by asphyxiation. **Near-drowning** is defined as recovery after submersion. Victims are typically children or adolescents. Males—more often engaged in risk-taking behavior—have a significantly greater incidence of drowning/near-drowning episodes than females.

HEALTH PROMOTION/ILLNESS PREVENTION

Prevention is key to avoiding near-drowning events. Common sense health teaching should include the following points:

- Maintain constant surveillance of children in or around water.
- Do not swim alone.
- Test the water depth before diving in head first; never dive into shallow water.
- Avoid alcoholic beverages when swimming, boating or while in proximity to water.
- Assure that water rescue equipment, such as life jackets, floatation devices, and rope, is immediately available when around water.

CHART 13-6

BEST PRACTICE for
Preventing, Recognizing, and Treating Altitude-Related Illnesses

- Plan a slow ascent to allow for acclimatization.
- Learn to recognize clinical manifestations of altitude-related illnesses.
- Avoid overexertion and overexposure to cold; rest at present altitude.
- Ensure adequate hydration and nutrition.
- Avoid alcohol and sleeping pills when at high altitude.
- For progressive or advanced acute mountain sickness (AMS), recognize symptoms and implement an immediate descent; provide oxygen at high concentration.
- To prevent the occurrence of AMS, discuss the use of acetazolamide (Diamox) with your health care provider.
- Protect skin and eyes from the sun's harmful ultraviolet rays at high altitude. Wear sunscreen (at least SPF 30) and high quality wraparound sunglasses or goggles.

COLLABORATIVE MANAGEMENT

Assessment

When water is aspirated into the lungs, the composition of the water is a key factor in the pathophysiology of the near-drowning event. Aspiration of fresh water causes surfactant to wash out of the lungs. Surfactant reduces surface tension within the alveoli, increases lung compliance and alveolar radius, and decreases the work of breathing. Loss of surfactant from fresh water aspiration destabilizes the alveoli and leads to increased airway resistance. Conversely, salt water—a hypertonic fluid—creates an osmotic gradient that draws protein-rich fluid from the vascular space into the alveoli. The consequences of both types of aspiration include impaired alveolar ventilation and resultant intrapulmonary shunting, which further compound the hypoxic state. Another concern is water quality during the near-drowning event. Client outcome may be negatively impacted by contaminants in the water such as chemicals, algae, microbes, sand, and mud. These substances can worsen lung injury and cause a lung infection.

Factors that help predict outcome for victims of near-drowning include the length of time submerged underwater, the degree of damage to the brain caused by hypoxia, the water temperature, client age, and health status. Very cold water seems to have a protective effect—especially for children. Successful resuscitations have been reported even after prolonged arrest intervals. Hypothermia offers some protection to the hypoxic brain by reducing cerebral metabolic rate. The diving reflex is a physiologic response to asphyxia, which produces bradycardia, a reduction in cardiac output, and vasoconstriction of vessels in the intestine, skeletal muscles, and kidney. These physiologic effects reduce myocardial oxygen consumption and enhance blood flow to the heart and cerebral tissues. Survival may be linked to some combination of the effects of hypothermia and the diving reflex.

The cause of the submersion should also be discerned if possible. The client may have suffered a medical condition or injury that precipitated the near-drowning event such as a seizure, myocardial infarction, stroke, or spinal cord injury while in the water. Injuries sustained from diving into shallow water or body surfing such as cervical spine trauma can also increase the difficulty of rescue and resuscitation efforts.

Interventions

FIRST AID. Immediate emergency care should focus on a safe rescue of the victim. Potential rescuers must consider their own swimming abilities and limitations as well as any natural or man-made hazards before attempting to save the victim; failure to do so could place additional lives in jeopardy. Once rescuers gain access to the victim, priorities include safe removal from the water while maintaining spine stabilization with a board or floatation device, and initiating airway clearance and ventilatory support measures. If hypothermia is a concern, gentle handling of the victim is essential to prevent ventricular fibrillation. There is no indication for attempts to get the water out of the victim's lungs. Abdominal thrusts should only be delivered if airway obstruction is suspected.

HOSPITAL CARE. Once the victim is safely removed from the water, airway and cardiopulmonary support interventions should ensue including oxygen administration, endotracheal intubation, and CPR if necessary. In the clinical setting, gastric decompression with a nasogastric or orogastric tube is indicated to prevent aspiration of gastric contents and improve ventilatory function. After a period of artificial ventilation by mask, the client typically has a distended abdomen, which impairs movement of the diaphragm and inhibits lung ventilation if it is not decompressed as described. Clients who experience near-drowning require complex care to support their body systems. The full spectrum of critical care technology may be needed to manage the physiologic derangements and sequelae of near-drowning, including pulmonary infection, acute respiratory distress syndrome (ARDS) and central nervous system impairment. The client's outcome may be difficult to predict in the early stages of care.

GET READY for the NCLEX Examination!

KEY POINTS

- Heat-related injuries can be mild (heat exhaustion) to severe (heat stroke), and can be easily prevented (see Chart 13-1).
- The priority for first aid for heat stroke, after a patent airway is established, is to cool the client as quickly as possible.
- North American pit vipers can be characterized by the triangular-shaped head and retractable fangs; nonpoisonous snakes do not have these features.
- The management of a client who has a snakebite depends on the severity of envenomation (see Table 13-1); both local and systemic manifestations can occur.
- The priority for first aid when a client has a snakebite is to decrease the venom circulation; do *not* use a tourniquet.
- Antivenom drugs are available for most types of poisonous snakebites; monitor for an allergic response when these medications are given.
- The bite of a brown recluse spider can cause tissue necrosis; in rare cases systemic manifestations can occur, including death.
- Cold applications, such as ice, should be used as first aid for poisonous spider bites.
- The venom of a bark scorpion is neurotoxic; monitor the client for signs of respiratory failure that may require mechanical ventilation.
- Single bee and wasp stings cause local reactions unless the person is allergic to them or received multiple stings.
- Arthropod bites and stings may be prevented through client education (see Chart 13-4).
- Epinephrine is the drug of choice for bee and wasp sting allergic reactions, followed by an antihistamine drug.
- The best way to prevent lightning injuries is to avoid places where lightning is likely to strike (see Chart 13-5).
- Lightning causes central nervous system and cardiovascular complications, as well as skin burns.
- Two common cold injuries are hypothermia and frostbite; both can be prevented by selecting appropriate layered clothing; cotton should not be worn.
- In moderate to severe cases of hypothermia, coagulopathy (abnormal clotting) or cardiac failure can occur.
- The priority for care of a client with a cold injury is warming; alcohol should be avoided.
- Frostbite can be mild (frostnip) to serious (fourth degree); severe frostbite can result in amputation due to tissue necrosis and gangrene.
- High altitude can cause a range of physiologic consequences in the body, primarily due to hypoxia.
- The priority for care of the client with illness related to high altitude is descent to a lower altitude.
- Acetazolamide (Diamox, Apo-Acetazolamide✱) is the drug of choice for prevention of mild altitude-related illness.
- Chart 13-6 outlines best practice strategies for preventing, recognizing, and treating altitude-related illnesses.
- Near-drowning victims often require cardiopulmonary support, including CPR.
- The client who has nearly drowned is at risk for pulmonary infection, ARDS, and central nervous system impairment.

ADDITIONAL STUDY RESOURCES

Go to your Student CD-ROM for Review Questions for the NCLEX Examination.

evolve Go to http://evolve.elsevier.com/Iggy/ for Integrated Management of Care Questions for the NCLEX Examination.

SELECTED BIBLIOGRAPHY

Asterisk indicates a classic or definitive work on this subject.

*American College of Surgeons Committee on Trauma. (1997). *Advanced trauma life support.* Chicago: Author.

Auerbach P.S. (2001). *Wilderness medicine: Management of wilderness and environmental emergencies* (4th ed.). St. Louis: Mosby.

Auerbach, P.S., Donner, H.J., & Weiss, E.A. (2003). *Field guide to wilderness medicine.* (2nd ed.). St. Louis: Mosby.

Bowman, W.D., et al. (Eds.). (2003). *Outdoor emergency care: Comprehensive prehospital care for nonurban settings* (4th ed.). Boston: Jones and Bartlett.

Boyer, L.V., McNally, J.T., & Binford, G.J. (2001). Spider bites. In P.S. Auerbach (Ed.), *Wilderness medicine* (4th ed., pp. 807-838). St. Louis: Mosby.

*Cacy, J., & Mold, J.W. (1999). The clinical characteristics of brown recluse spider bites treated by family physicians. *Journal of Family Practice, 48*(7), 536-542.

Cherington, M. (2003). Neurologic manifestations of lightning strike. *Neurology, 60,* 182-185.

Cooper, M.A., et al. (2001). Lightning injuries. In P.S. Auerbach (Ed.), *Wilderness medicine* (4th ed., pp. 73-110). St. Louis: Mosby.

Cummins, R.O. (Ed.). (2003). *ACLS: Principles and practice.* Dallas: American Heart Association.

*Dematte, J.E., et al. (1998). Near-fatal heat stroke during the 1995 heat wave in Chicago. *Annals of Internal Medicine, 129*(3), 173-181.

*Dinakaran, S., Desai, S.P., & Elsom, D.M. (1998). Telephone-mediated lightning injury causing cataract. *Injury, 29*(8), 645-646.

*Espaillat, A., Janigian, R., & To, K. (1999). Cataracts, bilateral macular holes, and rhegmatogenous retinal detachment induced by lightning. *American Journal of Ophthalmology, 127*(2), 216-217.

*Fahmy, S.F., et al. (1999). Lightning: The multisystem group injuries. *Journal of Trauma, 46*(5), 937-940.

First new management for poisonous snakebites in more than 50 years is now available: Biotechnology product provides safe and effective therapy for poisonous snake bites. (2001). *Clinical Nurse Specialist, 15*(3):121-123.

*Gentilello, L.M. (1999). Hypothermia in trauma. In D.D. Trunkey & F.R. Lewis (Eds.), *Current therapy of trauma* (4th ed., pp. 325-328). St. Louis: Mosby.

*Gold, B.S., & Wingert, W.A. (1994). Snake venom poisoning in the United States: A review of therapeutic practice. *Southern Medical Journal, 87*(6), 579-589.

Hackett, P.H., & Roach, R.C. (2001). High-altitude medicine. In P.S. Auerbach (Ed.), *Wilderness medicine* (4th ed., pp. 2-43). St. Louis: Mosby.

*Hoey, J. (1998). Hypothermia. *Canadian Medical Association Journal, 158*(2), 237.

*Holstege, C.P., et al. (1997). Crotalid snake envenomation. *Critical Care Clinics, 13*(4), 889-921.

Hutchinson, T.A., & Shahan, D.R. (Eds.). (2002). Polyvalent crotalid antivenin ovine Fab, *DRUGDEX(R) System.* Greenwood Village, CO: *MICROMEDEX.*

*Kanzenbach, T.L., & Dexter, W.W. (1999). Cold injuries. *Postgraduate Medicine, 105,*(1), 72-78.

*Krider, E.P., & Uman, M.A. (1995). Cloud-to-ground lightning: Mechanisms of damage and methods of protection. *Seminars in Neurology, 15*, 227-232.

*Laskowski-Jones, L. (1999). Responding to winter emergencies. *Dimensions of Critical Care Nursing, 18*(6), 13-21.

Laskowski-Jones L. (2000). Responding to summer emergencies. *Dimensions of Critical Care Nursing, 19*(4):2-12.

*Lazar, H.L. (1997). The treatment of hypothermia. *The New England Journal of Medicine, 337,* 1545-1547.

*Lee, R.C. (1997). Injury by electrical forces: Pathophysiology, manifestations, and therapy. *Current Problems in Surgery, 34*(9), 677-764.

*Lee, S. (1997). Envenomations II: Reptiles. *Toxtalk: A Publication of the Poison Control Center, 8(*1/2), 1-8. Philadelphia: Poison Control Center.

*Lewis, A.M.E. (1997). Understanding the principles of lightning injuries. *Journal of Emergency Nursing, 23*(6), 535-541.

*Lopez, R.E., & Holle, R.L. (1995). Demographics of lightning casualties. *Seminars in Neurology, 15*, 286-295.

**Morbidity & Mortality Weekly Report(MMWR)* (1998, May 22). Lightning-associated deaths–United States. *47*(19), 391-394.

Morris, J. (2003). Environmental emergencies. In L. Newberry (Ed.). *Sheehy's Emergency Nursing Principles and Practice* (5th ed., pp. 612-632). St. Louis: Mosby.

Norris, R.L., & Bush, S.P. (2001). North American venomous reptile bites. In P.S. Auerbach (Ed.), *Wilderness medicine* (4th ed., pp. 896-951). St. Louis: Mosby.

*Project Team of the Resuscitation Council (UK). (1999). Consensus guidelines: Emergency medical treatment of anaphylactic reactions. *Resuscitation, 41*, 93-99.

*Resnik, B.I., & Wetli, C.V. (1996). Lichtenberg figures. *American Journal of Forensic Medicine and Pathology, 17*(2), 99-102.

Suchard, J.R., & Connor, D.A. (2001). Scorpion envenomation. In P.S. Auerbach (Ed.), *Wilderness Medicine* (4th ed., pp. 839-862). St. Louis: Mosby.

Tisherman, S.A. (2002). Hypothermia, cold injury and drowning. In Peitzman, A.B., et al. (Eds.), *The trauma manual* (2nd ed., pp. 404-410). Philadelphia: Lippincott-Raven.

*van Zomeren, A.H., et al. (1998). Lightning stroke and neuropsychological impairment: cases and questions. *Journal of Neurology, Neurosurgery & Psychiatry, 64*(6), 763-769.

*Visscher, P.K., Vetter, R.S., & Camazine, S. (1996). Removing bee stings. *Lancet, 348*(9023), 301-302.

*Walpoth, B., et al. (1997). Outcome of survivors of accidental deep hypothermia and circulatory arrest treated with extracorporeal blood warming. *New England Journal of Medicine, 337*(21), 1500-1505.

*Watts, D.D. (1998). Hypothermic coagulopathy in trauma: Effect of varying levels of hypothermia on enzyme speed, platelet function, and fibrinolytic activity. *Journal of Trauma, 44*, 846-854.

UNIT **FOUR**

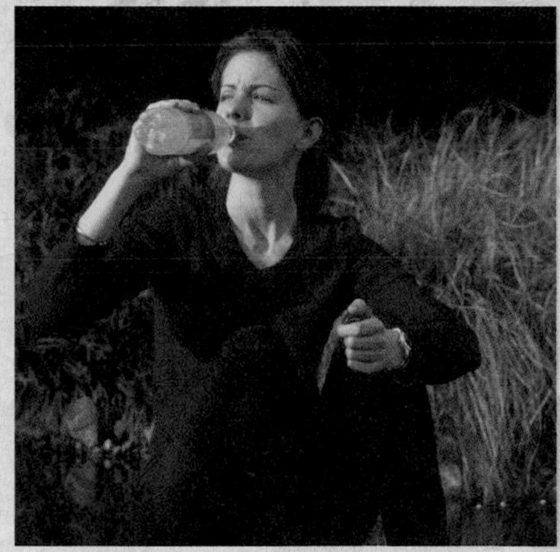

MANAGEMENT of CLIENTS with FLUID, ELECTROLYTE, and ACID-BASE IMBALANCES

CHAPTER

14 Fluid and Electrolyte Balance

M. LINDA WORKMAN

LEARNING OUTCOMES

After studying this chapter, you should be able to:

1. Explain why women and older adults have less total body water than do men and younger adults.
2. Interpret whether a client's serum electrolyte values are normal, elevated, or low.
3. Describe the expected blood volume responses when isotonic, hypertonic, or hypotonic intravenous fluids are infused.
4. Describe the expected blood osmolarity responses when isotonic, hypertonic, or hypotonic intravenous fluids are infused.
5. Explain the relationships between antidiuretic hormone, urine output volume, and osmolarity.
6. Analyze a client's hydration status on the basis of physical assessment findings.
7. Evaluate a client's food choices for sodium content.
8. Evaluate a client's food choices for potassium content.
9. Evaluate a client's food choices for calcium content.

Go to your Student CD-ROM for Review Questions for the NCLEX Examination keyed to these Learning Outcomes.

HOMEOSTASIS

The human body works best when some conditions are kept within a narrow range of normal. Examples of such conditions include body temperature, blood electrolyte values (e.g., sodium, potassium, and calcium), blood pH, and blood volume. No body system works well if 2 liters of blood volume are gained or lost. To keep conditions as close to normal as possible (a situation called **homeostasis**), the body has many safeguards or control mechanisms **(homeostatic mechanisms)** to prevent dangerous changes. For example, if a person is in a hot room (e.g., 110° F) and does not have good homeostatic mechanisms, his or her body temperature could go as high as 110° F, resulting in death. The homeostatic mechanisms of sweating to cool by evaporation and dilating blood vessels to expel body heat help to prevent body temperature from rising much more than 1° F above the normal 98.6° F, keeping body temperature in the normal range.

One very important area for homeostasis is maintaining the body's normal fluid volume and composition. Water is the most common substance in the body, making up about 55% to 60% of total adult body weight. This water (fluid) is divided into two spaces or compartments, the **extracellular fluid (ECF)** and the fluid inside the cells, the **intracellular fluid (ICF).** The ECF space contains about one third (15 L) of total body water. This space includes **interstitial fluid** (fluid between cells, sometimes called the "third space"), blood, lymph, bone, and connective tissue water, and the transcellular fluids. **Transcellular fluids** are the fluids in special body spaces and include cerebrospinal fluid, synovial fluid, peritoneal fluid, and pleural fluid. ICF contains the remaining two thirds (25 L) of total body water. Figure 14-1 shows the normal distribution of total body water.

Water is needed to deliver dissolved nutrients, electrolytes, and other substances to all organs, tissues, and cells. Most physiologic processes occur only in a watery environment. In the healthy adult, the volume of water in the fluid compartments remains within the normal range although the water moves constantly between compartments. Changes in either the amount of water or the amount of electrolytes in body fluids can affect the functioning of all cells, tissues, and organs. For proper function, the volume of all body fluids and the types and amount of dissolved substances must be carefully controlled.

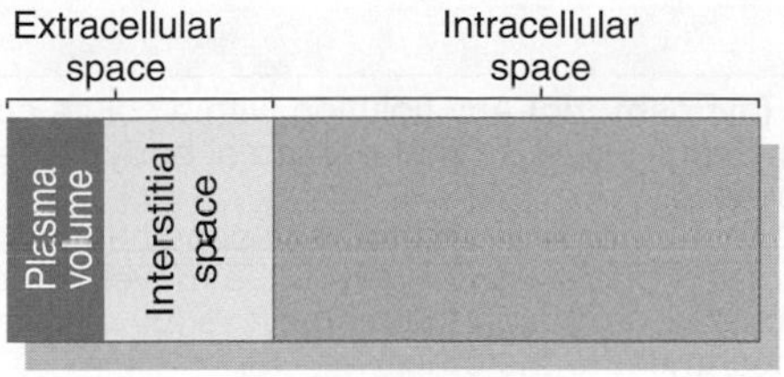

Figure 14-1 ■ Normal distribution of total body water.

ANATOMY AND PHYSIOLOGY REVIEW

Physiologic Influences on Fluid and Electrolyte Balance

Many processes control normal fluid and electrolyte balance. These processes work together to maintain balance so the internal environment remains stable even when the external environment changes.

Knowing the terms related to solutions helps to understand the processes involved in fluid and electrolyte balance (Table 14-1). Body fluids are composed of water and particles dissolved or suspended in water. The **solvent** is the water portion of fluids. **Solutes** are the particles dissolved or suspended in the water. Solutes vary in type and amount from one fluid space to another. Proper function is dependent on keeping the correct balance of fluid and electrolytes within each body fluid space.

Important processes involved in fluid and electrolyte balance include filtration, diffusion, osmosis, and active transport. These processes determine how, when, and where fluids and particles move across cell membranes.

FILTRATION

Definition

Filtration is the movement of fluid through a cell or blood vessel membrane because of hydrostatic pressure differences on both sides of the membrane. Basically, filtration depends on differences in water volume pressing against confining walls.

All fluid has weight. Fluid weight in a confined space is related to the amount of fluid present in that area. Water molecules in a confined space constantly press outward against the confining walls. **Hydrostatic pressure** is the force of the weight of water molecules pressing against the confining walls of a space. Hydrostatic pressure is a "water-pushing" pressure, because it is the force that pushes water outward from a confined space through a membrane (Figure 14-2).

Physiologic Activity

Water is the largest part of any body fluid. The amount of water in any body fluid space determines the hydrostatic pressure of that space. The amount of water in a fluid is inversely (negatively) related to the **viscosity** (thickness) of that fluid. Thus more water and less solute decrease viscosity, and less water with more solute increases viscosity. Blood, a viscous fluid ("thicker" than water), is confined within the blood vessels. Blood has hydrostatic pressure because of its weight and volume and because the heart is pumping blood into the arterial circulation.

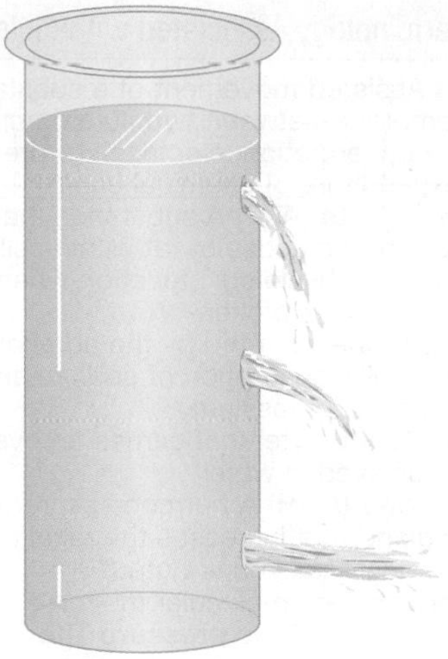

Figure 14-2 ■ Hydrostatic pressure. The pressure that water molecules exert against the sides of the container is highest where the weight of the water is greatest. (From Nave, C., & Nave, B. [1985]. Hydrostatic pressure. In *Physics for health sciences* [3rd ed.]. Philadelphia: W.B. Saunders.)

The hydrostatic pressures of two fluid spaces can be compared whenever a **permeable** (porous) membrane separates the two spaces. If the hydrostatic pressure is the same in both fluid spaces, a state of **equilibrium** (no difference between the two spaces) exists for hydrostatic pressure. If the hydrostatic pressure is not the same in both spaces, **disequilibrium** exists. This means that the two spaces have a **gradient,** or a graded difference, of hydrostatic pressure: one space has a higher hydrostatic pressure than the other. Because the human body constantly seeks equilibrium, a gradient forces movement on both sides of the membrane until an equilibrium exists (Figure 14-3).

In most instances, substances move from the greater amount of pressure or concentration to the lesser amount. Thus when a hydrostatic pressure gradient exists between two fluid spaces, fluid from the space with the higher hydrostatic pressure moves **(filters)** through the membrane into the space with the lower hydrostatic pressure. This filtration continues only as long as the hydrostatic pressure gradient exists. Equilibrium is reached when enough fluid leaves one space and enters the other space to make the hydrostatic pressure in both spaces equal.

When the two spaces are in equilibrium for hydrostatic pressure, a gradient no longer exists between them. Although water molecules may be exchanged evenly between two spaces in equilibrium, no net filtration of fluid occurs. In equilibrium, neither space gains nor loses water molecules, and the hydrostatic pressure in both spaces remains the same.

Clinical Function and Significance

Blood pressure is a hydrostatic filtering force measured in millimeters of mercury (mm Hg). It moves whole blood from the heart to tissue areas where filtration can occur. Filtration is important for the exchange of water, nutrients, and waste products when blood arrives at the tissue capillaries. One factor that determines whether or not fluid leaves the

TABLE 14-1 Terminology Associated with Fluid and Electrolyte Balance

active transport Assisted movement of a substance through a permeable membrane between two fluid compartments; occurs against a concentration, electrical, or pressure gradient; requires the expenditure of chemical energy
adenosine triphosphate (ATP) A substance that is generated by the metabolism of glucose or fat within cells and releases chemical energy for physiologic function when a high-energy phosphate bond (~P) is broken
aldosterone A hormone secreted by the adrenal cortex that stimulates the renal reabsorption of sodium and water and the renal excretion of potassium
anion A molecule (electrolyte) that carries an overall negative charge when dissolved in water
antidiuretic hormone (ADH) A hormone secreted from the posterior pituitary gland that increases the renal reabsorption of pure water and decreases urine output
brownian motion Inherent molecular motion
capillary (plasma) hydrostatic pressure The force generated by fluid within a capillary that tends to move fluid out from the capillary and into the interstitial space
capillary (plasma) osmotic pressure The force generated by the concentration of plasma solutes (osmotic and oncotic pressures) that tends to retain fluid within the capillary or move fluid from the interstitial space into the capillary
cation A molecule (electrolyte) that carries an overall positive charge when dissolved in water
cofactor A substance required to enhance the activity of an enzyme or a physiologic reaction
colloidal oncotic pressure The osmotic pressure exerted by the concentration of colloids (proteins) within a solution
diffusion Unimpeded movement of a substance through a permeable membrane between two fluid compartments; occurs down a concentration gradient; does not require the expenditure of chemical energy
disequilibrium A state in which two fluid compartments are unequal in at least one characteristic
electrolytes Substances that carry an electrical charge when dissolved in water
electroneutrality A state in which a body fluid has an equal number of cations and anions so that the fluid does not express an electrical charge
equilibrium A state in which two fluid compartments are equal in one or more characteristics
extracellular fluid (ECF) Body fluid present outside of cells; includes plasma, interstitial fluid, and transcellular fluid
facilitated diffusion Assisted movement of a substance through a permeable membrane between two fluid compartments; occurs down a concentration gradient; does not require the expenditure of chemical energy
filtration The movement of fluid through a biologic membrane as a result of hydrostatic pressure differences on the two sides of the membrane
gradient A graded difference in some characteristic between two fluid compartments
hydrostatic pressure The force of pressure exerted by static water in a confined space—"water-pushing" pressure
hypertonic (hyperosmotic) Any solution with a solute concentration (osmolarity) greater than that of normal body fluids (>310 mOsm/L)
hypotonic (hyposmotic) Any solution with a solute concentration (osmolarity) less than that of normal body fluids (<270 mOsm/L)
impermeable membrane A membrane separating two fluid compartments that does not permit the movement of one or more substances through the membrane (by diffusion) from one compartment to the other
insensible fluid loss Unregulated fluid losses from the skin, gastrointestinal tract, wounds, and pulmonary epithelium
interstitial fluid Fluid present in tissues between cells
intracellular fluid (ICF) Fluid found inside cells
isotonic (isosmotic) Any solution with a solute concentration equal to the osmolarity of normal body fluids or normal saline (0.9% NaCl), about 300 mOsm/L
natriuretic peptide (NP) A hormone secreted by cardiac atrial cells that increases the renal excretion of sodium and water
obligatory urine output The minimal amount of urine output necessary to ensure the excretion of metabolic wastes (about 400 mL/day)
osmolality The concentration of solute within a solution as measured by the amount of solute osmoles per kilogram of solvent
osmolarity The concentration of solute within a solution as measured by the amount of solute osmoles per liter of solution
osmoreceptor Specialized sensory nerve cells in the thalamus or hypothalamus that are sensitive to changes in the osmolarity of extracellular fluid
osmosis Diffusion of water (no other substance) through a selectively permeable membrane from an area of lower osmotic pressure to an area of greater osmotic pressure
osmotic pressure The pressure exerted by a solution that contains a relatively high concentration of solute; this pressure draws water from areas or compartments with lower concentrations of solute into the areas or compartments with higher concentrations of solute—"water-pulling" pressure
permeable membrane A membrane separating two fluid compartments that permits the movement of one or more substances through the membrane (by diffusion) from one compartment to the other
solubility The degree to which any given solute completely dissolves (dissociates) in water
solute The solid particles dissolved in a solution
solvent The fluid (water) portion of a solution
tissue hydrostatic pressure (THP) The force generated by fluid within the interstitial spaces that tends to move fluid into the capillary from the interstitial space
tissue osmotic pressure (TOP) The force generated by the concentration of interstitial fluid solutes that tends to retain fluid in the interstitial space or move fluid from the capillary into the interstitial space
transcellular fluid Extracellular fluid confined to a specific area or region of the body (cerebrospinal fluid, pericardial fluid, visceral fluid, aqueous humor, peritoneal fluid, and pleural fluid)
viscosity Gumminess or thickness of the molecules in a solution, causing friction within that solution

blood vessels and enters the tissue spaces **(interstitial fluid)** is the difference between the hydrostatic pressure of capillary blood and that of the interstitial fluid.

The lining of the capillaries is only one cell layer thick. Therefore the "wall" that holds blood in the capillaries is thin. Large spaces **(pores)** between the cells in the capillary membrane help water filter freely through capillary membranes in either direction if a hydrostatic pressure gradient is present (Figure 14-4).

Edema (tissue swelling with fluid collection) develops with changes in normal hydrostatic pressure differences, such as in clients with right-sided heart failure. In this con-

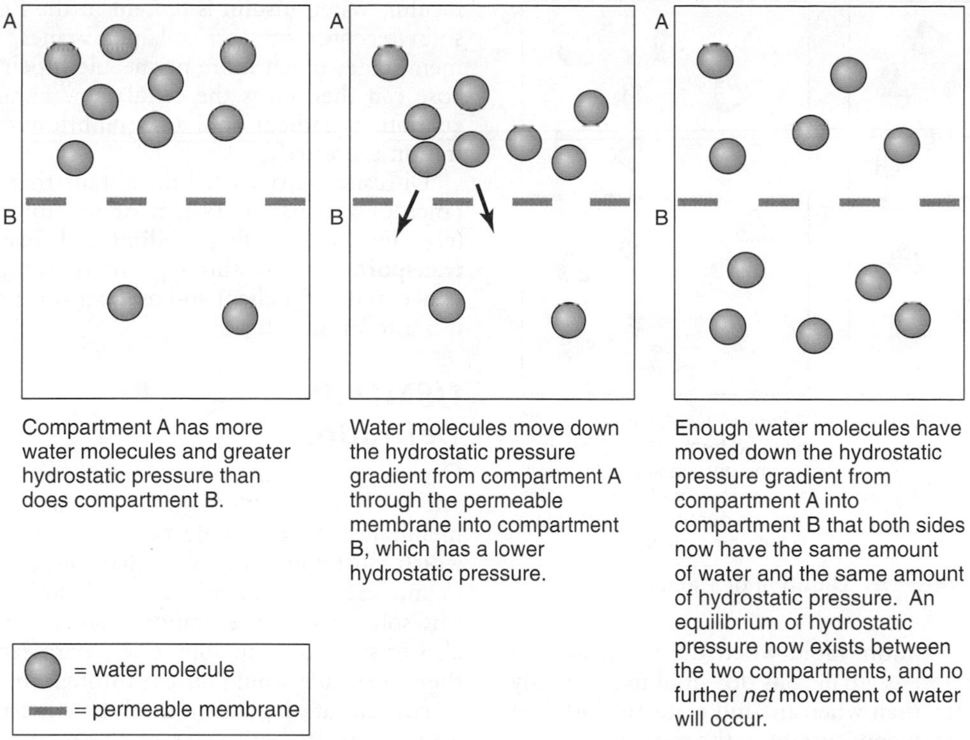

Figure 14-3 ■ The process of filtration. (© 1992. M. Linda Workman. All rights reserved.)

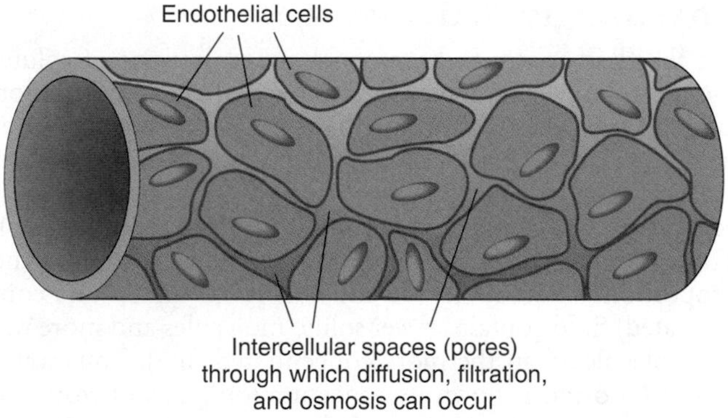

Figure 14-4 ■ The basic structure of a capillary.

dition, the volume of blood in the right side of the heart increases greatly because the right ventricle is too weak to pump blood efficiently into the pulmonary blood vessels. As blood backs up into the venous system, venous hydrostatic pressure rises. The increased venous pressure causes capillary hydrostatic pressure to increase until it is higher than the hydrostatic pressure in the interstitial space. Excess filtration of fluid from the capillaries into the interstitial tissue space occurs, forming visible edema.

DIFFUSION

Definition

Diffusion is the free movement of particles (solute) across a permeable membrane down a **concentration gradient,** that is, from an area of higher concentration to an area of lower concentration. Diffusion controls the movement of solute particles in solution across various body membranes.

Physiologic Activity

The diffusion of particles into and out of cells and body fluid spaces occurs via **brownian motion,** the kinetic energy of molecular motion. Brownian motion is the vibration of single molecules caused by electrons orbiting at the core of each molecule. Such motion causes totally random movement of molecules, which collide or bump into each other within a confined space. Each collision increases the speed of molecular movement.

As a result of the collisions, molecules in a solution spread out evenly through the available space. They move from an area of higher amounts (concentration) of molecules to an area of lower amounts until equal amounts are present in all areas. The number of collisions is related to the concentration of molecules in a confined space. Spaces with many molecules have more collisions and faster molecule movement than spaces with fewer molecules.

A concentration gradient exists when two fluid spaces have different amounts of the same type of molecules. Brownian motion of the molecules causes them to move down the concentration gradient. As a result of brownian motion, any membrane that separates two spaces is struck repeatedly by molecules. When the molecule strikes a pore in the membrane that is large enough for it to pass through, diffusion occurs (Figure 14-5). The chance of any single molecule colliding with the membrane and going through a pore is much greater on the side of the membrane with a higher molecule concentration.

The speed of diffusion is related to the concentration gradient (difference in amount) between the two sides of the membrane. The degree of concentration difference is known as the *steepness* of the gradient: The larger the concentration difference between the two sides, the steeper the

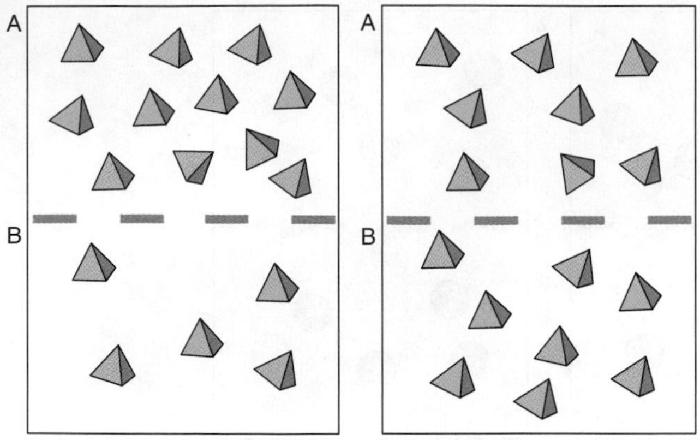

The concentration of solute is greater on side A than on side B, with a permeable membrane separating the two compartments.

Solute molecules have diffused from side A through the membrane into side B until an equilibrium of solute exists and the concentration of solute is the same on both sides.

Figure 14-5 ■ Diffusion of a solute.

gradient. Diffusion is more rapid when the concentration gradient is steeper (just as a ball rolls downhill more rapidly when the hill is steep than when the hill is nearly flat). The greater the difference in concentration, the more rapidly diffusion occurs from the area of higher concentration to the area of lower concentration.

Diffusion of solute particles continues through the membrane as long as a concentration gradient exists between the two sides of the membrane. *When the concentration of solute is the same on both sides of the membrane, an equilibrium exists and only an equal exchange (not a net movement) of solute continues.*

Clinical Function and Significance

Diffusion is important in the transport of gases and in the movement of most electrolytes, atoms, and molecules through cell membranes. Unlike capillary membranes, which permit the diffusion of most small-sized substances down a concentration gradient, cell membranes are *selective.* They permit the movement of some substances and inhibit the movement of other substances. Some molecules cannot move across a cell membrane, even when a steep "downhill" gradient exists, because the membrane is **impermeable** (not porous) to that molecule. Thus the concentration gradient is maintained across the membrane.

Impermeability and special transport systems cause differences in the concentrations of specific substances from one fluid compartment to another. For example, usually the fluid outside of the cells, the **extracellular fluid (ECF),** contains almost 10 times more sodium ions than the fluid inside the cell, the **intracellular fluid (ICF).** This extreme concentration difference is caused by the impermeability of the cell membrane to sodium and from a special "sodium pump" that moves any extra sodium out of the cell "uphill" against its concentration gradient and back into the ECF.

In some instances diffusion cannot occur without help, even down steep concentration gradients, because of membrane selectivity. A clinical example is the fact that, even though the amount of glucose is much higher in the ECF than in the ICF (creating a steep gradient for glucose), glucose cannot cross most cell membranes without the help of insulin. When insulin is present in the ECF, it binds to insulin receptor sites on cell membranes, which makes the membranes much more permeable (open) to glucose. Glucose can then cross the cellular membrane down its concentration gradient until an equilibrium of glucose concentration is created.

Diffusion across a cell membrane that requires the assistance of a transport system or membrane-altering system (e.g., insulin) is called **facilitated diffusion** or **facilitated transport.** Because this type of transport occurs down a concentration gradient and requires no energy from the cell, it is a form of diffusion.

OSMOSIS

Definition

Osmosis is the movement of water only (solvent) through a selectively permeable membrane. For osmosis to occur, a membrane must separate two fluid spaces, at least one of which must contain a solute that cannot move through the membrane. (The membrane is therefore impermeable to this solute.) A concentration gradient of this solute must also exist. If the membrane was permeable to this solute, then the solute would diffuse through the membrane down its concentration gradient until the concentrations of solute were equal on both sides of the membrane. Because the membrane is impermeable to the solute, these particles cannot cross the membrane, but water molecules can.

Physiologic Activity

For the fluid spaces to have equal concentrations of solute, the water molecules must move down their concentration gradient from the side with the higher concentration of water molecules (and thus a lower concentration of solute molecules) to the side with the lower concentration of water molecules (and thus a higher concentration of solute molecules). This movement continues until both spaces contain the same proportions of solute to solvent. The more dilute (less concentrated) fluid contains fewer solute molecules and more water molecules than the more concentrated fluid. Thus water moves by osmosis down its concentration gradient from the area of more dilute solute to the area of more concentrated solute until a new equilibrium occurs (Figure 14-6).

At this point, the concentrations of solute in the fluid spaces (the proportion of solute to solvent) on both sides of the membrane are equal, even though the total numbers of solute and volume of water may be different. This equilibrium occurs by the movement of water molecules rather than the movement of solute molecules.

Factors that determine whether and how fast osmosis occurs include the overall concentration of particles (solute) in solution, how easily the solute dissolves in water **(solubility),** and the amount of membrane available for osmosis.

CONCENTRATION OF SOLUTE

The concentration of particles in body fluids is expressed in milliequivalents per liter (mEq/L), millimoles per liter (mmol/L), and milliosmoles per liter (mOsm/L). Osmoles and milliosmoles are used to describe the total amount of solute particles (including electrolytes) contained in a solution. The number of milliosmoles present in body fluids is expressed as either osmolarity or osmolality.

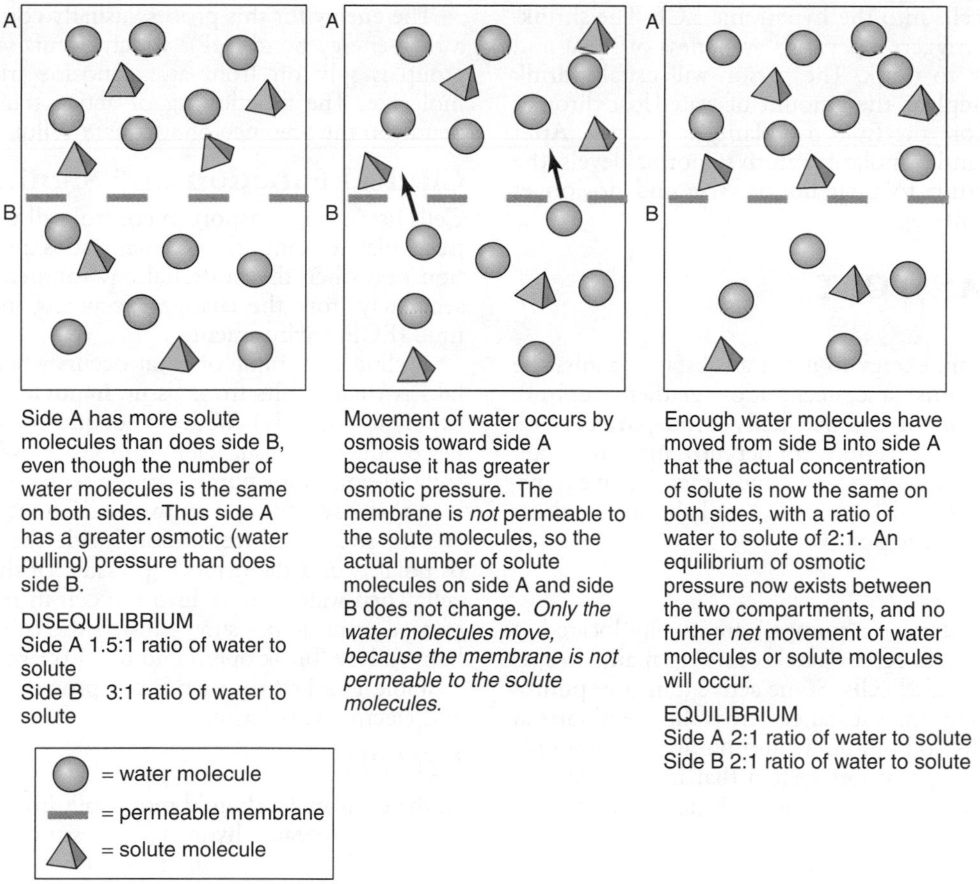

Figure 14-6 ■ The process of osmosis.

Osmolarity is the number of milliosmoles in a *liter* of solution; **osmolality** is the number of milliosmoles in a *kilogram* of solution. The normal osmolarity value for plasma and other body fluids ranges from 270 to 300 mOsm/L.

The body functions best when the osmolarity of the fluids in all body fluid spaces is close to 300 mOsm/L. Many mechanisms work to keep the solute concentration at or near optimum levels. When all body fluids have this solute concentration, the osmotic pressures (water-pulling) of the two fluid compartments are equal, and no *net* water movement occurs. In this situation, the body fluids are **isosmotic** to each other. Another term with the same meaning is **isotonic** (sometimes called **normotonic**). Examples of specific intravenous (IV) solutions with overall solute concentrations equaling 270 to 300 mOsm/L include 0.9% sodium chloride in water and Ringer's lactate in water. Because these solutions are isotonic (or isosmotic) to plasma, their addition to plasma does not change the osmolarity or osmotic pressure of the plasma.

Fluids with osmolarities (solute concentrations) greater than 300 mOsm/L are **hyperosmotic,** or **hypertonic,** compared with isosmotic fluids. Hyperosmotic fluids have a greater osmotic pressure than do isosmotic fluids and tend to pull water from the isosmotic fluid space into the hyperosmotic fluid space until an osmotic balance occurs.

Fluids with osmolarities of less than 270 mOsm/L are **hypo-osmotic,** or **hypotonic,** compared with isosmotic fluids. Hypo-osmolar fluids have a lower or smaller osmotic pressure than isosmotic fluids. As a result, water tends to be pulled from the hypo-osmotic fluid space into the isosmotic fluid space until an osmotic balance occurs.

SOLUBILITY OF SOLUTE

Solubility is the degree to which a solute dissolves in water. Solubility is related to osmotic pressure: The greater the solubility of the solutes in a fluid, the higher the osmotic pressure of that fluid.

AMOUNT OF AVAILABLE MEMBRANE

The greater the amount of membrane available for osmosis, the faster the rate of osmosis. More membrane increases the chances that water molecules will hit the membrane at a point where penetration is possible.

Clinical Function and Significance

Osmosis and filtration act together in capillary fluid dynamics to control both extracellular fluid (ECF) and intracellular fluid (ICF) volumes. The thirst mechanism is an example of how osmosis helps maintain homeostasis. The feeling of thirst is caused by the activation of cells in the brain that respond to changes in extracellular fluid (ECF) osmolarity. These cells are so sensitive to changes in ECF osmolarity that they are called *osmoreceptors.* When a person loses body water but most of the solute remains, such as through excessive sweating during exercise, ECF volume is decreased and osmolarity is increased (hypertonic conditions exist). The cells in the thirst center shrink as water moves from the cells into the hypertonic ECF. The shrinking of these cells triggers a person's awareness of thirst and increases the urge to drink. The person will usually drink enough fluid to replace the amount of water lost through sweating and restore the ECF osmolarity to normal. After the ECF volume and osmolarity return to normal levels, the osmoreceptors return to their normal size and no longer send stimulatory messages.

ACTIVE TRANSPORT

Definition

A cell must use extra energy to move a substance across the cell membrane against a concentration gradient (uphill). This type of movement is called **active transport** because the cell must make active efforts for net movement to occur. Because of its energy use and uphill movement, active transport is sometimes called "pumping," and the mechanisms are known as membrane pumps.

Physiologic Activity

Active transport systems or "pumps," are usually located in the cell membrane and act as "gatekeepers" to maintain special environments inside cells. Some active transport pumps can carry more than one substance across the membrane at the same time. The sodium-potassium pump is an example of a common active transport system that moves two substances at the same time in opposite directions against concentration gradients.

Sodium diffuses slightly down its concentration gradient into the intracellular fluid (ICF) because it has such a high extracellular fluid (ECF) concentration compared with its ICF concentration. Similarly, because potassium has such a high concentration inside the cells compared with its concentration in ECF, it diffuses slightly down its concentration gradient into the ECF. The action of the sodium-potassium pump moves the extra sodium out of the cell and returns the lost potassium back into the cell. The sodium-potassium pump requires the use of cellular energy.

The energy for this process usually comes from breaking a high-energy bond ($\sim$P), which occurs when a phosphate group is split off from an adenosine triphosphate (ATP) molecule. The functioning of active transport pumps depends on the presence of adequate cellular ATP.

Clinical Function and Significance

Cells use active transport to control cell volume and the intracellular concentration of many substances. All cells function best when their internal environments are maintained separately from the changes occurring in the extracellular fluid (ECF) environment.

A clinical example of what occurs when active transport fails is what results from tissue **hypoxia** (decreased oxygen supply in the body). Without adequate oxygen, ATP cannot be produced in sufficient amounts. Without ATP, the sodium-potassium pump cannot remove the extra sodium ions that have diffused from the ECF into the cell. The increased sodium concentration inside the cell increases the osmolarity and the osmotic pressure of the fluid inside the cell. Then water moves into the cell in response to the increased osmotic pressure, causing the cell to swell and perhaps to **lyse** (break open) and die if oxygen is not provided.

Table 14-2 lists the membrane processes involved in fluid and electrolyte balance.

LYMPH

At the capillary level, fluid moves out from the capillary at its arterial end (because hydrostatic pressure is greater there) into the interstitial space, and moves from the interstitial space back into the capillary at the venous end. In most cases, not all of the fluid that leaves the capillary at the arterial end and enters the interstitial space is returned to the capillary at the venous end. A small amount remains in the tissues. If this situation is not balanced by another mechanism to return the fluid to the systemic circulation, blood volume would become depleted and the interstitial areas would constantly be edematous. Instead, this extra fluid leaking out from the capillaries is returned to the systemic circulation as **lymph.**

TABLE 14-2 Summary of Membrane-Fluid Actions

Action	Definition	Specific Characteristics
Filtration	The movement of fluid through a biologic membrane as a result of hydrostatic pressure differences on both sides of the membrane	Does not require energy Is limited to solvent and low–molecular weight solute Usually occurs from capillaries to the interstitial fluid Depends on hydrostatic pressure differences Occurs more rapidly with steep gradients
Diffusion	The free movement of substances across a permeable membrane and down a concentration gradient	Does not require energy Is not pressure dependent Moves solute and solvent down their individual gradients Occurs more rapidly with steep gradients Is directly related in speed to the amount of membrane available Occurs in both directions across capillary and cell membranes Is responsible for maintaining tissue nutrition
Osmosis	The process by which only the *solvent* diffuses through a selectively permeable membrane	Does not require energy Involves movement of water only Depends on hydrostatic and osmotic pressures Occurs more rapidly with steep gradients
Active transport	The movement of a substance across a selectively permeable membrane and against a concentration, electrical, or pressure gradient	Requires energy Requires a transport system (pump) Helps to maintain a special intracellular environment

Lymph fluid is similar to blood plasma (from which it is formed) but contains far less protein. It is returned to the circulation by lymph vessels, or **lymphatics.** Lymphatics begin as small, thin-walled, veinlike vessels that join to form larger lymphatic vessels. Two large groups of lymphatic vessels connect the entire lymph system with the general circulatory system. The left thoracic lymph duct drains lymph from the abdomen, gastrointestinal tract, pelvis, lower extremities, left side of the thorax, left arm, and left side of the head and neck into the left subclavian vein at the point where it joins the left internal jugular vein (Figure 14-7). Lymph from the right arm, right side of the chest, and right side of the head and neck drains into the right subclavian vein through three lymph ducts. Lymph nodes are situated along the lymphatic paths and filter the lymph fluid.

Lymphatics carry lymph fluid in one direction: toward the heart. Lymph flow is slower than blood flow because lymph has no pump. Lymph flow is enhanced by skeletal muscle contractions, intrathoracic pressure changes during breathing, and a peristalsis-like motion in the lymph vessels.

Hormonal Regulation of Fluid and Electrolyte Balance

The endocrine system helps control fluid and electrolyte balance. Three hormones that help control these critical balances are aldosterone, antidiuretic hormone (ADH), and natriuretic peptide (NP).

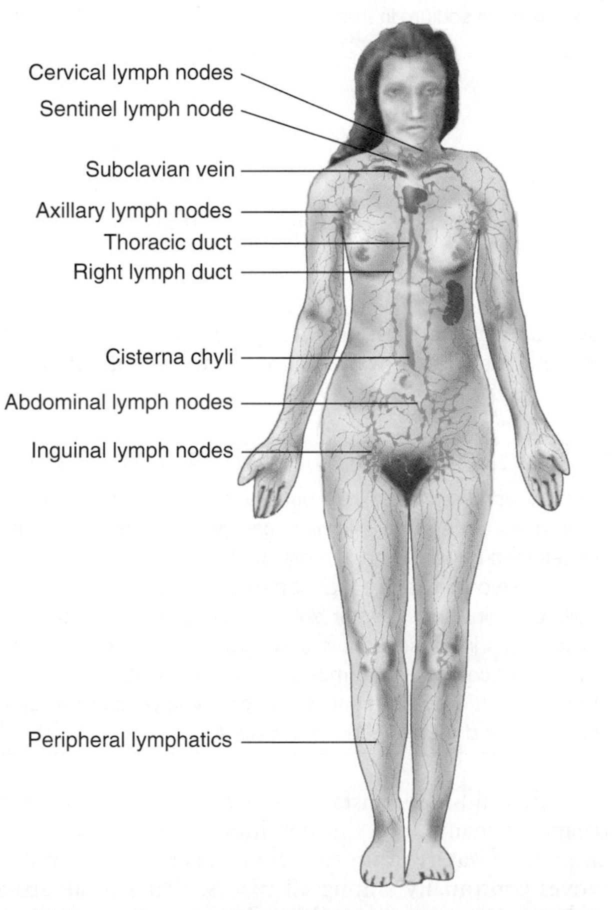

Figure 14-7 ■ Patterns of lymph drainage. (From Guyton, A., & Hall, J. [1996]. *Textbook of medical physiology* [9th ed.]. Philadelphia, W.B. Saunders.)

ALDOSTERONE

Aldosterone is a hormone secreted by the adrenal cortex. Aldosterone secretion is stimulated by either a decreased sodium level in the extracellular fluid (ECF) or an increased sodium level in urine. The secretion and function of aldosterone, angiotensinogen, and angiotensin are outlined in Figure 14-8. Aldosterone protects sodium balance by preventing sodium loss. Because sodium in body fluids exerts osmotic (water-pulling) pressure, water attempts to follow sodium in proportionate amounts. As a result of this sodium-water relationship, aldosterone secretion also helps regulate water balance.

In the kidney, blood is supplied to the nephrons via the afferent arteriole. Specialized cells **(juxtaglomerular cells)** inside the afferent arteriole near the nephron glomerulus are sensitive to changes in blood sodium levels. This area of the afferent arteriole touches a special area of the distal convoluted tubule (the **macula densa**). Together, the juxtaglomerular cells and the macula densa form the **juxtaglomerular complex.** When this complex senses that blood sodium levels are lower than normal or that the total blood volume is low, the macula densa triggers juxtaglomerular cells to secrete **renin.**

Renin acts on a plasma protein called **renin substrate** (formerly called **angiotensinogen),** converting it to angiotensin I. Angiotensin I is then further converted into angiotensin II by an enzyme called angiotensin-converting enzyme (ACE). **Angiotensin II** constricts many blood vessels and stimulates aldosterone secretion from the adrenal cortex.

Aldosterone acts on the distal tubules of the nephrons, triggering these areas to reabsorb sodium from the urine back into the blood. This action increases blood osmolarity. Aldosterone secretion increases when blood osmolarity or sodium levels are low, and its presence is normally needed to prevent excessive renal excretion of sodium. Aldosterone secretion also helps prevent blood potassium levels from becoming too high. Aldosterone secretion is stopped when blood osmolarity or serum sodium levels are greater than normal.

ANTIDIURETIC HORMONE

Antidiuretic hormone (ADH), or **vasopressin,** is produced in the brain and stored in the posterior pituitary gland. ADH release from the posterior pituitary gland is controlled by the hypothalamus in response to changes in blood osmolarity. The hypothalamus contains specialized cells **(osmoreceptors)** that are sensitive to changes in blood osmolarity. Increased blood osmolarity, especially an increase in the level of plasma sodium, results in a slight shrinkage of these cells and triggers ADH release from the posterior pituitary gland.

ADH acts directly on kidney tubules and collecting ducts, making them more permeable to water. As a result, more water is reabsorbed by these tubules and returned to the blood, decreasing blood osmolarity by making it more dilute. When blood osmolarity decreases, especially when the plasma sodium level is below normal, the osmoreceptors swell slightly and inhibit ADH release. Less water is then reabsorbed and more is lost from the body in the

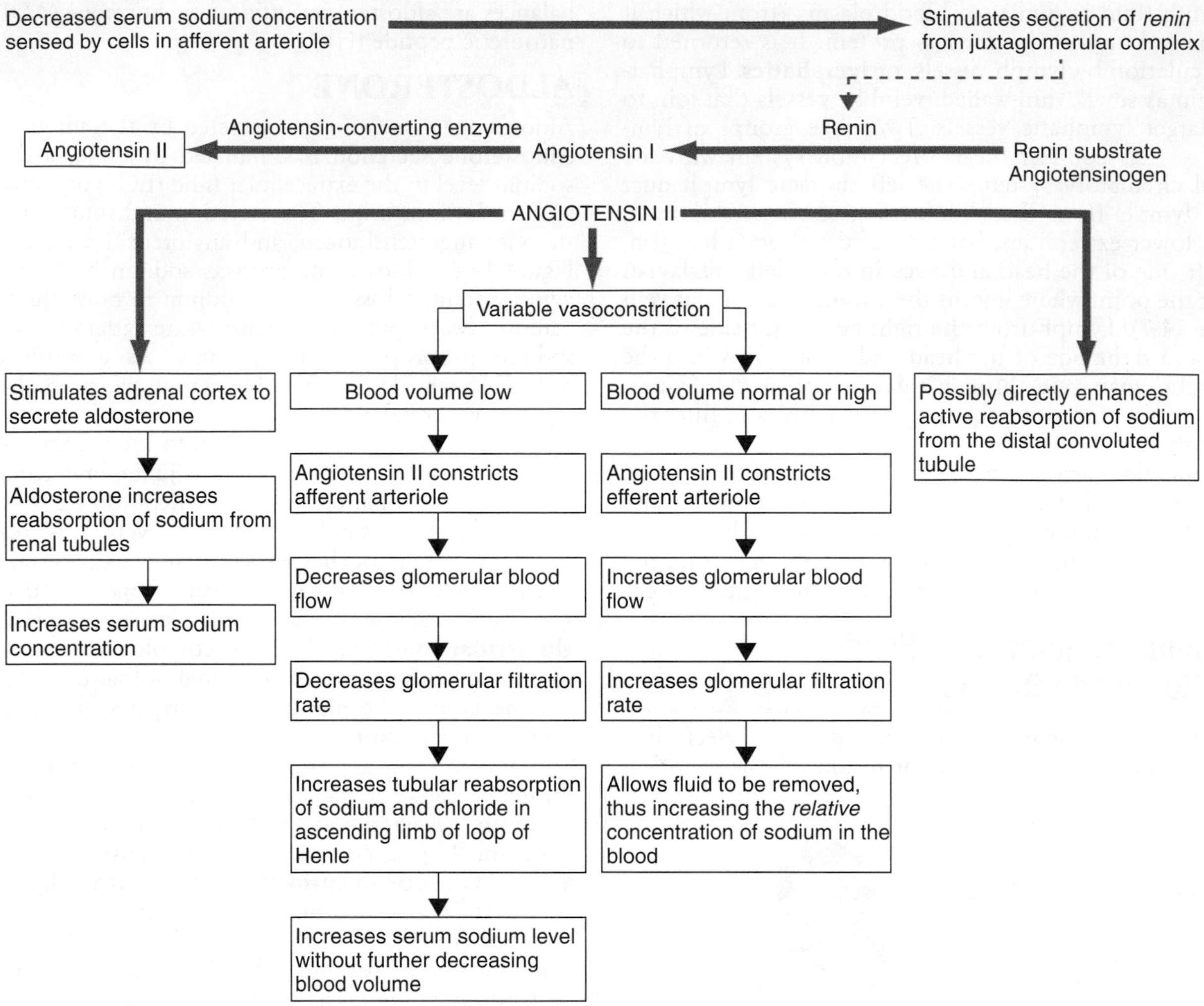

Figure 14-8 ■ The role of aldosterone, angiotensinogen, angiotensin I, and angiotensin II in the renal regulation of water and sodium.

urine. As a result, the amount of water in the extracellular fluid (ECF) decreases, bringing osmolarity to normal.

NATRIURETIC PEPTIDES

Natriuretic peptides (NPs) are hormones secreted by special cells that line the atria of the heart (atrial natriuretic peptide, or ANP) and the ventricles of the heart (brain natriuretic peptide, or BNP). They are secreted in response to increased blood volume and blood pressure, which stretch the heart tissue. NP binds to receptor sites in the nephrons, creating effects that oppose the renin-angiotensin system. When either ANP or BNP is secreted, kidney reabsorption of sodium is inhibited at the same time that glomerular filtration is increased. The outcome is increased output of urine with a high sodium content, which results in decreased circulating blood volume and decreased blood osmolarity.

Body Fluids

A person's age, gender, and ratio of lean mass to body fat affect the amount and distribution of body fluids. An older adult has less total body water than a younger adult. Because fat cells contain practically no water, an obese person has less total body water than a lean person of the same body weight.

WOMEN'S HEALTH CONSIDERATIONS

A woman of any age usually has less total body water than does a man of similar size and age. This difference is because men generally have more muscle mass than women and because women have a higher percentage of body fat. (Muscle cells contain mostly water and fat cells have very little water.) Differences in muscle mass and body fat are partly a result of the influence of sex hormones. This difference in fat to lean body weight may be responsible for some differences seen in women's and men's responses to drugs.

Body fluids are constantly purified and replaced as fluid balance is maintained through intake and output. The total amount of water within each fluid space is stable, but water moves continually among all spaces. Water in all spaces is exchanged continually while maintaining constant fluid volume. Table 14-3 lists the key points regarding fluid and electrolyte balance.

TABLE 14-3 Summary of Key Points Regarding Fluid and Electrolyte Balance

- All plasma electrolyte values must remain within a narrow range for proper physiologic functioning.
- The plasma is the entrance and exit site for all fluids and electrolytes.
- The primary organs or tissues of fluid and electrolyte regulation are the hypothalamus, kidney, adrenal glands, posterior pituitary gland, thyroid gland, and parathyroid glands.
- The total number of positive charges within a solution must be balanced by an equal number of negative charges to maintain electroneutrality.
- Although the specific types and concentrations of substances (solute) dissolved in body fluid vary from one fluid compartment to another, the total concentration of all solutes is the same in all fluid compartments (270 to 300 mOsm/L).
- Whenever possible, the body's regulatory mechanisms attempt to create or maintain an osmolar equilibrium in all body fluid compartments.
- A fluid compartment that is hyposmolar (hypotonic) to normal body fluids expels water from the compartment.
- A fluid compartment that is hyperosmolar (hypertonic) to normal body fluids draws water into it.

SOURCES OF FLUID INTAKE

Fluid intake is regulated through the thirst drive. Fluids enter the body primarily as liquids (Table 14-4). Because solid foods contain up to 85% water, some fluid also enters the body with ingested solid foods. In addition, water is a by-product of metabolism. This metabolic water accounts for about 300 mL of the daily water requirement. A rising blood osmolarity or a decreasing blood volume triggers the sensation of thirst. Sensations such as mouth dryness or the thought that a person has not had a drink recently also trigger the thirst drive. An adult drinks an average of 1500 mL of fluid per day and ingests an additional 800 mL of fluid from food.

ROUTES OF FLUID LOSS

The body has several ways to remove excess water and waste products (see Table 14-4). Of all the water loss pathways, the kidney is the most important and the most sensitive. Water loss by the kidney is closely regulated and is adjustable. The volume of urine excreted daily varies depending on the amount of fluid intake and the body's need to conserve fluids.

The minimum amount of urine per day needed to dissolve and excrete toxic waste products is 400 to 600 mL. This minimal volume is called the **obligatory urine output.** If the 24-hour urine output falls below the obligatory output amount, wastes are retained and can cause lethal electrolyte imbalances, acidosis, and a toxic buildup of nitrogen. This urine is maximally concentrated, with a **specific gravity** (the weight of the liquid compared with the weight of pure water) of 1.032 or higher and an osmolarity of at least 1400 mOsm/L.

Urine can also become very dilute, with a specific gravity of 1.005 and an osmolarity of 200 mOsm/L. Dilution normally results from a large fluid intake and is reflected in a large volume of urine output. The ability of the kidneys to make either concentrated or very dilute urine helps maintain fluid and electrolyte balance. With the influence of aldosterone, antidiuretic hormone (ADH), and natriuretic peptides, the kidney is able to respond when extracellular fluid concentrations, volumes, or pressures change.

TABLE 14-4 Routes of Fluid Ingestion and Excretion

Intake	Output
Measurable	
Oral fluids	Urine
Parenteral fluids	Emesis†
Enemas*	Feces†
Irrigation fluids*	Drainage from body cavities
Not Measurable	
Solid foods	Perspiration
Metabolism	Vaporization through the lungs

*Measured by subtracting the amount returned from the amount instilled.
†Measurement is accurate only when these substances are excreted in liquid form.

Other normal water loss occurs through the skin, the lungs, and the gastrointestinal tract. Additional water losses can occur via salivation, drainage from fistulas and drains, and gastrointestinal suction.

Water loss from the skin, lungs, and stool—called **insensible water loss,** because it cannot be controlled—can be significant. In a healthy adult, insensible water loss is about 15 to 20 mL/kg/day. Insensible water loss increases dramatically in hypermetabolic states such as thyroid crisis, trauma, burns, states of extreme stress, and fever. For every degree increase in body temperature, insensible water loss increases by about 10%. Insensible water loss also increases when the environment is hot and dry. Examples of clients at risk for increased insensible water loss include those being mechanically ventilated and those with rapid respirations (tachypnea). Insensible water loss (not including sweat) is pure water and does not contain electrolytes. Therefore excessive insensible water loss results in a more hypertonic extracellular fluid (ECF) with a smaller volume. If this loss is not balanced by intake, the hypertonic ECF and dehydration can lead to **hypernatremia** (elevated serum sodium level).

Loss by sweating is variable and can reach a maximum rate of about 2 L/hr. Although it contains electrolytes, sweat is slightly hypotonic compared to blood. The amount of sweating is controlled by the autonomic nervous system, body temperature, and blood flow in the skin.

Water loss through stool is normally minimal. However, this loss can increase greatly with severe diarrhea or excessive fistula drainage. Clients with ulcerative colitis can have a diarrheal fluid loss of several liters per day. Diarrheal fluid contains water, potassium, sodium, bicarbonate, and chloride. Thus with diarrhea, fluid and some electrolytes are lost.

Electrolytes

Electrolytes, or **ions,** are substances in body fluids that carry an electrical charge. **Cations** have positive charges; **anions** have negative charges. Body fluids are electrochemically neutral, which means that the number of positive ions is balanced by an equal number of negative ions. However, the distribution of ions differs between the extracellular fluid (ECF) and the intracellular fluid (ICF) (Figure 14-9).

Most electrolytes have different concentrations in the ICF and ECF. This concentration difference helps maintain membrane excitability and allows nerve impulse transmission. The

Plasma volume	Interstitial fluid	Intracellular fluid
Volume 3.5-5.5 L	Volume ~10 L	Volume ~30 L
Osmolarity 270-310 mOsm	Osmolarity 270-310 mOsm	Osmolarity 270-310 mOsm
Sodium 135-145 mEq/L	Sodium 135-145 mEq/L	Sodium 14 mEq/L
Potassium 3.5-5.0 mEq/L	Potassium 3.5-5.0 mEq/L	Potassium 140 mEq/L
Chloride 96-109 mEq/L	Chloride ~118 mEq/L	Chloride ~4-6 mEq/L
Calcium 8.5-10.0 mEq/L	Calcium 7.0-9.0 mEq/L	Calcium 1.0-8.0 mEq/L
Magnesium ~1.6 mEq/L	Magnesium ~1.3 mEq/L	Magnesium 6-30 mEq/L
Protein 7-8 g/L	Protein ~2 g/L	Protein 16 g/L

Figure 14-9 ■ The composition of various body fluids.

TABLE 14-5 Major Serum Electrolyte Concentrations and Functions

Electrolyte	Reference Range	International Recommended Units	Functions
Sodium (Na^+)	136-145 mEq/L	136-145 mmol/L	Maintenance of plasma and interstitial osmolarity Generation and transmission of action potentials Maintenance of acid-base balance Maintenance of electroneutrality
Potassium (K^+)	3.5-5.0 mEq/L	3.5-5.0 mmol/L	Regulation of intracellular osmolarity Maintenance of electrical membrane excitability Maintenance of plasma acid-base balance
Calcium (Ca^{2+})	9.0-10.5 mg/dL	2.25-2.75 mmol/L	Cofactor in blood-clotting cascade Excitable membrane stabilizer Adds strength/density to bones and teeth Essential element in cardiac, skeletal, and smooth muscle contraction
Chloride (Cl^-)	98-106 mEq/L	98-106 mmol/L	Maintenance of plasma acid-base balance Maintenance of plasma electroneutrality Formation of hydrochloric acid
Magnesium (Mg^{2+})	1.3-2.1 mEq/L	0.66-1.07 mmol/L	Excitable membrane stabilizer Essential element in cardiac, skeletal, and smooth muscle contraction Cofactor in blood-clotting cascade Cofactor in carbohydrate metabolism Cofactor in DNA and protein synthesis
Phosphorus (P*i*)	3.0-4.5 mg/dL	0.97-1.45 mmol/L	Activation of B-complex vitamins Formation of adenosine triphosphate and other high-energy substances Cofactor in carbohydrate, protein, and lipid metabolism

Data from Pagana, K., & Pagana, T. (2002). *Mosby's manual of diagnostic and laboratory tests* (2nd ed). St. Louis: Mosby.

normal ranges of electrolyte concentration are very narrow. Thus even small changes in these concentrations can cause major problems.

Table 14-5 lists major electrolytes, their normal serum concentrations, and main functions. Most electrolytes enter the body in ingested food.

Electrolyte homeostasis is controlled by balancing the dietary intake of electrolytes with the renal excretion or reabsorption of electrolytes. For example, the plasma level of potassium is maintained between 3.5 and 5.0 mmol/L. In theory, the potassium in common foods could greatly increase the ECF potassium level and lead to major problems. Usually, however, the kidney excretion of potassium keeps pace with potassium intake and prevents major changes in the blood potassium level.

SODIUM

Sodium (Na^+) is the major cation in the extracellular fluid (ECF) and is responsible for maintaining ECF osmolarity. The activity of the sodium-potassium pump keeps the sodium level of the intracellular fluid (ICF) low (about 14 mmol/L) while maintaining high sodium levels in blood and other extracellular fluids. Maintaining this difference in sodium levels is vital for the following functions:

- Skeletal muscle contraction
- Cardiac contractions

TABLE 14-6 Sodium Values of Common Foods*

Food Source	Amount (mg)
Table salt (1 tsp)	2000
Cheddar cheese (1 oz)	176
Cottage cheese (4 oz)	457
American cheese (1 oz)	439
Whole milk (8 oz)	120
Skim milk (8 oz)	126
Butter (1 tsp)	123
White bread (1 slice)	123
Whole-wheat bread (1 slice)	159
Soy sauce (1 tbsp)	1029
Ketchup (1 tbsp)	156
Mustard (1 tbsp)	188
Beef, lean (4 oz)	60
Pork, lean, fresh (4 oz)	60
Pork, cured (4 oz)	850
Chicken, light meat (4 oz)	70
Chicken, dark meat (4 oz)	70

Data from Pennington, J. (2004). *Bowe's and Church's food values of portions commonly used* (18th ed.). Philadelphia: J.B. Lippincott.

*U.S. Department of Agriculture recommended daily allowance for adults: 1100-3300 mg.

- Nerve impulse transmission
- Normal ECF osmolarity
- Normal ECF volume

The ECF sodium level determines whether water is retained, excreted, or moved from one fluid space to another.

To maintain electrical balance, the sodium (a cation) level within a body fluid must be matched by an equal number of anions (negatively charged substances). Each positive charge in the ECF must be balanced by a negative charge so the fluid does not carry either an overall positive or an overall negative charge. When this balance is present, a state of **electroneutrality** exists in that fluid. Changes in the plasma sodium level seriously change fluid volume and the distribution of other electrolytes.

The normal plasma sodium level ranges between 136 and 145 mEq/L or mmol/L (see Table 14-5). Sodium enters the body through the ingestion of many foods and fluids (Table 14-6). The average dietary intake of sodium is about 6 to 14 g/day. Sodium is also stored deep within the kidney tissues and can be released to the ECF as needed. Despite variation in sodium intake from one day to the next, the serum sodium level usually remains within the normal range. Serum sodium balance is regulated by the kidney under the influences of aldosterone, antidiuretic hormone (ADH), and natriuretic peptide (NP).

Low serum sodium levels inhibit the secretion of ADH and NP and trigger aldosterone secretion. Together these actions increase serum sodium levels by increasing kidney reabsorption of sodium and enhancing kidney loss of water.

High serum sodium levels inhibit aldosterone secretion and directly stimulate secretion of ADH and NP. Together these hormones increase kidney excretion of sodium and kidney reabsorption of water.

POTASSIUM

Potassium (K^+) is the major cation of the intracellular fluid (ICF). The normal plasma potassium level ranges from 3.5 to 5.0 mEq/L or mmol/L (see Table 14-5). The normal ICF potassium level is about 140 mEq/L (mmol/L). Because of its high concentration inside cells, potassium has some control over intracellular osmolarity and volume. Keeping this large difference in potassium concentration between the ICF and the extracellular fluid (ECF) is critical for excitable tissues to generate action potentials and transmit impulses. Functions of potassium include the following:

- Regulation of protein synthesis
- Regulation of glucose use and storage
- Maintenance of action potentials in excitable membranes

Because potassium levels in the blood and interstitial fluid are so low, any change seriously affects physiologic activities. For example, a decrease in blood potassium of only 1 mEq/L (from 4 mEq/L to 3 mEq/L) is a 25% difference in total ECF potassium concentration. In contrast, a 1-mEq/L decrease in blood sodium level (from 140 mEq/L to 139 mEq/L) is, overall, a much smaller change (less than 1%) in total ECF sodium concentration.

Potassium drifts out of cells down its concentration gradient into the ECF. Almost all foods contain potassium (Table 14-7). Potassium intake is about 2 to 20 g/day. Despite heavy potassium intake and the drifting of potassium from cellular storage sites into the ECF, the healthy adult keeps plasma potassium levels within the narrow range of normal values needed for physiologic function.

The main controller of ECF potassium level is the sodium-potassium pump within the membranes of all body

TABLE 14-7 Potassium Values of Common Foods*

Food Source	Amount (mg)
Corn flakes (1¼ c)	26
Cooked oatmeal (¾ c)	99
Egg (1 large)	66
Codfish, raw (4 oz)	400
Salmon, pink, raw (3½ oz)	306
Tuna fish (4 oz)	375
Apple, raw with skin (1 medium)	159
Banana (1 medium)	451
Cantaloupe (1 c pieces)	494
Grapefruit (½ medium)	175
Orange (1 medium)	250
Raisins (½ c)	700
Strawberries, raw (1 c)	247
Watermelon (1 c pieces)	186
White bread (1 slice)	27
Whole-wheat bread (1 slice)	44
Beef (4 oz)	480
Beef liver (3½ oz)	281
Pork, fresh (4 oz)	525
Pork, cured (4 oz)	325
Chicken (4 oz)	225
Veal cutlet (3½ oz)	448
Ham (4 oz)	328
Whole milk (8 oz)	370
Skim milk (8 oz)	406
Avocado (1 medium)	1097
Carrot (1 large)	341
Corn (4-inch ear)	196
Cauliflower (1 c pieces)	295
Celery (1 stalk)	170
Green beans (1 c)	189
Mushrooms (10 small)	410
Onion (1 medium)	157
Peas (¾ c)	316
Potato, white (1 medium)	407
Spinach, raw (3½ oz)	470
Tomato (1 medium)	366

Data from Pennington, J. (2004). *Bowe's and Church's food values of portions commonly used* (18th ed.). Philadelphia: J.B. Lippincott.

*U.S. Department of Agriculture recommended daily allowance for adults: 1875-5625 mg.

cells. This pump removes three sodium ions from the fluid inside the cell for every two potassium ions that it returns to the cell. In this way, the levels of both serum sodium and cellular potassium remain high.

Some potassium control also occurs through kidney function. The kidney is the excretory route for ridding the body of ECF potassium (80% of potassium removed from the body occurs via the kidney). Unlike sodium, no hormone has been identified that directly controls kidney reabsorption of potassium; thus the kidney does not conserve potassium directly.

CALCIUM

Calcium (Ca^{2+}) is a mineral with functions closely related to those of phosphorus and magnesium. Calcium is a **divalent cation** (an ion having two positive charges) that exists in the body in two forms: bound and ionized (unbound or free).

Bound calcium is usually attached to serum proteins, especially albumin. Ionized calcium is present in the blood and other extracellular fluid (ECF) as free calcium. Free calcium is the active form and must be kept within a narrow range in the ECF. The body functions best when blood calcium levels are maintained between 9.0 and 10.5 mg/dL, or between 2.25 and 2.75 mmol/L (see Table 14-5). Because the amount of calcium in the intracellular fluid (ICF) is low, calcium has a steep gradient between ECF and ICF. Calcium is important in the following actions:

- Bone strength and density
- Activation of enzymes or reactions
- Skeletal muscle contraction
- Cardiac muscle contraction
- Nerve impulse transmission
- Blood clotting

Calcium enters the body by dietary intake and absorption through the intestinal tract (Table 14-8). Absorption of dietary calcium requires the active form of vitamin D. Calcium is stored in the bones. When both plasma calcium levels and stored calcium levels are adequate, intestinal absorption of dietary calcium is reduced and urine excretion of excess calcium increases. When more calcium is needed, **parathyroid hormone (PTH)** is released from the parathyroid glands (Table 14-9). PTH causes serum calcium levels to increase in the following ways:

- Releasing free calcium from bone storage sites directly into the ECF **(resorption)**
- Stimulating vitamin D activation, thus increasing intestinal absorption of dietary calcium
- Inhibiting kidney excretion of calcium and stimulating kidney reabsorption of calcium

When excess calcium is present in plasma, PTH secretion is inhibited and the secretion of **thyrocalcitonin (TCT),** a hormone secreted by the thyroid gland, is increased. TCT causes the plasma calcium level to decrease in the following ways:

- Inhibiting bone resorption of calcium
- Inhibiting activation of vitamin D, causing decreased gastrointestinal uptake of calcium
- Increasing kidney excretion of calcium in the urine

PHOSPHORUS

Phosphorus (P) is in the body in both inorganic and organic forms. Normal serum levels of phosphorus range from 3.0 to 4.5 mg/dL, or 0.97 to 1.45 mmol/L (see Table 14-5). Most phosphorus (80%) can be found in the bones. Phosphorus is the major anion in the intracellular fluid (ICF), and its concentration inside cells is much higher than in extracellular fluid (ECF). Phosphorus is needed for the following cellular activities:

- Activating B-complex vitamins
- Forming and activating adenosine triphosphate (ATP)

TABLE 14-8 Calcium Values of Common Foods*

Food Source	Amount (mg)
Cheddar cheese (1 oz)	204
Cottage cheese (4 oz)	68
American cheese (1 oz)	174
Whole milk (8 oz)	288
Skim milk (8 oz)	302
Yogurt, low-fat (1 c)	415
Broccoli, raw (½ c)	75
Carrot (1 large)	37
Collard greens, raw (3 oz)	200
Green beans (1 c)	62
Rhubarb (1 c)	266
Spinach, raw (3½ oz)	93
Tofu (3 oz)	100

Data from Pennington, J. (2004). *Bowe's and Church's food values of portions commonly used* (18th ed.). Philadelphia: J.B. Lippincott.

*U.S. Department of Agriculture recommended daily allowance for adults: 800-1200 mg.

TABLE 14-9 Hormonal Regulation of Calcium

Hormone	Action
Parathyroid Hormone (PTH) Secreted in response to low or low-normal serum calcium levels Secretion results in a rise in serum calcium concentration	Increases bone resorption of calcium (leaching of stored calcium) Increases the absorption of ingested calcium from the gastrointestinal tract into the extracellular fluid Increases the renal reabsorption of calcium at the proximal convoluted tubule
Thyrocalcitonin (TCT) Secreted by the thyroid gland in response to high or high-normal serum calcium levels Secretion results in a reduction of the serum calcium concentration	Increases bone uptake of calcium Inhibits the absorption of calcium from the gastrointestinal tract so that ingested calcium is excreted from the body in the feces Inhibits the renal reabsorption of calcium at the proximal convoluted tubule so that more calcium is excreted in the urine

- Assisting in cell division
- Cooperating in carbohydrate metabolism
- Cooperating in protein metabolism
- Cooperating in lipid (fat) metabolism

Other phosphorus functions include acid-base buffering and calcium homeostasis. The average North American diet is high in phosphorus (1 to 2 g/day). Table 14-10 lists food sources of phosphorus.

Phosphorus balance and calcium balance are intertwined. Normally, plasma levels of calcium and phosphorus exist in a balanced, reciprocal relationship, which means that the product of the plasma concentrations remains constant. Therefore a change in the amount of plasma phosphorus results in an equal and opposite change in the amount of plasma calcium (and vice versa).

The regulation of ECF phosphorus occurs through the activity of parathyroid hormone (PTH). Increased PTH levels cause a net loss of phosphorus. Reduced PTH levels enhance kidney reabsorption of phosphorus, resulting in increased plasma levels of phosphorus.

MAGNESIUM

Magnesium (Mg^{2+}) is a mineral that forms a cation when dissolved in water. Adults have an average total body level of 25 g of magnesium, most of which (60%) is stored in bones and cartilage. Little magnesium is present in the extracellular fluid (ECF). Plasma levels of free magnesium range from 1.3 to 2.1 mg/dL, or 0.65 to 1.05 mmol/L (see Table 14-5). Much more magnesium is present in the intracellular fluid (ICF), and it has more functions inside the cells than in the blood. Magnesium is critical for the following intracellular reactions or activities:

- Skeletal muscle contraction
- Carbohydrate metabolism
- Adenosine triphosphate (ATP) formation
- B-complex vitamin activation
- Deoxyribonucleic acid (DNA) synthesis
- Protein synthesis

Extracellular magnesium regulates blood coagulation and skeletal muscle contractility.

The daily magnesium requirement for adults is about 300 mg. Table 14-11 lists food sources of magnesium.

Magnesium regulation occurs through the kidney and the gastrointestinal tract although the exact mechanisms are not known. When blood magnesium levels are low, ingested magnesium is rapidly absorbed in the small intestine and kidney excretion of magnesium stops. When blood magnesium levels are high, little if any magnesium is absorbed from food and the kidney increases magnesium excretion.

CHLORIDE

Chloride (Cl^-) is the major anion of the extracellular fluid (ECF) and works with sodium to maintain ECF osmotic pressure. Chloride is important in the formation of hydrochloric acid in the stomach. The normal plasma concentration of chloride ranges from 98 to 106 mEq/L or mmol/L (see Table 14-5).

Only a small amount of chloride is present inside the cells because negative charges on the cell membrane repel chloride and prevent it from crossing the membrane. However, extracellular chloride can enter cells when exchanged for another anion that is leaving the cell. This situation, called a **chloride shift,** decreases plasma chloride without a net body loss of chloride. Bicarbonate (HCO_3^-) is the anion most commonly exchanged for chloride.

Chloride enters the body through dietary intake. Because chloride (along with sodium, potassium, and many other minerals) is a part of a salt, most diets contain enough chloride to meet the normal needs of the body.

Fluid and Electrolyte Changes Associated with Aging

Only 45% to 50% of the body weight of older adults is water, compared with 55% to 60% in younger adults. This decrease occurs because of a loss of muscle mass and a reduced ratio of

TABLE 14-10 Phosphorus Values of Common Foods*

Food Source	Amount (mg)
Rolled oats, cooked (¾ c)	133
Egg (1 large)	90
Codfish (3 oz)	175
Tuna fish, white, canned (6½ oz)	405
Raisins (½ c)	75
White bread (1 slice)	26
Whole-wheat bread (1 slice)	23
Cheddar cheese (1 oz)	145
American cheese (1 oz)	211
Whole milk (8 oz)	228
Skim milk (8 oz)	247
Yogurt, low-fat (8 oz)	326
Beef (4 oz)	215
Beef liver (4 oz)	375
Pork, fresh (4 oz)	325
Chicken (4 oz)	200
Almonds (1 oz)	141
Peanuts (1 oz)	110

Data from Pennington, J. (2004). *Bowe's and Church's food values of portions commonly used* (18th ed.). Philadelphia: J.B. Lippincott.

*U.S. Department of Agriculture recommended daily allowance for adults: 800 mg.

TABLE 14-11 Magnesium Values of Common Foods*

Food Source	Amount (mg)
Rolled oats, cooked (¾ c)	42
Tuna fish, white, canned (6½ oz)	59
Raisins (½ c)	25
Beef (4 oz)	24
Pork (4 oz)	30
Chicken (4 oz)	26
Whole milk (8 oz)	33
Skim milk (8 oz)	28
Yogurt, low-fat (8 oz)	40
Peanut butter (1 tbsp)	22
Avocado (1 medium)	70
Broccoli (1 stalk)	24
Cauliflower (1 c pieces)	24
Peas (¾ c)	35
Potato (1 medium)	34
Spinach, raw (3½ oz)	88

Data from Pennington, J. (2004). *Bowe's and Church's food values of portions commonly used* (18th ed.). Philadelphia: J.B. Lippincott.

*U.S. Department of Agriculture recommended daily allowance for adults: 300-350 mg.

CHART 14-1

NURSING FOCUS on the OLDER ADULT
Impact of Age-Related Changes on Fluid and Electrolyte Balance

System	Change	Result
Skin	Loss of elasticity	An unreliable indicator of fluid status
	Decreased turgor	Dry, easily damaged skin
	Decreased oil production	
Renal	Decreased glomerular filtration	Poor excretion of waste products
	Decreased concentrating capacity	Increased water loss
Muscular	Decreased muscle mass	Decreased total body water Greater risk of dehydration
Neurologic	Diminished thirst reflex	Decreased fluid intake, increasing the risk of dehydration
Endocrine	Adrenal atrophy	Poor regulation of sodium and potassium, predisposing the client to hyponatremia and hyperkalemia

CHART 14-2

NURSING FOCUS on the OLDER ADULT
Normal Plasma Electrolyte Values for People Older Than 60 Years of Age

Electrolyte	Reference Range	International Recommended Units
Calcium (Ca^{2+})	9.0-10.5 mg/dL	2.2-2.75 mmol/L
>90 years	8.2-9.6 mg/dL	2.05-2.40 mmol/L
Chloride (Cl^-)	98-106 mEq/L	98-106 mmol/L
>90 years	98-111 mEq/L	98-111 mmol/L
Magnesium (Mg^{2+})	1.2-2.1 mEq/L	0.65-1.5 mmol/L
Phosphorus (P*i*)	3-4.5 mg/dL	0.97-1.45 mmol/L
Potassium (K^+)	3.5-5.0 mEq/L	3.5-5.0 mmol/L
Sodium (Na^+)	136-145 mEq/L	136-145 mmol/L
>90 years	132-146 mEq/L	132-146 mmol/L

Data for adults <90 years from Pagana, K., & Pagana, T. (2002). *Mosby's manual of diagnostic and laboratory tests* (2nd ed). St. Louis: Mosby.
Data for adults >90 years from Tietz, N.W. (Ed.). (1995). *Clinical guide to laboratory tests* (3rd ed.). Philadelphia: W.B. Saunders.

lean body weight to total body weight. This decrease in total body water places older adults at greater risk for dehydration.

Skin **turgor** (the normal resiliency of a pinched fold of skin) is not always an accurate assessment of extracellular deficient fluid (ECF) volume (dehydration) in the older adult because the natural aging process decreases turgor (Chart 14-1). Also, the older adult may have a reduced thirst sense and decreased kidney function, both of which increase the risk for dehydration and make assessment more difficult. When working with older clients, it is important to accurately record intake and output and weight, because these measurements reflect hydration status more accurately than does skin turgor.

The normal concentration of blood electrolytes also changes with the aging process. Chart 14-2 lists the normal electrolyte values for people older than 60 years of age.

CHART 14-3

Fluid and Electrolyte Assessment
USING GORDON'S FUNCTIONAL HEALTH PATTERNS

Nutritional-Metabolic Pattern
- What is your typical daily food intake? Describe a day's meals, snacks, and vitamins.
- How much salt do you typically add to your food? Do you use salt substitutes?
- How is your appetite?
- Do you have any difficulty chewing or swallowing?
- What is your typical daily fluid intake? What types of fluids (water, juices, soft drinks, coffee, tea)? How much?
- Have you had any recent change in your weight? Weight gain? Weight loss? How much?
- Have you noticed a change in tightness of your rings or shoes? Tighter? Looser?

Elimination Pattern
- What is your usual bowel elimination pattern? Frequency? Character? Discomfort? Laxatives?
- What is your usual urinary elimination pattern? Frequency? Amount? Color? Odor? Control?
- Have you noticed a change in the amount of urine?
- Do you have any problem with excessive perspiration?
- Do you have any other type of drainage?

Based on Gordon, M. (2002). Manual of nursing diagnosis (10th ed.). St. Louis: Mosby.

Electrolyte balance may be more difficult to maintain in older adults. Small changes in the levels of potassium and calcium may have serious results. Although the ranges of electrolytes in plasma and intracellular fluid (ICF) may remain normal, the balance is fragile and more easily disturbed in an older adult. Part of this fragility is related to decreased regulatory functions that occur with aging. Age-related kidney changes include decreased blood flow, decreased filtration, and decreased numbers of working nephrons. Kidney and capillary changes from hypertension are more likely to be present in the older adult.

ASSESSMENT OF FLUID AND ELECTROLYTE BALANCE

History

One way of organizing history data to assess the client's fluid and electrolyte status is to use Gordon's Functional Health Patterns (Gordon, 2002). The patterns that most affect fluid and electrolyte status are the Nutritional-Metabolic Pattern and the Elimination Pattern (Chart 14-3).

The client's nutritional history can reveal problems that affect fluid and electrolyte balance. Obtain this information directly because the client may not understand the connection between dietary intake and the onset of fluid and electrolyte imbalances.

The guidelines for obtaining a thorough fluid and electrolyte history do not differ from those for assessing any other system; however, the information collected is more specific. For example, exact intake and output volumes are important, as are serial daily weight measurements. You may need to guide the client in reporting accurately the amount of fluid ingested and changes in urine patterns. Also assess the types of fluids and foods ingested to determine amount and osmolarity. Many clients do not know that solid foods contain liquid. Solid foods such as ice cream, gelatin, and ices are liquids at body temperature, and these must be included when calculating fluid intake.

Output includes losses not only as urine but also as sweat, diarrhea, and insensible loss during fevers. Ask specific questions about prescribed and over-the-counter drugs and check the dosage, the length of time taken, and the client's adherence with the drug regimen. A client who is taking diuretics can have an imbalance of fluid, potassium, sodium, or hydrogen ions when other water loss occurs through vomiting or excessive sweating.

Older adults often use laxatives, which can disturb fluid and electrolyte balance. Misuse and overuse of these drugs can lead to serious imbalances.

Other important areas of the client history include body weight changes, thirst or excessive drinking, exposure to hot environments, and the presence of other disorders, such as kidney or endocrine diseases (e.g., Cushing's disease, Addison's disease, diabetes mellitus, and diabetes insipidus). Assess the client's level of consciousness and mental status, because changes in mental status occur with fluid imbalance. In such cases, you may need to check the accuracy of information with family members.

Physical Assessment

Hydration is the state of fluid balance. A normally hydrated adult is alert, has moist eyes and mucous membranes, has a urine output nearly the same as the amount of fluid ingested (with a urine specific gravity of about 1.015), and good skin turgor.

Assess skin turgor by pinching a fold of skin. This pinched fold should return immediately to its original shape after release. Decreased turgor, a sign of dehydration, is present when the fold remains in a pinched shape after being released and rebounds slowly **(tenting)** (Figure 14-10). Skin turgor is best assessed in body areas that have little fat tissue, such as over the sternum, on the forehead, or on the back of the hand. An older person has poor skin turgor on the hands and feet because of the loss of tissue elasticity related to aging; thus state of hydration is more difficult to assess in an older adult than in a younger adult. The best areas for assessing turgor in the older adult are over the sternum and on the forehead.

Skin hydration assessment also includes an examination for dryness. The mucous membranes and the conjunctiva are normally moist. An assessment of fluid balance always includes an examination of the eyes, nose, and oral mucous membranes. A dry, sticky, "cottony" mouth; the absence of tearing; weight loss; and decreased urine output all indicate deficient fluid volume.

Accurate measurement of fluid intake and output is needed to assess fluid and electrolyte status. Use volumetric devices to accurately measure actual fluid intake and output.

Include behavioral and neurologic assessment in fluid assessment because fluid imbalance can change neurologic function. In hypertonic states, neuron shrinkage may induce serious nervous system excitability and hyperactivity, and convulsions may occur. Another variable to assess is the degree of thirst, but this may be difficult to gauge in a confused older client.

Estimate insensible water loss (e.g., sweat) in every client. Consider possible fluid loss from other routes, including the following:

- Fluid losses from wounds
- Gastric or intestinal drainage
- Blood loss from hemorrhage
- Drainage of body secretions, such as bile and pancreatic juices through fistulas

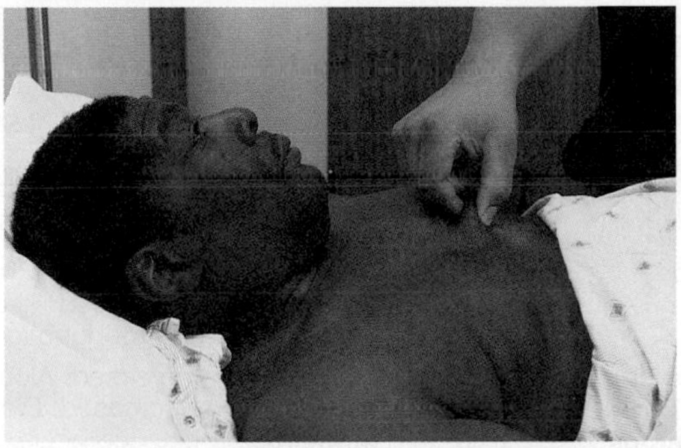

Figure 14-10 ■ Examining the skin turgor of an older client.

Electrolytes control the activity of excitable membranes, and electrolyte imbalances alter excitable membrane function. Electrolyte assessment includes a complete neuromuscular assessment of muscle tone and strength, movement, coordination, and tremors. Assessment of other systems, including the cardiac system (heart rate, the strength of contractions, and the presence of dysrhythmias) and gastrointestinal system (peristalsis), may indicate changes of excitable membrane function.

Your assessment must also focus on changes from previous findings (including mental status, physical examination data, and laboratory data). Fluid and electrolyte imbalances can occur quickly; therefore you must be familiar with the client's baseline assessment data to detect any changes.

Psychosocial Assessment

Psychosocial assessment related to fluid and electrolyte status includes both psychological and cultural factors that might influence balance. Depressed clients may refuse fluids or forget to drink adequate fluids. Clients with bulimia or anorexia nervosa (eating disorders) may abuse laxatives or may induce vomiting, causing fluid and electrolyte imbalances. Also assess social practices. For example, alcohol or drug abuse may cause fluid or electrolyte imbalance.

Diagnostic Assessment

Laboratory results help identify specific fluid and electrolyte imbalances or disorders that alter fluid and electrolyte status. Normal serum electrolyte values are listed in Table 14-5, and normal values for adults older than 60 years of age appear in Chart 14-2. Other laboratory values that are helpful in assessing fluid and electrolyte status include blood urea nitrogen level (BUN), blood glucose level, creatinine level, pH, bicarbonate level, osmolarity, hemoglobin, and hematocrit.

Urine test results may be helpful in assessing fluid status (Table 14-12). If a laboratory report is not available, you can perform some tests using a dipstick to help determine fluid and electrolyte status, including detecting substances normally not present in the urine, such as glucose, acetone, protein, and blood. Urine pH and specific gravity also can be determined in this way.

TABLE 14-12 Normal Urine Electrolyte Values

Electrolyte/ Characteristics	Normal Value*	Significance of Abnormal Value†
Calcium	2.5-7.5 mmol/day	Increased: Malignancy, thyrotoxicosis, hyperparathyroidism, osteoporosis, vitamin D intoxication Decreased: Hypoparathyroidism, rickets, kidney disease, hypothyroidism
Chloride	110-250 mEq/day 110-250 mmol/day	Increased: Increased salt intake, drug-induced diuresis, adrenocortical insufficiency Decreased: Reduced salt intake, water retention, vomiting, cerebral edema, adrenocortical hyperfunction
Magnesium	3.0-5.0 mmol/day	Increased: Alcohol intake, diuretics, corticosteroid therapy, cisplatin therapy Decreased: Dietary insufficiency
Phosphorus	12.9-42.0 mmol/day	Increased: Hyperparathyroidism, renal tubular damage, immobility, nonrenal acidosis Decreased: Hypoparathyroidism
Potassium	25-100 mmol/day (varies with diet)	Increased: Early starvation, hyperaldosteronism, metabolic acidosis Decreased: Addison's disease, renal disease
Sodium	40-220 mEq/day 40-220 mmol/day	Increased: Increased dietary intake, adrenal failure, diuretic therapy Decreased: Low sodium intake, sodium and water retention, adrenocortical hyperfunction, excessive diaphoresis, diarrhea
Osmolarity (osmolality) random	50-1200 mOsm/kg water	Increased: Dehydration, SIADH Decreased: Diabetes insipidus, primary polydipsia
Specific gravity	1.015-1.025	Increased: Dehydration, SIADH, diabetes mellitus, toxemia of pregnancy Decreased: Chronic renal insufficiency, diabetes insipidus, lithium toxicity, early renal disease

Data from Tietz, N. (Ed.). (1995). *Clinical guide to laboratory tests* (3rd ed.). Philadelphia: W.B. Saunders; & Pagana, K., Pagana, T. (2002). *Mosby's manual of diagnostic and laboratory tests* (2nd ed.). St. Louis: Mosby.
SIADH, Syndrome of inappropriate antidiuretic hormone.
*Based on a 24-hr total volume urine sample.
†Common conditions associated with abnormal values.

GET READY for the NCLEX Examination!

KEY POINTS

Safe Effective Care Environment

- Ensure access to adequate fluids for clients who are unable to talk or who have limited mobility.
- Evaluate the accuracy of intake and output measurements taken by unlicensed assistive personnel.

Health Promotion and Maintenance

- Encourage all clients to maintain an adequate fluid intake (minimum of 3 L per day) unless another condition requires fluid restriction.
- Teach all people to increase fluid intake when exercising, in hot or dry environments, or during conditions that increase metabolism (such as fever).
- Teach clients how to determine electrolyte content of processed foods by reading labels.

Psychosocial Integrity

- Check the hydration status of any client who has a sudden change in mental status.
- Identify changes in a client's mental status.

Physiological Integrity

- Use volumetric devices to measure intake and output for any client at risk for fluid volume deficits or excesses.
- Assess skin turgor on the forehead or the sternum of older clients.
- Use daily weights to determine fluid gains or losses.
- Ask clients about the use of drugs such as diuretics, laxatives, salt substitutes, and antihypertensives that may alter fluid and electrolyte status.
- Check the osmolarity, electrolyte composition, and flow rate of any intravenous solution.
- Correctly interpret laboratory electrolyte values.

ADDITIONAL STUDY RESOURCES

Go to your Student CD-ROM for Review Questions for the NCLEX Examination.

evolve Go to http://evolve.elsevier.com/Iggy/ for Integrated Management of Care Questions for the NCLEX Examination.

SELECTED BIBLIOGRAPHY

Asterisk indicates a classic or definitive work on this subject.

Berne, R., et al. (2004). *Physiology* (5th ed.). St. Louis: Mosby.
Call-Schmidt, T. (2001). Interpreting lab results: A primer. *MEDSURG Nursing, 10*(4), 179-184.
Ebersole, P., Hess, P., & Luggen, A. (2004). *Toward healthy aging: Human needs and nursing response* (6th ed.). St. Louis: Mosby.
Elgart, H. (2004). Assessment of fluids and electrolytes. *AACN Clinical Issues, 15*(4), 607-621.
Gordon, M. (2002). *Manual of nursing diagnosis* (10th ed.). St. Louis: Mosby.
Jarvis, C. (2004). *Physical examination and health assessment* (4th ed). Philadelphia: W. B. Saunders.
McConnell, E. (2002). Measuring fluid intake and output. *Nursing2002, 32*(7), 17.

Mead, M. (2000). Serum calcium. *Practice Nurse, 20*(2), 112.
*O'Donnell, M. (1995). Assessing fluid and electrolyte balance needs in elders. *American Journal of Nursing, 95*(1), 41-46.
Pagana, K., & Pagana, T. (2002). *Mosby's manual of diagnostic and laboratory tests* (2nd ed). St. Louis: Mosby.
Pennington, J. (2004). *Bowe's and Church's food values of portions commonly used* (18th ed.). Philadelphia: J.B. Lippincott.
*Stark, J. (1998). A comprehensive analysis of the fluid and electrolytes system. *Critical Care Nursing Clinics of North America, 10*(4), 471-475.
Trissel, L. (2003). *Handbook on injectable drugs* (12th ed.). Bethesda, MD: American Society of Health-System Pharmacists.

CHAPTER

15 Interventions for Clients with Fluid Imbalances

M. LINDA WORKMAN

LEARNING OUTCOMES

After studying this chapter, you should be able to:

1. Identify clients at risk for fluid imbalances.
2. Use laboratory data and clinical manifestations to assess fluid balance and imbalance.
3. Apply appropriate nursing techniques to promote comfort and safety in the client with dehydration.
4. Prioritize nursing care for the client with dehydration.
5. Explain why different types of intravenous fluids are used to treat different types of dehydration.
6. Develop a community-based teaching plan to prevent dehydration in the older client at continuing risk for fluid loss.
7. Analyze changes in clinical manifestations to determine the effectiveness of therapy for the client with dehydration.
8. Prioritize nursing care for the client with overhydration.
9. Analyze changes in clinical manifestations to determine the effectiveness of therapy for the client with overhydration.

Go to your Student CD-ROM for Review Questions for the NCLEX Examination keyed to these Learning Outcomes.

Proper body fluid balance is needed for normal functioning. All clients are at risk for some degree of fluid imbalance because many health problems can disrupt fluid intake or output. Fluid imbalances can occur in any setting. Although imbalances of fluid can involve electrolyte imbalances, this chapter focuses on client problems related to fluid imbalances.

DEHYDRATION

PATHOPHYSIOLOGY

In **dehydration,** fluid intake is less than what is needed to meet the body's fluid needs, resulting in a **fluid volume deficit.** Three basic types of dehydration are possible (Figure 15-1):

- **Isotonic dehydration,** in which water and dissolved electrolytes are lost in equal proportions
- **Hypertonic dehydration,** in which water loss is greater than electrolyte loss
- **Hypotonic dehydration,** in which electrolyte loss is greater than water loss

Dehydration is a condition rather than a disease and can be caused by many factors. Dehydration may be an *actual* decrease in total body water caused by either too little intake of fluid or too great a loss of fluid. Dehydration also can occur without an actual loss of total body water, such as when water shifts from the plasma into the interstitial space. This condition is called *relative* dehydration.

The actual incidence of dehydration is not known; however every ill client is at risk and the cost of treating dehydration is significant. (See the Resource Management box on p. 213.) Older clients are at high risk because they have less total body water than younger adults. Conditions affecting fluid intake in the older adult include decreased thirst sensation and difficulty with walking or other motor skills needed for ingesting fluids. Many older clients also take drugs such as diuretics and antihypertensives that increase fluid excretion.

Isotonic Dehydration

Isotonic dehydration is the most common type of fluid volume deficit. It involves loss of isotonic fluids from the extracellular fluid (ECF) space, including both the plasma and the interstitial spaces. Because isotonic fluid is lost, plasma osmolarity remains normal while volume is reduced. This type of dehydration does not cause a shift of fluids between spaces, so the intracellular fluid (ICF) volume remains normal. Isotonic dehydration decreases circulating blood volume **(hypovolemia)** and leads to inadequate tissue perfusion. Problems caused by isotonic dehydration result from loss of plasma volume. The body's defenses compensate during dehydration to maintain adequate blood flow to vital organs in spite of decreased vascular volume (Figure 15-2).

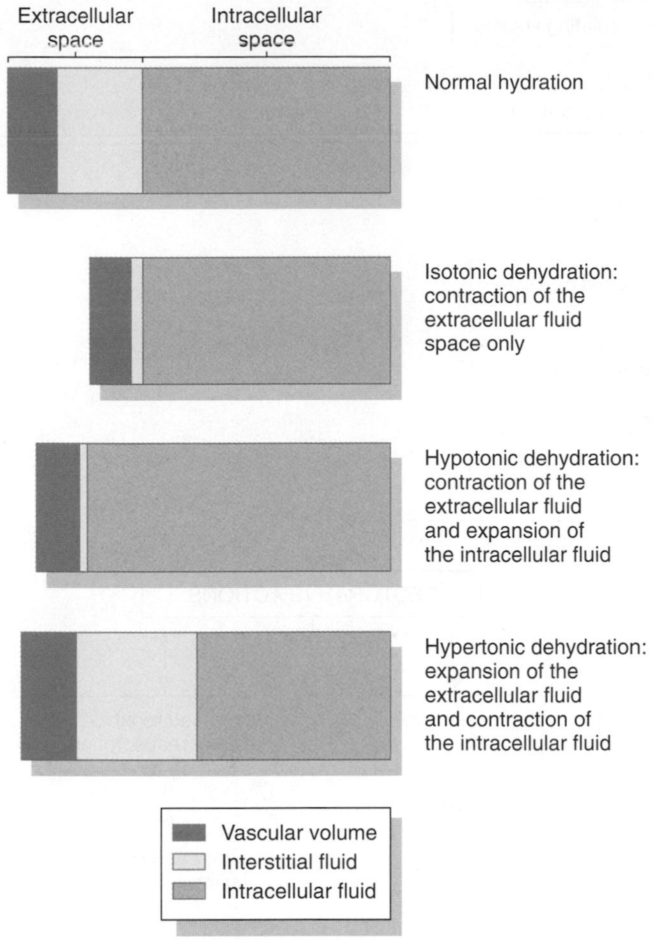

Figure 15-1 ■ Three types of dehydration. (© 1992 M. Linda Workman. All rights reserved.)

RESOURCE MANAGEMENT

PREVENTION OF DEHYDRATION

Cost of Care

- Dehydration is a common occurrence among older adults (in the community and in nursing home environments), clients who are somewhat cognitively impaired, and clients who have mobility problems.
- Dehydration is among the 10 most frequently reported diagnoses for Medicare hospitalizations.
- Treatment of dehydration and dehydration associated complications among clients older than 65 years of age accounts for nearly 2 million hospital days per year in the United States alone, with an estimate cost of $1.2 billion.
- Complications of dehydration can lead to increased morbidity and mortality rates.
- Most cases of dehydration are totally preventable.
- Most strategies to promote hydration require minimal costs.
- Awareness of dehydration as a health risk is under emphasized by health care personnel and family members.
- Time is a critical factor in ensuring adequate oral intake among older or impaired adults.

Implications for Nursing

Due to the high cost of treating problems associated with dehydration, nurses need to develop individualized plans in conjunction with clients to increase the availability and assistance needed to support adequate hydration, especially among older adults. The issue is not so much that nurses don't believe that hydration is important, it is in finding the time to ensure it happens. Educating unlicensed assistive personnel in the importance of taking the time to encourage older clients to drink fluids with and between meals is crucial in this time of nursing shortage. Using the time of medication administration to ensure that clients receiving oral medications drink 100 to 200 mL with oral medications is a simple way to promote hydration.

Data from Bennett, J. (2000). Dehydration: Hazards and benefits. *Geriatric Nursing, 21*(2), 84-88; Culp, K., Mentes, J., & Wakefield, B. (2003). Hydration and acute confusion in long-term care residents. *Western Journal of Nursing Research, 25*(3), 251-266; and Robinson, S., & Rosher, R. (2002). Can a beverage cart help improve hydration? *Geriatric Nursing, 23*(4), 208-211.

Isotonic dehydration has many causes (Table 15-1). These include poor intake of fluids and solutes, fluid shifts between fluid spaces, and heavy losses of isotonic body fluids.

Hypertonic Dehydration

Hypertonic dehydration is the second most common type of fluid volume deficit. It occurs when water loss from the extracellular fluid (ECF) is greater than electrolyte loss. This water loss increases the osmolarity of the remaining plasma, making it *hypertonic* or *hyperosmolar* compared with normal ECF. The hyperosmolar plasma has an increased osmotic pressure that causes water to move from the intracellular fluid (ICF) into the plasma and interstitial fluid spaces. The fluid shift leads to cellular dehydration and shrinkage. The fluid shift also causes the plasma volume to increase to normal or greater than normal levels. *Thus the compensatory mechanisms and symptoms of hypovolemic shock are not present.* The problems caused by hypertonic dehydration result from changes in the levels of specific electrolytes affecting excitable membrane activity. Compensation mechanisms for hypertonic dehydration occur in response to the increased ECF osmolarity (Figure 15-3).

Hypertonic dehydration is caused by the loss of water or any hypotonic body fluid (low osmolarity, or decreased level of solute particles compared with isotonic body fluid). Common causes of hypertonic dehydration include excessive sweating, hyperventilation, ketoacidosis, prolonged fevers, diarrhea, early-stage renal failure, and diabetes insipidus (see Table 15-1).

Hypotonic Dehydration

Hypotonic dehydration is the least common type of fluid volume deficit. The problems caused by hypotonic dehydration result from fluid shifts between spaces, causing a decrease in plasma volume.

Hypotonic dehydration involves excessive loss of sodium and potassium from the ECF. This loss leads to decreased blood and interstitial fluid osmolarity, making them hypotonic compared with normal ECF. The decreased ECF osmolarity lowers the osmotic pressure of plasma and interstitial fluids to below that of the fluid inside the cells, the ICF. As a result of this difference in osmotic pressure, water moves from the plasma and interstitial spaces into the cells, creating a plasma volume deficit and causing the cells to swell.

Cell swelling causes widespread problems and symptoms. Because brain cells are more sensitive to swelling than the cells of other tissues, neurologic problems often occur with

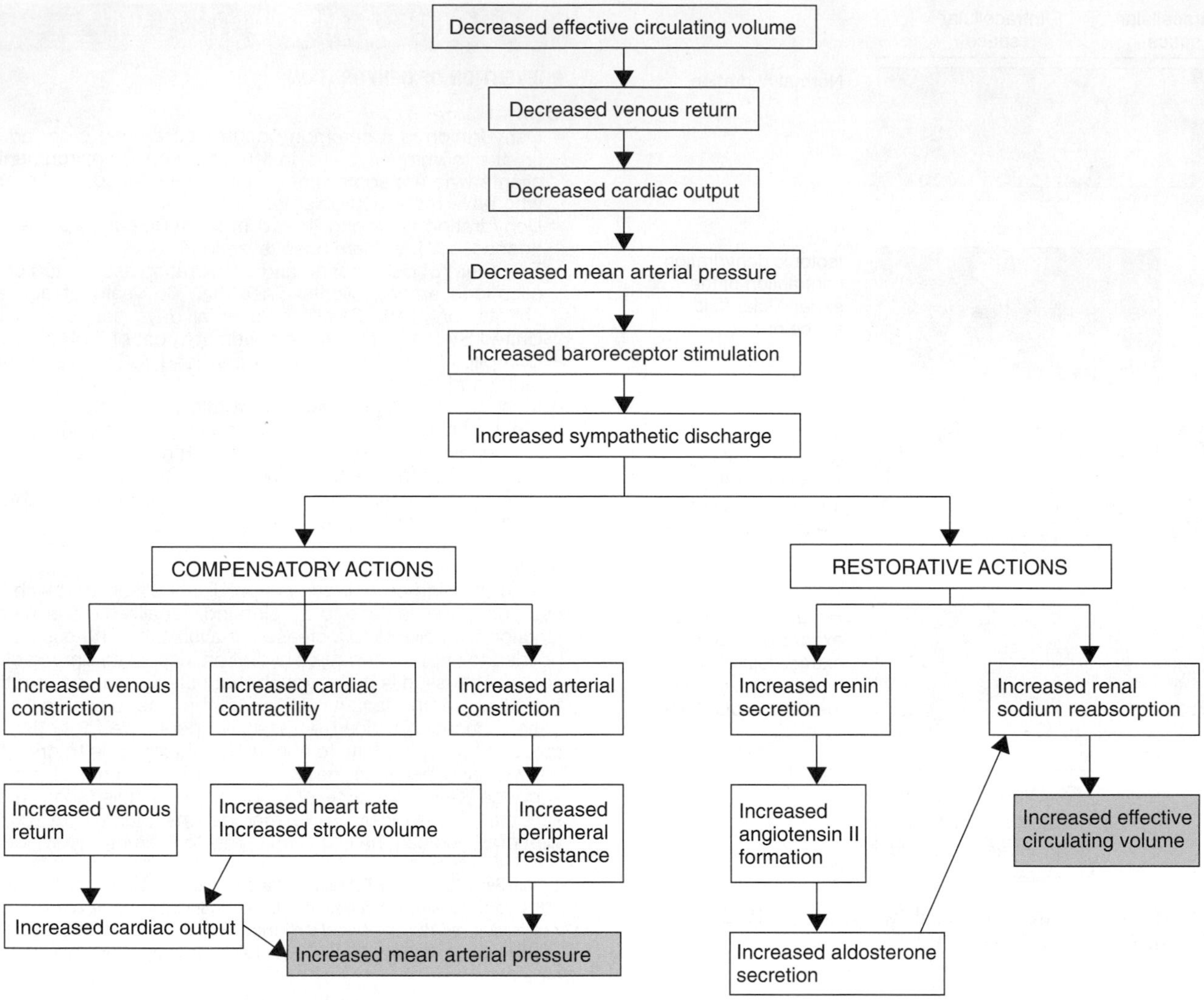

Figure 15-2 ■ Compensatory mechanisms associated with isotonic dehydration.

TABLE 15-1 Common Causes of Dehydration

Isotonic Dehydration
- Hemorrhage
- Vomiting
- Diarrhea
- Profuse salivation
- Fistulas
- Abscesses
- Ileostomy
- Cecostomy
- Frequent enemas
- Profuse diaphoresis
- Burns
- Severe wounds
- Long-term NPO (nothing by mouth)
- Diuretic therapy
- Gastrointestinal suction

Hypertonic Dehydration
- Hyperventilation
- Watery diarrhea
- Renal failure
- Ketoacidosis
- Diabetes insipidus
- Excessive fluid replacement (hypertonic)
- Excessive sodium bicarbonate administration
- Tube feedings
- Dysphagia
- Impaired thirst
- Unconsciousness
- Fever
- Impaired motor function
- Systemic infection

Hypotonic Dehydration
- Chronic illness
- Excessive fluid replacement (hypotonic)
- Renal failure
- Chronic or severe malnutrition

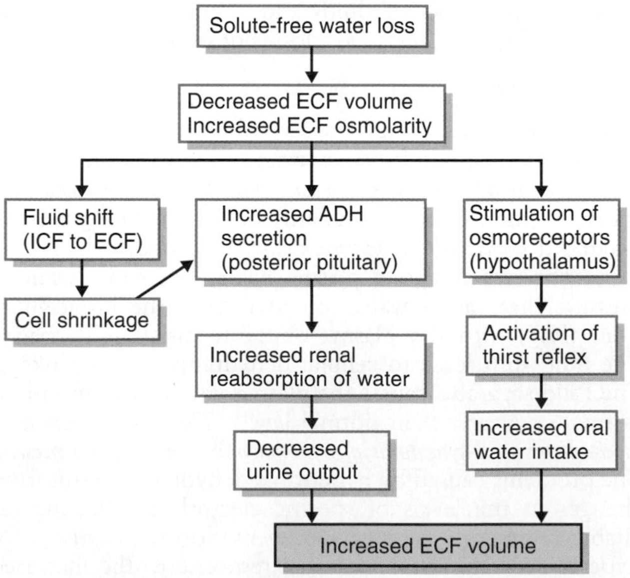

Figure 15-3 ■ Compensatory mechanisms associated with hypertonic dehydration. *ADH,* Antidiuretic hormone; *ECF,* extracellular fluid; *ICF,* intracellular fluid.

hypotonic dehydration. Hypotonic fluid also dilutes the normal electrolyte levels and causes sodium and potassium imbalances.

Hypotonic dehydration occurs more often with chronic illness. Chronic renal failure with sodium wasting leads to hypotonic dehydration. Malnutrition and ingesting excessive amounts of hypotonic fluids also cause hypotonic dehydration.

HEALTH PROMOTION/ILLNESS PREVENTION

Mild dehydration is common among healthy adults and is corrected or prevented easily by matching fluid intake with fluid output. Problems occur when people perform heavy exercise, especially in warm environments, without taking the time to replace excessive fluid losses. Teach all clients to drink more fluids whenever they engage in heavy physical activity.

Moderate to severe dehydration is more likely to occur in people who are unable to obtain fluids without help. Older adults living in long-term care facilities and those adults with cognitive or motor problems are dependent upon others for hydration. Dehydration in this population can be prevented with purposeful hydration programs (see the Evidence-Based Practice for Nursing box at right).

◆COLLABORATIVE MANAGEMENT

◆Assessment

HISTORY

Collect data on risk factors and factors causing dehydration (Table 15-2).

AGE. The client's age is important because dehydration in older adults develops quickly in response to small fluid losses. In addition, older people are more likely to have chronic illnesses or to be taking drugs, such as diuretics, that can lead to fluid and electrolyte imbalances.

HEIGHT AND WEIGHT. Measuring height and weight is important for calculating fluid needs. If possible, take these measurements directly. *Because 1 L of water weighs about 2.2 pounds (1 kg), changes in daily weights are the best indicators of fluid losses or gains.* A weight change of 1 pound corresponds to a fluid volume change of about 500 mL.

OTHER CHANGES. Ask the client about changes in ring or shoe tightness. A sudden decrease in tightness may indicate dehydration; an increase may reflect edema. Other related changes include palpitations or light-headedness on moving from a lying or a sitting position to a standing position caused by orthostatic hypotension. **Orthostatic hypotension** (also called **postural hypotension**) is a large drop in blood pressure during the first few seconds to minutes after changing from a sitting or lying position to a standing position.

Ask about any abnormal or excessive fluid losses, such as sweating, diarrhea, bleeding, vomiting, urination, salivation, and wound drainage. Other important information to collect includes history of chronic illnesses, recent acute illnesses, recent surgery, and drug regimens.

Ask specific questions about urine output, including the frequency and amount of voidings. Also ask about the client's usual fluid intake and the intake during the previous 24 hours. It is just as important to assess the *types* of fluids ingested as it is to assess the *amount* of fluids ingested, because fluids vary widely in osmolarity. Ask whether the client has recently engaged in strenuous physical activity and, if so, whether the activity took place in hot or dry environmental conditions.

EVIDENCE-BASED PRACTICE for Nursing

If you come, they will drink it

Robinson, S., & Rosher, R. (2002). Can a beverage cart help improve hydration? *Geriatric Nursing, 23*(4), 208-211.

This study compared the indicators of dehydration in older adults before, during, and after implementation of a dehydration prevention strategy. The dehydration prevention strategy was the use of a beverage cart and a designated "hydration assistant" to increase the fluid intake among 51 nursing home residents. The purpose of the study was to determine the effectiveness of a hydration program to increase fluid intake to a minimum of 1500 mL/day in preventing conditions associated with dehydration (delirium, urinary tract infections, respiratory infections, falls, skin breakdown, and constipation). The study used a quasiexperimental, prospective design. A hydration assistant was educated in the problems associated with dehydration and the techniques for oral fluid administration. A specific hydration needs assessment was performed for each resident to determine special fluid needs (e.g., sugar-free fluids, thickened fluids). A beverage cart was created using colorful pitchers and glasses. The intervention involved offering each resident who participated in the study an 8-oz drink at mid-morning and mid-afternoon. Each resident was offered at least four choices of beverages at each encounter.

Participants served as their own controls. Data regarding indicators of hydration were collected weekly for 9 weeks. These data included bioimpedence analysis of body water, and documentation of the number of bowel movements, laxatives, enemas, falls, episodes of mental status changes, urinary tract infections, respiratory tract infections, and skin breakdown. Additionally, the amount of fluid ingested with the intervention was recorded. Two weeks of data collection occurred before implementing the intervention. The intervention was implemented for the next 5 weeks. Data collection continued for 2 weeks after the intervention was stopped.

Fifty-three percent of the participants consistently achieved the goal of consuming an extra 8 oz of fluid twice each day. During the intervention, the participants had greater total body water volumes and fewer indicators of dehydration than they did before or after the intervention.

Level of Evidence: 3—Well-designed trial without randomization.

Critique. This study demonstrated that an extra 500 mL of fluid intake per day among nursing home residents could provide enough hydration to meet minimal fluid needs and prevent some problems of dehydration. Measuring the utility of a "hydration assistant" was not a stated purpose of this study but may be one of the most important study outcomes. Although it is useful to have participants serve as their own controls, a true control group would have strengthened the study. Additionally, examining daily weights of all participants during the data collection period could have validated the use of this measure as an outcome indicator for adequate hydration.

Implications for Nursing. This study demonstrated the usefulness of purposeful hydration in a nursing home population. Although the study pointed out that having a "hydration assistant" may not be feasible, the costs associated with the prevention of problems associated with dehydration could offset the cost of a hydration assistant. One of the benefits of having a hydration assistant is the amount of time this person could spend with each participant to encourage intake.

TABLE 15-2 Risk Factors for Dehydration

Illnesses
- Vomiting
- Diarrhea
- Burns
- Large, draining wounds
- Liver dysfunction
- Diabetes mellitus
- Diabetes insipidus
- Renal disease
- Hemorrhage
- Major venous obstruction
- Prolonged febrile state

Other Situations
- Extremes of age: older adults, infants
- Unconsciousness
- Motor limitations

Therapies
- Surgery
- Diuretics
- Nothing by mouth
- Excessive hypertonic enemas
- Nasogastric suction

PHYSICAL ASSESSMENT/CLINICAL MANIFESTATIONS

The clinical manifestations of dehydration depend on which body fluid spaces lose fluid, although all body systems are affected to some degree (Chart 15-1). The most obvious and life-threatening problems are seen when dehydration decreases the plasma volume.

CARDIOVASCULAR MANIFESTATIONS. Cardiovascular changes are good indicators of plasma volume changes. Heart rate increases with plasma volume deficits in an attempt to maintain blood pressure with less blood. Peripheral pulses are weak, difficult to find, and easily blocked with light pressure. If interstitial edema occurs with dehydration, the peripheral pulses may not be palpable. The blood pressure also decreases, as does the pulse pressure, with a greater decrease in the systolic blood pressure. Hypotension is more severe with the client in the standing position than with the client in the sitting or lying position (orthostatic or postural hypotension). Because the blood pressure with the client standing may be much lower than in other positions, first measure blood pressure with the client lying down, then sitting, and finally standing. These measures are also called "ortho checks" or "ortho changes."

Another indicator of hydration status is the degree of neck vein and hand vein filling. Normally, hand veins fill and become engorged when the hands are lower than the level of the heart. As the hands are raised above the level of the heart, the veins flatten or collapse (Figure 15-4). Neck veins are normally distended when a client is in the supine position. These veins flatten when the client moves to a sitting position. When dehydration causes a plasma volume deficit, neck and hand veins are flat, even when the neck and hands are not raised above the level of the heart. These cardiovascular changes are not seen in hypertonic dehydration.

RESPIRATORY MANIFESTATIONS. The respiratory rate increases with the degree of fluid loss from plasma volume. The decreased blood volume is perceived by the body as decreased oxygen levels **(hypoxia),** and increased respiratory rate is an attempt to maintain oxygen delivery.

CHART 15-1

KEY FEATURES of Dehydration

Manifestations of Dehydration in General*

Cardiovascular
- Increased pulse rate
- Thready pulse quality
- Decreased blood pressure
- Postural (orthostatic) hypotension
- Flat neck and hand veins in dependent positions
- Diminished peripheral pulses
- Weight loss

Respiratory
- Increased respiratory rate
- Increased depth of respirations

Neuromuscular
- Decreased central nervous system activity (lethargy to coma)
- Fever

Renal
- Decreased urine output
- Increased urine specific gravity

Integumentary
- Skin dry and scaly
- Turgor poor, tenting present
- Mouth dry and fissured, pastelike coating present

Gastrointestinal
- Decreased motility
- Diminished bowel sounds
- Constipation
- Thirst

Manifestations of Hypotonic Dehydration
- Skeletal muscle weakness

Manifestations of Hypertonic Dehydration
- Hyperactive deep tendon reflexes
- Increased sensation of thirst
- Pitting edema

*These manifestations are most severe with hypotonic dehydration.

SKIN MANIFESTATIONS. Changes in skin may indicate a change in hydration. Assess for changes in the skin and mucous membranes that may indicate dehydration, including skin color, moisture, skin turgor, and edema. In older clients this information is less reliable because of poor skin turgor resulting from the loss of elastic tissue and the loss of tissue fluids with aging. Assess skin turgor by checking the following:

- How easily the skin over the back of the hand and arm can be gently pinched between the thumb and the forefinger to form a "tent"
- How soon the pinched skin resumes its normal position after release
- Whether depressions (pits) remain in the skin after a finger is pressed firmly but gently (over the shin, over the sternum, and over the sacrum)
- How deep the depression is (in millimeters)
- How long the depression remains

In generalized dehydration, skin turgor is poor, with the tenting remaining for minutes after pinching the skin, and no skin depressions occur with gentle pressure. The skin is dry and scaly.

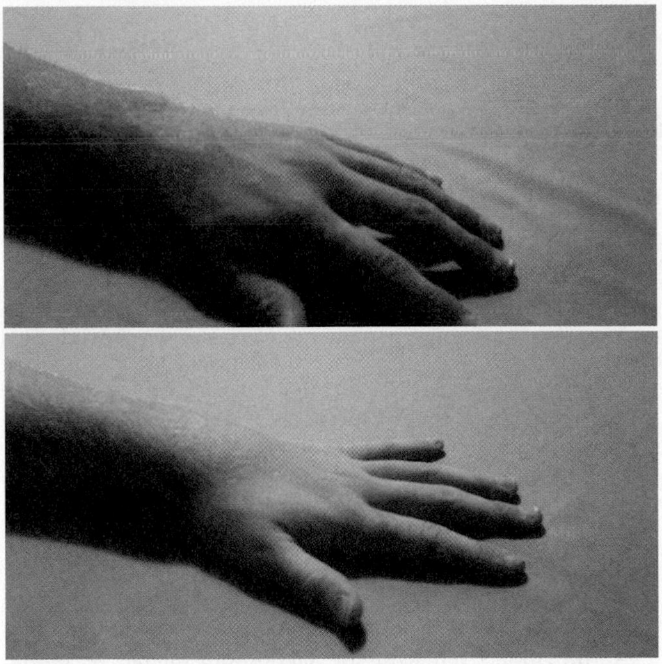

Figure 15-4 ■ Hand veins full and bulging in the dependent position *(top)*. Hand veins collapsed *(bottom)*.

CHART 15-2

BEST PRACTICE for
Brief Check of Mental Status

- Is the client awake?
- If the client is not awake, what type of stimulation is needed to wake the client?
  - Calling the client's name in a normal voice volume
  - Calling the client's name in a louder voice volume
  - Touching the client's arm or face while calling the client's name
  - Gently tapping or shaking an arm
  - Vigorously shaking a hand or arm
  - Applying a painful stimulus
- If the client is awake, ask questions that require more than a "yes" or "no" response to establish orientation to time and place.
- Avoid the use of nonsense questions (e.g., "Do helicopters eat their young?").
- Ask questions that are reasonable and likely to be known by the client, such as "When is your birthday?" Avoid questions such as "Who was vice president under Truman?"
- Is it necessary to repeat questions to obtain a response?
- Does the response answer the question asked?
- Does the client have difficulty with word choices in forming responses?
- Is the client irritated or upset by the questions?
- Can the client concentrate on a question long enough to provide an appropriate response, or is the attention span short?
- Can the client count by threes?
- Can the client count backward from 100 by threes?
- Does the client know the names of immediate family members?
- Does the client know who the questioner is (not necessarily the questioner's name but that person's role in the client's care, such as nurse, doctor, chaplain, therapist)?
- Does the client know his or her immediate location (e.g., home, hospital, clinic)?
- Does the client know the year?

CONSIDERATIONS FOR OLDER ADULTS

Assess skin turgor in an older adult by pinching the skin over the sternum or the forehead, rather than the back of the hand, because these areas more reliably indicate hydration (see Figure 14-10). As a person ages, the skin loses elasticity and tents on hands and arms even when the person is well hydrated.

In dehydration, oral mucous membranes are not moist. They may be covered with a thick, sticky, pastelike coating and may have cracks and fissures. The surface of the tongue may have deep furrows.

NEUROLOGIC MANIFESTATIONS. Dehydration may cause changes in mental status and body temperature status because blood flow in the brain is reduced. Mental status changes, especially confusion, with dehydration are more common among older adults and may be the first indication of a fluid balance problem. Chart 15-2 outlines how to assess mental status quickly. The client with dehydration often has a low-grade fever. One cause of the fever is the blood vessel constriction that occurs as a compensation for hypovolemia. The blood vessel constriction makes heat dissipation more difficult.

Fever can also cause dehydration. A client with a temperature greater than 102° F (39° C) for longer than 6 hours is especially at risk. Older adults, who normally have a body temperature range of 96° to 98° F (35.4° to 36.6° C), are at greater risk for dehydration during episodes of fever.

RENAL MANIFESTATIONS. The volume and the composition of urine output indicate hydration status. Monitor urine output, comparing total output with total fluid intake and daily weights. Accurate intake and output measurement is a major nursing responsibility. Urine output below 500 mL/day for any client without renal disease is cause for concern. Weigh the client each day at the same time and on the same scale. When possible, have the client wear the same amount and type of clothing for each weigh-in. Metabolic weight loss (even in starvation) usually accounts for only about ½ pound of weight loss per day. Any weight loss in excess of this amount is fluid loss.

PSYCHOSOCIAL ASSESSMENT

Observe the client for behavioral changes that occur with dehydration. At first, a dehydrated client may have a flat affect and may seem unconcerned about his or her health and possible treatment regimens. As dehydration worsens, the client may become anxious, restless, lethargic, and confused (especially an older adult client). These changes are more obvious in hypertonic and hypotonic dehydration because of intracellular fluid (ICF) shifts in brain cells, resulting in shrinkage or swelling of the cells. If dehydration continues, blood flow to the brain becomes so impaired that delirium and coma can occur.

LABORATORY ASSESSMENT

No single laboratory test result confirms or rules out dehydration. Instead, dehydration is determined by laboratory findings along with clinical manifestations. Laboratory findings depend on the type of dehydration present (Chart 15-3). Isotonic and hypotonic dehydration with plasma volume deficits show **hemoconcentration** (elevated levels of hemoglobin,

CHART 15-3

LABORATORY PROFILE
Dehydration

Values*	Isotonic Dehydration	Hypotonic Dehydration	Hypertonic Dehydration
Blood Values			
BUN	Normal or increased	Increased	Increased
Creatinine	Normal or increased	Increased	Increased
Sodium	Normal	<120 mEq/L (mmol)	>150 mEq/L (mmol)
Osmolarity	Normal	Decreased	Increased
Hematocrit	Increased	Increased	Normal or decreased
Hemoglobin	Increased	Increased	Normal or decreased
WBCs	Increased	Increased	Normal or decreased
Protein	Increased	Increased	Increased
Urine Values			
Specific gravity	>1.010	<1.010	>1.030
Osmolarity	Increased	Increased	Increased
Volume	Decreased	Decreased	Decreased

BUN, Blood urea nitrogen; *WBC*, white blood cell.
*All values reflect dehydration states alone and not the underlying pathologic changes or disease states contributing to the dehydration.

hematocrit, serum osmolarity, glucose, protein, blood urea nitrogen, and various electrolytes) because only the water is lost and other substances remain. Hemoconcentration is not present when dehydration is caused by hemorrhage, because loss of all blood and plasma products occurs together.

Specific urine laboratory values can help confirm dehydration if the client does not have renal dysfunction. Usually the urine of the client with dehydration is concentrated, with a specific gravity greater than 1.030. Volume is decreased, and osmolarity is greatly increased. The color is dark amber and has a strong odor.

Critical Thinking Challenge

The client is a 45-year-old, obese woman with type 1 diabetes who is brought to the emergency department in a coma. Her daughter tells you that the client has had pain and burning on urination for the past 3 days and that she has stopped drinking fluids so that she would not have to go to the bathroom as often. The daughter also tells you that the client has not taken her insulin for at least 2 days. The client's laboratory results are as follows: Blood glucose level is 540 mg/dL, white blood cell count (WBC) is 22,000/mm^3, hematocrit is 52%, serum potassium is 7 mmol/L, serum sodium is 140 mmol/L, blood osmolarity is 380 mOsm/L, and urine is positive for ketones.

1. What type of dehydration does she have?
2. What is the relationship between this type of dehydration and diabetes? (See Chapter 68.)
3. Would you expect her to have poor skin turgor or pitting edema? Why or why not?
4. Would you expect her to have hypotension? Why or why not?

evolve For suggested answer guidelines, go to http://evolve.elsevier.com/Iggy/.

Analysis

COMMON NURSING DIAGNOSES AND COLLABORATIVE PROBLEMS

The following are priority nursing diagnoses for clients with dehydration:

1. Deficient Fluid Volume related to excessive fluid loss or inadequate fluid intake
2. Decreased Cardiac Output related to decreased plasma volume
3. Impaired Oral Mucous Membrane related to inadequate oral secretions

The primary collaborative problem is Potential for Dysrhythmias.

ADDITIONAL NURSING DIAGNOSES AND COLLABORATIVE PROBLEMS

In addition to the common nursing diagnoses and collaborative problems, clients with dehydration may have one or more of the following:

- Constipation related to decreased body fluids
- Risk for Falls related to orthostatic (postural) hypotension
- Deficient Knowledge (medication regimen and preventive measures) related to lack of exposure or lack of interest in learning
- Risk for Impaired Skin Integrity related to deficiencies of interstitial fluid and inadequate tissue perfusion
- Ineffective Airway Clearance related to thick, sticky secretions
- Potential for Hypovolemic Shock
- Potential for Electrolyte Imbalances

Planning and Implementation

DEFICIENT FLUID VOLUME

NOC **PLANNING: EXPECTED OUTCOMES.** The client with dehydration is expected to have body fluid levels restored to normal as indicated by:

- Maintaining blood pressure and pulse (rate and quality) within normal limits
- Having 24-hour fluid intake balance with 24-hour fluid output
- Having urine specific gravity <1.030
- Having good skin turgor (no tenting when skin is pinched up)

INTERVENTIONS. Management of dehydration aims to prevent further fluid losses and increase fluid compartment volumes to normal ranges.

NIC **Fluid Management.** Diet therapy, oral rehydration therapy, and drug therapy are used to correct fluid volume deficit (Chart 15-4).

CHART 15-4

NIC INTERVENTION ACTIVITIES for The Client with Deficient Fluid Volume

Fluid Monitoring: *Collection and analysis of client data to regulate fluid balance*
- Monitor serum and urine electrolyte values, as appropriate.
- Monitor blood pressure, heart rate, and respiratory status.
- Monitor orthostatic blood pressure and change in cardiac rhythm, as appropriate.
- Monitor weight.
- Monitor intake and output.
- Note presence or absence of vertigo on rising.
- Monitor color, quantity, and specific gravity of urine.

Fluid Management: *Promotion of fluid balance and prevention of complications resulting from abnormal or undesired fluid levels*
- Administer IV therapy, as prescribed.
- Give fluids, as appropriate.
- Promote oral intake (e.g., provide a drinking straw, offer fluids between meals, change ice water routinely), as appropriate.
- Distribute the fluid intake over 24 hours, as appropriate.
- Encourage significant other to assist client with feedings, as appropriate.
- Offer snacks (e.g., frequent drinks and fresh fruits/fruit juice), as appropriate.

Oral Health Restoration: *Promotion of healing for a client who has an oral mucosa or dental lesion*
- Encourage frequent rinsing of mouth with any of the following: sodium bicarbonate solution, warm saline, or hydrogen peroxide solution.
- Monitor lips, tongue, mucous membranes, tonsillar fossae, and gums for moisture, color, texture, presence of debris, and infection, using good lighting and a tongue blade.
- Instruct client to avoid commercial mouthwashes.
- Monitor client every shift for dryness of the oral mucosa.
- Increase mouth care to every 2 hours and twice at night, if stomatitis is not controlled.
- Avoid use of lemon-glycerin swabs.
- Increase liquids on the meal tray.

NIC intervention activities selected from Dochterman, J.M., & Bulechek, G.M. (Eds.). (2004). *Nursing interventions classification (NIC)* (4th ed.). St. Louis: Mosby.

Diet Therapy. Mild to moderate dehydration is corrected with oral fluid replacement if the client is alert enough to swallow and can tolerate oral fluids. Encourage and measure fluid intake. The specific type of fluid needed for replacement varies with the type of dehydration.

Gain the client's cooperation in drinking oral replacement fluids by using fluids he or she enjoys and by carefully timing the intake schedule. Dividing the total amount of fluids needed by nursing shifts helps to meet fluid needs more evenly over 24 hours with less danger of overhydration. Offer the conscious client small volumes of fluids every hour to increase intake.

Oral Fluid Rehydration Therapy. Oral rehydration therapy (ORT) is the most cost-effective way to replace fluids for the client with dehydration. Specifically formulated solutions containing glucose and electrolytes are absorbed even when the client is vomiting or has diarrhea. Fluid losses from diarrhea are usually 2 to 3 L/day and should be replaced liter for liter, especially in older clients. A typical prescription might be "Resol 1 L every 8 hours." Table 15-3 lists commercially available ORT solutions.

Drug Therapy. Drug therapy for dehydration is directed at restoring fluid balance and controlling the causes of dehydration. Whenever possible, fluids are replaced by the oral route. When dehydration is severe or life threatening, or the client is unconscious, intravenous (IV) fluid replacement is needed. Calculation of how much fluid to replace is based on the client's weight loss and clinical manifestations. The rate of fluid replacement depends on the degree of dehydration and the presence of other cardiac, pulmonary, or renal problems.

The type of fluid prescribed by the health care provider varies with the type of dehydration and the client's cardiovascular status. Usually the client receives IV infusions of water with whatever solutes (especially electrolytes) are needed on the basis of laboratory values. Table 15-4 lists the osmolarity, caloric content, and tonicity of common IV fluids. Generally, isotonic dehydration is treated with isotonic fluid solutions, hypertonic dehydration is treated with hypotonic fluid solutions, and hypotonic dehydration is treated with hypertonic fluid solutions. The two most important areas to monitor during rehydration are pulse rate and quality and urine output.

Drug therapy corrects the causes of the dehydration. Antidiarrheal drugs are prescribed when diarrhea causes dehydration. Antimicrobial therapy may be used in clients with bacterial diarrhea. Antiemetics to control vomiting may be needed when vomiting induces dehydration. Antipyretics to reduce temperature are helpful when fever makes dehydration worse.

DECREASED CARDIAC OUTPUT

NOC **PLANNING: EXPECTED OUTCOMES.** The client with dehydration is expected to have cardiac output restored to normal levels and to maintain adequate oxygenation to vital organs as indicated by:
- Having blood pressure and pulse (rate and quality) within the client's normal range
- Maintaining a urine output of at least 30 mL/hr

INTERVENTIONS. Interventions of drug and oxygen therapy aim to increase circulating fluid volume, support compensatory mechanisms, and prevent complications.

Drug Therapy. Drug therapy to increase body fluid volume and prevent excessive fluid loss is the same as that for the client with fluid volume deficit. Drugs to increase venous return or improve cardiac contractility are used only when a cardiac problem also is present.

TABLE 15-3 Commercial Solutions for Oral Rehydration Therapy

Brand Name	Na^+ (mEq/L)	K^+ (mEq/L)	Cl^- (mEq/L)	Citrate (mEq/L)	Sugar or Starch	Calories (kcal/L)
Ricelyte (Mead-Johnson)	50	25	45	34	Rice syrup (30 g)	126
Resol (Wyeth-Ayerst)	50	20	50	34	Dextrose (20 g)	84
Rehydralyte (Ross Labs)	75	20	65	30	Dextrose (25 g)	100
Pedialyte (Ross Labs)	45	20	35	30	Dextrose (25 g)	100
Gastrolyte (Rorer)	60	20	60	10	Dextrose (17.8 g)	75
Rapolyte (Richmond)	90	20	80	30	Dextrose (20 g)	84
Lytren (Mead-Johnson)	50	25	45	30	Dextrose (20 g)	84
Oralyte (Rugby)	45	20	25	48	Dextrose (25 g)	100
Kao Lectrolyte (Pharmacia & UpJohn)	50	20	—	30	Dextrose (20 g)	84

Data from United States Pharmacopeia Dispensing Information (USP DI): Vol I. (2000). *Drug information for the health care professional* (20th ed.). Englewood, CO: Micromedix.

TABLE 15-4 Characteristics of Common Intravenous Therapy Solutions

Solution	Osmolarity (mOsm/L)	pH	Calories* (kcal)	Tonicity
0.9% saline	308	5	0	Isotonic
0.45% saline	154	5	0	Hypotonic
5% dextrose in water (D_5W)	272	3.5-6.5	170	Isotonic†
10% dextrose in water ($D_{10}W$)	500	3.5-6.5	340	Hypertonic†
5% dextrose in 0.9% saline	560	3.5-6.5	170	Hypertonic†
5% dextrose in 0.45% saline	406	4	170	Hypertonic†
5% dextrose in 0.225% saline	321	4	170	Isotonic†
Ringer's lactate	273	6.5	9	Isotonic
5% dextrose in Ringer's lactate	525	4-6.5	179	Hypertonic†

Data from Trissel, L. (2003). *Handbook on injectable drugs* (12th ed.). Bethesda, MD: American Society of Hospital-System Pharmacists.

*Calories are calculated on the basis of a volume of 1000 mL.

†*Solution tonicity at the time of administration.* Within a short time after administration, the dextrose is metabolized, and the tonicity of the infused solution decreases in proportion to the osmolarity or tonicity of the nondextrose components (electrolytes) within the water.

Oxygen Therapy. Oxygen is delivered by mask or nasal cannula to the client with dehydration. Give the client water-nebulized oxygen at the rate or amount specified by the health care provider's prescription.

NIC **Fluid Monitoring.** Monitoring vital signs and level of consciousness is important when caring for clients with dehydration (see Chart 15-4). Monitor the pulse, blood pressure, pulse pressure, central venous pressure, respiratory rate, and skin and mucous membrane color every 15 minutes. Monitor urine output at least every hour until the fluid imbalance is resolved.

Critical Thinking Challenge

The client with diabetic ketoacidosis and dehydration is prescribed to receive intravenous normal saline (0.9% sodium chloride) at 1000 mL/hr for the first 2 hours. Ten (10) units of regular insulin are given immediately IV push and a continuous insulin infusion of 10 units/hr is prescribed until the ketosis has stopped.

1. What is the osmolarity of the normal saline solution? Is this considered hypotonic, isotonic, or hypertonic?
2. What would be the rationale for giving this client saline when her serum sodium level is in the normal range?
3. Why is the client not prescribed oral replacement fluids?
4. Should the care of this client be assigned to an RN, LPN/LVN, or assistive nursing personnel? (Explain your rationale for the caregiver assignment.)
5. What criteria would you use to determine whether the fluid replacement is adequate?
6. How often should this client be assessed? Why?

evolve For suggested answer guidelines, go to http://evolve.elsevier.com/Iggy/.

IMPAIRED ORAL MUCOUS MEMBRANE

NOC **PLANNING: EXPECTED OUTCOMES.** With appropriate intervention, the client with dehydration is expected to have moist mucous membranes as indicated by:

- Absence of cracks or fissures on lips and tongue
- Absence of coating on tongue

INTERVENTIONS. Interventions for oral health include drug therapy, fluid replacement, and good oral hygiene, as well as the early diagnosis and prevention of complications (see Chart 15-4).

Drug Therapy. Drug therapy to increase fluid volume and prevent fluid loss is the same as that discussed earlier for deficient fluid volume (p. 218). Saliva substitutes, such as

Salivart, can reduce the sensation of mouth dryness. *To prevent aspiration, do not use such agents in an unconscious client.*

Oral Hygiene. Nursing actions to promote oral hygiene can increase the client's comfort. Keep the lips clean and moist. Offer mouth care at least every 8 hours to reduce the thick, sticky coating on the tongue and mouth during dehydration.

Mouth care includes gentle toothbrushing several times a day and rinsing hourly. Teach the client to avoid mouthwashes and swabs that contain alcohol or glycerin because these products dry the oral mucosa further and may sting open areas of the mucosa. Rinsing the mouth with dilute solutions of hydrogen peroxide two times per day is a good form of oral hygiene; however, when used more often, it increases oral dryness. Tap water and normal saline rinses can be used safely as often as the client wishes.

Prevention of Complications. A dry mouth can cause sores and fissures in the mucosa, increasing the risk for infection. The thick, sticky coating also is an excellent breeding ground for organisms. A complication of mouth dryness is a wide variety of oral infections. Chart 15-4 lists NIC interventions for mouth care.

POTENTIAL FOR DYSRHYTHMIAS

NOC **PLANNING: EXPECTED OUTCOMES.** The client with dehydration is expected to maintain his or her normal cardiac rhythm.

INTERVENTIONS. Interventions are aimed at correcting the dehydration and recognizing dysrhythmias so that appropriate drug therapy can be initiated.

Drug Therapy. Drug therapy to increase body fluid volume and prevent excessive fluid loss is the same as that discussed earlier for deficient fluid volume (p. 218).

Elevated potassium or calcium levels can cause life-threatening dysrhythmias. Drug therapy to reduce these electrolytes may be prescribed. If potassium levels are high, a combination of 20 units of regular insulin in 100 mL of 20% dextrose may be prescribed to promote movement of potassium from the blood into the intracellular fluid (ICF). Drugs such as etidronate (Didronel) and plicamycin (Mithracin) may be prescribed to reduce high serum calcium levels.

Monitoring. Monitor the client for signs and symptoms of cardiac dysrhythmias every 15 minutes until he or she is fully rehydrated. Assess the rate, rhythm, and quality of the apical pulse and compare those findings with the client's baseline measurements. Assess for fatigue, chest discomfort or pain, and shortness of breath. Assess hand grasps and deep tendon reflexes, and record changes from baseline.

Clients at risk for dysrhythmias are monitored using electrocardiography (ECG). The pattern may show tall T waves or a shortened ST segment. Immediately report any change from the client's baseline ECG to the health care provider.

Community-Based Care

No extensive home care preparations are necessary for clients with mild dehydration or for those with dehydration of sudden onset. The imbalance is corrected before discharge from the facility and is unlikely to recur. Clients who are most likely to be discharged before the imbalance is completely corrected and who are susceptible to recurrent episodes are those with chronic problems, such as renal disease, diabetes, cancer, adrenal insufficiency, and many endocrine disorders. These clients often need long-term diet and drug therapy.

CHART 15-5

HOME CARE ASSESSMENT of
The Client at Risk for Dehydration

Assess cardiovascular status.
- Vital signs, including apical pulse, pulse pressure, presence or absence of orthostatic hypotension, and quality and rhythm of peripheral pulses
- Presence or absence of peripheral edema
- Hand vein filling in the dependent position
- Neck vein filling in the recumbent and sitting positions
- Weight gain or loss

Assess cognition and mental status.
- Level of consciousness
- Orientation to time, place, and person
- Can the client accurately read a seven-word sentence containing no words greater than three syllables?

Assess condition of skin and mucous membranes.
- Presence or absence of skin tenting over the sternum or the forehead
- Moistness of skin, most reliable on chest and back
- Presence or absence of coating on tongue or teeth
- Can the client spit?

Assess neuromuscular status.
- Reactivity of patellar and biceps reflexes
- Oral temperature
- Handgrip strength
- Steadiness of gait

Assess renal system.
- Observe urine specimen for color, odor, cloudiness, and amount

Ask about the following:
- 24-hour fluid intake and output
- 24-hour diet recall
- 24-hour activity recall
- Over-the-counter and prescribed medications the client has taken

Assess client's understanding of illness and compliance with treatment.
- Signs and symptoms to report to health care provider
- Medication plan (correct timing and dose)

Perform a focused assessment (Chart 15-5) and a mental status check at every home visit to a client at risk for dehydration. Review drugs, manifestations of dehydration, and health care resources with the client and family.

Education is important in the prevention and early detection of dehydration. Teach the client at risk for dehydration about diet, drug regimens, and the manifestations of dehydration. Explain the meaning of changes found on assessment.

Stress the importance of recording accurate daily weights in assessing hydration status. Instruct clients to weigh themselves on the same scale daily, close to the same time each day, and with about the same amount of clothing on each time. Keeping a chart comparing the recorded weights from one day to the next can help the client recognize early-stage dehydration.

Instruct clients to take drugs as prescribed and not increase the use of diuretics. Explain that if a diuretic is not taken one day, the next day's dose should not be doubled. Teach clients how and where to assess skin turgor. Teach them how to measure their own peripheral pulse and obtain a return demonstration.

If the client has any mobility impairment, instruct the family to keep fluids in places that the client can access. Teach them to modify containers, such as opening zip-top cans and covering them with foil, to ensure that the client can easily open container lids. "Sipper" containers not only provide easy access but also are unbreakable and reduce spillage.

Critical Thinking Challenge

Your diabetic client has had her dehydration and diabetic ketoacidosis corrected. She is going home and will be managed at the diabetes clinic.

1. What specific areas of teaching will you emphasize to her?
2. What fluids would be most useful in preventing a recurrence of the dehydration?

evolve For suggested answer guidelines, go to http://evolve.elsevier.com/Iggy/.

Evaluation: Outcomes

Evaluate the care of the client with dehydration on the basis of the identified nursing diagnoses and collaborative problems. The expected outcomes include that the client should:

- Ingest at least 1500 mL of hypotonic fluids each day
- Maintain a fluid output approximately equal to fluid intake
- Have urine output volumes and specific gravity within normal limits
- State that oral mucosal discomfort is relieved
- Experience no oral mucosal complication

Specific indicators for these outcomes are listed for each nursing diagnosis and collaborative problem under the Planning and Implementation section (see earlier).

OVERHYDRATION

PATHOPHYSIOLOGY

Overhydration, also called fluid overload, is an excess of body fluid. It is not a disease but rather a clinical sign of a problem in which fluid intake or retention is greater than the body's fluid needs. Overhydration may be either an actual excess of total body fluid or a relative fluid excess in one or more body fluid spaces. The three basic types of fluid volume excess are isotonic overhydration, hypotonic overhydration, and hypertonic overhydration (Figure 15-5).

Most problems caused by overhydration are related to fluid volume excess in the vascular space or to dilution of specific electrolytes and blood components. Clinical manifestations vary with the type and degree of overhydration (Chart 15-6). The conditions leading to overhydration (fluid overload) are related to excessive intake or inadequate excretion of fluid. Table 15-5 lists common causes of overhydration.

Isotonic Overhydration

Isotonic overhydration is also called **hypervolemia** because the problems result from excessive fluid in the extracellular fluid (ECF) space. In isotonic overhydration, isotonic fluids are ingested or retained, so that osmolarity remains normal. Only the ECF compartment expands, and fluid does not shift between the spaces. The problems caused by severe isotonic overhydration are circulatory overload and edema. Figure 15-6 outlines the compensation that occurs in response to mild or moderate isotonic overhydration. When isotonic overhydration is severe, or when it occurs in a person with poor cardiac function, overhydration can lead to heart failure and pulmonary edema.

Hypotonic Overhydration

In hypotonic overhydration (water intoxication), the excess fluid is hypotonic to normal body fluids. Thus the osmolarity of the ECF decreases, and hydrostatic pressure increases. Fluid moves into the intracellular space because of the decreased plasma osmotic pressure, and all fluid spaces expand (see Figure 15-5). Because the excess fluid is hypotonic, electrolyte imbalances caused by dilution occur with hypotonic overhydration.

Hypertonic Overhydration

Hypertonic overhydration is rare and is caused by an excessive sodium intake. The hyperosmolarity of the plasma and interstitial compartments draws fluid from the intracellular fluid (ICF) compartment. Thus the ECF volume expands, and the ICF volume contracts (see Figure 15-5).

COLLABORATIVE MANAGEMENT

Assessment

Manifestations of overhydration vary with the specific type, the body fluid spaces involved, and the degree of overhydration. Clients with isotonic overhydration or hypertonic overhydration have circulatory overload and pitting edema (Figure 15-7). Clients with hypotonic overhydration have problems

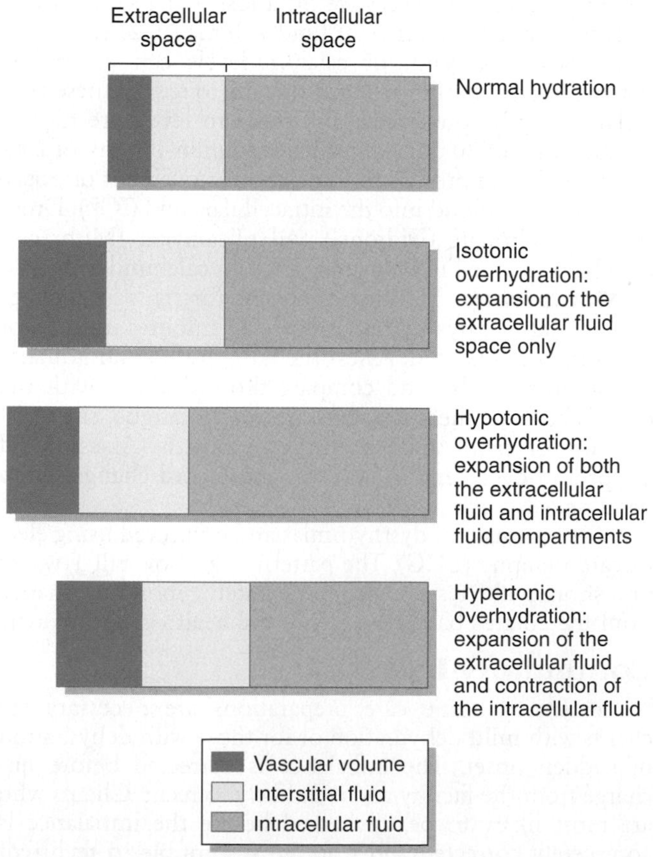

Figure 15-5 ■ Three types of overhydration. (© 1992 M. Linda Workman. All rights reserved.)

CHART 15-6

KEY FEATURES of Overhydration

Manifestations of Overhydration in General

Cardiovascular
- Increased pulse rate
- Bounding pulse quality
- Peripheral pulses full
- Elevated blood pressure
- Decreased pulse pressure
- Elevated central venous pressure
- Distended neck and hand veins
- Engorged venous varicosities
- Weight gain

Respiratory
- Respiratory rate increased
- Shallow respirations
- Dyspnea increases with exertion or in the supine position
- Moist crackles present on auscultation

Integumentary
- Pitting edema in dependent areas
- Skin pale and cool to touch

Neuromuscular
- Altered level of consciousness
- Headache
- Visual disturbances
- Skeletal muscle weakness
- Paresthesias

Gastrointestinal
- Increased motility

Manifestations of Isotonic Overhydration
- Liver enlargement
- Ascites formation

Manifestations of Hypotonic Overhydration
- Polyuria
- Diarrhea
- Nonpitting edema
- Cardiac dysrhythmias associated with electrolyte dilution
- Projectile vomiting

with cellular swelling and electrolyte dilution. Chart 15-6 lists the common manifestations of overhydration.

A diagnosis of overhydration is based on assessment findings and the results of laboratory tests. In isotonic overhydration, serum electrolyte values are normal, but decreased hemoglobin, hematocrit, and serum protein levels may result from **hemodilution** (excessive water in the vascular space). In hypertonic overhydration caused by kidney failure, electrolytes, blood urea nitrogen (BUN), and creatinine levels are elevated. Hypotonic overhydration decreases the complete blood count, serum proteins, and electrolyte levels.

Common Nursing Diagnoses and Collaborative Problems

Nursing diagnoses and collaborative problems that may apply to clients with overhydration include the following:

- Excess Fluid Volume related to compromised regulatory mechanisms (inability of the kidneys to maintain body fluid balance)

TABLE 15-5 Common Causes of Overhydration

Isotonic Overhydration
- Poorly controlled IV therapy
- Renal failure
- Long-term corticosteroid therapy

Hypotonic Overhydration
- Early renal failure
- Congestive heart failure
- Syndrome of inappropriate antidiuretic hormone
- Poorly controlled IV therapy
- Replacement of isotonic fluid loss with hypotonic fluids
- Psychogenic polydipsia
- Irrigation of wounds and body cavities with hypotonic fluids

Hypertonic Overhydration
- Excessive sodium ingestion
- Rapid infusion of hypertonic saline
- Excessive sodium bicarbonate therapy

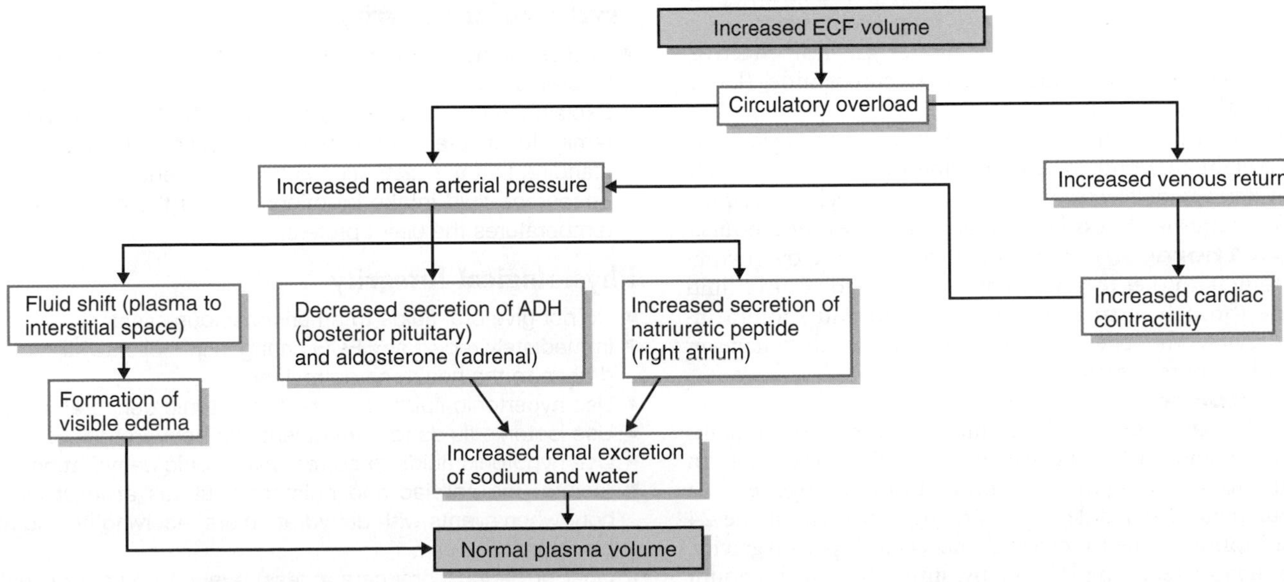

Figure 15-6 ■ Compensatory mechanisms associated with hypervolemia. *ADH,* Antidiuretic hormone; *ECF,* extracellular fluid.

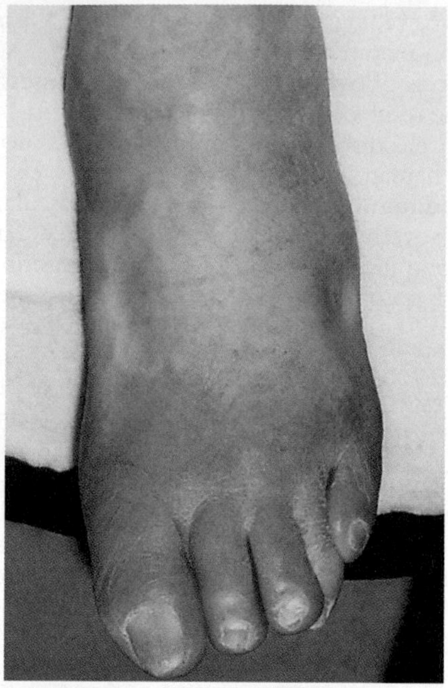

Figure 15-7 ■ Pitting edema.

- Deficient Knowledge (fluid restrictions, drug therapy, and manifestations of fluid excess) related to lack of exposure or lack of interest in learning
- Potential for Electrolyte Imbalances
- Potential for Hypertension
- Potential for Pulmonary Edema

Interventions

Interventions for clients with fluid volume excess aim to restore normal fluid balance, provide supportive care until the imbalance is resolved, and prevent future fluid overload. Drug and diet therapies are the basis of intervention.

Drug Therapy. Diuretics may be prescribed for clients with overhydration if renal failure is not the cause. Diuretics work on the kidneys to increase the water or sodium excretion. Osmotic diuretics, such as mannitol (Osmitrol), are often prescribed first to prevent severe electrolyte imbalances. If osmotic diuretics are not effective, high-ceiling (loop) diuretics, such as furosemide (Lasix, Furoside✱), may be prescribed.

Monitor the client for response to drug therapy, especially weight loss and increased urine output. Observe for manifestations of electrolyte imbalance, especially changes in ECG patterns. Assess laboratory findings every 8 hours.

Diet Therapy. For the client with chronic overhydration, long-term diet therapy may be needed to control fluid volume through restrictions of both fluid and sodium intake. Review the client's serum sodium levels whenever overhydration is present.

Monitoring

Intake and Output. Accurately measure fluid intake and output and explain the reason for any fluid restriction. In addition to regulating the total amount of fluid ingested in a 24-hour period, schedule fluid offerings throughout the 24 hours. Monitor urine for color, character, and specific gravity. If the client is receiving IV therapy, infuse the exact amount prescribed. Monitor for indicators of increased fluid overload (increased pulse quality, increasing neck vein distention, presence of crackles in lungs, increasing peripheral edema).

Weight. Fluid retention may not be visible. A sudden weight gain, however, indicates fluid retention. Metabolism can account for no more than a half pound of weight gain in one day. Each pound of weight gained (after the first half pound) equates to 500 mL of retained water. Weigh the client at the same time every day (before breakfast), using the same scale. Whenever possible, have the client wear the same type of clothing for each weigh-in.

GET READY for the NCLEX Examination!

KEY POINTS

Safe Effective Care Environment

- Monitor all intravenous infusions at least once per hour.
- Use a pump or controller to deliver intravenous fluids to clients with overhydration.
- Assess the oral mucous membranes at least every shift for clients with dehydration.

Health Promotion and Maintenance

- Instruct clients at risk for fluid imbalance to weigh themselves on the same scale daily, close to the same time each day, and with about the same amount of clothing on each time, and to monitor these daily weights for changes or trends.
- Encourage all clients to maintain an adequate fluid intake (minimum of 3 L/day) unless another condition requires fluid restriction.
- Instruct clients who exercise heavily (athletes) to take scheduled fluid replacement breaks.
- Instruct caregivers of older adults who have cognitive impairments or mobility problems to schedule offerings of fluids at regular intervals throughout the day.
- Teach people who are concerned about incontinence that reducing fluid intake does not help incontinence.

Psychosocial Integrity

- Assess the hydration status of any client with altered mental status.
- Explain the purpose of fluid restriction to the client and the family to ensure cooperation and prevent the misunderstanding that the restriction is a punishment.
- Encourage fluid intake by offering fluids the client likes at temperatures the client prefers.

Physiological Integrity

- Do not give oral fluids to an unconscious client.
- Immediately report any ECG changes in a client with dehydration to the health care provider.
- Use hypertonic fluids to correct hypotonic dehydration.
- Use isotonic fluids to correct isotonic dehydration.
- Use hypotonic fluids to correct hypertonic dehydration.
- Monitor the cardiac and pulmonary status at least every hour when clients with dehydration are receiving IV fluid replacement therapy.
- Offer or perform oral care at least every 4 hours for clients with dehydration.

ADDITIONAL STUDY RESOURCES

Go to your Student CD-ROM for Review Questions for the NCLEX Examination.

evolve Go to http://evolve.elsevier.com/Iggy/ for Integrated Management of Care Questions for the NCLEX Examination.

SELECTED BIBLIOGRAPHY

Asterisk indicates a classic or definitive work on this subject.

Ackley, B., & Ladwig, G. (2002). *Nursing diagnosis handbook: A guide to planning care* (5th ed.). St. Louis: Mosby.

Bennett, J. (2000). Dehydration: Hazards and benefits. *Geriatric Nursing, 21*(2), 84-88.

Brown, J., & Marland, G. (2002). Hydration in older people with mental health problems. *Nursing Times, 98*(3), 38-39.

Call-Schmidt, T. (2001). Interpreting lab results: A primer. *MEDSURG Nursing, 10*(4), 179-184.

Cannon, J. (2004). Recognizing chronic renal failure. *Nursing2004, 34*(1), 50-53.

Culp, K., Mentes, J., & Wakefield, B. (2003). Hydration and acute confusion in long-term care residents. *Western Journal of Nursing Research, 25*(3), 251-266.

Dochterman, J.M., & Bulechek, G.M. (Eds.). (2004). *Nursing interventions classification (NIC)* (4th ed.). St. Louis: Mosby.

Ebersole, P., Hess, P., & Luggen, A. (2004). *Toward healthy aging: Human needs and nursing response* (6th ed). St. Louis: Mosby

Hamilton, S. (2001). Detecting dehydration and malnutrition in the elderly. *Nursing2001, 31*(12), 56-57.

Kraft, P. (2000). The osmotic shift. *Journal of Intravenous Nursing, 23*(4), 220-224.

Krantz, M., & Baker, W. (2002). ECG challenge: Test your interpretive skills. *Consultant, 42*(14), 1757-1763.

Maintaining oral hydration in older people. (2001). *Best Practice, 5*(1), 1-6.

McCance, K., & Huether, S. (2002). *Pathophysiology: The biologic basis for disease in adults and children* (4th ed). St. Louis: Mosby.

McConnell, E. (2002). Measuring fluid intake and output. *Nursing2002, 32*(7), 17.

Mentes, J., Lyon, S., & Titler, M. (2000). Hydration management protocol. *Journal of Gerontological Nursing, 26*(10), 6-14.

Moorhead, S., Johnson, M., & Maas, M. (Eds.). (2004). *Nursing outcomes classification (NOC)* (3rd ed.). St. Louis: Mosby.

Pagana, K., & Pagana, T. (2002). *Mosby's manual of diagnostic and laboratory tests* (2nd ed.). St. Louis: Mosby.

Robinson, S., & Rosher, R. (2002). Can a beverage cart help improve hydration? *Geriatric Nursing, 23*(4), 208-211.

Suhayda, R., & Walton, J. (2002). Preventing and managing dehydration. *MEDSURG Nursing, 11*(6), 267-279.

*Stark, J. (1998). A comprehensive analysis of the fluid and electrolytes system. *Critical Care Nursing Clinics of North America, 10*(4), 471-475.

*Tietz, N.W. (Ed.). (1995). *Clinical guide to laboratory tests* (3rd ed.). Philadelphia: W.B. Saunders.

Trissel, L. (2003). *Handbook on injectable drugs* (12th ed.). Bethesda, MD: American Society of Health-System Pharmacists.

Yen, P. (2000). Focus on fluids. *Geriatric Nursing, 21*(4), 222-223.

CHAPTER

16 Interventions for Clients with Electrolyte Imbalances

M. LINDA WORKMAN

LEARNING OUTCOMES

After studying this chapter, you should be able to:

1. Identify clients at risk for imbalances of potassium.
2. Use laboratory data and clinical manifestations to assess potassium balance and imbalance.
3. Prioritize nursing care for the client with potassium imbalance.
4. Develop a community-based teaching plan to prevent deficiencies or excesses of potassium in the older adult client at risk for potassium imbalance.
5. Explain the effects of potassium imbalances on the activity of digoxin.
6. Differentiate diuretics that increase potassium loss from those that reduce potassium loss.
7. Analyze changes in clinical manifestations to determine the effectiveness of therapy for the client with potassium imbalance.
8. Identify clients at risk for imbalances of sodium.
9. Use laboratory data and clinical manifestations to assess sodium balance and imbalance.
10. Identify drugs that contain large amounts of sodium.
11. Prioritize nursing care for the client with sodium imbalance.
12. Develop a community-based teaching plan to prevent deficiencies or excesses of sodium in the older adult client at risk for sodium imbalance.
13. Analyze changes in clinical manifestations to determine the effectiveness of therapy for the client with sodium imbalance.
14. Identify clients at risk for imbalances of calcium.
15. Use laboratory data and clinical manifestations to assess calcium balance and imbalance.
16. Prioritize nursing care for the client with calcium imbalance.
17. Develop a community-based teaching plan to prevent deficiencies or excesses of calcium in the older adult client at risk for calcium imbalance.
18. Analyze changes in clinical manifestations to determine the effectiveness of therapy for the client with calcium imbalance.

Go to your Student CD-ROM for Review Questions for the NCLEX Examination keyed to these Learning Outcomes.

Electrolyte imbalances can occur in healthy people as a result of changes in fluid intake and output. These imbalances are usually mild and are easily corrected. Severe electrolyte imbalances are life threatening and can occur in any setting. People at greatest risk for severe imbalances are older clients, clients with chronic renal or endocrine disorders, clients who are mentally impaired, and clients who are taking drugs that alter fluid and electrolyte levels. Ill people are at some risk for electrolyte imbalances.

POTASSIUM IMBALANCES

Hypokalemia

PATHOPHYSIOLOGY

Because 98% of total body potassium (K^+) is inside cells, minor changes in extracellular potassium levels cause major changes in cell membrane excitability and in other cellular processes. **Hypokalemia** is a serum potassium level below

3.5 mEq/L (mmol/L). A common electrolyte imbalance, hypokalemia can be life threatening because every body system is affected.

Low serum potassium levels increase the difference in the amount of potassium between the fluid inside the cells **(intracellular fluid [ICF])** and the fluid outside the cells **(extracellular fluid (ECF])**. This increased difference reduces the excitability of cells. As a result, the cell membranes of all excitable tissues, such as nerve and muscle, are less responsive to normal stimuli.

The severity of problems caused by hypokalemia is related to how rapidly the serum potassium level drops. When the loss of ECF potassium is gradual, cells adjust and cellular potassium decreases in proportion to the ECF potassium level. In this situation, the potassium difference between the two fluid compartments remains unchanged and symptoms of hypokalemia may not appear until the potassium loss is extreme. Rapid reduction of serum potassium levels can cause dramatic changes in function.

Etiology

Hypokalemia may result either from an *actual* total body potassium loss or from the movement of potassium from the ECF to the ICF, causing a *relative* decrease in extracellular potassium level. Table 16-1 lists the common causes of hypokalemia.

Actual potassium depletion occurs when potassium loss is excessive or when potassium intake is not adequate to match normal potassium loss. Relative hypokalemia occurs when total body potassium levels are normal but the potassium distribution between fluid spaces is abnormal. Conditions that increase cell uptake of potassium, leading to hypokalemia, include metabolic alkalosis and insulin use.

Incidence/Prevalence

The actual incidence of hypokalemia is not known, although it is a common occurrence in acute care and long-term care settings. Mild hypokalemia, caused by dilution when a person drinks a large amount of fluid that does not contain potassium, occurs often but is corrected easily and quickly by diet.

TABLE 16-1 Common Causes of Hypokalemia

Actual Potassium Deficits

Excessive Potassium Loss

- Inappropriate or excessive use of drugs
  - Diuretics
  - Digitalis
  - Corticosteroids
- Increased secretion of aldosterone
  - Cushing's syndrome
- Diarrhea
- Vomiting
- Wound drainage (especially gastrointestinal)
- Prolonged nasogastric suction
- Heat-induced excessive diaphoresis
- Renal disease impairing reabsorption of potassium

Inadequate Potassium Intake

- Nothing by mouth

Relative Potassium Deficits

Movement of Potassium from Extracellular Fluid to Intracellular Fluid

- Alkalosis
- Hyperinsulinism
- Hyperalimentation
- Total parenteral nutrition

Dilution of Serum Potassium

- Water intoxication
- IV therapy with potassium-poor solutions

COLLABORATIVE MANAGEMENT

PHARM e-REVIEW

Assessment

HISTORY

Collect data from clients at risk as well as from those with actual hypokalemia.

AGE. Age is important because renal urine concentration decreases with aging, which increases potassium loss. Older adults are more likely to use drugs that lead to potassium loss.

DRUGS. Ask the client about drugs, especially diuretics, corticosteroids, and beta-adrenergic agonists or antagonists. These drugs increase potassium loss through the kidneys. A common cause of hypokalemia is the use and misuse of diuretics. In clients taking digoxin (Lanoxin, Novodigoxin✱), hypokalemia increases the sensitivity of the cardiac muscle to the drug and may result in digoxin toxicity, even when the digoxin level is within the therapeutic range.

Ask whether the client takes a potassium supplement, such as potassium chloride (KCl). The client may not be taking the supplement as prescribed because of its unpleasant taste.

OTHER FACTORS. Any acute or chronic disease may lead to potassium loss. Ask the client about recent illnesses and medical or surgical interventions. A thorough diet history, including a typical day's food and beverage intake, helps identify clients at risk for hypokalemia.

PHYSICAL ASSESSMENT/CLINICAL MANIFESTATIONS

The clinical manifestations of hypokalemia are seen as altered function of many systems (Chart 16-1).

MUSCULOSKELETAL MANIFESTATIONS. Skeletal muscles become weak in response to hypokalemia, and a stronger stimulus is needed to begin muscle contraction. A client may be so weak that he or she is unable to stand. Hand grasps are weak, and **hyporeflexia** (a decreased response to deep tendon reflex stimulation) may be seen. Severe hypokalemia causes flaccid paralysis. Assess for muscle weakness and determine the client's ability to perform activities of daily living (ADLs).

RESPIRATORY MANIFESTATIONS. The respiratory system can be seriously affected by hypokalemia through weakness of the muscles needed for breathing. Skeletal muscle weakness results in shallow respirations. *Thus respiratory status should be assessed first in any client who might have hypokalemia.* Assess the client's breath sounds, ease of respiratory effort, color of nail beds and mucous membranes, and rate and depth of respiration. Assess respiratory status at least every 2 hours because respiratory insufficiency is a major cause of death.

CARDIOVASCULAR MANIFESTATIONS. Assess the cardiovascular system by first palpating the peripheral pulses. In the client with hypokalemia, the pulse is usually thready and weak. Palpation is difficult, and the pulse is easily blocked with light pressure. The pulse rate can range from very slow to very rapid, depending on whether a **dysrhythmia** (irregular heartbeat) also is present. Measure blood pressure with the client in the lying, sitting, and standing positions because orthostatic (postural) hypotension occurs with hypokalemia.

NEUROLOGIC MANIFESTATIONS. The neurologic manifestations of hypokalemia include changes in mental status. The client may have short-term irritability and anxiety followed by lethargy that progresses to confusion and coma as hypokalemia worsens. Severe hypokalemia decreases sensory awareness. For example, the client may not be able to identify mild pain, touch, heat, and cold.

GASTROINTESTINAL MANIFESTATIONS. Hypokalemia decreases smooth muscle contractions within the gastrointestinal (GI) system, which leads to decreased peristalsis. The client has hypoactive bowel sounds and may have nausea, vomiting, constipation, and abdominal distention. Assess distention by measuring abdominal girth. Auscultate for bowel sounds in all four abdominal quadrants to assess the extent of decreased peristalsis. Severe hypokalemia can cause **paralytic ileus** (the absence of peristalsis).

PSYCHOSOCIAL ASSESSMENT

Behavioral changes caused by hypokalemia can occur quickly. You may need to obtain information about the client's behavior from close family members or friends if the client is confused.

Collect data about the onset and duration of behavioral changes as well as their association with any physical change. The client may be lethargic and unable to perform simple problem-solving tasks such as counting backward from 100 by threes. As hypokalemia progresses, the client may become more confused, especially to time and place. In severe hypokalemia, coma may develop.

LABORATORY ASSESSMENT

Hypokalemia is confirmed by a serum potassium value below 3.5 mEq/L (mmol/L). However, this value alone does not determine whether potassium loss has occurred or whether potassium has moved from the blood into the cells.

OTHER DIAGNOSTIC ASSESSMENTS

A baseline electrocardiogram (ECG) and continuous cardiac monitoring may be prescribed for a client with severe hypokalemia. Hypokalemia causes electrical conduction changes in the heart, including ST-segment depression, flat or inverted T waves, and increased U waves. Dysrhythmias can lead to death, particularly in older adults who are taking digoxin.

CHART 16-1

KEY FEATURES of Hypokalemia

Cardiovascular Manifestations
- Variable pulse rate, more often rapid
- Pulse quality thready and weak
- Peripheral pulses difficult to palpate
- Orthostatic (postural) hypotension
- Electrocardiographic abnormalities
  - ST depression
  - Inverted T wave
  - Prominent U wave
  - Heart block

Respiratory Manifestations
- Shallow, ineffective respirations resulting from profound weakness of the skeletal muscles of respiration
- Diminished breath sounds

Neuromuscular Manifestations
- Anxiety, lethargy, confusion, coma
- Loss of tactile discrimination
- General skeletal muscle weakness
- Deep tendon hyporeflexia
- Eventual flaccid paralysis

Gastrointestinal Manifestations
- Decreased motility
- Hypoactive to absent bowel sounds
- Nausea
- Vomiting
- Abdominal distention
- Paralytic ileus
- Constipation

Renal Manifestations
- Decreased ability to concentrate urine
- Polyuria
- Decreased specific gravity

Critical Thinking Challenge

The client is a 75-year-old woman who fell when she attempted to get up during intermission while attending a concert with a friend. When asked whether she takes any drugs, she tells you that she has been taking Diuril for 20 years to manage her high blood pressure. The only other drugs she takes are an aspirin each day and a multivitamin. She is alert and just a little anxious. Her vital signs are as follows: T 98.4; P 102, thready, slightly irregular; R 30 and shallow; BP 98/50; O_2 saturation 95%.

1. What other assessment data should you obtain?
2. What question should you ask about her drug regimen?
3. Should you apply oxygen? Why or why not?
4. Should she be monitored by electrocardiography? Why or why not?

evolve For suggested answer guidelines, go to http://evolve.elsevier.com/Iggy/.

Analysis

COMMON NURSING DIAGNOSES AND COLLABORATIVE PROBLEMS

The following are priority nursing diagnoses for clients with hypokalemia:

1. Risk for Falls related to skeletal muscle weakness
2. Constipation related to smooth muscle atony

The primary collaborative problem is Potential for Respiratory Insufficiency.

ADDITIONAL NURSING DIAGNOSES AND COLLABORATIVE PROBLEMS

In addition to the common nursing diagnoses and collaborative problems, clients with hypokalemia may have one or more of the following:

- Impaired Physical Mobility related to skeletal muscle weakness
- Total Self-Care Deficit related to skeletal muscle weakness
- Decreased Cardiac Output related to dysrhythmia

Critical Thinking Challenge

The 75-year-old client with hypokalemia tells you that she took two doses of Diuril today because she and her friend were going to a Chinese restaurant after the concert and she was afraid the salty food would make her hypertension worse. She has not eaten in the last 7 hours and has only had one cup of coffee in the past 4 hours. She says she last saw her doctor 6 months ago and that the blood work done at that time was "okay."

1. Is she at risk for any other fluid or electrolyte imbalance?
2. If so, what specific imbalance is she at risk for and why?

evolve For suggested answer guidelines, go to http://evolve.elsevier.com/Iggy/.

Planning and Implementation

RISK FOR FALLS

NOC **PLANNING: EXPECTED OUTCOMES.** The client with hypokalemia is expected to avoid falls and have a return to a normal serum potassium level.

INTERVENTIONS. Interventions for hypokalemia aim to prevent potassium loss, increase serum potassium levels, and provide a safe environment for the client. (See Chart 16-2 for NIC interventions for hypokalemia.) Drug and diet therapies help restore normal serum potassium levels.

Drug Therapy. Drug therapies for the treatment and prevention of hypokalemia include additional potassium and drugs to prevent potassium loss.

Potassium Supplements. Most potassium supplements are potassium chloride, potassium gluconate, potassium citrate, or a combination of these salts. The amount and the route of potassium replacement depend on the degree of potassium loss. A client with a serum potassium level of 3 mEq/L needs 100 to 200 mEq of potassium supplement; a client with a serum potassium level of 2.0 mEq/L needs 500 to 600 mEq.

Potassium is given intravenously for severe hypokalemia. A dilution of no more than 1 mEq/10 mL of solution is recommended. *The maximum recommended infusion rate is 5 to 10 mEq/hr; this rate is never to exceed 20 mEq/hr under any circumstances.* Older clients may not be able to handle this rate. Because rapid infusion of potassium can cause cardiac arrest, potassium is not given by intravenous (IV) push.

Potassium is a severe tissue irritant and is never given by intramuscular or subcutaneous injection. Tissues damaged by potassium can become necrotic and slough, causing loss of function and requiring reconstructive surgery. IV potassium solutions irritate veins and can cause phlebitis. Check the orders carefully to ensure that the client receives the correct amount of potassium. Assess the IV site every 2 hours and ask the client whether he or she feels burning or pain at the site. *Stop the IV solution immediately if infiltration occurs.*

Oral potassium preparations may be taken as liquids or solids. Potassium has a strong, unpleasant taste that is difficult to mask. Because potassium chloride can cause nausea and vomiting, advise clients not to take it on an empty stomach.

Potassium-Sparing Diuretics. Diuretics that increase the renal excretion of potassium can cause hypokalemia. These classes of diuretics include high-ceiling (loop) diuretics (e.g., furosemide [Lasix, Furoside✱], bumetanide [Bumex], and ethacrynic acid [Edecrin]) and the thiazide diuretics (chlorothiazide [Diuril], hydrochlorothiazide [Esidrix, HydroDIURIL, Urozide✱], and quinethazone [Hydromox]). Avoid these drugs in clients with actual hypokalemia and in those who are at risk for hypokalemia. A potassium-sparing diuretic may be prescribed for clients with hypokalemia who need diuretic therapy. Potassium-sparing diuretics increase urine output without increasing potassium loss. Potassium-sparing diuretics include spironolactone (Aldactone, Novospiroton✱), triamterene (Dyrenium), and amiloride (Midamor).

Diet Therapy. Consult with the dietitian in teaching the client how to increase dietary potassium intake. Eating foods that are naturally rich in potassium helps to restore normal potassium levels and prevent further loss. Table 14-7 lists the potassium content of common foods.

CHART 16-2

NIC **INTERVENTION ACTIVITIES for The Client with Hypokalemia**

Electrolyte Management: Hypokalemia: *Promotion of potassium balance and prevention of complications resulting from serum potassium levels lower than desired*

- Monitor lab values associated with hypokalemia (e.g., elevated glucose, metabolic alkalosis, reduced urine osmolality, urine potassium, hypochloremia, and hypocalcemia).
- Administer prescribed supplemental potassium (PO, NG, or IV), per policy.
- Prevent/reduce irritation from potassium supplement (e.g., administer PO or NG potassium supplements during or after meals to minimize GI irritation, dilute IV potassium adequately, administer IV supplement slowly, and apply topical anesthetic to IV site), as appropriate.
- Administer potassium-sparing diuretics (e.g., spironolactone [Aldactone] or triamterene [Dyrenium]), as appropriate.
- Avoid administration of alkaline substances (e.g., IV sodium bicarbonate and PO or NG antacids), as appropriate.
- Monitor neurologic manifestations of hypokalemia (e.g., muscle weakness, altered level of consciousness, drowsiness, apathy, lethargy, confusion, and depression).
- Monitor cardiac manifestations of hypokalemia (e.g., hypotension, broad T wave, U wave, ectopy, tachycardia, and weak pulse).
- Monitor renal manifestations of hypokalemia (e.g., acidic urine, reduced urine osmolality, nocturia, polyuria, and polydipsia).
- Monitor GI manifestations of hypokalemia (e.g., anorexia, nausea, cramps, constipation, distention, and paralytic ileus).
- Monitor pulmonary manifestations of hypokalemia (e.g., hypoventilation and respiratory muscle weakness).
- Monitor for symptoms of respiratory failure (e.g., low Pa_{O_2} and elevated Pa_{CO_2} levels and respiratory muscle fatigue).
- Monitor for rebound hyperkalemia.

NIC intervention activities selected from Dochterman, J.M., & Bulechek, G.M. (Eds.). (2004). *Nursing interventions classification (NIC)* (4th ed.). St. Louis: Mosby. No part of this work is to be altered without prior written permission from the Publisher.

GI, Gastrointestinal; Pa_{O_2}, partial pressure of arterial oxygen; Pa_{CO_2}, partial pressure of arterial carbon dioxide.

Safety. For a client with muscle weakness from hypokalemia, use safety measures, eliminate hazards, and assist with ambulation. Remove obstacles or slippery areas from the ambulation path, and make certain the client wears nonslip footgear. Be sure to have the client wear a gait belt when ambulating with assistance.

CONSTIPATION

NOC **PLANNING: EXPECTED OUTCOMES.** The client with hypokalemia is expected to have a normal bowel elimination pattern as indicated by:

- Stool amount appropriate for the diet
- Stools are soft and formed
- No discomfort when stool is passed

INTERVENTIONS. Interventions aim to restore normal serum potassium levels and induce gastric motility. Interventions include drug and diet therapies to restore serum potassium levels to normal values (discussed earlier under Drug Therapy and Diet Therapy [Risk for Falls], p. 229, stimulate intestinal peristalsis, and prevent constipation.

Drug Therapy. Laxatives that add bulk or fiber may be used to stimulate peristalsis. Other drugs that enhance gastric emptying and stimulate gastrointestinal (GI) motility, such as metoclopramide (Reglan, Maxeran✱), are used to treat constipation associated with hypokalemia.

Diet Therapy. Provide high-fiber foods and plenty of liquids for the client who is not on fluid restrictions. To ensure cooperation, prepare a list of foods that contain high concentrations of fiber and ask the client to select favorite items from that list.

Comfort Measures. Provide privacy when the client uses the toilet or bedpan. Close the door, draw the privacy curtains, and ask visitors to step out of the room. Because physical activity promotes gastric motility, encourage the client to walk whenever his or her condition permits. A bedridden client can benefit from frequent position changes and mild bed exercises.

POTENTIAL FOR RESPIRATORY INSUFFICIENCY

NOC **PLANNING: EXPECTED OUTCOMES.** The client with hypokalemia is expected to have a breathing pattern adequate to maintain gas exchange as indicated by:

- Pulse oximetry within the normal range
- Absence of cyanosis or pallor

INTERVENTIONS. Monitor the client's respiratory rate and depth at least once per hour, noting in particular increased rate and decreased depth. Assess respiratory muscle effectiveness by checking the client's ability to cough. Examine the face, oral mucosa, and nail beds for pallor or cyanosis. Evaluate arterial blood gas values for **hypoxemia** (decreased blood oxygen levels) and **hypercapnia** (increased arterial carbon dioxide levels). See Chapter 30 for respiratory assessment techniques.

Critical Thinking Challenge

Your client's serum potassium level is 2.4 mEq/L and her serum sodium is 142 mEq/L. In addition, her hematocrit is 47%. She is prescribed to receive 1 L of normal saline (0.9% sodium chloride) with 40 mEq of potassium added. The rate of administration prescribed is 200 mL/hr.

1. What vein should you choose to start this IV? Why?
2. How many mEq of potassium will she be receiving per hour at this infusion rate?
3. What safety precautions should you take with this prescription and why?
4. Should the care of this client be assigned to an RN, LPN/LVN, or assistive nursing personnel? (Explain your rationale for the caregiver assignment.)
5. What assessment data would you need to determine whether the interventions are effective?

evolve For suggested answer guidelines, go to http://evolve.elsevier.com/Iggy/.

Community-Based Care

No special home care preparations are needed for clients with mild hypokalemia or sudden-onset hypokalemia. The imbalance is corrected before discharge and, with teaching, is unlikely to recur. Clients with chronic diseases are more likely to be discharged before the imbalance is completely corrected and are at risk for recurrence. These clients often need long-term diet and drug therapy. Health teaching for prevention and early detection is a major nursing responsibility.

Instruct the at-risk client (especially one using diuretics or corticosteroids) about the proper use of drugs, the symptoms of hypokalemia, when to seek medical help, and which foods are rich in potassium. Teach the client to assess the rate, rhythm, and quality of the peripheral pulses at least once each day and whenever any symptoms of hypokalemia appear. For clients at chronic risk for hypokalemia, stress how often serum potassium levels should be checked.

A home care aide may be needed to assist with hygiene and ensure a safe environment. Weekly visits by a nurse may also be needed to assess changes and ensure adherence with the drug regimen. Perform a focused assessment at every home visit to a client at risk for hypokalemia (Chart 16-3). Review drugs, the symptoms of hypokalemia, and health care resources with the client and family.

Critical Thinking Challenge

After restoration of fluid volume and serum potassium levels, your client with hypokalemia is discharged to home and advised to make an appointment with her usual health care provider. She tells you that years ago she tried taking potassium supplements but found the taste too unpleasant to continue.

1. What should you teach this client to prevent a recurrence of the imbalance?
2. What should you teach this client to reduce her risk for falling?
3. How could this client increase her intake of potassium without using potassium supplements?

evolve For suggested answer guidelines, go to http://evolve.elsevier.com/Iggy/.

Evaluation: Outcomes

Evaluate the care of the client with hypokalemia on the basis of the identified nursing diagnoses and collaborative problems. The expected outcomes are that the client should:

- Return to and maintain a normal serum potassium level (between 3.5 and 5.0 mEq/L)
- Adhere to prescribed drug and diet therapies
- Identify the early manifestations of hypokalemia
- Avoid falls

CHART 16-3

HOME CARE ASSESSMENT of
The Client at Risk for Hypokalemia

Assess respiratory status.
- Rate, depth, rhythm of respiration
- Color of lips, tongue, nail beds
- Can the client complete a sentence without taking a breath?

Assess cardiovascular status.
- Vital signs, including apical pulse, pulse pressure, presence or absence of orthostatic hypotension, and quality and rhythm of peripheral pulses
- Presence or absence of peripheral edema
- Hand vein filling in the dependent position
- Neck vein filling in the recumbent and sitting positions
- Weight gain or loss

Assess cognition and mental status.
- Level of consciousness
- Orientation to time, place, and person
- Can the client accurately read a seven-word sentence containing no words greater than three syllables?

Assess condition of skin and mucous membranes.
- Presence or absence of skin tenting over the sternum or the forehead
- Moistness of skin (most reliable on chest and back)
- Presence or absence of coating on tongue or teeth
- Can the client spit?

Assess neuromuscular status.
- Reactivity of patellar and biceps reflexes
- Oral temperature
- Handgrip strength
- Steadiness of gait

Assess renal system.
- Observe urine specimen for color, odor, cloudiness, and amount.

Ask about the following:
- 24-hour fluid intake and output
- 24-hour diet recall
- 24-hour activity recall
- What over-the-counter and prescribed medications has the client taken?
- Has the client experienced any dizziness or lightheadedness?
- Does the client have a headache (what time of day, associated with what activities)?
- Muscle twitches, cramps, pain, or spasms

Assess the client's understanding of illness and adherence to treatment.
- Signs and symptoms to report to health care provider
- Medication plan (correct timing and dose)

- Have normal bowel elimination patterns
- Maintain adequate gas exchange
- Maintain regular cardiac rate and rhythm

Specific indicators for these outcomes are listed for each nursing diagnosis and collaborative problem under the Planning and Implementation section (see earlier).

Hyperkalemia

PATHOPHYSIOLOGY

Hyperkalemia is a serum potassium level greater than 5.0 mEq/L (mmol/L). Because the range of normal serum potassium values is narrow, even slight increases above normal values can affect excitable tissues, especially the heart.

A high serum potassium level decreases the potassium difference between the intracellular fluid (ICF) and the extracellular fluid (ECF). This decreased difference increases cell excitability; as a result, excitable tissues respond to less intense stimuli and may even discharge spontaneously.

TABLE 16-2 Common Causes of Hyperkalemia

Actual Potassium Excesses

Excessive Potassium Intake
- Overingestion of potassium-containing foods or medications
  - Salt substitutes
  - Potassium chloride
- Rapid infusion of potassium-containing IV solution
- Bolus IV potassium injections
- Transfusions of whole blood or packed cells

Decreased Potassium Excretion
- Adrenal insufficiency (Addison's disease, adrenalectomy)
- Renal failure
- Potassium-sparing diuretics

Relative Potassium Excesses

Movement of Potassium from Intracellular Fluid to Extracellular Fluid
- Tissue damage
- Acidosis
- Hyperuricemia
- Uncontrolled diabetes mellitus

Hyperkalemia alters the function of all excitable membranes to some degree. The excitable membrane in the heart is very sensitive to serum potassium increases and the most serious complications of hyperkalemia are altered cardiac function.

The problems that occur with hyperkalemia are related to how rapidly ECF potassium levels increase. Sudden rises in serum potassium cause severe problems at potassium levels between 6 and 7 mEq/L. When serum potassium rises slowly, problems may not occur until potassium levels reach 8 mEq/L or higher.

Hyperkalemia may result from an actual increase in total body potassium or from the movement of potassium from the cells into the blood. Table 16-2 lists common causes of hyperkalemia.

Hyperkalemia is rare in people with normal kidney function. Most cases of hyperkalemia occur in hospitalized clients and in those undergoing medical treatment. Those at greatest risk for hyperkalemia are chronically ill clients, debilitated clients, and older adults.

COLLABORATIVE MANAGEMENT

Assessment

HISTORY

Age is important because renal function decreases with aging. Ask about chronic illnesses (particularly renal disease and diabetes mellitus), recent medical or surgical treatment, and urine output, including frequency and amount of voidings. Ask about drug use, particularly potassium-sparing diuretics and angiotensin-converting enzyme (ACE) inhibitors. Obtain a diet history to determine the intake of potassium-rich foods or the use of salt substitutes (which contain potassium).

Collect data regarding symptoms related to hyperkalemia. Ask if the client has had palpitations, skipped heartbeats, other cardiac irregularities, muscle twitching, weakness in the leg muscles, or unusual tingling or numbness in the hands, feet, or face. Ask about recent changes in bowel habits, especially diarrhea.

CHART 16-4

KEY FEATURES of
Hyperkalemia

Cardiovascular Manifestations
- Irregular heart rate, usually slow
- Decreased blood pressure
- Electrocardiographic abnormalities
  - Tall T waves
  - Widened QRS complexes
  - Prolonged PR intervals
  - Flat P waves
- Ectopic beats
- Late; dysrhythmias, ventricular fibrillation, cardiac arrest in diastole

Respiratory Manifestations
- Unaffected until late, when profound weakness of the skeletal muscles causes respiratory failure

Neuromuscular Manifestations
- Early phase, or mild, hyperkalemia
  - Muscle twitches, cramps
  - Paresthesias
- Late phase, or severe, hyperkalemia
  - Profound weakness
  - Ascending flaccid paralysis in distal to proximal direction; involves the arms and legs

Gastrointestinal Manifestations
- Increased motility
- Hyperactive bowel sounds
- Diarrhea

PHYSICAL ASSESSMENT/CLINICAL MANIFESTATIONS

The manifestations of hyperkalemia are listed in Chart 16-4. Cardiovascular changes are the most severe problems from hyperkalemia and are the most common cause of death in clients with hyperkalemia. Cardiac manifestations of hyperkalemia include bradycardia, hypotension, and electrocardiographic (ECG) changes of tall, peaked T waves, prolonged PR intervals, flat or absent P waves, and wide QRS complexes (Figure 16-1). As serum potassium levels rise, **ectopic beats** (beats generated outside the normal conduction system in the ventricles) may appear. Complete heart block, asystole, and ventricular fibrillation are life-threatening complications of severe hyperkalemia.

The neuromuscular response to hyperkalemia has two phases. Skeletal muscles twitch in the early stages of hyperkalemia, and the client may be aware of unusual nerve sensations (e.g., tingling and burning) that are followed by numbness in the hands and feet and around the mouth **(paresthesia).** As hyperkalemia worsens, muscle twitching changes to weakness followed by flaccid paralysis. The weakness moves up from the hands and feet and first affects the muscles of the arms and legs. Trunk, head, and respiratory muscles are not affected until serum potassium levels reach lethal levels.

The smooth muscle of the gastrointestinal (GI) tract has increased motility. As a result, the client may have diarrhea and spastic colonic activity. Listen to bowel sounds and observes stools. Bowel sounds are hyperactive, with audible rushes and gurgles. Bowel movements are frequent and watery.

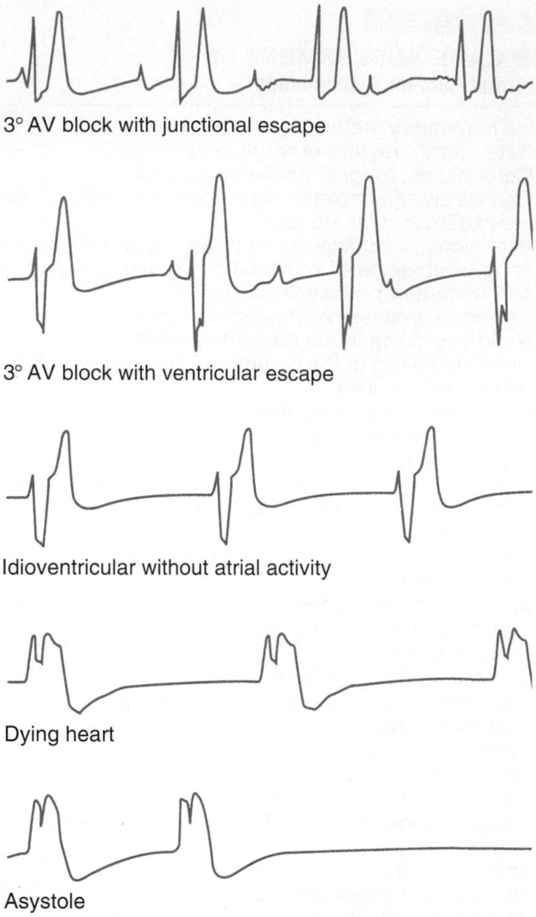

Figure 16-1 ■ Electrocardiographic (ECG) changes associated with hyperkalemia. (Modified with permission from John M. Clochesy.)

LABORATORY ASSESSMENT

A serum potassium level over 5.0 mEq/L confirms hyperkalemia. If hyperkalemia results from dehydration, levels of other electrolytes, hematocrit, and hemoglobin also are elevated. Hyperkalemia caused by renal failure occurs with elevated serum creatinine and blood urea nitrogen, decreased blood pH, and normal or low hematocrit and hemoglobin levels.

◆Interventions

Interventions for hyperkalemia are aimed at rapidly reducing the serum potassium level. Drug therapy can restore normal potassium balance by enhancing potassium excretion and promoting the movement of potassium from the extracellular fluid (ECF) into the cells. Monitoring the client's response to intervention is another major nursing responsibility. (See Chart 16-5 for NIC interventions for hyperkalemia.)

Eliminate extra potassium by stopping potassium-containing infusions. Keeping the IV catheter open is useful in managing hyperkalemia. Withhold oral potassium supplements and provide a potassium-restricted diet.

Increasing potassium excretion helps reduce hyperkalemia if renal function is normal. Potassium-excreting diuretics, such

CHART 16-5

NIC **INTERVENTION ACTIVITIES for**
The Client with Hyperkalemia

Electrolyte Management: Hyperkalemia: *Promotion of potassium balance and prevention of complications resulting from serum potassium levels higher than desired*

- Administer electrolyte-binding and electrolyte-excreting resins (e.g., Kayexalate) as prescribed, if appropriate.
- Monitor lab values for changes in oxygenation or acid-base balance, as appropriate.
- Administer prescribed medications to shift potassium into the cell (e.g., 50% dextrose and insulin, sodium bicarbonate, calcium chloride, and calcium gluconate), as appropriate.
- Avoid potassium-sparing medications (e.g., spironolactone [Aldactone] and triamterene [Dyrenium]), as appropriate.
- Maintain potassium restrictions.
- Administer prescribed diuretics, as appropriate.
- Monitor fluid status, including intake and output, as appropriate.
- Monitor potassium levels after diuresis.
- Monitor cardiac manifestations of hyperkalemia (e.g., decreased cardiac output, heart blocks, peaked T waves, fibrillation, or asystole).
- Respond to cardiac arrest.

NIC intervention activities selected from Dochterman, J.M., & Bulechek, G.M. (Eds.). (2004). *Nursing interventions classification (NIC)* (4th ed). St. Louis: Mosby. No part of this work is to be altered without prior written permission from the Publisher.

as furosemide, are prescribed. For a client with renal problems, drug therapy to increase potassium excretion includes cation exchange resins that promote intestinal sodium absorption and potassium excretion, such as sodium polystyrene sulfonate (Kayexalate). However, this therapy may take many hours to reduce potassium levels. If potassium levels are dangerously high, additional measures, such as dialysis, are needed.

Movement of potassium from the extracellular fluid (ECF) to the intracellular fluid (ICF) can help reduce serum potassium levels temporarily. Potassium movement into the cells is enhanced by insulin. Insulin increases the activity of the sodium-potassium pumps, which move potassium from the ECF into the cell (see Chapter 14). IV fluids containing glucose and insulin are prescribed to help decrease serum potassium levels (usually 100 mL of 10% to 20% glucose with 10 to 20 units of regular insulin). These IV solutions are hypertonic and are infused through a central line or in a vein with a high blood flow to avoid local vein inflammation. Observe the client for manifestations of hypokalemia and hypoglycemia during this therapy.

Cardiac monitoring allows for the early recognition of dysrhythmias and other manifestations of hyperkalemia on cardiac muscle. Compare recent ECG tracings with the client's baseline tracings or with tracings obtained when the client's serum potassium level was close to normal.

Health teaching is key to the prevention of hyperkalemia and the early detection of complications. The teaching plan for the client at risk for hyperkalemia includes diet, drugs, and recognition of the manifestations of hyperkalemia. Diet education includes knowledge of foods to avoid (those high in potassium) and permissible foods containing little potassium (Chart 16-6). Instruct the client to read the labels on drug and food packages to determine the potassium content. Warn clients to avoid salt substitutes, which contain potassium.

CHART 16-6

CLIENT EDUCATION GUIDE
Dietary Management of Hyperkalemia

You Should Avoid

- Meats, especially organ meat and preserved meat
- Dairy products
- Dried fruit
- Fruits high in potassium
  - Bananas
  - Cantaloupe
  - Kiwi
  - Oranges
- Vegetables high in potassium
  - Avocados
  - Broccoli
  - Dried beans or peas
  - Lima beans
  - Mushrooms
  - Potatoes (white or sweet)
  - Seaweed
  - Soybeans
  - Spinach

You May Eat

- Eggs
- Breads
- Butter
- Cereals
- Sugar
- Fruits low in potassium (fresh, frozen, or canned)
  - Apples
  - Apricots
  - Berries
  - Cherries
  - Grapefruit
  - Peaches
  - Pineapple
  - Cranberries
- Vegetables low in potassium
  - Alfalfa sprouts
  - Cabbage
  - Carrots
  - Cauliflower
  - Celery
  - Eggplant
  - Green beans
  - Lettuce
  - Onions
  - Peas
  - Peppers
  - Squash

Data from Pennington, J. (2004). *Bowe's and Church's food values of portions commonly used* (18th ed.). Philadelphia: Lippincott-Raven.

SODIUM IMBALANCES

Hyponatremia

PATHOPHYSIOLOGY

Hyponatremia is a serum sodium (Na^+) level below 136 mEq/L (mmol/L). Because sodium is the major cation of the blood and interstitial fluid and maintains the osmolarity of these fluids, sodium imbalances often occur with fluid volume imbalances.

The problems caused by hyponatremia involve two mechanisms. The first mechanism is a change in cell excitability. As the sodium level in the blood and other extracellular fluid

TABLE 16-3 Common Causes of Hyponatremia

Actual Sodium Deficits

Increased Sodium Excretion
- Excessive diaphoresis
- Diuretics (high-ceiling diuretics)
- Wound drainage (especially gastrointestinal)
- Decreased secretion of aldosterone
- Hyperlipidemia
- Renal disease (scarred distal convoluted tubule)

Inadequate Sodium Intake
- Nothing by mouth
- Low-salt diet

Relative Sodium Deficits

Dilution of Serum Sodium
- Excessive ingestion of hypotonic fluids
- Psychogenic polydipsia
- Freshwater drowning
- Renal failure (nephrotic syndrome)
- Irrigation with hypotonic fluids
- Syndrome of inappropriate antidiuretic hormone secretion
- Hyperglycemia
- Congestive heart failure

(ECF) decreases, the difference in sodium levels between the ECF and the cellular fluid also decreases. Less sodium is present to move across the excitable membrane, resulting in slower membrane depolarization. The second mechanism is the movement of water from the ECF space into the cells. Cells swell, and their functions are impaired.

Many conditions can lead to hyponatremia (Table 16-3). Hyponatremia can result from the loss of total body sodium, the movement of sodium from the blood to other fluid spaces, or the dilution of serum sodium from excessive water in the plasma.

COLLABORATIVE MANAGEMENT

Assessment

The manifestations of hyponatremia are caused by its effects on excitable cellular activity. The cells especially affected are those involved in cerebral, neuromuscular, and gastric smooth muscle functions (Chart 16-7).

CEREBRAL MANIFESTATIONS. Changes in cerebral function are the most obvious problems of hyponatremia. Because these changes may be seen as either depressed activity or excessive activity (and sometimes both), establishing the client's usual cognitive and behavioral patterns is essential. Behavioral changes result from cerebral edema and increased intracranial pressure. Closely observe and document the client's behavior and level of consciousness.

NEUROMUSCULAR MANIFESTATIONS. Assess the client's neuromuscular status during each nursing shift for changes from baseline. The neuromuscular response to hyponatremia is general muscle weakness. Muscle tone and deep tendon reflexes diminish.

Muscle weakness occurs bilaterally and is worse in the legs and arms. Assess deep tendon reflexes by lightly tapping the patellar (knee) tendons and Achilles (heel) tendons with a reflex hammer and document the degree of reflex movement. The technique for assessing motor strength and reflexes is described in depth in Chapter 44.

CHART 16-7

KEY FEATURES of Hyponatremia

Cardiovascular Manifestations*
- Normovolemic
  - Rapid pulse rate
  - Normal blood pressure
- Hypovolemic
  - Rapid pulse rate
  - Pulse quality thready and weak
  - Hypotension
  - Central venous pressure normal or low
  - Flat neck veins in supine position
- Hypervolemic
  - Rapid, bounding pulse
  - Central venous pressure normal or elevated
  - Blood pressure normal or elevated

Respiratory Manifestations
- Late manifestations related to skeletal muscle weakness
  - Shallow, ineffective respiratory movements
- Hypervolemia
- Pulmonary edema
  - Rapid, shallow respiration
  - Moist crackles

Neuromuscular Manifestations
- Generalized skeletal muscle weakness
- Diminished deep tendon reflexes

Cerebral Manifestations
- Personality changes
- Headache

Renal Manifestations
- Increased urine output
- Decreased urine specific gravity

Gastrointestinal Manifestations
- Increased motility
- Nausea
- Hyperactive bowel sounds
- Diarrhea

*Symptoms vary with changes in vascular volume.

GASTROINTESTINAL MANIFESTATIONS. The smooth muscle of the gastrointestinal (GI) system responds to decreased serum sodium levels with increased motility, causing nausea, diarrhea, and abdominal cramping. Assess the GI system by listening to bowel sounds and observing stools. Bowel sounds are hyperactive, with rushes and gurgles over the splenic flexure and in the lower left quadrant. Bowel movements are frequent and watery. Peristaltic movements may be palpated through the abdominal wall and may even be visible on the abdominal surface.

CARDIOVASCULAR MANIFESTATIONS. Hyponatremia has little direct effect on cardiac muscle contractility; however, cardiac output is changed with hyponatremia. When hyponatremia occurs with changes in blood volume, these fluid changes alter cardiac function. The cardiac responses to hyponatremia and **hypovolemia** (decreased plasma volume, or fluid deficit) are a rapid, weak, thready pulse. Peripheral pulses are difficult to palpate and are easily blocked with light pressure. Neck veins are flat when the client is in the supine position. Blood pressure, especially diastolic pressure, is decreased. The client may have severe hypotension when moving from a

CHART 16-8

NIC INTERVENTION ACTIVITIES for The Client with Sodium Imbalances

Electrolyte Management: Hyponatremia: *Promotion of sodium balance and prevention of complications resulting from serum sodium levels lower than desired*

- Monitor for electrolyte imbalances associated with hyponatremia (e.g., hypokalemia, metabolic acidosis, and hypoglycemia), as appropriate.
- Monitor for renal loss of sodium (oliguria).
- Monitor intake and output.
- Weigh client daily and monitor trends.
- Monitor for indications of fluid overload/retention (e.g., crackles, elevated CVP or PCWP, edema, neck vein distention, and ascites), as appropriate.
- Administer hypertonic (3% to 5%) saline at 3 mL/kg/hr or per policy for rapid correction of hyponatremia, as appropriate.
- Maintain fluid restriction, as appropriate.
- Monitor for neurologic and/or neuromuscular manifestations of hyponatremia (e.g., lethargy, increased ICP, confusion, headache, seizures, coma, fatigue, tremors, apprehension, muscle weakness, and hyperreflexia).
- Monitor for cardiovascular manifestations of hyponatremia (e.g., elevated blood pressure, cold and clammy skin, and hypo- or hypervolemia).

Electrolyte Management: Hypernatremia: *Promotion of sodium balance and prevention of complications resulting from serum sodium levels higher than desired*

- Monitor for indications of dehydration (e.g., decreased sweating, decreased urine, decreased skin turgor, and dry mucous membranes).
- Monitor vital signs, as appropriate.
- Weigh client daily and monitor trends.
- Provide comfort measures to decrease thirst.
- Maintain patent IV access.
- Monitor intake and output.
- Provide frequent oral hygiene.
- Administer isotonic (0.9%) saline, hypotonic (0.45%) saline, hypotonic (5%) dextrose, or diuretics, as appropriate, based on fluid status and urine osmolality.
- Maintain sodium restrictions.

NIC intervention activities selected from Dochterman, J.M., & Bulechek, G.M. (Eds.). (2004). *Nursing interventions classification (NIC)* (4th ed.). St. Louis: Mosby. No part of this work is to be altered without prior written permission from the Publisher.
CVP, Central venous pressure; *ICP*, intracranial pressure.

lying or sitting position to a standing position. The central venous pressure is low.

When hyponatremia occurs with **hypervolemia** (increased plasma volume or fluid excess), cardiac changes include a full pulse with normal or high blood pressure. Central venous pressure is normal or high depending on how well the left ventricle handles the extra fluid. Peripheral pulses are full and difficult to block; however, they may not be palpable if edema is present.

Interventions

Interventions with drug therapy and diet therapy aim to restore serum sodium levels to normal and prevent complications. Chart 16-8 lists NIC interventions for electrolyte management of hyponatremia.

Drug Therapy. Drug therapy can restore serum sodium levels to normal. Drug therapy regimens vary depending on whether or not fluid imbalance occurs with hyponatremia and how fast the imbalance has developed. In chronic hyponatremia, sodium is replaced slowly.

When hyponatremia occurs with a fluid deficit (hypovolemia), IV saline infusions are prescribed to restore both sodium and fluid volume. Severe hyponatremia may be treated with small-volume infusions of hypertonic (2% to 3%) saline. The infusions are delivered through a controller to prevent accidental increases in infusion rate. Monitor the infusion rate and the client's response.

When hyponatremia occurs with fluid excess, drug therapy includes giving osmotic diuretics that promote the excretion of water rather than sodium, such as mannitol (Osmitrol). Assess the client hourly for signs of excessive fluid loss, potassium loss, and increased sodium levels.

Drug therapy for hyponatremia caused by inappropriate secretion of antidiuretic hormone (ADH) includes agents that antagonize ADH, such as lithium and demeclocycline (Declomycin).

Diet Therapy. Diet therapy can help restore normal sodium balance in mild hyponatremia. Table 14-6 lists the sodium content of common foods. Collaborate with the dietitian to teach the client about which foods to increase in the diet. Therapy involves increasing oral sodium intake and restricting oral fluid intake. Fluid restriction may be needed long-term when overhydration is the cause of the hyponatremia or when renal fluid excretion is impaired. Measure fluid intake and output and reinforce the purpose of the fluid restriction.

Hypernatremia

PATHOPHYSIOLOGY

Hypernatremia is a serum sodium level over 145 mEq/L. High serum sodium levels can be caused by or can cause changes in fluid volumes. Table 16-4 lists common causes of hypernatremia.

As serum sodium level rises, a larger difference in sodium levels occurs between the extracellular fluid (ECF) and the intracellular fluid (ICF). More sodium is present

TABLE 16-4 Common Causes of Hypernatremia

Actual Sodium Excesses
Decreased Sodium Excretion
- Hyperaldosteronism
- Renal failure
- Corticosteroids
- Cushing's syndrome or disease

Increased Sodium Intake
- Excessive oral sodium ingestion
- Excessive administration of sodium-containing IV fluids

Relative Sodium Excesses
Decreased Water Intake
- Nothing by mouth

Increased Water Loss
- Increased rate of metabolism
- Fever
- Hyperventilation
- Infection
- Excessive diaphoresis
- Watery diarrhea
- Dehydration

CHART 16-9

KEY FEATURES of Hypernatremia

Cardiovascular Manifestations
- Decreased myocardial contractility
- Diminished cardiac output
- Heart rate and blood pressure respond to vascular volume

Respiratory Manifestations
- Problems associated with pulmonary edema when hypernatremia is accompanied by hypervolemia

Central Nervous System Manifestations*
- Hypernatremia and normovolemia or hypovolemia
  - Increased neural activity
  - Agitation, confusion, seizures
- Hypernatremia and hypervolemia
  - Decreased neural activity
  - Lethargy, stupor, coma

Neuromuscular Manifestations
- Mild or early hypernatremia
  - Spontaneous muscle twitches
  - Irregular contractions
- Severe or late hypernatremia
  - Skeletal muscle weakness
  - Diminished or absent deep tendon reflexes

Renal Manifestations
- Decreased urine output
- Increased urine specific gravity

Integumentary Manifestations
- Dry, flaky skin
- Presence or absence of edema related to accompanying fluid volume changes

*Upper neural function changes are related to volume changes as well as sodium increases.

to move rapidly across cell membranes during depolarization. With mild hypernatremia, most excitable tissues are excited more easily. This condition is called **irritability** and excitable tissues overrespond to stimuli. In addition, the osmolarity of the ECF increases as the level of sodium increases. This problem causes water to move from the cells into the ECF to dilute the hyperosmolar ECF. Therefore when hypernatremia persists or worsens, compensatory actions cause severe cellular dehydration. The dehydrated excitable tissues may no longer be able to respond to stimuli.

COLLABORATIVE MANAGEMENT

Assessment

The manifestations of hypernatremia vary with the severity of imbalance and whether a fluid imbalance is also present. Rapid increases in serum sodium cause more obvious and severe symptoms. Gradual increases in serum sodium may produce no observable physical changes, even when sodium levels increase to ranges that are well above normal. The manifestations of hypernatremia involve changes in excitable membrane activity, especially cerebral, neuromuscular, and cardiac function (Chart 16-9).

CENTRAL NERVOUS SYSTEM MANIFESTATIONS. Altered cerebral function is the most common problem of hypernatremia. Assess the client's mental status for attention span, recall of recent events, and cognitive function. In hypernatremia with normal or decreased fluid volumes, the client may have a short attention span and be agitated or confused about recent events. Manic episodes or seizures may occur if serum sodium continues to rise. When hypernatremia occurs with blood volume overload, the client may be lethargic, drowsy, stuporous, and even comatose.

NEUROMUSCULAR MANIFESTATIONS. Skeletal muscles responses vary with the degree of sodium increases. Mild rises cause muscle twitching and irregular muscle contractions. As hypernatremia worsens, the muscles and nerves are less able to respond to a stimulus. The muscles become progressively weaker with rigid paralysis. Deep tendon reflexes are reduced or absent. Muscle weakness occurs bilaterally and has no specific pattern. Assess neuromuscular status by observing for twitching in muscle groups. Assess muscle strength by having the client perform handgrip and arm flexion against resistance. Assess peripheral nerve responses by lightly tapping the patellar (knee) tendons and Achilles (heel) tendons with a reflex hammer and measuring the movement.

CARDIOVASCULAR MANIFESTATIONS. Increased serum sodium slows the movement of calcium into the heart cells, which decreases contractility. Assess cardiac status by measuring blood pressure and the rate and quality of the apical and peripheral pulses. Pulse rate and blood pressure may be normal, above normal, or below normal, depending on the fluid volume and how rapidly the imbalance occurred.

Pulse rate is increased in clients with hypernatremia and hypovolemia. Peripheral pulses are difficult to palpate and are easily blocked. Hypotension and severe orthostatic (postural) hypotension are present, and pulse pressure is reduced.

Clients with hypernatremia and hypervolemia have slow to normal bounding pulses. Peripheral pulses are full and difficult to block. Neck veins are distended, even with the client in the upright position. Blood pressure, especially diastolic blood pressure, is increased.

Common Nursing Diagnoses and Collaborative Problems

Nursing diagnoses and collaborative problems that may apply to clients with hypernatremia include the following:

- Excess Fluid Volume related to excess sodium intake
- Decreased Cardiac Output related to poor cardiac contractility
- Risk for Falls related to skeletal muscle weakness
- Impaired Memory related to fluid and electrolyte imbalances
- Readiness for Enhanced Nutrition related to the need for dietary sodium restrictions
- Potential for Pulmonary Edema

Interventions

Drug and diet therapies aim to prevent further increases in serum sodium and decrease high serum sodium levels. Chart 16-8 lists NIC interventions for electrolyte management of hypernatremia. Other interventions used when sodium levels become life threatening include hemodialysis and blood ultrafiltration.

Drug Therapy. When hypernatremia is caused by fluid loss, drug therapy is used to restore fluid balance. Hypotonic IV infusions, usually 0.225% or 0.45% sodium chloride, are prescribed. Hypernatremia caused by fluid and sodium losses require fluid replacement with IV infusions of isotonic sodium chloride (NaCl) solutions. Hypernatremia caused by poor renal excretion of sodium requires drug therapy with diuretics that promote sodium loss, such as furosemide (Lasix, Furoside✱), bumetanide (Bumex), and ethacrynic acid (Edecrin). Assess the client hourly for symptoms of excessive fluid, sodium or potassium losses.

Diet Therapy. Mild hypernatremia can be prevented or corrected by ensuring adequate water intake among older adults or those who may not have self-access to water. Dietary sodium restriction may be needed to prevent sodium excess when renal problems are present. In addition, fluids must often be restricted. Collaborate with the dietitian to teach the client how to determine the sodium content of foods, beverages, and drugs. Stress the importance of adhering to the diet.

CALCIUM IMBALANCES

Hypocalcemia

PATHOPHYSIOLOGY

Hypocalcemia is a total serum calcium (Ca^{2+}) level below 9.0 mg/dL or 2.25 mmol/L. Calcium is stored in bone, with only a small amount of total body calcium present in extracellular fluid (ECF). Because the normal blood level of calcium is so low, any change in calcium levels has major effects on function.

Calcium is an excitable membrane stabilizer, regulating depolarization and the generation of action potentials. Calcium decreases sodium movement across excitable membranes, decreasing the rate of depolarization. Low serum calcium levels increase sodium movement across excitable membranes, allowing depolarization to occur more easily and at inappropriate times.

TABLE 16-5 Common Causes of Hypocalcemia

Actual Calcium Deficits

Inhibition of Calcium Absorption from the Gastrointestinal Tract

- Inadequate oral intake of calcium
- Lactose intolerance
- Malabsorption syndromes
  - Celiac sprue
  - Crohn's disease
- Inadequate intake of vitamin D
- End-stage renal disease

Increased Calcium Excretion

- Renal failure—polyuric phase
- Diarrhea
- Steatorrhea
- Wound drainage (especially gastrointestinal)

Relative Calcium Deficits

Conditions That Decrease the Ionized Fraction of Calcium

- Hyperproteinemia
- Alkalosis
- Calcium chelators or binders
  - Citrate
  - Mithramycin
  - Penicillamine
  - Sodium cellulose phosphate (Calcibind)
  - Aredia
- Acute pancreatitis
- Hyperphosphatemia
- Immobility

Endocrine Disturbances

- Removal or destruction of parathyroid glands
  - Thyroidectomy
  - Irradiation of thyroid
  - Strangulation
  - Neck injuries

Hypocalcemia is caused by many chronic and acute conditions as well as medical or surgical treatments. Table 16-5 lists the common causes of hypocalcemia.

Actual calcium loss (a reduction in total body calcium) occurs when the absorption of calcium from the gastrointestinal (GI) tract slows or when calcium is lost from the body. Relative calcium loss causes total body calcium amounts to remain normal while serum calcium levels are low. This type of hypocalcemia occurs when the free or ionized (unbound) calcium in the body is reduced or when parathyroid gland function is decreased.

CULTURAL CONSIDERATIONS

Many black and Asian clients have a lactose intolerance caused by a deficiency of the enzyme lactase. These clients cannot use the nutrients in milk and have cramping, diarrhea, and abdominal pain after ingesting dairy products. Dairy products, especially milk, are common and rich source of both calcium and vitamin D. Clients with lactose intolerance may, therefore, have difficulty obtaining enough calcium and vitamin D from other sources to maintain normal calcium levels in the blood and bones.

WOMEN'S HEALTH CONSIDERATIONS

Postmenopausal women are at risk for calcium loss. This problem is related to reduced weight-bearing activities and a decrease in estrogen levels. In general, women are

Continued

smaller framed than men and the female skeleton does not bear as much weight as the male skeleton. As they age, many women decrease weight-bearing activities such as running and walking. Osteoporosis occurs when weight-bearing activity decreases or is limited. In addition, the estrogen secretion that protects against osteoporosis diminishes. All of these factors increase the risk for calcium loss in postmenopausal women.

CONSIDERATIONS FOR OLDER ADULTS

Older adults are at risk for most electrolyte imbalances as a result of age-related organ changes. For example, older adults have less total body water than younger adults, and therefore are more at risk for fluid imbalances. Older adults are more likely to be taking drugs that affect fluid or electrolyte balance. Some older adults have dietary calcium or vitamin D deficits because of reduced income or problems with obtaining, preparing, or eating food.

COLLABORATIVE MANAGEMENT

Assessment

The diet history is important to assess for the risk of hypocalcemia. Ask the client about his or her intake of calcium-containing foods and whether a calcium supplement is taken regularly (see Table 14-8).

One indicator of hypocalcemia is a report of frequent, painful muscle spasms ("charley horses") in the calf or foot during rest or sleep. Other information that indicates possible hypocalcemia is a history of recent orthopedic surgery or bone healing. Endocrine disturbances and treatments are risk factors for hypocalcemia. A history of thyroid surgery, therapeutic irradiation of the upper middle chest and neck area, or a recent anterior neck injury increase the risk for hypocalcemia. The most common manifestations of hypocalcemia are caused by overstimulation of the nerves and muscles (Chart 16-10).

NEUROMUSCULAR MANIFESTATIONS. The client usually notices symptoms in the limbs, with changes occurring first in the hands and feet. Paresthesias occur at first, with sensations of tingling and numbness. If hypocalcemia continues or worsens, actual muscle twitching or painful cramps and spasms occur. Paresthesias may also affect the lips, nose, and ears. These problems may signal the onset of neuromuscular overstimulation and tetany.

Assess for hypocalcemia by testing for **Trousseau's** and **Chvostek's signs.** To test for Trousseau's sign, place a blood pressure cuff around the upper arm, inflate the cuff to greater than the client's systolic pressure, and keep the cuff inflated for 1 to 4 minutes. Under these hypoxic conditions, a positive Trousseau's sign occurs when the hand and fingers go into spasm in palmar flexion (Figure 16-2). To test for Chvostek's sign, tap the face just below and in front of the ear (over the facial nerve) to trigger facial twitching of one side of the mouth, nose, and cheek (Figure 16-3).

CARDIOVASCULAR MANIFESTATIONS. With hypocalcemia, the heart rate may be slower or slightly faster than normal, with a weak, thready pulse. Severe hypocalcemia causes severe hypotension and electrocardiographic (ECG) changes, including a prolonged ST interval and a prolonged QT interval.

INTESTINAL MANIFESTATIONS. Hypocalcemia increases peristaltic activity. Auscultate the abdomen for hyperactive bowel sounds. The client may report painful abdominal cramping and diarrhea.

Common Nursing Diagnoses and Collaborative Problems

Nursing diagnoses and collaborative problems that may apply to clients with hypocalcemia include the following:

- Acute Pain related to hypocalcemia-induced muscle spasms and hyperactive gastric motility
- Decreased Cardiac Output related to hypocalcemia-induced dysrhythmias or reduced myocardial contractility

CHART 16-10

KEY FEATURES of Hypocalcemia

Cardiovascular Manifestations
- Decreased heart rate
- Decreased myocardial contractility
- Diminished peripheral pulses
- Hypotension
- Electrocardiographic abnormalities
  - Prolonged ST interval
  - Prolonged QT interval

Respiratory Manifestations
- Not directly affected
- Respiratory failure or arrest can result from decreased respiratory movement because of muscle tetany or seizure activity

Neuromuscular Manifestations*
- Anxiety, irritability, psychosis
- Paresthesias followed by numbness
- Irritable skeletal muscles—twitches, cramps, tetany, seizures
- Hyperactive deep tendon reflexes
- Positive Trousseau's sign
- Positive Chvostek's sign

Gastrointestinal Manifestations
- Increased gastric motility
- Hyperactive bowel sounds
- Abdominal cramping
- Diarrhea

*The neuromuscular system is most profoundly affected by hypocalcemia.

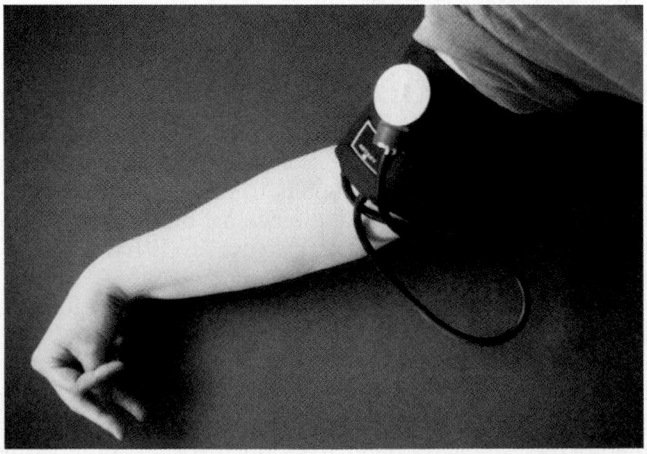

Figure 16-2 ■ Palmar flexion–positive Trousseau's sign in hypocalcemia.

- Deficient knowledge (dietary calcium) related to lack of exposure
- Risk for Injury related to bone density loss
- Readiness for Enhanced Nutrition related to the need to increase oral calcium intake

Interventions

Interventions aim to restore normal calcium levels and prevent complications. Chart 16-11 lists NIC interventions for electrolyte management of hypocalcemia. Interventions include drug therapy, diet therapy, reducing environmental stimuli, and preventing injury.

Drug Therapy. Drug therapy for hypocalcemia includes direct calcium replacement, drugs that enhance the absorption of calcium, and drugs that decrease nerve and muscle responses. Chart 16-12 lists the different drug types used to manage hypocalcemia.

Diet Therapy. A high-calcium diet is needed for clients with mild hypocalcemia and for those with chronic conditions that cause them to be at continuous risk for hypocalcemia. Collaborate with the dietitian to assist the client in selecting calcium-rich foods. The calcium content of common foods is listed in Table 14-8.

Environmental Management. The excitable membranes of the nervous system and the skeletal system are overstimulated in hypocalcemia. Therefore you must reduce the stimulation of these systems.

Use seizure precautions for the client with hypocalcemia. Such precautions include padding the siderails of the bed and keeping emergency equipment (e.g., oxygen and suction) at the bedside. Keep an emergency cart equipped with emergency drugs and an endotracheal tray just outside the client's room.

Injury Prevention. The client with long-standing calcium loss may have brittle, fragile bones that fracture easily and cause little pain. When lifting or moving a client with fragile bones, use a lift sheet rather than pulling the client. Observe for normal range of joint motion and for any unusual surface bumps or depressions over bony areas.

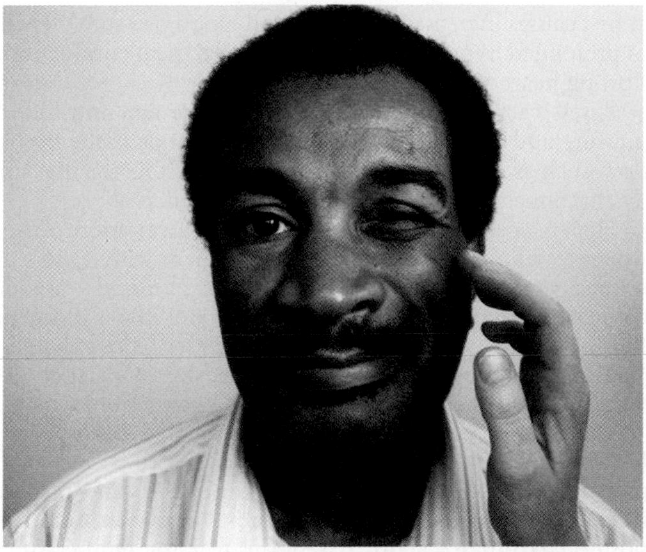

Figure 16-3 ■ Facial muscle response–positive Chvostek's sign in hypocalcemia.

Hypercalcemia

PATHOPHYSIOLOGY

Hypercalcemia is a total serum calcium level above 10.5 mg/dL or 2.75 mmol/L. Because the normal range for serum calcium is so narrow, even small increases have severe effects. Although the effects of hypercalcemia occur first in excitable tissues, all systems are affected to some degree.

Hypercalcemia means either that the amount of serum calcium is so great that the normal calcium-controlling mechanisms cannot keep pace or that at least one mechanism is not functioning properly. Hypercalcemia causes excitable tissues to be less sensitive to normal stimuli thus requiring a stronger stimulus to function. The excitable tissues affected most by hypercalcemia are the heart, muscles, nerves, and intestinal smooth muscles.

CHART 16-11

NIC INTERVENTION ACTIVITIES for The Client with Calcium Imbalances

Electrolyte Management: Hypocalcemia: *Promotion of calcium balance and prevention of complications resulting from serum calcium levels lower than desired*

- Monitor trends in serum levels of calcium (e.g., ionized calcium), as available.
- Monitor fluid status, including intake and output, as appropriate.
- Administer appropriate prescribed calcium salt (e.g., calcium carbonate, calcium chloride, and calcium gluconate), as indicated.
- Monitor for side effects of IV administration of ionized calcium (e.g., calcium chloride), such as thrombophlebitis, soft tissue damage with extravasation, clotting, and thrombus formation, as appropriate.
- Encourage intake of calcium (e.g., dairy products, seafood, nuts, broccoli, spinach, and supplements), as appropriate.
- Provide adequate intake of vitamin D (e.g., vitamin supplement and organ meats) to facilitate GI absorption of calcium, as appropriate.
- Monitor for neuromuscular manifestations of hypocalcemia (e.g., tetany, muscle twitching, cramping, grimacing, seizure, altered deep tendon reflexes, and spasm).
- Monitor for cardiovascular manifestations of hypocalcemia (e.g., decreased contractility, decreased cardiac output, hypotension, lengthened ST segment, and prolonged QT interval).
- Monitor for overcorrection and hypercalcemia.

Electrolyte Management: Hypercalcemia: *Promotion of calcium balance and prevention of complications resulting from serum calcium levels higher than desired*

- Monitor intake and output.
- Monitor trends in serum levels of calcium (e.g., ionized calcium), as available.
- Monitor for fluid overload resulting from hydration therapy (e.g., daily weight, urine output, jugular vein distention, lung sounds, and right atrial pressure), as appropriate.
- Monitor for neuromuscular manifestations of hypercalcemia (e.g., weakness, malaise, paresthesias, myalgia, hypotonia, decreased deep tendon reflexes, and poor coordination).
- Administer indomethacin (Indocin), calcitonin, or plicamycin (Mithracin), as appropriate.
- Encourage mobilization to prevent bone resorption.
- Monitor for recurring hypercalcemia 1 to 3 days after cessation of therapeutic measures.

NIC intervention activities selected from Dochterman, J.M., & Bulechek, G.M. (Eds.). (2004). *Nursing interventions classification (NIC)* (4th ed.). St. Louis: Mosby. No part of this work is to be altered without prior written permission from the Publisher.
GI, Gastrointestinal.

CHART 16-12

DRUG THERAPY for Hypocalcemia

Drug	Precautions
Oral Calcium Supplements	
Calcium carbonate Calcium citrate Calcium gluconate Calcium lactate	Dose must be increased in older clients because of decreased intestinal absorption. Use with thiazide diuretics can increase the risk for hypercalcemia. Use with phenytoin decreases the bioavailability of both drugs; phenytoin should not be given within 3 hours of calcium administration.
Intravenous Calcium	
Calcium acetate Calcium chloride Calcium gluconate	All must be administered slowly, not to exceed 27 g/min. Clients should be monitored for electrocardiographic changes during administration. Observe the client for infiltration; calcium is a severe tissue irritant/vesicant. There is a potential for hypercalcemia and hypomagnesemia. The injection should be warmed to body temperature before administration.
Agents That Increase Calcium Absorption	
Aluminum hydroxide	This agent reduces serum phosphorus levels, causing the countereffect of increasing calcium levels; there is a potential for hypophosphatemia. Signs and symptoms include bradycardia, decreased deep tendon reflexes, shortness of breath, and confusion.
Vitamin D Alfacalcidol✱ Calcifediol Calcitriol Dihydrotachysterol	This agent increases the intestinal absorption of calcium; there is a potential for hypercalcemia. This is a fat-soluble vitamin and is stored to some degree; there is a risk for vitamin D toxicity resulting in renal failure and/or cardiac failure.
Agents That Reduce Nerve and Skeletal Muscle Excitability	
Magnesium sulfate	This agent is a tissue irritant; the preferred route of administration is intravenous. There is a potential for hypermagnesemia; signs and symptoms of toxicity include bradycardia, flushing, headache, nausea, vomiting, shortness of breath, hypotension.
Methocarbamol Robaxin Carbacot Metaxalone Skelaxin Orphenadrine Banflex Flexoject Myolin Diazepam Valium Vivol✱ E-Pam✱ Carisoprodol Soma Vanadom	These agents act at the level of the central nervous system to decrease skeletal muscle activity. All have some sedative effect. All have some risk for psychological dependency and abuse.

Calcium is needed by many of the enzymes involved in blood-clotting. Hypercalcemia causes faster clotting times. Clots may form when they are not needed to control bleeding. Excessive clotting related to hypercalcemia occurs more easily in vessels with slow or blocked blood flow.

Causes of hypercalcemia include increased absorption of calcium, decreased excretion of calcium, and increased bone resorption of calcium (Table 16-6).

◆COLLABORATIVE MANAGEMENT

◆Assessment

The manifestations of hypercalcemia are related to both the severity of the imbalance and how quickly the imbalance occurred. The client with a mild but rapidly occurring calcium excess usually has more severe problems than the client whose hypercalcemia is severe but has developed slowly. Chart 16-13 lists the common manifestations of hypercalcemia.

CARDIOVASCULAR MANIFESTATIONS. The most serious and life-threatening problems of hypercalcemia are changes in cardiac function. Mild hypercalcemia at first causes increased heart rate and blood pressure. Severe or prolonged hypercalcemia depresses electrical conduction, slowing heart rate.

Assess cardiac status by measuring pulse rate and blood pressure and observing for indications of poor tissue blood flow, such as cyanosis and pallor. Examine ECG tracings for dysrhythmias, especially a shortened QT interval.

Hypercalcemia allows blood clots to form more easily whenever blood flow is poor. Thus the client with hypercalcemia is at risk for clot formation in areas of blood vessel or tissue damage and in vessels in which blood flow is blocked. Blood clotting is more likely in the lower legs, the pelvic region, areas where blood flow is blocked by internal or external constrictions, and where venous obstruction occurs.

Assess each client for slowed or impaired blood flow. Measure and record calf circumferences with a soft tape measure. Ask the client to alternately dorsiflex and plantar flex the ankles and state whether calf pain occurs in either position **(Homan's sign).** Assess the feet for temperature, color, and capillary refill to determine the blood flow to and from the area.

TABLE 16-6 Common Causes of Hypercalcemia

Actual Calcium Excesses

Increased Calcium Absorption
- Excessive oral intake of calcium
- Excessive oral intake of vitamin D

Decreased Calcium Excretion
- Renal failure
- Use of thiazide diuretics

Relative Calcium Excesses

Increased Bone Resorption of Calcium
- Hyperparathyroidism
- Malignancy
  - Direct invasion (cancers of breast, lung, prostate, and osteoclastic bone and multiple myeloma)
  - Indirect resorption (liver cancer, small cell lung cancer, and cancer of the adrenal gland)
- Hyperthyroidism
- Immobility
- Use of glucocorticoids

Hemoconcentration
- Dehydration
- Use of lithium
- Adrenal insufficiency

NEUROMUSCULAR MANIFESTATIONS. The neuromuscular manifestations include severe muscle weakness and decreased deep tendon reflexes without paresthesia. Central nervous system manifestations include an altered level of consciousness that can range from confusion and lethargy to coma. Psychiatric problems also can occur.

INTESTINAL MANIFESTATIONS. Decreased peristalsis is an early manifestation of hypercalcemia. The client may have constipation, anorexia, nausea, vomiting, and abdominal pain. Bowel sounds are hypoactive or absent. Assess the intestinal tract by listening for bowel sounds in all four abdominal quadrants. The abdomen increases in size because the intestinal contents remain in the tract instead of being moved forward. Assess abdominal size by measuring abdominal girth with a soft tape measure in a line circling the abdomen at the umbilicus.

RENAL MANIFESTATIONS. Hypercalcemia causes increased urine output and leads to dehydration. Chronic hypercalcemia may cause renal **calculi** (stones) to form in the kidney, because the excess calcium precipitates out of solution. Measure intake and output, assess voided urine for blood or cloudiness, and strain the urine for stones.

◆Interventions

Interventions for hypercalcemia aim to reduce serum calcium levels through drug therapy and dialysis. Chart 16-11 lists NIC interventions for electrolyte management of hypercalcemia.

Drug Therapy. IV solutions containing calcium are stopped. Discontinue giving oral drugs containing calcium or vitamin D (e.g., calcium-based antacids).

Fluid volume replacement can help restore normal serum calcium levels. IV normal saline (0.9% sodium chloride) is usually prescribed because sodium increases the excretion of calcium in the urine.

Thiazide diuretics are discontinued and are replaced with diuretics that enhance the excretion of calcium, such as furosemide (Lasix, Furoside✱). Calcium chelators (calcium binders) help lower serum calcium levels. Such drugs include plicamycin (Mithracin) and penicillamine (Cuprimine, Pendramine✱).

CHART 16-13

KEY FEATURES of
Hypercalcemia

Cardiovascular Manifestations
- Increased heart rate (early phase)
- Increased blood pressure
- Bounding, full peripheral pulses
- Electrocardiographic abnormalities
  - Shortened ST segment
  - Widened T wave
- Potentiation of digoxin-associated toxicities
- Decreased clotting time
- Late phase
  - Bradycardia
  - Cardiac arrest, sinus arrest

Respiratory Manifestations
- Ineffective respiratory movement related to profound skeletal muscle weakness

Neuromuscular Manifestations
- Disorientation, lethargy, coma
- Profound muscle weakness
- Diminished or absent deep tendon reflexes

Renal Manifestations
- Increased urine output
- Dehydration
- Formation of renal calculi

Gastrointestinal Manifestations
- Decreased motility
- Hypoactive bowel sounds
- Anorexia, nausea
- Abdominal distention
- Constipation

Drugs to prevent hypercalcemia include agents that inhibit calcium resorption from bone, such as phosphorus, calcitonin (Calcimar), bisphosphonates (etidronate), and prostaglandin synthesis inhibitors (aspirin, nonsteroidal anti-inflammatory drugs).

Dialysis. When severe hypercalcemia causes life-threatening cardiac problems, drug therapy may not reduce serum calcium levels fast enough to prevent death. Dialysis (either hemodialysis or peritoneal dialysis) or blood ultrafiltration may be necessary.

Cardiac Monitoring. Continuously monitor clients with hypercalcemia to identify dysrhythmias and decreased cardiac output. Compare recent electrocardiogram (ECG) tracings with the client's baseline tracings. Especially look for changes in the T waves and the QT interval as well as changes in rate and rhythm.

PHOSPHORUS IMBALANCES

Hypophosphatemia

PATHOPHYSIOLOGY

Hypophosphatemia is a serum phosphorus level below 3.0 mEq/L. Even though the serum phosphorus level has a narrow range of normal (3.0 to 4.5 mEq/L), body functions are not usually impaired with rapid, wide changes in serum phosphorus levels. Reduced function occurs more often with chronic hypophosphatemia.

Most of the effects of hypophosphatemia are related to decreased energy metabolism and imbalances of other electrolytes and body fluids. Because of the reciprocal relationship between phosphorus and calcium, decreases in serum phosphorus levels cause increases in serum calcium levels.

Three main processes lead to decreased serum phosphorus levels: decreased absorption of phosphorus, increased excretion of phosphorus, and intracellular phosphorus shift (Table 16-7).

COLLABORATIVE MANAGEMENT

Assessment

The manifestations of hypophosphatemia occur when low serum phosphorus levels are severe or prolonged. Acute manifestations of hypophosphatemia are related to the decreased amounts of high-energy compounds (e.g., adenosine triphosphate [ATP]) needed to perform normal metabolic functions. Manifestations are most apparent in the cardiac, musculoskeletal, hematologic, and central nervous systems (Chart 16-14).

CARDIOVASCULAR MANIFESTATIONS. Cardiac changes include decreased stroke volume and decreased cardiac output. Peripheral pulses are slow, difficult to find, and easy to block. Cardiac depression is caused by low stores of intracellular energy. Without sufficient energy in myocardial cells, contractions are weak and ineffective. Prolonged hypophosphatemia causes progressive but reversible cardiac muscle damage.

MUSCULOSKELETAL MANIFESTATIONS. Hypophosphatemia weakens skeletal muscles and may cause acute muscle breakdown **(rhabdomyolysis).** The weakness is generalized, and paresthesias usually are not present. When skeletal muscle weakness becomes profound, respiratory movements are ineffective, leading to respiratory failure. Assess for muscle strength and observe respiratory effort.

The manifestations of chronic hypophosphatemia are most evident in the skeletal system. Bone density is decreased, which leads to fractures and changes in bone shape. These changes are caused by the bone calcium loss that occurs with hypophosphatemia. Assess the client for unusual lumps or depressions over bony areas that indicate bone fractures.

CENTRAL NERVOUS SYSTEM MANIFESTATIONS. Central nervous system manifestations are not apparent until hypophosphatemia is severe. These first appear as irritability and may progress to seizure activity followed by coma.

Interventions

Discontinue drugs that promote hypophosphatemia (e.g., antacids, osmotic diuretics, and calcium supplements). Oral replacement of phosphorus along with a vitamin D supplement may correct moderate hypophosphatemia or prevent hypophosphatemia in at risk clients. IV phosphorus is given only when serum phosphorus levels fall below 1 mg/dL and the client has serious manifestations. Infuse IV phosphorus slowly because the problems caused by hyperphosphatemia are equally serious.

Diet therapy involves increasing the intake of phosphorus-rich foods while decreasing the intake of calcium-rich foods (Chart 16-15).

TABLE 16-7 Common Causes of Phosphorus Imbalance

Hypophosphatemia

Insufficient Phosphorus Intake
- Malnutrition
- Starvation
- Use of aluminum hydroxide-based antacids
- Use of magnesium-based antacids

Increased Phosphorus Excretion
- Hyperparathyroidism
- Hypercalcemia
- Renal failure
- Malignancy

Intracellular Shift
- Hyperglycemia
- Hyperalimentation
- Respiratory alkalosis
- Uncontrolled diabetes mellitus
- Alcohol abuse

Hyperphosphatemia
- Decreased renal excretion resulting from renal insufficiency
- Tumor lysis syndrome
- Increased intake of phosphorus
- Hypoparathyroidism

CHART 16-14

KEY FEATURES of Hypophosphatemia

Cardiovascular Manifestations
- Decreased contractility
- Cardiomyopathy (reversible)

Respiratory Manifestations
- Shallow respirations

Musculoskeletal Manifestations
- Weakness
- Rhabdomyolysis
- Decreased deep tendon reflexes

Central Nervous System Manifestations
- Irritability
- Confusion
- Seizures

Hematologic Manifestations
- Increased bleeding
- Decreased platelet aggregation
- Immunosuppression

CHART 16-15

CLIENT EDUCATION GUIDE
Dietary Management of Hypophosphatemia

You Should Avoid	You May Eat
Milk	Fish
Cheese	Beef
Yogurt	Chicken
Collard greens	Pork
Rhubarb	Organ meats
	Nuts
	Whole-grain breads and cereals

Hyperphosphatemia

PATHOPHYSIOLOGY

Hyperphosphatemia is a serum phosphorus level above 4.5 mEq/L. Serum phosphorus levels above normal are well tolerated by most body systems.

The problems caused by hyperphosphatemia center on the hypocalcemia that results when serum phosphorus levels increase. These problems include increased membrane excitability to the extent that membranes depolarize spontaneously.

Causes of increased serum phosphorus levels include renal insufficiency, certain cancer treatments, increased phosphorus intake, and hypoparathyroidism. Table 16-7 lists specific common causes of hyperphosphatemia.

◆COLLABORATIVE MANAGEMENT

Hyperphosphatemia causes few direct problems with body function. However, hypocalcemia is usually present because calcium and phosphorus ions exist in the blood in a balanced reciprocal relationship: when one increases, the other decreases. The hypocalcemia greatly alters many body system functions and can cause life-threatening side effects. Thus the management of hyperphosphatemia entails the management of hypocalcemia.

MAGNESIUM IMBALANCES

Hypomagnesemia

PATHOPHYSIOLOGY

Hypomagnesemia is a serum magnesium (Mg^{2+}) level below 1.2 mEq/L. Most problems leading to hypomagnesemia are caused by decreased magnesium intake or increased magnesium loss. As a result, hypomagnesemia reflects a decrease in the total body magnesium content.

The effects of hypomagnesemia are caused by increased membrane excitability and the accompanying serum calcium and potassium imbalances. Excitable membranes, especially nerve cell membranes, may depolarize spontaneously.

Hypomagnesemia is caused by decreased absorption of dietary magnesium or increased renal magnesium excretion. Table 16-8 lists the specific causes of hypomagnesemia.

TABLE 16-8 Common Causes of Magnesium Imbalance

Hypomagnesemia

Insufficient Magnesium Intake
- Malnutrition
- Starvation
- Diarrhea
- Steatorrhea
- Celiac disease
- Crohn's disease

Increased Magnesium Excretion
- Drugs (diuretics, aminoglycoside antibiotics, cisplatin, amphotericin B, cyclosporine)
- Citrate (blood products)
- Ethanol ingestion

Intracellular Movement of Magnesium
- Hyperglycemia
- Insulin administration
- Sepsis
- Alkalosis

Hypermagnesemia
- Increased magnesium intake
  - Magnesium-containing antacids and laxatives
  - IV magnesium replacement
- Decreased renal excretion of magnesium resulting from renal insufficiency

◆COLLABORATIVE MANAGEMENT

◆Assessment

Common clinical manifestations of hypomagnesemia are seen in the neuromuscular, central nervous, and intestinal systems (Chart 16-16).

NEUROMUSCULAR MANIFESTATIONS. The neuromuscular manifestations cause increased nerve impulse transmission. Normally, magnesium inhibits nerve impulse transmission at synapse areas. Decreased magnesium levels increase impulse transmission from nerve to nerve or from nerve to skeletal muscle. The client with hypomagnesemia has hyperactive deep tendon reflexes (+4), painful paresthesia (numbness and tingling), and tetanic muscle contractions. Positive Chvostek's and Trousseau's signs may be present because hypomagnesemia may occur with hypocalcemia (see the earlier discussion of these assessment signs under Neuromuscular Manifestations [Hypocalcemia], p. 238). Skeletal muscle weakness is present if intracellular magnesium levels

CHART 16-16

KEY FEATURES of Hypomagnesemia

Cardiovascular Manifestations
- Electrocardiographic changes
  - Tall T waves
  - Depressed ST segments
- Dysrhythmias
  - Ectopic beats
  - Ventricular tachycardia
  - Ventricular fibrillation
- Hypertension

Gastrointestinal Manifestations
- Decreased motility
- Anorexia
- Nausea
- Abdominal distention
- Decreased bowel sounds

Respiratory Manifestations
- Shallow respirations

Neuromuscular Manifestations
- Fasciculations
- Twitches
- Paresthesias
- Positive Trousseau's sign
- Positive Chvostek's sign
- Hyperreflexia
- Tetany
- Seizures

Central Nervous System Manifestations
- Irritability
- Confusion
- Psychosis

are also decreased. The client may have tetany and seizures as hypomagnesemia worsens.

CENTRAL NERVOUS SYSTEM MANIFESTATIONS. Central nervous system (CNS) manifestations are caused by increased nerve impulse transmission. Increased CNS irritability may present as psychological depression, psychosis, and confusion.

INTESTINAL MANIFESTATIONS. Intestinal manifestations are intestinal smooth muscle contraction. Clients have decreased gastric motility, anorexia, nausea, constipation, and abdominal distention. A paralytic ileus may occur when hypomagnesemia is severe.

Interventions

Interventions for hypomagnesemia aim to correct the magnesium imbalance and manage the specific problem that caused the hypomagnesemia. In addition, because hypocalcemia often occurs with hypomagnesemia, interventions also aim to restore normal serum calcium levels.

Discontinue drugs that promote magnesium loss, such as high-ceiling (loop) diuretics, osmotic diuretics, aminoglycoside antibiotics, and drugs containing phosphorus. Magnesium is replaced intravenously with magnesium sulfate ($MgSO_4$) when hypomagnesemia is severe. The IV route is used because $MgSO_4$ causes pain and tissue damage when injected intramuscularly. Assess deep tendon reflexes at least hourly in the client receiving IV magnesium to monitor effectiveness and prevent hypermagnesemia. Oral magnesium often causes diarrhea and can increase magnesium loss. If hypocalcemia is also present, drug therapy to increase serum calcium levels is prescribed.

Diet therapy consists of increasing the intake of foods that contain high amounts of magnesium (see Table 14-11).

Hypermagnesemia

PATHOPHYSIOLOGY

Hypermagnesemia is a serum magnesium level above 2.1 mEq/L. Magnesium is a membrane stabilizer. When magnesium excess occurs, excitable membranes are less excitable and need a stronger-than-normal stimulus to respond. With severe hypermagnesemia, excitable membranes may not respond to any stimulus.

Hypermagnesemia results from increased intake of magnesium coupled with decreased renal excretion of magnesium. Table 16-8 lists the specific causes of hypermagnesemia.

COLLABORATIVE MANAGEMENT

Assessment

Most manifestations of hypermagnesemia occur as a result of reduced membrane excitability. Manifestations usually are not apparent until serum magnesium levels exceed 4 mEq/L. The most common manifestations are seen in the cardiac, central nervous, and neuromuscular systems.

The cardiac manifestations include bradycardia, peripheral vasodilation, and hypotension. These problems become more severe as serum magnesium levels increase. Electrocardiographic (ECG) changes show a prolonged PR interval with a widened QRS complex. Bradycardia can be severe and cardiac arrest is possible. Hypotension with a wide pulse pressure is also severe, with a diastolic pressure lower than normal. *Clients with severe hypermagnesemia are in grave danger of cardiac arrest.*

Central nervous system manifestations result from depressed nerve impulse transmission. Clients may be drowsy or lethargic. Coma may occur if the hypermagnesemia is prolonged or severe.

Neuromuscular manifestations result from decreased nerve impulse transmission to the skeletal muscles. Deep tendon reflexes are reduced or even absent. Voluntary skeletal muscle contractions become progressively weaker and finally stop.

Hypermagnesemia has no direct effect on the lungs; however, when the respiratory muscles are weak, respiratory insufficiency can lead to respiratory failure and death.

Interventions

Interventions for hypermagnesemia aim to reduce the serum magnesium level and correct the underlying problem that caused the hypermagnesemia.

All oral and parenteral magnesium are discontinued. When renal failure is not present, giving magnesium-free IV fluids can reduce serum magnesium levels. High-ceiling (loop) diuretics such as furosemide (Lasix, Furoside✱) can further reduce serum magnesium levels. When cardiac problems are severe, giving calcium may reverse the cardiac effects of hypermagnesemia.

Diet therapy can prevent hypermagnesemia when other chronic conditions increase the risk for excess serum magnesium. Dietary restrictions involve limiting meat, nuts, legumes, fish, vegetables, and whole-grain cereal products. To prevent the recurrence of hypermagnesemia, teach the client to avoid drugs that increase magnesium, such as magnesium-containing antacids, laxatives, or enemas.

GET READY for the NCLEX Examination!

KEY POINTS

Safe Effective Care Environment

- Do not give intravenous potassium at a rate greater than 20 mEq/hr.
- Never give potassium supplements by the intramuscular or subcutaneous routes.
- Use a pump or controller when giving intravenous potassium-containing solutions.
- Use a gait belt when assisting a client with muscle weakness to walk.
- Collaborate with the dietitian to teach clients about diets that are restricted in potassium, sodium, or calcium.
- Use a lift sheet to move or reposition a client with hypocalcemia.

Health Promotion and Maintenance

- Teach all clients to take drugs as prescribed, especially diuretics, antihypertensives, and cardiac drugs.
- Teach clients who are taking digoxin to measure their pulse for rate, rhythm, and quality.
- Teach clients who are taking diuretics to measure their pulse for rate, rhythm, and quality.

- Include the person who prepares the client's meals when teaching about dietary electrolyte restrictions.

Psychosocial Integrity

- Assess clients who have a sudden change in cognition for electrolyte imbalances.
- Determine the client's food preferences and dislikes when planning an electrolyte restricted diet.

Physiological Integrity

- Clearly mark the IV bag that contains potassium.
- Assess the IV site of a person receiving IV solutions containing potassium at least every 2 hours.
- Document the condition of the IV site of a person receiving intravenous potassium infusions at least every 2 hours.
- Immediately stop the infusion of potassium-containing solutions if infiltration or extravasation is suspected.
- Avoid administering magnesium sulfate by the intramuscular route.
- Assess all clients with hyperkalemia for cardiac dysrhythmias and ECG abnormalities, especially tall T waves, conduction delays, and heart block.
- Assess the respiratory status of all clients with hypokalemia.
- Monitor the hydration status of clients who have hypernatremia, hyperkalemia, or hypercalcemia.
- Assess the bowel sounds; deep tendon reflexes; heart rate, rhythm and quality; and hand grasps to evaluate the client's responses to therapy for an electrolyte imbalance.

ADDITIONAL STUDY RESOURCES

Go to your Student CD-ROM for Review Questions for the NCLEX Examination.

evolve Go to http://evolve.elsevier.com/Iggy/ for Integrated Management of Care Questions for the NCLEX Examination.

SELECTED BIBLIOGRAPHY

Asterisk indicates a classic or definitive work on this subject.

Adams, M., & Pelter, M. (2004). Electrolyte imbalances. *American Journal of Critical Care, 13*(1), 85-86.

Adrogue, H., & Madias, N. (2000). Primary care: Hypernatremia. *The New England Journal of Medicine, 342*(20), 1492-1499.

*Ahern-Gould, K., & Stark, J. (1998). Quick resource for electrolyte imbalance. *Critical Care Nursing Clinics of North America, 10*(4), 477-490.

Burger, C. (2004). Emergency: Hypokalemia. *American Journal of Nursing, 104*(11), 61-65.

Call-Schmidt, T. (2001). Interpreting lab results: A primer. *MEDSURG Nursing, 10*(4), 179-184.

Call-Schmidt, T., & Williams-Evans, S. (2000). How to recognize hypokalemia. *Nursing2000, 30*(2), 22.

Castiglione, K. (2000). Hyperkalemia. *American Journal of Nursing, 100*(1), 55.

*Chmielewski, C. (1998). Hyperkalemic emergencies: Mechanisms, manifestations, and management. *Critical Care Clinics of North America, 10*(4), 449-457.

Collins, N. (2002). Take the guesswork out of sodium restrictions. *Nursing2002, 32*(8), 32hn7-32hn8.

Criner, J., et al. (2002). Rhabdomyolysis: The hidden killer. *MEDSURG Nursing, 11*(3), 138-143.

Dochterman, J.M., & Bulechek, G.M. (Eds.). (2004). *Nursing interventions classification (NIC)* (4th ed). St. Louis: Mosby.

Ebersole, P., Hess, P., & Luggen, A. (2004). *Toward healthy aging: Human needs and nursing response* (6th ed). St. Louis: Mosby.

Francis, J. (2001). ECG challenge–hypocalcemia. *Emergency Medicine, 33*(8), 41-42.

*Gosling, P. (1999). Fluid balance in the critically ill: The sodium and water audit. *Care of the Critically Ill, 15*(1), 11-16.

Guyton, A., & Hall, J. (2000). *Textbook of medical physiology* (10th ed.). Philadelphia: W.B. Saunders.

Hadaway, L. (2001). How to safeguard delivery of high-alert drugs. *Nursing2001, 31*(2), 36-41.

Held-Warmkessel, J. (2000). Test your knowledge: Altered calcium metabolism. *Clinical Journal of Oncology Nursing, 4*(3), 139-140.

Incredibly easy! Understanding hypokalemia. (2002). *Nursing2002, 32*(3), 65.

Innerity, S. (2000). Hypomagnesemia in acute and chronic illness. *Critical Care Nursing Quarterly, 23*(2), 1-19.

Jordan, K. (2000). Fluid resuscitation in acutely injured patients. *Journal of Intravenous Nursing, 23*(2), 81-87.

Kraft, P. (2000). The osmotic shift. *Journal of Intravenous Nursing, 23*(4), 220-224.

Krantz, M., & Baker, W. (2002). ECG challenge: Test your interpretive skills. *Consultant, 42*(14), 1757-1763.

Kugler, J., & Hustead, T. (2000). Hyponatremia and hypernatremia in the elderly. *American Family Physician, 61*(12), 3623-3630.

McCance, K., & Huether, S. (2002). *Pathophysiology: The biologic basis for disease in adults and children* (4th ed). St. Louis: Mosby.

Moorhead, S., Johnson, M., & Maas, M. (Eds.). (2004). *Nursing outcomes classification (NOC)* (3rd ed). St. Louis: Mosby.

*O'Donnell, M. (1995). Assessing fluid and electrolyte balance needs in elders. *American Journal of Nursing, 95*(1), 41-46.

Pagana, K., & Pagana, T. (2002). *Mosby's manual of diagnostic and laboratory tests* (2nd ed). St. Louis: Mosby.

Ruholl, L. (2002). Managing medications for older patients. *Nursing2002, 32*(3), 32hn6-32hn8.

*Stark, J. (1998). A comprehensive analysis of the fluid and electrolytes system. *Critical Care Nursing Clinics of North America, 10*(4), 471-475.

Trissel, L. (2003). *Handbook on injectable drugs* (12th ed.). Bethesda, MD: American Society of Health-System Pharmacists.

Webster, A., Brady, W., & Morris, F. (2002). Recognizing signs of danger: ECG changes resulting from an abnormal serum potassium concentration. *Emergency Medicine Journal, 19*(1), 74-77.

CHAPTER

17 Infusion Therapy

LYNN C. HADAWAY

LEARNING OUTCOMES

After studying this chapter, you should be able to:

1. Categorize the purpose and types of intravenous (IV) infusion therapy.
2. Identify the types and characteristics of vascular access devices (VADs).
3. Evaluate clients for vascular access needs.
4. Distinguish the components of an infusion system.
5. Differentiate the types of rate control devices and nursing considerations for their use.
6. Prioritize nursing interventions for maintaining an infusion system.
7. Assess, prevent, and manage complications related to infusion therapy and VADs.
8. Determine special needs of older adults receiving IV therapy.
9. Identify nursing considerations for intra-arterial, intraperitoneal, subcutaneous, intraosseous, epidural, and intrathecal infusion therapy.

Go to your Student CD-ROM for Review Questions for the NCLEX Examination keyed to these Learning Outcomes.

Infusion therapy is the delivery of parenteral medications and fluids through a wide variety of catheter types and locations using multiple techniques and procedures. Intravenous (IV) and intra-arterial therapy delivers the solution into the vascular system. The peritoneal cavity can be used for infusion of certain types of oncology medications. Subcutaneous therapy and hypodermoclysis slowly infuse certain fluids and medications into the subcutaneous tissue; other medications can be delivered to the central nervous system through the epidural or intrathecal space. The intraosseous space can be used for emergency access in infants, children, and adults. This chapter focuses on access for and administration of all types of infusion therapy.

INTRODUCTION TO INFUSION THERAPY

Virtually all clients will require some type of infusion therapy during their hospital stay. Although less common, infusion therapy is also seen in community-based settings, including the client's home. The number of vascular access devices (VADs) inserted annually in the United States now exceeds seven million. Infusion therapy is also delivered in all health care settings, including home care, ambulatory clinics, physician's offices, and long-term care facilities. Infusion therapy is the center of the treatment plan for many clients, and it spans all age groups from birth to death.

The services of a specialized team of infusion nurses has the highest recommendation from the Centers for Disease Control as a strategy to reduce complications and improve client outcomes (O'Grady et al., 2002). This specialty practice encompasses the management of infusion therapy services for a facility or agency, including the following:

- Policy and procedure development
- Insertion of several types of peripheral and central venous catheters
- Monitoring clinical outcomes
- Serving as an educational resource for staff nurses
- Consulting on a variety of clinical and management issues, such as product selection and purchasing decisions

The rapid advances in technology for infusion therapy have driven the need for nurses specializing in vascular access and infusion therapy; however, not all health care agencies have an infusion therapy team. All nurses who provide direct client care are expected to perform basic infusion therapy procedures, although there are wide variations in responsibilities among facilities.

Several professional organizations strive to improve clinical outcomes with infusion therapy and vascular access through educational opportunities and publications. The Infusion Nurses Society (INS), formerly the Intravenous Nurses Society, publishes standards of practice intended to serve as the framework for policy and procedure development in all health care settings. These standards establish the performance criteria for all nurses delivering infusion therapy (Intravenous

Nurses Society, 2000). The Infusion Nurses Certification Corporation (INCC) offers a written certifying examination. Nurses who successfully complete this examination have mastered an advanced body of knowledge in this specialty and may use the initials *CRNI,* which stand for "certified registered nurse infusion." The Association for Vascular Access (AVA) is a multidisciplinary organization focusing on advanced practices with vascular access. The Oncology Nursing Society (ONS) writes guidelines about chemotherapy and biotherapy administration, and the American Society of Parenteral and Enteral Nutrition (ASPEN) writes standards and guidelines for all types of nutrition.

TYPES OF INFUSION THERAPY FLUIDS

Infusion therapy encompasses many types of parenteral fluids for multiple purposes. These fluids may be administered through several routes, but the most common route is via a vein (IV route). The primary goals of infusion therapy include the following:

- Achieving normal fluid and electrolyte balance
- Achieving optimal nutrition status
- Maintaining hemostasis through blood and blood component administration
- Treating numerous conditions with medications

Intravenous Fluids

Currently more than 200 IV fluids are available from commercial manufacturers that meet the requirements established by the United States Pharmacopeia (USP). Each solution is classified by its tonicity and pH. Tonicity is categorized by comparison to normal blood plasma. Normal plasma osmolarity is about 290 mOsm/L. Parenteral fluids close to this value are considered **isotonic;** those above 350 mOsm/L are considered **hypertonic;** and those below 250 mOsm/L are considered **hypotonic.** The pH of the IV fluids measures the acidity or alkalinity and usually ranges from 3.5 to 6.2. Extremes of both osmolarity and pH can cause vein damage leading to phlebitis and thrombosis. Therefore fluids and medications with a pH value less than 5 and greater than 9 and osmolarity greater than 500 mOsm/L should not be infused through a peripheral vein (Intravenous Nurses Society, 2000).

Parenteral Nutrition

Parenteral nutrition formulas include dextrose, protein, fat, vitamins, and numerous trace elements tailored to the specific metabolic needs of their client. Parenteral nutrition should be used *only* when the gastrointestinal (GI) tract cannot be used. The GI tract produces a better physiologic response and is less expensive and easier to manage. The osmolarity of all parenteral nutrition fluids is greater than 500 mOsm/L, requiring a central venous catheter for infusion of all formulas. Infusion of low-dextrose formulas through a peripheral vein leads to high rates of vein damage and subsequent phlebitis, thrombosis, and extravasation injury. Repeated peripheral venipunctures are usually needed when short peripheral catheters are used, thus increasing the rate of complications and the cost of therapy. (See Chapter 64 for a complete discussion of parenteral nutrition.)

Blood Transfusion and Other Components

Blood transfusion is accomplished using packed red blood cells, created by removing a large portion of the plasma from whole blood leaving the oxygen carrying red blood cells. Other blood components include platelets, fresh frozen plasma, albumin, and several specific clotting factors. Each component has detailed requirements for blood-type compatibility and infusion techniques. Facilities that are accredited by the Joint Commission on Accreditation of Healthcare Organizations (JCAHO) are required to ensure that blood components are properly ordered, handled and dispensed, and administered along with appropriate client monitoring. Positive client identification is essential before any blood component is administered. An acute hemolytic transfusion reaction due to an incompatible blood transfusion is a sentinel event requiring an intense analysis of the cause and corrective action. Established policies and procedures must be rigidly followed to ensure a safe transfusion and reduce the risk of complications. (See Chapter 43 for a complete discussion of blood transfusions.)

Medications

IV medications provide a rapid therapeutic effect but can also lead to immediate serious reactions. Hundreds of medications are available for infusion by a variety of techniques, mandating easy access to a reliable nursing reference written specifically for IV administration of medications. As with all drug administration, you must be knowledgeable about drug indications, proper dosage, contraindications, and precautions. However, IV administration also requires knowledge of appropriate dilution, rate of infusion, pH and osmolarity, compatibility with other IV medications, and specific aspects of client monitoring because of the immediate effect. Regardless of familiarity with the drug, never assume that IV administration is the same as giving that drug by other routes. New information is continuously being published, and new drugs are rapidly being introduced.

Medication safety is of paramount importance in all health care settings today. JCAHO now produces client safety goals annually. One major goal is improving the safety of high-alert medications. An example is concentrated electrolyte solutions (e.g., potassium chloride), which require restricted access, prominent warnings about the concentration, and storage in a secured location. Other strategies to reduce medication errors include limiting available concentrations of drugs and dispensing all drugs, including catheter flush solutions, in single-dose containers.

PRESCRIBING INFUSION THERAPY

An order for infusion therapy written by a physician or authorized prescriber is necessary before you begin IV therapy. To be complete, the order for infusion fluids must include the following:

- Specific type of fluid
- Rate of administration written in milliliters per hour, or the total amount of fluid and the total number of hours for infusion (e.g., 125 mL/hr or 1000 mL/8 hr)

- Medications and the specific dose to be added to the fluid such as electrolytes or vitamins

A medication order must include the following:

- Medication name, preferably by generic name
- Specific dose and route
- Frequency of administration

Some continuously infused medications, such as those for pain management, are prescribed as milligrams per hour. The type and volume of dilution for infusion medications may be included in the order; however, the infusion pharmacist may determine these factors for medication admixture.

You are responsible for determining that the order is appropriate for the client and clarifying any questions before administration. An example is an order for 5% dextrose in water to keep vein open (KVO). This order does not specify the rate of infusion and is not considered complete (Intravenous Nurses Society, 2000).

VASCULAR ACCESS DEVICES

A catheter, also known as a **vascular access device (VAD),** is a plastic tube placed in a blood vessel to deliver fluids and medications. Therapy characteristics determine whether the infusion can be given safely through peripheral veins or if the large central veins of the chest are needed. Advances in catheter materials and insertion techniques have radically expanded the types of VADs currently used. This discussion includes the description and uses for seven types: short peripheral catheters, midline catheters, peripherally inserted central catheters (PICC), nontunneled percutaneous central catheters, tunneled catheters, implanted ports, and hemodialysis catheters.

Technologic improvements have caused a change in how we approach vascular access. Repeated venipunctures with short peripheral catheters should not be done. Instead the goal is to assess the client's needs for vascular access and choose the device that has the best chance of infusing the prescribed therapy for the required length of time while using the minimal number of catheters.

Short Peripheral Catheters

Short peripheral catheters are composed of a plastic cannula built around a sharp stylet extending slightly beyond the cannula (Figure 17-1). The stylet allows for the venipuncture, and the cannula is advanced into the vein. These catheters are designed with a safety mechanism to house or cover the sharp end of the stylet after it is removed from the client. These stylets are hollow-bore, blood-filled needles that carry the highest risk of exposure to bloodborne pathogens if needle stick injury occurs. A federal law enacted in 2000 amended the Bloodborne Pathogen Standards from the Occupational Safety and Health Administration (OSHA) requiring the use of catheters with an engineered safety mechanism.

INSERTION

Short peripheral catheters are inserted into superficial veins of the hand and forearm. In emergent situations, these catheters can also be used in the external jugular vein of the neck. In infants the feet can be used, although the use of veins in the feet of adults should be avoided because of an increased risk of deep vein thrombosis.

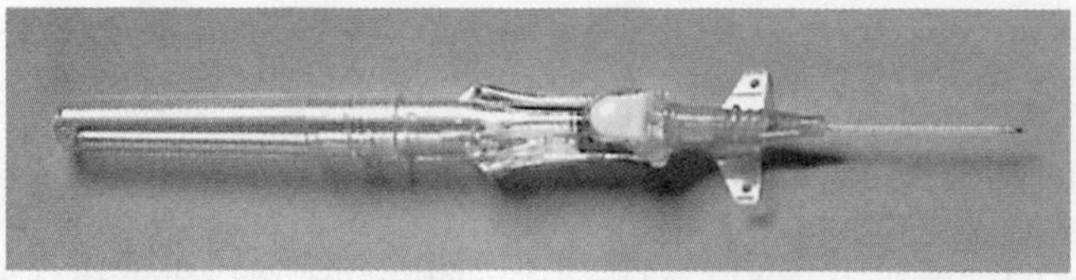

Figure 17-1 ■ Insyte AutoGuard IV catheters. With the push of a button, the needle instantly retracts, reducing the risk of accidental needle stick injuries. (Courtesy Becton Dickinson Infusion Therapy Systems, Sandy, UT.)

These catheters range in length from ¾ inch to 1¼ inch with gauge sizes from 26 gauge (the smallest) to 14 gauge (the largest). The smallest gauge catheter capable of delivering the prescribed therapy should be chosen. Current design allows for a thin-wall construction, providing a larger lumen without increasing the outer diameter. This design improves the capacity for fluid flow through the catheter while using a smaller gauge and thereby decreasing the possibility of vein irritation from a large catheter. For example, a thin-walled 24-gauge Insyte (BD Medical, Sandy, UT) catheter has about the same flow-rate capabilities as a 22-gauge non–thin-walled Angiocath (BD Medical, Inc.) Larger gauge sizes will always allow for faster flow rates but also cause phlebitis more often. Table 17-1 lists each gauge size and its common uses.

Short peripheral catheters are allowed to dwell for 72 to 96 hours and then require removal and insertion at another venous site. If the length of the client's therapy is expected to be longer than six days, a midline catheter or PICC should be chosen (O'Grady et al., 2002). When selecting the site for insertion of a peripheral catheter, consider the client's age, history, and diagnosis; the type and duration of the prescribed therapy; and, whenever possible, the client's preference. Chart 17-1 lists the major criteria for the placement of peripheral VADs.

PLACEMENT

The most appropriate veins for peripheral catheter placement include the dorsal venous network, basilic, cephalic, and median veins, as well as their branches (Figure 17-2). Veins on the hand may not be appropriate in older clients with a loss of skin turgor and poor vein condition or for active clients receiving infusion therapy in an ambulatory clinic or home care. Mastectomy, axillary lymph node dissection, lymphedema, paralysis of the upper extremity, and the presence of dialysis grafts or fistulas alter the normal pattern of blood flow through the arm. Cannulation of veins in the extremity affected by these conditions requires a physician's order. Short peripheral catheters are not recommended for obtaining routine blood samples (Intravenous Nurses Society, 2000).

Veins on the palm side of the wrist should be avoided because the median nerve is located close to veins in this area, making the venipuncture more painful and difficult to stabilize. The cephalic vein begins above the thumb and extends up the entire length of the arm. This vein is usually large and prominent, appearing as a prime site for catheter insertion. Research has shown, however, that the sensory branch of the median nerve can intersect with the cephalic vein up to three times from its origin to about 4 to 5 inches up the lateral aspect of the arm (Vialle et al., 2001). Transection of the nerve can result in permanent loss of function, and local nerve

TABLE 17-1 Choosing the Gauge Size for Peripheral Catheters

24- and 26-gauge	Use for neonates, pediatric, and older clients Recommended when extremely small-diameter veins are the only choice Blood return in the flash chamber may be slower Suitable for most infusions, but flow rates are slower May be used for blood transfusion ***without an infusion pump;*** a unit of packed red blood cells should be divided into two bags to accommodate the extended infusion time
22-gauge	Used for all infusions including blood and blood products Infusion rates will be slightly slower Recommended for most adults, especially those with small or fragile veins Not appropriate when rapid flow rates are required such as trauma or surgery
20-gauge	Used for all infusions including blood and blood products suitable for minor surgical procedures Most commonly used size
18-gauge	Trauma and surgery Rapid flow rates Requires a large vein to allow room for blood to flow in the vein around the catheter Irritation to the vein wall and phlebitis results when the catheter is too large for the chosen vein
16- and 14-gauge	High-risk surgical procedures and trauma Large volumes and rapid flow Requires a large vein Mechanical irritation and phlebitis are likely

CHART 17-1

BEST PRACTICE for
Placement of Short Peripheral Venous Catheters

- Verify that the order for infusion therapy is complete and appropriate for infusion through a short peripheral catheter.
- For adults, choose a site for placement in the upper extremity.
- Choose the client's nondominant arm when possible.
- Choose a distal site and make all subsequent venipunctures proximal to previous sites.
- Do not use the arm on the side of a mastectomy, lymph node dissection, arteriovenous shunt or fistula, or paralysis.
- Avoid choosing a site in an area of joint flexion.
- Avoid choosing a site in a vein that feels hard or cordlike.
- Avoid choosing a site close to areas of cellulitis, dermatitis, or areas of complications from previous catheter sites.

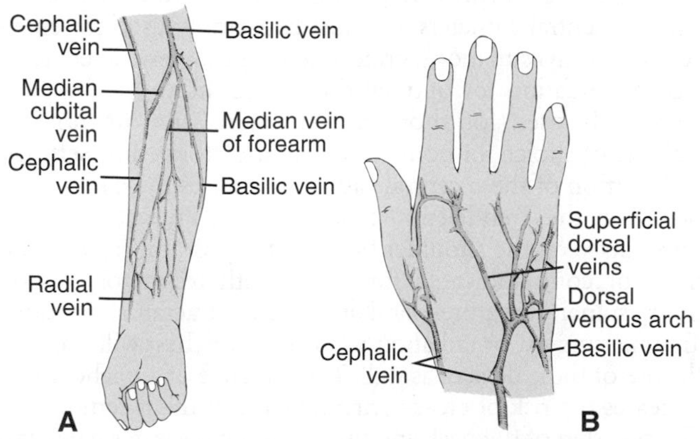

Figure 17-2 ■ Common IV sites. **A,** Inner arm. **B,** Dorsal surface of hand.

damage can become a chronic systemic pain syndrome. Complaints of tingling, feeling "pins and needles" in the extremity, or numbness during the venipuncture procedure can indicate nerve puncture. The procedure should be stopped immediately, the catheter removed, and a new site chosen.

Winged needles may be placed in the veins of the hand and forearm. Although these devices are easy to insert, they are associated with a high frequency of infiltration. They are most commonly used for injection of single-dose medications or for drawing blood samples. Like a short peripheral catheter, winged needles should also have an engineered safety mechanism to house the needle when removed.

Midline Catheters

INDICATIONS

Midline catheters are 6 to 8 inches long and are inserted through the veins of the antecubital fossa. The basilic vein is preferred over the cephalic vein because of its larger diameter, and it will allow greater hemodilution of the fluids and medications being infused. The catheter tip is located in the upper-arm level with the axilla. These catheters are used for therapies lasting from 1 to 4 weeks; however, there are no recommendations for the optimal dwell time (O'Grady et al., 2002). Because of the extended dwell time, sterile technique is used for insertion of a midline catheter. Additional education and skill assessment are required for the nurse to be considered qualified to insert midline catheters.

A midline catheter can be used when skin integrity or limited peripheral veins make it difficult to maintain a short peripheral catheter. Other indications include the following:

- Fluids for hydration
- Five to 10 days of antibiotics to treat urosepsis or pneumonia
- Heparin infusions for deep vein thrombosis
- Bronchodilators, such as aminophylline
- Steroids

Limiting venipunctures in clients who have received anticoagulation agents is desirable to avoid excessive bruising and hematoma formation. Metabolic changes in steroid-dependent clients results in changes in the skin and vein conditions, making repeated venipuncture difficult.

The fluids and medications infused through a midline catheter should have a pH between 5 and 9 and a final osmolarity of less than 500 mOsm/L (Intravenous Nurses Society, 2000). The pH and osmolarity outside these parameters increase the risk of complications like phlebitis and thrombosis.

Midline catheters should not be used for infusion of **vesicant medications,** which are drugs that will cause tissue damage if they escape into the subcutaneous tissue **(extravasation).** At this tip location, larger amounts of the drug can extravasate before the problem is detected. All parenteral nutrition formulas, including those with low concentrations of dextrose, have an osmolarity greater than 500 mOsm/L and should not be infused through a midline catheter. Blood sampling from a midline catheter should not be routinely performed (Intravenous Nurses Society, 2000). Midline catheters should not be placed in extremities affected by mastectomy with lymphedema, paralysis, or dialysis grafts and fistulas.

Midline catheters may be designed with pressure-sensitive valves located near the internal catheter tip (e.g., Groshong, made by Bard Access Systems, Salt Lake City, UT) or in the external catheter hub (e.g., PASV, made by Boston Scientific, Natick, MA). These valves open when pressure is applied, allowing for infusion and aspiration; however, when no pressure is applied, they are closed to prevent blood refluxing into the lumen or air entering the bloodstream. The manufacturers of both catheters state that saline only can be used to flush these lines, eliminating the need for heparin to maintain lumen patency.

Peripherally Inserted Central Catheters

PLACEMENT

A peripherally inserted central catheter (PICC) is a long catheter inserted through the veins of the antecubital fossa or the middle of the upper arm. In adults the catheter length ranges from 40 to 65 cm, with the tip residing in the superior vena cava (SVC). Placement of the catheter tip in veins distal to the SVC should be avoided. This inappropriate tip location, often called mid-clavicular catheters, are associated with much higher rates of thrombosis than when the tip is located in the SVC (Kearns, Coleman, & Wehner, 1996). Mid-clavicular tip locations should be used only when anatomic or pathophysiologic changes prohibit advancement of the catheter into the SVC (National Association of Vascular Access Networks, 1998).

PICCs should be inserted early in the course of therapy, before veins of the extremity have been damaged from multiple venipunctures and infusions. Insertion methods using guidewires and ultrasound greatly improve insertion success. The basilic vein is the preferred site for insertion; however, the cephalic vein can be used if necessary. Sterile technique is used for insertion to reduce the risk of bloodstream infections. A chest radiograph indicating that the tip resides in the lower SVC is required before the catheter can be used for infusion. PICCs are available in single-, dual-, or triple-lumen configurations and are available with both Groshong and PASV valves.

PICCs have lower complication rates because of the insertion site in the upper extremity. The dry skin of the arm has fewer types and numbers of microorganisms, leading to lower rates of infection. Inadvertent arterial puncture or excessive bleeding can be controlled by direct pressure. Insertion complications such as pneumothorax associated with other central venous catheters do not occur with PICCs. In addition, PICC lines are less expensive than central catheters (Smelling et al., 2001).

INDICATIONS

PICCs can accommodate the infusion of all types of therapy because the tip resides in the SVC where the rapid blood flow will quickly dilute the fluids being infused. Therefore, there are no limitations on the pH or osmolarity of fluids that can be infused through a PICC. Clients requiring lengthy courses of antibiotics, antineoplastic agents, parenteral nutrition formulas, vasopressor agents, and numerous other fluids can benefit from a PICC. PICCs have been reported to dwell successfully for months or even years; however, the optimal dwell time is not known (O'Grady et al., 2002).

PICCs can be used for blood sampling; however, lumen sizes of 4F or larger are recommended. Using lumens with small diameters may not yield a sample capable of producing the needed test results. Transfusion of blood through a PICC usually requires the use of an infusion pump. Packed red blood cells are cold and viscous. The length of the PICC adds resistance and may prevent the blood from infusing within the 4-hour limitation.

Teach clients with a PICC to perform normal activities of daily living; however, they should avoid excessive physical activity. Muscle contractions in the arm from physical activity like heavy lifting can lead to catheter dislodgment and possible lumen occlusion.

PICC insertion is commonly performed in the client's hospital room, an outpatient treatment facility, or the radiology department. Nurses placing these catheters require a high level of skill with venipuncture and central venous catheter management. Additional education, along with documented competency assessment, is required.

Nontunneled Percutaneous Central Catheters

Nontunneled percutaneous central catheters are inserted through the subclavian vein in the upper chest or the jugular veins in the neck using sterile technique. They are usually 15 to 20 cm long and have dual or triple lumens. The tip resides in the SVC, confirmed by a chest x-ray. Nontunneled percutaneous central catheters are most commonly used for emergent or trauma situations, critical care, and surgery. There is no recommendation for optimal dwell time; however, these are commonly used for short-term situations and are not the catheter of choice for home care or ambulatory clinic settings.

Insertion of these central catheters requires the client to be placed in the Trendelenburg position, usually with a rolled towel between the shoulder blades. This position may be difficult or contraindicated for clients with respiratory conditions, spinal curvatures, and increased intracranial pressure. Trauma, surgery, or radiation in the neck or chest will prohibit the use of these devices as well. The presence of a tracheotomy increases the risk of cross-contamination of the insertion site. The oily skin of the neck and upper chest has greater types and numbers of microorganisms, resulting in greater numbers of bloodstream infections with this type of catheter.

Tunneled Central Catheters

Tunneled central venous catheters have a portion of the catheter lying in a subcutaneous tunnel, separating the points where the catheter enters the vein from where it exits the skin. This separation is intended to prevent the organisms on the skin from reaching the bloodstream (Figure 17-3). The catheter has a cuff made of a rough material that is positioned inside the subcutaneous tunnel. The tissue granulates into this cuff, providing a mechanical barrier to microorganisms and anchoring the catheter in place. This design requires surgical techniques for insertion. Single, dual, and triple lumens are available. These catheters were originally named for the physicians who designed them, including Broviac, Hickman, and Leonard catheters. These names are now trade names and should be used when referring to those particular brands.

Tunneled catheters are used primarily when the need for infusion therapy is frequent and long-term. Clients needing parenteral nutrition for months, years, or the remainder of their life commonly choose a tunneled catheter. Tunneled catheters are also chosen when several weeks or months of infusion therapy are needed and a PICC is not a good choice. For example, paraplegic clients needing 6 to 8 weeks of antibiotics are not good candidates for a PICC because of the excessive use of the upper extremities for mobility. Some oncology clients may prefer a tunneled catheter instead of an implanted port because they cannot tolerate the needle sticks required for accessing those devices.

Implanted Ports

Implanted ports consist of a portal body, a dense septum over a reservoir, and a catheter (Figure 17-4). A subcutaneous pocket is surgically created to house the port body. The catheter is inserted into the vein and attached to the portal body. The septum is made of self-sealing silicone and is located in the center of the port body over the reservoir. The catheter extends from the side of the port body. The incision is closed, and no part of the catheter is visible externally; therefore this device has the least impact on body image.

PLACEMENT

Venous ports may be placed on the upper chest or the upper extremity. The venous catheter may enter either the subclavian or internal jugular vein and is available as a single- or double-lumen device. Although an implanted port is most commonly used in the venous system, the catheter may be placed in arteries, the epidural space, or the peritoneal cavity, with the port pocket located over a bony prominence.

MAINTENANCE

Implanted ports are accessed by using a noncoring needle specially designed with a deflected tip. This design slices through the dense septum without coring out a small piece of it, thus preserving the integrity of the septum. Port bodies placed in the chest have a larger septum and will usually tolerate about 2000 punctures. Port bodies placed in the upper extremity are smaller and are rated to tolerated about 750 punctures. Before puncture, the port is palpated to locate the septum. Carefully palpate to feel the shape and depth of the port body to ensure puncture of the septum, not the attached catheter. Noncoring port access needles, also called **Huber needles,** may have a straight shaft or may be bent at a right angle. Some have attached extension sets and wings to stabilize the needle. One important feature is an engineered safety mechanism to contain the needle when it is removed from the septum. Because the dense septum holds tightly to the needle, there can be a rebound when it is pulled from the septum, often resulting in needle stick injury to the nurse (Figure 17-5).

An implanted port needs to be flushed after each use and at least once a month between courses of therapy. When not accessed, there is no external catheter requiring a dressing. Puncture of the skin over the port is required to gain access to the port body, causing pain for some clients. Topical anesthetic creams can be used to make the access procedure more tolerable for the client.

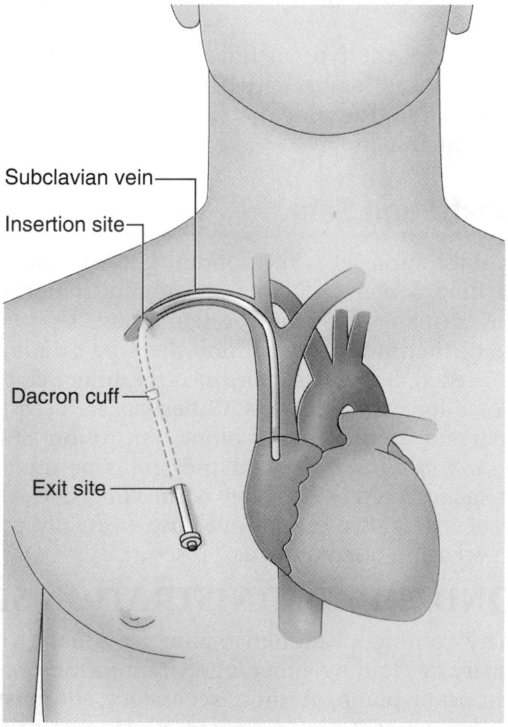

Figure 17-3 ■ Tunneled catheter. A portion of this catheter lies in a subcutaneous tunnel, separating the points where the catheter enters the vein from where it exits the skin.

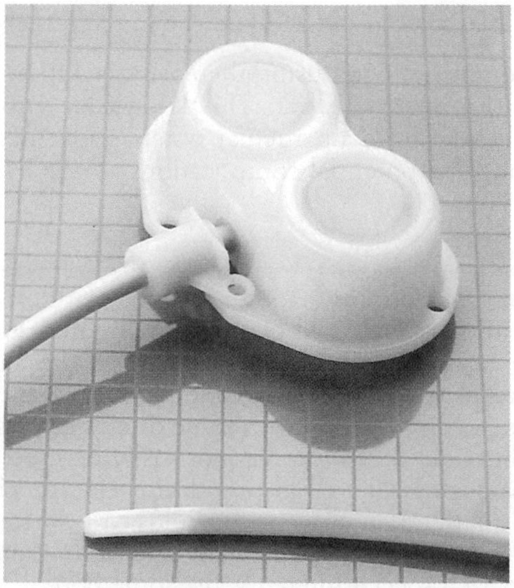

Figure 17-4 ■ A dual-lumen implanted port for venous access. (Courtesy of HMP-Horizon Medical Products Inc., Manchester, GA.)

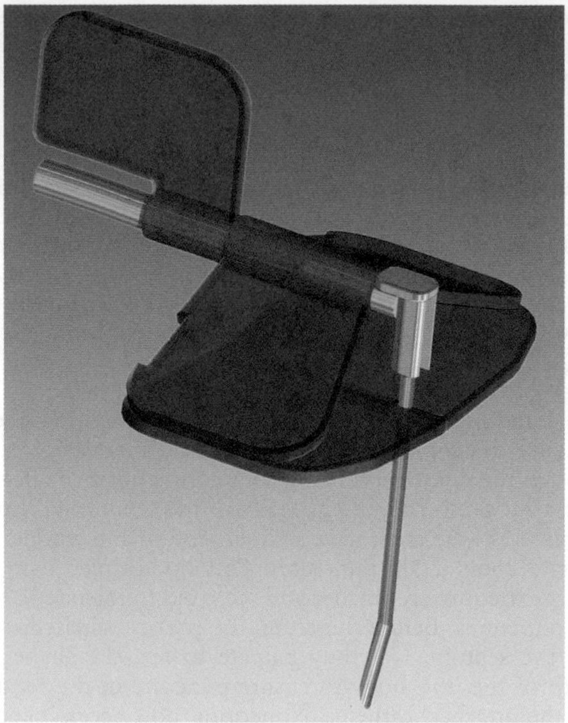

Figure 17-5 ■ Huber Plus Noncoring Needle. The safety mechanism traps the needle to prevent needle stick injury. (Courtesy of NowMedical, Chadds Ford, PA.)

Dialysis Catheters

Dialysis catheters have very large lumens to accommodate the hemodialysis procedure or a pheresis procedure that harvests specific blood cells. They may be tunneled for long-term needs or nontunneled for short-term needs. A dialysis catheter is critical to the client's management of renal failure and must function well. Bloodstream infection and vein thrombosis are common problems; therefore this catheter should not be used for administration of other fluids or medications, except in an emergency.

INFUSION SYSTEMS

Nurses administering infusion therapies need to understand how infusion systems work. This knowledge ensures that you can benefit from a particular system's advantages while minimizing any potential complications.

Containers

Infusion containers are made of glass or plastic. *Glass* bottles were the original fluid container to be mass produced. They are easily sterilized; it is easy to read the amount of fluid remaining in the bottle; and they do not have the problems of compatibility with some drugs like plastic does. Glass bottles are heavy and cannot easily be used in many situations, such as client transport during emergencies. Glass bottles do require an air vent for fluids to flow freely from them. The most common method is to use an administration set with a special filtered vent. Some bottles may have a straw tube open to the room air through the rubber stopper in the bottle and extending to above the level of the fluid. Bottles with a venting straw do not have a barrier to prevent contaminants in the air from entering the fluid.

Plastic containers are considered **closed systems** because they do not rely on outside air to allow the fluid to infuse. Instead, atmospheric pressure pushes against the flexible sides of the container, allowing the fluid to flow by gravity. For this reason, plastic containers do not require vented administration sets. These containers are lightweight, unbreakable, and easy to use in emergency conditions.

Plastic containers are commonly made of polyvinyl chloride (PVC). To increase flexibility and strength, PVC requires the addition of plasticizers. The most common chemical used as a plasticizer is di-2-ethylhexyl-phthalate or DEHP. There has been growing concern in the past few years over the exposure of clients to this chemical. DEHP does not chemically bind to the PVC and can leach from the plastic fluid container or tubing and can be infused to the client with the IV fluid or medication.

Plastic containers present incompatibility issues with insulin, nitroglycerin, lorazepam (Ativan), fat emulsions, and lipid-based drugs. Nitroglycerin and insulin adhere to the walls of the PVC container, making it impossible to know exactly how much medication the client is receiving.

Another concern with plastic bags is the accuracy of reading the amount of fluid remaining in the container. The middle graduations have been shown to be 10% above or below the actual amount of fluid, but the first and last markings could be inaccurate by as much as 40% (Perucca, 2001).

Semirigid containers are made of plastic but offer some of the benefits of glass, such as the absence of plasticizers and drug compatibility problems. These containers are lightweight and unbreakable but are more bulky and less flexible. They also require an air vent to allow the fluid to flow freely. Recent changes have led to a traditional flexible plastic bag made from materials other than PVC and do not require DEHP.

Regardless of the type of fluid container being used, it should be checked for cracks or pinholes before use. Always check the fluid for turbidity or any unusual color that could indicate contamination.

Administration Sets

The administration set is the conduit between the catheter and the fluid container. Numerous administration sets are available in many different configurations. The type and purpose of the infusion determine the type of administration set needed. Some sets are *generic,* meaning that they are appropriate for most infusions. Other sets are used for specific types of infusions, such as blood transfusion. Still other sets are *dedicated,* meaning that they must be used with a specific manufacturer's infusion controlling device. Information that describes their proper use is usually provided on the packaging of administration sets.

SECONDARY ADMINISTRATION SETS

A primary continuous administration set is used to infuse the primary IV fluid by either a gravity infusion or an electronic infusion pump. A short **secondary administration set,** also known as a **piggyback set,** is attached to the primary set at a Y-injection site and is used to deliver intermittent medications. Chart 17-2 shows the procedure for pig-

CHART 17-2

BEST PRACTICE for
Piggybacking an Intermittent Medication

1. Verify the order from the health care provider.
2. Check the compatibility between the medication and the large-volume parenteral (LVP) infusion and its additives.
3. Spike the medication minibag with the secondary set.
4. Prime the secondary set, close the roller clamp, and hang the mini-bag on the other arm of the IV pole.
5. Place the hanger that comes with the secondary set on the IV pole with the LVP.
6. Cleanse the Y-site injection port on the LVP administration set.
7. Attach the secondary set to the Y-site.
8. Lower the level of the LVP by hanging it from the hanger. Do not adjust the LVP roller clamp. (The rate will decrease and then stop when the secondary set is opened.)
9. Open the roller clamp on the secondary set and regulate the flow to the desired rate.
10. When the intermittent infusion completes, the LVP will automatically begin again. Hang the LVP from the IV pole, and adjust the roller clamp to deliver the prescribed rate.

CHART 17-3

BEST PRACTICE for
Backpriming Method for Infusing an Intermittent Medication

- The backpriming method allows multiple medications to be infused through the same secondary set.
- Assess the primary fluid container for admixed medications. If present, these medications *must* be compatible with the secondary medication.
- Lower the empty secondary container and allow fluid to flow into it from the primary container.
- Close the clamp and disconnect the secondary container.
- Attach the new secondary container with the next dose of medication.
- Hang and adjust the rate or set the infusion pump as indicated. If using an infusion pump, follow the specific manufacturer's guidelines to backprime the secondary set.

gybacking an intermittent medication. Once attached, these sets should remain connected together as an infusion system. If multiple intermittent medications are required, it may be possible to use only one secondary set rather than a secondary set for each medication. This depends on the compatibility of the medications. Chart 17-3 explains the sets to use one secondary set to infuse multiple medications using the backpriming method. This process eliminates the costs of using multiple secondary sets and allows you to adhere to the Infusion Nurses Society (INS) standards of practice. These sets are changed every 72 to 96 hours (Intravenous Nurses Society, 2000; O'Grady et al., 2002).

INTERMITTENT ADMINISTRATION SETS

An intermittent administration set is used to infuse multiple doses of medications when no primary continuous fluid is being infused through a catheter that has been capped with a needleless connection device. The medication container from the previous dose is removed and the new one attached. The sterile cap covering the distal end of the set is removed, and the set is attached to the catheter. Because both ends of the set are being manipulated with each dose, the INS standards of practice state that this set should be changed every 24 hours. If a secondary administration set is detached from the primary set, it should be considered an intermittent set and changed every 24 hours (Intravenous Nurses Society, 2000).

Administration sets are sterile in the fluid pathway and under the sterile caps on each end of the set. The set is not packaged as a completely sterile product and cannot be added to a sterile field. Careful attention is required to maintain the sterility of the spike and the connection end of the tubing to prevent introduction of microorganisms into the catheter and bloodstream.

ADD-ON DEVICES

Several other types of add-on devices include short extension sets, injection caps, and filters. Extension sets may be packaged as a sterile product for adding to a sterile field; however, you should always check the product label to ascertain this information.

Administration sets have two ways to connect to the catheter hub: a slip lock or a Luer-Lok. The *slip lock* is a male end that slips into the female catheter hub. A *Luer-Lok* connection has the same male end with a threaded collar that requires twisting onto the corresponding threads of the catheter hub. All set connections should have a Luer-Lok design to ensure that the set remains firmly connected. Loose connections lead to fluid leakage and increase the risk of contamination and subsequent bloodstream infection. When using a central venous catheter, a Luer-Lok connection is critical to reduce the risk of air embolism. Tape is not considered an adequate mechanism for securing set connections.

Filters may be integral to the administration set or may be separate add-on pieces. Their purpose is to remove particulate matter, microorganisms, and air from the infusion system. Filter sizes depend on the pore size, with common sizes being 5 microns intended to remove gross particles, 1.2 microns used to filter lipid-containing parenteral nutrition, and 0.22 microns intended to remove all particles and microorganisms. Filters should be placed as close to the catheter hub as possible.

Particulate matter in the IV fluid, a primary reason to use filters, comprises undissolved, unintended substances and may include rubber pieces, glass particles, cotton fibers, drug particles, paper, and metal fibers. These particles become trapped in the small circulation of the lungs. A red blood cell is about 5 microns in diameter and is the largest size that can pass through the pulmonary capillary bed, and yet IV fluids may contain particles larger than this. For clients receiving infusion therapy for long periods, there could be a significant amount of particles that block the blood flow through the pulmonary circulation (Weinstein, 2001). Microcirculation in the spleen, kidneys, and liver could also be affected. Particulate matter has also been implicated in the development of phlebitis in peripheral veins (O'Grady et al., 2002).

Other concerns with using filters include the possibility for filter rupture, their use with certain drugs that bind to the filter surface, using the correct size of filter for drugs with large molecules, and choosing a filter that will tolerate the pressure exerted by infusion pumps. Rupture of the filter is most commonly associated with the exertion of high pressure exceeding the limit tolerated by the specific filter. Some drugs cannot be filtered because they are retained inside the filter because of their chemical nature or molecule size. For these reasons, medication filtration during the process of admixing is now used as an alternative to final filtration at the bedside. Drugs of a very small quantity should be administered below the filter.

Filters used on blood administration sets have much larger pore size and are not interchangeable with filters used for fluids and medications. A standard blood filter ranges from 170 to 220 microns and removes microclots and other debris caused by blood collection and storage. Microaggregate filters have a pore size of 20, 40, or 80 microns and are used to remove degenerating platelets, white blood cells, and fibrin strands present in blood within 5 days of storage. Leukocyte removal filters are used to remove white blood cells that cause febrile and allergic blood transfusion reactions, cytomegalovirus, and some herpes viruses. They are measured by efficiency rather than pore size (Weir, 2001).

NEEDLELESS CONNECTION DEVICES

In July 1992 the Occupational Safety and Health Administration (OSHA) published guidelines entitled *Occupational Exposure to Bloodborne Pathogens, Final Rule.* This document requires health care organizations to initiate engineering controls "that isolate or remove the bloodborne pathogen hazard from the workplace." This standard was amended in 2000 with the passage of the Needlestick Safety and Prevention Act, which requires the use of devices engineered with safety mechanisms and mandates the involvement of staff performing these tasks directly with selecting products. It also requires each employer to maintain a sharps injury log with details of each incident. Many products are designed to minimize health care workers' exposure to contaminated needles. Blunt cannulas injected through a pre-slit septum and luer-activated valves are the prevailing designs of these products.

Although these devices have reduced the incidence of accidental needle sticks for health care professionals, concern remains about a possible increase in the risk of infection to the client. Several early studies compared these needleless devices with the conventional use of needles to connect tubing together. Also, studies have been done that compare the infection risk of various designs of needleless devices. According to the Centers for Disease Control, when these systems are used according to the manufacturer's instructions, they do not increase the risk of bloodstream infection to your client. All injection sites must be adequately cleaned with an alcohol pad before connecting an IV set or syringe (O'Grady et al., 2002).

The original needleless injection devices have become a source of concern because of their tendency to promote blood reflux into the catheter lumen when the administration set or syringe is disconnected. Over time this small amount of blood can lead to lumen occlusion from a thrombus (Hadaway, 1998). To overcome this blood reflux or negative fluid displacement, positive pressure flushing techniques must be used. This can be accomplished by one of two methods:

- As you flush the last 0.5 mL of fluid into the catheter, withdraw the blunt cannula from the injection port or
- After flushing all fluid into the catheter, continue to hold your thumb on the syringe plunger while closing a clamp on the catheter or extension set and then disconnect the syringe.

New designs of needleless systems overcome this problem by causing a positive fluid displacement within the catheter lumen (Figure 17-6). The device holds a small amount of fluid in a reservoir. When the syringe or administration set is disconnected, this fluid is automatically pushed out to the catheter tip to prevent blood moving into the catheter lumen. When a positive fluid displacement needleless connector is used, positive pressure flushing techniques cannot be used because these techniques defeat the internal mechanism. Some of these devices allow for the elimination of heparinized saline as the final catheter flush; therefore the catheter can be flushed with normal saline only.

Rate-Controlling Devices

The ability to regulate the rate and volume of infusions is critical to the safe and accurate administration of medications and fluids to clients. Nurses have a choice of numerous devices designed to regulate infusions. Infusion devices can be mechanically or electronically regulated.

Mechanically regulated systems include elastomeric balloons, spring-coiled syringes and containers, and a multichambered fluid container placed in a mechanical roller. These devices are commonly used to deliver intermittent medications such as antibiotics in alternative care settings. They are powered by positive pressure from the collapsing balloon or roller returning to its coiled position. Fluid volume is determined by the size of the fluid container; however, most hold 50 to 100 mL. They deliver a preset infusion rate determined by the size of the opening in the tubing connected to the fluid container; therefore additional tubing is not required. These small, portable devices do not require power sources such as batteries or electricity.

Electronic infusion devices fall into two categories: controllers and pumps, based on the mechanism of operation.

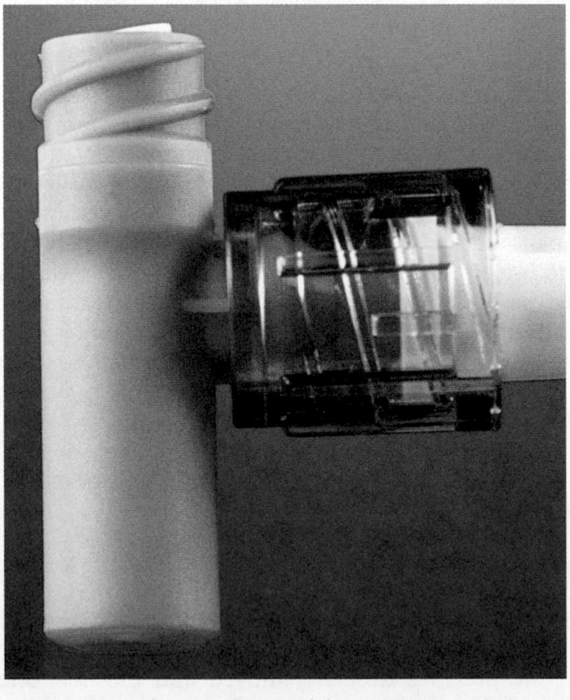

Figure 17-6 ■ The new design of the CLC2000 causes a positive fluid displacement within the catheter lumen. (Courtesy of ICU Medical, San Clemente, CA.)

Nurses and clients who use these electronic infusion devices reap the benefits of some of the latest computer technology. Electronic infusion devices can save nursing time, prevent clients from receiving too much infusion solution, and keep infusion access devices patent; however, the nurse must remember that the use of these devices does not decrease the practitioner's responsibility to monitor carefully the client's infusion site and the infusion rate.

A **controller** is a stationary, pole-mounted electronic device that uses a sensor to monitor fluid flow and to detect when flow has been interrupted. Controllers rely completely on gravity to create fluid flow and do not create pressure. Because controllers rely on counting drops, which vary in size and therefore volume, controllers are not as accurate as pumps.

Pumps may be either large and pole-mounted or ambulatory and portable. As their name indicates, these devices actually pump medications or fluids under pressure. They accurately measure the volume of fluid being infused by using one of three mechanisms:

- A syringe-type mechanism that fills and empties
- A wavelike, peristaltic action that pushes fluid along the tubing
- A series of microchambers that fill and empty

Regardless of the pumping mechanism, these devices require dedicated cassette tubing designed to match the pump.

Syringe pumps use a battery-powered piston to push the plunger continuously at a selected milliliter-per-hour rate. The use of syringe pumps is limited to small-volume continuous or intermittent infusions and is dependent on the syringe size. Antibiotics and patient-controlled analgesia are frequently delivered with syringe pumps. Pediatric clients and those requiring fluid restrictions can also benefit from using a syringe pump because smaller yet accurate volumes can be used to dilute medications. Syringe pumps are generally not appropriate for continuous administration of larger volumes because they require frequent syringe changes.

Ambulatory pumps are generally used for home care clients and allow them to return to their usual activities while receiving infusion therapy. They have a wide range of sizes, with some requiring a backpack, but they usually weigh less than 6 pounds. They are used to deliver accurately continuous infusions such as parenteral nutrition or many programmable medication schedules. Frequent battery recharging or replacement is usually necessary.

Electronic infusion devices can be programmed in many different ways and require a thorough knowledge of the specific brand being used. Infusion rate and the volume to be infused are usually entered in single milliliter increments, but some can be programmed as fractions of a milliliter for use in infants. Some pumps allow the rate to be programmed to taper or ramp up and down at the beginning and ending of the infusion. Secondary syringe infusion, secondary infusion rate, remote site programming, adjustable infusion pressure, and integration into the nurse call system are also possible.

Electronic infusion devices have a variety of alarms, such as air-in-line, upstream and downstream occlusion, infusion complete, and low-battery or power warnings. All devices must have some mechanism to prevent free flow of the infusing fluid or medication. When the cassette or tubing is removed from the pump, this mechanism will automatically stop fluid flow until it is properly replaced in the pump. This prevents accidental rapid infusion of large amounts of fluid or medication leading to serious clinical problems.

CATHETER CARE AND MAINTENANCE

Educating the Client

Before catheter insertion, educate the client about the following:

- The type of catheter to be used
- The therapy required
- Alternatives to the catheter and therapy
- Client activity limitations
- Any signs or symptoms of complications that should be reported to a health care professional

Whereas written information should be provided before placement of a long-term catheter, you should continue to assess the client's understanding of the information and provide more information or answers as needed. Most manufacturers of PICCs, tunneled catheters, and implanted ports provide information booklets written for clients; however, specific information about the chosen procedures and supplies may be required. The booklets may be useless to clients who cannot read or have a low reading level.

Confirming Tip Location

All central venous catheters require a postinsertion chest radiograph to document the tip location. The initial verbal and subsequent written report should contain specific information about the catheter tip location in relation to anatomic structures. Your knowledge of accurate tip location is required before beginning infusion through the catheter. Repeating the chest radiograph during catheter use may be necessary if the client complains of unusual pain or sensation.

Performing the Nursing Assessment

Nursing assessment of all infusion systems should be systematic. Begin with the insertion site and work upward. Know the type of catheter your client has in place. Complications are frequently seen at or near the catheter; however, you will need to know the length of catheter, the insertion site, and tip location to do a complete assessment. Assess the insertion site by looking for redness, swelling, hardness, or drainage. Lightly palpate the area over the dressing. When a midline catheter or PICC is used, assess the entire extremity and upper chest of signs of phlebitis and thrombosis. When a tunneled catheter is used, assess the exit site, the entire length of the tunnel, and the point where the catheter enters the vein. For a well-healed catheter, it may not be possible to detect the vein entrance site; however, on newly inserted catheters there could be a small puncture site with a suture. For implanted ports, assess the incision and surgically created subcutaneous pocket.

Assess the integrity of the dressing, making sure it is clean, dry, and adherent to the skin on all sides. Check all connections on the administration set and ensure that they are secure. Check the rate of infusion for all fluids by either counting drops or checking the electronic infusion pump.

Assess the amount of fluid that has infused from the container. Is it accurate, or is it infusing too fast or too slow? Adjust the rate to the prescribed flow rate. Check all labels on fluid containers for the client's name and fluid or medication.

Avoid taking blood pressures in an extremity with any type of catheter in place. If a short peripheral catheter is being used for continuous infusion, the compression while taking the blood pressure can increase venous pressure, causing fluid to overflow from the puncture site, resulting in an infiltration. When a midline catheter or PICC is being used, compression from the blood pressure cuff could increase vein irritation and lead to phlebitis.

Venipuncture for blood sampling should be performed in the extremity opposite from all catheters. Blood samples should not be drawn from a venipuncture site proximal to an infusing peripheral catheter because the infusing fluid could alter the results of the test to be performed. Venipuncture at or near the insertion site of a midline catheter or PICC could inadvertently damage the catheter and add to areas of venous inflammation.

A

B

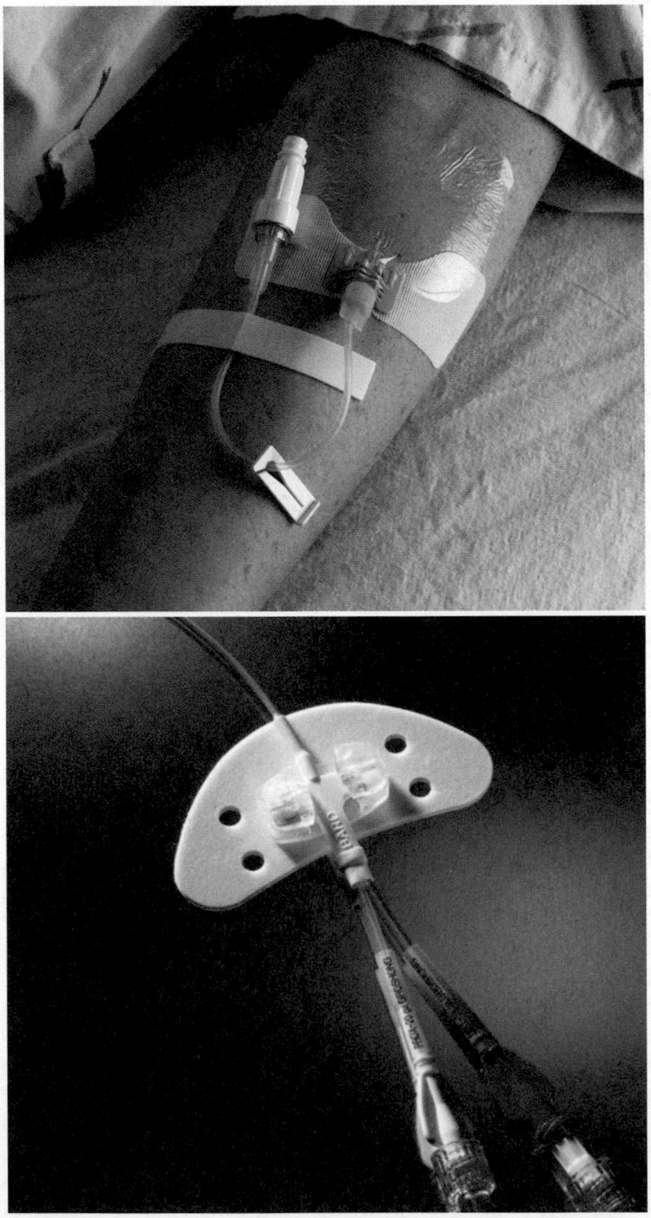

Figure 17-7 ■ The Statlock provides a standardized method to prevent catheter movement. (Courtesy of Venetec International, San Diego, CA.)

Securing and Dressing the Catheter

Adequate catheter securement is vital to prevent many complications. Tape, sutures, and specially designed securement devices can be used for this purpose. For a short peripheral catheter, tape strips are most common; however, the tape should be *clean*. Tape strips from a peripheral IV start kit are preferred. Strips of tape should not be taken from rolls of tape moved between client's rooms, from other procedures, or from uniform pockets. Precutting tape and placing it on the client's bedrails or other object should also be avoided.

Securement devices are designed for all catheter types and provide a standardized method to prevent catheter movement (Figure 17-7). PICCs and nontunneled percutaneous central catheters may be sutured in place; however, this creates additional breaks in the skin that could become infected. If these sutures are loose or broken, the physician must be notified to replace them or some additional securement method must be used. Tunneled catheters usually have sutures placed near the skin exit site that are removed after the tunnel has healed. The incision over a port pocket will have sutures until it has healed also.

Dressings used over the insertion site protect the skin and puncture site. For a short peripheral catheter, the transparent membrane dressings do not require routine changes but rather may remain until the catheter is removed. Tape and gauze or a transparent membrane dressing can be used for midline catheters and all types of central venous dressings. Tape and gauze dressings should be changed every 48 hours. Transparent membrane dressings are changed once or twice weekly. The initial dressing on a midline catheter or PICC is usually tape and gauze changed within 24 hours after insertion because some bleeding is likely. Transparent membrane dressings can be used for subsequent dressing.

Site protection may be needed for short peripheral catheters or for port access needles. Plastic shields can be placed over the site to prevent accidental bumping or pressure from clothing (Figure 17-8).

Remove the dressing by pulling laterally from side to side. It can also be removed by holding the external catheter

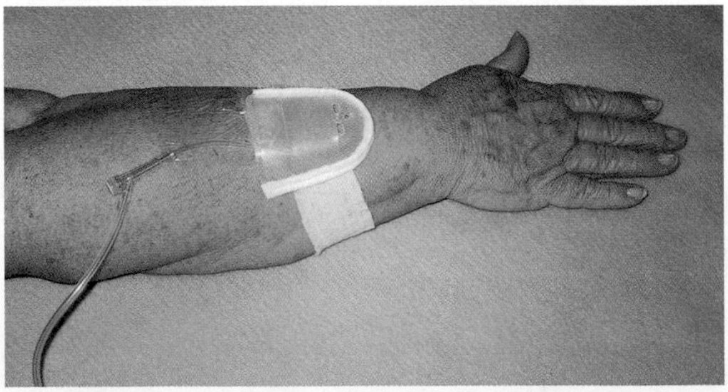

Figure 17-8 ■ I.V. House, a commercially available safety device used for IV site protection, guards the integrity of the older adult's skin while helping to secure the site. (Courtesy I.V. House, Hazelwood, MO.)

and pulling it off toward the insertion site. Never pull it off by pulling away from the insertion site because this could dislodge the catheter.

After removing the dressing from a midline catheter or any central venous catheter, take note of the external catheter length. Compare this length with the original length at insertion. If this length has changed, the catheter tip location has also changed and may no longer be in a vein appropriate for infusion. This situation may require a repeat chest radiograph and careful assessment of the type of therapy and remaining length of therapy required.

The external catheter, dressing, and all attached tubing must be protected from water because water is a source of contamination. While bathing, the extremity should be covered. Plastic trash bags can be taped over the extremity; however, devices specially designed for this purpose are usually more convenient for your client to use.

Changing Administration Sets and Needleless Connectors

Primary and secondary administration sets are usually changed every 72 or 96 hours; however, certain types of fluids require more frequent change. These include lipid emulsion, blood products, and drugs such as propofol.

All connections must be secured by using a luer-locking device. Do not rely on tape to secure connections. Tape residue attracts organisms and increases the risk of infection.

Plan the change of administration sets and fluid containers to occur at the same time, if possible, to minimize the number of times the system is opened. For short peripheral catheters, the administration set and catheter should also be changed at the same time to avoid excessive manipulation of the catheter.

Needleless connector devices can be changed when the administration set is changed. If it is being used for intermittent infusions, the device should be changed at least once per week. Fluid leakage from the device indicates the integrity has been compromised, and it should be changed immediately.

Precautions to prevent air emboli are required when changing the set or connectors attached to any catheter; however, central venous catheters require special attention. The client should be lying flat to ensure that the catheter exit site is at or below the level of the heart. Some catheters may have a pinch clamp that can be closed during this procedure. Ask the client to perform a Valsalva maneuver by holding his or her breath and bearing down while you disconnect the old set and reconnect the new. This will prevent air from entering the lumen, the heart, and pulmonary circulation.

Controlling Infusion Pressure

Fluid flow through the infusion system requires that the pressure on the external side be greater than the pressure at the catheter tip. Fluid flow can be slowed or obstructed by many causes. At or above the catheter hub, kinked tubing, tubing or syringe diameter, and fluid temperature or viscosity could create resistance to flow. Inside the catheter lumen, resistance is created by the catheter length and diameter or by deposits of fibrin, thrombus, or drug precipitate. Near the catheter tip, resistance to flow comes from the catheter tip impinging on the vein wall, thrombus, or venous spasm.

All catheter manufacturers have warnings about the use of excessive pressure. Gravity and infusion pumps do not exert pressure too high for the catheter to handle; however, excessive pressure from syringes can lead to catheter damage. For this reason, use of 10-mL syringes is often recommended for use with central venous catheters. Although these larger syringes will generate less pressure, it is still possible to reach excessive pressure levels if great force is applied against a syringe attached to a catheter that is partially occluded. Catheter patency must be carefully assessed before each use. Attach a 10-mL syringe filled with saline and attempt to flush the catheter without excessive force. If resistance is felt, *always stop the flush! Never forcefully flush any catheter with any size of syringe.* Catheter rupture or forcing a blood clot into circulation could result.

Flushing the Catheter

Catheter flushing prevents contact between incompatible drugs and maintains patency of the lumens. Normal saline alone or normal saline followed by heparinized saline may be used. When using valved catheters and certain positive fluid-displacement needleless devices, normal saline alone is acceptable because these devices have mechanisms that prevent the backflow of blood into the catheter lumen. When one of these products is not being used, the final flush should be normal saline followed by heparinized saline.

Before using any catheter, you should flush with normal saline to remove the heparinized saline left from the previous use and to determine lumen patency. Apply slow, gentle pressure to the syringe plunger. *If you feel any resistance, stop the procedure immediately.* During the flushing procedure, always aspirate for a brisk blood return from the catheter lumen. If the catheter will not yield a blood return, further diagnostic studies may be needed to determine the cause of the problems. Heparin is incompatible with many other medications, and the normal saline prevents contact between drugs and prevents drug precipitate from forming.

For short peripheral catheters, usually 3 mL normal saline is adequate to flush the catheter. For all other catheters, 5 to 10 mL of preservative-free normal saline is needed. Bacteriostatic normal saline is limited to no more than 30 mL in a 24-hour period in adults. By using 10 mL before and after each dose of medication, it is easy to exceed this limitation.

The concentration of heparinized saline ranges from 10 to 100 units/mL. The chosen concentration should not affect the client's clotting factors. Lower concentrations are used when the catheter is needed for frequent intermittent infusions; however, for infrequent use, 100 units/mL is preferred. Be sure that you know the policy and procedure established by your facility. Hemodialysis catheters may have larger concentrations of heparin used, such as 5000 units/mL; however, the heparin is aspirated before catheter use.

The volume of heparinized saline for catheter flushing should be a quantity that is twice the volume of the catheter lumen and the extension set or connectors added on, usually 3 to 5 mL.

Heparin use for catheter flushing is the cause of growing concern. It is often difficult for clients to remember the sequence of multiple flush solutions, adding to the need for repeated education of clients in home care. As mentioned previously, heparin is incompatible with many other drugs. Heparin may also interfere with obtaining blood samples taken from the catheter lumen, especially when coagulation studies are needed. Heparin-induced thrombocytopenia can also result from small doses used to flush catheters, resulting in loss of an extremity from blood clots and even death.

Catheters should be flushed immediately following each use. Delay in disconnecting the intermittent administration set and flushing the catheter could cause lumen occlusion from blood that backflows into the lumen when the infusion pressure is lower than venous pressure.

All fluids used to flush catheters should be obtained from single-dose containers or prefilled syringes. Vials used for multiple doses contribute to medication errors and increase the risk of contamination.

Obtaining Blood Samples from the Catheter

Short peripheral and midline catheters should not be routinely used for obtaining blood samples. This additional manipulation could lead to vein irritation that requires removal of the catheter. Central venous catheters can be used for obtaining blood samples after a careful assessment of the risk versus the benefits. If your client has no peripheral venipuncture sites or is fearful of needles, using the central venous catheter may be appropriate. The risks associated with obtaining blood samples from a central venous catheter are numerous. This procedure calls for additional hub manipulation, which is a major cause of bloodstream infection. Consider the laboratory tests needed and the types of fluids that have recently been infused. Heparin interferes with coagulation studies; electrolytes in the fluid may alter the results of serum electrolytes; and antibiotics such as vancomycin may interfere with measuring the peak serum levels of the drug.

If blood sampling from a central venous catheter is the best alternative, use methods that do not require the use of needles. Vacuum tubes attached directly to the catheter hub eliminate the need to transfer the blood from a syringe into the tubes. For small-diameter catheters, the vacuum in the tube may cause the catheter to temporarily collapse, preventing the backflow of blood into the tube. In this situation, small syringes should be used because they create less pressure on aspiration, the opposite of what small syringes do on injection. Transfer of the blood from the syringe to the vacuum tube requires the use of a special transfer device to avoid the use of needles.

Removing the Catheter

Short peripheral catheters are usually removed 72 or 96 hours after insertion. If a complication develops, they should be removed immediately. Lift opposite sides of the transparent dressing and pull laterally to remove the dressing from the site while stabilizing the catheter. Slowly withdraw the catheter from the skin, and immediately cover the puncture site with dry gauze. Do not use an alcohol pad because this will interfere with coagulation. Hold pressure on the site until hemostasis is achieved.

Removal of midline catheters and PICCs must be performed with the same slow, gentle techniques used to insert the catheter. Veins can develop venospasms when rapid or forceful techniques are used. After explaining to the client that this procedure will not be painful, remove the dressing and withdraw the catheter in short segments by pulling from the insertion site. If you feel resistance, always stop and never apply force to the catheter. Extreme traction or force could cause the catheter to break and embolize to the heart or pulmonary circulation.

Simple distraction techniques and deep breathing may be sufficient to relax the client and remove the catheter. If these fail, replace the dressing and apply heat; allow time for the vein wall to relax. Keeping the extremity warm and dry and asking the client to drink warm liquids could facilitate removal. Use of medications to relax the vein wall may be required if the catheter cannot be removed after several hours. Radiographic studies may also be needed to determine whether the cause is a thrombosis instead of venospasm.

Nontunneled percutaneous central catheters are removed by clipping any sutures and withdrawing the catheter in short segments. Venospasm does not commonly occur when removing these catheters because the vein diameter is large.

For all catheters, immediately after the catheter comes out of the skin, apply digital pressure with a dry gauze dressing to stop any bleeding. Apply a sterile occlusive gauze dressing with an antiseptic ointment. When a central venous catheter is removed, a tract between the skin and vein creates a conduit for air to be pulled into the vein. The ointment seals off the tract. After removal, measure the catheter length and compare it with the length documented on insertion. If the entire catheter length was not removed, contact the physician immediately.

Removal of tunneled catheters and implanted ports requires surgical techniques and is usually performed by nurse practitioners or physicians.

COMPLICATIONS OF INFUSION THERAPY

Complications from infusion therapy can be minor and limited or life threatening. Serious life-altering or life-threatening complications are dramatically increasing in frequency and severity and present a tremendous financial burden to the U.S. health care system. Catheter-related bloodstream infections (CRBSIs) are an excellent example. In critical care units in U.S. hospitals, about 80,000 CRBSIs occur annually. When the entire hospital is included, that number escalates to 250,000, and if the entire health care system is considered, the number soars to 500,000. Using the 250,000 that occur in hospitals, studies have estimated that 12% to 25% of clients die from these infections. Estimates of the cost for treating one episode of CRBSI range from $34,000 to $56,000. The annual costs for treating all CRBSIs range from $296 million to $2.3 billion (O'Grady et al., 2002).

Local complications of IV therapy occur at or near the catheter. A priority for care of clients with intravenous therapy is to prevent, assess, and detect these complications. In some cases, nurses also manage these problems. Definitions, causes, signs and symptoms, treatment, and prevention of local complications are summarized in Table 17-2. **Systemic complications** of IV therapy involve the entire vascular system or multiple systems. Information on common systemic complications can be found in Table 17-3. For central venous catheters, complications can occur during the insertion procedure or during the dwell time; these problems are described in Tables 17-4 and 17-5.

Text continued on p. 266

TABLE 17-2 Local Complications of Intravenous Therapy

Complication	Definition	Cause	Signs and Symptoms	Treatment	Prevention
Infiltration	Leakage of a nonvesicant IV solution or medication into the extravascular tissue	Peripheral catheter has punctured the vein in a second location Obstruction of blood flow causing increased pressure and fluid overflow from peripheral puncture site Inflammatory process causing fluid leakage at the capillary level Fibrin sheath fully encasing a central venous catheter leading to retrograde flow and leakage from venipuncture site Damaged septum of implanted port Dislodged port access needle	IV rate slows down; increasing edema at or above the insertion site; client may complain of skin tightness; blanching or coolness of skin; burning, tenderness or general discomfort at the insertion site; fluid leaking from puncture site; presence or absence of a blood return is not reliable diagnostic tool on a short peripheral catheter	Stop infusion and remove short peripheral catheter immediately after identification of problem. Apply sterile dressing if weeping from tissue occurs. Apply cold compresses. Elevate extremity if it increases client comfort. Insert a new catheter in the opposite extremity. For all central venous catheters, obtain a dye study to determine the cause of the problem. For implanted port, remove and insert a new port access needle.	Stabilize short peripheral catheter well; use smallest catheter that will accomplish the infusion; avoid placement over area of flexion; use handboard if sites in an area of flexion must be used; avoid placing restraints in the area of an IV site; make successive venipunctures proximal to the previous site; monitor site frequently; educate client about activities and signs and symptoms. For all central venous catheters, always obtain a brisk blood return before using the catheter for infusion. Frequently assess proper positioning of port access needle. Stabilize it well and protect from clothing.
Extravasation	Leakage of a vesicant IV solution or medication into the extravascular tissue	Same as infiltration	Same as infiltration Tissue sloughing appears in 1 to 4 wk	Stop infusion and disconnect administration set. Aspirate drug from short peripheral catheter or port access needle. Leave short peripheral catheter or port access needle in place to deliver antidote, if indicated by established policy. If possible, aspirate residual drug from the exit site of a central venous catheter. Administer antidote according to established policy. Apply cold compresses for all drugs EXCEPT vinca alkaloids and epipodophyllotoxins. Photograph site. Monitor at 24 hr, 1 wk, 2 wk, and as needed. Surgical interventions may be required. Provide written instructions to client and family.	Same as infiltration. Know the vesicant potential before giving any IV medication.

Continued

TABLE 17-2 Local Complications of Intravenous Therapy—*cont'd*

Complication	Definition	Cause	Signs and Symptoms	Treatment	Prevention
Phlebitis and post-infusion phlebitis	Inflammation of the vein Post-infusion phlebitis presents within 48 to 96 hr after the catheter has been removed	Mechanical cause from insertion technique, catheter size, and lack of catheter securement Chemical cause from extremes of pH and/or osmolarity of the fluid or medication Bacterial cause from a break in aseptic technique, poor securement, and extended dwell time	Client may complain of pain at the IV site; nurse may observe that vein appears red and inflamed along the length; vein may become hard and cordlike (see Table 17-6)	Remove short peripheral catheter at the first sign of phlebitis; use warm compresses to relieve pain. Monitor frequently. Document using Phlebitis Scale. Restart a new catheter using the opposite extremity. Mechanical phlebitis occurring in the first week after PICC insertion may be treated without catheter removal. Apply continuous heat; rest and elevate the extremity. Significant improvement is seen in 24 hr and complete resolution is seen within 72 hr. Remove catheter if treatment is unsuccessful.	Choose the smallest gauge catheter for the required therapy. Avoid sites of joint flexion or stabilize with a handboard. Avoid infusing fluids or medications with a pH below 5 or above 9 through a peripheral vein. Avoid infusing fluids or medications with a final osmolarity above 500 mOsm/L through a peripheral vein. Rotate sites every 72 to 96 hr according to established policy. Adequately secure the catheter. Use aseptic technique. For PICCs, teach client to avoid excessive physical activity with the extremity.
Thrombosis	Blood clot inside the vein	Traumatic venipuncture Multiple venipuncture attempts Use of catheters too large for the chosen vein Contact between the catheter and the vein wall, especially at or near the central venous catheter tip Fluid volume deficits in clients with a central venous catheter	Slowed or stopped infusion rate Swollen extremity Tenderness and redness Engorged peripheral veins of the ipsilateral chest and extremity Difficulty moving the neck or jaw	Stop infusion and remove short peripheral catheter immediately. Apply cold compresses to decrease blood flow and stabilize the clot. Elevate extremity. Surgical intervention may be required. For central venous catheters, notify the physician and obtain orders for a diagnostic study. Low-dose thrombolytic agents can be used to lyse the clot.	Use good venipuncture technique. Make only 2 attempts to perform venipuncture. Choose the smallest-gauge catheter in the largest vein possible. Secure catheter adequately. Use handboards if short peripheral catheters are placed in areas of joint flexion. Ensure adequate hydration to avoid changes in blood composition and flow. Prophylactic low-dose warfarin (Coumadin, Warfilone✱) may be prescribed for clients with a central venous catheter.
Thrombophlebitis	The presence of a blood clot and vein inflammation	Same as phlebitis and thrombosis	Same as phlebitis and thrombosis	Same as phlebitis and thrombosis. Apply cold compresses initially followed by warm.	Same as phlebitis and thrombosis.
Ecchymosis and hematoma	Ecchymosis is the infiltration of blood into the surrounding tissue Hematoma is the uncontrolled bleeding from a venipuncture site creating a painful lump	Venipuncture by unskilled person Venipuncture attempts into veins that cannot be seen or palpated Anticoagulated and steroid-dependent clients are at the greatest risk Using fragile veins or areas of poor skin turgor Excessive pressure or failure to apply direct pressure for the required time when removing a catheter	Swelling usually seen first Bruising at the insertion site Pain or tenderness	Remove IV device and apply light pressure; excessive pressure could cause other fragile veins in the area to rupture. For hematoma, apply direct pressure until bleeding has stopped. See treatment for infiltration.	Avoid veins that cannot be easily seen or palpated. Know your client's history. Use good venipuncture technique. Apply direct pressure long enough to control bleeding.

Site infection	Localized redness and hardness at the IV site caused by invasion of microorganisms in the absence of simultaneous bloodstream infection	Break in aseptic technique during insertion or the handling of sterile equipment Lack of proper hand hygiene and skin antisepsis	Site appears red, swollen, and warm; client may complain of tenderness at the site; may observe purulent or malodorous exudate	Clean exit site with alcohol, expressing drainage if present. For short peripheral, midline catheter or PICC, remove using sterile technique and avoid contact between skin and catheter. Amputate catheter tip into a sterile container. Send catheter tip for culture, if ordered. Clean site with alcohol and cover with dry sterile dressing; physician to evaluate for septic phlebitis and need for antimicrobial therapy or surgical intervention.	Use strict aseptic technique when inserting, maintaining, or removing catheters. Practice good hand hygiene. Ensure dressing remains clean, dry and adherent to skin at all times.
Venous spasm	A sudden contraction of the vein or artery	Catheter advancement immediately after tourniquet removal Infusion of cold fluids such as blood Sudden changes in the infusion pressure Removal of a midline catheter or PICC	Cramping or pain at or above the insertion site Numbness in the area Slowing of the infusion rate Inability to withdraw midline catheter or PICC	Temporarily slow infusion rate. Apply warm compress. Does not require immediate removal of short peripheral catheter. If occurring during midline catheter or PICC removal, do not apply tension or attempt forceful removal. Reapply a dressing, apply heat, encourage client to drink warm liquids, and keep extremity covered and dry. 12 to 24 hr may be required before catheter can be removed.	Allow time for vein diameter to return to normal after tourniquet removal and before advancing catheter. Infuse fluids at room temperature, if possible. For a midline catheter or PICC, gently withdraw the catheter in short segments.
Nerve damage	Inadvertent piercing or complete transection of a nerve	Venipuncture near known nerve locations Unanticipated nerve locations	Complaints of tingling or feeling pins and needles at or below the insertion site Numbness at or near the insertion site	Immediately stop the insertion procedure if the client complains of extreme pain. Remove the catheter if complaints of discomfort do not improve when the catheter is secured.	Avoid using the cephalic vein near the wrist. Avoid using veins on the palm side of the wrist. Adequately secure the catheter but avoid tape that is too tight. Support areas of joint flexion with an armboard.

PICC, Peripherally inserted central catheter.

TABLE 17-3 Systemic Complications of Intravenous Therapy

Complication	Definition	Cause	Signs and Symptoms	Treatment	Prevention
Circulatory overload	Disruption of fluid homeostasis with excess fluid in the circulatory system	Infusion of fluids at a rate greater than the client's system can accommodate	Client may complain of shortness of breath and cough; client's blood pressure is elevated, and there is puffiness around the eyes and edema in dependent areas; client's neck veins may be engorged, and nurse may hear moist breath sounds.	Slow the IV rate and notify physician; raise client to an upright position; monitor vital signs and administer oxygen as ordered; administer diuretics as ordered.	Monitor intake and output carefully and notify physician as soon as an imbalance is noticed between the client's intake and output.
Speed shock	Systemic reaction to the rapid infusion of a substance unfamiliar to the client's circulatory system	Rapid infusion of drugs or bolus infusion, which causes the drug to reach toxic levels quickly	Client may complain of lightheadedness or dizziness and chest tightness; nurse may note that client has a flushed face and an irregular pulse; without intervention, client may lose consciousness and go into shock and cardiac arrest.	Immediately discontinue the drug infusion and hang D_5W to keep the vein open; monitor vital signs carefully and notify physician for further treatment orders.	Be aware of the appropriate infusion rate of medications and adhere to them; use of infusion control devices assists in prevention of speed shock.
Allergic reaction	Local or general response to an allergen	May be a response to tape, cleansing agent, drug, solution, or IV device	A client having a local reaction may exhibit a wheal, redness, or itching at the IV site; in the case of a general reaction, client may complain of itching, running nose, and tearing; nurse may note bronchospasm, wheezing, and a truncal rash; without treatment, client may experience anaphylaxis.		
Catheter embolism	A shaving or piece of catheter breaks off and floats freely in the vessel	May occur if the needle of an over-the-needle catheter is reinserted into the catheter or if the needle of a through-the-needle catheter is inadvertently pulled back through the catheter	Client will experience a decrease in blood pressure and complain of pain along the vein; pulse becomes weak, rapid, and thready, and nurse may note cyanosis of the nail beds and circumorally; client may lapse into unconsciousness.	Discontinue catheter and apply a tourniquet high on the limb of the catheter site; inspect catheter for any rough edges; an x-ray is taken to determine the presence of any catheter piece; surgical intervention may be necessary.	When inserting over-the-needle catheters, never reinsert the needle into the catheter; avoid pulling a through-the-needle catheter back through the needle during insertion.

TABLE 17-4 Insertion-Related Complications of Central Venous Catheter

Problem	Definition	Possible Causes	Signs and Symptoms	Treatment	Prevention
Pneumothorax	Collection of air in the pleural space (space between the lung and chest wall)	Puncture of the pleural covering of the lung by the introducer on insertion of a direct subclavian approach	Chest pain Dyspnea Apprehension Cyanosis Decreased breath sounds on the affected side Abnormal chest x-ray findings	Remove catheter or assist with removal. Assess client by monitoring vital signs, and assess breath sounds. Notify physician immediately if suspected after insertion. Administer oxygen as ordered. Assist with insertion of a chest tube.	Use jugular or upper extremity insertion sites instead of subclavian sites. Use ultrasound to locate veins.
Hemothorax	Collection of blood in the pleural cavity	Result of puncture or transection of the subclavian vein or artery	Similar to pneumothorax; usually see dyspnea first and then tachycardia Decreased hemoglobin because of blood pooling	Same as for pneumothorax. Apply pressure on insertion site after introducer needle and catheter are removed.	Use jugular or upper extremity insertion sites instead of subclavian sites. Use ultrasound to locate veins.
Chylothorax	Lymph (chyle) enters the pleural cavity	Transection of the thoracic duct on the left side	Same as in hemothorax Usually noted on insertion with withdrawal of a milklike substance	Same as for pneumothorax.	Use right side for subclavian insertion. Use jugular or upper extremity insertion sites. Use ultrasound to locate veins.
Hydrothorax	Infusion of IV fluids directly into the thoracic cavity	Transection of the subclavian vein and placement of the catheter into the thoracic cavity	Same as in pneumothorax with absence of vesicular breath sounds and a murmur with a flat sound over the location	Same as for pneumothorax with removal of the catheter and aspiration of fluid.	Use jugular or upper extremity insertion sites instead of subclavian sites. Use ultrasound to locate veins.
Air embolism	Air enters the central venous system	Air is introduced into the central venous system during catheter insertion, tubing changes, catheter rupture, and catheter removal	Chest pain, dyspnea, hypoxia Anxiety, tachycardia, hypotension Nausea Light-headed, dizzy Loud churning heard over the pericardium on auscultation is possible but not always heard	Clamp catheter immediately. Place client in lateral Trendelenburg position on left side. Notify physician immediately. Oxygen therapy. Arterial blood gases. Electrocardiogram.	Lie client flat when changing administration sets or needleless connectors. Close slide clamp on catheter extension, if present. Ask client to perform a Va -salva maneuver, if possible. Use Luer-Lok connections on all catheters. Apply occlusive dressing with antiseptic ointment when removing a central venous catheter. Allow to remain in place for at least 24 hr.
Arterial puncture	Cannulation of an artery	Accessed the artery instead of the vein	Pulsating of bright red blood from the introducer needle	Remove needle immediately and apply pressure to the site. Secure a pressure dressing for 5-10 min.	Use ultrasound to locate veins during insertion procedure.
Nerve injury	Damage to one of the ulnar, median, or radial cords	Ineffective cannulation of the vein	Tingling to sensory motor deficit to complete paralysis	Immediate removal of catheter.	Use ultrasound during cannulation.
Malpositioned catheters	Catheter has passed into the jugular vein, the right atrium, the azygos vein or several other tributary veins	Improper client positioning during insertion Insertion of catheter length that is too short or too long for client	No signs or symptoms may be experienced before detection on initial chest radiograph to confirm tip location Ear, neck, or back pain Palpitations or dysrhythmias Inability to irrigate	Place client in semi-Fowler's position and flush with 20 to 50 mL of saline. Notify physician to reposition catheter by guidewire exchange. Refer to radiology for repositioning under fluoroscopy.	Insertion under fluoroscopy. Proper client measurement for catheter length. Proper client positioning.

PICC, Peripherally inserted central catheter; *SVC,* superior vena cava.

TABLE 17-5 Complications During the Dwell of Central Venous Catheters

Complication	Definition	Possible Causes	Signs and Symptoms	Treatment	Prevention
Catheter migration	Movement of a properly placed catheter tip to another vein No change in the external catheter length	Changes in intrathoracic pressure caused by coughing, vomiting, sneezing, heavy lifting, and congestive heart failure	For migration to the jugular vein complaints of hearing a running stream or gurgling sound on the side of catheter insertion For migration to the azygos vein, back pain between the shoulder blades Neurologic complications if medications are infused	Stop all infusions and flush catheter. Notify physician. Obtain a chest radiograph to assess tip location. Spontaneous repositioning back to the SVC is possible. Repositioning by radiology may be required.	Catheter tip properly placed in the lower third of the SVC near the junction with the right atrium. Instruct client to perform normal activities of daily living but to avoid excessive physical activity.
Catheter dislodgment	Movement of catheter into or out of the insertion site	Inadequate catheter securement Excessive physical activity with a PICC	External catheter length has changed, also changing the internal tip location No other signs or symptoms may be immediately noticed	Stop all infusions and flush catheter. NEVER readvance the catheter into the insertion site. Determine the amount of external catheter length and compare with the length documented on insertion. Notify the physician or nurse inserting the catheter for further assessment.	Proper catheter securement. Instruct client to perform normal activities of daily living but to avoid excessive physical activity.
Catheter rupture	Catheter is broken, damaged, or separated from hub or port body	Forcefully flushing a catheter with any size syringe against resistance Using scissors to remove a dressing Catheter compression of a subclavian inserted catheter between the clavicle and first rib. Also known as pinch-off syndrome	Fluid leaking from insertion site Pain or swelling during infusion Reflux of blood into the catheter extension Inability to aspirate blood from catheter	Repair of the damaged segment; depends on the availability of a repair kit designed for the specific brand of catheter being used; repair may be considered a temporary measure instead of a permanent treatment. Catheter exchange using several special techniques. Remove catheter.	NEVER use excessive force when flushing a catheter, regardless of syringe size. On injection, small syringes generate more pressure than larger syringes. Use of a 10-mL syringe is generally recommended for flushing procedures. Catheter insertion through jugular or upper extremity sites instead of subclavian site.
Lumen occlusion	Catheter lumen is partially or totally blocked	Drug or mineral precipitate (calcium, diazepam, and phenytoin are common) Lipid sludge from long-term infusion of fat emulsion Blood clots and fibrin sheath caused by blood reflux into lumen Allowing administration sets to remain connected for extended periods after medication has infused	Infusion stops or pump alarm sounds Inability or difficulty administering fluids Inability or difficulty drawing blood Increased resistance to flushing of the catheter	Assess history of catheter use. A suddenly developing problem may indicate contact between incompatible medications. A problem that develops over an extended period may indicate a gradual clot formation. For drug precipitate, determine the pH of the precipitated drug. Use hydrochloric acid for acidic drug. Use sodium bicarbonate for alkaline drugs. For blood clot, use thrombolytic enzymes such as alteplase.	Always flush with normal saline between, before, and after each medication given through the catheter. Use positive-pressure flushing techniques when a negative fluid displacement needleless connector is being used. Use a positive fluid displacement needleless connector. Flush catheters immediately when medication infusion is complete.

Phlebitis	Inflammation of the vein wall	Mechanical phlebitis is common with PICC lines and will appear within 7 days after insertion Chemical phlebitis may be seen with catheter rupture	Pain, redness, slight swelling May progress to cellulitis and palpable cord or collateral circulation	Mechanical phlebitis: conservative measures, warm compresses applied for 20 min four times daily for about 48-72 hr. Mild exercise. Chemical: change catheter or medication.	
Thrombosis	Formation of a blood clot in a vessel within the neck, chest, or arms that occurs in the presence of a central venous catheter	Stasis, vessel wall injury, or hypercoagulability	Chest pain, earache, or jaw pain Edema of neck, supraclavicular area, or extremities Edema at puncture site Jugular distention Collateral circulation on the affected side	Anticoagulant therapy. Possible catheter removal.	
Exit, port pocket, or tunnel infection	Infection may be localized at the insertion site or in the catheter or may progress to systemic infection	Failure to maintain sterile technique during catheter insertion or care Wet or soiled dressing remaining on site Immunosuppression Contaminated catheter or solution	Redness, warmth, tenderness, swelling at the insertion site Cellulitis Possible exudate of purulent material Local rash or pustules Fever, chills, malaise Leukocytosis Nausea and vomiting Elevated urine glucose level	Monitor vital signs closely. Monitor culture site. Redress with sterile technique. Treat systemically with antibiotics or antifungals, depending on culture results. Blood cultures. Remove catheter.	
Bloodstream infection	Invasion of pathogenic organisms enter the client's circulation	Inadequate skin antiseptic agents and application techniques Manipulation of the catheter hub leading to intraluminal contamination Inadequate hand hygiene	Early symptoms include fever, chills, headache, and general malaise; if left, client may experience severe infection, which may lead to vascular collapse and death	Change the entire infusion system from solution to IV device; notify physician, obtain cultures, and administer antibiotics as prescribed; if the infusate is the suspected cause, send a specimen to the laboratory for evaluation.	Same as for local infection above.

PICC, Peripherally inserted central catheter; *SVC*, superior vena cava.

TABLE 17-6 Phlebitis Scale from INS Standards of Practice

Grade	Criteria
0	No symptoms
1	Erythema with or without pain
2	Pain at access site with erythema and/or edema
3	Pain at access site with erythema and/or edema Streak formation Palpable cord
4	Pain at access site with erythema and/or edema Streak formation Palpable venous cord >1 inch long Purulent drainage

Data from Intravenous Nurses Society: Infusion Nursing Standards of Practice (2000). *Journal of Intravenous Nursing, 23*(65), 556.

OLDER ADULT CARE

The aging process causes numerous changes in all body functions, and yet aging occurs differently in each person. Nutrition, environment, genetics, social factors, and education are just a few of the factors that influence the older adult's needs. Because all body functions are affected, infusion therapy can be affected by these changes.

Skin Care

Aging skin becomes thinner and loses subcutaneous fat, decreasing the skin's ability for thermal regulation. Fewer nerve endings mean the decreased ability to feel pain. Your client *may* not perceive pain from traumatic venipuncture requiring excessive probing or multiple attempts; however, this action increases the risk of fluid leakage and subsequent infiltration or extravasation injury. Inserting and removing a catheter and dressing could tear the skin layers.

Skin antisepsis is extremely important because of the possible compromised immune status of the older client. Lipids are normally found in skin as a protective agent, and alcohol easily dissolves lipids. Whereas greater numbers of organisms may be killed, the skin can also become excessively dry and cracked. Current recommendations call for using friction when cleaning the skin to penetrate the layers of the epidermis. Excessive friction may damage fragile skin. Chlorhexidine gluconate is now the preferred agent, and the product currently available contains alcohol. Check for allergies to iodine before using iodine or iodophors. Iodophors such as povidone-iodine require contact with the skin for a minimum of 2 minutes to be effective. All antiseptic solutions must be thoroughly dry before applying the dressing or tape.

Skin should never be shaved before venipuncture, but excessive amounts of hair can be clipped away. Shaving causes microabrasions that can lead to infection. Skin of an older client may be more delicate and therefore more easily nicked while shaving.

Skin integrity can easily be compromised by the application of tape or dressings. Use of skin protectant solutions puts a protective barrier between the skin and dressing and improves the adherence of the dressing to the skin. Removal of tape and dressings may require adhesive remover solutions or an alcohol pad may accomplish the same purpose.

Vein and Catheter Selection

Vein and catheter selection are of highest importance in older adults. Insertion sites must be chosen carefully after consideration of skin integrity, vein condition, and activities of daily living. The general principle of starting with the most distal sites usually indicates use of hand veins. Fragile skin and small tortuous veins on the back of the hand (dorsum) should be avoided, and the initial IV site should be higher on the arm.

Venous distention must be accomplished with a flat tourniquet; however, the veins may require longer to distend. Allowing a tourniquet to remain in place for extended periods causes an overfilling of the vein and can result in a hematoma when the vein is punctured. On extremely fragile skin, the tourniquet application can lead to ecchymotic areas. A tourniquet may not be required in veins that are already distended; however, these veins must be carefully palpated to determine their condition. Hard, cordlike veins should be avoided. Blood pressure cuffs can also be used for venous distention. Inflate the cuff and release until the pressure is slightly less than diastolic pressure. Other methods to distend veins include the following:

- Light tapping, but avoid forceful slapping
- Asking the client to open and close the fist so the muscles can force blood into the veins. Make sure the hand is relaxed when the venipuncture is attempted.
- Placing the extremity lower than the heart
- Heat applied to the entire extremity for 10 to 20 minutes and removed just before making the venipuncture

As with all clients, venipuncture technique requires adequate skin and vein stabilization during the puncture and complete catheter advancement. Veins of an older adult are more likely to roll away from the needle. Low angles of 10 to 15 degrees between the skin and catheter will improve your success with venipuncture.

As soon as the catheter enters the vein, it may be necessary to release the tourniquet. Release of venous pressure from the puncture can lead to ecchymosis. Allowing the tourniquet to remain in place during the complete catheter advancement could increase this problem.

Catheter securement may mean that the administration sets are placed out of easy reach of a confused client. Using flexible netting over the extremity may prevent the client from pulling at the dressing or tubing while allowing you easy assess to the site. Rolled bandages should not be used to cover the extremity because they will prevent easy visualization of the site, allowing complications to progress to an advanced state before recognition.

Choosing a midline catheter or PICC may be best in older clients with poor skin turgor, limited venous sites, or veins that are fragile, tortuous, or hard. These catheters are placed in the upper extremity, where venous distention techniques can be used. Inserting nontunneled percutaneous central catheters in older adults may be a great challenge. Venous distention for insertion requires the Trendelenburg position and a well-hydrated client. Fluid volume deficit prevents adequate distention of the subclavian or jugular veins. Respiratory conditions like chronic obstructive pulmonary disease, spinal curvatures, and increased intracranial pressure may contraindicate this position. Tunneled catheters and implanted ports may be appropriate after consideration of the surgical techniques required to insert these catheters.

Cardiac and Renal Changes

Because of changes in cardiac and renal status, the accuracy of infusion volume and flow rate measurements is very important in the older adult. The health care provider's order for infusion therapy should be assessed for appropriateness for the client's condition. Electronic controlling devices may be required to ensure the necessary accuracy. When fluid restrictions are required, medications could be diluted in small quantities and delivered using a syringe pump or a manual IV push. For instance, 1 g of an antibiotic could be diluted in 10 mL normal saline instead of the more common 50 mL. This would allow the client to have more fluid to drink. Serum sodium levels should be considered when normal saline is routinely used for dilution in clients with hypertension or cardiac problems. For a poorly controlled diabetic client, dextrose solutions for dilution may not be preferred, although well-controlled diabetic clients may not have a problem with the small amount of dextrose in the solution. Consultation with the pharmacist and prescriber may be needed to answer these questions.

ALTERNATIVE SITES FOR INFUSION

Many reasons drive the need for infusion through sites other than the venous circulation. Through numerous technologic advances, we are now capable of infusion into arteries, peritoneum, bone marrow, epidural and intrathecal space, and subcutaneous tissue.

Arterial Therapy

DESCRIPTION

Catheters are placed into arteries to obtain repeated arterial blood samples, to monitor various hemodynamic pressures continuously, and to infuse antineoplastic agents. Catheters placed in the radial, brachial, or femoral arteries are used for obtaining blood samples or arterial pressure monitoring. Pulmonary artery pressure measures the function of the left heart and is accomplished by advancing a catheter through the central venous system, through the right heart chambers, and into the pulmonary artery.

Arterial waveforms and pressures are converted to digital values displayed on attached monitors. Between the catheter and the monitor is a special administration set capable of handling high infusion pressure, a pressurized fluid container with heparinized solution, a continuous flush attachment, a three-way stopcock, and a transducer. The transducer is positioned at the level of the client's atrium and secured to an IV pole to enable correct arterial pressure measurements.

Catheters used for pressure monitoring are inserted percutaneously through veins of the upper extremity or the subclavian or jugular sites. Insertion procedures are similar to the procedures used for venous cannulation. Removal requires the deflation of arterial balloons, if used, and applying digital pressure for longer than when removing a venous catheter.

Antineoplastic agents administered arterially allow infusion of a high concentration of drug directly to the tumor site before it is diluted in the circulatory system or metabolized by the liver or kidneys. Drug infusion through the same blood supply feeding the tumor optimizes cell kill at the tumor site while minimizing systemic side effects. The most common arterial sites include the hepatic and celiac arteries for liver tumors, although the carotid artery for tumors of the head, neck, or brain and pelvic arteries for cervical tumors have been used. Necrotizing pancreatitis has also been treated with infusion of protease inhibitors and antibiotics (West, 1998).

Arterial catheter insertion can be either a surgical procedure or an interventional radiologic procedure. Implanted ports are commonly used for extended therapies. For short-term therapy, an external catheter may be used for 3 to 7 days, although longer periods result in high complication rates.

One other device used for arterial infusion of antineoplastic agents is an implanted pump with an attached catheter. These small devices hold 50 mL of fluid in an upper chamber. The lower chamber exerts pressure when the upper chamber is filled, causing the drug to flow at 1 to 2 mL/day. Changes in blood pressure, body temperature, and altitudes alter the flow rate. The client must return for refilling the fluid chamber every 14 days.

NURSING CONSIDERATIONS

All arterial catheters require close attention to securing all junctions on the administer sets with luer-locked devices. When an infusion pump is used, it should have a pumping pressure high enough to overcome arterial pressure. Observe the insertion site and involved extremity closely. Assess for warmth, sensation, capillary refill, and pulse. When the carotid artery is involved, perform neurologic assessments. When a femoral catheter is used, anti-embolic stockings or other measures are indicated.

Complications from arterial catheters are similar to those from venous catheters, including infection, bleeding from the insertion site, catheter migration, infiltration, and catheter lumen or arterial occlusion.

Intraperitoneal Infusion

DESCRIPTION

Intraperitoneal (IP) therapy is the administration of antineoplastic agents into the peritoneal cavity. IP therapy is used to treat intra-abdominal malignant tumors such as ovarian or colorectal tumors that have moved to the peritoneum after surgery.

Catheters used for IP therapy may be an implanted port for long-term treatment or an external catheter for temporary use. These catheters, including those attached to an implanted port, have large internal lumens with multiple side-holes along the catheter length to allow for delivery of large quantities of fluid. Administration of IP therapy includes three phases: the instillation phase; the dwell phase, usually 1 to 4 hours; and the drain phase. Because this treatment involves the delivery of biohazardous agents, additional competency is required to handle the infusion properly.

NURSING CONSIDERATIONS

The client is in the semi-Fowler's position for the infusion. Your client may experience nausea and vomiting caused by increasing pressure on the internal organs from the infusing fluid. Pressure on the diaphragm may cause respiratory distress. Reducing the flow rate and treatment with antiemetic drugs is indicated. Severe pain may indicate that the catheter has migrated and an abdominal radiograph is needed to determine its location.

During the dwell and drainage phases, your client may need assistance in frequently moving from side to side to distribute the fluid evenly around the abdominal cavity. After the fluid has drained, the catheter is flushed with normal saline, although heparinized saline may be used in implanted ports. Catheter lumen occlusion is caused by the formation of fibrous sheaths or fibrin clots or plugs inside the catheter or around the tip.

Exit site infection, indicated by redness, tenderness, and warmth of the tissue around the catheter and microbial peritonitis and inflammation of the peritoneal membranes from the invasion of microorganisms, can occur. The client may experience a fever and complain of abdominal pain. Abdominal rigidity and rebound tenderness may be present. This condition is preventable by using strict aseptic technique in the handling of all equipment and infusion supplies. Management includes antimicrobial therapy administered either intravenously or intraperitoneally.

Subcutaneous Infusion

DESCRIPTION

Subcutaneous (SC or **Sub Q) therapy** has rapidly expanded in the past few years, with many drugs being infused to treat numerous conditions (Table 17-7). SC therapy is often used in palliative care clients who cannot tolerate oral medications, when intramuscular injections are too painful, or when vascular access is not available or is too difficult to obtain. Other studies reveal that SC infusion therapy produces better outcomes compared with IV infusion. A survey of SC infusion practices in hospices in the United States found that 73% used continuous SC infusion, primarily for pain management (Herndon & Fike, 2001).

Hypodermoclysis involves the slow infusion of isotonic fluids into the client's subcutaneous tissue. In the early to mid-twentieth century, this was the acceptable method for infusing parenteral fluids; however, severe reactions related to misuse occurred in the 1950s, causing this method to lose favor with physicians. In the 1980s, hypodermoclysis gained acceptance again because of the growth of the specialties of geriatrics and palliative health care (Slesak et al., 2003).

Hypodermoclysis can be used for short-term fluid volume replacement. The client must have sufficient sites of intact skin without infection, inflammation, bruising, scarring, or edema. The most common sites are the front and sides of the thighs and hips, the upper abdomen, and the area under the clavicle. Unlike IV therapy, the upper extremity should not be used because fluid is absorbed more readily from sites on the torso with larger stores of adipose tissue. Hypodermoclysis should not be used if the fluid replacement needs exceed 3000 mL/day, in emergency situations, or if there are bleeding or coagulation problems (Brown & Worobec, 2000).

TABLE 17-7 Examples of Subcutaneous Infusion Therapy

Disease or Condition	Drug or Therapy
Chronic iron overload	Deferoxamine mesylate (Desferal)
Chronic pain management	Morphine (Morphitec✱) Hydromorphone (Dilaudid) Fentanyl Haloperidol (Haldol, Peridol✱) Midazolam (Versed)
Diabetes, type 1	Insulin
Rheumatoid arthritis	Etanercept (Enbrel)
Head and neck malignant tumors	Amifostine (Ethyol)
Pulmonary arterial hypertension	Treprostinil (Remodulin)
Chronic asthma	Terbutaline (Brethine)
Recurrent preterm labor	Terbutaline (Brethine)

Hyaluronidase 150 units may be mixed with each liter of infusion fluid. This is an enzyme that improves the absorption of the infusing fluids from the SC tissue. An intradermal test dose is required because of the possibility of an allergic reaction. If the enzyme is not used, the infusion may not be well absorbed and redness at the insertion site is more likely (Brown & Worobec, 2000).

A small-gauge winged infusion or "butterfly" needle, a small-gauge short peripheral catheter, or an infusion set specially designed for subcutaneous infusion can be chosen. The SC infusion sets have a small needle extending at a right angle from a flat disk that helps to stabilize the needle.

NURSING CONSIDERATIONS

When choosing the infusion site, consider the client's level of activity. The area under the clavicle or the abdomen may have the least interference with ambulation. Clip excess hair in the area, and clean the chosen site with the antiseptic solution, preferably chlorhexidine gluconate. Prime the infusion tubing and the attached SC infusion set or winged needle. Gently pinch an area of about 2 inches (1 cm) and insert the needle. After securing the needle, cover the site with a transparent dressing. Hydrocortisone cream can be applied to the skin to prevent irritation.

Flow rates for hydration fluids begin at 30 mL/hr. After 1 hour, the rate can be increased if the client has experienced no discomfort. The maximum rate is 75 to 80 mL/hr (Brown & Worobec, 2000). For pain medication infusion, the flow rate is usually 2 or 3 mL/hr. If required for adequate pain control, two subcutaneous sites may be needed (Pasero, 2002).

Assess the site at least twice daily. Redness, heat, leakage, bruising, swelling, and complaints of pain indicate tissue irritation and the infusion needle should be removed. Rotate the SC site at least once per week.

Other complications include pooling of the fluid at the insertion site and an uneven fluid drip rate. Both of these problems may be resolved by restarting the infusion in another location. An infusion pump may also be used. Small ambulatory infusion pumps can be used to allow for greater mobility.

Intraspinal Infusion

The spinal column is covered by three layers: the dura mater, or outermost covering; the arachnoid, or middle layer; and the pia mater, which is closest to the spinal cord. Two spaces used for infusion are the **epidural** space between the dura mater and vertebrae and the **subarachnoid** space. The epidural space consists of fat, connective tissue, and blood vessels that protect the spinal cord. Medications infused into the epidural space must diffuse through the dura mater, and there is the possibility that some drug will be absorbed systemically. **Intrathecal** medications are infused into the subarachnoid space closer to the spinal cord, allowing reduced doses.

DESCRIPTION

Postoperative and chronic pain management are the primary indications for epidural infusion. Opioids administered epidurally slowly diffuse across the dura mater to the dorsal horn of the spinal cord. They lock onto receptors and block pain impulses from ascending to the brain. The client receives pain relief from the level of the injection caudally (toward the toes). Local anesthetics administered epidurally work on the sensory nerve roots in the epidural space to block pain impulses. The physician administers the first dose of medication; then, depending on state law, the type of medication, and facility policies, nurses trained in epidural therapy may administer subsequent doses.

Intrathecal infusion is used for treating cancers that cross the blood-brain barrier and involve the central nervous system (CNS). Some medications used to treat CNS neoplasms, such as methotrexate and cytarabine, are not effective intravenously because they cannot cross the blood-brain barrier. Others must be administered in large doses to cross this natural protective mechanism. It may not be possible to administer large doses of chemotherapeutic agents intravenously because of the severe systemic side effects associated with them. Administration of medications via the intrathecal route eliminates this problem because the medication is administered directly into the cerebrospinal (CSF). Intrathecal infusion is also used to treat spasticity of neurologic diseases such as cerebral palsy, multiple sclerosis, reflex sympathetic dystrophy, or traumatic and anoxic acquired brain injuries.

Temporary catheters used for epidural therapy can be a percutaneous catheter that is secured at the site and extends up the back toward the shoulder. These catheters are used for postoperative pain management and usually dwell for only several hours or a few days. Infection and subsequent meningitis and catheter migration are the possible complications.

Epidural catheters used for longer periods include a tunneled catheter and implanted port. Tunneled catheters are tunneled toward the abdomen and have a subcutaneous cuff to act as a barrier to infection. The external catheter exists the skin on the abdomen, so it can be easily reached for use by the client or caregiver. An epidural implanted port is the same design as an IV implanted port and is accessed with the same noncoring needle. The catheter extends from the lumbar puncture site to the port pocket and is located over a bony prominence on the abdomen through a subcutaneous tunnel. Surgically implanted pumps, described earlier for intra-arterial infusion, can also be used to deliver epidural and intrathecal infusion.

NURSING CONSIDERATIONS

Intraspinal catheters are usually inserted in the lumbar region. The external portion of a temporary epidural catheter is laid along the back toward the head and usually extends over the shoulder. The entire catheter length is taped for added security. Dressings are usually not routinely changed because they are only used for short periods. If bleeding or fluid leakage requires dressing removal, extreme care is required to prevent dislodging the catheter.

For a tunneled catheter or implanted port, the entire subcutaneous tunnel and port pocket should be frequently assessed. Measurement of an external catheter segment could help identify catheter migration.

An in-line filter is used on all intraspinal infusions to block the infusion of particulate matter. Medications commonly contain preservatives such as alcohol, phenols, or sulfites; however, these are toxic to the CNS. All medications used for intraspinal infusion must be free of preservatives. Alcohol and products containing alcohol should not be applied to the insertion site because the solution could track along the catheter and cause nerve damage. Povidone iodine solutions are preferred for skin antisepsis before insertion and during catheter dwell, including tunneled catheter exit sites and implanted port pockets.

Complications from epidural and intrathecal infusion can be caused by the type of medication being infused or be related to the catheter. It is important to know the specific location of the intraspinal catheter because the doses of medications are quite different. When used for pain management, doses are usually 10 times greater for epidural than for intrathecal infusion. Your client should be assessed for response to the drugs being given, their level of alertness, respiratory status, and itching.

Catheter-related complications include infection, bleeding or leakage of CSF, occlusion of the catheter lumen, and catheter migration. Infection in the client receiving either epidural or intrathecal therapy could be the result of a lack of asepsis when handling the medication or during the administration. There may be local evidence of infection, such as redness or swelling at the catheter exit site. The client may also exhibit neurologic and systemic signs of infection, such as headache, stiff neck, or temperature higher than 101° F (38.3° C).

Intraosseous Therapy

DESCRIPTION

Intraosseous (IO) therapy allows access to the rich vascular network located in the long bones. This vascular network is more prominent in children younger than 6 years of age. Thus IO is typically regarded as a pediatric procedure, but it can be used in adults also. Victims of trauma, burns, cardiac arrest, and other life-threatening conditions benefit from this therapy because often clinicians are unable to access these clients' vascular systems for traditional IV therapy. Research indicates that absorption rates of large-volume parenteral (LVP) infusions and medications administered via the IO route are similar to those achieved with peripheral or central venous administration. IO should be used only during the immediate period of resuscitation and should not be used longer than 24 hours. After establishing IO access, efforts should continue to obtain IV access as well.

Theoretically, any needle can be used to provide therapy and access the medullary space. In children, an 18-gauge needle is chosen, whereas adults require a 15- or 16-gauge needle. Needles specifically designed for IO are preferred because they have the following:

- A needle with a removable stylet that screws into the cannula to keep the needle from retracting during insertion
- A short shaft to eliminate accidental dislodgment after placement
- An adjustable guard to stabilize the needle at skin level
- Graduations along the needle to guide the practitioner during insertion

Sites chosen include the distal or proximal tibia and the distal femur. The sternum is not recommended because it is too thin to accommodate a needle; it could lead to pneumothorax and may interfere with other resuscitation efforts.

NURSING CONSIDERATIONS

If IV access cannot be obtained within the first few minutes of resuscitation procedures, IO may be attempted. The leg is restrained, and the site is cleaned with an antiseptic agent. After successful insertion, the needle must be secured to prevent movement out of the bone. The same doses of fluids and medications can be infused IO as IV. An infusion pump may be used for rapid flow rates.

Improper needle placement is the most common complication of IO therapy. An accumulation of fluid under the skin at either the insertion site or on the other side of the limb indicates that the needle is either not far enough in to penetrate the bone marrow or is too far into the limb and has protruded through the other side of the shaft. Needle obstruction occurs when the puncture has been accomplished but there has been a delay in flushing. This delay may cause the needle to become clotted with bone marrow.

Osteomyelitis is a serious complication of IO therapy that occurs in fewer than 1% of clients. This bone infection is unusual but is generally caused by allowing the IO needle to remain in place for a lengthy period or by the use of hypertonic solutions (West, 1998).

Compartment syndrome is a condition in which increased tissue pressure in a confined anatomic space causes decreased blood flow to the area. The decreased circulation to the area leads to hypoxia and pain in the area. This is rare in IO therapy, but the nurse should monitor the site carefully and alert the physician promptly if the client exhibits any signs of decreased circulation to the limb, such as coolness, swelling, mottling, or discoloration. Without improvement in perfusion to the limb, the client may require amputation of the limb.

GET READY for the NCLEX Examination!

KEY POINTS

- Infusion therapy is the delivery of parenteral medications and fluids through a wide variety of catheters and locations.
- Infusion therapy is used for establishing fluid and electrolyte balance, achieving optimum nutrition, maintaining hemostasis, and treating or preventing illnesses with medications.
- Vascular access devices (VADs) are catheters that are used to deliver fluids and medications.
- Common types of VADs include short peripheral catheters, midline catheters, peripherally inserted central catheters (PICCs), nontunneled percutaneous and tunneled central catheters, implanted ports, and hemodialysis catheters.
- The type of VAD that is used depends on the reason for infusion therapy, the client's condition, and the length of therapy.
- PICCs, tunneled central catheters, and implanted ports are commonly used for long-term infusion therapy.
- Devices engineered with safety mechanisms are required by the Occupational Safety and Health Administration (OSHA) to prevent injuries from needles, thus preventing bloodborne pathogen hazards.
- Infusion controllers and pumps are electronic devices used to regulate the flow of infusion fluids and medications.
- Nursing care for clients receiving IV therapy includes using sterile technique when starting the therapy and when changing part of the infusion system, changing and securing the site dressing, and assessing the site for local complications (see Table 17-2).
- Most catheters are flushed with either normal saline or heparinized saline on a periodic basis per agency policy.
- Older adults present special challenges when infusion therapy is used; physiologic changes of the skin and cardiac/renal systems must be taken into consideration.
- Small catheters should be used for older adults and should be inserted using a 10- to 15-degree angle to prevent rolling of the vein.
- Nurses are also responsible for detecting and managing systemic complications of infusion therapy as outlined in Tables 17-3, 17-4, and 17-5.
- Arterial therapy is used primarily for the administration of antineoplastic agents directly into a tumor site; the liver is the most common arterial site for this purpose.
- Intraperitoneal therapy is used for antineoplastic agent administration into the peritoneal cavity, especially for ovarian and colorectal tumors that have metastasized into the peritoneum.
- Subcutaneous therapy of fluids (hypodermoclysis) involves a slow infusion for a short time; the thighs, hips, and abdomen are commonly used sites.
- Epidural and intrathecal administration of medications is the common use for intraspinal infusion. Epidural infusions are most commonly for pain management; intrathecal infusions are usually antineoplastic agents used for cancers that cross the blood-brain barrier into the central nervous system.
- Intraosseous therapy allows fluids and medications to be absorbed by the rich vascular network of the long bones; it is used most often in children, but it can be used for adults as well.

ADDITIONAL STUDY RESOURCES

Go to your Student CD-ROM for Review Questions for the NCLEX Examination.

evolve Go to http://evolve.elsevier.com/Iggy/ for Integrated Management of Care Questions for the NCLEX Examination.

SELECTED BIBLIOGRAPHY

Asterisk indicates a classic or definitive work on this subject.

Brown, M., & Worobec, F. (2000). Hypodermoclysis: Another was to replace fluids. *Nursing 2000, 30*(5), 58-59.

Brunelle, D. (2003). Impact of a dedicated infusion therapy team on the reduction of catheter-related nosocomial infections. *Journal of Infusion Nursing, 26*(6), 362-366.

CDRH. (2001). *Safety assessment of Di(2ethylhexyl)phthalate (DEHP) released from PVC medical devices.* Rockville, MD: Center for Devices and Radiological Health, Food and Drug Administration.

Chernecky, C., et al. (2003). Preferences in choosing venous access devices by intravenous and oncology nurses. *Journal of Vascular Access Devices, 8*(1), 35-40.

Crosby, C., & Mares, A. (2001). Skin antisepsis: Past, present and future. *Journal of Vascular Access Devices, 6*(1), 26-31.

Fong, N., et al. (2001). Peripherally inserted central catheters: Outcome as a function of the operator. *Journal of Vascular and Interventional Radiology, 12*, 723-729.

Galloway, M. (2002). Using benchmarking data to determine vascular access device selection. *Journal of Infusion Nursing, 25*(5), 320-325.

Gorski, L.A. (2003). Central venous access device occlusions. Part 2: Nonthrombotic causes and treatment. *Home Healthcare Nurse, 21*(3), 168-171.

*Hadaway, L.C. (1998). Thrombotic and nonthrombotic complications: Loss of patency. *Journal of Intravenous Nursing, 21*(5S), S143-S160.

*Hadaway, L.C. (1999a). I.V. Rounds: Choosing the right vascular access device, Part 1. *Nursing 99, 29*(2), 18.

*Hadaway, L.C. (1999b). IV Rounds: Choosing the right vascular access device, Part 2. *Nursing, 99, 29*(7), 28.

*Hadaway, L.C. (1999c). Vascular access devices: Meeting patient's needs. *MedSurg Nursing, The Journal of Adult Health, 8*(5), 296-303.

Hadaway, L.C. (2001). IV Rounds: Managing a vasovagal reaction. *Nursing 2001, 31*(4), 73.

Hadaway, L.C. (2003). Skin flora and infection. *Journal of Infusion Nursing, 26*(1), 44-48.

Herndon, C., & Fike, D. (2001). Continuous subcutaneous infusion practices of United States hospices. *Journal of Pain Symptom Management, 22*(6), 1027-1034.

Hunter, M.R. (2003). Development of a vascular access team in an acute care setting. *Journal of Infusion Nursing, 26*(92), 86-91.

Intravenous Nurses Society (INS). (2000). Infusion nursing standards of practice. *Journal of Intravenous Nursing, 23*(6S).

*Kearns, P.J., Coleman, S., & Wehner, J.H. (1996). Complications of long arm catheters: A randomized trial of central vs peripheral tip location. *Journal of Parenteral and Enteral Nutrition, 20*(1), 20-24.

Monarch, K. (2002). Legal aspects of infusion practice: Trends and issues. *Journal of Infusion Nursing, 25*(6 Suppl): S21-30.

*National Association of Vascular Access Networks (NAVAN). (1998). Position paper: Tip location of peripherally inserted central catheters. *Journal of Vascular Access Devices, 3*(2), 8-10.

O'Grady, N., et al. (2002). Guideline for the prevention of intravascular catheter-related infections. *Morbidity and Mortality Weekly Report, 51*(RR10), 1-26.

Pasero, C. (2002). Subcutaneous opioid infusion. *American Journal of Nursing, 102*(7), 61-62.

Perucca, R. (2001). Infusion therapy equipment: Types of infusion therapy equipment. In J. Hankins et al. (Eds.), *Infusion therapy in clinical practice* (2nd ed.). Philadelphia: W.B. Saunders.

Rosenthal, K. (2004). Where did this patient's I.V. therapy go awry? *Nursing 2004, 34*(5), 56-57.

Ryder, M. (2001). *The role of biofilm in vascular catheter-related infections.* Physicians & Scientists Publishing Co. Retrieved February 5, 2002, from http://www.medpub.com/cme.htm.

Santolucito, J.B. (2001). A retrospective evaluation of the timeliness of physician-initiated PICC referrals. *Journal of Vascular Access Devices, 6*(3), 20-26.

Slesak, G., et al. (2003). Comparison of subcutaneous and intravenous rehydration in geriatric patients: A randomized trial. *Journal of the American Geriatric Society, 51*(2), 155-160.

Smelling, R., et al. (2001). Central venous catheters for infusion therapy in gastrointestinal cancer. A comparative study of tunneled centrally placed catheters and peripherally inserted central catheters. *Journal of Intravenous Nursing, 24*(1), 38-47.

Trimble, T. (2003a). IV Rounds. Peripheral I.V. starts: Insertion techniques. *Nursing 2003, 33*(8), 17.

Trimble, T. (2003b). IV Rounds. Peripheral I.V. starts: Vein preparation tips. *Nursing 2003, 33*(7), 17.

Viale, P.H. (2003). Complications associated with implantable vascular access devices in the patient with cancer. *Journal of Infusion Nursing, 26*(2), 97-102.

Vialle, R., et al. (2001). Anatomic relations between the cephalic vein and the sensory branches of the radial nerve: How can nerve lesions during vein puncture be prevented? *Anesthesia and Analgesia, 93*, 1058-1061.

Weinstein, S. (2001). *Plumer's principles and practice of intravenous therapy* (7th ed.). Philadelphia: J.B. Lippincott.

Weir, J. (2001). Blood component therapy. In J. Hankins et al. (Eds.), *Infusion therapy in clinical practice* (2nd ed., pp. 156-175). Philadelphia: W.B. Saunders.

*West, V. (1998). Alternative routes of administration. *Journal of Intravenous Nursing, 21*(4), 221-231.

Zwicker, C.D. (2003). The elderly patient at risk. *Journal of Infusion Nursing, 26*(3), 137-143.

CHAPTER

18 Acid-Base Balance

M. LINDA WORKMAN

LEARNING OUTCOMES

After studying this chapter, you should be able to:

1. Describe the relationship between free hydrogen ion level and pH.
2. Explain the role of bicarbonate in the blood.
3. Explain the concept of compensation.
4. Compare the role of a buffer in conditions of acidosis and alkalosis.
5. Compare the roles of the respiratory system and the renal system in maintaining acid-base balance.
6. Describe the role of oxygen in maintaining acid-base balance.
7. Interpret whether the client's arterial blood gas values are normal, elevated, or low.

Go to your Student CD-ROM for Review Questions for the NCLEX Examination keyed to these Learning Outcomes.

Acid-base balance occurs through control of hydrogen ion (H^+) production and elimination. Body fluid **pH** is a measure of the body fluid's free hydrogen ion level. The free hydrogen ion level, or pH, has the narrowest range of normal and the tightest control mechanisms of all electrolytes. The level of free hydrogen ions, formed from acids, must be rigidly controlled for proper function. Even small changes in the free hydrogen ion level, or pH, of body fluids can cause major problems in function. Keeping the pH within the normal range involves balancing acids and bases in body fluids.

The normal free hydrogen ion level of blood and other body fluids is quite low (less than 0.0001 mEq/L) compared with the body fluid levels of other electrolytes (see Chapters 14 and 16). Because it is so low, free hydrogen ion level is measured in pH units, calculated as the negative logarithm of the concentration in milliequivalents per liter (Figure 18-1). Normal pH ranges from 7.35 to 7.45 for arterial blood and from 7.31 to 7.41 for venous blood.

Because pH is calculated in negative logarithm units, the value of pH is inversely related (negatively related) to the level of free hydrogen ions. In other words, the lower the pH value of a fluid, the higher the level of free hydrogen ions in that fluid. The pH of a solution may range from 1 (as acidic as possible) to 14 (as alkaline as possible), with 7 being neutral. *A change of 1 pH unit actually represents a 10-fold change in free hydrogen ion level.* Therefore even a pH unit change of one tenth (e.g., a change from 7.4 to 7.3) represents a large increase in the free hydrogen ion level. Table 18-1 lists terms used to describe acid-base balance.

Changes from normal blood pH (7.35 to 7.45) interfere with many normal physiologic functions by:

- Changing the shape of hormones and enzymes so that they may no longer perform their normal functions
- Changing the distribution of other electrolytes, causing fluid and electrolyte imbalances
- Altering the responses of excitable membranes so that the heart, nerves, skeletal muscles, and gastrointestinal tract are either less or more active than normal
- Decreasing the uptake, activity, and effectiveness of many hormones and drugs

Fortunately, the body has many mechanisms to ensure minimal changes in free hydrogen ion level.

INTRODUCTION TO ACID-BASE BALANCE

As discussed in Chapters 14 and 16, body fluids are electrically neutral even though they contain ions with overall positive charges (**cations** or **protons**) and ions with overall negative charges **(anions).** When fluids contain an equal number of positive and negative charges, the electrical charge of the fluid remains neutral. The body keeps blood pH between 7.35 and 7.45 in a similar manner; however, this value is not strictly neutral (7.0 is neutral) but rather is slightly alkaline. Normal body fluid pH remains at a near-neutral value when the acids and bases are nearly balanced, limiting the total number of free or unbalanced hydrogen ions. Acid-base balance occurs by matching the rate of hy-

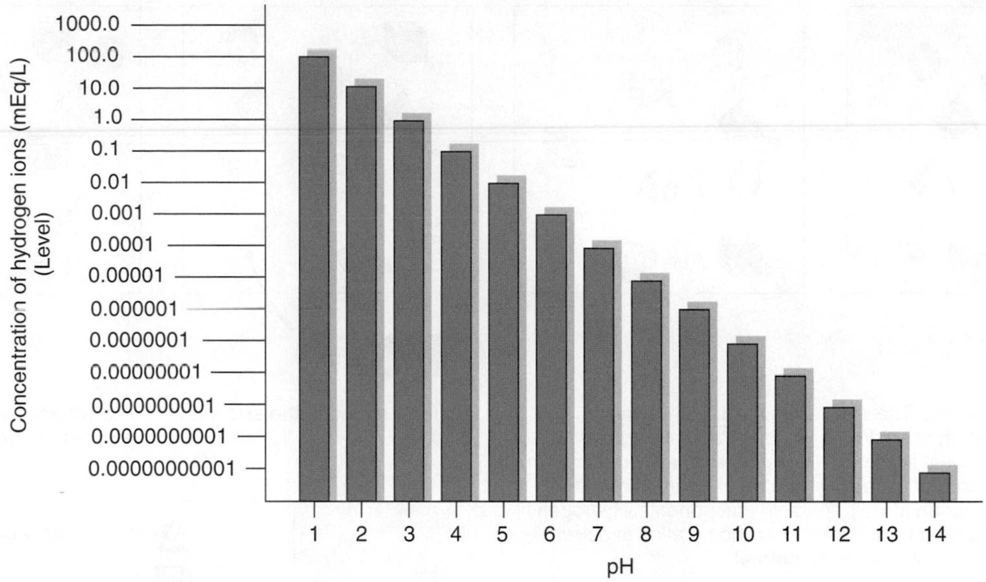

Figure 18-1 ■ Relationship between pH and concentration of hydrogen ions.

TABLE 18-1 Pertinent Acid-Base Balance Terminology

acid Any substance releasing a hydrogen ion when dissolved in water

anaerobic metabolism Cellular metabolism occurring without the presence of oxygen

base Any substance binding a hydrogen ion when dissolved in water

buffer A substance capable of binding a hydrogen ion from body fluids (acting as a base) or releasing a hydrogen ion into body fluids (acting as an acid)

chemoreceptors Special cells in the respiratory center of the brain sensitive to changes in the carbon dioxide concentration of extracellular fluid

pH The concentration of hydrogen ions in a solution, calculated as the negative logarithm of the milliequivalent concentration per liter

drogen ion production with activities for hydrogen ion removal or uptake.

Acid-Base Chemistry

ACIDS

Acids are substances that release hydrogen ions when dissolved in water (H_2O). An acid in solution *increases* the amount of free hydrogen ions in that solution. The strength of an acid is measured by how easily it releases a hydrogen ion in solution. A strong acid, such as hydrochloric acid (HCl), **dissociates** (separates) completely in water and readily releases all of its hydrogen ions:

HCl	+	H_2O	$\rightarrow$	H^+	+	Cl^-	+	H_2O
Hydrochloric acid		Water		Hydrogen ion		Chloride ion		Water

A weak acid does not completely separate in water; it releases only some of its hydrogen ions. In the following example, each molecule of acetic acid (CH_3COOH), a weak acid, contains a total of four hydrogen molecules. When acetic acid combines with water, it releases only one of its four hydrogen molecules. The other three hydrogen molecules remain bound to the acetic acid molecule:

$$CH_3COOH + H_2O \rightarrow H^+ + CH_3COO + H_2O$$

BASES

A **base** binds free hydrogen ions in solution. Thus bases are hydrogen acceptors that reduce the amount of free hydrogen ions in solution. Strong bases bind hydrogen ions easily. Examples of strong bases include sodium hydroxide (NaOH) and ammonia (NH_3).

Weak bases bind hydrogen ions less readily. Examples of weak bases include aluminum hydroxide ($AlOH_3$) and bicarbonate (HCO_3^-). Although bicarbonate is a weak base, bicarbonate ions in the body prevent major changes in body fluid pH.

BUFFERS

Buffers can either release a hydrogen ion into a fluid or bind a hydrogen ion from a fluid. Most substances, when dissolved in water, react by either releasing a hydrogen ion (an acid) or binding a free hydrogen ion (a base). Buffers dissolved in water can react in two ways: either as an acid (releasing a hydrogen ion) or as a base (binding a hydrogen ion).

How a buffer reacts when dissolved in water depends on the existing acid-base balance of that fluid. Buffers always try to bring the fluid as close as possible to the normal body fluid pH of 7.35 to 7.45. If the fluid is basic (with few free hydrogen ions), the buffer releases hydrogen ions into the fluid (Figure 18-2). If the fluid is acidic (with many free hydrogen ions), the buffer acts as a base, binding some hydrogen ions. Buffers act like hydrogen ion "sponges," soaking up hydrogen ions when too many are present and squeezing out hydrogen ions when too few are present. Because of this flexibility, buffers are important regulators of body fluid pH, or hydrogen ion level (acid-base balance).

Liquids with a pH of 7.0 are neutral; they have a free hydrogen ion level in which the number and strength of acids and bases are equal. Figure 18-3 represents the concept of

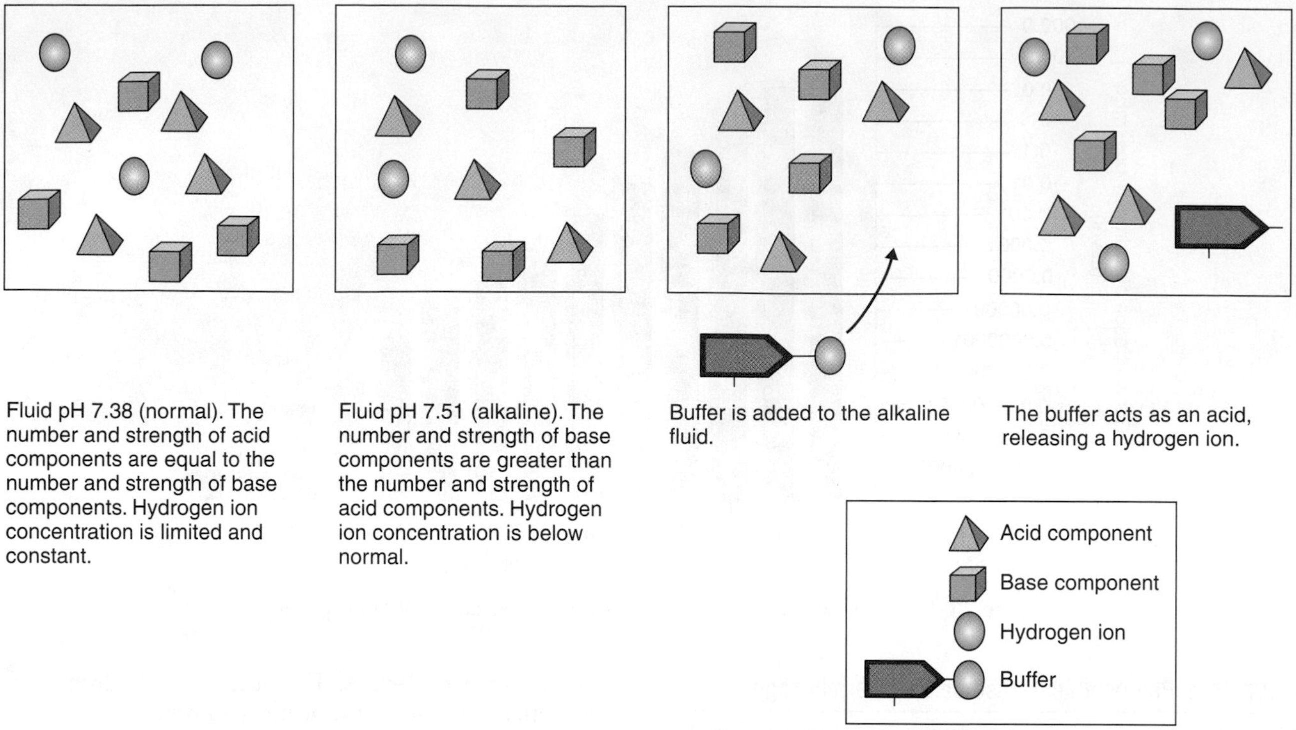

Figure 18-2 ■ Action of buffer in solution. (© 1992 by M. Linda Workman. All rights reserved.)

AAABBB	AAAABBB	AAABB
AAABBB	AAAABBB	AAABB
AAABBB	AAAABBB	AAABB
Neutral	Acidic (acid excess)	Acidic (base deficit)

Figure 18-3 ■ Concept of acidic versus normal pH. **A** = Acid; **B** = base.

AAABBB	AAABBBB	AABBB
AAABBB	AAABBBB	AABBB
AAABBB	AAABBBB	AABBB
Neutral	Alkaline (base excess)	Alkaline (acid deficit)

Figure 18-4 ■ Concept of alkaline versus normal pH. **A** = Acid; **B** = base.

neutral pH. This figure shows that the combined *strength* and *amount* of all acids are equal to the combined *strength* and *amount* of all bases in a given solution. This is not the actual case in human physiology. However, in acid-base homeostasis, the relative amounts and strengths of acids and bases are nearly equal, so the overall free hydrogen ion levels remain constant.

Liquids with a pH ranging from 1.0 to 6.99 have more or stronger (or both) acids compared with the amount or strength (or both) of bases. Such liquids are *acidic* (see Figure 18-3), which means that more free hydrogen ions are being released than bound, increasing the number of free hydrogen ions.

Liquids with a pH ranging from 7.01 to 14.0 have more or stronger (or both) bases compared with the amount or strength (or both) of acids. These liquids are *basic,* which means that more hydrogen ions are being bound than released, decreasing the number of free hydrogen ions (Figure 18-4).

Body Fluid Chemistry

BICARBONATE IONS

Body fluids contain many different types of acids and a few types of bases. The most common base in human body fluid is bicarbonate (HCO_3^-); the most common acid is carbonic acid (H_2CO_3). In health, the body keeps these substances within extracellular fluid (ECF) at a constant ratio of one molecule of carbonic acid to 20 free bicarbonate ions (1:20) (Figure 18-5). To maintain this ratio, both carbonic acid and bicarbonate must be carefully controlled. Both of these substances and their constant ratio are related to the production and elimination of carbon dioxide (CO_2) and hydrogen ions (H^+).

A key concept in understanding acid-base balance is the *carbonic anhydrase equation.* This equation, driven by the enzyme carbonic anhydrase, shows how hydrogen ion levels and carbon dioxide levels are directly related to one another, so that an increase in one causes an equal increase in the other:

$$\underset{\text{Carbon dioxide}}{CO_2} + \underset{\text{Water}}{H_2O} \Leftrightarrow \underset{\text{Carbonic acid}}{H_2CO_3} \Leftrightarrow \underset{\text{Hydrogen ion}}{H^+} + \underset{\text{Bicarbonate ion}}{HCO_3^-}$$

Carbon dioxide is a gas that forms carbonic acid when combined with water. Carbon dioxide is a changeable part

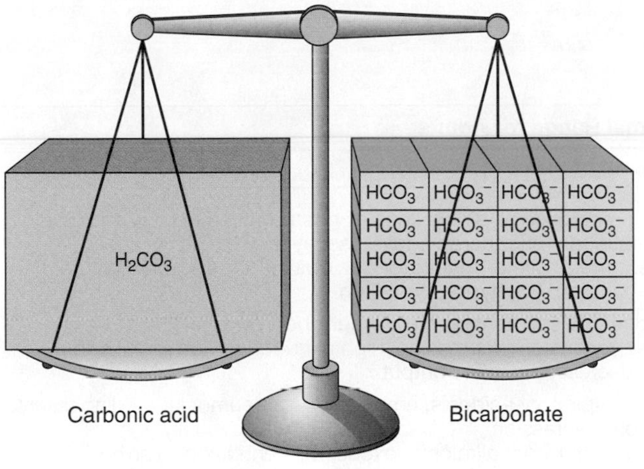

Figure 18-5 ■ Normal ratio of carbonic acid to bicarbonate is 1:20.

of carbonic acid. Carbonic acid is not stable, and the body needs to keep a 1:20 ratio of carbonic acid to bicarbonate. As soon as carbonic acid is formed from water and carbon dioxide, it immediately separates into free hydrogen ions and bicarbonate ions. *Therefore the carbon dioxide content of a fluid is directly related to the amount of hydrogen ions in that fluid. Whenever conditions cause carbon dioxide to increase, more free hydrogen ions are created. Likewise, whenever free hydrogen ion production increases, more carbon dioxide is produced.*

RELATIONSHIP BETWEEN CARBON DIOXIDE AND HYDROGEN IONS

When excess carbon dioxide is produced, the amount of carbon dioxide increases and the carbonic anhydrase equation shifts to the right, causing an increase in hydrogen ions (and a decrease in pH):

$$\mathbf{CO_2} + H_2O \rightleftharpoons H_2CO_3 \rightleftharpoons H^+ + HCO_3^-$$

When very little carbon dioxide is produced, no free hydrogen ions are created by the carbonic anhydrase equation.

When excess hydrogen ions are produced or brought into the body, the carbonic anhydrase equation shifts to the left, causing the creation of more carbon dioxide:

$$CO_2 + H_2O \leftrightharpoons H_2CO_3 \leftrightharpoons \mathbf{H^+} + HCO_3^-$$

When the amount of free hydrogen ions in body fluids is low, no extra carbon dioxide is produced.

CALCULATION OF FREE HYDROGEN ION LEVEL

The pH is a calculation of the free hydrogen ion level in body fluids. A formula is used because the actual number of free hydrogen ions is not easily measured. The pH calculations come from a mathematical formula (the Henderson-Hasselbalch equation) that shows how three factors are related: the level of free hydrogen ions, the amount of bases, and the strength of acids in a solution. In the body, if two of these three factors are known, the third factor can then be calculated.

Because the normal ratio of carbonic acid and bicarbonate level in ECF is 1:20, the only factor that changes is the carbon dioxide level. Whenever the carbon dioxide level changes, the pH changes to the same degree, in the opposite direction. Thus when the carbon dioxide level of a liquid increases, the pH drops, indicating more free hydrogen ions (more acidic). On the other hand, when the carbon dioxide level of a liquid decreases, the pH rises, indicating fewer free hydrogen ions (more alkaline).

An increase in bicarbonate causes the amount of hydrogen ions to decrease and the pH to increase, or become more alkaline (basic). Conversely, an increase in the carbon dioxide level causes the free hydrogen ion level to increase and the pH to decrease, or become more acidic.

Because the kidneys control bicarbonate levels and the lungs control carbon dioxide levels in the healthy person, pH is also described as the function of the kidneys divided by the function of the lungs:

$$\text{pH} = \frac{\text{Kidneys (bicarbonate)}}{\text{Lungs (carbon dioxide)}}$$

SOURCES OF ACIDS

Acids are formed as normal waste products of carbohydrate, protein, and fat metabolism. Carbohydrate metabolism forms carbon dioxide, which can then be converted to free hydrogen ions. Fat and protein metabolism directly create acids.

GLUCOSE METABOLISM (PRODUCTION OF CARBON DIOXIDE). Carbon dioxide is a waste product of glucose breakdown and other metabolic reactions. (The complete breakdown of one molecule of glucose forms 36 molecules of adenosine triphosphate [ATP], six molecules of water, and six molecules of carbon dioxide.) Because of the relationship between carbon dioxide and free hydrogen ions, any increase in carbon dioxide levels always leads to increased amounts of hydrogen ions. The result is a decrease in pH.

Carbon dioxide is exhaled by the lungs during breathing. One factor that determines blood pH is how much carbon dioxide is produced by body cells during metabolism versus how rapidly that carbon dioxide is removed by breathing.

FAT AND PROTEIN METABOLISM. The breakdown of food for energy results in the formation of *fixed acids*. Protein breakdown forms sulfuric acid. Fat breakdown forms fatty acids and ketoacids.

INCOMPLETE METABOLISM OF GLUCOSE AND FATS. Incomplete breakdown of glucose, which occurs whenever cells metabolize under **anaerobic** (no oxygen) conditions, forms lactic acid. Anaerobic conditions occur with hypoxia, sepsis, and shock. Incomplete breakdown of fatty acids, occurring when large amounts of fatty acids are being metabolized, forms ketoacids (Guyton & Hall, 2000).

DESTRUCTION OF CELLS. Whenever cells are damaged or destroyed, cell membranes are broken and cell contents are released. Some cell structures contain acids that are released into the extracellular fluid (ECF) when this occurs.

SOURCES OF BICARBONATE IONS

Bicarbonate is the primary buffer of the ECF. Bicarbonate comes from the breakdown of carbonic acid, intestinal absorption of ingested bicarbonate, pancreatic production of bicarbonate, movement of cellular bicarbonate into the ECF, and kidney reabsorption of filtered bicarbonate. Once bicarbonate is in the ECF, it is kept at a level 20 times greater than that of carbonic acid.

CHART 18-1

LABORATORY PROFILE
Acid-Base Assessment

Test	Normal Range for Adults: Arterial	Venous	Significance of Abnormal Findings
pH >90 yr	7.35-7.45 7.25-7.45	7.31-7.41	Increased: metabolic alkalosis, loss of gastric fluids, decreased potassium intake, diuretic therapy, fever, salicylate toxicity Decreased: metabolic or respiratory acidosis, ketosis, renal failure, starvation, diarrhea, hyperthyroidism
Pao_2 (mm Hg) >90 yr	80-100 >50		Increased: increased ventilation, oxygen therapy, exercise Decreased: respiratory depression, high altitude, carbon monoxide poisoning, decreased cardiac output
$Paco_2$ (mm Hg)	35-45	40-50	Increased: respiratory acidosis, emphysema, pneumonia, cardiac failure, respiratory depression Decreased: respiratory alkalosis, excessive ventilation, diarrhea
Bicarbonate (mEq/L or mmol/L)	22-26	24-29	Increased: bicarbonate therapy, metabolic alkalosis Decreased: metabolic acidosis, diarrhea, pancreatitis
Lactate	3-7 mg/dL 0.3-0.8 mmol/L	5-20 mg/dL 0.6-2.2 mmol/L	Increased: hypoxia, exercise, insulin infusion, alcoholism, pregnancy Decreased: fluid overload

Pao_2, Partial pressure of arterial oxygen; *$Paco_2$*, partial pressure of arterial carbon dioxide.

ACID-BASE HOMEOSTASIS

As long as body cells are healthy, they continually produce acids, carbon dioxide, and hydrogen ions. Despite this production, hydrogen ions, bicarbonate, oxygen, and carbon dioxide levels are kept within normal limits when physiologic function is normal. Chart 18-1 lists normal values for these substances in arterial and venous blood. This homeostasis depends on three factors:

- Hydrogen ion production is consistent and not excessive.
- Carbon dioxide loss from the body through breathing must keep pace with hydrogen ion production.
- The ratio between carbonic acid and bicarbonate must be kept at 1:20.

Acid-Base Regulatory Mechanisms

To keep the free hydrogen ion level (pH) of the ECF within the narrow range of normal, the body has chemical, respiratory, and renal mechanisms for acid-base balance (Table 18-2).

CHEMICAL ACID-BASE CONTROL MECHANISMS

Buffers are the first line of defense against changes in the amount of free hydrogen ions. Because they are always present in body fluids, buffers act fast to reduce or raise the amount of free hydrogen ions to normal. By acting as hydrogen ion "sponges," buffers can bind hydrogen ions when too many are present or release hydrogen ions when not enough are present. Buffers are composed of chemicals or proteins.

CHEMICAL BUFFERS. Chemical buffers are paired mixtures, usually a weak base and an acid salt. The two most common chemical buffer systems are bicarbonate buffers (which are active in both the extracellular fluid [ECF] and intracellular fluid [ICF]) and phosphate buffers (which are active in the ICF).

PROTEIN BUFFERS. Proteins are the largest source of buffers. Proteins in body fluids can either bind or release free hydrogen ions as needed. Both ICF and ECF proteins serve as buffers.

A major cell protein buffer is hemoglobin. Hemoglobin buffers hydrogen ions directly and also buffers acids formed during the production of carbon dioxide. When the amount of free hydrogen ions in the blood increases, some of the excess hydrogen ions cross the membranes of red blood cells and bind to the large numbers of hemoglobin molecules in each red blood cell.

Extracellular protein buffers are albumin and globulins. These proteins buffer carbonic acid and other acids present in the ECF as a result of catabolism.

RESPIRATORY ACID-BASE CONTROL MECHANISMS

When chemical buffers alone cannot prevent changes in blood pH, the respiratory system is the second line of defense against changes. Breathing controls the amount of free hydrogen ions by controlling the amount of carbon dioxide in arterial blood. Carbon dioxide is converted into hydrogen ions through the carbonic anhydrase reaction. Therefore the carbon dioxide level is directly related to the hydrogen ion level. Breathing rids the body of the excess carbon dioxide created through metabolism.

The amount of carbon dioxide in venous blood increases during normal metabolism. This carbon dioxide is moved in the blood to the lung capillaries. Because the amount (pressure) of carbon dioxide is far higher in capillary blood than in the air in the alveoli, carbon dioxide diffuses freely from the blood into the alveolar air. Once in the alveoli, carbon dioxide is exhaled during breathing and is lost from the body. Because the amount (pressure) of carbon dioxide in normal atmospheric air is nearly zero, carbon dioxide usually continues to be exhaled even when breathing is impaired to some degree.

HYPERVENTILATION. Respiratory regulation of acid-base balance is under the control of the central nervous system (Figure 18-6). Special receptors in the respiratory areas of the brain are sensitive to changes in the amount of carbon dioxide in brain tissues. As the amount of carbon dioxide begins to rise above normal in brain blood and tissues, these central receptors trigger the neu-

TABLE 18-2 Acid-Base Regulatory Mechanisms

Mechanism Type	Key Characteristics
Chemical	
Protein buffers	Very rapid response
Extracellular	Provide immediate response to changing conditions
Albumin	Can handle relatively small fluctuations in hydrogen ion production and elimination encountered under normal metabolic and health conditions
Globulins	
Intracellular	
Hemoglobin	
Chemical buffers	
Extracellular	
Bicarbonate	
Intracellular	
Phosphate	
Bicarbonate	
Respiratory	
Increased hydrogen ions	Primarily assist buffering systems when the fluctuation of hydrogen ion concentration is acute
Increased carbon dioxide	
Stimulates central respiratory neurons, leading to increased rate and depth of breathing, causing more carbon dioxide to be lost and decreasing the hydrogen ion concentration	
Decreased hydrogen ions	
Decreased carbon dioxide	
Inhibition of central respiratory neurons, leading to decreased rate and depth of breathing, causing normally produced carbon dioxide to be retained, increasing the hydrogen ion concentration	
Renal	
Mechanisms to decrease pH	The most powerful regulator of acid-base balance
Increased renal excretion of bicarbonate	Respond to large or chronic fluctuations in hydrogen ion production or elimination
Increased renal reabsorption of hydrogen ions	
Mechanisms to increase pH	Slowest response (hours to days)
Decreased renal excretion of bicarbonate	Longest duration
Decreased renal reabsorption of hydrogen ions	

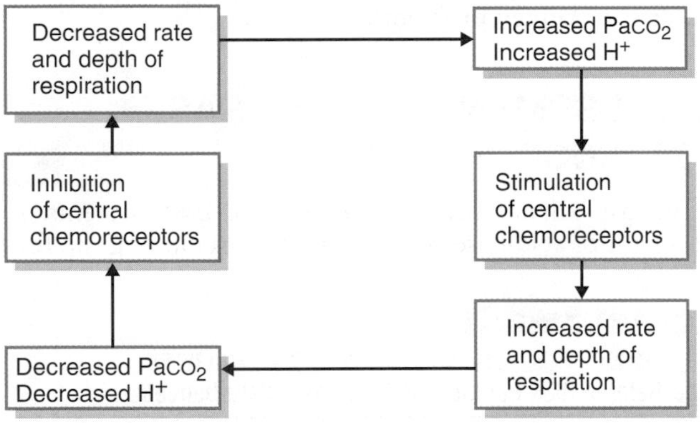

Figure 18-6 ■ Neural regulation of respiration and hydrogen ion concentration. *Pa_{CO_2}*, Partial pressure of arterial carbon dioxide; *H^+*, hydrogen ion.

rons to increase the rate and depth of breathing. As a result, more carbon dioxide is exhaled ("blown off") from the lungs and the amount carbon dioxide in the ECF decreases. When the amount of arterial carbon dioxide returns to normal, the rate and depth of breathing return to levels that are normal for the person.

HYPOVENTILATION. If the amount of ECF free hydrogen ions is too low, then the amount of carbon dioxide also is too low. Central receptors sense these low carbon dioxide levels and stop or slow the neuron activity in the respiratory centers, decreasing the rate and depth of breathing. As a result, less carbon dioxide is lost through the lungs and more carbon dioxide is retained in arterial blood. This retention of already-formed carbon dioxide, together with the normal production of carbon dioxide from metabolism, results in a rapid return of the arterial carbon dioxide levels (and hydrogen ion levels) to normal. When these levels are normal, the rate and depth of breathing also return to normal levels.

The respiratory system's response in regulating acid-base balance is rapid. Changes in the rate and depth of breathing occur within minutes after changes in the hydrogen ion level or carbon dioxide level of the ECF occur.

RENAL ACID-BASE CONTROL MECHANISMS

The kidneys are the third line of defense against wide changes in body fluid pH. Renal mechanisms are stronger for regulating acid-base balance but take longer than chemical and respiratory mechanisms to completely respond. (They take 24 to 48 hours to respond.) When blood pH changes are persistent, renal mechanisms that increase excretion and reabsorption rates of acids or bases (depending on the direction of the pH changes) begin to operate. These mechanisms are kidney movement of bicarbonate, formation of acids, and formation of ammonium.

KIDNEY MOVEMENT OF BICARBONATE. This first renal mechanism occurs in the kidney tubules in two ways: (1) kidney movement of bicarbonate produced elsewhere in the body and (2) kidney movement of bicarbonate produced in the kidneys. Much of the bicarbonate made in other body areas is excreted in the urine. When blood hydrogen ion levels are high, this bicarbonate is reabsorbed from the kidneys back into circulation, where it can help buffer excess hydrogen ions. When blood hydrogen ion levels are low, the bicarbonate remains in the urine and is excreted. When hydrogen ion excess occurs, the kidney tubules also can make additional bicarbonate that will be reabsorbed.

FORMATION OF ACIDS. The second renal mechanism occurs through the phosphate-buffering system inside the cells of the kidney tubules. When the newly created bicarbonate made in the kidney cells is reabsorbed into the blood along with sodium, the urine has an excess of anions, including phosphate (HPO_4^{2-}). This negatively charged fluid draws hydrogen ions (which carry a positive charge) into the urine. Once the hydrogen ion is in the urine, it binds to phosphate ions, forming an acid, H_2PO_4, which is then excreted in the urine.

FORMATION OF AMMONIUM. In the third renal mechanism, ammonia (NH_3), which is formed during normal protein breakdown, is converted into ammonium (NH_4^+). The ammonia is secreted into the urine, where it can combine with hydrogen ions to form ammonium, stays in the urine, and then is excreted from the body. This "trapping" of hydrogen ions in ammonium prevents the free hydrogen ion level in the urine from becoming so high that it inhibits movement of hydrogen ions from the blood into the urine. The overall result is a loss of hydrogen ions and an increase in blood pH.

COMPENSATION

In the process of *compensation,* the body attempts to correct changes in blood pH. A pH below 6.9 or above 7.8 is usually fatal. The normal pH range for human extracellular fluid (ECF) is 7.35 to 7.45. Both the kidneys and the lungs can compensate for acid-base imbalances, but they are not equal in their compensatory responses. The respiratory system is much more sensitive to acid-base changes and can begin compensation efforts within seconds to minutes after a change in pH. However, these efforts are limited and can be overwhelmed easily. The renal compensatory mechanisms are much more powerful and result in rapid changes in ECF composition. However, these more powerful mechanisms are not fully triggered unless the acid-base imbalance continues for several hours to several days.

RESPIRATORY COMPENSATION. The lungs can usually compensate for acid-base imbalances of a metabolic origin. For example, when prolonged running causes buildup of lactic acid, hydrogen ion levels in the ECF increase and the pH drops. To bring the pH back to normal, breathing is triggered in response to increased carbon dioxide levels. Both the rate and depth of respiration increase. These respiratory efforts cause the blood to lose carbon dioxide with each exhalation, so ECF levels of carbon dioxide and free hydrogen ions gradually decrease. When the lungs can fully compensate, the pH returns to normal.

RENAL COMPENSATION. A healthy kidney can correct or compensate for changes in blood pH when the respiratory system is either overwhelmed or is not healthy. For example, in a person with chronic obstructive pulmonary disease (COPD), the respiratory system cannot exchange gases adequately. Carbon dioxide is retained and the blood pH falls (becomes more acidic). To oppose this process, the kidney excretes more hydrogen ions and increases the reabsorption of bicarbonate back into the blood. As a result, the blood pH remains either within or closer to the normal range. When these backup mechanisms are completely effective, acid-base problems are fully compensated and the pH of the blood returns to normal, even though the levels of oxygen and bicarbonate may be abnormal.

Sometimes, however, the respiratory problem causing the acid-base imbalance is so severe that kidney actions can only partially compensate, and the pH is not quite normal. Even partial compensation is helpful because it prevents the acid-base imbalance from becoming severe or life threatening.

Age-Related Changes in Acid-Base Balance

Older adults are at greater risk for pH problems than are younger people because their lungs and kidneys are less able to respond to minor changes in hydrogen ion production or elimination. In addition, older adults often take drugs that alter normal pH-compensating mechanisms (Chart 18-2).

Gas exchange during breathing is reduced as a person ages. There is less alveolar membrane for gas exchange in older persons, and many also have some degree of blood vessel thickening, which further impairs gas movement through capillaries. These conditions can cause carbon dioxide retention, increasing the free hydrogen ion level.

Because kidney function decreases with age, older adults are less able to excrete hydrogen ions or produce bicarbonate ions. The kidneys may be able to handle ordinary changes resulting from normal metabolism but cannot compensate when health problems such as pneumonia, fever, or infection, interfere with acid-base balance.

Two drugs often prescribed for older clients are diuretics and digoxin. Both agents increase kidney excretion of hydrogen ions, which can result in an increased blood pH.

All older clients are at risk for acid-base disturbances. This risk is even greater for clients with pulmonary, vascular, cardiac, or kidney problems.

ASSESSMENT OF ACID-BASE BALANCE

Acid-base balance involves all cells and body systems. Assessment of acid-base balance involves examining the func-

CHART 18-2

NURSING FOCUS on the OLDER ADULT
Age-Related Risk Factors for Acid-Base Disturbances

Disturbance	Risk Factors

Increased hydrogen ion concentration	Pulmonary diseases
	  Chronic obstructive pulmonary disease (COPD)
	  Pneumonia
	Dehydration
	Infection
	Renal disease
	Vascular disease
	  Atherosclerosis
	  Arteriosclerosis
	  Angiitis

Decreased hydrogen ion concentration	Overhydration
	Congestive heart failure
	Drugs
	  Diuretics (loop and thiazide)
	  Digoxin
	  Insulin
	  Antibiotics
	  Chemotherapeutic agents

tioning of systems responsible for acid-base balance, especially the lungs and kidneys. Assessment also involves examining body responses to changes in the levels of acids or bases. Behavioral and neurologic assessments also are included in assessment of acid-base balance because changes in pH can alter neurologic function.

History

One way of organizing history data to assess the client's acid-base status is the use of Gordon's Functional Health Patterns (Gordon, 2002). The patterns that affect acid-base balance most are Activity-Exercise, Elimination, and Cognitive-Perceptual patterns (Chart 18-3), showing the effectiveness of lung and kidney function.

Physical Assessment

Hydration status can indicate fluid balance. A normally hydrated adult is alert, has moist eyes and mucous membranes, has a urine output nearly the same as the amount of fluid ingested (with a urine specific gravity between 1.010 and 1.030), and has good skin turgor (see Chapter 14). A dry, sticky, "cottony" mouth; the absence of tearing; weight loss; and decreased urine output all indicate either a problem with oral intake or excess fluid loss. Accurate assessment of fluid intake and output can help determine kidney function and acid-base balance.

Hydrogen ions affect the activity of excitable membranes, and acid-base imbalances alter the function of these membranes. Acid-base assessment includes assessment of muscle tone and strength, movement, coordination, and tremors. Assessment of other systems, including the cardiac (heart rate, rhythm, and strength of contractions) and gastrointestinal (motility) systems, may indicate changes in excitable membrane function.

Part of your assessment focuses on changes from previous findings, including mental status, physical examination data, and laboratory data. Acid-base imbalances can occur quickly and you must be familiar with the client's baseline assessment data to detect any changes.

CHART 18-3

Acid-Base Assessment
USING GORDON'S FUNCTIONAL HEALTH PATTERNS

Activity-Exercise Pattern
- Have you had any shortness of breath or difficulty breathing at rest or during activity?
- Have you noticed any changes in your breathing rate or depth?
- Do you have a hard time "catching" your breath?
- Do you have any difficulty clearing excretions?
- Do you feel the need for additional energy to accomplish routine tasks?
- Do you have any difficulty concentrating?
- Have you noticed any changes in your interest in normal daily activities?
- Have you noticed any changes in your leisure activities?

Elimination Pattern
- What is your usual urinary elimination pattern? Frequency? Amount? Color? Odor? Control?
- Have you noticed any changes in the amount of urine?
- Has your urine changed color or odor?
- What is your usual bowel elimination pattern? Frequency? Amount? Control?
- Have you noticed any changes in the number or consistency of your stools?

Cognitive-Perceptual Pattern
- Have you noticed any changes in memory lately?
- Have you noticed an increase in anxiety or feelings of apprehension?
- Are you sleeping more or sleeping less than usual for you?
- Have you noticed any changes in your attention span?
- Have your muscles seemed weak or "twitchy" lately?

Based on Gordon, M. (2002). *Manual of nursing diagnosis* (10th ed.). St. Louis: Mosby.

Diagnostic Assessment

Arterial blood gases (ABGs) are important in identifying specific acid-base imbalances and are discussed fully in Chapter 19 (see also Chart 18-1). Other laboratory values helpful in assessing acid-base balance include serum electrolyte levels, blood urea nitrogen (BUN) level, glucose level, creatinine level, and osmolarity.

Urine test results may be helpful in determining whether a kidney or metabolic problem is affecting acid-base balance. Such tests include glomerular filtration rate and detection of substances that should not be present in the urine, such as glucose, acetone, protein, or blood.

GET READY for the NCLEX Examination!

KEY POINTS

- The normal pH of the body's extracellular fluids (including blood) is 7.35 to 7.45.
- The normal pH of arterial blood is slightly higher (less acidic) than venous blood.
- The more hydrogen ions present, the more acidic the fluid.
- The less hydrogen ions present, the more alkaline the fluid.
- Lower pH values (below 7.35) mean acidosis is present.
- Higher pH values (above 7.45) mean alkalosis is present.
- The pH in the body can be described as the relationship of bicarbonate to carbonic acid, or a 20:1 ratio.
- Carbon dioxide is the most changeable component of carbonic acid.
- The concentration of carbon dioxide is directly related to the concentration of hydrogen ions. Anything that increases the carbon dioxide level in the blood, increases the hydrogen ion content and lowers the pH.
- An acid gives up hydrogen ions in solution; a base binds hydrogen ions in solution.
- Acids are normally formed in the body as a result of metabolism and incomplete oxidation of glucose and fats.
- Acid-base balance is regulated by chemical, respiratory, and renal mechanisms.
- Chemical buffers are the immediate way that acid-base imbalances are corrected.
- The lungs control the amount of carbon dioxide that is retained or exhaled.
- The kidneys regulate the amount of hydrogen and bicarbonate ions that are retained or excreted by the body.
- Compensation is the process in which the body uses its three regulatory mechanisms to correct for changes in the pH of body fluids.

- If a lung problem causes retention of carbon dioxide, the healthy kidney compensates by increasing the amount of bicarbonate that is produced and retained.
- The best way to determine acid-base balance is by analyzing arterial blood gases (ABGs).

ADDITIONAL STUDY RESOURCES

Go to your Student CD-ROM for Review Questions for the NCLEX Examination.

Go to http://evolve.elsevier.com/Iggy/ for Integrated Management of Care Questions for the NCLEX Examination.

SELECTED BIBLIOGRAPHY

Adrogue, H.E., & Adrogue, H.J. (2001). Acid-base physiology. *Respiratory Care, 46*(4), 328-341.

Berry, B., & Pinard, A. (2002). Assessing tissue oxygenation. *Critical Care Nurse, 22*(3), 22-24, 26-30, 32-36.

Call-Schmidt, T. (2001). Interpreting lab results: A primer. *MEDSURG Nursing, 10*(4), 179-184.

Capovilla, J. (2000). Noninvasive blood gas monitoring. *Critical Care Nursing Quarterly, 23*(2), 79-86.

Ebersole, P., Hess, P., & Luggen, A. (2004). *Toward healthy aging: Human needs and nursing response* (6th ed.). St. Louis: Mosby.

Gordon, M. (2002). *Manual of nursing diagnosis* (10th ed.). St. Louis: Mosby.

Guyton, A., & Hall, J. (2000). *Textbook of medical physiology* (10th ed.). Philadelphia: W.B. Saunders.

Jarvis, C. (2004). *Physical examination and health assessment* (4th ed.). Philadelphia: W.B. Saunders.

McCance, K., & Huether, S. (2002). *Pathophysiology: The biologic basis for disease in adults and children* (4th ed.). St. Louis: Mosby.

McConnell, E. (2002). Measuring fluid intake and output. *Nursing2002, 32*(7), 17.

Pagana, K., & Pagana, T. (2002). *Mosby's manual of diagnostic and laboratory tests* (2nd ed.). St. Louis: Mosby.

Simmons, J., & Assell, C. (2001). Acid-base basics. *Support Line, 23*(1), 6-11, 24, 28.

Trissel, L. (2003). *Handbook on injectable drugs* (12th ed.). Bethesda, MD: American Society of Health-System Pharmacists.

Wallace, L. (2000). Using color to simplify ABG interpretation. *MEDSURG Nursing, 9*(4), 205-207.

CHAPTER 19

Interventions for Clients with Acid-Base Imbalances

M. LINDA WORKMAN

LEARNING OUTCOMES

After studying this chapter, you should be able to:

1. Identify clients at risk for acidosis.
2. Use laboratory data and clinical manifestations to determine the presence of acidosis.
3. Analyze arterial blood gases to determine whether acidosis is respiratory or metabolic in origin.
4. Analyze arterial blood gases to determine whether respiratory acidosis is acute or chronic.
5. Prioritize nursing care for the client with acute acidosis.
6. Develop a community-based teaching plan to prevent acidosis in the client at continuing risk for acid-base imbalances.
7. Identify clients at risk for alkalosis.
8. Use laboratory data and clinical manifestations to determine the presence of alkalosis.
9. Analyze arterial blood gases to determine whether alkalosis is respiratory or metabolic in origin.
10. Prioritize nursing care for the client with alkalosis.
11. Develop a community-based teaching plan to prevent alkalosis in the client at continuing risk for acid-base imbalances.

Go to your Student CD-ROM for Review Questions for the NCLEX Examination keyed to these Learning Outcomes.

Acid-base imbalances are changes in the blood hydrogen ion level or pH. These changes are caused by problems with the acid-base regulatory mechanisms of the body or by exposure to dangerous conditions. Imbalances in which blood pH is below normal reflect **acidosis,** and imbalances in which blood pH is above normal reflect **alkalosis.** Acid-base imbalances impair the function of many organs and can be life threatening. Table 19-1 lists key points about acid-base imbalances.

ACIDOSIS

PATHOPHYSIOLOGY

In acidosis, the acid-base balance of the blood and other extracellular fluid (ECF) is disturbed by an excess of hydrogen ions (H^+). This problem is reflected as an arterial blood pH below 7.35. The amount or strength (or both) of acids is greater than normal compared with the amount or strength of bases.

Acidosis is not a disease; it is a condition caused by a disorder or pathologic process. Acidosis can be caused by metabolic problems, respiratory problems, or both. Clients at greatest risk for acute acidosis are those with problems that impair breathing. Older adults with chronic health problems are at greater risk for developing acidosis (Chart 19-1).

Acidosis can result from an actual or relative increase in the amount or strength of acids. An actual acid excess results in acidosis by either overproducing acids (and release of hydrogen ions) or undereliminating normally produced acids (retention of hydrogen ions). Examples of problems that increase acid production include diabetic ketoacidosis and seizures. Examples of problems that decrease acid elimination include respiratory or renal impairment.

In *relative* acidosis, the amount or strength of acids does not increase. Instead, the amount or strength (or both) of the bases decreases (to create a *base deficit*), which makes the fluid relatively more acidic than basic. A relative acidosis *(base deficit)* is caused by either overeliminating bases (bicarbonate ions [HCO_3^-]) or underproducing bases (Figure 19-1). Examples of problems that underproduce bases include pancreatitis and dehydration. A condition that overeliminates bases is diarrhea.

Regardless of its origin, acidosis causes major changes in body function. The main problems are related to the fact that hydrogen ions are **cations** (positively charged ions). An

TABLE 19-1 Key Points Related to Acid-Base Imbalances

- Acidosis is an increase in the hydrogen ion concentration (pH) of the blood and is reflected by an arterial blood pH below 7.35.
- Acidosis can result from an actual acid excess or a relative base deficit.
- Metabolic acidosis usually results from a lack of bicarbonate or from excess acid production in the body.
- Respiratory acidosis results from the retention of carbon dioxide in the body, causing increased carbonic acid production.
- Manifestations of acidosis are related to fluid and electrolyte imbalances that accompany acid-base imbalance, such as hyperkalemia.
- Chronic respiratory acidosis is common in the medical-surgical setting as a result of chronic obstructive pulmonary disease, such as emphysema.
- Alkalosis is a decrease in the hydrogen ion concentration of the blood, which is reflected by an arterial blood pH above 7.45.
- Alkalosis can result from an actual base excess or an acid deficit.
- Metabolic alkalosis most often occurs when body acids are lost, such as in prolonged vomiting or nasogastric suctioning.
- Respiratory alkalosis most often occurs when hyperventilation causes excessive loss of carbon dioxide.
- Dehydration and hypokalemia are associated with metabolic alkalosis and account for most of the clinical manifestations seen in this type of acid-base imbalance.
- The goal of management for any type of acid-base imbalance is to restore fluid, electrolyte, and acid-base balance to normal or near-normal.

increase in hydrogen ions creates imbalances of other electrolytes, especially potassium. These electrolyte imbalances then disrupt the functions of nerves, cardiac muscle, and skeletal muscle. The early manifestations of acidosis first appear in the musculoskeletal, cardiac, respiratory, and central nervous systems. Even slight increases in blood hydrogen ion levels reduce the activity of many hormones and enzymes, leading to death. Many drugs are less effective during acidosis.

Acidosis can be caused by metabolic problems, respiratory problems, or combined metabolic and respiratory problems. Specific causes of acidosis are listed in Table 19-2.

Metabolic Acidosis

Four processes can result in metabolic acidosis: overproduction of hydrogen ions, underelimination of hydrogen ions, underproduction of bicarbonate ions, and overelimination of bicarbonate ions.

OVERPRODUCTION OF HYDROGEN IONS

Metabolic processes that increase blood hydrogen ion levels are excessive breakdown of fatty acids, anaerobic glucose breakdown (lactic acidosis), and excessive intake of acids.

Excessive breakdown of fatty acids occurs with diabetic ketoacidosis or starvation. When glucose is not available for fuel, the body breaks down fats (lipids). The products of excessive fatty acid breakdown are strong acids *(ketoacids),* which release large amounts of hydrogen ions.

Anaerobic lactic acidosis occurs when cells are forced to use glucose without adequate oxygen (anaerobic metabolism); as a result, glucose is incompletely broken down and forms lactic acid. Lactic acid molecules leave the cell, enter the blood, and release hydrogen ions, causing acidosis. Lactic acidosis occurs whenever the body has too little oxygen.

CHART 19-1

NURSING FOCUS on the OLDER ADULT
The Older Client Experiencing Acid-Base Imbalance

When Obtaining a Client's History

- Assess risk factors for acid-base imbalance, including medications, chronic health problems (especially renal disease, pulmonary disease), and acute health problems.
- Obtain the history when the client is awake and more familiar with his or her surroundings.
- Ask the client to list all prescribed and over-the-counter medications (especially diuretics and antacids). If the client cannot recall this information or seems confused, ask the significant other to bring medications from home to show the nurse.
- Ask the client to recall what liquids he or she has taken in the past 24 hours and whether he or she has urinated as much as usual.

When Assessing the Client

- Compare the client's mental status with what the family, significant other, or health record states is the client's baseline.
- Observe the rate and depth of respiration.
  - Can the client complete a sentence without stopping to take a breath?
  - Examine the color of the client's nail beds and mucous membranes.
- Obtain a urine specimen and observe for color and character. Test for specific gravity and pH.
- Examine skin turgor for dehydration. Attempt to pinch the skin to form a tent over the sternum and on the forehead. If a tent forms, record how long it remains.
- Measure the rate and quality of the pulse.
- Observe the client's clinical responses and laboratory values carefully while the acid-base imbalance is being corrected.
- Administer IV therapy by pump or controller.

AAABBB	**AAAABBB**	**AAABB**
AAABBB	**AAAABBB**	**AAABB**
AAABBB	**AAAABBB**	**AAABB**
Acid-base balance	Actual acidosis (acid excess)	Relative acidosis (base deficit)

Figure 19-1 ■ Concepts of actual and relative acidosis. **A** = Acid; **B** = base.

Conditions that cause lactic acidosis include heavy exercise, seizure activity, fever, and tissue hypoxia.

Excessive intake of acidic substances floods the body directly with hydrogen ions. Common drugs or agents that cause acidosis when ingested in excess include alcoholic beverages, methyl alcohol (a poison), and acetylsalicylic acid (aspirin).

UNDERELIMINATION OF HYDROGEN IONS

Acidosis can occur when hydrogen ions are produced at the normal rate but are not removed at the same rate they are produced. Most hydrogen ion loss occurs through the lungs and the kidneys. Kidney failure causes acidosis when the kidney tubules cannot secrete hydrogen ions into the urine. As a result, too many hydrogen ions are retained.

UNDERPRODUCTION OF BICARBONATE IONS

As discussed in Chapter 18, bicarbonate is the most common base in the blood and buffers carbonic acid (H_2CO_3). A base-deficit state exists when blood levels of bicarbonate

TABLE 19-2 Common Causes of Acidosis

Pathology	Condition
Metabolic Acidosis	
Overproduction of hydrogen ions	Excessive oxidation of fatty acids ▪ Diabetic ketoacidosis ▪ Starvation Hypermetabolism ▪ Heavy exercise ▪ Seizure activity ▪ Fever ▪ Hypoxia, ischemia Excessive ingestion of acids ▪ Ethanol intoxication ▪ Methanol ingestion ▪ Salicylate intoxication
Underelimination of hydrogen ions	Renal failure
Underproduction of bicarbonate	Renal failure Pancreatitis Liver failure Dehydration
Overelimination of bicarbonate	Diarrhea Buffering of organic acids
Respiratory Acidosis	
Underelimination of hydrogen ions	Respiratory depression ▪ Anesthetics ▪ Drugs (especially opioids) ▪ Poisons ▪ Electrolyte imbalance ▪ Trauma Cerebral edema Spinal cord injuries ▪ Neurologic diseases Guillain-Barré Polio Myasthenia gravis Inadequate chest expansion ▪ Skeletal deformities ▪ Muscle weakness ▪ Nonpulmonary restriction Obesity Fluid Tumor Body casts Chest eschar Airway obstruction ▪ Asthma ▪ Cancer ▪ Bronchiolitis Alveolar-capillary block ▪ Thrombus or embolus ▪ Vascular occlusive disease ▪ Pneumonia ▪ Pulmonary edema ▪ Tuberculosis ▪ Cystic fibrosis ▪ Atelectasis ▪ Acute respiratory distress syndrome (ARDS) ▪ Emphysema ▪ Cancer

are too low. Base-deficit acidosis occurs when hydrogen ion production and removal are normal but too few bicarbonate ions are present to balance the hydrogen ions. Such base deficits occur when bicarbonate ions are not produced at the normal rate. Because bicarbonate is made in the kidneys and in the pancreas, renal failure and reduced hepatic or pancreatic function can cause a base-deficit acidosis (McCance & Huether, 2002).

OVERELIMINATION OF BICARBONATE IONS

Base-deficit acidosis occurs when hydrogen ion production and removal are normal but too many bicarbonate ions have been lost. A common cause of base-deficit acidosis is diarrhea.

Respiratory Acidosis

Respiratory acidosis results when any area of respiratory function is impaired, reducing the exchange of oxygen (O_2) and carbon dioxide (CO_2). This impairment causes carbon dioxide retention. Because any increase in carbon dioxide levels causes a corresponding increase in hydrogen ion levels, carbon dioxide retention leads to acidosis. This relationship is shown by the following carbonic anhydrase equation:

$$\mathbf{CO_2} + H_2O \Longrightarrow H_2CO_3 \Longrightarrow H^+ + HCO_3^-$$

An excess of carbon dioxide forces the equation to the right, first increasing the amount of carbonic acid. The carbonic acid then rapidly separates into hydrogen ions and bicarbonate ions. The increase in free hydrogen ions in the blood is acidosis.

Unlike metabolic acidosis, respiratory acidosis results from only one mechanism: retention of carbon dioxide, causing increased production of free hydrogen ions. All causes of respiratory acidosis lead to an acid-excess acidosis. Four types of problems can cause respiratory acidosis: respiratory depression, inadequate chest expansion, airway obstruction, and reduced alveolar-capillary diffusion.

RESPIRATORY DEPRESSION

Respiratory depression is reduced function of the brainstem neurons that trigger breathing movements. The result is a reduced rate and depth of breathing, which causes poor gas exchange and a retention of carbon dioxide. Respiratory depression may be chemical or physical in origin.

Chemical depression of respiration can occur with anesthetic agents, drugs (especially opioids), and poisons such as methyl alcohol, pesticides, and botulinus toxin that cross the blood-brain barrier. Specific electrolyte imbalances also slow or inhibit these neurons (see Chapter 16 for a discussion of electrolyte imbalances).

Physical depression of respiration occurs in response to many problems. Neurons can be damaged or destroyed by trauma or when problems in other areas of the brain increase the intracranial pressure. Such an increase causes edema, which leads to pressure on the respiratory centers located in the brainstem. Problems causing cerebral edema and respiratory depression include brain tumors, cerebral aneurysm, stroke, overhydration, and hyponatremia.

INADEQUATE CHEST EXPANSION

Any problem that restricts chest movement can reduce gas exchange. Chest expansion can be restricted by skeletal trauma or deformities, respiratory muscle weakness, or external constriction.

Skeletal problems restrict chest wall movement when broken or malformed bones distort the shape of the chest. Broken ribs restrict chest movement because they do not provide the rigid structure needed for chest pressure changes (as in flail chest). Pain from broken ribs may also cause the client to breathe more shallowly.

Respiratory muscle weakness reduces chest movement. This weakness can be caused by electrolyte imbalances, fatigue, muscular dystrophy, muscle damage or breakdown, and inflammatory myositis.

External conditions also can restrict the chest movement needed for full lung expansion. Causes of restricted chest movement include body cast enclosure of the chest, tight scar tissue around the chest, severe obesity, abdominal masses, ascites, and **hemothorax** (blood in the thoracic cavity).

AIRWAY OBSTRUCTION

Prevention of air movement into and out from the lungs through airway obstruction leads to poor gas exchange, carbon dioxide retention, and acidosis. The upper airway can be obstructed externally by clothing, neck edema, and local lymph node enlargement. Internal obstruction of the upper airway can be caused by aspiration of foreign objects, constriction of bronchial smooth muscles, and edema. Internal obstruction of the lower airways is caused by smooth muscle constriction, edema, and excessive mucus, all of which occur in asthma, bronchiolitis, and emphysema.

REDUCED ALVEOLAR-CAPILLARY DIFFUSION

Gas exchange in the lungs occurs by diffusion at the point where the alveolar membranes and capillary membranes meet. Any problem that prevents or slows diffusion causes carbon dioxide retention and acidosis. Some disorders that reduce diffusion include pneumonia, fluid aspiration, pneumonitis, tuberculosis, emphysema, acute respiratory distress syndrome, chest trauma, pulmonary emboli, and pulmonary edema.

Combined Metabolic and Respiratory Acidosis

Metabolic and respiratory acidosis can occur at the same time. Uncorrected acute respiratory acidosis always leads to **anaerobic** (lacking adequate oxygen) metabolism and lactic acidosis (McCance & Huether, 2002). Combined acidosis is more severe than either metabolic acidosis or respiratory acidosis alone. Cardiac arrest is an example of a problem leading to combined metabolic and respiratory acidosis.

◆ COLLABORATIVE MANAGEMENT

The Concept Map below addresses assessment and nursing care issues related to respiratory acidosis.

CONCEPT MAP Respiratory Acidosis (COPD Related)

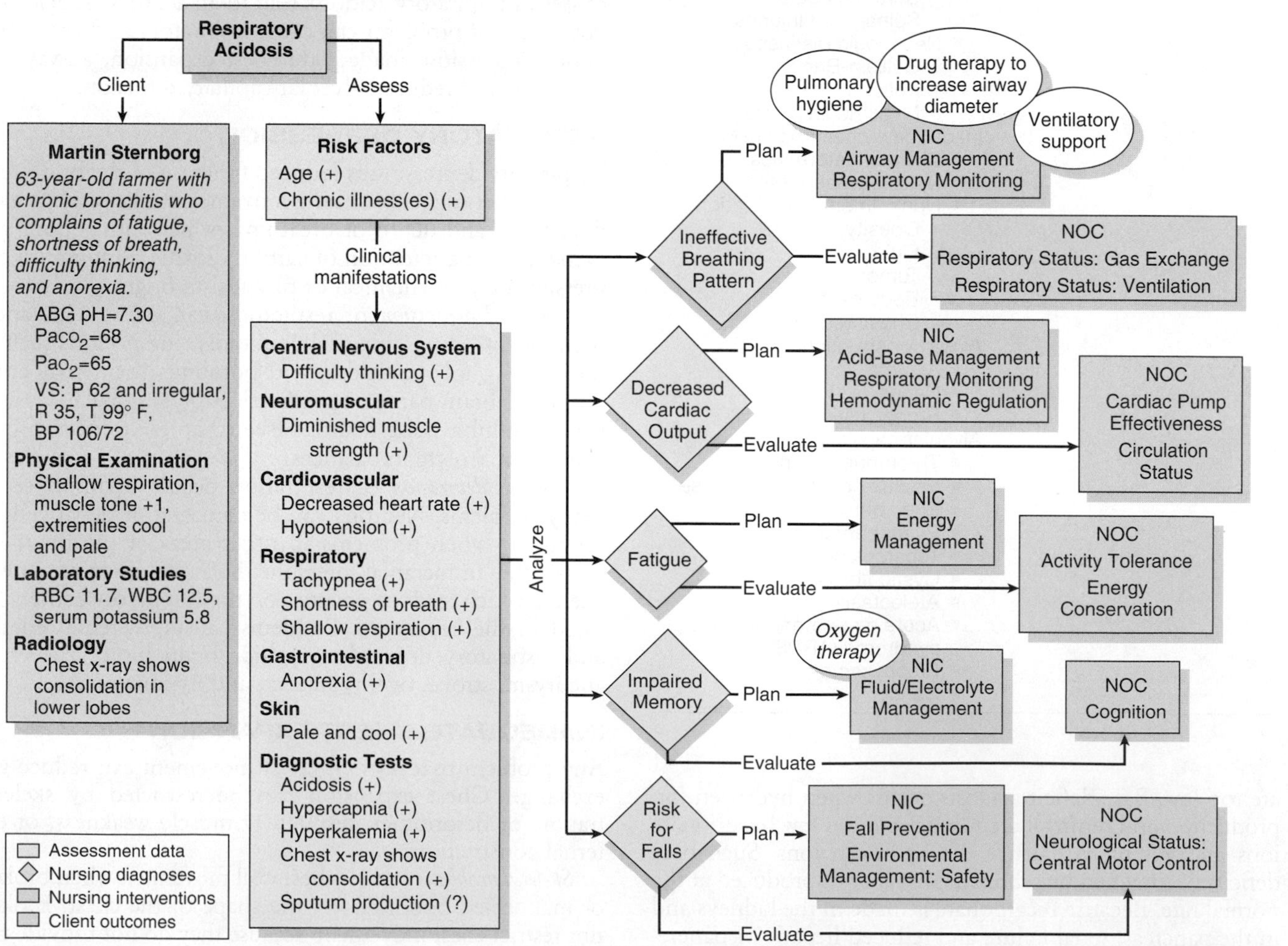

Concept Map by Elaine Bishop Kennedy, EdD, RN

Assessment

HISTORY

When taking the history from any client, collect data about risk factors related to the development of acidosis, specifically age, nutrition, and presenting symptoms.

Older adults are more at risk for problems leading to acid-base imbalance, including cardiac, renal, or pulmonary impairment. In addition, older adults are more likely to be taking drugs that disrupt acid-base, fluid, and electrolyte balance, especially diuretics and aspirin. Ask about specific risk factors, such as any type of breathing problem, kidney failure, diabetes mellitus, diarrhea, pancreatitis, and fever.

Obtain a detailed diet history to determine total caloric intake and the proportions of carbohydrates, fats, and proteins ingested. Ask the client specifically whether he or she has fasted or followed a strict diet within the past week.

Ask the client if he or she has had headaches, behavior changes, increased drowsiness, reduced alertness, reduced attention span, lethargy, anorexia, abdominal distention, nausea or vomiting, muscle weakness, or increased fatigue. Having the client relate activities of the previous 24 hours may help identify activity intolerance, behavior changes, and unexplained fatigue. Because the central nervous system is often depressed in acidosis, you may need to obtain this information from the client's family.

PHYSICAL ASSESSMENT/CLINICAL MANIFESTATIONS

The key clinical manifestations of acidosis are similar whether the cause is metabolic or respiratory (Chart 19-2). Clinical manifestations appear as changes in excitable membrane activity in neurons, skeletal muscle, and gastric smooth muscle.

CHART 19-2

KEY FEATURES of Acidosis

Central Nervous System Manifestations
- Depressed activity (lethargy, confusion, stupor, and coma)

Neuromuscular Manifestations
- Hyporeflexia
- Skeletal muscle weakness
- Flaccid paralysis

Cardiovascular Manifestations
- Delayed electrical conduction
  - Ranges from bradycardia to heart block
  - Tall T waves
  - Widened QRS complex
  - Prolonged PR interval
- Hypotension
- Thready peripheral pulses

Respiratory Manifestations
- Kussmaul respirations (in metabolic acidosis with respiratory compensation)
- Variable respirations (generally ineffective in respiratory acidosis)

Integumentary Manifestations
- Warm, flushed, dry skin in metabolic acidosis
- Pale to cyanotic and dry skin in respiratory acidosis

CENTRAL NERVOUS SYSTEM MANIFESTATIONS. Depression of central nervous system function is common and may range from lethargy to confusion, especially in older clients. As acidosis worsens, the client may become stuporous and unresponsive. Assess the client's mental status (see Chapter 44).

NEUROMUSCULAR MANIFESTATIONS. An increase in blood hydrogen ion levels, along with hyperkalemia, reduces muscle tone and deep tendon reflexes. Assess muscle strength by having the client do the following:
- Squeeze your hand
- Keep his or her arms flexed while you pull down on the lower arms
- Push both feet against a flat surface while you apply resistance

Muscle weakness from acidosis is bilateral and can progress to flaccid paralysis. Breathing is less effective when skeletal muscles become weak.

CARDIOVASCULAR MANIFESTATIONS. The early cardiac manifestations are increased heart rate and cardiac output. With worsening acidosis or with acidosis and hyperkalemia, electrical conduction through the heart is reduced and heart rate decreases. Peripheral pulses may be hard to find and are easily blocked. The client may have hypotension as a result of vasodilation.

RESPIRATORY MANIFESTATIONS. Assess the client's rate, depth, and ease of breathing. Use pulse oximetry to determine how well oxygen is delivered to the peripheral tissues.

If acidosis is metabolic in origin, the rate and depth of breathing increase in proportion to the rising hydrogen ion level. Breaths are deep, rapid, and not under voluntary control. This pattern is called **Kussmaul respiration.**

If acidosis is respiratory in origin, respiratory efforts are reduced. Respirations are usually shallow and rapid.

SKIN MANIFESTATIONS. With metabolic acidosis, breathing is unimpaired and the rate is increased. This increased gas exchange causes vasodilation and makes the client's skin and mucous membranes appear warm, dry, and pink. With respiratory acidosis, breathing is ineffective and skin and mucous membranes are pale to cyanotic.

PSYCHOSOCIAL ASSESSMENT

It is vital to complete a psychosocial assessment, because behavioral changes may be the first clinical manifestations of acidosis. Observe and document the client's behavior by description (objectively) rather than by interpretation (subjectively). For example, you should state that "the client does not recognize close family members" rather than "the client is confused" or state that "the client spit out the oral drugs" rather than "the client is uncooperative." Ask family members if the client's behavior is typical and establish a baseline for comparison with later assessment findings.

LABORATORY ASSESSMENT

Arterial blood pH is the laboratory value used to confirm acidosis. Acidosis is present when arterial blood pH is less than 7.35. However, this test alone does not indicate what is causing the acidosis or its origin. Manifestations of metabolic acidosis and respiratory acidosis are similar, but their treatments are different. Therefore it is critical to obtain and interpret other laboratory data, such as arterial blood gas (ABG) values and blood levels of electrolytes (Chart 19-3).

METABOLIC ACIDOSIS. The following laboratory data indicate metabolic acidosis:

ABGs

Low pH (<7.35)
Low bicarbonate level (<21 mEq/L)
Normal partial pressure of arterial carbon dioxide ($Paco_2$)

Electrolytes

Elevated serum potassium level
Normal chloride levels (acid excess or high anion gap acidosis)
Elevated chloride levels (base deficit or normal anion gap acidosis)

The pH is low because buffering and respiratory compensation are not adequate to keep the amount of free hydrogen ions at a normal level. The bicarbonate level is below normal for any or all of the following reasons.

- Bicarbonate has been lost, causing a base-deficit acidosis.
- Bicarbonate production is inadequate, causing a base-deficit acidosis
- Bicarbonate may be bound to other substances.

The carbon dioxide level is normal or even slightly decreased because gas exchange is adequate and carbon dioxide retention is not a factor. The oxygen level is normal because gas exchange is adequate.

The serum potassium level is often high in acidosis as the body attempts to maintain electroneutrality during buffering. Figure 19-2 shows the movement of potassium ions as serum pH changes. As the blood hydrogen ion level rises, some of the excess hydrogen ions enter red blood cells for intracellular buffering. The movement of hydrogen ions into the cells creates an excess of positive ions inside the cells. To balance these extra positive charges, an equal number of potassium ions move from the cells into the blood. This increases the blood potassium level, causing hyperkalemia.

RESPIRATORY ACIDOSIS. The following laboratory data indicate respiratory acidosis:

ABGs

Low pH (<7.35)
Elevated $Paco_2$
Low partial pressure of arterial oxygen (Pao_2)

Electrolytes

Elevated serum potassium levels
Variable serum bicarbonate levels

CHART 19-3

LABORATORY PROFILE
Acid-Base Imbalances

Imbalance	Laboratory Value Changes						
	pH	HCO_3^-	Pao_2	$Paco_2$	K^+	Ca^{2+}	Cl^-
Metabolic acidosis	↓	↓	Ø	Ø and ↓	↑	Ø	Ø and ↑
Respiratory acidosis	↓	↑	↓	↑	↑	Ø	↑↓
Combined acidosis	↓	↓↑	↓	↑	↑	Ø	↑
Metabolic alkalosis	↑	↑	Ø	Ø and ↑	↓	↓	↓
Respiratory alkalosis	↑	↓	Ø	↓↓	↓	↓	↑
Combined alkalosis	↑	↑	Ø	↓	↓	↓	↓

↑, Above normal; ↓, below normal; ↑↓, value can increase or decrease depending on other factors; Ø, normal; HCO_3^-, bicarbonate ions; Pao_2, partial pressure of arterial oxygen; $Paco_2$, partial pressure of arterial carbon dioxide; K^+, potassium ions; Ca^{2+}, calcium ions; Cl^-, chloride ions.

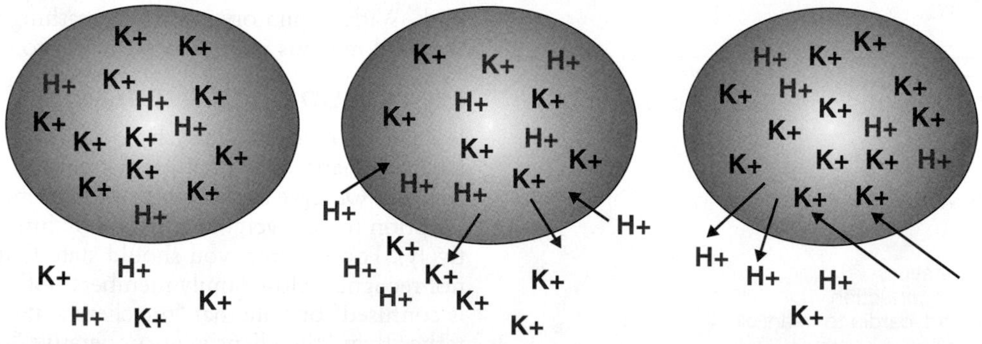

Under normal conditions, the intracellular potassium content is much greater than that of the extracellular fluid. The concentration of hydrogen ions is low in both compartments.

In acidosis, the extracellular hydrogen ion content increases, and the hydrogen ions move into the intracellular fluid. To keep the intracellular fluid electrically neutral, an equal number of potassium ions leave the cell, creating a relative hyperkalemia.

In alkalosis, more hydrogen ions are present in the intracellular fluid than in the extracellular fluid. Hydrogen ions move from the intracellular fluid into the extracellular fluid. To keep the intracellular fluid electrically neutral, potassium ions move from the extracellular fluid into the intracellular fluid, creating a relative hypokalemia.

Figure 19-2 ■ Movement of potassium in response to changes in the extracellular fluid hydrogen ion concentration. (© M. Linda Workman. All rights reserved.)

The pH is lowered by the increased amount of free hydrogen ions in the blood. If the kidneys partially compensate for this acidosis, pH is low but not as abnormal as could be expected with the degree of carbon dioxide retention. A client with rapid onset of respiratory acidosis usually has a normal bicarbonate level because kidney compensation has not started. When respiratory acidosis persists for 24 hours or longer, kidney compensation increases the production and retention of bicarbonate. Chronic respiratory acidosis is indicated by an elevated bicarbonate level and increased $Paco_2$.

$Paco_2$ is high and Pao_2 is low because the pulmonary problem impairs gas exchange, causing carbon dioxide retention and poor oxygenation. Carbon dioxide is 20 times more diffusible than is oxygen across the alveolar membrane. Therefore a decreased Pao_2 usually occurs before an increased $Paco_2$.

Serum potassium levels are elevated in acute respiratory acidosis. They are normal or low in chronic respiratory acidosis when renal compensation is present.

Critical Thinking Challenge

The client is a 65-year-old woman with type 1 diabetes mellitus and pneumonia. Her vital signs on admission are as follows: T 103.4; P 122, thready; R 34, shallow.

Her urine is positive for ketones. Her arterial blood gases (ABGs) are as follows: pH 7.21; HCO_3^- 22 mEq/L; $Paco_2$ 50 mm Hg; Pao_2 78 mm Hg.

1. What type of acid-base imbalance is present?
2. Is the origin of the imbalance metabolic or respiratory? Explain your answer.
3. Is compensation present or not present? Explain your answer.

evolve For suggested answer guidelines, go to http://evolve.elsevier.com/Iggy/.

Common Nursing Diagnoses and Collaborative Problems

Nursing diagnoses and collaborative problems that may apply to clients with acidosis include the following:

- Deficient Fluid Volume related to dehydration
- Decreased Cardiac Output related to poor cardiac contractility and decreased vascular volume
- Risk for Falls related to skeletal muscle weakness
- Impaired Memory related to fluid and electrolyte imbalances
- Ineffective Breathing Pattern related to reduced gas exchange
- Fatigue related to inadequate tissue oxygenation

Interventions

Interventions for acidosis focus on correcting the underlying problem, increasing aerobic metabolism, and monitoring for changes (Chart 19-4). To ensure appropriate interventions, the specific type of acidosis must first be identified.

METABOLIC ACIDOSIS. Interventions for metabolic acidosis include hydration and drugs or treatments to control the problem causing the acidosis. For example, if the acidosis is a result of diabetic ketoacidosis, insulin is given to correct the hyperglycemia and halt the production of ketone bodies. Rehydration and antidiarrheal drugs are given if the acidosis is a result of prolonged diarrhea. *Bicarbonate is administered only if serum bicarbonate levels are low.*

RESPIRATORY ACIDOSIS. Interventions aim to maintain a patent airway and enhance gas exchange. Such interventions can include drug therapy, oxygen therapy, pulmonary hygiene (positioning and breathing techniques), ventilatory support, and prevention of complications. (See Chapter 33 for a complete discussion of common disorders causing respiratory acidosis.)

Drug Therapy. Drug therapy includes agents to increase the diameter of upper and lower airways and to thin pulmonary secretions. Drug therapy is not aimed directly at altering arterial pH.

Drugs to Increase Airway Diameter. Drugs that relax bronchial smooth muscle increase airway diameter. Many of these agents are adrenergic agonists and methylxanthines. Examples of these drugs include albuterol (Novo-Salmol✱, Proventil, Ventolin), ephedrine, fenoterol (Berotec✱), isoproterenol (Isuprel), metaproterenol (Alupent), pirbuterol (Maxair), terbutaline (Brethine, Bricanyl),

CHART 19-4

NIC INTERVENTION ACTIVITIES for The Client with Acidosis

Acid-Base Management: Metabolic Acidosis: *Promotion of acid-base balance and prevention of complications resulting from serum bicarbonate levels lower than desired*

- Monitor ABG levels for decreasing pH level, as appropriate.
- Maintain patent IV access.
- Monitor intake and output.
- Monitor determinants of tissue oxygen delivery (e.g., Pao_2, Sao_2, and hemoglobin levels and cardiac output), if available.
- Monitor loss of bicarbonate through the GI tract (e.g., diarrhea, pancreatic fistula, small bowel fistula, and ileal conduit), as appropriate.
- Administer fluids as prescribed.
- Administer insulin and fluid hydration (isotonic and hypotonic) for diabetic ketoacidosis, causing metabolic acidosis, as appropriate.
- Prepare client for dialysis (e.g., assist with catheter placement for dialysis), as appropriate.
- Institute seizure precautions.

Acid-Base Management: Respiratory Acidosis: *Promotion of acid-base balance and prevention of complications resulting from serum pCO_2 levels higher than desired*

- Monitor ABG levels for decreasing pH level, as appropriate.
- Monitor determinants of tissue oxygen delivery (e.g., Pao_2, Sao_2, and hemoglobin levels and cardiac output), if available.
- Monitor for symptoms of respiratory failure (e.g., low Pao_2 and elevated $Paco_2$ levels and respiratory muscle fatigue).
- Monitor work of breathing (e.g., respiratory rate, heart rate, use of accessory muscles, and diaphoresis).
- Provide low-carbohydrate, high-fat diet (e.g., Pulmocare feedings) to reduce CO_2 production, if indicated.
- Monitor neurologic status (e.g., level of consciousness and confusion).

NIC intervention activities selected from Dochterman, J.M., & Bulechek, G.M. (Eds.). (2004). *Nursing interventions classification (NIC)* (4th ed.). St. Louis: Mosby. No part of this work is to be altered without prior written permission from the Publisher.

ABG, Arterial blood gas; *GI,* gastrointestinal; *Pao_2,* partial pressure of arterial oxygen; *Sao_2,* arterial oxygen saturation; *$Paco_2$,* partial pressure of arterial carbon dioxide.

aminophylline (Phyllocontin, Truphylline), and theophylline (Bronkodyl, Theo-Dur).

Some drugs increase bronchodilation by reducing the inflammation of bronchial luminal tissues. These agents are cortisol (steroid) based, such as beclomethasone (Vanceril, Beclovent), dexamethasone (Dexasone), flunisolide (Aero-Bid, Bronalide✱), and triamcinolone (Azmacort).

Drugs to Thin Bronchial Secretions. Some drugs can break up mucus when thick, sticky lung secretions obstruct airways. These agents are mucolytics; one example is acetylcysteine (Mucomyst, Mucosil). (See Chapter 33 for a discussion of drugs used for chronic airflow limitation [CAL].)

Oxygen Therapy. Oxygen therapy helps promote gas exchange for clients with respiratory acidosis. However, you must use caution when giving oxygen to clients with chronic obstructive pulmonary disease (COPD) and carbon dioxide retention as evidenced by a high $Paco_2$ level. The only breathing trigger for these clients is a decreased arterial oxygen level. Giving too much oxygen to these clients decreases their respiratory drive and may lead to respiratory arrest.

Pulmonary Hygiene. To promote effective gas exchange, use positioning techniques to enhance the removal of lung secretions, and specific breathing techniques to change airway resistance, keeping alveoli inflated. Help the client assume a Fowler's or semi-Fowler's position to increase lung expansion. Increasing fluid intake may reduce the thickness of lung secretions and assist in their removal.

Ventilation Support. Mechanical ventilation may be needed for clients who are unable to keep their oxygen saturation at 90% or who have respiratory muscle fatigue. Chapters 31 and 35 discuss the criteria for mechanical ventilation and the nursing care needs of clients who are being mechanically ventilated.

Prevention of Complications. Monitoring clients' breathing status is critical in preventing complications. For clients experiencing chronic respiratory acidosis, assess breathing status at least every 2 hours. Auscultate breath sounds and assess the ease with which air moves into and out of the lungs. Examine the client for any muscle retractions, the use of accessory muscles, and whether breathing produces a sound that can be heard without a stethoscope. Assess the color of the nail beds and mucous membranes for cyanosis (a late finding).

Critical Thinking Challenge

The diabetic client with ketoacidosis and respiratory acidosis caused by pneumonia is started on insulin therapy and antibiotic therapy.

1. Should this client receive oxygen therapy? Why or why not?
2. Should this client receive intravenous bicarbonate? Why or why not?
3. What electrolyte imbalance should you be alert for with this client?

evolve For suggested answer guidelines, go to http://evolve.elsevier.com/Iggy/.

TABLE 19-3 Common Causes of Alkalosis

Pathology	Condition
Metabolic Alkalosis	
Increase of base components	Oral ingestion of bases ▪ Antacids ▪ Milk-alkali syndrome Parenteral base administration ▪ Blood transfusion ▪ Sodium bicarbonate ▪ Total parenteral nutrition
Decrease of acid components	Prolonged vomiting Nasogastric suctioning Cushing's syndrome or disease (hypercortisolism) Hyperaldosteronism Thiazide diuretics
Respiratory Alkalosis	
Excessive loss of carbon dioxide	Hyperventilation ▪ Fear ▪ Anxiety ▪ Mechanical ventilation ▪ Central nervous system stimulation Salicylates Catecholamines Progesterone Hypoxemia ▪ Asphyxiation ▪ High altitudes ▪ Shock ▪ Early-stage pulmonary problems Pneumonia Asthma Pulmonary emboli

ALKALOSIS

PATHOPHYSIOLOGY

In clients with alkalosis, the acid-base balance of the blood is disturbed and has an excess of bases, especially bicarbonate (HCO_3^-). The amount or strength (or both) of the bases is greater than normal compared with the amount or strength of the acids. Alkalosis is a decrease in the free hydrogen ion level of the blood and is reflected by an arterial blood pH above 7.45. Like acidosis, alkalosis is not a disease but rather a manifestation of a problem. Alkalosis can be caused by metabolic problems, respiratory problems, or both (Table 19-3).

Alkalosis can result from an actual or relative increase in the amount or strength (or both) of bases. In an actual base excess, alkalosis occurs when base (usually bicarbonate) is either overproduced or undereliminated.

In *relative* alkalosis, the actual amount or strength of bases does not increase. Instead, the amount or strength (or both) of the acids decreases, creating an *acid deficit* and making the blood more basic than acidic. A relative base-excess alkalosis (acid deficit) results from an overelimination or underproduction of acids (Figure 19-3).

The problems of alkalosis are serious and potentially life threatening. Treatment is aimed at correcting the cause of alkalosis after identifying whether it is respiratory or metabolic in origin.

Whether metabolic, respiratory, or both, alkalosis greatly affects specific functions. The pathologic effects are caused by the electrolyte imbalances that occur in response to decreased blood cation levels. The most common problems of alkalosis are related to increased stimulation of the central nervous, neuromuscular, and cardiovascular systems.

Metabolic Alkalosis

Most conditions that result in metabolic alkalosis create the acid-base imbalance through either an increase of bases (base excess) or a decrease of acids (acid deficit).

AAABBB AAABBB AAABBB	AAABBBB AAABBBB AAABBBB	AABBB AABBB AABBB
Acid-base balance	Actual alkalosis (base excess)	Relative alkalosis (acid deficit)

Figure 19-3 ■ Concepts of actual and relative alkalosis. **A** = Acid; **B** = base.

BASE EXCESS

Increases in bases are caused by excessive intake of bicarbonates, carbonates, acetates, citrates, and lactates. Excessive use of oral antacids containing sodium bicarbonate or calcium carbonate can also cause a metabolic alkalosis. Other base excesses can occur during medical treatments, such as citrate excesses during massive blood transfusions, acetate and lactate excesses during hyperalimentation, and IV sodium bicarbonate given to correct acidosis.

ACID DEFICIT

Decreases in acids can be caused by disease processes or medical treatment. Other causes include prolonged vomiting, excess cortisol, and hyperaldosteronism. Medical treatments that promote acid loss causing metabolic alkalosis include thiazide diuretics and prolonged nasogastric suctioning.

Respiratory Alkalosis

The main problem that causes respiratory alkalosis is excessive loss of carbon dioxide through hyperventilation (rapid respirations). Clients may hyperventilate in response to anxiety, fear, or improper settings on mechanical ventilators. Hyperventilation can also result from direct stimulation of central respiratory centers because of fever, metabolic acidosis, central nervous system lesions, and drugs (e.g., salicylates, catecholamines, and progesterone).

◆COLLABORATIVE MANAGEMENT

◆Assessment

PHYSICAL ASSESSMENT/CLINICAL MANIFESTATIONS

Clinical manifestations are the same for metabolic or respiratory alkalosis. Many symptoms are the result of the hypocalcemia (low calcium levels) and hypokalemia (low potassium levels) that usually occur with alkalosis (see Figure 19-2). These problems change the function of the central nervous, neuromuscular, cardiovascular, and respiratory systems (Chart 19-5).

CENTRAL NERVOUS SYSTEM MANIFESTATIONS. Overexcitement of the central and peripheral nervous systems is the major cause of the symptoms associated with alkalosis. Clients have dizziness, agitation, confusion, and hyperreflexia, which may progress to seizure activity. Tingling or numbness around the mouth and in the toes may be present. Other indicators of alkalosis with hypocalcemia are positive Chvostek's and Trousseau's signs (see Chapter 16).

NEUROMUSCULAR MANIFESTATIONS. Alkalosis occurs with hypocalcemia and hypokalemia, both of which alter neuromuscular function. Hypocalcemia increases nervous system activity, causing muscle cramps, twitches, and charley horses. Deep tendon reflexes are hyperactive. **Tetany** (continuous contractions) of muscle groups also may be present. Tetany is painful and indicates a rapidly worsening condition.

CHART 19-5

KEY FEATURES of
Alkalosis

Central Nervous System Manifestations
- Increased activity
- Anxiety, irritability, tetany, seizures
- Positive Chvostek's sign
- Positive Trousseau's sign
- Paresthesias

Neuromuscular Manifestations
- Hyperreflexia
- Muscle cramping and twitching
- Skeletal muscle weakness

Cardiovascular Manifestations
- Increased heart rate
- Normal or low blood pressure
- Increased digitalis toxicity

Respiratory Manifestations
- Increased rate and depth of ventilation in respiratory alkalosis
- Decreased respiratory effort associated with skeletal muscle weakness in metabolic alkalosis

Skeletal muscles may contract as a result of nerve overstimulation, but they become weaker because of the hypokalemia. Handgrip strength decreases, and the client may be unable to stand or walk. Respiratory efforts become less effective as the skeletal muscles of respiration weaken.

CARDIOVASCULAR MANIFESTATIONS. Alkalosis increases myocardial irritability, especially when accompanied by hypokalemia. Heart rate increases and the pulse is thready. When hypovolemia (decreased blood volume) is also present, the client may have severe hypotension. The hypokalemia occurring with alkalosis increases myocardial sensitivity to digoxin, which increases the risk for digoxin toxicity.

RESPIRATORY MANIFESTATIONS. Increases in the rate and depth of breathing are the main causes of respiratory alkalosis. Tidal volume (the volume of air inhaled and exhaled with each breath) is nearly normal, but minute volume (the total volume of air inhaled and exhaled in 1 minute) rises with the increased respiratory rate. The increased minute volume may be caused by anxiety or physiologic changes.

LABORATORY ASSESSMENT

Arterial blood pH greater than 7.45 confirms alkalosis, but this test alone does not identify its cause. Because the manifestations of metabolic alkalosis and respiratory alkalosis are similar, it is critical to obtain additional laboratory data, especially arterial blood gas (ABG) values and specific serum electrolytes levels (see Chart 19-3).

METABOLIC ALKALOSIS. The following laboratory data indicate metabolic alkalosis:

ABGs

High pH (>7.45)
Elevated bicarbonate level (>28 mEq/L)
Rising partial pressure of arterial carbon dioxide ($Paco_2$)
Normal partial pressure of arterial oxygen (Pao_2)

Electrolytes

Decreased serum potassium levels
Decreased serum calcium levels

The pH is high because buffering and respiratory compensation are not adequate to maintain the free hydrogen ion level within the normal range. *The hallmark of metabolic alkalosis is an increased bicarbonate level with a rising* $PaCO_2$. The rising $PaCO_2$ compensates for the decreased hydrogen ion level. The serum potassium level decreases as hydrogen ions move out from cells and potassium from the blood moves into cells (see Figure 19-2). As the pH increases, calcium binding increases and the serum calcium level decreases, causing hypocalcemia. Most of the serious problems of alkalosis are caused by the resulting hypocalcemia.

RESPIRATORY ALKALOSIS. The following laboratory data indicate respiratory alkalosis:

ABGs

High pH
Low bicarbonate level
Low $PaCO_2$

Electrolytes

Low serum potassium level
Low serum calcium level

The pH is high because buffering and renal compensation cannot maintain the hydrogen ions at a normal level.

The classic respiratory alkalosis profile is a reduced bicarbonate level (not usually less than 15 mEq/L) along with a very low $PaCO_2$. The carbon dioxide level is low because it is being exhaled more rapidly than it is being produced. The bicarbonate level is low in response to the pH increase. Many blood and cellular buffers release hydrogen ions that combine with the blood bicarbonate ions and form carbonic acid, thus reducing the blood level of bicarbonate.

As in metabolic alkalosis, the blood potassium level is reduced as the body attempts to maintain electroneutrality. Again, as the pH increases, calcium binding increases and the blood level of calcium decreases, causing hypocalcemia.

Common Nursing Diagnoses and Collaborative Problems

Nursing diagnoses and collaborative problems that may apply to clients with alkalosis include the following:

- Acute Pain related to muscle spasms
- Acute Confusion related to excess central nervous system excitation
- Risk for Falls related to skeletal muscle weakness and hypotension

Interventions

Interventions are planned to prevent further losses of hydrogen, potassium, calcium, and chloride ions; to restore fluid balance; and to monitor changes (Chart 19-6).

Drug therapy is used for alkalosis. Drugs are prescribed to resolve the causes of alkalosis and to restore normal fluid, electrolyte, and acid-base balance. For example, the client with metabolic alkalosis caused by diuretic therapy receives fluid and electrolyte replacement. Antiemetic drugs are prescribed if the client is vomiting. Fluids and electrolytes are replaced orally or parenterally. Carefully monitor the client's progress and adjust fluid and electrolyte therapy. Serum electrolyte values are monitored daily until they return to normal or near normal.

CHART 19-6

NIC INTERVENTION ACTIVITIES for The Client with Alkalosis

Acid-Base Management: Metabolic Alkalosis: *Promotion of acid-base balance and prevention of complications resulting from serum* HCO_3 *levels higher than desired*

- Monitor ABG levels for increased pH level.
- Maintain patent IV access.
- Monitor intake and output.
- Monitor determinants of tissue oxygen delivery (e.g., PaO_2, SaO_2, and hemoglobin levels and cardiac output), if available.
- Avoid administration of alkaline substances (e.g., IV sodium bicarbonate and PO or NG antacids) as appropriate.
- Monitor for electrolyte imbalances associated with metabolic alkalosis (e.g., hypokalemia, hypocalcemia, and hypochloremia), as appropriate.
- Monitor for renal loss of acid (e.g., diuretic therapy), as appropriate.
- Replace extracellular fluid deficit with IV saline, as appropriate.
- Administer antiemetics to reduce loss of HCl in emesis, as appropriate.

Acid-Base Management: Respiratory Alkalosis: *Promotion of acid-base balance and prevention of complications resulting from serum* pCO_2 *levels lower than desired*

- Monitor ABG levels for increased pH level.
- Monitor for indications of impending respiratory failure (e.g., low PaO_2 level, respiratory muscle fatigue, low SaO_2/SvO_2 level).
- Monitor for hyperventilation resulting in respiratory alkalosis (e.g., hypoxemia, CNS injury, hypermetabolic states, GI distention, pain, and stress).
- Monitor for cardiopulmonary manifestations of respiratory alkalosis (e.g., arrhythmias, decreased cardiac output, and hyperventilation).
- Provide oxygen therapy, if necessary.
- Reduce oxygen consumption to minimize hyperventilation (e.g., promote comfort, control fever, and reduce anxiety), as appropriate.
- Provide mechanical ventilatory support, if necessary.

NIC intervention activities selected from Dochterman J.M., & Bulechek, G.M. (Eds.). (*2004*). *Nursing interventions classification (NIC)* (4th ed.). St. Louis: Mosby.

ABG, Arterial blood gas; *HCO_3*, bicarbonate; *PaO_2*, partial pressure of arterial oxygen; *SaO_2*, arterial oxygen saturation; *SvO_2*, venous oxygen saturation; *$PaCO_2$*, partial pressure of arterial carbon dioxide; *GI*, gastrointestinal.

GET READY for the NCLEX Examination!

KEY POINTS

Safe Effective Care Environment

- Use caution in giving oxygen to people who have COPD.
- Assess and document the condition of the site from which an arterial blood gas sample was obtained at least every 2 hours for the first 24 hours.

Health Promotion and Maintenance

- Teach all clients to take drugs as prescribed, especially diuretics, antihypertensives, and cardiac drugs.
- Instruct all clients at continuing risk for respiratory acidosis to stop smoking.
- Assist clients interested in smoking cessation to find an appropriate smoking cessation program.

Psychosocial Integrity

- Assess the oxygenation status of any client with acute confusion.
- Monitor the neurologic status at least every 2 hours in clients being treated for an acid-base imbalance.
- Assist clients who have anxiety-induced respiratory alkalosis to identify causes of anxiety.
- Teach clients who have anxiety-induced respiratory alkalosis to use stress management techniques.

Physiological Integrity

- Check the serum potassium level for any client who has acidosis.
- Assess heart rate and rhythm at least every 2 hours for any client with an acid-base imbalance.
- Assess the airway of any client who has acute respiratory acidosis.
- Monitor arterial blood gas values to evaluate the effectiveness of therapy for acid-base imbalances.
- Assess the oxygenation status of any client with acidosis.
- Provide a low carbohydrate, high-fat diet to the client with chronic respiratory acidosis.

ADDITIONAL STUDY RESOURCES

Go to your Student CD-ROM for Review Questions for the NCLEX Examination.

evolve Go to http://evolve.elsevier.com/Iggy/ for Integrated Management of Care Questions for the NCLEX Examination.

SELECTED BIBLIOGRAPHY

Banker, D., Whittier, F., & Rutecki, G. (2003). Acid-base disturbances: 5 rules that can simplify diagnosis. *Consultant, 43*(3), 381, 386-388.

Berry, B., & Pinard, A. (2002). Assessing tissue oxygenation. *Critical Care Nurse, 22*(3), 22-24, 26-30, 32-36.

Call-Schmidt, T. (2001). Interpreting lab results: A primer. *MEDSURG Nursing, 10*(4), 179-184.

Dochterman, J.M., & Bulechek, G.M. (Eds.). (2004). *Nursing interventions classification (NIC)* (4th ed.). St. Louis: Mosby.

Epstein, S., & Singh, N. (2001). Respiratory acidosis. *Respiratory Care, 46*(4), 366-383.

Foster, G., Vaziri, N., & Sassoon, C. (2001). Respiratory alkalosis. *Respiratory Care, 46*(4), 384-391.

Isenhour, J., Slovis, C. (2001). Arterial blood gas analysis: A simple, 3 step approach: Co-oximetry is required for patients with CO poisoning. *Journal of Respiratory Diseases, 22*(5), 289-292, 295-296.

Khanna, A., & Kurtzman, N. (2001). Metabolic alkalosis. *Respiratory Care, 46*(4), 354-365.

Kischner, M. (2002). Additional step in ABG analysis (letter to the editor in response to the Berry & Pinard article). *Critical Care Nurse, 22*(5), 16-17.

Kraut, J., & Madias, N. (2001). Approach to patients with acid-base disorders. *Respiratory Care, 46*(4), 392-403.

McCance, K., & Huether, S. (2002). *Pathophysiology: The biologic basis for disease in adults and children* (4th ed.). St. Louis: Mosby.

McConnell, E. (2002). Measuring fluid intake and output. *Nursing2002, 32*(7), 17.

O'Neill, D. (2001). Making sense of arterial blood gases. *Nursing Times, 97*(27), 36-37, 39.

Pagana, K., & Pagana, T. (2002). *Mosby's manual of diagnostic and laboratory tests* (2nd ed.). St. Louis: Mosby.

Paulson, W. (2000). Problem solving in acid-base diagnosis. Case study: From acid-base disorders to clinical diagnosis. *Journal of Critical Illness, 15*(2), 113-117.

Shoulders-Odom, B. (2000). Using an algorithm to interpret arterial blood gases. *DCCM - Dimensions of Critical Care Nursing, 19*(1), 36-41.

Swenson, E. (2001). Metabolic acidosis. *Respiratory Care, 46*(4), 342-353.

Trissel, L. (2003). *Handbook on injectable drugs* (12th ed.). Bethesda, MD: American Society of Health-System Pharmacists.

UNIT **FIVE**

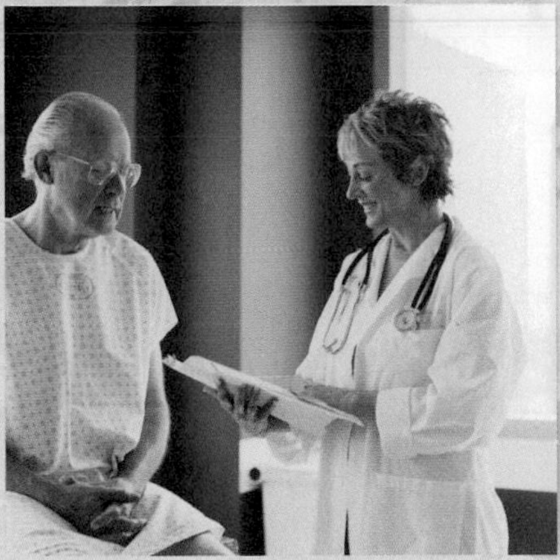

MANAGEMENT of PERIOPERATIVE CLIENTS

CHAPTER

20 Interventions for Preoperative Clients

REBECCA M. PATTON

LEARNING OUTCOMES

After studying this chapter, you should be able to:

1. Differentiate among the various types and purposes of surgery.
2. Identify personal factors that increase the client's risk for complications during and immediately following surgery.
3. Use effective communication when teaching clients and family members about what to expect during the surgical experience.
4. Assume the role of client advocate.
5. Perform an accurate preoperative assessment of the client's physical and psychosocial status.
6. Identify laboratory value changes that may affect the client's response to drugs, anesthesia, and surgery.
7. Describe the legal implications and proper procedures for obtaining informed consent.
8. Explain the purposes and techniques commonly used for client preoperative preparation.
9. Prioritize teaching needs for the client preparing for surgery.
10. Recognize client conditions or issues that need to be communicated to the surgical and postoperative teams.

Go to your Student CD-ROM for Review Questions for the NCLEX Examination keyed to these Learning Outcomes.

Any client undergoing surgery today receives the benefits of advances in surgical techniques, anesthesia, pharmacology, medical devices, and many supportive interventions. Research defining best practices has resulted in improved outcomes in all areas of the perioperative experience. The technology explosion is responsible for the development of new diagnostic and interventional devices for the use and refinement of new surgical techniques. Examples of such technical advances include the GAMMA knife for brain tumor resections, robotics, and other types of minimally invasive surgeries. Advances in anesthetic agents and techniques also have developed. These changes improve the ways that a surgical client is treated and has made anesthesia safer than ever before.

Cost reduction initiatives by third-party payers are also a driving force as to how the health care community manages the surgical client. Shortened stays and outpatient treatment have become the expected. Ambulatory surgical services are common, with more clients being admitted as inpatients *after* a procedure, rather than before. Some clients may only be observed after surgery and may not be admitted as an inpatient. In response to the ongoing health care delivery changes and the use of multiple settings, nurses have modified their interventions, remaining focused on client care before **(preoperative)**, during **(intraoperative)**, and after **(postoperative)** surgery.

OVERVIEW

The preoperative period begins when the client is scheduled for surgery and ends at the time of transfer to the surgical suite. As a nurse, you must act as an educator, an advocate, and a promoter of health. The surgical environment demands the use of knowledge, judgment, and skills based on the principles of nursing science. Perioperative nursing places special emphasis on safety and client education.

The client's readiness for surgery is critical to the outcome. Care before surgery focuses on client readiness. This care includes education and any intervention needed before surgery to reduce anxiety and complications and to promote cooperation in procedures after surgery. Use adult teaching and learning principles in teaching clients and families before surgery. It is important to validate and clarify information the client has received from the surgeon or other members of the surgical team. In addition, during assessment before surgery it is not uncommon to identify problems that warrant further client assessment and/or intervention before the procedure. Communication and collaboration with the surgical team is essential so that correct actions are taken to achieve the desired outcome.

Categories and Purposes of Surgery

Surgical procedures are categorized according to the following:

- The reason for the surgery
- The urgency of the procedure
- The degree of risk
- The anatomic location
- The extent of surgery required

The primary purposes, or reasons, for surgery can be divided into five general subcategories: diagnostic, curative, restorative, palliative, and cosmetic. **Palliative surgery** makes the client more comfortable, and **cosmetic surgery** reconstructs the skin and underlying structures. The urgency of the procedure can be elective, urgent, and emergent. The degree of risk is classified as minor or major.

Category by location is based on the area of the body on which the surgery occurs (e.g., abdominal surgery, intracranial surgery, or heart surgery). The extent can be simple, modified, or radical. Table 20-1 explains the categories and gives examples of surgical procedures.

Surgical Settings

The term **inpatient** refers to a client who is admitted to a hospital. The client may be admitted the day before or, more often, the day of surgery (often termed same-day admission [SDA]), or the client may already be an inpatient when surgery is needed. The terms **outpatient** and **ambulatory** refer to a client who goes to the surgical area the day of the surgery and returns home on the same day (i.e., same-day surgery [SDS]). Hospital-based ambulatory surgical centers,

TABLE 20-1 Selected Categories of Surgical Procedures

Category	Description	Condition or Surgical Procedure
Reasons for Surgery		
Diagnostic	Performed to determine the origin and cause of a disorder or the cell type for cancer	Breast biopsy Exploratory laparotomy Arthroscopy
Curative	Performed to resolve a health problem by repairing or removing the cause	Laparoscopic cholecystectomy Mastectomy Hysterectomy
Restorative	Performed to improve a client's functional ability	Total knee replacement Finger reimplantation
Palliative	Performed to relieve symptoms of a disease process, but does not cure	Colostomy Nerve root resection Tumor debulking Ileostomy
Cosmetic	Performed primarily to alter or enhance personal appearance	Liposuction Revision of scars Rhinoplasty Blepharoplasty
Urgency of Surgery		
Elective	Planned for correction of a nonacute problem	Cataract removal Hernia repair Hemorrhoidectomy Total joint replacement
Urgent	Requires prompt intervention; may be life threatening if treatment is delayed more than 24-48 hr	Intestinal obstruction Bladder obstruction Kidney or ureteral stones Bone fracture Eye injury Acute cholecystitis
Emergent	Requires immediate intervention because of life-threatening consequences	Gunshot or stab wound Severe bleeding Abdominal aortic aneurysm Compound fracture Appendectomy
Degree of Risk of Surgery		
Minor	Procedure without significant risk; often done with local anesthesia	Incision and drainage (I&D) Implantation of a venous access device (VAD) Muscle biopsy
Major	Procedure of greater risk, usually longer and more extensive than a minor procedure	Mitral valve replacement Pancreas transplant Lymph node dissection
Extent of Surgery		
Simple	Only the most overtly affected areas involved in the surgery	Simple/partial mastectomy
Radical	Extensive surgery beyond the area obviously involved; is directed at finding a root cause	Radical prostatectomy Radical hysterectomy

freestanding surgical centers, physicians' offices, and ambulatory care centers are common. About 70% to 90% of all surgical procedures in North America are performed in ambulatory centers (Bryant, 2002).

One advantage of outpatient surgery is that clients are not separated from the comfort and security of their home and family. With improvements in surgical techniques and anesthesia, more procedures are performed safely on an outpatient basis. Same-day surgery, however, presents new challenges for the client who does not have an adequate or available support system. An older spouse may be unable to assist in care before or after surgery. Clients who are responsible for others may be unable to perform their usual tasks within the family. They may try to continue their family role but jeopardize their own health by doing so. As a result, their stress, fears, and anxieties about the surgical experience and about returning home immediately after surgery may be increased.

COLLABORATIVE MANAGEMENT

PHARM REVIEW

Assessment

HISTORY

Data collection about the client before surgery begins in various settings (e.g., the surgeon's office, the preadmission or admission office, the inpatient unit, and over the telephone). Use privacy to increase the client's comfort with the interview process. Anesthesia and surgery are both physical and emotional stressors. Collect the following data:

- Age
- Use of tobacco, alcohol, or illicit substances, including marijuana
- Current medications
- Use of complementary or alternative medicines, such as herbal therapies, folk remedies, or acupuncture
- Medical history
- Prior surgical procedures and experiences
- Prior experience with anesthesia
- Autologous or directed blood donations
- Allergies, including sensitivity to latex products
- General health
- Family history
- Type of surgery planned
- Knowledge about and understanding of events during the perioperative period
- Adequacy of the client's support system

When taking a history, screen the client for problems that increase the risk for complications during and after surgery. Some problems that increase the surgical risk or increase the risk for complications after surgery are listed in Table 20-2.

AGE. Older clients are at increased risk for complications. The normal aging process decreases immune system functioning and delays wound healing. The frequency of chronic illness increases in older clients. See Chart 20-1 for other changes in older adults that may alter the operative response or risk.

DRUGS AND SUBSTANCE USE. The use of tobacco increases the risk for pulmonary complications because of changes it causes to the lungs and chest cavity. Excessive alcohol and illicit substance use can alter the client's responses to anesthesia and pain medication. Withdrawal of alcohol before surgery may lead to delirium tremens. Prescription and over-the-counter drugs may also affect how the client reacts to the operative experience.

TABLE 20-2 Selected Factors That Increase Surgical Risk or Increase the Risk of Postoperative Complications

Age
- Older than 65 years

Medications
- Antihypertensives
- Tricyclic antidepressants
- Anticoagulants
- Nonsteroidal anti-inflammatory drugs (NSAIDs)

Medical History
- Decreased immunity
- Diabetes
- Pulmonary disease
- Cardiac disease
- Hemodynamic instability
- Multisystem disease
- Coagulation defect or disorder
- Anemia
- Dehydration
- Infection
- Hypertension
- Hypotension
- Any chronic disease

Prior Surgical Experiences
- Less-than-optimal emotional reaction
- Anesthesia reactions or complications
- Postoperative complications

Health History
- Malnutrition or obesity
- Medication, tobacco, alcohol, or illicit substance use or abuse
- Altered coping ability

Family History
- Malignant hyperthermia
- Cancer
- Bleeding disorder

Type of Surgical Procedure Planned
- Neck, oral, or facial procedures (airway complications)
- Chest or high abdominal procedures (pulmonary complications)
- Abdominal surgery (paralytic ileus, deep vein thrombosis)

The potential effects of specific drugs are listed in Table 20-3. Another area of concern is the potential for reaction or serious adverse effects with some herbs, such as those listed in Table 20-4.

MEDICAL HISTORY. Ask the client about his or her medical history. Many chronic illnesses increase surgical risks and need to be considered when planning care. For example, a client with systemic lupus erythematosus may need additional drugs to offset the stress of the surgery. A diabetic client may need a more extensive bowel preparation because of decreased intestinal motility. An infection may need to be treated before surgery.

CARDIAC HISTORY. Ask the client specifically about cardiac disease because complications from anesthesia occur more often in clients with cardiac problems. Cardiac problems that increase surgical risks include coronary artery disease, angina, myocardial infarction (MI) within 6 months before surgery, heart failure, hypertension, and dysrhythmias. These problems impair the client's ability to withstand hemodynamic changes and alter the response to anesthesia. The risk for an MI during surgery is higher in clients with pre-existing heart problems.

CHART 20-1

NURSING FOCUS on the OLDER ADULT

Changes of Aging as Surgical Risk Factors

Physiologic Change	Nursing Interventions	Rationales
Cardiovascular System		
Decreased cardiac output Increased blood pressure	Determine normal activity levels and note when the client tires.	Knowing limits helps prevent fatigue.
Decreased peripheral circulation	Monitor vital signs, peripheral pulses, and capillary refill.	Having baseline data helps detect deviations.
Respiratory System		
Reduced vital capacity Loss of lung elasticity	Teach coughing and deep breathing exercises.	Pulmonary exercises help prevent pulmonary complications.
Decreased oxygenation of blood	Monitor respirations and breathing effort.	Having baseline data helps detect deviations.
Renal/Urinary System		
Decreased blood flow to kidneys Reduced ability to excrete waste products Decline in glomerular filtration rate	Monitor intake and output. Assess overall hydration. Monitor electrolyte status.	Ongoing assessment helps detect fluid and electrolyte imbalances and decreased renal function.
Nocturia common	Assist frequently with toileting needs, especially at night.	Frequent toileting helps prevent incontinence and falls.
Neurologic System		
Sensory deficits Slower reaction time	Orient the client to the surroundings. Allow extra time for teaching the client.	An individualized preoperative teaching plan is developed on the basis of the client's orientation and any neurologic deficits.
Decreased ability to adjust to changes in the surroundings	Provide for the client's safety.	Safety measures help prevent falls and injury.
Musculoskeletal System		
Increased incidence of deformities related to osteoporosis or arthritis	Assess the client's mobility. Teach turning and positioning. Encourage ambulation.	Interventions help prevent complications of immobility.
	Place on fall precautions, if indicated.	Safety measures help prevent injury.

TABLE 20-3 Effects of Routine Medications Taken Preoperatively

Drug	Implications for the Perioperative Experience	Nursing Interventions	Rationales
Antidysrhythmics			
Quinidine gluconate (Quinate✱, Quinaglute Dura-Tabs) Procainamide hydrochloride (Pronestyl, Procan SR)	Antidysrhythmic medications affect the client's tolerance of anesthesia and potentiate anesthetics that are neuromuscular blockers. Antidysrhythmics depress cardiac function by decreasing cardiac output and slowing pulse rate. Antidysrhythmics may cause peripheral vasodilation.	Communicate the use and type of antidysrhythmics to the anesthesia personnel. Monitor vital signs. Obtain a baseline electrocardiogram, as ordered. Assess the client's peripheral circulation.	Cardiac complications during surgery can be life threatening. Ongoing monitoring helps to detect deviations and potential complications.
Antihypertensives			
Methyldopa (Aldomet, Novomedopa✱) Captopril (Capoten) Clonidine hydrochloride (Catapres)	Antihypertensive agents alter the client's response to muscle relaxants and opioid analgesics by inhibiting synthesis and storage of norepinephrine. Antihypertensives may cause a hypotensive crisis intraoperatively and postoperatively.	Monitor blood pressure and pulse frequently. Assess for hypotension during transfer and turning.	Ongoing monitoring helps to detect deviations and potential complications. Hypotensive crisis can occur and may be prevented through timely assessments.
Corticosteroids			
Dexamethasone (Decadron, Dexasone) Hydrocortisone sodium (Solu-Cortef) Prednisone (Deltasone✱, Winpred)	Surgery increases the demand for corticosteroids in the client with no adrenal function. Steroids delay wound healing because of blockage of collagen formation. Steroids increase the serum glucose level and block fibroblast formation. Steroids increase the risk of hemorrhage. Steroids mask the signs and symptoms of infection.	Continue steroid therapy during surgery. Monitor vital signs. Assess for signs of hyperglycemia. Assess for subtle signs of infection and bleeding. Monitor wound healing, support the incision area with binders, and splint the wound when the client is turning, coughing, and deep breathing.	Continuation of steroid therapy avoids problems associated with abrupt withdrawal. Ongoing monitoring helps to detect deviations and potential complications. It is important to detect early signs and symptoms of infection. Specific wound and incision care helps to prevent complications.

aPTT, Partial thromboplastin time, activated; *INR,* International Normalized Ratio; *NPO,* nothing by mouth; *PT,* prothrombin time.

Continued

TABLE 20-3 Effects of Routine Medications Taken Preoperatively—*cont'd*

Drug	Implications for the Perioperative Experience	Nursing Interventions	Rationales
Anticoagulants			
Warfarin sodium (Coumadin, Warfilone sodium✱) Heparin sodium (Leo-Heparin, Hepalean✱) Aspirin (acetylsalicylic acid, Ancasal✱, Astrin✱, Coryphen✱)	Anticoagulant therapy increases the risk of hemorrhage intraoperatively and postoperatively.	Monitor coagulation studies (aPTT, PT, INR). Monitor for signs of bleeding. Gradually discontinue anticoagulants 24-48 hr before surgery, as ordered. Have an antidote (protamine sulfate for heparin and vitamin K [Mephyton] for warfarin sodium) available to reverse the effects of the anticoagulant.	Coagulation studies help detect bleeding disorders. Anticoagulant administration is discontinued to avoid hemorrhage. An antidote needs to be available to prevent complications of bleeding in an emergency situation.
Antiseizure Medications			
Phenobarbital (Luminal, Gardenal✱)	Seizure activity can cause injury to the surgical wound. Antiseizure medications alter the metabolism of anesthetic agents.	Maintain use of the drug. Inform the anesthesia provider to allow for adjustment of the dosage of the anesthetic. Assess for seizure activity. Pad the siderails of the bed. Place suction equipment at the bedside.	Antiseizure medications prevent seizures. Safety measures prevent injury.
Glaucoma Medications			
Demecarium bromide (Humorsol) Echothiophate (Phospholine iodide) Pilocarpine hydrochloride (Isopto Carpine, Pilocar, Miocarpine✱) Timolol maleate (Timoptic)	Glaucoma medications have cumulative systemic effects and can cause respiratory and cardiovascular collapse, especially during surgery.	Consult the physician about stopping Humorsol at least 2 wk before surgery. Monitor respiratory status and cardiac output. Assess for increased intraocular pressure.	Collaboration with the physician helps prevent complications. Ongoing monitoring helps to detect complications.
Antidiabetic Agent			
Insulin	Insulin needs decrease preoperatively when the client is on NPO status. Postoperative insulin demands increase because of IV administration of dextrose. Insulin levels may fluctuate during healing because of dietary and activity restrictions and the physical stress of surgery.	Monitor serum glucose levels. Administer antibiotics and other intermittent medications in normal saline instead of dextrose when possible, as prescribed, or as per facility policy.	Monitoring detects an increased or a decreased need for insulin. The use of normal saline prevents complications.

aPTT, Partial thromboplastin time, activated; *INR,* International Normalized Ratio; *NPO,* nothing by mouth; *PT,* prothrombin time.

PULMONARY HISTORY. Older clients, those with chronic respiratory problems, and smokers are at risk for pulmonary complications because of smoking- or age-related lung changes. Increased chest rigidity and loss of lung elasticity reduce anesthesia excretion. Smoking increases the blood level of **carboxyhemoglobin** (carbon monoxide on oxygen-binding sites of the hemoglobin molecule), which decreases oxygen delivery to organs. Action of cilia in pulmonary mucous membranes decreases, which leads to retained secretions and predisposes the client to infection (pneumonia) and **atelectasis** (collapse of alveoli). Atelectasis reduces gas exchange and causes intolerance of anesthesia.

Chronic lung problems such as asthma, emphysema, and chronic bronchitis also reduce the elasticity of the lungs, which reduces gas exchange. As a result, clients with these problems have reduced tissue oxygenation.

PREVIOUS SURGERY AND ANESTHESIA. The number and type of previous surgical procedures affect the client's readiness for surgery. Previous surgery, especially with complications, may increase fears and concerns about the scheduled surgery. Ask about the client's previous experience with anesthesia and all allergies. These data provide information about tolerance of and possible fears about the use of anesthesia. The family medical history and problems with anesthetics may indicate possible reactions to anesthesia, such as malignant hyperthermia (see Chapter 21).

A sensitivity or allergy to certain substances alerts you to a possible reaction to anesthetic agents or to substances that are used before or during surgery. For example, povidone-iodine used for skin cleansing contains the same allergens found in shellfish. Clients who are allergic to shellfish may have an adverse reaction to povidone-iodine. The client with an allergy to bananas often also has a latex allergy.

TABLE 20-4 Potential Effects of Herbs

Herb	Potential Effect
Black cohosh	Bradycardia, hypotension, joint pains
Bloodroot	Bradycardia, dysrhythmia, dizziness, impaired vision, intense thirst
Boneset	Liver toxicity, mental changes, respiratory problems
Coltsfoot	Fever, liver toxicity
Dandelion	Interactions with diuretics, increased concentration of lithium or potassium
Ephedra	Headache, dizziness, insomnia, tachycardia, hypertension, anxiety, irritability, dry mouth
Feverfew	Interference with blood-clotting mechanisms
Garlic	Hypotension, blood clotting inhibition, potentiation of diabetes drugs
Ginseng	Headache, anxiety, insomnia, hypertension, tachycardia, asthma attacks, postmenopausal bleeding
Goldenseal	Vasoconstriction
Hawthorn	Hypotension
Kava	Damage to the eyes, skin, liver, and spinal cord from long-term use
Licorice	Hyperkalemia, hypernatremia
Lobelia	Hearing and vision problems
Motherwort	Increased anticoagulation
Nettle	Hypokalemia
Senna	Potentiation of digoxin
St. John's Wort	Antidepressant, photosensitivity
Valerian root	Mild sedative or tranquilizer effect, hepatotoxicity

BLOOD DONATIONS. Clients may donate their own blood **(autologous donations)** for a few weeks just before the scheduled surgery date. If they need blood during or after surgery, an autologous blood transfusion can be given. This practice eliminates transfusion reactions and reduces the risk of acquiring bloodborne disease.

Clients can donate their own blood up to 5 weeks before surgery if they are infection free, have a hemoglobin level greater than 11 g/dL (110 g/L), and have a physician's recommendation. Clients with cardiac disease may need additional clearance from their cardiologist before making an autologous donation. The physician may prescribe supplemental iron before the first donation. Autologous donations can be made as often as every 3 days if other criteria are met. Usually a total of 2 to 4 units is donated. The last donation cannot be made within 72 hours before surgery.

A special tag is placed on the blood bag when an autologous blood donation has been made. The blood donor center gives the client a matching tag that he or she wears or brings to the surgical area before surgery. This procedure helps to ensure that clients receive only their own blood. If the blood is not used, it goes to the blood bank to be used as would any other unit of donated blood.

Clients may wish to have family and friends donate blood exclusively for their use, if needed. This practice (called **directed blood donation**) is possible only if the blood types are compatible and the donor's blood is acceptable. Clients may fear disease transmission from unknown blood and feel more comfortable knowing who gave the blood. Many centers do not accept directed blood, stating that it gives a false sense of security. As with autologous blood donations, a special tag is attached to the blood bag. This tag notes the names of the client and the donor and bears the client's signature.

Ask whether autologous or directed blood donations have been made and document this information in the chart. It is important to know the specific blood collection center where the donation was made and whether the blood has arrived before the client goes into surgery. The hospital receives and stores the blood units until they are used or are no longer needed. Unused blood is returned to the collection center.

PLANNING FOR BLOODLESS SURGERY. Increased use of "bloodless surgery," or minimally invasive surgery, provides alternatives for clients with religious or medical restrictions to blood transfusions. These programs reduce or eliminate the need for transfusion during and after surgery. Some techniques used include limiting blood samples (the number of samples, as well as the volume of blood drawn per sample) before surgery and stimulating the client's own red blood cell production with epoetin alpha (Epogen, Procrit) before, during, and after surgery. Supplemental iron, folic acid, vitamin B_{12}, and vitamin C may be prescribed before surgery to help red blood cell formation. Newer equipment and surgical techniques cause less blood loss than older techniques. Such advances include recycling blood suctioned during surgery and immediately transfusing it back into the client. Assess, monitor, teach, and support the client during the bloodless surgery process.

DISCHARGE PLANNING. Assess the client's home environment, self-care capabilities, and support systems and anticipate postoperative needs before surgery. *All clients, regardless of how minor the procedure or how often they have had surgery, should have discharge planning.* Older clients and dependent adults may need transportation referrals to and from the physician's office or the surgical setting. A home care nurse may be needed to monitor recovery and to provide instructions. All clients with few support systems may need follow-up care at home. Some clients need a planned direct admission to a rehabilitation hospital or center for physical therapy following surgery, such as after a total hip replacement. Shortened hospital stays require adequate discharge planning to achieve the desired outcomes after surgery.

PHYSICAL ASSESSMENT/CLINICAL MANIFESTATIONS

The preoperative client may be any age, with a health status that varies from well to debilitated. Perform a complete assessment before surgery to obtain baseline data. During assessment, identify current health problems, potential complications related to anesthesia, and possible complications that may occur after surgery.

When beginning the assessment, obtain a complete set of vital signs. You may need to obtain vital signs several times for accurate baseline values. Previous vital signs from another admission (if available in the medical record) are helpful to compare against current vital signs. Abnormal vital signs may require postponement of surgery until the problem is treated and the client's condition is stable. Also assess for anxiety, which could increase blood pressure, pulse, and respiratory rate. Document these findings as part of the overall assessment.

Throughout the physical assessment, focus on problem areas identified from the client's history and on all body systems affected by the surgical procedure. The older adult (Chart 20-2; see also Chapter 5) or chronically ill client is at

CHART 20-2

NURSING FOCUS on the OLDER ADULT

Specific Considerations When Planning Care for the Older Preoperative Client

- Greater incidence of chronic illness
- Greater incidence of malnutrition
- More allergies
- Increased incidence of impaired self-care abilities
- Inadequate support systems
- Decreased ability to withstand the stress of surgery and anesthesia
- Increased risk for cardiopulmonary complications after surgery
- Risk of a change in mental status when admitted (related to unfamiliar surroundings, change in routine, drugs given, and so forth)
- Increased risk of a fall and resultant injury

increased risk for complications during and after surgery. Morbidity and mortality during or after surgery are higher in older and chronically ill clients.

Report any abnormal assessment findings to the surgeon and to anesthesiology personnel. In this way, you are a proactive client advocate exercising professional legal responsibility. Often, established protocols or care maps identify what interventions are to be performed before surgery.

CARDIOVASCULAR SYSTEM. Cardiac problems may cause as many as 30% of surgery-related deaths. Check the client for hypertension, which is common, is often undiagnosed, and can affect the response to surgery. Cardiac assessment includes listening to heart sounds for rate, regularity, and abnormalities. Examine the client's hands and feet for temperature, color, peripheral pulses, capillary refill, and edema. Report any problems, such as absent peripheral pulses, pitting edema, or cardiac symptoms, such as chest pain, shortness of breath, and dyspnea, to the physician for further assessment and evaluation. (Cardiac assessment is discussed further in Chapter 36.)

RESPIRATORY SYSTEM. In assessing the client's respiratory status, consider the client's age, smoking history (including exposure to secondhand smoke), and any chronic illness. Observe the client's posture; respiratory rate, rhythm, and depth; overall respiratory effort; and lung expansion. Document any clubbing of the fingertips (swelling at the base of the nail beds caused by a chronic lack of oxygen) or cyanosis. Auscultate the lungs to assess for any abnormal breath sounds (crackles, wheezes, rubs). (More information on respiratory assessment is found in Chapter 30.)

RENAL/URINARY SYSTEM. Kidney function affects the excretion of drugs and waste products, including anesthetic and analgesic agents. If renal function is reduced, fluid and electrolyte balance can be altered, especially in older clients. Ask about problems such as urinary frequency, **dysuria** (painful urination), **nocturia** (awakening during nighttime sleep because of a need to void), difficulty starting urine flow, and **oliguria** (scant amount of urine). Ask the client about the appearance and odor of the urine. Equally important is an assessment of usual fluid intake and degree of continence. If the client has renal or urinary problems, consult with the physician about further workup. (Renal/urinary assessment is discussed further in Chapter 72.)

Kidney impairment decreases the excretion of drugs and anesthetic agents. As a result, drug effectiveness may be altered. Scopolamine (Buscopan✱), morphine, meperidine (Demerol), and barbiturates often cause confusion, disorientation, apprehension, and restlessness when given to clients with decreased kidney function.

NEUROLOGIC SYSTEM. Assess the client's overall mental status, including level of consciousness, orientation, and ability to follow commands, before planning preoperative teaching and care after surgery. A problem in any of these areas affects the type of care needed during the surgical experience. Determine the client's baseline neurologic status to be able to identify changes that may occur later. Also assess for any motor or sensory deficits. (See Chapter 44 for complete nervous system assessment.)

The usual neurologic status of a mentally impaired or older client may be difficult to assess. The client who has been independent and oriented at home may become disoriented in an unfamiliar hospital setting. Family members can often provide information about what the client was like at home.

Assess the client's risk for falling, especially in older clients. Evaluate factors such as mental status, muscle strength, steadiness of gait, and sense of independence to determine the client's risk. Document the client's ability to ambulate and the steadiness of gait as baseline data.

MUSCULOSKELETAL SYSTEM. Musculoskeletal problems may interfere with positioning during and after surgery. For example, clients with arthritis may be able to assume surgical positions but have discomfort after surgery from prolonged joint immobilization. Other anatomic features, such as the shape and length of the neck and the shape of the chest cavity, may interfere with respiratory and cardiac function or require special positioning during surgery.

Ask about a history of joint replacements and document the exact location of any prostheses. During surgery, ensure that electrocautery pads, which could cause an electrical burn, are not placed on or near the area of the prosthesis.

NUTRITIONAL STATUS. Malnutrition and obesity increase surgical risk. Surgery increases metabolic rate and depletes potassium, vitamin C, and B vitamins, all of which are needed for wound healing and blood clotting. In malnourished clients, decreased serum protein levels slow recovery. Negative nitrogen balance may result from depleted protein stores. This problem increases the risk for delayed wound healing, possible dehiscence or evisceration (see Chapter 22), dehydration, and sepsis.

Some older clients may have nutritional imbalances because of chronic illness, diuretic or laxative use, poor dietary planning or habits, anorexia, lack of motivation, or financial limitations. Indications of poor fluid or nutritional status include brittle nails, muscle wasting, dry or flaky skin, hair changes (e.g., dull, sparse, dry), decreased skin turgor, orthostatic (postural) hypotension, decreased serum protein levels, and abnormal serum electrolyte values.

The obese client is often malnourished because of an imbalanced diet. Obesity increases the risk for poor wound healing because of excessive **adipose** (fatty) tissue. Fatty tissue has few blood vessels, little collagen, and decreased nutrients, all of which are needed for wound healing. Obesity stresses the heart and reduces the lung volumes, which can affect the surgery and recovery. In addition, obese clients may need larger doses of drugs and may retain them longer after surgery.

PSYCHOSOCIAL ASSESSMENT

Perform a psychosocial assessment to determine the client's level of anxiety, coping ability, and support systems. Provide information and offer support as needed.

Most clients have some degree of anxiety and fear before surgery. The extent of these reactions varies according to the type of surgery, the perceived effects of the surgery and its potential outcome, and the client's personality. Surgery may be seen as a threat to life, body image, self-esteem, self-concept, or lifestyle. Clients may fear death, pain, helplessness, decreased socioeconomic status, a diagnosis of life-threatening conditions, possible disabling or crippling effects, or the unknown.

Anxiety and fear affect the client's ability to learn, cope, and cooperate with teaching and operative procedures. Anxiety and fear may also influence the amount and type of anesthesia needed and may slow recovery. Be aware of potential fears and anxieties when interviewing the client and planning teaching.

Assess coping mechanisms used by the client under similar situations or in the past when confronted with a stressful situation. Ask open-ended questions about the client's feelings about the entire surgical experience. Factors that influence coping include age; previous surgical or sick-role experiences; and emotional and physical signs of fear, anxiety, or discomfort. Signs of fear and anxiety include anger, crying, restlessness, profuse sweating, increased pulse rate, palpitations, sleeplessness, diarrhea, and urinary frequency.

LABORATORY ASSESSMENT

Laboratory tests before surgery provide baseline data about the client's health and help predict potential complications. The client scheduled for surgery in an ambulatory surgical center or admitted to the hospital on the morning of or day before surgery may have preadmission testing (PAT) performed from 24 hours to 28 days before the scheduled surgery. These test results are usually valid unless there has been a change in the client's condition that warrants repeated testing or the client is taking drugs that can alter laboratory values (such as warfarin [Coumadin], aspirin, or diuretics). Some facilities have time limits for tests, especially pregnancy testing or any other test results that would require altering the surgical plan.

The choice of laboratory testing before surgery varies among facilities and depends on the client's age, medical history, and the type of anesthesia planned. The most common tests are urinalysis, blood type and crossmatch, complete blood count or hemoglobin level and hematocrit, clotting studies (prothrombin time [PT], International Normalized Ratio [INR], activated partial thromboplastin time [aPTT], and platelet count), electrolyte levels, and serum creatinine level. Depending on a female client's age and the nature of the planned procedure, a pregnancy test may also be needed.

Urinalysis is performed to assess abnormal substances in the urine such as protein, glucose, blood, and bacteria. If renal disease is suspected or if the client is older, the physician may request other tests to determine the type and degree of disease present.

Report electrolyte imbalances or other abnormal results to the anesthesia team and the surgeon before surgery. **Hypokalemia** (decreased serum potassium level) increases the risk for toxicity if the client is taking digoxin, slows recovery from anesthesia, and increases cardiac irritability. **Hyperkalemia** (increased serum potassium level) increases the risk for dysrhythmias, especially with the use of anesthesia. *Hypokalemia and hyperkalemia must be corrected before the surgery.*

Other studies may be needed, depending on the client's medical history. For example, baseline arterial blood gas (ABG) values are assessed before surgery for clients with chronic pulmonary problems. Chart 20-3 lists abnormal laboratory findings and their possible causes.

RADIOGRAPHIC ASSESSMENT

A chest x-ray may be requested before surgery. Often, young healthy adults are not required to have a chest x-ray. A chest x-ray determines the size and shape of the heart, lungs, and major vessels and determines the presence of pneumonia or tuberculosis. A chest x-ray also provides baseline data in case of complications. Abnormal x-ray findings alert the surgeon to potential cardiac or pulmonary complications. Heart failure, cardiomyopathy, pneumonia, or infiltrates may cause the cancellation or delay of elective surgery. For emergency surgery, x-ray results assist the anesthesia provider in selecting anesthesia.

Other radiographic studies are based on client need, medical history, and the nature of the surgical procedure. For example, a client with back pain may have computed tomography (CT) or magnetic resonance imaging (MRI) examinations before a **laminectomy** (spinal surgery) to identify the exact location of the problem.

OTHER DIAGNOSTIC ASSESSMENTS

An electrocardiogram (ECG) may be required for all clients older than a specific age who are to have general anesthesia. The age varies among facilities but is often 40 to 45 years. An ECG may also be ordered for clients with a history of cardiac disease or those at risk for cardiac complications. An ECG provides baseline information on new or existing cardiac problems, such as an old myocardial infarction (MI). A client with a known cardiac problem may need a cardiology consultation before surgery. Prophylactic drugs, such as nitroglycerin and antibiotics, may be needed throughout the surgical period to reduce or prevent stress on the heart. Abnormal or potentially life-threatening ECG results may cause the cancellation of surgery until the client's cardiac status is stable.

A focused assessment of the preoperative client is shown in Chart 20-4.

◆Analysis

COMMON NURSING DIAGNOSES AND COLLABORATIVE PROBLEMS

The following are priority nursing diagnoses for preoperative clients:

1. Deficient Knowledge (specific experiences before, during, and after surgery) related to a lack of exposure.
2. Anxiety related to the threat of a change in health status or fear of the unknown

CHART 20-3

LABORATORY PROFILE
Perioperative Assessment

		Significance of Abnormal Findings	
Test	**Normal Range for Adults**	**Increased in**	**Decreased in**
Potassium (K^+) level	3.5-5.0 mEq/L, or 3.5-5.0 mmol/L	Dehydration Renal failure Acidosis Cellular/tissue damage Hemolysis of the specimen	NPO status when potassium replacement is inadequate Excessive use of non–potassium-sparing diuretics Vomiting Malnutrition Diarrhea Alkalosis
Sodium (Na^+)	≤90 yr: 136-145 mEq/L, or 136-145 mmol/L >90 yr: 132-146 mEq/L, or 132-146 mmol/L	Cardiac or renal failure Hypertension Excessive amounts of IV fluids containing normal saline Edema Dehydration (hemoconcentration)	Nasogastric drainage Vomiting or diarrhea Excessive use of laxatives or diuretics Excessive amounts of IV fluids containing water Syndrome of inappropriate antidiuretic hormone (SIADH)
Chloride (Cl^-)	≤90 yr: 90-110 mEq/L, or 98-106 mmol/L >90 yr: 98-111 mEq/L, or 98-111 mmol/L	Respiratory alkalosis Dehydration Renal failure Excessive amounts of IV fluids containing sodium chloride (NaCl)	Excessive nasogastric drainage Vomiting Excessive use of diuretics Diarrhea
Carbon dioxide (CO_2)	≤60 yr: 23-30 mEq/L, or 23-30 mmol/L 60-90 yr: 23-31 mEq/L, or 23-31 mmol/L >90 yr: 20-29 mEq/L, or 20-29 mmol/L	Chronic pulmonary disease Intestinal obstruction Vomiting or nasogastric suctioning Metabolic alkalosis	Hyperventilation Diabetic ketoacidosis Diarrhea Lactic acidosis Renal failure Salicylate toxicity
Glucose (fasting)	≤60 yr: 70-105 mg/dL, or 4.1-5.9 mmol/L 60-90 yr: 82-115 mg/dL, or 4.6-6.4 mmol/L >90 yr: 75-121 mg/dL, or 4.2-6.7 mmol/L	Hyperglycemia Excessive amounts of IV fluids containing glucose Stress Steroid use Pancreatic or hepatic disease	Hypoglycemia Excess insulin
Creatinine	*Females:* ≤60 yr: 0.5-1.1 mg/dL, or 44-97 µmol/L 60-90 yr: 0.6-1.2 mg/dL, or 53-106 µmol/L >90 yr: 0.6-1.3 mg/dL, or 53-115 µmol/L *Males:* <60 yr: 0.6-1.2 mg/dL, or 53-106 µmol/L 60-90 yr: 0.8-1.3 mg/dL, or 71-115 µmol/L >90 yr: 1.0-1.7 mg/dL, or 88-150 µmol/L	Renal damage with destruction of large number of nephrons Renal insufficiency Acute renal failure Chronic renal failure End-stage renal disease (ESRD)	Atrophy of muscle tissue
Blood urea nitrogen (BUN)	<60 yr: 10-20 mg/dL, or 2.1-7.1 mmol/L 60-90 yr: 8-23 mg/dL, or 2.9-8.2 mmol/L >90 yr: 10-31 mg/dL, or 3.6-11.1 mmol/L	Dehydration Renal failure Excessive protein in diet Liver failure	Overhydration Malnutrition
Prothrombin time (pro time, PT)	11-12.5 sec, 85%-100%, or 1:1.1 client-control ratio	Coagulation defect (bleeding disorder)	Coagulation (clotting) disorder, such as thrombophlebitis or pulmonary embolus
International Normalized Ratio (INR)	0.7-1.8	Anticoagulant therapy (aspirin, warfarin)	Extensive cancer
Partial thromboplastin time, activated (aPTT)	30-40 sec	Coagulation defect (bleeding disorder) Anticoagulant therapy (heparin) Liver disease	Coagulation (clotting) disorder, such as thrombophlebitis or pulmonary embolus Extensive cancer

IRU, International recommended unit; *NPO*, nothing by mouth.

CHART 20-3

LABORATORY PROFILE
Perioperative Assessment—*cont'd*

Test	Normal Range for Adults	Significance of Abnormal Findings: Increased in	Significance of Abnormal Findings: Decreased in
White blood cell (WBC) count (leukocyte count)	Total: 5000-10,000/mm³, or 7.4 IRU	Infection Inflammation Stress Tissue necrosis	Immune disorder Immunosuppressant therapy
Hemoglobin, total	*Females:* 18-44 yr: 12-16 g/dL, or 117-155 g/L 45-64 yr: 11.7-16.0 g/dL, or 117-160 g/L 65-74 yr: 11.7-16.1 g/dL, or 117-161 g/L *Males:* 18-44 yr: 14-18 g/dL, or 132-173 g/L 45-64 yr: 13.1-17.2 g/dL, or 131-172 g/L 65-74 yr: 12.6-17.4 g/dL, or 126-174 g/L	Dehydration Polycythemia Chronic pulmonary disease Congestive heart failure	Blood loss Anemia Renal failure
Hematocrit	*Females:* 18-44 yr: 35%-45% 45-74 yr: 37%-47% *Males:* 18-44 yr: 42%-52% 45-64 yr: 39%-50% 65-74 yr: 37%-51%	Dehydration Polycythemia High altitude	Blood loss Anemia Renal failure

IRU, International recommended unit; *NPO*, nothing by mouth.

CHART 20-4

FOCUSED ASSESSMENT of
The Preoperative Client

As part of the cardiopulmonary assessment, take and record vital signs; report the following:
- Hypotension or hypertension
- Heart rate of less than 60 or more than 120 beats/min
- Irregular heart rate
- Chest pain
- Shortness of breath or dyspnea
- Tachypnea
- Pulse oximetry reading of less than 94%

Assess for and report any signs or symptoms of infection, including the following:
- Fever
- Purulent sputum
- Dysuria or cloudy, foul-smelling urine
- Any red, swollen, draining IV or wound site
- Increased white blood cell count

Assess for and report signs or symptoms that could contraindicate surgery, including the following:
- Increased prothrombin time (PT), International Normalized Ratio (INR), or activated partial thromboplastin time (aPTT)
- Hypokalemia or hyperkalemia
- Client report of possible pregnancy or positive pregnancy test

Assess for and report other clinical conditions that may need to be evaluated by a physician or advanced nurse practitioner before proceeding with the surgical plans, including the following:
- Change in mental status
- Vomiting
- Rash
- Recent administration of an anticoagulant medication

ADDITIONAL NURSING DIAGNOSES AND COLLABORATIVE PROBLEMS

In addition to the common nursing diagnoses, preoperative clients may have one or more of the following:
- Disturbed Sleep Pattern related to internal sensory alterations (e.g., illness and anxiety)
- Ineffective Coping related to the impending surgery
- Anticipatory Grieving related to the effects of surgery
- Disturbed Body Image related to anticipated changes in the body's appearance or function
- Disabled Family Coping related to temporary family disorganization and role changes
- Powerlessness related to the health care environment, loss of independence, and loss of control of one's body

Planning and Implementation

DEFICIENT KNOWLEDGE

NOC **PLANNING: EXPECTED OUTCOMES.** The client is expected to know what to expect during and after surgery and participate in his or her recovery as indicated by:
- Explaining the purpose and expected results of the planned surgery
- Asking questions when a term or procedure is not known
- Adhering to the NPO (nothing by mouth) requirements
- Stating an understanding of preoperative preparations (e.g., skin preparation, bowel preparation)
- Demonstrating correct use of exercises and techniques to be used after surgery for the prevention of compli-

CHART 20-5

NIC INTERVENTION ACTIVITIES for The Preoperative Client

Preoperative Coordination: *Facilitating preadmission diagnostic testing and preparation of the surgical client*
- Review planned surgery.
- Obtain client history, as appropriate.
- Complete a physical assessment, as appropriate.
- Describe and explain preadmission treatments and diagnostic tests.
- Interpret diagnostic test results, as appropriate.
- Determine the client's expectations about the surgery.
- Provide time for the client and significant other to ask questions and voice concerns.
- Discuss postoperative discharge plans.
- Determine ability of caretakers.

NIC intervention activities selected from Dochterman, J.M., & Bulechek, G.M. (Eds.). (2004). *Nursing interventions classification (NIC)* (4th ed.). St. Louis: Mosby. No part of this work is to be altered without prior written permission from the Publisher.

TABLE 20-5 Preoperative Teaching Checklist

Consider the following items when planning individualized preoperative teaching for clients and families:
- Fears and anxieties
- Surgical procedure
- Preoperative routines (e.g., NPO, enemas, blood samples, showering)
- Invasive procedures (e.g., lines, catheters)
- Coughing, turning, deep breathing
- Incentive spirometer
  - How to use
  - How to tell when used correctly
- Lower extremity exercises
- Stockings and pneumatic compression devices
- Early ambulation
- Splinting
- Pain management

NPO, Nothing by mouth.

cations (e.g., splinting the incision, coughing/deep breathing, performing leg exercises, ambulating as early as permitted).

INTERVENTIONS. Interventions to increase the client's knowledge level are listed in Chart 20-5. Because the surgical experience is foreign to many people, focus on teaching the client and family members. Preoperative teaching may begin in the surgeon's office for planned or elective surgery. Pamphlets, written instructions, and videotapes may be given or sent to the client. More teaching may occur when the client has preadmission testing. Some facilities hold classes before surgery for groups of clients or show videos for those who are having the same or similar surgical procedures. A tour of the operating suite and the postanesthesia care unit (PACU) may be included.

Explore the client's level of knowledge and understanding. Increased access to information via the Internet may be helpful but is also a concern. Some Internet information may not be accurate or may not apply to a specific client's plan of care.

Information about informed consent, dietary restrictions, specific preparation for surgery (bowel and skin preparations), exercises after surgery, and plans for pain management promote clients' participation and help achieve the desired outcome. A sample educational checklist is shown in Table 20-5. Because education occurs in a variety of settings, coordination of client teaching efforts is challenging. When you care for the client just before surgery (same-day, ambulatory surgery [outpatient] unit or inpatient hospital unit), assess the client's and family members' knowledge and provide additional information as needed.

Ensuring Informed Consent. Surgery of any type involves invasion of the body and requires informed consent from the client or legal guardian (Figure 20-1). Clients deserve, and rightly demand, to be informed and involved in decisions affecting their health care. Consent implies that the client has been given sufficient information to understand the following:
- The nature of and reason for surgery
- Who will be performing the surgery and whether others will be present during the procedure (e.g., students)
- All available options and the risks associated with each option
- The risks associated with the surgical procedure and its potential outcomes
- The risks associated with the use of anesthesia

Informed consent helps protect the client from any unwanted procedures and protects the surgeon and the facility from lawsuit claims related to unauthorized surgery or uninformed clients. Written record of informed consent is documented on a "consent form," but can also be documented in the physician's notes. The consent form documents the client's consent and signature for the procedure listed.

As a competent adult, it is the client's right to refuse treatment for any reason, even when refusal might lead to death. For example, in the case of Jehovah's Witnesses, some clients will not accept blood transfusions because of their religious convictions.

The surgeon is responsible for having the consent form signed before sedation is given and before surgery is performed. *You, as a nurse, are not responsible for providing detailed information about the surgical procedure. Rather, your role is to clarify facts that have been presented by the physician and dispel myths that the client or family may have about the surgical experience.* You ensure that the consent form is signed and you serve as a witness to the signature, not to the fact that the client is informed. If you believe that the client has not been adequately informed, contact the surgeon and request that he or she see the client for clarification. Document this action in the chart.

Clients who cannot write may sign with an X, which must be witnessed by two persons. In an emergency, telephone or telegram authorization is acceptable and should be followed up with written consent as soon as possible. The number of witnesses (usually two) and the type of documentation vary according to the facility's policy. In a life-threatening situation in which every effort has been made to contact the person with medical power of attorney, consent is desired but not essential. In place of written or oral consent, written consultation by at least two physicians who are not associated with the case may be requested by the physician. This formal consultation legally supports the decision for surgery until the appropriate person can sign a consent form. If the client is not capable of giving consent and has no family, the court can appoint a legal guardian to represent the client's best interests.

Northwest Hospital Center

The hospital centered around its patients.

REQUEST AND AUTHORIZATION FOR MEDICAL AND/OR SURGICAL TREATMENT, BLOOD PRODUCTS ADMINISTRATION

1. I hereby request and authorize Dr.________________________ and/or his/her associates and whomever they may designate as their assistants, to administer such treatment as is necessary and to perform the following operation__________
____
and such additional operations or procedures as are considered necessary on the basis of conditions that may be revealed during the course of said operation or treatment.
2. The reasons why the above named surgery and/or treatment is considered necessary, its advantages, probability of success, possible complications, and risks, as well as possible alternative modes of treatment were explained to me by Dr.________________________.
3. I request and authorize the administration of such anesthetics and/or other medications as are necessary.
4. Final disposition of any tissues or parts surgically removed is to be handled in accordance with the customary practices of the hospital.
5. I am aware that the practice of medicine and surgery is not an exact science and I acknowledge that no guarantees have been made to me concerning the results of the operation or procedure.
6. I hereby acknowledge that I have read and fully understand the above request and authorization for medical and/or surgical treatment.
7. I consent to the admittance of permitted observers, the use of closed-circuit television, taking of photographs (including motion pictures), and the preparation of drawings and similar illustrative material, and I also consent to the use of such photographs and other material for scientific purposes, provided my identity is not revealed by the pictures or by the descriptive text accompanying them.
8. I consent to release of my social security number in accordance with the Safe Medical Device Act.

Date	Time	Signature of Patient or Patient Surrogate

Witness	Signature of Physician

CONSENT TO BLOOD/BLOOD PRODUCTS TRANSFUSION

After discussing the risks, benefits and alternatives to transfusion of blood (donor/autologous) (circle one or both) or blood products with my physician or his designee, I consent to the administration of these products.

Date	Time	Signature of Patient or Patient Surrogate

Witness	Signature of Physician

703/1019-3-R-8/97 (40-1331)

Figure 20-1 ■ A surgical consent form. (Courtesy of Northwest Hospital Center, Randallstown, MD.)

A blind client may sign his or her own consent form, which usually needs to be witnessed by two persons. Clients who speak a language other than the general language of the facility require a translator and a second witness. Some facilities have consent forms written in more than one language.

Some surgical procedures, such as intraocular lens implants, sterilization, and experimental procedures, may require a special permit in addition to the standard consent. National and local governing bodies and the individual facility determine which procedures require a separate permit. Separate consents for anesthesia and blood products also may be required.

Surgical procedures that are site specific, such as left, right, or bilateral, require client identification before surgery. The client is asked to mark the site with a marker to ensure the correct site is used and the wrong site is avoided.

Client Self-Determination. Clients receiving medical care have the right to have or to initiate advance directives, such as a living will or durable power of attorney, as mandated by the Patient Self-Determination Act. Advance directives provide legal instructions to the health care providers about the client's wishes and are to be followed. *Surgery does not provide an exception to a client's advance directives or living will.*

Implementing Dietary Restrictions. Regardless of the type of surgery and anesthesia planned, the client is restricted to **nothing by mouth (NPO)** for 6 to 8 hours before surgery. NPO means no eating, drinking (including water), or smoking (nicotine stimulates gastric secretions). It is common practice to begin NPO status at midnight on the night before surgery. This precaution ensures that the stomach contains a limited volume of gastric secretions, which decreases the risk for aspiration. Outpatients and clients who are scheduled for admission to the hospital on the same day that surgery is performed, must receive written and oral instructions about remaining NPO after midnight. *Emphasize the importance of adherence. Failure to adhere can result in cancellation of surgery or increase the risk for aspiration during or after surgery.*

The exact amount of time a client must be NPO before surgery is controversial. Clients, especially older adults, who fast for 8 or more hours may have imbalances of fluids, electrolytes, and blood glucose levels.

Administering Regularly Scheduled Medications. On the day of surgery, the client's usual drug schedule may need to be altered. Consult the medical physician and the anesthesia provider for instructions about drugs, such as those taken for diabetes, cardiac disease, or glaucoma, as well as regularly scheduled anticonvulsants, antihypertensives, anticoagulants, antidepressants, or corticosteroids. The physician may prescribe some drugs, including over-the-counter drugs, such as aspirin, to be stopped until after surgery. The physician may prescribe other drugs to be given by the intravenous (IV) route to maintain the drug level in the blood. *Drugs for cardiac disease, respiratory disease, seizures, and hypertension are commonly allowed with a sip of water before surgery.* Some antihypertensive or antidepressant drugs may be withheld on the day of surgery because of possible adverse effects on blood pressure during surgery.

The diabetic client who takes insulin may be given a reduced dose of intermediate- or long-acting insulin based on the blood glucose level, or may be given regular (fast-acting) insulin in divided doses on the day of surgery. Alternatively, an IV infusion of 5% dextrose in water may be given with the insulin to prevent low blood sugar during surgery. Because of the many treatment approaches to diabetes, clarify drug and IV prescriptions with the physician. (See Chapter 68 for more information about diabetes.)

Intestinal Preparation. Bowel or intestinal preparations are performed to prevent injury to the colon and to reduce the number of intestinal bacteria. Evacuation of the bowel is needed when a client is having major abdominal, pelvic, perineal, or perianal surgery. The surgeon's preference and the type of surgical procedure determine the type of bowel preparation. Table 20-6 shows common bowel preparation regimens and their complications. An enema ordered to be given until return flow is clear is a stressful procedure, especially for the older client. Repeated enemas can cause electrolyte imbalance, fluid volume imbalances, vagal stimulation, and postural (orthostatic) hypotension. Enemas also cause severe anorectal discomfort in clients with hemorrhoids. Some

TABLE 20-6 Complications of Common Bowel Preparations for the Surgical Client

Surgical Site	Preparation	Complications
Stomach, duodenum, and proximal jejunum	Oral laxative (e.g., castor oil preparation or bisacodyl [Dulcolax, Laxit✱]) Clear liquid diet the evening before surgery NPO after midnight	Abdominal cramping Dehydration Electrolyte imbalance Fatigue
Small intestine	Oral laxative (e.g., magnesium citrate) Clear liquid diet the evening before surgery Multiple-position enema the evening before surgery NPO after midnight	Abdominal cramping Dehydration Electrolyte imbalance Fatigue
Large intestine to rectum	Multiple or combination of oral laxatives 12-24 hr before surgery Multiple-position tap water or antibiotic (neomycin) enemas (three times or until the return flow is clear) the evening and morning before surgery Oral antibiotics to sterilize the bowel (e.g., neomycin and erythromycin) 24 hr before surgery Clear liquid diet the day before surgery NPO after midnight	Abdominal cramping Fatigue and weakness Fluid excess or deficit Potassium or sodium deficit Decreased cardiac output from vagal stimulation Irritation of bowel and rectal mucosa from enemas

NPO, Nothing by mouth.

physicians prescribe potent laxatives (e.g., polyethylene glycol electrolyte solution [GoLYTELY]) instead of enemas, especially for older clients. Bowel preparations can be exhausting, and you must take safety precautions to prevent falls.

Skin Preparation. The skin preparation may be embarrassing or uncomfortable for the client, especially if the surgical site is in a sensitive or private body area. Provide a warm, comfortable, and private environment during the procedure. The skin is the body's first line of defense against infection. A break in this barrier increases the risk for infection, especially for older clients. Skin preparation before surgery is the first step in the prevention of surgical wound infection.

EVIDENCE-BASED PRACTICE for Nursing

Gently remove hair at the surgical site

Kjonniken, I., et al. (2002). Preoperative hair removal: A systematic literature review. *AORN Journal, 75*(5), 928-936, 938, 940.

This study was performed in response to the 1999 guidelines of the Centers for Disease Control and Prevention (CDC), which strongly recommends that "hair should not be removed preoperatively unless the hair at or around the incision site will interfere with the surgical procedure. If hair is removed, however, it should be done immediately before surgery, preferably with clippers." This research is an analysis of the evidence regarding preoperative hair removal by shaving, clipping, and the use of depilatories. The authors performed an exhaustive review of the medical and nursing literature from 1966 to 1999 that examined whether or not hair was removed from the surgical site before surgery, the timing of the removal, the method of the removal, and the association of surgical site infections (SSIs). The studies cited as the basis for the CDC guidelines were included in the review, as were many additional randomized and observational studies performed during the designated timeframe.

Ten team members performed the analysis. More than 130 published studies were examined by the team. All members of the team assessed each article independently based on the scale provided by the U.S. Agency for Healthcare Research and Quality. In plenary sessions, all members of the team established the relevance and quality of each published study.

The analysis resulted in conclusions somewhat different from the guidelines recommended by the CDC. No strong evidence supported the decision not to remove hair. Wet or dry shaving the evening before the procedure has a higher rate of SSIs than did the use of either clipper or depilatories. Hair removed with clippers should be performed as close as possible to the surgical procedure.

Level of Evidence: 1—Quantitative systematic review.

Critique. The team used strong research procedures in the assessment and categorization of the existing data. The method used to determine the levels of evidence for categorizing the data was appropriate and applied equally. The review exposes the lack of well-controlled, randomized clinical trials to answer the questions surrounding preoperative hair removal from surgical sites.

Implications for Nursing. There is a lack of clarity regarding the "one best practice" for surgical site preparation with regard to hair removal. Clearly, cleanliness is important and so is the avoidance of skin injury. Shaving, especially dry shaving is known to nick or abrade skin. The degree of skin injury is also, in part, related to the skill of the person doing the shaving. Depilatories, while not nicking skin surfaces, can also cause chemical injury to sensitive skin, resulting in a nonintact skin surface. Whatever hair removal system is used, nurses must use careful handling to reduce or prevent skin injury. In addition, if nurses observe a skin injury at the intended surgical site, documentation is essential.

One or two days before the scheduled surgery, the surgeon may ask the client to shower using an antiseptic solution such as povidone-iodine (Betadine) or hexachlorophene. Instruct the client to be especially careful to clean around the proposed surgical site. If the client is hospitalized before surgery, showering and cleaning are repeated the night before surgery or in the morning before transfer to the surgical suite. This cleaning reduces contamination of the surgical field and reduces the number of organisms at the site. After the final cleaning procedure, especially for an orthopedic surgical procedure, the area may be covered with sterile towels or drapes to prevent contamination.

A controversial step in skin preparation after the cleaning is the shave. Many health care professionals believe that shaving contaminates the surgical area and traumatizes the skin around the area where the incision will be made. Thus whether or not to shave, the timing of the shave, and the equipment used remain controversial (see the Evidence-Based Practice for Nursing box at left).

Factors that predispose to wound contamination include bacteria found in hair follicles, disruption of the normal protective mechanisms of the skin, and nicks in the skin. Shaving of hair creates the potential for infection. Hair clipping with electrical clippers is often used to decrease the problems caused by traditional razors. The Centers for Disease Control and Prevention (CDC) recommend that if shaving is necessary, the hair should be removed using disposable sterile supplies and aseptic principles *immediately* before the start of the surgical procedure. Shaving is performed in the treatment room, the holding area of the operating suite, or the operating room (OR). Figure 20-2 shows areas shaved for various surgical procedures. Shaving, especially of the head or genital area, can be emotionally upsetting to the client, and regrowth of this hair can be uncomfortable.

Preparing the Client for Tubes, Drains, and Vascular Access. Prepare the client for possible placement of tubes, drains, and vascular access devices. Preparation reduces the client's anxiety and fear, and the family's negative reaction. Be careful not to scare the client while providing information about the purpose of each tube.

Tubes. The client may need an indwelling urinary (Foley) catheter before, during, or after surgery to keep the bladder empty and to monitor renal function. The client having abdominal or genitourinary surgery usually has a Foley catheter.

A nasogastric (NG) tube may be inserted before abdominal surgery to decompress or empty the stomach and the upper bowel. More often, however, the tube is placed after the induction of anesthesia, when insertion is less disturbing to the client and is easier to perform.

Drains. Drains are often placed during surgery to help remove fluid from the surgical site. Some drains are under the dressing; others are visible and require emptying. Drains come in various shapes and sizes (see Chapter 22). Inform the client that drains are often used routinely and that generally they are not painful but may cause some discomfort. Discuss the reasons drains should not be kinked or pulled.

Vascular Access. A vascular access (line) is placed for clients receiving a general anesthetic and most clients receiving other types of anesthetics. An access is needed to give drugs and fluids before, during, and after surgery. Clients who

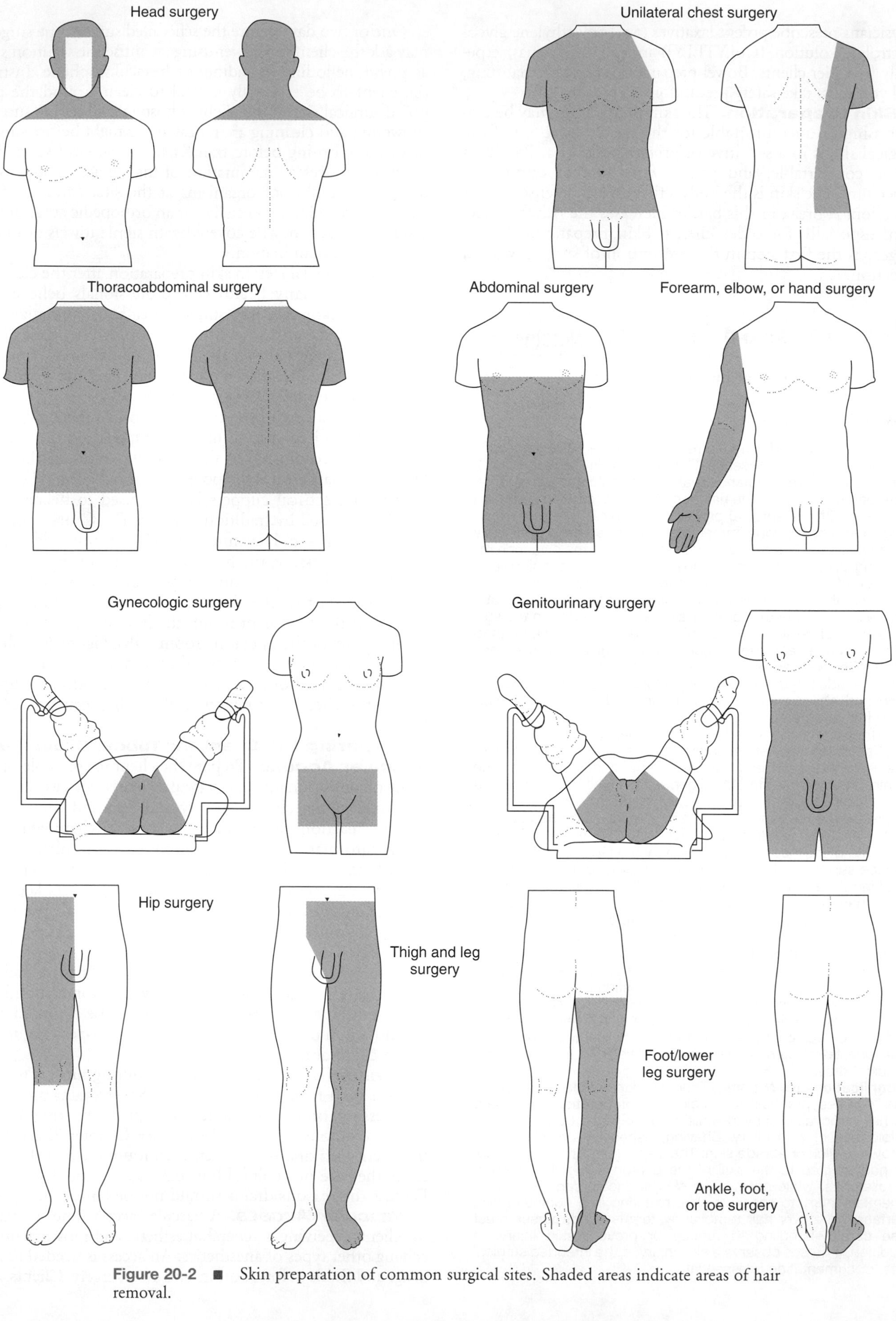

Figure 20-2 ■ Skin preparation of common surgical sites. Shaded areas indicate areas of hair removal.

are dehydrated or at risk for dehydration may receive fluids before surgery.

CONSIDERATIONS FOR OLDER ADULTS

Older adult clients are at greater risk for dehydration because their fluid reserves are lower than those of young or middle-aged adults. Carefully monitor the older adult client and clients with cardiac disease receiving IV fluids. (See Chapter 17 for more information on IV therapy.)

The IV access is usually placed in the arm or the back of the hand using a large, short catheter (e.g., 18-gauge, 1-inch catheter). This type of access provides the least resistance to fluid or blood infusion, especially in an emergency when rapid infusions may be needed. Depending on the client's needs and the facility's policies, the IV access can be placed before surgery when the client is in the hospital room, in the holding or admission area of the surgical suite, or in the OR.

Teaching About Postoperative Procedures and Exercises. Teach the client and family members about exercises and procedures (e.g., checking dressings and obtaining vital signs frequently) to be performed after surgery. Family members can be helpful in reminding clients to perform these exercises. Preoperative teaching reduces apprehension and fear, increases cooperation and participation in care after surgery, and decreases complications.

CHART 20-6

CLIENT EDUCATION GUIDE
Perioperative Respiratory Care

Deep (Diaphragmatic) Breathing
1. Sit upright on the edge of the bed or in a chair, being sure that your feet are placed firmly on the floor or a stool. (After surgery, deep breathing is done with the client in Fowler's position or in semi-Fowler's position.)
2. Take a gentle breath through your mouth.
3. Breathe out gently and completely.
4. Then take a deep breath through your nose and mouth, and hold this breath to the count of five.
5. Exhale through your nose and mouth.

Expansion Breathing
1. Find a comfortable upright position, with your knees slightly bent. (Bending the knees decreases tension on the abdominal muscles and decreases respiratory resistance and discomfort.)
2. Place your hands on each side of your lower rib cage, just above your waist.
3. Take a deep breath through your nose, using your shoulder muscles to expand your lower rib cage outward during inhalation.
4. Exhale, concentrating first on moving your chest, then on moving your lower ribs inward, while gently squeezing the rib cage and forcing air out of the base of your lungs.

Splinting of the Surgical Incision
1. Unless coughing is contraindicated, place a pillow, towel, or folded blanket over your surgical incision and hold the item firmly in place.
2. Take three slow, deep breaths to stimulate your cough reflex.
3. Inhale through your nose, then exhale through your mouth.
4. On your third deep breath, cough to clear secretions from your lungs while firmly holding the pillow, towel or folded blanket against your incision.

When the fear or anxiety level is high, explore the client's feelings before discussing procedures.

Discussion, demonstration with return demonstration, and practice by the client aid in the ability to perform various breathing (Chart 20-6) and leg (Chart 20-7) exercises after surgery. Emphasize the need to begin exercises early in the recovery phase and to continue them, with 5 to 10 repetitions each, every 1 to 2 hours after surgery for at least the first 48 hours. Explain that the client may need to be awakened for these activities.

Breathing Exercises. In deep, or diaphragmatic, breathing, the diaphragm flattens during inspiration, enlarging the chest cavity and expanding the lungs. After you demonstrate and explain the technique, urge the client to practice the five steps of deep breathing.

For clients with chronic lung disease or limited chest expansion, as seen in older clients because of the aging process, expansion breathing exercises are useful. For the client having chest surgery, expansion breathing exercises strengthen accessory muscles and are started before surgery. Expansion breathing may be used after surgery during chest physiotherapy (percussion, vibration, and postural drainage) to help loosen secretions and maintain an adequate air exchange.

Incentive Spirometry. Incentive spirometry is another way to encourage the client to take deep breaths. Its purpose is to promote complete lung expansion and to prevent pulmonary problems. Various types of incentive spirometers are available; some examples are shown in Figure 20-3. With all types, the client must be able to seal the lips tightly around the mouthpiece, inhale spontaneously, and hold his or her breath for 3 to 5 seconds for effective lung expansion. Goals (e.g., attaining specific volumes) can be set according to the client's ability and the type of incentive spirometer. Seeing a light move up a column or a bellows expanding reinforces and motivates the client to continue performance.

Coughing and Splinting. Coughing may be performed along with deep breathing every 1 to 2 hours after surgery. The purposes of coughing are to expel secretions, keep the lungs clear, allow full aeration, and prevent pneumonia and atelectasis. Coughing may be uncomfortable for the client, but when performed correctly, it should not harm the incision. Splinting (e.g., holding) the incision area provides support, promotes a feeling of security, and reduces pain during coughing. The proper technique for splinting the incision site and coughing is described in Chart 20-6. A folded bath blanket or pillow is helpful to use as a splint.

The use of routine coughing exercises after surgery is controversial. Some surgeons believe coughing may harm the surgical wound and that it would be better to use other, safer measures for pulmonary hygiene, such as deep breathing and incentive spirometer exercises. When routine coughing exercises should be avoided for a specific client, such as after a hernia repair, the surgeon usually writes a "do not cough" prescription.

Leg Procedures and Exercises. Antiembolism stockings (TED or Jobst stockings), elastic (Ace) wraps, or pneumatic compression devices (e.g., "sequentials" or "boots") may be used during and after surgery along with leg exercises and early ambulation to promote venous return. Venous stasis can lead to deep vein thrombosis (DVT) or a pulmonary embolus (PE) if the blood clot breaks off and travels to the lungs.

CHART 20-7

CLIENT EDUCATION GUIDE

Postoperative Leg Exercises

Exercise No. 1

1. Lie in bed with the head of your bed elevated to about 45 degrees.
2. Beginning with your right leg, bend your knee, raise your foot off the bed, and hold this position for a few seconds.
3. Extend your leg by unbending your knee, and lower the leg to the bed.
4. Repeat this sequence four more times with your right leg, then perform this same exercise five times with your left leg.

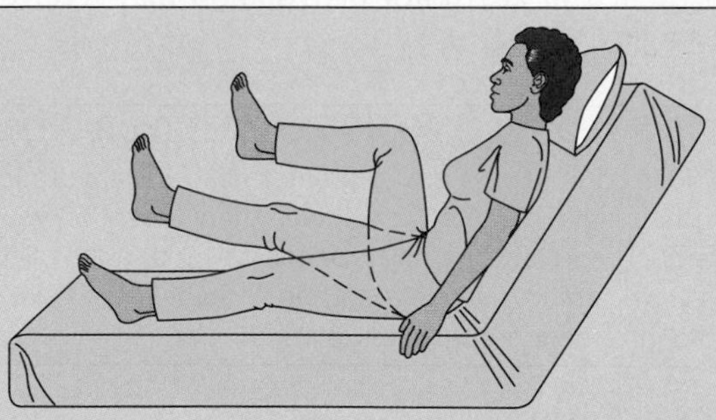

Exercise No. 2

1. Beginning with your right leg, point your toes toward the bottom of the bed.
2. With the same leg, point your toes up toward your face.
3. Repeat this exercise several times with your right leg, then perform this same exercise with your left leg.

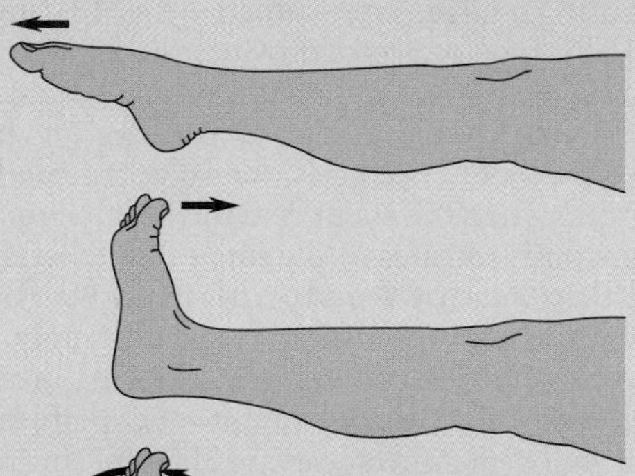

Exercise No. 3

1. Beginning with your right leg, make circles with your ankles, first to the left, then to the right.
2. Repeat this exercise several times with your right leg, then perform this same exercise with your left leg.

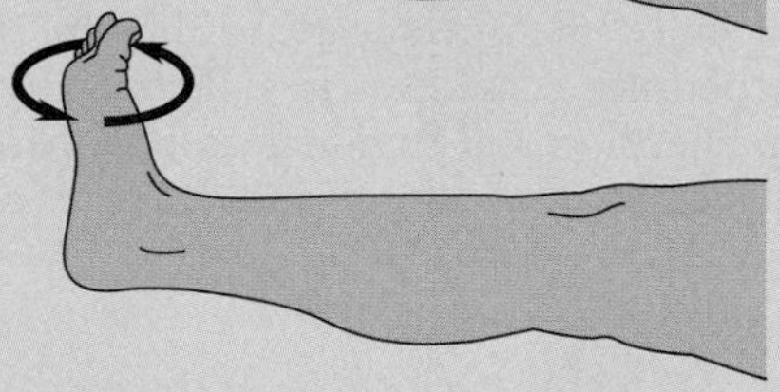

Exercise No. 4

1. Beginning with your right leg, bend your knee and *push* the ball of your foot into the bed or floor until you feel your calf and thigh muscles contracting.
2. Repeat this exercise several times with your right leg; then perform this same exercise with your left leg.

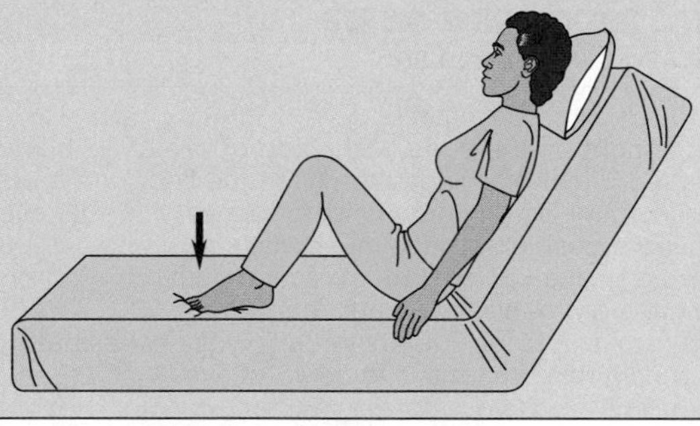

A

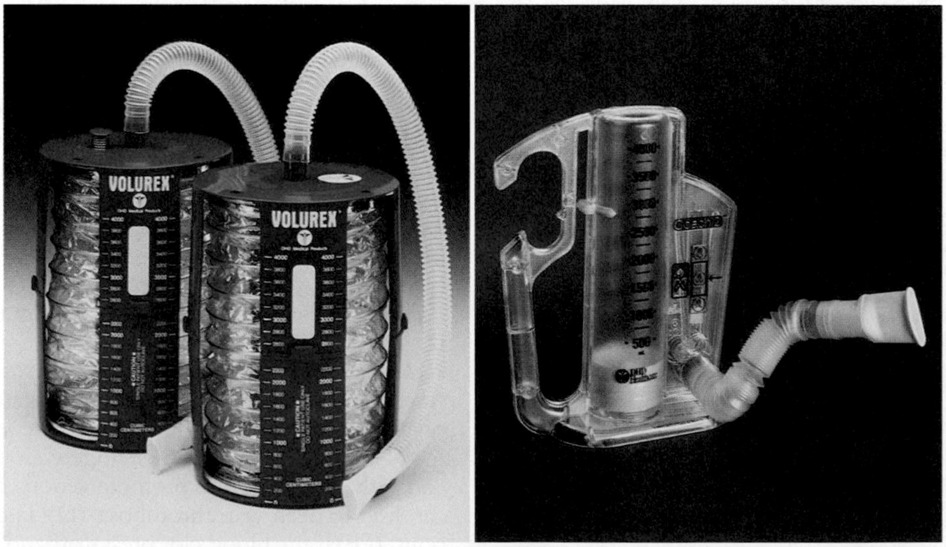

B

Figure 20-3 ■ Examples of volume incentive spirometers for lung expansion. **A,** A volume displacement incentive spirometer. **B,** A volumetric incentive spirometer. (Courtesy of DHD Healthcare, Canastota, NY.)

Specific interventions depend on the client's risk factors. Clients at greater risk for DVT:

- Are obese
- Are older than 40 years of age
- Have cancer
- Have decreased mobility or are immobile
- Have a leg fracture or leg trauma
- Have a history of DVT, PE, varicose veins, or edema
- Are taking oral contraceptives
- Smoke
- Have decreased cardiac output
- Are undergoing pelvic surgery

Antiembolism Stockings and Elastic Wraps. These stockings and elastic wraps provide graduated compression of the legs, starting at the end of the foot and ankle. Measure the client's leg length and circumference before ordering the stocking size. Elastic wraps are used when the legs are too large or too small for the stockings. Assist the client in applying the devices and ensure that they are neither too loose (are ineffective) nor too tight (inhibit blood flow). The devices need to be worn properly and should be removed one to three times per day for 30 minutes for skin care and inspection.

Pneumatic Compression Devices. Pneumatic compression devices enhance venous blood flow by providing intermittent periods of compression on the legs. Measure the client's legs and order the correct size. Place the boots on the client's legs, then set and check the compression pressures (usually 35 to 55 mm Hg). Figure 20-4 shows various types of sequential devices. Antiembolism stockings may be worn in addition to the boots and may reduce some of the uncomfortable sensations of the boots (e.g., itching, sweating, heat).

Leg Exercises. Leg exercises also promote venous return. Teach the leg exercises outlined in Chart 20-7 and then urge the client to practice these exercises before surgery. The exercises are important, even when other devices are used.

Early Ambulation. Mobility soon after surgery (early ambulation) stimulates intestinal motility, enhances lung expansion, mobilizes secretions, promotes venous return,

A

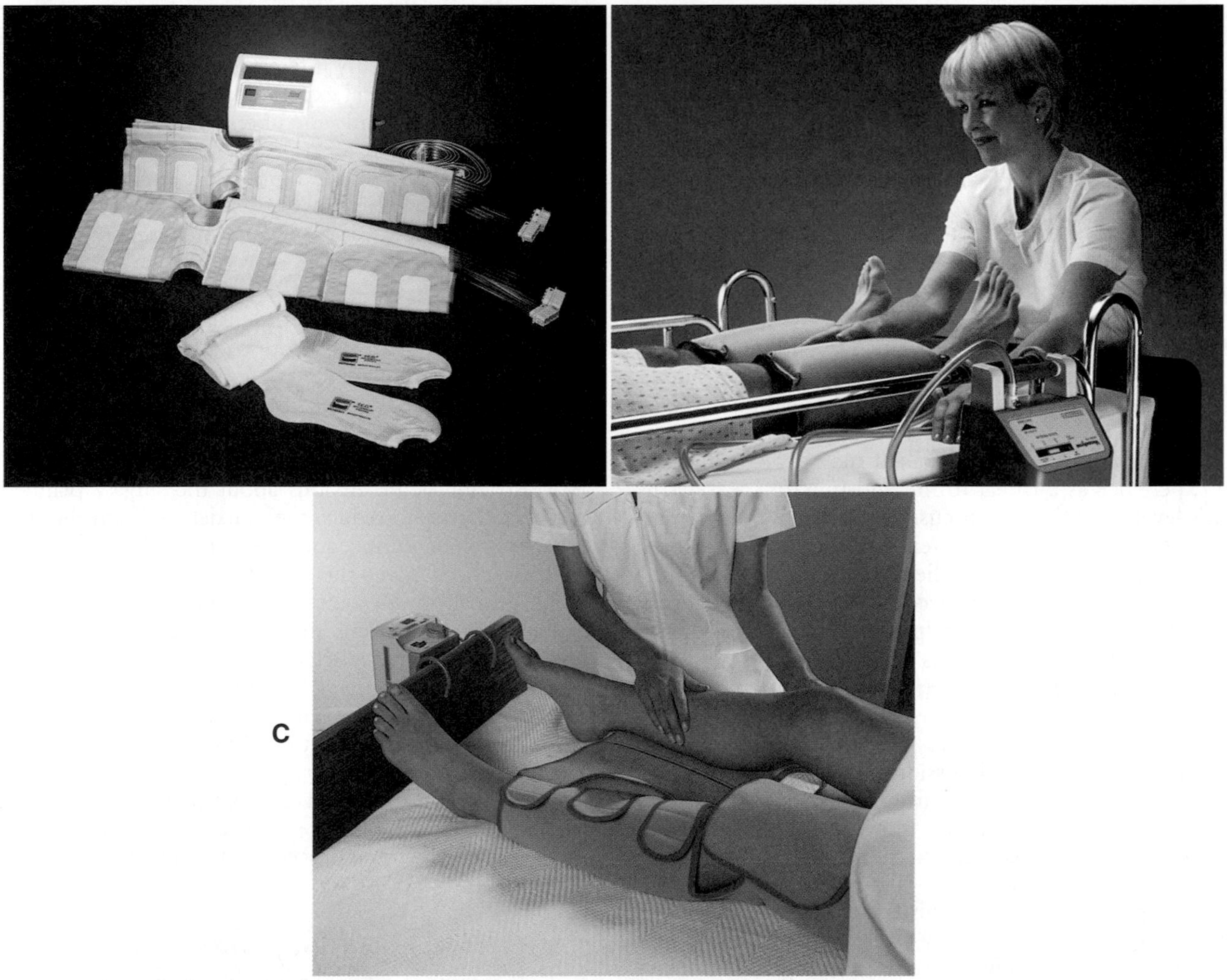

B

C

Figure 20-4 ■ Examples of external pneumatic compression devices used to promote venous return and prevent deep vein thrombosis (DVT). **A,** Kendall SCD machine, sleeves, and TED stockings. **B,** Venodyne pneumatic compression system. **C,** Flowtron DVT calf garments. (**A** courtesy of The Kendall Healthcare Company, Mansfield, MA; **B** courtesy of Venodyne, Inc., Norwood, MA; **C** courtesy of Huntleigh Healthcare, Eatontown, NJ.)

prevents joint rigidity, and relieves pressure. For most types of surgery, teach the client to turn at least every 2 hours after surgery while confined to bed. Teach clients how to use the bed siderails safely for turning and how to protect the surgical wound (splinting) when turning. Assure clients that assistance and pain medication will be given as needed to reduce any anxiety and pain they may have with this activity.

For certain surgical procedures, such as some brain, spinal, and orthopedic procedures, the surgeon may prescribe turning restrictions. Ask the surgeon about other interventions to prevent complications of immobility in clients with turning restrictions. Inform the client of anticipated turning restrictions during preoperative teaching.

Many clients are allowed and encouraged to get out of bed the day of or the day after surgery. Assist the client into a chair or with ambulation after the surgery, the next day, or when the surgeon specifies. If a client must remain in bed, help the client turn, deep breathe, and perform leg exercises at least every 2 hours to prevent complications from immobility.

Range-of-Motion Exercises. Passive or active range-of-motion (ROM) exercises help prevent joint rigidity and muscle contracture. The client should perform these exercises three to five times each, three to four times per day while bedridden. Teach the client these procedures and inform the client that he or she will receive help as needed after surgery. (Guidelines for ROM exercises are found in Chapter 22.)

ANXIETY

NOC **PLANNING: EXPECTED OUTCOMES.** Before surgery, the client is expected to have manageable preoperative anxiety as indicated by:

- Expressing a reduced level of anxiety
- Showing an absence of body language indicators of anxiety (e.g., hand wringing, facial tension, dilated pupils, sweating, elevated blood pressure, elevated pulse rate)

INTERVENTIONS. Anxiety often causes restlessness and sleeplessness. The surgical client may perceive the surgical experience as a threat to life and function. Assess the client's level of anxiety, as discussed earlier under Psychosocial Assessment on p. 301. Interventions such as teaching and communicating with the client before surgery, enabling the client to use previously successful coping mechanisms, and giving antianxiety drugs help reduce the anxiety. Incorporate available support systems into the plan of care.

Preoperative Teaching. Assess the client's knowledge about the surgical experience that has been acquired from prior surgical experiences and procedures and from other sources (see earlier discussion under Deficient Knowledge, p. 303). Provide factual information about the surgery and the perioperative experience to promote the client's understanding. Allow ample time for questions. Respond to the questions accurately and refer unanswered questions to the proper person. During the discussion, continually assess the client's responses and anxiety level. Be careful not to provide information that might increase anxiety. Clients have ranked psychosocial support as the most important part of preoperative teaching. The informed, educated client is better able to anticipate events and maintain self-control and is thus less anxious.

Encouraging Communication. Having the client state feelings, fears, and concerns is a technique to reduce anxiety. Develop a trusting relationship with the client so that he or she can express feelings freely without fear of ridicule or judgment. Keep the client informed by clarifying information, answering questions, and allaying fears about the surgery.

Promoting Rest. The stress and anxiety of impending surgery often interfere with the client's ability to sleep and rest the night before surgery. The period before surgery is physically and emotionally stressful. To help the client relax, determine what the client usually does to relax and fall asleep. If the client is able, urge him or her to continue these methods of relaxation. A back rub is relaxing and can be performed by a nurse or family member. The surgeon may prescribe a sedative or hypnotic drug to help the client be well rested for surgery.

Using Distraction. Distraction may be used as an intervention for anxiety, especially in the 24 hours immediately before surgery. Listening to music or audiotapes may decrease anxiety, as may watching television, reading, or visiting with family members.

Teaching Family and Significant Others. Assess the readiness and desire of the family to take an active part in the client's care. The involved family provides support, can assist with the care plan, and helps reduce anxiety. A positive sign of family interest is members' asking of questions about the surgical experience. After family readiness is determined, keep family members informed and encourage their involvement in all aspects of education. Emphasize the important role of the family before surgery but guide discussions and practice sessions so that family members do not dominate the sessions. Family members can encourage and help the client practice exercises to be performed after surgery.

Inform the family of the time for surgery, if known, and of any schedule changes. If the client is an outpatient, provide clear directions to the client and family regarding any specific night-before procedures, what time and where to report, and what to bring with them. Encourage the family to stay with the client before surgery for support.

Most families are anxious about the surgery planned for their loved one. To reduce their anxiety, explain the routines expected before, during, and after surgery. Tell the family that after the client leaves the hospital room or admission area, there is usually a 30- to 60-minute preparation period in the operating area (holding room, treatment area) before the surgery actually begins. After surgery, the client is taken to the postanesthesia care unit (PACU) for 1 to 2 hours before returning to the hospital room or discharge area. Tell the family about the best place to wait for the client or surgeon according to the facility's policy and the physician's preference. Many hospitals and surgical centers have surgical waiting areas so that families can wait in comfortable surroundings and be easily located when the procedure is completed.

Critical Thinking Challenge

The client, a 52-year-old single account executive, has been waiting for 45 minutes to go into surgery for an emergency open reduction with internal fixation of his left ankle. He is about 100 pounds overweight and fractured his ankle in multiple places when he slipped on a wet floor while at work. The client is anxious about having surgery and his ability to get back home to his dog. His constant focus is who will take care of his dog until he gets there. The medical record review documented that he minimized his preoperative teaching since "I only broke my ankle" and appeared disinterested in the cough and deep breathing exercises. During assessment, he told you that he is allergic to strawberries, bananas, tape, and roses. Although he told you he is a nonsmoker, you find him smoking a cigarette when you come back into the room.

1. As the preoperative nurse, how do you decrease this client's anxiety and assess his readiness for surgery?
2. Are any of his allergies important to document or communicate with the rest of the surgical team? Why or Why not?
3. What should you do about the disparity between his statement that he is not a smoker and the fact that you found him smoking?
4. What nursing diagnoses should be anticipated in this client's care?

evolve For suggested answer guidelines, go to http://evolve.elsevier.com/Iggy/.

PREOPERATIVE CHART REVIEW

Review the client's chart to ensure that all documentation, preoperative procedures, and orders are completed. Check the surgical informed consent form and, if indicated, any other special consent forms to see that they are signed and dated, and that they contain the witnesses' signatures. Confirm that the scheduled procedure, including the identification of left versus right when necessary, is what is listed on the consent form. Even though it might be obvious, have the client mark the correct area for surgery. Document allergies according to facility policy. Accurate documentation of height and weight is important for proper dosage calculation of the anesthetic agents. Ensure that the results of all laboratory, radiographic, and diagnostic tests are on the chart. Document any abnormal results and report them to the surgeon and the anesthesia provider. If the client is an autologous blood donor or has had directed blood donations made, those special slips must be included in the chart. Record a current set of vital signs (within 1 to 2 hours of the scheduled surgery time) and document any significant physical or psychosocial observations.

Report special needs, concerns, and instructions (advance directives) to the surgical team. For example, advise the surgical team whether the client is a member of Jehovah's Witnesses and does not accept blood products or whether the client is hard of hearing and does not have his or her hearing aid. This information assists the surgical team in providing continuity of care while the client is in the surgical area.

Critical Thinking Challenge

You are about to send the client, described earlier in the critical thinking exercise, to the surgical suite.

1. How should you communicate this client's allergies?
2. What risk factors does this client have for specific postoperative complications? Why?

evolve For suggested answer guidelines, go to http://evolve.elsevier.com/Iggy/.

PREOPERATIVE CLIENT PREPARATION

Facilities usually require the client to remove most clothing and wear a hospital gown into the operating room (OR); however, underwear may be worn in above-the-waist surgery, and socks may be worn, except in foot or leg surgery. If prescribed by the surgeon, apply antiembolism stockings before surgery. In some ambulatory settings, such as for cataract surgery, minimal clothes are removed.

Clients are advised to leave all valuables at home. If the client has valuables, including jewelry, money, or clothes, they are given to a family member or locked in a safe place, according to the facility's policy. If rings cannot be removed, tape them in place. Remove all pierced jewelry. Religious emblems may be pinned or fastened securely to the client's gown. Some facilities have paper emblems from a religious leader.

The client wears an identification band that clearly gives the first and last name, hospital number, physician, and birth date. An optional bracelet, usually red, identifies any allergies. A bracelet indicating that a blood sample for type and crossmatch has been drawn may be worn, depending on the facility's policy.

Dentures, including partial dental plates, are removed and placed in a labeled denture cup. Denture removal is a safety measure to prevent aspiration and obstruction of the airway. If a client has any capped teeth, document this finding on the checklist.

All prosthetic devices, such as artificial eyes and limbs, are removed and given to a family member or safely stored, as are contact lenses, wigs, and toupees. Check for hairpins and clips, which, if not removed, can conduct electrical current used during surgery and cause scalp burns.

Some facilities allow hearing aids in the surgical suite to help communication before and after surgery. If the client is sent to surgery with a hearing aid, communicate this to the surgical nurse to prevent accidental loss of or damage to the device. Some facilities allow dentures, wigs, and glasses to be worn into the operating suite to prevent embarrassment to the client. These items are removed when absolutely necessary.

The removal of fingernail polish or artificial nails is controversial. Polish is flammable, and artificial nails may affect the accuracy of pulse oximetry readings. In some facilities at least one artificial nail must be removed in order to monitor oxygen saturation by pulse oxymetry.

After the client is prepared for surgery and the operating suite is ready to receive him or her, ask the client to empty the bladder. This action prevents incontinence or overdistention and is a starting point for intake and output measurement. An overly full bladder may hinder access to the surgical site. Answer any questions, offer reassurance as needed, and give any prescribed drugs.

PREOPERATIVE MEDICATIONS

Preoperative drugs may be prescribed regardless of the type of planned anesthesia. Various drugs reduce anxiety, promote relaxation, reduce pharyngeal secretions, prevent laryngospasm, inhibit gastric secretions, and decrease the amount of anesthetic needed for the induction and maintenance of anesthesia. Drug selection is based on the client's age, physical and psychological condition, medical history, and height and weight; other drugs the client takes routinely; test results; and the type and extent of the planned surgical procedure. If more than one response is required, combination therapy may be prescribed. A typical combination consists of a sedative or tranquilizer, an opioid analgesic, and an anticholinergic agent.

Preoperative drugs are often given when the client is "on call" to the surgical suite. After positively identifying the

NORTHWEST HOSPITAL CENTER
PRE-OPERATIVE CHECKLIST

Date of Surgery________________

Addressograph Plate

ALLERGIES

CLINICAL DATA:	YES	NO	COMMENTS
Authorization for Surgical Treatment Completed			
Height & Weight Charted			
History and Physical			
Chest X-Ray			
EKG Report			
Urine Report			
Blood Sugar Within Range of (75-250mg%)			
Hematocrit Within Range of (27-55%)			
Potassium Within Range of (3.2-5.5mEq/L)			
Results Out of Range Reported to Dept. of Anesthesia			

Anesthesiologist Time: By:

PATIENT PREPARATION:	YES	NO	COMMENTS
Jewelry Removed			
Hair Piece, Wig, Hairpin, Barrettes, Beads, Rubberbands Removed			
Loose Teeth or Caps Noted			
Dentures Removed			
Artificial Eye, Contact Lenses, Glasses Removed			
Any Prosthetic Appliance Removed			
Voided or Catheterized - I&O Sheet on Chart			
Identification Bracelet in Place			
Parenteral Fluids Patent & Infusing at cc/hr			
B/P, T.P.R. Charted			
Premedication Given As Ordered			
Side Rails Up-Pt. Care Data & Care Plan on Chart			
Is Patient on Isolation - If Yes, What Type			

COMMUNICATION ASSESSMENT:	Normal	Abnormal	COMMENTS
Vision			
Hearing			
Mental			
Speech			
Other			

Patient's Preferred Name:

Limb For Burial ☐ Yes ☐ No Funeral Home:

R.N. Completing Checklist

702/1091-3-R-4/95 (40-1471) pl/3133N

Figure 20-5 ■ A preoperative checklist. (Courtesy of Northwest Hospital Center, Randallstown, MD.)

client (using the arm band and asking the client to state his or her name) and making sure the operative permit is signed, give the correct drugs. Then raise the siderails, place the call system within easy reach of the client while reminding him or her not to try to get out of bed. Place the bed in a low position. Tell the client that he or she may become drowsy and have a dry mouth as a result of the drugs.

A more common practice is for the preoperative drugs to be given *after* the client is transferred to the operating area. This practice permits the surgical team and anesthesia personnel to make more accurate assessments and have last-minute discussions with a client not yet affected by drugs. In addition, after the client is in the operating area, drugs can be given by the IV route. The oral or intramuscular (IM) route is used less often because of variable absorption rates.

CLIENT TRANSFER TO THE SURGICAL SUITE

In the immediate preoperative period, review and update the client's chart, reinforce teaching, ensure that the client is correctly dressed for surgery, and give prescribed preoperative drugs. Use a preoperative checklist for a smooth, efficient transfer to the surgical suite (Figure 20-5). The client, along with the signed consent form, the completed preoperative checklist, the chart, and the Addressograph plate, is transported to the surgical suite.

Most clients in the hospital setting are transferred to the surgical suite on a stretcher with the siderails up. In special circumstances (e.g., clients requiring traction, those having orthopedic surgery, and those who should be moved as little as possible), the client is transferred in the hospital bed. Other factors that influence the decision to transfer in a bed are the client's age, size, and physical condition. In ambulatory settings, clients either walk or are transferred to the surgical suite on a stretcher or in a wheelchair.

Evaluation: Outcomes

Evaluate the care of the preoperative client on the basis of the identified nursing diagnoses. The expected outcomes include that the client:

- States understanding of the informed consent and preoperative procedures
- Demonstrates postoperative exercises and techniques for prevention of complications
- Has reduced anxiety

Specific indicators for these outcomes are listed for each nursing diagnosis under the Planning and Implementation section (see earlier).

GET READY for the NCLEX Examination!

KEY POINTS

Safe Effective Care Environment

- Ask the client if an advance directive has been completed.
- Ask the client to explain in his or her own words what surgical procedure is being done and why.
- If the client's explanation of the scheduled surgery is not consistent with the documentation, notify the surgeon and request that the surgeon speak to the client.
- Ensure that the client is wearing proper identification.
- Ensure that the client is not asked to sign an operative permit or any other legal document after the preoperative drugs have been given.
- After the client has received preoperative drugs, keep the siderails up and the bed in the "low" position.

Health Promotion and Maintenance

- Teach clients about dietary restrictions and preoperative preparations.
- Teach the client specific interventions to perform after surgery to prevent complications (incision splinting, deep breathing exercises, range of motion exercises, as described in Charts 20-6 and 20-7).

Psychosocial Integrity

- Pace your interview to match the learning needs and style of the individual client.
- Allow the client the opportunity to express fear or anxiety regarding the surgical procedure or its possible outcome.
- Explain all diagnostic procedures, restrictions, and follow-up care to the client scheduled for a surgical procedure.
- Communicate any concerns or fears the client has to the surgeon and anesthesia personnel.

Physiological Integrity

- Communicate to the surgeon and anesthesia personnel any physical or laboratory change that may alter the client's response to drugs, anesthesia, or surgery.
- Check that documentation for any procedure to be performed on one of a paired organ or extremity clearly indicates which organ or extremity is involved.
- Ensure that dentures and any other personal items are removed from the client before the client is transferred to the surgical suite.

ADDITIONAL STUDY RESOURCES

Go to your Student CD-ROM for Review Questions for the NCLEX Examination.

evolve Go to http://evolve.elsevier.com/Iggy/ for Integrated Management of Care Questions for the NCLEX Examination.

SELECTED BIBLIOGRAPHY

Asterisk indicates a classic or definitive work on this subject.

*American Society of Anesthesiologists Task Force. (1999). Practice guidelines for preoperative fasting and the use of pharmacologic agents to reduce the risk of pulmonary aspiration: Application to healthy patients undergoing elective procedures. *Anesthesiology, 90*(3), 896-905.

American Society of PeriAnesthesia Nurses (2004). *Standards, recommended practices, and guidelines.* Denver: Author.

Association of Perioperative Registered Nurses. (2002). Recommended practices for skin preparation of patients. *AORN Journal, 75*(1), 184-187.

Association of Perioperative Registered Nurses. (2003a). ANA code for nurses with interpretive statements: Explications perioperative nursing. In *Standards, recommended practices and guidelines* (pp. 53-83). Denver: Author.

Association of Perioperative Registered Nurses. (2003b). AORN clinical path template. In *Standards, recommended practices and guidelines* (pp. 117-125). Denver: Author.

Beyea, S. (2002). Accident prevention in surgical settings: Keeping patients safe. *AORN Journal, 75*(2), 361-363.

Beyea, S. (2004). Evidence-based practice in perioperative nursing. *American Journal of Infection Control, 32*(2), 97-100.

Bryant, K. (2002). Ambulatory surgery industry takes steps forward. *OR Today, 2*(10), 34-35.

Cogliano, J., & Kisner, D. (2002). Bloodless medicine and surgery in the OR and beyond. *AORN Journal, 76*(5), 830, 832-837, 839.

Dochterman, J., & Bulechek, G. (eds). (2004). *Nursing interventions classification (NIC)* (4th ed.). St. Louis: Mosby.

*Dunn, D. (1998). Preoperative assessment criteria and patient teaching for ambulatory surgery patients. *Journal of PeriAnesthesia Nursing, 13*(5), 274-291.

Dunn, D. (2004). Preventing perioperative complications in an older adult. *Nursing 2004, 34*(11), 36-41.

Ebersole, P., Hess, P., & Luggen, A. (2004). *Toward healthy aging: Human needs and nursing response* (6th ed.). St. Louis: Mosby.

Fort, C. (2002). Get pumped to prevent DVT. *Nursing2002, 32*(9), 50-52.

George-Gay, B., & Parker, K. (2003). Understanding the complete blood count with differential. *Journal of PeriAnesthesia Nursing, 18*(2), 96-117.

Golembiewski, J. (2002). Allergic reactions to drugs: Implications for perioperative care. *Journal of PeriAnesthesia Nursing, 17*(6), 393-398.

Kjonniken, I., et al. (2002). Preoperative hair removal: A systematic literature review. *AORN Journal, 75*(5), 928-936, 938, 940.

McEwen, D. (2002). Ambulatory surgery. In M.H. Meeker & J.C. Rothrock (Eds.). *Alexander's care of the patient in surgery* (12th ed.). St. Louis: Mosby.

Meeker, M.H., & Rothrock, J.C. (2003). *Alexander's care of the patient in surgery* (12th ed.). St. Louis: Mosby.

Moorhead, S., Johnson, M., & Maas, M. (Eds.). (2004). *Nursing outcomes classification (NOC)* (3rd ed.). St. Louis: Mosby.

*Murphy, J. (1999). Preoperative consideration with herbal medicines. *AORN Journal, 69*(1), 173-183.

Pagana, K., & Pagana, T. (2002). *Mosby's manual of diagnostic and laboratory tests* (2nd ed.). St. Louis: Mosby.

Seal, L., & Paul-Cheadle, D. (2004). A systems approach to preoperative surgical patient skin preparation. *American Journal of Infection Control, 32*(2), 57-62.

Tappen, R., Muzic, J., & Kennedy, P. (2001). Preoperative assessment and discharge planning for older adults undergoing ambulatory surgery. *AORN Journal, 73*(2), 464-474.

Walton, J. (2001). Helping high-risk surgical patients beat the odds. *Nursing2001, 31*(5), 54-59.

Wood, B. (2002). Caring for a limited-English proficient patient. *AORN Journal, 75*(2), 305-308.

CHAPTER 21

Interventions for Intraoperative Clients

REBECCA M. PATTON

LEARNING OUTCOMES

After studying this chapter, you should be able to:

1. Discuss nursing interventions to reduce client and family anxiety.
2. Explain procedures to ensure the identity of the client and the accuracy of the planned surgical procedure.
3. Describe the roles and responsibilities of various intraoperative personnel.
4. Identify interventions to ensure the client's safety and dignity during an operative procedure.
5. Identify nursing responsibilities for management of clients receiving anesthesia.
6. Select nursing interventions to prevent skin breakdown for older adults clients during surgery.
7. Recognize the clinical manifestations of malignant hyperthermia.
8. List interventions for the client with malignant hyperthermia.
9. Discuss the potential adverse reactions and complications of specific anesthetic agents.
10. Assess clients for specific problems related to positioning during surgical procedures.

Go to your Student CD-ROM for Review Questions for the NCLEX Examination keyed to these Learning Outcomes.

Safety and advocacy for the client during surgery are the main concerns of perioperative nurses. Many hazards can be managed, prevented, reduced, and controlled by nursing actions and observations. The client entering the surgical suite (operating room, or OR) is at risk for infection, impaired skin integrity, increased anxiety, altered body temperature, and injury related to positioning and other hazards. The surgical phase is filled with unfamiliar experiences and uncertain outcomes. Nursing care during this period is critical, because the client's physical needs, spiritual needs, comfort, safety, dignity, and psychological status are dependent on the perioperative nurse. Specific procedures and policies may differ among agencies, but similarities reflect the standards and recommended practices for perioperative nursing, as published by AORN, the Association of periOperative Registered Nurses.

OVERVIEW

Members of the Surgical Team

The surgical team consists of the surgeon, one or more surgical assistants, the anesthesia provider, and the OR staff.

Perioperative, or operating room (OR), nurses include the holding area nurse, circulating nurse, scrub nurse, and specialty nurses. The number of assistants, circulating nurses, and scrub nurses depends on the complexity and projected length of the surgical procedure. For some minor procedures, only a circulating nurse may be needed in addition to the surgeon. More complex procedures may require additional nursing staff to either circulate or scrub.

SURGEON AND SURGICAL ASSISTANT

The **surgeon** is a physician who assumes responsibility for the surgical procedure and any surgical judgments about the client. The **surgical assistant** might be another surgeon (or physician, such as a resident or intern) or a physician's assistant, nurse, or surgical technologist. Under the direction of the surgeon and within the legal scope of practice for each state, the assistant may hold retractors, suction the wound (to improve viewing of the operative site), cut tissue, suture, and dress wounds.

ANESTHESIA PROVIDERS

The **anesthesiologist** is a physician who specializes in giving anesthetic agents. A **certified registered nurse anesthetist (CRNA)** is a registered nurse with additional credentials who delivers anesthetic agents under the supervision of an anesthesiologist, surgeon, dentist, or podiatrist. The anesthesia provider gives anesthetic drugs to induce and maintain anesthesia and delivers other drugs as needed to support the client during surgery.

The anesthesia provider monitors the client during surgery by assessing and monitoring the following:

- The level of anesthesia (i.e., by using a peripheral nerve stimulator or bispectral analysis)
- Cardiopulmonary function (using electrocardiographic [ECG] monitoring, pulse oximetry, end-tidal carbon dioxide monitoring, arterial blood gases [ABGs], and hemodynamic monitoring via arterial lines and/or pulmonary artery catheters)
- Vital signs
- Intake and output

Depending on the client's needs, anesthesia personnel give intravenous (IV) fluids, including blood and blood products.

PERIOPERATIVE STAFF

Perioperative, or OR, staff have several roles during surgery, depending on their education, experience, skill, and job responsibilities. Regardless of their role, the OR nurse uses the nursing process, develops a plan of nursing care, and coordinates care delivery to clients and their family members.

HOLDING AREA NURSE. Some operating suites have a presurgical holding area next to the main ORs. The client waits in this area until the OR is ready. The holding room nurse manages the care while the client is in this area. This nurse greets the client on arrival, reviews the medical record and preoperative checklist, and ensures that the operative consent forms are signed. The nurse assesses the client's physical and emotional status, gives emotional support, answers questions, and provides additional education as needed. The nurse begins documentation on a perioperative nursing record (Figure 21-1).

The holding area is busy, with many staff members performing different procedures before surgery (e.g., starting IV lines or inserting epidural catheters). The holding area nurse maintains an atmosphere to promote comfort, privacy, and confidentiality. Depending on the facility's policy, family members may be able to wait with the client.

CIRCULATING NURSE. The **circulating nurse,** or **circulator** is a registered nurse. This nurse coordinates, oversees, and is involved in the client's nursing care in the OR. The circulating nurse's actions are vital to the smooth flow of events before, during, and after surgery. This nurse is responsible for the activities within that particular OR. The circulator sets up the OR and ensures that supplies, including blood products and diagnostic support, are available as needed. All anticipated equipment is gathered and inspected by the circulator to make certain that it is safe and functional before the surgery. Depending on the procedure and position required, the circulator makes up the operating bed (OR table) with gel pads (to prevent pressure sores) and heating pads (to prevent hypothermia) under the sheets, as indicated.

If there is no holding area nurse, the circulator assumes the responsibilities of that nursing role as well. Even when there is a holding area nurse, the circulator also greets the client and reviews findings with the holding area nurse. The circulator is responsible for continuity of care.

Once the client is ready to be moved into the OR, the circulating nurse assists the OR team in the transfer to the operating bed. The nurse positions the client, protecting bony areas with extra padding while providing comfort and reassurance. While observing the client, the circulating nurse also assists the anesthesia provider with the induction of anesthesia. The circulator then may "prep" (scrub) the surgical site before the client is draped with sterile drapes.

Throughout the surgery, the circulating nurse:

- Monitors traffic in the room
- Assesses the amount of urine and blood loss
- Reports findings to the surgeon and anesthesia provider
- Ensures that the surgical team maintains sterile technique and a sterile field
- Anticipates the client's and surgical team's needs, providing supplies and equipment as needed
- Communicates information regarding the client's status with family members during long or unique procedures
- Documents care, events, interventions, and findings

Depending on facility policy, the circulating nurse may record drugs given, blood, and blood components. (This also may be a function of the anesthesia provider.)

Before the procedure is over, the circulating nurse completes documentation (Figure 21-2; see also Figure 21-1). The presence of drains or catheters, the length of the surgery, and a count of all sponges, "sharps" (needles, blades), and instruments are recorded in the nursing record. The nurse notifies the postanesthesia care unit (PACU) of the client's estimated time of arrival and any special needs.

SCRUB NURSE/SURGICAL TECHNOLOGIST. The **scrub nurse** and/or the surgical technologist sets up the sterile field (Figure 21-3), drapes the client, and hands sterile supplies, sterile equipment, and instruments to the surgeon and the assistant. Knowledge of the surgical procedure allows the scrub nurse to anticipate which instruments and types of sutures the surgeon will need. Anticipating these needs reduces the duration of anesthesia for the client. In addition, the surgeon's anxiety and tension are reduced when the scrub nurse is familiar with the procedure and can anticipate and respond accordingly. Throughout the surgical procedure, the scrub nurse (with the circulating nurse) maintains an accurate count of sponges, sharps, instruments, and amounts of irrigation fluid and drugs used.

A specially trained person who is not a nurse may perform the scrub role. Such people are called **operating room technicians (ORTs)** or **surgical technologists.** Often certified surgical technologists (CSTs) are used in the OR.

SPECIALTY NURSE. The **specialty nurse** is educated in a particular type of surgery (e.g., orthopedic, cardiac, ophthalmologic) and is responsible for nursing care specific to clients needing that type of surgery. The specialty nurse assesses, maintains, and recommends equipment, instruments, and supplies used in that specialty. During surgery the specialty nurse may act as the scrub or circulating nurse.

If the facility uses laser technology, nurses specially trained in the use, care, and maintenance of the laser are needed. This nurse may be called a laser specialty nurse or a laser nurse coordinator. (**Laser** is an acronym for *l*ight *a*mplification by the *s*timulated *e*mission of *r*adiation.) A laser gives off a high-powered beam of light that cuts tissue more cleanly than do scalpel blades. This process creates intense

Our Lady of Lourdes Medical Center
1600 Haddon Avenue Camden, N.J. 08103

PRE-OPERATIVE RECORD

PRE-OPERATIVE

Patient Name ________ Surgeon ________ Date ________

Procedure ________

Arrival ________ **ID** ☐ Verbal ☐ Nameband **Pt Verbalizes** ☐ Procedure Site ☐ Surgeon **NPO** Since ________

Allergies: ☐ NDA ☐ Latex ☐ Other ________ ☐ Drugs ________

Lab Data: ☐ CBC ☐ Urinalysis ☐ Chemistry ☐ Coag Studies ________ ☐ Pregnancy Test

Reports: ☐ EKG ☐ Chest ☐ H & P ☐ Other

Consents: ☐ Surgical ☐ Blood ☐ Anesthesia

Blood Products - # of units
In OR ________
Blood Bank ________
☐ Type and Screen ________
☐ Type and Cross ________
☐ Autologus ________
☐ Directed ________
☐ Homologus ________

Equipment: ☐ IV's ☐ Foley ☐ Ventilator ☐ Cardiac Monitor ☐ IABP ☐ Other ________

Prosthesis: ☐ None ☐ Opthalmic ☐ Otic ☐ Dental ☐ Jewelry Disposition of Prosthesis ________

Orientation: ☐ Awake ☐ Oriented ☐ Sedated ☐ Confused ☐ Agitated ☐ Crying

Implants / Other Comments: ________

________ RN SIGNATURE ________

INTRA-OPERATIVE

Identification: ☐ Verbal ☐ Nameband Scrub Nurse: ☐ Sees Permits ☐ Aware of Allergies

Skin Condition: ☐ Intact ☐ Presence of Lesions - Type / Location ________

Skin Prep: ☐ Betadine ☐ Hibiclens ☐ Other ________

Position: ☐ Supine ☐ Prone ☐ Lithotomy ☐ Lateral ☐ Jackknife ☐ Fracture Table

☐ Other ________ Positioned by ________

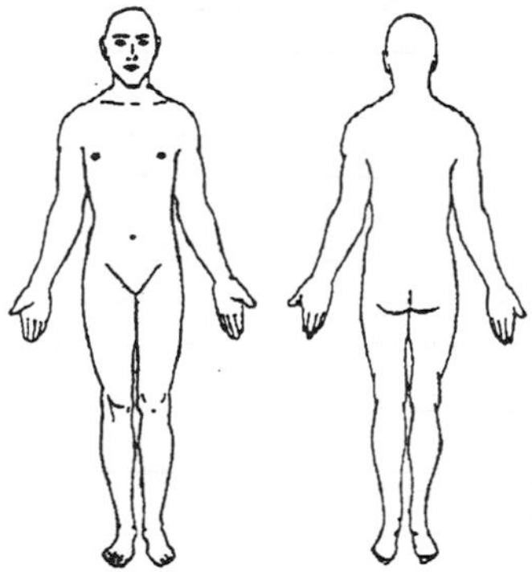

Equipment Codes:
= - Safety Strap applied by ________
X - Grounding Pad applied by ________
T - Tourniquet applied by ________
Δ - Pressure Pads applied by ________
S - Sandbag applied by ________
R - Roll applied by ________
A - Action Donut applied by ________
Z - Zoll Defib Pad applied by ________

Supports:
☐ Kidney Rest ________
☐ Stirrups ________
☐ Arms @ Side ________
☐ Arms on Armboard ________
☐ Action Pads ________
☐ Black Leg Positioner ________
☐ Bean Bag ________

Tourniquet Unit # ________ mm/Hg ________ Inflated ________ Deflated ________

Warming Blanket Unit # ________ Temp ________ On ________ Off ________

Electrocautery Unit # ________ Coag @ ________ Cut @ ________

Pad # ________ Exp. Date ________ ESU Pad Skin Site ________

Defibrillator # ________ Time / Joules ________

BiPolar Unit # ________ Setting ________ Other Equipment ________

Comments ________

________ RN SIGNATURE ________

FORM #PO1 (REV. 4/96)

Figure 21-1 ■ A perioperative nursing record with areas for charting preoperatively upon the client's arrival in the operating room (OR) suite and upon initial preparation intraoperatively. (Courtesy of Our Lady of Lourdes Medical Center, Camden, NJ.)

Our Lady of Lourdes Medical Center
1600 Haddon Avenue Camden, N.J. 08103

INTRA-OPERATIVE RECORD

Patient Name ____________ Date ________ Suite ________

☐ Scheduled ☐ Emergency ☐ Add On In Room ______ Began ______ End ______ Out ______

Surgeon ____________ Assistant ____________

Anesthesia ____________ Perfusion/Other ____________

Type of Anesthesia: ☐ General ☐ Spinal ☐ Epidural ☐ Regional Block ☐ Local ASB ☐ Local

Scrub ____________ Circulator ____________

Relief ____________ Relief ____________

Preoperative Diagnosis ____________

Postoperative Diagnosis ____________

Procedure ____________

Clamp/Bypass on ________ off________ EBL ________

Specimens: Cultures ☐ **Aerobic** ☐ **Anaerobic**________ Implant Log# ________

Irrigation: ________

Wound Classification:
Pre-Op I II III IV
Post-Op I II III IV
ASA Classification I II III IV

Medication Dispensed to OR Table (Include time, drug, amt used, site/route should be prepared by and given by)

Counts: ☐ Correct ________ ☐ Incorrect ________ Comments: ________

Intra-operative X-ray ☐ Yes ☐ No Type ________

Drains / Packing: ☐ None ☐ Foley Inserted by ________ ☐ Immediate urine output
☐ Jackson Pratt / Davol ______ ☐ Hemovac______ ☐ Penrose ______ ☐ Packing ______ Other ______
☐ Chest Tubes # and size ________ ☐ Pleuravac ☐ Auto transfusion pleuravac

Post Op Skin Condition: ________

ESU Pad Skin Site ________ Dressing Site ________

Receiving Unit ☐ PACU ☐ CVU ☐ ICU / CCU ☐ SDS ☐ Nursing Unit ________ Report given to ________

RN Signature ________ Surgeon Signature ________

FORM #PO2 (REV. 7/96) White - Original Copy Yellow - O.R. Copy Pink - Surgeon Copy Goldenrod - Pharmacy Copy

Figure 21-2 ■ An interdisciplinary intraoperative record. Names of all personnel involved are listed, and both the circulating nurse's and the surgeon's signatures are required for completion. (Courtesy of Our Lady of Lourdes Medical Center, Camden, NJ.)

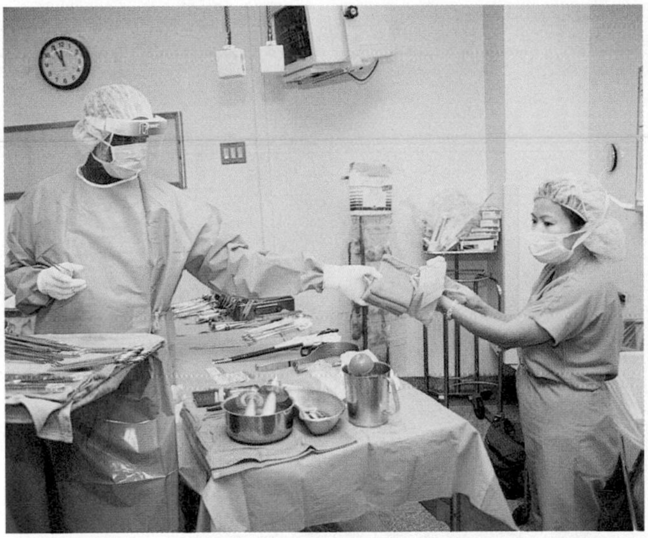

Figure 21-3 ■ Setting up the sterile table.

heat, rapidly clots blood vessels or tissue, and turns target tissue (such as a tumor) into vapor. All personnel must observe safety measures (e.g., wear eye shields, read door signs) during laser procedures to prevent injury to the client and staff.

Preparation of the Surgical Suite and Team Safety

During surgery, the client is unable to protect himself or herself, and all members of the surgical team must provide protection. The operating room (OR) layout prevents infection by reducing contaminants through air exchanges in the room and limiting the traffic and activities in the OR. Safety straps are used for the client, and the operating bed is locked in place. Heating pads are used to prevent hypothermia, and interventions are used to prevent skin breakdown.

The nurse ensures electrical safety through proper placement of grounding pads and use of electrical equipment that meets safety standards. All equipment used during surgery must be functional and in proper working condition as determined by the safety procedure of that facility. Equipment is cleaned and, when required, sterilized so that it can be used as a part of the procedure. The scrub and circulating nurses together ensure a correct count of surgical instruments, sharps, and sponges. Counts are performed before the beginning of the procedure, during the procedure as items are added or at the time personnel are relieved from that assignment, and immediately before complete skin closure.

Fire prevention and prevention of complications from the use of hazardous or toxic substances are concerns of all OR personnel. Ignition sources, oxidizers, and fuels are present in the OR and increase the risk for fires. Such events are rare but can occur during any kind of procedure. A cool room temperature (between 68° and 73° F [21° to 30° C]), with low humidity (30% to 60%) is optimal. The nurse is aware of emergency measures to take in the event of a fire or spill.

LAYOUT

The surgical suite is located out of the mainstream of the hospital and near the PACU and support services (e.g., blood bank, pathology and laboratory departments). Traffic flow is patterned to reduce contamination from outside the suite. Within the suite, clean and contaminated areas are separate. The surgical area is divided into three zones–unrestricted, semirestricted, and restricted–to ensure proper movement of clients and personnel.

The size of a surgical suite depends on the size and surgical capabilities of the facility. Most suites contain staff areas as well as areas related to client care, surgery, and surgical support. Staff areas include locker rooms and staff lounges. Client care areas include an admission or preoperative holding area and operating rooms. Surgical support areas include a number of ORs, cabinets for sterile supplies, separate utility rooms for clean and soiled equipment, and a clean linen room.

Figure 21-4 shows a typical OR. The exact number of tables and equipment used in a room is based on the needs of each client. A communication system links the OR and the main desk of the surgical suite. The system includes an intercom with separate systems for routine and emergency calls.

New OR designs use computers with the surgical equipment, lights, OR bed, and communications. These "hi-tech" rooms are similar to traditional ORs with the addition of computer equipment and panels. These rooms are more efficient for the surgical team with voice-activated commands operating some equipment that used to require manual operation.

HEALTH AND HYGIENE OF THE SURGICAL TEAM

People are a source of bacteria in the surgical setting. Everyone has bacteria on the skin, the hair, and in the airways. Because these organisms can be transmitted to the client, special health standards and dress are needed. Every surgical setting has policies and procedures regarding personnel and attire. Health standards require that all members of the surgical team and other support personnel in the surgical suite be free of communicable diseases. Anyone who has an open wound, cold, or any infection should not participate in surgery.

Good personal hygiene helps prevent and control infection, as does frequent handwashing. Shedding of organisms and skin debris is greatest immediately after showering, so surgical staff should bathe a few hours before changing into OR attire. Jewelry carries many organisms and should be minimal. All personnel must wash their hands between occasions of seeing clients and performing procedures, and more often when indicated. Hands of surgical personnel may be cultured on a regular basis to determine the potential for **nosocomial** (hospital-acquired) infections and to identify sources of pathogens. Further interventions or cultures are needed if quality reports (e.g., through the facility's quality improvement program) indicate a problem. Routine cultures are usually obtained every 3 to 6 months. Surgical attire and the surgical scrub help to prevent contaminations.

SURGICAL ATTIRE

All members of the surgical team and all OR personnel must wear scrub attire for use within the surgical suite. Scrub attire is clean, not sterile. It is worn to reduce contamination from home and areas outside of the surgical setting. Basic surgical attire is a shirt and pants, a cap or hood (Figure 21-5), and shoe

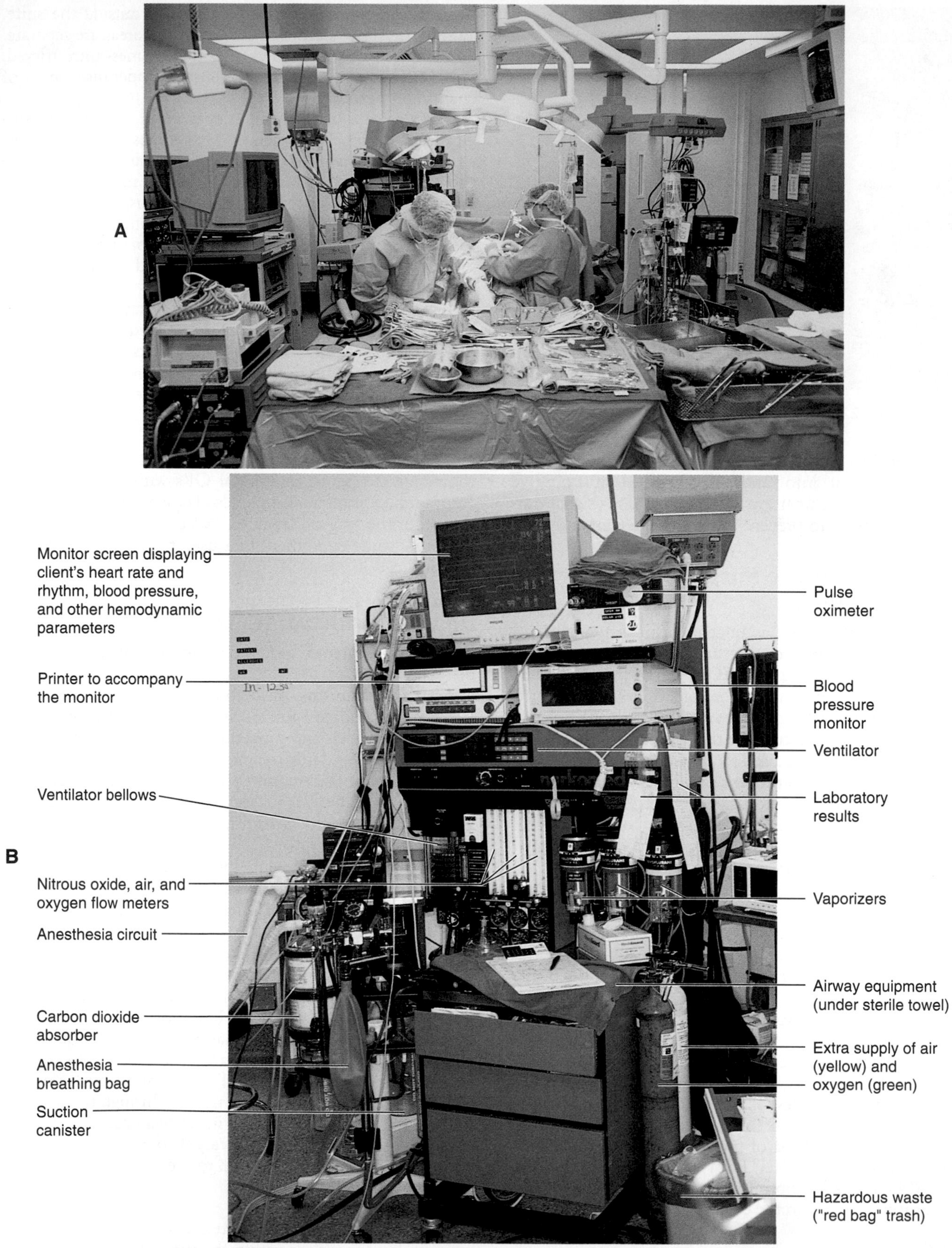

Figure 21-4 ■ **A,** A typical operating room. **B,** A typical anesthesia station with an anesthesia machine.

coverings. *Staff change into clean surgical attire in the OR suite locker rooms, not at home.* All members of the surgical team must cover their hair, including any facial hair.

In addition to basic attire, everyone must wear protective attire. This includes a mask, eyewear, gloves, gown, and shoe covers. Everyone who enters an OR where a sterile field is present must wear a mask. Surgical team members who are scrubbed and at the client's bedside during the surgery must also wear a sterile fluid-resistant gown, sterile gloves, and eye protectors (Figure 21-6). Team members who are *not* scrubbed (e.g., anesthesia provider and circulating nurse) may wear cover scrub jackets (to prevent shedding of organisms from bare arms) and eyewear, as warranted.

SURGICAL SCRUB

The surgeon, all assistants, and the scrub nurse perform a surgical scrub after putting on a mask and before putting on the sterile gown and gloves (Figure 21-7). *The scrub does not make the hands and forearms sterile.* When the scrub is performed correctly, it reduces the number of organisms from the hands, arms, and nails. Rings, watches, and bracelets are removed before scrubbing because they may harbor organisms. Fingernails are kept short, clean, and healthy. Artificial nails are not worn because they, too, can harbor organisms.

A surgical antimicrobial solution is used for the surgical scrub. Vigorous rubbing that creates friction is used from the fingertips to the elbow. The scrub continues for 3 to 5 minutes, followed by a rinse. During the rinse, hands and arms are positioned so that water runs off, rather than up or down, the arms. After scrubbing, personnel enter the OR with their hands held higher than the elbows and thoroughly dry their hands and forearms with a sterile towel. This person is then assisted into a sterile gown **("gowning")** and puts on sterile gloves **("gloving")**.

Gowns, gloves, and materials used at the operative field must be sterile. These items are changed between surgical procedures and as they become contaminated. The areas of the surgical gown considered sterile are the front of the gown from 2 inches below the neck to the waist area, and the elbow to the wrist area. Only when they are properly scrubbed and attired do members of the surgical team handle sterile drapes and equipment.

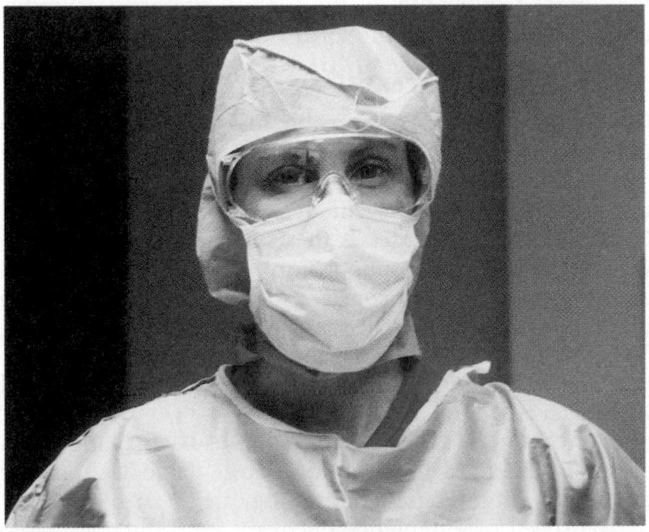

Figure 21-5 ■ An example of a hood-type hair covering that adequately covers facial and scalp hair.

Anesthesia

The word *anesthesia* means "negative sensation." Anesthesia delivery is a precise science. It requires the skill of an anesthesiologist, a certified registered nurse anesthetist (CRNA) working under the direction of an anesthesiologist or another physician, or an anesthesiologist's assistant (AA, similar to a physician's assistant) working under the direction of an anesthesiologist.

Anesthesia is an induced state of partial or total loss of sensation, occurring with or without loss of consciousness. The purpose of anesthesia is to block nerve impulse transmission, suppress reflexes, promote muscle relaxation, and, in some cases, achieve a controlled level of unconsciousness. Anesthesia providers use a separate anesthesia record for documentation (Figure 21-8).

Usually the anesthesia provider selects the anesthesia after consulting with the client and surgeon, and after considering specific client-related factors. The nurse and client communicate client preferences and fears about anesthesia to the anesthesia provider. Client health problems are major factors in the selection and dosage of anesthesia. Selection is also influenced by the following:

- Type and duration of the procedure
- Area of the body having surgery

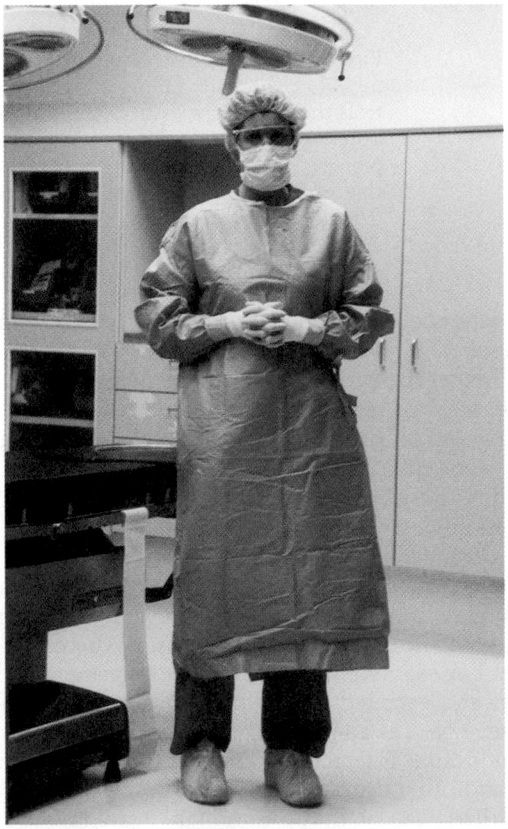

Figure 21-6 ■ Typical attire for all scrubbed personnel. Note complete hair covering, eye shields, mask, sterile gloves over the sleeves of the sterile gown, and shoe coverings. Note that when not in use, the hands are typically folded in front of the body, never below the waist.

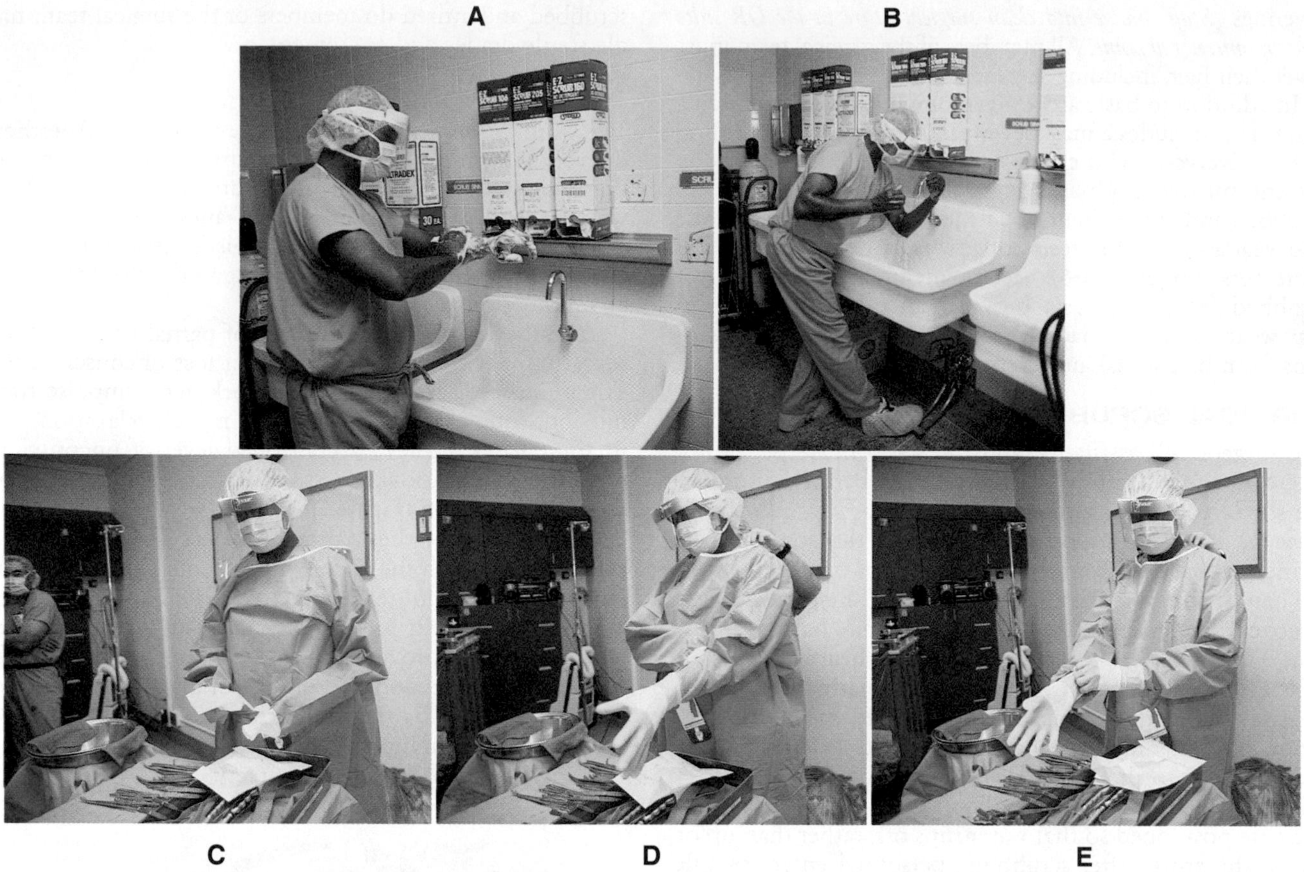

Figure 21-7 ■ The scrubbing, gowning, and gloving process. **A,** The surgical scrub. **B,** Rinsing. Note the water falling off the hands and arms. Also note the foot-operated handle that controls the water flow. (After scrubbing and rinsing, the scrub nurse dries his hands and arms with a sterile towel inside the operating room, then is assisted into a sterile gown.) **C,** The scrub nurse prepares sterile gloves. Note that the scrub nurse's hands are inside the sleeves of the gown and that he is touching the sterile gloves only with the sterile sleeves. **D,** The scrub nurse puts on his first sterile glove while the sterile gown is being tied in the back. Note again that his hand never emerges from under the sterile sleeve. **E,** The scrub nurse puts on his second sterile glove.

- Safety issues to reduce injury, such as airway management
- Whether the procedure is an emergency
- Options for management of pain after surgery
- How long it has been since the client ate, had any liquids, or any drugs
- Client position needed for the surgical procedure

Anesthesia delivery begins with selecting and giving preoperative drugs (see Chapter 20). The nurse must know the actions of commonly used drugs and their effects during and after surgery. Anesthesia affects many systems and can worsen other health problems, increasing the client's need for care. For example, most anesthetics are metabolized by the liver and excreted by the kidneys. Liver or kidney impairment increases anesthetic effects and the risk for toxicity. In addition, interactions may occur between the anesthetics and other drugs the client has received.

Anesthesia can be induced in many ways (Table 21-1):

- General or balanced anesthesia
- Local or regional anesthesia
- Hypnosis or hypnoanesthesia
- Cryothermia
- Acupuncture

Hypnosis or **hypnoanesthesia** (which induces a passive, trancelike state), **cryothermia** (use of cold [e.g., ice] reduces the surface temperature of the surgical site), and acupuncture are not often used in North America.

GENERAL ANESTHESIA

General anesthesia is a reversible loss of consciousness induced by inhibiting neuronal impulses in several areas of the central nervous system (CNS). This state can be achieved with a single agent or a combination of agents. General anesthesia depresses the CNS, resulting in **analgesia** (pain relief or pain suppression), **amnesia** (memory loss of the surgery), and unconsciousness, with loss of muscle tone and reflexes. The client is unconscious and unaware. This type of anesthesia is used most often in surgery of the head, neck, upper torso, and abdomen. It may also be used when clients are unable to cooperate.

STAGES OF GENERAL ANESTHESIA. Induction of general anesthesia involves four stages. Table 21-2 lists the expected client responses and nursing care for each stage.

The speed of **emergence** (recovery from the anesthesia) depends on the type of anesthetic agent, the length of time the client is anesthetized, and whether a reversal agent is

OUR LADY OF LOURDES MEDICAL CENTER
CAMDEN, NEW JERSEY

ANESTHESIA RECORD

DATE	ANESTHESIA RECORD NUMBER
CONSENT	PHYS. STATUS 1 2 3 4 E1 E2 E3 E4 5
PREMEDICATION (DRUG, DOSE, TIME, EFFECT)	

NAME
ADDRESS
ROOM
MEDICAL RECORDS NUMBER
SEX
AGE
BUSINESS DATA PLATE

15 30 45 15 30 45 15 30 45 15 30 45 15 30

AGENTS: N_2O, O_2
FLUIDS

B.P. V Λ
PULSE •
START ANES X
START OP ⊙
END ANES ⊗
TEMP Δ
SUCTION S
REC. ROOM R

°C: 38, 36, 34, 32, 30
240, 220, 200, 180, 160, 140, 120, 100, 80, 60, 40, 20, 10

RESP. O — SPON., ASST., CONT., VENT.

SYMBOLS

PREOPERATIVE DIAGNOSIS

AGENTS	TECHNIQUES	DOSAGE
A.		
B.		
C.		
D.		
E.		
F.		
G.		

REMARKS (INDUCTION, MAINTENANCE, EMERGENCE)

FLUID SUMMARY	RECOVERY (OR)
DEXTROSE - H_2O	REFLEX IN OR YES ______ NO ___
RING - LAC	CONSC. IN OR YES ______ NO ___
SALINE	NAUSEA ______ EMESIS ______
PLASMA	HYPOTENSION
BLOOD	
OTHER	
BLO. LOSS, HOW MEASURED	

1. OP NP OT NT (D - B)
2. CUFF-PACK TUBE SIZE______
3. TECHNICAL DIFFICULTY
4. MACHINE
VAPORIZER
MONITOR

POST OPERATIVE DIAGNOSIS

OPERATION

SURGEON	ANESTHETIST

OLLH FORM F20 (12/81)

Figure 21-8 ■ An anesthesia record. (Courtesy of Our Lady of Lourdes Medical Center, Camden, NJ.)

TABLE 21-1 Advantages and Disadvantages of Various Types of Anesthesia

Type	Advantages	Disadvantages
General		
Inhalation	Most controllable method Induction and reversal accomplished with pulmonary ventilation Few side effects	Must be used in combination with other agents for painful or prolonged procedures Limited muscle relaxant effects Postoperative nausea and shivering common Explosive
Intravenous	Rapid and pleasant induction Low incidence of postoperative nausea and vomiting Requires little equipment	Must be metabolized and excreted from the body for complete reversal Contraindicated in presence of hepatic or renal disease Increased cardiac and respiratory depression Retained by fat cells
Balanced	Minimal disturbance to physiologic function Minimal side effects Can be used with older and high-risk clients	Drug interactions can occur Pharmacologic effects on the body may be unpredictable
Regional or Local	Gag and cough reflexes stay intact Allows participation and cooperation by the client Less disruption of physical and emotional body functions Decreased chance of sensitivity to the agent Decreased intraoperative stress	Difficult to administer to an uncooperative or upset client No way to control agent after administration Absorbs rapidly into the blood and causes cardiac depression (hypotension) or overdose Increased nervous system stimulation (overdose) Not practical for extensive procedures because of the amount of drug that would be required to maintain anesthesia

TABLE 21-2 The Four Stages of General Anesthesia and Related Nursing Interventions

Stage	Description	Nursing Interventions	Rationales
Stage 1 (Analgesia and sedation, relaxation)	Begins with induction and ends with loss of consciousness. Client feels drowsy and dizzy, has a reduced sensation to pain, and is amnesic. Hearing is exaggerated.	Close operating room doors, dim the lights, and control traffic in the operating room. Position client securely with safety belts. Keep discussions about the client to a minimum.	Avoiding external stimuli in the environment promotes relaxation. Using safety measures in stage 1 prepares for stage 2. Being sensitive to the client maintains his or her dignity.
Stage 2 (Excitement, delirium)	Begins with loss of consciousness and ends with relaxation, regular breathing, and loss of the eyelid reflex. Client may have irregular breathing, increased muscle tone, and involuntary movement of the extremities during this stage. Laryngospasm or vomiting may occur. Client is susceptible to external stimuli.	Avoid auditory and physical stimuli. Protect the extremities. Assist the anesthesiologist or CRNA with suctioning as needed. Stay with client.	Sensory stimuli can contribute to the client's response. Safety measures help to prevent injury. Staying with the client is emotionally supportive.
Stage 3 (Operative anesthesia, surgical anesthesia)	Begins with generalized muscle relaxation and ends with loss of reflexes and depression of vital functions. The jaw is relaxed, and there is quiet, regular breathing. The client cannot hear. Sensations (i.e., to pain) are lost.	Assist the anesthesiologist or CRNA with intubation. Place client into operative position. Prep (scrub) the client's skin over the operative site as directed.	Providing assistance helps promote smooth intubation and prevent injury. Performing procedures as soon as possible promotes time management to minimize total anesthesia time for the client.
Stage 4 (Danger)	Begins with depression of vital functions and ends with respiratory failure, cardiac arrest, and possible death. Respiratory muscles are paralyzed; apnea occurs. Pupils are fixed and dilated.	Prepare for and assist in treatment of cardiac and/or pulmonary arrest. Document occurrence in the client's chart.	Teamwork and preparedness help decrease injuries and complications, and promote the possibility of a desired outcome for the client.

CRNA, Certified registered nurse anesthetist.

used. Retching, vomiting, and restlessness may occur during emergence although not all clients have these responses. Suction equipment must be available to prevent aspiration. During recovery, shivering, rigidity, and slight cyanosis may occur. These responses are caused by a temporary change in the body's temperature control. The nurse provides warm blankets, radiant light, and oxygen to decrease the effects of emergence.

ADMINISTRATION OF GENERAL ANESTHESIA. General anesthesia is administered by inhalation and IV injection.

INHALATION. Inhalation is an easily controlled method of giving general anesthesia because intake and excretion of the agent occur mainly by the lungs. The client inhales the anesthetic gas or vapor through a mask. The agent then crosses the alveolar membrane to the general circulation. The agent enters the bloodstream and is delivered to many tissues, where it is metabolized.

To improve gas exchange and control the anesthesia, respiration may be assisted or controlled. With **assisted respiration,** an endotracheal (ET) tube is inserted. The ET tube is then connected to the anesthesia machine (see Figure 21-4, *B*). The anesthesia provider overrides, or "assists," the client's own breathing effort and can manually start the breathing cycle.

Controlled respiration uses a mechanical ventilator to automatically inflate the lungs. Controlled ventilation is started after **apnea** (absence of spontaneous respiratory effort) is induced.

The anesthesia provider inserts the ET tube with the help of the circulating nurse. A laryngoscope is used to see the vocal cords, and the tube is placed in the trachea (Figure 21-9). With the ET tube in place, the client has an open airway (through the tube) for the inhaled anesthetic and oxygen.

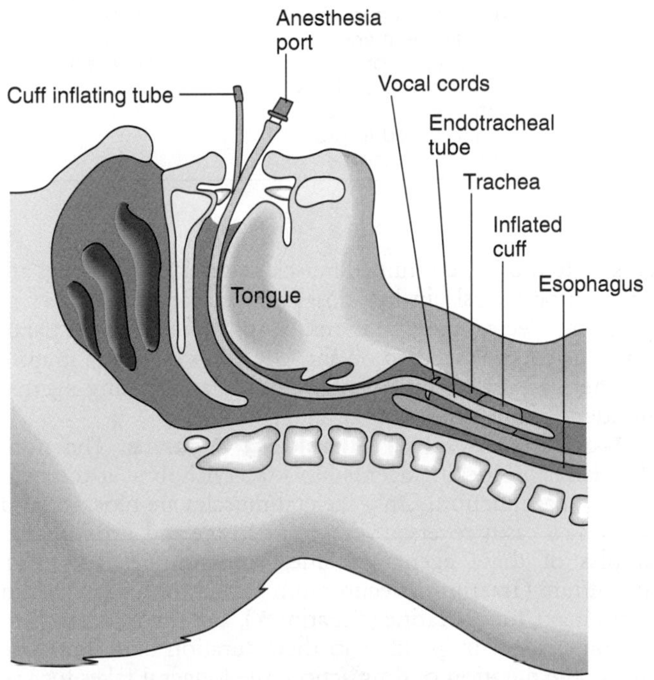

Figure 21-9 ■ An oral endotracheal tube in position. The cuff of the tube was placed just below the vocal cords, then inflated to seal off the airway.

Inhalation anesthetic agents are either gases or volatile agents. Table 21-3 lists the advantages, disadvantages, and nursing implications of inhalation agents.

Gaseous Agents. Nitrous oxide (N_2O) is the most commonly used agent and is usually given with oxygen. It is a colorless, odorless gas that provides analgesia.

Volatile Agents. Liquid agents vaporized for inhalation are "volatile" agents. Oxygen is the carrier, flowing over or bubbling through the liquid in the vaporizer system on the anesthesia machine. All volatile agents cause shivering after surgery because of their effect on the hypothalamus. Awakening is rapid, within 15 to 21 minutes. Table 21-3 lists features and interventions for volatile agents.

INTRAVENOUS INJECTION. IV anesthetic agents are injected, through an IV line, into the blood. The agent rapidly and smoothly spreads through the client's body. The drug is diluted by the blood, but is present at high enough levels in the brain, liver, and kidneys to induce anesthesia. Awakening is related to the client's metabolism. Table 21-4 lists advantages, disadvantages, and nursing implications of IV anesthetic agents.

Barbiturates. Barbiturates are often used for IV induction of anesthesia. These drugs act on the CNS, inducing reactions ranging from mild sedation to deep loss of consciousness. The barbiturate used most often is thiopental sodium (Pentothal). It acts rapidly, causing unconsciousness within 30 seconds. Because this agent depresses breathing and cardiac function, the client's vital signs are monitored continuously until the drug is eliminated.

Ketamine (Ketalar). Ketamine is a **dissociative anesthetic agent** (one that promotes a feeling of separation or dissociation from the environment). Rapid onset of a trancelike, analgesic state occurs. Ketamine is often used for diagnostic and short surgical procedures.

Emergence reactions are common during recovery from ketamine. The OR nurse reports the use of the drug to the PACU nurse so that precautions can be implemented. If the client is combative or restless, the siderails of the bed are padded to prevent injury. External stimuli are reduced until the client awakens. For severe reactions during recovery, small doses of diazepam (Valium, Vivol✱, Novo-Dipam✱) may be needed.

Propofol (Diprivan). Propofol is a short-acting anesthetic agent. Hypnosis occurs in less than 1 minute from the time of injection. The drug is eliminated rapidly and the client becomes responsive within 8 minutes after the infusion ends.

ADJUNCTS TO GENERAL ANESTHETIC AGENTS. Other drugs, such as hypnotics, opioid analgesics, and neuromuscular blocking agents, may be used as part of the anesthesia regimen.

HYPNOTICS. The benzodiazepines may be used for many effects. Common drugs in this class include midazolam (Versed), lorazepam (Ativan, Novolorazem✱), and diazepam (Valium, Vivol✱, Novo-Dipam✱). All have hypnotic, sedative, muscle relaxant, and amnesic effects. Lower doses may be used for sedation before surgery. These drugs also may be used as part of IV conscious sedation for short diagnostic procedures. Higher doses of midazolam can induce general anesthesia. These drugs may be used during surgery along with regional or local anesthesia. Adverse effects include respiratory depression, apnea, and oversedation.

TABLE 21-3 Advantages, Disadvantages, and Related Nursing Implications of Various General Inhalation Anesthetic Agents

Agent	Advantages	Disadvantages	Nursing Interventions	Rationales
Nitrous oxide (N_2O)	Rapid induction and recovery Useful for short procedures When used with other agents, reduces the required concentration of the other agents Minimal cardiovascular and respiratory depression	Relatively weak anesthetic agent May produce hypoxia if the concentration is high Needs addition of other agents for longer procedures	Assess oxygenation via pulse oximetry, physical assessment.	Ongoing assessment leads to early detection and treatment of potential complications.
Halothane (Fluothane)	Rapid and smooth induction Low incidence of postoperative nausea and vomiting Less irritating to the respiratory tract than other inhalation agents	Shivering common postoperatively Malignant hyperthermia possible in susceptible clients Metabolized by the liver Hypotension and bradycardia may occur Can sensitize the myocardium to dysrhythmias	Monitor heart rate for bradycardia. Monitor blood pressure for hypotension. Provide warm blankets, radiant heat.	Ongoing assessment leads to early detection and treatment of potential complications. Warmth helps promote client comfort and decrease shivering.
Enflurane (Ethrane)	Rapid induction and recovery Does not alter heart rate or rhythm	Respiratory depression and hypotension may occur Malignant hyperthermia possible in susceptible clients Lowers seizure threshold	Monitor respiratory rate and depth for hypoventilation. Assess oxygenation via pulse oximetry, physical assessment. Monitor blood pressure for hypotension.	Ongoing assessment leads to early detection and treatment of potential complications.
Isoflurane (Forane)	Rapid induction and recovery Has some muscle relaxant properties Stimulates the heart, which helps keep a stable heart rate Is not significantly metabolized; no renal or hepatic damage	Respiratory depression possible Malignant hyperthermia possible in susceptible clients	Monitor respiratory rate and depth for hypoventilation.	Ongoing assessment leads to early detection and treatment of potential complications.
Desflurane (Suprane)	Rapid induction, recovery, and awakening	May cause coughing and excitement during induction May increase heart rate and blood pressure with deep levels of anesthesia. Malignant hyperthermia possible in susceptible clients May cause changes in mental function	Monitor heart rate and blood pressure. Caution client and family that client should not drive or operate hazardous machinery until mental status has returned to preoperative baseline.	Ongoing assessment leads to early detection and treatment of potential complications. Specific instructions will help prevent other injuries or accidents.

CRNA, Certified registered nurse anesthetist.

OPIOID ANALGESICS. Common opioid analgesics used to enhance anesthesia include morphine sulfate (Statex✱), meperidine (Demerol), fentanyl (Sublimaze), and sufentanil (Sufenta). The use of opioids during surgery helps provide pain relief after surgery. *All opioid analgesics depress respiration.* Breathing is monitored and an open airway is maintained. Reduced dosages are used for older clients, clients with a circulatory problem (e.g., heart failure), and debilitated clients.

Fentanyl and sufentanil induce analgesia in lower doses, but at higher doses they are used to induce anesthesia. Fentanyl is 75 to 125 times more potent than morphine and sufentanil is five times more potent than fentanyl. It is often used in open heart surgery when the sternum must be opened. The client is monitored for bradycardia and decreased cardiac output.

NEUROMUSCULAR BLOCKING AGENTS. The neuromuscular blocking agents are used to relax the jaw and vocal cords immediately after induction so that the endotracheal tube can be placed. These drugs may be used during surgery to provide continued muscle relaxation. The drugs are given intravenously in low doses and may cause circulatory problems, decreased respirations, or apnea from muscle paralysis. The client is secured on the OR bed with safety straps.

There are two types of neuromuscular blocking agents: nondepolarizing and depolarizing.

Nondepolarizing Blocking Agents. The nondepolarizing blocking agents block acetylcholine at the neuromuscular junction. Only skeletal muscles are blocked, and the drug is easily reversed with neostigmine and atropine. Examples of these agents include pancuronium (Pavulon), atracurium (Tracrium), vecuronium (Norcuron), doxacurium (Nuromax), tubocurarine (Tubarine✱), and mivacurium (Mivacron). These drugs differ in their duration of action. The longer the duration of drug action, the longer it takes for the client to recover.

Depolarizing Blocking Agents. The depolarizing blocking agents overstimulate the motor end plate at the neuromuscular junction. In the process, potassium is forced out

TABLE 21-4 Advantages, Disadvantages, and Related Nursing Implications of Various General Intravenous Anesthetic Agents

Agent	Advantages	Disadvantages	Nursing Interventions	Rationales
Barbiturates				
Thiopental sodium (Pentothal) Methohexital sodium (Brevital)	Rapid, pleasant induction and recovery Acts directly on the central nervous system Short acting Low incidence of postoperative nausea and vomiting	Strong respiratory and cardiovascular depressant effect No antagonist medication available Mild to severe local tissue reaction with extravasation Poor analgesic, muscle relaxant effects	Monitor respiratory rate and depth for hypoventilation. Monitor heart rate for bradycardia. Monitor blood pressure for hypotension. Assess IV site.	Ongoing assessment leads to early detection and treatment of potential complications.
Nonbarbiturates				
Ketamine hydrochloride (Ketalar)	Rapid induction Short acting Can be given IM or IV No respiratory depression or loss of muscle tone (protects the airway) Protective reflexes remain intact Stimulates the cardiovascular system Can use for clients with respiratory or cardiac disorders Good amnesic effect Postoperative emergence reactions generally last only 24 hr	Emergence reactions—hallucinations, irrational behaviors, distorted images, unpleasant dreams, restlessness—are common Increased heart rate Increased blood pressure Increased cardiac output Poor muscle relaxant effect Nausea, vomiting, and aspiration possible	Minimize external stimuli: noise, light, touch, movement. Speak in a calm, soothing voice. Reassure client and family that emergence reactions are common and temporary. Have suction equipment near. Monitor blood pressure for hypertension. Monitor heart rate for tachycardia.	Stimuli increase the severity of the emergence reaction. Quiet promotes comfort, decreases anxiety. Reassurance decreases anxiety. Suction may be needed in the event of vomiting to prevent aspiration. Ongoing assessment leads to early detection and treatment of potential complications.
Propofol (Diprivan)	Short acting Rapidly metabolized Client becomes responsive quickly postoperatively Minimal postoperative nausea, vomiting, or sedation	Allergic skin reactions have occurred Client becomes aware of postoperative pain and discomfort sooner than with other anesthetics	Be prepared to administer analgesic medications as prescribed early in the postoperative period. Plan for nonpharmacologic pain interventions (see Chapter 7).	Awareness of pain very early in the postoperative period can be frightening. Pain can increase blood pressure and increase anxiety.
Opioids (As Adjunct)				
Fentanyl (Sublimaze)	Excellent postoperative analgesia Long-acting analgesia	Significant respiratory depression can occur several hours after administration Cardiovascular depression can occur	Monitor respiratory rate and depth for hypoventilation. Monitor blood pressure for hypotension. Have atropine, naloxone (Narcan), vasopressors, and resuscitative equipment nearby.	Ongoing assessment leads to early detection and treatment of potential complications. Having necessary supplies and equipment available provides for prompt response to an emergency.

CRNA, Certified registered nurse anesthetist.

of the muscle cells and into the blood, which can cause hyperkalemia. Clients often have brief muscle twitching, which causes muscle aches after awakening. Other side effects include increased salivation (increasing the risk for aspiration) and increased intraocular pressure (thus the agents may be not be used for clients with glaucoma). An example of a commonly used depolarizing blocking agent is succinylcholine (Anectine). There is no specific antidote for these agents.

BALANCED ANESTHESIA. **Balanced anesthesia** is a combination of IV drugs and inhalation agents used to obtain specific effects. A combination is used to provide hypnosis, amnesia, analgesia, muscle relaxation, and reduced reflexes with minimal disturbance of physiologic function. This method provides safe and controlled anesthetic delivery, especially for older and high-risk clients. An example of balanced anesthesia is the use of thiopental for induction, nitrous oxide for amnesia, morphine for analgesia, and pancuronium for muscle relaxation. Many combinations are possible, and selection is based on the individual client and the specific surgical procedure.

COMPLICATIONS FROM GENERAL ANESTHESIA. Complications can range from minor and annoying (sore throat) to death. Improvement in anesthesia delivery and surgical techniques has resulted in a decline in anesthesia-related deaths, even among higher-risk clients.

MALIGNANT HYPERTHERMIA. Malignant hyperthermia (MH) is an acute, life-threatening complication of certain drugs used for general anesthesia. The reaction begins in skeletal muscle exposed to specific agents, causing increased calcium levels in muscle cells and increased muscle metabolism. Serum calcium and potassium levels are increased, as is the metabolic rate, leading to acidosis, cardiac dysrhythmias, and a high body temperature.

Onset of MH may occur immediately after induction of anesthesia, several hours into the procedure, or, rarely, even after the anesthetic has been terminated. Clinical features reflect the increased muscle calcium level and the greatly increased body metabolism. Manifestations include tachycardia, dysrhythmias, muscle rigidity (especially of the jaw and upper chest), hypotension, tachypnea, skin mottling, cyanosis, and myoglobinuria (presence of muscle proteins in the urine). The most sensitive indication is an unexpected rise in the end-tidal carbon dioxide level with a decrease in oxygen saturation. Another early indication is sinus tachycardia. *Extremely elevated temperature, as high as 111.2° F (44° C), is a late sign of MH.* Survival depends on early diagnosis and the actions of the entire surgical team. Time is crucial when MH is diagnosed. Dantrolene sodium, a skeletal muscle relaxant, is the drug of choice along with other interventions.

For a known history or risk, the client can be treated before, during, and after surgery with dantrolene to prevent this problem. Chart 21-1 lists best practices for care of the client with MH.

Genetic Considerations

MH is a genetic disorder transmitted as an autosomal dominant trait. The client with a genetic predisposition for MH is at risk for this complication from halothane, enflurane, isoflurane, desflurane, sevoflurane, and succinylcholine. This rare syndrome is most common in young adults. Males are affected more often than females (despite the autosomal dominant pattern of inheritance) because of gender differences in muscle mass. Once a client or family history of MH is known, family members can have a muscle biopsy to determine whether they are at risk.

OVERDOSE. An anesthesia overdose can occur if the client's metabolism and drug elimination are slower than expected. Other drugs (e.g., antihypertensives) also alter metabolism, and interactions can occur between the anesthetic and the client's regular drugs. Accurate information about the client's height, weight, and history, is vital in determining the anesthetic type and dosage. Death during surgery is more often related to pre-existing health problems than to anesthesia overdose.

UNRECOGNIZED HYPOVENTILATION. The respiratory system is most often involved when the client has an anesthesia-induced complication. Failure to exchange gases adequately can lead to cardiac arrest, permanent brain damage, and death. Monitoring standards include the use of an end-tidal carbon dioxide monitor to confirm carbon dioxide in the client's expired gas and a breathing system disconnect monitor to detect any break in the breathing circuit equipment.

COMPLICATIONS OF SPECIFIC ANESTHETIC AGENTS. Specific complications are discussed earlier in the chapter. Older or debilitated clients are at greater risk for complications because of decreased metabolism or poor general physical condition. (For surgical risk factors, see Chapter 20.)

COMPLICATIONS OF INTUBATION. Many complications can occur from intubation (e.g., broken or injured teeth and caps, swollen lip, or vocal cord trauma). Intubation may be difficult because of anatomic variance or disease presence (e.g., small oral cavity, tight jaw joint, or presence of tumor). Improper neck extension during intubation also may cause injury. The surgeon should be in the operating room (OR) during the intubation process in case a tracheostomy is needed when the endotracheal (ET) tube is placed. ET placement causes tracheal irritation and edema. The client may have a sore throat after surgery.

CHART 21-1

BEST PRACTICE for
Care of the Client with Malignant Hyperthermia

- Stop all inhalation anesthetic agents and succinylcholine.
- If an endotracheal (ET) tube is not already in place, intubate immediately.
- Ventilate the client with 100% oxygen, using the highest possible flow rate.
- Administer dantrolene sodium (Dantrium) intravenously at a dose of 2 to 3 mg/kg.
- If possible, terminate surgery. If termination is not possible, continue surgery using anesthetic agents that do not trigger malignant hyperthermia (MH).
- Assess arterial blood gases (ABGs) and serum chemistries for metabolic acidosis and hyperkalemia.
  - If metabolic acidosis is evident by ABG analysis, administer sodium bicarbonate intravenously.
  - If hyperkalemia is present, administer 10 units of insulin in 50 mL of 20% dextrose intravenously.
- Use active cooling techniques.
  - Administer iced saline (0.9% NaCl) intravenously at a rate of 15 mL/kg every 15 minutes for three doses.
  - Apply a cooling blanket over the torso.
  - Wrap or rub extremities with cold, wet towels or ice wrapped in towels.
  - Lavage the stomach, bladder, rectum, and open body cavities (if appropriate) with sterile iced normal saline.
- Monitor core body temperature to assess effectiveness of interventions and avoid hypothermia.
- Monitor cardiac rhythm by electrocardiography (ECG) to assess for dysrhythmias.
- Insert a Foley catheter to monitor urine output.
- Treat any dysrhythmias that do not resolve on correction of hyperthermia and hyperkalemia with antidysrhythmic agents *other than calcium channel blockers*.
- Administer IV fluids at a rate and volume sufficient to maintain urine output above 2 mL/kg/hr.
- Monitor urine for presence of blood or myoglobin.
- If urine output falls below 2 mL/kg/hr, consider using osmotic or loop diuretics, depending on the client's cardiac and renal status.
- Contact the Malignant Hyperthermia Association of the United States (MHAUS) hotline for more information regarding treatment: (800) 644-9373.
- Transfer the client to the intensive care unit (ICU) when stable.
- Continue to monitor the client's temperature, ECG, ABGs, electrolytes, creatine kinase, coagulation studies, and serum and urine myoglobin levels until they have remained normal for 24 hours.
- Instruct the client and family about testing for MH risk.
- Refer the client and family to the Malignant Hyperthermia Association of the United States at (800) 986-4287 or http://www.mhaus.org.
- Report the incident to the North American Malignant Hyperthermia Registry at the University of Pittsburgh: (412) 692-5464.

Data from Malignant Hyperthermia Association of the United States; and Dunn, D. (1997). Malignant hyperthermia. *AORN Journal, 65*(4), 728-762.

LOCAL OR REGIONAL ANESTHESIA

Local or regional anesthesia briefly disrupts sensory nerve impulse transmission from a specific body area or region.

TABLE 21-5 Advantages, Disadvantages, and Related Nursing Implications of Local or Regional Anesthetic Agents

Agent	Advantages	Disadvantages	Nursing Interventions	Rationales
Procaine (Novocain) Tetracaine (Pontocaine) Lidocaine (Xylocaine) Mepivacaine (Carbocaine, Polocaine) Bupivacaine (Marcaine, Sensorcaine)	Easily administered Rapid onset (4-17 min) Can be administered topically or by injection Excellent muscle relaxant effects Protective reflexes (cough, gag) remain intact Client does not lose consciousness Many are available with epinephrine added	Absorbs into the bloodstream Can cause cardiac depression and dysrhythmias with absorption Difficult to control dosage Drug interactions with monoamine oxidase (MAO) inhibitors can cause hypertension Tremors, twitching, shivering, respiratory arrest can occur with absorption	Assess for return of movement and sensation in the area anesthetized.	Movement returns first, then sense of touch, pain, warmth, and cold, in that order.
			Monitor blood pressure and pulse.	Ongoing assessment leads to early detection and treatment of potential complications.
			Assess administration site for pallor, drainage.	Protection prevents injury to the area.
			Protect area anesthetized until full sensation has returned.	Duration of anesthetic is 3-6 hr.

Motor function may or may not be affected. The client remains conscious and able to follow instructions. Because the gag and cough reflexes remain intact, the risk for aspiration is low. Local or regional anesthesia is often supplemented with sedatives, opioid analgesics, or hypnotics to reduce anxiety and increase comfort.

The OR nurse provides the client with information, directions, and emotional support before, during, and after the procedure. Table 21-5 describes local and regional anesthetic agents and related nursing implications.

LOCAL ANESTHESIA. Local anesthesia is delivered topically and by local infiltration. Sometimes when the term *local* is used, it means *any* form of anesthesia that is not general anesthesia.

TOPICAL ANESTHESIA. Topical agents are applied *directly* to the area of skin or mucous membrane surface to be anesthetized. Often the anesthetic is an ointment or spray. This method is often used for respiratory intubation and for diagnostic procedures, such as bronchoscopy or cystoscopy. The onset of action is 1 minute, and the duration is 20 to 30 minutes. Cardiac depression is a potential complication of topical agents applied to the pulmonary tract.

LOCAL INFILTRATION. Local infiltration is the injection of an anesthetic agent directly *into* the tissue around an incision, wound, or lesion. Peripheral nerve function is blocked at its origin. This method is often used during superficial suturing.

REGIONAL ANESTHESIA. Regional anesthesia, a type of local anesthesia, may be used when:

- General anesthesia cannot be used because of medical problems (e.g., dysrhythmias and pulmonary disease)
- The client has had adverse reactions to general anesthesia
- The client has a preference and a choice is possible
- Pain management after surgery is enhanced by regional anesthesia

If the client has eaten and the surgery is an emergency, it may be possible to perform surgery with the client under regional anesthesia (depending on the procedure) to decrease the risk for aspiration. Types of regional anesthesia include field block, nerve block, spinal, and epidural.

FIELD BLOCK. A field block occurs with a series of injections *around* the operative field. Injecting around a specific nerve or group of nerves depresses sensation at a local area. This type of block is used for chest procedures, hernia repair, dental surgery, and some plastic surgeries.

NERVE BLOCK. A nerve block occurs with injection of the local anesthetic agent *into or around* a nerve or group of nerves in the involved area. Nerve blocks disrupt sensory and motor impulse transmission. They prevent pain during a procedure, are used diagnostically to identify the cause of pain, and can be used to relieve chronic pain.

Figure 21-10 shows common nerve block sites. Lidocaine (Xylocaine) or bupivacaine (Marcaine) is often the agent used. A nerve block takes effect within minutes after the injection, and lasts longer than with local infiltration. Epinephrine added to the agent prolongs the effect. Seizures, cardiac depression, dysrhythmias, and respiratory depression may occur if the nerve-blocking agent is injected (by accident) into the bloodstream. The nurse observes for signs of systemic absorption, sensitivity, or overdose.

SPINAL ANESTHESIA. Spinal anesthesia, also called intrathecal block, occurs by injecting an anesthetic agent into the cerebrospinal fluid in the subarachnoid space (Figure 21-11). The drug acts on the nerves as they emerge from the spinal cord and before they leave the spinal canal. This type of block inhibits the autonomic, sensory, and motor nervous systems. The drug is absorbed rapidly into the nerve fibers, producing analgesia with relaxation. This method often used for lower abdominal and pelvic surgery.

EPIDURAL ANESTHESIA. The anesthetic agent is injected into the epidural space and the spinal cord areas are never entered. Because the agent can diffuse or "float up" the spinal canal, the client can have anesthetic effects as high as the T4 level. Breathing problems may make injection at this high a level less desirable.

Epidural anesthesia is used for anorectal, vaginal, perineal, hip, and lower extremity surgeries. Two advantages of this type of anesthesia are:

- Decreased cardiac and pulmonary complications (especially important for the older client)
- Use of the epidural catheter for pain control after surgery (see Chapter 7)

COMPLICATIONS OF LOCAL OR REGIONAL ANESTHESIA. Complications of local or regional anesthesia are related to client sensitivity to the anesthetic agent (anaphylaxis), incorrect delivery technique, systemic absorption, and overdosage. The nurse observes for central nervous system (CNS) stimulation followed by CNS and cardiac depression, which are signs of a systemic toxic reaction. The nurse also assesses for restlessness, excitement, incoherent

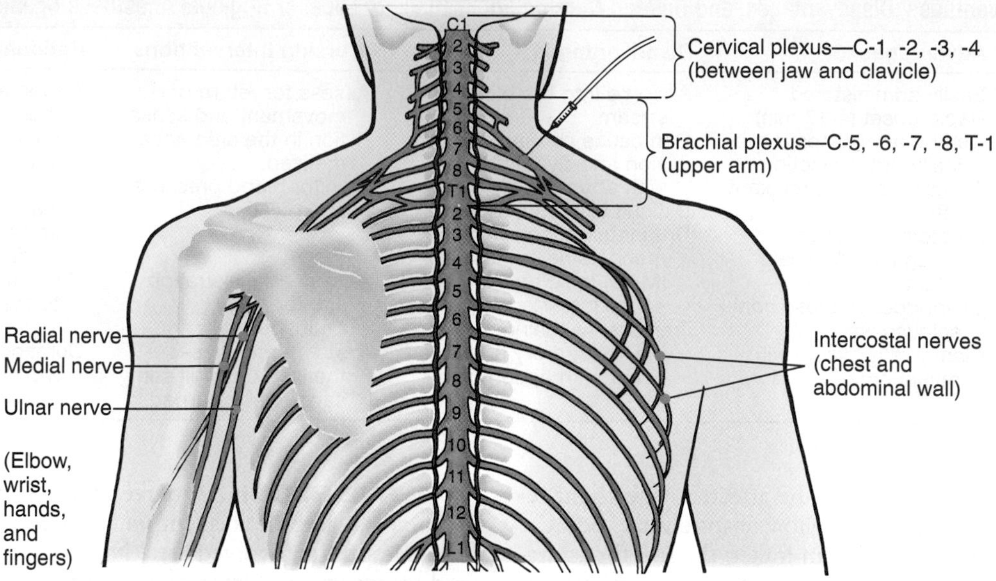

Figure 21-10 ■ Nerve block sites.

speech, headache, blurred vision, metallic taste, nausea, vomiting, tremors, seizures, and increased pulse, respirations, and blood pressure. Interventions include establishing an open airway, giving oxygen, and notifying the surgeon. Usually a fast-acting barbiturate is needed for treatment. If the toxic reaction is untreated, unconsciousness, hypotension, apnea, cardiac arrest, and death may result.

Cardiac arrest may occur as a rare complication of spinal anesthesia. Epinephrine is given to prevent cardiac arrest in clients in whom sudden, unexplained bradycardia develops.

Local complications include edema and inflammation as early problems. Abscess formation, tissue necrosis, and/or gangrene may occur later. Abscesses result from contamination during injection of the agent. Necrosis and gangrene are rare but may occur as a result of prolonged blood vessel constriction in the injected area.

The nurse's role in the delivery of regional anesthesia consists of the following:

- Assisting the anesthesia provider
- Observing for breaks in sterile technique
- Providing emotional support for the client
- Staying with the client
- Offering information and reassurance
- Positioning the client comfortably and safely

CONSCIOUS SEDATION

Conscious sedation is the IV delivery of sedative, hypnotic, and opioid drugs to reduce the level of consciousness but allow the client to maintain a patent airway and to respond to verbal commands. The amnesia action is short and the client usually has a rapid return to activities of daily living. Diazepam (Valium, Vivol✱, Novo-Dipam✱), midazolam (Versed), meperidine (Demerol), fentanyl (Sublimaze), alfentanil (Alfenta), and morphine sulfate are the most commonly used drugs. Conscious sedation is used for endoscopy, cardiac catheterization, closed fracture reduction, cardioversion, and other special but short procedures.

Selection of clients for conscious sedation is based on specific criteria. The physician determines whether the client is a candidate. In most states, a credentialed registered nurse may deliver conscious sedation under physician supervision and within the state-defined scope of nursing practice. Credentialing includes advanced training in IV drug delivery, airway management, and advanced cardiac life support (ACLS).

The nurse monitors the client during and after the procedure for response to the procedure and the drugs. The airway, level of consciousness, oxygen saturation, electrocardiographic (ECG) status, and vital signs are monitored every 15 to 30 minutes until the client is fully awake, oriented, and vital signs have returned to baseline levels.

The client receiving IV conscious sedation can be discharged to go home with a responsible adult. If the client returns to the general medical-surgical nursing unit, the unit staff nurses continue monitoring. The client is expected to be sleepy but arousable for several hours after the procedure. Oral intake is not permitted until 30 minutes after the client has received the sedation or according to the physician's prescription. When fluids are permitted, the nurse makes sure that the client is awake and positioned to avoid aspiration.

◆COLLABORATIVE MANAGEMENT

PHARM REVIEW

◆Assessment

HISTORY

On arrival in the surgical suite, the client is taken to the holding area or directly into the operating suite. The holding area nurse or the circulating nurse greets the client on arrival. *Correct identification of the client is the responsibility of every member of the health care team.* The nurse verifies the client's identity with two types of identifiers (name, birth date, medical record number, or social security number). For example, the nurse checks the client's identification bracelet and asks, "What is your name and when were you born?" This prac-

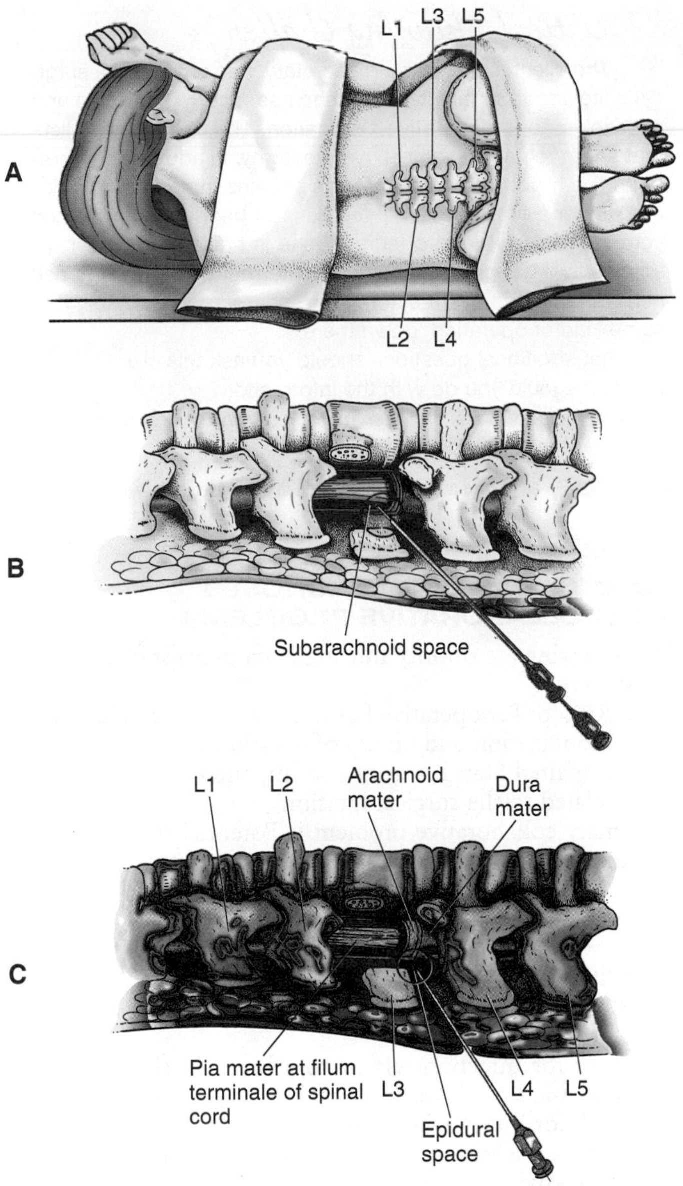

Figure 21-11 ■ Administration of spinal and epidural anesthesia. **A,** Spinal or epidural anesthesia is administered by inserting a spinal needle between the second and third or the third and fourth lumbar vertebrae (L2-3 or L3-4). The client is placed in the flexed lateral (fetal) position (shown here) or seated on the edge of the operating bed with the back arched and the chin tucked to the chest. **B,** Spinal anesthesia (viewed from the side). A large needle is inserted to the surface of the dura mater, and a second, smaller needle is passed through the first to penetrate the dura mater and arachnoid mater. An anesthetic is injected, sometimes through an indwelling catheter, directly into the cerebrospinal fluid in the subarachnoid space. **C,** Epidural anesthesia (viewed from the side). The needle is inserted to the surface of the dura mater, and the anesthetic is injected, usually through an indwelling catheter, into the epidural space.

tice prevents errors by drowsy or confused clients. For example, if a client is asked, "Are you Mr. Gates?" he may respond inappropriately if he is anxious or sedated. The nurse always validates identification using the medical record and identification bracelet, and by asking the client or family.

After completing the identification process, the nurse validates that the surgical consent form has been signed and witnessed. The nurse asks, "What kind of operation are you having today?" to ascertain that the client's perception of the procedure, the operative permit, and the operative schedule are the same. When the procedure involves a specific site, validating the side on which a procedure is to be performed (e.g., for amputation, cataract removal, or hernia repair) is the responsibility of each health care professional before and at the time of surgery. Facilities usually have the client and/or nurse initial the correct surgical site. Before proceeding, each health care professional thoroughly investigates *any* discrepancy and notifies the surgeon and anesthesia provider.

The nurse asks the client about any allergies and determines whether autologous blood was donated. A red allergy bracelet on the client's wrist and the medical record must be verified with what has been communicated.

The nurse checks the client's attire to ensure adherence with facility policy. Dentures and dental prostheses (e.g., bridges and retainers), jewelry (including body piercing), eyeglasses, contact lenses, hearing aids, wigs, and other prostheses are removed. The nurse pays special attention to the removal of dentures, because the denture plate could become loose and obstruct the airway during surgery. At times, the anesthesia provider may request that dentures be left in place to ensure a snug fit of the anesthesia mask. In some facilities, clients may wear eyeglasses and hearing aids until after anesthesia induction.

MEDICAL RECORD REVIEW

The circulating nurse and anesthesia provider review the client's medical record in the holding area or the operating room (OR). The medical record provides information needed to identify client needs during surgery and allows the circulating nurse to assess and plan specific care during and after surgery. The medical record is the main source of information on the type and location of the planned surgery. The nurse checks the medical record to ensure required data are present before surgery is started.

ADVANCE DIRECTIVES AND DO-NOT-RESUSCITATE ORDERS. Ethical dilemmas may occur during or after surgery. As a client advocate, the nurse may have to intervene on behalf of the client's rights and wishes. The nurse must be familiar with the advance directives and do-not-resuscitate (DNR) orders for each client. *These directives are to be honored in the surgical environment regardless of the situation.* It is difficult for some health care providers not to treat the client in the OR for an emergency situation, and they may ignore an advance directive or living will. Some surgical teams suspend DNR orders while a client is undergoing a surgical procedure. The position statement of Association of periOperative Registered Nurses, regarding the care of clients with DNR orders states that suspending a DNR order during surgery undermines a client's right to self-determination (AORN, 2003b).

ALLERGIES AND PREVIOUS REACTIONS TO ANESTHESIA OR TRANSFUSIONS. The nurse asks about allergies and previous reactions to anesthesia or blood transfusions. Allergies to iodine products or shellfish indicate a risk for a reaction to the agents used to clean the surgical area. Latex allergies must be assessed with all clients. Latex-induced anaphylaxis accounts for about 10% of the anaphylactic reactions that occur during surgery (see Chapters 23 and 26). Latex-free equipment and supplies must be used when the client has a latex allergy. The nurse documents the allergy in the medical record and notifies the OR team.

The client's previous experience with anesthesia helps the nurse and anesthesia provider anticipate needs and plan interventions. For example, if a client is restless or agitated as a reaction to anesthesia, the nurse can have padding for the siderails and protective restraints available. The use of blood and blood products during surgery may be influenced by the client's history, religious beliefs, preferences, and past transfusion reactions.

AUTOLOGOUS BLOOD TRANSFUSION. **Autologous blood transfusion** (reinfusing the client's own blood) may be used for surgery. Chapters 20 and 43 discuss autologous transfusion in more detail. Chart 21-2 outlines best practices for autologous blood transfusion during surgery.

LABORATORY AND DIAGNOSTIC TEST RESULTS. The OR nurse reviews the most recent laboratory findings and test results to inform the surgical team about the client's medical condition and to alert them for potential problems. The most recent results are usually obtained within 24 to 28 hours before surgery for hospitalized clients and within 4 weeks for ambulatory surgery clients. The nurse reports all abnormal findings or results to the surgeon and anesthesia provider. Laboratory values greater than or less than the normal range are potentially life threatening for clients having surgery (see Chapter 20). For example, if the hemoglobin level is less than 10 g/dL, oxygen transport capacity is reduced, affecting the amount and type of anesthesia used as well as the impact of blood loss during surgery.

MEDICAL HISTORY AND PHYSICAL EXAMINATION FINDINGS. The OR nurse checks that the medical history and examination findings, including usual pulse and blood pressure, are recorded. This information provides the circulating nurse, surgeon, anesthesia provider, and postanesthesia care unit (PACU) nurse with baseline data to assess the client's reaction to the surgery and anesthesia. Drugs taken before surgery may affect the client's reaction to surgery and wound healing. For example, aspirin reduces platelet action, increasing clotting time and the risk for hemorrhage.

Knowing the client's medical history and age (Chart 21-3) allows the nurse to plan interventions for the care and safety of high-risk clients. The nurse carefully monitors older clients and those with cardiac disease for potential fluid overload.

After completing the medical record review, the nurse may insert an IV catheter and perform a surgical shave. The circulating nurse provides emotional support and explains procedures to the client. *The client is never left unattended.* If the client is in the holding area, he or she is moved to the OR after the preoperative routine is completed.

CHART 21-2

BEST PRACTICE for
Intraoperative Autologous Blood Salvage and Transfusion

- Be aware of the cell-processing method to be used.
- Make sure that collection containers are labeled for the client.
- Assist with sterile setup as necessary.
- Assist with processing and reinfusing procedures as needed.
- Document the transfusion process.
- Monitor the client's vital signs during the transfusion procedure.

Critical Thinking Challenge

The client, a 62-year-old secretary, has entered the surgical suite about 30 minutes after she has received atropine and midazolam for preoperative medication. The OR schedule lists that she is to have a vaginal hysterectomy. In addition, the preoperative history indicates that she smokes three packs of cigarettes per day and drinks three cans of beer each day. When you ask her what kind of surgery she is having today, her response is "I am going to have a hemorrhoidectomy." You ask her if she means hysterectomy and she responds, "Well, it is some kind of operation 'down there.'"

1. What additional questions should you ask this client?
2. What should you do with the information?
3. What effect, if any, will her history of smoking and drinking have on her surgical experience?

evolve For suggested answer guidelines, go to http://evolve.elsevier.com/Iggy/.

Analysis

COMMON NURSING DIAGNOSES AND COLLABORATIVE PROBLEMS

The following are priority nursing diagnoses for clients during surgery:

1. Risk for Perioperative Positioning Injury related to immobilization and effects of anesthesia
2. Impaired Skin Integrity and Impaired Tissue Integrity related to the surgical incision

A primary collaborative problem is Potential for Hypoventilation.

ADDITIONAL NURSING DIAGNOSES AND COLLABORATIVE PROBLEMS

In addition to the common nursing diagnoses and collaborative problems, clients during surgery may have one or more of the following:

- Risk for Infection related to a break in skin integrity (i.e., incision, invasive lines)
- Risk for Injury related to client's inability to advocate for themselves and the exposure to hazards in the surgical environment
- Risk for Disuse Syndrome related to a decreased level of consciousness or to immobilization

CHART 21-3

NURSING FOCUS on the OLDER ADULT
Intraoperative Nursing Interventions

- Allow clients to retain eyeglasses and hearing aids until anesthesia has been administered.
- Use a small pillow under the client's head if his or her head and neck are normally bent slightly forward.
- Lift clients into position to prevent shearing forces on fragile skin.
- Position arthritic and artificial joints carefully to prevent postoperative pain and discomfort from strain on those joints.
- Pad bony prominences to prevent pressure sores.
- Provide extra padding for those clients with decreased peripheral circulation.
- Use head caps to prevent heat loss through the scalp.
- Place stockinette on extremities to conserve body heat.
- Warm prepping solutions and IV and irrigation fluids as indicated.
- Follow strict aseptic technique.
- Carefully monitor intake and output, including blood loss.

- Hypothermia related to evaporation from skin and exposed tissue in a cool environment, body heat loss, changes in the hypothalamus from anesthetic agents, or inadequate body covering
- Fear related to the threat of death, actual or perceived, or anticipation of events posing a threat to self-esteem
- Anxiety related to loss of control or the threat of death
- Deficient Fluid Volume related to decreased intake, evaporative fluid loss through the skin and exposed tissue, or blood loss
- Potential for Peripheral Neurovascular Dysfunction related to intraoperative positioning

Planning and Implementation

RISK FOR PERIOPERATIVE POSITIONING INJURY

NOC **PLANNING: EXPECTED OUTCOMES.** The client is expected to be free of injury as indicated by:

- Capillary refill and peripheral pulses are adequate in all extremities
- Sensory perception and motor function after surgery is at the same level as before surgery
- Absence of skin redness or open skin areas
- Absence of bruising

INTERVENTIONS. Interventions are used to prevent injury from positioning during surgery. Because of anesthesia and the narrow OR bed, the client's normal defense mechanisms cannot guard against nerve or joint damage and muscle stretch or strain. Thus proper positioning is important. The risk for pressure ulcer formation also is greater among clients having surgery than for those hospitalized clients who do not undergo surgery. (See the Evidence-Based Practice for Nursing box at right.) The circulating nurse pads the operating bed with foam and/or silicone gel pads, and properly places the grounding pads. This nurse coordinates the transfer to the operating bed and helps the client to a comfortable position. The nurse assesses the skin, especially of older clients, for bruising or injury, placing extra padding as indicated.

The client is usually in a supine position after transfer to the operating bed. Anesthesia may be given with the client supine, and he or she may then be repositioned for surgery (Figure 21-12).

The circulating nurse coordinates positioning of the client for surgery and modifies the position according to the client's safety and special needs. Factors influencing the *timing* of repositioning include the following:

- The surgical site
- The age and size of the client
- The anesthetic delivery technique
- Pain on movement (conscious client)

Factors influencing the actual *position* include the following:

- The specific procedure being performed
- The surgeon's request
- The client's age, size, and weight
- Any pulmonary, skeletal, or muscular limitations, such as arthritis, joint replacements, or emphysema

Table 21-6 lists complications related to prolonged immobility during surgery and some preventive nursing actions.

The dorsal recumbent, prone, lithotomy, and lateral positions are most often used for surgery. Figure 21-12 shows many surgical positions and the use of protective padding. When general anesthesia is used, the nurse positions the client slowly to prevent hypotension from blood vessel dilation. Proper positioning is ensured by assessing for the following:

- Anatomic alignment
- Interference with circulation and breathing
- Protection of skeletal and neuromuscular structures
- Optimal exposure of the operative site and IV line
- Adequate access to the client for the anesthesia provider
- The client's comfort and safety
- Preservation of the client's dignity

The nurse is aware of potential complications related to specific positions and modifies care as needed. For example, clients in the lithotomy position may develop leg swelling, pain in the legs or back, and reduced sensation or foot pulses. The nurse ensures proper padding and position changes at regular intervals. Throughout the surgery, the nurse prevents obstruction of circulation, respiration, or nerve conduction

EVIDENCE-BASED PRACTICE for Nursing

Pressure ulcers do occur in surgery

Schoonhoven, L., Defloor, T., Grypdonck, M. (2002). Incidence of pressure ulcers due to surgery. *Journal of Clinical Nursing, 11*(4), 479-487.

This descriptive, prospective study sought to determine the incidence of pressure ulcers caused by positioning during surgery. Two hundred and eight subjects from nine different surgical specialties were enrolled in the study as a convenience sample. The sample included 73 women and 136 men, with a mean age of 59 years. Study criteria included that the surgery was planned and expected to have a minimum duration of 4 hours. The population did not contain clients undergoing gynecologic procedures or surgery for trauma. The presence of a pressure ulcer before surgery did not exclude the subject; however, the preexisting ulcers were not included in the analysis. Mean length of the surgical procedures was 6 hours and 38 minutes.

The skin of the subjects was assessed before surgery and the findings documented. Skin was assessed immediately after surgery and daily for 14 days or until discharge. Skin lesions were described, categorized by a standard scale, and photographed. Subjects discharged before 14 days were contacted and asked to describe any skin lesions.

A total of 44 (21.2%) subjects developed one or more pressure ulcers (n = 70) within 48 hours after surgery. An additional 12 subjects developed pressure ulcers on day 3 or later after surgery. The majority of lesions were on the heels with about 15% of lesions forming on the sacral area. Some subjects developed ulcers on the chin and ears as a result of a specific surgical procedure for vertebral surgery that involved a face mask and traction. About 12% of subjects were impaired in some way as a result of their pressure ulcers.

Level of Evidence: 3—Well-designed trial without randomization.

Critique. The prospective nature of the study is a major strength as is the preoperative assessment. The data were collected by four persons trained in the assessment of pressure ulcers, with high inter-rater reliability. Randomization would have added strength to the study. No mention is made of racial or ethnic differences among the subjects. The study was conducted in The Netherlands, where there is a relatively homogeneous ethnic population. While homogeneity limits generalization to other populations, it strengthens the validity of findings within an ethnic population.

Implications for Nursing. Most health care professionals are under the false impression that pressure ulcer formation is a slow process seen in clients who are chronically immobile. This study reinforces the findings of other studies that complete immobility—even for short periods—is a major risk factor for pressure ulcer development. Nurses should take proactive, preventive measures for all clients who are immobilized for 2 hours or longer, no matter what their age or health status.

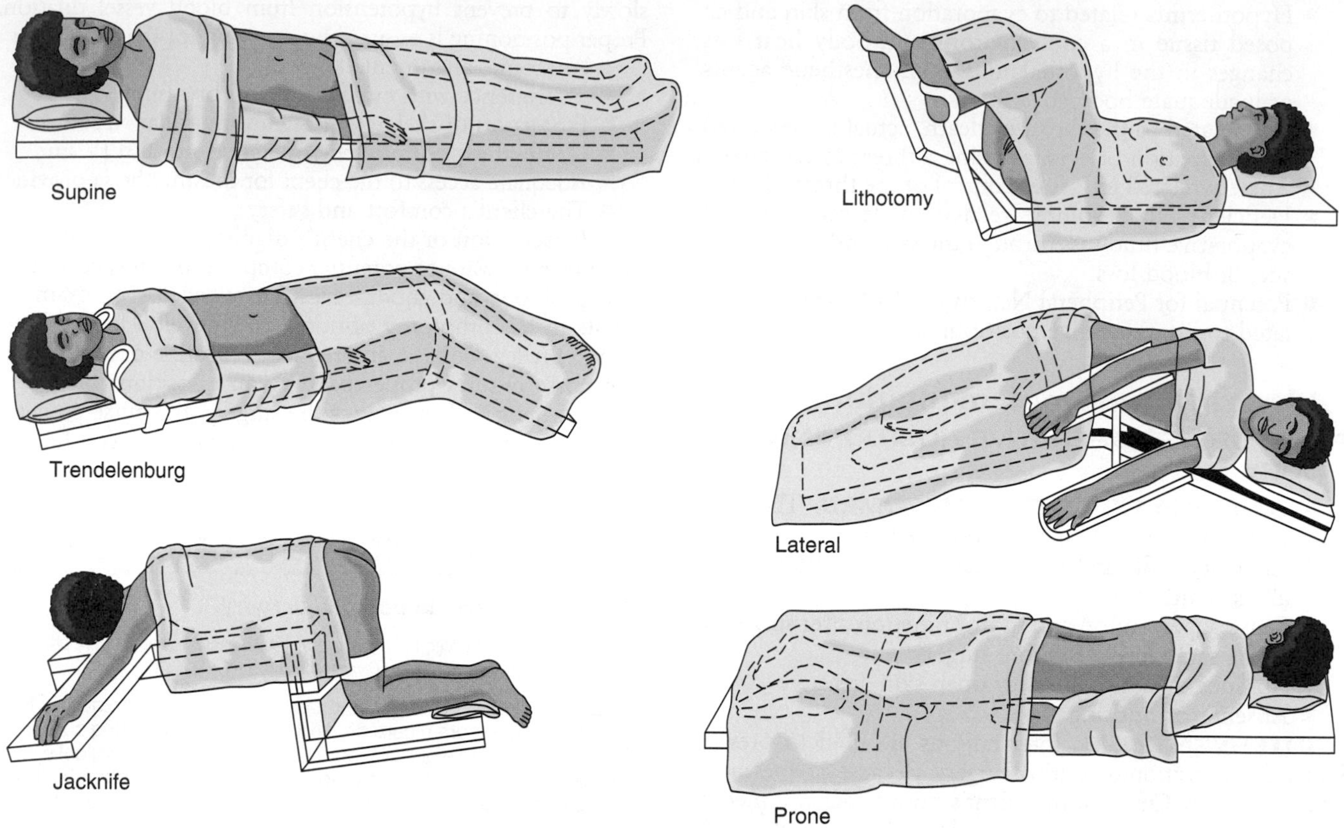

Figure 21-12 ■ Common surgical positions.

TABLE 21-6 Interventions to Prevent Neuromuscular Complications Related to Intraoperative Positioning

Anatomic Area	Complications	Interventions
Brachial plexus	Paralysis Loss of sensation in the arm and shoulder	Pad the elbow. Avoid excessive abduction. Secure the arm firmly on an arm board, positioned at shoulder level.
Radial nerve	Wrist drop	Support the wrist with padding. Do not overtighten wrist straps.
Medial or ulnar nerves	Hand deformities	Place a safety strap above or below the area.
Peroneal nerve	Foot drop	Place a pillow or padding under the knees. Support the lower extremities. Do not overtighten leg straps.
Tibial nerve	Loss of sensation on the plantar surface of the foot	Place a safety strap above the ankle. Do not place equipment on the lower extremities.
Joints	Stiffness Pain Inflammation	Place a pillow or foam padding under bony prominences. Maintain good body alignment. Slightly flex joints and support with pillows, trochanter rolls, or pads.

caused by tight straps, poorly placed pads and pillows, or the position of the bed.

Critical Thinking Challenge

The 62-year-old client about to have a vaginal hysterectomy is brought into the OR. She weighs 96 pounds.

1. In what position should you place this client for a vaginal hysterectomy?
2. What areas on this client are most likely to be injured as a result of poor positioning or inadequate padding?

evolve For suggested answer guidelines, go to http://evolve.elsevier.com/Iggy/.

IMPAIRED SKIN INTEGRITY AND IMPAIRED TISSUE INTEGRITY

NOC **PLANNING: EXPECTED OUTCOMES.** The client is expected to have minimal skin and tissue impairment or infection as a result of surgery as indicated by:

- Absence of inflammation, purulent drainage, or dehiscence of the incision
- Maintenance of a white blood cell count within normal limits

INTERVENTIONS. Surgery places the client at risk for wound complications (such as incisional tears and lacerations), infection, and loss of body fluids. Sterile surgical

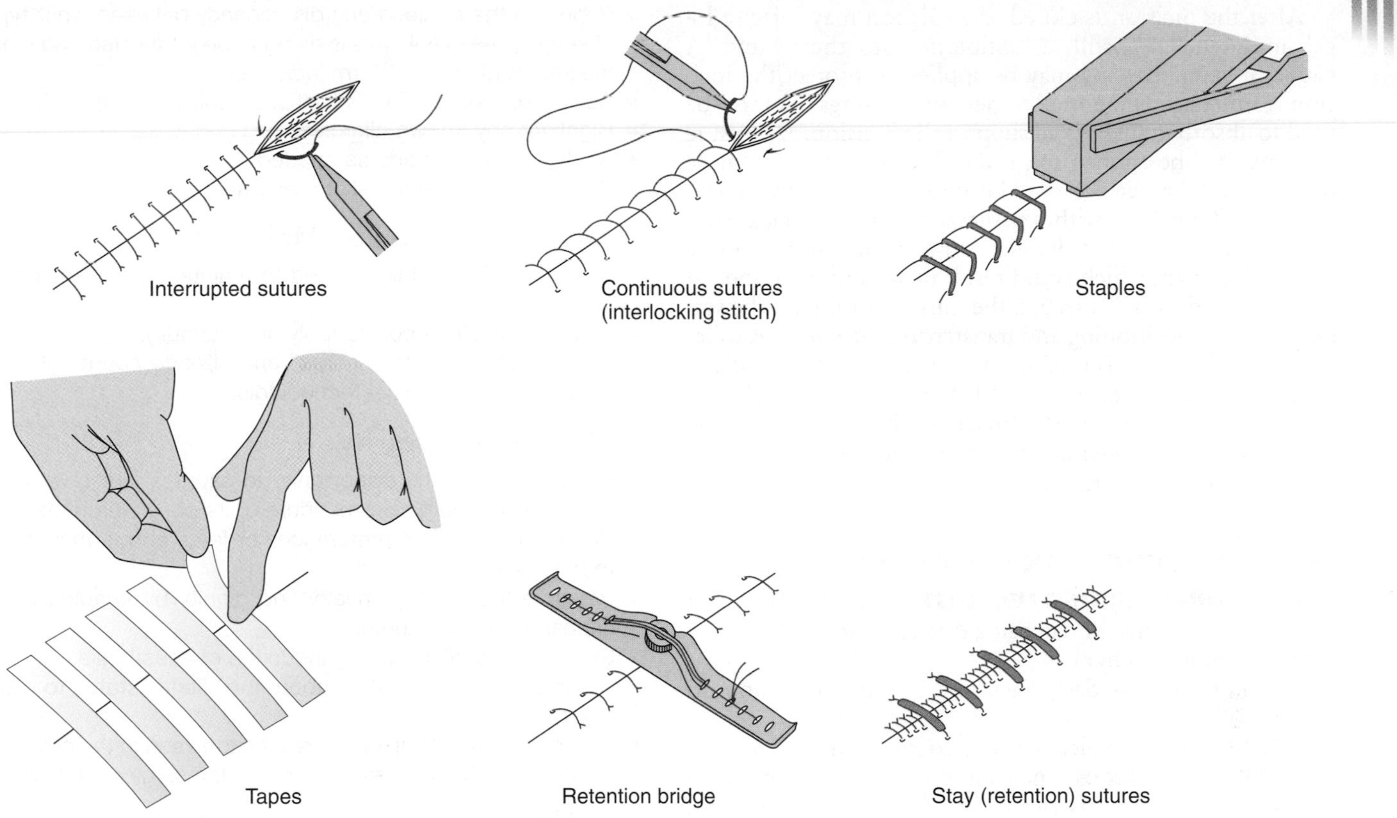

Figure 21-13 ■ Common skin closures.

technique and the use of protective drapes, skin closures, and dressings reduce complications and promote wound healing.

Plastic Adhesive Drape. If a sterile plastic adhesive drape is used, the scrub nurse helps the surgical assistant apply the drape after the surgical site has been cleaned and dried. The plastic drape is applied directly to the client's skin to prevent shifting and exposure of skin edges. *The surgeon makes the incision through the plastic drape.* The cut edge sticks to the skin and creates a seal to reduce bacterial movement into the wound. The scrub nurse and surgical assistant *gently* remove the drape after closure of the incision. Special attention is paid to older clients and those with fragile skin to prevent skin tearing when the adhesive drape is removed.

Skin Closures. Skin and tissue closures, such as sutures and staples, are used to:

- Hold wound edges in place until wound healing is complete
- Occlude blood vessels, preventing hemorrhage and fluid loss
- Prevent wound contamination

The quality of the wound edges and the type of closure material used determine the strength and integrity of the closure. The wound is usually closed in layers to keep tissues together and promote healing with minimal scarring. The surgeon selects the method and type of closures based on the surgical site, the tissue involved, the size and depth of the wound, and the age and medical history of the client. A combination of sutures and clips is commonly used for closure of internal layers of the wound. Staples, retention (stay) sutures, and skin closure tapes (Steri-Strips) are used for closure of superficial skin wounds. Figure 21-13 shows commonly used wound closures.

A suture is one or more strands of material and varies by size, or gauge. The size sequence, from largest diameter to smallest, is 5, 4, 3, 2, 1, 0, 00 (2-0), 000 (3-0), 0000 (4-0), and so forth, to 11-0. Size 0 is thick and often used to close the deep layers of an abdominal wound. The smaller diameter sutures (e.g., 11-0) are used in plastic surgery and eye surgery. Other suture material features, such as type (e.g., nylon, silk, Vicryl), color (e.g., green, blue, black, white, violet), and structure (e.g., twisted, braided), are listed on the package.

Sutures are absorbable or nonabsorbable. **Absorbable sutures** are digested over time by body enzymes. These sutures first lose strength and then gradually disappear from the tissue. Catgut suture, such as "plain gut" and "chromic gut," is a type of natural absorbable suture. Other absorbable sutures are made of synthetic materials. The client's health, the presence of inflammation, and the type of suture used all influence absorption time, which is usually about 2 weeks.

Nonabsorbable sutures become encapsulated in the tissue during the healing process and remain in the tissue unless they are removed. These sutures are made of silk, cotton, steel, nylon, polyester, or other synthetic material. *Body enzymes do not affect nonabsorbable sutures.* Nonabsorbable sutures are used for connecting blood vessels, "wiring" the sternum together after open heart surgery, and closing external wounds. The surgeon may use a double or interlocking stitch to increase closure integrity. Retention (stay) sutures (see Figure 21-13) may be used in addition to standard sutures for clients at high risk for impaired wound healing (those having major abdominal surgery, obese clients, clients with diabetes, and those taking steroids).

After the incision is closed, the surgeon may inject a local anesthetic or instill an antibiotic into the wound. A gauze or spray dressing may be applied to protect the incision from contamination. A variety of dressings may also be used to absorb drainage and support the incision. A pressure dressing may be applied to prevent bleeding. One or more drains (see Chapter 22) may be inserted to remove secretions and fluids from within tissues around the surgical area. These secretions, if not drained, slow healing and promote bacterial growth, which could result in wound infection.

After the dressing is secure, the nurse coordinates the surgical team in positioning and transferring the client. A roller board or a lift sheet is used to move the client from the operating bed to a stretcher or bed. Some clients are able to move themselves over to the stretcher. The circulating nurse and anesthesia provider go with the client to the PACU and report the client's surgical experience to the PACU nurse (see Chapter 22).

POTENTIAL FOR HYPOVENTILATION

NOC **PLANNING: EXPECTED OUTCOMES.** The client is expected to be free of damaging events related to hypoventilation as indicated by:

- Maintenance of SaO_2, PaO_2, and blood pH within normal limits
- Return to presurgical level of cognitive function

INTERVENTIONS. Interventions aim to prevent injury resulting from anesthesia (see earlier discussion). The nurse, surgeon, and anesthesia provider monitor the client according to official standards. These standards, adopted by both the American Society of Anesthesiologists and the American Association of Nurse Anesthetists, include continuous monitoring of breathing, circulation, and cardiac rhythms; blood pressure and heart rate recordings every 5 minutes; and the continuous presence of an anesthesia provider during the case.

Evaluation: Outcomes

The nurse evaluates the care of the client during surgery on the basis of the identified nursing diagnoses and collaborative problems. The expected outcomes are that the client:

- Is safely anesthetized without complications
- Does not experience any injury related to surgical positioning or equipment
- Is free of skin or tissue contamination during surgery
- Is free of skin tears, bruises, redness, abrasion, or maceration over pressure points and elsewhere

Specific indicators for these outcomes are listed for each nursing diagnosis and collaborative problem under the Planning and Implementation section (see earlier).

GET READY for the NCLEX Examination!

KEY POINTS

Safe Effective Care Environment

- Ensure that all personnel entering the OR are wearing proper OR attire for their role.
- Observe for and inform OR personnel of any break in sterile field or sterile technique.
- Check the identity of the client.
- Report to the surgeon any discrepancy between what type of surgery the client says is going to be performed and what the informed consent form indicates.
- Review preoperative checklist and informed consent forms.
- Highlight any known allergies.
- Apply grounding pads as needed.
- Complete any needed skin preparation.

Health Promotion and Maintenance

- Apply padding to the OR bed to maintain the client's skin integrity.
- Position the client comfortably and carefully.
- Perform an accurate "sharps" and sponge count with the scrub nurse or surgical technologist.

Psychosocial Integrity

- Allow the client the opportunity to express fear or anxiety regarding the surgical procedure or its possible outcome.
- Communicate client preferences or fears about anesthesia to the anesthesia provider.
- Preserve the client's privacy and dignity by keeping body exposure to a minimum.
- Stay with the client during induction of anesthesia.
- Communicate information about the client's status to waiting family members.
- Ensure that the client's wishes, as expressed in the advance directives statement, are honored in the surgical setting.

Physiological Integrity

- Ask the client when was the last time he or she had anything to eat or drink.
- Know the expected client responses and side effects to anesthesia induction and awakening produced by the various anesthetic agents.
- Assess the client for tachycardia, increased end-tidal carbon dioxide level, and increased body temperature as indicators of malignant hyperthermia.
- Keep dantrolene sodium available during and after surgery as drug therapy for malignant hyperthermia.
- Monitor the client's airway, level of consciousness, oxygen saturation, ECG, and vital signs during and immediately following conscious sedation.
- Assess all skin areas and document findings before transferring the client to the postanesthesia care unit.

ADDITIONAL STUDY RESOURCES

Go to your Student CD-ROM for Review Questions for the NCLEX Examination.

evolve Go to http://evolve.elsevier.com/Iggy/ for Integrated Management of Care Questions for the NCLEX Examination.

SELECTED BIBLIOGRAPHY

Asterisk indicates a classic or definitive work on this subject.

Agarwal, M., Hamilton-Stewart, P., & Dixon, R. (2002). Contaminated operating room boots: The potential for infection. *American Journal of Infection Control, 30*(3), 179-183.

Allen, G. (2002). Supplemental perioperative oxygen to reduce the incidence of surgical-wound infection. *AORN Journal, 76*(2), 330-331.

American Society of PeriAnesthesia Nurses. (2000). *Standards of perianesthesia nursing practice.* New Jersey: Author.
Association of PeriOperative Registered Nurses. (2002). Recommended practices for skin preparation of patients. *AORN Journal, 75*(1), 184-187.
Association of periOperative Registered Nurses. (2003a). Position statement: AORN official statement on RN first assistant. In *Standards, recommended practices and guidelines* (pp. 159-160). Denver: Author.
Association of periOperative Registered Nurses. (2003b). Position statement: Perioperative care of patients with do not resuscitate (DNR) orders. In *Standards, recommended practices and guidelines* (pp. 155-156). Denver: Author.
Association of periOperative Registered Nurses. (2003c). Recommended practices for the care and cleaning of surgical instruments and powered equipment. In *Standards, recommended practices and guidelines* (pp. 291-299). Denver: Author.
Association of periOperative Registered Nurses. (2003d). Recommended practices for disinfection. In *Standards, recommended practices and guidelines* (pp. 227-231). Denver: Author.
Association of periOperative Registered Nurses. (2003e). Recommended practices for documentation of perioperative nursing care. In *Standards, recommended practices and guidelines* (pp. 233-235). Denver: Author.
Association of periOperative Registered Nurses. (2003f). Recommended practices for environmental cleaning for the surgical practice setting. In *Standards, recommended practices and guidelines* (pp. 257-263). Denver: Author.
Association of periOperative Registered Nurses. (2003g). Recommended practices for hazards in the surgical environment. In *Standards, recommended practices and guidelines* (pp. 283-289). Denver: Author.
Association of periOperative Registered Nurses. (2003h). Recommended practices for laser safety in the practice setting. In *Standards, recommended practices and guidelines* (pp. 301-305). Denver: Author.
Association of periOperative Registered Nurses. (2003i). Recommended practices for managing the patient receiving conscious sedation/analgesia. In *Standards, recommended practices and guidelines* (pp. 213-220). Denver: Author.
Association of periOperative Registered Nurses. (2003j). Recommended practices for positioning the patient in the perioperative practice setting. In *Standards, recommended practices and guidelines* (pp. 323-331). Denver: Author.
Association of periOperative Registered Nurses. (2003k). Recommended practices for skin preparation. In *Standards, recommended practices and guidelines* (pp. 339-343). Denver: Author.
Association of periOperative Registered Nurses. (2003l). Recommended practices for sponge, sharp, and instrument counts. In *Standards, recommended practices and guidelines* (pp. 221-226). Denver: Author.
Association of periOperative Registered Nurses. (2003m). Recommended practices for sterile field-maintaining. In *Standards, recommended practices and guidelines* (pp. 351-355). Denver: Author.
Association of periOperative Registered Nurses. (2003n). Recommended practices for sterilization in the practice setting. In *Standards, recommended practices and guidelines* (pp. 357-366). Denver: Author.
Association of periOperative Registered Nurses. (2003o). Recommended practices for surgical attire. In *Standards, recommended practices and guidelines* (pp. 215-219). Denver: Author.
Association of periOperative Registered Nurses. (2003p). Recommended practices for surgical hand scrubs. In *Standards, recommended practices and guidelines* (pp. 277-281). Denver: Author.
Association of periOperative Registered Nurses. (2003q). Recommended practices for traffic patterns in the perioperative practice setting. In *Standards, recommended practices and guidelines* (pp. 373-375). Denver: Author.
Association of periOperative Registered Nurses. (2003r). Recommended practices for use and selection of barrier materials for surgical gowns and drapes. In *Standards, recommended practices and guidelines* (pp. 271-275). Denver: Author.
Bauer, J. (2002). Surgical tape. *RN, 65*(6), 63-65.
Beyea, S. (2002). Accident prevention in surgical settings: Keeping patients safe. *AORN Journal, 75*(2), 361-363.
*Curry, M. (1994). Perioperative nursing care of the elderly patient: A case study. *ACORN Journal, 7*(2), 23-26.
Denault, D. (2002). What counts most in the operating room. *Nursing2102, 32*(4), 32hn8.
Dochterman, J., & Bulechek, G. (Eds.). (2004). *Nursing interventions classification (NIC)* (4th ed.). St. Louis: Mosby.
Documenting postoperative transfer. (2002). *Nursing2102, 32*(3), 82.
Domanovic, M., et al. (2003). Using intraoperative radiation therapy: A case study. *AORN Journal, 77*(2), 412-417.
Dunn, D. (2004). Preventing perioperative complications in an older adult. *Nursing 2004, 34*(11), 36-41.
Ebersole, P., Hess, P., & Luggen, A. (2004). *Toward healthy aging: Human needs and nursing response* (6th ed.). St. Louis: Mosby.
ECRI. (2003). Health devices: Focus on surgical fire safety. 32(1), Plymouth Meeting, PA: Author.
*Entrup, M.H. (1991). Perioperative complications of anesthesia. *Surgical Clinics of North America, 71*(6), 1151-1173.
Flower, J. (2000). Beyond surgery: Predictions for surgery in the next century. *Surgical Services Management, 6*(1), 29-32.
Folin, A., Nyberg, B., & Nordstrom, G. (2000). Reducing blood exposures during orthopedic surgical procedures. *AORN Journal, 71*(3), 573-582.
Garvin, M. (2003). Perioperative hand hygiene: the challenge of integrating rinseless products in the OR. *Infection Control Today, 7*(4), 36-40.
Haslego, S. (2002). Malignant hyperthermia: How to spot it early. *RN, 65*(7), 31-36.
Homa, D., & Palfreyman, M. (2000). Infectious diseases in the O.R. *CRNA: The Clinical Forum for Nurse Anesthetists, 11*(1), 8-14.
Keating, E.M., & Meding, J. (2002). Perioperative blood management practices in elective orthopaedic surgery. *Journal of the American Academy of Orthopaedic Surgeons, 10*(6), 393-399.
Kjonniken, I., et al. (2002). Preoperative hair removal: A systematic literature review. *AORN Journal, 75*(5), 928-936, 938, 940.
Martyn, V., et al. (2002). The theory and practice of bloodless surgery. *Transfusion and Apheresis Science, 27*(1), 29-43.
McEwen, D. (2003). Ambulatory surgery. In M.H. Meeker & J.C. Rothrock (Eds.), *Alexander's care of the patient in surgery* (12th ed., pp. 1189-1210). St. Louis: Mosby.
Meckes, P.F. (2003). Geriatric surgery. In M.H. Meeker & J.C. Rothrock (Eds.), *Alexander's care of the patient in surgery* (12th ed., pp. 1295-1315). St. Louis: Mosby.
Meeker, M.H., & Rothrock, J.C. (2003). *Alexander's care of the patient in surgery* (12th ed.). St. Louis: Mosby.
Meltzer, B. (2003). Seven keys to fast-track anesthesia. *Outpatient Surgery, IV*(3), 52-62.
Mok, E., & Wong, K-Y. (2003). Effects of music on patient anxiety. *AORN Journal, 77*(2), 396-410.
Moorhead, S., Johnson, M., & Maas, M. (Eds.). (2004). *Nursing outcomes classification (NOC)* (3rd ed.). St. Louis: Mosby.
Nussbaum, R., McInnes, R., & Willard, H. (2001). *Thompson & Thompson: Genetics in medicine* (6th ed.). Philadelphia: W.B. Saunders.
Quinn, A. (2002). Cyberknife: A robotic radiosurgery system. *Clinical Journal of Oncology Nursing, 6*(3), 149, 156.
Schoonhoven, L., Defloor, T., Grypdonck, M. (2002). Incidence of pressure ulcers due to surgery. *Journal of Clinical Nursing, 11*(4), 479-487.
Schroeter, K. (2003). Ethics in perioperative practice: Principles and applications. *AORN Journal, 75*(4), 818-824.
Squires, A. (2003). Documenting surgical incision site care. *Nursing2003, 33*(1), 74.
Warnock, K. (2003). Preventing surgical errors: The role of the surgical technologist. *The Surgical Technologist, 35*(6), 15-29.

CHAPTER

22 Interventions for Postoperative Clients

REBECCA M. PATTON

LEARNING OUTCOMES

After studying this chapter, you should be able to:

1. Describe the ongoing head-to-toe assessment of the postoperative client.
2. Prioritize nursing interventions for the client recovering from surgery and anesthesia during the first 24 hours.
3. Prioritize nursing care for the client who has respiratory depression after surgery.
4. Discuss the criteria for determining readiness of the client to be discharged from the postanesthesia care unit.
5. Use proper technique for wound assessment and dressing changes.
6. Recognize wound complications after surgery.
7. Describe steps to take when a client has a surgical wound dehiscence or evisceration.
8. Compare the actions, side effects, and nursing implications for different types of drug therapy for pain management after surgery.
9. Develop a community-based teaching plan for clients after surgery.

Go to your Student CD-ROM for Review Questions for the NCLEX Examination keyed to these Learning Outcomes.

The postoperative period starts at the completion of surgery and transfer of the client to the postanesthesia care unit (PACU), same day surgery unit (ambulatory care unit), or the intensive care unit. Discharge from these areas is based on the stability of the client and the meeting of specific discharge criteria. Many clients are able to be discharged to home shortly after the surgery is completed. They are observed and monitored until discharge criteria are met and are then discharged. Some clients move from the specialized nursing care in the PACU to a hospital inpatient floor or critical care unit for additional nursing care.

The postoperative period continues after the client's condition is stabilized, as well as after the client is discharged from the ambulatory surgery facility or hospital. The actual time spent away from home after surgery varies according to age, physical health, self-care ability, support systems, type and length of surgical procedure, anesthesia, any complications, and community resources.

OVERVIEW

The purpose of a PACU or recovery room is the ongoing evaluation and stabilization of clients, to anticipate, prevent, and treat complications after surgery. The PACU is usually located close to the surgical suite for ease of access and client transfer. The unit is usually a large and open room to provide best observation of clients and easy access to supplies and emergency equipment. Usually, adults are separated from children. The client area may be divided into individual cubicles. Privacy curtains or screens are closed only during bedside procedures. Each cubicle has equipment to monitor and care for the client, such as oxygen, suction equipment, cardiac monitors, airway equipment, and emergency drugs.

After the surgery is completed, the circulating nurse and the anesthesia provider accompany the client to the PACU. When the client is in critical condition, transfer may be directly from the operating room (OR) to the intensive (critical) care unit. On arrival, the anesthesia provider and the circulating nurse give the PACU nurse a verbal report (Table 22-1).

The PACU nurse is skilled in the care of clients with multiple medical and surgical problems immediately after a surgical procedure. This area requires in-depth knowledge of anesthetic agents, pharmacology, pain management, and surgical procedures. The PACU nurse is skilled in assessment and can make quick decisions if emergencies or complications occur. The client is monitored closely. The anesthesia provider and surgeon are consulted as needed.

TABLE 22-1 Report Guidelines on Arrival in the Postanesthesia Care Unit

The anesthesia providers explain the following:

- Type and extent of the surgical procedure
- Type of anesthesia
- Client's tolerance of anesthesia and the surgical procedure
- Client's allergies
- Pathologic condition
- Status of vital signs
- Type and amount of IV fluids and medications administered
- Estimated blood loss (EBL)
- Any intraoperative complications, such as a traumatic intubation

The circulating nurse adds information related to the following:

- Client's primary language and any sensory impairments
- Client's anxiety level before receiving anesthesia
- Special requests that were verbalized by the client preoperatively
- Client's preoperative and intraoperative respiratory function and dysfunction
- Pertinent medical history
- Location and type of incisions, dressings, catheters, tubes, drains, or packing
- Intake and output, including current IV fluid administration and estimated blood loss
- Joint or limb immobility while in the operating room, especially in the older client
- Other intraoperative positioning that may be relevant in the postoperative phase
- Any other important intraoperative occurrences

COLLABORATIVE MANAGEMENT

The Concept Map on p. 356 uses a client who is recovering from abdominal surgery as an example for addressing the common assessment and nursing care issues for clients in the postoperative period.

Assessment

HISTORY

Use the surgical team's report to plan the care for an individual client. After receiving the report and assessing the client, review the medical record for information about the client's history, presurgical physical condition, and emotional status. If possible, review this information *before* the client arrives in the PACU. If the client remains as an inpatient, the surgical and postanesthesia information is incorporated into the postoperative plan of care. Chapter 20 identifies situations that increase a client's risk for the following complications:

- Allergic reactions
- Hypothermia
- Hyperthermia
- Hypertension
- Hypotension
- Hypovolemic shock
- Renal failure
- Electrolyte imbalances
- Dysrhythmias
- Chronic heart failure
- Paralytic ileus
- Acute urinary retention
- Deep vein thrombosis (DVT)
- Pulmonary embolism (PE)
- Atelectasis or pneumonia
- Laryngeal edema
- Ventilator dependence
- Gastrointestinal (GI) bleeding
- Disseminated intravascular coagulation (DIC)
- Anemia
- Wound evisceration

PHYSICAL ASSESSMENT/CLINICAL MANIFESTATIONS

Assess the client and record data on a PACU record form (Figure 22-1). Assessment data include level of consciousness, temperature, pulse, respiration, and blood pressure. *The most important area to assess is respiration.* Examine the surgical area for bleeding. Monitor vital signs as often as your facility's policy states, the client's condition warrants, and the surgeon prescribes. Once the client is discharged from the PACU, vital signs are often measured every 15 minutes for four times, every 30 minutes for four times, every 2 hours for four times, and then every 4 hours for 24 to 48 hours if the client's condition is stable. Thereafter, vital signs are assessed according to the facility's policy, the client's condition, and the nurse's judgment.

The health care team determines the client's readiness for discharge from the PACU by the presence of a recovery score rating of at least 10 on the recovery scale (see Figure 22-1). Other criteria for discharge (e.g., stable vital signs; normal body temperature; no overt bleeding; return of gag, cough, and swallow reflexes; and the ability to take liquids) may be specific to the facility. After you determine that all criteria have been met, the client is discharged by the anesthesia provider to the hospital unit or to home. If an anesthesia provider has not been involved, which may be the case with local anesthesia or conscious sedation, the surgeon or nurse discharges the client once the discharge criteria have been met.

Assessment continues from the PACU to the intensive care or medical-surgical nursing unit. If the client is to be discharged from the PACU to home, assessment is continued by home care nurses or by the client or family members after instruction.

RESPIRATORY SYSTEM

AIRWAY ASSESSMENT. *When the client is admitted to the PACU, immediately assess for a patent airway and adequate gas exchange.* An artificial airway, such as an endotracheal (ET) tube, a nasal trumpet, or an oral airway, may be in place. If the client is receiving oxygen, document the type of delivery device and the concentration or liter flow of the oxygen. Continuously monitor pulse oximetry for oxygen saturation while the client is in the PACU.

Assess the rate, pattern, and depth of breathing to determine adequacy of air exchange. A respiratory rate of less than 10 breaths/min indicates anesthetic- or opioid analgesic–induced depression. Rapid, shallow respirations signal cardiac problems, increased metabolic rate, or pain.

BREATH SOUNDS. Listen to the lungs over all lung fields to assess breath sounds. Also check symmetry of breath sounds. If, for example, the client has an ET tube, it could move down into the right mainstem bronchus and prevent left lung expansion. In this case, lung sounds on the left are absent or decreased and only the right chest wall rises and falls with breathing.

OTHER RESPIRATORY ASSESSMENTS. Respiratory assessment includes ongoing inspection of the chest wall for accessory muscle use, sternal retraction, and diaphragmatic breathing. These signs could indicate an excessive anesthetic effect, airway obstruction, or paralysis,

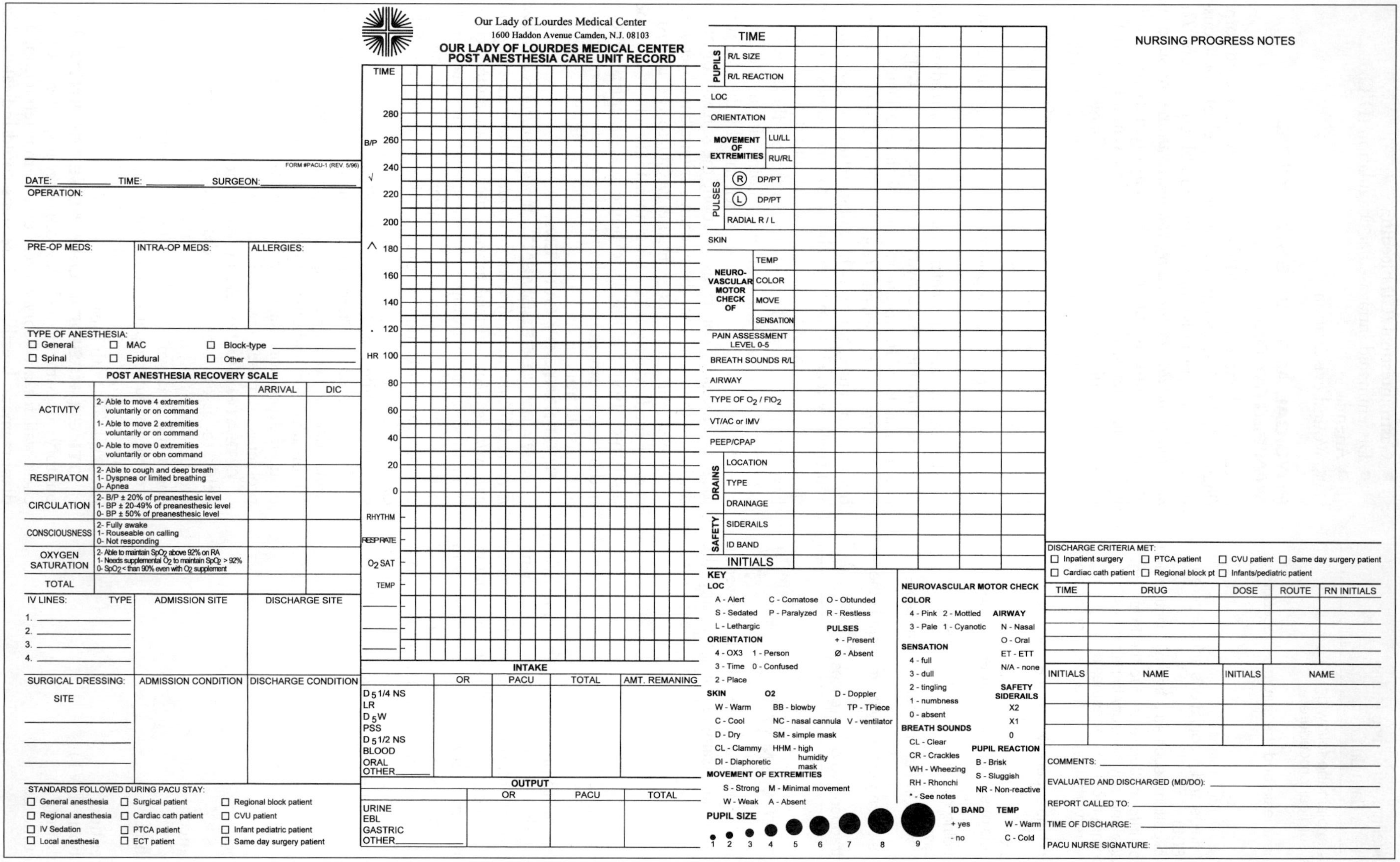

Our Lady of Lourdes Medical Center
1600 Haddon Avenue Camden, N.J. 08103

OUR LADY OF LOURDES MEDICAL CENTER
POST ANESTHESIA CARE UNIT RECORD

FORM #PACU-1 (REV. 5/96)

DATE: ________ TIME: ________ SURGEON: ________
OPERATION:

PRE-OP MEDS:	INTRA-OP MEDS:	ALLERGIES:

TYPE OF ANESTHESIA:
☐ General ☐ MAC ☐ Block-type ________
☐ Spinal ☐ Epidural ☐ Other ________

POST ANESTHESIA RECOVERY SCALE		ARRIVAL	DIC
ACTIVITY	2- Able to move 4 extremities voluntarily or on command 1- Able to move 2 extremities voluntarily or on command 0- Able to move 0 extremities voluntarily or obn command		
RESPIRATON	2- Able to cough and deep breath 1- Dyspnea or limited breathing 0- Apnea		
CIRCULATION	2- B/P ± 20% of preanesthesic level 1- BP ± 20-49% of preanesthesic level 0- BP ± 50% of preanesthesic level		
CONSCIOUSNESS	2- Fully awake 1- Rouseable on calling 0- Not responding		
OXYGEN SATURATION	2- Able to maintain SpO_2 above 92% on RA 1- Needs supplemental O_2 to maintain SpO_2 > 92% 0- SpO_2 < than 90% even with O_2 supplement		
TOTAL			

IV LINES:	TYPE	ADMISSION SITE	DISCHARGE SITE
1.			
2.			
3.			
4.			

SURGICAL DRESSING:	ADMISSION CONDITION	DISCHARGE CONDITION
SITE		

STANDARDS FOLLOWED DURING PACU STAY:
☐ General anesthesia ☐ Surgical patient ☐ Regional block patient
☐ Regional anesthesia ☐ Cardiac cath patient ☐ CVU patient
☐ IV Sedation ☐ PTCA patient ☐ Infant pediatric patient
☐ Local anesthesia ☐ ECT patient ☐ Same day surgery patient

TIME
B/P √ 280 260 240 220 200
^ 180 160 140 120
HR 100 80 60 40 20 0
RHYTHM
RESP RATE
O_2 SAT
TEMP

INTAKE	OR	PACU	TOTAL	AMT. REMANING
D_5 1/4 NS LR D_5W PSS D_5 1/2 NS BLOOD ORAL OTHER____				

OUTPUT	OR	PACU	TOTAL
URINE EBL GASTRIC OTHER____			

	TIME						
PUPILS	R/L SIZE						
	R/L REACTION						
LOC							
ORIENTATION							
MOVEMENT OF EXTREMITIES	LU/LL						
	RU/RL						
PULSES	Ⓡ DP/PT						
	Ⓛ DP/PT						
	RADIAL R / L						
SKIN							
NEURO-VASCULAR MOTOR CHECK OF	TEMP						
	COLOR						
	MOVE						
	SENSATION						
PAIN ASSESSMENT LEVEL 0-5							
BREATH SOUNDS R/L							
AIRWAY							
TYPE OF O_2 / FIO_2							
VT/AC or IMV							
PEEP/CPAP							
DRAINS	LOCATION						
	TYPE						
	DRAINAGE						
SAFETY	SIDERAILS						
	ID BAND						
INITIALS							

KEY
LOC
A - Alert C - Comatose O - Obtunded
S - Sedated P - Paralyzed R - Restless
L - Lethargic
PULSES
+ - Present
Ø - Absent
ORIENTATION
4 - OX3 1 - Person
3 - Time 0 - Confused
2 - Place
SKIN
W - Warm
C - Cool
D - Dry
CL - Clammy
DI - Diaphoretic
O2
BB - blowby
NC - nasal cannula
SM - simple mask
HHM - high humidity mask
D - Doppler
TP - TPiece
V - ventilator
MOVEMENT OF EXTREMITIES
S - Strong M - Minimal movement
W - Weak A - Absent
PUPIL SIZE
1 2 3 4 5 6 7 8 9

NEUROVASCULAR MOTOR CHECK
COLOR
4 - Pink 2 - Mottled
3 - Pale 1 - Cyanotic
AIRWAY
N - Nasal
O - Oral
ET - ETT
N/A - none
SENSATION
4 - full
3 - dull
2 - tingling
1 - numbness
0 - absent
SAFETY SIDERAILS
X2
X1
0
BREATH SOUNDS
CL - Clear
CR - Crackles
WH - Wheezing
RH - Rhonchi
* - See notes
PUPIL REACTION
B - Brisk
S - Sluggish
NR - Non-reactive
ID BAND
+ yes
- no
TEMP
W - Warm
C - Cold

NURSING PROGRESS NOTES

DISCHARGE CRITERIA MET:
☐ Inpatient surgery ☐ PTCA patient ☐ CVU patient ☐ Same day surgery patient
☐ Cardiac cath patient ☐ Regional block pt ☐ Infants/pediatric patient

TIME	DRUG	DOSE	ROUTE	RN INITIALS

INITIALS	NAME	INITIALS	NAME

COMMENTS: ________
EVALUATED AND DISCHARGED (MD/DO): ________
REPORT CALLED TO: ________
TIME OF DISCHARGE: ________
PACU NURSE SIGNATURE: ________

Figure 22-1 ■ Example of a postanesthesia care unit record. (Courtesy of Our Lady of Lourdes Medical Center, Camden, NJ.)

which could result in hypoxia. Listen for snoring and **stridor** (a high-pitched crowing sound). Snoring and stridor are signs of airway obstruction resulting from tracheal or laryngeal spasm or edema, mucus in the airway, or blockage of the airway from edema or tongue relaxation. When neuromuscular blocking agents are retained, the client has muscle weakness, which could affect gas exchange. Indicators of muscle weakness include the inability to maintain a head lift, weak hand grasps, and an abdominal breathing pattern.

When the client returns to an inpatient unit, complete an initial assessment on arrival (Chart 22-1) and then continue to assess for indications of respiratory depression or hypoxemia. Auscultate the lungs to check for effective expansion and for abnormal breath sounds. Listen to the lungs at least every 4 hours during the first 24 hours after surgery and then during every nursing shift, or more often, as indicated. Older clients, smokers, and clients with a history of pulmonary disease are at greater risk for respiratory complications after surgery and need more frequent assessment.

CARDIOVASCULAR SYSTEM

VITAL SIGNS. Assess blood pressure, pulse, and heart sounds on admission to the PACU and then at least every 15 minutes until the client's condition is stabile. Automated blood pressure cuffs and cardiac monitoring assist in continuous assessment.

Review vital signs after surgery for upward or downward trends and compare them to those taken before surgery. Report blood pressure changes of more or less than 25% of values obtained before surgery (15- to 20-point difference, systolic or diastolic) to the anesthesia provider or the surgeon. Decreased blood pressure, pulse pressure, and heart sounds indicate possible cardiac depression, fluid volume deficit, shock, hemorrhage, or the effects of drugs (see Chapters 7, 15, and 40). Bradycardia could indicate an anesthesia effect or hypothermia. Older clients are at risk for hypothermia because of age-related changes in the hypothalamus (the temperature regulation center), loss of subcutaneous tissue, and coolness of the operating room (OR) suite. An increased pulse rate could indicate hemorrhage, shock, or pain.

CARDIAC MONITORING. Cardiac monitoring is maintained until the client is discharged from the PACU. For clients at risk for dysrhythmias, monitoring may continue either on telemetry units or on general medical-surgical units. In assessing the vital signs of a client who is not being monitored continuously, compare the rate, rhythm, and quality of the apical pulse with the rate, rhythm, and quality of a peripheral pulse, such as the radial pulse. A **pulse deficit** (a difference between the apical and peripheral pulses) could indicate a dysrhythmia.

PERIPHERAL VASCULAR ASSESSMENT. Anesthesia and positioning during surgery (e.g., the lithotomy position for genitourinary procedures) may impair the peripheral circulation. Compare distal pulses on both feet for the quality of pulsation, observe the color and temperature of extremities, evaluate sensation, and determine the speed of capillary refill. Palpable dorsalis pedis pulses indicate adequate circulation and perfusion of the legs.

Assess the feet and legs for redness, pain, warmth, swelling, and **Homans' sign** (calf pain on dorsiflexion of the foot), which may occur with deep vein thrombosis (DVT). Foot and leg assessment may be performed once during a nursing shift, once daily, or once per visit, depending on the client's risk for complications and the facility's or agency's policy. (See Chapters 20 and 39 for more information on DVT.)

NEUROLOGIC SYSTEM

CEREBRAL FUNCTIONING. Assess cerebral function and the level of consciousness or awareness for *all* clients who have received general anesthesia (Table 22-2) or any type of sedation. Observe for lethargy, restlessness, or ir-

CHART 22-1

FOCUSED ASSESSMENT of
The Client on Arrival at the Medical-Surgical Unit After Discharge from the Postanesthesia Care Unit

Airway
- Is it patent?
- Is the neck in proper alignment?

Breathing
- What is the quality and pattern of the breathing?
- What is the respiratory rate and depth?
- Is the client receiving oxygen? At what setting? What is the pulse oximetry result?

Mental Status
- Is the client awake, able to be aroused, oriented, and aware?
- Does the client respond to verbal stimuli?

Surgical Incision Site
- How is it dressed?
- Mark the amount of drainage on the dressing immediately.
- Is there any bleeding or drainage under the client?
- Are there any drains present?
- Are the drains set properly (e.g., compressed if they should be compressed, not kinked, client not lying on them)?
- How much drainage is present in the drainage container?

Temperature, Pulse, and Blood Pressure
- Are these values within the client's baseline range?
- Are these values significantly different from when the client was in the postanesthesia care unit (PACU)?

Intravenous Fluids
- What type of solution is infusing and with what additives?
- How much solution was remaining on arrival?
- How much solution infused in the transport time from PACU?
- What is the infusion rate supposed to be set at? Is it?

Other Tubes
- Is there a nasogastric or other intestinal tube?
- What is the color, consistency, and amount of drainage?
- Is it set on suction if it is supposed to be? Is it on the right amount of suction?
- Is there a Foley catheter?
- Is the Foley draining properly?
- What is the color, clarity, and volume of urine output?

TABLE 22-2 Immediate Postoperative Neurologic Assessment: Return to Preoperative Level

Order of Return to Consciousness After General Anesthesia
1. Muscular irritability
2. Restlessness and delirium
3. Recognition of pain
4. Ability to reason and control behavior

Order of Return of Motor and Sensory Functioning After Local or Regional Anesthesia
1. Sense of touch
2. Sense of pain
3. Sense of warmth
4. Sense of cold
5. Ability to move

ritability, and test coherence and orientation. Determine awareness by observing responses to calling the client's name, touching the client, and giving simple commands such as "Open your eyes" and "Take a deep breath." Eye opening in response to a command indicates wakefulness or arousability but not necessarily awareness. Determine the degree of orientation to person, place, and time by asking the conscious client to answer questions such as "What is your name?" (person), "Where are you?" (place), and "What day is it?" (time).

CONSIDERATIONS FOR OLDER ADULTS

For an older adult, a rapid return to his or her level of orientation before surgery may not be realistic. Drugs and anesthetics often delay the older client's return of orientation (see Chapters 20 and 21).

Compare the client's baseline neurologic status (obtained before surgery) with the findings after surgery. Clients who had altered cerebral functioning before surgery as a result of another condition continue to have that alteration after surgery. After the client has a satisfactory level of consciousness (and all other criteria have been met), he or she is discharged from the PACU. On the medical-surgical nursing unit, assess the level of consciousness every 4 to 8 hours or as indicated by the client's condition and the facility's policy.

MOTOR AND SENSORY ASSESSMENT. Assess motor and sensory function for all clients who received general or regional anesthesia. General anesthesia depresses all voluntary motor function. Regional anesthesia alters the motor and sensory function of only part of the body. (See Chapter 21 for more information on anesthesia.) *Motor and sensory assessment is very important after epidural or spinal anesthesia.* Evaluate motor function by asking the client to move each extremity. The client who had epidural or spinal anesthesia remains in the PACU until sensory function (feeling) and voluntary motor movement of the legs have returned (see Table 22-2). Also assess the strength of each limb and compare the results on both sides.

Test for the return of sympathetic nervous system tone by gradually elevating the client's head and monitoring for hypotension. Begin this evaluation after the client's sensation has returned to at least the spinal dermatome level of T10. (See Chapter 44 for further neurologic assessment.) After the client is transferred to the nursing unit, continue neurologic assessment as indicated.

FLUID, ELECTROLYTE, AND ACID-BASE BALANCE. Fasting before and during surgery, the loss of fluid during the procedure, and the type and amount of blood or fluid given affect the client's fluid and electrolyte balance after surgery. Fluid volume deficit or fluid volume overload may occur after surgery. Sodium, potassium, chloride, and calcium imbalances also may result, as may changes in other electrolyte levels. Fluid and electrolyte imbalances occur more often in older or debilitated clients and in clients with health problems such as diabetes mellitus, Crohn's disease, or heart failure.

INTAKE AND OUTPUT. Intake and output measurement is part of the operative record and part of the circulating nurse's report to the PACU nurse. Record any intake or output, including intravenous (IV) fluid intake, vomitus, urine, and nasogastric (NG) tube drainage. You must know the total intake and output from both the OR and the PACU to assess fluid balance accurately and to complete the 24-hour intake and output record.

HYDRATION ASSESSMENT. The client's hydration status is assessed in the PACU and the medical-surgical unit. To determine hydration status, inspect the color and moisture of mucous membranes; the turgor, texture, and "tenting" of the skin (test over the sternum or forehead of an older client); the amount of drainage on dressings; and the presence of axillary sweat. Measure and compare total output (e.g., NG tube drainage, urine output, and wound drainage) with total intake to identify a possible fluid imbalance. Consider insensible fluid loss, such as sweat, when reviewing total output. Continue to assess intake and output as long as the client is at risk for fluid imbalances. Some facilities require intake and output to be measured if the client receives IV fluids or has a catheter, drains, or an NG tube.

INTRAVENOUS FLUIDS. Closely monitor IV fluids to promote fluid and electrolyte balance. Isotonic solutions such as lactated Ringer's (LR) and 5% dextrose with lactated Ringer's (D_5/LR) are used for IV fluid replacement in the PACU. After the client returns to the medical-surgical unit, the type and rate of IV infusions are based on need. A typical IV solution for the client being admitted to the nursing unit is 5% dextrose with 0.45% normal saline (D_5 0.45% NS). (See Chapters 15 and 17 for further discussion of IV fluids, electrolyte balance, and hydration assessment.)

ACID-BASE BALANCE. Acid-base balance is affected by the client's respiratory status before and during surgery; metabolic changes during surgery; and losses of acids or bases in drainage. For example, NG tube drainage or vomitus causes a loss of hydrochloric acid and leads to alkalosis. Examine arterial blood gas values and other laboratory values. (See Chapter 19 for more detailed information on acid-base imbalances.)

RENAL/URINARY SYSTEM. Control of urination may return immediately after surgery or may not return for hours after general or regional anesthesia. The effects of drugs, anesthetic agents, or manipulation during surgery can cause urine retention. Assess for urine retention by inspection, palpation, and percussion of the lower abdomen for bladder distention. Assessment may be difficult to perform after lower abdominal surgery. Urine retention is common early after surgery and requires intervention, such as intermittent (straight) catheterization, to empty the bladder.

When the client has an indwelling urinary (Foley) catheter, assess the urine for color, clarity, and amount. If the client is voiding, assess the frequency, amount per void, and any symptoms. Urine output should be close to the total intake for a 24-hour period. Consider other sources of output, such as sweat, vomitus, or diarrhea stools. Report a urine output of less than 30 mL/hr (240 mL per 8-hour nursing shift) to the physician. Decreased urine output may indicate hypovolemia or renal complications. (See Chapter 72 for renal/urinary assessment.)

GASTROINTESTINAL SYSTEM

NAUSEA AND VOMITING. One of the most common reactions after surgery is nausea and vomiting. About 30% of clients who receive general anesthesia have some form of gastrointestinal (GI) upset within the first 24 hours after surgery. Preventive therapy is effective in reducing the incidence. A drug often used is droperidol (Inapsine). Clients with a history of motion sickness are more likely to develop nausea and vomiting after surgery. Obese clients may be at risk because many anesthetics are retained by fat cells and remain in the body longer. Abdominal surgery and the use of opioid analgesics reduce intestinal peristalsis after surgery. These problems increase the risk for prolonged nausea and vomiting after surgery.

Nausea and vomiting can stress and irritate abdominal and GI wounds, increase intracranial pressure in clients who had head and neck surgery, elevate intraocular pressure in clients who had eye surgery, and increase the risk for aspiration. Assess the client continuously for nausea and vomiting. Often clients have nausea as the head of the bed is raised early after surgery. This symptom may occur with or without dizziness. You can help reduce this distressing symptom by having the client in a side-lying position before raising the head slowly.

GASTROINTESTINAL PERISTALSIS. In the PACU and later on the medical-surgical unit, assess for the return of peristalsis. Peristalsis may be delayed because of long anesthesia time, the amount of bowel handling during surgery, and opioid analgesic use. Clients who have abdominal surgery often have decreased peristalsis for at least 24 hours. This problem may persist for several days for those who have GI surgery.

Assessment. Auscultate for bowel sounds in all four abdominal quadrants and at the umbilicus. If NG suction is being used, turn off the suction before listening to prevent mistaking the sound of the suction for bowel sounds. In addition, ask the client whether flatus has been passed. Bowel sounds and flatus passage indicate active peristalsis. Abdominal cramping denotes trapped, nonmoving gas, not peristalsis.

Complications. Decreased peristalsis occurs in clients who have a paralytic ileus. The intestine wall is distended, and there is no movement of the intestinal wall. Assess for the manifestations of paralytic ileus (few or absent bowel sounds, a distended abdomen, abdominal discomfort, vomiting, and no passage of flatus or stool).

The client may also have constipation after surgery as a result of anesthesia, analgesia (especially opioid analgesics), decreased activity, and decreased oral intake. Assess the abdomen by inspection, auscultation, palpation, and percussion and record the elimination pattern to determine whether interventions are needed. Increased dietary fiber intake, the use of mild laxatives or bulk-forming agents, or the use of enemas may be needed.

NASOGASTRIC TUBE DRAINAGE. A nasogastric (NG) tube may be inserted during surgery to decompress and drain the stomach, to promote GI rest, to allow the lower GI tract to heal, and to provide an enteral feeding route. It may also be used to monitor any gastric bleeding and to prevent intestinal obstruction. The Levin tube and the Salem sump tube are two common tubes used. The Salem tube is a double-lumen tube with an air vent to keep the tube from sucking the gastric mucosa. This feature allows easy drainage of the stomach and prevents mucosal damage. The Levin tube is a single-lumen tube with no air vent. To promote drainage, suction (high, medium, or low) is applied to the NG tube. Suction is either continuous (recommended for the Salem tube) or intermittent.

TABLE 22-3 Calculating Nasogastric Tube Drainage

Formula

Drainage in collection device − Amount of irrigant = True (actual) amount of drainage

Example

A client's drainage container was marked at 150 mL at 7 AM. At 3 PM, there was 525 mL in the container. During the nursing shift, the nurse instilled 30 mL of saline as an irrigant into the tube four times, as prescribed by the physician.

525 mL − 150 mL = 375 mL of drainage

30 mL × 4 = 120 mL of irrigant

375 mL − 120 mL = 255 mL of actual drainage

Assessment. Record the color, consistency, and amount of the drained material every 8 hours (Table 22-3). In some instances, an occult blood test (Gastroccult) may be performed. Normal NG drainage fluid is greenish yellow. Red drainage fluid indicates active bleeding, and brown liquid or drainage with a "coffee-ground" appearance indicates old bleeding.

Complications. Assess the client for complications related to NG tube use, such as fluid and electrolyte imbalances, aspiration, and nares discomfort. To prevent aspiration, check the tube placement every 4 to 8 hours and before instilling any liquid into the tube. (See Chapter 59 for information on tube placement and care.) *After gastric surgery, do not move or irrigate the tube without an order from the surgeon.* Fluid and electrolyte imbalances can result from NG drainage and tube irrigation with water instead of saline. Imbalances include fluid volume deficit (see Chapter 15), hypokalemia and hyponatremia (see Chapter 16), hypochloremia, and metabolic alkalosis (see Chapter 19).

SKIN ASSESSMENT. The clean surgical wound heals at skin level in about 2 weeks in the absence of trauma, connective tissue disease, malnutrition, or the use of some drugs, such as steroids. Smokers, older clients, obese clients, diabetic clients, and those with reduced immunity have delayed wound healing. Complete healing of all tissue to presurgical integrity may take 6 months to 2 years. The physical health and age of the client, size and location of the wound, and stress on the wound all affect healing time. Because of the rich blood supply, head and facial wounds heal more quickly than abdominal and leg wounds.

NORMAL WOUND HEALING. During the first few days of normal wound healing, the incised tissue regains blood supply and begins to bind together. Fibrin and a thin layer of epithelial cells seal the incision. After 1 to 4 days, epithelial cells continue growing in the fibrin and strands of collagen begin to fill in the wound gaps. This process continues for 2 to 3 weeks. *At that time, the wound appears to be healed; however, healing is not complete for up to 2 years, until the scar is strengthened.* (See Chapter 70 for discussion of wound healing and wound infection.)

When the client is an inpatient, the surgeon usually removes the original dressing on the first or second day after surgery. Assess the incision on a regular basis, at least every 8 hours, for redness, increased warmth, swelling, tenderness or pain, and the type and amount of drainage. Some drainage, changing from **sanguineous** (bloody) to serosanguineous to

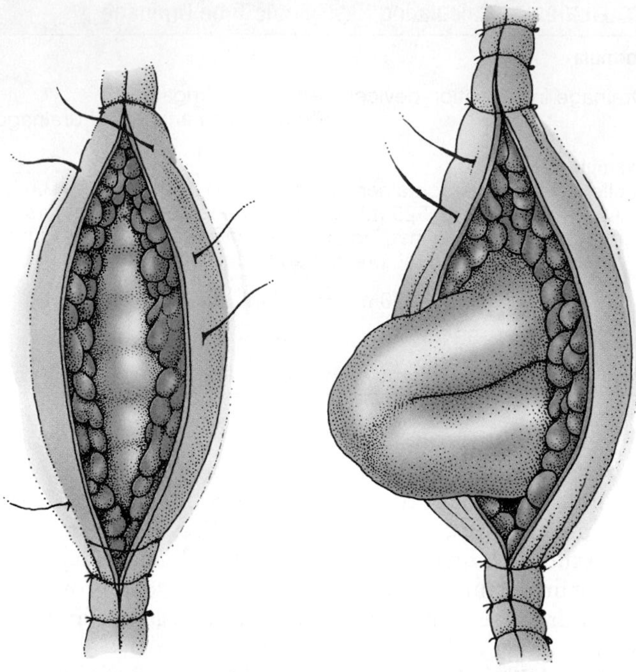

Figure 22-2 ■ Complications of wound healing.

serous (serum-like, or yellow), is normal during the first few days. Serosanguineous drainage continuing beyond the fifth day after surgery alerts you to the possibility of dehiscence, and the surgeon should be notified. Slight crusting on the incision line is normal, as is a pink color to the line itself, which is caused by inflammation from the surgical procedure. Slight swelling under the sutures or staples is also normal. Redness or swelling of or around the incision line, excessive tenderness or pain on palpation, and purulent or odorous drainage indicate wound infection and must be reported to the surgeon.

INEFFECTIVE WOUND HEALING. Ineffective wound healing may be caused by infection, distention from edema or paralytic ileus, stress at the surgical site, and health problems that cause delayed wound healing (such as diabetes). Wound **dehiscence** is a partial or complete separation of the outer wound layers, sometimes described as a "splitting open of the wound." **Evisceration** is the total separation of all wound layers and protrusion of internal organs through the open wound (Figure 22-2). Both of these problems occur most often between the fifth and tenth days after surgery. Wound separation occurs more often in obese clients and those with diabetes or who are using steroids. Dehiscence or evisceration may follow forceful coughing, vomiting or straining, and when not splinting the surgical site during movement. The client may state "Something gave way" or "I feel as if I just split open."

DRESSINGS AND DRAINS. Assess all dressings, including casts and elastic (Ace) bandages, for bleeding or other drainage on admission to the PACU and then hourly thereafter. When the client is on the nursing unit, assess the dressing each time vital signs are taken (at least every shift). During dressing inspection, check for drainage and record its amount, color, consistency, and odor. If drainage is present on a dressing or cast, monitor its progression by outlining it with a pen and indicating the date and time. Check the area underneath the client also, because drainage or blood may leak from the side of the dressing and not appear on the dressing itself. Ensure that the dressing does not restrict circulation or sensation.

The surgeon inserts a drain into or close to the wound if more than a minimal amount of drainage is expected. A Penrose drain (a single-lumen, soft, open, latex tube) is a gravity-type drain under the dressing. Drainage on the dressing is expected with open tube drains but is not expected with closed drainage systems. Assess closed-suction drains, such as Hemovac, VacuDrain, and Jackson-Pratt drains, for maintenance of suction. A T-tube may be placed after abdominal cholecystectomy to drain bile. Figure 22-3 shows commonly used drains.

Assess all drains for patency when the client is admitted to the PACU and every time vital signs are taken. Monitor the amount, color, and type of drainage while the client is in the PACU and at least every 8 hours after the client is transferred to the medical-surgical nursing unit. Large amounts of sanguineous drainage may indicate internal bleeding.

DISCOMFORT/PAIN ASSESSMENT. The client almost always has pain or discomfort after surgery. Pain is a subjective experience and may be more intense than the health care professional can appreciate. Pain after surgery is related to the surgical wound, tissue manipulation, drains, positioning during surgery, presence of an endotracheal (ET) tube, and the client's experience with pain. In assessing the client's discomfort and need for medication, consider the type, extent, and length of the surgical procedure. Assess for physical and emotional signs of acute pain, such as increased pulse and blood pressure, increased respiratory rate, profuse sweating, restlessness, increased confusion (in the older adult), wincing, moaning, and crying. When possible, ask the client to rate the pain before and after drugs are given (e.g., on a scale of 1 to 10, with 1 being no pain and 10 being extreme pain). Plan the client's activities around the timing of analgesia to improve mobility. Observe for a return of normal (baseline) physical behaviors. (See Chapter 7 for further discussion of pain assessment.)

Pain assessment is started by the PACU nurse. After transfer from the PACU, the medical-surgical nurse continues to assess the client's comfort level. Pain usually reaches its peak on the second day after surgery, when the client is more awake, is more active, and the anesthetic agents and drugs given during surgery have been excreted.

PSYCHOSOCIAL ASSESSMENT

Consider the psychological, social, and cultural issues of the client after surgery as you provide physical care. This assessment may be delayed or difficult to perform in the postanesthesia care unit (PACU) when the client is drowsy or incoherent. Consider the client's age and medical history, the surgical procedure, and the impact of surgery on recovery, body image, roles, and lifestyle.

Physical signs of anxiety include restlessness; increased pulse, blood pressure, and respiratory rate; and crying. The client may be anxious and ask questions about the results or findings of the surgical procedure. Reassure the client that the surgeon will speak with him or her after the client is

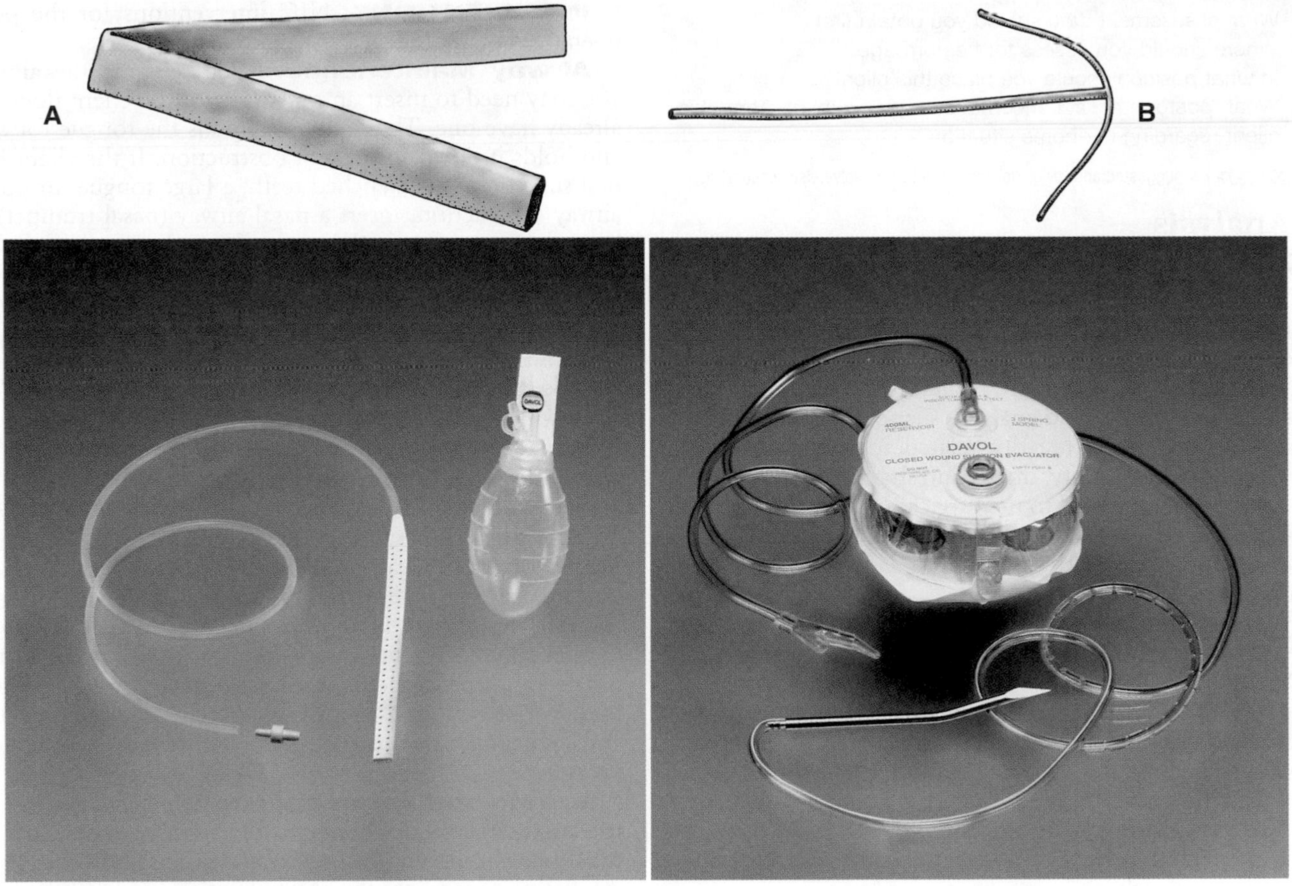

Figure 22-3 ■ Types of surgical drains. Gravity drains, such as the Penrose **(A)** and the T-tube **(B),** drain directly through a tube from the surgical area. In closed wound drainage systems, such as the Jackson-Pratt **(C)** and Hemovac **(D),** drainage collects in a collecting vessel by means of compression and reexpansion of the system. (**C** and **D** courtesy of C.R. Bard, Inc., Covington, GA.)

fully awake. If the surgeon has already spoken with the client, reinforce what was said.

After the client returns to the medical-surgical unit, continue the psychosocial assessment and also assess significant others for psychological discomfort.

LABORATORY ASSESSMENT

Laboratory tests are performed after surgery to monitor for complications. Tests are based on the surgical procedure, the client's medical history, and clinical manifestations after surgery. Common tests include analysis of electrolytes and a complete blood count (see Chart 20-3). A change in laboratory test results (e.g., electrolyte levels, hematocrit, and hemoglobin levels) often occurs during the first 24 to 48 hours after surgery because of blood and fluid loss and the body's reaction to the surgical process. Fluid loss with minimal blood loss may cause hemoconcentration of laboratory values. Such test results are reported as increased, but actually represent a concentrated normal value.

An early indication of infection is an increase in the band cells (immature neutrophils) in the white blood cell differential count. This increase is termed a **left-shift** (sometimes called "bandemia"). The source of infection may be the respiratory system, urinary tract, wound, or IV site. Obtain specimens for culture and sensitivity testing and monitor the culture reports at 24, 48, and 72 hours. Notify the surgeon of positive culture results. (See Chapters 23 and 29 for information on infection and assessment of immune function.)

Arterial blood gas (ABG) tests may be needed for clients who have respiratory or cardiac disease, those undergoing mechanical ventilation after surgery, and those who had chest surgery. Review ABG results and notify the surgeon of any acid-base imbalance or hypoxemia. (For more discussion on arterial blood gases and acidosis, see Chapters 18 and 19.)

Urine and renal laboratory tests also may be obtained (e.g., urinalysis, urine electrolyte levels, and serum creatinine levels). Other laboratory tests depend on the diagnosis, type of surgical procedure, and other health problems. Examples are a serum amylase level for a client who had pancreatic surgery and a blood glucose level for a client with diabetes.

Critical Thinking Challenge

The client is a 62-year-old woman with chronic gallbladder disease who developed biliary obstruction and required an emergency abdominal cholecystectomy. The client is single and lives next door to her 85-year-old mother, for whom she prepares meals and assists with activities of daily living. Her last vital signs before leaving the OR were BP 150/110, P 100, R 12.

She has a Foley catheter, an NG tube to continuous low suction, and a Penrose drain in her wound.

Continued

1. What assessment data should you obtain first?
2. Where should you assess for hemorrhage?
3. In what position should you place this client?
4. What postoperative concerns can you expect from this client regarding her home situation?

evolve For suggested answer guidelines, go to http://evolve.elsevier.com/Iggy/.

Analysis

COMMON NURSING DIAGNOSES AND COLLABORATIVE PROBLEMS

The following are priority nursing diagnoses for the client after surgery:

1. Impaired Gas Exchange related to the effects of anesthesia, pain, opioid analgesics, and immobility
2. Impaired Skin Integrity related to surgical wounds, decreased mobility, drains and drainage, and tubes
3. Acute Pain related to the surgical incision, positioning during surgery, and endotracheal (ET) tube irritation

The primary collaborative problem is Potential for Hypoxemia.

ADDITIONAL NURSING DIAGNOSES AND COLLABORATIVE PROBLEMS

In addition to the common nursing diagnoses and collaborative problems, clients may have one or more of the following problems after surgery:

- Risk for Aspiration related to decreased mobility, anesthesia, and opioid analgesic use
- Ineffective Airway Clearance related to ineffective or absent cough
- Constipation related to decreased mobility, anesthesia, and opioid analgesic use
- Risk for Infection related to surgery and invasive lines, catheters, and tubes
- Urinary Retention related to anesthesia, surgical procedures, and decreased mobility
- Delayed Surgical Recovery related to presence of other health problems (diabetes, obesity), or complications of surgery
- Bathing/Hygiene Self-Care Deficit related to surgical procedures, pain, and decreased mobility
- Disturbed Body Image related to surgical procedures, loss of a body part or function, and pain
- Interrupted Family Processes related to the impact of surgery and illness on the family system
- Potential for Hypovolemic Shock
- Potential for Deep Vein Thrombosis and Pulmonary Embolism

Planning and Implementation

IMPAIRED GAS EXCHANGE

NOC **PLANNING: EXPECTED OUTCOMES.** The client is expected to attain or maintain optimal lung expansion and breathing patterns after surgery as indicated by:

- Partial pressure of arterial oxygen (PaO_2) within normal range
- Partial pressure of arterial carbon dioxide ($PaCO_2$) within normal range
- Oxygen saturation values within normal range

INTERVENTIONS. NIC interventions for the postoperative client are listed in Chart 22-2.

Airway Maintenance. After assessing the airway, you may need to insert an oral airway if the client does not already have one. The oral airway pulls the tongue forward and holds it down to prevent obstruction. If the client had oral surgery or has clenched teeth, a large tongue, or upper airway obstruction, insert a nasal airway (nasal trumpet) to keep the airway open. Keep the manual resuscitation bag and emergency equipment for intubation or tracheostomy nearby. For clients whose only airway is a tracheostomy or laryngectomy stoma, alert other staff members by posting signs in the room and notes on the chart.

Positioning. *In the PACU, immediately position the client in a side-lying position or turn his or her head to the side to prevent aspiration.* Suction the mouth, nose, and throat to keep the airway clear of mucus or vomitus as needed.

Keep the client's head flat to prevent hypotension and possible shock, unless this position is contraindicated by the condition or surgical procedure. (For example, after intracranial surgery, the head of the bed or stretcher is elevated to promote ventilation and prevent cerebral edema.) Apply oxygen via a face tent, nasal cannula, or mask to eliminate inhaled anesthetic agents, increase oxygen levels, and raise the level of consciousness. After the client is fully reactive and stable, raise the head of the bed to promote respiratory function.

Breathing Exercises. After the client regains the gag and cough reflex and meets the agency's criteria for extubation (if intubated), remove the airway or ET tube. Usual extubation criteria are the ability to raise and hold the head up and evidence of thoracic breathing. Help the client to cough (with the incision splinted) and deep breathe to expand the lungs, promote gas exchange, and eliminate inhalation anesthetic agents. Chart 20-6 reviews breathing exercises and splinting of the surgical area. As soon as the

CHART 22-2

NIC INTERVENTION ACTIVITIES for The Postoperative Client

Postanesthesia Care: *Monitoring and management of the client who has recently undergone general or regional anesthesia*

- Administer oxygen, as appropriate.
- Monitor oxygenation.
- Ventilate, as appropriate.
- Monitor quality and number of respirations.
- Encourage client to deep breathe and cough.
- Monitor and record vital signs and perform pain assessment every 15 minutes or more often, as appropriate.
- Monitor urinary output.
- Monitor return of sensorium and motor function.
- Monitor neurologic status.
- Monitor level of consciousness.
- Monitor surgical site, as appropriate.
- Administer narcotic antagonists, as appropriate, per agency protocol.
- Determine client's status for discharge
- Provide client report to the postoperative nursing unit.
- Discharge client to next level of care.

NIC intervention activities selected from Dochterman, J.M., & Bulechek, G.M. (Eds.). (2004). *Nursing interventions classification (NIC)* (4th ed.). St. Louis: Mosby.

client is awake enough to follow commands, urge him or her to cough, use the incentive spirometer, and take deep breaths. Remind the client to continue these activities through out the postoperative period. The client who is unable to remove mucus or sputum requires oral or nasal suctioning. Perform mouth care after removing secretions.

Mobilization. Assist the client out of bed and to ambulate as soon as possible to help remove secretions and promote lung expansion. Even when the client has had extensive surgery, the goal may be to get out of bed the same day of or the first day after surgery. If this is not possible, assist the client to turn at least every 2 hours (side to side) and ensure that breathing exercises and leg exercises are performed (see Charts 20-6 and 20-7). Early ambulation reduces the risk for pulmonary complications, especially after abdominal, pelvic, or spinal surgery. The client may report pain and resist getting up, but you need to stress the importance of activity to prevent complications. When indicated, offer pain medication 30 to 45 minutes before the client gets out of bed.

IMPAIRED SKIN INTEGRITY

NOC **PLANNING: EXPECTED OUTCOMES.** The client is expected to have incision healing without wound complications as indicated by:

- Wound edges remaining together
- Absence of purulent drainage, induration or redness in, from or around the incision

INTERVENTIONS. Nursing assessment of the surgical area is critical (see the discussion of skin assessment on p. 345). Although most wound complications do not require additional surgical intervention, emergency surgical procedures may be needed.

NONSURGICAL MANAGEMENT. Wound care includes changing the dressing, assessing the wound for signs of infection, and caring for drains, including emptying, measuring, and documenting drainage features. Emphasize the importance of early deep breathing exercises to prevent forceful coughing. Encourage hip flexion when the client is in the supine position to reduce tension on a chest or abdominal wound. Remind the client to always splint the incision when coughing. Promote wound healing and protection of the skin in general, especially for the older client. Chart 22-3 lists best practices for skin care of the older client after surgery.

Dressings. The surgeon usually performs the first dressing change to assess the wound, remove any packing, and advance (pull partially out) or remove drains. Before the first dressing change, reinforce the dressing (add more dressing material to the existing dressing) if it becomes wet from drainage. Document the added material, as well as the color, type, amount, and odor of drainage fluid and time of observation. Assess the surgical site every shift and report any unexpected findings to the surgeon.

After removal of the dressing, the surgeon may leave the suture or staple line open to the air, which allows easy assessment of the wound and early detection of poor wound edge adherence, drainage, swelling, or redness. Some surgeons believe that air-drying promotes healing. A draining wound, however, is always covered with a dressing.

Dressing changes are prescribed by the surgeon; however, the facility or unit may have standards or policies that dictate specific protocols for dressing changes and incision care. An unchanged wet or damp dressing is a source of infection. Perform dressing changes using aseptic technique until the sutures or staples are removed.

Dressings vary with the surgical procedure and the surgeon's preference. Common dressings for large incisions consist of gauze or nonadherent pads covered with a larger absorbent pad held in place by tape or by Montgomery straps (Figure 22-4). Some incisions may be covered with a transparent plastic surgical dressing (such as Op-Site) or a spray in the operating room. This type of dressing stays intact for 3 to 6 days and allows direct observation of the wound. It also prevents contamination and eliminates the need for dressing changes.

Wound or suture line care consists of changing gauze dressings at least once during a nursing shift or daily and may include cleaning the area with sterile saline or some other solution. Some suture lines are left open to air without any dressing to cover the incision. The hospital's policy, the unit's standards, and the surgeon's preference determine what solution, if any, is used to clean the wound and how often dressings are changed. For large dressing changes or drain removal, offer the client a prescribed analgesic before the procedure.

Skin sutures or staples are usually removed 6 to 8 days after surgery, and the incision is secured with Steri-Strips. The surgeon or the nurse removes the sutures or staples, depending on the agency's policy. Before removing sutures, examine the condition and healing stage of the wound. If

CHART 22-3

NURSING FOCUS on the OLDER ADULT
Best Practices in Postoperative Skin Care

Improve perfusion to the wound to promote wound healing:
- Keep the client adequately hydrated to maintain cardiac output
- Keep the airway patent and provide adequate oxygenation.
- Keep the client's oxygen saturation on pulse oximetry at greater than 93%.

Conserve the client's energy:
- Allow the client to sleep in a darkened, quiet room.
- Administer medication to combat pain and sleeplessness, as prescribed.
- Provide rest periods throughout the day.
- Control the client's room temperature.
- Assist in activities of daily living.

Place the client on a safety program to prevent falls, if indicated.

Maintain strict aseptic technique in caring for breaks in the integument (IV or other catheters, indwelling urethral catheter, wound).

Maintain the client's psychosocial health:
- Prevent unnecessary stressors.
- Allow the client liberal visitation of supportive others.
- Enable the client to use individual successful coping mechanisms.
- Keep the client well groomed and bathed.

Protect fragile skin:
- Minimize the use of tape on the skin.
- Use hypoallergenic tape or Montgomery straps.
- Change dressings as soon as they become wet.
- Lift the client during transfer or repositioning.

Data from Jones, P.L., & Millman, A. (1990). Wound healing and the aged patient. *Nursing Clinics of North America, 25*(1), 263-277.

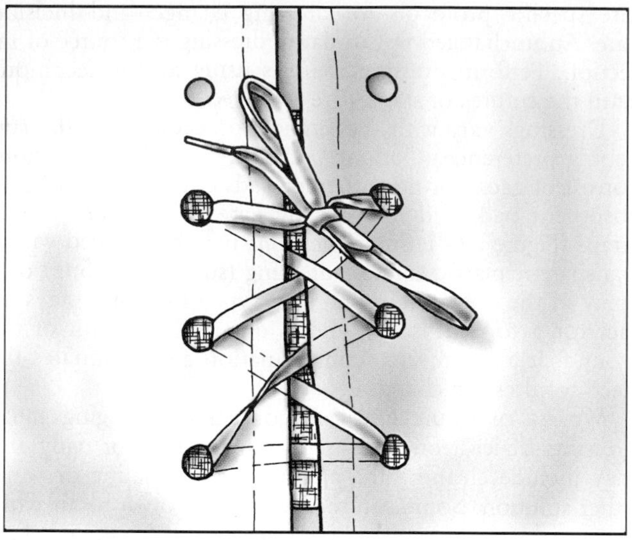

Figure 22-4 ■ Montgomery straps may be used when frequent dressing changes are anticipated. They help prevent skin irritation from frequent tape removal.

the wound does not appear to be healing well, notify the surgeon before removing sutures.

Drains. Drains (see Figure 22-3) may be placed in the wound or through a separate small incision (known as a "stab" wound) close to the incision during surgery. Drains provide an exit route for air, blood, and bile. Drains also help prevent deep infections and abscess formation during healing.

The Penrose drain is placed into the external aspect of the incision and drains directly onto the dressing and skin around the incision. Change a damp or soiled dressing and carefully clean under and around the Penrose drain. Then place absorbent pads distal to the drain to prevent skin irritation and wound contamination. Whether sutured in place or not, the drain can be dislodged or pulled out accidentally during a dressing change. As the wound heals, the surgeon shortens (advances) the drain by pulling it out and cutting the excess external portion until drainage stops.

Jackson-Pratt and Hemovac drains are two self-contained drainage systems that drain wounds directly through a tube via gravity and vacuum. These drains are sutured in place with a suture that seals the area when the drain is removed. Empty the reservoir and record the amount and color of drainage during every nursing shift or more often if prescribed. After emptying and compressing the reservoir, secure the drain to the client's gown (never to the sheet or mattress) to prevent pulling and stress on the surgical wound.

Drug Therapy. Wound infection is a major complication after surgery. It usually results from contamination during surgery, preoperative infection, debilitation, or immunosuppression. A client at risk for wound infection may receive antibiotic therapy with drugs that are effective against organisms common to the specific surgical site. These antibiotics are usually continued for 24 to 72 hours after surgery. The first dose may be given intravenously before or during surgery.

Wounds that become infected and open are treated with dressing changes and systemic antibiotic therapy. Depending on the surgeon's prescription, irrigate the wound (e.g., with sterile saline, hydrogen peroxide, povidone-iodine, or acetic acid), loosely pack it with solution-soaked gauze (e.g., neomycin, gentamicin, iodoform, povidone-iodine, saline, or acetic acid), and cover the wound with dry, sterile dressings. This procedure (wet-to-dry dressings) may be done one to three times daily. The packing promotes healing from within the wound and **debridement** (removal) of the infected tissue as the wound heals.

CHART 22-4

BEST PRACTICE for
Emergency Care of the Client with Surgical Wound Evisceration

EMERGENCY CARE

1. Call for help! Instruct the person who responds to notify the surgeon immediately and to bring any needed supplies into the client's room.
2. Stay with the client.
3. Cover the wound with a nonadherent dressing premoistened with warmed sterile normal saline. **NOTE:** The supplies needed for this emergency should be in the client's room, especially if the client is at high risk.
4. If premoistened dressings are not available, moisten sterile gauze or sterile towels in a sterile irrigation tray with sterile saline, then cover the wound.
5. If saline is not immediately available, cover the wound with gauze and then moisten with sterile saline using a sterile irrigation tray as soon as someone brings saline.
6. Do not attempt to reinsert the protruding organ or viscera.
7. While covering the wound, note the client's response and assess for manifestations of shock.
8. Place the client in a supine position with the hips and knees bent.
9. Take vital signs and document them. **NOTE:** If the person who answered the call for help is back in the room before this, instruct that individual to take vital signs while you focus on covering the wound and repositioning the client.
10. Provide support and reassurance to the client.
11. Continue assessing the client, including vital signs assessment, every 5 to 10 minutes until the surgeon arrives.
12. Keep dressings continuously moist by adding warmed sterile saline to the dressing as often as necessary. Do not let the dressing become dry.
13. When the surgeon arrives, report your finding and your interventions. Then follow the surgeon's directions.
14. Document the incident, the activity the client was engaged in at the time of the incident, your actions, and your assessments.

SURGICAL MANAGEMENT

Management of Dehiscence. *If dehiscence (wound opening) occurs, apply a sterile nonadherent (such as Telfa) or saline dressing to the wound and notify the surgeon.* A wound that becomes infected dehisces by itself, or it may be opened by the surgeon through an **incision and drainage (I&D)** procedure. In either case, the wound is left open rather than re-sutured and is treated as described previously.

Management of Evisceration. *An evisceration (a wound opening with protrusion of internal organs or viscera) is a surgical emergency. One nurse tends to the client while another nurse immediately notifies the surgeon.* Chart 22-4 lists best practices for emergency care of the client with surgical wound evisceration. Provide emotional support by explaining what happened and reassuring the client that the emergency will be handled competently.

The surgeon may prescribe a nasogastric (NG) tube to decompress the stomach and relieve internal pressure or to remove the stomach's contents if the client has been eating and general anesthesia is needed. Prepare the client for surgery (see Chapter 20) to close the wound. Regional or local anesthesia may be used, depending on the location and type of the wound. Nausea and vomiting, which stress the already fragile incision, are reduced when regional or local anesthesia is used. To increase the incision's integrity, stay or retention sutures of wire or nylon are used instead of standard sutures or staples (see Figure 21-13).

Prevention. Clients also are at risk for developing pressure ulcers from positioning during surgery, prolonged contact with damp surgical linens, and contact with unpadded surfaces. Pressure ulcers acquired during the surgical period increase lengths of stay and the risk for complications. Addressing early-stage pressure ulcers can prevent progression and limit complications.

Examine the client's skin for areas of redness or lost integrity. Document and report any abnormalities. Use padding and positioning to relieve pressure. Treat any open areas according to facility guidelines and the surgeon's prescription. Ensure that information about the client's skin condition in the PACU is communicated to the medical-surgical nurse.

ACUTE PAIN

NOC **PLANNING: EXPECTED OUTCOMES.** The postoperative client is expected to attain or maintain optimal comfort levels after surgery as indicated by:

- Reporting that pain is controlled
- Absence of physiologic indicators of acute pain (increased heart rate and blood pressure)
- Absence of facial grimacing, teeth clenching
- Willingness to move and participate in self care

INTERVENTIONS. Pain management after surgery includes drug therapy and other methods of management, such as positioning, massage, relaxation techniques, and diversion. Often the client has better pain relief from a combination of approaches. Assess the client's comfort level and the effectiveness of the therapies. See Chapter 7 for discussion of pain assessment and management. The client who has optimal pain control is better able to cooperate with the therapies and exercises to prevent complications and promote rehabilitation. Pain can be a factor in the risk for pulmonary complications after abdominal surgery. (See the Evidence-Based Practice for Nursing Box above.)

Drug Therapy. *The use of opioids or other analgesics for pain management may mask or increase the severity of symptoms of an anesthesia reaction. Therefore give these drugs with caution, especially in the PACU when the client's condition is not stabile.* Pain medication in the PACU is usually given intravenously in small doses. After receiving medication for pain, the client remains in the PACU for a defined period (often 30 to 45 minutes). Assess for hypotension, respiratory depression, and other side effects. Within 5 to 10 minutes after an IV injection, assess the effectiveness of the drug (i.e., on a rating scale) in relieving pain.

Opioid analgesics are given during the first 24 to 48 hours after surgery to control acute pain. Around-the-clock scheduling is more effective than "on demand" scheduling because more constant blood levels are achieved. Drugs commonly used include meperidine (Demerol), morphine (Statex✱), hydromorphone (Dilaudid), ketorolac (Toradol), codeine, butorphanol (Stadol), and oxycodone with aspirin (Percodan) or oxycodone with acetaminophen (Tylox, Percocet).

EVIDENCE-BASED PRACTICE for Nursing

Reduce pulmonary complications among older clients after abdominal surgery by managing pain

Shea, R., et al. (2002). Pain intensity and postoperative pulmonary complications among the elderly after abdominal surgery. *Heart & Lung, 31*(6), 440-449.

The purpose of this study was to examine whether pain after abdominal surgery in older adult clients influenced the development of postoperative pulmonary complications (PPCs). This exploratory study is a secondary analysis of data collected as part of a larger prospective study examining factors contributing to PPCs after abdominal or cardiothoracic surgery. The subgroup of subjects for which initial data were reanalyzed consisted of a convenience sample of clients over 60 years of age having open abdominal surgery with general anesthesia and a minimum postoperative stay of 48 hours. Clients with a preexisting pulmonary problem and those requiring more than 10 hours of mechanical ventilation after surgery were excluded from the analysis. PPCs were defined as the presence of any two of the following: new sputum/cough production, new onset of abnormal breath sounds, fever, chest x-ray showing infiltrate or atelectasis, or physician documentation of atelectasis/pneumonia. Pain was defined by self-report and the use of a numeric rating scale.

Data were analyzed for 86 subjects (49 men, 37 women; mean age of 70 years). Two groups were examined: those with a PPC (70 subjects) and those with no PPC (16 subjects). Statistically significant differences between the groups (as determined by analysis of variance) were found for mean pain scores at rest and pain with deep breathing, with the PPC group experiencing greater pain. Pain scores with coughing, movement, and walking were all greater in the PPC group, although these differences did not meet statistical significance. An additional finding was that subjects with a PPC had significantly longer lengths of stay than did subjects in the no PPC group.

Level of Evidence: 3—Well-designed trial without randomization.

Critique. Overall, the methods and analyses were appropriate for the purpose of the study. The criteria for PPC is a strength of the study. The study would be strengthened by randomization and a prospective approach.

Implications for Nursing. Postoperative pulmonary complications after abdominal surgery are costly in terms of morbidity, length of stay, and delayed recovery. Pain may inhibit the client from adequately performing interventions for prevention of pulmonary problems. Additionally, pain triggers the stress response, which reduces immune function, increasing the risk for PPC. Many nurses are hesitant to give opioid analgesics to older clients for fear of increasing confusion or depressing cardiopulmonary function. Ensuring that older clients have adequate pain management in the early postoperative period after abdominal surgery can enhance their participation in preventive interventions and may reduce the incidence of PPC in this population.

Assess the type, location, and intensity of the pain before and after giving medication (see also Discomfort/Pain Assessment on p. 346). Monitor the client's vital signs for hypotension and hypoventilation, after giving opioid drugs. Chart 22-5 lists more information about analgesics used after surgery.

Patient-controlled analgesia (PCA) via IV infusion or internal pump (the catheter is sutured into or near the surgical area) and epidural analgesia are often used for better pain control. In PCA, the client adjusts the dosage of the analgesic on the basis of the pain level and response to the drug. This method allows more consistent pain relief and more control by the client. The maximum dose per hour is "locked

CHART 22-5

DRUG THERAPY for Management of Postoperative Pain

Drug	Usual Dosage	Nursing Interventions	Rationales
Meperidine hydrochloride (Demerol)	50-150 mg PO or IM q3-4h 12.5-25 mg IV Maximum 6-8 doses	Monitor blood pressure. Move and ambulate the client slowly. Monitor pulse rate. Assess for decreased GI motility or GI upset.	Common side effects include decreased blood pressure, orthostatic (postural) hypotension, and bradycardia. Constipation, nausea, and vomiting can occur.
[1]Morphine sulfate (Epimorph✱, Statex✱)	2-15 mg IM or IV incrementally 10-30 mg PO q4h Maximum 6 doses	Monitor respiratory status.	Respiratory depression can be severe and require medical intervention.
		Monitor blood pressure. Assess for GI motility and urine output.	Hypotension, constipation, and urinary retention can occur.
Hydromorphone hydrochloride (Dilaudid)	1-4 mg IV or IM q3-4h 2-4 mg PO q3-4h	Monitor respirations. Monitor blood pressure. Monitor for food intolerance. Monitor fluid and electrolyte balance. Assess GI motility.	Respiratory depression, hypotension, anorexia, nausea, vomiting, and constipation can occur.
Codeine sulfate, codeine phosphate (Paveral✱)	15-60 mg IM or PO q4h Maximum 6 doses	Monitor respiratory status. Monitor for food intolerance. Monitor fluid and electrolyte balance.	Respiratory depression, nausea, and vomiting can occur.
		Assess GI motility.	Constipation is common; prophylactic interventions may be indicated.
Butorphanol tartrate (Stadol)	1-4 mg IM q3-4h 0.5-2 mg IV Maximum 6-8 doses	Monitor neurologic status and changes in level of consciousness. Monitor respiratory status.	Butorphanol can cause increased intracranial pressure and respiratory depression.
Oxycodone hydrochloride and aspirin (Percodan, Endodan✱, Oxycodan✱)	1-2 tablets (5-10 mg) PO q3-4h Maximum 80 mg	Assess GI tolerance of medication. Assess for GI bleeding. Monitor GI motility.	The aspirin component can irritate the stomach and could cause GI bleeding.
		Monitor coagulation studies (PT, aPTT).	Bleeding times and other coagulation study results may be increased because of the aspirin component.
		Monitor respiratory status.	Respiratory depression and constipation can be caused by the oxycodone component.
Oxycodone hydrochloride and acetaminophen (Tylox, Percocet, Endocet✱, Oxycocet✱)	1-2 tablets PO q3-4h Maximum 12 tablets	Monitor blood pressure and respiratory status. Assess for GI motility.	Respiratory depression, hypotension, and constipation can occur.
Ketorolac tromethamine [2](Toradol)	15-60 mg IM or IV q6h Maximum 120 mg 5-day administration maximum	Monitor for GI bleeding.	GI bleeding, ulceration, and perforation can occur.
		Monitor for renal effects, especially in older adults.	Decreased urine output, increased serum creatinine, hematuria, and proteinuria can occur. Ketorolac is cleared more slowly in older adults. Older persons are more sensitive to the renal effects of NSAIDs.
Ibuprofen (Motrin, Amersol✱, Novoprofen✱)	300-800 mg PO q4-6h Maximum 2400 mg daily	Monitor upper GI tolerance of medication. Give with food or milk.	Food or milk helps decrease irritation of the stomach.
		Monitor coagulation studies (PT, aPTT).	Bleeding times and other coagulation study results may be increased.
		Assess for signs of bleeding or delayed clotting.	Monitoring leads to early detection of complications.

PT, Prothrombin time; aPTT, activated partial thromboplastin time; NSAID, nonsteroidal anti-inflammatory drug; GI, gastrointestinal.

[1]**Med Error Alert!** Watch dosage; the dosage of morphine is only one-tenth that of meperidine.

[2]**Med Error Alert!** Do not confuse with Tramadol, a drug used for central analgesia.

CHART 22-6

DRUG THERAPY for
Management of Opioid Overdose

Drug	Usual Dosage	Nursing Interventions	Rationales
Naloxone hydrochloride (Narcan)	0.1-2 mg IV, SC, and IM; repeat every 2-3 min PRN on the basis of the client's response up to 10 mg	Maintain an open airway.	A patent airway maximizes respiratory effort.
		Administer oxygen as prescribed.	Oxygen helps prevent hypoxemia.
		Have suction available.	Vomiting can occur with administration of naloxone; suction prevents aspiration.
		Closely monitor vital signs and pulse oximetry readings until the client responds.	The threat of hypoxemia and respiratory depression or arrest is a concern until the naloxone becomes effective.
		Do not leave the client unattended until he or she is fully responsive.	Staying with the client promotes safety.
		Observe for significant reversal of analgesia.	With reversal of the narcotic's respiratory-depressive effects, analgesic effects will also be reversed.
		Continue to monitor the client for effects of the naloxone for at least 1 hr.	Continued monitoring leads to early detection of hypertension, hypotension, tachycardia, and dysrhythmias, which can be effects of naloxone.

SC, Subcutaneous.

in" to the pump so that the client cannot accidentally overdose. Drugs given by the PCA method include morphine, meperidine, and hydromorphone.

Epidural analgesia can be given intermittently by the anesthesia provider or by continuous drip through an epidural catheter left in place after epidural anesthesia. Drugs given by epidural catheter include the opioids fentanyl (Sublimaze), preservative-free morphine (Duramorph), and bupivacaine (Marcaine).

Take care not to overmedicate or undermedicate, especially with older clients. In assessing for overmedication, monitor vital signs, especially blood pressure and respiratory rate, and level of consciousness. Complications from the use of opioid analgesics include respiratory depression, hypotension, nausea, vomiting, and constipation. An opioid antagonist, such as naloxone (Narcan), may be needed to reverse the acute effects of opioid depression. Because of the short effect of the opioid antagonist, monitor the client's blood pressure and respirations every 15 to 30 minutes until the full effect of the opioid analgesic has passed. You may need to give more doses of the opioid antagonist during this time. (See Chart 22-6 for more information on opioid antagonists.) In addition, the client has breakthrough pain after the opioid antagonist is given, so other interventions to promote comfort are needed.

Assess for undermedication by asking the client about the effects of the drug and observing for nonverbal cues of pain or discomfort (e.g., restlessness, increased confusion, "picking" at bedcovers, and aggressive behaviors). Offer pain medication after checking for hypotension and respiratory depression.

As recovery progresses, reduce the doses and frequency of pain medications. Drugs are changed from injectable or PCA to oral as soon as the client can tolerate oral agents. Nonopioid analgesics, such as acetaminophen (Tylenol, Atasol✱), and nonsteroidal anti-inflammatory drugs (NSAIDs), such as ibuprofen (Motrin, Novo-Profen✱, Amersol✱) and ketorolac (Toradol), are used alone or with an opioid analgesic. Antianxiety drugs, such as hydroxyzine (Vistaril, Novo-Hydroxyzin✱), may be given with an opioid analgesic. This combination decreases pain-related anxiety, reduces muscle tension, and controls nausea.

Complementary and Alternative Therapies. Provide other comfort measures that may lower the amount of pain medication needed. These measures reduce anxiety and allow the client to relax and rest.

Positioning. In positioning the client, consider the position during surgery, the location of the surgical incision and drains, and problems such as arthritis and chronic lung disease. Assist the client to a position of comfort. Support the extremities with pillows. *Place no pillows under the knees, and do not raise the knee gatch, because this position could restrict circulation and increase the risk for thrombophlebitis.* Turn or help the client turn at least every 2 hours while he or she is bedridden to prevent complications caused by immobility.

On the basis of the surgeon's prescription and your assessment of the client's tolerance, encourage the client to increase activity progressively. Activity decreases stiffness, promotes lung expansion, and promotes venous blood return. When the client is first allowed out of bed, assist him or her to the side of the bed and into a chair. Teach the client to splint the surgical wound for support and comfort during the transfer.

Massage. Use gentle massage on stiff joints or a sore back to decrease discomfort. Assist the client to a side-lying position, and apply lotion with smooth, gentle strokes to increase blood flow to the area and promote relaxation. *Do not*

CHART 22-7

BEST PRACTICE for
Nonpharmacologic Interventions to Reduce Postoperative Pain and Promote Comfort

- Control or remove noxious stimuli.
- Cushion and elevate painful areas; avoid tension or pressure on those areas.
- Provide adequate rest to increase pain tolerance.
- Encourage the client's participation in diversional activities.
- Instruct the client in relaxation techniques; use audiotapes and breathing exercises.
- Provide opportunities for meditation.
- Help the client to stimulate sensory nerve endings near the painful areas to inhibit ascending pain impulses.
- Use ice to reduce and prevent swelling, as indicated.
- Find a general position of comfort for the client.
- Help the client stimulate the area contralateral (opposite) to the painful area.

massage the calves, because of the risk of loosening a clot and causing a life-threatening pulmonary embolus.

Relaxation and Diversion. Relaxation and diversion are also used to control acute episodes of pain that may occur during dressing changes and injections. Chapters 4 and 7 discuss how to instruct and guide the client through these pain control methods. Music and noise reduction have also been shown to decrease awareness of discomfort. Chart 22-7 lists other interventions that may help reduce pain and promote comfort.

Critical Thinking Challenge

The client described earlier (a 62-year-old woman who has undergone an abdominal cholecystectomy) has just arrived on the medical-surgical nursing unit. As soon as she is moved to the bed, she vomits a large amount of greenish-yellow liquid. You note that her dressing is completely soaked with serosanguineous drainage. Her vital signs are as follows: BP 102/78, P 132, R 24; pulse oximetry is 95% on room air. She is restless, diaphoretic, and has pulled on her NG tube twice. She received 2 mg of morphine IV about 45 minutes before she was discharged from the PACU.

1. What additional assessment data should you obtain?
2. Should you change her dressing? Why or why not?
3. How should you intervene for her vomiting?
4. Does this client require more frequent or less frequent monitoring than the every 2 hours specified by the facility's policy? Why or why not?

evolve For suggested answer guidelines, go to http://evolve.elsevier.com/Iggy/.

POTENTIAL FOR HYPOXEMIA

NOC **PLANNING: EXPECTED OUTCOMES.** The client is expected to attain or maintain preoperative baseline partial pressure of arterial oxygen ($Pa{O_2}$) values.

INTERVENTIONS. The key to preventing hypoxemia is to follow the interventions for the nursing diagnoses of Impaired Gas Exchange (p. 348), Ineffective Airway Clearance, and Ineffective Breathing Pattern. After surgery, monitor the client's arterial blood gas (ABG) and pulse oximetry values. A client who received conscious sedation with midazolam (Versed) or lorazepam (Ativan, Nu-Loraz✱) may be overly sedated or have pulmonary depression sufficient to need reversal with flumazenil (Romazicon) (Chart 22-8). Hypothermia after surgery causes shivering that increases oxygen demand and can induce hypoxemia. Many rewarming methods can be used, although prevention is more important. The highest incidence of hypoxemia after surgery occurs on the second postoperative day. Clients who normally have a low $Pa{O_2}$, such as those with lung disease or older adults, are at higher risk for hypoxemia.

Hypoxemia is treated with oxygen therapy. Depending on the surgeon's preference and established guidelines, oxygen therapy may continue through the second day after surgery. When hypoxemia occurs despite preventive care, interventions to manage the cause of the hypoxemia are prescribed. These may include respiratory treatments and mechanical ventilation (if needed).

Community-Based Care

Many clients are discharged after a brief hospital stay or directly from the PACU to home. Because of the shortened length of hospital stays, discharge planning, teaching, and referral begin before surgery and continue after surgery.

HOME CARE MANAGEMENT

If the client is discharged directly to home, assess information about the home environment for safety, cleanliness, and availability of caregivers. Use the database obtained on admission before surgery to determine the client's needs. For example, if the client is unable or not allowed to climb stairs and lives in a two-story house with only one bathroom, advise the client to rent a bedside commode. Collaborate with the social worker or discharge planner to identify needs related to care after surgery, including meal preparation, dressing changes, and personal hygiene. A referral to a home care nursing agency may be indicated.

The client is usually concerned about complications, pain, changes in the usual activity level, or payment of the hospital bill. The more extensive the surgical procedure is, the more fearful the client is of assuming self-care. Support the client and family members as they make discharge plans. The client with visible scars after surgery may need more emotional support from and acceptance of his or her family. He or she may be angry about the surgical outcome or about role changes. He or she may be concerned about financial matters and work. The surgical outcome may not have met the client's expectations, and further interventions may be necessary to assist in resolving his or her feelings. Ensure that referrals are made for additional counseling as indicated.

HEALTH TEACHING

The teaching plan for the client and family after surgery includes the following:

- Prevention of infection
- Care and assessment of the surgical wound
- Diet therapy
- Pain management
- Drug therapy
- Progressive increase in activity

If dressing changes are needed, instruct the client and family members on the importance of proper handwashing to prevent infection. Explain and demonstrate wound care to

CHART 22-8

DRUG THERAPY for Management of Benzodiazepine Overdose

Drug	Usual Dosage	Nursing Interventions	Rationales
Flumazenil (Romazicon)	0.2-1 mg IV at rate of 0.2 mg/min; repeat every 2-3 min PRN up to 3 mg in any 1 hr	Maintain an open airway.	A patent airway maximizes respiratory effort.
		Administer oxygen as prescribed.	Oxygen helps prevent hypoxemia.
		Have suction available.	Vomiting can occur with administration of flumazenil; suction prevents aspiration.
		Closely monitor the client's level of sedation, vital signs, and pulse oximetry readings until the client responds.	Hypoventilation may not be fully reversed with flumazenil; sedation, amnesia, and psychomotor effects of the benzodiazepines should be reversed.
		Do not leave the client unattended until fully responsive.	Seizures have occurred with reversal.
		Observe for significant reversal of sedation.	With reversal of the benzodiazepine's sedative and amnesia effect, the client will become more aware of pain/discomfort.
		Observe for up to 2 hr for re-sedation and respiratory depression.	The duration of action of the benzodiazepines is longer than that of flumazenil.

the client and family, who then perform a return demonstration. During teaching sessions, evaluate learning and promote adherence after discharge. At the same time, teach about the manifestations of complications such as wound infection. Also instruct the client and family about what to do if complications occur.

A diet high in protein, calories, and vitamin C promotes wound healing. Supplemental vitamin C, iron, and other vitamins are often prescribed after surgery to aid in wound healing and red blood cell formation. Instruct the client who needs dietary restrictions about the importance of following the prescribed diet while recovering from surgery. Encourage the older adult or debilitated client to continue using dietary supplements, if prescribed, between meals until the wound is completely healed and the energy levels are restored.

Teach the client about drugs for pain, especially about the proper dosage and frequency. Instruct the client to notify the surgeon if pain is not controlled or if the pain suddenly increases. If antibiotics or other drugs are prescribed, stress the importance of completing the entire prescription.

Surgery stresses the body, and time and rest are needed for healing. Teach the client to increase activity level slowly, rest often, and avoid straining the wound or the surrounding area. The surgeon decides when the client may climb stairs, return to work, drive, and resume other usual activities, such as sexual intercourse. The amount of weight that the client can lift safely after surgery is specifically defined by the surgeon (i.e., in pounds or kilograms). Remind clients of the weights of grocery bags, laundry baskets, children, and books.

Instruct the client in the use of proper body mechanics. A client whose work involves a moderate amount of physical labor may return to work about 6 weeks after abdominal surgery. However, he or she may be eager to return to normal activities and may not follow restrictions. Stress the importance of adherence to prevent complications or disability. *The client must receive written discharge instructions to follow at home.* A referral for a visiting nurse may be needed for follow-up.

HEALTH CARE RESOURCES

After returning home, the client may need equipment and assistance with dressing changes, activities of daily living (ADLs), and meal preparation. Referral to a home care agency is made, if needed. Home care may be paid for by third-party insurance payers, including Medicare, if the client is homebound and requires skilled care such as dressing changes or physical therapy. The home care nurse provides skilled nursing assessments, dressing supplies, education in self-care, and referrals for services as needed. Such referrals include Meals on Wheels, support groups, and homemaker services (e.g., for housekeeping and food shopping).

Critical Thinking Challenge

The 62-year-old client who had an abdominal cholecystectomy is getting ready for discharge. After her staples are removed, a 2-cm area of the incision opened and is draining small amounts of serous fluid. She is very upset about this development and is afraid to go home.

1. Is this a major complication? Why or why not?
2. How could you allay her fears?
3. What care for this wound would you recommend?

evolve For suggested answer guidelines, go to http://evolve.elsevier.com/Iggy/.

Evaluation: Outcomes

Evaluate the care of the client after surgery on the basis of the identified nursing diagnoses and collaborative problems. The expected outcomes include that the client:

- Attains and maintains adequate lung expansion and respiratory function.
- Has complete wound healing without complications.
- Has an acceptable comfort level after surgery.

Specific indicators for these outcomes are listed for each nursing diagnosis and collaborative problem under the Planning and Implementation section (see earlier).

CONCEPT MAP Postoperative Abdominal Surgery

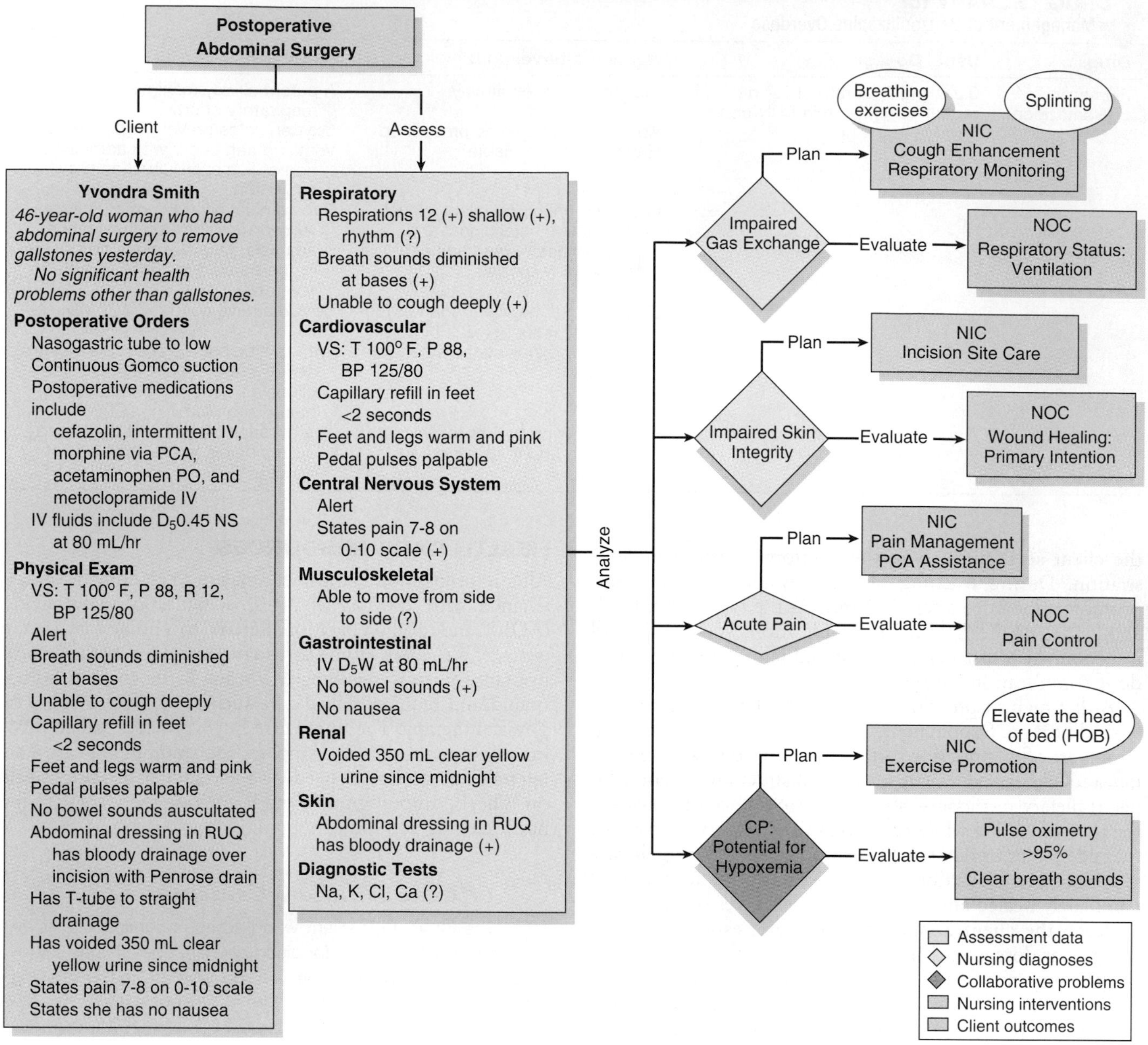

Concept Map by Elaine Bishop Kennedy, EdD, RN

GET READY for the NCLEX Examination!

KEY POINTS

Safe Effective Care Environment

- Use aseptic technique during all dressing changes.
- Use established criteria to determine when a client is ready to leave the postanesthesia care unit (PACU) for discharge to home or a medical-surgical nursing unit.
- Keep suction equipment, oxygen, and artificial breathing equipment near the client in the PACU.

Health Promotion and Maintenance

- Reinforce to the client after surgery the specific interventions to use to prevent complications (incision splinting, deep breathing exercises, range of motion exercises, as described in Chart 20-6).
- Encourage early ambulation.
- Stress the need for following the activity restrictions prescribed by the surgeon.

Psychosocial Integrity

- Explain all procedures, restrictions, drugs, and follow-up care to the client and family.

- Allow the client to verbalizes feelings about any change in physical appearance or lifestyle as a result of surgery.
- Reassure clients that taking pain medication when needed, even opioids, does not make them drug abusers.
- Remain with the client if wound dehiscence or evisceration occurs.
- Offer alternative therapies for relaxation, pain reduction, and distraction, such as massage, music therapy, and guided imagery.

Physiological Integrity

- Begin every assessment of the client after surgery by checking the airway and breathing effectiveness.
- Assess the incision site each shift (on the medical-surgical nursing unit).
- In the event of wound dehiscence or evisceration, have the client lie flat (supine); apply sterile, nonadherent dressing materials to the wound; and follow the steps outlined in Chart 22-4.
- Teach the client about any drugs to be continued after discharge from the facility setting.
- Instruct the client and family about the clinical manifestations of complications and when to seek assistance.

ADDITIONAL STUDY RESOURCES

Go to your Student CD-ROM for Review Questions for the NCLEX Examination.

evolve Go to http://evolve.elsevier.com/Iggy/ for Integrated Management of Care Questions for the NCLEX Examination.

SELECTED BIBLIOGRAPHY

Asterisk indicates a classic or definitive work on this subject.

*Acute Pain Management Guideline Panel. (1992). *Acute pain management in adults: Operative procedures.* AHCPR Publication No. 92-0022. Rockville, MD: Agency for Health Care Policy and Research, Public Health Service, U.S. Department of Health and Human Services.

Allen, G. (2002). Supplemental perioperative oxygen to reduce the incidence of surgical-wound infection. *AORN Journal, 76*(2), 330-331.

American Society of PeriAnesthesia Nurses. (2000). *Standards of perianesthesia nursing practice.* Cherry Hill, NJ: Author.

Aragon, D., Ring, C.A., & Covelli, M. (2003). The influence of diabetes mellitus on postoperative infections. *Critical Care Nursing Clinics of North America, 15*(1), 125-135.

Arnstein, P. (2002). Optimizing perioperative pain management. *AORN Journal, 76*(5), 812-817.

Bryan, S. (2002). Hemolytic transfusion reaction: Safeguards for practice. *Journal of PeriAnesthesia Nursing 17*(6), 399-402.

Bush, N., & Griffin-Sobel, J. (2003). Acute postoperative pain management and malfunctioning epidural catheter. *Oncology Nursing Forum, 30*(2), 227-228.

Candido, L. (2002). Treatment of surgical wound dehiscence. *Dermatology Nursing, 14*(3), 177-178, 181.

Collins, M., & McDonald, V. (2000). Managing postoperative pain at home. *Canadian Nurse, 96*(7), 26-29.

Dang, D., et al. (2002). Postoperative complications: Does intensive care unit staff nursing make a difference? *Heart & Lung, 31*(3), 219-228.

Dixon, L. (2002). Postoperative complications and the older adult. *Geriatric Nursing, 23*(11), 203.

Dochterman, J., & Bulechek, G. (Eds.). (2004). *Nursing interventions classification (NIC)* (4th ed.). St. Louis: Mosby.

Dunn, D. (2004). Preventing perioperative complications in an older adult. *Nursing 2004, 34*(11), 36-41.

Ebersole, P., Hess, P., & Luggen, A. (2004). Toward healthy aging: Human needs and nursing response (6th ed.). St. Louis: Mosby.

Facts and Comparisons. (2001). *Drug facts and comparisons* (55th ed.). St. Louis: Author.

Fort, C. (2002). Get pumped to prevent DVT. *Nursing2002, 32*(9), 50-52.

Golembiewski, J. (2003). Morphine and hydromorphone for postoperative analgesia: Focus on safety. *Journal of PeriAnesthesia Nursing, 18*(2), 120-122.

Golembiewski, J., & O'Brien, D. (2002). A systematic approach to the management of postoperative nausea and vomiting. *Journal of PeriAnesthesia Nursing, 17*(6), 364-376.

Griffis, C., & Gierat, S. (2003). Acute postoperative pain management and malfunctioning epidural catheter. *Oncology Nursing Forum, 30*(2), 227-228.

Hayes, J., Lehman, C., & Castonguay, P. (2002). Graduated compression stockings: Updating practice, improving compliance. *MEDSURG Nursing, 11*(4), 163-167, 191.

Hess, D. (2000). Detection and monitoring of hypoxemia and oxygen therapy. *Respiratory Care, 45*(1), 65-83.

Hrouda, B. (2000). How to remove surgical sutures and staples. *Nursing2000, 30*(2), 54-55.

Jacobs, V. (2000). Informational needs of surgical patients following discharge. *Applied Nursing Research, 13*(1), 12-18.

Kowalczyk, T. (2002). A low-tech approach to venous congestion. *RN, 65*(10), 26-30.

Letizia, M., O'Leary, J., & Vodvarka, J. (2003). Laryngeal edema: Perioperative nursing considerations. *MEDSURG Nursing, 12*(2), 111-115.

*Lusis, S.A. (1996). The challenges of nursing elderly surgical patients. *AORN Journal, 64*(6), 954-955, 957-962.

Mamaril, M. (2003). Standards of perianesthesia nursing practice: Advocating patient safety. *Journal of PeriAnesthesia Nursing, 18*(3), 168-172.

McGaffigan, P. (2002). Advancing sedation assessment to promote patient comfort. *Critical Care Nurse, 22*(1), Supplement 29-36.

Moorhead, S., Johnson, M., & Maas, M. (Eds.). (2004). *Nursing outcomes classification (NOC)* (3rd ed.). St. Louis: Mosby.

Morris, B., Morrison, R., & Yetsko, C. (2002). Venous thromboembolism: Prevention and treatment. *RN, 65*(10), 24hf3-24hf8.

Moz, T. (2004). Wound dehiscence and evisceration. *Nursing 2004, 34*(5), 88.

Pullen, R. (2003). Removing sutures and staples. *Nursing 2003, 33*(10), 18.

Shea, R., Brooks, J., Dayhoff, N., & Keck, J. (2002). Pain intensity and postoperative pulmonary complications among the elderly after abdominal surgery. *Heart & Lung, 31*(6), 440-449.

Sherwood, G., et al. (2003). Changing acute pain management outcomes in surgical patients. *AORN Journal, 77*(2), 374-393.

Squires, A. (2003). Documenting surgical incision site care. *Nursing2003,* 33(1), 74.

Tappen, R., Muzic, J., & Kennedy, P. (2001). Preoperative assessment and discharge planning for older adults undergoing ambulatory surgery. *AORN Journal, 73*(2), 464-474.

Tittle, M., McMillan, S., & Hagan, S. (2003). Validating the Brief Pain Inventory for use with surgical patients with cancer. *Oncology Nursing Forum, 30*(2), 325-330.

Walton, J. (2001). Helping high-risk surgical patients beat the odds. *Nursing2001, 31*(3), 54-59.

Wilson, M. (2000). Giving postanesthesia care in the critical care unit. *Dimensions of Critical Care Nursing, 21*(2), 38-43.

Wood, B. (2002). Caring for a limited-English proficient patient. *AORN Journal, 75*(2), 305-308.

UNIT **SIX**

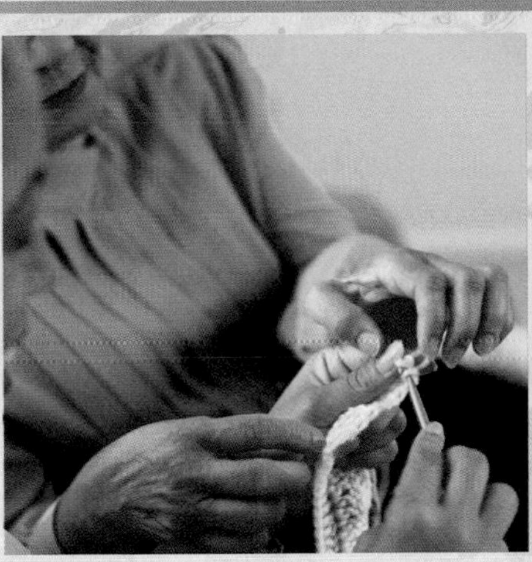

PROBLEMS of PROTECTION

Management of Clients with Problems of the Immune Response

CHAPTER

23 Concepts of Inflammation and the Immune Response

M. LINDA WORKMAN

LEARNING OUTCOMES

After studying this chapter, you should be able to:

1. Describe the concept of self-tolerance.
2. Explain the differences between inflammation and infection.
3. Compare and contrast the cells, purposes, and features of inflammation and immunity.
4. Describe the basis for the five cardinal manifestations of inflammation.
5. Interpret a white blood cell count with differential to indicate no immune problems, an acute bacterial infection, a chronic bacterial infection, or an allergic reaction.
6. Explain how complement activation and fixation assists in protection from infection.
7. Compare the cells, function, and protective actions of antibody-mediated immunity and cell-mediated immunity.
8. Compare the different types of antibody-mediated immunity for their protection effectiveness and duration of immunity.
9. Describe how the immune system responds to the presence of transplanted tissues or organs.
10. Explain the actions and short- and long-term side effects of immunosuppressive drugs.

Go to your Student CD-ROM for Review Questions for the NCLEX Examination keyed to these Learning Outcomes.

Injury and infectious diseases are common. Most people, however, are healthy more often than they are ill. Inflammation and immunity are the two major defenses that protect a person against diseases and other problems when the body is invaded by organisms. These same defenses also help the body recover after injury or tissue damage. Thus inflammation and immunity are critical to maintaining health and preventing disease. When these defenses are working well, the person is **immunocompetent.**

Immune function is reduced by many diseases, injuries, and medical therapies. Reduction of immune function may be temporary or permanent, but always endangers the client's health.

OVERVIEW

Immunity is composed of many cell functions that protect people against the effects of injury or microscopic invasion. People interact with many other living organisms in the environment. The size of these organisms varies from large (other humans and animals) to microscopic (bacteria, viruses, molds, spores, pollens, protozoa, and cells from other people or animals). As long as organisms do not enter the body's internal environment, they pose no threat to health. The body has some defenses to prevent organisms from gaining access to the internal environment. These defenses are not perfect, and invasion of the body's internal environment by organisms occurs often. Invasion occurs much more often than does an actual disease or illness because of proper immune functioning.

Purpose of Inflammation and Immunity

The purpose of inflammation and immunity is to neutralize, eliminate, or destroy organisms that invade the internal environment. To accomplish this purpose without harming the body, immune system cells use defensive actions only against non-self proteins and cells. Immune system cells can distinguish between the body's own healthy self cells and other, non-self proteins and cells.

Self versus Non-Self

Non-self proteins and cells include infected body cells, cancer cells, and all invading cells and organisms. This ability to recognize self versus non-self, which is necessary to prevent healthy body cells from being destroyed along with the invaders, is called **self-tolerance.** The immune system cells are the only body cells capable of determining self from non-self. Self-tolerance is possible because of the different kinds of proteins present on cell membranes.

All organisms are made up of cells. Each cell is surrounded by a plasma membrane (Figure 23-1). Many different proteins protrude through the cell's membrane. For example, in liver cells, many different proteins are present on the cell membrane surface. The amino acid sequence of each protein type differs from that of all other protein types. Some of these proteins are found on the liver cells of all animals (including humans) that have livers, because these protein types are specific to the liver and serve as a marker for liver tissues. Other protein types are found only on the liver cells of humans, because these protein types are specific markers for humans. Still other protein types are found only on the liver cells of humans with a specific blood type. In addition, each person's liver cells have surface protein types that are specific to that person. These proteins are unique to the person and would be identical only to the proteins of an identical twin. These unique proteins, found on the surface of all body cells of that individual, serve as a "universal product code" or a "cellular fingerprint" for that person. The proteins that make up the universal product code for one person are recognized as "foreign," or non-self, by the immune system of another person. Because the cell-surface proteins are non-self to another person's immune system, they are **antigens,** proteins capable of stimulating an immune response.

Human leukocyte antigens (HLAs) make up this unique universal product code for each person. "Leukocyte antigen" is not a correct term, because these antigens are also present on the surfaces of nearly all body cells, not just on leukocytes. HLAs are a normal part of the person and act as antigens only if they enter another person's body. These antigens specify the **tissue type** of a person. Other names for these personal cellular fingerprints are *human transplantation antigens, human histocompatibility antigens, major histocompatibility antigens,* and *class I antigens.*

Humans have about 40 major HLAs that are determined by a set of genes called the major histocompatibility complex (MHC). The exact number of *minor* HLAs that any person has is not known. The specific antigens that any person has (of a large number of possible antigens) are genetically determined by which MHC genes were inherited from his or her parents.

This universal product code (HLA) is key for recognition and self-tolerance. The immune system cells constantly come into contact with other body cells and with any invader that happens to enter the body. At each encounter, the immune system cells compare the surface protein universal product codes (HLAs) to determine whether or not the encountered cell belongs in the body (Figure 23-2). If the encountered cell's universal product code (HLA) perfectly matches the HLA of the immune system cell, the encountered cell is "self" and is not attacked by the immune system cell. If the encountered cell's universal product code (HLA) does not perfectly match the HLA of the immune system cell, the encountered cell is non-self, or foreign. The immune system cell takes action to neutralize, destroy, or eliminate the foreign invader.

Immune function changes during a person's life, according to nutritional status, environmental conditions, drugs, the presence of disease, and age. Immune function is most efficient when people are in their 20s and 30s and slowly declines with increasing age. Older adults have decreased immune function, increasing their risk for many health problems (Chart 23-1).

Organization of the Immune System

The immune system is not confined to any one organ or area of the body. Most immune system cells come from the bone marrow. Some of these cells mature in the bone mar-

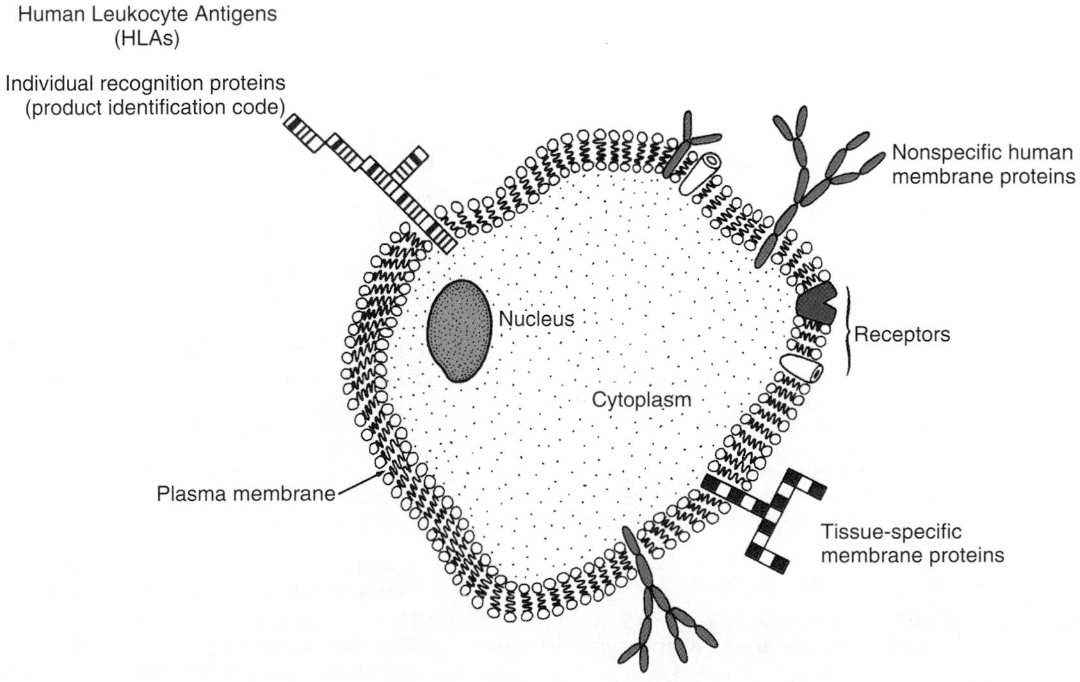

Figure 23-1 ■ Properties of human cell membranes.

row; others leave the bone marrow and mature in different body sites. When mature, most immune system cells are released into the blood, where they circulate to most body areas and have specific effects.

The bone marrow is the source of all blood cells, including immune system cells. The bone marrow produces an immature, undifferentiated cell called a **stem cell** (Abbas & Lichtman, 2003). This immature stem cell is also described as *pluripotent, multipotent,* and *totipotent.* These terms describe the potential future of the stem cell. When the stem cell is first created in the bone marrow, it is undifferentiated. The cell is not yet committed to maturing into a specific blood cell type. At this stage, the stem cell is flexible and could become any one of many mature blood cells. Figure 23-3 shows the possible outcomes for maturation of the pluripotent stem cell. The type of mature cell that the stem cell becomes depends on which pathway it follows.

The maturational pathway of any stem cell depends on body needs at the time, as well as on the presence of specific hormones (cytokines, factors) that direct maturation. For example, **erythropoietin** is made in the kidney. When immature stem cells are exposed to erythropoietin, they commit to the erythrocyte pathway and become mature red blood cells.

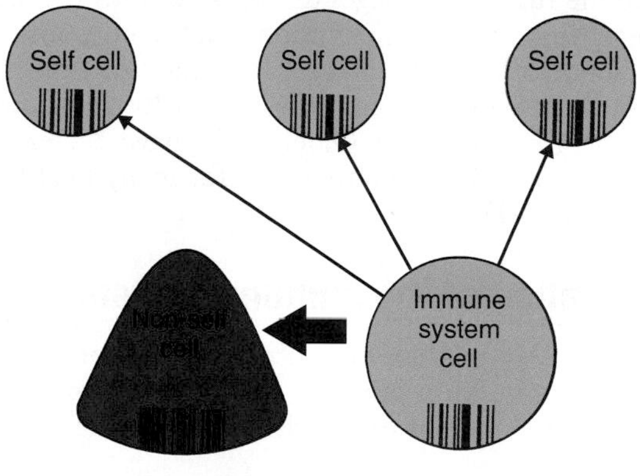

Figure 23-2 ■ Determination of self versus non-self cells.

White blood cells **(leukocytes)** protect the body from the effects of invasion by organisms. These cells are the immune system cells. Table 23-1 lists the functions of different immune system cells. The leukocytes provide protection through many defensive actions (Abbas & Lichtman, 2003). These actions include the following:

- Recognition of self versus non-self
- Phagocytic destruction of foreign invaders, cellular debris, and unhealthy or abnormal self cells
- Lytic destruction of foreign invaders and unhealthy self cells
- Production of antibodies directed against invaders
- Complement activation
- Production of cytokines that stimulate increased formation of leukocytes in bone marrow
- Production of cytokines that increase specific leukocyte growth and activity

The three processes needed for immunity are (1) inflammation, (2) antibody-mediated immunity (AMI), also known as humoral immunity, and (3) cell-mediated immunity (CMI). These processes use different defensive actions, and each process influences or requires assistance from the other two processes (Figure 23-4). *Therefore full immunity **(immunocompetence)** requires the function and interaction of all three processes.*

INFLAMMATION

Inflammation, sometimes called "natural" immunity, provides immediate protection against the effects of tissue injury and invading foreign proteins. The ability to produce an inflammatory response is critical to health and well-being. Inflammation differs from AMI and CMI in two important ways:

1. Inflammatory protection is immediate but short term against the effects of injury or invading organisms. It

CHART 23-1

NURSING FOCUS on the OLDER ADULT
Changes in Immune Function Related to Aging

Immune Component	Functional Change	Nursing Implications
Inflammation	There is a probable defect in neutrophil function.	Neutrophil counts may be normal, but activity is reduced or impaired.
	Leukocytosis does not occur during episodes of acute infection.	Clients may have an infection but not show expected changes in white blood cell counts.
	Older persons may not have a fever during inflammatory or infectious episodes.	Not only is there potential loss of protection through inflammation, but minor infections may be overlooked until the client becomes severely infected or septic.
Antibody-mediated immunity	The total number of colony-forming B-lymphocytes and the ability of these cells to mature into antibody-secreting cells are diminished.	Older adults are less able to make new antibodies in response to the presence of new antigens. Thus they should receive immunizations, such as "flu shots" and the pneumococcal vaccination.
	There is a decline in natural antibodies, decreased response to antigens, and reduction in the amount of time the antibody response is maintained.	Older adults may not have sufficient antibodies present to provide protection when they are re-exposed to microorganisms against which they have already generated antibodies. Thus older clients need to avoid people with viral infections and to receive "booster" shots for old vaccinations and immunizations.
Cell-mediated immunity	Thymic activity decreases with aging, and the number of circulating T-lymphocytes decreases.	Skin tests for tuberculosis may be falsely negative. Older clients are more at risk for bacterial and fungal infections, especially on the skin and mucous membranes, in the respiratory tract, and in the genitourinary tract.

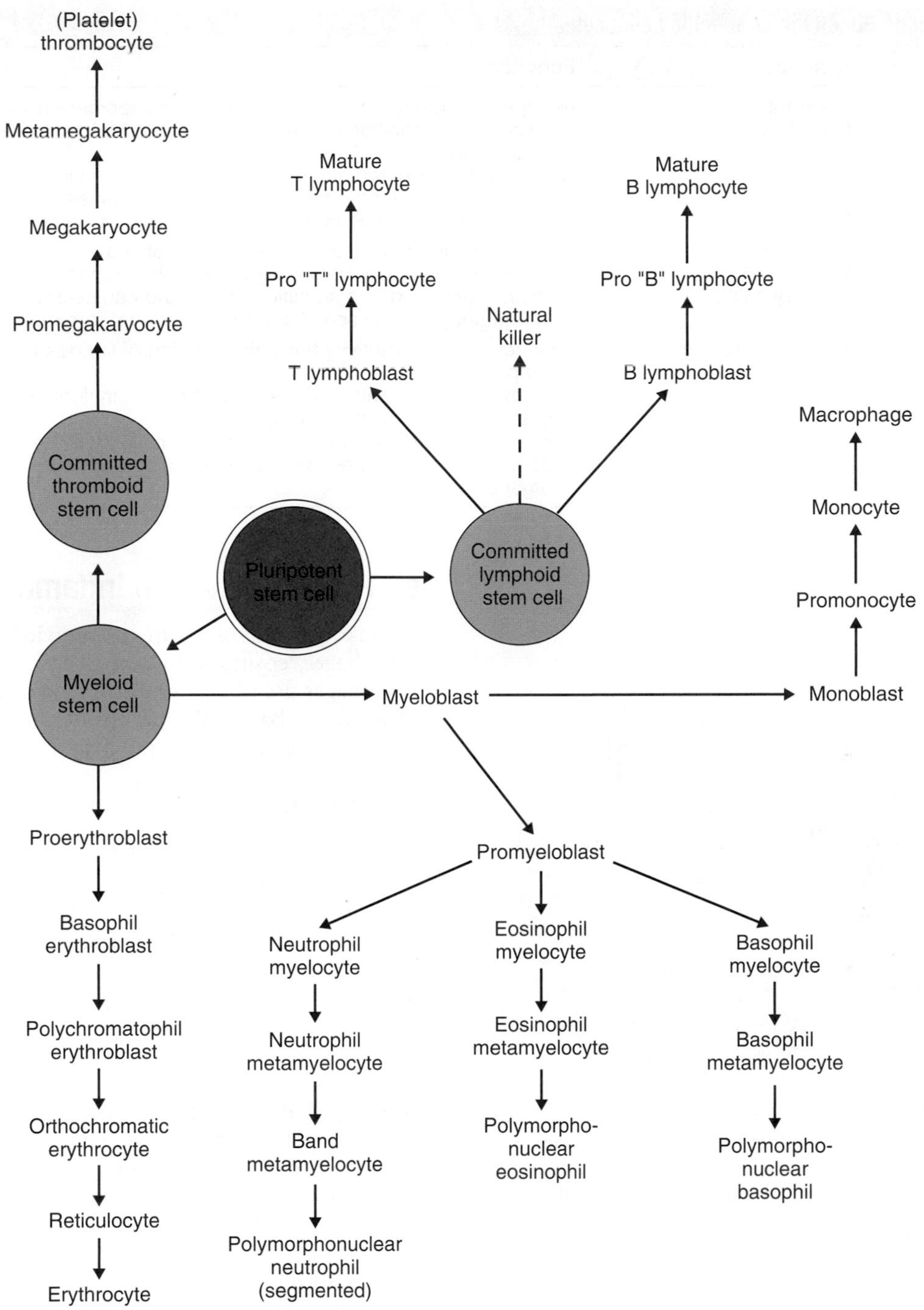

Figure 23-3 ■ Stem cell differentiation and maturation.

does not provide sustained, long-term immunity on repeated exposure to the same organisms.

2. Inflammation is a nonspecific body defense to invasion or injury and can be started quickly by almost any event.

Inflammation is nonspecific; the same tissue responses occur with any type of injury or invasion, regardless of the location on the body or the specific initiating agent. Thus inflammation triggered by a scald burn to the hand is the same as inflammation triggered by excess stomach acid or bacteria in the middle ear. How widespread the symptoms of inflammation are in the body depends on the intensity, severity, duration, and extent of exposure to the initiating injury or invasion. For example, a splinter in the finger triggers inflammation only at the splinter site, whereas a burn injuring 60% of the skin surface results in an inflammatory response involving the entire body.

Purpose

Inflammatory responses start tissue actions that cause visible and uncomfortable symptoms. Despite the discomfort, these actions are important in ridding the body of harmful organisms. However, if the inflammatory response is excessive, tissue damage may result. Inflammatory responses also help start both antibody-mediated and cell-mediated actions to activate a full immune response.

TABLE 23-1 Immune Functions of Specific Leukocytes

Variable	Leukocyte	Function
Inflammation	Neutrophil	Nonspecific ingestion and phagocytosis of microorganisms and foreign protein
	Macrophage	Nonspecific recognition of foreign proteins and microorganisms; ingestion and phagocytosis
	Monocyte	Destruction of bacteria and cellular debris; matures into macrophage
	Eosinophil	Weak phagocytic action; releases vasoactive amines during allergic reactions
	Basophil	Releases histamine and heparin in areas of tissue damage
Antibody-mediated immunity	B-lymphocyte	Becomes sensitized to foreign cells and proteins
	Plasma cell	Secretes immunoglobulins in response to the presence of a specific antigen
	Memory cell	Remains sensitized to a specific antigen and can secrete increased amounts of immunoglobulins specific to the antigen on re-exposure
Cell-mediated immunity	T-lymphocyte helper/ inducer T-cell	Enhances immune activity through secretion of various factors, cytokines, and lymphokines
	Cytotoxic/cytolytic T-cell	Selectively attacks and destroys non-self cells, including virally infected cells, grafts, and transplanted organs
	Natural killer cell	Nonselectively attacks non-self cells, especially body cells that have undergone mutation and become malignant; also attacks grafts and transplanted organs

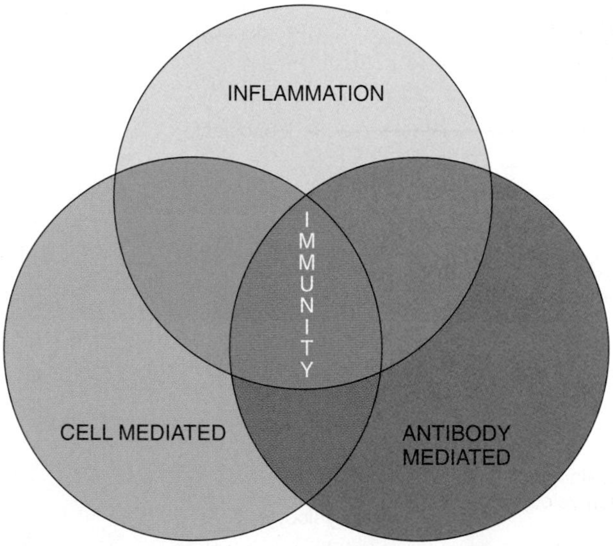

Figure 23-4 ■ The three divisions of immunity. Each division (inflammation, antibody-mediated immunity, and cell-mediated immunity) has an important independent function. In addition, the function of each division of immunity is profoundly influenced by the other two divisions. Most important, optimal function of all three divisions is necessary for complete immunity.

Infection

A confusing issue about inflammation is that this process occurs in response to tissue injury, as well as to invasion by organisms. *Infection is usually accompanied by inflammation; however, inflammation can occur without invasion by organisms.* Examples of inflammation without infection include sprain injuries to joints, myocardial infarction, sterile surgical incisions, thrombophlebitis, and blister formation. Examples of inflammation caused by noninfectious invasion by foreign proteins include allergic rhinitis, contact dermatitis, and other allergic reactions. Inflammations caused by infection include otitis media, appendicitis, bacterial peritonitis, viral hepatitis, and bacterial myocarditis, among many others. *Thus inflammation does not always mean that an infection is present.*

Cell Types Involved in Inflammation

The leukocytes involved in inflammation are neutrophils, macrophages, eosinophils, and basophils. Neutrophils and macrophages use phagocytosis to destroy and eliminate foreign invaders. Basophils and eosinophils act on blood vessels to cause tissue-level responses.

NEUTROPHILS

Description and Origin

Mature neutrophils make up between 55% and 70% of the normal total white blood cell (WBC) count. **Neutrophils** come from the stem cells and complete the maturation process in the bone marrow (Figure 23-5). They are called **granulocytes** because of the large number of granules present inside each cell. Other names for neutrophils are based on their appearance and maturity. Mature neutrophils are also called *segmented neutrophils* ("segs") or *polymorphonuclear cells* ("polys," PMNs,) because of their segmented nucleus. Less mature neutrophils are called *band neutrophils* ("bands" or "stabs") because of their nuclear shape.

Usually, maturation of a stem cell to a functional segmented neutrophil requires 12 to 14 days. This time is shortened by conditions that trigger the body to produce specific cytokines, such as granulocyte-macrophage colony-stimulating factor (GM-CSF) and granulocyte colony-stimulating factor (G-CSF). The purpose and action of cytokines are described later in this chapter under Cytokines, p. 374.

In the immunocompetent healthy person, more than 100 billion fresh, mature neutrophils are released from the bone marrow into the circulation daily (Abbas & Lichtman, 2003). This huge production is needed because the life span of a circulating neutrophil is short, about 12 to 18 hours.

Function

Although the neutrophils are the largest group of circulating leukocytes, each cell is small. This powerful army of small cells is the first internal line of defense against invaders (especially bacteria) in blood and extracellular fluid. It is the granules inside the neutrophils that destroy invaders by phagocytosis.

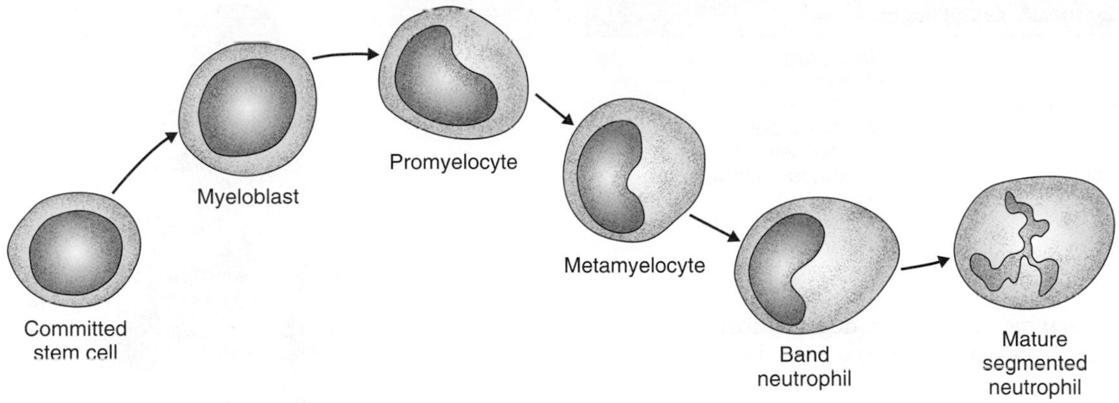

Figure 23-5 ■ Neutrophil maturation.

The mature neutrophil has many granules containing different enzymes that can degrade invaders.

Neutrophils have a small energy supply and no way of replenishing it; neither do they have a way of replenishing the enzymes used in phagocytosis. As a result, each neutrophil can take part in only one episode of phagocytosis before supplies are exhausted.

Mature neutrophils are the only neutrophil stage capable of phagocytosis. Because this cell type is responsible for continuous, instant, nonspecific protection against organisms, the percentage and actual number of mature circulating neutrophils is used to measure a client's risk for infection: the higher the numbers, the greater the resistance to infection. This measurement is the **absolute neutrophil count** (also called the absolute granulocyte count or total granulocyte count).

The differential of a normal white blood cell count shows the number and percent of all the different types of circulating leukocytes (Figure 23-6). This test indicates that most of the neutrophils released into the blood from the bone marrow are segmented neutrophils; only a small percentage are band neutrophils. The less mature neutrophil forms should not be in the blood. Some problems cause the neutrophils in the blood to change from being mostly segmented neutrophils to being less mature forms. This situation is termed a **left shift** or "bandemia" because the segmented neutrophil, which is seen at the far right of the neutrophil pathway (see Figure 23-5), is no longer the greatest number of circulating neutrophils. Instead, more of the circulating cells are "bands," the less mature cell type found farther left on the neutrophil pathway.

A left shift indicates that the client's bone marrow cannot produce enough mature neutrophils to keep pace with the continuing infection and is releasing immature neutrophils into the blood. Unfortunately, most of these immature cells are of no benefit, because they are not capable of phagocytosis.

Differential	%	/mm^3
Total WBC	100	10,000
segs	62	6200
bands	5	500
monos	3	300
lymphs	28	2800
eosin	1.5	150
baso	0.5	50

Figure 23-6 ■ Example of a laboratory slip showing the differential of a normal white blood cell (WBC) count.

MACROPHAGES

Description and Origin

Macrophages come from the committed myeloid stem cells in the bone marrow and form the mononuclear-phagocyte system. The stem cells first form monocytes and are released into the blood at this stage. Until they mature, monocytes have limited activity. Most monocytes move from the blood into body tissues, where they mature into macrophages. Some macrophages become "fixed" in position within the tissues, whereas others can move within and between tissues. Macrophages in various tissues have slightly different appearances and different names. Table 23-2 lists the tissue macrophages. Figure 23-7 shows the distribution of tissue macrophages throughout the body. The liver and spleen contain the greatest numbers of these cells.

Macrophages have long life spans, lasting from months to years. They are large and contain many lytic enzymes.

Function

Macrophages play more than one role in protecting against invasion and tissue injury. These cells are important in immediate inflammatory responses and also stimulate the longer-lasting immune responses of antibody-mediated immunity (AMI) and cell-mediated immunity (CMI). Specific macrophage functions include phagocytosis, repair of injured tissues, antigen presenting/processing, and secretion of cytokines that help control the immune system.

The inflammatory function of macrophages is phagocytosis. Macrophages can easily distinguish between self and non-self and are very effective at trapping invading cells. Unlike neutrophils, macrophages are able to renew their energy

TABLE 23-2 Tissue Macrophages

Tissue	Macrophage
Lung	Alveolar macrophage
Connective tissue	Histiocyte
Brain	Microglial cell
Liver	Kupffer cell
Peritoneum	Peritoneal macrophage
Bone	Osteoclast
Joints	Synovial type A cell
Kidney	Mesangial cell

supplies and enzymes needed to degrade foreign protein. Therefore each macrophage can take part in many phagocytic events.

BASOPHILS

Description and Origin

Basophils come from myeloid stem cells and make up only about 1% of the total circulating WBC count. They are released from the marrow after a short maturation period. These cells cause the manifestations of inflammation.

Function

Basophils have granules containing many chemicals (vasoactive amines) that act on blood vessels. These chemicals include heparin, histamine, serotonin, kinins, and leukotrienes. When released into the blood, most of these chemicals act on smooth muscle and blood vessel walls. Heparin inhibits blood and protein clotting. Histamine constricts small veins and respiratory smooth muscles. Constriction of respiratory smooth muscle narrows airways and restricts breathing. Constriction of veins inhibits blood flow and decreases venous return. This effect causes blood to collect in capillaries and small arterioles. Kinins dilate arterioles and increase capillary permeability. These actions cause blood plasma to leak into the interstitial space **(vascular leak syndrome).**

EOSINOPHILS

Description and Origin

Eosinophils come from the myeloid line and contain many vasoactive chemicals. Usually, only 1% to 2% of the total white blood cell (WBC) count is composed of eosinophils.

Function

Eosinophils act against infestations of parasitic larvae. Eosinophil granules contain many different substances. Some substances induce inflammation when released. In addition, enzymes from eosinophils degrade the vasoactive chemicals released by other leukocytes and can limit inflammatory reactions. This is why the number of circulating eosinophils increases during an allergic response.

Phagocytosis

A key process of inflammation is phagocytosis. **Phagocytosis** is the engulfing and destruction of invaders. This action also rids the body of debris after tissue injury. Neutrophils and macrophages are most efficient at phagocytosis. Phagocytosis involves the seven steps shown in Figure 23-8.

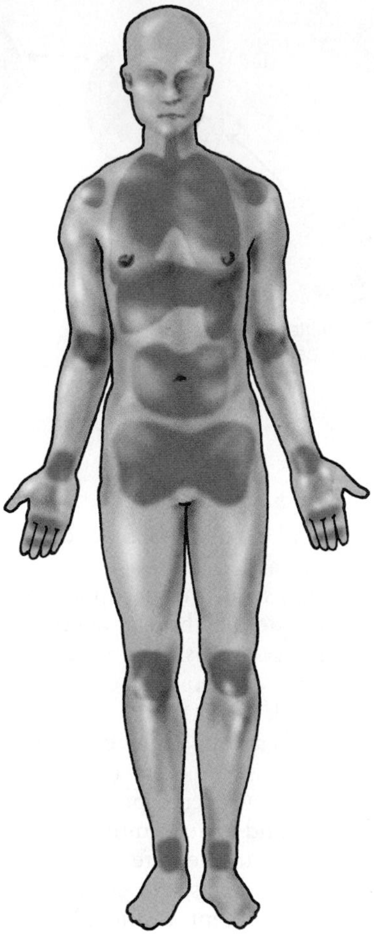

Figure 23-7 ■ Areas of highest concentration of tissue macrophages.

EXPOSURE AND INVASION

Leukocytes that engage in phagocytosis and stimulate inflammation are present in the blood and other extracellular fluids. For phagocytosis to start, leukocytes must first be exposed to organisms, foreign proteins, or debris from damaged tissues. Phagocytosis is triggered by injury or invasion.

ATTRACTION

Phagocytosis can only occur when the WBC comes into direct contact with the target (antigen, invader, or foreign protein). Some substances act as chemical magnets that attract neutrophils and macrophages. These substances are called **chemotaxins** or **leukotaxins.** Damaged tissues and blood vessels secrete chemotaxins. In addition, substances that combine with the surface of invading foreign proteins serve as chemotaxins. This combining (and attracting) mechanism is described next.

ADHERENCE

Because phagocytosis requires direct contact of the leukocyte with its intended target, the phagocytic cell must first bind to the surface of the target. A process called opsonization increases contact of the cell with its target.

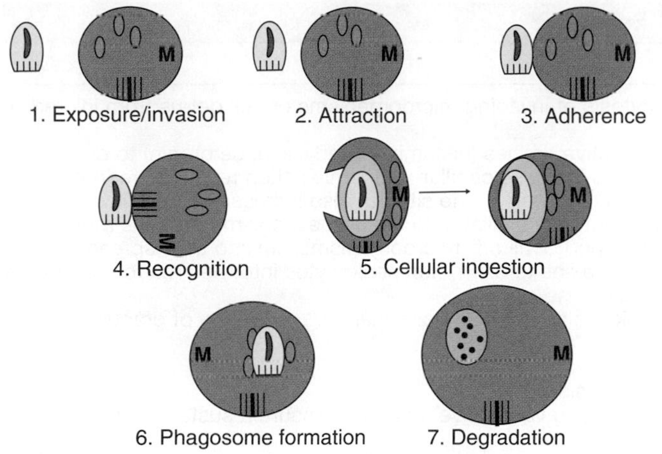

Figure 23-8 ■ Steps of phagocytosis.

Opsonization

The word *opsonin* means "to cover food with a sauce before eating." In inflammation, opsonins coat a target cell (antigen or organism). Coating the target makes it easier for phagocytic cells to stick to it. Many substances can act as opsonins. Some are particles from dead neutrophils, antibodies, and activated (fixated) complement components.

Complement Activation and Fixation

One type of opsonization is complement activation and fixation. Twenty different types of inactive complement proteins are present in the blood. These proteins are made by the liver. With proper stimulation, each complement protein is activated, joins other activated complement proteins, surrounds an antigen, and "fixes" or sticks to the antigen. Complement fixation occurs quickly as a cascade or chain reaction.

RECOGNITION

When the phagocytic cell sticks to the surface of the target cell, it "recognizes" the non-self. The phagocytic cells examine the universal product codes (human leukocyte antigens [HLAs]) of whatever they encounter. Recognition of non-self is made easier by opsonins on the target cell surface. Phagocytic cells start phagocytosis only if the target cell is recognized either as non-self or as debris from damaged self cells.

CELLULAR INGESTION

Because phagocytic destruction occurs inside the cell, the target cell is brought inside the phagocytic cell. The phagocytic cell bends its membrane around to enclose (engulf) the target cell. Once the target is enclosed in the phagocytic cells, a vacuole is formed.

PHAGOSOME FORMATION

When the phagocyte's granules are inside the vacuole, the structure is called a **phagosome (phagolysosome).** These granules break and release enzymes to destroy the ingested target.

DEGRADATION

The enzymes in the phagosome digest the engulfed target. The target is broken into smaller pieces until only small particles of debris remain.

Sequence of Inflammatory Responses

Inflammatory responses occur in a predictable sequence. The sequence is the same regardless of the triggering event. Responses at the tissue level cause the **five cardinal manifestations of inflammation:** warmth, redness, swelling, pain, and decreased function. Inflammatory responses occur in three stages and the timing of the stages may overlap (Table 23-3).

STAGE I (VASCULAR)

In stage I of the inflammatory response, the early effects involve changes in blood vessels. When inflammation results from tissue injury, this stage has two phases.

Phase I

The first phase is rapid but short-term blood vessel constriction caused by trauma to blood vessel smooth muscle. This phase lasts only seconds and may be so short that the person is unaware of it.

Phase II

In the second phase, blood flow to the area increases **(hyperemia)** and swelling **(edema)** forms at the site of injury or invasion. Injured tissues and the leukocytes in this area secrete histamine, serotonin, and kinins that constrict the small veins and dilate the arterioles in the area of injury. These blood vessel changes cause redness and warmth of the tissues. This increased blood flow increases delivery of nutrients to injured tissues.

Capillary leak also occurs, allowing blood plasma to leak into the tissues. This response causes swelling and pain. Edema at the site of injury or invasion protects the area from further injury by creating a cushion of fluid. The extra fluid also can dilute any toxins or organisms that have entered the area. The duration of these responses depends on the severity of the initiating event.

The macrophage is the major cell involved in stage I of inflammation. The action is rapid because macrophages are already in place at the site of injury or invasion. This action is limited because the number of macrophages is so small. To enhance the inflammatory response, the tissue macrophages secrete several cytokines. One cytokine is colony-stimulating factor (CSF), which triggers the bone marrow to increase the rate of white blood cell (WBC) production from 14 days to a matter of hours. Some of the cytokines also increase the release of neutrophils from the bone marrow and attract them to the site of injury or invasion, which leads to the next stage of inflammation.

STAGE II (CELLULAR EXUDATE)

In stage II, **neutrophilia** (increased number of circulating neutrophils) occurs, along with the formation of exudate, commonly called **pus.**

The most active cell in this stage is the neutrophil. Under the influence of cytokines, the neutrophil count can increase up to five times within 12 hours after the onset of inflammation. At the site of inflammation, neutrophils attack and destroy organisms and remove dead tissue through phagocytosis.

In acute inflammation, the healthy person produces enough mature neutrophils to keep pace with invasion and

TABLE 23-3 Stages of Inflammation

Onset	Cells Involved	Actions
Stage I: Vascular		
Minutes after injury or invasion	Tissue macrophages	Limited phagocytosis of invading microorganisms or cell debris from injured tissues Secretion of vasoactive amines (histamine, bradykinin, serotonin) to dilate blood vessels and increase capillary leak; this action results in redness, warmth, swelling, and pain at the site but also increases blood flow to the area; more nutrients are available to the tissues; plasma proteins move into the tissues, clot, and "wall off" microorganisms, limiting their spread Secretion of chemotaxins to draw more leukocytes into the area to sustain the inflammatory response Secretion of cytokines to increase bone marrow production of granulocytes
Stage II: Cellular Exudate		
Hours after injury or invasion	Granular myeloid cells ▪ Neutrophils ▪ Basophils ▪ Eosinophils	Increased phagocytosis Secretion of slow-acting vasoactive amines to ensure a sustained inflammatory response Secretion of substances to increase the rate of neutrophil maturation and macrophage maturation
Stage III: Tissue Repair and Replacement		
Begins at initial injury and continues until new tissues are formed and mature or are functional	Neutrophils Macrophages	Stimulation of mitotically active cells to divide; stimulation of fibroblasts in blood vessels to grow and release collagen to form scaffold on which to build scar tissue

prevent the organisms from growing. At the same time, the WBCs and inflamed tissues secrete cytokines, which allow tissue macrophages to increase and trigger bone marrow production of monocytes. This reaction begins slowly but its effects are long lasting.

During this phase, the arachidonic acid cascade starts to increase the inflammatory response. This action begins by the conversion of fatty acids in plasma membranes into arachidonic acid (AA). Then, enzymes (including cyclooxygenase) convert AA into many chemicals that are further processed into the substances that continue the inflammatory response in the tissues. These substances include histamine, leukotrienes, prostaglandins, serotonin, and kinins. Many anti-inflammatory drugs stop this cascade by preventing cyclooxygenase from converting AA into inflammatory substances.

When an infection stimulating inflammation lasts longer than just a few days, the bone marrow cannot produce and release enough mature neutrophils into the blood to keep pace with the growth of organisms. In this situation, the bone marrow begins to release immature neutrophils, reducing the number of circulating mature neutrophils. This reduction of functional neutrophils limits the helpful effects of inflammation and increases the risk for sepsis.

STAGE III (TISSUE REPAIR AND REPLACEMENT)

Although stage III is completed last, it begins at the time of injury and is critical to the final function of the inflamed area.

Some of the WBCs involved in inflammation start the replacement of lost tissues or repair of damaged tissues by inducing the remaining healthy cells to divide. In tissues that are unable to divide, WBCs trigger new blood vessel growth and scar tissue formation. Because scar tissue does not behave like normal tissue, loss of function occurs wherever damaged tissues are replaced with scar tissue. The degree of function lost is determined by how much tissue is replaced by scar tissue.

Inflammation alone cannot provide immunity. Inflammatory cells must interact with lymphocytes to provide long-lasting immunity. Long-lasting immune actions develop through antibody-mediated immunity (AMI) and cell-mediated immunity (CMI).

ANTIBODY-MEDIATED IMMUNITY

Antibody-mediated immunity (AMI), also known as humoral immunity, involves antigen-antibody interactions to neutralize, eliminate, or destroy foreign proteins. Antibodies are produced by B-lymphocytes (also known as B-cells).

Purpose

The main functions of B-cells are to become sensitized to a specific foreign protein **(antigen)** and to produce antibodies directed specifically against that protein. The antibody (rather than the actual B-cell) causes one of several actions to neutralize, eliminate, or destroy that antigen.

Cell Types Involved in Antibody-Mediated Immunity

The cells with the most direct role in AMI are the B-cells. Macrophages and T-lymphocytes (discussed later under Cell-Mediated Immunity, p. 373) work with B-cells to start and complete antigen-antibody interactions. Therefore, for optimal AMI, the entire immune system must function adequately.

B-cells start as stem cells in the bone marrow, the primary lymphoid tissue. Those stem cells destined to become B-cells commit early to the lymphocyte pathway (see Figure 23-3). At the point of commitment, these stem cells are restricted to lymphocyte development. The lymphocyte stem cells are

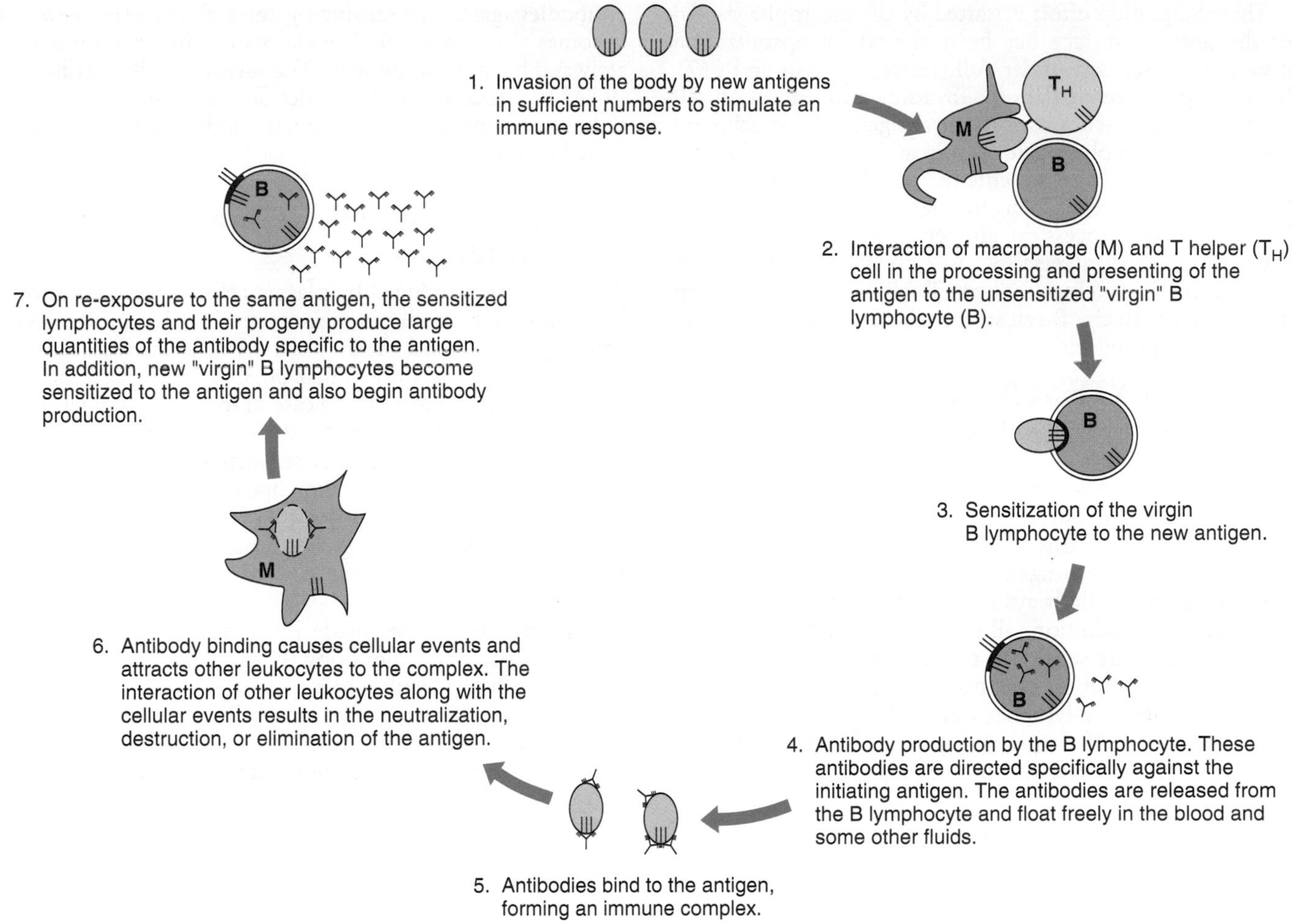

Figure 23-9 ■ Sequence of events stimulating antibody-mediated immunity.

released from the bone marrow into the blood. They then migrate into many secondary lymphoid tissues, where maturation is completed.

The secondary lymphoid tissues for B-cell maturation are the spleen, parts of lymph nodes, tonsils, and Peyer's patches of the intestinal tract.

Antigen-Antibody Interactions

The body learns to make enough of any specific antibody to provide long-lasting immunity against specific organisms or toxins. Seven steps are needed to produce a specific antibody directed against a specific antigen whenever the person is exposed to that antigen. These steps are exposure (invasion), antigen recognition, lymphocyte sensitization, antibody production and release, antigen-antibody binding, antibody-binding reactions, and sustained immunity, or memory (Figure 23-9).

EXPOSURE (INVASION)

Antibody actions occur inside the body or on a few body surfaces. For a person to make an antibody that can exert its effects on a specific antigen, the antigen must first enter the person. Not all exposures or invasions result in antibody production. Invasion by the antigen must occur in such large numbers that some of the antigen evades detection by the body's natural nonspecific defenses or overwhelms the ability of the inflammatory response to get rid of the invader.

Take, for example, a person who has never been exposed to the childhood viral disease chickenpox. This person baby-sits for three children who develop chickenpox lesions within the next 10 hours. These children, in the pre-eruption stage, shed many millions of live chickenpox virus particles via droplets from the upper respiratory tract. Because small children are often unconcerned about the finer points of infection control, they drink out of the baby-sitter's cup, kiss the baby-sitter directly (and wetly) on the lips, and sneeze and cough directly into the baby-sitter's face. During the 5 hours spent with the children at close range, the baby-sitter is heavily invaded by the chickenpox virus (varicella-zoster) and will become sick with this disease within 14 to 21 days. While the virus is growing and the disease is developing, the baby-sitter's white blood cells are taking part in antibody-antigen actions to prevent the baby-sitter from having chickenpox more than once.

ANTIGEN RECOGNITION

To begin making antibodies against an antigen, the "naive," or "virgin," unsensitized B-cell must first recognize the antigen as non-self. B-cells need the help of macrophages and helper/inducer T-cells to recognize an antigen.

This recognition effort is started by the macrophages. After the antigen surface has been altered by opsonization (previously discussed under Adherence, pp. 366 and 367), the macrophage recognizes the invading antigen as non-self and physically attaches itself to the antigen. This attachment does not result in phagocytosis or in antigen destruction. Instead, the macrophage presents the attached antigen to the helper/inducer T-cell. Then, the helper/inducer T-cell and the macrophage process the antigen to expose the antigen's recognition sites (universal product code). After processing the antigen, the helper/inducer T-cell brings the antigen into contact with the B-cell so that the B-cell can recognize the antigen as non-self.

LYMPHOCYTE SENSITIZATION

Once the B-cell recognizes the antigen as non-self, the B-cell is "sensitized" to this antigen. A single naive B-cell can become sensitized only once. *Therefore each B-cell can be sensitized to only one type of antigen.*

Sensitizing allows this B-cell to respond to any substance that carries the same antigens (codes) as the original antigen. The sensitized B-cell always remains sensitized to that specific antigen. In addition, all cells produced by that sensitized B-cell also are sensitized to that same specific antigen.

Immediately after it is sensitized, the B-cell divides and forms two types of B-lymphocytes, each one remaining sensitized to that specific antigen (Figure 23-10). One new cell becomes a **plasma cell** and immediately starts to produce antibodies against the sensitizing antigen. The other new cell becomes a memory cell. The plasma cell functions immediately and has a short life span. The **memory cell** remains sensitized but does not start to function until the next exposure to the same antigen (discussed later under Sustained Immunity: Memory, p. 372).

ANTIBODY PRODUCTION AND RELEASE

Antibodies are produced by plasma cells. When fully stimulated, each plasma cell can make as much as 300 molecules of antibody per second. Each plasma cell produces antibody specific only to the antigen that originally sensitized the parent B-cell. For example, in the case of the baby-sitter who was exposed to and invaded by the chickenpox virus, the plasma cells derived from the B-cells sensitized to the chickenpox virus can make only anti-chickenpox antibodies. The antibody class (e.g., immunoglobulin G [IgG] or immunoglobulin M [IgM]) that the plasma cell produces may vary, but the antibody can only be forever directed against the chickenpox virus.

Antibody molecules made by plasma cells are released into the blood and other body fluids as free antibody. Each free antibody molecule remains in the blood for 3 to 30 days. Because the antibody is in body fluids (or body "humors") and is separate from the B-cells, this type of immunity is sometimes called **humoral immunity.** *Circulating an-*

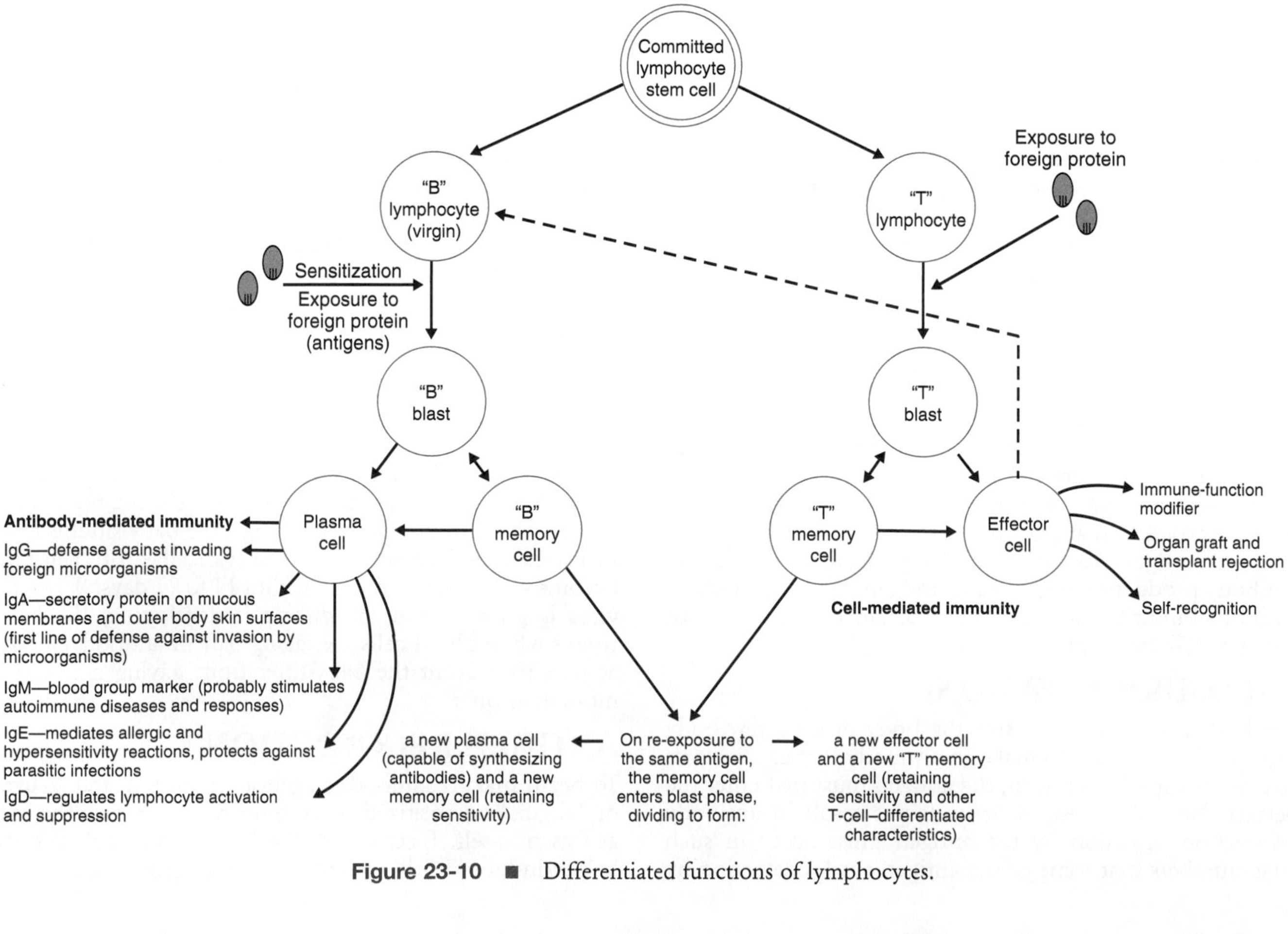

Figure 23-10 ■ Differentiated functions of lymphocytes.

tibodies can be transferred from one person to another to provide the receiving person with immediate immunity of short duration.

ANTIBODY-ANTIGEN BINDING

Antibodies are Y-shaped molecules (Figure 23-11). The tips of the short arms of the Y recognize the specific antigen and bind to it. Because each antibody molecule has two tips (Fab fragments, or arms), each antibody can bind either to two separate antigens or to two areas of the same antigen.

The stem of the Y forms the "Fc fragment." This area can bind to Fc receptor sites on white blood cells (WBCs). The WBC then has not only its own means of attacking antigens, but also has the added power of having surface antibodies that stick to antigens (Figure 23-12).

The actual binding of antibody to antigen is usually not lethal to the antigen. Instead, antibody-antigen binding starts other actions that neutralize, eliminate, or destroy the antigen.

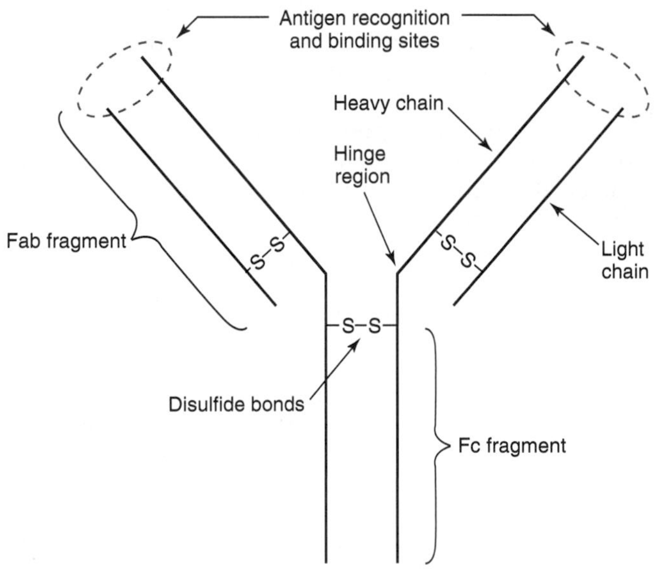

Figure 23-11 ■ Basic antibody structure.

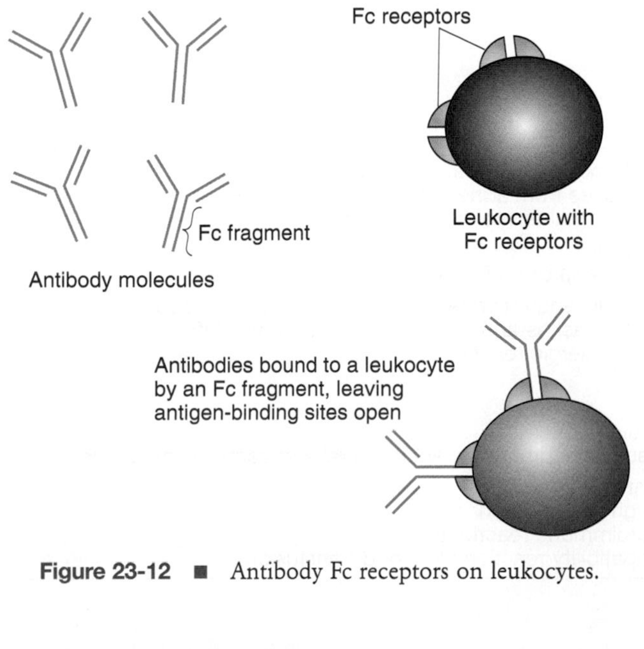

Figure 23-12 ■ Antibody Fc receptors on leukocytes.

ANTIBODY-BINDING ACTIONS

The binding of antibody to antigen triggers reactions that neutralize, eliminate, or destroy the bound antigen. These actions include agglutination, lysis, complement fixation, precipitation, and inactivation or neutralization.

Agglutination

Agglutination is a clumping action that results from the antibody linking antigens together, forming large and small immune complexes (Figure 23-13). Agglutination alone does not directly destroy the antigen. This action starts other defensive effects. First, it slows the movement of the antigen through body fluids. Second, the irregular shape of the antigen-antibody complex (see Figure 23-13) increases the chances of the complex being attacked by other WBCs (e.g., macrophages, neutrophils).

Lysis

Lysis, cell membrane destruction, occurs because of antibody binding to membrane-bound antigens of some invaders. The actual binding makes holes in the invader's membrane, weakening the invader. This response usually requires that complement be activated and "fixed" to the immune complex. Bacteria and viruses are the non-self cells that are damaged most through lysis caused by the binding of antibody to antigens.

Complement Fixation

Some classes of antibodies can remove or destroy antigen through complement activation and complement fixation. (The mechanism by which complement assists in immunity is discussed earlier under Adherence, pp. 366 and 367.) The two classes of antibody that can activate the complement system are IgG and IgM. Binding of antibody from either of these classes to antigen provides a binding site for the first component of complement (C1q). Once C1q is activated, other proteins of the complement system are activated in a cascade.

Precipitation

Precipitation is similar to agglutination. With precipitation, however, antibody molecules bind so much antigen that large, insoluble, antigen-antibody complexes are formed. These complexes cannot stay in suspension in the blood.

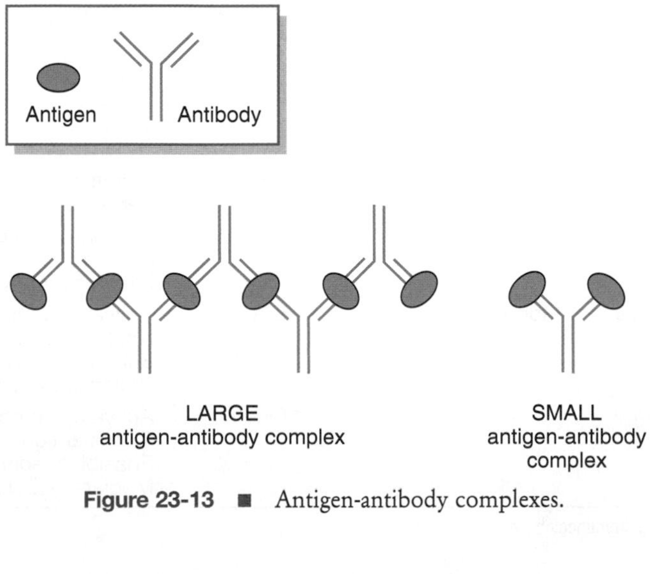

Figure 23-13 ■ Antigen-antibody complexes.

Instead, they form a large precipitate, which can be acted on and removed by neutrophils and macrophages.

Inactivation-Neutralization

Inactivation (neutralization) does not result in the immediate destruction of the antigen. Usually only a small area of the antigen, the **active site,** causes the harmful effects. The rest of the antigen may not be harmful to the host. When an antibody binds to an antigen and covers up the antigen's active site, the antigen is made harmless without destroying it.

SUSTAINED IMMUNITY: MEMORY

The sustained immunity, or memory, function of antibody-mediated immunity (AMI) provides us with long-lasting immunity to a specific antigen. Sustained immunity results from memory B-cells made during the lymphocyte sensitization stage. These memory cells remain sensitized to the specific antigen to which they were originally exposed. On re-exposure to the same antigen, the memory cells rapidly respond. First, the memory cells divide and form new sensitized blast cells and new sensitized plasma cells. The blast cells continue to divide, producing many more sensitized plasma cells. The sensitized plasma cells rapidly make large amounts of the antibody specific for the sensitizing antigen.

This ability of the memory cells to respond on re-exposure to the same antigen that originally sensitized the B-cell allows a rapid and large immune (anamnestic) response to the antigen. So much antibody is made that usually the invading organisms are removed completely, so that the person does not become ill. Because of this process, most people do not become ill with chickenpox or other infectious diseases more than once, even though they are exposed many times to the causative organism. Without the action of memory, people would remain susceptible to specific diseases on subsequent exposure to the organisms, and no sustained immunity would be generated.

General Antibody Classification

All antibodies are **immunoglobulins,** also called **gamma globulins.** These names are based on the structure and function of antibodies. A globulin is a protein that is globular rather than straight. Because antibodies are globular proteins, they are "globulins." The term *immunoglobulin* is used for antibodies because they are globular proteins that provide immunity. Antibodies also are called "gamma globulins" because all free antibodies in the plasma separate out in the gamma fraction of plasma proteins during electrophoresis. The five antibody types are classified by differences in size, timing, and association (Table 23-4).

Acquiring Antibody-Mediated Immunity

Two broad categories of immunity are innate-native immunity and adaptive (acquired) immunity.

INNATE-NATIVE IMMUNITY

Innate-native immunity (sometimes called "natural immunity") is a natural feature of a person. It can be a barrier to prevent organisms from entering the body or can be an attacking force that eliminates organisms that have already entered the body. This type of immunity cannot be developed or transferred from one person to another and is not an adaptive response to exposure or invasion by foreign proteins.

The inflammatory responses are part of innate immunity. Other parts of innate immunity include skin, mucosa, antimicrobial chemicals, complement, and natural killer cells (Abbas & Lichtman, 2003).

ADAPTIVE IMMUNITY

Adaptive immunity is the immunity that a person's body makes (or can receive) as an adaptive response to invasion by organisms or foreign proteins. For example, antibody-mediated immunity is an acquired immunity. Adaptive immunity occurs either naturally or artificially through lymphocyte responses and can be either active or passive.

Active Immunity

Active immunity occurs when antigens enter the body and the body responds by making specific antibodies against the antigen. This type of immunity is active because the body takes an active part in making the antibodies. Active immunity can occur under natural or artificial conditions.

TABLE 23-4 Classification and Characterization of Antibodies

Type	Configuration	Content in Blood	Function
IgA	Dimer	<15%	"Secretory"; present in body secretions, such as tears, mucus, saliva Inhibits bacteria and viruses from adhering to skin and mucous membranes, making penetration into the internal environment more difficult
IgD	Monomer	<1%	Modification of IgM activity Serves as an activated receptor on B-lymphocytes
IgE	Monomer	<1%	Degranulation of basophils and mast cells during inflammatory responses Assists in clearance of parasites and prevention of pulmonary infections Mediates many types of allergic reactions
IgG	Monomer	75%	Activates complement Neutralizes toxins Enhances phagocytosis Provides significant sustained immunity against viral and bacterial infections
IgM	Pentomer	10%	Activates complement Clears antigens through precipitation Possibly mediates autoimmune reactions Mediates ABO incompatibility reactions in blood transfusions

Ig, Immunoglobulin.

NATURAL ACTIVE IMMUNITY

Natural active immunity occurs when an antigen enters the body without human assistance and the body responds by actively making antibodies against that antigen (e.g., chickenpox virus). Most of the time, the invasion that triggers antibody production usually also causes the disease. However, processes occurring in the body at the same time as infection create immunity to that antigen. Thus the person will not become ill after a second exposure to the same antigen. *This type of immunity is the most effective and the longest lasting.*

ARTIFICIAL ACTIVE IMMUNITY

Artificial active immunity is the protection developed by vaccination or immunization. This type of immunity is used to prevent infections or illnesses (e.g., tetanus, diphtheria, polio) that have such serious consequences that avoiding the disease altogether is most desirable. Small amounts of specific antigens are placed as a vaccination into a person. The person's immune system responds by actively making antibodies against the antigen. Because antigens used for this procedure have been specially processed **(attenuated)** to make them less likely to grow in the body, this exposure does not cause the disease. Artificial active immunity lasts many years, although repeated but smaller doses of the original antigen are required as a "booster" to retain the protection.

Passive Immunity

Passive immunity occurs when antibodies against an antigen are in a person's body but were not created there. Rather, these antibodies are transferred to the person's body after being made in the body of another person or animal. Because these antibodies are foreign to the receiving person, the antibodies are recognized as non-self and eliminated quickly. For this reason, passive immunity only provides immediate, short-term protection against a specific antigen.

Natural passive immunity occurs when antibodies are passed from the mother to the fetus via the placenta or to the infant through colostrum and breast milk.

Artificial passive immunity involves injecting a person with antibodies that were produced in another person or animal. This type of immunity is used when a person is exposed to a serious disease for which he or she has little or no actively acquired immunity. Instead, the injected antibodies are expected to inactivate the antigen. This type of immune protection is temporary, lasting only days to a few weeks. Some of the problems in which artificial passive immunity may be used include exposure to rabies, tetanus, and poisonous snake bites.

AMI works with inflammation to protect against infection. However, AMI can provide the most effective, long-lasting immunity only when its actions are combined with those of cell-mediated immunity (CMI).

CELL-MEDIATED IMMUNITY

Cell-mediated immunity (CMI), or cellular immunity, involves many white blood cell (WBC) actions and interactions. This type of immunity is provided by lymphocyte stem cells that mature in the secondary lymphoid tissues of the thymus and pericortical areas of lymph nodes. Certain CMI responses influence and regulate the activities of antibody-mediated immunity (AMI) and inflammation by producing and releasing cytokines. For total immunocompetence, then, CMI must function optimally.

Cell Types Involved in Cell-Mediated Immunity

The WBCs with the most important roles in CMI include several specific T-lymphocytes (T-cells) along with a special population of cells known as natural killer (NK) cells. T-cells have a variety of subsets, each of which has a specific function.

One way of identifying different T-cell subsets is to examine certain "marker proteins" (antigens) on the cell membrane's surface. More than 200 different T-cell proteins have been identified on the cell membrane, and 11 of these (named T1 through T11) are commonly used clinically to identify specific cells. Antibodies have been made against each of these 11 proteins. Thus each T-cell subset can be identified by its reaction to the commercial antibodies. Most T-cells have more than one antigen on their cell membrane. For example, all mature T-cells contain T1, T3, T10, and T11 proteins. Certain T-cells also contain other specific T-cell membrane antigens.

The names used to identify specific T-cell subsets include the specific membrane antigen and the overall actions of the cells in a subset. The three T-lymphocyte subsets that are critically important for the development and continuation of CMI are helper/inducer T-cells, suppressor T-cells, and cytotoxic/cytolytic T-cells.

HELPER/INDUCER T-CELLS

The cell membranes of helper/inducer T-cells contain the T4 protein. These cells are usually called T4+ cells or T_H cells. The most correct name for helper/inducer T-cells is CD4+ (cluster of differentiation 4). The T4 cells may also be referred to as cells that are OKT4 positive or Leu-3 positive because of the specific antigens on the membrane surface.

Helper/inducer T-cells easily recognize self cells versus non-self cells. In response to the recognition of non-self (antigen), helper/inducer T-cells secrete lymphokines that can enhance the activity of other WBCs.

Most lymphokines secreted by the helper/inducer T-cells increase immune function. These lymphokines increase bone marrow production of stem cells and speed up their maturation. Thus helper/inducer T-cells act as organizers in "calling to arms" various squads of WBCs involved in inflammatory, antibody, and cellular defensive actions to destroy or neutralize antigens.

SUPPRESSOR T-CELLS

The membranes of suppressor T-cells contain the T8-lymphocyte antigen; these cells are commonly called T8+ cells or T_S-cells. Suppressor T-cells help regulate CMI.

Suppressor T-cells prevent continuous overreactions **(hypersensitivity)** when a person is exposed to non-self cells or proteins. This function is important in preventing the formation of autoantibodies directed against normal, healthy self cells, which is the basis for many autoimmune diseases.

The suppressor T-cells secrete lymphokines that have an overall *inhibitory* action on most cells of the immune system. These lymphokines inhibit both the growth and activation of immune system cells.

Suppressor T-cells have the opposite action of helper/inducer T-cells. For optimal function of CMI, then, a balance between helper/inducer T-cell activity and suppressor T-cell activity must be maintained. This balance occurs when the helper/inducer T-cells outnumber the suppressor T-cells by a ratio of 2:1. When this ratio increases, overreactions can occur, some of which are tissue damaging as well as unpleasant. When the helper-suppressor ratio decreases, immune function is suppressed, and the person's risk for infections increases.

CYTOTOXIC/CYTOLYTIC T-CELLS

Cytotoxic/cytolytic T-cells are also called T_C-cells. Because they have the T8 protein present on their surfaces, they are a subset of suppressor cells. Cytotoxic/cytolytic T-cells destroy cells that contain a processed antigen's major histocompatibility complex (MHC). This activity is most effective against self cells infected by parasites, such as viruses or protozoa.

Parasite-infected self cells have both self MHC proteins (universal product code) and the parasite's antigens on the cell surface. This allows the person's immune system cells to recognize the infected self cell as abnormal, and the cytotoxic/cytolytic T-cell can bind to it.

When the cytotoxic/cytolytic T-cell binds to the infected cell's MHC complex, the cytotoxic/cytolytic T-cell makes holes in the membrane of the infected cell and delivers a "lethal hit" of enzymes to the infected cell, causing it to lyse and die. Once the lethal hit has been delivered to the infected cell, the cytotoxic/cytolytic T-cell releases the dying infected cell and can then attack and destroy other infected cells that carry the same antigen MHC complex.

NATURAL KILLER CELLS

Natural killer (NK) cells are also known as CD16+ cells and are very important in providing CMI. The actual site of NK cell differentiation and maturation is unknown. Although this cell type has some T-cell features, it is not a true T-cell subset (Abbas & Lichtman, 2003).

NK cells have direct cytotoxic effects on some non-self cells. Unlike cytotoxic/cytolytic T-cells, NK cells can exert these cell killing effects without first being sensitized. Nor do they need to share any of the MHC proteins in common with the non-self cell. The cell killing actions of NK cells are independent of the interactions of other white blood cells. NK cells conduct "seek and destroy" missions in the body to eliminate non-self cells.

NK cells are most effective in destroying unhealthy or abnormal self cells. The non-self cells most often harmed by NK cells are cancer cells and virally infected body cells.

Cytokines

CMI regulates the immune system by the production and activity of cytokines. **Cytokines** are small protein hormones produced by the many WBCs (and some other tissues). Cytokines made by the macrophages, neutrophils, eosinophils, and monocytes are **monokines;** cytokines produced by T-cells are **lymphokines.**

Cytokines work like other types of hormone: one cell produces a cytokine, which in turn exerts its effects on other cells of the immune system. The cells responding to the cytokine may be located close to or remote from the cytokine-secreting cell. The cells that change their activity when a cytokine is present are "responder" cells. For a responder cell to respond to the presence of a cytokine, the responder cell must have a specific receptor to which the cytokine can bind. Once the cytokine binds to its receptor, the responder cell changes its activity (Figure 23-14).

Cytokines control many inflammatory and immune responses (Corwin, 2000a; Corwin, 2000b). Some cytokines are **pleiotropic,** in that the effects are widespread within the immune system, setting into motion many different immune actions. Other cytokines have specific actions limited to only one type of cell. Cytokines include the interleukins, interferons, colony stimulating factors, and tumor necrosis factor. The interleukins are the largest group of cytokines, with interleukin-25 (IL-25) being the most recently defined. Although there are many cytokines, not all are clinically useful at this time. Table 23-5 lists the cytokines that have current clinical importance.

Protection Provided by Cell-Mediated Immunity

Cell-mediated immunity (CMI) helps protect the body through the ability to differentiate self from non-self. The non-self cells most easily recognized by CMI are cancer cells and those self cells infected by organisms that live within host cells. CMI watches for and rids the body of self cells that might potentially harm the body. *CMI is important*

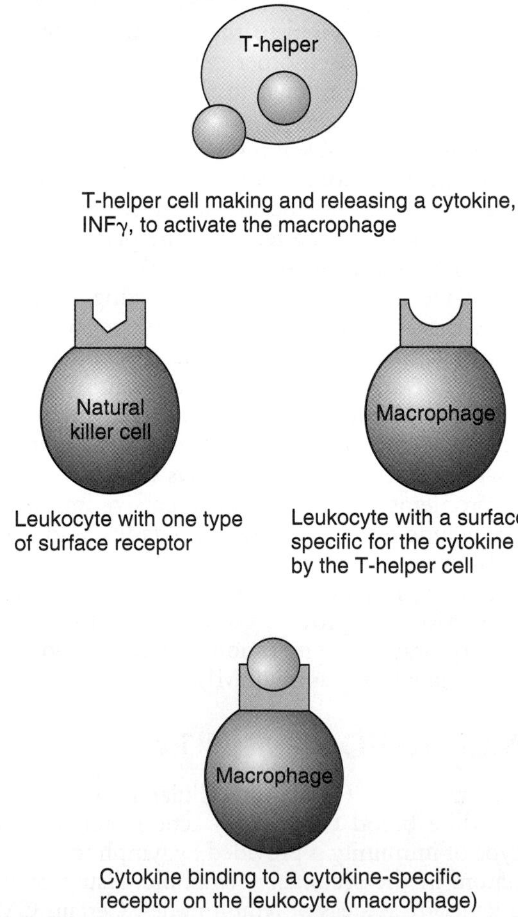

Figure 23-14 ■ Cytokine receptors on leukocytes.

TABLE 23-5 Activity of Selected Cytokines

Cytokine	Cellular Origin	Inducing Event	Cytokine Action
IL-1 (Proinflammatory)	Macrophages Monocytes Natural killer cells	Contact with gram-negative bacterial products Contact with CD4+ cell Presence of TNF	Stimulates increased production of prostaglandins Induces fever Increases proliferation of CD4+ cells Stimulates growth and differentiation of B-lymphocytes Induces further secretion of IL-1 and IL-6
IL-2 (Proinflammatory)	T-helper cells (CD4+ T-cells) CD8+ T-cells	T-cell activation by antigens	Increases growth and differentiation of T-lymphocytes Stimulates increased production of IL-2 from activated lymphocytes Enhances NK activity and activity of tumor-infiltrating lymphocytes
IL-3 (Multilineage CSF)	T-helper cells (CD4+ T-cells)	Infection or antigen invasion	Pluripotent (pleiotropic) stimulation of bone marrow stem cells
IL-4 (B-cell stimulatory factor)	T-helper cells (CD4+ T-cells) Activated mast cells	Presence of anti-Ig antibody	Stimulates growth and differentiation of B-lymphocytes Stimulates increased production of IgG and IgE Induces further secretion of IL-4, IL-5, and IL-6 Suppresses inflammation
IL-5 (B-cell growth factor)	T-helper cells (CD4+ T-cells) Activated mast cells	Helminth infection Pulmonary infection	Stimulates growth and differentiation of eosinophils Stimulates increased production of IgA and IgE
IL-6 (Proinflammatory)	Activated T-cells Fibroblasts Vascular endothelial cells Macrophages Monocytes	Infection or inflammation Presence of IL-1 TNF	Stimulates liver to produce fibrinogen, macroglobulin, C-protein Stimulates growth of activated B-lymphocytes Increases production of bone marrow stem cells
IL-8 (Monocyte chemotactic factor)	Activated T-cells Macrophages Platelets Fibroblasts Endothelial cells	Infection or inflammation	Chemotactic factor for neutrophils, basophils and eosinophils Stimulates neutrophil activation
IL-9	T-helper cells (CD4+ T-cells)	Infection or inflammation	Stimulates mast cell growth Induces IL-4 production Stimulates lymphocyte activation
IL-10	Mature lymphocytes Macrophages Monocytes	Infection or inflammation	Enhances activity of cytotoxic/cytolytic T-cells Suppresses inflammatory response
Interferon-alpha (INF-α)	Macrophages	Viral infection	Decreases viral proliferation
Interferon-beta (INF-β)	Fibroblasts	Viral infection	Decreases viral proliferation
Interferon-gamma (INF-γ)	T-helper cells (CD4+ T-cells) T-suppressor cells (CD8+ T-cells) NK cells	Viral infection	Decreases viral proliferation Activates macrophages Induces differentiation of committed lymphoid stem cells Activates neutrophils Activates NK cells
TNF (Proinflammatory)	Activated macrophages Activated mast cells Activated NK cells Activated T-cells	Infection or inflammation (especially infection with gram-negative microorganisms)	Increases leukocyte adhesion Induces fever Stimulates production of CSF Induces cytolysis of virally infected cells Induces secretion of IL-1 and IL-6
GM-CSF	Activated T-cells Macrophages Fibroblasts Vascular endothelial cells	Infection or inflammation	Increases growth and differentiation of committed myeloid stem cells Slightly activates macrophages
Monocyte-macrophage CSF (M-CSF)	Fibroblasts Vascular endothelial cells	Infection or inflammation	Increases growth and differentiation of committed monocyte-macrophage progenitor cells
G-CSF	Macrophages Vascular endothelial cells Fibroblasts	Infection or inflammation	Increases proliferation and maturation of neutrophils
Erythropoietin	Renal parenchymal cells	Hypoxia	Increases growth and differentiation of erythrocytes

CSF, Colony-stimulating factor; *G,* granulocyte; *GM,* granulocyte-macrophage; *Ig,* immunoglobulin; *IL,* interleukin; *INF,* interferon; *M,* macrophage; *NK,* natural killer; *TNF,* tumor necrosis factor.

in preventing the development of cancer and metastasis after exposure to carcinogens.

Transplant Rejection

Natural killer (NK) cells and cytotoxic/cytolytic T-cells also destroy cells from other people or animals. Although this action is usually helpful, it is also responsible for rejection of grafts and transplanted organs. Because the solid organ transplanted into the host is seldom a perfectly identical match of universal product codes (human leukocyte antigens [HLAs]) between the donated organ and the recipient host, the client's immune system cells recognize a newly transplanted organ as non-self. Without intervention, the host's immune system starts inflammatory and immunologic actions to destroy or eliminate these non-self cells. This activity causes rejection of the transplanted organ. Graft rejection is a result of a complex series of responses that change over time and involve different components of the immune system. Graft rejection can be hyperacute, acute, or chronic.

HYPERACUTE REJECTION

Hyperacute graft rejection begins immediately on transplantation and is an antibody-mediated response. Antigen-antibody complexes form in the blood vessels of the transplanted organ. The host's blood has pre-existing antibodies to one or more of the antigens (including blood group antigens) present in the donated organ. The antigen-antibody complexes adhere to the lining of blood vessels and activate complement. The activated complement in the blood vessel linings triggers the blood clotting cascade, causing small clots to form throughout the new organ. Widespread clotting occludes blood vessels and leads to ischemic necrosis, inflammation with phagocytosis of the necrotic blood vessels, and release of lytic enzymes into the new organ. These enzymes cause massive cellular destruction and graft loss.

Hyperacute rejection occurs mostly in transplanted kidneys. The following clients are at greatest risk for hyperacute rejection:

1. Those who have received donated organs of an ABO blood type different from their own
2. Those who have received multiple blood transfusions at any time in life before transplantation
3. Those who have a history of multiple pregnancies
4. Those who have received a previous transplant

The manifestations of hyperacute rejection are apparent within minutes of attachment of the donated organ to the host's blood supply. The process cannot be stopped once it has started, and the rejected organ is removed as soon as hyperacute rejection is diagnosed.

ACUTE REJECTION

Acute graft rejection occurs within 1 week to 3 months after transplantation. Two mechanisms are responsible. The first mechanism is antibody mediated and results in vasculitis within the transplanted organ. This reaction differs from that of hyperacute rejection in that blood vessel necrosis (rather than thrombotic occlusion) leads to the organ's destruction.

The second mechanism is cellular. Host cytotoxic/cytolytic T-cells and NK cells enter the transplanted organ through the blood, penetrate the organ cells, start an inflammatory response, and cause lysis of the organ cells (Abbas & Lichtman, 2003).

Diagnosis of acute rejection is made by laboratory tests that show impaired function of the donated organ, along with biopsy of the donated organ. Symptoms of acute rejection vary with each client and with the specific organ transplanted. For example, when acute rejection occurs in a transplanted kidney, the client usually has some tenderness in the kidney area and may have other general symptoms of inflammation.

An episode of acute rejection after solid organ transplantation does not automatically mean that the client will lose the new organ. Drug management of host immune responses at this time may limit the damage to the organ and allow the graft to be maintained.

CHRONIC REJECTION

The origin of **chronic rejection** is not clear, but it is similar to chronic inflammation and scarring. The smooth muscles of blood vessels overgrow and occlude the vessels. Functional tissue of the donated organ is replaced with fibrotic, scarlike tissue. Because this fibrotic tissue is not organ tissue, the transplanted organ's function is reduced in proportion to the amount of normal tissue that is replaced by fibrotic tissue. This type of reaction is long-standing and occurs continuously as a response to chronic ischemia caused by blood vessel injury. The results of chronic rejection are unique to different transplanted organs. For example, in transplanted lungs, chronic rejection thickens small airways. In transplanted livers, chronic rejection destroys bile ducts. In transplanted hearts, this process is called **accelerated graft atherosclerosis (AGA)** and is the major cause of death in clients who have survived 1 or more years after heart transplantation (Augustine, 2000).

Although good control over host immune function can delay this type of rejection, the process probably occurs to some degree with all transplanted solid organs. Because the fibrotic changes are permanent, there is no cure for chronic graft rejection. When the fibrosis increases to the extent that the transplanted organ can no longer function, the only recourse is retransplantation.

TREATMENT OF TRANSPLANT REJECTION

Rejection of transplanted solid organs involves all three components of immunity, although cell-mediated immune (CMI) responses are most significant in the rejection process.

Maintenance

The drugs used for routine immunosuppressive therapy after solid organ transplantation are combinations of specific immunosuppressants (cyclosporine [Sandimmune, Neoral, Gengraf]), less specific immunosuppressants (azathioprine [Imuran] or mycophenolate [CellCept, Myfortic]), and one of the corticosteroids, such as prednisone (Apo-Prednisone✱, Deltasone✱) or prednisolone (Delta-Cortef) (Table 23-6). Cyclosporine induces the specific and effective suppression of rejection. This drug, however, induces major long-term adverse actions and is expensive (see the Resource Management box on p. 378.) The dosage of all immunosuppressive agents is ad-

TABLE 23-6 Drugs Used to Prevent or Treat Transplant Rejection

Drug	Action	Problems/Precautions
Immunosuppressants		
Cyclosporine (Sandimmune, Neoral, Gengraf)	Reduces T-lymphocyte production of cytokines important in stimulating T-lymphocyte proliferation and activation (especially interleukin-2)	Has nephrotoxic, neurotoxic, and hepatotoxic properties. Stimulates hyperglycemia—may cause diabetes mellitus. Increases body and facial hair. Causes gingival hyperplasia. Blood levels are sensitive to the presence of other drugs. Must be mixed following strict manufacturer guidelines. Do not administer to clients receiving tacrolimus.
Azathioprine (Imuran)	Converts to an antimetabolite that inhibits DNA synthesis and cell division in T- and B-lymphocytes and myeloid cells	Has hepatotoxic properties. Has high incidence of nausea and vomiting. Suppresses hematologic functions. Use is less frequent compared to mycophenolate mofetil.
Mycophenolate mofetil (CellCept)	Selectively inhibits T- and B-lymphocyte proliferation by interfering with purine synthesis and cell division	Has fewer side effects than azathioprine. Has been demonstrated more effective as part of triple therapy in clients after kidney transplantation. Is less selective than cyclosporine.
Mycophenolate sodium (Myfortic)	Similar to mycophenolate mofetil	Is a different formulation of mycophenolate mofetil. Has fewer gastrointestinal effects than mycophenolate mofetil.
Tacrolimus FK506 (Prograf)	Suppresses T-cell growth and production of interleukin-2	Do not administer with cyclosporine. Has nephrotoxic and neurotoxic properties. Induces hyperglycemia. Has a frequent incidence of nausea, vomiting, and weight loss. May be used as rescue agent in kidney rejection.
Sirolimus (Rapamune)	Suppresses lymphocyte production and B-cell synthesis of antibodies	Induces liver changes, toxicity occurs at lower doses in people with liver impairment. Do not give with grapefruit juice. Increases the risk for infection.
Corticosteroids (prednisone, prednisolone, Decadron, among others)	Directly cytotoxic to circulating lymphocytes Suppresses bone marrow stem cell proliferation	Induces general immunosuppression. Immunosuppression more profound than with other agents. Suppresses adrenal cortical activity. Numerous metabolic and endocrine side effects.
Antibodies		
Interleukin-2 receptor antagonists: Basiliximab (Simulect) Daclizumab (Zenapax)	Binds to interleukin-2 receptors on activated lymphocytes, especially helper/inducer T-cells, preventing proliferation and limiting activation	Used as initial induction therapy, not as continuing therapy. IV administration only. Approved as prophylaxis for kidney transplant only. Synthesized through recombinant DNA technology and contains both human (90%) and mouse (10%) DNA sequences. May induce anaphylaxis. High incidence of flu-like symptoms.
Antithymocyte globulin (Atgam)	Depletes existing T-lymphocytes through antigen-antibody binding actions	Is a polyclonal antibody raised in horses. May induce anaphylaxis or other immune side effects. Side effects increase on re-exposure. Has limited duration of action.
Muromonab-CD3 (Orthoclone OKT3)	Binds to the OKT3 receptor on lymphocytes, down-regulating the receptor action Depletes circulating T-lymphocytes through antigen-antibody binding actions May induce programmed cell death (apoptosis) of bound T-lymphocytes	Is a monoclonal antibody raised in a mouse model. May induce anaphylaxis or other immune side effects. Has limited duration of action. May be inactivated by human antimouse antibodies. Induction of capillary leak syndrome is common. May require premedication with corticosteroids.

justed to the immune response of each client. Treatment with these agents increases the risk for bacterial and fungal infections and for cancer development.

Tacrolimus (Prograf) is used in maintenance therapy and rescue therapy. It is similar to erythromycin and specifically suppresses T-cell actions, including production of interleukin-2 (IL-2). These effects occur through several mechanisms. Without continuous stimulation by IL-2, helper/inducer T-cells and cytotoxic/cytolytic T-cells are slow to reproduce and do not perform their usual functions. Suppression of these two cell populations allows the donated organ to remain free from immunologic destruction. The general immunosuppression is not as profound and the host's risk for infection is not greatly increased. Tacrolimus also prevents activation of unsensitized cytotoxic/cytolytic T-cells.

A newer approach to prevent transplant rejection for clients undergoing kidney transplantation is the use of monoclonal antibodies directed against the IL-2 receptor site on activated T-cells (especially helper/inducer T-cells). These antibodies, basiliximab (Simulect) or daclizumab (Zenapax), are given intravenously within 2 hours before the transplant surgery and within the first few days after the surgery. By binding the antibodies to the IL-2 receptor site, T-cell growth and activation are reduced for several months.

RESOURCE MANAGEMENT

TRANSPLANT REJECTION PROPHYLAXIS

Cost of Care

- The most useful agent in preventing rejection of transplanted solid organs is cyclosporin.
- Cost of maintaining therapeutic levels of this drug for an average-sized adult ranges between $1100 and $1500 per month.
- Clients must take this drug daily for the life of the transplanted organ.
- The effectiveness of this drug is highly dependent on following manufacturer's directions for mixing and administering.
- An antifungal agent, ketoconazole, when taken orally has been demonstrated to slow metabolism of cyclosporin and maintain therapeutic blood levels at lower doses (about 40% to 50% of cyclosporin dose needed when taken without ketoconazole).
- The cost of ketoconazole daily maintenance therapy is about $100 per month.

Implications for Nursing

Because of the high cost of medications to prevent transplant rejection, nurses need to incorporate proper medication administration into their client teaching plans and reinforce this information frequently. Nurses can assist in cost reductions by observing for sustained therapeutic blood levels of cyclosporin in clients and exploring what factors may be contributing to this effect.

Data from Augustine, S. (2000). Heart transplantation: Long-term management related to immunosuppression, complications, and psychosocial adjustments. *Critical Care Clinics of North America, 12*(1), 69-77; Drug Facts and Comparisons. (2004). *Drug facts and comparisons* (58th ed.). St. Louis: Wolters Kluwer; and Personal communication, with CVS Pharmacies, January 2004.

Rescue Therapy

Certain agents are used only to reduce the host's immunologic responses during rejection episodes, especially acute rejection. These agents may be used in addition to or in place of the maintenance drugs in the host's normal treatment regimen.

ANTILYMPHOCYTE GLOBULIN

Antilymphocyte globulin (ALG) is an antibody (or group of antibodies) produced in an animal after the animal has been exposed to human lymphocytes. The globulin can be made more specific by exposing the animal to human T-cells instead of mixed lymphocytes. When these antihuman lymphocyte antibodies are given to humans, the antibodies selectively attack and clear lymphocytes from body fluids, blood, and the transplanted organ. These agents are given only for a short time to combat the acute rejection episode.

Most clients receiving ALG have some immunologic side effects, ranging from low-grade fever and malaise to serum sickness and anaphylaxis. The side effects usually increase in intensity on repeated exposure to ALG.

MUROMONAB-CD3 (ORTHOCLONE OKT3)

Muromonab-CD3 is an antibody directed specifically against the human T-cell cell-surface antigen CD3. This antibody is generated in mice rather than in horses. Because the agent is generated in mice, the clients receiving it rapidly develop antimouse antibodies. These antimouse antibodies attack the CD3 and prevent its anti–T-cell activities. This antibody is most effective against rejection during the first episode in which it is used. Its effect in combating graft rejection decreases with each use.

Antibodies made in other animals, especially mice, cause side effects in humans because the animal proteins in the antibodies are recognized as "foreign" by the human immune system. The incidence of side effects is decreasing because newer antibodies have been "humanized." This process removes most of the mouse-specific proteins from the antibody and replaces them with human specific proteins. The "humanized" antibodies made by mice now contain up to 95% human proteins rather than mouse proteins.

GET READY for the NCLEX Examination!

KEY POINTS

- Inflammation and immunity are provided through the actions and products of white blood cells (WBCs).
- Different types of WBCs provide different types of immune or inflammatory protection.
- The differential of the WBC count can be used to determine the client's risk for infection, the presence or absence of infection, the presence or absence of an allergic reaction, and whether an infection is bacterial or viral.
- WBCs are the only body cells able to recognize non-self cells and try to attack or destroy them.
- Self-tolerance is the special ability of WBCs to recognize healthy self cells and not attempt to attack or destroy them.
- Human leukocyte antigens (HLAs) are an individual's tissue type and are inherited from parents.
- Immunocompetence requires that all three parts of inflammation and immunity have optimal functioning.
- Inflammation is a general, nonspecific protective response.
- The five cardinal manifestations of inflammation are redness, warmth, swelling, pain, and loss of function.
- Inflammation and infection are not the same thing. Infection almost always is accompanied by inflammation but inflammation often occurs without infection.
- The tissue responses to inflammation are helpful if confined to the area of invasion or infection and do not extend beyond the acute phase.
- Chronic inflammation can damage tissues and reduce function.
- The cells and actions of cell-mediated immunity control and coordinate the entire inflammatory and immune responses.
- Inflammation cannot be transferred from one person to another.
- Immune function declines with age, making the older adult at increased risk for infection and cancer development.
- Antibody-mediated immunity (also known as "humoral" immunity) can be transferred from one person (or animal) to another.
- Antibodies transferred from one person into another person have a short-term effect.
- Natural, active immunity is the most beneficial and long-lasting type of immunity.
- Vaccinations cause artificial active immunity and require "boosting" for best long-term effects.
- An individual's normal membrane proteins would be antigens in another person.

- Transplant rejection is a normal response of the immune system that can damage or destroy the transplanted organ.
- Clients who receive transplanted organs (unless from an identical sibling) must take immunosuppressive drugs daily to prevent transplant rejection.
- Clients who take immunosuppressive drugs have an increased risk for infection and for cancer development.

ADDITIONAL STUDY RESOURCES

Go to your Student CD-ROM for Review Questions for the NCLEX Examination.

evolve Go to http://evolve.elsevier.com/Iggy/ for Integrated Management of Care Questions for the NCLEX Examination.

SELECTED BIBLIOGRAPHY

Abbas, A., & Lichtman, A. (2003). *Cellular and molecular immunology* (5th ed.). Philadelphia: W.B. Saunders.

Augustine, S. (2000). Heart transplantation: Long-term management related to immunosuppression, complications, and psychosocial adjustments. *Critical Care Clinics of North America, 12*(1), 69-77.

Bauer, S. (2002). Psychoneuroimmunology Part I: Physiology. *Clinical Journal of Oncology Nursing, 6*(3), 167-170.

Banchereau, J. (2002). The long arm of the immune system. *Scientific American, 287*(5), 52-59.

Corwin, E. (2000a). Understanding cytokines part II: Implications for nursing research and practice. *Biological Research for Nursing, 2*(1), 41-48.

Corwin, E. (2000b). Understanding cytokines part I: Physiology and mechanism of action. *Biological Research for Nursing, 2*(1), 30-40.

Facts and Comparisons. (2004). *Drug facts and comparisons* (58th ed.). St. Louis: Author.

Incredibly easy! (2003). Reviewing the immune system. *Nursing2003, 33*(3), 70-71.

McCance, K., & Huether, S. (2002). *Pathophysiology: The biologic basis for disease in adults and children* (4th ed.). St. Louis: Mosby.

Nussbaum, R., McInnes, R., & Willard, H. (2001). *Thompson & Thompson: Genetics in medicine* (6th ed.). Philadelphia: W.B. Saunders.

Otto, S. (2003). Understanding the immune system. *Journal of Infusion Nursing, 26*(2), 79-85.

Parkin, J., & Cohen, B. (2001). An overview of the immune system. *The Lancet, 357*(9270), 1777-1789.

Pierce, J., Cackler, A., & Arnett, M. (2004). Why should you care about free radicals? *RN, 67*(1), 38-42.

Workman, M.L. (2003). The cellular basis of bacterial infection. *Critical Care Clinics of North America, 15*(1), 1-11.

CHAPTER

24

Interventions for Clients with Connective Tissue Disease and Other Types of Arthritis

DONNA D. IGNATAVICIUS • CYNTHIA KINDLER MATZKO

LEARNING OUTCOMES

After studying this chapter, you should be able to:

1. Compare and contrast the pathophysiology and clinical manifestations of osteoarthritis (OA) and rheumatoid disease (RA).
2. Prioritize collaborative interventions for clients with OA and RA.
3. Determine common nursing diagnoses for postoperative clients having total joint replacement surgery.
4. Evaluate the expected outcomes for clients having total joint replacement surgery.
5. Interpret laboratory findings for clients with rheumatoid disease.
6. Identify the nursing implications associated with drug therapy for clients with rheumatoid arthritis.
7. Identify educational needs for clients with arthritis.
8. Differentiate between discoid lupus erythematosus and systemic lupus erythematosus.
9. Describe the priority nursing interventions for clients who have progressive systemic sclerosis.
10. Discuss the treatment of gout based on knowledge of pathophysiology.
11. Explain the differences between polymyositis, systemic necrotizing vasculitis, polymyalgia rheumatica, ankylosing spondylitis, Reiter's syndrome, and Sjögren's syndrome.
12. Describe interventions that clients can use to prevent Lyme disease.
13. Identify the primary concern in care for clients with Marfan syndrome.
14. Describe current treatment strategies for clients with fibromyalgia.

Go to your Student CD-ROM for Review Questions for the NCLEX Examination keyed to these Learning Outcomes.

Connective tissue disease (CTD) is the major focus of *rheumatology,* the study of rheumatic disease. A **rheumatic disease** is any disease or condition involving the musculoskeletal system. In this text, CTDs are discussed separately from other musculoskeletal conditions because most CTDs are classified as autoimmune disorders.

Most common CTDs are characterized by chronic pain and progressive joint deterioration, which results in decreased function. Some of these disorders have additional localized clinical manifestations, whereas others are systemic. The economic and social costs of these diseases are staggering and will increase steadily as "baby boomers" continue to age. Client management requires an interdisciplinary approach, including medicine, surgery, nursing, and physical and occupational therapy.

More than 40 million people in the United States (1 in 6) have at least one of more than 100 types of arthritis. **Arthritis** means inflammation of one or more joints. In clinical practice, however, arthritis often refers to either **noninflammatory arthritis** or **inflammatory arthritis.** Noninflammatory arthritis such as OA is not systemic. Systemic autoimmune diseases, such as RA and systemic lupus erythematosus, are connective tissue diseases that are inflammatory.

OSTEOARTHRITIS

PATHOPHYSIOLOGY

Osteoarthritis is the most common arthritis and the second most common cause of disability among adults in the United States. It is also a common cause of disability worldwide (Kee, 2000). **Osteoarthritis (OA)** may be called degenerative joint disease (DJD); however, this term is no longer current. Joint pain and loss of function are common problems with OA.

Osteoarthritis is characterized by the progressive deterioration and loss of cartilage in one or more joints. Weight-bearing joints (hips and knees), the vertebral column, and the hands are primarily affected because they are used most often and, except for the hands, bear the mechanical stress of body weight. Most clients have the *primary (idiopathic)* form of the disease; *secondary* OA can result from other musculoskeletal conditions or from trauma. OA can also be classified as *nodal* (with hand involvement) or *non-nodal* (without hand involvement) (Kee, 2000).

In affected joints, the normal bluish-white, translucent cartilage becomes soft, opaque, and yellow. Fissures, pitting, and ulcerations develop, and the cartilage thins. As cartilage and the bone beneath the cartilage begin to erode, the joint space narrows and **osteophytes** (bone spurs) form (Figure 24-1). Inflammatory enzymes enhance tissue deterioration as a result of altered cartilage metabolism. The repair process is then unable to overcome the rapid process of degeneration. Bone cysts and secondary **synovitis** (synovial inflammation) are common in advanced disease. **Subluxation** (partial joint dislocation) and joint deformities eventually cause marked immobility, pain, muscle spasm and, possibly, inflammation.

Etiology and Genetic Risk

Although the causative mechanisms of *primary* OA at the cellular level have not been well identified, the disease may be initiated by developmental, genetic, metabolic, and traumatic factors. Age is the strongest risk factor, but research does not support that aging is the only cause of the disease. OA is thought to derive from defective chondrocyte metabolism, which explains the lack of a systemic response. Some clients report a family history of OA, which supports a possible genetic cause, especially for women who have the nodal type. Obesity also contributes to the likelihood of degeneration, particularly in the knees.

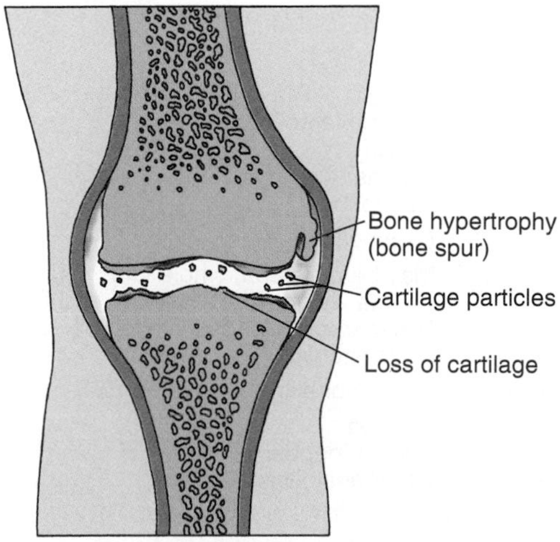

Figure 24-1 ■ Joint changes in degenerative joint disease.

Trauma to the joints from excessive use or abuse predisposes a person to OA. Certain heavy manual occupations (e.g., carpet installation, construction, farming) cause high-intensity or repetitive stress to the joints. The risk of hip and knee OA is also increased in professional athletes, especially football and soccer players, runners, and gymnasts. Lack of exercise can contribute to muscle loss, or **sarcopenia.** Muscle tissue helps to support joints, particularly those that bear weight (e.g., hips and knees).

In a small percentage of people, congenital anomalies, trauma, and joint sepsis can result in *secondary* OA. For example, injuries from motor vehicle accidents can cause OA in later years. Certain metabolic diseases (e.g., diabetes mellitus, Paget's disease of the bone) and blood disorders (e.g., hemophilia, sickle cell disease) can also cause joint degeneration. Inflammatory joint diseases, such as rheumatoid arthritis, can lead to secondary OA.

Incidence/Prevalence

The prevalence of OA varies among different populations but is a universal problem. About three-fourths of people older than 55 years of age have joint changes that can be seen on x-ray examination, although not all of those individuals actually develop OA.

WOMEN'S HEALTH CONSIDERATIONS

Before 50 years of age, more men than women have OA. The disease is much more common in women, especially black women, after 50 years of age; the reason for this difference is not known. Women are more prone to hand involvement, especially in the distal and proximal interphalangeal joints of the fingers, which often produces painful, bony nodes. Women also have a greater number of affected joints compared with men, but men have more hip involvement.

HEALTH PROMOTION/ILLNESS PREVENTION

Several lifestyle considerations can help prevent or slow joint degeneration and subsequent OA. These practices include the following:

- Keep weight within normal limits; obesity causes excess wear on joints, especially hips and knees.
- Avoid or limit activities that promote stress on joints, such as jogging.
- Limit participation in recreational sports that can damage joints, such as football.
- Avoid risk-seeking activities to prevent trauma that can result in OA later in life.

◆COLLABORATIVE MANAGEMENT

PHARM REVIEW

◆Assessment

HISTORY

Ask questions about the course of the disease. Collect information specifically related to osteoarthritis OA, such as the nature and location of joint pain and how much pain is the client experiencing. Use a 0-to-10 scale to assess pain intensity on the day of the interview. Chapter 7 discusses pain assessment in detail.

Other questions to ask include the following:

- If joint stiffness has occurred, where and for how long?
- When and where has any joint swelling occurred?
- What relieves the pain or stiffness?
- Is there any loss of function or difficulty in accomplishing activities of daily living?

Because this disease is observed more often in older women, age, gender, and ethnicity are important factors for the nursing history. Ask clients about their occupation, nature of work, history of trauma, weight history, exercise, and current or previous involvement in sports. A history of obesity is significant, even for clients currently within the ideal range for body weight. A family history of arthritis is also noted. Determine whether the client has a current or previous medical condition that may cause joint manifestations.

PHYSICAL ASSESSMENT/CLINICAL MANIFESTATIONS

In the early stage of the disease, the clinical manifestations of OA may appear similar to those of rheumatoid arthritis (RA). The distinction between OA and RA becomes more evident as the disease progresses. Table 24-1 differentiates the major characteristics of both diseases and their treatments.

JOINT INVOLVEMENT. The typical client with OA is a middle-aged or older woman who complains of chronic joint pain and stiffness. Early in the course of the disease, the pain diminishes after rest and intensifies after activity. Later the pain occurs with slight motion or even when the client is at rest. Because cartilage has no nerve supply, the pain is probably due to joint and soft-tissue involvement and to spasms of the surrounding muscles. During examination of the joints, the nurse can often elicit pain or tenderness by palpation or by putting the joint through range of motion. **Crepitus,** a continuous grating sensation caused by irregular cartilage, may be felt or heard as the joint is put through passive range of motion. One or more joints are affected. The client may also complain of joint stiffness that usually lasts less than 30 minutes after a period of inactivity.

On inspection, the joint is often enlarged because of bony hypertrophy; rarely does a joint appear to be hot and inflamed. The presence of inflammation in clients with OA usually indicates a secondary synovitis. Approximately 50% of clients with hand involvement display the characteristic **Heberden's nodes** (at the distal interphalangeal joints) and **Bouchard's nodes** (at the proximal interphalangeal joints). Although OA is not a bilateral, symmetric disease, these large bony nodes appear on both hands, especially in women. The nodes may be painful and red. Some clients experience pain in developing nodes, which stops once the nodes are fully developed. Others, however, report no nodal pain unless bumped. These nodes tend to be familial and are often a cosmetic concern to clients. The nodes feel hard and cause tenderness when palpated.

OTHER CLINICAL MANIFESTATIONS. Joint effusions are common when the knees are involved. When trying to differentiate the presence of fluid from subcutaneous tissue, you may be able to move fluid from the **infrapatellar notch** (the area directly below the knee) into the **suprapatellar area** (directly above the knee). Other ways to detect fluid in the knee involve grasping the medial and lateral aspect of the knee between the thumb and third finger and pushing down on the top surface of the patella with the forefinger **(ballottement).** If fluid is present, the patella will be able to be pressed down a distance and then rise back up when the forefinger is removed. Subcutaneous tissue cannot be relocated.

Observe any atrophy of skeletal muscle from disuse. The vicious pain cycle of the disease discourages the movement of painful joints, which may result in contractures, muscle atrophy, and further pain. Loss of function may result, depending on which joints are involved. Hip or knee pain may cause the client to limp and restrict walking distance.

TABLE 24-1 Differential Features of Rheumatoid Arthritis and Degenerative Joint Disease

Characteristic	Rheumatoid Arthritis	Osteoarthritis
Typical onset (age)	35-45 yr	>60 yr
Gender affected	Female (3:1)	Female (2:1)
Risk factors or cause	Autoimmune (genetic) Emotional stress (triggers exacerbation)	Aging Genetic factor Obesity Trauma Occupation
Disease process	Inflammatory	Degenerative
Disease pattern	Bilateral, symmetric, multiple joints Usually affects upper extremities first Distal interphalangeal joints of hands spared Systemic	May be unilateral, single joint Affects weight-bearing joints and hands, spine Metacarpophalangeal joints spared Nonsystemic
Laboratory findings	Elevated rheumatoid factor, antinuclear antibody, ESR	Normal or slightly elevated ESR
Common drug therapy	NSAIDs Methotrexate Leflunomide (Arava) Corticosteroids Biological response modifiers Other immunosuppressive agents	NSAIDs Acetaminophen Other analgesics

ESR, Erythrocyte sedimentation rate; *NSAIDs*, nonsteroidal anti-inflammatory drugs.

Osteoarthritis (OA) can often affect the spine, especially the lumbar region at the L3-4 level or the cervical region at C4-6. Compression of spinal nerve roots may occur as a result of vertebral facet bone spurs. The client typically complains of radiating pain, stiffness, and muscle spasms in one or both extremities. Spinal and vertebral arteries may also become compressed.

Severe pain and deformity interfere with ambulation and self-care. In addition to performing a musculoskeletal assessment, conduct a functional assessment of the client with OA to determine mobility and the ability to perform activities of daily living (ADLs). Chapter 10 describes ADLs and functional assessment in depth.

PSYCHOSOCIAL ASSESSMENT

Osteoarthritis (OA) is a chronic condition that may cause permanent changes in lifestyle. An inability to care for oneself in advanced disease prevents socialization and results in role changes and other losses. Therefore the client may exhibit a variety of behaviors indicative of the grieving process, such as anger and depression.

The client may experience a role change in the family, workplace, or both. To identify changes that have been or need to be made, ask the client about his or her roles before the disease developed. Coping strategies to help in living with the disease should also be identified. Kee (1998) found four themes that help people cope with OA. In addition to role changes, joint deformities and bony nodules often cause an alteration in body image and self-esteem. Observe the client's response to body changes. Does the client ignore them or seem overly occupied with them? How does he or she refer to the changes–with anger, degradation, or humor? These clues help to assess the client's acceptance of body alterations.

LABORATORY ASSESSMENT

The health care provider uses the history and physical examination to make the diagnosis of OA The results of routine laboratory tests are usually normal but can be helpful in screening for associated conditions. The erythrocyte sedimentation rate (ESR) and high-sensitivity C-reactive protein (hsCRP) may be slightly elevated when secondary synovitis (synovial inflammation) occurs. ESR also tends to rise with age and infection.

RADIOGRAPHIC ASSESSMENT

Routine x-rays are useful in determining structural joint changes. Specialized views are obtained when the disease cannot be visualized on standard x-ray film but is suspected. A computed tomography (CT) scan may be used to determine vertebral involvement.

OTHER DIAGNOSTIC ASSESSMENTS

The health care provider may order magnetic resonance imaging (MRI) or computed tomography (CT) studies to detect degenerative bony changes, especially in the spine.

Critical Thinking Challenge

You are assigned to care for an older adult in an assisted-living facility. She has long-standing OA of both the hips and knees and a history of diabetes mellitus, heart failure, and hypertension. She is able to care for herself but uses a walker for ambulation because of chronic joint pain and deterioration.

1. How would you perform a physical assessment of this client?
2. What might you expect to find during the physical assessment?
3. How might her other medical diagnoses affect the findings of the physical assessment?

evolve For suggested answer guidelines, go to http://evolve.elsevier.com/Iggy/.

Analysis

COMMON NURSING DIAGNOSES AND COLLABORATIVE PROBLEMS

The following are priority nursing diagnoses for clients with osteoarthritis (OA):

1. Chronic Pain related to muscle spasm, cartilage deterioration, or joint inflammation
2. Impaired Physical Mobility related to pain and muscle atrophy

ADDITIONAL NURSING DIAGNOSES AND COLLABORATIVE PROBLEMS

In addition to the common nursing diagnoses, clients may have secondary problems caused by the pain and immobility common in OA, including one or more of the following:

- Activity Intolerance related to pain and fatigue
- Self-Care Deficit (Partial) related to pain, fatigue, and immobility
- Disturbed Body Image related to the effects of loss of body function
- Impaired Walking related to joint pain
- Ineffective Coping related to chronic pain and decreased function
- Imbalanced Nutrition: More Than Body Requirements related to decreased activity and mobility

Planning and Implementation

CHRONIC PAIN

NOC **PLANNING: EXPECTED OUTCOMES.** The major concern of the client with OA is pain control. Therefore the client is expected to take personal actions to control pain. Indicators include that the client will consistently demonstrate the ability to:

- Recognize pain onset
- Use previous measures that were effective
- Use analgesics appropriately
- Use non-analgesic relief measures
- Report changes in pain symptoms or sites to health care professional
- Report that pain is controlled

INTERVENTIONS. Pain control may be accomplished at home with drug and nonpharmacologic measures. If these measures become ineffective, surgery may be performed to reduce pain. A comprehensive pain assessment should be performed before and after implementing interventions (Chart 24-1).

NONSURGICAL MANAGEMENT. Management of chronic joint pain is difficult for both the client and the health care professional. A combination of modalities is often used, including analgesics, rest, positioning, thermal modalities,

CHART 24-1

NIC INTERVENTION ACTIVITIES for The Client with Osteoarthritis

Analgesic Administration: *Use of pharmacologic agents to reduce or eliminate pain*

- Determine pain location, characteristics, quality, and severity before medicating client.
- Check medical order for drug, dose, and frequency of analgesic prescribed.
- Attend to comfort needs and other activities that assist in relaxation to facilitate response to analgesia.
- Administer analgesics around-the-clock to prevent peaks and troughs of analgesia, especially with severe pain.
- Set positive expectations regarding the effectiveness of analgesics to optimize client response.
- Document response to analgesic and any untoward effects.

Pain Management: *Alleviation of pain or a reduction in pain to a level of comfort that is acceptable to the client*

- Observe for nonverbal cues of discomfort, especially in those unable to communicate effectively.
- Consider cultural influences on pain response.
- Determine the impact of the pain experience on quality of life (e.g., sleep, appetite, activity, cognition, mood, relationships, performance of job, and role responsibilities).
- Evaluate, with the client and the health care team, the effectiveness of past pain control measures that have been used.
- Consider the client's willingness to participate, ability to participate, preference, support of significant others for method, and contraindications when selecting a pain relief strategy.
- Teach the use of nonpharmacologic techniques (e.g., biofeedback, TENS, hypnosis, relaxation, guided imagery, music therapy, distraction, activity therapy, acupressure, hot/cold application, and massage) before, after and, if possible, during painful activities; before pain occurs or increases; and along with other pain relief measures.
- Promote adequate rest/sleep to facilitate pain relief.
- Utilize a multidisciplinary approach to pain management, when appropriate.
- Consider referrals for client, family, and significant others to support groups, and other resources, as appropriate.
- Monitor client satisfaction with pain management at specified intervals.

NIC intervention activities selected from Dochterman, J.M., & Bulechek, G.M. (Eds.). (2004). *Nursing interventions classification (NIC)* (4th ed.). St. Louis: Mosby.

weight control, and integrative therapies. Chapter 7 elaborates on methods of pain control for chronic pain.

NIC **Analgesic Administration.** The purpose of drug therapy is to reduce pain and secondary joint inflammation if present. Acetaminophen (Tylenol, Atasol✱) is the primary drug of choice for pain relief; it is not an anti-inflammatory medication. Clients are at risk for liver damage if they take more than 4000 mg daily, have concurrent alcoholism, or have pre-existing liver disease.

Topical salicylates, such as over-the-counter (OTC) Aspercreme, are useful for some clients as a temporary pain reliever. Topical capsaicin products may also be used. This expensive OTC drug works by blocking substance P, a neurotransmitter for pain (Kee, 2000). Tell the client to expect a burning sensation for a short time after applying capsaicin. Recommend the use of plastic gloves for application. To prevent burning of eyes or other body areas, wash hands immediately after applying capsaicin.

If acetaminophen or topical agents are not successful in relieving pain, the analgesic drug class of choice is usually **nonsteroidal anti-inflammatory drugs (NSAIDs)** (see Chart 24-9 later in this chapter). Most NSAIDs work by inhibiting both forms of the enzyme cyclooxygenase, COX-1 and COX-2. COX-1 produces prostaglandins that help regulate normal cell activity, including protecting the lining of the gastrointestinal (GI) tract. COX-2 produces prostaglandins mainly at the sites of inflammation. A subgroup of NSAIDs has been developed to inhibit only the COX-2 enzyme. COX-2–inhibiting medications, such as celecoxib (Celebrex), meloxicam (Mobic), and valdecoxib (Bextra), appear to manage pain and inflammation with fewer adverse side effects of GI distress or bleeding. Clients allergic to sulfa drugs may also be allergic to celecoxib and therefore should not take it. All of the COX-2 inhibiting drugs are thought to cause cardiovascular disease, such as myocardial infarction, and may soon be unavailable on the market.

For temporary relief of pain in a single joint, the health care provider may inject an individual joint with cortisone. Frequently injected joints include the knee, base of the thumb, shoulder, and the trochanteric bursa, which people often identify as the hip.

Other local agents, such as hyaluronate (Hyalgan) and hylan GF 20 (Synvisc), are used as joint injections for OA of the knee. These synthetic joint fluid implants replace or supplement the body's natural hyaluronic acid, which is broken down by inflammation. Muscle relaxants, such as cyclobenzaprine hydrochloride (Flexeril), are sometimes given for painful muscle spasms, especially those occurring in the back. Remind the client not to drive or operate dangerous machinery when taking muscle relaxants. Potent analgesics are not usually appropriate for the client with OA because of the chronic nature of the pain.

NIC **Pain Management.** In addition to analgesics, many nonpharmacologic measures can be used for clients with OA.

Rest. Several types of rest are used to treat clients with OA:

- *Local* rest involves immobilizing a joint with a splint or brace. If a joint becomes acutely inflamed, the joint is rested until inflammation subsides. Rest the joint when painful, but exercise it to maintain mobility and tone. Balance rest and activity. Consult the occupational therapist (OT), who fits the client for the appropriate device and explains its use.
- *Systemic* rest refers to immobilizing the entire body, such as during a nap. Teach the client about the importance of sleeping about 8 to 10 hours and, if possible, resting an additional 1 to 2 hours each day.
- *Psychological* rest is equally important because it allows relief from the daily stresses that can enhance pain.

Positioning. Joints should be placed in their functional position. When the client is in a supine position (recumbent), he or she should use a small pillow under the head or neck but avoid the use of other pillows. The use of large pillows under the knees or head may result in flexion contractures. If needed, the legs may be elevated 8 to 12 inches (20.3 to 30.5 cm) to reduce back discomfort. Remind the client to use proper posture when standing and sitting to reduce undue strain on the vertebral column.

Thermal Modalities. In general, the client with OA uses heat instead of cold to reduce pain. Heat often helps to decrease the muscle tension around the tender joint and thereby decreases pain. Heat is a temporary relief measure that may be used by the client as often as desired. The application of cold is usually reserved for acutely inflamed joints.

Suggest hot showers and baths, hot packs or compresses, and moist heating pads. Regardless of treatment, teach the client to check that the heat source is not too heavy or so hot that it causes burns. A temperature just above body temperature is adequate to promote comfort.

A physical therapist may provide special heat treatments, such as paraffin dips, diathermy (electrical current), and ultrasonography (sound waves). A 15- to 20-minute heat application usually is sufficient to temporarily reduce pain, spasm, and stiffness. Collaborate with the physical therapist to provide comprehensive care.

Weight Control. Contrary to what has been proposed by the media and uninformed authors, there is no "arthritis diet." According to the National Arthritis Foundation, there is no one food that causes or cures arthritis. A well-balanced diet is recommended. Gradual weight loss for obese clients may lessen the stress on weight-bearing joints, decrease pain, and perhaps slow joint degeneration. If needed, collaborate with the dietitian to provide more in-depth teaching about nutrition and meal planning.

Transcutaneous Electrical Nerve Stimulation. Transcutaneous electrical nerve stimulation (TENS) may be particularly helpful for vertebral involvement. The physician or health care provider collaborates with the nurse and physical therapist to determine whether this pain management modality would be beneficial. The client must be able to control the TENS unit for pain relief.

Complementary and Alternative Therapies. Clients may also use acupuncture, acupressure, tai chi, therapeutic touch, hypnosis, magnets, music therapy, and imagery for pain relief (see Chapters 4 and 7). A study by McCaffrey and Freeman (2003) found that music was an effective intervention for controlling pain in community-dwelling older adults (see the Evidence-Based Practice for Nursing box at right).

Cayenne pepper (the source of capsaicin products) and other dietary supplements, gamma-linolenic acid (GLA, Efamol), glucosamine, and chondroitin complement traditional therapies. GLA can be found in evening primrose oil, borage seed oil, and black currant seed oil. GLA is an omega-6 fatty acid, one of the body's essential fatty acids, and is used for both OA and rheumatoid arthritis (RA). Omega-3 fatty acids are found in certain types of fish (e.g., salmon) or may be taken in fish oil capsules. Glucosamine and chondroitin are natural products (also known as nutraceuticals) found in bone cartilage that may help reduce pain and possibly slow the progression of OA. Many clients have reported positive results, especially decreased pain and inflammation, from these dietary supplements and topical analgesics.

Topical creams have gained increased popularity for short-term pain relief. A study by Cohen (2003) found that topical applications of glucosamine and chondroitin sulfate were effective in relieving knee pain due to OA. Other studies have examined herbal ointments and formulas and found improvement in hand and knee pain (Gemmell, Jacobson, & Hayes, 2003).

Stem Cell Therapy. In certain degenerative disorders, such as OA, stem cells are depleted and have decreased the ability to multiply and differentiation. Ongoing research is exploring methods for delivering mesenchymal stem cell preparations from bone marrow to affected knee joints. This treatment has the potential to stimulate regeneration of cartilage and inhibit joint destruction (Barry, 2003).

EVIDENCE-BASED PRACTICE for Nursing

How does music therapy impact pain perception in clients with osteoarthritis?

McCaffrey, R., & Freeman, E. (2003). Effect of music on chronic osteoarthritis in older people. *Journal of Advanced Nursing, 44*(5), 517-524.

The purpose of this clinical trial was to examine the effect of music as a nursing intervention on osteoarthritis (OA) pain in community-dwelling older adults. The control group sat quietly for 20 minutes each day, and the experimental group listened to music for 20 minutes each day. All 66 subjects completed the Short Form McGill Pain Questionnaire on day 1, 7, and 14. The subjects in the experimental group experienced significantly less OA pain that the control group, demonstrating the value of music as an intervention to control pain.

Level of Evidence: 3—This study was a well-designed trial without randomization of the overall sample, but the sample was randomly assigned.

Critique. This study used random assignment of a selected sample for an experimental design. Although the sample was small, it illustrated the importance of the intervention to nursing practice. The study needs to be repeated with larger samples of various cultures and in various settings where older adults reside.

Implications for Nursing. Interventions for pain control other than medication are needed for clients with chronic pain, such as that experienced by clients with OA. Nurses can use this measure in the community when working with older adults or in long-term care, rehabilitation, and assisted living settings. In some cases, clients who are hospitalized may be candidates for music as an intervention.

SURGICAL MANAGEMENT. Surgery may be indicated when all other measures are inadequate to provide pain control for clients with OA. The most common surgical procedure performed for these clients is **total joint arthroplasty (TJA)** (surgical creation of a joint), also know as total joint replacement (TJR). Almost any synovial joint of the body can be replaced with a prosthetic system that consists of at least two parts, one for each joint surface.

A less invasive procedure using arthroscopy may be used to remove damaged cartilage (see Chapter 54). An **osteotomy** (bone resection) may be performed to correct joint deformity, but this procedure is less common because of the success rate of TJR.

Indications. Total joint arthroplasty is a procedure of last resort for pain management; it is used when all other methods of pain relief have been unsuccessful. The hips and knees are the joints most commonly replaced, but replacements of finger and wrist joints, elbows, shoulders, toe joints, and ankles have become more popular in the past 20 years.

Although TJAs are performed most often for clients with OA, other conditions causing joint damage may also require surgery. These disorders include RA, congenital anomalies, trauma, and osteonecrosis. **Osteonecrosis** is bony necrosis secondary to lack of blood flow, usually from trauma or chronic steroid therapy.

Contraindications. The primary contraindications for TJA are infection anywhere in the body, advanced osteoporosis, and severe inflammation. An infection elsewhere in the body or from the joint being replaced can result in an infected TJA and subsequent prosthetic failure. Therefore if a client has a urinary tract infection, for example, the physician treats the infection before surgery. Advanced osteoporosis can cause bone shattering during insertion of the prosthetic device. Acute joint inflammation is treated before surgery because the mechanical stress of the procedure may promote further inflammation and prosthetic failure.

As a group, TJAs are very successful. Many clients who have lived with chronic, unbearable pain for years and could not function independently at home or in the workplace no longer experience pain in the diseased joint. The pain relief and psychological benefit often outweigh the perioperative risks and costs, but the surgeon and client must make that decision with the case manager. When the client is of advanced age, this decision may become an ethical issue in addition to a physical risk and cost-versus-benefit decision (see the Legal/Ethical Issues box below).

Total Hip Arthroplasty. The most commonly replaced joint is the hip. More than 80% of hip replacements last 20 years as a result of improvements in prosthetic design and surgical technology (Branson & Goldstein, 2003). Although clients of any age can undergo total hip replacement (THA), the procedure is performed most often in clients older than 60 years of age. The special needs and normal physiologic changes of older clients often complicate the perioperative period and may result in additional postoperative complications. (See Chapters 20 to 22 for routine perioperative care and the special considerations needed for care of the older client.)

Preoperative Care. As with any procedure, preoperative care begins with assessing the client's level of understanding about the impending surgery. The surgeon explains the procedure and realistic postoperative care expectations during the office visit, but this education may have occurred weeks or months before the scheduled surgery. Older clients in particular may forget some of the information or may not know what questions to ask. Many orthopedic surgeons employ nurses who follow up and address client concerns. An interdisciplinary clinical pathway that outlines expectations during pre-admission, hospitalization, and post-hospitalization phases of care should be reviewed with the client and family or significant other.

In addition, nurse educators or orthopedic nurses may lead formal classes in the hospital or clinic several weeks before surgery to answer questions and clarify information. Pre-admission sessions are an excellent way for nurses to provide education and support and to improve customer satisfaction. During the class, the client sees the prosthesis or a picture of the device and receives written instructions or a teaching booklet to reinforce the information.

In some hospitals or orthopedic office practices, the physical therapist may meet the client before surgery to explain transfers, precautions, ambulation, and postoperative exercises. An occupational therapist may be available to demonstrate assistive/adaptive devices that facilitate independent activities of daily living (ADLs).

Because venous thromboembolism is a serious postoperative complication, especially for hip surgery, the client's risk factors for clotting problems are determined, including history of previous clotting, obesity, and advanced age. Medications that increase the risk of clotting, such as NSAIDs and hormone replacement therapy (HRT), are discontinued before surgery.

Because TJAs are elective procedures, **autologous blood transfusions** are appropriate. The client may donate blood before surgery to be used as needed during and after surgery. This pre-deposit autologous blood donation is a cost-effective blood replacement alternative for clients who are undergoing elective surgeries. It also avoids the risk of blood transfusion reaction.

Operative Procedures. For both total hip and knee arthroplasty, the client is given a dose of intravenous (IV) antibiotics, usually a cephalosporin such as cefazolin (Ancef), at least 1 hour before the initial surgical incision is made or during surgery. Vancomycin (Vancocin) or clindamycin (Cleocin) may be used for clients who are allergic to cephalosporins.

The anesthesiologist or nurse anesthetist places the client having hip or knee replacement under general or **neuroaxial** (epidural/spinal) anesthesia. Neuroaxial induction reduces blood loss and the incidence of deep vein thrombosis. Intraoperative blood loss with hypotensive neuroaxial anesthesia is usually less than that for general anesthesia, thereby decreasing the need for postoperative blood transfusions.

Two types of incisions for hip replacement may be used. The more traditional 8- to 10-inch (20.3 to 24.5 cm) incision is usually longitudinal on the anterolateral thigh. A posterior incision may be used instead to preserve muscle, depending on the surgeon's preference. Some clients are candidates for a minimally invasive two-incision technique, which is gaining popularity. One small incision is used for the acetabular component, and the other is used for the femoral component. Berger (2003) reported that this newer procedure decreased postoperative complications, including hip dislocation. Wenz, Gurkan, and Jibodh (2002) found that their postoperative clients had earlier ambulation and needed less transfer assistance compared with clients who underwent traditional hip surgery. Therefore, hospital stay is shorter.

If the prosthesis is cemented, polymethyl methacrylate (an acrylic fixating substance) is used. During the surgical

LEGAL/ETHICAL ISSUES

QUALITY OF LIFE FOR CLIENTS HAVING TOTAL JOINT REPLACEMENT

Quality of life (QOL) or quality of well-being (QWB) is a difficult concept to define. In general, it is determined by the client's opinion about the importance of certain elements of his or her life and satisfaction with those elements. Few studies have compared the high cost of surgery with QOL following total joint replacement. This *utilitarian* ethical approach is based on the belief that a person deserves resources based on the real or potential productivity that he or she offers to society.

Health economists consider a resource or intervention a bargain for society if it costs less than $30,000 per quality of well year. Lavernia, Guzman, and Gachupin-Garcia (1999) calculated the cost per quality of well year for 100 clients undergoing a total knee replacement. The clients completed the QWB Index before surgery and at 3 months, 6 months, 1 year, and 2 years after surgery. The differences in the scores before and after surgery were multiplied by the client's life expectancy to obtain the cost per quality of well year. The calculated costs were about $30,700 at 3 months but steadily decreased to about $6,600 by 2 years postsurgery. Based on this study, total knee replacement meets the utilitarian approach to ethical decision making and should be considered an appropriate investment by society.

From Lavernia, C.J., Guzman, J.F., & Gachupin-Garcia, A. (1999). Cost effectiveness and quality of life in knee arthroplasty. *Clinical Orthopaedics, 345,* 134-139.

procedure, the operative area is irrigated with a cool solution. To help prevent infection, the surgeon may mix an antibiotic with the cement or plant antibiotic-impregnated beads deep into the wound. The surgeon also inserts one or two wound drains to remove exudate from the tissues, which might serve as a medium for pathogenic growth and cause wound infection.

Although polymethyl methacrylate is an excellent initial fixative, it has a finite life span and deteriorates over time, which loosens the implant and causes pain. When a prosthesis eventually loosens and causes pain, it is replaced in a procedure called a **revision arthroplasty.** Bone grafts **(allografts)** can be placed to fill in the bony defects that result from removing the old prosthesis. During the healing process, the essentially dead bone revascularizes and grafts with the client's own bone. To prevent prosthetic loosening, a number of noncemented devices that do not require a fixating substance are commonly used instead.

Postoperative Care. In addition to providing the routine postoperative care discussed in Chapter 22, assess for and assist in the prevention of possible postoperative complications following a joint replacement. Table 24-2 summarizes common postoperative complications of total hip replacement surgery, including nursing measures for prevention, assessment, and intervention. Chart 24-2 highlights special concerns for the care of older adults in the postoperative period.

Prevention of Dislocation. A common complication of total hip replacement is **subluxation** (partial dislocation) or total dislocation. Therefore correct positioning is maintained at all times. When the client returns from the postanesthesia care unit (PACU), place him or her in a supine position with the head slightly elevated. Place a trapezoid-shaped abduction pillow, wedge, sling, or splint (with or without straps) between the client's legs to prevent adduction beyond the midline of the body. In some hospitals this device is no longer used because it is uncomfortable and unnecessary in most cases. Abduction devices are usually reserved for clients who are restless or are unable to follow instructions, especially older adults. One or two regular bed pillows are used in most cases. For devices with straps, be sure to loosen the straps every 2 hours and check the client's skin for irritation or breakdown.

Place and support the affected leg in neutral rotation. Keep the client's heels off the bed to prevent skin breakdown, particularly likely to occur in older adults. Turning the client is controversial and is dictated by agency policy or surgeon preference. In most cases you are safe to turn the client toward either side as long as the abduction device or other pillow is in place. Some surgeons allow only turning directly onto one side or the other.

Observe for possible signs of hip dislocation, which include increased hip pain, shortening of the affected leg, and leg rotation. If any of these clinical manifestations occur, keep the client in bed and notify the surgeon immediately. The surgeon manipulates and relocates the affected hip after the client receives an analgesic or is anesthetized. The hip is then immobilized by an abduction splint or other device until healing occurs, usually in about 6 weeks.

Prevention of Thromboembolic Complications. The most potentially *life-threatening* complication following THA is venous thromboembolism (VTE), which includes deep venous thrombosis (DVT) and pulmonary embolism (PE). Older clients are especially at increased risk for VTE because of age and compromised circulation before surgery. Obese clients and those with a history of DVT are also at high risk for thrombi. In clients with TJA, thrombi usually develop in the thigh; these thrombi become life-threatening emboli more readily than thrombi in the calf and other areas. For this reason, thigh-high stockings and sequential

TABLE 24-2 Nursing Interventions to Prevent Complications of Total Joint Replacement Surgery

Complication	Prevention/Intervention
Dislocation	Position correctly. For hip, keep legs slightly abducted. For hip, prevent hip flexion beyond 90 degrees. Assess for pain, rotation, and extremity shortening. Report immediately to physician.
Infection	Use aseptic technique for wound care and emptying of drains. Wash hands thoroughly when caring for client. Culture drainage fluid, if change. Monitor temperature. Report excessive inflammation or drainage to physician.
Venous thromboembolism	Have client wear elastic stockings and/or sequential compression device. Teach leg exercises to client. Encourage fluid intake. Observe for signs of thrombosis (redness, swelling, or pain). Observe client for changes in mental status. Administer anticoagulant as prescribed. Do not massage legs. Do not use knee gatch on bed.
Hypotension, bleeding, or infection	Take vital signs at least every 4 hours. Observe client for bleeding. Report excessively low blood pressure or bleeding to physician.

CHART 24-2

NURSING FOCUS on the OLDER ADULT
Total Hip Replacement

- Use an abduction pillow or splint to prevent adduction after surgery if the client is very restless or has an altered mental state.
- Keep the client's heels off the bed to prevent pressure ulcers.
- Do not rely on fever as a sign of infection; older clients often have infection without fever. Decreasing mental status typically occurs when the client has an infection.
- When assisting the client out of bed, move him or her slowly to prevent orthostatic (postural) hypotension.
- Encourage the client to deep breathe and cough, and use the incentive spirometer every 2 hours to prevent atelectasis and pneumonia.
- As soon as permitted, get the client out of bed to prevent complications of immobility.
- Anticipate the client's need for pain medication, especially if he or she is unable to verbalize the need for pain control.
- Expect a temporary change in mental state immediately after surgery as a result of the anesthetic and unfamiliar sensory stimuli. Reorient the client frequently.

compression devices (SCDs) are typically used during the hospital stay (see Chapter 22). Foot-sole pumps (A-V Impulse System) may also be used.

Anticoagulants, such as aspirin (Ecotrin, buffered aspirin), warfarin (Coumadin, Warfilone*), subcutaneous low-molecular-weight (LMW) heparin, and fondaparinux (Arixtra), are prescribed to prevent VTE. Aspirin may be given to clients with a low risk for VTE. Warfarin may be used for clients who are predisposed to VTE or for those already on the drug for another condition.

During the past decade, the use of LMW heparins has markedly increased for clients with total hip and knee replacements. Examples include enoxaparin (Lovenox), dalteparin (Fragmin), and tinzaparin (Innohep), approved for use in the United States. Other LMW heparins, such as bemiparin (Zibor), are approved for use in other countries. These drugs work to maximize anti-factor Xa and antithrombin to decrease clotting. Given in a low prophylactic dose, they do not affect prothrombin time or activated partial thromboplastin time. However, monitor complete blood count and platelet count because LMW heparins can cause **thrombocytopenia** (decreased platelets). Assess for bleeding, including occult blood in stool and bruising. Protamine can be given as an antidote for all heparins. Be especially alert for signs and symptoms of neurologic dysfunction because spinal and epidural hematomas can occur in clients who received neuroaxial anesthesia.

Fondaparinux (Arixtra) is the first antithrombotic agent that may be prescribed for clients undergoing hip and knee arthroplasty. Its action is similar to that of LMW heparins, and it also has no effect on coagulation tests. Like other drugs, however, the client is at risk for bleeding. No antidote exists at this time for fondaparinux. A complete discussion of nursing care associated with clients taking anticoagulants and VTE can be found in Chapter 39.

The physical therapist (PT) teaches leg exercises, which are begun in the immediate postoperative period and continue until the client is fully ambulatory. These exercises include plantar flexion and dorsiflexion (heel pumping), circumduction (circles) of the feet, gluteal and quadriceps muscle setting, and straight-leg raises (SLRs). The client performs gluteal exercises by pushing the heels into the bed and achieves **quadriceps-setting exercises** ("quad sets") by straightening the legs and pushing the back of the knees into the bed. In addition to preventing clots, these exercises improve muscle tone, which aids restoring the function of the extremity.

Prevention of Infection. Another common potential complication of hip replacement is infection. Infection can occur during hospitalization or for months or years later. Most infections are caused by contamination during surgery.

Monitor the surgical incision and vital signs carefully—every 4 hours for the first 24 hours and every 8 hours thereafter. Observe for signs of infection, such as an elevated temperature and excessive or foul-smelling drainage from the incision. An older client may not have a fever with infection but instead may experience an altered mental state. Obtain a sample of the drainage for culture and sensitivity to determine the offending organisms and the antibiotics that may be needed for treatment.

Assessment of Bleeding and Management of Anemia. Observe the surgical hip dressing for bleeding or other type of drainage at least every 4 hours or when vital signs are taken. Empty and measure the bloody fluid in the drain every shift. The total amount of drainage is usually less than 50 mL/8 hr (possibly more if the client has received a plasma expander such as dextran). The surgeon usually removes the drains and operative dressing 48 to 72 hours after surgery. Clients who have the "mini-incision" surgery may not have a drain. Care must be taken to prevent tape burns when the surgical dressing is removed, especially in older adults.

The surgeon also orders periodic hemoglobin and hematocrit assessments to determine whether the client is anemic and requires blood transfusions. Although some clients receive several units of blood during surgery, the hematocrit and hemoglobin levels may fall below the normal level, in which case additional blood is needed 1 to 2 days after surgery. Blood pressure may be lower than usual because of blood loss during surgery or because cement was used during surgery. (Cement tends to dilate blood vessels and cause hypotension.)

If the client did not donate his or her own blood, another method for blood replacement is intraoperative or postoperative **blood salvage.** The shed blood is collected intraoperatively via aspiration from the surgical site. Using a cell saver, about 50% of the red blood cells are saved for reinfusion. This procedure is used most commonly for bilateral joint replacements or revision surgeries. Blood can be replaced postoperatively by collecting shed blood via suction into a reservoir, filtering the blood, and re-infusing it within a few hours.

Postoperative blood replacement has been standard practice until recently. A preventive alternative is the use of epoetin alfa (Epogen, Procrit, Eprex*), an approved treatment for anemia that may prevent the necessity of postoperative blood transfusion when given to clients undergoing TJA.

Assessment for Neurovascular Compromise. As with other bone surgery, frequent neurovascular assessments are necessary to monitor for a possible compromise in circulation to the distal extremity. Check and document color, temperature, distal pulses, capillary refill, movement, and sensation. Remember to compare the operative leg with the nonoperative one. Such assessments are performed at the same time the vital signs are checked.

Management of Pain. Although hip arthroplasty is performed to relieve joint pain, the client does experience pain related to the surgical procedure. Many clients state that they have pain after surgery but that it is of a different type and is less excruciating than the pain before surgery. Pain control may be achieved by epidural analgesia, patient-controlled analgesia (PCA), intramuscular opioid analgesia, or a combination of techniques. Chapter 7 contains a chart of commonly used opioid analgesics used for acute pain and related nursing interventions. Keep in mind that the client may also receive other analgesics or anti-inflammatory drugs for chronic arthritic pain in other joints.

Another device for pain control after TJA is a small pump called the Pain Buster. This pump continuously infuses a local anesthetic, such as bupivacaine, directly into the surgical site. The local infusion decreases the amount of opioids that the client needs (e.g., morphine), thus reducing the risk of adverse drug reactions. The device is also ideal for ambulatory surgical clients, who may go home with the device (Kettelman, 2000). After the catheter is removed in 24 to 48 hours, the entire device is discarded and the site is covered with a sterile dressing.

CONSIDERATIONS FOR OLDER ADULTS

Anticipate the older client's need for pain medication if he or she cannot verbalize the need. Many older adults experience several days of increased disorientation or delirium as a result of surgery and anesthesia.

Regardless of the pain management method used, most clients do not require parenteral analgesia after the first 2 days. Oral opioids, such as oxycodone (Supeudol✱) or oxycodone plus acetaminophen (Percocet, Tylox), are then commonly prescribed until the pain can be controlled by NSAIDs such as ketorolac (Toradol, Acular) or ibuprofen (Motrin, Apo Ibuprofen✱); however, these NSAIDs can impair bone healing (Hutchinson, 2004). Current recommendations are that clients who have orthopedic surgery take NSAIDs on a short-term basis, up to 14 days. More information on pain medication can be found in Chapter 7.

Progression of Activity. The client with a THA is usually allowed to get out of bed the day after surgery, and physical therapy is initiated. Permitted activities differ among surgeons and hospitals, but prolonged bedrest can cause numerous complications (e.g., atelectasis and pneumonia), especially in the older adults. When getting the client out of bed, stand on the same side of the bed as the client's affected leg. After achieving a sitting position, the client stands on the unaffected leg and pivots to the chair with assistance. To prevent hip dislocation, ensure that the client does not flex the hips beyond 90 degrees (Figure 24-2). Raised toilet seats, straight-back chairs, and reclining wheelchairs help prevent hyperflexion.

The surgeon, the type of prosthesis, and the surgical approach determine the resumption of weight bearing on the affected leg. A client with a cemented implant is usually allowed immediate partial weight bearing (PWB) or full weight bearing (FWB) to tolerance. A client with an uncemented prosthesis cannot tolerate FWB until bony ingrowth occurs. Typically, only PWB is permitted for the first few weeks or until there is x-ray evidence of bony ingrowth.

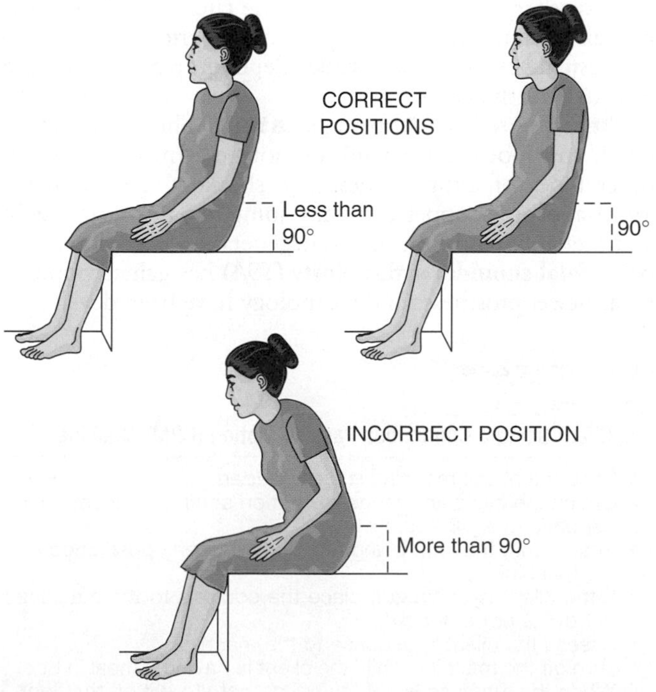

Figure 24-2 ■ Correct and incorrect hip flexion after a total hip replacement.

The physical therapist (PT) teaches the client how to follow these weight-bearing restrictions and helps the client progress to FWB status, if possible. Most clients use a walker, but younger clients may use crutches. Clients are usually advanced to a single cane or crutch if they can walk without a severe limp by 1 month after surgery. When the limp disappears, they no longer need an ambulatory/assistive device and are permitted to sit in chairs of normal height, use regular toilets, and drive a car.

Promotion of Self-Care. The hospital's occupational therapy department often supplies assistive/adaptive devices to help with activities of daily living (ADLs). Particularly important for clients are devices designed for reaching to prevent them from bending or stooping and flexing the hips more than 90 degrees. Extended handles on shoehorns and dressing sticks are particularly useful for helping clients achieve independence in ADLs.

For clients who have traditional surgery, the length of stay in the acute care hospital is typically 3 days, but older clients or those experiencing postoperative complications may stay longer. Discharge may be to the home, a rehabilitation unit, transitional care unit, or long-term care facility for rehabilitation or custodial care. For clients who have the "mini-incision" approach, discharge on the surgical day or the next day is typical. The interdisciplinary team provides written instructions for post-hospital care and reviews them with clients and their family members

CHART 24-3

CLIENT EDUCATION GUIDE
Total Hip Replacement

Hip Precautions
- Do not sit or stand for prolonged periods.
- Do not cross your legs beyond the midline of your body.
- Do not bend your hips more than 90 degrees.
- Use an ambulatory aid, such as a walker, when walking.
- Use assistive/adaptive devices for dressing, such as for putting on shoes and socks.
- Resume sexual intercourse as usual upon the advice of your surgeon.

Pain Management
- Report increased hip pain to the physician immediately.
- Take oral analgesics as prescribed and only as needed.
- Do not overexert yourself; take frequent rests.

Incisional Care
- Inspect your hip incision every day for redness, heat, or drainage; if any of these are present, call your physician immediately.
- Cleanse your hip incision with a mild soap and water every day; be sure to dry it thoroughly.

Other Care
- Continue walking and performing the leg exercises as you learned in the hospital.
- Report pain, redness, or swelling in your legs to your physician immediately.
- Report chest pain or shortness of breath to your physician immediately.
- If you are taking an anticoagulant for 4 to 6 weeks, follow the precautions learned in the hospital to prevent bleeding; avoid using a straight razor, avoid injuries, and report bleeding or excessive bruising to your surgeon immediately.

(Chart 24-3). A copy of the post-hospital instructions is sent with clients who are transferred to a facility. Rehabilitation usually takes about 6 weeks, although this time frame depends on the client's age and tolerance as well as the type of prosthesis used.

Total Knee Arthroplasty. After total hip arthroplasty, the second most common total joint arthroplasty procedure involves the knee (total knee arthroplasty, or TKA). The knee is not a simple hinged joint; it is a condylar joint that rotates slightly when flexed and extended. The expected use of a TKA is about 10 to 15 years, but the time is variable depending on the age of the client, type of prosthesis, and activity of the client postoperatively.

Preoperative Care. Only severe symptoms and disability justify TKA in clients with osteoarthritis (OA). Like hip arthroplasty, TKAs are typically avoided in people younger than 60 years of age. The preoperative care for clients undergoing a TKA is similar to that for total hip replacement. The major difference is the teaching, which depends on the postoperative protocol used by the orthopedic surgeon.

Operative Procedures. As with the hip, the knee can be replaced with the client under general or neuroaxial (epidural or spinal) anesthesia. The surgeon typically makes a central longitudinal incision about 8 inches (20.3 cm) long. Osteotomies of the femoral and tibial condyles and of the posterior patella are performed, and the surfaces are prepared for the prosthesis. Noncemented implants are used less for the knee than they are for the hip. The surgeon inserts one or two surgical drains and applies a pressure dressing to prevent bleeding. Some clients have bilateral knee replacements as part of one surgery.

Postoperative Care. Postoperative nursing care of the client with a TKA is similar to that for the client with a total hip arthroplasty; however, maintaining abduction is not necessary. The surgeon usually prescribes a continuous passive motion (CPM) machine, which can be applied in the postanesthesia care unit (PACU) or not used until 1 to 2 days after surgery (Figure 24-3). The CPM keeps the prosthetic knee in motion and prevents the formation of scar tissue, which could impede mobility of the knee and exacerbate postoperative pain. In the immediate postoperative period, the surgeon may also order ice packs or a Hot/Ice Machine to decrease swelling at the surgical site. Swelling and bruising are common with this type of surgery.

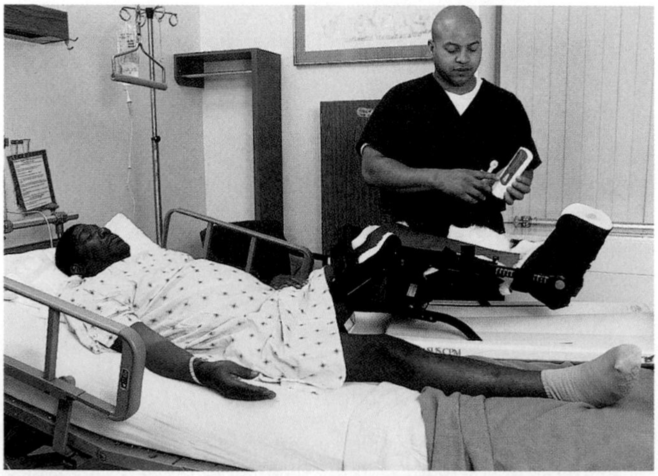

Figure 24-3 ■ A continuous passive motion machine in use.

The surgeon, PT, or technician presets the CPM machine for the appropriate range of motion and cycles per minute. A typical initial setting is 20 to 30 degrees of flexion and full extension (0 degrees) at two cycles per minute, but this setting varies according to surgeon preference. The CPM machine is generally used for 8 to 12 hours per day, with the range of motion increased gradually. The current trend is intermittent use for several hours at a time. Note the client's response to the device and follow the surgeon's protocol for settings.

Some machines do not allow the leg to achieve full extension, thus promoting flexion contractures. One solution is for the client to use the CPM machine during the day and sleep in a knee immobilizer at night to achieve the desired extension. Chart 24-4 outlines the nurse's responsibility when caring for a client using the CPM machine.

In general, pain-control measures for clients with TKA are similar to clients with total hip arthroplasty. Intra-articular morphine for the first 24 hours after surgery is a safe and effective alternative for pain management.

Because dislocation is a rare problem for a client with total knee replacement (TKR), special positioning is usually not required. The knee should be maintained in a neutral position and not rotated internally or externally. Other complications that affect clients with THA may also affect clients with TKA, such as venous thromboembolism, infection, and bleeding. Monitor neurovascular status frequently to check for compromise to the distal operative leg. The preventive and treatment measures described earlier for total hip arthroplasty are also used for TKA (see earlier discussion of postoperative care for total hip arthroplasty, p. 387).

The goal for discharge from the acute hospital unit is that the client should walk independently with a cane or walker and have close to 90 degrees of flexion in the operative knee. The use of a stationary bicycle can help gain flexion. After discharge from the hospital, the client should not hyperflex the knee or kneel for prolonged periods. Rehabilitation usually takes about 6 weeks, depending on the age and tolerance of the client.

Other Joint Arthroplasties. Shoulder, elbow, hand, and foot replacements are not performed as often as other types of arthroplasties. The shoulder (glenohumeral joint) and other upper extremity joints do not bear weight and therefore tend to have less degeneration and subsequent pain. **Total shoulder arthroplasty (TSA)** has gained popularity as newer prostheses and technology have been developed.

CHART 24-4

BEST PRACTICE for
The Client Using a Continuous Passive Motion (CPM) Machine

- Ensure that the machine is well padded.
- Check the cycle and range-of-motion settings at least once per shift (every 8 hours).
- Ensure that the joint being moved is properly positioned on the machine.
- If the client is confused, place the controls to the machine out of his or her reach.
- Assess the client's response to the machine.
- Turn off the machine while the client is having a meal in bed.
- When the machine is not in use, do not store it on the floor.

These procedures usually decrease arthritic pain and increase the client's ability to perform activities of daily living (ADLs). Because the glenohumeral joint is complex and has many **articulations** (joint surfaces), subluxation (or dislocation) can be a complication. A Neer-type prosthesis is commonly used, with or without cement. A **hemiarthroplasty** (replacement of part of the joint), typically the humeral component, may be performed as an alternative to TSA.

The client's operative arm may be placed in a CPM machine shortly after surgery (see Chart 24-4). As an alternative, passive exercises are done to begin shoulder mobilization. As for other total joint arthroplasties, frequent neurovascular assessments are important. Major complications are rare, although a few cases of pulmonary embolism (PE) have occurred. Monitor the client's respiratory rate and rhythm carefully to detect early indications of a PE. The hospital stay is shorter than for a total hip replacement or total knee replacement, usually 1 to 2 days until pain is controlled. Rehabilitation with physical therapy generally takes 2 to 3 months.

Total elbow arthroplasty (TEA) is performed most commonly for clients with rheumatoid arthritis (RA). It is usually successful in increasing range of motion, but infection and loosening may occur because of extensive tissue cutting during surgery. A CPM device may be used postoperatively, or passive exercises are prescribed. In general, elbow motion is allowed as tolerated. Physical therapy may not be necessary, but the need depends on the individual client. Generalized swelling usually resolves in 3 to 6 months.

Any joint of the hand or foot can be replaced **(finger or metatarsal arthroplasties),** often for clients with RA. Flexible, silicone prostheses are implanted without the use of polymethyl methacrylate because the devices are not ceramic or metal.

For the hand, a bulky dressing is used temporarily after surgery and is then replaced with a dynamic splint, brace, cast, or very small CPM machine. Edema formation is controlled if the client elevates the arm as much as possible. The rehabilitation program for finger arthroplasties may last for weeks, until normal function and strength return. These procedures are typically performed in specialized hand centers. Toe replacements typically require less rehabilitation.

Any bone of the wrist can also be replaced, including the heads of the radius and ulna. The postoperative pressure dressing is removed in 2 to 3 days, and a splint is applied. The client usually regains full function within 6 to 12 weeks, but lifting may be restricted for a longer period. Occupational therapists are usually involved with upper-extremity rehabilitation.

Because the ankles support about 25% of the body's weight and are complex joints, developing an implant that is both small enough and strong enough has been difficult. When a **total ankle arthroplasty (TAA)** is performed, an **arthrodesis** (bone fusion) is usually performed for added stability. Although TAAs have been problematic for more than three decades, newer noncemented prosthetic systems have renewed interest in ankle replacements. Ankle replacements have better client outcomes for clients with RA and OA than has arthrodesis alone.

Postoperative complications include infection, delayed wound healing, nerve injuries, and loosening. Therefore, TAA is not as successful as total hip or knee replacements. Noncemented prostheses seem to be preferred over cemented ones to prevent loosening. The client is allowed to begin weight bearing at about 6 weeks, and rehabilitation continues for about 3 months.

IMPAIRED PHYSICAL MOBILITY

NOC **PLANNING: EXPECTED OUTCOMES.** The client with osteoarthritis (OA) is expected to move purposefully in his or her own environment independently, with or without an assistive device. Indicators include that the client will have noncompromised:

- Balance and coordination
- Gait
- Joint movement
- Transfer performance
- Walking

INTERVENTIONS. Management of the client with OA is an interdisciplinary effort. Collaborate with physical (PT) and occupational therapists (OT) to meet the goal of independent function. Major interventions include therapeutic exercise and the promotion of ADLs and ambulation by teaching about health and the use of assistive devices.

Exercise. Two types of exercise are recommended for the client with OA: recreational and therapeutic. **Recreational exercise** includes hobbies and sports, with no planned purpose other than relaxation. **Therapeutic exercise** includes carefully planned activities that are designed to improve muscle strength, muscle tone, and joint range of motion. Therapeutic exercise can also reduce pain and improve the client's psychological health.

Certain recreational activities may also be therapeutic, such as doing the breaststroke during swimming to enhance chest and arm muscles. Aerobic exercises (e.g., walking, biking, swimming, aerobic dance) are recommended. Usually the PT prescribes exercises for the client with OA, but the nurse reinforces their techniques and principles. The ideal time for exercise is immediately after the application of heat. To prevent further joint damage, clients should rigorously follow the instructions for exercise outlined in Chart 24-5.

Use of Assistive Devices. The PT evaluates the client's need for ambulatory aids such as canes, walkers, or platform crutches. Although many clients do not like to use

CHART 24-5

CLIENT EDUCATION GUIDE
Exercises for Clients with Osteoarthritis or Rheumatoid Arthritis

- Follow the exercise instructions that have been prescribed specifically prescribed for you. There are no universal exercises; your exercises have been specifically tailored to your needs.
- Do your exercises on both "good" and "bad" days. Consistency is important.
- Respect pain. If pain increases as you exercise, stop and report this to your health care provider.
- Use active rather than active-assist or passive exercise whenever possible.
- Reduce the number of repetitions when the inflammation is severe and you have more pain.
- Do not substitute your normal activities or household tasks for the prescribed exercises.
- Avoid resistive exercises when your joints are severely inflamed.

these aids or may forget how to use them, they do help prevent further joint deterioration and pain. An OT evaluates the client's ability to perform ADLs and can provide ideas and devices for assistance.

Community-Based Care

The client with OA is not usually hospitalized for the disease itself but for surgical management. The cost of medical and surgical care for clients with OA has been evaluated (see the Resource Management box below).

HOME CARE MANAGEMENT

If weight-bearing joints are markedly involved, the client may have difficulty going up or down stairs. Making arrangements to live on one floor with accessibility to all rooms is often the best solution. A home care nurse, PT, or OT assesses the need for structural alterations to the home to accommodate ambulatory aids and enable the client to perform activities. For example, a kitchen counter may need to be lowered, or a seat and handrails may need to be installed in the shower. If the client has undergone a total hip replacement, an elevated toilet seat is necessary for several weeks postoperatively to prevent excessive hip flexion.

HEALTH TEACHING

Learning how to protect the joint is the most important feature of client education. Preventing further damage to joints slows the progression of OA and minimizes pain. Explain the general rules of joint protection and cite examples (Chart 24-6).

As with other diseases in which drugs and diet therapy are used, teach the medication protocol, desired and potential side effects, and toxic effects to the client and family. Emphasize the importance of reducing weight and eating a well-balanced diet to promote tissue healing.

Many clients with "arthritis" look for a cure after becoming frustrated and desperate about the course of the disease and treatment. Better control of arthritis is possible, but cure is not yet available. Unfortunately tabloids, books, and the media often cite "curative" remedies. People spend billions of dollars each year on quackery, including liniments, special diets, and copper bracelets. More hazardous substances, such as snake venom and industrial cleaners, are also advertised as remedies. Refer the client to the Arthritis Foundation for up-to-date information about new "cures." The practice of wearing a copper bracelet will not cure arthritis, but it will not hurt the client. If the client is doing something that can be potentially harmful, however, instruct the client to avoid that modality and provide the rationale.

With most types of arthritis and connective tissue disease (CTD), clients must live with a chronic, unpredictable, and painful disorder. Their roles, self-esteem, and body image may be affected by these diseases. Body image is often not as devastating in OA as in the inflammatory arthritic diseases, such as RA. The psychosocial component is discussed in more detail under Psychosocial Assessment (Rheumatoid Arthritis) on p. 395.

HEALTH CARE RESOURCES

The client who has undergone surgery is most likely to need help from community resources. After an arthroplasty, he or she needs extensive assistance with mobility. The client may be discharged to home, a long-term care facility, a transitional care unit, or a rehabilitation unit. Collaborate with the case manager and physician to find the best placement. If the client is discharged to home, home care nurses may be approved for several visits, depending on the concurrent systemic diseases. A nursing assistant may visit the home to help with hygiene-related needs, and a physical therapist may work with ambulatory and mobility skills. A client who has undergone a total hip or knee replacement should not be discharged to home alone. A family member, significant other, or other caregiver

RESOURCE MANAGEMENT

OSTEOARTHRITIS

Cost of Care

- The cost of medical care for older clients with osteoarthritis (OA) is about twice that of older clients with no symptomatic OA.
- The average individual cost of arthritis-related care for clients with rheumatoid arthritis (RA) is about $2200 per year. Medications account for almost two thirds of the cost, and hospital care accounts for 16%. By contrast, the average individual cost for clients with OA is about $550 per year. Medications account for about one third of the cost, and hospital care accounts for close to one half of the cost (most due to total joint arthroplasty).
- Although the individual cost of care for clients with OA is about one fourth of that for clients with RA, the total cost for OA is about seven times greater because the higher prevalence of OA.
- One half of the costs for OA is due to sick days from work: $15.5 billion in the United States.
- Clinical pathways for total hip replacement reduce the length of stay and hospital costs.

Implications for Nursing

Because of the high cost of medications for OA and RA, nurses need to become more familiar with the use of integrative therapies for pain management. Research has shown that some modalities are as effective as analgesics and others serve as excellent adjuncts for pain control. For clients undergoing total joint replacement, extensive staff and client education is needed to follow clinical pathways and ensure positive clinical and cost outcomes.

CHART 24-6

CLIENT EDUCATION GUIDE
Evidence-Based Instructions for Joint Protection

- Use large joints instead of small ones; for example, place your purse strap over your shoulder instead of grasping the purse with your hand.
- Do not turn a doorknob clockwise. Turn it counterclockwise to avoid twisting your arm and promoting ulnar deviation.
- Use two hands instead of one to hold objects.
- Sit in a chair that has a high, straight back.
- When getting out of bed, do not push off with your fingers; use the entire palm of both hands.
- Do not bend at your waist; instead, bend your knees while keeping your back straight.
- Use long-handled devices, such as a hairbrush with an extended handle.
- Use assistive/adaptive devices, such as Velcro closures and built-up utensil handles, to protect your joints.
- Do not use pillows in bed, except a small one under your head.
- Avoid twisting or wringing your hands.

must be in the home at all times for at least the first 4 to 6 weeks—when the client needs the most assistance.

Provide written instructions about the required care, regardless of whether the client goes home or to another inpatient facility. Communication with the new care provider is essential for seamless continuity of care. Arrangements are made for the client to return to the same acute care hospital if needed.

The Arthritis Foundation is an important community resource for all clients with arthritis and CTD. This organization provides information to lay people and health care professionals and refers clients and their families to other resources as needed. Local support groups can help clients and their families cope with these diseases.

Critical Thinking Challenge

Your older client is unable to obtain pain control for OA of the hip and knee and therefore undergoes a left cemented total hip replacement. She returns to the assisted living facility for rehabilitation following a 3-day hospital stay. She is able to ambulate with a walker in her room and wears thigh-high elastic stockings. Her discharge medication orders include Coumadin and Tylox for pain.

1. What teaching should you reinforce with her related to Coumadin?
2. What weight-bearing allowance will she most likely have?
3. What surgical complications is she still at risk for, and how can you help prevent them?

evolve For suggested answer guidelines, go to http://evolve.elsevier.com/Iggy/.

Evaluation: Outcomes

Evaluate the care of the client with OA on the basis of the identified nursing diagnoses. The expected outcomes are that the client:

- Takes personal actions to control pain
- Moves purposefully in his or her own environment independently with or without an assistive device

Specific indicators for these outcomes are listed for each nursing diagnosis under the Planning and Implementation section (see earlier).

RHEUMATOID ARTHRITIS

PATHOPHYSIOLOGY

Rheumatoid arthritis (RA) is one of the most common connective tissue diseases and is the most destructive to the joints. It is a chronic, progressive, systemic inflammatory autoimmune disease process that primarily affects the synovial joints. **Systemic** means this disease affects the body system, affecting many joints and other tissues.

In RA, autoantibodies (rheumatoid factors [RFs]) are formed that attack healthy tissue, especially synovium, causing inflammation. RFs consist mainly of immunoglobulin M and G, and they bind with antigens forming immune complexes. Phagocytes attempt to engulf these complexes and, as a result, release powerful enzymes, such as cytokines. The B- and T-lymphocytes of the immune system are also stimulated and increase the inflammatory response.

Inflammation occurs first in the synovial membrane, which lines the joint cavity. It then begins to involve the articular cartilage, joint capsule, and surrounding ligaments and tendons. Three processes cause cartilage damage in clients with RA (McCance & Huether, 2002):

1. Neutrophils and other cells in synovial fluid are activated and break down the joint cartilage
2. Cytokines, especially interleukin-1 (IL-1) and tumor necrosis factor–alpha (TNFA), cause chondrocytes to attack cartilage. TNF has effects on lipid metabolism, coagulation, insulin resistance, and endothelial function.
3. Synovium digests cartilage, releasing inflammatory substances, such as IL-1 and TNFA. (See Chapter 23 for a complete discussion of the inflammatory response.)

The synovium then thickens and becomes hyperemic, fluid accumulates in the joint space, and a pannus forms. The **pannus** is vascular granulation tissue composed of inflammatory cells; it erodes articular cartilage and eventually destroys bone. As a result, fibrous adhesions, bony ankylosis, and calcifications occur; bone loses density and secondary osteoporosis occurs.

Permanent joint changes can be avoided if RA is diagnosed early. Early, aggressive treatment to suppress synovitis may cause a remission. RA is a disease characterized by natural remissions and exacerbations. Medical treatment helps control the disease to decrease the intensity and number of exacerbations. Preventing RA flares helps prevent joint erosion and permanent joint damage. Advancement of knowledge regarding the disease process and immune system provides many newer treatment options that better control this disease.

Rheumatoid arthritis is a systemic disease; that is, areas of the body besides the synovial joints can be affected. Inflammatory responses similar to those occurring in synovial tissue may be seen in any organ or body system in which connective tissue is prevalent. If blood vessel involvement **(vasculitis)** occurs, the organ supplied by that vessel can be affected. The result is malfunction and eventual failure of the organ or system. These pathologic changes may occur late in the disease process and cause life-threatening problems.

The etiology of RA remains unclear, but research suggests a combination of environmental and genetic factors.

Genetic Considerations

Rheumatoid arthritis shows some familial clustering, suggesting either a genetic predisposition or gene-environment interaction. Gene mutations are associated with RA, especially if they are present in a person with varieties of the tissue type human leukocyte antigen (HLA)-DRB, HLA-DR4, or HLA-DP (McCance & Huether, 2002). For example, the risk for developing the disease in a person with HLA-DRB tissue type who is homozygous for mutations in any one of three susceptibility genes is 30% to 40% for men and 45% to 55% for women (Online Mendelian Inheritance in Man, 2004).

Some researchers suspect that female reproductive hormones influence the development of RA because it affects women more often than men—usually young- to middle-aged women. Others suspect that infectious organisms may play a role, particularly the Epstein-Barr virus (McCance & Huether, 2002). Physical and emotional stresses have been linked to exacerbations of the disorder and may be contributing factors in its development.

CULTURAL CONSIDERATIONS

Despite the common lay belief that warm, dry climates can be beneficial to people with RA, there are no significant differences in its prevalence among geographic locations. The incidence of RA in China is somewhat lower than elsewhere in the world (about 0.3%) and substantially higher among the Pima Indians in North America (about 5%) (Harris, 2001). The cause for these differences is not known.

COLLABORATIVE MANAGEMENT

Assessment

The onset of rheumatoid arthritis (RA) may be acute and severe or slow and insidious; clients may have vague complaints that last for several months before diagnosis. The onset of the disease is more common in the winter months than in the warmer months. The manifestations of RA can be categorized as early or late disease and as articular (joint) or extra-articular (Chart 24-7).

PHYSICAL ASSESSMENT/CLINICAL MANIFESTATIONS

EARLY DISEASE MANIFESTATIONS. The client with RA typically complains of joint stiffness, swelling, pain, fatigue, and may complain of generalized weakness and morning stiffness. Anorexia and a weight loss of about 2 or 3 pounds (1 kg) may occur early in the disease process. Persistent low-grade fever may accompany these complaints. In clients with early disease, the upper-extremity joints are often involved initially, typically the proximal interphalangeal (PIP) and metacarpophalangeal (MCP) joints of the hands. These joints may be slightly reddened, warm, stiff, swollen, and tender or painful, particularly on palpation **(synovitis).** The typical pattern of joint involvement in RA is bilateral and symmetric (e.g., both wrists), and the number of joints involved usually increases as the disease progresses. In early disease, the client may complain of migrating symptoms known as **migratory arthritis.** The presence of only *one* hot, swollen, painful joint (out of proportion to the other joints) may mean the joint is infected. Refer the client to the health care provider (generally the rheumatologist) immediately. Single hot, swollen joints are considered infected until proven otherwise and require immediate long-term antibiotic treatment.

CHART 24-7

KEY FEATURES of
The Client with Rheumatoid Arthritis

Early Manifestations
Joint
- Inflammation

Systemic
- Low-grade fever
- Fatigue
- Weakness
- Anorexia
- Paresthesias

Late Manifestations
Joint
- Deformities (e.g., swan neck or ulnar deviation)
- Moderate to severe pain and morning stiffness

Systemic
- Osteoporosis
- Severe fatigue
- Anemia
- Weight loss
- Subcutaneous nodules
- Peripheral neuropathy
- Vasculitis
- Pericarditis
- Fibrotic lung disease
- Sjögren's syndrome
- Renal disease

LATE DISEASE MANIFESTATIONS. As the disease worsens, the joints become progressively inflamed and quite painful. The client complains of morning stiffness (also called the **gel phenomenon**), which lasts between 45 minutes and several hours after awakening. On palpation, the joints feel soft and look puffy because of synovitis and **effusions** (joint swelling with fluid, especially the knees). The fingers often appear spindle-like. Note any muscle atrophy (which can result from disuse secondary to joint pain) and a decreased range of motion in the affected joints.

Most or all synovial joints are eventually affected. The temporomandibular joint (TMJ) may be involved in severe disease, but such involvement is uncommon. When the TMJ is affected, the client typically complains of pain when chewing or opening the mouth.

When the spinal column is involved, the cervical joints are most likely to be affected. During clinical examination, gently palpate the posterior cervical spine and identify it as cervical pain, tenderness, or loss of motion. Cervical disease may result in subluxation, especially with the first and second vertebrae. This complication may be life threatening because branches of the phrenic nerve that supply the diaphragm can be compressed, and respiratory function may be subsequently compromised. The client is also in danger of becoming quadriparetic or quadriplegic. If you identify cervical pain or loss of range of motion in the cervical spine of a person with RA, report this information to the client's physician, generally the rheumatologist. Collaboration of such information will assist the physician or other provider to obtain the necessary cervical spine x-ray and may save that client's life. Surgical stabilization is sometimes necessary.

JOINT INVOLVEMENT. Joint deformity occurs as a late, articular manifestation, and secondary osteoporosis can cause bone fractures. Observe common deformities, especially in the hands and feet (Figure 24-4). Extensive wrist involvement can result in carpal tunnel syndrome (see Chapter 54 for assessment and management of carpal tunnel syndrome).

Palpate the tissues around the joints to elicit pain or tenderness associated with other rheumatoid complications. For example, **Baker's cysts** (enlarged popliteal bursae) may occur and cause tissue compression and pain. Tendon rupture is also possible, particularly rupture of the Achilles tendon.

SYSTEMIC COMPLICATIONS. Numerous extra-articular clinical manifestations are associated with advanced disease. Assess other body systems to ascertain systemic involvement. In addition to increased joint swelling and tenderness, moderate to severe weight loss, fever, and extreme fatigue are common in late disease **exacerbations,** often called "flares." Approximately 25% of clients have the

A
B
C

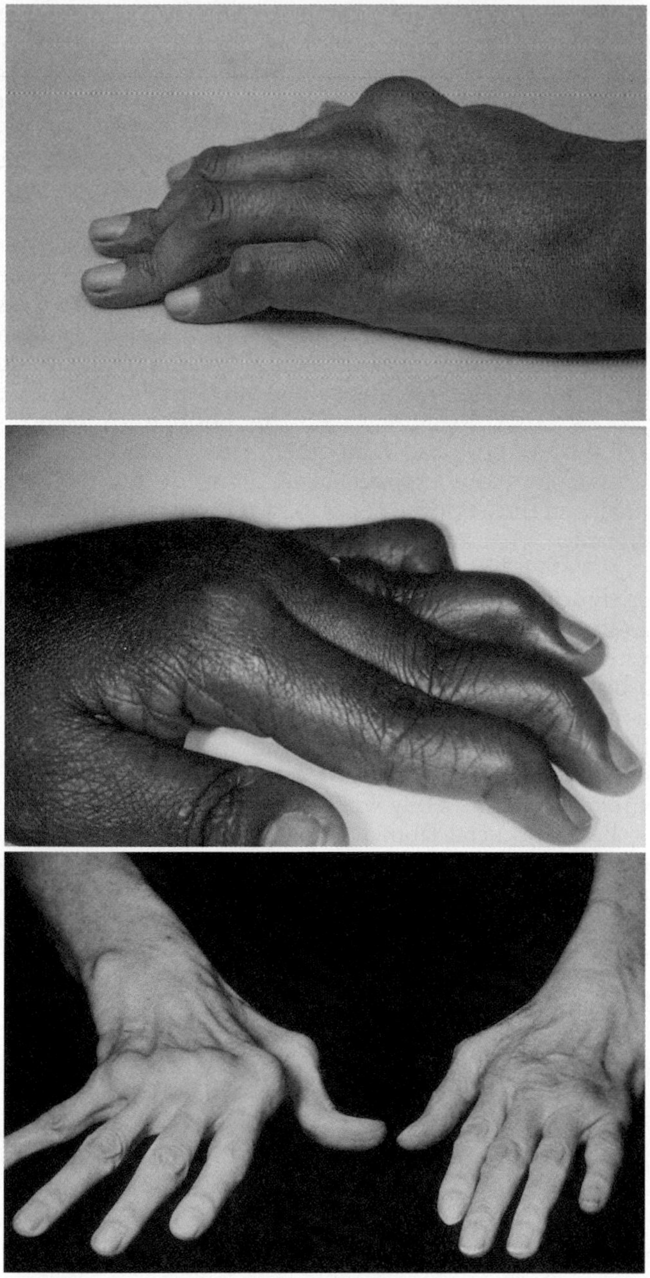

Figure 24-4 ■ Common joint deformities seen in rheumatoid arthritis. **A,** Boutonniere, or buttonhole. **B,** Swan neck. **C,** Ulnar deviation *(on left).* (From the Arthritis Teaching Slide Collection, copyright 1980. Used by permission of the Arthritis Foundation.)

characteristic round, movable, nontender **subcutaneous nodules,** which most often appear on the ulnar surface of the arm, on the fingers, or along the Achilles tendon. These nodules can disappear and reappear at any time and are associated with severe, destructive disease. Rheumatoid nodules are not generally a problem themselves; however, they occasionally open and become infected, and they may interfere with activities of daily living (ADLs). Bumping nodules may cause discomfort or pain. Occasionally nodules are identified within the lungs.

Inflammation of the blood vessels results in vasculitis, particularly of small- to medium-sized vessels. When arterial involvement occurs, major organs and body systems become ischemic and malfunction. Ischemic skin lesions appear in groups as small, brownish spots, most commonly around the nail bed **(periungual lesions).** Monitor the number of lesions, note their location each day, and report vascular changes to the health care provider. An increased number of lesions indicates increased vasculitis, and a decreased number indicates decreased vasculitis. Also carefully assess any larger lesions that appear on the lower extremities; such lesions often lead to ulceration, which heal slowly as a result of decreased circulation. Peripheral neuropathy associated with decreased circulation can cause foot drop and paresthesias (burning and tingling sensations), most often in older adults.

Respiratory complications manifest as pleurisy, pneumonitis, diffuse interstitial fibrosis, and pulmonary hypertension. Cardiac complications include pericarditis and myocarditis. Assess for ocular involvement, which typically manifests as iritis and scleritis. If either of these complications is present, the sclera of one or both eyes is reddened and the pupils have an irregular shape.

ASSOCIATED SYNDROMES. Several syndromes are seen in clients with advanced RA. The most common is **Sjögren's syndrome,** which includes a triad of the following:

- Dry eyes (keratoconjunctivitis sicca [KCS], or the sicca syndrome)
- Dry mouth **(xerostomia)**
- Dry vagina (in some cases)

In Sjögren's syndrome, immune complexes and inflammatory cells are thought to obstruct secretory glands and ducts. The syndrome is usually associated with connective tissue diseases such as RA but may occur alone. Note the client's complaint of dry mouth or dry eyes. Some clients state that their eyes feel "gritty," as if sand is in their eyes. Inspect the mouth for dry, sticky membranes and the eyes for redness and lack of tearing.

Less commonly observed is **Felty's syndrome,** which is characterized by RA, hepatosplenomegaly (enlarged liver and spleen), and leukopenia. **Caplan's syndrome** is characterized by the presence of rheumatoid nodules in the lungs and pneumoconiosis, which is noted primarily in coal miners and asbestos workers. The health care provider diagnoses these syndromes by physical examination and diagnostic testing.

PSYCHOSOCIAL ASSESSMENT

Rheumatoid arthritis (RA) and other inflammatory types of arthritis are chronic diseases that can be crippling if not well controlled. Fear of becoming disabled and dependent, uncertainty about the disease process, altered body image, devaluation of self, frustration, and depression are common psychosocial problems (Smedstad & Liang, 2001). Physical limitations caused by disease may limit activities of daily living (ADLs). These physical limitations result in role changes in the family and society. For example, the person may not be able to cook for the family or be an active sexual partner. In addition, extreme fatigue often causes clients to desire an early bedtime and may result in a reluctance to socialize.

Body changes may also cause poor self-esteem and body image. Because many societies value people with physically fit, attractive bodies, the client with RA may be embarrassed to be seen in public places. The client may grieve or experience degrees of depression. The potential exists for the client to experience a feeling of helplessness accompanied by a loss of control over a disease that can "consume" the body. Fortunately, newer medications have significantly improved the treatment of RA and provide the client with hope and better control of the disease.

Living with a chronic disease and the pain that results may be difficult for the client, family, and significant others. The client may experience a loss of control and independence, especially if he or she is over 65 years of age (Ignatavicius, 2001). Chronic suffering affects quality of life. Assess the client's emotional and mental status in relation to the disease and its problems and evaluate the client's support systems and resources. Help each client gain control of his or her disease. Clients who are knowledgeable about their disease and treatment options will feel emotionally stronger to cope with their disease and better able to discuss treatment options with their physician.

LABORATORY ASSESSMENT

Laboratory tests help to support a diagnosis of RA, but no single test or group of tests can confirm it. Chart 24-8 summarizes the common laboratory tests that the health care provider uses for diagnosing connective tissue diseases.

RHEUMATOID FACTOR. The test for **rheumatoid factor (RF)** measures the presence of unusual antibodies of the immunoglobulin G (IgG) and IgM type that develop in a number of connective tissue diseases. Two methods may be used to ascertain the degree to which these antibodies are present in the body: Rose-Waaler and latex agglutination. In both procedures, values are reported as titers.

The Rose-Waaler test is more specific for a diagnosis of RA than the latex agglutination test, but it is not as sensitive. A client with a positive Rose-Waaler result probably has RA and is seropositive; a client with a negative test result may or may not have the disease or has seronegative inflammatory polyarthritis. Approximately 60% of individuals with RA are seropositive and have a positive titer.

ANTINUCLEAR ANTIBODY TITER. The antinuclear antibody (ANA) test measures the titer of unusual antibodies that destroy the nuclei of cells and cause tissue death. The fluorescent method is sometimes referred to as FANA. If this test result is positive (a value higher than 1:8), various subtypes of this antibody are identified and measured. ANA is often negative until later in the disease process. ANA does not have to be positive to diagnosis RA. ANA can be positive in other rheumatic diseases, such as systemic lupus erythematosus. It is also positive in a small percentage of the population without any underlying disease.

ERYTHROCYTE SEDIMENTATION RATE. The erythrocyte sedimentation rate (ESR) or "sed rate," when it is elevated, can confirm inflammation or infection anywhere in the body. An elevation in the ESR helps point to a diagnosis of an inflammatory connective tissue disease; however, a high ESR does not always relate to severity of inflammatory disease. The high-sensitivity C-reactive protein, or hsCRP, is another useful test to measure inflammation and may be done along with or instead of the ESR.

Because several laboratory procedures are used to measure ESR, normal values will vary; women have higher normal values than men. In general, a value of 20 to 40 mm/hr

CHART 24-8

LABORATORY PROFILE
Connective Tissue Disease

Test	Normal Range for Adults	Significance of Abnormal Findings
Rheumatoid factor		
Rose-Waaler	Negative	Elevations of either titer (increase in number at right of colon) indicative of possible CTD Increased Rose's titer indicative of RA (seropositive); not a sensitive test
Latex agglutination	<1:16	Latex titer not as specific to one disease, but quite a sensitive test
ANA (total)	Negative (if positive, types of ANA identified [e.g., anti-DNA, anti-DNP, anti-RNA] to indicate what part of cells are involved)	Elevations common in SLE, PSS, RA, and other inflammatory CTDs (5% of healthy adults have positive ANA results)
Serum complement (C′ or CH_{50})	Varies greatly among laboratories	Decreased value indicative of active autoimmune disease such as SLE
LE preparation	Negative	A type of ANA (anti-DNP); not reliable because negative result does not rule out SLE; can be used as screening test
SPEP		
Albumin	3.5-5.0 g/dL	Increased levels of gamma globulins indicative of CTD (inflammatory type)
Globulin		
$Alpha_1$ globulin	0.1-0.3 g/dL	Increased level of alpha globulins possible in RA
$Alpha_2$ globulin	0.6-1.0 g/dL	
Beta globulin	0.7-1.1 g/dL	
Gamma globulin	0.8-1.6 g/dL	
HLA testing (HLA-B27)	None	Presence of HLA-B27 indicative of Reiter's syndrome or ankylosing spondylitis

ANA, Antinuclear antibody; *CTD*, connective tissue disease; *DNP*, dinitrophenol; *ESR*, erythrocyte sedimentation rate; *HLA*, human leukocyte antigen; *LE*, lupus erythematosus; *PSS*, progressive systemic sclerosis; *RA*, rheumatoid arthritis; *SLE*, systemic lupus erythematosus; *SPEP*, serum protein electrophoresis.

indicates mild inflammation; 40 to 70 mm/hr, moderate inflammation; and 70 to 150 mm/hr, severe inflammation.

The ESR is not always a reliable indicator but may sometimes be used to monitor a client's response to anti-inflammatory drug therapy. This value should decrease if the drug dosage is effective. The ESR may also be elevated with infection and in older adults.

OTHER LABORATORY TESTS. Serum complement attaches to immune complexes in an attempt to destroy them. If a large amount of complement is used in this lytic process, the concentration of free-floating complement in the blood diminishes. Normal values vary considerably, depending on the laboratory technique used. An abnormal finding is indicated by a decrease in serum complement and is seen primarily in clients with vasculitis.

In **serum protein electrophoresis,** the protein fractions of the plasma are measured, and an electrical current is used to separate them. The level of alpha globulin is raised in acute inflammation; in chronic inflammatory conditions such as RA, the level of gamma globulin is increased because of the increase in immunoglobulins.

The **serum immunoglobulins** can be separated into subtypes. In chronic inflammation, IgG is needed to combine with RF. Thus in RA the IgG value is typically elevated.

The presence of most chronic diseases usually causes mild to moderate anemia, which contributes to the client's fatigue. Therefore the client's complete blood count (CBC) is monitored for a low hemoglobin, hematocrit, and red blood cell (RBC) count. An increase in white blood cell (WBC) count is consistent with an inflammatory response. A decrease in the WBC count may indicate Felty's syndrome. Thrombocytosis (increased platelets) is common in clients with RA. Additional laboratory tests may be performed depending on the body systems and organs that may be affected by the disease. For example, if heart involvement is suspected, the health care provider may order cardiac enzymes.

OTHER DIAGNOSTIC ASSESSMENTS

A standard x-ray is used to visualize the joint changes and deformities typical of RA. A computed tomography (CT) scan may help to determine the presence and degree of cervical spine involvement.

An **arthrocentesis** is a diagnostic procedure that may be used for clients with joint involvement. It may be performed at the bedside or in a physician's office or clinic. After administering a local anesthetic, the physician inserts a large-gauge needle into the joint (usually the knee) to aspirate a sample of synovial fluid; this procedure may also relieve pressure. The fluid is analyzed for inflammatory cells and immune complexes, including RF. Fluid from clients with RA shows increased WBCs, turbidity, and volume. After the procedure, monitor the insertion site for bleeding or leakage of synovial fluid. Notify the physician if either of these problems occurs. Teach the client to use ice and rest the affected joint for 24 hours. Often the health care provider will recommend acetaminophen as needed for pain. If increased pain or swelling occurs, have the client notify the health care provider.

A bone scan or joint scan can also assess the extent of joint involvement. Magnetic resonance imaging (MRI) may be performed to assess spinal column disease.

Because RA can affect multiple body systems, tests to diagnose specific systemic manifestations are performed as necessary. For example, electromyography helps to confirm peripheral neuropathy. Pulmonary function tests help to determine the presence of lung involvement.

Interventions

As in other types of arthritis, the health care team manages pain by using a combination of pharmacologic and nonpharmacologic measures. Total joint arthroplasty may be indicated when these measures are no longer effective (see earlier discussion of this surgery in the section on Osteoarthritis, p. 385). The Plan of Care on pp. 398 to 402 highlights the most important interdisciplinary interventions for the client with rheumatoid arthritis (RA).

Drug Therapy. Some medications prescribed for RA have analgesic, antipyretic, and anti-inflammatory actions. Other drugs are immunosuppressive and disease modifying, which may cause remission of the illness and prevent erosive joint changes. Biological response modifiers are the newest class of disease-modifying drugs that help reduce signals for the immune system to cause inflammation and thereby reduce the amount of inflammation that the joint receives (see Chart 24-9 on pp. 403-404). These medications have demonstrated superior performance, giving clients additional benefits never before imagined. Clients with inflammatory diseases other than RA are also using various biological response modifying medications successfully. Future genetic research will further advance these medications to give even better control of autoimmune diseases. Although RA is a chronic disease and no cure is yet available, medications now used are better able to control the disease and prevent further deterioration.

Management of Mild Disease. The health care provider, usually a rheumatologist, makes decisions about appropriate drug therapy for clients with rheumatoid disease based on the severity of the disease. Mild disease is usually managed with nonsteroidal anti-inflammatory drugs (NSAIDs) or disease-modifying agents.

Nonsteroidal Anti-Inflammatory Drugs. The NSAIDs are often an initial drug category of choice for inflammatory arthritis to relieve pain and inflammation (see Chart 24-9). The choice of which one to administer depends on the client's needs and the physician's preference. To minimize gastrointestinal (GI) problems, the NSAID may be given with an H2-blocking agent, such as ranitidine (Zantac) or misoprostol (Cytotec). If there is no clinical change after 6 to 8 weeks, the health care provider may discontinue the current NSAID and try another one. This process may be repeated until an effective drug is found for that client. Celecoxib (Celebrex), and valdecoxib (Bextra) are COX-2 inhibiting NSAIDs that are usually preferred over older NSAIDs. COX-2 inhibitors have a decreased incidence of GI side effects associated with older NSAIDs (for further information, see Analgesic Administration [Osteoarthritis], p. 384). However, all COX-2 inhibiting drugs have recently been associated with cardiovascular disease, such as myocardial infarction, and may soon be unavailable on the market.

Salicylates are an older type of NSAID and were previously the drug of choice for pain and inflammation. Within the United States, they are no longer the drug of choice to treat RA because of toxicities, mainly GI bleeding. Salicylates are excellent anti-inflammatory drugs and relatively inexpensive, and therefore they are still used

Text continued on p. 404.

PLAN of CARE MEDICAL DIAGNOSIS: RHEUMATOID ARTHRITIS

NURSING DIAGNOSIS NO. 1 ■ Impaired Physical Mobility

	Expected Outcomes	Nursing Interventions	Rationales
RELATED FACTORS Discomfort Pain Musculoskeletal impairment Intolerance to activity **DEFINING CHARACTERISTICS** Limited ability to perform gross motor skills Limited ability to perform fine motor skills Limited range of motion Difficulty turning	Has full or improved range of motion in all joints Able to turn without assistance Has stable posture during performance of activities of daily living Able to perform fine motor skills Able to perform gross motor skills	NIC **Exercise Therapy: Joint Mobility** Collaborate with physical therapy in developing and executing an exercise program.	Physical therapists are the primary health care professionals responsible for developing and executing an exercise program.
		Initiate pain control measures before beginning joint exercise.	Initiating pain control measures before joint exercise increases the likelihood of client comfort and willingness to engage in the exercise.
		D Dress the client in nonrestrictive clothing.	Nonrestrictive clothing permits full range of joint motion.
		D Protect the client from trauma during exercise.	Stretching exercises may cause the client to be off balance.
		D Assist the client to an optimal body position for passive/active joint movement.	Neutral alignment is optimal positioning for joint movement.
		D Encourage active range-of-motion exercises, according to regular, planned schedule.	Regular active range-of-motion exercise periods maximize the exercise benefit to joints.
		Assist the client to develop a schedule for active range-of-motion exercises.	Regular exercise maximizes the benefit of the exercise.
		D Encourage ambulation, if appropriate.	Ambulation is a form of active joint exercise and also improves cardiovascular tone.
		NIC **Positioning** Provide a firm mattress.	A firm mattress offers support.
		D Encourage the client to get involved in positioning changes, as appropriate.	Involving the client in positioning changes actively exercises the muscles and joints and permits him or her a measure of control in the positioning process.
		Premedicate the client before turning, as appropriate.	Premedicating the client before turning will increase comfort and decrease resistance to repositioning from fear of pain.
		D Position in proper body alignment.	Proper body alignment preserves the functionality of the muscles and bony skeleton.
		Immobilize or support the affected body part, as appropriate.	Immobilization or support of the affected body part will permit healing and decrease further injury.
		D Elevate the affected body part, as appropriate.	Elevation of the affected body part may decrease edema by using gravity to assist with fluid drainage.
		D Avoid placing the client in a position that increases pain.	Repositioning should provide the client with a measure of comfort. Pain may indicate improper body positioning.

D Indicates tasks that can be delegated to unlicensed assistive personnel at the discretion of the nurse.

PLAN of CARE MEDICAL DIAGNOSIS: RHEUMATOID ARTHRITIS—*cont'd*

NURSING DIAGNOSIS NO. 1 ■ Impaired Physical Mobility—*cont'd*

	Expected Outcomes	Nursing Interventions	Rationales
		D Minimize friction and shearing forces when positioning and turning the client.	Friction and shearing forces will cause damage to the skin and underlying tissues.
		Develop a written schedule for repositioning, as appropriate.	A written schedule for repositioning permits all health care workers to participate in repositioning.
		D Use a hand roll or a trochanter roll, as appropriate.	Hand rolls and trochanter rolls are devices to support limbs.
		D Place frequently used objects within reach.	Placing frequently used objects within reach permits the client safe, convenient access.
		D Place the bed-positioning switch within easy reach.	Placing the bed-positioning switch within easy reach permits the client to change position safely and conveniently.
		Other Interventions	
		Instruct in the use of assistive devices.	The client will need instruction in the proper use of canes, crutches, walkers, splints, or other assistive devices.
		Continuing Care Considerations	
		Refer the client to rehabilitative services, as appropriate.	Ongoing support from physical therapists, occupational therapists, and others may be needed to help the client resume activities of daily living.
		Refer the client to a vocational counselor, as appropriate.	Long-term physical impairment may require the client to change employment.
		Collaborate with community organizations to inform the public about injury prevention.	Injury prevention saves the individual and society as a whole an enormous economic burden.

NURSING DIAGNOSIS NO. 2 ■ Chronic Pain

	Expected Outcomes	Nursing Interventions	Rationales
RELATED FACTORS		NIC **Pain Management**	
Chronic physical/psychological disability	Denies fatigue	Perform a comprehensive assessment of pain to include location, characteristics, onset/duration, frequency, quality, intensity or severity of pain, and precipitating factors.	A plan for pain management must be based on the client's unique responses to pain.
DEFINING CHARACTERISTICS	Weight remains within ±5 pounds of desired weight		
Atrophy of involved muscle group	No verbal report or observation of alteration in sleep patterns		
Sleep patterns: Change in			
Fatigue	No verbal report or observation of alteration in activity level		
Reduced interaction with people		Reduce or eliminate factors that precipitate or increase the pain experience.	Preventing a pain experience is preferred to trying to control or eliminate pain.
Altered ability to continue previous activities	No verbal report or observation of guarding or protective gestures		
Protective gestures			
Irritability	No verbal report or observation of restlessness	Select and implement a variety of measures to facilitate pain relief, as appropriate.	Pharmacologic, nonpharmacologic, and interpersonal strategies may provide pain relief depending on the client's unique responses to the therapeutic interventions.
Self-focus			
Depression	No verbal report or observation of irritability		

Continued

PLAN of CARE MEDICAL DIAGNOSIS: RHEUMATOID ARTHRITIS—*cont'd*

NURSING DIAGNOSIS NO. 2 ■ Chronic Pain—*cont'd*

Expected Outcomes	Nursing Interventions	Rationales
No verbal report or observation of self-focusing behavior	Encourage the client to monitor his or her own pain and to intervene appropriately.	The client is the best person to manage his or her own pain.
No verbal report or observation of depression No verbal report or observation of impaired socialization	Use pain control measures before pain becomes severe.	Medicating the client in a timely manner prevents pain from reaching acutely unpleasant levels.
Denies experiencing pain greater than a 5 on a 0 to 10 pain scale	Teach the use of nonpharmacologic techniques before, after and, if possible, during painful activities; before pain occurs or increases; and along with other pain relief measures.	Nonpharmacologic techniques help the client establish a sense of control over his or her pain experience.
	NIC **Analgesic Administration**	
	Administer analgesics around-the-clock.	Administration around-the-clock prevents peaks and troughs of analgesia, especially with severe pain.
	Evaluate the effectiveness of analgesics at regular frequent intervals after each administration, but especially after the initial dose; also observe for any signs and symptoms of untoward effects.	Frequent evaluation of analgesic effectiveness permits the nurse to adjust the dose and timing interval to the client's need and provides an early warning of adverse responses.
	Implement actions to decrease the untoward effects of analgesics.	Actions taken to prevent predictable but unwanted effects of narcotic analgesics (e.g., constipation) increase client comfort.
	NIC **Progressive Muscle Relaxation**	
	Have the patient tense, for 5 to 10 seconds, each of 8 to 16 major muscle groups.	Tensing the foot muscles for no longer than 5 seconds helps avoid cramping.
	Terminate the session gradually.	Gradual termination maintains the sense of well-being and relaxation.
	Instruct the client to wear comfortable, nonrestrictive clothing.	The client's personal comfort will facilitate relaxation.
	Instruct the client to breathe deeply and to slowly release the breath and tension.	Proper breathing will help the client focus on relaxation rather than external stimuli.
	Instruct the client to focus on the sensations in the muscles both while they are relaxed and while they are tense.	Focusing on the muscle sensations will help build memory that can be called on at later times for relaxation.
	Other Interventions	
	Consider the use of hypnosis, biofeedback, magnetic field therapy, and/or acupuncture to aid in the control of chronic pain.	Cognitive and behavioral strategies may serve as adjuncts to or replacements for pharmacologic or surgical interventions for chronic pain. Each therapy has differing modes of action that may or may not benefit the patient.

D Indicates tasks that can be delegated to unlicensed assistive personnel at the discretion of the nurse.

PLAN of CARE MEDICAL DIAGNOSIS: RHEUMATOID ARTHRITIS—*cont'd*

NURSING DIAGNOSIS NO. 2 ■ Chronic Pain—*cont'd*

	Expected Outcomes	Nursing Interventions	Rationales
		Consider the use of herbals (e.g., ginseng, St. John's wort) after consultation with the client's physician and pharmacist.	Herbals may provide relief from symptoms that often accompany pain, such as fatigue and depression.
		Refer the client to the Pain Advisory Committee.	The Pain Advisory Committee is a multidisciplinary committee with wide expertise in pain relief interventions.
		Continuing Care Considerations	
		Refer the client to an advanced practice nurse pain specialist, social worker, home care nurse, and/or psychologist, as appropriate.	Health team members are able to provide continuing support for the client facing chronic pain.
		Collaborate with health team members to secure a referral to a pain management clinic.	Pain management clinics combine many health care disciplines to focus on the management of chronic pain. The client's individual needs and responses to pain are evaluated, and a unique pain management program is initialed and adjusted.

NURSING DIAGNOSIS NO. 3 ■ Fatigue

	Expected Outcomes	Nursing Interventions	Rationales
RELATED FACTORS Stress Anxiety Depression Disease states: Rheumatoid arthritis **DEFINING CHARACTERISTICS** Energy: Lack of Inability to maintain usual level of physical activity Rest requirements: Increased Inability to maintain usual routines Concentration: Compromised Perceived need for additional energy to accomplish routine tasks Decreased performance Feelings of guilt for not keeping up with responsibilities	No verbal report or observation of being lethargic or listless Denies feeling tired No verbal report or observation of lack of energy Able to maintain usual routines	NIC **Energy Management** Monitor the client for evidence of excess physical and emotional fatigue.	Extended periods of inactivity may place the client at risk for excessive fatigue when carrying out desired activities.
		Monitor nutritional intake.	Ensure that the client has adequate energy resources.
		Arrange physical activities (e.g., avoid activity immediately after meals).	Such an arrangement reduces competition for oxygen supply to vital body functions.
		Encourage alternate rest and activity periods.	This avoids extended periods of either activity or exercise.
		Assist the client to schedule rest periods and avoid care activities during scheduled rest periods.	Rest periods should help restore the client's energy levels.
		D Use passive and/or active range-of-motion exercises.	Exercise relieves muscle tension, and stretching helps diminish muscle spasm.
		Encourage physical activity (e.g., ambulation or performance of activities of daily living, consistent with client's energy resources).	Physical exercise helps build muscle mass and endurance.

Continued

PLAN of CARE MEDICAL DIAGNOSIS: RHEUMATOID ARTHRITIS—*cont'd*

NURSING DIAGNOSIS NO. 3 ■ Fatigue—*cont'd*

	Expected Outcomes	Nursing Interventions	Rationales
		Teach activity organization and time management techniques (e.g., assigning priority to activities to accommodate energy levels, establishing realistic activity goals).	Activity organization and time management techniques are used to prevent fatigue.
		Continuing Care Considerations	
		Avoid overexertion, stress, extremes of temperature, and people with upper respiratory tract infection.	Stressors exacerbate fatigue.

NURSING DIAGNOSIS NO. 4 ■ Disturbed Body Image

	Expected Outcomes	Nursing Interventions	Rationales
RELATED FACTORS Biophysical Psychosocial Illness Illness treatment **DEFINING CHARACTERISTICS** Verbal report of feelings that reflect an altered view of one's body in appearance, structure, or function Nonverbal response to actual or perceived change in body structure and/or function Actual change in structure and/or function Change in social involvement Not looking at body part Preoccupation with change or loss Verbal report: Negative feelings about body (e.g., feelings of helplessness, hopelessness, or powerlessness)	Views, monitors, and acknowledges body Acknowledges loss of significant objects Does not verbalize self-negating statements Denies alteration in relationship with significant other	NIC **Body Image Enhancement**	
		Assist the client to discuss changes caused by illness or surgery, as appropriate.	The client who experiences changes caused by illness or surgery may be reluctant to verbalize his or her feelings.
		Assist the client to separate physical appearance from feelings of personal worth, as appropriate.	The client's feeling of personal worth may be strongly tied to physical appearance so that negative changes in appearance trigger feelings of low self-worth.
		Determine the client's and family's perceptions of the alteration in body image versus reality.	The client's and family's perceptions of the alteration in body image may vary significantly from the reality of the change.
		Determine if a change in body image has contributed to increased social isolation.	A client who experiences a negative change in body image may withdraw from social contact.
		Identify means of reducing the impact of any disfigurement.	The use of clothing, wigs, or cosmetics may reduce the impact of any disfigurement.
		Assist the client to identify actions that will enhance appearance.	Assisting the client to enhance his or her appearance will improve his or her self-concept.
		Other Interventions	
		Provide an atmosphere of caring and acceptance.	A client with traumatic changes in body parts or functioning may be especially sensitive to cues that indicate an aversive reaction.
		Continuing Care Considerations	
		Refer the client to restorative specialists, as appropriate.	Restorative specialists have expertise in body enhancement and techniques to maximize appearance to improve self-concept.
		Refer the client to a support group of others who have experienced the same loss.	The client may receive useful information and support from others who are experiencing the same circumstances.

CHART 24-9

DRUG THERAPY for Arthritis and Connective Tissue Disease*

Drug	Usual Dosage	Nursing Interventions	Rationales
NSAIDs	Dosage varies depending on which drug is being used.	Observe for fluid retention, increased blood pressure, and changes in renal function.	Most NSAIDs cause sodium retention, which can lead to edema, hypertension, renal damage, and congestive heart failure. Drugs should be used with caution in older adults.
		Monitor electrolyte and complete blood count values.	Most NSAIDs cause increased sodium levels and can cause bone marrow suppression.
		Observe for CNS changes (e.g., dizziness or confusion).	Most NSAIDs can cause CNS effects, especially in older adults.
Hydroxychloroquine sulfate (Plaquenil)	Dosage is 200 mg PO daily.	Instruct client to have frequent (every 6-12 mo) ophthalmologic examination.	Drug can cause retinal damage.
Immunosuppressive agents, e.g., azathioprine (Imuran), cyclophosphamide (Cytoxan, Procytox✱), methotrexate (Rheumatrex) (most commonly used)	Dosage varies depending on disease activity and route of drug administration.	Monitor for side effects and toxic effects, including but not limited to nausea/vomiting, bone marrow suppression, alopecia, and increased liver enzymes.	The side effects and toxic effects of these drugs can be devastating.
		Instruct client to avoid crowds and people with infections such as influenza. If ill, seek medical attention.	Bone marrow suppression or immune suppression increases the risk of infection.
Prednisone (Deltasone, Apo-Prednisone✱)	Dosage is 10-150 mg PO daily. For maintenance, attempt to give dose every other day (to allow client's adrenal glands to function).	Observe for cushiongoid changes, such as moonface, buffalo hump, striae, acne, thin skin, bruising, fluid retention, and increased blood pressure.	These changes are expected and tend to be dose related. Changes diminish as dose decreases.
		Monitor electrolyte and glucose levels. Monitor weight.	Chronic steroid therapy can cause sodium or fluid retention, potassium depletion, and elevated glucose level.
		Observe for long-term effects of chronic steroid therapy, such as osteoporosis, cataracts, hypertension, diabetes, and impaired healing.	These complications may need to be treated with other drugs or modalities.
		Teach client to increase dietary calcium and vitamin D and to take a supplement.	
		Instruct client to avoid crowds and individuals with infections such as influenza.	Drug suppresses immune system (lymphocytes) and increases risk of infection or decreased healing.
Sulfasalazine (Azulfidine)	500 to 3000 mg daily in 2 to 4 doses.	Check for sulfa allergy, or kidney or liver disease.	Drug is a sulfa medication that has potential renal/liver toxicities.
		Teach client to drink adequate fluids.	Failure to drink fluids may cause formation of urine crystals.
		Teach men that the drug can lower sperm count.	Low sperm count may interfere with ability to conceive.
Leflunomide (Arava)	10 to 20 mg daily.	Teach client to get prescribed laboratory tests, usually every 6 to 8 weeks.	Increased liver enzymes and decreased blood count have been reported.
		Remind client to use strict birth control.	Drug can cause birth defects.

CBC, Complete blood count; *CNS*, central nervous system; *COX-2*, cyclooxygenase-2; *CTDs*, connective tissue diseases; *MS*, multiple sclerosis; *NSAIDs*, nonsteroidal anti-inflammatory drugs; *SC*, subcutaneously; *TB*, tuberculosis.

*This is not a comprehensive list; this chart lists only the common drugs used for arthritis and connective tissue disease.

Continued

CHART 24-9

DRUG THERAPY for
Arthritis and Connective Tissue Disease*—*cont'd*

Drug	Usual Dosage	Nursing Interventions	Rationales
Biological response modifiers (BRMs)	Dose typically depends on body weight or response to medication.	Do not give BRMs if client has a serious infection, TB, or MS.	Drugs may exacerbate infections, MS, or lupus.
Etanercept (Enbrel)	Usually 25 mg SC twice weekly	Teach client to report site reaction.	Site reactions can be painful.
Infliximab (Remicade)	Varies from 200 to 400 mg IV each treatment	Refrigerate all BRMs except Remicade.	Refrigeration prevents drug decomposition.
Adalimumab (Humira)	Typically 40 mg SC every 2 wk		
Anakinra (Kineret)	Typically 100 mg SC daily		

CBC, Complete blood count; *CNS,* central nervous system; *COX-2,* cyclooxygenase-2; *CTDs,* connective tissue diseases; *MS,* multiple sclerosis; *NSAIDs,* nonsteroidal anti-inflammatory drugs; *SC,* subcutaneously; *TB,* tuberculosis.
*This is not a comprehensive list; this chart lists only the common drugs used for arthritis and connective tissue disease.

within some countries or when a client has specific needs or restrictions. Salicylates must be taken with food and are sometimes given with GI-acid lowering agents providing GI protection such as proton pump inhibitors. Monitor the client for heartburn, indigestion, stomach discomfort, or black, tarry bowel movements (signs and symptoms of ulceration or GI bleeding). Report such symptoms to the health care provider.

Disease-Modifying Anti-Rheumatic Drugs. **Disease-modifying antirheumatic drugs (DMARDs)**, such as hydroxychloroquine (Plaquenil), sulfasalazine, or minocycline, may be prescribed to slow the progression of mild rheumatoid disease before it worsens (see Chart 24-9).

Hydroxychloroquine (Plaquenil) is an antimalarial drug that helps decrease joint and muscle pain and often helps clients with early RA or other inflammatory autoimmune diseases such as systemic lupus erythematosus (SLE), described later in this chapter. Some health care providers may use Plaquenil as one of the initial treatments for mild disease. The client usually takes 400 mg each evening with a light snack. Occasionally the dose is divided into 200 mg twice daily with food.

Clients generally tolerate Plaquenil quite well. In a few cases, mild stomach discomfort, light-headedness or headache have been reported. The most serious adverse effect of the drug is retinal damage. Teach clients to report blurred vision or headache. Remind clients to have an eye examination every 6 to 12 months to detect changes in the cornea, lens, or retina. If this complication occurs, the health care provider discontinues the drug. Eye complications are rare, but prevention safety is the reason for the recommendation.

Sulfasalazine (Azulfidine) is a medication that may be prescribed for mild to moderate inflammatory arthritis conditions such as RA or psoriatic arthritis (an inflammatory arthritis variant described later). The usual dosage is 1000 mg twice daily taken with breakfast and supper. Starting doses may be less, such as 500 mg once or twice daily, gradually building up to the standard adult dose. Minimization of such GI side effects as sulfa taste, bloating, stomach discomfort, and gas occurs by gradually increasing drug dosing. Monitor the complete blood count (CBC), paying special attention for a decrease in white blood cells (WBCs) or platelet count. Changes in blood counts are rare but severe potential side effects for which the medication must be discontinued. Clients with an allergy to sulfa drugs or aspirin should not take sulfasalazine.

Minocycline (Minocin, a form of the antibiotic tetracycline) is sometimes used to treat mild RA symptoms. Although its mechanism of action is not known, it has both antimicrobial and anti-inflammatory effects. It is also an immune modifier, inhibiting certain chemicals that cause bone and cartilage damage.

Minocycline differs from other agents used for RA in that it has a low incidence of adverse effects. In addition, the client does not develop a resistance to the drug after prolonged use (Sears & Ganger, 2000).

Management of Moderate to Severe Disease. The health care provider selects medications that can slow progression of moderate to severe rheumatoid arthritis (RA). The client may take several of these drugs together, but not in the same drug class. For example, the provider may prescribe methotrexate and infliximab at the same time, along with a NSAID to help relieve pain and inflammation (see Chart 24-9).

Methotrexate (Rheumatrex). Methotrexate, an immunosuppressive medication, in a low, once-a-week dosage (generally 25 mg or less per week), has become the mainstay of therapy for advancing and sustaining RA because it is effective and relatively inexpensive. It is a slow-acting drug, taking 4 to 6 weeks to begin to control inflammatory joint symptoms. Observe for desired drug effects, such as a decrease in joint pain and swelling.

Monitor the client for potential side effects of decreasing WBCs and platelets (as a result of bone marrow suppression) or elevations in liver enzymes or serum creatinine. Remind clients to avoid alcoholic beverages while taking methotrexate to prevent liver toxicity. Teach the client to observe and report other side and toxic effects, which include mouth sores and acute dyspnea from pneumonitis. Rarely, lymph node tumor (lymphoma) has been associated in people who have RA and are taking methotrexate. Folic acid, one of the B vitamins, is often given to clients who are taking methotrexate to help decrease some of the drug's side effects.

Pregnancy is not recommended while taking methotrexate because birth defects are possible. Strict birth control is recommended for childbearing women who are in need of methotrexate to control their RA. If pregnancy is ever desired, the client is informed to consult the rheumatologist as well as their OB/GYN health care provider. Generally, the physician will discontinue the drug at least 3 months before planned pregnancy. Methotrexate may be restarted after birth if the client does not breast feed.

Leflunomide (Arava). Leflunomide is a slow-acting immune-modulating medication that helps diminish inflammatory arthritis symptoms of joint swelling, stiffness, and improves mobility. It is generally prescribed as follows: a loading dose of 100 mg daily for 3 days followed by 20 mg daily thereafter. Inform the client that the drug generally takes 4 to 6 weeks and sometimes up to 3 months before maximum benefit is realized.

Arava is a potent medication that is generally tolerated, but side effects of hair loss, diarrhea, decreased WBCs and platelets, or increased liver enzymes have been reported. Teach clients to report these changes and monitor laboratory results carefully. Remind them to avoid alcohol. Inform them that Arava can cause birth defects, and therefore recommend strict birth control to women of childbearing age. Tell clients to contact the health care provider immediately if pregnancy occurs while taking the drug. Cholestyramine (Questran) is available to help block the drug's action.

Critical Thinking Challenge

A 57-year-old woman has had RA for nearly 10 years. Although she is independent in her activities of daily living (ADLs), she complains of constant pain. She is taking Rheumatrex, Celebrex, Arava, and prednisone, but her disease continues to progress slowly. Because of diabetes mellitus, she can only take a low dose of prednisone. Her husband died 3 years ago, but she has no family who live nearby. When her daughter calls her, the client seems negative, hopeless, and depressed.

1. What are this client's priority nursing diagnoses?
2. What factors are contributing to her emotional state?
3. What outcomes are desired for this client?

evolve For suggested answer guidelines, go to http://evolve.elsevier.com/Iggy/.

Biological Response Modifiers. As a group, biological response modifiers (BRMs) are classified as the newest antiarthritic drugs that neutralize the biologic activity of tumor necrosis factor (TNF) by inhibiting its binding with TNF receptors. Any one of the BRMs may be tried. If one drug is not effective, the health care provider prescribes another drug in the same class. All these medications are extremely expensive at this time, and insurance companies may not completely pay for their use.

Clients with multiple sclerosis or tuberculosis are not given TNF inhibitors. Determine whether the client has had a recent negative purified protein derivative (PPD) test. If not, a PPD skin test is typically administered, and the selected BRM is not started until the results are known to be negative. Collaborate with the client's health care provider to ensure that this process is complete.

Etanercept (Enbrel) is given subcutaneously by injection either as 50 mg once weekly or as 25 mg twice weekly. Immunosuppression with medications such as methotrexate is generally tried before using Enbrel or other biological response modifiers. Methotrexate may also be continued in combination with biologic therapies because the combination may be more effective than either drug alone. Most clients tolerate Enbrel or Enbrel and methotrexate together; however, laboratory monitoring is important. Combination therapy requires complete blood count (CBC), serum creatinine, and a liver panel to be drawn regularly, generally every 4 to 8 weeks. In general, clinical outcomes with Enbrel have been excellent.

Teach the client or family member how to self-administer Enbrel injections. Injection site reactions and infections (especially respiratory) are possible adverse effects. Ice and hydrocortisone 1% cream can be used if the client develops a red itchy rash at the site of an injection. The drug manufacturer cannot yet predict long-term potential side effects regarding severity of infection or cancer risk. To date what has been seen is mild increase in upper respiratory infections with occasional serious infections. The health care provider should be notified if infection or a delay in wound healing occurs.

Infliximab (Remicade), first approved to treat Crohn's disease, is given in a single IV infusion over several hours. The initial dose generally used for RA is 3 mg/kg of body weight. Following the first few weeks of therapy, the drug is repeated at intervals between 2 and 8 weeks, depending on the response of the client. Clients typically take methotrexate before starting Remicade and continue on combination therapy.

Teach the client to report symptoms of infusion reaction: chest discomfort, tachycardia, shortness of breath, or lightheadedness. If any of these symptoms are reported, decrease the IV rate or discontinue it. These symptoms generally subside, but the physician must be notified in case medical assistance is needed. Dose, rate, and interval changes may be needed. Acetaminophen and Benadryl are medications often given to each client before the start of Remicade, and are often used at the time of reported infusion reaction. Clients who experience serious adverse effects, such as hypertension or anaphylaxis, may require permanent discontinuation of the drug.

Adalimumab (Humira) is the first fully human TNF inhibitor and was approved by the federal Food and Drug Association (FDA) in January 2003. Humira is a 40-mg once every 2 weeks subcutaneous injection. Symptoms of inflammatory arthritis tend to decrease with the use of Humira, including less joint swelling, less stiffness, and better movement.

Injection site reactions and adverse effects similar to the other TNF inhibitors have been reported. Careful monitoring, especially with combination therapy of Humira and methotrexate or other immunosuppressive medication, is important and similar to combination therapy with other BRMs.

Anakinra (Kineret) is another biological response modifier. Instead of affecting tumor necrosis factor (TNF), however, it works to inhibit a different protein signal of the immune system called interleukin-1 (IL-1). IL-1 is also a pro-inflammatory protein that signals the immune system to increase inflammation. It is thought that IL-1 is a weaker protein than TNF, but having an alternative medication that targets a different receptor site is helpful when a client is unable to take other biologics. Clients who have multiple sclerosis or tuberculosis can not take TNF inhibitors, but Kineret can be used with this population.

Injection site reactions occur more often with Kineret compared with other BRMs. Ice and hydrocortisone 1% cream are recommended. Remind clients to rotate injection sites. Kineret is administered with a simple jet that the client can use for self-administration. The client has the option to eliminate the simple jet or administer the subcutaneous injection traditionally.

Adjunctive Treatment. Some drugs are given as adjuncts to the previously described medications. It is not unusual for a client to be taking several disease-modifying drugs, such as methotrexate, a BRM, and an adjunct medication. Each drug works differently to relieve symptoms and slow the progression of the disease.

Glucocorticoids (steroids)–usually Prednisone (Deltasone, Medrol)–are given for their fast-acting anti-inflammatory and immunosuppressive effects. Prednisone may be given in high dose for short duration **(pulse therapy)** or as a low chronic dose. Moderate-dose, short-term tapering bridge therapy is commonly used when inflammation is symptomatic and other RA medications are insufficient or have not yet had an effect.

Chronic steroid therapy can result in numerous complications, such as diabetes mellitus, infection, fluid and electrolyte imbalances, hypertension, osteoporosis, and glaucoma. Some drug effects are dose related, whereas others are not. Observe the client for complications associated with chronic steroid therapy and report them to the health care provider. For example, if blood pressure becomes elevated or significant laboratory values change, notify the physician.

Instruct clients taking chronic steroids to take calcium 1200 to 1500 mg daily plus vitamin D 800 mg daily to help prevent osteoporosis. Bisphosphonate medications such as Fosamax or Actonel are often prescribed as well. Bone density measurements are recommended.

Clients with RA may experience one or a few joints that have more pain and inflammation than the others. Cortisone injections in single joints may be used to relieve local pain and inflammation. Have the client ice and rest the joint for 24 hours following the procedure. Oral analgesia is sometimes also needed during that time.

Other Drugs. Other immunosuppressive agents that may be used are azathioprine (Imuran) and cyclophosphamide (Cytoxan). Cyclophosphamide is sometimes given specifically to control RA vasculitis. Such immunosuppressive medications may cause bone marrow suppression and occasionally leukemia or lymphoma. White blood cells are expected to decrease 7 to 14 days following the administration of IV cyclophosphamide; therefore laboratory results are closely monitored to ensure safe limits. Hemorrhagic cystitis is a concern more with oral cyclophosphamide. Instruct the client to drink water and void frequently (about every 2 hours while awake), which dilutes the urine and empties the bladder, thus decreasing opportunity for bladder irritation from residual drug. Hair thinning or loss can be seen with immunosuppressive medications. Cyclophosphamide may also cause sterility; strict birth control is recommended.

Clients should be well informed of each medication's desired and specific potential side effects, the method for taking the medication correctly, and recommended monitoring methods. When taken correctly and monitored, these immunosuppressive medications help control severe autoimmune inflammatory diseases.

Gold therapy is less frequently used to treat RA now that methotrexate and the newer biologic medications are available; however, gold may still sometimes be used to modify RA disease and reduce pain and inflammation. Some clients take gold if they are unable to use other immunosuppressive or biologic medications. The most commonly used parenteral preparation is gold sodium thiomalate (Myochrysine). For intramuscularly administered gold, a test dose of 10 mg is given to detect an allergy to the drug, and weekly gold injections are given thereafter. The dosage increases from 25 to 50 mg weekly. Blood tests must be monitored before each injection. The client's urine is tested for protein level and a CBC is taken. Report any laboratory results outside the normal range to the physician, and hold the gold injection.

If the client responds to gold without having toxic effects (e.g., rash, blood dyscrasias, renal involvement), the injections are slowly tapered to every 2 weeks, then every 3 weeks, and then once a month. If remission does not occur after a total of 1000 mg has been given, the drug is usually discontinued.

Auranofin (Ridaura) is different from IM gold in that it is a form of oral gold that is occasionally used to treat mild RA. Three milligrams twice-daily dosing is generally prescribed. Its major side effects are GI symptoms, especially diarrhea, nausea, and vomiting. Teach the client to report any GI problems to the health care provider.

Analgesic drugs may be prescribed to supplement the pain relief property in anti-inflammatory drugs specific for RA. Some analgesics include acetaminophen (Tylenol), propoxyphene (Darvon), and propoxyphene napsylate (Darvocet-N). Propoxyphene and its associated products can cause headache, dizziness, and drowsiness. In clients with decreased metabolic rates, this slowly excreted drug may accumulate in the body over a long period and can cause death, especially in older adults. Teach the client about the side effects and toxic effects of these drugs and advise the client to report any unusual symptoms or complaints to the physician.

Nonpharmacologic Modalities. Adequate rest, proper positioning, and ice and heat applications are important in pain management (see Pain Management [Osteoarthritis], p. 384). If acute inflammation is present, the physical therapist (PT) or assistive nursing personnel applies ice to the "hot" joints for pain relief until the inflammation lessens. The ice pack should not be too heavy. Heated paraffin (wax) dips may help decrease pain and increase comfort of arthritic hands. Finger and hand exercises are often done more easily following paraffin treatment.

To relieve morning stiffness or the pain of late-stage disease, recommend a hot shower rather than a sponge bath or a tub bath. It is often difficult for the client with RA to get into and out of a bathtub, although special hydraulic lifts and tub chairs may be available. Grab bars and nonskid tread in the tub floor are important safety features to discuss with all clients.

Hot packs applied directly to involved joints may be beneficial. Most physical therapy departments have machines that keep hot packs ready anytime they are needed (Figure 24-5). At home, the client may use the microwave or stovetop heating instructions to warm the heat pack. Teach the client to follow the instructions given with each heating device used.

Plasmapheresis. Plasmapheresis (sometimes called plasma exchange) is an in-hospital procedure prescribed by a health care provider in which the client's plasma is treated to remove the antibodies causing the disease. This procedure may be combined with pulse therapy for clients with severe, life-threatening disease.

Complementary and Alternative Therapies. Some clients may have pain relief from hypnosis, acupuncture, magnet therapy, imagery, or music therapy. Stress management is also popular as a pain relief intervention. Chapters 4 and 7 discuss these therapies in detail.

Good nutrition is an important part of the management of RA. The inflammatory state may place a greater burden on the metabolism of some essential nutrients. This catabolic state may be related to increased cytokine production, specifically tumor necrosis factor (Kremer, 2001). Further research will contribute to future nutritional recommendations. Some attention has been given to specific foods:

- Omega-3 fatty acids (found in coldwater fish such as salmon, sea bass, and tuna) may help decrease inflammation; however, the amount needed may be impractical for human consumption.
- Fish oil capsules containing omega-3 fatty acids at 2.5 to 5 g daily (should not be taken if the client is taking anticoagulant therapy) may be recommended in areas in which coldwater fish are not available.

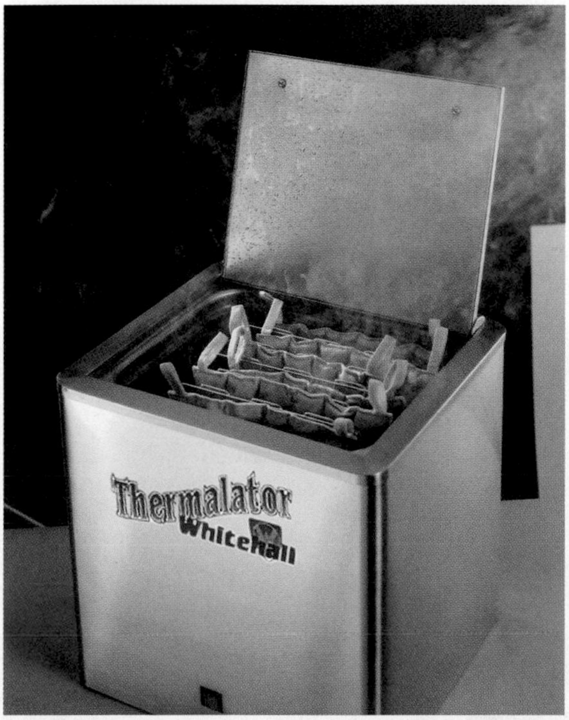

Figure 24-5 ■ Heating units used to keep hot packs warm. (Courtesy Whitehall Manufacturing, City of Industry, CA.)

- Antioxidant vitamins (A,C, E) may help maintain the normal function of the immune system.
- Trace elements such as zinc, selenium, copper, and iron may be needed in sufficient amounts for joint health.

According to the Arthritis Foundation, there is no one food that causes or cures RA; however, healthy nutrition in general is supported. Refer the client to the Arthritis Foundation's pamphlet regarding diet and arthritis. Refer the client to the health care provider or dietitian for vitamin- and nutrition-specific questions or recommendations.

Promotion of Self-Care. Although the physical appearance of a client with severe RA may create the image that independence in activities of daily living (ADLs) is not possible, a number of alternative methods can be used to perform these activities. Do not automatically perform these activities for the client; clients with RA do not want to be dependent. For example, hand deformities often prevent a client from opening packages of food, such as a box of crackers; however, he or she may prefer to use his or her teeth to open the crackers rather than depend on someone else.

In the hospital or long-term care facility, a client may not eat because of the barriers of heavy plate covers, milk cartons, small packages of condiments, and heavy containers. Styrofoam or paper cups may bend and collapse as the client attempts to hold them. A china or heavy plastic cup with handles may be easier to manipulate. Collaborate with the dietitian to allow access to food and total independence in eating.

When fine motor activities (e.g., squeezing a tube of toothpaste) become impossible, larger joints or body surfaces can substitute for smaller ones. For example, teach the client to use the palm of the hand to press the paste onto the brush. Devices such as long-handled brushes can allow clients to brush their hair; dressing sticks can facilitate putting on pants. These examples illustrate the need to assess the problem area, suggest alternative methods, and refer the client to an occupational or physical therapist for special assistive and adaptive devices if necessary.

Management of Fatigue. Nursing interventions depend in part on identifying the factors contributing to fatigue. For example, increases in pain, sleep disturbances, and weakness are positively associated with increased fatigue. Anemia may also be a contributing factor and may be treated with iron (if an iron deficiency anemia is present), folic acid, or vitamin supplements prescribed by the health care provider. Chronic normochromic or chronic hypochromic anemia often occurs in most chronic, systemic diseases. Assess for drug-related blood loss, such as that caused by salicylate therapy or other NSAIDs, by checking the stool for gross or occult blood. Older white women are the most likely clients to experience GI bleeding as a result of taking these medications.

When fatigue results from muscle atrophy, the physician prescribes an aggressive physical therapy program to strengthen muscles and prevent further atrophy. Clients experience increased fatigue when pain prevents them from getting adequate rest and sleep. Measures to facilitate sleep include promoting a quiet environment, giving warm beverages, and administering hypnotics or relaxants as prescribed, if necessary.

In addition to identifying and managing specific reasons for fatigue, determine the client's usual daily activities and teach principles of **energy conservation,** including the following:

- Pacing activities
- Allowing rest periods
- Setting priorities
- Obtaining assistance when needed

Chart 24-10 lists specific suggestions for conserving energy and thus increasing activity tolerance.

Enhancement of Body Image. Body image may be affected by both the disease process and drug therapy. Steroids can cause a moon-faced appearance, acne, striae, "buffalo humps," and weight gain. Determine the client's perception of these changes and the impact of the reactions of family and significant others. The most important intervention is communicating acceptance of the client. When a trusting relationship is established, encourage the client to express his or her feelings.

Another way to improve body image while in the hospital or nursing home is to use personal items. A hospital gown reinforces the sick role. Encourage clients to wear their own clothes, to brush their hair, and to use makeup if desired. Assist the client as needed. The use of colored hair accessories, nail polish, and perfume may improve a female client's image and self-concept.

As a reaction to body image disturbance and the presence of a chronic, painful disease, clients may display behaviors indicative of loss. They may use coping strategies that range from denial or fear to anger or depression. In an attempt to regain control over the effects of the disease process, they may appear to be manipulative and demanding and sometimes may be referred to as having an "arthritis personality." This personality, which has negative connotations, is a myth. Clients are trying to cope with the effects of their illness and should be treated with patience and understanding. Continually assess and accept these behaviors, but remain realistic in discussing goals to improve self-esteem. Emphasize clients' strengths and help them identify previously successful coping strategies.

Community-Based Care

Clients with rheumatoid arthritis (RA) are usually managed at home but may be institutionalized in a long-term care setting if they become restricted to bed or a wheelchair. Some clients may be discharged to a rehabilitation facility for several weeks to aid in developing strategies, techniques, and skills for independent living at home.

HOME CARE MANAGEMENT

The amount of home care preparation depends on the severity of the disease. Structural changes may be necessary if there are deficits in activities of daily living (ADLs) or mobility. Doors must be wide enough to accommodate a wheelchair or walker if one is used. Ramps are needed to prevent the client in a wheelchair from becoming homebound. If the client cannot negotiate stairs, he or she must have access to facilities for all ADLs on one floor. Handrails should be available in the bathroom and halls.

To promote continued homemaking functions, countertops and appliances may require structural changes. The client may also require handrails and elevated chairs and toilet seats, which facilitate transfers (Figure 24-6).

CHART 24-10

CLIENT EDUCATION GUIDE
Energy Conservation for the Client with Arthritis

- Balance activity with rest. Take one or two naps each day.
- Pace yourself; do not plan too much for one day.
- Set priorities. Determine which activities are most important, and do them first.
- Delegate responsibility and tasks to your family and friends.
- Plan ahead to prevent last-minute rushing and stress.
- Learn your own activity tolerance and do not exceed it.

HEALTH TEACHING

Health teaching is a vital role for nurses in the diagnosis and management of arthritis. Many people have signs and symptoms of joint inflammation but do not seek medical attention. Teach clients to seek professional health care to reduce pain and disability (see the Meeting Healthy People 2010 Objectives box below).

Meeting HEALTHY PEOPLE 2010 Objectives

ARTHRITIS AND OTHER RHEUMATIC CONDITIONS

Objective 2.7: Increase the proportion of adults who have seen a health care provider for their chronic joint symptoms.

- Teach clients with suspected arthritis the importance of seeing a health care provider for initial evaluation and follow-up care.
- Educate clients that maintaining functional ability and managing pain can reduce arthritis pain and disability.
- Remind older adults that arthritis is not a normal part of the aging process.
- Assist the client in locating local health care providers who specialize in arthritis management (e.g., rheumatologists, internists).
- Teach clients about the availability of community support groups for people with arthritis.

Objective 2.8: Increase the proportion of persons with arthritis who have had effective evidence-based arthritis education as an integral part of the management of their condition.

- Teach clients about community education programs at local hospitals or through the Arthritis Foundation, such as the Arthritis Self-Help course.
- Educate clients about the value of evidence-based education programs (reduces pain and visits to the health care provider).
- Provide client and family education about arthritis and its management, as needed.

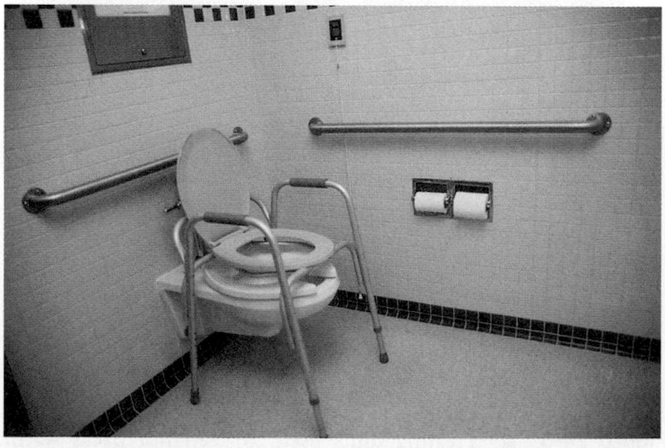

Figure 24-6 ■ Handrails and an elevated toilet seat make transfers easier for the client.

Health teaching is also important for promoting compliance with a treatment plan. A client who understands the disease process and the treatment rationale can better follow and ask questions about the treatment plan.

Teach clients to discuss any questions with their health care provider before trying any over-the-counter or home remedies. Some remedies may be harmful. Check with the Arthritis Foundation for the latest information on arthritis myths and quackery.

Information about drug therapy, joint protection, energy conservation, rest, and exercise should be taught to client, family, and significant others. This information is summarized in Charts 24-5, 24-6, 24-9, and 24-10.

The client with RA often complains of being on an "emotional roller coaster" from coping with a chronic illness every day. Control over one's life is an important human need. The client with an unpredictable chronic disease may lose this control, and this lowers self-esteem. Health care providers must allow the client to make decisions about care. Families and significant others must also include the client in decision-making. Although the client's behavior may be perceived as demanding or manipulative, his or her self-esteem cannot be improved without this important aspect of interpersonal relationships.

Increased dependency also affects a sense of control and self-esteem. Some clients ignore their health needs and portray a tough image for others by insisting that they need no assistance. Emphasize to the client and family that asking for help may be the best decision at times to prevent further joint damage and disease progression.

Rheumatoid arthritis (RA) may also affect work and social roles. The client may have physical difficulty doing tasks that require lifting, climbing, grasp, gross or fine motor activities. The severity of RA disease may cause difficulty with total number of hours worked. Some people with RA are able to do their jobs well without problem; others may have varying degrees of difficulty. Clients who are no longer able to do their job at work may need to discuss having a lighter workload with their employer, but some may need to file for disability with their company and social security.

Arthritis support groups and self-help courses provide the education and the support that clients, families, and friends need; however, refer the client to a psychological counselor or religious or spiritual leader for emotional support and guidance during times of crisis or as needed. Identify and recommend other support systems within the family and community when necessary.

HEALTH CARE RESOURCES

The need for health care resources for the client with RA is similar to that for the client with osteoarthritis. A home care nurse or aide, physical therapist, or occupational therapist may be needed. In collaboration with the discharge planner, the nurse in the hospital or nursing home identifies these resources and makes sure they are available before discharge.

Critical Thinking Challenge

The 57-year-old woman with RA decides to see a new rheumatologist. After a thorough examination and consultation, he wants her to try Enbrel. She is concerned that she will not be able to self-administer the injections and is worried that Medicare and her supplemental insurance will not pay for it. She lives on monthly disability checks for her and her deceased husband.

1. What health teaching will this client require?
2. As her home care nurse, what outcomes would you observe for to determine the effectiveness of the new medication?
3. Why do you think the physician prescribed the new medication?

evolve For suggested answer guidelines, go to http://evolve.elsevier.com/Iggy/.

LUPUS ERYTHEMATOSUS

PATHOPHYSIOLOGY

The word *lupus* is the Latin term for "wolf." In the mid-nineteenth century, the facial rash accompanying this disease was thought to look like bites caused by a wolf. The rash was usually red, and thus the term *erythematosus,* a Latin word meaning "reddened," was added to describe the disease.

There are two main classifications of lupus: **discoid lupus erythematosus (DLE)** and **systemic lupus erythematosus (SLE).** A small percentage of clients with lupus have the DLE type, which affects only the skin.

SLE is a chronic, progressive, inflammatory connective tissue disorder that can cause major body organs and systems to fail. It is characterized by spontaneous remissions and **exacerbations** ("flare-ups"), and the onset may be acute or insidious. The condition is potentially fatal, but the survival rate has improved dramatically most recently in countries where SLE is diagnosed early and treated adequately. Today more than 90% of clients with SLE are living 10 years after diagnosis (Edworthy, 2001). Improvements in determining the cause, diagnosis, and treatment of lupus account for the prolonged survival of these clients.

Lupus is thought to be an autoimmune process; that is, abnormal antibodies are produced and react with the client's tissues. Antinuclear antibodies (ANAs) primarily affect the deoxyribonucleic acid (DNA) within the cell nuclei. As a result, immune complexes form in the serum and organ tissues, which causes inflammation and damage. These complexes invade organs directly or cause **vasculitis** (vessel inflammation), which deprives the organs of arterial blood and oxygen.

Many clients with SLE have some degree of kidney involvement–the leading cause of death. Other causes of death from SLE are cardiac and central nervous system involvement.

In kidney disease, renal biopsies show the following progressive changes within the glomeruli:

- In minimal lupus nephritis, the glomeruli are slightly irregular; immunoglobulins and complement are seen by electron microscopy.
- Focal, or mild, lupus nephritis is characterized by further glomerular changes, and immune complex deposits are common. In this type of lupus, the client begins to show clinical signs of renal impairment.
- In diffuse, severe proliferative nephritis, more than 50% of the glomeruli are affected, and the client is in renal failure.

Lupus affects women between the ages of 15 and 40 years at a rate 8 to 10 times more often than men. Black women have the disease more than white women, but the reason is unknown. The onset of the disease occurs most often during the childbearing years, but it has been reported in young children and older adults. A genetic predisposition is likely based on the trend to develop the disease in twins and the occurrence of autoimmune disease in families of clients who have lupus.

A genetic link between lupus, rheumatoid arthritis, and psoriatic arthritis involves a protein called Runx-1, which helps the thymus gland train cells of the immune system. Research indicates that clients with these diseases have an altered Runx-1 binding site on one of three chromosomes. The interpretation of this finding is not clear, but it demonstrates, in part, the genetic etiology of these autoimmune diseases (Wade, 2003).

A transient lupus-like syndrome can occur in some clients taking selected medications, especially procainamide (Pronestyl) and hydralazine (McCance & Huether, 2003). When these drugs are discontinued, the syndrome usually resolves.

◆COLLABORATIVE MANAGEMENT

◆Assessment

It is impossible to describe a typical textbook picture of a client with lupus because of the extreme variability of symptoms. When the disease is in remission, the client may appear healthy and have no activity limitations. When the disease flares, the client may be so ill that admission to a critical care unit is required. Chart 24-11 highlights the clinical manifestations that occur with systemic lupus.

CHART 24-11

KEY FEATURES of Systemic Lupus Erythematosus and Progressive Systemic Sclerosis

Systemic Lupus Erythematosus	Progressive Systemic Sclerosis
Skin Manifestations	
■ Inflamed, red rash ■ Discoid lesions	■ Inflamed ■ Fibrotic ■ Sclerotic ■ Edematous
Renal Manifestations	
■ Nephritis	■ Renal failure
Cardiovascular Manifestations	
■ Pericarditis ■ Raynaud's phenomenon	■ Myocardial fibrosis ■ Raynaud's phenomenon
Pulmonary Manifestations	
■ Pleural effusions	■ Interstitial fibrosis ■ Pulmonary hypertension
Neurologic Manifestations	
■ CNS lupus	■ Not common
Gastrointestinal Manifestations	
■ Abdominal pain	■ Esophagitis ■ Ulcers
Musculoskeletal Manifestations	
■ Joint inflammation ■ Myositis	■ Joint inflammation ■ Myositis
Other Manifestations	
■ Fever ■ Fatigue ■ Anorexia ■ Vasculitis	■ Fever ■ Fatigue ■ Anorexia ■ Vasculitis

CNS, Central nervous system.

PHYSICAL ASSESSMENT/CLINICAL MANIFESTATIONS

SKIN INVOLVEMENT. The major skin manifestation of SLE is a dry, scaly, raised rash on the face **("butterfly" rash)** (Figure 24-7). This rash may also appear on the sun exposed upper body. The rash of systemic lupus is generally nonscarring, but it may increase in a lupus flare and disappear when the disease is in remission.

Individual round **discoid** (coinlike) **lesions** are the scarring lesions of discoid lupus. The lesions are especially evident when the client is exposed to sunlight or ultraviolet light.

Alopecia is common in lupus. Observe all skin changes and monitor them daily while the client is in an acute care setting.

MUSCULOSKELETAL CHANGES. In addition to skin changes, **polyarthritis** occurs in 90% of clients with SLE. The initial joint changes are similar to those seen in rheumatoid arthritis (RA), but severe deformities are not common. Small joints and the knees are most commonly involved. **Osteonecrosis** (bone necrosis from lack of oxygen) is often seen in clients with SLE who have been treated for at least 5 years, usually with steroids. Chronic steroid therapy may cause the constriction of small blood vessels supplying the joint, which causes the tissue to die. The hip is most commonly affected, and complaints of pain and decreased mobility result.

Observe for muscle atrophy, which can result from disuse or from skeletal muscle invasion by the immune complexes **(myositis).** Myalgia (muscle pain) may also occur. Inspect and palpate the major muscles, especially those in the extremities.

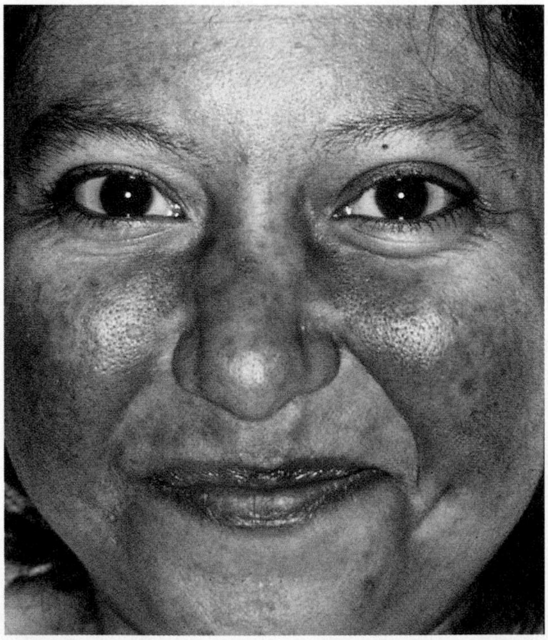

Figure 24-7 ■ The characteristic "butterfly" rash of systemic lupus erythematosus.

SYSTEMIC MANIFESTATIONS. Because SLE is an inflammatory condition, fever and fatigue are common findings. Fever is the classic sign of a flare, or exacerbation. Various degrees of generalized weakness, fatigue, anorexia, and weight loss occur. These signs may be the only evidence of impending disease, which makes diagnosis by the health care provider difficult. Consequently, some clients have a diagnosis of "probable SLE."

Any or all body systems may be affected by SLE. Because lupus nephritis is the leading cause of death, carefully assess for signs of renal involvement (e.g., changes in urine output, proteinuria, hematuria, and fluid retention). Approximately 50% of clients with SLE have some type of nephritis.

Pleural effusions or pneumonia are found in almost half of all cases of SLE, but **this** complication is usually not life threatening. Pulmonary restrictive or obstructive changes may not result in overt clinical signs; however, progressive involvement can lead to dyspnea and arterial blood gas abnormalities. Perform a complete respiratory assessment to determine any abnormalities in respiratory pattern or breath sounds.

Pericarditis is the most common cardiovascular manifestation and causes tachycardia, chest pain, and myocardial ischemia. Monitor the vital signs at least every 4 hours while the client is in the hospital, and report chest pain immediately to the physician.

Raynaud's phenomenon is noted in 15% of cases of lupus. On exposure to cold or extreme stress, the client with Raynaud's phenomenon complains of the characteristic red, white, and blue color changes and severe pain in the digits; these changes are caused by arteriolar vasospasm. Ask clients whether color changes occur when their hands or feet are exposed to cold or when they are extremely stressed.

Neurologic manifestations are varied. Central nervous system effects include psychoses, paresis, seizures, migraine headaches, and cranial nerve palsies. Peripheral neuropathies are also common. Perform a neurologic assessment as described in Chapter 44.

Monitor abdominal pain, which most often result from serositis (peritoneal involvement). Mesenteric arteritis, pancreatitis from arteritis of the pancreatic artery, and colonic ulcers also can cause abdominal pain with lupus. Note liver enlargement on assessment of the abdomen. Jaundice is rare. More than 50% of clients have lymph enlargement, and 10% have splenomegaly. Palpate the lymph nodes and document findings. Vasculitis affecting any major or small vessels can lead to organ failure.

PSYCHOSOCIAL ASSESSMENT

The psychosocial results of lupus can be devastating. With either DLE or SLE, the rash can be disfiguring and embarrassing. Young adult women who never had a blemish are confronted with a rash that cannot be completely covered with makeup. If chronic steroid therapy is used, side effects such as acne, striae, fat pads, and weight gain intensify the problem of an already altered body image.

Chronic fatigue and generalized weakness may prevent the client from being as active as in the past. He or she may avoid social gatherings and may withdraw from family activities. The unpredictability and chronicity of SLE can cause fear and anxiety. Fear may increase if the client knows another person with the disease, particularly if the other person has more advanced, severe disease. Unfortunately, the myth that lupus is fatal is still common. Inform the client that control of lupus is generally possible with regular medical monitoring, medications, and healthy practices, such as limiting sun exposure to prevent exacerbation of the disease.

Assess the client's feelings about the illness to identify areas requiring intervention. Determine the client's usual coping mechanisms and support systems before developing a plan of care. See Psychosocial Assessment (Rheumatoid Arthritis), p. 395, for additional information about the psychosocial assessment of clients with chronic illness.

LABORATORY ASSESSMENT

Because discoid lupus erythematosus (DLE) is not a systemic condition, the only significant test is a skin biopsy. The physician gently scrapes skin cells from the rash for microscopic evaluation. The characteristic lupus cell and a number of inflammatory cells confirm the diagnosis.

Some of the immunologic-based laboratory tests used to diagnose SLE are the same as those performed for rheumatoid arthritis (RA): rheumatoid factor, antinuclear antibody, erythrocyte sedimentation rate, serum protein electrophoresis, serum complement (especially C_3 and C_4), and immunoglobulins (see Chart 24-8). A false-positive Venereal Disease Research Laboratory (VDRL) syphilis test is common with lupus.

Newer and more specific immunologic tests, such as anti-Ro (SSA), anti-La (SSB), anti-RNP, anti-Smith (anti-Sm), anti-DNA, and anti-phospholipid antibodies (AP) are also performed. High titers of some of these antibodies are associated with lupus (Kuper & Failla, 2000). The rheumatologist generally orders and interprets immunologic tests for clients suspected of having lupus.

In addition to immunologic testing, several tests are performed to evaluate the possible involvement of major organs and body systems. A complete blood count (CBC) commonly shows **pancytopenia** (a decrease of all cell types), probably caused by direct attack of the blood cells or bone marrow by immune complexes. Serum electrolyte levels, renal function, cardiac and liver enzymes, and clotting factors are also routinely assessed to determine other body system functioning.

Interventions

The health care provider often prescribes potent drugs that are used topically and systemically. In addition, precautions are taken to prevent further skin impairment and exacerbations. Many of the skin lesions do not disappear, even with treatment, but they usually fade when the disease is in remission.

Drug Therapy. With DLE, the client's major concern is the rash or discoid lesions. Clients with systemic lupus erythematosus (SLE) may also be concerned about skin changes. Topical cortisone preparations help to reduce inflammation and promote fading of the skin lesions. In addition, the health care provider may prescribe the antimalarial agent hydroxychloroquine (Plaquenil) for some clients to decrease the inflammatory response; other systemic medications are usually not used (see Chart 24-9).

The aim of management of SLE is to treat the disease aggressively until remission. In addition to medications for skin lesions, the health care provider often prescribes chronic steroid therapy to treat the systemic disease process. For renal or central nervous system lupus, the health care provider may also prescribe immunosuppressive agents (e.g., azathioprine [Imuran]), which are sometimes used for clients with RA (see Chart 24-9). Although clinical manifestations improve during remission, maintenance doses of these drugs are usually continued to prevent further exacerbations of the disease. Observe for side effects and toxic effects of these medications and report their occurrence to the physician.

For severe renal involvement, azathioprine or cyclophosphamide (Cytoxan) may be given in combination with steroids. For clients who do not respond to this regimen, IV pulse (high-dose) glucocorticoids, cyclophosphamide, and plasmapheresis may be tried (see discussion under Rheumatoid Arthritis on p. 407). Renal transplantation has been successful for some clients. Recent advances in allogenic stem cell transplantation have improved symptoms in clients who respond poorly to steroids or immunosuppressive drugs (Kuper & Failla, 2000).

Skin Protection. Clients with lupus should avoid prolonged exposure to sunlight and other forms of ultraviolet lighting, including certain types of fluorescent light. Instruct clients that they may need to wear long sleeves and a large-brimmed hat when outdoors. They should use sun-blocking agents with an SPF (sun protection factor) of 30 or higher on exposed skin surfaces.

In addition, teach the client to clean the skin with mild soap (e.g., Ivory) and to avoid harsh, perfumed substances. The skin is rinsed and dried well, and lotion is applied. Excess powder and other drying substances should be avoided. Cosmetics must be carefully selected and should include moisturizers and sun protectors. Consider referring a client to a medical cosmetologist who specializes in applying makeup for skin lesions of all types.

The client's hair should receive special attention because alopecia (hair loss) is common. Recommend the use of mild protein shampoos and the avoidance of harsh treatments (e.g., permanents or highlights) until the hair regrows during remission.

Critical Thinking Challenge

A 32-year-old African-American female visits her physician's office (where you are a nurse) with complaints of a facial rash. On further questioning, you find that she has been more fatigued than usual and has an achy left ankle. Her infant son is 2 months old, and she has just stopped bleeding from her traumatic vaginal delivery (the infant weighed 10 pounds, and she was in labor for 18 hours, causing extended postpartum bleeding).

1. When obtaining a complete history, what other questions should you ask the client?
2. What risk factors does she have for SLE?
3. What laboratory tests will the health care provider most likely order?
4. If the client is diagnosed with SLE, what type of health teaching will she need?

evolve For suggested answer guidelines, go to http://evolve.elsevier.com/Iggy/.

Community-Based Care

Community-based care for the client with lupus is similar to that for RA. In general, the client is home but may need repeated hospitalizations during exacerbations of disease. The client usually does not need rehabilitation or a long-term care facility because severe joint deformity and prolonged immobility are not common.

Two major differences exist between SLE and RA in terms of education of the client and family or significant others. First, teach the client with SLE how to protect the skin (Chart 24-12). Second, body temperature is monitored carefully with SLE. Fever is the major sign of an exacerbation, during which the client can become seriously ill. Teach the client to report any other unusual or new clinical manifestations to the health care provider immediately.

Many clients become frustrated that family members, significant others, and lay people do not have a good understanding of lupus. When lupus is in complete remission, the client appears to be healthy; however, an exacerbation can necessitate rapid admission to a critical care unit. This unpredictability disrupts the client's life and can cause fear and anxiety. Help the client identify coping strategies and support systems that can help with functioning in the community.

Teach the possible effects of the disease on lifestyle, including fatigue. Women of childbearing age need to know that pregnancy can be a stressor and can cause an exacerbation of the disease, either during pregnancy or after delivery. The pregnant client also has an increased risk of miscarriage, stillbirth, or premature birth. Pregnancy is not recommended for those with cardiac, renal, or central nervous system involvement. Sexual counseling regarding contraception options may be necessary.

Although the Arthritis Foundation is a general resource for all clients with connective tissue disease, the Lupus Foundation is a national organization and has chapters in every state to provide information and assistance for clients with lupus. Local support groups and services are offered free of charge.

CHART 24-12

CLIENT EDUCATION GUIDE

Evidence-Based Practice for Skin Protection in Clients with Lupus Erythematosus

- Cleanse your skin with a mild soap, such as Ivory.
- Dry your skin thoroughly by patting rather than rubbing.
- Apply lotion liberally to dry skin areas.
- Avoid powder and other drying agents, such as rubbing alcohol.
- Use cosmetics that contain moisturizers.
- Avoid direct sunlight and any other type of ultraviolet lighting, including tanning beds.
- Wear a large-brimmed hat, long sleeves, and long pants when in the sun.
- Use a sun-blocking agent with a sun protection factor (SPF) of at least 30.
- Inspect your skin daily for open areas and rashes.

PROGRESSIVE SYSTEMIC SCLEROSIS

PATHOPHYSIOLOGY

Progressive systemic sclerosis (PSS), one of a family of diseases, is often referred to as **systemic scleroderma.** *Scleroderma* means hardening of the skin, which is only one clinical manifestation of PSS. Some clients have only skin involvement, or localized scleroderma. As the name implies, PSS is a generalized, systemic disease. It is less common than systemic lupus erythematosus (SLE) but is associated with a higher mortality rate. Chart 24-11 shows a comparison of the clinical manifestations of these two diseases.

Progressive systemic sclerosis is a chronic connective tissue disease characterized by inflammation, fibrosis, and sclerosis of the skin and vital organs. The inflammatory process is so similar to that of lupus that clients are often diagnosed as having probable SLE until the disease progresses or until antibody testing supports the diagnosis. The inflamed tissue undergoes fibrotic and then sclerotic changes. The tissue most obviously affected is the skin, but renal involvement is the leading cause of death. Respiratory involvement and hypertension are also common. Clients with PSS do not respond well to the steroids and immunosuppressants used for lupus, and therefore the mortality rate is higher.

The classification for systemic sclerosis is as follows:

- **Diffuse cutaneous scleroderma**–skin thickening on the trunk, face, proximal and distal extremities.
- **Limited cutaneous scleroderma–**thick skin limited to sites distal to the elbow and knee but also involve the face and neck. Clients have the **CREST syndrome:**

*C*alcinosis (calcium deposits)
*R*aynaud's phenomenon
*E*sophageal dysmotility
*S*clerodactyly (scleroderma of the digits)
*T*elangiectasia (spiderlike hemangiomas)

- **Sine scleroderma**–internal organ manifestations, vascular, and serologic abnormalities, but without clinically detectable skin changes
- **Overlap scleroderma**–any of the preceding three types of scleroderma occurring with lupus, inflammatory muscle disease, or RA
- **Undifferentiated connective tissue disease**–without skin thickening or internal organ abnormalities seen in PSS but with serologic abnormality, Raynaud's phenomenon, or other clinical features of systemic sclerosis (Siebold, 2001)

Little is known about the cause of PSS, but autoimmunity is suspected. The occurrence of more than one case per family is uncommon, but other connective tissue diseases may be noted in the family history.

Progressive systemic sclerosis has been described in people of all races and in all geographic areas. Women are affected three to four times more often than men. The onset of the disease is usually between 30 and 50 years of age. The incidence is higher in coal miners, who have a high incidence of silicosis, a possible predisposing or contributing factor to PSS. Prolonged exposure to other toxins, such as vinyl chloride and epoxy resins, may also predispose an individual to PSS.

◆COLLABORATIVE MANAGEMENT

◆Assessment

PHYSICAL ASSESSMENT/CLINICAL MANIFESTATIONS

Arthralgia (joint pain) and stiffness are common manifestations that you can elicit during the musculoskeletal examination. The acute inflammation that occurs with rheumatoid arthritis (RA) is not common, and deformities are rare.

Findings on inspection of the skin depend on the stage of the scleroderma. Typically there is a painless, symmetric, pitting edema of the hands and fingers; this edema may progress to include the entire upper and lower extremities and face. In this edematous phase, the fingers are described as sausage-like. The skin is taut, shiny, and free of wrinkles. If diffuse scleroderma occurs, swelling is replaced by tightening, hardening, and thickening of skin tissue; this phase is sometimes called the *indurative phase* (Figure 24-8). The skin loses its elasticity, and range of motion is markedly decreased; ulcerations may occur. Joint contractures may develop, and the client may be unable to perform activities of daily living (ADLs) independently.

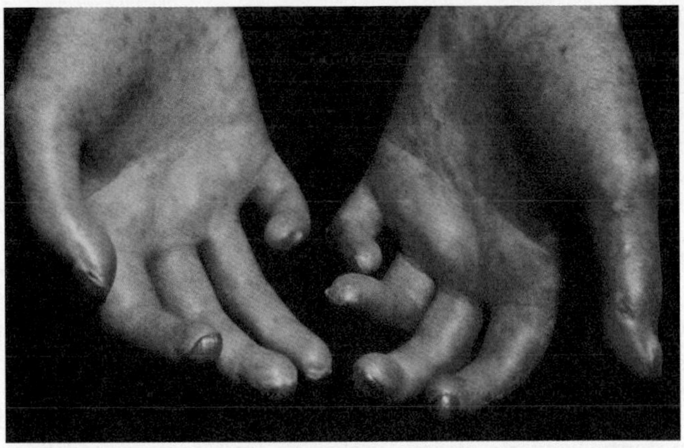

Figure 24-8 ■ Late-stage skin changes seen in clients with progressive systemic sclerosis. (From the Arthritis Teaching Slide Collection, copyright 1980. Used by permission of the Arthritis Foundation.)

Major organ damage is likely to develop with diffuse scleroderma, specifically affecting the following areas:

- Gastrointestinal tract
- Cardiovascular system
- Pulmonary system
- Renal system

Involvement of the gastrointestinal (GI) tract, particularly the esophagus, is common. The esophagus loses its motility, resulting in dysphagia and esophageal reflux. A small, sliding hiatal hernia may be present, and swallowing may be difficult. Reflux of the gastric contents can cause esophagitis and subsequent ulceration, particularly in the lower two thirds of the esophagus. Intestinal changes are similar to those of the esophagus. Peristalsis is diminished, which causes clinical manifestations similar to a partial bowel obstruction. Malabsorption is a common complication, causing malodorous diarrheal stools.

In addition to assessing problems of the digestive tract, observe for cardiovascular manifestations. Raynaud's phenomenon occurs in various degrees in most clients with PSS. On exposure to cold or emotional stress, the small arterioles in the digits of both hands and feet rapidly constrict, which causes decreased blood flow. In severe cases, the client experiences digit necrosis, excruciating pain, and autoamputation of the distal digits (the tips of the digits fall off spontaneously). (See Chapter 39 for a complete discussion of this disorder.) In many clients, vasculitic lesions, often around the nail beds **(periungual lesions),** are evident. Myocardial fibrosis, another common problem, is evidenced by electrocardiographic (ECG) changes, cardiac dysrhythmias, and chest pain.

Lung involvement in the client with PSS may go undetected until late in the disease or sometimes until autopsy.

Fibrosis of the alveoli and interstitial tissues is present in almost all cases of the disease, but clinical manifestations may not be present. Clients with scleroderma and pulmonary arterial hypertension have a more serious prognosis. Recently, bosentan (Tracleer), the first of a new class of drugs called *endothelin receptor antagonists,* demonstrated (in clinical trials) improved walk tests for clients with class III-IV pulmonary arterial hypertension. Various doses improved clients' breathing during exercise, but the potential for liver injury at the highest dose caused recommended doses to be lowered. The client usually takes 62.5 mg twice daily for 4 weeks and then increases the dose to 125 mg twice daily. In clinical practice, clients seem to tolerate bosentan and demonstrate improved breathing. Teach the client the desired and potential adverse effects, including liver toxicity and birth defects.

Renal involvement is an important aspect of the overall disease process and often causes malignant hypertension and death. Assess for signs of impending organ failure, such as changes in urine output and increased blood pressure.

LABORATORY ASSESSMENT

The laboratory findings for PSS are similar to those for SLE. Clinical findings and the client's response to drug therapy help the health care provider differentiate between the two diseases. Additional tests depend on which organs seem to be affected. Upper and lower gastrointestinal series are commonly performed because of the frequency of GI clinical manifestations.

Interventions

The medical management of progressive systemic sclerosis (PSS) aims to force the disease into remission and thus slow disease progression. The health care provider uses drug therapy primarily for this purpose, but it is often unsuccessful. Systemic steroids and immunosuppressants are used in large doses and often in combination (see Chart 24-9).

Local skin protective measures can help to maintain skin integrity. Teach the client to use mild soap and lotions and gentle cleaning techniques. The skin should be inspected daily for further changes or open lesions. Skin ulcers are treated according to their type and location.

In addition to drug therapy to control the overall disease process, specific measures can provide comfort. The client with PSS not only experiences chronic joint pain but also has severe, acute pain during episodes of Raynaud's phenomenon. A bed cradle and footboard keep bed covers away from the skin in severe cases. Adjust the room temperature to prevent chilling, which can precipitate digit vasospasm. The client who can tolerate touching of the affected areas can wear gloves and socks to increase warmth. Because cigarette smoking and extreme emotional stress can also cause symptoms to recur, the client should try to avoid or minimize these factors as much as possible. Chapter 39 describes the management of clients with Raynaud's phenomenon in more detail.

The client with esophageal involvement may need small, frequent meals rather than the traditional three meals daily. He or she should minimize the intake of foods and liquids that stimulate gastric secretion (e.g., spicy foods, caffeine, alcohol). Instruct the client to keep his or her head elevated for 1 to 2 hours after meals. The client may need to be in this position continuously. Histamine antagonists and antacids help to reduce and neutralize gastric acid. To help prevent choking, collaborate with the dietitian for dietary changes (Chart 24-13).

CHART 24-13

BEST PRACTICE for
The Client with Progressive Systemic Sclerosis and Esophagitis

- Keep the client's head elevated at least 60 degrees during meals and for at least 1 hour after each meal.
- Provide small, frequent meals rather than three large meals each day.
- Give the client small amounts of food for each bite, and explain the importance of chewing each bite carefully before swallowing.
- Provide semisoft foods, such as mashed potatoes and pudding or custard; liquids are most likely to cause choking.
- Collaborate with the dietitian about the client's diet.
- Teach the client to avoid foods that increase gastric secretion, such as caffeine, pepper, and other spices.
- Give antacids if the health care provider prescribes them.

Nursing care for the client with joint pain and decreased mobility is very similar to that for the client with rheumatoid arthritis (see Interventions [Rheumatoid Arthritis], p. 397). Nonsteroidal anti-inflammatory drugs are given for inflammation and pain. Joint protection and energy conservation are also important for these clients.

Community-Based Care

Community-based care for the client with PSS is similar to that for the client with lupus. The client is treated at home but may need frequent hospitalizations if major organ involvement occurs during exacerbations. The Arthritis Foundation and Scleroderma Foundation are excellent resources for more information about the disease and how to manage it.

GOUT

PATHOPHYSIOLOGY

Gout, or gouty arthritis, is a systemic disease in which urate crystals deposit in the joints and other body tissues, causing inflammation. The cause and treatment of gout have been firmly established. The classic case of well-advanced disease is seldom seen today unless the client does not comply with the therapeutic regimen. There are two major types of gout: primary and secondary.

Primary gout is the most common type and results from one of several inborn errors of purine metabolism. An end product of purine metabolism is uric acid, which is usually excreted by the kidneys. In primary gout, the production of uric acid exceeds the excretion capability of the kidneys; sodium urate is deposited in synovium and other tissues, resulting in inflammation. Primary gout is inherited as an X-linked trait; males are affected through female carriers. Approximately 25% of clients have a family history of gout. Primary gout affects middle-aged and older men (85% to 90% of clients with gout) and postmenopausal women. The peak time of onset is during a person's 30s and 40s.

Secondary gout involves hyperuricemia (excessive uric acid in the blood) caused by another disease. Secondary gout affects people of all ages. Renal insufficiency, diuretic therapy, and certain chemotherapeutic agents decrease the normal excretion of uric acid and other waste products. Disorders such as multiple myeloma and certain carcinomas result in increased production of uric acid because of a greater turnover of cellular nucleic acids. Treatment involves management of the underlying disorder.

There are four phases of the primary disease process: asymptomatic hyperuricemic, acute, intercritical (intercurrent), and chronic. The client is usually unaware of the **asymptomatic hyperuricemic phase** unless he or she has had a serum uric acid level determination. The serum level is elevated, but no overt signs of the disease are present.

The first "attack" of gouty arthritis begins the **acute phase.** The client experiences excruciating pain and inflammation in one or more small joints, usually the metatarsophalangeal joint of the great toe. Of all clients with gout, 75% experience inflammation of this joint **(podagra)** as the initial manifestation. The erythrocyte sedimentation rate (ESR) and white blood cell count are increased as a result of the inflammatory process.

Months or perhaps years can pass before additional attacks occur; this is the **intercritical,** or intercurrent, **phase** of the disease. The client is asymptomatic, and no abnormalities are found during examination of the joints.

After repeated episodes of acute gout, deposits of urate crystals develop under the skin and within the major organs, particularly in the renal system. The client is then classified as having **chronic tophaceous gout.** In chronic gout, urate kidney stone formation is more common than renal insufficiency.

COLLABORATIVE MANAGEMENT

Assessment

Collect historical data, including age, gender, and a family history of gout. Gout affects more men than women, particularly men who have relatives with gout. A complete medical history is needed to determine whether gout has been caused by another problem. There is a tendency to overuse diuretics, especially among women, which can lead to secondary gout.

ACUTE GOUT

Overt manifestations are present in the acute and chronic phases of gout. You most likely will encounter a client with acute gout; chronic gout is not common in the United States today. Joint inflammation is the most common finding and is usually so painful that the client seeks medical care. Inspect the inflamed area. It is usually too painful and swollen to be touched or moved.

CHRONIC GOUT

With chronic gout, inspect the skin for **tophi,** or deposits of sodium urate crystals (Figure 24-9). Although tophi may occur anywhere, they commonly appear on the outer ear. Other common sites for tophi are the arms and fingers near the joints. The tophi are hard on palpation and are irregular in shape. When the skin over the tophi is irritated, it may break open, and a yellow, gritty substance is discharged. Infection may result.

Other manifestations of chronic gout include signs of renal calculi (stones) or renal dysfunction. Stones develop in about 20% of clients with gout. In some cases, urate kidney stones occur before the arthritis is present.

The health care provider orders determinations of serum uric acid levels to validate hyperuricemia. Because the serum uric acid level can be altered by food intake, serial measurements are usually obtained. A consistent level of more than 8 mg/100 mL is generally considered abnormal. Urinary uric acid levels are also measured; an overproduction of uric acid is confirmed by an excretion of more than 600 mg/24 hr after a 5-day restriction of purine intake.

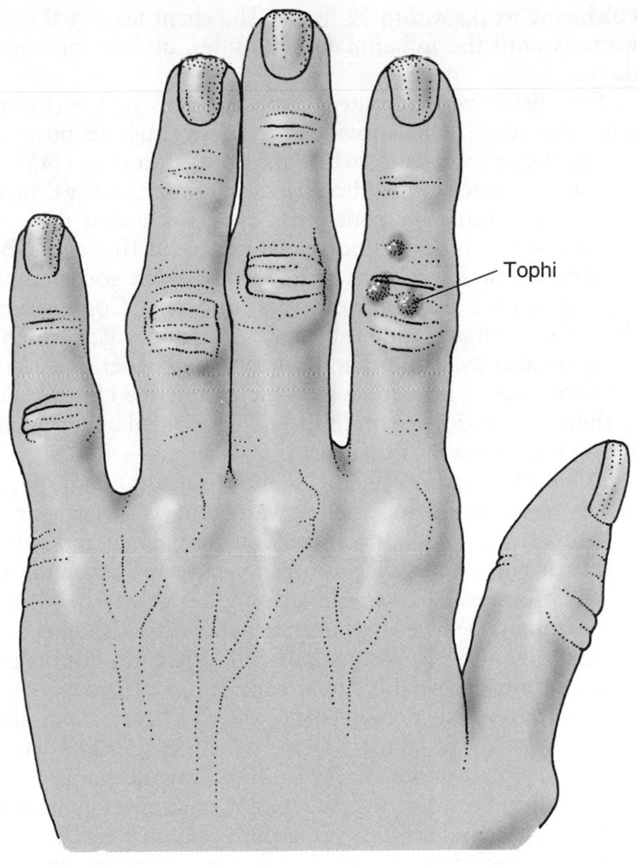

Figure 24-9 ■ Typical appearance of tophi, which may occur in chronic gout, on an index finger.

The health care provider may order renal function tests, such as blood urea nitrogen (BUN) and serum creatinine levels, to monitor possible kidney involvement. A definitive diagnostic test for the disease is synovial fluid aspiration (arthrocentesis) to detect the needle-like crystals that are characteristic of the disorder.

Interventions

Gout is one of the easiest diseases for the health care provider to diagnose and treat in its early phases. If the client receives treatment and complies with drug therapy, he or she should experience no further symptoms and no change in body image or lifestyle. The client with gout is usually treated on an ambulatory basis.

Drug Therapy. Drug therapy is the primary component of management for clients with gout. In acute gouty "attacks," the inflammation subsides spontaneously within 3 to 5 days; however, most clients cannot tolerate the pain for that long. The drugs used for acute gout are different from those used for chronic gout. The health care provider typically prescribes a combination of colchicine (Colsalide, Novo-colchicine✱) and a nonsteroidal anti-inflammatory drug (NSAID), such as indomethacin (Indocin, Novomethacin✱) or ibuprofen (Motrin, Amersol✱), for acute gout. IV colchicine works within 12 hours. The client takes oral medications until the inflammation subsides, usually for 4 to 7 days.

For clients with repeated acute episodes or for chronic gout, the health care provider prescribes drugs to promote uric acid excretion or to reduce its production on a continuous, maintenance basis. Allopurinol (Zyloprim) is the drug of choice. As a xanthine oxidase inhibitor, it prevents the conversion of xanthine to uric acid. Probenecid (Benemid, Benuryl✱) is also effective as a uricosuric drug in gout because it promotes the excretion of excess uric acid. Combination drugs that contain probenecid and colchicine (e.g., ColBenemid) are also available. The health care provider and nurse monitor serum uric acid levels to determine the effectiveness of these medications. Aspirin should be avoided because it inactivates the effects of the drug.

Diet Therapy. Whether or not to recommend special dietary restrictions for clients with gout is controversial. Some physicians advocate a strict low-purine diet and advise clients to avoid foods such as organ meats, shellfish, and oily fish with bones (e.g., sardines). Some health care providers and dietitians believe that limiting protein foods, especially red and organ meats, is sufficient. Still others do not believe that diet restrictions affect treatment. It is well known, however, that excessive alcohol intake and fad "starvation" diets can cause a gouty attack. Clients usually determine which foods precipitate acute attacks and try to avoid them.

In addition to food and beverage restrictions, clients with gout should avoid all forms of aspirin and diuretics because they may precipitate an attack. Likewise, excessive physical or emotional stress can exacerbate the disease. Stress-management techniques may be helpful for the client with gout.

Having the client drink more fluids is one of the best measures to prevent the formation of urinary stones. Increasing fluid intake helps to dilute urine and prevent sediment formation. Uric acid is more soluble in urine with a high pH and therefore is less likely to form urinary stones in that environment. The client's urinary pH can be increased with an intake of alkaline ash foods, such as citrus fruits and juices, milk, and certain dairy products. The value of adhering to a strict diet rich in these foods is questionable, however.

The client with a diagnosis of gout is seldom hospitalized unless renal complications develop. If the client follows the prescribed interventions, chronic tophaceous gout should not develop.

OTHER CONNECTIVE TISSUE DISEASES

The care of clients with connective tissue diseases (CTDs) is often similar regardless of the specific diagnosis. This section describes other fairly common diseases that are classified as CTDs.

Polymyositis/Dermatomyositis

Polymyositis is a diffuse inflammatory disease of skeletal (striated) muscle that causes symmetric weakness and atrophy. When a rash accompanies polymyositis, the disease is called **dermatomyositis.** Both diseases vary in their mode of onset and progression and are characterized by spontaneous remissions and exacerbations. Women are affected twice as often as men, and men and women between 30 and 60 years of age are most susceptible to either disease.

In addition to proximal muscle and possible skin involvement, clients typically have polyarthritis, **polyarthralgia** (aching around multiple joints), and Raynaud's phenomenon (see Chapter 39). Clients with dermatomyositis have the characteristic heliotrope (lilac) rash and periorbital (around the eyes) edema. Malignant neoplasms are more common in these clients than in the rest of the population; as many as 30% of clients older than 55 years of age have malignancies. Many clients have difficulty swallowing or talking because of severe muscle weakness.

These conditions are treated with high-dose steroids, immunosuppressive agents, and supportive care. Particular attention is given to nutrition.

Systemic Necrotizing Vasculitis

Necrotizing vasculitis is a term for a group of diseases whose primary manifestation is **arteritis** (inflammation of arterial walls), which causes ischemia in the tissues usually supplied by the involved vessels. The drug of choice for most types of vasculitis is chronic steroid therapy (prednisone), although immunosuppressive drugs may also be used.

Polyarteritis nodosa affects middle-aged men most often and involves every body system. Treatment is similar to that for systemic lupus, but the prognosis is not as promising. Renal disorders and cardiac involvement are the most common causes of death. **Hypersensitivity vasculitis** is the most common form of vasculitis and primarily causes skin lesions as an allergic response to drugs, infections, or tumors. **Takayasu's arteritis,** or the **aortic arch syndrome,** is also called the "pulseless" disease. Women in their 20s, particularly those of Japanese descent, are affected most often. Cerebral ischemia is manifested by visual changes, syncope, and vertigo.

Polymyalgia Rheumatica and Temporal Arteritis

Polymyalgia rheumatica (PMR) is a clinical syndrome characterized by stiffness, weakness, and aching of the proximal musculature (i.e., the shoulder and pelvic girdles). Systemic manifestations such as low-grade fever, arthralgias (aching around joints) and stiffness, fatigue, and weight loss occur in the majority of cases. The most common joints affected are the neck, shoulder, and hip joints. Stiffness is worse in the morning.

Most clients have an increased erythrocyte sedimentation rate (ESR) and a normochromic, normocytic anemia (see Chart 24-8). The disease commonly occurs in women over 50 years of age and typically responds to low-dose steroid therapy in 1 to 3 days (Mikanowicz & Leslie, 2000).

Giant cell arteritis (GCA), or **temporal arteritis (TA),** occurs in as many as 20% of people with PMR. GCA is a systemic vasculitis that affects large and midsized arteries. Clinical manifestations may be classified as systemic, myalgic, and arteritic (Chart 24-14).

The cause of both PMR and GCA is unknown, but a genetic predisposition related to HLA-DRB1 is likely. The dis-

CHART 24-14

KEY FEATURES of
Giant Cell (Temporal) Arteritis

Systemic Manifestations
- Fatigue, malaise
- Fever
- Weight loss
- Night sweats

Myalgic Manifestations (if client has polymyalgia rheumatica [PMR])
- Proximal, symmetric muscle pain
- Stiffness

Arteritic Manifestations
- Erythema
- Pain (especially localized temporal headache)
- Swelling
- Tenderness (especially scalp)
- Amaurosis fugax (temporary vision loss in one eye)
- Diplopia or any vision change (requires urgent management)

order is easy to miss because most clients are older women who complain of declining vision (also an age-related change). GCA is treated *urgently* with high doses of corticosteroids, often as high as 40 to 80 mg daily (Mikanowicz & Leslie, 2000). Taking calcium and vitamin D is important for preventing osteoporosis that can result from steroid therapy, especially in middle-aged women.

Ankylosing Spondylitis

Ankylosing spondylitis (AS) is also known as *Marie-Strümpell disease* or *rheumatoid spondylitis.* The disease affects the vertebral column and causes spinal deformities. Although this disorder is present in both men and women at any age in adulthood, young white men under 40 years of age are most commonly affected. Other features include **iritis** (inflammation of the iris), arthritis or arthralgia (joint aching), and nonspecific systemic manifestations such as malaise and weight loss.

Although the exact cause is unknown, ankylosing spondylitis is associated with the HLA-B27 antigen. Compromised respiratory function caused by a rigid chest wall is the major threat to health. Most clients function normally but live with chronic discomfort. As in other times of inflammatory arthritis, anti-inflammatory drugs, heat applications, and physical therapy are the key components of management (see earlier discussion of pain management for rheumatoid arthritis, p. 397).

Disease-modifying antirheumatic drugs (DMARDs), such as methotrexate (Rheumatrex), have been successful in slowing disease progress. Biological response modifiers (TNF inhibitors), such as infliximab (Remicade), have also been approved for managing ankylosing spondylitis.

Reiter's Syndrome

As with ankylosing spondylitis, **Reiter's syndrome** is associated with the HLA-B27 antigen. This disease most often affects young white men. The complete syndrome is a triad of arthritis, conjunctivitis, and **urethritis** (inflammation of the urethra) resulting from exposure to sexually transmitted disease or dysentery (infectious diarrhea). Urethritis is often the first clinical manifestation.

Although the disease is characterized by this triad of manifestations, other conditions such as **balanitis circinata** (ringlike inflammation of the glans penis) and skin lesions are equally significant for confirmation of the diagnosis.

Management is symptomatic and may be complex if there is organ involvement. NSAIDs and physical therapy are generally prescribed.

Sjögren's Syndrome

With **Sjögren's syndrome,** inflammatory cells and immune complexes obstruct secretory ducts and glands. As a result, the client has dry eyes *(sicca syndrome),* a dry mouth *(xerostomia),* and a dry vagina. Severe cases involve swelling of the parotid and lacrimal areas and systemic manifestations (e.g., fever, fatigue). Of clients with the syndrome, 50% have an associated disease, such as rheumatoid arthritis (RA) or progressive systemic sclerosis (PSS).

Local management includes meticulous care of the mouth, eyes, and perineal areas and the use of artificial tears and saliva. Systemic steroids (prednisone) may also be administered. Pilocarpine is sometimes useful for the eyes. Without treatment, the client can lose vision, and oral ulcerations, dental caries, and difficulty in swallowing or talking may ensue.

Marfan Syndrome

Marfan syndrome is inherited as an autosomal, dominant trait with equal prevalence in males and females. Clients with this syndrome have abnormalities of the skeletal, ocular, cardiopulmonary, and central nervous systems as a result of a basic defect in extracellular microfibrils. Microfibrils are very small fibers within cells.

Clients with the classic form of Marfan syndrome tend to be excessively tall and have elongated hands and feet. The diagnosis of milder forms of Marfan syndrome is often missed in young men, especially athletes involved in sports such as basketball.

Other skeletal abnormalities include scoliosis, a funnel-shaped chest, loss of the normal cervical curve, and hyperextensibility of the joints. Subluxation of the lens is usually bilateral and occurs by the age of 5 years, causing decreased visual acuity or glaucoma.

Cardiovascular problems are responsible for most deaths resulting from Marfan syndrome. The average life span is 32 years. Mitral valve prolapse with regurgitation as well as aortic aneurysm with regurgitation and aortic rupture are common. The client is closely monitored by echocardiography (Holcomb, 2000).

Management is both palliative and preventive and includes careful monitoring, cardiovascular medications, and orthopedic surgery if needed. Genetic counseling should also be part of the treatment plan, especially for women of childbearing age.

Infectious Arthritis

Any infectious agent can invade the joint space and cause inflammation and tissue destruction. Certain pathogens, such as *Staphylococcus aureus,* destroy tissue rapidly; others, especially viruses, do not cause irreversible damage. The cornerstone of management is local or systemic antibiotic therapy for 6 to 8 weeks.

Lyme Disease

Lyme arthritis is a reportable systemic infectious disease caused by the spirochete ***Borrelia burgdorferi*** and results from the bite of an infected deer tick. Signs and symptoms of Lyme disease generally begin with identification of a large "bull's-eye" circular rash along with malaise, fever, headache, and muscle or joint aches. More than 85% of the disease in the United States is seen in New England; the mid-Atlantic states, including Maryland and Virginia; the upper mid-West, including Wisconsin and Minnesota; and northern California, especially during the summer months (Sigal, 2001).

In the early and localized stage I, the client appears with flu-like symptoms, rash (erythema migrans, the "bull's-eye" rash), and pain and stiffness in the muscles and joints. Symptoms begin within 3 to 32 days of the tick bite. Doxycycline, amoxicillin, or cefuroxime is prescribed for 10 to 21 days.

Stage II (early disseminated stage) occurs 2 to 12 weeks after the tick bite. The client experiences carditis with dysrhythmias, dyspnea, dizziness, or palpitations as well as central nervous system disorders such as meningitis, facial paralysis (often misdiagnosed as Bell's palsy), and peripheral neuritis. For severe disease, IV antibiotics (e.g., ceftriaxone or cefotaxime) are given.

If Lyme disease is not diagnosed and treated in the earlier stages, later chronic complications (e.g., arthralgias, fatigue, and memory/thinking problems) can result. This late stage III (chronic persistent stage) occurs weeks to years after the tick bite. For some clients, the first and only sign of Lyme disease is arthritis. In other cases the disease may not respond to antibiotics, and the client develops permanent damage to joints and the nervous system (Sigal, 2001). Prevention is the best strategy for Lyme disease (Chart 24-15).

CHART 24-15

CLIENT EDUCATION GUIDE

Prevention and Early Detection of Lyme Disease

- Avoid heavily wooded areas or areas with thick underbrush.
- Walk in the center of the trail.
- Avoid dark clothing. Lighter-colored clothing makes spotting ticks easier.
- Use an insect repellent on your skin and clothes when in an area where ticks are likely to be found.
- Wear long-sleeved tops and long pants.
- Wear closed shoes and a hat or cap.
- Bathe immediately after being in an infested area, and inspect your body for ticks (about the size of a pinhead); pay special attention to your arms, legs, and hairline.
- Gently remove with tweezers or fingers any tick that you find. Dispose of the tick by flushing it down the toilet (burning a tick could spread infection).
- Wait 4 to 6 weeks after being bitten by a tick before being tested for Lyme disease (testing before this time is not reliable).
- Report symptoms, such as a rash or influenza-like illness, to your physician.
- Obtain a vaccine to prevent disease if you live in a high-risk area.

Pseudogout

Pseudogout is a disease that mimics the clinical manifestations of gout. In this disease, however, the crystals deposited in the joints are calcium pyrophosphate, not sodium urate. These crystals usually migrate to cartilage, but they can also deposit in tendons, ligaments, and synovium.

The client most susceptible to pseudogout is an older hospitalized male. Although the cause is not certain, the incidence is highest in men with metastatic cancer or endocrine imbalances such as hypothyroidism. Nonsteroidal anti-inflammatory drugs (NSAIDs) usually control manifestations of the disease.

Psoriatic Arthritis

Psoriatic arthritis (PsA) affects about 5% to 10% of people who have psoriasis, a skin condition characterized by a scaly, itchy rash, usually on the elbows, knees, and scalp. Fingernail and toenail lifting and pitting may also occur (see Chapter 70 for discussion of this disease). The joint pain associated with psoriasis is often associated with stiffness, especially in the morning. Neck and back pain are particularly common, but various forms of the disease can cause small joint arthritis or involvement of the sacroiliac joints of the spine.

TABLE 24-3 Common Disorders Associated with Arthritis

▪ Crohn's disease	▪ Hyperparathyroidism
▪ Ulcerative colitis	▪ Hyperthyroidism
▪ Tuberculosis	▪ Diabetes mellitus
▪ Hemophilia	▪ Sickle-cell anemia crisis
▪ Whipple's disease	▪ Psoriasis
▪ Intestinal bypass surgery	▪ Infection

Psoriatic arthritis (PsA) occurs most often in people between 20 and 50 in men and women of all races. Nail symptoms are common in clients who have the associated arthritis. Causes may include genetic and environmental factors, infectious agents, and immune system dysfunction.

Although most clients do not experience destructive and deforming arthritis, those who do suffer a major impact on their quality of life. Treatment is focused on managing joint pain and inflammation, controlling skin lesions, and slowing the progression of the disease. Health teaching for skin care is similar to that for lupus. Management of joint inflammation is similar to that for rheumatoid arthritis. Methotrexate (Rheumatrex), sulfasalazine (Azulfidine), and biological response modifiers have been used with success. Further discussion regarding management of psoriasis can be found in Chapter 70.

Other Disease-Associated Arthritis

A number of other diseases can cause secondary arthritis. Tuberculosis, Crohn's disease, ulcerative colitis, hemophilia, and sickle-cell anemia are typical examples. To manage joint involvement, the primary disease is treated. For example, when a client with Crohn's disease is in remission, joint manifestations also subside. Conditions in which joint involvement can occur are presented in Table 24-3.

Fibromyalgia Syndrome

Fibromyalgia syndrome (FMS), also referred to as simply fibromyalgia, was previously known as fibrositis. The name was changed because FMS is now understood to be a

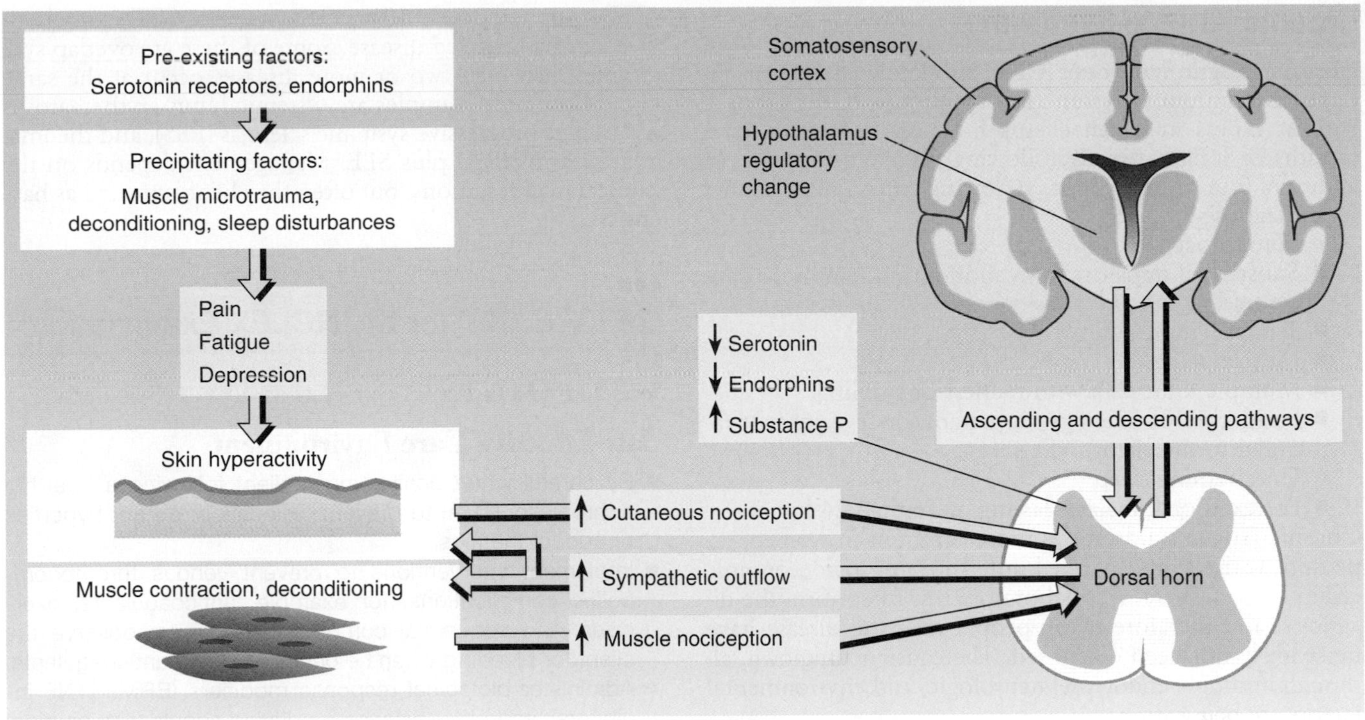

Figure 24-10 ■ Theoretic pathophysiologic model of fibromyalgia.

chronic pain syndrome, not an inflammatory disease. Pain and tenderness are located at specific sites in the back of the neck, upper chest, trunk, low back, and extremities. These tender points are also known as **trigger points** and can typically be palpated to elicit pain in a predictable, reproducible pattern. The pain is typically described as burning and gnawing. As seen in the theoretic pathophysiologic model in Figure 24-10, increased muscle tenderness may be due to the inability to tolerate pain, possibly related to dysfunction in the brain, especially the thalamus and hypothalamus (McCance & Huether, 2002).

The pain and tenderness tend to come and go but typically worsen in response to stress, increased activity, and weather conditions. The client complains of mild to severe fatigue, and sleep disturbances are common. Some clients note numbness or tingling in their extremities, and others are sensitive to noxious odors, loud noises, and bright lights. Headaches and jaw pain are also common.

Other symptoms include the following:

- Gastrointestinal (GI), including abdominal pain, diarrhea and constipation, and heartburn
- Genitourinary, including dysuria, urinary frequency, urgency, and pelvic pain
- Cardiovascular, including dyspnea, chest pain, and dysrhythmias
- Visual, including blurred vision and dry eyes

Many clients with these symptoms become frustrated because they are not properly diagnosed and are in constant pain and discomfort. Some clients are diagnosed as having chronic fatigue syndrome (CFS). CFS, migraine headache, irritable bowel syndrome (IBS), and myofascial pain are often present in clients with FMS. As a result, clients can become depressed and anxious.

Most clients are women between 30 and 50 years of age. It is unlikely that the disease is caused by one factor. Possible precipitating factors include CFS, Lyme disease, trauma, medications, and flu-like illness (McCance & Huether, 2002). FMS may also be aggravated by deep-sleep deprivation. Instruct clients to limit caffeine, alcohol, or other unnecessary substances that could interfere with deep sleep. Establish a regular sleep pattern.

Secondary FMS can accompany any connective tissue disease (CTD), particularly lupus and rheumatoid disease, and may not necessarily be related to sleep patterns. Antidepressive agents such as amitriptyline (Elavil, Apo-Amitriptyline✱) or nortriptyline (Pamelor) may promote sleep and reduce pain or muscle spasm. These drugs should be used with caution in older adults because they can cause confusion and orthostatic hypotension. Trazodone (Desyrel) may be preferred for this population because of its minimal side effects. Selective serotonin reuptake inhibitors (SSRIs), such as sertraline (Zoloft) and escitalopram oxalate (Lexapro), may be prescribed to manage depression. Observe for side effects. Monitor for postural blood pressure changes. Instruct clients to observe for drowsiness and not to operate dangerous machinery or drive if drowsy.

Physical therapy, along with nonsteroidal anti-inflammatory drugs (NSAIDs) and muscle relaxants may be prescribed to help decrease fibromyalgia pain. Instruct the client to exercise at home regularly. Home exercise should include stretching, strengthening, and low-impact aerobic exercise. Walking, swimming, rowing, biking, and water exercise are good examples of low-impact exercise. Complementary and alternative therapies, such as tai chi, acupuncture, hypnosis, and stress management, may help some clients with symptom relief (Taggart, et al., 2003). Refer the client to the land, water, and walking exercise pamphlets produced by the Arthritis Foundation. Inform clients about the National Chronic Fatigue Syndrome and Fibromyalgia Association for additional information.

Chronic Fatigue Syndrome

Chronic fatigue syndrome (CFS), also known as chronic fatigue and immune dysfunction syndrome (CFIDS), is a chronic illness in which clients have severe fatigue for 6 months or longer, usually following flu-like symptoms. In addition, four or more of the following criteria must be met for a diagnosis of CFS:

- Sore throat
- Substantial impairment in short-term memory or concentration
- Tender lymph nodes
- Muscle pain
- Multiple joint pain with redness or swelling
- Headaches of a new type, pattern, or severity (not familiar to the client)
- Unrefreshing sleep
- Postexertional malaise lasting more than 24 hours

Chronic fatigue syndrome is most common in women, especially Latinos, and is not limited to any socioeconomic group or age. There is no laboratory test to confirm the diagnosis, and therefore many people with the disease have most likely not been diagnosed. The cause is unknown, although immune, endocrine, neurologic, and environmental factors are being studied.

Management of the client is challenging in that there is no cure for FMS. Treatment is supportive and focuses on alleviation or reduction of symptoms. For example, NSAIDs may help with body aches and pain. Low-dose antidepressants may also be effective in promoting sleep and preventing or treating depression. Teach the client to follow good health practices, such as adequate sleep, proper nutrition, regular exercise (but not excessive to increase fatigue), stress management, and energy conservation. Complementary and alternative therapies, such as acupuncture, tai chi, massage, and herbal supplements may be helpful for some clients.

Refer the client to the National Chronic Fatigue Syndrome and Fibromylagia Association, American Association for Chronic Fatigue Syndrome, and the Chronic Fatigue and Immune Dysfunction Syndrome Association of America.

Local Inflammatory Disorders

Two of the most common inflammatory conditions, bursitis and tendinitis, are localized to specific connective tissues. Both problems are caused by repetitive motion and overuse related to aging, sports, or work injuries. **Bursitis** is an irritation of subcutaneous tissues and inflammation of the underlying bursae. **Tendinitis** is inflammation of one or more tendon sheaths.

Tight shoes often irritate the heel and cause bursitis. Higher impact aerobic exercise and diseases such as rheumatoid arthritis (RA) and gout can lead to bursitis and tendinitis.

The conservative management for both inflammatory conditions includes rest, ice, and NSAIDs to relieve pain. More aggressive treatment may include corticosteroid injections or surgery to remove the inflamed tissue.

Mixed Connective Tissue Disease

A diagnosis of mixed CTD is made when a client presents with clinical manifestations that are not typical of any one CTD. Approximately 10% of clients with CTDs are classified as having mixed disease. Some of these are overlap syndromes, in which two or more diseases occur at the same time. Common examples are systemic lupus erythematosus (SLE) plus progressive systemic sclerosis (PSS), and rheumatoid arthritis (RA) plus SLE. Management depends on the clinical manifestations, but often the client is treated as having SLE.

GET READY for the NCLEX Examination!

KEY POINTS

Safe Effective Care Environment

- Be careful when positioning a client following a total hip arthroplasty (THA) to prevent dislocation; do not hyperflex or adduct the legs.
- Implement interventions to prevent venous thromboembolitic complications, for example, anticoagulants, exercises, and sequential compression devices; observe the client for bleeding when he or she is taking anticoagulants.
- Administer biological response modifiers (BRMs [TNF inhibitors]) and other disease-modifying agents with caution; do not give TNF inhibitors to clients with tuberculosis or multiple sclerosis.
- Prioritize care for clients with systemic lupus erythematosus (SLE) by monitoring for life-threatening complications, such as renal failure.

Health Promotion and Maintenance

- Teach clients who have osteoarthritis (OA) or are prone to the disease to lose weight (if obese), avoid trauma, and limit strenuous weight-bearing activities.
- Instruct clients with arthritic pain to use multiple modalities for pain relief, including ice/heat, rest, positioning, complementary and alternative therapies, and medications as prescribed.
- Remind clients with arthritis and connective tissue diseases to contact local chapters of the Arthritis Foundation and other disease-specific national groups for information and support groups.
- Teach clients to monitor and report side and adverse effects of drugs used to treat OA and connective tissue diseases.
- Teach clients who are taking hydroxychloroquine (Plaquenil) to have frequent (every 6 months) eye examinations to monitor for retinal changes.
- Reinforce the importance of good health practices, such as adequate sleep, proper nutrition, regular exercise, and stress-management techniques.
- Teach clients with arthritis what exercises to do (Chart 24-5), joint protection techniques (Chart 24-6), and energy conservation guidelines (Chart 24-10).

Psychosocial Integrity

- Recognize that clients with rheumatoid arthritis (RA) may have body image disturbance as a result of potentially deforming joint involvement and nodules.
- Encourage clients with arthritis and connective tissue diseases to "ventilate" about their chronic illness and identify coping strategies that have previously been successful.

- Be aware that chronic, painful diseases affect the client's quality of life and role performance.
- Accept behaviors of clients that may seem manipulative or demanding and emphasize the clients' strengths.
- Teach clients with SLE to avoid sunlight; exacerbations of the disease may be triggered.
- Remind clients with gout to avoid factors that trigger an attack, such as aspirin, organ meats, and alcohol.
- Teach people ways to avoid Lyme disease as listed in Chart 24-15.
- Recognize that clients with fibromyalgia syndrome (FMS) and chronic fatigue syndrome (CFS) are often frustrated because they have not been diagnosed or have been misdiagnosed.
- Teach clients with FMS and CFS that antidepressant drugs can promote sleep and decrease pain as well as prevent or treat the depression that is common with these illnesses.

Physiological Integrity

- Be aware that most of the connective tissue diseases and arthritic disorders have a genetic basis as part of their etiology; most are also classified as autoimmune diseases and have remissions and exacerbations.
- Differentiate that OA is primarily a degenerative joint problem, whereas rheumatoid arthritis RA is a systemic disease.
- Realize that older clients have OA more than younger clients; younger clients have RA more than older adults; other differences between the two diseases are summarized in Table 24-1.
- Monitor laboratory test results for clients with autoimmune connective tissue diseases as highlighted in Chart 24-8.
- Assess for side and adverse effects of medications used for arthritis and connective tissue diseases as specified in Chart 24-9.
- Be aware that disease-modifying antirheumatic drugs (DMARDs) and BRMs slow the progression of connective tissue diseases, especially RA and SLE.
- Assess clients with rheumatoid arthritis for early or late clinical manifestations as listed in Chart 24-7.
- Differentiate clinical manifestations and prognosis for clients with SLE versus progressive systemic sclerosis (PSS), as listed in Chart 24-11.
- Plan interdisciplinary care for clients with arthritis and other diseases in which arthritis is a major manifestation.
- Assess for swallowing ability in clients who have PSS; collaborate with the dietitian for food modifications if needed.
- Monitor for acute joint inflammation for clients with a history of gout; the great toe and other small joints are most typically affected.
- Assess for visual complaints (indicating possible giant cell arteritis) in clients with polymyalgia rheumatica; report changes immediately to the health care provider.
- Be aware that arthritis often accompanies other diseases, such as psoriasis, Crohn's disease, and hemophilia.

ADDITIONAL STUDY RESOURCES

Go to your Student CD-ROM for Review Questions for the NCLEX Examination.

evolve Go to http://evolve.elsevier.com/Iggy/ for Integrated Management of Care Questions for the NCLEX Examination.

SELECTED BIBLIOGRAPHY

Asterisk indicates a classic or definitive work on this subject.

Abelson, A.G., et al. (2002). A common sense guide to rheumatologic tests. *Patient Care for the Nurse Practitioner, 6(Apr).*

Amado, J.A., & Thomas, D.J. (2002). Early Recognition of Marfan's syndrome. *Journal of the American Academy of Nurse Practitioners, 14*(5), 201-204.

American College of Rheumatology Subcommittee on Rheumatoid Arthritis Guidelines. (2002). Guidelines for the management of rheumatoid arthritis. *Arthritis & Rheumatism, 46*(2), 328-342.

Arthritis Foundation. (2003). 2003 Drug guide. *Supplement to Arthritis Today, 1-26.*

Barry, F.P. (2003). Mesenchymal stem cell therapy in joint disease. *Novartis Foundation Symposium, 249*, 86-96.

Berger, R.A. (2003). Total hip arthroplasty using the minimally invasive two-incision approach. *Clinical Orthopedics, 417,* 232-241.

Branson, J.J., & Goldstein, W.M. (2003). Primary total hip arthroplasty. *AORN Journal, 78*(6), 956-969.

Cohen, M., Wolfe, R., Mai, T., & Lewis, D. (2003). A randomized, double blind, placebo controlled trial of a topical cream containing glucosamine sulfate, chondroitin sulfate, and camphor for osteoarthritis of the knee. *Journal of Rheumatology, 30*(3), 523-528.

D'Arcy, Y. (2002). How to treat arthritis pain. *Nursing 2002, 32*(7), 30-31.

*Eaton, L., & Meiner, S.E. (1999). Marfan syndrome: Identification and management. *MEDSURG Nursing, 8*(2), 113-117.

Edworthy, S.M. (2001). Clinical manifestations of systemic lupus erythematosus. In W.N. Kelley et al. (Eds.), *Textbook of rheumatology* (6th ed., pp. 1105-1123). Philadelphia: W.B. Saunders.

*Geier, K. (1998). Perioperative blood management. *Orthopaedic Nursing, 17*(Suppl 1), 6-36.

Gemmell, H.A., Jacobson, B.H., & Hayes, B.M. (2003). Effect of a topical herbal cream on osteoarthritis of the hand and knee: A pilot study. *Journal of Manipulative Physiologic Therapy, 26*(5), 15.

Gever, M.P. (2002). Infliximab: Test your drug IQ. *Critical Care, 33*(1), 32cc6-32cc7.

Goolsby, M.J. (2002). Guidelines for the management of rheumatoid arthritis: 2002 Update. *Journal of the American Academy of Nurse Practitioners, 14*(10), 432-437.

Hahn, B.H. (2001). Management of systemic lupus erythematosus. In W.N. Kelley et al. (Eds.), *Textbook of rheumatology* (6th ed., pp. 1125-1143). Philadelphia: W.B. Saunders.

Harris, E.D. (2001). Treatment of rheumatoid arthritis. In W.N. Kelley et al. (Eds.), *Textbook of rheumatology* (6th ed., pp. 1001-1022). Philadelphia: W.B. Saunders.

Hawke, M. (2002). Scleroderma–conquering the unknown. *Nursing Spectrum,* 12(19DC):10-11.

Holcomb, S.S. (2000). Reviewing Marfan syndrome. *Nursing 2000, 30*(5), 32cc10-32cc12.

Hussar, D. (2002). New drugs 2002–Part III. *Nursing 2002, 32*(7), 60.

Hutchinson, R. (2004). Pain control: COX-2-selective NSAIDs. *American Journal of Nursing, 104*(3), 52-56.

Ignatavicius, D.D. (2001). Rheumatoid arthritis and the older adult. *Geriatric Nursing, 22*(3), 139-142.

Kajs-Wyllie, M. (2002). Lupus cerebritis: A case study. *Journal of Neuroscience Nursing, 34*(4), 176-182.

Karch, A.M., & Karch, F.E.(2003). A Weekly Dosage Taken Daily: Drugs available in new once-weekly formulations require extra vigilance. *American Journal of Nursing, 103*(4), 64.

Kastanek, L. (2002). Using Anakinra for adult rheumatoid arthritis. *The Nurse Practitioner. 27*(4), 62-65.

*Kee, C.C. (1998). Living with osteoarthritis: Insiders' views. *Applied Nursing Research, 11*(1), 19-26.

Kee, C.C. (2000). Osteoarthritis: Manageable scourge of aging. *Nursing Clinics of North America, 35*(1), 199-208.

Kerr, K.L., & Johnson, D.A. (2000). Advanced practice nurses in rheumatology. *Practice View–American College of Rheumatology, 1*(7), 1-8.

Kettelman, K. (2000). Soothing the ache of joint surgery. *Nursing 2000, 30*(7), 14.

Klippel, J.H. (2001). *Primer on the rheumatic diseases* (12th ed.). Atlanta: The Arthritis Foundation.

Kremer, J.M. (2001). Nutrition and rheumatic diseases. In W.N. Kelley, et al. (Eds.), *Textbook of rheumatology* (6th ed., pp. 713-727). Philadelphia: W.B. Saunders.

Kuper, B.C., & Failla, S. (2000). Systemic lupus erythematosus: A multisystem autoimmune disorder. *Nursing Clinics of North America, 35*(1), 253-266.

*Lash, A.A. (1998). Quality of life in systemic lupus erythematosus. *Applied Nursing Research, 11*(3), 130-137.

*Lavernia C.J., Guzman, J.F., & Gachupin-Garcia, A. (1999). Cost effectiveness and quality of life in knee arthroplasty. *Clinical Orthopaedics, 345,* 134-139.

Litton, K.A. (2003). Defenses gone awry. *RN, 66* (3), *53-59.*

Loeser, R.F. (2003). A stepwise approach to the management of osteoarthritis. *Bulletin on the Rheumatic Diseases, 52*(5), 1-4.

Mankin, H.J., & Brandt, K.D. (2001). Pathogenesis of osteoarthritis. In W.N. Kelley, et al. (Eds.), *Textbook of rheumatology* (6th ed., pp. 1391-1407). Philadelphia: W.B. Saunders.

*Matula, P.A., & Shollenberger, D. (1999). Total joint project: Acute care to home care. *MEDSURG Nursing, 8*(2), 92-98.

McCaffrey, R., & Freeman, E. (2003). Effect of music on chronic osteoarthritis pain in older people. *Journal of Advanced Nursing, 44*(5), 517-524.

McCance, K.L., & Huether, S.E. (2002). *Pathophysiology* (4th ed.). St. Louis: Mosby.

*McGrath, A. (1997). Clinical snapshot: Raynaud's syndrome. *American Journal of Nursing, 97*(1), 34-35.

Medication Update Department. (2003). Rheumatoid arthritis treatment approved. *The Nurse Practitioner, 28*(4), 51.

Mikanowicz, C.K., & Leslie, M. (2000). Polymyalgia rheumatica and temporal arteritis: A case presentation. *Nursing Clinics of North America, 35*(1), 245-252.

*Morris, B.A., Colwell, C.W., & Hardwick, M.E. (1998). The use of low molecular weight heparins in the prevention of venous thromboembolic disease. *Orthopaedic Nursing, 17*(6), 23-29.

Pepper, G.A. (2000). Nonsteroidal anti-inflammatory drugs: New perspectives on a familiar class. *Nursing Clinics of North America, 35*(1), 223-244.

Petruzzi, L.M. & Vivino, F.B. (2003). Sjögren's syndrome–implications for perioperative practice. *AORN Journal 77*(3), 611-612, 614, 616-621, 624-628.

*Ritter, M.A., et al. (1999). Intra-articular morphine and/or bupivacaine after total knee replacement. *Journal of Bone and Joint Surgery, 81*(2), 301-303.

Sears, J.R., & Ganger, P.M. (2000). Antibiotics to treat RA. *RN, 63*(1), 41-42.

Sharkey, N.A., Williams, N.I., & Guerin, J.B. (2000). The role of exercise in the prevention and treatment of osteoporosis and osteoarthritis. *Nursing Clinics of North America, 35*(1), 209-222.

Siebold, J.R. (2001). Scleroderma and mixed connective tissue diseases In W.N. Kelley, et al. (Eds.), *Textbook of rheumatology* (6th ed., pp. 1211-1239). Philadelphia: W.B. Saunders.

Sigal, L.H. (2001). Lyme disease. In W.N. Kelley, et al. (Eds.), *Textbook of rheumatology* (6th ed., pp. 1485-1492). Philadelphia: W.B. Saunders.

Sledge, C.B., et al. (2001). The hip. In W.N. Kelley, et al. (Eds.), *Textbook of rheumatology* (6th ed., pp. 1743-1759). Philadelphia: W.B. Saunders.

Smedstad, L.M., & Liang, M.H. (2001). Psychosocial management of rheumatic diseases. In W.N. Kelley et al. (Eds.), *Textbook of rheumatology* (6th ed., pp. 729-734). Philadelphia: W.B. Saunders.

Solomon, L. (2001). Clinical features of osteoarthritis. In W.N. Kelley et al. (Eds.), *Textbook of rheumatology* (6th ed., pp. 1409-1418). Philadelphia: W.B. Saunders.

Strand, C.V., & Keystone, E. (2001). Biologic agents for the treatment of rheumatoid arthritis. In W.N. Kelley et al. (Eds.), *Textbook of rheumatology* (6th ed., pp. 899-911). Philadelphia: W.B. Saunders.

Taggert, H.M., et al. (2003). Effects of t'ai chi exercise on fibromyalgia symptoms and health-related quality of life. *Orthopaedic Nursing, 22*(5), 353-360.

Wade, N. (2003). Autoimmune diseases share a genetic defect, scientists find. Accessed April 18, 2004, from http://www.immunesupport.com/library/showarticle.cfm/ID/1575.

Weinblatt, M.E., et al. (2003). Adalimumab, a fully human antitumor necrosis factor (monoclonal antibody, for the treatment of rheumatoid arthritis in patients taking concomitant methotrexate–the Armada Trial. *Arthritis & Rheumatism, 49*(1), 35-45.

Wenz, J.F., Gurkan, I., & Jibodh, S.R. (2002). Mini-incision total hip arthroplasty: A comparative assessment of perioperative outcomes. *Orthopedics, 25*(10), 1031-1043.

Windsor, R.E.M., & Insall, J.N. (2001). The knee. In W.N. Kelley, et al. (Eds.), *Textbook of rheumatology* (6th ed., pp. 1759-1769). Philadelphia: W.B. Saunders.

Wise, C. (2003). The rational use of steroid injections in arthritis and nonarticular musculoskeletal pain syndromes. *Bulletin on the Rheumatic Diseases, 52*(1), 1-4.

CHAPTER 25

Interventions for Clients with HIV/AIDS and Other Immunodeficiencies

JAMES G. SAMPSON

LEARNING OUTCOMES

After studying this chapter, you should be able to:

1. Compare primary and secondary immunodeficiencies for cause and onset of problems.
2. Explain the differences in nursing care required for a client with a pathogenic infection versus a client with an opportunistic infection.
3. Distinguish between the conditions of human immunodeficiency virus (HIV) infection and acquired immunodeficiency syndrome (AIDS) for clinical manifestations and risks for complications.
4. Describe the ways in which HIV is transmitted.
5. Identify techniques to reduce the risk for infection in an immunocompromised client.
6. Develop a teaching plan for condom use among sexually active, non–English-speaking adults.
7. Prioritize nursing care for the client with AIDS who has impaired gas exchange.
8. Identify teaching priorities for the HIV-positive client receiving highly active antiretroviral therapy.
9. Develop a community-based teaching plan for the client with immune deficiency living at home.
10. Plan a week of meals for the client who has protein-calorie malnutrition.
11. Identify drug therapy categories that have the potential to reduce immune function.
12. Describe the infections that adult clients with congenital immunodeficiencies are at greatest risk for developing.
13. Describe the nursing actions and responsibilities for administration of IV immunoglobulin.

Go to your Student CD-ROM for Review Questions for the NCLEX Examination keyed to these Learning Outcomes.

Immune system function is concerned with helping the body prevent infection. The immune system assists the body to monitor and maintain those cells and substances that are considered "self," belonging to the body. Such things as newly made cells and compatible blood transfusions are deemed self and safe by the immune system. However, when the immune system detects something that does not belong to the body and represents a potential threat, its job is then to attack and destroy the "non-self" or "foreign" substance. Infection is a major threat. We are exposed to many organisms every day. The efficiency of the immune system prevents disease despite this exposure.

When the immune system fails to recognize infectious threats, disaster can soon follow. Immune system failure can be the result of a primary (congenital) immunodeficiency in which one or more parts of the system are not functioning properly from birth. These problems are usually genetic mutations that are discovered in the infant or child who is repeatedly sick. Immune system failure can also be secondary (acquired after birth) as the result of viral infection, contact with a toxin, or medical therapy. These problems can cause a normal immune system to stop functioning. In either case, the immune system is no longer able to distinguish what should be in the body from a foreign invader. The consequences for the immunodeficient client can range from mild, localized health problems to total immune system failure, leaving the body open to attack from any foreign pathogen.

Acquired (Secondary) Immunodeficiencies

ACQUIRED IMMUNODEFICIENCY SYNDROME

PATHOPHYSIOLOGY

Acquired immunodeficiency syndrome (AIDS) is the most common secondary immunodeficiency disease in the world. First identified in 1981, HIV/AIDS is now a serious worldwide epidemic.

Etiology and Genetic Risk

The cause of HIV infection is a virus–the human immunodeficiency virus. Like most viruses, HIV is a parasite looking for a way into a cell, to take over the cell, and to force the cell into making more copies of itself. These new virus particles then look for additional cells to infect, repeating the cycle as long as there are new host cells to infect.

THE HIV INFECTIOUS PROCESS

VIRAL FEATURES. The virus particle has an outer envelope with special "docking proteins," known as gp41 and gp120, that assist in finding a host (Figure 25-1). Inside, the virus has two protein coatings and the genetic material with reverse transcriptase (RT) attached. The first challenge is for the HIV particle to get inside a host cell. HIV accomplishes this task by finding a way into the host's bloodstream. One of the cells that it "hijacks" is the CD4+ lymphocyte, also known as the CD4+ cell, helper/inducer T-cell, or T4-cell (see Chapter 23). This cell directs immune system defenses and regulates the activity of all immune system cells. If the HIV successfully enters a CD4+ cell, it can then create more virus particles.

VIRUS-HOST INTERACTIONS. When a person is infected with HIV, the virus randomly "bumps" into many cells. The docking proteins on the outside of the virus try to find special receptors on a host cell that will allow the virus to bind and then enter the cell. The CD4+ cell has receptors on its surface known as CD4 and CCR5 (Figure 25-2). Proteins on the HIV particle surface recognize the CD4 and CCR5 receptors on the CD4+ cell. These HIV proteins are gp120 and gp41. When the HIV gp120 binds to the CD4 receptor and the gp41 binds to the CCR5 receptor, the virus then enters CD4+ cell (Figure 25-3). *Viral binding to both receptors is needed to enter the cell.*

Viruses, like human cells, have genetic material. After entering a host cell, the HIV must get its genetic material into the host cell's DNA. HIV belongs to a family of viruses called **retroviruses.** Viruses, like human cells, have genetic material. The genetic material of the human cell is double-stranded DNA (ds-DNA). The genetic material of HIV is single-stranded RNA (ss-RNA). To infect and take over a human cell, the genetic material must be the same. HIV overcomes this problem by bringing along an enzyme at the time of infection, *reverse transcriptase (RT).* RT takes HIV's ss-RNA and converts it into ds-DNA, which makes the viral genetic material the same as human DNA. Then HIV must get its DNA into the nucleus of the CD4+ cell and place it within the human DNA. HIV also makes an enzyme called *integrase.* This enzyme allows the viral ds-DNA to be inserted into the host ds-DNA, which completes the infection of CD4+ cell.

HIV particles are made within the infected CD4+ cell, using all the metabolic machinery of the host. The new virus particle is made in the form of one long protein strand. The strand is clipped, using chemical scissors called HIV protease, into several small functional pieces. These pieces are formed into a new finished viral particle. (The drug class known as protease inhibitors work here to inhibit HIV protease.) Once the new virus particle is finished, it fuses with

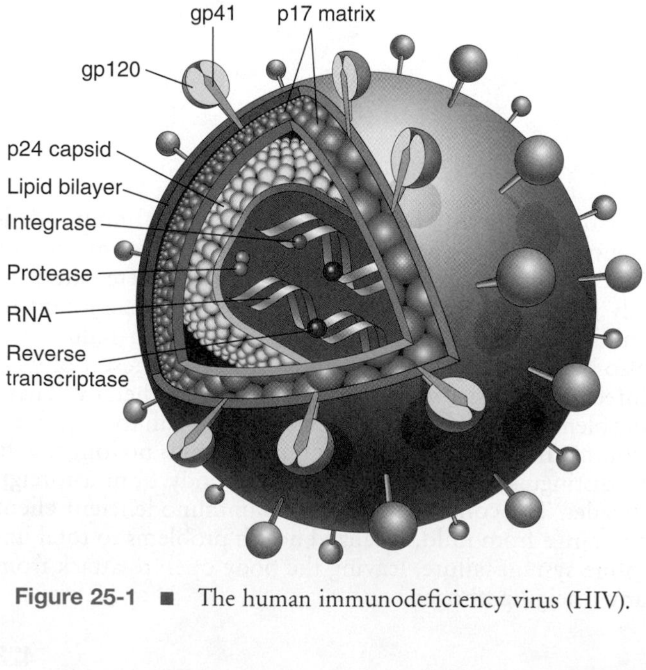

Figure 25-1 ■ The human immunodeficiency virus (HIV).

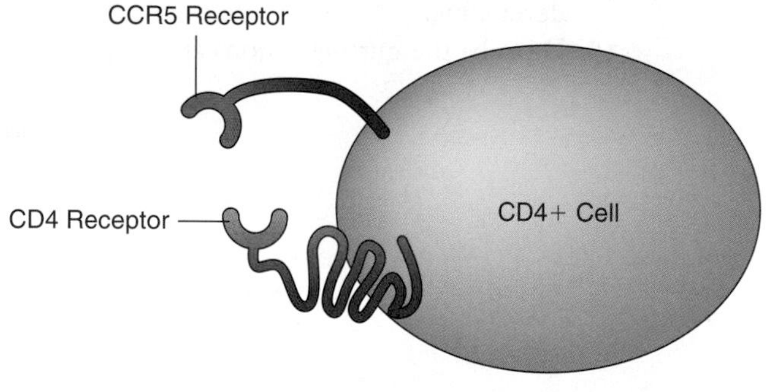

Figure 25-2 ■ The CD4+ cell receptors for the HIV "docking" proteins.

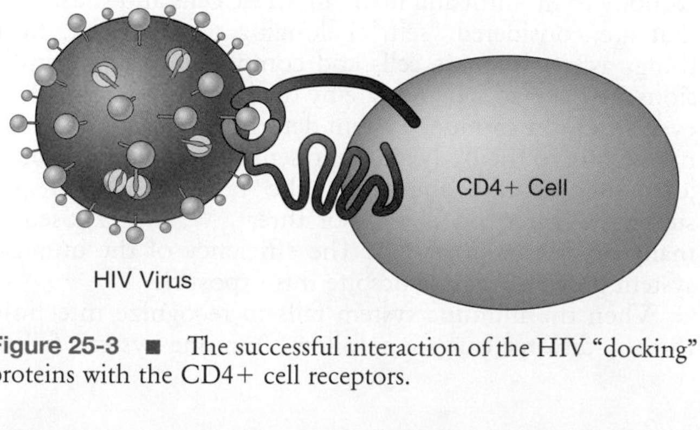

Figure 25-3 ■ The successful interaction of the HIV "docking" proteins with the CD4+ cell receptors.

the CD4+ cell membrane and buds off from the host cell in search of another CD4+ cell to infect (Figure 25-4).

EFFECTS OF HIV INFECTION. The new genetic instructions now direct CD4+ cells to change their role in immune system defenses. The new role is to be an "HIV factory." Not only is the immune system made weaker by removing some CD4+ cells from circulation, but also the most important cell in the immune system becomes an HIV factory. Up to 10 billion virus particles are made daily. In early HIV infection, the immune system can still attack and destroy most of the newly created virus particles. With time, however, the number of HIV particles overwhelms the immune system. Gradually, CD4+ cell counts fall, viral numbers (viral load) rise, and the client eventually dies of opportunistic infections or cancer.

Everyone who has AIDS has HIV infection; however, not everyone who has HIV infection has AIDS. The distinction rests with the number of CD4+ cells the client has and whether any opportunistic infections have occurred. A healthy adult usually has at least 800 to 1000 CD4+ cells/mm^3 of blood.

When a person is infected with HIV, the first manifestations are fever, night sweats, chills, headache and muscle aches. All of these problems can be caused by exposure to almost any virus, such as influenza–not just to HIV. With time, the symptoms go away, and the person feels well again. In actuality, there is a war going on in the body between HIV and the immune system.

As time passes, with more CD4+ cells infected and taken out of service, the CD4+ cell count drops to below normal levels and those that remain may not function normally. Poor CD4+ cell function as a result of HIV infection leads to the following immune system abnormalities:

- Lymphocytopenia (decreased numbers of lymphocytes)
- Increased production of incomplete and nonfunctional antibodies
- Abnormally functioning macrophages

As the CD4+ cell level drops, the client is at risk for bacterial, fungal, and viral infections, as well as for some opportunistic cancers (Figure 25-5). **Opportunistic infections** are those caused by organisms that are present as part of the normal environment and are kept in check by normal immune function.

Opportunistic infections occur because of the profound immune suppression of the person with AIDS. These infections may result from primary infection or reactivation of an old infection.

A diagnosis of AIDS requires that the person be HIV positive and have either a CD4+ cell count of less than 200 cells/mm^3 or an opportunistic infection. Once AIDS is diagnosed, even if the client's CD4+ cell count goes higher than 200 cells/mm^3 or if the infection is successfully treated, the AIDS diagnosis remains and the client never reverts to being just HIV positive.

HIV CLASSIFICATION

The Centers for Disease Control and Prevention (CDC) classifies HIV infection by combining clinical conditions that occur with HIV infection and three ranges of CD4+ cell counts (Table 25-1). The classification begins with acute HIV infection (clinical category A) and spans a continuum that ends with AIDS (clinical category C). The classifications are further divided into 1, 2, and 3 based on the client's CD4+ cell count. *The person with HIV infection can transmit the virus to others at all stages of disease.*

CLINICAL CATEGORY A. A person in clinical category A is HIV positive. The person might not have symptoms at this stage, may have persistently enlarged lymph nodes **(lymphadenopathy),** or may have acute but temporary "flu-like" symptoms as the only disease manifestations. Clients have the additional classification of A1, A2, or A3 depending on their CD4+ cell counts. When the count is at least 500/μL, the disease is classified as A1. When the count is between 200

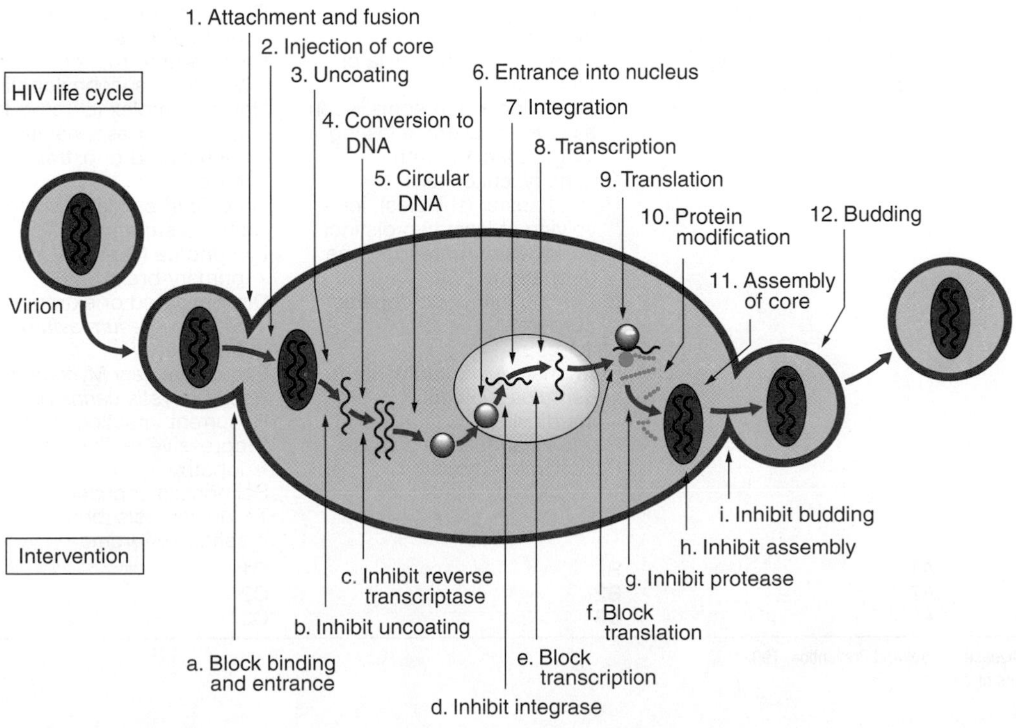

Figure 25-4 ■ The life cycle of HIV.

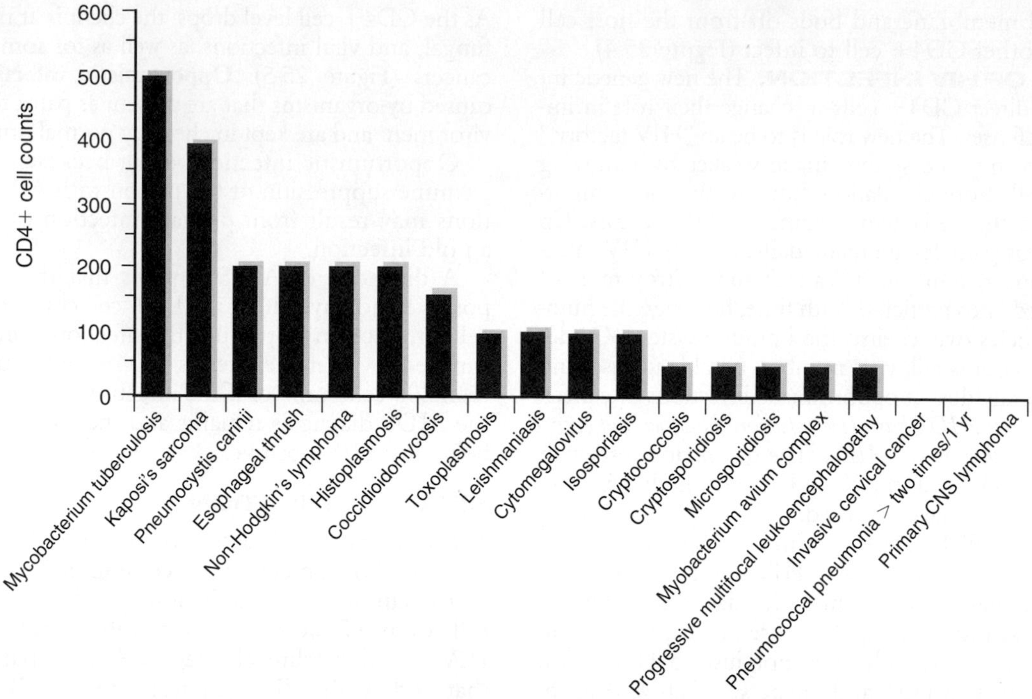

Figure 25-5 ■ Frequency of opportunistic infections among clients with AIDS.

TABLE 25-1 Centers for Disease Control and Prevention Classification System for HIV Infection and AIDS Case Definition

	Clinical Categories		
CD4+ Cell Categories	**A**	**B**	**C***
	HIV positive, asymptomatic *or* Persistent generalized lymphadenopathy *or* Acute (primary) HIV infection with accompanying illness or history of acute infection as the only manifestations	Bacterial endocarditis, meningitis, pneumonia, or sepsis Vulvovaginal candidiasis that is persistent for more than 1 month or poorly responsive to therapy Oropharyngeal candidiasis (thrush) Severe cervical dysplasia or carcinoma Constitutional symptoms, such as fever or diarrhea lasting longer than 1 month Oral hairy leukoplakia Herpes zoster (shingles), involving at least two distinct episodes or more than one dermatome Idiopathic thrombocytopenic purpura Listeriosis Pulmonary *Mycobacterium tuberculosis* infection Nocardiosis Pelvic inflammatory disease Peripheral neuropathy	Bronchial, tracheal, pulmonary, or esophageal candidiasis Invasive cervical cancer Disseminated or extrapulmonary coccidioidomycosis Chronic intestinal cryptosporidiosis Cytomegalovirus disease other than that of the liver, spleen, or lymph nodes Cytomegalovirus retinitis with vision loss HIV-related encephalopathy Herpes simplex (chronic; bronchitis, pneumonitis; or esophagitis) Disseminated or extrapulmonary histoplasmosis Chronic intestinal isosporiasis Kaposi's sarcoma Lymphoma (Burkitt's, immunoblastic, or primary brain) Disseminated or extrapulmonary *Mycobacterium avium* complex or *M. kansasii* Extrapulmonary *Mycobacterium tuberculosis* *Pneumocystis carinii* pneumonia Recurrent infectious pneumonia Progressive multifocal leukoencephalopathy Salmonella septicemia Toxoplasmosis (brain) Wasting syndrome
1 ≥ (500/μL	A1	B1	C1
2 200-499/μL	A2	B2	C2
3 <200/μL*	A3	B3	C3

Data from Centers for Disease Control and Prevention, 1992.
*AIDS indicator conditions or counts.

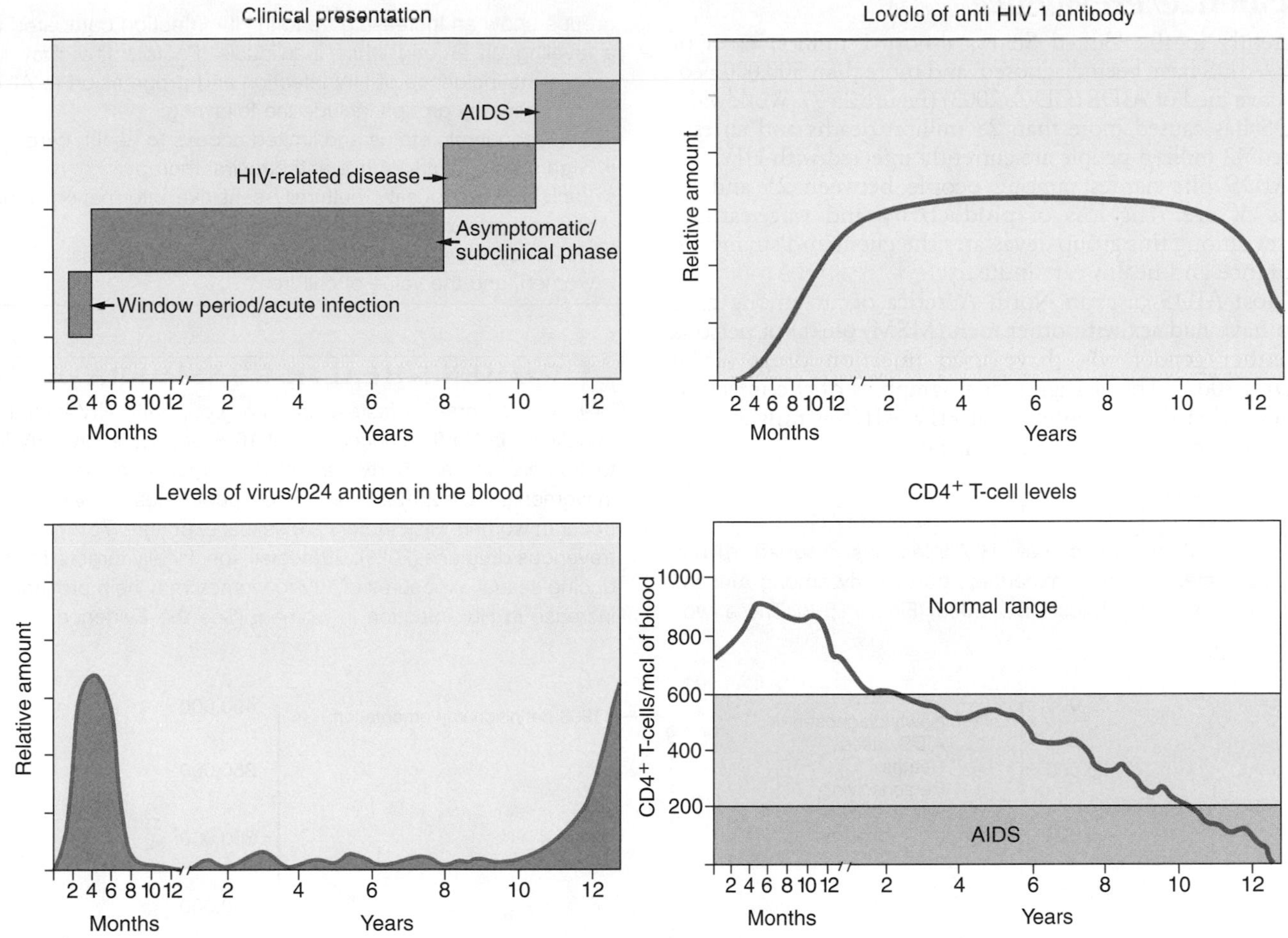

Figure 25-6 ■ Correlation of HIV infection stages, levels of HIV antibodies, levels of HIV, and levels of T4 (CD4+) cells over time.

and 499/μL, the disease is classified as A2. When the count is less than 200/μL, the disease is classified as A3.

CLINICAL CATEGORY B. The client with HIV infection is in clinical category B if one or more of the problems listed in Table 25-1, column B, are present and are (1) caused by HIV infection or indicate a deficiency in cell-mediated immunity, or (2) are complicated by HIV infection. The list gives examples of category B clinical conditions but is not comprehensive. Clients have the additional classification of B1, B2, or B3 depending on their CD4+ cell count. When the count is at least 500/μL, the disease is classified as B1. When the count is between 200 and 499/μL, the disease is classified as B2. When the count is less than 200/μL, the disease is classified as B3.

CLINICAL CATEGORY C. The HIV-positive client in clinical category C has AIDS if any one of the health problems listed on Table 25-1, column C, is present. These problems meet the CDC case definition for AIDS. Clients have the additional classification of C1, C2, or C3 depending on their CD4+ cell counts. When the count is at least 500/μL, the disease is classified as C1. When the count is between 200 and 499/μL, the disease is classified as C2. When the count is less than 200/μL, the disease is classified as C3.

HIV PROGRESSION

The time from the beginning HIV infection to development of AIDS ranges from months to years (Figure 25-6). The range depends on how HIV was acquired, personal factors, and interventions. For people who have been transfused with HIV-contaminated blood, for example, AIDS develops quickly. For those who become HIV positive as a result of a single sexual encounter, there is usually a longer period before progression to AIDS. Other personal factors that may influence progression to AIDS include frequency of re-exposure to HIV, presence of other sexually transmitted diseases (STDs), nutritional status, pregnancy, and stress.

Genetic Considerations

About 1% of people with HIV infection are **long-term nonprogressors (LTNPs).** These people have been infected with HIV for at least 10 years and have remained asymptomatic, with CD4+ cell counts within a normal range.

A genetic difference for this population is that their CCR5 receptors are abnormal and nonfunctional. Most LTNPs have mutations in both pairs of the CCR5 gene allele. The mutation creates a defective receptor called CCR5Δ32. This defective receptor does not bind to the HIV docking proteins. Cells with this defective receptor successfully resist the entrance of the HIV. People who have only one mutated CCR5 gene allele have fewer normal CCR5 receptors. Although these people can be infected with HIV, disease progression is slow compared with that in people who have normal CCR5 gene alleles.

Incidence/Prevalence

Currently in the United States, almost 1 million cases of HIV/AIDS have been diagnosed, and more than 500,000 people have died of AIDS (CDC, 2003) (Figure 25-7). Worldwide, AIDS has caused more than 28 million deaths and an estimated 42 million people are currently infected with HIV.

AIDS hits hardest among people between 25 and 44 years of age. The loss of productivity and wage-earning power among this group devastates the client and strains the insurance and health care industry.

Most AIDS cases in North America occur among men who have had sex with other men (MSM) (46%) or persons of either gender who have used injection drugs (25%) (CDC, 2003). The changing demographics of the infection indicate that the perception that HIV/AIDS is only a problem for homosexual white men is false.

CULTURAL CONSIDERATIONS

More than 73% of new HIV infections reported in the United States occurs in minorities, particularly among African Americans and Hispanics (CDC, 2003) (Figure 25-8). These two groups show an increasing trend in HIV infection compared to a leveling off among white individuals. Factors that may increase the incidence of HIV infection and progression to AIDS among minority groups include the following:

- Socioeconomic status and limited access to health care
- High cost of highly active antiretroviral therapy
- Lack of good quality, culturally sensitive information about risk and prevention
- Health beliefs about HIV treatment, sexual practices, roles of women, and the value of children

WOMEN'S HEALTH CONSIDERATIONS

Women are the fastest growing group with HIV infection and AIDS. In North America, about 16% of people with HIV infection are women. Thirty percent of new cases are diagnosed in women (Figure 25-9). In less affluent countries, 50% of cases occur in women. Risk factors are sexual exposure (75%) and intravenous drug use (25%). Strategies specifically targeted to reducing sexual exposures of HIV to women may help prevent an increase in HIV infection in women. (See the Evidence-Based

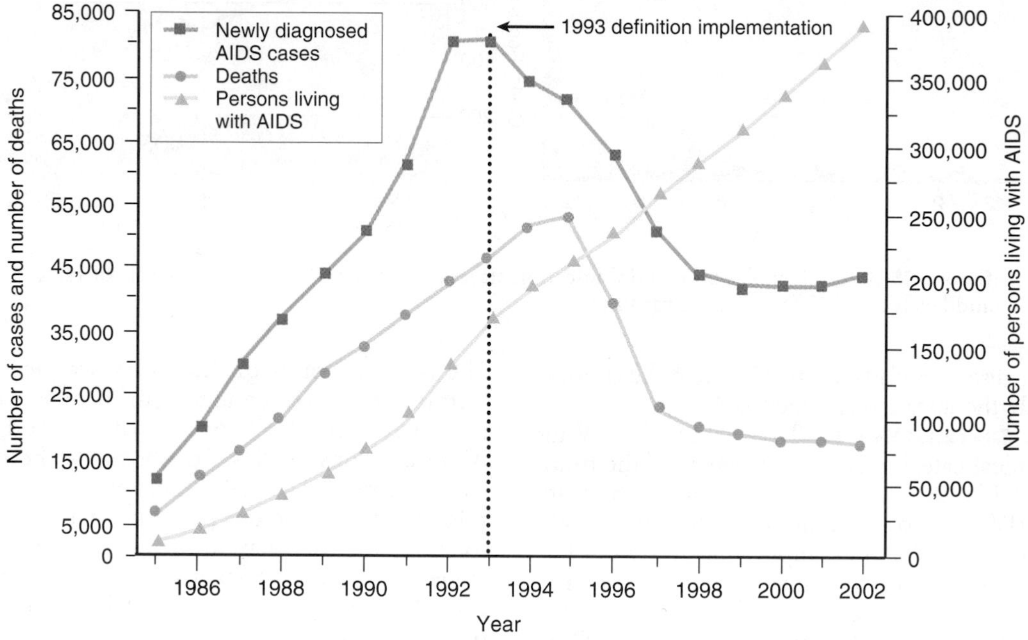

Figure 25-7 ■ AIDS cases, deaths, and persons living with AIDS by year, 1985-2002 (adjusted for reporting delays).

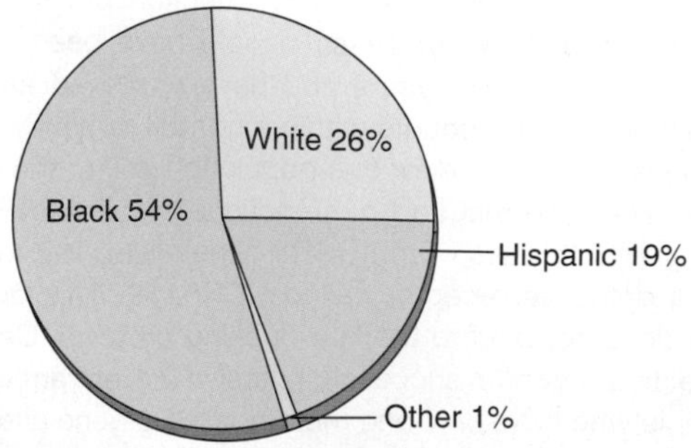

Figure 25-8 ■ Estimates of annual new HIV infections in the United States by ethnicity and race.

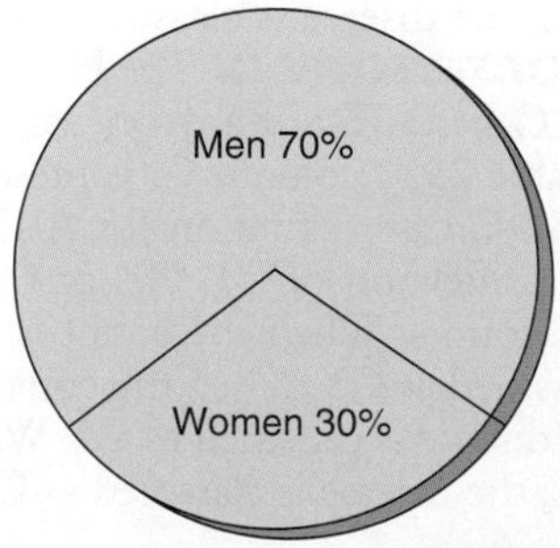

Figure 25-9 ■ Estimates of annual new HIV infections in the United States by gender.

Practice for Nursing box below.) Women with HIV infection have a poorer outcome with shorter mean survival time than men. This outcome may be the result of late diagnosis and social or economic factors that reduce access to medical care.

Gynecologic problems, especially persistent or recurrent vaginal candidiasis, may be the first signs of HIV infection in women. Other common problems include genital herpes, pelvic inflammatory disease, and cervical neoplasia.

Most women with HIV are of childbearing age. The effect of pregnancy on the course of HIV infection is not known. There is conflicting evidence that pregnancy may or may not speed up the progression of disease.

CONSIDERATIONS FOR OLDER ADULTS

Infection with HIV can occur at any age. Assess the older client for risk behaviors, including a sexual and drug use history. Decline in immune function increases the risk for HIV infection after exposure in this population. In the older woman, changes in vaginal tissue as a result of aging may increase susceptibility to sexually transmitted HIV infection.

AIDS is a disease with a high mortality rate. The fatality rate is at least 60% for adults and, to date, there is no cure. Thus a major focus for health care in North America and worldwide is prevention of HIV infection. The United States has defined several goals related to HIV and AIDS prevention, as shown in the Meeting Healthy People 2010 Objectives box on p. 430.

HEALTH PROMOTION/ILLNESS PREVENTION

The most important aspect for prevention of HIV transmission is education. All people, regardless of age, gender, ethnicity, or sexual orientation, are susceptible to HIV infection. HIV infection is preventable because of the modes of viral transmission and the fragile nature of the virus.

HIV has been found in most body fluids of infected clients, including blood, semen, vaginal secretions, breast milk, amniotic fluid, urine, feces, saliva, tears, cerebrospinal fluid, lymph nodes, cervical cells, corneal tissue, and brain tissue. HIV is transmitted most often in the following three ways:

- Sexual: genital, anal, or oral sexual contact with exposure of mucous membranes to infected semen or vaginal secretions
- Parenteral: sharing of needles or equipment contaminated with infected blood or receiving contaminated blood products
- Perinatal: from the placenta, from contact with maternal blood and body fluids during birth, or from breast milk from an infected mother to child

HIV is not transmitted by casual contact in the home, school, or workplace. Sharing household utensils, towels and linens, and toilet facilities does not transmit HIV. In addition, HIV is not spread by mosquitos or other insects.

Sexual Transmission

Abstinence and mutually monogamous sex with a noninfected partner are the only absolutely safe methods of preventing HIV infection through sexual contact. These practices may not be feasible because of personal, cultural, or economic factors.

Many forms of sexual expression can spread HIV infection if one partner is infected. The risk for becoming infected from a partner who is HIV positive is always present, although some sexual practices are more risky than others. The virus concentrates most heavily in blood and seminal fluid, although it is also present in vaginal secretions. Thus risk differs by gender, sexual act, and the viral load of the infected partner.

GENDER

HIV is most easily transmitted when infected body fluids come into contact with mucous membranes or nonintact skin. The vagina has much more mucous membrane than does the penis. Thus HIV, like all other sexually transmitted diseases (STDs), is more easily transmitted from infected male to uninfected female than vice versa.

EVIDENCE-BASED PRACTICE for Nursing

Gender-sensitive interventions are effective in changing behavior

Ehrhardt, A., et al. (2002). A gender-specific HIV/STD risk reduction intervention for women in a health care setting: Short- and long-term results of a randomized clinical trial. *AIDS Care, 14*(2), 147-161.

This study sought to determine whether a gender-specific group intervention had short-term and/or long-term effects in helping women to reduce their number of unsafe sexual encounters and enhance their implementation of sexual alternatives. The study included 360 subjects who received either an eight-session group intervention, a four-session group intervention, or no specific intervention. Subjects were followed up at 1 month, 6 months, and 12 months after intervention for an assessment of sexual practices/activities using a structured format with closed and open-ended items. The items assessed such variables as total number of sexual activities, activity by type, partner type, use of condoms, and other protection. Variables of age, work status, ethnicity, education levels, and number of children were similar for all three groups. The level of participation by the subjects in both intervention groups was similar and the percentage of participants who were available for follow-up at 12 months was high.

The results indicated that participants in the eight-session intervention were more than twice as likely to reduce unsafe sexual encounters as women in the control group. Women in the four-session intervention group overall had fewer unsafe sexual encounters compared with control subjects but the difference did not meet statistical significance.

Level of Evidence: 1—At least one properly designed randomized controlled clinical trial (RCT) of appropriate size (more than 100 subjects).

Critique. The study methods were appropriate for the purpose and study questions. The study limitations include that the subjects were drawn from a population that self-selected for a clinical trial on HIV/STD prevention, thus their overall motivation may have been different than that of the general population would be. Additionally, data regarding number of sexual encounters, safe or otherwise, was obtained by self-report and recall.

Implications for Nursing. With HIV infection increasing among American women and women worldwide, more interventions are needed that specifically target women. The results of this study indicate a positive "dose" effect, in that with each additional session attended, participants were better able to make changes in unsafe sexual practices. This finding may have represented an increasing level of confidence associated with more specific education on alternative sexual practices and means of protection.

Meeting HEALTHY PEOPLE 2010 Objectives

HIV/AIDS

Objective 21.10: Confine annual incidence of diagnosed AIDS cases among adolescents and adults to no more than 12 per 100,000 population.

- Include questions regarding sexual activity and use of safer sex practices whenever obtaining a health history from a client of any age, gender, occupation, socioeconomic status, religion, or educational background.
- Assess all clients for current and past exposures to bloodborne or sexually transmitted diseases.
- Encourage clients to know their own and their partners' HIV status.
- Teach clients safer sex practices.
- Direct clients who are IV drug users to drug rehabilitation programs and support groups.
- Direct clients who abuse alcohol to alcohol rehabilitation programs and support groups.
- Develop culturally sensitive and age-appropriate education materials of various literacy levels for HIV prevention.
- Enlist the assistance of educational, religious, and civic groups and institutions in the dissemination of information regarding prevention of HIV infection.
- Encourage people who are HIV positive to:
  - Avoid sharing toothbrushes, razors, or other items that could become contaminated with blood.
  - Not donate sperm, blood, plasma, or body organs or other body tissues.
  - Inform his or her physician, dentist, and eye doctor about the client's HIV status.
  - Clean blood or other body fluid spills on household or other surfaces with freshly diluted household bleach: 1 part bleach to 10 parts water. (Do not use bleach on wounds.)

Objective 21.11: Increase years of healthy life of an individual infected with HIV by extending the interval of time between an initial diagnosis of HIV infection and AIDS diagnosis and between AIDS diagnosis and death.

- Teach HIV-positive persons who have no signs or symptoms of immunodeficiency to seek regular medical evaluation and follow-up.
- Encourage HIV-positive persons to adhere to drug regimen, especially highly active antiretroviral therapy (HAART).
- Teach HIV-infected persons to begin or maintain behaviors known to assist in maintaining or improving immune function (e.g., diet appropriate in number of calories for the client's individual metabolic needs that is high in protein and vitamins and low in fat; regular exercise; adequate rest; and reduction of physical, emotional, or spiritual stress).
- Encourage HIV-positive persons to use safer sex practices for their own protection as well as for partner protection.
- Encourage HIV-positive women to avoid pregnancy.

SPECIFIC SEXUAL ACTS

Sexual acts or practices that permit infected seminal fluid to come into contact with mucous membranes or nonintact skin are the most risky for sexual transmission of HIV. Such practices include oral sex and anal intercourse.

In oral sex, the risk increases when the penis and seminal fluid of an infected person come into contact with the mucous membranes of the mouth and throat (fellatio) of a noninfected person. Oral sex in which the uninfected partner's oral mucous membranes and tongue come into contact with infected vaginal secretions (cunnilingus) also places the uninfected person at risk. This risk is increased if sores or other open areas are present in the mouth.

In anal intercourse, the risk increases when the penis and seminal fluid of an infected person come into contact with the mucous membranes of the uninfected partner's rectum. *Anal intercourse in which the semen depositor is infected is a risky sexual practice regardless of whether the semen receiver is male or female.* Anal intercourse not only allows seminal fluid contact with the mucous membranes of the rectum, but also causes tearing of the mucous membranes, making infection more likely.

CHART 25-1

CLIENT EDUCATION GUIDE
Condom Use to Prevent Sexually Transmitted Diseases

- Use latex condoms rather than natural membrane condoms.
- Store condoms in a cool, dry place.
- Do not use condoms that were in damaged packages or those that show signs of age, such as those that are brittle, sticky, or discolored.
- Handle condoms carefully to avoid puncturing them.
- Put a condom on before making any genital contact.
- Hold the tip of the condom and unroll it onto the erect penis, making sure that no air is trapped in the tip. Leave space at the tip to collect semen.
- Use adequate lubrication. Use water-based lubricants only. Petroleum or oil-based lubricants such as petroleum jelly, cooking oil, shortening, and lotions can damage the condom.
- Replace a broken condom immediately. If ejaculation occurs after the condom breaks, there may be some protection in the immediate use of a spermicide.
- After ejaculation, the condom must remain on until the penis is withdrawn. While the penis is still erect, hold the condom against the base of the penis while withdrawing.
- Never reuse condoms.

From Centers for Disease Control. (1988). Condoms for prevention of sexually transmitted diseases. *Morbidity and Mortality Weekly Report, 37*(9), 133-137.

VIRAL LOAD

The higher the blood level of HIV **(viremia),** the greater the risk for sexual and perinatal transmission. Current highly active antiretroviral therapy (HAART) has caused the viral load of some infected clients to drop below detectable levels. Although it is assumed that there is far less virus in seminal or vaginal fluids of these individuals, the risk for disease transmission is presumed to still exist.

Safer sex practices are those that reduce the risk of nonintact skin or mucous membranes coming in contact with infected body fluids and blood. Such practices include using the following:

- A latex condom for genital and anal intercourse (Chart 25-1)
- A condom or latex barrier (dental dam) over the genitals or anus during oral-genital or oral-anal sexual contact
- Latex gloves for finger or hand contact with the vagina or rectum

Parenteral Transmission

Preventive practices to reduce transmission among injection drug users include the use of proper cleaning of "works" (needles, syringes, and other drug paraphernalia). Instruct clients to clean a used needle and syringe by first filling and flushing with clear water. Next, the syringe should be filled with ordinary household bleach. The bleach-filled syringe should be shaken for 30 to 60 seconds. Advise drug users to carry a small container with this solution whenever sharing needles. Some communities have a needle exchange program in which needles and syringes are used only once and exchanged for clean ones.

CHART 25-2

BEST PRACTICE for
Postexposure Prophylaxis (PEP) for Occupational HIV Exposure

PEP is not recommended in the following scenarios:
- Percutaneous injury, source HIV negative
- Mucosal exposure, small volume (a few drops), source HIV negative

PEP should be considered in the following scenarios:
- Percutaneous injury or mucosal contact, source HIV status unknown, recommend two-drug PEP, until source client's HIV status is determined. If negative, discontinue PEP.
- Percutaneous injury, *source HIV positive, asymptomatic, viral load (VL) <1500*, solid needle, superficial injury, recommend two-drug PEP. Mucosal contact, small volume (a few drops), consider two-drug PEP.
- Percutaneous injury, *source HIV positive, symptomatic, AIDS or opportunistic infections (OIs), recent seroconverter, high VL*, solid needle, superficial injury, recommend three-drug PEP. Mucosal contact, small volume (a few drops), recommend two-drug PEP.
- Percutaneous injury, *source HIV positive, asymptomatic, VL <1500*, large-bore hollow needle, visible blood on device, needle used in source client's vein or artery, recommend three-drug PEP. Mucosal contact, large volume (major blood splash), recommend two-drug PEP.
- Percutaneous injury, *source HIV positive, symptomatic, AIDS or OIs, recent seroconverter, high VL*, large-bore hollow needle, visible blood on device, needle used in source client's vein or artery, recommend three-drug PEP. Mucosal contact, large volume (major blood splash), recommend three drug PEP.

PEP uses two or three drugs, generally from one, two, or three classes of antiretroviral agents:

NRTI Class
- ZVD + 3TC
- 3TC + d4T
- ddl + d4T

NNRTI Class
- Efavirenz

PI Class
- Indinavir
- Nelfinavir
- Lopinavir/ritonavir

Start PEP as soon as possible after exposure.
Standard therapy is to use these medications for 4 weeks.

NRTI, Nucleoside analog reverse transcriptase inhibitors; NNRTI, non-nucleoside analog reverse transcriptase inhibitors; PI, protease inhibitors.

The risk for AIDS transmission through blood and blood products has been reduced to a national average of 0.02%. Several measures are used to protect the nation's blood supply. All donated blood in North America is screened for the HIV antibody, and blood that is positive for HIV antibodies is discarded. Because of the time lag in antibody production (seroconversion) after exposure to HIV, infected blood can test negative for HIV antibodies. False-negative results also can occur. The small but real possibility of HIV transmission through blood and blood products has resulted in more stringent indications for transfusion and an increase in autologous transfusion.

Perinatal Transmission

The risk for perinatal transmission in pregnant clients with AIDS ranges between 14% and 45% for each pregnancy. Pregnant women who receive zidovudine have an 8.3% transmission rate to their babies compared with 25.5% in women who do not receive antiretroviral therapy. A single dose of nevirapine, given during labor to the mother, and a single dose given to the baby at 48 to 72 hours is an alternative therapy for infected women who have not received other antiretroviral therapy.

HIV transmission can occur across the placenta during pregnancy, with infant exposure to blood and vaginal secretions during birth or after birth through breast milk. Inform women of childbearing age with HIV infection about the risks for perinatal transmission. Consult a maternal-child textbook for more information about reducing perinatal transmission of HIV.

TABLE 25-2 Recommendations for Preventing HIV Transmission by Health Care Workers

- Workers should adhere to standard precautions.
- Workers with exudative lesions or weeping dermatitis should not perform direct client care or handle client care equipment and devices used in invasive procedures.
- Workers must follow guidelines for disinfection and sterilization of reusable equipment used in invasive procedures.
- Workers infected with HIV are not restricted from practice of non–exposure-prone procedures, as long as they comply with standard precautions and sterilization/disinfection recommendations.
- Workers should identify exposure-prone procedures by institutions where they are performed.
- Workers who perform exposure-prone procedures should know their HIV antibody status.
- Workers who are infected with HIV should seek advice from an expert review panel before performing exposure-prone procedures to determine under what circumstances they may continue to practice these procedures. These circumstances would include notification of prospective clients of HIV positivity.

Modified from Centers for Disease Control. (1991). Recommendations for preventing transmission of human immunodeficiency virus and hepatitis B virus to patients during exposure-prone invasive procedures. *Morbidity and Mortality Weekly Report, 40*(RR-8), 1-9.

Transmission and Health Care Workers

Needle stick or "sharps" injuries are the primary means of HIV infection for health care workers. In addition, health care workers can be infected through exposure of nonintact skin and mucous membranes to blood and body fluids. Because there is a time lag between the time of infection with HIV and the production of serum antibodies (seroconversion), infected people can test negative for HIV and still transmit the virus. *The best prevention for health care providers is the consistent use of standard precautions for all clients as recommended by the Centers for Disease Control and Prevention (CDC)* (see Chapter 29). Chart 25-2 lists the recommended actions for prevention of HIV infection after a needle stick or other occupational exposure (postexposure prophylaxis [PEP]).

The public may be alarmed about HIV transmission by health care workers. It is recommended that HIV-infected health care workers wear gloves when in contact with clients' mucous membranes or nonintact skin. Infected workers with weeping dermatitis or open lesions should not perform direct care activities. The CDC (1991) has recommended guidelines for preventing HIV transmission by health care workers during exposure-prone invasive procedures (Table 25-2). These include any procedure in which there is a risk for broken skin injury to the health care worker and the worker's blood is likely to make contact with

CHART 25-3

CLIENT EDUCATION GUIDE
CDC Recommendations for HIV Testing

You should be tested for AIDS if you fall within one or more of the following groups:

- People with sexually transmitted disease
- Injection drug users
- People who consider themselves at risk
- Women of childbearing age with identifiable risks, including the following:
  - Used injection drugs
  - Engaged in prostitution
  - Had sexual partners who were infected or at risk
  - Had contact with men from countries with high HIV prevalence
  - Received a transfusion between 1978 and 1985
- People planning to get married
- People undergoing medical evaluation or treatment for manifestations that may be HIV related
- People admitted to hospitals
- People in correctional institutions such as jails and prisons
- Prostitutes and their customers

Modified from Centers for Disease Control. (1987). Public Health Service guidelines for counseling and antibody testing to prevent HIV infection and AIDS. *Morbidity and Mortality Weekly Report, 36*(31), 509-515.

the client's body cavity, subcutaneous tissues, or mucous membranes. These recommendations aim to reduce the risk of HIV transmission to clients.

Testing

Testing for HIV antibodies or other features of the virus is complex, requiring interpretation, counseling, and confidentiality. Testing plays a role in prevention because tests are a way of diagnosing HIV infection before immune changes or symptoms develop. Those who test positive can be educated and encouraged to modify their behaviors to prevent transmission to others. Chart 25-3 lists conditions for which HIV antibody testing is advised.

Pretest and post-test counseling must be performed by trained personnel. Counseling helps the client make an informed decision about testing and provides an opportunity to teach risk reduction behaviors. Post-test counseling is needed to interpret the results, discuss risk reduction, and provide psychological support and health promotion information for the client with a positive test result. Testing methods, their accuracy, and indications are presented under the heading "Laboratory Assessment" on p. 436.

Recommendations for people who test positive for antibody to HIV are presented in the Meeting Healthy People 2010 Objectives box on p. 430. People who test positive should also be counseled on how to inform sexual partners and those with whom they have shared needles.

COLLABORATIVE MANAGEMENT

The care of the client with HIV disease or AIDS is complex, affecting all body systems. The Concept Map on p. 433 addresses assessment and nursing care issues related to clients who have HIV disease or AIDS.

Assessment

The person who has HIV disease is monitored on a regular basis for changes in immune function or health status that indicate disease progression and warrant prophylaxis or intervention. Continuous, comprehensive assessment of the client with AIDS is crucial, because he or she may have problems related to disease in many organ systems. Assess subtle changes so that infections and other problems can be found early and treated.

HISTORY

Collect information about age, gender, occupation, and residence. Thoroughly assess the current illness, including its nature, when it started, the severity of symptoms, associated problems, and any interventions to date. Ask the client about when AIDS was diagnosed and what clinical symptoms led to that diagnosis. Ask the client to give a chronology of infections and clinical problems since the diagnosis. Assess the client's health history, including whether he or she received a blood transfusion between 1978 and 1985. (Since 1985, donated blood in the United States has been routinely tested for HIV contamination.)

Ask the client about sexual practices, any sexually transmitted diseases (STDs), and any major infectious diseases, including tuberculosis and hepatitis. If the client has hemophilia, ask about treatment with clotting factors. Determine whether the client has engaged in past or present injection drug use, including needle exposure and sharing. Assess the client's level of knowledge regarding the diagnosis, symptom management, diagnostic tests, treatments, community resources, and modes of HIV transmission. Also assess the client's understanding and use of safer sex practices.

PHYSICAL ASSESSMENT/CLINICAL MANIFESTATIONS

HIV disease and AIDS are a progression continuum. The client with HIV disease may either have few manifestations and problems or may have problems that are acute rather than chronically present. The client with AIDS, however, usually has more problems of long duration and greater severity. Look for many possible manifestations. These include shortness of breath or cough, fever, night sweats, fatigue, nausea and vomiting, weight loss, swollen lymph nodes, diarrhea, visual changes, headache, memory loss, confusion, seizures, personality changes, dry skin, rashes, skin lesions, and pain (Chart 25-4).

OPPORTUNISTIC INFECTIONS. The client with HIV/AIDS can develop pathogenic infections and opportunistic infections. Pathogenic infections are caused by virulent organisms and occur even among people whose immune systems are functioning normally. Opportunistic infections are those caused by organisms that are present as part of the normal environment and are kept in check by normal immune function. Only when immune function is depressed are such organisms capable of causing infection.

Opportunistic infections occur because of the profound immune suppression of the person with AIDS (see Figure 25-5). They may result from primary infection or reactivation of a latent infection. Opportunistic infections account for many of the clinical symptoms observed in AIDS and can be protozoan, fungal, bacterial, or viral. More than one infection may be present in a client with AIDS.

Opportunistic infections do not pose a threat to the immunocompetent health care worker caring for a client with HIV infection or AIDS. When the client with HIV infection or AIDS has a pathogenic infection, however, such as tuberculosis at a transmissi-

CONCEPT MAP Acquired Immunodeficiency Syndrome

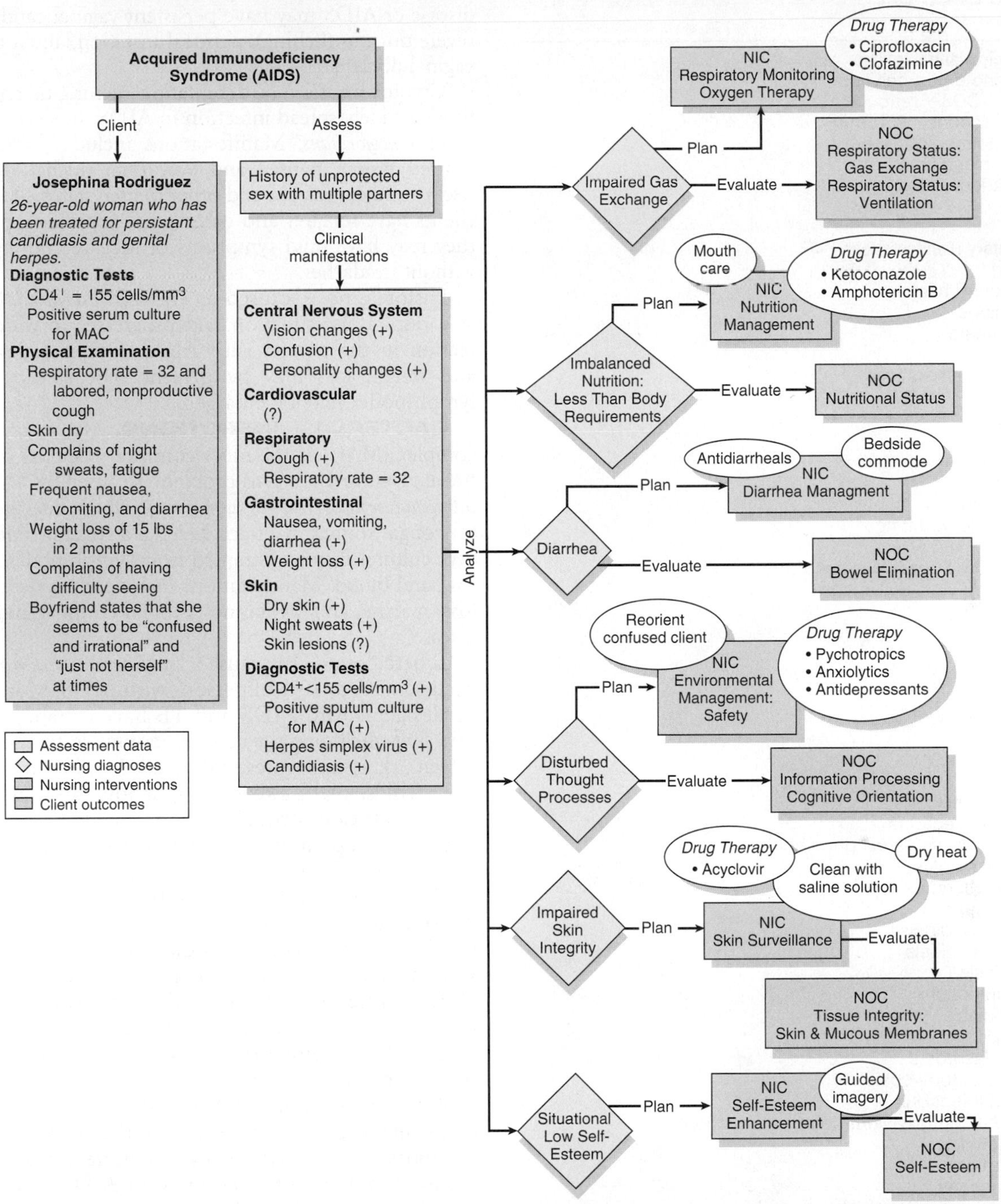

Concept Map by Elaine Bishop Kennedy, EdD, RN

ble stage, health care personnel must use appropriate precautions to prevent disease spread.

PROTOZOAL INFECTIONS. *Pneumocystis carinii* pneumonia (PCP) is the most common opportunistic infection in persons infected with HIV. Dyspnea on exertion, tachypnea, a persistent dry cough, and fever may be observed. The client with PCP has fatigue and weight loss. Crackles may be present on lung auscultation.

Toxoplasmosis encephalitis, caused by *Toxoplasma gondii,* is acquired through contact with contaminated cat feces or by ingesting infected, undercooked meat. The client may have subtle changes in mental status, neurologic deficits, headaches, and fever. Other symptoms include difficulties with speech, gait, and vision; seizures; lethargy; and confusion. Perform a comprehensive baseline mental status examination and monitor the client to detect subtle changes.

Cryptosporidiosis is an intestinal infection caused by *Cryptosporidium* organisms. In AIDS, this illness ranges from a mild diarrhea to a severe wasting with electrolyte imbalance. Diarrhea may result in fluid loss of up to 15 to 20 L/day.

FUNGAL INFECTIONS. *Candida albicans* is part of the natural flora of the gastrointestinal tract. In the person with AIDS, candidiasis (overgrowth of the *Candida* fungus) occurs because the weakened immune system can no longer

CHART 25-4

KEY FEATURES of AIDS

Immunologic Manifestations
- Low white blood cell counts:
  - CD4+/CD8+ ratio <2
  - CD4+ count <200/mm^3
- Hypergammaglobulinemia
- Opportunistic infections
- Lymphadenopathy
- Fatigue

Integumentary Manifestations
- Dry skin
- Poor wound healing
- Skin lesions
- Night sweats

Respiratory Manifestations
- Cough
- Shortness of breath

Gastrointestinal Manifestations
- Diarrhea
- Weight loss
- Nausea and vomiting

Central Nervous System Manifestations
- Confusion
- Dementia
- Headache
- Fever
- Visual changes
- Memory loss
- Personality changes
- Pain
- Seizures

Opportunistic Infections
- Protozoal infections
  - *Pneumocystis carinii* pneumonia
  - Toxoplasmosis
  - Cryptosporidiosis
  - Isosporiasis
  - Microsporidiosis
  - Strongyloidiasis
  - Giardiasis
- Fungal infections
  - Candidiasis
  - Cryptococcosis
  - Histoplasmosis
  - Coccidioidomycosis
- Bacterial infections
  - *Mycobacterium avium* complex infection
  - Tuberculosis
  - Nocardiosis
- Viral infections
  - Cytomegalovirus infection
  - Herpes simplex virus infection
  - Varicella-zoster virus infection

Malignancies
- Kaposi's sarcoma
- Non-Hodgkin's lymphoma
- Hodgkin's lymphoma
- Invasive cervical carcinoma

control fungal growth. *Candida* stomatitis or esophagitis is a frequent finding in AIDS. Clients may report food tasting "funny," mouth pain, difficulty in swallowing, and retrosternal pain (pain behind the ribs). On examination of the mouth and the back of the throat, you may see cottage cheese–like, yellow-white plaques and inflammation. Esophagitis is diagnosed by endoscopic biopsy and culture. Women with HIV disease or AIDS may have persistent vaginal candidiasis with severe pruritus (itching), perineal irritation, and a thick, white vaginal discharge.

Cryptococcosis is a debilitating meningitis and is sometimes a widely spread infection in AIDS. It is caused by *Cryptococcus neoformans.* Manifestations include fever, headache, blurred vision, nausea and vomiting, nuchal rigidity (stiff neck), mild confusion, and other mental status changes. Some clients have seizures and other focal neurologic problems or they may have mild symptoms of malaise and fever with or without headaches.

Histoplasmosis, caused by *Histoplasma capsulatum,* begins as a respiratory infection and progresses to widespread infection in the person with AIDS. Dyspnea, fever, cough, and weight loss may be present. The spleen, liver, and lymph nodes may be enlarged.

BACTERIAL INFECTIONS. *Mycobacterium avium* complex (MAC) is the most common bacterial infection associated with AIDS. This problem is caused by *Mycobacterium intracellulare* or *Mycobacterium avium,* which infects the respiratory or gastrointestinal tract. MAC is a systemic infection. Positive cultures may be obtained from lymph nodes, bone marrow, and blood. Manifestations include fever, debility, weight loss, malaise, and sometimes swollen lymph glands or organ disease.

Tuberculosis (TB), caused by *Mycobacterium tuberculosis,* occurs in 2% to 10% of persons with AIDS. More than 50% of all clients with AIDS and TB have extrapulmonary disease sites, including the central nervous system, bones, liver, spleen, skin, and intestinal tract. Manifestations include fever, chills, night sweats, weight loss, and anorexia. Pulmonary TB causes cough, dyspnea, and chest pain. Symptoms of extrapulmonary infection vary with the site. The person with TB and a CD4+ count below 200/mm^3 may not have a positive TB skin test (PPD) because of an inability to mount an immune response to the antigen, a condition known as **anergy.** Other diagnostic tests include a chest x-ray, acid-fast sputum smear, and sputum culture.

The nurse or respiratory therapist who gives cough-inducing aerosol treatments, such as pentamidine isethionate, to clients with AIDS should be screened with a PPD skin test every 6 months.

Recurrent pneumonia from bacterial infections occurs often among clients with AIDS. In the current CDC classification system for AIDS, two or more episodes of pneumonia in a 12-month period is an AIDS case definition. Manifestations include chest pain, productive cough, fever, and dyspnea.

VIRAL INFECTIONS. Cytomegalovirus (CMV) can infect many sites in persons with AIDS, including the eye (CMV retinitis), respiratory and gastrointestinal tracts, and central nervous system. CMV infection can also cause many nonspecific problems such as fever, malaise, weight loss, fatigue, and swollen lymph nodes. CMV retinitis impairs vision, ranging from slight to total blindness.

CMV infection also causes colitis, with diarrhea, abdominal bloating and discomfort, and weight loss. In addition, CMV can cause encephalitis, pneumonitis, adrenalitis, hepatitis, and disseminated infection.

Herpes simplex virus (HSV) infections in people with HIV disease or AIDS occur in the perirectal, oral, and genital areas. The manifestations are more widespread and of longer duration among clients with HIV/AIDS than among those who are immunocompetent. Numbness or tingling at the site of infection occur up to 24 hours before vesicle (blister) formation. Lesions are painful, with chronic ulcerative lesions after vesicle rupture. Clients may have fever, pain, bleeding, and lymph node enlargement in the affected area. Other manifestations include headache, myalgia, and malaise.

Varicella-zoster virus (VZV) infection (shingles) is usually not a new infection for people with AIDS. This virus, present in the nerve ganglia of many people, causes chickenpox. When people who have had the chickenpox previously are immunocompromised, VZV leaves the nerve ganglia and enters body fluids and other tissue areas, causing shingles. Manifestations begin with pain and burning along sensory nerve tracts. Large fluid-filled blisters form and crust over. Other problems include headache and low-grade fever.

MALIGNANCIES. The AIDS-weakened immune response increases the risk for cancer. Cancers occurring with AIDS include Kaposi's sarcoma, Hodgkin's lymphoma, non-Hodgkin's lymphoma, and invasive cervical cancer (CDC, 2003).

KAPOSI'S SARCOMA. Kaposi's sarcoma (KS) is the most common AIDS-related malignancy, occurring in 1% to 21% of clients with AIDS. The risk for KS appears to be related to co-infection with some types of herpes virus.

KS develops as small, purplish brown, raised lesions that are usually not painful or itchy. The lesions can occur anywhere on the body. Most clients with KS have skin or mucous membrane lesions. In some clients, lesions develop in the lymph nodes, intestinal tract, or lungs. KS is diagnosed by biopsy and histologic examination of the lesion. Assess KS lesions for number, size, and location, and monitor their progression.

MALIGNANT LYMPHOMAS. Malignant lymphomas occurring with AIDS are non-Hodgkin's B-cell lymphomas, such as Burkitt's lymphoma, immunoblastic lymphoma, and primary brain lymphoma. Manifestations include weight loss, fever, and night sweats.

ENDOCRINE COMPLICATIONS. Clients with HIV disease may have disease-related endocrine problems, such as gonadal dysfunction, body shape changes, adrenal insufficiency, diabetes mellitus, and elevated triglycerides and cholesterol (Table 25-3).

Many HIV-positive men have low testosterone levels and HIV-positive women often have irregular menstrual cycles. With this gonadal dysfunction comes a decrease in body muscle mass for both genders and a change in libido.

Body shape changes from fat redistribution or lipodystrophy are common in clients receiving antiretroviral therapies, especially protease inhibitors. Manifestations include "buffalo humps" or cervical (neck) fat development and large abdominal fat accumulations. Other body areas, such as the face, arms, and legs, have a wasted appearance.

Adrenal dysfunction can result from the glands being infected by opportunistic infections (cytomegalovirus, *Mycobacterium avium*, or tuberculosis), resulting in adrenal insufficiency. This problem manifests as fatigue, weight loss, nausea, vomiting, low blood pressure, and electrolyte disturbances, and can be life threatening.

Clients taking protease inhibitors have a higher than expected incidence of type 1 diabetes and hyperlipidemia. These problems are seen even among clients who have no other risks for these problems or the associated heart disease.

TABLE 25-3 Endocrine Complications of HIV Infection or Treatment

Endocrine Gland	Problems/Dysfunction

Gonads	Decreased testosterone
	  Reduced libido
	  Reduced fertility
	  Decreased muscle mass
	Decreased estrogen
	  Reduced libido
	  Premature menopause
	  Decreased muscle mass

Adrenal cortex	Increased cortisol
	  Fat redistribution
	  Decreased muscle mass
	Decreased cortisol
	  Adrenal insufficiency
	    Hypoglycemia
	    Hyperkalemia
	    Hypotension
	    Fatigue
	    Weight loss

Pancreas	Reduced exocrine function
	  Fatty food intolerance
	  Cholelithiasis
	  Pancreatitis
	Reduced endocrine function
	  Diabetes mellitus
	  Hyperlipidemia

OTHER CLINICAL MANIFESTATIONS. All body systems are affected to some degree in AIDS.

AIDS DEMENTIA COMPLEX. HIV-associated dementia complex, or AIDS dementia complex (ADC), refers to the manifestations of central nervous system involvement. ADC occurs in about 70% of people with AIDS. It is a result of infection of cells within the central nervous system by HIV. ADC causes cognitive, motor, and behavioral impairments. Manifestations range from barely noticeable to severe dementia.

Some neurologic complications may be due to HIV infection or drug side effects, including peripheral neuropathies and myopathies. Symptoms of peripheral neuropathies include paresthesias and burning sensations, pain, and gait changes. Myopathies are accompanied by leg weakness, ataxia, and muscle pain.

WASTING SYNDROME. AIDS wasting syndrome is not due to any single factor. It may be a result of altered metabolism from malignancy or opportunistic infection. Diarrhea, malabsorption, anorexia, and oral and esophageal lesions can all contribute to persistent and sometimes extreme weight loss, and the client may appear quite emaciated.

SKIN CHANGES. Many clients have dry, itchy, irritated skin and many types of skin rashes. Folliculitis, eczema, or psoriasis may also be present. When the platelet count is low, petechiae or bleeding gums may be present.

PSYCHOSOCIAL ASSESSMENT

Psychosocial data collection for a client with AIDS is very important. Ask about the client's social support system, including family, significant others, and friends. To protect confidentiality, learn who in this support system is aware of the client's diagnosis so that it is not inadvertently mentioned.

Some clients, because of fear of discrimination, are quite selective about whom they tell. Health care professionals must respect the client's choices as much as possible without compromising care. Offer resources to help with disclosure to sexual partners or significant others.

The client may be closest to a lover or a friend who is not legally recognized as next of kin. Obtain the name and telephone number of that person and learn whether a health care proxy or durable power-of-attorney document has been signed.

Ask about the client's activities of daily living (ADLs), as well as any changes that may have occurred since the diagnosis. Also assess the client's employment status and occupation, social activities and hobbies, living arrangements, and financial resources, including health insurance.

To plan care and monitor changes, assess the client's anxiety level, mood, and cognitive ability. Ask about any experiences with discrimination and how they were handled. After assessing the client's level of self-esteem and changes in body image, work with him or her to identify strengths and coping strategies. Gather information about any suicidal ideation, depression, or other psychological problems. Also ask about the client's use of support groups or other community resources.

LABORATORY ASSESSMENT

LYMPHOCYTE COUNTS. A lymphocyte count is performed as part of a complete blood count (CBC) with differential (see Chapter 23). The normal white blood cell (WBC) count is between 4500 and 11,000 cells/mm^3, with a differential of about 30% to 40% lymphocytes (an absolute number of 1500 to 4500). Clients with AIDS are often leukopenic, with a WBC count of less than 3500 cells/mm^3, and lymphopenic (less than 1500 lymphocytes/mm^3).

CD4+/CD8+ COUNTS. The percentage and number of CD4+ (T4) and CD8+ (T8) cells are an important part of an immune profile. People with HIV disease usually have a lower than normal number of CD4+ cells. Some clients with AIDS have fewer than 100 cells/mm^3 (normal: 500 to 1600 cells/mm^3), whereas the number of CD8+ cells remains normal. The normal ratio of CD4+ to CD8+ cells is 2:1. In HIV disease and AIDS, because of a low number of CD4+ cells, this ratio is low. Low CD4+ cell counts and a low CD4+/CD8+ ratio are associated with increased manifestations of disease.

ANTIBODY TESTS. When the body is infected with HIV, the normal response is to make an antibody to the infecting agent. This antibody is usually made 3 weeks to 3 months after the infection first occurs, although in some people antibodies are not made until 36 months after initial infection.

Thus antibody tests measure the client's response to the virus (the antigen) rather than measuring parts of the virus. HIV antibody can be measured by enzyme-linked immunosorbent assay (ELISA) and Western blot analysis. False-negative results (incorrectly indicating the absence of HIV infection) have been reported early in the infection, in people with cancer, and in people receiving long-term immunosuppressive therapy.

ENZYME-LINKED IMMUNOSORBENT ASSAY (ELISA). The ELISA test is inexpensive and accurate. The client's serum is mixed with HIV grown in culture. If the client has antibodies to HIV, they bind to the HIV antigens and can be detected (a positive test). However, this test can be negative even when the person has HIV infection if the test is performed before antibodies are made in sufficient amounts. The period of time between when a person is first infected with the virus and when viral replication is occurring but the immune system has not yet started making antibodies is called the "window period." This means that if the client has an episode of unprotected sex with an HIV positive person one night and comes in for testing a week later, the ELISA will be negative even though the client may have active HIV. Thus testing during the window does not provide useful information

False-positive test results (incorrectly indicating HIV infection) occur in about 0.1% (1 of 1000) of those tested with ELISA. False-positive results sometimes occur in pregnant women and women who have had children, injection drug users, people who have had malaria, clients with lymphomas, and those with reactivity to the HLA-DR4 leukocyte antigen.

WESTERN BLOT. If the results of an ELISA are positive, they are confirmed by Western blot analysis. This test is more sophisticated and expensive than the ELISA. The Western blot detects serum antibodies to four specific major HIV antigens. A positive Western blot result is based on the presence of antibodies to at least two of the major HIV antigens.

The result is considered inconclusive if two of the major antibodies are not detected but other antibodies to HIV are. The person should then be retested. If a person has a positive test result for HIV antibodies, it does not mean that he or she has AIDS, only that he or she has been infected with the virus.

Both the ELISA and Western blot are blood-based tests. This means special equipment and trained personnel must be used to test for HIV infection. Some HIV testing is more simplified, using techniques that are not blood-based so that testing can be done anywhere, even at home. Two such tests involve oral testing for HIV antibody. The test uses a device that is placed against the gum and cheek for 2 minutes. Fluid (not saliva) is drawn into an absorbable pad, which, in an HIV-positive person, contains antibodies. The pad is placed in a solution, if the result is positive, a change is observed similar to a positive result in a urine pregnancy test. Total testing time is about 15 minutes. If results are positive for HIV, a blood test is needed to confirm the result. The oral tests have the same accuracy as blood testing, and can provide results quickly. A urine test to detect HIV antibodies is also available, but it is not a rapid test.

Home test kits require that a drop of blood be placed upon a test card with a special code number. The card is mailed to a laboratory where the blood is tested for HIV antibodies. A special telephone number is called and the code entered. Test results are then given.

VIRAL CULTURE. Virus cultures also can determine the presence of HIV. This test is rarely used because of the time involved.

VIRAL LOAD TESTING. Viral load testing (also called viral burden testing) measures the presence of HIV viral genetic material (ribonucleic acid [RNA]) or other viral proteins in the client's blood rather than the body's response to the virus. These tests are quantitative and indicate the level of viral burden or viral load. Such tests are useful in monitoring disease progression and treatment effectiveness.

QUANTITATIVE RNA ASSAYS. Currently, three quantitative assays are used for viral load testing: the reverse transcriptase-polymerase chain reaction (RT-PCR), the branched deoxyribonucleic acid method (bDNA), and the nucleic acid sequence–based assay (NASBA). All three assays use gene amplification to determine the amount of HIV RNA present in a client's serum, and all have a specificity of 100%. Even if only a few infected cells are present in a serum sample, tiny amounts of the HIV RNA are amplified by these methods to allow detection. Such tests are useful in the clinical management of disease and in diagnosing HIV infection in people who have no indication of infection. These tests are used to monitor therapy effectiveness and as indicators of the need to change drug regimens.

p24 ANTIGEN ASSAY. The p24 antigen assay quantifies the amount of p24 (HIV viral core protein) in the client's serum. Because this assay is not as sensitive as antibody tests or assays of viral genetic material, it is used mostly to determine treatment efficacy.

OTHER LABORATORY TESTS. Other laboratory tests monitor the overall health of the client and detect or diagnose any infections or other problems related to HIV disease. Such tests include blood chemistries, a complete blood count (CBC) with differential and platelets, prothrombin time and partial thromboplastin time, a serologic test for syphilis (STS), and antigens to hepatitis A, hepatitis B, and hepatitis C. Tests to further evaluate the immune profile of a client may include bone marrow aspiration with biopsy and cultures.

OTHER DIAGNOSTIC ASSESSMENTS

Other diagnostic tests are performed on the basis of the client's manifestations. Such tests may include testing stool for ova and parasites; biopsies of the skin, lymph nodes, lungs, liver, gastrointestinal tract, or brain; a chest x-ray; gallium scans; bronchoscopy, endoscopy, or colonoscopy; liver and spleen scans; computed tomography scans; pulmonary function tests; and arterial blood gas analysis.

Critical Thinking Challenge

Your client is a 32-year-old white man who is new to your outpatient clinic. He complains of fatigue, abdominal pain, mild fever, nausea, and anorexia for almost 2 months. His most worrisome symptoms are a yellowing of his eyes and a darkening of his urine for the past week. He has tried to eat right, take vitamins, and get more rest, but he feels that he is getting worse, not better. A social history reveals that he was in a monogamous gay relationship for 6 years, which recently broke up. He has been dating and occasionally has had unprotected sexual relations with his dates. His most recent HIV test was 1 year ago and was negative. His last episode of unprotected anal receptive intercourse was 2 weeks ago.

1. He asks if his current symptoms are related to his recent sexual encounters. How should you respond?
2. Would you counsel this man to have an HIV test? Why or why not?
3. Should you teach this client about safer sex practices? Why or why not?

evolve For suggested answer guidelines, go to http://evolve.elsevier.com/Iggy/.

Analysis

COMMON NURSING DIAGNOSES AND COLLABORATIVE PROBLEMS

The following are the most common nursing diagnoses for clients with AIDS:

1. Risk for Infection related to immunodeficiency
2. Impaired Gas Exchange related to anemia, respiratory infection (*Pneumocystis carinii* pneumonia [PCP], cytomegalovirus [CMV] pneumonitis, pulmonary Kaposi's sarcoma [KS]), anemia, fatigue, or pain
3. Acute Pain or Chronic Pain related to neuropathy, myelopathy, malignancy, or infection
4. Imbalanced Nutrition: Less Than Body Requirements related to high metabolic need, nausea and vomiting, diarrhea, difficulty chewing or swallowing, or anorexia
5. Diarrhea related to infection, food intolerance, or drugs
6. Impaired Skin Integrity related to KS, infection, altered nutritional state, incontinence, immobility, hyperthermia, or malignancy
7. Disturbed Thought Processes related to AIDS dementia complex (ADC), central nervous system infection, or malignancy
8. Chronic Low Self-Esteem related to changes in body image, decreased self-esteem, or helplessness
9. Social Isolation related to stigma, virus transmissibility, infection control practices, or fear

The primary collaborative problem is Potential for Infection (processed under Risk for Infection, below).

ADDITIONAL NURSING DIAGNOSES AND COLLABORATIVE PROBLEMS

In addition to the common nursing diagnoses and collaborative problems, clients with AIDS may have one or more of the following:

- Activity Intolerance related to fatigue, discomfort, central nervous system defect, weakness, or anemia
- Risk for Injury related to central nervous system defect, mental status changes, depression, or thrombocytopenia
- Disturbed Sensory Perception (Visual) related to CMV retinitis or blindness
- Disturbed Sleep Pattern related to pain, discomfort, anxiety, or depression
- Ineffective Coping related to the diagnosis of AIDS
- Disabled Family Coping related to the diagnosis of AIDS
- Anticipatory Grieving related to potential loss of role and function or impending death

Planning and Implementation

RISK FOR INFECTION

The client with AIDS is susceptible to opportunistic infections because of immunodeficiency secondary to HIV infection.

NOC **PLANNING: EXPECTED OUTCOMES.** The client is expected to remain free of opportunistic diseases. Indicators include the following:

- Absence of chills, fever, or temperature instability
- Absence of purulent drainage or sputum
- Absence of diarrhea
- Absence of chest x-ray infiltration
- Maintenance of white blood cell (WBC) count within the client's normal range

NIC **INTERVENTIONS.** NIC interventions that can help the client minimize the chances of acquiring an infection are provided in Chart 25-5. Chart 25-6 outlines best practices for prevention of infection in a hospitalized immunocompromised client. Some strategies are investigational, including drug therapy and immune function enhancement.

CHART 25-5

NIC **INTERVENTION ACTIVITIES for**
The Client at Risk for Infection

Infection Protection: *Prevention and early detection of infection in a client at risk*
- Monitor for systemic and localized signs and symptoms of infection.
- Monitor vulnerability to infection.
- Monitor absolute granulocyte count, WBC count, and differential results.
- Follow neutropenic precautions, as appropriate.
- Screen all visitors for communicable disease.
- Maintain asepsis for client at risk.
- Inspect skin and mucous membranes for redness, extreme warmth, or drainage.
- Obtain cultures, as needed.
- Promote sufficient nutritional intake.
- Monitor for change in energy level/malaise.
- Instruct client to take antibiotics as prescribed.
- Teach client and family members how to avoid infections.

NIC intervention activities selected from Dochterman, J.M., & Bulechek, G.M. (Eds.). (2004). *Nursing interventions classification (NIC)* (4th ed.). St. Louis: Mosby. No part of this work is to be altered without prior written permission from the Publisher.
WBC, White blood cell.

CHART 25-6

BEST PRACTICE for
Prevention of Infection in an Immunocompromised Client

- Place the client in a private room whenever possible.
- Use good handwashing technique before touching the client or any of his or her belongings.
- Ensure that the client's room and bathroom are cleaned at least once each day.
- Do not use supplies from common areas for immunosuppressed clients. For example, keep a sleeve or box of paper cups in the client's room, and do not share this box with any other client. Other articles include drinking straws, plastic knives and forks, dressing materials, gloves, and bandages.
- Limit the number of health care personnel entering the client's room.
- Monitor vital signs every 4 hours; note minor temperature elevation, which may suggest early sepsis.
- Inspect the client's mouth at least every 8 hours.
- Inspect the client's skin and mucous membranes (especially the anal area) for the presence of fissures and abscesses at least every 8 hours.
- Inspect open areas, such as IV sites, every 4 hours for manifestations of infection.
- Change wound dressings daily.
- Obtain specimens of all suspicious areas for culture, and promptly notify physician.
- Assist the client in performing coughing and deep-breathing exercises.
- Encourage activity at appropriate level for the client's current health status.
- Change IV tubing daily.
- Keep frequently used equipment in the room for use by the client only (e.g., blood pressure cuff, stethoscope, thermometer).
- Limit visitors to healthy adults.
- Use strict aseptic technique for all invasive procedures.
- Monitor the white blood cell count, especially the absolute neutrophil count (ANC), daily.
- Avoid the use of indwelling urinary catheters.
- Keep fresh flowers and potted plants out of the client's room.

Drug Therapy. Chart 25-7 lists treatments for opportunistic infections. Some medications have demonstrated antiretroviral effects; however, *it is important to remember that antiretroviral therapy only inhibits viral replication and does not kill the virus.* Treatment with only one antiretroviral agent, known as monotherapy, promotes drug resistance and does not improve the duration or quality of life for the client with HIV/AIDS. Instead, multiple drugs are used together in regimens popularly called "cocktails." These regimens consist of combinations of different types of antiretroviral agents. Such a therapeutic approach is termed highly active antiretroviral therapy (HAART) and is showing good results as measured by reduced viral load and improved CD4+ lymphocyte counts.

The main actions of each drug category are explained below. The specific drugs, dosages, and nursing implications are presented in Chart 25-8. Drawbacks to HIV/AIDS drug therapy include the expense of the drugs, side effects, food and timing requirements, and the number of daily drugs. The daily regimen is lifelong and burdensome.

Nucleoside Analog Reverse Transcriptase Inhibitors. Nucleoside analogs have a similar structure to the four nucleoside bases of DNA. These drugs are converted in the virally infected cell into a "counterfeit" form of a nucleotide base and compete with the actual nucleotide for placement in DNA. Thus they suppress production of reverse transcriptase (RT) and inhibit viral DNA synthesis and replication. This class of anti-HIV agents includes zidovudine (Retrovir, AZT), didanosine (ddI, Videx), zalcitabine (ddC, HIVID), lamivudine (Epivir, 3TC✱), stavudine (d4T, Zerit), tenofovir (Viread), emtricitabine (Emtriva), and abacavir (Ziagen).

Non-Nucleoside Analog Reverse Transcriptase Inhibitors. Non-nucleoside analog reverse transcriptase inhibitors also inhibit synthesis of reverse transcriptase. These drugs suppress viral replication but do not kill the virus. These drugs include nevirapine (Viramune), delavirdine (Rescriptor), and efavirenz (Sustiva) (see Chart 25-8).

Protease Inhibitors. Protease inhibitors block the HIV protease enzyme, preventing viral replication and release of viral particles. The HIV initially produces all of its proteins, including the ones needed to move viral particles out of a cell, in one long strand. For the proteins to be active, this large protein must be broken down into separate smaller proteins through the action of the viral enzyme HIV protease. The protease inhibitor drugs, when taken into an HIV-infected cell, make the protease enzyme work on the drug rather than on the initial large protein. Thus active proteins are not produced and the viral particles cannot leave the cell to infect other cells. Drugs include ritonavir (Norvir), indinavir (Crixivan), saquinavir (Invirase), nelfinavir (Viracept), amprenavir (Agenerase), lopinavir (Kaletra), atazanavir (Reyataz), and fosamprenavir (Lexiva).

Fusion Inhibitors. Fusion inhibitors are the newest class of antiretroviral medications. Enfuvirtide (Fuzeon) was recently approved for treatment of advanced, drug-resistant HIV infection. After gp120 and the CD4+ cell interact, the next step is for gp41 to fuse HIV and the host cell together for transfer of genetic information. Enfuvirtide works by blocking the fusion of HIV with a host cell by blocking the ability of gp41 to fuse with the host cell. Without fusion, infection of new cells does not occur.

Immune Enhancement. Research is being conducted to evaluate treatments that may enhance or replenish the immune system of clients with AIDS. Some of these

CHART 25-7

DRUG THERAPY for AIDS-Related Opportunistic Infections

Drug	Indication	Usual Dosage	Nursing Interventions	Rationales
Trimethoprim (TMP)/ sulfamethoxazole (SMX) (Apo-Sulfatrim ✱, Bactrim, Cotrim, Septra)	*Pneumocystis carinii* pneumonia	160 mg TMP and 800 mg SMX PO q12h	Monitor I&O. Encourage fluids. Monitor CBC, urinalysis, bilirubin, creatinine, alkaline phosphatase. Assess for sore throat, pallor, purpura, jaundice, weakness.	I&O are monitored because TMP/SMX is nephrotoxic. These values are monitored because TMP/SMX suppresses the immune system. These signs are assessed for because TMP/SMX is hepatotoxic.
Pentamidine isethionate (Pentam)	*P. carinii* pneumonia	4 mg/kg IM or IV once daily for 14-21 days	Monitor blood pressure, heart rate, and rhythm. Administer with client lying down. Monitor for hypoglycemia. Administer IV over 1 hr. Monitor liver function, CBC.	BP and heart rate are monitored because pentamidine causes hypotension when administered rapidly. Monitoring is necessary because pentamidine causes severe hypoglycemia that may be fatal. Liver function and CBC are monitored because pentamidine is hepatotoxic and immunosuppressive.
Pentamidine isethionate (Pentam, Pentacarinat✱)	*P. carinii* pneumonia	Inhalant 300 mg via nebulizer every 4 wk	See above.	See above.
Pyrimethamine (with sulfadoxine) (Daraprim)	Toxoplasmosis	50-75 mg PO daily for 1-3 wk, then 25 mg daily for 4-5 wk	Administer with food or milk. Monitor CBC and platelets.	Pyrimethamine irritates the GI tract. The CBC and platelets are monitored because pyrimethamine suppresses bone marrow activity.
Sulfadiazine	Toxoplasmosis Nocardiasis	500-2000 mg PO q6h daily for 3-4 wk	Monitor urine output, CBC. Encourage fluids. Advise client to avoid sun. Assess for sore throat, pallor, purpura, jaundice, weakness.	Urine output and the CBC are monitored because sulfadiazine causes renal toxicity. Fluids are necessary because sulfadiazine suppresses bone marrow activity. Clients should avoid the sun because sulfadiazine increases photosensitivity.
Dapsone (Avlosulfon✱, DDS)	Toxoplasmosis	50-100 mg PO daily	Monitor CBC. Assess for fever, sore throat, purpura, jaundice.	The CBC is monitored because dapsone suppresses bone marrow activity.
Metronidazole (Flagyl, Novonidazole✱)	Cryptosporidiosis Giardiasis	7.5 mg/kg PO q6h; 15 mg/kg IV initial dose, then 7.5 mg/kg PO q6h	Administer with food or milk. Teach client to avoid alcohol during treatment. Assess for dry mouth, dizziness, fungal infection.	Food or milk is recommended because metronidazole irritates the GI tract. Alcohol causes formation of acetaldehyde and headache, nausea, vomiting, and diarrhea.
(!)[1] Ketoconazole (Nizoral)	Candidiasis Coccidioidomycosis Histoplasmosis	200-400 mg PO daily, single dose	Administer with food or milk. Avoid antacids for 2 hr. Teach client to avoid sun and alcohol during treatment. Monitor hepatic function.	Ketoconazole irritates the GI tract. Gastric acid is needed to activate drug. Ketoconazole increases photosensitivity. Hepatic function is monitored because ketoconazole is hepatotoxic.

(!)[1] ***Med Error Alert!*** *Do not confuse with Neoral, an immunosuppressant.*

I&O, Intake and output; *CBC,* complete blood count; *GI,* gastrointestinal; *MAO,* monoamine oxidase.

Continued

CHART 25-7

DRUG THERAPY for
AIDS-Related Opportunistic Infections—*cont'd*

Drug	Indication	Usual Dosage	Nursing Interventions	Rationales
Fluconazole (Diflucan)	Candidiasis Cryptococcal meningitis	200-400 mg PO or IV initially, then 100-200 mg daily for 2-4 wk	Monitor hepatic function. Assess for abdominal pain, fever, diarrhea.	Hepatic function is monitored because fluconazole is hepatotoxic.
Rifampin (Rifadin, Rofact✱)	*Mycobacterium avium* complex Tuberculosis	10 mg/kg/day PO	Assess breath sounds, sputum.	Assessment of breath sounds and sputum determines treatment effectiveness.
			Monitor hepatic function, CBC.	Rifampin is hepatotoxic.
			May turn body secretions orange.	
Ethambutol (Myambutol, Etibi✱)	*Mycobacterium avium* complex Tuberculosis	25-30 mg/kg PO 2-3 times/wk	Assess vision changes.	Vision changes are assessed because ethambutol causes retrobulbar neuritis and decreased visual acuity (reversible).
			Assess hepatic and renal function, CBC, urinalysis.	This assessment is necessary because ethambutol increases uric acid concentrations. Ethambutol suppresses bone marrow activity.
Amphotericin B (Fungizone)	Candidiasis Other fungal infections	0.3-1 mg/kg/day IV, maximum 50 mg daily	Assess renal function.	Renal function is assessed because amphotericin B is nephrotoxic.
			Assess infusion site.	Amphotericin B causes thrombophlebitis.
			Assess CBC.	The CBC is checked because amphotericin B suppresses bone marrow activity. Amphotericin B is *very* toxic.
Azithromycin (Zithromax)	*Mycobacterium avium* complex	600 mg PO daily plus ethambutol 15 mg/kg/day	Give with food.	Drug induces nausea and vomiting on an empty stomach.
			Assess for visual disturbances.	Azithromycin in combination with ethambutol can cause optic neuritis.
Ciprofloxacin (Cipro)	*Mycobacterium avium* complex Urinary tract infections	250-750 mg PO q12h; 200-400 mg IV q12h	Monitor I&O. Encourage fluids.	
			Administer on empty stomach (1 hr before or 2 hr after meals) if tolerated.	An empty stomach is recommended for best absorption.
			Teach client to avoid sun.	Client should avoid the sun because ciprofloxacin increases photosensitivity.
			Assess for dizziness, fungal infection. Infuse over 1 hr.	
Clarithromycin (Biaxin)	*Mycobacterium avium* complex	500 mg PO twice daily, given with 15 mg/kg/day ethambutol	Give with food.	Drug induces nausea and vomiting on an empty stomach.
			Assess for visual disturbances.	Clarithromycin in combination with ethambutol can cause optic neuritis.
Clofazimine (Lamprene)	*Mycobacterium avium* complex	50-300 mg PO daily	Assess vision changes, dizziness, drowsiness.	Vision changes and dizziness are assessed because clofazimine increases sedation.
			Instruct client to avoid sun.	Clofazimine increases photosensitivity (especially of eyes).
			Use lotions for dry skin.	Clients should use lotions because clofazimine causes dry, scaly skin.
			Monitor hepatic and renal function.	

I&O, Intake and output; *CBC*, complete blood count; *GI*, gastrointestinal; *MAO*, monoamine oxidase.

CHART 25-7

DRUG THERAPY for AIDS-Related Opportunistic Infections—*cont'd*

Drug	Indication	Usual Dosage	Nursing Interventions	Rationales
Pyrazinamide (Tebrazid ✱)	Tuberculosis	20-30 mg/kg/day PO	Monitor hepatic function, uric acid.	Pyrazinamide is hepatotoxic and increases uric acid concentration.
			Assess temperature q4h.	The client's temperature is assessed because pyrazinamide stimulates fever.
Isoniazid ![2] (Laniazid, Isotamine)	Tuberculosis	5-10 mg/kg/day PO or IM, or 15 mg/kg PO or IM 2-3 times/wk	Administer on empty stomach.	Taking isoniazid on an empty stomach enhances absorption.
			Monitor hepatic function.	Isoniazid is hepatotoxic.
			Assess for vision changes.	Vision changes are assessed because isoniazid is neurotoxic.
			Instruct client to avoid alcohol and tyramine-containing foods.	Isoniazid is an MAO inhibitor.
Ganciclovir (Cytovene)	Cytomegalovirus retinitis	5 mg/kg IV q12h for 14-21 days 1000 mg PO q8h	Monitor neutrophil and platelet count. Infuse over 1 hr. Give with food.	Neutrophil and platelet counts are monitored because ganciclovir suppresses bone marrow activity.
Acyclovir (Zovirax)	Herpes simplex Herpes zoster Varicella zoster	200-800 mg PO five times daily; 5-10 mg/kg IV q8h for 7-10 days	Monitor renal function. Encourage fluids.	Acyclovir is nephrotoxic.
			Rotate infusion site.	Various infusion sites are used because acyclovir is a blood vessel irritant.

[2]***Med Error Alert!*** *Do not confuse with Lamisil, an antifungal agent.*

CHART 25-8

DRUG THERAPY for HIV Infection

Drug	Usual Dosage	Nursing Interventions	Rationales
Nucleoside Analog Reverse Transcriptase Inhibitors			
Zidovudine (Retrovir)	300 mg twice daily	Assess for dizziness.	Drug crosses the blood-brain barrier, causing dizziness.
		Monitor CBC, hepatic and renal function.	Zidovudine induces bone marrow suppression, hepatotoxicities, and nephrotoxicities.
Didanosine (ddI, Videx) (Videx EC)	125-300 mg twice daily 250-400 mg daily	Administer on an empty stomach.	Enhances drug absorption.
		Assess vision, hearing, touch, and balance.	Drug induces peripheral neuropathy.
		Monitor CBC.	Drug induces bone marrow suppression.
		Assess for abdominal pain.	Drug can cause severe pancreatitis.
Zalcitabine (ddC, HIVID)	0.75 mg PO q8h	Assess vision, hearing, touch, and balance.	Drug induces peripheral neuropathy.
		Tell client to avoid alcoholic beverages.	Elevates liver enzymes.
Lamivudine (Epivir, 3TC ✱)	150 mg PO twice daily or 300 mg PO daily	Teach client to avoid fatty foods. Assess abdominal pain.	Can cause severe pancreatitis.
		Assess vision, hearing, touch, and balance.	Induces peripheral neuropathy.
Emtricitabine (Emtriva)	200 mg PO daily	Same as for lamivudine.	Same as for lamivudine.
Stavudine (d4T, Zerit)	40 mg twice daily	Assess vision, hearing, touch, and balance.	Induces peripheral neuropathy.
		Assess for generalized pain.	Induces arthralgias.

CNS, Central nervous system; *SC*, subcutaneous.
*Many drug interactions often occur with protease inhibitors.

Continued

CHART 25-8

DRUG THERAPY for HIV Infection—*cont'd*

Drug	Usual Dosage	Nursing Interventions	Rationales
Nucleoside Analog Reverse Transcriptase Inhibitors—*cont'd*			
Abacavir (Ziagen)	300 mg twice daily	Assess for flu-like symptoms (fever, rash, headache, nausea, sore throat, fatigue, shortness of breath).	Manifestations of a hypersensitivity reaction.
		If flu-like symptoms are present, stop drug permanently.	Hypersensitivity can progress to life-threatening emergency.
Tenofovir (Viread)	250 mg PO daily	If also taking ddI, Videx, didanosine, must take these drugs at least 2 hr apart.	Can boost ddI levels into the toxic range in some people.
		Monitor liver and renal function.	Can cause high creatinine and transaminase levels.
Combivir (zidovudine 300 mg + lamivudine 150 mg)	1 tab PO twice daily	Same as with zidovudine and lamivudine individually.	A combination agent containing both drugs.
Trizivir (3 drugs in one) (zidovudine 300 mg + lamivudine 150 mg + abacavir 300 mg)	1 tab PO twice daily	Same as with zidovudine, lamivudine, and abacavir individually.	A combination agent containing all 3 drugs.
Epzicom (abacavir 600 mg + lamivudine 300 mg)	1 tab PO daily	Same as with abacavir and lamivudine individually.	A combination agent containing both drugs.
Truvada (tenofovir 300 mg + emtricitabine 200 mg)	1 tab PO daily	Same as with tenofovir and emtricitabine individually.	A combination agent containing both drugs.
Non-Nucleoside Analog Reverse Transcriptase Inhibitors			
Nevirapine (Viramune)	200 mg twice daily	Assess for rash. Assess for headache. Assess for abdominal pain.	Allergic reactions are common. Most common side effect. Drug may induce liver toxicity.
Efavirenz (Sustiva)	600 mg once daily	Assess for headaches, dysphoria, dizziness, insomnia, and nightmares.	Drug crosses blood-brain barrier and can induce CNS manifestations.
		Avoid contact with medication during pregnancy.	Drug is mutagenic and can induce birth defects.
Delavirdine (Rescriptor)	400 mg three times daily	Store at room temperature. Assess for headache or rash. Give 1 hr before or after antacids.	Recommended storage. Common side effects. Absorption is inhibited by antacids.
Protease Inhibitors*			
Saquinavir (Invirase)	600 mg q8h	Tell client to take with or just after a high-fat, high-calorie meal.	Drug is best absorbed with a fatty meal.
		Instruct client to wear sunscreen.	Drug increases photosensitivity.
Indinavir (Crixivan)	800 mg q8h	Administer on an empty stomach. Assess for jaundice. Assess for flank or back pain or hematuria.	Enhances drug absorption. Induces hyperbilirubinemia. Induces nephrolithiasis.
Ritonavir (Norvir)	600 mg q12h	Administer with a light meal. Monitor serum lipid levels.	Enhances drug absorption. Can elevate serum lipid levels.
Nelfinavir (Viracept)	625 mg q12h	Administer with food.	Causes diarrhea, which is lessened when taken with food.
		Monitor blood glucose levels.	Can induce hyperglycemia.
Amprenavir (Agenerase)	200-800 mg daily	Monitor blood glucose levels.	Can induce hyperglycemia.
Lopinavir (Kaletra) (now available as combination: 133 mg lopinavir + 33 mg ritonavir)	3 capsules twice daily	Administer with food. Avoid giving to clients with known sulfonamide allergy.	Enhances drug absorption. Cross-reactivity possible.
Atazanavir (Reyataz)	400 mg PO daily	Monitor blood bilirubin levels. Administer with food. Check sclera and skin at each clinic visit.	Can induce hyperbilirubinemia. Enhances drug absorption. Icterus and jaundice are signs of high bilirubin levels.
Fosamprenavir (Lexiva)	1400 mg twice daily	Monitor serum lipid levels.	Can elevate serum lipid levels.
Fusion Inhibitors			
Enfuvirtide (Fuzeon)	90 mg SC twice daily	Monitor for skin reactions at injection site.	Infection risks and lipodystrophy if injection site is not rotated.

CNS, Central nervous system; *SC*, subcutaneous.
*Many drug interactions often occur with protease inhibitors.

TABLE 25-4 Complementary and Alternative Therapies for HIV/AIDS

Agents with Antiviral Effects	Immune-Enhancing Agents
■ Shark cartilage	■ Astragalus
■ Curcumin	■ Echinacea
■ Hypercin	■ Ascorbic acid
■ Compound Q	
■ SPV-30	
■ Aloe vera	

methods include bone marrow transplantation, lymphocyte transfusion, and infusions of lymphokines, particularly interleukin-2, and other biological response modifiers.

Complementary and Alternative Therapies. Complementary therapies are often used by people with HIV/AIDS. Such therapies include vitamins, shark cartilage, and botanical products available at health food stores. The usefulness of these products has yet to be established through well-controlled clinical trials. In addition, some botanicals alter the effects of prescription drugs. Ask the client which botanicals are being used and check with the pharmacist to determine known drug interactions. Table 25-4 lists the botanical agents often used by clients to enhance immune function or slow viral replication.

Health Maintenance. HIV can remain latent inside a cell for long periods and only cause active infection when the cell is stimulated. The specific signals for the cell to become activated are not known, but concurrent viral or parasitic infections are suspected. Teach the client to avoid exposure to infection (Chart 25-9).

IMPAIRED GAS EXCHANGE

NOC **PLANNING: EXPECTED OUTCOMES.** The client is expected to maintain adequate oxygenation and perfusion and to experience minimal dyspnea. Indicators include the following:

- Rate and depth of respiration within the normal range
- Pulse oximetry within the normal range
- Absence of cyanosis or pallor

INTERVENTIONS. The nurse or respiratory therapist uses drug therapy, respiratory support and maintenance, comfort, and rest.

Drug Therapy. Appropriate drug therapy is started after identification of an infectious or other cause for respiratory difficulty (see Chart 25-7). A common respiratory infection among people with HIV disease or AIDS is *Pneumocystis carinii* pneumonia (PCP). The treatment of choice for PCP is trimethoprim/sulfamethoxazole (Apo-Sulfatrim✱, Bactrim, Cotrim, Septra), given intravenously or orally, depending on the severity of infection. Many clients with AIDS have adverse reactions to this medication, including nausea, vomiting, hyponatremia, rashes, fever, leukopenia, thrombocytopenia, and hepatitis.

Pentamidine isethionate (Pentacarinat✱, Pentam), usually given IV or IM, is also used to treat PCP. Aerosolized pentamidine isethionate is used for clients with CD4+ counts below 200 and for those who have already had PCP.

Other drug therapies include dapsone (Avlosulfon) and atovaquone (Mepron), which can be used as therapy for existing PCP or as prophylaxis. For moderate to severe PCP, steroids may be used to reduce the inflammation.

CHART 25-9

CLIENT EDUCATION GUIDE

Prevention of Infection Among Immunocompromised Clients

- Avoid crowds and other large gatherings of people who might be ill.
- Do not share personal toilet articles, such as toothbrushes, toothpaste, washcloths, or deodorant sticks, with others.
- If possible, bathe daily.
- Wash the armpits, groin, genitals, and anal area at least twice a day with an antimicrobial soap.
- Clean your toothbrush daily by either running it through the dishwasher or rinsing it in liquid laundry bleach.
- Wash your hands thoroughly with an antimicrobial soap before you eat or drink, after touching a pet, after shaking hands with anyone, as soon as you come home from any outing, and after using the toilet.
- Eat a low-bacteria diet, and avoid salads, raw fruit and vegetables, undercooked meat, pepper, and paprika.
- Wash dishes between use with hot, sudsy water or use a dishwasher.
- Do not drink water that has been standing for longer than 15 minutes.
- Do not reuse cups and glasses without washing.
- Avoid changing pet litter boxes. If unavoidable, use gloves or wash hands immediately.
- Avoid turtles and reptiles as pets.
- Do not feed pets raw or undercooked meat.
- Take your temperature at least once a day.
- Report any of the following signs or symptoms of infection to your physician immediately:
  - Temperature greater than 100° F (38° C)
  - Persistent cough (with or without sputum)
  - Pus or foul-smelling drainage from any open skin area or normal body opening
  - Presence of a boil or abscess
  - Urine that is cloudy or foul smelling or that causes burning on urination
- Take all prescribed medications as prescribed.
- Do not dig in the garden or work with houseplants.
- Avoid travel to areas of the world with poor sanitation or less-than-adequate health care facilities.

Respiratory Support and Maintenance. The client also needs care to maintain respiratory function and avoid complications. Assess the respiratory rate, rhythm, and depth; breath sounds; and vital signs and monitor for cyanosis at least every 8 hours. Apply oxygen and humidify the room as prescribed. Also monitor mechanical ventilation, perform suctioning and chest physical therapy as needed, and evaluate blood gas results.

Comfort. Assess the client's comfort. The client with respiratory difficulties may be more comfortable with the head of the bed elevated. Pace activities to reduce shortness of breath and exhaustion. Provide psychological support during periods of respiratory distress.

Rest and Activity. Most clients with HIV/AIDS have fatigue, especially when respiratory problems also are present. Fatigue can be made worse by certain therapies. Consult with the client to pace activities to conserve energy. Guide the client in active and passive range-of-motion (ROM) exercises. Schedule non–time-critical activities, such as bathing, so that he or she is not fatigued at mealtime.

PAIN

The client with severe HIV disease or AIDS often has pain from a variety of causes. Pain can result from enlarged organs stretching the viscera or compressing nerves. Tumor invasion of bone and other tissues can cause pain. Many clients with AIDS have peripheral neuropathy-induced pain from the disease or drug therapies. Many have generalized joint and muscle pain.

NOC **PLANNING: EXPECTED OUTCOMES.** The client is expected to achieve an acceptable level of comfort and pain reduction. Indicators include the following:

- Reporting that pain is controlled
- Absence of physiologic indicators of acute pain (increased heart rate and blood pressure)
- Absence of facial grimacing, teeth clenching
- Willingness to move and participate in self-care

INTERVENTIONS. Pharmacologic and nonpharmacologic approaches are used to manage pain in the client with HIV/AIDS, depending on the cause of the pain.

Comfort Measures. The use of pressure-relieving mattress pads, warm baths or other forms of hydrotherapy, massage, and applying heat or cold to painful areas may reduce pain levels, with or without drug therapy. Take care when moving or assisting the client. Use lift sheets to avoid pulling or grasping the client with joint pain. The client may be thin and have poor circulation, contributing to pain and discomfort. Help the client change positions often.

Drug Therapy. The type of drugs used depends on what is causing the pain. For arthralgia and myalgia, nonsteroidal anti-inflammatory drugs (NSAIDs) may reduce inflammation and increase comfort without inducing drowsiness. The neuropathic pain of peripheral neuropathy may respond best to tricyclic antidepressants such as amitriptyline (Elavil) or to anticonvulsant medication such as phenytoin (Dilantin) or carbamazepine (Tegretol). Drugs for neuropathic pain may take from several days to weeks before a full effect is seen. During this time, opioids may be needed to control pain.

When opioids are used, assess the client for pain intensity. Mild to moderate pain is treated with weaker opioids such as oxycodone or codeine. More intense pain is treated with stronger opioids such as morphine, hydromorphone (Dilaudid), or fentanyl transdermal (Duragesic). Combinations of weak and strong opioids along with non-opioid medications may be used to provide the best sustained pain relief and allow the client to participate in activities to the extent that he or she wishes.

Complementary and Alternative Therapies. Many clients with pain from HIV/AIDS use therapies such as guided imagery, distraction, progressive relaxation, body-talk, and biofeedback to help control pain. Such therapies can be used with more traditional and pharmacologic measures to improve comfort.

IMBALANCED NUTRITION: LESS THAN BODY REQUIREMENTS

Many clients with AIDS have difficulty maintaining their weight and nutritional status. This problem may be caused by fatigue, anorexia, nausea and vomiting, difficult or painful swallowing, diarrhea, or wasting syndrome.

NOC **PLANNING: EXPECTED OUTCOMES.** The client is expected to maintain optimal weight through adequate nutrition and hydration. Indicators include the following:

- Selecting foods high in calories and protein
- Maintaining current weight or gaining weight
- Drinking at least 3 L of oral fluids per day
- Maintaining blood levels of albumen, prealbumin, and hemoglobin within normal ranges

INTERVENTIONS. Because there are multiple factors for poor nutrition in AIDS, diagnostic procedures are needed to determine the cause. Once the cause is determined, appropriate therapy is initiated. For example, in the client who has candidal esophagitis, nutrition is affected because of swallowing difficulties.

Drug Therapy. Therapy can include ketoconazole (Nizoral) or fluconazole (Diflucan) orally, or intravenous (IV) amphotericin B (Fungizone). Administer the medication as prescribed and monitor for side effects such as nausea and vomiting, which further alter nutritional status. Provide mouth care and ice chips and keep unpleasant odors out of the client's environment. Antiemetics are used as needed.

Diet Therapy. Monitor the client's weight, intake and output, and calorie count. Assess food preferences and any dietary cultural or religious practices. Instruct the client about a high-calorie, high-protein, nutritionally sound diet. Encourage the client to avoid dietary fat, because fat intolerance often occurs as a result of the disease and as a side effect of some antiretroviral medications. In collaboration with the dietitian, provide an appropriate diet, including small, frequent meals (better tolerated than large meals). Supplemental vitamins and fluids are indicated in some cases. For the client who cannot achieve adequate nutrition through food, tube feedings or total parenteral nutrition may be needed.

Mouth Care. Provide frequent mouth care for clients susceptible to oral ulceration or infection. Rinses of sodium bicarbonate with normal saline every 2 hours or several times a day are helpful. Give the client a soft toothbrush and advise him or her to drink plenty of fluids. For oral pain, analgesics or viscous lidocaine may be needed.

DIARRHEA

Clients with AIDS often suffer from diarrhea. Sometimes an infectious cause (e.g., *Giardia* or amoeba) can be determined and treated, or the cause is determined but no effective therapy is available. Many clients are lactose intolerant, and HIV disease makes this condition worse. Diarrhea may occur as a side effect of therapy with protease inhibitors. In some cases, clients with AIDS have diarrhea and no cause can be identified.

NOC **PLANNING: EXPECTED OUTCOMES.** The client is expected to have decreased diarrhea; maintain fluid, electrolyte, and nutritional status; and reduce incontinence. Indicators include the following:

- Stool amount is appropriate for the diet
- Stools are formed and soft
- Recognizes urge to defecate
- Maintains control of stool passage

INTERVENTIONS. For most clients with AIDS and diarrhea, symptom management is all that is available. Antidiarrheals, such as diphenoxylate hydrochloride (Diarsed✱, Lomotil) or loperamide (Imodium), given on a regular schedule, provide some relief. Consult with the dietitian and offer dietary counseling about appropriate foods. Recommended dietary changes include less roughage; less fatty, spicy, and sweet food; and no alcohol or caffeine. Some clients obtain relief when they eliminate dairy products from the diet or eat smaller amounts of food more often and drink plenty of fluids, especially between meals.

Provide the client with a bedside commode or a bedpan if needed. Some clients cannot reach the bathroom in time because of immobility or anal sphincter weakness, others because of the urgency to defecate. Provide privacy, support, and understanding.

IMPAIRED SKIN INTEGRITY

The most common skin lesion in AIDS is Kaposi's sarcoma (KS). Lesions may be localized or widespread. Large lesions can cause pain and restrict movement. They can impede circulation, causing open, weeping, painful lesions. Another cause of impaired skin integrity is herpes simplex virus (HSV) infection.

NOC **PLANNING: EXPECTED OUTCOMES.** The client is expected to have healing of any existing lesions and avoid increased skin breakdown or secondary infection. Indicators include the following:

- Absence of new lesions or open skin areas
- Existing lesions become smaller in diameter
- Absence of purulent drainage, induration or redness in, from, or around skin lesions

INTERVENTIONS. KS can be treated with local radiation, intralesional chemotherapy, or cryotherapy. Systemic therapy is used in clients with rapidly progressive disease or with major involvement of the intestinal tract, lungs, or other organs. Therapies include chemotherapy (single agent or combination), interferon-alpha, and interferon-alpha plus zidovudine.

Treatment of painful KS lesions includes analgesics and comfort measures. Keep open, weeping KS lesions clean and dressed to reduce the risk for secondary infection. Many clients with skin KS are concerned about their appearance and the risk of being identified as HIV positive. Makeup (if lesions are not open), long-sleeved shirts, and hats may help in maintaining a normal appearance.

For the client with an HSV abscess, provide good skin care. Clean abscesses at least once per shift with normal saline and allow them to air-dry or dry with a heat lamp. This infection is painful and requires analgesics, assistance with position, and other comfort measures. Modified Burow's solution (Domeboro) soaks promote healing for some clients. HSV infection is treated with acyclovir (Zovirax) given intravenously, orally, or in some cases, topically, depending on the severity of the infection.

DISTURBED THOUGHT PROCESSES

Neurologic changes with disturbed thought processes are major areas of concern for clients with HIV infection or AIDS. These changes may be due to psychological stressors accompanying the disease or to organic disorders caused by opportunistic infections, cancer, or HIV encephalitis.

NOC **PLANNING: EXPECTED OUTCOMES.** The client is expected to show improved mental status. Indicators include that the client demonstates the following behaviors:

- Identifies self and significant others
- Identifies correct month and year
- Recalls immediate, recent, and remote information accurately

INTERVENTIONS. Clients with AIDS suffer from enormous loss and psychological stress, which complicates the assessment of any changes in behavior or affect. Assess baseline neurologic and mental status by using neurologic assessment tools (see Chapter 44) to compare any changes. Evaluate the client for subtle changes in memory, ability to concentrate, affect, and behavior. It is important to determine whether the cause of the neurologic changes is treatable.

Orientation. Reorient the confused client to person, time, and place as needed, reminding the client of your identity and explaining what is to be done at any given time. Using calendars, clocks, and radios and putting the bed close to a window also may help keep the client oriented. Give simple directions; use short, uncomplicated sentences; explain activities in simple language; and involve the client in planning the daily schedule. Ask relatives or significant others to bring in familiar items from home. Arrange all items in the client's environment in the same location as at home.

Drug Therapy. Various agents are used as appropriate for different conditions contributing to altered thought processes in the person with AIDS. Psychotropic drugs are used to treat ongoing behavioral problems or emotional disorders. Antidepressants and anxiolytics are often prescribed.

Safety Measures. Attention to safety is crucial to the well-being of the neurologically impaired client with AIDS. He or she may not be aware of activities or surroundings and may need help with bathing, dressing, eating, ambulating, and other activities of daily living (ADLs). Make the environment, whether a hospital room or long-term care facility, safe and comfortable.

Some clients are susceptible to seizures. Institute seizure precautions, including using padded siderails and having an artificial oral airway available. Anticonvulsants may be added to the medications.

Assess the client with neurologic manifestations for increased intracranial pressure. Report immediately any changes in level of consciousness, vital signs, pupil size or reactivity, or limb strength to the physician for appropriate intervention. Corticosteroids may be given to reduce intracranial pressure.

Support. Work closely with the family and significant others of the neurologically impaired client. There is great trauma in seeing a loved one unable to care for himself or herself or demonstrating unusual or childlike behavior. Answer questions honestly and sensitively. Teach the family and significant others how to reorient the client. Encourage them to continue to provide the client with news of family happenings or current events. Collaborate with the social worker to identify community resources for the client and family.

CHRONIC LOW SELF-ESTEEM

The client with AIDS may have changes in self-esteem and self-concept. Contributing to this are dramatic changes in appearance that alter the person's body image. Many clients also have abrupt, significant changes in their relationships with others and in day-to-day activities, including a job or other productive activities. All changes can disrupt the self-concept.

NOC **PLANNING: EXPECTED OUTCOMES.** The client is expected to identify positive aspects of himself or herself and accept himself or herself. Indicators include that the client often or consistently demonstrates the following behaviors:

- Verbalizes self-acceptance
- Maintains eye contact
- Accepts compliments from others
- Expresses feelings of self-worth

INTERVENTIONS. Provide a climate of acceptance for clients with AIDS by promoting a trusting relationship and by helping clients express feelings and identify positive aspects of themselves. Allow for privacy but do not avoid or isolate the client. Encourage self-care, independence, control, and decision making by helping the client set short-term, attainable goals and offering praise when these are achieved.

Complementary therapy in the form of guided imagery is used by many clients to increase their sense of control and enhance self-esteem. Imagery can focus on helping clients cope with distressing side effects or painful procedures. Other uses of imagery include picturing battle scenes in which the virus is killed by immune system cells.

SOCIAL ISOLATION

Many clients with AIDS face discrimination, rejection, and isolation. Friends or health care workers sometimes avoid or refuse to have anything to do with them. Misunderstanding and fear lead to misuse of proper infection control procedures, and clients are inappropriately isolated.

NOC **PLANNING: EXPECTED OUTCOMES.** The client is expected to identify behaviors that cause social isolation and demonstrate behaviors that reduce social isolation. Indicators include that the client often or consistently demonstrates the following behaviors:

- Interacts with close friends, significant others, and family members
- Demonstrates cooperation with others
- Uses assertive behaviors as appropriate

INTERVENTIONS. Interventions for social isolation focus on promoting interactions and on education to reduce fear of AIDS transmission.

Promotion of Interaction. Establish a therapeutic nurse-client relationship and do not isolate the client. Show understanding and concern while helping the client find ways to reduce feelings of rejection and isolation. Reduce barriers to social contact. Assess the client's social support resources. Teach family and significant others about HIV transmission and the use of standard precautions to reduce anxiety and increase contact with the client (see Chapter 29).

Encourage the client to verbalize feelings about self, coping skills, and a sense of control over the situation. Help the client to identify support systems, including those already in place and those that need to be arranged.

Education. The most important aspect for prevention of HIV transmission is education. All people, regardless of age, gender, ethnicity, or sexual orientation, are susceptible to HIV infection. HIV infection is preventable because of the mode of viral transmission and the fragile nature of the virus.

Critical Thinking Challenge

You are the new charge nurse on a busy medical-surgical floor at a community hospital. On a particularly busy day, one of the "new hires" tells you that she had a needle stick injury, at the start of shift, today. She was giving her 78-year-old diabetic client insulin and accidentally stuck herself, trying to put the needle into an overflowing sharps container. In talking with other nurses, she doubts that this is a high-risk needle stick since it was with an insulin syringe, and the client is an older woman, who is obviously at low risk for HIV. She washed off the blood thoroughly from her finger, applied Betadine, and covered it with a Band-Aid. Because it is almost change of shift, the nurse wants to fill out an incident report and go home.

1. How will you counsel this nurse about the needle stick injury?
2. What rights and obligations does she have?
3. For what other bloodborne diseases has this incident placed her at risk?
4. Should postexposure prophylaxis be started? Why or why not?
5. Should this nurse inform her sexual partner(s) of this incident? Why or why not?

evolve For suggested answer guidelines, go to http://evolve.elsevier.com/Iggy/.

Community-Based Care

The usual course of illness is one of intermittent acute infections and periods of relative wellness over months or years. Often, this period is followed by chronic, progressive debilitation. Because of the cyclic nature of HIV disease and AIDS, the client often spends long periods at home between hospital admissions or clinic visits. In some instances, especially as the illness becomes more severe, he or she may need referral to a long-term care facility, home care agency, or hospice. In collaboration with the social worker, dietitian, and other available resources, work with clients to plan what will be needed and how they will manage at home with self-care and activities of daily living (ADLs).

HOME CARE MANAGEMENT

When the client is discharged to home, assess the client's status, ability to function, and actual or potential needs for care. Some clients do not need home care but do need to maintain a link with primary care providers. Home care can range from help with ADLs for clients with weakness, debility, or limited function to around-the-clock nursing care, medications, and nutritional support for severely or terminally ill clients. Assess available resources, including family members and significant others willing and able to be caregivers. Help the family make arrangements for outside caregivers or respite care, if needed. Clients may need referrals or help in planning housing, finances, insurance, legal services, funeral arrangements, and spiritual counseling.

Home care aides may be involved in daily or weekly care of the client with AIDS in the home. Usually a home care nurse makes routine visits for assessment purposes, especially as the client becomes increasingly debilitated. Chart 25-10 lists focused assessment areas for the client with AIDS at home.

HEALTH TEACHING

Educating the client, family, and significant others is a high priority when preparing for discharge. Instruct about modes of transmission and preventive behaviors (guidelines for safer sex; not sharing toothbrushes, razors, and other potentially blood-contaminated articles). Caregivers also need instruction about best practices for infection control precautions to prevent transmission while caring for the client in the home (Chart 25-11), nursing techniques to use in the home, and coping or support strategies.

Teach the client, family, and significant others how to protect the client from infection, to identify manifestations of potential infections, and what to do if these appear. Teach

CHART 25-10

FOCUSED ASSESSMENT of
The Person with AIDS

Assess cardiovascular and respiratory status.
- Vital signs
- Presence of acute chest pain or dyspnea
- Presence of cough
- Presence of fever
- Activity tolerance

Assess nutritional status.
- Food intake
- Weight loss or gain
- General condition of skin
- Financial resources

Assess neurologic status.
- Cognitive changes
- Motor changes
- Sensory disturbances

Assess gastrointestinal status.
- Mouth and oropharynx
- Presence of dysphagia
- Presence of abdominal pain
- Presence of nausea, vomiting, diarrhea

Assess psychological status.
- Presence of anxiety
- Presence of depression

Assess activity and rest.
- Activities of daily living (ADLs)
- Mobility and ambulation
- Fatigue
- Sleep pattern
- Presence of pain

Assess home environment.
- Safety hazards
- Structural barriers affecting functional ability

Assess client's and caregiver's adherence and understanding of illness and treatment, including the following:
- Manifestations to report to nurse
- Medication schedule and side or toxic effects

Assess client's and caregiver's coping skills.

CHART 25-11

BEST PRACTICE for
Infection Control for Home Care of the Person with AIDS

Direct Care
- Follow standard precautions and good handwashing techniques.
- Do not share razors or toothbrushes.

Housekeeping
- Wipe up feces, vomitus, sputum, urine, or blood or other body fluids and the area with soap and water. Dispose of solid wastes and solutions used for cleaning by flushing them down the toilet. Disinfect the area by wiping with a 1:10 solution of household bleach (1 part bleach to 10 parts water). Wear gloves during cleaning.
- Soak rags, mops, and sponges used for cleaning in a 1:10 bleach solution for 5 minutes to disinfect them.
- Wash dishes and eating utensils in hot water and dishwashing soap or detergent.
- Clean bathroom surfaces with regular household cleaners, then disinfect them with a 1:10 solution of household bleach.

Laundry
- Rinse clothes, towels, or bedclothes if they become soiled with feces, vomitus, sputum, urine, or blood. Then dispose of the soiled water by flushing it down the toilet. Launder these clothes with hot water and detergent with 1 cup of bleach added per load of laundry.
- Keep soiled clothes in a plastic bag.

Waste Disposal
- Dispose of needles and other "sharps" in a labeled puncture-proof container such as a coffee can with a lid, using standard precautions to avoid needle stick injuries. Decontaminate full containers by adding a 1:10 bleach solution. Then seal the container with tape and place it in a paper bag. Dispose of the container in the regular trash.
- Remove solid waste from contaminated trash such as paper towels or tissues, dressings, disposable incontinence pads, and disposable gloves, then flush the waste down the toilet. Place these items in tied plastic bags and dispose of them in the regular trash.

about the use of self-care strategies, such as good hygiene, balanced rest and exercise, skin care, mouth care, and safe administration of any prescribed drugs (including potential side effects). During dietary teaching, stress the following:
- Good nutrition
- Avoidance of raw or rare fish, fowl, or meat
- Thorough washing of fruits and vegetables
- Proper food handling and refrigeration practices

Teach the client to avoid large crowds, especially in enclosed areas, not to travel to countries with poor sanitation, and to avoid cleaning pet litter boxes.

PSYCHOSOCIAL PREPARATION

Clients with AIDS are often concerned about the possible social stigma and rejection. Be aware that this fear is realistic and help identify ways to avoid problems, as well as identify coping strategies for difficult situations. Support family members and significant others in efforts to help the client and provide protection from discrimination.

Encourage clients to continue as many usual activities as possible. Except when too ill or too weak, they can continue to work and participate in most social activities. Support clients in their selection of friends and relatives with whom to discuss the diagnosis. Stress that sexual partners and care providers should be informed; beyond that, it is up to the client. Some clients have severe depression or anxiety about the future. Almost all feel the burden of having a fatal disease widely considered unacceptable and feel compelled to maintain some secrecy about the illness. Referrals to community resources, mental health/behavioral health professionals, and support groups can help the client verbalize fears and frustrations and cope with the illness.

HEALTH CARE RESOURCES

In many cities, community organizations have been set up to assist people with AIDS. Often composed of volunteers, they offer excellent services to the community. The types and number of services vary by agency and city, but many include HIV testing and counseling, clinic services, buddy systems, support groups, respite care, education and outreach, referral services, and even housing. Clients may also need referrals to other local resources, such as home care agencies, companies that provide home IV therapy, community mental health/behavioral health agencies, Meals on Wheels, and others. In addition, educational materials and support groups are available through Internet access.

Evaluation: Outcomes

The overall goals for care of clients with AIDS are to maintain the maximum possible level of function for as long as possible, minimize infections, and maintain quality of life and dignity during the course of progressive illness. Evaluate the care of the client with AIDS on the basis of the identified nursing diagnoses and collaborative problems. Expected outcomes include that the client should:

- Remain free from opportunistic infections
- Have adequate respiratory function
- Achieve an acceptable level of physical comfort
- Attain adequate weight, nutritional, and fluid status
- Maintain skin integrity
- Remain oriented
- Maintain self-esteem
- Maintain a support system and involvement with others
- Adhere to the prescribed therapy regimen

Specific indicators for these outcomes are listed for each nursing diagnosis and collaborative problem under the Planning and Implementation section (see earlier).

NUTRITION-RELATED IMMUNODEFICIENCIES

Good nutrition is needed for proper immune function. White blood cells (WBCs) are highly active cells that constantly shed surface proteins and need nutrients to remake these components. Immunodeficiency related to nutrition results from biologic, political, economic, and cultural factors. Immunodeficiency from poor nutrition can be prevented and treated.

Malnutrition is a major cause of global immunodeficiency, seen most often in less affluent countries, in the urban and rural poor of North America, and in the chronically ill. Hospitalized adult medical-surgical clients also are at high risk for malnutrition. Four points should be kept in mind:

- Anorexia occurring with chronic disease, acute infection, or treatment often leads to reduced oral intake.
- Absorption or utilization of nutrients is sometimes impaired because of gastrointestinal diseases or absorption problems.
- Host defenses during infection increase the demand for nutrients, which is met at the expense of the body's stores.
- Hospitalized clients are often undernourished because of many hours of nothing by mouth and because of IV fluid infusions that lack essential nutrients.

Malnutrition can impair any aspect of immune function. The degree of impairment is related to the severity of malnutrition. Nutrient excess, especially fats and carbohydrates, also have detrimental effects on immune function. Nutritional problems are often a complex of deficiency or excess of one or more nutrients.

Protein-Calorie Malnutrition

PATHOPHYSIOLOGY

Protein-calorie malnutrition (PCM) affects all aspects of immune function. The greatest impairment occurs in cell-mediated immunity, with decreased numbers of T-lymphocytes and thymic changes. The result is anergy and an increased risk for infection. The estimated incidence of PCM ranges from 25% to 50% of hospitalized clients. PCM causes reduced energy and protein synthesis. The following are manifestations of PCM in adults:

- Leanness and cachexia
- Decreased effort tolerance and lethargy
- Intolerance to cold
- Ankle and shin edema
- Dry, flaking skin and various types of dermatitis
- Poor wound healing
- A higher than usual incidence of postoperative infection

◆COLLABORATIVE MANAGEMENT

The management of clients with PCM is to treat the precipitating event and supply protein and calories, sometimes with nutrient supplements. In clients with severe PCM, any infection is treated first and then fluid and electrolyte imbalances are corrected. Then a gradual but steady replacement of protein and energy is undertaken. Often this refeeding begins parenterally, because a severely malnourished gut may be unable to absorb food. Replenishment of protein and calories is accompanied by vitamin supplementation as needed, nutrition education, and a progressive increase in physical activity.

PCM is easier to prevent than to treat. Be aware of hospitalized clients at risk for PCM. Chart 25-12 lists practices to reduce the risk for PCM in hospitalized clients.

Obesity

PATHOPHYSIOLOGY

The incidence and severity of infectious disease increase among obese people. Impaired cell-mediated immunity and decreased neutrophil activity occur with obesity, making obese people at greater risk for infection. Excess dietary fats suppress all aspects of immune function. The obese client also may have a coexisting PCM.

Often the obese client is not recognized as malnourished because of the excessive weight. For these clients, nutritional status is assessed by laboratory measurements and diet history.

◆COLLABORATIVE MANAGEMENT

Good nutrition is important to maintain and improve immune defenses. Consult with the physician and dietitian to provide a diet that is sufficient in calories and protein but is low in fat.

Protect the obese client by maintaining a safe environment. Use good handwashing before all contact with the

CHART 25-12

BEST PRACTICE for
Reducing the Risk for Protein-Calorie Malnutrition in the Hospitalized Client

- Measure height and weight when the client is admitted to the agency, reweighing at least weekly.
- Monitor the client's ability to eat the prescribed diet and the amounts eaten.
- Obtain dietary consultation when needed.
- Evaluate whether nutrients consumed are sufficient to meet basal and stress-related energy needs.
- Avoid prolonged use of standard IV fluids that provide less than 200 calories/L.
- Assess and monitor laboratory values for serum albumin, prealbumin, and leukocyte counts.
- Schedule tests and procedures so that the client spends minimal time fasting.

client. Ensure that strict aseptic techniques are used for all invasive procedures. Assess the client every shift for manifestations of local or systemic infection and notify the physician of any suspected infection.

THERAPY-INDUCED IMMUNODEFICIENCIES

PATHOPHYSIOLOGY

Some secondary immunodeficiencies may be related to other conditions that cause the loss of immunoglobulins or destruction of lymphocytes. The most common cause of secondary immunodeficiency is the use of drugs and other treatment modalities for various diseases. Sometimes immunosuppression is a desired effect, as in organ transplantation or for the treatment of autoimmune disorders. Often immunosuppression is an undesirable, complicating side effect of therapy that is used for another intent, such as cancer chemotherapy, and may even require changing the therapeutic regimen. Various therapies cause different types and degrees of immunosuppression. The challenge is to have maximal therapeutic effect without leaving the client overly immunosuppressed and susceptible to serious complications.

Drug-Induced Immunodeficiencies

Several drug classes have major immunosuppressive effects. Some induce general immunosuppression; others are more specific and target one part of the immune system more than another.

CYTOTOXIC DRUGS

Most cytotoxic drugs interfere with all rapidly dividing cells. White blood cells (WBCs), including lymphocytes and phagocytes, rapidly divide and are susceptible to this type of destruction. The result is a decrease in the number of lymphocytes and phagocytic cells. Cytotoxic drugs interfere with the ability of lymphocytes to produce and release products such as lymphokines and antibodies, causing general immunosuppression. Most cytotoxic drugs are used for cancer and autoimmune disorders.

CORTICOSTEROIDS

Corticosteroids are hormones used to treat many autoimmune diseases, neoplasms, and endocrine disorders. Corticosteroids have both anti-inflammatory and immunosuppressive effects. They inhibit inflammation by stabilizing blood vessel membranes and decreasing permeability, blocking the movement of neutrophils and monocytes. These drugs disrupt the synthesis of arachidonic acid, the main precursor for a variety of inflammatory chemicals.

Corticosteroids keep T-cells in the bone marrow, reducing the number of circulating T-cells and resulting in lymphopenia and suppressed cell-mediated immunity.

Corticosteroids interfere with immunoglobulin G (IgG) production and reduce antibody-antigen binding. These drugs have many effects that alter disease activity, and numerous side effects, including the following:

- Central nervous system changes, such as euphoria, insomnia, or psychosis
- Cardiovascular changes, such as hypertension or edema
- Gastrointestinal effects, such as gastric irritation, ulcers, and increased appetite (with weight gain)
- Other changes (e.g., hyperglycemia, muscle weakness, delayed wound healing, osteoporosis, and body fat redistribution)

CYCLOSPORINE

Cyclosporine (Sandimmune, Neoral) is a specific immunosuppressant that selectively suppresses the helper-inducer T-lymphocytes by blocking their growth and development. Cyclosporine is used to prevent organ transplant rejection and graft-versus-host disease. This drug is occasionally used for disorders, such as uveitis, rheumatoid arthritis, and other autoimmune diseases.

Radiation-Induced Immunodeficiencies

Radiation is toxic to dividing and resting cells. Because most lymphocytes are sensitive to radiation, exposure can induce profound lymphopenia, causing general immunosuppression. Whether or not immunodeficiency occurs after radiation therapy depends on the location and dose of radiation. Exposure to the iliac and femur in adults can cause generalized immunosuppression because these bone areas are the primary blood cell–producing sites.

COLLABORATIVE MANAGEMENT

Management of the client with treatment-induced immunodeficiency aims to improve immune function and protect him or her from infection. The most severe immunosuppression occurs while he or she is receiving the immunosuppressive drugs or during radiation treatment. The severity and duration of the immunosuppression are related to the dosage of specific drugs. Although this impairment is usually temporary, with good recovery of immune and inflammatory responses within weeks or months of therapy completion, the potential for severe infections makes this problem a major treatment concern. Common infections occurring during this period include those of fungal origin, yeast, residual viral breakthrough, and a variety of bacteria.

Work closely with clients and other health care professionals to provide safe care to those at risk for infection. Chart 25-6 lists specific nursing actions to prevent infection among clients with drug-induced or any type of immunosuppression. Good handwashing by all health care personnel before contact with the client is essential for infection prevention. Health care professionals must use aseptic technique with any invasive procedure.

In some instances, drug-induced immunosuppression can be reduced or avoided by giving biological response modifiers (BRMs) to stimulate bone marrow production of immune system cells. Although not appropriate for all types of disorders, this treatment can reduce the client's risk for infection during drug therapy. BRMs are expensive, however, and not consistently covered by insurance. See Chapters 28 and 43 for further discussion about this treatment.

Many clients remain at home during periods of immunosuppression. Teach the client and family best practices to reduce the client's risk for infection (see Chart 25-9).

For clients receiving chronic therapy with immunosuppressive drugs, drug dosages are altered according to their responses. The lowest dose that achieves the desired effect is given.

Congenital (Primary) Immunodeficiencies

Congenital, or primary, immunodeficiencies are disorders in which the immunodeficient person is born with a defect in the development or function of one or more immune components. As a result, the immune response does not adequately protect the client from infection, cancer, or other disease. Most congenital immunodeficiencies are rare.

Some congenital immunodeficiencies are inherited as an X-linked trait (such as Bruton's agammaglobulinemia or Wiskott-Aldrich syndrome), and some are recessive (such as ataxia-telangiectasia). For many congenital immunodeficiencies, however, the genetic defect and inheritance pattern have not been clearly identified. Examples of congenital immunodeficiencies are listed in Table 25-5.

Congenital immunodeficiencies are classified according to the type of immune function that is impaired: antibody mediated, cell mediated, or combined. Because cell-mediated and combined immunodeficiencies are so severe that the affected person usually does not survive childhood, only antibody-mediated problems (seen in adults) are discussed in this chapter.

BRUTON'S AGAMMAGLOBULINEMIA

PATHOPHYSIOLOGY

A classic congenital antibody-mediated immunodeficiency is Bruton's disease or Bruton's agammaglobulinemia. Boys born with this disease usually start to have problems at about 6 months of age, after maternal antibodies, transferred through the placenta, have been lost. The first manifestations are recurrent otitis, sinusitis, pneumonia, furunculosis, meningitis, and septicemia with organisms such as *Pneumococcus, Streptococcus,* and *Haemophilus.* Laboratory assessment shows an absence of circulating immunoglobulin (antibodies).

COLLABORATIVE MANAGEMENT

Except for clients with poliomyelitis, chronic echovirus infection, or a lymphoreticular malignancy, the overall prognosis for Bruton's disease is good if antibody replacement is started early. Immune serum globulin is regularly given to these clients, usually about 100 to 400 mg/kg IV every 3 to 4 weeks (Table 25-6). The dosage and schedule are individualized. Antibiotics are used for specific infections. Long-term prophylactic antibiotic therapy may also be used. Often, severe sinopulmonary disease later develops in some clients.

TABLE 25-5 Congenital Immunodeficiencies

Antibody-Mediated Immunodeficiencies
- X-linked agammaglobulinemia (Bruton's)
- Acquired hypogammaglobulinemia (common variable immunodeficiency)
- Selective IgA deficiency

Cell-Mediated Immunodeficiencies
- Congenital thymic aplasia (DiGeorge syndrome)
- Chronic mucocutaneous candidiasis

Combined Immunodeficiencies
- Severe combined immunodeficiencies
- Wiskott-Aldrich syndrome
- Immunodeficiency with ataxia-telangiectasia
- Nezelof syndrome

COMMON VARIABLE IMMUNODEFICIENCY

PATHOPHYSIOLOGY

The client with common variable immunodeficiency, or hypogammaglobulinemia, has recurrent bacterial infections similar to those seen with Bruton's disease. The client has low levels of circulating antibodies (immunoglobulins) of all classes.

Hypogammaglobulinemia differs from Bruton's disease in that it usually first appears later (in adolescence or young adulthood), occurs almost equally in males and females, and the infections are less severe. Common complications include giardiasis (intestinal infection with *Giardia lamblia*), gastric cancer, bronchiectasis, and cholelithiasis (gallbladder stones).

COLLABORATIVE MANAGEMENT

Treatment is similar to that for Bruton's disease. Regular infusions of immune serum globulin and regular or intermittent use of antibiotics protect the affected person against infection.

SELECTIVE IMMUNOGLOBULIN A DEFICIENCY

PATHOPHYSIOLOGY

Selective immunoglobulin A (IgA) deficiency is the most common congenital immunodeficiency seen in adults, occurring in 1 per 600 to 800 individuals (McCance & Huether, 2002). The client may be asymptomatic or have chronic recurrent upper respiratory tract infections, skin infections, urinary tract infections, vaginal infections, and diarrhea. Selective IgA deficiency does not reduce life span. Because IgA is the major antibody in secretions, bacterial infections are seen mostly in the respiratory, gastrointestinal, and urogenital tracts. Some clients with IgA deficiency also have malabsorption syndrome.

COLLABORATIVE MANAGEMENT

Therapy for IgA deficiency is limited to vigorous treatment of infections. *Unlike other immunoglobulin deficiencies, IgA deficiency should never be treated with exogenous immune globulin for two reasons. First, exogenous immune globulin contains very little IgA and would not help boost IgA levels. Second, because clients with IgA deficiency make normal amounts of all other antibodies, they are at high risk for severe allergic reactions to exogenous immune globulin.* If malabsorption syndrome occurs with IgA deficiency, the client needs nutritional supplements (e.g., partial or total enteral or parenteral nutrition).

TABLE 25-6 Administration of Intravenous Immune Serum Globulin

Indications	Dosage	Nursing Interventions	Rationales
B cell or humoral immunodeficiencies ▪ Bruton's hypogammaglobulinemia ▪ Common variable immunodeficiency ▪ Combined immunodeficiencies: severe combined immunodeficiencies	Gamimune 100-200 mg/kg or 2-4 mL/kg IV once monthly *or* Sandoglobulin 0.2-0.3 g/kg IV once monthly Gammagard 200-400 mg/kg IV once monthly Iveegam 200-800 mg/kg IV once monthly	Observe client closely and monitor vital signs during infusion and for 30-60 min thereafter. Slow the rate of infusion or stop it temporarily if side effects occur.	Monitoring detects signs of anaphylaxis and routine side effects. Side effects occur in 10% of clients and include skeletal pain, back pain, nausea, chills, headache, chest tightness, and abdominal cramps. Side effects appear to be related to the rate of infusion.

GET READY for the NCLEX Examination!

KEY POINTS

Safe Effective Care Environment

- Use standard precautions for all clients regardless of age, gender, race or ethnicity, sexual orientation, education level, and profession.
- Ask clients about Advance Directives and document the status.
- Use good handwashing techniques before providing any care to a client who is either immunocompromised or immunodeficient.

Health Promotion and Maintenance

- Identify clients at high risk for infection as a result of work environment or leisure activities.
- Encourage all clients who are HIV positive to use condoms and other precautions during sexual intimacy even if the partner is also HIV positive.
- Inform all clients who smoke that smoking decreases overall immune function.
- Assist clients interested in smoking cessation to find an appropriate smoking cessation program.
- Teach clients with protein-calorie malnutrition what foods to include in the diet.
- Teach the client and family about the clinical manifestations of infection and when to seek medical advice.

Psychosocial Integrity

- Treat all clients, regardless of diagnosis, with dignity.
- Do not assume that any visitor or family member knows the client's diagnosis.
- Pace your interview to match the learning needs and style of the individual client.
- Allow the client the opportunity to express fear or anxiety regarding a change in health status.
- Refer clients newly diagnosed with HIV infection to local resources and support groups.
- Encourage all clients who are HIV positive to inform their sexual partners of their HIV status.
- Explain all diagnostic procedures, restrictions, and follow-up care to the client scheduled for tests.
- Allow clients who experience a change in physical appearance to mourn this change.

Physiological Integrity

- Encourage clients to adhere to their antiviral drug regimen.
- Pace nonurgent health care activities to reduce the risk for fatigue among clients with AIDS.
- Teach clients the expected side effects and possible adverse reactions to prescribed drugs.
- Assess the immunodeficient client every shift for manifestations of infection.
- Assess the skin integrity of the perianal region of a client with AIDS-related diarrhea after every bowel movement.

ADDITIONAL STUDY RESOURCES

Go to your Student CD-ROM for Review Questions for the NCLEX Examination.

evolve Go to http://evolve.elsevier.com/Iggy/ for Integrated Management of Care Questions for the NCLEX Examination.

SELECTED BIBLIOGRAPHY

Asterisk indicates a classic or definitive work on this subject.

*Abbas, A., Lichtman, A., & Pober, J. (1997). *Cellular and molecular immunology* (3rd ed.). Philadelphia: W.B. Saunders.

Ackley, B., & Ladwig, G. (2002). *Nursing diagnosis handbook: A guide to planning care* (5th ed.). St. Louis: Mosby.

AIDS: Its prevalence and treatment in the United States. (2001). *The American Journal for Nurse Practitioners, 5*(3), 58.

Barroso, J. (2002). HIV-related fatigue. *American Journal of Nursing, 102*(5), 83-85.

Bradley-Springer, L. (2001). HIV prevention: What works? *American Journal of Nursing, 101*(6) 45-50.

Brooke, P. (2001). The legal realities of HIV exposure. *RN, 64*(12), 71-73.

Bursaw, M., Keenan, K., & Ehrhart, M. (2001). HIV update. *Nursing 2001, 31*(2), 62-63.

*Centers for Disease Control. (1987). Public Health Service guidelines for counseling and antibody testing to prevent HIV infection and AIDS. *Morbidity and Mortality Weekly Report, 36*(31), 509-515.

*Centers for Disease Control. (1991). Recommendations for preventing transmission of human immunodeficiency virus and hepatitis B virus to clients during exposure-prone invasive procedures. *Morbidity and Mortality Weekly Report, 40*(RR-8), 1-9.

*Centers for Disease Control and Prevention. (1998a). Public Health Service guidelines for the management of health-care worker exposure to HIV and recommendations for postexposure prophylaxis. *Morbidity and Mortality Weekly Report, 47* (RR-7), 1-32.

*Centers for Disease Control and Prevention. (1998b). Public Health Service taskforce recommendations for the use of anti-retroviral drugs in pregnant women infected with HIV-1 for maternal health and reducing perinatal HIV-1 transmission in the U.S. *Morbidity and Mortality Weekly Report, 47*(RR-2), 1-30.

Centers for Disease Control and Prevention (2003). *HIV/AIDS surveillance report* 2002, *14*(10), 1-48. Rockville, MD: Author. Available at http://www.cdc.gov/hiv/stats/hasr1302.pdf.

Coyne, P., Lyne, M., & Watson, A. (2002). Symptom management in people with AIDS. *American Journal of Nursing, 102*(9), 48-57.

Daughtry, L., Bankston, J., & Deshotels, J. (2002). HIV meds: Keeping trouble at bay. *RN, 65*(2), 31-36.

Dochterman, J., & Bulechek, G. (Eds.). (2004). *Nursing interventions classification (NIC)* (4th ed.). St. Louis: Mosby.

Ebersole, P., Hess, P., & Luggen, A. (2004). *Toward healthy aging* (6th ed.). St. Louis: Mosby.

Ehrhardt, A., et al. (2002). A gender-specific HIV/STD risk reduction intervention for women in a health care setting: Short- and long-term results of a randomized clinical trial. *AIDS Care, 14*(2), 147-161.

Facts and Comparisons. (2004). *Drug facts and comparisons* (58th ed.). St. Louis: Author.

Godwin, C. (2004). What's new in the fight against AIDS? *RN, 67*(4), 46-52.

Goldrick, B. (2004). HIV advances. *American Journal of Nursing, 104*(5), 37-38.

Haddad, A. (2003). Ethics in action: HIV patient wants "natural therapy." *RN 66*(3), 27-30.

Holzemer, W. (2002). HIV and AIDS: The symptom experience. *American Journal of Nursing, 102*(4), 48-52.

Holzemer, W. (2002). The symptom experience: What cell counts and viral loads won't tell you. *American Journal of Nursing. 102*(4):48-52.

Holzemer, W., et al. (2000). The patient adherence profiling-intervention tailoring (CAP-IT) intervention for enhancing adherence to HIV/AIDS medications: A pilot study. *Journal of the Association of Nurses in AIDS Care, 11*(1) 36-44.

Jagger, J., & Perry, J. (2003). Lab workers: Small group, big risk. *Nursing2003, 33*(1), 72.

Jones, S. (2004). Taking HAART. *Nursing 2004, 34*(6), 6-11.

Kemppainen, J.K. (2001). Prediction of quality of life in AIDS patients. *Journal of the Association of Nurses in AIDS Care, 12*(1), 61-70.

Lactic acidosis a threat for HIV clients. (2002). *Nursing2002, 32*(7), 28.

McCance, K., & Huether, S. (2002). *Pathophysiology: The biologic basis for disease in adults and children* (4th ed.). St. Louis: Mosby.

New HIV test: Accurate results in 20 minutes flat. (2003). *Nursing 2003, 33*(1), 34.

Nussbaum, R., McInnes, R., & Willard, H. (2001). *Thompson & Thompson: Genetics in medicine* (6th ed.). Philadelphia: W.B. Saunders.

On-and-off therapy works and cuts costs too. (2002). *Nursing 2002, 32*(2), 33.

Pagana, K., & Pagana, T. (2002). *Mosby's manual of diagnostic and laboratory tests* (2nd ed.). St. Louis: Mosby.

Randolph, S. (2002). When candida turns deadly. *RN, 65*(3), 41-45.

Sande, M.A., & Volberding, P.A. (2002). *The medical management of AIDS* (6th ed.). Philadelphia: W.B. Saunders.

Sankar, A., et al. (2002). Adherence discourse among African-American women taking HAART. *AIDS Care, 14*(2), 203-218.

Sellers, C., & Angerame, M. (2002). HIV/AIDS in older adults: A case study and discussion. *AACN Clinical Issues, 13*(1), 5-21.

Trzcianowska, H., & Mortensen, E. (2001). HIV and AIDS: Separating fact from fiction. *American Journal of Nursing, 101*(6), 53-59.

Trzynka, S., & Erlen, J. (2004). HIV disease susceptibility in women and the barriers to adherence. *MEDSURG Nursing, 13*(2), 97-104.

Welch, K. (2002). Predictors of survival in older men with AIDS. *Geriatric Nursing, 23*(2), 62-68.

Williams, A. (2001). Adherence to HIV regimens: 10 vital lessons. *American Journal of Nursing, 101*(6), 37-44.

CHAPTER 26

Interventions for Clients with Immune Function Excess: Hypersensitivity (Allergy) and Autoimmunity

M. LINDA WORKMAN

LEARNING OUTCOMES

After studying this chapter, you should be able to:

1. Compare the bases and manifestations of allergy and autoimmunity.
2. Discuss anaphylaxis prevention measures.
3. Discuss the nursing responsibility for a client with anaphylaxis.
4. Identify the common drugs, dosages, and side effects used as therapy for anaphylaxis.
5. Describe allergy testing techniques.
6. List the defining characteristics of type I, type II, type III, type IV, and type V hypersensitivity reactions.
7. Explain the differences in mechanisms of action between antihistamines and mast cell stabilizers.
8. Develop a community-based teaching plan for the client who has severe allergic reactions.

Go to your Student CD-ROM for Review Questions for the NCLEX Examination keyed to these Learning Outcomes.

The inflammatory and immune responses are normally helpful, protecting the body against infection and cancer development. These responses also stimulate tissue growth and repair after injury. When inflammation or immune responses are prolonged, excessive, or occur at an inappropriate time, however, normal tissues are damaged. These responses are "overreactions" to invaders and foreign antigens, and are known as hypersensitivity or allergic responses. In addition, inflammatory and immune responses can fail to recognize self cells and attack normal body tissues. This type of reaction is known as an autoimmune response. Hypersensitivity and autoimmune responses can severely damage cells, tissues, and organs.

Hypersensitivities/Allergies

Hypersensitivity or allergy is an increased or excessive response to the presence of an **antigen** (foreign protein or allergen) to which the client has been previously exposed. These responses cause problems that range from uncomfortable (e.g., itchy, watery eyes or sneezing) to life-threatening (e.g., allergic asthma, anaphylaxis, bronchoconstriction, or circulatory collapse). The terms hypersensitivity and allergy are used interchangeably. Hypersensitivity reactions are classified into five basic types, determined by differences in timing, pathophysiology, and clinical manifestations (Table 26-1). Each type may occur alone or along with one or more other types.

TYPE I: RAPID HYPERSENSITIVITY REACTIONS

Type I, or rapid, hypersensitivity, also called *atopic allergy*, is the most common type of hypersensitivity. This type results from the increased production of the immunoglobulin E (IgE) antibody class. Acute inflammation occurs when IgE responds to an antigen, such as pollen, and causes the release of histamine and other vasoactive amines from basophils, eosinophils, and mast cells. Examples of type I reactions include anaphylaxis, allergic asthma (discussed in Chapter 33); atopic allergies such as hay fever, allergic rhinitis; and allergies to specific allergens such as latex, bee venom, peanut, iodine,

TABLE 26-1 Mechanisms and Examples of Types of Hypersensitivities

Mechanism	Clinical Examples
Type I: Immediate	
Reaction of IgE antibody on mast cells with antigen, which results in release of mediators, especially histamine	Hay fever Allergic asthma Anaphylaxis
Type II: Cytotoxic	
Reaction of IgG with host cell membrane or antigen adsorbed by host cell membrane	Autoimmune hemolytic anemia Goodpasture's syndrome Myasthenia gravis
Type III: Immune Complex–Mediated	
Formation of immune complex of antigen and antibody, which deposits in walls of blood vessels and results in complement release and inflammation	Serum sickness Vasculitis Systemic lupus erythematosus Rheumatoid arthritis
Type IV: Delayed	
Reaction of sensitized T-cells with antigen and release of lymphokines, which activate macrophages and induce inflammation	Poison ivy Graft rejection Positive TB skin tests Sarcoidosis
Type V: Stimulated	
Reaction of autoantibodies with normal cell-surface receptors, which stimulates a continual overreaction of the target cell	Graves' disease B-cell gammopathies

IgE, Immunoglobulin E; *IgG*, immunoglobulin G; *TB*, tuberculosis.

shellfish, drugs, and thousands of other environmental antigens. Allergens can be contacted in the following ways:

- Inhaled (plant pollens, fungal spores, animal dander, house dust, grass, ragweed)
- Ingested (foods, food additives, drugs)
- Injected (bee venom, drugs, biologic substances such as contrast dyes and adrenocorticotropic hormone)
- Contacted (pollens, foods, environmental proteins)

Some reactions occur just in the areas exposed to the antigen, such as the mucous membranes of the nose and eyes, causing symptoms of rhinorrhea, sneezing, and itchy red, watery, eyes. Other reactions may involve all blood vessels and bronchiolar smooth muscle causing widespread blood vessel dilation, decreased cardiac output, and bronchoconstriction. This condition is known as **anaphylaxis.**

Allergic Rhinitis

PATHOPHYSIOLOGY

Allergic rhinitis, also called "hay fever," is triggered by reactions to airborne allergens, especially plant pollens, molds, dust, animal dander, wool, food, and air pollutants. Some acute episodes are "seasonal," tending to recur at the same time each year. They often coincide with the timing of large environmental exposure and last only a few weeks. Chronic rhinitis, or perennial rhinitis, tends to occur intermittently (with no predictable seasonal pattern) or continuously when a person is exposed to certain allergens. In "nonallergic

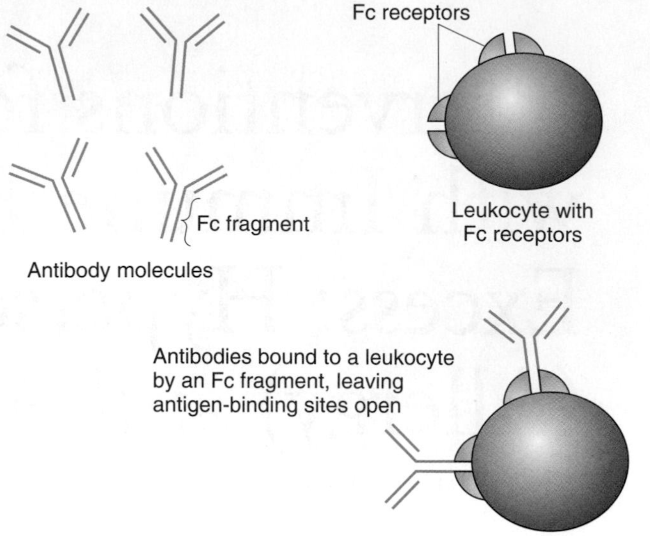

Figure 26-1 ■ Antibody Fc receptors on the basophils and mast cells.

rhinitis," the same manifestations are present although no allergic cause is identified and the immune system does not appear to be involved.

On first exposure to an **allergen** (an antigen that provokes allergic sensitization), the person responds by making antigen-specific IgE. This antigen-specific IgE binds to the surface of basophils and mast cells (Figure 26-1). These cells have many granules containing vasoactive amines (including histamine) that are released when stimulated. Once the antigen-specific IgE is formed, the person is sensitized to that allergen.

In a type I allergic reaction, the previously sensitized person is re-exposed to the provoking allergen. The resulting response has a primary phase and a secondary phase. In the primary phase, the allergen binds to two adjacent IgE molecules on the surface of a basophil or mast cell, which breaks or distorts the cell membrane. These membrane changes cause the cell to degranulate, releasing the vasoactive amines within the granules into the tissue fluids (Figure 26-2).

The most common vasoactive amine is *histamine,* a short-acting biochemical. Histamine causes capillary leak, nasal and conjunctival mucous secretion, and itching (pruritus), often occurring with erythema (redness). These symptoms last for about 10 minutes after histamine is first released. When the allergen is continuously present, mast cells continuously release histamine and other proteins, prolonging the response.

The secondary phase results from the release of other proteins. These other proteins draw more white blood cells to the area and stimulate a more general inflammatory reaction through actions of leukotriene and prostaglandins. This reaction occurs in addition to the allergic reaction stimulated in the primary phase. The resulting inflammation increases the clinical manifestations and is probably responsible for continuing the response.

Etiology and Genetic Risk

The tendency to produce IgE in response to antigen exposure is based on genetic inheritance, but no single gene has been found to be responsible. Specific allergies are *not* in-

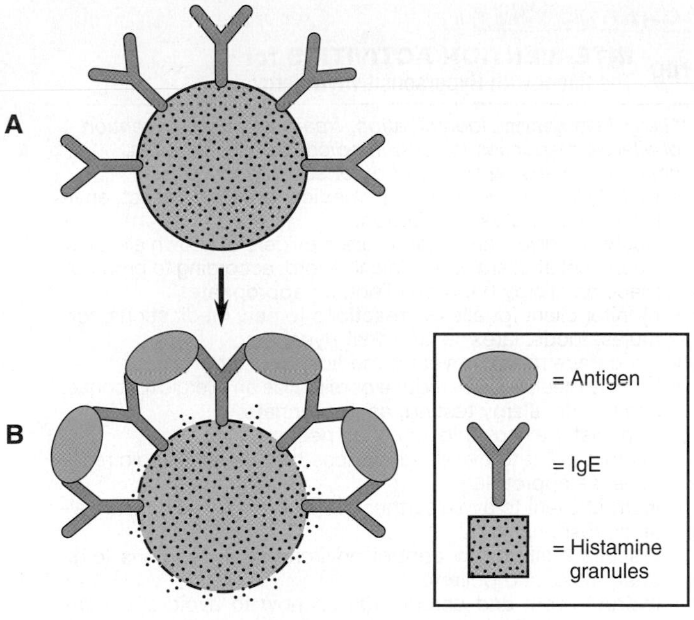

Figure 26-2 ■ Degranulation and histamine release. **A,** Mast cell with IgE. **B,** Mast cell degranulation and histamine release when allergen binds to IgE.

herited. About 50% of clients with allergic rhinitis have one parent with type I allergies.

Incidence/Prevalence

Atopic allergies, including allergic rhinitis, affect about 10% of the population in North America (McCance & Huether, 2002). Men and women are affected equally. Racial differences have not been documented.

COLLABORATIVE MANAGEMENT

Assessment

HISTORY

An accurate and detailed history may provide insight into the possibility of allergic rhinitis. Ask the client to describe the onset and duration of problems in relation to possible allergen exposure. Ask about work, school, and home environments, and possible exposures through hobbies, leisure time or sports activities. Because a tendency toward type I allergic responses can be inherited, ask about the presence of allergies among close relatives.

PHYSICAL ASSESSMENT/CLINICAL MANIFESTATIONS

The client with allergic rhinitis usually has **rhinorrhea** (a "runny" nose), a "stuffy" nose, and itchy, watery eyes. The client may breathe through his or her mouth and the voice has a nasal sound. Drainage from the nose is usually clear or white. The nasal mucosa appears swollen and pink. The client may have a headache or feel pressure over the frontal and maxillary sinuses. Transillumination of the sinuses may be decreased. If nasal secretions drip posteriorly, the client may have a dry, scratchy throat and pharyngitis. The client often feels as though he or she has a cold that has lasted longer than a week. Fever is rare unless an infection occurs with the rhinitis.

LABORATORY ASSESSMENT

A complete blood count and differential indicate the presence of an allergic response by an increase in eosinophils. A client with severe seasonal allergic rhinitis may have an eosinophil count as high as 12% (normal being 1 to 2%). Some clients have an increased total white blood count, but the percentage of neutrophils remains normal (55% to 70%). If an acute infection occurs with allergic rhinitis, both the total white blood cell count and the number of neutrophils increase.

Other laboratory tests that indicate the presence of an allergic reaction include serum immunoglobulin E (IgE) levels and the radioallergosorbent test (RAST). A normal level of IgE for adults is about 39 IU/mL (or less than 100 IU/mL). This level can increase greatly with allergies. The usual IgE test does not indicate the specific allergen, only the tendency to have allergic responses. The RAST test shows the blood level of IgE directed against a specific antigen and thus can determine specific allergies. However, the expense of this study limits its use in allergy testing.

ALLERGY TESTING

SKIN TESTING. With most type I reactions, skin testing can show which specific allergens are causing the reaction. Skin testing can be performed as scratch testing and intradermal testing. Patch testing is often reserved for contact dermatitis and other manifestations of type IV hypersensitivities.

Scratch Testing. A scratch or prick test can show an *immediate* hypersensitivity reaction to an allergen. Scratch tests are used in routine allergy testing to determine the cause of allergic rhinitis, asthma, urticaria (hives) or any other type I reactions. Allergens introduced through a scratch or prick cause a localized reaction (wheal) when the test result is positive. Results are usually determined after 15 to 20 minutes.

Client Preparation. For best results, systemic glucocorticoids and antihistamines are discontinued for 5 days before the test to avoid suppressing an allergic response during the test. Nasal sprays to reduce mucous membrane swelling are permitted, except for sprays that contain an antihistamine. Some allergists recommend that aspirin and other nonsteroidal anti-inflammatory agents be withheld before allergy testing.

Procedure. The best sites for scratch testing are the inside of the arm or on the back. Other sites are used if a rash or skin problem is present on the arms or back. Gently clean the skin with soap and water, and remove surface oils with alcohol.

Small drops of sera containing different known allergens are placed on the skin. The skin is scratched or pricked through the drop with a bifurcated skin testing needle. Control drops are also applied; normal saline drops are negative controls and histamine drops are positive controls. The reactions of the allergen-tested areas are examined for the presence and size of a reaction. These areas are then compared to the control areas. Areas showing erythema and wheal formation are considered positive for that antigen. Degree of sensitivity is estimated by the size of the response.

Serious reactions in response to scratch testing are rare. Ensure that emergency equipment is readily available during a scratch test.

Follow-up Care. After testing is completed for the day, wash the solution from the skin. Topical steroids and oral antihistamines may be given to reduce itching and increase client comfort. If an antihistamine that causes sedation is given, the client will need to have another person drive him or her home.

Intradermal Testing. Intradermal testing is reserved for substances that are strongly suspected of causing allergy but did not test positive with scratch testing. Intradermal testing increases the risk for an adverse reaction, including anaphylaxis, but it is usually a safe procedure. Ensure that emergency equipment is in the room with the client. Small amounts of testing sera (0.1 mL) are injected intradermally on the client's upper arm and the area is observed for erythema and wheal formation. The degree of allergy is estimated by the size of the response. Client preparation and follow-up care are the same as for scratch testing.

ORAL FOOD CHALLENGE. Some clients have allergic rhinitis even when the allergen does not come into contact with the nasal mucosa but is ingested orally. The oral food challenge is used to identify specific allergens if skin testing is not conclusive and if keeping a food diary has failed to determine the offending food items. This test requires the client to eliminate suspected foods for 7 to 14 days before testing. After this time, the client is directed to eat defined food for at least 1 day and to monitor for manifestations of allergy. When many food allergies are present, the client may have to eat only one food type per day of testing.

Interventions

Chart 26-1 lists NIC interventions for allergy management. Common interventions include avoidance therapy, desensitization therapy, and symptomatic therapy. Many clients use a combination of all three types of therapy for management of allergic rhinitis and other manifestations of type I allergy.

AVOIDANCE THERAPY. When specific allergens have been identified, urge the client to avoid direct or close contact with these agents. Some allergens, such as certain foods or drugs, may be easy to avoid. Other substances, such as pollen, mold, or dust mites, may require environmental changes.

Many airborne allergens can be reduced by air-conditioning and air-cleaning units. Removing cloth drapes, upholstered furniture, and carpeting reduces air-borne allergens. Covering mattresses and pillows with plastic or an ultra fine mesh cover also reduces exposure to dust mites and mold.

Pet-induced allergies pose special challenges. Sometimes simple interventions, such as keeping pets out of the bedroom and thorough cleaning of the room to remove animal hair and dander, may reduce symptoms. Frequent bathing of the pet or keeping the pet outdoors can decrease allergen exposure. Depending on the severity of the allergy and how well other methods provide relief, pets with fur, feathers, or dander may need to be removed from the household.

SYMPTOMATIC THERAPY. When avoidance therapy is impractical, symptomatic therapy can be effective in reducing the allergic response and making the client more comfortable.

CHART 26-1

NIC INTERVENTION ACTIVITIES for The Client with Hypersensitivity/Allergy

Allergy Management: *Identification, treatment, and prevention of allergic responses to food, medications, insect bites, contrast material, blood, and other substances*

- Identify known allergies (e.g., medication, food, insect, environmental) and usual reaction.
- Notify caregivers and health care providers of known allergies.
- Document all allergies in clinical record, according to protocol.
- Place an allergy band on client, as appropriate.
- Monitor client for allergic reactions to new medications, formulas, foods, latex, and/or test dyes.
- Encourage client to wear a medical alert tag.
- Provide medication to reduce or minimize an allergic response.
- Assist with allergy testing, as appropriate.
- Administer allergy injections, as needed.
- Instruct client to avoid substances that cause allergic reactions, as appropriate.
- Instruct client to avoid further use of substances causing allergic responses.
- Discuss methods to control environmental allergens (e.g., dust, mold, and pollen).
- Instruct client and caregiver(s) on how to avoid situations that put the client at risk and how to respond if an anaphylactic reaction should occur.
- Instruct client and caregiver on use of epinephrine pen.

Anaphylaxis Management: *Promotion of adequate ventilation and tissue perfusion for a client with a severe allergic (antigen-antibody) reaction*

- Place individual in a comfortable position.
- Apply tourniquet per protocol immediately proximal to the allergen point of entry (e.g., injection site, IV site, insect bite, etc.), when possible, as appropriate.
- Establish and maintain a patent airway.
- Administer oxygen at high flow rate (10-15 L/min).
- Start an IV infusion of normal saline, lactated Ringer's, or a plasma volume expander, as appropriate.
- Reassure the individual and family members.
- Monitor for signs of shock (e.g., respiratory difficulty, cardiac arrhythmias, seizures, and hypotension).
- Administer spasmolytics, antihistamines, or corticosteroids as indicated if urticaria, angioedema, or bronchspasm present.
- Monitor for recurrence of anaphylaxis within 24 hours.

NIC interventions selected from Dochterman, J.M., & Bulechek, G.M. (Eds.). (2004). *Nursing interventions classification (NIC)* (4th ed.). St. Louis: Mosby.

Drug Therapy. Drug therapy involves the use of steroidal and nonsteroidal agents (to reduce inflammation), vasoconstrictors, antihistamines, mast cell stabilizers, and drugs that inhibit the release or action of leukotrienes. Some drugs reduce the response and other drugs prevent the response. Chart 26-2 lists common drugs used for symptomatic relief of allergic rhinitis.

Decongestants. Decongestants are available as systemic oral drugs or nasal sprays. These drugs do not clear the allergen or prevent the release of mediators such as histamine. They have actions similar to adrenergic drugs and work by causing vasoconstriction in the inflamed tissue, thereby reducing the edema. Decongestants often contain ephedrine, phenylephrine, or pseudoephedrine. Secretions are reduced when vasoconstricting drugs are combined with an anticholinergic drug, such as scopolamine or atropine. Many combination decongestants are available by prescription and as over-the-counter cold and allergy drugs. Side ef-

CHART 26-2

DRUG THERAPY for Allergic Rhinitis

Drug	Usual Dosage	Nursing Implications	Rationales
Antihistamines			
Diphenhydramine (Benadryl, Allerdryl✱, Hyrexin)	25-50 mg q4-6h	Instruct client not to drive or operate heavy machinery.	Drug can cause significant sedation.
		Do not give during an acute asthma attack.	Sedation decreases the voluntary muscle contractions needed for breathing.
Chlorpheniramine (Chlor-Trimeton, Telachlor, Teldrin, Phenetron)	2-8 mg 1-3 times daily	Avoid alcoholic beverages. Same as for diphenhydramine.	Drug potentiates the effects of alcohol.
Loratadine (Claritin)	10 mg daily	Give every other day to clients with renal or hepatic dysfunction.	Renal or hepatic dysfunction reduces drug clearance.
Desloratadine (Clarinex, Neoclarityn✱)	10 mg daily	Same as for loratadine.	Same as for loratadine.
Cetirizine (!) (Zyrtec)	5-10 mg daily	Reduce dose for clients with renal or hepatic dysfunction.	Same as for loratadine.
Fexofenadine (Allegra)	60 mg twice daily or 180 mg daily	Same as for loratadine.	Same as for loratadine.
Ebastine (Ebastel)	5-10 mg daily	Instruct clients not to drive or operate heavy machinery.	Induces drowsiness.
		Do not take with erythromycin.	Erythromycin inhibits elimination.
Mizolastine (Mistamine, Mizollen)	10 mg daily	Do not give to clients with cardiac disease, bradycardia, or dysrhythmias.	Increases the QT interval; may provoke fatal dysrhythmias.
Corticosteroids (Oral) *(may be given as a "taper" or "short-term burst")*			
Prednisolone (Cotolone, Delta-Cortef)	5-40 mg daily	Not recommended unless symptoms are severe or debilitating.	Systemic side effects are common and serious: ▪ GI ulceration ▪ Poor wound healing ▪ Decreased immune function ▪ Increased risk for infections ▪ Weight gain ▪ Hyperglycemia ▪ Personality changes ▪ Fluid retention
Prednisone (Deltasone, Prednicot, Orasone, Pred-Pak)	5-60 mg daily	Same as for prednisolone.	Same as for prednisolone.
Leukotriene Antagonists			
Zafirlukast (Accolate)	20 mg twice daily	Take 1 hr before or 2 hr after eating.	Drug absorption is slowed by the presence of food.
		There is an increased incidence of upper respiratory infections when co-administered with inhaled corticosteroids.	Drugs reduce local inflammatory and immune responses.
		Reduce dose in clients who are also taking aspirin.	Aspirin increases plasma concentration of drug.
Zileuton (Zyflo)	600 mg four times daily	Do not take with terfenadine or theophylline.	Drug increases plasma concentrations of terfenadine and theophylline.
Corticosteroids (Nasal)*			
Beclomethasone (Beconase)	1-2 metered sprays per nostril, 1-2 times daily (about 50 mcg/metered spray)	Use daily as directed.	Effectiveness depends on regular use.
		Symptoms may persist for 2-3 days after initial administration.	Maximum effectiveness requires continued use for 48-72 hr.
Fluticasone (Flonase)	2 metered sprays per nostril daily (about 50 mcg/metered spray)	Same as for beclomethasone.	Same as for beclomethasone.

(!) ***Med Error Alert!** Do not confuse with Zantac, a histamine blocker for gastric acidity.*

Data from Facts and Comparisons. (2004). *Drug facts and comparisons* (58th ed.). St. Louis: Author.
GI, Gastrointestinal.
*Additional drugs include Nasacort, Nasonex, and many others.

Continued

CHART 26-2

DRUG THERAPY for Allergic Rhinitis—*cont'd*

Drug	Usual Dosage	Nursing Interventions	Rationales
Mast Cell Stabilizers (Nasal)			
Cromolyn sodium (Nasalcrom)	1 spray/nostril 4-6 times daily	Use daily as directed.	Effectiveness depends on regular use.
		Start therapy 3-4 wk before expected allergy season.	Requires regular use for prophylactic effect.
Decongestants (Nasal)			
Phenylephrine (Neo-Synephrine, dozens of others)	1 spray/nostril 4-6 times daily	Caution client not to use more frequently than directed or for longer than 4 days.	Overuse or continued use causes a rebound nasal congestion and worsens symptoms.
Oxymetazoline (Afrin, many others)	1 spray/nostril twice daily	Same as for phenylephrine.	Same as for phenylephrine.

Data from Facts and Comparisons. (2004). *Drug facts and comparisons* (58th ed.). St. Louis: Author.

fects include dry mouth, increased blood pressure, and sleep difficulties. Because effects are systemic, instruct clients with high blood pressure, glaucoma, or urinary retention to consult with a health care professional before taking any decongestant.

Antihistamines. Antihistamines compete with histamine at its receptor site and block histamine from binding to the receptor. This action prevents vasodilation and capillary leak. Many antihistamines also decrease secretions. Older antihistamines, such as diphenhydramine (Allerdryl✱, Benadryl) and chlorpheniramine (Allergy, Aller-Chlor, Chlor-Trimeton), often induce sedation. Newer antihistamines, such as desloratadine (Clarinex), cetirizine (Zyrtec), and fexofenadine (Allegra), are less sedating. Not every client responds to each drug in the same way.

Corticosteroids. Corticosteroids decrease inflammatory and immune responses in many ways, one of which is by preventing the synthesis of mediators. Corticosteroid nasal sprays can prevent the symptoms of rhinitis. Systemic corticosteroids can produce severe side effects. These drugs are avoided for rhinitis and are used only on a short-term basis for other problems associated with type I reactions.

Mast Cell Stabilizers. Mast cell stabilizing nasal sprays, such as cromolyn sodium (Nasalcrom), prevent mast cell membranes from opening when an allergen binds to IgE. Thus these drugs prevent the symptoms of allergic rhinitis but are not useful during an acute episode.

Leukotriene Antagonists. Leukotriene antagonists may be used to treat allergic rhinitis. Zileuton (Zyflo) prevents leukotriene synthesis. Zafirlukast (Accolate) blocks the leukotriene receptor. Both are oral agents and work best in the prevention of allergic rhinitis.

Complementary and Alternative Therapies. Some clients with rhinitis obtain relief through the use of aromatherapy. Possible mechanisms of action include competition and desensitization. Clients with pollen allergies report decreased problems after eating unprocessed honey.

DESENSITIZATION THERAPY. Desensitization therapy, commonly called "allergy shots," may be needed when allergens are identified and cannot be avoided easily. Desensitization commonly involves subcutaneous injections of small amounts of the allergen. After the allergen has been identified, a very dilute injection solution (1:100,000 or 1:1,000,000) of the allergen is compounded. A 0.05-mL dose of this solution is injected subcutaneously. Usually an increasing dose is given weekly (or more often) until the client is receiving a 0.5-mL dose. The client is then started on the lowest dose of the next higher concentration of allergen solution. The process is repeated with increasing concentrations of allergen solutions until the client is receiving the maximum dose of the greatest concentration (usually 1:100), depending on his or her response. Injections are usually given at weekly intervals during the first year, every other week for the second year, and then every 3 to 4 weeks for the third year. The recommended course of treatment is about 5 years.

Desensitization appears to reduce allergic responses by competition. In theory, the very small amounts of allergen first injected are too low to bind to the IgE already present but are enough to induce immunoglobulin G (IgG) production against that allergen. Because IgG is not associated with either mast cells or basal cells, allergens that bind to IgG do not trigger allergic responses. IgG removes the allergen from the body by precipitation (see Chapter 23). By gradually increasing the allergen injection, large amounts of IgG are produced against the allergen. When the client is then exposed to the allergen in the environment, the IgG binds to it and clears it from the body before IgE can bind to it and trigger an allergic reaction. Because so much more IgG can be produced compared with IgE, IgG is successful in the competition to bind the allergen.

Desensitization can also be accomplished orally with sublingual immunotherapy (SLIT). Instead of injections, the allergen is introduced through sublingual absorption. The allergen is absorbed directly into the circulatory system through the blood vessels under the tongue. Two major drawbacks of SLIT are the difficulty of dose control and the expense. This method requires higher levels of the allergen (compared to subcutaneous injections), which increases the cost.

Anaphylaxis

PATHOPHYSIOLOGY

Anaphylaxis, the most dramatic and life-threatening example of a type I hypersensitivity reaction, occurs rapidly and systemically. It affects many organs within seconds to minutes after allergen exposure. Anaphylaxis is not common,

TABLE 26-2 Common Agents That Cause Anaphylaxis

Drugs/Foreign Proteins
Antibiotics (penicillin, cephalosporins, tetracycline, sulfonamides, streptomycin, vancomycin, chloramphenicol, amphotericin B, others)
Adrenocorticotropic hormone, insulin, vasopressin, protamine*
Allergen extracts, muscle relaxants, hydrocortisone, vaccines, local anesthetics (lidocaine, procaine)*
Whole blood, cryoprecipitate, immune serum globulin*
Radiocontrast media*
Opiates

Foods	Other Agents
Shellfish	Pollens
Eggs	Exercise
Legumes, nuts	Heat/cold
Grains	Other
Berries	
Preservatives	
Bananas	

Insects/Animals
Hymenoptera: bees, wasps, hornets
Fire ants
Snake venom

*Anaphylaxis caused by these substances is probably a result of direct mast cell degranulation rather than an IgE-mediated hypersensitivity event.

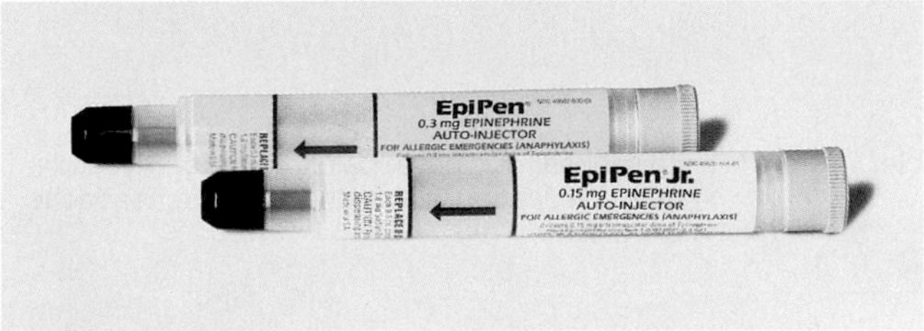

Figure 26-3 ■ EpiPen and EpiPen Jr. self-injectors for epinephrine (Courtesy of Dey, Napa, CA).

and the episodes can vary in severity. *It can be fatal.* Many substances can trigger anaphylaxis in a susceptible person (Table 26-2).

HEALTH PROMOTION/ILLNESS PREVENTION

Because anaphylaxis has a rapid onset and a potentially fatal outcome (even with appropriate medical intervention), prevention is critical. Teach the client with a history of allergic reactions to avoid allergens whenever possible, to wear a medical alert bracelet, and to alert health care personnel about specific allergies. Some clients must carry an emergency anaphylaxis kit (e.g., a bee sting kit with injectable epinephrine), or an epinephrine injector, such as the EpiPen automatic injector (Dey, Napa, CA). The EpiPen device is an easy-to-use, spring-loaded injector that delivers 0.3 mg of epinephrine per 2-mL dose (Figure 26-3).

The medical records of clients with a history of anaphylaxis should prominently display the list of specific allergens. Ask the client about drug allergies before giving any drug or therapeutic agent. Skin tests should be performed before giving any substance that has a high incidence of causing anaphylactic reactions, such as iodine-containing dyes. Be aware of common cross-reacting agents. For example, a client who is allergic to penicillin is also likely to react to cephalosporins because both have a similar chemical structure. People who have an allergy to bananas are likely to have a latex allergy.

Take precautionary measures if an agent must be used despite a history of allergic reactions. Start an IV solution and place intubation equipment and a tracheostomy set at the bedside. The client is often premedicated with diphenhydramine (Benadryl, Allerdryl✱). The substance is given first intradermally, then subcutaneously, and then intramuscularly in increasing doses at 20- to 30-minute intervals so the initial dose by the next route does not exceed the final dose by the previous route.

COLLABORATIVE MANAGEMENT

Assessment

A client having an anaphylactic reaction first has feelings of uneasiness, apprehension, weakness, and impending doom. Often the client is anxious and frightened. These feelings are followed, often quickly, by generalized itching and urticaria (hives). Erythema and sometimes **angioedema** (diffuse swelling) of the eyes, lips, or tongue occur next. Intensely itchy skin wheals or hives may appear and sometimes merge to form large, red blotches.

Histamine and other biochemicals cause bronchoconstriction, mucosal edema, and excess mucus production. Respiratory symptoms include congestion, rhinorrhea, dyspnea, and increasing respiratory distress with audible wheezing.

On auscultation, crackles, wheezing, and reduced breath sounds are heard. Clients may have laryngeal edema as a "lump in the throat," hoarseness, and stridor (a crowing sound). Distress increases as the tongue and larynx swell and more mucous is produced. Stridor and anxiety increase as the airway begins to close. Respiratory failure may follow from laryngeal edema, suffocation, or lower airway constriction causing hypoxemia (insufficient oxygenation of blood).

The client is usually hypotensive and has a rapid, weak, irregular pulse. These findings are due to vasodilation and extensive capillary leak. The client is faint and diaphoretic with increasing anxiety and confusion. If the client is not treated immediately, he or she may lose consciousness. Dysrhythmias, shock, and cardiac arrest may occur within minutes as intravascular volume is lost and the heart becomes hypoxic. Seventy percent of deaths are caused by respiratory failure or by shock and cardiac dysrhythmias.

Interventions

NIC interventions for clients with anaphylaxis are listed in Chart 26-1.

Assess respiratory function first. Emergency respiratory management is critical during an anaphylactic reaction, because the severity of the reaction increases with time. An airway must be established or stabilized immediately. Cardiopulmonary resuscitation may be needed. Epinephrine (1:1000) 0.3 to 0.5 mL is given subcutaneously as soon as symptoms of systemic anaphylaxis appear. This drug constricts blood vessels, improves cardiac contraction, and dilates the bronchioles. The same dose may be repeated every 15 to 20 minutes if needed. Other drugs used to treat anaphylaxis are listed in Chart 26-3.

Antihistamines, such as diphenhydramine (Allerdryl✱, Benadryl) 25 to 100 mg are usually given IV, IM, or orally to treat angioedema and urticaria. If needed, an endotracheal

CHART 26-3

DRUG THERAPY for Anaphylaxis

Drug	Mechanism	Side Effects
Sympathomimetics		
Epinephrine (Adrenalin)	Rapidly stimulates alpha- and beta-adrenergic receptors of autonomic nervous system (alpha: vasoconstriction; beta: bronchodilation).	Pallor, tachycardia and palpitations, nervousness, muscle twitching, sweating, anxiety, insomnia, hypertension, headache, hyperglycemia.
Isoproterenol (Isuprel)	Stimulated beta-adrenergic receptors, relaxing bronchial muscle and dilating vessels.	Same as for epinephrine.
Ephedrine sulfate (Vatronol)	Similar to isoproterenol, but with longer duration of action.	Same as for epinephrine.
Antihistamines		
Diphenhydramine HCl (Allerdryl ✱, Benadryl)	Competes with histamine for H_1 receptors on effector cells, thus blocking effects of histamine on bronchioles, gastrointestinal tract, and blood vessels.	Drowsiness, confusion, insomnia, headache, vertigo, photosensitivity, diplopia, nausea, vomiting, dry mouth.
CORTICOSTEROIDS		
Prednisone (PO) Hydrocortisone sodium succinate (Solu-Cortef) (IV/IM) Methylprednisolone sodium succinate (Solu-Medrol) (IV/IM) Beclomethasone (inhalant)	Anti-inflammatory; inhibits mast cell degranulation.	Fluid and sodium retention, hypertension, cushingoid state, gastric distress, adrenal suppression, psychosis, osteoporosis, susceptibility to infection.
Methylxanthines		
Aminophylline (Truphylline)	Relaxes bronchial smooth muscle.	Restlessness, dizziness, palpitations, tachycardia, nausea, vomiting, epigastric distress, headache, convulsions.
Vasopressors		
Norepinephrine (Levophed)	Raises blood pressure and cardiac output in severely decompensated states.	Headache, tachycardia, fibrillation, decreased urine output, hypertension, metabolic acidosis
Dopamine (Intropin)	Raises blood pressure and cardiac output in severely decompensated states.	Dysrhythmias, tachycardia, hypertension, dyspnea, nausea and vomiting, azotemia, headache.
Inhaled Beta-Adrenergic Agonists		
Metaproterenol (Alupent, Metaprel)	Rapidly stimulates $beta_2$-receptor sites in pulmonary smooth muscle, causing bronchodilation.	Palpitations, tachycardia, dysrhythmias, hypokalemia.
Albuterol (Proventil, Ventolin)	Same as for metaproterenol.	Same as for metaproterenol, plus painful urination, flushing of the face.

tube may be inserted or an emergency tracheostomy may be performed.

If the client can breathe independently, give oxygen to reduce hypoxemia. Start oxygen therapy via nasal cannula at 2 to 6 L/min or via face mask at 40% to 60% before arterial blood gas results are obtained. Monitor pulse oximetry to determine oxygenation adequacy, with the goal of maintaining oxygen saturation greater than 90%. Arterial blood gases may be ordered to determine therapy effectiveness. Use suction to remove excess mucous secretions, if indicated. Continually assess the client's respiratory rate and depth. Assess breath sounds continually for bronchospasm and other abnormal breath sounds. Elevate the bed to 45 degrees unless severe hypotension is also present.

For severe bronchospasm, the client is given theophylline 6 mg/kg IV over 20 to 30 minutes. If the client is taking aminophylline regularly, no more than 3 mg/kg is given. Maintenance aminophylline (0.3 to 0.5 mg/kg/hr) is initiated. The client may be given an inhaled beta-adrenergic agonist such as metaproterenol (Alupent) or albuterol (Proventil) via high-flow nebulizer every 2 to 4 hours. Corticosteroids are added to emergency interventions, but they are not effective immediately. Oral steroids are continued (at lower doses) after the anaphylaxis is under control to prevent the late recurrence of symptoms.

Continually assess for changes in any body system or for adverse effects of drug therapy. For severe anaphylaxis, the client is admitted to a critical care unit for cardiac, pulmonary arterial, and capillary wedge pressure monitoring. Observe the client for fluid overload from the rapid drug and IV fluid infusions and report changes to the physician immediately. The client is discharged from the hospital when respiratory and cardiovascular systems have returned to baseline.

Critical Thinking Challenge

The client is a 75-year-old woman with hypertension who comes to an urgent care center with a swollen lower face. Her lips and tongue are so swollen that she can hardly talk. She tells you (in response to your question about drugs) that she was started on a new blood pressure drug one week ago. When she gives you the drug bottle, you see that it is benazepril, an angiotensin-converting enzyme (ACE) inhibitor. She also tells you she has diabetes and did not take her insulin yet today.

1. What is your first action?
2. What additional assessment data should you obtain?
3. Is it likely that her new antihypertensive drug is responsible for this reaction since she has been taking it for a week?
4. Why should you or should you not start oxygen on this client?
5. Would epinephrine be helpful in this situation? Why or why not? Where, how much, and by what route would you administer it?
6. Would diphenhydramine (Benadryl) be helpful in this situation? Why or why not?
7. What other drugs should you be prepared to give?
8. Is this client's history of pollen allergies and diabetes an important factor in her immediate care?

evolve For suggested answer guidelines, go to http://evolve.elsevier.com/Iggy/.

Latex Allergy

PATHOPHYSIOLOGY

Latex allergy is a type I hypersensitivity reaction in which the specific allergen is a protein found in processed natural latex rubber products. When the allergen enters the body through inhalation or direct contact with blood vessels (such as might occur during surgery), interaction with IgE occurs, leading to a type I reaction. For some people, latex allergen contact is limited to the skin or mucous membranes, causing contact dermatitis, a type IV delayed hypersensitivity reaction (see p. 462). Others may have a "mixed" allergic response to latex, with symptoms of both type I and type IV hypersensitivities. Others may have only one or the other type of reaction.

The incidence of latex hypersensitivity is increasing (Becker, 2000; Floyd, 2000). People at greatest risk are those with a high exposure to natural latex products, such as health care workers, clients with spina bifida, and people who routinely use latex condoms.

COLLABORATIVE MANAGEMENT

Ask all clients about their use of and known reactions to natural latex products. In addition, consider your own exposure and risk for reactions to natural latex products.

Avoiding products that contain natural latex proteins can prevent reactions and initial sensitivity. More products, such as surgical gloves, tubing, and vial closures, are now being made from synthetic substances that do not contain latex proteins. One such product is the glove, ElastyLite. *It is essential to use latex-free products in the care of a client with a known latex allergy.* Interventions for the client who has a type I or a type IV reaction to latex are the same as for reactions caused by other allergens.

TYPE II: CYTOTOXIC REACTIONS

PATHOPHYSIOLOGY

In a type II (cytotoxic) reaction, the body makes special autoantibodies directed against self cells that have some form of foreign protein attached to them. The autoantibody binds to the self cell and forms an immune complex (Figure 26-4). The self cell is then destroyed along with the attached protein by phagocytosis or lysis (see Chapter 23). Clinical examples of type II reactions include hemolytic anemias, thrombocytopenic purpura, hemolytic transfusion reactions (when a client receives the wrong blood type during a transfusion), Goodpasture's syndrome, and drug-induced hemolytic anemia.

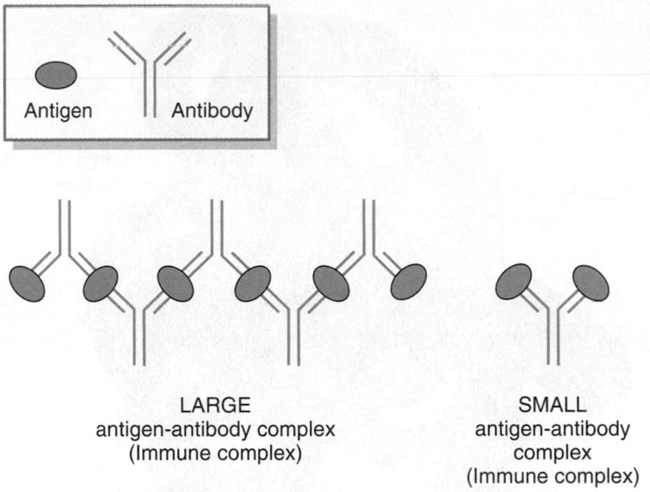

Figure 26-4 ■ Antibody-antigen complexes.

COLLABORATIVE MANAGEMENT

Treatment of type II cytotoxic reactions begins with discontinuation of the offending drug or blood product. Plasmapheresis (filtration of the plasma to remove specific substances) to remove autoantibodies may be beneficial. Otherwise, treatment is symptomatic. Complications such as hemolytic crisis and renal failure can be life threatening.

TYPE III: IMMUNE COMPLEX REACTIONS

PATHOPHYSIOLOGY

In a type III reaction, excess antigens cause immune complexes to form in the blood (Figure 26-5). These circulating complexes usually lodge in small blood vessel walls. Common sites include the kidneys, skin, joints, and other small blood vessels. The deposited complexes trigger inflammation, and tissue or vessel damage results.

There are many immune complex disorders (mostly connective tissue disorders) caused by type III reactions. For example, the manifestations of rheumatoid arthritis are caused by immune complexes that lodge in joint spaces followed by destruction of tissue and, later, scarring and fibrous changes. Systemic lupus erythematosus (SLE) has immune complexes lodged in the vessels (vasculitis), the glomeruli (nephritis), the joints (arthralgia, arthritis), and other organs and tissues. (See Chapter 24 for a discussion of SLE.)

Serum sickness is a group of symptoms that occurs after receiving serum or certain drugs. It is caused by a collection of immune complexes deposited in blood vessel walls of the skin, joints, and kidney. The most common causes of serum sickness today are penicillin, other antibiotics, and some animal serum-based drugs. Serum sickness is less common now

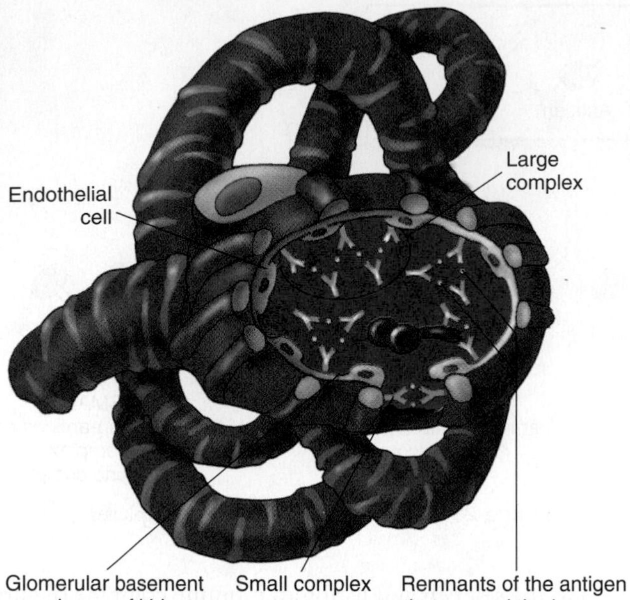

Figure 26-5 ■ An immune complex in a type III hypersensitivity reaction.

that vaccines are made with human proteins. Agents known to cause serum sickness include antilymphocyte globulin and antithymocyte globulin, used to treat organ transplant rejection.

COLLABORATIVE MANAGEMENT

The client with serum sickness has fever, **arthralgia** (achy joints), rash, lymphadenopathy (enlarged lymph nodes), malaise, and possibly polyarthritis and nephritis, about 7 to 12 days after receiving the causative agent. Alert the client to the possibility of serum sickness and what symptoms to look for whenever you give a foreign serum. Also keep emergency equipment and drugs close at hand in case the client has an anaphylactic reaction.

Serum sickness is usually self-limiting, and symptoms subside after several days. Treatment is usually symptomatic; antihistamines are given for itching and aspirin for arthralgias. Prednisone is given if symptoms are severe.

TYPE IV: DELAYED HYPERSENSITIVITY REACTIONS

PATHOPHYSIOLOGY

In a type IV reaction, the reactive cell is the T-lymphocyte (T-cell). Antibodies and complement are not involved. Sensitized T-cells (from a previous exposure) respond to an antigen by releasing chemical mediators and triggering macrophages to destroy the antigen. Unlike a type I reaction, which occurs immediately, a type IV response typically occurs hours to days after exposure. A type IV reaction consists of a local collection of lymphocytes and macrophages, causing edema, induration, ischemia, and tissue damage at the site.

An example of a small type IV reaction is a positive purified protein derivative (PPD) test for tuberculosis. In a client previously exposed to tuberculosis, an intradermal injection of this agent causes sensitized T-cells to clump at the injection site, release lymphokines, and activate macrophages. Induration and erythema at the site of the injection appear after about 24 to 72 hours.

Other examples of type IV reactions include contact dermatitis, poison ivy skin rashes, local response to insect stings, tissue transplant rejections, and sarcoidosis.

COLLABORATIVE MANAGEMENT

Interventions

Removal of the offending antigen is the major focus of management. The reaction is self-limiting in 5 to 7 days, and the client is treated symptomatically. Monitor the reaction site and sites distal to the reaction for circulation adequacy. Diphenhydramine (Benadryl) is of minimal benefit for type IV reactions because histamine is not the main mediator. In addition, IgE does not cause this type of reaction, and desensitization does not reduce the response. Corticosteroids or other anti-inflammatory agents can reduce the discomfort and help resolve the reaction more quickly.

Identification of Allergen. Patch testing can be used to identify the allergens. This type of testing involves skin contact with potential allergens. Contact with a specific allergen causes a delayed hypersensitivity reaction that develops in 48 to 96 hours.

Test chemicals are applied to intact skin under occlusive tape patches. After the patches are removed, the skin areas in contact with the chemical are examined closely for the presence of localized redness, swelling, and blisters. For a positive patch test result to have clinical relevance, the client must have a history of exposure to substances containing the allergen.

Client Preparation. To prevent suppression of a response to a potential allergen, systemic corticosteroids or antihistamines are discontinued for at least 48 hours before the test. Topical steroids may be used as long as the agent is not applied on the area to be tested. Explain that patch testing does not involve pricking the skin with needles. Inform the client that testing will involve three separate visits to the allergist or dermatologist; one to apply the test patches, a second for an initial reading, and a third for detection of delayed reactions.

Procedure. The upper back is the best site to apply test patches. After the client has undressed, inspect the back for a rash and the presence of hair. If rash is present, use other test sites such as the flanks, the lower back, or the upper arms. Shave any hair to prevent poor patch contact and false-negative results. Remove skin oils with alcohol to promote adhesion of the patches.

Small quantities of chemicals and solutions in standardized concentrations are placed in separate metal chambers that are backed with hypoallergenic adhesive tape. Carefully apply the tape to the skin so that each chemical is held in contact with the skin surface. Mark each chamber for later identification. As many as 60 or more chemicals may be tested at the same time.

Instruct the client to keep the test sites dry at all times. Baths are substituted for showers until testing is complete. Instruct the client to use caution when washing the hair to avoid getting the patches wet. Discourage the client from engaging in activity that will result in sweating. Tell the client not to reapply patches that come loose, because this interferes with interpretation of the test results. Reinforce the need to remove loose or nonadherent test patches for reapplication.

The initial reading is performed 2 days after application. The tape containing the chemical-filled chambers is peeled away from the skin, and each area of contact is marked with indelible ink for future reading. Document any initial allergic or irritant reactions in the client's medical record. The final reading of the test results is 2 to 5 days later.

Follow-up Care. If a potential allergen is identified, the client is given a list of items containing that chemical to be avoided.

Critical Thinking Challenge

The client is a 26-year-old man who crawled through poison ivy during a paint ball game 3 days ago. He now has poison ivy rash and blisters over his face, neck, hands, and arms. He said that he began itching yesterday and took oral Benadryl 25 mg six times yesterday. He is distressed that the rash is spreading even after using Benadryl. He is worried that the rash and blisters on his face and neck will make breathing difficult.

1. What additional assessment data should you obtain?
2. Why should you or should you not start oxygen on this client?
3. Would epinephrine be helpful in this situation? Why or why not? Where, how much, and by what route would you administer it?
4. Would more Benadryl be helpful in this situation? Why or why not?
5. What should you tell this client about potential respiratory problems?
6. What additional drugs should you be prepared to give and what should you teach this client about his medications?

evolve For suggested answer guidelines, go to http://evolve.elsevier.com/Iggy/.

TYPE V: STIMULATORY REACTIONS

PATHOPHYSIOLOGY

This type of reaction involves inappropriate stimulation of a normal cell surface receptor by an autoantibody, resulting in a continuous "turned-on" state for the cell. An example of this type of reaction is Graves' disease, a form of hyperthyroidism. In Graves' disease, an autoantibody binds to the thyroid-stimulating hormone (TSH) receptor sites on the thyroid gland. This binding continually stimulates thyroid cells to produce thyroid hormones, causing the client to have severe hyperthyroidism (see Chapter 67). The manifestations occur even though the thyroid gland itself is completely normal. In a sense, the tissue responding to the autoantibody is "out of control" from the body's normal feedback system of checks and balances.

COLLABORATIVE MANAGEMENT

For type V reactions involving only one organ, the management focuses on removing enough of the responding (stimulated) tissue to return the function to normal. With Graves' disease, thyroid tissue is either surgically removed or destroyed with radiation. For type V reactions in which antibody stimulation is more widespread, treatment focuses on reducing the production of autoantibodies through immunosuppression.

Autoimmunity

Autoimmunity is a process whereby a person develops an inappropriate immune response. In this response, antibodies and/or lymphocytes are directed against healthy normal cells and tissues. For unknown reasons, the immune system fails to recognize certain body cells or tissues as self and thus triggers immune reactions. The responses, both antibody- and cell-mediated, are similar to normal immune responses against invading organisms, but these reactions are now directed against normal body cells. Causes of loss of recognition of self cells are not known.

Examples of diseases that have an autoimmune cause include systemic lupus erythematosus (SLE), polyarteritis nodosa, scleroderma, rheumatoid arthritis, autoimmune hemolytic anemia, rheumatic fever, and Hashimoto's thyroiditis (Table 26-3). Other diseases, such as type 1 diabetes mellitus, may have multiple causes, one of which is autoimmune.

Management of autoimmunities depends on the organ or organs affected. Anti-inflammatory drugs and immunosuppressive drugs are commonly used along with symptomatic treatment.

TABLE 26-3 Known or Probable Autoimmune Disorders

Disorder	Autoantigen
Systemic Or Non–Organ Specific	
Systemic lupus erythematosus	DNA, DNA proteins
Rheumatoid arthritis	IgG, possibly cartilage
Progressive systemic sclerosis	DNA proteins
Mixed connective tissue disorder	DNA proteins
Organ Specific	
Autoimmune hemolytic anemia	Erythrocytes
Autoimmune thrombocytopenic purpura	Platelets
Diabetes mellitus, type I	Islet cells, insulin, insulin receptor
Dermatomyositis	Unknown
Glomerulonephritis	Glomerular basement membranes
Goodpasture's syndrome	Glomerular basement membranes, pulmonary basement membranes
Graves' disease	Thyroid-stimulating hormone receptor
Hashimoto's thyroiditis	Thyroid cell surface
Idiopathic Addison's disease	Adrenal cell
Myasthenia gravis	Acetylcholine receptor, acetylcholine
Pernicious anemia	Intrinsic factor, parietal cell, B_{12} complexes
Psoriasis	Stratum corneum
Reiter's syndrome	Possibly collagen, conjunctival cells
Sjögren's syndrome	Salivary gland cells, vaginal mucous cells, lacrimal gland cells
Uveitis	Uveal tract cells (eye)
Vasculitis	Unknown, possibly collagen or endothelial cells

IgG, Immunoglobulin G.

WOMEN'S HEALTH CONSIDERATIONS

Virtually all autoimmune disorders, especially rheumatic disorders, occur much more commonly among women than men (McCance & Huether, 2002; Workman, 2000). The risk for autoimmune disease among women compared to men ranges from 5:1 to 20:1. In addition, most autoimmune disorders occur more frequently among white women compared to women of any other ethnicity.

SJÖGREN'S SYNDROME

PATHOPHYSIOLOGY

Sjögren's syndrome (SS) is a group of problems that often appear with other autoimmune disorders. Problems include dry eyes, dry mucous membranes of the nose and mouth (xerostomia), and vaginal dryness. These problems are caused by autoimmune destruction of the lacrimal, salivary, and vaginal mucous producing glands. Often, the client with SS also has rheumatoid arthritis. Fibromyalgia often accompanies SS.

Most clients with SS are women between 35 and 45 years old. SS occurs more frequently among clients with certain tissue types, specifically HLA-DRW52, HLA-DR3, and HLA-B8. Although an exact triggering agent has not been identified, viral infection is strongly suspected. The three viruses thought to be triggers for the autoimmune changes leading to SS are the human immunodeficiency virus type 1 (HIV-1), human T-cell lymphotrophic virus type 1 (HTLV-1), and Epstein-Barr Virus (EBV).

Insufficient tears cause inflammation and ulceration of the cornea. Insufficient saliva decreases digestion of carbohydrates, promotes tooth decay, and increases the incidence of oral and nasal infections. Vaginal dryness increases the incidence of infection and may cause pain during sexual intercourse.

◆COLLABORATIVE MANAGEMENT

◆Assessment

The client with Sjögren's syndrome (SS) usually has blurred vision, burning and itching of the eyes, and thick mattering in the conjunctiva. Difficulty swallowing food is common and the client often has changes in taste sensation. Ask the client about nosebleeds **(epistaxis)** and frequent upper respiratory infections.

Physical examination reveals enlarged lymph nodes. If rheumatoid arthritis (RA) accompanies SS, the client has swollen, painful joints and limited joint mobility (see Chapter 24 for a complete discussion of RA). Laboratory assessment may show increased presence of general antinuclear antibodies, anti-SS-A or anti-SS-B antibodies, and elevated levels of IgM rheumatoid factor.

◆Interventions

IMMUNOMODULATION. Currently, there is no cure for SS. The intensity and the progression of the disorder can be slowed by suppressing immune and inflammatory responses. Drugs used to modulate the immune system in clients with SS include low-dose chemotherapy with methotrexate (Rheumatrex) or cyclophosphamide (Cytoxan). Both drugs have serious long-term side effects, especially on liver and bone marrow function. Other immunosuppressive drugs used to manage SS are corticosteroids, cyclosporine (Neoral, Sandimmune), and hydroxychloroquine (Plaquenil).

SYMPTOMATIC THERAPY. A variety of artificial tears and artificial saliva can help reduce the dry eye and dry mouth symptoms. Teach clients to use humidifiers in the home to increase environmental moisture. Use of water-soluble vaginal lubricants and moisturizers can increase client comfort and reduce the incidence of vaginitis. Some clients relieve dry mouth with systemic pilocarpine (Salagen). This agent mimics the effects of the parasympathetic nervous system, causing increased salivation.

Another intervention for dry eyes is to block the tear outflow channel (nasal punctum). The punctum can be blocked temporarily with small plugs or can be closed surgically. Either method allows the tears produced to remain in contact with the eye longer.

Pain control is an issue for clients who also have either rheumatoid arthritis or fibromyalgia. Nonsteroidal anti-inflammatory drugs (NSAIDs) rather than pure analgesics are commonly used to decrease the inflammation and reduce the associated pain. Many different types and strengths of NSAIDs are available by prescription and over-the-counter. The mechanism of action and side effects are similar for all NSAIDs although the duration of action and cost vary.

GOODPASTURE'S SYNDROME

PATHOPHYSIOLOGY

Goodpasture's syndrome is an autoimmune disorder in which autoantibodies are made against the glomerular basement membrane and neutrophils. The two organs with the most damage are the lungs and the kidney. Lung damage is manifested as pulmonary hemorrhage. Kidney damage manifests as glomerulonephritis that may rapidly progress to complete renal failure (see Chapters 74 and 75). Unlike other autoimmune disorders, Goodpasture's syndrome occurs most often in adolescent or young adult men (McCance & Huether, 2002). The exact cause or triggering agent is unknown.

◆COLLABORATIVE MANAGEMENT

Goodpasture's syndrome usually is not diagnosed until serious lung and/or kidney problems are present. Manifestations include shortness of breath, hemoptysis (bloody sputum), decreased urine output, weight gain, generalized nondependent edema, hypertension, and tachycardia. Chest x-rays show areas of consolidation. The most common cause of death is uremia as a result of renal failure.

Spontaneous resolution of Goodpasture's syndrome has occurred but is rare. Interventions focus on reducing the immune-mediated damage and performing some type of renal supportive therapy.

IMMUNOMODULATION

Drug Therapy. The mainstay of drug therapy for Goodpasture's syndrome is high-dose corticosteroids. Other drug therapy to suppress the autoimmune response is the same as that for Sjögren's syndrome (SS).

Other Therapy. Additional therapy to reduce immune responses involves plasmapheresis (filtration of the plasma to remove some proteins) to remove the autoantibodies. If the lungs and kidneys do not have permanent damage, clients undergoing plasmapheresis have shown clinical improvement. Some clients using plasmapheresis need infusions of intravenous immunoglobulin (IVIG) to maintain antibody protection against infection.

RENAL SUPPORT THERAPY. Depending upon the level of renal function remaining, the client may need ongoing dialysis. Therapy usually begins with hemodialysis. For long-term therapy, peritoneal or hemodialysis may be used depending on the client's health status, ability to self-manage the infusion and drainage systems, and lifestyle (see Chapter 75).

Renal transplantation is an option for some clients with Goodpasture's syndrome. After transplantation, renal function is normal. In rare instances, clients have been disease-free after transplantation. In others, the renal problems are improved but the lung destruction continues. Some of the drugs used to prevent kidney rejection also suppress the autoimmune response.

GET READY for the NCLEX Examination!

KEY POINTS

Safe Effective Care Environment

- Ensure that only latex-free products are used for a client who has a known latex allergy.
- Ensure that all allergies are documented in a prominent place in the client's medical record.
- Keep emergency equipment and drugs (epinephrine, Benadryl, and cortisol) in or near the room of a client with known severe allergies or a history of anaphylaxis.

Health Promotion and Maintenance

- Encourage all adult clients with severe allergies or those who have a history of anaphylaxis to wear a medical alert bracelet.
- Identify clients at high risk for allergic reactions as a result of home, work environment, or leisure activities.
- Teach the client and family about the clinical manifestations of allergic reactions and when to seek medical advice.

Psychosocial Integrity

- Stay with the client in anaphylaxis.
- Allow the client the opportunity to express fear or anxiety during an allergic response.
- Explain all diagnostic procedures, restrictions, and follow-up care to the client scheduled for tests.
- Reassure clients who are in anaphylaxis that the appropriate interventions are being instituted.

Physiological Integrity

- Assess the client receiving immunosuppressive drugs as treatment of an autoimmune disorder every shift for clinical manifestations of infection.
- Immediately assess the respiratory status and airway of clients who show any symptom of an allergic reaction.
- Immediately discontinue the IV medication of a client having an anaphylactic reaction to that medication. **Do not** discontinue the IV, but change the IV tubing and hang normal saline.
- Hold the dose of any prescribed medication when a client develops angioedema.
- Give oxygen to any client in anaphylaxis.
- Teach the client who has a known drug allergy, which other drugs are likely to stimulate the same reactions.
- Teach the client who carries an EpiPen, how to assemble and use the device. Obtain a return demonstration.

ADDITIONAL STUDY RESOURCES

Go to your Student CD-ROM for Review Questions for the NCLEX Examination.

Go to http://evolve.elsevier.com/Iggy/ for Integrated Management of Care Questions for the NCLEX Examination.

SELECTED BIBLIOGRAPHY

Abbas, A., & Lichtman, A. (2003). *Cellular and molecular immunology* (5th ed.). Philadelphia: W. B. Saunders.

Ackley, B., & Ladwig, G. (2002). *Nursing diagnosis handbook: A guide to planning care* (5th ed.). St. Louis: Mosby.

Avella, P., & Walker, M. (2000). Goodpasture's syndrome: A nursing challenge. *Nursing2000, 30*(3), 32cc1-2, 32cc4, 32cc6.

Becker, H. (2000). An analysis of the epidemiology of latex allergy: Implications for primary prevention. *MEDSURG Nursing, 9*(3), 135-143.

Cohen, S. (2001). About latex allergy. *Nursing 2001, 31*(2), 76.

D'Epiro, N. (2000). Deciphering autoimmune disease in women. *Patient Care, 34*(7), 49-52, 54, 59, 63-66.

DeRaps, P., & Lynch, J. (2003). Focus on solutions for allergic rhinitis. *CE-Today for Nurse Practitioners, 2*(2), 15-23.

Dochterman, J., & Bulechek, G. (Eds.). (2004). *Nursing interventions classification (NIC)* (4th ed.). St. Louis: Mosby.

Facts and Comparisons. (2004). *Drug facts and comparisons* (58th ed.). St. Louis: Author.

Floyd, P. (2000). Latex allergy update. *Journal of Perianesthesia Nursing, 15*(1), 25-30.

Gelfand, E. (2000). The clinical use of intravenous immunoglobulin in immunodeficiency and allergic disorders. *Journal of Intravenous Nursing, 23*(5S), S14-S17.

Goldrick, B. (2003). Emerging infections: Allergic aspergillosis. *American Journal of Nursing, 103*(4), 89.

Gonzales, F. (2004). How will your patient respond to contrast media? *Nursing 2004, 34*(1), 32hn1-32hn3.

Green, S., & Martin, D. (2003). Is every sneeze an allergy? Diagnosing and treating allergic vs nonallergic rhinitis. *The American Journal for Nurse Practitioners, 7*(5), 9-18.

Hathaway, L. (2005). Patient-education guide: Anaphylaxis. *Nursing 2005, 35*(1), 46-47.

Hayden, M.L. (2003). Assessing and improving quality of life in allergic rhinitis. *CE-Today for Nurse Practitioners, 2*(2), 7-13.

Lenehan, G. (2002). Latex allergy: Separating fact from fiction. *Nursing2002, 32*(3), 58-63.

LoBuono, C. (2000). Eliminating allergy triggers. *Patient Care for the Nurse Practitioner, 3*(4), 45-52.

Lynch, J. (2003). An examination of severe, intractable, allergic rhinitis. *CE-Today for Nurse Practitioners, 2*(2), 25-28.

McCance, K., & Huether, S. (2002). *Pathophysiology: The biologic basis for disease in adults and children* (4th ed.). St. Louis: Mosby.

Moorhead, S., Johnson, M., & Maas, M. (Eds.). (2004). *Nursing outcomes classification (NOC)* (3rd ed.). St. Louis: Mosby.

Myers, J. (2000). Emergency: Chemotherapy-induced hypersensitivity reaction. *American Journal of Nursing, 100*(4), 53-54.

Nussbaum, R., McInnes, R., & Willard, H. (2001). *Thompson & Thompson: Genetics in medicine* (6th ed.). Philadelphia: W. B. Saunders.

Pagana, K., & Pagana, T. (2002). *Mosby's manual of diagnostic and laboratory tests* (2nd ed.). St. Louis: Mosby.

Pepper, G. (2000). Nonsteroidal anti-inflammatory drugs: New perspectives on a familiar drug class. *Nursing Clinics of North America, 35*(1), 223-244.

Swenson, M. (2000). Autoimmunity and immunotherapy. *Journal of Intravenous Nursing, 23*(5S), S8-S13.

Vale, D. (2000). Recognition and management of Sjögren's syndrome: Strategies for the advanced practice nurse. *Nursing Clinics of North America, 35*(1), 267-278.

van Steekelenburg, J., Clement, P., & Beel, M. (2002). Comparison of five new antihistamines (H1-receptor antagonists) in patients with allergic rhinitis using nasal provocation studies and skin tests. *Allergy, 57*(4), 346-350.

Wilburn, S. (2001). When latex allergies limit employment. *American Journal of Nursing, 101*(8), 88.

Workman, M.L. (2000). Immune mechanisms in rheumatic disease. *Nursing Clinics of North America, 35*(1), 175-188.

CHAPTER

27

Altered Cell Growth and Cancer Development

M. LINDA WORKMAN

LEARNING OUTCOMES

After studying this chapter, you should be able to:

1. Explain why causes of cancer can be hard to establish.
2. Compare the features of benign and malignant tumors.
3. List three cancer types associated with tobacco use.
4. Identify cancer types for which primary prevention is possible.
5. Compare the cancer development processes of initiation and promotion.
6. Describe the TNM system for cancer staging.
7. Explain the differences between a "low-grade" cancer and a "high-grade" cancer.
8. Discuss the roles of oncogenes and suppressor genes in cancer development.
9. Identify four common sites of distant metastasis for cancer.
10. Discuss the role of immunity in protection against cancer.
11. Identify which cancer types arise from connective tissues and which types arise from glandular tissues.
12. Describe how genetic predisposition can increase a person's risk for cancer development.
13. Identify behaviors that reduce the risk for cancer development and cancer death.
14. Identify specific issues about genetic testing for cancer predisposition.

Go to your Student CD-ROM for Review Questions for the NCLEX Examination keyed to these Learning Outcomes.

Many people have some type of altered cell growth such as a mole or a skin tag. Most types of altered cell growth are harmless (benign) and do not require intervention. Malignant cell growth or cancer, however, is serious and, without intervention, leads to death. Cancer is a common health problem in the United States and Canada. Nearly 1.5 million people are newly diagnosed with cancer each year (American Cancer Society, 2005). Some types of cancer can be prevented; others have better cure rates if diagnosed early. As a nurse, you can have a vital impact in educating the public about cancer prevention and early detection methods.

HISTORICAL PERSPECTIVE

Although cancer is common today, it is not a new disorder. Even prehistoric humans developed cancer. Some types of cancer are more common today, especially among more affluent societies, than in centuries past. Two reasons for this increase are the long life expectancy of people in more affluent countries and increased exposure to substances that cause cancer.

Cancer will occur in about 1 of every 3 persons currently living in North America (American Cancer Society, 2005), although cancer risk differs for each person. Cancer prevention is a major health focus for the United States (see the Meeting Healthy People 2010 Objectives box on p. 468). More than 10 million Americans with a history of cancer are alive today, nearly 5 million of whom are considered cured (American Cancer Society, 2005). Terms used to describe abnormal cell growth and cancer are listed in Table 27-1.

PATHOPHYSIOLOGY

Growth of cells and tissues is expected during infancy and childhood, and many human body cells continue to "grow" by cell division **(mitosis)** long after maturation is complete. Such cells are located in tissues where constant damage or wear is likely and continued cell growth is

Meeting HEALTHY PEOPLE 2010 Objectives

CANCER

Objective 17.1: Reduce cancer deaths to a rate of no more than 103 per 100,000 people.

- Assess all clients for current and past exposures to carcinogens.
- Assist clients to identify personal cancer risks.
- Assist clients to avoid known environmental carcinogens.
- Assess all clients for a family history of cancer to identify clients at genetic high risk for cancer.
- Refer identified clients at genetic high risk for cancer to an appropriate level genetic counselor.
- Teach clients to avoid excessive sun exposure and to use protective clothing, hats, and sun-screening agents when sun exposure is not avoidable.
- Teach client about tobacco-related cancers.
- Assist clients who smoke to reduce or quit smoking.
- Teach clients about alcohol-related cancers.
- Teach clients about the importance of limiting dietary fat, smoked meats, and red meats.
- Teach clients about the importance of increasing dietary fiber.
- Encourage clients to see a health care provider at least once per year for cancer screening.
- Teach clients the correct technique for breast self-examination or testicular self-examination.
- Encourage client to engage in self-screening measures, such as whole body skin examination, breast self-examination, or testicular self-examination, on a monthly basis.
- Instruct clients who have any of the seven warning signs of cancer to follow up with their primary care provider as soon as possible.
- Encourage female clients to follow American Cancer Society guidelines for cervical, breast, and colorectal cancer screening appropriate for age and risk categories.
- Encourage male clients to follow American Cancer Society guidelines for prostate and colorectal cancer screening appropriate for age and risk categories.

needed to replace dead tissues. Cells of the skin, hair, mucous membranes, bone marrow, and linings of organs such as the lungs, stomach, intestines, bladder, and uterus, among others, have the ability to divide throughout a person's life span. The growth of these cells is well controlled, ensuring that only the right number of cells is always present in any tissue or organ.

Some tissues and organs stop growing by cell division after development is complete. For example, heart muscle cells no longer divide after fetal life; the number of heart muscle cells is fixed at birth. The size of the heart increases as the person grows because each cell gets larger, but the number of heart muscle cells does not increase. Growth that causes tissue to increase in size by enlarging each cell is **hypertrophy.** Growth that causes tissue to increase in size by increasing the number of cells is **hyperplasia** (Figure 27-1).

Any new or continued cell growth not needed for normal development or replacement of dead and damaged tissues is called **neoplasia.** This cell growth is always abnormal even if it causes no harm. Whether the new cells are benign or malignant, neoplastic cells develop from normal cells (parent cells). Thus cancer cells were once normal cells but changed to no longer look, grow, or function normally. The strict processes controlling normal growth and function have been lost. To understand how cancer cells grow, it is helpful to first understand the regulation and function of normal cells.

Biology of Normal Cells

Many different normal cells work together to make the whole person function at an optimal level. For optimal function, each cell must perform in a predictable manner.

TABLE 27-1 Terminology Commonly Associated with Abnormal Cell Growth

anaplastic Without shape or differentiation, small and round
aneuploid More or less than the normal number of chromosomes
apoptosis The finite life span of normal cells; "programmed cell death"
benign New, nonmalignant cell growth not needed for normal growth or replacement
carcinogenesis The transformation of a normal cell into a cancer cell
doubling time The amount of time it takes for a tumor to double in size by mitotic cell divisions
euploid The normal chromosome number
fibronectin A large, extracellular, transformation-sensitive cell-surface protein present on normal cells that allows normal cells to adhere tightly together
gene expression The activation, or "turning on," of a specific gene to the extent that it synthesizes a specific protein that influences the activity of a cell or group of cells
gene suppression The deactivation, or "turning off," of a specific gene so that it is silent and does not synthesize a protein
generation time The period of time necessary for one cell to enter and complete one round of cell division by mitosis
initiation The damage of a normal cell's DNA by a carcinogen
latency The period of time between when a carcinogenic agent or substance damaged the DNA of a normal cell (initiated it) and when an overt cancer is present
malignant Cancerous, new growth of cells by invasion that is not needed for normal development or tissue replacement
metastasis Invasive growth of cancer cells from the original tumor into distant areas
mitosis Cell division by exact duplication
morphology Appearance or shape
multipotent An undifferentiated cell that has multiple potentials for maturation and differentiation (also called totipotent and pluripotent)
neoplasia New cell growth not needed for normal body growth or replacement of dead or missing tissue
oncogene A developmental gene (proto-oncogene) expressed at an inappropriate time, capable of transforming a normal cell into a cancer cell
ploidy The chromosome content of a cell
  aneuploid ploidy The chromosome content of a cell that is greater or lesser than the normal chromosome number for the species
  diploid (euploid) ploidy The normal chromosome content of a cell for the species (e.g., human cells have 46 chromosomes [23 pairs] per cell)
primary tumor A tumor formed in a specific tissue as a result of a carcinogenic agent or event
promotion Enhancement of cell division in a cell initiated by a carcinogen
proto-oncogene A developmental gene expressed during early embryonic development
secondary tumor A tumor formed as a result of breaking off from a primary tumor and spreading to distant sites (metastasis)
suppressor gene A gene that suppresses the expression of an oncogene
transformation The changing of a normal cell into a cancer cell by a carcinogenic agent or event

CHARACTERISTICS OF NORMAL CELLS

HAVE LIMITED CELL DIVISION. Normal cells divide (undergo mitosis) for one of two reasons: (1) to develop normal tissue or (2) to replace lost or damaged normal tissue. Even when they are capable of mitosis, normal cells divide only when body conditions and nutrition are just right.

UNDERGO APOPTOSIS. Normal cells have a finite life span. With each round of cell division, the telomeric DNA at the ends of the chromosomes shorten (see Chapter 11). When this DNA is gone, the cell responds to signals for programmed cell death, **apoptosis.** The purpose of apoptosis is to ensure each organ has adequate number of cells at their functional peak.

SHOW SPECIFIC MORPHOLOGY. Each normal cell type has a distinct and recognizable appearance, size, and shape, as shown in Figure 27-2.

HAVE A SMALL NUCLEAR-CYTOPLASMIC RATIO. As shown in Figure 27-2, the size of the normal cell nucleus is small compared with the size of the rest of the cell, including the cytoplasm.

PERFORM SPECIFIC DIFFERENTIATED FUNCTIONS. Every normal cell has at least one special function to contribute to whole-body homeostasis. For example, skin cells make keratin, liver cells make bile, cardiac muscle cells contract, nerve cells conduct impulses, and red blood cells make hemoglobin to carry oxygen.

ADHERE TIGHTLY TOGETHER. Normal cells make proteins that protrude from the cell surface, allowing cells to bind closely and tightly together. One such protein is fibronectin, which keeps most normal tissues bound tightly to each other. Exceptions are blood cells. Red blood cells and white blood cells produce no fibronectin and do not usually adhere together.

ARE NONMIGRATORY. Because normal cells are tightly bound together, they do not wander from one tissue into the next (with the exception of red blood cells and white blood cells).

GROW IN AN ORDERLY AND WELL-REGULATED MANNER. Normal cells do not divide unless body conditions are optimal for cell division. These conditions include the need for more cells, adequate space, and sufficient nutrients and other resources. Cell division, occurring in a well-recognized pattern, is described by the cell cycle. Figure 27-3 shows the phases of the cell cycle.

Living cells not actively reproducing are in a reproductive resting state termed G_0. During the G_0 period, cells actively carry out their functions but do not divide. Normal cells spend most of their lives in the G_0 state, just like most humans spend most of their lives in a nonpregnant state.

Mitotic cell division makes one cell divide into two cells. These two cells are identical to each other and to the original cell that started the mitotic cell division. The steps of entering and completing the cell cycle are tightly controlled.

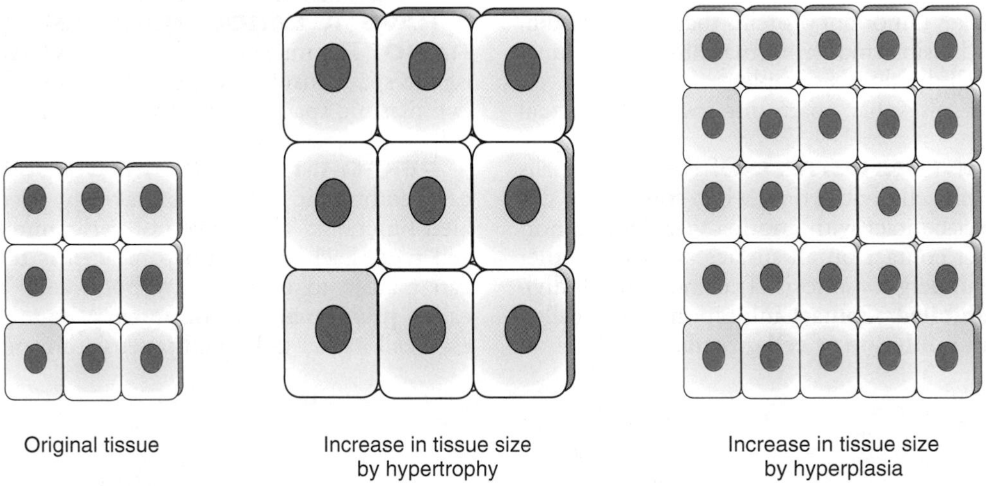

Figure 27-1 ■ Tissue growth by hypertrophy and hyperplasia.

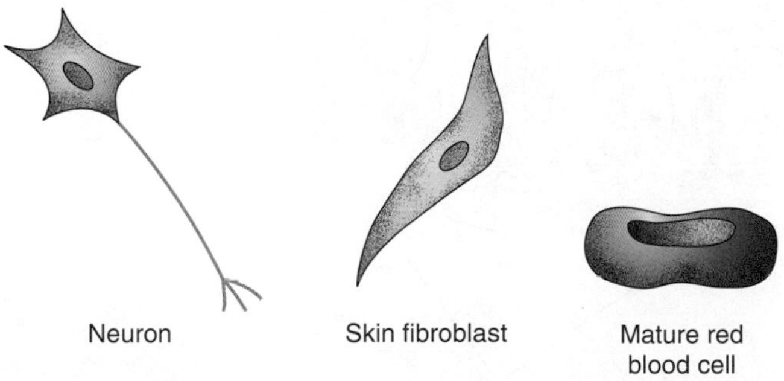

Figure 27-2 ■ Distinctive morphology of some normal cells.

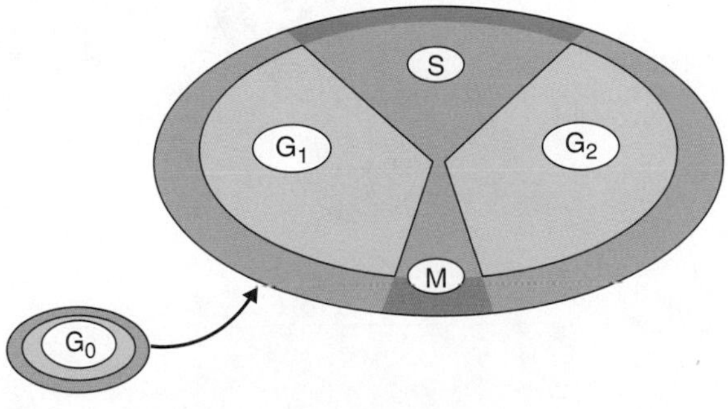

Figure 27-3 ■ The cell cycle.

Much of this control is regulated by proteins produced by "suppressor genes."

Control of whether or not a cell enters the cell cycle and completes the cycle to form two new cells is dependent on the presence and absence of specific proteins. Proteins that promote cells to enter and complete cell division belong to a family of proteins known as "cyclins." When cyclins are activated, they first allow a cell to leave the G_0 state and enter the cycle. These activated cyclins then permit the cell to move through the different phases of the cell cycle and actually divide. The cyclins are the products of proto-oncogenes (see later discussion under Oncogene Activation on p. 476). Proteins produced by suppressor genes regulate the amount of cyclins present in a cell and ensure that cell division occurs only when it is needed. Thus normal cell division represents a balance between the proteins that promote cell division (cyclins) and the proteins that limit cell division (suppressor gene products).

Figure 27-4 shows the activities of the phases of the cell cycle:

- **G_1.** The cell is getting ready for division by taking on extra nutrients, making more energy, and growing extra membrane. The amount of cell fluid (cytoplasm) also increases.
- **S.** Because making one cell into two cells requires twice as much of everything, including deoxyribonucleic acid (DNA), the cell must double its DNA content through DNA synthesis. This process occurs in S phase.
- **G_2.** The cell makes important proteins that will be used in actual cell division and in normal physiologic function after cell division is complete.
- **M.** The single cell splits apart into two cells (actual mitosis).

ARE CONTACT INHIBITED. Of the normal cells that can divide, each cell divides only when some of its surface is not in direct contact with another cell. Once a normal cell is in direct contact on all surface areas with other cells, it no longer undergoes mitosis. Thus normal cell division is **contact inhibited.** Contact inhibition is also called **density-dependent inhibition of cell growth.**

ARE EUPLOID. Most normal human cells have 23 pairs of chromosomes, the correct number for human beings.

Each normal, mature cell has a specific structure and function. The fact that normal mature cells have many different shapes and functions is interesting, considering that all humans started life as a single cell. The function and behavior of that first single cell and its daughter cells are quite different from those of normal adult human cells. Knowledge about these differences has helped in understanding how cancer develops.

CHARACTERISTICS OF EARLY EMBRYONIC CELLS

HAVE RAPID AND CONTINUOUS CELL DIVISION. Early embryonic cells (from conception to the eighth day) spend most of their time within the cell cycle, actively reproducing. The time it takes one cell to divide into two cells **(generation time)** ranges from 2 to 8 hours.

DO NOT RESPOND TO SIGNALS FOR APOPTOSIS. Early embryonic cells have long telomeres that do not shorten with each cell division. Although some cells during fetal life undergo apoptosis for development of specific structures, this is not a feature of embryonic cells.

SHOW ANAPLASTIC MORPHOLOGY. Anaplasia means "without specific shape or differentiation." Early embryonic cells do not look like the mature cells they will eventually become. They all have the same anaplastic appearance–small and rounded (Figure 27-5).

HAVE A LARGE NUCLEAR-CYTOPLASMIC RATIO. The nucleus of these cells is large, taking up most of the space inside the cell. The ratio of nuclear space to cytoplasmic space is larger than that for a normal mature cell.

PERFORM NO SPECIFIC FUNCTIONS. These early embryonic cells do not have any specific or differentiated functions. They have not yet committed to a specific cell type. Each early embryonic cell is totally flexible and can mature to become any body cell. This flexibility is called **pluripotency, multipotency,** or **totipotency** because each cell has an unlimited potential for maturation.

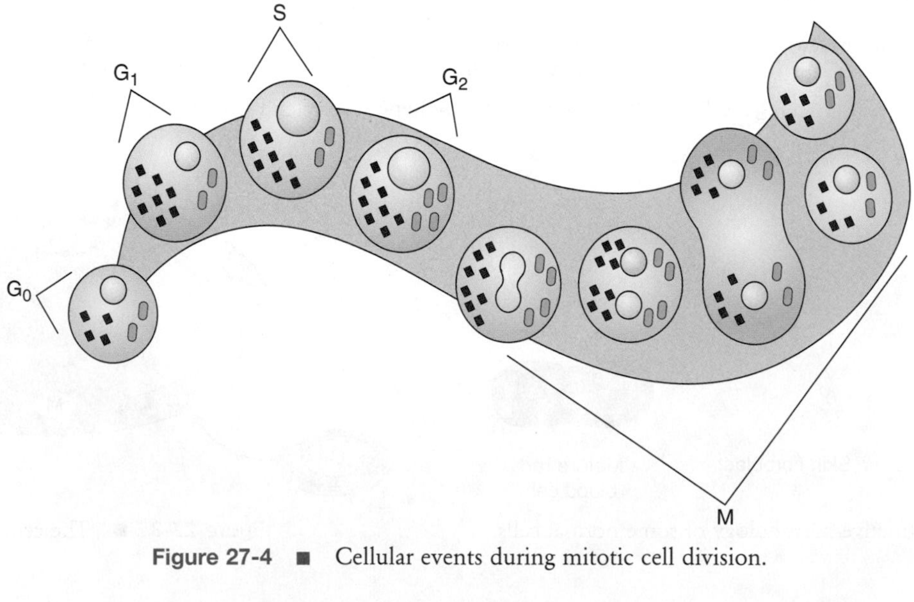

Figure 27-4 ■ Cellular events during mitotic cell division.

ADHERE LOOSELY TOGETHER. Early embryonic cells do not make fibronectin and are not tightly bound together.

ARE ABLE TO MIGRATE. Because early embryonic cells are not tightly bound together, they do not remain in one place within the embryo but migrate throughout the early embryo.

ARE NOT CONTACT INHIBITED. Having all sides of an early embryonic cell in continuous contact with the surfaces of other cells does not inhibit embryonic cell division.

ARE EUPLOID. Although early human embryonic cells differ from mature cells in many ways, they have 23 pairs of chromosomes.

COMMITMENT. At about day 8, early embryonic cells start changing into differentiated cells. In response to unknown signals, each cell commits itself to a specific outcome. The cell has not yet taken on any differentiated features; rather, it positions itself within a group of cells that will eventually become only one specific organ or tissue.

Commitment involves turning off specific early embryonic genes that controlled or regulated early rapid growth. These genes, called **proto-oncogenes,** remain as normal cellular genes but have limited function after early embryonic life. These genes are usually either "turned off," suppressed with little expression, or expressed but tightly controlled.

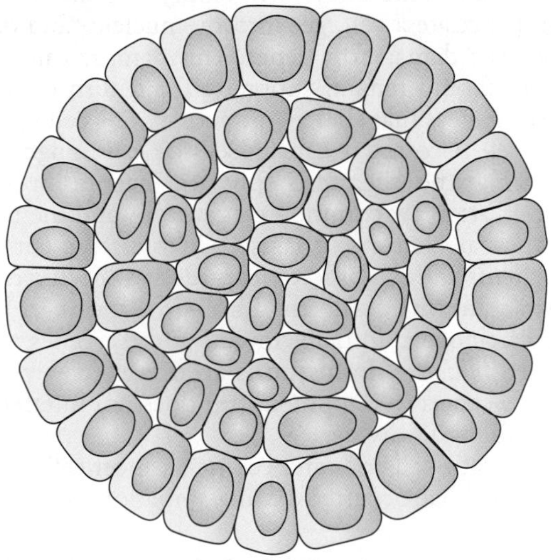

Figure 27-5 ■ Embryonic cells at about 5 days after conception.

After the early embryonic regulatory genes are "turned off" **(suppressed),** other specific genes that control the expression of differentiated functions must be "turned on" **(expressed)** selectively in different cell types. For example, the gene for insulin is actively expressed only in pancreatic beta cells and is suppressed in all other cells. This selective gene expression directs the normal growth and differentiation of specific body cells.

Biology of Abnormal Cells

Body cells are exposed to personal and environmental conditions that can alter how the cells grow or function. When either cell growth or cell function is changed, the cells are considered abnormal. Table 27-2 compares features of normal, embryonic, benign tumor, and cancer cells.

CHARACTERISTICS OF BENIGN TUMOR CELLS

Benign tumor cells are normal cells growing in the wrong place or at the wrong time. Examples include moles, uterine fibroid tumors, skin tags, endometriosis, and nasal polyps. Benign tumor cells:

HAVE CONTINUOUS OR INAPPROPRIATE CELL GROWTH. Benign tumors are tissues not needed for normal function, growing too much or in the wrong place.

SHOW SPECIFIC MORPHOLOGY. Benign tumors look like the tissues they come from, retaining the specific morphology of parent cells.

HAVE A SMALL NUCLEAR-CYTOPLASMIC RATIO. Just like completely normal cells, benign tumor cells have a small nucleus compared with the rest of the cell.

PERFORM SPECIFIC DIFFERENTIATED FUNCTIONS. Not only do benign tumors look like their parent cells, but they also perform the same differentiated functions. For example, in endometriosis, one type of benign tumor, the normal lining of the uterus (endometrium) grows in an abnormal place (such as on an ovary, on the peritoneum, or in the chest cavity). This displaced endometrium acts just like normal endometrium by changing each month under the influence of estrogen. When the hormone level drops and the

TABLE 27-2 Characteristics of Normal and Abnormal Cells

Characteristic	Normal Cell	Embryonic Cell	Benign Tumor Cell	Malignant Cell
Cell division	None or slow	Rapid, continuous	Continuous or inappropriate	Rapid or continuous
Appearance	Specific morphologic features	Anaplastic	Specific morphologic features	Anaplastic
Nuclear-cytoplasmic ratio	Small	Large	Small	Large
Differentiated functions	Many	None	Many	Some or none
Adherence	Tight	Loose	Tight	Loose
Migratory	No	Yes	No	Yes
Growth	Well regulated	Well regulated	Expansion	Invasion
Chromosomes	Diploid (euploid)	Diploid (euploid)	Diploid (euploid)	Aneuploid*
Mitotic index	Low	High	Low	High*

*Depends on the degree of malignant transformation.

normal endometrium sheds from the uterus, the displaced endometrium, wherever it is, also sheds.

ADHERE TIGHTLY TOGETHER. Benign tumor cells make fibronectin and bind tightly to one another. In addition, many benign tissues are "encapsulated," or surrounded with fibrous connective tissue, helping to hold the benign tissue together.

ARE NONMIGRATORY. Benign tissues do not wander but remain tightly bound and do not invade other body tissues.

GROW IN AN ORDERLY MANNER. Benign tumor cells follow normal cell growth patterns even though their growth is not needed. Growth may continue beyond an appropriate time, but the rate of growth is normal. The benign tumor grows by hyperplastic expansion. *They do not invade.*

ARE EUPLOID. Benign tumor cells have 23 pairs of chromosomes, the correct number for human beings.

CHARACTERISTICS OF CANCER CELLS

Cancer (malignant) cells are abnormal, serve no useful function, and are harmful to normal body tissues. Malignant tumors commonly:

HAVE RAPID OR CONTINUOUS CELL DIVISION. Some cancer cells have a short generation time (2 to 4 hours), but most cancer cells have a generation time similar to that of the parent cells. Cancer cells divide nearly continuously. Almost as soon as one round of mitosis is complete, the daughter cells begin a new round.

DO NOT RESPOND TO SIGNALS FOR APOPTOSIS. Most cancer cells have long telomeres and a lot of the enzyme, telomerase, which maintains telomeric DNA. As a result, cancer cells do not respond to apoptotic signals and have an unlimited life span (are "immortal").

SHOW ANAPLASTIC MORPHOLOGY. Cancer cells lose the specific appearance of their parent cells, becoming **anaplastic.** As a cancer cell becomes even more malignant, it becomes smaller and rounded. This loss of specific appearance can make diagnosis of cancer type difficult, because many types of cancer cells look alike.

HAVE A LARGE NUCLEAR-CYTOPLASMIC RATIO. The nucleus of a cancer cell is larger than that of a normal cell, and the cancer cell is small. The nucleus occupies much of the space within the cancer cell, creating a large nuclear-cytoplasmic ratio.

LOSE SOME OR ALL DIFFERENTIATED FUNCTIONS. Along with losing the appearance of the parent cell, cancer cells lose some functions that the parent cells performed. *Cancer cells serve no useful purpose.*

ADHERE LOOSELY TOGETHER. Cancer cells do not make fibronectin. As a result, they adhere poorly to each other, and cancer cells easily break off from the main tumor.

ARE ABLE TO MIGRATE. Because cancer cells do not bind tightly together and have many enzymes on their cell surfaces, they are able to slip through blood vessels and tissues, spreading from the main tumor site to many other body sites. This ability to spread **(metastasize)** is a key feature of cancer cells and a major cause of death among people with cancer.

GROW BY INVASION. Cancer cells expand and extend into other tissues, both close by and more remote from the original tumor, by invasion. Invasion and persistent growth make untreated cancer deadly.

ARE NOT CONTACT INHIBITED. Cancer cells continue to divide even when touched on all surface areas by other cells; thus their growth is not contact inhibited. The persistence of cancer cell division is one factor making the disease so difficult to control.

ARE ANEUPLOID. As cancer cells become more malignant, they lose or gain chromosomes. Thus they can have more than 23 pairs or less than 23 pairs.

CANCER DEVELOPMENT

Carcinogenesis/Oncogenesis

Carcinogenesis and **oncogenesis** are other names for cancer development. Table 27-3 lists key concepts about cancer development. The process of changing a normal cell into a cancer cell is called **malignant transformation.** This process occurs through the steps of *initiation, promotion, progression,* and *metastasis.*

INITIATION

The first step in carcinogenesis is **initiation.** Normal cells can become cancer cells if their proto-oncogenes are turned back on at any time after early embryonic life. Anything that can penetrate a cell, get into the nucleus, and damage the DNA can damage the genes. This damage can turn on genes that should remain suppressed and turn off normal genes. Substances that change the activity of a cell's genes so that the cell becomes a cancer cell are **carcinogens.** Carcinogens may be chemicals, physical agents, or viruses. Table 27-4 lists a few common carcinogens and the types of cancer they are known to cause. Chapters presenting the care of clients with specific cancers discuss specific carcinogens (when known) within the Etiology sections.

Pure carcinogens initially mutate a cell's genes and are thus called *initiators.* Initiation is an irreversible event that can lead to cancer development if it does not interfere with the cell's ability to divide.

After initiation, a cell can become a cancer cell if the cellular changes that occurred during initiation are enhanced

TABLE 27-3 Key Concepts Related to Cancer Development

- Neoplastic cells originate from normal body cells.
- Transformation of a normal cell into a cancer cell involves mutation of the genes (DNA) of the normal cell.
- Early embryonic genes that are overexpressed can cause a cell to develop into a tumor.
- Only one cell has to undergo malignant transformation for cancer to begin.
- Benign tumors grow by expansion, whereas malignant tumors grow by invasion.
- Most tumors arise from cells that are capable of cell division.
- A key feature of cancer cells is the loss of apoptosis. These cells have an "infinite" life span.
- Primary prevention of cancer involves avoiding exposure to known causes of cancer.
- Secondary prevention of cancer involves screening for early detection.
- Tobacco use is a causative or permissive factor in 30% of all malignant neoplasms.
- Tumors that metastasize from the primary site into another organ are still designated as tumors of the originating tissue.

by **promotion.** A cancer cell is not a health threat unless it can divide. If it cannot divide, it cannot form a tumor. *If growth conditions are right, however, widespread metastatic disease can develop from just one cancer cell.*

PROMOTION

Once a normal cell has been initiated by a carcinogen and is a cancer cell, it can become a tumor if its growth is enhanced. The time between a cell's initiation and the development of an overt tumor is called the **latency period,** which can range from months to years.

Promoters are substances that promote or enhance growth of the initiated cancer cell. They can also shorten the latency period. Promoters may be hormones, drugs, or a wide variety of chemicals.

PROGRESSION

After cancer cells have grown to the point that a detectable tumor is formed (a 1-cm tumor has at least 1 billion cells in it), other events must occur for this tumor to become a health problem. First, the tumor must develop its own blood supply. In the early stages, the tumor receives nutrition only by diffusion. After the tumor reaches 1 cm, however, diffusion is not efficient, and cells in the center of the tumor become hypoxic and start to die. To continue to grow and survive, the tumor makes **tumor angiogenesis factor (TAF).** TAF triggers capillaries and other blood vessels in the area to grow new branches into the tumor. These blood vessels ensure the tumor's continued nourishment.

As tumor cells continue to divide, some of the new cells change features from the original, initiated cancer cell. Actual colonies or subpopulations within the tumor begin to appear. These cell groups differ from the original cancer cell. Some of the differences provide these cell groups with advantages that allow them to live and divide no matter how the conditions around them change; these differences are thus called "selection advantages." Changes that a tumor undergoes at this time can allow it to become more malignant. Over time, the tumor cells have fewer and fewer normal cell features.

The original tumor is called the **primary tumor.** It is usually identified by the tissue from which it arose (parent tissue), such as in breast cancer or lung cancer. When primary tumors are located in vital organs, such as the brain or lungs, they can grow excessively and either lethally damage the vital organ or "crowd out" healthy organ tissue and interfere with that organ's ability to perform its vital function. At other times, the primary tumor is located in soft tissue that can expand without damage as the tumor grows. One such site is the breast. The breast is not a vital organ, and even if it had a large tumor in it, the primary tumor alone would not cause the client's death. When the tumor spreads from the original site into vital areas, life functions can be disrupted.

TABLE 27-4 Known Environmental Carcinogens*

Carcinogen	Associated Cancer Site or Neoplasm
Alcoholic beverages	Liver, esophagus, mouth, pharynx, breast, colon, and rectum
Anabolic steroids	Liver
Arsenic	Lung, skin
Asbestos	Lung, pleura, peritoneum, pericardium
Benzene	Myelogenous leukemia
Chemotherapy drugs Alkylating agents Anthracycline antibiotics Antimetabolites	Acute leukemia, lymphoma
Cyclosporine	Non-Hodgkin's lymphoma
Diesel exhaust	Lung
Formaldehyde	Nasopharynx
Hair dyes	Bladder
Ionizing radiation	Bone marrow, thyroid, many organs
Mineral oils	Skin
Pesticides	Lung
Polycyclic hydrocarbons	Lung, skin, scrotum
Polychlorinated biphenyls	Liver, skin
Sunlight	Skin, eyes
Tobacco	Lung, esophagus, mouth, pharynx, larynx, pancreas, bladder, kidney, liver, stomach, colon, rectum, leukemia

Data from U.S. Department of Health and Human Services, Public Health Service, National Toxicology Program. (December 2002). *Report on Carcinogens* (10th ed.). Author.
*This is a partial list selected from over 200 substances listed by the above source.

METASTASIS

In metastasis, cancer cells move from the primary location by breaking off from the original group and establishing remote colonies. These additional tumors are called **metastatic** or **secondary tumors.** *Even though the tumor is now in another organ, it is still a cancer from the original altered tissue. For example, when breast cancer spreads to the lung and the bone, it is breast cancer in the lung and bone, not lung cancer and not bone cancer.* Metastasis occurs through many steps, as shown in Figure 27-6.

EXTENSION INTO SURROUNDING TISSUES. Tumors secrete enzymes that open up areas of surrounding tissue. Pressure, created as the tumor increases in size, forces tumor cells to invade new territory.

BLOOD VESSEL PENETRATION. Enzymes also make large pores in the client's blood vessels, allowing tumor cells to enter the blood and circulate throughout the body.

RELEASE OF TUMOR CELLS. Because tumor cells are loosely held together, clumps of cells break off of the primary tumor into blood vessels for transport.

INVASION. Tumor cells circulate through the blood and enter tissues at remote sites. When conditions in the remote site can support tumor cell growth, the cells stop circulating (arrest) and invade the surrounding tissues, creating secondary tumors. Table 27-5 lists the common sites of metastasis for specific tumor types. Three routes of spread are local seeding, bloodborne metastasis, and lymphatic spread.

Local Seeding. Local seeding is the shedding of cancer cells in the local area of the primary tumor. In ovarian cancer, for example, cells often spill from the primary tumor into the peritoneal cavity and set up multiple secondary sites.

Bloodborne Metastasis. Bloodborne metastasis (tumor cell release into the blood) is the most common cause of cancer spread. Clumps of cancer cells can become

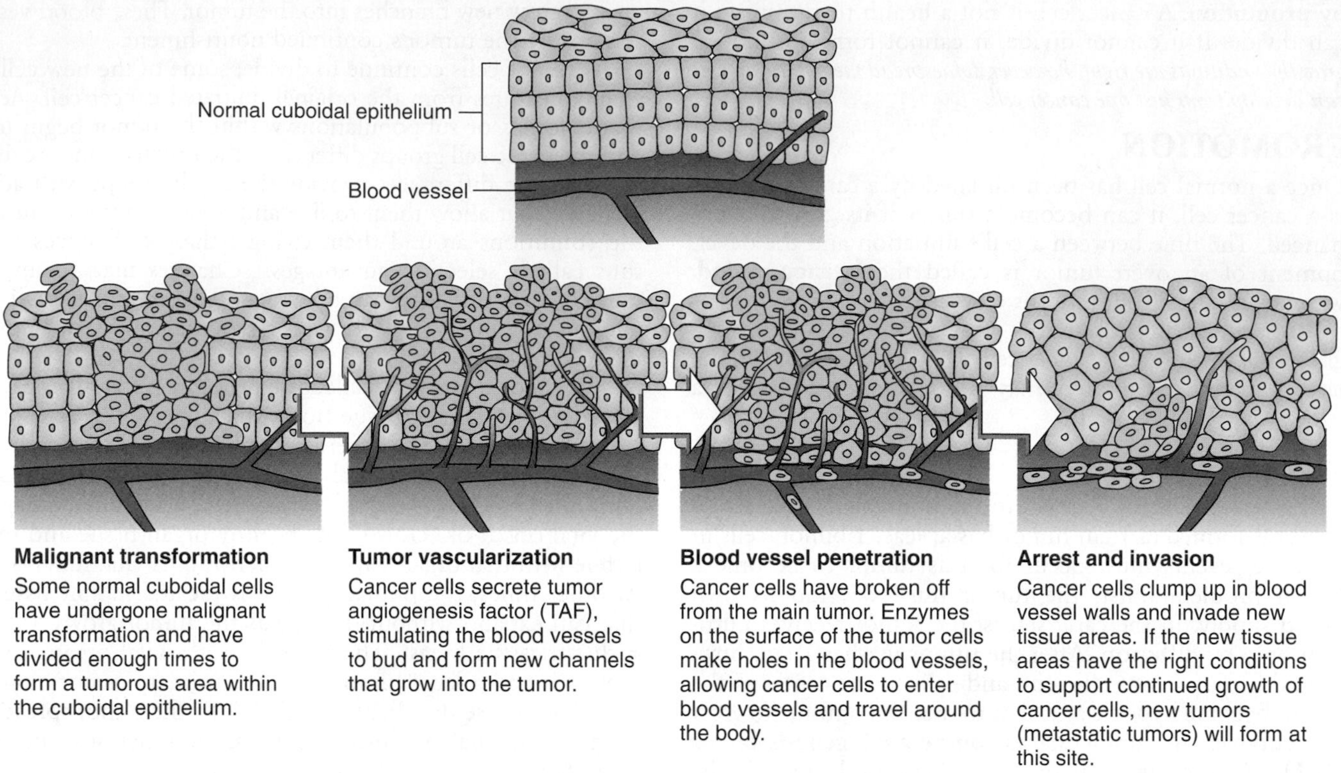

Figure 27-6 ■ The steps of metastasis.

TABLE 27-5 Common Sites of Metastasis for Different Cancer Types

Breast Cancer Bone* Lung* Liver Brain	**Prostate Cancer** Bone (especially spine and legs)* Pelvic nodes
Lung Cancer Brain* Bone Liver Lymph nodes Pancreas	**Melanoma** Gastrointestinal tract Lymph nodes Lung Brain
Colorectal Cancer Liver* Lymph nodes Adjacent structures	**Primary Brain Cancer** Central nervous system

*Most common site of metastasis for the specific malignant neoplasm.

trapped in capillaries. These clumps damage the capillary wall and allow cancer cells to enter the surrounding tissue.

Lymphatic Spread. Lymphatic spread is related to the number, structure, and location of lymph nodes and vessels. Primary sites that are rich in lymphatics have more early metastatic spread than areas with few lymphatics.

Cancer Classification

Cancers are classified by the type of tissue from which they arise (e.g., glandular, connective). Terms that describe cancer by tissue origin are listed in Table 27-6. Other ways to classify cancer include biologic behavior, anatomic site, and degree of differentiation.

About 100 different types of cancer arise from various tissues or organs. Figure 27-7 compares cancer distribution by site and gender. Cancers are divided into two major categories: solid and hematologic.

Solid tumors develop from specific tissues (e.g., breast cancer and lung cancer). Hematologic cancers (e.g., leukemias and lymphomas) arise from blood cell–forming tissues.

Cancer Grade and Stage

Systems of grading and staging have been developed to help standardize cancer diagnosis, prognosis, and treatment. Grading of a tumor classifies cellular aspects of the cancer. Staging classifies clinical aspects of the cancer.

GRADING

Some cancer cells are "more malignant" than others, varying in their aggressiveness and sensitivity to treatment. Some cancer cells barely resemble the tissue from which they arose, are aggressive, and spread rapidly. These cells are a "high-grade" cancer. On the basis of cell appearance and activity, grading compares the cancer cell with the normal parent tissue from which it arose.

Different clinical groups have established different grading systems for different types of cancer cells, but overall they resemble the standard system listed in Table 27-7. This system rates cancer cells with the lowest rating given to those cells that closely resemble normal cells, and the highest rating given to cancer cells that barely resemble normal cells.

TABLE 27-6 Classification of Tumors by Tissue of Origin

Prefix	Tissue of Origin	Benign Tumor	Malignant Tumor*
Adeno	Epithelial glands	Adenoma	Adenocarcinoma
Chondro	Cartilage	Chondroma	Chondrosarcoma
Fibro	Fibrous connective	Fibroma	Fibrosarcoma
Glio	Glial cells (brain)	Glioma	Glioblastoma
Hemangio	Blood vessel	Hemangioma	Hemangiosarcoma
Hepato	Liver	Hepatoma	Hepatocarcinoma Hepatoblastoma
Leiomyo	Smooth muscle	Leiomyoma	Leiomyosarcoma
Lipo	Fat/adipose	Lipoma	Liposarcoma
Lympho	Lymphoid tissues		Malignant lymphomas Hodgkin's lymphoma Non-Hodgkin's lymphoma Burkitt's lymphoma Cutaneous T-cell
Melano	Pigment-producing skin		Melanoma
Meningio	Meninges	Meningioma	Malignant meningioma Meningioblastoma
Neuro	Nerve tissue	Neuroma Neurofibroma	Neurosarcoma Neuroblastoma
Osteo	Bone	Osteoma	Osteosarcoma
Renal	Kidney		Renal cell carcinoma
Rhabdo	Skeletal muscle	Rhabdomyoma	Rhabdomyosarcoma
Squamous	Epithelial layer of skin, mucous membranes, and organ linings	Papilloma	Squamous cell carcinoma of skin, bladder, lungs, cervix

*Carcinomas are tumors of glandular tissue; sarcomas are tumors of connective tissue; blastomas are tumors of less differentiated, embryonal tissues.

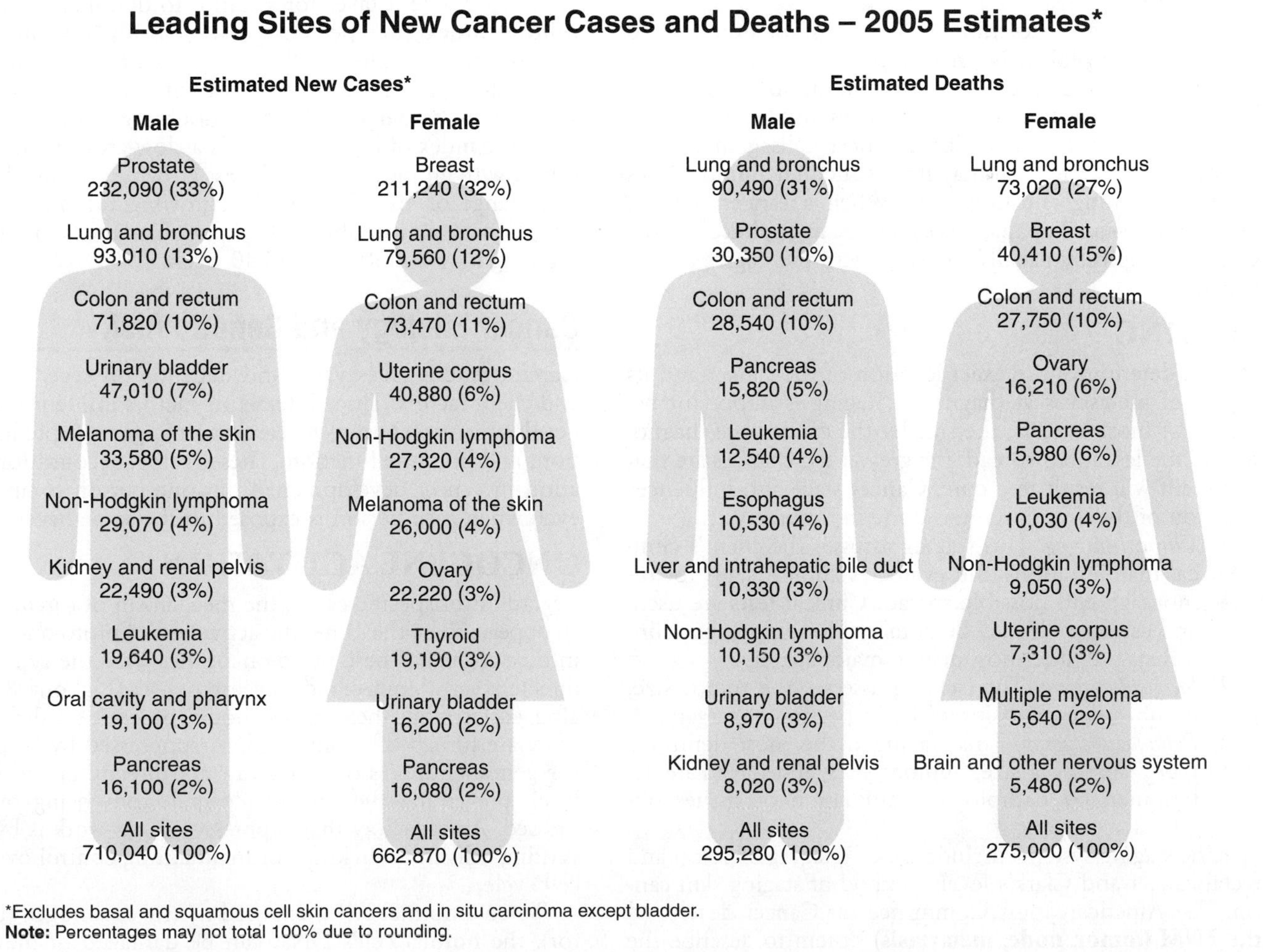

Figure 27-7 ■ Cancer incidence and death by site and gender. (Courtesy American Cancer Society, Atlanta, GA.)

TABLE 27-7 Grading of Malignant Tumors

Grade	Cellular Characteristics
G_x	Grade cannot be determined.
G_1	Tumor cells are well differentiated and closely resemble the normal cells from which they arose. This grade is considered a low grade of malignant change. These tumors are malignant but are relatively slow growing.
G_2	Tumor cells are moderately differentiated; they still retain some of the characteristics of normal cells but also have more malignant characteristics than do G_1 tumor cells.
G_3	Tumor cells are poorly differentiated, but the tissue of origin can usually be established. The cells have few normal cell characteristics.
G_4	Tumor cells are poorly differentiated and retain no normal cell characteristics. Determination of the tissue of origin is difficult and perhaps impossible.

TABLE 27-8 Staging of Cancer—TNM Classification

	Primary Tumor (T)
T_x	Primary tumor cannot be assessed
T_0	No evidence of primary tumor
T_{is}	Carcinoma in situ
T_1, T_2, T_3, T_4	Increasing size and/or local extent of the primary tumor
	Regional Lymph Nodes (N)
N_x	Regional lymph nodes cannot be assessed
N_0	No regional lymph node metastasis
N_1, N_2, N_3	Increasing involvement of regional lymph nodes
	Distant Metastasis (M)
M_x	Presence of distant metastasis cannot be assessed
M_0	No distant metastasis
M_1	Distant metastasis

Modified from American Joint Committee on Cancer. (1988). In O.H. Beahrs, et al. (Eds.). *Manual for staging of cancer* (3rd ed., p. 7). Philadelphia: J. B. Lippincott.

Grading the cells is one of the first steps in confirming cancer. Grading is a means of evaluating the client with cancer for prognosis and appropriate therapy. It also allows health care professionals to evaluate the results of management and compare local, regional, national, and international statistics.

PLOIDY

Cancer cells can be described by chromosome number and appearance, or **ploidy.** Normal human cells have 46 chromosomes (23 pairs), the normal diploid number. When malignant transformation occurs, changes in the genes and chromosomes also occur. Some cancer cells gain or lose whole chromosomes and may have structural abnormalities of the remaining chromosomes. When a cancer cell has more or less than 23 pairs, it is said to be **aneuploid.** The degree of aneuploidy usually increases with the degree of malignancy.

STAGING

Staging determines the exact location of the cancer and its degree of metastasis at diagnosis. Staging is important because, for most cancers, the smaller the cancer is at diagnosis and the less it has spread, the greater the chances are that treatment will result in a cure. Cancer stage also influences selection of therapy. Staging is done in three ways:

1. *Clinical staging.* This staging assesses the client's clinical manifestations and evaluates clinical signs for tumor size and possible spread. Clinical tests are used, and cancer cells may be obtained for biopsy, but clinical staging does not include major surgery.
2. *Surgical staging.* This staging assesses the tumor size, number, sites, and spread by inspection at surgery.
3. *Pathologic staging.* This staging is the most definitive type. The tumor size, number, sites, and spread are determined by pathologic examination of tissues obtained at surgery.

Specific staging systems include Dukes' staging of colon and rectal cancer and Clark's levels method of staging skin cancer. The American Joint Committee on Cancer developed the **TNM (tumor, node, metastasis)** system to describe the anatomic extent of cancers. The stages guide treatment and are useful for prognosis and comparison of treatment results. The TNM staging systems have specific prognostic value for each solid tumor type. Table 27-8 shows a basic TNM staging system. TNM staging is not useful for leukemia or lymphomas. Staging for these cancers is discussed in Chapter 43.

Tumor growth is discussed in terms of **doubling time** (the amount of time it takes for a tumor to double in size) and **mitotic index** (the percentage of actively dividing cells within a tumor). The smallest detectable tumor is about 1 cm in diameter and contains 1 billion cells. To reach this size, a must undergo at least 30 doublings. A tumor with a mitotic index of less than 10% is a slow-growing tumor; a tumor with an index of 85% is fast growing. Tumors have a wide range of growth rates. Fast-growing tumors, such as lymphomas, may double in 4 weeks; an adenocarcinoma of the lung may double in 21 to 40 weeks.

Cancer Etiology and Genetic Risk

Carcinogenesis takes years and depends on several tumor and client factors. Three interacting factors influence cancer development: exposure to carcinogens, genetic predisposition, and immune function. These factors account for variation in cancer development from one person to another, even when each person is exposed to the same hazards.

ONCOGENE ACTIVATION

Regardless of specific cause, the mechanism of carcinogenesis appears to be the same: the activation of proto-oncogenes into oncogenes. These proto-oncogenes were the genes that directed early embryonic development. At about 8 days after conception, these genes should be controlled forever. They are turned off, controlled, or suppressed by "suppressor genes." Suppressor genes can act directly at the DNA level, preventing the proto-oncogene from being overexpressed. Another way that suppressor genes work is by preventing cells from dividing, or maintaining control over the cell cycle.

When a normal cell is exposed to any carcinogen (initiator), the normal cell's DNA can be damaged or mutated.

TABLE 27-9 Example Malignancies Associated with Altered Oncogene Activity

Oncogene	Malignancies
ABL1	Chronic myelogenous leukemia, other leukemias
BRAF	Gastric
CCND1	Breast
ERBB-1	Glioblastomas, squamous cell carcinoma
ERBB-2 (HER-2/neu)	Breast, salivary gland, ovarian carcinomas
FES	Acute promyelocytic leukemia, lung, bladder
HRAS	Breast, melanoma, lung, kidney, bladder, colon
JUN	Lung
Ki-RAS	Colorectal
MYC	Burkitt's lymphoma, T-cell and B-cell neoplasms, breast, gastric, lung
MYCL	Lung
MYCN	Small cell lung cancer
NRAS	Ovarian, thyroid, melanoma, leukemia
PRAD-1	Breast, squamous cell cancers
RET	Thyroid, multiple endocrine neoplasias
TRK	Colorectal, thyroid

The mutations damage suppressor genes, preventing them from controlling the expression of proto-oncogenes. As a result, the proto-oncogenes are turned on or overexpressed. When proto-oncogenes are turned on, they are then called **oncogenes** and can cause the cell to change from normal cells to cancer cells. When oncogenes are overexpressed in a cell, excessive amounts of cyclins are produced and upset the balance between cell growth enhancement and cell growth limitation. The effect of these excessive cyclins is greater than the effect of the suppressor gene products, thus allowing uncontrolled cell division.

About 70 different proto-oncogenes that can be activated into oncogenes have been identified. *These oncogenes are not abnormal genes but are part of every cell's normal makeup and were important in early development.* Oncogenes become a problem only if they are activated after development is complete, as a result of exposure to carcinogenic agents or events. Activation of some specific oncogenes causes specific cancers. Table 27-9 lists known oncogenes and the cancers they cause. External and personal factors are associated with oncogene activation.

EXTERNAL FACTORS CAUSING CANCER

Between 78% and 80% of cancer in North America may be the result of environmental, or external, factors (American Cancer Society, 2005). Environmental carcinogens are chemical, physical, or viral agents that cause cancer. Table 27-4 lists known environmental causes of human cancer.

Chemical Carcinogenesis

Many chemicals, drugs, and other products used in everyday life are known to be carcinogenic, and hundreds more are suspected of being carcinogenic.

TABLE 27-10 Malignancies Associated with Tobacco Use

■ Lung	■ Oral cavity
■ Pharyngeal	■ Laryngeal
■ Esophagus	■ Pancreatic
■ Cervical	■ Kidney
■ Bladder	■ Liver
■ Stomach	■ Myeloid leukemia

Data from American Cancer Society. (2005). *Cancer facts and figures—2005.* Report No. 00-300M-No. 5008.05. Atlanta: Author.

Some chemicals are complete carcinogens that can both initiate and promote cancer. Others are pure initiating agents, or incomplete carcinogens. Still others are only promoting agents. Some substances, such as tobacco and alcohol, appear to be only mildly carcinogenic; it takes long-term exposure to large amounts of these substances before a cancer develops. However, these two substances can act as co-carcinogens; when taken together, they enhance each other's carcinogenic activity.

Cells are not susceptible to chemical carcinogenesis to the same degree. Normal cells that have the ability to divide are at greater risk for cancer development than are normal cells that are not capable of cell division. For example, cancers commonly arise in bone marrow, skin, lining of the gastrointestinal tract, ductal cells of the breast, and lining of the lungs. All of these cells normally undergo cell division. Cancers of nerve tissue, cardiac muscle, and skeletal muscle are rare. These cells do not normally undergo cell division.

About 30% of cancers diagnosed in North America are related to tobacco use (American Cancer Society, 2005). Tobacco is the single most important source of preventable carcinogenesis. It contains many different carcinogens and co-carcinogens. Tobacco use both initiates and promotes cancer. The risk for cancer development from tobacco use depends on a person's immune function, amount of tobacco exposure, type of tobacco exposure, and tobacco tar content.

Tissues with the greatest risk for tobacco-induced cancer are those that have direct contact with tobacco or tobacco smoke. Cigarette smoking and tobacco use also promote the development of other cancers. Table 27-10 lists the specific cancers that appear to be associated with tobacco use.

Physical Carcinogenesis

Physical agents or events cause cancer by the same mechanism as for chemical carcinogens (i.e., DNA damage). Two physical agents that cause cancer are radiation and chronic irritation.

RADIATION

Even small doses of radiation affect cells. Some effects are temporary and can be repaired. Other effects cannot be repaired and either may be lethal to the damaged cell or induce cancer in the damaged cell. The two types of radiation that cause cancer are ionizing and ultraviolet (UV). Some ionizing radiation is found naturally in such elements as radon, uranium, and radium. Most rocks and soil contain various amounts of uranium and radium. Other sources of ionizing radiation include x-rays for diagnosis and treatment of disease, as well as cosmic radiation. UV radiation is a type of solar radiation, coming from the sun. Other sources of UV radiation include tanning beds and germicidal lights.

UV rays do not penetrate deeply and the most common cancer type caused by UV exposure is skin cancer.

Both ionizing and UV radiation mutate genes. Although radiation exposure induces cancers more often among cells that can divide, it can cause cancer among nondividing cells as well.

CHRONIC IRRITATION

Chronic irritation and tissue trauma are suspected to cause cancer. The incidence of skin cancer is higher in people with burn scars or other types of severe skin injury. Chronically irritated tissues undergo frequent cell division and thus are at an increased risk for spontaneous DNA mutation.

Viral Carcinogenesis

Few viruses have been proven to be carcinogenic to humans, although more are suspected to play major roles in cancer development. When viruses infect body cells, they break the DNA chain and insert their own genetic material into the human DNA chain. Breaking the DNA, along with viral gene insertion, mutates the normal cell's DNA and can either activate an oncogene or damage suppressor genes. Viruses that cause cancer are **oncoviruses.** Table 27-11 lists cancers of known viral origin.

Dietary Factors Related to Cancer Development

Cancer development may be related to many dietary practices. However, the relationship of diet to cancer is poorly understood. Because dietary factors are rarely independent of other possible carcinogenic agents, evidence of dietary contributions to cancer development is clouded. Suspected dietary factors include low fiber intake, high intake of red meat, and high animal fat intake. Preservatives, contaminants, preparation methods, and additives (dyes, flavorings, and sweeteners) may have cancer-promoting effects. Chart 27-1 lists foods that have carcinogenic potential.

PERSONAL FACTORS AND CANCER DEVELOPMENT

Personal factors, including immune function, age, and genetic risk, also affect whether a person is likely to develop cancer.

Immune Function

The immune system protects the body from foreign invaders and non-self cells (see Chapter 23). Non-self cells include cells that are no longer normal, such as cancer cells. The part of the immune system that protects against cancer is cell-mediated immunity. Natural killer (NK) and helper T-cells provide immune surveillance.

The role of the immune system in protecting against cancer is supported by cancer incidence in immunosuppressed people. Adults older than 60 years of age have immune systems that function at less than optimal levels, and this group has a higher incidence of cancer compared with that of the general population. Organ transplant recipients taking immunosuppressive drugs to prevent organ rejection also have a higher incidence of cancer. In clients with acquired immunodeficiency syndrome (AIDS), incidence may be as high as 70%.

Age

Advancing age is the single most important risk factor for cancer (American Cancer Society, 2005).

CONSIDERATIONS FOR OLDER ADULTS

Seventy-seven percent of cancer occurs in people older than 55 years of age (American Cancer Society, 2005). This higher incidence reflects lifelong accumulation of DNA mutations that result in cell changes and cancer. Older adults may not be able to repair these mutations as they once did. Immune function, especially cell-mediated immunity, is also reduced in the older adult. Cancer assessment considerations for the older adult are listed in Chart 27-2.

Manifestations of cancer in older clients may be overlooked as changes of normal aging. Older adults must be aware of and report symptoms such as the seven warning signs of cancer (Table 27-12) to health care providers. Health care providers need to investigate all manifestations suggestive of disease.

Genetic Risk

As previously discussed, oncogenes are risk factors related to carcinogenesis. Proto-oncogenes, precursors of oncogenes, are passed on from generation to generation. The development of cancer, however, depends on more than these genes. The proto-oncogene must be overexpressed to an oncogene

TABLE 27-11 Malignancies Associated with a Known Viral Origin

Virus	Malignancies
Epstein-Barr virus	Burkitt's lymphoma, B-cell lymphoma, nasopharyngeal carcinoma
Hepatitis B virus	Primary liver carcinoma
Human papillomavirus	Cervical carcinoma, vulvar carcinoma, and other anogenital carcinomas
Human lymphotrophic virus type I	Adult T-cell leukemia
Human lymphotrophic virus type II	Hairy cell leukemia

Data from Cooper, G. (1995). *Oncogenes* (2nd ed.). Boston: Jones & Bartlett.

CHART 27-1

CLIENT EDUCATION GUIDE
Dietary Habits to Reduce Cancer Risk

- Avoid excessive intake of animal fat.
- Avoid nitrites (prepared lunch meats, sausage, bacon).
- Minimize your intake of red meat.
- Keep your alcohol consumption to no more than one or two drinks per day.
- Eat more bran.
- Eat more cruciferous vegetables, such as broccoli, cauliflower, Brussels sprouts, and cabbage.
- Eat foods high in vitamin A (such as apricots, carrots, and leafy green and yellow vegetables) and vitamin C (such as fresh fruits and vegetables, especially citrus fruits).

for cancer to occur. In some people, the sequence of a specific proto-oncogene is different, which may allow it to be activated more easily. In other people, the proto-oncogene is normal, but the gene controlling proto-oncogene activity, the suppressor gene, may be abnormal.

These variations in gene sequence may be small single nucleotide polymorphisms (SNPs), or may be large areas of mutations. Both types of gene problems can be inherited or can occur as a result of exposure to carcinogens. Table 27-9 lists specific cancers associated with altered oncogene activity; Table 27-13 lists specific cancers associated with altered suppressor gene activity.

CHART 27-2

NURSING FOCUS on the OLDER ADULT
Cancer Assessment Considerations

Cancer Type	Assessment Consideration
Colorectal cancer	Ask the client whether bowel habits have changed over the past year (e.g., in consistency, frequency, or color). Is there any obvious blood in the stool? Test at least one stool specimen for occult blood during the client's hospitalization. Encourage the client to have a baseline colonoscopy. Encourage the client to reduce dietary intake of animal fats, red meat, and smoked meats. Encourage the client to increase dietary intake of bran, vegetables, and fruit.
Bladder cancer	Ask the client about the presence of: Pain on urination Blood in the urine Cloudy urine Increased frequency or urgency
Prostate cancer	Ask the client about: Hesitancy Change in the size of the urine stream Pain in the back or legs History of urinary tract infections
Skin cancer	Examine skin areas for moles or warts. Ask the client about changes in moles (e.g., color, edges, or sensation).
Leukemia	Observe the skin for color, petechiae, or ecchymosis. Ask the client about: Fatigue Bruising Bleeding tendency History of infections and illnesses Night sweats Unexplained fevers
Lung cancer	Observe the skin and mucous membranes for color. How many words can the client say between breaths? Ask the client about: Cough Hoarseness Smoking history Exposure to inhalation irritants Shortness of breath Activity tolerance Frothy or bloody sputum Pain in the arms or chest Difficulty swallowing

Patterns of genetic risk for cancer have also been identified, including the following:

- Inherited predisposition for specific cancers
- Inherited conditions associated with cancer
- Familial clustering
- Chromosomal aberrations

Table 27-14 lists conditions associated with an increased genetic risk for cancer development.

Genetic Testing for Cancer Predisposition

Genetic testing is available to confirm or rule out a person's genetic risk for a few specific cancers. Most tests are performed on peripheral blood. These tests are expensive and often not covered by insurance. Genetic testing should not

TABLE 27-12 The Seven Warning Signs of Cancer

C	Changes in bowel or bladder habits
A	A sore that does not heal
U	Unusual bleeding or discharge
T	Thickening or lump in the breast or elsewhere
I	Indigestion or difficulty swallowing
O	Obvious change in a wart or mole
N	Nagging cough or hoarseness

TABLE 27-13 Malignancies Associated with Altered Suppressor Gene Activity (Selected)

Suppressor Gene	Malignancies
APC	Colorectal, stomach, pancreatic
ATM	Leukemia, lymphoma, breast, ovarian
BRCA1	Breast, ovarian
BRCA2	Breast, ovarian
CDK4	Melanoma
CDKN2A	Mesothelioma, melanoma
DCC	Colorectal
DPC4	Pancreatic, colon
FUS1	Lung
Ink4a	Melanoma
MEN1	Parathyroid, pituitary, adrenal, carcinoid, pancreatic islet cell
MLH1	Colorectal
MSH2	Colorectal
MTS1	Melanoma, brain tumors, leukemia, sarcomas, breast, bladder, ovarian, lung, kidney
NF1	Neurofibroma, colon, astrocytoma
NF2	Neurofibroma, meningioma, schwannoma
NKX3.1	Prostate
PTEN	Breast, prostate, endometrial
RB1	Retinoblastoma, sarcomas, breast, bladder, esophageal, small cell lung
SMAD3	Prostate
Tp53	Breast, bladder, colorectal, esophageal, liver, lung, ovarian, brain tumors, sarcomas, leukemia, lymphoma
VHL	Renal cell carcinoma, pheochromocytoma, hemangioblastoma

TABLE 27-14 Conditions Associated with a Genetic Predisposition for Cancer

Condition	Specific Cancer Type
Inherited cancers*	Breast cancer Prostate cancer Ovarian cancer
Familial clustering	Breast cancer Melanoma
Bloom syndrome	Leukemia
Familial polyposis	Colorectal cancer
Chromosomal aberrations	
Down syndrome (47 chromosomes)	Leukemia
Klinefelter syndrome (47, XXY)	Breast cancer
Turner's syndrome (45, XO)	Leukemia Gonadal carcinoma Meningioma Colorectal cancer

*Not all breast, prostate, or ovarian cancers are inherited.

TABLE 27-15 Racial Differences in Cancer Development

White	Asian
Common Cancer Types	*Common Cancer Types*
1. Lung	1. Breast
2. Breast	2. Colorectal
3. Colorectal	3. Prostate
4. Prostate	4. Lung
	5. Stomach
African American	**Hispanic**
Common Cancer Types	*Common Cancer Types*
1. Lung	1. Prostate
2. Prostate	2. Breast
3. Breast	3. Colorectal
4. Colorectal	4. Lung
5. Uterine	

Data from American Cancer Society. (2005). *Cancer facts and figures—2005.* Report No. 00-300M-No. 5008.05. Atlanta: Author.

be performed unless a family history clearly indicates the possibility of increased genetic risk. *These tests do not diagnose the presence of cancer.*

A variety of issues and potential problems exist with genetic testing for cancer risk. Correct interpretation of the results is critical. Ideally, a genetic counselor is involved in giving the client information before, as well as after, testing is performed. *When a client tests positive for a cancer-causing gene mutation, his or her risk for cancer development is greatly increased, but the cancer may never develop.*

Other issues regarding genetic testing include who will have access to the information and whether or not to share the test results with family members. Many clients fear that if they test positive for a cancer-causing gene, they may face discrimination for insurance coverage or in the workplace. Some states have confidentiality safeguards and others do not. Genetic testing has implications for the entire family, not just the client being tested. For more information on genetic testing, see Chapter 11.

CULTURAL CONSIDERATIONS

The incidence of cancer varies among races. American Cancer Society data (2003a) show that African Americans have a higher incidence of cancer than white individuals do, and the death rate is higher for African Americans. Since 1960 the overall incidence among African Americans has increased 27%, whereas for white individuals it has increased 12%. Cancer sites and cancer-related mortality vary along racial lines as well. Table 27-15 shows common cancers among white, African American, Asian, and Hispanic populations. Understanding these variations can help in planning prevention and early detection strategies that are ethnically specific.

When risks for cancer development are assessed, however, ethnicity and genetic predisposition cannot be considered alone. Behavior and socioeconomic factors must also be assessed. The American Cancer Society (2005) reports that cancer incidence and survival are often related to socioeconomic factors. These factors include the availability of health care services or the belief that seeking early health care has a positive effect on the outcome of cancer diagnosis. (See the Evidence-Based Practice for Nursing box on p. 481.)

CANCER PREVENTION

Cancer prevention activities can focus on primary prevention or secondary prevention. **Primary prevention** is the use of strategies to prevent the actual occurrence of cancer. This method of cancer prevention is most effective when there is a known cause for a cancer type. **Secondary prevention** is the use of screening strategies to detect cancer early, at a time when cure or control is more likely.

Primary Prevention

AVOIDANCE OF KNOWN OR POTENTIAL CARCINOGENS

An effective primary prevention strategy is to avoid known or potential carcinogens. This method is effective when a cause of cancer is known and avoidance is easily accomplished. Examples are using skin protection during sun exposure, avoiding tobacco, and eliminating environmental asbestos. As more cancer causes are identified, avoidance may become even more effective.

MODIFICATION OF ASSOCIATED FACTORS

Absolute causes are not known for many cancers, but some conditions appear to increase risk. Example are the increased incidence of cancer among people who consume alcohol; the association of a diet high in fat and low in fiber with colon cancer, breast cancer, and ovarian cancer; and a greater incidence of cervical cancer among women with many sexual partners. Modifying behavior to reduce the associated factor may decrease the risk for cancer development.

REMOVAL OF "AT RISK" TISSUES

When a person has a known high risk for developing a specific type of cancer, removal of the tissue reduces the risk. Examples include removing moles to prevent conversion to skin cancer,

EVIDENCE-BASED PRACTICE for Nursing

Limited access to health care is not the only factor in ethnicity-based differences in breast cancer outcomes

Bibb, S. (2001). The relationship between access and stage at diagnosis of breast cancer in African American and Caucasian women. *Oncology Nursing Forum, 28*(4), 711-719.

The purpose of this secondary analysis was to examine the influence of various factors on screening and early detection practices for breast cancer between African-American and Caucasian women using a Department of Defense military health system for primary care. The use of this health care system eliminated the bias of differences in consumer costs for preventive care.

The study examined the tumor registry records of 635 clients (62 African-American women and 573 Caucasian women) in whom breast cancer was diagnosed over a 10-year period at a specific military health system. Data were collected regarding stage at diagnosis, use of breast cancer screening techniques, age at diagnosis, means of discovery, and socioeconomic status.

Overall, diagnosis was made at later stages of the disease in African-American women than in Caucasian women. The age at diagnosis was younger among the African-American women and fewer tumors were discovered by mammography than for Caucasian women. Although socioeconomic status was different for the two groups, the health care consumer costs and access were not different. No significant difference between the time of disease diagnosis and the initiation of treatment was noted for the two groups.

The findings of an earlier age of disease onset and a higher stage of disease at diagnosis for African-American women are consistent with the findings from studies not confined to a military health system. The authors speculate that barriers to earlier diagnosis are personal rather than related to economic access to appropriate services. The investigators suggest that breast health care interventions for African-American women need to focus at least as much on increasing awareness of the need for adhering to recommended screening guidelines as it does on reducing economic access barriers.

Level of Evidence: 3—Well-designed trial without randomization (large cohort study).

Critique. The study examined differences in breast cancer diagnosis between African-American women and Caucasian women when equal economic access to health care was available. The study has some limitations based on the retrospective nature of a secondary analysis. Socioeconomic status was not directly measured in the initial data; instead, the surrogate of military rank was used as the economic indicator. The level of education for the individual women also was not collected. While the percentage of study participants who were African American (≈10%) reflects the national distribution, the small number (62) limits the generalizability of the study results.

Implications for Nursing. African-American women may have an average age of onset for breast cancer at an age younger than when annual mammography screenings are recommended. Therefore the importance of monthly breast self-examination (BSE) and yearly clinical breast examinations (CBE) must be stressed. The development and testing of culturally appropriate teaching tools for BSE are needed.

removing colon polyps to prevent colon cancer, and removing breasts to prevent breast cancer. Not all "at risk" tissues can be removed (e.g., those that are part of essential organs).

CHEMOPREVENTION

A newer form of cancer prevention, **chemoprevention,** is being tried. This strategy uses drugs, chemicals, natural nutrients, or other substances to disrupt one or more steps important to cancer development. These agents may be able to reverse existing gene damage or halt the progression of the transformation process. Chemopreventive agents work in one of the following ways to disrupt at least one step in the process of cancer:

- Blocking an inactive compound from becoming an active carcinogen
- Blocking the direct action of a carcinogen on DNA
- Enhancing the rate of elimination of a carcinogen from the body
- Suppressing the activity of a carcinogen
- Suppressing the promoting activity of a carcinogen
- Suppressing the progression of a premalignant or early-stage malignancy into a more malignant state

Table 27-16 lists agents under investigation for chemoprevention. At this time, only a few agents have been found effective and are commonly prescribed.

The goal of chemopreventive strategies is prevention of cancer development. Target populations for whom chemoprevention might be effective include the following:

- Healthy people with no known specific cancer risk
- People at greater than normal risk because of increased environmental exposure or decreased immune function
- People with precancerous lesions
- People with a history of cancer

TABLE 27-16 Agents Under Investigation for Chemoprevention of Cancer

Category of Prevention	Specific Agents
Prevention of carcinogen formation	Ascorbic acid (vitamin C) Tocopherol (type of vitamin E) Selenium Caffeic acid
Blocking the action of a carcinogen on DNA ("antimutagens")	Carotenoids (vitamin A derivative) Retinoids (vitamin A derivative) Ellagic acid Flavones Oltipraz Butylated hydroxyanisole
Enhancing the elimination of a carcinogen	Isothiocyanate Indole-3-carbinol
Suppression of carcinogenic action	Aspirin Retinoids Indomethacin Selenium Steroidal anti-inflammatory agents Protease inhibitors
Antipromotion activity	Carotenoids Retinoids Selenium Coumarin Piroxicam Indomethacin Calciferol (vitamin D) Hormone antagonists Tamoxifen Finasteride Evista
Suppression of progression	Danazol Interferon Cysteamine Vorozole

Secondary Prevention

SCREENING PROGRAMS

Regular screening for cancer does not reduce cancer incidence but can greatly reduce some types of cancer deaths. For most adults, specific routine screening techniques are encouraged annually as part of health maintenance. General screening recommendations are listed in chapters discussing cancers by organ system. The age and type of participation in specific screening tests are different for people who have an identified increased risk for a specific cancer type. Examples of recommended screenings include the following (American Cancer Society, 2003b):

- Yearly mammography for women older than age 40 years
- Yearly clinical breast examination for women older than age 40 years
- Colonoscopy at age 50 years and then every 10 years
- Yearly fecal occult blood in adults of all ages
- Yearly prostate specific antigen (PSA) test and digital rectal examination (DRE) for men over age 50 years

GENE THERAPY FOR CANCER PREVENTION

Because cancer development clearly involves gene changes (either inherited gene mutations or acquired gene damage), researchers have suggested that altering damaged genes could prevent cancer development. Currently, people can be screened for some gene mutations that increase the risk for cancer. Examples of these gene mutations include the BRCA-1 gene, which increases the risk for both breast and ovarian cancer; the BRCA-2 gene, which increases the risk for breast cancer; and the APC gene, which increases the risk for colon cancer. Screening can help a person at increased genetic risk for cancer to alter lifestyle factors, participate in early detection methods, or even have at-risk tissue removed. Although it is not yet possible to "fix" or remove an abnormal gene in humans, gene therapy in the future is not out of the realm of possibility.

GET READY for the NCLEX Examination!

KEY POINTS

Safe Effective Care Environment

- Ensure that clients in hospitals and other inpatient settings are not exposed to environmental chemicals.
- Position shields properly when clients in inpatient settings are having x-ray examinations taken at the bedside.

Health Promotion and Maintenance

- Teach clients to use sunscreen and to wear protective clothing during sun exposure.
- Encourage clients to participate in the recommended cancer screening activities for their age group and cancer risk category.
- Inform all clients who smoke that smoking increases the risk for development of many cancer types.
- Assist clients interested in smoking cessation to find an appropriate smoking cessation program.

Psychosocial Integrity

- Assess the client's knowledge about causes of cancer and his or her screening/prevention practices.
- Assist clients who fear a cancer diagnosis to understand that finding cancer at an early stage increases the chances for cure.
- Educate clients who undergo genetic testing for cancer predisposition about the risks to confidentiality of the test results.

Physiological Integrity

- Ask all clients about their exposures to environmental agents that are known or suspected to increase the risk for cancer.
- Obtain a detailed family history (at least three generations) to assess the client's risk for familial or inherited cancer.
- Teach clients the "seven warning signs of cancer" (see Table 27-12).

ADDITIONAL STUDY RESOURCES

Go to your Student CD-ROM for Review Questions for the NCLEX Examination.

evolve Go to http://evolve.elsevier.com/Iggy/ for Integrated Management of Care Questions for the NCLEX Examination.

SELECTED BIBLIOGRAPHY

Asterisk indicates a classic or definitive work on this subject.

American Cancer Society. (2003a). *Cancer facts and figures for African Americans-2003.* Report No. 8614.03. Atlanta: Author.

American Cancer Society. (2003b). *Cancer prevention and early detection. Facts & Figures-2003.* Report No. 8600.03. Atlanta: Author.

American Cancer Society. (2005). *Cancer facts and figures–2005.* Report No. 00-300M-No. 5008.05. Atlanta: Author.

Bargonetti, J., & Manfredi, J. (2002). Multiple roles of the tumor suppressor *p53*. *Current Opinion in Oncology, 14*(1), 86-91.

Bibb, S. (2001). The relationship between access and stage at diagnosis of breast cancer in African American and Caucasian women. *Oncology Nursing Forum, 28*(4), 711-719.

Calzone, K., & Biersecker, B. (2002). Genetic testing for cancer predisposition. *Cancer Nursing, 25*(1), 15-25.

Clark, P., & Gomez, E. (2001). Details on demand: Consumers, cancer information, and the internet. *Clinical Journal of Oncology Nursing, 5*(1), 19-24.

Frank-Stromborg, M., & Olsen, S. (2001). *Cancer prevention in diverse populations: Cultural implications for health care professionals.* Pittsburgh: Oncology Nursing Society.

Hanahan, D., & Weinberg, R. (2000). The hallmarks of cancer. *Cell, 100*(1), 57-70.

Hawkins, R. (2001). Mastering the intricate maze of metastasis. *Oncology Nursing Forum, 28*(6), 959-965.

Houftek, J., & Atwood, J. (2003). Genetic susceptibility to lung cancer: Implications for smoking cessation. *MEDSURG Nursing, 12*(1), 45-49.

Jegathesean, J. et al. (2005). Apoptosis: Understanding the new molecular pathway. *MEDSURG Nursing, 13*(6), 371-376.

Jennings-Dozier, K., & Lawrence, D. (2000). Sociodemographic predictors of adherence to annual cervical cancer screening in minority women. *Cancer Nursing, 23*(5), 350-356.

Lessick, M., et al. (2001). Advances in genetic testing for cancer risk. *MEDSURG Nursing, 10*(3), 123-127.

Likes, W., & Itano, J. (2003). Human papillomavirus and cervical cancer: Not just a sexually transmitted disease. *Clinical Journal of Oncology Nursing, 7*(3), 271-275.

Loescher, L. (2003). The biology of cancer. In A. Tranin, A. Masny, & J. Jenkins (Eds.). *Genetics in oncology practice: Cancer risk assessment.* Pittsburgh: Oncology Nursing Society.

Loud, J., et al. (2002). Applications of advances in molecular biology and genomics to clinical cancer care. *Cancer Nursing, 25*(2), 110-122.

Machia, J. (2001). Breast cancer: Risk, prevention, and tamoxifen. *American Journal of Nursing, 101*(4), 26-35.

Macleod, K. (2000). Tumor suppressor genes. *Current Opinion in Genetics and Development, 10*(1), 81-93.

Maes, S. (2004). Geriatric oncology comes of age. *ONS News, 19*(2), 1, 4-5, 7.

O'Rourke, J., & Mahon, S. (2003). A comprehensive look at the early detection of ovarian cancer. *Clinical Journal of Oncology Nursing, 7*(1), 41-47.

Peltomaki, P. (2003). Role of DNA mismatch repair defects in the pathogenesis of human cancer. *Journal of Clinical Oncology, 21*(6), 1174-1179.

Peters, J., et al. (2001). Cancer genetics fundamentals. *Cancer Nursing, 24*(6), 446-461.

*Singh, D., & Lippman, S. (1998). Cancer chemoprevention: Part 1. Retinoids, carotenoids and other classic antioxidants. *Oncology, 12*(11), 1643-1658.

Tranin, A., Masny, A., & Jenkins, J. *Genetics in oncology practice: Cancer risk assessment.* Pittsburgh: Oncology Nursing Society.

United States Preventive Services Task Force. (2003). Chemoprevention of breast cancer: Recommendations and rationale. *American Journal of Nursing, 103*(5), 107-113.

U.S. Department of Health and Human Services, Public Health Service, National Toxicology Program. (December 2002). *Report on Carcinogens* (10th ed.). Author.

Volker, D. (2001). Carcinogenesis: Application to clinical practice. *Clinical Journal of Oncology Nursing, 5*(5), 225-226, 229.

Workman, M.L. (2004). The biology of cancer. In C. Varrichio (Ed.). *A cancer source book for nurses* (8th ed., pp. 13-28). Boston: Jones & Bartlett.

Zimmerman, V. (2002). Gene mutations and cancer. *American Journal of Nursing, 1028*), 28-37.

CHAPTER

28 General Interventions for Clients with Cancer

M. LINDA WORKMAN

LEARNING OUTCOMES

After studying this chapter, you should be able to:

1. Identify the goals of cancer therapy.
2. Distinguish between cancer surgery for cure and cancer surgery for palliation.
3. Discuss how the nursing care needs for the client undergoing cancer surgery compare to those for the client undergoing any other type of surgery.
4. Compare the purposes and side effects of radiation therapy and chemotherapy for cancer.
5. Prioritize nursing care for the client with radiation-induced skin problems.
6. Develop a community-based teaching plan for the client receiving external beam radiation.
7. Compare the personnel safety issues for working with clients receiving teletherapy radiation versus those receiving brachytherapy radiation.
8. Identify nursing interventions to promote safety for the client experiencing chemotherapy-induced anemia or thrombocytopenia.
9. Develop a community-based teaching plan for the client receiving chemotherapy.
10. Prioritize nursing care for the client with chemotherapy-induced neutropenia.
11. Prioritize nursing care for the client with mucositis.
12. Explain the rationale for hormonal manipulation therapy.
13. Discuss the uses of biological response modifiers as supportive therapy in the treatment of cancer.
14. Explain the basis of targeted therapy for cancer.
15. Identify clients at risk for oncologic emergencies.
16. Prioritize nursing care needs for clients experiencing oncologic emergencies.

Go to your Student CD-ROM for Review Questions for the NCLEX Examination keyed to these Learning Outcomes.

Most people fear cancer and consider a cancer diagnosis to involve suffering and death. In affluent countries, more than 50% of people diagnosed with cancer are cured, and thousands of others live 5 years or longer after the diagnosis (American Cancer Society, 2005). Regardless of treatment type, cancer always affects a person's physical and psychological functioning.

Providing care to clients and families experiencing cancer is complex and challenging. This chapter describes the general interventions for cancer and the problems associated with cancer treatment. For specific treatment regimens and client problems that occur with specific cancer types, consult the chapters in which the cancer is described. Table 28-1 lists common cancer types and the specific locations within this text where the interventions are presented.

GENERAL DISEASE-RELATED CONSEQUENCES OF CANCER

Cancer can develop in any organ or tissue but tends to occur more commonly in some tissues than in others. Cancer destroys normal tissue, decreasing function in that tissue or organ. Even when cancers occur in nonvital tissues or organs, they can cause death by **metastasizing** (spreading) into vital organs and disrupting critical physiologic processes (see Chapter 27). Cancers that are left untreated cause the following:

- Impaired immune and hematopoietic (blood-producing) function
- Altered gastrointestinal (GI) tract structure and function
- Motor and sensory deficits
- Decreased respiratory function

These impairments cause great physical and emotional distress. Without intervention, cancer invasion of normal tissues leads to death.

Impaired Immune and Hematopoietic Function

Impaired immune and hematopoietic function occurs most often in clients with leukemia and lymphoma, but also can occur with any cancer that invades the bone marrow. Tumor cells enter the bone marrow and reduce the production of healthy white blood cells, which are needed for normal immune function (see Chapter 23). Thus clients who have cancer, especially leukemia, are at an increased risk for infection.

When cancer invades the bone marrow, it also decreases the number of red blood cells **(anemia)** and platelets **(thrombocytopenia).** These changes may be caused by the cancer itself, such as in leukemia, or by the cancer treatment. In either case, the client is anemic and is at risk for excessive bleeding.

TABLE 28-1 Text Location of Specific Cancer Content

Cancer Type	Chapter	Patho/ Etiol	Treatment and Nursing Interventions
Bladder	73	1701	1702-1704
Brain	48	1055-1056	1056-1066
Breast	77	1794-1796	1802-1820
Cervical	78	1845-1846	1846-1849
Colorectal	60	1317-1319	1320-1325
Esophageal	58	1274	1276-1280
Head and Neck	32	571-572	573-580
Kidney	74	1722-1723	1723-1724
Leukemia	43	897-898	900-908
Lung	33	613-614	614-625
Lymphoma	43	908-909	909-910
Ovarian	78	1849	1850
Prostate	79	1864-1865	1865-1870
Skin	70	1608	1610
Stomach	59	1306	1308-1310

Altered Gastrointestinal Structure and Function

Cancer can alter gastrointestinal (GI) function and impair nutrition. For example, tumors may obstruct or compress structures anywhere along the GI tract, reducing the client's ability to absorb nutrients and eliminate wastes. Tumors also increase metabolic rate and increase the need for protein, carbohydrates, and fat at a time when the client has less energy for meal preparation or eating.

Many tumors spread to the liver, profoundly damaging this organ. The liver has many important functions in metabolism. Reduced liver function leads to malnutrition and death among clients with cancer.

Many clients with cancer have anorexia that often interferes with their ability to meet energy needs. **Cachexia** (extreme body wasting and malnutrition) develops from an imbalance between food intake and energy use. This problem may occur even when nutritional intake appears adequate. Changes in taste can result from the cancer or the treatment and reduce appetite. Cancer-related causes of malnutrition are listed in Table 28-2.

TABLE 28-2 Causes of Malnutrition in Clients with Cancer

Anorexia

Local causes
- Pelvic or abdominal tumors
- Hepatic metastases
- Intestinal compression or obstruction
- Others

Remote causes
- Food aversions
- Early satiety

Treatment-related causes
- Postsurgical small stomach or stasis
- Drugs, including chemotherapy
- Radiation—local and systemic effects

Systemic illness
- Infection
- Hepatitis or pancreatitis
- Endocrinopathies

Taste disorders
- Drugs (e.g., metronidazole)
- Remote effects of neoplasm and its treatment
- Local disease and its treatment (e.g., stomatitis, nasopharyngeal tumor, radiation, and surgery)
- Nausea and vomiting

Psychogenic causes
- Depression
- Anxiety
- Conditioned aversions

Intolerance of institutional food

Difficulty in Eating

Head and neck tumors and their treatment
Xerostomia
Stomatitis
Loss of teeth and dental problems
Dysphagia and odynophagia

Maldigestion or Malabsorption

Pancreatic insufficiency
Bile salt deficiency
Hypersecretory syndrome
- Zollinger-Ellison syndrome
- Pancreatic cholera
- Bowel infiltration
- Diffuse invasion (e.g., lymphoma)
- Local blockage
- Fistula

Postsurgical causes
- Esophageal surgery (with vagotomy, gastric statis, diarrhea, and steatorrhea)
- Gastrectomy—dumping, achlorhydria, or afferent loop syndrome
- Small intestine resections

Postirradiation causes
- Enteritis (may occur as late sequelae)
- Fistula
- Stenosis
- Obstruction

Protein-Losing Enteropathy Malutilization

Cancer cachexia
Steroids
- Nitrogen wasting
- Hyperglycemia
- Calcium loss

Nutritional support for the client with cancer, especially one undergoing cancer therapy, is complex and controversial. A diet high in protein and carbohydrates is often prescribed to help the client maintain weight and to provide the nutrients for energy and cellular repair. However, some scientists believe that an excessive intake of protein and vitamins increases the nutrition of the cancer cells and contributes to cancer progression. Clients often believe their cancers can be cured more easily if weight is gained or maintained. Currently no one nutritional plan meets the needs of all clients with cancer (Wilson, 2000).

Motor and Sensory Deficits

Motor (movement) and sensory deficits occur when cancers invade bone or the brain, or compress nerves. In clients with bone metastases, the primary cancer started in another organ (e.g., the prostate, breast, or lung). The bone sites most often affected are the vertebrae, ribs, pelvis, and femur. The humerus, scapula, sternum, skull, and clavicle are also common sites of cancer spread. Bone metastases cause fractures, spinal cord compression, and hypercalcemia, each of which reduces mobility.

The client may have sensory changes if the spinal cord is damaged by tumor pressure or if nerves are compressed. Sensory, motor, and cognitive functions are severely impaired when cancer spreads to the brain.

The client with cancer may also have pain. Pain does not always accompany cancer, but it can be a significant problem for clients with terminal cancer. Chapter 7 provides an in-depth discussion of the causes and management of cancer pain.

Decreased Respiratory Function

Cancer can disrupt gas exchange in several ways and often results in death. For example, tumors in the airways cause airway obstruction. If lung tissue is involved, lung capacity is decreased. Tumors can also press on blood and lymph vessels in the chest, blocking blood flow through the chest and lungs and resulting in pulmonary edema and dyspnea. Tumors also can thicken the alveolar membrane and damage pulmonary blood vessels, reducing gas exchange.

TREATMENT-RELATED CONSEQUENCES OF CANCER

The purpose of cancer treatment is to prolong survival time or improve quality of life (see the Meeting Healthy People 2010 Objectives box above). Although a few spontaneous regressions of cancer have been reported, most clients would die within months of diagnosis without cancer therapy. Therapies for cancer include surgery, radiation, chemotherapy, hormonal manipulation, immunotherapy, gene therapy, and targeted therapy. These therapies may be used separately or in combination to kill cancer cells. The type and amount of therapy depends on the specific type of cancer, whether or not the cancer has spread, and the health of the client. One or more regimens (protocols) have been established for most types of cancer. These regimens are based on experiments with cancer cells and animals and on experience with other clients with cancer.

> **Meeting HEALTHY PEOPLE 2010 Objectives**
>
> **CANCER**
>
> *Objective 17.16: Increase the number of cancer survivors who are living 5 years or longer after diagnosis.*
>
> - Encourage clients to seek early health care advice whenever one of the seven warning signs of cancer is present.
> - Teach clients being treated for cancer the importance of compliance with the scheduled treatment regimen.
> - Teach the client to follow up with health care visits after cancer treatment is completed.
> - Teach the client with cancer to continue with recommended screening practices.
> - Encourage the client who has been treated for cancer to avoid known environmental carcinogens.
> - Assist clients who smoke to reduce or quit smoking.
> - Teach clients about the importance of limiting dietary fat, smoked meats, and red meats.

Surgery

RATIONALE FOR CANCER TREATMENT

Surgery is the oldest form of cancer treatment and was the first method to cure cancer. Surgery for cancer involves the removal of diseased tissue. If cancer is confined to the removed tissue, surgery alone can result in a "cure" for that cancer. Although many cancers have spread too far at the time of diagnosis for surgery alone to cure, it may still be a useful part of diagnosis, treatment, follow-up, and rehabilitation.

MECHANISM OF ACTION

Cancer surgery may be used for any of the following purposes: prophylaxis, diagnosis, cure, control, palliation, determination of therapy effectiveness, and reconstruction.

PROPHYLAXIS. Prophylactic surgery is performed when a client has either an existing "premalignant" condition or a known family history that strongly predisposes the person to the development of cancer. The "at-risk" tissue or organ is removed to prevent cancer development. An example of prophylactic surgery for a premalignant condition is removing a benign mole from a location where continuous irritation or exposure to sunlight occurs.

DIAGNOSIS (BIOPSY). Diagnostic surgery provides proof of cancer. All or part of a suspected lesion is removed for examination and testing. Specific types of biopsies are listed Table 28-3.

CURE. Surgery alone can result in a cure rate of 27% to 30% when all visible and microscopic tumor is removed or destroyed. Types of curative surgeries are described in Table 28-4.

CONTROL (CYTOREDUCTIVE SURGERY). Cancer control, or cytoreductive surgery, "debulks" by removing part of the tumor and leaving a known amount of gross tumor. This type of surgery alone cannot result in a cure, but decreases the number of cancer cells and increases the chances that other therapies can be successful.

PALLIATION. The goal of palliative surgery is to improve quality of life during the survival time. Tumor tissue

TABLE 28-3 Diagnostic/Biopsy Surgeries for Cancer

Biopsy Type	Description	Problem/Limitations
Needle	Aspirating cells in a fluid or in very soft tissue Boring a "core" of solid tissue by using a long needle or making a punch, scrape, or bite	Sample error—may biopsy only noncancerous cells in a tissue or organ Sample size may not be adequate for accurate testing Procedure may spread cancer by seeding it into surrounding tissues Procedure may damage healthy tissue
Incisional	Removing a wedge of suspected tissue from a larger tissue mass, leaving some tumor cells in the tissue	Sample error Tumor seeding Damage to healthy tissue
Excisional	Completely removing an entire lesion without removing any adjacent normal tissues	Tumor seeding Leaving micrometastasis Damage to healthy tissue
Staging	Performing multiple needle or incisional biopsies in tissues where metastasis is suspected or likely	Tumor seeding Sample error Damage to healthy tissue

TABLE 28-4 Curative Surgeries for Cancer

Surgery Type	Description	Purpose/Use
Local excision	Removal of all identifiable tumor along with a small margin of normal tissues	Small, localized tumors
Wide local excision (radical)	Removal of identifiable tumor plus immediate tissue or adjacent tissue	Small tumors with only local tissue invasion
Wide excision	Removal of tumor, surrounding tissue, adjacent structures, and usual lymph channels draining the area	Small to moderate-size tumors with known local invasion
Extended radical excision	Removal of tumor, lymphatics, adjacent organs, and all tissues in the region	Tumor infiltrate in a wide area but with no known distant metastasis

that is causing pain, obstruction, or difficulty swallowing is removed. The specific procedure used depends on the client's specific problem.

DETERMINATION OF THERAPY EFFECTIVENESS ("SECOND LOOK"). Second-look surgery is a "rediagnosis" after treatment. The purpose is to assess the disease status in clients who have been treated and have no symptoms of remaining tumor. The results of this surgery are used to determine whether a specific therapy should be continued or discontinued.

RECONSTRUCTIVE OR REHABILITATIVE SURGERY. This type of surgery increases function, enhances appearance, or both. Examples include breast reconstruction after mastectomy, replacement of the esophagus after radiation damage, bowel reconstruction, revision of scars, release of contractures, and placement of penile implants.

SIDE EFFECTS OF SURGICAL THERAPY

Unlike surgery performed for many other reasons, cancer surgery involves the loss of a specific body part or its function. Sometimes whole organs are removed, such as the kidney, lung, breast, testes, arm, or tongue. Any organ loss reduces function. The amount of function lost and how much the loss affects clients depends on the location and extent of the surgery. Some cancer surgery results in major scarring or disfigurement. Clients may be anxious about the chances of surviving the cancer and may be grieving about a loss of body image or a change in lifestyle.

NURSING CARE OF CLIENTS UNDERGOING SURGICAL THERAPY

The physical care needs of the client having surgery for cancer are similar to those related to surgery for other reasons (see Chapters 20 to 22). Consider the client's ability (and the ability of family and significant others) to cope with the uncertainty of cancer and its treatment and with the changes in body image and role. For example, surgery involving the genitals, urinary tract, colon, and rectum may permanently damage these organs. Surgical procedures to create a urinary or fecal diversion (e.g., a colostomy) may damage nerves, causing erectile dysfunction in men and painful intercourse in women.

Radiation

RATIONALE FOR CANCER TREATMENT

The purpose of radiation therapy for cancer is to destroy cancer cells with minimal exposure of the normal cells to the damaging actions of radiation. The effects of radiation are seen only in the tissues in the path of the radiation beam. Some effects are apparent within days or weeks, whereas other effects may not be apparent for months to years after radiation therapy is completed.

MECHANISM OF ACTION

Most radiation therapy for cancer is ionizing radiation. When cells are exposed to this type of radiation, atoms within the cell are "kicked out" of orbit, resulting in a tremendous release of intracellular energy. Ionizing radiation is given off naturally by radium and cobalt, and can also be generated by linear accelerators. Naturally occurring radiation is called **gamma radiation;** radiation that is generated by machine is called **roentgen radiation.** Their effect on cells is the same.

Cells damaged by radiation either die outright or become unable to divide. Radiation damage can occur any time a cell is exposed to radiation and is not confined to cells actively dividing. However, cells in the cell cycle have more damage when exposed to radiation than do nondividing cells.

Three different types of energy, or rays, are produced by gamma radiation: gamma, beta, and alpha rays. These rays vary in their ability to penetrate tissues and damage cells. Table 28-5 lists the features of these three types of gamma radiation, and Figure 28-1 shows the penetrating ability of each.

TABLE 28-5 Characteristics of Different Types of Gamma Radiation

Gamma Ray
Gamma rays are very light and have a low energy-transfer potential. They travel at the speed of light, allowing them to be concentrated and penetrate deeply into tissues.
This is the most common type of radiation used for the treatment of cancer.
This type of radiation can also cause serious, irreversible harm to tissues.
Exposure to this type of radiation must be avoided or severely limited.
Beta Ray
Beta rays are heavier and travel at a moderate to high speed. They have a high linear energy-transfer potential and do not penetrate tissues or other substances well.
Some beta rays are used inside the body for specific radiation therapy.
Beta rays are used in some diagnostic tests.
Beta rays pose health hazards to humans exposed to them, but exposure must be considerable for damage to occur.
Alpha Ray
Alpha rays are very heavy and slow. They easily transfer energy to their surroundings and quickly lose their ability to penetrate tissues (0.04 mm into tissue).
Currently, alpha rays are used in laboratory tests rather than as treatment for cancer.
This type of radiation is harmful to humans only if it is ingested chronically.

The amount of radiation delivered to a tissue is called the **exposure;** the amount of radiation absorbed by the recipient tissue is called the **dose.** The dose is always less than the exposure. Three factors determine the absorbed dose: intensity of exposure, duration of exposure, and closeness of the radiation source to the cells.

The intensity of the radiation decreases with the distance from the radiation source (Figure 28-2). This factor is known as the **inverse square law.** For example, the radiation dose received at a distance of 2 feet from the radiation source is only one fourth of the dose received at a distance of 1 foot from the radiation source; the dose of radiation received at 3 feet is only one ninth of the dose received at 1 foot.

KILLING EFFECTS OF RADIATION. If the dose of radiation is high enough, all cells are killed immediately. This does not usually happen because all cells within a tumor absorb the radiation dose slightly differently. Therefore their overall response to the radiation is slightly different. A few cells die immediately, and more die within the next 24 hours as they attempt to divide. Some cells become sterile as a result of this single treatment. Still other cells repair the radiation-induced damage and recover.

Because of the varying responses of all cancer cells within a given tumor, radiation is given as a series of divided doses. Small doses of radiation are given on a daily basis for a set period of time to allow greater destruction of cancer cells while reducing the damage to normal tissues. This dose division is called **fractionation.** Standard radiotherapy is usually fractionated between 180 and 280 rad/day, multiplied by as many days as needed to achieve the total prescribed dose (rad is an acronym meaning "radiation absorbed dose").

The total dose of radiation needed depends on the size and location of the tumor and on the radiation sensitivity of the tumor and surrounding normal tissues. Some normal tissues are more sensitive than others to radiation. For example, healthy breast tissue can tolerate much higher doses of radiation than can the liver. A total dose of 1200 rad might be prescribed for a primary liver tumor, but a total dose of 5000 to 6000 rad might be needed for a breast cancer (delivered over 28 to 30 separate days). A 6000-rad dose delivered to the liver would destroy the liver as well as the tumor.

Two types of radiation delivery are usually used for cancer therapy: teletherapy and brachytherapy. The type used depends on the client's general health and on the site, size, and location of the tumor to be irradiated. The optimum

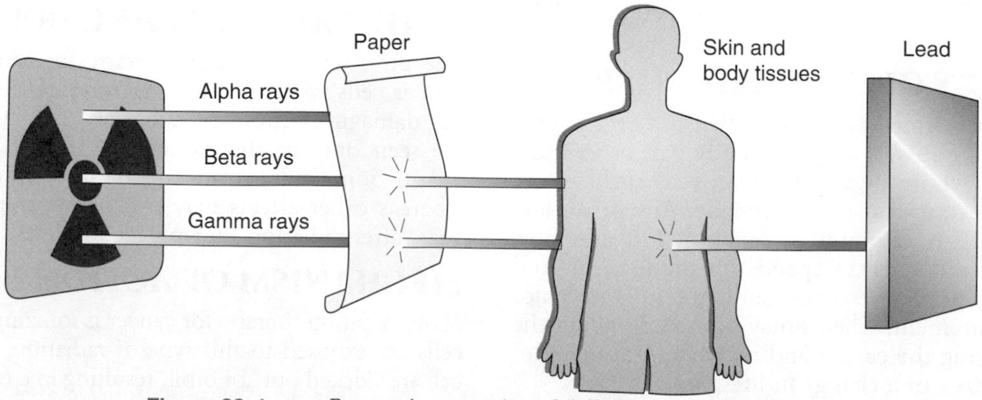

Figure 28-1 ■ Penetrating capacity of different types of radiation.

dose of radiation is one that can kill the cancer cells with an acceptable level of damage to normal tissues (some damage to normal tissues cannot be avoided).

TELETHERAPY. **Teletherapy** means distant treatment. In teletherapy, the radiation source is external to the client. Because the source is external, the client is not radioactive and poses no hazard to anyone. This type of therapy is also called **beam radiation.**

The exact location of the tumor is determined for greater accuracy of radiation therapy. Once the pattern of radiation delivery is determined, the client must always be in exactly the same position for all treatments. Ensure that the client can get into and maintain this position. Position-fixing devices and markings, either on the client's body or on the devices, ensure the proper position each day of treatment.

BRACHYTHERAPY. **Brachytherapy** means "short" or "close" therapy. With brachytherapy, the radiation source comes into direct, continuous contact with the tumor tissues for a specific period of time. This method provides a high dose of radiation in tumor tissues and a limited dose in surrounding normal tissues. Brachytherapy radiation has the same tissue effects as radiation delivered by external sources.

Brachytherapy uses radioactive isotopes either in solid form or within body fluids. Isotopes can be delivered to the tumor tissues in several ways. *With all types of brachytherapy, the radiation source is within the client. Therefore the client emits radiation for a period of time and is a hazard to others.*

Unsealed Radiation Sources. Isotopes that can be suspended in a fluid are unsealed and given via the oral or intravenous (IV) routes or as an instillation into body cavities, such as the peritoneal cavity and the spinal fluid space. Because the isotopes are unsealed, they are not completely confined to any one body area. Usually, they concentrate more in some body tissues than in others. These soluble isotopes enter body fluids and eventually are eliminated in waste products, which are radioactive and can be harmful to other people.

An example of brachytherapy with soluble isotopes is the ingestion or injection of the radionuclide iodine^{131} (an iodine base with a half-life of 8.05 days) to treat some thyroid cancers. The radioactive iodine concentrates in the thyroid gland and destroys the thyroid cancer cells. Most of this isotope is eliminated within 48 hours. Once the isotope is eliminated, neither the client nor the body wastes are radioactive.

Sealed Radiation Sources. Solid or sealed radiation sources are implanted within or very near the tumor. These radiation sources can be temporary or permanent. Most of the implants emit continuous, low-energy radiation to tumor tissues. Some devices (e.g., seeds or needles) can be placed into the tissues and stay in place by themselves. Other sources must be held in place with special applicators. Needles and seeds are preloaded with the radioactive isotope and are radioactive at the time of insertion into the tumor ("hot implantation"). Some of these devices are so small and the half-life of the isotope so short that the device is permanently left in place (most often for prostate cancer). Other devices are removed and reused in other clients.

In "afterloading," the implant is placed within the cavity without the radioactive isotope. Special applicators hold the implant in position. When placement is correct and the client is in the proper environment, the implant is loaded with the radioisotope. After the prescribed dose has been delivered, the implant, radioisotopes, and position-holding applicators are removed. *With solid implants, the client emits radiation while the implant is in place, but the excreta are not radioactive.*

Traditional implants deliver "low-dose rates" (LDR) of radiation continuously and clients are hospitalized for several days. A new variation on this therapy is radiation delivery at "high-dose rates" (HDR). For this type of delivery, the client comes into the radiation therapy department several times a week and the stronger radiation device is placed for only an hour or so each time. The client goes home between treatments and is only radioactive when the implant is in place. Chart 28-1 lists the best practices for care of the client with sealed implant radiation sources.

SIDE EFFECTS OF RADIATION THERAPY

The immediate and long-term side effects of all types of radiation are limited to the tissues exposed to the radiation. Therefore the side effects vary according to the site. Skin

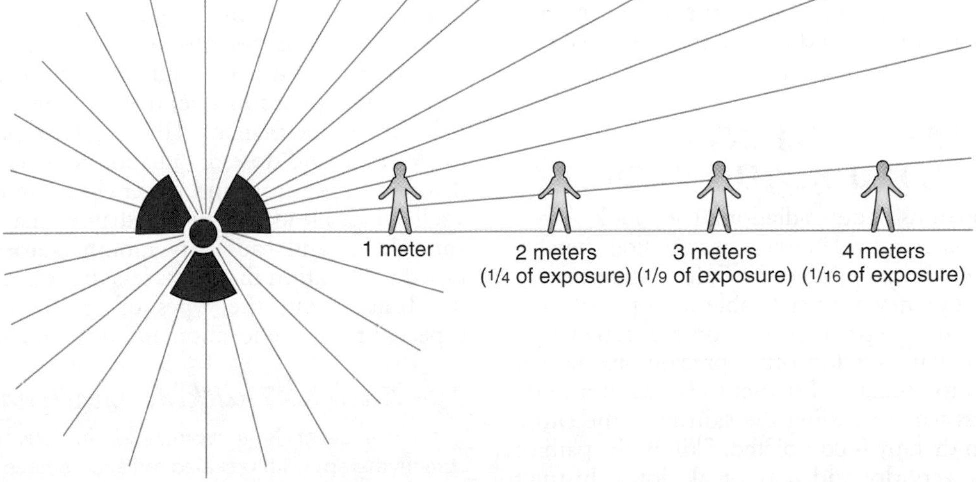

Figure 28-2 ■ The inverse square law of radiation exposure.

CHART 28-1

BEST PRACTICE for
Care of the Client with Sealed Implants of Radioactive Sources

- Assign the client to a private room with a private bath.
- Place a "Caution: Radioactive Material" sign on the door of the client's room.
- Wear a dosimeter film badge at all times while caring for clients with radioactive implants. The badge offers no protection but measures an individual's exposure to radiation and should be used by only one individual.
- Pregnant nurses should not care for these clients; do not allow pregnant women or children younger than 16 years of age to visit.
- Limit each visitor to one-half hour per day. Be sure visitors are at least 6 feet from the source.
- Never touch the radioactive source with bare hands. In the rare instance that it is dislodged, use a long-handled forceps to retrieve it. Deposit the radioactive source in the lead container kept in the client's room.
- Save all dressings and bed linens until after the radioactive source is removed. After the source is removed, dispose of dressings and linens in the usual manner. Other equipment can be removed from the room at any time.

changes and hair loss are local but are likely to be permanent depending on the total absorbed dose.

Depending on the dose, altered taste sensations and fatigue are two systemic side effects often noted by clients receiving external beam radiation, regardless of the radiation site. Taste changes are thought to be caused by metabolites released from dead and dying cells. Many clients develop an aversion to the taste of red meats. Fatigue may be related to the increased energy demands needed to repair damaged cells. Regardless of the cause, radiation-induced fatigue can be debilitating and may last for weeks to months. Many clients are surprised by the degree of fatigue they have and adjust their lifestyle to manage this symptom. Although clinicians have suggested that clients increase rest time to reduce fatigue, early research indicates exercise may help reduce radiation-related fatigue (see the Evidence-Based Practice for Nursing box at right).

Radiation damage to normal tissues during cancer therapy can start the inflammatory responses that cause tissue fibrosis and scarring. These effects may not be apparent for many years after radiation treatment. For example, women who receive high-dose radiation (HDR) therapy for uterine cancer may develop radiation-induced changes in the colon years later, resulting in constipation and obstruction.

NURSING CARE OF CLIENTS UNDERGOING RADIATION THERAPY

Most clients are anxious about radiation. They look to you to explain the purpose and side effects of radiation therapy. When clients receive accurate, objective information regarding radiation therapy, they are better able to cope with the treatment and continue to participate in normal activities.

Chart 28-2 lists skin care and other precautions needed with external radiation therapy. Instruct the client not to remove the markings when cleaning the skin until the entire course of radiation therapy is completed. Skin in the path of radiation becomes very dry and may break down. Instruct clients not to use lotions or ointments in these areas unless the radiologist prescribes them. Because skin in the radiation path is more sensitive to sun damage, advise against direct skin exposure to the sun during treatment and for at least 1 year after completing radiation therapy.

The normal tissues most sensitive to external radiation are bone marrow cells, skin, mucous membranes, hair follicles, and gonadal (reproductive) tissues. Some changes caused by radiation are permanent. The long-term problems vary with the location and dose of radiation received. For example, radiation to the throat and upper chest can cause difficulty in swallowing. Head and neck radiation may damage the salivary glands and cause dry mouth **(xerostomia).** Bone exposed to radiation therapy is less dense and breaks more easily. Teach about the types of symptoms that might be expected from the location and dose of radiation received.

EVIDENCE-BASED PRACTICE for Nursing

Exercise may reduce radiation-related fatigue

Sarna, L., & Conde, F. (2001). Physical activity and fatigue during radiation therapy: A pilot study using Actigraph monitors. *Oncology Nursing Forum, 28*(6), 1043-1046.

This prospective, descriptive pilot study sought to explore the effect of purposeful exercise on the experience of radiation-induced fatigue. Seven subjects who were receiving a 5-week course of external beam radiation therapy for cancer participated in this repeated measures study. Activity and fatigue were measured at the beginning and end of the second and fifth weeks of therapy. Activity was determined by Actigraph watch recordings and self-reports with the use of activity diaries. Fatigue was measured using the Profile of Mood States (POMS) vigor-activity and fatigue-inertia subscales, a Linear Analogue Scales for Fatigue (LAS-F), and the Symptom Distress Scale (SDS).

The data indicated that subjects who participated in purposeful exercise had an overall increase in activity at the end of the second and fifth weeks of therapy compared to the beginnings of the same weeks of therapy. Fatigue scores decreased at the ends of the same weeks compared to the beginnings of those weeks. Additionally, the subjects reported less fatigue by the fifth week of therapy compared to the second week of therapy. These findings are different from the levels of activity and perceptions of fatigue typically reported by clients receiving radiation therapy who do not participate in purposeful exercise activity. The findings do, however, support those of recent research examining the effects of exercise in clients receiving chemotherapy for cancer.

Level of Evidence: 6—Uncontrolled case series.

Critique. The study represented pilot work in the area of the effects of exercise on side effects for clients receiving radiation therapy for cancer. The sample size was small and no control group was used for comparison. The investigators used appropriate data collection techniques. Although the results of this study cannot be generalized at this time, they indicate that more study of an exercise intervention for ameliorating side effects of radiation therapy is needed.

Implications for Nursing. Fatigue is a distressing and often debilitating side effect of radiation therapy. Current interventions have included more frequent rest periods and reduction of nonessential activity. The results of this study suggest that activity not only may not worsen the perception of fatigue among clients undergoing radiation therapy, but might actually decrease the fatigue.

Critical Thinking Challenge

The client is a woman in her 60s who is receiving brachytherapy with a sealed radiation source for 49 hours. She is concerned about being radioactive and the side effects of therapy, especially alopecia.

1. What precautions will you teach this client to prevent radiation exposure to others?
2. What precautions should you take when you provide direct care to this client?
3. How should you handle her excrement?
4. What should you tell her about the possibility of alopecia?
5. What immediate and long-term side effects of therapy could this client expect to have?

evolve For suggested answer guidelines, go to http://evolve.elsevier.com/Iggy/.

CHART 28-2

CLIENT EDUCATION GUIDE
Radiation Therapy for Cancer

- Wash the irradiated area gently each day with either water alone or with a mild soap and water.
- Use your hand rather than a washcloth to be more gentle.
- Rinse soap thoroughly from your skin.
- Take care not to remove the markings that indicate exactly where the beam of radiation is to be focused.
- Dry the irradiated area with patting motions rather than rubbing motions; use a clean, soft towel or cloth.
- Use no powders, ointments, lotions, or creams on your skin at the radiation site unless they are prescribed by your *radiologist*.
- Wear soft clothing over the skin at the radiation site.
- Avoid wearing belts, buckles, straps, or any type of clothing that binds or rubs the skin at the radiation site.
- Avoid exposure of the irradiated area to the sun.
- Avoid heat exposure.

Chemotherapy

Chemotherapy, the treatment of cancer with chemical agents, has a major role in cancer therapy. Chemotherapy is used to cure and to increase survival time.

RATIONALE FOR CANCER THERAPY

As described in Chapter 27, cancer cells are able to separate from the original tumor, spread to new areas, and establish new cancers at distant sites **(metastasize).** Clients with metastatic cancer will die unless treatment eliminates the metastatic cancer cells and the original cancer cells.

Chemotherapy is useful in treating cancer because its effects are systemic, providing the opportunity to kill metastatic cancer cells that may have escaped local treatment. Chemotherapy used along with surgery or radiation is termed **adjuvant** therapy.

MECHANISM OF ACTION

Chemotherapy is used as cancer treatment because it has some selectivity for killing cancer cells over normal cells. This killing effect on cancer cells is related to the ability of chemotherapy to damage DNA and interfere with cell division. Thus the tumors most sensitive to chemotherapy are those that have rapid growth.

Chemotherapy drugs usually are given systemically and exert their cell-damaging **(cytotoxic)** effects against healthy cells as well as cancer cells. The normal cells most affected by chemotherapy are those that divide rapidly, including skin, hair, intestinal tissues, spermatocytes, and blood-forming cells.

Chemotherapy drugs are classified by the specific types of action they exert in the cancer cell. Table 28-6 lists categories and specific agents.

ANTIMETABOLITES. Antimetabolites are similar to normal metabolites needed for vital cell processes. Most cell reactions require metabolites in order to begin or continue the reaction. Antimetabolites closely resemble normal metabolites and are "counterfeit" metabolites that fool cancer cells into using the antimetabolites in cellular reactions. Because antimetabolites cannot function as proper metabolites, their presence impairs cell division.

ANTITUMOR ANTIBIOTICS. Antitumor antibiotics damage the cell's DNA and interrupt DNA or ribonucleic acid (RNA) synthesis. Exactly how the interruptions occur varies with each agent.

ALKYLATING AGENTS. All alkylating agents cross-link DNA, making the two DNA strands bind tightly together. This tight binding prevents proper DNA and RNA synthesis, inhibiting cell division.

ANTIMITOTIC AGENTS. Antimitotic agents are usually made from plant sources. They interfere with the formation of microtubules so cells cannot complete mitosis during cell division. As a result, the cancer cell either does not divide at all or divides only once, resulting in two daughter cells that cannot continue to divide.

TOPOISOMERASE INHIBITORS. Topoisomerase is an enzyme needed for DNA synthesis and cell division. It nicks and straightens the DNA helix, allowing the DNA to be copied, and then reattaches the DNA together. Topoisomerase inhibitors prevent these processes, causing DNA breakage and cell death.

MISCELLANEOUS CHEMOTHERAPEUTIC AGENTS. The actions of other chemotherapeutic agents do not fit any of the chemotherapy categories and include the following:

- Inhibition of important enzyme systems
- Competition for important substances in metabolic pathways

COMBINATION CHEMOTHERAPY. Successful cancer chemotherapy involves giving more than one specific anticancer drug in a timed manner. This technique is called **combination chemotherapy.** Using more than one drug is much more effective in killing cancer cells than using a single agent. However, the damage caused to normal tissues also increases with combination chemotherapy.

The selection of drugs is based on known tumor sensitivity to the drugs and the degree of side effects expected. For example, most chemotherapy drugs suppress bone marrow activity and immune function to some degree, but some agents cause more immunosuppression than others. There is also variation in the timing of drug-induced immunosuppression.

The time when bone marrow activity and white blood cell counts are at their lowest levels after chemotherapy is the **nadir.** The nadir occurs at different times for different drugs (see Table 28-6). For instance, the expected nadir for cytarabine is 5 to 7 days and for mitomycin C is about 4 weeks. To reduce immunosuppression, combination chemotherapy avoids using drugs with nadirs that occur at or near the same time.

TREATMENT ISSUES

DRUG DOSAGE. The doses of most chemotherapy agents are calculated according to the type of cancer and the client's size. Most commonly, calculations are based on milligrams per square meter of total body surface area (TBSA). This measure uses the client's height and weight

TABLE 28-6 Categories of Chemotherapeutic Agents

Generic Name	Usual Dose	Nadir
Antimetabolites		
Capecitabine (Xeloda)	2500 mg/m^2	Not reported
Cladribine (Leustatin)	0.09 mg/kg/day	10-14 days
**Cytarabine (Cytosar, ara-C)	100-300 mg/m^2	4-7 days
Floxuridine (FUDR)	0.1-0.6 mg/kg	4-7 days
*5-Fluorouracil (Adrucil, Efudex, Fluoroplex)	300-750 mg/m^2	9-14 days
Fludarabine (Fludara)	25 mg/m^2	3-25 days
*Gemcitabine (Gemzar)	1000-1250 mg/m^2	7-12 days
6-Mercaptopurine (Purinethol)	80-100 mg/m^2	5-40 days
**Methotrexate (Mexate, Folex)	3.3 mg/m^2	10-14 days
Pentostatin (Nipent)	4 mg/m^2	3-10 days
Raltitrexed (Tomudex)	3 mg/m^2	7-10 days
6-Thioguanine (Lanvis)	2-3 mg/kg	1-4 wk
Trimetrexate (Neutrexin)	45 mg/m^2	10-14 days
Antitumor Antibiotics		
Bleomycin (Blenoxane)	10-20 units/m^2	7-14 days
**Dactinomycin (Cosmegen)	0.4-0.6 mg/m^2	14-21 days
**Daunorubicin (Cerubidine)	30-60 mg/m^2	10-14 days
**Doxorubicin (Adriamycin, Rubex)	50-80 mg/m^2	10-15 days
**Epirubicin (Ellence)	100-120 mg/m^2	10-14 days
**Idarubicin (Idamycin)	12-25 mg/m^2	10-14 days
*Mitomycin C (Mutamycin)	10-20 mg/m^2	21-50 days
*Mitoxantrone (Novantrone)	12-14 mg/m^2	7-10 days
**Plicamycin (Mithracin)	0.025-0.03 mg/m^2	10-12 days
Alkylating Agents		
Altretamine (Hexalen)	260 mg/m^2	3-4 weeks
**Busulfan (Myleran)	1-8 mg	14-21 days
**Carboplatin (Paraplatin)	360 mg/m^2	21-28 days
**Carmustine (BiCNU)	200-250 mg/m^2	4-6 weeks
Chlorambucil (Leukeran)	1-4 mg/m^2	28 days
**Cisplatin (Platinol)	25-120 mg/m^2	10-20 days
Cyclophosphamide (Cytoxan, Procytox)	50-500 mg/m^2	7-14 days
Alkylating Agents—cont'd		
Estramustine (Emcyt)	14 mg/kg/day	≈4 wk
**Ifosfamide (IFEX)	1.2 g/m^2	10 days
**Lomustine (CCNU, CeeNU)	130 mg/m^2	4-6 wk
**Mechlorethamine (Mustargen)	0.2-0.3 mg/kg	10-14 days
**Melphalan (Alkeran)	1-6 mg/m^2	14-21 days
Oxaliplatin (Eloxatin)	50-85 mg/m^2	5-14 days
**Streptozocin (Zanosar)	500-1500 mg/m^2	14 days
Temozolomide (Temodar)	150-200 mg/m^2	21-28 days
Thiotepa (Thioplex)	0.3-0.8 mg/kg	15-30 days
Antimitotics		
*Docetaxel (Taxotere)	60-100 mg/m^2	8-10 days
*Paclitaxel (Taxol)	100-250 mg/m^2	8-11 days
Vinblastine (Velban, Velbe, Velsar)	5-10 mg/m^2	5-11 days
Vincristine (Oncovin, leurocristine, VCR)	0.5-2 mg/m^2	7 days
Vindesine (DAVA, Eldisine)	2 mg/m^2	2-7 days
Vinorelbine (Navelbine)	30 mg/m^2	7-10 days
Topoisomerase Inhibitors		
*Etoposide (VP16, VePesid)	50-100 mg/m^2	8-10 days
*Irinotecan (Camptosar)	125-150 mg/m^2	18-25 days
*Teniposide (Vumon, VM-26)	100-180 mg/m^2	8-10 days
*Topotecan (Hycamtin)	1.5 mg/m^2	7-14 days
Other Agents		
*Asparaginase (Elspar, Kidrolase)	200-1000 International Units/kg	4-10 days
Bexarotene (Targretin)	300 mg/m^2	4-8 wk
Dacarbazine (DTIC)	75-250 mg/m^2	10-14 days
Hydroxyurea (Hydrea)	25 mg/kg	4-7 days
Leucovorin (Wellcovorin)	10 mg/m^2	N/A
Levamisole (Ergamisol)	50 mg	N/A
**Procarbazine (Matulane, Natulan✱)	100-300 mg	14-28 days
Thalidomide (Thalomid)	100-300 mg	N/A

Facts and Comparisons. (2004). *Drug facts and comparisons* (58th ed.). St. Louis: Author.
*, Moderately emetogenic; **, highly emetogenic

and is calculated as follows: the height of the client (in centimeters) is multiplied by his or her weight (in kilograms), and the result is divided by 10,000 (moving the decimal point four spaces to the left). For example, a woman who is 68 inches tall (173 cm) and weighs 143 pounds (65 kg) has a TBSA of 11,245 cm^2, or 1.12 m^2.

DRUG SCHEDULE. Chemotherapy drugs are given on a regular basis and are timed to maximize cancer cell kill and minimize damage to normal cells. The schedule may vary somewhat to accommodate a client's response to therapy, but chemotherapy is usually scheduled every 3 to 4 weeks for a specified number of times (on average, 6 to 12 times). The entire planned schedule is the *course* of chemotherapy.

DRUG ADMINISTRATION. Most chemotherapy drugs are given IV, although other routes may be used for specific cancers (Table 28-7). The techniques and care needs for different routes are described with the specific cancer type most commonly associated with the specific administration route. Chapter 17 describes the types of venous access devices, many of which are used for chemotherapy.

TABLE 28-7 Routes of Chemotherapy Administration

Route	Typical Cancer
Oral	Hodgkin's lymphoma Leukemia (maintenance phase) Small cell lung cancer
Intravenous	Most solid tumors, leukemias Lymphomas
Intra-arterial	Hepatic tumors (primary and metastatic) Head and neck cancers
Isolated limb perfusion	Cancers confined to a limb ▪ Osteogenic sarcoma ▪ Ewing's sarcoma ▪ Rhabdomyosarcoma ▪ Regional melanoma
Intracavitary	
▪ Intraperitoneal	Ovarian cancer
▪ Intraventricular	Brain tumors
▪ Intrathecal	Brain tumors Prophylaxis for acute lymphocytic leukemia
▪ Intravesical	Bladder tumors

TABLE 28-8 Chemotherapy Tissue Vesicants and Irritants

Vesicants	Irritants
Amsacrine	Bleomycin
Dactinomycin	Carmustine
Daunorubicin	Cisplatin
Doxorubicin	Dacarbazine
Epirubicin	Etoposide
Esorubicin	Fluorouracil
Idarubicin	Mitoxantrone
Mechlorethamine	Paclitaxel
Menogaril	Plicamycin
Mitomycin C	Streptozocin
Pyrazofurin	Teniposide
Vinblastine	
Vincristine	
Vindesine	
Vinorelbine	

The IV route is the most preferred route for chemotherapy because the effects of the drugs are rapid and because many of these agents are irritating or damaging to tissues. A major complication of IV infusion is **extravasation,** or the movement of the IV needle so the drug leaks into the surrounding tissues. When the drugs given are **vesicants** (chemicals that cause tissue damage on direct contact), the results of extravasation can include pain, infection, and tissue loss. Surgical intervention is sometimes needed. Table 28-8 lists known vesicant and irritant chemotherapy drugs.

The most important nursing intervention for extravasation is prevention. Small extravasations resolve without extensive treatment if less than 0.5 mL of the drug has leaked into the tissues. If a larger amount has leaked, extensive tissue damage occurs and surgical intervention may be necessary. Immediate treatment depends on the specific drug. With some drugs, cold compresses to the area are prescribed; for other agents, warm compresses are used. Antidotes may be injected into the site of extravasation. Consult with the oncologist and pharmacist to determine the specific antidote needed for the extravasated drug. Chart 28-3 outlines the best practices for documenting an extravasation event.

Most chemotherapy drugs are absorbed through the skin and mucous membranes. As a result, the health care workers who prepare or give these drugs (especially nurses and pharmacists) are at risk for absorbing them. Even at low doses, long-term exposure to chemotherapy drugs can affect health. Use extreme caution and wear protective clothing whenever preparing, giving, or disposing of chemotherapy drugs. The Occupational Safety and Health Administration (OSHA) and the Oncology Nursing Society have established practice guidelines and protective standards.

CHART 28-3

BEST PRACTICE for
Documentation of Extravasation

- Document the date and time when extravasation was suspected or identified.
- Document the date and time when the infusion was started.
- Record the time when the infusion was stopped.
- Document the exact contents of the infusion fluid and the volume of fluid infused.
- Document the estimated amount of fluid extravasated.
- Document the needle type and size.
- Diagram the exact insertion site.
- Indicate on the diagram the location and number of venipuncture attempts.
- Record the time between the extravasation and the last full blood return.
- Identify all agents administered in the previous 24 hours through this site (list agent administered, dosage and volume, and order of administration).
- Take and record the client's vital signs.
- Take a photograph of the site.
- Document the administration of neutralizing or antidote agents.
- Document the application of compresses.
- Document other nursing interventions.
- Record the client's responses to nursing interventions.
- Document the physician notification (including the time).
- Document the written and oral instructions given to the client about follow-up care.
- Document any consultation request.
- Sign the documentation.

SIDE EFFECTS OF CHEMOTHERAPY

Serious side effects occur with aggressive chemotherapy, including **alopecia** (hair loss), nausea and vomiting, open sores on mucous membranes **(mucositis),** and many skin changes. Other distressing side effects include anxiety, sleep disturbance, altered bowel elimination, and decreased mobility.

Drug therapy is used to reduce the severity of these symptoms. Nonpharmacologic nursing interventions include massage, guided imagery, Reiki, aromatherapy, and other forms of complementary therapy. Many clients have found these interventions to be helpful in reducing distressing side effects (see the Evidence-Based Practice for Nursing Box below).

EVIDENCE-BASED PRACTICE for Nursing

Massage helps manage cancer treatment symptoms

Smith, M., et al. (2002). Outcomes of therapeutic massage for hospitalized cancer patients. *Journal of Nursing Scholarship, 34*(3), 257-263.

This prospective, quasiexperimental study examined the effect of therapeutic massage on the perception of pain, sleep quality, anxiety, and treatment-related symptom distress among clients hospitalized for cancer treatment. The study used a two-group design with one group of 20 subjects receiving the therapeutic massage intervention of 15 to 30 minutes of light Swedish massage techniques performed by a registered nurse who was also a certified massage therapist. Each subject in the intervention group received three massages during 1 week of hospitalization. The control group of 21 subjects received a nurse interaction of 20 minutes of deliberate focused communication with the same nurse who provided massage to the treatment group. Pre- and post-testing of the subjects' perceptions of pain (numerical rating scale; 4-point Likert-type scale), sleep patterns (Verran and Snyder-Halpern Sleep Scale), symptom distress (Symptom Distress Scale), and anxiety (State-Trait Anxiety Inventory) were performed for all subjects and analyzed using a repeated measures factorial analysis of variance.

The mean scores for pain, symptom distress, and anxiety improved from baseline for subjects in the treatment group. Only anxiety improved over baseline for subjects in the nursing interaction group. Neither group experienced improvement in sleep quality.

Level of Evidence: 5—Well-conducted case control study.

Critique. The study provides data to support nonpharmacologic interventions to improve the comfort of clients undergoing cancer therapy. The sample was small, nonrandomized, and mostly male (95%), limiting generalizability. Except for the dimension of pain, the measurement instruments used had well-established validity and reliability. Several strengths of the study included that the intervention was performed by one individual and the study controlled for the issue of attention.

Nursing Implications. The nursing shortage has reduced the amount of time available for nurses to use massage as an intervention. Few well-designed studies have been performed to examine the benefit of therapeutic massage as an intervention for clients with cancer. This study supports the use of this intervention by nurses in the hospital setting.

TABLE 28-9 Agents Used for Chemoprotection

Agent	Cytotoxic Problem Prevented
Amifostine (Ethyol)	Xerostomia
Dexrazoxane (Zinecard)	Cardiomyopathy
Mesna (MESNEX)	Hemorrhagic cystitis
Pamidronate (Aredia)	Skeletal complications

The side effects on the hematopoietic (blood-producing) system can be life threatening and are the most common reason for changing the dosage or schedule. The suppressive effects on the blood-forming cells of bone marrow cause anemia, immunosuppression, and **thrombocytopenia** (decreased numbers of platelets).

One approach to decrease the impact of chemotherapy on normal tissues is to give the agents with drugs that protect specific healthy cells. These drugs, called **cytoprotectants,** have little effect on cancer cells but do protect some normal cells (Table 28-9).

NURSING CARE OF CLIENTS UNDERGOING CHEMOTHERAPY

The major care issue during chemotherapy is managing the distressing symptoms occurring with therapy. For some clients, the symptoms are so unpleasant that they stop treatment. Chart 28-4 lists NIC interventions for clients undergoing chemotherapy.

ALOPECIA. Clients receiving cancer chemotherapy often have whole-body hair loss. Some drugs may cause only thinning of the scalp hair. Others cause a more complete hair loss.

Reassure clients that hair loss is temporary. Hair regrowth usually begins about 1 month after completion of chemother-

CHART 28-4

NIC INTERVENTION ACTIVITIES for The Client with Cancer

Chemotherapy Management: *Assisting the client and family to understand the action and minimize side effects of antineoplastic agents*

- Monitor for side effects and toxic effects of chemotherapeutic agents.
- Provide information to client and family on how antineoplastic drugs work on cancer cells.
- Instruct client and family on ways to prevent infection, such as avoiding crowds and using good hygiene and handwashing techniques.
- Instruct client to promptly report fever, chills, nosebleeds, excessive bruising, and tarry stools.
- Instruct client and family to avoid the use of aspirin products.
- Administer antiemetic drugs for nausea and vomiting.
- Teach the client relaxation and imagery techniques to use before, during, and after treatments, as appropriate.
- Ensure adequate fluid intake to prevent dehydration and electrolyte imbalance.
- Monitor the effectiveness of measures to control nausea and vomiting.
- Teach client and family to monitor for signs and symptoms of stomatitis.
- Instruct client on proper oral hygiene techniques.
- Inform client that hair loss is expected, as determined by type of chemotherapeutic agent used.
- Assist client in obtaining a wig or other head-covering device, as appropriate.
- Provide nutritious, appetizing foods of client's choice.
- Monitor nutritional status and weight.
- Discuss with client the possibility of sterility and other reproductive system impairments, as appropriate.
- Instruct long-term survivors and their families of the possibility of second malignancies and the importance of reporting increased susceptibility to infection, fatigue, or bleeding.

NIC intervention activities selected from Dochterman, J.M., & Bulechek, G.M. (Eds.). (2004). *Nursing interventions classification (NIC)* (4th ed.). St. Louis: Mosby.

apy. Inform the client that the new hair may differ from the original hair in color, texture, and thickness. No known treatment completely prevents alopecia.

Assist clients in selecting a type of head covering that suits their income and lifestyle. High-quality wigs are expensive but can look very much like the client's own hair. Many local units of the American Cancer Society offer wigs that other clients have used and then donated to be lent to other clients with cancer. Clients can disguise hair loss with caps, scarves, and turbans.

NAUSEA AND VOMITING. Chemotherapy-induced nausea and vomiting arises from a variety of local and central nervous system mechanisms. Most chemotherapy drugs are **emetogenic** (vomiting inducing) to some degree, depending on the dose. Most drugs induce nausea and vomiting when the drug is given and for 1 to 2 days afterward. Some drugs, such as cisplatin, induce delayed nausea and vomiting that can continue as long as 5 to 7 days after receiving it. Clients who have chemotherapy-related nausea and vomiting during one round of chemotherapy may begin to have the same symptoms before the next round as a result of sheer anticipation.

CONSIDERATION FOR OLDER ADULTS

At times, older clients have received lower doses of chemotherapy drugs because it was thought the older person would not be able to tolerate the side effects of nausea and vomiting. Research indicates that older clients do not have greater nausea and vomiting than do younger clients. Therefore their chemotherapy regimens should not be altered on this basis alone.

Drug Therapy. Many antiemetics are available to relieve nausea and vomiting. These drugs vary in the side effects they produce and how well they control chemotherapy-induced nausea and vomiting. One or more antiemetics are usually given before and after chemotherapy. Antiemetic drugs commonly used to control chemotherapy-induced nausea and vomiting are listed in Chart 28-5. Client response to antiemetic therapy is highly variable, and the drug combinations must be individualized for best effect. Antiemetic drugs vary in cost.

CHART 28-5

DRUG THERAPY for Chemotherapy-Induced Nausea and Vomiting

Drug	Usual Dosage	Side Effects
Serotonin Antagonists		
Ondansetron (Zofran)	8 mg q8h	Constipation, diarrhea, fever, light-headedness, drowsiness
Granisetron Kytril)	1 mg q12h	Fever, dysrhythmias, chest pain, fainting
Dolasetron (Anzemet)	1.8 mg/kg	
Palonosetron (Aloxi)	0.25 mg	
CNS Depressants		
Trimethobenzamide (Tigan, Benzacot, Arrestin, T-Gen)	200 mg three or four times daily	Drowsiness, blurred vision, dizziness, diarrhea, headache, mental depression, tremors
Benzodiazepines		
Lorazepam (Ativan)	1-3 mg twice or three times daily	Amnesia, bradycardia, hypotension, muscle weakness, anemia
Phenothiazines		
Prochlorperazine (Compazine, Stemetil✱)	10-20 mg four times daily	Hypotension, CNS depression, extrapyramidal reactions, dry mouth, blurred vision
Chlorpromazine (Thorazine, Ormazine)	25-50 mg four times daily	Hypotension, CNS depression, extrapyramidal reactions, dry mouth, blurred vision
Antihistamines		
Diphenhydramine (Benadryl)	25-50 mg four times daily	Drowsiness, dry mouth, hypotension
Corticosteroids		
Dexamethasone (Decadron)	5-10 mg daily	Fluid and electrolyte imbalances, immunosuppression, GI bleeding, bruising, cushingoid symptoms
Prokinetic Agents		
Metoclopramide (Reglan)	20-40 mg four times daily	Drowsiness, dry mouth, diarrhea, depression, dysrhythmias
Cannabinoids		
Dronabinol (Marinol)	2.5-10 mg twice or three times daily	Potential dependency mood changes, drowsiness, tachycardia, increased appetite

CNS, Central nervous system; *GI*, gastrointestinal.

Complementary and Alternative Therapies. Assist the client with nausea and vomiting to achieve comfort through nonpharmacologic means along with antiemetics. Music, progressive muscle relaxation, guided imagery, acupressure, or distraction may help reduce anxiety and relieve nausea and vomiting. Assess the client for complications resulting from excessive vomiting, such as dehydration and electrolyte imbalances.

MUCOSITIS. Clients undergoing chemotherapy often develop *mucositis* (sores in mucous membranes) of the entire gastrointestinal (GI) tract, especially in the mouth (stomatitis). Normally, the lining of the GI tract undergoes rapid cell division and quickly replaces cells. In chemotherapy, mucous membrane cells are killed more rapidly than they are replaced, resulting in sore formation. Mouth sores are painful and interfere with eating. Chart 28-6 lists the best practices for clients with mucositis.

Frequent mouth assessment and oral hygiene are key in managing stomatitis and mucositis. Stress the importance of good and frequent oral hygiene, including tooth cleaning and mouth rinsing. Because most clients with mucositis also have bone marrow suppression and are at risk for bleeding, they must take care to avoid traumatizing the oral mucosa. Instruct clients to use a soft-bristled toothbrush or disposable mouth sponges and to avoid using dental floss and water pressure gum cleaners (e.g., a WaterPik). Encourage clients to rinse the mouth with plain water or saline every hour while awake. Teach them to avoid mouthwashes that contain alcohol or other drying agents that may further irritate the mucosa.

Oral hygiene equipment must be kept clean. Remind clients not to share toothbrushes with anyone. Toothbrushes can be cleaned daily by running them through a home dishwasher or by rinsing them with a concentrated solution of liquid bleach or hydrogen peroxide.

Many compounds are available for pain relief from stomatitis or mucositis. Many hospitals offer their own special "swish and spit" mixtures, which contain a local anesthetic combined with anti-inflammatory agents. Tell the client that these mixtures are not to be swallowed.

CHART 28-6

BEST PRACTICE for
Mouth Care for Clients with Mucositis

- Examine the client's mouth (including the roof, under the tongue, and between the teeth and cheek) every 4 hours.
- Document the location, size, and character of fissures, blisters, sores, or drainage.
- Get an order to obtain specimens of sores or drainage for culture.
- Brush the teeth and tongue with a soft-bristled brush or sponges every 8 hours.
- Rinse the mouth with a solution of one-half peroxide and one-half normal saline every 12 hours.
- Avoid the use of alcohol or glycerin-based mouthwashes.
- Administer antimicrobial medications as prescribed.
- Administer topical analgesic medications as prescribed or as needed.
- Help the conscious client to "swish and spit" room-temperature tap water or normal saline as needed.
- Apply petrolatum jelly to the client's lips after each episode of mouth care and as needed.
- Assist the client in using "artificial saliva" as needed, if prescribed.
- Assist the client in menu choices to avoid spicy or hard food.
- Offer complete mouth care before and after every meal.

BONE MARROW SUPPRESSION. Bone marrow suppression reduces the circulating number of leukocytes, erythrocytes, and platelets. Decreased leukocyte numbers, especially neutrophils **(neutropenia),** cause immunosuppression. Decreased erythrocytes and platelets cause hypoxia, fatigue, and an increased tendency to bleed.

Immunosuppression places the client at extreme risk for infection and is the major dose-limiting side effect of cancer chemotherapy. Most chemotherapy drugs suppress bone marrow function to some degree and contribute to the life-threatening complication of neutropenia. This problem decreases the client's protective responses to organism invasion. The severity and duration of the impairment are related directly to the dosage of specific chemotherapeutic agents. This impairment is temporary, with good recovery of protection within weeks after therapy completion. However, the seriousness of potential infection complications makes this problem a major treatment concern. The infectious processes that occur most commonly are fungal, bacterial, and some residual viral breakthrough. *Most of the infections that develop in a client with neutropenia result from overgrowth of the client's own normal flora.*

Decreased numbers of circulating erythrocytes **(anemia)** and platelets **(thrombocytopenia)** also result from the bone marrow suppression caused by some chemotherapy drugs. Anemia causes clients to feel fatigued, and some tissues are hypoxic. The cardiac and respiratory systems may not be able to maintain adequate oxygenation. Thrombocytopenia increases the risk for excessive bleeding. When the platelet count is less than 50,000/mm^3, any small trauma can lead to prolonged bleeding. Clients with fewer than 20,000 platelets/mm^3 may have spontaneous and uncontrollable bleeding requiring transfusion therapy.

Drug Therapy. Immunosuppression can be managed with the use of biological response modifiers (BRMs) to stimulate bone marrow production of immune system cells. Although not appropriate for all types of cancer, this supportive treatment can reduce the risk for infection during chemotherapy. However, BRMs are expensive and not consistently covered by insurance. This treatment is discussed under Immunotherapy on p. 499.

Complementary and Alternative Therapies. Many clients with cancer use complementary and alternative therapies to boost immune function and prevent infection. Common therapies include shark cartilage, Echinacea, and megadoses of vitamin C. Although benefit has not yet been determined in clinical trials, the use of these therapies does not appear to have harmful effects.

Protection from Infection. Chart 28-7 lists the best practices for infection prevention among immunosuppressed clients. Good handwashing before contact with the client is essential for prevention of infection. Health care workers must use aseptic technique when performing any invasive procedure.

Many clients remain at home during periods of immunosuppression. Teach clients and family members precautions to reduce the risk for infection (Chart 28-8).

Provide a safe hospital environment for clients with thrombocytopenia. Teach them how to avoid excessive bleeding when they are discharged before the platelet count has returned to normal. Chart 28-9 lists the best practices for bleeding precautions during hospitalization. Teach clients how to prevent bleeding and what to do if bleeding occurs (Chart 28-10).

Critical Thinking Challenge

The client is a 65-year-old man receiving combination chemotherapy for cancer. He is a very active man who works in his garden daily, plays tennis three times each week, bowls weekly, works at his church as a counselor, and tutors second graders in reading. He will receive six rounds of cyclophosphamide, doxorubicin, vincristine, and prednisone. He is concerned about his appearance, especially alopecia, and what activities he can continue to perform throughout his course of chemotherapy. He also wants to know if he can still have sex with his wife during the months he will be receiving treatment.

1. What will you tell this client about hair loss?
2. Which activities should this client **not** perform during the week of nadir? Why?
3. Which activities are safe for this client to perform during the week in which nadir is reached? Why?
4. What modifications should this client make (if any) for sexual intercourse? Why?

evolve For suggested answer guidelines, go to http://evolve.elsevier.com/Iggy/.

CHART 28-7

BEST PRACTICE for
Care of the Client with Neutropenia

- Place the client in a private room whenever possible.
- Use good handwashing technique before touching the client or any of the client's belongings.
- Ensure that the client's room and bathroom are cleaned at least once each day.
- Do not use supplies from common areas for immunosuppressed clients. For example, keep a sleeve or box of paper cups in the client's room, and do not share this box with any other client. Other articles include drinking straws, plastic knives and forks, dressing materials, gloves, and bandages.
- Limit the number of health care personnel entering the client's room.
- Monitor vital signs every 4 hours; note minor temperature elevation, which may suggest early sepsis.
- Inspect the client's mouth at least every 8 hours.
- Inspect the client's skin and mucous membranes (especially the anal area) for the presence of fissures and abscesses at least every 8 hours.
- Inspect open areas, such as IV sites, every 4 hours for manifestations of infection.
- Change wound dressings daily.
- Obtain specimens of all suspicious areas for culture, and promptly notify the physician.
- Assist the client in performing coughing and deep-breathing exercises.
- Encourage activity at a level appropriate for the client's current health status.
- Change IV tubing daily.
- Keep frequently used equipment in the room for use with this client only (e.g., blood pressure cuff, stethoscope, thermometer).
- Limit visitors to healthy adults.
- Use strict aseptic technique for all invasive procedures.
- Monitor the white blood cell count, especially the absolute neutrophil count (ANC), daily.
- Avoid the use of indwelling urinary catheters.
- Keep fresh flowers and potted plants out of the client's room.
- Teach the client to eat a low-bacteria diet.

CHART 28-8

CLIENT EDUCATION GUIDE
Prevention of Infection

- Avoid crowds and other large gatherings of people who might be ill.
- Do not share personal toilet articles, such as toothbrushes, toothpaste, washcloths, or deodorant sticks, with others.
- If possible, bathe daily.
- Wash the armpits, groin, genitals, and anal area at least twice a day with an antimicrobial soap.
- Clean your toothbrush daily by either running it through the dishwasher or rinsing it in liquid laundry bleach.
- Wash your hands thoroughly with an antimicrobial soap before you eat or drink, after touching a pet, after shaking hands with anyone, as soon as you come home from any outing, and after using the toilet.
- Eat a low-bacteria diet, and avoid salads, raw fruit and vegetables, undercooked meat, pepper, and paprika.
- Wash dishes between use with hot, sudsy water, or use a dishwasher.
- Do not drink water that has been standing for longer than 15 minutes.
- Do not reuse cups and glasses without washing.
- Do not change pet litter boxes.
- Take your temperature at least once a day.
- Report any of the following signs or symptoms of infection to your physician immediately:
    - Temperature greater than 100° F (38° C)
    - Persistent cough (with or without sputum)
    - Pus or foul-smelling drainage from any open skin area or normal body opening
    - Presence of a boil or abscess
    - Urine that is cloudy or foul smelling or that causes burning on urination
- Take all prescribed medications.
- Do not dig in the garden or work with houseplants.

CHART 28-9

BEST PRACTICE for
Care of the Client with Thrombocytopenia

- Handle the client gently.
- Use a lift sheet when moving and positioning the client in bed.
- Avoid intramuscular injections and venipunctures.
- When injections or venipunctures are necessary, use the smallest-gauge needle for the task.
- Apply firm pressure to the needle stick site for 10 minutes or until the site no longer oozes blood.
- Apply ice to areas of trauma.
- Test all urine and stool for the presence of occult blood.
- Observe IV sites every 2 hours for bleeding.
- Avoid trauma to rectal tissues:
    - Do not take temperatures rectally.
    - Do not administer enemas.
    - Administer well-lubricated suppositories and with caution.
    - Advise the client not to have anal intercourse.
- Measure the client's abdominal girth daily.
- Use an electric razor.
- Teach the client to avoid mouth trauma by:
    - Using soft-bristled toothbrush or tooth sponges
    - Not flossing
    - Avoiding dental work, especially extractions
    - Avoiding hard foods
    - Making certain that dentures fit and do not rub
- Encourage the client not to blow the nose or insert objects into the nose.
- Instruct the client to avoid contact sports.
- Advise the client to wear shoes with firm soles whenever he or she is ambulating.

CHART 28-10

CLIENT EDUCATION GUIDE
The Client at Risk for Bleeding

- Use an electric razor.
- Use a soft-bristled toothbrush, and do not floss.
- Do not have dental work performed without consulting your doctor.
- Do not take aspirin or any aspirin-containing products. Read the label to be sure that the product does not contain aspirin or salicylates.
- Do not participate in contact sports or any activity likely to result in your being bumped, scratched, or scraped.
- If you are bumped, apply ice to the site for at least 1 hour.
- Notify your doctor if you:
  - Experience an injury and persistent bleeding results
  - Have excessive menstrual bleeding
  - See blood in your urine or bowel movement
- Avoid anal intercourse.
- Take a stool softener to prevent straining during a bowel movement.
- Do not use enemas or rectal suppositories.
- Avoid bending over at the waist.
- Do not wear clothing or shoes that are tight or that rub.
- Avoid blowing your nose or placing objects in your nose. If you must blow your nose, do so gently without blocking either nasal passage.

Hormonal Manipulation

RATIONALE FOR CANCER TREATMENT

Hormones are naturally occurring chemicals secreted by endocrine (ductless) glands and picked up by capillaries. Once in the bloodstream, hormones circulate to all body areas but exert their effects only on their specific target tissues. Some hormones make hormone-sensitive tumors grow more rapidly. Some tumors require specific hormones to divide. Thus decreasing the amount of these hormones to hormone-sensitive tumors can slow the cancer growth rate.

MECHANISM OF ACTION

HORMONE AGONISTS. Hormonal manipulation can help control some types of cancer for many years. Usually, this therapy does not lead to a cure. The endocrine system usually maintains a delicate hormone balance. When a large amount of one hormone is given, it upsets the balance and disturbs the uptake of other hormones. If a tumor depends on hormone A for growth and a large quantity of hormone B (similar to A) is given to the client, hormone B will interfere with the tumor's uptake of hormone A or will limit the amount of hormone A produced. As a result, tumor growth is slowed and survival time increases. Table 28-10 lists the drugs commonly used in hormonal manipulation for cancer therapy.

HORMONE ANTAGONISTS. Some drugs are hormone antagonists that compete with natural hormones at the receptor sites. Often, they are antibodies specific to the receptor. When hormone antagonists are given, they bind to the specific hormone receptor on or in the tumor cell and prevent the needed hormone from binding to the receptor. If a tumor needs a certain hormone to grow and the hormone can enter or activate the cell only through a receptor, hormone antagonists can slow down tumor growth.

TABLE 28-10 Common Agents Used for Hormonal Manipulation of Cancer

Type of Agent	Example
Hormone Agonists	
Androgen	Calusterone Danocrine Fluoxymesterone Testosterone Testolactone
Estrogen	Conjugated estrogens Diethylstilbestrol Ethinyl estradiol
Progestin	Medroxyprogesterone Megestrol
Luteinizing-hormone releasing hormone (LHRH)	Leuprolide Goserelin
Hormone Antagonists	
Antiandrogens	Bicalutamide Nilutamide Fluoxymesterone Flutamide Cyproterone acetate
Antiprogestins	Mifepristone
Antiestrogens	Droloxifene Idoxifene Tamoxifen Toremifene Trioxifene mesylate Zindoxifene
Gonadotropin-releasing hormone (GnRH)	Abarelix
Aromatase Inhibitors	Anastrozole Exemestane Fulvestrant Letrozole

HORMONE INHIBITORS. A new class of drugs used for hormonal therapy in breast cancer is the aromatase inhibitors. Aromatase is an enzyme that leads to the production of estrogen in the adrenal gland. Aromatase inhibitors prevent this production and reduce blood levels of estrogens (see Table 28-10).

SIDE EFFECTS OF HORMONE THERAPY

Androgens and the antiestrogen receptor drugs cause masculinizing effects in women. Chest and facial hair may develop, menstrual periods stop, and breast tissue shrinks. Clients may have some fluid retention. For men and women receiving androgens, acne may develop, hypercalcemia is common, and liver dysfunction may occur with prolonged therapy. Women receiving estrogens or progestins have irregular but heavy menses, fluid retention, and breast tenderness. Male and female clients who take estrogen or progestins are at increased risk for deep vein thrombosis.

Feminine manifestations often appear in men who take estrogens, progestins, or antiandrogen receptor drugs. Facial hair thins or disappears, facial skin becomes smoother, body fat is redistributed, and **gynecomastia** (breast development in men) can occur. Testicular and penile atrophy also occurs to some degree. Although sexual function may continue, achieving and maintaining an erection is much more difficult.

Immunotherapy: Biological Response Modifiers

Biological response modifiers (BRMs) modify the client's biologic responses to tumor cells. The BRMs in current use as cancer therapy are cytokines, which are small protein hormones made by white blood cells. Cytokines made by macrophages, neutrophils, eosinophils, and monocytes are *monokines*; cytokines produced by lymphocytes (especially the T-lymphocytes) are *lymphokines*. Cytokines generally make the immune system work better (see Chapter 23).

RATIONALE FOR CANCER TREATMENT

Cytokines enhance the immune system. Immune function plays an important role in cancer prevention (see Chapters 23 and 27). Cytokines and other BRMs work as a cancer treatment by stimulating the immune system to recognize cancer cells and take actions to eliminate or destroy them. Some BRMs may also be useful in a supporting role. Other BRMs (colony-stimulating factors) stimulate faster recovery of bone marrow function after treatment-induced suppression.

MECHANISM OF ACTION

The activity of cytokines is similar to that of any other peptide hormone in that one cell produces and secretes a cytokine, which then exerts its effects on other cells of the immune system. The cells responding to the cytokine may be right next to the cytokine-secreting cell or quite remote from it. Cells that change their activity in response to the cytokine are *responder* cells. For a responder cell to respond to a cytokine, the membrane of the responder cell must have a specific receptor for the cytokine. The cytokine binds to this receptor and changes the activity of the responder cell.

BIOLOGICAL RESPONSE MODIFIERS FOR CANCER THERAPY. Two types of BRMs are used as cancer therapy: interleukins (ILs) and interferons (INFs). Some agents can stimulate specific immune system cells to attack and destroy cancer cells; other agents block cancer cell access to an essential function or nutrient.

Interleukins. More than 25 ILs have been identified. Some are produced through recombinant DNA technology. ILs help different immune system cells recognize and destroy abnormal body cells. In particular, IL-1, -2, and -6 appear to "charge up" the immune system and enhance attacks on cancer cells by macrophages, natural killer (NK) cells, and tumor-infiltrating lymphocytes.

Interferons. Interferons are cell-produced proteins that can protect noninfected cells from viral infection and replication. There are many types of INFs. Although all of them are similar, each type has unique functions. The most completely characterized INF is INF alfa-2b.

Different body cells can produce INF, with leukocytes producing the most. INFs also are commercially produced by recombinant DNA technology. Cancer-related functions of INF include the ability to do the following:

- Slow down tumor cell division
- Stimulate the growth and activation of NK cells

TABLE 28-11 Colony-Stimulating Factors

Agent	Cell Type Affected	Indications
Sargramostim (Leukine, Prokine)	All granulocytes ▪ Neutrophils ▪ Eosinophils Monocytes Macrophages	Chemotherapy-induced leukopenia
Filgrastim (Neupogen) Pegfilgrastim (Neulasta)	Neutrophils	Chemotherapy-induced neutropenia
Epoetin alfa (Epogen, Procrit) Darbepoetin alfa (Aranesp)	Erythrocytes	Chemotherapy-induced anemia Chemotherapy-induced fatigue Anemia induced by renal failure
Oprelvekin (Neumega)	Platelets	Chemotherapy-induced thrombocytopenia

- Help cancer cells resume a more normal appearance and revert to their previous normal cell features
- Inhibit the expression of oncogenes

INFs have been effective to some degree in the treatment of malignant melanoma, hairy cell leukemia, renal cell carcinoma, ovarian cancer, and cutaneous T-cell lymphoma.

BIOLOGICAL RESPONSE MODIFIERS FOR CANCER SUPPORT. BRMs used for supportive therapy during cancer treatment are the colony-stimulating factors (Table 28-11). These factors induce more rapid recovery of the bone marrow after suppression by chemotherapy. This effect has two benefits. First, when bone marrow suppression is shortened or less severe, clients are less at risk for life-threatening infections and anemia. Second, because the colony-stimulating factors allow more rapid bone marrow recovery, clients can receive their chemotherapy on time and may even be able to tolerate higher doses, improving the curative outcome of chemotherapy. These agents must be used cautiously in clients with leukemia or lymphoma.

SIDE EFFECTS OF BIOLOGICAL RESPONSE MODIFIER THERAPY

Clients receiving interleukins have generalized and sometimes severe inflammatory reactions. Fluid shifts and capillary leak are widespread with edema forming in most tissues. Tissue swelling affects the function of all organs and can be life threatening. Clients receiving high-dose BRM therapy should receive care in an intensive care or monitoring unit. The effects of BRM therapy are limited to the period of acute drug infusion and resolve when treatment is completed.

Many BRMs induce symptoms of mild inflammation during and immediately after receiving the drug, including fever, chills, rigors, and flu-like general malaise. Problems are worse when higher doses are given, and they seem to become less severe over time. Fever is treated with acetaminophen. Clients with severe rigors are managed with meperidine (Demerol).

Interferon therapy causes peripheral neuropathy similar to that found in clients who have long-standing diabetes mellitus. Some of the problems resulting from the neuropathy include decreased sensory perception, visual disturbances, decreased hearing, unsteady balance and gait, and orthostatic hypotension. It is not known whether the neuropathy is temporary or permanent.

Skin rashes, dryness, itching, and peeling occur with many types of BRM therapy. The skin problems are more severe at higher doses and when more than one type of BRM is used at the same time. These reactions are temporary but can cause much discomfort and distress to the client. Advise clients to apply moisturizers (perfume-free) to the skin and to use mild soap to clean the skin. Involved areas must be protected from the sun with clothing or the use of sunscreen agents. Inform clients to avoid swimming and to refrain from using topical steroid creams on affected areas.

Interferon therapy has been reported to increase depression. It is not known whether this symptom is more intense among clients who have pre-existing depression.

Gene Therapy

Gene therapy as a cancer treatment is experimental. Although response rates have been limited, these successes indicate the potential for gene therapy as a form of cancer treatment.

MECHANISM OF ACTION

INCREASED TUMOR CELL SUSCEPTIBILITY. One method of using gene therapy for cancer is to render the tumor cells more susceptible to damage or death by other treatments. Inserting a viral enzyme gene into brain tumor cells makes them more susceptible to being killed by antiviral agents. Other techniques involve inserting human leukocyte antigen (HLA) genes different from the client's own HLAs into the tumor cells. This technique makes the client's immune system cells better able to recognize the cancer cells as foreign and take steps to eliminate or destroy them. Both methods of gene therapy for cancer have shown some success in early-phase clinical trials.

INCREASED IMMUNE SYSTEM CELL ACTIVITY. Some immune system cells are capable of attacking and killing cancer cells (see Chapter 23). This ability is increased when more of certain cytokines, such as IL-2, are present. Some gene therapy involves inserting additional genes for cytokines into the client's own immune system cells. These "charged-up" cancer-fighting immune system cells remain active for up to 6 months and can participate in cancer cell–killing episodes.

POTENTIAL USES OF GENE THERAPY FOR CANCER TREATMENT. Because cancer is caused by one or more changes in the genes of a normal cell, it is reasonable to think that planned gene changes could influence a cancer cell to become normal. Research for gene therapy against cancer includes the following areas:

- Inserting additional or healthy suppressor genes into cancer cells
- Inserting chemotherapy resistance genes into normal cells so higher doses of chemotherapy can be given without affecting normal cells
- Removing damaged, mutated, or activated oncogenes
- Inserting multiple genes into cancer cells to make them more easily recognized by immune system cells and more susceptible to other treatment modalities

TABLE 28-12 Agents Used for Targeted Cancer Therapy

Agent	Cancer Type
Antibodies	
Alemtuzumab (MabCampath)	Chronic myelogenous leukemia
Campath-1H	Chronic lymphocytic leukemia
CD22 (LymphoCide)	B-cell leukemia
Cetuximab (Erbitux)	Colorectal cancer, non–small cell lung cancer
Gemtuzumab ozogamicin (Mylotarg)	Acute myelocytic leukemia
Imatinib mesylate (Gleevec)	Chronic myelogenous leukemia
Lym-1 (Oncolym)	Lymphoma
Rituximab (Rituxan)	Non-Hodgkin's lymphoma
Tositumomab (Bexxar)	Non-Hodgkin's lymphoma
Trastuzumab (Herceptin)	Breast cancer
Antisense Agents	
AP 12009	Brain tumors
GEM 231	Multiple types of cancer
ISIS 2503	Lymphomas; multiple types of cancer
ISIS 3521/LY900003	Lung cancer
MG98	Bladder cancer; head and neck cancer
Oblimersen sodium (Genasense)	Pancreatic cancer

Targeted Therapy

Targeted therapies combine biologic therapy and gene therapy. These therapies take advantage of one or more differences in a cancer cell that is either not present or only slightly present in normal cells. Agents used as targeted therapies are either antibodies that "target" a cellular element of the cancer cell or "antisense" drugs that work at the gene level. These differences are a result of specific gene expression in cancer cells. Table 28-12 lists some agents used for targeted therapy.

MECHANISM OF ACTION

MONOCLONAL ANTIBODIES. Usually, antibodies are specific to a protein, receptor, or a cellular substance needed by the cancer cell for growth. When the antibody binds to the target within a cancer cell, some process important to cancer cell survival does not take place.

Many antibodies for cancer treatment have recently been approved and are currently in use. Trastuzumab (Herceptin) binds to a receptor for a protein made by some breast cancer cells. Binding this receptor prevents the division of cancer cells and makes them more easily killed by immune system cells. Another monoclonal antibody, rituximab (Rituxan) has a similar effect in some types of lymphoma.

In certain types of colorectal carcinoma, epidermal growth factor binds to the epidermal growth factor receptor (EGFR) site and activates it, leading to the generation of signals that increase the growth potential of the cancer cell. Blocking the EGFR reduces this potential. Anti-EGFR antibodies are a targeted therapy that bind to the EGFR receptor and prevent it from binding to epidermal growth factor. Another approach that targets the EGFR is a chemical that inhibits an enzyme, tyrosine kinase, which is important in the signaling pathway. Another targeted therapy drug is imatinib mesylate (Gleevec). This drug binds to the energy site of tyrosine kinase and prevents its activation. The drug is most useful in cancers that over-express the ABL1 oncogene, such as Philadelphia-chromosome positive chronic myeloid leukemia.

ANTISENSE DRUGS. Antisense drugs are a new form of cancer therapy that targets the process of making proteins important to the cancer development pathway. Genes for these proteins first make messenger RNA (mRNA). See Chapter 11 for a discussion of the steps of protein synthesis. Normally, the mRNA is then translated into protein. Some of these proteins then either enhance the growth of tumor cells or convert normal cell into cancer cells. The antisense drugs bind to the mRNA made by specific cancer genes, preventing them from making the cancer causing protein.

Currently, most antisense drugs are in the experimental stage but have the potential for great future benefit. They are given by continuous IV infusion.

SIDE EFFECTS OF TARGETED THERAPY

Allergic reactions are an issue in clients receiving monoclonal antibodies. Most of these antibodies were developed in animals and may express some animal proteins. More recently, much of the animal portion of these antibodies was removed. Thus the risk for allergic reactions is reduced but not eliminated. Clients receiving antibodies over time may develop their own antibodies to the drugs, making them less effective and possibly causing severe inflammatory or allergic reactions.

ONCOLOGIC EMERGENCIES

Cancer is a chronic disease. However, a number of acute conditions associated with cancer and its treatment can occur. These conditions, or complications, often require immediate intervention and are thus *oncologic emergencies.* Early diagnosis of such conditions is essential to avoid life-threatening situations.

Sepsis and Disseminated Intravascular Coagulation

PATHOPHYSIOLOGY

Sepsis, or septicemia, is a condition in which organisms enter the bloodstream. Septic shock is a life-threatening result of sepsis and a common cause of death in clients with cancer. Clients with cancer are at risk for infection and sepsis because their white blood cell counts are often low and their immune function is usually impaired. Chapter 40 describes the pathophysiology of sepsis and septic shock.

Disseminated intravascular coagulation (DIC) is a problem with the blood-clotting process. DIC is triggered by many severe illnesses, including cancer. In clients with cancer, DIC is caused by sepsis (often a gram-negative infection), by the release of thrombin or thromboplastin (clotting factors) from cancer cells, or by blood transfusions. DIC is most often seen in leukemia and in adenocarcinomas of the lung, pancreas, stomach, and prostate.

Extensive, abnormal clotting occurs throughout the small blood vessels of clients with DIC. This widespread clotting uses up the existing clotting factors and platelets. This process is followed by extensive bleeding. Bleeding from many sites is the most common problem and ranges from minimal to fatal hemorrhage. Clots block blood vessels and decrease blood flow to major body organs and results in pain, strokelike manifestations, dyspnea, tachycardia, oliguria (decreased urine output), and bowel necrosis (tissue death). Chapter 40 describes in-depth the collaborative management of sepsis-induced DIC.

◆COLLABORATIVE MANAGEMENT

DIC is a life-threatening problem and has a mortality rate greater than 70% even when proper therapies are instituted. Thus the best treatment plan for sepsis and DIC is prevention. Identify those clients at greatest risk for sepsis and DIC. Practice strict adherence to aseptic technique during invasive procedures and during contact with nonintact skin and mucous membranes in immunocompromised clients. Teach clients and family members the early manifestations of infection and sepsis and when to seek medical assistance.

When sepsis is present and DIC is likely, treatment focuses on reducing the infection and halting the DIC process. IV antibiotic therapy is initiated. During the early phase of DIC, anticoagulants (especially heparin) are given to limit clotting and prevent the rapid consumption of circulating clotting factors. Cryoprecipitated clotting factors are given when DIC has progressed and hemorrhage is the primary problem.

Syndrome of Inappropriate Antidiuretic Hormone

PATHOPHYSIOLOGY

In healthy people, antidiuretic hormone (ADH) is secreted by the posterior pituitary gland only when more fluid (water) is needed in the body, such as when plasma volume is decreased (see Chapter 14). Certain health problems induce ADH secretion when not needed by the body.

Cancer is the most common cause of the syndrome of inappropriate antidiuretic hormone (SIADH). The cancer most commonly causing SIADH is carcinoma of the lung (especially small cell lung cancer), but SIADH may occur in other types of cancer, especially when tumors are present in the brain. Some tumors actually make and secrete ADH, whereas others stimulate the brain to make and secrete ADH. Drugs often used in clients with cancer also can cause SIADH (e.g., morphine sulfate, cyclophosphamide).

In SIADH, water is reabsorbed to excess by the kidney and put into systemic circulation. The increased water causes hyponatremia (decreased serum sodium levels) and fluid retention. Mild manifestations include weakness, muscle cramps, loss of appetite, and fatigue. Serum sodium levels range from 115 to 120 mEq/L (normal range is 135 to 145 mEq/L). More serious problems occur when even more water is retained, including weight gain, nervous system changes, personality changes, confusion, and extreme muscle weakness. As the sodium level drops toward 110 mEq/L, seizures, coma and death may follow.

◆COLLABORATIVE MANAGEMENT

SIADH is managed by treating the condition and the cause. Treatment includes fluid restriction (sometimes total fluid intake is reduced to 1 L/day), increased sodium intake, and drug therapy. The drug most often used is demeclocycline, which is taken orally. This drug, an antibiotic, works in opposition to ADH. Monitor serum sodium levels closely, because hypernatremia can develop suddenly as a result of this treatment.

A second method for managing SIADH is to reduce or eliminate the underlying cause. Immediate cancer therapy, usually either radiation or chemotherapy, can cause such tumor regression that ADH production returns to normal.

Spinal Cord Compression

PATHOPHYSIOLOGY

Spinal cord compression and damage occur either when a tumor directly enters the spinal cord or when the vertebrae collapse from tumor degradation of the bone. Tumors may begin in the spinal cord but more often spread from other areas of the body, such as the lung, prostate, breast, and colon. Spinal cord compression often causes back pain before neurologic deficits occur. Neurologic problems are specific to the level of spinal compression and include numbness; tingling; loss of urethral, vaginal, and rectal sensation; and muscle weakness. If paralysis occurs, it is usually permanent.

◆COLLABORATIVE MANAGEMENT

Early recognition and treatment of spinal cord compression are key to a good outcome. Assess the client for neurologic changes consistent with spinal cord compression. Teach clients and families to recognize the manifestations of early spinal cord compression and to seek help as soon as problems are apparent.

Treatment is often palliative. Usually, high-dose corticosteroids are given first to reduce swelling around the spinal cord and relieve symptoms. High-dose radiation may be given to reduce the size of the tumor in the area and relieve compression. Radiation also may be used along with chemotherapy to treat the total disease. Surgery may be performed to remove the tumor from the area and rearrange the bony tissue so less pressure is placed on the spinal cord. External back or neck braces may be used to reduce the weight borne by the spinal column and to reduce pressure on the spinal cord or spinal nerves.

Hypercalcemia

PATHOPHYSIOLOGY

Hypercalcemia (increased serum calcium level) occurs most often in clients with bone metastasis. Cancer in bone causes the bone to release calcium into the bloodstream. In clients with cancer in other parts of the body (especially the lung, head and neck, kidney, or lymph nodes), the tumor secretes parathyroid hormone, causing bone to release calcium. Decreased mobility and dehydration worsen hypercalcemia.

Early manifestations of hypercalcemia include fatigue, loss of appetite, nausea, vomiting, constipation, and polyuria (increased urine output). More serious problems include severe muscle weakness, loss of deep tendon reflexes, paralytic ileus, dehydration, and electrocardiographic (ECG) changes. The severity of manifestations depends on how high the serum calcium level is and how quickly it developed (see also Chapter 16).

◆COLLABORATIVE MANAGEMENT

Cancer-induced hypercalcemia develops very slowly for many clients, which allows the body time to adapt to this electrolyte change. As a result, symptoms of hypercalcemia may not be evident until the serum calcium level is greatly elevated. Because adaptation does occur, cancer-induced hypercalcemia is treated only when manifestations are present.

Oral hydration alone may be enough to reduce the serum calcium and relieve symptoms. Normal saline is used when parenteral hydration is needed.

Many drugs lower serum calcium levels. Some agents, such oral glucocorticoids, calcitonin, diphosphonate, gallium nitrate, and mithramycin, lower levels quite dramatically. These drugs do not cure hypercalcemia but instead reduce serum calcium levels temporarily. When cancer-induced hypercalcemia is life threatening or occurs with renal impairment, dialysis can temporarily reduce serum calcium levels.

Superior Vena Cava Syndrome

PATHOPHYSIOLOGY

Superior vena cava (SVC) syndrome occurs when the SVC is compressed or obstructed by tumor growth (Figure 28-3). SVC compression can lead to a painful and life-threatening emergency, most often in clients with lymphomas and lung cancer. Clients with cancer of the breast, esophagus, colon, and testes may also be affected.

The manifestations of SVC syndrome result from the blockage of blood flow in the venous system of the head, neck, and upper trunk. Early manifestations occur when the client arises after a night's sleep and include edema of the face, especially around the eyes, and tightness of the shirt or blouse collar (Stokes' sign). As the compression worsens, the client develops edema in the arms and hands, dyspnea, erythema of the upper body, and epistaxis (nosebleeds). Late manifestations include hemorrhage, cyanosis, mental status changes from lack of blood to the brain, decreased cardiac output, and hypotension. Death results if compression is not relieved.

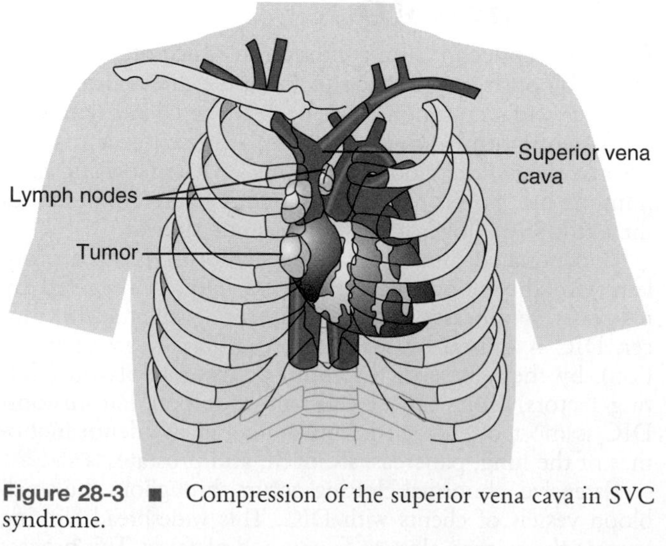

Figure 28-3 ■ Compression of the superior vena cava in SVC syndrome.

COLLABORATIVE MANAGEMENT

SVC syndrome is a late-stage manifestation; the tumor is usually widespread. High-dose radiation therapy to the mediastinal area may be used to provide temporary relief. Surgery is rarely performed for this condition because the tumor may have increased intrathoracic pressure to such a level that it may be impossible to close the chest after the procedure. A metal stent can be placed in the vena cava in an interventional radiation department to relieve swelling. Follow-up angioplasty can keep this stent open for a longer period of time. (See Chapter 39 for more information on stenting procedures.)

The best treatment results occur when SVC syndrome is in the early stages. Assess each client for manifestations of SVC syndrome and notify the physician.

Tumor Lysis Syndrome

PATHOPHYSIOLOGY

In tumor lysis syndrome (TLS), large numbers of tumor cells are destroyed rapidly. Their intracellular contents, including potassium and purines (DNA components), are released into the bloodstream faster than the body can eliminate them (Figure 28-4). Unlike other oncologic emergencies, TLS is a positive sign that cancer treatment is effective.

Severe or untreated TLS can cause severe tissue damage and death. Serum potassium levels can increase to the point of hyperkalemia, causing severe cardiac dysfunction (see Chapter 16). The large amounts of released purines are converted in the liver to uric acid and released into the blood, causing hyperuricemia. These uric acid crystals precipitate in the kidney, forming a sludge in the kidney tubules; this effect blocks the tubules and leads to acute renal failure.

TLS is most often seen in clients receiving radiation or chemotherapy for cancers that are very sensitive to these therapies, including leukemia, lymphoma, small cell lung cancer, and multiple myeloma.

COLLABORATIVE MANAGEMENT

Prevention through hydration is the best management for TLS. Hydration alone can dilute the serum potassium level and increases the kidney filtration rate. As a result, urine flows through the kidney at a greatly increased rate. This action prevents the precipitation of uric acid crystals, increases the excretion of potassium, and mechanically flushes any renal tubular sludge.

With tumors known to be very sensitive to cancer therapy, instruct clients to drink at least 3000 mL (5000 mL is more desirable) of fluid the day before, the day of, and for 3 days after treatment. Some fluids should be alkaline (sodium bicarbonate) to help prevent uric acid precipitation. Stress the importance of keeping fluid intake consistent throughout the 24-hour day and help clients draw up a schedule of fluid intake.

Because some clients have nausea and vomiting after cancer therapy and may not feel like drinking fluids, stress the importance of following the antiemetic regimen. Instruct clients to contact their health care provider or cancer clinic immediately if nausea and vomiting prevent adequate fluid intake so they can be started on parenteral fluids.

Treatment becomes more aggressive for clients who become hyperkalemic or hyperuricemic. In addition to increased fluid intake (oral or parenteral), diuretics (especially osmotic types) are given to increase urine flow through the kidney. These agents are given with caution because clients must not become dehydrated. Drugs that increase the excretion of purines, such as allopurinol (Aloprim, Zyloprim) or rasburicase (Elitek), are given. To reduce serum potassium levels for mild to moderate hyperkalemia, sodium polystyrene sulfonate can be given orally or as a retention enema. This treatment does not immediately reduce serum potassium level. For more severe hyperkalemia, IV infusions containing glucose and insulin may be given. Clients who have severe hyperkalemia and hyperuricemia may need dialysis.

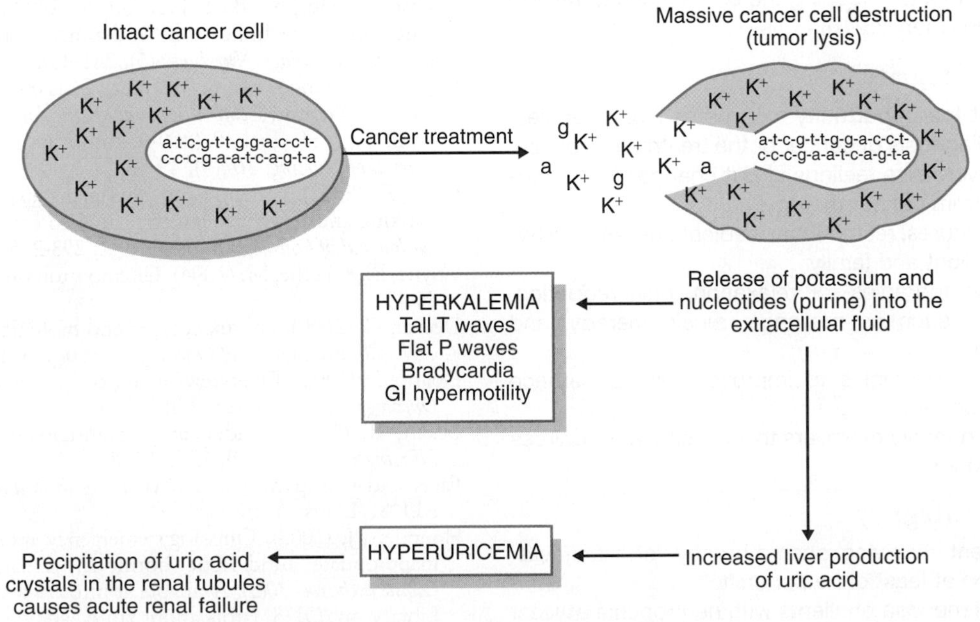

Figure 28-4 ■ Pathology of tumor lysis syndrome.

CANCER TREATMENT FAILURE

More than 50% of people diagnosed with cancer in North America each year are cured of their disease, and many others live 5 years or longer. However, some will have cancer treatment failure and die. With cancer, the process of dying is usually long, lasting weeks or months. Clients and families need special support and assistance during this time. Chapter 9 addresses hospice care and important physical, emotional, social, and spiritual needs of clients and families during and after the dying process.

GET READY for the NCLEX Examination!

KEY POINTS

Safe Effective Care Environment

- Use aseptic technique during all central line dressing changes or any invasive procedure.
- Ask all clients about Advance Directives and document their status.
- Use good handwashing techniques before providing any care to a client who is immunosuppressed.
- Use bleeding precautions for any client with thrombocytopenia or pancytopenia (see Chart 28-9).
- Position shields properly when clients in inpatient settings are receiving brachytherapy.
- Use appropriate personal protection (gowns, gloves, masks) when mixing or administering chemotherapeutic agents.

Health Promotion and Maintenance

- Teach clients receiving radiation therapy how to care for the skin in the radiation path (see Chart 28-2).
- Identify clients at high risk for infection because of disease or therapy.
- Teach the client and family about the clinical manifestations of infection and when to seek medical advice.
- Teach clients at risk for bleeding the precautions to take to avoid injury (see Chart 28-10).

Psychosocial Integrity

- Allow the client the opportunity to express fear or anxiety regarding the diagnosis of cancer or the treatment regimen.
- Allow client to verbalize feelings about changes in appearance resulting from cancer therapy.
- Explain all procedures, restrictions, medications, and follow-up care to the client and family.
- Offer alternative therapies for relaxation, pain reduction, and distraction, such as massage, music therapy, and guided imagery.
- Help clients use strategies to improve their appearance when alopecia occurs.
- Refer clients and family members to local cancer resources and support groups.

Physiological Integrity

- Assess the client receiving chemotherapy for manifestations of infection at least once per shift.
- Inspect the oral mucosa of clients with neutropenia at least once per shift.
- Report any temperature over 100° F in a client with neutropenia.
- Teach the client about any medications to be continued after discharge from the hospital.
- Instruct the client and family in the clinical manifestations of complications and when to seek assistance.
- Pace nonurgent health care activities to reduce the risk for fatigue among clients with anemia or pancytopenia.

ADDITIONAL STUDY RESOURCES

Go to your Student CD-ROM for Review Questions for the NCLEX Examination.

evolve Go to http://evolve.elsevier.com/Iggy/ for Integrated Management of Care Questions for the NCLEX Examination.

SELECTED BIBLIOGRAPHY

American Cancer Society. (2005). *Cancer facts and figures–2005.* Report No. 00-300M-No. 5008.05. Atlanta: Author.

Anastasia, P. (2001). Nursing considerations for managing topotecan-related hematologic side effects. *Clinical Journal of Oncology Nursing, 5*(1), 9-13.

Bedell, C. (2003) Pegfilgrastim for chemotherapy-induced neutropenia. *Clinical Journal of Oncology Nursing, 7*(1),55-64.

Bender, C., et al. (2002). Chemotherapy-induced nausea and vomiting. *Clinical Journal of Oncology Nursing, 6*(2), 94-102.

Birner, A. (2003). Safe administration of oral chemotherapy. *Clinical Journal of Oncology Nursing, 7*(2), 158-162.

Brandt, J. (2002). Rasburicase: An innovative new treatment for hyperuricemia associated with tumor lysis syndrome. *Clinical Journal of Oncology Nursing, 6*(1), 12-16.

Bremerkamp, M. (2000). Mechanism of action of 5-HT3 receptor antagonists: Clinical overview and nursing implications. *Clinical Journal of Oncology Nursing, 4*(5), 201-207.

Brown, C., & Yoder, L. (2002). Stomatitis: An overview. *American Journal of Nursing, 102*(4), 20-23.

Bruce, S. (2004). Radiation-induced xerostomia: How dry is your patient? *Clinical Journal of Oncology Nursing, 8*(1), 61-67.

Buchsel, P. (2003). Gelclair7 oral gel. *Clinical Journal of Oncology Nursing, 7*(1), 109-112.

Buchsel, P., Murphy, B., & Newton, S. (2002). Epoetin Alfa: Current and future indications and nursing implications. *Clinical Journal of Oncology Nursing, 6*(5), 261-267.

Cagen, D., Franco, M., & Vasquez, D. (2002). The ABCs of low blood cell count. *Clinical Journal of Oncology Nursing, 6*(1), 34-36.

Cantril, C., & Haylock, P. (2004). Tumor lysis syndrome. *American Journal of Nursing, 104*(4), 49-56.

Cope, D. (2002). Patients' and physicians' experiences with sperm banking and infertility issues related to cancer treatment. *Clinical Journal of Oncology Nursing, 6*(5), 293-295, 309.

Coyne, B., & Leslie, M. (2004). Chemo's toll on memory. *RN, 67*(4), 40-43.

Decker, G. (2000). Pharmacologic and biologic therapies in cancer care. *Clinical Journal of Oncology Nursing, 4*(5), 242-244.

Doane, L. (2002). Overview of tumor lysis syndrome. *Seminars in Oncology Nursing, 18*(3), 2-3.

Eckert, R. (2001). Understanding anticipatory nausea. *Oncology Nursing Forum, 28*(10), 1553-1558.

Facts and Comparisons. (2004). *Drug facts and comparisons* (58th ed.). St. Louis: Author.

Flounders, J. (2003). Oncology emergency modules: Syndrome of inappropriate antidiuretic hormone. *Oncology Nursing Forum–Online exclusive, 30*(3). Available at http://www.ons.org/xp6/ONS/Library.xml/ONS_Publications.xml/ONF.xml Digital object identifier is 10.1188/03.ONF.E63-E70

Flounders, J., & Ott, B. (2003). Oncology emergency modules: Spinal cord compression. *Oncology Nursing Forum–Online exclusive, 30*(1). Available at http://www.ons.org/xp6/ONS/Library.xml/ONS_Publications.xml/ONF.xml Digital object identifier is 10.1188/03.ONF.E17-E23

Gillespie, T. (2003). Anemia in cancer: Therapeutic implications and interventions. *Cancer Nursing, 26*(2), 119-128.

Gobel, B. (2002). Management of tumor lysis syndrome: Prevention and treatment. *Seminars in Oncology Nursing, 18*(3), 12-16.

Golant, M., Altman, T., & Martin, C. (2003). Managing cancer side effects to improve quality of life. *Cancer Nursing, 26*(1), 37-43.

Gosselin, T., & Waring, J. (2001) Nursing management of patients receiving brachytherapy for gynecologic malignancies. *Clinical Journal of Oncology Nursing, 5*(2), 59-63.

Held-Warmkessel, J. (2005). Managing 3 critical cancer complications. *Nursing 2005, 35*(1), 58-63.

Hellerstedt, B., & Pienta, K. (2002). The current state of hormonal therapy for prostate cancer. *CA A Cancer Journal for Clinicians, 52*(3), 154-179.

Hendrix, C., deLeon, C., & Dillman, R. (2002). Radioimmunotherapy for non-Hodgkin's lymphoma with yttrium 90 ibritumomab tiuxetan. *Clinical Journal of Oncology Nursing, 6*(3), 144-148.

Hodgson, N., & Given, C. (2004). Determinants of functional recovery in older adults surgically treated for cancer. *Cancer Nursing, 27*(1), 10-16.

Hood, L. (2003). Chemotherapy in the elderly: Supportive therapy for chemotherapy-induced myelotoxicity. *Clinical Journal of Oncology Nursing, 7*(2), 185-190.

Jenkins, M., & Ashley, J. (2002). Sex and the oncology patient. *American Journal of Nursing, 102*(4 Suppl.), 13-15.

Kaplow, R. (2002). Pathophysiology, signs, and symptoms of acute tumor lysis syndrome. *Seminars in Oncology Nursing, 18*(3), 6-11.

Lengacher, C., et al. (2002). Frequency of use of complementary and alternative medicine in women with breast cancer. *Oncology Nursing Forum, 29*(10), 1445-1452.

Marek, C. (2003). Antiemetic therapy in patients receiving cancer chemotherapy. *Oncology Nursing Forum, 30*(2), 259-269.

McCance, K., & Huether, S. (2002). Pathophysiology: The biologic basis for disease in adults and children (4th ed.). St. Louis: Mosby.

McGrath, P. (2002). Reflections on nutritional issues associated with cancer therapy. *Cancer Practice, 10*(2), 94-101.

McGuire, D. Mucosal tissue injury in cancer therapy. (2002) *Cancer Practice, 10*(4), 179-191.

Moran, A., & Camp-Sorrell, D. (2002). Maintenance of venous access devices in patients with neutropenia. *Clinical Journal of Oncology Nursing, 6*(3), 126-130.

Ott, M. (2002). Complementary and alternative therapies in cancer symptom management. *Cancer Practice, 10*(3), 162-166.

Peterson, K. (2003). Central line sepsis. *Clinical Journal of Oncology Nursing, 7*(2), 218-221.

Phillips, M. (2003). Pegfilgrastim. *Clinical Journal of Oncology Nursing, 7*(2), 238-239.

Plaisance, L., & Ellis, J. (2002). Opioid-induced constipation. *American Journal of Nursing, 102*(3), 72-73.

Rittenberg, C. (2002). A new class of antiemetic agents on the horizon. *Clinical Journal of Oncology Nursing, 6*(2), 103-104.

Robbins, M., & Gosselin, T. (2002). Symptom management in radiation oncology. *American Journal of Nursing, 102*(4 Suppl.), 32-36.

Sarna, L., & Conde, F. (2001). Physical activity and fatigue during radiation therapy: A pilot study using Actigraph monitors. *Oncology Nursing Forum, 28*(6), 1043-1046.

Schneider, S., Prince-Paul, M., & Allen, M. (2004). Virtual reality as a distraction intervention for women with breast cancer. *Oncology Nursing Forum, 31*(1), 81-88.

Seeley, K., & DeMeyer, E. (2002). Nursing care of patients receiving Campath. *Clinical Journal of Oncology Nursing, 6*(3), 138-143.

Shih, A., et al. (2003). Mechanisms for radiation-induced oral mucositis and the consequences. *Cancer Nursing, 26*(3), 222-229.

Smith, M., et al. (2002). Outcomes of therapeutic massage for hospitalized cancer patients. *Journal of Nursing Scholarship, 34*(3), 257-263.

Sorokin, P. (2002). New agents and future directions in biotherapy. *Clinical Journal of Oncology Nursing, 6*(1), 19-26.

Spencer-Cisek, P. (2002). The role of growth factors in malignancy: A focus on the epidermal growth factor receptor. *Seminars in Oncology Nursing, 18*(2, Suppl. 2), 13-19.

Sweeney, C. (2002). Understanding peripheral neuropathy in patients with cancer: Background and patient assessment. *Clinical Journal of Oncology Nursing, 6*(3), 163-167.

Tan, S. (2002). Recognition and treatment of oncologic emergencies. *Journal of Infusion Nursing, 25*(3), 182-188.

Tariman, J. (2003). Thalidomide: Current therapeutic uses and management of its toxicities. *Clinical Journal of Oncology Nursing, 7*(2), 143-147.

Tasota, F., & Tate, J. (2001). Interpreting the highs and lows of platelet counts. *Nursing2001, 31*(2), 25.

Tuinstra, N. (2003). Outpatient administration of radiolabeled monoclonal antibodies. *Clinical Journal of Oncology Nursing, 7*(1), 106.

Viele, C. (2002). Gemtuzumab ozogamicin. *Clinical Journal of Oncology Nursing, 6*(5), 298-299, 304.

Waxman, E., & Herbst, R. (2002). The role of the epidermal growth factor receptor in the treatment of colorectal carcinoma. *Seminars in Oncology Nursing, 18*(2, Suppl. 2), 20-29.

West, C., et al. (2003). The PRO-SELF: Pain control program–An effective approach for cancer pain management. *Oncology Nursing Forum, 30*(1), 65-73.

White, C. (2002). Painful lesions in a pancytopenic patient. *Clinical Journal of Oncology Nursing, 6*(1), 47-49, 51.

Whitman, M. (2001). Understanding the perceived need for complementary and alternative nutraceuticals: Lifestyle issues. *Clinical Journal of Oncology Nursing, 5*(5), 190-194.

Wilkes, G. (2002). New therapeutic options in colon cancer: Focus on oxaliplatin. *Clinical Journal of Oncology Nursing, 6*(3), 131-137.

Wilson, R. (2000). Optimizing nutrition for patients with cancer. *Clinical Journal of Oncology Nursing, 4*(1), 23-28.

Witt, J. (2002). Living with fatigue. *American Journal of Nursing, 102*(4), 28-31.

Workman, M.L. (2002). Breast cancer: New strategies to beat an old enemy. *Nursing2002, 32*(10), 58-63.

CHAPTER

29 Interventions for Clients with Infection

FRANK EDWARDS MYERS • GAYLE K. GILMORE

LEARNING OUTCOMES

After studying this chapter, you should be able to:

1. Explain the chain of infection.
2. Describe the principles of infection control in inpatient and community-based settings.
3. Identify the Centers for Disease Control and Prevention (CDC) hand hygiene recommendations for health care workers.
4. Differentiate the four types of transmission-based precautions.
5. Identify the major causes and results of inadequate antimicrobial therapy.
6. Assess the common clinical manifestations of infection.
7. Interpret laboratory test findings related to infections and infectious diseases.
8. Evaluate nursing interventions for management of the client with an infection.
9. Develop a teaching plan for clients who have an infection or infectious disease.

Go to your Student CD-ROM for Review Questions for the NCLEX Examination keyed to these Learning Outcomes.

Infections and infectious diseases have been the major cause of millions of deaths worldwide for centuries. Today threats of bioterrorism have been added to the concerns about drug-resistant and re-emerging infections. Appropriately used, antibiotics and vaccines prevent many types of infection, but their utility is limited by misuse, cost, and distribution issues. World trade and people traveling and interacting with each other and their diversified environments cause exposure to a wider variety of infectious agents than in the past. Advancing technology and invasive procedures introduce microorganisms into the body, resulting in infection, even though in other environments these microorganisms are harmless. This chapter provides an overview of infection and general principles for prevention and management. Specific infections are described throughout this text.

OVERVIEW

Definitions

The infection process requires the following:

- Pathogen (agent)
- Portal of exit for the agent
- Means of transmission
- Portal of entry to the host
- Susceptible **host** (infection recipient)

A **pathogen** is any microorganism capable of producing disease. Infections can be **communicable** (transmitted from person to person, such as influenza) or not communicable (e.g., peritonitis). Microorganisms with differing levels of **pathogenicity** (ability to cause disease) surround everyone. **Virulence** is a term often used as a synonym for pathogenicity; however, virulence is related more to the frequency with which a pathogen causes disease (degree of communicability) and its ability to invade and damage a host. Virulence can also indicate the severity of the disease.

Many microorganisms live in or on the human host without causing disease. Some microbes are beneficial. Each body location harbors its own characteristic bacteria, or **normal flora.** Normal flora often functions to compete with and prevent infection from unfamiliar microorganisms attempting to invade a body site. In some instances, microorganisms that are often pathogenic may be present in the tissues of the host and yet not cause symptomatic disease; this process is called **colonization.**

In the United States, the Centers for Disease Control and Prevention (CDC) collect epidemiologic information about the occurrence and nature of infectious diseases. The CDC then makes recommendations to health care agencies for infection control and prevention. Certain diseases, such as tuberculosis, must be reported to health departments and the CDC. The Infection Control (IC) Officer for each health care agency is responsible for tracking infections and ensuring compliance with federal and local requirements.

Chain of Infection

The development of infection depends on a series of factors noted as the **chain of infection** (Figure 29-1). To prevent the spread of infection, the chain of infection must be broken at any point. Eliminating microorganisms, establishing host immunity, and interrupting transmission are examples of ways to break this chain.

RESERVOIR

Reservoirs (sources of infectious agents) are numerous. Animate reservoirs include people, animals, and insects. Inanimate reservoirs include soil, water, other environmental sources, or medical equipment (e.g., intravenous [IV] solutions and urine collection devices). The host's body can be a reservoir; pathogens colonize skin and body substances (e.g., feces, sputum, saliva, wound drainage). A person with an active infection or an asymptomatic **carrier** (one who harbors an infectious agent without active disease) is a reservoir. Examples of community reservoirs include sewage, stagnant or contaminated water, and improperly handled foods.

PATHOGEN

Several classes of microorganisms produce infection (Table 29-1). Bacteria like *Neisseria meningitidis* can exist in the respiratory tract while causing no illness, but if the bacteria invade the bloodstream or cerebrospinal fluid, the bacteria become extremely pathogenic. Another example is *Enterococcus,* which lives as normal flora in our gastrointestinal system, where it is nonpathogenic and assists in the digestive process; but if it enters the bloodstream, *Enterococcus* can cause disease.

Continued multiplication of a pathogen is sometimes accompanied by toxin production. **Toxins** are protein molecules released by bacteria to affect host cells at a distant site. **Exotoxins** are produced and released by certain bacteria into the surrounding environment. Botulism, tetanus, diphtheria, and *Escherichia coli* 0157:H7–related systemic diseases are attributed to exotoxins. **Endotoxins** are produced in the cell walls of certain bacteria and released only with cell lysis. Typhoid and meningococcal diseases are caused by endotoxins.

HOST

Host factors influence the development of infection (Table 29-2). Host defenses provide the body with an efficient system for protection against pathogens. Breakdown of these defense mechanisms may increase the **susceptibility** (risk) of the host to infection.

IMMUNITY. The client's immune status plays a large role in determining risk for infection. Congenital abnormalities, as well as acquired health problems (e.g., renal failure, steroid dependence, cancer, acquired immunodeficiency syndrome [AIDS]), can result in numerous immunologic deficiencies. Depression of the immune system may render the host more susceptible to infection or cripple the host's ability to combat organisms that have gained entry.

Immunity is resistance to infection; it is usually associated with the presence of antibodies or cells that act on specific microorganisms. **Passive immunity** is of short duration (days or months) and either natural by transplacental transfer from the mother or artificial by injection of antibodies (e.g., immune globulin). **Active immunity** lasts for years and is natural by infection or artificial by stimulation (e.g., vaccine) of the body's immune defenses. Chapter 23 discusses the immune system and immunity in detail.

Environmental factors can also influence clients' immune status and thus their susceptibility to or ability to fight infection. Examples include alcohol consumption,

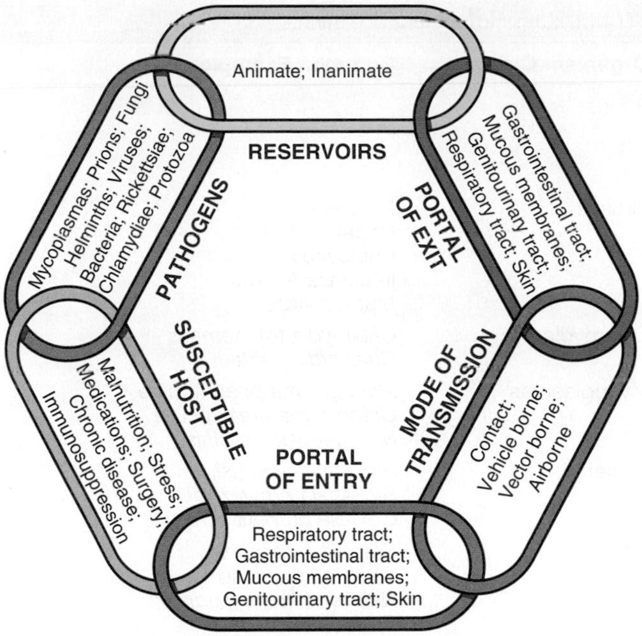

Figure 29-1 ■ The chain of infection: the process by which pathogens are transmitted from the environment to a host, invade the host, and cause infection.

nicotine use, inhalation of bone marrow–suppressing toxic chemicals, and certain vitamin deficiencies. Malnutrition, especially protein-calorie malnutrition, places clients at increased risk for infection.

Medical and surgical interventions may impair normal immune response. Steroid therapy, chemotherapy for malignant neoplasms, and cytotoxic therapy intended to suppress the immune response (e.g., cyclosporine in organ transplant recipients) increase the risk of infection. Medical devices (e.g., intravascular or urinary catheters, endotracheal tubes) may also interfere with normal host defense mechanisms. Surgery, trauma, and burns result in non-intact skin. *The body's skin is the best barrier or defense against infection.* When this barrier is broken, infection often results.

OTHER FACTORS. Hormonal factors play a role in the incidence and mortality rate of many infectious diseases. People with diabetes mellitus and adrenal insufficiency experience increased numbers of acute and chronic bacterial infections.

PORTAL OF ENTRY

Microorganisms may enter the body in a variety of ways (Table 29-3), and some specific sites of infection have key features.

RESPIRATORY TRACT. Pathogens may enter the body through the respiratory tract. Microbes in droplets are sprayed into the air when people with infected oral or nasal tissue talk, cough, or sneeze. A susceptible host then inhales droplets, and pathogens localize in the lungs or are distributed via the lymphatic system or bloodstream to other areas of the body. Microorganisms that enter the body by the respiratory tract and produce distant infection include influenza virus, *Mycobacterium tuberculosis,* and *Streptococcus pneumoniae.*

GASTROINTESTINAL TRACT. Some pathogens enter the body by ingestion through the gastrointestinal

TABLE 29-1 Infectious Organisms*

Organism Class	Common Examples	Common Disease Manifestations
Prions		Bovine spongiform encephalitis (BSE),† Creutzfeldt-Jakob disease, Kuru†
		Possible role in Alzheimer's disease, Parkinson disease, and amyotrophic lateral sclerosis (ALS)‡
Viruses	Poliovirus	Poliomyelitis
	Hepatitis A virus	Hepatitis
	Rhinovirus	Common cold
	Influenza A virus	Influenza
	Mumps virus	Mumps
Chlamydiae	*Chlamydia trachomatis*	Trachoma, lymphogranuloma venereum, conjunctivitis
	Chlamydia psittaci	Psittacosis (parrot fever)
Mycoplasmas	*Mycoplasma pneumoniae*	Pneumonia
	Ureaplasma urealyticum	Urethritis
	Mycoplasma hominis	Pyelonephritis, pelvic inflammatory disease
Rickettsiae	*Rickettsia rickettsii*	Rocky Mountain spotted fever
	Rickettsia prowazekii	Typhus
	Coxiella burnetii	Q fever
Bacteria	*Staphylococcus* sp.	Superficial skin infections, osteomyelitis, pneumonia, bacteremia
	Streptococcus sp.	Pharyngitis, skin infections, pneumonia
	Neisseria meningitidis	Meningitis
	Escherichia coli	Urinary tract infection
	Pseudomonas aeruginosa	Skin infection, otitis, urinary tract infection
Fungi	*Candida albicans*	Thrush, vaginitis
	Aspergillus sp.	Sinusitis, brain abscess
	Cryptococcus neoformans	Meningitis, pneumonia
	Histoplasma capsulatum	Pneumonia
	Coccidioides immitis	Pneumonia
Protozoa	*Entamoeba histolytica*	Diarrhea, colitis
	Plasmodium sp.	Malaria
	Leishmania sp.	Fever, weight loss, cutaneous lesions
	Toxoplasma gondii	Chorioretinitis, encephalitis
	Pneumocystis carinii	Pneumonia
Helminths	*Ancylostoma duodenale* (hookworm)	Anemia
	Ascaris lumbricoides (roundworm)	Intestinal obstruction
	Enterobius vermicularis (pinworm)	Anal pruritus
	Schistosoma sp. (blood flukes)	Hydronephrosis
	Taenia solium (pork tapeworm)	Epilepsy from cysticercosis

*Organisms are presented in order of increasing complexity.

†Prusiner, S. Nobelist believes prions may be at root of Alzheimer's, Parkinson's, ALS. *Reuter's health*, October 20, 1999; available at http://www.reutershealth.com. (Dr. Stanley Prusiner is a 1997 Nobel Prize winner for the discovery of prions.)

‡Mastrianni, J.A., & Roos, R.P. (2000). The prion diseases. *Seminars in Neurology, 20*(3), 337-352.

TABLE 29-2 Host Factors That Influence the Development of Infection

Host Factor	Increased Risk of Infection
Natural immunity	Congenital or acquired immunodeficiencies
Normal flora	Alteration of normal flora by antibiotic therapy
Age	Infants and older clients
Hormonal factors	Pregnancy, diabetes, corticosteroid therapy, and adrenal insufficiency
Phagocytosis	Defective phagocytic function, circulatory disturbances, and neutropenia
Skin/mucous membranes/ normal excretory secretions	Break in skin or mucous membrane integrity; interference with flow of urine, tears, or saliva; interference with cough reflex or ciliary action; changes in gastric secretions
Nutrition	Malnutrition or dehydration
Environmental factors	Smoking, alcohol consumption, and inhalation of toxic chemicals
Medical interventions	Invasive therapy, chemotherapy, radiation therapy, and steroid therapy; surgery

(GI) tract. Some stay in the GI tract and produce disease (e.g., *Shigella* causing self-limited disease). Others invade the GI tract to produce local and distant infection (e.g., *Salmonella enteritidis*). Some produce limited GI symptoms, causing systemic infection (e.g., *Salmonella typhi*) or profound involvement of organs (e.g., hepatitis A virus). An estimated 76 million cases of foodborne illness in the United States occur each year. This type of illness results in 325,000 hospitalizations and 1,800 deaths every year (Centers for Disease Control and Prevention [CDC], 2003).

TABLE 29-3 Portals of Entry of Selected Disease-Producing Organisms

Infecting Organisms	Resultant Diseases
Respiratory Tract	
Neisseria meningitidis	Meningococcal pneumonia, meningococcal meningitis, meningococcemia
Cryptococcus neoformans	Cryptococcal meningitis, cryptococcal pneumonia
Mycobacterium tuberculosis	Tuberculosis
Influenza A virus	Influenza
Streptococcus pneumoniae	Pneumococcal pneumonia
Measles virus (rubeola)	Measles
Legionella pneumophila	Legionnaires' disease
Varicella-zoster virus	Chickenpox
Gastrointestinal Tract	
Salmonella enteritidis	Gastroenteritis
Salmonella typhi	Typhoid fever
Clostridium botulinum	Botulism
Poliovirus	Poliomyelitis
Hepatitis A virus	Hepatitis A
Escherichia coli 0157:H7	Possibly, hemolytic uremic syndrome
Genitourinary Tract	
Neisseria gonorrhoeae	Gonorrhea
Chlamydia trachomatis	Lymphogranuloma venereum, cervicitis, urethritis, endometritis
Enterobacteriaceae *(E. coli, Klebsiella sp., Serratia sp., Proteus sp.)*	Urinary tract infections
Intact Skin or Mucous Membranes	
Rhinovirus	Common cold
Respiratory syncytial virus	Pneumonia, bronchiolitis, tracheobronchitis
Schistosoma sp.	Schistosome dermatitis (swimmer's disease)
Herpes simplex virus	Oral or genital herpes
Bloodstream	
Hepatitis B or C viruses	Hepatitis B or C
Plasmodium sp.	Malaria
Clostridium tetani	Tetanus
Human immunodeficiency virus	Acquired immunodeficiency syndrome

GENITOURINARY TRACT. Microorganisms also enter through the genitourinary tract. Urinary tract infection (UTI) is one of the most common **health care–associated infections** (HAIs). More than 55% of clients in adult intensive care units (ICU) have urinary catheters in place. Indwelling urinary catheters are a primary cause of UTIs (National Nosocomial Infectious Surveillance, 2002a). The use of urinary catheters coated with silver alloy may reduce the risk of urinary tract infections (Saint et al., 2000).

WOMEN'S HEALTH CONSIDERATIONS

Women have a higher risk for UTIs than men because they have shorter urethras. Microorganisms (often colonic flora) colonize the perineal area, the urethral meatus and, potentially, the bladder. Older women are at even a greater risk because of decreased resistance to infection, stress incontinence, decreased thirst (causing dehydration), and in some cases the inability to use proper hygiene.

SKIN/MUCOUS MEMBRANES. While intact skin is the best barrier to prevent most infections, some pathogens, such as *Treponema pallidum,* can enter the body through intact skin or mucous membranes. Most enter through breaks in these normally effective surface barriers. Sometimes a medical procedure creates a break in cutaneous or mucocutaneous barriers, as in catheter-acquired **bacteremia** (bacteria in the bloodstream) and surgical-wound infections. Fragile skin of older clients and of those receiving prolonged steroid therapy increases infection risk.

BLOODSTREAM. Microorganisms can gain direct access to the bloodstream, especially when invasive devices or tubes are used. The National Nosocomial Infection Surveillance (NNIS) reported that for every 1000 days that central venous catheters are in place in medical/surgical and intensive care unit (ICU) clients, 4.8 infections result (NNIS, 2002b). As technology changes, improvements such as new materials for catheters reduce the risk of acquiring bloodstream infections. In the community setting, biting insects can inject organisms into the bloodstream, causing infection (e.g., Lyme disease and West Nile viral encephalitis).

MODE OF TRANSMISSION

For infection to be transmitted from an infected source to a susceptible host, a transport mechanism is required. Microorganisms are transmitted by several routes. The following are four common routes:

- Contact transmission
- Droplet transmission
- Airborne transmission
- Vector-borne transmission

CONTACT TRANSMISSION. Contact transmission is the usual mode of transmission of all infections. Many infections are spread by direct or indirect contact. With **direct contact,** the source and host have physical contact; microorganisms are transferred directly from skin to skin or from mucous membrane to mucous membrane. Often called person-to-person transmission, direct contact is best illustrated by the spread of the "common cold."

Indirect contact transmission involves the transfer of microorganisms from a source to a host by passive transfer from an inanimate object (a fomite). Contaminated articles may serve as sources of infection (e.g., the transfer of hepatitis B virus to a susceptible via a shared contaminated glucometer). **Fecal-oral transmission** is another route of transmitting infection. Ingestion of enteric pathogens (e.g., eating food prepared by a hepatitis A–infected person with unwashed hands) can result in disease transmission.

DROPLET TRANSMISSION. Indirect transmission may involve contact with infected secretions or **droplets.** Droplets are produced when a person talks or sneezes. These droplets travel short distances (less than 1 m). Susceptible hosts may acquire infection by contact with droplets deposited on the nasal, oral, or conjunctival membranes. An example of droplet-spread infection is influenza. Droplets, unlike airborne droplet nuclei, discussed below, do not stay suspended in the air.

AIRBORNE TRANSMISSION. Airborne transmission occurs when small airborne particles containing pathogens leave the infected source and enter a susceptible host. These pathogens can be suspended in the air for a prolonged time. The particles carrying pathogens are usually contained in droplet nuclei or dust; they are most often propelled from the respiratory tract by coughing or sneezing. A susceptible person then inhales the particles directly into the respiratory tract. Tuberculosis is communicated via airborne transmission.

VECTOR-BORNE TRANSMISSION. Vector-borne transmission of infection involves insects and animals as intermediaries between two or more hosts (e.g., ticks transmit Rocky Mountain spotted fever and Lyme disease; mosquitoes spread malaria). In these cases, the vector usually bites an infected source that has the pathogen. The vector then carries the pathogen and injects it into its new host.

PORTAL OF EXIT

The portal of exit completes the chain of infection. Exit of the microbe from the host often occurs through the portal of entry. An organism, such as *Mycobacterium tuberculosis,* enters the respiratory tract and then exits the respiratory tract as the infected host coughs. Some organisms can exit from the infected host by several routes. For example, varicella-zoster virus can spread through direct contact with infective fluid in vesicles and by airborne transmission.

Physiologic Defenses Against Infection

Strong and intact host defenses can prevent microbes from entering the body or destroy a pathogen that has entered. Conversely, impaired host defenses may be unable to defend against microbial invasion, allowing entry of microbes that can destroy cells and cause infection. Host defense mechanisms may be classified as nonspecific or specific.

NONSPECIFIC DEFENSES

Nonspecific mechanisms, usually representing the first encounter an invading pathogen has with its human host, include invasion of body tissues, such as skin and mucous membranes; phagocytosis; and inflammation.

BODY TISSUES. Intact skin forms the first and most important physical barrier to the entry of microorganisms. In addition to providing a mechanical barrier, the skin's slightly acidic pH (resulting from breakdown of lipids into fatty acids), together with normal skin flora, creates an unfriendly environment for many bacteria.

Mucous membranes' mucociliary action provides some mechanical protection against pathogenic invasion. More important, however, mucous membranes are bathed in secretions that inactivate many microorganisms. **Lysozymes,** which dissolve the cell walls of some bacteria, are present in large quantities in many body secretions, particularly in tears and nasal mucus.

Other body systems provide natural barriers to infection. The healthy respiratory tract clears about 90% of all inhaled material by upper airway filtration, humidification, mucociliary transport, and expulsion by coughing. Peristaltic action mechanically empties the gastrointestinal (GI) tract of pathogenic organisms. Stomach acid, intestinal secretions, pancreatic enzymes, and bile, together with the competition from normal bowel flora, provide an environment that protects the GI tract from invasion by harmful organisms. In the genitourinary tract, the flushing action of urine eliminates pathogenic organisms. The low pH of urine also maintains a sterile environment, although some microorganisms, such as *E. coli,* thrive in an acid medium.

PHAGOCYTOSIS. **Phagocytosis** occurs when a foreign substance evades the first-line mechanical barriers and enters the body. Various leukocyte types function differently in the immune reaction, but neutrophils bear primary responsibility for phagocytosis. This process of engulfing, ingesting, killing, and disposing of an invading organism is an essential mechanism in host defense. Phagocytic dysfunction dramatically increases a client's risk for infection.

INFLAMMATION. Inflammation is another important nonspecific defense mechanism in preventing the spread of infection. Inflammation occurs when tissue becomes damaged. Damaged cells release enzymes, and polymorphonuclear leukocytes are attracted to the infected site from the bloodstream. One important enzyme, histamine, increases the permeability of the capillaries in inflamed tissues, thus allowing fluid, proteins, and white blood cells to enter an inflamed area. Other enzymes activate fibrinogen, which causes leaked fluid to clot and prevents its flow away from the damaged site into unaffected tissue, essentially "walling off" the inflamed tissue. The process of phagocytosis disposes of the invading microorganism and often dead tissue. If inflammation is caused by infection, the end products of inflammation form pus, which is subsequently absorbed or exits the body through a break in the skin. Chapter 23 discusses the process of inflammation in more detail.

SPECIFIC DEFENSES

Specific defense responses to specific microorganisms are provided by the antibody- and cell-mediated immune systems. The **antibody-mediated immune system** produces antibodies directed against certain pathogens. These antibodies inactivate or destroy invading microorganisms as well as protect against future infection from that microorganism. Resistance to other microorganisms is mediated by the action of specifically sensitized T-lymphocytes and is called **cell-mediated immunity.** The components of the immune system work both independently and together to protect against infection. Chapter 23 describes the function of the immune system in detail.

HEALTH PROMOTION/ILLNESS PREVENTION

Infection Control in Inpatient Health Care Agencies

Infections occur most often in high-risk clients, such as older adults and those who have inadequate immune systems (immunocompromised). Physiologic and other factors contribute to infection risk in older adults (Chart 29-1). Implement interventions to prevent infection and detect signs and symptoms as early as possible. Chart 29-2 summarizes nursing interventions for Infection Protection.

Infection acquired in the inpatient health care setting (not present or incubating at admission) is termed **nosocomial,** or **health care–associated infection (HAI).** HAIs can be **endogenous** (from a client's flora) or **exogenous** (from outside the client, often from the hands of health care workers). Therefore, use of the term *nosocomial infection* does

CHART 29-1

NURSING FOCUS on the OLDER ADULT

Factors That May Increase Risk of Infection in the Older Client

Factor	Aging-Associated Changes or Conditions
Immune system	Decreased antibody production, lymphocytes, and fever response
Integumentary system	Thinning skin, decreased subcutaneous tissue, decreased vascularity, slower wound healing
Respiratory system	Decreased cough and gag reflexes
Gastrointestinal system	Decreased gastric acid and intestinal motility
Chronic illness	Diabetes mellitus, chronic obstructive pulmonary disease, neurologic impairments
Functional/cognitive impairments	Immobility, incontinence, dementia
Invasive devices	Urinary catheters, feeding tubes, IV devices, tracheostomies
Institutionalization	Increased person-to-person contact and transmission

CHART 29-2

NIC INTERVENTION ACTIVITIES for The Client at Risk for Infection

Infection Protection: *Prevention and early detection of infection in a client at risk*

- Monitor for systemic and localized signs and symptoms of infection.
- Monitor vulnerability to infection.
- Monitor absolute granulocyte count, WBC count, and differential results.
- Screen all visitors for communicable disease.
- Inspect skin and mucous membranes for redness, extreme warmth, or drainage.
- Obtain cultures, as needed.
- Promote sufficient nutritional intake.
- Encourage fluid intake, as appropriate.
- Teach the client and family about signs and symptoms of infections and when to report them to the health care provider.
- Teach client and family members how to avoid infections.

NIC intervention activities selected from Dochterman, J.M., & Bulechek, G.M. (Eds.). (2004). *Nursing interventions classification (NIC)* (4th ed.). St. Louis: Mosby. No part of this work is to be altered without prior written permission from the Publisher.
WBC, White blood cell.

not imply that an infection was caused by health care (or poor health care delivery) but only that it occurred while receiving health care. HAIs are acquired by about two million inpatients yearly, causing 88,000 deaths with a cost of about $4.6 billion annually (CDC, 2000). Clients who develop nosocomial surgical site infection (SSI) have longer and more costly hospitalizations, are 60% more likely to spend time in an intensive care unit (ICU) and are twice as likely to die as those who do not have an SSI (Kirkland et al., 1999). Although the exact causes of HAIs are difficult to identify, it is estimated that about one third of them could be prevented using the recommended CDC infection control interventions (Harbarth, Sax, & Gastmeier, 2003).

Infection control within a health care facility is designed to reduce the risk of HAIs and thus reduce morbidity and mortality. Infection control and prevention programs include the following:

- Facility- and department-specific infection control policies and procedures
- Surveillance and analysis
- Client and staff education
- Community and multidisciplinary networking
- Product evaluation with an emphasis on quality and cost savings

Monitoring HAIs promotes client safety, as evidenced by the decreased rate in ICUs during 1990 and 1999 (CDC, 2000). The program is usually coordinated and implemented by a health care professional certified in infection control (CIC) who has varied clinical and administrative experience.

Infection Control in Community-Based Settings

The Association for Professionals in Infection Control and Epidemiology (APIC) and the Society for Healthcare Epidemiology of America (SHEA) consensus panel have published requirements for activities of infection control and epidemiology in community-based settings (Friedman et al., 1999). Three primary goals were noted:

- To protect the client
- To protect health care providers, visitors, and others in the health care environment
- To accomplish these goals in a timely, efficient, and cost-effective manner

Of special note are the CDC guidelines for pregnant health care personnel.

The goals for infection control and epidemiology are the same for all health care settings. Functions of infection control and epidemiology, including the following principal functions, were summarized by the APIC and SHEA consensus report:

- To obtain and manage critical data, including infection surveillance
- To develop and recommend policies and procedures
- To intervene directly to prevent infections
- To educate and train health care workers, clients, and nonmedical caregivers

Methods of Infection Control

All health care workers who come in contact with clients or care areas are involved in some aspect of the infection control program of the agency. Infections can be prevented or controlled in at least three ways:

- Hand hygiene
- Disinfection/sterilization
- Barriers (e.g., gloves; see discussion of transmission precautions)

HAND HYGIENE

Health care workers' hands are the primary way in which disease is transmitted from client to client. In 2002 the Centers for Disease Control and Prevention (CDC) released a document entitled "CDC Hand Hygiene Recommendations." These recommendations are summarized in Chart

29-3. Handwashing is still an important part of hand hygiene, but it is recognized that in some health care settings, sinks may not be readily available. Despite years of education, health care workers often find it difficult to leave the client care setting to wash their hands. Effective **handwashing** includes wetting, soaping, lathering, applying friction under running water for at least 15 seconds, rinsing, and adequate drying. Friction is essential to emulsify skin oils and to disperse transient bacteria and soil from hand surfaces. The time it takes for health care workers to leave the client care area, find a sink, get the water temperature correct, wash their hands, and dry them was one reason why poor hand hygiene existed long after definitive evidence showed that it was essential to quality care. Handwashing can also cause dry skin, and therefore hand lotions are essential to maintain good hand health and hygiene.

Alcohol-based hand rubs have allowed care providers to spend less time seeking out sinks and more time delivering care. Nevertheless, hand rubs have their limitations. If your hands are visibly dirty, soiled, or feel sticky or you have just toileted, wash your hands instead of using alcohol-based rubs. Alcohol-based hands rubs are also ineffective against spore-forming organisms such as *Clostridium difficile,* a common cause of health care–associated diarrhea, especially in older adults taking antibiotics.

The CDC recommends the use of antiseptic solutions such as chlorhexidine, povidone-iodine, or PCMX, for handwashing in the care of clients who are at high risk (e.g., immunocompromised clients). The use of these solutions is also recommended after caring for clients who are infected with multiply resistant or other virulent organisms.

ARTIFICIAL FINGERNAILS. The CDC guidelines (2002) also addressed the issue of artificial fingernails, which have been linked to a number of outbreaks due to poor fingernail health and hygiene. The guidelines recommended that artificial fingernails and extenders not be worn during the provision of caring for clients at high risk for infections, such as those in ICUs or operating suites. Some health care agencies have banned artificial nails for all health care workers in any client care unit or clinical department. The Joint Commission on Accreditation of Healthcare Organizations has incorporated the CDC guidelines into their 2004 National Patient Safety Goals.

GLOVES. Gloves are an essential part of infection control and should be worn as part of Standard Precautions. However, gloves are not impervious barriers. Either handwashing or use of alcohol-based hand rubs should be done after removing gloves.

Most health care settings in the United States and Canada have switched from latex to non-latex gloves. The National Institute of Occupational Safety and Health (NIOSH) issued a public warning about potential allergic reactions to those exposed to latex in gloves and other medical products. Reactions include rashes, nasal or eye symptoms, asthma, and (rarely) shock (NIOSH, 1998). People with **latex allergy** usually have an allergy to foods such as bananas, kiwis, and avocados. Hands should be washed after removal of latex gloves to minimize contact time between the skin and proteins in the gloves that may cause allergic reactions.

CHART 29-3

BEST PRACTICE for Hand Hygiene

- When hands are visibly soiled or contaminated with proteinaceous material or are visibly soiled with blood or other body fluids, wash hands with soap and water.
- If hands are not visibly soiled, use an alcohol-based hand rub for decontaminating hands or wash hands with soap and water.
- Use either alcohol-based hand rub or wash with soap and water (decontaminate hands) before having direct contact with clients.
- Decontaminate hands before donning sterile gloves to perform a procedure, such as inserting an invasive device (e.g., indwelling urinary catheter).
- Decontaminate hands after contact with a client's intact skin (e.g., taking a pulse) or with body fluids or excretions/secretions.
- Decontaminate hands after removing gloves.
- Decontaminate hands after contact with inanimate objects (including medical equipment) in the immediate vicinity of the client.

Data from CDC Hand Hygiene Recommendations (2002).

DISINFECTION/STERILIZATION

Sterilization and disinfection have allowed invasive procedures to become much more common and safe. **Sterilization** means destroying all living organisms and bacterial spores. All items that invade human tissue where bacteria are not commonly found should be sterilized. **Disinfection** does not kill spores and only ensures a reduction in the level of disease-causing organisms. High-level disinfection is adequate when an item is going into an internal area of the body where the client has resident bacteria or normal flora (e.g., GI and respiratory tracts). As with sterilization, no high-level disinfection can occur without first cleaning the item. This can be especially difficult with items that have narrow lumens where organic debris can become trapped and are not easily visible. For example, endoscopes have been especially challenging to clean and have been linked to a number of infectious outbreaks.

CENTERS FOR DISEASE CONTROL AND PREVENTION TRANSMISSION-BASED GUIDELINES

PRECAUTIONS. The isolation guidelines from the Centers for Disease Control and Prevention (CDC) focus on transmission mechanisms and combine the best aspects of previous guidelines. Included in these guidelines are standard, airborne, droplet, and contact precautions.

Standard precautions acknowledge that all body excretions, secretions, and moist membranes and tissues, excluding perspiration, are potentially infectious. The protective measures from universal precautions and body-substance isolation are combined. Table 29-4 outlines the guidelines for standard precautions. Table 29-5 notes which body fluids have the highest risk for transmission of bloodborne disease.

Airborne precautions are used for clients known or suspected to have infections transmitted by the airborne transmission route; such infections are caused by organisms that can be suspended in air for prolonged periods. Negative airflow rooms are required to prevent airborne spread of microbes. Enclosed booths with high-efficiency particulate air (HEPA) filtration or ultraviolet light may be used for sputum induction procedures. Tuberculosis, measles (rubeola), and chickenpox (varicella) are examples of airborne diseases (Table 29-6).

Droplet precautions are used for clients known or suspected to have infections transmitted by the droplet transmission route. Such infections are caused by organisms in droplets that may travel 3 feet but are not suspended for long time periods. Examples of infectious conditions requiring droplet precautions include influenza, mumps, pertussis, and meningitis caused by either *Neisseria meningitidis* or *Haemophilus influenzae* type B (see Table 29-6).

Contact precautions are used for clients known or suspected to have infections transmitted by direct contact or contact with items in the client's environment. Clients with significant multidrug-resistant organism infection or colonization, such as methicillin-resistant *Staphylococcus aureus* [MRSA] or vancomycin-resistant *Enterococcus* [VRE], are placed on contact precautions. Other infections requiring contact precautions include pediculosis, scabies, respiratory syncytial virus (RSV), and *Clostridium difficile* (see Table 29-6).

MULTIDRUG-RESISTANT INFECTIONS. It is important to note that MRSA and VRE are no more transmissible than their drug-sensitive counterparts, *S. aureus* and *Enterococcus* organisms. The precautions in these cases are due to the implications for clients if they acquire these infections. Containment of drug-resistant organisms is an area in which there is currently much debate.

The CDC suggests a 12-step program to control antimicrobial resistance in health care settings. Those steps are based on preventing infections, diagnosing and treating infections effectively, using antimicrobials wisely, and preventing transmission of these microbes. In addition to infection control measures to prevent infection transmission, the CDC recommends that nurses educate clients about protection against influenza and pneumonia through immunization. Specific interventions for caring for clients with indwelling urinary catheters were also included in the 12-step program.

TABLE 29-4 Standard Precautions

These precautions are to be used with all clients to protect all health care workers from contracting or transmitting communicable disease:

- *Gloves* should be worn for contact with all body fluids, moist body tissues and mucous membranes, and nonintact skin of all clients; for handling *o*ther *p*otentially *i*nfectious *m*aterials (OPIM), items, or surfaces; and for performing venipuncture and other vascular access procedures. Gloves should be changed after each client contact.
- *Masks and/or protective eyewear* should be worn during procedures that are likely to cause splashes of body fluids.
- *Gowns or aprons* should be worn during procedures likely to result in splashes of blood or body fluids.
- *Handwashing* should be done immediately on contact with body fluids or OPIM. Hands should be washed as soon as gloves are removed.
- *Needles and sharp instruments* should be placed in puncture-resistant containers for disposal to prevent injuries from needles or other sharp items. Needles should not be recapped, bent, or removed from syringe.
- *Mouth-to-mouth resuscitation* should be performed with use of mouthpieces or other ventilation devices.

Modified from Garner, J.S., & Hospital Infection Control Practices Advisory Committee (HICPAC). (1996). Guidelines for isolation precautions in hospitals. *American Journal of Infection Control, 24*, 24-52.

TABLE 29-5 Transmission of Bloodborne Disease by Various Body Fluids

Body Fluids Likely to Transmit Bloodborne Disease

- Blood and other body fluids containing visible blood
- Semen and vaginal/cervical secretions
- Tissues
- Cerebrospinal fluid
- Amniotic fluid
- Synovial fluid
- Pleural fluid
- Peritoneal fluid
- Pericardial fluid
- Breast milk—from mother to child

Body Fluids Not Likely to Transmit Bloodborne Disease Unless Blood is Visible

- Feces
- Nasal secretions
- Sputum
- Vomitus
- Sweat
- Tears
- Urine
- Saliva, except in oral surgery or dentistry

Occupational Exposure to Sources of Infection

The Occupational Safety and Health Administration (OSHA) is a federal agency that protects workers from injury or illness at their place of employment. Unlike the voluntary guidelines developed by the CDC, OSHA regulations are law. Employers can be fined or disciplined for noncompliance with OSHA regulations. The regulation for prevention of exposure to bloodborne pathogens, such as hepatitis B and C or the human immunodeficiency virus (HIV), is one example of an OSHA regulation.

Reduction of skin and soft tissue injuries (e.g., needle sticks) is of utmost importance to reduce bloodborne pathogen transmission to health care personnel. OSHA mandates that sharp objects ("sharps") and needles be handled with care. Availability and consistency in the use of protective devices are vital. Almost half of contaminated sharp-object exposures involve nurses. Needleless devices have helped to decrease these exposures, especially when caring for clients receiving infusion therapy (see Chapter 17).

Problems from Inadequate Antimicrobial Therapy

Inadequate antimicrobial therapy may range from an incorrect choice of antibiotics to poor compliance. Some infections relapse in a subtle fashion. Drug regimen **noncompliance** (deliberate failure to take medication) or **nonadherence** (accidental failure to take medication) prevents contact of harmful microorganisms with sufficient concentrations of antibiotics and contributes to resistant-organism development.

Some diseases have legal sanctions that compel a client to complete treatment. Tuberculosis (TB) is the most common disease that has such a requirement. Clients who are at risk for noncompliance with an anti-TB drug regimen may be placed on **directly observed therapy** (DOT). This means that a health care worker must observe and validate client compliance with the drug regimen. DOT has been very effective at reducing the spread of multidrug resistant TB.

TABLE 29-6 Transmission-Based Infection Control Precautions*

Precautions (In Addition to Standard Precautions)	Examples of Diseases in Category
Airborne Precautions 1. Private room with monitored negative airflow (with appropriate number of air exchanges and air discharge to outside or through HEPA); keep door(s) closed 2. Special respiratory protection: N-95† or HEPA† respirator for known or suspected TB Susceptible persons not to enter room of client with known or suspected measles or varicella unless immune caregivers are not available Susceptible persons who must enter room must wear N-95 or HEPA 3. Transport: client to leave room only for essential clinical reasons, wearing surgical mask	Diseases that are known or suspected to be transmitted by air: Measles (rubeola) *M. tuberculosis*, including multidrug-resistant TB (MDRTB) Varicella (chickenpox)‡; disseminated zoster (shingles)‡
Droplet Precautions 1. Private room: if not available, may cohort with client with same active infection with same microorganisms if no other infection present; maintain distance of at least 3 feet from other clients if private room not available 2. Mask: required when working within 3 feet of client 3. Transport: as above	Diseases that are known or suspected to be transmitted by droplets: Diphtheria (pharyngeal) Streptococcal pharyngitis Pneumonia Scarlet fever (in infants or young children) Influenza Rubella Invasive disease (meningitis, pneumonia, sepsis) caused by *Haemophilus influenzae* type B or *Neisseria meningitidis* Mumps Pertussis
Contact Precautions 1. Private room: if not available, may cohort with client with same active infection with same microorganisms if no other infection present 2. Wear gloves when entering room 3. Wash hands with antimicrobial soap before leaving client's room 4. Wear gown to prevent contact with client or client-contaminated items or if client has uncontrolled body fluids; remove gown before leaving room 5. Transport: client to leave room only for essential clinical reasons; during transport, use needed precautions to prevent disease transmission 6. Dedicated equipment for this client only (or disinfect after use before taking from room)	Diseases that are known or suspected to be transmitted by direct contact: *Clostridium difficile* Colonization or infection caused by multidrug-resistant organisms (e.g., MRSA, VRE) Pediculosis Respiratory syncytial virus Scabies Viral hemorrhagic infections (Ebola, Lassa, or Marburg)

Modified from Garner, J.S., & Hospital Infection Control Practices Advisory Committee (HICPAC). (1996). Guidelines for isolation precautions in hospitals. *American Journal of Infection Control, 24*, 24-52.

HEPA, High-efficiency particulate air filter; *MRSA*, methicillin-resistant *Staphylococcus aureus; TB*, tuberculosis; *VRE*, vancomycin-resistant *Enterococcus*.

*Modification by facilities: The Centers for Disease Control and Prevention encourages facilities to adapt these guidelines, still following sound epidemiologic principles (e.g., some have removed TB transmission prevention guidelines from the airborne precautions category and added a separate category).

†Before use: training and fit testing required for personnel.

‡Add contact precautions for draining lesions.

Serious complications of infection may also result from incomplete or inadequate antibiotic therapy. Local infections that could be cured without complications, such as cellulitis and pneumonia, may progress to abscess formation if appropriate drug therapy is not continued. Although antibiotics do not always prevent abscess, early therapy may prevent or limit the size of an abscess.

In addition to abscess formation, inadequate therapy may promote systemic complications. If the infection is not resolved, or if it is treated with drugs that are ineffective for the offending microorganism, the pathogen may enter the bloodstream. Inadequately treated small local infections may also spread to produce complications, such as **septicemia** (systemic sepsis) with leukocytosis (increased white blood cell count) or leukopenia (decreased white blood cell count) and disseminated intravascular coagulation (DIC). After pathogens invade the bloodstream, no site is protected from invasion.

Systemic sepsis may progress to **septic shock,** more accurately called sepsis-induced distributive shock. In septic shock, insufficient cardiac output is compounded by hypovolemia; inadequate blood supply to vital organs leads to hypoxia (lack of oxygen) and metabolic failure. Chapter 40 describes this type of shock and its management in detail.

◆COLLABORATIVE MANAGEMENT

◆Assessment

HISTORY

Careful attention to the history of a client with a possible infectious disease will help you determine risk factors for infection. The age of the client, a history of cigarette smoking or alcohol use, current illness or disease (such as diabetes), past and current medication use (such as steroids), familial predisposition, and poor nutritional status may place him or her at increased risk for a number of infectious diseases. Ask the client about previous vaccinations or immunizations, including the dates of administration.

Determine whether the client has been exposed to infectious agents. A history of recent exposure to someone with similar clinical symptoms or to contaminated food or water, as well as the time of exposure, assists in identifying a possible source of infection. This information will be helpful in determining the incubation period for the disease and thus for providing a clue to its cause.

Contact with animals, including pets, may facilitate exposure to infection. Question the client about recent animal contact at home or work or in leisure activities (e.g., hunting). Insect bites should be documented.

A travel history should also be obtained. Travel to areas both within and outside the client's home country may expose a susceptible client to infectious organisms not encountered in the local community.

A thorough sexual history may reveal behavior associated with an increased risk of sexually transmitted diseases. Obtain a history of IV drug use and a transfusion history to assess the client's risk for hepatitis B, hepatitis C, and HIV infections.

Identifying the type and location of symptoms may point to affected organ systems. The onset order of symptoms gives clues to the specific problem. Gathering a history of past infection or colonization with multidrug-resistant organisms will allow for proper initiation of isolation.

PHYSICAL ASSESSMENT/CLINICAL MANIFESTATIONS

Disorders caused by pathogens vary, depending on the infection cause and site. Common clinical manifestations are associated with specific sites of infection. Carefully inspect the skin for symptoms of local infection at any site (pain, swelling, heat, redness, or pus). Wounds can become infected because the integrity of the skin is violated.

Fever (generally a temperature above 101° F [38° C]), chills, and malaise are primary indicators of a systemic infection. Fever may accompany other noninfectious disorders, and infection can be present without fever. The older adult, whose normal temperature may be 1° to 2° lower than the normal temperature in younger adults, may manifest fever at 99° F (37° C). In a client with an infection, fever (hyperthermia) is a normal immune response that can help eliminate the pathogen. Assess the client for these symptoms and carefully ask about the history and pattern of symptoms.

Lymphadenopathy, photophobia, pharyngitis, and gastrointestinal (GI) disturbance (usually diarrhea or vomiting) are often associated with infection. To detect enlargement, palpate the cervical, axillary, and other lymph nodes; examine the throat for redness.

PSYCHOSOCIAL ASSESSMENT

The client with an infectious disease often has psychosocial concerns. Delay in diagnosis because of the need to await clinical test results produces anxiety. Assess the client's level of understanding about various diagnostic procedures and the time required to obtain test results. Plan education on risk reduction or harm minimization for a time in which the client is receptive to education and motivated.

Feelings of malaise and fatigue often accompany infection. Assess the client's current level of activity and the impact of these symptoms on family, occupational, and recreational activities.

The potential spread of infection to others is an additional stress associated with the diagnosis of infection. The client may curtail family and social interactions for fear of spreading the illness. Determine the client's and family's understanding of the infection, the mode of transmission, and mechanisms that may limit or prevent transmission. Isolation, although sometimes necessary for preventing transmission of the organism, can be emotionally difficult for the client and family. Loss of contact with job and social gatherings can lead to depression, which may result in a weakening of the immune system.

Finally, a number of transmissible infectious diseases, especially those identified with socially stigmatized behaviors (such as IV drug abuse), are associated with some degree of social labeling. The client may feel socially isolated and may experience guilt related to behavior that increased the risk for infection. Observe the client carefully for signs of the client's reaction to social labels and how these feelings further affect socialization.

LABORATORY ASSESSMENT

The definitive diagnosis of an infectious disease requires identification of a microorganism in the tissues of an infected client in the presence of symptoms of the disease caused by that organism. Direct examination of blood, body fluids, and tissues under a microscope in the laboratory may not yield a definitive identification; however, laboratory assessment usually provides helpful information about microorganisms, such as shape, motility, and reaction to staining agents. Even when direct microscopy does not provide a conclusive specific diagnosis, often enough information is gathered for initiating appropriate antibiotic therapy.

CULTURE AND SENSITIVITY. The most definitive procedure for identification of a microorganism is **culture,** or isolation of the pathogen by cultivation in tissue cultures or artificial media. Specimens for culture can be obtained from almost any body fluid or tissue. The health care provider usually decides when and where the specimen for culture is taken. It is important to note, however, that sometimes a well-intentioned specimen acquisition can result in poor client care.

Proper collection and handling of specimens for culture, following standard precautions, are essential for obtaining accurate results. Specimens collected must be appropriate for the suspected infection. Material must be of adequate quantity, freshly obtained and placed in a sterile container to preserve the specimen and microorganism, and properly labeled.

After isolation of a microorganism in culture, antibiotic **sensitivity** testing is usually performed to determine the effects of various antibiotics on that particular microorganism. A microorganism that is killed by acceptable levels of an antibiotic is considered sensitive to that drug. An organism that is not killed by tolerable levels of an antibiotic is considered resistant to that drug. Preliminary results are usually available in 24 to 48 hours, but the final results generally take 72 hours. Antibiotic therapy should not begin until after the culture specimen is obtained.

COMPLETE BLOOD COUNT. A complete blood count (CBC) is often done for the client with a suspected infection. Five types of leukocytes (white blood cells) have been identified:

- Neutrophils
- Lymphocytes
- Monocytes
- Eosinophils
- Basophils

In most active infections, especially those caused by bacteria, the total leukocyte count is elevated. Various diseases are characterized by changes in the percentages of the different types of leukocytes. The differential count most often shows an increased number of immature neutrophils, or a **shift to the left.** A few infectious diseases, however, such as malaria and infectious mononucleosis, are associated with neutropenia (decreased neutrophils).

ERYTHROCYTE SEDIMENTATION RATE. The erythrocyte sedimentation rate (ESR) measures the rate at which red blood cells fall through plasma. This rate is most significantly affected by an increased number of acute-phase reactants, which occurs with inflammation. Thus an elevated ESR (>20 mm/hr) indicates inflammation or infection somewhere in the body. Chronic infection, most notably osteomyelitis, and chronic abscesses are commonly associated with an elevated ESR. The ESR is chronically elevated with arthritis as well. The effectiveness of therapy is often monitored by a decrease in this value.

SEROLOGIC TESTING. Serologic testing is performed to identify pathogens by detecting antibodies to the organism. The antibody titer tends to increase during the acute phase of infectious diseases such as hepatitis B. The titer decreases as the client improves.

RADIOGRAPHIC ASSESSMENT

X-ray films are often obtained to determine activity or destruction by an infectious microorganism. Radiologic studies (such as chest films, sinus films, joint films, GI studies, and renal films) are typically done for diagnosis of infection in a specific body site.

OTHER DIAGNOSTIC ASSESSMENTS

More sophisticated techniques for infection diagnosis include computed tomography (CT) scans and magnetic resonance imaging (MRI). Tomography is helpful in assessing for abscesses. CT scans help identify suspected osteomyelitis and fluid collections that point to possible infection. MRI scans provide a cross-sectional assessment for infection.

Another diagnostic tool for the evaluation of a client with an infectious disease is ultrasonography. This noninvasive procedure is particularly helpful in detecting infection involving the heart valves.

Scanning techniques using radioactive substances, such as gallium, can determine the presence of inflammation. Inflammatory tissue is identified by its increased uptake of the injected radioactive material.

Biopsy of the infected site may be needed for tissue culture. Biopsy sites may include the liver, bone marrow, skin, pleura, lymph nodes, kidney, bone, or even the brain. To obtain specimens, invasive procedures (e.g., bronchoscopy or endoscopy) or surgery (e.g., open lung biopsy or laparotomy) may be necessary.

◆Analysis

COMMON NURSING DIAGNOSES AND COLLABORATIVE PROBLEMS

The following are priority nursing diagnoses for clients with an infection or infectious disease:

1. Hyperthermia related to an increased metabolic state
2. Risk for Social Isolation related to altered state of wellness

The inclusion of other nursing diagnoses depends on the type and extent of the infection. For example, a client with pneumonia might experience Ineffective Airway Clearance and Fatigue; a client with a sexually transmitted disease may have Altered Sexuality Patterns.

ADDITIONAL NURSING DIAGNOSES AND COLLABORATIVE PROBLEMS

In addition to the priority nursing diagnoses, clients with an infection or infectious disease may have one or more of the following:

- Acute Pain related to physical injury
- Fatigue related to disease state
- Risk for Deficient Fluid Volume related to hypermetabolic state

The primary additional collaborative problem is Risk for Sepsis, Septic Shock, and Disseminated Intravascular Coagulation (DIC).

◆Planning and Implementation

HYPERTHERMIA

NOC **PLANNING: EXPECTED OUTCOMES.** The client with an infection or infectious disease is expected to have a balance of heat production, heat gain, and heat loss. Indicators include that the client will have noncompromised:

- Sweating when hot
- Shivering when cold
- Apical heart rate
- Respiratory rate
- Reported thermal comfort

INTERVENTIONS. The primary concern is to provide measures to eliminate the underlying cause of hyperthermia (fever) and to destroy the causative microorganism. In collaboration with the health care team, nurses use a variety of methods to manage fever.

Drug Therapy. Drug therapy plays a major role in collaborative management of clients with infection. Antimicrobials, also called anti-infective agents, are the cornerstone of drug therapy. Antipyretics are used to decrease client discomfort and prevent fever from worsening.

Antimicrobial Therapy. Antibiotics, antiviral agents, and antifungals are common types of antimicrobials. The sulfonamides, the first antibiotic group, were used in the mid-1930s. Shortly thereafter, in the 1940s, penicillin became the primary antibiotic used systemically. Since then, a wide variety of antimicrobial drugs have been developed for treatment, as well as prevention, of infection associated with virtually every class of microorganism. Effective antibiotics are available to treat nearly all bacterial infections, but misuse of antibiotics has contributed to the development of antibiotic-resistant bacteria. A few effective antifungal agents have been developed, but these drugs generally exhibit more toxicity than antibacterial agents. Effective agents are currently available for the treatment of influenza type A virus infection and HIV, but some viruses, such as HIV, mutate rapidly; thus these agents have a limited duration of effectiveness.

Effective antimicrobial therapy requires delivery of an appropriate agent, sufficient dosage, proper administration route, and sufficient therapy duration. These four requirements ensure delivery of a concentration of drug sufficient to inhibit or kill infecting microorganisms. Health care providers collaborate on selecting drugs and dosing. Teach the drug's actions, side effects, and toxic effects to your clients. Antimicrobials act on susceptible pathogens by doing the following:

- Inhibiting cell wall synthesis (penicillins and cephalosporins)
- Injuring the cytoplasmic membrane (antifungal agents)
- Inhibiting biosynthesis, or reproduction (erythromycin, tetracycline, and gentamicin)
- Inhibiting nucleic acid synthesis (actinomycin)

Observe and report side effects and toxic effects. These adverse reactions vary according to the specific classification of the drug. Most antibiotics can cause nausea, vomiting, and rashes. Before administering an antimicrobial agent, check to see that the prescribed drug is not one to which the client is allergic (Table 29-7). An accurate allergy history before drug therapy begins is essential.

Antipyretic Therapy. Antipyretic drugs, such as aspirin (ASA, Ancasal✱) and acetaminophen (Tylenol, Ace-Tabs✱), are given to reduce hyperthermia. Because antipyretics mask fever, monitoring the course of the disease may be difficult. Therefore, unless the client is extremely uncomfortable or if hyperthermia presents a significant risk (e.g., in the client with heart failure, febrile seizures, or head injury), antipyretics are not always prescribed.

Be alert for waves of sweating after each dose. Sweating may be accompanied by a fall in blood pressure followed by return of fever. These unpleasant side effects of antipyretic therapy can often be alleviated by liberal administration of fluids and by regular scheduling of drug administration.

NIC **Fever Treatment.** Other interventions to reduce fever may include external cooling and fluid administration. Performing a thorough assessment before and after interventions are implemented is essential (Chart 29-4).

External Cooling. Cooling or hypothermia blankets, or ice bags and packs, can be effective external mechanisms for reducing fever. Alternative cooling methods may be used. Sponging the client's body with tepid water or saline solution or applying cool compresses to the skin and pulse points to reduce body temperature is sometimes helpful. Observe the client for shivering during any form of external cooling. Shivering may indicate that the client is being cooled too quickly.

The use of fans is discouraged because they can disperse airborne- or droplet-transmitted pathogens. Fans can also disturb air balance in negative pressure rooms, making them positive pressure rooms and allowing possible transmission of the agent to those outside the room.

Fluid Administration. In clients with fever, fluid volume loss is increased from rapid evaporation of body fluids and increased perspiration. As body temperature increases, fluid volume loss increases. Therefore the client may be at risk for deficient fluid volume, or *dehydration.* Monitor carefully for signs of dehydration, such as increased thirst, decreased skin turgor, dry mucous membranes, and disorientation, especially in older adults. Increase oral fluid intake and provide IV fluids as prescribed. Chapter 15 discusses interventions for dehydration in detail.

TABLE 29-7 Allergic Reactions to Antibiotic Therapy

- Flushing
- Wheezing
- Sneezing
- Pruritus
- Urticaria
- Rashes
- Maculopapular to exfoliative dermatitis
- Vascular eruptions
- Erythema multiforme (Stevens-Johnson syndrome)
- Angioneurotic edema
- Serum sickness (headache, fever, chills, hives, malaise, and conjunctivitis)
- Anaphylaxis (laryngeal edema, bronchospasm, hypotension, vascular collapse, and cardiac arrest)
- Death

RISK FOR SOCIAL ISOLATION

PLANNING: EXPECTED OUTCOMES. The client with an infection or infectious disease is expected to cope with feelings of social isolation and to interact with others.

INTERVENTIONS. Education is the major intervention for meeting this goal. Develop an educational program to instruct the client and family about the mode of transmission of infection and mechanisms that prevent spread to others. Assess coping mechanisms that the client has used in the past.

As part of the health care team, ensure that the client and family understand the disease process and its cause. Explain the mode of transmission of the infecting microorganism, risk for transmission to others, and mechanisms that may prevent transmission. If necessary, ensure that the client and

CHART 29-4

NIC INTERVENTION ACTIVITIES for The Client with Infection

Fever Treatment: *Management of a client with hyperpyrexia caused by nonenvironmental factors*

- Monitor temperature as frequently as is appropriate.
- Monitor blood pressure, pulse, and respiration, as appropriate.
- Monitor skin color and temperature.
- Monitor for decreasing levels of consciousness.
- Monitor for intake and output.
- Monitor for seizure activity.
- Monitor WBC, hemoglobin, and hematocrit values.
- Administer antipyretic medication, as appropriate.
- Cover the client with a sheet only, as appropriate.
- Administer a tepid sponge bath, as appropriate.
- Encourage increased intake of oral fluids, as appropriate.
- Administer IV fluids, as appropriate.
- Encourage or administer oral hygiene, as appropriate.
- Place client on hypothermia blanket, as appropriate.
- Monitor temperature closely to prevent treatment-induced hypothermia.

NIC intervention activities selected from Dochterman, J.M., & Bulechek, G.M. (Eds.). (2004). *Nursing interventions classification (NIC)* (4th ed.). St. Louis: Mosby. No part of this work is to be altered without prior written permission from the Publisher.
WBC, White blood cell.

family can state specific ways in which precautions will be instituted in the home after discharge from the hospital.

Because the client requiring precautions may feel secluded, health care workers, as well as family members and friends, are encouraged to maintain contact with the client. Personnel caring for the client are reminded that the pathogen, not the client, requires isolation. Encourage family members and friends to visit and to use appropriate infection control measures. Communication by telephone or Internet is often effective for continuing contact with loved ones. Television, Internet, and radio help bring the outside world into the life of the client confined to the room.

In the long-term care setting, an outbreak of respiratory or gastrointestinal (GI) infection usually requires limiting visitors, activities, and admissions to the facility. Nurses working in a nursing home need to be familiar with state regulations regarding managing infections in this type of setting.

Community-Based Care

Clients with infections may be cared for in the home, hospital, nursing home, or an ambulatory setting, depending on the type and severity of the infection. Infections among older adults in nursing homes are common. Residents often have meals together in a communal dining room and participate in group activities. Immunizing residents against respiratory infections is highly recommended because these illnesses can cause severe complications or death in older adults. Other sources of infection, such as indwelling urinary catheters, are removed when possible to prevent urinary tract infections.

HOME CARE MANAGEMENT

The client with an infectious disease, such as osteomyelitis, who is discharged from the hospital to home may require continued, long-term antibiotic therapy. Emphasizing the importance of a clean home environment, especially for the client who continues to be immunocompromised or who is uniquely susceptible to **superinfection** (i.e., reinfection or a second infection of the same kind) helps to reduce the chance of infection. Medications often need to be refrigerated. Ensure that the client has access to proper storage facilities and instruct him or her to check for signs of improper storage, such as discoloration of the medication.

Inquire about the availability of handwashing facilities in the home, and check that supplies and instructions are provided as needed. Most individuals do not know how to wash hands correctly, so demonstration with the client and requesting a repeat demonstration may be necessary.

HEALTH TEACHING

INFECTION CONTROL. Explaining the disease and making certain that the client understands what is causing the illness is the primary goal of health teaching. Discuss whether the pathogen causing the infection can be spread to others and the modes of transmission.

If the client has an infectious disease that is potentially transmissible, teach the client, family, or home caregivers transmission prevention precautions. Explain whether any special household cleaning is necessary and, if so, what those special steps include. If syringes with needles are used to administer medication, explain how to dispose safely and legally of needles in the community. Clothing soiled with blood or other body fluids can be washed with bleach or disinfectant (e.g., Lysol). Recommended cleaning measures should be based on actual available equipment and facilities.

DRUG THERAPY. For the client who is discharged to the home setting to complete a course of antibiotic therapy, the importance of compliance with the planned drug regimen needs to be stressed. Explain the importance of both the timing of doses and the completion of the planned number of days of therapy. The client (and family as appropriate) should also be taught how the agents need to be taken (e.g., before meals, with meals, and without other agents) and the possible side effects. Side effects include those that are expected (such as gastric distress after oral administration of erythromycin) as well as more severe adverse reactions (such as rash, fever, or other systemic signs and symptoms of an acute adverse drug reaction). Emphasis should be placed on teaching about allergic manifestations and the need for notifying a health care provider if an adverse reaction occurs (see Table 29-7). Also discuss what to do if a drug dose is missed (e.g., doubling the dosage, waiting until the next dose time).

In the past, many clients with severe infection were hospitalized for several weeks or longer, simply to receive IV antibiotic therapy. Since the implementation of managed care, many clients have been discharged with an IV device to continue parenteral antibiotics at home or in the nursing home. The client, family member, or home care nurse administers the drugs. Chapter 17 describes infusion therapy in the community setting.

PSYCHOSOCIAL SUPPORT. The client with an infection is often anxious and fearful that the infection will be transmitted to family members or friends. Teaching the client and the family ways of preventing the spread of disease allays these fears. Careful attention is paid to the client's concerns. Making concrete suggestions (e.g., "Your wife can wear gloves when changing your dressing") to address specific concerns reduces these fears.

The client with an infectious disease associated with lifestyle behaviors, such as sexual activity or IV drug abuse, may experience guilt related to the disease. Encourage verbalization of feelings associated with the illness, and assist in locating support systems that may help alleviate these feelings.

HEALTH CARE RESOURCES

In unusual instances, a client who has been hospitalized for an infectious disease may not be able to return to the home setting immediately. In such circumstances, temporary placement in a long-term care facility may be advantageous. Care requirements, client history of infection or colonization with multidrug-resistant organisms, medication schedules, and personal needs and preferences are carefully noted on transfer documents. When possible, person-to-person communication between the two facilities will facilitate a smooth transition from the hospital to the intermediate care setting.

Home care services are often used to ensure appropriate administration of antibiotics in the client's home. Health teaching and wound care may also be needed. These services have proved efficient, effective, psychologically supportive, and less expensive than hospitalization or intermediate care facilities.

Evaluation: Outcomes

Evaluating the care of the client with an infection or infectious disease on the basis of the identified nursing diagnoses

TABLE 29-8 Sample Bioterrorism Agents and Clinical Management

Pathogen or Agent and Disease Information	Clinical Management*
Anthrax (Bacillus anthracis) ▪ **Cutaneous:** 1-7 days after contact, exposed skin itching progressing to papular and vesicular lesions, eschar, edema, ulceration, and sloughing. If untreated, may spread to lymph nodes and bloodstream. Fatality 5%-20%. ▪ **Inhalation:** 48 hr after organism or spore inhalation, flu-like illness with possible brief improvement. 2-4 days from initial symptoms, abrupt onset of severe cardiopulmonary illness (dyspnea, tachycardia, fever, diaphoresis, thoracic edema, shock, and respiratory failure). If antibiotics delayed until onset of cardiopulmonary symptoms, mortality high. May be confused with common upper respiratory infection (URI). ▪ **Other forms:** Gastrointestinal, meningeal, and sepsis.	**For cutaneous and inhaled anthrax:** No person-to-person spread. Contact precautions are not needed unless client presents directly from exposure. Standard precautions for: ▪ Prescribed wound cleansing and management of lesions ▪ Ventilator support for respiratory failure ▪ Postmortem care
Botulism (*Clostridium botulinum* and Neurotoxin) ▪ Toxin ingestion results in dysphasia, dry mouth, drooping eyelids, and blurred or double vision. Vomiting and constipation or diarrhea may be present initially, extending to symmetric flaccid paralysis in an alert person. Acute bilateral cranial nerve impairment and descending weakness or paralysis follow. ▪ Neurologic symptoms after 12-36 hr for foodborne botulism and in 24-72 hr after aerosol exposure. Case fatality up to 10%. Recovery may take months.	Standard precautions: decontamination of client is not required. No person-to-person spread. Consider outbreak with suspicion of a single case. Consult with Centers for Disease Control and Prevention (CDC) and health departments. Advise careful cleanup and disposal of suspected contaminated food source *after* consultation with health department about any needed laboratory sampling. Interdisciplinary planning for nutrition and rehabilitation support during lengthy neuromuscular and respiratory recovery.
Plague (*Yersinia pestis*) ▪ **Lymphatic infection:** 2-8 days after bites from fleas of an infected rodent (rarely after infected tissue or body fluid contact), onset of fever and chills, painful lymphadenopathy (or bubo—usually inguinal, axillary, or cervical lymph nodes), headache, gastrointestinal (GI) symptoms, and rapidly progressive weakness. 50%-60% fatality if untreated. ▪ **Pneumonic:** 1-3 days after aerosolized organism inhalation, fever and chills, productive cough, hemoptysis, rapidly progressive weakness. GI symptoms and bronchopneumonia. Survival unlikely if not treated within 18 hr of symptom onset. ▪ **Other forms:** Sepsis with coagulopathy, rarely meningitis.	Droplet precautions: required for pneumonic plague (until 72 hr of antibiotic therapy). Contact precautions until decontamination is complete: ▪ For any suspected gross contamination. See documentation information listed under Anthrax—above. Standard precautions: ▪ For prescribed management of bubo(s) if incised to drain. Community and other environmental modifications: ▪ Apply insecticide to infested environment and pets (to kill fleas). ▪ Reduce food and water supply for rodents. ▪ Avoid sick or dead animals.
Smallpox (Variola Virus) (Variola Major and Minor) ▪ 10-17 days after droplet or airborne virus inhalation or contact with bleeding lesions, onset of severe myalgias, headache, and high fever. 2-3 days later, a papular rash appears on face and spreads to extremities (and palms and soles). The rash quickly (simultaneously) becomes vesicular, then painful and pustular (contrasted to varicella rash that crops and concentrates more on trunk with various stages of macules to vesicles seen at one time). Clients are infectious at onset of rash until scabs separate (3 wk). Historically, variola major kills 20%. ▪ May be confused with varicella.	Standard, contact, and airborne precautions for clients with vesicular rash pending diagnosis. Same for varicella and variola. ▪ Also, avoid contact with organism while handling contaminated clothes and bedding. Wear protective attire (gloves, gown, and N-95 respirator). One case is a public health emergency—highly communicable. Consult CDC and health departments at earliest suspicion. Vaccine does not give reliable lifelong immunity. Previously vaccinated persons are considered susceptible. *Following exposure:* Initiate airborne precautions and observe for unprotected contacts (from days 10-17). Vaccinate within 2-3 days of exposure.

Other Key Points

Other agents besides the preceding may be used (e.g., salmonella, shigella, tularemia, brucellosis, and various bacterial toxins).

Assessment: Include account of symptoms, client's incident (what, where, when, how, others exposed or ill, and officials aware).

Treatment: Antibiotic-resistance possible. Vaccine and postexposure prophylaxis are subject to change. If any of the above diseases are suspected, consult infection control practitioner for coordination with community health officials and CDC about current recommendations and specimen collection. *If terrorism suspected*, Federal Bureau of Investigation (FBI) will coordinate evidence collection and delivery.

Multiple exposures planning: Emergency and critical care managers must address availability and acquisition of stocks of medications, vaccines, equipment (e.g., ventilators), and communications with officials, as well as public information needs.

Data from *CDC Emerging Infectious Diseases Journal, 5*(4), July-August 1999, available at http://www.cdc.gov/ncidod/eid/; and English, J., et al. (1999). *Bioterrorism readiness plan: A template for healthcare facilities* (pp. 11-26). APIC Bioterrorism Task Force and CDC Hospital Infections Program Bioterrorism Working Group (http://www.apic.org/bioterror/).

*See CDC transmission precautions.

and collaborative problems is important. The expected outcomes include that the client:

- Have a balance of heat production, heat gain, and heat loss
- Copes with feelings of social isolation
- Interacts with others as appropriate

Specific indicators for these outcomes are listed for each nursing diagnosis under the Planning and Implementation section (see earlier).

CRITICAL ISSUES FOR THE NEXT DECADE

In 1969 the U.S. Surgeon General, testifying to the U.S. Congress, made the following historic statement, "The time has come to close the book on infectious disease." Thirty-five years later, infections and infectious diseases are stronger than any time in the past 40 years. Predicting the critical issues for the next decade can be difficult, but certain critical issues internationally, nationally, and locally in some cases stand out. Critical issues for the next 5 to 10 years include bioterrorism (Table 29-8), pandemic influenza, emerging and re-emerging infectious diseases, and multidrug-resistant pathogens.

If left unchecked, multidrug resistance may bring us to a post-antibiotic era. Some microbes formerly treatable with antibiotics have become resistant to all but rarely used antibiotics. *Enterococcus, Yersinia pestis, Mycobacterium tuberculosis, and Staphylococcus aureus* are among these organisms. More information can be obtained on these critical issues from the *Emerging Infectious Diseases Journal* (see http://www.cdc.gov/ncidod/eid/).

GET READY for the NCLEX Examination!

KEY POINTS

- The chain of infection includes pathogen, portal of exit for the pathogen, means of transmission, portal of entry to the host, and susceptible host.
- Nonspecific defenses against infection include body tissues, phagocytosis, and inflammation; specific defenses rely on the immune system.
- Health care–associated infection, also called nosocomial infection, is acquired in a health care setting and is not present or incubating on admission to the facility.
- Infections can be prevented or controlled through hand hygiene, disinfection/sterilization, and barriers; proper hand hygiene is the most important intervention because health care workers' hands are the primary way in which disease is transmitted from client to client.
- Handwashing and alcohol-based hand rubs are two methods of hand hygiene (see Chart 29-3).
- The Centers for Disease Control and Prevention (CDC) recommend a ban on artificial fingernails for health care professionals when they are caring for clients at high risk for infection.
- Standard precautions are used with all clients in health care settings, assuming that all body excretions and secretions are potentially infectious.
- Airborne precautions are used for clients who have infections transmitted through the air, such as tuberculosis.
- Droplet precautions are used for clients who have infections transmitted by droplets, such as influenza and certain types of meningitis.
- Contact precautions are used for clients who have infections transmitted by direct contact or contact with items in the client's environment.
- Examples of multiple-resistant organisms include methicillin-resistant *Staphylococcus aureus* (MRSA) and vancomycin-resistant *Enterococcus* organisms.
- If infections are not treated or are inadequately treated, systemic sepsis (septicemia), septic shock, and disseminated intravascular coagulation (DIC) may result.
- A culture is the most definitive way to confirm and identify microorganisms; sensitivity testing determines which antibiotics will destroy the identified microbes.
- The differential count usually shows a shift to the left (increased number of immature neutrophils) during active infections.
- Antimicrobials and antipyretics are the most common types of drugs used when infection is accompanied by hyperthermia (fever).
- Antipyretics are used only when the fever presents a significant risk or the client is extremely uncomfortable because they may mask the disease.
- Nursing interventions for fever management are listed in Chart 29-4.
- Health teaching about clinical manifestations of infection and drug therapy is important for the client with an infection being managed at home; some clients may need health care nursing services for IV antibiotic therapy.
- Critical issues for the next decade include bioterrorism, pandemic influenza, emerging and re-emerging infectious diseases, and multidrug-resistant pathogens.

ADDITIONAL STUDY RESOURCES

Go to your Student CD-ROM for Review Questions for the NCLEX Examination.

evolve Go to http://evolve.elsevier.com/Iggy/ for Integrated Management of Care Questions for the NCLEX Examination.

SELECTED BIBLIOGRAPHY

Asterisk indicates a classic or definitive work on this subject.

Antimicrobial Resistance Interagency Task Force. (2002). Antimicrobial Resistance Interagency Task Force 2002 annual report on a public health action plan to combat antimicrobial resistance. Available at http://www.cdc.gov/drugresistance/actionplan/index.htm.

*Binder, S., & Levitt, A. Centers for Disease Control and Prevention (CDC). (1998). *Preventing emerging infectious diseases: A strategy for the 21st century.* Atlanta: Author.

Celia, F. (2002). Cutaneous anthrax: An overview. *Dermatology Nurse, 14*(2), 89-92.

*Centers for Disease Control and Prevention. (1994). Guidelines for preventing the transmission of *Mycobacterium tuberculosis* in health-care facilities, 1994. *Morbidity and Mortality Weekly Report, 43*(RR-13), 1-132.

*Centers for Disease Control and Prevention. (1998). Guidelines for infection control in health care personnel, 1998. *American Journal of Infection Control, 26,* 322.

Centers for Disease Control and Prevention. (2000). Monitoring hospital-acquired infections to promote patient safety, 1990-1999. *Morbidity and Mortality Weekly Report, 49*(8), 149-153.

Centers for Disease Control and Prevention. (2001). Management of occupational exposures to hepatitis B, hepatitis C, and HIV and recommendations for postexposure prophylaxis. *Morbidity and Mortality Weekly Report,* 50 (RR-11), 1-42.

Centers for Disease Control and Prevention. (2001). Recognition of illness associated with the intentional release of biologic agent. *Morbidity and Mortality Weekly Report, 50*(41), 893-897.

Centers for Disease Control and Prevention (CDC). (2002). Guideline for hand hygiene in health-care settings: recommendations of the Healthcare Infection Control Practices Advisory Committee and the HICPAC/SHEA/APIC/IDSA Hand Hygiene Task Force. *Morbidity and Mortality Weekly Report, 51*(RR-16), 1-44.

Centers for Disease Control and Prevention (2002). Guidelines for the prevention of intravascular catheter-related infections, 2002. *Morbidity and Mortality Weekly Report, 51*(RR-10), 1-36.

Centers for Disease Control and Prevention (2002). Smallpox response plan and guidelines, Draft 3.0 available at http://www.bt.cdc.gov/agent/smallpox/response-plan/index.asp#guidec.

Centers for Disease Control and Prevention. Food Safety Office (2003). Available at http://www.cdc.gov/foodsafety/.

Centers for Disease Control and Prevention (2003). Guideline for environmental infection control in health-care facilities: 2003 recommendations of CDC and the Healthcare Infection Control Practices Advisory Committee (HICPAC). *Morbidity and Mortality Weekly Report, 52* (RR-10), 1-48.

*Centers for Disease Control and Prevention & Hospital Infection Control Practices Advisory Committee (HICPAC). (1999). Guidelines for prevention of surgical site infection. *Infection Control and Hospital Epidemiology, 20*(4), 254-255, 257.

Chin, J. (Ed.) (2000). *Control of communicable diseases manual* (17th ed.). Washington, DC: American Public Health Association.

*Crabtree, T.D., et al. (1999). Gender-dependent differences in outcome after the treatment of infection in hospitalized patients. *Journal of the American Medical Association, 282*(22), 2143-2148.

*English, J., et al. (1999). *Bioterrorism readiness plan: A template for healthcare facilities* (pp. 11-26). APIC Bioterrorism Task Force and CDC Hospital Infections Program Bioterrorism Working Group; available at http://www.cdc.gov/ncidod/hip/Bio/13apr99APIC-CDC Bioterrorism PDF.

*Friedman, C., et al. (1999). Requirements for infrastructure and essential activities of infection control and epidemiology in out-of-hospital settings: A Consensus Panel report. *American Journal of Infection Control, 27*(5), 418-430.

*Garner, J.S., & Hospital Infection Control Practices Advisory Committee (HICPAC). (1996). Guidelines for isolation precautions in hospitals. *American Journal of Infection Control, 24,* 24-52.

*Gehring, L.L., & Ring, P. (1999). Latex allergy: Creating a safe environment. *MEDSURG Nursing, 8*(6), 358-362.

Harbarth, S., Sax, H., & Gastmeier, P. (2003). The preventable proportion of nosocomial infections. *Journal of Hospital Infections, 54,* 258-266.

*Henderson, D.A. (1999). Consensus statement of smallpox: Clinical and epidemiologic features. *Emerging Infectious Diseases Journal, 5*(4), 2127-2137.

*Herwaldt, L.A., Smith, S.D., & Carter, C.D. (1998). Infection control in the outpatient setting. *Infection Control and Hospital Epidemiology, 19*(1), 41-73.

Kahn, A.S., et al. (2000). Biological and chemical terrorism: Strategic plan for preparedness and response: Recommendations of the CDC Strategic Planning Workgroup. *Morbidity and Mortality Weekly Report, 49*(RR-4), 1-14.

*Kaufmann, A.F., Meltzer, M.I., & Schmid, G.P. (1997). The economic impact of a bioterrorism attack: Are prevention and postattack intervention programs justifiable? *Emerging Infectious Diseases Journal, 3*(2), 4.

*Kirkland, K.B., et al. (1999). The impact of surgical site infections in the 1990's: Attributable mortality, excess length of hospitalization, and extra costs. *Infection Control and Hospital Epidemiology, 20*(11), 725-730.

*McGuckin, M., et al. (1999). Patient education model for increasing hand washing compliance. *American Journal of Infection Control, 27*(4), 309-314.

*Meltzer, M.I., Cox, N.J., & Fukuda, K. (1999). The economic impact of pandemic influenza in the United States: Priorities for intervention. *Emerging Infectious Diseases Journal, 5*(5), 659-670.

*Miller, J.M. (1998) *A guide to specimen management in clinical microbiology* (2nd ed.). Washington, DC: American Society for Microbiology.

Muto, C.A., et al. (2003). SHEA guideline for preventing nosocomial transmission of multidrug-resistant strains of *Staphylococcus aureus* and *Enterococcus. Infection Control and Hospital Epidemiology 24*(5), 362-386

*National Institute for Occupational Safety and Health. (1998). *NISOH alert: Preventing allergic reactions to natural rubber latex in the workplace* (updated September 1998, pp. 1, 3, 5-7). Atlanta: U.S. Government Printing Office. No. 97-135. Available at http://www.cdc.gov/niosh/latexalt.html.

National Nosocomial Infections Surveillance System. (2002a). *National nosocomial infections surveillance (NNIS) system report, data summary from January 2002-June 2002, issued August 2002.* Atlanta: Hospital Infection Program, National Center for Infectious Diseases, Centers for Disease Control and Prevention.

National Nosocomial Infections Surveillance System. (2002b). *NNIS antimicrobial resistance report of selected antimicrobial resistant pathogens associated with nosocomial infections in intensive care unit patients.* Atlanta: Hospital Infection Program, National Center for Infectious Diseases, Centers for Disease Control and Prevention; available at http://www.cdc.gov/ncidod/hip/surveill/nnis.htm.

Osterholm, M.T. (2000). Emerging infections–Another warning. *New England Journal of Medicine, 342*(17), 1280-1281.

Parker, P.J., & Jagger, G.J. (2003). 2001 Percutaneous injury rates. *Advances in Exposure Prevention, 6*(3), 32-36.

*Rhinehart, E., & Friedman, M. (1999) Infection control in home care. Gaithersburg, MD: Association for Professionals of Infection Control and Epidemiology.

Saint S., et al (2000a). Are physicians aware of which of their patients have indwelling urinary catheters? *American Journal of Medicine 109*(6) 476-480.

Saint, S., et al. (2000b). The potential clinical and economic benefits of silver alloy urinary catheters in preventing urinary tract infections. *Archives of Internal Medicine, 160,* 2670-2675.

*Smith, P.W., & Rusnak, P.G. (1997). Infection prevention and control in the long-term-care facility. *American Journal of Infection Control, 25*(6), 488-512.

*Steed, C.J. (1999). Common infections in the hospital: The nurse's role in prevention. *Nursing Clinics of North America, 34*(2), 443-461.

UNIT **SEVEN**

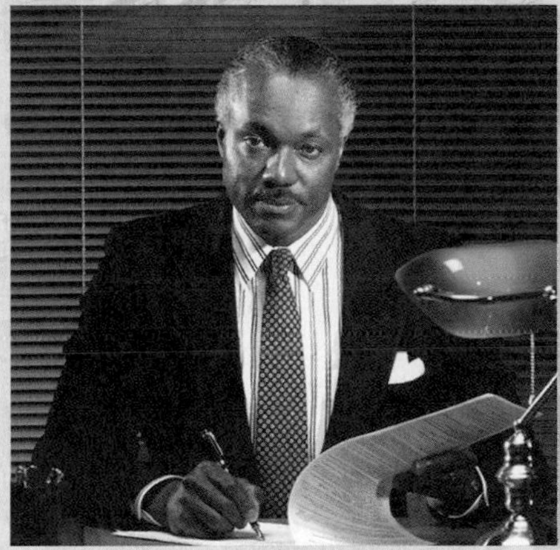

PROBLEMS of OXYGENATION

Management of Clients with Problems of the Respiratory Tract

CHAPTER

30 Assessment of the Respiratory System

CHRISTINE A. GATES • M. LINDA WORKMAN

LEARNING OUTCOMES

After studying this chapter, you should be able to:

1. Compare the structures and functions of the upper airways to those of the lower airways.
2. Distinguish between normal and abnormal (adventitious) breath sounds.
3. Describe the respiratory changes associated with aging.
4. Calculate the pack-year smoking history for the client who smokes or who has ever smoked cigarettes.
5. Demonstrate proper technique when using observation and auscultation to assess the respiratory system.
6. Demonstrate proper technique when using palpation and percussion to assess the respiratory system.
7. Interpret arterial blood gas values to assess the client's respiratory status.
8. Prioritize educational needs for the client undergoing pulmonary function tests.
9. Prioritize nursing care needs for the client after bronchoscopy or open lung biopsy.

Go to your Student CD-ROM for Review Questions for the NCLEX Examination keyed to these Learning Outcomes.

Respiratory problems are common and are the fifth leading cause of death in the United States. Some respiratory problems are chronic, and the client has physical and lifestyle limitations. Many acute health problems, medical therapies, and surgeries adversely affect respiratory function temporarily or permanently. Knowledge of anatomy, physiology, pathophysiology, and pulmonary diagnostic tests is needed to assess the client with respiratory problems.

ANATOMY AND PHYSIOLOGY REVIEW

The two purposes of breathing are to provide oxygen for tissue metabolism and to remove carbon dioxide, the major waste product of metabolism. The respiratory system also influences the following functions:

- Acid-base balance
- Speech
- Sense of smell
- Fluid balance
- Temperature control

Upper Respiratory Tract

The upper airways consist of the nose, the sinuses, the **pharynx** (throat), and the **larynx** ("voice box") (Figure 30-1).

NOSE AND SINUSES

The nose is the organ of smell, with receptors from cranial nerve I (olfactory) located in the upper areas. This organ is rigid and contains two passages separated in the middle by the **septum.** The upper one third of the nose is composed of bone; the lower two thirds is composed of cartilage, allowing limited movement. The septum and interior walls of the nasal cavity are lined with mucous membranes that have a rich blood supply. The **anterior nares** (nostrils or external openings into the nasal cavities) are lined with skin and hair, which help keep foreign particles or organisms from entering the lungs. The posterior nares are openings from the nasal cavity into the nasopharynx.

Three bony projections **(turbinates)** protrude into the nasal cavities from the walls of the internal portion of the nose (see Figure 30-1). Turbinates increase the total surface area for filtering, heating, and humidifying inspired air before it passes into the nasopharynx. Inspired air entering the nose is first filtered in the nares. Particles not filtered out in the nares are trapped in the mucous layer of the turbinates. These particles are moved by **cilia** (hairlike projections) to the oropharynx, where they are either swallowed or expectorated. Inspired air is humidified by contact with the mucous membrane and is warmed by heat from the vascular network.

Animation: Location of Sinuses

The **paranasal sinuses** are air-filled cavities within the bones that surround the nasal passages (Figure 30-2). Lined with ciliated membrane, the purposes of the sinuses are to

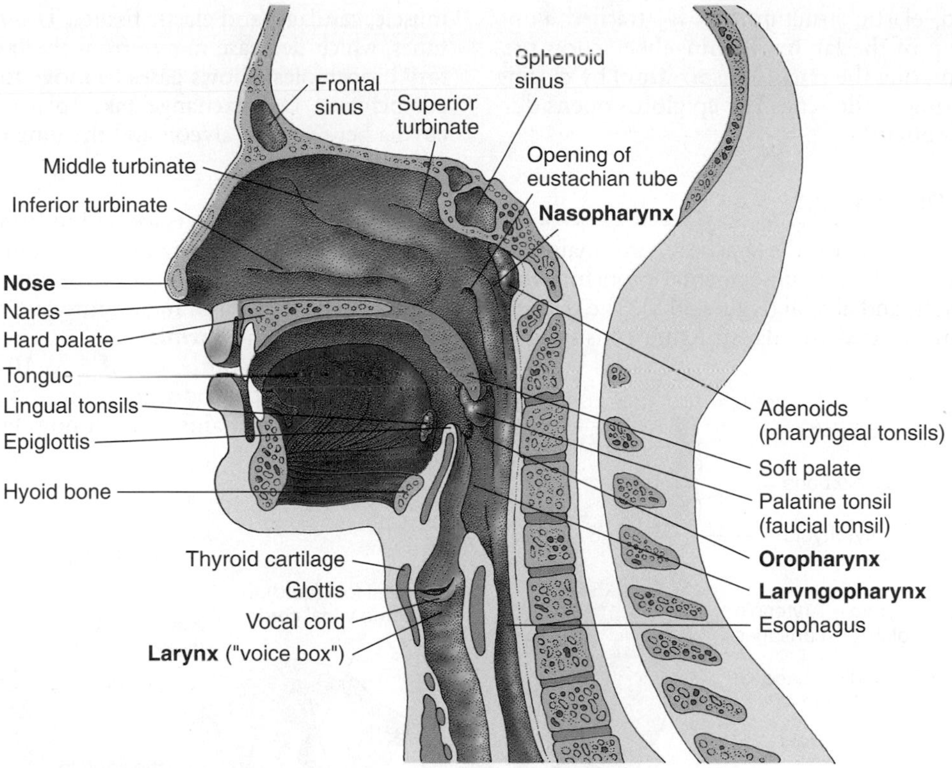

Figure 30-1 ■ Structures of the upper respiratory tract.

provide resonance during speech and to decrease the weight of the skull.

PHARYNX

The **pharynx,** or throat, is a passageway for both the respiratory and digestive tracts. It is located behind the oral and nasal cavities. The throat is divided into the nasopharynx, the oropharynx, and the laryngopharynx (see Figure 30-1).

The **nasopharynx** is located behind the nose, above the soft palate. It contains the adenoids and the opening of the eustachian tube. The **adenoids** (pharyngeal tonsils) trap organisms that enter the nose or mouth. The *eustachian tube* connects the nasopharynx with the middle ear and opens during swallowing to equalize pressure within the middle ear.

The oropharynx is located behind the mouth, below the nasopharynx. It extends from the soft palate to the base of the tongue and is used for breathing and swallowing. The *palatine tonsils* (also known as *faucial tonsils*) are located on the side borders of the oropharynx. These tonsils also guard the body against invading organisms.

The laryngopharynx is located behind the larynx and extends from the base of the tongue to the esophagus. It is the critical dividing point where solid foods and fluids are separated from air. At this point, the passageway divides into the larynx and the esophagus.

LARYNX

The **larynx** is located above the trachea, just below the throat at the base of the tongue. It is innervated by the recurrent laryngeal nerves. The larynx is composed of several cartilages (Figure 30-3). The *thyroid cartilage* is the largest and is commonly called the "Adam's apple." The *cricoid cartilage,* which contains the vocal cords, lies below the thyroid cartilage. The *cricothyroid membrane* is located below the level of the vocal cords and joins the thyroid and cricoid cartilages. This site is used in an emergency for access to the lower airways. In this procedure, called a **cricothyroidotomy** (or cricothyrotomy), an opening is made between the thyroid and cricoid cartilage and results in a tracheostomy. The two *arytenoid cartilages,* which attach at the back ends of the vocal cords, work with the thyroid cartilage in vocal cord movement.

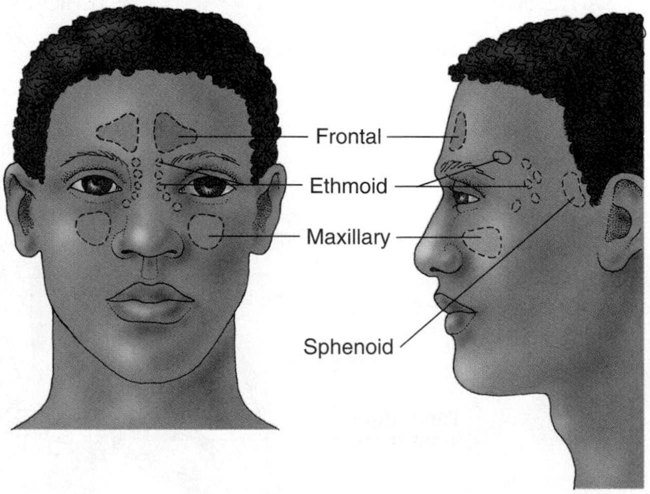

Figure 30-2 ■ The paranasal sinuses.

Inside the larynx are two pairs of vocal cords: the false vocal cords and the true vocal cords. The opening between the true vocal cords is the **glottis** (Figure 30-4). The **epiglot-**

tis is a leaf-shaped, elastic structure that is attached along one edge to the top of the larynx. Its hingelike action prevents food from entering the trachea **(aspiration)** by closing over the glottis during swallowing. The epiglottis opens during breathing and coughing.

Lower Respiratory Tract

The lower airways consist of the trachea; two mainstem bronchi; lobar, segmental, and subsegmental bronchi; bronchioles; alveolar ducts; and alveoli (Figure 30-5). The tracheobronchial tree is an inverted treelike structure consisting of muscle, cartilage, and elastic tissues. This system of branching tubes, which decrease in size from the trachea to the respiratory bronchioles, allows gases to move to and from the lung parenchyma. Gas exchange takes place in the lung parenchyma between the alveoli and the lung capillaries.

TRACHEA

The **trachea** (windpipe) is located in front of the esophagus. It begins at the lower edge of the cricoid cartilage of the larynx and extends to the level of the fourth or fifth thoracic vertebra. The trachea branches into the right and left mainstem bronchi at the **carina.**

The trachea is composed of 6 to 10 C-shaped cartilaginous rings. The open portion of the C is the back portion of the trachea and contains smooth muscle that is shared with the esophagus.

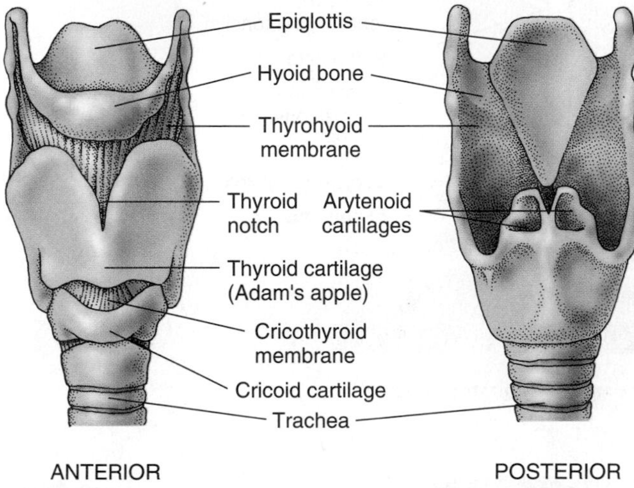

Figure 30-3 ■ Structures of the larynx.

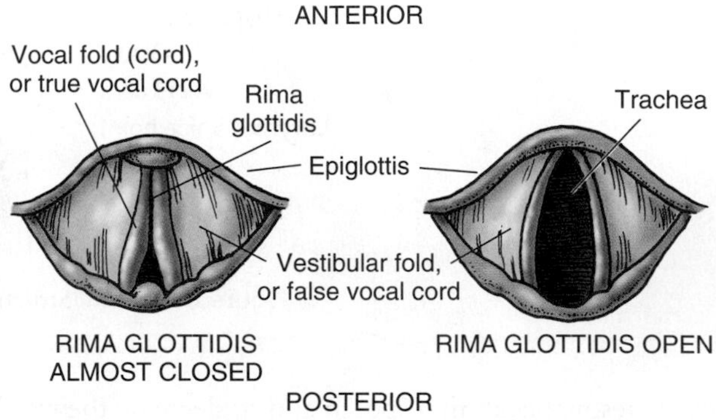

Figure 30-4 ■ Detail of the glottis (two vocal folds and the intervening space, the rima glottidis).

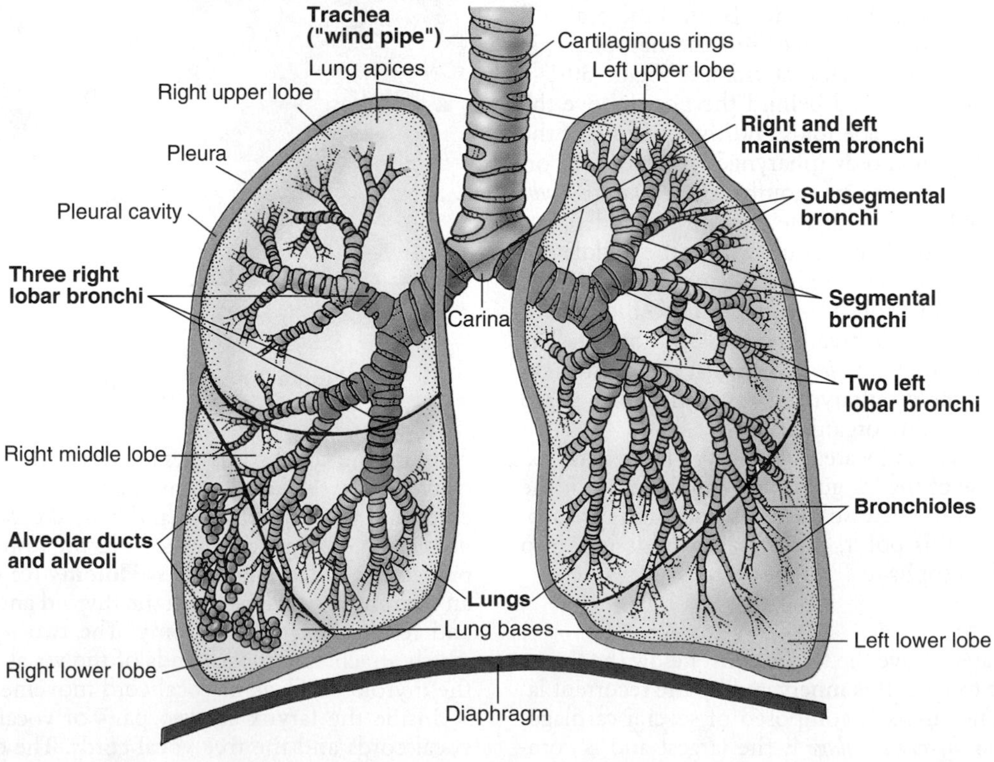

Figure 30-5 ■ Structures of the lower respiratory tract (structural size and proportions not drawn to scale).

MAINSTEM BRONCHI

The mainstem, or primary, bronchi begin at the carina. The bronchus is similar in structure to the trachea. The right bronchus is slightly wider, shorter, and more vertical than the left bronchus. Because of the more vertical line of the right bronchus, it can be accidentally intubated when an endotracheal tube is passed. Similarly, when a foreign object is aspirated from the throat, it most often enters the right bronchus.

LOBAR, SEGMENTAL, AND SUBSEGMENTAL BRONCHI

The mainstem bronchi each branch into the five secondary (lobar) bronchi that enter each of the five lobes of the lung. Each lobar bronchus is surrounded by connective tissue, blood vessels, nerves, and lymphatics, and each branches into segmental and subsegmental divisions. The cartilage of these lobar bronchi is ring-shaped and resists collapse. The bronchi are lined with a ciliated, mucus-secreting membrane. The cilia move mucus up and away from the lower airway to the trachea, where the mucus is either spit out or swallowed.

BRONCHIOLES

The bronchioles branch from the secondary bronchi and divide into smaller and smaller tubes: the terminal and respiratory bronchioles (Figure 30-6). These tubes are less than 1 mm in diameter. They have no cartilage and depend entirely on the elastic recoil of the lung to remain open **(patent).** The terminal bronchioles do not participate in gas exchange.

ALVEOLAR DUCTS AND ALVEOLI

Alveolar ducts branch from the respiratory bronchioles and resemble a bunch of grapes. Alveolar sacs arise from these ducts. The alveolar sacs contain groups of alveoli, which are the basic units of gas exchange (see Figure 30-6). A pair of healthy adult lungs has about 300 million alveoli, which are surrounded by lung capillaries. These small alveoli are numerous and share common walls, making a large surface area for gas exchange. In a healthy adult, this surface area is about the size of a tennis court. **Acinus** is a term for the structural unit consisting of a respiratory bronchiole, an alveolar duct, and an alveolar sac.

In the walls of the alveoli, specific cells **(type II pneumocytes)** secrete **surfactant,** a fatty protein that reduces surface tension in the alveoli. Without surfactant, **atelectasis** (collapse of the alveoli) occurs. In atelectasis, gas exchange is reduced because the alveolar surface area is reduced.

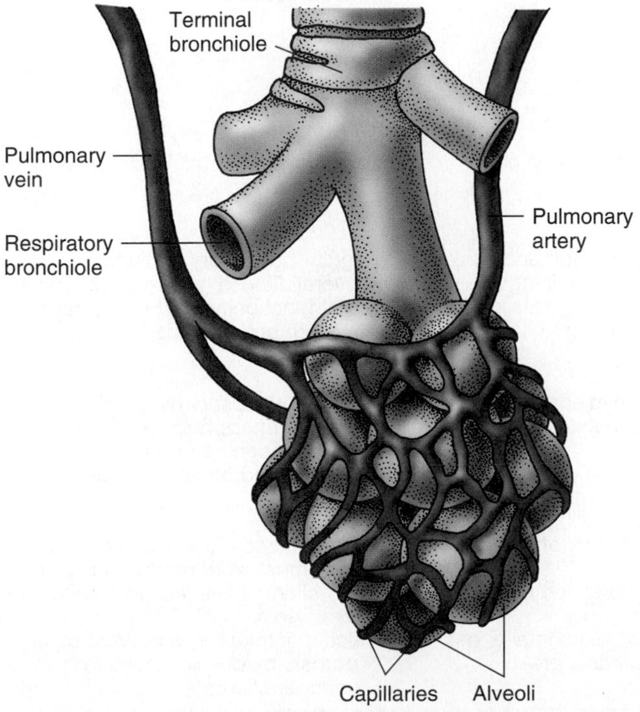

Figure 30-6 ■ The terminal bronchioles and the acinus.

LUNGS

The lungs are spongelike, elastic, cone-shaped organs located in the pleural cavity in the chest. The apex (top) of each lung extends above the clavicle; the base (bottom) of each lung lies just above the **diaphragm** (the major muscle of inspiration). The lungs are composed of millions of alveoli and their related ducts, bronchioles, and bronchi. The right lung, which is larger than the left, is divided into three lobes: upper, middle, and lower. The left lung, which is somewhat narrower than the right lung to make room for the heart, is divided into two lobes.

The hilum is the point at which the primary bronchus, blood vessels, nerves, and lymphatics enter each lung. The chest wall is innervated by the phrenic (diaphragm) and intercostal (pleura, ribs, and muscles) nerves. The bronchi are innervated by the vagus nerve. The lung parenchyma is not innervated.

The **pleura** is a continuous smooth membrane composed of two surfaces that totally enclose the lungs. The **parietal pleura** lines the inside of the chest cavity and the upper surface of the diaphragm. The **visceral pleura** covers the lung surfaces. These two surfaces are lubricated by a thin fluid that is produced by the cells lining the pleura. This fluid allows the surfaces to glide smoothly and painlessly during respirations.

Animation: Pulmonary Circulation ◀

Blood flow in the lungs occurs through two separate systems: bronchial and pulmonary. The bronchial system carries the blood needed to meet the metabolic demands of the lungs. The bronchial arteries, which arise from the thoracic aorta, are part of the systemic circulation and do not participate in gas exchange.

The pulmonary circulation is a highly vascular capillary network. Oxygen-poor blood travels from the right ventricle of the heart into the pulmonary artery, which eventually branches into arterioles that form the capillary networks. The capillaries are meshed around and through the alveoli, the site of gas exchange (see Figure 30-6). Freshly oxygenated blood travels from the capillaries and through the venules to the pulmonary veins and then to the left atrium. From the left atrium, oxygenated blood flows into the left ventricle, where it is pumped throughout the systemic circulation.

Accessory Muscles of Respiration

Breathing occurs through changes in the size of and pressure within the chest cavity. Contraction and relaxation of specific skeletal muscles (and the diaphragm) cause changes in the size and pressure of the chest cavity. Accessory muscles that help in this process include the scalene muscles, which lift the first two ribs; the sternocleidomastoid muscles, which raise the sternum; and the trapezius and pectoralis muscles, which fix the shoulders. At times, various back and abdominal muscles are used when the work of breathing is increased.

Respiratory Changes Associated with Aging

The respiratory changes that occur with aging are described in Chart 30-1. Many changes in older clients result from heredity and a lifetime of exposure to environmental stimuli (e.g., cigarette smoke, bacteria, air pollutants, and industrial fumes and irritants). Table 30-1 shows the age-related changes in the partial pressure of arterial oxygen (PaO_2).

Respiratory disease is a major cause of illness and chronic disability in older clients. Although respiratory function normally declines with age, there is usually no problem keeping pace with the demands of ordinary activ-

CHART 30-1

NURSING FOCUS on the OLDER ADULT

Changes in the Respiratory System Related to Aging

Physiologic Change	Nursing Interventions	Rationales
Alveoli		
Alveolar surface area decreases. Diffusion capacity decreases. Elastic recoil decreases. Bronchioles and alveolar ducts dilate. Ability to cough decreases.	Encourage vigorous pulmonary hygiene (i.e., encourage the client to turn, cough, and deep breathe), especially if he or she is confined to bed or has had surgery.	There is increased potential for mechanical or infectious respiratory complications in these situations.
Airways close early.	Encourage upright position.	The upright position minimizes ventilation-perfusion mismatching.
Lungs		
Residual volume increases. Vital capacity decreases. Efficiency of oxygen and carbon dioxide exchange decreases. Elasticity decreases.	Include inspection, palpation, percussion, and auscultation in lung assessments.	Inspection, palpation, percussion, and auscultation are needed to detect normal age-related changes.
	Help client in actively maintaining health and fitness.	Health and fitness helps to keep losses in respiratory functioning to a minimum.
	Assess the client's respirations for abnormal breathing patterns.	Periodic breathing patterns (e.g., Cheyne-Stokes) can occur.
	Encourage frequent oral hygiene.	Oral hygiene aids in the removal of secretions.
Pharynx and Larynx		
Muscles atrophy. Vocal cords become slack. Laryngeal muscles lose elasticity and cartilage.	Have face-to-face conversations with client when possible.	Client's voice may be soft and difficult to understand.
Pulmonary Vasculature		
Increased vascular resistance to blood flow through pulmonary vascular system occurs. Pulmonary capillary blood volume decreases. Risk of hypoxia increases.	Assess the client's level of consciousness.	Client can become confused during acute respiratory conditions.
Exercise Tolerance		
Body's response to hypoxia and hypercarbia decreases.	Assess for subtle manifestations of hypoxia.	Early assessment helps to prevent complications.
Muscle Strength		
Respiratory muscle strength, especially the diaphragm and the intercostals, decreases.	Encourage pulmonary hygiene and help the client in actively maintaining health and fitness.	Regular pulmonary hygiene and overall fitness help maintain maximal functioning of the respiratory system and prevent illness.
Susceptibility to Infection		
Effectiveness of the cilia decreases. Immunoglobulin A decreases. Alveolar macrophages are altered.	Encourage pulmonary hygiene, and help the client in actively maintaining health and fitness.	Regular pulmonary hygiene and overall fitness help maintain maximal functioning of the respiratory system and prevent illness.
Chest Wall		
Anteroposterior diameter increases. Thorax becomes shorter.	Discuss the normal changes of aging.	Clients may be anxious because they must work harder to breathe.
Progressive kyphoscoliosis occurs. Chest wall compliance (elasticity) decreases.	Discuss the need for increased rest periods during exercise.	Older clients have less tolerance for exercise.
Mobility may decrease. Osteoporosis is possible.	Encourage adequate calcium intake (especially during a woman's premenopause phase).	Calcium intake helps prevent osteoporosis by building bone in younger clients.

ity. The sedentary older adult, however, often feels breathless during exercise.

It is difficult to determine which respiratory changes in older adults are related to normal aging and which changes are caused by respiratory disease or exposure to pollutants. Age-related neuromuscular and cardiovascular changes also may cause abnormal breathing, even if the lungs are normal.

ASSESSMENT TECHNIQUES

History

Obtaining accurate information from the client is important for identifying the type and severity of breathing problems. Chart 30-2 lists questions to ask clients (based on Gordon's Functional Health Patterns) to assess the impact of pulmonary function.

DEMOGRAPHIC DATA

Age, gender, and race can affect the physical and diagnostic findings related to breathing. Many of the diagnostic studies for respiratory disorders (e.g., pulmonary function tests) use these data for determining predicted normal values.

WOMEN'S HEALTH CONSIDERATIONS

Women, especially smokers, have greater bronchial responsiveness (i.e., bronchial hyperreactivity) and larger airways than men. This factor increases the risk for a more rapid decline in lung function as an older adult, especially in people who were or are smokers.

CULTURAL CONSIDERATIONS

The largest chest volumes are found in white individuals; the smallest volumes are found in Native Americans/American Indians. The chest volumes of black individuals are significantly larger than those of Asian Americans but not as large as those of whites (Jarvis, 2004). Compared with whites, black individuals and other people with dark skin usually show a lower oxygen saturation rate (3% to 5% lower) as measured by pulse oximetry; this results from deeper coloration of the nail bed and does not reflect true oxygen status.

TABLE 30-1 Age Distributions and Partial Pressure of Arterial Oxygen (Pao_2) Values (Mean)

Age (yr)	Pao_2 (mm Hg)
40-44	95
45-49	88.6
50-54	87.1
55-59	85.1
60-64	84.8
65-69	82.3
70-74	79.1
75-79	82.9
80-84	83.4
85-90	83.2

Modified with permission from Cerveri, I., et al. (1995). Reference values of arterial oxygen tension in the middle-aged and elderly. *American Journal of Respiratory and Critical Care Medicine, 152,* 934-941.

FAMILY HISTORY AND GENETIC RISK

Obtain a family history to assess for respiratory disorders with a genetic component, such as cystic fibrosis, some lung cancers, and $alpha_1$-antitrypsin deficiency (one risk factor for emphysema). Clients with asthma often have a family history of allergic symptoms and reactive airways. Ask about a history of infectious disease, such as tuberculosis, because family members may have similar environmental or occupational exposures.

PERSONAL HISTORY

Ask clients about their own respiratory history (Table 30-2).

Smoking History

Ask the client about the use of cigarettes, cigars, pipe tobacco, marijuana, and other controlled substances. Assess whether the client has passive exposure to smoke in the home or workplace. If the client smokes, ask for how long, how many packs a day, and whether the client has quit smoking (and how long ago). Document the smoking history in **pack-years** (number of packs smoked per day multiplied by number of years). Because the client may have guilt or denial about this habit, assume a nonjudgmental attitude during the interview.

Smoking induces changes in the airways, and these changes lead to varying degrees of airway obstruction. Men who continue to smoke have a more rapid decline in their pulmonary function than do nonsmokers. The pulmonary function of clients who have quit smoking for 2 or more

CHART 30-2

Respiratory Assessment
USING GORDON'S FUNCTIONAL HEALTH PATTERNS

Health Perception–Health Management Pattern
- How has your general health been?
- Have you had any colds this past year?
- Have you missed work or school because of illness this past year?
- Do you use cigarettes? For how many years? How many packs per day?

Activity-Exercise Pattern
- Do you feel you have sufficient energy to perform tasks or routines that are required of you?
- Do you feel you have sufficient energy to do what you would like to do?
- Do you exercise? How often? For how long each time? What type(s) of exercise do you perform?
- What activities do you perform in your spare time?
- What is your ability to perform the following tasks?

Feeding______	Grooming______
Bathing______	General mobility______
Toileting______	Cooking______
Bed mobility______	Home maintenance______
Dressing______	Shopping______

Functional Levels Code
Level 0: Full self-care
Level I: Requires use of equipment or device
Level II: Requires assistance or supervision of another person
Level III: Requires assistance or supervision of another person and the use of equipment or devices
Level IV: Is dependent and does not participate

Based on Gordon, M. (2002). *Manual of nursing diagnosis* (10th ed.). St. Louis: Mosby.

TABLE 30-2 Important Aspects to Assess in a Respiratory System History

Smoking history
Childhood illnesses
- Asthma
- Pneumonia
- Communicable diseases
- Hay fever
- Allergies
- Eczema
- Frequent colds
- Croup
- Cystic fibrosis

Adult illnesses
- Pneumonia
- Sinusitis
- Tuberculosis
- HIV and AIDS
- Lung disease such as emphysema and sarcoidosis
- Diabetes
- Hypertension
- Heart disease

Influenza, pneumococcal (Pneumovax) and BCG vaccinations
Surgeries of the upper or lower respiratory system
Injuries to the upper or lower respiratory system
Hospitalizations
Date of last chest x-ray, pulmonary function test, tuberculin test, or other diagnostic tests and results
Recent weight loss
Night sweats
Sleep disturbances
Lung disease and condition of family members
Geographic areas of recent travel
Occupation and leisure activities

AIDS, Acquired immunodeficiency syndrome; *BCG,* bacille Calmette-Guérin; *HIV,* human immunodeficiency virus.

years appears to decline less rapidly than in clients who continue to smoke.

Drug Use

Ask about drugs taken for breathing problems and about drugs taken for other conditions. For example, a cough can be a side effect of some antihypertensive drugs (angiotensin-converting enzyme [ACE] inhibitors). Determine which over-the-counter drugs (e.g., cough syrups, antihistamines, decongestants, inhalants, nasal sprays) the client is using. Also assess the use of home remedies. Ask about past drug use and the reason for its discontinuation. For example, the client may have used many bronchodilator inhalers but may prefer one particular drug for relieving breathlessness. Some drugs for other conditions can cause permanent changes in lung function. For example, clients may have pulmonary fibrosis if they received bleomycin (Blenoxane) as chemotherapy for cancer or amiodarone (Cordarone) for cardiac problems.

Allergies

Information about allergies is important to the respiratory history. Ask whether the client has any known allergies to substances such as foods, dust, molds, pollen, bee stings, trees, grass, animal dander and saliva, or any drugs. Ask the client to describe specific allergic responses. For example, does he or she wheeze, have trouble breathing, cough, sneeze, or have rhinitis after exposure to the allergen? Has he or she ever been treated for an allergic response? If the client has received treatment for allergies, ask about what caused the need for treatment, the type of treatment, and the response to treatment.

Document any known allergies and the specific type of allergic response in a prominent place in the client's medical record.

Travel and Area of Residence

Travel and area of residence may be relevant for a history of exposure to certain diseases. For example, *histoplasmosis,* a fungal disease caused by inhalation of contaminated dust, is found in the central United States and Central America. *Coccidioidomycosis,* another fungal disease, is found mostly in the western and southwestern United States, Mexico, and portions of Central America.

DIET HISTORY

Assess the client's diet history to determine allergic reactions to certain foods or preservatives. Manifestations range from rhinitis, chest tightness, weakness, shortness of breath **(dyspnea),** urticaria, and severe wheezing to loss of consciousness. Ask about his or her usual food intake and whether any breathing problems occur with eating. Malnutrition may occur if the client has difficulty breathing during eating or while preparing food.

OCCUPATIONAL HISTORY AND SOCIOECONOMIC STATUS

Explore the home, community, and workplace for environmental factors that could cause or worsen lung disease. Occupational lung diseases include pneumoconiosis, which results from the inhalation of dust (e.g., coal dust, stone dust, silicone dust); toxic lung injury; and hypersensitivity disease (e.g., hypersensitivity to latex). The occupational history includes the exact dates of employment and a brief job description. Exposure to industrial dusts of any type or to the chemicals found in smoke and fumes may cause breathing disorders. Bakers, coal miners, stone masons, cotton handlers, woodworkers, welders, potters, plastic and rubber manufacturers, printers, farm workers, and steel foundry workers are at risk for breathing problems.

Ask the client about the home and living conditions, such as the type of heat used (e.g., gas heater, wood-burning stove, fireplace, kerosene heater). Determine exposure to environmental irritants (e.g., noxious fumes, chemicals, animals, birds, air pollutants). Ask about hobbies and leisure activities. Pastimes such as painting, working with ceramics, model airplane building, furniture refinishing, or woodworking may have exposed the client to harmful chemical irritants.

CURRENT HEALTH PROBLEMS

Whether the breathing problem is acute or chronic, the current health problem usually includes cough, sputum production, chest pain, and shortness of breath at rest or on exertion. During the interview, explore the present illness in chronologic order. This analysis of the problem(s) includes the following:

- Onset
- Duration
- Location
- Frequency
- Progressing and radiating patterns

- Quality and number of symptoms
- Aggravating and relieving factors
- Associated manifestations
- Treatments

Cough

Cough is the main sign of lung disease. Ask the client how long the cough has been present (e.g., 1 week, 3 months) and whether it occurs at a specific time of day (e.g., on awakening in the morning, which is common in smokers) or in relation to any physical activity. Determine whether the cough is productive or nonproductive, congested, dry, tickling, or hacking.

Sputum Production

Sputum production is an important symptom associated with coughing. Check the duration, color, consistency, odor, and amount of sputum. Sputum may be clear, white, tan, gray or, if infection is present, yellow or green.

Describe the consistency of sputum as thin, thick, watery, or frothy. Smokers with chronic bronchitis have mucoid sputum. Excessive pink, frothy sputum common occurs with pulmonary edema. Pneumococcal pneumonia often produces rust-colored sputum, and foul-smelling sputum often occurs with a lung abscess. Blood in the sputum **(hemoptysis)** is most often seen in clients with chronic bronchitis or lung cancer. Clients with tuberculosis, pulmonary infarction, bronchial adenoma, or lung abscess may have grossly bloody sputum.

Quantify sputum by describing its volume in terms such as teaspoon, tablespoon, and cups or fractions of cups. Normally, the bronchial tree can produce up to 3 ounces (90 mL) of sputum per day. Determine whether sputum production is increasing, possibly from external stimuli (e.g., an irritant in the work setting) or an internal cause (e.g., chronic bronchitis or a pulmonary abscess).

Chest Pain

A detailed description of chest pain helps distinguish whether pain is pleural, musculoskeletal, cardiac, or gastrointestinal in origin. Ask the client whether the pain is continuous or made worse by coughing, deep breathing, or swallowing.

Dyspnea

The perception of **dyspnea** (difficulty in breathing or breathlessness) is subjective and varies among clients. A client's feeling of dyspnea may not be consistent with the severity of the presenting problem. Determine the type of onset (slow or abrupt); the duration (number of hours, time of day); relieving factors (changes of position, drug use, activity cessation); and whether wheezing, crackles, or stridor occurs with the breathlessness.

Try to quantify dyspnea by asking whether this symptom interferes with **activities of daily living (ADLs)** and, if so, how severely. For example, is the client breathless while dressing, showering, shaving, or eating? Does dyspnea occur after walking one block or climbing one flight of stairs? Table 30-3 classifies dyspnea with changes in ADL performance. A dyspnea assessment scale may be used to assess dyspnea (see Chapter 33).

Ask about **paroxysmal nocturnal dyspnea (PND),** which is intermittent dyspnea during sleep, and about **orthopnea,** which is a shortness of breath that occurs when lying down but is relieved by sitting up. These two conditions often occur with chronic lung disease and left-sided heart failure. In PND, the client has a sudden onset of breathing difficulty that is severe enough to awaken the client from sleep.

TABLE 30-3 Correlation of Dyspnea Classification with Performance of Activities of Daily Living

Classification	Activities of Daily Living Key
Class I: No significant restrictions in normal activity. Employable. Dyspnea occurs only on more than normal or strenuous exertion.	*4:* No breathlessness, normal.
Class II: Independent in essential ADLs but restricted in some other activities. Dyspneic on climbing stairs or on walking on an incline but not on level walking. Employable only for sedentary job or under special circumstances.	*3:* Satisfactory, mild breathlessness. Complete performance is possible without pause or assistance but not entirely normal.
Class III: Dyspnea commonly occurs during usual activities, such as showering or dressing, but the client can manage without assistance from others. Not dyspneic at rest; can walk for more than a city block at own pace but cannot keep up with others of own age. May stop to catch breath partway up a flight of stairs. Is probably not employable in any occupation.	*2:* Fair, moderate breathlessness. Must stop during activity. Complete performance is possible without assistance, but performance may be too debilitating or time consuming.
Class IV: Dyspnea produces dependence on help in some essential ADLs such as dressing and bathing. Not usually dyspneic at rest. Dyspneic on minimal exertion; must pause on climbing one flight, walking more than 100 yards, or dressing. Often restricted to home if lives alone. Has minimal or no activities outside of home.	*1:* Poor, marked breathlessness. Incomplete performance; assistance is necessary.
Class V: Entirely restricted to home and often limited to bed or chair. Dyspneic at rest. Dependent on help for most needs.	*0:* Performance not indicated or recommended; too difficult.

ADLs, Activities of daily living.

Physical Assessment

ASSESSMENT OF THE NOSE AND SINUSES

Video Clip: Inspection of the Nose

Inspect the client's external nose for deformities or tumors, and inspect the nostrils for symmetry of size and shape. Nasal flaring may indicate increased respiratory effort. To observe the interior nose, ask the client to tilt the head back for a penlight examination. Use a nasal speculum and nasopharyngeal mirror for a more thorough inspection of the nasal cavity.

Inspect for color, swelling, drainage, and bleeding. The mucous membrane of the nose normally appears redder than the oral mucosa, but it is usually pale, engorged, and bluish-gray

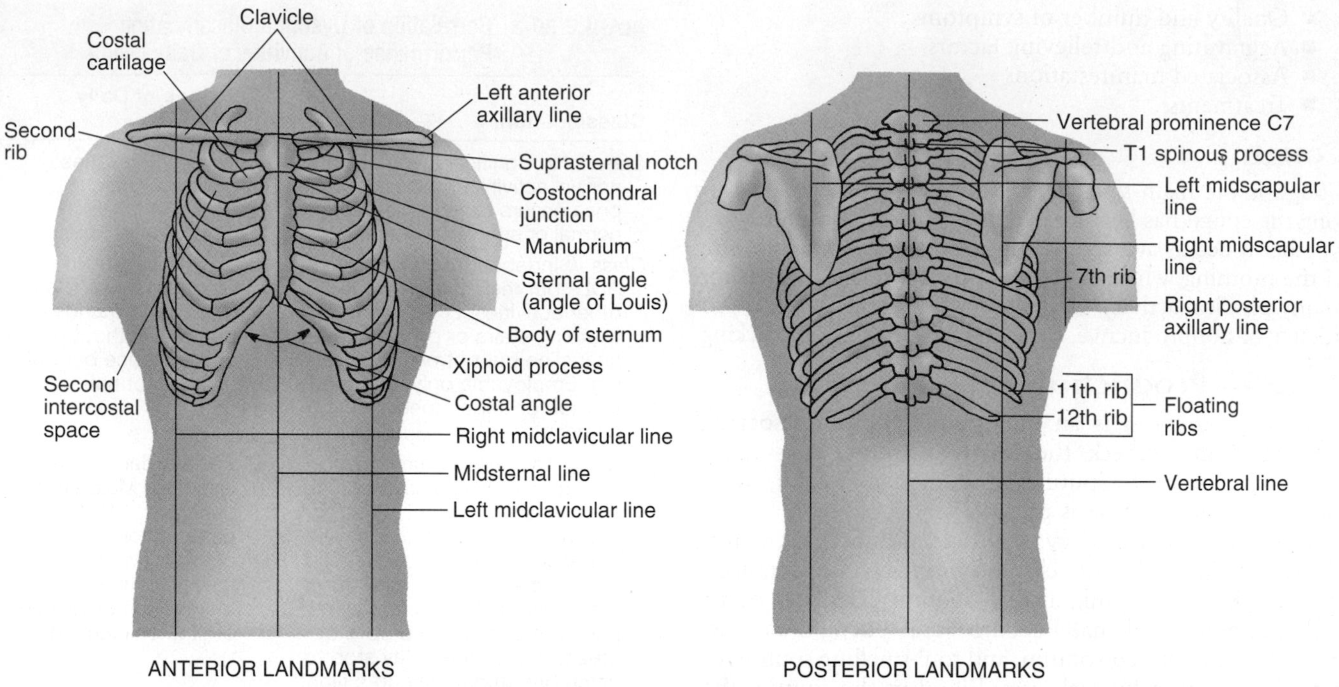

Figure 30-7 ■ Anterior and posterior thoracic landmarks.

in clients with allergic rhinitis. Check the nasal septum for bleeding, perforation, or deviation. Some degree of septal deviation is common in most adults and appears as an S shape, inclining toward one side or the other. A perforated septum is present if the light shines through the perforation into the opposite nostril; this condition is often found in cocaine users. Nasal polyps, a common cause of obstruction, are pale, shiny, gelatinous lumps or "bags" attached to the turbinates.

Occlude one naris at a time to check whether air moves through the nonoccluded side easily. Palpate the nose and paranasal sinuses to detect tenderness or swelling. Only the frontal and maxillary sinuses are easily examined because the ethmoid and sphenoid sinuses lie deep within the skull (see Figure 30-2). Using your thumbs, check for sinus tenderness by pressing upward on the frontal and maxillary areas. Assess both sides at the same time. Tenderness in these areas suggests inflammation or acute sinusitis. Tenderness in response to tapping a finger over these areas also indicates inflammation.

Transillumination of the sinuses may be used to detect sinusitis. In a darkened room, place the bulb of a penlight on the client's cheek (just under the corner of the eye) and observe for light penetration through the roof of the mouth. Normally a faint glow of light through the bone outlines the sinus. Transillumination is absent or decreased in sinusitis; however, this test is not conclusive for sinusitis.

ASSESSMENT OF THE PHARYNX, TRACHEA, AND LARYNX

Assessment of the pharynx begins with inspection of the external structures of the mouth. To examine the posterior pharynx, use a tongue depressor to press down one side of the tongue at a time (to avoid stimulating the gag reflex). As the client says "ah," observe the rise and fall of the soft palate and uvula and inspect for color and symmetry, evidence of discharge (postnasal drainage), edema or ulceration, and tonsillar enlargement or inflammation.

Inspect the neck for symmetry, alignment, masses, swelling, bruises, and the use of accessory neck muscles in breathing. Palpate lymph nodes for size, shape, mobility, consistency, and tenderness. Tender nodes are usually movable and suggest inflammation. Malignant nodes are often hard and are fixed to the surrounding tissue.

Gently palpate the trachea for position, mobility, tenderness, and masses. Firm palpation may trigger coughing or gagging. The space on either side of the trachea should be equal. Many lung disorders cause the trachea to deviate from the midline. Tension pneumothorax, large pleural effusion, mediastinal mass, and neck tumors push the trachea away from the affected area. Pneumonectomy, fibrosis, and atelectasis pull the trachea toward the affected area. Decreased tracheal mobility may occur with cancer or fibrosis of the mediastinum.

The larynx is usually examined by a specialist with a laryngoscope. An abnormal voice, especially hoarseness, may be heard when there are problems of the larynx.

ASSESSMENT OF THE LUNGS AND THORAX

Inspection

Video Clip: Respiratory Excursion

Begin inspection of the chest by assessing the anterior and posterior thorax. Normal landmarks of the chest and thorax are shown in Figure 30-7. If possible, have the client sit up during the assessment. He or she should be undressed to the waist and draped for privacy and warmth. Observe the chest and compare one side with the other. Work from the top (apex) and move downward toward the base while inspecting for discoloration, scars, lesions, masses, and spinal deformities such as kyphosis, scoliosis, and lordosis.

Observe the rate, rhythm, and depth of inspirations as well as the symmetry of chest movement. Impaired movement or unequal expansion may indicate disease of the lung or the pleura. Observe the type of breathing (e.g., pursed-lip or diaphragmatic breathing) and the use of accessory muscles. While observing respiration, document the duration of the inspiratory (I) and expiratory (E) phases. The ratio of these phases (the I-E ratio) is normally 1:2. A prolonged expiratory phase indicates an obstruction of air outflow and is often seen in clients with asthma or chronic obstructive pulmonary disease (COPD).

Animation: Patterns of Respiration

Examine the shape of the client's chest and compare the anteroposterior (AP) diameter with the lateral diameter. This ratio normally ranges from 1:2 to about 5:7, depending on body build. The ratio increases to 1:1 in clients with emphysema, which results in the typical barrel-chest appearance.

Normally the ribs slope downward. Clients with air trapping in the lungs caused by chronic asthma or emphysema, however, have little or no slope to the ribs (i.e., the ribs are more horizontal).

Check for abnormal retractions of the intercostal spaces during inspiration, which indicate airflow obstruction. These retractions may be due to lung fibrosis, severe acute asthma, emphysema, or tracheal or laryngeal obstruction.

Palpation

Video Clip: Respiratory Excursion, Tactile Fremitus

Palpate the chest after inspection. Palpation is performed to assess respiratory movement symmetry and observable abnormalities, to identify areas of tenderness, and to check vocal or tactile **fremitus** (vibration).

Assess chest expansion by placing your thumbs on the client's spine at the level of the ninth ribs and extending the fingers laterally around the rib cage. As the client inhales, both sides of the chest should move upward and outward together in one symmetric movement and move your thumbs apart. On exhalation, the thumbs should come back together as they return to the midline. Decreased movement on one side (unilateral or unequal expansion) may be a result of pain, trauma, or **pneumothorax** (air in the pleural cavity). Respiratory lag or slowed movement on one side occurs with the presence of a pulmonary mass, pleural fibrosis, atelectasis, pneumonia, or a lung abscess.

Palpate any abnormalities found on inspection (e.g., masses, lesions, bruises, swelling). Also palpate for tenderness, particularly if the client has reported pain. **Crepitus** (subcutaneous emphysema) is felt as a crackling sensation beneath the fingertips. Document this finding, especially if it occurs around a wound site or if a pneumothorax is suspected. Crepitus indicates that air is trapped within the tissues.

Video Clip: Tactile Fremitus

Tactile (vocal) fremitus is a vibration of the chest wall produced when the client speaks. This vibration can be palpated on the chest wall. To check tactile fremitus, place the palm or the base of your fingers against the client's chest wall and instruct him or her to say the number *99*. Using the same hand and moving from the apices to the bases, compare vibrations from one side of the chest with those from the other side. Palpable vibrations are transmitted from the tracheobronchial tree, along the solid surface of chest wall, to your hand.

Check the symmetry of the vibrations and areas of enhanced, diminished, or absent fremitus. Fremitus is decreased if the transmission of sound waves from the larynx to the chest wall is slowed. This situation can occur when the pleural space is filled with air **(pneumothorax)** or fluid **(pleural effusion)** or when the bronchus is obstructed.

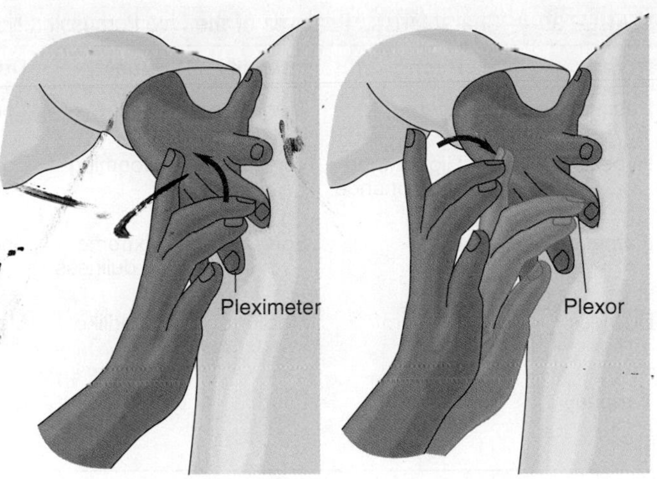

Figure 30-8 ■ Percussion technique.

Fremitus is increased over large bronchi because of their proximity to the chest wall. Diseases such as pneumonia and abscesses increase the density of the thorax and enhance transmission of the vibrations.

Percussion

Video Clip: Diaphragmatic Excursion

Use percussion to assess for pulmonary resonance, the boundaries of organs, and diaphragmatic excursion. Percussion involves tapping the chest wall, which sets the underlying tissues into motion and produces audible sounds. Place the distal joint of the middle finger of the less dominant hand firmly over the intercostal space to be percussed. No other part of your hand should touch the client's chest wall because doing so will absorb the vibrations. Then deliver a quick, sharp strike with the middle finger of your dominant hand to the distal joint of the positioned finger (Figure 30-8). Maintain a loose, relaxed wrist while delivering the taps with the tip of your finger, not the finger pad. Repeat this technique two or three times to determine the intensity, pitch, quality, and duration of the sound produced. Long fingernails limit the ability to percuss.

Animation: Percussion Tones

Percussion produces five distinguishable notes (Table 30-4). These sounds assist in determining the density of the underlying structures (i.e., whether the lung tissue contains air or fluid or is solid). Percuss over the intercostal spaces only because percussing the sternum, ribs, or scapulae yields bone sound. Percussion penetrates only 2 to 3 inches (5 to 7 cm), and therefore deeper lesions are not detected using this technique.

Begin percussion with the client sitting in an upright position. Assess the posterior thorax first and proceed systematically, beginning at the apex and working toward the base. The apex of the lung extends about $\frac{3}{4}$ to $1\frac{1}{2}$ inches (2 to 4 cm) above the clavicle. Posteriorly there is about a 2-inch (5-cm) width of lung tissue at the apex.

Assess diaphragmatic excursion by instructing the client to "take a deep breath and hold it" while you percuss downward until dullness is heard at the lower lung border. Normal resonance of the lung stops at the diaphragm, where the sound becomes dull; mark this site. Repeat the process after instructing the client to "let out all your breath and hold." The difference between the two markings or sounds is the **diaphragmatic excursion.** Normal excursion ranges from 1 to 2 inches (3 to 5 cm). The diaphragm is normally higher on the right because of the location of the liver. Diaphragmatic

TABLE 30-4 Characteristic Features of the Five Percussion Notes

Note	Pitch	Intensity	Quality	Duration	Findings
Resonance	Low	Moderate to loud	Hollow	Long	Resonance is characteristic of normal lung tissue.
Hyperresonance	Higher than resonance	Very loud	Booming	Longer than resonance	Hyperresonance indicates the presence of trapped air, so it is commonly heard over an emphysematous or asthmatic lung and occasionally over a pneumothorax.
Flatness	High	Soft	Extreme dullness	Short	An example location is the sternum. Flatness percussed over the lung fields may indicate a massive pleural effusion.
Dullness	Medium	Medium	Thudlike	Medium	An example location is over the liver and the kidneys. Dullness can be percussed over an atelectatic lung or a consolidated lung.
Tympany	High	Loud	Musical, drumlike	Short	Examples are the cheek filled with air and the abdomen distended with air. Over the lung, a tympanic note usually indicates a large pneumothorax.

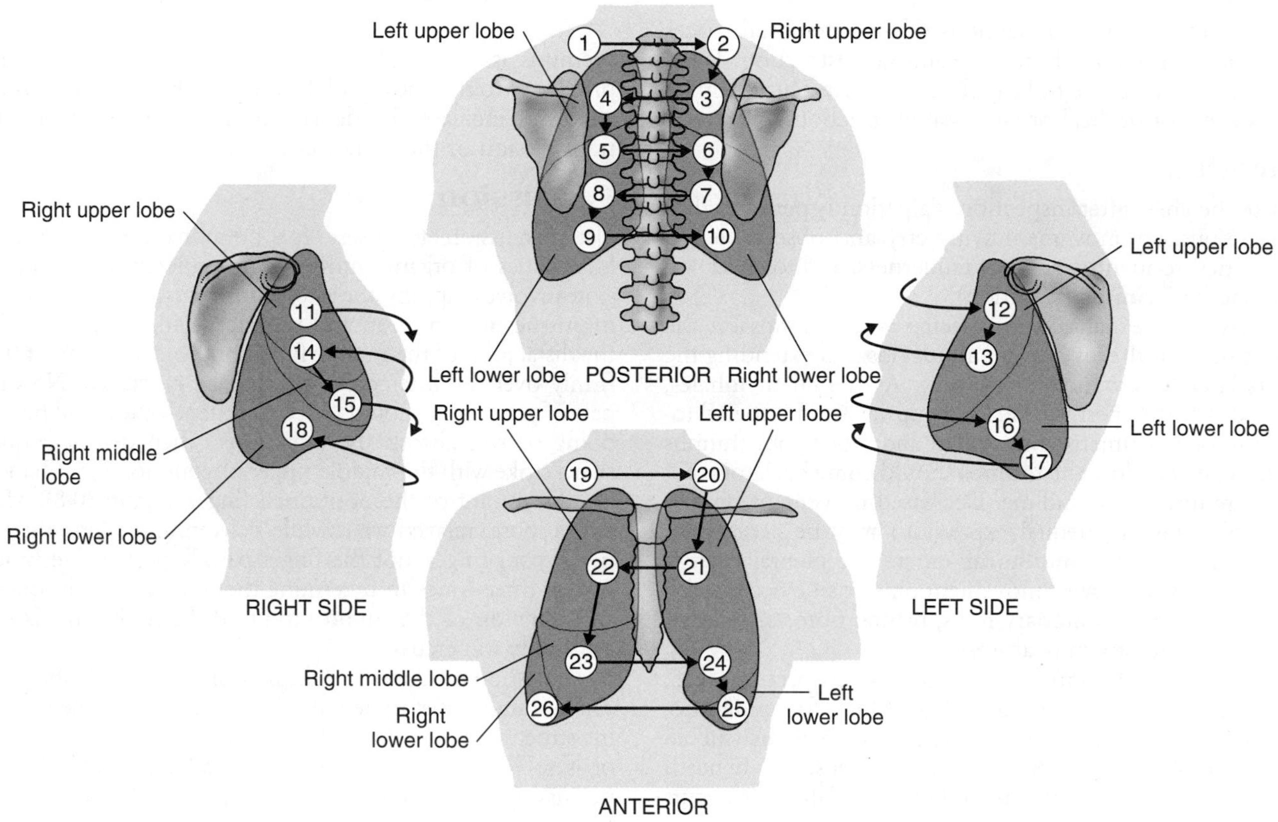

Figure 30-9 ■ Sequence for percussion and auscultation.

excursion may be decreased or absent in clients with pleurisy, diaphragm paralysis, or emphysema.

▶ Video Clip: Anterior Thorax

Continue to assess the thorax with percussion of the anterior and lateral chest. The percussion note changes from resonance of the normal lung to dullness at the borders of the heart and liver. The presence of fluid or solid material (e.g., pneumonia, pleural effusion, fibrosis, atelectasis, and tumors) is indicated by a dull percussion note over lung tissue.

Auscultation

Auscultation includes listening for normal breath sounds, adventitious sounds, and voice sounds. This technique provides information about the flow of air through the tracheobronchial tree and helps to identify fluid, mucus, or obstruction in the respiratory system. The diaphragm of the stethoscope is designed to detect high-pitched sounds.

Begin auscultation with the client sitting in an upright position. With the stethoscope pressed firmly against the chest wall (clothing can distort or muffle sounds), instruct the client to breathe slowly and deeply through an open mouth. (Breathing through the nose would set up turbulent sounds that are transmitted to the lungs.) Use a systematic approach, beginning at the apices and moving down through the intercostal spaces to the bases (Figure 30-9). Avoid listening over bony structures while auscultating the thorax posteriorly, laterally, and anteriorly. Listen to a full respiratory cycle, noting the quality and intensity of the breath sounds. Observe the client for dizziness caused by

TABLE 30-5 Characteristics of Normal Breath Sounds

	Pitch	Amplitude	Duration	Quality	Normal Location
Bronchial (tubular, tracheal) 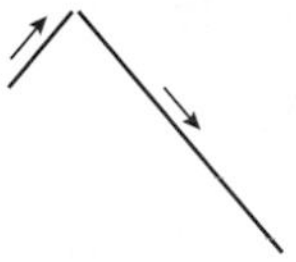	High	Loud	Inspiration < expiration	Harsh, hollow, tubular, blowing	Trachea and larynx
Bronchovesicular 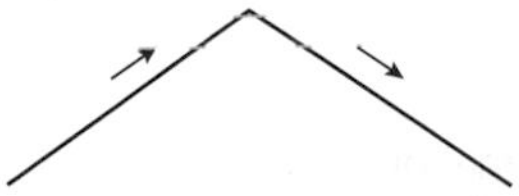	Moderate	Moderate	Inspiration = expiration	Mixed	Over major bronchi where fewer alveoli are located; posterior, between scapulae (especially on right); anterior, around upper sternum in first and second intercostal spaces
Vesicular 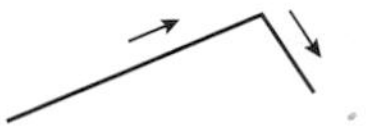	Low	Soft	Inspiration > expiration	Rustling, like the sound of the wind in the trees	Over peripheral lung fields where air flows through smaller bronchioles and alveoli

From Jarvis, C. (2000). *Physical examination and health assessment* (3rd ed.). Philadelphia: W.B. Saunders. Used with permission.

hyperventilation during auscultation. If dizziness occurs, tell the client to breathe normally for a few minutes.

NORMAL BREATH SOUNDS

Normal breath sounds are produced as air vibrates while moving through the respiratory passages from the larynx to the alveoli. Breath sounds are identified by their location, intensity, pitch, and duration within the respiratory cycle (e.g., early or late inspiration and expiration). Normal breath sounds are known as **bronchial** or tubular (harsh hollow sounds heard over the trachea and mainstem bronchi), **bronchovesicular** (heard over the branching bronchi), and **vesicular** (a soft rustling sound heard in the periphery over small bronchioles) (Table 30-5). Describe these sounds as normal, increased, decreased (diminished), or absent.

When bronchial breath sounds are heard peripherally, they are abnormal. This increased sound occurs when the bronchial sounds are transmitted to an area of increased density, such as in clients with atelectasis, tumor, or pneumonia. When audible in an abnormal location, bronchovesicular breath sounds may indicate normal aging or an abnormality such as pulmonary consolidation and chronic airway disease.

ADVENTITIOUS BREATH SOUNDS

Adventitious sounds are additional breath sounds superimposed on normal sounds, and they indicate pathologic changes in the lung. Table 30-6 describes adventitious sounds: crackle, wheeze, rhonchus, and pleural friction rub. Adventitious sounds vary in pitch, intensity, duration, and the phase of the respiratory cycle in which they occur. Document exactly what you hear on auscultation.

VOICE SOUNDS

If abnormalities are found during the physical assessment of the lungs and thorax, assess the client for vocal resonance. Voice sounds through the normally air-filled lung produce a muffled, unclear sound because sound vibrations travel poorly through air. Vocal resonance is increased when the sound travels through a solid or liquid medium. The presence of a consolidated area of the lung, pneumonia, atelectasis, pleural effusion, tumor, or abscess causes increased vocal resonance.

BRONCHOPHONY. Bronchophony is the abnormally loud and clear transmission of voice sounds through an area of increased density. To assess bronchophony, ask the client to repeat the number *99* while you systematically auscultate the thorax.

WHISPERED PECTORILOQUY. Whispered pectoriloquy is the enhanced voice heard through the chest wall. It is much more sensitive than bronchophony. Ask the client to whisper the number sequence *one, two, three* while you listen with a stethoscope. Whispered words normally sound faint and indistinct. If they are heard loudly and distinctly, consolidation of lung tissue may be present.

EGOPHONY. Egophony is another abnormally enhanced vocal resonance and has a high-pitched, bleating, nasal quality. Auscultate the thorax while the client repeats the letter *E*. Egophony exists when this letter is heard as a flat, nasal sound of *A* through the stethoscope. This abnormal sound occurs in areas of consolidation, pleural effusion, or abscess.

OTHER INDICATORS OF RESPIRATORY ADEQUACY

Assess other indicators of respiratory adequacy because gas exchange affects all body systems. Some indicators (e.g., cyanosis) indicate immediate oxygenation problems. Other changes (e.g., clubbing, weight loss, unevenly developed muscles) reflect long-term oxygenation problems.

Skin and Mucous Membranes

Assess the skin and mucous membranes for the presence of pallor or cyanosis, which could indicate inadequate oxygenation. Areas to assess include the nail beds and the mu-

TABLE 30-6 Characteristic Features of Adventitious Breath Sounds

Adventitious Sound	Occurrence in the Respiratory Cycle	Character	Association
Discontinuous			
Fine crackles Fine rales High-pitched rales	Either early or late inspiration	Popping, discontinuous sounds caused by air moving into previously deflated airways; sounds like hair being rolled between fingers near the ear "Velcro" sounds late in inspiration usually associated with restrictive disorders	Asbestosis Atelectasis Interstitial fibrosis Bronchitis Pneumonia Chronic pulmonary diseases
Coarse crackles Low-pitched crackles	More common on expiration but may be present early in inspiration	Lower pitched, coarse, discontinuous rattling sounds caused by fluid or secretions in large airways; likely to change with coughing or suctioning	Bronchitis Pneumonia Tumors Pulmonary edema
Continuous			
Wheeze	Audible during either inspiration, expiration, or both	Squeaky, musical, continuous sounds associated with air rushing through narrowed airways; may be heard without a stethoscope Arise from the small airways Usually do not clear with coughing	Inflammation Bronchospasm Edema Secretions Pulmonary vessel engorgement (as in cardiac "asthma")
Rhonchus (rhonchi)	Audible during both inspiration and expiration but commonly more prominent on expiration	Lower-pitched, coarse, continuous snoring sounds Arise from the large airways	Thick, tenacious secretions Sputum production Obstruction by foreign body Tumors
Pleural Friction Rub	Heard during both inspiration and expiration, generally at the end of inspiration and the beginning of expiration	Loud, rough, grating, scratching sounds caused by the inflamed surfaces of the pleura rubbing together; often associated with pain on deep inspirations Heard in lateral lung fields	Pleurisy Tuberculosis Pulmonary infarction Pneumonia Lung cancer

cous membranes of the oral cavity. Examine the fingers for clubbing (see Figure 33-10), which indicates hypoxia of long duration.

General Appearance

Observe the client for muscle development and general body build. Long-term respiratory problems limit the ability to maintain body weight and lead to a loss of general muscle mass. Arms and legs may appear thin or poorly muscled. The muscles of the neck and chest may be hypertrophied, especially in the client with chronic obstructive pulmonary disease (COPD).

Endurance

Observe how easily the client moves and whether he or she is short of breath while resting or becomes short of breath when walking 10 to 20 steps. As the client speaks, note how often he or she pauses for breath between words.

Psychosocial Assessment

Assess those aspects of the client's lifestyle that either can affect respiratory function or are affected by it. Some respiratory problems may be worsened by stress. Ask about present life stresses and usual coping mechanisms.

Chronic respiratory disease may cause changes in family roles and relationships, social isolation, financial problems, and unemployment or disability. Discuss coping mechanisms to assess the client's reaction to these psychosocial stressors and discover strengths and ineffective behaviors. For example, the client may react to stress with dependence on family members, withdrawal, or nonadherence with interventions. After completing the psychosocial assessment, assist the client in determining the support systems available to help cope with changes resulting from breathing problems.

Critical Thinking Challenge

The client is a 68-year-old female homemaker who comes to the emergency department with shortness of breath and cough. She had been a smoker for 45 years until the last 5 years, when she quit successfully with family support. She is anxious, as are her daughter and husband, who have accompanied her.

1. What specific family information should you obtain?
2. Is the client's socioeconomic status relevant? Why or why not?
3. What other assessment questions should you ask?

evolve For suggested answer guidelines, go to http://evolve.elsevier.com/Iggy/.

Diagnostic Assessment

LABORATORY TESTS

Blood Tests

Several laboratory tests (Chart 30-3) are useful in assessing respiratory problems. A red blood cell (RBC) count provides data about the transport of oxygen. The hemoglobin molecule, found in RBCs, transports oxygen to the tissues. A deficiency of hemoglobin could cause hypoxemia.

CHART 30-3

LABORATORY PROFILE

Respiratory Assessment

Test	Normal Range for Adults	Significance of Abnormal Findings
Blood Studies		
Complete Blood Count		
Red blood cells	*Females:* 18-44 yr: 3.8-5.1 million/mm^3 45-64 yr: 3.8-5.3 million/mm^3 65-74 yr: 3.8-5.2 million/mm^3 *Males:* 18-44 yr: 4.3-5.7 million/mm^3 45-64 yr: 4.2-5.6 million/mm^3 65-74 yr: 3.8-5.8 million/mm^3	*Elevated levels* (polycythemia) may be due to the excessive production of erythropoietin, which occurs in response to a hypoxic stimulus, as in COPD, and from living at a high altitude. *Decreased levels* indicate possible anemia, hemorrhage, or hemolysis.
Hemoglobin, total	*Females:* 18-44 yr: 11.7-15.5 g/dL, or 117-155 g/L 45-64 yr: 11.7-16 g/dL, or 117-160 g/L 65-74 yr: 11.7-16.1 g/dL, or 117-161 g/L *Males:* 18-44 yr: 13.2-17.3 g/dL, or 132-173 g/L 45-64 yr: 13.1-17.2 g/dL, or 131-172 g/L	Same as for red blood cells.
Hematocrit	*Females:* 18-44 yr: 35%-45% 45-74 yr: 35%-47% *Males:* 18-44 yr: 39%-49% 45-64 yr: 39%-50% 65-74 yr: 37%-51%	Same as for red blood cells.
White blood cell count (leukocyte count, WBC count)	*Total:* 4.5-11.0 $\times 10^3$ cells/μL, or 7.4 IRU *Black clients:* 3.6-10.2 $\times 10^3$ cells/μL	*Elevations* indicate possible acute infections or inflammations, pneumonia, meningitis, tonsillitis, or emphysema. *Decreased levels* may indicate an overwhelming infection, an autoimmune disorder, or immunosuppressant therapy.
Differential White Blood Cell (Leukocyte) Count		
Neutrophils	1.8-7.7 $\times 10^3$ cells/μL; 18%-77% of total *Black clients:* slightly lower	*Elevations* indicate possible acute bacterial infection (pneumonia), COPD, or inflammatory conditions (smoking). *Decreased levels* indicate possible viral disease (influenza).
Eosinophils	0-0.7 $\times 10^3$ cells/μL; 0%-7% of total	*Elevations* indicate possible COPD, asthma, or allergies. *Decreased levels* indicate pyogenic infections.
Basophils	0-0.15 $\times 10^3$ cells/μL; 0%-1.5% of total	*Elevations* indicate possible inflammation; seen in chronic sinusitis, hypersensitivity reactions. *Decreased levels* may be seen in an acute infection.
Lymphocytes	1.5-4.0 $\times 10^3$ cells/μL; 15%-40% of total	*Elevations* indicate possible viral infection, pertussis, and infectious mononucleosis. *Decreased levels* may be seen during corticosteroid therapy.
Monocytes	0-0.8 $\times 10^3$ cells/μL; 0%-8% of total	*Elevations:* see Lymphocytes; also may indicate active tuberculosis. *Decreased levels:* see Lymphocytes.
Arterial Blood Gases		
Pao$_2$	83-100 mm Hg *Older adults:* values may be lower	*Elevations* indicate possible excessive oxygen administration. *Decreased levels* indicate possible COPD, asthma, chronic bronchitis, cancer of the bronchi and lungs, cystic fibrosis, respiratory distress syndrome, anemias, atelectasis, or any other cause of hypoxia.
Paco$_2$	*Females:* 32-45 mm Hg *Males:* 35-48 mm Hg	*Elevations* indicate possible COPD, asthma, pneumonia, anesthesia effects, or use of opioids (respiratory acidosis). *Decreased levels* indicate hyperventilation/respiratory alkalosis.
pH	Up to 60 yr: 7.35-7.45 60-90 yr: 7.31-7.42 >90 yr: 7.26-7.43	*Elevations* indicate metabolic or respiratory alkalosis. *Decreased levels* indicate metabolic or respiratory acidosis.
HCO_3^-	22-26 mEq/L	*Elevations* indicate possible respiratory acidosis as compensation for a primary metabolic alkalosis. *Decreased levels* indicate possible respiratory alkalosis as compensation for a primary metabolic acidosis.
Sao$_2$	94%-98% *Older adults:* values may be slightly lower	*Decreased levels* indicate possible impaired ability of hemoglobin to release oxygen to tissues.

COPD, Chronic obstructive pulmonary disease; *HCO_3^-*, bicarbonate ion; *IRU*, international recommended unit; *Paco$_2$*, partial pressure of arterial carbon dioxide; *Pao$_2$*, partial pressure of arterial oxygen; *Sao$_2$*, arterial oxygen saturation; *WBC*, white blood cell count.

Continued

CHART 30-3

LABORATORY PROFILE
Respiratory Assessment—*cont'd*

Test	Normal Range for Adults	Significance of Abnormal Findings
Sputum Studies		
Gram stain	Negative	Presence of gram-positive or gram-negative bacteria indicates the type of microorganism causing the respiratory infection.
Culture and sensitivity	Negative	Presence of microorganisms indicates possible respiratory infections (e.g., pneumonia or bronchitis).
Acid-fast stain	No acid-fast bacilli	Presence of bacilli indicates possible tuberculosis.
Cytologic tests	Negative	Presence of abnormal cells indicates possible malignancy.

Arterial blood gas (ABG) analysis assesses oxygenation (partial pressure of arterial oxygen [PaO_2]), alveolar ventilation (partial pressure of arterial carbon dioxide [$PaCO_2$]), and acid-base balance. Blood gas studies provide information for monitoring treatment results, adjusting oxygen therapy, and evaluating the client's responses.

Sputum Tests

Sputum specimens obtained by expectoration or tracheal suctioning assist in the identification of organisms or abnormal cells, such as in cancer or an allergy. Sputum culture and sensitivity analyses identify bacterial infection and determine which specific antibiotics will be most effective. Sputum cytologic examination helps diagnose malignant lesions by identifying cancer cells. Benign conditions, such as allergy or autoimmunity, may also be identified by cytologic testing. Eosinophils and Curschmann's spirals (a mucous form) are often found by cytologic study in clients with allergic asthma.

RADIOGRAPHIC EXAMINATIONS

Standard X-rays

Chest x-rays are used for clients with respiratory tract disorders to evaluate the status of the chest and to provide a baseline for comparison with future changes. Standard chest x-rays are performed from **posteroanterior** (PA; back to front) and left lateral (LL) positions. Portable chest x-rays (taken anteroposterior [AP], front to back) cost more, and the films are of lower quality and are more difficult to interpret.

Chest x-rays are used to assess pathologic changes in the lung, such as with pneumonia, atelectasis, pneumothorax, and tumor. Chest x-rays also can be used to detect the presence of pleural fluid and the position and placement of an endotracheal tube or other invasive catheters. These films have limitations, however, and may appear normal, even when severe chronic bronchitis, asthma, or emphysema is present.

Sinus and facial x-rays are used to assess fluid levels in the sinus cavities to assist in the diagnosis of acute or chronic sinusitis.

Digital Chest Radiography

Digital imaging, which uses less radiation, has started to replace most film images. Digital imaging is especially useful to assess lung and chest lesions. A computer enhances the image to give the greatest amount of detail. The image can be adjusted to emphasize a specific area.

Computed Tomography

When an x-ray reveals a suspicious lesion, computed tomography (CT) is useful because pulmonary soft tissue densities, tumors, and blood clots can be seen. Chest CT is usually performed with consecutive 5- to 10-mm cross-sectional views of the entire thorax. Then, using higher resolution, 1-mm scans are taken of suspicious areas.

Usually CT scans require a contrast agent injected intravenously. The contrast enhances the visibility of structures such as tumors, blood vessels, and chambers of the heart. These scans assist in making a diagnosis. Your role in this diagnostic test is to provide information to the client and to determine whether the client has any sensitivity to the contrast material. Ask the client whether he or she has a known allergy to iodine or shellfish.

Ventilation and Perfusion Scanning

A ventilation and perfusion scan ($\dot{V}/\dot{Q}$ scan) identifies the areas of the lung being ventilated and the distribution of blood within the lungs. It is one of the tests used to support or rule out a diagnosis of pulmonary embolism.

The physician first injects a radionuclide with the client in a supine position and then takes six perfusion views: anterior, posterior, right and left lateral, and two obliques. If the perfusion scan is normal, there is no reason to continue with the ventilation scan. Otherwise, the client inhales a radioactive gas or radioaerosol, and the lung is scanned continuously as the gas makes its way into the lungs (the "wash-in" phase) once the gas has reached equilibrium within the lungs, and then while the gas is leaving the lungs (the "wash-out" phase).

Teach the client about the procedure, and explain that the radioactive substance clears from the body in about 8 hours.

OTHER NONINVASIVE DIAGNOSTIC TESTS

Pulse Oximetry

Pulse oximetry identifies hemoglobin saturation. Usually hemoglobin is almost 100% saturated with oxygen. The pulse oximeter uses a wave of infrared light and a sensor placed on the client's finger, toe, nose, earlobe, or forehead. Ideal normal pulse oximetry values are 95% to 100%. Normal values are a little lower in older clients and in clients with dark skin. To avoid confusion with the PaO_2 values from arterial blood gases, pulse oximetry readings are recorded as the SaO_2 (arterial oxygen saturation), or SpO_2.

Pulse oximetry can detect desaturation before manifestations (e.g., dusky skin, pale mucosa, nail beds) occur. Causes for low readings include client movement, hypothermia, decreased peripheral blood flow, ambient light (sunlight, infrared lamps), decreased hemoglobin, edema, and fingernail polish. Covering the sensor or changing its position may help accuracy if too much ambient light is present.

Results lower than 91% (and certainly below 86%) are an emergency and require immediate treatment. When the SaO_2 is below 85%, body tissues have a difficult time becoming oxygenated. An SaO_2 less than 70% is usually life threatening, but in some cases values below 80% may be life threatening. *Pulse oximetry is less accurate at lower values.*

Pulmonary Function Tests

Pulmonary function tests (PFTs) evaluate lung function and breathing problems. These studies include lung volumes and capacities, flow rates, diffusion capacity, gas exchange, airway resistance, and distribution of ventilation. The results are interpreted by comparing the client's data with expected findings for age, gender, race, height, weight, and smoking status.

The PFTs are useful in screening clients for lung disease even before the onset of manifestations. Serial testing provides objective data that may be used as a guide to treatment (e.g., changes in lung function can support a decision to continue, change, or discontinue a specific therapy). PFTs performed before surgery may identify the client at risk for lung complications after surgery. One of the most common reasons for performing such tests is to determine the cause of dyspnea. When performed while the client exercises, PFTs help to determine whether dyspnea is caused by lung or cardiac dysfunction or by muscle weakness. These tests are also useful for determining the effect of occupation on lung function and any related disability.

CLIENT PREPARATION. Explain the purpose of the tests for planning care. Advise the client not to smoke for 6 to 8 hours before testing. According to institutional policy and procedure, bronchodilator drugs may be withheld for 4 to 6 hours before the test. The client with breathing problems often fears further breathlessness and is anxious before these "breathing" tests. Help reduce anxiety by describing what will happen during and after the testing.

PROCEDURE. Pulmonary function tests (PFTs) can be performed at the bedside or in the respiratory laboratory. The client is asked to breathe through the mouth only. A nose clip may be used to prevent air from escaping. The client performs different breathing maneuvers while measurements are obtained (Figure 30-10). Table 30-7 describes the most commonly used PFTs and their purpose.

FOLLOW-UP CARE. Because many breathing maneuvers are performed during PFTs, observe the client for increased dyspnea or bronchospasm after these studies. Document whether drugs were given during testing.

Exercise Testing

Exercise increases metabolism and gas transport as energy is used. Reasons for exercise testing are listed in Table 30-8. These tests are performed on a treadmill or bicycle or by a self-paced 12-minute walking test. The normal client's exercise is limited by hemodynamic factors, whereas the pulmonary client is limited by breathing capacity, gas exchange compromise, or both. Explain exercise testing and assure the client of close monitoring by trained professionals throughout the test.

Skin Tests

Skin tests are used with other diagnostic data to identify various infectious diseases (e.g., tuberculosis), viral diseases (e.g., mononucleosis and mumps), and fungal diseases (e.g., coccidioidomycosis and histoplasmosis). Allergies and the status of the immune system also can be demonstrated through skin

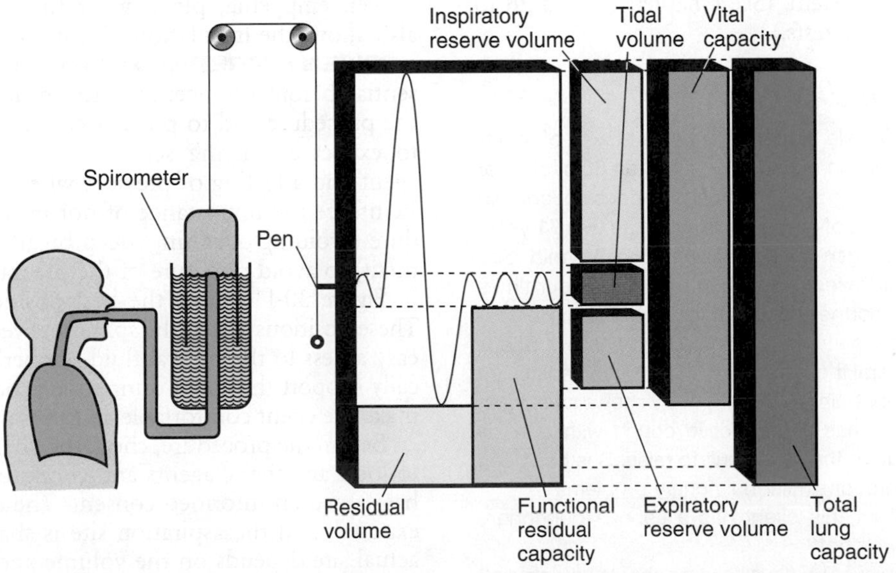

Figure 30-10 ■ Common measurements in pulmonary function testing. (Modified from Luce, J.M., Pierson, D.J., & Tyler, M.L. [1993]. *Intensive respiratory care* [2nd ed.]. Philadelphia: W.B. Saunders.)

TABLE 30-7 Characteristics and Purposes of Pulmonary Function Tests

Test	Purpose
FVC (forced vital capacity) records the maximum amount of air that can be exhaled as quickly as possible after maximum inspiration.	*FVC* gives an indication of respiratory muscle strength and ventilatory reserve. FVC is often reduced in obstructive disease (because of air trapping) and in restrictive disease.
FEV_1 (forced expiratory volume in 1 sec) records the maximal amount of air that can be exhaled in the first second of expiration.	*FEV_1* is effort dependent and declines normally with age. It is reduced in certain obstructive and restrictive disorders.
FEV_1/FVC is the ratio of expiratory volume in 1 sec to FVC.	This ratio provides a much more sensitive indication of obstruction to airflow. This ratio is the hallmark of obstructive pulmonary disease. It is normal or increased in restrictive disease.
$FEF_{25\%-75\%}$ records the forced expiratory flow over the 25%-75% volume (middle half) of the FVC.	This measure provides a more sensitive index of obstruction in the smaller airways.
FRC (functional residual capacity) is the amount of air remaining in the lungs after normal expiration. FRC test requires use of the helium dilution, nitrogen washout, or body plethysmography technique.	Increased FRC indicates hyperinflation or air trapping, which may result from obstructive pulmonary disease. FRC is normal or decreased in restrictive pulmonary diseases.
TLC (total lung capacity) is the amount of air in the lungs at the end of maximum inhalation.	Increased TLC indicates air trapping associated with obstructive pulmonary disease. Decreased TLC indicates restrictive disease.
RV (residual volume) is the amount of air remaining in the lungs at the end of a full, forced exhalation.	RV is increased in obstructive pulmonary disease such as emphysema.
DLCO (diffusion capacity of carbon monoxide) reflects the surface area of the alveolocapillary membrane. The client inhales a small amount of CO, holds for 10 sec, and then exhales. The amount inhaled is compared with the amount exhaled.	DLCO is reduced whenever the alveolocapillary membrane is diminished, such as occurs in emphysema, pulmonary hypertension, and pulmonary fibrosis. It is increased with exercise and in conditions such as polycythemia and congestive heart disease.

TABLE 30-8 Indications for Exercise Testing

- To assess a client's functional capacity (ability to work and perform activities of daily living)
- To determine the reason for exercise limitation: cardiac, pulmonary, or poor conditioning
- To evaluate changes in exercise capacity related to disease or treatment
- To determine the basis for the development of a pulmonary rehabilitation program
- To determine whether supplemental oxygen is required during exercise

testing. Exposure to the allergen or organism used in testing produces a specific reaction (delayed hypersensitivity reaction) of the client's immune system. (See Chapters 23 and 26 for further discussion of these tests.)

Critical Thinking Challenge

The 68-year-old female homemaker has a history of shortness of breath, especially on exertion. She was an 80 pack-year smoker until she quit 5 years ago. Her husband does not and did not smoke. Her father died of emphysema when he was 71 years old. She is on home oxygen continuously at 2 to 3 L/min. She uses an albuterol and Atrovent solution in a nebulizer four times daily and PRN to treat shortness of breath and wheezing. Her respiratory rate (RR) is 24 breaths/min, labored, and shallow. She is pale, anxious, has bilateral though limited chest movement, slight retractions, and digital clubbing. Pulse oximetry shows an oxygen saturation of 87%. She has a productive cough with a small amount of mucoid sputum that is difficult to raise. She has been hospitalized twice before for similar pulmonary problems.

1. Can you assume that this client has a serious pulmonary problem? Why or why not?
2. What additional, noninvasive physical data should you obtain?
3. How could you determine whether the data you have already obtained accurately reflect the client's respiratory status?

evolve For suggested answer guidelines, go to http://evolve.elsevier.com/Iggy/.

OTHER INVASIVE DIAGNOSTIC TESTS

Endoscopic Examinations

Endoscopic studies to assess breathing problems include bronchoscopy, laryngoscopy, and mediastinoscopy (Table 30-9). The most common complications are related to the anesthetic agents and bleeding.

Thoracentesis

Thoracentesis is the aspiration of pleural fluid or air from the pleural space. It can be used for diagnosis or treatment. Microscopic examination of the pleural fluid helps in making a diagnosis. Pleural fluid may be drained to relieve pulmonary compression and the respiratory distress caused by cancer, empyema, pleurisy, or tuberculosis. Thoracentesis also allows the instillation of drugs into the pleural space.

CLIENT PREPARATION. Client preparation is essential before thoracentesis to ensure cooperation during the procedure and to prevent complications. Tell the client to expect a stinging sensation from the local anesthetic agent and a feeling of pressure when the needle is inserted. Reinforce the importance of not moving during the procedure (avoiding coughing, deep breathing, or sudden movement) to avoid puncture of the pleura or lung.

Figure 30-11 shows the best positions for thoracentesis. These positions widen the spaces between the ribs and permit easy access to the pleural fluid. Properly position and physically support the client during the procedure. Use pillows to make the client comfortable and to provide physical support.

Before the procedure, check the client's history for allergy to local anesthetic agents and check to make sure the client has signed an informed consent. The entire chest or back is exposed, and the aspiration site is shaved if necessary. The actual site depends on the volume and location of the effusion (determined by x-rays, sonography, and percussion).

PROCEDURE. Thoracentesis is often performed at the bedside, although sonography or computed tomography may be used to guide it. After draping the client and

TABLE 30-9 Care of the Client Undergoing Endoscopic Tests for Respiratory Disorders

Purpose and Description	Nursing Interventions	Rationales
Bronchoscopy		
To assess airway anatomy for tumors, obstruction, and atelectasis.	Allow the client nothing by mouth for several hours before the test.	The client may aspirate gastric contents if vomiting occurs.
To assist in the diagnosis of infection or cancer by biopsy of lesions; biopsy techniques include the brush biopsy and needle aspiration.	Assess for allergies to iodine, local anesthetics, or pretest medications.	A knowledge of allergies helps prevent allergic reactions.
	Place pulse oximeter.	Pulse oximetry allows continuous monitoring throughout the procedure.
To remove thick secretions, mucus plugs, or foreign bodies.	Administer pretest medications (atropine, diazepam) as prescribed.	Pretest medications help decrease secretions, prevent bradycardia, and reduce anxiety.
A flexible fiberoptic bronchoscope is inserted through the mouth, nose, endotracheal tube, or tracheostomy tube. The procedure may be performed in the operating room or radiology department. Oxygen administration and blood pressure monitoring are standard procedures.	Prepare the client for topical anesthetic administration into the oropharynx.	Explanations about the effects of the anesthetic agent (numbness and gagging) help to decrease anxiety.
	Remove the client's dentures if present.	Injury may occur if dentures are left in place.
	After the procedure, monitor the client's vital signs for 15 min until stable, and monitor for hemoptysis.	Assessment helps detect respiratory distress and signs of complications related to the procedure.
	After the procedure, allow the client nothing by mouth until the gag reflex returns.	Allowing the client nothing by mouth reduces the possibility of aspiration.
	Discourage smoking, talking, and coughing for several hours.	Throat irritation is decreased by avoiding these activities.
Laryngoscopy		
Direct: To detect or remove lesions or foreign bodies in the larynx or to diagnose cancer by removing tissue for biopsy or samples for culture. A fiberoptic laryngoscope is used.	Allow the client nothing by mouth for several hours before the test.	Aspiration is possible if vomiting occurs.
	Assess the client for allergies to iodine, contrast media, or local anesthetics.	A knowledge of allergies helps prevent allergic reactions.
Indirect: To assess the function of the vocal cords or to obtain tissue for biopsy. Observations are made during rest and phonation by using a laryngeal mirror, head mirror, and light source.	Administer pretest medications (atropine, diazepam) as prescribed.	Pretest medications help decrease secretions, prevent bradycardia, and reduce anxiety.
	Assess the client for fears concerning the procedure. Assure the client that he or she will be monitored for any respiratory problems.	Reassurance helps decrease fears about not being able to breathe during the procedure.
	For indirect laryngoscopy, assist the client to sit in an upright position, and encourage normal breathing.	An upright sitting position facilitates the passage of the laryngeal mirror into the mouth.
	After the procedure, allow the client nothing by mouth until the gag reflex returns.	The client may aspirate gastric contents if vomiting occurs.
	Encourage coughing and fluid intake.	Hydration and coughing promote the expectoration of secretions.
	Assess vital signs every 15 min for at least 2 hr after procedure and then every 2 hr for the first 24 hr. Assess the client for bleeding.	Frequent monitoring of vital signs enables the nurse to detect changes such as dyspnea.
	After the procedure, administer lozenges or gargles as prescribed.	Lozenges and gargles help to relieve a sore throat.
Mediastinoscopy		
To inspect and remove samples for biopsy of lymph nodes that drain the lung.	Explain preoperative measures and the procedure to the client.	Explanations about the anticipated procedure help to decrease anxiety.
To detect metastasis of lung cancer.	Assess the client postoperatively for bleeding, pneumothorax, and vocal cord paralysis.	Ongoing assessment for complications helps to ensure prompt treatment.
To obtain tissue for biopsy for diagnosis of tuberculosis or sarcoidosis.	Assess the client for pain, and administer analgesics as prescribed.	Medication decreases the discomfort associated with the procedure.
The procedure is performed in the operating room with the client under local or general anesthesia; a suprasternal incision is used.	Assess vital signs every 15 min for at least 2 hr after procedure and then every 2 hr for the first 24 hr.	Frequent monitoring of vital signs helps to detect changes such as dyspnea.

cleaning the skin with an antiseptic agent, a local anesthetic is injected into the selected site. Keep the client informed of the procedure while observing for shock, pain, nausea, pallor, diaphoresis, cyanosis, tachypnea, and dyspnea.

The short 18- to 25-gauge thoracentesis needle (with an attached syringe) is advanced into the pleural space. Gentle suction is applied as the fluid in the pleural space is slowly aspirated. A vacuum collection bottle is sometimes needed to remove larger volumes of fluid. To prevent re-expansion pulmonary edema, usually no more than 1000 mL of fluid is removed at one time. If a pleural biopsy is to be performed, a second, larger needle with a cutting edge and collection chamber is used. After the needle is withdrawn, pressure is applied to the puncture site, and a small sterile dressing is applied.

FOLLOW-UP CARE. After thoracentesis, a chest x-ray is performed to rule out possible pneumothorax and subsequent **mediastinal shift** (shift of center thoracic structure toward one side). Monitor vital signs and auscultate breath

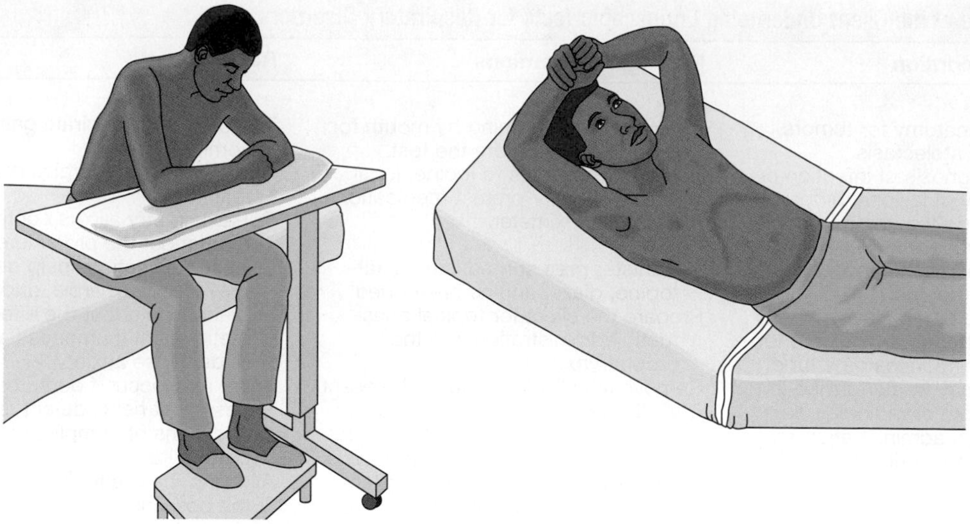

Figure 30-11 ■ Positions for thoracentesis.

sounds for absent or reduced sounds on the affected side. Observe the puncture site and dressing for leakage or bleeding. Also assess for complications, such as reaccumulation of fluid in the pleural space, subcutaneous emphysema, infection, and tension pneumothorax. Encourage the client to breathe deeply to promote re-expansion of the lung. Document the procedure, including the client's response; the volume and character of the fluid removed; any specimens sent to the laboratory; the location of the puncture site; and respiratory assessment findings before, during, and after the procedure.

Lung Biopsy

A lung biopsy is performed to obtain tissue for histologic analysis, culture, or cytologic examination. The tissue samples are used to make a definite diagnosis about the type of cancer, infection, inflammation, or lung disease. There are several types of lung biopsies. The site and extent of the lesion determine which one is used. Transbronchial biopsy (TBB) and transbronchial needle aspiration (TBNA) are performed during bronchoscopy. Transthoracic needle aspiration is a percutaneous approach for areas not accessible by bronchoscopy. An open lung biopsy is performed in the operating room.

CLIENT PREPARATION. The client may worry about the outcome of the biopsy and may associate the term *biopsy* with *cancer.* Explain what to expect before and after the procedure and explore the client's feelings and fears. To reduce discomfort and anxiety, an analgesic or sedative may be prescribed before the procedure. Inform the client undergoing percutaneous biopsy that discomfort is reduced with a local anesthetic agent but that pressure may be felt during needle insertion and tissue aspiration. Open lung biopsy is performed in the operating room with the client under general anesthesia, and the usual preoperative preparations apply (see Chapter 20).

PROCEDURE. Percutaneous lung biopsy may be performed in the client's room or in the radiology department after an informed consent has been obtained. Fluoroscopy, CT, or ultrasonography is often used to visualize more clearly the area undergoing biopsy and to guide the procedure. Positioning of the client is similar to that for thoracentesis. The skin is cleansed with an antiseptic agent and a local anesthetic is given. Under sterile conditions, a spinal-type 18- to 22-gauge needle is inserted through the skin into the desired area (e.g., tissue, nodule, lymph node) and tissue needed for microscopic examination is obtained. Apply a dressing after the procedure.

An open lung biopsy is performed in the operating room. The client undergoes a thoracotomy where lung tissue is exposed. At least two tissue specimens are taken (usually from an upper lobe and a lower lobe site). A chest tube is placed to remove air and fluid so the lung can reinflate, and then the chest is closed.

FOLLOW-UP CARE. Monitor the client's vital signs and breath sounds at least every 4 hours for 24 hours, and assess for signs of respiratory distress (e.g., dyspnea, pallor, diaphoresis, tachypnea). Pneumothorax is a serious complication of needle biopsy and open lung biopsy. Report reduced or absent breath sounds immediately. Monitor for hemoptysis (which may be scant and transient) or, in rare cases, for frank bleeding from vascular or lung trauma.

GET READY for the NCLEX Examination!

KEY POINTS

Safe Effective Care Environment

- When using aerosolized drugs or other chemicals, close the door to the room where they are being used.
- Use gloves when obtaining a sputum specimen.

Health Promotion and Maintenance

- Teach clients who come into contact with inhalation irritants in their workplaces or for leisure time activities to use a mask to avoid respiratory contact with these substances.
- Inform all clients who smoke that smoking increases the risk for development of many pulmonary problems.
- Assist clients interested in smoking cessation in finding an appropriate smoking cessation program.

- Encourage older adults who are confined to bed for any reason or who are recovering from surgery to turn, cough, and deep breathe at least every 2 hours.
- Encourage all clients over 50 years of age and anyone with a respiratory problem to receive a yearly influenza vaccination.

Psychosocial Integrity

- Assess the degree to which breathing problems interfere with the client's ability to perform activities of daily living.
- Pace your interview to match the learning needs and style of the individual client.
- Explain all diagnostic procedures, restrictions, and follow-up care to the client scheduled for tests.

Physiological Integrity

- Document any known specific allergies that have respiratory manifestations.
- Ask the client about recent travel.
- Assess the airway and breathing effectiveness for any client who experiences shortness of breath or any change in mental status.
- Assess the client's respiratory status every 15 minutes for at least the first 2 hours after undergoing an endoscopic test for respiratory disorders.

ADDITIONAL STUDY RESOURCES

Go to your Student CD-ROM for Review Questions for the NCLEX Examination.

Go to http://evolve.elsevier.com/Iggy/ for Integrated Management of Care Questions for the NCLEX Examination.

SELECTED BIBLIOGRAPHY

Berne, R., et al. (2004). *Physiology* (5th ed.). St. Louis: Mosby.

Carroll, P. (2002). Procedural sedation: Capnography's heightened role. *RN, 65*(10), 54-62.

Ebersole, P., Hess, P., & Luggen, A. (2004). *Toward healthy aging: Human needs and nursing response* (6th ed.). St. Louis: Mosby.

Finesilver, C. (2001). Perfecting your skills: Respiratory assessment. *RN,* April suppl., 16-28.

Frakes, M. (2001). Measuring end-tidal carbon dioxide: Clinical applications and usefulness. *Critical Care Nurse, 21*(5), 23-35.

Gordon, M. (2002). *Manual of nursing diagnosis* (10th ed.). St. Louis: Mosby.

Hess, D. (2000). Detection and monitoring of hypoxemia and oxygen therapy. *Respiratory Care, 45*(1), 65-83.

Interpreting pulmonary function test results. (2002). *Nursing2002, 32*(2), 78.

Jarvis, C. (2004). *Physical examination and health assessment* (4th ed.). Philadelphia: W.B. Saunders.

Mahler, D., Fierro-Carrion, G., & Baird, J. (2003). Evaluation of dyspnea in the elderly. *Clinics in Geriatric Medicine, 19*(1), 19-33.

Moore, A. (2000). Tips for getting a more reliable O_2 sat reading. *RN, 63*(2), 73.

Nussbaum, R., McInnes, R., & Willard, H. (2001). *Thompson & Thompson: Genetics in medicine* (6th ed.). Philadelphia: W.B. Saunders.

Pagana, K., & Pagana, T. (2002). *Mosby's manual of diagnostic and laboratory tests* (2nd ed.). St. Louis: Mosby.

Petty, T. (2002). Spirometry: A key tool for every office. *Consultant, 42*(14), 1753.

Pruitt, W., & Jacobs, M. (2004). Interpreting arterial blood gases: Easy as ABC. *Nursing 2004, 34*(8), 50-53.

Schallom, L., & Aherns, T. (2002). Will my patient survive this cardiac arrest? *Nursing2002, 32*(2), 32cc1-32cc2.

Villars, P., Kanusky, J., & Levitzky, M. (2002). Functional residual capacity: The human windbag. *American Association of Nurse Anesthetist Journal, 70*(5), 399-407.

Zeleznik, J., (2003). Normative aging of the respiratory system. *Clinics in Geriatric Medicine, 19*(1), 1-18.

CHAPTER

31 Interventions for Clients Requiring Oxygen Therapy or Tracheostomy

CHRISTINE A. GATES • M. LINDA WORKMAN

LEARNING OUTCOMES

After studying this chapter, you should be able to:

1. Compare the uses and nursing care issues of oxygen delivery by nasal cannula with oxygen delivery by mask.
2. Explain the problems of oxygen therapy for those clients whose respiratory efforts are controlled by the hypoxic drive.
3. Analyze changes in clinical manifestations to determine the effectiveness of therapy for the client receiving oxygen.
4. Use laboratory data and clinical manifestations to determine the presence of hypoxemia or hypercarbia.
5. Develop a community-based teaching plan for the client receiving supportive oxygen therapy at home.
6. Prioritize nursing care needs for the client with a new tracheostomy.
7. Identify techniques to reduce the risk for aspiration when helping the client with a tracheostomy to eat.
8. Develop a community-based teaching plan for the client with a tracheostomy living at home.

Go to your Student CD-ROM for Review Questions for the NCLEX Examination keyed to these Learning Outcomes.

OXYGEN THERAPY

OVERVIEW

Oxygen (O_2) is a gas that is essential for life, as well as a potent drug used for relief of **hypoxemia** (low levels of oxygen in the blood) and **hypoxia** (decreased tissue oxygenation). The oxygen content of atmospheric air is about 21%. Therapeutic oxygen is prescribed when the oxygen needs of the client cannot be met by atmospheric or "room air" alone. Oxygen is used for both acute and chronic breathing problems that cause decreased blood and tissue oxygen levels as indicated by decreased partial pressure of arterial oxygen (PaO_2) levels or by decreased arterial oxygen saturation (SaO_2). Conditions outside the respiratory system that increase oxygen demand, decrease oxygen-carrying capability of the blood, or decrease cardiac output also are indications for oxygen therapy. Such conditions include sepsis, fever, some poisons, and decreased hemoglobin levels or poor hemoglobin quality.

The goal of oxygen therapy is to use the lowest *fraction of inspired oxygen (FIO_2)* to have an acceptable blood oxygen level without causing harmful side effects. Although oxygen improves the PaO_2 level, it does not cure the problem or stop the disease process. The average client requires an oxygen flow of 2 to 4 L/min via nasal cannula or up to 40% via Venturi mask. The client who is hypoxemic and has chronic **hypercarbia** (increased partial pressure of arterial carbon dioxide [$PaCO_2$] levels) needs lower levels of oxygen delivery, usually 1 to 2 L/min via nasal cannula, to prevent decreased respiratory effort. (A low PaO_2 level is this client's primary drive for breathing.)

◆COLLABORATIVE MANAGEMENT

◆Assessment

Arterial blood gas (ABG) analysis is the best measure for determining the need for oxygen therapy and for evaluating its effects. Oxygen need can also be determined by noninvasive monitoring, such as pulse oximetry.

Common Nursing Diagnoses and Collaborative Problems

Nursing diagnoses and collaborative problems that may apply to clients requiring oxygen therapy include the following:

- Anxiety related to hypoxemia
- Acute Confusion related to hypoxemia
- Risk for Impaired Spontaneous Ventilation related to oxygen therapy.

Critical Thinking Challenge

The client is an 87-year-old man who is currently in the ICU after a CABG repair. He has been weaned from the ventilator and is currently using a 40% Venturi mask for O_2 delivery. You note that his Sao_2 is dropping gradually from 98% to 90% over the last 30 minutes and he appears short of breath. The physician and respiratory therapist have been notified.

1. What additional assessment data should you obtain?
2. What interventions might you initiate until the doctor or RT arrives?

evolve For suggested answer guidelines, go to http://evolve.elsevier.com/Iggy/.

Interventions

Before starting oxygen therapy and while caring for a client receiving oxygen therapy, you must be knowledgeable about oxygen hazards and complications. You should also know the rationale and the expected outcome related to oxygen therapy for each client receiving oxygen. Chart 31-1 lists NIC interventions for clients using oxygen therapy.

HAZARDS AND COMPLICATIONS OF OXYGEN THERAPY

COMBUSTION. Oxygen itself does not burn, but it supports and enhances combustion. Therefore a fire burns more readily in the presence of oxygen. Take special precautions during oxygen delivery, including posting a sign on the door of the client's room. Smoking is prohibited in the client's room, including at home, when oxygen is in use. All electrical equipment must be grounded (i.e., with three prongs having a green or red dot on the plate). Frayed cords must be repaired because they can cause a spark that can ignite a flame. Flammable solutions (containing alcohol or oil) are not used in rooms where oxygen is in use.

OXYGEN-INDUCED HYPOVENTILATION. Assess for oxygen-induced hypoventilation in the client whose main respiratory drive is hypoxia (hypoxic drive), such as in the client with chronic lung disease who also has hypercarbia. The arterial carbon dioxide ($Paco_2$) level for these clients gradually rises over time. The central chemoreceptors in the brain (medulla) are normally sensitive to increased $Paco_2$ levels. When these receptors are active, they stimulate breathing and cause an increased respiratory rate. When the $Paco_2$ increases gradually to above 60 to 65 mm Hg, this normal mechanism no longer functions. The central chemoreceptors lose sensitivity to increased levels of $Paco_2$ and do not respond by increasing the rate and depth of respiration. This loss of sensitivity to high levels of $Paco_2$ is called **CO_2 narcosis**. For these

CHART 31-1

NIC INTERVENTION ACTIVITIES for The Client with Respiratory Problems

Oxygen Therapy: *Administration of oxygen and monitoring of its effectiveness*

- Clear oral, nasal, and tracheal secretions, as appropriate.
- Maintain airway patency.
- Set up oxygen equipment and administer through a heated, humidified system.
- Monitor the oxygen liter flow.
- Monitor position of oxygen delivery device.
- Periodically check oxygen delivery device to ensure that the prescribed concentration is being delivered.
- Monitor the effectiveness of oxygen therapy (e.g., pulse oximetry, ABGs), as appropriate.
- Ensure replacement of oxygen mask/cannula whenever the device is removed.
- Observe for signs of oxygen-induced hypoventilation.
- Monitor for signs of oxygen toxicity and absorption atelectasis.
- Monitor oxygen equipment to ensure that it is not interfering with the client's attempts to breathe.
- Monitor client's anxiety related to need for oxygen therapy.
- Monitor for skin breakdown from friction of oxygen device.
- Provide for oxygen when client is transported.
- Instruct client and family about use of oxygen at home.
- Arrange for use of oxygen devices that facilitate mobility and teach client accordingly.

Artificial Airway Management: *Maintenance of endotracheal and tracheostomy tubes and prevention of complications associated with their use*

- Provide 100% humidification of inspired gas/air.
- Provide adequate systemic hydration via oral or intravenous fluid administration.
- Inflate endotracheal/tracheostomy cuff using minimal occlusive volume technique or minimal leak technique.
- Suction the oropharynx and secretions from the top of the tube cuff before deflating cuff.
- Monitor cuff pressures every 4 to 8 hours during expiration using a three-way stopcock, calibrated syringe, and mercury manometer.
- Change endotracheal tapes/ties every 24 hours, inspect the skin and oral mucosa, and move ET tube to the other side of the mouth.
- Monitor for presence of crackles and rhonchi over large airways.
- Institute measures to prevent spontaneous decannulation: secure artificial airway with tape/ties; administer sedation and muscle paralyzing agent, as appropriate, and use arm restraints, as appropriate.
- Provide additional intubation equipment and Ambu bag in a readily available location.
- Provide trachea care every 4 to 8 hours as appropriate: clean the inner cannula, clean and dry the area around the stoma, and change tracheostomy ties.
- Inspect skin around tracheal stoma for drainage, redness, and irritation.
- Maintain sterile technique when suctioning and providing tracheostomy care.
- Shield the tracheostomy from water.
- Tape the tracheostomy obturator to head of bed.
- Tape a second tracheostomy tube (same type and size) and forceps to head of bed.
- Institute chest physiotherapy, as appropriate.
- Elevate head of the bed or assist client to a sitting position in a chair during feedings, as appropriate.
- Add food coloring to enteral feedings as appropriate.

NIC intervention activities selected from Dochterman, J.M., & Bulechek, G.M. (Eds.). (2004). *Nursing interventions classification (NIC)* (4th ed.). St. Louis: Mosby. No part of this work is to be altered without prior written permission from the Publisher.
ABG, Arterial blood gas.

clients, the stimulus to breathe is a decreased arterial oxygen level. The low oxygen levels are sensed by peripheral chemoreceptors in the carotid sinus areas and aortic arch. When arterial oxygen (PaO_2) levels drop (hypoxemia), these receptors signal the brain to increase the respiratory rate and depth—this is known as the **hypoxic drive** to breathe.

The hypoxic drive occurs only in the presence of severely elevated $PaCO_2$ levels (i.e., in the client who has hypoxemia and hypercarbia). When the client with low PaO_2 levels and high $PaCO_2$ levels receives oxygen therapy, the PaO_2 level increases, removing the stimulation for breathing, and the client has respiratory depression. (The client being ventilated mechanically is not at risk for this complication.)

Oxygen therapy is prescribed at the lowest liter flow (usually 1, 2, or 3 L/min) needed to treat the hypoxemia. A system that delivers precise oxygen levels (e.g., a Venturi mask) is preferred for this client. However, a client with chronic obstructive pulmonary disease may not tolerate a face mask.

Closely monitor the respiratory rate and depth while the client is receiving oxygen. This monitoring is especially important when it is the first time the client receives oxygen or when the $PaCO_2$ levels are not known. Manifestations of hypoventilation are seen during the first 30 minutes of oxygen therapy. The client's color improves (from ashen or gray to pink) because of an increase in the PaO_2 level before the apnea or respiratory arrest occurs from loss of the hypoxic drive. Therefore carefully monitor the level of consciousness, respiratory pattern and rate, and pulse oximetry for clients at risk for oxygen-induced hypoventilation, apnea, and respiratory arrest. *Although oxygen-induced hypoventilation is a serious concern, untreated or inadequately treated hypoxemia is a greater threat to life.*

OXYGEN TOXICITY. Oxygen toxicity is related to the concentration of oxygen delivered, duration of oxygen therapy, and degree of lung disease present. In general, an oxygen level greater than 50% given continuously for more than 24 to 48 hours may damage the lungs. *Although oxygen toxicity is a serious concern, inadequately treated hypoxemia is a greater threat to life.*

The causes and manifestations of lung injury from oxygen toxicity are the same as those for acute respiratory distress syndrome (ARDS) (see Chapter 35). Initial symptoms include nonproductive cough, substernal chest pain, gastrointestinal (GI) upset, and dyspnea. As exposure to high levels of oxygen continues, the symptoms become more severe with decreased vital capacity, decreased compliance (which results in more dyspnea), crackles, and hypoxemia. Prolonged exposure to high oxygen levels damages lung tissues. Atelectasis, pulmonary edema, hemorrhage, and hyaline membrane formation result. Surviving this critical condition depends on correcting the underlying disease process and decreasing the oxygen amount delivered.

The toxic effects of oxygen are difficult to treat, making prevention a priority. The lowest level of oxygen needed to maintain oxygenation and prevent oxygen toxicity is prescribed. Closely monitor arterial blood gases (ABGs) during oxygen therapy and notify the physician of PaO_2 levels greater than 90 mm Hg. Also monitor the prescribed oxygen level and length of therapy to identify the client at higher risk. High oxygen levels are avoided unless absolutely necessary. The use of continuous positive airway pressure (CPAP) with an oxygen mask, bilevel positive airway pressure (BiPAP), or positive end-expiratory pressure (PEEP) on the mechanical ventilator (see Chapter 35) may reduce the amount of oxygen needed. As soon as the client's condition allows, the prescribed amount of oxygen is decreased.

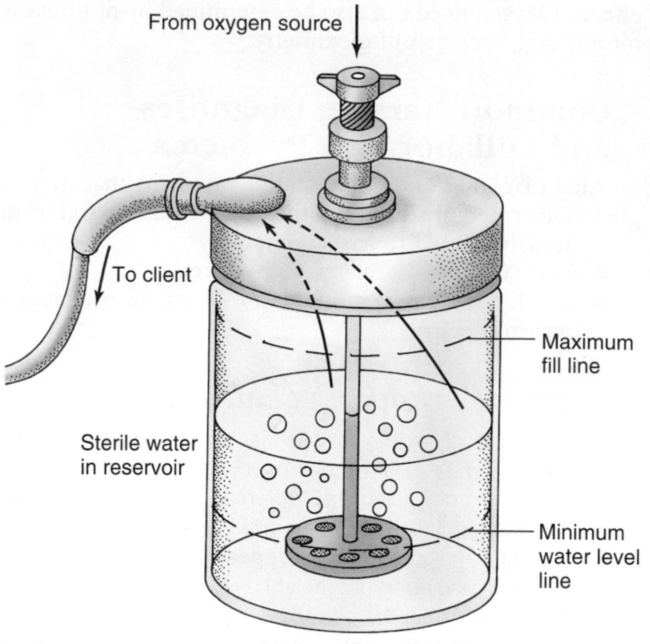

Figure 31-1 ■ A bubble humidifier bottle used with oxygen therapy.

ABSORPTION ATELECTASIS. Nitrogen in the air normally helps maintain patent airways and alveoli. Making up 79% of room air, nitrogen prevents alveolar collapse. When high oxygen levels are delivered, nitrogen is diluted, oxygen diffuses from the alveoli into the circulation, and the alveoli collapse. Collapsed alveoli cause atelectasis (called absorption atelectasis), which is detected by auscultation. Monitor the client closely for crackles and decreased breath sounds every 1 to 2 hours when oxygen therapy is started and as often as needed thereafter.

DRYING OF MUCOUS MEMBRANES. When an oxygen flow rate higher than 4 L/min is needed, humidity is added to the delivery system (Figure 31-1). Ensure that oxygen can be seen bubbling through the water in the humidifier.

Oxygen can also be humidified via a large-volume jet nebulizer (LVN) in mist form (aerosol) (Figure 31-2). A heated nebulizer raises the humidity even more and is used when oxygen is delivered through an artificial airway. Usually the upper airway passages warm the air during breathing, but these passages are bypassed when an artificial airway is in use.

For the client to receive properly humidified oxygen, the humidifier or LVN must have a sufficient amount of sterile water and the flow rate must be adequate. Condensation often forms in the tubing. Remove this condensation as it collects by disconnecting the tubing and emptying the water. Some humidifiers and LVNs have a water trap that hangs from the tubing so that the condensation can be drained without disconnecting. *To prevent bacterial contamination, never drain the fluid back into the humidifier or LVN.* Check the water level and change the humidifier as needed.

INFECTION. The humidifier or LVN may be a source of bacteria, especially if it is heated. The LVN is more likely to be a bacterial source because it uses room air. *Pseudomonas aeruginosa* is often the organism involved. Oxygen delivery

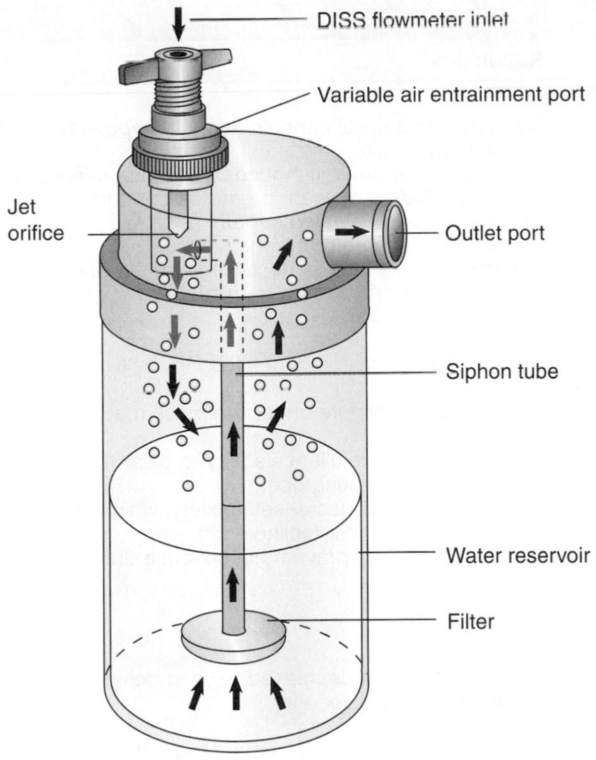

Figure 31-2 ■ An all-purpose large-volume jet nebulizer (LVN).

CHART 31-2

BEST PRACTICE for
Oxygen Therapy

- Check the physician's order with the type of delivery system and liter flow or percentage of oxygen actually in use.
- Obtain an order for humidification if oxygen is being delivered at 4 L/min or more.
- Be sure the oxygen and humidification equipment is functioning properly.
- Check the skin around the client's ears, back of the neck, and face every 4 to 8 hours for pressure points and signs of irritation.
- Provide mouth care every 8 hours and as needed; assess nasal and oral mucous membranes for cracks or other signs of dryness.
- Pad the elastic band and change its position frequently to prevent skin breakdown.
- Pad tubing in areas that put pressure on the skin.
- Cleanse the cannula or mask by rinsing with clear, warm water every 4 to 8 hours or as needed.
- Cleanse skin under the tubing, straps, and mask every 4 to 8 hours or as needed.
- Lubricate the client's nostrils, face, and lips with nonpetroleum cream to relieve the drying effects of oxygen.
- Position the tubing so it does not pull on the client's face, nose, or artificial airway.
- Ensure that there is no smoking and that no candles or matches are lit in the immediate area.
- Assess and document the client's response to oxygen therapy.
- Provide the client with ongoing teaching and reassurance to enhance the client's adherence with oxygen therapy.

equipment such as cannulas and masks can also harbor organisms. Change equipment as per policy or protocol, which ranges from every 24 hours for humidification systems to every 7 days or whenever necessary for cannulas and masks.

OXYGEN DELIVERY SYSTEMS

Oxygen can be delivered by many systems. Regardless of the type of delivery system used, it is important to understand its indications, advantages, and disadvantages. Use the equipment properly and ensure appropriate equipment maintenance. Consult a respiratory therapist whenever there is a question or concern about an oxygen delivery system.

The type of delivery system used depends on the following:

- Oxygen concentration required by the client
- Oxygen concentration achieved by a delivery system
- Importance of accuracy and control of the oxygen concentration
- Client comfort
- Expense to the client
- Importance of humidity
- Client mobility

Oxygen delivery systems are classified by the rate of oxygen delivery. There are two systems: low-flow systems and high-flow systems. Low-flow systems do not provide enough flow of oxygen to meet the total oxygen need and air volume of the client. Part of the tidal volume is supplied by breathing room air. The total level of oxygen received depends on the respiratory rate and tidal volume. High-flow systems have a flow rate that meets the entire oxygen need and tidal volume regardless of the client's breathing pattern. High-flow systems are used for critically ill clients and when delivery of precise levels of oxygen is needed.

If the client needs a mask but is able to eat, request a prescription for a nasal cannula to be used at mealtimes only. Reapply the mask after the meal is completed. To increase mobility, up to 50 feet of connecting tubing can be used with connecting pieces. Best nursing practices for clients receiving oxygen therapy are listed in Chart 31-2.

LOW-FLOW OXYGEN DELIVERY SYSTEMS. Low-flow delivery systems include the nasal cannula, simple face mask, partial rebreather mask, and non-rebreather mask (Table 31-1). These systems are inexpensive, easy to use, and fairly comfortable. A disadvantage is that the actual amount of oxygen delivered is variable and depends on the client's breathing pattern. The oxygen is diluted with room air (21% oxygen), which lowers the amount of oxygen actually received.

NASAL CANNULA. The nasal cannula, or nasal prongs (Figure 31-3), is used at flow rates of 1 to 6 L/min. Oxygen concentrations of 24% (at 1 L/min) to 44% (at 6 L/min) can be achieved. Flow rates greater than 6 L/min do not increase oxygenation because the **anatomic dead space** (places where air flows but the structures are too thick for gas exchange) is full. In addition, high flow rates increase mucosal irritation. With the use of a nasal cannula, an effective oxygen level can be delivered to clients who are nose breathers and those who are mouth breathers.

The nasal cannula is often used for clients with chronic lung disease and for any client requiring long-term oxygen therapy. The client who retains carbon dioxide rarely receives oxygen at a rate higher than 2 to 3 L/min because of the risk for losing the drive to breathe, thereby increasing the risk for apnea or respiratory arrest. Place the nasal prongs in the nostrils, with the openings facing the client.

SIMPLE FACE MASK. A simple face mask is used to deliver oxygen concentrations of 40% to 60% for short-term oxygen therapy or in an emergency (Figure 31-4). A minimum flow rate of 5 L/min is needed to prevent the re-

TABLE 31-1 Comparison of Low-Flow Oxygen Delivery Systems

FIO_2 Delivered	Nursing Interventions	Rationales
Nasal Cannula		
24%-40% FIO_2 at 1-6 L/min ≈24% at 1 L/min ≈28% at 2 L/min ≈32% at 3 L/min ≈36% at 4 L/min ≈40% at 5 L/min ≈44% at 6 L/min	Ensure that prongs are in the nares properly.	A poorly fitting nasal cannula leads to hypoxemia and skin breakdown.
	Provide water-soluble jelly to nares PRN.	This substance prevents mucosal irritation related to the drying effect of oxygen; promotes comfort.
	Assess the patency of the nostrils.	Congestion or a deviated septum prevents effective delivery of oxygen through the nares.
	Assess the client for changes in respiratory rate or depth.	The respiratory pattern affects the amount of oxygen delivered. A different delivery system may be needed.
Simple Face Mask		
40%-60% FIO_2 at 5-8 L/min; flow rate must be set at least at 5 L/min to flush mask of carbon dioxide ≈40% at 5 L/min ≈45%-50% at 6 L/min ≈55%-60% at 8 L/min	Be sure mask fits securely over nose and mouth.	A poorly fitting mask reduces the FIO_2 delivered.
	Assess skin and provide skin care to the area covered by the mask.	Pressure and moisture under the mask may cause skin breakdown.
	Monitor the client closely for risk of aspiration.	The mask limits the client's ability to clear the mouth, especially if vomiting occurs.
	Provide emotional support to the client who feels claustrophobic.	Emotional support decreases anxiety, which contributes to a claustrophobic feeling.
	Suggest to the physician to switch the client from a mask to the nasal cannula during eating.	Use of the cannula prevents hypoxemia during eating.
Partial Rebreather Mask		
60%-75% at 6-11 L/min, a liter flow rate high enough to maintain reservoir bag two thirds full during inspiration and expiration	Make sure that the reservoir does not twist or kink, which results in a deflated bag.	Deflation results in decreased oxygen delivered and rebreathing of exhaled air.
	Adjust the flow rate to keep the reservoir bag inflated.	The flow rate is adjusted to meet the pattern of the client.
Non-Rebreather Mask		
80%-95% FIO_2 at liter flow to maintain reservoir bag two-thirds full	Interventions as for partial rebreather mask; this client requires close monitoring.	Rationales as for partial rebreather mask. Monitoring ensures proper functioning and prevents harm.
	Make sure that valves and rubber flaps are patent, functional, and not stuck. Remove mucus or saliva.	Valves should open during expiration and close during inhalation to prevent dramatic decrease in FIO_2. Suffocation can occur if the reservoir bag kinks or if the oxygen source disconnects.
	Closely assess the client on increased FIO_2 via non-rebreather mask. Intubation is the only way to provide more precise FIO_2.	The client may require intubation.

FIO_2, Fraction of inspired oxygen.

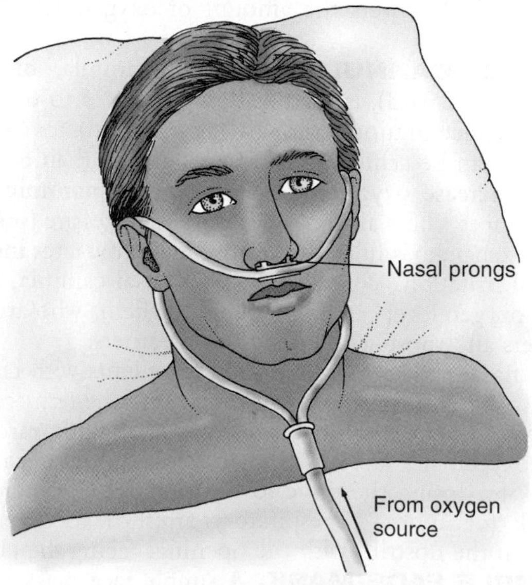

Figure 31-3 ■ A nasal cannula (prongs).

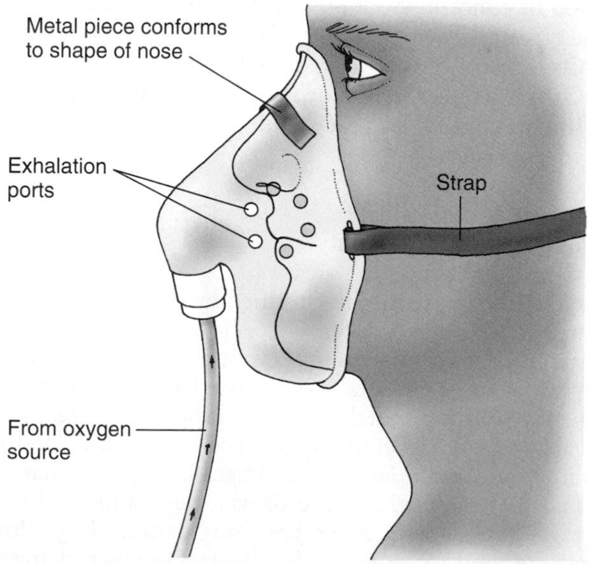

Figure 31-4 ■ A simple face mask used to deliver oxygen.

breathing of exhaled air. Give special attention to skin care and to the proper fitting of the mask so that inspired oxygen levels are maintained.

PARTIAL REBREATHER MASK. A partial rebreather mask provides oxygen concentrations of 60% to 75%, with flow rates of 6 to 11 L/min. It is a mask with a reservoir bag but no flaps (Figure 31-5). The client first rebreathes with each breath, one third of the exhaled tidal volume, which is high in oxygen and provides a high fraction of inspired oxygen (FIO_2). Ensure that the bag remains slightly inflated at the end of inspiration; otherwise, the client will not be getting the desired amount of oxygen. If needed, call the respiratory therapist for assistance.

NON-REBREATHER MASK. A non-rebreather mask provides the highest oxygen level of the low-flow systems and can deliver an FIO_2 greater than 90%, depending on the client's breathing pattern. This type of mask is often used with clients whose respiratory status is unstable and who may require intubation.

The non-rebreather mask has a one-way valve between the mask and the reservoir and two flaps over the exhalation ports (Figure 31-6). The valve allows the client to draw all needed oxygen from the reservoir bag, and the flaps prevent room air from entering through the exhalation ports. During exhalation, air leaves through these exhalation ports while the one-way valve prevents exhaled air from re-entering the reservoir bag. *It is crucial to ensure that the valve and flaps are intact and functional during each breath.* Some models include only one flap on the mask, or one of the exhalation flaps may be removed for safety purposes. *If the oxygen source should fail or be depleted when both flaps are in place, the client would not be able to inhale room air.* The flow rate is kept at a level high enough to keep the bag inflated during inhalation, usually 10 to 15 L/min. Assess for this safety feature at least hourly.

HIGH-FLOW OXYGEN DELIVERY SYSTEMS. High-flow systems (Table 31-2) include the Venturi mask, aerosol mask, face tent, tracheostomy collar, and T-piece. These devices deliver an accurate oxygen level that meets the client's oxygen needs when properly fitted. A high-flow system provides oxygen concentrations of 24% to 100% at 8 to 15 L/min.

VENTURI MASK. The Venturi mask (commonly called Venti mask) delivers the most accurate oxygen concentration. It works by pulling in a proportional amount of room air for each liter flow of oxygen. An adaptor is located between the bottom of the mask and the oxygen source (Figure 31-7). Adaptors with holes of different sizes allow specific amounts of air to mix with the oxygen. Precise delivery of oxygen results. Each adaptor also determines the needed flow rate. For example, to deliver 24% of oxygen, the flow rate must be 4 L/min. Another type of Venturi mask has one adaptor with a dial that is used to select the amount of oxygen desired. Humidification is not needed with the Venturi mask. This system is best for the client with chronic lung disease because it delivers a precise oxygen concentration.

OTHER HIGH-FLOW SYSTEMS. The face tent, aerosol mask, tracheostomy collar, and T-piece are often used to provide high humidity with oxygen delivery. A dial on the humidification source regulates the oxygen level being delivered. A face tent fits over the chin, with the top extending halfway across the face. The oxygen level delivered varies, but the face tent, instead of a tight-fitting mask, is useful for facial trauma or burns. An aerosol mask is used when high humidity is needed after extubation or upper airway surgery, or for thick secretions. The tracheostomy collar is used to deliver high humidity and the desired oxygen to the client with a tracheostomy. A special adaptor, called the T-piece, is used to deliver any desired FIO_2 to the client with a tracheostomy, laryngectomy, or endotracheal tube (Figure 31-8). Adjust the

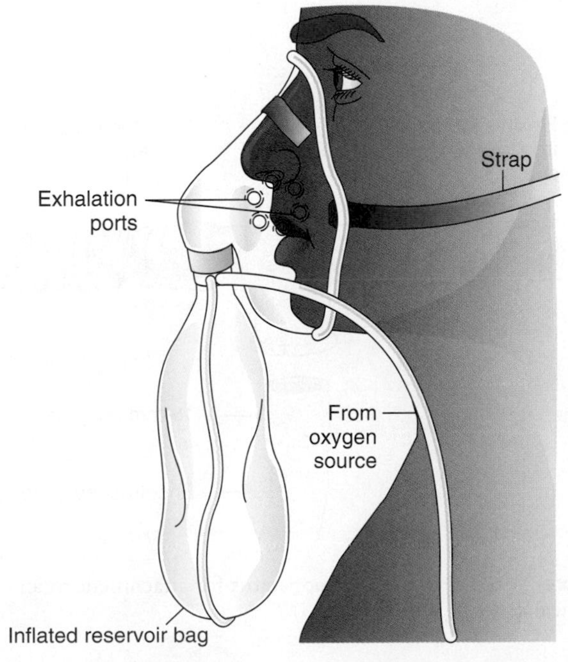

Figure 31-5 ■ A partial rebreather mask.

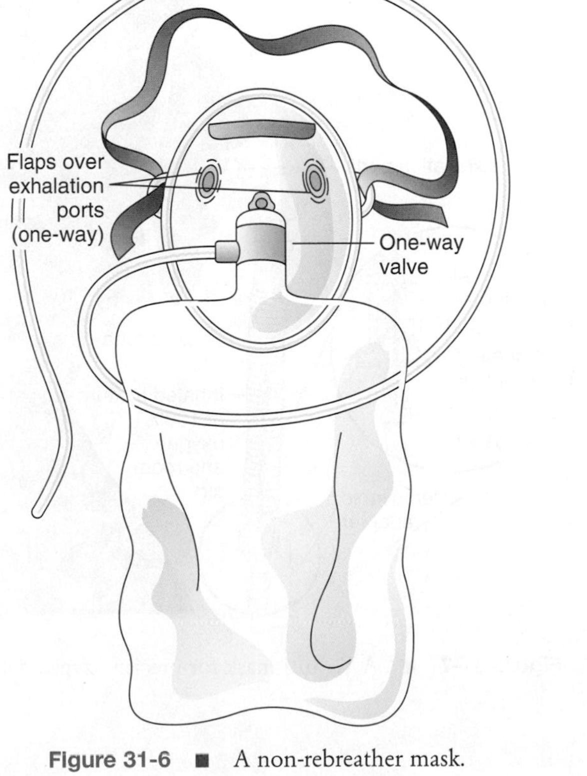

Figure 31-6 ■ A non-rebreather mask.

TABLE 31-2 Comparison of High-Flow Oxygen Delivery Systems

FIO_2 Delivered	Nursing Interventions	Rationales
Venturi Mask (Venti Mask)		
24%-55% FIO_2 with flow rates as recommended by the manufacturer, usually 4-10 L/min; provides high humidity	Perform constant surveillance to ensure an accurate flow rate for the specific FIO_2.	An accurate flow rate ensures FIO_2 delivery.
	Keep the orifice for the Venturi adaptor open and uncovered.	If the Venturi orifice is covered, the adaptor does not function and oxygen delivery varies.
	Provide a mask that fits snugly and tubing that is free of kinks.	FIO_2 is altered if kinking occurs or if the mask fits poorly.
	Assess the client for dry mucous membranes.	Comfort measures may be indicated.
	Change to a nasal cannula during mealtimes.	Oxygen is a drug that needs to be given continuously.
Aerosol Mask, Face Tent, Tracheostomy Collar		
24%-100% FIO_2 with flow rates of at least 10 L/min; provides high humidity	Assess that aerosol mist escapes from the vents of the delivery system during inspiration and expiration.	Humidification should be delivered to the client.
	Empty condensation from the tubing.	Emptying prevents the client from being lavaged with water, promotes an adequate flow rate, and assures a continued prescribed FIO_2.
	Change the aerosol water container as needed.	Adequate humidification is ensured only when there is sufficient water in the canister.
T-Piece		
24%-100% FIO_2 with flow rates of at least 10 L/min; provides high humidity	Empty condensation from the tubing.	Condensation interferes with flow rate delivery of FIO_2 and may drain into the tracheostomy if not emptied.
	Keep the exhalation port open and uncovered.	If the port is occluded, the client can suffocate.
	Position the T-piece so that it does not pull on the tracheostomy or endotracheal tube.	The weight of the T-piece pulls on the tracheostomy and causes pain or erosion of skin at the insertion site.
	Make sure the humidifier creates enough mist. A mist should be seen during inspiration and expiration.	An adequate flow rate is needed to meet the inspiration effort of the client. If not, the client will be "air-hungry."

FIO_2, Fraction of inspired oxygen.

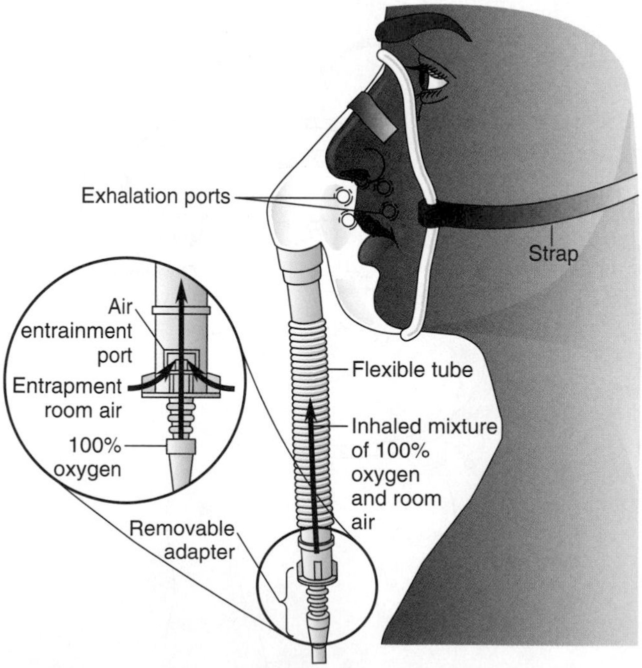

Figure 31-7 ■ A Venturi mask for precise oxygen delivery.

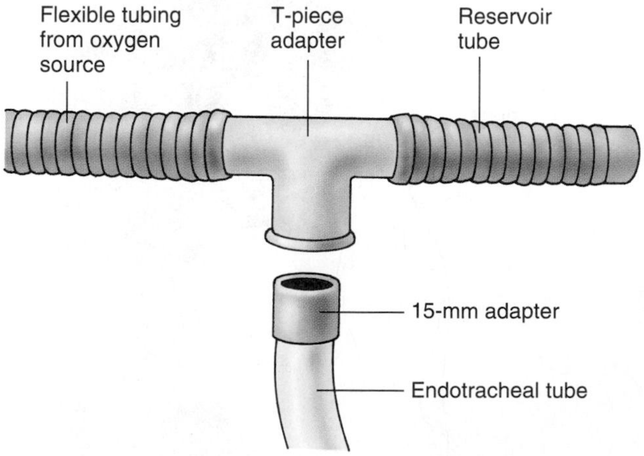

Figure 31-8 ■ A T-piece apparatus for attachment to an endotracheal or tracheostomy tube.

flow rate so that the aerosol appears on the exhalation side of the T-piece.

NONINVASIVE POSITIVE-PRESSURE VENTILATION. Noninvasive positive-pressure ventilation (NPPV) is a technique using positive pressure to keep alveoli open and improve gas exchange without the need for airway intubation. This type of ventilation can deliver oxygen or may just use room air. A nasal mask or full face mask delivery system allows mechanical delivery of either bi-level positive airway pressure (BiPAP) or continuous nasal positive airway pressure (CPAP).

For BiPAP, a cycling machine delivers a set inspiratory positive airway pressure each time the client begins to inspire. As the client begins to exhale, the machine delivers a lower set end-expiratory pressure. Together, these two pressures improve tidal volume.

Nasal continuous positive airway pressure delivers a set positive airway pressure throughout each cycle of inhalation and exhalation. The effect is to open collapsed alveoli. Clients who may benefit from this form of oxygen or air delivery include those with atelectasis after surgery or cardiac-induced pulmonary edema. This technique is also used for sleep apnea. The effect of this use is to hold open the upper airways.

TRANSTRACHEAL OXYGEN THERAPY. Transtracheal oxygen (TTO) is a long-term method of delivering oxygen directly into the lungs. A small, flexible catheter is passed into the trachea via a small incision (Figure 31-9) under local anesthesia. TTO avoids the irritation that nasal prongs cause. Clients also report it to be more cosmetically acceptable. A TTO team provides formal client education, including the purpose of TTO and care of the catheter. A TTO flow rate is prescribed for rest and for activity. A flow rate also is prescribed for the nasal cannula, which is to be used when the TTO catheter is being cleaned. Most clients using this delivery method have a 55% reduction in required oxygen flow at rest and a 31% decrease with activity.

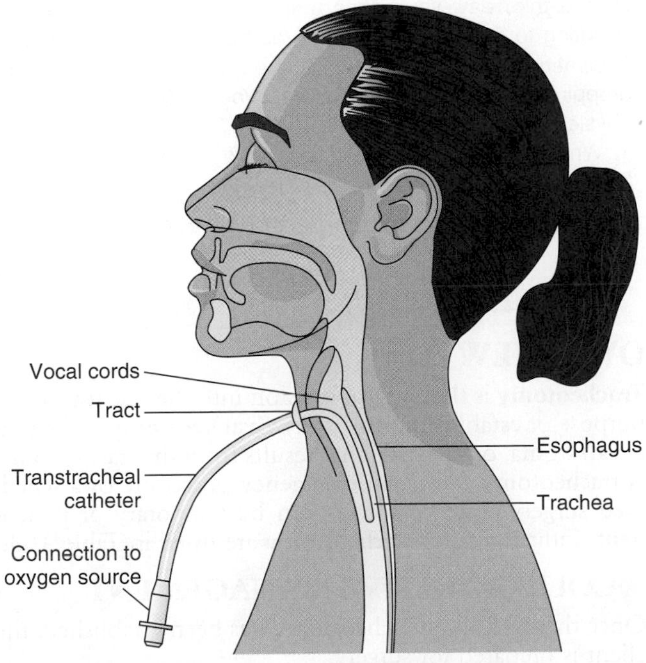

Figure 31-9 ■ Example of transtracheal oxygen delivery.

Community-Based Care

HOME CARE MANAGEMENT

CRITERIA FOR HOME OXYGEN THERAPY. The client must be stable and optimally treated before the need for home oxygen is considered. For Medicare to cover the cost of continuous oxygen therapy, the client must have severe hypoxemia defined as a partial pressure of arterial oxygen (PaO_2) level of less than 55 mm Hg or an arterial oxygen saturation (SaO_2) of less than 88% on room air and at rest. The criteria vary when hypoxemia is caused by cardiac rather than pulmonary problems, or when oxygen is needed only at night or with exercise.

CLIENT EDUCATION. After the need for home oxygen therapy is verified, begin a teaching plan about oxygen therapy. Assist the client to select a durable medical equipment (DME) company to deliver oxygen equipment and a community health nursing agency for follow-up care in the home. The client is re-evaluated for the need for oxygen therapy about 6 months after discharge from the health care facility and yearly thereafter.

While providing discharge planning and teaching, be sensitive to the client's psychological adjustment to oxygen therapy. Encourage the client to share feelings and concerns. The client may be concerned about social acceptance. Help the client realize that adherence to oxygen therapy is important for being able to participate in activities of daily living (ADLs) and other events that bring enjoyment.

HOME CARE PREPARATION

EQUIPMENT FOR HOME OXYGEN THERAPY. The nurse or respiratory therapist teaches the client about the equipment needed for home oxygen therapy:

- Oxygen source
- Oxygen delivery device
- Humidification source
- Safety aspects of using and maintaining the equipment

Home oxygen therapy is provided in one of three ways: compressed gas in a tank or a cylinder, liquid oxygen in a reservoir, or an oxygen concentrator. Compressed gas in an oxygen tank (green) is the most often used oxygen source. An oxygen tank is economical, and pure oxygen can be delivered at a wide range of flow rates. The large H cylinder may be used as a stationary source and the small E tank is available for transporting the client (Figure 31-10). As a safety precaution, the tanks must always be in a stand or rack. A tank that is accidentally knocked over could suddenly decompress and move around in an uncontrolled manner. Smaller (and lighter) D or C cylinders are also available for the client to carry.

Liquid oxygen for home use is oxygen gas that has been liquefied. A concentrated amount of oxygen is available in a lightweight and easy-to-carry container similar to a Thermos bottle (Figure 31-11). The client is able to fill the portable tank from the large stationary liquid vessel. This type of oxygen lasts longer than gaseous oxygen in a conventional tank of the same size; however, it is expensive, and the oxygen evaporates if it is not used continuously.

The oxygen concentrator is a machine that removes nitrogen, water vapor, and hydrocarbons from room air. It is sometimes referred to as an *oxygen extractor*. Oxygen is concentrated from room air and is delivered at more than 90%.

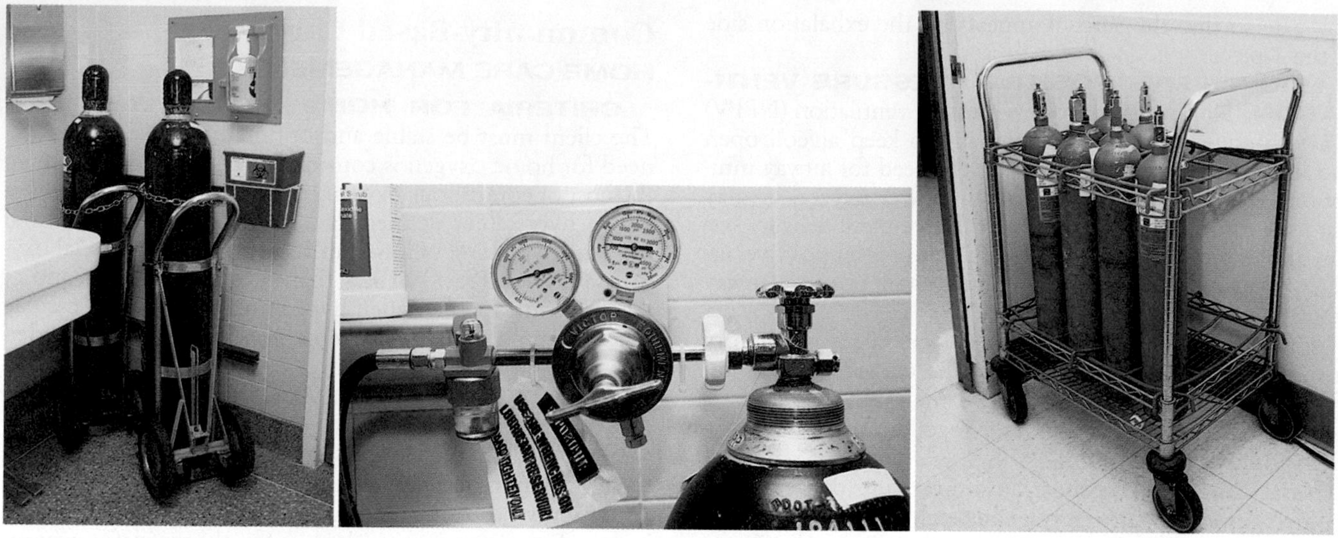

Figure 31-10 ■ Comparison of a large H oxygen cylinder, with a stand *(left)*, regulator, and flowmeter *(middle)*, and several small E cylinders *(right)*.

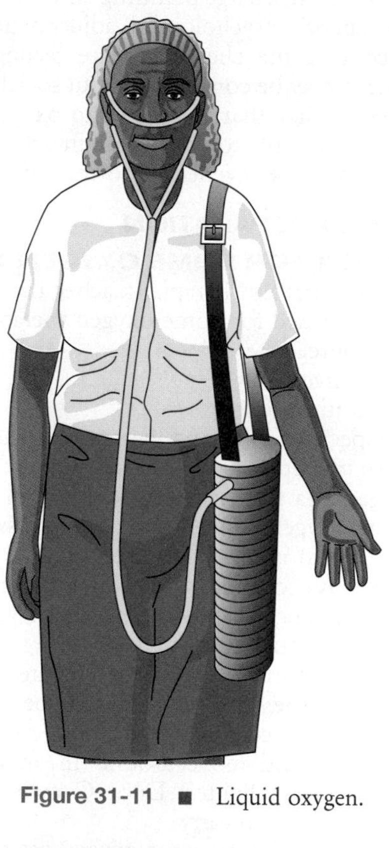

Figure 31-11 ■ Liquid oxygen.

The concentrator, although noisy and not portable, is often used in the home as a stationary system. Portable tanks are used when the client leaves home. The system is the least expensive and does not need to be filled.

Humidification is rarely needed for any of these oxygen systems. Humidification may be helpful, however, when the flow rate is higher than 4 L/min.

In any of the three home oxygen systems, an oxygen-conserving reservoir-type nasal cannula can be used to reduce oxygen flow needs by about 50%. Two types available are the mustache type and the pendant type. A reservoir for storage of exhaled oxygen is attached to the tubing. The stored oxygen is then delivered back to the client on the next inhalation. The reservoir sits on top of the upper lip (mustache type) or hangs around the neck (pendant type).

Critical Thinking Challenge

The 87-year-old, post-CABG repair male client is in the ICU. His respiratory rate is 28, heart rate is 100 to 110, BP is slightly elevated, and ABG shows hypoxemia and mild hypercarbia. Lungs have wheezes and mild crackles bilaterally with reduced breath sounds at the bases. The physician orders BiPAP started. The RT starts the client on the machine at the prescribed settings, with an 8 L/min bleed-in of oxygen to the circuit. The client remains on these settings for the next 2 days. On the third day, you notice that the client is no longer attempting to cough up secretions (as he had been before), his respirations are 36 to 40 and labored, and his Sa_{O_2} is again dropping to between 89% and 90%. You notify the RT and the physician.

1. What assessments should be made?
2. What interventions could be initiated?

evolve For suggested answer guidelines, go to http://evolve.elsevier.com/Iggy/.

TRACHEOSTOMY

OVERVIEW

Tracheotomy is the surgical incision into the trachea for the purpose of establishing an airway. **Tracheostomy** is the (tracheal) stoma, or opening, that results from the tracheotomy. A tracheotomy can be an emergency procedure or a scheduled surgery. Tracheostomies can be temporary or permanent. Indications for tracheostomy are listed in Table 31-3.

COLLABORATIVE MANAGEMENT

Once the need for a tracheostomy has been established, the client is prepared for surgery.

TABLE 31-3 Indications for Tracheostomy

- Acute airway obstruction when oral or nasal intubation is not feasible
- Airway protection (e.g., after head and neck cancer surgery)
- Prolonged intubation or need for mechanical ventilation
- Decreased airway dead space in combination with other indicators
- Control of pulmonary secretions refractory to conventional methods
- Airway reconstruction after laryngeal trauma or laryngeal cancer surgery
- Obstructive sleep apnea refractory to conventional therapy

Common Nursing Diagnoses and Collaborative Problems

Nursing diagnoses and collaborative problems that may apply to clients requiring tracheostomy include the following:

- Impaired Verbal Communication related to physical barrier (tracheostomy; intubation)
- Imbalanced Nutrition: Less Than Body Requirements related to presence of endotracheal tube
- Risk for Infection related to invasive procedures
- Impaired Oral Mucous Membrane related to mechanical factors (endotracheal tube)
- Impaired Social Interaction related to communication barriers

Interventions

PREOPERATIVE CARE

The care for the client having a tracheostomy is similar to that for a laryngectomy (see Chapter 32). Focus on the client's knowledge deficits through teaching, and discuss tracheostomy care, communication, and speech.

OPERATIVE PROCEDURES

Initially, the neck is extended and an endotracheal (ET) tube is placed by the anesthesia provider to maintain the airway. An incision is then made through the anterior skin of the neck, exposing the tracheal rings and moving other tissues out of the surgical path. A second incision is made through the tracheal rings to enter the trachea (Figure 31-12). The types of incisions and specific techniques vary, depending on the surgeon's preference and the reason for the surgery.

After the trachea is entered, the ET tube is removed while the tracheostomy tube is inserted. The tracheostomy tube is secured in place with sutures and tracheostomy ties (or Velcro tube holders). A chest x-ray is obtained to ensure proper placement of the tube. If intubation is not possible, a tracheotomy can be done with the client awake under local anesthesia.

POSTOPERATIVE CARE

Immediately after surgery, focus care on ensuring a patent airway. Confirm the presence of bilateral breath sounds. Assess the client for complications from the procedure.

COMPLICATIONS

Major complications can arise after surgery. Table 31-4 lists the manifestations, management, and prevention of other serious complications of tracheostomy.

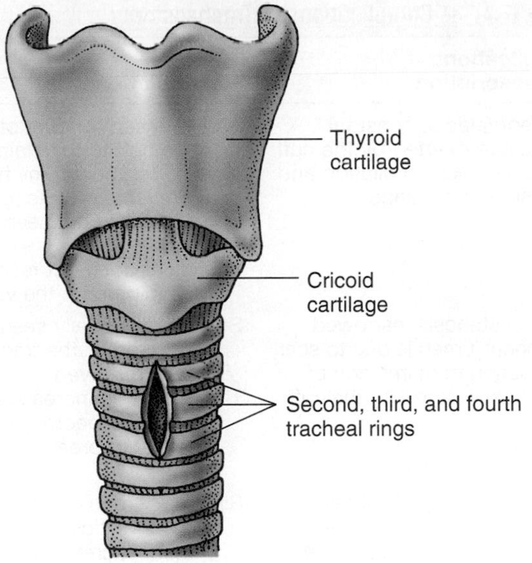

Figure 31-12 ■ A vertical tracheal incision for a tracheostomy.

TUBE OBSTRUCTION. The tube can be obstructed by secretions or by cuff displacement. Indicators of obstruction include difficulty breathing; noisy respirations; difficulty inserting a suction catheter; thick, dry secretions; and unexplained peak pressures (if a mechanical ventilator is in use). Assess the client at least hourly for tube patency. Prevent obstruction by helping the client to cough and deep breathe, providing inner cannula care, humidifying the oxygen source, and suctioning. If tube obstruction occurs as a result of cuff prolapse over the end of the tracheostomy tube, the physician repositions or replaces the tube.

TUBE DISLODGMENT AND ACCIDENTAL DECANNULATION. Prevent tube dislodgment and decannulation by securing the tube in place. This intervention reduces movement and traction on the tube from oxygen or ventilator tubing or accidental pulling by the client. *Tube dislodgment in the first 72 hours after surgery is an emergency because the tracheostomy tract has not matured and replacement is difficult.* The tube may end up in the subcutaneous tissue instead of in the trachea. If this occurs, first ventilate the client using a manual resuscitation bag and face mask while another nurse calls for help.

Ensure that a tracheostomy tube of the same type (including an obturator) and size (or one size smaller) is at the bedside at all times, along with a tracheostomy insertion tray. If decannulation occurs after 72 hours, extend the client's neck and open the tissues of the stoma to secure the airway. With the obturator inserted into the tracheostomy tube, quickly and gently replace the tube and remove the obturator. Check for airflow through the tube and for bilateral breath sounds. If you are unable to secure the airway, notify a more experienced nurse, respiratory therapist, or physician for assistance. Ventilate via a bag-valve mask. If the client is in distress and further attempts to secure the airway fail, call the resuscitation team, including an anesthesiologist, for assistance.

PNEUMOTHORAX. Pneumothorax (air in the chest cavity) can develop during the tracheotomy procedure if the thoracic cavity is accidentally entered. When pneumothorax

TABLE 31-4 Complications of Tracheostomy

Complications and Description	Manifestations	Management	Prevention
Tracheomalacia: constant pressure exerted by the cuff causes tracheal dilation and erosion of cartilage.	An increased amount of air is required in the cuff to maintain the seal. A larger tracheostomy tube is required to prevent an air leak at the stoma. Food particles are seen in tracheal secretions. The client does not receive the set tidal volume on the ventilator.	No special management is needed unless bleeding occurs.	Use an uncuffed tube as soon as possible. Monitor cuff pressure and air volumes closely and detect changes.
Tracheal stenosis: narrowed tracheal lumen is due to scar formation from irritation of tracheal mucosa by the cuff.	Stenosis is usually seen after the cuff is deflated or the tracheostomy tube is removed. The client has increased coughing, inability to expectorate secretions, or difficulty in breathing or talking.	Tracheal dilation or surgical intervention is used.	Prevent pulling of and traction on the tracheostomy tube. Properly secure the tube in the midline position. Maintain proper cuff pressure. Minimize oronasal intubation time.
Tracheoesophageal fistula (TEF): excessive cuff pressure causes erosion of the posterior wall of the trachea. A hole is created between the trachea and the anterior esophagus. The client at highest risk also has a nasogastric tube present.	Similar to tracheomalacia: ▪ Food particles are seen in tracheal secretions. ▪ Increased air in cuff is needed to achieve a seal. ▪ The client has increased coughing and choking while eating. ▪ The client does not receive the set tidal volume on the ventilator.	Manually administer oxygen by mask to prevent hypoxemia. Use a small soft feeding tube instead of a nasogastric tube for tube feedings. A gastrostomy or jejunostomy may be performed. Monitor the client with a nasogastric tube closely; assess for TEF and aspiration.	Maintain cuff pressure. Monitor the amount of air needed for inflation and detect changes. Progress to a deflated cuff or cuffless tube as soon as possible.
Trachea-innominate artery fistula: a malpositioned tube causes its distal tip to push against the lateral wall of the tracheostomy. Continued pressure causes necrosis and erosion of the innominate artery. ***This is a medical emergency.***	The tracheostomy tube pulsates in synchrony with the heartbeat. There is heavy bleeding from the stoma. ***This is a life-threatening complication.***	Remove the tracheostomy tube immediately. Apply direct pressure to the innominate artery at the stoma site. Prepare the client for immediate repair surgery.	Correct the tube size, length, and midline position. Prevent pulling or tugging on the tracheostomy tube. Immediately notify the physician of the pulsating tube.

occurs during tracheotomy, it usually does so at the apex of the lung. Chest x-rays after placement are used to assess for pneumothorax.

SUBCUTANEOUS EMPHYSEMA. When there is an opening (rent) in the trachea, air escapes into fresh tissue planes of the neck, causing subcutaneous emphysema. Air can also progress throughout the chest and axillary tissues into the face. Inspect and palpate for air under the skin around the new tracheostomy.

BLEEDING. A small amount of bleeding from the tracheotomy incision can be expected for the first few days, but constant oozing is abnormal. Wrap gauze around the tube and pack gauze gently into the wound to apply pressure to the bleeding sites.

INFECTION. In the hospital, use sterile technique to prevent infection during suctioning and tracheostomy care. Assess the stoma site at least once per shift for purulent drainage, redness, pain, or swelling. Tracheostomy dressings may be used to keep the stoma clean and dry. Change these dressings often because moist dressings provide a medium for bacterial growth. Careful wound care prevents most local infections.

TRACHEOSTOMY TUBES

Many types of tracheostomy tubes are available (Table 31-5 and Figure 31-13). The one chosen depends on the specific needs of the client. Tracheostomy tubes are available in many sizes and are made of various types of materials, such as plastic or metal. The tubes may be disposable or reusable. A tracheostomy tube may or may not have a cuff. It also may have an inner cannula that can be either disposable or reusable. For clients receiving mechanical ventilation, a cuffed tube is used in acute care settings. A noncuffed tube is used for airway maintenance when mechanical ventilation is not required.

For tubes with a reusable inner cannula, inspect, suction, and clean the inner cannula. During the first 24 hours after surgery, perform cannula care as often as needed, perhaps every 30 to 60 minutes. Thereafter, care is determined by the client's needs and agency policy. In planning for self-care, teach the client to remove the inner cannula and check for cleanliness. Also instruct the client about suctioning and tracheostomy cleaning.

Because breathing and swallowing move the tube, a cuffed tube is not protective against aspiration. Having a cuffed tube inflated may give a false sense of security that aspiration cannot occur during feeding or mouth care. In addition, the pilot balloon does not reflect whether the correct amount of air is present in the cuff.

A fenestrated tube can function in many different ways. When the inner cannula is in place, the fenestration is covered over (closed), and the tube functions as a double-lumen tube. With the inner cannula removed and the plug or red de-

TABLE 31-5 Types of Tracheostomy Tubes

Double-Lumen Tube
The double-lumen tube has three major parts:
- Outer cannula—fits into the stoma and keeps the airway open. The faceplate indicates the size and type of tube and has small holes on both sides for securing the tube with tracheostomy ties.
- Inner cannula—fits snugly into the outer cannula and locks into place. Provides the universal adaptor for use with the ventilator and other respiratory therapy equipment. Some may be removed, cleaned, and reused; others are disposable.
- Obturator—is a stylet with a blunt end used to facilitate the direction of the tube when inserting or changing a tracheostomy tube. It is removed immediately after tube placement and is always kept with the client and at the bedside in case of accidental decannulation.

Single-Lumen Tube
The single-lumen tube is a long tube used for clients with long or extra-thick necks. Often called a "bull neck trach" because of the long distance from the skin to the trachea or the longer length of the trachea in large people. More intensive nursing care is required with this tube because there is no inner cannula to ensure a patent lumen.

Cuffed Tube
A cuff, when inflated, seals the airway. Used with mechanical ventilation to prevent aspiration of oral or gastric secretions, or for tube feeding. A pilot balloon attached to the outside of the tube indicates the presence or absence of air in the cuff.

Cuffless Tube
The cuffless tube is a plastic, silicone-like (Silastic) tube or a metal tube, usually double lumen, used for long-term airway management in clients who require a tracheostomy, who can protect themselves from aspiration, and who do not require mechanical ventilation. Many people can speak with this tube in place.

Fenestrated Tube
The fenestrated tube has a precut opening (fenestration) in the upper posterior wall of the outer cannula. It is used to wean the client from a tracheostomy by ensuring that the client can tolerate breathing through his or her natural airway before the entire tube is removed. This tube allows the client to speak.

Cuffed Fenestrated Tube
The cuffed fenestrated tube facilitates mechanical ventilation and speech. It is often used for clients with spinal cord paralysis or neuromuscular disease who do not require ventilation all the time. When not being mechanically ventilated, the client can have the cuff deflated and the tube capped for speech. A cuffed fenestrated tube is never used in weaning from a tracheostomy because the cuff, even fully deflated, may partially obstruct the airway.

Metal Tracheostomy Tube
The metal tracheostomy tube is used for permanent tracheostomy. It is a cuffless double-lumen tube and can be cleaned and reused indefinitely. A special adaptor attaches a manual resuscitation bag. Popular types are the Jackson and Holinger tubes.

Talking Tracheostomy Tube
The talking tracheostomy tube provides a means of communication for the client who is using a ventilator on a long-term basis. An extra air channel allows air to flow up through the vocal cords so that the client can speak with the cuff inflated. The air can cause drying of the vocal cords from constant dry airflow. Examples are the Pitt Trach Speaking Tube (National Catheter Corporation) and Communitrach (Implant Technologies, Inc.).

cannulation stopper locked in place, air can pass through the fenestration, as well as around the tube and up through the natural airway. The client can cough and speak, adjusting to breathing through the upper air passages. If the client has trouble with any of these actions, he or she should be evaluated for proper tube placement, patency, size, and fenestration. *Do not cap the tube until the problem is identified and corrected.* A fenestrated tube may or may not have a cuff.

With a cuffed fenestrated tube, some air flows through the natural airway when the client is not being mechanically ventilated. *Always deflate the cuff before capping the tube with the decannulation cap; otherwise, the client has no airway* (Figure 31-14).

Clients with metal tracheostomy tubes scheduled for magnetic resonance imaging (MRI) need to change to a plastic tube. Metal tubes could be dislodged or heat up with exposure to the magnetic field during the scan.

Care Issues for the Client with a Tracheostomy

PREVENTION OF TISSUE DAMAGE

Tissue damage can occur at the point where the inflated cuff presses against the tracheal mucosa. Mucosal ischemia occurs when the pressure exerted by the cuff on the mucosa exceeds the capillary perfusion pressure. To reduce the risk for tracheal damage, keep the cuff pressure between 14 and 20 mm Hg or 20 and 28 cm H_2O (ideally, 25 cm H_2O or less).

Most cuffs are designed to use a high volume of air while maintaining a low pressure on the tracheal mucosa. Inflate the cuff to form a seal between the trachea and the cuff while creating the least amount of pressure. If the cuff cannot be inflated to seal well enough, a larger-diameter tube may be needed. The two methods of cuff inflation are (1) the *minimal leak technique* (for cuffs without pressure relief valves) and (2) the *occlusive technique* (for cuffs with pressure relief valves). A pressure cuff inflator can be used to inflate the cuff to a specified pressure or to check the cuff pressure (Figure 31-15).

Check the cuff pressure at least once during each shift, especially with the minimal leak technique, and keep the pressure at 14 to 20 mm Hg or 20 to 28 cm H_2O. In rare situations, the cuff pressure is increased to maintain ventilator volumes when peak pressures are greater than 50 mm Hg (65 cm H_2O) and positive end-expiratory pressure (PEEP) is greater than 10 mm Hg (14 cm H_2O). High PEEP values can deflate the cuff over time and more air may need to be added periodically to maintain a proper seal. Manufacturers provide guidelines for the recommended volumes for each tracheostomy cuff size. Most cuffs are adequately inflated with less than 10 mL of air.

Although a high cuff pressure causes tracheal damage, other factors may make the damage worse. The client who is malnourished, hypotensive, dehydrated, hypoxic, older, or receiving corticosteroids has poor tissue healing and is at risk for greater tissue damage. Tube friction and movement are important factors that contribute to tracheal mucosa damage. Reduce local airway damage by maintaining proper cuff pressures, stabilizing the tube, suctioning judiciously, and preventing and treating malnutrition, hemodynamic instability, or hypoxia.

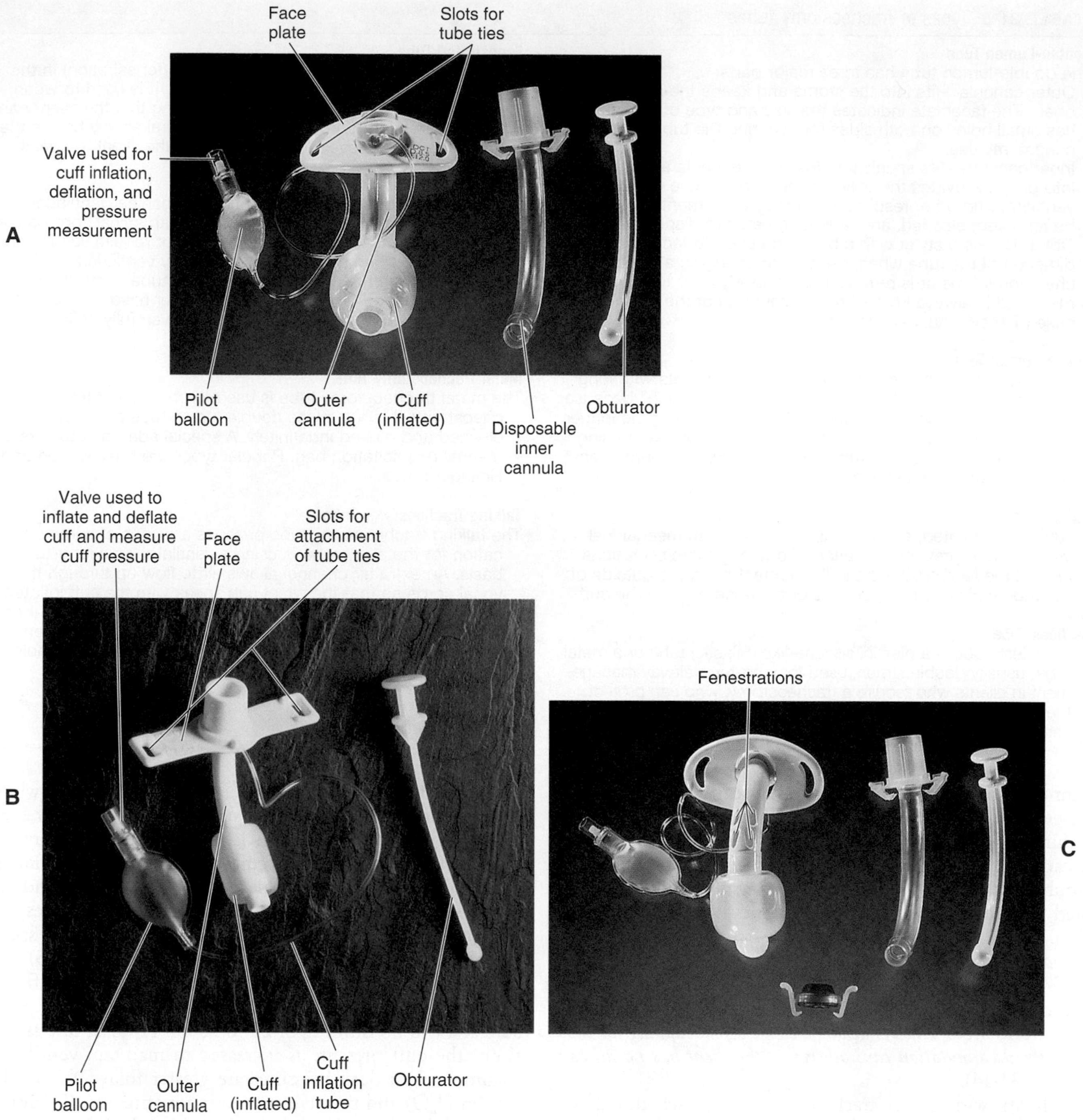

Figure 31-13 ■ Tracheostomy tubes. **A,** Dual-lumen cuffed tracheostomy tube with disposable inner cannula. **B,** Single-lumen cannula cuffed tracheostomy tube. **C,** Dual-lumen cuffed fenestrated tracheostomy tube. (Courtesy of Mallinckrodt, Inc., Shiley Tracheostomy Products, St. Louis, MO.)

AIR WARMING AND HUMIDIFICATION

The tracheostomy tube bypasses the nose and mouth, which normally humidify, warm, and filter the air before it reaches the lower respiratory tract. If humidification and warming are not adequate, tracheal damage can occur. Thick, dried secretions can occlude the airways.

To prevent these complications, humidify the air as prescribed. On an ongoing basis, assess for a fine mist emerging from the tracheostomy collar or T-piece during inspiration and expiration. To increase the amount of humidity delivered, a warming device can be attached to the humidification source. At the same time, a temperature probe is placed in the tubing circuit. *The temperature is kept between 98.6° and 100.4° F (37° and 38° C). It should never exceed 104° F (40° C).* Monitor the circuit temperature at least hourly by feeling the tubing and by checking the temperature probe. Ensure adequate hydration, which also helps to liquefy secretions. Increasing the flow rate at the flowmeter also increases the amount of delivered humidity.

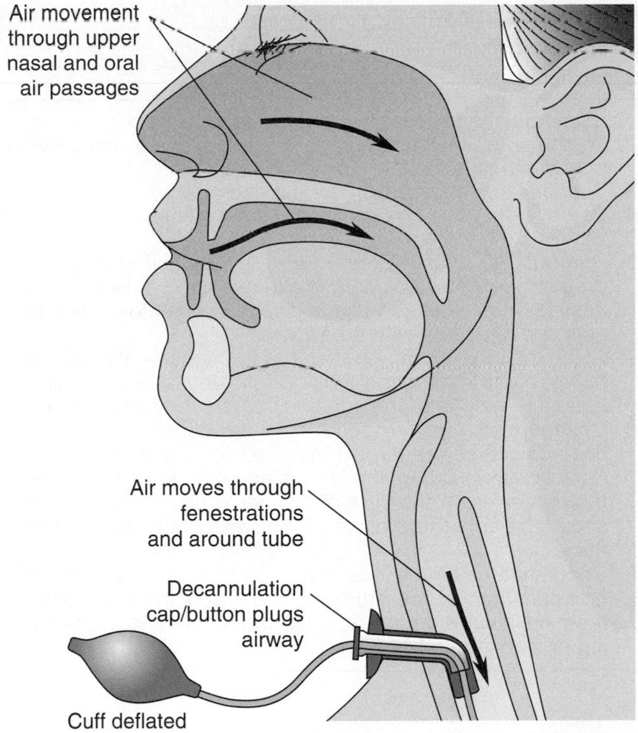

Figure 31-14 ■ Breathing through a fenestrated tracheostomy tube with a cap in place and the cuff deflated.

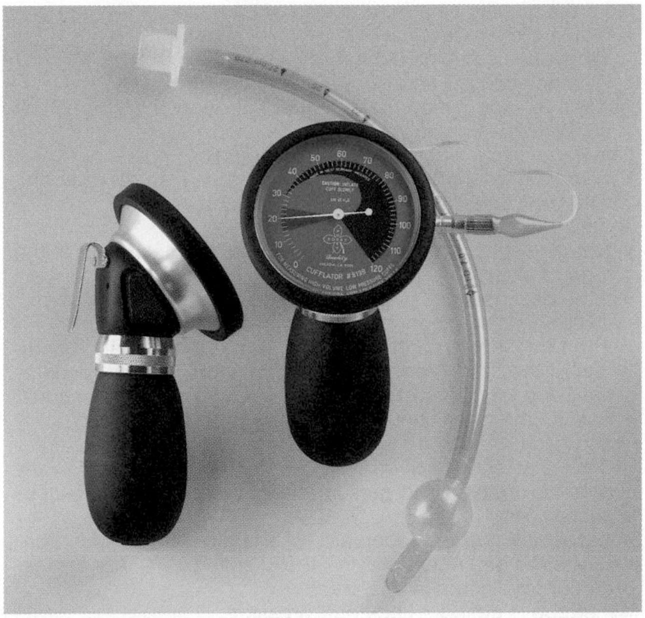

Figure 31-15 ■ An aneroid pressure manometer for cuff inflation and measuring cuff pressures. (Courtesy of J.T. Posey Company, Arcadia, CA.)

SUCTIONING

Suctioning maintains a patent airway and promotes gas exchange by removing secretions from the client who cannot cough adequately. Chart 31-3 lists best practices for suctioning. Assess the client's need for suctioning. Suctioning is indicated when audible or noisy secretions, crackles or wheezes on auscultation, restlessness, increased pulse or respiratory rates, or mucus in the artificial airway is present. Other indications include client requests for suctioning or an increase in the peak airway pressure on the ventilator.

Suctioning is performed most often through an artificial airway but can be accomplished either through the nose or the mouth. Suctioning of both routes is considered routine for the client with retained secretions.

Suctioning through the nose has similar complications as suctioning through an artificial airway. Entry through the nasal vault into the throat can be painful. Slow, careful placement of the catheter, with a good understanding of the nasopharyngeal anatomy, can make the procedure less traumatic. Placing a nasopharyngeal airway and suctioning through it helps prevent trauma to the nasal mucosa. Advance the catheter through the nasopharynx and into the laryngopharynx while the client receives oxygen by mask or nasal cannula. Once the catheter enters the larynx, the client may cough. On inhalation, insert the catheter through the vocal cords and into the trachea. Occasionally, the catheter can be disconnected from suction and attached to an oxygen source, with the client receiving oxygen via the catheter.

Suctioning can cause hypoxia, tissue (mucosal) trauma, infection, vagal stimulation, bronchospasm, and cardiac dysrhythmias.

HYPOXIA. The following are causes of hypoxia in the client with a tracheostomy:

- Ineffective oxygenation before, during, and after suctioning
- Use of a catheter that is too large for the artificial airway
- Prolonged suctioning time
- Excessive suction pressure
- Too frequent suctioning

CHART 31-3

BEST PRACTICE for Suctioning the Artificial Airway

1. Assess the need for suctioning (routine unnecessary suctioning causes mucosal damage, bleeding, and bronchospasm).
2. Wash hands. Don protective eyewear. Maintain standard precautions or body substance precautions.
3. Explain to the client that sensations such as shortness of breath and coughing are to be expected but that any discomfort will be very short in duration.
4. Check the suction source. Occlude the suction source, and adjust the pressure dial to between 80 and 120 mm Hg to prevent hypoxemia and trauma to the mucosa.
5. Set up a sterile field.
6. Preoxygenate the client with 100% oxygen for 30 seconds to 3 minutes (at least three hyperinflations) to prevent hypoxemia. Keep hyperinflations synchronized with inhalation.
7. Quickly insert the suction catheter until resistance is met. *Do not apply suction during insertion.*
8. Withdraw the catheter 0.4 to 0.8 inch (1 to 2 cm), and begin to apply suction. Use intermittent suction and a twirling motion of the catheter during withdrawal. *Never suction longer than 10 to 15 seconds.*
9. Hyperoxygenate for 1 to 5 minutes or until the client's baseline heart rate and oxygen saturation are within normal limits.
10. Repeat as needed for up to three total suction passes.
11. Suction mouth as needed, and provide mouth care.
12. Describe secretions, and document client's responses.

Prevent hypoxia by hyperoxygenating the client with 100% oxygen with a manual resuscitation bag attached to an oxygen source. If the client is able to take deep breaths, instruct him or her to do so three or four times with the existing oxygen delivery system before suctioning. If possible, monitor the heart rate or use a pulse oximeter while suctioning to assess tolerance of the procedure. Assess for hypoxia (e.g., increased heart rate and blood pressure, oxygen desaturation, cyanosis, restlessness, anxiety, and cardiac dysrhythmias). Oxygen saturation below 90% by pulse oximetry indicates hypoxemia. If hypoxia occurs, stop the suctioning procedure. Using the 100% oxygen delivery system, reoxygenate the client until baseline parameters are achieved.

Use a catheter of the correct size to reduce the risk for hypoxia. The size should not exceed half of the size of the tracheal lumen. In adults, the standard catheter size is 12 Fr or 14 Fr. Correct catheter size allows efficient removal of secretions without causing hypoxemia.

TISSUE TRAUMA. The respiratory tract mucosa is fragile, and frequent suctioning, prolonged suctioning time, excessive suction pressure, and nonrotation of the catheter cause damage. Prevent trauma by suctioning only when needed. Lubricate the catheter with sterile water or saline before insertion. *Apply suction only during the withdrawal of the catheter.* Use a twirling motion during withdrawal to prevent grabbing of the mucosa.

Apply suction intermittently for only 10 to 15 seconds. Estimate this time frame by holding your own breath and counting to 10 or 15 during suctioning. At the end of the 15 seconds, end the suctioning procedure. Fifteen seconds does not seem long to a healthy person, but most clients who need suctioning have respiratory compromise and cannot tolerate more than 15 seconds of suctioning.

INFECTION. Each catheter pass introduces bacteria into the trachea. In the hospital, use sterile technique for suctioning and for all suctioning equipment, including suction catheters, gloves, and saline or water. Suction the mouth after suctioning the artificial airway. *Never use oral suction equipment for suctioning an artificial airway, because the mouth contains bacteria, which could be introduced into the lungs.* Use clean technique with home suctioning procedures because the number of virulent organisms in the home environment is lower than in the hospital.

VAGAL STIMULATION AND BRONCHOSPASM. Vagal stimulation results in severe bradycardia, hypotension, heart block, ventricular tachycardia, asystole, or other dysrhythmias. *If vagal stimulation occurs, stop suctioning immediately and oxygenate the client manually with 100% oxygen.* Bronchospasm sometimes occurs when the catheter passes into the airway. The client may need a bronchodilator to relieve bronchospasm and respiratory distress. In addition, hypoxia caused by suctioning can stimulate a variety of cardiac dysrhythmias. If the client has cardiac monitoring in place, check the monitor during suctioning.

TRACHEOSTOMY CARE

Tracheostomy care keeps the tube free of secretions, maintains a patent airway, and provides wound care. This procedure is performed whether or not the client is able to clear secretions. Perform tracheostomy care according to agency policy, usually every shift and as needed. Charts 31-3 and 31-4 outline best practices for tracheostomy care.

CHART 31-4

BEST PRACTICE for Tracheostomy Care

1. Assemble the necessary equipment.
2. Wash hands. Maintain standard precautions or body substance precautions.
3. Suction the tracheostomy tube if necessary.
4. Remove old dressings and excess secretions.
5. Set up a sterile field.
6. Remove and clean the inner cannula. Use half-strength hydrogen peroxide to clean the cannula and sterile saline to rinse it. If the inner cannula is disposable, remove the cannula and replace it with a new one.
7. Clean the stoma site and then the tracheostomy plate with half-strength hydrogen peroxide followed by sterile saline. Ensure that none of the solutions enters the tracheostomy.
8. Change tracheostomy ties if they are soiled. Secure new ties in place before removing soiled ones to prevent accidental decannulation. If a knot is needed, tie a square knot that is visible on the side of the neck. One or two fingers should be able to be placed between the tie tape and the neck.
9. Document the type and amount of secretions and the general condition of the stoma and surrounding skin. Document the client's response to the procedure and any teaching or learning that occurred.

CHART 31-5

FOCUSED ASSESSMENT of The Client with a Tracheostomy

Note the quality, pattern, and rate of breathing:
- Within client's baseline?
  Tachypnea can indicate hypoxia.
  Dyspnea can indicate secretions in the airway.

Assess for any cyanosis, especially around the lips, which could indicate hypoxia.
Check the client's pulse oximetry reading.
If oxygen is ordered, is the client receiving the correct amount, with the correct equipment and humidification?
Assess the tracheostomy site:
- Note the color, consistency, and amount of secretions in the tube or externally.
- If the tracheostomy is sutured in place, is there any redness, swelling, or drainage from suture sites?
- If the tracheostomy is secured with ties, what is the condition of the ties? Are they moist with secretions or perspiration? Are the secretions dried on the ties? Is the tie secure?
- Assess the condition of the skin around the tracheostomy and neck. Be sure to check underneath the neck for secretions that may have drained to the back. Check for any breakdown related to pressure from the ties or from excess secretions.
- Assess behind the faceplate for the size of the space between the outer cannula and the client's tissue. Are any secretions collected in this area?

If the tube is cuffed, check cuff pressure.
Auscultate the lungs.
Is a second (emergency) tracheostomy tube and obturator available?

Before proceeding with tracheostomy care, assess the client as shown in Chart 31-5. The need for suctioning and tracheostomy care is determined by the amount and consistency of secretions, medical diagnosis (specifically pulmonary diseases), ability of the client to cough and deep breathe, need for mechanical ventilation, and wound care required. Inspect the inner lumen of a single-lumen tube

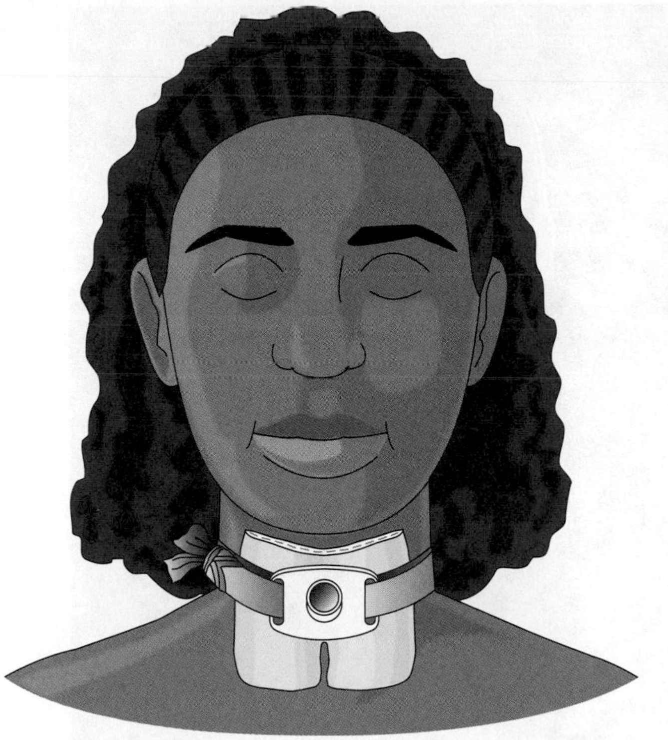

Figure 31-16 ■ Placement of precut gauze and tie around a tracheostomy tube.

with a flashlight or penlight to assess for the presence of secretions.

Secure tracheostomy tubes in place using either twill tape ties or Velcro tracheostomy tube holders. Both devices require changing when soiled to keep them clean and to avoid having them act as a medium for infection. A properly secured tie or holder allows space for only one or two fingers to be placed between the tie or holder and the neck. Tube movement causes irritation and coughing, which in turn may cause decannulation. *Keeping the tube secure while changing the ties or holder to prevent accidental decannulation is critical.* One way to accomplish this safely is to keep the old ties or holder on the tube while changing tubes, but a secure hand on the tube is the most reliable method of tube stabilization. Include the client in this process as a step toward self-care. Figure 31-16 shows correct technique for applying a tracheostomy dressing. Figure 31-17 shows the use of Velcro tracheostomy tube holders.

BRONCHIAL AND ORAL HYGIENE

Bronchial hygiene promotes a patent airway and prevents infection. Turn and reposition the client every 1 to 2 hours, support out-of-bed activities, and encourage ambulation. These actions promote lung expansion and gas exchange, and help remove secretions. Coughing and deep breathing, combined with the chest percussion, vibration, and postural drainage, promote pulmonary care (see Chapter 33).

Oral hygiene is important to ensure a patent airway, prevent bacterial overgrowth and dental caries, and to promote comfort. Maintain standard or body substance precautions during the procedure. Avoid using glycerin swabs or mouthwash that contains alcohol to clean the mouth because these products dry the mouth, change its pH, and promote

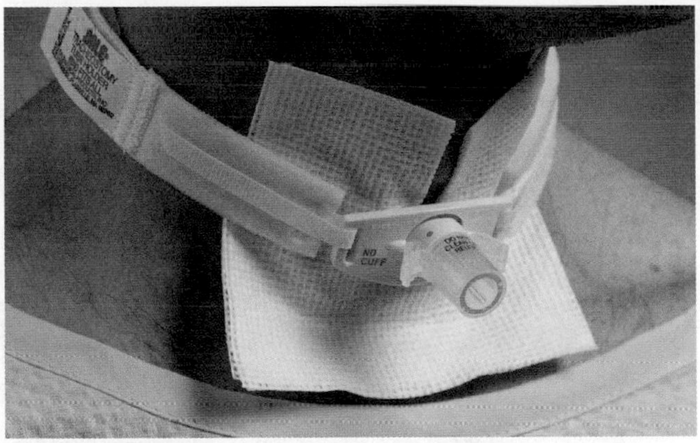

Figure 31-17 ■ Velcro tracheostomy tube holder. (Courtesy of Dale Medical Products, Inc., Plainville, MA.)

bacterial growth. Instead, use a toothette or soft-bristled toothbrush moistened in water for mouth care. Hydrogen peroxide solutions can help remove crusted matter but may break down healing tissue. Use these agents only with a physician's prescription.

During oral care, examine the mouth for any change in mucosal integrity or dental problems. Ulcers, bacterial or fungal *(Candida)* growth, and other infections are treated medically. Apply lip balm or water-soluble jelly to prevent cracked lips or skin breakdown and to promote client comfort. Mouth care is a simple method of promoting oral health, comfort, and aesthetic appearance. Offering an opportunity for the client or family member to perform mouth care encourages participation in care and increases self-esteem.

Oral secretions can move down the trachea and collect above the inflated cuff of the endotracheal tube. When the cuff is deflated, the secretions can move into the lungs. The Hi-Lo Evac endotracheal tube has an additional lumen open to the area above the cuff and can help prevent aspiration of oral secretions (Figure 31-18). The additional lumen allows suctioning of the airway above the cuff before deflating, thus preventing movement of oral secretions deeper into the airway.

NUTRITION

Swallowing can be a major problem for the client with a tracheostomy tube in place. In a normal swallow, the larynx lifts and moves forward to protect itself from the passing stream of food and saliva. Laryngeal lift also opens the upper esophageal sphincter. The tracheostomy tube sometimes tethers the larynx in place, making it unable to move efficiently. The result is difficulty in swallowing. Also, when the tracheostomy tube cuff is inflated, it can balloon backward and interfere with the passage of food through the esophagus. The common wall of the posterior trachea and the anterior esophagus is very thin, allowing this pushing problem. Instruct the client to keep the head of the bed elevated for at least 30 minutes after eating. Chart 31-6 outlines best practices to prevent aspiration during swallowing.

SPEECH AND COMMUNICATION

The client can speak when there is a cuffless tube, when a fenestrated tracheostomy tube is in place, and when the fenestrated tube is capped or covered. Until natural speech is fea-

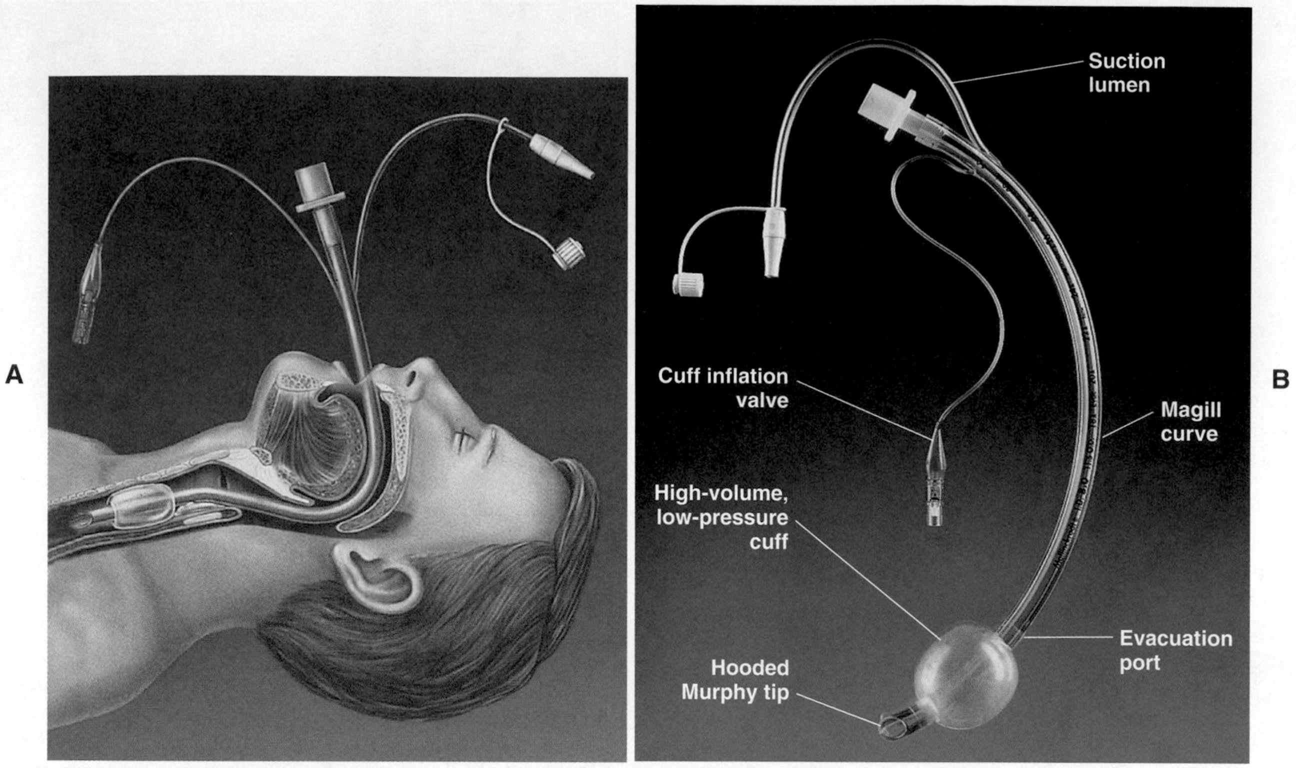

Figure 31-18 ■ The Hi-Lo Evac endotracheal tube system. **A,** The system positioned within a client. **B,** The Hi-Lo Evac tube. (Courtesy of Mallinckrodt, Inc., Shiley Tracheostomy Products, St. Louis, MO.)

sible, teach the client and family about other communication means. A writing tablet, Magic Slate, communication board with pictures and letters, hand signals, or a computer, as well as a call light within reach, are used to promote communication and decrease frustration from not being able to speak or be understood. Phrase questions for "yes" or "no" answers to help the client respond efficiently. Move the client closer to the nurses' station and mark the central call light system to indicate that the client cannot speak.

The inability to talk is a major stressor for the client. Helping communication is an important nursing function. When the client can tolerate cuff deflation, he or she places a finger over the tracheostomy tube on exhalation. This forces air up through the larynx, vocal cords, and mouth and allows speech. During the process of decannulation, when the fenestrated tube is "capped," the client has the benefit of speech without the need to cover the tube.

A device to increase speech for the client with a tracheostomy is a special one-way valve that fits over the tube and replaces the need for finger occlusion (Figure 31-19). The valve allows the client to breathe in through the tracheostomy tube. On exhalation, the valve closes so that air is forced through the vocal cords, allowing speech. For this valve to assist in speech, the client must not be connected to a ventilator, must have the cuff deflated, and must be able to breathe around the tube. Some valves have an extra port for supplemental oxygen without impairing the ability to speak.

EMOTIONAL CARE

Addressing psychological concerns is an important aspect of nursing care of clients recovering from a tracheostomy. While providing physical care, keep in mind the emotional impact of an artificial airway. Acknowledge the client's frustration in communication and allow sufficient time for communication. When speaking to the client, use a normal tone of voice. The tracheostomy tube does not alter hearing or comprehension.

BODY IMAGE

The client may have a change in body image because of deformity, the presence of a stoma or artificial airway, speech changes, a change in the method of eating, or difficulty with speech. Help the client set realistic goals, starting with involvement in self-care.

Work with the family to ease the client into a more normal social environment. Provide encouragement and positive reinforcement while demonstrating acceptance and caring behaviors. Assess the family for the need for counseling.

After surgery, the client may feel shy and socially isolated. He or she can wear loose-fitting shirts, decorative collars, or scarves to cover the tracheostomy tube.

WEANING

Weaning the client from a tracheostomy tube entails a gradual decrease in the tube size and ultimate removal of the tube. Carefully monitor this process, especially after each change. The physician, nurse practitioner, or respiratory advanced-practice nurse performs the steps in the process.

CHART 31-6

BEST PRACTICE for
Preventing Aspiration During Swallowing

- Avoid having meals when the client is fatigued.
- Provide smaller and more frequent meals.
- Provide adequate time; do not "hurry" the client.
- Provide close supervision if the client is self-feeding.
- Keep emergency suctioning equipment close at hand.
- Avoid water and other "thin" liquids.
- Thicken liquids.
- Avoid foods that generate thin liquids during the chewing process, such as fruit.
- Position the client in the most upright position possible.
- When possible, completely (or at least partially) deflate the tube cuff during meals.
- Suction after initial cuff deflation to clear the airway and allow maximal comfort during the meal.
- Feed each bite or encourage the client to take each bite slowly.
- Encourage the client to "dry swallow" after each bite to clear residue from the throat.
- Avoid consecutive swallows by cup or straw.
- Provide controlled small volumes of liquids, using a spoon.
- Encourage the client to "tuck" his or her chin down and forward while swallowing.
- Allow the client to indicate when he or she is ready for the next bite.
- If the client coughs, stop the feeding until the client indicates that the airway has been cleared.
- Continuously monitor tolerance to oral food intake by assessing respiratory rate, ease, pulse oximetry, and heart rate.

First, the cuff is deflated as soon as the client can manage secretions and does not need mechanical ventilation. This change allows him or her to breathe through the tube and through the upper airway. Next, the tube is changed to an uncuffed tube. If this is tolerated, the size of the tube is gradually decreased. When a small fenestrated tube is placed (No. 4 or 6, depending on the size of the airway), the tube is capped so that all air passes through the upper airway and the fenestra, with none passing through the tube. Assess the client to ensure adequate airflow around the tube when it is capped. The tube may be removed after he or she tolerates more than 24 hours of capping. Place a dry dressing over the stoma (which gradually heals on its own). Usually, a small scar remains.

Another device used for the transition from tracheostomy to natural breathing is a *tracheostomy button*. The button maintains stoma patency and assists spontaneous breathing. The Kistner tracheostomy tube and Olympic tracheostomy button are examples of this type of device. To function, they must fit properly. A disadvantage is the possibility of decannulation: the tube can dislodge from the trachea but remain in the neck tissues.

Critical Thinking Challenge

The 87-year-old post-CABG repair client has been reintubated due to respiratory failure. The client went to surgery 7 days later for a tracheotomy and returned to the ICU, where he remained on the ventilator.

1. What indications for a tracheotomy did this client meet?
2. What factor is foremost in determining this client's ability to be weaned from the ventilator?

evolve For suggested answer guidelines, go to http://evolve.elsevier.com/Iggy/.

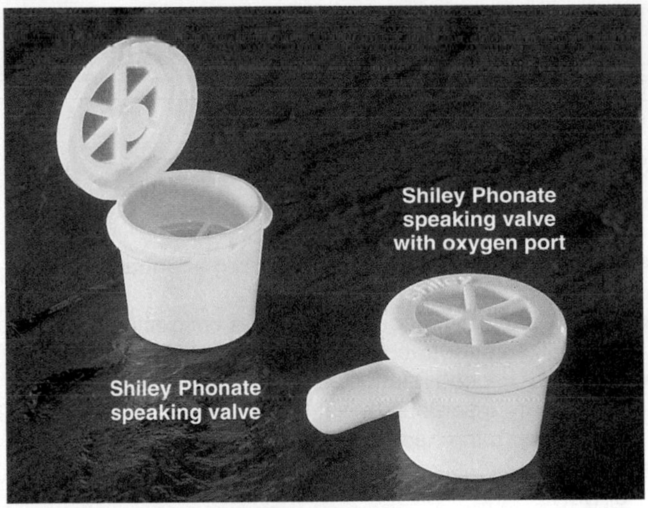

Figure 31-19 ■ The Shiley Phonate Speaking Valve. *Left,* The valve in place over a tracheostomy tube. *Right,* The valve up close. (Courtesy of Mallinckrodt, Inc., Shiley Tracheostomy Products, St. Louis, MO.)

Community-Based Care

By the time of discharge from the hospital, the client should be able to provide self-care, which may include tracheostomy care, nutritional care, suctioning, and methods of communication. Although education begins before surgery, most self-care is taught in the hospital. Teach the client and family how to care for the tracheostomy tube. Review airway care, including cleaning and inspecting for signs of infection. Teach clean suction technique and review the plan of care.

Instruct the client to use a shower shield over the tracheostomy tube when bathing to prevent water from entering the airway. Teach the client to cover the airway with cotton or foam to protect it during the day. Covering the permanent opening filters the air entering the stoma, keeps humidity in the airway, and enhances appearance. Attractive coverings are available in the form of cotton scarves, decorative collars, crocheted bibs, and jewelry. Using colored seam binding for tracheostomy ties after the stoma has matured may enhance overall body image. Shirt or dress color can be matched or coordinated with seam bindings.

Teach the client to increase humidity in the home. Instruct him or her to instill normal saline into the artificial airway 10 to 15 times a day, as prescribed. The client should continue the selected method of communication that began in the hospital and should wear a medical alert bracelet.

The health care team assesses specific discharge needs and makes referrals to home care agencies and durable medical equipment (DME) companies (for suction equipment and tracheostomy supplies). Clinic or physician follow-up visits occur early after discharge, but the home care nurse also is an important resource for the client and family. The home care nurse initiates (with a physician's prescription) and coordinates the services of nutritionists, nurses, speech pathologists, and social workers. The home care or hospital nurse informs the client and family of community resources that can offer support and friendships.

GET READY for the NCLEX Examination!

KEY POINTS

Safe Effective Care Environment

- Never allow water condensation in an oxygen delivery system to drain back into the system.
- Use sterile technique when performing endotracheal or tracheal suctioning.
- Inspect the oral mucous membranes each shift for anyone who has an endotracheal tube.
- Keep a tracheostomy tube (and obturator) and tracheostomy insertion tray at the bedside for the first 72 hours after a tracheostomy has been performed.
- Never use oral suctioning equipment to suction an artificial airway.

Health Promotion and Maintenance

- Monitor the rate and depth of respiration at least every hour for any client with hypercarbia and CO_2 narcosis who is receiving oxygen by mask or nasal cannula.
- Use aspiration precautions for any client with an altered level of consciousness or who has an endotracheal tube (see Chart 31-6).
- Teach the client and family how to perform tracheostomy care (see Chart 31-4).

Psychosocial Integrity

- Allow the client and family members the opportunity to express fear or anxiety regarding a change in breathing status or the possibility of intubation and mechanical ventilation.
- Teach family members ways to communicate with a client who is intubated or being mechanically ventilated.
- Reassure clients who are intubated that the loss of speech is temporary.
- Encourage clients with permanent tracheostomies to become involved in self care.

Physiological Integrity

- Apply oxygen to anyone who is hypoxemic.
- Ensure that all oxygen therapy delivered to the client is humidified (and warmed, when possible).
- Monitor arterial blood gases (ABGs) and oxygen saturation of all clients receiving oxygen therapy.
- Assess the skin under the mask and under the plastic tubing every shift for clients receiving oxygen by mask.
- Assess the skin of the nares and under the elastic band every shift for clients receiving oxygen by nasal cannula.
- Observe any client receiving oxygen at greater than a 50% concentration for early symptoms of oxygen toxicity (i.e., nonproductive cough, substernal chest pain, gastrointestinal [GI] upset, and dyspnea).
- Use a manual resuscitation bag to ventilate the client if the tracheostomy tube has dislodged or been decannulated.
- Assess the new tracheostomy stoma site at least once per shift for purulent drainage, redness, pain, and swelling as indicators of infection.
- Keep the tracheal cuff pressure between 14 and 20 mm Hg to prevent tissue injury.
- Secure new tracheostomy ties or tube holders in place before removing the soiled ones to prevent accidental decannulation.

ADDITIONAL STUDY RESOURCES

Go to your Student CD-ROM for Review Questions for the NCLEX Examination.

evolve Go to http://evolve.elsevier.com/Iggy/ for Integrated Management of Care Questions for the NCLEX Examination.

SELECTED BIBLIOGRAPHY

Asterisk indicates a classic or definitive work on this subject.

Brook, A., et al. (2000). Early versus late tracheostomy in patients who require prolonged mechanical ventilation. *American Journal of Critical Care, 9*(5), 352-359.

Dixon, B., & Tasota, F. (2003). Action stat: Inadvertent tracheal decannulation. *Nursing2003, 33*(1), 96.

Frakes, M. (2001). Measuring end-tidal carbon dioxide: Clinical applications and usefulness. *Critical Care Nurse, 21*(5), 23-35.

Francois, B., et al. (2003). Complications of tracheostomy performed in the ICU: Subthyroid tracheostomy vs surgical cricothyroidotomy. *Chest, 123*(1), 151-158.

Harkin, H., & Russell, C. (2001a). Preparing the patient for tracheostomy tube removal. *Nursing Times, 97*(26), 34-36.

Harkin, H., & Russell, C. (2001b). Tracheostomy patient care. *Nursing Times, 97*(25), 34-36.

Hess, D. (2000). Detection and monitoring of hypoxemia and oxygen therapy. *Respiratory Care, 45*(1), 65-83.

McConnell, E. (2002). Clinical dos & don'ts: Providing tracheostomy care. *Nursing2002, 32*(1), 17.

Mahler, D., Fierro-Carrion, G., & Baird, J. (2003). Evaluation of dyspnea in the elderly. *Clinics in Geriatric Medicine, 19*(1), 19-33.

Moore, A. (2000). Tips for getting a more reliable O_2 sat reading. *RN, 63*(2), 73.

Pagana, K., & Pagana, T. (2002). *Mosby's manual of diagnostic and laboratory tests* (2nd ed.). St. Louis: Mosby.

Paul-Allen, J., & Ostrow, L. (2000). Survey of nursing practices with closed-system suctioning. *American Journal of Critical Care, 9*(1), 9-19.

Perkins, L., & Shortall, S. (2000). Ventilation without intubation. *RN, 63*(1), 34-38.

Pruitt, W., & Jacobs, M. (2003). Basics of oxygen therapy. *Nursing 2003, 33*(10), 43-45.

Richmond, A., Jarog, D., & Hanson, V. (2004). Unplanned extubation in adult critical care. *Critical Care Nurse, 24*(1), 32-37.

Schreiber, D. (2001). Trach care at home: A how-to guide. *RN, 64*(7), 43-46.

Seay, S., Gay, S., & Strauss, M. (2002). Emergency: Tracheostomy emergencies: Correcting accidental decannulation or displaced tracheostomy tube. *American Journal of Nursing, 102*(3), 61-63.

Sell, S., & Tasota, F. (2004). Action stat: Tracheostomy mucus plug. *Nursing 2004, 34*(10), 88.

Simmons, P., & Simmons, M. (2004). Informed nursing practice: The administration of oxygen to patients with COPD. *MEDSURG Nursing, 13*(2), 82-85.

*St. John, R. (1999). Advances in artificial airway management. *Critical Care Clinics of North America, 11*(1), 7-17.

St. John, R. (2004). Airway management. *Critical Care Nurse, 24*(2), 93-96.

Woodrow, P. (2002). Managing patients with a tracheostomy in acute care. *Nursing Standard, 16*(44), 17-23.

CHAPTER 32

Interventions for Clients with Noninfectious Problems of the Upper Respiratory Tract

M. LINDA WORKMAN

LEARNING OUTCOMES

After studying this chapter, you should be able to:

1. Prioritize nursing care needs for the client after a nasoseptoplasty.
2. Compare the manifestations and care needs of a client with an anterior nosebleed with those of a client with a posterior nosebleed.
3. Prioritize nursing care needs for a client with facial trauma.
4. Describe the pathophysiology and the potential complications of sleep apnea.
5. Develop a plan of communication for a client who has a disruption of speech and cannot read.
6. Use clinical manifestations and laboratory data to determine airway adequacy in a client with laryngeal or neck injury.
7. Identify the risk factors for head and neck cancer.
8. Explain the psychosocial consequences of surgery for head and neck cancer.
9. Develop a community-based teaching plan for the client who is getting ready to go home after undergoing a complete laryngectomy.

Go to your Student CD-ROM for Review Questions for the NCLEX Examination keyed to these Learning Outcomes.

The upper airway structures include the nose, sinuses, oropharynx, larynx, and trachea. These areas may have specific health problems and also may be affected by other common acute and chronic disorders. Clients with upper respiratory problems are found in the community and many health care settings. The major nursing priority with disorders of the upper respiratory tract is maintaining a patent airway.

NONINFECTIOUS DISORDERS OF THE NOSE AND SINUSES

Fracture of the Nose

PATHOPHYSIOLOGY

Nasal fractures often result from injuries received during falls, sports activities, motor vehicle accidents, or physical assaults. If the bone or cartilage is not displaced, serious complications usually do not result from the fracture, and treatment may not be needed. Displacement of either the bone or cartilage, however, can cause airway obstruction or cosmetic deformity and is a potential source of infection.

COLLABORATIVE MANAGEMENT

Assessment

Document any nasal problem, including deviation, malaligned nasal bridge, a change in nasal breathing, crepitus on palpation, midface bruising, and pain. Blood or clear (cerebrospinal) fluid rarely drains from one or both nares. The presence of drainage could indicate a skull fracture. Although important in evaluating general facial fractures, x-rays are not always useful in the diagnosis of nasal fractures.

Interventions

The physician performs a simple closed reduction of the nasal fracture (using local or general anesthesia) within the first 24 hours after injury. After 24 hours the fracture is more difficult to reduce because of edema and scar formation. Simple closed fractures need not be surgically treated. Treatment focuses on pain relief and local cold compresses to decrease swelling.

Rhinoplasty. Reduction and surgery may be needed for severe fractures or for those that do not heal properly. **Rhinoplasty** is a surgical reconstruction of the nose for cosmetic purposes and to improve airflow. The client returns from surgery with packing in both nostrils; this packing prevents bleeding and provides support for the reconstructed nose. The gauze packing is usually treated with an antibiotic ointment, such as bacitracin (Bacitin✱) to reduce the risk for infection. A "moustache" dressing (or drip pad), often a folded 2 × 2 gauze pad, is usually placed under the nose (Figure 32-1). A splint or cast may cover the nose for additional alignment and protection. The nurse or client changes the drip pad as necessary.

After surgery, observe for edema and bleeding. Check vital signs every 4 hours until the client is discharged. Assessing how often the client swallows is a priority. Repeated swallowing may indicate posterior nasal bleeding. Use a penlight to examine the throat for bleeding, and notify the surgeon if bleeding is present. The client with uncomplicated rhinoplasty is usually discharged the day of surgery. Instruct the client and family about routine care.

Place the client in a semi-Fowler's position and instruct him or her to move slowly and to rest as much as possible. Apply cool compresses to the nose, eyes, or face to reduce swelling and discoloration. If a general anesthetic was used, the client may eat soft foods once he or she is alert and the gag reflex has returned. Urge the client to drink at least 2500 mL/day.

To prevent bleeding, teach the client to limit Valsalva maneuvers (e.g., forceful coughing or straining during a bowel movement) for the first few days after the packing is removed. Laxatives or stool softeners may be prescribed to ease bowel movement. Instruct the client to avoid aspirin and nonsteroidal anti-inflammatory drugs (NSAIDs) to prevent bleeding. Prophylactic antibiotics may be prescribed to prevent infection. Recommend the use of a humidifier at home to prevent excessive drying of the mucosa. Explain that edema and discoloration may last for weeks and that the final surgical result will be evident in 6 to 12 months.

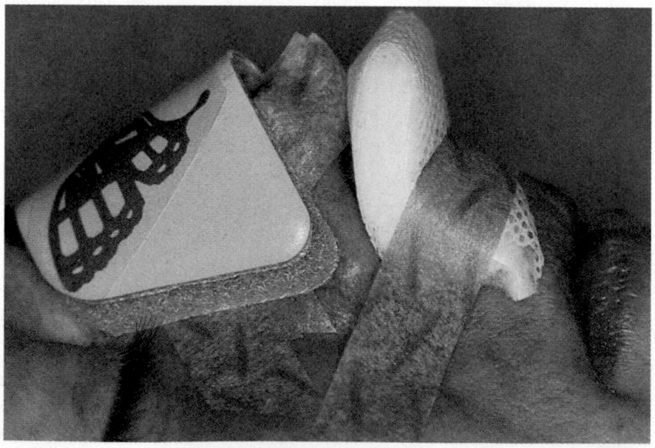

Figure 32-1 ■ Immediate postoperative appearance of a client who has undergone rhinoplasty. Note the splint and gauze drip pad (moustache dressing). (From Tardy, M.E. [1997]. *Rhinoplasty: The art and science* [p. 207]. Philadelphia: W.B. Saunders. Used with permission.)

Nasoseptoplasty. Nasoseptoplasty, or **submucous resection (SMR),** may be needed to straighten a deviated septum when chronic symptoms (e.g., a "stuffy" nose) or discomfort occur. Most adults have a slight nasal septum deviation with no symptoms. Major deviations, however, may obstruct the nasal passages or interfere with airflow and sinus drainage. The deviated section of the cartilage and bone is removed as an outpatient surgical procedure. The amount resected depends on the type and degree of deformity. Nursing care is similar to that for a rhinoplasty.

Epistaxis

PATHOPHYSIOLOGY

Epistaxis (nosebleed) is a common problem because of the rich capillary network within the nose. Nosebleeds may occur as a result of trauma, hypertension, blood dyscrasia (e.g., leukemias), inflammation, tumor, decreased humidity, nose blowing, nose picking, chronic cocaine use, and procedures such as nasogastric suctioning. Men are usually affected more often than women. Older adults tend to bleed most often from the posterior portion of the nose.

◆COLLABORATIVE MANAGEMENT

◆Assessment

The client often reports that the bleeding started after sneezing or blowing the nose. Document the amount and color of the blood and take the vital signs. Ask the client about the number, duration, and causes of previous bleeding episodes. Record this information in the client's medical record.

◆Interventions

Chart 32-1 lists the best practices for emergency care of the client with a nosebleed. Medical attention is needed if the nosebleed does not respond to these interventions. In such cases the affected capillaries may be cauterized with silver nitrate or electrocautery and the nose packed. Anterior packing controls bleeding from the anterior nasal cavity.

Posterior nasal bleeding is an emergency. Posterior packing or nasal pressure tubes are used to stop bleeding that originates in the posterior nasal region. With packing, a string is attached to a large gauze pack and then threaded through the nose and out the mouth. The physician positions the pack in the posterior nasal cavity above the pharynx and then tapes the string to the client's cheek to prevent movement of the pack. Balloon pressure catheter tubes or stents look like very short (about 6 inches) urinary catheters. These tubes have an exterior balloon along the tube length in addition to an anchoring balloon on the end. The tubes are inserted into both nares. The physician first inflates the anchoring balloon to keep the tubes in place. Then the pressure balloons are inflated carefully for both tubes at the same time to compress bleeding vessels (Figure 32-2). Placement of posterior packing or pressure tubes is uncomfortable, and the airway may be obstructed if the pack slips. Most clients who have posterior nasal bleeding are hospitalized.

Observe the client for respiratory distress and for tolerance of the packing or tubes. Humidification, oxygen, bedrest, and antibiotics may be prescribed. Opioid pain medication may be prescribed. Assess clients receiving opioids at least hourly for gag and cough reflexes. Oral care and adequate hydration are important because of mouth breathing. Use pulse oximetry to monitor for hypoxemia. The tubes or packing are usually removed after 1 to 5 days.

After the tubes or packing are removed, teach the client interventions to use at home for comfort and safety. Petroleum jelly can be applied to the nares for lubrication and comfort. Nasal saline sprays and humidification add moisture and prevent rebleeding. Instruct the client to avoid vigorous nose blowing, the use of aspirin or other NSAIDs, and strenuous activities such as heavy lifting.

Nasal Polyps

PATHOPHYSIOLOGY

Nasal polyps are benign grapelike clusters of mucous membrane and connective tissue. They often occur bilaterally and are caused by irritation to the nasal mucosa or sinuses, allergies, or infection (chronic sinusitis). If polyps become too large, airway obstruction may result.

CHART 32-1

BEST PRACTICE for
Emergency Care of a Client with an Anterior Nosebleed

EMERGENCY CARE

- Position the client upright and leaning forward to prevent blood from entering the stomach and possible aspiration.
- Reassure the client and attempt to keep him or her quiet to reduce anxiety and blood pressure.
- Apply direct lateral pressure to the nose for 5 minutes, and apply ice or cool compresses to the nose and face if possible.
- Maintain standard or body substance precautions.
- If nasal packing is necessary, loosely pack both nares with gauze or nasal tampons.
- To prevent rebleeding from dislodging clots, instruct the client not to blow the nose for several hours after the bleeding stops.
- Seek medical assistance if these measures are ineffective or if the bleeding occurs frequently.

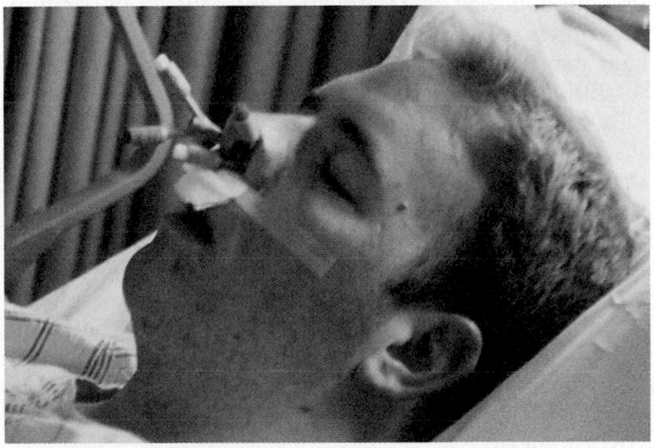

Figure 32-2 ■ Client with balloon stents in place to control a posterior nasal bleed.

◆COLLABORATIVE MANAGEMENT

◆Assessment

Manifestations of nasal polyps include obstructed nasal breathing, a change in the character of nasal discharge, and a change in speech quality. Clients who have had polyps are at risk for recurrence.

◆Interventions

Surgery is the treatment of choice for nasal polyps. The extent of the surgery required depends on the location and type of polyp present.

Benign nasal polyps are treated with nasally inhaled steroids and surgical removal **(polypectomy).** A polypectomy can be performed using either local or general anesthesia. Observe the client for bleeding after surgery. The nostrils are usually packed with gauze for 24 hours after surgery. Nasal polyps often recur if they are not completely removed.

Inverting papilloma is a rare, benign lesion that erodes nasal and facial bones and is often first diagnosed as a benign polyp. Inverting papillomas grow by pressure into adjacent structures. Extensive sinus and nasal surgery is needed for complete removal and prevention of regrowth.

Juvenile angiofibromas are cellularly different from other polyps. These tumors often occur in adolescent males and may resolve spontaneously when adulthood is reached. When the lesions are local, they can be removed by nasal surgery. Invasive tumors may require removal by skull-base resection.

Cancer of the Nose and Sinuses

PATHOPHYSIOLOGY

Tumors of the nasal cavities and sinuses are rare and may be either benign or malignant. Malignant tumors can occur at all ages, but the peak incidence is 40 to 45 years of age in men and 60 to 65 years of age in women. Asian Americans have a higher incidence of nasopharyngeal cancer.

◆COLLABORATIVE MANAGEMENT

◆Assessment

The onset of sinus cancer is slow, and manifestations resemble sinusitis. Thus the client may have advanced disease at diagnosis. Manifestations of nasal or sinus cancer include persistent nasal obstruction, drainage, bloody discharge, and pain that does not improve after treatment of sinusitis. Local lymph node enlargement often occurs on the side with tumor mass.

◆Interventions

Radiation therapy is the main treatment for nasopharyngeal cancers. Chart 32-2 lists some NIC interventions for clients having radiation therapy. Surgical removal is performed if radiation therapy is not successful.

The specific surgery depends on tumor size and location and the degree of invasion. Problems after surgery include a change in body image or speech and altered nutrition. These problems are most common when the maxilla and floor of the nose are involved in the surgery. Clients often also have changes in taste and smell.

CHART 32-2

NIC **INTERVENTION ACTIVITIES for**
The Client with Noninfectious Disorders of the Nose and Sinus

Radiation Therapy Management: *Assisting the client to understand and minimize the side effects of radiation treatments*

- Monitor for alterations in skin integrity and treat appropriately.
- Avoid use of adhesive tapes and other skin-irritating substances.
- Avoid application of deodorants and aftershave lotion to treated area.
- Discuss the need for skin care, such as maintenance of dye markings, avoidance of soap and other ointments, and protection during sunbathing or heat application.
- Monitor for indications of infection of oral mucous membranes.
- Encourage good oral hygiene with use of dental floss or WaterPik, as appropriate.
- Initiate oral health restoration activities, such as use of artificial saliva, mouth sprays, and use of sugarless mints, as appropriate.
- Monitor client for anorexia, nausea, vomiting, changes in taste, esophagitis, and diarrhea, as appropriate.
- Promote adequate fluid and nutritional intake.
- Assist client in managing fatigue by planning frequent rest periods, spacing activities, and limiting daily demands, as appropriate.
- Encourage rest immediately after radiation treatment.
- Facilitate expression of fears about prognosis or success of radiation treatments.

Communication Enhancement: *Speech Deficit: Assistance in accepting and learning alternate methods for living with impaired speech*

- Provide verbal prompts/reminders.
- Listen attentively.
- Refrain from shouting at the client with communication disorders.
- Use picture board, if appropriate.
- Use hand gestures, as appropriate.
- Perform prescriptive speech-language therapies during informal interactions with client.
- Teach esophageal speech, as appropriate.
- Instruct client and family on use of speech aids (e.g., tracheal-esophageal prosthesis and artificial larynx).
- Encourage client to repeat words.
- Provide positive reinforcement and praise, as appropriate.
- Carry on one-way conversations, as appropriate.
- Reinforce need for follow-up with speech pathologist after discharge.

NIC intervention activities selected from Dochterman, J.M., & Bulechek, G.M. (Eds.). (2004). *Nursing interventions classification (NIC)* (4th ed.). St. Louis: Mosby.

Provide general postoperative care (see Chapter 22), including maintaining a patent airway, monitoring for hemorrhage, providing wound care, assessing nutritional status, and performing tracheostomy care (if needed). (See Chapter 31 for tracheostomy care.) Perform meticulous mouth and maxillary cavity care with saline irrigations using a water pick (e.g., WaterPik) or a syringe. Assess the client for pain and infection. Optimal nutrition is essential after surgery to promote healing.

Facial Trauma

PATHOPHYSIOLOGY

Facial trauma is described by the specific bones (e.g., mandibular, maxillary, orbital, or nasal fractures) and the side of the face involved. Mandibular (lower jaw) fractures can occur at any point on the mandible and are the most common facial fractures. **Le Fort I** is a nasoethmoid complex fracture. **Le Fort II** is a maxillary *and* nasoethmoid complex fracture. **Le Fort III** is a combination of I and II plus an orbital-zygoma fracture, often called "craniofacial disjunction" because it leaves the midface with no connection to the skull. The rich blood supply of the face leads to extensive bleeding with facial trauma.

COLLABORATIVE MANAGEMENT

Assessment

The first action to take with facial trauma is airway assessment. Manifestations of an airway obstruction include stridor, shortness of breath, dyspnea, anxiety, restlessness, hypoxia, hypercarbia, decreased oxygen saturation, cyanosis, and loss of consciousness. After establishing the airway, assess the amount and site of soft-tissue trauma, bleeding, and possible fractures. Check for soft-tissue edema, facial asymmetry, pain, or leakage of spinal fluid through the ears or nose, indicating a temporal bone or basilar skull fracture. Assess vision and eye movement because orbital and maxillary fractures can entrap the eye. Because facial trauma can occur with spinal cord trauma and skull fractures, cranial computed tomography, facial series, and cervical spine films also are obtained.

Interventions

The priority action is to establish and maintain a patent airway. Anticipate the need for emergency intubation, tracheotomy, or cricothyroidotomy. When the client arrives at a trauma center, care focuses on establishing an airway, controlling hemorrhage, and assessing for the extent of injury. If shock is present, fluid resuscitation and identification of bleeding sites are started immediately.

Time is critical in stabilizing the client who has head and neck trauma. Early response and treatment by the following appropriate services, including the trauma team, maxillofacial surgeon, general surgeon, otolaryngologist, plastic surgeon, and dentist, optimize the client's recovery.

Stabilization of the fractured segment of a *mandibular fracture* allows the teeth to heal in proper alignment. The client remains in fixed occlusion for 6 to 10 weeks. Antibiotic therapy may be prescribed because of oral wound contamination. Delay in treatment, tooth infection, or poor oral care may result in mandibular bone infection. The client may then require surgical debridement, intravenous (IV) antibiotic therapy, and an extended period in fixation.

Facial fractures often are repaired with microplating surgical systems such as BoneSource. These shaping plates hold the bone fragments in place until **osteoneogenesis** (new bone growth) occurs. Large areas of skull can be replaced with BoneSource. Bone cells grow into the BoneSource and rematrix into a stable bone support. The plates may remain in place permanently or may be removed after healing has occurred.

If the mandibular fracture is repaired with titanium plates, teach the client about oral care, soft-diet restrictions, and follow-up care with a dentist. These plates are permanent and do not interfere with magnetic resonance imaging (MRI) studies.

Fixation methods may use resorbable devices (plates and screws) to hold tissues in place. These devices are made from a plastic-like material that retains its integrity for about

8 weeks and then slowly biodegrades. Resorbable devices are not used when the area has previously been irradiated or for clients who smoke, have drug or alcohol dependence, uncontrolled diabetes mellitus, immunosuppression, or impaired cardiac function.

Inner maxillary fixation (IMF) is another common method of securing a mandibular fracture. The bones are realigned and then wired in place with the bite closed. The physician can repair nondisplaced aligned fractures in a clinic or office using local dental anesthesia. General anesthesia is used to repair displaced or complex fractures or fractures that occur with other facial bone fractures.

After surgery teach the client about oral care with an irrigating device, such as a WaterPik. If the client is undergoing inner maxillary fixation, teach self-care with wires in place, including a dental liquid diet. There is a risk for aspiration if vomiting occurs because of the inability to open the jaws to allow ejection of the emesis. Teach the client how to cut the wires if emesis occurs. *Instruct the client to keep wire cutters with him or her at all times in case this emergency arises.* If the wires are cut, instruct the client to return to the physician for rewiring as soon as possible to reinstitute fixation.

Nutrition is important for any client with fractures. Oral needs may be difficult to meet because of oral fixation, pain, and surgery. Consult with the dietitian for client teaching and support.

NONINFECTIOUS DISORDERS OF THE ORAL PHARYNX AND TONSILS

Obstructive Sleep Apnea

PATHOPHYSIOLOGY

Sleep apnea is a breathing disruption during sleep that lasts at least 10 seconds and occurs a minimum of 5 times in an hour. Although sleep apnea can have a neurologic origin, the most common form occurs as a result of upper-airway obstruction by the soft palate or tongue. Factors that contribute to sleep apnea include obesity, a large uvula, a short neck, smoking, enlarged tonsils or adenoids, and oropharyngeal edema. Men are affected more often than women, and the risk increases with age.

During sleep, the muscles relax and the tongue and neck structures are displaced. As a result, the upper airway is obstructed even though chest-wall movement is unimpaired. The apnea increases the arterial carbon dioxide level and decreases the pH. These blood-gas changes stimulate neural activity. The sleeper is aroused spontaneously after 10 seconds or longer of apnea and corrects the obstruction, and respiration resumes. After the client goes back to sleep, the cycle begins again, sometimes as often as every 5 minutes.

This cyclic pattern of disrupted sleep prevents the state of deep sleep needed for maximum rest. As a result, the person may have excessive daytime sleepiness, an inability to concentrate, and irritability.

COLLABORATIVE MANAGEMENT

Assessment

Clients are often unaware that they have sleep apnea. The disorder should be suspected for any person who has persistent daytime sleepiness or complains of "waking up tired," particularly if he or she snores heavily. Other manifestations include irritability and personality changes. In some cases sleep apnea is diagnosed by family members who observe the problem while the client sleeps in a supine position. A complete health assessment should be performed when excessive daytime sleepiness is a problem.

The most accurate test for sleep apnea is polysomnography (PSG) performed during an overnight sleep study. The client is directly observed while wearing a variety of monitoring equipment, including an electroencephalograph (EEG), an electrocardiograph (ECG), a pulse oximeter, and an electromyograph (EMG). This test determines the depth of sleep, type of sleep, respiratory effort, oxygen saturation adequacy, and muscle movement. Nursing diagnoses that may apply to clients with sleep apnea include the following:

- Sleep Deprivation related to disrupted sleep cycle
- Ineffective Breathing pattern related to obesity, musculoskeletal issues, and soft tissue position
- Fatigue related to sleep deprivation
- Risk for Injury related to decreased mental awareness

Interventions

NONSURGICAL MANAGEMENT. A change in sleeping position or weight loss may be all that is needed to reduce or correct mild sleep apnea. Position-fixing devices that prevent subluxation of the tongue and neck structures also may be effective in preventing obstruction. For more severe sleep apnea, nonsurgical or surgical methods to prevent obstruction may be needed.

A common nonsurgical method to prevent airway collapse is the use of noninvasive positive-pressure ventilation (NPPV) to hold open the upper airways. A nasal mask or full-face mask delivery system allows mechanical delivery of either bilevel positive airway pressure (BiPAP) or nasal continuous positive airway pressure. With BiPAP, a cycling machine delivers a set inspiratory positive airway pressure at the beginning of each inspiration. As the client begins to exhale, the machine delivers a lower set end expiratory pressure. These two pressures improve tidal volume and hold open the upper airways.

Nasal continuous positive airway pressure (CPAP) delivers a set positive airway pressure continually during each cycle of inhalation and exhalation. For CPAP ventilation through a face mask during sleep, a small electric compressor delivers positive pressure at an individually determined setting. Proper fit of the mask over the nose and mouth is key to successful treatment. Although intrusive, these methods are well accepted by most clients after an initial adjustment period.

Two drugs have been approved to treat sleep apnea. One drug, Xyrem (sodium oxybate), a CNS depressant, induces a deep sleep state. This action does not treat the cause of sleep apnea but works by improving the sleep cycle and thus increasing daytime wakefulness. This drug has been widely abused as a "date rape" agent, and many health care providers are reluctant to prescribe it. Provigil (modafinil) is helpful for clients who have *narcolepsy* (uncontrolled daytime sleep) from sleep apnea by promoting daytime wakefulness.

SURGICAL MANAGEMENT. Surgical intervention for sleep apnea may involve a simple adenoidectomy, uvulectomy, or remodeling of the entire posterior oropharynx (**uvulopalatopharyngoplasty [UPP]**). Both conventional and laser surgeries are used for this purpose. A tracheostomy may be needed for very severe sleep apnea that is not relieved by more moderate interventions.

Oropharyngeal Cancer

Clients with cancer of the mouth, tongue, tonsils, and pharynx have many nursing needs related to airway maintenance, communication, nutrition, and self-image. Chapter 57 provides an in-depth discussion of the management of clients with oropharyngeal cancer.

NONINFECTIOUS DISORDERS OF THE LARYNX

Vocal Cord Paralysis

PATHOPHYSIOLOGY

Vocal fold (cord) paralysis may result from injury, trauma, or disease that affects the larynx, laryngeal nerves, or vagus nerve. Prolonged intubation with an endotracheal (ET) tube may cause temporary or, rarely, permanent paralysis. Laryngeal paralysis may occur in clients with neurologic disorders. Damage to the vagus nerve (by chest injury) or brainstem may lead to nerve dysfunction. The laryngeal nerves may be damaged from trauma or disorders that involve the chest, esophagus, or thyroid. Paralysis of both vocal cords may result from direct injury, stroke involving the brainstem, or total thyroidectomy.

COLLABORATIVE MANAGEMENT

Assessment

Vocal fold paralysis may be unilateral or bilateral. When only one vocal cord is involved (most common), the airway remains patent but the voice is affected. Manifestations of **abducted** (open) bilateral vocal cord paralysis include hoarseness; a breathy, weak voice; and aspiration of food. Bilateral **adducted** (closed) vocal cord paralysis causes airway obstruction and is a medical emergency if the symptoms are severe and the client is unable to compensate. Stridor is the major manifestation. The client with vocal cord paralysis is at risk for aspiration because airway may not close during swallowing.

Interventions

Securing a patent airway is the primary intervention. Place the client in a high Fowler's position to aid in breathing and proper alignment of airway structures. Assess for upper airway obstruction. *Immediately notify the physician if dyspnea with stridor occurs.* Emergency endotracheal intubation or tracheostomy may be needed.

Various surgical procedures can improve the voice. One procedure for abducted vocal cord paresis involves injecting polytef (Teflon) into the affected cord so it enlarges toward the unaffected cord. This technique improves closure during speaking and eating.

Teach the client to hold his or her breath during swallowing. This action allows the larynx to rise, close, and divert food back into the esophagus during swallowing. Also teach the client to tuck his or her chin down and forward during swallowing to prevent aspiration. Indications of aspiration include immediate coughing on swallowing of liquids or solids, a "wet"-sounding voice, and "tearing up" or watery eyes on swallowing. Chest x-rays and laryngeal and chest auscultation are also useful to diagnose aspiration pneumonia.

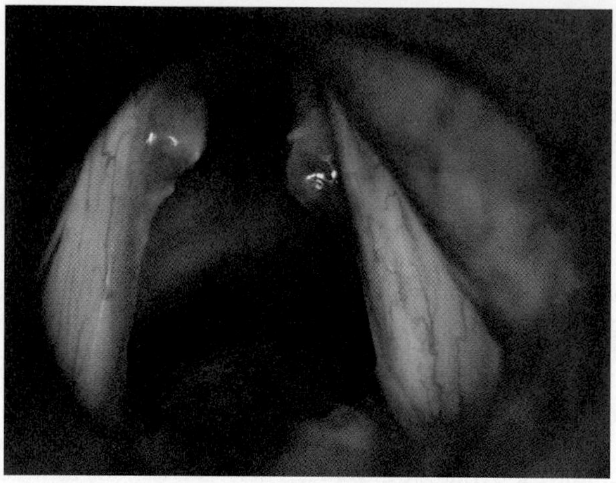

Figure 32-3 ■ Unilateral left vocal cord nodule caused by contact and voice abuse, often seen after viral illnesses. Differential diagnosis includes cancer and trauma. The origin of the nodule may be scar tissue, bacteria, or viruses.

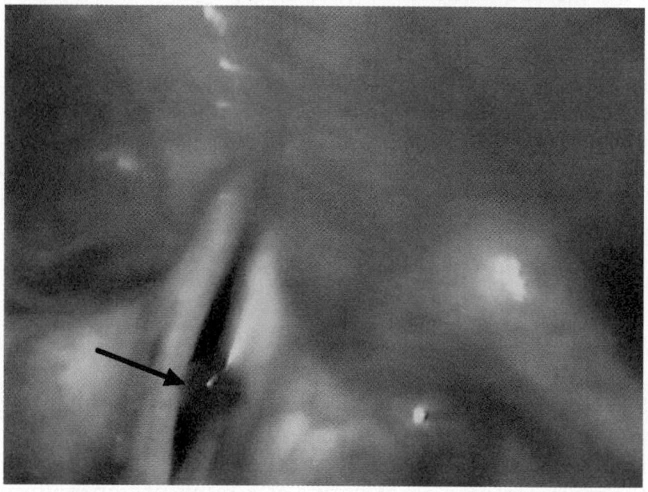

Figure 32-4 ■ A hemorrhagic vocal cord polyp.

Vocal Cord Nodules and Polyps

PATHOPHYSIOLOGY

Nodules often appear at the point at which the vocal cords touch during speech. **Nodules** are enlarged fibrous tissues (Figure 32-3) caused by infectious processes or overuse of the voice. People most affected are teachers, coaches, sports fans, singers, and those who use their voices in noisy environments.

Vocal cord polyps (Figure 32-4) are chronic, edematous masses. They occur most often in smokers, people with allergies, or those who live in dry climates. Vocal cysts also may occur.

COLLABORATIVE MANAGEMENT

Nodules and polyps are painless. The main manifestation is hoarseness because of the loss of coordinated closure of the vocal cords and vocal wave (Figure 32-5).

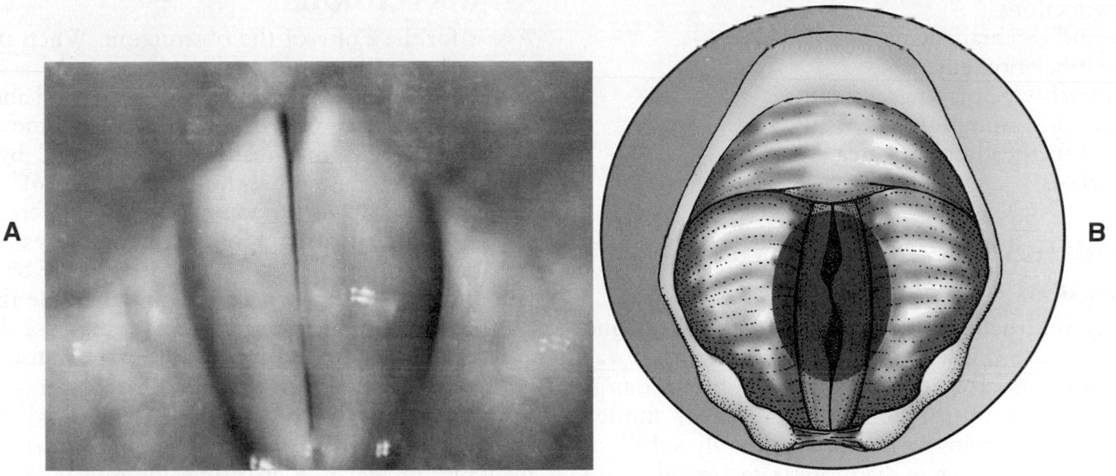

Figure 32-5 ■ **A,** Close-up view of normal vocal cords in phonation. Saying the letter *E* in a high pitch allows the examiner to evaluate the total movement of the cords in all pitch ranges and evaluate the membrane contact. **B,** Vocal cord nodules and polyps prevent approximation of the vocal cords. Hoarseness results.

Management of cord nodules or polyps is aimed at educating the client and family. Instruct the client about tobacco use hazards, smoking-cessation programs, and the importance of voice rest. Treatment includes not whispering and avoiding heavy lifting. Stool softeners are used to avoid bearing down during elimination **(Valsalva maneuvers),** which would cause the glottis to close. Humidifying inspired air may soothe the vocal cords and prevent overdrying.

Speech therapy is used for behavioral voice changes and helps the client learn to reduce speech intensity. Speech therapy may make surgery unnecessary.

If hoarseness is not relieved by voice rest or speech therapy, the surgeon may remove the nodules or polyps under direct laryngoscopy. Laser and surgical resection are used to remove the mucous membrane of the affected cord. If both cords are involved, one cord is usually allowed to heal before surgery is performed on the other cord. These procedures are often performed as outpatient surgery. Thus, client education must be performed before surgery and before the client goes home.

After surgery the client must maintain complete voice rest for about 14 days to promote healing. Chart 32-2 on p. 566 lists NIC interventions for communication enhancement. Teach about alternative methods of communication such as a slate board, pen and paper, "magic slate," or alphabet board. While the client is an inpatient, place a sign on the client's door, over the bed, and on the intercom system to help implement voice rest.

Laryngeal Trauma

PATHOPHYSIOLOGY

Laryngeal trauma occurs with a crushing or direct blow injury, fracture, or injury such as that induced by prolonged endotracheal intubation.

◆COLLABORATIVE MANAGEMENT

Manifestations of laryngeal trauma include **dyspnea** (difficulty breathing), **aphonia** (inability to produce sound), hoarseness, and **subcutaneous emphysema** (air present in the subcutaneous tissue). Bleeding from the airway **(hemoptysis)** may, occur depending on the location of the trauma. The physician performs a direct visual examination by laryngoscopy or fiberoptic laryngoscopy of the larynx to determine the nature and extent of the injury.

Management of clients with laryngeal injuries consists of airway assessment and monitoring vital signs (including respiratory status and pulse oximetry) every 15 to 30 minutes. *Maintaining a patent airway is a priority.* Apply oxygen and humidification as prescribed to maintain adequate oxygen saturation. If the client is experiencing respiratory difficulty, stay with him or her and instruct other trauma team members to prepare for an emergency intubation or tracheostomy. Manifestations of respiratory difficulty include increasing tachypnea, nasal flaring, anxiety, sternal retraction, shortness of breath, dyspnea, restlessness, decreased oxygen saturation, decreased level of consciousness, and stridor.

Surgical intervention is necessary for lacerations of the mucous membranes, cartilage exposure, and paralysis of the cords. Laryngeal repair is performed as soon as possible to prevent laryngeal stenosis and to cover any exposed cartilage. An artificial airway may be needed.

OTHER UPPER AIRWAY DISORDERS

Upper Airway Obstruction

PATHOPHYSIOLOGY

Upper airway obstruction is a life-threatening emergency in which there is an interruption in airflow through the nose, mouth, pharynx, or larynx. Early recognition is essential to prevent further complications, including respiratory arrest. Causes of upper airway obstruction include the following:

- Tongue edema (surgery, trauma)
- Occlusion by the tongue (e.g., with loss of gag reflex, loss of pharyngeal muscle tone, unconsciousness, and coma)
- Laryngeal edema
- Peritonsillar and pharyngeal abscess
- Head and neck cancer

- Thick secretions
- Stroke and cerebral edema
- Smoke inhalation edema
- Facial, tracheal, or laryngeal trauma
- Foreign-body aspiration
- Burns of the head or neck area
- Anaphylaxis

COLLABORATIVE MANAGEMENT

Assessment

Upper airway obstruction is frightening to the client and family. Prompt care is essential to prevent a partial airway obstruction from progressing to a complete obstruction. A client with a partial obstruction (e.g., caused by limited edema or a small foreign body) may have only subtle or general manifestations such as diaphoresis, tachycardia, and elevated blood pressure. Unexplained or persistent recurrent symptoms warrant evaluation even though the symptoms are vague. To rule out any potentially life-threatening condition (e.g., tumor, foreign body, or infection), diagnostic procedures, such as a chest x-ray, lateral neck films, direct laryngoscopic examination, and computed tomography, are performed.

Observe for hypoxia and hypercarbia, restlessness, increasing anxiety, sternal retractions, a "seesawing" chest, abdominal movements, or a feeling of impending doom related to actual air hunger. Use pulse oximetry for ongoing monitoring of oxygen saturation. Continually assess for stridor, cyanosis, and changes in level of consciousness.

Interventions

Assess for the cause of the obstruction. When the obstruction is due to the tongue falling back or the accumulation of secretions, slightly extend the client's head and neck and insert a nasal or an oral airway. Suction to remove obstructing secretions. If the obstruction is caused by a foreign body, perform abdominal thrusts (Figure 32-6).

Upper airway obstruction may require emergency procedures such as cricothyroidotomy, endotracheal intubation, or a tracheostomy. Direct laryngoscopy may be performed before or with these procedures to determine the cause of obstruction. The health care provider may use direct laryngoscopy in a controlled situation to remove foreign bodies.

Cricothyroidotomy. Cricothyroidotomy is an emergency procedure that is often performed outside the hospital by emergency medical personnel or in the emergency department by a physician. A **cricothyroidotomy** is a stab wound at the cricothyroid membrane between the thyroid cartilage and the cricoid cartilage ring (see Figure 30-3). Any hollow tube–but preferably a tracheostomy tube–can be placed through this opening to keep the new airway open until a formal tracheotomy can be performed. This procedure is used when it is the *only* way to secure an airway. Another emergency procedure to bypass an obstruction involves the physician inserting a 14-gauge needle directly into the cricoid space to allow air into and out of the lungs.

Endotracheal Intubation. Endotracheal intubation is performed by inserting a tube into the trachea via the nose **(nasotracheal)** or mouth **(orotracheal)** by a physician, nurse anesthetist, or other specially trained personnel.

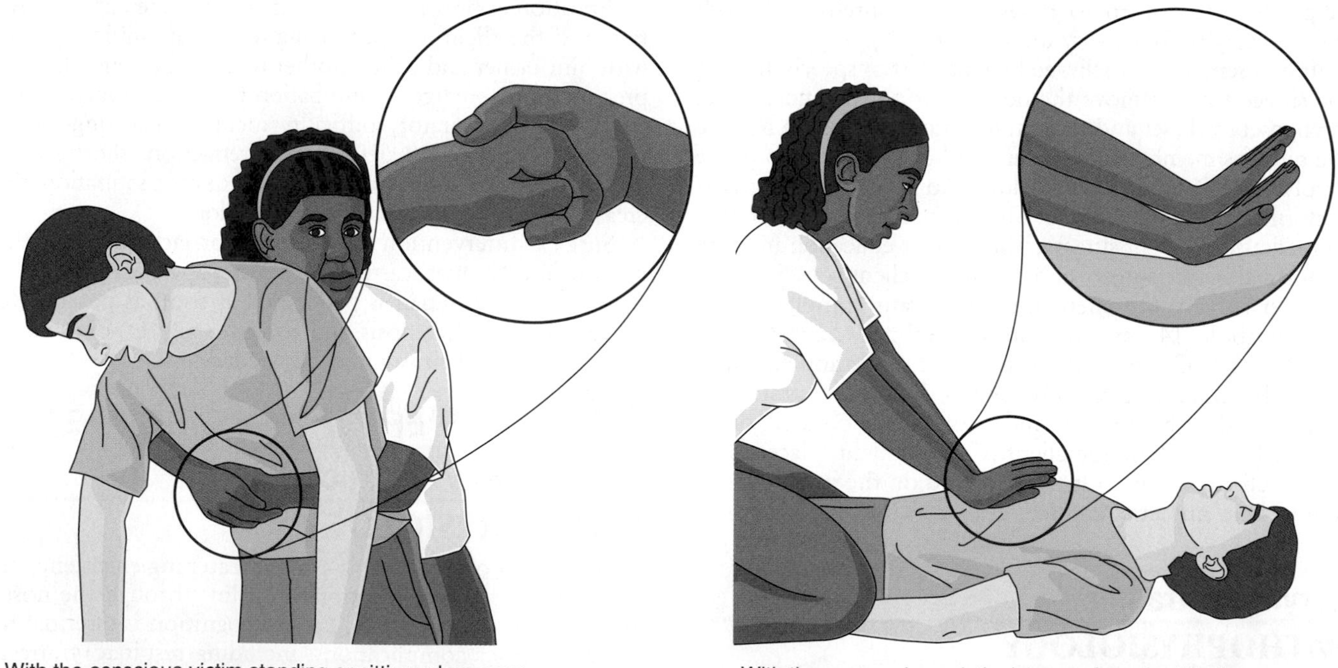

With the conscious victim standing or sitting, place your fist between the victim's lower rib cage and navel. Wrap the palm of your hand around your fist. A quick inward, upward thrust expels the air remaining in the victim's lungs, and with it the foreign body. If the first thrust is unsuccessful, repeat several thrusts in rapid succession until the foreign body is expelled or until the victim loses consciousness.

With the unconscious victim lying supine, straddle the victim's thighs. Place one hand on top of the other as shown, with the heel of the bottom hand just above the victim's navel. Quickly thrust inward and upward, toward the victim's head.

Figure 32-6 ■ The abdominal thrust maneuver (formerly known as the Heimlich maneuver) for relief of upper airway obstruction caused by a foreign body.

Tracheostomy. A tracheostomy is a surgical procedure that takes about 5 to 10 minutes to perform. Ideally it is performed in the operating room with the client under local or general anesthesia. It can be performed at the bedside. A tracheostomy can be performed with the client under local anesthesia if there is concern that the airway will be lost during the induction of anesthesia. An emergency tracheostomy is reserved for the client who cannot be easily intubated with an endotracheal tube. The emergency tracheostomy can establish an airway in less than 2 minutes. Care of the client with a tracheostomy is discussed in detail in Chapter 31.

Clients receiving mechanical ventilation as part of the treatment for upper airway obstruction or respiratory failure may require a tracheostomy after 7 or more days of continuous oral or nasal intubation. In such cases the procedure is performed to prevent laryngeal injury by the endotracheal tube.

Neck Trauma

PATHOPHYSIOLOGY

Neck injuries may be caused by a knife, gunshot, or traumatic accident. The client with neck trauma may have more than one injury, including cardiovascular, respiratory, intestinal, and neurologic damage. The final outcome of this type of injury depends on the initial assessment and care. Consult a critical care or emergency textbook and see Chapter 48 for more in-depth information.

COLLABORATIVE MANAGEMENT

Assessment

The priority in caring for a client with neck trauma is assessment for a patent airway. After airway patency is assured, then assess for manifestations of bleeding or impending shock.

Perform a baseline neurologic assessment for mental status, sensory level, and motor function. Injury to the carotid artery may result in death, stroke, or paralysis related to disruption of blood flow to the brain (see Chapter 44). A carotid angiogram may be performed to rule out vascular injuries.

Esophagus injury may occur with neck trauma. Assess for chest pain and tenderness, oral bleeding, and **crepitus** (crackling sounds when palpating the skin). A barium or meglumine diatrizoate (Gastrografin) swallow may be needed to rule out an esophageal perforation injury.

Interventions

Cervical spine injuries often occur at the same time as a neck injury (see Chapter 46). Health care personnel must take great care not to make these injuries worse by causing neck movement while establishing the airway. Prepare to assist in emergency intubation, cricothyrotomy, or tracheostomy to establish a patent airway. Interventions for clients in shock are detailed in Chapter 40.

Head and Neck Cancer

PATHOPHYSIOLOGY

Head and neck cancer can disrupt breathing, eating, facial appearance, self-image, speech, and communication. This form of cancer can be devastating, even when treated successfully. The care needs for clients with these problems are complex, requiring a comprehensive team approach. The client can receive appropriate care only after the location and size of the tumor are accurately identified.

Head and neck cancer is curable when treated early. The prognosis for those who have more advanced disease at diagnosis depends on the extent and location of the tumor. Untreated cancer of the head and neck is a fatal disease within 2 years of diagnosis.

Most head and neck cancers (80%) are squamous cell (mucosal epithelial) carcinomas that are slow growing, usually requiring several years to develop (Figure 32-7). Many head and neck tumors first appear as infiltrating ulcerations.

The cancer begins when the mucosa is chronically irritated and changes into a tougher mucosa **(squamous metaplasia)**. This tougher mucosa occurs by increasing the mucosal thickness (**acanthosis** or hyperplasia) or by developing a keratin layer **(keratosis).** At the same time, changes at the gene level enhance the growth of abnormal epithelial cells that eventually become malignant. These lesions may then take the form of white, patchy lesions **(leukoplakia)** or red, velvety patches **(erythroplasia).**

The growth and spread **(metastasis)** of head and neck cancer first occur into nearby structures, such as mucosa, muscle, and bone. Systemic spread through the blood and lymphatic systems may also occur. Distant metastasis occurs most often to the lungs or liver.

At diagnosis, the degree of malignancy is determined by cellular analysis. Earlier stage cancers are described as *carcinoma in situ* and *well differentiated.* Without treatment, cancers progress to be *moderately differentiated* and, finally, *poorly differentiated.* Most head and neck cancers arise from squamous tissue, but they also can start from salivary glands or

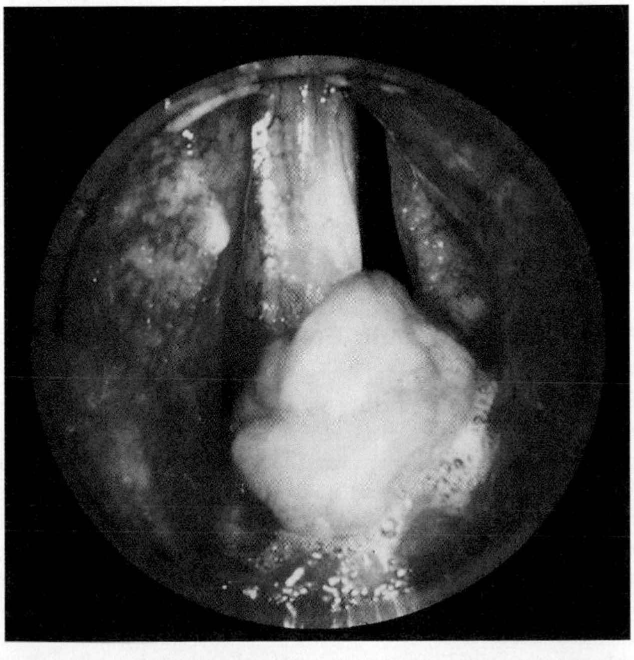

Figure 32-7 ■ Laryngeal cancer is frequently caused by the combination of alcohol and tobacco. This laryngoscopic photograph shows a large granular cell tumor of the true vocal cord. (From Wenig, B.M. [1993]. *Atlas of the head and neck pathology.* Philadelphia: W.B. Saunders. Used with permission.)

thyroid cells. Less common head and neck tumors are malignant melanomas and adenocarcinomas. Treatment is based on tumor cell type and degree of spread at diagnosis.

Etiology

Many risk factors contribute to the development of head and neck cancer, but the actual cause is unknown. The two most important risk factors are tobacco and alcohol use, especially in combination. Other risk factors include chewing tobacco, pipe smoking, marijuana, voice abuse, chronic laryngitis, exposure to industrial chemicals or hardwood dust, and poor oral hygiene.

Incidence/Prevalence

The frequency of occurrence of head and neck carcinoma is increasing. The American Cancer Society (ACS) estimates 47,000 newly diagnosed cases of *oral* and *laryngeal* cancers occur in the United States each year. This cancer type accounts for more than 4% of all carcinomas and more than 11,000 deaths per year (ACS, 2005). Men are affected three times more often than women. Most head and neck cancers occur in people over 60 years of age.

◆COLLABORATIVE MANAGEMENT

PHARM REVIEW

◆Assessment

HISTORY

The client with head and neck cancer may have difficulty speaking because of hoarseness, shortness of breath, tumor bulk, and pain. It is important to be sensitive to these difficulties during the interview.

Ask about tobacco and alcohol use, history of recurrent acute or chronic laryngitis or pharyngitis, oral sores, and lumps in the neck. Calculate the client's smoking history in **pack-years** (the number of packs smoked per day times the number of years the client has smoked). Ask about alcohol intake (how many drinks per day and for how many years). These questions may be uncomfortable for both you and the client but are an important part of the history. Also ask about exposure to environmental or occupational pollutants.

Assess problems related to risk factors. For example, nutrition may be poor because of alcohol intake and impaired liver function. Assess dietary habits and any weight loss. Ask about any chronic lung disease, which may have an impact on the client's breathing pattern.

PHYSICAL ASSESSMENT/CLINICAL MANIFESTATIONS

Table 32-1 lists the warning signs of head and neck cancer. With *laryngeal* cancer, hoarseness may occur because of tumor size and an inability for the vocal cords to come together for normal phonation. Figure 32-8 shows the common sites of laryngeal cancer. Lesions of the true vocal cords are the earliest form of laryngeal cancer. Any person who has a history of hoarseness, mouth sores, or a lump in the neck for 3 to 4 weeks or longer should be evaluated for laryngeal cancer.

Inspection and palpation of the head and neck are important parts of the physical examination. A nurse practitioner may perform a laryngeal examination using a laryngeal mirror or fiberoptic laryngoscope. Lesions may be seen on inspection. The neck is palpated to assess for enlarged lymph nodes.

TABLE 32-1 Warning Signs of Head and Neck Cancer

- Pain
- Lump in the mouth, throat, or neck
- Difficulty swallowing
- Color changes in the mouth or tongue to red, white, gray, dark brown, or black
- Oral lesion or sore that does not heal in 2 weeks
- Persistent or unexplained oral bleeding
- Numbness of the mouth, lips, or face
- Change in the fit of dentures
- Burning sensation when drinking citrus juices or hot liquids
- Persistent, unilateral ear pain
- Hoarseness or change in voice quality
- Persistent or recurrent sore throat
- Shortness of breath
- Anorexia and weight loss

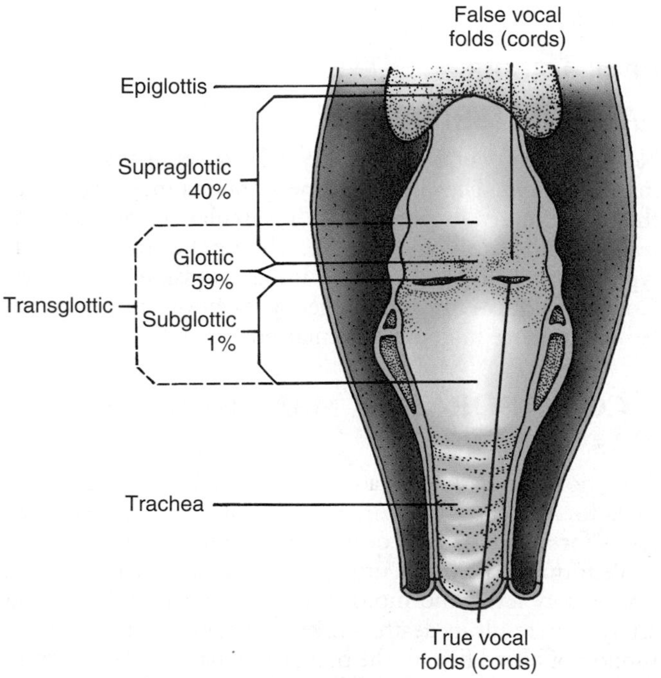

Figure 32-8 ■ Sites and incidence of primary laryngeal tumors.

PSYCHOSOCIAL ASSESSMENT

Often the client with head and neck cancer has a long-standing history of cigarette or alcohol use or both. The client or family may feel denial, guilt, blame, or shame once the diagnosis is suspected. Assess the adequacy of support systems and coping mechanisms. Documentation of social and family support is needed because the client often needs extensive assistance at home after treatment. Consult with a social worker as needed. Evaluate the cognitive functioning (see Chapter 44) and the level of education or literacy of the client and family to plan important teaching before and after surgery.

Document any family history of cancer as well as the client's age, gender, occupation, and ability to perform the activities of daily living (ADLs). Ask the client whether his or her occupation requires continual oral communication. Job retraining may be needed if treatment affects speech.

LABORATORY ASSESSMENT

Diagnostic laboratory tests include a complete blood count, bleeding times, urinalysis, and blood chemistries. The client with chronic alcoholism may have low protein and albumin levels from poor nutrition. Renal and liver function tests are performed to rule out cancer spread and to evaluate the client's ability to metabolize drugs and chemotherapeutic agents.

RADIOGRAPHIC ASSESSMENT

Many types of radiographic studies, including x-rays of the skull, sinuses, neck, and chest, are useful in diagnosing cancer spread, second primary tumors, and the extent of tumor invasion. Computed tomography (CT) of the head and neck, with or without contrast media, helps to evaluate the tumor's exact location.

OTHER DIAGNOSTIC ASSESSMENTS

Magnetic resonance imaging (MRI) can help differentiate normal from diseased tissue. An MRI is more sensitive than a CT in defining the extent of soft-tissue invasion.

The brain, bone, and liver are evaluated with nuclear imaging, bone scans, SPECT (single-photon emission computerized tomography) scans, and PET (positron emission tomography) scans. These tests help locate additional tumor sites.

Other helpful tests include direct and indirect laryngoscopy, tumor mapping, and biopsy. Panendoscopy is performed with general anesthesia to define the extent of the tumor. This procedure includes laryngoscopy, nasopharyngoscopy, esophagoscopy, and bronchoscopy. Tumor-mapping biopsies are performed to identify tumor location. Biopsy tissues taken at the time of the panendoscopy confirm the diagnosis and determine the tumor type, cell features, and location. Tumor staging by the TNM (tumor, nodes, metastasis) method (see Chapter 27) is performed at this time.

Analysis

COMMON NURSING DIAGNOSES AND COLLABORATIVE PROBLEMS

The primary collaborative problem is Potential for Respiratory Obstruction.

The following are priority nursing diagnoses for clients with head and neck carcinomas:

1. Risk for Aspiration related to edema, anatomic changes, or alteration of protective oropharyngeal reflexes
2. Anxiety related to threat of death, change in role status, change in economic status
3. Disturbed Body Image related to tumor and treatment modalities

ADDITIONAL NURSING DIAGNOSES AND COLLABORATIVE PROBLEMS

In addition to the common nursing diagnoses and collaborative problems, clients with head and neck carcinomas may have one or more of the following:

- Acute Pain or Chronic Pain related to tumor invasion of tissues and nerves and surgical intervention
- Imbalanced Nutrition: Less Than Body Requirements related to dysphagia, anxiety, tumor process, surgical resection, or chronic alcohol intake
- Impaired Verbal Communication related to tumor invasion, hoarseness, pain, or surgical resection
- Impaired Skin Integrity related to altered circulation, nutritional deficit, tumor invasion, radiation, chemical factors (body secretions or substances), or surgical wound
- Ineffective Coping related to altered body image, communication method, or ineffective social support
- Impaired Social Interaction related to body image disturbance and lifestyle practices
- Impaired Adjustment related to self-care of the tracheostomy and nasogastric tubes, alternative communication methods, and body-image disturbance
- Deficient Knowledge (treatment regimen and resources) related to lack of exposure to or lack of interest in learning

Critical Thinking Challenge

The client is a 65-year-old man who recently retired from his job as a laborer in a steel mill for 47 years. He has just been diagnosed with laryngeal cancer. He started smoking at 15 years of age and smoked three packs per day until he was 60 years of age, when he was able to quit successfully. He drinks two beers every evening. His hobbies include bowling, playing poker with his friends weekly, refinishing furniture, and singing in his church choir. His other health problems include seasonal asthma and hypertension. He once had a deep vein thrombosis in his right calf. His current over-the-counter and prescribed drugs include aspirin 81 mg daily, hydrochlorothiazide, and Primatene Mist oral inhaler. He is angry about the diagnosis, saying that he might as well take up smoking again for all the good it did him to quit.

1. Calculate this client's smoking history in pack-years.
2. What risk factors does this client have for head and neck cancer?
3. Should you encourage him to refrain from smoking now? Why or why not?
4. What activities are likely to be affected by the disease or its treatment?

evolve For suggested answer guidelines, go to http://evolve.elsevier.com/Iggy/.

Planning and Implementation

POTENTIAL FOR RESPIRATORY OBSTRUCTION

NOC PLANNING: EXPECTED OUTCOMES. The client with head and neck cancer is expected to attain and maintain adequate tissue oxygenation. Indicators include the following:

- Arterial blood gas values within the normal range
- Rate and depth of respiration within the normal range
- Pulse oximetry within the normal range
- Absence of cyanosis or pallor

INTERVENTIONS. The goal of treatment is to remove or eradicate the cancer while preserving as much normal function as possible. The physician presents the available treatment options. Surgery, radiation, or chemotherapy may each be used alone or in combination. In planning treatment options, the client's general physical condition, nutritional status, and age; the effects of the tumor on body function; and the client's personal choice are all considered. Treatment for laryngeal cancer may range from radiation therapy (for a small specific area or tumor) to total laryngopharyngectomy, with bilateral neck dissections followed by radiation therapy. The specific treatment depends on the extent and location of the lesion. Voice-conservation procedures are used only if they do not risk incomplete removal of the tumor. Nursing care focuses on the client's total needs, including preoperative preparation, competent in-hospital care, discharge planning and teaching, and extensive outpatient rehabilitation.

NONSURGICAL MANAGEMENT. Monitor the respiratory system by assessing respiratory rate, breath sounds, pulse oximetry, arterial blood gas values, and the results of pulmonary function tests. Respiratory distress may indicate narrowing of the airway related to tumor growth, edema, or both. Position the client for optimal air exchange. Teach client and family about the use of Fowler's and semi-Fowler's positions. Sitting upright in a reclining chair may promote more comfortable breathing. Chapters 7 and 9 provide additional information on palliation and pain control for clients who elect not to have therapy and for those whose therapy has not been effective.

Radiation Therapy. Radiation treatment of small cancers in specific locations has a cure rate of at least 80%. The cure rate for larger cancers is lower when radiation is used as the only therapy. Standard therapy uses 5000 to 7500 rad (radiation absorbed dose), usually over 6 weeks and in daily or twice-daily doses. The physician may recommend radiation alone or in combination with surgery. Because radiation therapy slows tissue healing, it might *not* be recommended before surgery. Radiation therapy is an outpatient treatment (see Chapter 28). Most clients have uncomfortable side effects during and for a few weeks following radiation therapy (see Chart 32-2).

Hoarseness may become worse. Reassure the client and family that voice improves within 4 to 6 weeks after completion of radiation therapy. Urge the client to use voice rest and alternate means of communication until the effects of radiation therapy have passed.

Most clients have a sore throat and difficulty swallowing during radiation therapy to the neck. Gargling with saline or sucking ice may decrease discomfort. Mouthwashes and throat sprays containing a local anesthetic agent such as lidocaine or diphenhydramine can provide temporary relief. Alert the physician to the client's pain so that analgesic drugs can be prescribed.

The skin at the site of irradiation becomes red and tender and may peel during therapy. Instruct the client to avoid exposing this area to sun, heat, cold, and abrasive treatments such as shaving. Teach the client to wear protective clothing made of soft cotton and to wash this area gently with a mild soap, such as Dove. Stress that only the lotions or powders prescribed by the radiologist should be used until the area has healed.

If the salivary glands are in the path of irradiation, the client has a dry mouth **(xerostomia)**. This side effect is long-term and may be permanent. Some of the consequences of reduced saliva include increased risk for dental caries, increased risk for oral infections, halitosis (bad breath), and changes in taste sensation. Although there is no cure for xerostomia, interventions can help reduce the discomfort. Heavy fluid intake, particularly water, and humidification can help ease the discomfort. Some clients benefit from the use of artificial saliva, such as Salivart, or saliva stimulants, such as Salagen and cevimeline (pilocarpine-based cholinergic drugs). Additional interventions for dry mouth include chewing gum and sucking hard candy.

Chemotherapy. Chemotherapy can be used alone or in addition to surgery or radiation for head and neck cancer. Chapter 28 discusses the general care needs of clients receiving chemotherapy.

SURGICAL MANAGEMENT. Tumor size and location (TNM classification) determines the type of surgery needed for the specific head and neck cancer. Reconstruction is also determined by the tumor size and amount of tissue to be resected and reconstructed. Surgical procedures for head and neck cancers include laryngectomy (total and partial), tracheostomy, and oropharyngeal cancer resections.

Laryngectomy and Related Surgery. The major types of surgery for laryngeal cancer include cordal stripping, **cordectomy** (excision of a vocal cord), partial laryngectomy, and total laryngectomy. If cancer is in the lymph nodes in the neck or if the tumor has a high rate of nodal spread, the surgeon performs a nodal neck dissection along with removal of the primary tumor ("radical neck"). A pathologist evaluates the resected lymph nodes for tumor invasion.

Preoperative Care. Teach the client and family about the tumor. The surgeon explains the surgical procedure and obtains informed consent. Discuss and interpret the implications of such consent with the client and family.

Explain about self-care of the airway, alternate methods of communication, suctioning, pain control methods, the critical care environment (including ventilators and critical care routines), nutritional support, feeding tubes, and goals for discharge. The client will need to learn new methods of speech. Help the client prepare for this change through preoperative teaching and the use of an alternate form of communication (e.g., pen and pencil, "magic slate," picture or alphabet board). Assess which communication method is most preferred by the client before surgery.

A team approach for planning care and rehabilitation is critical for the best outcome. The team should include nurses, physicians, speech pathologists, social workers, dietitians, respiratory therapists, and occupational and physical therapists. Professionals from all these disciplines help to evaluate and prepare the client who has head and neck cancer. Chapter 20 describes general preoperative assessment and education in detail.

Operative Procedures. Hemilaryngectomy (vertical or horizontal) and supraglottic laryngectomy are types of partial voice conservation laryngectomies. Table 32-2 lists specific information about the various surgical procedures for laryngeal cancer.

To protect the airway, a tracheostomy is needed. With a partial laryngectomy, the tracheostomy is usually temporary. With a total laryngectomy, the upper airway is separated from the pharynx and esophagus, and the trachea is brought out through the skin in the neck and sutured in place, creating a stoma. This airway opening is *always* permanent and is referred to as a laryngectomy stoma.

Neck dissection includes the removal of lymph nodes, the sternocleidomastoid muscle, the jugular vein, the 11th cranial nerve, and surrounding soft tissue. Because the 11th cranial nerve (spinal accessory nerve) is cut during this procedure, shoulder drop will be present after surgery. Physical therapy exercises are needed after surgery to help the client ease the shoulder drop by using other muscle groups.

Postoperative Care. Head and neck surgery often lasts 8 hours or longer. Usually the client spends the immediate period after surgery in the surgical intensive care unit. Monitor airway patency, vital signs, hemodynamic status,

TABLE 32-2 Surgical Procedures for Laryngeal Cancer and Their Effect on Voice Quality

Procedure	Description	Resulting Voice Quality
Laser surgery	Tumor reduced or destroyed by laser beam through laryngoscope	Normal/hoarse
Transoral cordectomy	Tumor (early lesion) resected through laryngoscope	Normal/hoarse (high cure rate)
Laryngofissure	No cord removed (early lesion)	Normal (high cure rate)
Supraglottic partial laryngectomy	Hyoid bone, false cords, and epiglottis removed Neck dissection on affected side performed if nodes involved	Normal/hoarse
Hemilaryngectomy or vertical laryngectomy	One true cord, one false cord, and one half of thyroid cartilage removed	Hoarse voice
Total laryngectomy	Entire larynx, hyoid bone, strap muscles, one or two tracheal rings removed Nodal neck dissection if nodes involved	No natural voice

and comfort level. Monitor for hemorrhage and other general complications of anesthesia and surgery (see Chapter 22). Take vital signs hourly for the first 24 hours and then every 2 hours until the client is stable. After the client is transferred from the critical care unit, monitor vital signs every 4 hours or according to agency policy. The client is generally out of bed by the second postoperative day.

Complications after head and neck cancer surgery include airway obstruction, hemorrhage, wound breakdown, and tumor recurrence. The first priorities after head and neck surgery are airway maintenance and ventilation. Other priorities include wound, flap, and reconstructive tissue care; pain management; nutrition; and psychological adjustment, including speech therapy.

Airway Maintenance and Ventilation. Immediately after surgery, the client may need ventilatory assistance because of a long-term smoking history, chronic lung disease, and a long duration of anesthesia. Most clients wean easily from the ventilator after this type of surgery because the thoracic and abdominal cavities are not entered. When weaned from the ventilator, the client usually uses a tracheostomy collar (over the artificial airway or open stoma) with oxygen and humidification to help mobilize mucus secretions. Secretions may remain blood-tinged for 1 to 2 days. Use body substance precautions, and report any increase in bleeding to the surgeon. Humidifying the air helps to remove crusts and prevent obstruction of the tube with secretions. Some surgeons prescribe instillations of 5 to 10 mL of sterile saline into the airway every 2 hours; however, this practice is controversial.

A laryngectomy tube is used for clients who have undergone a *total laryngectomy* and need an appliance to prevent scar tissue contracture at the skin-tracheal border. This tube is similar to a standard tracheostomy tube but is shorter and fatter with a larger lumen and more acute angle (Figure 32-9). Laryngectomy tube care is similar to tracheostomy tube care (see Chapter 31) except that the client can change the laryngectomy tube daily or as needed. A laryngectomy button is similar to a laryngectomy tube but is made of Silastic, has a single lumen, and is very short. A button is comfortable for the client, is easily removed for cleaning, and is available in various sizes and lengths for a custom fit. Provide a "magic slate" or paper and pencil for communication because the client cannot create speech other than mouthing words.

Coughing, deep breathing, and saline instillation are usually effective in clearing secretions. The lack of a surgical incision in the chest or abdomen improves the ability to cough. Instruct the client in the proper techniques for coughing and deep breathing to clear secretions (see Chapter 22).

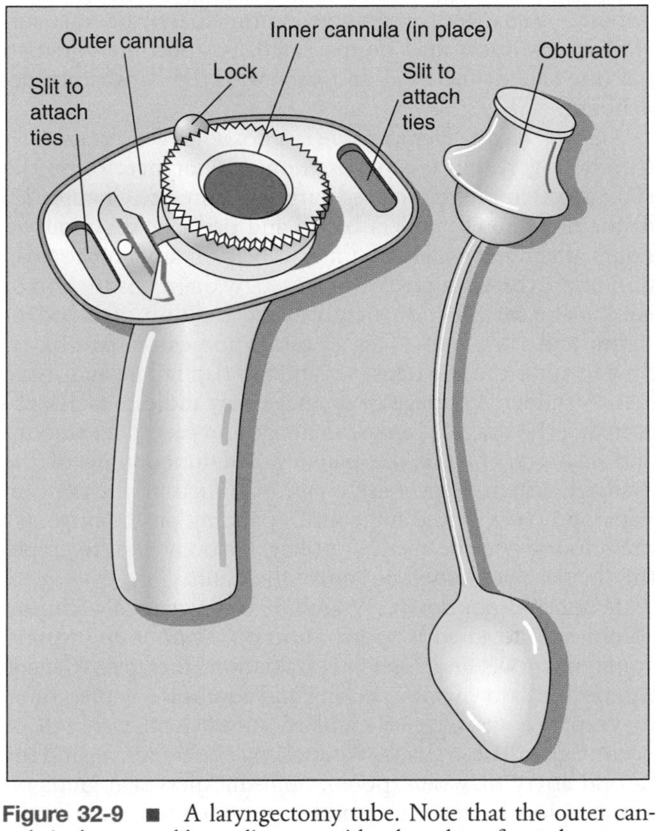

Figure 32-9 ■ A laryngectomy tube. Note that the outer cannula is shorter and has a diameter wider than that of a tracheostomy tube.

Oral secretions can be suctioned by the client using a Yankauer or tonsillar suction or with a soft red latex catheter. Teach the client to suction away from the side of the surgery to prevent wound opening immediately after surgery. Clients can participate in their own care by using a table mirror for visibility. Provide a clean environment for the catheter.

Stoma care following a total laryngectomy is a combination of wound care and airway care. Inspect the stoma with a flashlight. Clean the suture line with half-strength hydrogen peroxide to prevent secretions from forming crusts and obstructing the airway. Perform suture line care every 1 to 2 hours during the first few days after surgery and then every 4 hours thereafter. The mucosa of the stoma and trachea should be bright and shiny and without crusts, similar to the appearance of the oral mucosa.

Wound, Flap, and Reconstructive Tissue Care. Tissue "flaps" may be used to close the wound and improve appearance. Commonly used reconstructive flaps are pectoralis major myocutaneous flaps, island flaps, rotation flaps, trapezius flaps, split-thickness skin grafts (STSGs), and free flaps with microvascular anastomosis (scapula, fibula, or radial forearm free flaps). These flaps may be used for reconstruction after any type of head and neck resection. After neck dissection, the surgeon places an STSG over the exposed carotid artery before covering it with skin flaps or reconstructive flaps.

The first 24 hours after surgery are critical. Evaluate all flaps every hour for the first 72 hours. Monitor capillary refill, color, and Doppler activity of the major feeding vessel. Report any changes to the surgeon immediately because surgical intervention may be indicated. Position the client so that the side of the head and neck with the flaps is not dependent.

Hemorrhage. Hemorrhage is a possible complication after any surgery, but it is uncommon with laryngectomy. The surgeon often places a closed surgical drain (see Chapter 22) in the neck area to collect blood and drainage for about 72 hours after surgery. The drain also helps maintain the position of the reconstructed skin flaps. Any drain obstruction or equipment malfunction may cause a buildup of blood or serum under the flaps. This accumulation can impair blood flow to and from the flaps, resulting in flap failure and tissue loss. A sudden stoppage of drainage may indicate a clot obstructing the drain. Monitor drainage and record its amount and character. Check the patency and functioning of the drainage system. Report any drain malfunction or change in flap appearance to the surgeon. Depending on the surgeon's prescription and the agency's policy, you may need to empty the drainage contained or "milk" the drain.

Wound Breakdown. Wound breakdown is a common complication caused by poor nutrition, alcohol use, wound contamination, and previous radiation therapy. Manage wound breakdown with packing and local care as prescribed to keep the wound clean and to stimulate the growth of healthy granulation tissue. Wounds may be extensive, and the carotid artery may be exposed. Split-thickness skin grafts often are placed over the carotid artery for protection in the event of wound dehiscence. As the wound heals, granulation tissue covers the artery and prevents rupture. If granulation is slow and the carotid artery is at risk, another surgical flap may be made to cover the carotid artery and close the wound.

If the carotid artery ruptures because of drying or infection, place *immediate constant pressure* over the site and secure the airway. Maintain direct manual pressure on the carotid artery and *immediately* transport the client to the operating room for carotid resection. *Carotid artery rupture has a high risk of stroke and death.* An immediate nursing response can save the client's life.

Pain Management. After surgery, pain should be controlled and the client should still be able to participate in his or her care. Morphine (Statex✱) often is given by IV bolus and continuously for the first days after surgery. As the client progresses, acetaminophen with codeine, then acetaminophen alone, can be given by feeding tube. Oral drugs for pain and discomfort are started only after the client can tolerate oral nutrition. After discharge, the client still requires pain management, especially if he or she is receiving radiation therapy. An adjunct to the pain regimen may be liquid nonsteroidal anti-inflammatory drugs (NSAIDs). These drugs provide excellent pain relief and can be used along with opioid analgesics (see also Chapter 7). Amitriptyline (Elavil) or other tricyclic antidepressants may also be used for the lancinating pain of nerve-root involvement.

Nutrition. A nasogastric, gastrostomy, or jejunostomy tube is placed during surgery for nutritional support while the head and neck heal. Initially the client receives IV fluids or parenteral nutrition until the intestinal tract has recovered from the effects of anesthesia. After that, nutrients can be given via the feeding tube. The nutritional support team or dietitian assesses the client before surgery and is available for consultation after surgery. The common nutrition goal is to provide 35 to 40 kcal/kg of body weight. Replacement of protein and water loss is calculated carefully.

The nasogastric tube (the most commonly used type of tube) usually remains in place for 7 to 10 days after surgery. Before removing the tube, assess the client's ability to swallow if nutrition is to be given by mouth. Aspiration *cannot* occur following a total laryngectomy because the airway and esophagus have been completely separated. Reassure the client that aspiration will not occur, and stay with him or her during the first few swallowing attempts. Swallowing may be uncomfortable at first, and the prescribed analgesics may be needed.

Speech Rehabilitation. The client's voice quality and speech are altered after surgery. Although this problem has enormous effects on the client's ability to maintain social interactions, continue employment, and maintain a desired quality of life, it is often poorly addressed while he or she is hospitalized (see the Evidence-Based Practice for Nursing box on p. 577). Working with the client and family toward developing an acceptable communication method during the inpatient period is essential for a satisfactory outcome.

Together with the speech pathologist, discuss the principles of speech therapy with the client and family early in the course of the treatment plan (see Chart 32-2). Voice and speech differences depend on the type of surgical resection (see Table 32-2). Speech production varies with client practice, amount of tissue removed, and radiation effects, but the speech can be very understandable.

The speech rehabilitation plan for clients who have a total laryngectomy at first consists of writing or using a picture board. The client then uses an artificial larynx and eventually learns esophageal speech. For success, the client needs support and encouragement from the speech pathologist, hospital team, and family while relearning to speak. This process can be time consuming and requires concentration each time the client speaks. Having a **laryngectomee** (person who has had a laryngectomy) from one of the local self-help organizations visit the client and family is often beneficial. The International Association of Laryngectomees is very active and supportive, as is the American Cancer Society (ACS) Visitor Program.

Common means of speech communication after laryngectomy include esophageal speech, the use of mechanical devices, and the use of a tracheoesophageal fistula (TEF).

ESOPHAGEAL SPEECH. Most clients who have a total laryngectomy attempt esophageal speech. Sound can be produced this way by "burping" the air swallowed or injected into

EVIDENCE-BASED PRACTICE for Nursing

Silence is not golden

Happ, M.B., Roesch, T., & Kagan, S. (2004). Communication needs, methods, and perceived voice quality following head and neck surgery: A literature review. *Cancer Nursing, 27*(1), 1-9.

The authors sought to examine the problems associated with loss of speech as a result of temporary or permanent changes induced by medical or surgical intervention for head and neck cancer. Although numerous articles in both the nursing and medical literature discussed issues related to temporary speech loss through intubation, mechanical ventilation, and chemical paralysis in the critical care setting, only one study targeted the inpatient postoperative recovery period for clients with head and neck cancer. The authors then expanded their search to include the first 12 months after head and neck surgery. The search of relevant literature from 1968 through 2002 revealed a total of only 10 published studies and one clinical case report specifically addressing the communication needs, methods, or perceived voice quality of clients with head and neck cancer surgery during the postoperative period.

The 11 studies varied considerably in sample size, timing of data collection (postoperative stage of clients), and study design, but three common themes consistently emerged. These themes were information needs (of the client and family), communication methods and perceived voice quality, and quality-of-life perceptions that included disfigurement and socialization. Overwhelmingly, the studies indicated that the education needs and preparation for postoperative communication impairment were unaddressed or poorly addressed for this client population.

Level of Evidence: 4—Well-conducted qualitative systematic review (integrative review on nonexperimental design studies).

Critique. The authors used the appropriate methods of searching the literature for an exhaustive review on the topic. This review highlights the need for additional studies to understand the dimensions of information needed among these clients and their families.

Implications for Nursing. Whereas all cancer surgeries result in some degree of tissue loss and potential function reduction, surgery for head and neck cancer is the most obviously disfiguring and often results in a permanent speech change or loss. These results are obvious to anyone who interacts with the client and are a constant reminder to the client of the cancer diagnosis.

Adjustment to the changes require much time and work. Nursing care can be key to this adjustment but must begin during the perioperative time. Nurses need to help the client and family learn exactly what to expect after surgery. Presenting accurate information in a matter-of-fact but sensitive way before surgery can reduce anxiety and help the client and family to have realistic and optimistic expectations. Working with a client for whom speech has been lost is frustrating to the client, nurse, and family. Talking for the client does not help, nor does pretending to understand what the client is trying to communicate. Nurses must allow whatever time it takes to ensure that the client's needs and wishes are accurately understood. The in-hospital time for these clients after surgery is longer than are most other hospital stays and therefore represents an opportune time for nurses to implement interventions for symptom management, client education for self-care and communication, stress and anxiety reduction, and resocialization.

the esophageal pharynx and shaping the words in the mouth. The voice produced is a monotone; it cannot be raised or lowered and carries no pitch. In the English language, the vocal cords are necessary for 15 consonants; the remaining 10 consonants can be formed by shaping the mouth. Clients must have adequate hearing, or esophageal speech will be difficult because they will use their mouth to shape the words as they hear them. Hearing-impaired clients may require hearing aids.

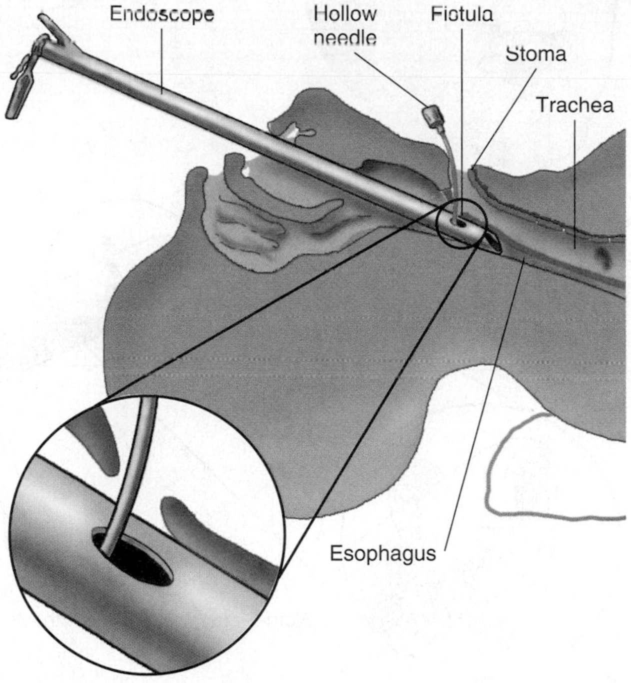

Figure 32-10 ■ One method of creating a tracheoesophageal fistula.

Some clients have intestinal bloating as a result of swallowing air for esophageal speech. Antacids may help to reduce bloating sensations. Esophageal speech also helps to strengthen the respiratory and abdominal muscles, which aids in clearing secretions and in breathing.

MECHANICAL DEVICES. The client who cannot attain esophageal speech can use mechanical devices called **electrolarynges.** Most are battery-powered devices placed against the side of the neck or cheek. The air inside the mouth and throat is vibrated, and the client moves his or her lips and tongue as usual. Another external device (Cooper-Rand), also battery powered, consists of a plastic tube that is placed in the client's mouth and vibrates during speech. The quality of speech generated with these devices is robot-like and does not sound natural.

TRACHEOESOPHAGEAL FISTULA. A tracheoesophageal fistula (TEF) may be used if esophageal speech is ineffective and if the client meets strict criteria. A surgical fistula is created between the trachea and the esophagus either at the time of the laryngectomy or later (Figure 32-10). The surgeon places a catheter into the laryngectomy stoma and surgically creates a fistula into the esophagus. The catheter is usually sutured to the neck to prevent accidental dislodgment. After the fistula heals, a silicone prosthesis (e.g., the Blom-Singer prosthesis) is inserted in place of the catheter (Figure 32-11). The client covers the stoma and the opening of the prosthesis with a finger or opens and closes the opening with a special valve to divert air from the lungs, through the trachea, into the esophagus, and out of the mouth. Lip and tongue movement, not the prosthesis itself, produces speech.

Surgical Procedures for Other Head and Neck Cancers. The major types of resections, defined by the tumor location of the *oropharyngeal cancer,* are called composite resections. **Composite resections** are a combina-

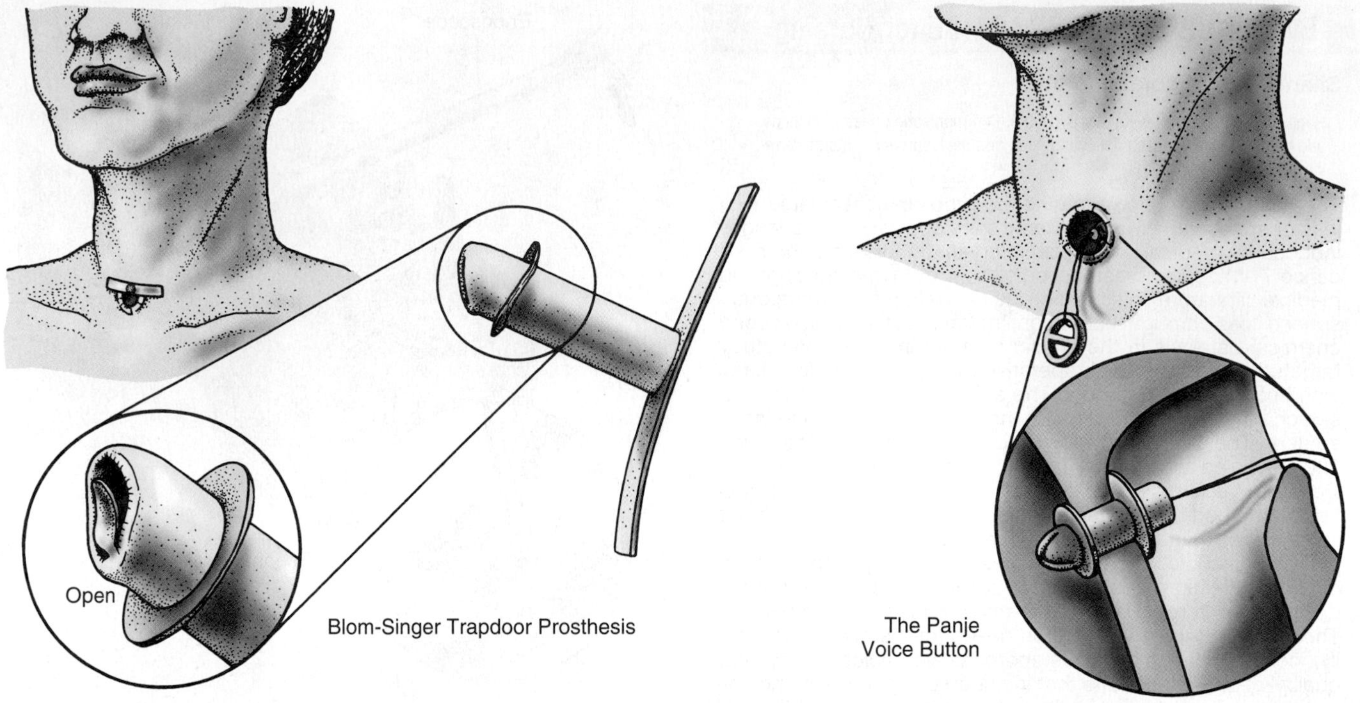

Figure 32-11 ■ Examples of tracheoesophageal prostheses.

tion of surgical procedures that include partial or total glossectomies, partial mandibulectomies and, if needed, nodal neck dissections. Tracheostomy may be planned to provide an adequate airway. (See Chapter 57 for more information about oral cancer.)

Tracheotomy. A **tracheotomy** is a surgical incision into the trachea for the purpose of establishing an airway (tracheostomy). It can be performed as an emergency procedure or as a scheduled surgical procedure. A tracheostomy can be temporary or permanent. Chapter 31 discusses the nursing care of a client with a tracheostomy.

RISK FOR ASPIRATION

NOC **PLANNING: EXPECTED OUTCOMES.** The client with head and neck cancer is expected not to aspirate food, gastric contents, or oral secretions into the lungs. Indicators include that the client often or consistently demonstrates the following behaviors:

- Positions self upright for eating or drinking
- Selects foods according to swallowing ability
- Chooses liquids and foods of proper consistency

INTERVENTIONS. The surgical changes in the upper respiratory tract and altered swallowing mechanisms increase the client's risk for aspiration. Aspiration can result in life-threatening pneumonia, weight loss, prolonged hospitalization, and increased costs. Chart 32-3 lists NIC interventions for aspiration prevention.

The presence of a nasogastric (NG) feeding tube may further increase the potential for aspiration because of the incompetent lower esophageal sphincter (LES). The one exception is the client who has undergone a total laryngectomy. In these cases the airway is separated from the esophagus, making aspiration impossible; such a client is *not* at risk.

A dynamic swallow study, such as a barium swallow under fluoroscopy, evaluates a client's ability to protect the airway from aspiration and helps determine the appropriate method of swallow rehabilitation. In many cases enteral feedings are used either because of the client's inability to swallow or because of continued aspiration potential.

When an NG tube is in place, help prevent aspiration through the use of routine reflux precautions. These precautions include elevating the head of the bed and strictly adhering to tube feeding regimens, including no bolus feedings at night. Check residual feeding before each bolus feeding (or every 4 to 6 hours with continuous feeding), and evaluate the client's tolerance of the tube feeding. If the residual volume is too high (above 100 mL or as otherwise prescribed by the physician), withhold the feeding and notify the physician. Check the pH of pulmonary secretions. Because residual volume cannot be checked with micropore feeding tubes, use other techniques to assess tube placement. (See Chapter 64 for other interventions related to NG tubes and tube feedings.)

Swallowing can be a major problem for the client who has a tracheostomy tube. Swallowing can be normal if the cranial nerves and anatomic structures are intact. In a normal swallow, the larynx elevates and moves forward to protect itself from the passing stream of food and saliva. Laryngeal elevation also assists in opening the upper esophageal sphincter. The tracheostomy tube sometimes fixes the larynx in place, making it unable to perform this motion efficiently. The result is difficulty in swallowing.

The tracheostomy tube cuff can balloon backward when inflated and interfere with the passage of food through the esophagus. The common wall of the posterior trachea and the anterior esophagus is very thin, which allows this pushing phenomenon. The client with head and neck cancer who

CHART 32-3

NIC INTERVENTION ACTIVITIES for The Client with Head and Neck Cancer

Aspiration Precautions: *Prevention or minimization of risk factors in the client at risk for aspiration*

- Monitor level of consciousness, cough reflex, gag reflex, and swallowing ability.
- Monitor pulmonary status.
- Maintain an airway.
- Position upright 90 degrees or as far as possible.
- Keep suction setup available.
- Feed in small amounts.
- Check NG or gastrostomy tube placement before feeding.
- Check NG or gastrostomy tube residual before feeding.
- Avoid liquids or use thickening agent.
- Offer foods or liquids that can be formed into a bolus before swallowing.
- Cut food into small pieces.
- Request medication in elixir form.
- Break or crush pills before administration.
- Keep head of bed elevated 30 to 45 minutes after feeding.

Smoking Cessation Assistance: *Helping another to stop smoking*

- Give smoker clear, consistent advice to quit smoking.
- Help choose best method for giving up cigarettes, when client is ready to quit.
- Refer to group programs or individual therapists, as appropriate.
- Assist client with any self-help methods.
- Help client plan specific coping strategies and resolve problems that result from quitting.
- Inform client that dry mouth, cough, scratchy throat, and feeling on edge are symptoms that may occur after quitting; the patch or gum may help with cravings.
- Advise client to keep a list of "slips" or near-slips, what causes them, and what he or she learned from them.
- Advise client to avoid smokeless tobacco, dipping, and chewing as these can lead to addiction and/or health problems including oral cancer, gum problems, loss of teeth, and heart disease
- Manage nicotine replacement therapy.
- Contact national and local resource organizations for resource materials.
- Follow client for 2 years after quitting, if possible, to provide encouragement.
- Help client deal with any lapses (e.g., reassure client that he or she is not a "failure," reassure that much can be learned from this temporary regression, assist client in identifying reasons for the relapse).
- Support client who begins smoking again by helping to identify what has been learned.
- Encourage the relapsed client to try again.
- Serve as a nonsmoking role model.

NIC intervention activities selected from Dochterman, J.M., & Bulechek, G.M. (Eds.). (2004). *Nursing interventions classification (NIC)* (4th ed.). St. Louis: Mosby. No part of this work is to be altered without prior written permission from the Publisher.

is cognitively intact may adapt to eating normal food when the tracheostomy tube is small and the cuff is not inflated.

The client who has had a subtotal, vertical, or supraglottic laryngectomy *must* be observed for aspiration. It is critical to teach the client to use alternate methods of swallowing without aspirating. The "supraglottic" method of swallowing is especially effective after a partial laryngectomy or base-of-tongue resection (Chart 32-4). To reinforce teaching and learning, place a chart in the client's room detailing the steps. A dynamic swallow study is performed to guide rehabilitation therapy for swallowing and to evaluate the client's ability to protect the airway.

CHART 32-4

CLIENT EDUCATION GUIDE The Supraglottic Method of Swallowing

1. Place yourself in an upright, preferably out-of-bed, position.
2. Clear your throat.
3. Take a deep breath.
4. Place ½ to 1 teaspoon of food into your mouth.
5. Hold your breath or "bear down" (Valsalva maneuver).
6. Swallow twice.
7. Release your breath, and clear your throat.
8. Swallow twice again.
9. Breathe normally.

This method exaggerates the normal protective mechanisms of cessation of respiration during the swallow. The double swallow attempts to clear food that may be pooling in the pharynx, vallecula, and piriform sinuses. This method is used only after a dynamic radiographic swallow study has demonstrated that it is appropriate and safe for the client.

ANXIETY

NOC **PLANNING: EXPECTED OUTCOMES.** The client with head and neck cancer is expected to have decreased anxiety. Indicators include that the client often or consistently demonstrates the following behaviors:

- Verbalization of reduced anxiety
- Absence of distress, irritability, and facial tension
- Effective use of coping strategies

INTERVENTIONS. Conferences with the physician, clinical nurse specialist, dietitian, speech pathologist, physical therapist, psychologist, social worker, and general nursing staff may be beneficial. Explore the reason for anxiety (e.g., fear of the unknown, lack of preoperative teaching, fear of pain, fear of airway compromise, fear of hospitalization, loss of control). The client and family often benefit from further information. Before the client is scheduled for surgery (and while still at home), home care nurses or community-sponsored associations (e.g., ACS) may be able to decrease fears about the disease process and surgical interventions.

Give prescribed antianxiety drugs, such as diazepam (Valium, Meval✱), with caution because of the possibility of respiratory depression. The location of the tumor and the presence of any other lung disease may cause some degree of airway obstruction. For anxiety in these clients, the physician prescribes drug therapy judiciously and may choose lorazepam (Ativan, Novo-Lorazem✱) rather than a sedating agent.

DISTURBED BODY IMAGE

NOC **PLANNING: EXPECTED OUTCOMES.** The client with head and neck cancer is expected to accept body image changes. Indicators include that the client often or consistently demonstrates the following behaviors:

- Willingness to touch the affected body part
- Willingness to use strategies to enhance appearance
- Participation in self-care
- Interaction with visitors, staff, and family members

INTERVENTIONS. The client with head and neck cancer may have a permanent change in body image because of deformity, the presence of a stoma or artificial airway, speech changes, and a change in the method of eating.

The client may not be able to speak at all or have permanent hoarseness or speech deficits. Help the client set realistic goals, starting with involvement in self-care. Teach the client alternate communication methods so he or she can functionally communicate in the hospital and after discharge.

Teach the family to ease the client into a more normal social environment. Provide encouragement and positive reinforcement while demonstrating acceptance and caring behaviors. The family also may benefit from counseling sessions initiated while the client is still in the hospital.

After surgery the client may feel reserved and socially isolated because of the change in voice and facial appearance. Loose-fitting, high-collar shirts or sweaters (e.g., turtleneck), scarves, and jewelry can be worn to cover the laryngectomy stoma, tracheostomy tube, and physical changes related to surgery. Cosmetics may aid in covering any disfigurement. Most surgeons try to place the surgical incisions in the natural skin fold lines if doing so does not pose a risk for cancer recurrence.

Critical Thinking Challenge

The client, a 65-year-old man 7 days postoperative after a laryngectomy and radical neck dissection, is being discharged to home. After hearing the discharge order, he starts to cry and shake his head in a "no" gesture. His wife, who has been saying throughout the postoperative period that "everything will be all right," is amazed that he does not want to come home today, especially because she has planned a little get-together with their grown children, minister, and the neighbors to welcome him back.

1. Should you try to get this client's discharge orders changed?
2. What question(s) should you ask the wife? The client?
3. What might be causing the client's anxiety?
4. What teaching priorities are needed?

evolve For suggested answer guidelines, go to http://evolve.elsevier.com/Iggy/.

CHART 32-5

HOME CARE ASSESSMENT of Clients After Laryngectomy

Assess respiratory status.
- Observe rate and depth of respiration.
- Auscultate lungs.
- Check patency of airway.
- Examine the tracheostomy exudate for amount, color, and character.
- Examine nail beds and mucous membranes for evidence of cyanosis.
- Obtain a pulse oximetry reading.

Assess condition of wound.
- Remove dressings (noting condition of dressings).
- Cleanse the wound.
- Compare with previous notations of wound condition:
  - Presence, amount, and nature of exudate
  - Presence/absence of cellulitis
  - Presence/absence of odor

Assess client's psychosocial functioning.
- Ask the client about passing the time, visitors, and trips outside the house.
- Observe whether the client communicates responses directly or whether a family member speaks for the client.
- Observe client and family member interactions.
- Determine what method of communication the client has selected, and observe the client's skill with it.
- Is the client wearing pajamas, or is the client dressed?

Take the client's temperature.

Assess the client's understanding of illness and compliance with treatment.
- Manifestations to report to the health care provider
- Medication plan (correct timing and dose)
- Ambulation or positioning schedule
- Dressing changes/skin care
- Diet modifications (24-hour diet recall)
- Skill in tracheostomy or dressing care

Assess client's nutritional status.
- Change in muscle mass
- Lackluster nails/sparse hair
- Recent weight loss greater than 10% of usual weight
- Impaired oral intake
- Difficulty swallowing
- Generalized edema

Community-Based Care

If no complications occur, the client is usually ready to be discharged home or to an extended care facility within 2 weeks. At the time of discharge, he or she should be able to provide self-care, which may include tracheostomy or stoma care, nutrition, wound care, and methods of communication.

The client and family may feel more secure about discharge if they receive a referral to selected support groups or a community health agency familiar with the care of clients recovering from head and neck cancer. The health care team assesses the specific discharge needs and makes the appropriate referrals to home care agencies, including professionals such as nutritionists, nurses, physical therapists, speech pathologists, and social workers. Coordinate the scheduling for chemotherapy or radiation therapy with the client and family.

HOME CARE MANAGEMENT

Extensive home care preparation is needed after a laryngectomy for cancer. The convalescent period is long, and airway management is complicated. The client or family must be able to take an active role in care.

General cleanliness of the home is assessed. If the client has severe or long-standing respiratory problems, adjustments in the home to allow for one-floor living may be needed. Increased humidification is needed. A humidifier add-on to a forced-air furnace can be obtained. If the cost of this add-on is not manageable or if the home is heated by radiators, a room humidifier or vaporizer may be appropriate.

A home care nurse is involved with care after discharge and is an important resource for the client and family. The home care nurse assesses the client and home situation for problems in self-care, complications, adjustment, and adherence to the medical regimen. Chart 32-5 lists assessment areas for the client in the home following a laryngectomy. This nurse reinforces health care teaching, self-care teaching, and smoking-cessation regimens.

HEALTH TEACHING

Although education begins before surgery, most self-care is taught in the hospital. Teach the client and family how to care for the stoma or tracheostomy or laryngectomy tube, depending on the type of surgery performed. Review incision and airway care, including cleaning and inspecting for signs of infection. Chart 32-6 lists the highlights of self-care for the client who is discharged after laryngeal cancer surgery. Many of these actions also apply to any surgery for head and neck cancer.

CHART 32-6

CLIENT EDUCATION GUIDE
Home Laryngectomy Care

- Avoid swimming, and use care when showering or shaving.
- Lean slightly forward and cover the stoma when coughing or sneezing.
- Wear a stoma guard or loose clothing to cover the stoma.
- Clean the stoma with mild soap and water. Lubricate the stoma with a non–oil-based ointment as needed.
- Increase humidity by using saline in the stoma as instructed, a bedside humidifier, pans of water, and houseplants.
- Obtain and wear a MedicAlert bracelet and emergency care card for life-threatening situations.

STOMA CARE. Instruct the client to use a shower shield over the tracheostomy tube or laryngectomy stoma when bathing to prevent water from entering the airway. Suggest that the client wear a protective cover or stoma guard to protect the stoma during the day. For clients with permanent stomas following laryngectomy or for those with permanent tracheostomies, covering the permanent opening has a double benefit: (1) filtering the air entering the stoma while keeping humidity in the airway and (2) enhancing aesthetic appearance. Attractive coverings are available in the form of cotton scarves, crocheted bibs, and jewelry. Using colored seam binding for tracheostomy ties after the stoma has matured may enhance overall body image. Shirt or dress color can be matched or coordinated with seam bindings of various colors.

Instruct the client how to increase humidity in the home. If prescribed, teach the client to instill normal saline into the artificial airway 10 to 15 times a day.

COMMUNICATION. The client continues the selected method of alternate communication that began in the hospital. Instruct him or her to wear a medical alert (MedicAlert) bracelet and carry a special identification card (Figure 32-12). For clients who have a laryngectomy, this card is available from the local chapters of the International Association of Laryngectomees. The card instructs the reader about providing an emergency airway or resuscitating someone who has a stoma.

SMOKING CESSATION. A difficult but important issue after head and neck cancer surgery is smoking cessation. Smoking is a major risk factor for head and neck cancer. Stress that smoking cessation can reduce the risk for developing other cancers and can increase the rate of healing from surgery.

Smoking cessation is not an easy task, and most clients require continuing support and reinforcement to sustain this action. Chemical and psychological assistance are available for smoking cessation (see Chart 32-3).

PSYCHOSOCIAL PREPARATION

The many changes resulting from a laryngectomy influence physical, social, and emotional functioning. Many clients perceive changes in their quality of life. Begin preparing the client and family for these changes by scheduling a visit from a person who has adjusted to these changes.

The client who is discharged to home with a permanent stoma, tracheostomy tube, nasogastric (NG) tube, and wounds has an altered body image. Stress the importance of returning to as normal a lifestyle as possible. Most clients can resume

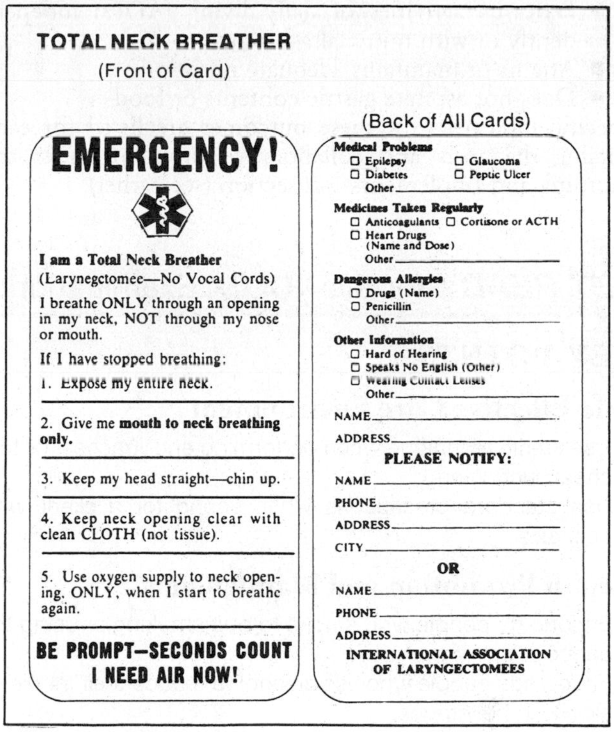
TOTAL NECK BREATHER
(Front of Card)

EMERGENCY!

I am a Total Neck Breather
(Larynegctomee—No Vocal Cords)
I breathe ONLY through an opening in my neck, NOT through my nose or mouth.
If I have stopped breathing:
1. Expose my entire neck.
2. Give me **mouth to neck breathing only.**
3. Keep my head straight—chin up.
4. Keep neck opening clear with clean CLOTH (not tissue).
5. Use oxygen supply to neck opening, ONLY, when I start to breathe again.

BE PROMPT—SECONDS COUNT
I NEED AIR NOW!

(Back of All Cards)

Medical Problems
☐ Epilepsy ☐ Glaucoma
☐ Diabetes ☐ Peptic Ulcer
Other ______

Medicines Taken Regularly
☐ Anticoagulants ☐ Cortisone or ACTH
☐ Heart Drugs (Name and Dose)
Other ______

Dangerous Allergies
☐ Drugs (Name)
☐ Penicillin
Other ______

Other Information
☐ Hard of Hearing
☐ Speaks No English (Other)
☐ Wearing Contact Lenses
Other ______

NAME ______
ADDRESS ______

PLEASE NOTIFY:

NAME ______
PHONE ______
ADDRESS ______
CITY ______

OR

NAME ______
PHONE ______
ADDRESS ______

INTERNATIONAL ASSOCIATION OF LARYNGECTOMEES

Figure 32-12 ■ Emergency wallet card for identification of laryngectomy.

many of their usual activities within 4 to 6 weeks after surgery. A longer time is required after a combination of radiation therapy and surgery. The client may be frustrated at times while trying to adjust to changes in smell, taste, and communication.

The client with a total laryngectomy cannot produce sounds during laughing and crying, and mucous secretions may appear unexpectedly when these emotions arise or when coughing or sneezing occur. The mucus can be embarrassing, and the client needs to be prepared to cover the stoma with a handkerchief or gauze. The client who has undergone composite resections has difficulty with speech *and* swallowing. He or she may need to deal with tracheostomy and feeding tubes in public places.

HEALTH CARE RESOURCES

Inform the client and family of community organizations (e.g., ACS) and local laryngectomee clubs, which can offer support, information, and friendships. When the client has problems paying for health care services, equipment, and prescriptions, a visiting nurse agency may be helpful in directing him or her to available resources.

In many areas the local unit of the ACS or Canadian Cancer Society can help provide dressing materials and nutritional supplements to clients in need. This organization may also provide transportation to and from follow-up visits or radiation therapy.

◆Evaluation: Outcomes

Evaluate the care of the client with head and neck carcinomas on the basis of the identified nursing diagnoses and collaborative problems. The expected outcomes are that the client:

- Maintains a patent airway
- Performs self-care of the artificial airway and wound

- Performs activities of daily living (ADLs) independently or with minimal assistance
- Attains or maintains adequate nutrition
- Does not aspirate gastric contents or food

Specific indicators for these outcomes are listed for each nursing diagnosis and collaborative problem under the Planning and Implementation section (see earlier).

GET READY for the NCLEX Examination!

KEY POINTS

Safe Effective Care Environment

- Use sterile technique when performing endotracheal or tracheal suctioning.
- Use standard precautions when caring for a client with epistaxis.

Health Promotion and Maintenance

- Encourage people who smoke to quit smoking or using tobacco in any way.
- Encourage people who use alcohol to reduce their intake of alcoholic beverages.
- Teach clients how to blow the nose without closing off one nostril.
- Use aspiration precautions for any client with an altered level of consciousness or who has an endotracheal tube (see Chart 31-6).
- Teach the client and family how to perform tracheostomy care (see Chart 31-4)
- Teach clients who have had radiation therapy to the neck or oral cavity to have dental examinations at least every 6 months.

Psychosocial Integrity

- Allow the client and family members the opportunity to express fear or anxiety regarding a cancer diagnosis or a change in breathing status.
- Teach family members ways to communicate with a client who is unable to speak after surgery for head and neck cancer.
- Encourage clients with permanent tracheostomies to become involved in self-care.
- Encourage the client who has had head and neck surgery for cancer to look at the wound and touch the affected area.
- Allow the client and family to grieve about the loss of function and change in body image.
- Allow time to communicate with the client who has voice loss as a result of disease or treatment.
- Refer clients and families to the ACS after surgery for head and neck cancer.

Physiological Integrity

- Assess airway patency for any client who experiences facial or nasal trauma.
- Notify the emergency team when a client experiences a posterior nasal bleed.
- Check the airway and packing at least every hour for a client who has posterior nasal packing placed after nasal surgery or posterior nasal epistaxis.
- Instruct clients who have had mandibular immobilization or fixation after a mandibular fracture to keep wire cutters with them at all times.
- Apply oxygen to any client who develops stridor.
- Ensure that oxygen therapy delivered to the client is humidified (and warmed, when possible).
- Use a manual resuscitation bag to ventilate the client if the tracheostomy tube has dislodged or been decannulated.
- Assess the new tracheostomy stoma site at least once per shift for purulent drainage, redness, pain, and swelling, as indicators of infection.
- Keep the tracheal cuff pressure between 14 and 20 mm Hg to prevent tissue injury.
- Teach clients receiving radiation therapy how to care for the skin in the radiation path (see Chart 28-2).

ADDITIONAL STUDY RESOURCES

Go to your Student CD-ROM for Review Questions for the NCLEX Examination.

evolve Go to http://evolve.elsevier.com/Iggy/ for Integrated Management of Care Questions for the NCLEX Examination.

SELECTED BIBLIOGRAPHY

Abernathy, W., et al. (2000). Nonmetallic fixation in elective maxillofacial surgery. *AORN Journal, 71*(1), 193-198.

American Cancer Society. (2005). *Cancer facts and figures, 2005.* 01-300M-No.5008.05. Atlanta: Author.

Astle, A., & Caufield, E. (2003). Bedside tracheostomy: A step by step guide. *RN, 66*(10), 41-45.

Bhattacharyya, N. (2002). Cancer of the nasal cavity. *Archives of Otolaryngology Head and Neck Surgery, 128,* 1079-1083.

Bruce, S. (2004). Radiation-induced xerostomia: How dry is your patient? *Clinical Journal of Oncology Nursing 8*(1), 61-67.

Cady. J. (2002). Laryngectomy: Beyond loss of voice–caring for the patient as a whole. *Clinical Journal of Oncology Nursing, 6*(6), 347-353.

Carr, M., et al. (2000). Communication after laryngectomy: An assessment of quality of life. *Otolaryngology C Head and Neck Surgery, 122*(1), 39-43.

Chasens, E., & Umlauf, M. (2003). Nocturia: A problem that disrupts sleep and predicts obstructive sleep apnea. *Geriatric Nursing, 24*(2), 76-81, 105.

Dochterman, J., & Bulechek, G. (Eds.). (2004). *Nursing interventions classification (NIC)* (4th ed.). St. Louis: Mosby.

Ebersole, P., Hess, P., & Luggen, A. (2004). *Toward healthy aging: Human needs and nursing response* (6th ed.). St. Louis: Mosby.

Edwards, S., & Metheny, N. (2000). Measurement of gastric residual volume: State of the science. *MEDSURG Nursing, 9*(3), 125-128.

Facts and Comparisons. (2004). *Drug facts and comparisons* (58th ed.). St. Louis: Author.

Happ, M.B., Roesch, T., & Kagan, S. (2004). Communication needs, methods, and perceived voice quality following head and neck surgery: A literature review. *Cancer Nursing, 27*(1), 1-9.

Harrahill, M. (2002). Tracheobronchial injuries. *Journal of Emergency Nursing, 28*(3), 265-266.

Jagim, M. (2003). Airway management: Rapid-sequence intubation in trauma patients. *American Journal of Nursing, 103*(10), 32-35.

Koliha, C. (2003). Obstructive sleep apnea in head and neck cancer patients post-treatment...Something to consider? *ORL Head and Neck Nursing, 21*(1), 10-14.

Lennie, T., Christman, S., & Jadack, R. (2001). Educational needs and altered eating habits following a total laryngectomy. *Oncology Nursing Forum, 28*(4), 667-674.

Levin, W., & Parraga, M. (2002). The current management of epistaxis. *The Clinical Advisor November/December 2002*, 33-40.
Marchiondo, K. (2000). Pickwickian syndrome: The challenge of severe sleep apnea. *MEDSURG Nursing, 9*(4), 183-188.
McCance, K., & Huether, S. (2002). *Pathophysiology: The biologic basis for disease in adults and children* (4th ed.). St. Louis: Mosby.
Merritt, S., & Berger, B. (2004). Obstructive sleep apnea-hypoapnea syndrome. *American Journal of Nursing, 104*(7), 49-52.
Metheny, N., & Titler, M. (2001). Assessing placement of feeding tubes. *American Journal of Nursing, 101*(5), 36-45.
Moorhead, S., Johnson, M., & Maas, M. (Eds.). (2004). *Nursing outcomes classification (NOC)* (3rd ed.). St. Louis: Mosby.
Pagana, K., & Pagana, T. (2002). *Mosby's manual of diagnostic and laboratory tests* (2nd ed.). St. Louis: Mosby.
Perkins, L., & Shortall, S. (2000). Ventilation without intubation. *RN, 63*(1), 34-38.
Prettyman, A. (2001). Obstructive sleep apnea: Diagnosis and management. *The American Journal for Nurse Practitioners, 5*(8), 27-32.
Pruitt, W., & Jacobs, M. (2003). Basics of oxygen therapy. *Nursing 2003, 33*(10), 43-45.
Pullen, R. (2003). Caring for a patient on pulse oximetry. *Nursing 2003, 33*(9), 30.
Pullen, R. (2004). Measuring gastric residual volume. *Nursing 2004, 34*(4), 18.
Schoem, S. (2000). Oral appliances for the treatment of snoring and obstructive sleep apnea. *Otolaryngology C Head and Neck Surgery, 122*(2), 259-262.
Shellenbarger, T. (2000). Nosebleeds: Not just kids = stuff. *RN, 63*(2), 50-54, 56.
Stansberry, T. (2001). Narcolepsy: Unveiling a mystery. *American Journal of Nursing, 101*(8), 50-53.
St. John, R. (2004). Airway management. *Critical Care Nursing,* 24(2), 93-96.
Tate, J., & Tasota, F. (2002). More than a snore: Recognizing the danger of sleep apnea. *Nursing2002, 32*(8), 46-49.
Yantis, M. (2002). Obstructive sleep apnea syndrome. *American Journal of Nursing, 102*(6), 83-85.

CHAPTER 33

Interventions for Clients with Noninfectious Problems of the Lower Respiratory Tract

M. LINDA WORKMAN

LEARNING OUTCOMES

After studying this chapter, you should be able to:

1. Explain the differences in pathophysiology between asthma from bronchospasm, and asthma from inflammation.
2. Prioritize educational needs for the client at step III of stepped therapy for asthma.
3. Interpret peak expiratory rate flow (PERF) readings for the need for intervention.
4. Discuss the complications of chronic oral steroid therapy for treatment of chronic airflow limitation (CAL).
5. Compare the pathophysiology and clinical manifestations of asthma, bronchitis, and emphysema.
6. Identify risk factors for chronic obstructive pulmonary disease (COPD).
7. Prioritize educational needs for the client with COPD who is receiving oxygen therapy at home.
8. Describe the mechanisms of action, side effects, and nursing implications for pharmacologic management of COPD.
9. Describe interventions for energy conservation for the client with COPD.
10. Prioritize nursing care needs for the client immediately following lung volume reduction surgery.
11. Explain the nutritional needs for the client with COPD.
12. Use laboratory data and clinical manifestations to determine the effectiveness of therapy for impaired gas exchange in a client with obstructive or restrictive breathing problems.
13. Identify the risk factors for lung cancer.
14. Compare the side effects of radiation treatment for lung cancer with those of chemotherapy for lung cancer.
15. Explain how to troubleshoot the chest tube drainage system in a client 1 day after a thoracotomy.
16. Develop a community-based teaching plan for a client getting ready to go home after a pneumonectomy.

Go to your Student CD-ROM for Review Questions for the NCLEX Examination keyed to these Learning Outcomes.

Lower airway problems directly affect gas exchange and have serious consequences. Many of these problems are chronic and progressive, requiring major changes in a person's lifestyle. The older client with an airway problem may need special help even before the disorder becomes severe. Chart 33-1 lists nursing issues for the older client with a respiratory problem.

CHRONIC AIRFLOW LIMITATION

Chronic airflow limitation (CAL) is group of chronic lung diseases that includes asthma, chronic bronchitis, and pulmonary emphysema. Emphysema and chronic bronchitis, termed **chronic obstructive pulmonary disease (COPD),** are characterized by bronchospasm and dyspnea (Figure 33-1).

CHART 33-1

NURSING FOCUS on the OLDER ADULT
Respiratory Disorders

- Provide rest periods between such activities as bathing, meals, and ambulation.
- Place the client in an upright position for meals to prevent aspiration.
- Encourage nutritional fluid intake after the meal to promote increased calorie intake.
- Schedule medications around routine activities to increase medication adherence.
- Arrange chairs in strategic locations to allow the client with dyspnea to walk and rest as needed.
- Encourage prompt access to a health care facility for any manifestation of infection.
- Ensure that the client has received the pneumococcal vaccine.
- Encourage the client to have an annual flu vaccination.

The tissue damage is not reversible and increases in severity, eventually leading to respiratory failure. Asthma, unlike COPD, is an intermittent disease with *reversible* airflow obstruction and wheezing.

More than 40 million Americans suffer from some form of CAL, and 1 million people between the ages of 40 and 65 years have moderate to severe disability from CAL. Although some problems are not reversible, good management strategies can help maintain optimal functioning and improve overall health (see the Meeting Healthy People 2010 Objectives box at right).

Meeting HEALTHY PEOPLE 2010 Objectives

RESPIRATORY DISEASES

Objective 24.2: Reduce the overall asthma morbidity, as measured by a reduction in asthma hospitalization rates to 10 per 10,000 people.

- Teach the client with asthma to develop an asthma action plan in conjunction with their primary health care provider.
- Assist clients with asthma who smoke to reduce or quit smoking.
- Instruct the client with asthma in the correct technique for use of an inhaler.
- Educate clients with asthma that taking asthma medications as prescribed can reduce asthma exacerbations and morbidity.
- Teach the client with asthma to correctly use a peak flow meter.
- Assist the client with asthma to identify personal triggers for asthma attacks.
- Instruct the client with asthma how to adjust medications based on peak flow readings and expected exposures to environments or activities likely to trigger an asthma attack.
- Instruct clients with asthma to obtain annual vaccinations against influenza
- Remind clients to avoid secondhand smoke.

Objective 24.14: Reduce to no more than 3% the proportion of adults 45+ with chronic obstructive pulmonary disease.

- Educate clients who smoke cigarettes to reduce or quit smoking.
- Teach clients who have occupations or hobbies that cause exposure to inhalation irritants to use respiratory protection.
- Encourage clients with a family history of emphysema to be tested for $alpha_1$ antitrypsin deficiency.
- Teach clients the importance of seeing a health care provider promptly for any new or persistent respiratory symptoms.

Asthma

PATHOPHYSIOLOGY

Bronchial asthma is an intermittent and reversible airflow obstruction affecting only the airways, not the alveoli (see Figure 33-1). Airway obstruction can occur in two ways: (1) inflammation, and (2) airway hyperresponsiveness (sometimes called "twitchy airways"). Inflammation obstructs the **lumen** (i.e., the inside) of airways. Airway hyperresponsiveness obstructs airways by constricting bronchial smooth muscle causing a narrowing of the airway from the outside. Airway inflammation can trigger bronchiolar hyperresponsiveness, and many people with asthma have both problems at the same time. Severe airway obstruction can be fatal. More than 5000 deaths from acute asthma occur in the United States each year (Centers for Disease Control and Prevention, 2003).

Etiology and Genetic Risk

Asthma may be classified into different types based on the events known to trigger the attacks; however, the pathophysiology is similar for all types of asthma. Inflammation of the mucous membranes lining the airways is a key event in triggering an asthma attack. Inflammation occurs in response to the presence of specific allergens; nonallergenic general irritants such as cold air, dry air, or fine airborne particles; microorganisms; and aspirin. Airway hyperresponsiveness can occur with exercise, an upper respiratory illness, and for unknown reasons. Asthma from inflammation or hyperresponsive airways may have a genetic component, although a specific gene or mutation has not yet been identified.

When asthma is well controlled, the airway changes are temporary and reversible. With poor control, chronic inflammation can lead to damage and hyperplasia of the bronchial epithelial cells and of the bronchial smooth muscle. When asthma attacks are frequent, even exposure to low levels of the triggering agent or event may stimulate an attack.

INFLAMMATION

For some people, allergens bind to specific antibody molecules (especially immunoglobulin E [IgE]). These molecules are attached to tissue cells called mast cells and white blood cells called basophils. These cells are filled with granules containing chemicals that can start local inflammatory responses (see Chapters 23 and 26). Some of these chemicals, such as histamine, start an immediate inflammatory response. Others, such as leukotriene, interleukin-4, and eotaxin, are slower and cause later, prolonged inflammatory responses. These chemicals also attract more white blood cells (eosinophils, macrophages, and basophils) to the area, which then release even more inflammatory-inducing chemicals **(mediators).**

When allergens bind to the IgE molecules on mast cells, chemicals are released that start inflammatory responses in the airway mucous membranes (see Figure 26-2). Responses include blood vessel dilation and capillary leak, leading to tissue swelling with increased secretions and mucus production. This is the most common cause of asthma and is termed **atopic asthma** (McCance & Huether, 2002).

Inflammation can also occur through general irritation rather than allergic responses. Although some of the same

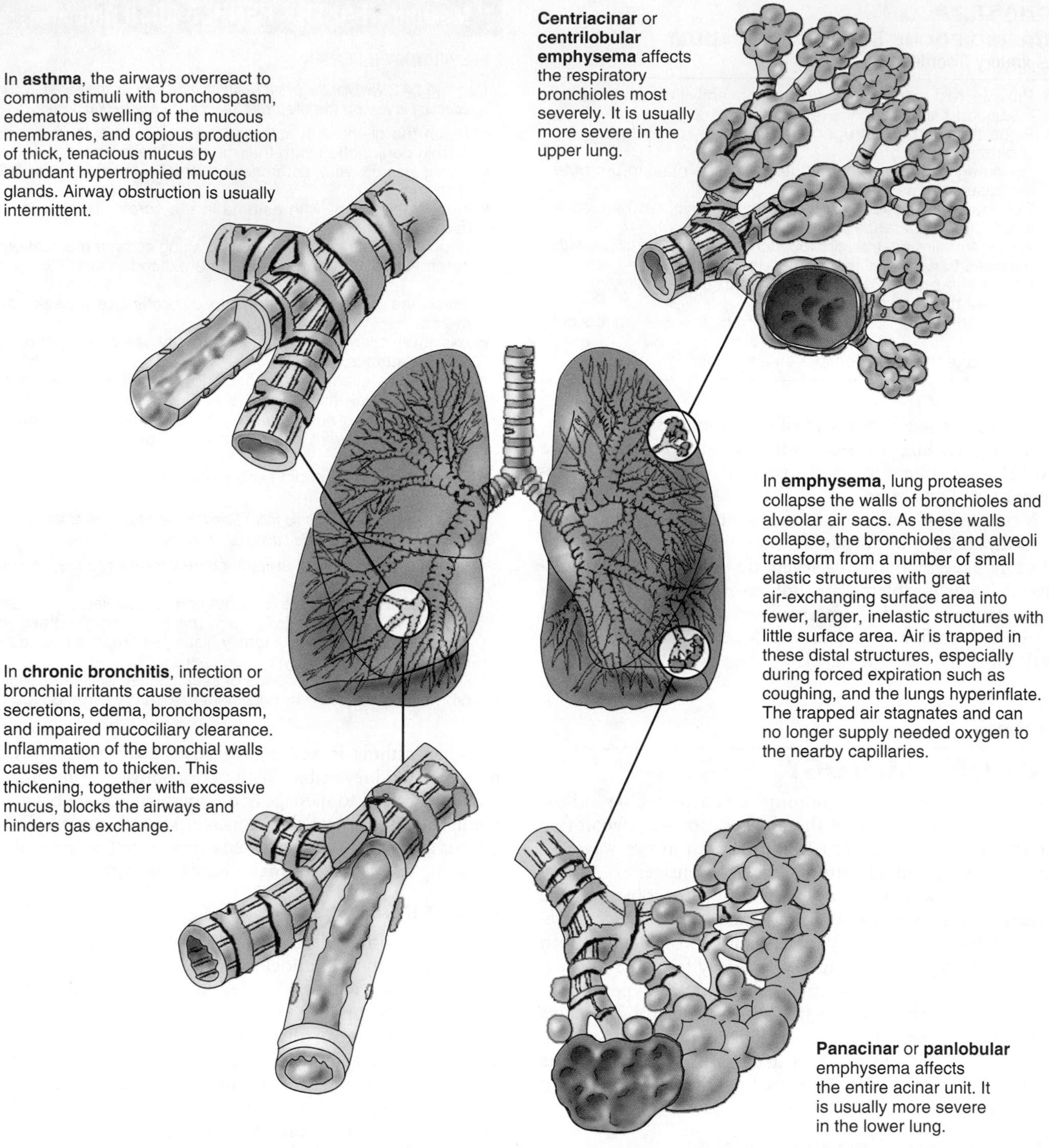

Figure 33-1 ■ The pathophysiology of chronic airflow limitation (CAL).

cells and chemicals cause this response, allergy therapy is not useful for general irritation-induced asthma.

BRONCHOSPASM

Hyperresponsive airways cause **bronchospasms,** narrowing of the bronchial tubes through constriction of the smooth muscle around and within the bronchial walls. In some people, small amounts of pollutants or respiratory viruses stimulate nerve fibers, causing constriction of bronchial smooth muscle. If these substances also stimulate an inflammatory response at the same time, the chemicals released during inflammation bind to smooth muscle receptors and cause constriction. Severe bronchospasm alone, especially in smaller bronchioles, can profoundly limit airflow to the alveoli.

ASPIRIN AND OTHER NONSTEROIDAL ANTI-INFLAMMATORY DRUGS

Some clients have asthma after taking aspirin and other nonsteroidal anti-inflammatory drugs (NSAIDs). This response is not a true allergy. It results from increased production of

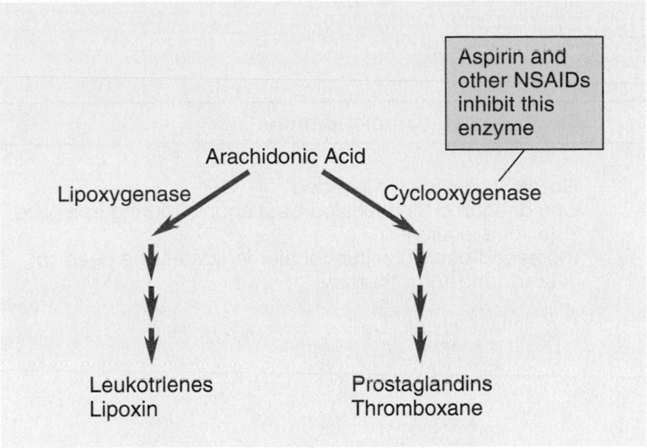

Figure 33-2 ■ Production pathways of inflammatory biochemicals.

leukotriene when other inflammatory pathways are suppressed. One chemical, arachidonic acid, can be converted into different substances when it is acted on by different enzymes. Aspirin and other NSAIDs inhibit the cyclooxygenase enzyme pathway. When this pathway is blocked, more arachidonic acid is available to be acted on by another enzyme, lipoxygenase, and changed to leukotriene (Figure 33-2).

Incidence/Prevalence

Asthma can occur at any age. About half of adults with asthma also had the disease in childhood. Asthma is more common in urban settings than in rural settings.

CONSIDERATIONS FOR OLDER ADULTS

Asthma occurs as a new disorder in about 3% of people older than 55 years of age. Another 3% of people older than 60 years of age have asthma as a continuing chronic disorder. Lung and airway changes as a part of aging make any breathing problem more serious in the older adult. One problem related to aging is a change in the sensitivity of beta-adrenergic receptors. When stimulated, these receptors relax smooth muscle and cause bronchodilation. As these receptors become less sensitive, they no longer respond as quickly or as strongly to agonists (epinephrine, dopamine) and beta-adrenergic drugs.

COLLABORATIVE MANAGEMENT

Assessment

Asthma is diagnosed and classified on the basis of the frequency and severity of the manifestations, as well as on the client's response to asthma drugs. These classes are the basis for current asthma therapy (Chart 33-2).

HISTORY

The client with asthma usually has a pattern of episodes of shortness of breath **(dyspnea),** chest tightness, coughing, wheezing, and increased mucus production. Ask whether the manifestations occur continuously, seasonally, in association with specific activities or exposures, or more frequently at night. Some clients notice these manifestations lasting 4 to 8 weeks after a chest cold or other upper respiratory tract infection. The client with atopic or allergic asthma may also have other allergic symptoms such as rhinitis, skin rash, or pruritus. Ask whether any other family members have asthma or respiratory problems. Ask about the client's current or previous smoking habits. Wheezing in nonsmokers is an important symptom in the diagnosis of asthma.

PHYSICAL ASSESSMENT/CLINICAL MANIFESTATIONS

The client with mild to moderate asthma may have no manifestations between asthma attacks. During an acute episode the most common manifestations are an audible wheeze and increased respiratory rate. The wheeze is louder on exhalation. When inflammation occurs with asthma, coughing may increase.

The client may use accessory muscles to help breathe during an attack. Observe for muscle retraction at the sternum, the suprasternal notch, and between the ribs. The client with long-standing, severe asthma may have a "barrel chest," caused by air trapping (Figure 33-3). The anteroposterior (AP) diameter (diameter between the front and the back of the chest) increases with air trapping, giving the chest a rounded rather than an oval shape. The normal chest is nearly twice as wide as it is thick. In the client with severe, chronic asthma, the AP diameter may equal or exceed the lateral diameter. Compare the AP diameter of the chest with the lateral diameter. Air trapping also increases the space between the ribs.

Along with an audible wheeze, the breathing cycle is longer and requires more effort. The client may be unable to complete a sentence of more than five words between breaths. Examine the oral mucosa and nail beds for cyanosis. Pulse oximetry shows poor oxygen saturation related to the degree of dyspnea. Other indicators of hypoxemia include changes in the level of consciousness and tachycardia.

LABORATORY ASSESSMENT

Laboratory tests can help determine the type of asthma and the degree of breathing impairment. Arterial blood gas (ABG) levels show how well the client is obtaining oxygen (see Chapter 19 for discussion of ABGs). The arterial oxygen level ($Pa{O_2}$) may decrease during an asthma attack. Early in the attack, the arterial carbon dioxide level ($Pa{CO_2}$) may be decreased as the client increases respiratory effort. Later in an asthma episode, $Pa{CO_2}$ rises, indicating carbon dioxide retention and poor gas exchange. Atopic asthma often occurs with an elevated serum eosinophil count and immunoglobulin E (IgE) levels. The sputum may contain eosinophils and mucous plugs with shed epithelial cells (Curschmann spirals).

PULMONARY FUNCTION TESTS

The most accurate tests for asthma are the pulmonary function tests (PFTs) measured using spirometry. Baseline PFTs are obtained for all clients diagnosed with asthma. The most important PFTs for a client with asthma are the **forced vital capacity (FVC)** (volume of air exhaled from full inhalation to full exhalation), **forced expiratory volume in the first second (FEV_1)** (volume of air blown out as hard and fast as possible during the first second of the most forceful exhalation after the greatest full inhalation), and **peak expiratory**

CHART 33-2

KEY FEATURES of
Asthma: The Step System

Clinical Manifestations	Treatment Recommendations
I. Mild Intermittent Symptoms or episodes occur twice per week or less. Client is symptom free between episodes/exacerbations. Episodes/exacerbations are short, lasting only a few hours. Symptoms are present at night no more frequently than twice per month. PFTs are normal between episodes. During episodes/exacerbations, FEV_1 or PEF is at least 80% of normal. PEF variability is less than 20%.	No daily medication needed Use of short-acting inhaled beta agonist during episodes (rescue inhaler) Increased use of rescue inhaler indicates the need to start long-term therapy
II. Mild Persistent Symptoms or episodes occur more than twice per week but not daily. Symptoms are present at night more than twice per month. During episodes/exacerbations, FEV_1 or PEF is at least 80% of normal. PEF variability is 20% to 30%. Activity is affected during episodes/exacerbations.	Use of a daily anti-inflammatory: Inhaled corticosteroid (CSC) Inhaled cromolyn Leukotriene antagonist Use of a rescue inhaler for relief during episodes
III. Moderate Persistent Symptoms occur daily. Symptoms or episodes occur more than twice per week and may persist for days. Client uses short-acting inhaled bronchodilator daily. Symptoms are present at night at least once per week. PEF variability is greater than 30%.	Daily use of inhaled CSC (low to moderate dose) Use of long-acting inhaled beta agonist (bronchodilator) Use of a rescue inhaler for relief during episodes (daily use means the client should be evaluated for progression to step IV)
IV. Severe Persistent Symptoms are continuously present. Episodes/exacerbations are frequent. During episodes/exacerbations, FEV_1 or PEF is less than 60% of normal. Physical activity is limited. Symptoms are frequently present at night. PEF variability is greater than 30%.	Daily use of inhaled CSC (high dose) Daily use of long-acting inhaled bronchodilator Frequent courses of systemic corticosteroids May include systemic methylxanthines

Modified from National Institutes of Health. (1997). *Guidelines for the diagnosis and management of asthma.* Expert panel report 2(97 4051). Bethesda, MD: U.S. Department of Health and Human Services.

PFTs, Pulmonary function tests; *PEF*, peak expiratory flow; *FEV_1*, volume of air blown out as hard and fast as possible during the first second of the most forceful exhalation after the greatest full inhalation.

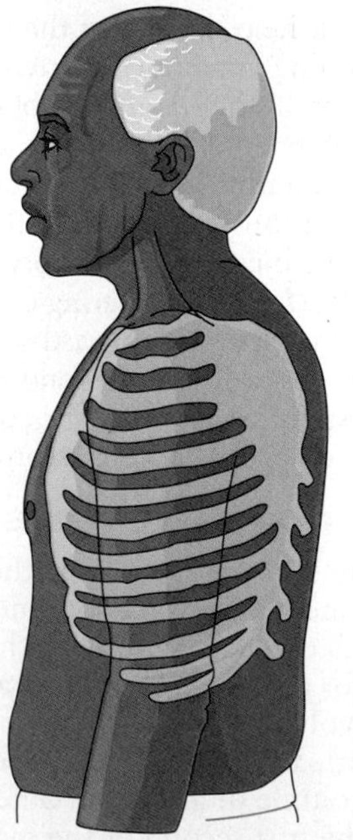

Figure 33-3 ■ Typical barrel chest in a client with chronic airflow limitation (CAL).

rate flow (PERF) (fastest airflow rate reached at any time during exhalation). A decrease in either the FEV_1 or the PERF of 15% to 20% below the expected value for age, gender, and size is common for the client with asthma. An increase of 12% in these values after treatment with bronchodilators is diagnostic for asthma. Airway responsiveness is tested by measuring the PERF and FEV_1 before and after the client inhales the drug methacholine, which induces bronchospasm in susceptible people.

OTHER DIAGNOSTIC ASSESSMENTS

Chest x-rays may be used to rule out other causes of dyspnea or to track changes in chest structure over time. For the client taking theophylline, blood drug levels are used to determine whether a therapeutic level is being maintained.

Interventions

The goals of asthma therapy are to improve airflow, relieve symptoms, and prevent episodes. Adult asthma is best managed when the client is an active partner in the management plan. The successful management plan includes client education, drug therapy, and lifestyle management, including exercise. Chart 33-3 lists NIC intervention activities for the client with asthma.

CHART 33-3

NIC **INTERVENTION ACTIVITIES for**
The Client with Asthma

Asthma Management: *Identification, treatment, and prevention of reactions to inflammation/constriction in the airway passages.*

- Determine baseline respiratory status to use as a comparison point.
- Document baseline measurements in clinical record.
- Compare current status with previous status to detect changes in respiratory status.
- Monitor peak expiratory flow rate (PERF), as appropriate.
- Educate client about the use of PERF meter at home.
- Determine client/family understanding of disease and management.
- Instruct client/family on antiinflammatory and bronchodilator medications and their appropriate use.
- Teach proper techniques for using medication and equipment (e.g., inhaler, nebulizer, peak flow meter).
- Determine compliance with prescribed treatments.
- Assist in the recognition of signs/symptoms of impending asthmatic reaction and implementation of appropriate response measures.
- Monitor rate, rhythm, depth, and effort of respiration.
- Observe chest movement, including symmetry, use of accessory muscles, and supraclavicular and intercostal muscle retractions.
- Administer medications as appropriate and/or per policy and procedural guidelines.
- Auscultate lung sounds after treatment to determine results.
- Use a calm reassuring approach during asthma attack.

NIC intervention activities selected from Dochterman, J.M., & Bulechek, G.M. (Eds.). (2004). *Nursing interventions classification (NIC)* (4th ed.). St. Louis: Mosby. No part of this work is to be altered without prior written permission from the Publisher.

CHART 33-4

CLIENT EDUCATION GUIDE
Asthma

- Avoid potential environmental asthma triggers, such as smoke, fireplaces, dust, mold, and weather changes (especially warm to cold or sudden barometric changes).
- Avoid medications that could trigger asthma (e.g., aspirin, nonsteroidal anti-inflammatory drugs [NSAIDs], and beta blockers).
- Avoid food that has been prepared with monosodium glutamate (MSG) or metabisulfite.
- If you experience symptoms of exercise-induced asthma, use your bronchodilator inhaler 30 minutes before exercise to prevent or reduce bronchospasm.
- Be sure you know the proper technique and correct sequence when you use metered dose inhalers.
- Be sure to get adequate rest and sleep.
- Reduce stress and anxiety; learn relaxation techniques; adopt coping mechanisms that have worked for you in the past.
- Wash all bedding with hot water to destroy dust mites.
- Monitor your peak expiratory flow rates as you were instructed.
- Seek immediate emergency care if you experience any of the following:
  - Gray or blue fingertips or lips
  - Difficulty breathing, walking, or talking
  - Retractions of the neck, chest, or ribs
  - Nasal flaring
  - Failure of medications to control worsening symptoms
  - Peak expiratory rate flow declining steadily after treatment, or a flow rate 50% below your usual flow rate

Client Education. Asthma is often an intermittent disease. With guided self-care, clients can co-manage this disease, increasing symptom-free periods and decreasing the number and severity of attacks. Such management decreases the number of hospital admissions and increases participation in client-chosen pleasure, work, and family activities. Overall improved management through guided self-care has been shown to decrease health care costs. Self-care requires extensive education for the client to be able to self-treat (including adjusting the frequency and dosage of prescribed drugs) and determine when to consult the health care provider. Teach the client to assess symptom severity at least twice daily with a peak flow meter and adjust drugs to manage inflammation and bronchospasms to prevent or relieve symptoms. Education involves a specified drug therapy plan that is tailored to meet the personal pattern of asthma for the client. The client keeps a symptom and intervention diary to learn his or her triggers of asthma symptoms, early cues for impending attacks, and personal response to drugs. Proper use of an asthma action plan is helpful for any severity of asthma. Chart 33-4 lists areas to emphasize when teaching the client with asthma.

Drug Therapy. Pharmacologic management of adult clients with asthma is based on the step category for severity and treatment (see Chart 33-2). Some may need drug therapy only during an asthma episode. For others, daily drugs are needed to keep asthma episodic rather than a more frequent problem. This therapy involves the use of bronchodilators, steroidal and nonsteroidal agents to reduce inflammation, mast cell stabilizers, monoclonal antibodies, and drugs that inhibit the release or action of leukotrienes. Thus some drugs reduce the response, and other drugs actually prevent the response. Some drugs combine two agents from different classes for better response. Chart 33-5 lists common agents used for preventive and symptomatic therapy of asthma.

Bronchodilators. Bronchodilators increase bronchiolar smooth muscle relaxation. They have no effect on inflammatory processes. Thus when a client with asthma has airflow obstruction by both bronchospasm and inflammation, at least two types of drug therapy are needed. Bronchodilators work by stimulating the beta$_2$-adrenergic receptors on bronchial smooth muscle in the same way that the sympathetic nervous system transmitters, epinephrine and norepinephrine, do. These drugs include beta$_2$ agonists, cholinergic antagonists, and methylxanthines

Beta$_2$ Agonists. Beta$_2$ agonists bind to the beta$_2$-adrenergic receptors and cause an increase in the intracellular level of a substance called cyclic adenosine monophosphate (cAMP). This substance triggers smooth muscle relaxation.

SHORT-ACTING BETA$_2$ AGONISTS. Short-acting beta$_2$ agents provide rapid but short-term relief. These inhaled drugs are most useful when an attack begins or as premedication when the client is about to begin an activity that is likely to induce an asthma attack. Such agents include albuterol (Proventil, Ventolin), bitolterol (Tornalate), and pirbuterol (Maxair). When inhaled from either a metered dose inhaler (MDI) or a dry powder inhaler (DPI), the drug is delivered directly to the site of action and systemic effects are minimal (unless the agent is overused or abused). Teach the client the correct technique to use with an inhaled drug to

CHART 33-5

DRUG THERAPY for Asthma

Drug	Usual Dosage	Nursing Interventions	Rationales
Bronchodilators			
Short-Acting Beta$_2$ Agonists			
Albuterol (Proventil, Ventolin)	1-2 inhalations q4-6h (90 mcg/inhaled dose)	Teach client to monitor heart rate.	Excessive use causes systemic symptoms, especially tachycardia.
		Increase water/fluid intake.	Chronic use increases mouth and throat dryness.
		Instruct client to use bronchodilator at least 5 min before other inhaled drugs.	Bronchodilation allows better penetration of other inhaled drugs.
		Teach client the correct technique for using the inhaler and obtain a return demonstration.	Correct technique is essential in getting the medication to the site of action. If the client does not inhale during medication delivery, drug exits the nose or is swallowed.
Bitolterol (Tornalate)	2 inhalations q8h (370 mcg/inhalation)	Same as for albuterol.	Same as for albuterol.
Pirbuterol (Maxair)	1-2 inhalations q4-6h (200 mcg/inhalation)	Same as for albuterol.	Same as for albuterol.
Long-Acting Beta$_2$ Agonists			
Salmeterol (Serevent)	2 inhalations q12h (≈25 mcg/inhalation with an aerosol inhaler) (50 mcg/inhalation with a dry powder inhaler)	Do not use to relieve acute symptoms.	Drug has slow onset of action.
		Shake inhaler well before using.	Drug separates easily.
		Teach client not to exhale into device.	Exhaling into device moistens the drug and causes clumping.
Formoterol fumarate (Foradil Aerolizer)	1 inhalation q12h (12 mcg/inhalation with dry powder inhaler)	Same as for salmeterol.	Same as for salmeterol.
Methylxanthines			
Theophylline (Theo-Dur, Uniphyl, Theolair, Bronkodyl)	10-12 mg/kg/day PO (loading dose)	Monitor drug levels.	Drug has narrow therapeutic range and many toxicities.
	Maintenance dose is usually 200-800 mg daily	Space doses equally throughout the 24-hr day.	Maintains more even blood drug levels.
		Observe client for nausea, vomiting, diarrhea, tachycardia, dysrhythmias, restlessness.	These are symptoms of toxicity.
		Teach client to avoid caffeine intake while on this drug.	Caffeine potentiates side effects.
		Encourage client to take as prescribed daily.	Efficacy is related to continued correct use.
		Teach client to take oral dose with meals.	Food reduces GI irritation.
		Administer IV doses using a pump or controller.	A pump or controller prevents accidental overdose.
Aminophylline (Truphylline)	Loading dose: 5-7 mg/kg IV Maintenance dose: 0.5-1.2 mg/kg/hr	Observe for skin rash or sloughing.	A drug component, ethylenediamine, can cause severe skin reactions.
		Same as for theophylline.	Drug is 80% theophylline.
Oxtriphylline (Apo-Oxtriphylline✱, Choledyl)	75-150 mg PO four times daily	Same as for theophylline.	Drug contains significant amounts of theophylline.
Cholinergic Antagonists			
Ipratropium (Atrovent, Apo-Ipravent✱)	2-4 inhalations 4-6 times daily 18 mcg/inhalation	Shake container well.	Drug separates on standing.
		Increase water/fluid intake.	Drug causes mouth dryness.
		Teach client to observe for blurred vision, eye pain, headache, nausea, nervousness, palpitations.	These are systemic symptoms of overdose.

Data from Facts and Comparisons. (2004). *Drug facts and comparisons* (58th ed.). St. Louis: Wolters Kluwer.
SC, Subcutaneous.

CHART 33-5

DRUG THERAPY for Asthma—*cont'd*

Drug	Usual Dosage	Nursing Interventions	Rationales
Anti-Inflammatories			
Corticosteroids—Oral			
Prednisolone (Cotolone, Delta-Cortef)	5-40 mg daily	Not recommended unless symptoms are severe or debilitating.	Systemic side effects are common and serious: ▪ GI ulceration ▪ Poor wound healing ▪ Decreased immune function ▪ Increased risk for infections ▪ Weight gain ▪ Hyperglycemia ▪ Personality changes ▪ Fluid retention
Prednisone (Deltasone, Prednicot, Orasone, Pred-Pak)	5-60 mg daily	Same as for prednisolone.	Same as for prednisolone.
Corticosteroids—Inhaler			
Budesonide (Pulmicort)	200 mcg/inhalation (dry powder inhaler)	Use daily as directed.	Effectiveness depends on regular use.
		Symptoms may persist for 2-3 days after initial administration.	Maximum effectiveness requires continued use for 48-72 hr.
		Observe mouth and throat for lesions.	Excessive use decreases local immune response and increases susceptibility to oral infections, especially candidiasis.
Fluticasone (Flovent)	2 metered sprays daily (50 mcg/metered spray) (100-250 mcg per Rotadisk dry powder inhaler)	Same as for budesonide.	Same as for budesonide.
Beclomethasone (Vanceril, Beclovent, Qvar ✱, Becloforte ✱)	2-4 inhalations three to four times daily (42 mcg/inhalation)	Same as for budesonide.	Same as for budesonide.
Triamcinolone (Azmacort)	2 inhalations three to four times daily (100 mcg/inhalation)	Same as for budesonide.	Same as for budesonide.
Flunisolide (AeroBid, Bronalide ✱)	2 inhalations twice daily (250 mcg/inhalation)	Same as for budesonide.	Same as for budesonide.
Leukotriene Antagonists			
Zafirlukast (Accolate)	20 mg twice daily	Take 1 hr before or 2 hr after eating.	Drug absorption is slowed by presence of food.
		Incidence of upper respiratory infections is increased when co-administered with inhaled corticosteroids.	Drugs reduce local inflammatory and immune responses.
		Reduce dose in clients also taking aspirin.	Aspirin increases plasma concentration of drug.
Zileuton (Zyflo)	600 mg four times daily	Do not take with terfenadine or theophylline.	Drug increases plasma concentrations of terfenadine and theophylline.
Montelukast (Singulair)	10 mg daily	Do not abruptly substitute for oral or inhaled steroids.	Drug requires time to peak action.
		Reduce dose in clients with hepatic impairment.	Hepatic impairment prolongs blood levels of drug.
Inhaled Anti-Inflammatory			
Nedocromil (Tilade)	2 inhalations q6h (2 mg/inhalation)	Not for use during acute attack.	Drug has slow onset to peak action.
		Instruct client to use daily even when no symptoms are present.	Efficacy is related to continued correct use.
		Discontinue use if symptoms worsen with drug.	Client may be sensitive to propellants.

Continued

CHART 33-5

DRUG THERAPY for Asthma—*cont'd*

Drug	Usual Dosage	Nursing Interventions	Rationales
Combination Agents			
Fluticasone and salmeterol (Advair Diskus)	1 inhalation q12h 250/50 (250 mcg of fluticasone with 50 mcg of salmeterol) 500/50 (500 mcg of fluticasone with 50 mcg of salmeterol)	Same as for each agent alone.	Same as for each agent alone.
Ipratropium and albuterol (Combivent)	2 inhalations four times daily (18 mcg ipratropium with 103 mcg albuterol)	Same as for each agent alone.	Same as for each agent alone.
Mast Cell Stabilizers			
Cromolyn sodium (Intal)	1-2 inhalations four times daily	Use daily as directed.	Effectiveness depends on regular use.
		Start therapy 3-4 wk before expected allergy season.	Requires regular use for prophylactic effect.
Monoclonal Antibodies			
Omalizumab (Xolair)	150-375 mg SC every 3-4 wk	Assess client for anaphylaxis for the first 2 hr after injection.	Some clients have allergies to the mouse parts of the antibody.
		Not for use during acute attack.	Drug has slow onset to peak action.
		Roll vial gently for 10-20 min until drug is no longer gel-like.	Drug is slow to dissolve.

Data from Facts and Comparisons. (2004). *Drug facts and comparisons* (58th ed.). St. Louis: Author.
SC, Subcutaneous.

achieve the greatest benefit from the drug. Chart 33-6 describes the proper way to use an MDI. Figure 33-4 shows a client using a "spacer" with an MDI inhaler. Chart 33-7 describes the proper care and use of a DPI. Figure 33-5 shows a client using a DPI.

LONG-ACTING BETA$_2$ AGONISTS. Long-acting beta$_2$ agonists are also delivered by inhaler directly to the site of action: the bronchioles. Unlike short-acting agonists, long-acting drugs need time to build up an effect, but the effects are longer lasting. Thus these drugs are useful in preventing an asthma attack but have no value during an acute attack. Proper use of the long-acting agonists can decrease reliance on short-acting agonists.

Cholinergic Antagonists. Cholinergic antagonists, sometimes called anticholinergic drugs, are similar to atropine and block the parasympathetic nervous system. This blockade allows the sympathetic nervous system to dominate, resulting in increased bronchodilation and decreased pulmonary secretions. The most common drug in this class is ipratropium (Atrovent), which is used as an inhalant. Most cholinergic antagonists are short acting and must be used several times a day. Tiotropium is a new long-acting drug for use once a day (Boyle & Locke, 2004).

Methylxanthines. Methylxanthines are used when other types of management are ineffective. The classic drug in this class is theophylline (Theo-Dur). Other drugs include aminophylline (Truphylline), oxtriphylline (Choledyl✱), and dyphylline (Dilor, Lufyllin). These drugs are given systemically, have narrow therapeutic ranges, and have many side effects. Blood levels of these drugs need to be monitored closely because the drug level that causes dangerous side effects is not much higher than the level needed to dilate the bronchioles. The most dangerous side effects result from excessive cardiac and central nervous system stimulation.

Anti-Inflammatory Agents. Anti-inflammatory agents decrease the inflammatory responses in the airways. Some are given systemically and have more side effects. Others are used as inhalants and have few systemic side effects.

Corticosteroids. Corticosteroids decrease inflammatory and immune responses in many ways, including by preventing the synthesis of mediators. Local corticosteroids in inhaled sprays can be helpful in preventing the manifestations of asthma. Newer high-potency steroid inhalers, such as fluticasone (Flovent) and budesonide (Pulmicort), may be used once per day for maintenance. Systemic corticosteroids, because of severe side effects, are avoided for mild to moderate asthma and are used on a short-term basis for moderate asthma. For some clients with severe asthma, daily systemic corticosteroids may be needed.

Inhaled Anti-Inflammatory Agents. A newer category of nonsteroidal inhaled anti-inflammatory agent is nedocromil (Tilade). This agent inhibits the release of inflammatory mediators from respiratory cells and white blood cells. In addition, it reduces nerve stimulation in the lung. These actions prevent asthma episodes rather than reversing an episode.

Mast Cell Stabilizers. Inhaled sprays containing mast cell stabilizers, such as cromolyn sodium (Intal), prevent mast cell membranes from opening when an allergen binds to IgE. Thus these drugs help prevent atopic asthma attacks but are not useful during an acute episode.

Monoclonal Antibodies. This new drug class was approved in 2003. Omalizumab (Xolair) binds to the IgE re-

CHART 33-6

CLIENT EDUCATION GUIDE
How to Use an Inhaler Correctly*

Without a Spacer (Preferred Technique)
1. Before each use, remove the cap and shake the inhaler according to the instructions in the package insert.
2. Tilt your head back slightly and breathe out fully.
3. Open your mouth and place the mouthpiece 1 to 2 inches away.
4. As you begin to breathe in deeply through your mouth, press down firmly on the canister of the inhaler to release one dose of medication.
5. Continue to breathe in slowly and deeply (usually over 3 to 5 seconds).
6. Hold your breath for at least 10 seconds to allow the medication to reach deep into the lungs, then breathe out slowly.
7. Wait at least 1 minute between puffs.
8. Replace the cap on the inhaler.
9. At least once a day, remove the canister and clean the plastic case and cap of the inhaler by thoroughly rinsing in warm, running tap water.

Without a Spacer (Alternative Method)
1. Follow steps 1 and 2 above.
2. Place the mouthpiece into your mouth, over your tongue, and seal your lips tightly around it.
3. Follow steps 4 to 9 above.

With a Spacer
1. Before each use, remove the caps from the inhaler and the spacer.
2. Insert the mouthpiece of the inhaler into the non-mouthpiece end of the spacer.
3. Shake the whole unit vigorously three or four times.
4. Place the mouthpiece into your mouth, over your tongue, and seal your lips tightly around it.
5. Press down firmly on the canister of the inhaler to release one dose of medication into the spacer.
6. Breathe in slowly and deeply. If the spacer makes a whistling sound, you are breathing in too rapidly.
7. Remove the mouthpiece from your mouth and, keeping your lips closed, hold your breath for at least 10 seconds, then breathe out slowly.
8. Wait at least 1 minute between puffs.
9. Replace the caps on the inhaler and the spacer.
10. At least once a day, clean the plastic case and cap of the inhaler by thoroughly rinsing in warm, running tap water; at least once a week, clean the spacer in the same manner.

*Avoid spraying in the direction of the eyes.

ceptor sites on mast cells and basophils. This action prevents allergens from triggering the release of mediators from mast cells and basophils. Thus these drugs help prevent atopic asthma attacks but are not useful during an acute episode.

Leukotriene Antagonists. Leukotriene antagonists work in several ways to prevent an asthma episode. Zileuton (Zyflo) prevents leukotriene synthesis. Zafirlukast (Accolate) and montelukast (Singulair) block the leukotriene receptor. All are oral drugs.

Exercise/Activity. Regular exercise, including aerobic exercise, is a recommended part of asthma therapy. Aerobic exercise assists in maintaining cardiac health, enhancing skeletal muscle strength, and promoting ventilation and perfusion. Clients with asthma need to examine the conditions that trigger an attack and adjust the exercise routine as needed. Some may need to premedicate with inhaled beta agonists before beginning activity. For others, adjusting the environment may be needed. For example, outdoor ice-skating

CHART 33-7

CLIENT EDUCATION GUIDE
How to Use a Dry Powder Inhaler (DPI)

For Inhalers Requiring Loading
First load the drug by:
- Turning the device to the next dose of drug, or
- Inserting the capsule into the device, or
- Inserting the disk or compartment into the device.

After Loading the Drug and for Inhalers That Do Not Require Drug Loading
- Read your doctor's instructions for how fast you should breathe for your particular inhaler.
- Place your lips over the mouthpiece and breathe in forcefully. (There is no propellant in the inhaler; only your breath pulls the drug in.)
- Remove the inhaler from your mouth as soon as you have breathed in.
- Never exhale (breathe out) into your inhaler. Your breath will moisten the powder, causing it to clump and not be delivered accurately.
- Never wash or place the inhaler in water.
- Never shake your inhaler.
- Keep your inhaler in a dry place at room temperature.
- If the inhaler is preloaded, discard the inhaler after it is empty.
- Because the drug is a dry powder and there is no propellant, you may not feel, smell, or taste it as you inhale.

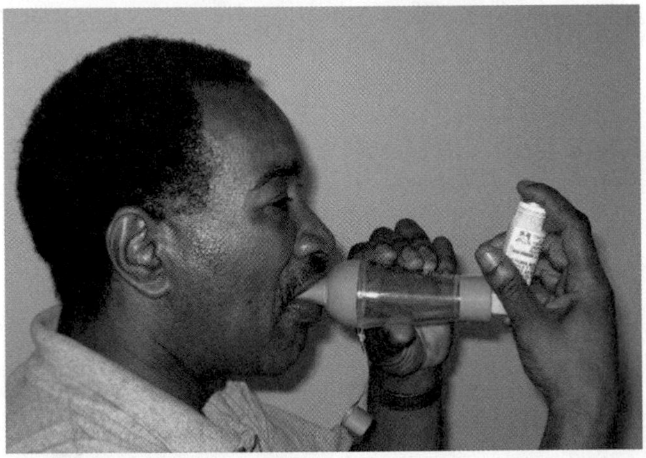

Figure 33-4 ■ Client using an aerosol inhaler with a spacer.

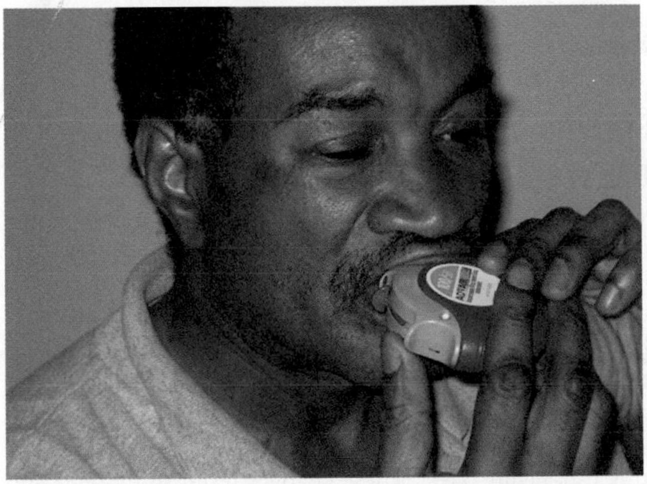

Figure 33-5 ■ Client using a dry powder inhaler (DPI).

in cold, dry air can trigger an attack; indoor ice-skating may be less of a problem. Sports that involve more "rest" action, such as baseball, are less likely to trigger symptoms than "nonrest" action sports, such as basketball.

Oxygen Therapy. Supplemental oxygen is often used during an acute asthma attack. Oxygen is delivered by mask, nasal cannula, or endotracheal tube. High flow rates or concentrations may be needed when bronchospasms are severe and limit flow of oxygen through the bronchiole tubes. Heliox, a mixture of helium and oxygen (often 50% helium and 50% oxygen) can help improve oxygen delivery to the alveoli. This gas mixture is lower in density than oxygen alone or oxygen with atmospheric air (which contains nitrogen) and flows even when airway resistance is high.

Status Asthmaticus. Status asthmaticus is a severe, life-threatening acute episode of airway obstruction that intensifies once it begins and often does not respond to common therapy. The client arrives in the emergency department with extremely labored breathing and wheezing. Use of accessory muscles for breathing and distention of neck veins are observed. If the condition is not reversed, the client may develop pneumothorax, and cardiac or respiratory arrest. The physician immediately prescribes intravenous (IV) fluids, potent systemic bronchodilators, steroids (to decrease inflammation), epinephrine, and oxygen in an attempt to reverse the acute condition. Prepare for emergency intubation. When wheezing decreases, management is similar to that for any client with asthma.

Critical Thinking Challenge

It is March in Minnesota. The client is a 22-year-old female college athlete who comes to the health clinic with audible wheezes on exhalation. She explains, between breaths, that she was running her normal 5 miles on the outdoor track when she started wheezing. She does have asthma and usually carries an albuterol inhaler with her when she runs. Today, she forgot her "rescue" inhaler but did take Advair one puff by DPI, 2 hours ago. Her vital signs are as follows: BP 132/92, P 68, R 34.

1. What additional assessment data should you obtain?
2. Should you start oxygen on this client? Why or why not?
3. Should she take another dose of Advair? Why or why not?
4. What is the probable cause of this client's asthma attack?
5. What should you teach her to help her avoid another episode?

evolve For suggested answer guidelines, go to http://evolve.elsevier.com/Iggy/.

Chronic Obstructive Pulmonary Disease

PATHOPHYSIOLOGY

Most clients with emphysema have chronic bronchitis at the same time, but each condition has its own pathophysiologic process (Figure 33-6).

Emphysema

ANATOMIC AND FUNCTIONAL CHANGES

The two major changes that occur with pulmonary emphysema are loss of lung elasticity and hyperinflation of the lung (see Figure 33-1). These changes result in dyspnea and the need for an increased respiratory rate.

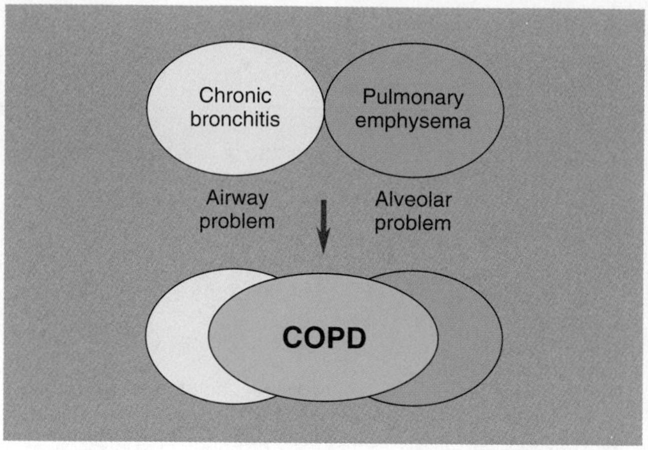

Figure 33-6 ■ The interaction of chronic bronchitis and emphysema in COPD.

Enzymes that degrade protein (proteases) damage the alveoli and the small airways by breaking down elastin. This causes the alveolar sacs to lose their elasticity and the small airways to collapse or narrow. Some alveoli are destroyed, and others become large and flabby, with decreased area for gas exchange.

An increased amount of air becomes trapped in the lungs. Causes of air trapping are loss of elastic recoil in the alveolar walls, overstretching and enlargement of the alveoli into air-filled spaces called bullae, and collapse of small airways (bronchioles). These changes greatly increase the work of breathing. The hyperinflated lung flattens the diaphragm (Figure 33-7), weakening the effect of this muscle. As a result, the client with emphysema needs to use additional muscles (accessory muscles) in the neck, chest wall, and abdomen to inhale and exhale. This increased effort increases the need for oxygen, making the client work harder and have an "air hunger" sensation. Often, inhalation starts before exhalation is completed, resulting in an uncoordinated pattern of breathing.

Gas exchange is affected by the increased work of breathing and the loss of alveolar tissue. Although some alveoli enlarge, the curves of alveolar walls decrease and there is less surface area available for gas exchange. Often the client adjusts by increasing the respiratory rate, so arterial blood gas (ABG) values may not show gas exchange problems until the client has advanced disease. Then carbon dioxide is produced faster than it can be eliminated, resulting in carbon dioxide retention and chronic respiratory acidosis (see Chapter 19). The client with late-stage emphysema also has a low arterial oxygen (PaO_2) level, because it is difficult for oxygen to move from diseased lung tissue into the bloodstream.

EMPHYSEMA CLASSIFICATION

Emphysema is classified as panlobular, centrilobular, or paraseptal depending on the pattern of destruction and dilation of the gas-exchanging units (acini) (see Figure 33-1). Each type can occur alone or in combination in the same lung.

Panlobular (panacinar) emphysema (PLE) has destruction of the entire alveolus uniformly. This type is diffuse and more severe in the lower lung areas.

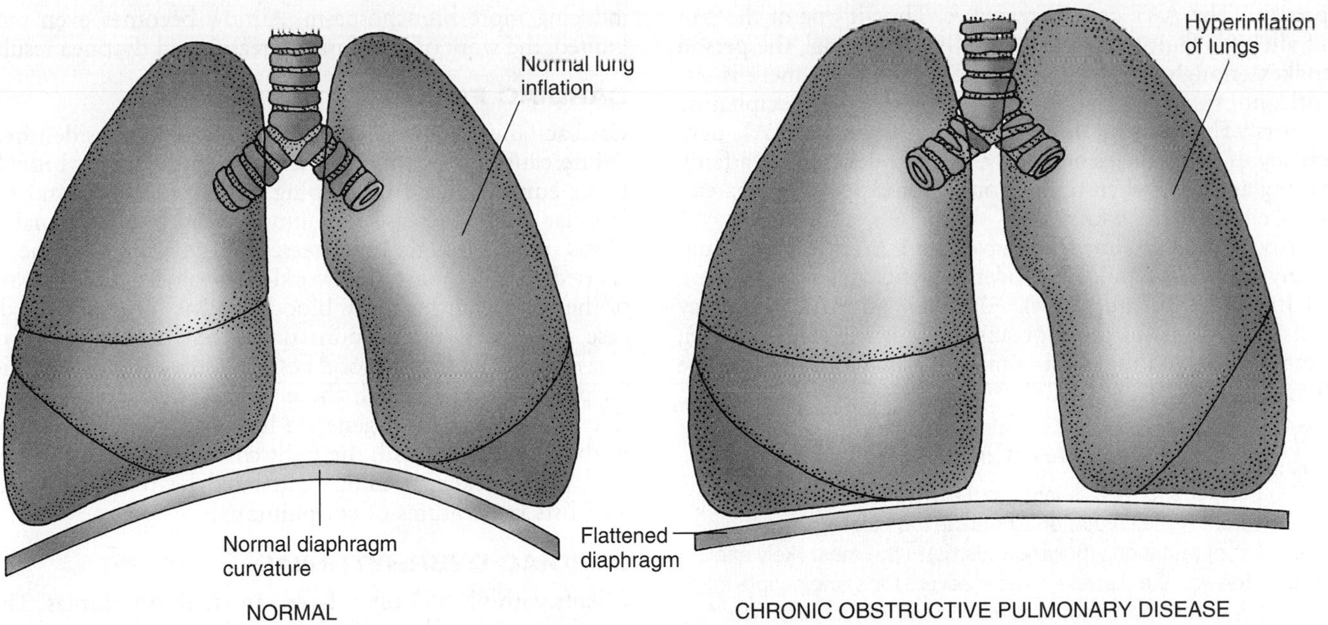

Figure 33-7 ■ Diaphragm shape and lung inflation in the normal client and in the client with chronic airflow limitation (CAL).

In centrilobular (centriacinar) emphysema (CLE), openings occur in the bronchioles and allow spaces to develop as tissue walls break down. Although this is a diffuse disease, the upper lung sections are most severely affected. This type of emphysema is often seen in long-standing cigarette smokers.

In paraseptal or distal acinar emphysema, the disease is confined to only the alveolar ducts and alveolar sacs. This type forms bullae and often affects the upper half of the lungs.

Chronic Bronchitis

Bronchitis is an inflammation of the bronchi and bronchioles caused by chronic exposure to irritants, especially tobacco smoke. The irritant triggers inflammation, with vasodilation, congestion, mucosal edema, and bronchospasm. Unlike emphysema, bronchitis affects only the airways rather than the alveoli.

Chronic inflammation causes an increase in the number and size of mucous glands, which produce large amounts of thick mucus. The bronchial walls thicken (often to twice the normal thickness) and impair airflow. This thickening, along with excessive mucus, blocks some of the smaller airways and narrows larger ones. Small airways are affected before large airways become involved.

Chronic bronchitis hinders airflow and gas exchange because of mucous plugs and infection narrowing the airways. As a result, the PaO_2 decreases (hypoxemia) and the arterial blood carbon dioxide level ($PaCO_2$) increases (respiratory acidosis).

Etiology and Genetic Risk

CIGARETTE SMOKING

Smoking is the most important risk factor for COPD. The client with an 8-pack-year history usually has obstructive lung changes but no manifestations of disease. The client with a 20-pack-year history or longer often has early stage COPD found as changes in pulmonary function tests (PFTs).

The harmful effects of tobacco result in part because inhaled smoke triggers the release of excessive amounts of the enzyme elastase protease from cells in the lungs. The elastase protease breaks down elastin, the major component of alveoli. By impairing the action of cilia, smoking also inhibits the cilia from clearing the bronchi of mucus, cellular debris, and fluid.

In addition to the increased risk for COPD from active smoking, passive smoking (or secondhand smoke) contributes to upper and lower respiratory problems. The risk is greater when exposure occurs in small, confined spaces.

> **CULTURAL CONSIDERATIONS**
>
> The prevalence of smoking remains higher among African-Americans, blue-collar workers, and less educated people than in the overall population of the United States. Smoking prevalence is highest among Northern Plains American Indians/Native Americans and Alaskan Natives. The overall prevalence of smoking for both men and women has decreased over the past two decades, but the decrease for women has been less than it has for men (American Cancer Society, 2005). Development of culturally appropriate smoking cessation programs as well as research examining barriers to cessation in these populations may help reduce this disparity.

ALPHA$_1$-ANTITRYPSIN DEFICIENCY

A special enzyme, alpha$_1$-antitrypsin (AAT), is made by the liver and is normally present in the lungs. One purpose of AAT is to regulate the other enzymes (proteases) that are present to break down inhaled pollutants and microorganisms. AAT prevents the proteases from working on lung structures.

The production of normal amounts of AAT is dependent on the inheritance of a pair of normal gene alleles for this protein. The AAT gene is recessive. Thus if one of the pair of alleles is faulty and the other allele is normal, the person makes enough AAT to prevent COPD unless there is significant exposure to cigarette smoke and other precipitating factors. This person, however, is a carrier for AAT deficiency. If both alleles are faulty, COPD develops at a fairly young age even when the person is not exposed to cigarette smoke or other irritants.

About 100,000 Americans have severe AAT deficiency, and many more have mild to moderate deficiencies (Nussbaum, McInnes, & Willard, 2001). Although an AAT deficiency causes problems in other organs, such as the skin and liver, lung diseases are the most common problem caused by the deficiency.

Genetic Considerations

The gene for AAT is large and many mutations have been discovered. Not all mutations increase the risk for emphysema. Variation of mutations (polymorphisms) is the most likely explanation for why the disease is more severe for some people than for others. The most serious mutation for an increased risk for emphysema is at the Z allele, although other mutations also increases the risk but to a lesser degree.

Replacement of the deficient enzyme is a promising new treatment. Currently, the enzyme can be replaced intravenously, with one dose maintaining blood levels for about a week. Delivery of the enzyme by aerosol inhaler is also being tried.

AIR POLLUTION

Air pollution alone plays only a relatively small role in the client with emphysema and chronic bronchitis. The effect of air pollution is additive to tobacco exposure.

Incidence/Prevalence

The prevalence of chronic bronchitis and emphysema in the United States has been estimated at about 13.5 million (for chronic bronchitis) and 2 million (for emphysema). Chronic obstructive pulmonary disease/chronic airflow limitation (COPD/CAL) is the fourth leading cause of death for women of all ages and is the fifth for men (Centers for Disease Control and Prevention, 2002).

Complications

COPD affects the delivery of oxygen to all tissues. Complications of the disorder can result in organ anoxia and tissue death. Major problems occur, such as hypoxemia, acidosis, respiratory infection, cardiac failure, and dysrhythmias.

HYPOXEMIA AND ACIDOSIS

As the client with COPD is less able to exchange gas, oxygenation decreases and carbon dioxide levels increase, leading to hypoxemia and acidosis. Thus most tissues have decreased function.

RESPIRATORY INFECTIONS

The client with COPD is at risk for respiratory infections from the increased mucus and poor oxygenation. The organisms most often causing bacterial infections include *Streptococcus pneumoniae, Haemophilus influenzae,* and *Moraxella catarrhalis.* Acute respiratory infections make COPD manifestations worse by increasing inflammation and mucus production, and inducing more bronchospasm. Airflow becomes even more limited, the work of breathing increases, and dyspnea results.

CARDIAC FAILURE

Cardiac failure, especially **cor pulmonale** (right-sided heart failure caused by pulmonary disease), occurs with bronchitis or emphysema. Air trapping, airway collapse, and stiff alveolar walls increase the lung tissue pressure, making blood flow through lung vessels more difficult. The increased pressure makes the workload heavy on the right side of the heart, which pumps blood into the lungs. As the disease progresses, the amount of oxygen in the blood decreases, causing major blood vessels in the lung to constrict. To pump blood through these narrowed vessels, the right side of the heart must generate high pressures. In response to this heavy workload, the right chambers of the heart enlarge and thicken, causing right-sided heart failure. Chart 33-8 lists key features of cor pulmonale.

CARDIAC DYSRHYTHMIAS

Clients with COPD often have cardiac dysrhythmias. They may be a result of hypoxemia (from decreased oxygen to the heart muscle), other cardiac disease, drug effects, or acidosis.

HEALTH PROMOTION/ILLNESS PREVENTION

Health experts agree that the incidence and severity of COPD would be drastically reduced by smoking cessation. COPD is rare among people who have never smoked cigarettes. Disease progression can be slowed by smoking cessation. Other measures to reduce the incidence of COPD are to avoid inhalation irritants in all environments. Using masks when working in areas with high levels of particulate matter can reduce individual exposure. Proper venting of workplaces and recreation areas that have airborne or particulate matter also reduces exposure.

◆COLLABORATIVE MANAGEMENT

PHARM REVIEW

◆Assessment

HISTORY

RISK FACTORS. Consider age, gender, occupational history, and ethnic-cultural background when taking a history from a client who may have chronic obstructive pul-

CHART 33-8

KEY FEATURES of
Cor Pulmonale

- Hypoxia and hypoxemia
- Increasing dyspnea
- Fatigue
- Weakness
- Enlarged and tender liver
- Warm, cyanotic extremities with bounding pulses
- Cyanotic lips
- Distended neck veins
- Right ventricular enlargement (hypertrophy)
- Lower sternal or epigastric pulsations
- Gastrointestinal disturbances, such as nausea or anorexia
- Dependent edema
- Metabolic and respiratory acidosis
- Pulmonary hypertension

monary disease (COPD). COPD is seen more often in older men. Some types of COPD, particularly panlobular emphysema, occur in families, especially those with alpha$_1$ antitrypsin (AAT) deficiency.

Obtain a thorough smoking history, because tobacco use is a major risk factor. Ask about the length of time the client has smoked and the number of packs smoked daily. Use these data to determine the pack-year smoking history.

CURRENT PROBLEM. Ask the client to describe his or her breathing problems. Assess whether the client has any difficulty breathing while talking. Can he or she speak in complete sentences, or is it necessary to take a breath between every one or two words? Ask about the presence, duration, or worsening of wheezing, coughing, and shortness of breath. Determine what activities trigger these problems. Assess the client's cough pattern. If the cough is productive, ask whether sputum is clear or colored and how much is produced each day. Ask the client to recall the time of day when the sputum production is greatest. Smokers often have a productive cough when they get up in the morning; nonsmokers generally do not. Ask whether sputum production has increased or changed during the past year.

Check the relationship between activity tolerance and dyspnea by asking the client to compare his or her activity level and shortness of breath now with those of a month ago and a year ago. Likewise, ask about any difficulty with eating and sleeping. Many clients sleep in a semi-sitting position because breathlessness is worse when lying down **(orthopnea).** Ask about usual daily activities and any difficulty with sleeping, bathing, dressing, or sexual activity.

WEIGHT AND DIET. Weigh the client and compare this weight with previous weights. Unplanned weight loss occurs with an increase in COPD severity. The client with COPD has increased metabolic needs as a result of the increased work of breathing. Dyspnea and mucus production often result in poor food intake and inadequate nutrition. Ask the client to recall a typical day's meals and fluid intake.

PHYSICAL ASSESSMENT/CLINICAL MANIFESTATIONS

GENERAL APPEARANCE. Observe the client's general appearance, including weight in proportion to height, posture, mobility, muscle mass, and overall hygiene. The client with increasingly severe COPD is thin, with loss of muscle mass in the extremities, although the neck muscles may be enlarged. The client tends to be slow moving and slightly stooped. Usually he or she will sit with a forward-bending posture, sometimes with the arms held forward (Figure 33-8). When dyspnea becomes severe, the client may have such activity intolerance that bathing and general grooming are neglected.

RESPIRATORY CHANGES. Inspect the chest to assess the breathing rate and pattern. The client with respiratory muscle fatigue breathes with rapid, shallow respirations and may have paradoxical respirations or use accessory muscles in the abdomen or neck. The respiratory rate could be as high as 40 to 50 breaths/min. Three breathing patterns often seen with respiratory muscle fatigue are abdominal paradox, respiratory alternans, and asynchronous breathing (Table 33-1).

Palpate the client's chest for areas of tenderness and abnormal retractions and for symmetric chest expansion. The client with emphysema has limited diaphragmatic movement (excursion) because the diaphragm is flattened and below its usual resting state. Decreased vibration (fremitus) may be felt when the client says "ninety-nine" because vibrations are not transmitted through obstructed airways. On percussion the chest is hyperresonant because of the presence of trapped air.

Auscultate the chest to assess the depth of inspiration and any abnormal breath sounds. Crackles occur with emphysema and chronic bronchitis. Note the pitch and location of the sound, and the point in the respiratory cycle at which the sound is heard. A silent chest may indicate obstruction or pneumothorax.

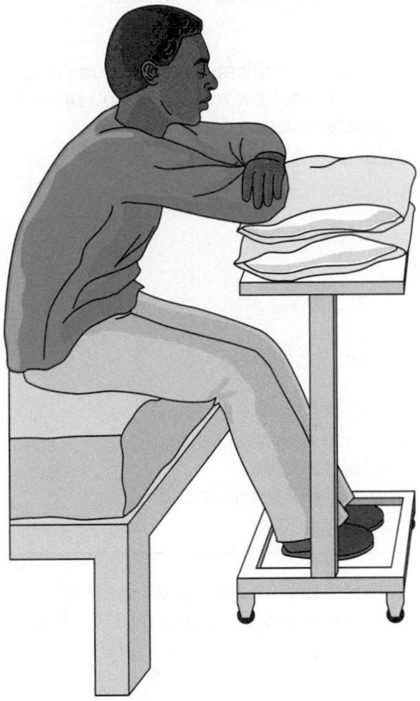

Sitting on the edge of a bed with the arms folded and placed on two or three pillows positioned over a nightstand.

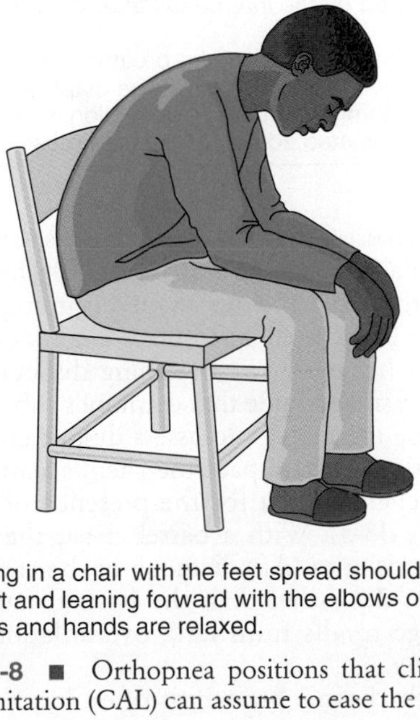

Sitting in a chair with the feet spread shoulder-width apart and leaning forward with the elbows on the knees. Arms and hands are relaxed.

Figure 33-8 ■ Orthopnea positions that clients with chronic airflow limitation (CAL) can assume to ease the work of breathing.

Dyspnea Assessment Guide

Direct Measure of Dyspnea

Indicate the amount of shortness of breath you are having at this time by marking the line.

shortness of breath as bad as can be

no shortness of breath

Subjective Symptoms

On a scale of 0–4 with 0 indicating no distress and 4 indicating much distress, how much are you presently distressed by: *(circle answer)*.

poor appetite	0	1	2	3	4
worn out or weak	0	1	2	3	4
suffocation	0	1	2	3	4
tightness	0	1	2	3	4
congestion	0	1	2	3	4
a feeling of panic or anxiety	0	1	2	3	4

Objective Sign

Rise of the clavicle during inspiration:
ABSENT = not detected
MILD = seen but not pronounced
SEVERE = pronounced

Figure 33-9 ■ A dyspnea assessment tool. (Redrawn from Gift, A.G. [1989]. A dyspnea assessment guide. *Critical Care Nurse,* 9[8], 79.)

TABLE 33-1 Breathing Patterns Commonly Seen in Clients with Respiratory Muscle Fatigue

Abdominal paradox. The diaphragm is nonfunctional; inspiration is accomplished by the intercostal and abdominal accessory muscles.
Respiratory alternans. Diaphragmatic breathing alternates with abdominal paradox; may serve to rest the diaphragm.
Asynchronous breathing. The chest wall motion is unorganized; reflects the uncoordinated activity of fatigued muscles.

Assess the degree of dyspnea using an assessment tool called a Visual Analog Dyspnea Scale (VADS). The VADS is a straight line with verbal anchors at the beginning and end of a 100-mm line. Ask the client to place a mark on the line to indicate his or her perceived breathing difficulty. Figure 33-9 shows an assessment guide that combines subjective and objective data. Use these scales to assess dyspnea, determine the therapy effectiveness, and pace the client's activities.

Examine the client's chest for the presence of a "barrel chest" (see Figure 33-3). With a barrel chest, the ratio between the anteroposterior (AP) diameter of the chest and its lateral diameter is 2:2 rather than the normal ratio of 1:2. This shape change results from lung overinflation and diaphragm flattening.

The client with chronic bronchitis often has a cyanotic, or blue-tinged, dusky appearance and has excessive sputum production. Assess the client for cyanosis, delayed capillary refill, and clubbing of the fingers (Figure 33-10), which indicate chronically decreased arterial oxygen levels.

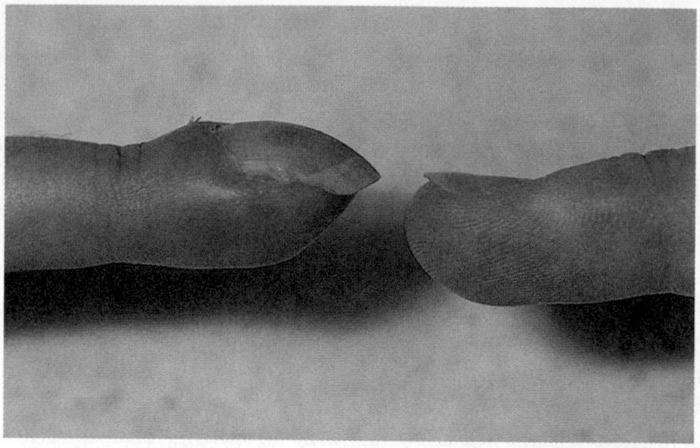

Figure 33-10 ■ Late digital clubbing *(left)* compared to a normal digit *(right)*. (From Swartz, M.H. [1998]. *Textbook of physical diagnosis: History and examination.* Philadelphia: W.B. Saunders.)

CARDIAC CHANGES. Assess the client's heart rate and rhythm. Check for swelling of the feet and ankles (dependent edema) or other manifestations of right-sided heart failure. Examine nail beds and oral mucous membranes. The client with later-stage emphysema may have pallor or frank cyanosis.

PSYCHOSOCIAL ASSESSMENT

COPD affects all aspects of a person's life. Socialization may be reduced when friends avoid the client with COPD because of annoying coughs, excessive sputum, or dyspnea. The client may choose to be isolated because dyspnea causes fatigue or because of embarrassment from coughing and excessive sputum production. In addition, because of the association with cigarette smoking and disease development, the client may feel a social stigma (see the Evidence-Based Practice for Nursing box on p. 599).

Ask the client about interests and hobbies to assess whether socialization has decreased or whether hobbies cause exposure to inhalation irritants. Ask about home conditions for exposure to smoke or crowded living conditions that promote transmission of respiratory infections.

The client's economic status may be affected by the disease through changes in income and health insurance coverage. If the client is the head of the household, severe COPD may require role changes that have a negative impact on self-image. Drugs, especially the metered dose inhalers (MDIs) and dry powder inhalers (DPI), are expensive, and many clients with limited incomes may use them only during exacerbations and not as prescribed on a scheduled basis.

Anxiety and fear related to dyspnea and feelings of breathlessness may reduce the client's ability to participate in a full life. Work, family, social, and sexual roles can be affected. Assess the client's awareness and use of support groups and services.

LABORATORY ASSESSMENT

Arterial blood gas (ABG) values identify abnormal oxygenation, ventilation, and acid-base status. Compare serial or repeated ABG values to assess changes in the client's respiratory status. Once baseline ABG values are obtained, pulse oximetry

EVIDENCE-BASED PRACTICE for Nursing

Women with COPD need social support and specific guidelines for management of dyspnea and fatigue to cope well with the disease.

O'Neill, E. (2002). Illness representations and coping of women with chronic obstructive pulmonary disease: A pilot study. *Heart & Lung, 31*(4), 295-302.

The purpose of this qualitative study was to determine how women with chronic obstructive pulmonary disease (COPD) recognize and respond to symptoms. A total of 21 participants were interviewed and kept symptom diaries.

The most difficult physical problems for the subjects were fatigue and dyspnea. Other important findings included the high level of depression and stigma felt by the subjects. They also perceived a loss of social support and intimacy.

Level of Evidence: 6—Uncontrolled descriptive qualitative study.

Critique. The study designed followed acceptable procedures for qualitative research. Data were collected until redundancy was apparent. Information was obtained by audiotaping direct interviews using an open guide with questions and probes to allow for flexibility of response. The interviewer also took notes. A professional transcriptionist transcribed the tapes. Feedback from participants was used to verify the data. An independent researcher analyzed selective portions of the transcripts for reliability. A drawback of the study was that all participants were also participating in a pulmonary rehabilitation program. Thus the sample may have different motivations and perceptions compared to women with COPD who do not choose or are unable to participate in a pulmonary rehabilitation program.

Implications for Nursing. Nurses must provide more practical information on ways to manage dyspnea and fatigue. These physical problems have a large impact on the client's quality of life and degree of continued socialization. Nurses must individualize energy conservation plans to meet each client's needs rather than just provide a general listing of energy conservation measures.

can gauge the response to treatment. As COPD worsens, the amount of oxygen in the blood decreases **(hypoxemia)** and the amount of carbon dioxide in the blood increases **(hypercarbia).** Chronic respiratory acidosis (increased arterial carbon dioxide [Pa_{CO_2}]) then results; metabolic alkalosis (increased arterial bicarbonate) occurs as compensation. Not all clients with COPD are carbon dioxide retainers, even when hypoxemia is present. Carbon dioxide diffuses more easily across lung membranes than does oxygen. Hypercarbia is a problem in advanced emphysema (because the alveoli are affected) rather than in bronchitis (wherein the airways are affected).

Sputum samples are obtained for culture from hospitalized clients with an acute respiratory infection. In the community, sputum cultures are rarely obtained. The infection is treated on the basis of manifestations and the common bacterial organisms. A white blood cell count helps to confirm the presence of infection.

Other blood tests include hemoglobin and hematocrit to determine polycythemia (a compensatory increase in red blood cells in the chronically hypoxic client). Serum electrolyte levels are examined because hypophosphatemia, hyperkalemia, hypocalcemia, and hypomagnesemia reduce muscle strength. In clients suspected of alpha$_1$-antitrypsin (AAT) deficiency, serum AAT levels are drawn.

RADIOGRAPHIC ASSESSMENT

Chest x-rays are obtained to rule out other chest diseases and to check the progress of clients with respiratory infections or chronic disease. With advanced emphysema, chest x-rays show hyperinflation and a flattened diaphragm. Chest x-rays may not be helpful in the diagnosis of early or moderate disease.

TABLE 33-2 Classification of COPD Severity

Stage	Manifestations	Pulmonary Function Test Results
0 (At risk)	Chronic cough Chronic sputum production Exposure to environmental risk factors	Normal
I (Mild)	±Chronic cough ±Sputum production	FEV_1/FVC <70% FEV_1 <80% of predicted
II (Moderate)	±Dyspnea ±Chronic cough ±Sputum production	FEV_1/FVC <70% FEV_1 <80% but at least 50% of predicted
III (Severe)	±Dyspnea ±Chronic cough ±Sputum production	FEV_1/FVC <70% FEV_1 <50% but at least 30% of predicted
IV (Very severe)	±Dyspnea ±Chronic cough ±Sputum production	FEV_1/FVC <70% FEV_1 <30% of predicted OR FEV_1 <50% of predicted **with either** respiratory failure or heart failure

Data from National Heart, Lung, and Blood Institute. (2003). *Global initiative for chronic obstructive pulmonary disease: Global strategy for the diagnosis, management, and prevention of chronic obstructive pulmonary disease.* (NIH Publication No. 2701A.) Rockville, MD. Author.

OTHER DIAGNOSTIC ASSESSMENTS

COPD is classified from mild to severe on the basis of manifestations and pulmonary function test (PFT) changes (Table 33-2; see Table 30-7). Airflow rates and lung volume measurements help distinguish airway disease (obstructive disease) from interstitial lung disease (restrictive diseases). PFTs determine lung volumes, flow volume curves, and diffusion capacity. Each test is performed before and after the client inhales a bronchodilator agent.

The lung volumes measured for COPD are vital capacity (VC), residual volume (RV), and total lung capacity (TLC). RV is most profoundly affected, although all volumes and capacities change to some degree in COPD. The RV increase reflects the trapped, stale air remaining in the lungs.

Flow volume curves measure the client's ability to move air into and out of the lung. The rate of airflow out of the lungs during a rapid, forceful, and complete exhalation from TLC to RV (forced expiratory volume [FEV]) indirectly measures the flow resistance of the lung. A diagnosis of COPD is based mostly on the FEV_1 (the FEV in the first second of exhalation). FEV_1 can also be expressed as a percentage of the forced vital capacity (FVC). As the disease progresses, the ratio of FEV_1 to FVC becomes smaller.

The diffusion test measures how well a test gas (carbon monoxide) diffuses across the alveolar-capillary membrane and combines with the hemoglobin of red blood cells. In emphysema, alveolar wall destruction causes a large decrease in surface area for diffusion of gas into the blood, leading to a decreased diffusion capacity. In bronchitis, even though lung volumes are increased, the diffusion capacity is usually normal.

The client with COPD has decreased oxygen saturation, often as low as 91%. Pulse oximetry results lower than 90% require medical attention.

Peak expiratory flow meters are used to monitor the effectiveness of the prescribed drugs to relieve obstruction. Peak flow rates increase as obstruction resolves. Teach the client to self-monitor the peak expiratory flow rates at home and adjust drugs as needed.

Analysis

COMMON NURSING DIAGNOSES AND COLLABORATIVE PROBLEMS

The following are priority nursing diagnoses for clients with chronic obstructive pulmonary disease (COPD):

1. Impaired Gas Exchange related to alveolar-capillary membrane changes, reduced airway size, ventilatory muscle fatigue, and excessive mucus production
2. Ineffective Breathing Pattern related to airway obstruction, diaphragm flattening, fatigue, and decreased energy
3. Ineffective Airway Clearance related to excessive secretions, fatigue, decreased energy, and ineffective cough
4. Imbalanced Nutrition: Less Than Body Requirements related to dyspnea, excessive secretions, anorexia, and fatigue
5. Anxiety related to dyspnea, a change in health status, and situational crisis
6. Activity Intolerance related to fatigue, dyspnea, and an imbalance between oxygen supply and demand

A primary collaborative problem for clients with COPD is Potential for Pneumonia or Other Respiratory Infections.

ADDITIONAL NURSING DIAGNOSES AND COLLABORATIVE PROBLEMS

In addition to the common nursing diagnoses and collaborative problems, clients with COPD may have one or more of the following:

- Fatigue related to a change in metabolic energy or hypoxemia
- Deficient Knowledge (disease process, prescribed treatments, activity limitations) related to unfamiliarity with information resources
- Sexual Dysfunction related to extreme fatigue
- Impaired Spontaneous Ventilation related to ventilatory muscle fatigue
- Disturbed Sleep Pattern related to dyspnea or an unfamiliar environment (hospitalization)
- Disturbed Thought Processes related to hypoxemia or sleep deprivation
- Ineffective Coping related to high degree of threat, inadequate level of perception of control, changes in lifestyle, situational crisis, or knowledge deficit
- Ineffective Role Performance related to a change in health status or role loss

Other collaborative problems for clients with COPD include Potential for Respiratory Failure and Potential for Right-Sided Heart Failure.

> **Critical Thinking Challenge**
>
> The client is a 54-year-old secretary who is newly diagnosed with emphysema after having two episodes of pneumonia this year. She is currently a smoker and has smoked two packs of cigarettes per day since age 16 years. She is divorced and lives in an apartment in the same city as her three grown children. Her COPD is classified as II—moderate (see Table 33-2). She is crying and blaming herself for this disease. Although she says she would like to quit smoking, she thinks it will not help because "the damage has already been done." She also tells you that her father died with COPD at the age of 62. She worries that her smoking may have harmed her children.
>
> 1. What is the priority nursing responsibility for this client?
> 2. Explain your rationale for its priority.
> 3. Calculate this client's smoking history in pack-years.
> 4. Would smoking cessation at this time help this client? Why or why not?

evolve For suggested answer guidelines, go to http://evolve.elsevier.com/Iggy/.

Planning and Implementation

IMPAIRED GAS EXCHANGE

NOC **PLANNING: EXPECTED OUTCOMES.** The client with COPD is expected to attain and maintain gas exchange at a level within his or her chronic baseline values. Indicators include the following:

- Maintenance of SpO_2 of at least 88%
- Absence of cyanosis
- Maintenance of cognitive orientation

INTERVENTIONS. NIC interventions for the client with COPD are listed in Chart 33-9. Most clients with COPD use nonsurgical management to improve or maintain gas exchange. Surgical management requires that the client meet strict criteria.

NONSURGICAL MANAGEMENT. The mainstays of COPD management include airway maintenance, monitoring, drug therapy, and oxygen therapy.

Airway Maintenance. The most important intervention to improve gas exchange is to maintain a patent airway. Keep the client's head, neck, and chest in alignment. Assist him or her to liquefy secretions and clear the airway of secretions.

Monitoring. Assess the hospitalized client with COPD at least every 2 hours, even when the purpose of hospitalization is not COPD management. Provide the prescribed oxygen, assess the client's response to treatment, and prevent complications.

If the client's condition continues to worsen despite treatment, more aggressive therapy is needed. Intubation and mechanical ventilation may be needed for clients in respiratory failure, including those who are unable to sustain spontaneous breathing patterns.

NIC **Oxygen Therapy.** Oxygen is prescribed for relief of hypoxemia (decreased blood oxygen levels) and hypoxia (decreased tissue oxygenation). The need for oxygen therapy and its effectiveness can be determined by arterial blood gas values and oxygen saturation by pulse oxymetry. The client with COPD may need an oxygen flow of 2 to 4 L/min via nasal cannula or up to 40% via Venturi mask. The client who is hypoxemic and also has chronic hypercarbia requires lower levels of oxygen delivery, usually 1 to 2 L/min via nasal cannula.

CHART 33-9

NIC INTERVENTION ACTIVITIES for
The Client with Chronic Obstructive Pulmonary Disease

Airway Management: *Facilitation of patency of air passages*
- Position client to maximize ventilation potential.
- Perform chest physical therapy, as appropriate.
- Remove secretions by encouraging coughing or by suctioning.
- Instruct how to cough effectively.
- Assist with incentive spirometer, as appropriate.
- Auscultate breath sounds, noting areas of decreased or absent ventilation and presence of adventitious sounds.
- Administer bronchodilators, as appropriate.
- Teach client how to use prescribed inhalers, as appropriate.
- Administer aerosol treatments, as appropriate.
- Administer ultrasonic nebulizer treatments, as appropriate.
- Administer humidified air or oxygen, as appropriate.
- Regulate fluid intake to optimize fluid balance.
- Position to alleviate dyspnea.
- Monitor respiratory and oxygenation status, as appropriate.

Cough Enhancement: *Promotion of deep inhalation by the client with subsequent generation of high intrathoracic pressures and compression of underlying lung parenchyma for the forceful expulsion of air*
- Monitor results of pulmonary function tests, particularly vital capacity, maximal inspiratory force, forced expiratory volume in 1 second (FEV_1), and FEV_1/FVC, as appropriate.
- Assist client to a sitting position with head slightly flexed, shoulders relaxed, and knees flexed.
- Encourage client to take several deep breaths.
- Encourage client to take a deep breath, hold it for 2 seconds, and cough two or three times in succession.
- Instruct client to inhale deeply several times, to exhale slowly, and to cough at the end of exhalation.

Oxygen Therapy: *Administration of oxygen and monitoring of its effectiveness*
- Clear oral, nasal, and tracheal secretions, as appropriate.
- Maintain airway patency.
- Set up oxygen equipment and administer through a heated, humidified system.
- Monitor the oxygen liter flow.
- Monitor position of oxygen delivery device.
- Periodically check oxygen delivery device to ensure that the prescribed concentration is being delivered.
- Monitor the effectiveness of oxygen therapy (e.g., pulse oximetry, ABGs), as appropriate.
- Ensure replacement of oxygen mask/cannula whenever the device is removed.
- Monitor client's ability to tolerate removal of oxygen while eating.
- Observe for signs of oxygen-induced hypoventilation.
- Monitor for signs of oxygen toxicity and absorption atelectasis.
- Monitor oxygen equipment to ensure that it is not interfering with the client's attempts to breathe.
- Monitor client's anxiety related to need for oxygen therapy.
- Monitor for skin breakdown from friction of oxygen device.
- Provide for oxygen when client is transported.
- Instruct client and family about use of oxygen at home.
- Arrange for use of oxygen devices that facilitate mobility and teach client accordingly.

Energy Management: *Regulating energy use to treat or prevent fatigue and optimize function*
- Determine client's physical limitations.
- Encourage verbalization of feelings about limitations.
- Monitor nutritional intake to ensure adequate energy resources.
- Consult with dietitian about ways to increase intake of high-energy foods.
- Monitor cardiorespiratory response to activity (e.g., tachycardia, other dysrhythmias, dyspnea, diaphoresis, pallor, hemodynamic pressures, and respiratory rate).
- Limit environmental stimuli (e.g., light and noise) to facilitate relaxation.
- Promote bedrest/activity limitation (e.g., increase number of rest periods).
- Arrange physical activities to reduce competition for oxygen supply to vital body functions (e.g., avoid activity immediately after meals).
- Assist client to schedule rest periods.
- Avoid care activities during scheduled rest periods.
- Plan activities for periods when the client has the most energy.
- Assist with regular physical activities (e.g., ambulation, transfers, turning, and personal care), as needed.
- Monitor client's oxygen response (e.g., pulse rate, cardiac rhythm, and respiratory rate) to self-care or nursing activities.
- Teach client and significant other techniques of self-care that will minimize oxygen consumption (e.g., self-monitoring and pacing techniques for performance of activities of daily living).
- Assist the client to identify tasks that family and friends can perform in the home to prevent/relieve fatigue.
- Assist the client in assigning priority to activities to accommodate energy levels.
- Assist client to identify preferences for activity.
- Evaluate programmed increases in levels of activities.

NIC intervention activities selected from Dochterman, J.M., & Bulechek, G.M. (Eds.). (2004). *Nursing interventions classification (NIC)* (4th ed.). St. Louis: Mosby.
ABG, Arterial blood gas.

A low arterial oxygen level is this client's primary drive for breathing. The use of continuous low-flow oxygen for the client with stage III or IV COPD has been shown to increase life span (Boyle & Locke, 2004; Wong, 2001). More information on oxygen therapy is found in Chapter 31.

Drug Therapy. Drug therapy for COPD involves the same inhaled and systemic drugs as for asthma. These drugs include beta-adrenergic agents, cholinergic antagonists, methylxanthines, corticosteroids, cromolyn sodium/nedocromil, and leukotriene modifiers (see Chart 33-5). The client with COPD is more likely to be taking systemic agents (in addition to inhaled drugs) than is the client with asthma. An additional drug class for COPD is the mucolytics, which thin secretions, making them easier to expectorate.

Mucolytic agents are prescribed for the client with thick, tenacious (sticky) mucous secretions. Nebulizer treatments with normal saline or with a mucolytic agent such as acetylcysteine (Mucosil, Mucomyst✱) or dornase alfa (Pulmozyme) and normal saline help thin secretions and facilitate expectoration. Guaifenesin (Organidin, Naldecon Senior EX) is a systemic mucolytic that is taken orally.

Stepped therapy is recommended for clients with chronic bronchitis or emphysema (Table 33-3). The key elements of stepped therapy include drug therapy, monitoring, and control of environmental irritants and allergens. The expected outcomes of stepped therapy are for the client to have more awareness of the disease and to participate in symptom management.

SURGICAL MANAGEMENT. Lung transplantation is performed for select clients with end-stage COPD. (See the lung transplantation section under Surgical Management [Cystic Fibrosis] on p. 608.) The more common surgical procedure for clients with COPD is lung reduction surgery.

TABLE 33-3 The Stepped Approach of Drug Therapy for COPD

Step	COPD Stage*	Drug Recommendations
1	I	Ipratropium 3-6 puffs four times daily by MDI with spacer. Beta$_2$ agonist for rescue as needed by MDI with spacer. (If symptoms are not well controlled, proceed to next step.)
2	II	Add beta$_2$ agonist (short-acting) 2-6 puffs q3-6h by MDI with spacer. Consider use of long-acting beta$_2$ agonist once daily. (If symptoms are not well controlled, proceed to next step.)
3	III	Add long-acting theophylline 200-400 mg PO twice daily for a therapeutic blood level of 8 to 12 mcg/mL. (If response is unsatisfactory, discontinue theophylline and proceed to the next step.)
4	IV	Add prednisone 40 mg PO daily. If client improves, taper dose to the lowest dose that manages symptoms. At lowest prednisone dose, consider an inhaled steroid.

MDI, Metered dose inhaler.
*Although the steps of therapy are correlated to COPD stage, client response is the best indicator for maintaining or changing steps.

Lung reduction surgery can improve gas exchange in the client with COPD. The goal of this surgery is improvement of gas exchange through removal of hyperinflated lung tissue. These areas of the lungs are filled with stagnant air that is not renewed with some atmospheric air (containing oxygen) during each respiratory cycle. Instead, this stagnant air continues to receive carbon dioxide until the level of carbon dioxide in the hyperinflated alveolus is the same as that in the capillary. Hyperinflated lung areas are useless for gas exchange. After successful lung reduction, most clients have at least a 75% improvement in FEV_1, decreased TLC and RV, and increased activity tolerance. Oxygen therapy may no longer be needed.

Preoperative Care. Clients are selected for this procedure on the basis of having end-stage emphysema, minimal chronic bronchitis, and stable cardiac function; being ambulatory and not dependent on a ventilator; not having pulmonary fibrosis, asthma, or late-stage cancer; and having been a nonsmoker for at least 6 months. The client must complete pulmonary rehabilitation before surgery to maximize lung and muscle function. The client must reach a state in which he or she is able to walk, without stopping, for 30 minutes at 1 mile/hr and maintain a 90% or better oxygen saturation level.

In addition to standard preoperative testing, the client having lung reduction surgery has tests to determine the location of greatest lung hyperinflation and poorest lung blood flow. These tests include pulmonary plethysmography, gas dilution, and perfusion scans.

Operative Procedures. Usually, lung reduction is performed on both lungs through either a large midline incision or a transverse anterior thoracotomy. Each lung is deflated separately and examined for color and texture differences. Normal lung tissue darkens to purple or gray when deflated and becomes more dense or rubbery in texture. Hyperinflated areas do not deflate, and they remain pink with a spongy texture. After areas to remove have been identified, the surgeon removes as much of this tissue as possible, sealing off and reinforcing the remaining normal lung tissue.

Postoperative Care. After lung reduction surgery, the client needs close monitoring for continuing respiratory problems as well as for usual postoperative complications. In addition to the usual care required after thoracotomy (see Surgical Management [Lung Cancer], p. 617), bronchodilator and mucolytic therapies are maintained initially. Pulmonary hygiene includes incentive spirometry 10 times per hour while awake, chest physiotherapy starting on the first day after surgery, and hourly pulmonary assessment.

Pain is usually managed by epidural delivery of opioids during the early period after surgery. This type of analgesic delivery reduces pain, limits sedation and cognitive dysfunction, and allows the client to more fully participate in pulmonary hygiene measures.

INEFFECTIVE BREATHING PATTERN

NOC **PLANNING: EXPECTED OUTCOMES.** The client with COPD is expected to achieve an effective breathing pattern that decreases the work of breathing. Indicators include the following:

- Respiratory rhythm within normal limits for the client's age
- Presence of synchronous thoracoabdominal movement
- Use of accessory muscles appropriate to the client's activity level
- Increased activity tolerance

INTERVENTIONS. Before any intervention, assess the client to determine the breathing pattern, especially the rate, rhythm, depth, and use of accessory muscles. The client with COPD relies more on accessory muscles than on the diaphragm for breathing. These muscles, however, are less efficient than the diaphragm, and the work of breathing increases. Determine whether there are any contributing factors to the increased work of breathing, such as respiratory infection. Most clients with COPD can benefit from some degree of pulmonary rehabilitation therapy. These interventions aim to improve the client's breathing efforts and decrease the work of breathing through the use of specific breathing techniques, positioning, exercise conditioning, and energy conservation.

Breathing Techniques. Diaphragmatic or abdominal and pursed-lip breathing techniques may be helpful for managing dyspneic episodes. The client uses these techniques, shown in Chart 33-10, during all activities. The amount of stale air in the lungs is reduced, and the client gains confidence and control in managing dyspnea. Teach these techniques when the client is free of dyspnea.

Diaphragmatic or Abdominal Breathing. In diaphragmatic breathing, the client consciously increases movement of the diaphragm. Lying on the back allows the abdomen to relax.

Pursed-Lip Breathing. Breathing through pursed lips uses the mild resistance of partially closed lips to prolong exhalation and to increase airway pressure. This technique delays airway compression and reduces air trapping.

CHART 33-10

CLIENT EDUCATION GUIDE
Breathing Exercises

Diaphragmatic or Abdominal Breathing
- Lie on your back with your knees bent.
- Place your hands or a book on your abdomen to create resistance.
- Begin breathing from your abdomen while keeping your chest still. You can tell if you are breathing correctly if your hands or the book rises and falls accordingly.

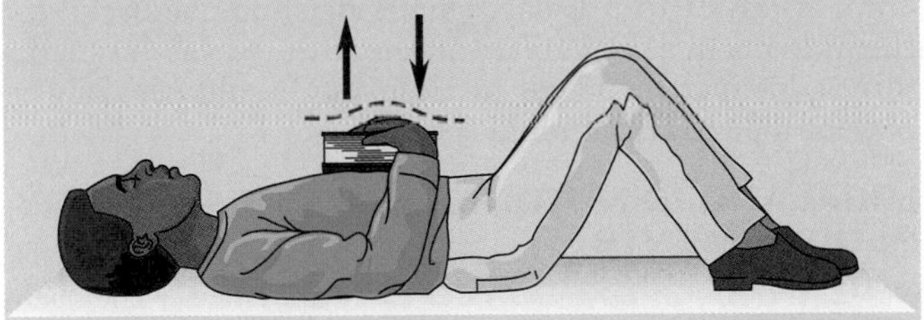

Pursed-Lip Breathing
- Close your mouth and breathe in through your nose.
- Purse your lips as you would to whistle. Breathe out slowly through your mouth, without puffing your cheeks. Spend at least twice the amount of time it took you to breathe in. Use your abdominal muscles to squeeze out every bit of air you can.
- Remember to use pursed-lip breathing during any physical activity. Always inhale before beginning the activity and exhale while performing the activity. Never hold your breath.

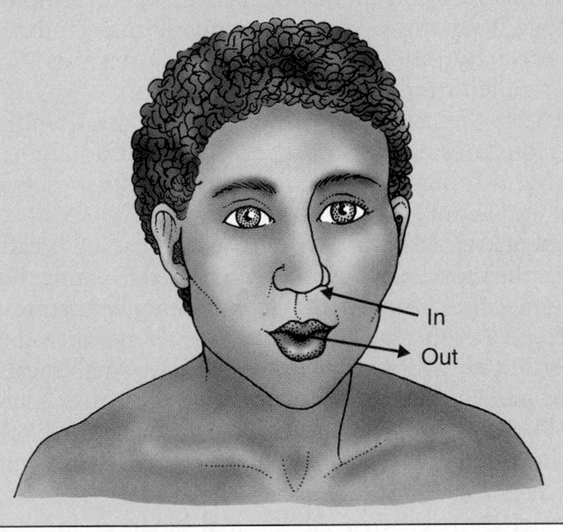

Pursed-lip breathing can be used during diaphragmatic or abdominal breathing.

Positioning. Assist the client to an upright position, with the head of the bed elevated. Various positions help alleviate dyspnea by increasing chest expansion, relaxing the chest muscles, and placing the diaphragm in the proper position to contract. These positions conserve energy by supporting the client's arms and upper body.

The client uses the standing position when there is no place to sit (Figure 33-11). Clients with COPD rely on use of accessory muscles for breathing. Supporting the thorax allows these muscles to work better.

Exercise Conditioning. Clients with exercise-induced shortness of breath respond to dyspnea by limiting their activity, even basic activities of daily living (ADLs). Over time, the muscles of ventilation and other large muscle groups weaken and are less efficient in the use of oxygen. The result is increased dyspnea with lower activity levels.

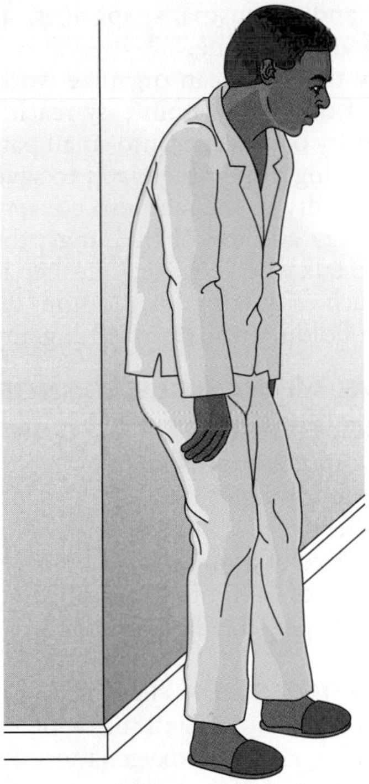

Figure 33-11 ■ The standing position that is used to help clients with chronic airflow limitation (CAL) to breathe. The client stands with back and hips against a wall and with the feet about 30 cm (12 inches) from the wall. The shoulders are relaxed and bent slightly forward.

Exercise conditioning of the large muscle groups or retraining of the ventilatory muscles may be part of a pulmonary rehabilitation program. Two techniques are isocapneic hyperventilation and resistive breathing. Isocapneic hyperventilation increases endurance. The client hyperventilates into a machine that controls the levels of oxygen and carbon dioxide. In resistive breathing, the client breathes against a set resistance. Resistive breathing increases ventilatory muscle strength and endurance.

Energy Conservation. Energy conservation is the planning and pacing of activities for maximal tolerance and minimal discomfort. Once the FEV_1 falls below 50% predicted, the client's ability to perform ADLs is limited. Ask the client to describe a typical daily schedule. Each activity is divided into its smaller parts to determine whether that task can be performed in a different way or at a different time of the day. Assist the client to plan and pace daily activities. Rest periods are paced between activities. Development of a personal chart outlining the day's activities and planned rest periods is helpful (see Chart 33-9).

Instruct the client to avoid working with the arms raised. Activities involving the arms decrease exercise tolerance because the accessory muscles of ventilation are then used to stabilize the arms and shoulders. Many activities involving the arms can be done sitting at a table leaning on the elbows. Teach the client to adjust work heights to reduce back strain and fatigue. Remind him or her to keep arm motions smooth and flowing to prevent jerky motions that waste energy. The use of adaptive tools for housework, such as long-handled dustpans, sponges, and dusters, reduces bending and reaching.

Suggest how the client can organize work spaces so that items used most often are within easy reach. Measures such as dividing laundry or groceries into small parcels that can be handled easily, using disposable plates to save washing time, and letting dishes dry in the rack also conserve energy. Talking requires energy and use of the lungs; therefore instruct the client not to talk when engaged in other activities that require energy, such as walking. In addition, teach him or her to avoid breath-holding while performing any activity.

INEFFECTIVE AIRWAY CLEARANCE

NOC **PLANNING: EXPECTED OUTCOMES.** The client with COPD is expected to maintain a patent airway. Indicators include the following:

- Coughs effectively
- No occurrence of aspiration
- Maintenance of SpO_2 of at least 88%
- Uses the stepped therapy approach to control manifestations

INTERVENTIONS. The client with COPD often has difficulty with removal of secretions, which results in compromised breathing and poor oxygenation. Excessive mucus also increases the risk for respiratory infections. Assess breath sounds routinely as part of physical assessment and before and after interventions. Careful use of drugs combined with controlled coughing, hydration, and postural drainage may help in airway clearance. If these measures fail, a tracheostomy may be needed on a temporary or permanent basis.

Controlled Coughing. Because the client with COPD has excessive mucus, coughing at specific times of the day is helpful. Teach the client to cough on arising in the morning to eliminate mucus that collected during the night. Coughing to clear mucous before mealtimes may facilitate a more pleasant meal. Coughing before bedtime may ensure clear lungs for a less interrupted night's sleep.

To cough effectively, the client sits in a chair or on the side of a bed with feet placed firmly on the floor. Instruct him or her to turn the shoulders inward and to bend the head slightly downward, hugging a pillow against the stomach. The client then takes a few deep breaths. After the third to fifth deep breath (in through the nose, out through pursed lips), instruct the client to bend forward slowly while coughing two or three times from the same breath. Observe the color, consistency, odor, and amount of secretions. On return to a sitting position, the client takes a comfortable deep breath. The entire coughing procedure is repeated at least twice. After coughing exercises, allow the client to rest; provide mouth care.

Chest Physiotherapy and Postural Drainage. Chest physiotherapy (PT) with postural drainage (Figure 33-12) helps move secretions into central airways, reexpand lung tissue, and promote efficient use of the ventilatory muscles. Chest PT combines chest percussion with vibration to loosen secretions. Postural drainage uses specific positions and gravity to help remove secretions. Postural drainage with chest PT, although helpful for some clients, is not used routinely on all clients with COPD.

Suctioning. Suctioning is performed only when abnormal breath sounds are present, not on a routine schedule. For the client with a weak cough, weak pulmonary muscles, and inability to expectorate effectively, the nurse or respiratory therapist performs nasotracheal suctioning. Assess the client for dyspnea, tachycardia, and dysrhythmias during the procedure. Assess for improved breath sounds after suctioning. Suctioning is discussed in detail in Chapter 31.

Positioning. Assist the client who can tolerate sitting in a chair out of bed for 1-hour periods two to three times a day. This position helps move secretions and keeps the diaphragm in a better position for ventilation.

Hydration. Unless hydration needs to be avoided for other health problems, instruct the client with COPD to drink at least 2 to 3 L/day. Humidifiers may be useful for clients living in a dry climate or who use dry heat during the winter. Instruct the client to clean the humidifier daily to prevent the growth of mold spores.

IMBALANCED NUTRITION: LESS THAN BODY REQUIREMENTS

NOC **PLANNING: EXPECTED OUTCOMES.** The client with COPD is expected to achieve and maintain a body weight within 10% of ideal. Indicators include the following:

- Maintains an appropriate weight/height ratio
- Maintains serum albumin or prealbumin within the normal range

INTERVENTIONS. The client with COPD often has food intolerance, nausea, early satiety, loss of appetite, and meal-related dyspnea. The increased work of breathing raises calorie and protein needs. These conditions lead to protein-calorie malnutrition for many clients. Malnourished clients lose total body mass, ventilatory muscle mass and strength, lung elasticity, and alveolar-capillary surface area. All of these problems reduce effective breathing.

Identify clients at risk for or who have this complication and request dietary consultation. Monitor the client's weight and other indicators of nutrition, such as skin condition and serum prealbumin levels.

Dyspnea Management. Shortness of breath (dyspnea) is the most common problem related to eating. Dyspnea during mealtimes can be reduced by resting before meals. The biggest meal of the day is planned for the time when the client is most hungry and well rested. Four to six small meals a day may be preferred to three larger ones. Instruct the client to use pursed-lip and abdominal breathing to alleviate dyspnea. A bronchodilator used 30 minutes before the meal may be helpful to reduce dyspnea due to bronchospasm.

Food Selection. Abdominal bloating and a feeling of fullness often prevent the client from eating a complete meal. Teach about foods that are easy to chew and not gas forming. Dry foods stimulate coughing, and foods such as milk and chocolate may increase the thickness of saliva and secretions. Advise the client to avoid these foods when symptomatic. Inform the client that caffeinated beverages should be avoided because they increase urine output and may lead to dehydration.

Urge the client to eat high-calorie, high-protein foods. Dietary supplements, such as Pulmocare, provide nutrition with reduced carbon dioxide production. If early satiety (feeling too "full" to eat) is a problem, advise the client to avoid drinking fluids before and during the meal.

Assistance with Feeding. Help the client who tires easily. Many clients do not have the energy to feed themselves when they are working hard to breathe and may not have the urge to eat. Oral hygiene before meals may increase appetite.

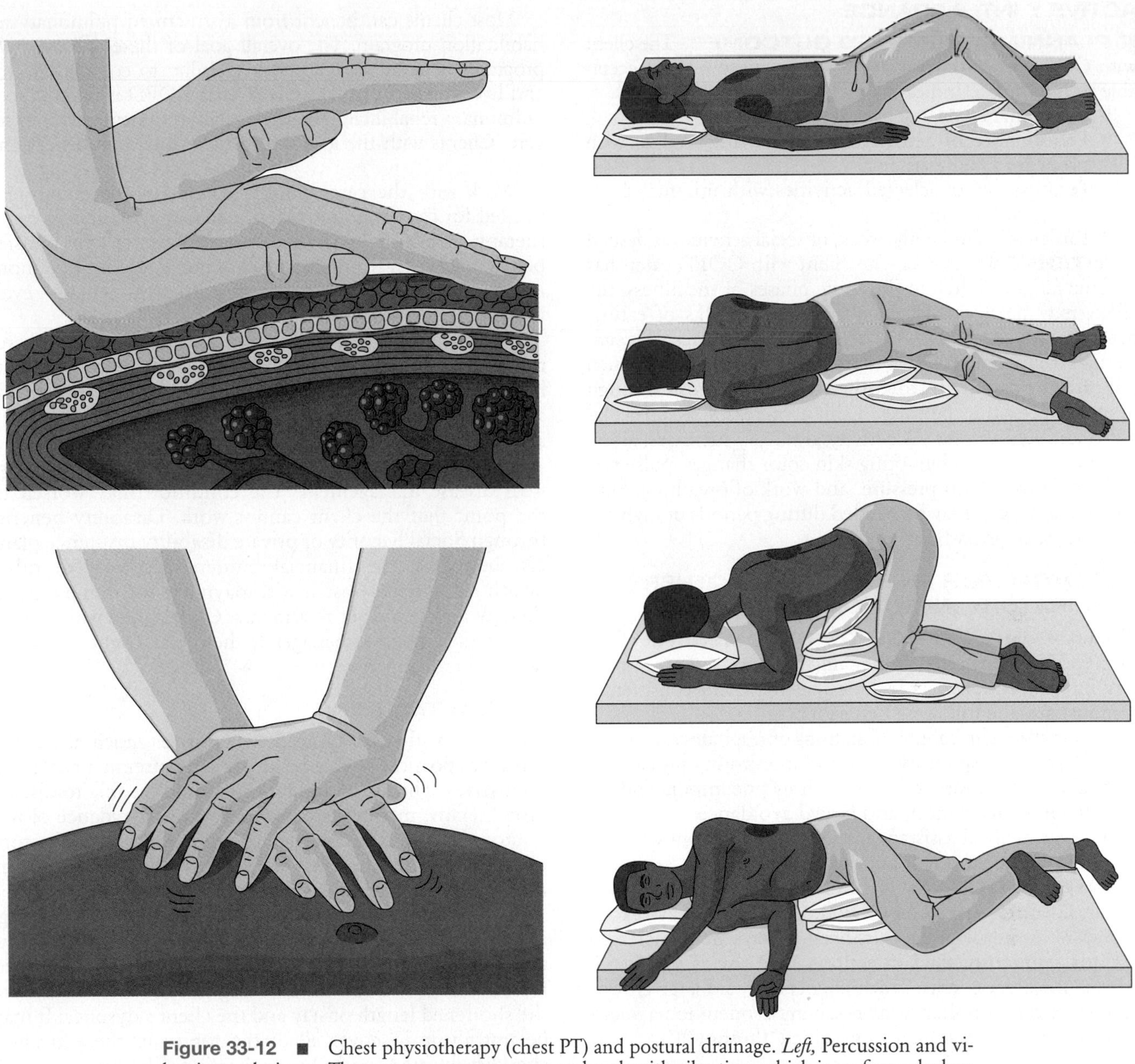

Figure 33-12 ■ Chest physiotherapy (chest PT) and postural drainage. *Left,* Percussion and vibration techniques. The nurse may use one or two hands with vibration, which is performed when the client exhales or coughs. *Right,* Positions for postural drainage of respiratory secretions.

ANXIETY

NOC **PLANNING: EXPECTED OUTCOMES.** The client with COPD is expected to have decreased anxiety. Indicators include that the client consistently demonstrates the following behaviors:

- Identifying factors that contribute to anxiety
- Identifying activities to decrease anxiety
- Verbalizing anxiety is reduced or absent

INTERVENTIONS. Clients with COPD often have increased anxiety during acute dyspneic episodes, especially if they feel as though they are choking on excessive secretions. Also, anxiety has been shown to cause dyspnea.

Psychological Interventions. If symptoms are worsened because of anxiety, it is important that the client understand this effect and has a plan for dealing with anxiety. Together with the client, develop a written plan that states exactly what the client should do if symptoms flare. Having a plan provides confidence and control in knowing what to do, which often helps reduce anxiety. Stress the use of pursed-lip and diaphragmatic breathing techniques during periods of anxiety or panic.

Family, friends, and support groups can be helpful. Recommend professional counseling, if needed, as a positive suggestion and in no way suggest that this need represents a failure of the client to cope. Stress that talking with a counselor can help identify techniques to maintain control over the dyspnea and feelings of panic.

Complementary and Alternative Therapy. Explore other approaches to help the client control dyspneic episodes and panic attacks. Examples include progressive relaxation, hypnosis therapy, and biofeedback. Biofeedback helps the client determine the impact of various stimuli on symptoms. Ultimately the client learns to relax and control these stimuli to avoid the aggravating symptoms.

ACTIVITY INTOLERANCE

NOC **PLANNING: EXPECTED OUTCOMES.** The client with COPD is expected to increase activity to a level acceptable to him or her. Indicators include the following:

- Maintenance of baseline SaO_2 with activity
- Performance of activities of daily living (ADLs) with no or minimal assistance
- Performance of selected activities with minimal dyspnea or tachycardia
- Participation in family, work, or social activities as desired

INTERVENTIONS. The client with COPD often has chronic fatigue. While in the acute phases of the illness, the client may need extensive help with the ADLs of eating, bathing, and grooming. As the acute problem resolves, encourage the client to pace activities and provide as much self-care as possible. Instruct the client not to rush through morning activities, because rushing increases dyspnea, fatigue, and hypoxemia. As activity gradually increases, assess the client's response by noting skin color changes, pulse rate and regularity, blood pressure, and work of breathing. Supplemental oxygen may be needed during periods of high energy use, such as bathing or walking.

POTENTIAL FOR PNEUMONIA OR OTHER RESPIRATORY INFECTIONS

NOC **PLANNING: EXPECTED OUTCOMES.** The client with COPD is expected to remain free from serious respiratory infection. Indicators include that the client consistently demonstrates the following behaviors:

- Verbalizes clinical manifestations of respiratory infection
- Describes respiratory infection monitoring procedures
- Uses prevention activities such as pneumonia and influenza vaccination, and crowd avoidance
- Seeks medical assistance when manifestations of respiratory infection first appear

INTERVENTIONS. Pneumonia is one of the most common complications of COPD. Clients who have excessive secretions or who have artificial airways are at increased risk for respiratory tract infections. The risk is greatly increased for older clients. Teach clients to avoid large crowds and stress the importance of receiving a pneumonia vaccination and a yearly influenza vaccine ("flu shot").

Community-Based Care

HOME CARE MANAGEMENT

Most clients with chronic obstructive pulmonary disease (COPD) are treated in the ambulatory care setting and cared for at home. When pneumonia or a severe exacerbation of the disease develops, the client usually returns home after treatment. For clients with advanced disease, however, 24-hour care may be needed for ADLs and for monitoring for acute episodes or progression of the illness. Clients may not be able to enjoy work or recreational activities because of severe dyspnea and fatigue. If home care is not possible, placement in a long-term care setting may be needed.

Hypoxemic clients can benefit from long-term use of oxygen at home. Home oxygen may be needed only during periods of exercise or sleep if hypoxemia occurs only during these times. Continuous, long-term oxygen therapy can reverse tissue hypoxia and decrease pulmonary vascular resistance. It can also improve cognitive ability and well-being. For more information on oxygen therapy, see Chapter 31.

Most clients can benefit from a structured pulmonary rehabilitation program. The overall goal of these collaborative programs is to increase a person's ability to compensate for and live with COPD. The client with COPD is referred to a pulmonary rehabilitation program before illness becomes severe. Clients with the least severe functional loss benefit the most.

Work with the case manager to obtain the equipment needed for care at home. Client needs may include oxygen therapy, a hospital-type bed, a nebulizer, a tub transfer bench, and visits from a home care nurse to continue monitoring the health status, review the drug regimen, and evaluate home care needs.

The client with COPD faces a lifelong disease with remissions and exacerbations. Explain to the client and family that he or she may have periods of anxiety, depression, and ineffective coping. The client who was a smoker may also have self-directed anger.

Financial concerns often increase anxiety and interfere with disease management. The condition may worsen to the point that the client cannot work. Disability benefits through Social Security or private disability insurance plans can help ease the financial burden. Medicare or other health insurers may assist with payment for home oxygen therapy and nebulizer treatments. Collaborate with the social worker or case manager to help the client make the needed arrangements.

HEALTH TEACHING

The client with COPD needs to know as much about the disease as possible so that he or she can better manage it and themselves. The client and family should be able to discuss drug therapy, manifestations of infection, avoidance of respiratory irritants, the diet therapy regimen, and activity progression. Instruct the client to identify and avoid stressors that can worsen the disease.

Instruct the client in techniques of pursed-lip breathing, diaphragmatic breathing, positioning, relaxation therapy, energy conservation, and coughing and deep breathing. Two factors that interfere with teaching hospitalized clients are the shortened length of stay and the client's dyspnea. It may be unrealistic to cover all of the topics in the education checklist during a single hospitalization. The primary nurse or case manager must coordinate teaching with the home care or clinic staff.

HEALTH CARE RESOURCES

Provide appropriate referrals as needed. Home care visits may be warranted, particularly if the client must use home oxygen therapy for the first time. Chart 33-11 lists assessment areas for the client with COPD at home. Referral to assistance programs, such as Meals on Wheels, can be helpful. Provide a list of support groups, as well as Better Breathing groups sponsored by the American Lung Association. If the client is having difficulty with smoking cessation and indicates the desire for assistance, make the referrals.

Critical Thinking Challenge

The client is a 68-year-old man with stage III COPD. He is being discharged to home on newly prescribed supplemental oxygen and is to start using a spacer with his inhaled drugs. He has concerns that the use of oxygen means that he is dying and that he will no longer be able to leave the house. He asks you if he should try to use the oxygen only when he feels severely breathless. Upon hearing that her husband is about to be discharged, his wife says "Not today. Home isn't ready for him yet."

1. What is your priority nursing interventions for this client and his wife?
2. Are this client's fears justified? Why or why not?
3. What will you teach this client about the use of oxygen therapy?
4. How will you address the wife's concerns?

evolve For suggested answer guidelines, go to http://evolve.elsevier.com/Iggy/.

Evaluation: Outcomes

Evaluate the care of the client with COPD on the basis of the identified nursing diagnoses and collaborative problems. The expected outcomes are that the client should:

- Attain and maintain gas exchange at a level within his or her chronic baseline values
- Achieve an effective breathing pattern that decreases the work of breathing.
- Maintain a patent airway
- Achieve and maintain a body weight within 10% of his or her ideal weight
- Have decreased anxiety

CHART 33-11

HOME CARE ASSESSMENT of The Client with Chronic Obstructive Pulmonary Disease

Assess respiratory status and adequacy of ventilation.
- Measure rate, depth, and rhythm of respirations.
- Examine mucous membranes and nail beds for evidence of hypoxia.
- Determine use of accessory muscles.
- Examine chest and abdomen for paradoxical breathing.
- Count number of words client can speak between breaths.
- Determine need and use of supplemental oxygen. (How many liters per minute is the client using?)
- Determine level of consciousness and presence/absence of confusion.
- Auscultate lungs for abnormal breath sounds.
- Measure oxygen saturation by pulse oximetry.
- Determine sputum production, color, and amount.
- Ask about activity level.
- Observe general hygiene.
- Measure body temperature.

Assess cardiac status.
- Measure rate, quality, and rhythm of pulse.
- Check dependent areas for edema.
- Check neck veins for distention with the client in a sitting position.
- Measure capillary refill.

Assess nutritional status.
- Weight maintenance, loss, or gain
- Food and fluid intake
- Use of nutritional supplements
- General condition of the skin

Assess client's and caregiver's adherence and understanding of illness and treatment, including the following:
- Correct use of supplemental oxygen
- Correct use of inhalers
- Medication schedule and side effects
- Manifestations to report to the health care provider
- Use of pursed-lip and diaphragmatic breathing techniques
- Scheduling of rest periods and priority activities
- Participation in rehabilitation activities

- Increase activity to a level acceptable to him or her
- Avoid serious respiratory infections

Specific indicators for these outcomes are listed for each nursing diagnosis and collaborative problem under the Planning and Implementation section (see earlier).

CYSTIC FIBROSIS

PATHOPHYSIOLOGY

Cystic fibrosis (CF) is a genetic disease that affects many organs and lethally impairs pulmonary function. Although this disorder is present from birth and is first seen in early childhood, many clients now live into adulthood.

The underlying problem of CF is blocked chloride transport in the cell membranes. The error in chloride transport causes the formation of mucus that has little water content. The thick, sticky mucus causes problems in the lungs, pancreas, liver, salivary glands, and testes. The mucus plugs up glands in these organs, causing atrophy and organ dysfunction. Nonpulmonary problems include pancreatic insufficiency with malnutrition and intestinal obstruction, poor growth, male sterility, and cirrhosis of the liver. These primary problems cause a multitude of secondary problems. The primary cause of death in the client with CF is respiratory failure.

The pulmonary problems of CF result from the constant presence of thick, sticky mucus and are the most serious complications of the disease. The mucus narrows airways, reducing airflow. The constant presence of mucus results in chronic respiratory tract infections, chronic bronchitis, and chronic dilation of the bronchioles (bronchiectasis). Lung abscesses are common. Over time, the bronchioles distend and have increased numbers (hyperplasia) of mucus-producing cells and increased mucus-producing cell size (hypertrophy). Complications include pneumothorax, arterial erosion and hemorrhage, and respiratory failure.

Etiology and Genetic Risk

CF is an autosomal recessive disorder in which both gene alleles must be mutated for the disease to be expressed. The CF gene is located on chromosome 7 and produces a protein that controls chloride movement across cell membranes. There is great variation in the severity of CF; however, life expectancy is always considerably reduced, with an average of 33 years. People with one mutated allele are carriers and have few or no symptoms of CF but can pass the abnormal allele on to their children. Currently, more than 1000 different mutations have been identified. The inheritance of different mutations is thought to be responsible for the wide variation in disease severity.

Incidence/Prevalence

The disorder is most common among white individuals, and about 4% are carriers. CF is very rare among African Americans or Asians. Males and females are affected equally.

COLLABORATIVE MANAGEMENT

Assessment

Usually cystic fibrosis (CF) is diagnosed in childhood. The major diagnostic test is sweat chloride analysis. The defect in chloride movement prevents absorption of sodium chloride in the sweat glands; thus more chloride than normal is present in the sweat. The sweat chloride test is positive for CF when the chloride level in the sweat ranges between 60 and 200 mEq/L (mmol/L), compared with the normal value of 5 to 35 mEq/L.

NONPULMONARY MANIFESTATIONS

The adult client with CF is usually smaller and thinner than average. Other manifestations include abdominal distention, gastroesophageal reflux, rectal prolapse, foul-smelling stools, and **steatorrhea** (excessive fat in stools). The client may be malnourished and have many vitamin deficiencies. As pancreatic function decreases, the client has symptoms of diabetes mellitus from loss of insulin production.

PULMONARY MANIFESTATIONS

The pulmonary problems caused by CF are progressive. The respiratory infections are frequent or chronic with periods of exacerbations. Clients usually have chest congestion, limited exercise tolerance, cough, sputum production, use of accessory muscles, and decreased pulmonary function (especially FVC and FEV_1). Chest x-rays show persistent infiltrate and an increased anteroposterior (AP) diameter.

During an acute exacerbation or when the disease progresses to end stage, the client has increased chest congestion, reduced activity tolerance, increased crackles, increased cough, increased sputum production (often with hemoptysis), and severe dyspnea. Fatigue increases in proportion with the dyspnea. Arterial blood gas (ABG) studies show acidosis with greatly reduced partial pressure of arterial oxygen (PaO_2), increased partial pressure of arterial carbon dioxide ($PaCO_2$), increased bicarbonate levels, and low pH.

When infection is present, the client has fever, an elevated white blood cell count, and decreased oxygen saturation. Other manifestations of infection include tachypnea, tachycardia, intercostal retractions, weight loss, and increased fatigue.

Interventions

The client with CF needs daily therapy to slow disease progress and enhance gas exchange. There is no cure for CF.

NONSURGICAL MANAGEMENT. The management of the client with CF is complex and lifelong. Nutritional management focuses on weight maintenance, vitamin supplementation, diabetes management, and pancreatic enzyme replacement. Pulmonary management is focused on preventive maintenance and management of pulmonary exacerbation.

Preventive/Maintenance Therapy. The client with CF uses a regimen of chest physiotherapy, positive expiratory pressure, active cycle breathing technique, and an individualized regular exercise program. Pulmonary function tests (PFTs), especially FEV_1, are monitored regularly. Maintenance drugs include bronchodilators, anti-inflammatory agents, mucolytics, and antibiotics.

Exacerbation Therapy. Exacerbation therapy is needed when the client with CF has a change in manifestations from baseline. Such changes include increased chest congestion, decreased activity tolerance, increased or new-onset crackles, and at least a 10% decrease in FEV_1. Other manifestations occurring with exacerbation include increased sputum production with bloody or purulent sputum, increased frequency and duration of coughing, decreased appetite, weight loss, fatigue, decreased SaO_2, and ventilatory muscle retractions. Often infection is present and the client also has fever, increased lung infiltrate on chest x-ray, and an elevated white blood cell count.

Every attempt is made to avoid having the client with CF mechanically ventilated. Treatment focuses on airway clearance, increased oxygenation, and antibiotic therapy. Supplemental oxygen is prescribed on the basis of SaO_2 levels. Heliox delivery of 50% oxygen and 50% helium may improve gas exchange and oxygen saturation. The respiratory therapist initiates airway clearance techniques (ACTs) four times a day. Bronchodilator and mucolytic therapies are intensified (higher doses given more frequently than for maintenance). Steroidal anti-inflammatory agents are started or increased.

Depending on the severity of the exacerbation, a 10- to 14-day course of oral antibiotics may be prescribed. If the exacerbation is more severe, aerosolized tobramycin is prescribed. If oral/inhaled antibiotics are not effective, or if the exacerbation is very severe, IV antibiotics are used, usually an aminoglycoside, such as tobramycin and colistin or meropenem (Merrem).

As specialized treatment for CF improves and life span increases, other problems may occur. Clients may have bronchiole bleeding from lung arteries. Interventional radiology may be needed to embolize the bleeding arterial branches. Clients with CF may undergo this procedure repeatedly to control hemoptysis. See Chapter 39 for information on interventional radiology vascular procedures.

SURGICAL MANAGEMENT. The surgical management of the client with CF involves lung and/or pancreatic transplantation. *These procedures do not cure the disease, because the genetic defect in chloride transport and production of thick, sticky mucus remains.* Rather, the client has reduced manifestations initially and then has gradual progression of the disease. Transplantation extends life by 10 to 20 years, depending on other factors.

Fewer lung transplants are performed compared with transplantation of other solid organs. The problem is related to the scarcity of available lungs. In addition, many of the people who could benefit from lung transplantation have serious problems in other organs that make extended surgical procedures dangerous.

Lung transplant procedures include a lobe or a single lung transplantation, as well as double-lung transplantation. The type of procedure is determined by the client's age and overall condition, the cause of the lung problem, and the life expectancy after transplantation. Usually, the client with CF has a unilateral or bilateral lobe transplant from a living-related donor.

Preoperative Care. Many factors are considered before lung transplantation surgery. Recipient and donor criteria vary from one program to another, but some criteria are universal.

Recipient Criteria. The person who will receive the transplant, the **recipient,** must have severe, irreversible lung damage. It is important, however, that the client be well enough to survive the surgery. Usually clients must be younger than 55 years of age, although transplantation is considered on an individual basis. The following are exclusion criteria:

- Severe psychiatric disorders or self-destructive tendency
- Proven history of noncompliance or poor compliance with medical regimens

- Current cancer or cancer within the last 5 years
- Systemic infection
- Irreversible heart, kidney, or liver damage/disease
- Presence of any problem that would be made worse by immunosuppression

Donor Criteria. The following are donor criteria, regardless of whether the lung tissue is obtained from a cadaver or from a living-related donor:

- Infection free
- Cancer free
- Healthy lung tissue
- Close tissue match with the recipient
- Same blood type as the recipient

When the donor is living-related, the following are additional criteria:

- Age is younger than 55 years.
- Donor has normal cardiac function.
- Pulmonary function will remain adequate after tissue removal.
- The donor has had no previous chest surgery.
- Donor is psychologically stable.
- Donor has not been coerced into this situation.

Teaching. Regardless of the disease process that led to the need for lung transplantation, two activities are important before surgery. These activities are teaching the client the expected regimen of pulmonary hygiene to be used in the period immediately after surgery and assisting the client in a pulmonary muscle strengthening/conditioning regimen.

Operative Procedures. The client may or may not need to be placed on cardiopulmonary bypass, depending on the exact procedure. The client having single-lung or lobe transplantation usually does not need bypass. The client having double-lung transplantation needs cardiopulmonary bypass.

The most common incision used for lung transplantation is a transverse thoracotomy ("clamshell") for best access. The diseased lung or lungs are removed. The new lobes, lung, or lungs are placed in the chest cavity with **anastomoses** (connections) made to the proper airways (trachea, mainstem bronchus, or secondary bronchus) and blood vessels. Usually, lung transplantation surgery is completed within 4 to 6 hours.

Postoperative Care. The client is intubated for at least 48 hours. In addition, chest tubes and arterial lines are in place. Much of the care needed is the same as that for any thoracic surgery.

Major problem areas after lung transplantation are bleeding, infection, and transplant rejection. Bleeding is most common in clients who had cardiopulmonary bypass with anticoagulation. Usually the client remains in the intensive care unit for several days following transplantation.

Immunosuppressive drug regimens must be started immediately after surgery, which increases the risk for infection. The drugs generally used for routine long-term immunosuppressive therapy after organ transplantation are combinations of very specific immunosuppressants (cyclosporine [Sandimmune]), less specific immunosuppressants (azathioprine [Imuran] or mycophenolate mofetil [CellCept]), and one of the corticosteroids, such as prednisone (Apo-Prednisone✱, Deltasone✱) or prednisolone (Delta-Cortef). Corticosteroids are avoided in the first 10 to 14 days after surgery because of their negative impact on the healing process. (See Chapter 23 for more information on antirejection therapy.)

PRIMARY PULMONARY HYPERTENSION

PATHOPHYSIOLOGY

Pulmonary hypertension can occur as a complication of other lung disorders. Primary pulmonary hypertension (PPH) occurs in the absence of other lung disorders, and its cause is unknown although exposure to some drugs increases the risk. This disorder is rare and occurs mostly in women between the ages of 20 and 40 years.

The pathologic problem in PPH is blood vessel constriction with increasing vascular resistance in the lung. Pulmonary blood pressure rises and blood flow decreases, leading to poor perfusion and hypoxemia. Eventually, the right side of the heart fails **(cor pulmonale)** from the continuous workload of pumping against the high pulmonary pressures. Without treatment, death usually occurs within 2 years after diagnosis.

Genetic Considerations

Although most cases of primary pulmonary hypertension (PPH) are sporadic with no known cause, about 6% of people who develop PPH also have a close relative with the disorder. This type of PPH is considered to be "familial," in that genetics probably play a role but no single gene has been identified. In performing a pulmonary assessment for any client with breathing problems, especially young women, ask whether any family members have PPH. It is suggested that these relatives have baseline pulmonary function tests performed.

◆COLLABORATIVE MANAGEMENT

◆Assessment

The most common early manifestations are dyspnea and fatigue in an otherwise healthy adult. Some clients also have angina-like chest pain. Table 33-4 lists the classification of PPH.

Diagnosis is made from the results of right-sided heart catheterization showing elevated pulmonary pressures. Other test results suggesting pulmonary hypertension include abnormal ventilation-perfusion scans and pulmonary function tests (PFTs) showing reduced functional pulmonary volumes with reduced diffusion capacity, and spiral computed tomography (CT).

◆Interventions

Nonsurgical interventions that reduce pulmonary pressures and slow the development of cor pulmonale involve drugs that dilate pulmonary vessels and prevent clot formation. Warfarin (Coumadin) therapy is taken daily to achieve an International Normalized Ratio (INR) of 1.5 to 2.0. Calcium channel blockers, such as nifedipine (Procardia) and diltiazem (Cardizem) have been used to dilate blood vessels. These agents, however, cause general vessel dilation and some degree of hypotension. Prostacyclin agents provide the best specific dilation of pulmonary

TABLE 33-4 Severity Classification for Pulmonary Hypertension

Class	Manifestations
I	Pulmonary hypertension diagnosed by pulmonary function tests and right-sided cardiac catheterization No limitation of physical activity Moderate physical activity does not induce dyspnea, fatigue, chest pain, or light-headedness
II	No manifestations at rest Mild to moderate physical activity induces dyspnea, fatigue, chest pain, or light-headedness
III	No or slight manifestations at rest Mild (less than ordinary) activity induces dyspnea, fatigue, chest pain, or light-headedness
IV	Dyspnea and fatigue present at rest Unable to carry out any level of physical activity without manifestations Manifestations of right-sided heart failure apparent (dependent edema, engorged neck veins, enlarged liver)

Data from Eells, P. (2004). Advances in prostacyclin therapy for pulmonary arterial hypertension. *Critical Care Nurse, 24*(2), 42-54.

blood vessels. Continuous infusion of a naturally occurring prostacyclin agent, epoprostenol (Flolan), through a small IV pump reduces pulmonary pressures and increases lung blood flow. An alternate therapy is the delivery of a synthetic prostacyclin, treprostinil (Remodulin) by subcutaneous infusion through a microinfusion pump is also effective.

When the heart has undergone some hypertrophy and cardiac output has fallen, the client may be started on a regimen of digoxin (Lanoxin) and diuretics. Oxygen therapy is used when dyspnea is continuous or uncomfortable. These therapies do not cure the disorder; they just improve function and reduce symptoms.

Surgical management of primary pulmonary hypertension involves whole-lung transplantation. When cor pulmonale also is present, the client may need a combined heart-lung transplantation. It is not known whether the process of pulmonary vasoconstriction can begin again in the transplanted lungs or if the transplant is a "cure."

INTERSTITIAL PULMONARY DISEASES

The category of interstitial pulmonary diseases contains a variety of lung disorders, also called **fibrotic lung** diseases, that have some features in common. All affect the alveoli, blood vessels, and surrounding support tissue of the lungs rather than the airways. Thus these disorders are **restrictive** (preventing good expansion and recoil of the gas exchange unit) rather than obstructive. With restrictive disease, the lung tissues thicken, causing reduced gas exchange and "stiff" lungs that do not expand well. Unlike obstructive problems, air trapping does not occur and the client does not develop a "barrel chest." Often the onset of these disorders is slow and dyspnea is the most common manifestation.

Sarcoidosis

PATHOPHYSIOLOGY

Sarcoidosis is a granulomatous disorder of unknown cause that can affect any organ, but the lung is involved most often. Sarcoidosis develops over time with growths called **granulomas** forming in the lungs. Granulomas contain lymphocytes, macrophages, epithelioid cells, and giant cells.

Pulmonary sarcoidosis involves autoimmune responses in which the normally protective T-lymphocytes increase and cause damaging actions in lung tissue. Alveolar cells are the targets of the damaging actions. No single cause for T-lymphocyte activation has been identified, although infection and genetic predisposition appear to play a role. Alveolar inflammation **(alveolitis)** occurs from the presence of immune cells in the alveoli. Chronic inflammation causes **fibrosis** (scar tissue formation in the lungs). The fibrosis reduces **lung compliance** (elasticity) and the ability to exchange gases. **Cor pulmonale** (right-sided cardiac failure) is often present, because the heart can no longer pump effectively against the stiff, fibrotic lung.

The disease usually affects young adults. Manifestations include enlarged lymph nodes in the hilar area of the lungs, lung infiltrate on chest x-ray, skin lesions, and eye lesions. The first indication of disease may be an abnormal chest x-ray in an otherwise healthy client. The most common symptoms include cough, dyspnea, hemoptysis, and chest discomfort. In many clients, the illness resolves permanently. Others may have progressive pulmonary fibrosis and severe systemic disease.

COLLABORATIVE MANAGEMENT

Assessment

Sarcoidosis is suspected in the client who has a cough, dyspnea, and abnormal chest x-ray but is otherwise asymptomatic. Other conditions to rule out before diagnosing sarcoidosis are lung infections and cancer. Fiberoptic bronchoscopy may also be used in the diagnosis of this disorder (see Chapter 30).

Sarcoidosis is staged on the basis of x-ray findings. Higher stages have greater damage and more widespread disease. Pulmonary function studies often show a restrictive pattern of decreased lung volumes and impaired diffusing capacity. Irreversible lung changes develop in 10% to 15% of clients. Clients who develop severe restrictive disease may also develop secondary pulmonary hypertension.

Interventions

The goal of therapy is to lessen symptoms and prevent fibrosis. Management varies. If the client is asymptomatic and has normal pulmonary function, no treatment is given. The presence of manifestations; decreased total lung capacity (TLC), diffusing capacity, or forced vital capacity (FVC); involvement of other organs; and hypercalcemia are indicators for treatment.

Corticosteroids are the main type of therapy. Dosages vary from 40 to 60 mg daily with tapering doses over 6 to 8 weeks, to a maintenance dose of 10 to 15 mg for 6 months. Further therapy may occur over 12 months. Follow-up and monitoring include assessment of symptom severity, pulmonary function studies, chest x-rays, a complete blood count, serum creatinine, serum calcium, and urinalysis. Teach the client about side effects of steroid therapy and other aspects of physical care as indicated.

Idiopathic Pulmonary Fibrosis

PATHOPHYSIOLOGY

Idiopathic pulmonary fibrosis is a common restrictive lung disease. The typical client is an older adult with a history of cigarette smoking or chronic exposure to inhalation irritants such as metal particles, dust, organic chemicals, and wood fires. Unlike sarcoidosis, pulmonary fibrosis is highly lethal. Most clients have progressive disease with few remission periods. Even with proper treatment, clients usually survive less than 5 years after diagnosis.

Pulmonary fibrosis is an example of excessive wound healing. Once lung injury occurs, an inflammatory process begins tissue repair. The inflammation continues beyond normal healing time, causing extensive fibrosis and scarring. These changes thicken alveolar tissues, making gas exchange difficult.

COLLABORATIVE MANAGEMENT

Assessment

The onset of disease is slow, with early symptoms of mild dyspnea on exertion. Pulmonary function tests show decreased FVC. As the fibrosis progresses, the client becomes more dyspneic and hypoxemia becomes severe. Eventually, the client needs high levels of oxygen and often is still hypoxemic. Respirations are rapid and shallow.

Interventions

The goal of therapy is to slow the fibrotic process and manage dyspnea. Corticosteroids and other immunosuppressants are the mainstays of therapy. Immunosuppressant drugs include cytotoxic drugs such as cyclophosphamide (Cytoxan, Neosar, Procytox✱), azathioprine (Imuran), chlorambucil (Leukeran), or methotrexate (Folex). These drugs have many side effects, including immunosuppression, nausea, and lung and liver damage. Starting drug therapy early is critical, even though not all clients respond to therapy. Even among those who have a response to therapy, the disease continues to progress and leads to death by respiratory failure.

Lung transplantation is a curative therapy; however, the selection criteria, cost, and availability of organs make this option unlikely for most clients.

The client and family need support and help with community resources after diagnosis. The health care team assists the client and family in understanding the disease process and maintaining hope for control of the fibrosis. It is important to prevent respiratory infections. Teach the client and family about the manifestations of infection and encourage them to avoid respiratory irritants, crowds, and those with known infections.

Home oxygen is needed by the time the client becomes symptomatic because significant fibrosis has already occurred. Instruct him or her about oxygen use as a continuous therapy. Fatigue is a major problem. Instruct the client and family about energy conservation measures (see Energy Conservation [Chronic Obstructive Pulmonary Disease] on p. 603). Activity limitations and rest help reduce the work of breathing and oxygen consumption (see Chart 39-9).

Support the client's need to be as independent as possible and encourage him or her to pace activities and accept assistance as needed. The disease is costly because the client is often unable to work and may need home care.

Meeting HEALTHY PEOPLE 2010 Objectives

TOBACCO USE

Objective 3.1: Reduce to 13%, the proportion of adults (18 and older) who use tobacco.

Teach the client who smokes cigarettes the following techniques to quit smoking:

- Make a list of the reasons you want to stop smoking (e.g., your health and the health of those around you, saving money, social reasons).
- Set a date to stop smoking and keep it. Decide whether you are going to begin to cut down on the amount you smoke or are going to stop "cold turkey." Whatever way you decide to do it, keep this important date!
- Ask for help from those around you. Find someone who wants to quit smoking and "buddy up" for support. Look for assistance in your community, such as formal smoking cessation programs, counselors, and certified acupuncture specialists or hypnotists.
- Consult your health care provider about nicotine replacement therapy (i.e., patch, gum, etc.).
- Remove ashtrays and lighters from your view.
- Talk to yourself! Remind yourself of all the reasons you want to quit.
- Think of a way to reward yourself with the money you save from not smoking for a year.
- Avoid places that might tempt you to smoke. If you are used to having a cigarette after meals, get up from the table as soon as you are finished eating. Think of new things to do at times when you used to smoke.
- Find activities that keep your hands busy: needlework, painting, gardening, even holding a pencil.
- Take five deep breaths of clean, fresh air through your nose and out your mouth if you feel the urge to smoke.
- Keep plenty of healthy, low-calorie snacks, such as fruit and vegetables, on hand to nibble on. Try sugarless gum or mints as a substitute for tobacco.
- Drink at least eight glasses of water each day.
- Begin an exercise program with the approval of your health care provider. Be aware of the positive, healthy changes in your body since you stopped smoking.
- List the many reasons why you are glad that you quit. Keep the list handy as a reminder of the positive things you are doing for yourself.
- Think of each day without tobacco as a major accomplishment. It is!!

In the later stages of the disease, the focus is to reduce the sensation of dyspnea. This is often accomplished with the use of oral, parenteral, or nebulized morphine. Provide information about hospice, which supports and coordinates resources to meet the needs of the client and family when the prognosis for survival is less than 6 months.

OCCUPATIONAL PULMONARY DISEASE

PATHOPHYSIOLOGY

Exposure to occupational or environmental fumes, dust, vapors, gases, bacterial or fungal antigens, and allergens can result in a variety of respiratory disorders. Depending on the degree, frequency, and intensity of exposure, and on the specific disease, clients may have acute reversible effects or chronic lung disease. All occupational pulmonary diseases are made worse by cigarette smoking. Thus smoking cessation efforts are very important (see the Meeting Healthy People 2010 Objectives box above).

CHART 33-12

KEY FEATURES of
Common Occupational Pulmonary Diseases

Disease and Category	Causes and Manifestations
Occupational Asthmas	
Latency (allergic) asthma	Airway narrowing related only to workplace exposures Atopic allergic response to industrial irritants Develops after a period of exposure (from several weeks to several years) Characterized by airflow limitation Usually resolves when exposure ceases Obstructive disease
Irritant-induced asthma	Manifestations only in the workplace First onset usually within 24 hours of exposure Common irritants: chlorine, ammonia, and phosgene Characterized by sloughing of epithelium, thickening of the basement membranes, and mucosal inflammation Early manifestations: cough, wheeze, and dyspnea High exposures can lead to pulmonary edema, acute respiratory distress syndrome, and death Permanent tissue changes in most cases Obstructive and restrictive disease
Pneumoconiosis	
Silicosis	Chronic fibrosis from long-term inhalation of silica dust Found among people working in mines, stone quarries, foundries, and in the following industries: glass-making, pottery, sandblasting, tile and brick making, soap and polishes, and manufacture of filters Characterized by nodule formation between alveoli, leading to fibrosis Manifestations: dyspnea on exertion, fatigue, weight loss, reduced lung volume, and upper lobe fibrosis Restrictive disease
Coal miner's disease (black lung disease)	Massive deposits of coal dust in the lungs leading to diffuse fibrosis Develops earlier among miners who smoke Early manifestations are similar to bronchitis Emphysema is a late development Restrictive disease
Diffuse Interstitial Fibrosis	
Asbestosis	Occurs among people who work in asbestos mines, building construction/remodeling, and shipyards Characterized by diffuse pleural thickening and diaphragmatic calcification Restrictive disease
Talcosis	Occurs among people who work in industries that manufacture paint, ceramics, roofing materials, cosmetics, and rubber goods Restrictive disease
Berylliosis	Occurs among people who work in industries where metal is heated (steel mills, welding) or metal is machined, creating dust Has a genetic component for increased susceptibility to disease after beryllium exposure Restrictive disease
Extrinsic Allergic Alveolitis	
"Farmer's lung" "Bird fancier's lung" "Machine operator's lung"	Hypersensitivity pneumonitis as an immunologic response to inhaling dust or chemical that contains bacterial or fungal antigens Characterized by formation of granulomas with central necrosis in the alveoli and surrounding blood vessels Restrictive disease

Many occupational diseases have an onset of symptoms long after the initial exposure to the offending agent. The client's personal history can provide clues about the presence and cause of occupational pulmonary diseases. Common occupational pulmonary diseases include occupational asthma, pneumoconiosis, diffuse interstitial fibrosis, and extrinsic allergic alveolitis. Chart 33-12 lists the key features of these disorders.

COLLABORATIVE MANAGEMENT

Assessment

Consider an occupational cause for all clients with new-onset asthma or dyspnea. Obtain a thorough history of occupational exposure and onset of symptoms because there may or may not be a latency period between exposure and onset of symptoms. Determine whether the symptoms are acute or chronic. Ask the client about the use of inhalation protection and about cigarette smoking.

Interventions

Prevention is important to avoiding disability from occupationally related disease. Stress the importance of using special respirators and ensuring adequate ventilation when working in potentially harmful environments.

The client with occupational asthma with a latency period should be removed from the site of exposure, transferred to a job without exposure, and treated with medications for asthma. Nursing care is similar to the care for

TABLE 33-5 Features of the Major Types of Lung Cancer

Category and Type	Characteristics
Small cell lung cancer (SCLC)	20% of all lung cancers 99% association with cigarette smoking Fast growing Usually metastatic at time of diagnosis Paraneoplastic syndromes common Surgical resection not helpful Treatment regimen: combination chemotherapy
Non–small cell lung cancer (NSCLC)	Surgical resection helpful for stage I and II disease Combination chemotherapy helpful Targeted therapy helpful Radiation used for cure if disease is confined to the chest
Epidermoid carcinoma	30% of all lung cancers Strongly associated with cigarette smoking Slower growing, less invasive Found in bronchi and peripheral lung tissue
Adenocarcinoma	30%-35% of all lung cancers Incidence similar for smokers and nonsmokers Most common lung cancer in women Metastasis occurs early Found in peripheral lung tissue
Large cell	≈10% of all lung cancers Slow growing Found in peripheral lung tissue

TABLE 33-6 Endocrine Paraneoplastic Syndromes Associated with Lung Cancer

Ectopic Hormone	Manifestation
Adrenocorticotropic hormone (ACTH)	Cushing's syndrome
Antidiuretic hormone	Syndrome of inappropriate antidiuretic hormone (SIADH) ■ Weight gain ■ General edema ■ Dilution of serum electrolytes
Follicle-stimulating hormone (FSH)	Gynecomastia
Parathyroid hormone	Hypercalcemia
Ectopic insulin	Hypoglycemia

asthma not caused by the workplace environment. Refer the client to a social worker, who provides information regarding compensation and pensions.

Nursing interventions for clients with occupational lung restrictive disease are the same as for those with emphysema. Hypoxemic clients require supplemental oxygen. In addition, respiratory therapies to promote sputum clearance are essential.

LUNG CANCER

PATHOPHYSIOLOGY

Lung cancer is a leading cause of cancer-related deaths worldwide. In the United States, more deaths from lung cancer occur each year than from prostate cancer, breast cancer, and colon cancer combined. The American Cancer Society estimates that more than 186,000 new cases of lung cancer are diagnosed each year and that more than 165,000 deaths occur each year from lung care. The overall 5-year survival rate for all clients with lung cancer is only 14%. This poor long-term survival rate is due to the fact that most lung cancers are diagnosed at a late stage, when metastasis is present. Only 15% of clients have small tumors and localized disease at the time of diagnosis (American Cancer Society, 2005).

Despite many advances in cancer treatment, the prognosis for lung cancer remains poor unless the tumor can be removed completely by surgery. Treatment of lung cancer is often aimed toward relieving symptoms **(palliation)** rather than cure, because of the presence of metastasis.

More than 90% of all primary lung cancers arise from the bronchial epithelium. These cancers are collectively called bronchogenic carcinomas. Lung cancers can be classified according to their histologic cell type as small cell lung cancer (SCLC), epidermoid (squamous cell) cancer, adenocarcinoma, and large cell cancer (Table 33-5). The last three types are now referred to as non–small cell lung cancer (NSCLC) because of their similar responses to treatment. Chapter 27 discusses the general mechanisms and processes of cancer development.

Metastasis

Lung cancers **metastasize** (spread) by direct extension, through the blood and invading lymph glands and vessels. Tumors in the bronchial tubes can grow and obstruct the bronchus partially or completely. Tumors in other areas of lung tissue can grow so large that they can cause airway obstruction by compressing the airway. Tumors in the edges of the lungs spread and can compress the alveoli, nerves, blood vessels, and lymph vessels.

The patterns of metastasis depend on the type of tumor cell and the location of the tumor. Lung lymph nodes, as well as more distant lymph nodes, can be invaded.

Hematogenous (bloodborne) metastasis of lung cancer is due to invasion of blood vessels in the lungs. Tumor pieces **(emboli)** spread to distant body areas. These sites of metastasis include the bone, liver, brain, and adrenal glands.

Additional manifestations, known as **paraneoplastic syndromes,** complicate certain lung cancers. The paraneoplastic syndromes are caused by hormones secreted by tumor cells. Paraneoplastic syndrome commonly occurs with SCLC. Tables 33-6 and 33-7 list the endocrine and nonendocrine paraneoplastic syndromes, respectively, that may occur with lung cancer.

Staging

Lung cancer is staged at diagnosis to assess the size and extent of the disease. These factors are correlated to survival rate. The staging of lung cancer is based on the TNM system (T, primary *t*umor; N, regional lymph *n*odes; M, distant *m*etastasis). Table 33-8 shows the TNM system for lung cancer staging. Higher numbers represent later stages and less chance for cure or long-term survival.

Etiology and Genetic Risk

Lung cancers occur as a result of repeated exposure to inhaled substances that cause chronic tissue irritation or inflammation. Cigarette smoking is the major risk factor and

TABLE 33-7 Nonendocrine Paraneoplastic Syndromes Associated with Lung Cancer

Tissue/System	Manifestation
Connective tissue	Arthralgia Digital clubbing
Hematologic system	Anemia Leukocytosis Thrombocytopenia purpura Polycythemia Thrombocytosis
Neuromuscular system	Peripheral neuropathy Carcinomatous myopathy Cortical cerebellar degeneration Seizure Polymyositis Myasthenia-like syndrome
Integumentary system	Dermatomyositis Scleroderma Acanthosis nigricans
Vascular system	Thrombophlebitis Nonbacterial endocarditis
Renal system	Arterial thrombosis Nephrotic syndrome Proteinuria

TABLE 33-8 TMN Stage Grouping for Lung Cancer

Stage	Tumors	Nodes	Distant Metastasis
Occult carcinoma	T_x	N_0	M_0
Stage 0	T_{IS}	Carcinoma in situ	
Stage I	T_1 T_2	N_0 N_0	M_0 M_0
Stage II	T_1 T_2	N_1 N_1	M_0 M_0
Stage IIIa	T_3 T_3 $T_{1\text{-}3}$	N_0 N_1 N_2	M_0 M_0 M_0
Stage IIIb	Any T T_4	N_3 Any N	M_0 M_0
Stage IV	Any T	Any N	M_1

From Mountain, C.F., Greenberg, M.D., & Fraire, A.E. (1991). Tumor stages in non–small cell carcinoma of the lung. *Chest, 99*(5), 1258-1260.

is responsible for 85% of all lung cancer deaths (American Cancer Society, 2004). The risk for lung cancer is directly related to the total exposure to cigarette smoke as determined by the number of years of smoking and number of cigarettes smoked per day. Pipe and cigar smoking also increase risk. The incidence of lung cancer decreases when smoking stops, and after 15 years of smoking cessation, it approaches that of those who have never smoked. About 50,000 ex-smokers, however, develop lung cancer in the United States each year.

Nonsmokers exposed to "passive," or "secondhand," smoke also have a greater risk for lung cancer than do nonsmokers who are minimally exposed to cigarette smoke. Passive smoke has many of the carcinogens found in inhaled, or "mainstream," tobacco smoke.

Other risk factors for lung cancer include chronic exposure to asbestos, beryllium, chromium, coal distillates, cobalt, iron oxide, mustard gas, petroleum distillates, radiation, tar, nickel, and uranium. Air pollution that contains benzopyrenes and hydrocarbons also increase the risk for lung cancer.

Genetic Considerations

Variation is seen in lung cancer development among people with similar smoking histories, suggesting that genetic factors can influence susceptibility. Differences in two different genes are associated with differences in personal susceptibility to lung cancer. One of the P450 enzymes, CYP2D6, activates carcinogens present in tobacco. People who have a mutated CYP2D6 gene do not activate the tobacco carcinogen and are less susceptible to lung cancer even if they smoke. About 10% of the U.S. population has this "resistance to lung cancer" gene. Another enzyme, glutathione S transferase, detoxifies and clears carcinogens from the body. Women who are missing this active enzyme are less able to clear carcinogens and are thus at greater risk for lung cancer if they are exposed to tobacco smoke. Men missing this enzyme do not have a greater risk for lung cancer.

Incidence/Prevalence

Lung cancer is a major health problem throughout the world. It represents 13% of new cancers in both men and women.

HEALTH PROMOTION/ILLNESS PREVENTION

Primary prevention for lung cancer is directed at reducing tobacco smoking. Educational strategies start with elementary school children to discourage them from beginning to smoke. Nurses are actively involved in encouraging nonsmokers not to begin to smoke, in promoting smoking cessation programs, and in establishing a smoke-free environment. Such educational strategies have been successfully used in the United States (see the Meeting Healthy People 2010 Objectives box on p. 611). Encourage nonsmokers to avoid passive, or secondhand, smoke by avoiding environmental exposure.

Teach workers in industrial settings about safety precautions, such as wearing specialized masks and protective clothing, to reduce occupational hazards. Encourage people who are at high risk for lung cancer development to seek frequent health examinations.

Urge clients being treated for lung cancer to quit smoking. The actual diagnosis of the disease and its treatment time represent "teachable moments." Nearly 80% of lung cancer survivors (those who live 5 years or longer after diagnosis) who quit smoking remain nonsmokers. Many survivors also engage in other healthy lifestyle changes. (See the Evidence-Based Practice for Nursing box on p. 615.)

◆COLLABORATIVE MANAGEMENT

◆Assessment

HISTORY

Ask the client about risk factors, including smoking, hazards in the workplace, and warning signals (Table 33-9). Have the client describe how many packs of cigarettes per day have been smoked for how many years to determine the pack-year smoking history.

Ask about the presence of lung cancer manifestations, such as hoarseness, cough, sputum production, hemoptysis, shortness of breath, or change in endurance. Many mani-

EVIDENCE-BASED PRACTICE for Nursing

Lung cancer survivors participate in healthy behaviors

Evangelista, L., Sarna, L., Brecht, M., Padilla, G., & Chen, J. (2003). Health perceptions and risk behaviors of lung cancer survivors. *Heart & Lung, 32*(2), 131-139.

This study sought to determine to what degree lung cancer survivors maintain the healthy lifestyle changes started at the time of diagnosis. Survivorship was defined as a minimum of 5 disease-free years after the initial cancer treatment. One hundred and forty-two survivors of non–small cell lung cancer (NSCLC) were asked to complete a battery of questionnaires to determine their perceptions of their own health status, their maintenance of healthy lifestyle changes, and exposure to high-risk environments. The reported smoking status was confirmed by urinary cotinine biomarker. This test measures the presence of a nicotine metabolite in the urine. Ingestion of nicotine in any form results in the formation of cotinine as a metabolite.

Participants ranged from 5 to 21 years of survival after initial diagnosis with a mean survival of 10 years. The majority of participants (70%) perceived their overall health status to be in the good to excellent range. Most participants who used tobacco had quit at diagnosis and were able to maintain this important lifestyle change. Only 19 participants (13%) continued to use tobacco after diagnosis. More than one fourth of the participants reported continued exposure to secondhand smoke.

Level of Evidence: 3—Well-designed trial without randomization—cohort study.

Critique. The study was well designed and implemented for its purpose. Using multiple tools with established validity and reliability increase the credibility of the findings. Major strengths include the large sample size, use of a highly sensitive biomarker to confirm smoking status, and the direct collection of physical parameters to establish body mass index.

Implications for Nursing. The overall 5-year survival rate for clients with NSCLC is only 20%. About 2% of these clients develop a second primary lung cancer. Smoking cession is linked to longer survivorship after a lung cancer diagnosis and treatment. Lung cancer diagnosis represents a "teachable moment" when the benefits of smoking cessation are perceived as high. Even though it is gratifying to find that most of the participants who stopped smoking were able to maintain this lifestyle change, a substantial number continued to smoke. Even more disturbing was the number of participants who remain exposed to secondhand smoke. Nurses need to stress the benefits of smoking cessation and of avoiding secondhand smoke in this population.

festations are common and may have been present for years. Ask the client to describe any recent changes in symptoms or if position affects symptoms.

Assess for chest pain or discomfort, which can occur at any stage of tumor development. Chest pain may be localized or on just one side and can range from mild to severe. Ask about any sensation of fullness, tightness, or pressure in the chest, which may suggest obstruction. A piercing chest pain or pleuritic pain may occur on inspiration. Pain radiating to the arm results from tumor invasion of nerve plexuses in advanced disease.

PHYSICAL ASSESSMENT/CLINICAL MANIFESTATIONS—PULMONARY

OBSERVATION. Manifestations of lung cancer are often nonspecific and appear late in the disease process. Specific manifestations depend on the type and location of the tumor. Chills, fever, and cough may be related to pneumonitis or bronchitis that occur with obstruction. Assess sputum quantity and quality. Blood-tinged sputum may occur with bleeding from a tumor. Hemoptysis is a later finding in the course of the disease. If infection or necrosis is present, sputum may be purulent and copious.

TABLE 33-9 Warning Signals Associated with Lung Cancer

- Hoarseness
- Change in respiratory pattern
- Persistent cough or change in cough
- Blood-streaked sputum
- Rust-colored or purulent sputum
- Frank hemoptysis
- Chest pain or chest tightness
- Shoulder, arm, or chest wall pain
- Recurring episodes of pleural effusion, pneumonia, or bronchitis
- Dyspnea
- Fever associated with one or two other signs
- Wheezing
- Weight loss
- Clubbing of the fingers

Breathing patterns may be labored or painful. An obstructive breathing pattern may occur as prolonged exhalation alternating with periods of shallow breathing. Rapid, shallow breathing occurs with pleuritic chest pain and an elevated diaphragm. Inspiratory efforts are reduced in advanced disease. Look for abnormal retractions, the use of accessory muscles, flared nares, stridor, and asymmetric diaphragmatic movement on inspiration. Dyspnea and wheezing may be present with airway obstruction. Ask about the client's level of dyspnea at rest, with activity, and in the supine position (orthopnea).

PALPATION. You may find areas of tenderness or masses when palpating the chest wall. Increased vibrations felt on the chest wall **(fremitus)** indicate areas of the lung where airspaces are replaced with tumor or fluid. Fremitus is decreased or absent when the bronchus is obstructed. The trachea may be displaced from midline if a mass is present in the area.

PERCUSSION. Lung areas with masses sound dull or flat rather than hollow or resonant on chest percussion.

AUSCULTATION. Breath sounds may change with the presence of a tumor. Wheezes indicate partial obstruction of airflow in passages narrowed by tumors. Decreased or absent breath sounds indicate complete obstruction of an airway by a tumor or fluid. Increased loudness or sound intensity of the voice while listening to breath sounds indicates increased density of lung tissue from tumor compression. A pleural friction rub is heard when inflammation also is present.

PHYSICAL ASSESSMENT/CLINICAL MANIFESTATIONS—NONPULMONARY

Many other systems can be affected by lung cancer and have changes at the time of diagnosis. Heart sounds may be muffled by a tumor or fluid around the heart (cardiac tamponade). Dysrhythmias may occur as a result of hypoxemia or direct pressure of the tumor on the heart. Cyanosis of the lips and fingertips or clubbing of the fingers may be present (see Figure 33-10).

Bones become thin with tumor invasion and break easily. The client may have bone pain or pathologic fractures.

Late manifestations of lung cancer usually include fatigue, weight loss, anorexia, dysphagia, and nausea and vomiting. Superior vena cava syndrome may result from tumor pressure in or around the vena cava. This syndrome is an emergency (see Chapter 28). Lethargy and somnolence may develop, and the client may have confusion or personality changes as a result of brain metastasis. Bowel and bladder tone or function may be affected by tumor spread to the spine and spinal cord.

PSYCHOSOCIAL ASSESSMENT

The poor prognosis for lung cancer has made it a much-feared disease. Lung cancer manifestations, especially dyspnea, add to the client's fear and anxiety. The client with a history of cigarette smoking may feel guilt and shame. Convey acceptance and interact with the client in a nonjudgmental way.

Few clients with lung cancer are cured or live 5 years after diagnosis. Many are given limited palliative treatment for symptom relief. Fear of pain and death is common.

DIAGNOSTIC ASSESSMENT

The diagnosis of lung cancer is made by direct examination of cancer cells. Cytologic examination of early morning sputum specimens may identify tumor cells; however, cancer cells may not be present in the sputum. When pleural effusion is present, fluid can be obtained by thoracentesis for cytology.

Lung lesions may be first identified on chest x-rays. Computed tomography (CT) examinations are then used to identify the lesions more clearly. Usually, the entire chest is scanned at 5- to 10-mm slices and the suspicious areas are then scanned at 1- to 2-mm slices for the highest resolution.

Fiberoptic bronchoscopy provides direct visibility of the tracheobronchial tree. Specimens and bronchial brushings can be obtained with this technique, especially when lesions are located within or close to an airway. Needle biopsy during bronchoscopy also may be used to obtain cancer cells.

A thoracoscopy may be performed through a video-assisted thoracoscope entering the chest cavity via small incisions through the chest wall. This procedure allows direct visualization of the lung tissue. To identify metastasis in mediastinal lymph nodes, a mediastinoscopy may be performed through a small chest incision.

Other diagnostic studies may be needed to determine how widely the cancer has spread. Such tests include needle biopsy of lymph nodes, direct surgical biopsy, and thoracentesis with pleural biopsy. Magnetic resonance imaging (MRI) and radionuclide scans of the liver, spleen, brain, and bone help determine the location of metastatic tumors. Pulmonary function tests and arterial blood gas (ABG) analysis help determine the overall respiratory status. Positron emission tomography (PET) scanning is becoming the most thorough way to find metastases. Together, these tests help determine the extent of the cancer and the best methods to treat it.

Interventions for Cure

Interventions for the client with lung cancer can be aimed at curing the disease, increasing the client's survival time, and enhancing the client's quality of life through palliation. Both nonsurgical and surgical interventions are used to achieve these aims. Some clients with lung cancer may undergo interventions for all three aims at different stages in the disease process.

NONSURGICAL MANAGEMENT

Chemotherapy. Chemotherapy is often the treatment of choice for lung cancers, especially small cell lung cancer (SCLC). It may be used alone or as adjuvant therapy in combination with surgery for non–small cell lung cancer (NSCLC). Table 33-10 lists common agents used in combination for treatment of lung cancer. The exact combination of drugs used may vary depending on the response of the tumor and the overall health of the client.

TABLE 33-10 Common Chemotherapy Agents Used in the Treatment of Lung Cancer*

Generic Name	Trade Name
Carboplatin	Paraplatin
Cisplatin	Platinol
Docetaxel	Taxotere
Gemcitabine	Gemzar
Irinotecan	Camptosar
Paclitaxel	Taxol
Vinorelbine	Navelbine

*This listing is not comprehensive and only lists the most commonly used current agents. Regimens vary. Combinations usually include a platinum-based drug with an antimitotic. See Table 28-6 for more information on chemotherapeutic agents.

Side effects that occur with chemotherapy for lung cancer include **alopecia** (hair loss), nausea and vomiting, open sores on mucous membranes **(mucositis),** immunosuppression, anemia, and **thrombocytopenia** (decreased numbers of platelets).

Reassure clients that hair loss is temporary. Hair regrowth begins about 1 month after chemotherapy is completed. Hair loss can be disguised by the use of wigs, scarves, turbans, and caps.

The chemotherapy agents used for lung cancer treatment are **emetogenic** (inducing nausea and vomiting). Many effective antiemetic drugs are available. Usually one or more antiemetics are given before and after chemotherapy. Drugs used to control chemotherapy-induced nausea and vomiting are listed in Chart 28-5. Client response to antiemetic therapy varies, and the drug combinations are individualized for best effect.

Frequent mouth assessment and oral hygiene are key in managing mucositis. Stress the importance of good, frequent oral hygiene, including tooth cleaning and mouth rinsing. Instruct clients to use a soft-bristled toothbrush or disposable mouth sponges and to avoid using dental floss and water-pressure gum cleaners (such as a WaterPik).

Immunosuppression, which greatly increases the risk for infection, is the major dose-limiting side effect of chemotherapy for lung cancer. Immunosuppression can be managed by the use of biological response modifiers (BRMs) to stimulate bone marrow production of immune system cells. Teach the client and family about precautions to take to reduce the client's chances of developing an infection (see Chart 28-8). (See Chapter 28 for more information about chemotherapy and associated nursing care.)

Genetic Considerations

An experimental treatment for advanced NSCLC takes advantage of genetic differences in cancer cells. A "targeted therapy" is erlotinib (Tarceva). This once-a-day tablet inhibits the enzyme tyrosine kinase from activating the epidermal growth factor receptors on lung cancer cells. With the receptor inactivated, cancer cell growth is slowed significantly. Although this drug is too new to know whether its use will cure NSCLC, it is extending the life spans of some clients by as much as 2 years. Because this drug targets the cancer cell receptors, the side effects on normal cells are minimal.

Radiation Therapy. Radiation therapy can be an effective treatment for locally advanced lung cancers confined to the chest. Best results are seen when radiation is used in addition to surgery or chemotherapy. Radiation may be performed before surgery to shrink the tumor and make resection easier.

Usually radiation therapy for lung cancer is performed daily for a 5- to 6-week period. Only the areas thought to have cancer are in the radiation path. The immediate side effects of this treatment are skin irritation and peeling, fatigue, nausea, and taste changes. Some clients have esophagitis during therapy. Narrowing of the esophagus can occur as a late response to radiation therapy for lung cancer.

Skin care in the radiation-treated area can be difficult. If the area has been marked with a dye to outline the areas for radiation, instruct the client not to wash off the markings. The use of ink or dye markings is rare, with most cancer centers using small permanent tattoos to mark the area. Instruct clients not to use lotions or ointments on the skin of the chest unless the radiologist prescribes them. Because skin in the radiation path is more sensitive to sun damage, advise clients to avoid direct skin exposure to the sun during treatment and for at least 1 year after radiation is completed.

SURGICAL MANAGEMENT. Surgery is the main treatment for stage I and stage II NSCLC. Total removal of a non–small cell primary lung cancer is undertaken in hope of achieving a cure. If complete resection is not possible, the surgeon removes the bulk of the tumor. The specific surgery depends on the stage of the cancer and the client's overall health and functional status. The procedure may involve only a thoracotomy with tumor removal. More often, lung cancer surgery involves removal of a lung segment, lobe **(lobectomy),** or entire lung **(pneumonectomy).**

Preoperative Care. The goals of care before surgery are to relieve anxiety and promote the client's participation (see Chapter 20 for routine preoperative care). Encourage the client to express fears and concerns, reinforce the surgeon's explanation of the surgical procedure, and provide education related to what is expected after surgery. Teach about the probable location of the surgical incision, shoulder exercises, and about the chest tube and drainage system (except after pneumonectomy).

Operative Procedures. Three types of incisions can be made depending on the location of the cancer: posterolateral, anterolateral, and median sternotomy (Figure 33-13). The incisions are large and are held open with retractors during surgery, contributing to pain after surgery.

A segmental resection **(segmentectomy)** is a lung resection that includes the bronchus, pulmonary artery and vein, and tissue of the involved lung segment or segments, which are divisions of lobes. A **wedge resection** is removal of the peripheral portion of small, localized areas of disease. A **lobectomy** is the removal of an entire lung lobe. A **pneumonectomy** is the removal of an entire lung, including all blood vessels. The bronchus to that lung is severed and sutured.

Postoperative Care. General care of the client after thoracotomy is reviewed in the Plan of Care on pp. 618 to 622. Care after surgery for clients who have undergone thoracotomy (except for pneumonectomy) requires closed-chest drainage to drain air and blood that accumulate in the pleural space. A **chest tube,** a drain placed in the pleural space to restore intrapleural pressure, allows re-expansion of

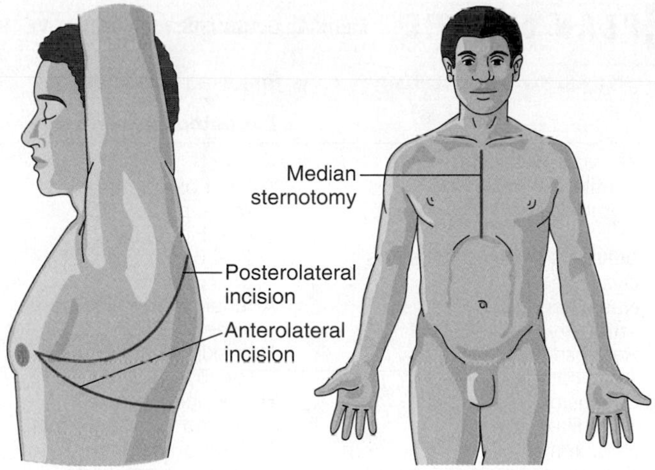

Figure 33-13 ■ Common incision locations for partial or total pneumonectomy.

the lung (Figure 33-14). The chest tube also prevents air and fluid from returning to the chest. The drainage system consists of one or more chest tubes or drains, a collection container placed below the chest level, and a water seal to keep air from entering the chest. The drainage system may use actual bottles (Figure 33-15) or, more often, a disposable self-contained system (Figure 33-16). The basic principles of gravity and pressure are the same with both systems.

Chest Tube Placement. The tip of the tube used to drain air is placed near the front lung apex (see Figure 33-14). The tube that drains liquid is placed on the side near the base of the lung. After lung surgery, two tubes, anterior and posterior, are used. The puncture wounds are covered with airtight dressings.

The chest tube is connected to about 6 feet of tubing that leads to a collection device or bottle placed several feet below the chest. The tubing allows the client to turn and move easily. Keeping the collection device below the chest allows gravity to drain the pleural space. When two chest tubes are inserted, they are joined by a Y-connector near the client's body; the 6 feet of tubing are attached to the Y-connector.

Drainage System. The chest drainage system uses a water seal mechanism that acts as a one-way valve to prevent air or liquid from moving back into the chest cavity. Earlier chest drainage consisted of one-, two-, and three-bottle systems. These bulky glass bottle systems have been replaced with one-piece disposable chest drainage devices. The Pleur-Evac system is a common device using a one-piece disposable plastic unit with three chambers. It duplicates the three-bottle system.

The three-bottle system (see Figure 33-15) is used to explain the principles and actions of water-seal chest drainage. The three bottles are connected to one another. The tube(s) from the client is(are) connected to the first bottle (or chamber) in the series of three. This bottle (chamber) is the collection container. The second bottle (chamber) in the series is the water seal to prevent air from moving back up the tubing system and into the chest. The third bottle (chamber), when suction is applied, is the suction regulator.

BOTTLE ONE. In setting up the system, bottle one (nearest to the client) does not at first have fluid in it. The tubing

Text continued on p. 623.

PLAN of CARE — MEDICAL DIAGNOSIS: POSTOPERATIVE THORACOTOMY

NURSING DIAGNOSIS NO. 1 ■ Impaired Gas Exchange

	Expected Outcomes	Nursing Interventions	Rationales
RELATED FACTORS Ventilation-perfusion imbalance **DEFINING CHARACTERISTICS** Dyspnea Nasal flaring Irritability Restlessness Tachycardia Confusion Skin: Pale, dusky Hypoxemia Breathing: Abnormal rate; abnormal depth Arterial blood gases: Abnormal	Arterial blood gases remain: pO_2 80-100 mm Hg; $pHCO_3$ 22-26 mm Hg; pCO_2 35-45 mm Hg Arterial pH remains between 7.35 and 7.45 Has skin with warm undertones Has a pulse between 60 and 100 beats/min No verbal report or observation of irritability No verbal report or observation of restlessness Has a respiratory rate that remains between 11 and 22 breaths/min Has respirations that remain regular and deep	NIC **Airway Management** D Place the client in semi-Fowler's position, if possible.	Semi-Fowler's position ensures that abdominal contents do not press against the diaphragm and restrict chest expansion.
		Encourage the client to cough frequently, or suction the client as necessary.	Coughing or suction will rid the airway of secretions.
		D Encourage the client to take slow, deep breaths; to turn; and to cough.	Effective aeration and cough will help rid the body of secretions. Frequent position changes will prevent secretions from pooling in one area.
		Assist the client with an incentive spirometer, as appropriate.	Incentive spirometry encourages the client to deep breathe.
		Administer humidified air or oxygen, as appropriate.	Humidified air will soothe respiratory passages. Increased oxygen will elevate the amount of oxygen in the alveoli available for exchange.
		Regulate fluid intake to optimize fluid balance.	Fluids will help keep lung secretions thin and easier to cough out of the airways.
		NIC **Respiratory Monitoring** D Monitor rate, rhythm, depth, and effort of respirations.	Changes in respiratory rate, rhythm, depth, or effort may signal a descent into respiratory failure.
		Note chest movement, watching for symmetry, use of accessory muscles, and supraclavicular and intercostal muscle retractions.	The use of accessory muscles indicates increased respiratory effort.
		Note location of trachea.	A deviated trachea may indicate a tension pneumothorax.
		Auscultate breath sounds, noting areas of decreased/absent ventilation and the presence of adventitious sounds.	Absent breath sounds or adventitious breath sounds indicate poor gas exchange or poor movement of air through the airways.
		Monitor for increased restlessness, anxiety, and air hunger.	A change in the client's level of consciousness is the earliest sign of deterioration in effective oxygenation.
		Note changes in SaO_2, SvO_2, end tidal CO_2, and ABG values, as appropriate.	These tests are indicators of the effectiveness of gas exchange or gas transport.
		D Monitor for dyspnea and the events that improve and worsen it.	Events that improve dyspnea should be encouraged, and events that worsen dyspnea need to be avoided.
		NIC **Oxygen Therapy** Maintain airway patency.	Oxygen requires free passage to the lungs.
		Monitor the effectiveness of oxygen therapy, as appropriate.	Pulse oximetry and ABGs reflect oxygen concentrations in the blood or attached to red blood cells.

D Indicates tasks that can be delegated to unlicensed assistive nursing personnel at the discretion of the nurse.

PLAN of CARE MEDICAL DIAGNOSIS: POSTOPERATIVE THORACOTOMY—*cont'd*

NURSING DIAGNOSIS NO. 1 ■ Impaired Gas Exchange—*cont'd*

	Expected Outcomes	Nursing Interventions	Rationales
		Monitor the client's anxiety related to the need for oxygen therapy.	Oxygen deprivation causes the sympathetic nervous system to secrete stress hormones, which are interpreted subjectively as anxiety.
		Provide for oxygen when the client is transported.	Portable oxygen should be provided when transporting a client who requires supplemental oxygen.
		Other Interventions	
		Advise the client to limit caffeine intake.	Caffeine causes diuresis and increases the risk of dehydration.
		Check chest tubes hourly.	Tube connections must be checked to ensure sterility and patency.
		Tape tubing junctions.	Taping prevents accidental disconnections.
		Position the drainage tube to prevent kinks and large loops of tubing.	Kinks and large loops of tubing can block drainage and prevent lung re-expansion.
		Observe the type and amount of drainage hourly, and mark the fluid level and time on the drainage system.	Notify the physician if more than 100 mL/hr drains. Excessive drainage may indicate hemorrhage.
		Check the water seal chamber for unexpected bubbling.	Bubbling may indicate an air leak in the system.
		Administer antibiotics as prescribed.	Infection of the lung tissue causes inflammation and exudate, which interferes with oxygen diffusion into the vascular system.
		Encourage the client to have a pneumococcal vaccination and to be revaccinated if the original vaccination is 5 to 10 years old.	The vaccine will lower the severity of illness and reduce the risk of serious complications or death.

NURSING DIAGNOSIS NO. 2 ■ Acute Pain

	Expected Outcomes	Nursing Interventions	Rationales
RELATED FACTORS Injury agents (biologic, chemical, physical, psychological) **DEFINING CHARACTERISTICS** Verbal or coded report of pain Observed evidence of pain Behavior: Guarding	Denies experiencing pain greater than a 5 on a 0 to 10 pain scale No verbal report or observation of guarding or protective gestures No verbal report or observation of alteration in sleep patterns No verbal report or observation of alteration in activity level	NIC **Pain Management** Perform a comprehensive assessment of pain to include location, characteristics, onset/duration, frequency, quality, intensity or severity of pain, and precipitating factors.	A plan for pain management must be based on the client's unique responses to pain.
		Reduce or eliminate factors that precipitate or increase the pain experience.	Preventing a pain experience is preferred to trying to control or eliminate pain.
		Select and implement a variety of measures to facilitate pain relief, as appropriate.	Pharmacologic, nonpharmacologic, and interpersonal strategies may provide pain relief depending on the client's unique responses to the therapeutic interventions.

Continued

PLAN of CARE MEDICAL DIAGNOSIS: POSTOPERATIVE THORACOTOMY—*cont'd*

NURSING DIAGNOSIS NO. 2 ■ Acute Pain—*cont'd*

Expected Outcomes	Nursing Interventions	Rationales
	Use pain control measures before pain becomes severe.	Medicating the client in a timely manner prevents pain from reaching acutely unpleasant levels.
	Teach the use of nonpharmacologic techniques before, after and, if possible, during painful activities; before pain occurs or increases; and along with other pain relief measures.	Nonpharmacologic techniques help the client establish a sense of control over his or her pain experience.
	NIC **Analgesic Administration**	
	Monitor vital signs before and after administering narcotic analgesics with first-time dose or if unusual signs are noted.	Narcotic analgesics may depress respirations or cause other adverse effects.
	Choose the IV rather than the IM route for frequent pain medication injections, when possible.	The IV route avoids tissue trauma and unpredictable absorption of medication.
	Administer analgesics around-the-clock.	Administration around-the-clock prevents peaks and troughs of analgesia, especially with severe pain.
	D Evaluate the effectiveness of analgesics at regular frequent intervals after each administration, but especially after the initial dose; also observe for any manifestations of untoward effects.	Frequent evaluation of analgesic effectiveness permits the nurse to adjust the dose and timing interval to the client's need and provides an early warning of adverse responses.
	Implement actions to decrease the untoward effects of analgesics.	Actions taken to prevent predictable but unwanted effects of narcotic analgesics (e.g., constipation) increase client comfort.
	Instruct the client to request PRN pain medication before the pain is severe.	Pain may be managed with lower doses of analgesics and fewer untoward effects if PRN drugs are used before pain becomes severe.
	Teach about the use of analgesics, strategies to decrease side effects, and expectations for involvement in decisions about pain relief.	Information about analgesics and the expectation for client involvement increase the client's sense of control over his or her pain.
	NIC **Patient-Controlled Analgesia (PCA) Administration**	
	Validate that the client can use a PCA device.	To use a PCA device, the client must be able to communicate, comprehend explanations, and follow directions.
	Document the client's pain, amount and frequency of drug dosing, and response to pain treatment in a pain flow sheet.	Information on the pain flow sheet will assist the health care team to adjust the analgesic regimen to the client's needs.

D Indicates tasks that can be delegated to unlicensed assistive nursing personnel at the discretion of the nurse.

PLAN of CARE MEDICAL DIAGNOSIS: POSTOPERATIVE THORACOTOMY—*cont'd*

NURSING DIAGNOSIS NO. 2 ■ Acute Pain—*cont'd*

Expected Outcomes	Nursing Interventions	Rationales
	Teach the client and family how to use the PCA device.	The device will not be used if the client and/or family do not know how to use or are afraid of the device.
	Teach the client how to titrate doses up or down depending on respiratory rate, pain intensity, and pain quality.	The client may prevent severe pain and untoward effects by judicious use of the PCA.
	NIC **Environmental Management: Comfort**	
	Determine sources of discomfort, such as damp dressings, positioning of tubing, constrictive dressings, wrinkled bed linens, and environmental irritants.	Control of environmental discomforts may decrease the need for pharmacologic intervention.
	D Position the client to facilitate comfort.	The nurse may decrease sources of discomfort by using principles of body alignment, supporting with pillows, supporting joints during movement, splinting over incisions, and immobilizing painful body parts.
	Other Interventions	
	Refer the client to the Pain Advisory Committee.	The Pain Advisory Committee is a multidisciplinary committee with wide expertise in pain relief interventions.
	Consider the use of alternative therapies such as yoga, meditation, spirituality, and/or religion.	The experience of meditation and prayer and the reflection on meaning may help the patient to relax, thereby easing the muscle tension that contributes to pain sensation.
	Consider the use of alternative therapies such as imagery, aromatherapy, music, touch, and laughter/humor.	Cognitive and behavioral strategies may serve as adjuncts to or replacements for pharmacologic or surgical interventions for chronic pain. Each therapy has a differing mode of action that may or may not benefit the patient.
	Manage continuous cutaneous opioid analgesia, neuraxial analgesia, intraspinal analgesia, or transdermal analgesia, as needed.	Methods of delivering analgesia other than the traditional IV route may provide substantial pain relief in a form that the client may tolerate with fewer untoward effects.
	Continuing Care Considerations	
	Refer the client to an advanced practice nurse pain specialist, social worker, home care nurse, and/or psychologist, as appropriate.	Health care team members are able to provide continuing support for the client facing chronic pain.

Continued

PLAN of CARE MEDICAL DIAGNOSIS: POSTOPERATIVE THORACOTOMY—*cont'd*

NURSING DIAGNOSIS NO. 3 ■ Activity Intolerance

	Expected Outcomes	Nursing Interventions	Rationales
RELATED FACTORS Imbalance between oxygen supply/demand **DEFINING CHARACTERISTICS** Verbal report: Fatigue Abnormal heart rate or blood pressure response to activity Exertional discomfort Dyspnea	Denies discomfort with exertion No verbal report or observation of dyspnea with exertion Has no electrocardiographic evidence of dysrhythmias or ischemia Denies fatigue Denies weakness Has a heart rate that remains regular and strong with activity	NIC **Energy Management** Monitor the client for evidence of excess physical and emotional fatigue.	Extended periods of inactivity may place the client at risk for excessive fatigue when carrying out desired activities.
		Monitor cardiorespiratory response to activity.	Tachycardia, other dysrhythmias, dyspnea, diaphoresis, pallor, hemodynamic pressures, and respiratory rate increases may result from increased activity.
		Monitor nutritional intake.	Ensure that the client has adequate energy resources.
		D Reduce physical discomforts.	Physical discomforts could interfere with cognitive function and self-monitoring/regulation of activity.
		Arrange physical activities (e.g., avoid activity immediately after meals).	Such an arrangement reduces competition for oxygen supply to vital body functions.
		D Encourage alternate rest and activity periods.	This avoids extended periods of either activity or exercise.
		Plan activities for periods when the client has the most energy.	The client will be better able to manage activities during peak energy periods.
		D Assist the client to sit on the side of the bed ("dangle") if unable to transfer or walk.	Sitting on the edge of the bed helps the client avoid orthostatic hypotension during transfer.
		Instruct the client to recognize manifestations of exercise tolerance/intolerance during and after exercise sessions.	Light-headedness; shortness of breath; more than the usual muscle, skeletal, or joint pain; weakness; extreme fatigue; angina; profuse sweating; and palpitations indicate that the exercise program is more taxing than the client can undertake.
		Establish a follow-up schedule.	Follow-up schedules should assist in maintaining motivation, assist in problem solving, and monitor progress.
		Other Interventions Instruct the client/significant other to recognize manifestations of fatigue.	Symptoms of undue fatigue require a reduction in activity.
		Provide assistive devices, as appropriate.	Splints, special hand tools, or other devices may assist the client to carry out desired activities with less energy expenditure.
		Consider the use of complementary and alternative therapies.	Complementary and alternative therapies may be used to cope with chronic disease and disability, especially if chronic pain is a problem.
		Continuing Care Considerations Collaborate with the client/family and the rehabilitation team.	Effective interdisciplinary interventions facilitate the client's ability to manage his or her life.

D Indicates tasks that can be delegated to unlicensed assistive nursing personnel at the discretion of the nurse.

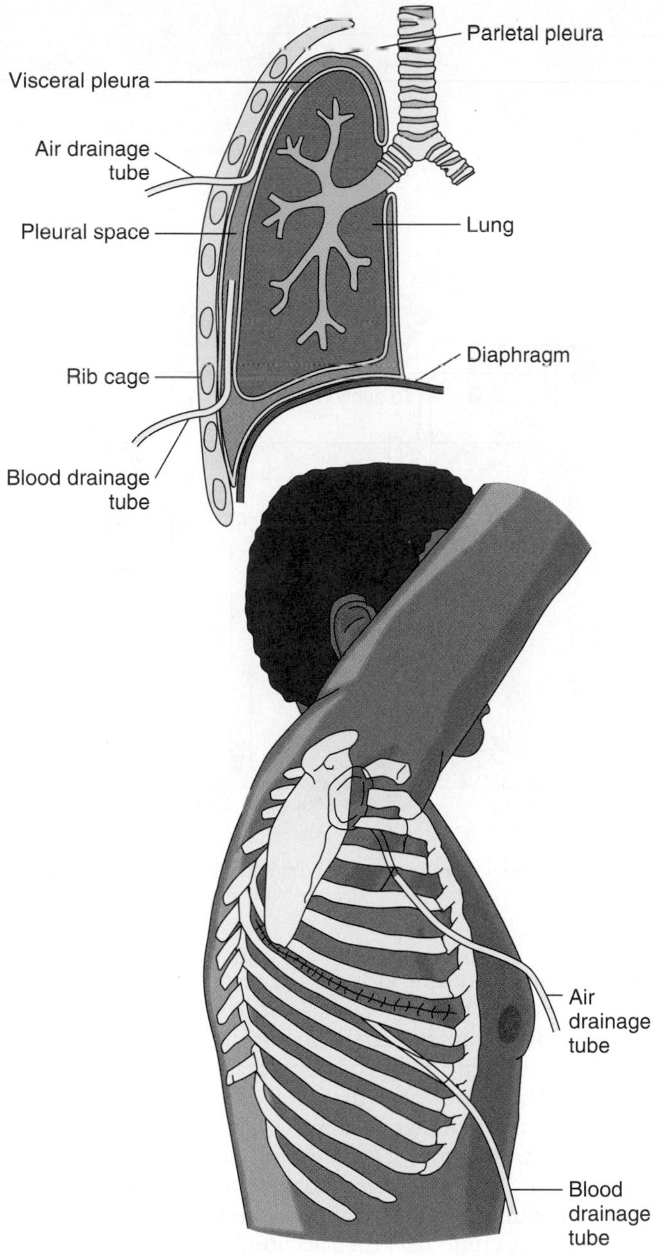

Figure 33-14 ■ Chest tube placement.

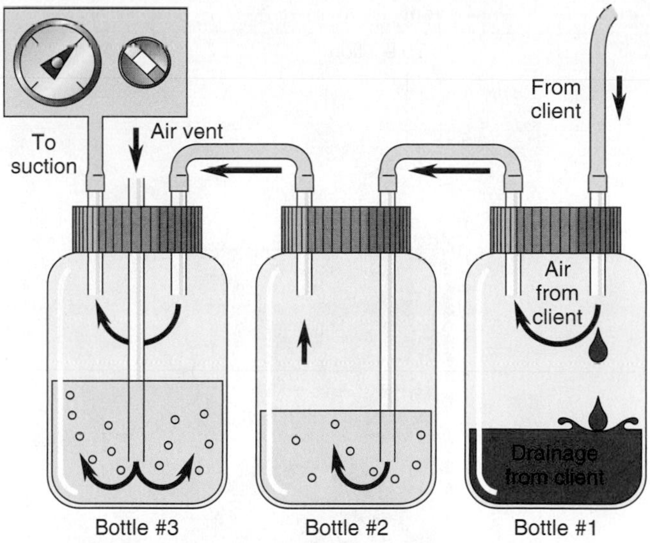

Figure 33-15 ■ Three-bottle chest drainage system.

from the client penetrates shallowly into the bottle, as does the tube connecting with bottle two. *It is critical that the stopper remain tightly connected to the bottle to maintain a closed system. If the stopper loosens and the chest tube is unclamped, the negative pressure in the pleural space will pull air into the space and cause a pneumothorax.*

Bottle (chamber) one collects the fluid draining from the client. This fluid is measured hourly during the first 24 hours. *The fluid must never come into direct contact with either the tube draining from the client or the tube connecting this bottle to bottle two.* If the tubing from the client enters the fluid, drainage stops.

BOTTLE TWO. Bottle two is the water seal that prevents air from entering the client's pleural space. Air from the pleural space also enters bottle one but moves immediately to bottle two through the connecting tube. This tube must always be under the water level in bottle two to prevent air from returning to the client. The bubbling of the water in bottle two indicates air drainage from the client. Bubbling is usually seen when intrathoracic pressure is greater than atmospheric pressure, such as when the client exhales, coughs, or sneezes. When the air in the pleural space has been removed, bubbling stops. A blocked or kinked chest tube also can cause bubbling to stop. Excessive bubbling in the second bottle may indicate an air leak. The water in the long tube of the second bottle rises and falls slightly with the client's respiratory cycle. A rise of 2 to 4 inches during inhalation and a fall during exhalation are normal. An absence of fluctuation may mean that the chest tube is obstructed, the expanded lung has blocked the eyelets of the chest tube, or no more air is leaking into the pleural space.

If the system consisted only of two bottles, drainage could occur only by gravity. Then, the second tube in the second bottle would be open to the air to prevent a buildup of pressure that could hinder air drainage.

BOTTLE THREE. The third bottle is the suction control bottle of the system. This stopper has three tubing connections: a short tube from the second bottle, a long open tube dipped into the water, and a short tube connecting to the suction unit. Suction enhances the pressure difference between the pleural space and the drainage system, causing the pressure to drop inside the system by 15 to 20 cm. Although the amount of suction generated by the suction unit can be increased, the amount of suction in the system is determined not by the suction unit but by the depth of the open tube in the water. While suction is applied, gentle bubbling is seen in the chamber.

COMMERCIAL CHEST DRAINAGE UNITS. Chest drainage units are self-contained units that work in exactly the same way that the three-bottle system does. From right to left, the system contains chambers for drainage, a water seal, and suction control (see Figure 33-16). The plastic devices reduce the risk of breakage or contamination of the drainage system and allow the client increased mobility.

Check hourly to ensure the sterility and patency of any chest drainage system. Tape tubing junctions to prevent ac-

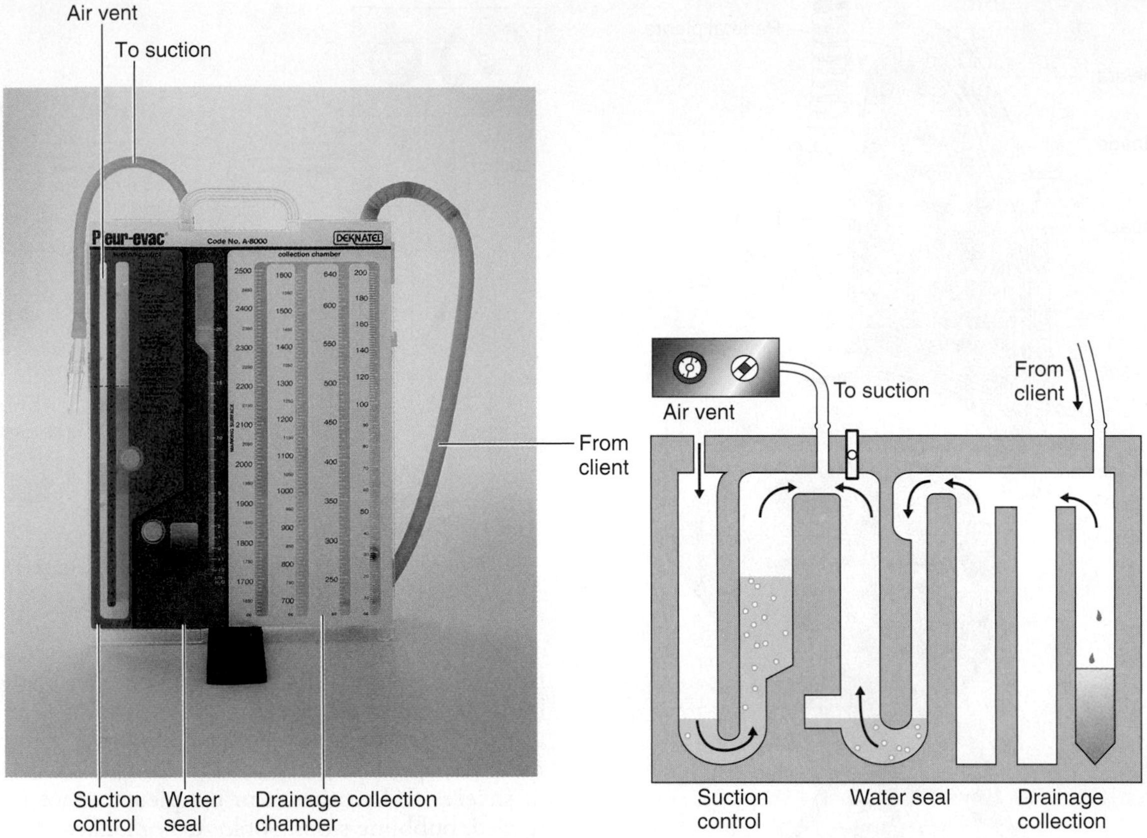

Figure 33-16 ■ *Left,* The Pleur-Evac drainage system, a commercial three-bottle chest drainage device. *Right,* Schematic of the drainage device.

cidental disconnections, and keep an occlusive dressing at the chest tube insertion site. Keep sterile gauze at the bedside to cover the insertion site immediately if the chest tube becomes dislodged. Also keep padded clamps at the bedside for use if the drainage system is interrupted. Position the drainage tubing to prevent kinks and large loops of tubing, which can block drainage and prevent lung re-expansion. Avoid vigorous stripping of the chest tube. Use gentle milking of the tube to move blood clots and prevent obstruction.

Assess the client's respiratory status and document the amount and type of drainage hourly. Usually the drainage in bottle one or chamber one is not emptied unless the container is so full that the fluid is in danger of coming into contact with the chest drainage tube. For the bottle system, place a tape marking for volume on the side of the bottle. When you check the volume, mark the fluid level and the time on the tape. The self-contained systems have calibrations on the collection chamber. Record the amount of hourly drainage. Notify the physician of drainage if more than 100 mL/hr occurs. After the first 24 hours, assess drainage at least every 8 hours.

Check the water seal chamber for unexpected bubbling created by an air leak in the system. Bubbling is normal during forceful expiration or coughing because air in the chest is being expelled. Continuous bubbling indicates an air leak that must be identified. Notify the physician if bubbling occurs continuously in the water seal bottle or chamber. On the physician's prescription, gently apply a padded clamp on the drainage tubing close to the occlusive dressing. If the bubbling stops, the air leak may be at the chest tube insertion site or within the chest, requiring physician intervention. Air bubbling that does not cease when you apply a padded clamp indicates that the air leak is between the clamp and the drainage system.

Pneumonectomy Care. After pneumonectomy, the pleural cavity on the affected side is an empty space. The surgeon sometimes inserts a clamped chest tube for only a day because serous fluid may then accumulate in the empty space and create adhesions, which reduce mediastinal shift toward the affected side. Closed-chest drainage is not usually used.

Complications of a pneumonectomy can include empyema and the development of a bronchopleural fistula. Positioning of the client after pneumonectomy varies according to surgeon preference and the client's comfort. Some surgeons want the client placed on the nonoperative side immediately after a pneumonectomy to reduce stress on the bronchial stump incision. Others prefer that the client be placed on the operative side to allow fluids to fill in the space formerly taken up by the lungs.

Interventions for Palliation

Oxygen Therapy. If the client is hypoxemic, supplemental oxygen is provided. Even if the client is not overtly hypoxemic, the physician may prescribe oxygen to relieve dyspnea and anxiety. Humidification is used with oxygen therapy for the client with lung cancer. (See Chapter 31 for issues related to home oxygen therapy.)

Drug Therapy. Bronchodilators and corticosteroids are prescribed for the client with bronchospasm to decrease bronchospasm, inflammation, and edema. Mucolytics may be of use to ease removal of thick mucus and sputum. Bacterial infections are treated with the appropriate antibiotic therapy.

Radiation Therapy. Radiation therapy can help relieve hemoptysis, obstruction of the bronchi and great veins (superior vena cava syndrome), **dysphagia** (difficulty swallowing) from esophageal compression, and pain resulting from bone metastasis. Usually radiation for palliation uses higher doses for shorter periods of time. Skin care issues and fatigue are the same as those occurring with radiation therapy for cure.

Laser Therapy. Lasers may be used to remove bronchial obstruction when tumors are accessible by bronchoscopy. The obstruction is debulked, and the airway is reopened. Laser therapy does not cause systemic or toxic effects and is usually well tolerated.

Thoracentesis and Pleurodesis. Pleural effusion can be a problem for the client with lung cancer. The excess fluid increases dyspnea, discomfort, and the risk for infection. The goal of treatment is to remove pleural fluid and prevent its formation. Fluid can be removed rapidly through suction after the placement of a large needle or catheter into the intrapleural space **(thoracentesis).** Fluid removal temporarily relieves hypoxia; however, the fluid can rapidly reform in the pleural space.

Another technique to relieve pleural effusion is to insert a chest tube to drain the fluid and to instill a **sclerosing** agent. The agent is an irritant that causes inflammation. The aim of thoracentesis and sclerosis is to create a **pleurodesis,** an inflammation that causes the pleura to stick to the chest wall and prevent formation of effusion fluid.

The procedure can be performed under local anesthesia at the bedside or in an operating room. Usually the client is also given an analgesic or sedative. Once the sclerosing agent is instilled, the chest tube is clamped to prevent drainage of the agent. Chart 33-13 reviews best practices for care of the client undergoing pleurodesis.

Dyspnea Management. The client with lung cancer tires easily and is often most comfortable resting in a semi-Fowler's position. Dyspnea is reduced with oxygen, use of a morphine drip, and positioning for comfort. The severely dyspneic client may be most comfortable sitting in a lounge chair or reclining chair.

Pain Management. The client with lung cancer may have chest pain and pain radiating to the arm. With bone metastasis, the client may also have bone pain. Perform a complete pain assessment with attention to onset, intensity, quality, duration, and the client's description of the pain. The goal of therapy is to help the client to be as pain free and as comfortable as possible.

Pharmacologic management with opioid drugs as oral, parenteral, or transdermal preparations is needed. Nonpharmacologic measures, such as positioning, hot or cold compresses, distractions, and guided imagery, may also be helpful. Prescribed analgesics are most effective when given around-the-clock. Additional PRN analgesics are used for breakthrough pain. Ongoing assessment and evaluation of the effectiveness of the pain control regimen is a primary nursing responsibility.

Hospice and End-of-Life Issues. For the client in the terminal phase of lung cancer, a referral to a hospice program can be beneficial. Hospice programs provide support to the terminally ill client and the family by meeting physical and psychosocial needs, adjusting the palliative care regimen as needed, making home visits, and providing volunteers for errands and respite care. (See Chapter 9 for a more complete discussion of end-of-life issues.) The American Cancer Society may also be able to provide assistance through support groups for clients and families or through the use of equipment, such as a hospital bed or bedside commode.

CHART 33-13

BEST PRACTICE for
The Client Undergoing Pleurodesis

- Reinforce explanation of the pleurodesis and inform the client that medication will be provided to promote comfort before the procedure. (The physician may administer IV analgesia/sedation immediately before the procedure.)
- Ensure that the chest tube is clamped after instillation of the sclerosing agent.
- Monitor vital signs and respiratory status at the completion of the procedure and then at least every 30 minutes until the effects of the IV medication have dissipated.
- Thereafter, monitor vital signs every 4 hours for 24 hours. (The client may experience a low-grade fever. Pleurodesis creates pleuritis between the visceral and parietal layers, thus preventing reaccumulation of fluid.)
- If a rotation schedule is ordered, assist the client to the correct position for appropriate time frames and provide reassurance.
- Unclamp the chest tube after completion of the rotation schedule or at the specified time ordered by the physician.
- Assess chest tube drainage and document the amount and character of the drainage.
- Perform a complete respiratory assessment every 2 hours and observe for manifestations of distress, including those of pneumothorax.
- Analgesics may be administered as needed to promote the client's comfort.
- When drainage has decreased (<150 mL in 12 to 24 hours), the physician may remove the chest tube. Maintain an occlusive dressing at the insertion site for a minimum of 48 hours.

GET READY for the NCLEX Examination!

KEY POINTS

Safe Effective Care Environment

- When using aerosolized drugs or other chemicals, close the door to the room where they are being used.
- Use gloves when obtaining a sputum specimen.
- Ensure there are no open flames or combustion hazards in rooms where oxygen is in use.

Health Promotion and Maintenance

- Teach clients who come into contact with inhalation irritants in their workplaces or for leisure time activities, to use a mask to avoid respiratory contact with these substances.
- Inform all clients who smoke that smoking increases the risk for development of many pulmonary problems.
- Assist clients interested in smoking cessation to find an appropriate smoking cessation program.
- Encourage older adults who are confined to bed for any reason or who are recovering from surgery to turn, cough, and deep breathe at least every 2 hours.

- Encourage all clients older than 50 years of age and anyone with a respiratory problem to receive a yearly influenza vaccination.
- Teach all clients who smoke the warning signs of lung cancer.

Psychosocial Integrity

- Assess the degree to which breathing problems interfere with the client's ability to perform activities of daily living.
- Pace your interview to match the learning needs and style of the individual client.
- Allow the client the opportunity to express fear or anxiety regarding the diagnosis of cancer or the treatment regimen.
- Allow clients to verbalize feelings about changes in appearance resulting from cancer therapy.
- Explain all diagnostic procedures, restrictions, and follow-up care to the client scheduled for tests.
- Help clients use strategies to improve their appearance when alopecia occurs.
- Refer clients and family members to local cancer resources and support groups.

Physiological Integrity

- Monitor the rate and depth of respiration at least every hour for any client with hypercarbia and CO_2 narcosis who is receiving oxygen by mask or nasal cannula.
- Document any known specific allergies that have respiratory manifestations.
- Assess the airway and breathing effectiveness for any client who experiences shortness of breath or any change in mental status.
- Assess the client's respiratory status every 15 minutes for at least the first 2 hours after undergoing an endoscopic test for respiratory disorders.
- Apply oxygen to anyone who is hypoxemic.
- Ensure that oxygen therapy delivered to the client is humidified (and warmed, when possible).
- Monitor arterial blood gases and oxygen saturation of all clients receiving oxygen therapy.
- Teach clients receiving radiation therapy how to care for the skin in the radiation path (see Chart 28-2).

ADDITIONAL STUDY RESOURCES

Go to your Student CD-ROM for Review Questions for the NCLEX Examination.

evolve Go to http://evolve.elsevier.com/Iggy/ for Integrated Management of Care Questions for the NCLEX Examination.

SELECTED BIBLIOGRAPHY

Asterisk indicates a classic or definitive work on this subject.

Aberle, M., & McLeskey, S. (2003). Biology of lung cancer with implications for new therapies. *Oncology Nursing Forum, 30*(2), 273-280.

Ackley, B., & Ladwig, G. (2002). *Nursing diagnosis handbook: A guide to planning care* (5th ed.). St. Louis: Mosby.

Adiutori, D. (2000). Primary pulmonary hypertension: A review for advanced practice nurses. *MEDSURG Nursing, 9*(5), 255-264.

American Cancer Society. (2005). *Cancer facts and figures-2005.* Report No. 01-300M-No. 5008.05. Atlanta: Author.

Asch-Goodkin, J. (2000). Eliminating disparities in asthma management. *Patient Care for the Nurse Practitioner, 3*(5), 68-83.

Ayes, D.M., & Lappin, J.S. (2004). Act fast when your patient has dyspnea. *Nursing 2004, 34*(7), 36-41.

Bernier, M., & Leonard, B. (2001). Pulmonary rehabilitation after acute COPD exacerbation. *Critical Care Clinics of North America, 13*(3), 375-387.

Boyle, A., & Locke, D. (2004). Update on chronic obstructive pulmonary disease. *MEDSURG Nursing, 13*(1), 42-48.

Brubacher, S., Gobel, B. (2003). Use of the Pleurx Pleural catheter for the management of malignant pleural effusions. *Clinical Journal of Oncology Nursing, 7*(1), 35-38.

*Centers for Disease Control and Prevention. (1998). Forecasted state-specific estimates of self-reported asthma prevalence-United States, 1998. *Morbidity and Mortality Weekly Report, 47*(47), 1022-1025.

Centers for Disease Control and Prevention. (2003). Asthma prevalence, health care use, and mortality, 2000-2001. National Center for Health Statistics. Available at http://www.cdc.gov/nchs/products/pubs/pubd/hestats/asthma/asthma.htm.

Chatila, W., et al. (2003). Respiratory failure after lung transplantation. *Chest, 123*(1), 165-173.

Cody, M. (2001). Is there help for a smoker? Understanding nicotine replacement therapy. *The American Journal for Nurse Practitioners, 5*(4), 32-41.

Cordes, M.E., & Brueggen, C. (2003). Diffuse malignant pleural mesothelioma: Part II. Symptom management. *Clinical Journal of Oncology Nursing, 7*(5), 545-552.

Dabbs, A., et al. (2003). Pattern and predictors of early rejection after lung transplantation. *American Journal of Critical Care, 12*(6), 497-507.

Dochterman, J., & Bulechek, G. (Eds.). (2004). *Nursing interventions classification (NIC)* (4th ed.). St. Louis: Mosby.

Dunn, N. (2001). Keeping COPD patients out of the ED. *RN, 64*(2), 33-37.

Duquette, S., LaLonde, L.C., & Traiger, G. (2000). Living-donor lobar lung transplantation: A case study. *Critical Care Nurse, 20*(1), 69-80.

Eells, P. (2004). Advances in prostacyclin therapy for pulmonary arterial hypertension. *Critical Care Nurse, 24*(2), 42-54.

Evangelista, L., et al. (2003). Health perceptions and risk behaviors of lung cancer survivors. *Heart & Lung, 32*(2), 131-139.

Facts and Comparisons. (2004). *Drug facts and comparisons* (58th ed.). St. Louis: Author.

Fehrenbach, C. (2002). Chronic obstructive pulmonary disease. *Nursing Standard, 17*(10), 45-52.

*Gazarian, P.K. (1997). Teaching your patient to use a metered-dose inhaler: The direct route for asthma therapy. *Nursing97, 27*(10), 52-54.

Gift, A., et al. (2004). Symptom clusters in elderly patients with lung cancer. *Oncology Nursing Forum, 31*(2), 203-210.

Goodfellow, L., & Jones, M. (2002). Bronchial hygiene therapy. *American Journal of Nursing, 102*(1), 37-43.

Goodwin, J., & Coleman, E. (2003). Exploring measures of functional dependence in the older adult with cancer. *MEDSURG Nursing, 12*(6), 359-366.

Green, F. (2002). Overview of pulmonary fibrosis. *Chest, 122*(6), 334S-339S.

Halpern, M., et al. (2003). Asthma: Resource use and costs for inhaled corticosteroid vs leukotriene modifier treatment–a meta-analysis. *Journal of Family Practice, 52*(5), 382-389.

Houfek, J., & Atwood, J. (2003). Genetic susceptibility to lung cancer: Implications for smoking cessation. *MEDSURG Nursing, 12*(1), 45-49.

Jablonski, R. (2000). Discovering asthma in the older adult. *Nurse Practitioner, 25*(3), 14, 24-25, 29-39.

Janson, S. (2000). Biologic markers of airway inflammation in asthma. *AACN Clinical Issues: Advanced Practice in Acute and Critical Care, 11*(2), 232-240.

Jones, A., & Rowe, B. (2000). Bronchopulmonary hygiene physical therapy and chronic obstructive pulmonary disease: A systematic review. *Heart and Lung, 29*(2), 125-135.

Judson, M. (2000). Clinical aspects of pulmonary sarcoidosis. *Journal of the South Carolina Medical Association, 96*(1), 9-17.
Kreamer, K. (2003). Getting the lowdown on lung cancer. *Nursing2003, 33*(11), 36-42.
Lanuza, D., Lefaiver, C., & Farcas, G. (2000). Research on the quality of life of lung transplant candidates and recipients: An integrative review. *Heart and Lung, 29*(3), 180-195.
Lindell, K., & Jacobs, S. (2003). Idiopathic pulmonary fibrosis, *American Journal of Nursing, 103*(4), 32-42.
Maliski, S., et al. (2003). The aftermath of lung cancer. *Cancer Nursing, 26*(3), 237-244.
McCance, K., & Huether, S. (2002). *Pathophysiology: The biologic basis for disease in adults and children* (4th ed.). St. Louis: Mosby.
McConnell, E. (2002). Teaching your patient to use a metered-dose inhaler. *Nursing2002, 32*(2), 73.
McHale, J., & Barth, M. (2000). Nursing care after pneumonectomy in patients with invasive pulmonary aspergillosis. *Critical Care Nurse, 20*(1), 37-44.
Meek, P. (2000). Influence of attention and judgment on perception of breathlessness in healthy individuals and patients with chronic obstructive pulmonary disease. *Nursing Research, 49*(1), 11-19.
Miracle, V. (2001). Taking the wind out of asthma. *Dimensions in Critical Care Nursing, 20*(1), 2-9.
Moorhead, S., Johnson, M., & Maas, M. (Eds.). (2004). *Nursing outcomes classification (NOC)* (3rd ed.). St. Louis: Mosby.
National Heart, Lung, and Blood Institute. (2003). *Global initiative for chronic obstructive pulmonary disease: Global strategy for the diagnosis, management, and prevention of chronic obstructive pulmonary disease.* NIH Publication No. 2701A. Rockville, MD. Author.
Nield, M. (2000). Dyspnea self-management in African-Americans with chronic lung disease. *Heart and Lung, 29*(1), 50-55.
Nussbaum, R., McInnes, R., & Willard, H. (2001). *Thompson & Thompson: Genetics in medicine* (6th ed.). Philadelphia: W.B. Saunders.
O'Neill, E. (2002). Illness representations and coping of women with chronic obstructive pulmonary disease: A pilot study. *Heart & Lung, 31*(4), 295-302.
Petty, M. (2003). Lung and lung-heart transplantation: Implications for nursing care when hospitalized outside the transplant center. *MEDSURG Nursing, 12*(4), 250-259.
Petty, T. (2003). Helping patients with COPD breathe easier. *Consultant, 43*(6), 687-688.
Phillip, M. (2000). Primary pulmonary hypertension. *MEDSURG Nursing, 9*(1), 17-20.
Pope, B. (2004). Chronic obstructive pulmonary disease. *Nursing2004, 34*(3), 56-57.
Puntillo, K., & Ley, J. (2004). Appropriately timed analgesics control pain due to chest tube removal. *American Journal of Critical Care, 13*(4), 292-301.
Reinke, L., & Hoffman, L. (2000). Asthma education: Creating a partnership. *Heart and Lung, 29*(3), 225-236.
Rogers, P., & Armstrong, I. (2002). Pulmonary hypertension. *Nursing Standard, 16*(24), 45-54.
Rosenberg, H., & Resnick, B. (2003). Exercise intervention in patients with chronic obstructive pulmonary disease. *Geriatric Nursing, 24*(2), 91-95.
Sabo, J., & Nord, P. (2000). Intravenous epoprostenol: A new therapy for primary pulmonary hypertension. *Critical Care Nurse, 20*(6), 31-40.
Sarna, L., et al. (2001). Barriers to tobacco cessation in clinical practice: Report from a national survey of oncology nurses. *Nursing Outlook, 49*(4), 166-172.
Silverman, E., et al. (2003). Current management of bronchiectasis: Review and 3 cases. *Heart & Lung, 32*(1), 59-64.
Simmons, P., & Simmons, M. (2004). Informed nursing practice: The administration of oxygen to patients with COPD. *MEDSURG Nursing, 13*(2), 82-85.
Smaha, D. (2001). Asthma emergency care: National guidelines summary. *Heart & Lung, 30*(6), 472-474.
Thomas, M. (2003). Epidermal growth factor receptor tyrosine kinase inhibitors: Application in non-small cell lung cancer. *Cancer Nursing, 26*(6S), 21S-25S.
Tishelman, C., Degner, L., & Mueller, B. (2000). Measuring symptom distress in patients with lung cancer. *Cancer Nursing, 23*(2), 82-90.
Togger, D., & Brenner, P. (2001). Metered dose inhalers. *American Journal of Nursing, 102*(10), 26-38.
Walker, A. (2003). Updates in small cell lung cancer treatment. *Clinical Journal of Oncology Nursing, 7*(5), 563-568.
Wong, D. (2001). COPD: Overview and update. *The American Journal for Nurse Practitioners, 5*(5), 9-25.
Wu, C., et al. (2001). Coping behaviors of individuals with chronic obstructive pulmonary disease. *MEDSURG Nursing, 10*(6), 315-320.

CHAPTER

34 Interventions for Clients with Infectious Problems of the Lower Respiratory Tract

M. LINDA WORKMAN

LEARNING OUTCOMES

After studying this chapter, you should be able to:

1. Explain the consequences of an untreated streptococcal infection of the upper respiratory tract.
2. Identify adults at highest risk for contracting influenza.
3. Develop a teaching plan to prevent influenza in the older adult.
4. Identify clients at risk for developing community-acquired or hospital-acquired pneumonia.
5. Compare the manifestations of pneumonia in the younger adult with those exhibited by the older adult client with pneumonia.
6. Describe the mechanisms of action, side effects, and nursing implications of drug therapy for pneumonia.
7. Identify adults at risk for tuberculosis (TB).
8. Interpret correctly the TB test results for a person with normal immune function and a person with human immunodeficiency virus/acquired immunodeficiency syndrome (HIV/AIDS).
9. Describe the mechanisms of action, side effects, and nursing implications of drug therapy for TB.
10. Develop a community-based teaching plan for continuing care of the client with active TB.
11. Compare the early and late manifestations of inhalation anthrax with those of other lower respiratory infections.

Go to your Student CD-ROM for Review Questions for the NCLEX Examination keyed to these Learning Outcomes.

DISORDERS OF THE NOSE AND SINUSES

Rhinitis

PATHOPHYSIOLOGY

Rhinitis, an inflammation of the nasal mucosa, is the most common problem of nose and sinuses. Inflammation can be caused by infection (viral or bacterial) or contact with allergens. Often an allergic rhinitis will make the mucous membranes more susceptible to invasion, and an infection will accompany the allergy.

Allergic rhinitis, often called *hay fever* or *allergies,* is triggered by hypersensitivity reactions to airborne allergens, especially plant pollens or molds (see Chapter 26). Some episodes are "seasonal" in that they tend to recur at the same time each year and last only a few weeks. *Chronic rhinitis* occurs either intermittently with no seasonal pattern or continuously whenever the person is exposed to allergens such as dust, animal dander, wool, and foods (e.g., seafood). Other causes of rhinitis include a "rebound" nasal congestion from overuse of nose drops or sprays **(rhinitis medicamentosa)** and chronic nasal inhalation of cocaine.

Acute viral rhinitis (**coryza,** or the common cold) is caused by any one of at least 200 viruses. It spreads from person to person by droplets from sneezing or coughing. Colds are most contagious in the first 2 to 3 days after symptoms appear. Colds are self-limiting unless a bacterial infection occurs at the same time. Complications occur most often in immunosuppressed people and older adults, especially if they live or work in crowded conditions or in group settings (e.g., long-term care facility).

COLLABORATIVE MANAGEMENT

Assessment

In both acute and chronic allergic rhinitis, the presence of the **allergen** (offending substance) causes a release of natural chemicals, such as histamine, from white blood cells in the nasal mucosa. These chemicals bind to blood vessel receptor sites, causing local blood vessel dilation and capillary leak, leading to edema and swelling of the nasal mucosa. The resulting symptoms include headache, nasal irritation, sneezing, nasal congestion, **rhinorrhea** (watery drainage from the nose), and itchy, watery eyes.

Viral or bacterial invasion of the nasal passages causes the same local tissue responses as allergic rhinitis. Often the client also has systemic manifestations, including a sore, dry throat and a low-grade fever.

Interventions

Management of the client with any type of rhinitis focuses on symptom relief and client education. Instruct the client in the correct use of the drug therapy prescribed.

Drug Therapy. Drugs, including antihistamines and decongestants, are prescribed but must be used with caution in the older adult because of side effects such as vertigo, hypertension, urinary retention, and insomnia. Antihistamines block the chemicals released by white blood cells from binding to receptor sites on blood vessels and nasal tissues, preventing local edema and itching. Decongestants work by constricting blood vessels, thus decreasing edema. Antipyretics are given if fever is present. Antibiotics are prescribed only for bacterial rhinitis. Rhinitis caused by overuse of nose drops or sprays is treated by discontinuing the offending drug. Steroid nasal sprays may be used to decrease the rebound nasal congestion during the time immediately after discontinuing the drug.

Complementary and Alternative Therapies. Some people are able to decrease the severity of acute viral rhinitis with the use of complementary and alternative therapy early in the course of the problem. Agents often used are Echinacea, large doses of vitamin C, and zinc preparations such as COLD-EEZE or Zicam. It is not clear how these agents reduce symptom severity or duration of illness, but it is believed they may help increase nonspecific immune function.

Supportive Therapy. Instruct the client about the importance of rest (8 to 10 hours a day) and fluid intake of at least 2000 mL/day (about eight glasses) unless other health problems (e.g., heart failure, chronic renal failure) limit this amount. Humidifying the air helps to relieve congestion. Ways to increase humidity include using a room humidifier, inhaling steam from a pan of boiled water after removing it from the heat, or breathing steamy air in the bathroom after running hot shower water.

The client is most likely to spread the infection during the first 2 to 3 days after symptoms begin. Teach the client to reduce the risk of spreading the cold by thoroughly washing hands, especially after nose blowing or sneezing. Instruct the client to avoid close contact with people who are more susceptible to infection, such as older adults, infants, and anyone who has a chronic respiratory problem. An uncomplicated cold typically subsides within 7 to 10 days.

The client with recurrent allergic rhinitis can have allergy testing to determine the cause. The client may prevent further episodes by avoiding the allergen or using desensitization therapy (see Chapter 26).

Sinusitis

PATHOPHYSIOLOGY

Sinusitis is an inflammation of the mucous membranes of one or more of the sinuses. Swelling can obstruct the flow of secretions from the sinuses, which may then become infected. The disorder often follows rhinitis. Other conditions leading to sinusitis include deviated nasal septum, polyps, tumors, inhaled air pollutants or cocaine, facial trauma, nasal intubation, dental infection, or decreased immune function. In chronic sinusitis, the mucous membrane is permanently thickened from repeated inflammation.

The most common organisms causing sinus infection are *Streptococcus pneumoniae, Haemophilus influenzae, Diplococcus,* or *Bacteroides.* Sinusitis most often develops in the maxillary and frontal sinuses. Complications include cellulitis, abscess, and meningitis.

Diagnosis is made on the basis of the client's history and manifestations. Transillumination of the affected sinus is decreased. Other diagnostic tests for sinusitis include sinus x-rays, endoscopic examination, and computed tomography (CT).

COLLABORATIVE MANAGEMENT

Assessment

The manifestations of sinusitis include nasal swelling and congestion, headache, facial pressure, pain (usually worse when the head is in a dependent position), tenderness to touch over the involved area, low-grade fever, cough, and purulent or bloody nasal drainage.

Interventions

NONSURGICAL MANAGEMENT. Treatment includes the use of broad-spectrum antibiotics (e.g., amoxicillin), analgesics for pain and fever (e.g., acetaminophen [Tylenol, Atasol✱]), decongestants (e.g., phenylephrine [Neo-Synephrine]), steam humidification, hot and wet packs over the sinus area, and nasal saline irrigations. Instruct the client to increase fluid intake to more than 10 glasses of water or juice per day unless another medical problem requires fluid restriction. If this treatment plan is not successful, the client may need to be evaluated with sinus films and CT. Surgical intervention may be needed.

SURGICAL MANAGEMENT

Antral Irrigation. Antral irrigation, also known as *maxillary antral puncture* and *lavage,* is an outpatient procedure. With the client under local anesthesia, a large-gauge needle is inserted into the maxillary sinus on the affected side. Fluid or pus is drained from the sinus. The sinus is then irrigated with saline solution, an antibiotic solution, or both.

Other Surgical Procedures. If antral irrigation is not successful, other surgical procedures may be used to open the sinus cavities. In the Caldwell-Luc procedure, the surgeon makes an incision under the upper lip into the maxillary sinus. The infected mucosa is then removed. With the

CHART 34-1

BEST PRACTICE for
Postoperative Care for Clients with Sinus Surgery

- Place the client in the semi-Fowler's position to promote drainage and prevent swelling.
- Perform gentle oral hygiene to promote healing and prevent injury to the surgical incision.
- Use ice compresses as prescribed for 24 hours.
- Change the "mustache" dressing under the nose as needed, and record the type and amount of drainage.
- Instruct the client to eat soft foods and increase fluid intake.
- Instruct the client to limit the Valsalva maneuver (no coughing, blowing the nose, or straining at stool) for at least 2 weeks postoperatively to prevent bleeding and tissue damage.

nasal antral window procedure, the surgeon makes an opening in the front portion of the lower nasal bone to improve drainage through the nares. After either procedure, the client may have difficulty eating for a few days because of pain and swelling. Chart 34-1 describes the best practices for postoperative care for clients undergoing these procedures. When the ethmoid sinuses need to be opened, the surgeon uses an external incision along the side of the nose from the middle of the eyebrow (Weber-Ferguson incision).

Endoscopic Sinus Surgery. Endoscopic sinus surgery is a common method of diagnosing and treating sinus disorders. Direct inspection of the sinuses through a sinus endoscope is completed with the client under general anesthesia in an outpatient surgical center. The procedure takes only minutes, although the nasal mucosa may take from 4 to 6 weeks to heal. The client goes home the same day and can return to work in 4 to 5 days. Instruct the client to use saline nasal sprays frequently (every 2 to 4 hours) to prevent mucosal crusting and promote healing.

DISORDERS OF THE ORAL PHARYNX AND TONSILS

Pharyngitis

PATHOPHYSIOLOGY

Pharyngitis, or "sore throat," is a common inflammation of the mucous membranes of the pharynx. It accounts for more than 15 million office visits each year in the United States. This condition often occurs with acute rhinitis and sinusitis.

Acute pharyngitis has many causes (Table 34-1). The most common bacteria causing pharyngitis is group A beta-hemolytic *Streptococcus*, but most adult cases are caused by a virus. The incidence of infection is highest between late fall and spring, especially in colder climates.

COLLABORATIVE MANAGEMENT

Assessment

The client with pharyngitis has throat soreness and dryness, throat pain, pain on swallowing **(odynophagia),** difficulty in swallowing **(dysphagia),** and fever. Viral and bacterial pharyngitis are often difficult to distinguish on physical assessment. When inspecting a throat infected with either virus or bacteria, you may see mild to severe **hyperemia** (redness) with or without enlarged tonsils and with or without exudate. Ask the about nasal discharge, which can vary from thin and watery to thick and purulent. Lymph node enlargement in the neck occurs with both viral and bacterial pharyngitis. When a tonsillar abscess occurs with pharyngitis, the client may have a "hot potato" voice, a thickened voice of poor quality.

TABLE 34-1 Causes of Pharyngitis

Bacterial Causes
- *Streptococcus*
- *Staphylococcus*
- *Haemophilus influenzae*
- Pneumococcus
- *Corynebacterium diphtheriae*
- *Neisseria gonorrhoeae*

Viral Causes
- Adenovirus
- Rhinovirus
- Epstein-Barr virus
- Cytomegalovirus (CMV)
- Influenza virus
- Parainfluenza virus
- Herpesvirus
- Coxsackievirus A
- Echovirus

Other Causes
- *Chlamydia*
- *Mycoplasma pneumoniae*
- *Candida*
- Physical and chemical causes
  - Alcohol
  - Tobacco
  - Heat
  - Irritants
  - Dehydration
  - Trauma

Bacterial infections are more often associated with enlarged red tonsils, exudate, purulent nasal discharge, and local lymph node enlargement. Chart 34-2 compares the manifestations of viral and bacterial pharyngitis. Viral pharyngitis is contagious for 2 to 3 days. Symptoms usually subside within 3 to 10 days after onset, and the disease is usually self-limiting.

Bacterial pharyngitis, such as group A streptococcal infection, can lead to serious medical complications (Table 34-2), including acute glomerulonephritis (Chapter 74) and rheumatic fever carditis. Acute glomerulonephritis may occur 7 to 10 days after the acute infection, and rheumatic fever may develop 3 to 5 weeks after the acute infection.

Throat cultures are important in distinguishing viral from a group A beta-hemolytic streptococcal infection; however, the results are not entirely accurate. False-negative cultures can occur, some of which are due to incorrect throat culture technique. The organisms are not uniformly distributed throughout the throat and can be missed during swabbing. To obtain a specimen, rub a cotton swab first over the right tonsillar area, moving across the right arch, the uvula, and then across the left arch to the left tonsillar area. The cotton swab is streaked on a blood agar plate, which is then incubated for 24 to 48 hours.

Many types of rapid tests and screens for group A beta-hemolytic streptococcal antigen are available. These tests vary in specificity and sensitivity and cost about the same as a culture and sensitivity, but the results are available more quickly than standard cultures. Two common tests are the GenProbe and the OIA (Optical Immunoassay).

A complete blood count (CBC) is performed when the client's condition is severe or does not improve. Clients who need a CBC are those who have high fevers, lethargy, or manifestations of complications. A CBC may indicate other causes of pharyngitis.

When taking a history, ask about the client's recent contacts (within the last 10 days) with people who have been ill. Specifically ask whether the client has been ill with symptoms of a cold or upper respiratory tract infection recently. Document any previous history of streptococcal infections,

CHART 34-2

KEY FEATURES of
Acute Viral and Bacterial Pharyngitis

Feature	Viral Pharyngitis	Bacterial Pharyngitis
Temperature	Low-grade or no fever	High temperature (>101° F [38° C], and usually 102°-104° F [38.5°-40° C])*
Ear manifestations	Retracted or dull tympanic membrane	Retracted or dull tympanic membrane
Throat manifestations	Scant or no tonsillar exudate Slight erythema of pharynx and tonsils	Severe hyperemia of pharyngeal mucosa, tonsils, and uvula Erythema of tonsils with yellow exudate
Neck manifestations	Possible lymphadenopathy	Anterior cervical lymphadenopathy and tenderness
Skin manifestations	No rash	Possible scarlatiniform rash Possible petechiae on chest or abdomen or both
Dysphagia, odynophagia	Present	Present
Other symptoms	No cough Rhinitis Mild hoarseness Headache	No cough Voice characterized by pain on voicing and slurred speech Headache Arthralgia Myalgia
Laboratory data	Complete blood count usually normal White blood cell count usually lower than 10,000/mm³ Negative throat culture results	Complete blood count abnormal White blood cell count usually >12,000/mm³* Throat culture results positive for beta-hemolytic streptococcus
Onset	Gradual	Abrupt

*May not be present in adults over 65 years of age.

TABLE 34-2 Complications of Group A Streptococcal Infection

Rheumatic fever	Sinusitis
Acute glomerulonephritis	Mastoiditis
Peritonsillar abscess	Bronchitis
Retropharyngeal abscess	Pneumonia
Otitis media	Scarlet fever

rheumatic fever, valvular heart disease, or penicillin allergy. Because diphtheria (*Corynebacterium diphtheriae*) can cause pharyngitis, ask about and document whether the client has had a diphtheria immunization.

Interventions

Most sore throats in adults are viral and do not require antibiotic therapy. Treatment includes rest, increased fluid intake, humidifying the air, analgesics for pain, warm saline gargles, and throat lozenges containing mild anesthetics.

The management of bacterial pharyngitis involves the use of antibiotics and the same supportive care provided for viral pharyngitis. For streptococcal infection, an oral penicillin or cephalosporin is prescribed. Drugs from the macrolide class (e.g., azithromycin or erythromycin) are recommended if the client is allergic to penicillin. *Stress the importance of completing the entire antibiotic prescription, even when symptoms improve or subside.* If the client cannot tolerate the drug, notify the physician so that the antibiotic can be changed. If adherence is a concern or if the client cannot swallow pills, long-acting penicillin can be given intramuscularly in a single dose.

The client should be re-evaluated if there is no improvement in 3 days or if manifestations are still present after completion of the antibiotic course. Persistent bacterial pharyngitis may occur with immunosuppression. Any client whose bacterial pharyngitis does not improve with antibiotics should consider HIV testing.

A rare complication of pharyngitis in adults is infection of the epiglottis and supraglottic structures **(epiglottitis).** The epiglottis is a flaplike structure that closes over the trachea during swallowing to prevent aspiration. An inflamed epiglottis can swell and obstruct the airway, causing a medical emergency. *Any client with pharyngitis who has stridor or indications of airway obstruction should be immediately evaluated by a health care provider in a setting in which intubation or tracheostomy can be performed quickly and safely.*

Teach the client how to take his or her oral temperature accurately every morning and evening until the infection resolves. The client is not contagious after 24 hours of antibiotic therapy. Family members or close contacts who also have a sore throat should be evaluated, and a throat culture may be indicated.

Tonsillitis

PATHOPHYSIOLOGY

Tonsillitis is an inflammation and infection of the tonsils and lymphatic tissues located on each side of the throat. The tonsils are lymphatic tissue shaped like a small almond. Each tonsil is covered by a mucous membrane and has small valleys **(crypts)** across the surface. Tonsils filter organisms and protect the respiratory tract from infection.

Tonsillitis is a contagious airborne infection. Acute or chronic tonsillitis can occur in any age group, but it is less common in adults. The infection is usually more severe when it occurs in adolescents or adults.

Acute tonsillitis usually lasts 7 to 10 days and is usually caused by bacteria. The most common organism is *Streptococcus.* Other bacterial causes include *Staphylococcus aureus, H. influenzae,* and *Pneumococcus.* Viruses also cause tonsillitis. Chronic tonsillitis may result from an unresolved acute infection or recurrent infections.

COLLABORATIVE MANAGEMENT

Assessment

Chart 34-3 lists the manifestations of acute tonsillitis. Diagnostic tests often used to rule out other causes of the sore throat and fever include a complete blood count (CBC), throat culture and sensitivity (C&S) studies, and Monospot test. If respiratory symptoms are present, chest x-rays may be needed. The white blood cell count is elevated in bacterial infections. Throat C&S studies identify the causative organism and direct the choice of drug therapy.

Interventions

The health care provider prescribes antibiotics (usually penicillin or azithromycin) for 7 to 10 days. Warm saline throat gargles, analgesics, antipyretics, and lozenges with topical anesthetic agents may provide symptom relief.

Surgical intervention for tonsillitis may be needed for recurrent acute infections (especially group A beta-hemolytic streptococcal infections), chronic infections that have not responded to antibiotic therapy, a peritonsillar abscess, and enlarged tonsils or adenoids that obstruct the airway.

Surgery is usually performed after the client has recovered from an acute tonsillitis and no infection is present (except with an acute peritonsillar abscess).

Surgery may involve complete tonsil removal (for chronic infection) or a partial tonsil removal for obstruction without infection. A common procedure to remove the tonsils is dissection and snare, although laser tonsillectomy, radiothermal ablation tonsillectomy, and tonsil "shaving" are being used increasingly. The adenoids may be removed at the same time. A tonsillectomy and adenoidectomy (T&A) is usually performed with the adult client under general anesthesia. After surgery, assess for airway clearance, provide pain relief, and monitor for excessive bleeding.

Peritonsillar Abscess

PATHOPHYSIOLOGY

Peritonsillar abscess (PTA), or *quinsy*, is a complication of acute tonsillitis. The infection spreads from the tonsil to the surrounding tissue, which forms an abscess. The most common cause of PTA is group A beta-hemolytic streptococcus.

CHART 34-3

KEY FEATURES of Acute Tonsillitis

- Sudden onset of a mild to severe sore throat
- Fever
- Muscle aches
- Chills
- Dysphagia, odynophagia (painful swallowing of food)
- Pain in the ears
- Headache
- Anorexia
- Malaise
- "Hot potato" voice (thickened voice of poor quality)
- Tonsils visually swollen and red with pus
- Tonsils may be covered with a white or yellow exudate
- Purulent drainage may be expressed by pressing a tonsil
- Uvula visually edematous or inflamed
- Cervical lymph nodes usually tender and enlarged

COLLABORATIVE MANAGEMENT

Signs of infection are pronounced on examination. Pus forms behind the tonsil and causes one-sided swelling with deviation of the uvula. The swelling may cause the client to drool, have severe throat pain radiating to the ear, have a voice change, and have difficulty swallowing. The client may also have a tonic contraction of the muscles of chewing **(trismus)** and have difficulty breathing.

Outpatient management with antibiotic therapy and percutaneous needle aspiration of the abscess is usually needed. The client usually improves in 36 hours. *Stress the importance of completing the antibiotic regimen and of coming to the emergency department quickly if symptoms of obstruction appear (drooling and stridor).* Instruct the client about comfort measures (e.g., warm saline gargles or irrigations, an ice collar, analgesics). Hospitalization is required when the client's airway is in jeopardy or when the infection does not respond to antibiotic therapy. Incision and drainage **(I&D)** of the abscess, plus additional antibiotic therapy, may be needed. A tonsillectomy may be performed to prevent recurrence.

DISORDERS OF THE LARYNX AND LUNGS

Laryngitis

PATHOPHYSIOLOGY

Laryngitis is an inflammation of the mucous membranes lining the larynx and may or may not include edema of the vocal cords. It can occur as a single problem or occur with upper respiratory infections. Laryngitis also can be a manifestation of a related disease process, such as throat or lung cancer. Common causes include exposure to irritating inhalants and pollutants (chemical agents, tobacco, alcohol, and smoke), overuse of the voice, inhalation of volatile gases (e.g., glue, paint thinner, butane), or intubation. An increasingly common cause of recurrent laryngitis is gastroesophageal reflux disease (GERD).

COLLABORATIVE MANAGEMENT

Assess the client for acute hoarseness, dry cough, and difficulty swallowing. Complete but temporary voice loss **(aphonia)** also may occur. A laryngeal mirror is used to examine the larynx visually and to identify inflammation, polyps, edema, or tumor. If suspicious lesions are present, an x-ray, computed tomography (CT), or fiberoptic laryngoscopic examination may be needed. Clients who may have a disorder other than acute laryngitis are referred to an ear, nose, and throat (ENT) specialist.

Nursing management is aimed toward symptom relief and prevention. Treatment consists of voice rest, steam inhalations, increased fluid intake, and throat lozenges. The health care provider may prescribe antibiotic therapy and bronchodilators when sinusitis, bronchitis, or a bacterial infection is also present. Inform the client and family about relief measures; infection prevention; and avoidance of alcohol, tobacco, and pollutants.

Preventive therapy is aimed toward increasing the client's and family's awareness of the hazards of tobacco and alcohol use. Emphasize the activities that place an added strain on the larynx, such as singing, cheering, public speaking, heavy lifting, and whispering. Speech therapy is used when vocal cord injury occurs with laryngitis and for any voice disorder. For recurrent bouts of laryngitis, further medical and voice evaluation is indicated.

Influenza

PATHOPHYSIOLOGY

Influenza, or "flu," is a highly contagious acute viral respiratory infection that can occur in adults of all ages. Epidemics are common and lead to complications of pneumonia or death, especially in older adults or debilitated or immunocompromised clients. Hospitalization may be required. Influenza may be caused by one of several viruses, usually referred to as A, B, and C.

The client with influenza usually has a severe headache, muscle aches, fever, chills, fatigue, weakness, and anorexia. Manifestations of sore throat, cough, and rhinorrhea (watery discharge from the nose) generally follow the initial symptoms for a week or longer. Most clients continue to feel fatigued for 1 to 2 weeks after the acute episode has resolved.

HEALTH PROMOTION/ILLNESS PREVENTION

Vaccinations for the prevention of influenza are widely available. The vaccine is changed every year on the basis of which specific viral strains are most likely to pose a problem during the influenza season (i.e., late fall and winter). Influenza vaccinations can be taken as an intramuscular injection (Fluviron, Fluzone) or as an intranasal spray (FluMist). People recommended to receive the vaccine each year include those older than 50 years of age, people with chronic illness or immune compromise, those living in institutions, and health care personnel providing direct care to clients (Centers for Disease Control and Prevention [CDC], 2000).

◆COLLABORATIVE MANAGEMENT

Viral infections do not respond to traditional antibiotic therapy. Antiviral agents may be effective for prevention and treatment of some types of influenza. Amantadine (Symmetrel) and rimantadine (Flumadine) have been effective in the prevention and treatment of influenza A. Ribavirin (Virazole) has been used for severe influenza B. Newer antivirals include zanamivir (Relenza), which is used as an oral inhalant, and oseltamivir (Tamiflu), which is an oral tablet. Both these antivirals prevent viral spread in the respiratory tract by inhibiting a viral enzyme (neuraminidase) that allows the virus to penetrate respiratory cells. These agents shorten the duration of influenzas A or B if taken within 24 to 48 hours after the onset of manifestations. Both agents also may be used for prevention.

Advise the client to stay in bed for several days and drink large amounts of fluids unless another medical problem requires fluid restriction (e.g., kidney disease or heart failure). Saline gargles may ease sore throat pain. Antihistamines may reduce the rhinorrhea. Other supportive and comfort measures are the same as those for acute rhinitis.

Pneumonia

PATHOPHYSIOLOGY

Pneumonia is an excess of fluid in the lungs resulting from an inflammatory process. The inflammation is triggered by many infectious organisms and by inhalation of irritating agents. Infectious pneumonias are categorized as community-acquired (CAP) or hospital-acquired **(nosocomial),** depending on where the client was exposed to the infectious agent. This distinction is important because nosocomial pneumonias are more likely to be resistant to antibiotics than are CAPs.

The inflammation occurs in the interstitial spaces, the alveoli, and often the bronchioles. The process begins when organisms penetrate the airway mucosa and multiply in the alveolar spaces. To do this, they must survive the lung's many defenses against microbial invasion, including the inflammatory response. White blood cells migrate to the area of infection, causing local capillary leak, edema, and exudate. These fluids collect in and around the alveoli, and the alveolar walls thicken. Both events reduce gas exchange and lead to hypoxemia. Red blood cells and fibrin also move into the alveoli. The capillary leak spreads the infection to other areas of the lung. If the organisms move into the bloodstream, sepsis results; if the infection extends into the pleural cavity, empyema results.

The fibrin and edema of inflammation stiffen the lung, reducing compliance and decreasing the vital capacity (VC). Alveolar collapse **(atelectasis)** further reduces the ability of the lungs to oxygenate the blood moving through it. As a result, arterial oxygen tension falls, causing **hypoxemia** (insufficient oxygen in the blood).

Pneumonia may occur as lobar pneumonia with **consolidation** (solidification, lack of air spaces) in a segment or an entire lobe of the lung or as bronchopneumonia with diffusely scattered patches around the bronchi. The extent of lung involvement after the organism invades depends on the host defenses. Bacteria multiply quickly in a person whose immune system is compromised. Tissue necrosis results when organisms form an abscess that perforates the bronchial wall.

Etiology

In general, people develop pneumonia when their immune systems are unable to combat the virulence of the invading organisms. Organisms from the environment, invasive devices, equipment and supplies, staff, or from other people can invade the body. Risk factors are listed in Table 34-3. Pneumonia can be caused by bacteria, viruses, mycoplasmas, fungi, rickettsiae, protozoa, and helminths (worms) (Table 34-4). Noninfectious causes of pneumonia include inhalation of toxic gases, chemicals, smoke, and aspiration of water, food, fluid, and vomitus.

Incidence/Prevalence

In the United States, two to four million cases of pneumonia occur each year, and it is the fifth leading cause of death (CDC, 2003b). The highest incidence among adults occurs in older adults, nursing home residents, hospitalized clients, and those being mechanically ventilated. Community-acquired pneumonia (CAP) is more common than nosocomial pneumonia and occurs in late fall and winter as a complication of

TABLE 34-3 Risk Factors Associated with Pneumonia

Community-Acquired Pneumonias
- Older adult
- No history of pneumococcal vaccination
- No history of having received the influenza vaccine in the previous year
- Chronic or other coexisting condition
- Recent history of or exposure to viral or influenza infections
- History of tobacco or alcohol use

Nosocomial Pneumonias
- Older adult
- Chronic lung disease
- Gram-negative colonization of the oropharynx and stomach
- Altered level of consciousness
- Aspiration
- Endotracheal, tracheostomy, or nasogastric tube
- Poor nutritional status
- Immunocompromised status (from disease, medications)
- Medications that increase gastric pH (histamine [H_2] blockers, antacids) or alkaline tube feedings
- Mechanical ventilation (ventilator acquired pneumonia [VAP])

TABLE 34-4 Common Organisms Causing Pneumonia*

Community-Acquired Pneumonias
- *Streptococcus pneumoniae* (Gram positive)
- *Staphylococcus aureus* (Gram positive)
- *Haemophilus influenzae* (Gram negative)
- *Legionella pneumophila* (Gram negative)
- *Mycoplasma pneumoniae* (smallest free-living organism)
- *Chlamydia pneumoniae* (parasite)

Nosocomial Pneumonias
- *Staphylococcus aureus* (Gram positive)
- *Pseudomonas aeruginosa* (Gram negative)
- *Enterobacter* organisms (Gram negative)
- *Klebsiella* organisms (Gram negative)
- *Haemophilus influenzae* organisms (Gram negative)
- *Acinetobacter* organisms (Gram negative)
- *Candida albicans* (fungus)

*Because of various factors that influence the incidence of the pathogenic causes of pneumonia, these organisms are listed loosely in order of incidence.

influenza. Hospital-acquired pneumonia is a common nosocomial infection. Nosocomial pneumonia has a 20% to 50% mortality; the highest incidence is in those clients infected with *Pseudomonas aeruginosa*, *Acinetobacter*, other "high-risk" organisms, or secondary bacteremia. Mortality also is higher in clients who have complications (Table 34-5).

CONSIDERATIONS FOR OLDER ADULTS

Pneumonia and influenza are the third leading cause of death for clients older than 85 years of age. The death rate for clients older than 64 years of age is steadily increasing (CDC, 2003b).

HEALTH PROMOTION/ILLNESS PREVENTION

Of the different types of pneumonia organisms, the most common are 6B, 23F, 14, 9V, 19A, and 19F. All these types are included in the pneumococcal vaccine. Client education is important in the prevention of pneumonia (Chart 34-4),

TABLE 34-5 Common Complications of Pneumonia

Complication	Definition
Hypoxemia	Arterial oxygen <80 mm Hg
Ventilatory failure	Lungs unable to move gas in and out of lungs mechanically, resulting in hypoxemia and hypercarbia
Atelectasis	Collapse of the affected alveoli and associated lobes of the lungs
Pleural effusion	Collection of fluid in the pleural space (usually sterile fluid that resolves)
Pleurisy	Pain caused by friction between layers of pleura

CHART 34-4

CLIENT EDUCATION GUIDE
Preventing Pneumonia

- Know whether you are at risk for pneumonia.
- Have the annual influenza vaccine after discussing appropriate timing of the vaccination with your primary health care provider.
- Discuss the pneumococcal vaccine with your primary health care provider, and have the vaccination as recommended.
- Avoid crowded public areas during flu and holiday seasons.
- Cough, turn, move about, and perform deep-breathing exercises as directed by your nurse or other health care professional.
- If you are using respiration equipment at home, clean the equipment as you have been taught.
- Avoid indoor pollutants, such as dust, secondhand (passive) smoke, and aerosols.
- If you do not smoke, do not start.
- If you smoke, seek professional help on how to stop (or at least decrease) your habit.
- Be sure to get enough rest and sleep on a daily basis.
- Eat a healthy, balanced diet and take in a sufficient amount of nonalcoholic fluids each day.

as is making the vaccines readily available to those most at risk.

Other prevention techniques include strict handwashing to avoid the spread of organisms. Respiratory therapy equipment must be well maintained and decontaminated or changed as recommended. Use sterile water rather than tap water in gastrointestinal tubes, and institute aspiration precautions as indicated. Specific interventions to prevent aspiration are discussed in Chapter 31.

COLLABORATIVE MANAGEMENT

PHARM e-REVIEW

The Concept Map on p. 635 addresses assessment and nursing care issues related to clients who have pneumonia.

Assessment

HISTORY

In taking the history from the client who may have pneumonia, consider the risk factors for infection (see Table 34-3). Obtain the information from a family member if the client is confused or too dyspneic. Document age; living, work, or school environment; diet, exercise, and sleep routines; swallowing problems; presence of a nasogastrointestinal tube; tobacco and alcohol use; past and current use of drugs; and his-

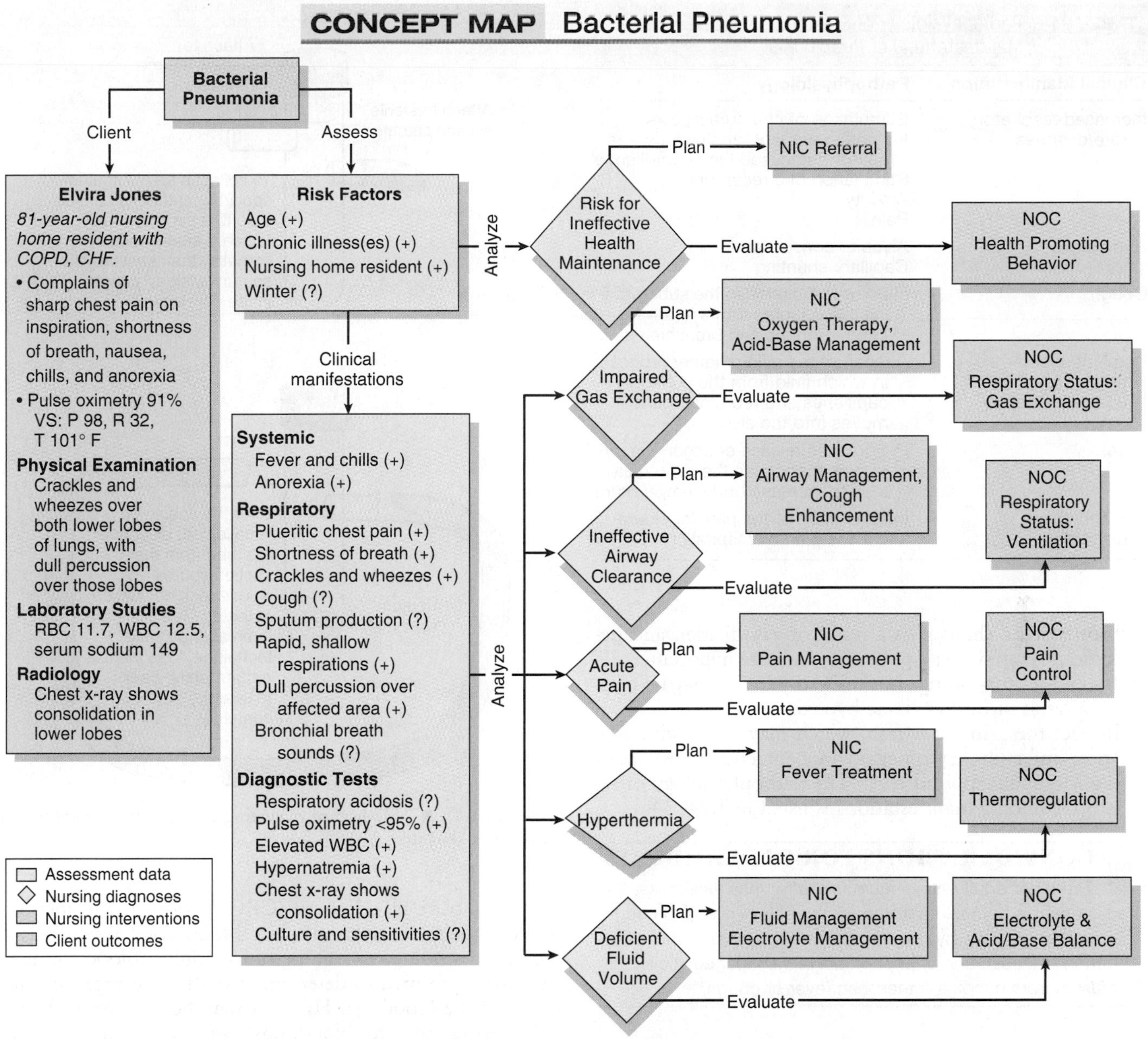

Concept Map by Elaine Bishop Kennedy, EdD, RN

tory of drug addiction or injection drug use. Ask the client about past respiratory illnesses and whether he or she has been exposed to influenza or pneumonia or has had a recent viral infection. Ask about recent skin rashes, insect bites, or exposure to animals.

If the client has chronic respiratory problems, ask whether respiratory equipment is used in the home. Assess whether the client's home cleaning level is adequate to prevent infection. Ask the client when the last influenza or pneumococcal vaccine was taken.

PHYSICAL ASSESSMENT/CLINICAL MANIFESTATIONS

First observe the client's general appearance. Many clients with pneumonia have flushed cheeks, bright eyes, and an anxious expression. The client may have chest or pleuritic pain or discomfort, myalgia, headache, chills, fever, cough, tachycardia, dyspnea, tachypnea, and sputum production. Severe chest muscle weakness also may be present from sustained coughing.

Observe the client's breathing pattern, position, and use of accessory muscles. The hypoxic client may be uncomfortable in a lying position and sit upright, balancing with the hands. Assess the client's cough and the amount, color, consistency, and odor of sputum produced.

Crackles are heard with auscultation when there is fluid in interstitial and alveolar areas. Wheezing may be heard as a result of inflammation and exudate in the airways. Bronchial breath sounds are heard over areas of density or consolidation. Tactile fremitus is increased over areas of pneumonia, and percussion is dulled in these areas. Chest expansion may be diminished or unequal on inspiration.

In evaluating vital signs, compare the results with baseline values. The client with pneumonia is likely to be hypotensive

TABLE 34-6 Pathophysiology of Selected Clinical Manifestations of Pneumonia

Clinical Manifestation	Pathophysiology
Increased respiratory rate/dyspnea	Stimulation of chemoreceptors Increased work of breathing as a result of decreased lung compliance Stimulation of J receptors Anxiety Pain
Hypoxemia	Alveolar consolidation Capillary shunting
Cough	Fluid accumulation in the subepithelial mechanoreceptors in the trachea, bronchi, and bronchioles
Purulent, blood-tinged, or rust-colored sputum	A result of the inflammatory process in which fluid from the pulmonary capillaries and red blood cells moves into the alveoli
Fever	Phagocytes release endogenous pyrogens that cause the hypothalamus to increase body temperature
Pleuritic chest discomfort	Inflammation of the parietal pleura causes pain on inspiration

with orthostatic changes as a result of vasodilation and dehydration. A rapid, weak pulse may indicate hypoxemia, dehydration, or impending shock. Dysrhythmias may be present as a result of cardiac tissue hypoxia.

Inspect the skin for a rash, which may occur with *Mycoplasma* infection, cytomegalovirus infection (CMV), or Rocky Mountain spotted fever. The pathophysiology of selected pneumonia manifestations is listed in Table 34-6.

CONSIDERATIONS FOR OLDER ADULTS

The older adult with pneumonia often has weakness, fatigue, lethargy, confusion, and poor appetite. Fever and cough may be absent, but hypoxemia is usually present. The most common manifestation of pneumonia in the older adult client is confusion from hypoxia rather than fever or cough.

PSYCHOSOCIAL ASSESSMENT

The client with pneumonia often has pain, fatigue, and dyspnea, all of which promote anxiety. Assess anxiety by looking at the client's facial expression and general tenseness of facial and shoulder muscles. Listen to the client carefully and use a calm, slow approach to assessment. Because of airway obstruction and muscle fatigue, the client with dyspnea speaks in broken sentences. Keep the interview short if the client has significant dyspnea or breathing discomfort.

LABORATORY ASSESSMENT

Sputum is obtained and examined by Gram stain, culture, and sensitivity testing; however, the responsible organism is not identified about 50% of the time. A sputum sample is easily obtained from the client who can cough into a specimen container. Extremely ill clients may need suctioning to obtain a sputum specimen. In these situations, a sputum specimen is obtained by sputum trap (Figure 34-1) during suctioning.

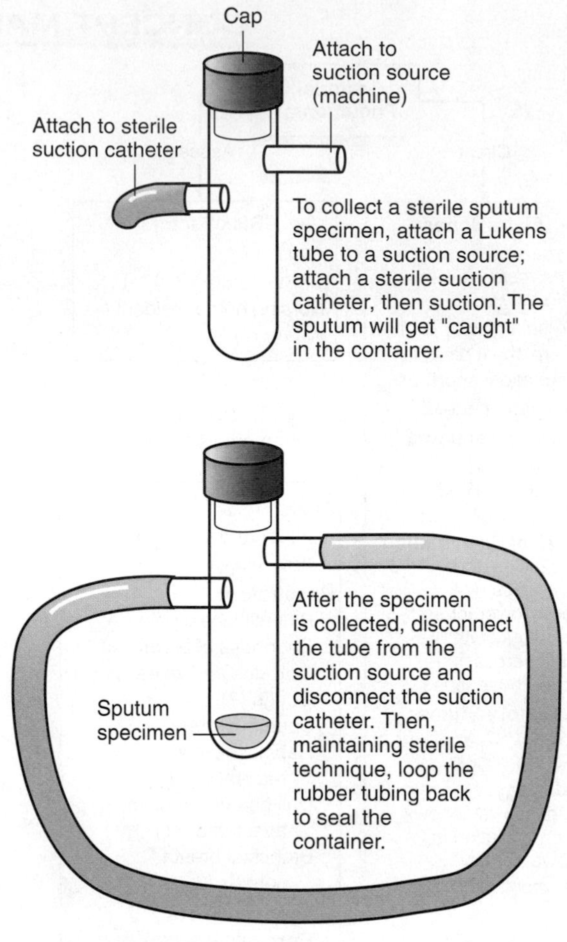

Figure 34-1 ■ Method of collecting a sterile sputum specimen using a Lukens tube.

A complete blood count (CBC) is obtained to identify **leukocytosis** (an elevated white blood count), which is a common finding, except in older adults. Blood cultures may be performed to determine whether the organism has invaded the blood. An HIV test may be performed. Urine may be examined for blood, pus, or protein, which may occur in the septic client with pneumonia.

Arterial blood gases (ABGs) determine baseline arterial oxygen and carbon dioxide levels and help identify a need for supplemental oxygen. Serum electrolyte, blood urea nitrogen (BUN), and creatinine levels also are assessed. A high BUN level may occur as a result of dehydration. Hypernatremia occurs with dehydration as a result of fever and decreased fluid intake.

RADIOGRAPHIC ASSESSMENT

Pneumonia usually appears on chest x-ray as an area of increased density. It may involve a lung segment, a lobe, one lung, or both lungs. In the older adult, the chest x-ray is essential for early diagnosis of pneumonia because symptoms are often vague.

OTHER DIAGNOSTIC ASSESSMENTS

Pulse oximetry is used to assess for hypoxemia. More invasive tests may be needed, such as transtracheal aspiration, bronchoscopy, or direct needle aspiration of the lung to obtain lower airway specimens. Thoracentesis is most often used in clients who have an accompanying pleural effusion.

Critical Thinking Challenge

When you bring the morning medications to your 86-year-old male client in the long-term care facility, he does not know who you are. This problem is a change from yesterday, when he told you all about the visit 4 days earlier from his daughter, who teaches kindergarten, and his three grandchildren. You note that he has not eaten or had anything to drink from his breakfast tray. Because he is diabetic, you hold the morning dose of his oral antidiabetic agent. Concerned, you check his vital signs, which are as follows: T 99.0, P 110 and thready, R 34, BP 96/60. All these values are different from his usual morning vital sign values. You are concerned that he may either have pneumonia or urosepsis.

1. What additional assessment data should you obtain?
2. What risk factors does he have for urosepsis?
3. What risk factors does he have for pneumonia?
4. Should you notify his physician or nurse practitioner?
5. What should you do about his oral antidiabetic medication and other morning medications (Lasix, multivitamin, captopril)?
6. Should you apply oxygen? If so, how?

evolve For suggested answer guidelines, go to http://evolve.elsevier.com/Iggy/.

Analysis

COMMON NURSING DIAGNOSES AND COLLABORATIVE PROBLEMS

The following are priority nursing diagnoses for clients with pneumonia:

1. Impaired Gas Exchange related to effects of alveolar-capillary membrane changes
2. Ineffective Airway Clearance related to effects of infection, excessive tracheobronchial secretions, fatigue and decreased energy, chest discomfort, and muscle weakness

A primary collaborative problem for the client with pneumonia is Potential for Sepsis.

ADDITIONAL NURSING DIAGNOSES AND COLLABORATIVE PROBLEMS

In addition to the common nursing diagnoses and collaborative problems, clients with pneumonia may have one or more of the following:

- Acute Pain related to effects of inflammation of parietal pleura, coughing
- Deficient Fluid Volume related to increased respiratory rate.
- Deficient Fluid Volume related to fever, infection, and increased metabolic rate
- Disturbed Sleep Pattern related to pain, dyspnea, unfamiliar environment (hospitalization)
- Potential for Pleural Effusion

Planning and Implementation

IMPAIRED GAS EXCHANGE

NOC **PLANNING: EXPECTED OUTCOMES.** The client with pneumonia is expected to have adequate gas exchange. The following are indicators of adequate gas exchange:

- Maintenance of SaO_2 of at least 95%
- Absence of cyanosis
- Maintenance of cognitive orientation

INTERVENTIONS. NIC interventions for the client with pneumonia are listed in Chart 34-5. Interventions to treat and manage impaired gas exchange are similar to those for the client with chronic airflow limitation (CAL) (see Chapter 33). In pneumonia, oxygen is the gas exchange affected most; therefore, hypoxemia is the primary problem. Carbon dioxide retention is not common in pneumonia.

Incentive spirometry, also referred to as **sustained maximal inspiration,** is a type of bronchial hygiene used in pneumonia. The objective is to improve inspiratory muscle performance and to prevent or reverse **atelectasis** (alveolar collapse). Instruct the client to exhale fully; then place the mouthpiece in his or her mouth; and take a long, slow, deep breath for 3 to 5 seconds. Evaluate technique, and record the volume of air inspired. Instruct the client to perform 5 to 10 breaths per session every hour while awake.

INEFFECTIVE AIRWAY CLEARANCE

NOC **PLANNING: EXPECTED OUTCOMES.** The client with pneumonia is expected to maintain a patent airway. Indicators are the following:

- Effective cough
- Absence of pallor or cyanosis
- Absence of crackles and wheezes on auscultation
- Decreased tactile fremitus

INTERVENTIONS. For the client with pneumonia, interventions for ineffective airway clearance are similar to those for COPD or asthma. Because of fatigue, muscle weakness, chest discomfort, and excessive secretions, the client with pneumonia often has difficulty clearing secretions. Help the client to cough and deep breathe at least every 2 hours. The alert client may use an incentive spirometer to facilitate deep breathing and stimulate coughing. Chest physiotherapy (CPT or chest PT) is no longer recommended for uncomplicated pneumonia. Dehydration should be avoided, but there is no evidence that hydration helps to clear secretions. Adequate hydration may help to thin secretions and make them easier to remove. Monitor intake and output to ensure adequate hydration when fever and tachypnea are present.

The health care provider prescribes bronchodilators, especially beta-2 agonists (see Chart 33-5), when bronchospasm is part of the disease process. They are initially given by aerosol nebulizer and then by metered-dose inhaler (see Chart 33-5). Inhaled steroids are rarely used with acute pneumonia except when the client also has bronchial asthma or respiratory failure.

POTENTIAL FOR SEPSIS

NOC **PLANNING: EXPECTED OUTCOMES.** The client with pneumonia is expected to be free of the invading organism and to return to a pre-pneumonia health status. Indicators are the following:

- Absence of fever
- Absence of pathogens in blood and sputum cultures
- White blood cell count and differential within normal limits

INTERVENTIONS. The key to effective treatment of pneumonia is eradication of the organism causing the infection. Anti-infectives are given for all types of pneumonias

CHART 34-5

NIC **INTERVENTION ACTIVITIES for**
The Client with Pneumonia

Cough Enhancement: *Promotion of deep inhalation by the client with subsequent generation of high intrathoracic pressures and compression of the underlying lung parenchyma for the forceful expulsion of air*
- Assist client to a sitting position with neck slightly flexed, shoulders relaxed, and knees flexed.
- Encourage client to take several deep breaths.
- Encourage client to take a deep breath, hold it for 2 seconds, and cough two or three times in succession.
- Instruct client to inhale deeply, bend forward slightly, and perform three or four huffs (against an open glottis).
- Instruct client to inhale deeply several times, to exhale slowly, and to cough at the end of exhalation.
- Initiate lateral chest wall rib spring techniques during the expiration phase of the cough maneuver, as appropriate.
- Instruct client to follow coughing with several maximal inhalation breaths.
- Encourage use of incentive spirometry, as appropriate.
- Promote systemic fluid hydration, as appropriate.

Oxygen Therapy: *Administration of oxygen and monitoring of its effectiveness*
- Clear oral, nasal, and tracheal secretions, as appropriate.
- Restrict smoking.
- Maintain airway patency.
- Set up oxygen equipment and administer through a heated, humidified system.
- Administer supplemental oxygen as ordered.
- Monitor the oxygen liter flow.
- Monitor position of oxygen delivery device.
- Instruct client about importance of leaving oxygen delivery device on.
- Periodically check oxygen delivery device to ensure that the prescribed concentration is being delivered.
- Monitor the effectiveness of oxygen therapy (e.g., pulse oximetry, ABGs), as appropriate.
- Ensure replacement of oxygen mask/cannula whenever the device is removed.
- Monitor client's ability to tolerate removal of oxygen while eating.
- Change oxygen delivery device from mask to nasal prongs during meals, as tolerated.
- Observe for signs of oxygen-induced hypoventilation.
- Monitor for signs of oxygen toxicity and absorption atelectasis.
- Monitor client's anxiety related to need for oxygen therapy.
- Monitor for skin breakdown from friction of oxygen device.
- Provide for oxygen when client is transported.

Respiratory Monitoring: *Collection and analysis of client data to ensure airway patency and adequate gas exchange*
- Monitor rate, rhythm, depth, and effort of respirations.
- Note chest movement, watching for symmetry, use of accessory muscles, and supraclavicular and intercostal muscle retractions.
- Monitor breathing patterns: bradypnea, tachypnea, hyperventilation, Kussmaul respirations, Cheyne-Stokes respirations, apneustic Biot's respiration, and ataxic patterns.
- Palpate for equal lung expansion.
- Monitor for diaphragmatic muscle fatigue (paradoxical motion).
- Auscultate breath sounds, noting areas of decreased/absent ventilation and presence of adventitious sounds.
- Determine the need for suctioning by auscultating for crackles and rhonchi over major airways.
- Auscultate lung sounds after treatments to note results.
- Monitor for increased restlessness, anxiety, and air hunger.
- Note changes in Sao_2, Svo_2, end tidal CO_2, and ABG values, as appropriate.
- Monitor client's ability to cough effectively.
- Note onset, characteristics, and duration of cough.
- Monitor client's respiratory secretions.
- Monitor for dyspnea and events that decrease and worsen it.
- Monitor chest x-ray reports.
- Place the client on side, as indicated, to prevent aspiration; log roll if cervical aspiration is suspected.
- Institute respiratory treatments (e.g., nebulizer), as needed.

NIC intervention activities selected from Dochterman, J.M., & Bulechek, G.M. (Eds.). (2004). *Nursing interventions classification (NIC)* (4th ed.). St. Louis: Mosby. No part of this work is to be altered without prior written permission from the Publisher.
ABG, Arterial blood gas; Sao_2, arterial oxygen saturation; Svo_2, venous oxygen saturation; CO_2, carbon dioxide.

except those caused by viruses. The health care provider prescribes anti-infective therapy. The exact drug or drugs are determined by the organism suspected or identified, whether the pneumonia is community-acquired (CAP) or hospital-acquired, and whether the client has other conditions or factors that increase the risk for complication (Table 34-7). Initial treatment is based on the manifestations, prior experience, and the most common organisms causing pneumonia in that geographic region. The initial therapy may be continued if the specific organism is not identified.

The client may be able to be switched from intravenous (IV) to oral therapy in 2 or 3 days, depending on the response (e.g., stable clinical condition, afebrile). The course of anti-infective therapy varies with the drug used and the organism(s) involved. Usually anti-infectives are used for 7 to 10 days for a client with uncomplicated CAP and up to 21 days for an immunocompromised client.

Drug resistance is becoming increasingly common, especially for infections with *Streptococcus pneumoniae*. This problem is known as drug-resistant *S. pneumoniae,* or DRSP. DRSP is most common among people over 65 years of age and among those who became infected as a result of exposure to young children from a day-care environment.

For pneumonia resulting from aspiration of food or stomach contents, interventions focus on prevention of lung damage and treating the infection. Aspiration of acidic substances (e.g., vomitus or stomach contents) can cause widespread inflammation, leading to acute respiratory distress syndrome (ARDS) and permanent lung damage. In these conditions, steroids and nonsteroidal anti-inflammatory agents are used with antibiotics to reduce the inflammatory response.

Community-Based Care

The client needs to continue the anti-infective drugs as prescribed. An important nursing role is to reinforce, clarify, and provide information to the client and family as indicated.

HOME CARE MANAGEMENT

No special changes are needed in the home. If the home consists of more than one story, the client may prefer to stay on one floor for a few weeks because stair climbing may increase fatigue and dyspnea. Bath and hygiene needs may be met by using a bedside commode if a bathroom is not located on the level the client is using. Home care needs will depend on the client's level of fatigue, dyspnea, and family and social support.

TABLE 34-7 Recommended Drug Categories for the Treatment of Pneumonia

Pneumonia Type	Recommended Drug Categories with Alternatives
Community-Acquired Pneumonias	
Age <60 yr with no comorbidity	Cefuroxime (add erythromycin if concern for *Mycoplasma, Chlamydia*, or *Legionella* is high) Azithromycin (alternative if client is allergic to penicillin/cephalosporin or is erythromycin intolerant) Levofloxacin (if client is macrolide* intolerant or pneumonia fails to resolve)
Age >60 or <60 yr with comorbidity	Ceftriaxone and azithromycin (or erythromycin) Levofloxacin (alternative if macrolide intolerant or pneumonia fails to resolve) Trovafloxacin
Aspiration pneumonia	Ampicillin/sulbactam and clindamycin Trovafloxacin (alternative if penicillin/cephalosporin allergy) Ceftriaxone and clindamycin
Hospital-Acquired (Nosocomial) Pneumonias	
Gram-positive infections	Ticarcillin/clavulanate Vancomycin Imipenem/cilastatin Piperacillin/tazobactam Cefepime and metronidazole
Gram-negative infections	Ciprofloxacin Aminoglycoside (amikacin, gentamicin) if renal function is stable Ceftazidime Aztreonam Ticarcillin

*Macrolides include erythromycin, azithromycin, clarithromycin, and dirithromycin.

CHART 34-6

FOCUSED ASSESSMENT of The Client Recovering from Pneumonia

Ascertain whether the client has had any of the following:
- Chills
- Fever
- Persistent cough
- Dyspnea
- Wheezing
- Hemoptysis
- Increased sputum production
- Chest discomfort
- Increasing fatigue
- Any other symptoms that have failed to resolve

Assess the client for the following:
- Fever
- Diaphoresis
- Cyanosis, especially around the mouth or conjunctiva
- Dyspnea, tachypnea, or tachycardia
- Adventitious or abnormal breath sounds
- Weakness

The long recovery phase of pneumonia, especially in the older client, can be frustrating and perhaps depressing. Fatigue, weakness, and a residual cough can last for weeks. Some clients fear they will never return to a "normal" level of functioning. It is important to prepare the client for the course of the disease and to offer reassurance that complete recovery will occur. Early after discharge, a home health nursing assessment may be helpful (Chart 34-6).

HEALTH TEACHING

Review all drugs with the client and family and emphasize completing anti-infective therapy. Instruct the client to notify the health care provider if chills, fever, persistent cough, dyspnea, wheezing, hemoptysis, increased sputum production, chest discomfort, or increasing fatigue recurs or if symptoms fail to resolve. Emphasize the importance of getting plenty of rest and gradually increasing exercise.

An important aspect of education for the client and family is the avoidance of upper respiratory tract infections and viruses. Instruct the client to avoid crowds (especially in the fall and winter when viruses are prevalent), people who have a cold or flu, and exposure to irritants such as smoke. An annual influenza vaccine is recommended, and the pneumococcal vaccine is currently recommended once every 5 years (possibly more often for clients at high-risk). A balanced diet and adequate fluid intake are essential.

HEALTH CARE RESOURCES

Inform clients who smoke that smoking is a risk factor for pneumonia. Provide them with information on smoking-cessation classes through the American Lung Association (ALA) and American Cancer Society. The health care provider may prescribe nicotine patches. *Warn the client of the danger of myocardial infarction if smoking is continued while using the patches.* Urge the client to enroll in a smoking-cessation program to assist in the nicotine withdrawal process in conjunction with nicotine patches. Give him or her information booklets on pneumonia provided by the ALA. Urge the client who has not already been vaccinated against influenza or pneumonia to take this preventive measure when the pneumonia has resolved.

◆Evaluation: Outcomes

Evaluate the care of the client with pneumonia on the basis of the identified nursing diagnoses and collaborative problems. The expected outcomes are that the client:
- Attains or maintains adequate gas exchange
- Maintains patent airways
- Is free of the invading organism
- Returns to his or her pre-pneumonia health status

Specific indicators for these outcomes are listed for each nursing diagnosis and collaborative problem under the Planning and Implementation section (see earlier).

Severe Acute Respiratory Syndrome (SARS)

A new respiratory infection was first identified in China early in November 2002. At first appearing as an atypical pneumonia, the infection has been termed **severe acute respiratory syndrome,** or **SARS.** As of July 2003, more than 8400 cases of SARS had been reported to the World Health Organization, 325 cases in North America. In more affluent countries, the mortality rate is 8%. This rate is higher in less affluent countries.

PATHOPHYSIOLOGY

The cause of SARS is a new virus from a family of virus types known as *coronaviruses.* These viruses have ribonucleic acid (RNA) as their genetic material and have many projections that look like a halo or "corona" when examined by electron microscopes. This family of viruses causes many forms of the common cold. The new virus is a mutated form of the coronavirus and is more virulent than most members of this virus family. The virus infects cells of the respiratory tract, triggering an inflammatory response. It stays in the respiratory passageways rather than spreading into the blood because it grows best at temperatures slightly lower than the normal core body temperature.

The virus is easily spread by airborne droplets from infected people through sneezing, coughing, and talking. It can contaminate surfaces and objects, although it does not survive on nonliving surfaces for long periods. People at greatest risk for SARS are those in close direct contact with an infected person. The portals of entry for infection with the virus are the mucous membranes of the eyes, nose, and mouth.

COLLABORATIVE MANAGEMENT

Assessment

The manifestations of SARS are the same as those of any respiratory infection. Usually, the client has a fever higher than 100.4° F (38.0° C), a headache, and general body aches. Mild cold symptoms of a runny nose, sore throat, and watery eyes may also be present. Within 2 to 7 days, the client develops a dry cough and has difficulty breathing. Hypoxia, with cyanosis, low oxygen saturation, and a feeling of breathlessness, indicates more severe illness. Chest x-rays show a pattern similar to pneumonia or other respiratory distress syndromes.

Diagnosis is made by the manifestations and by ruling out other causes of the symptoms. No rapid test specific for this disorder exists at this time. About 28 days after the infection starts, a blood test for antibodies to the virus or pieces of the RNA from the virus can confirm the diagnosis (usually the client is well by this time).

Interventions

No known effective treatment for this infection exists at this time. Standard antibiotic agents and antiviral drugs are not able to kill the virus or prevent its replication. Interventions are supportive to allow the client's own immune system to fight the infection. Oxygen is given when hypoxia or breathlessness is present. Respiratory treatments to dilate the bronchioles and move respiratory secretions are used. If gas exchange is not improved with oxygen therapy alone, intubation and mechanical ventilation may be needed. Antibiotics are used to treat a bacterial pneumonia that may occur with SARS.

PREVENTION OF INFECTION SPREAD

A major nursing responsibility is the prevention infection spread. Handwashing is a key prevention intervention. Gloves may be used but are not a replacement for good handwashing. Use airborne and contact precautions with clients who are suspected to have SARS. Use gowns and eye protection when coming into direct contact with the client. Airborne isolation is recommended. When the client is out of the isolation environment, he or she must wear a mask. If for some reason the client cannot wear a mask, all other people in the environment should wear a mask.

When performing procedures that normally induce coughing or promote aerosolization of particles (e.g., suctioning, using a positive-pressure face mask, obtaining a sputum culture, or giving aerosolized treatments), be sure to protect yourself and other health care workers. Wear a disposable particulate mask respirator (e.g., N-95, N-99, or N-100) and protective eyewear during such procedures. Keep the door to the client's room closed. Avoid touching your face with contaminated gloves. Wash your hands after you remove the gown, gloves, eyewear, and face shield and whenever you leave the client's room. Wear clean gloves when disinfecting contaminated surfaces or equipment.

Pulmonary Tuberculosis

PATHOPHYSIOLOGY

Tuberculosis (TB) is a highly communicable disease caused by *Mycobacterium tuberculosis.* It is the most common bacterial infection worldwide. The organism is transmitted via **aerosolization** (i.e., an airborne route). When a person with active TB coughs, laughs, sneezes, whistles, or sings, droplets become airborne and may be inhaled by others. Far more people are infected with the bacillus than actually develop active TB.

The bacillus multiplies freely when it reaches a susceptible site (bronchi or alveoli). An exudative response occurs, causing a nonspecific pneumonitis. With the development of acquired immunity, further growth of bacilli is controlled in most initial lesions. These lesions usually resolve and leave little or no residual bacilli. Only a small percentage of people initially infected will develop active TB (5% to 15%). The greatest risk for active TB among people who are HIV negative is during the first 2 years after infection.

Cell-mediated immunity develops 2 to 10 weeks after infection and is manifested by a positive reaction to a tuberculin test. The primary infection may be so small that it does not appear on a chest x-ray. The process of infection occurs in the following order:

1. The granulomatous inflammation created by the tubercle bacillus in the lung becomes surrounded by collagen, fibroblasts, and lymphocytes.
2. **Caseation necrosis** (necrotic tissue being turned into a granular mass) occurs in the center of the lesion. If this area shows on x-ray, it is called **Ghon tubercle,** or the primary lesion.

Areas of caseation then undergo resorption, degeneration, and fibrosis. These necrotic areas may calcify **(calcification)** or liquefy **(liquefaction).** If liquefaction occurs, the liquid

TABLE 34-8 American Lung Association Classification of Tuberculosis

Class	Criteria
0	No TB exposure, not infected
1	TB exposure, no evidence of infection
2	TB infection, no disease
3	TB clinically active (clients with completed diagnostic evidence of TB—both a significant reaction to TB skin test and clinical or x-ray evidence of TB)
4	TB: not clinically active (clients with history of TB or abnormal chest x-ray film but no significant TB skin test reaction or clinical evidence)
5	TB. suspect (diagnosis pending); used during diagnostic testing of suspect clients for no longer than 3 mo

material then empties into a bronchus, and the evacuated area becomes a cavity **(cavitation).** Bacilli continue to grow in the necrotic cavity wall and spread via lymph channels into new areas of the lung.

A lesion also may progress by direct extension if bacilli multiply rapidly during inflammation. The lesions may extend through the pleura, resulting in pleural or pericardial effusion. **Miliary** or **hematogenous TB** is the spread of TB throughout the body when a large number of organisms enter the blood. Many tiny, discrete nodules scattered throughout the lung are seen on chest x-ray. The brain, meninges, liver, kidney, or bone marrow can become infected as a result of spread through the blood.

Initial infection is seen more often in the middle or lower lobes of the lung. The local lymph nodes are infected and enlarged. An asymptomatic period usually follows the primary infection and can last for years or decades before clinical symptoms develop. *An infected individual is not infectious to others until manifestations of disease occur.*

Secondary TB is a reactivation of the disease in a previously infected person. Reactivation is more likely when defenses are lowered, which may be part of the reason older adults and people with HIV disease are at greater risk for TB. The upper lobes are the most common site of reactivation and are referred to as **Simon's foci.** The ALA's TB classification is shown in Table 34-8.

Etiology

Mycobacterium tuberculosis is a nonmoving, slow-growing, acid-fast rod transmitted via the airborne route. People who are most often infected are those having repeated close contact with an infectious person who has not yet been diagnosed with TB. The risk of transmission is reduced after the infectious person has received proper medication for 2 to 3 weeks, clinical improvement occurs, and acid-fast bacilli [AFB] in the sputum are reduced.

Incidence/Prevalence

The incidence of TB has been steadily increasing in the United States and worldwide for two decades. The increase is related to the onset of HIV infection. In the United States, the following people are at greatest risk for development of TB:

- Those in constant, frequent contact with an untreated individual
- Those who have immune dysfunction or HIV
- Individuals who live in crowded areas such as long-term care facilities, prisons, and mental health facilities
- Older and homeless people
- Abusers of injection drugs or alcohol
- Lower socioeconomic groups
- Foreign immigrants (especially from Mexico, the Philippines, and Vietnam)

COLLABORATIVE MANAGEMENT

Assessment

Early detection of tuberculosis (TB) depends on subjective findings rather than on observable symptoms. TB has a slow onset, and many clients are not aware of symptoms until the disease is advanced. *A diagnosis of TB should be considered for any client with a persistent cough or other symptoms compatible with TB, such as weight loss, anorexia, night sweats, hemoptysis, shortness of breath, fever, or chills.*

HISTORY

Assess the client's past exposure to TB. Ask about the client's country of origin and travel to foreign countries where there is a high incidence of TB. It is important to ask about the results of any previous tests for TB. Also ask whether the client has had bacillus Calmette-Guérin (BCG) vaccine. The BCG vaccine contains attenuated tubercle bacilli and is used in many countries to produce increased resistance to TB. *Anyone who has received BCG vaccine within the previous 10 years will have a positive skin test that can complicate interpretation.* Usually the size of the skin response decreases each year after BCG vaccination. These clients should be evaluated for TB with a chest x-ray. The effectiveness of BCG vaccine in preventing TB is controversial, and it is not used for this purpose in the United States.

PHYSICAL ASSESSMENT/CLINICAL MANIFESTATIONS

The client with TB has progressive fatigue, lethargy, nausea, anorexia, weight loss, irregular menses, and a low-grade fever. Manifestations may have been present for weeks or months. Night sweats may occur with the fever. The client has a cough and mucopurulent sputum, which may be streaked with blood. Chest tightness and a dull, aching chest pain occur with the cough.

Physical examination of the chest does not provide conclusive evidence of TB. You may hear dullness with percussion over involved the lung fields, bronchial breath sounds, crackles, and increased transmission of spoken or whispered sounds. Partial obstruction of a bronchus from endobronchial disease or compression by lymph nodes may produce localized wheezing.

DIAGNOSTIC ASSESSMENT

A diagnosis of TB is suggested by the manifestations and a positive smear for acid-fast bacillus. Sputum is obtained, smeared on a slide, and stained with a red dye. After the slide has dried, it is treated with an acid alcohol to remove the stain. TB does not destain with this procedure and remains red. The acid-fast bacillus test is not specific for TB (other organisms are also acid-fast), but it is used as a quick method to determine whether TB treatment and precautions should be started until more definitive testing can be completed.

Sputum culture of *M. tuberculosis* confirms the diagnosis. Traditional cultures are slow growing, requiring weeks to determine a positive or negative result. Newer techniques (BACTEC) enhance culture growth and allow identification 1 to 3 weeks instead of 4 to 6 weeks. After drugs are started, sputum samples are obtained again to determine therapy effectiveness. Cultures are usually negative after 3 months of treatment.

The polymerase chain reaction (PCR) assay is used for rapid identification of mycobacteria in selected situations. This test amplifies the organism's genetic material (DNA) and identifies the organism within hours instead of weeks. Although highly accurate, its high cost and limited availability limit the widespread use of this test as a TB screening or diagnostic tool.

The tuberculin test (Mantoux test) result is the most commonly used reliable test of TB infection. A small amount (0.1 mL) of purified protein derivative (PPD) is given intradermally in the forearm. An area of induration (not just redness) measuring 10 mm or greater in diameter 48 to 72 hours after injection indicates exposure to and infection with TB. Recent studies indicate that a reading after 72 hours rather than after just 48 hours is more accurate. The incidence of false-negative readings is greater at 48 hours. (See the Evidence-Based Practice for Nursing box at right). *A positive reaction does not mean that active disease is present but indicates exposure to TB or the presence of inactive (dormant) disease.* A reaction of 5 mm or greater is considered positive in people with HIV infection. A reduced skin reaction or a negative skin test does not rule out TB disease or infection of the very old or anyone who is severely immunocompromised. This condition is called **anergy.**

Screening is performed yearly for anyone at high risk for coming into contact with people infected with TB. Screening is particularly important for foreign-born people and migrant workers. Participation in screening programs is enhanced when programs are delivered in a culturally sensitive and nonthreatening manner.

Once a person's skin test is positive for TB, a chest x-ray is needed to detect clinically active TB or old, healed lesions. Caseation and inflammation may be seen on the x-ray if the disease is active. Clients are instructed to seek medical attention if they have manifestations of TB.

The chest x-rays of HIV-infected clients may be normal or may show infiltrates in any lung zone along with hilar lymph node enlargement.

Common Nursing Diagnoses and Collaborative Problems

Nursing diagnoses and collaborative problems that may apply to clients with TB include the following:

- Impaired Gas Exchange related to disease progression
- Ineffective Airway Clearance related to increased secretions or fatigue
- Deficient Knowledge (Infection Control, Therapeutic Regimen, Nutrition) related to lack of exposure or information misinterpretation
- Fatigue related to poor tissue oxygenation and increased metabolism
- Imbalanced Nutrition: Less Than Body Requirements related to increased metabolism, poor appetite, drug regimen, or fatigue
- Social Isolation related to altered state of wellness or changed appearance

EVIDENCE-BASED PRACTICE for Nursing

Time makes a difference

Singh, D., Sutton, C., & Woodcock, A. (2002). Tuberculin test measurement: Variability due to the time of reading. *Chest, 122*(4), 1299-1301.

This study sought to compare the 48-hour results of the Mantoux purified protein derivative (PPD) testing for tuberculosis (TB) with those obtained at 72 hours after intradermal injection. The Mantoux test is the most frequently used method to identify latent TB infection worldwide. Historically, test results are recommended to be read at either 48 hours or 72 hours after the initial intradermal injection; however, it is not known whether the timing of these two readings are truly comparable.

A total of 116 healthy adult volunteers were injected with 10 units of the PPD, and the skin test results were read at both 48 hours and 72 hours for all subjects. None of the subjects had a history of tuberculosis, HIV disease, IV drug use, or recent exposure to tuberculosis. Among the 116 subjects, 106 had a history of vaccination with bacillus Calmette-Guérin (BCG) and would be expected to have a positive PPD test result, defined as an area of induration greater than 15 mm. Areas of induration were significantly greater at the 72-hour reading than at the 48-hour reading. The number of subjects considered to have a positive PPD test at 48 hours was 28 and the number of subjects considered to have a positive PPD test at 72 hours was 36. Thus, the 48 hour reading yielded a false negative result in 8 subjects (22%).

Level of Evidence: 3—Well-designed trial without randomization; time series.

Critique. The major problem with this study was a failure to control inter-rater reliability among the observers/readers of the PPD test.

Implications for Nursing. Nurses are often responsible for conducting mass TB screening programs in schools, student health services, inpatient and outpatient settings, health fairs, and places of employment. With an option of evaluating the test at either 48 or 72 hours, the scheduling of tested persons to return for evaluation in 48 hours may result in a significant number of false-negative results. Such people would not be further evaluated and would pose a public health risk. Thus, when planning TB screenings, nurses should either schedule test readings at 72 hours or, if readings show any induration at 48 hours, the person should return for a second evaluation at 72 hours.

Critical Thinking Challenge

You are the outpatient nurse in the infectious disease clinic. The client is a 62-year-old registered nurse who works at a prison clinic/hospital. She has type 2 diabetes, hypertension, and gastroesophageal reflux disease (GERD), and she had a mastectomy 7 years ago for breast cancer. She has smoked since she was 17 years of age (two packs per day). Her prescribed drugs include lisinopril (Zestril), tamoxifen (Nolvadex, Tamofen✱), omeprazole (Prilosec, Losec✱), and metformin (Glucophage). On screening last week, her PPD had an indurated area of 5 mm 48 hours after the injection and 20 mm 72 hours after the injection.

1. Does this woman have active TB?
2. What are her risk factors for TB?
3. Calculate her smoking history in pack years.
4. What assessment data should you obtain?

evolve For suggested answer guidelines, go to http://evolve.elsevier.com/Iggy/.

Interventions

Combination drug therapy is the most effective method of treating TB and preventing transmission. Increasing the

CHART 34-7

DRUG THERAPY for Tuberculosis*

Drug	Usual Dosage	Nursing Interventions	Drug Action/Rationale for Use
Isoniazid (INH)	5 mg/kg PO, IM (maximum 300 mg) daily; 15 mg/kg (maximum 900 mg) biweekly	Observe for drug interactions, which may inhibit drug metabolism of phenytoin, carbamazepine, primidone, and warfarin. Instruct the client to take on empty stomach and avoid antacids. Monitor for signs of hepatitis and neurotoxicity effects.	Isoniazid inhibits the synthesis of mycolic acids and acts to kill actively growing organisms in the extracellular environment and inhibits the growth of dormant organisms in the macrophages and caseating granulomas.
Rifampin (RIF)	10 mg/kg PO (maximum 600 mg) daily or biweekly	Instruct the client that secretions, including urine, will be orange colored and that the drug will permanently discolor soft contact lenses. Observe for drug interactions, which may enhance elimination of theophylline, steroids, opioids, oral hypoglycemics, warfarin, and occasionally vitamin D. Observe for hepatotoxic effects. RIF decreases effectiveness of oral contraceptives.	RIF has the unique ability to kill slower growing organisms that reside in the caseating granuloma and macrophage.
Pyrazinamide (PZA)	15-30 mg/kg PO (maximum 2000 mg) daily; 50 mg/kg biweekly	Observe for hepatotoxic effects.	Pyrazinamide is the most active drug at killing mycobacteria present in macrophages. The acidic environment in the macrophage inhibits most agents.
Ethambutol (EMB)	15 mg/kg daily PO; 50 mg/kg biweekly	Obtain baseline visual acuity and color discrimination, especially to the color green. Repeat testing every 1-2 mo.	Ethambutol inhibits bacterial ribonucleic acid (RNA) synthesis. It is slow acting and must be used in combination with other bactericidal agents.
Streptomycin (SM)	1000 mg IM, IV over 1 hr, daily for 2 mo followed by biweekly injections until treatment is completed	Obtain baseline audiometric test every 1-2 mo. It can impair the eighth cranial nerve. Older clients are especially susceptible.	Streptomycin is an aminoglycoside antibiotic that is active against extracellular organisms only.
Amikacin	15 mg/kg daily IM, IV (usual dose 1 g)	Ensure adequate hydration, monitor renal function and hearing. Amikacin can lead to renal toxicity and ototoxicity.	Amikacin is an aminoglycoside antibiotic that can be used if streptomycin is not available.
Rifapentine (Priftin)	600 mg twice weekly	Doses must be separated by at least 72 hr. Instruct the client that metabolism of other drugs may be faster, causing lower blood concentrations and a need for higher doses (especially for antidiabetic drugs, barbiturates, and antibiotics). Instruct female clients to use additional forms of birth control, because this drug decreases the effectiveness of oral contraceptives. Observe for hepatotoxic effects.	Rifapentine has high bacteriostatic and bactericidal action against slow-growing intracellular bacteria.

*Newer drugs contain combinations of rifampin and isoniazid (Rifamate) or of rifampin, isoniazid, and pyrazinamide (Rifater).

number of clients with TB who complete curative therapy is a major focus for Healthy People 2010 (see the Meeting Healthy People 2010 Objectives box on p. 644). Active TB is treated with a combination of drugs to which the organism is sensitive. Therapy continues until the disease is under control. The use of multiple-drug regimens destroys organisms as quickly as possible and reduces the emergence of drug-resistant organisms. Current therapy uses isoniazid (INH) and rifampin throughout the therapy; pyrazinamide is added for the first 2 months (Chart 34-7). This protocol shortens the therapy from 6 to 12 months to 6 months. Ethambutol or streptomycin may be added to the regimen as the fourth drug.

Strict adherence to the prescribed drug regimen is crucial for suppressing the disease. Thus your major role is teaching the client about drug therapy. Accurate information provided

Meeting HEALTHY PEOPLE 2010 Objectives

TUBERCULOSIS

Objective 22.25: Increase to at least 90% the proportion of all tuberculosis patients who complete curative therapy within 12 months.

- Teach all clients to have yearly TB skin tests.
- Assist clients who have a positive TB skin test to have follow-up screening for a definitive diagnosis.
- Develop culturally appropriate education materials.
- Ensure that education materials are written or presented at no greater than a fourth-grade literacy level.
- Educate those clients who are diagnosed with TB to:
  - Take all medication as prescribed
  - Keep all follow-up appointments
  - Identify contacts
- Implement a direction observation therapy (DOT) program for those clients who have not consistently taken medication as prescribed.
- Refer clients who do not have money for medications to the appropriate resource for obtaining low-cost or no-cost TB drugs.

in multiple formats (e.g., pamphlets, videos, drug-schedule worksheets) can be of value in client education. An anxious client may not absorb information well. You may need to repeat the information and obtain the help of family members. To determine whether the client understands how to take the drugs, ask him or her to describe the treatment regimen, major side effects, and when to call the health care agency and physician.

TB is often treated outside the acute care setting, with the client convalescing in the home setting. Airborne precautions are not necessary in this setting because family members have already been exposed; however, all members of the household need to undergo TB testing. Instruct the client to cover the mouth and nose when coughing or sneezing, to place used tissues in plastic bags, and to wear a mask when in contact with crowds until the drugs suppress infection.

Tell the client sputum specimens are needed every 2 to 4 weeks once drug therapy is initiated. When the results of three sputum cultures are negative, the client is no longer infectious and may return to former employment. Remind him or her to avoid exposure to any inhalation irritants because they can cause further lung damage.

The hospitalized client with active TB is placed under Airborne Precautions (see Chapter 29) in a well-ventilated room. The room should have at least six exchanges of fresh air per minute and should be ventilated to the outside if possible. All health care workers must wear a N95 or high-efficiency particulate air (HEPA) respirator when caring for the client (Figure 34-2). When there is risk of hand and clothing contamination, implement standard precautions by using appropriate barrier protection (i.e., gowns and gloves). Perform thorough handwashing before and after client care. Precautions are discontinued when the client is no longer considered infectious.

The TB drugs may cause the client to have nausea. Teach him or her to prevent nausea by taking the daily dose at bedtime. Antiemetics may also prevent this problem. Instruct the client about the need for a well-balanced diet to promote healing. An increased intake of foods that are rich in iron, protein, and vitamin C is recommended for the client with TB. Consult with the nutritionist for specialized needs.

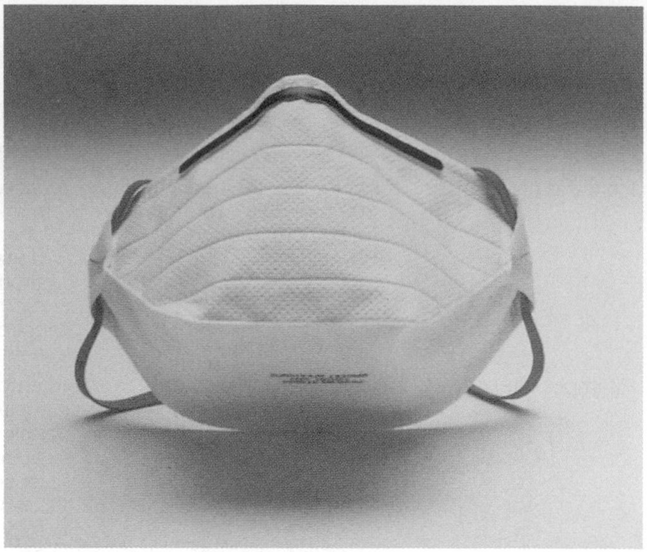

Figure 34-2 ■ A high-efficiency particulate air (HEPA) respirator used in the care of clients with active or "rule-out" tuberculosis. (Courtesy of Uvex Safety, Smithfield, RI.)

The client with TB may have changes in physical stamina and also faces concerns about the prognosis of the disease. Be realistic in offering a positive outlook for the client who adheres to the drug regimen. Tell him or her that fatigue will diminish as the treatment progresses. With current resistant strains of TB, however, you must emphasize that not taking the drugs as prescribed could lead to an infection that is difficult to treat or has total drug resistance.

Community-Based Care

HOME CARE MANAGEMENT

Most clients with TB are managed outside the hospital; however, clients may be diagnosed with TB while in the hospital if pneumonia is suspected or other complications exist. Discharge may be delayed if the living situation is high risk or if nonadherence is likely. Consult with the social service worker in the hospital or the community health nursing agency to ensure that the client is discharged to the appropriate environment with continued supervision.

HEALTH TEACHING

Instruct the client to follow the drug regimen exactly as prescribed and always to have a supply on hand. Teach about side effects and ways of reducing them to ensure adherence. Remind the client that the disease is usually no longer contagious after drugs have been taken for 2 to 3 consecutive weeks and clinical improvement is seen; however, he or she must continue with the prescribed drugs for 6 months or longer as prescribed. Directly observed therapy (DOT), in which the nurse or other health care provider watches the client swallow the drugs, may be indicated in some situations. This practice contributes to more treatment successes, fewer relapses, and less drug resistance.

The client who has weight loss and severe lethargy should gradually resume his or her usual activities. Proper nutrition must be maintained to prevent recurrence of infection.

To help with concerns about the contagious aspect of the infection, provide the client with information about TB. A key to preventing transmission is identifying those in close contact with the infected person so that they can be tested and treated if needed. Health care professionals have an important role in this aspect of care. Identified contacts are assessed with a TB test and possibly a chest x-ray to determine TB infection status. Multidrug therapy may be indicated. In addition, certain high-risk contacts receive prophylactic therapy, usually with INH.

HEALTH CARE RESOURCES

Instruct the client to receive follow-up care by a health care provider for at least 1 year during active treatment. The American Lung Association (ALA) can provide free information to the client about the disease and its treatment. In addition, Alcoholics Anonymous and other health care resources for clients with alcoholism are available if needed. Assist the client who uses illicit drugs to locate a drug treatment program. Urge smokers to quit, and assist them in finding an appropriate smoking-cessation program.

Critical Thinking Challenge

The client (a 62-year-old registered nurse) is confirmed to have active TB. She lives at home with her husband, who is 70 years old and has moderate heart failure. She is the sole support of the family and is concerned about when she can go back to work. Her prescribed drug regimen for the first 2 months includes the following:

- Isoniazid (INH) 250 mg taken orally (PO) daily
- Rifampin (RIF) 500 mg PO daily
- Pyrazinamide (PZA) 750 mg PO daily
- Ethambutol (EMB) 750 mg PO daily

If her cultures indicate that the organism causing her infection is not drug resistant and if the sputum culture at 2 months is negative, the PZA and EMB will be discontinued and she will continue to take the INH and RIF daily for an additional 4 months.

1. When can this client go back to work?
2. Should this client's husband be tested? Why or why not?
3. Are there any issues or special considerations for the prescribed TB drug therapy and the client's other drug regimen?
4. Is this client a candidate for DOT? Why or why not?
5. What specific precautions or actions will you recommend that this client make in her home care?

evolve For suggested answer guidelines, go to http://evolve.elsevier.com/Iggy/.

Lung Abscess

PATHOPHYSIOLOGY

A lung abscess is a localized area of lung destruction caused by liquefaction necrosis, which is usually related to pyogenic bacteria. Clients with this problem often have a history of pneumonia, aspiration of oropharyngeal contents, or obstruction as a result of a tumor or foreign body. Other causes of aspiration leading to lung abscess formation include any condition that alters the ability to swallow, such as alcoholic blackouts, seizure disorders, other neurologic deficits, and swallowing disorders. Bronchial obstruction may cause a necrotizing process in the lung that eventually becomes an abscess.

Multiple abscesses and cavities form in clients with tuberculosis (TB) or fungal infections of the lung. Immunosuppressed clients, such as those receiving chemotherapy or those with a disease such as leukemia or AIDS, are at high risk for fungal infections. Most common organisms are anaerobic bacteria, *Staphylococcus* or other gram-positive organisms, or gram-negative or opportunistic infections such as fungi.

COLLABORATIVE MANAGEMENT

Assessment

Ask the client about any recent history of influenza, pneumonia, febrile illness, cough, and foul-smelling sputum production. Ask about the sputum color and odor and about any **pleuritic chest pain** (a stabbing pain on taking a deep breath). Often the client is febrile, pale, fatigued, and cachectic. Auscultation may reveal decreased breath sounds, and there is dullness on percussion in the involved area. Bronchial breath sounds and crackles are often heard over the site of the lesion. A chest x-ray and sputum samples are needed for the diagnosis.

Interventions

Nursing diagnoses and interventions for the client with pneumonia also apply to the client with a lung abscess. Treatment involves antibiotics and drainage of the abscess. More than one antibiotic may be prescribed. Provide frequent mouth care and observe for oral overgrowth of *Candida albicans.*

Inhalation Anthrax

PATHOPHYSIOLOGY

Inhalation anthrax (also known as respiratory anthrax) is a bacterial infection caused by the gram-positive, rod-shaped organism *Bacillus anthracis,* which lives as a spore in contaminated soil. Infection with this organism can occur through the skin, the intestinal tract, or the lungs. Inhalation anthrax is a rare natural occurrence in the United States, but it has a fatality rate of nearly 100% without treatment. It is not spread by person-to-person contact. Because the inhalation form of the disease is so rare, any occurrence is considered unnatural or an intentional act of bioterrorism.

This organism first forms a **spore,** an encapsulated organism that is inactive. When many spores are inhaled into the deep parts of the lungs, macrophages engulf them. Once inside the macrophage, the organism leaves its capsule and replicates. The active bacteria produce several toxins that they release into the infected tissues and the blood. These toxins increase the virulence of the organism by creating massive edema in infected tissues, suppressing neutrophil action, causing hemorrhage, and destroying both lung cells and white blood cells. The infected macrophages carry the organisms to the hilar and mediastinal lymph nodes. From these nodes, the organisms can enter the blood and spread rapidly, causing sepsis and meningitis.

COLLABORATIVE MANAGEMENT

Assessment

Inhalation anthrax is a two-stage illness, and manifestations may not begin until as long as 8 weeks after exposure to the organism. Manifestations are listed in Chart 34-8.

CHART 34-8

KEY FEATURES of
Inhalation Anthrax

Prodromal Stage (Early)	Fulminant Stage (Late)
Fever Fatigue Mild chest pain Dry cough No manifestations of upper respiratory infection Mediastinal "widening" on chest x-ray	Sudden onset of breathlessness Dyspnea Diaphoresis Stridor on inhalation and exhalation Hypoxia High fever Mediastinitis Pleural effusion Hypotension Septic shock

PRODROMAL STAGE

The first stage, the "prodromal" stage, is difficult to differentiate from influenza or pneumonia. Manifestations are nonspecific. In this stage, clients have a fever, some fatigue, mild chest pain, and a dry, harsh cough. *A special feature of inhalation anthrax is that it is* ***not*** *accompanied by upper respiratory manifestations of rhinitis, headache, watery eyes, or sore throat.* Usually, the client starts to feel better, and symptoms improve in 2 to 4 days.

Although diagnosis is difficult at this stage, if the client begins appropriate antibiotic therapy, the likelihood of survival is high. Diagnostic tests may show a slightly elevated white blood cell count with increasing numbers of band neutrophils. Other indicators of inhalation anthrax that may be detectable at this time are positive Gram stain of the serum and a mediastinal "widening" on chest x-ray as the lymph nodes in the area greatly enlarge. After several days, blood cultures may be positive for the organism and the genetic material of the bacteria may be detected through the amplification process of the polymerase chain reaction (PCR). These more definitive diagnostic tests may not be evident, however, until the disease has progressed to the fulminant stage.

FULMINANT STAGE

The second or "fulminant" stage begins after the client feels a little better. Usually there is a sudden onset of a feeling of breathlessness. This sensation rapidly progresses to severe respiratory distress, dyspnea, diaphoresis, stridor on inhalation and exhalation, and cyanosis. The client has a high fever. Mediastinitis and pleural effusions develop. As the disease spreads through the blood, causing septic shock and meningitis, death often occurs within 24 to 36 hours after the onset of breathlessness even if antibiotics are started in this stage.

Interventions

The naturally occurring organism has a cell wall and is sensitive to many antibiotics, including the penicillins and the cephalosporins; however, it is thought that organisms grown for bioterrorism may have been altered to be resistant to these antibiotics. Therefore the antibiotics used for suspected or diagnosed inhalation anthrax include combination therapy with ciprofloxacin, doxycycline, and amoxicillin (Chart 34-9). The same drugs are used individually in oral form for prophylaxis when people have been exposed to inhalation anthrax.

CHART 34-9

DRUG THERAPY for
Prophylaxis and Treatment of Inhalation Anthrax

Prophylaxis	Treatment
Ciprofloxacin (Cipro) 500 mg PO twice daily *Or* Doxycycline (Vibramycin) 100 mg PO twice daily *Or* *(if organism is proven susceptible to penicillin)*	Ciprofloxacin (Cipro I.V.) 400 mg IV q12h *Or* Doxycycline (Doxy 100) 100 mg IV q12h *Plus one or two of the following secondary agents (parenteral form; dosage based on client's weight and age)*
Amoxicillin (Amoxil, Trimox) 500 mg q8h	Rifampin (RIF) Clindamycin (Cleocin) Vancomycin (Vancocin, Vancoled)
Prophylaxis must continue for 60 days (or longer if exposure was heavy)	**Treatment with intravenous drugs continues for at least 7 days. When the response is good and the client improves, IV drugs are changed to oral agents and are continued for at least 60 days.**

Teach clients with any type of lower respiratory infection to be especially vigilant for changes after they think they are getting well. They need to seek medical attention immediately on having a setback that starts with breathlessness.

Pulmonary Empyema

PATHOPHYSIOLOGY

Empyema is a collection of pus in the pleural space. The most common cause of empyema is pulmonary infection, lung abscess, or infected pleural effusion. Pneumonia or lung abscess can spread across the pleura. Lymph node obstruction can cause a **retrograde** (backward) flood of infected lymph into the pleural space. In addition, a liver abscess or abdominal abscess can spread through the lymphatic system into the lung area. Thoracic surgery and chest trauma can introduce bacteria directly into the pleural space, leading to empyema. Blood from trauma may collect in the pleural space. Poor drainage of this blood promotes infection.

COLLABORATIVE MANAGEMENT

Assessment

Important history findings include recent febrile illness (including pneumonia), chest pain, dyspnea, cough, and trauma. Observe and document the character of the sputum. Chest wall motion may be reduced on physical examination. If a pleural effusion is present, fremitus may be decreased or absent on palpation, percussion may sound flat, and breath sounds are decreased on auscultation. With compression of lung tissue near the effusion, abnormal breath sounds include bronchial breath sounds, egophony, and whispered pectoriloquy (see Chapter 30).

Some clients have fever, chills, night sweats, and weight loss. If there is cardiac compromise, the client may be hypotensive because of a mediastinal deviation. The PMI (point of maximal impulse) may be displaced on cardiac palpation.

A chest x-ray is ordered, and a sample of the pleural fluid is obtained via thoracentesis for help in making the diagnosis (see Chapter 30). Empyema fluid is thick, opaque, exudative, and foul smelling. The pleural fluid is sent to the laboratory and is analyzed for color, red blood cell count, white blood cell count and differential, glucose and protein levels, lactate dehydrogenase (LDH), and pH. Gram stains, acid-fast stains, and cytology studies are also performed. A protein level higher than 3 g/100 mL indicates an exudative process.

Interventions

Therapy for empyema is focused on emptying the empyema cavity, re-expanding the lung, and controlling the infection. Antibiotics appropriate for the identified organism are prescribed. Closed-chest drainage (see Chapter 33) is used to promote lung expansion. The health care provider places one or more chest tubes in the lower parts of the empyema sac. Underwater seal drainage is used without suction initially, but suction may be added if the lung fails to expand with gravity drainage alone. The tube is removed when the lung is fully expanded and the infection is under control. Open thoracotomy and removal of a portion of the pleura may be needed for thick pus or marked pleural thickening. Nursing considerations are the same as those for clients with a pleural effusion, pneumothorax, or infection.

GET READY for the NCLEX Examination!

KEY POINTS

Safe Effective Care Environment

- Teach clients with respiratory infections to limit infection spread by washing hands after blowing the nose or using a tissue.
- Instruct clients that colds are most easily spread to others during the first 2 to 3 days after symptoms begin.
- Ask clients from other countries whether or not they have had BCG as a vaccination against TB. Clients who have had BCG usually have a large, positive reaction to a PPD skin test, making the test less reliable as an indicator of active TB disease.
- Use airborne precautions for any client who has TB or SARS manifestations until proven otherwise.
- Keep the door to the room of any client with a respiratory infection closed until the cause of the infection is identified.

Health Promotion and Maintenance

- Receive a yearly influenza vaccination because you come into contact more frequently with infected people and also because you can have a mild or subclinical case of influenza and spread it to people who are immunocompromised.
- Urge all adults over 50 years of age, anyone who has a chronic respiratory problem, and anyone who is immunocompromised to any degree to receive yearly influenza vaccinations.
- Urge all adults over 50 years of age, anyone who has a chronic respiratory problem, and anyone who is immunocompromised to any degree to receive the pneumonia vaccination.
- Stress to clients that they should complete the medication regimen for any respiratory infection for which anti-infective therapy has been prescribed.
- Urge all people to quit smoking or using tobacco in any form.
- Encourage family members of clients with TB who live at home to ensure good ventilation of the home with open windows whenever possible.

Psychosocial Integrity

- Assess any older client who has acute confusion for pneumonia (remembering that they may not have a cough or fever).
- Assure the family of an older adult client with pneumonia who is confused that the new-onset confusion is temporary.
- Reassure the client who feels depressed by the degree of fatigue felt and the activity intolerance experienced that the recovery times for influenza and pneumonia are long (weeks to months), especially for the older adult.
- Inform clients who may be afraid of contracting inhalational anthrax that this disease is not transmitted by person-to-person contact.
- Inform clients who have a positive TB test that far more people are infected with the bacillus than have active TB disease.
- Assess the likelihood of adherence to the drug regimen for clients with TB.
- Identify clients who may require a directly observed therapy (DOT) program in which they must be directly observed by a health care professional while swallowing the drug.
- Assess the degree of social interaction for clients receiving drug therapy for active TB on an outpatient basis.

Physiological Integrity

- Teach all clients with a respiratory infection of bacterial origin to complete all anti-infective therapy as prescribed.
- Urge clients to limit the use of decongestant nasal sprays to no more than 4 days.
- Teach clients with allergic rhinitis to avoid contact with the offending allergen(s).
- Caution older adults using antihistamines that these drugs may make hypertension worse.
- Treat epiglottitis in an adult as an emergency because it can lead to complete respiratory obstruction.
- Assess the client receiving rifampin or rifapentine as drug therapy for TB for any manifestation of liver impairment (dark urine, clay-colored stools, anorexia, jaundiced sclera or hard palate).
- Inform women taking rifampin or rifapentine as drug therapy for TB that these drugs reduce the effectiveness of oral contraceptives and that another form of birth control should be considered while on this therapy.

ADDITIONAL STUDY RESOURCES

Go to your Student CD-ROM for Review Questions for the NCLEX Examination.

evolve Go to http://evolve.elsevier.com/Iggy/ for Integrated Management of Care Questions for the NCLEX Examination.

SELECTED BIBLIOGRAPHY

Asterisk indicates a classic or definitive work on this subject.

Ackley, B., & Ladwig, G. (2002). *Nursing diagnosis handbook: A guide to planning care* (5th ed). St. Louis: Mosby.

Baek, C., et al. (2000). Polymerase chain reaction detection of *Mycobacterium tuberculosis* from fine-needle aspirate for the diagnosis of cervical tuberculosis lymphadenitis. *Laryngoscope, 110*(1), 30-34.

Bhattacharyya, N., Kepnes, L., & Shapiro, J. (2001). Efficacy and quality of life impact on adult tonsillectomy. *Archives of Otolaryngology & Head and Neck Surgery, 127*(11), 1347-1350.

Bridges, C., et al. (2002). Prevention and control of influenza: Recommendations of the Advisory Committee on Immunization Practices (ACIP). *Morbidity & Mortality Weekly Report, 51*(RR03), 1-31.

Brooks, J. (2001). Postoperative nosocomial pneumonia: Nurse sensitive interventions. *AACN Clinical Issues for Advanced Practice in Acute and Critical Care, 12*(2), 305-323.

*Centers for Disease Control and Prevention. (1999). Progress toward the elimination of tuberculosis–United States, 1998. *Morbidity and Mortality Weekly Report, 48*(33), 732-736.

Centers for Disease Control and Prevention. (2001). Notice to readers: Considerations for distinguishing influenza-like illness from inhalational anthrax. *Morbidity and Mortality Weekly Report, 50*(44), 984-986.

Centers for Disease Control and Prevention. (2003a). *Guidelines and recommendations: Interim domestic infection control precautions for aerosol-generating procedures on patients with severe acute respiratory syndrome (SARS).* Department of Health and Human Services, May 20, 2003.

Centers for Disease Control and Prevention. (2003b). *Health, United States, 2003.* Department of Health and Human Services, March 11, 2004.

Centers for Disease Control and Prevention. (2003c). Update: Influenza activity–United States, 2002-03 season. *Morbidity and Mortality Weekly Report, 52*(02),26-28.

Centers for Disease Control and Prevention. (2003d) *Updated interim U.S. case definition for severe acute respiratory syndrome (SARS).* Department of Health and Human Services, July 11, 2003.

Connally, M. (2001). Black, white, and shades of gray: Common abnormalities in chest radiographs. *AACN Clinical Issues for Advanced Practice in Acute and Critical Care, 12*(2), 259-269.

Dochterman, J., & Bulechek, G. (Eds). (2004). *Nursing interventions classification (NIC)* (4th ed). St. Louis: Mosby.

Dreher, M., et al. (2004). What you need to know about SARS now! *Nursing 2004, 34*(1), 58-63.

Ebersole, P., Hess, P., & Luggen, A. (2004). *Toward healthy aging: Human needs and nursing response* (6th ed). St. Louis: Mosby.

Eckler, J. (2002). Keeping pulmonary tuberculosis at bay. *Nursing 2002, 32*(12), 70.

Facts and Comparisons. (2004). *Drug facts and comparisons* (58th ed). St. Louis: Author.

Frakes, M. & Evans, T. (2004). TB: Your vigilance is vital. *RN, 67* (11), 30-35.

Goldrick, B. (2003). Adult respiratory infections. *American Journal of Nursing, 103*(10), 65.

Goldrick, B. (2004a). Is SARS reemerging? *American Journal of Nursing, 104*(7), 28-29.

Goldrick, B. (2004b). 21st-century emerging and reemerging infections: Where do we go from here? *American Journal of Nursing, 104*(1), 67-70.

Goolsby, M. (2001). Viral upper respiratory infections. *Journal of the American Academy of Nurse Practitioners, 13*(2), 50-54.

Harris, J., & Miller, T. (2000). Preventing nosocomial pneumonia: Evidenced-based practice. *Critical Care Nurse, 20*(1), 51-67.

Harris, J., et al. (2000). Risk factors for nosocomial pneumonia in critically ill trauma patients. *AACN Clinical Issues, 11*(2), 198-231.

Havas, T. (2002). Obstructive adenoid tissue: An indication for power-shaver adenoidectomy. *Archives of Otolaryngology & Head and Neck Surgery, 128*(7), 789-791.

Hodnicki, D. (2001). Anthrax. *The American Journal for Nurse Practitioners, 5*(10), 21-24.

Johnson, J., & Force, R. (2000). Oseltamivir for flu prevention. *Journal of Family Practice, 49*(2), 183-184.

Kearney, K. (2001). Epiglottitis. *American Journal of Nursing, 101*(8), 37-38.

*Krouse, J. (1999). Introduction to sinus disease: I, Anatomy and physiology. *ORL–Head and Neck Nursing, 17*(2), 7-12.

*Krouse, J., & Krouse, H. (1999). Introduction to sinus disease: II, diagnosis and treatment. *ORL–Head and Neck Nursing, 17*(3), 6-17.

Leiner, S. (2000). Acute pharyngitis with lifelong implications. *The Nurse Practitioner, 25*(4), 119-122.

McCance, K., & Huether, S. (2002). Pathophysiology: *The biologic basis for disease in adults and children* (4th ed), St. Louis: Mosby.

Meredith, P. (2001). Community acquired pneumonia. *The American Journal for Nurse Practitioners, 5*(6), 9-17.

Moorhead, S., Johnson, M., & Maas, M. (Eds.). (2004). *Nursing outcomes classification (NOC)* (3rd ed). St. Louis: Mosby.

Orgill. R., Krempl, G., & Medina, J. (2002). Acute pain management following laryngectomy. *Archives of Otolaryngology & Head and Neck Surgery, 128*(7), 829-832.

Patel, N., & Criner, G. (2003). Community-acquired pneumonia in the elderly: Update on treatment strategies. *Consultant, 43*(6), 689-701.

Schultz, R. (2002). Straight talk about community-acquired pneumonia. *Nursing 2002, 32*(1), 46-49.

Singh, D., Sutton, C., & Woodcock, A. (2002). Tuberculin test measurement: Variability due to the time of reading. *Chest, 122*(4), 1299-1301.

Spencer, D., Whitman, K., & Morton, P. (2001). Inhalational anthrax. *MEDSURG Nursing, 10*(6), 308-312.

Spiegel, J., et al. (2000). Acute laryngitis. *Ear, Nose, and Throat Journal, 79*(7), 488.

Tasota, F., Henker, R., & Hoffman, L. (2002). Anthrax as a biological weapon: An old disease that poses new threats. *Critical Care Nurse, 22*(5), 21-34.

Thaler, E. (2002). Postoperative care after endoscopic sinus surgery. *Archives of Otolaryngology & Head and Neck Surgery, 128*(10), 1204-1208.

U.S. Department of Health and Human Services (2001). Update: Investigation of bioterrorism-related anthrax and adverse events from antimicrobial prophylaxis. *Morbidity and Mortality Weekly Report, 50*(44), 973-976.

Vergis, E., et al. (2000). Azithromycin vs cefuroxime plus erythromycin for empirical treatment of community-acquired pneumonia in hospitalized patients. *Archives of Internal Medicine, 160*(9), 1294-1300.

Wan, G.W., Lu, S., & Tsai, Y. (2004). Polymerase chain reaction used for the detection of airborne *Mycobacterium tuberculosis* in health care settings. *American Journal of Infection Control, 32*(1), 17-22.

West, J. (2002). Acute upper airway infections. *British Medical Journal, 61*(1), 215-230.

Woods, A. (2002). Anthrax: New threat from an ancient microbe. *Nursing 2002, 32*(1), 44-45.

Workman, M.L. (2003). The cellular basis of bacterial infection. *Critical Care Clinics of North America, 15*(1), 1-11.

World Health Organization (WHO). Epidemic surveys–Severe acute respiratory syndrome (SARS). July 10, 2003.

CHAPTER 35

Interventions for Critically Ill Clients with Respiratory Problems

JOHN M. CLOCHESY

LEARNING OUTCOMES

After studying this chapter, you should be able to:

1. Identify clients at risk for development of pulmonary embolism.
2. Describe the clinical manifestations of pulmonary embolism.
3. Use laboratory data and clinical manifestations to determine the presence of acidosis.
4. Describe the precautions to use for clients receiving heparin or warfarin.
5. Develop a community-based teaching plan for the client who has had a pulmonary embolism.
6. Compare the features of respiratory failure of ventilatory origin with those of respiratory failure of oxygenation origin.
7. Use laboratory data and clinical manifestations to determine the adequacy of ventilatory interventions.
8. Describe the indications for intubation.
9. Prioritize nursing care for the conscious client being mechanically ventilated.
10. Develop interventions to communicate effectively with a client who is unable to talk as a result of intubation.
11. Identify clients at risk for development of pneumothorax.

Go to your Student CD-ROM for Review Questions for the NCLEX Examination keyed to these Learning Outcomes.

Acute or chronic respiratory problems can progress to a life-threatening emergency and death, even with prompt treatment. Anyone can have an acute injury or problem that results in severe respiratory impairment. Older adults, however, are more at risk for developing critical respiratory problems or complications. The client who is short of breath is also anxious and fearful. You must therefore be prepared to manage both the physical and emotional needs of the client during any respiratory emergency.

PULMONARY EMBOLISM

PATHOPHYSIOLOGY

A **pulmonary embolism (PE)** is a collection of particulate matter (solids, liquids, or gaseous substances) that enters venous circulation and lodges in the pulmonary vessels. Large emboli obstruct pulmonary blood flow, leading to decreased systemic oxygenation, pulmonary tissue hypoxia, and potential death. Any substance can cause an embolism, but a blood clot is the most common.

Pulmonary embolism is the most common acute pulmonary disease (90%) among hospitalized clients. In most people with PE, a blood clot from a deep vein thrombosis (DVT) breaks loose from one of the veins in the legs or the pelvis. The thrombus breaks off, travels through the vena cava and right side of the heart, and then lodges in a smaller blood vessel in the lung. Platelets collect with the embolus, triggering the release of substances that cause blood vessel constriction. Widespread pulmonary vessel constriction and pulmonary hypertension impair gas exchange. Deoxygenated blood shunts into the arterial circulation, causing hypoxemia. About 12% of clients with PE do *not* have hypoxemia.

Etiology

The following are major risk factors for DVT leading to PE:

- Prolonged immobilization
- Central venous catheters
- Surgery
- Obesity
- Advancing age
- Hypercoagulability
- History of thromboembolism
- Cancer diagnosis

In addition, smoking, pregnancy, estrogen therapy, heart failure, stroke, cancer (particularly lung or prostate), Trousseau's syndrome, and trauma increase the risk for DVT and PE.

Fat, oil, air, tumor cells, amniotic fluid, foreign objects (e.g., broken intravenous [IV] catheters), injected particles, and infected fibrin clots or pus can enter the venous system and cause PE. Fat emboli from fracture of a long bone and oil emboli from diagnostic procedures do not impede blood flow; instead, they cause blood vessel injury and acute respiratory distress syndrome (ARDS). Amniotic fluid embolus has a mortality rate of 80% to 90% and occurs as a rare complication childbirth, abortion, or amniocentesis. Septic emboli often arise from a pelvic abscess, an infected IV catheter, and nonsterile injections of illegal drugs. The problem with septic emboli lies in the toxic effects of the infection more than in the vascular occlusion.

Incidence/Prevalence

Pulmonary embolism affects at least 500,000 people a year in the United States, about 10% of whom die. Many die within 1 hour of the onset of symptoms or before the diagnosis has even been suspected.

HEALTH PROMOTION/ILLNESS PREVENTION

Although pulmonary embolism (PE) can occur in healthy people and may give no warning, it occurs more often in some situations. Thus prevention of conditions contributing to PE is a major nursing concern. Preventive actions for PE are those that also prevent venous stasis and DVT. Best practices for PE prevention are outlined in Chart 35-1.

CHART 35-1

BEST PRACTICE for
Prevention of Pulmonary Embolism

- Initiate passive and active range-of-motion exercises for the extremities of immobilized and postoperative clients.
- Ambulate postoperative clients soon after surgery.
- Use antiembolism and pneumatic compression stockings and devices postoperatively.
- Avoid the use of tight garters, girdles, and constricting clothing.
- Prevent pressure under the popliteal space (such as with a pillow).
- Perform a comprehensive appraisal of peripheral circulation.
- Elevate the affected limb 20 degrees or greater, above the level of the heart, to improve venous return, as appropriate.
- Change client position every 2 hours or ambulate as tolerated.
- Prevent injury to the vessel lumen by preventing local pressure, trauma, infection, or sepsis.
- Refrain from massaging or compressing leg muscles.
- Instruct client not to cross legs.
- Administer prophylactic low-dose anticoagulant and antiplatelet medication.
- Instruct the client to avoid activities that result in the Valsalva maneuver.
- Administer medications that will prevent episodes of the Valsalva maneuver as appropriate.
- Instruct the client and family on appropriate precautions.
- Encourage smoking cessation.

Lifestyle changes can help reduce the risk for PE. Urge clients to stop smoking cigarettes, especially women who take oral contraceptives. Reducing weight and becoming more physically active, such as walking one or more miles each day, can dramatically reduce risk for PE. Teach clients who are traveling for long periods to drink plenty of water, change positions often, avoid crossing the legs, and get up from the sitting position at least 5 minutes out of every hour. Actions to prevent DVT and PE during the perioperative period are described in Chapters 20, 21, and 22.

For clients with a known risk for PE, small doses of prophylactic subcutaneous heparin may be prescribed every 8 to 12 hours. Heparin prevents excessive coagulation in clients immobilized for a prolonged period, after trauma or surgery, or when restricted to bedrest. Occasionally, a drug to reduce platelet aggregation, such as clopidogrel (Plavix), is used in place of heparin.

COLLABORATIVE MANAGEMENT

Assessment

HISTORY

Ask any client with sudden onset of breathing difficulty about the risk factors for PE, especially a history of DVT, recent surgery, or prolonged immobilization.

PHYSICAL ASSESSMENT/CLINICAL MANIFESTATIONS

RESPIRATORY MANIFESTATIONS. Chart 35-2 outlines the key features of PE. Assess the client for dyspnea occurring with tachypnea, tachycardia, and pleuritic chest pain (sharp, stabbing-type pain on inspiration). These symptoms are found in 80% of clients who have PE. Other symptoms vary depending on the severity and the type of embolism. Breath sounds may be normal, but crackles occur in 50% of clients with PE. Often a dry cough is present. **Hemoptysis** (blood sputum) may result from pulmonary infarction.

CARDIAC MANIFESTATIONS. Assess for distended neck veins, **syncope** (fainting or loss of consciousness), cyanosis, and hypotension. Hypotension associated with massive emboli results from acute pulmonary hypertension and impeded forward blood flow. Often abnormal heart sounds, such as an S_3 or S_4 sound occur. Electrocardiogram findings are abnormal, nonspecific, and transient. T-wave changes and

CHART 35-2

KEY FEATURES of Pulmonary Embolism

Symptoms
- Dyspnea, sudden onset
- Pleuritic chest pain
- Apprehension, restlessness
- Feeling of impending doom
- Cough
- Hemoptysis

Signs
- Tachypnea
- Crackles
- Pleural friction rub
- Tachycardia
- S_3 or S_4 heart sound
- Diaphoresis
- Fever, low-grade
- Petechiae over chest and axillae
- Decreased arterial oxygen saturation (Sao_2)

ST-segment abnormalities develop in 50% of clients, but left- and right-axis deviations occur with equal frequency.

MISCELLANEOUS MANIFESTATIONS. A low-grade fever may be present. Petechiae may be present on the skin over the chest and in the axillae. Some clients have more vague symptoms resembling the flu, such as nausea, vomiting, and general malaise.

LABORATORY ASSESSMENT

The hyperventilation triggered by hypoxia and pain first leads to respiratory alkalosis, indicated by low partial pressure of arterial carbon dioxide ($Paco_2$) values on arterial blood gas (ABG) analysis. The alveolar-arterial (A-a) gradient is increased. The "friendlier" Pao_2-Fio_2 (fraction of inspired oxygen) ratio is commonly used to assess shunt because it does not require use of the complex A-a gradient formula. As blood is shunted without picking up oxygen from the lungs, the $Paco_2$ level starts to rise, indicating respiratory acidosis. Later metabolic acidosis results from accumulation of lactic acid due to tissue hypoxia.

Even if ABG studies and pulse oximetry show hypoxemia, these results alone are not sufficient for the diagnosis of PE. A client with a small embolus may not be hypoxemic, and PE is not the only cause of hypoxemia.

RADIOGRAPHIC ASSESSMENT

A chest x-ray may show evidence of a PE if it is large. Some lung infiltration may be present around the embolism site. However, the chest x-ray may not show any acute changes. Spiral computed tomography (CT) scans are often used to diagnose PE.

In a few clients the physician performs a transesophageal echocardiography (TEE) (see Chapter 36) for help in detecting PE. Doppler ultrasound studies or impedance plethysmography (IPG) may be used to document the presence of DVT and to support a diagnosis of PE.

PSYCHOSOCIAL ASSESSMENT

The onset of symptoms is usually abrupt, making the client with PE anxious and fearful. Hypoxemia may cause the client to have a sense of impending doom and increased restlessness. The emergency nature of the disorder and admission to an intensive care unit (ICU) increase the client's anxiety and fear of death.

Critical Thinking Challenge

The client is a 36-year-old woman who had a laminectomy yesterday for a ruptured lumbar disk. She has had pain for several months and has been unable to participate in her usual exercise program. She smokes one pack of cigarettes per day and drinks about two glasses of wine per week. Her other medications include oral contraceptives, ibuprofen PRN for joint and muscle pain, and sumatriptan (Imitrex) several times a month for migraine headaches. When you go to assess her this morning, she tells you that she is nauseated and having some chest pain.

1. What risk factors does she have for a pulmonary embolism?
2. For what other clinical manifestations should you assess?
3. Is oxygen by mask appropriate for this client? Why or Why not?
4. What other actions should you initiate?

evolve For suggested answer guidelines, go to http://evolve.elsevier.com/Iggy/.

◆Analysis

COMMON NURSING DIAGNOSES AND COLLABORATIVE PROBLEMS

The primary collaborative problem for clients with PE is Hypoxemia. The following are priority nursing diagnoses for clients with PE:

1. Decreased Cardiac Output related to acute pulmonary hypertension
2. Anxiety related to hypoxemia and life-threatening illness
3. Risk for Injury (Bleeding) related to anticoagulation or fibrinolytic therapy

ADDITIONAL NURSING DIAGNOSES AND COLLABORATIVE PROBLEMS

In addition to the common nursing diagnoses and collaborative problems, clients with PE may have one or more of the following:

- Impaired Gas Exchange related to disrupted pulmonary perfusion and increased dead space
- Fatigue related to hypoxemia
- Impaired Oral Mucous Membrane related to oxygen therapy
- Acute Confusion related to hypoxemia
- Disturbed Sleep Pattern related to the ICU environment

◆Planning and Implementation

HYPOXEMIA

When a client has a sudden onset of dyspnea and pleuritic chest pain, notify the physician. Reassure the client and assist him or her to a position of comfort with the head of the bed elevated. Prepare for oxygen therapy and blood gas analysis while continuing to monitor and assess for other manifestations.

NOC **PLANNING: EXPECTED OUTCOMES.** The client with PE is expected to have adequate tissue perfusion in all major organs. The following are indicators of adequate perfusion:

- ABGs within normal limits
- Pulse oximetry above 95%
- Cognitive status not compromised
- Absence of pallor or cyanosis

INTERVENTIONS. Nonsurgical management of PE is most common. In some cases, surgery may be needed in addition to drug therapy. NIC intervention activities for the client with PE are listed in Chart 35-3.

NONSURGICAL MANAGEMENT. Goals of management for PE are to increase alveolar gas exchange, improve pulmonary perfusion, minimize risk for further thromboembolism, and prevent complications. Interventions include oxygen therapy, monitoring, and anticoagulation or fibrinolytic therapy.

Oxygen Therapy. Oxygen therapy is important for the client with PE (see Chapter 31). The severely hypoxemic client may need mechanical ventilation and close monitoring with arterial blood gas (ABG) studies. In less severe cases, oxygen may be applied by nasal cannula or mask. Use pulse oximetry to monitor oxygen saturation and determine the degree of hypoxemia.

Monitoring. Assess the client continually for any changes in status. Check vital signs, lung sounds, and cardiac and respiratory status at least every 1 to 2 hours. Document increasing dyspnea, dysrhythmias, distended neck veins, and pedal or sacral edema. Assess for crackles and other abnormal sounds on auscultation of the lungs along with cyanosis of the lips, conjunctiva, oral mucosa, and nail beds.

Anticoagulation/Fibrinolytic Therapy. The health care provider may prescribe anticoagulation to keep the embolus from enlarging and to prevent the formation of new clots. Active bleeding, stroke, and recent trauma are relative contraindications for this therapy. Before proceeding, each client is evaluated to determine the risk versus the benefit of therapy.

Heparin is usually used unless the PE is massive or is accompanied by hemodynamic instability. A fibrinolytic drug may then be used to break up the existing clot. Review the client's partial thromboplastin time (PTT)–also called activated partial thromboplastin time (aPTT)–before therapy is started, every 4 hours when therapy begins, and daily thereafter. Therapeutic PTT values usually range between 1.5 and 2.5 times the control value.

Some fibrinolytic drugs, such as alteplase (Activase, tPA) and urokinase (Abbokinase), are approved for use in treatment of PE. Specific criteria for use of these drugs are massive PE (those that obstruct blood flow to a lobe or multiple segments) and emboli that induce hemodynamic instability that includes failure to maintain blood pressure without supportive measures. *In addition to greatly increased risk for bleeding with the use of fibrinolytic drugs, urokinase use can induce allergic responses and anaphylaxis. Such reactions usually occur within the first hour of starting the urokinase infusion. If a reaction occurs, stop the infusion and prepare to give IV antihistamine, corticosteroids, or adrenergic agonists.*

Heparin therapy usually continues for 5 to 10 days. Most clients are started on a regimen of oral anticoagulants, such as warfarin (Coumadin, Warfilone✱), on the third day of heparin use. Therapy with both heparin and warfarin continues until the client has an International Normalized Ratio (INR) of 2.0 to 3.0. To facilitate early discharge, a low-molecular-weight heparin (e.g., dalteparin or enoxaparin) is often used along with the warfarin. Monitor the INR daily. Warfarin use continues for 3 to 6 weeks, but some clients at high risk may take warfarin indefinitely. Charts 35-4 and 35-5 list drugs used and laboratory tests monitored. Anticoagulants and associated nursing care are also discussed in Chapters 39, 41, and 42.

CHART 35-3

NIC INTERVENTION ACTIVITIES for The Client with Pulmonary Embolism

Embolus Care: Pulmonary: *Limitation of complications for a client experiencing, or at risk for, occlusion of pulmonary circulation*

- Evaluate chest pain (e.g., intensity, location, radiation, duration, and precipitating and alleviating factors).
- Auscultate lung sounds for crackles or other adventitious sounds.
- Monitor respiratory pattern for symptoms of respiratory difficulty (e.g., dyspnea, tachypnea, and shortness of breath).
- Monitor determinants of tissue oxygen delivery (e.g., Pao_2, Sao_2, and hemoglobin levels and cardiac output), if available.
- Monitor for symptoms of inadequate tissue oxygenation (e.g., pallor, cyanosis, and sluggish capillary refill).
- Monitor for symptoms of respiratory failure (e.g., low Pao_2 and elevated $Paco_2$ levels and respiratory muscle fatigue).
- Encourage good ventilation (e.g., incentive spirometry and cough and deep breathe every 2 hours).
- Monitor lab values for changes in oxygenation or acid-base balance, as appropriate.
- Instruct the client and/or family regarding diagnostic procedures (e.g., $\dot{V}/\dot{Q}$ scan), as appropriate.
- Encourage the client to relax.
- Monitor side effects of anticoagulant medications, if appropriate.

NIC intervention activities selected from Dochterman, J.M., & Bulechek, G.M. (Eds.). (2004). *Nursing interventions classification (NIC)* (4th ed.). St. Louis: Mosby. No part of this work is to be altered without prior written permission from the Publisher.

Pao_2, partial pressure of arterial oxygen; *Sao_2*, arterial oxygen saturation; *$Paco_2$*, partial pressure of arterial carbon dioxide.

SURGICAL MANAGEMENT. Two surgical procedures for the management of PE are embolectomy and inferior vena cava interruption.

Embolectomy. When fibrinolytic therapy is contraindicated in a client with massive or multiple large pulmonary emboli with shock, surgical embolectomy may be needed. **Embolectomy** is the removal of the embolus or emboli from the pulmonary blood vessels.

Inferior Vena Cava Interruption. The physician considers placing a vena cava filter as a lifesaving measure by preventing further embolus formation for some clients. Candidates for this procedure include clients with an absolute contraindication to anticoagulation, recurrent or major bleeding while receiving anticoagulants, septic PE, and those undergoing pulmonary embolectomy. Placement of a vena cava filter is detailed in Chapter 38.

DECREASED CARDIAC OUTPUT

NOC **PLANNING: EXPECTED OUTCOMES.** The client with PE is expected to have adequate circulation. The following are indicators of adequate circulation:

- Maintenance of pulse rate and blood pressure within the normal ranges
- Maintenance of a urine output of at least 30 mL/hr
- Absence of cyanosis

INTERVENTIONS. In addition to the interventions used for hypoxemia, IV fluid therapy and drug therapy are used to increase cardiac output.

Intravenous Fluid Therapy. Place and maintain IV access for fluid and drug therapy. Fluid therapy involves giving crystalloid solutions to restore plasma volume and prevent shock (see Chapter 40). Continuously monitor the electrocardiogram (ECG), pulmonary artery,

CHART 35-4

DRUG THERAPY for Pulmonary Embolism

Drug	Usual Dosage	Nursing Interventions	Rationales
Heparin sodium (Hepalean✱)	5000-10,000 units IVP initially; then dose adjustment is based on PTT, 1300 units/hr on continuous drip or, less preferably, intermittent infusion	Monitor PTT. Know expected therapeutic PTT range for each client.	Ongoing assessment helps detect side effects and prevent complications.
		Report PTT results. Monitor client for bleeding or bruising. Rebolus every time infusion is increased.	Reporting enables the physician to begin early treatment of a prolonged PTT.
		Do not use with salicylates.	An increased anticoagulation effect can occur with salicylates.
		Monitor platelets daily for thrombocytopenia.	Heparin-induced thrombocytopenia (HIT) a type of arterial thrombosis, can occur.
		Have the antidote, protamine sulfate, available.	Being prepared for an emergency helps prevent further complications.
		Avoid puncture sites and apply pressure to venipuncture and IM injection sites.	Pressure at puncture sites helps promote clotting.
		Avoid use of firm toothbrushes, straight razors, and rectal thermometers.	Safety measures help prevent bleeding.
Enoxaparin (Lovenox)	1 mg/kg SC q12h	Same as with unfractionated heparin.	Same as with unfractionated heparin.
Warfarin sodium (Coumadin, Warfilone sodium✱)	10-15 mg PO for 3 days initially; then dose adjustment is based on INR, usually 5-10 mg PO daily	Monitor INR. Know expected therapeutic INR range for each client.	Ongoing assessment helps detect side effects and prevent complications.
		Report INR results. Monitor the client for bleeding or bruising.	Reporting enables the physician to begin early treatment of a prolonged INR.
		Monitor for fever and skin rash.	Adverse drug reaction can occur.
		Consult the pharmacist about potential drug interactions.	There are many drug interactions with warfarin.
		Have the antidote, vitamin K, available.	Being prepared for an emergency helps prevent further complications.
		Apply pressure to venipuncture and IM injection sites.	Pressure at puncture sites helps promote clotting.
		Avoid use of firm toothbrushes, straight razors, and rectal thermometers.	Safety measures help prevent bleeding.
		Teach the client which foods are high in vitamin K.	Food sources of vitamin K will alter INR.
Alteplase (tissue plasminogen activator, recombinant; tPA; Activase)	100 mg IV infusion over 2 hr	Assess for internal and external bleeding.	Bleeding is the most common adverse effect.
		Reconstitute with sterile water without preservative immediately before use.	Recommended preparation ensures drug stability.
		Administer with caution to clients who have been receiving aspirin, dipyridamole, heparin, or other anticoagulants.	Other drugs with anticoagulation effects increase the risk of bleeding.

***Med Error Alert!** Enoxaparin can be given only subcutaneously, NOT intravenously or intramuscularly.*

IVP, Intravenous push, or bolus; *PTT*, partial thromboplastin time; *INR*, International Normalized Ratio; *SC*, subcutaneously.

and central venous/right atrial pressures of the client receiving IV fluids because increased fluids can worsen pulmonary hypertension and contribute to right-sided heart failure.

Drug Therapy. When IV therapy alone is not effective in improving cardiac output, drug therapy with agents that increase myocardial contractility **(positive inotropic agents)** may be prescribed. Such agents include milrinone (Primacor) and dobutamine (Dobutrex). Assess the client's cardiac status hourly during therapy with inotropic agents. Vasodilators, such as nitroprusside (Nipride, Nitropress), may be used to decrease pulmonary artery pressure if it is impeding cardiac contractility.

ANXIETY

NOC **PLANNING: EXPECTED OUTCOMES.** The client with PE is expected to have a reduction in the level of anxiety. Indicators include that the client consistently demonstrates the following behaviors:

- Verbalization of reduced anxiety

CHART 35-5

LABORATORY PROFILE

Blood Tests Used to Monitor Anticoagulation Therapy

Test	Normal Range	Significance of Abnormal Findings
Partial thromboplastin time (PTT, aPTT [APTT])	Normal values for each local laboratory may vary. When activator reagents are used by the laboratory, the normal clotting time is shortened. Common normal ranges are 20-30 sec in some laboratories and 30-40 sec in others. Therapeutic range for PE is 1.5-2.5 times the normal value (e.g., if normal is 20-30 sec, then therapeutic range is 40-75 sec).	*Subtherapeutic times* may signify that the client is not receiving enough heparin to prevent extension of the blood clot. An increase in the dosage or rate of infusion is usually indicated. *Therapeutic times* mean that the clotting time is increased from normal, but this increase is indicated in the case of PE. *Prolonged times* in clients with PE (i.e., >75 sec) indicate that the client is at risk of serious spontaneous bleeding. Heparin is usually held or decreased unit the PTT drops back into the therapeutic range.
Prothrombin time (protime, PT)	11-12.5 sec Therapeutic range for anticoagulant therapy in PE is 1.5-2 times the normal or control value in seconds. Control values can vary day to day because reagents used may vary. If INR values are reported with the PT, therapeutic range for PE is 2.5-3.0, or, 3.0-4.5 for recurrent PE.	*Subtherapeutic values* may signify that the client is not receiving enough warfarin. An increase in the dosage is usually indicated. *Therapeutic values* mean that the protime is increased from normal, but this increase is indicated in the case of PE. *Prolonged values* in the treatment of PE indicate that the client is at risk for bleeding. The warfarin dose is usually decreased or held, the client is instructed to eat foods high in vitamin K, or an injection of vitamin K may be given.

PE, Pulmonary embolism; *INR*, International Normalized Ratio; *aPTT* or *APTT*, activated partial thromboplastin time.

- Absence of distress, irritability, and facial tension
- Effective use of coping strategies

INTERVENTIONS. The client with PE is anxious and fearful for many reasons. Interventions for reducing anxiety in clients with PE include oxygen therapy (see the interventions for hypoxemia, p. 652), communication, and drug therapy.

Communication. Acknowledge the anxiety and the client's perception of a life-threatening situation. Speaking calmly and clearly, assure him or her that appropriate measures are being taken. When giving drugs, changing position, taking vital signs, or assessing the client, explain the rationale and share information.

Drug Therapy. If the client's anxiety increases or prevents adequate rest, an antianxiety drug may be prescribed. Unless the client is intubated and mechanically ventilated, agents that have a sedating effect are avoided.

RISK FOR INJURY (BLEEDING)

NOC **PLANNING: EXPECTED OUTCOMES.** The client with PE is expected to remain free from bleeding. Indicators are the following:

- Absence of bruising or petechiae
- Maintenance of hematocrit and hemoglobin within the normal range

INTERVENTIONS. As a result of anticoagulation or fibrinolytic therapy, the client's ability to start and continue the blood-clotting cascade when injured is seriously impaired, and the risk for bleeding is high. Your major objectives are to protect the client from situations that could lead to bleeding and to monitor closely the amount of bleeding that is occurring.

Assess often for evidence of bleeding in the form of oozing, confluent ecchymoses, petechiae, or purpura. Examine all stools, urine, nasogastric drainage, and vomitus visually for the appearance of blood, and test for occult blood. Measure any blood loss as accurately as possible. Measure the client's abdominal girth every 8 hours. Increases in abdominal girth can indicate internal hemorrhage. Best practices to prevent bleeding are outlined in Chart 35-6.

Monitor laboratory values daily. Review the complete blood count (CBC) results to determine the client's risk for bleeding and whether actual blood loss has occurred. If the client has severe blood loss, packed red blood cells may be prescribed (see the discussion of transfusion therapy in Chapter 43). Monitor the platelet count. A decreasing count may indicate ongoing clotting or development of heparin-induced thrombocytopenia (HIT) caused by the formation of anti-heparin antibodies.

Community-Based Care

The client with PE is discharged after the hemodynamic consequences of embolism have been resolved. Anticoagulation therapy usually continues after discharge.

HOME CARE MANAGEMENT

Some clients are discharged to home with minimal risk for recurrence and no permanent physiologic changes. Others may have extensive lung damage and need home and lifestyle modifications.

Clients with extensive lung damage may have activity intolerance and become fatigued easily. The living arrangements may need to be modified so that clients can spend all or most of the time on one floor and avoid stair climbing. Depending on the degree of impairment, clients may require some or much assistance with activities of daily living.

HEALTH TEACHING

The client with PE may continue anticoagulation therapy for weeks, months, or years after discharge, depending on

CHART 35-6

BEST PRACTICE for
Bleeding Precautions

- Handle the client gently.
- Use a lift sheet when moving or positioning the client in bed.
- Avoid IM injections and venipunctures.
- When injections are necessary, use the smallest gauge needle appropriate for the task.
- Apply firm pressure to the needle stick site for 10 minutes or until the site no longer oozes blood.
- Apply ice to areas of trauma.
- Test all urine and stool for the presence of occult blood.
- Check IV sites every 2 hours for bleeding.
- Avoid trauma to rectal tissue:
  - Do not take temperatures rectally.
  - Do not give enemas.
  - Administer well-lubricated suppositories with caution.
- Measure abdominal girth daily.
- If the client is to be shaved, use an electric shaver.
- Use a soft-bristled toothbrush or tooth sponge for oral care.
- Inspect the mouth and gums for bleeding every 4 hours.
- Pad the side rails of the bed.
- Encourage the client not to blow the nose or insert objects into the nose.
- If the client is to ambulate, ensure that the footwear has a firm sole.

the risks for PE. Teach the client and family about bleeding precautions, activities to reduce the risk for deep vein thrombosis (DVT) and recurrence of PE, complications, and the need for follow-up care (Chart 35-7).

HEALTH CARE RESOURCES

For clients continuing with anticoagulation therapy, a home care nurse usually visits at least once per week to draw blood and perform an assessment (see Chart 35-8 for a focused assessment guide). Clients with severe dyspnea may need home oxygen therapy. Respiratory therapy treatments can be performed in the home. The nurse or case manager coordinates arrangements for oxygen and other respiratory therapy to be available if needed at home.

Critical Thinking Challenge

The client described earlier with a PE is going home. She will continue warfarin therapy for at least 1 month.

1. What will you tell this client about warfarin therapy?
2. Is this client still at risk for a PE? Why or why not?
3. How can this client reduce her risk for PE?

evolve For suggested answer guidelines, go to http://evolve.elsevier.com/Iggy/.

Evaluation: Outcomes

Evaluate the care of the client with PE on the basis of the identified nursing diagnoses and collaborative problems. The expected outcomes are that the client:

- Attains and maintains adequate gas exchange and oxygenation
- Does not experience hypovolemia and shock
- Remains free from bleeding episodes
- States that levels of anxiety are reduced
- Uses effective coping strategies

Specific indicators for these outcomes are listed for each nursing diagnosis and collaborative problem under the Planning and Implementation section (see earlier).

CHART 35-7

CLIENT EDUCATION GUIDE
The Client After Pulmonary Embolism

- Use an electric shaver.
- Use a soft-bristled toothbrush, and do not floss.
- Do not have dental work done without consulting your health care provider.
- Do not take aspirin or aspirin-containing products. Read the labels of all over-the-counter medications to be sure that the product does not contain aspirin or salicylates.
- Do not participate in contact sports or in any activity in which you might be bumped, scraped, or scratched.
- Apply ice immediately to any site of injury.
- Avoid anal intercourse.
- Take a stool softener to prevent straining during a bowel movement.
- Do not use enemas or rectal suppositories.
- Do not wear clothing that is tight or rubs.
- Avoid bending over at the waist.
- Avoid positions in which your knees are bent for any length of time.
- Wear elastic stockings as prescribed.
- Avoid prolonged sitting or standing.
- Avoid blowing your nose or placing objects in your nose. If you must blow your nose, do so gently without blocking either nasal passage.
- Take the prescribed dosage of medication at the precise time it was prescribed to be taken.
- Do not stop taking the medication abruptly or without a physician's prescription.
- Notify your doctor if you:
  - Have an injury and persistent bleeding results.
  - Have excessive menstrual bleeding.
  - See blood in your urine or bowel movement.
  - Notice large bruises or areas of small red or purple marks over the skin.

ACUTE RESPIRATORY FAILURE

PATHOPHYSIOLOGY

Acute respiratory failure is classified by blood gas abnormalities. The critical values are partial pressure of arterial oxygen ($Pa{O_2}$) less than 60 mm Hg, arterial oxygen saturation ($Sa{O_2}$) less than 90%, or partial pressure of arterial carbon dioxide ($Pa{CO_2}$) greater than 50 mm Hg occurring with acidemia (pH <7.30). Acute respiratory failure is further defined as *ventilatory failure, oxygenation failure,* or a *combination of both ventilatory and oxygenation failure.* Whatever the underlying problem, the client in acute respiratory failure is always hypoxemic.

Ventilatory Failure

Ventilatory failure is the type of ventilation-perfusion ($\dot{V}/\dot{Q}$) mismatch in which perfusion is normal but ventilation is inadequate. Ventilatory failure occurs when the thoracic pressure does not change sufficiently to permit air movement into and out from the lungs. As a result, too little oxygen reaches the alveoli and carbon dioxide is retained. Both problems lead to hypoxemia.

Ventilatory failure is often the result of any of the following three problems: a mechanical abnormality of the lungs or chest wall, a defect in the respiratory control center in the brain, or impaired ventilatory muscle function, especially the diaphragm. Ventilatory failure is defined by a $Pa{CO_2}$ level above 45 mm Hg in clients who have otherwise healthy lungs.

CHART 35-8

HOME CARE ASSESSMENT of
The Client After Pulmonary Embolism

Assess respiratory status.
- Observe rate and depth of ventilation.
- Auscultate lungs.
- Examine nail beds and mucous membranes for evidence of cyanosis.
- Take a pulse oximetry reading.
- Ask the client if chest pain or shortness of breath is experienced in any position.
- Ask the client about the presence of sputum and its color and character.

Assess cardiovascular status.
- Take vital signs, including apical pulse, pulse pressure; assess for presence or absence of orthostatic hypotension and quality and rhythm of peripheral pulses.
- Take blood pressure in both arms.
- Note presence or absence of peripheral edema.
- Examine hand vein filling in the dependent position.
- Examine neck vein filling in the recumbent and sitting positions.

Assess lower extremities for deep vein thrombosis.
- Examine lower legs and compare with each other for the following:
  - General edema
  - Calf swelling
  - Surface temperature
  - Presence of red streaks or cordlike palpable structure
- Measure calf circumference.
- Ask the client to dorsiflex and plantarflex each foot. Note the ease with which the client can do this, and ask whether pain is experienced in either position.
- Gently squeeze the calf of each leg laterally and from front to back. Ask the client whether pain or tenderness is experienced with either maneuver.

Assess for evidence of bleeding.
- Examine the mouth and gums for oozing or frank bleeding.
- Examine all skin areas for bruising or petechiae.
- If the client voids during the visit, test the urine for occult blood.

Assess cognition and mental status.
- Level of consciousness
- Orientation to time, place, and person
- Can the client accurately read a seven-word sentence containing no words greater than three syllables?

Assess the client's understanding of illness and compliance with treatment.
- Manifestations to report to health care provider
- Medication plan (correct timing and dose)
- Bleeding precautions
- Prevention of deep vein thrombosis

Oxygenation Failure

In oxygenation failure, thoracic pressure changes are normal, and air moves in and out without difficulty but does not oxygenate the pulmonary blood sufficiently. Oxygenation failure occurs in the type of $\dot{V}/\dot{Q}$ mismatch in which air movement *(ventilation)* is normal but lung perfusion is decreased.

Combined Ventilatory and Oxygenation Failure

Combined ventilatory and oxygenation failure involves poor respiratory movements **(hypoventilation).** Gas exchange at the alveolar-capillary membrane is inadequate so that too little oxygen reaches the blood and carbon dioxide is retained. The condition may or may not include poor lung perfusion. When lung perfusion is not adequate, $\dot{V}/\dot{Q}$ mismatch occurs and both ventilation and perfusion are inadequate. This type of respiratory failure leads to a more profound hypoxemia than either ventilatory failure or oxygenation failure alone.

TABLE 35-1 Common Causes of Ventilatory Failure

Extrapulmonary Causes

Neuromuscular disorders
- Multiple sclerosis
- Myasthenia gravis
- Guillain-Barré syndrome
- Poliomyelitis

Spinal cord injuries affecting nerves to intercostal muscles

Central nervous system dysfunction
- Stroke
- Cerebral edema
- Increased intracranial pressure
- Meningitis

Chemical depression
- Opioid analgesics
- Sedatives
- Anesthetic agents

Kyphoscoliosis

Massive obesity

Sleep apnea

External obstruction/constriction

Intrapulmonary Causes

Airway disease
- Chronic obstructive pulmonary disease
- Asthma

Ventilation-perfusion ($\dot{V}/\dot{Q}$) mismatch
- Pulmonary embolism
- Pneumothorax
- Acute respiratory distress syndrome (ARDS)
- Amyloidosis
- Pulmonary edema
- Interstitial fibrosis

Etiology

VENTILATORY FAILURE

Many diseases and conditions can result in ventilatory failure. Causes of ventilatory failure are categorized as either **extrapulmonary** (involving nonpulmonary tissues but affecting respiratory function) or **intrapulmonary** (disorders of the respiratory tract). Table 35-1 lists common causes of ventilatory failure.

OXYGENATION FAILURE

Many lung diseases and problems can cause oxygenation failure. Problems include impaired diffusion of oxygen at the alveolar level, right-to-left shunting of blood in the pulmonary vessels, $\dot{V}/\dot{Q}$ mismatch, breathing air with a low partial pressure of oxygen (a rare problem), and abnormal hemoglobin that fails to bind oxygen. In one type of $\dot{V}/\dot{Q}$ mismatch, areas of the lungs are still being perfused, but gas exchange is unable to occur, which leads to hypoxemia. An extreme example of $\dot{V}/\dot{Q}$ mismatch is a right-to-left shunt. A normal shunt is less than 5% of cardiac output. With a right-to-left shunt, even more venous blood is not oxygenated, and applying 100% oxygen does not correct the

TABLE 35-2 Common Causes of Oxygenation Failure

- Low atmospheric oxygen concentration
  - High altitudes
  - Smoke inhalation
  - Carbon monoxide poisoning
- Pneumonia
- Congestive heart failure with pulmonary edema
- Pulmonary embolism (PE)
- Acute respiratory distress syndrome (ARDS)
- Interstitial pneumonitis-fibrosis
- Abnormal hemoglobin
- Hypovolemic shock
- Hypoventilation
- Complications of nitroprusside therapy
  - Thiocyanate toxicity
  - Methemoglobinemia

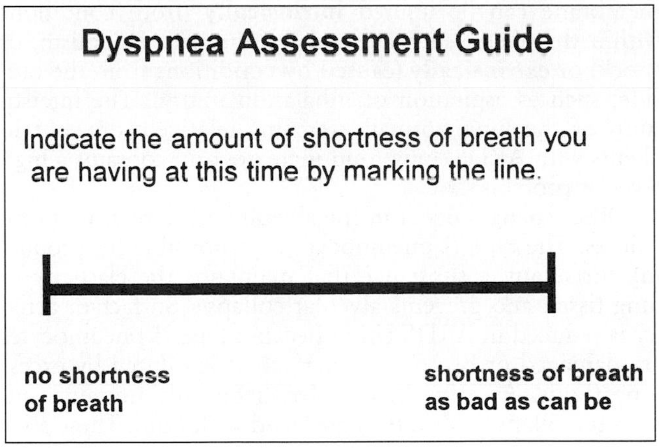

Figure 35-1 ■ A dyspnea assessment tool. (Modified from Gift, A. [1989]. A dyspnea assessment guide. *Critical Care Nurse, 9*[8], 79. Used with permission.)

problem. A classic cause of such a $\dot{V}/\dot{Q}$ mismatch is acute respiratory distress syndrome (ARDS). Table 35-2 lists specific causes of oxygenation failure.

COMBINED VENTILATORY AND OXYGENATION FAILURE

A combination of ventilatory failure and oxygenation failure occurs in clients who have abnormal lungs, such as those who have any form of **chronic airflow limitation (CAL),** such as chronic bronchitis, emphysema, or asthma. The bronchioles and alveoli are diseased (causing oxygenation failure), and the work of breathing increases until the respiratory muscles are unable to function effectively (causing ventilatory failure). Acute respiratory failure results. This process can also occur in clients who have cardiac failure along with respiratory failure. This problem is serious because the cardiac system cannot compensate for the hypoxia by increasing the cardiac output.

COLLABORATIVE MANAGEMENT

Assessment

Assess for **dyspnea** (perceived difficulty breathing), the hallmark of respiratory failure. Evaluate dyspnea with the use of a dyspnea assessment guide (Figure 35-1). Depending on the process, nature, and course of the underlying problem, the client may or may not be aware of changes in the work of breathing. In addition, the client needs to be alert enough to perceive the sensation of breathlessness.

Dyspnea is more intense when it develops rapidly. Slowly progressive respiratory failure may first be noticed as dyspnea on exertion (DOE) or when lying down. The client may have **orthopnea,** finding it is easier to breathe in an upright position. In the client with chronic respiratory problems, a minor increase in dyspnea from baseline may represent severe gas exchange problems.

Assess for a change in the client's respiratory rate or pattern, a change in lung sounds, and manifestations of hypoxemia and hypercarbia. Pulse oximetry may show decreased oxygen saturation, but an arterial blood gas (ABG) analysis is needed for the most accurate assessment of oxygenation. The health care provider reviews the ABG studies to identify the degree of hypercarbia and hypoxemia.

Interventions

Oxygen therapy is prescribed in acute respiratory failure to keep the partial pressure of arterial oxygen (PaO_2) level above 60 mm Hg while treating the underlying cause of the respiratory failure. Oxygen therapy is discussed in detail in Chapter 31. If supplemental oxygen does not maintain acceptable PaO_2 levels, mechanical ventilation may be needed.

Help the client find a position of comfort that allows easier breathing. To decrease the anxiety occurring with dyspnea, assist the client in using relaxation, diversion, and guided imagery. Start energy-conserving measures, such as minimal self-care and no unnecessary procedures. Pulmonary drugs given systemically or by metered dose inhaler (MDI) may be prescribed to widen the bronchioles and decrease inflammation to promote gas exchange. Teach the client how to use the inhaler and about the drugs. Encourage deep breathing and other breathing exercises.

ACUTE RESPIRATORY DISTRESS SYNDROME

PATHOPHYSIOLOGY

Acute respiratory distress syndrome (ARDS) is acute respiratory failure with the following indicators:

- Hypoxemia that persists even when 100% oxygen is given
- Decreased pulmonary compliance
- Dyspnea
- Noncardiac-associated bilateral pulmonary edema
- Dense pulmonary infiltrates on x-ray (ground-glass appearance)

Often ARDS occurs after an acute traumatic event in people with no previous pulmonary disease. The mortality rate is 50% to 60% even when intensive interventions are used. Other terms for ARDS include **noncardiogenic pulmonary edema, adult respiratory distress syndrome**, and the former term **shock lung.**

Despite different causes of lung injury in ARDS, a systemic inflammatory response is the common pathway in its development. Thus the manifestations of ARDS are similar regardless of the cause. The major site of injury in the lung is the alveolar-capillary membrane, which is normally permeable to only small molecules. The alveolar-capillary membrane can be injured **intrinsically** (from conditions within the client, such as sepsis, pulmonary embolism, or shock) or **extrinsically** (caused by conditions from the outside, such as aspiration or inhalation injury). The interstitium of the lung normally remains relatively dry, but in clients with ARDS, lung fluid increases and contains a high level of proteins.

Other changes occur in the alveoli and respiratory bronchioles. The type II pneumocyte is responsible for producing surfactant, a substance that maintains the elasticity of lung tissue and prevents alveolar collapse. Surfactant activity is reduced in ARDS either because type II pneumocytes are damaged or because the surfactant is diluted by excess lung fluids. As a result, the alveoli become unstable and tend to collapse unless they are filled with fluid. These alveoli can no longer participate in gas exchange. As a result, edema forms around terminal airways, which are compressed, closed, and can be destroyed. Lung volume is further reduced, and there is even less **compliance** (elasticity). As fluid continues to leak in more lung areas, fluid, protein, and blood cells collect in the alveoli and the interstitial space between the alveoli. Lymph channels are compressed and ineffective. Poorly ventilated alveoli receive blood but cannot oxygenate it, increasing the shunt. Hypoxemia and ventilation-perfusion ($\dot{V}/\dot{Q}$) mismatch result.

Etiology

Acute respiratory distress syndrome (ARDS) has many causes (Table 35-3). Some causes involve direct injury to lung tissue; others do not directly involve the respiratory system. Serious nervous system injury, such as head or spinal trauma, strokes, tumors, and sudden increases in cerebrospinal fluid pressure, may cause massive sympathetic discharge. Systemic blood vessel constriction results, with movement of large volumes of blood into lung circulation. Lung hydrostatic pressure increases and probably causes lung injury. Any problems that cause cerebral hypoxia can lead to the same type of lung injury.

Some factors produce ARDS by direct injury to the lung. For example, aspiration of gastric contents may obstruct or burn the airway when the gastric contents are highly acidic (pH less than 2.5). In such a direct injury, type I pneumocytes are destroyed. Injured capillaries allow protein and cells to escape from the blood vessels into lung tissues. Radiation, near-drowning, and inhalation of toxic gases all injure the alveolar and capillary tissue layers. Trauma, sepsis, drowning, and burns also cause the release of thromboplastins, which form fibrin clots in the peripheral blood. The clots, together with platelets and leukocytes, are filtered out in the lung. In many cases of ARDS, especially after trauma, clot production is increased and clot breakdown **(fibrinolysis)** is reduced. As a result, small emboli remain in the lung. Disseminated intravascular coagulation (DIC) plays a role in some clients.

TABLE 35-3 Common Causes of Acute Respiratory Distress Syndrome

- Shock
- Trauma
- Serious nervous system injury
- Pancreatitis
- Fat and amniotic fluid emboli
- Pulmonary infections
- Sepsis
- Inhalation of toxic gases (smoke, oxygen)
- Pulmonary aspiration
- Drug ingestion (e.g., heroin, opioids, aspirin)
- Hemolytic disorders
- Multiple blood transfusions
- Cardiopulmonary bypass
- Near-drowning (especially in fresh water)

Incidence/Prevalence

The actual incidence of ARDS is unknown, although a 2003 estimate suggested that 150,000 cases of ARDS occur yearly in the United States.

HEALTH PROMOTION/ILLNESS PREVENTION

A major goal in the prevention of ARDS is early recognition of clients at high risk for the syndrome. Because clients who aspirate gastric contents are at great risk, you must closely assess and monitor clients receiving tube feeding and those with neurologic problems that impair swallowing and gag reflexes. Follow meticulous infection control guidelines, including handwashing, invasive catheter and wound care, and body substance precautions. In addition, carefully observe clients who are being treated for any health problem associated with ARDS.

◆COLLABORATIVE MANAGEMENT

◆Assessment

PHYSICAL ASSESSMENT/CLINICAL MANIFESTATIONS

Assess the client's breathing and determine whether increased work of breathing is evident, as indicated by hyperpnea, grunting respiration, cyanosis, pallor, and retraction **intercostally** (between the ribs) or **substernally** (below the ribs). Document sweating and any change in mental status. No abnormal lung sounds are present on auscultation because the edema of ARDS occurs first in the interstitial spaces and not in the airways. Monitor vital signs at least hourly to assess for hypotension, tachycardia, and dysrhythmias.

DIAGNOSTIC ASSESSMENT

The diagnosis of ARDS is established by a lowered partial pressure of arterial oxygen ($Pa{O_2}$) value, determined by arterial blood gas (ABG) measurements. Because a widening alveolar oxygen gradient (increased fraction of inspired oxygen [$F{IO_2}$] does not yield corresponding increased $Pa{O_2}$ levels) develops with increased shunting of blood, the client has a progressive need for higher concentrations of oxygen. The client with ARDS is poorly responsive to high concentrations of oxygen **(refractory hypoxemia),** however, and often needs intubation and mechanical ventilation. A large difference between the predicted and actual alveolar oxygen tension indicates shunting. Sputum cultures obtained through bronchoscopy with protective brushings and by transtracheal aspiration are performed to determine if a lung infection also is present.

The chest x-ray usually shows diffuse haziness or a "whited-out" (ground-glass) appearance of the lung. An electrocardiogram (ECG) rules out cardiac problems and usually reveals no specific changes. Pulmonary artery (Swan-Ganz) catheter placement and hemodynamic monitoring is a diagnostic tool. In the client with ARDS, the pulmonary capillary wedge pressure (PCWP) is usually low to normal. This pressure differs from that in the client with cardiac-induced pulmonary edema, where the PCWP is above 18 mm Hg.

Common Nursing Diagnoses and Collaborative Problems

Nursing diagnoses and collaborative problems that may apply to clients with ARDS include the following:

- Anxiety related to hypoxemia, life-threatening illness, and loss of control
- Impaired Gas Exchange related to disrupted pulmonary ventilation and perfusion
- Fatigue related to hypoxemia and systemic inflammation
- Disturbed Sleep Pattern related to the intensive care unit (ICU) environment
- Imbalanced Nutrition: Less than Body Requirements related to presence of endotracheal tube, chemical paralysis, increased metabolic rate
- Risk for Injury related to elevated F_{IO_2} or barotrauma
- Potential for Ventilator-Associated Pneumonia (VAP)

Interventions

The client with ARDS often needs endotracheal intubation and mechanical ventilation with positive end-expiratory pressure (PEEP) or continuous positive airway pressure (CPAP). Sedation and paralysis may be needed for adequate ventilation and for reducing oxygen requirements. Because one of the side effects of PEEP is tension pneumothorax, you must assess lung sounds hourly and suction as needed to maintain a patent airway. Positioning may be important in promoting gas exchange.

Drug and Fluid Therapy. Corticosteroids may be used in the treatment of ARDS because they decrease white blood cell movement and stabilize the capillary membrane. Their effectiveness, however, has not been determined. It is thought that they may help minimize the fibrosis that occurs in late ARDS. Antibiotics are used to treat infections when organisms are identified.

Many interventions are under investigation, but none has been effective in decreasing mortality. Some of these interventions include agents that modify the inflammatory responses and oxidative stress (vitamins C and E, *N*-acetylcysteine), nitric oxide, surfactant replacement, and prone positioning.

The optimal fluid therapy for the client with ARDS remains unknown. Red blood cell transfusion may expand vascular volume. Fluid volume is titrated to maintain adequate cardiac output and tissue perfusion. Diuretics may help to decrease lung edema, but care should be taken to prevent dehydration and hypotension.

Nutrition Therapy. The client with ARDS is at risk for malnutrition, which further compromises the respiratory system and the immune response. Diaphragm function is also reduced. Therefore enteral nutrition (tube feeding) or parenteral nutrition (hyperalimentation) is started as soon as possible.

Case Management. Case management of the client with ARDS focuses on the phases of ARDS rather than day-to-day care. The course of ARDS and its management are divided into four phases:

Phase 1. This phase includes early changes with the client having dyspnea and tachypnea. Early interventions focus on supporting the client and providing oxygen.

Phase 2. Patchy infiltrates form from increasing pulmonary edema. Interventions include mechanical ventilation and prevention of complications.

Phase 3. This phase occurs over days 2 to 10, and the client has progressive hypoxemia that responds poorly to high levels of oxygen. Interventions focus on maintaining adequate oxygen transport, preventing complications, and supporting the failing lung until it has had time to heal.

Phase 4. Pulmonary fibrosis with progression occurs after 10 days. This phase is irreversible and is often called "late" or "chronic" ARDS. Clients who survive this stage will have some permanent lung changes. Interventions focus on preventing sepsis, pneumonia, and multiple organ dysfunction syndrome (MODS) as well as weaning the client from the ventilator. The client in this phase may be ventilator dependent for weeks to months. Care may occur in specialized units or facilities that focus on rehabilitation and long-term weaning. Some clients may not be weanable and may go home or to long-term care dependent on mechanical ventilation.

THE CLIENT REQUIRING INTUBATION AND VENTILATION

PATHOPHYSIOLOGY

With mechanical ventilation, the client who has severe problems of gas exchange may be supported until the underlying problem resolves or improves. Usually mechanical ventilation is a temporary life-support technique. The need for this support may be lifelong, especially for clients with chronic, progressive neuromuscular diseases that reduce effective ventilation.

Mechanical ventilation is most often used for clients with hypoxemia and progressive alveolar hypoventilation with respiratory acidosis. The hypoxemia is usually due to pulmonary shunting of blood when other methods of oxygen delivery do not provide a sufficiently high fraction of inspired oxygen (F_{IO_2}). Mechanical ventilation may be used for clients who need respiratory support after surgery, who are barely maintaining adequate gas exchange at the cost of expending energy with the high work of breathing, or who require general anesthesia or heavy sedation to allow diagnostic or therapeutic interventions.

COLLABORATIVE MANAGEMENT

Assessment

Assess the client about to be intubated in the same way as for other breathing problems. Once mechanical ventilation has been started, assess the respiratory system on an ongoing basis. Monitor and assess for complications related to the artificial airway or ventilator as well as for those related to mechanical ventilation.

Common Nursing Diagnoses and Collaborative Problems

Nursing diagnoses and collaborative problems that may apply to clients requiring mechanical ventilation include the following:

- Impaired Verbal Communication related to physical barrier.

- Disturbed Sleep Pattern related to interruptions for monitoring, noisy environment.
- Death Anxiety related to loss of independent breathing ability.
- Impaired Oral Mucous Membrane related to presence of endotracheal tube.
- Potential for Ventilator-Associated Pneumonia

Interventions

Endotracheal Intubation. The client who needs mechanical ventilation must have an artificial airway. The most common type of artificial airway for a short-term basis is the endotracheal (ET) tube. A tracheostomy is usually considered if the client requires an artificial airway for longer than 10 to 14 days, (see Chapter 31) to reduce tracheal and vocal cord damage.

The goals of intubation are to maintain a patent airway, provide a means to remove secretions, and provide ventilation and oxygen. Indications for intubation are listed in Table 35-4.

Endotracheal Tube. An ET tube is a long polyvinyl chloride tube that is passed through the mouth or nose and into the trachea (Figure 35-2). When properly positioned, the tip of the ET tube rests about 0.8 to 1.2 inches (2 to 3 cm) above the **carina** (the point at which the trachea divides into the right and left mainstem bronchi). Oral intubation is the easiest and quickest method of establishing an airway and is often performed as an emergency procedure. Because of increased problems with sinusitis, the nasal route is reserved for facial or oral traumas and surgeries and when oral intubation is not possible. The nasal route is not used if the client has a blood dyscrasia. An anesthesiologist, nurse anesthetist, or pulmonologist usually performs the intubation.

An ET tube has several parts (see Figure 35-2). The shaft of the tube has a radiopaque line running the length of the tube.

TABLE 35-4 Major Indications for Intubation

- Airway protection when the client loses reflexes because of anesthesia, medications, disease, or decreased level of consciousness
- To provide positive pressure or high oxygen concentration
- To bypass airway obstruction
- Facilitating pulmonary hygiene and suctioning of secretions when the client cannot handle secretions (as in diseases of chronic airflow limitation)

This line shows on x-ray and is used to determine correct tube placement. Short horizontal lines (depth markings) are used to place the tube correctly at the nares or mouth (at the incisor tooth) and to identify how far the tube has been inserted.

The cuff at the distal end of the tube is inflated after placement and can create a seal between the trachea and the cuff. The seal ensures delivery of a set tidal volume when mechanical ventilation is used. When the cuff is inflated to an adequate sealing volume, no air can pass around the cuff to the vocal cords, nose, or mouth. Thus the client is not able to talk when the cuff is inflated. The cuff should be inflated using minimal-leak or no-leak techniques.

The pilot balloon with a one-way valve permits air to be inserted into the cuff and prevents air from escaping. This balloon is a guide for determining whether air is present in the cuff, but it does not show how much or how little air is present.

The universal adaptor connects the ET tube to ventilator tubing or to other types of oxygen delivery systems. The endotracheal tube size is listed on the shaft of the tube. Adult tube sizes range from 7 to 9 mm. Tube size selected is based on the size of the client.

Preparing for Intubation. You must know the proper procedure for summoning intubation personnel in your facility to the bedside in an emergency situation. Explain the procedure to the client as clearly as possible. Basic life support measures, such as the establishment of a patent airway and the delivery of 100% oxygen by a manual resuscitation bag with a face mask, are crucial to the client's survival until help arrives.

In an emergency, bring the code (or "crash") cart, airway equipment box, and suction equipment (often already on the code cart) to the bedside. Maintain a patent airway through positioning and the insertion of an oral or nasopharyngeal airway until the client is intubated. During intubation, continuously monitor for changes in vital signs, signs of hypoxia or hypoxemia, dysrhythmias, and aspiration. Ensure that each intubation attempt lasts no longer than 30 seconds, preferably less than 15 seconds. After 30 seconds, provide oxygen by means of a mask and manual resuscitation bag to prevent hypoxia and cardiac arrest. Suction as necessary.

Verifying Tube Placement. Immediately after an ET tube is inserted, placement must be verified. The most accurate way to verify placement is by checking end-tidal carbon

A

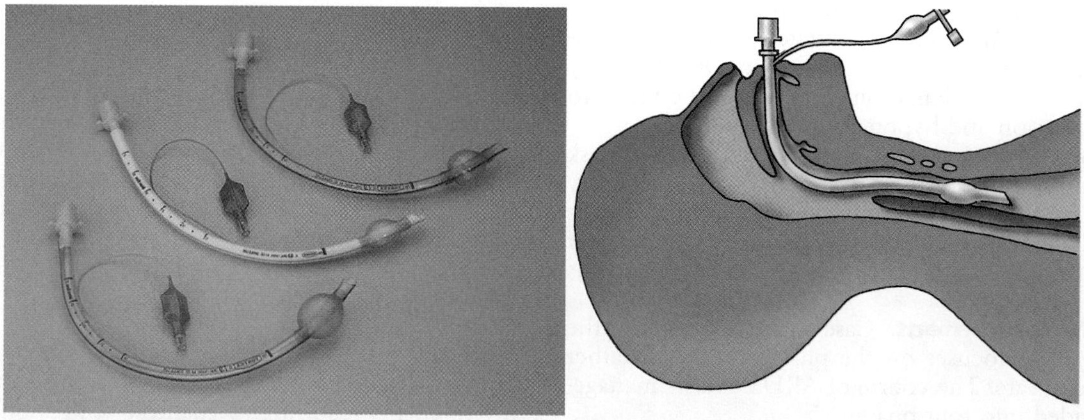

B

Figure 35-2 ■ **A,** Endotracheal tubes. (Courtesy of Sims Porter, Inc.) **B,** Correct placement of an oral endotracheal tube.

dioxide level. Assess for breath sounds bilaterally, symmetrical chest movement, and air emerging from the ET tube. If breath sounds and chest wall movement are absent on the left side, the tube may be in the right mainstem bronchus. The person intubating the client should be able to reposition the tube without repeating the entire intubation procedure.

Auscultate over the stomach to rule out esophageal intubation. If the tube is in the stomach, louder breath sounds are heard over the stomach than over the chest, and the abdomen may be distended. Continuously monitor chest wall movement and breath sounds until tube placement is verified by chest x-ray.

Stabilizing the Tube. The nurse, respiratory therapist, or anesthesia personnel stabilize the ET tube at the mouth or nose. The tube is marked at the level where it touches the incisor tooth or naris. Two people working together use a head halter technique to secure the tube. Chart 35-9 outlines best practices for securing an oral or nasal ET tube.

An oral airway may be inserted to keep the client from biting an oral tube. One person stabilizes the tube at the correct position and prevents head movement while a second person applies the tape. After the procedure is completed, verify and document the presence of bilateral and equal breath sounds and the level of the tube.

Nursing Care. Assess tube placement, minimal cuff leak, breath sounds, and chest wall movement regularly. Prevent pulling or tugging on the tube by the client to prevent dislodgment or "slipping" of the tube, and check the pilot balloon to ensure that the cuff is inflated. Suctioning, coughing, and speaking attempts can cause dislodgment. Neck flexion moves the tube away from the carina; neck extension moves the tube closer to the carina. Rotation of the head also causes the tube to move. Mouth secretions and tongue movement can loosen the tape and malposition the tube. When other measures fail, apply soft wrist restraints, as prescribed, for the client who is pulling on the tube. *Restraints are used as a last resort to prevent accidental extubation.* Adequate sedation (chemical restraint) may be needed to decrease agitation or prevent extubation. Obtain permission for restraints from the client or family. More information on airway management is found in Chapter 31.

Complications of an ET or nasotracheal tube can occur during placement, while in place, during extubation, or after extubation (either early or late). Trauma and complications can occur to the face; eye; nasal and paranasal areas; oral, pharyngeal, bronchial, tracheal, and pulmonary areas; esophageal and gastric areas; and cardiovascular, musculoskeletal, and neurologic systems.

Mechanical Ventilation. Mechanical ventilation to support and maintain respiratory function is widely used on medical-surgical units, in nursing homes, and in the home setting as well as in critical care units. The nurse plays a pivotal role in the coordination of care and the prevention of complications. Chart 35-10 reviews best practices for care of the client during mechanical ventilation.

The goals of mechanical ventilation are to improve oxygenation and ventilation and to decrease the work needed for an effective breathing pattern. Mechanical ventilation is used to support the client until lung function is adequate or until the acute episode has passed. *A ventilator does not cure diseased lungs; it provides ventilation until the client is able to resume the process of breathing.* It is important to remember why the client is using the ventilator so that management efforts also focus on correcting the causes of the respiratory failure. If normal oxygenation, ventilation, and respiratory muscle strength are achieved, mechanical ventilation can be discontinued.

Types of Ventilators. A wide variety of ventilators are available. The ventilator selected depends on the severity of the disease process and the length of time ventilator support is needed. Two major types of ventilators are negative-pressure and positive-pressure ventilators.

Negative-Pressure Ventilators. The negative-pressure ventilator is noninvasive and works by changing pressures in the chest cavity rather than by forcing air directly into the lungs (Figure 35-3). The iron lung, widely used during the poliomyelitis epidemic in the 1940s, is the classic negative-pressure ventilator. The client is placed in an airtight tube that surrounds either the chest area or the entire body and leaves the head exposed. During inspiration, with the expansion of the chest wall, negative pressure is generated in the chest cavity. Because of the pressure gradient, air moves from the atmosphere *(higher pressure)* into the thoracic cavity *(lower pressure).* At a preset time, negative pressure ceases and expiration occurs. Thus negative-pressure ventilators create pressure gradients that mimic normal ventilation.

Newer negative-pressure ventilators include the cuirass, poncho, and body wrap. These ventilators, which encase only the body trunk, are used for clients with neuromuscular disease, central nervous system problems, spinal cord injuries, and chronic obstructive pulmonary disease (COPD). Clients may use negative-pressure ventilation for home nighttime breathing support so that their muscles can rest. An artificial airway is not required. Newer models are lightweight and easy to use. The enclosing ventilator makes some direct nursing care more difficult. The client must be able to clear oral secretions and must have compliant (elastic) lungs to benefit from this mode of ventilation.

Positive-Pressure Ventilators. The positive-pressure ventilator is widely used in the acute care setting. During inspiration, pressure is generated that pushes air into the lungs and expands the chest. In most instances, an endotracheal (ET) tube or tracheostomy is needed. Positive-pressure ventilators are classified by the mechanism that ends inspiration and starts expiration. Inspiration is terminated or cycled in three major ways: pressure cycled, time cycled, or volume cycled.

PRESSURE-CYCLED VENTILATORS. Pressure-cycled ventilators (now rarely used) push air into the lungs until a preset airway pressure is reached. Tidal volumes and inspiratory time vary. Pressure-cycled ventilators are used for short periods, such as just after surgery and for respiratory therapy.

TIME-CYCLED VENTILATORS. Time-cycled ventilators push air into the lungs until a preset time has elapsed. Tidal volume and pressure vary, depending on the needs of the client and the type of ventilator.

VOLUME-CYCLED VENTILATORS. Volume-cycled ventilators push air into the lungs until a preset volume is delivered. A constant tidal volume is delivered regardless of the pressure needed to deliver the tidal volume. A set pressure limit, however, prevents excessive pressure from being exerted on the lungs. The advantage of this type of ventilator is that a constant tidal volume is delivered regardless of the

CHART 35-9

BEST PRACTICE for
Securing an Oral and Nasal Endotracheal Tube

Little evidence is available to provide clinical direction on the best method to secure endotracheal (ET) and nasotracheal tubes; however, adhesive tape is the easiest, cheapest, and most frequently used.

Adhesive tape may be irritating to the skin, and frequent tape changes may disrupt the skin integrity. An additional reported complication is nosocomial cutaneous mucomycosis occurring around the surgical tape securing the ET tube. Protecting the skin, especially on the face, is a high priority for clients and nurses. This must be balanced against making sure the ET tube is not dislodged. A simple yet effective method of securing the oral and nasotracheal tube is demonstrated here:

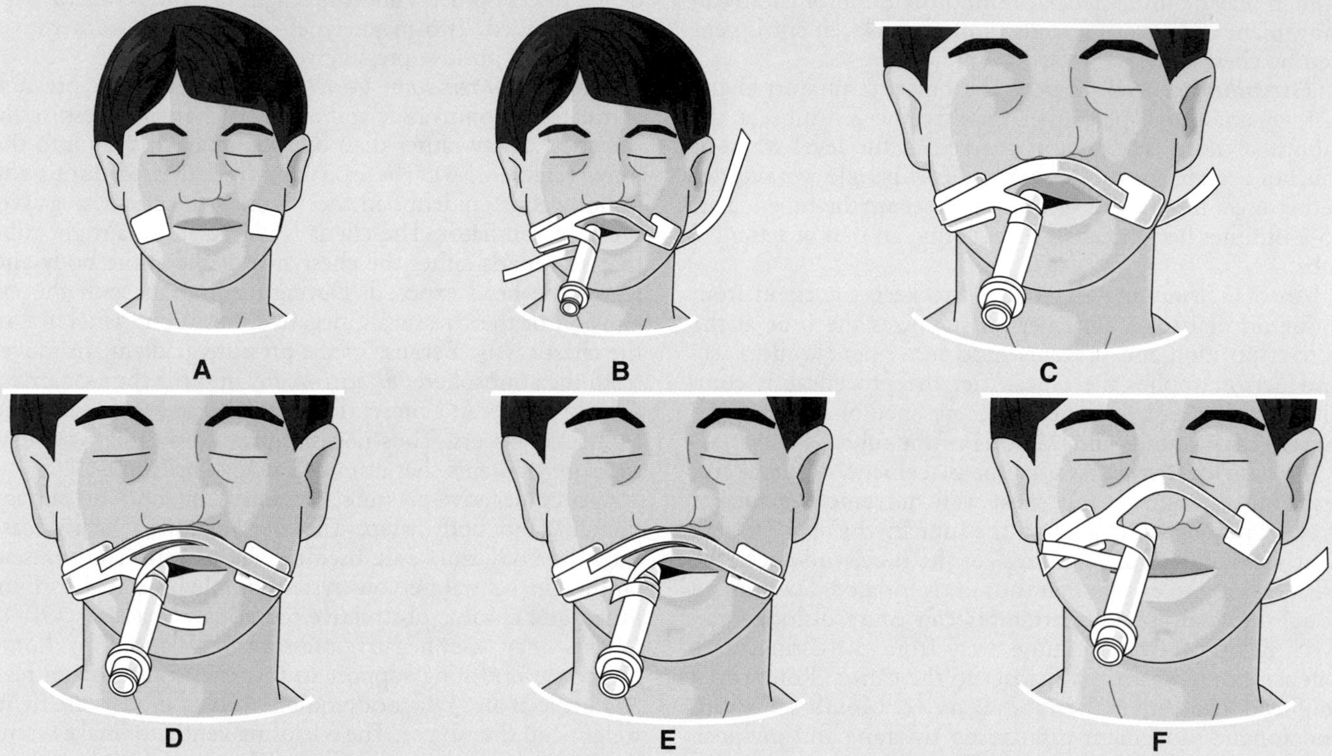

1. Prepare the skin by shaving the cheeks and upper lip, if possible.
2. Protect the skin by applying tincture of benzoin to the skin and ET tube and allow to dry (Mastisol may also be used, but Detachol must be used before removing the tape); then apply a 1 × 3-inch piece of thin DuoDerm or other protective or hydrocolloid membrane to the skin on the cheeks *(A)*.
3. Take a 30-inch (about 2½-foot) piece of adhesive tape and lay it on a flat surface, sticky side up. Take another piece of tape (about 10 inches), and cover the middle portion of the tape (sticky side to sticky side) to protect the back of the client's neck. A tongue blade on each end folded over can keep it from getting tangled or sticking prematurely.
4. Place the tape behind the client's neck. Remove the tongue blades, and place the tape on the protective membrane up to the end of the mouth on each side. Trim the tape as needed and split each end of the tape.
5. Take the upper part of one end of the tape, and place it on the upper lip. Take the lower part of the tape and wrap it securely around the tube *(B, C)*. Take the upper part of the other end of the tape, place it on the upper lip, and wrap the lower part securely around the tube *(D, E)*. Do not have the tube too far to either side of the mouth, or it can cause skin breakdown in the corner of the mouth or lips.
6. The same method can be used for nasal tubes, but do not tape the tube too tightly to the nose or skin breakdown will occur on the nares *(F)*.
7. Always tape the tube to the upper lip; never the lower. The lower jaw moves too much with attempts to speak or oral care, which will move the tube and cause irritation and discomfort for the client. The tape should be inspected at least every shift for signs of loosening or skin irritation or breakdown, especially with increased oral secretions. Tightness of the tape should also be checked each shift if swelling in the face and neck occurs or if there is an increase in fluid retention (as in anasarca, sepsis, or acute respiratory distress syndrome).

An additional technique for securing tubing that can decrease ET tube movement and provide a fulcrum for pulling on ventilator tubing is to attach a 6-inch (50-mL) piece of flexible ventilator tubing between the ET tube adaptor and the Y-connector of the ventilator tubing. The procedure for this technique is as follows:

1. Shave the chest or clean with alcohol a portion of the chest at right angles to the angle of Louis. Apply tincture of benzoin and allow to dry.
2. Prepare Montgomery straps by taking two 6-inch pieces of 2-inch wide adhesive tape. Double-back one end of each piece of tape, and cut a small hole in the ends that are doubled over.
3. Apply the tape to the prepared chest with the ends with the hole over each other. Take a 12-inch piece of twill (trach) tape, and thread through both holes. Position the tubing with the Y-connector over the holes and tie into place. This procedure allows all pulling on the tubing to place strain on the tape (straps) and not on the face or the tube. Caution should be taken if clients have increased partial pressure of arterial carbon dioxide retention, and end-tidal carbon dioxide monitoring may be useful when weaning.

CHART 35-10

BEST PRACTICE for
Care of the Client Receiving Mechanical Ventilation

- At least once every shift check to be sure the ventilator settings are set as prescribed.
- Check to be sure alarms are set (especially low-pressure and low-exhaled volume).
- Observe the exhaled volume digital display to be sure the client is receiving the prescribed tidal volume.
- Empty ventilator tubings when moisture collects. Never empty fluid in the tubing back into the cascade.
- Ensure adequate humidity by keeping delivered air temperature maintained at body temperature.
- If the client is on PEEP, observe the peak airway pressure dial to determine the proper level of PEEP.
- Assess the client's respiratory status each shift and as needed:
  - Observe the client's color (especially lips and nail beds).
  - Observe the client's chest for bilateral expansion.
  - Auscultate the lungs for crackles, rhonchi, wheezes, equal breath sounds, and decreased or absent breath sounds.
  - Obtain pulse oximetry reading.
  - Evaluate ABGs as indicated.
- Take vital signs at least every 4 hours.
- Be sure the tracheostomy cuff (or the endotracheal cuff) is adequately inflated to ensure tidal volume.
- Administer mouth care every 2 to 4 hours.
- Observe the client's need for tracheal/oral/nasal suctioning every 2 hours. Provide adequate suctioning as needed.
- Provide tracheostomy care every shift.
- Change tracheostomy tape or endotracheal tube tape as needed. Observe the client's mouth around the endotracheal tube for pressure sores.
- Move the oral endotracheal tube to the opposite side of the mouth once every 24 hours to prevent ulcers.
- Maintain accurate intake and output records to monitor fluid balance.
- Turn the client at least every 2 hours, and get the client out of bed as prescribed to promote pulmonary hygiene and prevent complications of immobility.
- Schedule treatments and nursing care at intervals to provide rest.
- Explain all procedures and treatments; provide access to a call bell; visit the client frequently.
- Include the client and his or her family in care whenever possible (especially suctioning and tracheostomy care).
- Provide a letter board or pencil and paper for communication. Request consultation with a speech therapist for assistance, if necessary.
- Observe ventilated clients for gastrointestinal distress (diarrhea, constipation, tarry stools).
- Document pertinent observations in the client's medical record (chart).
- Administer muscle-paralyzing agents, sedatives, and narcotic analgesics, as appropriate.
- Monitor the effectiveness of mechanical ventilation in terms of the client's physiologic and psychological status.
- Initiate relaxation techniques as appropriate.
- Monitor the client's progress on current ventilator settings and make appropriate changes as indicated.
- Monitor for adverse effects of mechanical ventilation: infection, barotrauma, reduced cardiac output.
- Position to facilitate ventilation/perfusion matching ("good lung down"), as appropriate.
- Monitor the effects of ventilator changes on oxygenation and the client's subjective response.
- Monitor readiness to wean.

Courtesy Our Lady of Lourdes Medical Center, Camden, NJ.
PEEP, Positive end-expiratory pressure; *ABGs*, arterial blood gases.

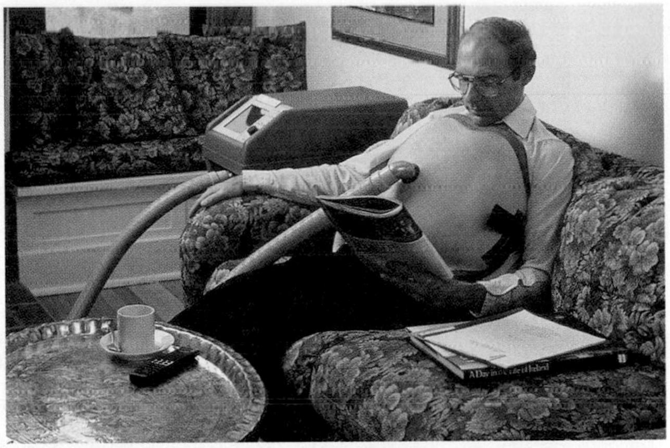

Figure 35-3 ■ A negative-pressure ventilator. Lifecare Chest Shell. (From Hill, N. [1986]. Clinical application of body ventilators. *Chest,* 90[6], 900. Used with permission.)

changing compliance of the lungs and chest wall or the airway resistance.

MICROPROCESSOR VENTILATORS. Microprocessor ventilators are computer-managed, positive-pressure ventilators. A microprocessor is built into the ventilator to allow ongoing monitoring of ventilatory functions, alarms, and client conditions. It often has components of volume-, time-, and pressure-cycled ventilators. The microprocessor ventilator is more responsive to clients who have severe lung disease and those who need prolonged weaning trials. Examples include the Draeger Evita XL and Puritan-Bennett 840.

Modes of Ventilation. The mode of ventilation is the way in which the client receives breaths from the ventilator.

Assist-Control Ventilation. Assist-control (AC) ventilation is the mode used most often and is mainly a resting mode. The ventilator takes over the work of breathing for the client. The tidal volume and ventilatory rate are preset. If the client does not trigger spontaneous breaths, a minimal ventilatory pattern is established. The ventilator is programmed to respond to the client's inspiratory effort if he or she does initiate a breath. In this case, the ventilator delivers the preset tidal volume while allowing the client to control the rate of breathing.

A disadvantage of the AC mode is that if the client's spontaneous ventilatory rate increases, the ventilator continues to deliver a preset tidal volume with each breath. The client may then hyperventilate, and respiratory alkalosis occurs. Causes of hyperventilation, such as pain, anxiety, or acid-base imbalances, must be corrected.

Synchronized Intermittent Mandatory Ventilation. Synchronized intermittent mandatory ventilation (SIMV) is similar to AC ventilation in that tidal volume and ventilatory rate are preset. If the client does not breathe, a minimal ventilatory pattern is established. Unlike the AC mode, SIMV allows spontaneous breathing at the client's own rate and tidal volume between the ventilator breaths. SIMV can be used as a main ventilatory mode or as a weaning mode. When used for weaning, the number of mechanical breaths (SIMV breaths) is gradually decreased (e.g., from 12 to 2), and the client gradually resumes spontaneous breathing.

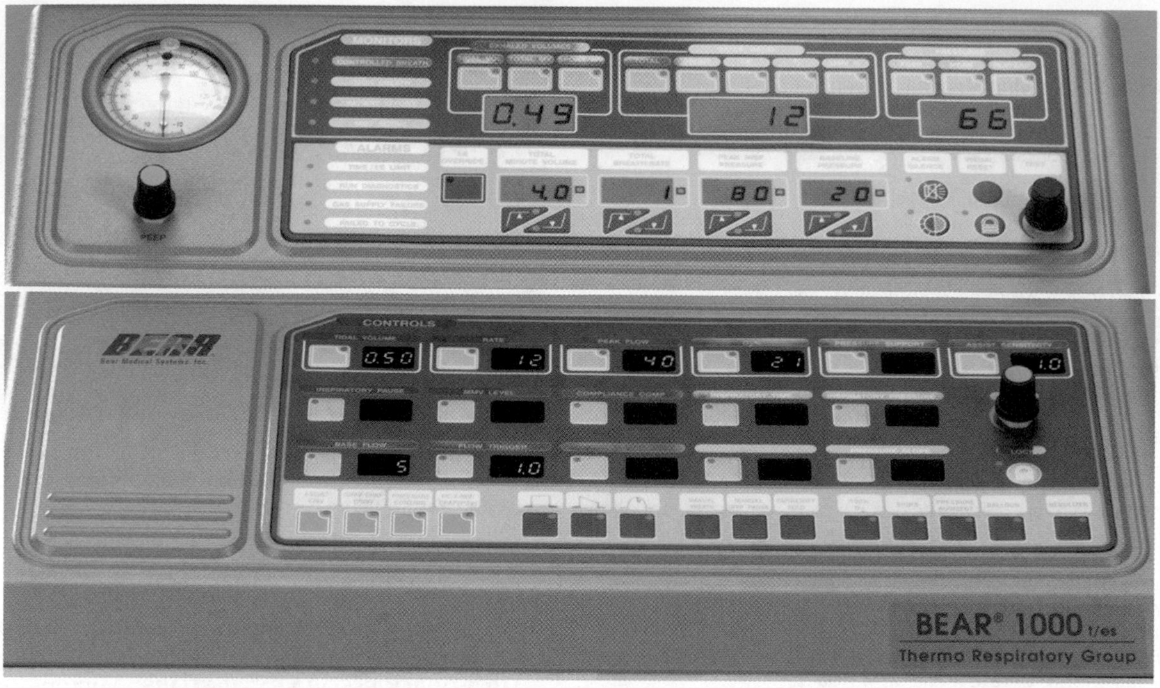

Figure 35-4 ■ Display signals and alarms *(top)* and control panel *(bottom)* of a typical volume-cycled ventilator. (Bear 1000t/es Adult Volume Ventilator. Courtesy Bear Medical Systems, Thermo Respiratory Group, Palm Springs, CA.)

The mandatory ventilator breaths are delivered when the client is ready to inspire. This action promotes synchrony between the ventilator and the client.

Bi-level Positive Airway Pressure. Bi-level positive airway pressure (BiPAP) provides noninvasive pressure support ventilation by nasal or face mask. Whereas BiPAP is most often used for clients with sleep apnea, it may be used for clients with ventilatory muscle fatigue to avoid the more invasive endotracheal intubation or tracheostomy.

Other Modes of Ventilation. Newer modes of ventilation, such as pressure support and continuous flow (flow-by), are part of most microprocessor ventilators. Both types decrease the work of breathing and are often used for weaning clients from mechanical ventilation. Other modes are maximum mandatory ventilation (MMV), inverse inspiration-expiration (I/E) ratio, permissive hypercarbia, airway pressure–release ventilation, proportional assist ventilation, high-frequency ventilation, and high-frequency oscillation. Many of these modes use special ventilators, tubing, or airways.

Ventilator Controls and Settings. The volume-cycled ventilator is the most widely used ventilator in the acute care setting. Regardless of the type of volume-cycled ventilator used, the controls and types of settings are universal (Figure 35-4). The physician prescribes the ventilator settings, and usually the ventilator is readied or set up by the respiratory department. The nurse assists in connecting the client to the ventilator and monitors the ventilator settings.

Tidal Volume. Tidal volume (V_T) is the volume of air the client receives with each breath. It can be measured on either inspiration or expiration. The average prescribed V_T ranges between 7 and 10 mL/kg of body weight (see the Evidence-Based Practice for Nursing box at right). Adding a zero to the weight of clients in kilograms gives an estimate of tidal volume.

EVIDENCE-BASED PRACTICE for Nursing

Less is better for tidal volumes

The Acute Respiratory Distress Syndrome Network. (2000). Ventilation with lower tidal volumes as compared with traditional tidal volumes for acute lung injury. *The New England Journal of Medicine, 342*(18), 1301-1308.

Traditionally, tidal volumes from 10 to 15 mg/kg body weight are used in mechanical ventilation; however, these volumes may cause stretch-induced lung injury in clients with acute lung injury and acute respiratory distress syndrome (ARDS; so-called volu-trauma). The purpose of this study was to compare these volumes with a lower tidal volume and evaluate clinical outcomes.

Clients were enrolled in a multicenter, randomized clinical trial. The trial compared traditional treatment (tidal volume of 12 mL/kg and plateau pressure of ≤50 cm water) with the treatment group (tidal volume of 6 mL/kg and plateau pressure of ≤30 cm of water or less). The outcomes were death before discharge or breathing without assistance and number of days without ventilator use from day 1 to day 28. The trial was stopped prematurely because mortality was lower in the treatment group as well as because of the greater number of days without ventilator use during the first 28 days.

Level of Evidence: 2—At least one properly designed randomized control trial of appropriate size (multisite).

Critique. This study has major implications for decreasing complications related to use of mechanical ventilation. Lessening the effect of volu-trauma can impact costs and length of stay as well functional status post-hospitalization. The study has limitations however, in that volume-assist control mode was used until the client was weaned. This is not consistently used in clinical practice; synchronized intermittent mandatory ventilation (SIMV) is more commonly used.

Implications for Nursing. Decreasing complications is a major role for nurses in critical care. Clients on mechanical ventilation are vulnerable to numerous insults and diligent care is required to assess and intervene when an untoward event occurs. This treatment change is simple yet may impact the survival of clients with acute lung injury and ARDS.

Rate, or Breaths per Minute. Rate, or breaths/min, is the number of ventilator breaths delivered per minute. The rate is usually set between 10 and 14 breaths/min.

Fraction of Inspired Oxygen. The **fraction of inspired oxygen** (FIO_2) is the oxygen level delivered to the client. The prescribed FIO_2 is determined by the arterial blood gas (ABG) value and the client's condition. Ventilators can provide 21% to 100% oxygen, depending on need.

The oxygen delivered to the client is warmed to body temperature (98.6° F [37° C]) and humidified to 100%. Humidification and warming are needed because upper air passages of the respiratory tree, which normally warm, humidify, and filter air, are bypassed. Humidification and warming prevent mucosal damage and ease clearance of secretions.

Sighs. **Sighs** are volumes of air that are 1.5 to 2 times the set tidal volume, delivered 6 to 10 times/hr. These may be used to prevent atelectasis in special circumstances. Sighs are rarely used, however, because they can cause **barotrauma** (lung damage from excessive pressure) and have not been shown to be useful.

Peak Airway (Inspiratory) Pressure. Peak airway (inspiratory) pressure (PIP) indicates the pressure needed by the ventilator to deliver a set tidal volume at a given dynamic compliance. The PIP value appears on the display on the front or top of the ventilator. Peak pressure is the highest pressure reached during inspiration. Monitoring trends in PIP reflect changes in resistance of the lungs and resistance in the ventilator. An increased PIP reading means increased airway resistance in the client or the ventilator tubing (bronchospasm, or pinched tubing), increased amount of secretions, pulmonary edema, or decreased pulmonary compliance (the lungs or chest wall are "stiffer" or harder to inflate). An upper pressure limit is set on the ventilator to prevent barotrauma. When the limit is reached, the high-pressure alarm sounds, and the remaining volume is not given.

Continuous Positive Airway Pressure. Continuous positive airway pressure (CPAP) applies positive airway pressure throughout the entire respiratory cycle for spontaneously breathing clients. Sedating drugs are given cautiously or not at all when the client is receiving CPAP so that respiratory effort is not suppressed. CPAP keeps the alveoli open during inspiration and prevents alveolar collapse during expiration. This process increases functional residual capacity (FRC), improves gas exchange, and improves oxygenation.

The most common use of CPAP is to help in the weaning process. During CPAP, no ventilator breaths are delivered. The ventilator just delivers oxygen and provides monitoring and an alarm system. The respiratory pattern is determined by the client's efforts. Normal levels of CPAP are 5 to 15 cm H_2O, adjusted to promote adequate oxygenation. If no pressure is set on the ventilator, the client receives no positive pressure. Thus, the client is then using the ventilator as a T-piece with alarms.

Modifications of CPAP include nasal CPAP and bi-level positive airway pressure (BiPAP). These modifications are used for select problems.

Positive End-Expiratory Pressure. Positive end-expiratory pressure (PEEP) is positive pressure exerted during the expiratory phase of ventilation. PEEP improves oxygenation by enhancing gas exchange and preventing atelectasis. It is used to treat persistent hypoxemia that does not improve with an acceptable oxygen delivery level. PEEP is often added when the partial pressure of arterial oxygen (PaO_2) remains low with an FIO_2 of 50% to 70% or greater.

The need for PEEP indicates a severe gas-exchange problem. It is important to lower the FIO_2 delivered whenever possible. Prolonged use of a high FIO_2 can damage lungs from the toxic effects of oxygen. PEEP prevents alveoli from collapsing because the lungs are kept partially inflated so that alveolar-capillary gas exchange is promoted throughout the ventilatory cycle. The effect should be an increase in arterial blood oxygenation so that the FIO_2 can be decreased.

Positive end-expiratory pressure (PEEP) is "dialed in" with the PEEP dial on the control panel. The amount of PEEP is usually 5 to 15 cm H_2O and is read (monitored) on the peak airway pressure dial, the same dial used to read the PIP. When PEEP is added, the dial does not return to zero at the end of exhalation; rather, it returns to a baseline that has been increased from zero by the amount of PEEP applied.

Flow. **Flow** is how fast the ventilator delivers each breath. It is usually set at 40 L/min. *If a client is agitated, is restless, has a widely fluctuating pressure reading on inspiration, or has other signs of air hunger, the flow may be set too low. Increasing the flow should be tried before using chemical restraints.*

Other Settings. Other settings may be used, depending on the type of ventilator and mode of ventilation. Examples include inspiratory and expiratory cycle, waveform, expiratory resistance, and plateau.

Nursing Management. The use of mechanical ventilation involves a complex decision-making process for both the client/family and the interdisciplinary health care team. The physical and psychological concerns of the client and family must be addressed because the mechanical ventilator often causes them anxiety. You must carefully explain the purpose of the ventilator and acknowledge that the client might feel some different sensations. Encourage the client and family to express their concerns. Act as the coach to help and support the client and family through this experience. In an emergency, explanations may not occur until the emergency has been controlled. Clients undergoing mechanical ventilation in intensive care units (ICUs) often experience delirium, or "ICU psychosis." These clients need frequent, repeated explanations and reassurance.

When caring for a ventilated client, you must be concerned with the client first and the ventilator second. It is vital that you understand why mechanical ventilation is needed. Causes such as excessive amounts of secretions, sepsis, and trauma require different interventions to allow ventilator independence. In addition, you must understand the client's chronic health problems, especially chronic obstructive pulmonary disease (COPD), left-sided heart failure, anemia, and malnutrition. These problems may slow weaning from mechanical ventilation and warrant close monitoring and intervention.

Three nursing goals in caring for the client with mechanical ventilation are to monitor and evaluate the response to the ventilator, manage the ventilator system safely, and prevent complications.

Monitoring the Client's Response. A major nursing responsibility is to monitor and evaluate the client's response to the ventilator. Assess vital signs and listen to breath sounds every 30 to 60 minutes at first. Monitor respiratory parameters (e.g., capnography and pulse oximetry), and check arterial blood gas (ABG) values. Vital signs change during hypercarbia and hypoxemia.

Assess the breathing pattern in relation to the ventilatory cycle to determine whether the client is tolerating or fighting the ventilator. Assess and record breath sounds, including bilateral equal breath sounds to ensure proper endotracheal (ET) tube placement. To determine the need for suctioning, observe secretions for type, color, and amount.

Assess the area around the ET tube or tracheostomy site at least every 4 hours for color, tenderness, skin irritation, and drainage. This monitoring provides information to guide the client's activities, such as weaning, physical or occupational therapy, and self-care. Pace activities so that oxygenation and ventilation are adequate. Interpret ABG values to evaluate ventilation and suggest ventilator settings that help the client.

Because you as the nurse spend the most time with the client, you are most likely to be the first person to recognize slight changes in vital signs or ABG values, fatigue, or distress. Promptly confer with the physician and implement the appropriate interventions.

While monitoring and evaluating the client's clinical status, also serve as a resource for the psychological needs of the client and family. Anxiety can reduce the tolerance of mechanical ventilation. Skilled and sensitive nursing care promotes psychological well-being and promotes synchrony with the ventilator. Because the client cannot speak, communication can be frustrating and anxiety producing. The client and family may panic because they believe that the voice has been lost. Reassure them that the ET tube prevents speech temporarily.

Plan methods of communication to meet the client's needs. Magic Slates, writing paper, computers, and tracheostomy tubes that permit talking are ways to facilitate communication. Finding a successful means for communication is important because the client often feels isolated as a result of the inability to speak. Try to anticipate the client's needs and provide easy access to frequently used belongings. Visits from family, friends, and pets and keeping a call light within reach are some ways of giving clients a sense of control over the environment. Urge the client to participate in self-care.

Managing the Ventilator System. Ventilator settings are prescribed by the physician. These settings include tidal volume, respiratory rate, fraction of inspired oxygen (FIO_2), mode of ventilation (assist-control [AC] ventilation, synchronized intermittent mandatory ventilation [SIMV]), and adjunctive modes, such as positive end-expiratory pressure (PEEP), pressure support, or continuous flow.

Perform and document ventilator checks according to the standards of the unit or facility. Respond promptly to alarms. During a ventilator check, compare the prescribed ventilator settings with the actual settings. Check the level of water in the humidifier and the temperature of the humidifying system to ensure that they are not too high. Temperature extremes damage the airway mucosa. Remove any condensation in the ventilator tubing by draining water into drainage collection receptacles, and empty them every shift. To prevent bacterial contamination, do not allow tubing moisture and water to enter the humidifier.

Mechanical ventilators have alarm systems that warn of a problem with either the client or the ventilator. *Alarm systems must be activated and functional at all times.* If the cause of the alarm cannot be determined, ventilate the client manually with a resuscitation bag until the problem is corrected by another health care professional. The two major alarms on a ventilator indicate either a high pressure or a low exhaled volume. Table 35-5 lists nursing interventions for various causes of ventilator alarms.

Provide proper care of the ET or tracheostomy tube. Maintain a patent airway by suctioning as needed. The following are indications for suctioning in the ventilated client:

- Presence of secretions
- Increased peak airway (inspiratory) pressure (PIP)
- Presence of rhonchi (wheezes)
- Decreased breath sounds

Careful maintenance of the ET or tracheostomy tube also ensures a patent airway. Assess the tube's position at least every 2 hours, especially for the client whose airway is attached to heavy ventilator tubing that may pull on the tracheostomy or ET tube. Position the ventilator tubing in such a way that the client can move without pulling on the ET or tracheostomy tube. The ET tube can move and slip into the right mainstem bronchus. To detect changes in the tube's position, mark the level at which the tube touches the client's teeth or nose. Give mouth care at least every shift for oral hygiene and to prevent loosening of the tape that holds the tube.

Preventing Complications. Most complications are due to the positive pressure from the ventilator. Nearly every body system is affected.

CARDIAC COMPLICATIONS. Cardiac problems from mechanical ventilation include hypotension and fluid retention. Hypotension is caused by positive pressure that increases thoracic pressure and inhibits blood return to the heart. The decreased venous return decreases cardiac output, reflected as hypotension. Hypotension is most often seen in clients who are dehydrated or need high PIP for ventilation. Teach the client to avoid a **Valsalva maneuver** (bearing down while holding the breath) and to prevent constipation, which could result in a Valsalva maneuver.

Fluid is retained because of decreased cardiac output. The kidneys receive less blood flow, which then stimulates the renin-angiotensin-aldosterone system to retain fluid. Also, humidified air in the ventilator system contributes to fluid retention. If humidification is not adequate, the airways become dehydrated and the secretions solidify. Monitor the client's fluid intake and output, weight, hydration, and signs of hypovolemia.

LUNG COMPLICATIONS. The lungs can experience **barotrauma** (damage to the lungs by positive pressure), **volutrauma** (damage to the lung by excess volume delivered to one lung over the other), and acid-base imbalance. Barotrauma includes pneumothorax, subcutaneous emphysema, and pneumomediastinum. Clients at highest risk for barotrauma have chronic airflow limitation (CAL), have blebs, are on PEEP, have dynamic hyperinflation, or require high pressures to ventilate the lungs (because of decreased compliance or "stiff" lungs, as seen in acute respiratory distress syndrome [ARDS]). Blood gas abnormalities can be corrected by ventilator changes and adjustment of fluid and electrolyte imbalances.

GASTROINTESTINAL AND NUTRITIONAL COMPLICATIONS. Gastrointestinal (GI) alterations result from the stress of mechanical ventilation. Stress ulcers occur in about

TABLE 35-5 Nursing Interventions for Various Causes of Ventilator Alarms

Cause	Nursing Interventions
High-Pressure Alarm (sounds when peak inspiratory pressure reaches the set alarm limit [usually set 10-20 mm Hg above the client's baseline PIP])	
There is an increased amount of secretions in the airways or a mucous plug.	Suction as needed.
The client coughs, gags, or bites on the oral ET tube.	Insert oral airway to prevent biting on the ET tube.
The client is anxious or fights the ventilator.	Provide emotional support to decrease anxiety. Increase the flow rate. Explain all procedures to the client. Provide sedation or paralyzing agent per the physician's prescription.
Airway size decreases related to wheezing or bronchospasm.	Auscultate breath sounds. Consult with the physician for management of bronchospasm.
Pneumothorax occurs.	Auscultate breath sounds. Consult with the physician about a new onset of decreased breath sounds or unequal chest excursion, which may be due to pneumothorax.
The artificial airway is displaced; the ET tube may have slipped into the right mainstem bronchus.	Assess the chest for unequal breath sounds and chest excursion. Obtain a chest x-ray as ordered to evaluate the position of the ET tube. After the proper position is verified, tape the tube securely in place.
Obstruction in tubing occurs because the client is lying on the tubing or there is water or a kink in the tubing.	Assess the system, moving from the artificial airway toward the ventilator. Empty water from the ventilator tubing, and remove any kinks.
There is increased PIP associated with deliverance of a sigh.	Consult with respiratory therapist or physician to adjust the pressure alarm.
Decreased compliance of the lung is noted; a trend of gradually increasing PIP is noted over several hours or a day.	Evaluate the reasons for the decreased compliance of the lungs. Increased PIP occurs in ARDS, pneumonia, or any worsening of pulmonary disease.
Low Exhaled Volume (or Low-Pressure) Alarm (sounds when there is a disconnection or leak in the ventilator circuit or a leak in the client's artificial airway cuff)	
A leak in the ventilator circuit prevents breath from being delivered.	Assess all connections and all ventilator tubings for disconnection.
The client stops spontaneous breathing in the SIMV or CPAP mode or on pressure support ventilation.	Evaluate the client's tolerance of the mode.
A cuff leak occurs in the ET or tracheostomy tube.	Evaluate the client for a cuff leak. A cuff leak is suspected when the client is able to talk (air escapes from the mouth) or when the pilot balloon on the artificial airway is flat (see section on tracheostomy tubes in Chapter 31).

ARDS, Acute respiratory distress syndrome; *CPAP*, continuous positive airway pressure; *ET*, endotracheal; *PIP*, Peak inspiratory pressure; *SIMV*, synchronized intermittent mandatory ventilation.

25% of clients receiving mechanical ventilation. Antacids, sucralfate (Carafate, Sulcrate✱), and histamine blockers such as ranitidine (Zantac) or proton-pump inhibitors such as esomeprazole (Nexium) are often prescribed as soon as the client is intubated. Changes in thoracic and abdominal cavity pressure can lead to a paralytic ileus. This problem affects absorption of nutrients through the GI system, requiring short-term parenteral nutritional support.

Malnutrition is a common problem in clients receiving mechanical ventilation. Because many other acute or life-threatening events occur at the same time, nutrition is often neglected. Malnutrition is an extreme problem for these clients and is a major reason why they cannot be weaned from the ventilator. In malnourished clients the respiratory muscles lose mass and strength. The diaphragm, the major muscle of inspiration, is affected early in this process. When the diaphragm and other respiratory muscles are weakened, ineffective breathing results, fatigue occurs, and the client cannot be weaned from the ventilator.

A balanced diet is essential whenever a ventilator is used. Furthermore, nutrition for the client with chronic obstructive pulmonary disease (COPD) requires that special attention be given to the percentage of carbohydrates in the diet. During metabolism, carbohydrates are broken down to glucose, which then produces energy, carbon dioxide, and water. Excessive carbohydrate loads increase carbon dioxide production, which the client with COPD may be unable to exhale. Hypercarbic respiratory failure results. Nutritional formulas with a higher fat content (e.g., Pulmocare, Nutri-Vent, intralipids) are calorie sources to combat this problem.

Electrolyte replacement is also important. Electrolytes have a major impact on ventilatory muscle function. Closely monitor potassium, calcium, magnesium, and phosphate levels, and replenish deficits as prescribed.

INFECTION. Infections are always a potential threat for the client using a ventilator. The ET or tracheostomy tube bypasses the body's normal process of filtering air and provides a direct access for bacteria to the lower parts of the respiratory system. Often within 48 hours the artificial airway is colonized with bacteria, which promotes pneumonia development. Aspiration of colonized fluid from the mouth or the stomach can be a source of infection. Pneumonia pro-

RESOURCE MANAGEMENT

THE CLIENT BEING MECHANICALLY VENTILATED

Cost of Care

Long-term mechanical ventilation is associated with 47% in-hospital mortality, with only 35% of clients surviving at 1 year. Many of the survivors of long-term mechanical ventilation have a need for continued care in an extended care facility. Many report a poor quality of life.

Caregivers of those who have required long-term mechanical ventilation report poor physical health and depression with those whose family member require extended institutional care reporting greater depression than those living at home.

Implications for Nursing

The likelihood of the need for continued care in an extended care facility and the risk of death during the first year following hospital discharge are common features of the population requiring prolonged mechanical ventilation. These factors need to be included in discussions of treatment options that the nurse and other members of the health care team have with clients and their families.

Data from Douglas, S.L., et al. (2002). Survival and quality of life: Short-term versus long-term ventilator patients. *Critical Care Medicine, 30*(12), 2655-2662; and Douglas, S.L., & Daly, B.J. (2003). Caregivers of long-term ventilator patients: Physical and psychological outcomes. *Chest, 123*(4), 1073-1081.

longs hospital stay and increases morbidity. *Infection prevention through strict adherence to infection control, especially handwashing, during suctioning and care of the tracheostomy or ET tube is essential.* To prevent pneumonia, implement ongoing oral care and pulmonary hygiene, including chest physiotherapy, postural drainage, and turning and positioning. More information on pneumonia can be found in Chapter 34.

MUSCULAR COMPLICATIONS. Muscle deconditioning can occur because of immobility. Having the client get out of bed, ambulate with assistance, and perform exercises not only improve muscle strength but also boost morale, facilitate gas exchange, and promote oxygen delivery to all muscles.

VENTILATOR DEPENDENCE. Another complication of mechanical ventilation is ventilator dependence, or inability to wean. Ventilator dependence can be psychological or physiologic, but more often it has a physiologic basis. The longer a client uses a ventilator, the more difficult is the weaning process because the ventilatory muscles fatigue and cannot assume breathing. The cost of maintaining a client with long-term ventilation is great in terms of both actual direct costs and the personal cost of caregivers (see the Resource Management box above). The health care team uses every method of weaning before a client is declared unweanable.

Along with the physician, social worker or psychologist, and a member of the clergy, discuss with the family and the client, as able, the client's quality of life, goals, and values. In accordance with this discussion, make arrangements for home ventilation, nursing home placement, or withdrawal of life support (in terminal cases). Family members who are responsible for providing care to clients receiving long-term mechanical ventilation are at risk for decline in physical health and for depression. These problems occur among caregivers of clients who are placed in care facilities as well as those who are cared for in the home (see the Evidence-Based Practice for Nursing box at right). Special units and facilities are available to maximize the rehabilitation and weaning of ventilator-dependent clients.

EVIDENCE-BASED PRACTICE for Nursing

Caregivers do not care for themselves

Douglas, S., & Daly, B. (2003). Caregivers of long-term ventilator patients: Physical and psychological outcomes. *Chest, 123*(4), 1073-1081.

This prospective, longitudinal, descriptive study examined the physical and psychosocial responses of caregivers of clients requiring long-term ventilation (LTV) either in the home or in a nonacute institutional setting. The purpose of the study was to describe the effects of caring for a client receiving LTV on depression, burden, role overload, and the physical health of caregivers at the time of hospital discharge and 6 months after discharge. This study was part of a larger study to examine the outcomes of clients receiving continuous mechanical ventilation after hospital discharge.

Study participants were caregivers of 135 clients who required LTV after discharge from an acute care setting. *Caregiver* was defined as the adult person who gives the majority of needed care to the client receiving LTV. Caregivers were either self-identified or identified by the client receiving LTV. Caregivers were interviewed both at the time of the client's discharge from the hospital and again 6 months later. Of the clients in the study, 77 had the same caregiver at 6 months as they did at discharge. Interview and data collection instruments used in the study were well-established and had acceptable levels of reliability and validity. Interviewers were trained to use the instruments appropriately, and interrater reliabilities remained at 90% or higher throughout the study period.

The results of the study showed that caregivers overall, experienced a decline in physical health, an increase in depression, and an increase in perceived role overload. About 15% of the subjects had manifestations of severe depression. Interestingly, subjects who were caregivers of clients in institutions had greater depression than did the caregivers of clients residing at home. The results of this study were consistent with those of studies examining caregiver responses for other populations, although the subjects in this study had higher depression scores than those reported among other caregiver groups.

Level of Evidence: 3—Well-designed study without randomization.

Critique. The study was well-designed and well-implemented. The methods and instruments used were appropriate for the questions posed by the study. Study limitations include self-identification and varied definition of the term *caregiver,* the high rate of "false-negative" results of one instrument in assessing depression compared with clinical manifestations, and a limited sample size.

Implications for Nursing. The ongoing care needs of a client requiring LTV place stress and burden on family member caregivers. This burden is still present even when the client is cared for in a long-term care facility. Nurses need to urge caregivers to care for themselves physically and emotionally. Assisting caregivers to find and use respite resources, to share the burden of care with others, and to participate in support groups are all actions that nurses can use to reduce the caregiver's stress and burden. An important intervention for nursing is to assess the caregiver on an ongoing basis for manifestations of depression and to identify caregivers who are at risk for severe depression.

Weaning. *Weaning* is the process of going from ventilatory dependence to spontaneous breathing. The weaning process is prolonged if complications develop. Many complications can be avoided through skillful nursing care. For example, turning and positioning the client not only promote comfort and prevent skin breakdown but also improve gas exchange and prevent pneumonia and atelectasis. Table 35-6 lists various weaning techniques.

TABLE 35-6 Weaning Methods

Synchronous Intermittent Mandatory Ventilation
- The client breathes between the machine's preset breaths/min rate.
- The machine is initially set on an SIMV rate of 12, meaning the client receives a minimum of 12 breaths/min by the ventilator.
- The client's respiratory rate will be a combination of ventilator breaths and spontaneous breaths.
- As the weaning process ensues, the physician prescribes gradual decreases in the SIMV rate, usually at a decrease of 1 to 2 breaths/min.

T-Piece Technique
- The client is taken off the ventilator for short periods (initially 5 to 10 minutes) and allowed to breathe spontaneously.
- The ventilator is replaced with a T-piece (see Chapter 31) or CPAP, which delivers humidified oxygen.
- The prescribed FIO_2 may be higher for the client on the T-piece than on the ventilator.
- Weaning progresses as the client is able to tolerate progressively longer periods off the ventilator.
- Nighttime weaning is not usually attempted until the client is able to maintain spontaneous respirations most of the day.

Pressure Support Ventilation
- PSV allows the client's respiratory effort to be augmented by a predetermined pressure assist from the ventilator.
- As the weaning process ensues, the amount of pressure applied to inspiration is gradually decreased.
- Another method of weaning with PSV is to maintain the pressure but gradually decrease the ventilator's preset breaths/min rate.

CPAP, Continuous positive airway pressure; *FIO_2*, fraction of inspired oxygen; *PSV*, pressure support ventilation; *SIMV*, synchronized intermittent mandatory ventilation.

CONSIDERATIONS FOR OLDER ADULTS

The older client, especially one who has smoked or who has a chronic lung problem such as COPD, is at risk for ventilator dependence and failure to wean. Age-related changes, such as increased chest wall stiffness, reduced ventilatory muscle strength, and decreased lung elasticity, reduce the likelihood of weaning. The usual manifestations of ventilatory failure—hypoxemia and hypercarbia—may be less obvious in the older adult, and other clinical measures of oxygenation, such as a change in mental status, must be used.

Extubation. **Extubation** is the removal of the endotracheal (ET) tube. The tube is removed when the need for intubation has been resolved. Before removal, explain the procedure. Set up the prescribed oxygen delivery system at the bedside, and bring in the equipment for emergency reintubation. Hyperoxygenate the client and thoroughly suction both the ET tube and the oral cavity. Then rapidly deflate the cuff of the ET tube and remove the tube at peak inspiration. Immediately instruct the client to cough. It is normal for large amounts of oral secretions to collect. Give oxygen by face mask or nasal cannula. The fraction of inspired oxygen (FIO_2) is usually prescribed at 10% higher than the level used while the ET tube was in place.

Monitoring after extubation is essential. Monitor the vital signs every hour initially, assessing the ventilatory pattern and for manifestations of respiratory distress. It is common for clients to be hoarse and have a sore throat for a few days after extubation. Instruct the client to sit in a semi-Fowler's position, take deep breaths every half-hour, use an incentive spirometer every 2 hours, and limit speaking in the immediate period after extubation. These measures help gas exchange, decrease laryngeal edema, and reduce vocal cord irritation. Observe closely for respirator fatigue and airway obstruction (see Chapter 31).

Early manifestations of obstruction are mild dyspnea, coughing, and the inability to expectorate secretions. Notify the physician at the onset of these problems. The physician then evaluates the need for reintubation. ***Stridor** is a high-pitched, crowing noise during inspiration caused by laryngospasm or edema above or below the glottis. This sound is a late manifestation of a narrowed airway and requires prompt attention.* Racemic epinephrine, a topical aerosol vasoconstrictor, is given, and reintubation may be needed.

CHEST TRAUMA

Chest injuries are responsible for about 25% of all civilian traumatic deaths. More than 50% of the injured die before arriving at health care facilities. Only 5% to 15% of all chest injuries require thoracotomy. The remainder can be treated with basic resuscitation, intubation, or chest tube placement. The initial emergency approach to all chest injuries is ABC (*a*irway, *b*reathing, *c*irculation) followed by rapid assessment and treatment of life-threatening conditions.

Pulmonary Contusion

PATHOPHYSIOLOGY

Pulmonary contusion, a potentially lethal injury, is the most common chest injury seen in the United States. After a contusion, respiratory failure develops over time rather than immediately. This condition most often follows injuries caused by rapid deceleration during vehicular accidents. Hemorrhage occurs in and between the alveoli. The resulting edema decreases pulmonary compliance and reduces the area for gas exchange. The client becomes hypoxemic and dyspneic. The bronchial mucosa is irritated and secretions increase.

COLLABORATIVE MANAGEMENT

Assessment

Clients with pulmonary contusion may be asymptomatic at first and can later develop respiratory failure. These clients present with hemoptysis, decreased breath sounds, crackles, and wheezes. Initially, the chest x-ray may show no abnormalities. A hazy opacity in the lobes or parenchyma may develop over several days. If there is no disruption of the parenchyma, resorption of the lesion often occurs without treatment.

Interventions

Treatment includes maintenance of ventilation and oxygenation. Central venous pressure (CVP) is monitored closely, and fluid intake is restricted as needed. The client in obvious respiratory distress may need mechanical ventilation with positive end-expiratory pressure (PEEP) to inflate the lungs.

A vicious cycle occurs in which more muscle effort is needed for ventilating a lung with a contusion and the client becomes progressively hypoxemic. This situation causes the client to tire easily, have reduced gas exchange, and become more fatigued and hypoxemic. Flail chest may also occur when pulmonary contusion occurs with parenchymal damage.

This condition often leads to acute respiratory distress syndrome (ARDS).

Rib Fracture

PATHOPHYSIOLOGY

After chest-wall contusion, rib fractures are the next most common injury to the chest wall. Rib fractures most often result from direct blunt trauma to the chest. Direct force applied to the ribs fractures them and drives the bone ends into the thorax. Thus there is a risk for intrathoracic injury, such as pulmonary contusion or pneumothorax, which occurs most often if ribs one through four are fractured.

COLLABORATIVE MANAGEMENT

The client has pain on movement and splints the chest defensively. Splinting reduces breathing depth and leads to inadequate clearance of pulmonary secretions. If the client has pre-existing pulmonary disease, the risk for atelectasis and pneumonia increases. Clients with injuries to the first or second ribs, flail chest, seven or more fractured ribs, or expired volumes of less than 15 mL/kg often have an intrathoracic injury and a poor prognosis.

Treatment for uncomplicated rib fractures is nonspecific because the fractured ribs reunite spontaneously. The chest is usually not splinted by tape or other materials. The main focus is to decrease pain so that adequate ventilation is maintained. An intercostal nerve block may be used if pain is severe. Potent analgesics that cause respiratory depression are avoided.

Flail Chest

PATHOPHYSIOLOGY

Flail chest is the inward movement of the thorax during inspiration, with outward movement during expiration. It usually involves one side of the chest and results from multiple rib fractures caused by blunt chest trauma leaving a segment of the chest wall loose. Flail chest often occurs in high-speed vehicular crashes. It is more common in older clients and has a high mortality rate (40%).

The movement of this loose segment becomes paradoxic to the expansion and contraction of the rest of the chest wall. Flail chest can also occur from bilateral separations of the ribs from their cartilage connections to each other anteriorly, without an actual rib fracture. This condition can occur during cardiopulmonary resuscitation on an older adult. Other injuries to the lung tissue under the flail segment may be present. Gas exchange is impaired, as is the ability to cough and clear secretions. Defensive splinting further reduces the client's ability to exert the extra effort required for breathing and may contribute later to failure to wean.

COLLABORATIVE MANAGEMENT

Assessment

Assess the client with a flail chest for paradoxic chest movement, dyspnea, cyanosis, tachycardia, and hypotension. **Paradoxic chest movement** is the "sucking inward" of the loose chest area during inspiration and a "puffing out" of the same area during expiration. The client is often anxious, short of breath, and in pain.

Interventions

Interventions include humidified oxygen, pain management, promotion of lung expansion through deep breathing and positioning, and secretion clearance by coughing and tracheal aspiration.

The client with a flail chest may be treated conservatively with vigilant respiratory care. Mechanical ventilation may be needed if respiratory failure or shock occurs. Monitor arterial blood gas (ABG) values closely, along with vital capacity. With severe hypoxemia and hypercarbia, the client is intubated and mechanically ventilated with PEEP. With pulmonary contusion or an underlying pulmonary disease, the risk for respiratory failure increases. Flail chest is best stabilized by positive-pressure ventilation rather than surgical intervention. Surgical stabilization is used only in extreme cases of flail chest.

Monitor the client's vital signs and fluid and electrolyte balance closely so that hypovolemia or shock can be treated immediately. If the client has a pulmonary contusion, monitor central venous pressure (CVP) and give IV fluids as prescribed. Assess for pain and intervene to relieve the pain. Analgesic drugs by IV, epidural, or nerve block route may be prescribed.

Give psychosocial support to the extremely anxious client by explaining all procedures, talking slowly, and allowing time to verbalize feelings and concerns.

Pneumothorax

PATHOPHYSIOLOGY

Any chest injury that allows air to enter the pleural space results in a rise in intrathoracic pressure and a reduction in vital capacity. Severity depends on the amount of pulmonary collapse produced. Pneumothorax is often caused by blunt chest trauma and may occur with some degree of hemothorax. The pneumothorax can be open (pleural cavity is exposed to outside air, as through an open wound in the chest wall) or closed.

COLLABORATIVE MANAGEMENT

Assessment findings commonly include the following:

- Reduced breath sounds on auscultation
- Hyperresonance on percussion
- Prominence of the involved side of the chest, which moves poorly with respirations
- Deviation of the trachea away from (closed) or toward (open) the affected side

In addition, the client may have pleuritic pain, tachypnea, and **subcutaneous emphysema** (air under the skin in the subcutaneous tissues).

A chest x-ray is used for diagnosis. Chest tubes may be needed to allow the air to escape and the lung to reinflate.

Tension Pneumothorax

PATHOPHYSIOLOGY

Tension pneumothorax, a rapidly developing and life-threatening complication of blunt chest trauma, results from an air leak in the lung or chest wall. Air forced into the chest cavity causes complete collapse of the affected lung. Air that enters the pleural space during expiration does not exit during inspiration. As a result, air continues to accumulate under pressure, compressing blood vessels, and limiting venous return. Because this process leads to decreased filling of the heart, cardiac output is reduced. If not promptly detected and treated, tension pneumothorax is quickly fatal. Causes of tension pneumothorax are blunt chest trauma, mechanical ventilation with positive end-expiratory pressure (PEEP), closed-chest drainage (chest tubes), and insertion of central venous access catheters.

COLLABORATIVE MANAGEMENT

Assessment

Assessment findings with tension pneumothorax include the following:

- Asymmetry of the thorax
- Tracheal deviation to the unaffected side
- Respiratory distress
- Absence of breath sounds on one side
- Distended neck veins
- Cyanosis
- Hypertympanic sound on percussion over the affected side

Pneumothorax is detectable on a chest x-ray. ABG assays show hypoxia and respiratory alkalosis.

Interventions

A large-bore needle is inserted into the second intercostal space in the midclavicular line of the affected side as initial treatment for tension pneumothorax. After this measure is completed, a chest tube is placed into the fourth intercostal space, and the other end is attached to a water seal drainage system until the lung reinflates.

Hemothorax

PATHOPHYSIOLOGY

Hemothorax is a common problem occurring after blunt chest trauma or penetrating injuries. A *simple* hemothorax is a blood loss of less than 1500 mL into the chest cavity; a *massive* hemothorax is a blood loss of more than 1500 mL.

Bleeding is caused by injury to the lung tissue, such as pulmonary contusions or lacerations, that can occur with rib and sternal fractures. Massive intrathoracic bleeding in blunt chest trauma may stem from the heart, great vessels, or the intercostal arteries.

COLLABORATIVE MANAGEMENT

Assessment

Physical assessment findings vary with the size of the hemothorax. If the hemothorax is small, the client may be asymptomatic. If the hemothorax is larger, the client may have respiratory distress. In addition, breath sounds are reduced on auscultation. Percussion on the involved side results in a dull sound. Blood in the pleural space is visible on a chest x-ray and confirmed by diagnostic thoracentesis.

Interventions

Interventions are aimed at removing the blood in the pleural space to normalize pulmonary function and to prevent infection. Anterior and posterolateral chest tubes are inserted to evacuate the pleural space. Carefully monitor the chest tube drainage. The physician evaluates chest x-rays serially to determine treatment effectiveness.

An open thoracotomy may be needed when there is initial evacuation of 1500 to 2000 mL of blood or persistent bleeding at the rate of 200 mL/hr over 3 hours. Monitor the vital signs, blood loss, and overall intake and output. Assess the client's response to the chest tubes, and infuse IV fluids and blood as prescribed. Autotransfusion of the blood lost through chest drainage may be considered.

Tracheobronchial Trauma

PATHOPHYSIOLOGY

Most tears of the tracheobronchial tree result from severe blunt trauma or rapid deceleration. The tears often involve the mainstem bronchi. Injuries to the trachea usually occur at the junction of the trachea and cricoid cartilage. These injuries are often caused by striking the neck against the dashboard or steering wheel during a motor-vehicle crash. Clients with lacerations of the trachea develop massive air leaks, which cause air to enter the mediastinum and extensive subcutaneous emphysema. Upper-airway obstruction may also occur, causing severe respiratory distress and inspiratory stridor. Large tracheal tears are managed by cricothyroidotomy or tracheotomy below the level of injury. A client with a torn mainstem bronchus may develop a tension pneumothorax rapidly once he or she is intubated and ventilated with positive pressure.

COLLABORATIVE MANAGEMENT

Assess the client for hypoxemia by ABG assays. Apply oxygen as needed. Depending on the degree of injury, the client may need mechanical ventilation or surgical repair. Assess vital signs every 15 minutes because the client is likely to be hypotensive and in shock. Continue to assess for subcutaneous emphysema and auscultate the lungs every 1 to 2 hours. Decreased breath sounds or wheezing may indicate further obstruction, atelectasis, or pneumothorax. Care of the client with a tracheostomy is discussed in Chapter 31.

GET READY for the NCLEX Examination!

KEY POINTS

Safe Effective Care Environment

- Use aseptic technique when caring for a client requiring pulmonary suctioning.
- Identify clients in your setting who are at risk for developing a pulmonary embolism.
- Use bleeding precautions for any client receiving anticoagulant or fibrinolytic therapy (see Chart 35-6).
- Keep antidotes available when clients are receiving heparin (antidote is protamine) or warfarin (antidote is vitamin K).
- Inspect the oral mucous membranes each shift for anyone who has an endotracheal tube.
- Ensure that alarm systems on mechanical ventilators are activated and functional at all times.

Health Promotion and Maintenance

- Teach clients ways to promote venous return and avoid deep vein thrombosis (DVT), especially when traveling long distances (see Chart 35-1).
- Use aspiration precautions for any client with an altered level of consciousness, poor gag reflex, neurologic impairment, or who has an endotracheal tube.
- Check the client with ARDS hourly for oxygen saturation, vital sign changes, or any indication of increased work of breathing such as cyanosis, pallor, and retractions.
- Assess all clients with blunt chest trauma for position of the trachea and bilateral breath sounds.
- Encourage all people to use proper safety restraints when driving or riding in motor vehicles.

Psychosocial Integrity

- Allow the client and family members the opportunity to express fear or anxiety regarding a change in breathing status or the possibility of intubation and mechanical ventilation.
- Explain all diagnostic procedures, restrictions, and follow-up care to the client scheduled for tests.
- Teach family members ways to communicate with a client who is intubated or being mechanically ventilated.
- Reassure intubated clients that speech loss is temporary.
- Remember that clients who are receiving mechanical ventilation and are being chemically paralyzed may have sensations of all types (can hear and can feel pain).

Physiological Integrity

- Notify the physician immediately for any client who develops sudden-onset respiratory difficulty.
- Check oxygen saturation by pulse oximetry for any client who has respiratory difficulty or who develops acute confusion.
- Evaluate arterial blood gas values to determine the severity of hypoxia and the client's response to therapy.
- Apply oxygen to anyone who is hypoxemic.
- Ensure that oxygen therapy delivered to the client is humidified (and warmed, when possible).
- Assess lung sounds bilaterally each hour for clients who are receiving PEEP.
- Check all ventilator settings against the prescription at least once per shift.
- Administer pain medications to clients who have rib fractures and encourage deep breaths.
- Maintain a patent airway on all clients who experience trauma.

ADDITIONAL STUDY RESOURCES

Go to your Student CD-ROM for Review Questions for the NCLEX Examination.

evolve Go to http://evolve.elsevier.com/Iggy/ for Integrated Management of Care Questions for the NCLEX Examination.

SELECTED BIBLIOGRAPHY

Asterisk indicates a classic or definitive work on this subject.

The Acute Respiratory Distress Syndrome Network. (2000). Ventilation with lower tidal volumes as compared with traditional tidal volumes for acute lung injury. *New England Journal of Medicine, 352*(18), 1301-1308.

Andrews, C. (2002). Emergency: Preventing air embolism. *American Journal of Nursing, 102*(1), 35-36.

Austan, F. (2002). Management of respiratory failure with noninvasive positive pressure ventilation and heliox adjunct. *Heart & Lung, 31*(3), 214-218.

Ayers, D., & Lappin, J. (2004). Act fast when your patient has dyspnea. *Nursing 2004, 34*(7), 36-41.

Balas, M. (2000). Prone positioning of patients with acute respiratory distress syndrome: Applying research to practice. *Critical Care Nurse, 20*(1), 24-36.

*Baldwin-Myers, A., et al. (1994). *Standards of care for the ventilator-assisted individual: A comprehensive management plan from hospital to home.* Loma Linda, CA: Loma Linda University/Respiratory Nursing Society.

Behnia, M., & Garrett, K. (2004). Association of tension pneumothorax with use of small-bore chest tubes in patients receiving mechanical ventilation. *Critical Care Nurse, 24*(1), 64-66.

*Burns, S. (1998). Making weaning easier: Pathways and protocols that work. *Critical Care Nursing Clinics of North America, 11*(4), 465-479.

*Burns, S. (1999). The long-term mechanically ventilated patient: An outcomes management approach. *Critical Care Nursing Clinics of North America, 10*(1), 87-97.

*Burns, S.M. (1999). Weaning from long-term mechanical ventilation. In C.M. Chulay & S.M. Burns (Eds.), *Care of the mechanically ventilated patient series.* Aliso Viejo, CA: American Association of Critical Care Nurses.

Carroll, P. (2002). Procedural sedation: Capnography's heightened role. *RN, 65*(10), 54-63.

*Clochesy, J., Daly, B., & Montenegro, H. (1995). Weaning chronically critically ill adults from mechanical ventilatory support: A descriptive study. *American Journal of Critical Care, 4*(2), 93-99.

Connelly, B., Gunzerath, L., & Knebel, A. (2000). A pilot study exploring mood state and dyspnea in mechanically ventilated patients. *Heart & Lung, 29*(3), 173-179.

Davies, P. (2002). Guarding your patient against ARDS. *Nursing 2002, 32*(3), 36-42.

Dochterman, J., & Bulechek, G. (eds). (2004). *Nursing interventions classification (NIC)* (4th ed). St. Louis: Mosby.

Douglas, S., & Daly, B. (2003). Caregivers of long-term ventilator patients: Physical and psychological outcomes. *Chest, 123*(4), 1073-1081.

Douglas, S., et al. (2002). Survival and quality of life: Short-term versus long-term ventilator patients. *Critical Care Medicine, 30*(12), 2655-2662.

Ebersole, P., Hess, P., & Luggen, A. (2004). *Toward healthy aging: Human needs and nursing response* (6th ed). St. Louis: Mosby.

Ellstrom, K. (2000). Relationship of psychoneurological, physiological, and environmental constructs to risk of unplanned extubation and outcomes in medical ICU patients. Doctoral Disseration, University of California Los Angeles.

El-Masri, M., Williamson, K., & Fox-Wasylyshyn, S. (2004). Severe acute respiratory syndrome: Another challenge for critical care nurses. *AACN Clinical Issues: Advanced Practice in Acute and Critical Care, 15*(1), 150-159.

Facts and Comparisons. (2004). *Drug facts and comparisons* (58th ed). St. Louis: Author.

Frawley, P., & Habashi, N. (2001). Airway pressure release ventilation: Theory and practice. *AACN Clinical Issues: Advanced Practice in Acute and Critical Care, 12*(2), 235-246.

Giuliano, K., & Higgins, T. (2005). New generation pulse oximetry in the care of critically ill patients. *American Journal of Critical Care, 14*(1), 26-37.

Greifzu, S. (2002). Caring for the chronically critically ill. *RN, 65*(7), 42-44, 46, 48-49.

Hanneman, S. (2004). Weaning from short-term mechanical ventilation. *Critical Care Nurse, 24*(1), 70-73.

Happ, M.B. (2000). Preventing treatment interference: The nurse's role in maintaining technological devices. *Heart and Lung, 29*(1), 60-69.

Happ, M.B. (2001). Communicating with mechanically ventilated patients: State of the science. *AACN Clinical Issues: Advanced Practice in Acute and Critical Care, 12*(2), 247-258.

Howard, A., et al. (2004). Comparison of 3 methods of detecting acute respiratory distress syndrome: Clinical screening, chart review, and diagnostic coding. *American Journal of Critical Care, 13*(1), 59-64.

Kleinpell, R. (2003). The role of the critical care nurse in the assessment and management of the patient with severe sepsis. *Critical Care Clinics of North America, 15*(1), 27-34.

Marion, B. (2001). A turn for the better: "Prone positioning" of patients with ARDS. *American Journal of Nursing, 101*(5), 26-34.

Marini, J.J,, & Gattinoni, L. (2004). Ventilatory management of acute respiratory syndrome: A consensus of two. *Critical Care Medicine, 32*(1), 250-255.

McCance, K., & Huether, S. (2002). *Pathophysiology: The biologic basis for disease in adults and children* (4th ed). St. Louis: Mosby.

Mitchell, D. (2004). Vent injury: How to avoid it. *RN, 67*(7), 54-59.

Moorhead, S., Johnson, M., & Maas, M. (Eds.). (2004). *Nursing outcomes classification (NOC)* (3rd ed). St. Louis: Mosby.

O'Bryan, L., Von Rueden, K., & Malila, F. (2002). Evaluating ventilator weaning best practice: A long-term acute care hospital systemwide quality initiative. *AACN Clinical Issues, 13*(4), 567-576.

O'Keefe, G. et al. (2001). Indicators of fatigue and of prolonged weaning from mechanical ventilation in surgical patients. *World Journal of Surgery, 25*(1), 98-103.

Pfeifer, L., et al. (2001). Preventing ventilator-associated pneumonia. *American Journal of Nursing, 101*(8), 24AA-24GG.

Phelan, B., Cooper, D., & Sangkachand, P. (2002). Prolonged mechanical ventilation and tracheostomy in the elderly. *AACN Clinical Issues, 13*(1), 84-93.

Pierce, L. (2000). Traditional and nontraditional modes of mechanical ventilation. *Critical Care Nurse, 20*(1), 81-84.

Pruitt, W. (2004). Manual ventilation by one or two rescuers. *Nursing 2004, 34*(11), 43-45.

Richmond, A., Jarog, D., & Hanson, V. (2004). Unplanned extubation in adult critical care: Quality improvement and education payoff. *Critical Care Nurse, 24*(1), 32-37.

Seay, S., Gay, S., & Strauss, M. (2002). Emergency: Managing tracheostomy decannulation and displacement. *American Journal of Nursing, 102*(3), 59,61-63.

Spritzer, C. (2003). Unraveling the mysteries of mechanical ventilation: A helpful step-by-step guide. *Journal of Emergency Nursing, 29*(1), 29-36.

St. John, R. (2004). Airway management. *Critical Care Nurse, 24*(2), 93-96.

Veronesi, J. (2004). Blunt chest injuries. *RN, 67*(3), 48-54.

Winkelman, C. (2004). Inactivity and inflammation: Selected cytokines as biologic mediators in muscle dysfunction during critical illness. *AACN Clinical Issues: Advanced Practice in Acute and Critical Care, 15*(1), 74-82.

Woodruff, D. (2003). Protect your patient while he's receiving mechanical ventilation. *Nursing 2003, 33*(7), 32hn1-32hn4.

Yagan, M., White, D., & Staab, J. (2000). Sedation of the mechanically ventilated patient. *Critical Care Nursing Quarterly, 22*(4), 90-100.

Yantis, M.A. (2003). Assisting patients using positive airway pressure therapy. *Home Healthcare Nurse, 21*(3), 160-165.

Yosefy, C., et al. (2003). BiPAP ventilation as assistance for patients presenting with respiratory distress in the department of emergency medicine. *American Journal of Respiratory Medicine, 2*(4), 343-347.

UNIT **EIGHT**

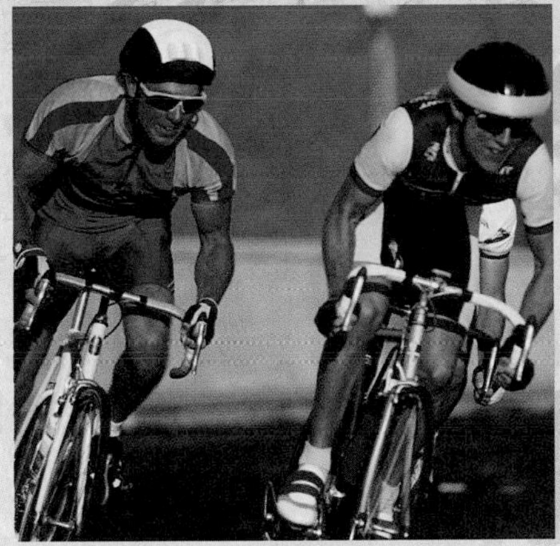

PROBLEMS of CARDIAC OUTPUT and TISSUE PERFUSION

Management of Clients with Problems of the Cardiovascular System

CHAPTER

36 Assessment of the Cardiovascular System

DEANNE A. BLACH

LEARNING OUTCOMES

After studying this chapter, you should be able to:

1. Review the anatomy and physiology of the cardiovascular system.
2. Describe cardiovascular changes associated with aging.
3. Identify factors that place clients at risk for cardiovascular problems.
4. Perform appropriate physical assessment for clients with cardiovascular problems.
5. Interpret laboratory test findings for clients with suspected or actual cardiovascular disease.
6. Explain and pre- and post-test care associated with diagnostic cardiovascular testing.
7. Explain the purpose of hemodynamic monitoring.

Go to your Student CD-ROM for Review Questions for the NCLEX Examination keyed to these Learning Outcomes.

In every year since 1900 (except 1918), cardiovascular disease (CVD) has been the number one cause of death in the United States. It remains the major cause of mortality in the twenty-first century, resulting in 42% of all deaths, or nearly one million deaths, each year in the United States. CVD kills more people than the next five causes of death combined, including cancer, chronic lower respiratory diseases, accidents, diabetes, influenza, and pneumonia. It is the leading cause of death for women. In addition, the American Heart Association (AHA) estimates that about one in five people has experienced, and is living with some form of CVD (AHA, 2002).

ANATOMY AND PHYSIOLOGY REVIEW

Heart

Structure

The human heart is a cone-shaped, hollow, muscular organ located in the mediastinum between the lungs (Figure 36-1). It is about the size of an adult fist. The heart rests on the diaphragm, tilting forward and to the left in the client's chest. Each beat of the heart pumps about 60 mL of blood, or 5 L/min. During strenuous physical activity, the heart can double the amount of blood pumped to meet the increased oxygen needs of the peripheral tissues.

The heart is encapsulated by a protective covering called the *pericardium* (see Figure 36-2). Cardiac muscle tissue is composed of three layers: epicardium, myocardium, and endocardium. The *epicardium,* the outer surface, is a thin, transparent tissue. The *myocardium,* the middle layer, is composed of striated muscle fibers interlaced into bundles. This layer is responsible for the contractile force of the heart. The innermost layer, the *endocardium,* is composed of endothelial tissue. This tissue lines the inside of the chambers of the heart and covers the four heart valves.

CHAMBERS OF THE HEART

A muscular wall (septum) separates the heart into two halves: right and left. Each half has an upper chamber (atrium) and a lower chamber (ventricle) (see Figure 36-2).

RIGHT SIDE. The right atrium (RA) is a thin-walled structure that receives deoxygenated venous blood (venous return) from all peripheral tissues by way of the superior and inferior venae cavae and from the heart muscle by way of the coronary sinus. Most of this venous return flows passively from the RA, through the opened tricuspid valve, and to the right ventricle during ventricular diastole, or filling. The remaining venous return is actively propelled by the RA into the right ventricle during atrial systole, or contraction.

The right ventricle is a flat muscular pump located behind the sternum. The right ventricle generates enough pressure (about 25 mm Hg) to close the tricuspid valve, open the pulmonic valve, and propel blood into the pulmonary artery and the lungs. The workload of the right ventricle is light compared with that of the left ventricle because the pulmonary system is normally a low-pressure system, which imposes less resistance to flow.

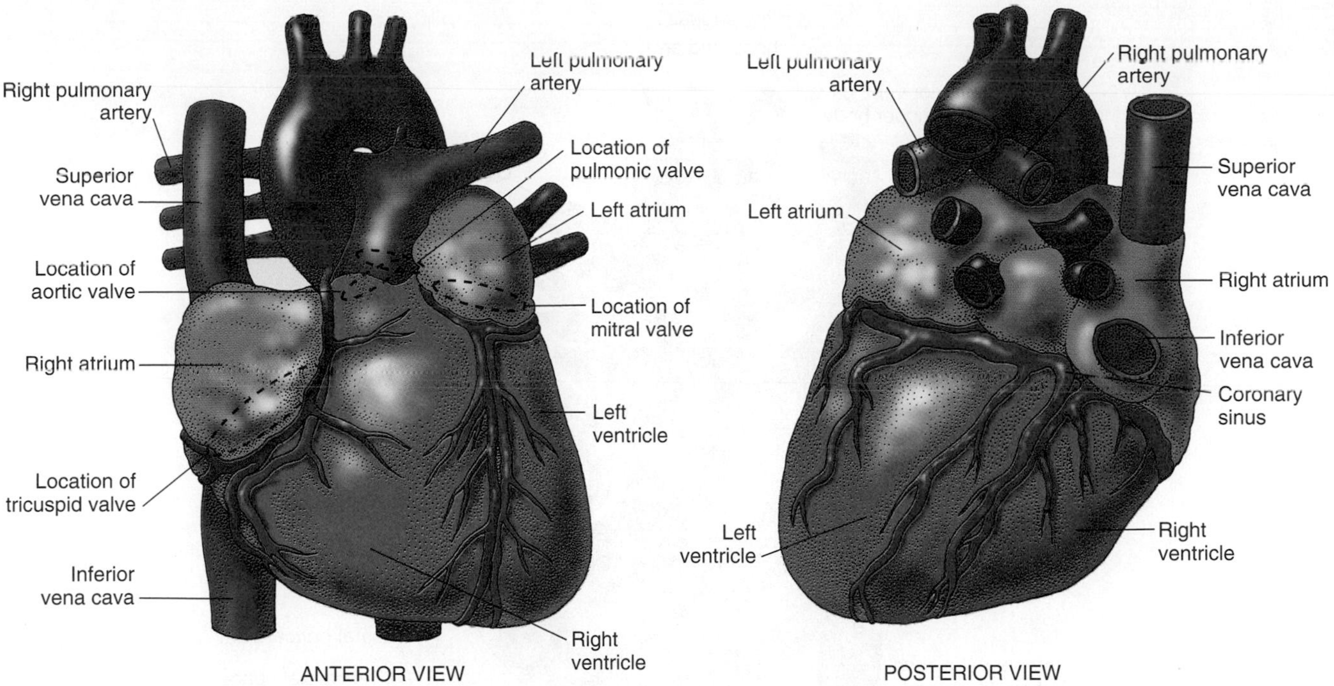

Figure 36-1 ■ Surface anatomy of the heart.

LEFT SIDE. After blood is reoxygenated in the lungs, it flows freely from the four pulmonary veins into the left atrium. Blood then flows through an opened mitral valve into the left ventricle during ventricular diastole. When the left ventricle is almost full, the left atrium contracts, pumping the remaining blood volume into the left ventricle. With systolic contraction, the left ventricle generates enough pressure (approximately 120 mm Hg) to close the mitral valve and open the aortic valve. Blood is propelled into the aorta and into the systemic arterial circulation. Blood flow through the heart is shown in Figure 36-2.

The left ventricle is ellipsoid in shape and is the largest and most muscular chamber of the heart. Its wall is two to three times the thickness of the right ventricular wall. The left ventricle must generate a higher pressure than the right ventricle because it must contract against a high-pressure systemic circulation, which imposes a greater resistance to blood flow.

Blood is propelled from the aorta throughout the systemic circulation to the various tissues of the body; blood returns to the RA because of pressure differences. The pressure of blood in the aorta of a young adult averages about 100 to 120 mm Hg, whereas the pressure of blood in the RA averages about 0 to 5 mm Hg. These differences in pressure produce a pressure gradient, with blood flowing from an area of higher pressure to an area of lower pressure. The heart and vascular structures are responsible for maintaining these pressures.

HEART VALVES

The four cardiac valves are responsible for maintaining the forward flow of blood through the chambers of the heart (see Figure 36-2). These valves open and close passively in response to pressure and volume changes within the cardiac chambers. The cardiac valves are classified into two types: atrioventricular (AV) valves and semilunar valves. Both AV valves are supported by chordae tendineae, which keep them from everting into the atria during systole.

ATRIOVENTRICULAR VALVES. The AV valves separate the atria from the ventricles. The tricuspid valve is composed of three leaflets and separates the RA from the right ventricle. The mitral (bicuspid) valve is composed of two leaflets and separates the left atrium from the left ventricle.

During ventricular diastole, the valves act as funnels and facilitate the flow of blood from the atria to the ventricles. During systole, the valves close to prevent the backflow (regurgitation) of blood into the atria.

SEMILUNAR VALVES. The two semilunar valves are the pulmonic valve and the aortic valve. The pulmonic valve separates the right ventricle from the pulmonary artery. The aortic valve separates the left ventricle from the aorta. Each semilunar valve consists of three cuplike cusps, or pockets, around the inside wall of the artery. These cusps prevent blood from flowing back into the ventricles during ventricular diastole. During ventricular systole, these valves are open to permit blood flow into the pulmonary artery and the aorta.

CORONARY ARTERIES

The heart muscle receives blood to meet its metabolic needs through the coronary arterial system (Figure 36-3). The coronary arteries originate from an area on the aorta just beyond the aortic valve. The two main coronary arteries are the left coronary artery (LCA) and the right coronary artery (RCA).

Coronary artery blood flow to the myocardium occurs primarily during diastole, when coronary vascular resistance is minimized. To maintain adequate blood flow through the coronary arteries, **mean arterial pressure (MAP)** must be at least 60 mm Hg. A MAP of between 60 and 70 mm Hg is necessary to maintain perfusion of major body organs, such as the kidneys and brain.

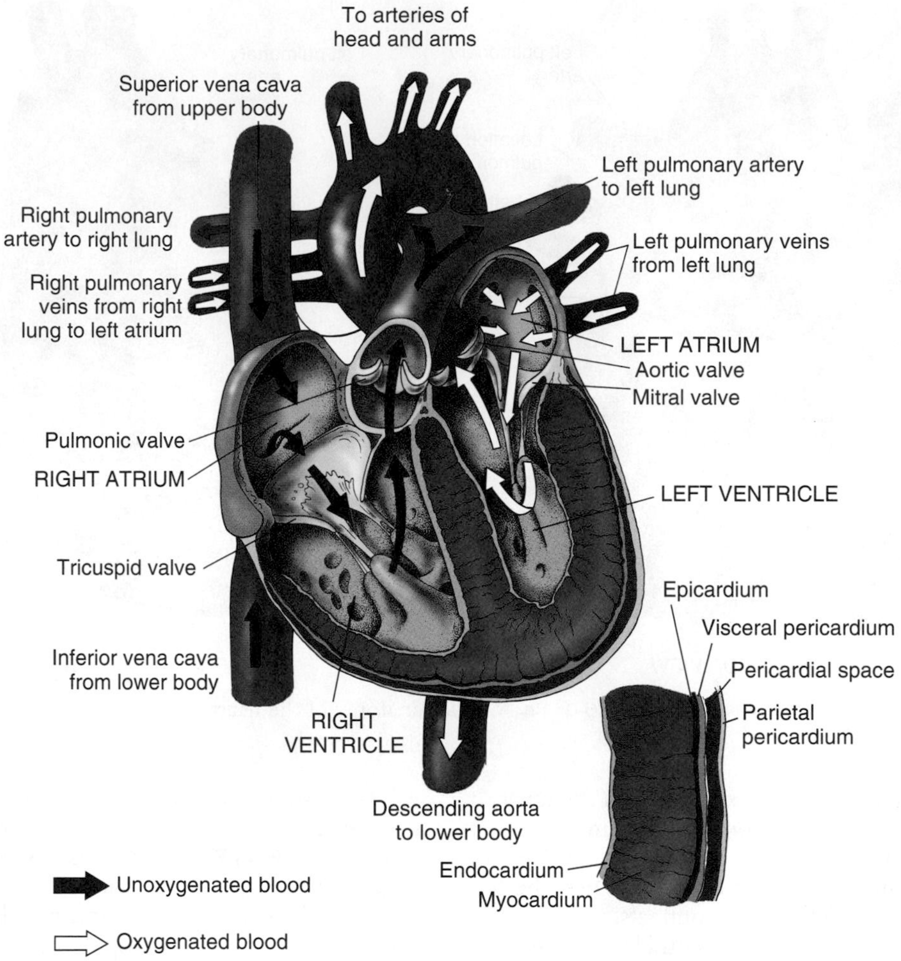

Figure 36-2 ■ Blood flow through the heart.

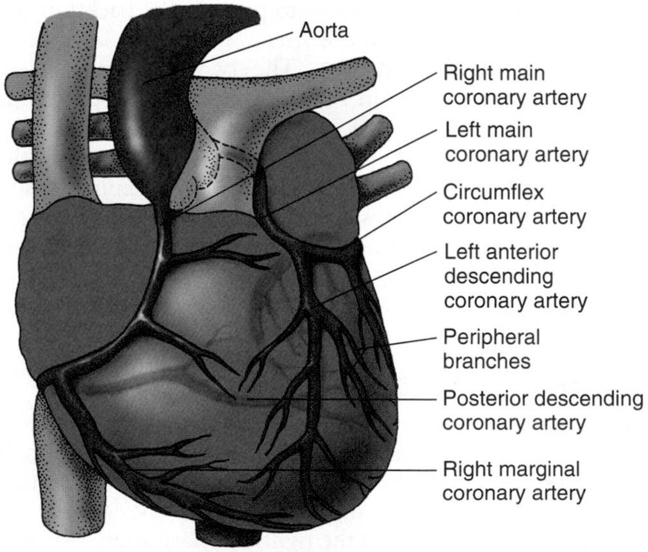

Figure 36-3 ■ Coronary arterial system.

LEFT MAIN ARTERY. The left main artery divides into two branches: the left anterior descending (LAD) and the circumflex coronary artery (LCX). The LAD branch descends toward the anterior wall and the apex of the left ventricle. It supplies blood to portions of the left ventricle, ventricular septum, chordae tendineae, papillary muscle, and, to a lesser extent, the right ventricle.

The LCX descends toward the lateral wall of the left ventricle and apex. It supplies blood to the left atrium, the lateral and posterior surfaces of the left ventricle, and sometimes portions of the interventricular septum. In 45% of people, the LCX supplies the sinoatrial (SA) node, and in 10% of people it supplies the AV node. Peripheral branches (diagonal and obtuse marginal) arise from the LAD and LCX and form an abundant network of vessels throughout the entire myocardium.

RIGHT CORONARY ARTERY. The RCA originates from the right sinus of Valsalva, encircles the heart, and descends toward the apex of the right ventricle. The RCA supplies the RA, right ventricle, and inferior portion of the left ventricle. The branching pattern of the coronary arteries varies considerably among individuals.

Function

ELECTROPHYSIOLOGIC PROPERTIES OF THE HEART

The electrophysiologic properties of heart muscle are responsible for regulating heart rate (HR) and rhythm. Cardiac muscle cells possess the characteristics of automaticity, excitability, conductivity, contractility, and refractoriness.

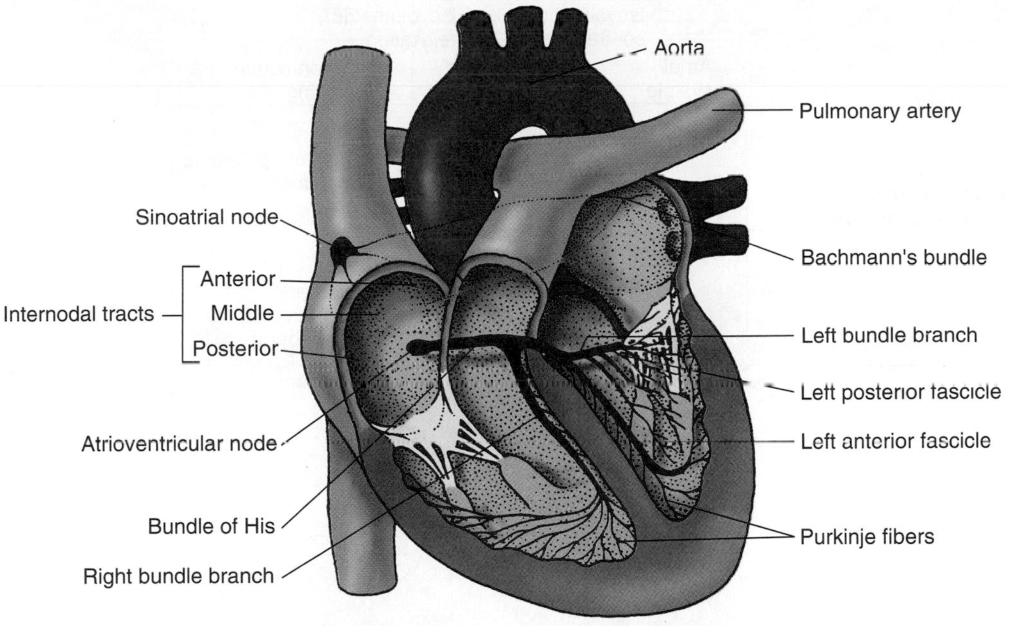

Figure 36-4 ■ Conduction system of the heart.

Automaticity refers to the ability of all cardiac cells to initiate an impulse spontaneously and repetitively. **Excitability** is the ability of the cells to respond to a stimulus by initiating an impulse **(depolarization). Conductivity** means that cardiac cells transmit the electrical impulses they receive. Because the cells possess the property of **contractility,** they also contract in response to an impulse. **Refractoriness** means that cardiac cells are unable to respond to a stimulus until they have recovered (repolarized) from the previous stimulus. These properties are described more completely in Chapter 37.

CONDUCTION SYSTEM OF THE HEART

The cardiac conduction system is composed of specialized tissue capable of rhythmic electrical impulse formation (Figure 36-4). It can conduct impulses much more rapidly than other cells located in the myocardium. The SA node, located at the junction of the RA and the superior vena cava, is considered the main regulator of HR. The SA node is composed of pacemaker cells, which spontaneously initiate impulses at a rate of 60 to 100 times/min, and myocardial working cells, which transmit the impulses to the surrounding atrial muscle.

An impulse from the SA node initiates the process of depolarization and hence the activation of all myocardial cells. The impulse travels through both atria to the atrioventricular (AV) node located in the junctional area. After the impulse reaches the AV node, conduction of the impulse is delayed briefly. This delay allows the atria to contract completely before the ventricles are stimulated to contract. The intrinsic rate of the AV node is 40 to 60 beats/min.

The bundle of His is a continuation of the AV node and is located in the interventricular septum. It divides into the right and left bundle branches. The bundle branches extend downward through the ventricular septum and fuse with the Purkinje fiber system. The Purkinje fibers are the terminal branches of the conduction system and are responsible for carrying the wave of depolarization to both ventricular walls. Purkinje fibers can act as an intrinsic pacemaker, but their discharge rate is only 20 to 40 beats/min.

Animation: Cardiac Cycle

SEQUENCE OF EVENTS DURING THE CARDIAC CYCLE

The phases of the cardiac cycle are generally described in relation to changes in pressure and volume in the left ventricle during filling (diastole) and ventricular contraction (systole) (Figure 36-5). **Diastole,** normally about two thirds of the cardiac cycle, consists of relaxation and filling of the atria and ventricles, whereas **systole** consists of the contraction and emptying of the atria and ventricles.

Cardiac-muscle contraction results from the release of large numbers of calcium ions from the sarcoplasmic reticulum. These ions diffuse into the **myofibril sarcomere** (the basic contractile unit of the myocardial cell). Calcium ions promote the interaction of actin and myosin protein filaments, causing these filaments to link and overlap. Cross-bridges, or linkages, are formed as the protein filaments slide over or overlap each other. These cross-bridges act as force-generating sites. The sliding of these protein filaments of multiple myofibril sarcomeres shortens the sarcomeres, producing myocardial contraction.

Cardiac muscle relaxes when calcium ions are pumped back into the sarcoplasmic reticulum, causing a decrease in the number of calcium ions around the myofibrils. This reduced number of ions causes the protein filaments to disengage or dissociate, the sarcomere to lengthen, and the muscle to relax.

MECHANICAL PROPERTIES OF THE HEART

The electrical and mechanical properties of cardiac muscle determine the function of the cardiovascular system. The heart is able to adapt to various pathophysiologic conditions (e.g., stress, infections, hemorrhage) to maintain adequate blood flow to the various body tissues. Blood flow from the heart into the systemic arterial circulation is measured clinically as cardiac output (CO), the amount of blood pumped from the

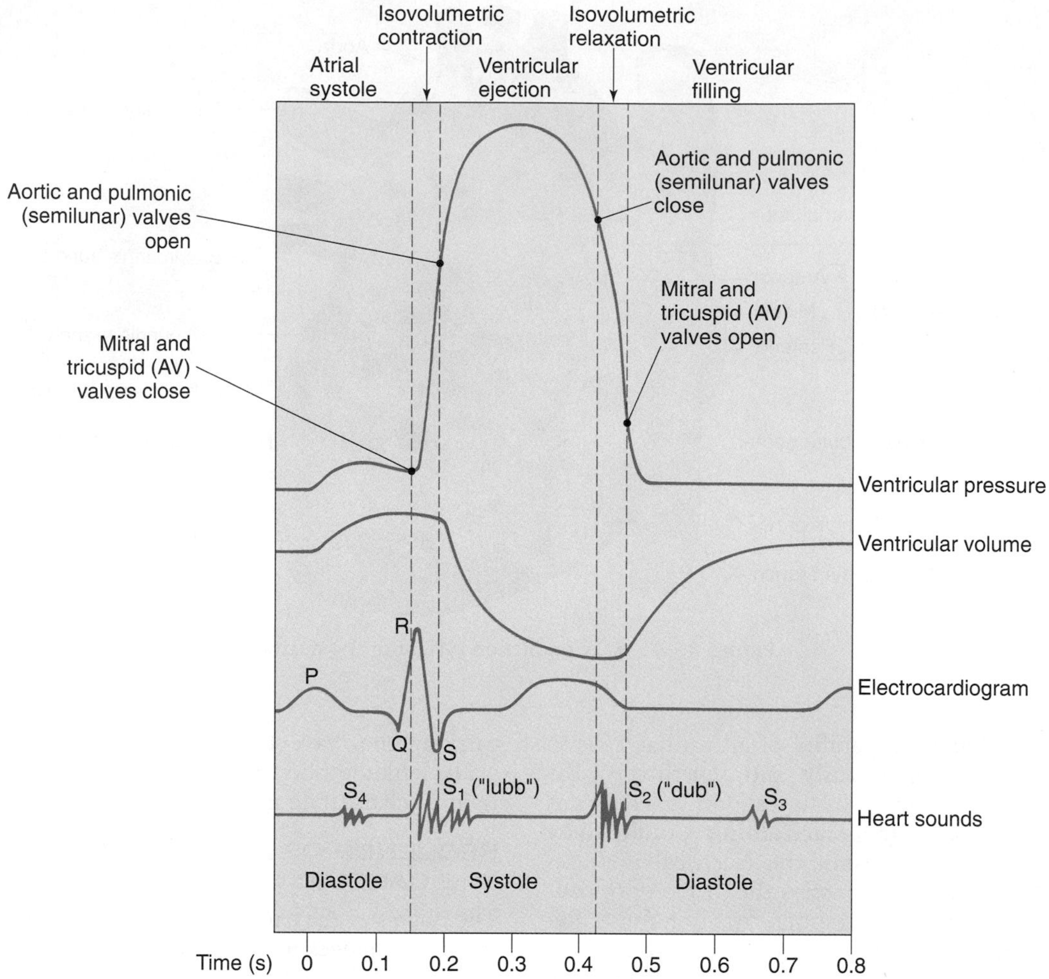

Figure 36-5 ■ Events of the cardiac cycle.

left ventricle each minute. CO depends on the relationship between heart rate (HR) and stroke volume (SV); it is the product of these two variables:

Cardiac output = Heart rate × Stroke volume

CARDIAC OUTPUT AND CARDIAC INDEX. **Cardiac output (CO)** is the volume of blood (in liters) ejected by the heart each minute. In adults the CO ranges from 4 to 7 L/min. Because cardiac output requirements vary according to body size, the cardiac index is calculated to adjust for differences in body size. The **cardiac index** can be determined by dividing the CO by the body surface area. The normal range is 2.7 to 3.2 L/min/m² of body surface area.

HEART RATE. Heart rate (HR) refers to the number of times the ventricles contract each minute. The normal resting HR for an adult is between 60 and 100 beats/min. Increases in HR increase myocardial oxygen demand. The HR is extrinsically controlled by the autonomic nervous system (ANS), which adjusts rapidly when necessary to regulate cardiac output. The parasympathetic (vagus nerve) system slows the HR, whereas sympathetic stimulation has an excitatory effect. An increase in circulating endogenous catecholamines (e.g., epinephrine and norepinephrine) usually causes an increase in HR and vice versa. Many cardiovascular drugs, including beta blockers and calcium channel blockers, mimic this pattern by decreasing the HR.

Other factors, such as the central nervous system (CNS) and baroreceptor (pressoreceptor) reflexes, influence the effects of the ANS on HR. Pain, fear, and anxiety can increase the HR. The baroreceptor reflex acts as a negative-feedback system. If a client experiences hypotension, the baroreceptors in the aortic arch sense a lowered pressure in the blood vessels. A signal is then relayed to the parasympathetic system to have less of an inhibitory effect on the sinoatrial (SA) node; this results in a reflex increase in HR.

STROKE VOLUME. **Stroke volume** (SV) is the amount of blood ejected by the left ventricle during each systole. Several variables influence stroke volume and, ultimately, CO. These variables include HR, preload, afterload, and contractility.

PRELOAD. **Preload** refers to the degree of myocardial fiber stretch at the end of diastole and just before contraction. The stretch imposed on the muscle fibers results from the volume contained within the ventricle at the end of diastole. Preload is determined by the amount of blood returning to the heart from both the venous system (right heart) and the pulmonary system (left heart) (left ventricular end-diastolic volume (LVED).

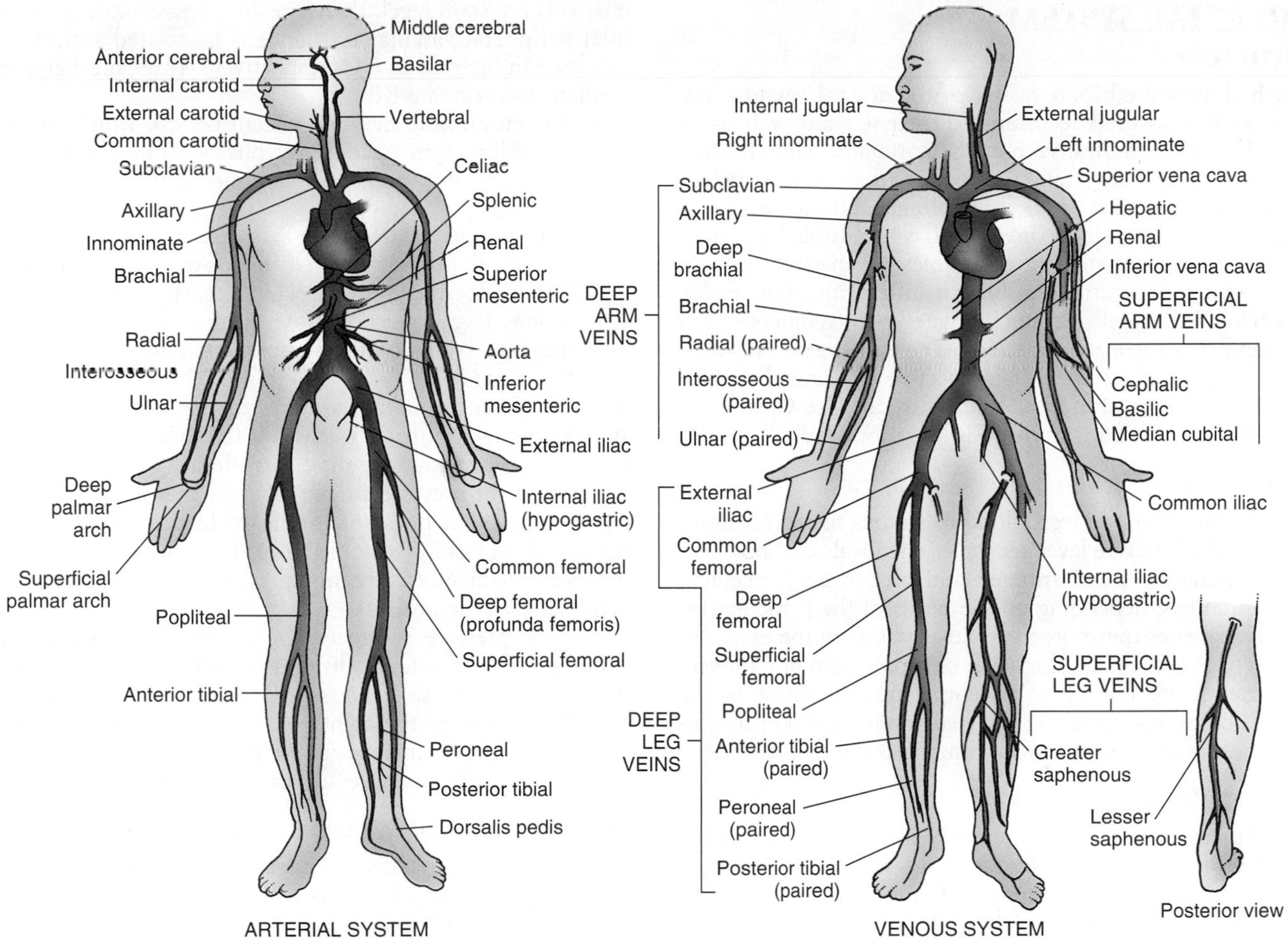

Figure 36-6 ■ Anatomy of the arterial and venous systems.

Animation: Blood Flow ◀

An increase in ventricular volume increases muscle-fiber length and tension, thereby enhancing contraction and improving stroke volume. This statement is derived from Starling's law of the heart: The more the heart is filled during diastole (within limits), the more forcefully it contracts. Excessive filling of the ventricles results in excessive LVED volume and pressure, however, and may result in decreased cardiac output.

AFTERLOAD. Another determinant of stroke volume, **afterload,** is the pressure or resistance that the ventricles must overcome to eject blood through the semilunar valves and into the peripheral blood vessels. The amount of resistance is directly related to arterial blood pressure and the diameter of the blood vessels.

Impedance, the peripheral component of afterload, is the pressure that the heart must overcome to open the aortic valve. The amount of impedance depends on aortic compliance and total systemic vascular resistance, a combination of blood viscosity and arteriolar constriction. A decrease in stroke volume can result from an increase in afterload without the benefit of compensatory mechanisms.

CONTRACTILITY. Contractility also affects stroke volume and CO. Myocardial contractility is the force of cardiac contraction independent of preload. Contractility is increased by factors such as sympathetic stimulation, calcium release, and positive inotropic drugs. Factors such as hypoxia and acidemia decrease contractility.

Vascular System

The vascular system serves several purposes:

- To provide conduits for blood to travel from the heart to nourish the various tissues of the body
- To carry cellular wastes to the excretory organs
- To allow lymphatic flow to drain tissue fluid back into the circulation
- To return blood to the heart for recirculation

This system of conduits depends on an efficient heart and patent blood vessels to regulate and maintain systemic and regional blood flow and temperature.

The vascular system is divided into the arterial system and the venous system (Figure 36-6). In the arterial system, blood moves from the larger conduits to a network of smaller blood vessels, called arterioles, that meet the capillary bed. In the venous system, blood travels from the capillaries to the venules and to the larger system of veins, eventually returning in the venae cavae to the heart for recirculation.

ARTERIAL SYSTEM

Structure

The high-pressure blood vessels of the arterial vascular system can be classified according to their size and wall structure. The large arteries, such as the aorta and femoral arteries, follow relatively straight routes and have few branches. Smaller arteries, such as the internal iliac and mesenteric arteries, divide from larger ones and have multiple branches.

Arteries may branch into arterioles or anastomose with other arteries. The arterioles branch into terminal arterioles, which join with capillaries and ultimately with venules to form the capillary network (Figure 36-7). The exchange of nutrients across the capillary membrane occurs primarily by three processes: osmosis, filtration, and diffusion. (See Chapter 14 for detailed discussions of osmosis, filtration, and diffusion.)

Function

The arterial system delivers blood to various tissues for nourishment. At the tissue level, nutrients, chemicals, and body defense substances are distributed and exchanged for cellular waste products, depending on the needs of the particular tissue. The arteries transport the cellular wastes to the excretory organs (e.g., kidneys and lungs) to be reprocessed or removed. The arteries also contribute to temperature regulation in the tissues. Blood can be either directed toward the skin to promote heat loss or diverted away from the skin to conserve heat.

Blood Pressure

Blood pressure (BP) is the force of blood exerted against the vessel walls. Pressure in the larger arterial blood vessels is greater (about 80 to 100 mm Hg) and decreases as blood flow reaches the capillaries (about 25 mm Hg). By the time blood enters the RA, the BP is about 0 to 5 mm Hg.

INDIRECT MEASUREMENT OF BLOOD PRESSURE

The BP in the arterial system is determined primarily by the quantity of blood flow or cardiac output (CO) as well as by the resistance in the arterioles:

Blood pressure = Cardiac output × Peripheral vascular resistance

Any factor that increases CO or total peripheral vascular resistance increases the BP. In general, BP is maintained at a relatively constant level; therefore an increase or decrease in total peripheral vascular resistance is associated with a decrease or an increase in CO, respectively. Three mechanisms mediate and regulate BP:

- The autonomic nervous system (ANS), which excites or inhibits sympathetic nervous system activity in response to impulses from chemoreceptors and baroreceptors
- The kidneys, which sense a change in blood flow and activate the renin-angiotensin-aldosterone mechanism
- The endocrine system, which releases various hormones (e.g., catecholamine, kinins, serotonin, histamine) to stimulate the sympathetic nervous system at the tissue level

Systolic BP represents the amount of pressure/force generated by the left ventricle to distribute blood into the aorta with each contraction of the heart; diastolic BP represents the amount of pressure/force sustained by the arteries during the relaxation phase of the heart. In the adult, systolic pressure is normally 90 to 135 mm Hg, and diastolic pressure is normally 60 to 85 mm Hg. BP is expressed as systolic pressure/diastolic pressure.

Systolic pressure is affected by a number of factors, including CO and arterial distention. When CO decreases, systolic pressure also decreases. Diastolic pressure is determined primarily by the ability of the heart to rest while filling with blood. An increase in peripheral vascular resistance increases diastolic pressure and cardiac workload.

REGULATION OF BLOOD PRESSURE

The ANS and the renal system are primarily responsible for regulating BP. External factors can also affect BP.

AUTONOMIC NERVOUS SYSTEM. Blood pressure (BP) is regulated by balancing the sympathetic and parasympathetic nervous systems of the ANS. Changes in sympathetic and parasympathetic activity are responses to messages sent by the sensory receptors in the various tissues of the body. These receptors, including the baroreceptors, chemoreceptors, and stretch receptors, respond differently to the biochemical and physiologic changes of the body.

Baroreceptors in the arch of the aorta and at the origin of the internal carotid arteries are stimulated when the arterial walls are stretched by an increased BP. Impulses from these baroreceptors inhibit the vasomotor center, which is located in the pons and the medulla. Inhibition of this center results in a drop in BP.

Several 1- to 2-mm collections of tissue have been identified in the bifurcations of the carotid arteries and along the aortic arch. These carotid and aortic bodies contain specialized **chemoreceptors** that are sensitive primarily to hypoxemia (a decrease in the partial pressure of arterial oxygen [PaO_2]). When stimulated, the carotid chemoreceptors send impulses along Hering's nerves, and the aortic chemoreceptors send impulses along the vagus nerves to activate a vasoconstrictor response.

The chemoreceptors are also stimulated by hypercapnia (an increase in partial pressure of arterial carbon dioxide [$PaCO_2$]) and acidosis. The direct effect of carbon dioxide on the CNS, however, is 10 times stronger than the effect it produces by stimulating the chemoreceptors.

Stretch receptors found in the venae cavae and the right atrium (RA) are sensitive to pressure or volume changes.

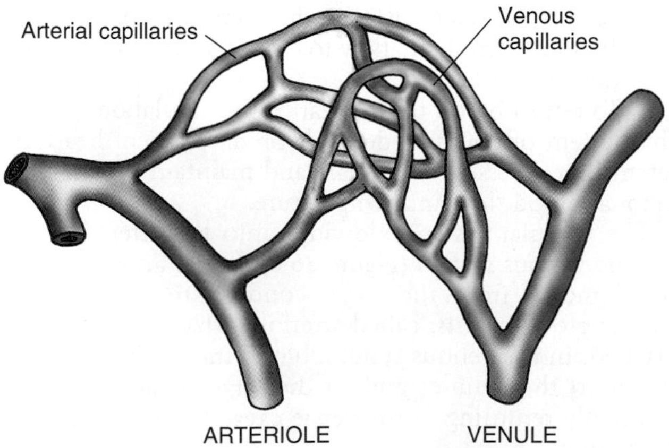

Figure 36-7 ■ Structure of the capillary bed.

When a client is hypovolemic, the stretch receptors in the blood vessels sense a reduced volume or pressure and send fewer impulses to the CNS. This reaction stimulates the sympathetic nervous system to increase the heart rate (HR) and constrict the peripheral blood vessels.

RENAL SYSTEM. The renal system also helps to regulate cardiovascular activity. When renal blood flow or pressure decreases, the kidneys retain sodium and water. BP tends to rise because of fluid retention and activation of the renin-angiotensin-aldosterone mechanism. This mechanism results in vasoconstriction and sodium retention (and thus fluid retention). Vascular volume is also regulated by the release of antidiuretic hormone (vasopressin) from the posterior pituitary gland (see Chapter 14).

EXTERNAL FACTORS. Other factors can influence the activity of the cardiovascular system. Emotional behaviors (e.g., excitement, pain, anger) stimulate the sympathetic nervous system to increase BP and HR. Increased physical activity such as exercise increases BP and pulse rate. Body temperature can affect the metabolic needs of the tissues, thereby influencing the delivery of blood. In hypothermia, tissues require fewer nutrients and blood pressure falls. In hyperthermia, the metabolic requirement of the tissues is greater, and BP and pulse rate rise.

VENOUS SYSTEM

Structure

The venous system is composed of a series of veins that are located adjacent to the arterial system (see Figure 36-6). A second superficial venous circulation runs parallel to the subcutaneous tissue of the extremity. These two venous systems are connected by communicating veins that provide a means for blood to travel from the superficial veins to the deep veins. Blood flow is directed toward the deep venous circulation.

The venules collect blood from the capillaries and the terminal arterioles. White blood cells also enter and exit the body tissues at the venules. Venules branch into veins, which are low-pressure blood vessels. Veins have the ability to accommodate large shifts in volume with minimal changes in venous pressure. This flexibility allows the venous system to accommodate the administration of intravenous (IV) fluids and blood transfusions, blood loss, and dehydration. All veins in the superficial and deep venous systems in the legs (except the smallest and the largest veins) have valves that direct blood flow back to the heart; this prevents retrograde flow (backflow). The force that propels the blood forward in the veins is skeletal muscle in the extremities.

Function

The primary function of the venous system is to complete the circulation of blood by returning blood from the capillaries to the right side of the heart. The venous system also acts as a reservoir for a large portion of the blood volume. In contrast to the arterial system, which consists of a high-pressure, continuous flow system through relatively rigid conduits, the venous system consists of a low-pressure, intermittent flow system through collapsible tubes that work against the effects of gravity.

Gravity exerts an increase in hydrostatic pressure (capillary blood pressure) when the client is in an upright position, which delays venous return. Hydrostatic pressure is lessened when the client is lying down, and thus there is less hindrance of venous return to the heart.

Cardiovascular Changes Associated with Aging

A number of physiologic changes in the cardiovascular system occur with advancing age (Chart 36-1). Many of these changes result in a loss of cardiac reserve. Thus these changes are usually not evident when the older adult is resting. They become apparent only when the person is physically or emotionally stressed and the heart cannot meet the increased metabolic demands of the body.

ASSESSMENT TECHNIQUES

History

A thorough history must be obtained, including demographic data, personal and family history, diet, socioeconomic status, and a functional assessment. The focus of the history is on obtaining information relative to client's risk factors and symptoms of cardiovascular disease (Chart 36-2).

DEMOGRAPHIC DATA

Demographic data include the client's age, gender, and ethnic origin. The incidence of conditions such as coronary artery disease (CAD) and valvular disease increases with age (AHA, 2002). The incidence of CAD also varies with the client's gender. Men have a higher baseline risk for CAD than women of all ages, except in the oldest age group of 80 years and older (National Cholesterol Education Program [NCEP], 2002). Postmenopausal women are two to three times more likely than premenopausal women to have CAD. The incidence for CAD in women is about 10 years later than for men and 20 years later for myocardial infarction (MI) and death to occur (AHA, 2002). After an acute MI, women tend to die more frequently and have survival disadvantages compared with men.

White women with abdominal obesity (greater waist circumference than hip circumference) are more likely to experience cardiovascular disease (CVD) than are white women with fat distributed in their buttocks, hips, and thighs (greater hip circumference than waist circumference). Clients with an early onset of obesity (during adolescence) and an elevated waist-hip ratio appear to be at especially high risk for cardiovascular disease. Diabetes mellitus is also a major risk factor, especially in women.

Age, gender, ethnic background, and family history of CVD are considered nonmodifiable or uncontrollable risk factors for CVD. Modifiable risk factors (e.g., high blood pressure, smoking, excessive blood cholesterol), if controlled, can reduce the risk of heart disease. These factors are discussed under Modifiable Risk Factors beginning on p. 685.

FAMILY HISTORY AND GENETIC RISK

Review the family history, and obtain information about the age, health status, and cause of death of immediate family members. A positive family history for CAD in a first-degree relative (parent, sibling, or child) is a major risk factor. This risk factor is more significant than other risk factors such as hy-

CHART 36-1

NURSING FOCUS on the OLDER ADULT
Changes in the Cardiovascular System Related to Aging

Change	Nursing Interventions	Rationales
Cardiac Valves Calcification and mucoid degeneration occur, especially in mitral and aortic valves.	Assess heart rate and rhythm and heart sounds for murmurs. Question clients about dyspnea.	Murmurs may be detected before other symptoms. Valvular abnormalities may result in rhythm changes.
Conduction System Pacemaker cells decrease in number. Fibrous tissue and fat in the sinoatrial node increase. Few muscle fibers remain in the atrial myocardium and bundle of His. Conduction time increases.	Assess the electrocardiogram (ECG) and heart rhythm for dysrhythmias or a heart rate less than 60 beats/min.	The sinoatrial (SA) node may lose its inherent rhythm. Atrial dysrhythmias occur in 50%-90% of older adults; 80% of older adults experience premature ventricular contractions (PVCs).
Left Ventricle The size of the left ventricle increases. The left ventricle becomes stiff and less distensible. Fibrotic changes in the left ventricle decrease the speed of early diastolic filling by about 50%.	Assess the ECG for a widening QRS complex and a longer QT interval. Assess the heart rate at rest and with activity. Assess for activity intolerance.	Ventricular changes result in decreased stroke volume, ejection fraction, and cardiac output during exercise; the heart is less able to meet increased oxygen demands. Maximum heart rate with exercise is decreased. The heart is less able to meet increased oxygen demands.
Aorta and Other Large Arteries The aorta and other large arteries thicken and become stiffer and less distensible. Systolic blood pressure increases to compensate for the stiff arteries. Systemic vascular resistance increases as a result of less distensible arteries; therefore the left ventricle pumps against greater resistance, contributing to left ventricular hypertrophy.	Assess blood pressure. Note increases in systolic, diastolic, and pulse pressures. Assess for activity intolerance and shortness of breath. Assess the peripheral pulses.	Hypertension may occur and must be treated to avoid target organ damage.
Baroreceptors Baroreceptors become less sensitive.	Assess the client's blood pressure with the client lying and then sitting or standing. Assess for dizziness when the client changes from a lying to a sitting or standing position. Teach the client to change positions slowly.	Orthostatic (postural) and postprandial changes occur because of ineffective baroreceptors. Changes may include blood pressure decreases of 10 mm Hg or more, dizziness, and fainting.

pertension, obesity, diabetes, or sudden cardiac death. The younger the age of onset and the more first-degree relatives are affected, the greater the risk for CAD (NCEP, 2002).

Heart disease has many contributory factors, including a genetic tendency. Researchers have found a gene mutation called *R1141X,* which appears in a gene called *ABCCG.* The mutation causes pseudoxanthoma elasticum (PXE), a rare connective tissue disorder that causes the cardiac muscle fibers to calcify in the coronary arteries and contributes to high BP. People with CAD are four times more likely to have the mutation (Trip et al., 2001). Genetic screening for PXE and aggressive strategies to reduce modifiable risk factors may help reduce the incidence of heart disease.

PERSONAL HISTORY

Review the client's history, noting any major illnesses such as diabetes mellitus, renal disease, anemia, high BP, stroke, bleeding disorders, connective tissue diseases, chronic pulmonary diseases, heart disease, and thrombophlebitis. These conditions can influence the client's cardiovascular status.

Ask about previous treatment for CVD, identify previous diagnostic procedures (e.g., electrocardiography, cardiac catheterization), and request information about any medical or invasive treatment of CVD. It is important to ask specifically about recurrent tonsillitis, streptococcal infections, and rheumatic fever because these conditions may lead to valvular abnormalities of the heart. In addition, inquire about any known congenital heart defects. Many clients with congenital heart problems are living into adulthood because of improved treatment and surgical modalities.

Clients are asked in detail about their medication history, beginning with any current or recent use of prescription or over-the-counter (OTC) medications or herbal/natural products (e.g., ginseng). Inquire about known sensitivities to any drug and the nature of the reaction (e.g., nausea, rash). Clients should be asked whether they have recently used cocaine or any IV "street" drugs because these substances may be associated with chest pain or endocarditis.

Ask female clients whether they are taking oral contraceptives or an estrogen replacement. There is an increased

CHART 36-2

Cardiovascular Assessment
USING GORDON'S FUNCTIONAL HEALTH PATTERNS

Health Perception-Health Management
- What advice has your health care provider offered you about exercise, diet, or smoking?
- Are you able to follow that advice?
- What medications (both over-the-counter and prescription) are you supposed to be taking?
- Are you taking them as suggested or prescribed?
- What problems have you had with the medications?

Nutrition-Metabolic
- What is your usual daily diet? (Analyze the diet for saturated fat, cholesterol, total calorie, and sodium content.)
- How much fluid do you drink daily? Are you thirsty?
- What do you weigh? When did you last weigh yourself?
- How often do you weigh yourself?
- What is your height?
- Do you know your cholesterol level? What is it?
- How often do you feel nauseated or not interested in eating?
- Do your feet/ankles swell during the day? At night, too?

Elimination
- How often do you urinate in the daytime?
- How often do you wake up at night to urinate?

Activity/Exercise
- What is the most strenuous exercise you did last week?
- How active are you compared with 6 months ago? 1 year ago?
- How often do you feel fatigued or tired?
- Can you climb a flight of stairs and walk a block without feeling short of breath or experiencing chest pain?
- Do you experience leg cramps when you walk or climb stairs?

Sleep/Rest
- Where do you sleep? (In bed? In a lounge chair?)
- How many pillows do you sleep on?
- Do you ever wake up at night short of breath?
- What happens when you wake up short of breath?
- Do you ever wake up at night with pain or cramps in your legs? How do you relieve that sensation?

Cognitive/Perceptual
- How is your memory? What does your family say about your memory?
- How often do you feel dizzy, disoriented, or faint?
- Do you ever have chest discomfort? How often? What precipitates it? What is it like? How do you relieve it? What is its level on a scale of 0 to 10?
- Do you ever have leg or buttock pain? What are its characteristics?
- How do you learn best?

Role/Relationship
- What is your job?
- What does a day's work entail?
- What are your family responsibilities?
- With whom do you live?
- Who is available to help you?

Sexuality/Reproductive
- Has your ability to engage in sexual activity changed in the past year?
- If so, how?
- Do you take any medications that affect your sexual response? If so, what?

Coping/Stress Tolerance
- What do you think has been happening to you?
- How do you respond to being caught in a traffic jam or meeting a deadline?
- What do you do to relax?
- What do you do when you feel stressed?

Based on Gordon, M. (2002). *Manual of nursing diagnosis* (10th ed.). St. Louis: Mosby.

incidence of myocardial infarction (MI) and stroke in women over the age of 35 who take oral contraceptives, but only if they smoke, have diabetes, or have hypertension.

DIET HISTORY

A diet history includes the client's recall of food and fluid intake during a 24-hour period, self-imposed or medically prescribed dietary restrictions or supplementations, and the amount and type of alcohol consumption. The dietitian reviews the type of foods selected by the client for the amount of sodium, sugar, cholesterol, fiber, and fat. Working with the dietitian, explore the client's attitude toward food, knowledge level of essential and nonessential dietary elements, and willingness to make changes in the diet. Cultural beliefs and economic status can influence the choice of food items and therefore must be reviewed. Family members or significant others who are responsible for shopping and cooking are included in this discussion.

SOCIOECONOMIC STATUS

The social history includes information about the client's domestic situation, such as marital status, number of children, household members, living environment, and occupation. Identification of support systems is especially important in exploring the possibility that the client might have difficulty paying for medications or treatment.

Ask about the client's occupation, including the type of work performed and the requirements of the specific job. For instance, does the job involve lifting of heavy objects? Is the job emotionally stressful? What does a day's work entail? Does the client's job require him or her to be outside in extreme weather conditions?

MODIFIABLE RISK FACTORS

Personal habits that are risk factors for heart disease include cigarette smoking, physical inactivity, obesity, psychological variables, and certain chronic diseases. These factors are considered modifiable or controllable risk factors. Inquire about each of the following modifiable risk factors.

Cigarette Smoking

Cigarette smoking is a major risk factor for cardiovascular disease (CVD), specifically coronary artery disease (CAD) and peripheral vascular disease (PVD) (AHA, 2002). According to the U.S. Department of Health and Human Services (DHHS), cigarette smoking is directly responsible for 21% of all deaths from CAD. Three compounds in cigarette smoke have been implicated in the development of CAD: tar, nicotine, and carbon monoxide. Smoking costs

Americans more than $157 billion each year in medical care (AHA, 2002).

The risks to the cardiovascular system from cigarette smoking appear to be dose related, noncumulative, and transient. The smoking history should include the number of cigarettes smoked daily, the duration of the smoking habit, and the age of the client when smoking started. A person who smokes fewer than four cigarettes per day has twice the risk of CVD disease of a person who does not smoke; a person who smokes more than 20 cigarettes per day has four times the risk. Typically the smoking history is recorded in **pack-years,** which is the number of packs per day multiplied by the number of years the client has smoked.

Inquire about the client's desire to quit, past attempts to quit, and the methods used. Ascertain nicotine dependence by asking questions such as the following:

- How soon after you wake up in the morning do you smoke?
- Do you find it difficult not to smoke in places where smoking is prohibited?
- Do you smoke when you are ill?

Clients should be directed to smoking-cessation programs through the support of group meetings and new behavioral and pharmacologic approaches (including nicotine replacement patches and bupropion). Few physicians are trained to implement these programs. Identifying experienced health care providers who can implement smoking cessation programs for clients is a priority. A structured program is essential to provide the support necessary to quite smoking.

Three to four years after a client has stopped smoking, his or her cardiovascular risk appears to be similar to that of a person who has never smoked. Be sure to ask clients who do not currently smoke whether they have ever smoked and when they quit. Passive smoke significantly reduces the blood flow velocity in health young adults' coronary arteries (JAMA, 2001), and the risk of dying increases by 30% among those who are exposed to secondhand smoke (AHA, 2002).

Physical Inactivity

A sedentary lifestyle is also considered a significant risk factor in the development of heart disease. Regular physical activity promotes cardiovascular fitness and produces beneficial changes in blood pressure and levels of blood lipids and clotting factors. Unfortunately few people in the United States engage in the recommended exercise guidelines: 30 minutes daily of light to moderate exercise, which is equivalent to a 30-minute brisk walk. According to the American Heart Association (AHA), only 22% of Americans engage in this much exercise five times a week, and only 15% engage in vigorous physical activity (enough to promote cardiopulmonary fitness) three times a week (AHA, 2002). Increased physical exercise should be encouraged in accordance with a person's overall health status as part of a lifestyle change to reduce the risk for CAD (NCEP, 2002). Ask clients about the type of exercise they perform, how long a period they have participated in the exercise, and the frequency and intensity of the exercise.

Obesity

About 64% of American adults are **overweight** when defined as a body mass index (BMI) of 25 to 30 compared with 56% in 1994. **Obesity,** defined as a BMI greater than 30, increased from 23% in 1994 to 31% in 2002 (JAMA, 2002). It is particularly a problem for African-American women, Mexican Americans, and native Hawaiians (AHA, 2002). The Framingham Heart Study confirmed that obesity is a strong indicator of cardiovascular disease (CVD), especially when abdominal obesity is present (D'Agostino et al., 2001). It is also associated with hypertension, hyperlipidemia, and diabetes; all are known contributors to CVD.

Psychological Factors

A variety of psychological factors are more vulnerable to the development of heart disease. People who are highly competitive, overly concerned about meeting deadlines, and often hostile or angry are at higher risk for heart disease. Psychological stress, anger, depression, and hostility are all closely associated with risk of developing heart disease.

You might ask the client, "Have you ever experienced road rage?" or "How do you respond when you have to wait for an appointment?" Chronic anger and hostility appear to be closely associated with CVD. The constant arousal of the sympathetic nervous system (ANS) as a result of anger may influence blood pressure, serum fatty acids and lipids, and clotting mechanisms. Observe the client and determine his or her response to stressful situations.

Critical Thinking Challenge

Your client is a middle-aged African-American man, an accountant with a 20-year history of hypertension treated with a beta blocker and diuretic. He works long hours, his eating habits are poor, and he is 35 pounds overweight. He smoked a pack of cigarettes every day for 23 years but recently quit. His father died at age 55 of a myocardial infarction (MI). The client's total cholesterol is 242 mg/dL, his low-density lipoprotein (LDL) is 150 mg/dL, and his high-density lipoprotein (HDL) is 30 mg/dL. He was recently told at work that layoffs are likely; he is supporting two children in college and has one child with an addiction problem living at home. His mother has been living with the family since the loss of her husband 2 years ago.

1. How could this client modify his lifestyle further to help decrease his risk of cardiac disease?
2. What is the significance of his nonmodifiable risk factors?
3. What cultural and age-related variables should be considered in health teaching for this client?
4. What psychosocial issues need to be addressed?

evolve For suggested answer guidelines, go to http://evolve.elsevier.com/Iggy/.

CURRENT HEALTH PROBLEMS

Inquiring about major concerns helps to establish priorities in nursing care and management. The client is asked to describe his or her health concerns. Expand on the description of these concerns by obtaining information about their onset, duration, chronology, frequency, location, quality, intensity, associated symptoms, and precipitating, aggravating, and relieving factors. Major symptoms identified by clients with CVD include chest pain or discomfort, dyspnea, fatigue, palpitations, weight gain, syncope, and extremity pain.

Chronic Disease

Clients who have diabetes mellitus, hyperlipidemia, or hypertension are also at risk for cardiovascular problems. Those who are not diagnosed or are not compliant with the treatment plan have a much higher risk than those who are following the direction of a health care provider. These chronic illnesses are discussed elsewhere in this text.

Pain or Discomfort

Pain or discomfort, a common symptom of heart disease, can result from ischemic heart disease, pericarditis, and aortic dissection. Chest pain can also be due to noncardiac conditions such as pleurisy, pulmonary embolus, hiatal hernia, and anxiety. Thoroughly evaluate the nature and characteristics of the chest pain. Because pain resulting from myocardial ischemia is life threatening and can lead to serious complications, its cause should be considered ischemic (reduced or obstructed blood flow to the myocardium) until proven otherwise.

When assessing for pain, use alternative terms such as "discomfort," "heaviness," "pressure," and "indigestion." Some clients, especially women, do not experience pain in the chest but instead feel discomfort or indigestion. The client may also describe the sensation as aching, choking, strangling, tingling, squeezing, constricting, or viselike.

> **WOMEN'S HEALTH CONSIDERATIONS**
>
> Women respond uniquely to heart disease, often differing from the classic symptoms presented by men. Men typically have substernal pain occurring with activity or stress; the pain is often relieved by rest. Subtle symptoms and atypical chest pain are more common in women, who may not respond to rest or medication. Women report more back pain, indigestion, nausea, vomiting, and anorexia. Therefore, antacids, rather than nitroglycerin, may relieve their pain (DeVon & Zerwic, 2003).

Ask the client to identify when the pain was first noticed (onset):

- Did the pain begin suddenly or develop gradually (manner of onset)?
- How long did it last (duration)?

If the client has repeated painful episodes, assess how often the pain occurs (frequency). Ask whether this pain is different from any other episodes of pain. Ask the client to describe what activities he or she was doing when it first occurred, such as sleeping, arguing, or running (precipitating factors). The client can be asked to point to the area where the chest pain occurred (location) and to describe how the pain spread (radiation).

In addition, the client describes how the pain feels and whether it is sharp or dull (quality). To understand the severity of the pain, ask the client to grade it from 0 to 10, with 0 indicating an absence of pain and 10 indicating severe pain (intensity). The client may also report other signs and symptoms that occur at the same time (associated symptoms), such as dyspnea, diaphoresis, nausea, and vomiting. Other factors that need to be addressed are those that may have made the chest pain worse (aggravating factors) or less intense (relieving factors). Chest pain can arise from a variety of sources (Table 36-1). By obtaining the appropriate information, you may assist in identifying the source of the chest discomfort.

Dyspnea

Dyspnea can occur as a result of both cardiac and pulmonary disease. Dyspnea is described as difficult or labored breathing and is experienced as uncomfortable breathing or shortness of breath. When obtaining the client's history, as-

TABLE 36-1 Assessment of Chest Discomfort: How Various Types of Chest Pain Differ

Onset	Quality and Severity	Location and Radiation	Duration and Relieving Factors
Angina Sudden, usually in response to exertion, emotion, or extremes, in temperature	Squeezing, vise-like pain	Substernal; may spread across the chest and the back and/or down the arms	Usually lasts less than 15 min; relieved with rest, nitrate administration, or oxygen therapy
Myocardial Infarction Sudden, without precipitating factors, often in early morning	Intense stabbing, viselike pain or pressure, severe	Substernal; may spread throughout the anterior chest and to the arms, jaw, back, or neck	Usually last 30 min or longer or is relieved with opioids
Pericarditis Sudden	Sharp, stabbing, moderate to severe	Substernal; usually spreads to the left side or the back	Intermittent; relieved with sitting upright, analgesia, or administration of anti-inflammatory agents
Pleuropulmonary Variable	Moderate ache, worse on inspiration	Lung fields	Continuous until the underlying condition is treated or the client has rested
Esophageal-Gastric Variable	Squeezing, heartburn, variable severity	Substernal; may spread to the shoulders or the abdomen	Variable; may be relieved with antacid administration, food intake, or taking a sitting position
Anxiety Variable, may be in response to stress or fatigue	Dull ache to sharp stabbing; may be associated with numbness in fingers	Usually the left side of chest without radiation	Usually lasts a few minutes

certain what factors precipitate and relieve dyspnea, what level of activity produces dyspnea, and the client's body position when dyspnea occurred.

There are several types of dyspnea. Dyspnea that is associated with activity, such as climbing stairs, is referred to as dyspnea on exertion (DOE). This is usually an early symptom of heart failure and may be the only symptom experienced by women.

The client with advanced heart disease may experience orthopnea, or dyspnea that appears when he or she lies flat. The client may use several pillows at night to elevate the head and chest or may sleep in a recliner to prevent nighttime breathlessness. The severity of orthopnea is measured by the number of pillows or the amount of head elevation needed to provide restful sleep. Orthopnea is usually relieved within a matter of minutes by sitting up or standing.

Paroxysmal nocturnal dyspnea (PND) develops after the client has been lying down for several hours. In this position, blood from the lower extremities is redistributed to the venous system, which increases venous return to the heart. A diseased heart is unable to compensate for the increased volume and is ineffective in pumping the additional fluid into the circulatory system. Pulmonary congestion results. The client awakens abruptly, often with a feeling of suffocation and panic. The client usually sits upright with the legs dangled over the bedside to relieve the dyspnea. This sensation may last for 20 minutes before disappearing.

Fatigue

Fatigue may be described as a feeling of tiredness or weariness resulting from activity. The client may complain that a certain activity takes longer to complete or that he or she tires easily after activity. Although fatigue in itself is not diagnostic of heart disease, many people with heart failure are limited by leg fatigue during exercise. Fatigue that occurs after mild activity and exertion usually indicates inadequate cardiac output (due to low stroke volume) and anaerobic metabolism in skeletal muscle. It can also accompany other symptoms or may be an early indication of heart disease in women.

Question the client to determine the time of day he or she experiences fatigue as well as the activities that he or she can perform. Fatigue resulting from decreased cardiac output is often worse in the evening. Ask whether the client can perform the same activities as he or she could perform a year ago or the same activities as others of the same age. Often the client limits activities in response to fatigue and unless questioned is unaware how much less active he or she has become.

Palpitations

A feeling of fluttering in the chest, an unpleasant awareness of the heartbeat, and an irregular heartbeat are referred to as **palpitations.** Palpitations may result from a change in heart rate or rhythm or from an increase in the force of heart contractions. Rhythm disturbances that may cause palpitations include paroxysmal supraventricular tachycardia, premature contractions, and sinus tachycardia. Those that occur during or after strenuous physical activity, such as running and swimming, may indicate overexertion or possibly heart disease. Noncardiac factors that may precipitate palpitations include anxiety, stress, fatigue, insomnia, hyperthyroidism, and the ingestion of caffeine, nicotine, or alcohol. Ask the client about specific factors that that precipitate the client's palpitations.

Weight Gain

A sudden weight increase of 2.2 pounds (1 kg) can result from an accumulation of excessive fluid (1 L) in the interstitial spaces. Weight gain is the best indicator of fluid retention. This condition is commonly known as **edema.** It is possible for weight gains of up to 10 to 15 pounds (4.5 to 6.8 kg, or 4 to 7 L of fluid) to occur before edema is apparent. Inquire whether the client has noticed a tightness of shoes, indentations from socks, or tightness of rings.

Syncope

Syncope refers to a transient loss of consciousness. The most common cause is decreased perfusion to the brain. Any condition that suddenly reduces cardiac output, resulting in decreased cerebral blood flow, can potentiate a syncopal episode. Conditions such as cardiac rhythm disturbances, especially ventricular dysrhythmias, and valvular disorders, such as aortic stenosis, may potentiate this symptom.

Near-syncope refers to dizziness with an inability to remain in an upright position. Explore the circumstances that lead to dizziness or syncope.

CONSIDERATIONS FOR OLDER ADULTS

Syncope in the aging individual may result from hypersensitivity of the carotid sinus bodies in the carotid arteries. Pressure applied to these arteries while turning the head, shrugging shoulders, or other performing a Valsalva maneuver (bearing down during defecation) may stimulate a vagal response. A decrease in blood pressure and heart rate can result, which can produce syncope. This type of syncopal episodes may also result from postural (orthostatic) or postprandial (after eating) hypotension as a result of this response.

Extremity Pain

Extremity pain may be caused by two conditions: ischemia from atherosclerosis and venous insufficiency of the peripheral blood vessels. Clients who report a moderate to severe cramping sensation in their legs or buttocks associated with an activity such as walking have intermittent claudication related to reduced arterial tissue perfusion. Claudication pain is usually relieved by resting or lowering the affected extremity to decrease tissue demands or to enhance arterial blood flow. Leg pain that results from prolonged standing or sitting is related to venous insufficiency from either incompetent valves or venous obstruction. This pain may be relieved by elevating the extremity.

FUNCTIONAL HISTORY

After the history of the client's cardiovascular status is obtained, he or she may be classified according to the New York Heart Association's Functional Classification (Table 36-2). The four classifications (I, II, III, and IV) depend on the degree to which ordinary physical activities (routine activities of daily living [ADLs]) are affected by heart disease. The Killip Classification provides a more objective description of the hemodynamics of heart failure and is described in Chapter 41.

Physical Assessment

A thorough physical assessment is the foundation for the nursing database and the formation of nursing diagnoses and collaborative problems. Any changes noted during the course of illness can be compared with this initial database. Evaluate the client's vital signs on admission to the hospital or during the initial visit to the clinic or health care provider's office.

GENERAL APPEARANCE

Physical assessment begins with the client's general appearance. Assess the following areas: general build and appearance, skin color, distress level, level of consciousness, shortness of breath, position, and verbal responses.

Clients can have left- or right-sided heart failure, or both. As a result, poor cardiac output and decreased cerebral perfusion may cause confusion, memory loss, and slowed verbal responses. Clients with chronic heart failure may also appear malnourished, thin, and cachectic. Late signs of severe right-sided heart failure are ascites, jaundice, and anasarca (generalized edema) as a result of prolonged congestion of the liver. Heart failure may also cause fluid retention and may be manifested by obvious generalized dependent edema. Chapter 38 differentiates right and left failure in detail.

INTEGUMENTARY SYSTEM

Assessment and evaluation of the integumentary system are determined primarily by the color and temperature of the skin. The best areas in which to assess circulation include the nail beds, mucous membranes, and conjunctival mucosa because small blood vessels are located near the surface of the skin.

TABLE 36-2 New York Heart Association Functional Classification of Cardiovascular Disability

Class I
- Clients with cardiac disease but without resulting limitations of physical activity
- Ordinary physical activity does not cause undue fatigue, palpitation, dyspnea, or anginal pain

Class II
- Clients with cardiac disease resulting in slight limitation of physical activity
- They are comfortable at rest
- Ordinary physical activity results in fatigue, palpitation, dyspnea, or anginal pain

Class III
- Clients with cardiac disease resulting in marked limitation of physical activity
- They are comfortable at rest
- Less than ordinary physical activity causes fatigue, palpitation, dyspnea, or anginal pain

Class IV
- Clients with cardiac disease resulting in inability to carry on any physical activity without discomfort
- Symptoms of cardiac insufficiency or of the anginal syndrome may be present, even at rest
- If any physical activity is undertaken, discomfort is increased

Excerpted from *Diseases of the heart and blood vessels—nomenclature and criteria for diagnosis* (6th ed.). Boston: Little, Brown; copyright 1964 by the New York Heart Association.

Skin Color

If there is normal blood flow or adequate perfusion to a given area in light-colored skin, it appears pink, perhaps rosy in color, and it is warm to the touch. Decreased perfusion is depicted as cool, pale, and moist skin. Pallor is characteristic of anemia and can be seen in areas such as the nail beds, palms, and conjunctival mucous membranes.

A bluish or darkened discoloration of the skin and mucous membranes in light-skinned individuals is referred to as **cyanosis.** This condition results from an increased amount of deoxygenated hemoglobin. It is not an early sign of decreased perfusion but occurs later with other symptoms. Dark-skinned individuals may experience cyanosis as a graying of the same tissues.

Central cyanosis involves decreased oxygenation of the arterial blood in the lungs and appears as a bluish tinge of the conjunctivae and the mucous membranes of the mouth and tongue. Central cyanosis may indicate impaired lung function or a right-to-left shunt found in congenital heart conditions. Because of impaired circulation, there is marked desaturation of hemoglobin in the peripheral tissues, which produces a bluish or darkened discoloration of the nail beds, earlobes, lips, and toes.

Peripheral cyanosis occurs when blood flow to the peripheral vessels is decreased by peripheral vasoconstriction. The clamping down of the peripheral blood vessels results from a low cardiac output or an increased extraction of oxygen from the peripheral tissues. Peripheral cyanosis localized in an extremity is usually a result of arterial or venous insufficiency. **Rubor** (dusky redness) that replaces pallor is a dependent foot suggests arterial insufficiency.

Skin Temperature

Skin temperature can be assessed for symmetry by touching different areas of the client's body (e.g., arms, hands, legs, feet) with the dorsal surface of the hand or fingers. Decreased blood flow results in decreased skin temperature. Skin temperature is lowered in several clinical conditions, including heart failure, peripheral vascular disease, and shock.

EXTREMITIES

Assess the client's hands, arms, feet, and legs for skin changes, vascular changes, clubbing, and edema. Skin mobility and turgor are affected by fluid status. Dehydration and aging reduce skin turgor, and edema decreases skin mobility. Vascular changes in an affected extremity may include paresthesia, muscle fatigue and discomfort, numbness, pain, coolness, and loss of hair distribution from a reduced blood supply.

Clubbing of the fingers and toes results from chronic oxygen deprivation in these tissue beds. Clubbing is characteristic in clients with advanced chronic pulmonary disease, congenital heart defects, and cor pulmonale. Clubbing can be identified by assessing the angle of the nail bed. The angle of the normal nail bed is 160 degrees. With **clubbing,** the nail straightens out to an angle of 180 degrees, and the base of the nail becomes spongy. Figure 36-8 describes assessment of clubbing using the Schamroth method.

Peripheral edema is a common finding in clients with cardiovascular problems. The location of edema helps to determine its potential cause. Bilateral edema of the legs may be

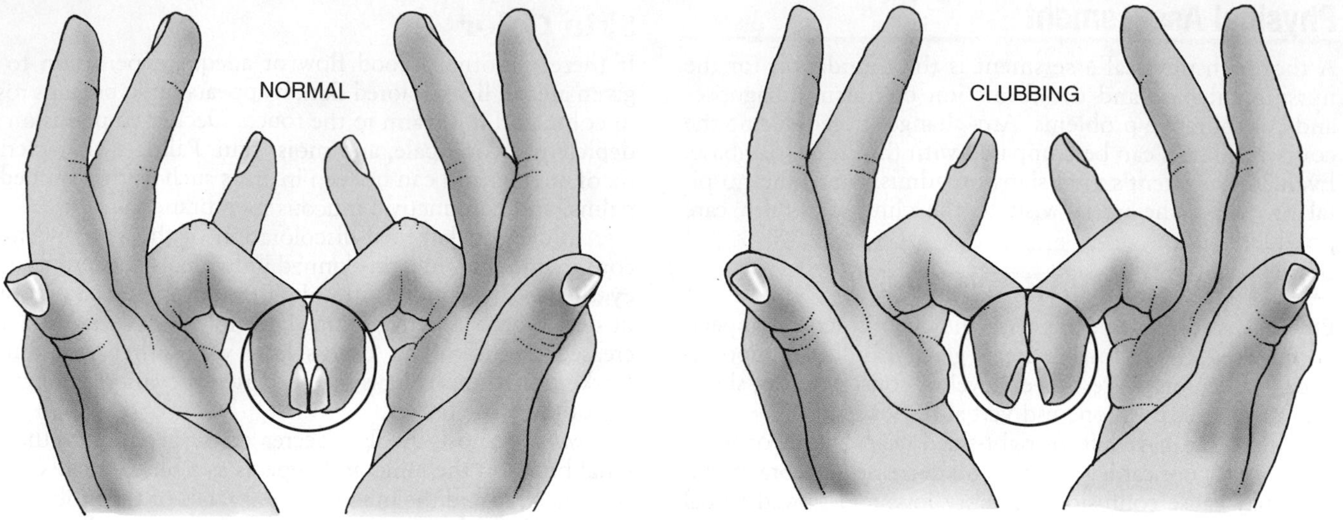

Figure 36-8 ■ Assessment of clubbing by the Schamroth method. The client places the fingernails of the ring fingers together and holds them up to a light. If the examiner can see a diamond shape between the nails, there is no clubbing. Clubbing is identified by the absence of the diamond shape.

seen in clients with heart failure or chronic venous insufficiency. Abdominal and leg edema can be seen in clients with heart disease and cirrhosis of the liver. Localized edema in one extremity may be the result of venous obstruction (thrombosis) or lymphatic blockage of the extremity (lymphedema). Edema may also be noted in dependent areas, such as the sacrum, when a client is confined to bed. In other clients, edema results from third spacing, such as when plasma proteins decrease.

Document the location of edema as precisely as possible (e.g., midtibial or sacral) and the number of centimeters from an anatomic landmark. The extent of edema can be characterized as mild, moderate, and severe (or 1, 2, 3, or 4). However, these values are not precise and are subjective. Determine whether the edema is pitting (the skin can be indented) or nonpitting.

Blood Pressure

Arterial blood pressure is measured indirectly by sphygmomanometry (Chart 36-3). This technique of measurement is described in greater detail in nursing skills textbooks.

The National High Blood Pressure Education Program Joint National Committee on Prevention, Detection, Evaluation, and Treatment of High Blood Pressure (2002) has recommended a new system of categorizing levels of blood pressure. High normal blood pressure is considered a systolic reading of 130 to 139 mm Hg or a diastolic pressure of 85 to 89. A blood pressure that exceeds 135/85 mm Hg increases the workload of the left ventricle and oxygen consumption of the myocardium. Approximately 50 million Americans (one out every five Americans) have **hypertension,** which is defined as a blood pressure greater than 140/90 mm Hg.

A new category has been designated **prehypertension.** This classification includes blood pressure (BP) readings of 120 to 139 mm Hg systolic or 80 to 89 mm Hg diastolic. Prehypertensive clients are at a higher risk to develop hypertension. Normal BP is classified as systolic pressure less than 120 mm Hg and diastolic blood pressure less than 80 mm Hg. Although the cause of hypertension is not known in 90% of people, it can be effectively controlled with lifestyle modification or medication. Hypertension is a cause of approximately five million deaths each year on its

CHART 36-3

BEST PRACTICE for
Accurate Blood Pressure Measurement

Select the proper cuff size.
- Adult cuff size is 12 to 14 cm wide and 30 cm long.
- Pediatric cuffs vary in width and length.
- Larger adult cuff size is 18 to 20 cm in width.

Ensure that equipment is properly assembled and calibrated.
- The cuff bladder should be intact inside the cuff.
- The sphygmomanometer should be calibrated to 0 mm Hg every few months to ensure reliability.

The cuff must be placed above the area to be auscultated (e.g., if the right arm is used, the cuff is placed above the brachial artery).

Follow these steps to ensure correct blood pressure measurement and recording:
- After palpating the brachial or radial pulse, inflate the cuff 30 mm Hg above the level at which those pulses disappear. Release the cuff slowly to palpate the systolic pressure. Reinflate the cuff, and auscultate the systolic and diastolic pressures. The auscultated pulses are referred to as the *Korotkoff sounds.*
- Record measurements on both arms to rule out dissecting aortic aneurysm, coarctation of the aorta, vascular obstruction, and possibly errors in measurement. Perform subsequent readings on the extremity with the highest pressure.
- If the client's arms are inaccessible (after amputation or mastectomy), you can obtain readings using the client's thigh or calf. Auscultate the popliteal artery or the posterior tibial artery, respectively.
- Obtain and record the client's blood pressure with the client in different positions, including supine, sitting, and standing positions.
- Record the position of the client and the site used to obtain the blood pressure.

own and is a major contributor to the development of CAD and heart failure.

A BP less than 90/60 mm Hg may be inadequate for providing proper and sufficient nutrition to body cells. In certain circumstances, such as shock and hypotension, the Korotkoff sounds are less audible or are absent. In these cases palpate the BP, use an ultrasonic device (Doppler device), or obtain a direct measurement by arterial catheter. When BP is palpated, the diastolic pressure is usually not obtainable. More information on direct measurement of arterial pressure is available under Hemodynamic Monitoring on p. 703.

POSTURAL BLOOD PRESSURE

Clients may report dizziness or light-headedness when they move from a flat, supine position to a sitting or a standing position at the edge of the bed. Normally these symptoms are transient and pass quickly; pronounced symptoms may be due to postural hypotension. **Postural (orthostatic) hypotension** occurs when the BP is not adequately maintained while moving from a lying to a sitting or standing position. It is defined as a decrease of more than 20 mm Hg of the systolic pressure or more than 10 mm Hg of the diastolic pressure as well as a 10% to 20% increase in heart rate. The causes of postural hypotension include medications, depletion of blood volume, prolonged bedrest, and age-related changes or disorders of the ANS.

To detect orthostatic changes in BP, first measure the BP when the client is supine. After remaining supine for at least 3 minutes, the client changes position to sitting or standing. Normally systolic pressure drops slightly or remains unchanged as the client rises, whereas diastolic pressure rises slightly. After the position change, a time delay of 1 to 5 minutes should be permitted before auscultating BP and palpating the radial pulse. The cuff should remain in the proper position on the client's arm. Observe and record any signs or symptoms of distress. If the client is unable to tolerate the position change, he or she is returned to the previous position of comfort.

PARADOXICAL BLOOD PRESSURE

Paradoxical blood pressure is defined as an exaggerated decrease in systolic pressure by more than 10 mm Hg during the inspiratory phase of the respiratory cycle (normal is 3 to 10 mm Hg). Certain clinical conditions that potentially alter the filling pressures in the right and left ventricles may produce a paradoxical BP. Such conditions include pericardial tamponade, constrictive pericarditis, and pulmonary hypertension. During inspiration the filling pressures normally decrease slightly; however, the decreased fluid volume in the ventricles resulting from these pathologic conditions produces an exaggerated or marked reduction in cardiac output. The procedure for assessing a paradoxical BP is found in Chapter 39, Chart 39-12.

PULSE PRESSURE

The difference between the systolic and diastolic values is referred to as pulse pressure. A normal pulse pressure for an adult is 30 to 40 mm Hg. This value can be used as an indirect measure of cardiac output.

Narrowed pulse pressure is rarely normal and results from increased peripheral vascular resistance or decreased stroke volume in clients with heart failure, hypovolemia, or shock. Narrowed pulse pressure can also be seen in clients who have mitral stenosis or regurgitation. An increased pulse pressure may be seen in clients with slow heart rates, aortic regurgitation, atherosclerosis, hypertension, and aging.

Ankle Brachial Index

The **ankle brachial index (ABI)** can be used to assess the vascular status of the lower extremities. A BP cuff is applied to the lower extremities just above the malleoli. The systolic pressure is measured by Doppler ultrasound at both the dorsalis pedis and posterior tibial pulses. The higher of these two pressures is then divided by the higher of the two brachial pulses to obtain the ABI.

Normal values for ABI are 1 or higher because BP in the legs is usually higher than BP in the arms. ABI values less than 0.80 usually indicate moderate vascular disease, whereas values less than 0.50 indicate severe vascular compromise.

A **toe brachial pressure index (TBPI)** may be performed instead of or in addition to the ABI to determine arterial perfusion in the feet and toes. It is defined as toe systolic pressure divided by brachial (arm) systolic pressure (Bonham, 2003).

VENOUS AND ARTERIAL PULSES

Venous Pulses

Observe the venous pulsations in the neck to assess the adequacy of blood volume and central venous pressure (CVP). Specially trained or critical care nurses can assess **jugular venous pressure (JVP)** to estimate the filling volume and pressure on the right side of the heart. An increase in JVP causes **jugular venous distention (JVD).**

Video Clip: Pulses, Lower Extremities ◀

Normally the JVP is 3 to 10 cm H_2O. Increases in JVP are usually caused by right ventricular failure. Other causes include tricuspid regurgitation or stenosis, pulmonary hypertension, cardiac tamponade, constrictive pericarditis, hypervolemia, and superior vena cava obstruction.

Arterial Pulses

Assessment of arterial pulses provides information about vascular integrity and circulation. For clients with suspected or actual vascular disease, all major peripheral pulses, including the temporal, carotid, brachial, radial, ulnar, femoral, popliteal, posterior tibial, and dorsalis pedis pulses, need to be assessed for presence or absence, amplitude, contour, rhythm, rate, and equality. Examine the peripheral arteries in a head-to-toe approach with a side-to-side comparison (Figure 36-9).

Animation: Pulse Variations ◀

A hypokinetic pulse is a weak pulse indicative of a narrow pulse pressure. It is seen in clients with hypovolemia, aortic stenosis, and decreased cardiac output. A hyperkinetic pulse is a large, "bounding" pulse caused by an increased ejection of blood. It is seen in clients with a high cardiac output (with exercise or thyrotoxicosis) and in those with increased sympathetic system activity (with pain, fever, or anxiety).

In **pulsus alternans,** a weak pulse alternates with a strong pulse despite a regular heart rhythm. It is seen in clients with severely depressed cardiac function. Clients may be asked to hold their breath to exclude any false readings. You can palpate the brachial or radial arteries to assess this condition, but it is more accurately assessed by auscultation of blood pressure.

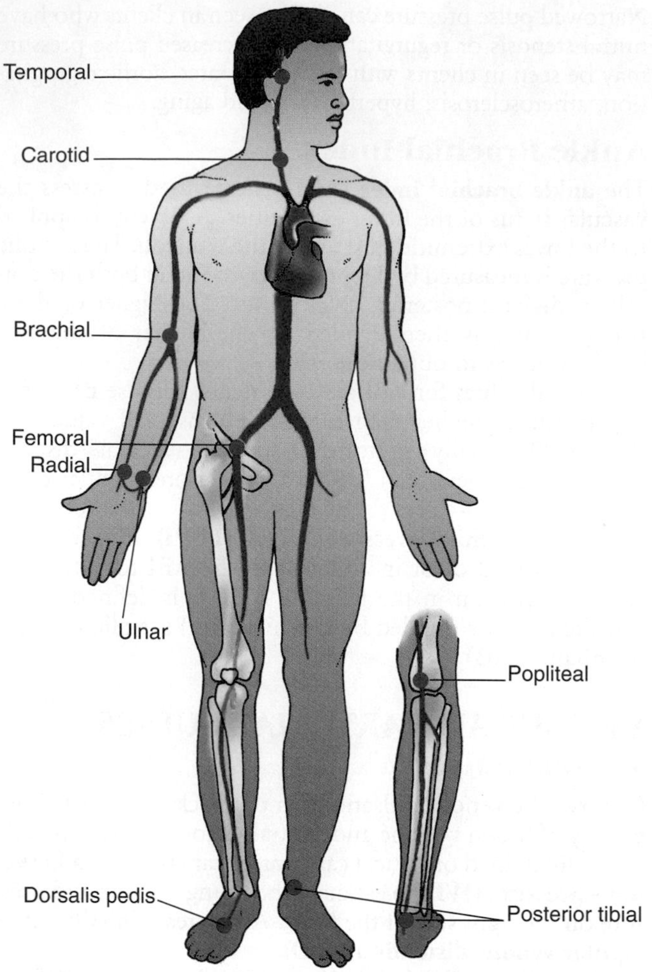

Figure 36-9 ■ Pulse points for assessment of arterial pulses.

▶ Video Clip: Carotid Artery

Auscultation of the major arteries (e.g., carotid and aorta) is necessary to assess for bruits. **Bruits** are swishing sounds that may develop in narrowed arteries and are usually associated with atherosclerotic disease. Assess for the absence or presence of bruits by placing the bell of the stethoscope over the skin of the carotid artery while the client holds his or her breath. Normally there are no sounds if the artery has uninterrupted blood flow. A bruit may develop when the internal diameter of the vessel is narrowed by 50% or more, but this does not indicate the severity of disease in the arteries.

PRECORDIUM

Assessment of the precordium (the area over the heart) involves inspection, palpation, percussion, and auscultation. In most settings the medical-surgical nurse seldom performs precordial palpation and percussion; however, the critical care nurse should perform a complete assessment. Place the client in a supine position, with the head of the bed slightly elevated for comfort. Some clients may require elevation of the head of the bed to 45 degrees for ease and comfort in breathing.

▶ Video Clip: Anterior Chest

Inspection

A cardiac examination is usually performed in a systematic order, beginning with inspection. Inspect the chest from the side, at a right angle, and downward over areas of the precordium where vibrations are visible. Cardiac motion is of low amplitude, and sometimes the inward movements are more easily detected by the naked eye.

Examine the entire precordium, focusing on the precordial areas (Figure 36-10) and noting any prominent precordial pulses. Movement over the aortic, pulmonic, and tricuspid areas is abnormal. Pulses in the mitral area (the apex of the heart) are considered normal and are referred to as the **apical impulse,** or the **point of maximal impulse (PMI).** The apical impulse should be located at the left fifth intercostal space (ICS) in the midclavicular line. If the apical impulse appears in more than one ICS and has shifted lateral to the midclavicular line, it may indicate left ventricular hypertrophy.

◀ Video Clip: Auscultatory Landmarks

Palpation

Palpate with the fingers and the most sensitive part of the palm of the hand to detect precordial motion and thrills, respectively. Continue to palpate by inching your hand in a Z pattern along the chest, starting with the aortic area and passing through all seven areas. Turning the client on his or her left side brings the heart closer to the surface of the chest. This may be helpful in achieving maximum tactile sensitivity during the assessment.

An abnormal forceful thrust accompanied by a sustaining outward movement over the left anterior side of the chest usually indicates left ventricular enlargement. An outward systolic lift along the left sternal border that extends from the fourth to the fifth ICS represents right ventricular enlargement.

Heaves and **lifts** are terms used to describe pulsations associated with valvular diseases or pulmonary hypertension. **Thrills** are vibrations associated with turbulent blood flow caused by abnormal heart valve function (mitral regurgitation, tricuspid regurgitation, and pulmonic stenosis). Specially trained nurses or primary care practitioners usually assess for these abnormalities.

◀ Animation: Auscultation of Heart Valves

Percussion

Cardiac size is determined most accurately by chest x-ray; percussion is now rarely used to determine the size of the heart. The size of the left ventricle, however, can be estimated by locating the apical impulse by inspection and palpation.

Auscultation

Auscultation evaluates heart rate and rhythm, cardiac cycle (systole and diastole), and valvular function. The technique of auscultation requires a good-quality stethoscope and extensive clinical practice. As a medical-surgical nurse, it is important to be familiar with normal heart sounds. Identifying common abnormal heart sounds becomes important when in critical care, telemetry, and advanced practice areas.

Evaluate heart sounds in a systematic order. Examination usually begins at the aortic outflow tract area and progresses slowly to the apex of the heart. The diaphragm of the stethoscope is pressed tightly against the chest to listen for high-frequency sounds and is useful in listening to the first and second heart sounds and high-frequency murmurs. Repeat the progression from the base to the apex of the heart using the bell of the stethoscope, which is held lightly against the chest. The bell is able to screen out high-frequency sounds and is useful in listening for low-frequency gallops (diastolic filling sounds) and murmurs.

◀ Video Clips: Auscultation with Diaphragm and Bell

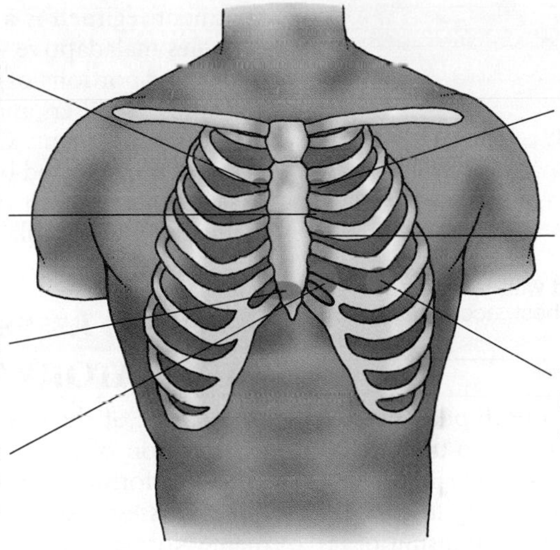

Figure 36-10 ■ Areas for myocardial inspection, palpation, and auscultation.

Attention is given to the areas in Figure 36-10 (except the epigastric area). Auscultation checks for heart rate and rhythm, murmurs, extrasystolic sounds, and rubs in the presence of a current or suspected cardiac problem.

NORMAL HEART SOUNDS

The first heart sound (S_1) is created by the closure of the mitral and tricuspid valves (atrioventricular valves) (see Figure 36-5). When auscultated, the first heart sound is softer and longer; it is of a low pitch and is best heard at the lower left sternal border or the apex of the heart. It may be identified by palpating the carotid pulse while listening. S_1 marks the beginning of ventricular systole and occurs right after the QRS complex on the electrocardiogram (ECG).

The first heart sound can be accentuated or intensified in conditions such as exercise, hyperthyroidism, and mitral stenosis. A decrease in sound intensity occurs in clients with mitral regurgitation and heart failure.

The second heart sound (S_2) is caused mainly by the closing of the aortic and pulmonic valves (semilunar valves) (see Figure 36-5). S_2 is characteristically shorter. It is higher pitched and is heard best at the base of the heart at the end of ventricular systole.

The splitting of heart sounds is often difficult to differentiate from diastolic filling sounds (gallops). A splitting of S_1 (closure of the mitral valve followed by closure of the tricuspid valve) occurs physiologically because left ventricular contraction occurs slightly before right ventricular contraction. Closure of the mitral valve is louder than closure of the tricuspid valve, however, so splitting is often not heard. Normal splitting of S_2 occurs because of the longer systolic phase of the right ventricle. Splitting of S_1 and S_2 can be accentuated by inspiration (increased venous return), and it narrows during expiration.

ABNORMAL HEART SOUNDS

PARADOXICAL SPLITTING. Abnormal splitting of S_2 is referred to as *paradoxical splitting* and is characteristic of a wider split heard on expiration. Paradoxical splitting of S_2 is heard in clients with severe myocardial depression that causes early closure of the pulmonic valve or a delay in aortic valve closure. Such conditions include myocardial infarction (MI), left bundle-branch block, aortic stenosis, aortic regurgitation, and right ventricular pacing.

GALLOPS AND MURMURS. Gallops and murmurs are common abnormal heart sounds that may occur with heart disease, but they can occur in some healthy individuals.

GALLOPS. Diastolic filling sounds (S_3) and (S_4) are produced when blood enters a noncompliant chamber during rapid ventricular filling. The third heart sound (S_3) is produced during the rapid passive filling phase of ventricular diastole when blood flows from the atrium to a noncompliant ventricle. The sound arises from vibrations of the valves and supporting structures. The fourth heart sound (S_4) occurs as blood enters the ventricles during the active filling phase at the end of ventricular diastole.

S_3 is termed **ventricular gallop,** and S_4 is referred to as **atrial gallop.** These sounds can be caused by decreased compliance of either or both ventricles. You can best hear left ventricular diastolic filling sounds with the client on his or her left side. The bell of the stethoscope is placed at the apex and at the left lower sternal border during expiration.

An S_3 heart sound is most likely to be a normal finding in children or young adults up to 30 years of age. An S_3 gallop in clients older than 35 years of age is considered abnormal and represents a decrease in left ventricular compliance. S_3 can be detected as an early sign of heart failure or as a ventricular septal defect.

An atrial gallop (S_4) may be heard in clients with hypertension, anemia, ventricular hypertrophy, MI, aortic or pulmonic stenosis, and pulmonary emboli. It may also be heard with advancing age because of a stiffened ventricle.

The auscultation of both S_3 and S_4, called a *summation* or a *quadruple gallop,* is an indication of severe heart failure. If the quadruple rhythm is present and the client has tachycardia (a shortened diastole), the two sounds may actually fuse to produce a rhythm that sounds like a horse galloping.

MURMURS. Murmurs reflect turbulent blood flow through normal or abnormal valves. They are classified according to their timing in the cardiac cycle: systolic murmurs (e.g., aortic stenosis and mitral regurgitation) occur between S_1 and S_2, whereas diastolic murmurs (e.g., mitral stenosis and aortic regurgitation) occur between S_2 and S_1. Murmurs can occur during presystole, midsystole, or late

TABLE 36-3 Grading of Heart Murmurs

Grade I	Very faint
Grade II	Faint but recognizable
Grade III	Loud but moderate in intensity
Grade IV	Loud and accompanied by a palpable thrill
Grade V	Very loud, accompanied by a palpable thrill, and audible with the stethoscope partially off the client's chest
Grade VI	Extremely loud, may be heard with the stethoscope slightly above the client's chest, accompanied by a palpable thrill

systole or diastole or can last throughout both phases of the cardiac cycle. They are also graded according to their intensity, depending on their level of loudness (Table 36-3).

Describe the location of a murmur according to where it is best heard on auscultation. Some murmurs transmit or radiate from their loudest point to other areas, including the neck, the back, and the axilla. The configuration is described as crescendo (increases in intensity) or decrescendo (decreases in intensity). The quality of murmurs can be further characterized as harsh, blowing, whistling, rumbling, or squeaking. They are also described by pitch, usually high or low.

PERICARDIAL FRICTION RUB. A **pericardial friction rub** originates from the pericardial sac and occurs with the movements of the heart during the cardiac cycle. Rubs are usually transient and are a sign of inflammation, infection, or infiltration. Pericardial friction rubs may be heard in clients with pericarditis resulting from MI, cardiac tamponade, or post-thoracotomy.

Psychosocial Assessment

To most people, the heart is a symbol of their ability to exist, survive, and love. A client with a heart-related illness, whether acute or chronic, usually perceives it as a major life crisis. The client, families, and significant others confront not only the possibility of death but also fears about pain, disability, lack of self-esteem, physical dependence, and changes in family dynamics. You may assess the meaning of the illness to the client and family members by asking, "What do you understand about what happened to you (or the client)?" and "What does that mean to you?" When the client or family members perceive the stressor as overwhelming, formerly adequate support systems may no longer be effective. In these circumstances, the client and family members attempt to cope to regain a sense or feeling of control.

Coping behaviors vary among clients. Those who feel helpless to meet the demands of the situation may exhibit behaviors such as disorganization, fear, and anxiety. You may ask the client or family members, "Have you ever encountered such a situation before?" "How did you manage that situation?" and "To whom can you turn for help?" The answers to these questions often reassure the client that he or she has encountered difficult situations in the past and has the ability and resources to cope with them.

A common and normal response is *denial,* which is a defense mechanism that enables the client to cope with threatening circumstances. The client may deny that he or she has the current cardiovascular condition, may state that it was present but is now absent, or may be excessively cheerful. Denying the seriousness of the illness while following the treatment regimen is a protective response; however, denial becomes maladaptive when the client is noncompliant with significant portions of medical and nursing care.

Family members and significant others may be more anxious than the client. Often they recall all events of the illness, are unprotected by denial, and are afraid of recurrence. Disagreements often occur between the client and family members over compliance with appropriate follow-up care.

Diagnostic Assessment

LABORATORY TESTS

Assessment of the client with cardiac dysfunction includes examination of the blood for abnormalities. The examination is performed to establish a diagnosis, detect concurrent disease, assess risk factors, and monitor response to treatment. Normal values for serum cardiac enzymes and serum lipids are listed in Chart 36-4.

Serum Markers of Myocardial Damage

Events leading to cellular injury cause a release of enzymes from intracellular storage, and circulating levels of these enzymes are dramatically elevated. Acute myocardial infarction (MI), also known as acute coronary syndrome, can be confirmed by abnormally high levels of enzymes or isoenzymes. These serum studies are commonly referred to as *cardiac markers.*

TROPONIN

Troponin is a myocardial muscle protein released into the bloodstream with injury to myocardial muscle. Troponin T and I are not found in healthy clients, so any rise in values indicates cardiac necrosis or acute MI. Specific markers of myocardial injury, troponin T and I have a wide diagnostic time frame, making them useful for clients who present several hours after the onset of chest pain. Even low levels of troponin T should be treated vigorously because of increased risk of death from cardiovascular disease (CVD). Obtaining cardiac markers at the bedside in the emergency department can be done as "point of care" (POC) testing for clients experiencing or at risk for acute MI with results available within 15 to 20 minutes. These markers are evaluated in addition to clinical signs and symptoms and ECG changes when identifying at-risk clients.

CREATINE KINASE (CK)-MB

Creatine kinase (CK) is an enzyme specific to cells of the brain, myocardium, and skeletal muscle. The appearance of CK in the blood indicates tissue necrosis or injury, with CK levels following a predictable rise and fall during a specified period. Cardiac specificity must be determined by measuring isoenzyme activity. There are three isoenzymes of CK: CK-MM is the predominant isoenzyme of skeletal muscle; CK-MB is found in myocardial muscle; and CK-BB occurs in the brain. CK-MB activity is most specific for MI and shows a predictable rise and fall during 3 days; a peak level occurs approximately 24 hours after the onset of chest pain.

Treatment modalities for early intervention after acute MI and acute ischemia require more rapid diagnosis of MI. An assay using monoclonal anti–CK-MB antibodies (stat CK) can detect myocardial necrosis accurately 3 hours after

CHART 36-4

LABORATORY PROFILE
Cardiovascular Assessment

Normal Range	Significance of Abnormal Findings
Serum Cardiac Enzymes	
Creatine kinase (CK) *Females*: 30-135 units/L *Males*: 55-170 units/L Values higher after exercise	Elevations indicate possible brain myocardial, and skeletal muscle necrosis or injury.
CK-MM (CK$_3$) 100% of total CK	Elevations occur with muscle injury.
CK-MB (CK$_2$) 0% of total CK	Elevations occur with myocardial injury or after percutaneous transluminal angioplasty and intracoronary streptokinase infusion.
CK-BB (CK$_1$) 0%	Elevations occur with brain tissue injury.
Serum Lipids	
Total lipids 400-1000 mg/dL	Elevation indicates increased risk of coronary artery disease (CAD).
Cholesterol 122-200 mg/dL, or 3.16-6.5 mmol/L *Older adult (>70 yr)*: 144-280 mg/dL	Elevation indicates increased risk of CAD.
Triglycerides *Females*: 35-135 mg/dL *Males*: 40-160 mg/dL *Older adult (>65 yr)*: 55-260 mg/dL	Elevation indicates increased risk of CAD.
Plasma high-density lipoproteins (HDLs) *Females*: mean 55-60 mg/dL *Males*: mean, 45-50 mg/dL Older adult range increases with age	Elevations protect against CAD.
Plasma low-density lipoproteins (LDLs) 60-180 mg/dL *Older adult (>65 yr)*: 92-221 mg/dL	Elevation indicates increased risk of CAD.
HDL: LDL ratio 3:1	Elevated ratios may protect against CAD.
VLDL 25%-50%	Elevated level indicates risk of CAD.
C-reactive protein (CRP) <1.0 mg/dL	Elevation may indicate tissue infarction or damage.
Serum Markers	
Troponins Cardiac troponin T <0.2 ng/mL Cardiac troponin I <0.03 ng/mL	Elevations indicate myocardial injury or infarction.
Myoglobin <90 mcg/L	Elevation indicates myocardial infarction.

VLDL, Very-low-density lipoproteins.

emergency department admission when examined with an electrocardiogram (ECG). Two subforms of CK-MB (CK-MB$_1$ and CK-MB$_2$) have also been identified. Abnormal elevations of these CK subforms may occur as early as 2 hours after MI. These subforms remain elevated for up to 12 hours after MI and appear to be very sensitive and specific early diagnostic markers of MI.

MYOGLOBIN

Another early marker of an MI is myoglobin. **Myoglobin**, a low-molecular-weight heme protein found in cardiac and skeletal muscle, is the earliest marker detected–as early as 2 hours after an MI with rapid decline after 7 hours. Because myoglobin is not cardiac specific, is found in skeletal and cardiac muscle, and is detected very early in the bloodstream makes its clinical usefulness more limited than troponin.

Serum Lipids

Elevated lipid levels are considered a risk factor for coronary artery disease (CAD). Cholesterol, triglycerides, and the protein components of high-density lipoproteins (HDL) and low-density lipoproteins (LDL) are evaluated to assess a client's degree of risk for CAD. The risk for CAD is three times greater in clients with a serum cholesterol level greater than 260 mg/dL than in clients with a serum level less than 200 mg/dL.

Each of the lipoproteins contains varying proportions of cholesterol, triglyceride, protein, and phospholipid. HDL contains mainly protein and 20% cholesterol, whereas LDL is predominantly cholesterol. Elevated LDL levels are positively correlated with CAD, whereas elevated HDL levels are negatively correlated and appear to be a protective factor.

A nonfasting blood sample for the measurement of serum cholesterol levels is acceptable. If triglycerides are to be evaluated with cholesterol, the health care provider requests the specimen after a 12-hour fast.

Homocysteine

Homocysteine is an amino acid that is produced when proteins breaks down. A certain amount of homocysteine is present in the blood, but elevated values may be an independent risk factor for the development of CVD. Although the relationship between homocysteine and CVD remains controversial, some studies suggest that elevated levels of homocysteine increase the risk of CVD as much as smoking and hyperlipemia, especially in women. A scientific advisory from the American Heart Association to reduce total homocysteine recommends screening for total homocysteine in high-risk clients who have a personal or family history of premature heart disease. Clients usually fast for 10 to 12 hours before the test, and the blood must be separated and frozen within 1 hour of collection. A level less than 12 mmol/dL is considered optimal.

Client education should emphasize the nutritional aspect in decreasing homocysteine levels. By eating foods rich in B complex vitamins, especially folic acid, homocysteine levels can be reduced and may decrease the risk for CVD. Some health care providers prescribe supplemental folic acid to clients with high homocysteine levels. Encourage the client to consume a diet high in folate, vitamin B$_6$, and vitamin B$_{12}$, such as in vegetables, fruits, legumes, meats, fish, and fortified grains and cereals.

C-Reactive Protein

Recent studies have shown that inflammation is a common and critical component to the development of atherothrombosis. **Highly sensitive C-reactive protein (hsCRP)** has been the most studied marker of inflammation. Any inflammatory process can produce CRP in the blood. Elevations are also seen with hypertension, infection, and smoking. A level less than 1 mg/dL is considered low risk; a level over 3 mg/dL places the client at high risk for heart disease. The most useful time to measure CRP appears to be for risk assessment in middle-aged or older persons. Cholesterol-lowering drugs known as *statins* are promoted because they may modify the anti-inflammatory process. Clients may reduce their CRP level with a low-fat, low-cholesterol diet; smoking cessation; exercise; statins; and aspirin.

Blood Coagulation Tests

Blood coagulation tests evaluate the ability of the blood to clot and are important in clients with a greater tendency to form thrombi (e.g., clients with atrial fibrillation, prosthetic valves, or infective endocarditis). They are also important for clients receiving anticoagulant therapy (e.g., during cardiac surgery, after thrombolytic therapy, and during treatment of an established thrombus).

PROTHROMBIN TIME AND INTERNATIONAL NORMALIZED RATIO

Prothrombin time (PT) and International Normalized Ratio (INR) are used when initiating and maintaining therapy with oral anticoagulants, such as sodium warfarin (Coumadin, Warfilone✱). They measure the activity of prothrombin, fibrinogen, and factors V, VII, and X. INR is the most reliable way to monitor anticoagulant status in warfarin therapy. The therapeutic ranges vary significantly based on the reason for the anticoagulation and the client's history.

PARTIAL THROMBOPLASTIN TIME

Partial thromboplastin time (PTT) is assessed in clients who are receiving heparin (Hepalean✱). It measures deficiencies in all coagulation factors except VII and XIII.

Arterial Blood Gases

Arterial blood gas (ABG) determinations are often obtained in clients with CVD. Determination of tissue oxygenation, carbon dioxide removal, and acid-base status is essential to appropriate intervention and treatment. (See Chapter 18 for a complete discussion of ABGs.)

Serum Electrolytes

Fluid and electrolyte balance is essential for normal cardiovascular performance. Cardiac manifestations often occur when there is an imbalance in either fluids or electrolytes in the body. For example, the cardiac effects of hypokalemia (low serum potassium level) include increased electrical instability, ventricular dysrhythmias, and an increased risk of digitalis toxicity. The effects of hyperkalemia on the myocardium include slowed ventricular conduction, peaked T waves on the ECG, and contraction followed by asystole (cardiac standstill).

Cardiac manifestations of hypocalcemia are ventricular dysrhythmias, a prolonged QT interval, and cardiac arrest. Hypercalcemia shortens the QT interval and causes AV block, digitalis hypersensitivity, and cardiac arrest.

Serum sodium values reflect fluid balance and may be decreased, indicating a fluid excess in clients with heart failure (dilutional hyponatremia).

Because magnesium regulates some aspects of myocardial electrical activity, hypomagnesemia has been implicated in some forms of rapid ventricular dysrhythmias. Another manifestation of hypomagnesemia is hypokalemia that is unresponsive to potassium replacement.

Complete Blood Count

The erythrocyte (red blood cell) count is usually decreased in rheumatic fever and infective endocarditis. It is increased in heart diseases characterized by inadequate tissue oxygenation.

Decreased hematocrit and hemoglobin levels (e.g., caused by hemorrhage or hemolysis from prosthetic valves) indicate anemia and can lead to angina or aggravate heart failure. Vascular volume depletion with hemoconcentration (e.g., hypovolemic shock and excessive diuresis) results in an elevated hematocrit.

The leukocyte (white blood cell) count is typically elevated after an MI and in various infectious and inflammatory diseases of the heart (e.g., infective endocarditis and pericarditis).

Critical Thinking Challenge

A middle-aged man, an accountant, with multiple cardiovascular risk factors comes to the emergency department with complaints of a dull, aching feeling in his shoulder and arm. His admission laboratory results include creatinine kinase of 190 units/L, troponin level of greater than 2.0 ng/mL, and C-reactive protein of 1.0 mg/dL.

1. What additional assessment should you perform for this client?
2. What is the significance of each of these test results?
3. How might the client's cardiac markers differ from hospital admission to discharge?

evolve For suggested answer guidelines, go to http://evolve.elsevier.com/Iggy/.

RADIOGRAPHIC EXAMINATIONS

Chest Radiography

Posteroanterior and left lateral x-ray views of the chest are routinely obtained to determine the size, silhouette, and position of the heart. In acutely ill clients, a simple anteroposterior (AP) view is obtained at the bedside. Cardiac enlargement, pulmonary congestion, cardiac calcifications, and placement of central venous catheters, endotracheal tubes, and hemodynamic monitoring devices are assessed by x-ray.

Angiography

Angiography of the arterial vessels, or **arteriography,** is an invasive diagnostic procedure that involves fluoroscopy and the use of contrast media. This procedure is performed when an arterial obstruction, narrowing, or aneurysm is suspected. The radiologist performs selective arteriography to evaluate specific areas of the arterial system. For example, a coronary arteriography, which is performed during left-sided cardiac catheterization, assesses arterial circulation within the heart. Angiography can also be performed on arteries in the extremities, mesentery, and cerebrum. Angiography is discussed under the appropriate associated diseases elsewhere in this text.

TABLE 36-4 Indications for Cardiac Catheterization

- To confirm suspected heart disease, including coronary artery disease, myocardial disease, valvular disease, and valvular dysfunction
- To determine the location and extent of the disease process
- To assess the following:
  - Stable, severe angina unresponsive to medical management
  - Unstable angina pectoris
  - Uncontrolled heart failure, ventricular dysrhythmias, or cardiogenic shock associated with acute myocardial infarction, papillary muscle dysfunction, ventricular aneurysm, or septal perforation
- To determine best therapeutic option (percutaneous transluminal coronary angioplasty, stents, coronary artery bypass graft, valvulotomy versus valve replacement)
- To evaluate effects of medical or invasive treatment on cardiovascular function, percutaneous transluminal coronary angioplasty, or coronary artery bypass graft patency

TABLE 36-5 Complications of Cardiac Catheterization

Right-Sided Heart Catheterization
- Thrombophlebitis
- Pulmonary embolism
- Vagal response

Left-Sided Heart Catheterization and Coronary Arteriography
- Myocardial infarction
- Stroke
- Arterial bleeding or thromboembolism
- Dysrhythmias

Right-Sided or Left-Sided Heart Catheterization*
- Cardiac tamponade
- Hypovolemia
- Pulmonary edema
- Hematoma or blood loss at insertion site
- Reaction to contrast medium

*In addition to those cited for each procedure.

Cardiac Catheterization

The most definitive, but most invasive, test in the diagnosis of heart disease is cardiac catheterization. **Cardiac catheterization** may include studies of the right or left side of the heart and the coronary arteries. Some of the most common indications for cardiac catheterization are listed in Table 36-4.

CLIENT PREPARATION. Assessment of the client's physical and psychosocial readiness and knowledge level is an important aspect of client preparation because many clients have anxiety and fear about cardiac catheterization. Most individuals are very anxious and fearful about the procedure.

Review the purpose of the procedure, inform the client about the length of the procedure, state who will be present, and describe the appearance of the catheterization laboratory. The client is also informed about the sensations that may be experienced during the procedure, such as palpitations (as the catheter is passed up to the left ventricle), a feeling of heat or a hot flash (as the medium is injected into either side of the heart), and a desire to cough (as the medium is injected into the right side of the heart). Written or illustrated materials or videotapes may be used, if available, to assist in the client's understanding.

The risks of cardiac catheterization are usually explained by the interventional cardiologist. The risks vary with the procedures to be performed and the client's physical status (Table 36-5). Several complications may follow coronary arteriography, such as the following:

- Myocardial infarction (MI)
- Stroke
- Arterial bleeding
- Thromboembolism
- Lethal dysrhythmias
- Death

The cardiologist or radiologist obtains a written informed consent from the client or responsible party prior to the procedure.

The client may be admitted to the hospital on the day of the catheterization procedure. Standard preoperative tests are performed, which usually include a chest x-ray, complete blood count, coagulation studies, and 12-lead ECG. The client receives nothing by mouth after midnight or has only a liquid breakfast if the catheterization is to take place in the afternoon. The catheterization site is shaved and antiseptically prepared according to the institution's policy.

Nursing assessment before the procedure includes measuring the client's vital signs, auscultating the heart and the lungs, and evaluating the peripheral pulses. Question the client about any history of allergy to iodine-based contrast agents. An antihistamine or steroid may be given to a client with a positive history or to prevent a reaction. A mild sedative is usually administered before the procedure. If the client normally takes a digitalis preparation or diuretic, it is usually withheld before the catheterization.

PROCEDURE. The client is taken to the cardiac catheterization laboratory (sometimes referred to as the "cath lab"), placed in the supine position on the x-ray table, and securely strapped to the table. Inform the client that this precaution is necessary because the table turns like a cradle during the procedure. The physician injects a local anesthetic at the insertion site. During the procedure, the client is instructed to report any chest pain, pressure, or other symptoms to the staff.

RIGHT-SIDED HEART CATHETERIZATION. The right side of the heart is catheterized first and may be the only side examined. The cardiologist inserts a catheter through the femoral vein to the inferior vena cava or through the basilic vein to the superior vena cava. The catheter is advanced through either the inferior or the superior vena cava and, guided by fluoroscopy, is advanced through the right atrium (RA), through the right ventricle and, at times, into the pulmonary artery (Figure 36-11). Intracardiac pressures (right atrial, right ventricular, pulmonary artery, and pulmonary artery wedge pressures) and blood samples are obtained. A contrast medium is usually injected to detect any cardiac shunts or regurgitation from the pulmonic or tricuspid valves.

LEFT-SIDED HEART CATHETERIZATION. In a left-sided heart catheterization, the cardiologist advances the catheter against the blood flow from the femoral or brachial artery up the aorta, across the aortic valve, and into the left ventricle. Alternatively the cardiologist may pass the catheter from the right side of the heart through the atrial septum, using a special needle to puncture the septum. Intracardiac pressures and blood samples are obtained. The pressures of the left atrium, left ventricle, and aorta, as well as mitral and aortic valve status, are evaluated. The cardiologist injects contrast dye into the ventricle; cineangiograms

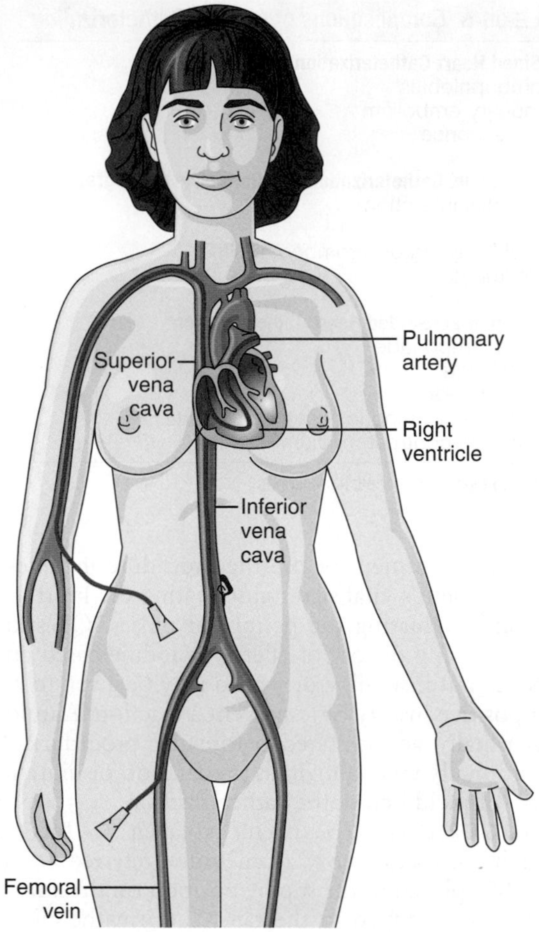

Figure 36-11 ■ Right-sided heart catheterization. The catheter is inserted into the femoral vein and advanced through the inferior vena cava (or, if into an antecubital or basilic vein, through the superior vena cava), right atrium, and right ventricle and into the pulmonary artery.

(rapidly changing films) evaluate left ventricular motion. Calculations are made regarding end-systolic volume, end-diastolic volume, stroke volume, and ejection fraction.

CORONARY ARTERIOGRAPHY. The technique for coronary arteriography is the same as for left-sided heart catheterization. The catheter is advanced into the aortic arch and positioned selectively in the right or left coronary artery. Injection of a contrast medium permits visualization of the coronary arteries. By assessing the flow of the medium through the coronary arteries, information about the site and severity of coronary lesions is obtained.

INTRAVASCULAR ULTRASONOGRAPHY. An alternative to injecting a medium into the coronary arteries is **intravascular ultrasonography (IVUS),** which introduces a flexible catheter with a miniature transducer at the distal tip to visualize the coronary arteries. The transducer emits sound waves, which reflect off the plaque and the arterial wall, creating an image of the blood vessel. IVUS is more reliable than angiography in indicating plaque distribution and composition, arterial dissection, and degree of stenosis of the occluded artery.

FOLLOW-UP CARE. After cardiac catheterization, the client is typically restricted to bedrest, and the insertion site extremity is kept straight. A soft knee brace can be applied to prevent bending of the affected extremity. Some cardiologists allow the head of the bed to be elevated up to 30 or 45 degrees during the period of bedrest, whereas other cardiologists prefer that the client remain supine. Current practice is for clients to remain in bed for 4 to 6 hours unless a special closure is used. Several arterial closure devices are available during the procedure to eliminate the need for manual compression or sandbags after the catheterization. Examples include arteriotomy sutures and collagen plugs to seal the insertion site.

There are many post-catheterization nursing responsibilities. Monitor vital signs every 15 minutes for 1 hour, then every 30 minutes for 2 hours or until vital signs are stable, and then every 4 hours or according to hospital policy. Assess the insertion site for bloody drainage or hematoma formation. Peripheral pulses in the affected extremity, as well as skin temperature and color, are monitored with every vital sign check.

Observe for complications of cardiac catheterization (see Table 36-5). Complaints of pain and discomfort at the insertion site, chest pain, nausea, or feelings of light-headedness should be reported. The client is recovered in the post-anesthesia care unit or other specialty area where monitored beds are located. Because the contrast medium acts as an osmotic diuretic, monitor urine output and ensure that the client receives sufficient oral and IV fluids for adequate excretion of the medium. Pain medication for insertion site or back discomfort may be given as prescribed.

If the client experiences chest pain, dysrhythmias, bleeding, hematoma formation, or a dramatic change in peripheral pulses in the affected extremity, contact the physician immediately and provide prompt intervention. Neurologic changes, such as visual disturbances, slurred speech, swallowing difficulties, and extremity weakness, should also be reported.

OTHER DIAGNOSTIC TESTS

Electrocardiography

The **electrocardiogram (ECG)** is a routine part of every cardiovascular evaluation and is one of the most valuable diagnostic tests. Various forms are available: resting ECG, continuous ambulatory ECG (Holter monitoring), exercise ECG (stress test), and signal-averaged ECG. The resting ECG provides information about cardiac dysrhythmias, myocardial ischemia, the site and extent of MI, cardiac hypertrophy, electrolyte imbalances, and the effectiveness of cardiac drugs. The normal ECG pattern of one cardiac cycle is illustrated in Figure 36-12. Further discussion of the interpretation and evaluation of normal and abnormal patterns is found in Chapter 37.

RESTING ELECTROCARDIOGRAPHY

The ECG graphically records the electrical current generated by the heart. This current is measured by electrodes that are placed on the skin and connected to an amplifier and strip chart recorder (Figure 36-13). In the standard 12-lead ECG, five electrodes attached to the arms, legs, and chest measure current from 12 different views or leads: three bipolar limb leads (Figure 36-14), three unipolar augmented leads (Figure 36-15), and six unipolar precordial leads (Figure 36-16). Placement of the leads allows the health care provider to view myocardial electrical conduction from different axes or positions, identifying sections of the heart in which electrical conduction is abnormal.

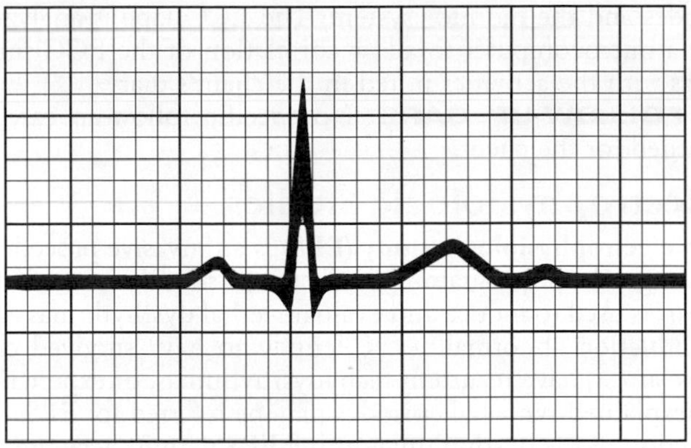

Figure 36-12 ■ A normal ECG pattern in lead II.

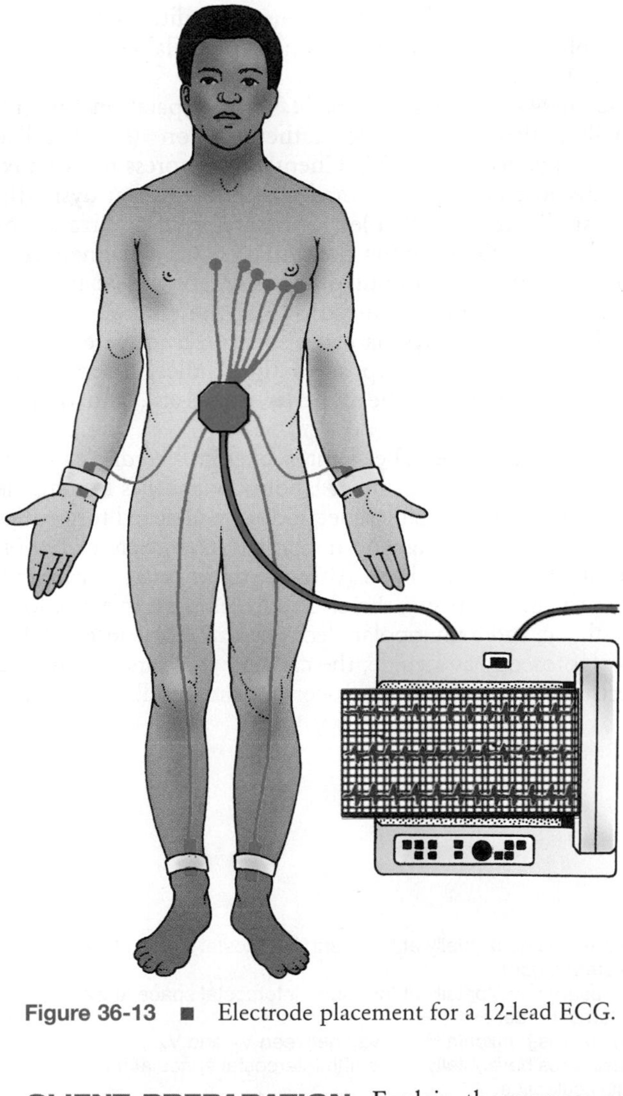

Figure 36-13 ■ Electrode placement for a 12-lead ECG.

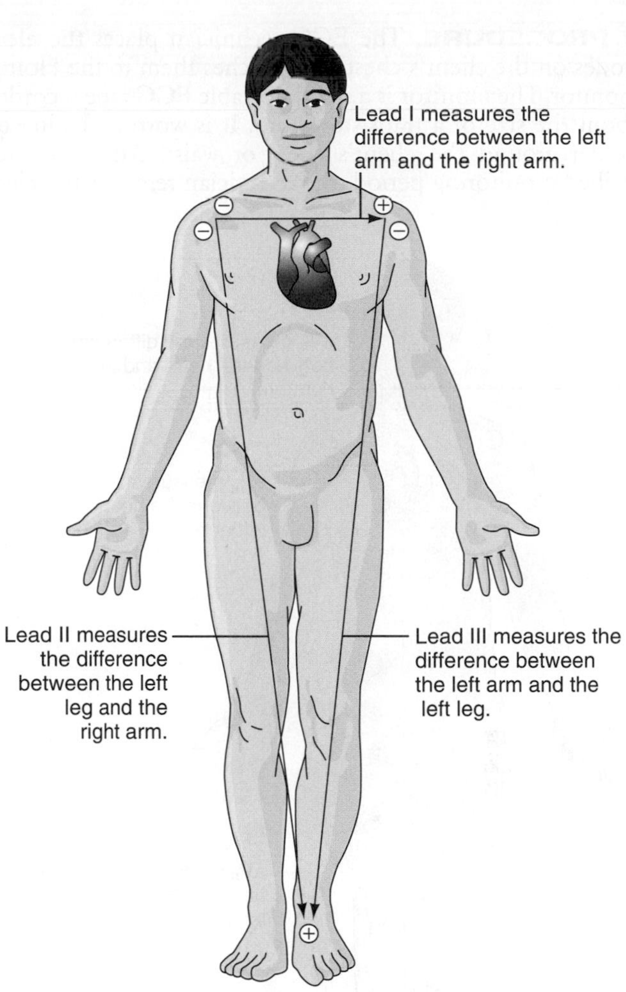

Figure 36-14 ■ Standard ECG limb leads.

CLIENT PREPARATION. Explain the purpose and procedure of the resting ECG, inform the client that the test is safe and painless, and remind him or her to lie as still as possible during the test.

PROCEDURE. The ECG is performed with the client in a supine position with the chest exposed. Before applying the electrodes, the nurse or the technician washes the skin to reduce skin oils and improve electrode contact. To ensure good contact between the skin and the electrodes for the limb leads, the electrodes should be placed on a flat surface above the wrists and the ankles. A total of 10 electrodes are used for a standard ECG and are attached to lead wires that connect to the ECG machine. The 12-lead ECG reading is obtained by selecting the indicators on the machine.

FOLLOW-UP CARE. No specific follow-up care is warranted.

AMBULATORY ELECTROCARDIOGRAPHY

Ambulatory ECG (also called *Holter monitoring*) allows continuous recording of cardiac activity during an extended period (usually 24 hours) while the client is performing his or her usual activities of daily living (ADLs). The ambulatory ECG allows the assessment and correlation of dyspnea, chest pain, CNS symptoms (e.g., light-headedness and syncope), and palpitations with actual cardiac events and the client's activities.

CLIENT PREPARATION. Encourage the client to maintain a normal day's schedule. He or she is instructed to keep a diary, or log, in which to note the time of activities (e.g., eating, sleeping, walking, working) and to record any symptoms such as chest pain, light-headedness, fainting, and palpitations. Instruct the client to avoid operating heavy machinery, using electric shavers and hair dryers, and bathing or showering because these activities may interfere with the ECG recorder. If the client is hospitalized, the nurse may need to make the diary entries.

PROCEDURE. The ECG technician places the electrodes on the client's chest and attaches them to the Holter monitor. The monitor is a small portable ECG tape recorder about the size of a transistor radio. It is worn in a sling or holder around the client's chest or waist. After the prescribed monitoring period, the technician removes the electrodes and the monitor system. The ECG tape is analyzed by a microcomputer to allow correlation of the ECG findings with the activities noted in the client's diary.

FOLLOW-UP CARE. No specific follow-up care is needed for the client.

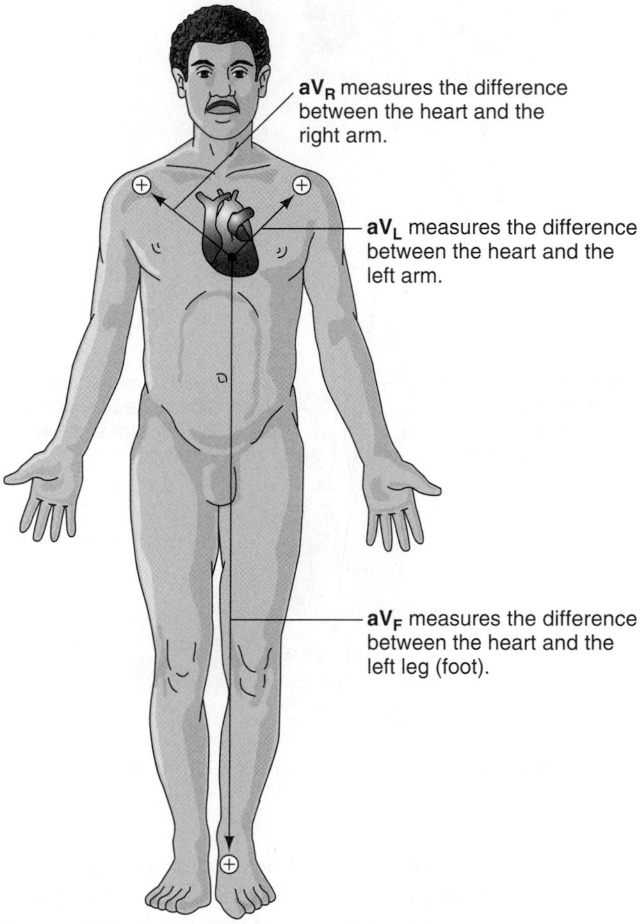

Figure 36-15 ■ Unipolar augmented ECG leads.

Electrophysiologic Studies

An **electrophysiologic study (EPS)** is an invasive procedure during which programmed electrical stimulation of the heart is used to induce and evaluate lethal dysrhythmias and conduction abnormalities. Clients who have survived cardiac arrest, have recurrent tachydysrhythmias, or experience unexplained syncopal episodes may be referred for EPS. Induction of the dysrhythmia during EPS permits accurate diagnosis of the dysrhythmia and aids in the search for an effective treatment. These procedures have risks similar to those for cardiac catheterization and are performed in a special catheterization laboratory, where conditions are strictly controlled and immediate treatment is available for any adverse effects.

CLIENT PREPARATION. The preparation for EPS parallels that for cardiac catheterization (see Cardiac Catheterization on p. 697). Clients may express fear or anxiety because attempts are made to induce lethal dysrhythmias similar to those that led to the initial hospitalization or resuscitation. Reassure the client that EPS is a planned, controlled event and that immediate treatment will be available for any dysrhythmia induced during the studies. An electrophysiologist (a physician who specializes in these studies) usually explains the purpose of the studies, describes the procedure (including the benefits and risks), and obtains written consent.

PROCEDURE. The client is taken to a cardiac catheterization laboratory or a similar laboratory and lies in a supine position on an x-ray table. Electrodes are attached for continuous ECG monitoring, and defibrillation pads are placed on the client's chest and back. After the nurse or technician prepares the insertion site, the electrophysiologist injects a local anesthetic, and a multipolar electrode catheter is inserted. Using fluoroscopy as a guide, the catheter is advanced until the electrodes rest in the RA, adjacent to the bundle of His, and

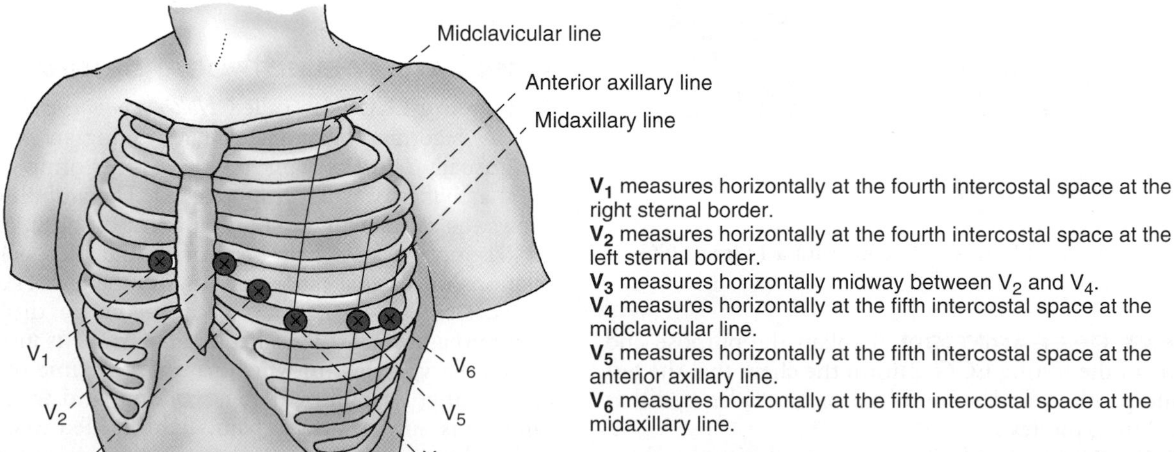

Figure 36-16 ■ Unipolar precordial ECG leads.

in the right ventricle. Additional electrodes may be placed for endocardial mapping.

During EPS, baseline conduction times can be measured: the AH interval (conduction time from the RA through the His bundle) and the HV interval (conduction time from the proximal His bundle to the ventricular myocardium). The catheter may be programmed to pace at varying rates to determine the function of the SA and AV node, or it may be programmed to deliver premature paced stimuli in an effort to initiate and evaluate tachydysrhythmia.

If the dysrhythmia is induced, it may terminate spontaneously or be treated by the physician. The physician might elect to use properly timed stimuli, rapid pacing, medications, or countershock to terminate the dysrhythmia.

The client is advised to inform the staff about any symptoms that he or she experiences. During rapid pacing, the client may be aware of the rapid heartbeat and state that he or she is experiencing palpitations. The client may also experience chest pain or loss of consciousness if he or she becomes hypotensive. The client often experiences back discomfort during the procedure because he or she must remain supine for 2 to 6 hours. Pain may develop at the insertion site as the anesthetic wears off.

FOLLOW-UP CARE. Follow-up care for EPS is the same as for cardiac catheterization. Comfort measures may be provided to alleviate back discomfort, including massage and position changes. If the client lost consciousness during the procedure and received electrical cardioversion or defibrillation, he or she may complain of chest discomfort over the area where the electrical current was applied. Assess the skin for any signs of redness, swelling, or burns. In addition, there may be memory loss for the events during the procedure; if so, provide reassurance and calmly explain the events of the procedure.

Exercise Electrocardiography (Stress Test)

The **exercise electrocardiography** test (also known as exercise tolerance, or **stress test**) assesses cardiovascular response to an increased workload. The stress test helps to determine the functional capacity of the heart and screens for asymptomatic coronary artery disease. Dysrhythmias that develop during exercise may be identified, and the effectiveness of antidysrhythmic drugs can be evaluated.

CLIENT PREPARATION. Because there are risks associated with exercising, the client must be adequately informed about the purpose of the test, the procedure, and the risks involved. Written consent must be obtained. Anxiety and fear are common before stress testing. Therefore assure the client that the procedure is performed in a controlled environment where prompt nursing and medical attention is available.

The client is instructed to get plenty of rest the night before the procedure. He or she may have a light meal 2 hours before the test but should avoid smoking or drinking alcohol or caffeine-containing beverages on the day of the test. The cardiologist decides whether the client should stop taking any cardiac medications. He or she is advised to wear comfortable, loose clothing and rubber-soled, supportive shoes. Instruct the client to tell the physician if symptoms such as chest pain, dizziness, shortness of breath, and an irregular heartbeat are experienced during the test.

Before the stress test, a resting 12-lead ECG, cardiovascular history, and physical examination are performed to check for any ECG abnormalities or medical factors that might interfere with the test.

Emergency supplies such as cardiac drugs, a defibrillator, and other necessary resuscitation equipment are available in the room in which the stress test is performed. It is important to be proficient in the use of resuscitation equipment when assisting the physician because chest pain, dysrhythmias, and other ECG changes may occur during this test.

PROCEDURE. The technician places electrodes on the client's chest and attaches them to a multilead monitoring system. Note baseline blood pressure (BP), heart rate (HR), and respiratory rate. The two major modes of exercise available for stress testing are pedaling a bicycle ergometer and walking on a treadmill. A bicycle ergometer has a wheel operated by pedals that can be adjusted to increase the resistance to pedaling. The treadmill is a motorized device with an adjustable conveyor belt; it can reach speeds of 1 to 10 miles/hr and can also be adjusted from a flat position to a 22-degree gradient.

After the client is shown how to use the bicycle or to walk on the treadmill, he or she begins to exercise. During the test, the BP and electrocardiogram (ECG) are closely monitored as the resistance to cycling or the speed and incline of the treadmill are increased. The client exercises until one of the following occurs:

- A predetermined HR is reached and maintained.
- Signs and symptoms such as chest pain, fatigue, extreme dyspnea, vertigo, hypotension, and ventricular dysrhythmias appear.
- Significant ST-segment depression occurs.

FOLLOW-UP CARE. After the test, the nurse continues to monitor the ECG and BP until the client has completely recovered. After the client has recovered, he or she can return home if the test was performed on an ambulatory basis. Advise the client to avoid a hot shower for 1 to 2 hours after the test because this may precipitate hypotension. If the client does not recover but continues to have pain or ventricular dysrhythmias or appears medically unstable, he or she is admitted to a telemetry unit for observation.

For clients who are unable to exercise because of conditions such as peripheral vascular disease or arthritis, pharmacologic stress testing with agents such as dobutamine may be indicated. The nursing considerations are similar to those for the client who has undergone an exercise electrocardiography.

Echocardiography

As a noninvasive, risk-free test, echocardiography is easily performed at the bedside or on an ambulatory care basis. **Echocardiography** uses ultrasound waves to assess cardiac structure and mobility, particularly of the valves. ECGs help to assess and diagnose cardiomyopathy, valvular disorders, pericardial effusion, left ventricular function, ventricular aneurysms, and cardiac tumors.

CLIENT PREPARATION. There is no special preparation for echocardiography. Inform the client that the test is painless and takes 30 to 60 minutes to complete. The client is instructed to lie quietly during the test and on his or her left side with the head elevated 15 to 20 degrees.

PROCEDURE. During an echocardiogram, a small transducer lubricated with gel to facilitate movement and conduction is placed on the client's chest at the level of the third or fourth intercostal space near the left sternal border. The transducer transmits high-frequency sound waves and receives them as they are reflected from different structures. These echoes are usually videotaped simultaneously with the echocardiogram and can be recorded on graph paper for a permanent record.

After the images are taped, cardiac measurements that require several images can be obtained. Routine measurements include chamber size, ejection fraction, and flow gradient across the valves.

FOLLOW-UP CARE. There is no specific follow-up care for a client who has undergone an echocardiogram.

Pharmacologic Stress Echocardiogram

A slightly more aggressive form of echocardiogram is a **pharmacologic stress echocardiogram** using either dobutamine or adenosine. This test is usually used when clients cannot tolerate exercise. Dobutamine (Dobutrex) increases the heart's contractility; adenosine (Adenocard) is a coronary artery dilator. Clients are required to have nothing by mouth (NPO status) for 3 to 6 hours before the test, except for sips of water with medications. The technician ensures that IV access is present before the procedure and monitors BP and pulse continuously throughout the procedure. After the procedure, vital signs are monitored until BP returns to baseline and the pulse rate slows to less than 100 beats/min.

Transesophageal Echocardiography

Echocardiograms may also be performed transesophageally (through the esophagus). **Transesophageal echocardiography (TEE)** examines cardiac structure and function with an ultrasound transducer placed immediately behind the heart in the esophagus or stomach. The transducer provides especially detailed views of posterior cardiac structures such as the left atrium, mitral valve, and aortic arch. Preparation and follow-up are similar to that for an upper gastrointestinal endoscopic examination (see Chapter 56).

Myocardial Nuclear Perfusion Imaging

The use of radionuclide techniques in cardiovascular assessment is called **myocardial nuclear perfusion imaging (MNPI).** Cardiovascular abnormalities can be viewed, recorded, and evaluated using radioactive tracer substances. These studies are useful for detecting myocardial infarction (MI) and decreased myocardial blood flow and for evaluating left ventricular ejection. Conducting myocardial nuclear imaging tests, in conjunction with exercise or the administration of vasodilating agents such as dipyridamole and adenosine, allow clearer identification of how the heart responds to stress.

CLIENT PREPARATION. Inform the client that the tests are relatively noninvasive. Because the amount of radioisotope is small, radiation exposure risks are minimal. If a dilating agent is to be used, the client is advised to abstain from cigarettes and caffeinated food or drinks for 4 hours before administration of the vasodilator.

PROCEDURE. Common tests in nuclear cardiology include technetium (^{99m}Tc) pyrophosphate scanning, thallium imaging, and multigated cardiac blood pool imaging.

TECHNETIUM PYROPHOSPHATE SCANNING. For this scan, a small dose of ^{99m}Tc pyrophosphate is injected into the antecubital vein. The client waits at least 2 hours while the renal system clears the unbound technetium. A gamma-scintillation camera scans the heart to identify the areas of increased uptake of the radioisotope. The radioisotope accumulates in damaged myocardial tissue and is referred to as a "hot spot." This test helps to detect an acute MI and define its location and size, but it does not show an old infarction.

THALLIUM IMAGING. For thallium imaging, a small dose of thallium-201 (^{201}Tl) is injected into the client's antecubital vein. A nuclear camera takes images of the heart 10 minutes later to detect areas of normal blood flow and intact cells, which rapidly take up the thallium. Necrotic or ischemic tissue does not take up the radioisotope and appears as "cold spots" on the scan. Scanning is repeated in 2 to 4 hours to evaluate thallium clearance.

Thallium imaging may be performed with the client at rest or during an exercise test. Dipyridamole (Persantine, Apo-Dipyridamole✱) is administered before the Persantine thallium test. Dobutamine hydrochloride (Dobutrex) or adenosine (Adenocard) may be given instead. By causing vasodilation, these drugs simulate the effects of exercise and are used for clients who are unable to exercise on a bike or treadmill. These medications may cause flushing, headache, dyspnea, and chest tightness for a few moments after injection.

Thallium imaging performed during an exercise test may demonstrate perfusion deficits not apparent at rest. First, the stress test procedure is performed (see Exercise Electrocardiography [Stress Test], p. 701). After the client reaches maximum activity level, a small dose of ^{201}Tl is injected intravenously. The client continues to exercise for approximately 1 to 2 minutes, after which the scanning is performed. Nuclear cardiologists often compare the resting and stress images to differentiate between fixed and reversible defects in the myocardium.

Thallium imaging is used to assess myocardial scarring and perfusion, to detect the location and extent of an acute or chronic MI, evaluate graft patency after coronary bypass surgery, and evaluate antianginal therapy, thrombolytic therapy, or balloon angioplasty.

CARDIAC BLOOD POOL IMAGING. Cardiac blood pool imaging is a noninvasive test for evaluating cardiac motion and calculating ejection fraction. It uses a computer to synchronize the client's electrocardiogram (ECG) with pictures taken by a gamma-scintillation camera. The technician attaches the client to an ECG and injects a small amount of ^{99m}Tc intravenously. The radioisotope is not taken up by tissue but remains "tagged" to red blood cells in the circulation. The camera may take pictures of the radioactive material as it makes its first pass through the heart.

During **multigated blood pool scanning,** the computer breaks the time between R waves on the ECG into fractions of a second, called "gates." The camera records blood flow through the heart during each of these gates. By analyzing the information from multiple gates, the computer can evaluate the ventricular wall motion and calculate ejection fraction (percentage of the left ventricular volume that is ejected with each contraction) and ejection velocity. Areas of decreased, absent, or paradoxical movement of the left ventricle may also be identified.

POSITRON EMISSION TOMOGRAPHY. Positron emission tomography (PED) scans are used to compare cardiac perfusion and metabolic function and differentiate normal from diseased myocardium. The technician administers the first radioisotope (nitrogen-13-ammonia) and then begins a 20-minute scan to detect myocardial perfusion. Next the technician administers a second radioisotope (fluoro-18-deoxyglucose). After a pause, a second scan is performed to detect the metabolically active myocardium, which is using glucose.

The two scans are compared. In a normal heart, performance and metabolic function will match. In an ischemic heart, there will be a mismatch: a reduction in perfusion and increased glucose uptake by the ischemic myocardium. The scanning procedure takes 2 to 3 hours, and the client may be asked to use a treadmill or exercise bicycle in conjunction with the scan.

FOLLOW-UP CARE. Depending on which test is performed, the client may complain of fatigue or discomfort at the antecubital injection site. If a stress test was paired with the study, the client will need follow-up care for the stress test.

Magnetic Resonance Imaging

Magnetic resonance imaging (MRI) is a noninvasive diagnostic option. An image of the heart or great vessels is produced through the interaction of magnetic fields, radio waves, and atomic nuclei showing hydrogen density. Simply put, the radio waves "bounce off" the body tissue being examined. Because each tissue has its own density, the computer image clearly differentiates between different types of tissues. MRI permits determination of cardiac wall thickness, chamber dilation, valve and ventricular function, and blood movement in the great vessels. Improved MRI techniques allow coronary artery blood flow to be mapped with nearly the accuracy of a cardiac catheterization.

Before an MRI, ensure that the client has removed all metallic objects, including watches, jewelry, clothing with metal fasteners, and hair clips. Clients with pacemakers should not undergo an MRI because the magnetic fields can deactivate the pacemaker. Approximately 5% of clients experience claustrophobia during the 15 to 60 minutes required to complete the scan.

Electronic-Beam Computed Tomography Scan

Electronic-beam computed tomography (EBCT) is a valuable tool in cardiovascular diagnostics. This test helps to determine whether calcifications are present in the arteries; calcifications are a common component of arterial plaque.

Hemodynamic Monitoring

Hemodynamic monitoring is an invasive system used in critical care areas to provide quantitative information about vascular capacity, blood volume, pump effectiveness, and tissue perfusion. Hemodynamic monitoring directly measures pressures in the heart and great vessels. These procedures are usually performed for more seriously ill clients and can provide more accurate measurements of blood pressure, heart function, and volume status.

Hemodynamic monitoring does involve significant risks, although complications are uncommon. Therefore informed consent is required. After obtaining consent, the nurse prepares a pressure-monitoring system. The components of this system are a catheter with an infusion system, a transducer, and a monitor. The catheter receives the pressure waves (mechanical energy) from the heart or the great vessels. The transducer converts the mechanical energy into electrical energy, which is displayed as waveforms or numbers on the monitor. Patency of the catheter is maintained with a slow continuous flush of normal saline, usually infused at 3 to 4 mL/hr under pressure to prevent the back up of blood and occlusion of the catheter.

To prepare the transducer, balance and calibrate it according to hospital policy and the manufacturer's specifications. Finally, identify the phlebostatic axis (Chart 36-5) and level the transducer to it. When the monitoring system is prepared, the physician inserts the catheter.

CHART 36-5

BEST PRACTICE for
Identification of the Phlebostatic Axis

1. Position the client supine.
2. Palpate the fourth intercostal space at the sternum.

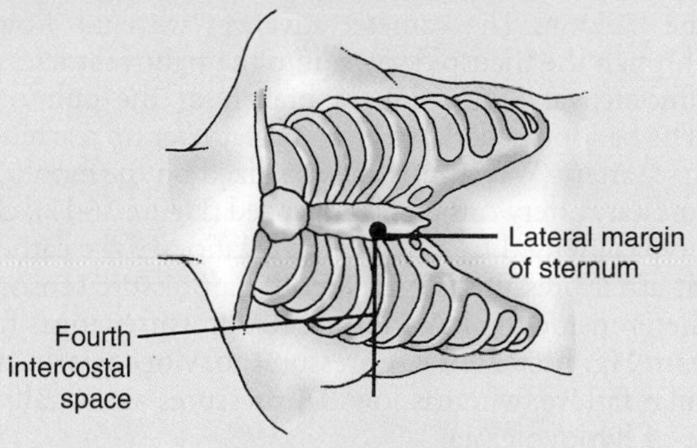

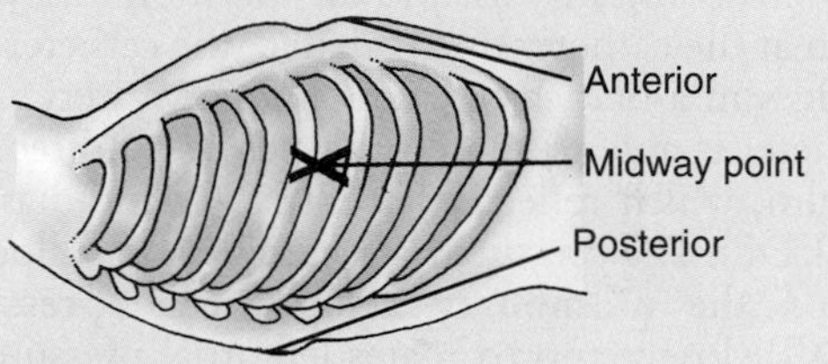

3. Follow the fourth intercostal space to the side of the client's chest.
4. Determine the midway point between anterior and posterior.
5. Find the intersection between the midway point and the line from the fourth intercostal space, and mark it with an X in indelible ink. This is the phlebostatic axis.

RIGHT ATRIAL, PULMONARY ARTERY, AND PULMONARY WEDGE PRESSURES

A pulmonary artery catheter is a multi-lumen catheter with the capacity to measure right atrial and indirect left atrial pressures or pulmonary artery wedge pressure (PAWP), also known as the **pulmonary artery occlusive pressure (PAOP).** A cardiac output measurement may also be obtained, as well as cardiac index and systemic and pulmonary vascular resistance.

CLIENT PREPARATION. The physician explains the procedure and advises the client and family members or significant others of the risks. The physician then obtains written consent for the procedure. The client and family should understand that the hemodynamic monitoring system represents an assessment tool. Although it is used to guide therapy, it is not itself a treatment. Ask the client to remain still and in the supine or Trendelenburg position for insertion of the catheter.

PROCEDURE. The physician inserts a balloon-tipped catheter percutaneously through a large vein, usually the internal jugular or subclavian, and directs it to the right atrium (RA). When the catheter tip reaches the RA, the physician inflates the balloon. The catheter advances with the flow of blood through the tricuspid valve, into the right ventricle, past the pulmonic valve, and into a branch of the pulmonary artery. The balloon is deflated after the catheter tip reaches the pulmonary artery. Waveforms are visualized on the monitor as the pulmonary artery catheter is advanced (Figure 36-17); chest x-ray is typically used to monitor the location of the catheter.

Right atrial pressure is measured by a pressure sensor on the catheter inside the RA. Normal RA pressure ranges from 1 to 8 mm Hg. Increased RA pressures may occur with right ventricular failure, whereas low RA pressures are usually indicative of hypovolemia.

Normal pulmonary artery pressure (PAP) ranges from 15 to 26 mm Hg systolic/5 to 15 mm Hg diastolic (mean, 15) and are constantly visible on the monitor. When the balloon at the catheter tip is inflated, the catheter advances and wedges in a branch of the pulmonary artery. The tip of the catheter is able to sense pressures transmitted from the left atrium, which reflect left ventricular end-diastolic pressure (LVEDP). The pressure measured during balloon inflation is called the **pulmonary artery wedge pressure (PAWP).** PAWP closely approximates left atrial pressure and LVEDP in clients with normal left ventricular function, normal heart rates, and no mitral valve disease. The PAWP is a mean pressure and normally ranges between 4 and 12 mm Hg.

Elevated PAWP measurements may indicate left ventricular failure, hypervolemia, mitral regurgitation, or intracardiac shunt. A decreased PAWP is seen with hypovolemia or afterload reduction. Individual values may be less important than the trend in values.

FOLLOW-UP CARE. The critical care nurse obtains and records RA pressure, PAP, and PAWP at appropriate intervals (usually every 1 to 4 hours). The trend of these pressures helps to guide medical therapy. During pressure recording, it is important that the transducer be at the level of the phlebostatic axis and that the client's position be appropriate. The client is usually supine with the head elevated up to 45 degrees during hemodynamic readings, although the client's position may not affect results (see the Evidence-Based Practice for Nursing box on p. 705). If the balloon remains in the wedge position after PAWP measurement, try to change the catheter's position by asking the client to cough or by changing the client's position. If these methods are not successful, notify the physician immediately.

Change the occlusive dressing over the catheter aseptically according to hospital policy. Inspect the insertion site for redness, induration, swelling, drainage, and intactness of the sutures. Detailed discussion of the management and care of clients with pulmonary artery catheters can be found in textbooks on critical care nursing.

Be sure to assess for a number of complications associated with pulmonary artery catheters. For example, pulmonary infarction or pulmonary rupture may occur if the catheter remains in the wedge position. Air embolism is possible if the balloon has ruptured and repeated attempts are made to inflate it. Ventricular dysrhythmias may occur during insertion or if the catheter tip slips back into the right ventricle and irritates the myocardium. Thrombus and embolus formation may occur at the catheter site. Infection may result, and bleeding may be pronounced if the infusion system becomes disconnected.

CARDIAC OUTPUT

Cardiac output can be measured using the thermodilution method when the client has a pulmonary artery catheter with a thermistor. A specified amount (5 or 10 mL) of iced

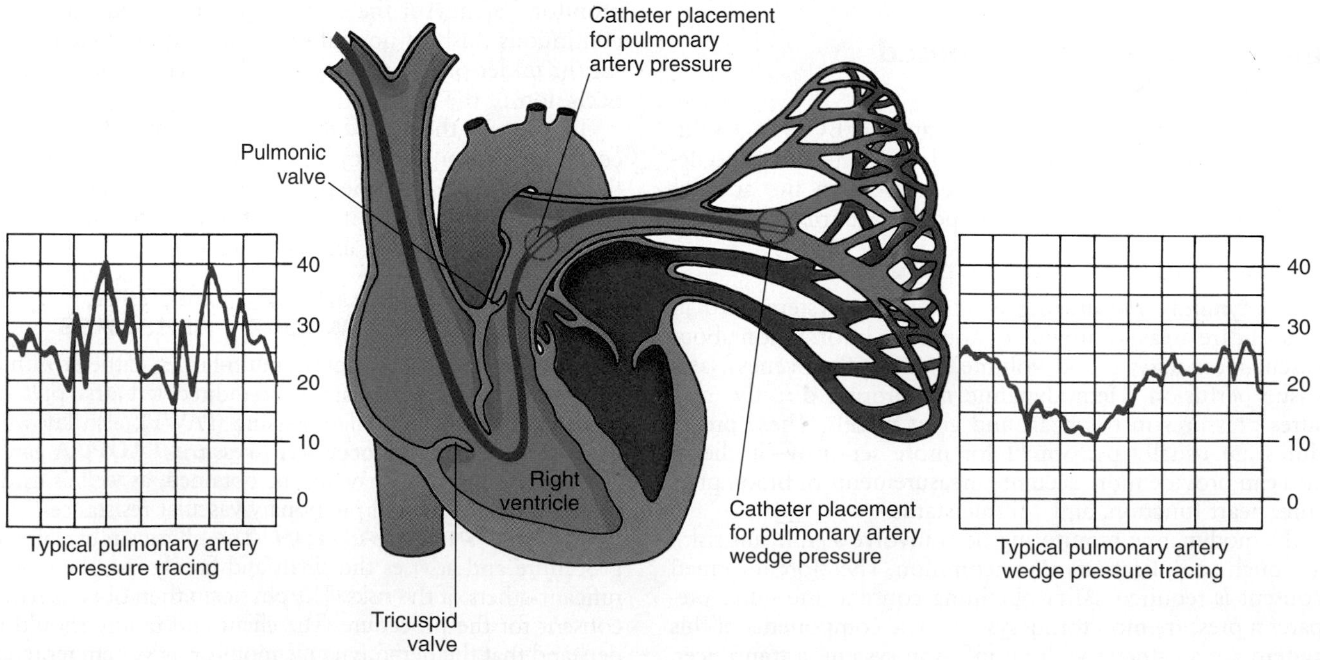

Figure 36-17 ■ Cardiac pressure waveforms can be visualized on the monitor.

or room-temperature IV solution (normal saline or dextrose in water) is injected into the proximal port of the catheter. The solution mixes with the blood in the RA and travels with the flow of blood through the heart. A temperature-sensitive device located on the tip of the catheter in the pulmonary artery registers and senses the change in blood temperature. This information is transmitted to a cardiac output computer, which displays a digital value. Nursing research continues to confirm that client positioning may not affect cardiac output readings (see the Evidence-Based Practice for Nursing box below).

MIXED VENOUS OXYGEN SATURATION MONITORING

Mixed venous oxygen saturation (SvO_2) reflects the balance between the client's oxygen supply and demand. SvO_2 may be measured with a pulmonary artery catheter with fiberoptics. Light travels down one optical fiber, is reflected by the red blood cells according to the oxygen saturation of the hemoglobin, and returns to an optical module for interpretation and continuous display. The normal range for SvO_2 is 60% to 80%. Using SvO_2 monitoring individualizes the plan of care so that the SvO_2 remains in the normal range and the client's oxygen supply and demand are in balance.

EVIDENCE-BASED PRACTICE for Nursing

What is the effect of the different positions on the accuracy of cardiac output readings?

Giuliano, K.K., et al. (2003). Backrest angle and cardiac output measurements in critically ill patients. *Nursing Research,* 52(4), 242-248.

The purpose of this study was to determine whether different position changes affect continuous cardiac output (CO) measurements in critical care clients with head elevation angles of 0 degrees, 30 degrees, and 45 degrees, at time intervals of 0 minutes, 5 minutes, and 10 minutes after changing positions.

The 26 adult critical care clients were recruited in an adult intensive care unit (ICU), and all had a cardiac output catheter in place for continuous CO measurements. Four repeated measures of analysis of variance (ANOVA) were done, one for each dependent variable: continuous cardiac index, stroke value, heart rate, and mean arterial pressure. No significant differences were found across the nine different measurement conditions. The lack of CO change in different positions was determined not to be due to compensatory changes within the CO determinants of stroke volume and heart rate.

Level of Evidence: 6—This study was small but was well-controlled research.

Critique. This study was conducted by a qualified nurse researcher and expert critical care nurses with critical care registered nurse (CCRN) status. The research question was answered using single-group, repeated-measures ANOVA with two participant factors: time and backrest angle. A repeated-measures ANOVA was used for this study because repeated measurements of cardiac index were done on each individual in the study. This allowed each person to serve as his or her own control. It also permitted a descriptive comparison to other studies, which used repeated measure ANOVA; however, the sample is small, and only one unit was used.

Implications for Nursing. These findings add to the growing body of evidence about positioning in current practice and support earlier research indicating that critically ill clients need not to be repositioned unnecessarily solely for the purpose of obtaining a cardiac output. It adds to other empirical data in demonstrating that CO measurements can be taken in different positions without significantly affecting the results.

SYSTEMIC INTRA-ARTERIAL MONITORING

Direct measurement of arterial BP is by invasive arterial catheter in critically ill clients. The physician or specially trained nurse inserts an intra-arterial catheter into the radial or femoral artery. After the physician has inserted the catheter, it is attached to pressure tubing. A normal saline flush solution is infused constantly under pressure to maintain the integrity of the system. A transducer attached to the tubing allows continuous direct monitoring of the arterial BP. Direct measurements of BP are usually 10 to 15 mm Hg greater than indirect (cuff) measurements. The arterial catheter may also be used to obtain blood samples for arterial blood gas values and other blood tests.

Because the arterial vasculature is a high-pressure system, frequent assessment of the arterial site and infusion system is essential. Note any bleeding around the intra-arterial catheter or any loose connections and correct the situation immediately. Collateral circulation must be assessed by Doppler or Allen's tests before and while the arterial catheter is in place. Color, pulse, and temperature distal to the insertion site should be scrupulously monitored for any early signs of circulatory compromise. Complications of systemic intra-arterial monitoring may include pain, infection, arteriospasm, or obstruction at the site with the potential for distal infarction, air embolism, and hemorrhage.

Impedance Cardiography

Unlike conventional hemodynamic monitoring, **impedance cardiography (ICG)** is a flexible and fast–acting noninvasive monitoring system that consists of four ICG electrodes, four electrocardiogram (ECG) electrodes, and a portable ICG monitor. Simply stated, it measures the total impedance (resistance) to the flow of electricity in the heart. ICG can be used in any setting: intensive care unit (ICU), emergency department (ED), and in the home. ICG is used to assess, plan, and individualize the treatment plan for clients with heart failure, severe trauma, or fluid management. It provides measures of thoracic fluid, left ventricular function (cardiac output and cardiac index), preload, afterload, and contractility of the heart.

GET READY for the NCLEX Examination!

KEY POINTS

Safe Effective Care Environment

- Assess the older adult for cardiovascular changes associated with aging as described in Chart 36-1.
- Assess clients for allergy to iodine-based contrast media before having diagnostic tests requiring a contrast agent.
- Following invasive cardiovascular diagnostic testing, such as angiography and cardiac catheterization, monitor the insertion site for bleeding and hematoma formation.
- Assess vital signs carefully in clients having invasive cardiovascular testing; report new dysrhythmias following testing.

Health Promotion and Maintenance

- Identify clients at risk for cardiovascular disease, especially those with hyperlipidemia, hypertension, excess weight, physical inactivity, smoking, psychological stress, a positive family history, and diabetes.

- Teach clients how to reduce the risk of heart disease through exercise, diet modification, smoking cessation, and medications, as needed.
- Inform clients that genetics and other nonmodifiable risk factors, such as family history and gender, contribute to the development of CAD.

Psychosocial Integrity

- Discuss with the client any feelings or concerns he or she might have about the stress of cardiac illness, diagnostic testing, or other issues and use therapeutic measures to decrease anxiety.
- Recognize that denial is a common and normal response to help clients cope with threatening circumstances.
- Be aware that coping behaviors of clients who have cardiovascular problems vary from client to client.
- Allow the client to express feelings about an actual or perceived loss of health or social status related to cardiovascular disease.

Physiological Integrity

- Assess the client's complaint of pain to differentiate between the pain of angina and myocardial infarction (MI) from other noncardiac causes; discomfort, indigestion, squeezing, heaviness, and "viselike" are common terms used to describe chest pain of cardiac origin.
- Recall that syncope is a transient loss of consciousness and is common in older adults.
- Use jugular venous pressure to assess the filling volume and pressure on the right side of the heart.
- Assess for bruits, which are swishing sounds that develop in narrowed arteries.
- Auscultate the heart for normal first and second sounds, as well as for abnormalities such as an S_3, S_4, murmur, or gallop.
- Monitor serum markers of myocardial damage and other cardiac related laboratory tests as listed in Chart 36-4.
- Assess clients having cardiac catheterizations for potential complications as listed in Table 36-5.
- Directly assess cardiac pressures and cardiac output when clients have invasive hemodynamic monitoring systems.

ADDITIONAL STUDY RESOURCES

Go to your Student CD-ROM for Review Questions for the NCLEX Examination.

evolve Go to http://evolve.elsevier.com/Iggy/ for Integrated Management of Care Questions for the NCLEX Examination.

SELECTED BIBLIOGRAPHY

Asterisk indicates a classic or definitive work on this subject.

American Heart Association. (2002). *Heart disease and stroke statistics–2003 update.* Dallas: Author.

Beyerle, K. (2002). Point of care testing of cardiac markers aids patient experiencing or at risk for acute myocardial infarction. *Nursing Management, 33*(9), 37-39.

Bonham, P.A. (2003). Determining the toe brachial pressure index. *Nursing 2003, 33*(9), 54-55.

Bridges, E.J., et al. (2000). Effect of the 30° lateral recumbent position in pulmonary artery and pulmonary artery wedge pressures in critically ill adult cardiac surgery patients. *American Journal of Critical Care, 9*(4), 262-275.

Burke, A.P., et al. (2002). Traditional risk factors and the incidence of sudden coronary death with and without coronary thrombosis in blacks. *Circulation, 105*(4), 419-424.

Cheek, D., & Cesan, A. (2003). What's different about heart disease in women? *Nursing 2003, 33*(8), 36-43.

Coffey, M., Crowder, G.K. & Cheek, D.J. (2003). Reducing coronary artery disease by decreasing homocysteine levels. *Critical Care Nurse, 23*(1), 25-30.

Critchley, J.A., & Capewell, S. (2003). Mortality risk reduction associated with smoking cessation in patients with coronary heart disease. *Journal of the American Medical Association, 290*(1), 86-97.

Crook, J., & Woody, F. (2003). Rapidly identify CHF with POC advances. *Nursing Management, 34*(1), 48-49.

D'Agostino, R.B., et al., for the CHS Risk Prediction Group (2001). Validation of the Framingham coronary heart disease prediction scores. *Journal of the American Medical Association, 286*(2), 180-187.

DeVon, H.A., & Zerwic, J.J. (2003). The symptoms of unstable angina: Do women and men differ? *Nursing Research, 52*(2), 108-118.

Fletcher, S.W., & Colditz, G.A. (2002). Failure of estrogen plus progestin therapy for prevention. *Journal of the American Medical Association, 288*(3), 366-368.

Funk, M., et al. (2002). Racial differences in the use of cardiac procedures in patients with acute myocardial infarction. *Nursing Research, 51*(3), 148-157.

Futterman, L., & Lemberg, L. (2002). High sensitivity C-reactive protein is the most effective prognostic measurement of acute coronary events. *American Journal of Critical Care, 11*(5), 482-486.

Gibbons, R.J., et al. (2002). *ACC/AHA 2002 guideline update for the management of patients with chronic stable angina: a report of the American College of Cardiology/American Heart Association Task Force on Practice Guidelines* (Committee to Update the 1999 Guidelines for the Management of Patient with Chronic Stable Angina). Accessed July 25, 2003, from http://www.acc.org/clinical/guidelines/stable/stable.pdf.

Giuliano, K.K, et al. (2003). Backrest angle and cardiac output measurement in critically ill patients. *Nursing Research, 52*(4), 242-248.

Groeneveld, P.W., Heidenreich, P.A., & Garber, A.M. (2003). Racial disparity in cardiac procedures and mortality among long-term survivors of cardiac arrest. *Circulation, 108*(3), 286-291.

Jarvis, C. (2004). *Physical examination and health assessment.* 4th ed. St. Louis: Elsevier Science.

Khattar, R.S., et al. (2001). Effect of aging on the prognostic significance of ambulatory systolic, diastolic, and pulse pressure in essential hypertension. *Circulation, 104*(7), 783-790.

Maas, M.L., et al. (2001). *Nursing care of older adults: Diagnoses, outcomes, and interventions.* St. Louis: Mosby.

Mehta, M. (2003). Assessing cardiovascular status. *Nursing 2003, 33*(1), 56-57.

Natarajan, et al. (2003). Sex differences in risk for coronary heart disease mortality associated with diabetes and established coronary heart disease. *Archives of Internal Medicine, 163*(14), 1735-1740.

National Cholesterol Education Program (2002). *Third report of the Expert Panel on Detection, Evaluation, and Treatment of High Blood Cholesterol in Adults (Adult Treatment Panel III).* Bethesda: National Heart, Lung, and Blood Institute, NIH Publication No. 02-5215.

National Heart, Lung, and Blood Institute (2002). *Postmenopausal hormone therapy: facts about postmenopausal hormone therapy.* Bethesda: NIH Publication No. 02-5200. Accessed August 8, 2003, from http://www.nhlbi.nih.gov/health/women/pht_facts.

National High Blood Pressure Education Program (2002). *Primary prevention of hypertension: clinical and public health advisory.* Bethesda: National Heart, Lung, and Blood Institute, NIH Publication No. 02-5076.

National High Blood Pressure Education Program (2003). *The seventh report of the Joint National Committee on Prevention, Detection, Evalua-*

tion, and Treatment of High Blood Pressure. Bethesda: National Heart, Lung, and Blood Institute, NIH Publication No. 03-5233.

*New York Heart Association Criteria Committee. (1964). *Diseases of the heart and blood vessels: Nomenclature and criteria for diagnosis* (6th ed.). Boston: Little, Brown.

Oliver-McNeil, S., & Artinian, N.T. (2003). Women's perceptions of personal cardiovascular risk and their risk-reducing behaviors. *American Journal of Critical Care, 11*(3), 221-227.

Otsuka, R., et al. (2001). Acute effects of passive smoking on the coronary circulation in healthy young adults. *Journal of the American Medical Association, 286*, 436-441.

Pagana, K.D., & Pagana, T.J. (2002). *Manual of diagnostic and laboratory tests* (2nd ed.). St. Louis: Mosby.

Paternak, R.C., et al. (2002). ACC/AHA/ NHLBI advisory on the use and safety of statins. *Journal of American College of Cardiology, 40*, 567-572.

Rauscher, F.M., et al. (2003). Aging, progenitor cell exhaustion, and atherosclerosis. *Circulation, 108*(4), 457-462.

Samara, J.N., & Popkin, B.M. (2003). Patterns and trends in food portion sizes, 1977-1998. *Journal of the American Medical Association, 290*, 450-453.

Sever, P.S., et al. (2003). Prevention of coronary and stroke events with atorvastatin in hypertensive patients who have average or lower than average cholesterol concentrations, in the Anglo-Scandinavian cardiac outcomes trial-lipid lowering arm (ASCOT-LLA): a multicentre randomized controlled trial. *The Lancet, 361*, 1149-1158.

Siomko, A.J. (2000). Demystifying cardiac markers. *American Journal of Nursing, 100*(1), 36-41.

*A Statement for Healthcare Professionals from the AHA Task Force on Risk Reduction. Primary Prevention of Coronary Heart Disease: Guidance from Framingham. (1998). AHA Scientific Statement. *Circulation, 97*(18), 1876-1887.

Turner, M.A. (2000). Monitoring hemodynamics noninvasively. *Nursing2000, 30*(5), 32cc1-32cc8.

Vakili, B.A., Kaplan, R.C., & Brown, D.L. (2001). Sex-based differences in early mortality of patients undergoing primary angioplasty for first acute myocardial infarction. *Circulation, 104*(25), 3034-3039.

Valli, G., & Giardina, E.G. (2002). Benefits, adverse effects and drug interactions of herbal therapies with cardiovascular effects. *Journal of American College of Cardiology, 39*, 1083-1095.

Writing Group for the Women's Health Initiative Investigators (2002). Risks and benefits of estrogen plus progestin in healthy postmenopausal women. *Journal of the American Medical Association-Express, 288*, 321-333.

Yeh, E.T.H., et al. (2001). C-reactive protein: Linking inflammation to cardiovascular complications. *Circulation, 104*(9), 974-979.

CHAPTER

37 Interventions for Clients with Dysrhythmias

PAMELA C. ZICKAFOOSE

LEARNING OUTCOMES

After studying this chapter, you should be able to:

1. Correlate the components of the electrocardiogram (ECG) with the cardiac conduction system.
2. Analyze a rhythm strip or ECG tracing to identify common cardiac dysrhythmias.
3. Identify typical physical assessment findings associated with common dysrhythmias.
4. Prioritize nursing diagnoses for clients experiencing dysrhythmias.
5. Plan care for clients experiencing common dysrhythmias.
6. Implement appropriate treatment modalities, including antidysrhythmic drugs, for common and lethal dysrhythmias.
7. Develop a teaching plan for clients experiencing common dysrhythmias.
8. Explain the purpose and types of pacing used as interventions for clients with dysrhythmias.
9. Differentiate between defibrillation and cardioversion, identifying the indications for the use of each.
10. Plan community-based care for a client after pacemaker or implantable cardioverter/defibrillator insertion.

Go to your Student CD-ROM for Review Questions for the NCLEX Examination keyed to these Learning Outcomes.

Cardiac dysrhythmias are abnormal rhythms of the heart's electrical system. Some dysrhythmias are life threatening, and others are benign. They are the result of disturbances of cardiac electrical impulse formation, conduction, or both. Many diseases (coronary artery disease [CAD] leading to ischemia and myocardial infarction [MI] are most common) as well as electrolyte imbalance, changes in oxygenation, and drug toxicity can affect the electrical activity of the heart, causing dysrhythmias. A dysrhythmia can markedly change the cardiac output and cause deterioration in vital signs. Although more common in older adults, dysrhythmias can occur in people of any age. To interpret and treat dysrhythmias correctly, an understanding of cardiac electrophysiology, the conduction system of the heart, and the principles of electrocardiography are needed.

REVIEW OF CARDIAC ELECTROPHYSIOLOGY

Electrophysiologic Properties

The electrophysiologic properties of cardiac cells regulate heart rate and rhythm. Specialized cardiac muscle cells possess unique properties: automaticity, excitability, conductivity, and contractility.

AUTOMATICITY

Automaticity (pacing function) is the ability of cardiac cells to generate an electrical impulse spontaneously and repetitively. Normally only primary pacemaker cells (SA node, AV junction) possess the ability to generate an electrical impulse. Under certain conditions, such as myocardial ischemia (decreased blood flow), electrolyte imbalance, hypoxia, drug toxicity, an abnormally configured electrical system, and infarction (cell death), any cardiac cell may generate electrical impulses independently and create dysrhythmias. Disturbances in automaticity may involve either an increase or a decrease in pacing function.

EXCITABILITY

Excitability is the ability of nonpacemaker myocardial cells to respond to an electrical impulse generated from pacemaker cells and to depolarize. Depolarization occurs when the normally negatively charged cells develop a positive charge.

CONDUCTIVITY

Conductivity is the ability to transmit an electrical stimulus from cell membrane to cell membrane. Consequently, excitable cells depolarize in rapid succession from cell to cell until all cells have depolarized. The wave of depolarization gives rise to the deflections of the electrocardiogram (ECG) waveforms that are recognized as the P wave and the QRS complex. Disturbances in conduction result when conduction is too rapid or too slow, when there is a total blockage of the pathway, or when there is an abnormal pathway that the electrical impulse travels. Re-entry is a situation in which a misdirected electrical impulse re-excites a conduction pathway through which it has already passed. Re-entry results in tachycardia.

CONTRACTILITY

Contractility is the ability of atrial and ventricular muscle cells to shorten their fiber length in response to electrical stimulation, generating sufficient pressure to propel blood forward. Contractility is the mechanical activity of the heart.

Action Potential

The cardiac cell membrane (sarcolemma) exhibits selective permeability to ions. An ion is an electrically charged particle. The selective permeability creates an electrical imbalance, known as an **action potential,** across the cell membrane. The cardiac cell at rest has an internal negative charge, whereas the charge outside the cell is positive. The state of electrical imbalance of the resting cell is called **resting membrane potential**.

Cardiac Conduction System

The cardiac conduction system consists of specialized cells (Figure 37-1). The conduction system is responsible for the generation and conduction of electrical impulses that cause atrial and ventricular depolarization. The conduction system consists of the sinoatrial node, atrioventricular junctional area, and bundle branch system.

SINOATRIAL NODE

The conduction system begins with the **sinoatrial (SA) node** (also called the sinus node), located close to the epicardial surface of the right atrium near its junction with the superior vena cava. The SA node is the heart's primary pacemaker. It can spontaneously and rhythmically generate electrical impulses at a rate of 60 to 100 beats/min, possessing the greatest degree of automaticity.

The SA node is richly supplied by the sympathetic and parasympathetic nervous systems, which accelerate and decelerate the rate of discharge of the sinus node, respectively. This process results in changes in the heart rate.

Impulses from the sinus node move directly through atrial muscle and lead to atrial depolarization, which is reflected in a P wave on the ECG. Atrial muscle contraction should follow. Within the atrial muscle are slow and fast conduction pathways leading to the atrioventricular (AV) node.

ATRIOVENTRICULAR JUNCTIONAL AREA

The **atrioventricular (AV) junctional** area consists of a transitional cell zone, the AV node itself, and the bundle of His. The AV node lies just beneath the right atrial endocardium, between the tricuspid valve and the ostium of the coronary sinus. Here T-cells (transitional cells) cause impulses to slow down or to be delayed in the AV node before proceeding to the ventricles. This delay is reflected in the PR segment on the ECG. This slow conduction provides a short delay, allowing the atria to contract and the ventricles to fill. The contraction is known as "atrial kick" and contributes additional blood volume for a greater cardiac output. The AV node is also controlled by both the sympathetic and the parasympathetic nervous systems. The bundle of His connects with the distal portion of the AV node and continues to perforate the interventricular septum.

BUNDLE BRANCH SYSTEM

The bundle of His extends as a right bundle branch down the right side of the interventricular septum to the apex of the right ventricle. On the left side it extends as a left bundle branch, which further divides into two fascicles.

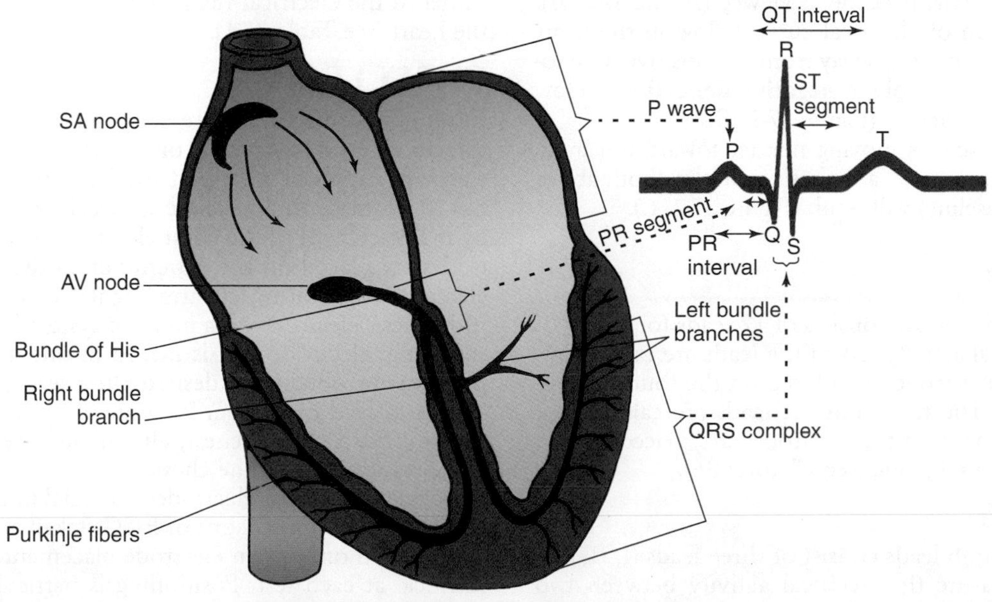

Figure 37-1 ■ The cardiac conduction system.

At the ends of both the right and left bundle branch systems are the Purkinje fibers. These fibers are an interweaving network located on the endocardial surface of both ventricles, from apex to base. The fibers then partially penetrate into the myocardium. **Purkinje cells** make up the bundle of His, bundle branches, and terminal Purkinje fibers. These cells are responsible for the rapid conduction of electrical impulses throughout the ventricles, leading to ventricular depolarization and the subsequent ventricular muscle contraction. A few nodal cells in the ventricles also occasionally demonstrate automaticity, giving rise to ventricular beats or rhythms.

ELECTROCARDIOGRAPHY

The **electrocardiogram (ECG)** provides a graphic representation, or picture, of cardiac electrical activity. The weak cardiac electrical currents are transmitted to the body surface. Electrodes, consisting of a conductive gel on an adhesive pad, are placed on specific sites on the body and attached to cables connected to an ECG machine or to a monitor. The cardiac electrical current is transmitted via the electrodes and through the lead wires to the machine or monitor, which displays the cardiac electrical activity.

A **lead** provides one view of the heart's electrical activity. Multiple leads, or views, can be obtained. Electrode placement is the same for male and female clients.

Lead systems are made up of a positive pole and a negative pole. An imaginary line joining these two poles is called the **lead axis**. The direction of electrical current flow in the heart is the **cardiac axis**. The relationship between the cardiac axis and the lead axis is responsible for the deflections seen on the ECG pattern:

- The baseline is the isoelectric line. It occurs when there is no current flow in the heart after complete depolarization and also after complete repolarization. Positive deflections occur above this line, and negative deflections occur below it. Deflections represent depolarization and repolarization of cells.
- If the direction of electrical current flow in the heart (cardiac axis) is toward the positive pole, a **positive deflection** (above the baseline) is viewed (Figure 37-2, *A*).
- If the direction of electrical current flow in the heart (cardiac axis) is moving away from the positive pole toward the negative pole, a **negative deflection** (below the baseline) is viewed (Figure 37-2, *B*).
- If the cardiac axis is moving neither toward nor away from the positive pole, a biphasic complex (both above and below baseline) will result (Figure 37-2, *C*).

Lead Systems

The standard 12-lead ECG consists of 12 leads (or views) of the heart's electrical activity. Six of the leads are called limb leads because the electrodes are placed on the four limbs in the frontal plane. The remaining six leads are called chest (precordial) leads because the electrodes are placed on the chest in the horizontal plane (see Chapter 36).

LIMB LEADS

Standard bipolar limb leads consist of three leads (I, II, and III) that each measure the electrical activity between two points and a fourth lead (right leg) that acts solely as a ground electrode (Table 37-1; see also Chapter 36). Of the three measuring leads, the right arm is always negative, the left leg is always positive, and the left arm can be either positive or negative. Bipolar leads can be obtained by using a monitor with either three or five electrode cables or a 12-lead ECG machine.

Unipolar limb leads consist of a positive electrode only. These leads can be obtained only by using a monitor with four or five electrode cables or a 12-lead ECG machine. The unipolar limb leads are aVR, aVL, and aVF, with *a* meaning augmented. *V* is a designation for a unipolar lead. The third letter denotes the positive electrode placement: *R* for right arm, *L* for left arm, and *F* for foot (left leg). The positive electrode is at one end of the lead axis. The other end is the center of the electrical field, at approximately the center of the heart (see Table 37-1).

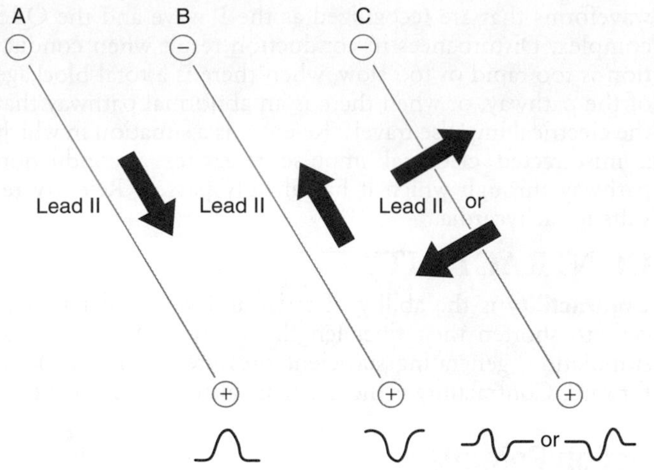

Figure 37-2 ■ **A,** The cardiac axis (bold arrow) is parallel to the lead axis (the line between the negative and the positive electrodes), going toward the positive electrode; a positive deflection is inscribed. **B,** The cardiac axis is parallel to the lead axis, going toward the negative electrode; a negative deflection is inscribed. **C,** The cardiac axis is perpendicular to the lead axis, going neither toward the positive electrode nor toward the negative electrode; a biphasic deflection is inscribed.

CHEST LEADS

Chest (precordial) leads are also unipolar (or V) leads and therefore can be obtained only from a monitor with five electrode cables or a 12-lead ECG machine, which usually has 10 electrode cables. There are six chest leads, determined by the placement of the chest electrode. The four limb electrodes are placed on the extremities, as designated on each electrode (right arm, left arm, right leg, and left leg). The fifth (chest) electrode on a monitor system is the positive, or exploring, electrode and is placed in one of six designated positions to obtain the desired chest lead (see Table 37-1). With a 12-lead ECG, four leads are placed on the limbs and six are placed on the chest, eliminating the need to move any electrodes about the chest.

Positioning of the electrodes is crucial in obtaining an accurate ECG. Comparisons of ECGs taken at different times will be valid only when electrode placement is accurate and identical at each test. Positioning is particularly important when serving clients with chest deformities or large breasts.

TABLE 37-1 Electrode Placement for 12 Leads

Lead	Negative Electrode	Positive Electrode	Ground Electrode
I	Right arm or under the right clavicle	Left arm or under the left clavicle	Right leg or lowest rib, left midclavicular line
II	Right arm or under the right clavicle	Left leg or lowest rib, left midclavicular line	Right leg or under the left clavicle
III	Left arm or under the left clavicle	Left leg or lowest rib, left midclavicular line	Right leg or under the right clavicle
aVR	Average potential of left arm (or under the left clavicle) and left leg (or lowest rib, left midclavicular line)	Right arm or under the right clavicle	Right leg or lowest rib, right midclavicular line
aVL	Average potential of right arm (or under the right clavicle) and left leg (or lowest rib, left midclavicular line)	Left arm or under the left clavicle	Same as for aVR
aVF	Average potential of right arm (or under the right clavicle) and left arm (or under the left clavicle)	Left leg or lowest rib, left midclavicular line	Same as for aVR
V_1	Average potential of right arm, left arm, and left leg	Fourth intercostal space (ICS), right sternal border	Same as for aVR
V_2	Same as for V_1	Fourth ICS, left sternal border	Same as for aVR
V_3	Same as for V_1	Midway between V_2 and V_4	Same as for aVR
V_4	Same as for V_1	Fifth ICS, left midclavicular line	Same as for aVR
V_5	Same as for V_1	Horizontal to V_4, left anterior axillary line	Same as for aVR
V_6	Same as for V_1	Horizontal to V_4, left midaxillary line	Same as for aVR

Clients may be asked to displace the breast to ensure proper electrode placement.

While obtaining a 12-lead ECG, the client should be as still as possible in a semi-reclined position, breathing normally. Any repetitive movement will cause artifact and could lead to inaccurate interpretation of the ECG.

Often nurses are responsible for obtaining 12-lead ECGs, but more commonly technicians are trained to take 12-lead ECGs in various health care settings. It is imperative that the technician notify the nurse or physician of any suspected abnormality. A nurse may direct a technician to take a 12-lead ECG on a client experiencing chest pain to observe for diagnostic changes, but it is ultimately the physician's responsibility to interpret the ECG.

Continuous Electrocardiographic Monitoring

PROCEDURE

For continuous electrocardiographic (ECG) monitoring, the electrodes are not placed on the limbs because movement of the extremities causes "noise," or motion artifact, on the ECG signal. Place the electrodes on the trunk, a more stable area, to minimize such artifacts and to obtain a clearer signal. If the monitoring system provides five electrode cables, place the electrodes as follows:

- Right arm electrode just below the right clavicle
- Left arm electrode just below the left clavicle
- Right leg electrode on the lowest palpable rib, on the right midclavicular line
- Left leg electrode on the lowest palpable rib, on the left midclavicular line
- Fifth electrode placed to obtain one of the six chest leads

With this placement, the monitor lead select control may be changed to provide lead I, II, III, aVR, aVL, or aVF or one chest lead. The monitor automatically alters the polarity of the electrodes to provide the lead selected.

If the monitoring system provides only three electrode cables, place the right arm, the left arm, and the left leg electrodes as described. In this case, the lead selected provides only lead I, II, or III.

The popular MCL_1 lead is a modified *(M)* bipolar chest *(C)* lead. It approximates the V_1 lead without requiring a five-electrode cable monitoring system because it is a bipolar lead system. To obtain MCL_1, place the negative electrode just below the left *(L)* midclavicle and the positive electrode in the V_1 position. The ground electrode can be placed anywhere but is usually placed under the right clavicle. Use this lead for bedside or telemetry monitoring to differentiate left from right electrical activity, such as left from right bundle branch block or left from right premature ventricular complexes, and to differentiate certain supraventricular beats from ventricular ectopic beats. Another bipolar lead, MCL_6, is frequently used. It can be achieved by placing the negative and ground electrodes as for MCL_1 and moving the positive electrode to the V_6 position. This approximates the V_6 lead. It is used for the same reasons as is the MCL_1.

The clarity of continuous ECG monitor recordings is affected by skin preparation and electrode quality. To ensure the best signal transmission and to decrease skin impedance, clean the skin and shave the area if needed. Make sure the area for electrode placement is dry. The gel on each electrode must be moist and fresh. Attach the electrode to the lead cable and then to the contact site. The contact site should be free of any lotion, tincture, or other substance that increases skin impedance. Electrodes cannot be placed on irritated skin or over scar tissue. The application of electrodes may be done by assistive nursing personnel, but the nurse must determine which lead to select and check for correct electrode placement. Assess the quality of the ECG rhythm transmission to the monitoring system, and assess and manage the client.

TELEMETRY

The ECG cables can be attached directly to a wall-mounted monitor (a hard-wired system) if the client's activity is restricted to bedrest and sitting in a chair, as in a critical care unit. For an ambulatory client, the ECG cable is attached to a battery-operated transmitter (a **telemetry** system) held in a pouch worn by the client. The ECG is transmitted via antennae located in strategic places, usually in the ceiling, to a remote monitor. Telemetry allows freedom of movement within a certain radius without losing transmission of the ECG.

Some acute care facilities employ monitor technicians who are educated in ECG rhythm interpretation and are responsible for the following:

- Watching a bank of monitors on a unit
- Printing ECG rhythm strips routinely and as needed
- Interpreting rhythms
- Communicating with the nurse to report the client's rhythm and significant changes

The technical support is particularly helpful on a telemetry unit that does not have monitors at the bedside. The nurse is reasonably assured that the ECG rhythm is being monitored "continuously," although some rhythms will not be observed by technicians. The nurse remains ultimately responsible for accurate ECG rhythm interpretation as well as for client assessment and management.

Some units have full-disclosure monitors, which continuously store ECG rhythms in memory up to a maximum amount of time, allowing nurses and physicians to access and print them for more thorough assessment and management of clients with dysrhythmias. Routine strips, as well as any changes in rhythm, are printed and documented in the client's record.

The physician is responsible for determining when monitoring can be suspended, such as when the client is showering. The health care provider also determines whether monitoring is needed during off-unit testing procedures and for transportation to other facilities. Collaborate with the physician in making these determinations.

Prehospital personnel, such as paramedics and emergency medical technicians (EMTs) with advanced training, frequently monitor a client's ECG rhythm at the scene and en route to a health care facility. They function under medical direction and protocols but may also be in communication with a nurse in the emergency department.

Electrocardiographic Paper

The electrocardiogram (ECG) strip is printed on graph paper (Figure 37-3), with each small block measuring 1 mm in height and width. ECG recorders and monitors are standardized at a speed of 25 mm/sec. Time is measured on the horizontal axis. At this speed, each small block represents 0.04 second. Five small blocks make up one large block, defined by darker bold lines and representing 0.20 second. Five large blocks represent 1 second, and 30 large blocks represent 6 seconds. Vertical lines in the top margin of the graph paper are usually 15 large blocks apart, representing 3-second segments.

Electrocardiographic Complexes, Segments, and Intervals

Complexes that make up a normal ECG consist of a P wave, a QRS complex, a T wave, and possibly a U wave. Segments include the PR segment, the ST segment, and the TP segment. Intervals include the PR interval, the QRS duration, and the QT interval (Figure 37-4).

P WAVE

The **P wave** is a deflection representing atrial depolarization. The shape of the P wave may be a positive, negative, or biphasic deflection, depending on the lead selected. When the electrical impulse is consistently generated from the sinoatrial (SA) node, the P waves have a consistent shape in a given lead. If an impulse is then generated from a different (ectopic) focus, such as atrial tissue, the shape of the P wave changes in that lead, indicating that an ectopic focus has fired.

PR SEGMENT

The **PR segment** is the isoelectric line from the end of the P wave to the beginning of the QRS complex, when the electrical impulse is traveling through the atrioventricular (AV) node, where it is delayed. It then travels through the ventricular conduction system to the Purkinje fibers.

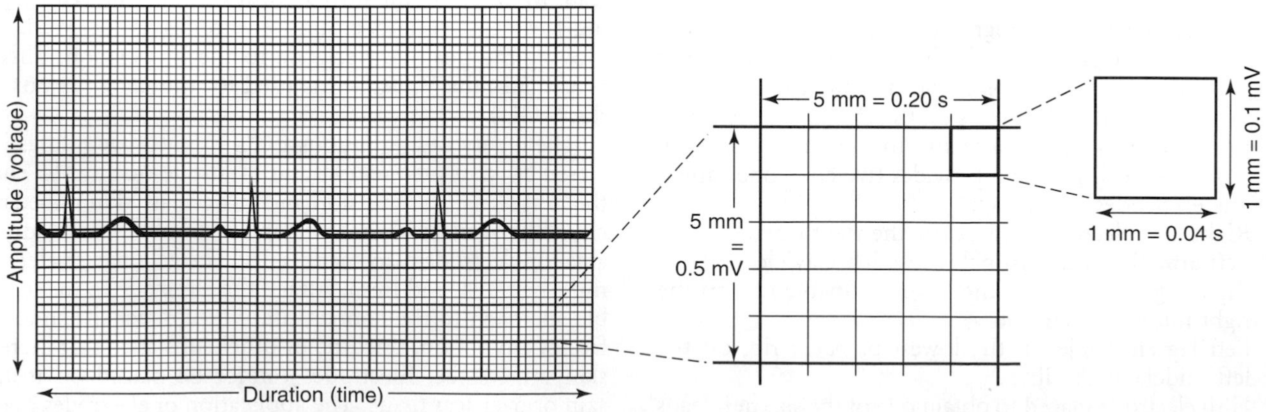

Figure 37-3 ■ Electrocardiographic waveforms are measured in amplitude (voltage) and duration (time).

PR INTERVAL

The **PR interval** is measured from the beginning of the P wave to the end of the PR segment. It represents the time required for atrial depolarization as well as the impulse delay in the AV node and the travel time to the Purkinje fibers. It normally measures from 0.12 to 0.20 second (five small blocks).

QRS COMPLEX

The **QRS complex** represents ventricular depolarization. The shape of the QRS complex depends on the lead selected. The Q wave is the first negative deflection and is not present in all leads. When present, it is small and represents initial ventricular septal depolarization. When the Q wave is abnormally present in a lead, it represents myocardial

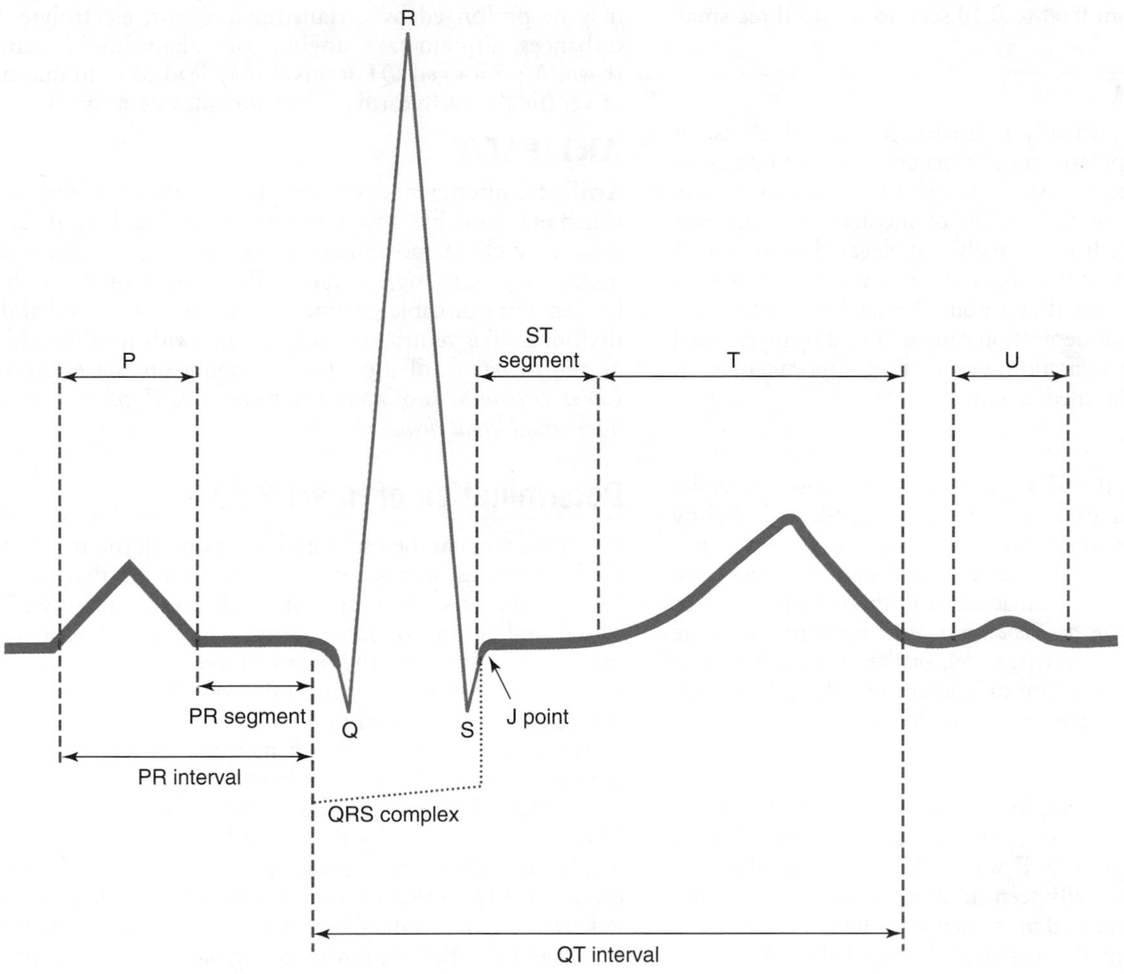

P wave:	Represents atrial depolarization.
PR segment:	Represents the time required for the impulse to travel through the AV node, where it is delayed, and through the bundle of His, bundle branches, and Purkinje fiber network, just before ventricular depolarization.
PR interval:	Represents the time required for atrial depolarization as well as impulse travel through the conduction system and Purkinje fiber network, inclusive of the P wave and PR segment. It is measured from the beginning of the P wave to the end of the PR segment.
QRS complex:	Represents ventricular depolarization and is measured from the beginning of the Q (or R) wave to the end of the S wave.
J point:	Represents the junction where the QRS complex ends and the ST segment begins.
ST segment:	Represents early ventricular repolarization.
T wave:	Represents ventricular repolarization.
U wave:	Represents late ventricular repolarization.
QT interval:	Represents the total time required for ventricular depolarization and repolarization and is measured from the beginning of the QRS complex to the end of the T wave.

Figure 37-4 ■ The components of a normal electrocardiogram.

necrosis (cell death). The R wave is the first positive deflection. It may be small, large, or absent, depending on the lead. The S wave is a negative deflection following the R wave and is not present in all leads.

QRS DURATION

The **QRS duration** represents the time required for depolarization of both ventricles. It is measured from the beginning of the QRS complex to the J point (the junction where the QRS complex ends and the ST segment begins). It normally measures from 0.04 to 0.10 second (up to three small blocks).

ST SEGMENT

The **ST segment** is normally an isoelectric line and represents early ventricular repolarization. It occurs from the J point to the beginning of the T wave. Its length varies with changes in the heart rate, the administration of medications, and electrolyte disturbances. It is normally not elevated more than 1 mm or depressed more than 0.5 mm from the isoelectric line. Its amplitude is measured at a point 1.5 to 2 mm after the J point. ST elevation or depression can be caused by myocardial injury, ischemia or infarction, conduction abnormalities, or the administration of medications.

T WAVE

The **T wave** follows the ST segment and represents ventricular repolarization. It is usually positive, rounded, and slightly asymmetric. If an ectopic stimulus excites the ventricles during this time, it may cause ventricular irritability, lethal dysrhythmias, and possible cardiac arrest in the vulnerable heart. This is known as the *R-on-T phenomenon.* T waves may become tall and peaked, inverted (negative), or flat as a result of myocardial ischemia, potassium or calcium imbalances, medications, or autonomic nervous system effects.

U WAVE

The **U wave,** when present, follows the T wave and may result from slow repolarization of ventricular Purkinje fibers. It is of the same polarity as the T wave, although generally it is smaller. It is not normally seen in all leads and is more common in lead V_3. Abnormal prominence of the U wave suggests an electrolyte abnormality (particularly hypokalemia) or other disturbance. Correct identification is important so that it is not mistaken for a P wave. If in doubt, notify the health care provider and request that a potassium level be obtained.

QT INTERVAL

The **QT interval** represents the total time required for ventricular depolarization and repolarization. The QT interval is measured from the beginning of the QRS complex to the end of the T wave. This interval varies with the client's age and gender and changes with the heart rate, lengthening with slower heart rates and shortening with faster rates. It may be prolonged by certain medications, electrolyte disturbances, Prinzmetal's angina, or subarachnoid hemorrhage. A prolonged QT interval may lead to a unique type of ventricular tachycardia called **torsades de pointes.**

ARTIFACT

Artifact is interference seen on the monitor or rhythm strip, which may look like a wandering or fuzzy baseline. It can be caused by client movement, loose or defective electrodes, improper grounding, or faulty ECG equipment, such as broken wires or cables. Some artifact can mimic lethal dysrhythmias like ventricular tachycardia (with toothbrushing) or ventricular fibrillation (with tapping on the electrode). *Client assessment is of utmost importance to distinguish artifact from actual lethal rhythms!*

Determination of Heart Rate

The heart rate can be estimated by counting the number of QRS complexes in 6 seconds and multiplying that number by 10 to calculate the rate for a full minute (Figure 37-5). This is called the 6-second strip method and is a quick method to determine the mean or average heart rate. This method is the least accurate; however, it is the method of choice for irregular rhythms.

For accuracy, the big block method is used if the QRS complexes are regular or evenly spaced. Count the number of big blocks between the same point in any two successive QRS complexes (usually R wave to R wave) and divide into 300 because there are 300 big blocks in 1 minute. It is easiest to use a QRS that falls on a dark line. If little blocks are left over when counting big blocks, count each little block as 0.2, add this to the number of big blocks, and then divide by 300 (Figure 37-6).

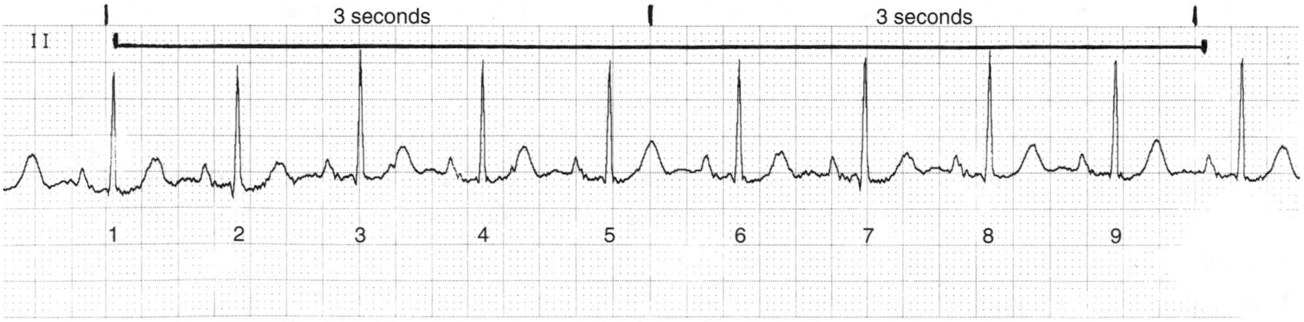

Figure 37-5 ■ Each segment between the dark lines (above the monitor strip) represents 3 seconds when the monitor is set at a speed of 25 mm/sec. To estimate the ventricular rate, count the QRS complexes in a 6-second strip and then multiply that number by 10 to estimate the rate for 1 minute. In this example, there are 9 QRS complexes in 6 seconds. Therefore the heart rate can be estimated to be 90 beats/min.

Count the number of large blocks in an interval and divide into 300 (the number of large blocks in 1 minute). For example, three large blocks equals a heart rate of 100 beats/min (300/3 = 100).

Another method (called the memory method) relies on memorization of the following sequence: 300, 150, 100, 75, 60, 50, 43, 37, 33, 30. This is the big block method with the math already done. Find a QRS complex that falls on the dark line representing 0.2 second or a big block, and count backwards to the next QRS complex. Each dark line is a memorized number. This is the method most widely used in hospitals for calculating heart rates for regular rhythms.

Commercially prepared electrocardiogram (ECG) rate rulers are based on these calculations and may be used for regular rhythms. Current monitoring systems will display a continuous heart rate and print the heart rate on the ECG strip. Use caution and confirm that the rate is correct by assessing the client's heart rate directly. Many factors can incorrectly alter the rate displayed by the monitor.

Electrocardiographic Rhythm Analysis

Analysis of an ECG rhythm strip requires a systematic approach using a five-step method facilitated by use of a measurement tool called an **ECG caliper** (Chart 37-1):

1. ***Determine the heart rate.*** If the atrial and ventricular rhythms are regular, the nurse may use any of the methods previously described to calculate the heart rate. If the rhythms are irregular, the nurse must use the 6-second strip method for accuracy. Normal heart rates fall between 60 and 100 beats/min. If the rate is less than 60 beats/min, this is **bradycardia.** If the rate is greater than 100 beats/min, this is **tachycardia.**
2. ***Determine the heart rhythm.*** Heart rhythms can be either regular or irregular. Irregular rhythms can be regularly irregular, occasionally irregular, or irregularly irregular. Check the regularity of the atrial rhythm by assessing the P-P intervals, placing one caliper point on a P wave, and placing the other point on the precise spot on the next P wave. Then move the caliper from P wave to P wave along the entire strip ("walking out" the P waves) to determine the regularity of the rhythm. P waves of a different shape (ectopic waves), if present, create an irregularity and do not walk out with the other P waves. A slight irregularity in the P-P intervals, varying no more than three small blocks, is considered essentially regular if the P waves are all of the same shape. This alteration is caused by changes in intrathoracic pressure during the respiratory cycle.

   Check the regularity of the ventricular rhythm by assessing the R-R intervals, placing one caliper point on a portion of the QRS complex (usually the most prominent portion of the deflection) and the other point on the precise spot of the next QRS complex. Move the caliper from QRS complex to QRS complex along the entire strip (walking out the QRS complexes) to determine the regularity of the rhythm. QRS complexes of a different shape (ectopic QRS complexes), if present, create an irregularity and do not "walk out" with the other QRS complexes. A slight irregularity of no more than three small blocks between intervals is considered essentially regular if the QRS complexes are all of the same shape.
3. ***Analyze the P waves.*** Check that the P-wave shape is consistent throughout the strip, indicating that atrial depolarization is occurring from impulses originating from one focus, normally the SA node. Determine whether there is one P wave occurring before each QRS complex, establishing that a relationship exists between the P wave and the QRS complex. This relationship indicates that

CHART 37-1

BEST PRACTICE for
Electrocardiographic Rhythm Analysis

1. Determine the heart rate.
2. Determine the heart rhythm.
3. Analyze the P waves.
4. Measure the P-R interval.
5. Measure the QRS duration.
6. Interpret the rhythm.

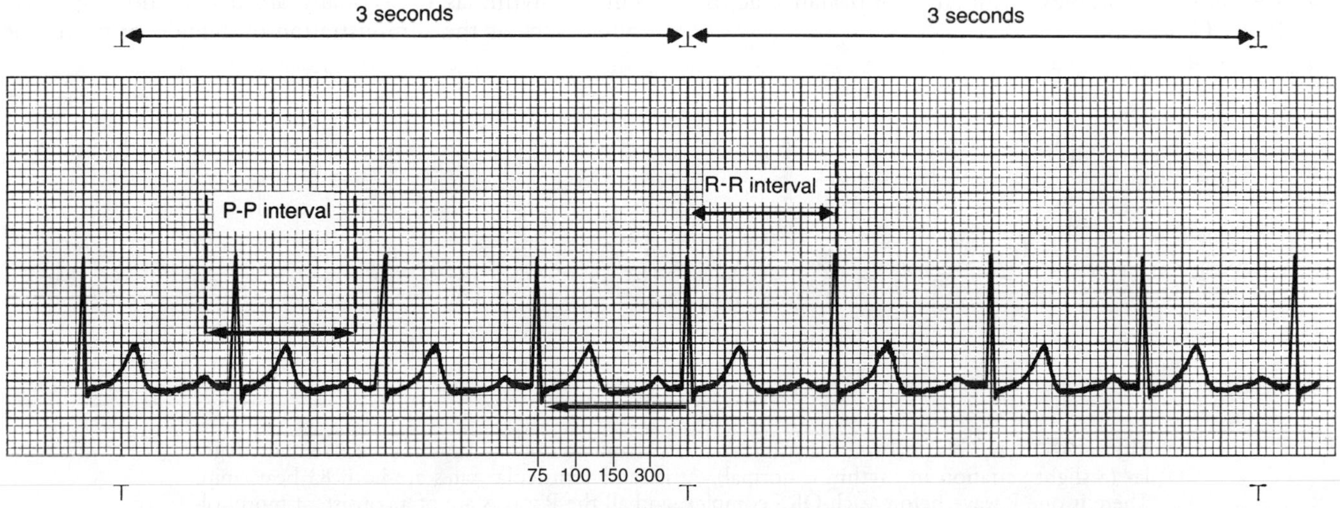

Figure 37-6 ■ In this example, the heart rate using the big block method is 300 ÷ 4 big blocks (between QRS complexes), or 75 beats/min. The memory method is also demonstrated with a heart rate of 75 beats/min.

an impulse from one focus is responsible for both atrial and ventricular depolarization. The nurse may observe more than one P wave shape, more P waves than QRS complexes, absent P waves, or P waves coming after the QRS, each indicating that a dysrhythmia exists. Ask these five questions when analyzing P waves:
- Are P waves present?
- Are the P waves occurring regularly?
- Is there one P wave for each QRS complex?
- Are the P waves smooth, rounded and upright in appearance, or are they inverted?
- Do all the P waves look similar?

4. ***Measure the PR interval.*** Place one caliper point at the beginning of the P wave and the other point at the end of the PR segment. The PR interval normally measures between 0.12 and 0.20 second. The measurement should be constant throughout the strip. The PR interval is unable to be determined if there are no P waves or if P waves occur after the QRS complex. Ask these three questions about the PR interval:
   - Are PR intervals greater than 0.20 second?
   - Are PR intervals less than 0.12 second?
   - Are PR intervals constant across the ECG strip?
5. ***Measure the QRS duration.*** Place one caliper point at the beginning of the QRS complex and the other at the J point, where the QRS complex ends and the ST segment begins. The QRS duration normally measures between 0.04 and 0.10 second. The measurement should be constant throughout the entire strip. Check that the QRS complexes are consistent throughout the strip. When the QRS is narrow (0.10 second or less), this indicates that the impulse was not formed in the ventricles and is referred to as supraventricular or "above the ventricles." When the QRS complex is wide (greater than 0.10 second), this indicates that the impulse is either of ventricular origin or of supraventricular origin with aberrant conduction, meaning deviating from the normal course or pattern. More than one QRS complex pattern or occasionally missing QRS complexes may be observed, indicating a dysrhythmia. Ask these questions to evaluate QRS intervals:
   - Are QRS intervals less than or greater than 0.12 second?
   - Are the QRS complexes similar in appearance across the ECG paper?
6. ***Interpret the rhythm.*** Using these rules, you can interpret the cardiac rhythm and differentiate normal and abnormal cardiac rhythms.

NORMAL RHYTHMS

Normal Sinus Rhythm

Normal sinus rhythm (NSR) is the rhythm originating from the sinoatrial (SA) node (dominant pacemaker) that meets the following electrocardiographic (ECG) criteria (Figure 37-7):
- *Rate:* Atrial and ventricular rates of 60 to 100 beats/min
- *Rhythm:* Atrial and ventricular rhythms regular
- *P waves:* Present, consistent configuration, one P wave before each QRS complex
- *PR interval:* 0.12 to 0.20 second and constant
- *QRS duration:* 0.04 to 0.10 second and constant

Sinus Arrhythmia

Sinus arrhythmia is a variant of NSR. It results from changes in intrathoracic pressure during breathing. In this context the term *arrhythmia* does not denote an absence of rhythm, as the term suggests. Instead, the heart rate increases slightly during inspiration and decreases slightly during exhalation. This irregular rhythm is frequently observed in healthy children as well as adults.

Sinus arrhythmia has all the characteristics of NSR except for its irregularity. The P-P and R-R intervals vary, with the difference between the shortest and the longest intervals being greater than 0.12 second (three small blocks):
- *Rate:* Atrial and ventricular rates are between 60 and 100 beats/min.
- *Rhythm:* Atrial and ventricular rhythms are irregular, with the shortest P-P or R-R interval varying at least 0.12 second from the longest P-P or R-R interval.
- *P waves:* One P wave before each QRS complex; consistent configuration.
- *PR interval:* Normal, constant.
- *QRS duration:* Normal, constant.

Sinus arrhythmias occasionally are due to nonrespiratory causes, such as the administration of digitalis or morphine.

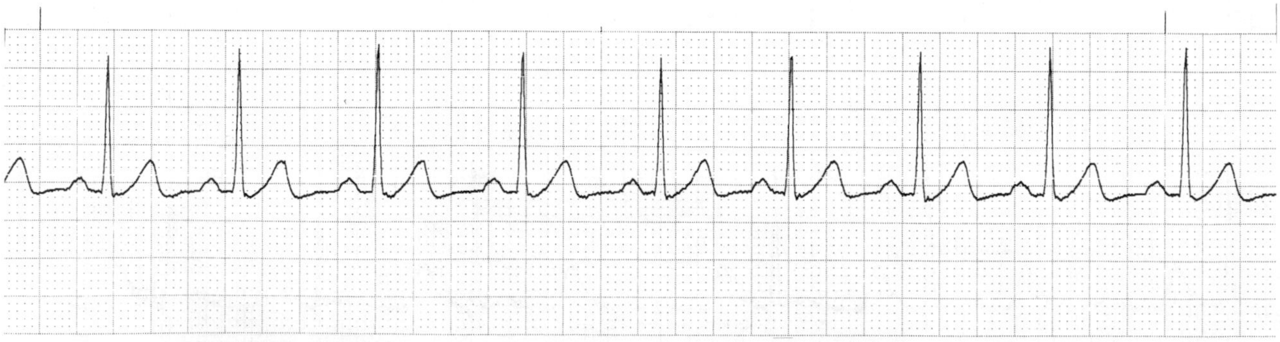

Figure 37-7 ■ Normal sinus rhythm. Both atrial and ventricular rhythms are essentially regular (a slight variation in rhythm is normal). Atrial and ventricular rates are both 83 beats/min. There is one P wave before each QRS complex, and all the P waves are of a consistent morphology, or shape. The PR interval measures 0.18 second and is constant; the QRS complex measures 0.06 second and is constant.

These drugs enhance vagal tone and cause decreased heart rate and irregularity unrelated to the respiratory cycle.

DYSRHYTHMIAS

OVERVIEW

Any disorder of the heartbeat uses the term *dysrhythmia.* Historically, the term **arrhythmia** has been used in the literature; however, it means an absence of cardiac rhythm. Although the terms are often used interchangeably, **dysrhythmia,** which means a disturbance in cardiac rhythm, is more accurate.

Dysrhythmias result from the following:

- A disturbance in the relationship between electrical conductivity and the mechanical response of the myocardium
- A disturbance in impulse formation (either from an abnormal rate or from an ectopic focus)
- A disturbance in impulse conduction (delays and blocks)
- The combination of several mechanisms

Although many dysrhythmias have no clinical manifestations, many others have serious consequences. A summary of key features is provided in Chart 37-2.

Dysrhythmia Terminology

TACHYDYSRHYTHMIAS

Tachydysrhythmias are heart rates greater than 100 beats/min. These rhythms may have serious hemodynamic consequences in the adult client with coronary artery disease (CAD). Coronary artery blood flow occurs predominantly during diastole, when the aortic valve is closed, and is determined by diastolic time and blood pressure in the root of the aorta. The following three points are important to understanding and appreciating the seriousness of tachydysrhythmias:

- Tachydysrhythmias shorten the diastolic time and therefore the coronary perfusion time (the amount of time available for blood to flow through the coronary arteries to the myocardium).
- Tachydysrhythmias initially increase cardiac output and blood pressure. However, a continued rise in heart rate decreases the ventricular filling time because of a shortened diastole, decreasing the stroke volume. Consequently, cardiac output and blood pressure will begin to decrease, reducing aortic pressure and therefore coronary perfusion pressure.
- Tachydysrhythmias increase the work of the heart, increasing myocardial oxygen demand.

The client with a tachydysrhythmia may have palpitations; chest discomfort; pressure or pain from myocardial ischemia or infarction; restlessness; anxiety; pale, cool skin; and syncope from hypotension. Tachydysrhythmias may also lead to heart failure. Presenting symptoms of heart failure may include dyspnea, orthopnea, pulmonary crackles, distended neck veins, fatigue, and weakness (see Chapter 38).

CHART 37-2

KEY FEATURES of Sustained Tachydysrhythmias and Bradydysrhythmias

- Chest discomfort, pressure, or pain, which may radiate to the jaw, the back, or the arm
- Restlessness, anxiety, nervousness, confusion
- Dizziness, syncope
- Palpitations (in tachydysrhythmias)
- Change in pulse strength, rate, and rhythm
- Pulse deficit
- Shortness of breath, dyspnea
- Tachypnea
- Pulmonary crackles
- Orthopnea
- S_3 or S_4 heart sounds
- Jugular venous distention
- Weakness, fatigue
- Pale, cool, skin; diaphoresis
- Nausea, vomiting
- Decreased urine output
- Delayed capillary refill
- Hypotension

BRADYDYSRHYTHMIAS

Bradydysrhythmias are characterized by a heart rate less than 60 beats/min. These rhythms can also have serious hemodynamic consequences. Consider the following three points:

- Myocardial oxygen demand is reduced from the slow heart rate, which is beneficial.
- Coronary perfusion time may be adequate because of a prolonged diastole, which is desirable.
- Coronary perfusion pressure may decrease if the heart rate is too slow to provide adequate cardiac output and blood pressure; this is a serious consequence.

Therefore the client may tolerate the bradydysrhythmia well if the blood pressure is adequate. If the blood pressure is not adequate, symptomatic bradydysrhythmias may lead to myocardial ischemia or infarction, dysrhythmias, hypotension, and heart failure.

PREMATURE COMPLEXES

Premature complexes are early complexes. They occur when a cardiac cell or cell group, other than the sinoatrial (SA) node, becomes irritable and fires an impulse before the next sinus impulse is generated. The abnormal focus is called an *ectopic focus* and may be generated by atrial, junctional, or ventricular tissue. Following the premature complex, there is a pause before the next normal complex, creating an irregularity in the rhythm. The client with premature complexes may be unaware of them or may feel palpitations or a "skipping" of the heartbeat. If premature complexes, especially those that are ventricular, become more frequent, the client may experience symptoms of decreased cardiac output.

REPETITIVE RHYTHMS

Premature complexes may occur repetitively in a rhythmic fashion:

- **Bigeminy** exists when normal complexes and premature complexes occur alternately in a repetitive two-beat pattern, with a pause occurring after each premature complex so that complexes occur in pairs.
- **Trigeminy** is a repetitive three-beat pattern, usually occurring as two sequential normal complexes followed by a premature complex and a pause, with the same pattern repeating itself in triplets.

- **Quadrigeminy** is a repetitive four-beat pattern, usually occurring as three sequential normal complexes followed by a premature complex and a pause, with the same pattern repeating itself in a four-beat pattern.

Such patterns may occur with atrial, junctional, or ventricular premature complexes. Clients may be unaware of the premature beats, or they may feel palpitations.

ESCAPE COMPLEXES AND RHYTHMS

Escape complexes or escape rhythms may occur when the SA node fails to discharge or is blocked or when a sinus impulse fails to depolarize the ventricles because of an atrioventricular (AV) nodal block. Escape complexes or rhythms serve as a secondary or escape pacemaker and are seen after a pause. Such impulses may originate from AV junctional or ventricular tissue. They cease when the SA node or the AV node regains the ability to function normally. If there are pauses followed by escape beats or rhythms, clients may feel light-headed, dizzy, or faint during the pause.

Classification of Dysrhythmias

Dysrhythmias are classified according to their site of origin. The sites include the SA node, atrial tissue, AV node, junctional tissue, and ventricular tissue. Dysrhythmias may be caused by a disturbance in impulse formation or by conduction delays or blocks. The incidence and the prevalence of dysrhythmias are not precisely known because they usually result from an underlying condition, such as heart disease. The incidence of dysrhythmias increases with age. A summary of the common dysrhythmias and their treatment is provided in Table 37-2.

SINUS DYSRHYTHMIAS

The sinus node is the **pacemaker** in all sinus dysrhythmias. Innervation from sympathetic and parasympathetic nerve fibers is normally in balance to ensure a normal sinus rhythm (NSR). An imbalance increases or decreases the rate of SA node discharge either as a normal response to activity or physiologic changes or as a pathologic response to disease.

SINUS TACHYCARDIA

PATHOPHYSIOLOGY. Dominant sympathetic nervous system stimulation of the heart or vagal inhibition results in an increased rate of SA node discharge, which increases the heart rate.

When the rate of SA node discharge exceeds 100 beats/min, the rhythm is called **sinus tachycardia** (Figure 37-8, *A*). Sinus tachycardia, with heart rates of 200 to 220 beats/min, is normal in infants and children. The rate gradually decreases until age 10 years. From age 10 years to adulthood, the heart rate normally does not exceed 100 beats/min except in response to activity and then usually does not exceed 160 beats/min. Rarely the heart rate reaches 180 beats/min. Sinus tachycardia initially enhances cardiac output and blood pressure. However, sustained increases in heart rate decrease coronary perfusion time, diastolic filling time, and coronary perfusion pressure while increasing myocardial oxygen demand.

Increased sympathetic stimulation is a normal response to physical activity but may also be caused by anxiety, pain,

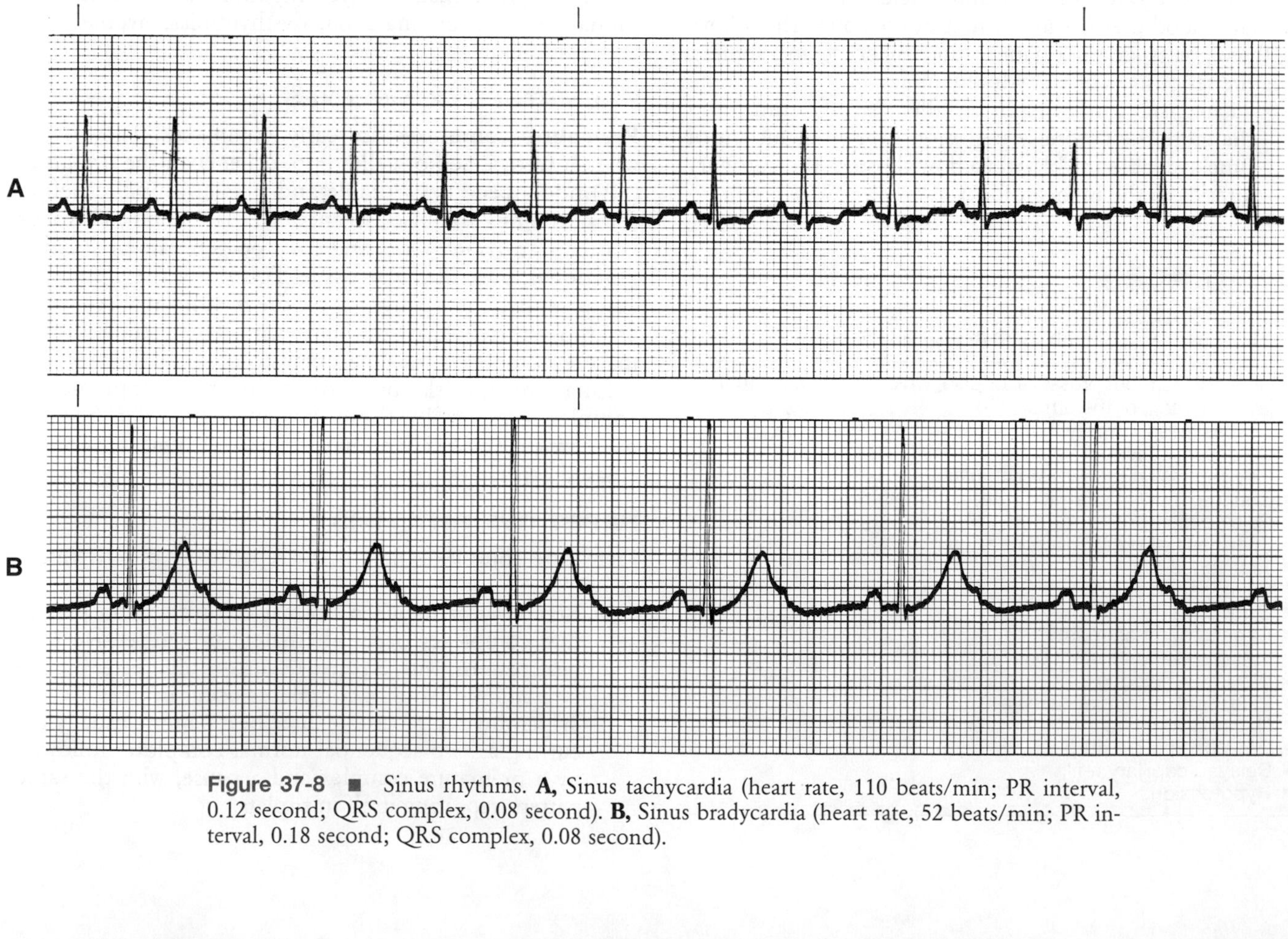

Figure 37-8 ■ Sinus rhythms. **A,** Sinus tachycardia (heart rate, 110 beats/min; PR interval, 0.12 second; QRS complex, 0.08 second). **B,** Sinus bradycardia (heart rate, 52 beats/min; PR interval, 0.18 second; QRS complex, 0.08 second).

TABLE 37-2 Common Dysrhythmias and Their Treatment

Dysrhythmia	Treatment
Sinus tachycardia	Correction of the underlying problem (e.g., fever, hypovolemia, pain, anxiety, or CHF) Beta-adrenergic blockade if increased catecholamine secretion is the underlying problem
Sinus bradycardia	Treatment is necessary only if the client is symptomatic (has hypotension, diaphoresis, chest discomfort or pain, pulmonary congestion, or altered level of consciousness) ▪ Atropine ▪ Pacemaker ▪ Avoidance of parasympathetic stimulation, such as prolonged suctioning or stimulation of the gag reflex
Premature Beats and Ectopic Rhythms	
Supraventricular beats (PACs, PJCs)	Correction of any underlying problem (e.g., anxiety, stress, caffeine or nicotine intake, CHF, effects of drugs, COPD, or asthma) Medication administration ▪ Propranolol ▪ Sedatives
Supraventricular rhythms	Correction of any underlying problem (e.g., CHF, COPD, asthma, stress, or drugs) Medication administration ▪ Diltiazem ▪ Adenosine ▪ Digitalis ▪ Propranolol ▪ Esmolol ▪ Amiodarone Vagal stimulation with carotid massage Valsalva maneuvers Overdrive atrial pacing Synchronized cardioversion if the above measures are unsuccessful
Premature ventricular complexes and ventricular tachycardia (not sustained)	Correction of any underlying problem (e.g., infection, electrolyte imbalance, effects of drugs, myocardial infarction, hypoxia CHF, stress, fatigue, or nicotine) Medication administration ▪ Lidocaine bolus and infusion ▪ Procainamide bolus and infusion ▪ Magnesium sulfate infusion ▪ Class I and II antidysrhythmics ▪ Amiodarone Restoration of electrolyte balance
Atrial flutter	Medication administration ▪ Diltiazem ▪ Amiodarone ▪ Propranolol ▪ Esmolol ▪ Ibutilide ▪ Digitalis Atrial overdrive pacing Cardioversion Catheter or surgical ablation
Atrial fibrillation	Medication administration ▪ Amiodarone ▪ Diltiazem ▪ Ibutilide ▪ Verapamil Anticoagulation Atrial overdrive pacing Cardioversion Surgery
Escape beats and rhythms	Correction of the underlying cause if the client is symptomatic Atropine administration Pacemaker Isoproterenol administration if pacemaker unavailable
Conduction Delays	
First-degree AV block	Treatment necessary only if the client is symptomatic Withhold digitalis (if the cause) Atropine administration if block is associated with symptomatic bradycardia
Second-degree AV block type I	Same as for first-degree AV block
Second-degree AV block type II	Pacemaker Isoproterenol administration if pacemaker unavailable
Third-degree AV block	Pacemaker Isoproterenol administration if pacemaker unavailable
Life-Threatening Dysrhythmias	
Sustained ventricular tachycardia	Medication administration ▪ Lidocaine bolus and infusion ▪ Procainamide bolus and infusion ▪ Amiodarone ▪ Magnesium sulfate infusion If unstable: synchronized cardioversion If pulseless: defibrillation, CPR
Ventricular fibrillation	Defibrillation CPR Medication administration ▪ Vasopressin ▪ Epinephrine ▪ Amiodarone ▪ Magnesium sulfate
Ventricular asystole	CPR Medication administration ▪ Epinephrine ▪ Atropine ▪ Pacemaker

AV, atrioventricular; *CHF*, congestive heart failure; *COPD*, chronic obstructive pulmonary disease; *CPR*, cardiopulmonary resuscitation; *PACs*, premature atrial complexes; *PJCs*, premature junctional complexes.

stress, fear, fever, anemia, hypoxemia, hyperthyroidism, and pulmonary embolism. Drugs such as catecholamines, atropine, caffeine, alcohol, nicotine, aminophylline, and thyroid medications may also increase the heart rate. In some cases, sinus tachycardia is a compensatory response to decreased cardiac output or blood pressure, as occurs in hypovolemia, shock, myocardial infarction (MI), and heart failure.

PHYSICAL ASSESSMENT/CLINICAL MANIFESTATIONS. The client may be asymptomatic except for the increased pulse rate. However, if the rhythm is not well tolerated, he or she may become symptomatic. Assess for fatigue, weakness, shortness of breath, orthopnea, neck vein distention, decreased oxygen saturation, and decreased blood pressure. Also assess for restlessness and anxiety from decreased cerebral perfusion and for decreased urine output from decreased renal perfusion. The adult client may also experience anginal pain and palpitations. The electrocardiographic (ECG) pattern may show T-wave inversion or ST-segment elevation or depression in response to myocardial ischemia.

INTERVENTIONS. Collaborate with the health care provider to identify the cause of sinus tachycardia and select the appropriate treatment. The goal is to decrease the heart rate to normal levels by treating the underlying cause. For example, if the client has angina, administer oxygen, help the client to rest, and administer nitroglycerin or morphine as prescribed. Diuretics and inotropic agents may be given for heart failure. Initiate intravascular volume replacement for hypovolemia, administer antipyretics and antibiotics to the client with fever and infection, or provide comfort measures and administer analgesics or opioids to the client with noncardiac pain, as prescribed. Maintain the client on bedrest if the tachycardia is causing hypotension or weakness.

Collaborate with the respiratory therapist, when indicated, to oxygenate and suction the client with hypoxemia from excessive airway secretions. Beta-adrenergic blocking agents may also be prescribed for the client with inappropriate sympathetic nervous system stimulation. Emotional support and relevant teaching are important for the client and family.

SINUS BRADYCARDIA

PATHOPHYSIOLOGY. Dominance of the parasympathetic nervous system, with excessive vagal stimulation to the heart, causes a decreased rate of sinus node discharge. This slows the heart rate and decreases the speed of conduction through the AV node and conduction system. When the rate of sinus node discharge is less than 60 beats/min in adults or lower, the normal range in infants and children, the rhythm is called **sinus bradycardia** (Figure 37-8, *B*). Sinus bradycardia increases coronary perfusion time, but it may decrease coronary perfusion pressure. However, myocardial oxygen demand is decreased.

Increased parasympathetic stimulation of the heart by the vagus nerve is a normal response to decreased physical activity. It also often occurs in well-conditioned athletes because the strong heart muscle is extremely efficient in providing an adequate stroke volume while not requiring a higher heart rate for a normal cardiac output. Excessive vagal stimulation may result from carotid sinus massage, vomiting, suctioning, Valsalva maneuvers (e.g., bearing down for a bowel movement or gagging), ocular pressure, or pain. Sinus bradycardia may also result from hypoxia, inferior wall MI, and the administration of drugs such as beta-adrenergic blocking agents, calcium channel blockers, and digitalis.

PHYSICAL ASSESSMENT/CLINICAL MANIFESTATIONS. The client may be asymptomatic except for the decreased pulse rate. At times, however, the rhythm may not be well tolerated. Assess the client for dizziness, weakness, syncope, confusion, hypotension, diaphoresis (excessive sweating), shortness of breath, ventricular ectopy (superficial beats), and anginal pain. T-wave inversion or ST-segment elevation or depression may occur in response to myocardial ischemia.

INTERVENTIONS. If the client is symptomatic and the underlying cause cannot be determined, the treatment of choice is atropine administration, given as prescribed to increase the heart rate to about 60 beats/min. Oxygen should be applied. If the heart rate does not increase sufficiently, an external pacemaker may be applied to increase the heart rate. However, if atropine administration succeeds in achieving an adequate heart rate but the client remains hypotensive, initiate intravascular volume replacement as prescribed rather than administering another dose of atropine. Excessive atropine may induce tachycardia and myocardial ischemia. If a medication is suspected to be the cause, withhold the drug and notify the physician.

Critical Thinking Challenge

During physical assessment class you find your female nursing student partner, who is on the track team, has an apical pulse of 44 beats/min with a regular heart rhythm. She states she sometimes has chest pain and shortness of breath after running.

1. What other assessment data are needed?
2. What cardiac dysrhythmia is expected on the ECG recording?
3. Does this dysrhythmia need treatment? Why or why not?

evolve For suggested answer guidelines, go to http://evolve.elsevier.com/Iggy/.

ATRIAL DYSRHYTHMIAS

With atrial dysrhythmias, the focus of impulse generation shifts away from the sinus node to the atrial tissue, which acts as an ectopic pacemaker for one or more beats. The shift changes the axis (direction) of atrial depolarization, resulting in a P-wave shape that differs from that of P waves with a sinus node origin. The most common atrial dysrhythmias are premature atrial complexes, supraventricular tachycardia, atrial flutter, and atrial fibrillation.

PREMATURE ATRIAL COMPLEXES

PATHOPHYSIOLOGY. A **premature atrial complex (PAC)** occurs when atrial tissue becomes irritable. This ectopic focus fires an impulse before the next sinus impulse is due, thus usurping the sinus pacemaker (Figure 37-9). The premature P wave from the atrial focus is early and has a shape different from that of the P wave generated from the sinus node. The premature P wave may not always be clearly visible because it can be hidden in the preceding T wave. The T wave must be closely examined for any change in shape and compared with other T waves to reveal a hidden P wave. A PAC is usually followed by a pause.

The causes of atrial irritability include stress; fatigue; anxiety; inflammation; infection; intake of caffeine, nicotine, or alcohol; and the administration of drugs such as cate-

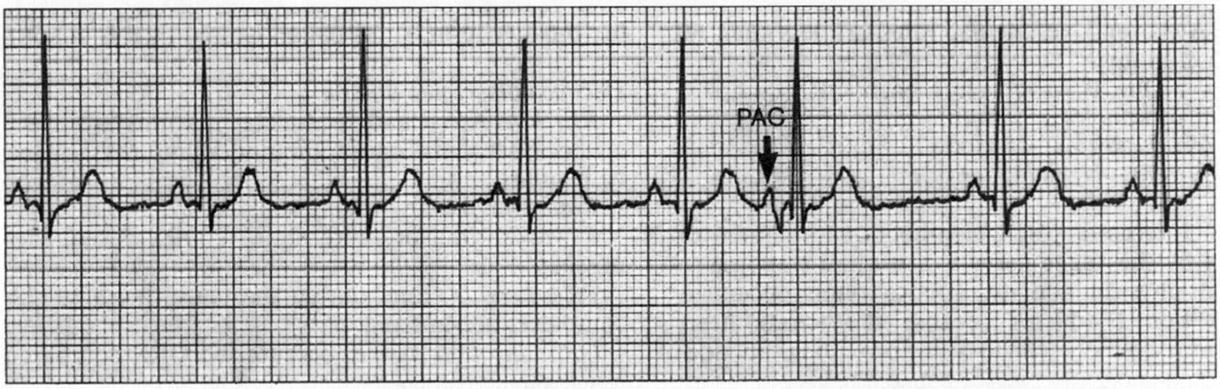

Figure 37-9 ■ Normal sinus rhythm with a premature atrial complex (PAC) at arrow.

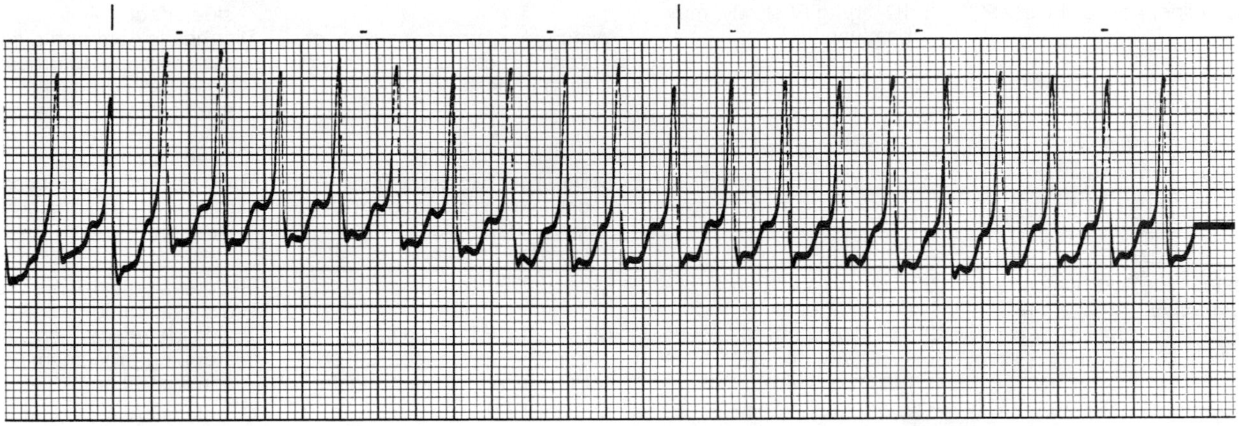

Figure 37-10 ■ Sustained supraventricular tachycardia in a client with Wolff-Parkinson-White syndrome. Heart rate is 200 beats/min.

cholamines, sympathomimetics, amphetamines, digitalis, or anesthetic agents. PACs may also result from myocardial ischemia, hypermetabolic states, electrolyte imbalance, or atrial stretch, as may occur with congestive heart failure, valvular disease, and pulmonary hypertension with cor pulmonale.

PHYSICAL ASSESSMENT/CLINICAL MANIFESTATIONS. The client is usually asymptomatic except for possible heart palpitations because PACs usually have no hemodynamic consequences.

INTERVENTIONS. No intervention is usually needed except to treat the cause, such as heart failure or valvular disease. If PACs occur frequently, they may signal the onset of more serious atrial tachydysrhythmias and therefore may warrant treatment. Administration of prescribed type IA antidysrhythmics or other drugs may be warranted. Teach the client measures to manage stress and substances to avoid that are known to increase atrial irritability.

SUPRAVENTRICULAR TACHYCARDIA

PATHOPHYSIOLOGY. Supraventricular tachycardia (SVT) involves the rapid stimulation of atrial tissue at a rate of 100 to 280 beats/min, with a mean of 170 beats/min in adults (Figure 37-10) and 200 to 300 beats/min in children. SVT is most often due to a re-entry mechanism in which one impulse circulates repeatedly throughout the atrial pathway, restimulating the atrial tissue at a rapid rate. The term **paroxysmal supraventricular tachycardia (PSVT)** is used when the rhythm is intermittent, initiated suddenly by a premature complex such as a PAC, and terminated suddenly with or without intervention.

During SVT the P waves have a shape different from that of sinus P waves. The P waves may not be visible, especially if there is a 1:1 conduction with rapid rates because the P waves are embedded in the preceding T wave.

The causes of SVT are the same as those for PACs. SVT may occur in healthy young people without evidence of heart disease, especially women under 40 years of age. The condition commonly occurs in clients with a pre-excitation syndrome, such as **Wolff-Parkinson-White (WPW) syndrome.**

PHYSICAL ASSESSMENT/CLINICAL MANIFESTATIONS. The clinical manifestations depend on the duration of the SVT and the rate of the ventricular response. In clients with a sustained rapid ventricular response, assess for palpitations, weakness, fatigue, shortness of breath, nervousness, anxiety, hypotension, and syncope. Hemodynamic deterioration may occur if the rate does not sustain adequate blood pressure. In that case SVT can result in angina, heart failure, and shock. With a nonsustained or slower ventricular response, the client may be asymptomatic except for transient palpitations.

INTERVENTIONS. If SVT occurs in a healthy person and terminates spontaneously, no intervention is necessary other than eliminating identified causative factors. If it is recurrent, the client should be studied in the electrophysiology laboratory. The preferred treatment for recurrent SVT is radiofrequency catheter ablation. In sustained SVT with a rapid ventricular response, the goals of treatment are to decrease the ventricular response, convert the dysrhythmia to a sinus rhythm, and treat the cause. Vagal stimulation (e.g., carotid massage) may be successful, but often only transiently, and must be performed only by a physician.

Administer oxygen and prescribed antidysrhythmic drugs, such as diltiazem (Cardizem), which slow the ventricular rate by increasing the AV block (Chart 37-3). Some may also succeed in converting the dysrhythmia. In the severely compromised client, the nurse may assist the physician in attempting atrial overdrive pacing or in delivering a synchronized electrical shock (cardioversion) to re-establish an organized rhythm and regain cardiac stability.

CHART 37-3

DRUG THERAPY for Dysrhythmias

Drug	Usual Dosage	Nursing Interventions	Rationales
Class I Drugs			
Type IA			
Quinidine sulfate (quinidine, Apo-Quinidine✱)	300-600 mg PO q8-12h 6-10 mg/kg IV slowly; may be given IM	Monitor BP.	Hypotension is a common side effect.
		Watch for diarrhea, nausea, or vomiting and administer with food if these occur.	Diarrhea is common during early therapy. Diarrhea and other gastrointestinal symptoms often decrease when quinidine is administered with food.
		Monitor for widening QRS complex, prolonged QT interval, heart block, onset or increase in number of PVCs.	Toxic side effects necessitate stopping quinidine administration.
Procainamide hydrochloride (Pronestyl)	50 mg/kg/day PO in 4 divided doses	Monitor BP.	Hypotension warrants drug discontinuation.
	20-30 mg IV, not to exceed 17 mg/kg, followed by infusion of 1-4 mg/min	Monitor for widening QRS complex, prolonged QT or PR interval, or heart block.	Toxic side effects necessitate stopping procainamide administration.
Disopyramide phosphate (Norpace)	100-200 mg PO q6h	Monitor BP.	Hypotension is a common side effect.
		Watch for shortness of breath and weight gain.	Disopyramide can cause heart failure in a client with CAD.
		Monitor for widening QRS complex, prolonged QT or PR interval, or heart block.	Toxic side effects necessitate stopping disopyramide administration.
Type IB			
Lidocaine (Xylocaine)	1-1.5 mg/kg IV bolus, then 0.5-0.75 mg/kg IV boluses q5-10min to a loading dose of 3 mg/kg, followed by 2-4 mg/min infusion. For VF or pulseless VT: 1-1.5 mg/kg IV bolus q3-5min to a loading dose of 3 mg/kg, followed by 2-4 mg/min infusion	Watch for confusion, paresthesias, slurring of speech, drowsiness, or seizure activity.	CNS adverse effects predominate; they may require a decrease in dosage or discontinuation of the infusion.
Mexiletine hydrochloride (Mexitil)	200-300 mg PO q8h with food	Monitor BP and heart rate.	Hypotension and bradycardia may occur.
	125-250 mg IV bolus for 5-10 min 0.5-1.5 mg/min infusion	Assess for tremors, blurred vision, dizziness, ataxia, or confusion.	CNS adverse reactions predominate.
Tocainide hydrochloride (Tonocard)	400 mg PO q8h initially 400-800 mg PO q8h Maximum of 2.4 g daily Take with food	Watch for tremors.	Tremors indicate that the maximum dose is being approached.
		Monitor heart rate and BP.	Bradycardia and hypotension may occur.
		Teach client to report shortness of breath, wheezing, chest pain, or cough as well as dyspnea and distended neck veins or swelling of the extremities.	Pulmonary fibrosis is a serious side effect, which necessitates discontinuation of the drug; the drug may also cause CHF.

AV, Atrioventricular; *BP*, blood pressure; *CAD*, coronary artery disease; *CHF*, congestive heart failure; *CNS*, central nervous system; D_5W, 5% dextrose in water; *EMD*, electromechanical dissociation; *PEA*, pulseless electrical activity; *PSVT*, premature supraventricular tachycardia; *PVC*, premature ventricular complex; *SVT*, supraventricular tachycardia; *VF*, ventricular fibrillation; *VT*, ventricular tachycardia.

CHART 37-3

DRUG THERAPY for Dysrhythmias—*cont'd*

Drug	Usual Dosage	Nursing Interventions	Rationales
Class I Drugs—*cont'd*			
Type IC			
Flecainide acetate (Tambocor)	100 mg PO twice daily Maximum dose of 400 mg daily	Monitor for an increase in frequency and severity of dysrhythmias.	Flecainide can induce dysrhythmias.
		Monitor heart rate and BP.	Bradycardia and hypotension may occur.
		Monitor for CHF dizziness, visual disturbances, paresthesias, and tremors.	Side effects may require a decrease in dosage or discontinuation of the drug.
Propafenone hydrochloride (Rythmol)	150-300 mg PO q8h	Monitor for an increase in dysrhythmias.	Propafenone can induce dysrhythmias.
		Monitor heart rate and BP.	Bradycardia and hypotension may occur.
		Monitor for CNS effects, dizziness, anxiety, ataxia, insomnia, confusion, and seizures, as well as CHF and gastrointestinal distress.	Side effects may require a decrease in dosage or discontinuation of the drug.
Class II Drugs			
Propranolol hydrochloride (Inderal, Apo-Propranolol✱)	10-80 mg PO four times daily before meals 0.1 mg/kg slow IV bolus divided into 3 equal doses given at intervals of 2-3 min at rate of 1 mg/min	Monitor heart rate and BP.	Bradycardia and decreased BP are expected effects.
		Assess for shortness of breath or wheezing.	$Beta_2$-blocking effects on the lungs can cause bronchospasm.
		Assess for insomnia, fatigue, and dizziness.	Side effects may require decrease in dosage or discontinuation of the drug.
Acebutolol hydrochloride (Sectral)	600-1200 mg PO daily	Monitor heart rate and BP.	Bradycardia and decreased BP are expected effects.
		Assess for shortness of breath or wheezing.	$Beta_2$-blocking effects on the lungs can cause bronchospasm.
		Assess for insomnia, fatigue, and dizziness.	Side effects may require a decrease in dosage or discontinuation of the drug.
Esmolol hydrochloride (Brevibloc)	Initially, 500 mcg/kg/min for 1 min, then 50 mcg/kg/min for 4 min IV Titrate up if necessary	Monitor heart rate and BP.	Bradycardia and decreased BP are expected effects.
		Assess for shortness of breath or wheezing.	$Beta_2$-blocking effects on the lungs can cause bronchospasm.
		Assess for insomnia, fatigue, and seizures.	Side effects may require a decrease in dosage or discontinuation of the drug.
Sotalol hydrochloride (Betapace)	Initial dose of 80 mg PO twice daily Dosage may be increased every 2-3 days, if necessary, to 240-320 mg daily in 2-3 divided doses	Assess ECG rhythm for torsades de pointes and other serious new ventricular dysrhythmias.	Sotalol may have proarrhythmic effects.
		Assess for fatigue, bradycardia, dyspnea, CHF, chest pain, hypotension, dizziness, hypoglycemia, nausea, and vomiting.	Adverse reactions may warrant drug discontinuation.
		Sotalol should not be administered to clients with hypokalemia or hypomagnesemia before correction of these imbalances.	Hypokalemia or hypomagnesemia may prolong the QT interval and cause torsades de pointes.
		Sotalol is contraindicated in clients with bronchial asthma, sinus bradycardia, or second- and third-degree AV block (unless a functioning pacemaker is present), prolonged QT syndrome, cardiogenic shock, or CHF.	Sotalol has beta-blocking (class II) effects and class III effects.

Continued

CHART 37-3

DRUG THERAPY for Dysrhythmias—*cont'd*

Drug	Usual Dosage	Nursing Interventions	Rationales
Class III Drugs Amiodarone hydrochloride (Cordarone)	800-1600 mg PO daily in divided doses for 1-3 wk, then 600-800 mg daily for 1 mo, then 200-600 mg daily (average of 400 mg daily) Rapid loading dose: 150 mg IV over first 10 min (15 mg/min); slow loading dose: 360 mg IV over next 6 hr (1 mg/min); maintenance infusion: 540 mg IV over next 18 hr (0.5 mg/min), then 720 mg/24 hr (0.5 mg/min)	Use volumetric infusion pump and PVC tubing with in-line filter and infuse via central line.	Drug is irritating to peripheral vasculature; drug is more stable in glass bottle.
		Rapid-loading IV dose must not be administered faster than 10 min. Must stay with client and monitor heart rate and BP.	Hypotension may occur. It should be treated by slowing the infusion and other standard therapy. Cordarone should not be discontinued unless necessary.
		Continually monitor ECG rhythm during IV infusion; measure QT and QT_c.	Bradycardia and AV block may occur and are treated by slowing the infusion rate and providing pacemaker therapy, if necessary. May cause a worsening of ventricular dysrhythmias.
		Assess the client's knowledge of the treatment regimen and side effects.	Drug has major side effects, which make noncompliance a problem; clients may take the drug for 1½-3 mo before full clinical effects are apparent.
		Monitor heart rate, BP, and cardiac rhythm when initiating therapy.	Bradycardia, hypotension, and worsening dysrhythmia can occur.
		Teach clients to report any muscle weakness, tremors, or difficulty with ambulation.	Muscle-related side effects usually develop during the first week of treatment.
		Teach clients to report shortness of breath, cough, pleuritic pain, or fever.	Pulmonary side effects may indicate drug-induced pulmonary toxicity.
		Teach clients to report any visual disturbances and to wear sunglasses outdoors in the daytime if they have photophobia.	Corneal pigmentation occurs in most clients but generally does not interfere with vision; if it does, the dosage is decreased.
		Teach clients to use barrier sunscreens.	Photosensitivity reactions may occur.
		Teach clients to report any signs of thyroid problems or hepatotoxicity.	Thyroid problems or hepatotoxicity may occur, necessitating a decrease in dosage or discontinuation of the drug.
Ibutilide fumarate (Corvert)	1 mg IV over 10 min for clients >60 kg; 0.01 mg/kg over 10 min for clients <60 kg May repeat dose 10 min after completion of first infusion if necessary	Stop infusion as soon as dysrhythmia is terminated, or in event of sustained or nonsustained VT, or marked prolongation of QT or QT_c.	Drug may cause potentially fatal dysrhythmias.
		Observe clients with continuous ECG monitoring and measure QT or QT_c for at least 4 hr following infusion or until QT_c has returned to baseline.	Acute ventricular dysrhythmias must be promptly identified and treated. Client may develop heart blocks.
		Clients with atrial fibrillation of >2-3 days' duration must be adequately anticoagulated for at least 2 wk.	Atrial fibrillation is associated with formation of thrombi in atrial chambers.
		Hypokalemia and hypomagnesemia must be corrected before Covert infusion.	This is important to reduce potential for proarrhythmia effects.

AF, Atrioventricular; *BP,* blood pressure; *CAD,* coronary artery disease; *CHF,* congestive heart failure; *CNS,* central nervous system; *D_5W,* 5% dextrose in water; *EMD,* electromechanical dissociation; *PEA,* pulseless electrical activity; *PSVT,* premature supraventricular tachycardia; *PVC,* premature ventricular complex; *SVT,* supraventricular tachycardia; *VF,* ventricular fibrillation; *VT,* ventricular tachycardia.

CHART 37-3

DRUG THERAPY for Dysrhythmias—*cont'd*

Drug	Usual Dosage	Nursing Interventions	Rationales
Class III Drugs—cont'd			
Dofetilide (Tikosyn)	125-500 mcg PO twice daily	Teach clients to change positions slowly.	Orthostatic hypotension is a common side affect of the drug.
		Inform clients that dosages will be adjusted, depending on the client's creatinine clearance level.	The client must have adequate creatinine clearance to prevent drug toxicity.
		Monitor clients on telemetry for several days; observe for and report bradycardia and hypotension.	Bradycardia and hypotension are common side effects.
Class IV Drugs			
Verapamil hydrochloride (Calan, Isoptin✱)	2.5-5 mg IV for 1-2 min for narrow-complex SVT or PSVT, after 15-30 min may give 5-10 mg IV for 1-2 min, if necessary, and repeat to a maximum of 20 mg 80-120 mg PO q6-8h	Monitor heart rate and BP.	Bradycardia and hypotension are common side effects.
		Teach clients to remain recumbent for at least 1 hr after IV administration.	Hypotension may occur; may be reversed with calcium chloride ($CaCl_2$), 0.5-1 g slow IV.
		Teach clients to change positions slowly when receiving oral therapy.	Dizziness and orthostatic hypotension often occur until tolerance develops.
		Teach clients to report dyspnea, orthopnea, distended neck veins, or swelling of the extremities.	Heart failure may occur, necessitating a decrease in dosage or discontinuation of the drug.
Diltiazem hydrochloride (Cardizem)	0.25 mg/kg IV for 2 min After 15 min, give 0.35 mg/kg IV for 2 min 5-15 mg/hr IV infusion	Monitor heart rate and BP.	Bradycardia and hypotension are common side effects.
		Teach clients to remain recumbent for at least 1 hr after IV administration.	Hypotension may occur.
		Teach clients to report dyspnea, orthopnea, distended neck veins, or swelling of the extremities.	Heart failure may occur, necessitating a decrease in dosage or discontinuation of the drug.
Other Drugs			
Digoxin (Lanoxin, Novodigoxin✱)	Rapid digitalization: 0.5-1 mg PO or IV initially; 0.125-0.5 mg PO q6h or IV until a total of 1-1.5 mg is reached Maintenance: 0.125-0.25 mg PO or IV daily or every other day (may be less for older adults)	Assess apical heart rate for 1 min before each dose.	Decreased heart rate is an expected response, but bradycardia may indicate toxicity.
		Assess for sudden increase in heart rate and change of rhythm from regular to irregular, or irregular to regular.	Changes in heart rate or rhythm may indicate toxicity.
		Teach clients to report anorexia, nausea, vomiting, diarrhea, paresthesias, confusion, or visual disturbances.	Side effect can indicate toxicity.
		Monitor serum potassium levels.	Hypokalemia increases the risk of toxicity and ventricular dysrhythmias.
		Monitor serum creatinine levels.	Impaired renal function can cause toxicity; the dosage is altered if this occurs.
Atropine sulfate	0.5-1 mg IV bolus may be repeated q3-5min, if necessary, to a maximum of 0.04 mg/kg For asystole, PEA, or EMD: 1 mg IV bolus q3-5min, if necessary, to a total of 0.04 mg/kg	Monitor heart rate and rhythm after administration.	Increased heart rate is expected.
		Assess for chest pain after administration.	Increased heart rate may cause ischemia in clients with CAD.
		Assess for urinary retention and dry mouth after administration.	Atropine is an anticholinergic agent.
		Avoid using in clients with angle-closure glaucoma.	Atropine increases intraocular pressure.

Continued

CHART 37-3

DRUG THERAPY for Dysrhythmias—*cont'd*

Drug	Usual Dosage	Nursing Interventions	Rationales
Other Drugs—cont'd Adenosine (Adenocard)	6 mg IV for 1-3 sec followed by 20-mL saline flush; may repeat in 1-2 min, if necessary, at 12 mg IV for 1-3 sec with 20-mL flush; may repeat 12 mg IV after 1-2 min if necessary	Monitor heart rate and rhythm after administration.	A short period of asystole is common after administration; bradycardia and hypotension may occur.
		Assess clients for facial flushing, shortness of breath, dyspnea, and chest pain.	These side effects commonly occur.
		Assess clients for recurrence of PSVT or ventricular ectopy.	Recurrence of PSVT is common; PVCs may occur.
Magnesium sulfate	1-2 g diluted in 100 mL of D_5W administered for 1-2 min for VF or VT 1-2 g in 50-100 mL of D_5W for 5-60 min for loading dose; 0.5-1 g/hr for 24 hr for supplementation	Assess ECG rhythm for conversion to sinus rhythm.	Hypomagnesemia may precipitate refractory VF.
		Assess clients for facial flushing, hypotension, and respiratory and CNS depression.	Magnesium sulfate causes vasodilation and respiratory and CNS depression.

AF, Atrioventricular; *BP,* blood pressure; *CAD,* coronary artery disease; *CHF,* congestive heart failure; *CNS,* central nervous system; *D_5W,* 5% dextrose in water; *EMD,* electromechanical dissociation; *PEA,* pulseless electrical activity; *PSVT,* premature supraventricular tachycardia; *PVC,* premature ventricular complex; *SVT,* supraventricular tachycardia; *VF,* ventricular fibrillation; *VT,* ventricular tachycardia.

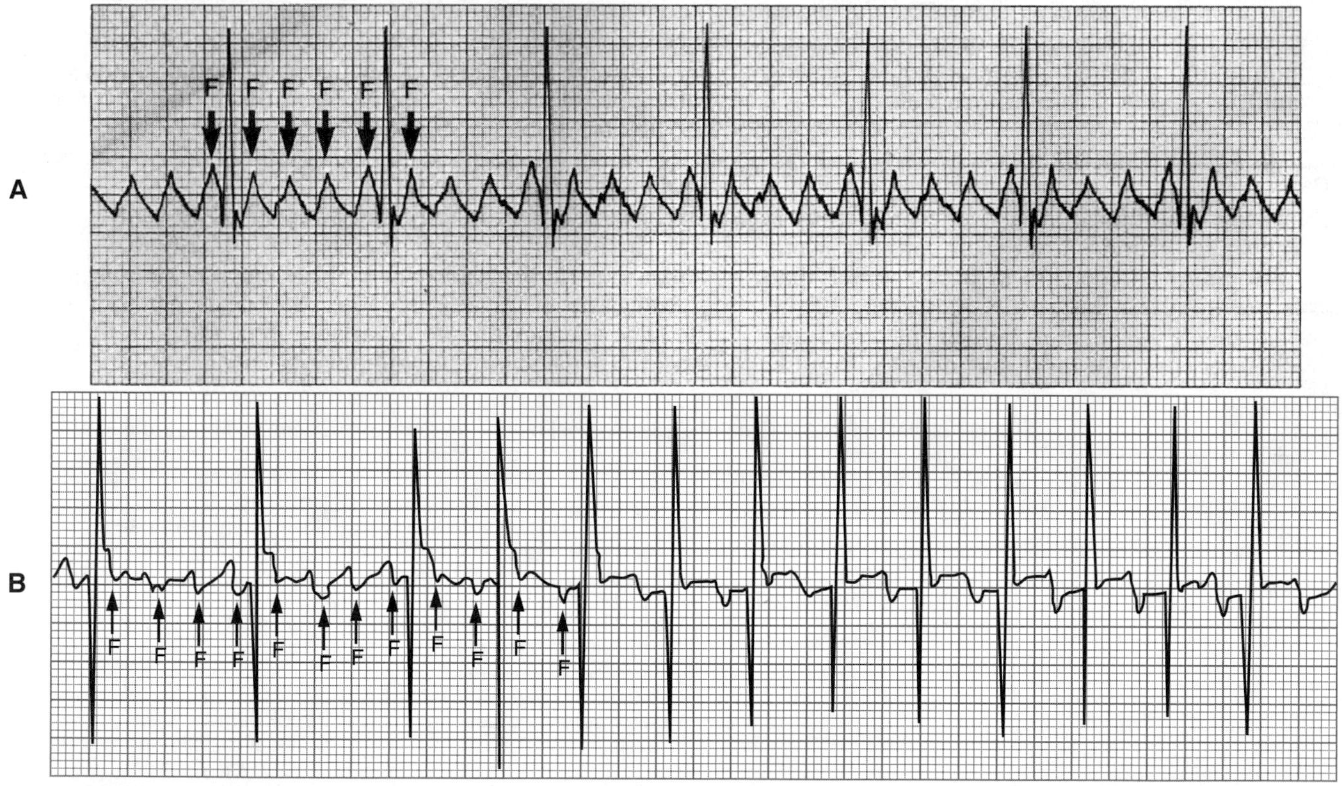

Figure 37-11 ■ Atrial dysrhythmias. **A,** Atrial flutter (F) with 4:1 block. The atrial rate is 280 beats/min; the ventricular rate is 70 beats/min. **B,** Atrial flutter with 4:1 conduction and then an 11-beat run with 2:1 conduction.

ATRIAL FLUTTER

PATHOPHYSIOLOGY. Atrial flutter is rapid atrial depolarization occurring at a rate of 250 to 350 times per minute. The most common rate is about 300 times per minute. An atrioventricular (AV) node blocks the number of impulses that reach the ventricles as a protective mechanism (Figure 37-11, *A*). When untreated, atrial flutter results in a 2:1 block (Figure 37-11, *B*). In general, when the ventricular rate is 150 beats/min, suspect atrial flutter with 2:1 block and carefully scrutinize the electrocardiographic (ECG) baseline for evidence of atrial flutter waves.

Atrial flutter may be caused by rheumatic or ischemic heart disease, heart failure (CHF), AV valve disease, pre-excitation syndromes, septal defects, pulmonary emboli, thyrotoxicosis, alcoholism, or pericarditis.

PHYSICAL ASSESSMENT/CLINICAL MANIFESTATIONS. The clinical manifestations depend on the rate of ventricular response. Assess the client for palpitations,

EVIDENCE-BASED PRACTICE for Nursing

Drug-induced QT prolongation in women during the menstrual cycle

Rodriquez, I., et al. (2001). Drug-induced QT prolongation in women during the menstrual cycle. *Journal of the American Medical Association, 285*(10), 1322-1326.

Ibutilide is an antiarrhythmic agent used for termination of atrial fibrillation and flutter. The purpose of this quantitative research study was to determine whether the degree of QT prolongation in response to ibutilide varies with the menstrual cycle phase and to compare QT prolongation between women and men.

Results indicated that the mean QT interval corrected for heart rate (QTc) after ibutilide infusion was greater for women during menses and the ovulatory phase compared with women during the luteal phase and compared with men. Menstrual cycle and gender differences exist in QTc responses to ibutilide, with the greatest increase in QTc corresponding to the first half of the menstrual cycle. Women are more likely than men to develop ibutilide-induced torsades de pointes.

Level of Evidence: 6—The study used a small sample, but it controlled for selected variables.

Critique. A sample of 38 men and 20 women were given a low dose of ibutilide. This dose was one third lower than normally given for rhythm conversion. Therefore the findings might be even greater when normal dosages are used in practice. Sample size was calculated to allow detection of a 30% difference in QTc prolongation between menstrual cycle phases and each gender, with an alpha of 0.05 and power of 0.80. One limitation is that this is the first study to compare QT-prolonging effects during the phases of the menstrual cycle. Differences in gender were the only statistically significant finding for QTc prolongation, although differences were noted among women in various life stages.

Implications for Nursing. Nurses are responsible for administering, monitoring, and reporting the results of ibutilide infusions. Prolonged QT intervals can lead to the development of serious ventricular dysrhythmias, such as ventricular tachycardia, ventricular fibrillation, and torsades de pointes. Dosages of antiarrhythmic medications may be adjusted or medications discontinued based on QT interval calculations. Nurses must know how to calculate the QTc accurately for client safety. It is generally accepted that a normal QTc is between 0.35 and 0.45 seconds. It is important to assess menstrual history as well as kidney function before the administration of antidysrhythmics that prolong the QT interval in women.

weakness, fatigue, shortness of breath, nervousness, anxiety, syncope (loss of consciousness), angina, and evidence of heart failure and shock. Carotid sinus massage transiently decreases the ventricular rate to facilitate rhythm interpretation, but it can be performed only by the physician. The client with a normal ventricular rate is usually asymptomatic. If the ventricular rate is below 100 beats/min, the term **controlled ventricular response** is used; above 100 bpm is called **rapid ventricular response.**

INTERVENTIONS. The treatment goals are the same as those for supraventricular tachycardia (SVT). Administer oxygen and prescribed drugs, such as ibutilide (Corvert), amiodarone (Cordarone), and diltiazem (Cardizem), to slow the rapid ventricular response. Studies on the effects of some of these drugs in women compared with men have been conducted to ensure their effectiveness and safety (see Evidence-Based Practice for Nursing box above).

If the client is hemodynamically compromised, cardioversion is the treatment of choice. Rapid atrial overdrive pacing may be attempted or radiofrequency catheter ablation may be necessary if the client does not respond to these therapies. These therapies are discussed later in this chapter.

RESOURCE MANAGEMENT

ATRIAL FIBRILLATION

Cost of Care

- The costs associated with the treatment of atrial fibrillation (AF) are enormous. Clients with AF make up the largest group of those hospitalized with *any* dysrhythmia, including all the life-threatening ventricular dysrhythmias combined.
- Hospital stays for AF are the longest of any hospitalizations wherein the principal diagnosis is a dysrhythmia.
- Economists estimate the annual cost of treating AF at a staggering one billion dollars.
- More than two million people in the United States have AF, requiring more than 365,000 hospitalizations each year.
- The estimated cost for each 4-day hospital stay is over $7,000 but may cost as much as $20,000.

Implications for Nursing

- Early detection and appropriate management of AF must be a priority; health promotion, especially for the older adult, is essential, and health teaching must target the components of treatment in a clear, concise manner that is individualized to the client.
- Evaluations of any older adult should include assessment for AF.
- Once AF is identified, restoration of normal sinus rhythm is crucial to prevent strokes and improve quality of life.

Data from Yee, C.A., & Rozewicz, B. (2003). Getting to the heart of atrial fibrillation. *Nursing Management, 34*(9), 21-27.

ATRIAL FIBRILLATION

PATHOPHYSIOLOGY. Atrial fibrillation (AF) is the most common dysrhythmia found in clinical practice. About 2.2 million Americans are affected with AF, and sustained AF increases with age. Ten percent of persons over the age of 80 years develop AF. Men are more likely to develop AF and women are more likely to die of AF (Josephson & McMullen, 2003). It is estimated that by the year 2050, the incidence of AF will increase to 5.6 million people, half of them females (Benson & Powless, 2003). With millions of cases of intermittent or sustained AF occurring each year in the United States, health care costs are soaring (see the Resource Management box above).

Multiple rapid impulses from many atrial foci, at a rate of 350 to 600 times per minute, depolarize the atria in a totally disorganized manner. The result is chaos, with no P waves, no atrial contractions, loss of the atrial kick, and an irregular ventricular response (Figure 37-12). The atria merely quiver in fibrillation (commonly called "A fib"). Recurrent episodes of AF eventually lead to sustained AF. Dilation and blood stagnation in the atria can lead to thrombus formation, and this increases the risk of stroke or other embolic events (Josephson & McMullen, 2003). In addition, AF causes a decrease in cardiac output, further compromising the heart's perfusion ability.

Atrial fibrillation occurs most commonly in clients with underlying cardiac disease. Cardiac damage may precede or cause AF. Of all acute myocardial infarctions (MIs), 10% to 15% are complicated by new onset of AF (Josephson & McMullen, 2003). It may also occur in clients with the following conditions:

- MI
- Rheumatic heart disease with mitral stenosis
- Atrial septal defect
- Heart failure
- Cardiomyopathy

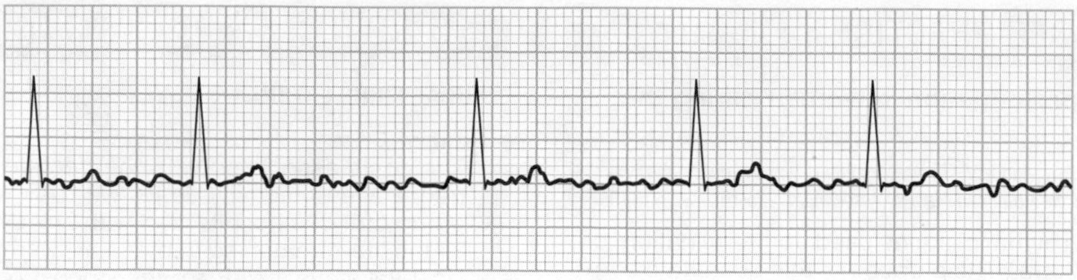

Figure 37-12 ■ Atrial dysrhythmias. Atrial fibrillation. (From Huszar, R.J. [2002]. *Pocket guide to basic dysrhythmias* [3rd ed.]. St. Louis: Mosby.)

- Hyperthyroidism
- Pulmonary emboli
- Wolff-Parkinson-White (WPW) syndrome
- Congenital heart disease
- Chronic constrictive pericarditis

Atrial fibrillation commonly occurs following cardiac surgery, in which case it is most often transient and usually responds well to treatment.

PHYSICAL ASSESSMENT/CLINICAL MANIFESTATIONS. Atrial fibrillation may be intermittent or chronic. Symptoms depend on the ventricular rate. If the ventricular rate is rapid, the presenting symptoms may be as described for supraventricular tachycardia (SVT). Because of loss of the atrial kick, however, the client in uncontrolled AF is at greater risk for an inadequate cardiac output. Assess the client for the presence of a pulse deficit, fatigue, weakness, shortness of breath, distended neck veins, dizziness, decreased exercise tolerance, anxiety, syncope, palpitations, chest discomfort or pain, and hypotension.

The client is also at risk for pulmonary embolism. Thrombi may accumulate within the right atrium and transported through the right ventricle to the lungs. Assess for shortness of breath, chest pain, hemoptysis, and a feeling of impending doom.

In addition, the client is at risk for systemic emboli, particularly an embolic stroke, which may cause severe neurologic impairment or death. Because about one third of clients with AF have thromboemboli, be sure to assess the client for evidence of embolic events. Changes in mentation, speech, sensory function, and motor function are particularly noted. Assess pulses, urine output, back pain, and complaints of gastrointestinal (GI) disturbances. Report any of these symptoms to the health care provider immediately. Clients with AF who have valvular disease are particularly at risk for thromboemboli.

INTERVENTIONS. Treatment is the same as for atrial flutter. In addition, the nurse may administer anticoagulants, such as heparin, enoxaparin (Lovenox), and sodium warfarin, as prescribed by the physician for clients considered at high risk for emboli. Before elective cardioversion, the health care provider prescribes anticoagulation therapy for about 6 weeks to prevent a thromboembolic event if the rhythm is successfully converted. To assess for the presence of atrial clots, a contraindication for cardioversion, the physician may order a transesophageal echocardiogram (TEE) before attempting emergency cardioversion (see Chapter 36). AF of greater than 12 months' duration is not likely to respond to attempts at conversion to sinus rhythm by drug therapies and may fail to respond to cardioversion. Cardioversion is discussed later in this chapter.

Clients with recurring, symptomatic AF resistant to medical therapies may be treated with radiofrequency catheter ablation to the bundle of His to interrupt all conduction between the atria and the ventricles. However, this treatment requires implantation of a permanent ventricular pacemaker and does not stop the atria from fibrillating. The atrial kick is not restored, and clients remain at risk for embolic events.

Clients in AF with decompensation may benefit from the **maze procedure,** an open chest surgical technique often performed with coronary artery bypass grafting (CABG). For the procedure, electrophysiologic mapping studies are done to confirm the diagnosis of AF. The surgeon places a maze of sutures in strategic places in the atrial myocardium, pulmonary artery, and possibly the superior vena cava to prevent electrical circuits from developing and perpetuating AF. Sinus impulses can then depolarize the atria before reaching the AV node and preserve the atrial kick. Postoperative care is similar to that after other open-heart surgical procedures (see Chapter 41).

JUNCTIONAL DYSRHYTHMIAS

Nodal cells in the atrioventricular (AV) junctional area can generate electrical impulses and are therefore secondary or latent pacemaker cells. They have a slower rate of discharge, usually 40 to 60 beats/min, and are usually suppressed. Occasionally these cells do generate impulses as an escape pacemaker when the sinus node is excessively slow, or the cells may do so inappropriately as irritable rhythms. These rhythms are most commonly transient, and clients usually remain hemodynamically stable.

VENTRICULAR DYSRHYTHMIAS

The ventricles have the fewest nodal cells and are the slowest pacemaker, generally being overcome by faster, higher pacemakers. However, irritable ventricular cells may generate electrical impulses and fire prematurely. Because the impulse originates in and depolarizes one ventricle first, then spreads to depolarize the other, the resultant QRS complex is wide, usually measuring greater than 0.12 second. The QRS complex is bizarre or oddly shaped, looking different from the normal QRS complexes. The repolarization sequence is also different so that the T wave is large and usually occurs in a direction opposite to the largest deflection of the QRS complex. The impulse most commonly is blocked in the AV node and cannot proceed further with retrograde conduction so that the atria and the sinoatrial (SA) node are usually not affected by the ventricular impulse. The atrial rhythm typically remains regular unless the underlying rhythm is sinus arrhythmia.

IDIOVENTRICULAR RHYTHM (VENTRICULAR ESCAPE RHYTHM)

PATHOPHYSIOLOGY. During an **idioventricular rhythm** (ventricular escape rhythm), the ventricular nodal cells pace the ventricles. Because their inherent rate of firing is slow, the rate is usually less than 40 beats/min. If P waves are seen, they are independent of the QRS complexes and are not related (AV dissociation).

Idioventricular rhythm is seen as a rhythm in the dying heart, where downward displacement of the pacemaker has occurred. Pulseless electrical activity (PEA) is characterized by no palpable pulse and therefore no perfusion, although electrical activity is displayed on the monitor. Common causes of PEA are hypovolemia, hypoxia, acidosis, hyperkalemia or hypokalemia, hypothermia, drug overdose, tension pneumothorax, coronary or pulmonary thrombosis, and cardiac tamponade.

PHYSICAL ASSESSMENT/CLINICAL MANIFESTATIONS. Because idioventricular pacemakers are unstable, unreliable, and slow, the client is hypotensive and in shock or, most typically, pulseless and therefore in cardiac arrest. Assess the client's airway, breathing, circulation, level of consciousness, and oxygenation.

EMERGENCY CARE: IDIOVENTRICULAR RHYTHMS. Usually idioventricular rhythms require immediate resuscitation measures, unless there is a do-not-resuscitate (DNR) order. Initiate cardiopulmonary resuscitation (CPR) and summon assistance. The team may initiate advanced cardiac life support (ACLS) measures, including epinephrine administration, intravascular volume replacement, and other measures. The physician may attempt pacemaker therapy or discontinue resuscitation efforts.

PREMATURE VENTRICULAR COMPLEXES

PATHOPHYSIOLOGY. Premature ventricular complexes (PVCs) result from increased irritability of ventricular cells. PVCs are early ventricular complexes followed by a pause. When multiple PVCs are present, the QRS complexes may be unifocal or uniform, meaning that they are of the same shape (Figure 37-13, *A*) or multifocal or multiform, meaning that they are of different shapes (Figure 37-13, *B*). PVCs frequently occur in repetitive rhythms, such as bigeminy, trigeminy, and quadrigeminy. Two sequential PVCs are a pair, or couplet. Three or more successive PVCs are usually called nonsustained ventricular tachycardia (NSVT) (Figure 37-13, *C*).

Premature ventricular contractions are common, and their frequency increases with age. PVCs may be insignificant or may occur with myocardial ischemia or MI, CHF, chronic hypoxemia, chronic airway limitation (CAL), anemia, hypokalemia, or hypomagnesemia. The administration of catecholamines, sympathomimetic drugs, and digitalis, as well as acidosis, anesthesia, stress, nicotine intake, ingestion of caffeine and alcohol, infection, trauma, or surgery, can also cause PVCs. Postmenopausal women often find that caffeine causes palpitations and PVCs.

PHYSICAL ASSESSMENT/CLINICAL MANIFESTATIONS. The client may be asymptomatic or may experience palpitations or chest discomfort caused by increased stroke volume of the normal beat after the pause. Peripheral pulses may be diminished or absent with the PVCs themselves because the decreased stroke volume of the premature beats may decrease peripheral perfusion. Because other rhythms also cause widened QRS complexes, it is essential that the nurse assess whether the premature complexes perfuse to the extremities. This is done by palpating the carotid, brachial, or femoral arteries while observing the monitor for widened complexes or auscultating for the apical heart sounds. With acute MI, PVCs may be considered warning dysrhythmias, possibly heralding the onset of ventricular tachycardia (VT) or ventricular fibrillation (VF). For a client with chest discomfort or pain, the nurse reports to the physician whether PVCs increase in frequency, are multiform, are R-on-T phenomena, or occur in runs of VT.

INTERVENTIONS. If there is no underlying heart disease, PVCs are not usually treated other than by eliminating any contributing cause (e.g., caffeine, stress). With acute myocardial ischemia or MI, the nurse treats significant PVCs by administering oxygen and amiodarone (Cordarone) as prescribed. If an MI occurs, administer other drugs as prescribed, including procainamide (Pronestyl), magnesium sulfate, and quinidine (see Chart 37-3). Potassium is administered as prescribed for replacement therapy if hypokalemia is the cause.

VENTRICULAR TACHYCARDIA

PATHOPHYSIOLOGY. Ventricular tachycardia (VT), sometimes referred to as "V tach," occurs with repetitive firing of an irritable ventricular ectopic focus, usually at a rate of 140 to 180 beats/min or more (Figure 37-14). VT may result from increased automaticity or a re-entry mechanism. It may be intermittent, as in three or more self-limiting beats (nonsustained VT), or sustained, lasting longer than 15 to 30 seconds. The sinus node may continue to discharge independently, depolarizing the atria but not the ventricles (atrioventricular [AV] dissociation), although P waves are seldom seen in sustained VT.

Ventricular tachycardia may occur in clients with ischemic heart disease, MI, cardiomyopathy, hypokalemia, hypomagnesemia, valvular heart disease, heart failure, drug toxicity, hypotension, or ventricular aneurysm. In clients who go into cardiac arrest, VT is commonly the initial rhythm before deterioration into ventricular fibrillation (VF) as the terminal rhythm. VT is not common in infants and children unless they have cardiac disease.

PHYSICAL ASSESSMENT/CLINICAL MANIFESTATIONS. Clinical manifestations of sustained VT partially depend on the ventricular rate. Slower rates are better tolerated. Clients may be hemodynamically compromised if the cardiac output decreases because of the shortened ventricular filling time and loss of the atrial kick. In some clients, VT causes cardiac arrest. Assess the client's airway, breathing, circulation, level of consciousness, and oxygenation.

INTERVENTIONS. For the *stable* client with sustained VT, administer oxygen, and confirm the rhythm via a 12-lead electrocardiogram (ECG). Amiodarone, lidocaine, or magnesium sulfate may be given. Current advanced cardiac life support (ACLS) guidelines state that elective cardioversion is highly recommended for stable VT. The physician may prescribe an oral antidysrhythmic agent, such as mexiletine (Mexitil) or sotalol (Betapace, Sotacor✱).

EMERGENCY CARE: VENTRICULAR TACHYCARDIA. For the client with unstable VT with a pulse, the physician or ACLS-qualified nurse administers emergency cardioversion followed by oxygen and antidysrhythmic therapy (Chart 37-4). Rapid atrial or ventricular overdrive pacing can be used if the VT is related to a significant bradydysrhythmia.

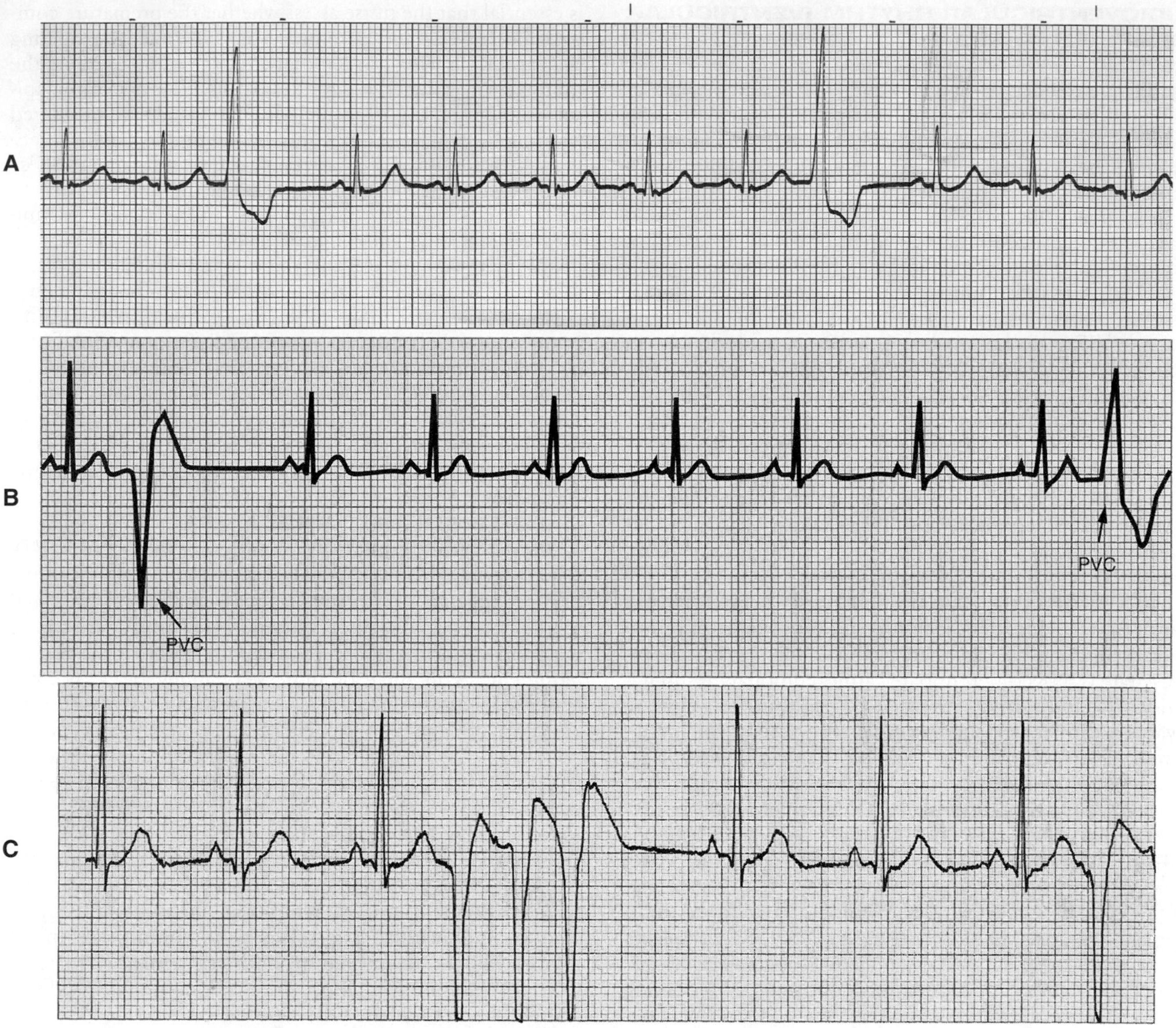

Figure 37-13 ■ Ventricular dysrhythmias. **A,** Normal sinus rhythm with unifocal premature ventricular complexes (PVCs). **B,** Normal sinus rhythm with multifocal PVCs (one negative and the other positive). **C,** Normal sinus rhythm with three consecutive PVCs (nonsustained ventricular tachycardia) and another unifocal PVC.

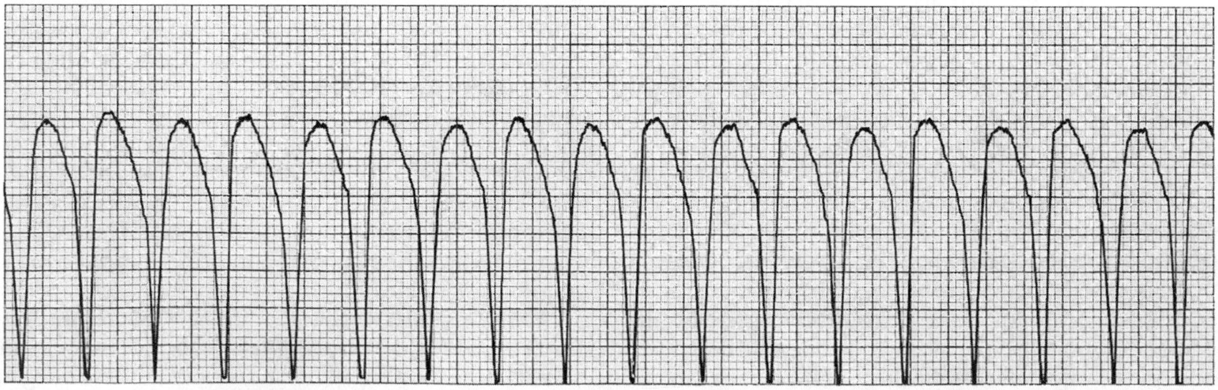

Figure 37-14 ■ Ventricular dysrhythmias. Sustained ventricular tachycardia at a rate of 166 beats/min.

CHART 37-4

BEST PRACTICE for
Emergency Care of Unstable Ventricular Tachycardia

EMERGENCY CARE

- Assist the physician with cardioversion.
- Provide oxygen and antidysrhythmic drugs as prescribed.
- Teach the client how to perform cough cardiopulmonary resuscitation (CPR), if ordered.
- Assist with or provide defibrillation (if you are certified in advanced cardiac life support [ACLS]).
- Initiate CPR if the client does not respond to the preceding measures.
- Maintain a patent airway at all times. Administer oxygen.
- Monitor airway, breathing, and circulation.
- Monitor the client for premature ventricular complexes (PVCs) and the recurrence of ventricular tachycardia (VT).
- Assess for manifestations of myocardial infarction, hypokalemia, or hypomagnesemia.

With pulseless VT, the physician or ACLS-qualified nurse or other health care provider must *immediately* defibrillate the client or initiate CPR and defibrillate as soon as possible. If the client remains pulseless, the nurse or other health care provider must resume CPR and full resuscitative measures following defibrillation. This includes airway management and administration of oxygen, epinephrine, vasopressin, and antidysrhythmic therapy with amiodarone (Cordarone), magnesium sulfate, and procainamide (Pronestyl).

If the rhythm has been successfully converted, attention is given to treating reversible causes of VT, such as myocardial ischemia, acidosis, hypokalemia, and hypomagnesemia. Ensure that oxygen therapy and antidysrhythmic agent administration are continued, and monitor the client closely for premature ventricular complexes (PVCs) and the recurrence of VT. The client with recurrent, medically refractory VT should be studied in the electrophysiology laboratory and may benefit from radiofrequency catheter ablation. Implantation of a cardioverter/defibrillator is often performed in clients who have experienced recurrent VT (see later).

VENTRICULAR FIBRILLATION

PATHOPHYSIOLOGY. Ventricular fibrillation (VF), sometimes called "V fib," is the result of electrical chaos in the ventricles. Impulses from many irritable foci fire in a totally disorganized manner so that ventricular contraction cannot occur. There are no recognizable deflections. Instead, there are irregular undulations of varying amplitudes, from coarse to fine (Figure 37-15, *A*). The ventricles merely quiver, consuming a tremendous amount of oxygen. There is no cardiac output or pulse and therefore no cerebral, myocardial, or systemic perfusion. This rhythm is *rapidly fatal* if not successfully terminated within 3 to 5 minutes.

Ventricular fibrillation may be the first manifestation of coronary artery disease (CAD). Clients with myocardial infarction (MI) are at great risk for VF, which may also occur in clients with myocardial ischemia, hypokalemia, hypomagnesemia, hemorrhage, antidysrhythmic therapy, rapid supraventricular tachydysrhythmias (SVTs), shock, asynchronous pacing with competition, or severe metabolic disease. VF also occurs following surgery or trauma.

PHYSICAL ASSESSMENT/CLINICAL MANIFESTATIONS. On initiation of VF, the client becomes faint, immediately loses consciousness, and becomes pulseless and apneic. There is no blood pressure, and heart sounds are absent. Respiratory and metabolic acidosis develop. Seizures

A
B

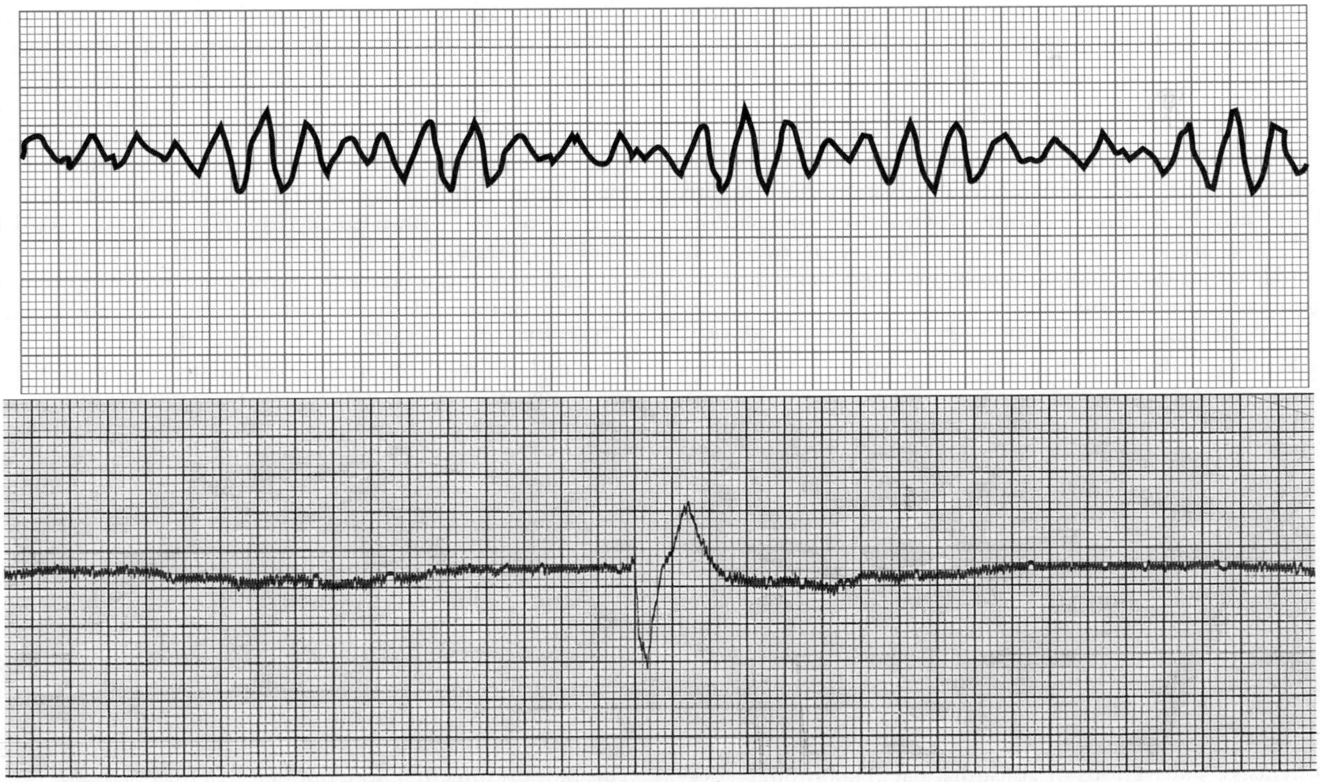

Figure 37-15 ■ Ventricular dysrhythmias. **A,** Coarse ventricular fibrillation. **B,** Ventricular asystole with one idioventricular complex.

may occur. Within minutes, the pupils become fixed and dilated, and the skin becomes cold and mottled. Death ensues without prompt restoration of an organized rhythm and cardiac output.

EMERGENCY CARE: VENTRICULAR FIBRILLATION. The goals of treatment are to terminate VF promptly and convert it to an organized rhythm. Therefore the priority is to defibrillate the client *immediately* according to ACLS protocol. If a defibrillator is not readily available, CPR must be continued until the defibrillator arrives.

If the VF does not terminate after three rapid successive shocks of increasing energy, the nurse and resuscitation team resume CPR and provide airway management. They also administer oxygen and antidysrhythmic therapy with vasopressin, epinephrine, amiodarone, procainamide (Pronestyl), lidocaine, and magnesium sulfate, along with attempting defibrillation frequently. If VF is successfully converted to an organized rhythm, the nurse continues supportive therapy and assists the physician in treating potential causes of VF and preventing its recurrence.

VENTRICULAR ASYSTOLE

PATHOPHYSIOLOGY. **Ventricular asystole,** sometimes called *ventricular standstill,* is the complete absence of any ventricular rhythm (Figure 37-15, *B*). There are no electrical impulses in the ventricles and therefore *no* ventricular depolarization, no QRS complex, no contraction, no cardiac output, and no pulse, respirations, or blood pressure. The client is in full cardiac arrest. The sinoatrial (SA) node, in some cases, may continue to fire and depolarize the atria, with only P waves seen on the electrocardiogram (ECG). The sinus impulses, however, do not conduct to the ventricles, and QRS complexes remain absent. In most cases, the entire conduction system is electrically silent, with no P waves seen on the ECG. There is only a mildly undulating line on the ECG. Fine ventricular fibrillation (VF) may resemble asystole in some leads. Because treatment of these two rhythms differs significantly, the nurse must assess two ECG leads for an accurate rhythm interpretation.

Ventricular asystole usually results from myocardial hypoxia, which may be a consequence of advanced heart failure. It may also be caused by severe hyperkalemia and acidosis. If P waves are seen, asystole is likely because of severe ventricular conduction blocks. Rarely, excessive vagal stimulation may cause asystole.

PHYSICAL ASSESSMENT/CLINICAL MANIFESTATIONS. Clients are in full cardiac arrest with a loss of consciousness and an absence of pulse, respirations, and blood pressure. Ventricular asystole is often unresponsive to resuscitation measures and fatal.

EMERGENCY CARE: VENTRICULAR ASYSTOLE. The goal of treatment is to restore cardiac electrical activity. The nurse or other health care provider initiates CPR immediately (unless there is a DNR order) and summons assistance. Another ECG lead is assessed to ensure that the rhythm is asystole and not fine VF, which warrants immediate defibrillation. Do NOT shock asystole. The nurse and resuscitation team manage the airway and administer oxygen, epinephrine, and atropine. The nurse assists the physician with the initiation of noninvasive pacing or invasive transvenous or epicardial pacing, although pacemaker therapy is generally not effective. The prognosis for clients with asystole is poor. Health care providers should consider termination of resuscitation efforts if there is no response after successful initiation of standard interventions when cessation is approved by an authorized physician. Nurses should know the criteria for termination of CPR and ACLS based on current facility and state legal policies.

An emerging clinical practice is allowing or encouraging family presence at resuscitation attempts. Interviews conducted with family members and significant others revealed this to be a positive experience. It allowed closure after the death of a loved one. Although there may be staff resistance and some limits to family presence, research shows a strong therapeutic effect from this practice (Eichhorn et al., 2001).

ATRIOVENTRICULAR BLOCKS

Atrioventricular (AV) blocks exist when supraventricular impulses are excessively delayed or totally blocked in the AV node or intraventricular conduction system. Conduction may be transiently or permanently abnormal for a number of reasons. The SA node continues to function normally, and atrial depolarizations and P waves occur regularly. Because of the conduction dysfunction, ventricular depolarizations and QRS complexes are either delayed or blocked.

The following are the different degrees of heart blocks:

- In *first-degree* AV block, all sinus impulses eventually reach the ventricles.
- In *second-degree* heart block, some sinus impulses reach the ventricles, but others do not because they are blocked.
- In *third-degree* heart block (complete heart block), none of the sinus impulses reaches the ventricles. The ventricles are therefore depolarized by a second, independent pacemaker.

AV blocks are differentiated by their PR intervals.

FIRST-DEGREE ATRIOVENTRICULAR BLOCK

PATHOPHYSIOLOGY. **First-degree AV block** is actually a conduction delay rather than a block. AV node conduction is slow, prolonging the PR interval to greater than 0.20 second. However, all sinus impulses eventually reach the ventricles. The underlying rhythm must still be identified (e.g., sinus rhythm with first-degree AV block (Figure 37-16, *A*).

PHYSICAL ASSESSMENT/CLINICAL MANIFESTATIONS. First-degree AV block has no hemodynamic consequences and produces no symptoms. Any symptoms are the result of the underlying rhythm (e.g., sinus bradycardia).

INTERVENTIONS. In the stable client, no treatment is needed. If the PR interval is particularly long or is getting progressively longer, the nurse must notify the physician. If the first-degree AV block is due to drug therapy, the nurse must withhold the offending drug and notify the physician. When first-degree AV block is associated with symptomatic bradycardia, oxygen is administered as prescribed to accelerate AV conduction.

SECOND-DEGREE ATRIOVENTRICULAR BLOCK TYPE I (WENCKEBACH OR MOBITZ TYPE I)

PATHOPHYSIOLOGY. In **second-degree AV block type I,** each successive sinus impulse takes a little longer to conduct through the impaired AV node, until one impulse is completely blocked and fails to depolarize the ventricles. This block results in a nonconducted or dropped beat (missing QRS complex). There is progressive prolongation of the PR interval, followed by a dropped beat and a pause (a char-

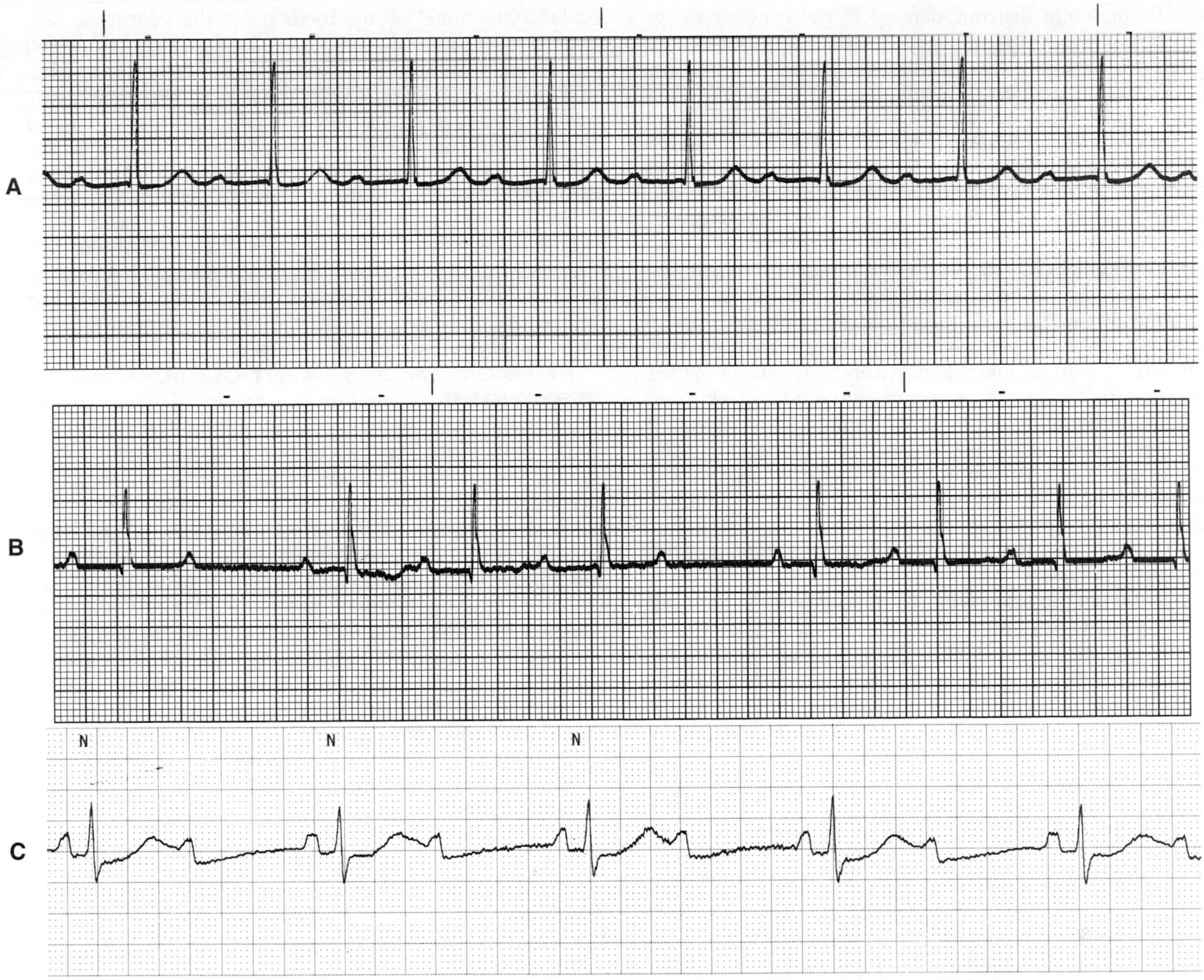

Figure 37-16 ■ Atrioventricular (AV) blocks. **A,** Normal sinus rhythm with first-degree AV block (PR interval, 0.36 second). **B,** Second-degree AV block type I (Wenckebach AV) with an irregular rhythm, grouped beating, and progressive prolongation of the PR interval until a P wave is completely blocked and not followed by a QRS complex. **C,** Second-degree AV block type II (Mobitz II) with 2:1 conduction, a constant PR interval, and wide QRS complex.

acteristic feature of this rhythm). Because of the dropped QRS complex, each group normally has one more P wave than QRS complexes (Figure 37-16, *B*).

PHYSICAL ASSESSMENT/CLINICAL MANIFESTATIONS. The client is usually asymptomatic if the frequency of dropped beats and the overall ventricular rate do not decrease the cardiac output. If the ventricular rate is too slow, decreasing the cardiac output, the client will have symptoms of a symptomatic bradydysrhythmia. This rhythm is usually transient and terminates spontaneously.

INTERVENTIONS. No intervention is required in the stable client because this rhythm rarely progresses to a more severe block. In the symptomatic client, administer oxygen and atropine as prescribed. If atropine is not successful in speeding AV nodal conduction time and increasing the heart rate, initiate pacemaker therapy as ordered and notify the physician.

SECOND-DEGREE HEART BLOCK TYPE II (MOBITZ TYPE II)

PATHOPHYSIOLOGY. In Mobitz type II block, the block is actually infranodal, occurring below the bundle of His. It involves a constant block in one of the bundle branches, resulting in a wide QRS complex in conducted beats and an intermittent block in the other bundle branch, resulting in dropped beats because both bundles are blocked (P waves are not followed by a QRS complex). Because the block is not in the AV node, sinus impulses that conduct to the ventricles always do so with a constant PR interval. Impulses may be blocked randomly, making the ventricular rhythm irregular. Alternatively, the impulses may be blocked at regular intervals, such as in 2:1 block, in which case the ventricular rhythm is regular (Figure 37-16, *C*).

Second-degree AV block type II is less common than type I. It may occur in the adult with an anterior wall MI because of severe ischemic damage to the conduction system. It may also be caused by rheumatic heart disease or degenerative disease of the conduction system. It is a serious block that may progress suddenly to a third-degree AV block (complete heart block) and an ominous prognosis.

PHYSICAL ASSESSMENT/CLINICAL MANIFESTATIONS. Symptoms depend on the frequency of dropped beats and the overall ventricular rate. If the cardiac output is inadequate, the client presents with a symptomatic bradydysrhythmia.

INTERVENTIONS. In the asymptomatic client, the nurse may assist the physician in initiating prophylactic pacing to avert the threat of sudden third-degree AV block. If slow ventricular rates are present, the nurse administers oxygen and atropine as prescribed. Atropine is usually ineffective because it does not reverse the infranodal block. Noninvasive (external) or invasive pacing is preferred. A permanent pacemaker may be required with recurrent Mobitz type II block. An isoproterenol (Isuprel) infusion may be administered with caution but may be dangerous in adults with ischemic heart disease.

THIRD-DEGREE HEART BLOCK (COMPLETE HEART BLOCK)

PATHOPHYSIOLOGY. In **third-degree heart block,** none of the sinus impulses conducts to the ventricles. The sinoatrial (SA) node is usually the pacemaker for the atria, producing P waves at a normal or even accelerated rate, while a separate, independent pacemaker paces the ventricles. Thus AV dissociation exists. If the block is in the AV node, a junctional escape focus paces the ventricles, producing normal QRS complexes at a rate of 40 to 60 beats/min. If the block is below the bundle of His (infranodal), a ventricular escape focus paces the ventricles, producing wide QRS complexes at a rate usually less than 40 beats/min (Figure 37-17, *A*). In either case, the atrial and ventricular rhythms are usually regular but independent of each other, with more P waves than QRS complexes.

Third-degree heart block in the adult may occur from ischemic injury with coronary artery disease (CAD) or MI, degenerative disease of the conduction system, hypoxia, or calcific aortic stenosis. Third-degree heart block may occur with congenital heart disease, the effects of drugs or electrolyte disturbances, or cardiac surgery.

PHYSICAL ASSESSMENT/CLINICAL MANIFESTATIONS. Clinical manifestations depend on the overall ventricular rate and cardiac output. Transient third-degree heart block may be well tolerated, particularly when the block is in the AV node. If the block is infranodal, it may have serious hemodynamic consequences. If cerebral perfusion is inadequate, clients may be confused and lightheaded or may experience episodes of syncope with or without seizures (Stokes-Adams attacks). Inadequate cardiac output may cause myocardial ischemia or MI, heart failure, or hypotension. Third-degree heart block may predispose to cardiac arrest, causing VT, VF, or asystole. Therefore it is regarded as a dangerous rhythm.

INTERVENTIONS. Third-degree AV block with a junctional escape pacemaker is often transient and well tol-

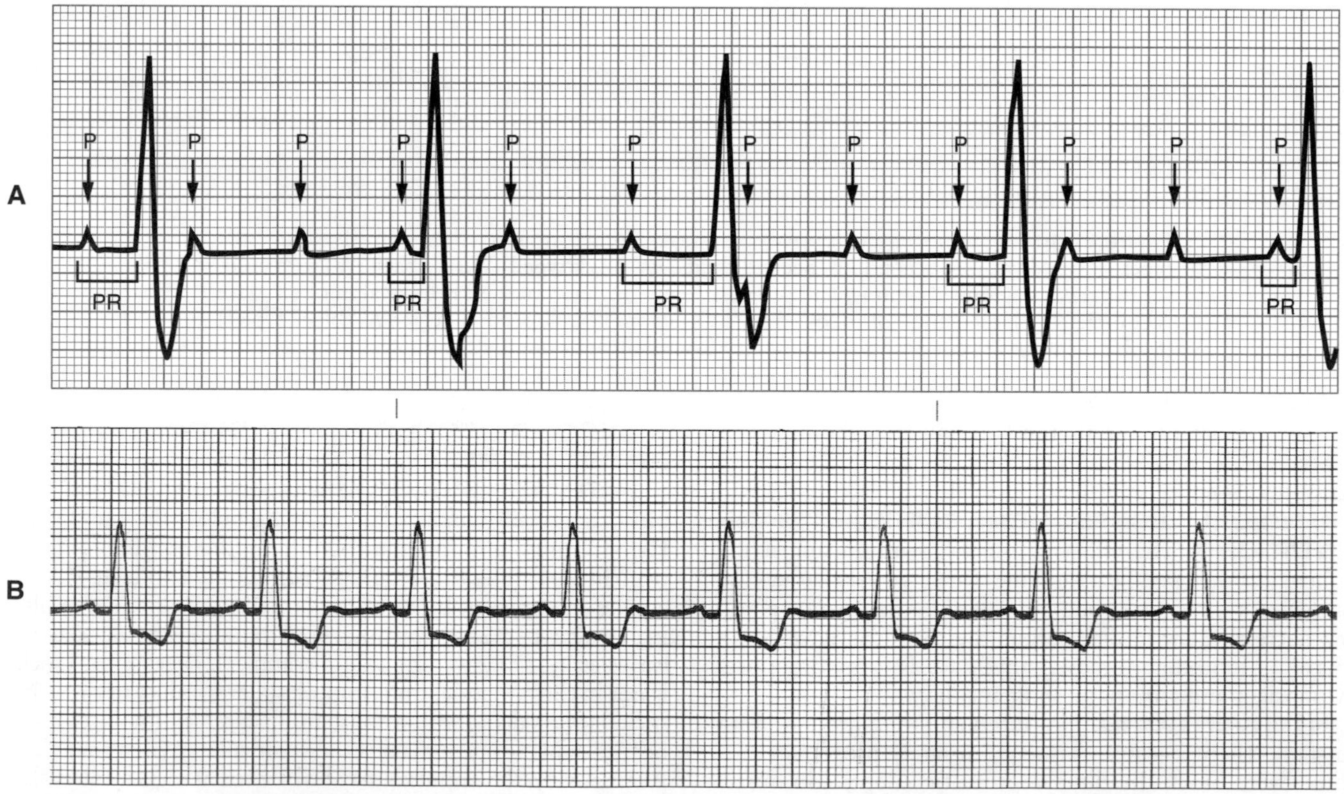

Figure 37-17 ■ Atrioventricular (AV) blocks. **A,** Third-degree AV block with regular atrial and ventricular rhythms, inconstant PR intervals (AV dissociation), and a ventricular escape focus pacing the ventricles at a rate of 38 beats/min, with wide QRS complexes. **B,** Normal sinus rhythm with bundle branch block (wide QRS complexes measuring 0.12 second).

erated. If the client is symptomatic, administer oxygen and atropine as prescribed. Clients with third-degree heart block with a ventricular escape pacemaker are frequently symptomatic. Administer oxygen and assist the physician in initiating pacing to avert the threat of cardiac arrest. Atropine is usually not successful in infranodal blocks with wide QRS complexes. Cautious use of isoproterenol (Isuprel) infusions may be necessary as a temporary measure while awaiting pacemaker therapy but is dangerous in clients with acute myocardial infarction. Implantation of a permanent pacemaker may be required for clients with recurrent third-degree infranodal block.

BUNDLE BRANCH BLOCKS

PATHOPHYSIOLOGY. Bundle branch block is a conduction delay or block within one of the two main bundle branches below the bifurcation of the bundle of His. When one bundle branch is blocked, the supraventricular impulse is able to descend only down the unblocked bundle branch and to depolarize that ventricle. The other ventricle is depolarized afterward as the wave of depolarization from the first ventricle proceeds from cell to cell to the other ventricle. Such slow depolarization prolongs the QRS duration to 0.12 second or longer. The underlying rhythm is usually sinus in origin (e.g., sinus rhythm with bundle branch block) (Figure 37-17, *B*).

Bundle branch block may be a temporary or a permanent conduction disorder. Right or left bundle branch blocks are occasionally seen in clients with normal hearts. More commonly they are seen in clients with cardiovascular disease, such as congenital heart disease, rheumatic heart disease, ventricular hypertrophy, cardiomyopathy, severe aortic stenosis, chronic degenerative disease of the conduction system, or fibrotic scarring of the conduction system. Transient bundle branch block may be seen with acute conditions such as coronary insufficiency, MI, or heart failure; during right-sided heart catheterization; or with rapid supraventricular rates.

PHYSICAL ASSESSMENT/CLINICAL MANIFESTATIONS. No clinical manifestations are specifically related to bundle branch block. Notify the physician when a new bundle branch block develops, especially in the client with an acute MI. The conduction disorder may deteriorate to a more significant block requiring pacemaker therapy.

INTERVENTIONS. No interventions are specifically related to bundle branch block. Assess the client during alterations in heart rate for symptoms of hemodynamic compromise, which are reported to the physician. Ensure that the client is resting and has adequate ventilation and oxygenation.

COLLABORATIVE MANAGEMENT

Analysis

COMMON NURSING DIAGNOSES AND COLLABORATIVE PROBLEMS

The following are priority nursing diagnoses for all clients with dysrhythmias:

1. Decreased Cardiac Output related to altered heart rate/rhythm
2. Ineffective Tissue Perfusion related to reduction of arterial blood flow

ADDITIONAL NURSING DIAGNOSES AND COLLABORATIVE PROBLEMS

In addition to the common nursing diagnoses, clients with dysrhythmias may have one or more of the following:

- Impaired Gas Exchange related to ventilation-perfusion imbalance
- Ineffective Coping related to uncertainty and situational crisis
- Activity Intolerance related to imbalance between oxygen supply/demand
- Deficient Knowledge related to cause and treatment of dysrhythmia

An additional collaborative problem is Potential for Pulmonary Edema.

Planning and Implementation

DECREASED CARDIAC OUTPUT AND INEFFECTIVE TISSUE PERFUSION

NOC **PLANNING: EXPECTED OUTCOMES.** The client with dysrhythmias is expected to have adequacy of blood flow ejected from the left ventricle to support systemic perfusion pressure. Indicators include that the following will not be compromised in the client:

- Apical heart rate
- Systolic and diastolic blood pressure
- Activity tolerance
- Cognitive status
- Skin color
- Peripheral pulses
- Ejection fraction

Additional indicators include that the client will not have any of the following:

- Dysrhythmias
- Abnormal heart sounds
- Angina
- Dyspnea
- Fatigue
- Pulmonary edema

INTERVENTIONS. The nurse's major role is to assess for complications and monitor the client for response to treatment (Chart 37-5). Interventions are specific to the type of dysrhythmia, the cause, the effect it has on cardiac output, and the risk it presents to the client. Interventions for specific dysrhythmias are summarized in Table 37-2.

NIC **CARDIAC CARE.** Monitor or direct assistive nursing personnel to monitor the client's electrocardiographic (ECG) rhythm or assess the client for manifestations associated with dysrhythmias, such as abnormal pulse rate and rhythm, palpitations, chest pain, syncope, decreased blood pressure, and dyspnea.

Assess the client's apical and radial pulses for a full minute for any irregularity, which may occur with premature beats, escape beats, atrial fibrillation (AF), or second-degree heart blocks. If the apical pulse rate differs from the radial pulse rate, a pulse deficit exists and suggests that not all beats are perfusing. Clinical manifestations of sustained tachydysrhythmias and bradydysrhythmias are summarized in Chart 37-2.

In a critical care setting, if the client has a pulmonary artery catheter and an arterial line, his or her hemodynamic profile is reviewed to determine the physiologic effects of

CHART 37-5

NIC **INTERVENTION ACTIVITIES for The Client with Dysrhythmias**

Cardiac Care: *Limitation of complications resulting from an imbalance between myocardial oxygen supply and demand for a client with symptoms of impaired cardiac function*

- Evaluate chest pain (e.g., intensity, location, radiation, duration, and precipitating and alleviating factors).
- Perform a comprehensive appraisal of peripheral circulation (e.g., check peripheral pulses, edema, capillary refill, color, and temperature of extremity).
- Monitor cardiovascular status.
- Document cardiac dysrhythmias.
- Monitor vital signs frequently.
- Evaluate the client's response to ectopy or dysrhythmias.
- Monitor appropriate laboratory values (e.g., cardiac enzymes, electrolyte levels).
- Provide antiarrhythmic therapy according to unit policy (e.g., antiarrhythmic medication, cardioversion, or defibrillation), as appropriate.
- Monitor client's response to antiarrhythmic medications.
- Arrange exercise and rest periods to avoid fatigue.
- Monitor the client's activity tolerance.
- Monitor for dyspnea, fatigue, tachypnea, and orthopnea.
- Promote stress reduction.
- Instruct the client on the importance of immediately reporting any chest discomfort.
- Offer spiritual support to the client and/or family (e.g., contact clergy), as appropriate.

NIC intervention activities selected from Dochterman, J.M., & Bulechek, G.M. (Eds.) (2004). *Nursing interventions classification (NIC)* (4th ed.). St. Louis: Mosby. No part of this work is to be altered without prior written permission from the Publisher.

the dysrhythmia. Also assess the psychosocial impact of dysrhythmias on clients and families and the effectiveness of their coping mechanisms.

Assessment of the client's past and current history is essential because dysrhythmias are associated with both acute and chronic disorders as well as with medical and surgical therapies. Review the interpretation of the client's 12-lead ECG and other ECG diagnostic tests, such as the Holter monitor, event monitor, or signal-averaged ECG.

NONSURGICAL MANAGEMENT. Nonsurgical management of dysrhythmias includes drug therapy, vagal maneuvers, temporary pacing, cardioversion, cardiopulmonary resuscitation (CPR), defibrillation, and catheter ablation.

Drug Therapy. Pharmacologic therapy administered for the control of dysrhythmias often includes drugs from one or more classes of antidysrhythmic agents (see Chart 37-3). The Vaughn-Williams classification is commonly used to classify drugs according to their effects on the action potential of cardiac cells. Other drugs also have antidysrhythmic effects but do not fit the Vaughn-Williams classification.

Vaughn-Williams Classification. Class I antidysrhythmics are membrane-stabilizing agents, stabilizing phase 4 to decrease automaticity. The three subclassifications in this group include type IA drugs, which moderately slow conduction and prolong repolarization, prolonging the QT interval. These drugs are used to treat or to prevent supraventricular and ventricular premature beats and tachydysrhythmias, but they are not as commonly used as other drugs. Examples include quinidine sulfate and procainamide hydrochloride (Pronestyl). Type IB drugs shorten repolarization. These drugs are used to treat or prevent ventricular premature beats, ventricular tachycardia (VT), and ventricular fibrillation (VF). Examples include lidocaine and mexiletine hydrochloride (Mexitil). Type IC drugs markedly slow conduction and widen the QRS complex. These drugs are used primarily to treat or to prevent recurrent, life-threatening ventricular premature beats, VT, and VF. Examples include flecainide acetate (Tambocor) and propafenone hydrochloride (Rythmol).

Class II antidysrhythmics control dysrhythmias associated with excessive beta-adrenergic stimulation by competing for receptor sites and thereby decreasing heart rate and conduction velocity. Beta-adrenergic blocking agents, such as propranolol (Lopressor) and esmolol hydrochloride (Brevibloc), are class II drugs. They are used to treat or to prevent supraventricular and ventricular premature beats and tachydysrhythmias. Sotalol hydrochloride (Betapace, Sotacor✱) is an antidysrhythmic agent with both noncardioselective beta-adrenergic blocking effects (class II) and action potential duration prolongation properties (class III). It is an oral agent recommended for the treatment of documented ventricular dysrhythmias, such as VT, that are life threatening.

Class III antidysrhythmics lengthen the absolute refractory period and prolong repolarization and the action potential duration of ischemic cells. Class III drugs include amiodarone (Cordarone) and ibutilide (Covert) and are used to treat or prevent ventricular premature beats, VT, and VF.

Class IV antidysrhythmics impede the flow of calcium into the cell during depolarization, thereby depressing the automaticity of the sinoatrial (SA) and atrioventricular (AV) nodes, decreasing the heart rate, and prolonging the AV nodal refractory period and conduction. Calcium channel blockers, such as verapamil hydrochloride (Calan, Isoptin✱) and diltiazem hydrochloride (Cardizem), are class IV drugs. They are used to treat supraventricular tachycardia (SVT), atrial flutter, and atrial fibrillation (AF) to slow down the ventricular response.

Other Antidysrhythmic Drugs. Other drugs, such as digoxin, atropine, adenosine, and magnesium sulfate, are frequently used to treat dysrhythmias. Digoxin (Lanoxin, Novodigoxin✱) increases vagal tone, slowing AV nodal conduction. It is useful in treating supraventricular tachydysrhythmias, particularly chronic AF, by controlling the rate of ventricular response. However, digoxin does not convert AF to sinus rhythm. Atropine is a parasympatholytic or vagolytic agent. It is used to treat vagally induced symptomatic bradydysrhythmias. Adenosine is an endogenous nucleoside that slows AV nodal conduction to interrupt re-entry pathways. It is effective in terminating paroxysmal SVT, a re-entrant tachydysrhythmia. Magnesium sulfate is an electrolyte administered to treat refractory VT or VF because these clients may be hypomagnesemic, with increased ventricular irritability.

Emergency Cardiac Drugs. In addition to antidysrhythmics, several other drugs are used during cardiac arrest (Chart 37-6). Epinephrine (Adrenalin) is a first-line agent in all cardiac arrests. It is given predominantly for its alpha-adrenergic effects to increase vasomotor tone for myocardial and cerebral perfusion. Its beta-adrenergic effects may stimulate the heart and increase myocardial contractility to improve cardiac output. Vasopressin has potent vasoconstricting effects and has been shown to be equivalent to epinephrine in VF and pulseless VT. It has a long half-life and is given one

CHART 37-6

DRUG THERAPY for Cardiac Arrest

Drug	Usual Dosage	Nursing Interventions	Rationales
Epinephrine (Adrenalin)	1-mg IV bolus followed by 20-mL saline flush q3-5min	Monitor for return of rhythm and pulse when used for asystole or VF.	Return of rhythm and pulse is the expected response.
	If this fails, consider 2-5 mg IV bolus q3-5min; 1-mg, 3-mg, and 5-mg IV boluses (3 min apart); or 0.1 mg/kg IV bolus q3-5 min	Assess for tachycardia, dysrhythmias, or hypertension.	Adverse reactions can occur with a dramatic response.
		Assess for the development of coarse VF when given during the VF.	This may improve the response to defibrillation.
	If necessary give endotracheally with dose at least 2-2½ times the IV dose		
Amiodarone hydrochloride (Cordarone)	300 mg IV push for cardiac arrest in VF/pulseless VT	Monitor for return of rhythm and pulse when used for recurrent unstable VT or VF.	Return of rhythm and pulse is the expected response.
	150 mg IVP over 10 min (15 mg/min), followed by 360 mg IV over next 6 hr (1 mg/min), followed by 540 mg IV over next 18 hr (0.5 mg/min)	Use with extreme caution in clients receiving other antidysrhythmics.	Amiodarone reduces the hepatic and renal clearance of certain antiarrhythmics, specifically procainamide, quinidine, and flecainide.
	After first 24 hr, continue maintenance infusion of 720 mg/24 hr (0.5 mg/min)	Use caution in clients with pulmonary, hepatic, or thyroid disease.	Amiodarone can cause fatal toxicity, especially in clients receiving more than 600 mg daily.
		Perform continuous cardiac monitoring while the client is receiving the loading dose.	There is a slow onset of antiarrhythmic effect and a high risk of life-threatening arrhythmias.
Dopamine hydrochloride (Intropin)	2.5-5 mcg/kg/min IV infusion; titrate to desired clinical response	Assess clients for increased BP.	Increased BP is the expected response.
	1-2 mcg/kg/min for renal and mesenteric vasodilation	Monitor for tachycardia, dysrhythmias, or hypertension.	Adverse reactions may occur.
		Monitor IV site for infiltration.	Extravasation of drug can occur, causing necrosis.
	2-10 mcg/kg/min for beta-adrenergic effects 10-20 mcg/kg/min for alpha-adrenergic effects	Assess for urine output <30 mL/hr, pallor, cyanosis, pain, or numbness in the extremities.	Dosages >10 mcg/kg/min cause vasoconstriction of renal and peripheral blood vessels; dosages of 2-5 mcg/kg/min may improve urine output by causing renal vasodilation and improving renal blood flow.
Dobutamine hydrochloride (Dobutrex)	2-20 mcg/kg/min IV infusion	Assess for increased BP.	Increased BP is the expected response.
		Assess for hypertension and dysrhythmias.	Adverse reactions may occur.
Norepinephrine (Levophed)	0.5-1 mcg/min IV infusion, titrate to desired effect, up to 8-30 mcg/min	Assess for increased BP.	Increased BP is the expected response.
		Monitor for bradycardia.	Reflex bradycardia may occur with a rise in BP.
		Monitor for hypertension and dysrhythmias.	Adverse reactions may occur with a dramatic response.
		Administer drug through central IV line.	Extravasation can occur.
		Assess for urine output <30 mL/hr, pallor, cyanosis, pain, or numbness in the extremities.	Norepinephrine is a powerful vasoconstrictor.
		Assess for chest pain after resuscitation.	Norepinephrine increases myocardial oxygen demand.

VF, Ventricular fibrillation; *VT*, ventricular tachycardia.

Continued

CHART 37-6

DRUG THERAPY for Cardiac Arrest—*cont'd*

Drug	Usual Dosage	Nursing Interventions	Rationales
Sodium bicarbonate	1 mEq/kg IV bolus given after the first 10 min of cardiac arrest if necessary 0.5 mEq/kg IV bolus q10min thereafter if necessary	Assess arterial blood gas values for metabolic acidosis.	Administration without evidence of metabolic acidosis can result in alkalosis, which can hinder resuscitation efforts.
Isoproterenol (Isuprel)	2-10 mcg/min IV infusion; titrate to desired clinical response	Assess for increased heart rate.	Increased heart rate is the expected response.
		Assess for tachycardia, hypotension, or hypertension.	Adverse reactions may occur with a dramatic response.
		Assess for chest pain after resuscitation.	Isoproterenol increases myocardial oxygen demand.
		Monitor for ventricular dysrhythmias.	Isoproterenol increases ventricular irritability, especially in clients who are hypokalemic or who are receiving digitalis.
Calcium chloride ($CaCl_2$)	2-4 mg/kg IV slowly; may repeat q10min if necessary	Calcium chloride is indicated only for cardiac arrest associated with hyperkalemia, hypocalcemia, or calcium channel blocker toxicity.	Calcium chloride may cause cellular damage and cerebrovascular spasm.
Vasopressin	40 units IV bolus, one time	Monitor for return of rhythm and pulse when used for VF or pulseless VT.	Return of rhythm and pulse is the expected response.

VF, Ventricular fibrillation; *VT*, ventricular tachycardia.

time as an intravenous (IV) bolus of 40 units. Dopamine hydrochloride (Intropin) is generally used for its beta-adrenergic effects after cardiac arrest but may be used for its alpha-adrenergic effects during resuscitation. Dobutamine hydrochloride (Dobutrex) is a beta-adrenergic agent used to improve myocardial contractility and increase cardiac output.

Norepinephrine (Levophed) or phenylephrine hydrochloride (Neo-Synephrine) may be used for their alpha-adrenergic effects to increase vasomotor tone and increase perfusion pressure. Sodium bicarbonate, along with regular insulin and calcium chloride, is administered during cardiac arrest for clients who are hyperkalemic. It may also be used, if necessary, to treat a documented bicarbonate metabolic acidosis, as occurs in diabetic ketoacidosis or tricyclic antidepressant overdose. In addition to hyperkalemia, calcium chloride is given for hypocalcemia or calcium channel blocker toxicity because it may cause cell damage and cerebrovascular vasospasm. Isoproterenol (Isuprel) is indicated to increase the heart rate in heart transplant clients, but pacing is preferred.

Vagal Maneuvers. **Vagal maneuvers** induce vagal stimulation of the cardiac conduction system, specifically the SA and AV nodes. Vagal maneuvers may be attempted to terminate supraventricular tachydysrhythmias and include **carotid sinus massage** and **Valsalva maneuvers.** The results of these interventions, however, are often temporary and further therapy must be initiated.

Carotid Sinus Massage. The physician massages over one carotid artery for a few seconds, observing for a change in cardiac rhythm. Massaging the carotid sinus causes vagal stimulation, slowing SA and AV nodal conduction. Prepare the client for the procedure, instruct him or her to turn the head slightly away from the side to be massaged, and observe the cardiac monitor for a change in rhythm. An electrocardiographic (ECG) rhythm strip is recorded before, during, and after the procedure. After the procedure, assess vital signs and the level of consciousness. Complications include bradydysrhythmias, asystole, VF, and cerebral damage. Because of these risks, carotid massage is *not* commonly performed. A defibrillator and resuscitative equipment must be immediately available during the procedure.

Valsalva Maneuvers. To stimulate a vagal reflex, the health care provider instructs the client to bear down as if straining to have a bowel movement. Prepare the client for the procedure, assess the heart rate, heart rhythm, and blood pressure; observe the cardiac monitor; and record an ECG rhythm strip before, during, and after the procedure to determine the effect of therapy.

Unintended vagal stimulation sometimes occurs, and the nurse must be cautious when performing procedures that may inadvertently cause vagal stimulation. For example, tracheal suctioning, enema administration, and rectal temperature checks can stimulate the vagus nerve and decrease the heart rate inappropriately. Instruct the client not to strain during bowel movements and to avoid constipation through proper diet and exercise. Stool softeners may be prescribed. Instruct the client to avoid inducing gagging during oral hygiene, which triggers a vagal response. Monitor the heart rate and rhythm of a client who is vomiting because a vagal reflex can result. Some clients experience a vagal response when raising their arms above their head and must be instructed to avoid this movement.

Temporary Pacing. **Temporary pacing** is a nonsurgical intervention that provides a timed electrical stimulus to the heart when either the impulse initiation or the intrinsic conduction system of the heart is defective. The electrical stimulus then spreads throughout the heart to depo-

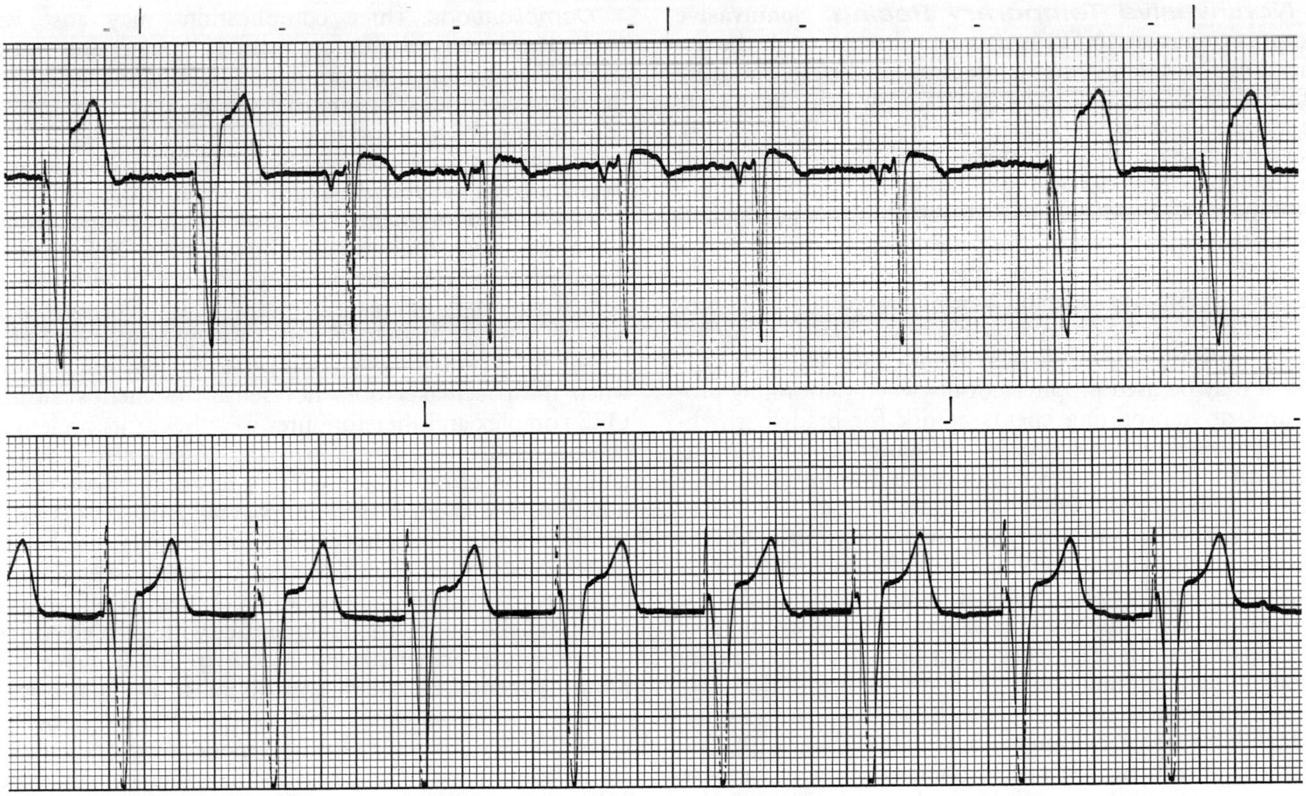

Figure 37-18 ■ Modes of pacing. **A,** Synchronous (demand) ventricular pacing. **B,** Asynchronous (fixed-rate) ventricular pacing at a rate of 70 beats/min.

larize the cells, which should be followed by contraction and cardiac output. Electrical stimuli may be delivered to the right atrium or right ventricle (single-chamber pacemakers) or to both (dual-chamber pacemakers).

When a pacing stimulus is delivered to the heart, a spike (or pacemaker artifact) is seen on the monitor or ECG strip. The spike should be followed by evidence of depolarization (i.e., a P wave, indicating atrial depolarization, or a QRS complex, indicating ventricular depolarization). This pattern is referred to as *capture,* indicating that the pacemaker has successfully depolarized, or captured, the chamber.

Temporary pacing is generally initiated in clients with symptomatic, atropine-refractory bradydysrhythmias, particularly second-degree heart block type II and third-degree heart block, or in clients with asystole. Temporary pacing may also be initiated prophylactically in hemodynamically stable clients with left bundle branch block in certain situations, such as insertion of a pulmonary artery catheter.

A different type of pacing may be used to terminate symptomatic tachydysrhythmias. Occasionally **atrial overdrive pacing** is attempted to terminate atrial tachydysrhythmias, such as atrial flutter or atrial fibrillation (AF). Overdrive pacing is accomplished by rapidly pacing the atrium to capture the heart and control depolarization, followed by no pacing, in the hope that the sinus node will regain control of the heart. Ventricular overdrive pacing may be done to terminate ventricular tachydysrhythmias in much the same way. Overdrive pacing is usually performed by the physician or advanced practice nurse who is specially trained. Have emergency equipment available in case the client becomes more unstable or goes into cardiac arrest.

Modes of Pacing. The two basic modes of pacing are synchronous (demand) pacing and asynchronous (fixed-rate) pacing.

Synchronous Pacing. Temporary pacing is most commonly done in the **synchronous (demand) mode.** The pacemaker's sensitivity is set to sense the client's own beats. When the client's intrinsic rate is above the rate set on the pulse generator, the pacemaker is inhibited from firing. When the client's rate is below that set on the generator, the pacemaker fires electrical impulses to stimulate depolarization (Figure 37-18, *A*).

Asynchronous Pacing. The **asynchronous (fixed-rate) mode** is used when the client is asystolic or profoundly bradycardic, as may occur after open-heart surgery. When the pulse generator is set in an asynchronous mode, it does not sense any intrinsic beats of the client. The pacemaker continues to fire at a fixed rate as set on the generator, regardless of the intrinsic rhythm. This continued firing is not a problem as long as the client remains asystolic or has a rate slower than the pacemaker rate because all beats come from the pacemaker and there is no competition from the client's beats (Figure 37-18, *B*). If the client's rate increases and equals or exceeds the pacemaker rate, however, competition (undersensing) is noted. The danger is that a pacemaker stimulus may reach the heart during the vulnerable period of repolarization (R-on-T phenomenon, with the pacer spike falling on the T wave) and possibly induce ventricular fibrillation (VF). Observe for pacemaker competition, and set the pacemaker to a synchronous mode to avert potential problems.

The two basic types of temporary pacing are noninvasive (external) temporary pacing and invasive temporary pacing.

Noninvasive Temporary Pacing. **Noninvasive temporary pacing (NTP)** is accomplished through the application of two large external electrodes. The electrodes are attached to an external pulse generator, which can operate on alternating current (AC) or battery power (Figure 37-19). The generator emits electrical pulses, which are transmitted through the electrodes and then transcutaneously to stimulate ventricular depolarization when the client's heart rate is slower than the rate set on the pacemaker.

Noninvasive temporary pacing is used as an emergency measure to provide demand ventricular pacing in a profoundly bradycardic or asystolic client until invasive pacing can be instituted or the client's intrinsic rate returns to normal. It may be used prophylactically when performing procedures or transporting clients at risk for bradydysrhythmias. However, it is used only as a temporary measure to maintain heart rate and perfusion until a more permanent method of pacing is used.

Procedure. In a nonemergent situation, explain NTP to the client and prepare the equipment. Wash the skin with soap and water. To prevent skin abrasion, the skin must not be shaved. Do not rub the skin or apply alcohol or tinctures on the skin because electrical current flows from the patches through the skin and causes discomfort. Apply the large posterior electrode on the client's back, between the spine and the left scapula, behind the heart (see Figure 37-19). The electrode should not be placed higher over bone because bone is a poor conductor of electrical current. The anterior electrode is then applied on the chest, between the V_2 and the V_5 positions, over the heart. The electrode cannot be placed over female breast tissue. Displace the breast tissue to position the electrode underneath the breast.

Set the pacing rate as ordered, and establish the stimulation threshold, the lowest current that achieves capture with each pacing spike followed by a QRS complex. The QRS complex is wide because one ventricle depolarizes first, followed by the other. The electrical current is then set 10% above threshold levels.

Palpate the right radial or carotid pulse, and assess the blood pressure using the client's right arm, ensuring that each paced beat is perfused. Vital signs are not taken on the left side of the body because they may not be accurate, particularly if a high milliamperage is used.

Complications. Three complications may arise with NTP. The first is discomfort from cutaneous and muscle stimulation and skin irritation as well as diaphoresis from the patch electrodes. Ensure that the electrodes are in good contact with the skin and in the best location to achieve the lowest threshold for consistent capture. Analgesics or sedatives are given as prescribed to provide comfort.

The second problem is loss of capture, which occurs when the pacing spike is not followed by a QRS complex. Ensure that the electrodes are in good contact with the skin and, if necessary, increase the current until capture is regained; however, higher currents cause more discomfort.

The third problem is inappropriate pacing, which occurs when the pacemaker does not sense the client's intrinsic QRS complex and therefore fires impulses at its preset rate, competing with the client's rhythm. Assess electrode contact and the effect of the client's position on pacemaker function. The client may need to avoid lying on his or her left side. If diaphoresis has caused poor contact and the electrodes must be replaced, first turn the pacemaker function off to avoid receiving electrical shocks when touching the gel side of the electrodes. Then replace with fresh electrodes.

Invasive Temporary Pacing. An **invasive temporary pacemaker** system consists of an external battery-operated pulse generator and pacing electrodes, or lead wires. These wires attach to the generator on one end and are in contact with the heart on the other end. Electrical pulses, or stimuli, are emitted from the negative terminal of the generator, flow through a lead wire, and stimulate the cardiac cells to depolarize. The current seeks ground by returning through the other lead wire to the positive terminal of the generator, thus completing a circuitous route. The intensity of electrical current is set by selecting the appropriate current output, measured in milliamperes.

The client does not usually feel invasive pacemaker stimuli; however, clients occasionally feel an uncomfortable sensation from the stimuli if strong electrical currents (high milliamperage) are delivered by the pacemaker. The discomfort may be alleviated by decreasing the current if possible.

Complications. Complications of invasive temporary pacing may be serious and include the following:

- Infection or hematoma at the pacemaker wire insertion site

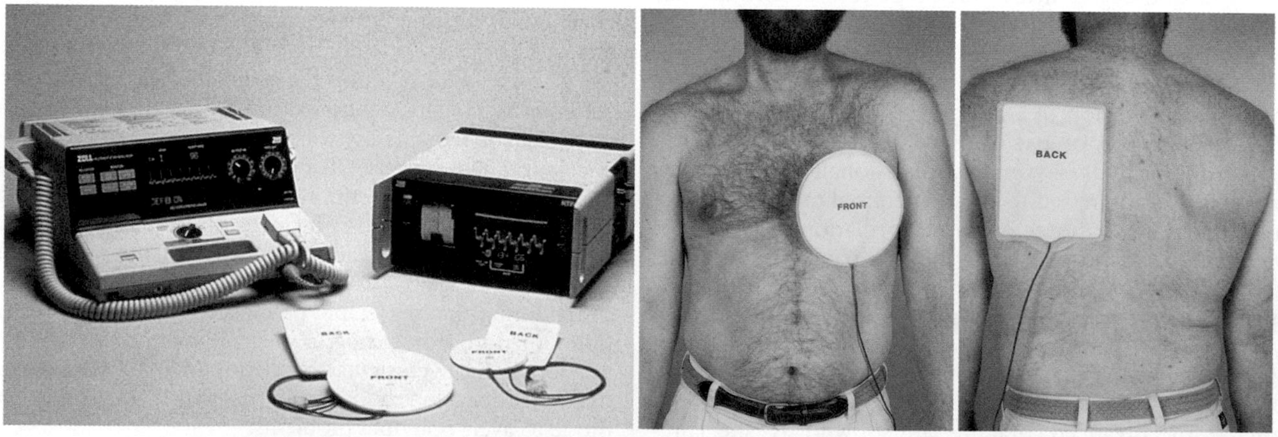

Figure 37-19 ■ Equipment and electrode placement for transcutaneous external pacing. (Courtesy Zoll Medical Corporation, Burlington, MA.)

- Ectopic complexes (usually premature ventricular complexes [PVCs]) caused by irritability from the pacing wire in the ventricle, use of high current, or undersensing with pacemaker competition
- Loss of capture, noted by the presence of a pacing stimulus or spike but no QRS complex
- Undersensing or pacemaker competition, noted when pacing stimuli occur at a fixed rate in the presence of an adequate intrinsic rhythm
- Oversensing, noted when the pacemaker fails to fire in the presence of an inadequate intrinsic rhythm
- Electromagnetic interference, noted by altered generator variables
- Stimulation of the chest wall or diaphragm, noted by rhythmic contraction of the chest-wall muscles or hiccups with the use of high current or from lead wire perforation, which could cause cardiac tamponade

Prevention of Microshock. When the metal external ends of lead wires are not attached to a pulse generator, insulate the wire ends to prevent microshock. The fingertips of rubber gloves work well for this purpose, and the wire ends may then be looped and covered with nonconductive tape. All electrical equipment in the room must be properly grounded using a three-pronged plug. Report faulty electrical equipment, such as frayed or broken electrical wires, to the biomedical engineering department. Neither the client nor the bed should be in contact with such equipment. The risk is that ungrounded electrical current may conduct through the lead wire, stimulate the heart, and induce ventricular fibrillation (VF). Remember to wear rubber gloves when touching any of the wires. Static electricity may be conducted from your hands to the client, causing dysrhythmias if gloves are not worn.

Cardiopulmonary Resuscitation. Management of the client in cardiac arrest depends on prompt recognition and therapeutic interventions for successful reversal of a potentially fatal event.

When cardiac arrest occurs, cardiac output ceases. The underlying rhythm is usually ventricular tachycardia (VT), ventricular fibrillation (VF), or asystole. In rare instances, cardiac arrest occurs in the presence of an organized electrocardiographic (ECG) rhythm but with no effectual mechanical response, a condition referred to as pulseless electrical activity (PEA). Without cardiac output, the client is pulseless and becomes unconscious because of inadequate cerebral perfusion. Shortly after cardiac arrest, respiratory arrest occurs.

Cardiopulmonary resuscitation (CPR) must be initiated immediately to help prevent brain damage and death. When finding an unresponsive client, confirm unresponsiveness and call 911 or the emergency response team before initiating CPR. The initial priorities are as follows:

- Maintenance of a patent airway
- Ventilation with a mouth-to-mask device
- Chest compressions

As soon as help arrives, a board is placed under the client who is not on a firm surface. To make room for the resuscitation team and the crash cart, the nurse commands that the area be cleared of movable items and unnecessary personnel.

Complications of CPR include rib fractures, fracture of the sternum, costochondral separation, lacerations of the liver and spleen, pneumothorax, hemothorax, cardiac tamponade, lung contusions, and fat emboli. The goal of resuscitation is the rapid return of a pulse, blood pressure, and consciousness. This is rarely achieved by CPR and basic measures alone. More definitive therapy must be initiated as soon as possible with advanced cardiac life support (ACLS) measures, including defibrillation, if warranted.

The goal is to be able to give a defibrillatory shock within 5 minutes of collapse outside of a hospital and within 3 minutes in a hospital. To help meet this goal, automated external defibrillators (AEDs) should be placed where there is a probability of at least one sudden cardiac arrest every 5 years, such as on airplanes.

Advanced Cardiac Life Support. When the crash cart arrives, apply ECG electrodes to the client's chest and turn on the monitor. Direct the team to continue CPR and continue to coordinate the personnel who respond to the emergency. If the client is found to be in VF or pulseless VT, the immediate priority is to defibrillate. Following defibrillation, CPR is resumed. An oropharyngeal airway is inserted to facilitate proper ventilation. A manual resuscitation bag (MRB) with mask is attached to an oxygen flowmeter set at 10 to 15 L/min. Direct the person managing the airway to ventilate the lungs with the MRB, maintaining the proper head-tilt, chin-lift position of the client. Initiate two large-bore IV lines if the client does not have any, infusing normal saline. These lines provide access for emergency drug administration. Suction equipment is also set up, with a tonsillar suction tube for suctioning vomitus and a suction catheter for endotracheal suctioning. Carotid or femoral pulse checks with or without chest compressions, blood pressure measurements, and pupil assessments are done at frequent intervals. Document all assessments and findings, therapeutic measures, and the client's responses throughout the resuscitation.

Additional measures include endotracheal intubation with ventilation and oxygenation, IV administration of emergency cardiac drugs, and occasionally external pacing. Chest compressions are continued as long as the client remains pulseless or until a physician decides to terminate resuscitation attempts.

Cardioversion. **Cardioversion** is a synchronized countershock that may be performed in emergencies for hemodynamically unstable ventricular or supraventricular tachydysrhythmias or electively for stable tachydysrhythmias that are resistant to medical therapies. If the client has been taking digitalis, the drug is withheld for up to 48 hours preceding an elective cardioversion, as prescribed. Digitalis increases ventricular irritability and puts the client at risk for VF after the countershock. For elective cardioversion for atrial flutter or fibrillation, the client must take anticoagulants for 4 to 6 weeks before the procedure to prevent embolization of clots from the heart to the brain or lungs.

The shock depolarizes a critical mass of myocardium simultaneously during intrinsic depolarization. It is intended to stop the re-entry circuit and allow the sinus node to regain control of the heart. Emergency equipment must be available during the procedure. The physician, advance practice nurse (e.g., nurse practitioner), or other qualified nurse explains the procedure to the client and assists him or her in signing a consent form unless the procedure is an emergency for a life-threatening dysrhythmia. Because the client is usually conscious, an anesthesiologist may administer a short-acting anesthetic agent as IV sedation.

The defibrillator should be set in the synchronized mode. This avoids discharging the shock during the vulnerable period (T wave), which may increase ventricular irritability, causing ventricular fibrillation (VF). Charge the defibrillator to the energy level requested, usually starting at a low rate. Ensure that the oxygen delivery device has been removed and turned away from the client. Oxygen supports combustion, and a fire may result if there is arcing from the paddles. One paddle is placed to the left of the precordium, and the other is placed on the right next to the sternum and just below the clavicle. Arcing is usually due to improper paddle contact on the chest. At least 25 pounds of pressure should be applied to each paddle to prevent arcing.

The health care provider loudly and clearly commands all personnel to clear contact with the client and the bed, as required for electrical safety. Ensure compliance of all personnel before delivering the shock. The buttons on the paddles are held down until a shock is delivered. There may be a short period before the energy is delivered while the defibrillator is synchronizing with the client's cardiac rhythm.

Another method of delivering synchronized cardioversion is known as the "hands off" method. Special patches are placed on the front and back of the client's thorax or upper right sternal area to deliver the shock. This procedure provides additional safety for the client as well as for the health care personnel.

After cardioversion, assess the client's response and heart rhythm. Therapy is repeated as ordered, if necessary, until the desired result is obtained or alternative therapies are considered. If the client's condition deteriorates into VF after cardioversion, ensure that the synchronizer is turned off so that immediate defibrillation can be administered. Most defibrillators have a dial to turn between synchronous and asynchronous modes.

Nursing care after cardioversion includes the following:

- Maintaining a patent airway
- Administering oxygen
- Assessing vital signs and the level of consciousness
- Administering antidysrhythmic drug therapy
- Monitoring for dysrhythmias
- Assessing for chest burns from paddle edges that may not have been on the conductive pad
- Providing emotional support
- Documenting the results of cardioversion

Defibrillation. **Defibrillation,** an asynchronous countershock, depolarizes a critical mass of myocardium simultaneously to stop the re-entry circuit, allowing the sinus node to regain control of the heart. Early defibrillation is critical in terminating pulseless VT or VF. It must not be delayed for any reason after the equipment and skilled personnel are present. The earlier defibrillation is performed, the greater the chance of survival.

If a defibrillator is not immediately available, an ACLS-qualified nurse may deliver a precordial thump to a pulseless client in VF. There is a slight chance that it may succeed in terminating the VF. A **precordial thump** is performed by striking the lower half of the sternum with a closed fist from a height of 8 to 12 inches (12 to 30 cm) above the sternum. If the client remains in VF, CPR is resumed and the nurse prepares for defibrillation. The defibrillator is charged to 200 Joules, 300 Joules, and 360 Joules for three successive countershocks on a monophasic defibrillator. More effective biphasic defibrillators that allow a lower DC shock and cause less damage to the myocardium are available in some facilities. Before defibrillation, loudly and clearly command all personnel to clear contact with the client and the bed, and ensure their compliance before delivering the shock. Depress the shock buttons on the defibrillator, and the energy is immediately released (see Figure 37-19). Repeat up to three times as needed for VF or pulseless VT. Then continue with the ACLS protocol. Nursing care for defibrillation is the same as for cardioversion.

Automatic External Defibrillation. The American Heart Association promotes the use of automatic external defibrillators (AEDs) for use by laypersons and health care providers responding to cardiac arrest emergencies. These devices are now found in public places such as malls and commercial jets. The client in cardiac arrest must be on a firm, dry surface. The rescuer places two large adhesive-patch electrodes on the client's chest in the same positions as for defibrillator paddles. The rescuer stops CPR and commands anyone present to move away, ensuring that no one is touching the client. This measure eliminates motion artifact when the machine analyzes the rhythm. The rescuer presses the "analyze" button on the machine. After rhythm analysis, which may take up to 30 seconds, the machine either advises that a shock is necessary or advises that a shock is not indicated. Shocks are recommended for VF or pulseless VT only.

After issuing a command to clear all contact with the client, the rescuer charges the defibrillator and presses both discharge buttons on the machine simultaneously, delivering the first shock at 200 Joules. The shock is delivered through the patches, so it is hands-off defibrillation, which is safer for the rescuer. The rescuer then presses the analyze button again, repeating the sequence. With sustained VF or VT, two more shocks may be delivered, with the third at 360 Joules. If the client remains in cardiac arrest, CPR is performed for 1 minute, and then another series of three shocks may be delivered, each at 360 Joules. It is imperative that ACLS be provided as soon as possible. Use of automatic external defibrillators (AEDs) results in earlier defibrillation of clients and therefore a greater chance of successful rhythm conversion and survival.

Critical Thinking Challenge

On the medical-surgical unit, there is a loud crash in the visitors lounge. You find a middle-aged visitor who is pulseless and without respiration on the floor.

1. What should you do first?
2. What actions will the cardiac arrest team take?
3. What cardiac rhythms could be present when the monitor is attached?
4. What treatment modalities should be anticipated for each possible rhythm?

evolve For suggested answer guidelines, go to http://evolve.elsevier.com/Iggy/.

Radiofrequency Catheter Ablation. **Radiofrequency catheter ablation** is an invasive procedure that may be used to abolish an irritable focus causing a supraventricular or ventricular tachydysrhythmia. The client must first undergo electrophysiologic studies and mapping procedures to locate the focus. Then radiofrequency waves are delivered to abolish the irritable focus. When ablation is performed in the AV nodal or His bundle area, damage may also occur to the normal conduction system, causing heart blocks and requiring implantation of a permanent pacemaker.

SURGICAL MANAGEMENT. Clients who experience life-threatening dysrhythmias may require surgical treatment for long-term management. The type of treatment depends on the nature of the dysrhythmia. Procedures include permanent pacing, coronary artery bypass grafting (CABG), aneurysmectomy, insertion of an implantable cardioverter/defibrillator, and open-chest cardiac massage.

Permanent Pacing. Permanent pacemaker insertion is performed for the resolution of conduction disorders that are not temporary, including complete heart block and sick sinus syndrome. Permanent pacemakers are usually powered by a lithium battery and have an average life span of 10 years. After the battery power is depleted, the generator must be replaced, a procedure done with the client under local anesthesia. Some pacemakers are nuclear powered and have a life span of 20 years or longer. Other pacemakers can be recharged externally.

A new type of pacemaker may be utilized to coordinate contractions between the right and left ventricles. In addition to pacing used in the right side of the heart, an additional lead is placed in the left lateral wall of the left ventricle through the coronary sinus. This procedure allows synchronized depolarization of the ventricles and is used in clients with moderate to severe heart failure to improve functional ability.

Surgical Procedures. The surgeon most commonly implants the pulse generator in a surgically made subcutaneous pocket at the shoulder in the right or left subclavicular area. The leads are introduced transvenously via the cephalic or the subclavian vein to the endocardium on the right side of the heart. After the procedure, the nurse monitors the client's electrocardiographic (ECG) rhythm to ensure that the pacemaker is functioning correctly. The implantation site is assessed for evidence of bleeding, swelling, redness, tenderness, or infection. The dressing over the site should remain clean and dry, and the client should be afebrile and have stable vital signs. The physician orders activity restrictions to enhance lead fixation. After 24 hours, activity is gradually increased. Complications of permanent pacemakers are similar to those for temporary invasive pacing.

Pacemaker checks are done on an ambulatory care basis at regular intervals. Reprogramming may be warranted if pacemaker problems develop. The pulse generator is interrogated using an electronic device to determine the pacemaker settings and battery life.

For clients who live far from the pacemaker clinic or physician's office, pacemaker information can be sent via transtelephonic transmission of data. The client attaches ECG electrodes to the wrists and places the telephone receiver in a transmitting unit. The sound signals are relayed via telephone lines to the clinic or office, where they are converted and recorded as the client's ECG rhythm strip and information about the pacemaker variables. The nurse stresses the need to keep clinic appointments for more detailed pacemaker checks and reprogramming, if necessary, as well as assessment.

Critical Thinking Challenge

Your client recently admitted from the ED with chest pain complains of nausea and suddenly develops third-degree heart block. The physician orders external cardiac pacing.

1. How should you prepare the client for this procedure?
2. How should the external pacer pads be applied?

External pacemaking fails, and the physician tells you to prepare for insertion of a temporary pacemaker.

3. What is the difference between a temporary pacemaker and external cardiac pacing?
4. What health teaching should you do in preparation for this treatment modality?

evolve For suggested answer guidelines, go to http://evolve.elsevier.com/Iggy/.

Coronary Artery Bypass Grafting. Coronary artery bypass grafting (CABG) is performed if the cause of the dysrhythmia is coronary artery insufficiency that is unresponsive to medical therapy. This procedure is described in Chapter 41.

Aneurysmectomy. Ventricular aneurysms are a complication of myocardial infarction (MI) and may be the source of intractable ventricular tachydysrhythmias. The surgeon resects the aneurysm, a dyskinetic or ballooning portion of the ventricular wall. Resection of the area eliminates the dangerous irritable focus and thus the cause of the dysrhythmias. Care of the client is similar to that for CABG, described in Chapter 41.

Insertion of Implantable Cardioverter/Defibrillator. The implantable cardioverter/defibrillator (ICD) is indicated for clients who have experienced one or more episodes of spontaneous sustained ventricular tachycardia (VT) or ventricular fibrillation (VF) unrelated to a MI or other causes amenable to correction.

Clients undergo electrophysiologic studies to assess the inducibility of VTs and their response to medication. If the dysrhythmias can be induced despite medical therapy, the client is considered a candidate for ICD implantation. Collaborate with the physician and the electrophysiology nurse to prepare the client for an ICD. A psychological profile is done to determine whether the client will be able to cope with the discomfort and fear associated with internal defibrillation from the ICD.

The leads are introduced percutaneously, and the generator is implanted in the left pectoral area, similar to a permanent pacemaker insertion procedure. This procedure is performed in the electrophysiology laboratory.

If the ICD therapies are not successful and the client remains in VF or pulseless VT, the qualified nurse or health care provider must promptly externally defibrillate the client.

The generator may be activated or deactivated by the physician's placing a magnet over the implantation site for a few moments. The client requires close monitoring in the postimplantation period for the occurrence of dysrhythmias and complications such as bleeding and cardiac tamponade. The nurse must know whether the ICD is activated or deactivated. Care of the client is similar to that following implantation of a permanent pacemaker.

Open-Chest Cardiac Massage. When external chest compressions and advanced cardiac life support measures are unsuccessful in resuscitating a client in cardiac arrest, the physician may decide whether to perform open-chest cardiac massage through a thoracotomy approach or through the median sternotomy incision in post–cardiac surgery clients. Internal defibrillation may also be performed. Open-chest cardiac massage is usually reserved for the client who goes into cardiac arrest during cardiac surgery, often because of cardiac tamponade. It may also be beneficial but is rarely indicated for hypothermia, crushing or penetrating chest injuries, penetrating abdominal trauma, or chest deformities prohibiting external chest compressions. This procedure is a drastic measure that frequently results in devastating consequences for the client.

Critical Thinking Challenge

The physician is performing an elective cardioversion on a client with symptomatic atrial flutter. Suddenly you note the cardiac rhythm on the monitor changes to ventricular fibrillation.

1. What electrical procedure should be used for ventricular fibrillation?
2. What is the difference between defibrillation and synchronized cardioversion?
3. What is the procedure for cardioversion/defibrillation, and what safety precautions should be used?

evolve For suggested answer guidelines, go to http://evolve.elsevier.com/Iggy/.

Community-Based Care

For many clients, dysrhythmias are a chronic disorder resulting from chronic cardiac and pulmonary diseases. Clients may be cared for in a variety of settings, including the acute care hospital, subacute unit, traditional nursing home, or their own home. They are admitted to the hospital when they experience life-threatening or potentially life-threatening dysrhythmias, often associated with an acute disorder. Others can be managed with office or clinic visits or in other settings.

HOME CARE MANAGEMENT

Clients discharged from the hospital may have considerable needs, often more related to their underlying chronic diseases than to their dysrhythmias, which should be essentially controlled by drug or device therapy. A case manager or care coordinator can assess the need for health care resources and coordinate access to services.

The focus of the home care nurse's interventions is assessment and health teaching. Clients and families often fear recurrence of a life-threatening dysrhythmia. Clients with an ICD may dread or fear the activation of the ICD. The community-based nurse provides the client and family members with an opportunity to verbalize their concerns and fears. Provide emotional support as well as information about support groups in the community, and make appropriate referrals. Assess the client for possible side effects of antidysrhythmic agents or complications from a pacemaker or ICD.

HEALTH TEACHING

PREVENTION OF RECURRENCE. Clients who have experienced a dysrhythmia associated with an acute disorder, such as electrolyte imbalance or ischemia related to an MI, are instructed in the prevention, early recognition, and management of that disorder. Teach the client and family about lifestyle modifications designed to prevent, decrease, or control the occurrence of dysrhythmias, as outlined in Chart 37-7. This teaching may be provided in the acute care setting, physician's office, health care clinic, or home setting.

CHART 37-7

CLIENT EDUCATION GUIDE
How to Prevent or Decrease Dysrhythmias

For Clients at Risk for Vasovagal Attacks Causing Bradydysrhythmias
- Avoid doing things that stimulate the vagus nerve, such as raising your arms above your head, applying pressure over your carotid artery, applying pressure on your eyes, bearing down or straining during a bowel movement, and stimulating a gag reflex when brushing your teeth or putting objects in your mouth.

For Clients with Premature Beats and Ectopic Rhythms
- Take the medications that have been prescribed for you, and report any adverse effects to your physician.
- Stop smoking, avoid caffeinated beverages as much as possible, and drink alcohol only in moderation.
- Learn ways to manage stress and avoid getting too tired.

For Clients with Ischemic Heart Disease
- If you have an angina attack, treat it promptly with rest and nitroglycerin administration as prescribed by your physician. This decreases your chances of experiencing a dysrhythmia.
- If chest pain is not relieved after taking the amount of nitroglycerin that has been prescribed for you, seek medical attention promptly. Also, seek prompt medical attention if the pain becomes more severe or you experience other symptoms, such as sweating, nausea, weakness, and palpitations.

For Clients at Risk for Potassium Imbalance
- Know the symptoms of decreased potassium levels, such as muscle weakness and cardiac irregularity.
- Eat foods high in potassium, such as tomatoes, beans, prunes, avocados, bananas, strawberries, and lettuce.
- Take the potassium supplements that have been prescribed for you.

DRUG THERAPY. Clients and designated caregivers must have a thorough understanding of the prescribed medications, including antidysrhythmic agents. Pharmacies provide written instructions with filled prescriptions. Teach clients and families the generic and trade names of their drugs as well as the drugs' purposes, using basic terms that are easily understood. Clear instructions regarding dosage schedules and common side effects are important (see Chart 37-3). Emphasize the importance of reporting these side effects and any dizziness, nausea, vomiting, chest discomfort, or shortness of breath to the health care provider. Chart 37-8 highlights special considerations for older adults receiving antidysrhythmic therapy.

PULSE CHECK. Teach all clients and their significant others or family members how to take a pulse. Instruct them to report any signs of a change in heart rhythm, such as a significant decrease in pulse rate, a rate greater than 100 beats/min, or increased rhythm irregularity.

PACEMAKER. Clients who have a permanent pacemaker are given written and verbal information about the type and settings of their pacemaker. They are taught to report any pulse rate lower than that set on the pacemaker. Review the proper care of the pacemaker insertion site and the importance of reporting any fever or any redness, swelling, or drainage at the pacemaker insertion site. If the surgical incision is near either shoulder, teach and demonstrate range-

CHART 37-8

NURSING FOCUS on the OLDER ADULT
Dysrhythmias

Older adults are at increased risk for dysrhythmias because of changes in their cardiac conduction system. The sinoatrial node has fewer pacemaker cells. There is a loss of fibers in the bundle branch system. Therefore older adults are at risk for sinus node dysfunction and may require pacemaker therapy. The most common dysrhythmias are premature atrial contractions, premature ventricular contractions, and atrial fibrillation. Dysrhythmias tend to be more serious in older clients because of underlying heart disease, causing cardiac decompensation. Consequently, blood flow to organs, which may already be decreased because of the aging process, is further compromised, leading to multisystem organ dysfunction. The following are special nursing considerations for the older client with dysrhythmias:

- Evaluate the client with dysrhythmias immediately for the presence of a life-threatening dysrhythmia or hemodynamic deterioration.
- Assess the client with a dysrhythmia for angina, hypotension, heart failure, and decreased cerebral and renal perfusion.
- Consider the following causes of dysrhythmias when taking the client's history: hypoxia, drug toxicity, electrolyte imbalances, heart failure, and myocardial ischemia or infarction.
- Assess the client's level of education, hearing, learning style, and ability to understand and recall instructions to determine the best approaches for teaching.
- Assess the client's ability to read written instructions.
- Teach the client the generic and trade names of prescribed antidysrhythmic drugs as well as their purposes, dosage, side effects, and special instructions for their use.
- Provide clear written instructions in basic language and easy-to-read print.
- Provide a written drug dosage schedule for the client, taking into account all the medications the client is taking and possible drug interactions.
- Assess the client for possible side effects or adverse reactions to drugs considering the client's age and health status.
- Teach the client to take his or her pulse and to report significant changes in heart rate or rhythm to the physician.
- Inform the client of available resources for blood pressure and pulse checks, such as blood pressure clinics, home health agencies, and cardiac rehabilitation programs.
- Instruct the client on the importance of keeping follow-up appointments with the physician and reporting symptoms promptly.
- Include the client's family members or significant other in all teaching whenever possible.
- Instruct the client to avoid drinking caffeinated beverages, to stop smoking, to drink alcohol only in moderation, and to follow his or her prescribed diet.

of-motion exercises to perform to prevent shoulder stiffness.

Clients with pacemakers are also instructed to keep handheld cellular phones at least 6 inches away from the generator, with the handset on the ear opposite the side of the generator. Teach them to avoid sources of strong electromagnetic fields, such as magnets and telecommunications transmitters. These may cause interference and could change the pacemaker settings, causing a malfunction. Magnetic resonance imaging (MRI) is contraindicated. Instruct clients to carry a pacemaker identification card and to wear a medical alert bracelet. Chart 37-9 outlines the major points for client and family teaching after the insertion of a permanent pacemaker.

IMPLANTABLE CARDIOVERTER/DEFIBRILLATOR. Clients with an implantable cardioverter/defibrillator (ICD) usually continue to receive antidysrhythmic drugs after discharge from the hospital. Provide clear instructions about the purposes of the medications, the dosage schedules, special instructions for taking the medications, and side effects that need to be reported. If clients experience an internal defibrillator shock, they must sit or lie down immediately and notify the physician. Some clients describe the experience of a shock as a quick thud or kick in the chest, whereas others relate severe pain similar to that of external defibrillation. Inform family members that they may feel an electrical shock if

CHART 37-9

CLIENT EDUCATION GUIDE
Permanent Pacemakers

- Follow the instructions for pacemaker site skin care that have been specifically prepared for you. Report any fever or redness, swelling, or drainage from the incision site to your physician.
- Keep your pacemaker identification card in your wallet, and wear a medical alert bracelet.
- Take your pulse for 1 full minute at the same time each day, and record the rate in your pacemaker diary. Take your pulse any time you feel symptoms of a possible pacemaker failure, and report your heart rate and symptoms to your physician.
- Know the rate at which your pacemaker is set and the basic functioning of your pacemaker. Know what rate changes to report to your physician.
- Do not apply pressure over your generator. Avoid tight clothing or belts.
- You may take baths or showers without concern for your pacemaker.
- Inform other physicians and dentists that you have a pacemaker. Certain tests they may wish to perform (such as magnetic resonance imaging) could affect or damage your pacemaker.
- Know the indications of battery failure for your pacemaker as you were instructed, and report these findings to your physician if they occur.
- Do not operate electrical appliances directly over your pacemaker site because this may cause your pacemaker to malfunction.
- Do not lean over electrical or gasoline engines or motors. Be sure that electrical appliances or motors are properly grounded.
- Avoid all transmitter towers for radio, television, and radar. Radio, television, other home appliances, and antennas do not pose a hazard.
- Be aware that antitheft devices in stores may cause temporary pacemaker malfunction. If symptoms develop, move away from the device.
- Inform airport personnel of your pacemaker before passing through a metal detector, and show them your pacemaker identification card. The metal in your pacemaker will trigger the alarm in the metal detector device.
- Stay away from any arc welding equipment.
- Be aware that it is safe to operate a microwave oven unless it does not have proper shielding (old microwave ovens) or is defective.
- Report any of the following symptoms to your physician if you experience them: difficulty breathing, dizziness, fainting, chest pain, weight gain, and prolonged hiccupping. If you have any of these symptoms, check your pulse rate and call your physician.
- If you feel symptoms when near any device, move 5 to 10 feet away from it and then check your pulse. Your pulse rate should return to normal.
- Keep all of your physician and pacemaker clinic appointments.
- Take all medications prescribed for you as instructed.
- Follow your prescribed diet.
- Follow instructions on restrictions on physical activity, such as no sudden, jerky movement for 8 weeks to allow the pacemaker to settle in place.

CHART 37-10

CLIENT EDUCATION GUIDE
Implantable Cardioverter/Defibrillator

- Follow the instructions for implantable cardioverter defibrillator (ICD) site skin care that have been specifically prepared for you.
- Report to your physician any fever or redness, swelling, soreness, or drainage from your incision site.
- Do not wear tight clothing or belts that could cause irritation over the ICD generator.
- Avoid activities that involve rough contact with the ICD implantation site.
- Keep your ICD identification card in your wallet and consider wearing a medical alert bracelet.
- Know the basic functioning of your ICD device and its rate cutoff as well as the number of consecutive shocks it can deliver.
- Avoid magnets directly over your ICD because they can inactivate the device. If beeping tones are coming from the ICD, move away from the electromagnetic field immediately (within 30 seconds) before the inactivation sequence is completed, and notify your physician.
- Inform all physicians and dentists caring for you that you have an ICD implanted because certain diagnostic tests and procedures must be avoided to prevent ICD malfunction. These include diathermy, electrocautery, and nuclear magnetic resonance tests.
- Avoid other sources of electromagnetic interference, such as devices emitting microwaves (not microwave ovens); transformers; radio, television, and radar transmitters; large electrical generators; metal detectors, including handheld security devices at airports; antitheft devices; arc welding equipment; and sources of 60-cycle (Hz) interference. Also avoid leaning directly over the alternator of a running motor of a car or boat.
- Report to your physician symptoms such as fainting, nausea, weakness, blackout, and rapid pulse rates.
- Take all medications prescribed for you as instructed.
- Follow instructions on restrictions on physical activity, such as not swimming, driving motor vehicles, or operating dangerous equipment.
- Follow your prescribed diet.
- Keep all physician and ICD clinic appointments.
- Sit or lie down immediately if you feel dizzy or faint to avoid falling if the ICD discharges.
- Postemergency telephone numbers.
- Know how to contact the local emergency medical services (EMS) systems in your community. Inform them in advance that you have an ICD so that they can be prepared if they need to respond to an emergency call for you.
- Know how to perform cough cardiopulmonary resuscitation (CPR) as instructed.
- Encourage family members to learn how to perform CPR. Family members should know that if they are touching you when the device discharges, they may feel a slight shock but that this is not harmful to them.
- Follow instructions on what to do if the ICD successfully discharges, after which you feel well. This may include maintaining a diary of the date, the time, activity preceding the shock, symptoms, the number of shocks delivered, and how you feel after the shock. The physician may wish to be notified each time the device discharges.
- Avoid strenuous activities that may cause your heart rate to meet or exceed the rate cutoff of your ICD because this causes the device to discharge inappropriately.
- Notify your physician if you are leaving town or are relocating for information regarding access to health care.

they are touching the client during delivery of the shock but that it is not harmful. Provide information about how to access the emergency medical services (EMS) system in the community. Recommend resources for the family to learn how to perform cardiopulmonary resuscitation (CPR).

Clients with an ICD are taught to avoid sources of strong electromagnetic fields, such as large electrical generators and radio or television transmitters. These may inhibit tachydysrhythmia detection and therapy or may cause inadvertent antitachycardial pacing or shocks. MRI is contraindicated for clients with ICDs. Handheld cellular phones must be at least 6 inches away from the generator, with the handset held to the ear opposite the side of the ICD. If the pulse generator emits a beeping sound or provides some other indicator, the client must move away from the area as quickly as possible to prevent deactivation of the device. The client with an ICD should carry an ICD identification card and wear a medical alert bracelet. Chart 37-10 highlights the important points for teaching clients and family members and significant others.

HEALTH CARE RESOURCES

The cardiac rehabilitation nurse typically provides written and oral information about dysrhythmias, antidysrhythmic drugs, pacemakers, and ICDs as well as information about cardiac exercise programs, educational programs, and support groups. The office or clinic nurse may also provide information about resources. Instruct the client on how to contact the local affiliate of the American Heart Association or the provincial affiliate of the Heart and Stroke Foundation in Canada for information about dysrhythmias, pacemakers, and CPR training.

Manufacturers of pacemakers and ICDs provide helpful booklets and videotapes to give clients and their families a better understanding of these therapies. Teach clients how to use transtelephonic systems for transmission of their rhythms to a clinic or health care provider's office. Stress the importance of keeping scheduled appointments for office visits with the cardiologist and pacemaker or ICD clinic. Instruct clients with an ICD to contact the local ambulance or paramedic services and emergency facilities to inform them that they have these devices implanted. The client and family are encouraged to attend pacemaker or ICD support groups.

Evaluation: Outcomes

Evaluate the care of the client with dysrhythmias on the basis of the identified nursing diagnoses and collaborative problems. The primary expected outcome is that the client will have adequacy of blood flow from the left ventricle to support systemic blood pressure. Specific indicators for these outcomes are listed for each nursing diagnosis under the Planning and Implementation section (see earlier).

GET READY for the NCLEX Examination!

KEY POINTS

Safe Effective Care Environment

- In collaboration with the health care team, assess clients at risk for dysrhythmias.
- Consult with other health care providers regarding a change in client status.
- Evaluate the effectiveness of medication administration and treatment modalities for clients with dysrhythmias.

- Utilize the correct procedure for electrical and client safety during use of a defibrillator for cardioversion/defibrillation.
- Use infection control precautions during resuscitation efforts for a client with a lethal dysrhythmia.

Health Promotion and Maintenance

- Teach clients with dysrhythmias the correct drug, dose, route, time, and side effects of prescribed medications, and to notify their physicians if adverse effects occur.
- Teach clients of all ages the importance of a balanced diet, regular exercise, caffeine limitation, and tobacco and alcohol cessation to prevent dysrhythmias.
- Teach family members cardiopulmonary resuscitation techniques to decrease their anxiety while living with a client with dysrhythmias.
- Teach clients the importance of adhering to their prescribed cardiac regimen, such as checking their pulse to ascertain pacemaker function.

Psychosocial Integrity

- Because dysrhythmias can be life threatening, assess clients' and family members' reactions to the diagnoses and their resources for coping.
- Allow the client opportunities to express feelings of anxiety and fear.
- Evaluate the effectiveness of clients/family members coping mechanisms with lifestyle changes associated with dysrhythmias.
- Provide age-appropriate care for clients with dysrhythmias.
- Explain emergency interventions to the client and family before performing them, if appropriate.
- Allow family members to be present during resuscitation efforts, if desired and allowed.

Physiological Integrity

- Assess clients with dysrhythmias for a decrease in cardiac output.
- Administer medications and evaluate/document their effectiveness.
- Monitor clients with dysrhythmias, including conducting a physical assessment and health history, as well as interpreting ECG rhythm strips. Report significant changes to the health care provider.
- Use Table 37-2 to provide appropriate interventions for clients with dysrhythmias.
- Identify and intervene in life-threatening situations by providing cardiopulmonary resuscitation, electrical therapy, or medication administration. Specifically, know the lethal rhythms of ventricular fibrillation, ventricular tachycardia without a pulse, and asystole.
- Use Charts 37-9 and 37-10 to educate clients with permanent pacemakers or ICDs.
- Evaluate the client's response to emergency interventions and recommend changes in treatment based on evaluation of his or her response.

ADDITIONAL STUDY RESOURCES

Go to your Student CD-ROM for Review Questions for the NCLEX Examination.

evolve Go to http://evolve.elsevier.com/Iggy/ for Integrated Management of Care Questions for the NCLEX Examination.

SELECTED BIBLIOGRAPHY

Ackley, B.J., & Ladwig, G.B. (2004). *Nursing diagnosis handbook. A guide to planning care* (6th ed.). St. Louis: Mosby.

Adams-Hamoda, M.G., et al. (2003). Factors to consider when analyzing 12-lead electrocardiograms for evidence of acute myocardial ischemia. *American Journal of Critical Care, 12*(1), 9-18.

American Heart Association. (2000). *2000 handbook of emergency cardiovascular care for healthcare providers.* Dallas, TX: American Heart Association.

American Heart Association. (2000). Guidelines 2000 for cardiopulmonary resuscitation and emergency cardiovascular care. *Circulation, 102*(8), 112-124.

American Heart Association. (2001). *ACLS provider manual.* Dallas, TX: American Heart Association.

American Heart Association. (2001). *Heart and stroke statistical update.* Dallas, TX: American Heart Association.

Beasley, B.M. (2003). *Understanding EKGs–a practical approach* (2nd ed.). Upper Saddle River, NJ: Prentice Hall.

Benson, L.M., & Powless, D. (2003). Dofetilide and atrial fibrillation. *American Journal of Nursing, 103*(2), 64AA-GG.

Bosen, D.M. (2002). Atrio-ventricular nodal reentry tachycardia. *Dimensions of Critical Care Nursing, 21*(4), 134-140.

Conover, M.B. (2003). *Understanding electrocardiography* (8th ed.). St. Louis: Mosby.

Doherty, J.U., Fuchs, S., & Tecce, M.A. (2000). Ventricular arrhythmias. *Geriatrics, 55*(8), 26-33.

Ehrat, K.S. (2002). *The art of EKG interpretation.* Dubuque, IA: Kendall/Hunt.

Eichhorn, D., et al. (2001). Family presence during invasive procedures and resuscitation: hearing the voice of the patient. *American Journal of Nursing, 101*(5), 48-55.

Ellis, K.M. (2002). *EKG plain and simple-from rhythm strips to 12-leads.* Upper Saddle River, NJ: Prentice Hall.

Futterman, L.G., & Lemberg, L. (2002). Ambulatory electrocardiographic monitoring: Use of the implantable loop recorder in the evaluation of syncope. *Journal of Cardiovascular Nursing, 16*(3), 24-33.

Geiter, H.B., Jr. (2004). Getting back to basics with permanent pacemakers, Part I. *Nursing 2004, 34*(10), 32cc1-32cc4.

Goodman, D. (2001). Automatic external defibrillation. *Medsurg Nursing, 10*(5), 251-255.

Gulanick, M., et al. (2003). *Nursing care plans: Nursing diagnosis and intervention* (5th ed.). St. Louis: Mosby.

Harris, J. (2002). Biphase defibrillation. *Emergency Nurse, 10*(7), 33-38.

Harvard Medical School. (2002). Delivering the shock of a lifetime. *Harvard Health Letter, 27*(11), 4.

Hebbar, A.K, & Hueston, W.J. (2002). Management of common arrhythmias: Part I. Supraventricular arrhythmias. *American Family Physician, 65*(12), 2479-2487.

Hebbar, A.K, & Hueston, W.J. (2002). Management of common arrhythmias: Part II. Ventricular arrhythmias and arrhythmias in special populations . *American Family Physician, 65*(12), 2491-2497.

Householder-Hughes, S.D. (2002). Advanced cardiac life support for the new millennium. *Journal of Cardiovascular Nursing, 16*(3), 9-23.

Josephson, L., & McMullen, M. (2003). Atrial fibrillation. Beyond irregularly irregular: Learn to recognize and manage atrial fibrillation in its various forms. *Critical Care Choices, Nursing 2003 (suppl), 33*(5), 4-10.

Madrid, P., & Sendelbach, S. (2001). Heart-smarter drugs for resuscitation. *American Journal of Nursing, May 2001 Suppl,* 42-44.

McCloskey, J.C., & Bulechek, G.M. (2000). *Nursing interventions classification (NIC)* (3rd ed.). St. Louis: Mosby.

McComb, J.M., & Camm, A.J. (2002). Primary prevention of sudden cardiac death using implantable cardioverter defibrillators. *British Medical Journal, 325*(7372), 1050-1051.

McConnell, E.A. (2002). Using an automated external defibrillator. *Nursing 2002, 32*(10), 18.

Myerburg, R.J., & Castellanos, A. (2002). Electrode positioning for cardioversion of atrial fibrillation. *The Lancet, 360,* 1263-1264.

Nacrelli, G., et al. (2000). Amiodarone: what have we learned from clinical trials? *Clinical Cardiology, 23,*73-82.

Newton, J.L. (2000). Action stat: Amiodarone overdose. *Nursing 2000, 30*(2), 33.

Pagana, K.D., & Pagana, T.J. (2003). *Mosby's diagnostic and laboratory test reference* (6th ed.). St. Louis: Mosby.

Paulus, K., et al. (2002). Anterior-posterior versus anterior-lateral electrode positions for cardioversion of atrial fibrillation: A randomised (sic) trial. *The Lancet, 360,* 1275-1279.

Rodriquez, I., et al. (2001). Drug-induced QT prolongation in women during the menstrual cycle. *Journal of the American Medical Association, 285*(10), 1322-1326.

Schott, R. (2002). Wearable defibrillator. *Journal of Cardiovascular Nursing, 16*(3), 44-52.

Schwertz, D.W. (2003). Forward. *Journal of Cardiovascular Nursing, 18*(1), 6-10.

Skidmore-Roth, L. (2003). *Mosby's nursing drug reference.* St. Louis: Mosby.

Squires, A. (2000). Critical care: Teaching patients about telemetry. *Nursing 2000, 30*(7), 32cc1-32cc4.

Stahl, M.A., & Richards, N.M. (2002). Ventricular assist devices: Developing and maintaining a training and competency program. *Journal of Cardiovascular Nursing, 16*(3), 34-43.

Swearingen, P.L. (2003). *Manual of medical-surgical nursing care. Nursing interventions and collaborative management* (5th ed.). St. Louis: Mosby.

Swearingen, P.L., & Keen, J.H. (2001). *Manual of critical care nursing. Nursing interventions and collaborative management* (4th ed.). St. Louis: Mosby.

Thaler, M.S. (2002). *The only EKG book you'll ever need* (4th ed.). Philadelphia: Lippincott, Williams & Wilkins.

Urden, L.D., Stacy, K.M., & Lough, M.E. (2002). *Thelan's critical care nursing: Diagnosis and management* (4th ed.). St. Louis: Mosby.

Urden, L.D., Stacy, K.M., & Lough, M.E. (2003). *Priorities in critical care nursing* (4th ed.). St. Louis: Mosby.

White, E. (2000). Patients with implantable cardioverter defibrillators: Transition to home. *Journal of Cardiovascular Nursing, 14*(3), 42-52.

White, M.M. (2002). Psychosocial impact of the implantable cardioverter defibrillator: Nursing implications. *Journal of Cardiovascular Nursing, 16*(3), 53-61.

Woods, A. (2001). Calling all pacemakers. *Nursing 2001, 31*(1), 46-47.

Wooten, J.M. (2002). Drug-induced arrhythmias. *RN, 65*(1), 37-44.

Yee, C.A., & Rozewicz, B. (2003). Getting to the heart of atrial fibrillation. *Nursing Management, 34*(9), 21-27.

CHAPTER 38

Interventions for Clients with Cardiac Problems

ELAINE BISHOP KENNEDY • DONNA D. IGNATAVICIUS

LEARNING OUTCOMES

After studying this chapter, you should be able to:

1. Explain the pathophysiology of heart failure.
2. Compare and contrast left-sided and right-sided heart failure.
3. Perform a comprehensive assessment of clients experiencing heart failure.
4. Identify common nursing diagnoses and collaborative problems for clients with heart failure.
5. Evaluate the effects of interventions for reducing preload and afterload.
6. Identify common drug therapies to improve cardiac output.
7. Describe special considerations for older adults with heart failure.
8. Discuss the prevention of complications for clients with heart failure.
9. Prioritize nursing care for clients experiencing heart failure.
10. Identify essential focused assessments used by the home care nurse for clients with heart failure.
11. Compare and contrast common valvular disorders.
12. Discuss surgical management for clients with valvular disease.
13. Develop a teaching/learning plan for clients with valvular disease.
14. Differentiate between common cardiac inflammations and infections–endocarditis, pericarditis, and rheumatic carditis.
15. Discuss the legal/ethical aspects related to heart transplantation, including resource management.

Go to your Student CD-ROM for Review Questions for the NCLEX Examination keyed to these Learning Outcomes.

Although most Americans do not consider heart disease an incurable illness, more people die of heart disease than from the next seven leading causes of death combined. ". . . About 250,000 people a year die of coronary heart disease (CHD) without being hospitalized. That's about half of all deaths from CHD–more than 680 Americans each day" (American Heart Association [AHA], 2003). These deaths are usually the result of heart failure. One in five clients who develop heart failure die within one year. Women have a poorer survival rate than men, with fewer than 15% of women surviving longer than 8 to 12 years.

Long-term survival of clients with heart disease depends on client compliance with therapy and a coordinated interdisciplinary approach to ensure the best management of the illness and the highest possible quality of life. Therefore, as described in Chapter 3, high-risk clients are often targeted for case management to coordinate their care through the health care continuum.

HEART FAILURE

Heart failure, sometimes referred to as **pump failure,** is a general term for the inadequacy of the heart to pump blood throughout the body. This deficit causes insufficient perfusion of body tissues with vital nutrients and oxygen. Heart failure results from a number of acute and chronic cardiovascular problems that are discussed elsewhere in this text.

PATHOPHYSIOLOGY

Types of Heart Failure

The following are the major types of heart failure:

- Left-sided heart failure
- Right-sided heart failure
- High-output failure

LEFT-SIDED HEART FAILURE

Because the two ventricles of the heart represent two separate pumping systems, it is possible for one to fail by itself for a short period. Most heart failure begins with failure of the left ventricle and progresses to failure of both ventricles. Typical causes of **left-sided heart (ventricular) failure** include hypertensive, coronary artery, and valvular disease involving the mitral or aortic valve. Decreased tissue perfusion from poor cardiac output and pulmonary congestion from increased pressure in the pulmonary vessels indicate left ventricular failure.

Left-sided heart failure was formerly referred to as **congestive heart failure (CHF);** it may be acute or chronic and mild to severe. CHF can be further divided into two subtypes: systolic heart failure and diastolic heart failure.

SYSTOLIC HEART FAILURE. **Systolic heart failure (systolic ventricular dysfunction)** results when the heart is unable to contract forcefully enough during systole to eject adequate amounts of blood into the circulation. Preload increases with decreased contractility, and afterload increases as a result of increased peripheral resistance (e.g., hypertension) (McCance & Huether, 2002). The **ejection fraction** (the percentage of blood ejected from the heart during systole) drops from a normal of 50% to 70% to below 40%. As the ejection fraction decreases, tissue perfusion diminishes and blood accumulates in the pulmonary vessels. Manifestations of systolic dysfunction may include symptoms of inadequate tissue perfusion or pulmonary and systemic congestion.

DIASTOLIC HEART FAILURE. In contrast, **diastolic heart failure (diastolic ventricular function)** occurs when the left ventricle is unable to relax adequately during diastole. Inadequate relaxation or "stiffening" prevents the ventricle from filling with sufficient blood to ensure an adequate cardiac output; however, the ejection fraction may remain near normal (Martin, 2003). Diastolic failure represents about 20% to 40% of all heart failure, primarily in older adults and in women following a myocardial infarction. Symptoms of diastolic failure are similar to those of systolic dysfunction.

RIGHT-SIDED HEART FAILURE

Right-sided heart (ventricular) failure may be caused by left ventricular failure, right ventricular myocardial infarction, or pulmonary hypertension. In right-sided heart failure, the right ventricle is unable to empty completely. Increased volume and pressure develop in the systemic veins, and systemic venous congestion develops with peripheral edema.

HIGH-OUTPUT FAILURE

High-output failure can occur when cardiac output remains normal or above normal, unlike left- and right-sided heart failure, which are typically low-output states. High-output failure is caused by increased metabolic needs or hyperkinetic conditions, such as septicemia (fever), anemia, and hyperthyroidism. This type of heart failure is not as common as other types.

Classifications of Heart Failure

Heart failure (HF) can be classified using two approaches: staging of the disease or functional classification.

DISEASE STAGING

Staging of the disease is centered on its risk, evolution, and progression in four stages. Stage A indicates a high risk for HF without any structural heart changes or disorders. In stage B, the client has a structural disorder but has not developed any symptoms of the disease. The client in stage C has a current or past history of HF with a structural disorder, and stage D indicates end-stage disease. The client with stage D illness requires ongoing, chronic support and treatments, including possible hospice care or heart transplantation (Artinian, 2003).

A more popular method for staging HF is the Killip Classification System, which is based on the heart's hemodynamic ability. Table 41-3 in Chapter 41 outlines this system.

FUNCTIONAL CLASSIFICATION

HF may also be categorized by its effect on the client's functional status. The client is categorized according to the relationship between symptoms and activity level. Class I and II are less severe. Class III and IV indicate severe limitations in activity level and functional ability. Table 36-2 in Chapter 36 summarizes the New York Heart Association (NYHA) categories.

Compensatory Mechanisms

When cardiac output is insufficient to meet the demands of the body, compensatory mechanisms operate to improve cardiac output (Figure 38-1). Although these mechanisms may initially increase cardiac output, they eventually have a damaging effect on pump function. Compensatory mechanisms include the following:

- Sympathetic nervous system stimulation
- Renin-angiotensin system (RAS) activation
- Other neurohumoral responses
- Myocardial hypertrophy

SYMPATHETIC NERVOUS SYSTEM STIMULATION

In heart failure (HF), stimulation of the sympathetic nervous system (i.e., increasing catecholamines) as a result of tissue hypoxia represents the most immediate compensatory mechanism. Stimulation of the adrenergic receptors causes an increase in heart rate (beta adrenergic) and blood pressure from vasoconstriction (alpha adrenergic).

Because cardiac output (CO) is the product of heart rate (HR) and stroke volume (SV)–CO = HR × SV)–an increase in HR results in an immediate *increase in cardiac output.* An increase in HR is limited in its ability to compensate for decreased CO. If HR becomes too rapid, diastolic filling time is limited and CO may start to decline. An increase in HR also significantly increases oxygen demand by the myocardium. If the heart is poorly perfused because of arteriosclerosis, HF may worsen.

Stroke volume (SV) is also *improved* by sympathetic stimulation. Sympathetic stimulation increases venous return to the

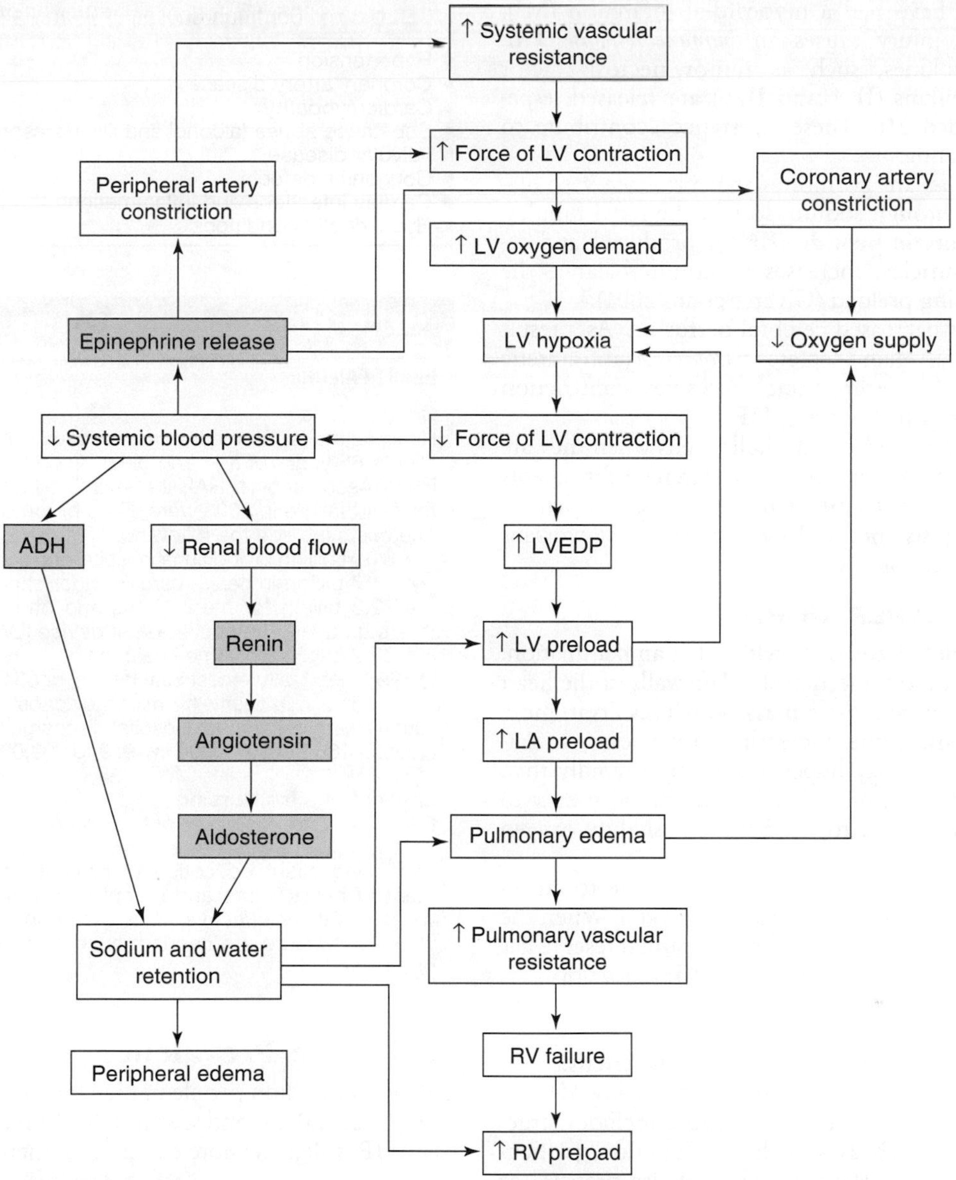

Figure 38-1 ■ Left-sided heart failure (congestive heart failure) from elevated systemic vascular resistance. Left heart failure leads to right heart failure. Systemic vascular resistance and preload are exacerbated by renal and adrenal mechanisms. *LV,* Left ventricular; *LVEDP,* left ventricular end-diastolic pressure; *LA,* left atrial; *ADH,* antidiuretic hormone; *RV,* right ventricular.

heart, which further stretches the myocardial fibers, causing dilation. In accordance with Starling's law of the heart, increased myocardial stretch results in more forceful contraction. More forceful contractions increase SV and CO. After a critical point is reached within the cardiac muscle, further volume and stretch will reduce the force of contraction and CO.

Sympathetic stimulation also results in *arterial vasoconstriction.* Constriction of the arteries has the benefit of maintaining blood pressure and improving tissue perfusion in low-output states; however, constriction of the arteries increases **afterload,** the resistance against which the heart must pump. Afterload is the major determinant of myocardial oxygen requirements. As afterload increases, the left ventricle requires more energy to eject its contents, and SV may decline.

RENIN-ANGIOTENSIN SYSTEM ACTIVATION

Reduced blood flow to the kidneys, a common occurrence in low-output states, results in activation of the renin-angiotensin system (RAS). Vasoconstriction becomes more pronounced in response to angiotensin II, and aldosterone secretion causes sodium and water retention. Preload and afterload increase; angiotensin II contributes to **ventricular remodeling,** resulting in progressive myocyte (myocardial cell) contractile dysfunction over time (McCance & Huether, 2002).

OTHER NEUROHUMORAL RESPONSES

In addition to the sympathetic nervous system and RAS responses, other mechanisms are activated when a client experiences heart failure (HF). Most of these actions contribute to worsening of the condition.

In clients who have had a myocardial infarction (MI), heart muscle cell injury causes an *immune response.* Proinflammatory cytokines, such as tumor necrosis factor (TNF) and interleukins (IL-1 and IL-6) are released, especially with left-sided HF. These substances contribute to ventricular remodeling.

Natriuretic peptides are hormones that promote vasodilation and diuresis through sodium loss in the renal tubules. The **B-type natriuretic peptide (BNP)**, produced and released by the ventricles, increases to counterbalance the RAS, thus decreasing preload (Givertz et al., 2001).

Low CO causes decreased cerebral perfusion. As a result the posterior pituitary gland secretes *vasopressin* (antidiuretic hormone, or ADH). The hormone causes vasoconstriction and fluid retention, which worsen HF.

Endothelin is secreted by endothelial cells when they are stretched. As the myocardial fibers are stretched in clients with HF, this potent vasoconstrictor is released, which increases peripheral resistance and hypertension. HF worsens as a result of these actions.

MYOCARDIAL HYPERTROPHY

Myocardial hypertrophy, with or without chamber dilation, is the final compensatory mechanism. The walls of the heart thicken to provide more muscle mass, which results in more forceful contractions, further increasing cardiac output. Cardiac muscle, however, may hypertrophy more rapidly than collateral circulation can provide adequate blood supply to the muscle. Often a hypertrophied heart is slightly oxygen deprived.

All the compensatory mechanisms contribute to an increase in the consumption of myocardial oxygen. When the demand for oxygen increases and the myocardial reserve has been exhausted, clinical manifestations of HF develop.

Etiology

Heart failure (HF) is caused by systemic hypertension in 75% of cases. About a third of clients experiencing MI also develop HF. The next most common cause includes structural heart changes, such as valvular dysfunction, particularly pulmonic or aortic stenosis, which cause pressure or volume overload on the heart. Common direct causes of HF are listed in Table 38-1.

CONSIDERATIONS FOR OLDER ADULTS

The use of certain drugs can also lead to heart failure (HF), especially in older adults. Long-term nonsteroidal anti-inflammatory drugs (NSAIDs), such as ibuprofen (Motrin), cause fluid and sodium retention. Many older adults take these drugs for arthritic pain and inflammation. Thiazolidinediones (TZDs) used for diabetics, such as pioglitazone (Actos) and rosiglitazone (Avandia), also cause fluid and sodium retention (Martin, 2003). These medications should be used with caution in the older adult population. These clients should be monitored closely by their health care provider.

Right-sided HF in the absence of left-sided HF is most often the result of pulmonary problems, such as chronic obstructive pulmonary disease (COPD) or cystic fibrosis. Acute respiratory distress syndrome (ARDS) may also cause right-sided HF.

TABLE 38-1 Common Causes of Heart Failure

- Hypertension
- Coronary artery disease
- Cardiomyopathy
- Substance abuse (alcohol and illicit/prescribed drugs)
- Valvular disease
- Congenital defects
- Cardiac infections and inflammations
- Hyperkinetic conditions

RESOURCE MANAGEMENT

HEART FAILURE

Cost of Care

Heart failure is the most common cause of hospitalization for clients 65 years of age and older. According to the American Heart Association (AHA), the estimated annual costs of care for heart failure in 2003 were $24.3 billion dollars (AHA, 2003). The costs include the following:

- $16.4 billion in additional hospital and nursing home charges
- $1.7 billion in health care provider charges
- $2.3 billion for medications and other medical durables (e.g., a left ventricular assist device [LVAD])
- $2.2 billion for home health care

In 1998, heart failure cost $3.6 million, or $5471 per hospital discharge. In 2000, nearly 1.4 million diagnostic cardiac catheterizations were performed. Hospital discharges for heart failure increased 165 from 377,000 in 1979 to 999,000 in 2000.

Implications for Nursing

Because of the high cost of hospitalization and nursing home care for clients with heart failure, nurses must be attuned to enhancing client education to promote client self-management of heart failure and compliance with therapy. Creative ways to deliver effective nursing care in the home to clients with heart failure are needed, such as disease management programs.

Incidence/Prevalence

Nearly five million people in the United States are living with HF (AHA, 2003), and about 550,000 new cases occur each year. HF is slightly more common in men than in women.

CONSIDERATIONS FOR OLDER ADULTS

The prevalence of heart failure (HF) steadily increases with aging. As many as 10% of people over 70 years of age have HF. About 80% of all hospital admissions for HF are clients older than 65 years of age (AHA, 2003). The cost of providing care for this number of people with HF is detailed in the Resource Management box above.

One of the Healthy People 2010 objectives for the United States is to reduce by 50% the number of hospitalizations of older adults with HF as the principal diagnosis. Interventions aimed at client and family education can help meet this objective (see the Meeting Healthy People 2010 Objectives box on p. 753).

◆COLLABORATIVE MANAGEMENT

◆Assessment

Manifestations of HF depend on the type of failure, the ventricle involved, and the underlying cause. Impaired tissue perfusion, pulmonary congestion, and edema dominate

Meeting HEALTHY PEOPLE 2010 Objectives

CARDIAC DISEASE

Objective 12.6: To reduce hospitalizations of older adults with heart failure as the principal diagnosis.

- For clients hospitalized for heart failure, collaborate with the case manager for discharge planning, including adequate support in the community.
- Provide a continuing plan of care for clients and their families or other caregivers when the client is discharged from the hospital.
- If the client is discharged to home, call the client to check that he or she has no impending signs and symptoms of heart failure (the case manager may make calls).
- Teach the client and family or other caregiver about when to call the health care provider for health changes so the client can be treated at home.
- Ensure that the interdisciplinary team provides the client with follow-up care in the home or nursing home.

CHART 38-1

KEY FEATURES of Left-Sided Heart Failure

Decreased Cardiac Output	Pulmonary Congestion
▪ Fatigue	▪ Hacking cough, worse at night
▪ Weakness	▪ Dyspnea/breathlessness
▪ Oliguria during the day	▪ Crackles or wheezes in lungs
▪ Angina	▪ Frothy, pink-tinged sputum
▪ Confusion, restlessness	▪ Tachypnea
▪ Dizziness	▪ S_3/S_4 summation gallop
▪ Tachycardia, palpitations	
▪ Pallor	
▪ Weak peripheral pulses	
▪ Cool extremities	

CHART 38-2

KEY FEATURES of Right-Sided Heart Failure

Systemic Congestion

- Jugular (neck vein) distention
- Enlarged liver and spleen
- Anorexia and nausea
- Dependent edema (legs and sacrum)
- Distended abdomen
- Swollen hands and fingers
- Polyuria at right
- Weight gain
- Increased blood pressure (from excess volume) or decreased blood pressure (from failure)

the picture of left ventricular failure (Chart 38-1). Conversely, systemic venous congestion and peripheral edema are associated with right ventricular failure (Chart 38-2).

HISTORY

When obtaining a history, keep in mind the many conditions that can lead to HF. Carefully question the client about his or her medical history, including high blood pressure, angina, MI, rheumatic heart disease, valvular disorders, endocarditis, and pericarditis. Ask about the client's perception of his or her activity tolerance, breathing pattern, urinary pattern, and fluid volume status as well as his or her knowledge about HF

LEFT-SIDED HEART FAILURE. With left ventricular systolic dysfunction, cardiac output (CO) is diminished, leading to impaired tissue perfusion, anaerobic metabolism, and unusual fatigue. Assess activity tolerance by asking whether the client can perform normal activities of daily living (ADLs) or climb flights of stairs without fatigue or dyspnea. Many clients with HF experience weakness or fatigue with activity or have a feeling of heaviness in their arms or legs. Ask about their ability to perform simultaneous arm and leg work (e.g., walking while carrying a bag of groceries). Such activity may place an unacceptable demand on the failing heart. Question the client to identify their most strenuous activity in the past week. Many clients unconsciously limit their activities in response to fatigue or dyspnea and may not realize how limited they have become.

Perfusion to the myocardium is often impaired with left ventricular failure, and especially with cardiac hypertrophy. The client may report chest discomfort or may describe palpitations, skipped beats, or a fast heartbeat.

As the amount of blood ejected from the left ventricle diminishes, hydrostatic pressure builds in the pulmonary venous system and results in fluid-filled alveoli and pulmonary congestion. Thus cough is often an early manifestation of HF. The client in early HF describes the cough as irritating, nocturnal (at night), and usually nonproductive. As HF becomes very severe, the client may begin expectorating frothy, pink-tinged sputum–a sign of pulmonary edema.

Dyspnea also results from rising pulmonary venous pressure and pulmonary congestion. Carefully question the client about the presence of dyspnea and when and how it developed. The client may refer to dyspnea as "trouble in catching my breath," "breathlessness," or "difficulty in breathing."

As **exertional dyspnea** develops (also called dyspnea upon exertion [DUE]), the client often discontinues previously tolerated levels of activity because of shortness of breath. Dyspnea at rest in the recumbent (lying flat) position is known as **orthopnea.** Ask the client how many pillows he or she usually uses to sleep or whether he or she sleeps in an upright position in a bed or a chair.

Clients who describe sudden awakening with a feeling of breathlessness 2 to 5 hours after falling asleep have **paroxysmal nocturnal dyspnea (PND).** Sitting upright, dangling the feet, or walking usually relieves this condition.

RIGHT-SIDED HEART FAILURE. Signs of systemic congestion occur as the right ventricle fails, fluid is retained, and pressure builds in the venous system. Edema develops in the lower legs and ascends to the thighs and abdominal wall. Clients may note that their shoes fit more tightly, or their shoes or socks may leave indentations on their swollen feet. They have removed their rings because of swelling in their fingers and hands. Ask about weight gain. An adult may retain 4 to 7 L of fluid (10 to 15 pounds [4.5 to 6.8 kg]) before pitting edema occurs.

Gastrointestinal complaints of nausea and anorexia may be a direct consequence of liver engorgement resulting from fluid retention. In advanced HF, ascites and an increased abdominal girth may develop from the pronounced liver congestion. Another finding related to fluid retention is diuresis at rest. At rest, fluid in the peripheral tissue is mobilized and excreted, and the client describes frequent awakening at night to urinate.

Obtain a careful nutritional history, questioning the client about the use of salt and the types of food consumed. Ask about daily fluid intake. Clients with HF may experience increased thirst and take in excessive fluid (4000 to 5000 mL) because of sodium retention.

PHYSICAL ASSESSMENT/CLINICAL MANIFESTATIONS

The signs and symptoms of HF can be considered in the context of these components of the syndrome:

- Failure of the left ventricle as a pump with decreased tissue perfusion and pulmonary venous congestion
- Failure of the right ventricle as a pump with systemic venous congestion

LEFT-SIDED HEART FAILURE. Left ventricular failure is associated with decreased cardiac output and elevated pulmonary venous pressure. Left ventricular failure may appear clinically as weakness, fatigue, dizziness, confusion, pulmonary congestion, breathlessness, oliguria (scant urine output), or death (see Chart 38-1). Decreased blood flow to the major body organs can cause organ failure, especially renal failure.

Obtain the client's vital signs. When obtaining blood pressure (BP), note the presence or absence of an auscultatory gap or orthostatic (postural) hypotension. The **proportional pulse pressure** is calculated as follows:

$$\frac{\text{Systolic BP} - \text{Diastolic BP}}{\text{Systolic BP}}$$

A proportional pulse pressure less than 25% indicates severely compromised cardiac output (CO). The pulse may be tachycardiac, or it may alternate in strength **(pulsus alternans).** Take the apical pulse for a full minute, noting any irregularity in heart rhythm. An irregular heart rhythm resulting from premature atrial contractions (PACs), premature ventricular contractions (PVCs), or atrial fibrillation (AF) is common in HF. The sudden development of an irregular rhythm may further compromise CO. Carefully monitor the client's respiratory rate, rhythm, and character as well as oxygen saturation. The respiratory rate typically exceeds 20 breaths/min.

Determine whether the client is oriented to person, place, and time. A short mental status examination may be used if there are concerns about orientation. Objective data are important because in daily conversation many people are skillful at covering up memory losses.

Palpate the precordium. Increased heart size is common, with a displacement of the apical impulse to the left. A third heart sound, **(S_3) gallop,** an early diastolic filling sound indicating an increase in left ventricular pressure, may be heard on auscultation. A fourth heart sound (S_4) can also occur; it is not a sign of failure but is a reflection of decreased ventricular compliance.

Crackles and wheezes may be present on auscultation of the lungs. Late inspiratory crackles and fine profuse crackles that repeat themselves from breath to breath and do not diminish with coughing indicate HF. Crackles are produced by intra-alveolar fluid and are often noted first in the dependent areas of the lungs. Crackles usually develop in the bases and spread upward as the condition worsens. Identify the precise location of the crackles. Wheezes indicate a narrowing of the bronchial lumen caused by engorged pulmonary vessels.

RIGHT-SIDED HEART FAILURE. Right ventricular failure is associated with increased systemic venous pressures and congestion. Signs and symptoms are listed in Chart 38-2.

On inspection, assess the neck veins for distention and measure abdominal girth (see Chapter 36). Hepatomegaly (liver engorgement), hepatojugular reflux, and ascites may also be assessed. Abdominal fluid can reach volumes of more than 10 L.

Examine the client for dependent edema. In ambulatory clients, edema is normally located in the ankles and legs. When the client is restricted to bedrest, the sacrum is dependent and edema accumulates there. Edema is an extremely unreliable sign of HF, and therefore accurate daily weights are needed to document fluid retention. *Weight is the most reliable indicator of fluid gain or loss.*

PSYCHOSOCIAL ASSESSMENT

HF is usually a chronic, debilitating disease. A number of studies have found that anxiety is common in clients with HF (Artinian, 2003). These clients are usually frustrated about dealing with a chronic illness. Symptoms such as dyspnea increase their anxiety level.

Clients with advanced HF, especially those with New York Heart Association (NYHA) class III or IV HF, are at high risk for depression. It is not certain whether the functional impairments contribute to the depression or depression affects functional ability (Artinian, 2003). Hospitalized clients may be depressed, particularly those who have been rehospitalized for an acute episode of HF. Some individuals, however, do not manifest depression until they are in the community. Lifestyle changes and quality of life issues can precipitate depression many months after the initial diagnosis of HF.

Assess clients and their families for anxiety and depression. Ask them about their usual methods of coping as well as any history of depression. If anxiety is present, notify the health care provider for further assessment using an anxiety assessment tool, such as the Beck Anxiety Inventory or the Hospital Anxiety and Depression Scale. If depression is suspected, perform a thorough assessment using a tool such as the Geriatric Depression Scale or the Zung Self-Rating Depression Scale. In many hospitals, social workers or psychologists administer these tools.

If anxiety or depression occurs, the client may require treatment with medications and nonpharmacologic modalities, such as cognitive behavior therapy, biofeedback, or relaxation training.

Hope is a major determinant of well-being for clients in HF. Clients who are hopeful tend to feel better and are more socially involved. Asking clients about their activities and the significant people in their life and how often they are able to interact with them will provide information about client and family coping.

LABORATORY ASSESSMENT

Electrolyte imbalance may occur from complications of HF or as side effects of drug therapy, especially diuretic therapy. Regular evaluations of a client's serum electrolytes, including sodium, potassium, magnesium, calcium, and chloride, are essential. Any impairment of renal function resulting from inadequate perfusion causes elevated blood urea nitrogen, serum creatinine, and creatinine clearance levels. Urinalysis may reveal proteinuria and high specific gravity. Hemoglobin and hematocrit tests should be performed to identify HF resulting from anemia. If the client has fluid volume excess, the hematocrit levels may appear low as a result of hemodilution.

A new laboratory test for B-type natriuretic peptide (BNP) is used for diagnosing HF in clients with acute dyspnea. As discussed earlier, BNP is part of the neurohormonal response to decreased CO from either left or right ventricular dysfunction. An increase in BNP best differentiates between the dyspnea of HF and that associated with lung dysfunction.

Arterial blood gas values often reveal hypoxia (low oxygen level) because oxygen does not diffuse easily through fluid-filled alveoli. Respiratory alkalosis may occur because of hyperventilation; respiratory acidosis may occur because of carbon dioxide retention. Metabolic acidosis may indicate an accumulation of lactic acid.

CONSIDERATIONS FOR OLDER ADULTS

Thyroxine (T_4) and thyroid-stimulating hormone (TSH) levels should be determined in clients who are over 65 years of age, have atrial fibrillation, or have evidence of thyroid disease. Heart failure (HF) may be caused or aggravated by hypothyroidism or hyperthyroidism.

RADIOGRAPHIC ASSESSMENT

Chest x-rays can be helpful in diagnosing left ventricular failure. Typically the heart is enlarged (cardiomegaly), representing hypertrophy or dilation. Pleural effusions develop less often and generally reflect biventricular failure.

OTHER DIAGNOSTIC ASSESSMENTS

An electrocardiogram (ECG) is also performed. The ECG may demonstrate ventricular hypertrophy, dysrhythmias, and any degree of myocardial ischemia, injury, or infarction. It is not helpful in determining the presence or extent of HF.

Echocardiography is useful in diagnosing cardiac valvular changes, pericardial effusion, chamber enlargement, and ventricular hypertrophy. It can also be used to determine ejection fraction. Radionuclide studies (thallium imaging or technetium pyrophosphate scanning) can also indicate the presence and cause of HF. Multigated angiographic (MUGA) scans provide information about left ventricular ejection fraction and velocity, which are typically low in clients with HF.

Pulmonary artery catheters allow the assessment of cardiac function and volume status in acutely ill clients. These measurements can confirm the diagnosis and guide the management of HF. Right atrial pressure may be normal or elevated in left ventricular failure and is elevated in right ventricular failure. Pulmonary artery pressure (PAP) and pulmonary artery wedge pressure (PAWP) are elevated in left-sided HF because volumes and pressures are increased in the left ventricle. (See Chapter 36 for a more detailed description of these diagnostic assessments.)

Analysis

COMMON NURSING DIAGNOSES AND COLLABORATIVE PROBLEMS

The following are priority nursing diagnoses for clients with HF:

1. Impaired Gas Exchange related to ventilation perfusion imbalance
2. Decreased Cardiac Output related to altered contractility, preload, and afterload
3. Activity Intolerance related to an imbalance between oxygen supply and demand

The primary collaborative problem is Potential for Pulmonary Edema.

ADDITIONAL NURSING DIAGNOSES AND COLLABORATIVE PROBLEMS

In addition to the common nursing diagnoses and collaborative problems, clients with HF may have one or more of the following:

- Excess Fluid Volume related to compromised regulatory mechanism
- Acute Confusion related to delirium
- Ineffective Therapeutic Regimen Management related to social support deficits, complexity of therapeutic regimen, or knowledge deficit
- Anxiety related to stress, change in health status and role function, or threat of death
- Ineffective Tissue Perfusion: Cerebral related to mechanical reduction of arterial blood flow
- Impaired Physical Mobility related to limited cardiovascular endurance
- Risk for Ineffective Tissue Perfusion: Renal related to hypovolemia

Some clients are also at risk for the following collaborative problems:

- Potential for Pneumonia
- Potential for Dysrhythmias

Planning and Implementation

IMPAIRED GAS EXCHANGE

NOC **PLANNING: EXPECTED OUTCOMES.** The client with HF is expected to have adequate pulmonary tissue perfusion. Indicators include noncompromised status of the following:

- Pulmonary artery pressure (PAP)
- Respiratory function
- Respiratory rate
- Arterial blood gases and pH
- Oxygen saturation

INTERVENTIONS. The purpose of care is to promote an optimal spontaneous breathing pattern that maximizes oxygenation and maintains a normal carbon dioxide level in the blood (Chart 38-3).

NIC **Ventilation Assistance.** Monitor, or have assistive personnel monitor, the client's respiratory rate, rhythm, and quality every 1 to 4 hours and auscultate breath sounds. The oxygen content of the blood is often markedly reduced in clients who are experiencing pulmonary congestion. The nurse may titrate the amount of supplemental oxygen delivered to the client within a range prescribed by the health care provider to maintain oxygen saturation at 92% or greater.

If the client is experiencing respiratory difficulty, place him or her in a high Fowler's position with pillows under each arm to maximize chest expansion and improve oxygenation. Repositioning and performing coughing and deep breathing exercises every 2 hours help to improve oxygenation and prevent atelectasis.

CHART 38-3

NIC **INTERVENTION ACTIVITIES for The Client with Heart Failure**

Ventilation Assistance: *Promotion of an optimal spontaneous breathing pattern that maximizes oxygen and carbon dioxide exchange in the lungs*

- Monitor respiratory and oxygenation status.
- Initiate and maintain supplemental oxygen, as prescribed.
- Position to alleviate dyspnea.
- Auscultate breath sounds, noting areas of decreased or absent ventilation and presence of adventitious sounds.
- Position to minimize respiratory efforts (e.g., elevate the head of the bed and provide overbed table for client to lean on).
- Monitor the effects of position change on oxygenation: ABG, Sao_2, Svo_2, end tidal CO_2, Q_{sp}/Q_t, A-aDO_2 levels.

Hemodynamic Regulation: *Optimization of heart rate, preload, afterload, and contractility*

- Monitor and document heart rate, rhythm, and pulses.
- Monitor peripheral pulses, capillary refill, and temperature and color of extremities.
- Monitor pulmonary capillary/pulmonary artery wedge pressure and central venous/right atrial pressure, if appropriate.
- Administer vasodilator and/or vasoconstrictor medication, as appropriate.
- Administer positive inotropic/contractility medications.
- Maintain fluid balance by administering IV fluids or diuretics, as appropriate.
- Monitor intake/output, urine output, and client weight, as appropriate.
- Monitor electrolyte levels.
- Auscultate heart sounds.

Energy Management: *Regulating energy use to treat or prevent fatigue and optimize function*

- Monitor cardiorespiratory response to activity (e.g., tachycardia, other dysrhythmias, dyspnea, diaphoresis, pallor, hemodynamic pressures, and respiratory rate).
- Determine client's physical limitations.
- Encourage alternate rest and activity periods.
- Arrange physical activities to reduce competition for oxygen supply to vital body functions (e.g., avoid activity immediately after meals).
- Encourage physical activity (e.g., ambulation or performance of activities of daily living, consistent with client's energy resources).
- Monitor client's oxygen response (e.g., pulse rate, cardiac rhythm, and respiratory rate) to self-care or nursing activities.
- Teach client and significant other techniques of self-care that will minimize oxygen consumption (e.g., self-monitoring and pacing techniques for performance of activities of daily living).

NIC intervention activities selected from Dochterman, J.M., & Bulechek, G.M. (Eds.) (2004). *Nursing interventions classification (NIC)* (4th ed.). St. Louis: Mosby.

ABG, Arterial blood gas, *CO_2*, carbon dioxide, *Sao_2*, saturation of arterial oxygen, *Svo_2*, saturation of venous oxygen, Q_{sp}/Q_t, physiologic blood flow per minute/cardiac output per minute; *A-aDO_2*, alveolar-arterial oxygen pressure difference.

DECREASED CARDIAC OUTPUT

NOC **PLANNING: EXPECTED OUTCOMES.** The client with HF is expected to have increased cardiac pump effectiveness. Indicators include noncompromised or mildly compromised:

- Systolic and diastolic blood pressure
- Apical pulse rate
- Ejection fraction
- Peripheral pulses
- Skin color
- Urine output
- Cognitive status

INTERVENTIONS. Interventions are directed at optimizing the two major components of cardiac output (CO): stroke volume (SV) (determined by preload, afterload, and contractility) and heart rate (HR).

NONSURGICAL MANAGEMENT. Nonsurgical management relies primarily on a variety of medications (Table 38-2). If drug therapy is ineffective, other nonsurgical options are available.

TABLE 38-2 Commonly Used Drug Classifications for Clients with Heart Failure

Angiotensin-converting enzyme (ACE) inhibitors
Diuretics
■ High-ceiling
■ Potassium-sparing
Human B-type natriuretic peptides
Nitrates
Inotropics
■ Beta-adrenergic agonists
■ Phosphodiesterase inhibitors
■ Calcium sensitizers
■ Digitalis
Beta-adrenergic blockers

NIC **Hemodynamic Regulation.** Interventions to improve stroke volume include reducing afterload, reducing preload, and improving cardiac muscle contractility. A major role of the nurse is to administer medications as prescribed, monitor for their therapeutic and adverse effects, and teach the client and family about drug therapy (see Chart 38-3).

Drugs That Reduce Afterload. By relaxing the arterioles, arterial vasodilators can reduce the resistance to left ventricular ejection (afterload) and improve CO. These drugs do not cause excessive vasodilation but reverse some of the inappropriate or excessive vasoconstriction common in HF.

Angiotensin-Converting Enzyme (ACE) Inhibitors. Clients with even mild heart failure (HF) resulting from left ventricular dysfunction should be given a trial of angiotensin-converting enzyme (ACE) inhibitors. ACE inhibitors are a group of arterial vasodilators such as enalapril (Vasotec), fosinopril (Monopril), and captopril (Capoten). In general, these drugs prolong and improve the quality of life for clients with HF. They enhance functional status, with 40% to 80% of clients showing an improvement in the NYHA class.

The ACE inhibitors suppress the renin-angiotensin system (RAS), which is activated in response to decreased renal blood flow. They prevent conversion of angiotensin I to angiotensin II, resulting in arterial resistance, arterial dilation, and increased SV. In addition, these drugs block aldosterone, which prevents sodium and water retention, thus decreasing fluid overload.

The health care provider usually starts doses of ACE inhibitors slowly and cautiously. The first dose of an ACE inhibitor is sometimes associated with a rapid drop in blood pressure (BP). Clients at risk for hypotension following ACE inhibitor administration have initial systolic BP less than 100 mm Hg, are older than 75 years of age, have a serum sodium level less than 137 mEq/L, or are volume depleted. Monitor BP for several hours after the initial dose and each time the dose is increased.

Clarify with the health care provider the guidelines for administering the vasodilator. For example, many clinicians maintain clients with HF at systolic BP ranging from 90 to 110 mm Hg. When such a BP is the maintenance level, assess the client for orthostatic hypotension, confusion, poor peripheral perfusion, and reduced urine output. Monitor serum potassium levels for hyperkalemia, serum creatinine for renal dysfunction, and the client for development of a cough while the client is receiving ACE inhibitors.

For clients with *acute* heart failure (HF), the health care provider may prescribe an intravenous (IV) push ACE inhibitor, such as Vasotec IV. Nursing implications for selected ACE inhibitors are described in Chapter 39 under Drug Therapy (Hypertension) and in Chart 39-3.

Human B-Type Natriuretic Peptides. Human B-type natriuretic peptides (hBNP) are one of the newest classes of drugs to treat *acute* HF. Endogenous BNP is released in response to decreased CO and causes *natriuresis*, or loss of sodium in the renal tubules, as well as vasodilation. Nesiritide (Natrecor) lowers PCWP and improves renal glomerular filtration. It is given as an IV bolus over 60 seconds, followed with a continuous infusion for up to 48 hours. When administering this drug, monitor BP and pulse carefully because it may cause dysrhythmias. Give Natrecor through a separate infusion line it because it is incompatible with heparin and most other parenteral medications.

Interventions That Reduce Preload. Ventricular fibers contract less forcefully when they are overstretched, such as in a failing heart. Interventions aimed at reducing preload attempt to decrease volume and pressure in the left ventricle, optimizing ventricular muscle stretch and contraction. Preload reduction is appropriate for HF accompanied by congestion with total body sodium and water overload.

Diet Therapy. In HF, diet therapy is aimed at reducing sodium and water retention.

In collaboration with the dietitian, the health care provider may restrict sodium intake in an attempt to decrease fluid retention. Many clients with HF need to omit only table salt (ingest no added salt) from their diet, thus reducing sodium intake to about 3 g daily.

If salt intake must be reduced further, the client may need to eliminate all salt in cooking as well as high-sodium foods, thus reducing sodium intake to 2 g daily. A dietitian is essential in helping to select foods that meet such a restricted therapeutic diet. About 25% of hospital admissions for clients with HF are due to excessive sodium intake. Therefore all clients must be advised to maintain an appropriate sodium restriction and avoid bingeing on high sodium foods (e.g., ham, bacon, pickles). Table 14-6 lists the sodium contents of some common foods.

Few clients are placed on severe fluid restrictions; however, clients with excessive aldosterone secretion may experience thirst and drink 3 to 5 L of fluid each day. As a result, their fluid intake may be limited to a more normal 2 L daily. Compliance with these simple strategies varies. When a fluid restriction is imposed on the hospitalized client, the nurse adjusts oral and IV therapy accordingly.

Weigh the client daily (1 kg of weight gain or loss equals 1 L of retained or lost fluid, respectively), and keep accurate records of fluid intake and output. The same scale should be used every morning before breakfast for the most accurate assessment of weight. The client's weight should decrease as excess fluid is excreted from the body.

Drug Therapy. Common drugs prescribed to reduce preload are diuretics and venous vasodilators. Chart 39-3 contains additional information about these medications.

Diuretics. The health care provider adds diuretics to the regimen when diet and fluid restriction have not been effective in managing the symptoms of systemic or pulmonary congestion associated with HF. Diuretics enhance the renal excretion of sodium and water by reducing circulating blood volume, decreasing preload, and reducing systemic and pulmonary congestion.

The type and dosage of diuretic prescribed depend on the degree of HF and renal function. High-ceiling (loop) diuretics, such as furosemide (Lasix, Furoside✱, Novosemide✱), torsemide (Demadex), and bumetanide (Bumex), are most effective for treating fluid volume overload. The practitioner may initially use a thiazide diuretic, such as hydrochlorothiazide (HydroDIURIL, Urozide✱) and metolazone (Zaroxolyn), for older clients with mild volume overload. Zaroxolyn is a long-acting agent and is therefore often given every second, third, or fourth day, depending on client need and tolerance.

The action of thiazide diuretics is self-limiting (i.e., diuresis decreases after edema fluid is lost); thus the excessive diuresis and dehydration that may occur with loop diuretics are uncommon occurrences with thiazide diuretics. Clients often prefer thiazide diuretics because of the gradual onset of diuresis.

Loop diuretics, nonetheless, are needed to ensure effective diuresis for many clients in HF. For clients with *acute* HF, Lasix or Bumex can be given by IV push (IVP). Lasix can be given in doses of 20 to 40 mg I, and increased by 20 mg every 2 hours until the desired response is obtained. The usual IV initial dose for Bumex is 1 to 2 mg once or twice daily, but it is more often given in a continuous infusion of 10 mg over 24 hours.

As HF progresses, many clients develop diuretic resistance with refractory edema. The health care provider may choose to treat this problem by administering two types of diuretics, most commonly a loop diuretic and a thiazide diuretic such as metolazone.

Monitor for and prevent potassium deficiency (hypokalemia) from diuretic therapy. The signs of hypokalemia are nonspecific neurologic and muscular complaints, such as generalized weakness, depressed reflexes, and irregular heart rate. Therefore the physician, nurse, and dietitian monitor serum potassium levels to accurately identify hypokalemia.

If the client's serum potassium level is less than 4.0 mEq/L, the health care provider has several alternatives:

- Add a potassium-sparing diuretic to the regimen (such as spironolactone [Aldactone])
- Request that clients further increase their dietary intake of potassium-rich foods
- Prescribe a potassium supplement

CONSIDERATIONS FOR OLDER ADULTS

Older clients receiving loop diuretics are particularly prone to dehydration, especially if they have type 2 diabetes mellitus. The nurse checks orthostatic blood pressures in the client receiving loop diuretics to detect volume depletion. The client is

Continued

weighed daily to detect the development of a slow, progressive weight loss despite an adequate diet. The nurse also looks for flat neck veins when the client is supine and for a loss of skin turgor. All these signs, plus disorientation in a very old client, may indicate excessive diuresis and volume depletion (Chart 38-4).

Clients being treated simultaneously with ACE inhibitors and diuretics may not experience hypokalemia. If their kidneys are not functioning well, they may develop hyperkalemia (elevated serum potassium level). Review the client's serum creatinine level. If the creatinine is greater than 1.8, notify the health care provider before administering supplemental potassium.

Venous Vasodilators. The health care provider may prescribe venous vasodilators (e.g., nitrates) for the client with HF with persistent dyspnea. Significant constriction of venous and arterial blood vessels occurs to compensate for reduced CO. Constriction reduces the volume of fluid that the vascular bed can hold and increases preload. Venous vasodilators may benefit from the following steps:

- Returning venous vasculature to a more normal capacity
- Decreasing the volume of blood returning to the heart
- Improving left ventricular function

Nitrates may be administered intravenously, orally, or topically. IV nitrates are used most often for *acute* HF. These drugs cause primarily venous vasodilation but also a significant amount of arteriolar vasodilation. It is essential to monitor the client's blood pressure when initiating nitrate therapy or increasing the dosage. Clients may initially report headache, but assure them that they will develop a tolerance to this effect and that the headache will cease or diminish. Acetaminophen (Tylenol, Exdol✱) can be given to help relieve discomfort.

Unfortunately, tolerance to the vasodilating effects develops when nitrates are uniformly administered during 24 hours. To prevent such tolerance, the health care provider may prescribe at least one 12-hour nitrate-free period out of every 24 hours (usually overnight). Nitrates, such as isosorbide (Imdur, Ismo) are prescribed to provide nitrate-free periods and reduce the problem of tolerance. Chapter 41 discusses nitrates in more detail.

Drugs That Enhance Contractility. Contractility of the heart can also be enhanced with drug therapy. Positive inotropic drugs are most commonly used, but vasodilators and beta adrenergic blockers may also be administered. For chronic HF, low-dose beta blockers are most commonly used. Digoxin (Lanoxin) may be prescribed to improve that client's symptoms, thereby decreasing dyspnea and improving activity. This older drug is very inexpensive. In some settings, nesiritide (Natrecor) may be administered for end-stage HF, although this medication is very expensive (see earlier discussion of Natrecor for acute HF).

Digitalis. Digoxin (Lanoxin, Novodigoxin✱), a cardiac glycoside, has been demonstrated to provide benefits for clients in heart failure (HF) with sinus rhythm and atrial fibrillation. "Dig" therapy reduces exacerbations of HF and hospitalizations when added to a regimen of angiotensin-converting enzyme (ACE) inhibitors, beta blockers, and diuretics. Digoxin increases functional capacity and improves hemodynamic parameters in clients with New York Heart Association (NYHA) class III and IV HF resulting from left systolic dysfunction. It may increase mortality, however, especially in older adults (McCance & Huether, 2002).

The potential benefits of digitalis derivatives include an increase in contractility, a reduction in heart rate (HR), a slowing of conduction through the atrioventricular node, and an inhibition of sympathetic activity while enhancing parasympathetic activity. Digitalis also may have a mild diuretic effect. Increased automaticity occurs with toxic digitalis levels or in the presence of hypokalemia (which increases sensitivity to digitalis), resulting in ectopic beats (premature ventricular contractions [PVCs]) may result.

Digoxin is erratically absorbed from the gastrointestinal tract. Many medications, especially antacids, interfere with its absorption. It is eliminated primarily by renal excretion.

The presentation of **digitalis toxicity** is often vague and nonspecific and includes anorexia, fatigue, and changes in mental status. Toxicity may cause nearly any dysrhythmia, but PVCs are most commonly noted. Carefully monitor the apical pulse rate and heart rhythm of clients receiving digoxin. The physician determines the desirable HR to achieve; many cardiologists prefer a rate less than 60 beats/min. Report the development of either an irregular rhythm in a client with a previously regular rhythm or a regular rhythm in a client with a previously irregular one. Monitor serum digoxin and potassium levels (hypokalemia potentiates digitalis toxicity) to identify toxicity.

Any medication that increases the workload of the failing heart also increases its oxygen requirement. Be alert for the possibility that the client may experience angina (chest pain) in response to digoxin.

CHART 38-4

NURSING FOCUS on the OLDER ADULT
Heart Failure

- Assess older clients with confusion for indications of heart failure. People older than 80 years of age often experience restlessness or confusion as the initial manifestation of heart failure.
- Auscultate the lungs carefully, recognizing that dependent crackles may not be an indication of heart failure in the older adult.
- Do not expect crackles to clear rapidly after treatment. Crackles may persist in the lung bases of older adults for an extended period after pulmonary congestion has decreased.
- Be especially alert for the signs of digitalis toxicity in the older client because it is common.
- If loop diuretics are used for diuresis, monitor the client closely for signs of excessive diuresis, dehydration, and hypokalemia.
- In older clients receiving drug therapy for heart failure, monitor for orthostatic hypotension. Cardiovascular changes associated with aging make this likely to develop.

CONSIDERATIONS FOR OLDER ADULTS

The half-life of digoxin in middle-aged adults is 36 hours; in older adults, who typically have diminished renal function, the half-life may be 48 hours or longer. Thus older clients are particularly susceptible to digoxin toxicity. Toxicity occurs in 10% to 20% of all clients taking digoxin, more commonly in older clients and clients with hypokalemia. Toxicity in older hypokalemic clients may be fatal, and therefore health teaching is essential.

Other Inotropic Drugs. Clients experiencing *acute* heart failure (HF) are candidates for IV medications that increase contractility, and these agents are often prescribed. For example, *beta-adrenergic agonists*, such as dobutamine (Dobutrex), are used for short-term treatment of acute episodes of HF. Dobutamine improves cardiac contractility and thus cardiac output and myocardial-systemic perfusion.

A more potent drug used for *acute* HF, milrinone (Primacor), functions as a vasodilator/inotropic medication with phosphodiesterase activity. Also known as a *phosphodiesterase inhibitor,* this drug increases cyclic adenosine monophosphate (cAMP), which enhances the entry of calcium into myocardial cells to increase contractile function. Like the beta-adrenergic drugs, Primacor is given intravenously.

Levosimendan (Simdax) is a calcium-sensitizing medication and a positive inotropic drug. It appears to bind to Troponin C in the heart muscle and therefore increases the contraction of the heart. Simdax is used most often in clients who have had or are at high risk for myocardial infarction. Chapter 41 discusses inotropic drugs in more detail.

Beta-Adrenergic Blockers. Beta blockers improve the condition of some clients in HF. It appears that prolonged exposure to increased levels of sympathetic stimulation and catecholamines worsens cardiac function. Beta-adrenergic blockade reverses this effect, improving morbidity, mortality, and quality of life for clients in HF.

Beta blockers must be started slowly for HF. In most cases, clients in HF should not be started on a beta blocker until their ACE inhibitor and diuretic doses have been stabilized for 2 weeks. Carvedilol (Coreg), metoprolol (Lopressor, Betaloc✱), and bisoprolol (Zebeta) are approved for treatment of HF. The first dose is extremely low, and the client is monitored either in the hospital or in the health care provider's office to detect bradycardia or hypotension.

Instruct the client to weigh daily while taking the beta blocker and to report any signs of worsening HF immediately. The health care provider gradually titrates the drug dose upward, and the client is evaluated at least weekly for changes in BP, pulse, activity tolerance, and orthopnea. A modest drop in BP is acceptable if the client remains asymptomatic and can stand without experiencing dizziness or a further drop in BP. The resting HR should remain between 55 and 60 and increase slightly with exercise. Activity tolerance improves, and less orthopnea is experienced. Most clients with mild and moderate HF demonstrate improved ejection fraction, decreased hospital admissions, and improvement in symptoms when beta blockers are added to their treatment regimens. The benefits of beta-blocker therapy accrue over a long period, not immediately.

For clients with *diastolic* HF, drug therapy has not been as effective. Calcium channel blockers, ACE inhibitors, and beta blockers have been used with various degrees of success.

Critical Thinking Challenge

You are a home care nurse visiting a 75-year-old widow with a long history of HF, myocardial infarction, pulmonary emphysema, hypertension, and type 2 diabetes mellitus. She is taking the following medications: Lasix, enalapril (Vasotec), digoxin, KCl, theophylline (Theo-Dur), and rosiglitazone (Avandia). She occasionally uses oxygen at night and sleeps sitting up in a lounge chair.

Today she complains that she "just doesn't feel right." Her pulse is 110, weak, and irregular, and her skin is pale and feels cooler than usual. She is dyspneic, has a respiratory rate of 34, and has crackles in her lung bases.

1. What additional information do you need to obtain?
2. What is the purpose of each of her medications?
3. What laboratory data would help diagnose her acute health problem?
4. What actions should you take at this time and why?

evolve For suggested answer guidelines, go to http://evolve.elsevier.com/Iggy/.

Other Nonsurgical Options. In addition to drug therapy, nonsurgical options, both noninvasive and invasive, may be used, including the following:

- Continuous positive airway pressure (CPAP)
- Cardiac resynchronization therapy (CRT)
- Investigative gene therapy

Continuous Positive Airway Pressure. **Continuous positive airway pressure (CPAP)** is a respiratory treatment that improves sleep apnea in clients with HF. It also improves cardiac output (CO) and ejection fraction (EF) by decreasing afterload and preload, blood pressure (BP), and dysrhythmias. Sleep apnea is directly correlated with coronary artery disease as a result of diminished oxygen supply to the heart during apneic episodes.

Cardiac Resynchronization Therapy. **Cardiac resynchronization therapy (CRT)** uses a permanent pacemaker alone or is combined with an implantable cardioverter-defibrillator to provide biventricular pacing. Electrical stimulation causes more synchronous ventricular contractions to improve EF, CO, and mean arterial pressure. This modality is indicated for clients with class III or IV HF and an EF of less than 35%. CRT improves the client's ability to perform activities of daily living (ADLs). Chapter 37 discusses pacing in more detail.

Gene Therapy. **Gene therapy** may be indicated for clients in end-stage HF who are not candidates for heart transplantation. This therapy replaces damaged genes with normal or modified genes by a series of injections of growth factor into the left ventricle. Although still investigative, this therapy has resulted in improved exercise tolerance and regrowth of cardiac cells (Bosen, 2003).

SURGICAL MANAGEMENT. Heart transplantation is still the ultimate choice for end-stage HF (see later). Several surgical procedures are available to improve CO in clients who are not candidates for a transplant or are awaiting transplant.

Ventricular Assist Devices. **Left ventricular assist devices (LVAD)** have been used for a number of years with varying success for clients awaiting heart transplantation. Recent studies have indicated that clients with end-stage HF who are ineligible for transplantation have shown improved survival rates with an LVAD compared with medical support alone (Bond et. al., 2003). Implantable, self-contained LVAD devices are now approved for long-term therapy. **Right ventricle assist devices (RVAD)** can be inserted for right ventricular failure as a result of pulmonary hypertension. Other clients require a bi-VAD as a "bridge to transplant" device. About 75% survive until a transplant is available (Bosen, 2003).

Newer Surgical Therapies. Several new therapies have been used to reshape the left ventricle in clients with heart failure (HF). Perioperative care is similar to the client experiencing a coronary artery bypass graft (CABG) (see Chapter 41). The procedures include the following:

- Partial left ventriculectomy (PLV)
- Endoventricular circular patch

- Acorn cardiac support device
- Myosplint

Also known as **heart reduction surgery,** PLV involves removing a triangle-shaped section of the weakened heart in the left lateral ventricle to reduce the ventricle's diameter and decrease wall tension. In **endoventricular circular patch** cardioplasty, the surgeon removes portions of the cardiac septum and left ventricular wall and grafts a circular patch (synthetic or autologous) into the opening. This procedure provides a more normal shape to the left ventricle to improve hemodynamics.

The **acorn cardiac support device** is a polyester mesh jacket that is placed over the ventricles to provide support and to avoid overstretching the myocardial muscle. The material for the jacket has been used for other procedures, such as vascular grafts. The mesh jacket appears to reduce hypertrophy of the heart muscle and assists with improvement of the EF.

The **Myosplint** is under investigation in Europe and the United States. Electrical stimulation of tension splints in the heart helps the ventricle change to a more normal shape.

ACTIVITY INTOLERANCE

NOC **PLANNING: EXPECTED OUTCOMES.** The client with HF is expected to take actions to manage energy for initiating and sustaining activity. Indicators include that the client consistently do the following:

- Balance activity and rest
- Use naps to restore energy
- Recognize energy limitations
- Organize activities to conserve energy
- Adapt lifestyle to energy level
- Report adequate endurance for activity

INTERVENTIONS. The purpose of interdisciplinary interventions is to regulate energy to prevent fatigue and optimize function (see Chart 38-3).

NIC **Energy Management.** The client in severe HF initially requires physical and emotional rest. On the first day of hospitalization, he or she may sit up in a chair for meals and perform basic leg exercises while out of bed. Nursing care should be organized to allow periods of rest. The interdisciplinary team observes and documents the client's physiologic response to activity.

As the client's condition improves, the physical therapist (PT) initiates ambulation, usually on hospital day 2. Check the blood pressure (BP), pulse, and oxygen saturation before and after the activity. A BP change of more than 20 mm Hg or a pulse increase of more than 20 beats/min may indicate that the activity is too stressful. Other indications of activity intolerance include dyspnea, fatigue, and chest pain. Ask a client displaying any of these symptoms to rate how hard he or she has been working on a scale of 1 to 20, with 20 being the maximum perceived exertion. If the client rates the exertion higher than 12, counsel him or her to slow down. If activity is tolerated, the PT steadily increases the activity level until the client is ambulating 200 to 400 feet several times per day.

If the client is able, the PT (or assistive nursing or PT personnel) might time him or her for 6 minutes while walking at a comfortable pace. The distance the client can walk can be used to determine his or her functional level and activity plan.

POTENTIAL FOR PULMONARY EDEMA

PLANNING: EXPECTED OUTCOMES. The client with HF is expected to be free of pulmonary edema. Indicators include that the client will have the following:

- No adventitious breath sounds
- Vital signs within normal limits
- Arterial blood gas values within normal limits

INTERVENTIONS. Monitor for manifestations of acute pulmonary edema, a life-threatening event that can result from severe HF. In pulmonary edema, the left ventricle fails to eject sufficient blood, and pressure increases in the lungs because of the accumulated blood. The increased pressure causes fluid to leak across the pulmonary capillaries and into the pulmonary interstitium.

Assess for early manifestations, such as crackles in the lung bases, dyspnea at rest, disorientation, and confusion, especially in older clients. Documentation of the precise location of the crackles is crucial because the level of the fluid ascends as the pulmonary edema worsens. The client in acute pulmonary edema is also extremely anxious, tachycardiac, and struggling for air. As pulmonary edema becomes more severe, he or she may have a moist cough productive of frothy, blood-tinged sputum, and his or her skin may be cold, clammy, or cyanotic.

The client diagnosed with pulmonary edema is admitted to the acute care hospital. The physician prescribes rapid-acting diuretics, such as Lasix or Bumex. Lasix is given intravenously over 1 to 2 minutes, usually at a starting dose of 40 mg, with another 40 mg repeated if needed in 30 minutes. Each increment of 40 mg of Lasix should be administered over 1 to 2 minutes to avoid ototoxicity. Bumex may be administered 1 to 2 mg IVP or as a continuous infusion to provide consistent fluid removal over 24 hours.

Oxygen is always used, and the client is placed in a high Fowler's position. IV morphine sulfate may be prescribed, 1 to 2 mg at a time, to reduce venous return (preload), decrease anxiety, and reduce the work of breathing. Monitor respiratory rate and BP closely. Nitroglycerin may be administered as a slow infusion to decrease preload and ease the oxygen demand on the heart. Monitor the client's BP closely while this medication is being given.

Insert a Foley catheter, if prescribed, to assess urine output after diuretic administration and to minimize exertion related to voiding. Diuresis normally begins within 5 minutes of the administration of IV Lasix and peaks at 30 minutes. Chart 38-5 summarizes the priority care for the client with acute pulmonary edema.

Clients often respond dramatically and quickly to these interventions, but their condition can also deteriorate rapidly because of pulmonary congestion and severe hypoxemia. Clients occasionally require bilateral positive airway pressure (biPAP) or intubation and ventilation to survive the acute episode (see Chapter 35 for a description of these modalities). A skilled nurse is needed to assist with intubation. If a client does not respond to other methods, vasodilators such as nitroglycerin or sodium nitroprusside may be administered intravenously, or inotropic support may be required. The client should be in an emergency department or intensive care unit (ICU), where the medications are carefully titrated via continuous infusion pumps and the client is closely assessed. Management of the client who is critically ill with HF is detailed in Chapter 41.

CHART 38-5

BEST PRACTICE for
Care of the Client with Pulmonary Edema

Emergency Care
- Identify the client's chief complaint.
- If the client's blood pressure is adequate, place the client in a high Fowler's position.
- Auscultate the client's lungs (posterior assessment).
- Ensure that vascular access is present, and check for patency.
- Provide oxygen as ordered.
- Provide an IV diuretic (usually furosemide) as prescribed.
- Anticipate urine output 5 to 15 minutes after diuretic administration; catheterize if ordered.

Continuing Care
- Monitor blood pressure, respiratory rate, pulse oximetry, pulse, cardiac rhythm, and the client's subjective report of ability to breathe.
- Provide additional medications as prescribed (usually morphine sulfate or nitroglycerin).
- Provide comfort measures and reassurance.
- Notify the health care provider if the client does not experience a rapid improvement and diuresis.

Community-Based Care

Clients who have not been adequately prepared for discharge or who do not have good community support and follow-up are at high risk for recurrent hospital admissions for heart failure (HF). In a case management system, the case manager or care coordinator assesses the client's needs for health care resources and facilitates appropriate placement. It is imperative that the case manager assess the available social supports. An inability to obtain help in activities such as food shopping and obtaining medications is a major contributor to hospital readmission. If home support is available, the client may be discharged home in the care of a family member or other caregiver. Home care nurses may direct the care, and aides may provide assistance with activities of daily living (ADLs).

Gorski and Johnson (2003) describe a collaborative approach between a case management and home health agency to manage clients with HF. The purpose of this disease management program was to improve clinical outcomes and decrease the cost of care through improved client education, evidence-based practice, and ongoing support. Results indicated that hospitalizations were reduced and clients were satisfied with their care.

If the client has multiple health problems or has been severely compromised by heart disease, he or she may require admission to a subacute unit or traditional nursing home for either transitional or long-term care. A variety of nontraditional approaches to the ambulatory care of clients with HF have been demonstrated to decrease rehospitalization rates. Costs involved in caring for the client with HF include a drug regimen that may be extensive. In one study, the overall mean monthly cost of medications for chronic HF was $440. Clients with class II and class III chronic HF had the highest costs of over $500 per month (Hussey et al., 2002).

HOME CARE MANAGEMENT

The focus of the home care nurse's interventions is assessment and health teaching, which is reimbursable by Medicare and other third-party payers. Chart 38-6 lists the major areas of assessment.

CHART 38-6

HOME CARE ASSESSMENT of
The Client with Heart Failure

Assess for signs of heart failure, including the following:
- Changes in vital signs (heart rate >100 beats/min at rest, new atrial fibrillation, blood pressure <90 or >150 systolic)
- Indications of poor tissue perfusion
  - Fatigue
  - Angina
  - Activity intolerance
  - Changes in mental status
  - Pallor or cyanosis
  - Cool extremities
- Indications of congestion
  - Presence of cough or dyspnea
  - Weight gain
  - Jugular venous distention and peripheral edema

Assess functional ability, including the following:
- Performance of activities of daily living
- Mobility and ambulation (review frequency and duration of walking, development of symptoms, and pulse rate)
- Cognitive ability

Assess nutritional status, including the following:
- Food and fluid intake
- Intake of sodium-rich foods
- Alcohol consumption
- Skin turgor

Assess home environment, including the following:
- Safety hazards, especially related to oxygen therapy
- Structural barriers affecting functional ability
- Social support (family, home health services)

Assess the client's compliance and understanding of illness and its treatment, including the following:
- Signs and symptoms to report to health care provider
- Dosages, effects, and side or toxic effects of medications
- When to report for laboratory and health care provider visits
- Ability to accurately weigh self on scale
- Presence of advanced directive
- Use of home oxygen, if appropriate

Assess client and caregiver coping skills

Clients with chronic HF must make many adjustments in their lifestyles. They must adhere to a medical regimen that includes dietary restrictions, activity prescriptions, and drug therapy. They need careful, concise explanations of the treatment plan. The community-based nurse in any setting encourages the client to verbalize fears and concerns about his or her illness and assists in exploring the appropriate coping skills. Client participation in treatment can help alleviate and control symptoms.

HEALTH TEACHING

Clients in HF and their nurses may have different priorities for health teaching. The Evidence-Based Practice for Nursing box on p. 762 describes a study that examined the perceived benefits of a home walking exercise program for clients with HF.

ACTIVITY SCHEDULE. For clients who qualify, Medicare usually provides reimbursement for assessment and teaching so that a home care nurse can continue teaching and assessment when the client returns home. Encourage clients with HF to stay as active as possible and to develop a regular exercise regimen. Those who are more active appear to have better outcomes. The primary outcome is development of a regular exercise routine (probably a home walking program) several times a week. Medicare and third-party payers typically

EVIDENCE-BASED PRACTICE for Nursing

Can a walk exercise program improve perceptions of well-being in clients with heart failure?

Corvera-Tindel, T., et al. (2002). Nurse-managed home walking program improves exercise duration and reduces symptoms in heart failure. VA HSR&D Annual Meeting, Washington, DC.

The purpose of this qualitative and quantitative research study was to compare the effects of a nurse-managed home walking exercise program on the functional status and quality of life in a group of advanced heart failure clients with a control group who carried out usual activities.

The progressive home walk exercise program was conducted over 12 weeks. The exercise periods progressed from once-a-day, 5 days a week, 10-minute periods to 60-minute periods five times a week with increasing exercise intensity. Clients were rated using a 6 Minute Walk Test (6MWT), Cardiac Quality of Life Index (C-QOL), Dyspnea-Fatigue Index (DFI), heart rate variability (HRV), as well as global ratings of symptoms and peak VO_2 and ventilatory threshold (CPX).

The sample (79 clients, all men, mean age 62.6) had a 79% (63) completion rate and a mean compliance rate of 74%. The 6MWT and the CPX showed that exercisers walked farther ($p = 0.001$) and longer ($p = 0.02$) than did the control group. Exercisers also reported improvement in dyspnea and fatigue scores ($t = 2.42$, $p = 0.02$) compared with the usual exercise group. The test measures were both objective and subjective and covered a range of issue associated with exercise and heart failure.

Level of Evidence: 5—The study used a randomized control sample of 79 clients.

Critique. The study used a randomized control sampling; however, all the subjects were men. One limitation, then, was that the study did not address women's response to a home walking exercise program. Another limitation was that racial or ethnic origins of the sample were not reported. The assumption is that all the subjects were white.

Implications for Nursing. Other studies have demonstrated that home exercise programs using stationary bicycles are effective in improving exercise tolerance. Such equipment may be expensive and thus pose a barrier to compliance. A home walking exercise program is a safe, low-cost alternative that appears to produce increases in exercise tolerance and decreases in dyspnea and fatigue.

do not reimburse for cardiac rehabilitation for HF, and paying for a cardiac rehabilitation program out of pocket is expensive.

Although most clients with HF appear to benefit from exercise programs, those with persistent crackles and uncontrolled edema despite medical therapy are not encouraged to exercise until their HF is stabilized. When exercise is indicated, teach the client to begin walking 200 to 400 feet per day. At home the client should try to walk at least three times a week and should slowly increase the amount of time walked (perhaps 10 minutes a week) over several months. If he or she experiences chest pain or pronounced dyspnea while exercising or experiences fatigue the next day, he or she is probably advancing the activity too quickly and should slow down. Encourage the client to keep an exercise diary that documents the time and duration of each exercise session as well as HR and any symptoms that occur with exercise.

INDICATIONS OF WORSENING HEART FAILURE. Many clients who are readmitted to hospitals for treatment of HF fail to seek medical attention promptly when symptoms recur. Instruct the client and caregiver to immediately report to the health care provider the occurrence of any of the following symptoms of worsening HF:

- Rapid weight gain (3 pounds in a week or 1 to 2 pounds overnight)
- Decrease in exercise tolerance lasting 2 to 3 days
- Cold symptoms (cough) lasting more than 3 to 5 days
- Excessive awakening at night to urinate
- Development of dyspnea or angina at rest or worsening angina
- Increased swelling in the feet, ankles, or hands

DRUG THERAPY. The health care provider or nurse provides oral and written instructions about the medication regimen. If digoxin is prescribed, teach the caregiver and client how to count a pulse rate. Assess their ability to accurately take and record the pulse rate. Chart 38-7 lists instructions for the client taking digoxin at home.

CHART 38-7

CLIENT EDUCATION GUIDE
Digoxin Therapy

- Establish one time of day to take this medication everyday.
- Continue taking this medication unless your health care provider tells you to stop.
- Do not take digoxin at the same time as antacids or cathartics (laxatives).
- Take your pulse rate before taking each dose of digoxin. Notify your health care provider of a change in pulse rate (60 to 100 beats/min is normal) or rhythm as well as increasing fatigue, muscle weakness, confusion, or loss of appetite (signs of digitalis toxicity).
- If you forget to take a dose, it may be delayed a few hours; however, if you do not remember it until the next day, you should take only your usual daily dose.
- Report for scheduled laboratory tests (such as potassium and digoxin levels).
- If potassium supplements are prescribed, continue the dose until told to stop by your health care provider.

Advise clients taking diuretics to take them in the morning to avoid waking during the night for voiding. After determining whether the client has a weight scale and can use it, emphasize the importance of weighing each morning. Although this simple intervention can greatly assist in managing HF, most clients do not weigh themselves regularly. Emphasize the relationship between weight gain, fluid retention, and HF. Daily weights indicate whether the client is losing or retaining fluid. Some motivated individuals are taught to use a sliding scale to adjust their daily diuretic dose depending on their daily weight, similar to the way a diabetic client adjusts an insulin dose based on the capillary glucose level. The home care nurse may reliably assess volume status by checking the pattern of daily weights.

Teach clients receiving angiotensin-converting enzyme (ACE) inhibitors to move slowly when changing positions, especially from a lying to a sitting position. Dizziness, lightheadedness, and cough need to be reported to the health care provider.

Clients taking diuretics and ACE inhibitors require that their serum potassium level and renal function be monitored at least every few months. Diuretics, especially loop diuretics such as Lasix and Bumex, deplete potassium and often cause hypokalemia. Conversely, ACE inhibitors may result in potassium retention. If potassium levels drop below 4.0 mEq/L, the primary care physician may prescribe potassium supplementation or add potassium-sparing diuretics such as spironolactone (Aldactone). Depending on the client's third-party payer, a dietitian may be consulted to provide information about potassium-rich foods to include in the diet.

DIET THERAPY. Clients with chronic HF are advised to restrict their dietary sodium. The home care nurse or dietitian provides written instructions on low- or restricted-sodium diets. A 3-g sodium diet is recommended for mild or moderate failure. Remind the client to avoid salty foods and table salt. Clients usually find this diet palatable and fairly easy to follow.

A 2-g sodium diet may be attempted for clients with severe HF. These clients are told not to add salt during or after meal preparation, to avoid milk and milk products, to use few canned or prepared foods, and to read food labels to determine sodium content. This diet is unpalatable, and for many clients the cost of low-sodium foods is a financial burden. Therefore the home care nurse or dietitian should assess the client for compliance.

Clients are instructed to confer with their health care provider if they want to use commercial salt substitutes. Most salt substitutes contain potassium, and the client's renal status and serum potassium level need to be considered before these products can be recommended. Clients may use lemon, garlic, and herbs to enhance the flavor of low-salt foods.

ADVANCE DIRECTIVES. About 50% of deaths from HF are sudden–many without any warning or worsening of symptoms. Because most of these deaths occur at home, it is important for the health care provider or home care nurse to discuss advance directives with the client and family. The family should be prepared to act in accordance with the client's wishes in the event of cardiac arrest. If resuscitation is desired, the family should know how to activate the Emergency Medical System (EMS) and how to provide cardiopulmonary resuscitation (CPR) until an ambulance arrives. If CPR is not desired, the client, family, and nurse should plan how the family will respond.

HEALTH CARE RESOURCES

A home care nurse may be needed to assess the client's adherence to medication and diet therapy and to monitor for worsening heart failure (HF). Clients with activity limitations benefit from the services of a home care aide. A dietitian might be consulted to assist with menu planning and teaching. Although participation in structured cardiac rehabilitation programs has been shown to be beneficial, referrals to such programs are not widespread because coverage is usually not provided by third-party payers.

In addition to home care support, other resources are available for client education and family support. The American Heart Association is an excellent community resource for pamphlets, books, cookbooks, and videotapes related to HF and heart disease. The organization also provides referrals to various local support groups for clients and their caregivers.

For equipment needs (e.g., home oxygen therapy, hospital bed), medical supply companies provide setup and maintenance services. Chapter 31 provides a detailed description of home oxygen therapy.

Evaluation: Outcomes

Evaluate the care of the client with HF on the basis of the identified nursing diagnoses and collaborative problems. The expected outcomes include that the client will:

- Have adequate pulmonary tissue perfusion
- Have increased cardiac pump effectiveness
- Take actions to manage energy
- Be free of pulmonary edema

Specific indicators for these outcomes are listed for each nursing diagnosis and collaborative problem under the Planning and Implementation section (see earlier).

Critical Thinking Challenge

Your 75-year-old home care client is admitted to the hospital with pulmonary edema. She is upset because her daughter and son-in-law are out of town and she does not know how to contact them to inform them of her hospital admission. Her best friend lives next door, but the friend does not drive.

1. What could you do to alleviate this client's anxiety?
2. What treatment do you anticipate for this client when she is hospitalized?
3. What options for follow-up care after discharge does she have?
4. What health teaching will she require?

evolve For suggested answer guidelines, go to http://evolve.elsevier.com/Iggy/.

VALVULAR HEART DISEASE

PATHOPHYSIOLOGY

Acquired valvular dysfunctions, in decreasing order of occurrence, are mitral stenosis, mitral regurgitation, mitral valve prolapse, aortic stenosis, and aortic regurgitation (Chart 38-8). The tricuspid valve is affected infrequently, primarily following endocarditis in IV drug abusers.

Mitral Stenosis

Mitral stenosis usually results from rheumatic carditis, which can cause valve thickening by fibrosis and calcification. Rheumatic fever is the most common cause of mitral stenosis. Nonrheumatic causes include atrial myxoma (tumor), calcium accumulation, and thrombus formation.

WOMEN'S HEALTH CONSIDERATIONS

Two thirds to three fourths of all clients with mitral stenosis are women. About two thirds of women with rheumatic mitral stenosis are younger than 45 years of age.

In mitral stenosis, the valve leaflets fuse and become stiff, and the chordae tendineae contract and shorten. The valve opening narrows, preventing normal blood flow from the left atrium to the left ventricle. As a result of these changes, left atrial pressure rises, the left atrium dilates, pulmonary artery pressures increase, and the right ventricle hypertrophies.

Pulmonary congestion and right-sided HF occur initially. Later, when the left ventricle receives insufficient blood volume, preload is decreased and cardiac output (CO) falls.

Clients with mild mitral stenosis are usually asymptomatic. As the valvular orifice narrows and pressure in the lungs increases, the client experiences dyspnea on exertion, orthopnea, paroxysmal nocturnal dyspnea (sudden dyspnea at night), and dry cough. Hemoptysis and pulmonary edema appear as pulmonary hypertension and congestion progress. Right-sided HF can cause hepatomegaly, neck vein distention, and pitting edema late in the disorder.

CHART 38-8

KEY FEATURES of Valvular Heart Disease

Mitral Stenosis	Mitral Insufficiency	Mitral Valve Prolapse	Aortic Stenosis	Aortic Insufficiency
Fatigue Dyspnea on exertion Orthopnea Paroxysmal nocturnal dyspnea Hemoptysis Hepatomegaly Neck vein distention Pitting edema Atrial fibrillation Rumbling, apical diastolic murmur	Fatigue Dyspnea on exertion Orthopnea Palpitations Atrial fibrillation Neck vein distention Pitting edema High-pitched holosystolic murmur	Atypical chest pain Dizziness, syncope Palpitations Atrial tachycardia Ventricular tachycardia Systolic click	Dyspnea on exertion Angina Syncope on exertion Fatigue Orthopnea Paroxysmal nocturnal dyspnea Harsh, systolic crescendo-decrescendo murmur	Palpitations Dyspnea Orthopnea Paroxysmal nocturnal dyspnea Fatigue Angina Sinus tachycardia Blowing, decrescendo diastolic murmur

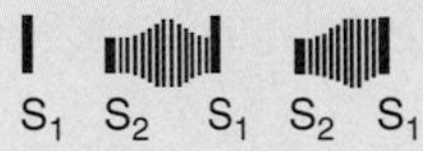

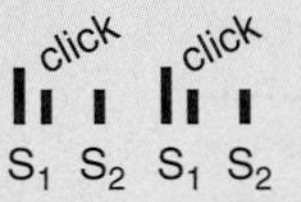

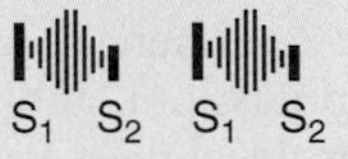

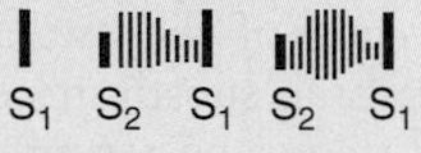

On palpation, the pulse may be normal, tachycardiac, or irregularly irregular (as in atrial fibrillation). Because the development of atrial fibrillation indicates that the client may decompensate, the physician should be notified immediately of the development of an irregularly irregular rhythm. A rumbling, apical diastolic murmur is noted on auscultation.

Mitral Regurgitation (Insufficiency)

The fibrotic and calcific changes occurring in **mitral regurgitation** (insufficiency) prevent the mitral valve from closing completely during *systole.* Incomplete closure of the valve allows the backflow of blood into the left atrium when the left ventricle contracts. During *diastole,* regurgitant output again flows from the left atrium to the left ventricle along with the normal blood flow. The increased volume must be ejected during the next systole. To compensate for the increased volume and pressure, the left atrium and ventricle dilate and hypertrophy.

Rheumatic heart disease is the predominant cause of mitral insufficiency. When it results from rheumatic heart disease, it usually coexists with some degree of mitral stenosis; it affects women more often than men. Nonrheumatic causes, more common in men, include papillary muscle dysfunction or rupture resulting from ischemic heart disease, infective endocarditis, and a congenital anomaly.

Mitral insufficiency usually progresses slowly; clients may remain symptom free for decades. Symptoms begin to occur when the left ventricle fails in response to increased blood volumes and include fatigue and chronic weakness as a result of reduced cardiac output (CO). Dyspnea on exertion and orthopnea develop later. A significant number of clients complain of anxiety, atypical chest pains, and palpitations. Assessment may reveal normal BP, atrial fibrillation (an irregularly irregular rhythm occurring in 75% of clients), or changes in respirations characteristic of left ventricular failure.

When right-sided HF develops, the neck veins become distended, the liver enlarges (hepatomegaly), and pitting edema is noted. A high-pitched systolic murmur at the apex, with radiation to the left axilla, is heard on auscultation. Severe regurgitation often exhibits a third heart sound (S_3).

Mitral Valve Prolapse

Mitral valve prolapse (MVP) occurs because the valvular leaflets enlarge and prolapse into the left atrium during systole. This abnormality is usually benign but may progress to pronounced mitral regurgitation.

Most clients with MVP are asymptomatic; however, they may report chest pain, palpitations, or exercise intolerance. Chest pain is usually atypical, with clients describing a sharp pain localized to the left side of the chest. Dizziness, **syncope** ("blackouts"), and palpitations may be associated with atrial or ventricular dysrhythmias.

A normal HR and BP is usually found on physical examination. A midsystolic click and a late systolic murmur may be audible at the apex. The intensity of the murmur is not related to the severity of the prolapse.

The etiology of MVP is variable and has been associated with conditions such as Marfan syndrome and other congenital cardiac defects (see Chapter 24 for a discussion on Marfan syndrome). Most often, however, no other cardiac abnormality is found. A familial occurrence is well established.

Mitral valve prolapse affects 5% to 10% of people. Although it is present in all age-groups, it is most common in women between 20 and 54 years of age.

Aortic Stenosis

In **aortic stenosis,** the aortic valve orifice narrows and obstructs left ventricular outflow during systole. This increased resistance to ejection or afterload results in ventricular hypertrophy. As stenosis progresses, cardiac output becomes fixed and unable to increase to meet the demands of the body during exertion, and symptoms develop. Eventually the left ventricle fails, volume backs up in the left atrium, and the pulmonary system becomes congested. Right-sided HF can occur late in the disease. *When the surface area of the valve becomes less than or equal to 1 cm, surgery is indicated on an urgent basis!*

The classic symptoms of aortic stenosis result from the fixed cardiac output: dyspnea, angina, and syncope occurring on exertion. When cardiac output falls in the late stages of the disease, the client experiences marked fatigue, debilitation, and peripheral cyanosis. A narrow pulse pressure is noted when the BP is examined. A diamond-shaped, systolic crescendo-decrescendo murmur is usually noted on auscultation.

Congenital valvular disease or malformation is the predominant etiologic factor in aortic stenosis. Bicuspid or unicuspid aortic valves are the primary reason for aortic stenosis in clients younger than 30 years and account for about 50% of the disease in clients 30 to 70 years of age. Rheumatic aortic stenosis is always concomitant with rheumatic disease of the mitral valve and develops in clients between 30 and 70 years of age. Atherosclerosis and degenerative calcification of the aortic valve are the predominant factors in people older than 70 years of age. Aortic stenosis has become the most common valvular disorder in countries with aging populations. Of clients with aortic stenosis, 80% are men.

Aortic Regurgitation (Insufficiency)

In clients with **aortic regurgitation,** the aortic valve leaflets do not close properly during diastole, and the *annulus* (the valve ring that attaches to the leaflets) may be dilated, loose, or deformed. This allows regurgitation of blood from the aorta back into the left ventricle during diastole. The left ventricle, in compensation, dilates to accommodate the greater blood volume and eventually hypertrophies.

Clients with aortic regurgitation remain asymptomatic for many years because of the compensatory mechanisms of the left ventricle. As the disease progresses and left ventricular failure occurs, the principal concerns are exertional dyspnea, orthopnea, and paroxysmal nocturnal dyspnea. Palpitations may be noted with severe disease, especially when the client lies on the left side. Nocturnal angina with diaphoresis often occurs.

On palpation, the nurse notes a "bounding" arterial pulse. The pulse pressure is usually widened, with an elevated systolic pressure and diminished diastolic pressure. The classic auscultatory finding is a high-pitched, blowing, decrescendo diastolic murmur.

Aortic insufficiency usually results from nonrheumatic conditions such as infective endocarditis, congenital anatomic aortic valvular abnormalities, hypertension, and Marfan syndrome (a rare, generalized, systemic disease of connective tissue). About 75% of clients with aortic regurgitation are men.

COLLABORATIVE MANAGEMENT

Assessment

A client with valvular disease may suddenly become ill or may slowly develop symptoms over many years. Information is collected about the client's family health history, including valvular or other forms of heart disease to which he or she may be genetically predisposed. Question the client about attacks of rheumatic fever and infective endocarditis, the specific dates when these occurred, and the use of antibiotic prophylaxis against the recurrence of rheumatic fever. Also question the client about a history of IV drug abuse. Discuss the client's fatigue level and tolerated activity level, the presence of angina or dyspnea, and the occurrence of palpitations, if present.

As part of the physical assessment, obtain the client's vital signs, inspect for signs of edema, palpate and auscultate the heart and lungs, and palpate the peripheral pulses. Findings consistent with valvular malformation are summarized in Chart 38-8.

In clients with mitral stenosis, the chest x-ray shows left atrial enlargement, prominent pulmonary arteries, and an enlarged right ventricle. In those with mitral regurgitation (insufficiency), the chest x-ray reveals an increased cardiac shadow, indicating left ventricular and left atrial enlargement.

In the later stages of aortic stenosis, the chest x-ray may show left ventricular enlargement and pulmonary congestion. Left atrial and left ventricular dilation appear on the chest x-ray of clients with aortic regurgitation (insufficiency). If HF is present, pulmonary venous congestion is also evident.

For valvular heart disease, echocardiography is the diagnostic procedure of choice because it is an excellent noninvasive tool for defining cardiac structure, movement of the valve leaflets, and size and function of the cardiac chambers. Exercise tolerance testing (ETT) and stress echocardiography are sometimes performed to evaluate symptomatic response, assess functional capacity, and enhance auscultatory findings. With either mitral or aortic stenosis, cardiac catheterization is often indicated to assess the severity of the stenosis and its other effects on the heart.

The health care provider also orders an electrocardiogram (ECG) to assess abnormalities such as left ventricular hypertrophy, as seen with mitral regurgitation and aortic regurgitation, or right ventricular hypertrophy, as seen in severe mitral stenosis. Atrial fibrillation is a common finding in both mitral stenosis and mitral regurgitation and may develop in aortic stenosis because of left atrial dilation.

Common Nursing Diagnoses and Collaborative Problems

Nursing diagnoses that may apply to clients with valvular heart disease include the following:

- Decreased Cardiac Output related to altered stroke volume
- Impaired Gas Exchange related to ventilation perfusion imbalance
- Activity Intolerance related to inability of the heart to meet metabolic demands during activity
- Acute Pain related to physiologic injury agent (hypoxia)

Interventions

Management of valvular heart disease depends on which valve is affected and the degree of valve impairment. Some clients can be managed with yearly monitoring and medications, whereas other clients require invasive procedures or heart surgery.

NONSURGICAL MANAGEMENT. Nonsurgical management focuses on drug therapy and rest. During the course of valvular disease, left ventricular failure with pulmonary or systemic congestion may develop. Diuretics, beta blockers, digoxin, and oxygen are often administered to improve the symptoms of heart failure (HF). Nitrates are administered cautiously to clients with aortic stenosis because of the potential for syncope associated with a reduction in left ventricular volume (preload). Vasodilators such as calcium channel blockers may be used to reduce the regurgitant flow for clients with aortic or mitral stenosis.

Prophylactic antibiotic therapy is required for all clients with valve disease before any invasive procedure. Procedures that require antibiotic coverage include bronchoscopy, endoscopy, sigmoidoscopy, colonoscopy, genitourinary instrumentation, surgery, and dental procedures of any type.

A major concern in valvular heart disease is maintaining cardiac output if atrial fibrillation develops. With mitral valvular disease, left ventricular filling is especially dependent on atrial contraction. When atrial fibrillation develops, there is no longer a single coordinated atrial contraction. Cardiac output can decrease by 25% to 30%, and HF may occur. Ineffective atrial contraction may also lead to the stasis of blood and thrombi in the left atrium. Monitor the client for the development of an irregular rhythm and notify the primary care provider if it develops. (See Chapter 37 for a detailed explanation of atrial fibrillation.)

The primary care provider usually institutes therapy to restore normal sinus rhythm or, if that is unsuccessful, to slow ventricular rate. The physician might elect to convert a client from atrial fibrillation to sinus rhythm using IV diltiazem (Cardizem, Apo-Diltiazem✱) or amiodarone (Cordarone, Pacerone). The client should be on a monitored unit where both cardiac rhythm and BP can be closely watched. Synchronized countershock (cardioversion) may be attempted if atrial fibrillation is rapid, the client decompensates, and the rhythm is unresponsive to medical treatment (see Chapter 37).

If the client remains in atrial fibrillation, low-dose amiodarone (Cordarone) or flecainide (Tambocor) is often prescribed to slow ventricular rate. Procainamide hydrochloride (Pronestyl hydrochloride, Procanbid) may be added to the regimen. A beta-blocking agent may also be considered to slow the ventricular response.

For valvular heart disease and chronic atrial fibrillation, anticoagulation with sodium warfarin (Coumadin, Warfilone✱) is usually a part of the medical treatment plan to prevent thrombus formation. A thrombus that forms on the wall of the heart is called a **mural thrombosis.** Thrombi may form in the atria or on defective valve segments, resulting in systemic emboli. If a portion breaks off and travels to the brain, one or more strokes may occur. Assess the client's baseline neurologic status and regularly reassess for neurologic changes.

Rest is often an important part of treatment. Activity may be limited because cardiac output (CO) cannot meet increased metabolic demands, and angina or HF can result. A balance of rest and exercise is needed to prevent muscle atrophy.

SURGICAL MANAGEMENT. Surgical repair or replacement of heart valves has a major effect on the prognosis of valvular heart disease. Correct timing is crucial. Repair or replacement of the valve is usually performed after symptoms of left ventricular failure have developed but before irreversible dysfunction occurs. Surgical therapy is the only definitive treatment of aortic stenosis and is recommended when angina, syncope, or dyspnea on exertion develops.

Reparative Procedures. Reparative procedures are gaining in popularity because of continuing problems with thrombi, endocarditis, and left ventricular dysfunction after valvular replacement. Reparative procedures do not result in a normal valve, but they usually "turn back the clock," resulting in a more functional valve and an improvement in cardiac output. Turbulent blood flow through the valve may persist, and degeneration of the repaired valve is possible.

Balloon Valvuloplasty. Balloon valvuloplasty, an invasive nonsurgical procedure, is possible for stenotic mitral and aortic valves; however, careful selection of clients is necessary. Valvuloplasty may be the initial treatment of choice for people with noncalcified, mobile mitral valves. Clients selected for aortic valvuloplasty are usually older and are at high risk for surgical complications or have refused operative treatment. The benefits of aortic valvuloplasty for aortic stenosis tend to be short lived, rarely lasting longer than 6 months.

When performing mitral valvuloplasty, the physician passes a balloon catheter from the femoral vein, through the atrial septum, and to the mitral valve. The balloon is inflated to enlarge the mitral orifice. For aortic valvuloplasty, the physician inserts the catheter through the femoral artery and advances it to the aortic valve, where it is inflated to enlarge the orifice. Valvuloplasty usually offers immediate relief of symptoms because the balloon has dilated the orifice and improved leaflet mobility. The results are comparable with those of surgical commissurotomy for appropriately selected clients.

After the procedure, observe the client closely for bleeding from the catheter insertion site and institute postangiogram precautions. Bleeding is likely after valvuloplasty because of the large size of the catheter. Also observe for signs of a regurgitant valve by closely monitoring heart sounds, CO, and heart rhythm. Because vegetations (thrombi) may have been dislodged from the valve, observe for any indication of systemic emboli (see Infective Endocarditis, p. 768).

Direct, or Open, Commissurotomy. Direct commissurotomy is accomplished with cardiopulmonary bypass during open heart surgery. The surgeon visualizes the valve, removes thrombi from the atria, incises the fused commissures (leaflets), and debrides calcium from the leaflets, widening the orifice.

Mitral Valve Annuloplasty. Mitral valve annuloplasty (reconstruction) is the reparative procedure of choice for most clients with acquired mitral insufficiency. To make the annulus (the valve ring that attaches to and supports the leaflets) smaller, the physician may suture the leaflets to an annuloplasty ring or take tucks in the client's annulus. Leaflet repair is often performed at the same time. Elongated leaflets may be shortened, and shortened leaflets may be repaired by lengthening the chordae that bind them in place. Perforated leaflets may be patched with synthetic grafts.

Annuloplasty and leaflet repair result in an annulus of the appropriate size and in leaflets that can close completely. Thus regurgitation is eliminated or markedly reduced.

Replacement Procedures. The development of *prosthetic* (synthetic) and *biologic* (tissue) valves has improved the surgical therapy and prognosis of valvular heart disease. Prosthetic valves come in a wide variety. Although prosthetic valves are durable, all clients must receive oral anticoagulation because of the possibility of clot formation.

Biologic valves may be **xenograft** (from other species), such as a porcine valve (from a pig) (Figure 38-2) or a bovine valve (from a cow). Because tissue valves are associated with little risk of clot formation, long-term anticoagulation is not indicated; however, xenografts are not as durable as prosthetic valves and usually must be replaced every 7 to 10 years. The durability of a xenograft is related to the age of the recipient. Calcium in the blood, which is present in larger quantities in younger clients, breaks down the valves.

A B C

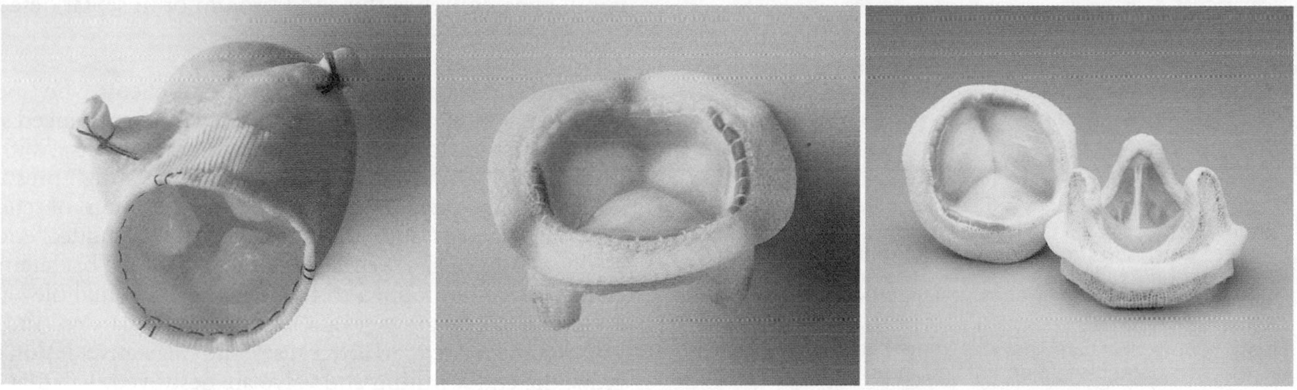

Figure 38-2 ■ Examples of biologic (tissue) heart valves. **A,** Freestyle, a stentless pig valve with no frame. **B,** Hancock II, a stented pig valve. **C,** Carpentier-Edwards pericardial bioprosthesis. (**A** and **B** courtesy of Medtronic, Inc., Minneapolis, MN; **C** courtesy of Baxter Healthcare Corporation, Edwards CVS Division, Santa Ana, CA.)

The older the client, the longer the xenograft will last. Valves donated from human cadavers and **pulmonary autographs** (relocation of the client's own pulmonary valve to the aortic position [Ross procedure]) are also being used for valve replacement.

An aortic valve is replaced with a mechanical valve for most symptomatic adults with aortic stenosis and aortic insufficiency. A tissue valve cannot be used because of the high pressure within the aorta.

Preoperative Care. Clients undergoing valve surgery have open heart surgery similar to the procedure for a coronary artery bypass graft (CABG) (see Chapter 41). Ideally, surgery is an elective and planned procedure. Instruct the client and family members or a significant other about the management of postoperative pain, incision care, and strategies to prevent respiratory complications (see Chapters 20 and 22). Teach clients receiving oral anticoagulants to stop taking them before surgery as the physician indicates, usually at least 72 hours before the procedure. Clients also need to have a preoperative dental examination. If dental caries or periodontal disease is present, these problems must be resolved before valve replacement.

Postoperative Care. Nursing interventions for open heart surgery for valve disorders are similar to those for a CABG (see Chapter 41); however, a few significant differences depend in part on the type of valvular surgery. Clients with mitral stenosis often have pulmonary hypertension and stiff lungs. Monitor respiratory status closely during weaning from the ventilator. Be especially vigilant for indications of bleeding in clients with aortic valve replacements because of a higher risk for postoperative hemorrhage.

Clients with valve replacements are also more likely to experience significant reductions in CO after surgery, especially those with aortic stenosis or left ventricular failure from mitral valve disease. Carefully monitor the client's CO and identifying any indications of pump failure. High filling pressures–pulmonary artery wedge pressure (PAWP) greater than 18 mm Hg–may be required to maintain an acceptable CO in the immediate postoperative period. Clients who have had valve replacements with prosthetic valves require lifetime prophylactic anticoagulation therapy to prevent thrombus formation.

Community-Based Care

The client with valvular heart disease may be discharged home on medical therapy or postoperatively after valve repair or replacement. Because fatigue is a common problem for clients, ensure that the home environment is conducive to providing rest while moving the client toward increased activity levels. Older clients with aortic stenosis may reside in long-term care.

HOME CARE MANAGEMENT

A home care nurse may be needed to help the client adhere to medication and activity schedules and to detect any problems, particularly with anticoagulant therapy. Clients who have undergone surgery may require a nurse for assistance with incision care. A home care aide may assist with activities of daily living if the client lives alone.

HEALTH TEACHING

The teaching plan for the client with valvular heart disease includes the following:

- The disease process
- Medications, including diuretics, vasodilators, beta blockers, calcium channel blockers, antibiotics, and anticoagulants
- The prophylactic use of antibiotics
- A plan of work, activity, and rest to conserve energy
- The purpose and nature of surgical intervention, if appropriate

Because clients with defective or repaired valves are at risk for infective endocarditis, teach them to adhere to the precautions described for endocarditis. Instruct clients to inform all health care providers of the valvular heart disease history; also tell them that they require antibiotic administration before all invasive procedures and tests. Instructions for the client are described in Chart 38-9.

Teach clients taking anticoagulants how to manage their drug therapy successfully, including dietary considerations (if taking warfarin) and the prevention of bleeding. For example, the client should be taught to avoid foods high in vitamin K and to use an electric razor to avoid skin cuts. In addition, the client should report any bleeding or excessive bruising to the health care provider.

CHART 38-9

CLIENT EDUCATION GUIDE
Valvular Heart Disease

- Notify all your health care providers that you have a defective heart valve.
- Remind the health care provider of your valvular problem when you have any dental work (cleaning, filling, or extraction), any examination by instrument (cystoscopy, endoscopy, or sigmoidoscopy), or any other invasive procedure (arteriogram, surgery).
- Request antibiotic prophylaxis before and after these procedures if the health care provider does not offer it.
- Clean all wounds and apply antibiotic ointment to prevent infection.
- Notify your health care provider immediately if you experience fever, petechiae (pinpoint red dots on your skin), or shortness of breath.

Teach clients who have undergone valve surgery how to care for the sternal incision and instruct them to watch for and report any fever, drainage, or redness at the site. Clients can usually return to normal activity after 6 weeks but should avoid heavy physical labor with their upper extremities for 3 to 6 months to allow the sternotomy incision to heal. Clients who have had valvular surgery should also avoid dental procedures for 6 months because of the potential for endocarditis. Some procedures may be done with caution but only if the client takes a course of antibiotic therapy. Those with prosthetic valves need to avoid any procedure using magnetic resonance technology.

Clients with valvular heart disease may have complicated medication schedules as well as long-term antibiotic or anticoagulant therapy. These circumstances potentially can lead to noncompliance. Provide clear, concise instructions about medication schedules, and discuss the risks associated with noncompliance.

The psychological response to valve surgery is similar to that following coronary artery bypass surgery. Clients may experience an altered self-image as a result of the required lifestyle changes or the visible medial sternotomy incision. In addition, clients with prosthetic valves may need to adjust to a soft but audible clicking sound of the prosthetic valve. Encourage clients to verbalize their feelings about the sternotomy incision and the prosthetic heart valve. It is common for clients to display a variety of emotions postoperatively, especially when they get home.

HEALTH CARE RESOURCES

The American Heart Association and the Mended Hearts Club is a community resource that provides information about valvular heart disease. A wallet-sized card can be obtained to identify the client as needing prophylactic antibiotics. An identification bracelet that states the name of the drug the client is taking should also be worn.

INFLAMMATIONS AND INFECTIONS

Infective Endocarditis

PATHOPHYSIOLOGY

Infective endocarditis (previously called *bacterial endocarditis*) refers to a microbial infection (e.g., viruses, bacteria, fungi) involving the endocardium. A healthy, defective, or prosthetic valve can be affected, but infection may also occur in apparently healthy endocardium or in septal defects.

Etiology

Infective endocarditis occurs primarily in clients who abuse IV drugs, have had valve replacements, have experienced systemic infection, or have structural cardiac defects. With a cardiac defect, blood may flow rapidly from a high-pressure area to a low-pressure zone, eroding a section of endocardium. Platelets and fibrin adhere to the denuded endocardium, forming a vegetative lesion. During bacteremia, bacteria become trapped in the low-pressure "sinkhole" and are deposited in the vegetation. Additional platelets and fibrin are deposited, which causes the vegetative lesion to grow; the endocardium and valve are destroyed. Valvular insufficiency may result when the lesion interferes with normal alignment of the valve. If vegetations become so large that blood flow through the valve is obstructed, the valve appears stenotic and then is very likely to *embolize* (i.e., cause emboli to be released).

Possible ports of entry for infecting organisms include the following:

- The oral cavity (especially if dental procedures have been performed)
- Skin rashes, lesions, or abscesses
- Infections (cutaneous, genitourinary, gastrointestinal, systemic)
- Surgery or invasive procedures, including IV line placement

Incidence/Prevalence

The incidence of infective endocarditis is estimated to be 1 per 1000 hospital admissions, with males and females equally affected. Mortality rates for infective endocarditis have remained high–up to 25% despite antibiotic therapy.

◆COLLABORATIVE MANAGEMENT

◆Assessment

Because mortality remains high, early detection of infective endocarditis is essential. Unfortunately, many clients (especially older adults) are misdiagnosed. Clinical manifestations usually occur within 2 weeks of a bacteremia (Chart 38-10).

Assessment usually reveals a recurrent fever. Most clients have temperatures from 99° to 103° F (37.2° to 39.4° C). As a result of physiologic changes associated with aging, however, many older adults remain afebrile. The severity of symptoms may depend on the virulence of the infecting organism.

PHYSICAL ASSESSMENT/CLINICAL MANIFESTATIONS

CARDIOVASCULAR MANIFESTATIONS. Assess the client's cardiovascular status. More than 90% of clients with infective endocarditis develop murmurs. Carefully auscultate the precordium, noting and documenting any new murmurs (usually regurgitant in nature) or any changes in the intensity or quality of an old murmur. An S_3 or S_4 heart sound may also be heard.

Heart failure (HF) is the most common complication of infective endocarditis. Assess for right-sided HF (as evidenced by peripheral edema, weight gain, and anorexia) and left-sided HF (as evidenced by fatigue, shortness of breath, and crackles on auscultation of breath sounds). See discussion of HF earlier in this chapter.

CHART 38-10

KEY FEATURES of Infective Endocarditis

- Fever associated with chills, night sweats, malaise, and fatigue
- Anorexia and weight loss
- Cardiac murmur (newly developed or change in existing)
- Development of heart failure
- Evidence of systemic embolization
- Petechiae
- Splinter hemorrhages
- Osler's nodes
- Janeway's lesions
- Positive blood cultures

EMBOLIC COMPLICATIONS. Arterial embolization is a major complication in up to 50% of clients with infective endocarditis. Fragments of vegetation break loose and travel randomly through the circulation. When the left side of the heart is involved, vegetation fragments are carried to the spleen, kidneys, gastrointestinal (GI) tract, brain, and extremities. When the right side of the heart is involved, emboli enter the pulmonary circulation.

Splenic infarction with sudden abdominal pain and radiation to the left shoulder can also occur. When performing an abdominal assessment, note rebound tenderness on palpation. The classic pain described with renal infarction is flank pain that radiates to the groin and is accompanied by hematuria or pyuria. Mesenteric emboli may result in the client complaining of diffuse abdominal pain, often after eating, and abdominal distention.

Whereas about a third of clients demonstrate neurologic changes, others have signs and symptoms of pulmonary problems. Emboli to the central nervous system cause either transient ischemic attacks (TIAs) or a stroke. Confusion, reduced concentration and aphasia, or dysphagia may occur. Pleuritic chest pain, dyspnea, and cough are symptoms of pulmonary infarction related to embolization.

PERIPHERAL MANIFESTATIONS. Petechiae (pinpoint red spots) occur in up to 40% of clients with endocarditis. Examine the mucous membranes, the palate, the conjunctivae, and the skin above the clavicles for small, red, flat lesions. Assess the distal third of the nail bed for **splinter hemorrhages,** which appear as black longitudinal lines or small red streaks.

DIAGNOSTIC ASSESSMENT

A positive blood culture is of prime diagnostic and therapeutic importance. Both aerobic and anaerobic specimens are obtained for culture. Some slow-growing organisms may take 3 weeks and require a specialized medium to isolate. Therefore cultures should be monitored by the laboratory for 3 to 4 weeks. Low hemoglobin and hematocrit levels may also be found.

Echocardiography has improved the ability to diagnose infective endocarditis accurately. Transesophageal echocardiography (TEE) allows visualization of cardiac structures that are difficult to see with transthoracic echocardiography (TTE). TEE provides good resolution and is very sensitive for discovering valvular abnormalities, thereby enabling the clinician to diagnose infective endocarditis more accurately (see Chapter 36).

The most reliable criteria for diagnosing endocarditis include positive blood cultures, a new regurgitant murmur, and evidence of endocardial involvement by echocardiography.

◆Interventions

Care of the client with endocarditis usually includes antimicrobials, rest balanced with activity, and supportive therapy for HF. If these interventions are successful, surgery is usually not required.

NONSURGICAL MANAGEMENT. The major component of treatment for endocarditis is drug therapy. Other interventions help to prevent the life-threatening complications.

Drug Therapy. Antimicrobials are the mainstay of treatment, with the choice of drug depending on the specific organism involved. Because vegetations surround and protect the offending microorganism, an appropriate medication must be given in a sufficiently high dose to ensure its destruction. Antimicrobials are most often given intravenously, with the course of treatment lasting 4 to 6 weeks. For most bacterial cases, the ideal antibiotic is one of the penicillins or cephalosporins.

Clients may be hospitalized for several days to institute IV therapy and then are discharged for continued IV therapy at home. After hospitalization, most clients who respond to therapy may continue therapy at home when they become afebrile, have negative blood cultures, and have no signs of HF or embolization.

Anticoagulants are of no value in preventing embolization from vegetations. Because they may result in bleeding, they are avoided unless they are required to prevent thrombus formation on a prosthetic valve.

Other Interventions. Complete bedrest need not be enforced unless clients are hemodynamically unstable; however, activities are balanced with adequate rest. Explain proper oral and general body hygiene and consistently use appropriate aseptic technique to protect the client from contact with potentially infective organisms. Nursing assessment for signs of HF (including rapid pulse, fatigue, cough, and dyspnea; new heart murmurs; and early signs of embolization) continues throughout the antimicrobial regimen.

SURGICAL MANAGEMENT. The cardiac surgeon may be consulted if antibiotic therapy is ineffective in sterilizing a valve, if refractory HF develops secondary to a defective valve, if large valvular vegetations are present, or if multiple embolic events occur. Current surgical interventions for infective endocarditis include the following:

- Removing the infected valve (either biologic or prosthetic)
- Repairing or removing congenital shunts
- Repairing injured valves and chordae tendineae
- Draining abscesses in the heart or elsewhere

Preoperative and postoperative care of clients having surgery involving the valves is similar to that described earlier for valve replacement (pp. 766 and 767).

Community-Based Care

Community-based care for clients with infective endocarditis is essential to resolve the problem, prevent relapse, and avoid complications. Clients and families need to be motivated and have the knowledge, physical ability, and resources to administer IV antibiotics at home. The home care nurse may be contacted to complete teaching started in the acute care institution and to monitor client compliance and health status.

The home care nurse and pharmacist arrange for appropriate supplies to be available to the client at home. Supplies include the prepared antibiotic, IV pump with tubing, alcohol wipes, IV access device, normal saline solution, and a heparin or saline lock flush solution drawn up in syringes. A saline lock, peripherally inserted central catheter (PICC line), or central catheter is positioned at a venous site that is easily accessible to the client or a family member.

Teach the client, family members, or a significant other how to administer the antibiotic and care for the infusion site while maintaining aseptic technique. The client or family member demonstrates this technique before the client is discharged from the hospital. Emphasize the importance of maintaining a blood level of the antibiotic by administering the antibiotics as scheduled. After stabilization at home, the health care provider contacts the client every 3 to 7 days to determine whether he or she is able to comply with and benefit from the IV antibiotic therapy.

Encourage proper hygiene, particularly oral hygiene. Clients are advised to use a soft toothbrush, to brush their teeth at least twice per day, and to rinse the mouth with water after brushing. They should not use irrigation devices or floss the teeth because bacteremia may result. Instruct clients to cleanse lacerations well and apply an antibiotic ointment.

Clients must remind health care providers (including their dentists) of their endocarditis and request prophylactic antibiotic coverage for every invasive procedure, including dental care. Such protection is essential because studies have documented low compliance with prophylaxis regimens by health care providers.

Teach self-monitoring for the manifestations of endocarditis, including the complications of HF and embolic phenomena. Instruct clients to monitor and record their temperature daily for up to 6 weeks. Teach clients to report fever, chills, malaise, weight loss, increased fatigue, sudden weight gain, or dyspnea to their primary care provider.

Pericarditis

PATHOPHYSIOLOGY

Acute pericarditis is an inflammation or alteration of the pericardium, the membranous sac that encloses the heart. Acute pericarditis may be fibrous, serous, hemorrhagic, purulent, or neoplastic. Acute pericarditis is most commonly associated with the following:

- Malignant neoplasms
- Idiopathic causes
- Infective organisms (bacteria, viruses, or fungi)
- Postmyocardial infarction (MI) syndrome (Dressler's syndrome)
- Postpericardiotomy syndrome
- Systemic connective tissue disease
- Renal failure

The cause of the pericarditis determines its presentation. Acute viral pericarditis commonly follows a respiratory infection and is more common in men between 20 and 50 years of age. In 5% to 15% of clients who experience an MI, **Dressler's syndrome** occurs from 1 to 12 weeks after the infarction. This syndrome is characterized by pericarditis, fever, and pericardial and pleural effusions. **Postpericardiotomy syndrome** occurs in 10% to 40% of clients after cardiac surgery.

Chronic constrictive pericarditis occurs when chronic pericardial inflammation causes a fibrous thickening of the pericardium. It is caused by tuberculosis, radiation therapy, trauma, renal failure, or metastatic cancer. In chronic constrictive pericarditis, the pericardium becomes rigid, preventing adequate filling of the ventricles and eventually resulting in cardiac failure.

COLLABORATIVE MANAGEMENT

Assessment

Assessment findings include substernal precordial pain that radiates to the left side of the neck, the shoulder, or the back. Pain is classically grating and oppressive and is aggravated by breathing (mainly on inspiration), coughing, and swallowing. The pain is worse when the client is in the supine position and may be relieved by sitting up and leaning forward. Ask all the questions to evaluate chest discomfort because it is important that the pain of pericarditis be differentiated from that of an acute MI (see Chapter 36).

A pericardial friction rub may be heard with the diaphragm of the stethoscope positioned at the left lower sternal border. This scratchy, high-pitched sound is produced when the inflamed, roughened pericardial layers create friction as their surfaces rub together.

Clients with chronic constrictive pericarditis show signs of right-sided HF, elevated systemic venous pressure with jugular distention, hepatic engorgement, and dependent edema. Exertional fatigue and dyspnea are common complications. Thickening of the pericardium is seen on echocardiography or a computed tomography (CT) scan.

Clients with acute pericarditis may have an elevated white blood cell count and usually have a fever. Therefore blood culture and sensitivity may be analyzed in the laboratory. The electrocardiogram (ECG) usually shows ST-T spiking with the onset of inflammation, which returns to baseline with treatment. Atrial fibrillation is also common. Echocardiograms may be used to determine a pericardial effusion.

Interventions

The client with acute pericarditis may be hospitalized for diagnostic evaluation, observation for complications, and symptom relief. The health care provider usually prescribes nonsteroidal anti-inflammatory drugs (NSAIDs) for the relief of pain. Clients who do not obtain pain relief within 48 to 96 hours and who do not have bacterial pericarditis may receive corticosteroid therapy. The nurse assesses for pain relief and assists the client to assume positions of comfort—usually sitting upright and leaning slightly forward. If the pain is not relieved within 24 to 48 hours, the nurse notifies the primary care provider.

The various causes of pericarditis require specific therapies. For example, bacterial pericarditis (acute) usually requires antibiotics and pericardial drainage. The usual clinical course of acute pericarditis is short term (2 to 6 weeks), but episodes may recur. Chronic pericarditis caused by malignant disease may be treated with radiation or chemotherapy, whereas uremic pericarditis is treated by hemodialysis.

The definitive treatment for chronic constrictive pericarditis is surgical excision of the pericardium **(pericardiectomy).**

Monitoring for Complications of Pericarditis. A significant complication of pericarditis is pericardial effusion, which occurs when the space between the parietal and

CHART 38-11

BEST PRACTICE for
Care of the Client with Pericarditis

- Assess the nature of the client's chest discomfort. (Pericardial pain is typically substernal; it is worse on inspiration and decreases when the client leans forward.)
- Auscultate for a pericardial friction rub.
- Assist the client to a position of comfort.
- Provide anti-inflammatory agents as prescribed.
- Explain that anti-inflammatory agents usually decrease the pain within 48 hours.
- Avoid the administration of aspirin and anticoagulants because these may increase the possibility of tamponade.
- Auscultate the blood pressure carefully to detect paradoxical blood pressure (pulsus paradoxus), a sign of tamponade.
  - Palpate the blood pressure and inflate the cuff above the systolic pressure.
  - Deflate the cuff gradually, and note when sounds are first audible on expiration.
  - Identify when sounds are also audible on inspiration.
  - Subtract the inspiratory pressure from the expiratory pressure to determine the amount of pulsus paradoxus (>10 mm Hg is an indication of tamponade).
- Inspect for other indications of tamponade, including jugular venous distention with clear lungs, muffled heart sounds, and decreased cardiac output.
- Notify the physician if tamponade is suspected.

visceral layers of the pericardium fills with fluid. Pericardial effusion puts the client at risk for cardiac tamponade, or excessive fluid within the pericardial cavity. Tamponade, which occurs in 15% of clients with acute pericarditis, restricts diastolic ventricular filling, and cardiac output drops. Findings of cardiac tamponade include the following:

- Jugular venous distention
- Paradoxical pulse (systolic blood pressure 10 mm Hg higher or more on expiration than on inspiration) (Chart 38-11)
- Decreased cardiac output
- Muffled heart sounds
- Circulatory collapse

Emergency Care: Acute Cardiac Tamponade. **Acute cardiac tamponade** may occur when small volumes (20 to 50 mL) of fluid accumulate rapidly in the pericardium. If the fluid accumulates slowly, the pericardium may stretch to accommodate several hundred milliliters of fluid. Report any suspicion of this complication to the physician immediately. *Cardiac tamponade is an emergency!* The physician may initially manage the decreased cardiac output (CO) with increased fluid volume administration while awaiting a chest x-ray or echocardiogram to confirm the diagnosis. Unfortunately, these tests are not always helpful because the fluid volume around the heart may be too small to visualize. Hemodynamic monitoring in a specialized critical care unit usually demonstrates compression of the heart, with all pressures (right atrial, pulmonary artery, and wedge) being similar and elevated (plateau pressures).

The physician may elect to perform a **pericardiocentesis** to relieve the pressure on the heart. Under echocardiographic or fluoroscopic and hemodynamic monitoring, the cardiologist inserts an 8-inch (20.3-cm), 16- or 18-gauge pericardial needle into the pericardial space. The physician and the nurse monitor the needle's position, recognizing that ST-wave and T-wave changes indicate myocardial injury and that the needle must be withdrawn slightly. When the needle is properly positioned, a catheter is inserted and all available pericardial fluid is withdrawn. Monitor the pulmonary artery, wedge, and right atrial pressures during the procedure. The pressures should return to normal as the fluid compressing the heart is removed, and the clinical manifestations of tamponade should resolve. In situations in which the cause of the effusion is unknown, pericardial fluid specimens may be sent to the laboratory for cell count, culture and sensitivity tests, and cytology.

After the pericardiocentesis, closely monitor the client for the recurrence of tamponade. Pericardiocentesis alone often does not resolve acute tamponade. Be prepared to provide adequate fluid volumes to increase CO and to prepare the client for emergency sternotomy if tamponade recurs.

If the client experiences a recurrence of tamponade or recurrent effusions or adhesions from chronic pericarditis, a portion or all of the pericardium may need to be removed to allow adequate ventricular filling and contraction. The surgeon may perform creation of a pericardial window, which involves removing a portion of the pericardium to permit excessive pericardial fluid to drain into the pleural space. In more severe cases, removal of the toughened encasing pericardium (pericardiectomy) may be necessary.

Rheumatic Carditis

PATHOPHYSIOLOGY

Rheumatic carditis, also called *rheumatic endocarditis,* is a sensitivity response that develops after an upper respiratory tract infection with group A beta-hemolytic streptococci, which occurs in about 40% of clients with rheumatic fever and affects more than one million Americans. The precise mechanism by which the infection causes inflammatory lesions in the heart is not established; however, inflammation is evident in all layers of the heart. The inflammation results in impaired contractile function of the myocardium, thickening of the pericardium, and valvular damage.

Rheumatic carditis is characterized by the formation of Aschoff's bodies, small nodules in the myocardium that are replaced by scar tissue. A diffuse cellular infiltrate also develops and appears to be responsible for the HF. The pericardium becomes thickened and covered with exudate, and a serosanguineous pleural effusion may develop. The most serious damage occurs to the endocardium, with inflammation of the valve leaflets developing. Hemorrhagic and fibrous lesions form along the inflamed surfaces of the valves, resulting in stenosis or regurgitation primarily of the mitral and aortic valves.

Rheumatic fever is a complication of about 3% of group A beta-hemolytic throat infections. Although the primary attacks occur most often in childhood, rheumatic fever may occur in adulthood. The incidence of rheumatic carditis had been decreasing consistently until the mid-1980s. At that time, a resurgence of rheumatic fever began in both the United States and Europe.

COLLABORATIVE MANAGEMENT

Rheumatic carditis is one of the major indicators of rheumatic fever. The following are common clinical manifestations:

- Tachycardia
- Cardiomegaly

- Development of a new murmur or a change in an existing murmur
- Pericardial friction rub
- Precordial pain
- Electrocardiogram (ECG) changes (prolonged PR interval)
- Indications of heart failure (HF)
- Evidence of an existing streptococcal infection

Primary prevention is extremely important. Teach all clients to consult their health care providers and receive appropriate antibiotic therapy if they develop the following indications of streptococcal pharyngitis: moderate to high fever, abrupt onset of a sore throat, a reddened throat with exudate, and enlarged and tender lymph nodes. Penicillin is the antibiotic of choice for treatment. Erythromycin (Eryc, Erythromid✱) is the alternative for penicillin-sensitive clients.

The signs of rheumatic carditis must be recognized promptly, and antibiotic therapy must be instituted immediately for secondary prevention. The client is urged to continue the antibiotic administration for the full 10 days to prevent reinfection. Suggest ways to manage the fever, such as maintaining hydration and administering antipyretics. Encourage the client to obtain adequate rest.

Emphasize tertiary prevention in client education, explaining that a recurrence of rheumatic carditis is probable with reinfection by streptococcus. Thus antibiotic therapy is essential for streptococcal infection. Antibiotic prophylaxis is necessary for the rest of his or her life to prevent infective endocarditis (see Infective Endocarditis, p. 768).

CARDIOMYOPATHY

Cardiomyopathy is a subacute or chronic disease of cardiac muscle. It is not common, occurring in only 10 to 20 per 100,000 population and resulting in about 30,000 deaths each year in the United States. The cause is usually unknown.

Cardiomyopathies are classified into three categories on the basis of abnormalities in structure and function: dilated cardiomyopathy, hypertrophic cardiomyopathy, and restrictive cardiomyopathy (Table 38-3).

Dilated Cardiomyopathy

Dilated cardiomyopathy (DCM) is the structural abnormality in 87% of cardiomyopathy cases. DCM involves extensive damage to the myofibrils and interference with myocardial metabolism. There is normal ventricular wall thickness but a dilation of both ventricles and impairment of systolic function. Decreased CO from inadequate pumping of the heart causes the client to experience dyspnea on exertion, decreased exercise capacity, fatigue, and palpitations. With the exception of peripartum cardiomyopathy, DCM is twice as common in men as in women and occurs most often in middle age. Causes may include alcohol abuse and chemotherapy.

Hypertrophic Cardiomyopathy

The cardinal features of **hypertrophic cardiomyopathy (HCM)** are asymmetric ventricular hypertrophy and disarray of the myocardial fibers. Left ventricular hypertrophy leads to a stiff left ventricle that results in diastolic filling abnormalities. Obstruction in the left ventricular outflow tract is seen in 75% to 80% of clients with HCM. In about 50% of clients, HCM is transmitted as a single-gene autosomal dominant trait. The American Heart Association (2002) reports that about 36% of young athletes who die suddenly probably had hypertrophic cardiomyopathy.

Restrictive Cardiomyopathy

Restrictive cardiomyopathy, the rarest of the three cardiomyopathies, results in restriction of filling of the ventricles. It is caused by endocardial or myocardial disease and produces a clinical picture similar to that of constrictive pericarditis.

◆COLLABORATIVE MANAGEMENT

◆Assessment

Findings in cardiomyopathy depend on the structural and functional abnormalities. Left ventricular or biventricular failure is characteristic of *dilated* cardiomyopathy (DCM). Some clients with DCM are asymptomatic for months to years and have left ventricular dilation confirmed on x-ray examination. Other clients experience sudden, pronounced symptoms of left ventricular failure, such as progressive dyspnea on exertion, orthopnea, palpitations, and activity intolerance. Right-sided HF develops late in the disease and is associated with a poor prognosis. Atrial fibrillation occurs in 25% of clients and is associated with embolism.

The clinical picture of *hypertrophic* cardiomyopathy (HCM) results from the hypertrophied septum, which in 80% of cases causes a mechanical obstruction and thereby reduces stroke volume (SV) and CO. Most clients are asymptomatic until late adolescence or early adulthood. The primary symptoms of HCM are exertional dyspnea (90% of clients), angina (75% of clients), and syncope. The chest pain is atypical in that it usually occurs at rest, is prolonged, has no relation to exertion, and is not relieved by the administration of nitrates. A high incidence of ventricular dysrhythmias is associated with HCM. Sudden death occurs and may be the first manifestation of the disease.

The earliest clinical finding in *restrictive* cardiomyopathy is exertional dyspnea. CO cannot increase during periods of exertion because of the fixed ventricular volume. The client also reports weakness, exercise intolerance, palpitations, and syncope.

Echocardiography, radionuclide imaging, and angiocardiography during cardiac catheterization are performed to diagnose and differentiate cardiomyopathies.

◆Interventions

The treatment of choice for the client with cardiomyopathy varies with the type of cardiomyopathy and may include both medical and surgical interventions.

NONSURGICAL MANAGEMENT. The care of clients with dilated or restrictive cardiomyopathy is initially the same as for HF. Drug therapy includes the use of diuretics, vasodilating agents, and cardiac glycosides to increase CO. Because clients are at risk for sudden death, the nurse urges them to report any palpitations, dizziness, or fainting, which might indicate a dysrhythmia. Antidysrhythmic drugs or implantable cardiac defibrillators may be used to control life-threatening dysrhythmias. To block inappropriate sympathetic stimulation and tachycardia, beta blockers (e.g., metoprolol) are used. If cardiomyopathy has developed in response to a toxin, further exposure to that

TABLE 38-3 Pathophysiology, Signs and Symptoms, and Treatment of Cardiomyopathies

	Hypertrophic Cardiomyopathy		
Dilated Cardiomyopathy	**Nonobstructed**	**Obstructed**	**Restrictive Cardiomyopathy**
Pathophysiology			
Fibrosis of myocardium and endocardium Dilated chambers Mural wall thrombi prevalent	Hypertrophy of all walls Hypertrophied septum Relatively small chamber size	Same as for nonobstructed except for obstruction of left ventricular outflow tract associated with the hypertrophied septum and mitral valve incompetence	Mimics constrictive pericarditis Fibrosed walls cannot expand or contract Chambers narrowed; emboli common
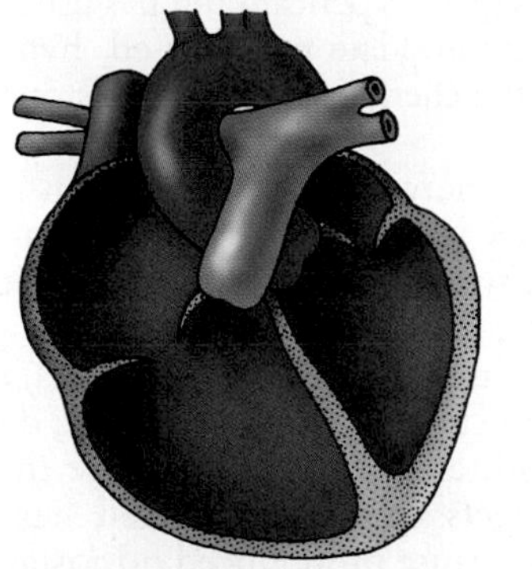		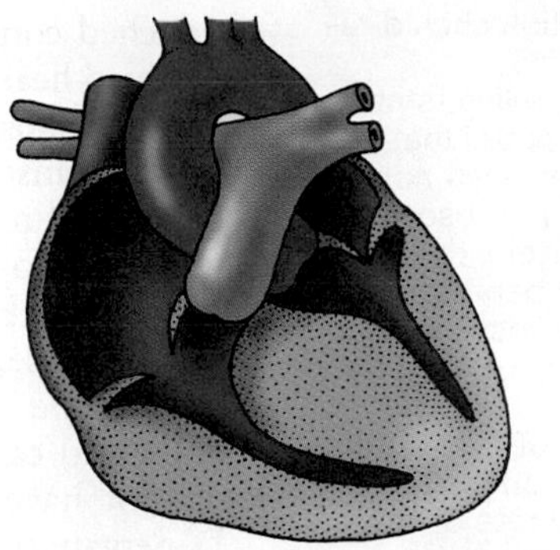	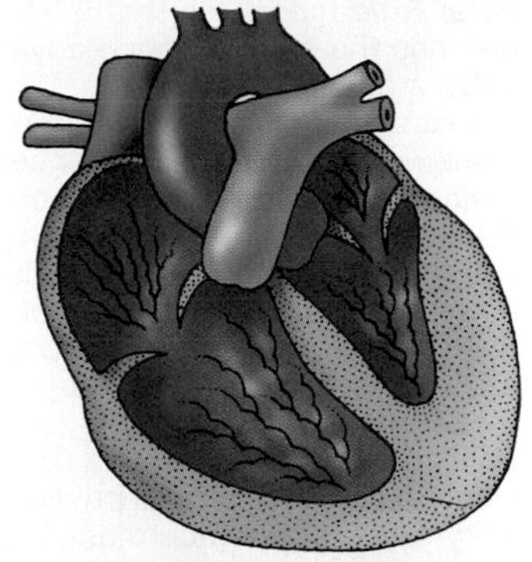
Signs and Symptoms			
Fatigue and weakness Heart failure (left side) Dysrhythmias or heart block Systemic or pulmonary emboli S_3 and S_4 gallops Moderate to severe cardiomegaly	Dyspnea Angina Fatigue, syncope, palpitations Mild cardiomegaly S_4 gallop Ventricular dysrhythmias Sudden death common Heart failure	Same as for nonobstructed except with mitral regurgitation murmur Atrial fibrillation	Dyspnea and fatigue Heart failure (right-sided) Mild to moderate cardiomegaly S_3 and S_4 gallops Heart block Emboli
Treatment			
Symptomatic treatment of heart failure Vasodilators Control of dysrhythmias Surgery: heart transplant	For both: Symptomatic treatment Beta blockers Conversion of atrial fibrillation Surgery: ventriculomyotomy or muscle resection with mitral valve replacement Digitalis, nitrates, and other vasodilators **contraindicated** with the obstructed form		Supportive treatment of symptoms Treatment of hypertension Conversion from dysrhythmias Exercise restrictions Emergency treatment of acute pulmonary edema

Data from Wynne, J., & Braunwald, E. (1992). The cardiomyopathies and myocarditis. In E. Braunwald (Ed.), *Heart disease: A textbook of cardiovascular medicine* (3rd ed.). Philadelphia: W.B. Saunders.

toxin must be avoided. Alcohol ingestion causes cardiac depressant effects and must also be avoided.

Management of obstructive HCM includes administering negative inotropic agents such as beta-adrenergic blocking agents (carvedilol) and calcium antagonists (diltiazem). They decrease the outflow obstruction that accompanies exercise and also decrease HR, resulting in less angina, dyspnea, and syncope. Vasodilators and cardiac glycosides are contraindicated in clients with obstructive HCM because vasodilating and positive inotropic effects may augment the obstruction. Strenuous exercise is also prohibited because it can increase the risk of sudden death.

SURGICAL MANAGEMENT. The type of surgery performed depends on the type of cardiomyopathy.

Excision of Hypertrophied Septum. Surgery may be considered for the small percentage of clients with obstructive HCM who do not respond to medical therapy. The most commonly used surgical treatment **(ventriculomyomectomy)** includes excising a portion of the hypertrophied ventricular septum to create a widened outflow tract. Surgery results in long-term improvement in exercise tolerance in most clients with HCM.

Cardiomyoplasty. Cardiomyoplasty is used when cardiac transplantation is not as option and the client is asymptomatic at rest. The latissimus dorsum muscle is dissected free of its distal insertion and is wrapped around the heart. For the next 2 months, the muscle is stimulated with increasing frequency until it can contract in synchrony with each heartbeat. Six months after surgery, effects of an enhanced cardiac output should be evident. This procedure has produced poor results.

Heart Transplantation. Heart transplantation is the treatment of choice for clients with severe DCM and may be considered for clients with restrictive cardiomyopathy.

LEGAL/ETHICAL ISSUES

TO WHOM SHOULD DONATED HEARTS BE ALLOCATED FOR TRANSPLANTATION?

In 2001, 4096 Americans were waiting for a heart transplant; however, only about 2200 heart transplants are performed each year because of a limited number of donor hearts. In the past, human organ allocation was both by recipient need and by region of the country. The Department of Health and Human Services (DHHS) has created the ***Final Rule,*** which mandates standardized criteria for placing clients on a transplantation list for defining a client's medical status. In addition, the ***Final Rule*** mandates that the person who is the best match and has the greatest need anywhere in the nation should receive a donated heart.

Critics temporarily blocked enactment of the ruling, stating there were serious ethical concerns. First, they noted that donating the heart to the most critically ill person does not always represent good stewardship of resources. In subsequent clarification, DHHS stated, "It is not the Department's intention to require transplantation of clients too ill to benefit; the final rule specifically prohibits policies that might result in such futile transplantations and organ wastage" (*Federal Register,* 42 CFR Part 121).

Critics also argued that a national allocation of transplants would result in less local publicity about transplant recipients. They expressed concern about the already low rate of donations when people are unable to perceive an immediate and local benefit. They feared that only the largest urban transplant centers would survive and that donation rates would drop still further, worsening the scarcity. DHHS responded by recognizing medical factors affecting organ movement, such as the limits of ischemic time. DHHS implemented a monitoring program to ensure that small and medium-sized transplant centers were not adversely affected by the final rule. Closure of such centers can adversely affect client access to transplant services.

The question of how best to allocate donated hearts remains controversial. Should donated hearts be allocated to the sickest person in the nation who is a match? Should the heart be provided to a person who lives in the region, matches the donor, and is most likely to benefit? What are the criteria for benefit? The ethical issue is, How do we decide what is a just or fair way to distribute scarce health care resources? Do we distribute to the person with the greatest need or to the person who is most likely to benefit? Should concerns about how to secure a continuing supply of the scarce resource deserve consideration when deciding how to allocate the resource?

Each year about 2300 clients in the United States receive cardiac transplants, most for DCM (see the Legal/Ethical Issues box above).

Preoperative Care. Criteria for candidate selection include the following:

- Life expectancy less than 1 year
- Age generally less than 65 years
- New York Heart Association (NYHA) class III or IV
- Normal or only slightly increased pulmonary vascular resistance
- Absence of active infection
- Stable psychosocial status
- No evidence of drug or alcohol abuse

Once the candidate is eligible and a heart is available, provide preoperative care as described in Chapter 20.

Operative Procedures. The surgeon transplants a heart from a donor with a comparable body weight and ABO compatibility into a recipient less than 6 hours after procurement. In the most common procedure **(orthotopic transplantation),** the surgeon removes the diseased heart and leaves the posterior walls of the client's atria. The remnant atria serve as the anchor for the donor heart. Anastomoses are made between the recipient and donor atria, aorta, and pulmonary arteries (Figure 38-3). Because the remaining remnant of the recipient's atria contains the sinoatrial node, two unrelated P waves are visible on the ECG.

Postoperative Care. The postoperative care of the heart transplant recipient is similar to that for conventional cardiac surgery; however, the nurse must be especially vigilant to identify occult bleeding into the pericardial sac with the potential for tamponade. The recipient's pericardium has usually stretched considerably to accommodate the diseased, hypertrophied heart, predisposing the client to concealed postoperative bleeding.

The transplanted heart is denervated and is unresponsive to vagal stimulation. The HR is about 100 beats/min and responds slowly to exercise, stress, or position change with increases in HR, contractility, and CO. In the early postoperative phase, the nurse may titrate isoproterenol (Isuprel) to support the HR and maintain cardiac output. Atropine, digitalis, and carotid sinus pressure are not used because they do not have their usual effects on the denervated heart. Denervation of the heart may cause pronounced orthostatic hypotension in the immediate postoperative phase, and the nurse cautions the client to change position slowly. Some clients also require a permanent pacemaker that is rate responsive to the client's activity level. The purpose is to increase CO and improve activity tolerance.

To suppress natural defense mechanisms (especially T- and B-cell function) and prevent transplant rejection, clients require immunosuppressants for the rest of their lives. The foundation of immunosuppressant therapy is large doses of glucocorticoids, such as methylprednisolone (Solu-Medrol) combined with several other drugs. These include monoclonal antibodies (such as OKT 3), tacrolimus (Prograf), and mycophenolate (CellCept). Nurses must be vigilant about handwashing and aseptic technique because clients are immunosuppressed and infection is the major cause of death. Infection usually develops in the immediate post-transplant period or during treatment for acute rejection.

Most clients experience their initial episode of acute rejection in the first 3 months after heart transplantation. Symptoms of rejection are often nonspecific and occur late in the rejection process. They include cardiac dysrhythmias (especially atrial dysrhythmias), hypotension, weakness, fatigue, and dizziness. To detect rejection, the surgeon performs right endomyocardial biopsies at regularly scheduled intervals and whenever symptoms occur.

About 75% of clients survive 3 years after transplantation; most return to NYHA class I or II status (AHA, 1998). Five years after transplantation, many of the surviving clients (20% to 40%) have a form of coronary artery disease (CAD) called **coronary artery vasculopathy (CAV),** which presents as diffuse plaque in the arteries of the donor heart. Because the heart is denervated, clients do not usually experience angina, and regularly scheduled exercise tolerance tests and angiography are required to identify CAV.

To delay the development of CAV, clients are encouraged to follow a prudent lifestyle similar to clients with CAD (see Chapter 41). The physician may prescribe a calcium channel blocker such as diltiazem (Cardizem) to prevent coronary

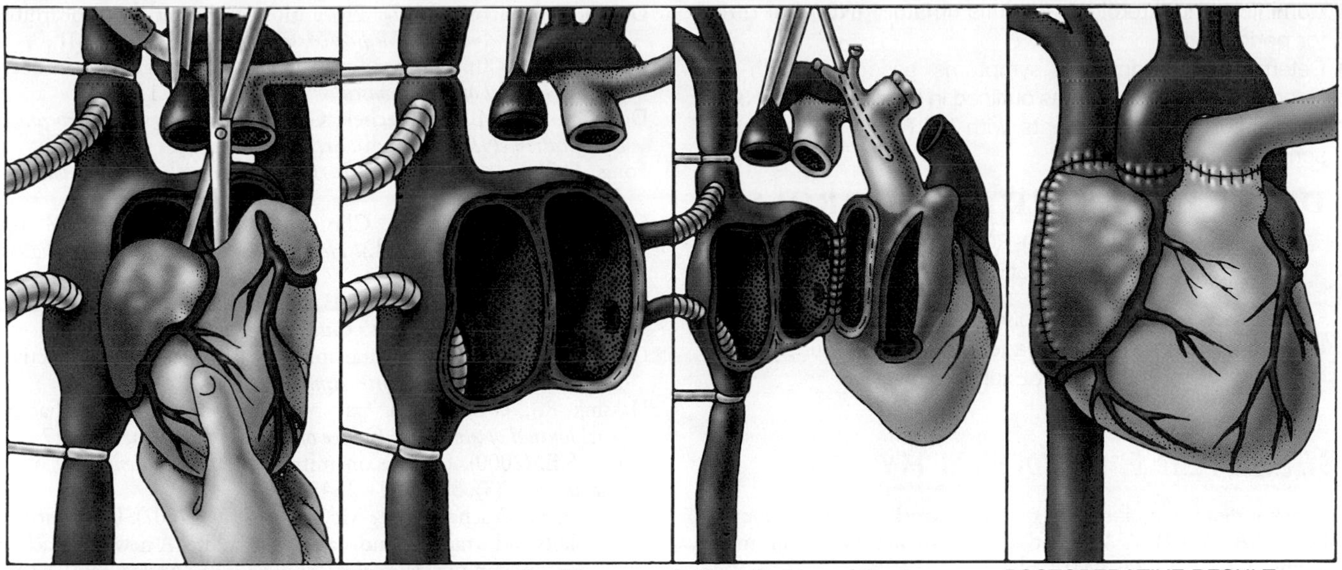

1. After the recipient is placed on cardiopulmonary bypass, the heart is removed.
2. The posterior walls of the recipient's left and right atria are left intact.
3. The left atrium of the donor heart is anastomosed to the recipient's residual posterior atrial walls, and the other atrial walls, the atrial septum, and the great vessels are joined.

POSTOPERATIVE RESULT

Figure 38-3 ■ Heart transplantation.

spasm and closure. Stress the importance of compliance with dietary modifications and medication regimens. The client is encouraged to participate in a regular exercise program but is cautioned to allow at least 10 minutes of warm up and cool down for the denervated heart to adjust to changes in activity level.

GET READY for the NCLEX Examination!

KEY POINTS

Safe Effective Care Environment

- Monitor the HF client on beta-blockers carefully for hypotension and bradycardia.
- Monitor the pulse of clients taking digitalis preparations before administration, and report a pulse that is not within the desired parameters to the health care provider.
- Monitor for evidence of digitalis toxicity, especially in older clients or in clients with known renal dysfunction (see Chart 38-7).
- Administer long-term antibiotic therapy to clients with valvular disease or cardiac infections.

Health Promotion and Maintenance

- Teach the HF client about a low sodium diet.
- In collaboration with the health care team, teach the HF client to exercise at least 10 minutes 3 to 5 times per week. Have them monitor their pulse and blood pressure. HR should remain within 20 beats/min and BP within 20 mm Hg of baseline.
- Teach clients taking ACE inhibitors to change positions slowly to avoid orthostatic hypotension.
- Teach clients the importance of avoiding respiratory or other infections.
- List foods high in potassium if the client is hypokalemic.
- Teach the client with valvular dysfunction, cardiac infection, or cardiomyopathy the necessity of taking preventive antibiotic therapy before any invasive procedure.

Psychosocial Integrity

- Assess the client for depression resulting from altered self-concept and anxiety.
- Assess the client's coping skills.
- Help the client with strategies for home maintenance to balance rest and activity.
- Help the client develop strategies to manage complex medication regimens.

Physiological Integrity

- Assess the client for symptoms of hypokalemia or hyperkalemia.
- Weigh daily and record.
- Assess for early signs and symptoms of pulmonary edema (e.g., crackles in the lung bases, dyspnea at rest, disorientation, confusion), especially in older adults.
- Assess for symptoms of worsening HF: rapid weight gain (3 pounds in a week), a decrease in exercise tolerance lasting 2 to 3 days, cold symptoms (cough) lasting more than 3 to 5 days, nocturia, development of dyspnea or angina at rest, or unstable angina.
- Monitor the client with valvular dysfunction for atrial fibrillation, which may lead to hemostasis and mural thrombi. Monitor for an irregularly irregular cardiac rhythm and administer warfarin as indicated.
- Assess neurovascular status regularly because emboli may cause strokes.

- Administer nonsteroidal anti-inflammatory (NSAIDs) drugs for pericarditis.
- Determine the signs and symptoms associated with left-sided and right-sided HF as outlined in Charts 38-1 and 38-2.
- Administer drugs for clients with HF (Table 38-2) as prescribed.

ADDITIONAL STUDY RESOURCES

Go to your Student CD-ROM for Review Questions for the NCLEX Examination.

evolve Go to http://evolve.elsevier.com/Iggy/ for Integrated Management of Care Questions for the NCLEX Examination.

SELECTED BIBLIOGRAPHY

Asterisk indicates a classic or definitive work on this subject.

Albert, N.A. (2004). A "current" choice for hemodynamic monitoring. *Nursing 2004, 34*(10), 58-60.

Alderman, L.M. (2000). Congenital heart disease: More than child's play. *Nursing 2000, 30*(5), 41-47.

American Heart Association. (2002). *Heart disease and stroke statistics–2003 update.* Dallas, Texas: American Heart Association.

Ammon, S. (2001). Managing patients with heart failure. *American Journal of Nursing, 101*(12), 34-40.

Artinian, N.T. (2003). The psychosocial aspects of heart failure. *American Journal of Nursing, 103*(12), 32-42.

Augustine, S.M. (2000). Heart transplantation: Long-term management related to immunosuppression, complications, and psychosocial adjustments. *Critical Care Clinics of North America, 12*(1),79-85.

Ayers, D.M.M. (2004). Heart failure. *Nursing 2004, 34*(11), 46-47.

Baker, S., & Graziano, J. (2003). A new device for heart failure. *RN, 66*(3), 32-36.

Bither, C. J., & Apple, S. (2001). Home management of the failing heart. *American Journal of Nursing, 101*(12): 41-47.

Bollinger, K., & Sadar, A.M. (2003). Care and management of the patient with right heart failure secondary to diastolic dysfunction: an advanced practice perspective and case review. *Critical Care Nursing Quarterly, 26*(1), 22-27.

Bond, A.E., et al. (2003). The left ventricular assist device. *American Journal of Nursing, 103*(1), 32-41.

Bosen, D.M. (2003). New strategies for treating patients with heart failure. *Nursing 2003, 33*(12), 44-47.

Buffolo, E., et al. (2003). End-stage cardiomyopathy and secondary mitral insufficiency surgical alternative with prosthesis implant and left-ventricular remodeling. *Journal of Cardiovascular Surgery, 18*(3): 201-205.

Carelock, J., & Clark, A.P. (2003). Heart failure: Pathophysiologic mechanisms. *American Journal of Nursing,* 101(12), 26-35.

Chachques, L.F., et al. (2003). Right ventricular cardiomyopathies: 10 year follow-up. *Annals of Thoracic Surgery, 75*(5), 1464-1468.

Christensen, D.M. (Fall 2004). Managing heart failure: What you need to know. *Med/Surg Insider,* 4-10.

Colbert, K., & Greene, M.H. (2003). Nesiritide (Natrecor): A new treatment for acutely decompensated congestive heart failure. *Critical Care Nursing Quarterly, 26*(1), 40-44.

Coughlin, A.M.C. (2004). Pump away with EECP. *Nursing 2004, 34*(1), 48-49.

Cupples, S.A., & Spruill, L.C. (2000). Evaluation criteria for the pretransplant patient. *Critical Care Clinics of North America, 12*(1), 37-47.

Dahl, J., & Penque, S. (2000). The effects of an advanced practice nurse-directed heart failure program. *Nurse Practitioner, 25*(3), 61-62, 65-66, 68.

*Dajani, A.S., et al. (1997). Prevention of bacterial endocarditis. *Journal of the American Medical Association, 277,* 1794-1801.

Deaton, C. (2000). Outcome measures: self-management in heart failure. *Journal of Cardiovascular Nursing, 14*(4), 116-118.

Dochterman, J.M., & Bulechek, G.M. (2004). *Nursing interventions classification (NIC)* (4th ed.). St. Louis: Mosby.

Fong, H.H.S., & Bauman, J.L. (2002). *Journal of Cardiovascular Nursing,* 16(4), 1-8.

Givertz, M., et al. (2001). Clinical aspects of heart failure (pp. 531-561). In P. Libby (Ed.). *Heart disease: A textbook of cardiovascular medicine.* Philadelphia: W.B. Saunders.

Gorski, L.A., & Johnson, K. (2003). A disease management program for heart failure. *Lippincott's Case Management, 8*(6), 265-273.

Guido, G.W. (2000). Heart transplant from an ethical perspective. *Critical Care Clinics of North America, 12*(1), 111-119.

Hassink, R.J., et al. (2003). Transplantation of cells for cardiac repair. *Journal of American College of Cardiology, 41*(5), 711-717.

Hines, S.E. (2000). Update on mitral prolapse. *Patient Care Nurse Practitioner, 3*(3), 37-37, 41-42, 45-46.

Hoercher, K.J., Vacha, C.J., & McCarthy, P. M. (2002). Left ventricular splints and wraps for end-stage heart failure: A new approach in the new millennium. *Journal of Cardiovascular Nursing, 16*(3), 82-86.

Hussey, C., Hardin, S., & Bla, C. (2002). Outpatient costs of medications for patients with chronic heart failure. *American Journal of Critical Care, 11*(5), 474-478.

Katz, A.M. (2003). Pathophysiology of heart failure: identifying targets for pharmacotherapy. *Medical Clinics of North America, 87*(2), 303-316.

Kearney, K. (2000). Emergency: Digitalis toxicity. *American Journal of Nursing, 100*(6), 51-52.

Khai, P.G., et al. (2000). Infective endocarditis. In T. Nguyen, et al. (Eds.). *Management of complex cardiovascular problems* (pp. 237-250). Armonk, NY: Futura Publishing.

Konick-McMahan, J., Bixby, J., & McKenna, C. (2003). Heart failure in older adults: Providing nursing care to improve outcomes. *Journal of Gerontological Nursing, 29*(12), 35-41.

Krau, S.D. (2000). The evolution of heart transplant. *Critical Care Clinics of North America, 12*(1), 1-9.

Levine, B.S. (2000). Intermittent positive inotrope infusion in the management of end-stage, low-output heart failure. *Journal of Cardiovascular Nursing, 14*(4): 76-93.

Liehr, P., et al. (2003). Addressing current challenges to cardiac rehabilitation care. *AACN Clinical Issues, 14*(1), 13-24.

Lindsey, M. R. (2003). Transmyocardial laser revascularization revisited. *Critical Care Nursing Quarterly, 26*(1), 69-75.

Martin, T. (2003). How heart failure complicates care. *Nursing Management, 34*(5), 27-32.

McCance, K.L., & Huether, S.E. (2002). *Pathophysiology: The biologic basis for disease in adults and children.* (4th ed.). St. Louis: Mosby.

Metra, M., et al. (2003). Marked improvement in left ventricular ejection fraction during long-term beta-blockade in patients with chronic heart failure: clinical correlates and prognostic significance. *American Heart Journal, 145*(2), 292-299.

Milfred-LaForest, S.K. (2000). Pharmacotherapy of systolic heart failure: A review of recent literature and practical applications, *Journal of Cardiovascular Nursing, 14*(4), 57-75.

Morbidity and mortality: 2002 chart book on cardiovascular, lung, and blood diseases. National Institutes of Health, National Heart, Lung, and Blood Institute.

Paul, S. (2000). Impact of a nurse-managed heart failure clinic: A pilot study. *American Journal of Critical Care, 9*(2), 140-146.

Popjes, E.D., & St. John Sutton, M. (2003). Hypertrophic cardiomyopathy. Pathophysiology, diagnosis, and treatment, *Geriatrics, 58*(3), 41-46.

Reeder, D.E., et al. (2000). The impact of angiotensin-converting enzyme inhibitors on managed care: Economic, clinical, and humanistic outcomes. *American Journal of Managed Care, 6*(3 Suppl), S112-131.

*Ritchie, J.L., et al. (1998). *ACC/AHA Guidelines for the management of patients with valvular heart disease–II. General principles: A report of the American College of Cardiology/American Heart Association Task Force on Practice Guidelines (Committee on Management of Patients with Valvular Heart Disease).* American Heart Association. Available at http://www.americanheart.org/reports.

Sanderson, J.E. (2000). Heart failure. In T. Nguyen, et al. (Eds.). *Management of complex cardiovascular problems* (pp. 237-250). Armonk, NY: Futura Publishing.

Saul, L., & Shatzer, M. (2003). B-type natriuretic peptide testing for detection of heart failure. *Critical Care Nursing Quarterly, 26*(1), 37-39.

Schall, M.B., & Flannery, J. (2004). Undertreatment of women with heart failure: A reversible outcome on hospital readmission. *Lippincott's Case Management: The Journal for Professional Practice, 9*(6), 250-253.

Sherrid M.V., Chaudhry, F.A., & Swistel, D.G. (2003). Obstructive hypertrophic cardiomyopathy: echocardiography, pathophysiology, and the continuing evolution of surgery for obstruction. *Annals of Thoracic Surgery, 75*(2), 620-632.

Smith, A.L., & Brown, C.S. (2003). New advances and novel treatments in heart failure. *Critical Care Nursing Quarterly, 26*(2), 3-15.

Strimike, C.L., & Wojcik, J. (2000). Getting the facts on heart failure treatment. *Nursing 2000, 30*(5), 32hn18-32hn20.

Tarolli, K.A. (2003). Left ventricular systolic dysfunction and nonischemic cardiomyopathy. *Critical Care Nursing Quarterly, 26*(1), 3-15.

Tasota, F.J., & Tate, J. (2000). Assessing digoxin levels. *Nursing 2000, 30*(3), 24.

Tedesco, C., Reigle, J., & Bergin, J. (2000). Sudden cardiac death in heart failure. *Journal of Cardiovascular Nursing, 14*(4), 40-56.

Tokarczyk, T.R. (2003). Cardiac transplantation as a treatment option for the heart failure patient. *Critical Care Nursing Quarterly,* 26(1), 61-68.

Wisniewski, A. (2004). Muscle up your knowledge of myocarditis. *Nursing 2004, 34*(10), 17.

Young, J.B. (2003). Combined cardiac resynchronization and implantable cardioversion defibrillation in advanced chronic heart failure: The MIRACLE ICD trial. *The Journal of the American Medical Association,* 189(20), 1003.

CHAPTER

39 Interventions for Clients with Vascular Problems

DEANNE A. BLACH • DONNA D. IGNATAVICIUS

LEARNING OUTCOMES

After studying this chapter, you should be able to:

1. Explain the pathophysiology of arteriosclerosis and atherosclerosis, including the factors that cause arterial injury.
2. Interpret essential laboratory data related to risk for atherosclerosis.
3. Discuss the role of diet therapy in the management of clients with arteriosclerosis.
4. Describe the differences between essential and secondary hypertension.
5. Develop a collaborative plan of care for a client with essential hypertension.
6. Explain the purpose, action, and nursing implications of drugs used to manage hypertension.
7. Identify cultural considerations that impact care for clients with hypertension.
8. Evaluate the effectiveness of interdisciplinary interventions to improve hypertension.
9. Compare and contrast assessment findings typically present in clients with peripheral arterial and peripheral venous disease.
10. Prioritize postoperative care for clients who have undergone peripheral bypass surgery.
11. Assess clients at risk for venous thromboembolism (VTE) and identify when VTE occurs.
12. Describe nursing interventions used to help prevent venous thromboembolism (VTE).
13. Describe the nurse's role in monitoring clients who are receiving anticoagulants.
14. Develop a continuing care plan for a client who has undergone an abdominal aortic aneurysm repair.
15. Compare and contrast Raynaud's and Buerger's disease.
16. Identify evidence-based practice for care of clients with venous leg ulcers.

Go to your Student CD-ROM for Review Questions for the NCLEX Examination keyed to these Learning Outcomes.

Disease associated with atherosclerosis is the leading cause of death in the United States. More than 1 million people die of heart and blood vessel diseases each year in the United States (American Heart Association, 2003). Atherosclerosis is often a major risk factor for cardiovascular disease, cerebrovascular disease, and peripheral vascular disease (PVD). People with atherosclerosis have an increased risk of developing one or more of these diseases.

Disorders of the vascular system cause many problems and may lead to complete shutdown of all body organs and eventually death. Although vascular disease can affect any portion of the human body, such as the heart, brain, and kidneys, the peripheral vascular system and its associated diseases are described here.

ARTERIOSCLEROSIS AND ATHEROSCLEROSIS

PATHOPHYSIOLOGY

Arteriosclerosis is a thickening, or hardening, of the arterial wall. **Atherosclerosis,** a type of arteriosclerosis, involves the formation of plaque within the arterial wall and is the leading contributor to coronary artery and cerebrovascular disease. The exact pathophysiology of atherosclerosis is not known, but the condition is thought to occur from vascular damage (Figure 39-1). After the vessel becomes inflamed, a fatty streak appears on the intimal surface (inner lining) of the artery. At this stage, the fatty streak may appear flattened

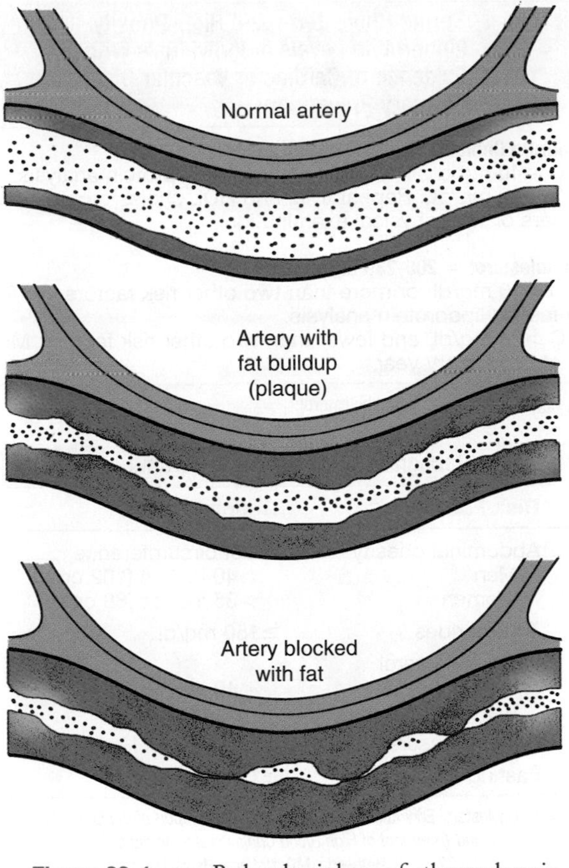

Figure 39-1 ■ Pathophysiology of atherosclerosis.

or elevated, but it generally does not affect the integrity of the arterial wall.

Next, a stable or unstable plaque develops. *Stable* plaque is a white, glistening, fibrous elevation that covers a lipid (primarily cholesterol) core. By contrast, *unstable* plaque has a liquid lipid core. At this stage, it is elevated enough to partially or completely occlude the blood flow of an artery.

In the final stage, the fibrous lesions become calcified, hemorrhagic, ulcerated, or thrombosed and affect all layers of the vessel. The rate of progression of the process may be influenced by genetic factors, certain chronic diseases (e.g., diabetes mellitus), and lifestyle habits, including smoking, eating habits, and level of exercise. When *stable* plaque ruptures, thrombosis and vasoconstriction obstruct the lumen causing inadequate perfusion to distal tissues. *Unstable* plaque rupture causes more severe damage, such as that seen in acute coronary syndrome (see Chapter 41).

Etiology and Genetic Risk

The exact etiology of atherosclerosis is unknown, but several theories attempt to explain its cause. One theory proposes that an injury to the **intimal** (innermost) **layer** of the artery may initiate the development of atherosclerosis. Another popular theory, known as platelet aggregation, proposes that after the intimal injury has occurred, platelets form a cluster at the arterial wall and produce a peptide that stimulates the proliferation of the smooth muscle cells of the intima. Eventually, this proliferation can narrow the artery enough to compromise the flow of blood or completely occlude arterial blood flow.

Another theory, the *lipid hypothesis*, assumes that after an intimal injury, a group of blood lipids (fats) accumulate. Again, fat accumulation can partially or completely occlude arterial blood flow. The principal lipids involved are cholesterol and triglyceride.

Many theorists believe that a combination of these two events provides the most appropriate explanation of the atherosclerotic process and that the process can occur in any arterial wall of the body. Usually the disease affects the larger arteries, such as the coronary artery beds, the aorta, carotid and vertebral arteries, renal, iliac, and femoral arteries, or any combination of these.

Intimal injury of the major arteries of the body can be attributed to many factors. Hypertension can cause a mechanical injury, whereas elevated levels of low-density lipoprotein cholesterol (LDL-C) and decreased levels of high-density lipoprotein cholesterol (HDL-C) can cause chemical injuries to the intimal wall. (See Chapter 36, which describes cholesterol in more detail.) Chemical injury can also be caused by elevated levels of toxins in the bloodstream, which may occur with renal failure or by carbon monoxide circulating in the bloodstream from cigarette smoking. The intimal wall can be weakened by the natural process of aging or by physiologic disorders, such as diabetes.

Genetic predisposition and diabetes have a fairly direct effect on the development of atherosclerosis. In general, studies have focused on the role of lipoproteins because of their role in the development of atherosclerosis. Some individuals have familial **hyperlipidemia,** an elevation of serum **lipid** (fat) levels. In these people, the liver makes excessive cholesterol and other fats, which accounts for the development of atherosclerosis. In some people with hereditary atherosclerosis, however, the blood cholesterol level is normal. The reason for the development and progression of plaque in these people is not understood.

Clients with severe diabetes mellitus frequently have premature and severe atherosclerosis from microvascular damage. The premature atherosclerosis occurs because diabetes promotes an increase in LDL-C and triglycerides in plasma. In addition, intimal arterial damage may result from the effect of hyperglycemia.

Factors indirectly related to atherosclerosis include obesity, a sedentary lifestyle, smoking, and stress. Clients who are obese or overweight are at greater risk, most often because of associated elevations in cholesterol levels. In general, obesity is defined as a body mass index (BMI) of greater than 30 kg/m^2, and overweight is defined as a BMI of greater than 25 kg/m^2.

CULTURAL CONSIDERATIONS

According to the American Heart Association (2003), African Americans and Hispanics have the highest percentage of people who are overweight and obese. Asian/Pacific Islanders have the smallest percentage. About two thirds of all Americans are overweight or obese.

Smoking causes vessel constriction, which decreases blood flow and tissue perfusion. African American and Native American/American Indian men smoke the most of all ethnic groups. Hispanics and Asian/Pacific Islanders smoke the least.

The causes for differences among groups are unknown. Environmental factors and genetic predisposition may help explain them.

Incidence/Prevalence

It is not known exactly how many people have atherosclerosis, but small plaques are almost always present in the arteries of young adults. The incidence can be better quantified by assessing diseases that result from atherosclerosis. Peripheral vascular disease (PVD) impacts 7 to 12 million people in the United States including many of the over-50 population (Ebersole, Hess, & Luggen, 2004). However, only 50% (5 million) have actual symptoms of the disease. Of the 2.5 million individuals diagnosed with PVD, 2.1 million are medically managed (Society of Interventional Radiology, 2003). Analysis of trends predicts that the number of people affected by atherosclerosis will increase as the population ages.

COLLABORATIVE MANAGEMENT

Assessment

PHYSICAL ASSESSMENT

Because of the high incidence of hypertension in clients with atherosclerosis, assess the blood pressure in both arms. The heart is also thoroughly assessed because associated cardiac disease is often present.

Palpate pulses at all of the major sites on the body and note any differences. Carotid arteries are palpated separately because of the risk of inadequate cerebral perfusion. Also palpate for temperature differences in the lower extremities and check capillary filling. Prolonged capillary filling (greater than 3 seconds in young to middle-aged adults; greater than 5 seconds in older adults) generally indicates poor circulation, although this indicator is not the most reliable. An extremity in a person with significant atherosclerotic disease may be cool or cold, with a diminished or absent pulse.

Many clients with vascular disease have a **bruit** in the larger arteries, which can be heard with a stethoscope or Doppler probe. A bruit is described as a turbulent, swishing sound, which can be soft or loud in pitch. The mere existence of a bruit is considered abnormal, but the role it plays in indicating the severity of vascular disease is not understood. Bruits often occur in the carotid, aortic, femoral, and popliteal arteries and usually indicate some degree of narrowing of the arterial wall. A decrease in intensity and audibility or a complete loss of a pulse may indicate an arterial occlusion.

LABORATORY ASSESSMENT

LIPID PROFILE. Clients with atherosclerosis often have elevated lipids, including cholesterol and triglycerides. Total serum cholesterol levels should be below 200 mg/dL. Elevated cholesterol levels must be validated by HDL and LDL determinations. Elevated low-density lipoprotein cholesterol (LDL-C) ("bad" cholesterol) levels indicate that a person is at an increased risk for atherosclerosis. Low high-density lipoprotein cholesterol ("good" cholesterol) (HDL-C) levels also indicate an increased risk. A desirable LDL-C level is one below 100 mg/dL for all individuals. A desirable HDL-C level is 40 mg/dL or above (Table 39-1).

WOMEN'S HEALTH CONSIDERATIONS

In some people, particularly women, an elevated cholesterol level may be due to an elevated HDL-C level, which is not considered a risk. However, the LDL-C level should also be below 100 to keep the risk of cardiovascular disease low.

TABLE 39-1 Serum Cholesterol and High-Density Lipoprotein Levels in Individuals Without Evidence of Cardiac or Vascular Disease (Primary Prevention)

Total Serum Cholesterol <200 mg/dL
HDL-C <40 mg/dL: Perform full fasting lipoprotein analysis.
HDL-C >40 mg/dL: Repeat total and HDL cholesterol testing in 5 years or with physical examination.

Total Cholesterol = 200-239 mg/dL
HDL-C <40 mg/dL or more than two other risk factors: Perform full fasting lipoprotein analysis.
HDL-C >40 mg/dL and fewer than two other risk factors: Monitor at least every year.

HDL-C, High-density lipoprotein cholesterol.

TABLE 39-2 Recognizing Metabolic Syndrome

Risk Factor	Defining Level
Abdominal obesity	Waist circumference
Men	>40 inches (102 cm)
Women	>35 inches (88 cm)
Triglycerides	≥150 mg/dL
HDL cholesterol	
Men	<40 mg/dL
Women	<50 mg/dL
Blood pressure	≥130/85 mm Hg
Fasting blood sugar	≥110 mg/dL

From National Cholesterol Education Program. (2002). *Third report of the Expert Panel on Detection, Evaluation, and Treatment of High Blood Cholesterol in Adults (Adult Treatment Panel III).* NIH Publication No. 02-5215. Bethesda, MD: National Heart, Lung, and Blood Institute.

Triglyceride levels may also be elevated with atherosclerosis and considered an emerging lipid risk factor by the Adult Treatment Panel (ATP III) Report No. 3 released by the National Heart, Lung, and Blood Institute (2002). A level of 150 mg/dL or above indicates **hypertriglyceridemia.** Elevated triglycerides are considered a marker for other atherogenic lipoproteins and an indicator for the **metabolic syndrome,** which increases the risk for coronary heart disease (Table 39-2).

HOMOCYSTEINE. Homocysteine is an essential sulfur-containing amino acid derived from dietary protein. Studies have shown a positive correlation between increased homocysteine levels and the development of peripheral vascular disease (PVD), coronary artery disease (CAD), stroke, and venous thrombosis. High serum levels of homocysteine can block production of nitric oxide on the vascular endothelium, making the cell walls less elastic and permitting plaque to build up. A serum homocysteine level greater than 15 mmol/L is considered a risk factor. Elevated homocysteine levels may be lowered by a diet enriched with B-complex vitamins, particularly folic acid. Usually, 1 mg or more of supplemental folic acid daily can improve endothelial function and lower homocysteine levels. The American Heart Association (2003) recommends homocysteine screening for high-risk clients who have a family history of premature cardiovascular disease, angina, CAD, or elevated cholesterol.

Interventions

Atherosclerosis progresses for years before clinical manifestations are evident. Adults with or at risk for atherosclerosis can often be identified through cholesterol screening and history.

Because of the high incidence of atherosclerosis in the United States, low-risk individuals 20 years of age and older are advised to have their total serum cholesterol level evaluated at least once every 5 years. More frequent measurements are suggested for individuals with multiple risk factors.

Interventions for individuals with atherosclerosis or who are at high risk for the disease focus on lifestyle changes. Teaching clients about the need for changes and how to make them is crucial. If lipoprotein levels do not improve, the health care provider prescribes medication to lower cholesterol and/or triglycerides.

Diet Therapy. The importance of nutrition should be emphasized for individuals with elevated homocysteine levels. Encourage a diet including enriched or fortified cereals that contain 100% of the daily requirement of folic acid, pyridoxine (vitamin B_6), and cyanocobalamin (vitamin B_{12}). If consumption of vegetables such as fruits, legumes, meats, fish, and fortified cereals and grains do not decrease homocysteine levels, multivitamins containing 0.4 mg of folic acid, 2 mg of pyridoxine, and 6 mcg of cyanocobalamin can be added.

Recent testing and management guidelines from the National Cholesterol Education Program (NCEP) have a major preventive focus for individuals with multiple risk factors (2002). In need of intensified lifestyle changes, these groups of high-risk clients, termed "coronary heart disease equivalents" include the following:

- Those with diabetes but without signs of vascular disease
- Individuals with a Framingham Heart Study 10-year absolute risk score of over 20% for CHD events
- Those identified with multiple metabolic risk factors

The new category groups these people at the same risk level as those who already have vascular disease. Therapeutic lifestyle change recommendations have also been broadened.

The focus of treatment remains on an aggressive approach to lowering LDL-C values and raising HDL-C levels. Having an LDL-C value of less than 100 mg/dL is optimal; values of 100 to 129 mg/dL are near or above optimal. Clients with LDL-C values of 130 to 159 mg/dL (borderline high) are advised to follow a fat-modified diet. In collaboration with the dietitian, instruct your clients with LDL-C values of 160 mg/dL or greater (high or very high) to follow a more structured diet aimed at decreasing saturated fat and cholesterol and, if appropriate, promoting weight loss. The HDL-C level should be greater than 40 mg/dL.

In the United States, 37% of the total caloric intake in the diets of many people is made up of fat. Overconsumption of fat and cholesterol leads to **hypercholesterolemia,** an elevated total blood cholesterol level. Elevated cholesterol levels can often be decreased if fat in the diet is limited to no more than 30% of the caloric intake.

To determine 30% of their caloric intake, clients first need to determine their ideal daily caloric intake. A dietitian can then calculate their fat limit in grams. In addition to tracking fat in grams, people need to assess the fatty acid content of foods.

Step One Diet. The Step One diet of the American Heart Association, often recommended to decrease the serum cholesterol level, calls for a total fat intake of less than 30% of total calories, with less than 10% of total caloric intake coming from saturated fat, up to 10% of total calories coming from polyunsaturated fat, and 10% to 15% coming from monounsaturated fat. The Step One diet limits its cholesterol intake to less than 300 mg daily.

In collaboration with the dietitian, educate the client about the fat content of foods in terms of the total amount of fat and saturation. Meats and eggs contain mostly saturated fats. Because canola (grapeseed) oil is rich in monounsaturated fat and safflower and sunflower oil are rich in polyunsaturated oils, they are recommended over highly saturated oils, such as palm or coconut oil. Cholesterol is found only in animal sources, such as meat and eggs, which are also high in saturated fats.

Step Two Diet. The client's serum cholesterol levels are retested 6 and 12 weeks after the initial dietary intervention. If the cholesterol level has not significantly decreased, the client may be referred to a registered dietitian for instruction on a more restricted diet, such as the Step Two diet. The Step Two diet limits saturated fat to less than 7% of total calories and cholesterol to less than 200 mg/day.

In addition to elevated LDL-C values, other variations of hyperlipidemias put clients at risk for atherosclerosis. A low-fat, low-cholesterol, high-fiber diet, however, can play a significant role in improving a lipid profile, regardless of the lipid alteration.

Smoking Cessation. Cigarette smoking lowers levels of high-density lipoprotein (HDL) cholesterol and dramatically increases the rate of progression of atherosclerosis.

Advise all clients who smoke to stop smoking and to avoid secondhand smoke. Describe the relationship of smoking to atherosclerosis, and assess his or her willingness to change the behavior. Health care providers can refer to the Agency for Healthcare Research and Quality's Practice Guidelines on Smoking Cessation (formerly the Agency for Health Care Policy and Research). This reference provides strategies to assist individuals in quitting smoking. A smoking cessation group, such as the American Cancer Society's Fresh Start, may help with this difficult process. Most formal programs encourage people to stop smoking "cold turkey."

Clients may consider using a nicotine patch (Nicoderm, Habitrol, ProStep), which helps relieve nicotine withdrawal symptoms. The patch is about 50% effective in helping clients to stop smoking and is available over the counter. The dose is determined by the client's weight and the extent to which he or she smokes. Clients are urged to stop smoking completely when the nicotine patch is initiated. Inform them that if they continue to smoke while using the patch, their risks for serious adverse effects are increased because the peak levels of nicotine are higher than those experienced from smoking alone. Serious cardiovascular effects, such as angina and dysrhythmias, may result from using the patch while still smoking, although the most common side effect is skin irritation. Many health insurance programs will not cover the costs associated with nicotine patches unless the client is enrolled in a smoking cessation program. In some areas of the country, tobacco settlement money is being used by states to fund cessation programs, provide counseling, patches, and oral medication at no charge to the smoker.

Nicotine gum (Nicorette) also may be used if a client feels the need to smoke. Clients should not chew more than 30 pieces of gum per day. Nicotine lozenges are also available as over-the-counter (OTC) aids. The nasal spray (e.g., Nicotrol) and inhaler forms of nicotine must be prescribed by a health care provider (Bialous & Sarna, 2004).

Some clients need an oral medication, such as bupropion (Wellbutrin, Zyban), to help decrease the urge to smoke. Because these drugs depress the central nervous system, clients taking them are carefully monitored by a health care provider.

Complementary and Alternative Therapies. Some individuals try other methods to help them stop smoking, including acupuncture, acupressure, hypnosis, and biofeedback. Many people have been successful using these methods, as discussed in Chapter 4.

Exercise. Regular exercise is recommended to promote optimal lipid levels and can actually prevent atherosclerosis. Exercise can also lead to regression of atherosclerotic plaque and the building of collateral circulation in people with atherosclerosis. The level of exercise required to provide protection from atherosclerotic disease has not been well established, but it is recommended that individuals get 30 minutes of moderate to vigorous exercise at least three to four times a week. Instruct clients with heart disease and other comorbid conditions, such as hypertension, vascular disease, or diabetes, to undergo an exercise tolerance (treadmill or stress) test before undertaking an exercise program (e.g., aerobics, walking, or running).

Drug Therapy. For clients with elevated total and LDL-C levels that do not respond adequately to dietary intervention, the health care provider prescribes one or more lipid-lowering agents (Chart 39-1). Drug choice is dependent on the lipid levels. Because most of these drugs can produce major side effects, they are generally given only when nonpharmacologic management has been unsuccessful. Bile acid–binding resins, such as cholestyramine (Questran) or colestipol (Colestid), were once given because of their low toxicity, but they are seldom used today.

In the 1980s, many studies reported that a potent and well-tolerated class of drugs called 3-hydroxy-3-methylglutaryl coenzyme A (HMG-CoA) reductase inhibitors (statins) successfully reduced total cholesterol by 20% when used for an extended time period. Medications such as pravastatin (Pravachol), lovastatin (Mevacor), simvastatin (Zocor), rosuvastatin (Crestor), and atorvastatin (Lipitor) lower both LDL-C and triglyceride levels. Statins reduce cholesterol synthesis in the liver and increase clearance of LDL-C from the blood. Therefore they are contraindicated in clients with active liver disease or during pregnancy, because they can cause muscle myopathies and marked decreases in liver function. Statin drugs are discontinued if the client has muscle cramping or elevated liver enzyme levels.

A different type of lipid-lowering agent, ezetimibe (Zetia), has been approved to be used in the place of or in combination with statin-type drugs. This medication inhibits the absorption of cholesterol through the small intestine. Vytorin has recently been approved as a combination drug containing ezetimibe and simvastatin. This medication reduces the absorption of cholesterol while reducing the amount of cholesterol synthesis in the liver.

Nicotinic acid or niacin (Niaspan), a B vitamin, lowers LDL-C and very-low-density lipoprotein (VLDL) cholesterol levels, and increases HDL-C levels. It is used as a single agent or in combination with an acid-binding resin drug or a statin.

CHART 39-1

DRUG THERAPY for Hyperlipidemia/Hypercholesterolemia

Drug	Usual Dosage (!)	Nursing Interventions	Rationales
HMG-CoA reductase inhibitors (statins)			
Lovastatin (Mevacor)	20 mg daily; may increase to 40-80 mg daily	Instruct clients to report muscle tenderness.	Although rare, myopathy has occurred as a side effect, especially when taken with fibric acid.
Simvastatin (Zocor)	5-10 mg daily; may increase to 40 mg daily		
Fluvastatin (Lescol)	20-40 mg daily; not to exceed 80 mg daily	Tell clients to take with evening meal.	Gastrointestinal (GI) disturbances, such as diarrhea, nausea, and vomiting, are common.
Atorvastatin (Lipitor)	10 mg daily; increased to 80 mg daily		
Pravastatin (Pravachol)	10-40 mg daily at bedtime	Monitor liver enzymes.	Minor liver enzyme elevations can occur but are rare.
Rosuvastatin (Crestor)	5-10 mg daily to start; increase to 20 mg daily for very high cholesterol levels; may increase to 40 mg daily	Teach clients to avoid grapefruit juice	Grapefruit juice alters drug metabolism and the drug's effects.
Nicotinic acid (Nicobid, Niaspan, Nia-Bid [niacin])	1.5-3 g daily, with maximum dose of 6 g daily	Encourage clients to take with meals.	Flushing of skin and pruritus are common side effects, which can be minimized when drug is taken with meals.
Fibric acid derivatives (fibrates)			
Gemfibrozil (Lopid)	600 mg twice daily	Instruct clients to take 30 minutes before meals or with meals if nausea or GI discomfort occurs.	Although drug is well tolerated, nausea and GI discomfort may occur and can be prevented if drug is taken with meals.
Fenofibrate (Tricor)	67 mg daily		
Ezetimibe (Zetia)	10 mg daily	Tell clients that they may take drug with or without food. Instruct clients that it is safe to take with HMG-CoA reductase inhibitors, but not with fibric acid derivatives.	GI disturbances are rare and do not depend on food intake.

(!) ***Med Error Alert!*** *Write "daily" rather than QD to prevent mistakes.*

Low doses are generally well tolerated, but higher doses can result in an elevation of hepatic enzymes and various other side effects. Gemfibrozil (Lopid) raises HDL-C and lowers triglyceride and VLDL levels, but it is not as effective in lowering LDL-C levels. Fenofibrate (Tricor) inhibits production of LDL-C, which is responsible for triglyceride development.

HYPERTENSION

PATHOPHYSIOLOGY

Hypertension is generally defined as a systolic blood pressure greater than or equal to 135 mm Hg and/or a diastolic blood pressure greater than or equal to 85 mm Hg in individuals who do not have diabetes.

In 2003, the Seventh Report of the Joint National Committee on Prevention, Detection, Evaluation, and Treatment of High Blood Pressure made significant changes in classifying blood pressure in adults. The new classification for **"normal" adult blood pressure** is less than 120 mm Hg systolic *and* less than 80 mm Hg diastolic. Adults with a blood pressure of 120 to 139 mm Hg systolic *or* 80 to 89 mm Hg diastolic, considered "normal" under previous guidelines, are now classified as prehypertensive and are in need of lifestyle changes to prevent cardiovascular complications (Table 39-3). The relationship between hypertension and cardiovascular events is direct and independent of other risk factors. The higher the blood pressure, the greater the chance for coronary, cerebral, renal, and peripheral vascular disease. Control of hypertension, however, has resulted in significant decreases in cardiovascular morbidity and mortality. (See the Meeting Healthy People 2010 Objectives box below.)

TABLE 39-3 Blood Pressure Classification

Classification	Blood Pressure Measurement	Blood Pressure Readings
Normal	Systolic *and* diastolic	<120 mm Hg <80 mm Hg
Prehypertension	Systolic *or* diastolic	120-139 mm Hg 80-89 mm Hg
Stage 1: Hypertension	Systolic *or* diastolic	140-159 mm Hg 90-99 mm Hg
Stage 2: Hypertension	Systolic *or* diastolic	≥160 mm Hg ≥100 mm Hg

From Joint National Committee. (2003). The seventh report of the Joint National Committee on Prevention, Detection, Evaluation, and Treatment of High Blood Pressure. NIH Publication No. 03-5233. Bethesda, MD: National Heart, Lung, and Blood Institute.

Meeting HEALTHY PEOPLE 2010 Objectives

BLOOD PRESSURE

Objective 12.11: Increase the proportion of adults with high blood pressure who are taking action to help control their blood pressure.

- Teach adults with high blood pressure the importance of controlling sodium intake, including reading food labels for sodium content and avoiding high-sodium foods, such as bacon, ham, and processed snacks.
- Refer overweight adults to a support group or weight reduction program.
- Teach about the importance of exercise and increased physical activity to reduce blood pressure.
- For the adult who smokes, teach about the relationship between cardiovascular disease and smoking; refer the individual to a smoking cessation program.
- Participate in community or health care agency health fairs to screen for hypertension and provide community education.
- Teach all adults to have their blood pressure taken at least once every 2 years; for those with hypertension, monitor blood pressure as recommended by the health care provider.

Several other changes were made in the national guidelines for blood pressure management. Thiazide-type diuretics are recommended for initial therapy in most clients with uncomplicated stage 1 hypertension. Stages 2 and 3 hypertension were combined into a single stage 2 category because most hypertensive clients need a combination of two or more drugs for optimal treatment.

The systemic arterial pressure is a product of cardiac output (CO) and total peripheral vascular resistance (PVR) (Figure 39-2). Cardiac output is determined by the stroke volume and heart rate ($CO = SV \times HR$). Control of peripheral vascular resistance, vessel constriction or dilation, is maintained by the autonomic nervous system and circulating hormones, such as norepinephrine and epinephrine. Consequently, any factor producing an increase in peripheral vascular resistance, heart rate, or stroke volume increases the systemic arterial pressure. Conversely, any factor that causes a decrease in peripheral vascular resistance, heart rate, or stroke volume decreases the systemic arterial pressure.

Stabilizing mechanisms exist in the body to exert an overall regulation of systemic arterial pressure and to prevent circulatory collapse. Four control systems play a major role in maintaining blood pressure: the arterial baroreceptor system, regulation of body fluid volume, the renin-angiotensin system, and vascular autoregulation.

Arterial Baroreceptors

The arterial baroreceptors are found primarily in the carotid sinus but also in the aorta and the wall of the left ventricle. The baroreceptors monitor the level of arterial pressure and counteract a rise in arterial pressure through vagally mediated cardiac slowing and vasodilation with decreased sympathetic tone. Therefore reflex control of circulation elevates the systemic arterial pressure when it falls and lowers it when it rises. Why baroceptor control fails in hypertension is unknown. There is evidence for upward resetting of baroreceptor sensitivity so that pressure measures are inadequately sensed even though pressure decreases are not.

Regulation of Body Fluid Volume

Changes in fluid volume also affect the systemic arterial pressure. If there is an excess of sodium and/or water in a person's body, the blood pressure rises through complex physiologic

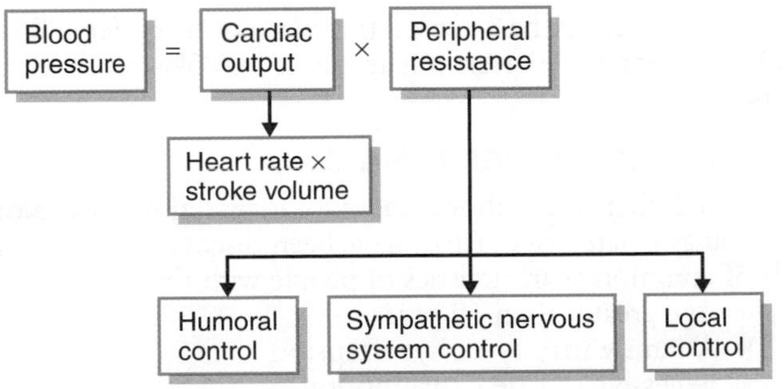

Figure 39-2 ■ The components of blood pressure.

mechanisms that change the venous return to the heart, producing a rise in cardiac output. If the kidneys are functioning adequately, a rise in systemic arterial pressure produces diuresis and a fall in pressure. Pathologic conditions change the pressure threshold at which the kidneys excrete sodium and water, thereby altering the systemic arterial pressure.

Renin-Angiotensin System

Renin, angiotensin, and aldosterone also regulate blood pressure (see discussion in Chapter 14). The kidney produces renin, an enzyme that acts on angiotensinogen (a plasma protein substrate) to split off angiotensin I, which is converted by an enzyme in the lung to form angiotensin II. Angiotensin II has strong vasoconstrictor action on blood vessels and is the controlling mechanism for aldosterone release. Aldosterone then works on the collecting tubules in the kidneys to reabsorb sodium. Sodium retention inhibits fluid loss, thus increasing blood volume and subsequent blood pressure.

Inappropriate secretion of renin may cause increased peripheral vascular resistance in essential (primary) hypertension. In high blood pressure, renin levels should fall because the increased renal arteriolar pressure should inhibit renin secretion. For most people with essential hypertension, however, renin levels are normal.

Vascular Autoregulation

The process of vascular autoregulation, which keeps perfusion of tissues in the body relatively constant, appears to be important in causing hypertension. This mechanism is poorly understood.

Sustained blood pressure elevation in clients with essential (primary) hypertension results in damage to blood vessels in vital organs. Essential hypertension produces medial hyperplasia (thickening) of the arterioles. As the blood vessels thicken and perfusion decreases, body organs are damaged; these changes can result in myocardial infarctions, strokes, peripheral vascular disease (PVD), or renal failure.

Malignant hypertension is a severe type of elevated blood pressure that rapidly progresses. A person with malignant hypertension usually has symptoms such as morning headaches, blurred vision, and dyspnea and/or symptoms of uremia (accumulation in the blood of substances ordinarily eliminated in the urine). Clients are often in their 30s, 40s, or 50s with their systolic blood pressure greater than 200 mm Hg. The diastolic blood pressure is greater than 150 mm Hg or greater than 130 mm Hg when there are pre-existing complications. Unless intervention occurs promptly, a client with malignant hypertension may experience renal failure, left ventricular failure, or stroke.

Etiology and Genetic Risk

Hypertension can be essential (primary) or secondary (Table 39-4). Essential hypertension accounts for 85% to 90% of all cases.

ESSENTIAL HYPERTENSION

Although there is no known cause for **essential hypertension,** several associated risk factors have been discovered on the basis of common characteristics of people with this disease:

- Age greater than 60 years
- A family history of hypertension
- Excessive calorie consumption
- Physical inactivity
- Excessive alcohol intake
- Hyperlipidemia
- African-American ethnicity
- High intake of salt or caffeine; reduced intake of potassium, calcium, or magnesium
- Obesity
- Smoking
- Stress

A family history of hypertension is a major risk factor. In families with hypertension, there may be a defect in renal secretion of sodium or a heightened sympathetic nervous system response to stress.

SECONDARY HYPERTENSION

Specific disease states and medications can increase a person's susceptibility to hypertension; a person with this type of elevation in blood pressure has **secondary hypertension.**

DISEASES. Renal vascular and renal parenchymal diseases are two of the most common causes of secondary hypertension. Hypertension can develop when there is any sudden damage to the kidneys. Renovascular hypertension is associated with narrowing of one or more of the main arteries carrying blood directly to the kidneys. Renal parenchymal diseases are related to infection, inflammation, and changes in kidney structure and function.

Dysfunction of the adrenal medulla or the adrenal cortex can cause secondary hypertension. Adrenal-mediated hypertension is due to primary excesses of aldosterone, cortisol, and catecholamines. In *primary aldosteronism,* excessive aldosterone causes hypertension and hypokalemia (low potassium levels). It usually arises from benign adenomas of the adrenal cortex. *Pheochromocytomas* originate most commonly in the adrenal medulla and result in excessive secretion of catecholamines. In *Cushing's syndrome,* excessive glucocorticoids are excreted from the adrenal cortex. The cause of Cushing's syndrome may be either adrenocortical hyperplasia or adrenocortical adenoma (Chapter 66).

Coarctation of the aorta is a congenital narrowing of the aorta that may cause hypertension. Occurring at any level of

TABLE 39-4 Etiology of Hypertension

Essential (Primary)
- No known cause
- Associated risk factors
  - Family history of hypertension
  - High sodium intake
  - Excessive calorie consumption
  - Physical inactivity
  - Excessive alcohol intake
  - Low potassium intake

Secondary
- Renal vascular and renal parenchymal disease
- Primary aldosteronism
- Pheochromocytoma
- Cushing's disease
- Coarctation of the aorta
- Brain tumors
- Encephalitis
- Psychiatric disturbances
- Pregnancy
- Medications
  - Estrogen (e.g., oral contraceptives)
  - Glucocorticoids
  - Mineralocorticoids
  - Sympathomimetics

the thoracic or abdominal aorta, the narrowing restricts blood flow through the aortic arch, resulting in an elevated blood pressure above the constriction. After surgical repair, the elevation in blood pressure eventually subsides.

Secondary hypertension is also associated with other neurogenic disturbances, such as brain tumors, encephalitis, and psychiatric disturbances.

MEDICATIONS. Medications that can cause secondary hypertension include estrogen, glucocorticoids, mineralocorticoids, sympathomimetics, cyclosporine, and erythropoietin. The use of estrogen-containing oral contraceptives is probably the most common cause of secondary hypertension in women. Discontinuation of medications capable of causing hypertension often reverses this problem.

Incidence/Prevalence

About 50 million Americans, or 1 in every 4 adults, have high blood pressure or are currently being treated for hypertension.

HEALTH PROMOTION/ILLNESS PREVENTION

Teach clients ways to decrease risk factors for hypertension. Risk factor prevention and lifestyle changes are discussed under the nursing diagnosis of Deficient Knowledge on p. 786.

◆COLLABORATIVE MANAGEMENT

PHARM e REVIEW

◆Assessment

HISTORY

During history taking, review the client's risk factors for hypertension. Ascertain the client's age; ethnic origin or race; family history of hypertension; average dietary intake of calories, sodium- and potassium-containing foods, and alcohol; and exercise habits. Also assess any past or present history of renal or cardiovascular disease and current use of medications.

PHYSICAL ASSESSMENT

When a diagnosis of hypertension is made, most clients have no symptoms; however, they may experience headaches, dizziness, or fainting as a result of the elevated blood pressure. Obtain blood pressure readings in both arms. Two or more readings are taken at each visit, with the average of the readings used as the value for the visit (Figure 39-3). To detect postural (orthostatic) changes, also take readings with the client in the supine (lying) or sitting position and at least 2 minutes later with the client standing. **Orthostatic hypotension** is a decrease in blood pressure (20 mm Hg systolic and/or 10 mm Hg diastolic) when the client changes position from lying to sitting.

Funduscopic examination of the eyes to observe vascular changes in the retina is done by a skilled practitioner. The appearance of the retina can be a reliable index of the severity and prognosis of hypertension.

Physical assessment is helpful in diagnosing several conditions that produce secondary hypertension. The presence of abdominal bruits is typical of clients with renovascular disease. Tachycardia, sweating, and pallor may suggest a pheochromocytoma or adrenal medulla tumor. Coarctation of the aorta is often characterized by elevation of blood pressure in the arms, with normal or low blood pressure in the lower extremities. Femoral pulses are also delayed or absent.

PSYCHOSOCIAL ASSESSMENT

Assess for psychosocial stressors that can worsen hypertension and that may affect the client's ability to collaborate in treatment. Job-related, economic, and other life stressors are evaluated, as well as the client's response to these stressors. Some clients may have difficulty coping with the lifestyle changes needed to control hypertension. Be sure to assess the client's past coping strategies.

DIAGNOSTIC ASSESSMENT

Although no laboratory tests are diagnostic of essential hypertension, several laboratory tests can assess possible causes of secondary hypertension. The presence of protein, red blood cells, pus cells, and casts in the urine; elevated levels of blood urea nitrogen (BUN); and elevated serum creatinine levels indicate renal disease. Urinary test results are positive for the presence of catecholamines in clients with a pheochromocytoma (tumor of the adrenal medulla). An elevation in levels of serum corticoids and 17-ketosteroids in the urine is diagnostic of Cushing's disease.

No specific x-ray studies can diagnose hypertension. Routine chest radiography may be of assistance in recognizing cardiomegaly (heart enlargement).

An electrocardiogram (ECG) is of value in determining the degree of cardiac involvement. Left atrial and ventricular hypertrophy is the first ECG sign of cardiac involvement resulting from hypertension. Left ventricular remodeling can be detected on the 12-lead ECG.

◆Analysis

COMMON NURSING DIAGNOSES AND COLLABORATIVE PROBLEMS

The following are priority nursing diagnoses for clients with hypertension:

1. Deficient Knowledge related to information misinterpretation or unfamiliarity with information resources
2. Risk for Ineffective Therapeutic Regimen Management related to noncompliance with or nonadherence to treatment

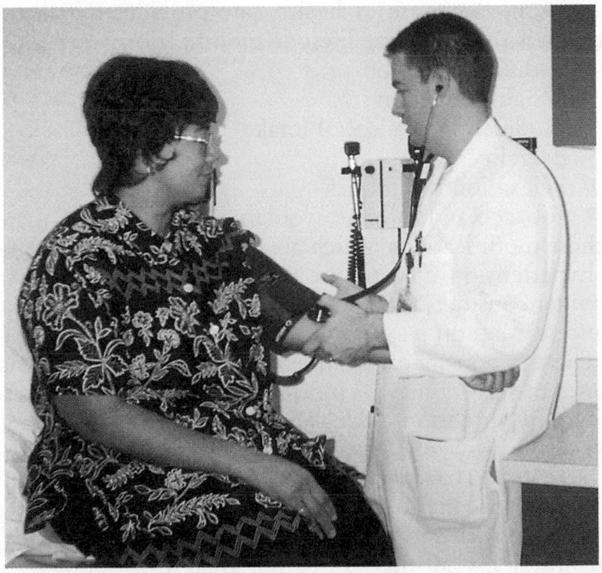

Figure 39-3 ■ Blood pressure screening during routine history and physical examination.

ADDITIONAL NURSING DIAGNOSES AND COLLABORATIVE PROBLEMS

In addition to the common nursing diagnoses, clients with hypertension may have one or more of the following:

- Ineffective Tissue Perfusion (Renal, Cerebral, Cardiopulmonary, and Peripheral) related to decreased blood flow
- Risk for Imbalanced Nutrition: More Than Body Requirements related to learned eating behaviors, ethnic and cultural values, lack of social support for weight loss, and/or imbalance between activity level and caloric intake
- Fatigue related to altered body chemistry (medications) and disease state
- Sexual Dysfunction related to altered body function from drug therapy
- Ineffective Coping related to inadequate level of perception of control
- Excessive Fluid Volume related to compromised regulatory mechanism
- Risk for Noncompliance related to knowledge and skill relevant to the regimen behavior

The following collaborative problems may also occur in some clients with hypertension:

- Potential for Cerebrovascular Hemorrhage
- Potential for Myocardial Infarction
- Potential for Retinal Hemorrhage

Planning and Implementation

DEFICIENT KNOWLEDGE

NOC **PLANNING: EXPECTED OUTCOMES.** The client with hypertension is expected to have an understanding about a specific treatment regimen. Indicators include that the client will be able to extensively describe:

- Specific disease process
- Rationale for treatment regimen
- Self-care responsibilities for ongoing treatment
- Self-monitoring techniques
- Expected effects of treatment
- Benefits of disease management

INTERVENTIONS. For the client with essential hypertension, the nurse or health care provider initially recommends the following lifestyle modifications:

- Sodium restriction
- Weight reduction
- Moderation of alcohol intake
- Exercise
- Relaxation techniques
- Tobacco and caffeine avoidance

If these modifications, which are considered the foundation of hypertension control, are unsuccessful, the health care provider considers the use of antihypertensive drugs (see the Concept Map on p. 787).

There is no surgical treatment for essential hypertension. However, surgery may be indicated for certain causes of secondary hypertension, such as renal vascular disease, coarctation of the aorta, and pheochromocytoma.

Sodium Restriction. In collaboration and consultation with the dietitian, advise all clients with hypertension to decrease their sodium chloride intake from the average of 150 mmol/L (150 mEq/L) to less than 100 mmol/L (100 mEq/L; less than 2.3 g of sodium) per day. To accomplish the goal, clients should avoid adding salt at the table, cooking with salt, or adding seasonings that contain sodium. Teach clients to avoid any food that comes from a factory, except for plain frozen vegetables and fruit.

A dietitian may review a 3-day dietary recall with the client to identify whether sodium intake has been excessive. In collaboration with the dietitian, suggest spices, herbs, fruits, and other non–salt-containing substances, such as powdered garlic and onion, to enhance the flavor of meat, chicken, seafood, and snacks. Instruct clients to read the labels on all food and to avoid those that are high in sodium. Salt substitutes are an alternative to salt. However, some substitutes are high in potassium, and therefore are contraindicated for some clients. Hyperkalemia can also occur in clients who are taking potassium-sparing diuretics, although it is unusual.

Weight Reduction. If a client's body mass index (BMI) is 25 or higher, weight loss is encouraged. Discuss the rationale for reducing or maintaining weight and help plan a weight reduction diet with the client. He or she may be referred to a group or organization for weight reduction. The cost of inactivity was $29 billion in 1987 and nearly $76 billion in 2000. Being active in some form of physical exercise is linked with taking fewer medications, having fewer hospitalizations, and fewer physician visits (CDC, 2003).

Because of the relationship of saturated fat and cholesterol to weight, a weight reduction plan is formulated with the following limits:

- Total fat: less than 30% of daily caloric intake
- Saturated fat: less than 10%
- Cholesterol: less than 300 mg/day

Moderation of Alcohol Intake. In general, instruct clients to limit alcohol intake to no more than 1 ounce of ethanol (2 ounces of liquor, 8 ounces of wine, or 24 ounces of beer) daily. Excessive alcohol consumption may elevate arterial blood pressure and can add "empty" calories.

Exercise. With the physician's approval and in collaboration with the physical therapist, help the client develop a regular exercise program. Exercise is critical for successful weight loss, lowered blood pressure, and increased endurance. The client should start an exercise program slowly and gradually work up to more rigorous activities, such as brisk walking, running, cycling, swimming, or stair climbing, 30 to 45 minutes three to five times a week. Teach the client to stop and notify the physician if severe shortness of breath, fainting, or chest pain occurs.

NIC **Smoking Cessation Assistance.** Although cigarette smoking is not directly related to hypertension, it is a major risk factor for cardiovascular disease. Therefore the client who smokes is strongly urged to stop (Chart 39-2). A smoking cessation program that best fits into his or her lifestyle should be planned. Explain use of nicotine patches and smoking cessation programs and implement follow-up to assess the client's plans for quitting. With the ability to reach many more people than traditional cessation programs, computer cessation programs have been shown to be effective in "precontemplators" who were otherwise not motivated to quit (Etter et al., 2001).

Complementary and Alternative Therapies. In addition to exercise, complementary modalities are often used by clients to reduce stress and thus decrease blood

CONCEPT MAP Hypertension

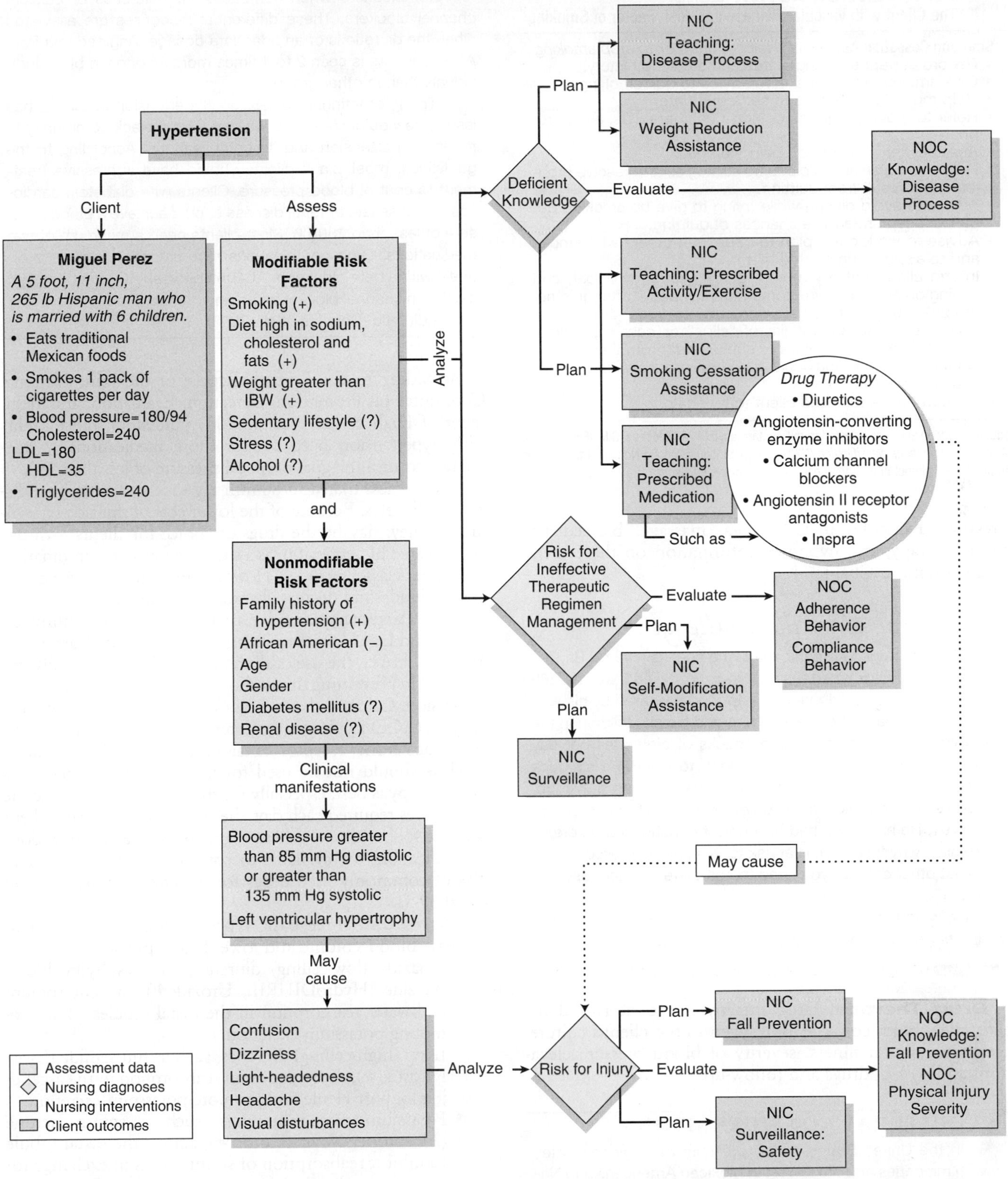

Concept Map by Elaine Bishop Kennedy, EdD, RN

CHART 39-2

NIC INTERVENTION ACTIVITIES for
The Client with Vascular Disease and Risk Factor of Smoking

Smoking Cessation Assistance: *Helping another to stop smoking*
- Record current smoking status and smoking history.
- Give smoker clear, consistent advice to quit smoking.
- Help motivated smokers to set a quit date.
- Refer to group programs or individual therapists, as appropriate.
- Assist client with any self-help methods.
- Help client plan specific coping strategies and resolve problems that result from quitting.
- Advise to avoid dieting while trying to give up smoking because it can undermine chances of quitting.
- Advise to work out a plan to cope with others who smoke and to avoid being around them.
- Inform client that dry mouth, cough, scratchy throat, and feeling on edge are symptoms that may occur after quitting; the patch or gum may help with cravings.
- Advise client to keep a list of "slips" or near slips, what causes them, and what he or she learned from them.
- Contact national and local resource organizations for resource materials.
- Encourage the relapsed client to try again.

pressure. Examples include yoga, massage, biofeedback, music therapy, and hypnosis. Information on these therapies is found in Chapter 4.

Critical Thinking Challenge

A middle-aged Hispanic man who speaks minimal English is diagnosed with hypertension. He is 5'10" and weighs 265 pounds. He eats traditional Mexican food prepared by his wife and mother-in-law who live with him and his six children in the inner city. He had smoked three packs of cigarettes per day (ppd) for 22 years and has now cut down to 1 ppd. He is a truck driver, but walking and loading boxes are also part of his job. He arrives at the clinic where you determine his blood pressure is 180/94. He has never had his cholesterol checked before.

1. Explain why this client is at risk for high blood pressure (BP).
2. What other data do you need to complete his initial assessment?
3. How would you obtain additional history for this client, keeping his cultural background in mind?

evolve For suggested answer guidelines, go to http://evolve.elsevier.com/Iggy/.

Drug Therapy. Drug therapy is individualized for each client, with consideration given to the client's culture, age, concomitant illness, severity of blood pressure elevation, and cost of drugs and follow-up.

CULTURAL CONSIDERATIONS

In the United States, blood pressure management rates vary in minorities and are lowest in Mexican Americans and Native Americans/American Indians. Socioeconomic and lifestyle factors may be significant barriers to control blood pressure in some minorities. There is a higher prevalence, incidence, and impact of hypertension among black individuals who also have a decreased treatment response with beta blockers, angiotensin-converting enzyme (ACE) inhibitors, or angiotensin receptor blockers when compared with diuretics or calcium channel blockers. These differential responses are alleviated when the diuretic is of an adequate dosage. Angioedema from ACE inhibitors is seen 2 to 4 times more as often in black individuals than in other groups.

The International Society on Hypertension in Blacks has issued new guidelines personalized for the black community to reduce hypertension and its complications. According to the guidelines, most black clients should have aggressive treatment to control blood pressure. Clients with diabetes, cardiovascular disease, or renal disease should achieve a blood pressure of less than 130/80. Most clients need a minimum of two medications. Drug combinations recommended include a diuretic with a beta blocker or ACE inhibitor, an ACE inhibitor with a calcium channel blocker, or an angiotensin II receptor blocker with a diuretic (Douglas et al., 2003).

According to the Seventh Report of the Joint National Committee on Prevention, Detection, Evaluation, and Treatment of High Blood Pressure 2003 guidelines, most clients with hypertension need two or more medications to adequately control the goal of blood pressure of less than 140/90 mm Hg, or less than 130/80 mm Hg for those with renal disease or diabetes. Because of the lower cost of thiazide-type diuretics, they may be the drugs of choice for clients with uncomplicated hypertension, as a single agent or in combination with other classes of drugs. However, men may experience decreased libido and decreased sexual performance.

In the largest hypertensive trial done to date, Antihypertensive and Lipid Lowering Treatment to Prevent Heart Attack Trial (ALLHAT), the use of diuretics have been practically unmatched in preventing the cardiovascular complications of hypertension. Calcium channel blockers, angiotensin-converting enzyme (ACE) inhibitors, angiotensin II receptor antagonists, and aldosterone receptor antagonists can be tried. Alpha blockers should not be used for initial therapy. Once-a-day drug therapy is best, especially for the older adult, because the more doses required each day, the higher the risk that a client will not follow the treatment regimen. Several classifications of medications are available to control hypertension. Examples of commonly used drugs for hypertension are listed in Chart 39-3.

Diuretics. Three basic types of diuretics are used to decrease blood volume and lower blood pressure:

- Thiazide (low-ceiling) diuretics, such as hydrochlorothiazide (HydroDIURIL, Urozide✱), prevent sodium and water reabsorption in the distal tubules while promoting potassium excretion.
- Loop (high-ceiling) diuretics, such as furosemide (Lasix, Furoside✱), depress sodium reabsorption in the ascending loop of Henle and promote potassium excretion.
- Potassium-sparing diuretics, such as spironolactone (Aldactone, Novospiroton✱), act on the distal tubule to inhibit reabsorption of sodium ions in exchange for potassium, thereby retaining potassium. When used, they are typically in combination with another type of diuretic to conserve potassium.

Diuretics are the drugs of choice for clients who have asthma, chronic airway limitation, and chronic renal disease and for selected clients with heart failure. They are particularly effective

CHART 39-3

DRUG THERAPY for Hypertension

Drug	Usual Dosage	Nursing Interventions	Rationales
Diuretics			
Thiazides (Low-Ceiling)			
Chlorothiazide (Diuril)	125-500 mg daily	Monitor potassium levels and watch for muscle weakness or irregular pulse.	Hypokalemia is a common occurrence.
Hydrochlorothiazide (Esidrix, HydroDIURIL)	12.5-50 mg daily	Encourage intake of foods high in potassium (e.g., bananas and orange juice).	Depleted potassium needs to be replaced.
Loop (High-Ceiling) Diuretics			
[1]Furosemide ([2]Lasix, Furoside✱)	20-80 mg PO daily 20-40 mg IV; increase by 20 mg every 2 hr until desired response	Same as for thiazide diuretics. Observe for dehydration, especially in older adults.	Same as for chlorothiazide. Loop diuretics can cause dehydration in older adults.
Bumetanide (Bumex)	0.5-2 mg PO daily or 0.5-1 mg IV; give 2nd or 3rd dose at 2- to 3-hr intervals not to exceed 10 mg daily	Same as for furosemide.	Same as for furosemide.
Potassium-Sparing Diuretics			
Spironolactone (Aldactone)	25-100 mg daily	Monitor potassium levels and watch for muscle weakness or irregular pulse.	Hypokalemia or hyperkalemia may occur.
Triamterene (Dyrenium)	50-100 mg daily		
Calcium Channel Blocking Agents			
[3]Verapamil (Apo-Verap✱, Calan, Calan SR, Isoptin, Isoptin SR)	80 mg q8h or 240 mg SR daily; may titrate upward	Monitor blood pressure (BP) and pulse; change positions slowly. Encourage intake of foods high in fiber.	Hypotension and decreased heart rate may occur. Constipation is a common side effect.
Amlodipine (Norvasc)	5-10 mg daily	Monitor BP and pulse; teach clients to change positions slowly. Use protective clothing or sunscreen when exposed to sun.	Same as verapamil. Photosensitivity is a common side effect.
[4]Diltiazem (Cardizem, Apo-Diltiaz✱, Cardizem CD, Cardizem SR)	30-360 mg daily in divided doses or in extended form	Monitor BP and pulse; teach clients to change positions slowly. Teach clients to avoid grapefruit juice.	Same as verapamil. Increased hypotensive effects may occur as a result of drug-food interaction.
Nicardipine (Cardene, Cardene SR, Cardene IV)	20-40 mg PO three times daily 0.5-2.2 mg/hr IV (for hypertensive crisis)	Do not give with grapefruit juice. Monitor digoxin level if the client is taking this drug.	Grapefruit juice increases drug level and hypotensive effect (applies to most calcium channel blockers). Nicardipine increases the effects of digoxin.
Angiotensin-Converting Enzyme (ACE) Inhibitors			
Captopril (Capoten, Novo-Captopril✱)	25-150 mg two to three times daily	Same as amlodipine. Teach client to report cough.	Same as amlodipine. Coughing is a common side effect of ACE inhibitors; drug is discontinued if this problem occurs.
Enalapril (Vasotec, Vasotec IV)	5-40 mg PO daily; 1.25 mg q6h over 5 min	Same as captopril.	Same as captopril.
Lisinopril (Zestril, Prinivil)	10-40 mg daily; increase to 80 mg daily if needed	Monitor BP and pulse; teach clients to change positions slowly. Monitor for and teach clients to report signs of heart failure (e.g., edema). Teach client to report cough.	Hypotension is a common side effect. This drug can cause heart and renal complications. Cough is a common side effect and requires discontinuation of the drug.

[1]*Med Error Alert!* Do not confuse furosemide with torsemide.

[2]*Med Error Alert!* Do not confuse Lasix with Lanoxin.

[3]*Med Error Alert!* Do not crush SR form of drug.

[4]*Med Error Alert!* Do not crush CD or SR forms of drug; do not confuse Cardizem CD and Cardizem SR. Do not confuse with Cardene IV.

Continued

CHART 39-3

DRUG THERAPY for Hypertension—*cont'd*

Drug	Usual Dosage	Nursing Interventions	Rationales
Angiotensin-Converting Enzyme (ACE) Inhibitors—*cont'd*			
Ramipril (Altace)	2.5-20 mg daily, or twice daily in divided doses	Same as lisinopril.	Same as lisinopril.
Angiotensin II Receptor Antagonists			
Candesartan (Atacand)	8-32 mg daily	Monitor BP and pulse; teach clients to change position slowly.	Hypotension is a common side effect.
		Observe for and teach client to report angioedema (swollen lips, face).	Angioedema is a serious but not common adverse effect of this drug.
Losartan (Cozaar)	25-50 mg daily	Monitor BP and pulse.	Same as above.
		Monitor for and report signs of heart failure, such as edema.	Heart failure can result from taking the drug.
Telmisartan (Micardis)	20-80 mg daily	Same as candesartan.	Same as candesartan.
Aldosterone Receptor Antagonists			
Eplerenone (Inspra)	50 mg daily initially, increased to 100 mg daily if response is not adequate.	Monitor renal function.	Risk of adverse effects increases with deteriorating renal function.
		Monitor triglycerides.	Dose-related adverse effect of hypertriglyceridemia occurred in 15% of study clients.
		Monitor sodium levels.	Hyponatremia may occur when taking this drug.
		Monitor potassium levels every 2 wk for the first few months then every 2 months thereafter.	Potassium imbalances may occur when taking this medication. ▪ Risk of hyperkalemia increases when using ACE inhibitors or angiotensin II receptor antagonists with Inspra. ▪ Do not give with potassium supplements and potassium-sparing diuretics. Client should not take salt substitutes with potassium and other foods rich in potassium.
		Teach client about potential drug and herbal interactions.	Grapefruit juice and St. John's wort, for example, can increase adverse effects.
		Caution client to be careful when getting out of bed, driving, and climbing stairs until the medication's effects are known.	Orthostatic hypotension may occur, especially in older adults.

for black individuals. Caution is indicated in using thiazide diuretics in hypertensive clients with gout or with a history of significant hyponatremia, because these problems can worsen.

Diuretics enhance the antihypertensive effectiveness when using multiple drug therapy combinations and are relatively inexpensive. Adherence to the medication regimen is enhanced because the drug can usually be prescribed on a once-a-day or, at most, twice-a-day schedule. However, the frequent voiding that occurs after a person takes a diuretic may interfere with daily activities. The most frequent side effect associated with diuretics is hypokalemia (low potassium levels). Monitor the serum potassium level and assess for irregular pulse and muscle weakness, which may indicate hypokalemia. Clients receiving potassium-depleting diuretics should eat foods high in potassium, such as bananas and orange juice. However, many individuals need a potassium supplement to maintain adequate serum potassium levels (see Chapter 14). Assess for hypokalemia and hyperkalemia in clients taking potassium-sparing diuretics. Both of these electrolyte disturbances are characterized by weakness and an irregular pulse, and are described in detail in Chapter 15.

Calcium Channel Blocking Agents. Calcium channel blockers, such as verapamil hydrochloride (Calan), amlodipine (Norvasc), and diltiazem (Cardizem), lower blood pressure by interfering with the transmembrane flux of calcium ions. This results in vasodilation and subsequent decrease in blood pressure.

Angiotensin-Converting Enzyme Inhibitors. Angiotensin-converting enzyme (ACE) inhibitors are also used as single or combination agents in the treatment of hyperten-

CHART 39-4

NURSING FOCUS on the OLDER ADULT
Hypertension

- Before initiating drug therapy, obtain blood pressure measurements with the client lying, sitting, and standing to assess for postural changes.
- Monitor the client's standing blood pressure during treatment.
- Instruct the client to avoid caffeine and nicotine for 1 hour before blood pressure measurements to obtain accurate readings.
- Teach the client that dizziness is a symptom of hypotension that should be reported.
- Instruct clients how to avoid orthostatic (postural) hypotension by avoiding sudden changes in position. Clients should arise from bed in three stages: sit in bed for 1 minute; sit on the side of the bed with legs dangling for 1 minute; and stand, holding onto a nonmovable object for 1 minute before walking. Clients should also be cautious about heat exposure (hot tub), alcohol intake, and exercise, which can lead to orthostatic hypotension.

sion. The angiotensin-converting enzyme converts angiotensin I to angiotensin II, one of the most powerful vasoconstrictors in the body, thereby preventing increased blood pressure. ACE inhibitors include captopril (Capoten), enalapril (Vasotec), and lisinopril (Prinivil).

Instruct the client receiving an ACE inhibitor for the first time to get out of bed slowly to avoid the severe hypotensive effect that can occur with initial use. Orthostatic hypotension may occur with subsequent doses, but it is less severe. If dizziness continues or there is a significant decrease in the systolic blood pressure (<20 mm Hg), notify the physician. The older client is at the greatest risk for postural hypotension because of the cardiovascular changes associated with aging. If a cough develops, the drug is discontinued.

CONSIDERATIONS FOR OLDER ADULTS

Seen more often in older adults, orthostatic (postural) hypotension is a decrease in systolic and diastolic blood pressure upon rising (Chart 39-4). When younger individuals stand, the body compensates for the change in gravitational forces when changing positions. Those most susceptible are older adults with systolic hypertension, diabetics, and those taking diuretics, vasodilators, or some psychotropic drugs. Orthostatic hypertension is often accompanied by dizziness, blurring or loss of vision, and syncope or fainting. For this reason, caution is needed to avoid volume depletion and too fast of dosage adjustment with antihypertensive drugs. Wearing elastic venous compression stockings is an effective strategy to reduce the risk of fainting and falls in older adults with postural hypotension.

Angiotensin II Receptor Antagonists. Angiotensin II receptor antagonists, also called angiotensin II receptor blockers (ARBs), make up a group of drugs that selectively block the binding of angiotensin II in the vascular and adrenal tissues by competing directly with angiotensin II but not inhibiting ACE. Examples of drugs in this group are candesartan (Atacand), losartan (Cozaar), and telmisartan (Micardis). Angiotensin II receptor antagonists can be used alone or in combination with other antihypertensive drugs. They are excellent options for clients who complain of cough associated with ACE inhibitors and for those with hyperkalemia. In addition, these drugs do not require initial adjustment of the dose for older adults or for clients with renal impairment.

Aldosterone Receptor Antagonists. In 2002, a new class of antihypertensive drugs was introduced to block the hypertensive effect of the mineralocorticoid hormone, aldosterone. Aldosterone increases sodium reabsorption by the kidney and is a significant contributor to hypertension, cardiac and vascular remodeling, and heart failure. Eplerenone (Inspra) lowers blood pressure by blocking aldosterone binding at the mineralocorticoid receptor sites in the kidney, heart, blood vessels, and brain. The recommended dosage is 50 mg daily, which can be increased to 100 mg daily. Generally well tolerated, eplerenone has dose-related adverse effects of hypertriglyceridemia, hyponatremia, and hyperkalemia. Using concurrent ACE inhibitors increases the risk of hyperkalemia. Monitor potassium levels carefully, initially every 2 weeks for the first few months then monthly thereafter.

When taking eplerenone, itraconazole (Sporanox) and ketoconazole (Nizoral) should not be taken. Drug interactions with these medications are common. Clients taking erythromycin, fluconazole (Diflucan), saquinavir (Fortovase), and verapamil (Isoptin) can take eplerenone but with a reduction in dosage by half to 25 mg daily. Grapefruit juice and the popular herb St. John's wort can also increase the chance of undesirable effects. Like all antihypertensives, clients need to be careful when getting up quickly, driving, or climbing stairs until they are familiar with the effects of the medication.

Other Drugs. *Beta-adrenergic blockers* are categorized as cardioselective (working only on the cardiovascular system) and noncardioselective. Cardioselective beta blockers may be prescribed to lower blood pressure by blocking beta receptors in the heart and peripheral vessels, reducing the cardiac rate and output. By blocking beta-adrenergic receptors in the heart, these drugs decrease heart rate and myocardial contractility. Common side effects of beta blockers include fatigue, weakness, depression, and sexual dysfunction, although the potential for side effects depends on the "selective" blocking effects of the drug.

Clients with diabetes who take beta blockers may not have the usual manifestations of hypoglycemia because the sympathetic nervous system is blocked. Counterregulatory responses to hypoglycemia, such as gluconeogenesis, may also be inhibited by certain beta blockers.

Beta blockers are the drug of choice for hypertensive clients with ischemic heart disease (IHD) because the heart is the most common target of end-organ damage with hypertension. If a beta blocker is not tolerated, a long-acting calcium channel blocker can be used. In clients with unstable angina or myocardial infarction (MI), beta blockers or calcium channel blockers should be used initially in combination with ACE inhibitors, with addition of other drugs if needed to control the blood pressure. Best practice for controlling hypertension in post-MI clients include a combination drug therapy of beta blockers, ACE inhibitors, and aldosterone antagonists plus intense management of lipids and the use of aspirin. Low-dose aspirin should only be considered once the blood pressure is controlled because of the increased risk for hemorrhagic stroke in the presence of uncontrolled hypertension.

Central alpha agonists act on the central nervous system, preventing reuptake of norepinephrine, resulting in lower peripheral vascular resistance and blood pressure. Clonidine (Catapres) is most commonly used in this drug classification, and is usually given as a transdermal patch, providing control of blood pressure for as long as 7 days. Side effects common to clonidine include sedation, postural hypotension, and impotence. This group of drugs is not indicated for first-line management of hypertension.

Alpha-adrenergic agonists, such as prazosin (Minipress), dilate the arterioles and veins. These drugs can lower blood pressure quickly, but their use is limited because of frequent and bothersome side effects.

RISK FOR INEFFECTIVE THERAPEUTIC REGIMEN MANAGEMENT

NOC **PLANNING: EXPECTED OUTCOMES.** The client with hypertension is expected to take personal actions to promote wellness, recovery, and rehabilitation based on professional advice. Indicators include that the client will consistently:

- Discuss prescribed treatment regimen with health care professional
- Perform treatment regimen as prescribed
- Monitor treatment and medication responses
- Keep appointments with health care professional

INTERVENTIONS. Clients who require pharmacologic treatment to control essential hypertension usually need to take medication for the rest of their lives. Frequently, however, some clients stop taking antihypertensive medications because they have no symptoms and experience troublesome side effects.

In the hospital setting, collaboration with the pharmacist is helpful to discuss the goals of therapy with the client, including potential side effects, to help identify potential problems. Assist the client in tailoring the therapeutic regimen to his or her activities of daily living (ADLs).

Clients who do not comply with antihypertensive treatment are at great risk for target organ damage and hypertensive crisis (malignant hypertension) (Chart 39-5). Clients in hypertensive crisis are admitted to critical care units, where they receive intravenous (IV) antihypertensive therapy, such as nitroprusside (Nipride), nicardipine (Cardene IV), fenoldopam (Corlopam), or labetalol (Normodyne). These drugs act quickly as vasodilators to decrease BP. Hospitalization for complications of hypertension can be costly in medical expenses, lost income, and deterioration in the quality of life.

Community-Based Care

HOME CARE MANAGEMENT

Many people do not successfully take medications as prescribed without some intervention designed to enhance adherence. There is no one cause of poor adherence. Clients often stop taking antihypertensive medications with the assumption that the hypertension is under control because they have no symptoms. Some just forget to take their doses. Others may think they are not sick enough. Many clients assume that if their blood pressure returns to normal levels with antihypertensives, they no longer need them. They may also stop taking antihypertensives because of adverse side effects or cost. Evidence-based approaches can be used to improve adherence to taking medications. Reviewing instructions and sending home written instructions appear to have the most impact on improving short-term adherence but less impact on long-term therapy. Self-administration of medications is a behavior that must be learned and most health care professionals have little training in how to assist others in behavior modification. Develop a plan with the client and identify what you will do to encourage adherence, and how other health care providers can also support the goal. Suggest adherence-improving approaches that can be easily incorporated into daily living.

If possible, the client should obtain an ambulatory blood pressure monitoring device (ABPM) for use at home so that the pressure can be checked periodically. Evaluate the client's ability to use this device. If the client cannot monitor the blood pressure, a family member or significant other may be taught how to perform this procedure. If weight reduction is a goal, suggest having a scale in the home for weight monitoring.

CHART 39-5

BEST PRACTICE for
Emergency Care of Clients with Hypertensive Crisis

EMERGENCY CARE

Assess
- Severe headache
- Extremely high blood pressure
- Dizziness
- Blurred vision
- Disorientation

Intervene
- Place client in a semi-Fowler's position.
- Administer oxygen.
- Administer IV nitroprusside (Nitropress), nicardipine (Cardene IV), or other infusion drug as prescribed (for nitroprusside, cover infusion bag to prevent drug breakdown by light).
- Monitor blood pressure every 5 to 15 minutes until the diastolic pressure is also below 90 and not less than 75; then monitor blood pressure every 30 minutes.
- Observe for neurologic or cardiovascular complications, such as seizures; numbness, weakness, or tingling of extremities; dysrhythmias; or chest pain.

HEALTH TEACHING

Instruct the client about sodium restriction, weight maintenance or reduction, alcohol restriction, stress management, and exercise (see Interventions [Arteriosclerosis and Atherosclerosis], p. 780). If necessary, also explain about the need to stop smoking. Provide oral and written information about the indications, dosage, times for administration, side effects, and drug interactions (see Chart 39-3) for antihypertensive medications. Stress that medications must be taken as prescribed and that when all of the medication has been consumed, the prescription must be renewed on a continual basis. Abrupt termination of medications such as beta blockers can result in angina (chest pain), myocardial infarction (MI), or rebound hypertension.

Also urge clients to report unpleasant side effects, such as excessive fatigue, cough, or sexual dysfunction. In many instances, an alternative medication can be prescribed to minimize certain side effects.

Hypertension is a chronic illness. Allow clients to verbalize feelings about the disease and its treatment. Advise them that their involvement in the treatment can lead to control of the disease and can prevent complications.

HEALTH CARE RESOURCES

A home care nurse may be needed for follow-up to monitor the blood pressure. Evaluate the client or family's ability to obtain accurate blood pressure measurements and assess compliance with treatment. The American Heart Association, the Red Cross, or a local pharmacy may be used for free blood pressure checks if clients cannot purchase equipment to monitor their blood pressure.

Evaluation: Outcomes

Evaluate the care of the client with hypertension on the basis of the identified nursing diagnoses and collaborative problems. The expected outcomes are that the client will:

- Understand a specific treatment regimen
- Take personal action to promote wellness, recovery, and rehabilitation based on professional advice

Specific indicators for these outcomes are listed for each nursing diagnosis under the Planning and Implementation section (see earlier).

Critical Thinking Challenge

On a return visit to the clinic, the 48-year-old client's blood pressure is now 166/90. His cholesterol level is 240, LDL-C is 180, and HDL-C is 35. His triglyceride level was 240. His weight is up to 275 pounds.

1. What questions would be important to ask in reviewing his history?
2. What lifestyle behaviors would you further analyze?
3. How can you help this client modify his behaviors?
4. What is the significance of these lipid values and what can be done about them?

evolve For suggested answer guidelines, go to http://evolve.elsevier.com/Iggy/.

RESOURCE MANAGEMENT

PERIPHERAL VASCULAR DISEASE

Cost of Care

- Each year, vascular disorders result in disability or death, and the financial impact on society is overwhelming.
- The cost of cardiovascular disease in 2003 was estimated at $352 billion according to the National Heart, Lung, and Blood Institute and the American Heart Association. This includes direct and indirect health care costs for expenditures such as health care provider fees, hospital care, nursing home services, medications, home care services, durable medical equipment, and loss of productivity to the client, family, and society.
- Case management and the use of critical care pathways by all health care providers decreases the cost of hospital care and helps decrease the length of stay for hospitalized clients.

Implications for Nursing

The medical and nursing management of clients with cardiovascular disease is costly. Research has identified certain risk factors that contribute to the development of cardiac and vascular disease. Be committed to identifying clients at risk and providing teaching and support toward reducing risk factors. Be involved in programs related to smoking cessation, weight reduction, lipid screening, stress reduction, and promoting healthy living behaviors.

PERIPHERAL ARTERIAL DISEASE

Peripheral vascular disease (PVD) includes disorders that alter the natural flow of blood through the arteries and veins of the peripheral circulation. PVD affects the lower extremities much more frequently than the upper extremities. Generally, a client with a diagnosis of PVD implies arterial disease (peripheral arterial disease [PAD]) rather than venous involvement. Some clients have both arterial and venous disease. The cost of PVD is staggering and is expected to rise as "baby boomers" age and obesity in the United States increases (see the Resource Management box above).

PATHOPHYSIOLOGY

PAD is a manifestation of systemic atherosclerosis and is a chronic condition in which partial or total arterial occlusion deprives the lower extremities of oxygen and nutrients. PAD of the lower extremities is sometimes referred to as lower extremity arterial disease (LEAD). Body tissues cannot live without an adequate oxygen and nutrient supply, and tissue eventually dies. Atherosclerosis is the most common cause of chronic altered blood flow. Fatty substances accumulate at the site of vessel wall injury and alter or totally occlude blood flow within the arteries. Tissue damage generally occurs below the arterial obstruction.

Obstructions are classified as inflow or outflow, according to the arteries involved and their relationship to the inguinal ligament (Figure 39-4). *Inflow* obstructions involve the distal end of the aorta and the common, internal, and external iliac arteries. They are located above the inguinal ligament. *Outflow* obstructions involve infrainguinal arterial segments (the femoral, popliteal, and tibial arteries) and are below the superficial femoral artery (SFA). Gradual inflow

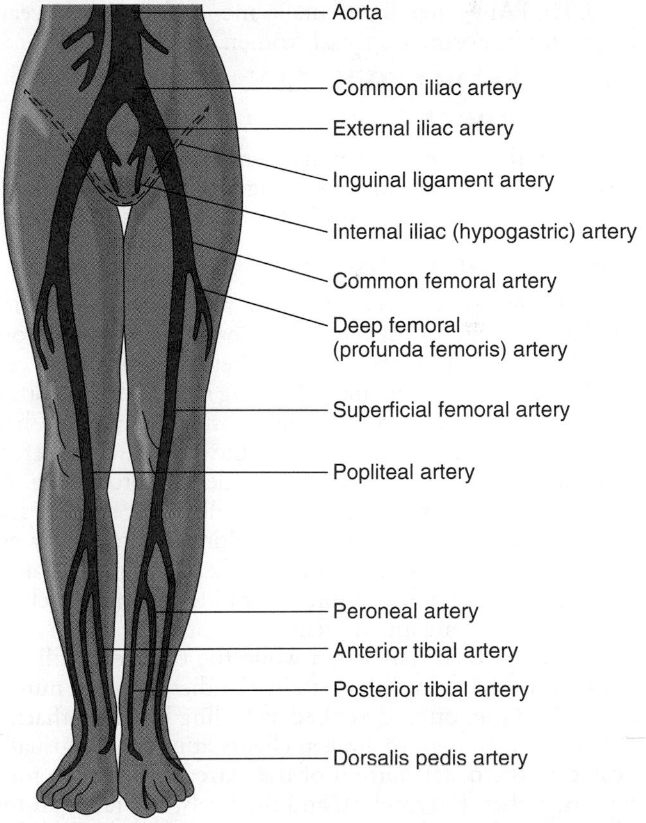

Figure 39-4 ■ Common locations of inflow and outflow lesions.

occlusions may not cause significant tissue damage; gradual outflow occlusions typically do.

Etiology and Genetic Risk

Because atherosclerosis is the most common cause of chronic arterial obstruction, the risk factors for atherosclerosis apply to PAD as well. Risk factors include hypertension, hyperlipidemia, diabetes mellitus, cigarette smoking, obesity, and familial predisposition. Advancing age also increases the risk of disease related to atherosclerosis. Clients with PAD have an increased risk for developing chronic angina, MI, or stroke and are 6 times as likely to die within 10 years compared to those without PAD.

Incidence/Prevalence

About 8 to 10 million people in the United States have PAD. The age-adjusted prevalence rate is 12% increasing to 20% in older adults age 70 years and older (Stewart et al., 2002). The presence of intermittent claudication in peripheral arterial disease is present in 15% to 40% of clients. Diagnosis of PAD is low because measurement of the ankle brachial index (ABI) is not a routine part of a clinic visit and many clients are not diagnosed unless they develop symptomatic leg pain. Black individuals appear to be affected more often than white individuals or Hispanics (Collins et al., 2003). PAD generally occurs in men older than 45 years of age and in postmenopausal women.

COLLABORATIVE MANAGEMENT

Assessment

The clinical course of chronic peripheral arterial disease (PAD) can be divided into four stages (Chart 39-6). Clients do not experience symptoms in the early stages of disease.

CHART 39-6

KEY FEATURES of Chronic Peripheral Arterial Disease

Stage I: Asymptomatic
- No claudication is present.
- Bruit or aneurysm may be present.
- Pedal pulses are decreased or absent.

Stage II: Claudication
- Muscle pain, cramping, or burning occurs with exercise and is relieved with rest.
- Symptoms are reproducible with exercise.

Stage III: Rest Pain
- Pain while resting commonly awakens the client at night.
- Pain is described as numbness, burning, toothache-type pain.
- Pain usually occurs in the distal portion of the extremity—toes, arch, forefoot, or heel—rarely in the calf or the ankle.
- Pain is relieved by placing the extremity in a dependent position.

Stage IV: Necrosis/Gangrene
- Ulcers and blackened tissue occur on the toes, the forefoot, and the heel.
- Distinctive gangrenous odor is present.

PHYSICAL ASSESSMENT

Most clients initially seek treatment for a characteristic leg pain known as **intermittent claudication** (a term derived from a word meaning "to limp"). Usually they can walk only a certain distance before a cramping, burning muscle discomfort or pain forces them to stop. The pain subsides after rest. When clients resume walking, they can walk the same distance before the pain returns; thus the pain is considered reproducible. As the disease progresses, clients can walk only shorter and shorter distances before pain recurs. Ultimately, pain may occur even while at rest. Question the client about the nature and characteristics of leg pain to determine whether the client may be experiencing intermittent claudication.

Rest pain, which may begin while the disease is still primarily in the stage of intermittent claudication, is a numbness or burning, often described as feeling like a toothache, that is severe enough to awaken clients at night. It is usually located in the distal portion of the extremities–in the toes, the foot arches, the forefeet, and the heels, but rarely in the calves or ankles. Clients can sometimes achieve pain relief by keeping the limb in a dependent position. Clients with rest pain often have advanced disease that may result in limb loss.

Clients with **inflow disease** experience discomfort in the lower back, buttocks, or thighs. Lower back or buttock discomfort indicates obstruction at or above the common iliac artery or abdominal aorta. Thigh discomfort indicates obstruction at or above the profunda femoris artery. Clients with *mild* inflow disease experience discomfort after walking about two blocks. This discomfort is not severe but causes the client to stop walking. It is relieved with rest. Clients with *moderate* inflow disease experience pain in these areas after walking about one or two blocks. The discomfort is described as being more like pain, but it subsides with rest most of the time. *Severe* inflow disease causes the client severe pain after walking less than one block. These clients usually have rest pain.

Clients with **outflow disease** describe burning or cramping in the calves, ankles, feet, and toes. Calf discomfort usually indicates arterial obstruction at or below the superficial femoral or popliteal artery. Instep or foot discomfort indicates an obstruction below the popliteal artery. Clients with *mild* outflow disease experience discomfort after walking about five blocks. This discomfort is relieved by rest. Clients with *moderate* outflow disease have pain after walking about two blocks. Intermittent rest pain may be present. Clients with *severe* outflow disease are usually unable to walk more than one-half block and usually experience rest pain. They may hang their feet off the bed at night for comfort. Clients with outflow disease complain more frequently of rest pain than do those with inflow disease.

Specific findings for PAD depend on the severity of the disease. Observe for loss of hair on the lower calf, ankle, and foot; dry, scaly, dusky, pale, or mottled skin; and thickened toenails. With severe arterial disease, the extremity is cold and gray-blue (cyanotic) or darkened. Pallor may occur when the extremity is elevated; dependent **rubor** may occur when the extremity is lowered. Muscle atrophy can accompany prolonged chronic arterial disease.

Palpate all pulses in both legs. The most sensitive and specific indicator of arterial function is the quality of the posterior tibial pulse because the pedal pulse is not palpable in a small percentage of people. The strength of the pulse should be compared bilaterally. Several scales are available for grading pulse strength.

CHART 39-7

KEY FEATURES of Lower Extremity Ulcers

Feature	Arterial Ulcers	Venous Ulcers	Diabetic Ulcers
History	Client complaints of claudication after walking approximately 1-2 blocks Rest pain usually present Pain at ulcer site Two or three risk factors present	Chronic nonhealing ulcer No claudication or rest pain Moderate ulcer discomfort Client complaints of ankle or leg swelling	Diabetes Peripheral neuropathy No complaints of claudication
Ulcer location and appearance	End of the toes Between the toes Deep Ulcer bed pale, with even edges Little granulation tissue	Ankle area Brown pigmentation Ulcer bed pink Usually superficial, with uneven edges Granulation tissue present	Plantar area of foot Metatarsal heads Pressure points on feet Deep Pale, with even edges Little granulation tissue
	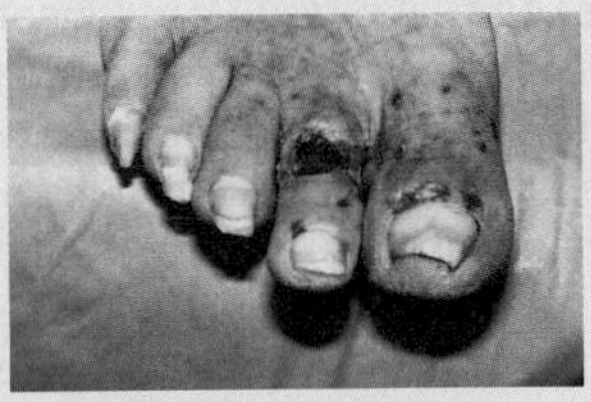	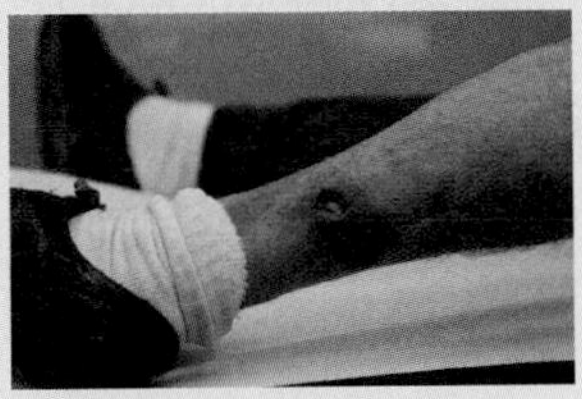	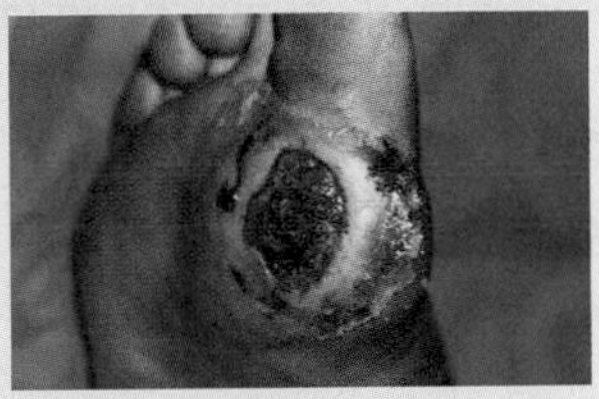
Other assessment findings	Cool or cold foot Decreased or absent pulses Atrophy of skin Hair loss Pallor with elevation Dependent rubor Possible gangrene When acute, neurologic deficits noted	Ankle discoloration and edema Full veins when leg slightly dependent No neurologic deficit Pulses present May have scarring from previous ulcers	Pulses usually present Cool or warm foot Painless
Treatment	Treat underlying cause (surgical, revascularization) Prevent trauma and infection Client education, stressing foot care	Long-term wound care (Unna boot, damp-to-dry dressings) Elevate extremity Client education Prevent infection	Rule out major arterial disease Control diabetes Client education regarding foot care Prevent infection

Photographs of arterial ulcer and diabetic ulcer from Callen, J.P., et al. (1993). *Color atlas of dermatology: Slide set.* Philadelphia: W.B. Saunders.

Note early signs of ulcer formation or complete ulcer formation, a complication of PAD. Arterial and venous stasis ulcers differ from diabetic ulcers (Chart 39-7).

Initially, **arterial ulcers** are painful and develop on the toes (often the great toe), between the toes, or on the upper aspect of the foot. With prolonged occlusion, the toes can become gangrenous. Typically, the ulcer is small, round, with a "punched out" appearance and well-defined borders. **Diabetic ulcers** develop on the plantar surface of the foot, over the metatarsal heads, and on the heel anywhere that pressure is exerted. Diabetic ulcers may not be painful because of diabetic neuropathy. **Venous stasis ulcers** cause minimal pain and occur in the ankle area. The foot is warm, and distal pulses are palpable. Note discoloration of the lower extremity at the ulcer site and stasis dermatitis. Skin lesions are discussed in further detail later in this chapter and in Chapter 70.

CULTURAL CONSIDERATIONS

Because only severe cyanosis is evident in the skin of dark-skinned clients, to detect cyanosis assess their skin and nail beds for a dull, lifeless color. The soles of the feet and the toenails are less pigmented and can enable detection of cyanosis or duskiness in the lower extremities.

RADIOGRAPHIC ASSESSMENT

Arteriography of the lower extremities is one x-ray for PAD, but it is not commonly performed today. This procedure involves injecting contrast medium into the arterial system and the risks, which include hemorrhage, thrombosis, embolus, and death, are serious.

OTHER DIAGNOSTIC ASSESSMENTS

The advent of noninvasive evaluation of arterial disease has become a popular method of diagnosis. Noninvasive testing provides information about the arterial system with minimal risk to the client.

SEGMENTAL SYSTOLIC BLOOD PRESSURE MEASUREMENTS. Using a Doppler probe, segmental systolic blood pressure measurements of the lower extremities at the thigh, calf, and ankle are an inexpensive, noninvasive method of assessing PAD. Normally, blood pressure readings in the thigh and calf are higher than those in the upper extremities. With the presence of arterial disease, these pressures are lower than the brachial pressure.

With *inflow* disease, pressures taken at the thigh level indicate the severity of disease. Mild inflow disease may cause a difference of only 10 to 30 mm Hg in pressure on the affected side compared with the brachial pressure. Severe inflow disease can cause a pressure difference of greater than 40 to 50 mm Hg. The ankle pressure is normally equal to or greater than the brachial pressure.

To evaluate *outflow* disease, compare ankle pressure with the brachial pressure, which provides a ratio known as the **ankle-brachial index (ABI).** The value can be derived by dividing the ankle blood pressure by the brachial blood pressure. An ABI of less than 0.9 in either leg is diagnostic of PAD.

EXERCISE TOLERANCE TESTING. Exercise tolerance testing (by stress test or treadmill) may give valuable information about claudication (muscle pain) without rest pain. The technician obtains resting pulse volume recordings and has the client walk on a treadmill until the symptoms are reproduced. At the time of symptom onset or after about 5 minutes, the technician obtains another pulse volume recording. Normally, there may be an increased waveform with minimal, if any, drop in the ankle pressure. In clients with arterial disease, the waveforms are decreased (dampened) and there is a decrease in the ankle pressure of 40 to 60 mm Hg for 20 to 30 seconds in the affected limb. If the return to normal pressure is delayed (longer than 10 minutes), the results suggest abnormal arterial flow in the affected limb.

PLETHYSMOGRAPHY. Plethysmography can also be performed to evaluate arterial flow in the lower extremities. The measurement provides graphs or tracings of arterial flow in the limb. If an occlusion is present, the waveforms are dampened to flattened, depending on the degree of occlusion.

Interventions

First determine whether the altered tissue perfusion is of arterial or venous origin. An accurate assessment often provides this information, but in some people both conditions may exist. In this case, each disease must be considered separately when appropriate interventions are planned.

NONSURGICAL MANAGEMENT. The interventions of exercise, position changes, promotion of vasodilation, drug therapy, and invasive nonsurgical procedures are used to increase arterial flow to the affected limb.

Exercise. Exercise may improve arterial blood flow to the affected limb through buildup of the *collateral* circulation. (Collateral circulation provides blood to the affected area through smaller vessels that develop and compensate for the occluded vessels.) Exercise is individualized for each client, but people with severe rest pain, venous ulcers, or gangrene should not participate. Other clients with peripheral arterial disease (PAD) can benefit from exercise that is initiated gradually and is slowly increased. Instruct the client to walk until the point of claudication, stop and rest, and then walk a little farther. Eventually, clients are able to walk longer distances as collateral circulation develops. Collaborate with the health care provider and physical therapist in determining an appropriate exercise program. Exercise rehabilitation has been used to relieve symptoms but requires a motivated client, and supervised sessions are generally not reimbursed by health care insurance.

Positioning. Positioning of the client to promote circulation has been somewhat controversial. Some clients have swelling in their extremities. Because swelling prevents arterial flow, feet should be elevated. Teach them to refrain from raising their legs above the heart level because extreme elevation *slows* arterial blood flow to the feet.

In severe cases, clients with PAD and swelling may sleep with the affected limb hanging from the bed, or they may sit upright in a chair for comfort. Instruct all clients with PAD to avoid crossing their legs and refrain from wearing restrictive clothing (e.g., garters to hold up hose, particularly common among older women), which interferes with blood flow.

Promoting Vasodilation. Vasodilation can be achieved by providing warmth to the affected extremity and preventing long periods of exposure to cold. Encourage the client to maintain a warm environment at home and to wear socks or insulated shoes at all times. Caution the client to *never* apply direct heat to the limb, such as with the use of heating pads or extremely hot water. Sensitivity is decreased in the affected limb, and the client may get burned without feeling it.

Encourage clients to prevent exposure of the affected limb to the cold because cold temperatures cause vasoconstriction (decreasing of the diameter of the blood vessels) and therefore decrease arterial blood flow. Clients should also drink adequate fluids to prevent increased blood viscosity.

Emotional stress, caffeine, and nicotine also can cause vasoconstriction. Emphasize that complete abstinence from smoking or chewing tobacco is the most effective method of preventing vasoconstriction. The vasoconstrictive effects of each cigarette may last up to 1 hour after the cigarette is smoked.

Drug Therapy. For clients with chronic PAD, prescribed drugs include hemorheologic and antiplatelet agents. Pentoxifylline (Trental) is a hemorheologic agent that increases the flexibility of red blood cells; it decreases blood viscosity by inhibiting platelet aggregation and decreasing fibrinogen, and thus increases blood flow in the extremities. Many clients report limited improvement in their daily lives after taking pentoxifylline. Moreover, clients with extremely limited endurance for walking have reported improvement to the point that they can perform some activities (e.g., walk to the mailbox or dining room) that were previously impossible.

Antiplatelet agents, such as aspirin (acetylsalicylic acid, Ancasal✱) and clopidogrel (Plavix), are commonly used for clients with PAD. Aspirin 325 or 81 mg daily is typically recommended for all clients with chronic PAD. However, in a trial of *c*lopidogrel versus *a*spirin in *p*atients at *r*isk of *i*schemic *e*vents (CAPRIE), clopidogrel demonstrated improvement over aspirin for risk reduction for myocardial infarction (MI), ischemic stroke, and vascular death, but the difference was slight. Therefore clients with peripheral vascular disease (PVD) with no contraindications to platelet therapy should receive either aspirin or clopidogrel.

Controlling hypertension can improve tissue perfusion by maintaining pressures that are adequate to perfuse the periphery but not constrict the vessels. Teach about the effect of blood pressure on the circulation and instruct in methods of control. For example, clients taking beta blockers may experience drug-related claudication or an exacerbation of symptoms. The health care provider closely monitors clients with PAD who are receiving beta blockers.

Percutaneous Transluminal Angioplasty. A nonsurgical but invasive method of improving arterial flow is **percutaneous transluminal angioplasty (PTA).** One or more arteries are dilated with a balloon catheter advanced through a cannula, which is inserted into or above an occluded or stenosed artery. When the procedure is successful, it opens the vessel lumen and improves arterial blood flow, creating a smooth inner-vessel surface. In addition, **stents** (wirelike devices) may be used along with the PTA to help keep the vessel open. Clients who are candidates for PTA must have occlusions or stenoses that are accessible to the catheter. The physician often uses PTA for those who are poor surgical candidates, who cannot withstand general anesthesia, or for whom amputation may be inevitable. Reocclusion may occur after this procedure, and the procedure may be repeated. Some clients are occlusion free for up to 3 to 5 years, whereas others may experience reocclusion within a year.

During PTA, intravascular stents may be placed to ensure adequate blood flow in a stenosed vessel. Candidates for intravascular stents are individuals with stenosis of the common or external iliac arteries. Intravascular stents are cost-effective and result in shorter hospital stays and earlier recoveries.

Laser-Assisted Angioplasty. Another invasive procedure is **laser-assisted angioplasty.** A laser probe is advanced through a cannula similar to that used for PTA. Laser-assisted angioplasty is usually reserved for clients with smaller occlusions in the distal superficial femoral, proximal popliteal, and common iliac arteries. Heat from the laser vaporizes the arteriosclerotic plaque to open the occluded or stenosed artery. If significant stenosis remains after the artery is opened, a balloon catheter may be inserted to further dilate the artery. Preparation of the client for PTA or laser-assisted angioplasty is similar to that for diagnostic angiography.

The *priority* for postprocedure nursing care is observing for bleeding at the puncture site. Closely observe vital signs and perform frequent checks of the distal pulses in both limbs. Clients are typically restricted to bedrest, with the limb straight for about 6 to 8 hours before ambulation, unless special collagen plugs are used to seal the vessel. Many receive anticoagulant therapy, such as heparin, during the procedure and for a short time after the procedure. Some type of antiplatelet drug is provided for 1 to 3 months after the procedure, however, clients usually take aspirin on a permanent basis.

Atherectomy. The technique of mechanical rotational abrasive **atherectomy** is used to improve blood flow to ischemic limbs in people with PAD. The rotational atherectomy device (Rotablator) is a high-speed rotary, metal burr ranging in size from 1.25 to 4.5 mm in diameter. The distal half of the burr is embedded with fine abrasive bits, which at rotational speeds of 100,000 to 120,000 rotations per minute result in fine-particle destruction of tissue. The Rotablator is designed to preferentially scrape "hard" surfaces (such as plaque) while minimizing damage to the vessel surface.

SURGICAL MANAGEMENT. Clients with severe rest pain or claudication that interferes with the ability to work or threatens loss of a limb become surgical candidates. **Arterial revascularization** is the surgical procedure most commonly used to increase arterial blood flow in an affected limb.

Surgical procedures are classified as inflow or outflow. Inflow procedures involve bypassing arterial occlusions above the superficial femoral arteries (SFAs). Outflow procedures involve surgical bypassing of arterial occlusions at or below the SFAs. For those who have both inflow and outflow problems, the inflow procedure (for larger arteries) is done before the outflow repair.

Inflow procedures include aortoiliac, aortofemoral, and axillofemoral bypasses. Outflow procedures include femoropopliteal and femorotibial bypasses. Inflow procedures are more successful, with less chance of reocclusion or postoperative ischemia. Outflow procedures are less successful in relieving ischemic pain and are associated with a higher incidence of reocclusion.

Graft materials for the bypasses are selected on an individual basis. For outflow procedures, the preferred graft material is an autogenous saphenous vein. However, these clients can experience coronary artery disease and may need this vein for coronary artery bypass. When the saphenous vein is not usable, the cephalic or basilic arm veins may be used.

Grafts made of synthetic materials, such as polytetrafluoroethylene (PTFE), Gore-Tex, and Dacron, have also been used when autogenous veins were not available. Although synthetic grafts have achieved adequate patency in arteries above the knee, they have failed to achieve satisfactory results in infrapopliteal outflow vessels. In addition, autogenous veins are often not long enough for use in these vessels. Composite grafts constructed from multiple vein segments offer even better patency to arteries below the knee.

Preoperative Care. Preparing the client for surgery is similar to procedures described for general or epidural anesthesia (see Chapter 20). Documentation of vital signs and peripheral pulses provides a baseline of information for comparison during the postoperative phase. Depending on the surgical procedure, the client may have an IV line, urinary catheter, central venous catheter, and/or arterial line. To prevent postoperative infection, antibiotic therapy is typically given before the procedure.

Operative Procedures. The anesthesiologist or nurse anesthetist places the client under general, epidural, or spinal anesthesia. Epidural or spinal induction is preferred for older adults to decrease the risk of cardiopulmonary complications in this age group. If arterial bypass is to be accomplished by autogenous grafts, the surgeon excises the appropriate veins through an incision. The occluded artery is then exposed through an incision, and the conduit veins or synthetic graft material is sutured above and below the occlusion to facilitate blood flow around the occlusion.

For *aortoiliac* and *aortofemoral* bypass surgery, the surgeon makes a midline incision into the abdominal cavity to expose the abdominal aorta, with additional incisions into each groin (Figure 39-5). Graft material is tunneled from the aorta to the groin incisions, where it is sutured in place.

In an *axillofemoral* bypass (Figure 39-6), the surgeon makes an incision beneath the clavicle and tunnels graft material sub-

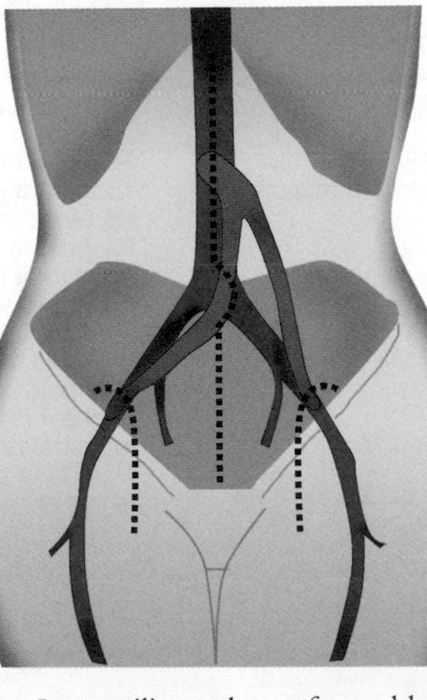

Figure 39-5 ■ In aortoiliac and aortofemoral bypass surgery, a midline incision into the abdominal cavity is required, with an additional incision in each groin.

cutaneously with a catheter from the chest to the iliac crest, into a groin incision, where it is sutured in place. Neither the thoracic nor the abdominal cavity is entered. For that reason, the axillofemoral bypass is used for high-risk clients who cannot tolerate a procedure requiring abdominal surgery.

Postoperative Care. Graft occlusion often occurs within the first 24 hours. Therefore astute nursing care is crucial. The Plan of Care below and on pp. 799-803 highlights the most important aspects of postoperative care.

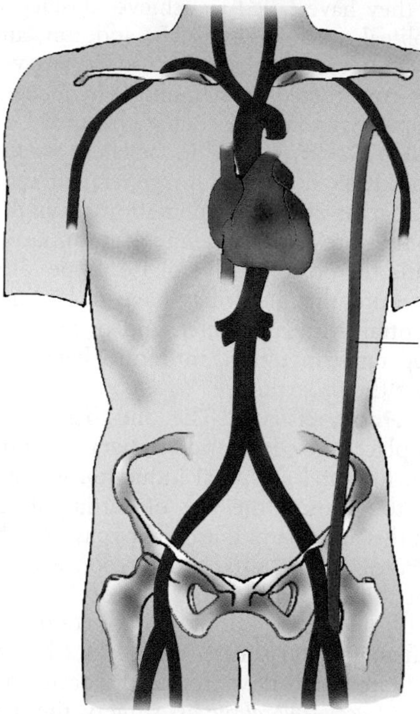

Figure 39-6 ■ An axillofemoral bypass graft.

Assessment for Graft Occlusion. Monitor the patency of the graft by checking the extremity every 15 minutes for the first hour, then hourly, for changes in color, temperature, and pulse intensity. Warmth, redness, and edema of the affected extremity are often expected outcomes of surgery as a result of increased blood flow. Immediately postoperatively, the operating room or postanesthesia care unit (PACU) nurse marks the site where the distal (dorsalis pedis or posterior tibial) pulse is best palpated or heard by Doppler ultrasonography. This information is communicated to the nursing staff on the critical care unit where the client will be sent.

Pain may be one of the first indicators of postoperative graft occlusion. Many people experience a throbbing pain caused by the increased blood flow to the extremity. Because this sensation is different from ischemic pain, be sure to assess the type of pain that the client is experiencing. Pain from occlusion may be masked by patient-controlled analgesia.

Promotion of Graft Patency. To promote graft patency, monitor the client's blood pressure and notify the surgeon if the pressure increases or decreases beyond normal limits. Hypotension may indicate hypovolemia, which can increase the risk of clotting. Range of motion of the affected limb is usually limited, with bending of the hip and knee contraindicated. Consult with the surgeon on a case-by-case basis regarding limitations of movement, including turning. Clients are restricted to bedrest for at least 24 hours postoperatively.

Coughing and deep breathing every 1 to 2 hours and using an incentive spirometer are essential. Clients who have undergone aortoiliac or aortofemoral bypass are allowed nothing by mouth (NPO) for at least 1 day postoperatively. Those who have undergone bypass surgery of the lower extremities not

Text continued on p. 804.

PLAN of CARE MEDICAL DIAGNOSIS: PERIPHERAL VASCULAR DISEASE

NURSING DIAGNOSIS NO. 1 ■ Chronic Pain

	Expected Outcomes	Nursing Interventions	Rationales
RELATED FACTORS Chronic physical/psychological disability **DEFINING CHARACTERISTICS** Atrophy of involved muscle group Fear of reinjury Altered ability to continue previous activities Protective gestures Irritability Depression	No verbal report or observation of alteration in activity level No verbal report or observation of guarding or protective gestures No verbal report or observation of restlessness No verbal report or observation of irritability No verbal report or observation of self-focusing behavior No verbal report or observation of depression Denies experiencing pain greater than 5 on a 0 to 10 pain scale	NIC **Pain Management** Perform a comprehensive assessment of pain to include location, characteristics, onset/duration, frequency, quality, intensity or severity of pain, and precipitating factors.	A plan for pain management must be based on the client's unique responses to pain.
		Determine the needed frequency of assessing client comfort and implement a monitoring plan.	Initial pain management strategies may require frequent evaluation to adjust dosing to maintain adequate comfort.
		Reduce or eliminate factors that precipitate or increase the pain experience.	Preventing a pain experience is preferred to trying to control or eliminate pain.
		Select and implement a variety of measures to facilitate pain relief, as appropriate.	Pharmacologic, nonpharmacologic, and interpersonal strategies may provide pain relief depending on the client's unique responses to the therapeutic interventions.

PLAN of CARE MEDICAL DIAGNOSIS: PERIPHERAL VASCULAR DISEASE—*cont'd*

NURSING DIAGNOSIS NO. 1 ■ Chronic Pain—*cont'd*

Expected Outcomes	Nursing Interventions	Rationales
	Use pain control measures before pain becomes severe.	Medicating the client in a timely manner prevents pain from reaching acutely unpleasant levels.
	Teach the use of nonpharmacologic techniques before, after and, if possible, during painful activities; before pain occurs or increases; and along with other pain relief measures.	Nonpharmacologic techniques help the client establish a sense of control over his or her pain experience.
	NIC **Analgesic Administration**	
	Administer analgesics around-the-clock.	Administration around-the-clock prevents peaks and troughs of analgesia, especially with severe pain.
	Evaluate the effectiveness of the analgesic at regular frequent intervals after each administration, but especially after the initial dose; also observe for any signs or symptoms of untoward effects.	Frequent evaluation of analgesic effectiveness permits the nurse to adjust the dose and timing interval to the client's need and provides an early warning of adverse responses.
	Document the client's response to the analgesic and any untoward effects.	Documentation provides the health care team with the information needed to evaluate accurately the client's response to the analgesic regimen.
	Implement actions to decrease the untoward effects of analgesics.	Actions taken to prevent the predictable but unwanted effects of narcotic analgesics (e.g., constipation) increase client comfort.
	Collaborate with the physician if drug, dose, route of administration, or interval changes are indicated, making specific recommendations based on equianalgesic principles.	The nurse working with the client is often in the best position to observe his or her response to the analgesic regimen.
	NIC **Progressive Muscle Relaxation**	
	Choose a quiet and comfortable setting, take precautions to prevent interruptions, and seat the client in a reclining chair or otherwise make him or her comfortable.	Ensuring the client's physical comfort and controlling environmental stimuli will aid relaxation efforts.
	Have the client tense, for 5 to 10 sec, each of 8 to 16 major muscle groups.	Tensing the foot muscles for no longer than 5 seconds prevents cramping.
	Terminate the session gradually.	Gradual termination maintains the sense of well-being and relaxation.
	Instruct the client to wear comfortable, nonrestrictive clothing.	The client's personal comfort will facilitate relaxation.

Continued

PLAN of CARE MEDICAL DIAGNOSIS: PERIPHERAL VASCULAR DISEASE—*cont'd*

NURSING DIAGNOSIS NO. 1 ■ Chronic Pain—*cont'd*

	Expected Outcomes	Nursing Interventions	Rationales
		Instruct the client to breathe deeply and to slowly release the breath and tension.	Proper breathing will help the client focus on relaxation rather than on external stimuli.
		Instruct the client to focus on the sensations in the muscles while they are relaxed and while they are tense.	Focusing on the muscle sensations will help build memory that can be called on at later times for relaxation.
		Other Interventions	
		Consider the use of hypnosis, biofeedback, magnetic field therapy, and/or acupuncture to aid in the control of chronic pain.	Cognitive and behavioral strategies may serve as adjuncts to or in place of pharmacologic or surgical interventions for chronic pain. Each therapy has different modes of action, which may or may not benefit the client.
		Refer the client to the Pain Advisory Committee.	The Pain Advisory Committee is a multidisciplinary committee with wide expertise in pain relief interventions.
		Continuing Care Considerations	
		Refer the client to an advanced practice nurse pain specialist, social worker, home care nurse, and/or psychologist, as appropriate.	Health care team members are able to provide continuing support for the client who is facing chronic pain.
		Collaborate with health care team members to secure a referral to a pain management clinic.	Pain management clinics combine many health care disciplines to focus on the management of chronic pain. The client's individual needs and responses to pain are evaluated, and a unique pain management program is initiated and adjusted.

NURSING DIAGNOSIS NO. 2 ■ Ineffective Tissue Perfusion: Peripheral

	Expected Outcomes	Nursing Interventions	Rationales
RELATED FACTORS Hypovolemia Hypervolemia Interruption of flow, arterial Mechanical reduction of venous and/or arterial blood flow Impaired transport of oxygen across the alveolar and/or capillary membrane **DEFINING CHARACTERISTICS** Capillary refill >3 sec Pulses absent or bilaterally unequal Claudication Delayed healing Skin: Pale	Has a pulse that remains strong and equal at all pulse points Has skin with warm undertones No verbal report or observation of delayed healing Denies extremity pain induced by activity No verbal report or observation of irritability	NIC **Circulatory Care: Arterial Insufficiency**	
		D Check peripheral pulses, edema, capillary refill, color, and temperature.	Perform a comprehensive appraisal of peripheral circulation to document arterial sufficiency.
		D Inspect skin for arterial ulcers or tissue breakdown.	Poor oxygenation and nutrition from arterial insufficiency leads to tissure necrosis.
		Monitor degree of discomfort or pain.	Hypoxia from poor oxygenation produces lactic acid, which stimulates pain fibers.
		D Place the extremity in a dependent position, as appropriate.	A dependent position uses gravity to encourage greater blood flow to the extremity.

D Indicates tasks that can be delegated to unlicensed assistive nursing personnel at the discretion of the nurse.

PLAN of CARE MEDICAL DIAGNOSIS: PERIPHERAL VASCULAR DISEASE—*cont'd*

NURSING DIAGNOSIS NO. 2 ■ Ineffective Tissue Perfusion: Peripheral—*cont'd*

	Expected Outcomes	Nursing Interventions	Rationales
		Administer antiplatelet or anticoagulant medications, as appropriate.	Antiplatelet and anticoagulant medications prevent the formation of blood clots, which further compromise peripheral circulation.
		D Change the client's position at least every 2 hours, as appropriate.	Position changes ensure that pressure does not impede circulation to the tissues.
		Encourage the client to exercise as tolerated.	Exercise causes muscle contraction, which improves blood flow.
		D Place sheepskin under the feet and lower legs, use a footboard/bed cradle at the foot of the bed, and have the client wear well-fitting shoes.	The client's extremity needs protection from injury, which might cause infection.
		D Use additional bed clothes and increase the room temperature, as appropriate.	Additional bed clothes and increased room temperature provide warmth to the extremities.
		Instruct the client regarding smoking, restrictive clothing, exposure to cold temperatures, and crossing of the legs and feet.	The client should avoid actions that interfere with circulation.
		Instruct the client regarding proper foot care.	Proper foot care protects the feet from tissue damage and subsequent infections that heal poorly.
		D Avoid applying direct heat to the extremity.	Poor peripheral circulation causes a diminished ability to determine heat and cold. The client could suffer burns without being aware of it.
		D Maintain adequate hydration.	Adequate hydration decreases blood viscosity, which lowers the risk of thromboembolus.
		Other Interventions	
		Teach the client/family the signs and symptoms of decreased tissue perfusion that need to be reported to the health care provider.	Early intervention may prevent loss of function due to poor tissue perfusion.
		Continuing Care Considerations	
		Monitor the client for adequate tissue perfusion.	Evidence of deteriorating tissue perfusion requires intervention.

NURSING DIAGNOSIS NO. 3 ■ Risk for Injury

	Expected Outcomes	Nursing Interventions	Rationales
RELATED FACTORS		NIC **Surveillance: Safety**	
Tissue hypoxia Biochemical, regulatory function (e.g., sensory dysfunction) Physical (e.g., broken skin, altered mobility)	Has a pulse that remains strong and equal at all pulse points No verbal report or observation of delayed healing Denies pain	Monitor the environment for potential safety hazards.	Removal or modification of the environment will prevent injuries from occurring.
		Communicate information about the client's risk to other nursing staff.	Caregivers in the environment are better able to prevent injury when high-risk clients are identified and monitored continuously.

Continued

PLAN of CARE — MEDICAL DIAGNOSIS: PERIPHERAL VASCULAR DISEASE—*cont'd*

NURSING DIAGNOSIS NO. 3 ■ Risk for Injury—*cont'd*

	Expected Outcomes	Nursing Interventions	Rationales
		Determine the client's health risk(s), as appropriate.	An appraisal and analysis of the client's risks provide the data for initiating prevention strategies.
		Retrieve and interpret laboratory data; contact the physician, as appropriate.	Laboratory data may provide an early warning of changes in the client's status.
		Compare the client's current status with his or her previous status.	Data comparisons provide ongoing feedback to detect improvements and deterioration in the client's condition.
		Obtain a consultation from the appropriate health care worker to initiate new treatment or to change existing treatments.	Collaboration with health care team members ensures prompt, accurate adjustments to the treatment regimen in an effort to prevent further injury to the client.
		Continuing Care Considerations	
		Educate the client and family about major risk factors and how to avoid/improve them.	The avoidance of injurious agents or activities prevents injury.

NURSING DIAGNOSIS NO. 4 ■ Risk for Peripheral Neurovascular Dysfunction

	Expected Outcomes	Nursing Interventions	Rationales
RELATED FACTORS Trauma or injury Vascular obstruction	Has a pulse that remains strong and equal at all pulse points Has a blood pressure that remains ±10 mm Hg of baseline No verbal report or observation of altered interpretation or response to stimuli No verbal report or observation of guarding or protective gestures Has skin with warm undertones Has a pulse that remains strong and equal at all pulse points No verbal report or observation of delayed healing Denies extremity pain induced by activity No verbal report of altered activity level Denies paresthesias or numbness	NIC **Peripheral Sensation Management** Monitor for paresthesia: numbness, tingling, hyperesthesia, and hypoesthesia.	Changes in sensation are clinical indicators of changes in circulation or nerve functioning.
		D Encourage the client to use the unaffected body part to determine the temperature of food, liquids, bathwater, and so on.	The client's unaffected body part is a better indicator of food or water temperature.
		D Encourage the client to use the unaffected body part to identify the location and texture of objects.	The client's unaffected body part has circulatory and nervous system competence and is better able to discriminate.
		Monitor the fit of bracing devices, prostheses, shoes, and clothing.	Constriction from clothing or abrasion from improperly fitting prostheses can cause skin breakdown.
		D Encourage the use of gloves or other protective clothing over the affected body part.	Protective gear should be worn when the affected body part is in contact with objects that may be potentially hazardous because of their thermal, textural, or other inherent characteristics.
		Avoid or carefully monitor the use of heat or cold, such as heating pads, hot water bottles, and ice packs.	The client/caregiver should monitor heat and cold with a thermometer to prevent thermal injury.
		Monitor for thrombophlebitis and deep vein thrombosis.	Pooling of blood from impaired circulation or impaired mobility facilitates the formation of thrombophlebitis and deep vein thrombosis.

D Indicates tasks that can be delegated to unlicensed assistive nursing personnel at the discretion of the nurse.

PLAN of CARE MEDICAL DIAGNOSIS: PERIPHERAL VASCULAR DISEASE—*cont'd*

NURSING DIAGNOSIS NO. 4 ■ Risk for Peripheral Neurovascular Dysfunction—*cont'd*

Expected Outcomes	Nursing Interventions	Rationales
	Instruct the client to use timed intervals, rather than the presence of discomfort, as a signal to alter position.	Using a time interval for repositioning is a safer standard, because sensation may be diminished.
	Instruct the client or family to examine skin daily for alterations in skin integrity.	Frequent skin inspection may prevent breaks in skin integrity.
	Instruct the client or family to monitor the position of body parts while bathing, sitting, lying, or changing position.	Improper positioning may increase damage to joints or place undue pressure over vulnerable areas of the skin.
	D Use pressure-relieving devices, as appropriate.	Cautious use of pressure-relieving devices may prevent pressure injury.
	Instruct the client to visually monitor the position of body parts.	If proprioception is impaired, the client will need to visually inspect the skin and monitor body position to prevent pressure injury or accidental injuries.
	Other Interventions	
	Assist the client to develop a plan to manage the stress in his or her life.	Emotional stress may cause vasoconstriction.
	Prepare the client for surgical intervention as ordered by the physician.	Procedures such as percutaneous transluminal angioplasty, laser-assisted angioplasty, atherectomy, or arterial revascularization may be needed to restore peripheral tissue perfusion.
	D Instruct the client to avoid crossing the legs.	Crossing the legs will interfere with blood flow.
	Instruct the client to completely abstain from tobacco products.	Nicotine causes vasoconstriction.
	Instruct the client to abstain from caffeine.	Caffeine causes vasoconstriction.
	Continuing Care Considerations	
	Teach the client/family how to assess tissue perfusion to the affected extremity.	Pain, pallor, paresthesias, pulselessness, paralysis, and poikilothermia are indicators of poor tissue perfusion.
	Instruct the client about the therapeutic regimen.	The client needs to follow foot care instructions, cease smoking, and avoid exposure of the affected extremity to heat/cold to prevent further injury to the extremity.
	D Remove safety hazards in the home.	Fall prevention and prevention of injury to the lower extremities is essential if the client has circulatory or nervous system impairments.

CHART 39-8

HOME CARE ASSESSMENT of
Clients with Peripheral Vascular Disease

Assess tissue perfusion to affected extremity(ies), including:
- Distal circulation, sensation, and motion
- Presence of pain, pallor, paresthesias, pulselessness, paralysis, poikilothermia (coolness)
- Ankle-brachial index

Assess adherence to therapeutic regimen, including:
- Following foot care instructions
- Quitting smoking
- Maintaining dietary restrictions
- Participating in exercise regimen
- Avoiding exposure to cold and constrictive clothing

Assess ability to manage wound care and prevent further injury, including:
- Use of compression stockings or compression pumps as directed
- Use of various dressing materials
- Signs and symptoms to report to nurse

Assess coping ability of client and family members.
Assess home environment, including:
- Safety hazards, especially related to falls

CHART 39-9

CLIENT EDUCATION GUIDE
Foot Care for the Client with Peripheral Vascular Disease

- Keep your feet clean by washing them with a mild soap in room-temperature water.
- Keep your feet dry, especially the ankles and between the toes.
- Avoid injury to your feet and ankles. Wear comfortable, well-fitting shoes. Never go without shoes.
- Keep your toenails clean and filed. Have someone cut them if you cannot see them clearly. Cut your toenails straight across.
- To prevent dry, cracked skin, apply a lubricating lotion to your feet.
- Prevent exposure to extreme heat or cold. Never use a heating pad on your feet.
- Avoid constricting garments.
- If a problem develops, see a podiatrist or physician.
- Avoid extended pressure on your feet or ankles, such as occurs when you lean against something.

involving the aorta or abdominal wall (femoropopliteal or femorotibial bypass) may remain NPO status until the first postoperative day when they are allowed clear liquids.

Treatment of Graft Occlusion. If manifestations of graft occlusion occur, notify the surgeon immediately. Perfusion through the graft must be resolved promptly to avoid ischemic injury to the limb. Emergency **thrombectomy** (removal of the clot), which the surgeon may perform at the bedside, is the most common treatment for acute graft occlusion. Thrombectomy is associated with excellent results in prosthetic grafts. Results of thrombectomy in autogenous vein grafts are not as successful and often necessitate graft revision and even replacement.

Local intra-arterial thrombolytic therapy with an agent such as tissue plasminogen activator (t-PA) or an infusion of a platelet inhibitor such as abciximab (ReoPro) may be used for acute graft occlusions in selected clients in settings wherein health care providers are experts on its use. Other antiplatelet drugs, such as the glycoprotein IIb/IIIa inhibitors tirofiban (Aggrastat) or eptifibatide (Integrilin) may be used as alternatives. The physician considers these therapies when the surgical alternative (e.g., thrombectomy with or without graft revision or replacement) carries high morbidity or mortality or when surgery for this type of occlusion has traditionally yielded poor results. When the physician prescribes thrombolytic therapy, closely assess the client for manifestations of bleeding.

Monitoring for Compartment Syndrome. Compartment syndrome occurs when tissue pressure within a confined body space becomes elevated and restricts blood flow. The resultant ischemia can lead to tissue damage and eventually tissue death. Assess the motor and sensory function of the affected extremity. The extremity should also be assessed for worsening pain, fullness, swelling, and tenseness. These symptoms should be reported to the health care provider immediately.

Assessment for Infection. Graft or wound infections can be life threatening and can endanger the client's limb. Use sterile technique when in contact with the incision and observe for symptoms of infection at or around the graft and incision sites. Assess the area for induration, erythema, tenderness, warmth, edema, or drainage. Also monitor for fever and leukocytosis (increased serum white blood cell count). Notify the surgeon if any of these symptoms occur.

Community-Based Care

HOME CARE MANAGEMENT

Peripheral arterial disease (PAD) is a chronic, long-term problem with frequent complications. Clients with PAD may benefit from a case manager who can follow them across the continuum of care. The goal is to maintain the client in the home environment.

Managing the client at home often requires an interdisciplinary team approach. Chart 39-8 outlines the assessment highlights for home care clients with peripheral vascular disease (PVD).

HEALTH TEACHING

Instruct all clients on methods to promote vasodilation. Teach clients to avoid raising their legs above the level of the heart unless venous stasis is also present. Provide written and oral instructions on foot care and methods to prevent injury and ulcer development for all clients (Chart 39-9).

Clients who have had surgery require additional instruction on incision care (see Chapter 22). Encourage all clients to avoid smoking and to limit dietary fat intake to less than 30% of the total daily calories. Remind clients to consume adequate fluids to prevent dehydration.

Clients with chronic arterial obstruction may fear recurrent occlusion or further narrowing of the artery. They often fear that they might lose a limb or become debilitated in other ways. Indeed, chronic PAD may worsen, especially in clients with diabetes mellitus. Reassure them that participation in prescribed exercise, diet, and pharmacologic therapy, along with cessation of smoking, can limit further formation of atherosclerotic plaques.

HEALTH CARE RESOURCES

Clients with arterial compromise may need assistance with activities of daily living (ADLs) if activity is limited by pain. They may need to limit or avoid stair climbing, depending on the severity of disease. Clients who have undergone surgery or need to limit activity usually need temporary help with ADLs.

Clients who must limit activity because of PAD may benefit from the assistance of a home care aide. Those who have undergone surgery may require a home care nurse to assist with incision care. The nurse or case manager arranges for home care resources before the client is discharged.

Critical Thinking Challenge

A 50-year-old African-American man develops diabetes a few years after an injury and is seeking pain relief because of a cramping, burning pain in his calf when he walks any great distance. He describes the pain to be "like a toothache." His blood pressure is 158/90 and his cholesterol is 210.

1. What impact does diabetes have on hypertension?
2. How does diabetes impact the development of peripheral vascular disease?
3. What diagnostic studies would be important for this client?
4. During assessment of this client, what findings would you expect?

evolve For suggested answer guidelines, go to http://evolve.elsevier.com/Iggy/.

ACUTE PERIPHERAL ARTERIAL OCCLUSION

PATHOPHYSIOLOGY

Although chronic peripheral arterial disease (PAD) progresses slowly, the onset of **acute arterial occlusions** may be sudden and dramatic. An embolus is the most common cause of peripheral occlusions, although a local thrombus may be the cause. Occlusion may affect the upper extremities, but it is more common in the lower extremities. Emboli originating from the heart are the most common cause of acute arterial occlusions. Most clients with an embolic occlusion have had an acute myocardial infarction (MI) and/or atrial fibrillation within the preceding weeks.

COLLABORATIVE MANAGEMENT

Clients with an acute arterial occlusion describe severe pain below the level of the occlusion that occurs even at rest. The affected extremity is cool or cold, pulseless, and mottled. Minute areas on the toes may be blackened or gangrenous. Those with acute arterial insufficiency often present with the "six *P*'s" of ischemia:

- *P*ain
- *P*allor
- *P*ulselessness
- *P*aresthesia
- *P*aralysis
- *P*oikilothermia (coolness)

The health care provider must initiate treatment promptly to avoid permanent damage or loss of an extremity. Anticoagulant therapy with unfractionated heparin (UFH; Hepalean✱) is usually the first intervention to prevent further clot formation. A bolus of up to 10,000 units may be prescribed. The client may also undergo angiography.

A surgical thrombectomy or embolectomy with local anesthesia may be performed to remove the occlusion. The physician makes an incision, which is followed by an **arteriotomy** (a surgical opening into an artery). The physician then inserts a Fogarty catheter into the artery and retrieves the embolus. It may be necessary to close the artery with a patch graft.

Postoperatively, monitor the affected extremity for improvement in color, temperature, and pulse, as well as other extremities for manifestations of new thrombi or emboli. Pain should significantly diminish after the surgical procedure, although mild incisional pain remains. Watch closely for complications caused by reperfusing the artery after thrombectomy or embolectomy, which include spasms and swelling of the skeletal muscle. Swelling of the skeletal muscles causing compartment syndrome is characterized by edema, pain on passive movement, poor capillary refill, numbness, and muscle tenseness. Fasciotomy (surgical opening into the tissues) may be necessary to prevent further injury and save the limb.

The use of systemic thrombolytic therapy for acute arterial occlusions has been disappointing because bleeding complications have outweighed the benefits obtained. Local intra-arterial thrombolytic therapy with alteplase (Activase) or t-PA and the use of platelet inhibitors, such as abciximab (ReoPro), have emerged as alternatives to surgical treatment in selected clients in settings where health care providers are familiar with their use and complications. When thrombolytics are given, monitor for manifestations of bleeding, bruising, or hematoma. When a client receives any platelet inhibitor, platelet counts need to be monitored for the first 3, 6, and 12 hours after the start of the infusion. If the platelet count decreases to below 100,000, the abciximab infusion needs to be readjusted or discontinued. If any of these complications occur, notify the physician immediately.

ANEURYSMS OF CENTRAL ARTERIES

PATHOPHYSIOLOGY

An **aneurysm** is a permanent localized dilation of an artery, which enlarges the artery to at least two times its normal diameter. An aneurysm may be described as *fusiform* (a diffuse dilation affecting the entire circumference of the artery) or *saccular* (an outpouching affecting only a distinct portion of the artery). Aneurysms may also be described as true or false. In true aneurysms the arterial wall is weakened by congenital or acquired problems. False aneurysms occur as a result of vessel injury or trauma to all three layers of the arterial wall.

Dissecting hematomas, traditionally called *dissecting aneurysms,* are more accurately described as *aortic dissections* (see the later discussion on p. 809). Aortic dissections differ from aneurysms in that they are formed when blood accumulates in the wall of an artery.

Aneurysms tend to occur at specific anatomic sites (Figure 39-7), most commonly in the abdominal aorta. Aneurysms often occur at a point where the artery is not supported by skeletal muscles or on the lines of curves or flexion in the arterial tree.

An aneurysm forms when the middle layer (media) of the artery is weakened, producing a stretching effect in the inner layer (intima) and outer layers (adventitia) of the artery. As the artery widens, tension in the wall increases and further widening occurs, thus enlarging the aneurysm. Hypertension (high blood pressure) produces more tension and enlargement within the artery. As the aneurysm grows, the risk of arterial rupture increases. When *dissecting* aneurysms occur, the aneurysm enlarges, blood is lost, and blood flow to organs is diminished.

Abdominal aortic aneurysms (AAAs) account for about 75% of all aneurysms. Most of these aneurysms are

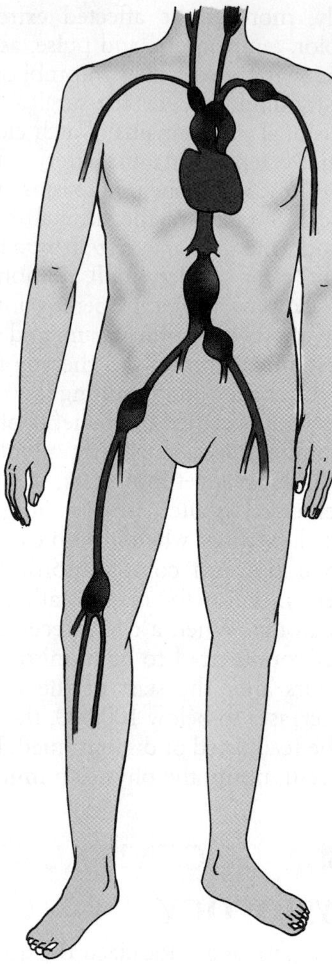

Figure 39-7 ■ Common anatomic sites of arterial aneurysms.

located between the renal arteries and the aortic bifurcation. Of all AAAs greater than 6 cm in diameter, 50% rupture within 1 year; of those aneurysms smaller than 6 cm in diameter, 15% to 20% rupture. Structural changes of the protein matrix in the aortic wall characterize AAAs. Plasma levels of specific biomarkers metalloproteinase-3 and -9 can determine whether AAA repair has been successful. When these markers reappear in the blood following surgery, they may signal a recurrence of the AAA (Sangiorgi et al., 2001).

Thoracic aortic aneurysms account for about 25% of all aneurysms and are frequently misdiagnosed. They are typically discovered when advanced imaging is intended to assess other conditions. Autopsies reveal the diagnosis is missed in about 10% of cases. Thoracic aortic aneurysms commonly develop between the origin of the left subclavian artery and the diaphragm. They are located in the descending, ascending, and transverse sections of the aorta. They can also occur in the aortic arch and are very difficult to manage surgically.

Aneurysms can cause symptoms by exerting pressure on surrounding structures or by rupturing. Rupture of an aneurysm is the most frequent complication and is life threatening because abrupt and massive hemorrhagic shock occurs with the rupture. Thrombi within the wall of an aneurysm can also be the source of emboli in distal arteries below the aneurysm.

Etiology

Atherosclerosis is the most common cause of all aneurysms, with hypertension and cigarette smoking being contributing factors. Syphilis (a sexually transmitted disease), Marfan syndrome (an autoimmune disease), and Ehlers-Danlos syndrome (a rare genetic disorder) are other causes of AAAs.

Incidence/Prevalence

The incidence of AAAs, estimated between 30 and 66 per 1000 persons, is increasing in the Western world. About 15,800 people in the United States die annually of abdominal aneurysms, making it the thirteenth leading cause of death in the United States. (National Heart, Lung, and Blood Institute, 2002). Thoracic aortic aneurysms occur most often in older adults and have a 50% mortality rate even with surgical intervention. AAAs are more common in men than in women (4:1).

◆COLLABORATIVE MANAGEMENT

◆Assessment

Most clients with abdominal or thoracic aneurysms are asymptomatic when their aneurysms are first discovered by routine examination or during radiographic study performed for another reason.

PHYSICAL ASSESSMENT

Because there may be symptoms, assess clients with a known or suspected *abdominal aortic aneurysm (AAA)* for abdominal, flank, or back pain. Pain related to an AAA is usually steady with a gnawing quality, is unaffected by movement, and may last for hours or days.

A pulsation in the upper abdomen slightly to the left of the midline between the xiphoid process and the umbilicus may be present. A detectable aneurysm is at least 5 cm in diameter. Auscultate for a bruit over the mass but avoid palpating the mass because it may be tender and there is a risk of rupture.

Although some clients have symptoms when the aneurysm is intact, many are asymptomatic until the time of rupture. If expansion and impending rupture of an AAA are suspected, assess for sudden and severe pain of sudden onset in the back or lower abdomen, which may radiate to the groin, buttocks, or legs.

Clients with a rupturing AAA are critically ill and in hemorrhagic (hypovolemic) shock. Signs include hypotension, diaphoresis, mental obtundation, oliguria, and dysrhythmias. Retroperitoneal hemorrhage is manifested by hematomas in the flanks. Rupture into the abdominal cavity causes abdominal distention.

When *a thoracic aortic aneurysm* is suspected, assess for back pain and manifestations of compression of the aneurysm on adjacent structures. Signs include shortness of breath, hoarseness, and difficulty swallowing. Thoracic aneurysms are not often detected by physical assessment, but occasionally a mass may be visible above the suprasternal notch. The client with suspected rupture of a thoracic aneurysm is assessed for sudden and excruciating back or chest pain. Rupture of a thoracic aneurysm is also indicated by hemorrhagic shock (see Chapter 40).

DIAGNOSTIC ASSESSMENT

An abdominal x-ray or a lateral x-ray of the spine often shows an AAA. The "eggshell" appearance of the aneurysm is essentially diagnostic.

Computed tomography (CT) scanning is the standard tool for assessing the size and location of an abdominal or thoracic aneurysm. A thoracic aneurysm can be diagnosed by chest x-ray. Aortic arteriography is usually performed for clients who are to undergo surgical repair of a thoracic aneurysm.

Ultrasonography is a noninvasive technique that provides an accurate diagnosis, as well as information about the size and location of an AAA.

Interventions

The size of the aneurysm and the presence of symptoms are the most important parameters in the determination of treatment.

NONSURGICAL MANAGEMENT. The goal of nonsurgical management is to monitor the growth of the aneurysm and maintain the blood pressure at a normal level to decrease the risk of rupture.

Because elevated blood pressure can increase the rate of aneurysmal enlargement, hypertension is an important risk factor for rupture. Clients with hypertension are treated with antihypertensives to decrease the rate of enlargement and the risk for early rupture.

For clients with small or asymptomatic aneurysms, frequent CT scans are necessary to monitor the growth of the aneurysm. Emphasize the importance of following through with scheduled tests to monitor the growth. Also explain the clinical manifestations of aneurysms that need to be promptly reported.

SURGICAL MANAGEMENT. Surgical management of an aneurysm may be an elective or an emergency procedure. For clients with either a *rupturing* abdominal aortic or a thoracic aneurysm, emergency surgery is performed.

Clients with an abdominal aortic aneurysm (AAA) 6 cm in diameter or wider usually undergo elective surgery. Some surgeons favor surgical treatment for clients with aneurysms 4 to 6 cm in diameter if the client is in good health. Clients in good health with aneurysms smaller than 4 cm and clients in poor health with aneurysms 4 to 6 cm in diameter undergo nonsurgical treatment until the aneurysm reaches 6 cm.

Clients with thoracic aortic aneurysms measuring 7 cm or more in diameter and clients with smaller aneurysms that are producing symptoms are advised to have elective surgery. Clients with aneurysms smaller than 7 cm in diameter that are not causing symptoms are treated nonsurgically until symptoms occur or the aneurysm enlarges to 7 cm.

The most common procedure performed for clients with an AAA has traditionally been an AAA resection or repair **(aneurysmectomy).** The mortality rate for elective AAA resection is 2% to 5%. The mortality rate for emergency surgery for expanding AAAs is 5% to 15% and 50% for those that have ruptured.

Newer technology, such as endothelial stent grafts, has improved mortality rates and shortened the hospital stay for selected clients who need aneurysm repair. The stents (wirelike devices) are inserted percutaneously (through the skin), avoiding abdominal incisions and therefore decreasing the risk of a prolonged postoperative recovery. Postoperative care is similar to care required following an arteriogram (angiogram).

Abdominal Aortic Aneurysm Resection. In an AAA resection, the physician excises the aneurysm from the abdominal aorta to prevent or repair the rupture. The goal is to secure stable aortic integrity and tissue perfusion throughout the body.

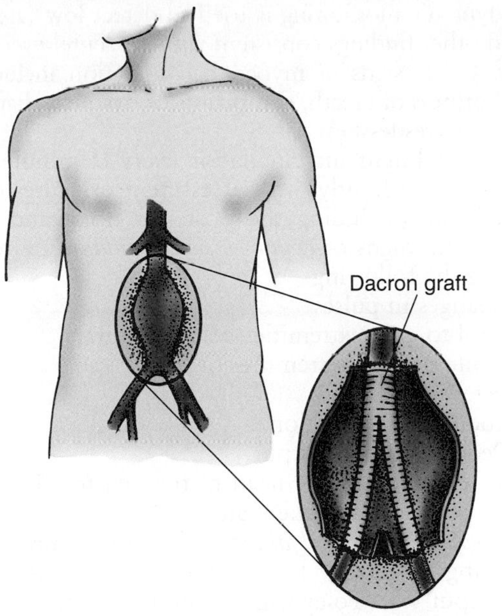

Figure 39-8 ■ Surgical repair of abdominal aortic aneurysm with a woven Dacron graft.

Preoperative Care. Interventions are similar to those for clients undergoing surgery with general anesthesia (see Chapter 20). A bowel preparation and emphasis on coughing and deep breathing are very important. Because significant blood loss may occur during AAA resection, clients planning elective surgery may be advised to bank their blood for autologous (self) transfusions postoperatively.

Assess all peripheral pulses to serve as a baseline for comparison postoperatively. Use a marker to note where the pulse is palpated or heard by Doppler ultrasonography to facilitate locating the pulse postoperatively.

Clients with ruptured aneurysms are brought to the operating suite directly from the emergency department. Preoperative care of clients with ruptured aneurysms involves administration of large volumes of IV fluids to maintain tissue perfusion.

Operative Procedures. The surgeon makes a midline abdominal incision from the xiphoid process to the symphysis pubis, or a wide transverse incision from flank to flank, to expose the aneurysm. Clamps are applied just above and just below the aneurysm, the aneurysm is excised, and a preclotted Dacron graft is sutured in an end-to-end fashion (Figure 39-8).

Postoperative Care. Immediately postoperatively, the client is typically admitted to a critical care unit for 24 hours, depending on his or her age and condition. In addition to providing the routine postoperative care discussed in Chapter 22, assess for and assist in prevention of the postoperative complications that can occur after an AAA repair. Complications include the following:

- Myocardial infarction
- Graft occlusion or rupture causing hemorrhage
- Hypovolemia and/or renal failure
- Respiratory distress
- Paralytic ileus

During the immediate postoperative period, the client's blood pressure is monitored with an arterial catheter. Continuous cardiac monitoring is used to detect any dysrhythmias.

Hemodynamic monitoring is used to detect low cardiac output and other findings consistent with an acute *myocardial infarction*. Other signs of myocardial infarction include chest pain, shortness of breath, complaints of dyspnea, diaphoresis, anxiety, and restlessness.

Assess vital signs and circulation every 15 minutes for the first hour, then hourly, with assessment of pulses distal to the graft site (including the posterior tibial and dorsalis pedis pulses). Signs of *graft occlusion or rupture* are reported, including the following:

- Changes in pulses
- Cool to cold extremities below the graft
- White or blue extremities or flanks
- Severe pain
- Abdominal distention
- Decreased urine output

Limit elevation of the head of the bed to 45 degrees or less to avoid flexion of the graft.

Hypovolemia and renal failure may occur because of blood loss during surgery or before if rupture occurred. Assess urine output via a Foley catheter hourly. If urine output is less than 50 mL/hr, notify the surgeon. Although advances in surgical technique have decreased the risk of renal failure after clamping during surgery, renal failure may occur. Renal failure caused by acute tubular necrosis is more common after emergency surgery. In addition to monitoring urine output, in collaboration with the physician, monitor serum creatinine and blood urea nitrogen (BUN) levels daily.

Assess respiratory rate and depth every hour and auscultate breath sounds every 4 hours to monitor for *respiratory complications*. The client may be maintained on a ventilator, however, early extubation is preferred if the client is stable. Opioids are administered for pain, as prescribed. If the client remains intubated, turning and suctioning are provided as needed. Firm abdominal support of the incision with a pillow or bath blanket during coughing exercises is needed for support. After extubation, assist the client to a bedside chair within 24 hours. Early mobility decreases the risk of atelectasis and deep vein thrombosis.

Paralytic ileus after AAA repair is expected for 2 to 3 days. Clients have a nasogastric tube set to low suction until bowel sounds return. Listen for bowel sounds every 8 hours and report their return to the physician. Prolonged absence of bowel sounds and distention may indicate a prolonged ileus or a bowel infarction.

Thoracic Aortic Aneurysm Repair. Repair of thoracic aneurysms is tailored to each client; the procedure depends on the type and location of the aneurysm. Total cardiopulmonary bypass (CPB) is necessary for excision of aneurysms in the ascending aorta, and partial bypass is often used during excision of aneurysms in the descending aorta.

Preoperative Care. The care of the client undergoing thoracic aneurysm resection is similar to that provided for the client having thoracic surgery.

Operative Procedures. The surgeon uses either a thoracotomy or a median sternotomy approach to enter the thoracic cavity. The surgeon exposes the aneurysm and excises it. After excising the aneurysm, the surgeon usually sews a Dacron graft or prosthesis onto the aorta. Saccular aneurysms, which have an outpouching from a distinct portion of the arterial wall, can sometimes be removed without resection of the aorta. Newer procedures do not remove the aneurysm. Instead, the surgeon cuts into the aneurysm and inserts a graft. The walls of the aneurysm are wrapped around the graft for stability.

Postoperative Care. The care of a client who has undergone thoracic aneurysm repair is similar to that of clients after other chest surgery. Clients who have undergone cardiopulmonary bypass (CPB) receive care similar to that described in Chapter 41. Assess for and assist in the prevention of postoperative complications that can occur after a thoracic aneurysm repair. Complications include:

- Hemorrhage
- Ischemic colitis
- Cerebral and spinal cord ischemia (causing paraplegia)
- Respiratory distress
- Cardiac dysrhythmias

Assess vital signs at least hourly, reporting any signs of *hemorrhage* (e.g., a decrease in blood pressure, an increase in pulse rate, rapid respirations, diaphoresis) to the physician immediately. Assess for bleeding or separation at the graft site by noting significant increases in chest drainage from the chest tubes.

Inadvertent interruption of the blood supply to the spinal cord during thoracic aneurysm repair can result in *paraplegia*. Assess the client hourly for sensation and motion in all extremities and report deficits immediately.

After thoracic aneurysm repair, clients are especially susceptible to *respiratory distress* from atelectasis or pneumonia. This problem occurs as a result of both CPB and incisional discomfort. Both atelectasis and pneumonia may cause shallow breathing and poor cough effort. These clients are often maintained on a ventilator, at least overnight, after surgery. For clients with a median sternotomy, the surgeon firmly splints the incision to prevent separation of the sternum.

Assess all clients recovering from thoracic aneurysm repair for cardiac *dysrhythmias*. The stress of the thoracic surgery, added to the increased incidence of arteriosclerosis in this group, may predispose these clients to a myocardial infarction, cardiac dysrhythmias, or heart failure.

Endovascular Repair of Abdominal Aortic Aneurysms. The repair of AAAs with **endovascular stent grafts** provides an alternative choice for some clients. Clients selected for endovascular repair of AAAs are generally at high risk for major abdominal surgery. Some clients with AAAs may be referred for endovascular repair before the aneurysm reaches the recommended diameter for elective surgery.

There are different designs of endovascular stent grafts for use, depending on the anatomic involvement of the aneurysm. The stent graft is flexible with either Dacron or polytetrafluoroethylene (PTFE) material. It is inserted through a skin incision into the femoral artery by way of a catheter-based system. The catheter is advanced to a level above the aneurysm, away from the renal arteries. The graft is released from the catheter, and the stent graft is deployed into place with a series of hooks. A defined proximal and distal neck is needed for tight seating of the stent to prevent leakage. This procedure is done in collaboration with the vascular surgeon, interventional radiologist, operating room team, and at some centers, vascular medicine physician.

The endovascular repair of AAAs has decreased the

length of hospital stay for clients requiring repair of abdominal aneurysms; however, the client needs to be closely monitored, in the hospital and at home, for the development of complications following the procedure. Expert nursing care is required to allow for early identification of problems and complications that can be resolved in a timely fashion. In addition, expert nursing skills are needed for the coordination and collaboration required for discharge planning and follow-up care for clients at home (see the Clinical Pathway on the Evolve website).

Endovascular stent repair is not without complications. Complications include the need for conversion from an endovascular repair to open surgical repair of the aneurysm, bleeding, aneurysm rupture, peripheral embolization, and misdeployment of the stent graft. All of these complications require surgical intervention.

Community-Based Care

Most clients are discharged to home after aneurysm repair. However, in the absence of family or other support systems, the postoperative client may be discharged to an extended (long-term) care facility for rehabilitation.

If discharged to home, the client must follow the instructions provided by the nurse regarding activity level and incisional care. Because stair climbing may be restricted initially, the client may need a bedside commode if the bathroom is inaccessible.

For clients who have not undergone surgical aneurysm repair, the teaching plan emphasizes the importance of compliance with the schedule of computed tomography (CT) scanning to monitor the size of the aneurysm. Educate the client receiving treatment for hypertension about the importance of continuing to take prescribed medication. Instruct the client and family or significant others about the signs and symptoms that must promptly be reported to the health care provider, which include the following:

- Abdominal fullness or pain, or back pain
- Chest or back pain, shortness of breath, difficulty swallowing, or hoarseness

Teach the client who has undergone repair of the aneurysm about activity restrictions, wound care, and pain management. Clients may not engage in activities that involve lifting heavy objects (usually more than 15 to 20 pounds [6.8 to 9.1 kg]) for 6 to 12 weeks postoperatively. Advise them to use discretion in activities that involve pulling, pushing, or straining. Clients who usually engage in vigorous activities should discuss them with their health care provider. Most individuals are restricted from driving a car for several weeks after discharge.

Clients who have not undergone aneurysm repair may fear rupture and subsequent death. Reinforce the rationales for CT monitoring of the size of the aneurysm and for controlling hypertension and encourages clients to verbalize their fears.

In collaboration with the case manager or social worker, assess the availability of transportation to and from appointments for clients needing CT monitoring. Clients who have undergone surgery may require the services of a home care nurse for assistance with dressing changes. A home care aide may be needed to assist with activities of daily living (ADLs).

ANEURYSMS OF THE PERIPHERAL ARTERIES

PATHOPHYSIOLOGY

Although femoral and popliteal aneurysms are relatively uncommon, they are often associated with an aneurysm in another location of the arterial tree. To detect a popliteal aneurysm, a pulsating mass is seen in the popliteal space. To detect a femoral aneurysm, observe a pulsatile mass over the femoral artery. Both extremities are evaluated because more than one femoral or popliteal aneurysm may be present.

COLLABORATIVE MANAGEMENT

The client may exhibit symptoms of limb ischemia, including diminished or absent pulses, cool to cold skin, and pain. Pain may also be present if an adjacent nerve is compressed. The recommended treatment for either type of aneurysm, regardless of the size, is surgery because of the risk of thromboembolic complications associated with their presence.

To treat a femoral aneurysm, the physician excises the aneurysm and restores circulation using a Dacron graft or an autogenous saphenous vein graft. Most surgeons prefer to bypass rather than resect a popliteal aneurysm.

Postoperatively, monitor for lower limb ischemia. Palpate pulses below the graft to assess graft patency. Often, Doppler ultrasonography is necessary to assess blood flow when pulses are not palpable. Sudden development of pain or discoloration of the extremity is reported immediately to the physician because it may indicate graft occlusion.

AORTIC DISSECTION

PATHOPHYSIOLOGY

Aortic dissection has traditionally been referred to as a dissecting aneurysm. However, because this condition is more accurately described as a dissecting hematoma, the term *aortic dissection* has gained favor.

Aortic dissection is thought to be caused by a sudden tear in the aortic intima, opening the way for blood to enter the aortic wall. Degeneration of the aortic media might be a prerequisite for this condition, with hypertension being an important contributing factor.

Aortic dissection is a relatively common event, occurring in at least 2000 people in the United States annually. It is often associated with connective tissue disorders such as Marfan syndrome (see Chapter 24). It also occurs in older people, peaking in adults in their 50s and 60s, and in women in their third trimester of pregnancy. Because the circulation of any major artery arising from the aorta can be impaired in clients with aortic dissection, this condition is highly lethal and represents an emergency situation.

Proximal dissections occur almost twice as often as distal dissections. Although the ascending aorta and descending thoracic aorta are the most common sites, dissections can also occur in the abdominal aorta and other arteries.

COLLABORATIVE MANAGEMENT

The most common presenting symptom is pain, with painless dissection occurring rarely. The pain is described as "tearing," "ripping," and "stabbing" and tends to move from its point of origin. Depending on the site of dissection, the client may feel pain in the anterior chest, back, neck, throat, jaw, or teeth.

Diaphoresis, nausea, vomiting, faintness, and apprehension are also common. Blood pressure is usually elevated unless complications, such as cardiac tamponade or rupture, have occurred. A decrease or absence of peripheral pulses is common, as is aortic regurgitation, which is characterized by a musical murmur better heard along the right sternal border. Neurologic deficits, such as an altered level of consciousness, paraparesis, and strokes, can also occur.

Chest x-ray, Doppler echocardiogram, computed tomography (CT), and aortic angiography may be used to confirm the diagnosis.

EMERGENCY CARE: AORTIC DISSECTION

The following are goals of emergency treatment:

- Elimination of pain
- Reduction of systolic blood pressure to 100 to 120 mm Hg
- Decrease in the velocity of left ventricular ejection

The physician prescribes IV sodium nitroprusside (Nitropress) or fenoldopam (Corlopam) by continuous drip initially to lower the blood pressure. If this regimen is ineffective, nicardipine hydrochloride (Cardene) may be used.

Subsequent treatment depends on the location of the dissection. Generally, clients receive continued medical treatment for uncomplicated distal dissections and surgical treatment for proximal dissections. For clients receiving long-term medical treatment, the systolic blood pressure must be maintained at or below 130 to 140 mm Hg. Beta blockers (propranolol) and calcium channel antagonists are indicated.

Clients receiving surgical intervention for a proximal dissection always require cardiopulmonary bypass (CPB) (see Chapter 41). The surgeon excises the intimal tear and obliterates entry in the false opening by suturing edges of the dissected aorta. Usually, a prosthetic graft is used.

Critical Thinking Challenge

A middle-aged client arrives at the emergency department complaining of a terrible pain described as a "ripping" sensation in his mid back. He is diaphoretic and very apprehensive. You note his blood pressure is 190/120 and have trouble finding any pedal pulses.

1. What additional assessment data should you collect at this time?
2. What are the priority nursing actions for this client?
3. What collaborative problems are priorities?
4. Should you delegate vital sign monitoring to unlicensed assistive personnel? Why or why not?

evolve For suggested answer guidelines, go to http://evolve.elsevier.com/Iggy/.

BUERGER'S DISEASE

PATHOPHYSIOLOGY

Buerger's disease (thromboangiitis obliterans) is a relatively uncommon occlusive disease limited to the medium and small arteries and veins. The distal upper and lower limbs are the most frequently affected. Typically, Buerger's disease is identified in young adult men who smoke. Larger arteries, such as the femoral and brachial, become involved in the late stages of the disease. The veins are less commonly involved.

The disease often extends into the perivascular tissues, resulting in fibrosis and scarring that binds the artery, vein, and nerve firmly together. For people who have this disease, cessation of cigarette smoking usually arrests the disease process, but persistence in smoking causes occlusion in the more proximal vessels.

The cause of Buerger's disease is unknown, although there is a strong association with tobacco smoking. A familial or genetic predisposition and autoimmune etiologic factors are also possible.

COLLABORATIVE MANAGEMENT

Assessment

The first clinical manifestation of Buerger's disease is usually claudication (pain in the muscles resulting from an inadequate blood supply) of the arch of the foot. Intermittent claudication may occur in the lower extremities. The pain may be ischemic, occurring in the digits while the client is at rest. Often, there is an aching pain that is more severe at night. Paroxysmal shocklike pain can be the result of ischemic neuropathy. Clients often experience increased sensitivity to cold and complain of coldness and numbness. On physical examination, pulses are often diminished in the distal extremities, and the extremities are cool and red or cyanotic in the dependent position.

A diagnosis of Buerger's disease is commonly based on a physical finding of peripheral ischemia, often in association with migratory superficial phlebitis. Ulcerations and gangrene may be seen in the digits. The ulcerations are usually sharply demarcated. The gangrenous lesion can be small or can affect the entire digit.

Arteriograms can be useful in delineating the degree of disease in the arteries. Commonly, arteriography reveals multiple segmental occlusions in the smaller arteries of the forearm, hand, leg, and foot. Plethysmographic studies of the fingers or toes may be diagnostic of the disease in the early stages. These studies can also be useful in following the progression of the disease in more proximal arteries.

Interventions

Nursing interventions are directed at the following:

- Preventing the progression of the disease
- Avoiding vasoconstriction
- Promoting vasodilation
- Relieving pain
- Treating ulceration and gangrene

To prevent the progression of Buerger's disease, complete abstinence from tobacco in all forms is essential. Extreme cold or prolonged exposure to cold should be avoided to prevent vasoconstriction. Instruct the client about medications that are prescribed for vasodilation. The treatment for Buerger's disease is similar to that for peripheral arterial disease (PAD) (see Interventions [Peripheral Arterial Disease], p. 796).

SUBCLAVIAN STEAL

PATHOPHYSIOLOGY

Subclavian steal occurs in the upper extremities from a subclavian artery occlusion or stenosis. The result is altered blood flow and ischemia in the arm. Subclavian steal can occur in people at any age but is more common in those with risk factors for atherosclerosis. Symptoms include tiredness in the arm with exertion, paresthesias, dizziness, and exercise-induced pain in the forearm when the arms are elevated.

COLLABORATIVE MANAGEMENT

Physical examination usually reveals a significant difference in the blood pressures between the arms. A difference greater than 20 mm Hg is considered significant. Another important finding is a subclavian bruit, which can occur on the affected side. The subclavian pulse may be decreased on the occluded side compared with the opposite side. The affected arm may also be discolored or cyanotic; however, this finding generally occurs only in severe cases.

Surgery is the recommended intervention for cyanosis or pain. One of three procedures may be used: endarterectomy of the subclavian artery, carotid-subclavian bypass, or dilation of the subclavian artery with placement of a vascular stent.

Postoperative nursing care of the client includes monitoring of the arterial flow in the affected arm. Check brachial and radial pulses frequently and observe for ischemic changes. Observe the arm for edema, redness, or any other signs.

THORACIC OUTLET SYNDROME

PATHOPHYSIOLOGY

Thoracic outlet syndrome is a compression of the subclavian artery at the thoracic outlet by anatomic structures, such as a rib or muscle. The arterial wall may be damaged, producing thrombosis or embolization to distal arteries of the arms. The three common sites of compression in the thoracic outlet are as follows:

- The interscalene triangle
- Between the coracoid process of the scapula and the pectoralis minor tendon
- Most commonly, the costoclavicular space

COLLABORATIVE MANAGEMENT

Thoracic outlet syndrome is more common in females and in people whose occupations require holding their arms up or leaning over, such as baseball players, golfers, or swimmers. It is also seen in clients who have had trauma such as whiplash or after clavicular fracture. Clients generally complain of neck, shoulder, and arm pain that may be intermittent. They may also have numbness and moderate edema of the extremity. The pain and numbness are worse when the arm is placed in certain positions, such as over the head or out to the side. Clients may have overdeveloped neck and shoulder muscles, and the affected arm may appear cyanotic.

Treatment includes physical therapy, exercises, and avoiding aggravating positions, such as elevating the arms. Surgical treatment involves resection of the anatomic structure that is compressing the artery. Surgery is performed only if a client has severe pain, has lost hand function, or is responding poorly to conservative treatment.

RAYNAUD'S PHENOMENON

PATHOPHYSIOLOGY

Raynaud's phenomenon is caused by vasospasm of the arterioles and arteries of the upper and lower extremities, usually unilaterally. *Raynaud's disease* occurs bilaterally. The two terms are sometimes used interchangeably, but although they are related, there are some differences. Raynaud's phenomenon usually occurs in people older than 30 years of age; Raynaud's disease can occur between the ages of 17 and 50 years of age. Raynaud's phenomenon can occur in either gender, but Raynaud's disease is more common in women.

The pathophysiology is the same for both entities. The etiology is unknown. Clients often have an associated systemic connective tissue disease, such as systemic lupus erythematosus or progressive systemic sclerosis (see Chapter 24).

As a result of vasospasm, the cutaneous vessels are constricted, and blanching of the extremity occurs, followed by cyanosis. When the vasospasm is relieved, the tissue becomes reddened or hyperemic. The client's extremities are numb and cold, and he or she may complain of pain and swelling. Ulcers may also be present. These attacks are intermittent and can be aggravated by cold or stress. In severe cases, the attack lasts longer and gangrene of the digits can occur.

COLLABORATIVE MANAGEMENT

Treatment involves relieving or preventing the vasoconstriction by drug therapy. Commonly prescribed drugs are nifedipine (Procardia), cyclandelate (Cyclospasmol), and phenoxybenzamine (Dibenzyline). These vasodilating agents may help to relieve the symptoms, but they can cause uncomfortable side effects, such as facial flushing, headaches, hypotension, and dizziness.

For severe symptoms that cannot be alleviated by drugs, a lumbar sympathectomy can be performed. The physician cuts the sympathetic nerve fibers that cause vasoconstriction of blood vessels in the lower extremities. This method is effective for foot symptoms. For the upper extremities, a similar procedure–sympathetic ganglionectomy–may provide symptom relief. The long-term effectiveness of these treatments is questionable.

Education of the client is important in prevention of complications. Explain methods to prevent vasoconstriction, such as minimizing exposure to cold, smoking cessation (if client smokes), and decreasing stress. The client is instructed to wear warm clothes, socks, or gloves when exposed to cool or cold temperatures. He or she should keep the home at a comfortably warm temperature and wear gloves to the grocery store. Help the client identify stressors and provide suggestions for reducing them. (See Chapter 24 for further discussion of Raynaud's disease as it relates to connective tissue disease.)

POPLITEAL ENTRAPMENT

Popliteal entrapment causes ischemic symptoms in the affected leg or foot because of anatomic compression of the popliteal artery. Popliteal entrapment occurs in young people, most often in men complaining of intermittent claudication of one or both extremities.

Physical examination may reveal ischemic changes of the affected extremity, with normal function of the unaffected limb. When the client is at rest, the nurse may note diminished distal pulses, although this is a rare finding. Diagnosis of popliteal entrapment is possible only after an accurate history, physical examination, and arteriography.

The recommended treatment is surgical repair of the anatomic compression. Reconstruction of the popliteal artery may be necessary to restore arterial blood flow to the limb. Nursing care involves preventing general postoperative complications and evaluating the patency of the graft or artery postoperatively. Observe for ischemic changes and evaluate distal pulses at frequent intervals postoperatively.

PERIPHERAL VENOUS DISEASE

To function properly, veins must be patent (unobstructed) with competent valves. Vein function also necessitates the assistance of the surrounding muscle beds to help pump blood toward the heart. If one or more veins are not operating efficiently, they become distended and clinical manifestations occur.

Three distinct phenomena alter the blood flow in veins:

- Thrombus formation *(venous thrombosis)* can lead to pulmonary embolism (PE), a life-threatening complication (see Chapter 35). **Venous thromboembolism (VTE)** is the current term that includes both deep vein thrombosis and PE.
- Defective valves lead to *venous insufficiency* and *varicose veins,* which are not life threatening but are problematic.
- Lack of skeletal muscle contractility

Venous Thromboembolism

PATHOPHYSIOLOGY

Venous thromboembolism (VTE) constitutes one of health care's greatest challenges, and includes both thrombus and embolus complications. A **thrombus** (also called a thrombosis) is a blood clot believed to result from an endothelial injury, venous stasis, or hypercoagulability. The thrombosis may not be specifically attributable to one element, or it may involve all three elements. It is often associated with an inflammatory process. When a thrombus develops, inflammation can occur around the clot, thickening the vein wall and consequently leading to embolization (the formation of an **embolus**).

Thrombophlebitis refers to a thrombus that is associated with inflammation; **phlebothrombosis** is a thrombus without inflammation. Thrombophlebitis can occur in superficial veins; however, it most frequently occurs in the deep veins of the lower extremities.

Deep vein thrombophlebitis, commonly referred to as **deep vein thrombosis (DVT),** not only is more common but also is more serious than superficial thrombophlebitis because it presents a greater risk for **pulmonary embolism (PE),** in which a dislodged blood clot travels to the pulmonary artery. DVT develops most often in the legs, but it is becoming more frequently seen due to increased use of central venous devices (Crowther & McCourt, 2004).

Thrombus formation has been associated with stasis of blood flow, endothelial injury, and/or hypercoagulability, known as **Virchow's triad.** The precise cause of these events remains unknown; however, a few predisposing factors have been identified. Thrombosis has commonly occurred in people undergoing certain surgical procedures.

Etiology

The highest incidence of clot formation occurs in clients who have undergone hip surgery, total knee replacement, or open prostate surgery. Other conditions that seem to promote thrombus formation are pregnancy, ulcerative colitis, heart failure, and immobility. Immobility occurs during prolonged bedrest, such as when a client is confined to bed during the perioperative period. Individuals who sit for long periods of time, such as on an airplane, are also at risk for VTE.

Phlebitis (vein inflammation) associated with invasive procedures, such as IV therapy, can predispose clients to thrombosis. Severe infections, systemic lupus erythematosus, polycythemia vera, oral contraceptives, and trauma have also been linked to thrombosis. Cancer, especially adenocarcinoma of the visceral organs, is the most common malignancy associated with DVT. Cancer has been discovered in nearly all people with fatal PEs who did not have other predisposing factors (Horlander et al., 2003).

Incidence/Prevalence

2.5 million individuals in the United States are affected by DVT each year (Day, 2003). It is estimated that 50,000 to 100,000 individuals die each year of pulmonary embolism (Horlander et al., 2003). The largest number of deaths occurred in the 75- to 84-year-old age-group. Black individuals have a high rate of death resulting from PE due to predisposing risk factors and coexisting diseases, such as certain cancers, chronic renal and cardiac failure, and an increased prevalence in smoking.

> **WOMEN'S HEALTH CONSIDERATIONS**
>
> The rate of diagnosis for DVT and PE is higher in women than in men. There have been suggestions that a possible diagnostic disparity exists among men and women for DVT and PE. However, in the United States, Stein and colleagues (2003) found a comparable effort was made to diagnose these venous disorders equally among genders. Duration of hospital stays was comparable with a primary discharge diagnosis of DVT and PE.

HEALTH PROMOTION/ILLNESS PREVENTION

In the community, if a person has a history of VTE, the following precautions should be taken:

- Avoid oral contraceptives.
- Drink adequate fluids to avoid dehydration.
- Exercise legs during long periods of bedrest or sitting.

In the inpatient setting, interventions to prevent VTE include the following:

- Client education
- Leg exercises
- Early ambulation
- Adequate hydration
- Graduated compression stockings (e.g., TEDs)
- Intermittent pneumatic compression, such as sequential compression devices (SCDs)
- Venous plexus foot pump

COLLABORATIVE MANAGEMENT

Assessment

People with DVT may have symptoms or may be asymptomatic. The classic signs and symptoms of DVT are calf or groin tenderness and pain, and sudden onset of unilateral swelling of the leg. Pain in the calf on dorsiflexion of the foot (positive Homan's sign) appears in only 10% of clients with DVT, and false-positive findings are common (Church, 2000). *Therefore checking a Homan's sign is not advised!* Examine the area described as painful, comparing this site with the contralateral limb. Gently palpate the site, observing for induration along the blood vessel, and for warmth and edema. Signs and symptoms, however, may be absent with thrombophlebitis. Because there are often silent clinical findings, have a high index of suspicion for this disorder especially for clients who are likely to develop VTE.

Localized edema in one extremity may suggest thrombophlebitis. Measure and compare right and left calf and thigh circumferences for changes over time as an indicator of DVT or venous insufficiency. However, serial leg measurements may not be the most reliable indicator of DVT.

DVT can also occur in the arm from an indwelling IV catheter or from compression injuries to the arm or subclavian vein by a rib. Although diagnostic tests for DVT are available, physical examination findings are often adequate for diagnosis. If a definitive diagnosis is lacking from physical examination alone, other diagnostic tests may be performed, such as contrast venography, duplex ultrasonography, Doppler flow studies, and impedance plethysmography.

Venography uses contrast medium to visualize clot formation in about 95% of people with DVT. Venography is not performed as frequently but is still considered the "gold standard" by many health care professionals for diagnosing DVT. Besides being painful for the client, complications to a venogram include hypersensitivity to the contrast dye, acute renal failure, extravasation of the medium, especially in those with arterial insufficiency, and precipitation of the thrombosis.

The preferred diagnostic test for DVT if a definitive diagnosis cannot be made by physical examination is **venous duplex ultrasonography**, a noninvasive test. Doppler flow studies may also be useful in the diagnosis of DVT, but they are more sensitive in detecting proximal rather than distal DVT. Normal venous circulation is characterized by audible signals, whereas thrombosed veins produce little or no flow. The accuracy of the duplex ultrasonographic scanning is dependent upon the technical skill of the health care professional performing the test. If the test is negative but a DVT is still suspected, a venogram may be needed to make an accurate diagnosis.

Impedance plethysmography assesses venous outflow and can detect more than 90% of DVTs that are located above the popliteal vein. However, it is not helpful in locating clots in the calf and is less sensitive than Doppler studies (Church, 2000).

Magnetic resonance direct thrombus imaging (MRI), another noninvasive test, is useful in finding a DVT in the proximal deep veins and is better than traditional venography in finding DVT in the inferior vena cava or pelvic veins.

A D-dimer test is a global marker of coagulation activation and measures fibrin degradation products produced from fibrinolysis. The test is widely used for the diagnosis of DVT when the client has few clinical signs and stratifies clients into a high-risk category for reoccurrence. Useful as an adjunct to noninvasive testing, a negative D-dimer test can exclude a DVT without an ultrasound.

Common Nursing Diagnoses and Collaborative Problems

Nursing diagnoses and collaborative problems that may apply to clients with DVT include the following:

1. Risk for Ineffective Tissue Perfusion (Peripheral) related to interruption of venous blood flow
2. Acute Pain related to physical injury agent (thrombus)

The most common collaborative problem is Potential for Embolism.

Interventions

The focus of treatment for thrombophlebitis is to prevent complications, such as pulmonary emboli, prevent further thrombus formation, and prevent an increase in size of the thrombus. Deep vein thrombophlebitis (thrombosis) is the most common type of thrombophlebitis. Clients with deep vein thrombosis (DVT) are often hospitalized for treatment, although this practice is changing as a result of the use of newer drugs.

NONSURGICAL MANAGEMENT. DVT is most often treated medically, using a combination of rest, drug therapy, and preventive measures.

Rest. Supportive therapy for DVT includes bedrest and elevation of the extremity. Some health care providers order intermittent or continuous warm, moist soaks to the affected area. *Do not massage the affected extremity to prevent the thrombus from dislodging and becoming an embolus.* All clients are evaluated for signs and symptoms of pulmonary embolism (PE), which include shortness of breath and chest pain. Emboli may also travel to the brain or heart, but these complications are not as common as PE.

Drug Therapy. Anticoagulants are the drugs of choice for a client with DVT and for clients at risk for DVT. The conventional treatment has been IV unfractionated heparin followed by oral anticoagulation with warfarin (Coumadin). However, unfractionated heparin can be problematic because each client's response to the drug is unpredictable, and hospital admission is usually required for laboratory monitoring and dose adjustments. Today the use of low-molecular weight heparin (LMWH) is changing the management of both DVT and PE.

Unfractionated Heparin Therapy. Many clients with a confirmed diagnosis of an existing blood clot are started on a regimen of IV unfractionated heparin (UFH; Hepalean✱) therapy. UFH is an anticoagulant agent that at low doses interacts with antithrombin III to produce selective inhibition of clotting factors IIa (thrombin) and Xa. At higher doses it inhibits practically all clotting factors. The ultimate result is inhibition of fibrin formation; the drug does nothing to the existing clot. The physician prescribes UFH to prevent the formation of other clots, which often develop in the presence of an existing clot, and to prevent enlargement of the existing clot. Over a long period of time, the existing clot is slowly absorbed by the body.

Before UFH administration, a baseline prothrombin time (PT), activated partial thromboplastin time (aPTT), International Normalized Ratio (INR), complete blood count (CBC) with platelet count, urinalysis, stool for occult blood, and creatinine level are required.

UFH is initially given in a bolus IV dose of about 100 units/kg of body weight, followed by constant infusion. The infusion is regulated by a reliable electronic infusion device that protects against accidental free flow of solution. The physician or clinical pharmacist prescribes concentrations of UFH (in 5% dextrose in water) and the number of units or milliliters per hour needed to maintain a therapeutic aPTT. Measurement of aPTT is obtained daily, or more frequently, and reported to the health care provider as soon as results are available to allow adjustment of heparin dosage. Therapeutic levels of aPTTs are usually 1½ to 2 times normal control levels. Assess clients for signs and symptoms of bleeding, which include hematuria, frank or occult blood in the stool, ecchymosis (bruising), petechiae, an altered level of consciousness, or pain.

UFH can also decrease platelet counts. Mild reductions are common and are resolved with continued heparin therapy. Severe platelet reductions, although rare, result from the development of antiplatelet bodies within 6 to 14 days after the beginning of treatment. Platelets aggregate into "white clots" that can cause thrombosis, usually in the form of an acute arterial occlusion. The provider discontinues heparin administration if severe **heparin-induced thrombocytopenia and thrombosis (HITT)** ($>$100,000 mm^3), or "white clot syndrome," occurs. LMWH is used more commonly today due to the complications involved with UFH.

Argatroban (Acova) or lepirudin (Refludan) are highly selective direct thrombin inhibitors that may be used as an alternative to heparin or for clients who have had HITT. Like heparin, these drugs increase the client's risk for bleeding. An oral anticoagulant may also be substituted for heparin if necessary.

Ensure that protamine sulfate, the antidote for heparin, is available, if needed, for excessive bleeding. Chart 39-10 highlights information important to nursing care and client education associated with anticoagulant therapy.

To *prevent* DVT, heparin may be given in low doses subcutaneously for high-risk clients, especially after orthopedic surgery. However, other pharmacologic agents are often used for prophylaxis:

- Low-molecular weight heparin (e.g., enoxaparin [Lovenox]) (drug class of choice after orthopedic surgery) (Crowther & McCourt, 2004)
- Selective factor Xa inhibitors (e.g., fondaparinux [Arixtra])
- Warfarin (Coumadin, Warfilone✱)

Prevention of DVT is crucial for clients at risk. Preventive measures are listed earlier under the Health Promotion/Illness Prevention section.

Low-Molecular Weight Heparin. Subcutaneous low-molecular weight heparins (LMWHs), such as enoxaparin (Lovenox), dalteparin (Fragmin), and ardeparin (Normiflo), have a consistent action and are approved for prevention and treatment of DVT. Danaparoid (Orgaran) is also classified as an LMWH but is actually a heparinoid. LMWHs bind less to plasma proteins, blood cells, and vessel walls, resulting in a longer half-life and more predictable response. These drugs inhibit thrombin formation due to reduced factor IIa activity and enhanced inhibition of factor Xa and thrombin.

Some clients may be safely managed at home with daily visits from a home care nurse. Candidates for home LMWH therapy must have stable DVT or PE, low risk for bleeding, adequate renal function, and normal vital signs. They must be willing to learn self-injection or have a family member, friend, or home care nurse administer the subcutaneous injections.

CHART 39-10

BEST PRACTICE for
The Client Receiving Anticoagulant Therapy

- Carefully check the dosage of anticoagulant to be administered, even if the pharmacy prepared the medication.
- Monitor the client for signs and symptoms of bleeding, including hematuria, frank or occult blood in the stool, ecchymosis, petechiae, altered mental status (indicating possible cranial bleeding), or pain (especially abdominal pain, which could indicate abdominal bleeding).
- Monitor vital signs frequently for decreased blood pressure and increased pulse (indicating possible internal bleeding).
- Have antidotes available as needed (e.g., protamine sulfate for heparin and vitamin K for warfarin [Coumadin, Warfilone✱]).
- Monitor activated partial thromboplastin time (aPTT) for clients receiving unfractionated heparin; monitor prothrombin time (PT) or International Normalized Ratio (INR) for clients receiving warfarin or low-molecular weight heparin (LMWH).
- Apply prolonged pressure over venipuncture sites and injection sites.
- When administering *subcutaneous* heparin, apply pressure over the site and do not massage.
- Teach the client going home while taking an anticoagulant to:
  - Use only an electric razor
  - Take precautions to avoid injury; for example, do not use tools such as hammers or saws, where accidents commonly occur
  - Report signs and symptoms of bleeding, such as blood in the urine or stool, nosebleeds, ecchymosis, or altered mental status
  - Take the prescribed dosage of medication at the precise time that it was prescribed to be given
  - Not stop taking the medication abruptly; the physician usually tapers the anticoagulant gradually

Some health care providers place the client on a regimen of IV unfractionated heparin (UFH) for several days, then follow up with an LMWH. In this case, the UFH is discontinued at least 30 minutes before the first LMWH injection. The usual dose of enoxaparin is 1 mg/kg of body weight, not to exceed 90 mg, and is repeated every 12 hours. If the client's creatinine level is greater than 2 mg/dL (indicating renal insufficiency), the health care provider lowers the dose. Dalteparin can be given once daily at 200 units/kg of body weight and does not require dose adjustment for renal insufficiency. The usual dose of ardeparin is 50 units/kg of body weight and is given every 12 hours.

Monitor the INR and stools daily for occult blood. The aPTTs are not checked on an ongoing basis because the doses of LMWH are not adjusted.

Warfarin Therapy. If the client is receiving continuous UFH, warfarin (Coumadin) may be added at least 5 days later. Clients receiving LMWH are placed on a regimen of warfarin after the first dose. Warfarin works in the liver to inhibit synthesis of the four vitamin K–dependent clotting factors and takes 3 to 4 days before it can exert therapeutic anticoagulation. The heparin continues to provide therapeutic anticoagulation until this effect is achieved with warfarin. IV heparin is then discontinued at that time.

Therapeutic levels of warfarin are monitored by measuring prothrombin time (PT) and/or the International Normalized Ratio (INR). Because PTs are often inconsistent and misleading, the INR was developed. Most laboratories report both results. Most clients receiving warfarin should have an INR between 1.5 and 2.0 to prevent recurrent DVT and minimizing the risk of stroke or hemorrhage (Ridker et al., 2003). Warfarin therapy should be started with low doses, at least 5 mg, and gradually titrated up according to the INR. Clients usually receive warfarin for 3 to 6 months after an episode of DVT or longer if no precipitating factors were discovered, with recurrence, or if there are continuing risk factors (Gallus et al., 2000).

Nursing assessment for bleeding is similar to that described for clients receiving heparin. Ensure that vitamin K, the antidote for warfarin, is available in case of excessive bleeding (see Chart 39-10). However, anticoagulation is not possible for 3 weeks after vitamin K administration.

Thrombolytic Therapy. The use of systemic thrombolytic therapy for DVT is effective in dissolving thrombi quickly and completely. The greatest advantage is thought to be the prevention of valvular damage and consequential venous insufficiency, or "postphlebitis syndrome." However, thrombolytic therapy is contraindicated postoperatively, during pregnancy, and after childbirth, trauma, strokes, or spinal injuries. To be most effective, thrombolytic therapy must be initiated within 5 days after the onset of symptoms.

Thrombolytic agents such as recombinant tissue plasminogen activator (t-PA), as well as platelet inhibitors such as abciximab (ReoPro), tirofiban (Aggrastat), and eptifibatide (Integrilin), may be effective in dissolving a clot or preventing new clots during the first 24 hours. Infusion can be given via a catheter so the thrombolytic agent can be injected directly into the thrombus. Compared to giving systemic thrombolytic dosing, this approach decreases the concentration needed and reduces the chance of bleeding. Thrombolytic agents, such as alteplase and reteplase, are used to treat peripheral vascular occlusion. Reteplase is a plasminogen activator that penetrates the clot and causes lysis. It is not compatible with heparin and should not be given in the same IV line. Reteplase has been used successfully in treating coronary thrombosis and use in peripheral vascular occlusion is experimental. The most serious complication from thrombolytic therapy is intracerebral bleeding. Be aware of the importance of thrombolytic therapy, its indications, and its implications for nursing care; closely monitor clients for signs and symptoms of bleeding.

Critical Thinking Challenge

An older adult who had a total hip replacement for osteoarthritis 3 days ago is diagnosed as having DVT of the operative leg calf. She lives alone, but plans to return home while receiving low–molecular weight heparin (LMWH) injections.

1. What health teaching will the client require?
2. What resources will she need at home during her recovery?
3. What laboratory tests will need to be monitored while she is receiving LMWH?

evolve For suggested answer guidelines, go to http://evolve.elsevier.com/Iggy/.

Prevention and Management of Peripheral Edema. The client's legs should be elevated when in bed and when in a chair. To help prevent chronic venous insufficiency, clients with active and resolving DVT are often instructed to wear knee- or thigh-high compression or elastic stockings for an extended period of time.

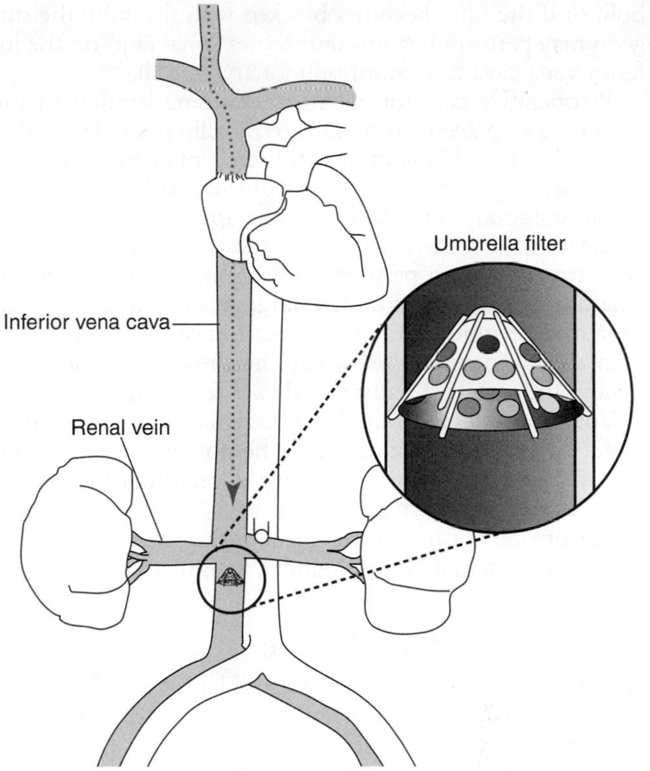

Figure 39-9 ■ An inferior vena caval filter.

SURGICAL MANAGEMENT. A deep vein thrombus is rarely removed surgically unless there is a massive occlusion that does not respond to medical treatment and the thrombus is of recent (1 to 2 days) onset. **Thrombectomy** is the most common surgical procedure for removing the thrombus. Preoperative and postoperative care of clients undergoing thrombectomy are similar to the care for clients undergoing arterial surgery (see earlier discussion under Acute Peripheral Arterial Occlusion, p. 805).

Inferior Vena Caval Interruption. Recurrent deep vein thrombosis (DVT) or pulmonary emboli that do not respond to medical treatment and for clients who cannot tolerate anticoagulation, **inferior vena caval interruption** may be indicated to prevent pulmonary emboli.

Preoperative care is similar to that provided for clients receiving local anesthesia (see Chapter 20). If clients have recently been taking anticoagulants, consult with the physician about interrupting this therapy in the preoperative period to avoid hemorrhage.

The surgeon inserts a filter device, or "umbrella," percutaneously into the inferior vena cava (Figure 39-9). The device is meant to trap emboli in the inferior vena cava before they progress to the lungs. Holes in the device allow blood to pass through, thus not significantly interfering with the return of blood to the heart. Popular inferior vena caval filters include the bird's nest filter and the Greenfield filter.

Postoperatively, inspect the incision on the right side of the chest for bleeding and signs or symptoms of infection. Other postoperative nursing care is similar to that for any client undergoing surgery (see Chapter 22).

Ligation or External Clips. If an inferior vena caval filter is not successful in preventing pulmonary emboli, or if the filter becomes blocked with thrombi, the surgeon may perform ligation or insert external clips on the inferior vena cava to prevent pulmonary emboli.

Preoperative care for clients undergoing ligation of the vena cava or placement of an external clip is similar to that for an abdominal laparotomy. If the client is receiving anticoagulation therapy, the nurse consults with the surgeon about temporary interruption of therapy.

Ligation and insertion of external clips in the inferior vena cava are often performed by means of an abdominal laparotomy. In a ligation, the surgeon ties off the inferior vena cava to block emboli. Application of an external clip, such as the Adams-DeWeese clip, narrows the inferior vena cava to four serrated transverse slits, 3 to 5 mm in diameter. If laparotomy is performed, the external clip procedure is preferred because there are fewer hemodynamic or venous complications and a low frequency of recurrent pulmonary emboli associated with its use.

Postoperative care for the client with inferior vena caval ligation or external clip placement is similar to that for an abdominal laparotomy.

Community-Based Care

Clients recovering from thrombophlebitis or deep vein thrombosis (DVT) are usually ambulatory when they are discharged from the hospital. The primary focus of planning for discharge is to educate the client about the hazards of anticoagulation therapy.

HOME CARE MANAGEMENT

Help the client identify situations and equipment that might cause trauma, such as the use of a straight-edged razor. Help the client and family or significant others to make arrangements to avoid hazardous situations and to procure alternative types of equipment if needed, such as an electric razor.

HEALTH TEACHING

Teach clients recovering from DVT to stop or avoid smoking and to avoid the use of oral contraceptives to decrease the risk of recurrence. Most clients are discharged on a regimen of warfarin (Coumadin, Warfilone✱) or low–molecular weight heparin (LMWH). Instruct clients and their families to avoid potentially traumatic situations, such as participation in contact sports. Provide written and oral information about the signs and symptoms of bleeding (see Chart 39-10). The client must report any of these manifestations to the health care provider immediately.

The anticoagulant effect of warfarin may be reversed by the omission of one or two doses of the drug or by the administration of vitamin K. In case of injury, clients are directed to apply pressure to bleeding wounds and to seek medical assistance immediately. Encourage them to carry an identification card or wear a medical alert bracelet that states that they are taking warfarin.

Also instruct clients to inform their dentist and other health care providers that they are taking warfarin before receiving treatment or prescriptions. Prothrombin times are affected by many prescription and over-the-counter medications, such as antacids, antihistamines, aspirin, mineral oil, oral contraceptives, and large doses of vitamin C. The action of warfarin is also affected by high-fat and vitamin K–rich foods, such as cabbage, cauliflower, broccoli, asparagus, turnips, spinach, kale, fish, and liver. Therefore instruct clients to eat a well-balanced diet with moderate amounts of vitamin K and to avoid taking additional medications without consulting a health care provider. Teach clients to also avoid hydration, alcohol, and sitting for prolonged periods of time. Arrange for clients to have prothrombin time (PT) and International Normalized Ratio (INR) determinations made 1 to 2 weeks after discharge.

Clients receiving subcutaneous LMWH injections at home need instruction on self-injection. Teach the appropriate caregiver and family members or friends, if necessary, to administer the injections

Clients who have experienced DVT may fear recurrence of a thrombus and may also be concerned about treatment with warfarin and the risk for bleeding. Assure them that participation in the prescribed treatment frequently helps in resolving this problem and that ongoing assessment of PTs and INRs should minimize the risks of bleeding.

HEALTH CARE RESOURCES

Clients discharged on a regimen of warfarin need access to a pharmacy to renew prescriptions and, if feasible, obtain a medical alert bracelet. They also need access to a laboratory for frequent monitoring of PTs and INRs.

Venous Insufficiency

PATHOPHYSIOLOGY

Venous insufficiency occurs as a result of prolonged venous hypertension, which stretches the veins and damages the valves. Valvular damage can lead to a backup of blood and further venous hypertension, resulting in edema. Edema occurs as the by-product of red blood cells as they break down and infiltrate the surrounding tissues. Because the client cannot eliminate waste products, they accumulate within the tissues. With time, this stasis (stoppage) results in venous stasis ulcers, swelling, and cellulitis.

Venous efficiency is altered when thrombosis occurs or when valves are not functioning correctly. Defective valves can result from prolonged venous hypertension, which stretches the veins and damages valves. Venous hypertension can occur in people who stand or sit in one position for long periods, such as teachers and office personnel. Pregnancy and obesity can also cause chronically distended veins, which lead to damaged valves. Thrombus formation can contribute to valve destruction. Chronic venous insufficiency often occurs in clients who have had thrombophlebitis.

Venous leg ulcer disease is a major cause of death, pain, and health care costs. The prevalence rate varies from 0.6 to 1.6 per 1000 for adults and increases to 10 to 30 per 1000 in persons older than 85 years of age. Because the ulcers take a great deal of time to heal and often reoccur, between $1.9 and $2.5 billion yearly is spent on venous disease in the United States. Greater than 80% of venous ulcer care is delivered in the community setting by home care nurses (Lorimer et al., 2003).

◆COLLABORATIVE MANAGEMENT

◆Assessment

Venous insufficiency may result in edema of both extremities. There may be **stasis dermatitis** or discoloration along the ankles, extending up to the calf. In people with long-term venous insufficiency, **stasis ulcers** often form. Ulcer formation can result from the edema or from minor injury to the limb. Venous ulcers typically occur over the malleolus, more often medially than laterally. The ulcer usually has irregular borders. In general, these ulcers are chronic and difficult to heal (see Chart 39-7). Many people live with ulcers for years, and recurrence is common. Some may lose one or both limbs if ulcers are not controlled.

Interventions

The focus of treating venous insufficiency is to decrease edema and promote venous return from the affected extremity. Clients are not usually hospitalized for venous insufficiency alone unless it is complicated by an ulcer or another disorder is occurring simultaneously.

NONSURGICAL MANAGEMENT. Treatment of chronic venous insufficiency is primarily nonsurgical, unless it is complicated by a venous stasis ulcer that requires surgical debridement. The goals of managing venous stasis ulcers are to heal the ulcer, prevent infection, and prevent stasis with recurrence of ulcer formation. A wound care specialist, such as a Wound, Ostomy, and Continence nurse, should be contacted to make recommendations for ulcer care. A dietitian can suggest dietary supplements, such as zinc and vitamins A and C, as well as high-protein foods to promote wound healing.

Management of Edema. Clients with chronic venous insufficiency wear elastic or compression stockings, which fit from the middle of the foot to just below the knee or to the thigh. Stockings should be worn during the day and evening. Legs should be elevated for at least 20 minutes four or five times per day. When the client is in bed, the legs should be elevated above the level of the heart (Chart 39-11).

Confer with the physician about the use of intermittent sequential pneumatic compression of the lower extremities or foot plexus pumps for clients with past or present venous stasis ulcers. If an open venous ulcer is present, the device may be applied over a dressing such as an Unna boot. Instruct the client to apply the pump as directed during the period of healing. Because of the high incidence of venous ulcer recurrence, clients with chronic venous insufficiency whose ulcers have healed are encouraged to continue compression therapy for life.

Management of Venous Stasis Ulcers. Venous stasis ulcers are slightly more manageable than ulcers resulting from arterial disease. They are chronic in nature, with some clients manifesting the same ulcer for years. Ulcers often heal, only to recur in the same area several years later.

Two types of occlusive dressings are used for venous stasis ulcers: oxygen permeable dressings and oxygen impermeable dressings. Because the role of atmospheric oxygen in wound healing is controversial, opinions vary with regard to which type of dressing is preferred. An oxygen-permeable polyethylene film and an oxygen-impermeable hydrocolloid dressing (e.g., DuoDerm) are common. Hydrocolloid dressings are left in place for a minimum of 3 to 5 days for best effect. Use strict aseptic technique when changing dressings. If the wound is infected, use contact precautions in addition to standard precautions.

Artificial skin products can be used for difficult-to-heal venous leg ulcers. These first-generation products are very expensive but are laying the foundation in the field with costs anticipated to come down in the future. Except for cultured epithelial autografts, artificial skins are only temporary. Artificial skin serves as a biologic cover to secrete growth factors to promote more growth factor secretion from the client's own skin to speed the wound healing process.

CONSIDERATIONS FOR OLDER ADULTS

The pedal pulses in older adults may be more difficult to find. Thin, shiny skin, thick ridged nails, and loss of hair on the lower legs are signs of arterial insufficiency associated with normal aging

If the client is ambulatory, an **Unna boot** may be used. An Unna boot dressing is constructed of gauze that has been moistened with zinc oxide. Apply the boot to the affected limb, from the toes to the knee, after the ulcer has been cleaned with normal saline solution. Povidone-iodine (Betadine) and hydrogen peroxide are not used, because they destroy granulation tissue. The Unna boot is then covered with an elastic wrap and hardens like a cast; this promotes venous return and prevents stasis. The Unna boot also forms a sterile environment for the ulcer. The physician or advanced-practice nurse should change the boot about once a week. Instruct the client about what to look for if arterial occlusion occurs from an Unna boot that is too tight.

Drug Therapy. The health care provider may prescribe topical agents, such as Accuzyme, to chemically debride the ulcer, eliminating necrotic tissue and promoting healing. If an infection or cellulitis develops, systemic antibiotics are necessary.

SURGICAL MANAGEMENT. Surgery for chronic venous insufficiency is not usually performed, because historically it has not been successful. Attempts at transplanting

CHART 39-11

CLIENT EDUCATION GUIDE
Venous Insufficiency

Elastic Stockings

- Wear elastic stockings as prescribed, usually during the day and evening.
- Put the stockings on upon awakening and before getting out of bed.
- When applying the stockings, do not "bunch up" and apply like socks. Instead, place your hand inside the stocking and pull out the heel. Then place the foot of the stocking over your foot and slide the rest of the stocking up. Be sure that rough seams on the stocking are on the outside, not next to your skin.
- Do not push stockings down for comfort, because they may function like a tourniquet and further impair venous return.
- Put on a clean pair of stockings each day. Wash them by hand (not in a washing machine) in a gentle detergent and warm water.
- If the stockings seem to be "stretched out," replace them with a new pair.

Do's and Don'ts

- Elevate your legs for at least 20 minutes four or five times a day. When in bed, elevate your legs above the level of your heart.
- Avoid prolonged sitting or standing.
- Do not cross your legs; crossing at the ankles is acceptable for short periods of time.
- Do not wear tight, restrictive pants; avoid girdles and garters.

vein valves have had limited success. Surgical debridement of venous ulcers is similar to that performed for arterial ulcers (see Chapter 70).

Community-Based Care

The goal for the client with chronic venous insufficiency is to be managed in the home. For clients with frequent acute complications and repeated hospital admissions, case management can help meet appropriate clinical and cost outcomes.

HOME CARE MANAGEMENT

Help clients with chronic venous insufficiency to plan for opportunities and facilities that allow for elevation of the lower extremities in and outside the home. In addition, clients with venous stasis ulcers need to plan for care of the ulcers.

HEALTH TEACHING

Instruct clients with chronic venous stasis to:

- Avoid standing still if possible
- Elevate their legs when sitting
- Avoid crossing their legs
- Avoid wearing tight girdles, tight pants, and narrow-banded knee-high socks

The physician prescribes support hose or antiembolism stockings. Teach clients to apply these stockings before they get out of bed in the morning and to remove them just before going to bed at night (see Chart 39-11). Also advise them that they will probably need to wear these stockings for the rest of their lives.

To improve circulation and aid in weight reduction, prescribe an exercise program on an individual basis with health care provider input. Encourage all clients to maintain an optimal weight and consult with the dietitian to plan a weight reduction diet. Instruct clients with venous stasis ulcers how to care for the ulcers at home.

Clients with venous stasis disease, especially those with venous stasis ulcers, may require long-term emotional support to assist them in meeting long-term needs. They may also need assistance in coping with necessary lifestyle adjustments, such as changes in occupation.

HEALTH CARE RESOURCES

Clients with venous stasis ulcers may need the assistance of a home care nurse to perform dressing changes. Clients with Unna boots need weekly transportation to their health care provider for dressing changes. Arrange for a sequential compression device in the home if the health care provider prescribes one.

VARICOSE VEINS

PATHOPHYSIOLOGY

Varicose veins are distended, protruding veins that appear darkened and tortuous. They can occur in anyone, but they are common in clients older than 30 years of age whose occupations require prolonged standing. Varicose veins are also frequently seen in pregnant women, clients with systemic problems (e.g., heart disease), obese clients, and clients with a family history of varicose veins.

As the vein wall weakens and dilates, venous pressure increases and the valves become incompetent (defective). The incompetent valves enhance the vessel dilation, and the veins become tortuous and distended. The client may complain of pain, especially after standing, and may experience a feeling of fullness in the legs. Nursing assessment reveals distended, protruding veins.

The Trendelenburg test assists with the diagnosis. The client is placed in a supine position with elevated legs. As the client sits up, the veins would normally fill from the distal end; however, if there are varicosities, the veins fill from the proximal end.

COLLABORATIVE MANAGEMENT

Conservative measures are the treatment of choice. Measures involve wearing elastic stockings and elevating the extremities as much as possible. Clients who continue to have pain or unsightly veins, despite this treatment, may opt for either sclerotherapy or surgical removal of the vein.

Sclerotherapy is performed on small or a limited number of varicosities. The physician injects a solution, such as sodium tetradecyl, directly into the vein, or he or she may use a laser device. A pressure dressing may be applied over the sclerosed vein to keep vessels free of blood for 24 to 72 hours. The surgeon performs an incision and drainage of trapped blood in the sclerosed vein 14 to 21 days after injection, followed by application of a second pressure dressing for 12 to 18 hours.

Varicose veins are surgically removed when they are larger than 4 mm in diameter or are in clusters. The stab avulsion technique may be used if the saphenous veins are competent. The surgeon exposes varices through 2- to 3-mm stab incisions, grasping the veins with hooks, and dividing and avulsing each vein.

The surgeon may need to strip (remove) affected veins if the saphenous vein is incompetent. The surgeon threads a long wire through an incision above an affected vein, pulling it down through the vein and out through an incision below the vein. After this procedure, the legs are bandaged with firm elastic (Ace) bandages.

Postoperatively, assess the groin and entire leg for bleeding through the elastic bandage. Instruct the client to keep the legs elevated and to perform range-of-motion exercises of the legs at least hourly. Clients are ambulatory and are often discharged from the hospital by the first postoperative day. At this time, instruct clients to continue to wear elastic stockings, walk, limit sitting, avoid standing in one place, and elevate their legs when sitting.

Application of RF (radio frequency) energy is a new technique done as an alternative to surgery. The vein is heated from the inside by the RF energy and shrinks. Collateral veins nearby take over.

Laser treatment is another alternative to surgery. Performed by interventional radiologists, the EndoVenous Laser Treatment uses a laser fiber to heat and close the main vessel that is contributing to the varicosity.

PHLEBITIS

Phlebitis is an inflammation of the superficial veins caused by an irritant, such as IV therapy (see Chapter 17). The client has a reddened, warm area radiating up an extremity, commonly an arm. Pain, soreness, and swelling of the extremity may also occur.

Management generally takes place at home and involves application of warm, moist soaks, which dilate the vein and promote circulation. Sometimes a heating unit is used to keep the soaks warm. Rarely, ice packs are used. Apply the soaks, making sure that the temperature is not hot enough to burn the client, and assess for complications, such as tissue necrosis, infection, or pulmonary embolus. After a few days of conservative therapy, the inflammation usually subsides. Elastic stockings may be prescribed.

VASCULAR TRAUMA

PATHOPHYSIOLOGY

Many types of trauma can result in vascular injury. Injuries to the blood vessels in the upper and lower extremities account for about 70% of all vascular injuries to the human body. Vascular injuries to the blood vessels include punctures, lacerations, and transections. Acute blunt or penetrating trauma may result in a false aneurysm or hematoma. Arteriovenous fistulas may be seen after penetrating injuries. The more common causes of penetrating injuries to the blood vessels are gunshot and knife wounds.

Blunt trauma, which is less common, can result from high-speed automobile accidents as a result of the shearing force of rapid deceleration. Vascular trauma can also occur during arterial puncture for arteriographic or hemodynamic studies in which a dissection, hematoma, or occlusive lesion occurs.

COLLABORATIVE MANAGEMENT

The history and physical examination aid in establishing the diagnosis in the client with vascular injury. Question the client or family about the mechanism of injury, the site of injury, the amount of blood loss, and symptoms present after the injury.

Assess for circulatory, sensory, or motor impairment but be aware that, despite significant trauma, impairment may not be apparent, especially if deep vessels have been injured. Arteriography provides essential information about the vascular injury. Emergency or urgent surgical intervention is needed for ischemia to maximize successful revascularization.

Management of vascular injuries is often initiated in a hospital emergency department. Careful triage of all clients is crucial. The most important principles in the management of vascular trauma are establishment of a patent airway, control of bleeding, and restoration of blood flow.

The method of repair varies with the type of vascular injury. Techniques include vein bypass grafting, lateral suture repair, thrombectomy (excision of blood clot), resection with end-to-end anastomosis, and vein patch grafting.

GET READY for the NCLEX Examination!

KEY POINTS

Safe Effective Care Environment

- In collaboration with the health care team, assess the home environment of the client with peripheral vascular disease for potential safety hazards, place high-risk clients on a fall prevention program.
- To reduce the risk of injury, caution clients about orthostatic hypertension when taking antihypertensive medications, especially diuretics.
- For clients with leg ulcers, initiate a consult with a Wound, Ostomy, and Continence Nurse or other wound specialist.
- Use contact precautions for infected, draining wounds.
- Use strict aseptic technique for changing dressings over open ulcers.
- Teach the client to report excessive drainage from the wound, development of redness, warmth, pain, or induration, and a temperature greater than 100° F.
- Insertion sites for IV lines, central line catheters, arterial lines, and Foley catheters should be cared for meticulously and observed for signs of infection.

Health Promotion and Maintenance

- In collaboration with the dietitian, assist the client to incorporate healthy eating behaviors to lower cholesterol and saturated fats, and increase fresh fruits, vegetables, and fiber in the diet. For overweight clients, assist in a weight reduction plan. Assist the diabetic client with maintaining normal blood glucose levels to enhance wound healing. For clients on warfarin, instruct on diet interaction, vitamin K moderation, and avoiding alcohol.
- Teach clients taking statin-type drugs to report adverse effects to their health care provider as described in Chart 39-1.
- For clients with wounds, collaborate with the dietitian to promote adequate intake of protein, vitamins C and A, and zinc to enhance wound healing.
- Teach clients ways to prevent deep vein thrombosis and subsequent embolism; in the hospital setting, provide measures, such as wearing compression stockings, to prevent or manage DVT.
- Encourage your client to stop smoking, take a daily walk, care for his or her feet and skin carefully, eat healthy, and drink plenty of fluids (also see Chart 39-2).
- For smoking or tobacco-chewing clients, initiate a consult to begin a tobacco cessation program.
- Assess the client for modifiable and nonmodifiable risk factors for cardiovascular disease and be ready to teach health promotion behaviors to the client and family. Pay particular attention to the client with a family history of cardiovascular disease.
- For clients with vascular disorders, teach them the importance of each medication, review the mechanism of action, potential side effects, and the duration for taking the medications. Instruct the client to report to the health care provider before stopping any medications.
- To prevent reoccurrence of leg ulcers, teach the client about avoiding trauma to the extremities, proper foot and skin care, proper clothing and footwear, applying prescribed compression stockings, and appropriate activity and extremity positioning.

Psychosocial Integrity

- Encourage the client to verbalize fears about facing sudden death and clarify misconceptions. Applying diversional activities if indicated for a prolonged hospital stay.
- Encourage biofeedback, relaxation therapy and assist clients with coping strategies to reduce stress.
- Monitor the client's response to stress to determine whether the behavior is a typical reaction or an unusual reaction to a

stressful situation. Report any unusual behavior immediately for appropriate intervention.
- Identify and address clients' concerns that could hinder learning.

Physiological Integrity

- Closely observe the client receiving anticoagulants or thrombolytics for signs of bleeding and monitor appropriate laboratory values.
- Assess respiratory, cardiovascular, gastrointestinal, renal, circulatory and neurovascular status closely on all postprocedure or postsurgical clients.
- Administer antihypertensives or vasopressors as prescribed to maintain sufficient pressure for adequate renal perfusion, graft patency, and cardiovascular status, including heart rate and blood pressure (see Chart 39-3).
- Monitor for indications of aneurysm rupture: diaphoresis, nausea, vomiting, pallor, hypotension, tachycardia, severe pain, and decreased level of consciousness, or a pulsating abdominal mass.
- Document assessment findings completely.
- Assess and manage pain effectively.

ADDITIONAL STUDY RESOURCES

Go to your Student CD-ROM for Review Questions for the NCLEX Examination.

evolve Go to http://evolve.elsevier.com/Iggy/ for Integrated Management of Care Questions for the NCLEX Examination.

SELECTED BIBLIOGRAPHY

ALLHAT Officers and Coordinators for the ALLHAT Collaborative Research Group. (2002a). Major outcomes in high-risk hypertensive patients randomized to Angiotensin-converting enzyme inhibitor or calcium channel blocker vs diuretic. The Antihypertensive and Lipid-Lowering Treatment to Prevent Heart Attack Trial (ALLHAT). *Journal of the American Medical Association, 288*(23), 2981-2997.

ALLHAT Officers and Coordinators for the ALLHAT Collaborative Research Group. (2002b). Major outcomes in moderately hypercholesterolemic, hypertensive patients randomized to pravastatin vs usual care. The Antihypertensive and Lipid-Lowering Treatment to Prevent Heart Attack Trial (ALLHAT-LLT). *Journal of the American Medical Association, 288*(23), 2998-3007.

American College of Chest Physicians. (2001). Sixth ACCP consensus conference on antithrombotic therapy. *Chest, 119*(1, suppl.)1S-370S.

American Heart Association. (2003). *Heart Disease and Stroke Statistics-2003 Update.* Dallas: American Heart Association.

Aquila, A. (2001). Deep venous thrombosis. *Journal of Cardiovascular Nursing, 15*(4), 25-44.

Ayello, E.A. (2000). On the lookout for peripheral vascular disease. *Nursing2000, 30*(6), 64hh1-64hh4.

Baumann, L.C., Chang, M.W., & Hoebeke, R. (2002). Clinical outcomes for low-income adults with hypertension and diabetes. *Nursing Research, 51*(3), 191-197.

Bialous, S.A., and Sarna, L. (2004). Sparing a few minutes for tobacco cessation. *American Journal of Nursing, 104*(12), 54-59.

Bussard, M.E. (2002). Reteplase: nursing implications for catheter-directed thrombolytic therapy for peripheral vascular occlusions. *Critical Care Nurse, 22*(3), 57-63.

Bussey, H. (2002). Traditional anticoagulant therapy: Why abandon half a century of success? *American Journal of Health-System Pharmacy, 59*(20), S3-S6.

Byrne, B. (2001). Deep vein thrombosis prophylaxis: the effectiveness and implications of using below-knee or thigh-length graduated compression stockings. *Heart and Lung,* 30(4), 277-284.

Church, V. (2000). Staying on guard for DVT and PE. *Nursing2000, 30*(2), 34-44.

Coffey, M., Crowder, G.K., & Check, D.J. (2003). Reducing coronary artery disease by decreasing homocysteine levels. *Critical Care Nurse, 23*(1), 25-30.

Collins, T.C., et al. (2003). The prevalence of peripheral arterial disease in a racially diverse population. *Archives of Internal Medicine, 163*(12), 1469-1474.

Crowther, M., & McCourt, K. (2004). Get the edge on deep vein thrombosis. *Nursing Management, 35*(1), 22-29.

Day, M.W. (2003). Recognizing and managing deep vein thrombosis. *Nursing2003, 33*(5), 36-42.

Douglas, J.G., et al. (2003). Consensus Statement of the Hypertension in African Americans Working Group of the International Society on Hypertension in Blacks. Management of high blood pressure in African Americans. *Archives of Internal Medicine, 163*(5) 525-541.

Ebersole, P., Hess, P., & Luggen, A.S. (2004). *Toward healthy aging* (6th ed.). St. Louis: Mosby.

Eichinger, S., et al. (2003). D-Dimer levels and risk of recurrent venous thromboembolism. *Journal of the American Medical Association, 290*(8), 1071-1074.

Etter, J.K., & Perneger, T.V. (2001). Effectiveness of a computer-tailored smoking cessation program. *Archives of Internal Medicine, 161*(21), 2696-2601.

Forette, F., et al. (2002). The prevention of dementia with antihypertensive treatment. New Evidence from the Systolic Hypertension in Europe (Syst-Eur) Study. *Archives of Internal Medicine, 162*(18), 2046-2052.

Gallus, A.S., et al. (2000). Consensus guidelines for warfarin therapy. An article published on the Internet by *The Medical Journal of Australia.* Available at http://www.mja.com.au.

Gerstein, H.C., et al. (2001). Albuminuria and risk of cardiovascular events, death, and heart failure in diabetic and nondiabetic individuals. *Journal of the American Medical Association,* 286(4), 421-426.

Heart Protection Study Collaborative Group (2003). MRC/BHF Heart Protection Study of cholesterol-lowering with simvastatin in 5963 people with diabetes: A randomized placebo-controlled trial. *Lancet 361,* 2005-2016.

Hess, C.T. (2003). Managing your patient's arterial ulcer. *Nursing2003, 33*(5), 17.

Horlander, K.T., Mannino, D.M., & Leeper, K.V. (2003). Pulmonary embolism mortality in the United States, 1979-1998. *Archives of Internal Medicine, 163*(14), 1711-1717.

Jarvis, C. (2004). *Physical examination and health assessment* (4th ed.). St. Louis: Mosby.

Joint National Committee. (2003). *The seventh report of the Joint National Committee on Prevention, Detection, Evaluation, and Treatment of High Blood Pressure.* NIH Publication No. 03-5233. Bethesda, MD: National Heart, Lung, and Blood Institute..

Kaatz, S. (2000). The venous side: Current directions in anticoagulant therapy. *J Am Osteopath Assoc,* 100(11), s17-s21.

Klompas, M. (2002). Does this patient have an acute thoracic aortic dissection? *Journal of the American Medical Association, 287*(17), 2262-2272.

Kuncl, N., & Nelson, K.M. (2000). Getting the skinny on lipid-lowering drugs. *Nursing2000, 30*(7), 52-53.

Lorimer, K.R., et al. (2003). Venous leg ulcer care: How evidence-based is nursing practice? *Journal of Wound, Ostomy, and Continence Nursing 30*(3), 132-142.

Luggen, A.S., & Meiner, S.E. (2001). *NGNA core curriculum for gerontological nursing* (2nd ed.). St. Louis: Mosby.

Maas, M.L., et al. (2001). *Nursing care of older adults: Diagnoses, outcomes, and interventions.* St. Louis: Mosby.

Malacaria, B., & Feloney, C.D.H. (2003). Going with the flow of anticoagulant therapy. *Nursing2003, 33*(3), 36-42.

McCance, K.L., & Huether, S.E. (2002). Pathophysiology: The biologic basis for disease in adults and children. St. Louis: Mosby.

National Cholesterol Education Program. (2002). *Third report of the Expert Panel on Detection, Evaluation, and Treatment of High Blood Cholesterol in Adults (Adult Treatment Panel III).* NIH Publication No. 02-5215. Bethesda, MD: National Heart, Lung, and Blood Institute.

National Heart, Lung, and Blood Institute. (2002). *Morbidity and mortality 2002 chartbook on cardiovascular, lung and blood diseases.* Washington, DC: National Institutes of Health, Public Health Service, U.S. Department of Health and Human Services.

National High Blood Pressure Education Program. (2002). Primary prevention of hypertension: Clinical and public health advisory. NIH Publication No. 02-5076. Bethesda, MD: National Heart, Lung, and Blood Institute.

Ridker, P.M., et al. (2003). Long term therapy, low-intensity warfarin therapy for the prevention of recurrent venous thromboembolism. *The New England Journal of Medicine, 348*(15), 1425-1434.

Sangiorgi, G., et al. (2001). Plasma levels of metalloproteinases-3 and -9 as markers of successful abdominal aortic aneurysm exclusion after endovascular graft treatment. *Circulation, 104*(suppl. 1), 288I-296I.

Sever, P.S., et al. (2003). Prevention of coronary and stroke events with atorvastatin in hypertensive patients who have average or lower than average cholesterol concentrations, in the Anglo-Scandinavian cardiac outcomes trial-lipid lowering arm (ASCOT-LLA): A multicentre randomized controlled trial. *The Lancet, 361,* 1149-1158.

Society of Interventional Radiology. (2003). Peripheral vascular disease statistics. Retrieved September 4, 2003, from http://www.sirweb.org.

Stein, P.D., et al. (2003). Venous thromboembolic disease. *Archives of Internal Medicine 163*(14), 1689-1694.

Stewart, K.J., et al. (2002). Exercise training for claudication. *The New England Journal of Medicine, 347*(24), 1941-1951.

White, W.B. (2003). Selective aldosterone blockage in hypertension: Clinical benefits across patient populations. Available at Medscape at http://www.medscape.com.

Woods, A. (2004). Loosening the grip of hypertension. *Nursing 2004, 34*(12), 36-43.

CHAPTER

40 Interventions for Clients with Shock

M. LINDA WORKMAN

LEARNING OUTCOMES

After studying this chapter, you should be able to:

1. Describe the clinical manifestations associated with the compensatory mechanisms for shock.
2. Identify clients at risk for hypovolemic shock.
3. Use laboratory data and clinical manifestations to determine the effectiveness of therapy for shock.
4. Explain the basis for intravenous therapy for shock.
5. Describe the mechanisms of action, side effects, and nursing implications for pharmacologic management of shock.
6. Prioritize nursing care for the client experiencing the nonprogressive stage of hypovolemic shock.
7. Compare the pathophysiology and clinical manifestations of the hyperdynamic and hypodynamic phases of septic shock.
8. Identify clients at risk for septic shock.
9. Identify nursing practices to reduce infection risk in an immunocompromised client.
10. Explain the rationale for the drug therapy for septic shock.
11. Prioritize nursing care for the client experiencing the hyperdynamic stage of septic shock.
12. Prioritize nursing care for the client experiencing the hypodynamic stage of septic shock.
13. Develop a community-based teaching plan for the client at risk for septic shock.

Go to your Student CD-ROM for Review Questions for the NCLEX Examination keyed to these Learning Outcomes.

Shock, the whole-body response to poor tissue oxygenation, is a condition rather than a disease. Any problem that impairs oxygen delivery to tissues and organs can start the syndrome of shock and lead to a life-threatening emergency. Clients in acute care settings are at higher risk, but shock can occur in any setting. When compensation or interventions are not effective and shock progresses, hypoxia can lead to multiple organ dysfunction syndrome (MODS) and death.

PATHOPHYSIOLOGY

Organs, tissues, and cells need a continuous supply of oxygen to function properly. The lungs first bring oxygen into the body. The cardiovascular system (heart, blood, and blood vessels) delivers oxygen to all tissues and removes cellular wastes. When any part of the cardiovascular system does not function properly for any reason, shock can result.

Shock begins with abnormal cellular metabolism, which occurs when too little oxygen is delivered to the tissues (McCance & Huether, 2002). In the past shock was classified as hypovolemic, cardiogenic, vasogenic, or septic, which indicated the origin of the problem causing the shock. Shock is now classified by the specific functional impairment caused: hypovolemic shock, cardiogenic shock, distributive shock, and obstructive shock (Effron & Chernow, 1992). Table 40-1 compares both classification systems and common problems leading to each shock category. The functional classification is used by researchers and guides clinicians and therefore is used in this chapter.

Many manifestations of shock are similar regardless of what starts the process or which tissues are affected first. These common manifestations are due to physiologic compensatory mechanisms. Manifestations unique to any one type of shock result from specific tissue dysfunction. The common features of shock are listed in Chart 40-1.

Review of Tissue Perfusion

Tissue oxygenation depends on how much oxygen from arterial blood perfuses the tissue. Organ perfusion is related to mean arterial pressure (MAP). Because the cardiovascular

TABLE 40-1 Comparison of New and Old Shock Classification Systems

Classification by Functional Impairment			
Hypovolemic	***Cardiogenic***	***Distributive***	***Obstructive***
Total body fluid decreased (in all fluid compartments) ■ Hemorrhage ■ Dehydration	Direct pump failure Fluid volume not affected ■ Myocardial infarction ■ Valvular problems Stenosis Incompetence ■ Myopathies ■ Dysrhythmias ■ Cardiac arrest	Fluid shifted from central vascular space Total body fluid volume normal or increased ■ Neural-induced loss of vascular tone ■ Chemical-induced loss of vascular tone Sepsis Anaphylaxis Capillary leak	Cardiac function decreased by non-cardiac factors Total body fluid volume not affected Central volume decreased ■ Pulmonary hypertension ■ Tension pneumothorax ■ Pericarditis ■ Thoracic tumor ■ Tamponade
Classification by Site of Origin			
Hypovolemic	***Cardiogenic***	***Vasogenic***	***Septic***
Central vascular volume decreased Total body fluid may or may not be decreased ■ Hemorrhage ■ Dehydration ■ Fluid shifts Trauma Burns Anaphylaxis	Direct pump failure Indirect pump failure Decreased cardiac output Total body fluid not decreased ■ Valvular problems Stenosis Incompetence ■ Myocardial infarction ■ Myopathies ■ Dysrhythmias ■ Cardiac arrest ■ Tamponade ■ Pericarditis ■ Pulmonary hypertension ■ Pulmonary emboli	Loss of vascular tone Total body fluid not decreased ■ Neurogenic Head trauma Vasovagal response ■ Vessel dilation Anaphylaxis Inflammation	Loss of vascular tone Eventual reduced cardiac output Seen as a more intense type of vasogenic shock ■ Infection

CHART 40-1

KEY FEATURES of Shock

Cardiovascular Manifestations
- Decreased cardiac output
- Increased pulse rate
- Thready pulse
- Decreased blood pressure
- Narrowed pulse pressure
- Postural hypotension
- Low central venous pressure
- Flat neck and hand veins in dependent positions
- Slow capillary refill in nail beds
- Diminished peripheral pulses

Respiratory Manifestations
- Increased respiratory rate
- Shallow depth of respirations
- Decreased $Paco_2$
- Decreased arterial Pao_2
- Cyanosis, especially around lips and nail beds

Neuromuscular Manifestations
- Early
  - Anxiety
  - Restlessness
  - Increased thirst
- Late
  - Decreased central nervous system activity (lethargy to coma)
  - Generalized muscle weakness
  - Diminished or absent deep tendon reflexes
  - Sluggish pupillary response to light

Renal Manifestations
- Decreased urine output
- Increased specific gravity
- Sugar and acetone present in urine

Integumentary Manifestations
- Cool to cold
- Pale to mottled to cyanotic
- Moist, clammy
- Mouth dry; pastelike coating present

Gastrointestinal Manifestations
- Decreased motility
- Diminished or absent bowel sounds
- Nausea and vomiting
- Constipation

$Paco_2$, Partial pressure of arterial carbon dioxide; *Pao_2*, partial pressure of arterial oxygen.

system is a closed but continuous circuit, the factors that influence MAP include the following:

- Total blood volume
- Cardiac output
- Size of the vascular bed

Total blood volume and cardiac output are directly related to MAP so that increases in either total blood volume or cardiac output raise MAP. Decreases in either total blood volume or cardiac output lower MAP.

The size of the vascular bed is inversely (negatively) related to MAP. This means that increases in the size of the vascular bed lower MAP and decreases raise MAP (Figure 40-1). Blood vessels, especially small arteries and veins connected to capillaries, can increase in diameter by relaxing the smooth muscle in vessel walls (dilating) or decrease in diameter by contracting the muscle **(vasoconstriction).** When blood vessels dilate and total blood volume remains the same, blood pressure decreases and blood flow is slower. When blood vessels constrict

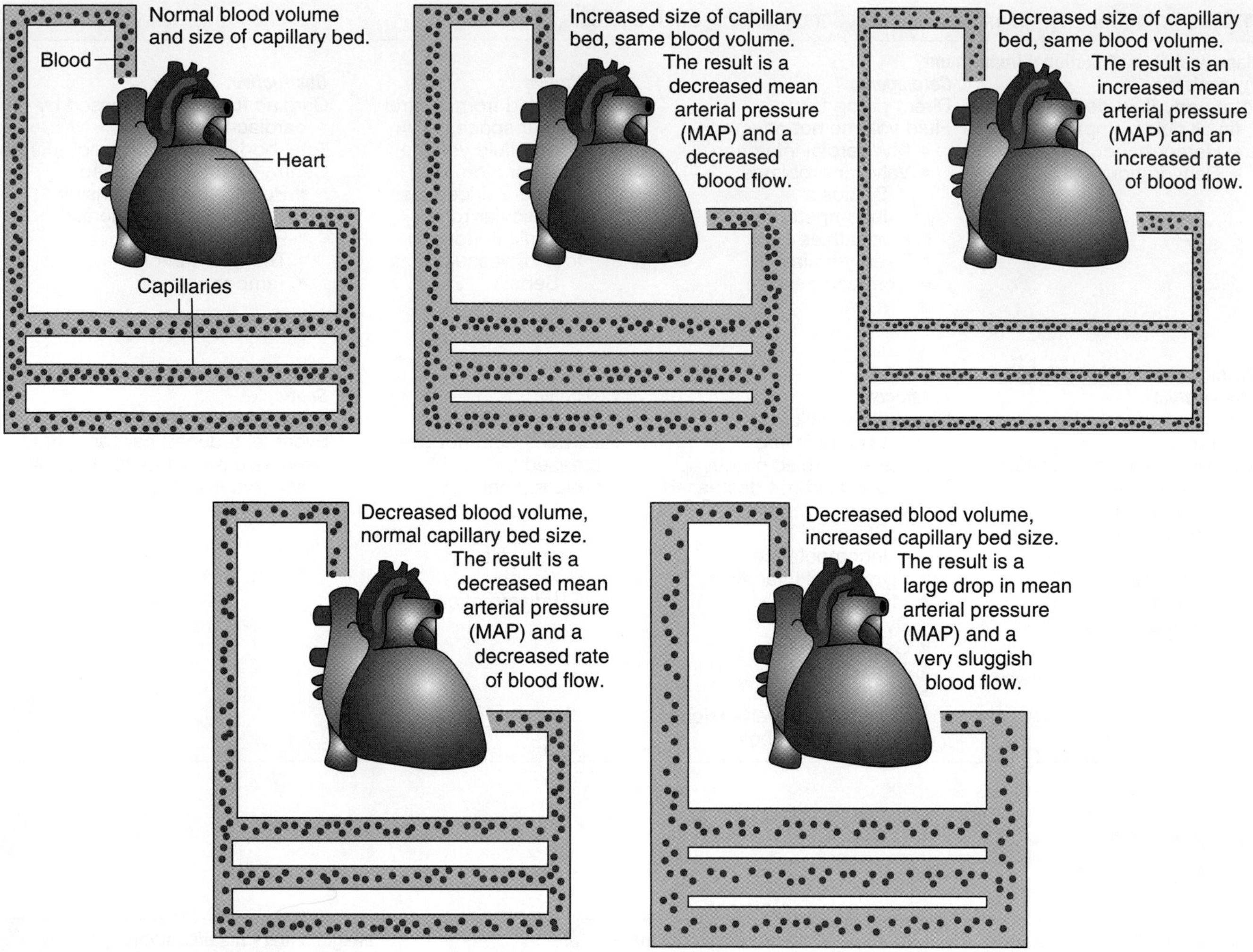

Figure 40-1 ■ Interaction of blood volume and the size of the capillary bed affecting mean arterial pressure.

and total blood volume remains the same, blood pressure increases and blood flow is faster.

Blood vessels contain nerves from the sympathetic division of the autonomic nervous system. Some nerves continuously stimulate vascular smooth muscle so that the blood vessels are normally partially constricted. This state of partial blood vessel constriction is called **sympathetic tone.** Increases in sympathetic stimulation constrict blood vessel smooth muscle even more, raising MAP. Decreases in sympathetic tone relax blood vessel smooth muscle, dilating them and lowering MAP.

Blood flow to organs varies and adjusts to changes in tissue oxygen needs. The body can selectively increase blood flow to some areas while reducing blood flow to others. Some organs, such as the skin and skeletal muscles, can tolerate low levels of oxygen for hours without dying or being damaged. Other organs (e.g., heart, brain, liver) tolerate **hypoxic** conditions (low levels of tissue oxygenation) poorly, and even just a few minutes without adequate oxygen results in serious or permanent damage.

The Processes of Shock

The problems common to all types of shock, regardless of cause, are the effects of **anaerobic cellular metabolism** (metabolism without oxygen). These effects are caused by inadequate tissue oxygenation and lead to impaired tissue function. The body begins to compensate to maintain or restore tissue perfusion and oxygenation even while the causes of shock are still present.

When the conditions that cause shock remain uncorrected, shock progresses through the following stages:

1. Initial stage
2. Nonprogressive stage
3. Progressive stage
4. Refractory stage

These stages of shock are classified on the basis of the following:

- How well compensatory mechanisms are working
- The severity of the clinical manifestations
- Whether tissue damage is reversible

The main trigger leading to shock is a sustained decrease in mean arterial pressure (MAP) that results from decreased cardiac output, decreased circulating blood volume, or expansion of the vascular bed. A decrease in MAP of 5 to 10 mm Hg below the client's baseline value is detected by pressure-sensitive nerve receptors **(baroreceptors)** in the aortic arch and carotid sinus (Berne, et al., 2004). These data are transmitted to brain centers, which stimulate compensatory mechanisms. These mechanisms ensure continued blood flow and oxygen delivery to vital organs while limiting blood

TABLE 40-2 Physiologic Events During Shock

Initial Stage
Decrease in baseline mean arterial pressure (MAP) of 5-10 mm Hg
Increased sympathetic stimulation
- Mild vasoconstriction
- Increase in heart rate

Nonprogressive Stage
Decrease in MAP of 10-15 mm Hg from the client's baseline value
Continued sympathetic stimulation
- Moderate vasoconstriction
- Increased heart rate
- Decreased pulse pressure

Chemical compensation
- Renin, aldosterone, and antidiuretic hormone secretion
    - Increased vasoconstriction
    - Decreased urine output
    - Stimulation of the thirst reflex

Some anaerobic metabolism in nonvital organs
- Mild acidosis
- Mild hyperkalemia

Progressive Stage
Decrease in MAP of >20 mm Hg from the client's baseline value
Anoxia of nonvital organs
Hypoxia of vital organs
Overall metabolism is anaerobic
- Moderate acidosis
- Moderate hyperkalemia
- Tissue ischemia

Refractory Stage
Severe tissue hypoxia with ischemia and necrosis
Release of myocardial depressant factor from the pancreas
Buildup of toxic metabolites
Multiple organ dysfunction syndrome (MODS)
Death

flow to less vital areas. Moving oxygenated blood into selected areas while bypassing others **(shunting)** causes the manifestations of shock.

If the events that caused the initial decrease in MAP are halted at this point, the compensatory mechanisms can return the body to a normal perfused and oxygenated state, even without outside intervention. If the initiating events continue and MAP decreases further, some tissues function under anaerobic conditions. This condition creates an increase in lactic acid levels and other harmful metabolites (e.g., protein-destroying enzymes and oxygen radicals). These substances cause electrolyte and acid-base imbalances with tissue-damaging effects and depressed heart muscle activity. Such effects are temporary and reversible if the cause of shock is corrected within 1 to 2 hours after onset. When such conditions continue for longer periods without help, the resulting acid-base imbalance, electrolyte imbalances, and increased metabolites cause so much cell damage in vital organs that multiple organ dysfunction syndrome (MODS) occurs and full recovery from shock is no longer possible. Table 40-2 lists the progression of shock.

INITIAL STAGE OF SHOCK (EARLY SHOCK)

The **initial** (early) stage of shock is present when the client's baseline MAP is decreased by less than 10 mm Hg. During this stage, compensatory mechanisms are so effective at returning MAP to normal levels that oxygenated blood flow to all vital organs is maintained. The cellular change in this stage is increased anaerobic metabolism with production of lactic acid, although overall cellular metabolism is still aerobic. Compensation (vascular constriction and increased heart rate) is effective, and both cardiac output and MAP are maintained within the normal range. Because vital organ function is not disrupted, the manifestations of shock are difficult to detect. *An increase in heart and respiratory rate from the client's baseline level or a slight increase in diastolic blood pressure may be the only objective manifestations of this early stage of shock.*

NONPROGRESSIVE STAGE (COMPENSATORY STAGE)

The **nonprogressive** (compensatory) stage of shock occurs when MAP decreases 10 to 15 mm Hg from baseline. Kidney and hormonal mechanisms are activated because cardiovascular compensation alone is not enough to maintain MAP and supply needed oxygen to the vital organs.

The kidneys and baroreceptors sense an ongoing decrease in MAP and trigger the release of renin, antidiuretic hormone (ADH), aldosterone, epinephrine, and norepinephrine. Kidney compensation occurs through the actions of renin, aldosterone, and ADH (see Chapter 14). Renin, secreted by the kidney, starts the reactions to decrease urine output, increase sodium reabsorption, and cause widespread blood vessel constriction (see Chapter 14, Figure 14-8). ADH is secreted by the posterior pituitary gland. ADH increases water reabsorption in the kidney and causes blood vessel constriction in the skin and other less vital tissue areas. Together these actions compensate for shock by keeping volume in the central blood vessels.

Tissue hypoxia occurs in nonvital organs and in the kidney, but it is not great enough to cause permanent damage. Because some metabolism is anaerobic, acid-base and electrolyte changes occur in response to the buildup of metabolites. Changes include **acidosis** (low blood pH) and **hyperkalemia** (increased blood potassium level) (see Chapters 16 and 19).

If the client is stable and compensatory mechanisms are supported by interventions, he or she can remain in this stage for hours without having permanent damage. Stopping the conditions that started the shock and providing supportive interventions can prevent the shock from progressing. The cellular effects of this stage are reversible with intervention.

PROGRESSIVE STAGE OF SHOCK (INTERMEDIATE STAGE)

The **progressive** stage of shock occurs when there is a sustained decrease in MAP of more than 20 mm Hg from baseline. In this stage compensatory mechanisms are functioning but no longer deliver sufficient oxygen, even to vital organs. Compensatory mechanisms use large amounts of oxygen in some tissues, which worsens the problem of general poor oxygenation. Vital organs develop hypoxia, and less vital organs become **anoxic** (no oxygen) and **ischemic** (cell dysfunction or death from lack of oxygen). As a result of poor oxygenation and a buildup of toxic metabolites, some tissues have severe cell damage and die.

The progressive stage of shock is a life-threatening emergency. Vital organs can tolerate this situation for only a short time before being damaged permanently. Immediate interventions are needed to reverse the effects of this stage of shock. Tolerance varies from person to person and depends on pre-existing health. The client's life usually can be saved if the conditions causing shock are corrected within 1 hour of the onset of the progressive stage.

REFRACTORY STAGE OF SHOCK (IRREVERSIBLE STAGE)

Formerly called the **irreversible stage,** the **refractory stage** of shock occurs when too much cell death and tissue damage results from too little oxygen reaching the tissues. Vital organs have overwhelming damage. This stage is termed *refractory* because the body is unable to respond effectively to interventions, and shock continues. The remaining cells metabolize anaerobically. *Therapy is not effective in saving the client's life, even if the cause of shock is corrected and MAP temporarily returns to normal.* So much tissue damage has occurred with widespread release of toxic metabolites and destructive enzymes that cell damage in vital organs continues.

MULTIPLE ORGAN DYSFUNCTION SYNDROME

The sequence of cell damage caused by the massive release of toxic metabolites and enzymes is termed **multiple organ dysfunction syndrome (MODS).** Once the damage has started, the sequence becomes a vicious cycle as more dead cells break open and release harmful metabolites. The metabolites trigger small clots *(microthrombi)* to form. The clots block tissue oxygenation and damage more cells, thus continuing the devastating cycle. MODS occurs first in the liver, heart, brain, and kidney. In septic shock, the lungs also are affected. The most profound change is damage to the heart muscle. One cause of this damage is the release of myocardial depressant factor (MDF) from the ischemic pancreas.

Etiology

Because shock is a manifestation of a pathologic condition rather than a disease state, its causes vary. Specific problems leading to different types of shock are listed in Table 40-3. *More than one type of shock can be present at the same time.* For example, trauma caused by a car accident may trigger hemorrhage (leading to hypovolemic shock) and a myocardial infarction (leading to cardiogenic shock).

TABLE 40-3 Causes of Shock

Hypovolemic Shock	**Distributive Shock**
Overall Cause Body fluid depletion	***Overall Cause*** Decreased vascular volume or tone
Hemorrhage ▪ Trauma ▪ Gastrointestinal ulcer ▪ Surgery ▪ Inadequate clotting Hemophilia Liver disease Malnutrition Bone marrow suppression Cancer Anticoagulation therapy Dehydration ▪ Vomiting ▪ Diarrhea ▪ Heavy diaphoresis ▪ Diuretic therapy ▪ Nasogastric suction ▪ Diabetes insipidus ▪ Hyperglycemia	***Specific Cause or Risk Factors*** Neural-induced ▪ Pain ▪ Anesthesia ▪ Stress ▪ Spinal cord injury ▪ Head trauma Chemical-induced ▪ Anaphylaxis ▪ Sepsis ▪ Capillary leak Burns Extensive trauma Hepatic dysfunction Hypoproteinemia
Cardiogenic Shock	**Obstructive Shock**
Overall Cause Direct pump failure	***Overall Cause*** Indirect pump failure
Specific Cause or Risk Factors Myocardial infarction Cardiac arrest Ventricular dysrhythmias ▪ Fibrillation ▪ Tachycardia Cardiac amyloidosis Cardiomyopathies ▪ Viral ▪ Toxic Myocardial degeneration	***Specific Cause or Risk Factors*** Cardiac tamponade Arterial stenosis Pulmonary embolus Pulmonary hypertension Constrictive pericarditis Thoracic tumors Tension pneumothorax

HYPOVOLEMIC SHOCK

Hypovolemic shock occurs when too little circulating blood volume causes a MAP decrease so that the body's total need for oxygen is not met. Common problems leading to hypovolemic shock are hemorrhage (external or internal) and dehydration.

Hypovolemic shock caused by external hemorrhage is common after trauma and surgery. Hypovolemic shock caused by internal hemorrhage occurs with blunt trauma, gastrointestinal (GI) ulcers, and poor control of surgical bleeding. External and internal hemorrhage can be caused by any problem that reduces the levels of clotting factors (see Table 40-3). Hypovolemia as a result of dehydration can be caused by any problem that decreases fluid intake or increases fluid loss (see Table 40-3).

CARDIOGENIC SHOCK

Cardiogenic shock occurs when the actual heart muscle is unhealthy and pumping is directly impaired. Table 40-3 lists the common causes of direct pump failure. These conditions decrease cardiac output and afterload, thus reducing MAP. Chapter 41 discusses cardiogenic shock resulting from myocardial infarction.

DISTRIBUTIVE SHOCK

Distributive shock is caused by a loss of sympathetic tone, blood vessel dilation, pooling of blood in venous and capillary beds, and increased blood vessel permeability (capillary leak). All these factors can decrease mean arterial pressure (MAP) and may be started by nerve changes (neural-induced) or the presence of chemicals (chemical-induced).

NEURAL-INDUCED DISTRIBUTIVE SHOCK. Neural-induced loss of MAP occurs when sympathetic nerve impulses controlling blood vessel smooth muscle are decreased and the smooth muscles of blood vessels relax, causing vasodilation. This blood vessel dilation can be a normal local response to injury, but shock results when the vasodilation is widespread or systemic. Common problems that can cause a systemic loss of sympathetic tone are listed in Table 40-3.

CHEMICAL-INDUCED DISTRIBUTIVE SHOCK. Chemical-induced distributive shock has three common origins: anaphylaxis, sepsis, and capillary leak syndrome. Chemical-induced distributive shock occurs when certain chemicals or foreign substances within the blood and blood vessels start widespread changes in blood vessel walls. The chemicals are usually **exogenous** (originate outside the body), but this type of shock also can be induced by substances normally found in the body **(endogenous)**.

ANAPHYLAXIS. **Anaphylaxis** is one result of type I allergic reactions (see Chapter 26). It begins within seconds to minutes after exposure to a specific allergen. It is termed *delayed,* however, because this type of reaction rarely occurs the first time a person encounters the allergen. It occurs on repeated exposure to the same allergen (McCance & Huether, 2002). Table 26-2 lists common allergens that can cause anaphylaxis.

Anaphylaxis is due to an antigen-antibody reaction that occurs in blood vessels throughout the body in response to contact with a substance to which the person has a severe allergy. This widespread reaction involves the interaction of the allergen, immunoglobulin E (IgE), basophils, and mast cells. It occurs within the walls of blood vessels, heart muscle cells, and bronchial tubes (see Chapters 23 and 26).

Anaphylaxis damages cells and causes the release of large amounts of histamine and other inflammatory chemicals. These natural chemicals move rapidly in the blood, causing massive blood vessel dilation and increased capillary leak. These responses result in severe hypovolemia and vascular collapse. Decreased cardiac contraction and dysrhythmias occur during anaphylaxis. These symptoms may be the result of heart-muscle changes induced by the antigen-antibody reaction, or they may result from the profound hypovolemia and resulting tissue hypoxia. Antigen-antibody reactions in the bronchial tissues cause severe edema and obstruction, which reduce gas exchange. The pulmonary problems, together with reduced circulation, cause extreme whole-body hypoxia. *Without intervention, this condition results in death.*

SEPSIS. Sepsis leading to distributive shock occurs when organisms are present in the blood. This form of shock is most commonly called **septic shock.** Sepsis often occurs with disseminated intravascular coagulation (DIC). Septic shock (sepsis-induced distributive shock) occurs most often with bacterial infection and has also been reported among clients with viral and yeast sepsis. Common organisms causing sepsis include gram-negative bacteria (*Pseudomonas aeruginosa, Escherichia coli,* and *Klebsiella pneumoniae*) and gram-positive bacteria (*Staphylococcus* and *Streptococcus*). Table 40-4 lists some of the health problems that increase the risk for septic shock.

Septic shock occurs when large amounts of toxins and endotoxins produced by bacteria are released into the blood, causing a whole-body inflammatory reaction. These substances react with blood vessels and cell membranes. Through the activity of white blood cells, the reactions start inflammatory and immune events known as the **systemic inflammatory response syndrome (SIRS).** These toxin-host actions activate complement, cause small clots to form within the capillaries of vital organs, increase capillary leakiness, injure cells (especially endothelial cells of blood vessels), and increase cell metabolism. Damage to endothelial cells reduces anticlotting actions and triggers the formation of small clots. Metabolism becomes anaerobic because of decreased MAP, clot formation in capillaries, and poor cell uptake of oxygen.

CAPILLARY LEAK SYNDROME. Capillary leak syndrome leading to distributive shock occurs when fluid shifts from the blood to the interstitial space. Such shifts are caused by increased size of capillary pores, loss of plasma osmolarity, and increased hydrostatic pressure in the blood. Problems causing fluid shifts include severe burns, liver disorders, ascites, peritonitis, paralytic ileus, severe malnutrition, large wounds, hyperglycemia, kidney disease, hypoproteinemia, and trauma.

TABLE 40-4 Conditions Predisposing to Sepsis-Induced Distributive Shock (Septic Shock)

- Malnutrition
- Immunosuppression
- Large, open wounds
- Mucous membrane fissures in prolonged contact with bloody or drainage-soaked packing
- Gastrointestinal ischemia
- Loss of gastrointestinal integrity
- Exposure to invasive procedures
- Malignancy
- Over 85 years of age
- Infection with resistant microorganisms
- Receiving cancer chemotherapy

OBSTRUCTIVE SHOCK

Obstructive shock is caused by problems that impair the ability of the normal heart muscle to pump effectively. The heart itself is normal, but conditions outside the heart prevent either adequate filling of the heart or adequate contraction of the healthy heart muscle. Common causes of obstructive shock are listed in Table 40-3.

Incidence/Prevalence

The exact incidence of shock is not known because it is a response rather than a disease. Shock is a common complication among hospitalized clients. Hypovolemic shock is most common among clients in emergency departments and after surgery or invasive procedures. Cardiogenic shock is the most common complication of myocardial infarction (MI) in clients who have damage to 40% or more of the heart muscle. Distributive shock from sepsis, which has a 40% to 85% mortality rate, is increasing among clients who are immunocompromised or have infections.

This chapter presents the collaborative management of clients with hypovolemic shock caused by hemorrhage and distributive shock caused by sepsis. Chapter 26 discusses anaphylaxis, and Chapter 41 discusses care of the client with cardiogenic shock as a result of MI.

HEALTH PROMOTION/ILLNESS PREVENTION

Hypovolemic Shock

Although hypovolemic shock often occurs as a complication of surgical intervention or trauma, primary prevention is possible. Chart 40-2 lists interventions to prevent shock. Teach all people to prevent dehydration by having an adequate fluid intake during exercise or when in hot, dry environments. Urge people to prevent trauma and hemorrhage by using proper safety equipment, seat belts, and being aware of hazards in the home or workplace.

Secondary prevention of hypovolemic shock is a major nursing responsibility. Keep in mind that just being a client

CHART 40-2

NIC INTERVENTION ACTIVITIES for Shock Prevention

Shock Prevention: *Detecting and treating a client at risk for impending shock*

- Monitor circulatory status: BP, skin color, skin temperature, heart sounds, heart rate and rhythm, presence and quality of peripheral pulses, and capillary refill.
- Monitor for signs of inadequate tissue oxygenation.
- Monitor for apprehension, increased anxiety, and changes in mental status.
- Monitor temperature and respiratory status.
- Monitor intake and output.
- Monitor laboratory values, especially hemoglobin and hematocrit levels, clotting profile, ABG and electrolyte levels, cultures, and chemistry profile.
- Note bruising, petechiae, and condition of mucous membranes.
- Note color, amount, and frequency of stools, vomitus, and nasogastric drainage.
- Test urine for blood, glucose, and protein, as appropriate.
- Monitor abdominal pain and girth.
- Monitor for early compensatory responses to fluid loss: increased heart rate, decreased BP, orthostatic hypotension, decreased urinary output, narrowed pulse pressure, decreased capillary refill, apprehension, pale and cool skin, and diaphoresis.
- Monitor for early signs of septic shock: warm, flushed, dry skin; increasing cardiac output and temperature; and declining SVR and PAP.
- Monitor for possible sources of fluid loss: chest tube, wound, and nasogastric drainage; diarrhea; vomiting; and increasing abdominal and extremity girth.
- Place client in supine position with legs elevated to increase preload, as appropriate.
- Administer IV and/or oral fluids, as appropriate.
- Initiate early administration of antimicrobial agents and closely monitor their effectiveness, as appropriate.

NIC intervention activities selected from Dochterman, J.M., & Bulechek, G.M. (Eds.). (2004). *Nursing interventions classification (NIC)* (4th ed). St. Louis: Mosby. No part of this work is to be altered without prior written permission from the Publisher.

PAP, Pulmonary artery pressure; *SVR,* systemic vascular resistance.

EVIDENCE-BASED PRACTICE for Nursing

Flowers and plants as sources of infection

LaCharity, L., & McClure, E. (2003). Are plants vectors for transmission of infection in acute care? *Critical Care Nursing Clinics of North America, 15*(1), 119-124.

This research is an analysis of the evidence regarding potted plants and cut flowers as infection sources in acute care settings, especially for clients at higher risk for infection. The authors reviewed current and historical nursing and medical literature. The review revealed that many health care professionals, hospitals, professional organizations, and the Centers for Disease Control and Prevention continue to recommend restriction of cut flowers and potted plants in rooms of clients at risk for infection and sepsis. These recommendations, however, were not based on clinical evidence. Few prospective clinical studies in which organisms were cultured from plants, soil, cut flowers, or vase water and compared with the organisms present in client wounds, drainage, or blood have been completed. Some recently published studies examined plant, soil, flower, and water environments under controlled conditions.

Soil of potted plants was found to contain bacteria and fungus. Standing vase water contained the largest variety and greatest quantities of microorganisms. Adding hydrogen peroxide to vase water reduced the number of organisms and did not adversely affect cut flowers. Using sterile or distilled water in vases did not reduce the growth of organisms.

Level of Evidence: 1—Quantitative systematic review.

Critique. Clinical studies are needed to compare organisms found in clients with infections who also have plants or flowers in the room to the organisms in the plant and flower environments. Studies are also needed that examine the presence of specific organisms on the hands of persons handling potted plants and flowers in the acute care setting and whether standard handwashing is effective in removing these organisms.

Implications for Nursing. Although no clear evidence links the actual transmission of infectious organisms from plants and flowers to clients, it seems reasonable for nurses to restrict these items from the rooms of clients who are immunocompromised or who have open wounds. Other precautionary recommendations include teaching the client to refrain from caring for plants or flowers, having personnel handling plants or flowers not have direct contact with clients, changing vase water at least every 3 days, and adding hydrogen peroxide to vase water. The use of good handwashing after handling flowers remains a major anti-infection strategy for nursing personnel and clients.

in the acute care setting is a risk factor. Identify clients at risk for dehydration and assess for early manifestations. This is especially important for those who have reduced cognition or reduced mobility or who are on nothing-by-mouth (NPO) status.

Assess all clients who have invasive procedures or trauma for obvious or occult bleeding. Compare pulse quality and rate to baseline. Compare urine output to fluid intake. Check vital signs for clients who have persistent thirst. Assess for shock in any client who develops a change in mental status, an increase in pain, or an increase in anxiety.

Septic Shock

Identify clients at risk for sepsis. Use aseptic technique during invasive procedures and when working with nonintact skin and mucous membranes in immunocompromised clients. Remove indwelling urinary catheters and intravenous (IV) access lines as soon as they are no longer needed. Contact with potted plants and cut flowers has been considered a source of potential infection and sepsis for susceptible clients. Restriction of these items in hospital units to prevent infection is controversial (see the Evidence-Based Practice for Nursing box above).

Early detection of septic shock is a major nursing responsibility. Because septic shock can be a complication of many conditions found in acute care settings, always consider the possibility of septic shock. Assess vital signs often (at least twice per shift) for changes from baseline levels. Review laboratory data for changes in total white blood cell count and in the differential. The hallmark of sepsis is a decreasing segmented neutrophil level with a rising band neutrophil level. This change is called a **left shift** (see Chapter 23).

COLLABORATIVE MANAGEMENT: HYPOVOLEMIC SHOCK

The Concept Map on p. 829 addresses assessment and nursing care issues related to clients with hypovolemic shock.

Assessment

HISTORY

Collect data on risk factors and causative factors related to hypovolemic shock. If the client is alert and stable, question him or her directly. If the client is not alert or if his or her

CONCEPT MAP Hypovolemic Shock

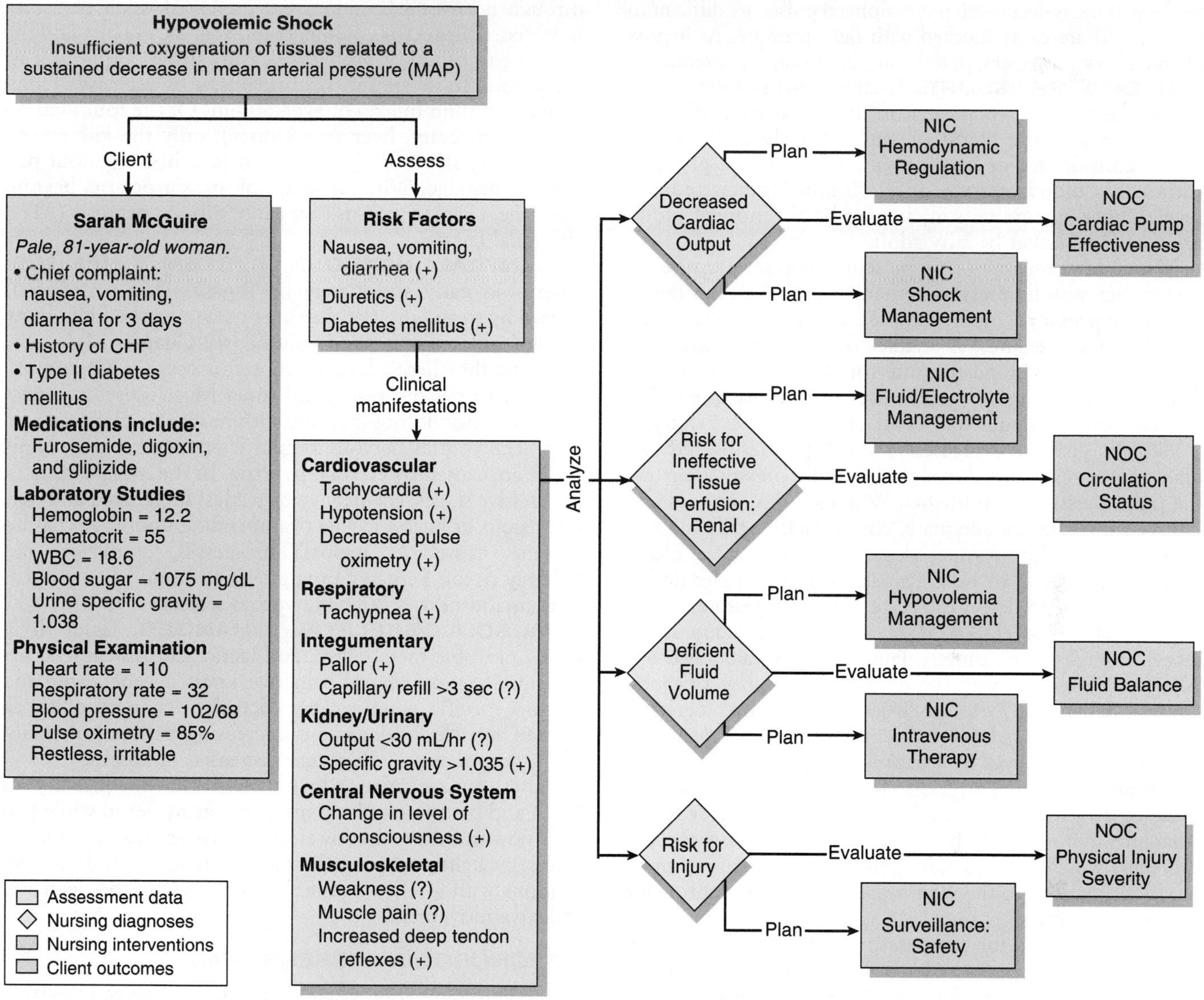

Concept Map by Elaine Bishop Kennedy, EdD, RN

condition is not stable, collect information from family members. *Age* is important because hypovolemic shock from trauma is more common in young adults, whereas sepsis is more common among older adults. Ask clients specific questions about recent illness, trauma, procedures, or chronic health problems that may lead to shock. Such problems include GI ulcers, general surgery, hemophilia, liver disorders, prolonged vomiting, and prolonged diarrhea. Ask about the use of drugs such as aspirin, diuretics, and antacids that may cause changes leading to hypovolemic shock or may indicate the presence of a problem that can contribute to shock.

Ask about fluid intake and output during the previous 24 hours. *Information about urine output is especially important because urine output is reduced during the first stages of shock, even when fluid intake is normal.*

Assess the client for obvious signs of factors that can lead to shock. Areas to examine for signs of hemorrhage include the gums, wounds, and sites of dressings, drains, and vascular accesses. Also check *under* the client for blood. Observe for any swelling or skin discoloration that may indicate an internal hemorrhage.

PHYSICAL ASSESSMENT/CLINICAL MANIFESTATIONS

Most manifestations of hypovolemic shock are caused by the changes resulting from compensatory efforts. **Compensation** or **compensatory mechanisms** are physiologic responses that try to keep an adequate blood flow to vital organs. Signs of shock are first evident as changes in cardiovascular function. As shock progresses, changes in the kidney, respiratory, integumentary, musculoskeletal, and central nervous systems become evident.

CARDIOVASCULAR CHANGES. Shock decreases mean arterial pressure (MAP), and the resulting early compensation is cardiovascular. Thus the earliest clinical signs of hypovolemic shock are cardiovascular.

PULSE. Assess the central and peripheral pulses for rate and quality. In the initial stage of hypovolemic shock, the pulse rate increases to keep cardiac output and MAP at normal levels, even though the actual **stroke volume** (amount of blood pumped out from the heart) per beat is decreased. Because stroke volume is decreased, the peripheral pulses are difficult to palpate and are easily blocked with light pressure. As hypovolemic shock progresses, peripheral pulses may be absent.

BLOOD PRESSURE. Changes in systolic blood pressure are not always present in the initial stage of shock. When assessing the blood pressure of a client at risk for shock, consider his or her normal baseline blood pressure. Although a blood pressure of 90/50 mm Hg may indicate severe shock in one person, it may be the normal blood pressure for another healthy adult.

When vasoconstriction is present, diastolic pressure increases but systolic pressure remains the same. As a result, the **pulse pressure,** or the difference between the systolic and diastolic pressures, is smaller (sometimes called "narrower"). Monitor blood pressure for changes from baseline levels and for changes from the previous measurement. For accuracy use the same equipment on the same extremity.

Systolic pressure decreases as shock progresses and cardiac output decreases. A reduced systolic pressure narrows the pulse pressure even further. When shock continues and interventions are not adequate, compensation fails and systolic and diastolic pressures decrease. At this stage, blood pressure is difficult to hear. Palpation or a Doppler device may be needed to detect the systolic blood pressure.

OXYGEN SATURATION. Oxygen saturation is assessed through pulse oximetry. Pulse oximetry values between 90% and 95% occur with the nonprogressive stage of shock, and values between 75% and 80% occur with the progressive stage of shock. *Any value below 70% is considered a life-threatening emergency and may signal the refractory stage of shock.*

SKIN CHANGES. Skin changes occur in shock because of decreased perfusion. An early compensatory mechanism for hypovolemic shock is blood vessel constriction in the skin, which reduces skin perfusion. This allows more blood to circulate to the vital organs, which cannot tolerate low oxygen levels.

Assess the skin for temperature, color, and degree of moisture. It feels cool or cold to the touch and is moist. As shock progresses, color changes are first evident in the mucous membranes and in the skin around the mouth. Pallor or cyanosis is best assessed in the oral mucous membranes in dark-skinned clients. Color changes in clients with lighter skin are noted first in the extremities and then in the central trunk area. The skin feels clammy or moist to the touch, not because sweating increases but because the normal fluid lost through the skin does not evaporate quickly on cold skin.

Evaluate capillary refill time by pressing on the client's fingernail until it blanches and then observing how fast the nail bed resumes color when pressure is released. Normally the nail bed capillaries resume color as soon as pressure is released. With shock, capillary refill is slow or is sometimes absent. Capillary refill may not be a reliable indicator for peripheral blood flow in older clients or those with anemia, diabetes mellitus, or peripheral vascular disease.

RESPIRATORY CHANGES. Assess the rate, depth, and ease of respiration and also auscultate the lungs for abnormal breath sounds. Respiratory rate increases during hypovolemic shock. This increase is a compensatory mechanism to provide oxygen to the critical tissues. When shock progresses to the stage at which lactic acidosis is present, the respiratory depth also increases.

RENAL/URINARY CHANGES. The renal system compensates for decreased MAP by saving body water through decreased filtration and increased water reabsorption. Assess urine for volume, color, specific gravity, and the presence of blood or protein. Measure urine output at least every hour. In severe shock, urine output is decreased (compared with fluid intake) or even absent. Of the four vital organs (heart, brain, liver, and kidney), only the kidney can tolerate hypoxia and anoxia for up to 1 hour without permanent damage. When hypoxia or anoxia persists beyond this time, clients are at risk for acute tubular necrosis (ATN) and renal failure.

CENTRAL NERVOUS SYSTEM CHANGES. Clients in early shock may be thirsty. This sensation is caused by stimulation of the thirst centers in the brain in response to decreased blood volume (see Chapter 14).

Assess the client's level of consciousness (LOC) and orientation to person, place, and time. Most causes of hypovolemic shock do not interfere with nerve impulse transmission. The central nervous system changes of hypovolemic shock are caused by cerebral hypoxia. In the initial and nonprogressive stages, clients may be restless or agitated and may be anxious or have a feeling of impending doom that has no obvious cause. As hypoxia progresses, confusion and lethargy occur. Lethargy progresses to somnolence and loss of consciousness as cerebral hypoxia worsens.

MUSCULOSKELETAL CHANGES. Tissue hypoxia, anaerobic metabolism, and lactic acidosis cause skeletal muscle weakness and pain. Weakness is generalized and has no specific pattern. The electrolyte changes of shock worsen muscle weakness by decreasing action potentials. Then deep tendon reflexes are decreased or absent.

Assess muscle strength by having the client squeeze your hand and by trying to keep his or her arms flexed while you pull downward on the lower arms. Assess deep tendon reflexes by lightly tapping the patellar tendons and Achilles tendons with a reflex hammer and observing the degree of reflexive movement.

PSYCHOSOCIAL ASSESSMENT

Changes in mental status and behavior may be early signs of shock. Observe the client closely and document behavior. Assess current mental status by evaluating LOC and noting whether the client is asleep or awake. If the client is asleep, attempt to awaken him or her and document how easily he or she is aroused. If the client is awake, determine whether he or she is oriented to person, time, and place. Avoid asking questions that can be answered with a "yes" or a "no" response. Consider the following points during assessment:

- Is it necessary to repeat questions to obtain a response?
- Does the response answer the question asked?
- Does the client have difficulty making word choices?
- Is the client irritated or upset by the questions?
- Can the client concentrate on a question long enough to answer appropriately, or is the attention span limited?

If possible, talk with family members to determine whether the client's behavior and mental status are typical or represent a change.

LABORATORY ASSESSMENT

Although no single laboratory finding confirms or rules out shock, changes in laboratory data may support the diagno-

CHART 40-3

LABORATORY PROFILE
Hypovolemic Shock

Test	Normal Range for Adults	Significance of Abnormal Findings
pH (arterial)	7.35-7.45	Decreased: insufficient tissue oxygenation causing anaerobic metabolism and acidosis
Pao_2	80-100 mm Hg	Decreased: anaerobic metabolism
$Paco_2$	35-45 mm Hg	Increased: anaerobic metabolism
Lactic acid (arterial)	0.3-0.8 mmol/L	Increased: anaerobic metabolism with buildup of metabolites
Hematocrit	*Females:* 37%-47% *Males:* 42%-52%	Increased: fluid shift, dehydration Decreased: hemorrhage
Hemoglobin	*Females:* 12-16 g/dL *Males:* 14-18 g/dL	Increased: fluid shift, dehydration Decreased: hemorrhage
Potassium	3.5-5.0 mEq/L or mmol/L	Increased: dehydration, acidosis

Data from Pagana, K., & Pagana, T. (2002). *Mosby's manual of diagnostic and laboratory tests* (2nd ed.). St. Louis: Mosby.
Pao_2, Partial pressure of arterial oxygen; *$Paco_2$*, partial pressure of arterial carbon dioxide.

sis of hypovolemic shock. (Chart 40-3 lists common laboratory findings occurring with hypovolemic shock.) As shock progresses, arterial blood gas values become abnormal. The pH decreases, the partial pressure of arterial oxygen (PaO_2) decreases, and the partial pressure of arterial carbon dioxide ($PaCO_2$) increases. Changes in other laboratory values may occur with specific causes of hypovolemic shock.

Hematocrit and hemoglobin levels decrease if shock is caused by hemorrhage. When shock is caused by dehydration or a fluid shift, hematocrit and hemoglobin levels are elevated.

Common Nursing Diagnoses and Collaborative Problems

Nursing diagnoses that may apply to clients with hypovolemic shock include the following:

- Anxiety related to potential for death
- Deficient Fluid Volume related to active fluid volume loss
- Decreased Cardiac Output related to hypovolemia
- Ineffective Tissue Perfusion (General) related to hypovolemia
- Disturbed Thought Processes related to decreased cerebral perfusion

Critical Thinking Challenge

Your client is a 33-year-old woman who is returned to your outpatient unit after having a surgical tubal ligation by colposcopy. After moving her from the stretcher to her bed, you take her vital signs. Her pulse is 110 and thready, blood pressure is 90/72, respiratory rate is 28, and pulse oximetry is 89%. When you shake her shoulder, she opens her eyes but does not answer any questions.

1. What should you do first?
2. What other assessment data should you obtain?
3. Given the type of surgery, where would you expect bleeding to occur and what manifestations would you expect to find?
4. She still has an IV in her left hand infusing dextrose 5% in 0.45% saline. The postsurgical orders indicate that it should be removed when she is stable. Should you remove it now? Why or why not?

evolve For suggested answer guidelines, go to http://evolve.elsevier.com/Iggy/.

CHART 40-4

BEST PRACTICE for
The Client in Hypovolemic Shock

- Ensure a patent airway.
- Start an IV catheter or maintain an established catheter.
- Administer oxygen.
- Elevate the client's feet, keeping his or her head flat or elevated to a 30-degree angle.
- Examine the client for overt bleeding.
- If overt bleeding is present, apply direct pressure to the site.
- Administer medications as prescribed.
- Increase the rate of IV fluid delivery.
- Do not leave the client.

CHART 40-5

NIC **INTERVENTION ACTIVITIES for**
The Client with Hypovolemic Shock

Shock Management: Volume: *Promotion of adequate tissue perfusion for a client with severely compromised intravascular volume*

- Monitor for signs and symptoms of persistent bleeding (e.g., check all secretions for frank or occult blood).
- Monitor the client closely for hemorrhage.
- Prevent blood volume loss (e.g., apply pressure to site of bleeding).
- Administer IV fluids, as appropriate.
- Note hemoglobin/hematocrit level before and after blood loss, as indicated.
- Administer blood products (e.g., platelets or fresh frozen plasma), as appropriate.
- Monitor coagulation studies, including prothrombin time (PT), partial thromboplastin time (PTT), fibrinogen, fibrin degradation/split products, and platelet counts, as appropriate.

NIC intervention activities selected from Dochterman, J.M., & Bulechek, G.M. (Eds.). (2004). *Nursing interventions classification (NIC)* (4th ed.). St. Louis: Mosby. No part of this work is to be altered without prior written permission from the Publisher.

Interventions

Interventions for clients in hypovolemic shock focus on reversing the shock, restoring fluid volume, and preventing complications through supportive and drug therapies. Surgery may be needed to correct the problem leading to hypovolemic shock. Chart 40-4 lists best practices for clients in hypovolemic shock. Chart 40-5 lists NIC interventions for clients with hypovolemic shock.

NONSURGICAL MANAGEMENT. The goals of shock management are to maintain tissue oxygenation, increase vascular volume to normal range, and support compensatory mechanisms. Oxygen therapy, fluid replacement therapy, and drug therapies are useful for this problem.

Oxygen Therapy. Oxygen therapy is useful whenever shock is present. Oxygen can be delivered by mask, hood, nasal cannula, nasopharyngeal tube, endotracheal tube, and tracheostomy tube. Oxygen is given in L/min (when using a cannula) or concentration by percentage (when using a mask).

Intravenous Therapy. Colloids and crystalloids are the two types of fluids used for volume replacement during hypovolemia. Colloid solutions contain large molecules (usually proteins or starches) (see Chapter 14). Crystalloid solutions contain nonprotein substances (e.g., minerals, salts, sugars).

Colloid Fluids. Protein-containing colloid fluids help restore osmotic pressure and fluid volume. Blood and blood products are often used for this purpose when shock is caused by blood loss. These fluids include whole blood, packed red blood cells, plasma, plasma fractions, and synthetic plasma expanders.

Whole blood and packed red blood cells increase hematocrit and hemoglobin levels along with fluid volume. Whole blood is used to replace large volumes of blood loss because it increases volume and improves the oxygen-carrying capacity of the blood. Packed red cells are given for moderate blood loss because they restore the red blood cell deficit and improve oxygen-carrying capacity without adding excessive fluid volume. Chapter 43 discusses nursing care issues when giving blood or blood products.

Human plasma, an acellular blood product containing some clotting factors, is given to restore osmotic pressure when hematocrit and hemoglobin levels are within normal ranges. Plasma protein fractions (e.g., Plasmanate) and synthetic plasma expanders (e.g., hetastarch [hydroxyethyl starch, Hespan]) increase plasma volume and are used as early treatment for hypovolemic shock before a cause has been established.

Crystalloid Fluids. Crystalloid fluids are given to help maintain an adequate fluid and electrolyte balance. Two common solutions are Ringer's lactate and normal saline. Ringer's lactate contains sodium, chloride, calcium, potassium, and lactate dissolved in water. This isotonic solution expands volume, and the lactate buffers any acidosis. Normal saline (0.9% sodium chloride in water) is a fluid replacement used to increase plasma volume when there has been no loss of red blood cells.

Drug Therapy. Drugs may be needed if the volume deficit is severe and the client does not respond sufficiently to the replacement of fluid volume and blood products. The actions of drugs for shock increase venous return, improve cardiac contractility, or improve cardiac perfusion by dilating the coronary vessels. Chart 40-6 lists the drugs used to treat hypovolemic shock.

Vasoconstricting Drugs. Many drugs stimulate venous return by constricting blood vessels and decreasing venous pooling of blood. These actions increase cardiac output and mean arterial pressure (MAP), which helps to improve tissue perfusion and oxygenation. Such agents include dopamine (Intropin, Revimine✱) and norepinephrine (Levophed). These drugs can produce serious side effects, and their dosages must be carefully calculated on the basis of the client's size and response to treatment (see Chart 40-6).

Drugs Enhancing Myocardial Contractility. Some drugs directly stimulate adrenergic receptor sites on the heart muscle ($beta_1$ receptors) and improve heart muscle cell contraction. Other drugs enhance cardiac contraction by slowing heart rate and allowing the left ventricle a longer filling time. When filling time is increased, more blood enters the left ventricle and stretches the muscle fibers. Thus greater recoil occurs, and more blood leaves the left ventricle during contraction. Some of these drugs also stimulate the ventricles. Drugs with these actions include dobutamine (Dobutrex) and milrinone (Primacor).

Drugs Enhancing Myocardial Perfusion. It is important to ensure that the heart is well perfused, especially when giving drugs to improve cardiac contraction, so that aerobic metabolism is maintained in the heart cells and maximum contractility can occur. Drugs that dilate coronary blood vessels while minimally dilating systemic vessels are used for this purpose. A common drug with this action is sodium nitroprusside (Nitropress, Nipride✱). *Care is taken because these drugs can cause systemic vasodilation and increase shock if the client is volume depleted.*

Monitoring. A major nursing action in caring for clients in hypovolemic shock is monitoring vital signs and level of consciousness (LOC). Monitor the following vital signs:

- Pulse
- Blood pressure
- Pulse pressure
- Central venous pressure (CVP)
- Respiratory rate
- Skin and mucosal color
- Oxygen saturation

Assess parameters at least every 15 minutes until the shock is controlled and the client's condition improves. Hemodynamic monitoring in critical care settings includes intra-arterial monitoring, mixed venous oxygen saturation (SvO_2), pulmonary artery monitoring, and pulmonary capillary wedge pressures. Table 40-5 compares the changes in hemodynamic patterns seen with different types of shock.

Insertion of a CVP catheter allows pressure to be monitored in the client's right atrium or superior vena cava while providing venous access. Changes in CVP reflect hypovolemic shock. As circulating volume decreases, the amount of blood returning to the right atrium also decreases, causing the CVP to decrease from baseline levels.

Intra-arterial catheters allow continuous monitoring of blood pressure and are an access for arterial blood sampling. Intra-arterial catheters are inserted into an artery (radial, brachial, femoral, or dorsalis pedis). The catheter is attached to pressure tubing and a transducer. The transducer converts pressure in the artery into an electrical signal that is seen as a visible waveform on an oscilloscope and as digital numeric value.

SURGICAL MANAGEMENT. The nonsurgical interventions described above are used to stabilize the client's hemodynamic status. After a cause has been established, surgical intervention may be needed to correct the cause of shock. Such procedures include vascular repair or revision, surgical hemostasis of major wounds, closure of bleeding ulcers, and chemical scarring (chemosclerosis) of varicosities.

CHART 40-6

DRUG THERAPY for Hypovolemic Shock

Drug	Usual Dosage	Nursing Interventions	Rationales
Vasoconstrictors			
Dopamine hydrochloride (Intropin, Revimine✱)	5-30 mcg/kg/min IV (for hypotension) 2-5 mcg/kg/min IV (for renal perfusion)	Assess the client for chest pain.	Dopamine increases myocardial oxygen consumption.
		Monitor urine output hourly.	Higher doses decrease renal perfusion and urine output.
		Assess blood pressure every 15 min.	Hypertension is a symptom of overdose.
		Assess the client for headache.	Headache is an early symptom of drug excess.
Epinephrine (Adrenalin)	0.5-1 mg IV initially, followed by 0.5 mg q5min May also be given by intracardiac injection	Monitor the client for dysrhythmias.	Epinephrine may cause ventricular tachydysrhythmias.
		Assess the client for chest pain.	Vasoconstriction may impair cardiac oxygenation.
Norepinephrine (Levophed)	0.5-1 mcg/kg/min continuous IV infusion to maintain blood pressure at 90-100 mm Hg	Assess for extravasation.	Norepinephrine can cause severe tissue damage and necrosis.
		Observe the client's extremities for color and perfusion.	Norepinephrine can cause such vasoconstriction that peripheral ischemia may result.
Phenylephrine (Neo-Synephrine)	80-200 mcg/min IV	Assess for chest pain.	Vasoconstriction may impair cardiac oxygenation.
Agents Enhancing Contractility			
Milrinone (Primacor)	50 mcg/kg bolus over 10 min; 0.3-0.75 mcg/kg/min continuous IV infusion	Assess blood pressure every 15 min.	Hypertension is a symptom of overdose.
Atropine sulfate	0.5-1 mg IV q5min, up to a total of 2 mg	Take pulse every 5 min.	Atropine sulfate may cause a rebound tachycardia.
		Monitor urine output every 30 min.	Atropine sulfate may cause urinary retention.
		Administer cautiously to clients with glaucoma.	Atropine sulfate may precipitate an episode of acute angle-closure glaucoma.
Dobutamine hydrochloride (Dobutrex)	2.5-20 mcg/kg/min continuous IV infusion	Assess the client for chest pain.	Dobutamine increases myocardial oxygen consumption.
		Assess blood pressure every 15 minutes.	Hypertension is a symptom of overdose.
Agents Enhancing Myocardial Perfusion			
Sodium nitroprusside (Nitropress, Nipride✱)	0.5-10 mcg/kg/min continuous IV infusion	Assess blood pressure every 15 min.	Hypotension may result from the systemic dilation of veins and arteries.

Med Error Alert! *Dopamine, norepinephrine, milrinone, dobutamine, and nitroprusside are all administered in doses of micrograms, not milligrams.*

Critical Thinking Challenge

Your client who had the tubal ligation by colposcopy has no external bleeding, but her abdomen is enlarging and you observe skin discoloration on her lower back.

1. Is oxygen an appropriate therapy for her? Why or why not?
2. Should you apply pressure to the abdominal-pelvic region? Why or why not?
3. What type(s) of IV solutions should you be prepared to give? Provide a rationale for your choice. (You may need to refer to the blood therapy section of Chapter 43.)

evolve For suggested answer guidelines, go to http://evolve.elsevier.com/Iggy/.

COLLABORATIVE MANAGEMENT: SEPSIS-INDUCED DISTRIBUTIVE SHOCK (SEPTIC SHOCK)

PHARM REVIEW

Assessment

Distributive shock caused by sepsis does not resemble other types of shock in that it has two distinctive phases (Figure 40-2). The first phase can be long, often lasting from hours to a day or longer. Manifestations during this phase are subtle. The chance for recovery is good when the client is recognized as being in the first phase of septic shock and appropriate interventions are started. The second phase of septic shock has a sudden onset and a rapid downhill course. If septic shock progresses to the second phase, chances for recovery are poor. Identifying clients in the first phase of septic shock can make the greatest difference in survival.

HISTORY

Collect data about risk factors and causative factors related to septic shock. Age is important because sepsis develops more easily among older, debilitated clients who are immunosuppressed. Chart 40-7 lists factors that increase the older adult's risk for shock. Ask about recent illness, trauma, invasive procedures, or chronic conditions that may lead to sepsis. Check which drugs the client has used in the past week. Some drugs may directly cause changes leading to shock. Also, a drug regimen may indicate a disease or problem that can contribute to septic shock. Such drugs include aspirin and aspirin-containing drugs, antibiotics, and cancer therapy drugs.

TABLE 40-5 Hemodynamic Pattern Changes Associated with Different Types of Shock

Type of Shock	Cardiac Output (CO)	Central Venous Pressure (CVP)	Pulmonary Artery Pressure (PAP)	Pulmonary Capillary Wedge Pressure (PCWP)
Hypovolemic	↓	↓	↓	↓
Cardiac	↓	↑	↑	↑
Obstructive	↓	↑	↑	↑
Distributive				
Anaphylactic	↓	↓	↓	↓
Sepsis (early)	↑	Ø	Ø or ↑	Ø or ↑
Sepsis (late)	↓	↓	↓	↓

Data from Jones, K. (1996). Shock. In J. Clochesy, et al. (Eds.). *Critical care nursing* (2nd ed., pp. 1371-1381). Philadelphia: W.B. Saunders.
↑, Increased; ↓, decreased; Ø, normal or unchanged.

PHYSICAL ASSESSMENT/CLINICAL MANIFESTATIONS

Manifestations of the first phase are unique to septic shock and are often opposite from those seen with all other types of shock. Chart 40-8 lists the manifestations of the first (hyperdynamic) phase of septic shock. These changes are caused by the body's response to endotoxins and affect most body systems.

CARDIOVASCULAR CHANGES. Endotoxins in the blood interact with white blood cells and blood vessel walls to trigger an inflammatory reaction. Some endotoxins also stimulate the heart muscle directly. As a result, cardiac output *increases* during the first phase of septic shock. This phase is hyperdynamic and also may be called the **high-output** or **warm-shock phase.** Increased cardiac output is reflected by tachycardia, increased stroke volume, a normal-to-elevated systolic blood pressure, and a normal CVP. Increased cardiac output and vasodilation make the skin color appear normal with pink mucous membranes and may feel warm to the touch. This situation is temporary and eventually the cardiac output is greatly reduced.

As septic shock progresses, disseminated intravascular coagulation (DIC) may occur. The endotoxins and inflamma-

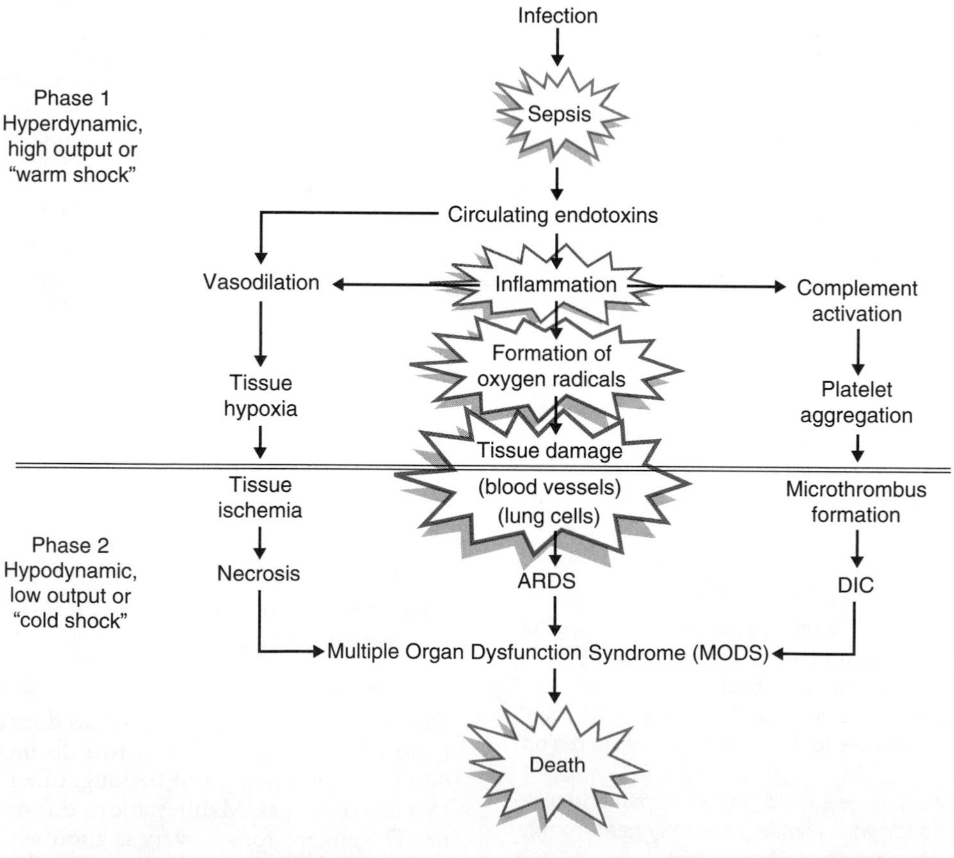

Figure 40-2 ■ The sequence of sepsis-induced distributive shock, septic shock. *ARDS,* Acute respiratory distress syndrome; *DIC,* disseminated intravascular coagulation.

CHART 40-7

NURSING FOCUS on the OLDER ADULT
Risk Factors for Shock

Hypovolemic Shock
- Diuretic therapy
- Diminished thirst reflex
- Immobility
- Use of aspirin-containing products
- Use of integrative therapies such as gingko biloba
- Anticoagulant therapy

Cardiogenic Shock
- Diabetes mellitus
- Presence of cardiomyopathies

Distributive Shock
- Diminished immune response
- Reduced skin integrity
- Presence of cancer
- Peripheral neuropathy
- Strokes
- Institutionalization (hospital or extended care facility)
- Malnutrition
- Anemia

Obstructive Shock
- Pulmonary hypertension
- Presence of cancer

tory reactions trigger complement activation (see Chapter 23). These actions damage endothelial cells of blood vessels, which then allows thousands of small clots to form in the tiny capillaries of the liver, kidney, brain, spleen, and heart. These small clots reduce oxygenation in those organs, causing hypoxia and ischemia and making overall metabolism anaerobic. This huge number of small clots uses clotting factors and fibrinogen faster than they can be produced by the liver. This problem makes clients much more susceptible to hemorrhage. Reduction of clotting factors and fibrinogen mark the beginning of the second phase of septic shock.

Because many small clots have formed, the clotting factors have been used and the blood vessels are dilated. Clients are hypovolemic in this phase of septic shock. Cardiac output, blood pressure, and pulse pressure decrease dramatically. This phase is called the **hypodynamic, low-output,** or **cold-shock phase** of septic shock. The manifestations of this phase are the same as those of the later stages of hypovolemic shock.

RESPIRATORY CHANGES. In the hyperdynamic phase of septic shock, respiratory rate and depth are increased, leading to respiratory alkalosis. When septic shock progresses to the hypodynamic phase, the life-threatening lung complication of acute respiratory distress syndrome (ARDS) may occur. ARDS in septic shock is caused by the continued systemic inflammatory response syndrome (SIRS)

CHART 40-8

KEY FEATURES of
Hyperdynamic Phase of Sepsis-Induced Distributive Shock (Septic Shock)

Assessment	Findings
General	
Assess the mental status and level of consciousness.	Irritability, restlessness, lethargy, disorientation, and inappropriate euphoria
Check the oral temperature.	Normal, subnormal, or elevated temperature
Cardiovascular System	
Check the pulse and blood pressure. Document the pulse pressure with each blood pressure reading.	Tachycardia: normal mean arterial blood pressure; widening pulse pressure
Check peripheral pulses.	"Bounding" peripheral pulses
Auscultate heart sounds at four valvular sites, and record the onset of murmur or gallop.	No murmur or gallop
Respiratory System	
Observe the rate, rhythm, and effort of breathing. Observe the symmetry of chest expansion.	Tachypnea, hyperventilation
Percuss and auscultate the lungs. Note the onset of adventitious sounds.	Crackles and decreased breath sounds
Check blood gas levels.	Respiratory alkalosis
Integumentary System	
Inspect and palpate the skin. Note color, vascularity, moisture, temperature, texture, thickness, mobility, and turgor. Assess the oral mucosa.	Warm, flushed skin and peripheral edema Pink oral mucous membranes
Immune System	
Check complete white blood count with differential and IL-6 levels.	Abnormal total white blood cell count "Left shift" (decreasing segmented neutrophils; rising band neutrophils) Rising IL-6 levels
Hematologic System	
Check platelets and clotting factors.	Decreasing fibrinogen levels Decreasing platelet levels Decreasing activated protein C Rising plasma D-dimer levels

IL-6, Interleukin-6.

increasing the formation of oxygen free radicals, which damage the lung cells. Oxygen free radicals also can form as a result of oxygen therapy and in response to release of oxidizing enzymes from damaged cells. *The presence of ARDS in a client with septic shock has a high mortality rate.*

SKIN CHANGES. It may be difficult to recognize the hyperdynamic phase of septic shock, often because the skin is warm and no cyanosis is evident. The normal appearance of the skin and mucous membranes leads health care professionals to believe circulation is unimpaired. When septic shock progresses so that circulation is compromised in the hypodynamic phase, the skin is cool and clammy, and pallor or cyanosis is present. In clients with DIC, petechiae and ecchymoses can occur anywhere. Blood may ooze from the gums, other mucous membranes, and venipuncture sites as well as around IV catheters.

PSYCHOSOCIAL ASSESSMENT

The indicator that clients may be in the beginning of septic shock is often a change in affect or behavior. Compare the client's current behavior, verbal responses, and general affect with those assessed earlier in the day or the day before. Clients may seem just slightly different in their reactions to greetings, comments, or jokes. They may be less patient than usual or act restless or fidgety. They may make statements such as, "I feel as if something is wrong, but I don't know what." If this behavior is a change from prior assessments, consider the possibility of sepsis and shock.

LABORATORY ASSESSMENT

The presence of bacteria in the blood supports the diagnosis of sepsis. Obtain specimens of urine, blood, sputum, and any drainage for culture to identify the causative organisms. Other abnormal laboratory findings that occur with septic shock include changes in the white blood cell count; the differential leukocyte count may show a left shift (see Chapter 23). Changes in hematocrit and hemoglobin levels usually are not present until late in septic shock. At that point, the hematocrit and hemoglobin levels, fibrinogen levels, and platelet count are low.

Another indicator of sepsis and septic shock is a reduction in the blood levels of **activated protein C.** This protein is an enzyme that helps prevent inappropriate clot formation. It is activated when it binds to healthy endothelial cells of blood vessels. In septic shock, the endothelial cells injured by endotoxins cannot activate protein C and thousands of small clots form in the capillaries of vascular organs. Decreasing levels of activated protein C indicate the beginning of septic shock even before other manifestations are evident (Kleinpell, 2003a).

Other biologic indicators of sepsis and septic shock are changes in plasma D-dimer levels and specific cytokine (interleukin-6 [IL-6] and interleukin-10 [IL-10]) levels. Plasma D-dimer levels rise during sepsis as the fibrin in clots is broken down. IL-6 is a proinflammatory cytokine and IL-10 is an anti-inflammatory cytokine. In sepsis, IL-6 levels rise and IL-10 levels either remain normal or decrease.

Analysis

A common collaborative problem for clients with septic shock is Potential for Multiple Organ Dysfunction Syndrome (MODS).

Planning and Implementation

POTENTIAL FOR MULTIPLE ORGAN DYSFUNCTION SYNDROME

NOC **PLANNING: EXPECTED OUTCOMES.** The client in septic shock is expected to have normal aerobic cellular metabolism. Indicators include the following:

- Arterial blood gases (pH, PaO_2, and $PaCO_2$) within the normal range
- Maintenance of a urine output of at least 20 mL/hr
- Maintenance of mean arterial blood pressure within 10 mm Hg of baseline
- Absence of multiple organ dysfunction syndrome (MODS)
- States measures to reduce the risk for sepsis

INTERVENTIONS. Interventions for septic shock focus on correcting the conditions causing shock and on preventing complications. Chart 40-9 lists the best practices for clients with septic shock.

Interventions for fluid volume deficit are the same as for hypovolemic shock.

Oxygen Therapy. Oxygen therapy is useful whenever poor tissue perfusion and poor oxygenation are present. Oxygen is delivered in the same ways as for hypovolemic shock.

Drug Therapy. The same drugs used to enhance cardiac output and restore vascular volume in hypovolemic shock are used for septic shock. A major focus of drug therapy is antibiotics to combat sepsis. In addition, drugs to counteract disseminated intravascular coagulation (DIC) may be needed. Septic shock and DIC have two distinctly different phases, and the drugs for each phase of septic shock are different. Drug therapy in the first phase is aimed at preventing coagulation by administering heparin. Drug therapy in the second, late phase of septic shock is aimed at increasing the blood's ability to clot. This therapy consists of clotting factors, plasma, platelets, or other blood products.

Antibiotics. Although septic shock can be caused by any organism, the most common agents are gram-negative

CHART 40-9

BEST PRACTICE for
The Client in Sepsis-Induced Distributive Shock (Septic Shock)

- Ensure a patent airway.
- Start or maintain an established IV catheter.
- Administer oxygen.
- Administer antibiotics.
- Obtain specimens of blood, urine, wound drainage, and sputum for culture.
- Increase the rate of IV fluid delivery.
- Use aseptic technique for any invasive procedure.
- Handle the client gently.
- Examine the client for overt bleeding, especially of gums, injection sites, and IV sites.
- Elevate the client's feet, keeping his or her head flat or elevated to a 30-degree angle.
- Take the client's vital signs every 5 minutes until they are stable.
- Administer medications as prescribed:
  Heparin during phase 1
  Clotting factors, platelets, and plasma during phase 2
- Do not leave the client.

bacteria. When blood cultures have identified specific bacteria, IV antibiotics with known activity against the bacteria are given. Multiple drugs with wide activity are prescribed when the causative organism is not known. Drugs and drug categories commonly used for septic shock include vancomycin, aminoglycosides, systemic penicillin or cephalosporins, macrolides, and quinolones.

Anticoagulants. When clients are in the early phase of septic shock and are beginning to form many small clots, heparin may be given to limit unneeded clotting and to prevent the consumption of clotting factors.

Clotting Factors and Blood Products. When septic shock progresses to the late phase and small clots have formed to such an extent that the client no longer has enough clotting factors to prevent hemorrhage, clotting factors are infused. These factors (cryoprecipitate) are obtained from pooled human serum. Infusing fresh frozen plasma (FFP) also helps to replace clotting factors. Platelets or other blood products also may be needed.

Activated Protein C. Synthetic activated protein C has been shown to stop the inflammatory responses and small clot formation of septic shock (Kleinpell, 2003a). This drug, drotrecogin alpha (Xigris), is given as a continuous infusion over 4 days.

Antibodies. Antibodies against the body's mediators for inflammation are being tested for their effectiveness in septic shock. Antibodies have been developed against the some proinflammatory cytokines, particularly interleukin-1 (IL-1), interleukin-6 (IL-6), and tumor necrosis factor (TNF). This experimental therapy shows promise in reducing the extensive mortality associated with septic shock.

CHART 40-10

HOME CARE ASSESSMENT of
Clients at Risk for Sepsis

Assess the client for any clinical manifestations of infection, including the following:
- Temperature, pulse, respiration, and blood pressure
- Color of skin and mucous membranes
- The mouth and perianal area for fissures or lesions
- Any nonintact skin area for the presence of exudates, redness, increased warmth, swelling
- Any pain, tenderness, or other discomfort anywhere
- Cough or any other symptoms of a cold or the flu
- Urine; or ask client whether urine is dark or cloudy, has an odor, or causes pain or burning during urination

Assess client's and caregiver's adherence to and understanding of infection prevention techniques.

Assess home environment, including the following:
- General cleanliness
- Kitchen and bathroom facilities, including refrigeration
- Availability and type of soap for handwashing
- Presence of pets, especially cats, rodents, or reptiles

CHART 40-11

CLIENT EDUCATION GUIDE
Infection Precautions

- Avoid crowds and other large gatherings of people, who might be ill.
- Do not share eating utensils or personal toilet articles (e.g., toothbrushes, toothpaste, washcloths, or deodorant sticks) with others.
- If possible, bathe daily.
- Wash the armpits, groin, genitals, and rectal area at least twice a day with an antimicrobial soap.
- Clean your toothbrush daily by either running it through the dishwasher or rinsing it in liquid laundry bleach.
- Wash your hands thoroughly with an antimicrobial soap before you eat or drink, after touching a pet, after shaking hands with anyone, as soon as you come home from any outing, and after using the toilet.
- Wash dishes between use with hot, sudsy water, or use a dishwasher.
- Do not drink water that has been standing for longer than 15 minutes.
- Do not reuse cups and glasses without washing them.
- Do not change pet litter boxes.
- Take your temperature at least once a day.
- Refrigerate and prepare food appropriately. Do not eat raw or undercooked meat, fish, poultry, or eggs.
- Report any of the following signs or symptoms of infection to your physician immediately:
  - Temperature greater than 100° F (38° C)
  - Persistent cough (with or without sputum)
  - Pus or foul-smelling drainage from any open skin area or normal body opening
  - Presence of a boil or abscess
  - Urine that is cloudy or foul-smelling or causes burning on urination
- Do not dig in the garden or work with houseplants.
- Use antibacterial cleansers to clean kitchen and bathroom surfaces at least twice each week. If you clean these areas yourself, wear rubber or vinyl work gloves while cleaning.
- Use a condom when having sex.
- Take all medications as prescribed.

Community-Based Care

Shock is a complication of another condition and is resolved before clients are discharged from the acute care setting. Because more clients are receiving treatment on an outpatient basis and are being discharged earlier from acute care settings, more clients at home are at increased risk for infection and septic shock.

HOME CARE MANAGEMENT

Evaluate the home environment for safety regarding infection hazards. Note the general cleanliness, especially in the kitchen and bathrooms. Chart 40-10 lists focused client and environmental assessment data to obtain during a home visit.

HEALTH TEACHING

Protecting vulnerable clients from infection and sepsis at home is an important nursing function. Instruct about the importance of self-care strategies, such as good hygiene, handwashing, balanced diet, rest, and exercise, skin care, and mouth care. If clients or family members do not know how to take a temperature or read a thermometer, teach them and obtain a return demonstration. Instruct clients to notify the health care provider immediately if fever or other signs of infection appear. Specific recommendations for infection precautions for clients at risk for sepsis are listed in Chart 40-11.

◆Evaluation: Outcomes

Evaluate the care of the client with sepsis-induced distributive shock. The expected outcome is that the client will maintain normal aerobic cellular metabolism.

Specific indicators for these outcomes are listed for the collaborative problem under the Planning and Implementation section (see earlier).

GET READY for the NCLEX Examination!

KEY POINTS

Safe Effective Care Environment

- Use strict aseptic techniques when performing invasive procedures, dressing changes, or handling nonintact skin.
- Use good handwashing techniques before providing any care to a client who is either immunocompromised or immunodeficient.

Health Promotion and Maintenance

- Encourage all adult clients to know their immunization history for tetanus.
- Identify clients at high risk for infection as a result of age, disease, work environment, or leisure activities.
- Teach the client and family about the clinical manifestations of infection and when to seek medical advice.
- Teach clients at risk for bleeding the precautions to take to avoid injury (see Chart 28-10).

Psychosocial Integrity

- Assess all clients at risk for shock for a change in affect, reduced cognition, altered level of consciousness, and increased anxiety.
- Stay with the client in shock.
- Explain all diagnostic procedures, restrictions, and follow-up care to the client scheduled for tests.
- Reassure clients who are in shock that the appropriate interventions are being instituted.

Physiological Integrity

- Assess the immunocompromised client every shift for infection.
- Assess the skin integrity of the client with reduced immune function at least every shift.
- Immediately assess vital signs of clients who have a change in level of consciousness, increased thirst, or anxiety.
- Assess for changes in pulse rate and quality rather than blood pressure as an indicator of shock.
- Give oxygen to any client in shock.
- Assess hourly urine output for adequacy of treatment for hypovolemic shock.

ADDITIONAL STUDY RESOURCES

Go to your Student CD-ROM for Review Questions for the NCLEX Examination.

evolve Go to http://evolve.elsevier.com/Iggy/ for Integrated Management of Care Questions for the NCLEX Examination.

SELECTED BIBLIOGRAPHY

Asterisk indicates a classic or definitive work on this subject.

Abbas, A., & Lichtman, A. (2003). *Cellular and molecular immunology* (5th ed.). Philadelphia: W.B. Saunders.

Ackley, B., & Ladwig, G. (2002). *Nursing diagnosis handbook: A guide to planning care* (5th ed.). St. Louis: Mosby.

Ahrens, T., & Vollman, K. (2003). Severe sepsis management: Are we doing enough? *Critical Care Nurse (Supplement October), 23*(5), 2-15.

Atassi, K., & Harris, M. (2001). Action stat: Disseminated intravascular coagulation. *Nursing 2001, 31*(3), 64.

Beery, T. (2003). Sex differences in infection and sepsis. *Critical Care Nursing Clinics of North America, 15*(1), 55-62.

Berne, R., et al. (2004). *Physiology* (5th ed.). St. Louis: Mosby.

Berry, B., & Pinard, A. (2002). Assessing tissue oxygenation. *Critical Care Nurse, 22*(3), 22-39.

Chavez, J., & Brewer, C. (2002). Stopping the shock slide. *RN, 65*(9), 30-35.

Cheek, D. et al. (2005). Sepsis: Taking a deeper look. *Nursing 2005, 35*(1), 38-42.

Dettenmeier, P., et al. (2003). Role of activated protein C in the pathophysiology of severe sepsis. *American Journal of Critical Care, 12*(6), 518-524.

Diehl-Oplinger, L. (2004). Choosing the right fluid to counter hypovolemic shock. *Nursing 2004, 34*(3), 52-54.

Dochterman, J., & Bulechek, G. (Eds.). (2004). *Nursing interventions classification (NIC)* (4th ed.). St. Louis: Mosby.

Dressler, D. (2004). DIC: Coping with a coagulation crisis. *Nursing 2004, 34*(5), 58-62.

Ebersole, P., Hess, P., & Luggen, A. (2004). *Toward healthy aging: Human needs and nursing response* (6th ed.). St. Louis: Mosby.

*Effron, M., & Chernow, B. (1992). Shock. In E. Rubenstein & D. Federman (Eds.), *Scientific American: Medicine* (pp. I card III Shock 1-12). New York: Scientific American.

Facts and Comparisons. (2004). *Drug facts and comparisons* (58th ed.). St. Louis: Author.

Felblinger, D. (2003). Malnutrition, infection, and sepsis in acute and chronic illness. *Critical Care Nursing Clinics of North America, 15*(1), 71-78.

Hadaway, L. (2003). Infusing without infecting. *Nursing 2003, 33*(10), 58-63.

Holcomb, S. (2002). Helping your patient conquer cardiogenic shock. *Nursing 2002, 32*(9), 32cc1-32cc6.

Kleinpell, R. (2003a). Advances in treating patients with severe sepsis: Role of drotrecogin alfa (activated). *Critical Care Nurse, 23*(3), 16-29.

Kleinpell, R. (2003b). The role of the critical care nurse in the assessment and management of the patient with severe sepsis. *Critical Care Nursing Clinics of North America, 15*(1), 27-34.

LaCharity, L., & McClure, E. (2003). Are plants vectors for transmission of infection in acute care? *Critical Care Nursing Clinics of North America, 15*(1), 119-124.

McCance, K., & Huether, S. (2002). *Pathophysiology: The biologic basis for disease in adults and children* (4th ed.). St. Louis: Mosby.

Mehta, M. (2003). Assessing cardiovascular status. *Nursing 2003, 33*(1), 56-58.

Moorhead, S., Johnson, M., & Maas, M. (Eds.). (2004). *Nursing outcomes classification (NOC)* (3rd ed.). St. Louis: Mosby.

Mower-Wade, D., & Kang, T. (2004). Sepsis: When defense turns deadly. *Nursing 2004, 34*(7), 32cc1-32cc4.

Mower-Wade, D., Bartley, M., & Chiari-Allwein, J. (2001). How to respond to shock. *Dimensions in Critical Care Nursing, 20*(2), 22-27.

O'Neill, D. (2001). The right plasma volume expander. *Nursing Times, 97*(27), 38-39.

Pagana, K., & Pagana, T. (2002). *Mosby's manual of diagnostic and laboratory tests* (2nd ed.). St. Louis: Mosby.

Paminter, S. (2001). Hands on detection of systemic circulatory deterioration. *Nursing Times, 97*(27), 40-42.

Ross, V. (2003). Uncertainty about the clinical detection of sepsis. *Journal of Infusion Nursing, 26*(1), 23-28.

Rudnicke, C. (2003). Transfusion alternatives. *Journal of Infusion Nursing, 26*(1), 29-33.

Sarvis, C. (2004). The role of bacterial toxins in wounds. *Nursing 2004, 34*(7), 68.

Sommers, M. (2003). The cellular basis of septic shock. *Critical Care Nursing Clinics of North America, 15*(1), 13-25.

*Stengle, J., & Dries, D. (1994). Sepsis in the elderly. *Critical Care Nursing Clinics of North America, 6*(2), 421-427.

Workman, M.L. (2003). The cellular basis of bacterial infection. *Critical Care Nursing Clinics of North America, 15*(1), 1-11.

CHAPTER

41

Interventions for Critically Ill Clients with Acute Coronary Syndromes

WADE HAGAN • DONNA D. IGNATAVICIUS

LEARNING OUTCOMES

After studying this chapter, you should be able to:

1. Describe the relationship between coronary artery disease (CAD) and acute coronary syndromes (ACS).
2. Explain the pathophysiology of ACS.
3. Compare and contrast stable angina, unstable angina, and myocardial infarction (MI).
4. Identify modifiable and nonmodifiable risk factors for ACS.
5. Interpret physical and diagnostic assessment findings in clients who have ACS.
6. Describe the psychosocial aspects of ACS.
7. Prioritize nursing care for clients who have ACS.
8. Identify the life-threatening complications of ACS.
9. Explain the advantages of thrombolysis for a client experiencing an MI.
10. Compare and contrast the drug classifications used to treat ACS.
11. Describe the appropriate nursing interventions for monitoring clients receiving drug therapy for ACS.
12. Develop a plan of care for the client who has undergone a percutaneous transluminal coronary angioplasty.
13. Manage care for the client who has undergone coronary artery bypass graft (CABG) surgery.
14. Discuss the differences between CABG surgery, minimally invasive direct coronary artery bypass, off-pump CABG, and transmyocardial laser revascularization.
15. Develop a discharge plan for the client with ACS.

Go to your Student CD-ROM for Review Questions for the NCLEX Examination keyed to these Learning Outcomes.

CORONARY ARTERY DISEASE

Coronary artery disease (CAD), also called coronary heart disease (CHD), is the single largest killer of American men and women in all cultural groups (American Heart Association [AHA], 2003). According to the AHA, CHD caused more than 1 of every 5 deaths in the United States in 2000. From 1990 to 2000, the death rate from CAD declined 25%. Multiple factors can be identified as contributing to the decline in CAD. These factors include more effective medical treatment and an increased awareness and emphasis on reducing the major modifiable cardiovascular risk factors (e.g., high blood pressure [BP], smoking, high cholesterol, obesity, diabetes).

PATHOPHYSIOLOGY

Coronary artery disease (CAD) is a broad term that includes stable angina pectoris and acute coronary syndromes. CAD affects the arteries that provide blood, oxygen, and nutrients to the myocardium. When blood flow through the coronary arteries is partially or completely blocked, ischemia and infarction of the myocardium may result. **Ischemia** occurs when insufficient oxygen is supplied to meet the requirements of the myocardium. **Infarction** (necrosis, or cell death) occurs when severe ischemia is prolonged and irreversible damage to tissue results.

CULTURAL CONSIDERATIONS

Several groups have a higher genetic risk for CAD than others. Black and Hispanic women have higher CAD risk factors than white women of comparable socioeconomic status. Of Native Americans/American Indians/Alaskan Natives 18 years of age and older, 63.7% of men and 81.4% of women have one or more CAD risk factors (hypertension [HTN], smoking, high cholesterol, excess weight, or diabetes mellitus). The leading cause of death for both men and women in the most prevalent ethnic groups is cardiac disease even though there are genetic predispositions to develop risk factors (AHA, 2003).

Stable Angina Pectoris

Angina pectoris means "strangling of the chest." Angina is a temporary imbalance between the coronary arteries' ability to supply oxygen and the cardiac muscle's demand for oxygen. Ischemia that occurs with angina is limited in duration, and it does not cause permanent damage of myocardial tissue.

Angina may be of two predominant types: stable angina and unstable angina. **Stable angina** is chest discomfort that occurs with moderate to prolonged exertion in a pattern that is familiar to the client. The frequency, duration, and intensity of symptoms remain stable over the preceding several months. Stable angina results in only slight limitation of activity and is usually associated with a stable atherosclerotic plaque. It is usually relieved by nitroglycerin or rest and often is managed medically with agents such as calcium channel blockers and beta-blocking medications. Rarely does stable angina require aggressive treatment. **Unstable angina** is discussed below under Acute Coronary Syndromes.

WOMEN'S HEALTH CONSIDERATIONS

More women than men have angina; many women experience **atypical angina.** Atypical angina can manifest itself as indigestion, pain between the shoulders, an aching jaw, or a choking sensation that occurs with exertion. Angina in women has often been diagnosed as panic disorder, stress, menopause-related problems, gastrointestinal disease, or hypochondriasis (*Harvard Heart Letter,* 2003).

Acute Coronary Syndromes

In **acute coronary syndromes,** it is believed that the atherosclerotic plaque in the coronary artery ruptures, resulting in platelet aggregation ("clumping"), thrombus (clot) formation, and vasoconstriction (Figure 41-1). The amount of disruption of the atherosclerotic plaque determines the degree of obstruction of the coronary artery and the specific disease process (unstable angina or myocardial infarction [MI]). Between 10% and 30% of clients with unstable angina progress to having an MI in 1 year, and 29% die of MI in 5 years (AHA, 2003).

UNSTABLE ANGINA PECTORIS

Unstable angina (as it is usually called), or USA, is chest pain or discomfort that occurs at rest or with exertion and causes marked limitation of activity. An increase in the

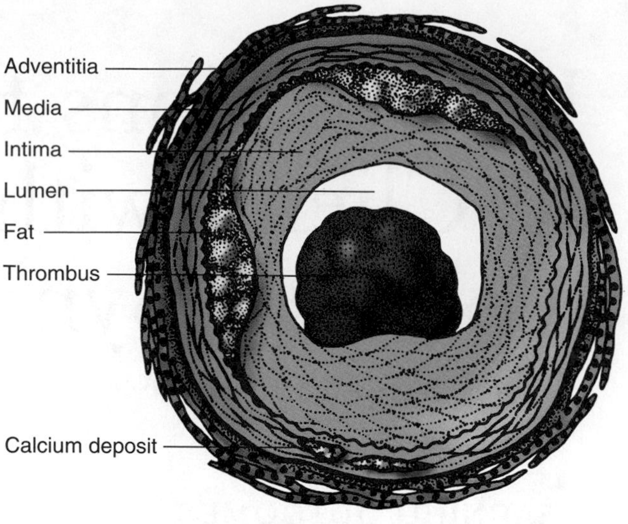

Figure 41-1 ■ A cross section of an atherosclerotic coronary artery.

number of attacks and an increase in the intensity of the pain characterize USA. The pain may last longer than 15 minutes, or it may be poorly relieved by rest or nitroglycerin. USA describes a broad spectrum of disorders, including *new-onset angina, variant (Prinzmetal's) angina, preinfarction angina,* and *crescendo angina.* The term used to describe the disorders that include unstable angina, subendocardial MI, and MI is **acute coronary syndromes.**

MYOCARDIAL INFARCTION

The most serious acute coronary syndrome is MI, often referred to as a "heart attack." Undiagnosed or untreated angina can lead to this very serious health problem.

Myocardial infarction (MI) occurs when myocardial tissue is abruptly and severely deprived of oxygen. When blood flow is acutely reduced by 80% to 90%, ischemia develops. Ischemia can lead to injury and necrosis **(infarction)** of myocardial tissue if blood flow is not restored. Most MIs are the result of atherosclerosis of a coronary artery, rupture of the plaque, subsequent thrombosis, and occlusion of blood flow. Other factors may be implicated, however, such as coronary artery spasm, platelet aggregation, and emboli from mural thrombi (thrombi lining the walls of the cardiac chambers).

Often MIs begin with infarction **(necrosis)** of the subendocardial layer of cardiac muscle. This layer has the longest myofibrils in the heart, the greatest oxygen demand, and the poorest oxygen supply. Around the initial area of infarction (zone of necrosis) in the subendocardium are two other zones: (1) the zone of injury, tissue that is injured but not necrotic, and (2) the zone of ischemia, tissue that is oxygen deprived. This pattern is illustrated in Figure 41-2.

PROCESS OF INFARCTION. Infarction is a dynamic process that does not occur instantly; rather, it evolves over a period of several hours. **Hypoxia** (decreased oxygen) from ischemia may lead to local vasodilation of blood vessels and acidosis. Potassium, calcium, and magnesium imbalances, as well as acidosis at the cellular level, may lead to suppression of normal conduction and contractile functions. Automaticity and ectopy are enhanced. Catecholamines (epinephrine and norepinephrine) released in

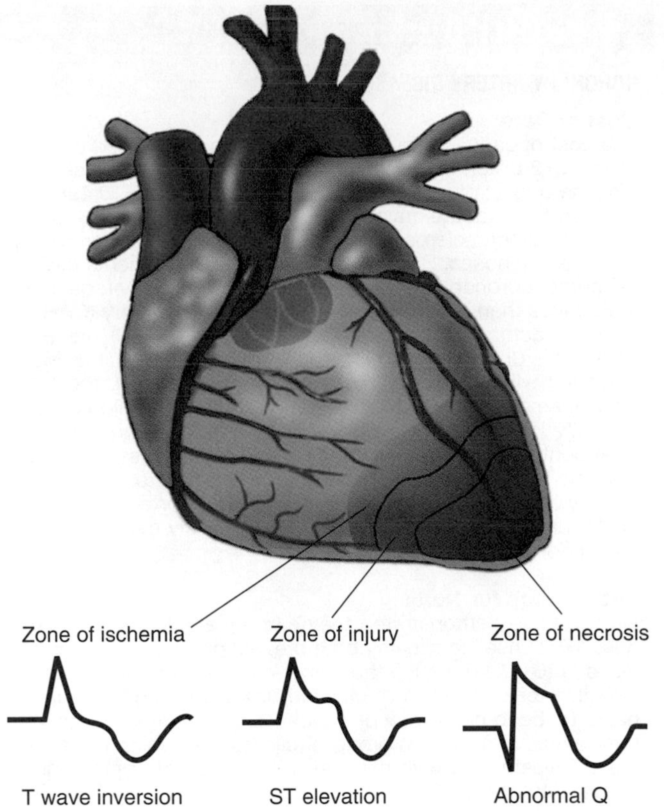

Figure 41-2 ■ Electrocardiographic changes and patterns associated with myocardial infarction.

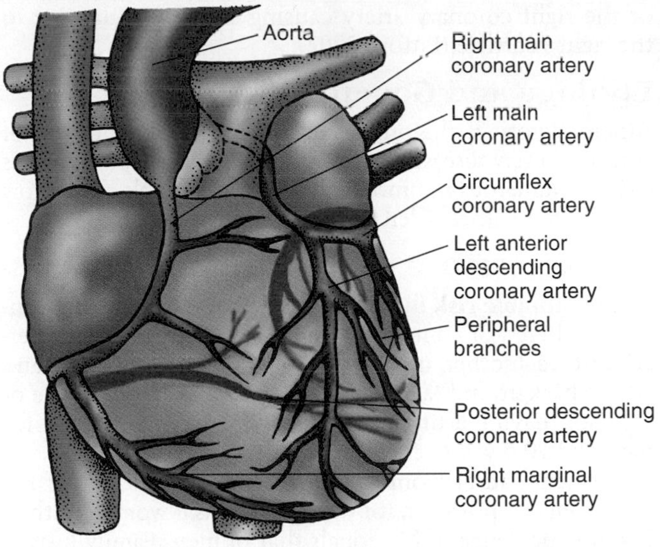

Figure 41-3 ■ Coronary arterial system.

TABLE 41-1 Major Coronary Vessels and the Structures They Perfuse

Left Anterior Descending Coronary Artery
- Most of the left ventricular muscle mass and septum

Left Circumflex Coronary Artery
- Posterior wall of the left ventricle
- SA node in 39% of clients
- AV node in 12% of clients
- Left ventricular muscle in 10% of clients

Right Coronary Artery
- Right ventricle
- Inferior portion of the left ventricle
- SA node in 59% of clients
- AV node in 88% of clients

SA, Sinoatrial; *AV*, atrioventricular.

response to hypoxia and pain may increase the heart's rate and contractility and afterload. These factors increase oxygen requirements in tissue that is already oxygen deprived. The area of infarction may extend into the zones of injury and ischemia. The actual extent of the zone of infarction depends on three factors: collateral circulation, anaerobic metabolism, and workload demands on the myocardium.

The infarction may involve only the subendocardium (called a **subendocardial MI**), or it may spread to the epicardium or to all three layers of cardiac muscle. When all three layers are involved, the MI is termed **transmural.** Subendocardial MIs have less effect on wall motion and cardiac output than do transmural infarctions.

PHYSIOLOGIC RESPONSE TO INFARCTION. Obvious physical changes do not occur in the heart until 6 hours after the infarction, when the infarcted region appears blue and swollen. After 48 hours, the infarct turns gray with yellow streaks as neutrophils invade the tissue and begin to remove the necrotic cells. By 8 to 10 days after infarction, granulation tissue forms at the edges of the necrotic tissue. Over a 2- to 3-month period, the necrotic area eventually develops into a shrunken, thin, firm scar. Scar tissue permanently changes the size and shape of the entire left ventricle **(ventricular remodeling).** Remodeling may decrease left ventricular function, cause heart failure, and increase morbidity and mortality.

CLASSIFICATION OF MYOCARDIAL INFARCTION BY LOCATION. The client's response to an MI also depends on which coronary artery or arteries were obstructed and which part of the left ventricle wall was damaged: anterior, lateral, septal, inferior, or posterior. Figure 41-3 details the major coronary arteries, and Table 41-1 describes the structures they perfuse.

Obstruction of the left anterior descending (LAD) artery causes anterior or septal MIs because the LAD artery perfuses the anterior wall and most of the septum of the left ventricle. Anterior wall MIs (AWMIs) account for 25% of all MIs and have the highest mortality rate. Clients with anterior MIs are most likely to experience left ventricular heart failure and ventricular dysrhythmias because a large segment of the left ventricle wall may have been damaged.

The circumflex artery supplies the lateral wall of the left ventricle and possibly portions of the posterior wall or the sinoatrial (SA) and atrioventricular (AV) nodes. Clients with obstruction of the circumflex artery may experience a posterior wall MI (PWMIs) or a lateral wall MI (LWMIs) and sinus dysrhythmias.

In most people, the right coronary artery perfuses the SA and AV nodes as well as the right ventricle and inferior or diaphragmatic portion of the left ventricle. Clients with obstruction of the right coronary artery often have **inferior wall MIs.** Inferior wall MIs (IWMIs) account for about 17% of all MIs and have a mortality rate of about 10%. Up to 50% of all inferior wall MIs are associated with an occlusion of the right coronary artery causing significant damage to the right ventricle (Litton, 2002).

Etiology and Genetic Risk

Atherosclerosis is the primary factor in the development of coronary artery disease (CAD) and acute coronary syndromes (ACS). Numerous nonmodifiable and modifiable risk factors contribute to atherosclerosis (also see Chapter 39).

NONMODIFIABLE RISK FACTORS

Nonmodifiable risk factors are personal elements that cannot be altered or controlled. These risk factors, which interact with each other, include age, gender, family history, and ethnic background (as discussed earlier). The average age of a person having a first heart attack is 65.8 years of age for men and 70.4 years of age for women (AHA, 2003).

Premenopausal women have a lower incidence of MI than men do; however, for postmenopausal women in their 70s, the incidence of MI equals that of men. Family history is also a risk factor; people whose parents had CAD are more susceptible.

Incidence/Prevalence

In 2000, the total mortality of those experiencing MI in the United States was 239,000. About every 29 seconds, an American suffers a coronary event, and about every minute someone will die of one. About half of the people who experience an MI in a given year will die of it.

Many people die from coronary heart disease without being hospitalized. Most of these are sudden deaths caused by cardiac arrest, usually resulting from ventricular fibrillation.

Ninety-five percent of sudden cardiac arrest victims die before reaching the hospital. To help combat this problem, automatic external defibrillators (AEDs) are found in many public places, such as in shopping centers and on airplanes. Employees are taught how to use these devices if a sudden cardiac arrest occurs.

> **WOMEN'S HEALTH CONSIDERATIONS**
>
> Twenty-five percent of men and 40% of women die within 1 year after having an initial recognized MI. Because women have heart attacks at older ages than men do, they are more likely to die from them within a few weeks.
>
> Studies have shown that women do not realize that heart disease is the number one killer among women (AHA, 2003). More disturbing are the recent findings that combined hormone replacement therapy (HRT) does not protect cardiac health in postmenopausal women; however, HRT has other protective effects, such as osteoporosis prevention. HRT is discussed in detail in Chapter 78.
>
> Causes of MI may be different in women, perhaps explaining the atypical presentations. Bursting plaques may not be as important for women as men because women distribute atherosclerosis more evenly through the arteries. Some women have narrow arteries that indicate, in general, a lower dose of blood thinning medications and the use of smaller catheters and stents. Women also tend to develop less collateral circulation than men. For more information, contact www.womenheart.org (Gorman et al., 2003).

Many clients who survive MIs are not able to return to work. CAD is the leading cause of premature, permanent disability in the United States Labor Force, accounting for 19% of disability allowances by the Social Security. The direct cost of cardiovascular disease and stroke in the United States in 2003 was estimated at $371.8 billion dollars (AHA, 2003) (see the Resource Management box above).

> **RESOURCE MANAGEMENT**
>
> **CORONARY ARTERY DISEASE**
>
> **Cost of Care**
>
> The cost of cancer care was $202.2 billion, compared with almost $372 billion spent to care for clients with cardiovascular disease and stroke (AHA, 2003). Medicare paid $10,428 per discharge for acute myocardial infarction (MI), $11,399 for coronary atherosclerosis, and $3617 for other coronary heart disease diagnoses. Becker (2003) reported that clients having off-pump coronary artery procedures had an average cost $1839 less than coronary artery bypass graft surgery (CABG).
>
> Risk factors for coronary artery disease (CAD) are also costly. It is unclear whether the AHA included these individual statistics with the $371.8 billion estimate. In 2000, the total cost of smoking cost Americans more than 157 billion dollars annually in medical care. In 1996, 31 billion dollars was the treatment cost of CAD for those who have excess weight or obesity. The annual cost for disease connected to physical inactivity is 76 billion dollars. Gentz (2000) reported that direct costs for testing clients with CAD are currently more than 150 billion dollars each year.
>
> **Implications for Nursing**
>
> Nurses have demonstrated they can save lives at a minimal cost by counseling clients about prevention of coronary artery disease (CAD). Because the same intervention may be cost-effective for one group of clients but not for another, nurses need to become aware of which cardiac interventions are cost-effective for which group of clients and which represent major investments with minimal expectation of improvement in client outcomes.

HEALTH PROMOTION/ILLNESS PREVENTION

MODIFIABLE RISK FACTORS

Modifiable risk factors include elevated serum cholesterol levels, cigarette smoking, hypertension, impaired glucose tolerance, obesity, physical inactivity, and stress. Individuals who have one or more of these risk factors should modify or eliminate them to decrease their chances of myocardial infarction (MI). For clients at risk for coronary artery disease (CAD), especially MI, assess which factors they have and teach ways that the factor(s) can be modified. A complete discussion of health teaching for decreasing risk factors may be found in Chapter 39 under the discussion of Arteriosclerosis/Atherosclerosis.

> **CULTURAL CONSIDERATIONS**
>
> Modifiable risk factors vary for people of different racial and ethnic backgrounds. A comparison of risk factors by racial/ethnic group is found in Table 41-2. Some of the differences may be explained by lack of access to health care for some groups or genetic factors. Native Americans/American Indians, for example, have the highest percentage of smokers among women and men; however, many of these individuals have poor access to care or language barriers in a predominantly English-speaking, white health care system. Dietary

preferences may also explain some of the differences. For instance, according to the AHA (2003), high cholesterol is more common in black and Hispanic populations. Diets higher in fat and cholesterol are often less expensive and may be a factor in explaining differences. Genetics may also contribute to the differences among ethnic groups. Obesity is also greater in these groups.

ELEVATED SERUM CHOLESTEROL LEVELS. The risk of CAD rises as serum cholesterol levels increase. It is estimated that around 97 million people have total cholesterol levels of greater than 200 mg/dL (Allen, 2000). In addition to measuring the total serum cholesterol, low-density lipoprotein (LDL) and high-density lipoprotein (HDL) levels are just as important in assessing risk for CAD and potential MI. LDL cholesterol has been termed "bad" and HDL cholesterol has been termed "good." Elevated levels of LDL combined with low levels of HDL increase the risk of MI. Total serum cholesterol levels put the individual at a higher risk of developing an MI. According to the AHA (2003), a 10% reduction in serum cholesterol may result in an estimated 30% reduction in the incidence of CAD and MI. The goal for LDL levels in clients who have existing CAD or diabetes mellitus is less than 100 mg/dL. HDL cholesterol levels should be above 40 mg/dL. Approaches to decrease cholesterol are focused on diet and medications that lower cholesterol levels.

CIGARETTE SMOKING. An estimated 25.7% of men and 21% of women smoke putting them at increased risk of MI (AHA, 2003). About five million American men and women are chewing tobacco, with the highest rates in the South and rural areas. **Passive smoking** from "second-hand smoke" substantially reduces blood flow velocity in the coronary arteries of healthy young adults, causing about 37,000 deaths annually (AHA, 2003).

Cigarette smoking accounts for 30% of the mortality rate from CAD. Smoking enhances the process of atherosclerosis through mechanisms that are still poorly understood. Nicotine initiates the release of catecholamines, resulting in an increased heart rate and peripheral vasoconstriction. This action causes increases in BP, cardiac afterload, and oxygen consumption. Cigarette smoking has also been found to cause endothelial dysfunction and increased vessel wall thickness. This process increases the risk for clot formation and vessel occlusion. Another factor of cigarette smoking is carbon monoxide, which has been found to decrease the oxygen content in arterial blood. The resulting hypertension may exacerbate the atherosclerotic process by increasing vessel wall permeability. The good news is that when cigarette smoking is stopped, the risk for CAD decreases. A person who stops smoking may decrease the risk of CAD by as much as 80% in 1 year. Reducing the tar and nicotine content of the cigarettes smoked does not reduce the risk of CAD (AHA, 2003).

PHYSICAL INACTIVITY. Physical inactivity may be the most important risk factor for the general population. Less active, less-fit persons have a 30% to 50% greater risk of developing high BP, which predisposes to CAD. Physical inactivity is more prevalent among women than men, among blacks and Hispanics than whites, among older than younger adults, and among the less affluent than the more affluent (AHA, 2003). Regular physical activity helps maintain body weight and muscle mass while optimizing BP and lipid values.

TABLE 41-2 Comparison of the Incidence of Smoking, Leisure Activity, Cholesterol Level, and Body Mass Index (BMI) Among Selected Racial/Ethnic Groups

	Men (%)	Women (%)
Smoking		
Hispanics	24.1	12.3
Asian/Pacific Islanders	24.3	7.1
Native Americans/American Indians	40.9	40.8
Blacks	26.1	20.8
Whites	25.8	21.6
No Leisure Activity		
Hispanics	48.9	57.4
Blacks	55.2	44.1
Asian/Pacific Islanders	30.9	45.5
Native Americans/American Indians	16.8	19.6
Whites	32.5	36.2
Cholesterol >200 mg/dL or higher*		
Hispanics	53	48
Blacks	45	45
Asian/Pacific Islanders	not reported	not reported
Native Americans/American Indians	35.7	35.6
Whites	52	49
BMI >30		
Hispanics	28.9	39.7
Blacks	28.1	49.7
Native Americans/American Indians	35.5	41.2
Asian/Pacific Islanders	36.7	27.1
Whites	27.3	30.1

Modified from the American Heart Association (2003).

*NOTE: A 10% decrease in total cholesterol levels may result in a 30% reduction in the incidence of coronary heart disease.

For women, studies have shown that moderate-intensity physical activity, such as walking, is associated with a substantial reduction in risk. Another study of men suggested, however, that intense exercising may contribute to plaque rupture and increase the number of cardiac episodes (Cadroy et al., 2003). Participating in physical exercise can reduce hypertension and increase secretions of endorphins, leading to less smoking and eating, improved metabolism, and a stronger feeling of well-being. Other benefits include decreased blood clotting and higher plasma HDL levels. Physical activity does not increase collateral circulation or reduce the size of existing plaques. Benefits include increased heart volume, increased cardiac capillary vascularity, and decreased heart rate.

The individual's response to stress may be associated with heart disease. Some evidence indicates that job stress may be associated with left ventricular hypertrophy.

OTHER FACTORS

One in five Americans has hypertension (HTN). *Hypertension* increases the workload of the heart, which increases the risk of myocardial infarction (MI). The cause of 90% to 95% of HTN is not known; however, it is easily detected and usually controllable. About 50% of clients having a first MI have a BP greater than 160/95 mm Hg.

CULTURAL CONSIDERATIONS

The prevalence of hypertension (HTN) among blacks and whites in the Southeastern United States is greater than among those in other regions of the country. Blacks have the highest prevalence in the United States and are among the highest in the world. They develop HTN earlier in life, and the average blood pressures (BP) are much higher than other groups (AHA, 2003). The causes for differences are not known but may be related to genetics or diet.

WOMEN'S HEALTH CONSIDERATIONS

For women, *impaired glucose tolerance* (e.g., diabetes) seriously increases the risk of CAD. *Obesity* is associated with increased serum cholesterol, elevated BP, and abnormal glucose tolerance. It may also have an independent effect on the risk of CAD. The distribution of adipose tissue seems to be important; women with fat deposited around the waist rather than the hips often have unfavorable lipid profiles and higher rates of CAD.

Elevated levels of serum *homocysteine,* an amino acid, are believed by some researchers to be associated with an increased risk of CAD. Clients with multiple risk factors have several times the risk of CAD as those without these characteristics. Although many factors place a person at risk for heart disease, there are well-documented, effective ways of promoting cardiovascular health. Some of these interventions, including health teaching, are described in Chart 41-1. Additional information is found in Chapter 39 under Arteriosclerosis/Atherosclerosis.

COLLABORATIVE MANAGEMENT

Assessment

HISTORY

If chest discomfort or other symptom is present at the time of the interview, collection of historical data is delayed until interventions for pain, vital sign instability, and dysrhythmias are initiated and the discomfort resolves. If possible, ask about how clients have managed the current episode of chest discomfort and which medications they are taking. When the client is *pain free,* information about family history and modifiable risk factors, including eating habits, lifestyle, and physical activity levels, is obtained.

PHYSICAL ASSESSMENT/CLINICAL MANIFESTATIONS

PAIN ASSESSMENT. Ask the client to describe his or her immediate concerns. The presence of chest, epigastric, jaw, back, or arm discomfort is noted. The client is asked to rate the discomfort on a scale of 0 to 10, with 10 being the highest level of discomfort. Clients often describe the discomfort as tightness, a burning sensation, pressure, or indigestion. Clients are asked what they have already done to try to relieve the pain. Pain management is described in detail in Chapter 7.

Rapid assessment of client with chest pain is crucial. It is important to differentiate among the types of chest pain and to identify the source. Question the client to determine the characteristics of the discomfort. Appropriate questions to ask concerning the discomfort include onset, location, radiation, intensity, duration, precipitating, and relieving factors.

CHART 41-1

CLIENT EDUCATION GUIDE
Prevention of Coronary Artery Disease

Smoking
- If you smoke, quit.
- If you don't smoke, don't start.

Diet
- Consume sufficient calories for your body:
  - 50% to 55% from carbohydrates
  - 30% to 35% from complex carbohydrates
  - 10% from simple sugars
  - Less than 30% from fat
  - 15% from monounsaturated fat
  - 10% from polyunsaturated fat
  - The remainder (5% to 10%) from saturated fat
  - 12% to 20% from protein
- Limit your cholesterol intake to less than 300 mg/day.
- Limit your sodium intake as specified by your health care provider.

Cholesterol
- Have your cholesterol and low-density lipoprotein (LDL) levels checked regularly.
- If your cholesterol and LDL levels are elevated, follow your health care provider's advice.

Physical Activity
- If you are middle-aged or older or have a history of medical problems, check with your health care provider before starting an exercise program.
- Appropriate exercise should be enjoyable, burn 400 calories per session, and sustain a heart rate of 120 to 150 beats/min, depending on your age.
- Exercise moderately at least three times each week, preferably five.
- Exercise periods should be at least 20 to 30 minutes long with 10-minute warm-up and 5-minute cool-down periods.
- If you are unable to exercise moderately three to five times each week, walk daily for 30 minutes at a comfortable pace.
- If you are unable to walk 30 minutes daily, walk any distance you can (e.g., park farther away from a site than necessary; use the stairs, not the elevator, to go one floor up or two floors down).

Diabetes
- Manage your diabetes with your health care provider.

Blood Pressure
- Have your blood pressure checked regularly.
- If your blood pressure is elevated, follow your health care provider's advice.
- Continue to monitor your blood pressure at regular intervals.

Obesity
- Avoid severely restrictive or fad diets.
- Consider a restriction in intake of saturated fats, simple sugars, and cholesterol-rich foods.
- Increase your physical activity.

Chart 41-2 compares and contrasts anginal and infarction pain. Because anginal pain is ischemic pain, it usually improves when the imbalance between oxygen supply and demand is resolved. For example, rest reduces tissue demands, and nitroglycerin improves oxygen supply. Discomfort from an MI does not usually resolve with such simple measures. Also noted is the presence of any associated symptoms, including nausea, vomiting, diaphoresis, dizziness, weakness, palpitations, and shortness of breath.

CHART 41-2

KEY FEATURES of
Angina and Myocardial Infarction

Angina	Myocardial Infarction
Substernal chest discomfort: ▪ Radiating to the left arm ▪ Precipitated by exertion or stress ▪ Relieved by nitroglycerin or rest ▪ Lasting <15 min Few associated symptoms	Substernal chest pressure: ▪ Radiating to the left arm, back, or jaw ▪ Occurring without cause, usually in the morning ▪ Relieved only by opioids ▪ Lasting 30 min or more Frequent associated symptoms: ▪ Nausea ▪ Diaphoresis ▪ Dyspnea ▪ Feelings of fear and anxiety ▪ Dysrhythmias ▪ Fatigue ▪ Epigastric distress ▪ Feeling "short of breath"

CULTURAL CONSIDERATIONS

Black individuals experience longer delays in seeking treatment for MI and higher mortality rates than white individuals. One factor thought to contribute to this delay is a greater incidence of dyspnea as an acute symptom of MI among both black males and black females rather than the more classic chest discomfort.

CONSIDERATIONS FOR OLDER ADULTS

The presence of the associated symptoms without chest discomfort is also significant. In 15% to 25% of all clients with MI, primarily older adults and clients with diabetes, chest pain or discomfort may be mild or absent, and clients may complain primarily of the associated symptoms. Some older clients may think they are experiencing indigestion and therefore not recognize that they are having an MI. Twenty-five percent of older adults experiencing an MI complain only of shortness of breath. The major manifestation of MI in people older than 80 years of age may be disorientation or confusion due to poor cardiac output.

CARDIOVASCULAR ASSESSMENT. Immediate assessment of BP, determination of heart rate, interpretation of cardiac rhythm, and presence of dysrhythmias is crucial. Sinus tachycardia with premature ventricular contractions (PVCs) frequently occurs in the first few hours after an MI.

Next assess distal peripheral pulses and skin temperature. The skin should be warm, with all pulses palpable. In the client with unstable angina or MI, poor cardiac output may be manifested by cool, diaphoretic skin, and diminished or absent pulses.

Auscultate for an S_3 gallop, which often indicates heart failure, a serious and common complication of MI. Also assess the respiratory rate and breath sounds for signs of heart failure. An increased respiratory rate is common because of anxiety and pain, but crackles or wheezes may indicate heart failure. Auscultation of an S_4 heart sound is a common finding in the client who has had a previous MI or hypertension.

The client with MI may experience a temperature elevation for several days after infarction. Temperatures as high as 102° F (40.9° C) may occur in response to myocardial necrosis.

PSYCHOSOCIAL ASSESSMENT

Denial is a common early reaction to chest discomfort associated with angina or MI. On average, the client with an acute MI waits more than 2 hours before seeking medical attention. Often the client rationalizes that symptoms are due to indigestion or overexertion. In some situations, denial is a normal part of adapting to a stressful event; however, denial that interferes with identification of a symptom, such as chest discomfort, can be harmful. Explain the significance of reporting any discomfort, emphasizing that the health care provider will immediately attempt to relieve the discomfort.

Fear, anxiety, and anger are other common reactions of clients and families. Nursing assessment focuses on assisting the client and family members in identifying these feelings. Allow the client and family time to explain their understanding of the event and clarify any misconceptions.

Critical Thinking Challenge

A 55-year-old female client visits an urgent care center with a complaint of burning epigastric pain. She states that she believes it is a bad case of persistent heartburn. Assessment findings show slight shortness of breath, diaphoresis, and nausea and vomiting. Vital signs are BP 122/78, P 82, R 20, T 98.2. She is 5 feet 2 inches tall and weighs 168 pounds. Her tentative diagnosis is to "r/o MI."

1. What additional data and assessments should you collect at this time?
2. What risk factors may have contributed to this health problem?
3. How do this client's initial symptoms differ from those of a male client who has an MI?

evolve For suggested answer guidelines, go to http://evolve.elsevier.com/Iggy/.

LABORATORY ASSESSMENT

At present no single ideal test to diagnose MI exists. Health care providers use a series of different blood tests to diagnose a MI. The most common diagnostic tests include troponin T and I, creatinine kinase-MB (CK-MB), and myoglobin. These tests are described in Chapter 36.

RADIOGRAPHIC ASSESSMENT

Unless there is associated cardiac dysfunction (e.g., valvular disease) or heart failure, a chest x-ray is not diagnostic for angina or MI.

OTHER DIAGNOSTIC ASSESSMENTS

ELECTROCARDIOGRAPHY. Twelve-lead electrocardiograms (ECGs) allow the health care provider to examine the heart from varying perspectives and to note both the occurrence and the location of ischemia (angina) or necrosis (infarction).

An ischemic myocardium does not repolarize normally. Thus 12-lead ECGs obtained during an anginal episode reveal ST depression, T-wave inversion, or both. **Variant angina,** caused by coronary vasospasm (vessel spasm), usually causes elevation of the ST segment during anginal attacks.

These ST- and T-wave changes usually subside when the ischemia is resolved and the pain is relieved; however, the T wave may remain flat or inverted for a period of time. If the client is not experiencing angina at the moment of the test, the ECG for the client with angina is usually normal unless the client has evidence of an old MI.

When infarction occurs, three ECG changes are usually observed: ST-segment elevation, T-wave inversion, and an abnormal Q wave (wider than 0.04 seconds or more than one third the height of the QRS complex). Women who have a myocardial infarction (MI), however, may not have an ST-segment elevation (Cheek & Cesan, 2003). Figure 41-2 shows the usual ECG changes seen in MI.

The **Q wave** develops because necrotic cells do not conduct electrical stimuli. Hours to days after the MI, the ST-segment and T-wave changes will return to normal, but the Q wave usually remains permanently. By identifying the lead in which the ECG changes are occurring, the health care provider can identify the location and extent of the infarction.

STRESS TEST. After the acute stages of an anginal episode or MI, the health care provider often orders an **exercise tolerance test (stress test)** to assess for ECG changes consistent with ischemia, evaluate medical therapy, and identify those who might benefit from referral for invasive therapy (see Chapter 36). Pharmacologic stress testing using agents, such as adenosine (Adenocard) or dobutamine (Dobutrex), may also be used. Women are better diagnosed using an echocardiography stress test rather than the thallium stress test (Cheek & Cesan, 2003).

MYOCARDIAL PERFUSION IMAGING (MPI). *Thallium* scans use radioisotope imaging to assess for ischemia or necrotic muscle tissue related to angina or myocardial infarction (MI). Areas of decreased or absent perfusion, referred to as *cold spots,* identify ischemia or infarction. Thallium may also be used with the exercise tolerance test. Dipyridamole thallium scanning (DTS) may also be used.

MAGNETIC RESONANCE IMAGING (MRI). Contrast-enhanced cardiovascular magnetic resonance (CMR) may also be used as a noninvasive approach to detect MI (Rademaker, 2003).

CARDIAC CATHETERIZATION. This procedure may be performed to determine the extent and exact location of obstructions of the coronary arteries. Cardiac catheterization allows the cardiologist and cardiac surgeon to identify clients who might benefit from percutaneous transluminal angioplasty (PCTA) or coronary artery bypass grafting (CABG). Each of the diagnostic tests in this section is described in detail in Chapter 36.

Analysis

The client with coronary artery disease (CAD) may have either angina or MI. If MI is suspected or cannot be completely ruled out, the client is admitted to a telemetry unit for continuous monitoring or to a critical care unit if hemodynamically unstable.

COMMON NURSING DIAGNOSES AND COLLABORATIVE PROBLEMS

The following are priority nursing diagnoses for clients with CAD:

1. Acute Pain related to biologic injury agents (imbalance between myocardial oxygen supply and demand)
2. Ineffective Tissue Perfusion (Cardiopulmonary) related to interruption of arterial blood flow
3. Activity Intolerance related to fatigue (caused by imbalance between oxygen supply and demand)
4. Ineffective Coping related to effects of acute illness and major changes in lifestyle

For the client experiencing an MI, the following are the most important collaborative problems:

1. Potential for Dysrhythmias
2. Potential for Heart Failure
3. Potential for Recurrent Symptoms and Extension of Injury

ADDITIONAL NURSING DIAGNOSES AND COLLABORATIVE PROBLEMS

In addition to the common nursing diagnoses and collaborative problems, clients with CAD may have one or more of the following:

- Ineffective Sexuality Patterns related to pain and effects of illness
- Impaired Physical Mobility related to pain or fear of movement
- Potential for Acute Renal Failure

Planning and Implementation

ACUTE PAIN

PLANNING: EXPECTED OUTCOMES. The client with CAD is expected to state that pain, if present, is relieved. Older women may not experience the characteristic chest pain and may have silent myocardial ischemia or silent MI (Chart 41-3).

INTERVENTIONS. The objective of management is to eliminate discomfort by providing pain relief modalities, decreasing myocardial oxygen demand, and increasing myocardial oxygen supply.

NIC **PAIN MANAGEMENT.** Evaluate chest or other complaints of pain, obtain vital signs, ensure the patency of IV accesses, and notify the health care provider of the client's condition. Chart 41-4 summarizes the appropriate interventions for the client with symptoms of CAD.

Drug Therapy. Pain relief helps to increase the oxygen supply and decrease myocardial oxygen demand. The Amer-

CHART 41-3

NURSING FOCUS on the OLDER ADULT
Silent Myocardial Ischemia/Silent Myocardial Infarction

Silent myocardial ischemia and silent myocardial infarction (MI), once believed relatively rare, are now recognized to affect 21% to 68% of older adults with coronary artery disease (CAD) (Aronow, 2003). Reasons for the frequent absence of chest pain in older adults with CAD may be due to cognitive impairment and inability to verbalize sensations of pain, has more collateral circulation, and a reduced sensitivity to pain. Older clients with acute MI also delay longer in seeking assistance.

Silent myocardial ischemia increases the incidence of new coronary events in older clients with CAD and should be treated aggressively. The prevalence of clinical unrecognized MI diagnosed by routine ECGs in older persons varies from 21% to 68%. Older persons with clinically unrecognized MI have a similar or higher incidence of new coronary events and mortality compared with those with unrecognized MI. They should be aggressively treated with antiplatelet drugs, beta blockers, angiotensin converting enzymes, and statins if necessary.

ican Heart Association (AHA) recommends several strategies, including morphine sulfate and oxygen. In addition, aspirin 325 mg may be administered orally (chewed) immediately to prevent future occlusions. At home or in the hospital, the client may use nitroglycerin to relieve anginal pain.

Nitroglycerin. **Nitroglycerin (NTG),** a nitrate often referred to as "nitro," increases collateral blood flow, redistributes blood flow toward the subendocardium, and causes dilation of the coronary arteries. Instruct the client to hold the tablet under the tongue and drink 5 mL of water, if necessary, to allow the tablet to dissolve. NTG spray is also available and is more quickly absorbed. Pain relief should begin within 1 or 2 minutes and should be clearly evident in 3 to 5 minutes. After 5 minutes, recheck the client's pain intensity and vital signs. If the blood pressure (BP) is less than 100 mm Hg systolic or 25 mm Hg lower than the previous reading, lower the head of the bed and notify the health care provider. If the client is experiencing some but not complete relief and vital signs remain stable, another NTG tablet or spray may be used. In 5-minute increments, a total of three doses may be administered in an attempt to relieve anginal pain.

Angina usually responds to NTG. The client typically states that the pain is relieved or markedly diminished. When simple measures, such as taking three sublingual nitroglycerin tablets one after the other, do not relieve chest discomfort, the client may be experiencing an MI. Immediately inform the health care provider and prepare the client for transfer to a specialized unit where close monitoring and appropriate management can be provided. If the client is at home or in the community, the client or family should call 911 for transfer to the closest emergency department.

In a specialized unit the health care provider may prescribe IV NTG for management of the chest pain. Begin the drug infusion slowly, checking the BP and pain level every 3 to 5 minutes. The nitroglycerin dose is increased until the pain is relieved, the BP falls excessively, or the maximum prescribed dose is reached. The BP is monitored continuously (Chart 41-5).

When the pain has subsided and the client is stabilized, the health care provider may change the medication to an oral or topical nitrate. During administration of long-term oral and topical nitrates, a 12-hour nitrate-free period should be maintained to prevent tolerance. The client may complain initially of headache. The health care provider may prescribe acetaminophen (Tylenol, Exdol✱) to be taken before the nitrate to ease some of this discomfort.

Morphine Sulfate. The health care provider usually prescribes morphine sulfate (MS) to relieve chest discomfort that is unresponsive to nitroglycerin. Morphine relieves MI pain, decreases myocardial oxygen demand, relaxes smooth muscle, and reduces circulating catecholamines. It is usually administered in 2- to 10-mg doses intravenously every 5 to 15 minutes until the maximum prescribed dose is reached or until the client experiences relief or signs of toxicity. Adverse effects of morphine include respiratory depression, hypotension, bradycardia, and severe vomiting. Treatment for morphine toxicity consists of administering naloxone (Narcan) 0.2 to 0.8 mg intravenously, vasopressors, administration of IV fluids, and oxygen therapy. Monitor the client's vital signs and cardiac rhythm every few minutes.

These strategies are often enough to relieve the pain. If these methods are not adequate, additional interventions, identified later under Ineffective Tissue Perfusion (Cardiopulmonary), may be attempted.

Other Interventions. Several interventions may assist in relieving chest pain. Supplemental oxygen may increase the amount of oxygen available to myocardial tissue. Therefore oxygen is often prescribed and administered at a flow of 2 to 4 L/min by nasal cannula titrated to maintain an arterial oxygen saturation (SaO_2) equal to or greater than 95%. If the BP is stable, assist the client in assuming any position of comfort. Placing the client in semi-Fowler's position often enhances comfort and tissue oxygenation. A quiet, calm environment and explanations of interventions often reduce anxiety and assist in relief of chest pain. If needed, instruct the client to take several deep breaths to increase oxygenation.

CHART 41-4

BEST PRACTICE for
Emergency Care of the Client with Chest Discomfort

EMERGENCY CARE

- Obtain the client's description of the chest discomfort.
- Obtain the client's vital signs (blood pressure, pulse, respiration).
- Assess the client's vascular access.
- Consult standing orders or notify the physician for specific intervention.
- Obtain a 12-lead electrocardiogram if indicated.
- Provide pain relief medication and aspirin as prescribed.
- Administer oxygen therapy as prescribed.
- Remain calm; stay with the client if possible.
- Assess the client's vital signs and intensity of pain 5 minutes after administration of medication.
- Remedicate with prescribed medications (if vital signs remain stable), and check the client every 5 minutes.
- Notify the physician if vital signs deteriorate or pain is not relieved after three doses of nitroglycerin.

Critical Thinking Challenge

Five hours ago, a 48-year-old African-American man becomes nauseated and short of breath while mowing his yard. His wife brings him to the emergency department with excruciating pain between his shoulders. He states that the pain is a 10 on a scale of 0 to 10 and radiates down his left arm.

1. What are four essential components you should include in your initial assessment of this client?
2. What diagnostic testing will most likely be done?
3. What are the priorities of care for this client over the next 4 hours?

evolve For suggested answer guidelines, go to http://evolve.elsevier.com/Iggy/.

INEFFECTIVE TISSUE PERFUSION (CARDIOPULMONARY)

NOC **PLANNING: EXPECTED OUTCOMES.** The client with coronary artery disease (CAD) is expected to have adequate blood flow through the coronary vasculature to maintain heart function. Indicators include the following uncompromised measurements in the client:

- Ejection fraction
- Pulmonary wedge pressure
- Cardiac enzymes
- Apical heart rate
- Systolic and diastolic blood pressure
- Additionally, the client will have no:
  Angina
  Profuse diaphoresis

CHART 41-5

DRUG THERAPY for Coronary Artery Disease

Drug	Usual Dosage	Nursing Interventions	Rationales
Nitrates			
Nitroglycerin (Nitrostat, NitroQuick)	0.3-0.4 mg sublingually q5min; up to 3 tablets over 15 min	Instruct the client to lie down with the head of the bed at a level of comfort when taking the sublingual form.	Hypotension can be dramatic, immediate, and intensified by the upright position.
Nitrolingual translingual spray	0.4 mg/metered spray	Monitor BP. Pay attention to orthostatic changes.	A decrease in BP occurs with vasodilation.
		Instruct the client to allow the sublingual tablet to dissolve and to avoid swallowing the tablet.	The sublingual dose is absorbed through the sublingual mucous membranes.
		Check the expiration date on sublingual tablets and sprays. Tablets should be replaced every 3-5 mo.	The efficacy of the tablets decreases with time.
		Determine whether pain is relieved.	Additional medication may be required to relieve pain.
		Monitor for headache.	Vasodilation is generalized.
Isosorbide dinitrate (Isordil, Iso-Bid)	2.5 mg sublingually q4-6h; 5-40 mg PO four times daily	Instruct the client taking sublingual forms to lie down before administration.	The hypotensive effect can be dramatic and immediate with sublingual administration.
	40 to 80 mg sustained-release tablet q8-12h	Monitor BP and assess for dizziness.	A decrease in BP occurs with vasodilation.
Isosorbide mononitrate (Imdur)	60-mg extended-release tablet daily	Schedule sustained-release form with an 8- to 12-hr dose-free interval.	Tolerance may develop.
Nitroglycerin patch (Minitran, Nitro-Dur, Nitrek)	Transdermally started at 5 mg/24 hr (10-cm² system)	Remove the patch from the client before defibrillation.	The client may develop a burn.
		Rotate application sites.	Rotation prevents skin irritation.
		Apply the patch to a clean, dry, hairless area.	The drug is better absorbed when the skin is clean, dry, and hairless.
		Remove patch after 12-14 hr each day.	Removal prevents drug tolerance.
Beta Blockers			
Propranolol (Inderal, Inderal LA, Novo-Pranol)	80-320 mg twice daily to four times daily	Assess heart rate before administration.	Beta-blocking effects cause a decrease in heart rate.
	1-3 mg IV at rate not to exceed 1 mg/min	Monitor BP.	The hypotensive effect is due to a decrease in cardiac output, suppressed renin activity, and beta-blocking effects.
		Observe for signs of heart failure.	Heart failure may occur as a result of a decrease in cardiac output.
		Assess for shortness of breath and wheezing.	$Beta_2$-blocking effects in the lungs can cause bronchoconstriction.
Metoprolol (Lopressor, Toprol XL, Betaloc✱), a cardioselective beta-adrenergic blocker	*Angina*: 100 mg daily *MI*: 100 mg twice daily; 5 mg IV over 2 min may be repeated twice for a total of 15 mg	Assess heart rate before administration; do not administer if heart rate <50 beats/min.	Beta blockers may cause further decreases in heart rate.
		Monitor BP and hold for systolic <90 mm Hg.	Decreased BP pressure is an anticipated effect.
		Assess client for cough, shortness of breath, edema, and weight gain.	These are indications of heart failure.
Calcium Channel Blockers			
Nifedipine (Adalat, Adalat CC, Adalat XL, Procardia, Procardia XL, Nu-Nifed✱)	10-30 mg PO three times daily	Monitor BP and assess for dizziness.	Vasodilation can cause dramatic hypotension, which occurs within minutes.
	30-60 mg daily for XL and CC	Assess for headache and edema of the lower extremities.	These are common side effects.
		Tell client that empty shell of med may be in stool (for XL drugs).	Shell encases active part of medication and is not absorbed by the body.
Verapamil (Calan, Isoptin)	40-80 mg PO four times daily or 120- to 240-mg sustained-release tablet once daily	Monitor heart rate.	This agent slows SA and AV node conduction.
		Monitor blood pressure and assess for dizziness.	Vasodilation decreases BP.
	5-10 mg IV over 2 min	Assess for constipation.	This is a common side effect.

SA, Sinoatrial; *AV*, atrioventricular.

CHART 41-5

DRUG THERAPY for Coronary Artery Disease—*cont'd*

Drug	Usual Dosage	Nursing Interventions	Rationales
Calcium Channel Blockers—*cont'd*			
Diltiazem (Cardizem, Cardizem CD, Cardizem SR, Dilacor-XR, Tiazac, Apo-Diltiaz✱)	30-60 mg PO four times daily or 120- to 480-mg sustained-release tablet once daily; increase dose slowly	Monitor BP and assess for dizziness.	Vasodilation decreases blood pressure.
		Monitor heart rate.	This drug slows SA and AV node conduction, but the decrease is not as great as that which occurs with verapamil.
		Teach client to avoid grapefruit juice.	Drug's hypotensive effects increase.
Amlodipine (Norvasc)	5-10 mg daily	Monitor BP and pulse.	Like all drugs in this class, SA node conduction is slower and vessels dilate.
		Teach client to observe for signs and symptoms of heart failure, such as sudden weight gain, dyspnea, edema.	Drug can cause heart failure.
[1] Bepridil (Vascor)	200-400 mg daily	Instruct client to avoid grapefruit juice.	This juice increases the hypotensive effects.
		Monitor liver function tests (LFTs).	Drug can increase LFTs.
		Do not break, chew, or crush tablet.	Drug is long-acting and releases slowly.
		Monitor BP and pulse.	Same as diltiazem.
Felodipine (Plendil, Renedil✱)	5-10 mg daily	Same as most calcium channel blockers.	Same as most calcium channel blockers
Isradipine (DynaCirc, DynaCirc CR)	2.5 mg twice daily, increase up to 10 mg twice daily	Do not break, chew, or crush CR form.	Same as bepridil.
		Notify health care provider if signs and symptoms of heart failure.	Same as bepridil.
		Monitor blood pressure and pulse.	Same as diltiazem.
[2] Nicardipine (Cardene, Cardene SR, Cardene IV)	20-40 mg PO three times daily 0.5-2.2 mg/hr IV	Same as isradipine.	Same as isradipine.
Antiplatelet Agents			
Aspirin (Empirin, Apo-ASA✱, Ecotrin)	81-650 PO daily	Suggest that the client take the daily dose with food.	Gastric irritation may occur.
		Question the client about ringing in the ears.	Tinnitus may occur with aspirin toxicity.
		Emphasize to the client that aspirin is an important cardiac medication and should be continued unless the client is told to stop.	Studies document significantly better survival rates for clients with coronary artery disease receiving aspirin.
Ticlopidine (Ticlid)	250 mg twice daily	Teach client to take drug with food.	Drug can cause diarrhea and other GI disturbances.
		Inform client to report any usual bleeding or bruising.	Drug prevents platelet aggregation, thus slowing down clot formation.
[3] Clopidogrel (Plavix)	*Recent MI:* 75 mg daily *Acute coronary syndrome:* 300 mg, then 75-150 mg daily	Same as ticlopidine.	Same as ticlopidine.

[1] ***Med Error Alert!*** *Do not confuse bepridil and prepidil.*
[2] ***Med Error Alert!*** *Do not confuse Cardene and Cardizem.*
[3] ***Med Error Alert!*** *Do not confuse Plavix with Paxil.*

INTERVENTIONS. Because myocardial infarction (MI) is a dynamic process, restoration of perfusion to the injured area often limits the amount of extension and improves left ventricular function. Complete, sustained reperfusion of coronary arteries in the first few hours after an MI has decreased mortality in clients with MI.

Thrombolytic Therapy. Fibrinolytics are used to dissolve thrombi in the coronary arteries and restore myocardial blood flow. Examples of these agents, which target the fibrin component of the coronary thrombosis, include tissue plasminogen activator (t-PA, alteplase [Activase]), anisoylated plasminogen-streptokinase activator complex (APSAC), and reteplase (Retavase). The health care provider may prescribe the administration of fibrinolytics intravenously or by the intracoronary route during cardiac catheterization. Thrombolytic agents are most effective when administered within the first 6 hours of a coronary event. Thrombolytics are underused nationwide in men and women, young and old.

Thrombolytic therapy should be given in a unit where the client can be continuously monitored. It is indicated for clients who have chest pain of greater than 30 minutes' duration that is unrelieved by nitroglycerin, with indications of transmural ischemia and injury as shown by the ECG. Contraindications include recent abdominal surgery or stroke because bleeding may occur when fresh clots are lysed (broken down). Table 41-3 lists the current contraindications to thrombolytic therapy.

Clients who weigh less than 65 kg may need to have their dose of thrombolytic weight adjusted to lessen the likelihood of bleeding. During administration, the nurse immediately reports any indications of bleeding to the health care provider. After administration, observe for signs of bleeding by doing the following:

- Documenting the client's neurologic status
- Observing all IV sites for bleeding and patency
- Monitoring clotting studies
- Observing for signs of internal bleeding (watching hemoglobin and hematocrit)
- Testing stools, urine, and emesis for occult blood

TABLE 41-3 Contraindications to Thrombolytic Therapy

Absolute
Active internal bleeding
Known allergy to streptokinase products
Recent head trauma
Known bleeding disorders
Suspected aortic dissection
Increased blood pressure 200/120 mm Hg
Pregnancy or recent delivery
Cerebrovascular processes: recent stoke (within 2 mo). Recent spinal or cerebral surgery, cranial neoplasm
Prolonged cardiopulmonary resuscitation
Relative
Endocarditis or pericarditis
Hemostatic defects
Severe uncontrolled hypertension
Trauma within last 10 days
Surgery within the last 10 days
Current use of oral anticoagulants
Active peptic ulcer disease

Data from Lapchak, P.A., et al. (2002). The nonpeptide glycoprotein IIb/IIIa platelet receptor antagonist SM-20302 reduces tissue plasminogen activator-induced intracerebral hemorrhage after thromboembolic stroke. *Stroke, 35*(1), 147-152.

Some concerns in thrombolytic administration are associated with the specific agent. For example, *streptokinase*, a first-generation thrombolytic agent, is not fibrin specific; thus it may create systemic bleeding problems. Therefore, it is not used as commonly as other agents.

Second- and third-generation fibrinolytics include tissue plasminogen activator (t-PA, alteplase [Activase]), reteplase (Retavase), tenecteplase (TNKase), and t-PA. These drugs are fibrin specific, have a short half-life (3 to 5 minutes), and lack antigenicity. Because some studies have associated t-PA with a more frequent occurrence of cerebrovascular bleeding, carefully document neurologic findings. Reteplase can be given in two boluses ½ hour apart, needs not be weight adjusted, and results in greater rates of reperfusion than t-PA.

Tenecteplase (TNKase) is a newer fibrinolytic to be approved for use in clients with MIs. This drug has some advantages over other fibrinolytics. First, it can be easily administered as a single bolus over 5 seconds. Tenecteplase also targets clots more specifically than other fibrinolytics, resulting in slightly less overall bleeding. Bleeding is still possible, however, and nursing considerations are similar to the other fibrinolytics. Dosage is based on the client's weight. Use the utmost caution in administering these agents to avoid administration errors and prevent complications. Research continues to investigate and develop new, improved thrombolytic agents.

Glycoprotein IIb/IIIa Inhibitors. Glycoprotein (GP) IIb/IIIa inhibitors target the platelet component of the thrombus. Abciximab (ReoPro), eptifibatide (Integrilin), and tirofiban (Aggrastat) are administered intravenously to prevent fibrinogen from attaching to activated platelets at the site of a thrombus. These medications have been used in acute coronary syndromes (especially unstable angina and non–Q-wave MI). They are also administered before and during percutaneous transluminal coronary angioplasty (PTCA) to ensure patency of the newly opened artery and in conjunction with fibrinolytic agents following MI. If the GP IIb/IIIa inhibitors are used with a fibrinolytic agent, then the dose of the thrombolytic should be reduced by 25% to 50% to decrease the likelihood of bleeding. During the administration of GP IIb/IIIa inhibitors, assess the client closely for indications of bleeding or hypersensitivity reactions. If either occurs, the health care provider is notified immediately regarding administration of the appropriate medications (e.g., antihistamines or corticosteroids) for a hypersensitivity response.

For some clients experiencing an MI, primary PTCA may be used to reopen the thrombosed coronary artery. PTCA has been associated with excellent return of blood flow through the coronary artery when it can be performed within 70 minutes of the onset of chest discomfort by an interventional cardiologist. Most community hospitals are now capable of performing emergent PTCA. When primary PTCA is not available, clients with MI should receive immediate thrombolytic agents if they are an appropriate candidate and then transferred to a facility that can perform PTCA. This procedure is described in detail later in this chapter.

Identification of Coronary Artery Reperfusion. Monitor the client for indications that the clot has been lysed and the artery reperfused. These indications include the following:

- Abrupt cessation of pain or discomfort
- Sudden onset of ventricular dysrhythmias

- Resolution of ST-segment depression
- A peak at 12 hours of markers of myocardial damage

After clot lysis with thrombolytics, large amounts of thrombin are released into the system, increasing the risk of vessel reocclusion. To maintain the patency of the coronary artery after thrombolytic therapy, the health care provider usually prescribes aspirin and IV heparin. Monitor the activated partial thromboplastin time (aPTT)–the usual appropriate range is $1\frac{1}{2}$ to $2\frac{1}{2}$ times the control sample)–and maintain the heparin infusion for 3 to 5 days as prescribed. Low-molecular-weight heparin (enoxaparin [Lovenox]) may be substituted for IV heparin.

Oral Drug Therapy. Clients who have had an MI, whether or not they are receiving thrombolytics, should begin aspirin therapy unless contraindicated. They may receive a chewable aspirin immediately and then an enteric-coated aspirin (Ancasal✱, Ecotrin) 80 to 325 mg daily or every other day to prevent platelet aggregation at the site of the obstruction.

Beta-adrenergic blocking agents (e.g., metoprolol [Lopressor, Toprol XL, Betaloc✱]) decrease the size of the infarct, ventricular dysrhythmias, and mortality rates in clients with MI. The physician usually prescribes a cardioselective beta-blocking agent within the first 24 hours after a myocardial infarction (MI). Beta blockers slow the heart rate and decrease the force of cardiac contraction (see Chart 41-5). Thus these agents prolong the period of diastole and increase myocardial perfusion while reducing the force of myocardial contraction. With beta blockade, the heart is capable of performing 25% to 30% more work without ischemia. During beta-blocking therapy, do the following:

- Monitor the heart rate (bradycardia is common)
- Check the BP
- Check the level of consciousness
- Monitor for any chest discomfort

Assess the lungs for crackles (indicative of heart failure) and wheezes (indicative of bronchospasm). Hypoglycemia, depression, nightmares, and forgetfulness are also problems with beta blockade, especially in older clients. Many of these side effects decrease with time, however.

Health care providers frequently prescribe angiotensin-converting enzyme (ACE) inhibitors within 48 hours of an MI to prevent ventricular remodeling and the development of heart failure. ACE inhibitors have been demonstrated to increase survival after an MI. Monitor the client for decreased urine output, hypotension, cough, and changes in serum potassium, creatinine, and blood urea nitrogen. (See Chapters 38 and 39 for a more detailed discussion of ACE inhibitors.)

For clients with angina, the health care provider may prescribe calcium channel blockers to enhance vasodilation and myocardial perfusion. Calcium channel blockers are indicated for clients with variant angina or for those who are hypertensive and continue to have angina despite therapy with beta blockers. They are not indicated after an MI. Monitor the client for hypotension and peripheral edema, and review the frequency of anginal episodes.

The recent Clopidogrel in Unstable Angina to Prevent Recurrent Ischemic Events (CURE) study showed that the combination of clopidogrel (Plavix) and aspirin was more effective in reducing death, MI, and stroke compared with aspirin alone. The risk of bleeding from using two antiplatelet agents together was not significantly increased (Palatnik, 2001).

Enhanced External Counterpulsation. Enhanced external counterpulsation (EECP) is a noninvasive procedure that may be used to manage the symptoms of chronic, stable angina. It works by increasing blood flow to the ischemic areas of the myocardium. The EECP device consists of a series of compressive cuffs that are placed around the client's calves and thighs (Figure 41-4). Teach clients that this procedure may be repeated as needed.

ACTIVITY INTOLERANCE

PLANNING: EXPECTED OUTCOMES. The client with coronary artery disease (CAD) is expected to walk at least 200 feet four times a day without chest discomfort or shortness of breath.

INTERVENTIONS. Activity intolerance is reduced by a planned program of cardiac rehabilitation implemented primarily by the nurse and physical therapist and continued after discharge.

NIC **Cardiac Care: Rehabilitative. Cardiac rehabilitation** is the process of actively assisting the client with cardiac disease in achieving and maintaining a vital and productive life while remaining within the limits of the heart's ability to respond to increases in activity and stress. It can be divided into three phases. *Phase 1* begins with the acute illness and ends with discharge from the hospital. *Phase 2* begins after discharge and continues through convalescence at home. *Phase 3* refers to long-term conditioning.

In the acute phase (phase 1), promote rest and ensure some limited mobility. Assistance may be needed for some activities of daily living (ADLs), such as assistance in ambulating to the bathroom. Clients progress at their own rate to increasing levels of activity, depending on their clinical status, age, and physical capabilities.

The next step in phase 1 is independent ambulation of the client in the room and to the bathroom. Encourage progressive ambulation in the hallway, usually 50, 100, and then 200 feet three times a day. In addition, the client may begin showering for 5 or 10 minutes with warm water; a stool should be available to facilitate rest and maintain balance.

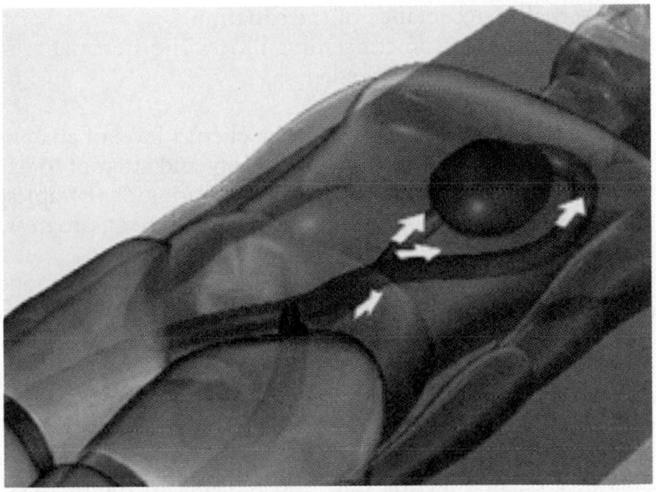

Figure 41-4 ■ Enhanced external counterpulsation device. This noninvasive procedure supplies blood and oxygen to the heart, reduces workload, and eases anginal symptoms.

CHART 41-6

NURSING FOCUS on the OLDER ADULT
Coronary Artery Disease

- Recognize that chest pain may not be evident in the older client; associated symptoms, such as unexplained dyspnea, confusion, or GI symptoms.
- Although older adults have a greater reduction in mortality from myocardial infarction (MI) with the use of thrombolytics, they also have the most severe side effects. Monitor older clients receiving thrombolytics extremely carefully.
- Dysrhythmia may be a normal age-related change rather than a complication of MI. Determine whether the dysrhythmia is causing significant symptoms, then notify the physician.
- If beta blockers are used, assess the client carefully for the development of side effects. Exacerbation of the depression already present in older adults is a significant problem with beta blockade.
- Plan slow, steady increases in activity. Older adults with minimal previous exercise show particular benefit from a gradual increase in activity.
- Older adults should plan longer warm-up and cool-down periods when participating in an exercise program. Their pulse rates may not return to baseline until 30 minutes or longer after exercise.

Assess the client's heart rate, blood pressure (BP), respiratory rate, and level of fatigue with each higher level of activity. Decreases greater than 20 mm Hg in the systolic BP, changes of 20 beats/min in the pulse rate, and complaints of dyspnea or chest pain indicate intolerance of activity. When such signs and symptoms develop, notify the health care provider and do not advance the client to the next level. Older adults with CAD often have needs and concerns different from those of younger adults, as described in Chart 41-6.

INEFFECTIVE COPING

NOC **PLANNING: EXPECTED OUTCOMES.** The client with CAD is expected to take personal actions to manage stressors related to CAD. Indicators include that the client will consistently be able to do the following:

- Identify effective coping patterns
- Verbalize a sense of control
- Report a decrease in stress
- Verbalize acceptance of the situation
- Seek information concerning illness and treatment
- Modify lifestyle as needed
- Adapt to life changes

INTERVENTIONS. Assess the client's level of anxiety while allowing expressions of any anxiety and attempt to define its origin. Simple, repeated explanations of therapies, expectations, and surroundings, as well as client progress, may help relieve anxiety.

NIC **Coping Enhancement.** Identify the client's current coping mechanisms; the most common are denial, anger, and depression. Denial allows the client to minimize a threat and use problem-focused coping mechanisms. The client may avoid discussing what has happened and yet comply with treatment regimens. This type of denial decreases anxiety and should not be discouraged; however, denial that results in a client's "acting out" and refusing to follow treatment regimens can be harmful. Because this behavior is usually due to extreme anxiety or fear, threats only worsen the behavior. Remain calm and avoid confronting the client.

CHART 41-7

NIC INTERVENTION ACTIVITIES for
Clients with Coronary Artery Disease

Pain Management: *Alleviation of pain or a reduction in pain to a level of comfort that is acceptable to the client*
- Perform a comprehensive assessment of pain to include location, characteristics, onset/duration, frequency, quality, intensity or severity of pain, and precipitating factors.
- Verify level of discomfort with client, note changes in the medical record, inform other health professionals working with the client.
- Ensure that client receives attentive analgesic care.
- Determine the needed frequency of making an assessment of client comfort and implement monitoring plan.
- Evaluate the effectiveness of the pain control measures used while performing thorough ongoing assessment of the pain experience.

Cardiac Care: Rehabilitative: *Promotion of maximum functional activity level for a client who has experienced an episode of impaired cardiac function that resulted from an imbalance between myocardial oxygen supply and demand*
- Monitor the client's activity tolerance.
- Maintain ambulation schedule, as tolerated.
- Instruct the client and family on the exercise regimen, including warm-up, endurance, and cool-down, as appropriate.
- Instruct the client and family on any lifting/pushing weight limitations, if appropriate.
- Encourage realistic expectations for the client and family.

Coping Enhancement: *Assisting a client to adapt to perceived stressors, changes, or threats that interfere with meeting life demands and roles*
- Appraise the client's understanding of the disease process.
- Use a calm, reassuring approach.
- Provide an atmosphere of acceptance.
- Assist the client in developing an objective appraisal of the event.
- Help client to identify the information he or she is most interested in obtaining.
- Provide factual information concerning diagnosis, treatment, and prognosis.
- Foster constructive outlets for anger and hostility.
- Explore with the client previous methods of dealing with life problems.
- Support the use of appropriate defense mechanisms.

NIC intervention activities selected from Dochterman, J.M., & Bulechek, G.M. (2004). *Nursing interventions classification (NIC)* (4th ed.). St. Louis: Mosby. No part of this work is to be altered without prior written permission from the Publisher.

Clearly indicate when a behavior is not acceptable and is potentially harmful as a result of noncompliance.

Anger may represent an attempt to regain control of life. Encourage the client to verbalize the source of frustration and provide opportunities for decision making and control.

Depression may be a client's response to grief and loss of function. Listen as the client verbalizes feelings of loss, being careful not to offer false or general reassurances. Depression is acknowledged, but the client is expected to perform ADLs and other activities within restrictions. Identify all improvements in the client's condition and share them. Chart 41-7 summarizes the major NIC intervention activities for clients with CAD.

POTENTIAL FOR DYSRHYTHMIAS

PLANNING: EXPECTED OUTCOMES. The client with CAD is expected to resume a normal sinus rhythm or normal rhythm and to be hemodynamically stable.

INTERVENTIONS. Dysrhythmias are the leading cause of death in most clients with myocardial infarction (MI) who die before they can be hospitalized. Even in the early period of hospitalization, 70% to 90% of clients with MI experience some abnormality of cardiac rhythm. Whenever a dysrhythmia develops in a client with CAD:

- Identify the dysrhythmia
- Assess hemodynamic status
- Evaluate for discomfort

Dysrhythmias are treated when they are causing hemodynamic compromise, are increasing myocardial oxygen requirements, or predispose to lethal ventricular dysrhythmias.

Typical dysrhythmias for the client with an *inferior* MI are bradycardias and second-degree AV blocks resulting from ischemia of the AV node. These rhythms tend to be transient. Monitor the cardiac rhythm and rate and the hemodynamic status. If the client becomes hemodynamically unstable, a temporary pacemaker may be necessary.

The client with an *anterior* MI is likely to exhibit ventricular irritability (premature ventricular contractions [PVCs]). Third-degree or bundle branch block is a serious complication in the client with an anterior MI because it indicates that a large portion of the left ventricle is involved. The health care provider may insert a pacemaker. Observe the client closely to detect the development of heart failure. Appropriate interventions for dysrhythmias are described in Chapter 37.

POTENTIAL FOR HEART FAILURE

PLANNING: EXPECTED OUTCOMES. The client with coronary artery disease (CAD) is expected to regain hemodynamic stability as evidenced by the following:

- BP and pulse rate within the client's acceptable range and adequate for metabolic demands
- Adequate urine output
- Mental alertness
- Clear lungs on auscultation
- Palpable peripheral pulses

INTERVENTIONS. Decreased cardiac output related to heart failure is a relatively common complication after an MI resulting from left ventricular dysfunction, rupture of the intraventricular septum, papillary muscle rupture with valvular dysfunction, or right ventricular infarction The most severe form of heart failure, *cardiogenic shock*, discussed on p. 854, accounts for most in-hospital deaths after an MI. The type of management used to increase cardiac output depends on the location of the MI and the type of heart failure that resulted from the infarction.

MANAGING LEFT VENTRICULAR FAILURE. When a client with MI experiences damage to the left ventricle, rupture of the intraventricular septum, or tear of a papillary muscle, a reduction occurs in the amount of blood that the heart can eject. When volume and pressure are markedly increased in the pulmonary vasculature, pulmonary complications develop.

Nursing Assessment and Monitoring. The development of left ventricular failure and pulmonary edema is assessed by auscultating for crackles and identifying their location in the lung fields. Wheezing, tachypnea, and frothy sputum may also occur with pulmonary edema. Auscultate the heart, paying particular attention to the presence of an S_3 heart sound.

Monitor for the following signs of poor organ perfusion that may result from decreased cardiac output:

- A change in orientation or mental status
- Urine output less than 1 mL/kg/hr or less than 30 mL/hr
- Cool, clammy extremities with decreased or absent pulses
- Unusual fatigue
- Recurrent chest pain

In specialized units, hemodynamic monitoring may be instituted to assess the client's preload, afterload, and cardiac output; however, hemodynamic monitoring in the hospital requires the insertion of a pulmonary artery catheter (see Chapter 36). Obtain and record hemodynamic measurements, which include the following:

- Right atrial pressure
- Pulmonary artery systolic and diastolic pressures
- Pulmonary artery wedge pressure (PAWP) (a measure of preload)
- Pulmonary vascular resistance
- Systemic vascular resistance (a measure of afterload)
- Cardiac output
- Central venous pressure (CVP)
- Cardiac index

Single values of these measurements are less significant than the trend of values combined with the client's clinical manifestations. These measurements help health care providers to identify heart failure and guide the administration of fluids and vasoactive drugs.

Classification of Postmyocardial Infarction Heart Failure. Killip categorized heart failure after an MI into four classes based on prognosis (Table 41-4).

Class I. Clients with class I heart failure often respond well to reduction in preload with IV nitrates and diuretics. Monitor the urine output hourly, check vital signs hourly, continue to assess for signs of heart failure, and review the serum potassium level.

Class II and Class III. Clients with class II and class III heart failure may require diuresis and more aggressive medical intervention, such as afterload reduction and contractility or enhancement of contractility. IV nitroprusside or nitroglycerin may be used to decrease both preload and afterload. These drugs are administered as continuous infusions in specialized units where the PAWP and BP can be closely monitored. The BP can drop in response to excessive vasodilation (see Chart 41-5).

Clients in class II and III are usually started on low dose beta blockers (usually Lopressor or Coreg). Dosing is titrated depending on goal achievement and drug tolerance. Other medications, including angiotensin-converting enzyme (ACE) inhibitors and angiotensin receptor blockers (ARBs), are commonly prescribed to promote ventricular remodeling. These medications are described in Chapter 38.

TABLE 41-4 Killip Classification of Heart Failure

Class	Description
I	Absent crackles and S_3
II	Crackles in the lower half of the lung fields and possible S_3
III	Crackles more than halfway up the lung fields and frequent pulmonary edema
IV	Cardiogenic shock

Positive inotropes, dobutamine (Dobutrex), and milrinone (Primacor), increase the force of cardiac contraction. They are administered by continuous IV infusion. The effects of these drugs on the vasculature and heart rate vary and may be dose dependent. An understanding of the anticipated effect of the drug and the desired dosage range is imperative. The infusions are titrated to optimize cardiac output. Use caution when administering these drugs because of the potential risk of increasing myocardial oxygen consumption and further decreasing cardiac output. The client is frequently monitored, paying particular attention to the development of chest pain (Chart 41-8).

Class IV: Cardiogenic Shock. Class IV heart failure is cardiogenic shock. In **cardiogenic shock,** necrosis of more than 40% of the left ventricle has occurred. Most clients have a stuttering pattern of chest pain, resulting in piecemeal extension of the MI. Manifestations of cardiogenic shock include the following:

- Tachycardia
- Hypotension
- BP less than 90 mm Hg or 30 mm Hg less than the client's baseline
- Urine output less than 30 mL/hr
- Cold, clammy skin with poor peripheral pulses
- Agitation, restlessness, or confusion
- Pulmonary congestion
- Tachypnea
- Continuing chest discomfort

Early detection is essential because established cardiogenic shock has a mortality rate of 65% to 100%.

Medical Management. Medical interventions aim to relieve pain and decrease myocardial oxygen requirements through preload and afterload reduction (see Charts 41-5 and 41-7). The health care provider prescribes IV morphine, which is used to decrease pulmonary congestion and relieve pain. Oxygen is administered; intubation and ventilation may be necessary.

Use the information gained from hemodynamic monitoring to titrate drug therapy. Preload reduction may be cautiously attempted with diuretics or nitroglycerin, as described for clients with Killip class III heart failure. (See Chapter 36 for a complete discussion of preload and afterload.) Monitor systolic pressure constantly, because vasodilation may result in a further decline in BP. Vasopressors and positive inotropes may be used to maintain organ perfusion, but such drugs increase myocardial oxygen consumption and can worsen ischemia. Use utmost caution in medication administration.

Use of an Intra-Aortic Balloon Pump. When clients do not respond to drug therapy with improved tissue perfusion, decreased workload of the heart, and increased cardiac contractility, an **intra-aortic balloon pump (IABP)** may be inserted. Insertion of an intra-aortic counterpulsation device, such as the IABP, is an invasive intervention that is used to improve myocardial perfusion during an acute MI, reduce preload and afterload, and facilitate left ventricular ejection.

The health care provider can insert an IABP percutaneously or through a surgical cutdown. Inflation of the IABP during diastole augments the diastolic pressure and improves coronary perfusion by increasing blood flow to the arteries. Deflation of the balloon just before systole reduces afterload at the time of systolic contraction. This action facilitates emptying of the left ventricle and improves cardiac output. The balloon catheter is attached to a pump console, which is triggered by an electrocardiogram (ECG) tracing and arterial waveform.

Immediate Reperfusion. Immediate reperfusion is an invasive intervention that shows some promise for clients with cardiogenic shock. The client is taken to the cardiac catheterization laboratory, and an emergency left-sided heart catheterization is performed. If the client has a treatable lesion or lesions, the surgeon performs an immediate percutaneous transluminal coronary angioplasty (PTCA or stent placement) in the catheterization laboratory, or the client is transferred to the operating suite for a coronary artery bypass graft (CABG).

MANAGING RIGHT VENTRICULAR FAILURE. Conditions other than left ventricular failure may result in decreased cardiac output after an MI. In about 30% of clients with inferior MIs, right ventricular infarction and failure develop. In this instance, the right ventricle fails independently of the left. Decreased cardiac output with a paradoxical pulse, clear lungs, and jugular venous distention results when the client is in semi-Fowler's position.

A right ventricular MI may be documented by echocardiography and by an ECG using right-sided precordial leads. The goal of medical management is to improve right ventricular stroke volume by increasing right ventricular fiber stretch or preload. To enhance right ventricular preload, the nurse administers sufficient fluids (as much as 200 mL/hr) to increase right atrial pressure to 20 mm Hg, as ordered. Monitor the pulmonary artery wedge pressure (PAWP) (attempting to maintain it below 15 to 20 mm Hg), and auscultate the lungs to ensure that left-sided failure is not developing. The client's cardiac output is monitored to ensure that fluid administration is having the desired effect.

POTENTIAL FOR RECURRENT SYMPTOMS AND EXTENSION OF INJURY

PLANNING: EXPECTED OUTCOMES. The client with coronary artery disease (CAD) is expected to experience minimal angina while engaging in activities of daily living (ADLs) and an exercise program.

INTERVENTIONS. Recurrent discomfort despite medical therapy is one of the major indications for surgical management of CAD. Clients who continue to have chest discomfort despite medical therapy or ischemia during a stress test may require invasive correction by PTCA or CABG to resolve angina or prevent myocardial infarction (MI). Before invasive treatment, a left-sided cardiac catheterization with coronary angiogram (see Chapter 36) is performed to document that the lesions are correctable and that left ventricular pump function is adequate.

Percutaneous Transluminal Coronary Angioplasty. **Percutaneous transluminal coronary angioplasty (PTCA)** is an invasive but nonsurgical technique. It is performed to reduce the frequency and severity of discomfort for clients with angina and to bridge clients to coronary bypass graft surgery.

Indications. Clients who are most likely to benefit from PTCA have single- or double-vessel disease with discrete, proximal, noncalcified lesions. This procedure often will not open complex lesions. When identifying which lesions are

CHART 41-8

DRUG THERAPY for
Commonly Used Intravenous Vasodilators and Inotropes

Drug	Usual Dosage	Nursing Interventions	Rationales
Nitrates			
Nitroprusside sodium (Nipride, Nitropress)	IV only by infusion device. Begin with 0.4-0.5 mcg/kg/min. May increase gradually to 10 mcg/kg/min.	Monitor BP q2-5 min when initiating therapy. If BP drops excessively, elevate the legs, decrease the dose, and increase fluids per unit policy. Monitor PAWP, SVR, BP, heart rate, urine output frequently. Titrate medication to obtain the desired effect.	This agent is a potent, rapidly reversible vasodilator acting on both peripheral venous and arterial musculature. BP may drop in 2 min.
		Protect from light.	This agent is light sensitive.
		Maintain dose at less than 3 mcg/min if possible.	Doses >3 mcg/min are associated with thiocyanate or cyanide toxicity.
		In clients requiring doses >3 mcg/min for >24-36 hr, monitor for metabolic acidosis, confusion, or hyperreflexia. Examine blood thiocyanate level.	These are indications of the toxic effects of cyanide.
Nitroglycerin (Tridil)	IV only by infusion device started at 5 mcg/min and gradually increased in increments of 5 q3-5min. If no response after 20 mcg/min, increase by 10-20 mcg until desired response.	Monitor BP q1-3 min when initiating therapy. If BP drops excessively, elevate the legs and decrease the dose according to unit policies. Monitor RAP, PAWP, SVR, BP, heart rate, and urine output frequently. Titrate medication to obtain the desired effect.	This agent dilates coronary arteries. It is a more potent systemic venodilator than an arterial vasodilator. BP may drop in 1 min.
		Intermittent administration of IV nitroglycerin should be considered.	Tolerance may develop rapidly to nitroglycerin administered by continuous IV.
		Monitor the client for headache.	Headache is a frequent side effect of initial nitroglycerin therapy.
Milrinone (Primacor)	IV bolus 50 mcg/kg given over 10 min; start infusion of 0.375-0.75 mcg/kg/min; reduce dose in renal impairment.	Assess BP and pulse q5min. If BP drops 30 mm Hg, stop infusion and call health care provider.	Hypotension is a common adverse effect.
		Monitor I&O and weight.	The drug causes diuresis.
Fenoldopam (Corlopam)	0.01-1.6 mcg/kg/min IV.	Assess BP and pulse q5min, then q1h × 2, then q4h, or according to agency policy. Monitor I&O and assess for signs of dehydration. Observe IV site for extravasation.	Same as milrinone.
Sympathomimetics			
Dopamine (Intropin)	IV only by infusion device. Starting dose 2-5 mcg/kg/min. Titrate up to 50 mcg/kg/min.	Determine the reason for use and the expected result. Observe the client's heart rate, ECG, BP, PAWP, SVR, cardiac output, and urine output q5min to q1h. Titrate the dose carefully to maintain the dose range and obtain the desired effect.	This agent is a dose-dependent activator of alpha, beta, and dopaminergic receptors. 2-5 mcg/kg/min stimulates dopaminergic receptors, which promotes renal and mesenteric blood flow. 5 mcg/kg/min stimulates beta receptors. This increases heart rate and contractility >10-15 mcg/kg/min, alpha effects predominate. This causes peripheral constriction.
		Infuse through a central catheter.	Extravasation can cause tissue necrosis and sloughing.
		Monitor the client for ectopy and angina.	These are adverse effects.
Dobutamine (Dobutrex)	IV only by infusion device, 2-10 mcg/kg/min. May increase to 40 mcg/kg/min.	Observe the client continuously during administration. Titrate the drug on the basis of heart rate, ECG findings, BP, PAWP, cardiac output, SVR, and urine output.	This agent is a very strong beta$_1$-receptor activator and a moderately strong beta$_2$-activator.
		Monitor for atrial and ventricular ectopy.	Dysrhythmias are an adverse effect.

ECG, electrocardiogram; *I&O*, input and output; *PAWP*, pulmonary artery wedge pressure; *RAP*, right atrial pressure; *SVR*, systemic vascular resistance.

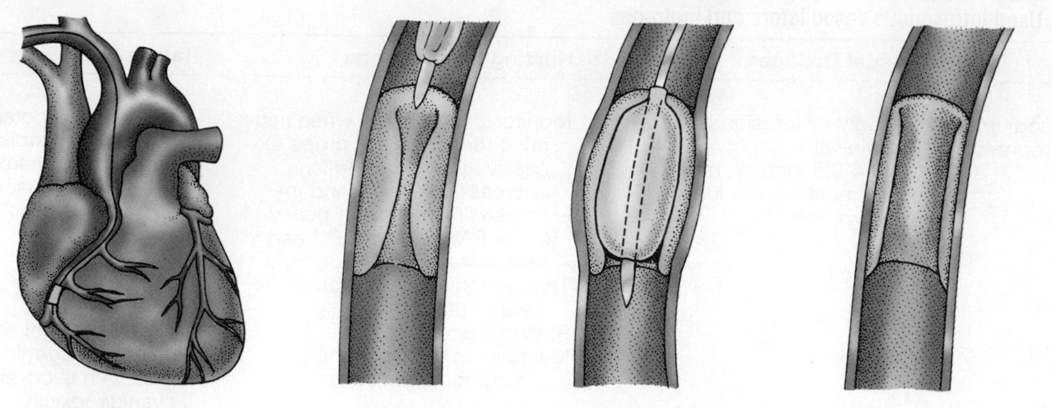

1. The balloon-tipped catheter is positioned in the artery.
2. The uninflated balloon is centered in the obstruction.
3. The balloon is inflated, which flattens plaque against the artery wall.
4. The balloon is removed, and the artery is left unoccluded.

Figure 41-5 ■ Percutaneous transluminal coronary angioplasty.

treatable with PTCA, the cardiologist considers the lesion's complexity and location as well as the amount of myocardium at risk. Treating lesions located in the left main artery would place a large amount of myocardial tissue at risk should the vessel close acutely; therefore these lesions are rarely treated with PTCA.

Percutaneous transluminal coronary angioplasty may also be used for the client with an evolving acute MI, either alone or in conjunction with thrombolytic therapy or glycoprotein (GP) IIb/IIIa inhibitor, to reperfuse the damaged myocardium. About 50% of clients needing revascularization are initially treated with PTCA.

Procedure. The physician performs PTCA under fluoroscopic guidance in the cardiac catheterization laboratory. A balloon-tipped catheter is introduced through a guidewire to the occlusion in the coronary artery. The physician activates a compressor that inflates the balloon at 4 to 14 atmospheres of pressure. This process compresses the plaque against the vessel wall, thus dilating the wall, and reduces or eliminates the occluding lesion (Figure 41-5). Balloon inflation may be repeated until angiography indicates a decrease in the stenosis (narrowing) to less than 50% of the vessel's diameter.

Following the procedure, IV heparin is administered in a continuous infusion to prevent thrombus formation. IV or intracoronary nitroglycerin or diltiazem (Cardizem) is given to prevent coronary vasospasm. PTCA initially reopens the vessel in more than 90% of appropriately selected clients. Within the first 24 hours, however, a small percentage of clients experience restenosis. At 6 months, restenosis or neointimal proliferation has an incidence of 20% to 50% (Grech, 2003c). GPIIb/IIIa inhibitors are also administered to prevent restenosis and maintaining the patency of the artery, reduce nonfatal MIs, and prevent deaths following PTCA.

Other techniques being used to ensure continued patency of the vessel are laser angioplasty, arthrectomy, and stents. Lasers may be used alone to remove atherosclerotic material from coronary arteries, or they may be used in conjunction with balloon angioplasty to create a smooth lumen about the size of the balloon. Arthrectomy devices can either excise and retrieve plaque or emulsify it. One of the advantages of arthrectomy is that it creates a less bulky vessel with better elastic recoil. **Stents** are used to maintain the

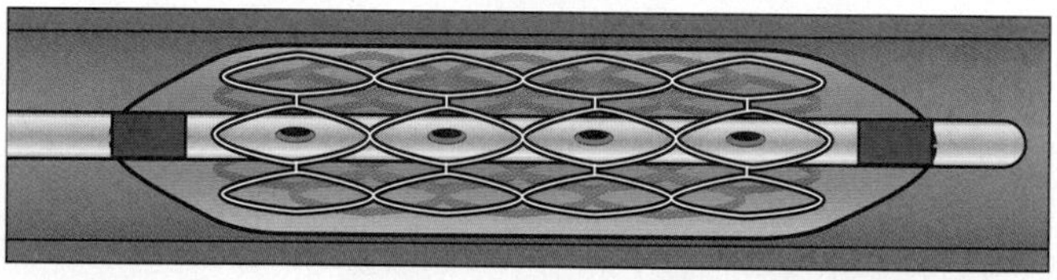

Figure 41-6 ■ A coronary stent open after balloon inflation.

patent lumen obtained by angioplasty or arthrectomy. By providing a supportive scaffold, stents prevent acute closure of the vessel from arterial dissection or vasospasm. Figure 41-6 depicts a stent positioned in a coronary artery.

Stents are an expandable mesh alloy tube placed at the site of the vessel lesion. The incidence of restenosis following placement of a stent is about 20% to 30%. Stents coated with drugs inhibit new cell and tissue growth and prevent neointimal hyperplasia are showing positive results. Sirolimus, paclitaxel, everolimus, and tacrolimus are some of the agents being used to reduce restenosis. Other therapies include brachytherapy (radiation) to prevent intimal artery hyperplasia (overgrowth) at the site of the stent. Rheolytic thrombectomy (e.g., AngioJet or Vortex) uses low-pressure, high-speed saline jets to disintegrate a thrombus. Endicor X-sizer lances and aspirates a clot simultaneously. Copper chelation, with the reagent tetrathiomolybdate (TTM), slows or stops cell proliferation, which can lead to restenosis.

Gene therapy has demonstrated that injecting vascular endothelial growth factor (VEGF) during angioplasty increased perfusion to the wall of the heart. Also, VEGF helps to initiate new blood vessel growth and development, which results in increased blood supply to cardiac muscle.

Postprocedure Care. Monitor for potential problems, which include acute closure of the vessel, bleeding from the insertion site, reaction to the dye used in angiography, hypotension, hypokalemia, and dysrhythmias.

The health care provider usually prescribes a long-term nitrate, calcium channel blocker, and aspirin therapy for clients after PTCA. A beta blocker and an angiotensin-converting enzyme (ACE) inhibitor may be added for clients who have had primary angioplasty following an MI. Many clients continue to have infusions of GPIIb/IIIa inhibitors during the initial hours after PTCA. Some clients may experience hypokalemia after the procedure and require careful monitoring and supplementation of potassium. Those who have intracoronary stents inserted may require clopidogrel (Plavix) for 6 to 9 months to prevent platelet aggregation. The nursing interventions for clients receiving these medications are described in Chart 41-5. Provide careful explanations of drug therapy and any recommended lifestyle changes.

Critical Thinking Challenge

Immediately following a PTCA and stent placement, the 48-year-old client admitted to your care arrives from the cardiology laboratory. The client denies any chest discomfort or shortness of breath. Heparin 1000 units/hr and normal saline 100 mL/hr are infusing. Laboratory results indicate an activated partial thromboplastin time (aPTT) value of 52 seconds.

1. What are three nursing priority assessments or interventions for a client following a PTCA or placement of a stent?
2. Which clients are most likely to benefit from a PTCA or stent?
3. What is the role of GPIIb/IIIa inhibitor administration following PTCA?

evolve For suggested answer guidelines, go to http://evolve.elsevier.com/Iggy/.

Coronary Artery Bypass Graft Surgery. Between 500,000 and 800,000 **coronary artery bypass graft** (CABG) surgeries were performed in the United States in 2001. It is the most common type of cardiac surgery and the most common procedure for older adults. Almost half of all CABGs are performed on clients older than 65 years of age. The occluded coronary arteries are bypassed with the client's own venous or arterial blood vessels or synthetic grafts. The internal mammary artery (IMA) is the current graft of choice because it has a 90% patency rate at 12 years after the procedure.

Coronary artery bypass graft is indicated when clients do not respond to medical management of CAD or when disease progression is evident. The decision for surgery is based on the client's symptoms and the results of cardiac catheterization. Candidates for surgery are clients who have the following:

- Angina with greater than 50% occlusion of the left main coronary artery
- Unstable angina with severe two-vessel or moderate three-vessel disease
- Ischemia with heart failure
- Acute MI
- Signs of ischemia or impending MI after angiography or PTCA
- Valvular disease
- Cardiogenic shock
- Coronary vessels unsuitable for PTCA

The vessels to be bypassed should have proximal lesions occluding more than 70% of the vessel's diameter but with good distal runoff. Bypass of less occluded vessels may result in poor perfusion through the graft and early obstruction. CABG is most effective when good ventricular function remains and the ejection fraction is more than 40% to 50%. Clients with lower ejection fractions are subject to develop more complications.

For most clients, the risk is low and the benefits of bypass surgery are clear. Surgical treatment of CAD does not appear to affect the life span. Early mortality rates are 1% to 2%. Left ventricular function is the most important long-term indicator of survival. CABG does improve the quality of life for most clients; 80% to 90% of clients are pain free at 1 year after CABG, and 70% remain pain free at 5 years after the procedure. The percentage of clients experiencing some pain increases sharply after 5 years.

LEGAL/ETHICAL ISSUES

IS INFORMED CONSENT POSSIBLE IN EMERGENT SITUATIONS?

Twenty-five years ago, physicians consistently provided care with a paternalistic "father knows best" approach. They decided what care was best for their clients and provided it with little input from them. For the past 15 years, however, there has been a movement toward client autonomy—the belief that clients should have the final say in their medical care. To ensure that they understand their options, many ethicists, lawyers, and health care providers have supported the concept of informed consent.

Informed consent has three important components: clients must be competent, must understand treatment options, and must make their choice freely without coercion by family or health care providers. The information provided to the client should include the following:

- Nature and purpose of the proposed treatment
- Expected outcome and likelihood of success
- Risks involved
- Alternatives to treatment
- Effect of not undergoing treatment

Unfortunately, health care is frequently provided in an emotionally charged atmosphere with clients in pain, hypoxic, or incapacitated. In addition, care to clients experiencing a myocardial infarction (MI) must be provided almost immediately, and there is little opportunity for them to weigh and evaluate options.

Some ethicists would argue that asking a client experiencing pain and anxiety to make a decision about care represents a distortion of informed consent. They might argue that clients presented themselves for emergent care and were therefore implying consent to standard treatment for that emergency. Benjamin and Curtis (1992) contended that it is appropriate for health care providers to act paternalistically and make health care decisions for clients in the following limited situations:

- If the client is incompetent or incapacitated and unable to make a rational decision
- If there is likely to be significant harm to the client if a decision is not made
- If clients are likely to approve of the decision when and if their capacity to make rational decisions is restored

Clients would meet Benjamin and Curtis's criteria for a paternalistic decision. In addition, *Heart Disease Weekly* (2003) presented research that would support clients at least remembering the details of informed consent. Six weeks after hospital discharge, 42% of clients who had angioplasty could not identify any risks and 41% could not identify any benefits. For coronary artery bypass graft (CABG) procedures, 45% could not identify any risks and 22% could not identify any benefits. However, in both groups, there was a high percentage (94%) of satisfaction with their decisions.

Implications for Nursing

In collaboration with the health care provider, it is the nurse's responsibility to be sure that the client desires and comprehends the medical and nursing care that is being provided. That usually entails ensuring that the client is fully informed and voluntarily consenting to the treatment. However, in some emergent situations or incapacitated clients, fully informed consent may not be reasonable or possible. In such situations, Benjamin and Curtis's criteria for making a paternalistic decision might be applied.

TABLE 41-5 Medication Administration Before Coronary Artery Bypass Graft Surgery

Medications Often Discontinued
- Digitalis 12 hr before surgery
- Diuretics 2 to 3 days before surgery
- Aspirin and anticoagulants 1 wk before surgery

Medications Often Administered
- Potassium chloride to maintain potassium between 3.5 and 4.0 mEq/L
- Scheduled beta blockers
- Scheduled calcium channel blockers
- Scheduled antidysrhythmics
- Scheduled antihypertensives
- Prophylactic antibiotic 20 to 30 min before surgery

Preoperative Care. CABG surgery may be planned as an elective procedure or performed on an emergency basis. (See the Legal/Ethical Issues box on p. 857 for a discussion of the dilemma of requiring a patient to provide informed consent under stressful conditions.) Clients undergoing elective surgery are often admitted on the morning of the surgery. Preoperative preparations and teaching are completed during prehospitalization interviews (see the Clinical Pathway on the Evolve website). Clients must understand that some medications will need to be adjusted because of the surgery. Ensure that appropriate medications have been discontinued preoperatively and that the necessary ones have been administered (Table 41-5).

Prehospital Preparation. Familiarize the client and family with the cardiac surgical critical care environment and prepare the client for postoperative care. If the procedure is elective, demonstrate and have the client return a demonstration of how to splint the chest incision, cough, deep breathe, and perform arm and leg exercises (see Chapter 20). Stress the following:

- The client should identify any pain to the nursing staff.
- Most of the pain will be in the site where the vein was harvested.
- Pain medication will be available.
- Coughing and deep breathing are important in preventing pulmonary complications.

Explain that the client should expect to have a sternal incision, possibly a leg incision, one or two chest tubes, a Foley catheter, pacemaker wires, and hemodynamic monitoring. An endotracheal tube will be connected to a ventilator for several hours postoperatively. The client and family must understand that the client will not be able to talk while the endotracheal tube is in place. The client should breathe with the ventilator and not fight it. When describing the postoperative course, emphasize that close monitoring and the use of sophisticated equipment are standard treatment.

Preoperative anxiety is common. An appropriate nursing assessment should identify the level of anxiety and the coping methods clients have used successfully in the past. Some clients may find it helpful to define their fears. Common sources of fear include fear of the unknown, fear of bodily harm, and fear of death.

In elective procedures, clients may benefit from detailed information about the surgery. Some may feel overwhelmed by so much material. Some need to discuss their feelings in detail or describe the experiences of people they know who have undergone CABG. Assess clients' anxiety level and helps them to cope.

Operative Procedures. Coronary artery bypass surgery is performed with the client under general anesthesia and for cardiopulmonary bypass or off-pump surgery. The anesthesiologist or nurse anesthetist administers anesthesia and intubates the client. The cardiac surgical team begins the procedure with a median sternotomy incision and visualization of the heart and great vessels. Another surgical team may begin harvesting the saphenous vein if it is to be used for the graft.

Cardiopulmonary bypass (CPB) is accomplished by cannulation of the inferior and superior venae cavae. The purpose of CPB is to provide oxygenation, circulation, and hypothermia during induced cardiac arrest. Blood is diverted from the heart to the bypass machine, where it is heparinized, oxygenated, and returned to the circulation through a cannula placed in the ascending aortic arch or femoral artery (Figure 41-7). During bypass, the client's core temperature is cooled to 90° F (32° C). Cooling decreases the rate of metabolism and demand for oxygen. The heart is perfused with a cardioplegic solution containing potassium, which decreases myocardial oxygen consumption and causes the heart to stop during diastole. This process ensures a motionless operative field and prevents myocardial ischemia.

Once the heart is arrested, the grafting procedure can begin. The surgeon uses the internal mammary artery (IMA), a saphenous vein, or both or a radial artery to bypass lesions in the coronary arteries (Figure 41-8). The distal end of the IMA is dissected and attached below the lesion on the coronary artery. If the surgeon uses a venous graft or the radial artery, it is anastomosed (sutured) proximally to the aorta and distally to the coronary artery just beyond the occlusion, thus improving myocardial perfusion. After flow rates through the grafts are measured, the heart is rewarmed slowly. The cardioplegic solution is flushed from the heart. The heart regains its rate and rhythm, or it may be defibrillated to return it to a normal rhythm. When the procedure is completed, the client is rewarmed by CPB and weaned from the bypass machine while the grafts are observed for patency and leakage. The surgeon may place atrial and ventricular pacemaker wires and mediastinal and pleural chest tubes. Finally, the surgeon closes the sternum with wire sutures.

Postoperative Care. After surgery the client is transported to a post–open heart surgery unit. There the client undergoes mechanical ventilation for 3 to 6 hours. The client requires highly skilled nursing care from a nurse qualified to provide post–cardiac surgery care, including routine postoperative care described in Chapter 22. The mediastinal tubes are connected to water-seal drainage systems and ground the epicardial pacer wires by connecting them to the pacemaker generator. Monitor pulmonary artery and arterial pressures as well as the heart rate and rhythm, which are displayed on a monitor (see the Clinical Pathway on the Evolve website).

Closely assess the client for dysrhythmias, such as ventricular ectopic rhythms, bradydysrhythmias, atrial fibrillation, or heart block. Treat symptomatic dysrhythmias according to unit protocol or the health care provider's order. Hypoxemia and hypokalemia are frequent causes of ventricular dysrhythmias. If the client has symptomatic bradydysrhythmias or heart block, turn on the pacemaker and adjust the pacemaker settings as ordered (see Chapter 37). Also,

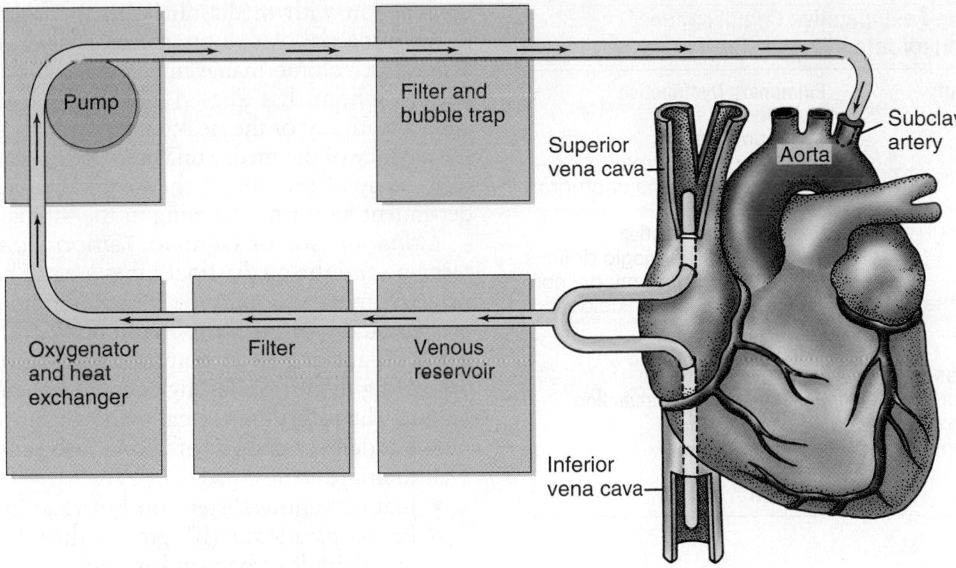

Figure 41-7 ■ Heart-lung bypass circuitry used during cardiopulmonary bypass.

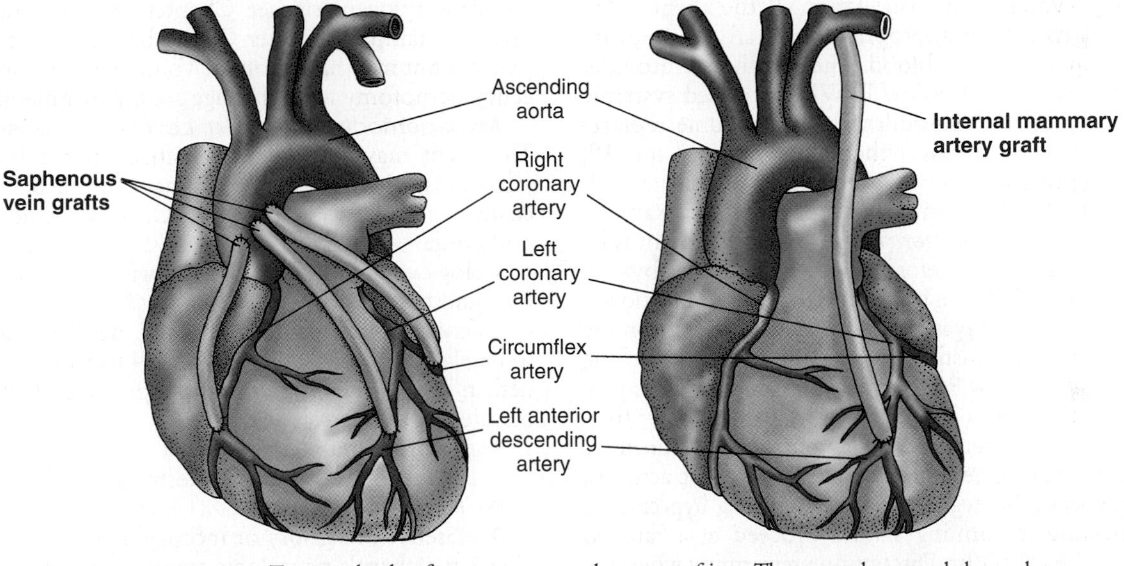

Figure 41-8 ■ Two methods of coronary artery bypass grafting. The procedure used depends on the nature of the coronary artery disease, the condition of the vessels available for grating, and the client's health status.

monitor for other complications of CABG, including fluid and electrolyte imbalance, hypotension, hypothermia, hypertension, bleeding, cardiac tamponade, and altered cerebral perfusion. Table 41-6 lists some of the possible postoperative complications of CABG.

Management of Fluid and Electrolyte Imbalance. Assessing fluid and electrolyte balance is a high priority in the early postoperative period. Edema is common; however, decisions concerning fluid administration are made on the basis of the blood pressure (BP), pulmonary artery wedge pressure (PAWP), right atrial pressure, cardiac output, cardiac index, systemic vascular resistance, blood loss, and urine output. An experienced nurse interprets the assessment findings and adjusts fluid administration on the basis of standing unit policies or specific orders from the physician.

Serum electrolytes (especially calcium, magnesium, and phosphorus) may be reduced postoperatively and are monitored carefully by both the physician and the nurse. Because the serum potassium level can fluctuate dramatically, electrolyte levels are checked frequently. Potassium and magnesium depletion is common and may result from hemodilution or diuretic therapy.

If the serum potassium level is depleted, the health care provider may order IV potassium replacement. The dose of potassium administered exceeds the usual recommended level of no more than 20 mEq of potassium per hour. For a potassium bolus, as much as 40 to 80 mEq may be mixed in 100 mL of IV solution and given at a rate as high as 40 mEq/hr. The drug must be given through a central catheter, and the rate of administration must be controlled by an infusion pump. The client must be placed on a cardiac monitor for intense, focused observation.

Management of Hypotension. Hypotension (systolic BP less than 90 mm Hg) is a significant problem because it

TABLE 41-6 Possible Postoperative Complications of Coronary Artery Bypass Graft Surgery

Decreased Cardiac Output	Pulmonary Dysfunction
▪ Reduced preload Hypovolemia Hemorrhage ▪ Increased preload Heart failure Cardiogenic shock ▪ Increased afterload Hypothermia Increased sympathetic activity ▪ Dysrhythmias Bradydysrhythmias Conduction defects Tachydysrhythmias ▪ Myocardial infarction	▪ Atelectasis ▪ Pneumonia ▪ Pulmonary edema ▪ Hemothorax/pneumothorax **Neurologic Dysfunction** ▪ Transient neurologic deficits ▪ Postpericardiotomy delirium ▪ Cerebrovascular accident **Acute Renal Failure** **Gastrointestinal Dysfunction** ▪ Stress ulcer ▪ Paralytic ileus **Infection**

may result in the collapse of a vein graft. Review the assessment parameters to identify what might be causing the hypotension. Decreased preload (decreased PAWP) can result from hypovolemia or vasodilation. If the client is hypovolemic, it might be appropriate to increase fluid administration or administer blood. The health care provider may treat the client with a low PAWP, decreased systemic vascular resistance, and vasodilation with volume replacement followed by vasopressor therapy to increase the BP; however, if hypotension is the result of left ventricular failure (increased PAWP), IV inotropes might be necessary.

Management of Hypothermia. Although the client is rewarmed to 98.6° F (35° C) before being removed from bypass, it is not uncommon for the body temperature to drift downward after the client leaves the surgical suite. Monitor the body temperature and institute rewarming procedures if the temperature drops below 96.8° F (36° C). Rewarming may be accomplished with warm blankets, rewarming lights, or thermal blankets. The danger of rewarming clients too quickly is that they may begin shivering, resulting in metabolic acidosis, increased myocardial oxygen consumption, and hypoxia. To prevent shivering, rewarming should proceed at a rate no faster than 1.8° F (1° C)/hr. Discontinue rewarming when the body temperature approaches 98.6° F (35° C) and the client's extremities feel warm.

Management of Hypertension. Hypothermia is a significant risk for the client following CABG surgery because it promotes vasoconstriction and hypertension. Other factors contributing to hypertension in the CABG client include CPB, medications, and the client's own sympathetic nervous system activity.

Postoperatively, many CABG clients experience hypertension (if hypertension is defined as a systolic BP greater than 140 to 150 mm Hg). Hypertension is dangerous because increased pressure promotes leakage from suture lines and may cause bleeding.

Management of Bleeding. Postoperative bleeding occurs to a limited extent in all clients. Mediastinal and pleural chest tube drainage is measured at least hourly, and drainage exceeding 150 mL/hr is reported to the surgeon. Clients with IMA grafts may have more chest drainage than those with saphenous vein grafts. To access the IMA, the pleural space has to be entered and will necessitate a pleural chest tube in conjunction with mediastinal tubes, making pulmonary assessment crucial. An autotransfusion of the chest drainage to assist with volume management when 500 mL has accumulated or 4 hours has elapsed may be done, depending on the clinical pathway or the health care provider's order. Maintain the patency of the mediastinal and pleural chest tubes. One effective way of promoting chest tube drainage is to prevent a dependent loop from forming in the tubing.

Management of Cardiac Tamponade. If the client is bleeding and the mediastinal tubes are not kept patent, blood may accumulate around the heart. The myocardium is compressed, and **cardiac tamponade** results. The fluid accumulating around the heart compresses the atria and ventricles, preventing them from filling adequately, and reduces cardiac output. The following are hallmarks of cardiac tamponade:

- Sudden cessation of previously heavy mediastinal drainage
- Jugular venous distention but clear lung sounds
- Pulsus paradoxus (BP greater than 10 mm Hg higher on expiration than on inspiration)
- An equalizing of PAWP and right atrial pressure
- Cardiovascular collapse

Tamponade can be confirmed by echocardiogram or chest x-ray. Pericardiocentesis (see Chapter 38) may not be appropriate for tamponade after CABG because the blood in the pericardium may have clotted. Volume expansion and emergency sternotomy with drainage are the treatments of choice.

Management of Altered Levels of Consciousness. The client may demonstrate changes in the level of consciousness, which may be permanent or transient. Transient changes related to anesthesia, CPB, air emboli, or hypothermia occur in as many as 75% of clients. Transient neurologic deficits may include slowness to arouse, memory loss, and confusion.

Clients with transient neurologic deficits usually return to baseline neurologic status within 4 to 8 hours. Permanent deficits associated with an intraoperative stroke may be manifested by the following:

- Abnormal pupillary response
- Failure to awaken from anesthesia
- Seizures
- Absence of sensory or motor function

Check the client's neurologic status every 30 to 60 minutes until the client has awakened from anesthesia; then check every 2 to 4 hours or per agency policy.

Pain Management. Differentiate between sternotomy pain, which is expected after CABG, and anginal pain, which might indicate graft failure. Typical sternotomy pain is localized, does not radiate, and often becomes worse when the client coughs or breathes deeply. The client may describe the pain as sharp, aching, or burning. Pain may stimulate the sympathetic nervous system, which increases the heart rate and vascular resistance while decreasing cardiac output. Administer the prescribed medication, in adequate doses, frequently enough to limit pain. During the process of weaning the client from mechanical ventilation, however, it may be necessary to use short-acting analgesics and to limit pain medication because of the respiratory depressant effects of analgesia.

Transfer from the Special Care Unit. Ventilation is usually provided for 3 to 6 hours postoperatively, until the client is breathing adequately and is hemodynamically stable. During the first day, the client usually has pacer wires, hemodynamic monitoring lines, and mediastinal tubes removed and is transferred to an intermediate care unit. All CABG clients, especially those with IMA grafts, are at high risk for atelectasis, the number one complication. Encourage clients to splint, cough, turn, and deep breathe to raise secretions. Guide them in a gradual resumption of activity. Two hours after extubation, clients should be dangled as tolerated and turned side to side. Within 4 to 8 hours after extubation, clients should be out of bed in a chair. By the first day after surgery, clients should be out of bed in a chair and ambulating 25 to 100 feet three times a day as tolerated. Continue to monitor for decreased cardiac output, pain, dysrhythmias, and infection.

Monitor the neurovascular status of the donor arm of clients who have had the radial artery used as a conduit in CABG. Assess the hand color, temperature (pulse both ulnar and radial stump), and capillary refill every hour initially. In addition, check the fingertips, hand, and arm for sensation and mobility at least every 4 hours. Intravenous nitroglycerin is often given for the first 24 hours postoperatively to promote vasodilation in the donor arm and therefore maintain circulation.

Many clients experience supraventricular dysrhythmias (especially atrial fibrillation) during the postoperative period, most commonly on the second or third postoperative day. Examine the monitor pattern for atrial fibrillation. When auscultating the heart, listen for an irregular rhythm. (See Chapter 37 for interventions for atrial fibrillation.)

Sternal wound infections develop between 5 days and several weeks postoperatively in about 3% of clients and are responsible for increased costs and longer length of stays. Be alert for the presence of **mediastinitis** (infection of the mediastinum) by the presence of the following:

- Fever continuing beyond the first 4 days after CABG
- Instability (bogginess or stepping) of the sternum
- Redness, induration, swelling, or drainage from suture sites
- An increased white blood cell count

The health care provider may perform a needle biopsy to confirm a sternal infection. Surgical debridement, antibiotic wound irrigation, and IV antibiotics are usually indicated. Four to 6 weeks of IV antibiotics are required if sternal osteomyelitis has developed. The mortality rate among clients with sternal surgical wound infections has been reported to range from 14% to 42% (Kohli et al., 2003). Prophylactic use of mupirocin (Bactroban) intranasally may be prescribed to decrease the incidence of sternal wound infection.

Postpericardiotomy syndrome is a source of chest discomfort in 10% to 40% of post–cardiac surgery clients. The syndrome is characterized by pericardial and pleural pain, pericarditis, a friction rub, an elevated temperature and white blood cell count, and dysrhythmias. Postpericardiotomy syndrome may occur days to weeks after surgery and seems to be associated with blood remaining in the pericardial sac. Observe for the development of pericardial or pleural pain. For most clients, the syndrome is mild and self-limiting; however, the client may require treatment similar to that for pericarditis. Be prepared to detect acute cardiac (pericardial) tamponade (see Chapter 38).

CONSIDERATIONS FOR OLDER ADULTS

Older adults may have different needs and experience slightly different problems after CABG. Special nursing concerns related to the older CABG client are detailed in Chart 41-9.

CHART 41-9

NURSING FOCUS on the OLDER ADULT
Coronary Artery Bypass Graft Surgery

- Be aware that perioperative mortality rates are higher for the older client (4% to 9%) than for the client younger than 60 years of age (1% to 2%).
- Monitor neurologic and mental status carefully because older adults are more likely to have transient neurologic deficits after coronary artery bypass graft (CABG) surgery than younger adults are.
- Observe for side effects of cardiac drugs because older clients are more likely to develop toxic effects from positive inotropes (dobutamine) and potent antihypertensives (nitroglycerin or nitroprusside).
- Monitor the client closely for dysrhythmias because older adults are more likely to have dysrhythmias, such as atrial fibrillation or supraventricular tachycardia, after CABG surgery.
- Be aware that recuperation after CABG surgery is slower for older clients and that their average length of hospital stay is longer.
- Teach the client and family that during the first 2 to 5 weeks after discharge, fatigue, chest discomfort, and lack of appetite may be particularly bothersome for older clients.
- Let someone know where you are when you are walking.

Minimally Invasive Direct Coronary Artery Bypass. The **minimally invasive direct coronary artery bypass (MIDCAB)** may be indicated for clients with a lesion of the left anterior descending (LAD) artery. In one of the most common MIDCAB procedures, after a 2-inch left thoracotomy incision is made and the fourth rib is removed, the left internal mammary artery (IMA) is dissected and attached to the still-beating heart below the level of the lesion in the LAD. Cardiopulmonary bypass (CPB) is not required. Postoperatively assess for chest pain and electrocardiogram (ECG) changes (Q waves and ST-segment and T-wave changes in leads V_2 to V_6) because occlusion of the IMA graft occurs acutely in 10% of clients. If there is any question of acute graph closure, immediately notify the health care provider. Clients tend to have more incisional pain after MIDCAB than after traditional CABG surgery, but the pain can usually be managed with oxycodone or codeine. Because they have a thoracotomy incision and a chest tube or smaller-lumen vacuum chest device, clients are encouraged to cough, deep breathe, and use an incentive spirometer for a week postoperatively. Most clients spend less than 6 hours in a critical care unit and are discharged in 2 or 3 days.

Transmyocardial Laser Revascularization. Transmyocardial laser revascularization is a new procedure for clients with unstable angina and inoperable CAD with areas of reversible myocardial ischemia. After a single-lung intubation, a left anterior thoracotomy is performed and the heart is visualized. A laser is used to create 20 to 24 long, narrow channels through the left ventricular muscle to the left ventricle. These channels will eventually allow oxygenated blood to flow during diastole from the left ventricle to nourish the muscle. After the surgery, the client is transported to a critical care unit, where hemodynamic monitoring is instituted for assessment of anginal episodes and bleeding disturbances. Although many clients report decreases in anginal episodes following the procedure, researchers have been unable to document why clients experience such an improvement.

Off-Pump Coronary Artery Bypass. Off-pump coronary artery bypass (OPCAB) is a procedure in which open heart surgery is performed without the use of a heart-lung bypass machine. Advantages include shorter hospital stays and decreased mortality, risk of infection, and cost. OPCAB does have some risk, for example, increased skill and steeper learning curve for surgeons to master the technique and inaccessible surgery sites.

Robotics. Robotic heart surgery is a new step toward less invasive open heart surgery. Surgeons operate endoscopically through 8- to 10-mm long incisions in the chest wall. Use of robotics provides surgeons with capabilities that simplify the surgical process, eliminates tremors that can exist with human hands, increases the ability to reach inaccessible sites, and improves depth perception and visual acuity.

Other advantages of robotic procedures include shorter hospital stays (average stay is 3 days), less pain due to smaller incisions, no need for heart-lung bypass machine, less anxiety for the client, and greater client acceptance. Also, the use of robotics will enable surgeons to perform telesurgery, performing heart procedures over long distances.

Disadvantages include computer failure, the skill and ability of the surgeon, and the length of surgery time (the time is about 50 minutes longer than the conventional surgery).

Community-Based Care

HOME CARE MANAGEMENT

Case management is most appropriate for clients who meet high-cost, high-volume, and high-risk criteria. Clients with coronary artery disease (CAD) clearly meet all these criteria. Clinical pathways and case management programs for clients who have CAD are in effect in most U.S. hospitals. By focusing on cardiovascular risk reduction and improving the continuity of care, health care professionals have reduced the length and cost of hospital stays. Posthospital case management should reduce hospital readmission rates and improve client health.

Clients who have experienced a myocardial infarction (MI), angina, or coronary artery bypass graft (CABG) surgery are usually discharged to home or to a subacute care setting with pharmacologic therapy and specific activity prescriptions. Depending on the procedure, hospital stays may be 4 to 7 days for clients with MI or those undergoing CABG and only 2 days for those undergoing percutaneous transluminal coronary angioplasty (PTCA); therefore clients are still recovering when they are discharged.

WOMEN'S HEALTH CONSIDERATIONS

A large number of middle-aged and older women who have had coronary artery bypass graft (CABG) surgery are living alone, and this number is expected to increase as baby boomers age. Few studies have been done to examine their special needs. Robinson (2002) conducted a qualitative descriptive study of 12 postoperative women in rural southwestern Louisiana living at home alone. All these women were white except one African American. Most reported educational levels ranging between the third and eighth grades. The researcher found four primary themes that described their at-home experience:

- Relief and gratitude that they had survived the surgery
- A need to continue living a full life
- A sense of vulnerability (feeling that they might have more heart problems)
- Regained independence, increasing self-worth and personal freedom

Robinson also noted that the knowledge of their surgery and heart disease was inadequate.

A home care nurse may be required for assessment and teaching following discharge and an aide for assistance with activities of daily living (ADLs) if clients are older or weaker (Chart 41-10). In addition, women, who tend to be older and living alone when coronary events occur, may have a greater need for home assistance after CABG surgery. Clients who were residents in long-term care may be returned there after hospitalization for unstable angina, MI, or CABG surgery.

Cardiac rehabilitation is available in many communities for clients after an MI or CABG surgery, but only 10% to 30% of clients participate in structured rehabilitation programs (Yates, Braklow-Whitton, & Agrawal, 2003). The most frequently cited reasons for nonparticipation are lack of insurance coverage, a physician's directive that it is unnecessary, and the client's decision that it is not necessary. Clients who participate in structured rehabilitation programs report greater improvement in exercise tolerance and improved ability to control stress. However, no difference in their return to work has been seen.

HEALTH TEACHING

The need for health teaching depends in part on the treatment plan or type of procedure that the client had. Cronin et al.

CHART 41-10

HOME CARE ASSESSMENT of
The Client Who Has Had a Myocardial Infarction

Assess cardiovascular function, including the following:
- Current vital signs (compare with previous to identify changes)
- Recurrence of discomfort (characteristics, frequency, onset)
- Indications of heart failure (weight gain, crackles, cough, or dyspnea)
- Adequacy of tissue perfusion (mentation, skin temperature, peripheral pulses, urine output)
- Indications of serious dysrhythmia (very irregular pulse, palpitations with fainting or near fainting)

Assess coping skills, including the following:
- Is client displaying denial, anger, or fear?
- Is the caregiver providing adequate support?
- Are the client and caregiver having disagreements about treatment?

Assess functional ability, including the following:
- Activity tolerance (examine the client's activity diary: review distance, duration, frequency, and symptoms occurring during exercise)
- Activities of daily living (is any assistance needed?)
- Household chores (who performs them?)
- Does client plan to return to work? When?

Assess nutritional status, including the following:
- Food intake (review client's intake of fats and cholesterol)

Assess client's understanding of illness and treatment, including the following:
- How to treat chest discomfort
- Signs and symptoms to report to health care provider
- Dosage, effects, and side effects of medications
- How to advance and when to limit activity
- Modification of risk factors for coronary artery disease

(2000) found that short hospital stays following a percutaneous transluminal coronary angioplasty (PTCA) did not allow enough time to educate adequately clients having the procedure (see the Evidence-Based Practice for Nursing box below). Because hospital stays are short and clients are quite ill during hospitalization, most in-hospital education programs concentrate on the skills essential for self-care after discharge.

As part of home visits or a cardiac rehabilitation program, identify the additional educational needs of the client and family as well as their readiness to learn. Develop a teaching plan, which usually includes education about the normal anatomy and physiology of the heart, the pathophysiology of angina and MI, risk factor modification, activity and exercise protocols, cardiac medications, and when to seek medical assistance. Clients are taught that myocardial healing after an MI begins early and is usually complete in 6 to 8 weeks. Those who have undergone CABG are told that the sternotomy should heal in about 6 to 8 weeks, but upper body exercise needs to be limited for several months.

Clients who have undergone CABG require instruction on incisional care for the sternum and the graft site. They should inspect the incisions daily for any redness, swelling, or drainage. The leg of a saphenous vein donor site is often edematous. Instruct clients to avoid crossing legs, to wear elastic stockings until the edema subsides, and to elevate the surgical limb when sitting in a chair. Clients who have had a radial artery graft are instructed to open and close the hand vigorously 10 times every 2 hours.

RISK FACTOR MODIFICATION. Modification of risk factors is a necessary part of a clients' management and involves changing their health maintenance patterns. Such modifications may include smoking cessation, altered dietary habits, regular exercise, BP control, and blood glucose control.

SMOKING CESSATION. For clients who smoke, explain the detrimental effects on the cardiovascular system of smoking tobacco, especially cigarettes. Many clients spontaneously quit smoking soon after an MI. Nurse counseling has been demonstrated to be a cost-effective way to assist clients to stop smoking. See Chapter 39 for more discussion. Other methods of smoking cessation include acupuncture, acupressure, and hypnosis.

DIET CONTROL. The mainstays of cholesterol control are diet therapy and administration of anti-hyperlipidemic agents. Research is being conducted to determine genetic implications for familial hypercholesterolemia. See Chapter 39 for a discussion of ways to lower cholesterol.

Also instruct clients not to add salt in food preparation or when beginning the meal. A reduction of 80 mg/day of sodium can reduce the systolic blood pressure (SBP) by 5 mm Hg and 3 mm Hg for the diastolic blood pressure (DBP). Maintain adequate dietary potassium, calcium, and magnesium intake. Increasing potassium to 80 mEq/day may reduce the SBP by 8 mm Hg (Zanabria & Welch, 2003). Booklets and cookbooks that can assist the client in learning to cook with reduced fats, oils, and salt are available from the American Heart Association (AHA).

Complementary and Alternative Therapies. The use of antioxidants (such as vitamin E) is an area of controversy. Some researchers report that the use of such agents counteracts the adverse effects of oxygen free radicals (derived from high cholesterol levels) on blood vessels and protects arteries. Other reports point out that excessive vitamin E increases the risk for liver damage and that the long-term effects of antioxidants are not known.

PHYSICAL ACTIVITY. Collaborate with the physical therapist to establish an activity and exercise schedule as part of client rehabilitation. Instruct the client to remain near home during the first week after discharge and to continue a walking program. Clients may engage in light housework or any activity done while sitting and that does not precipitate angina. During the second week, they are encouraged to increase social activities and possibly to return to work part-time. By the third week, they may begin to lift objects as

EVIDENCE-BASED PRACTICE for Nursing

What are the client's education needs in discharge teaching following PTCA?

Cronin, S.N., Freeman, L.H., Ryan, G., & Drake, D.M. (2000). Recovery after percutaneous transluminal coronary angioplasty: Assessment after discharge. *Critical Care Nurse, 20*(2), 70-76.

The concern that prompted this study was motivated by short hospital stays associated with percutaneous transluminal coronary angioplasty (PCTA), leaving insufficient time to assess the client's knowledge level, the need for teaching, and evaluating assimilation of the information. After discharge, clients may not respond appropriately to recurrences of chest pain. Clients may perceive that their hearts have been repaired and subsequent chest pain may be ignored as a result of client denial. The perception that their problem has been fixed may influence their reactions of modifying risk factors or making lifestyle changes. The purpose of the study was to examine these factors: prevalence and response to chest pain, the need for information, determination of concerns, and evaluation of lifestyle modifications.

The study was a descriptive, cross-sectional design that included the responses of 105 clients. Thirty-five subjects each were selected from clients who previously experienced PTCA at 1, 3, and 6 months. Clients had to be a minimum of 21 years of age, speak and understand English, able to participate in and respond to an interview format, have a home telephone, and first-time recipients of PTCA. A specific tool was used to obtain information about recurrent chest pain.

Level of Evidence: 5—This study used a cross-sectional design with an adequate sample size.

Critique. Demographics of the sample did not equally represent gender and race. Discrepancy in gender was greatest in groups 1 and 3. Group 1 was 1-month postprocedure, and group 3 was 6 months postprocedure. The most significant problem with the study was that the group's composition was 97.1% white and only 2.9% were African American. Ethnicity could play an important part in processing and acting on information. There could be a bigger impact on lifestyle changes in the African American group. Another limitation could be that the learning styles of the recipients were not assessed. Knowledge of specific learning styles could influence how instruction is delivered to the participants and impact retention.

Implications for Nursing

- Be aware that clients do experience chest pain following PTCA.
- Essential discharge teaching should include information regarding chest pain recurrence and specific instructions on necessary interventions.
- The number one learning need identified by clients was how to deal with feelings of depression and anxiety.
- Clients need information about taking over-the-counter medications.
- Be sure to include information on necessary modifications in diet, exercise, prescribed medications, and stress management.

CHART 41-11

CLIENT EDUCATION GUIDE
Activity for the Client with Coronary Artery Disease

- Begin by walking the same distance at home as in the hospital (usually 400 feet) three times each day.
- Carry nitroglycerin with you.
- Check your pulse before, during, and after the exercise.
- Stop the activity for a pulse increase of more than 20 beats/min, shortness of breath, angina, or dizziness.
- Exercise outdoors when the weather is good.
- Gradually increase the walking until the distance is $\frac{1}{4}$ mile twice daily (usually the end of the second week).
- After an exercise tolerance test and with your physician's approval, walk at least three times each week, increasing the distance by $\frac{1}{2}$ mile every other week, until the total distance is 2 miles.
- Avoid straining (lifting, pushups, pull-ups, and straining at bowel movements).

CHART 41-12

CLIENT EDUCATION GUIDE
Management of Chest Pain at Home

- Keep fresh nitroglycerin available for immediate use.
- At the first indication of chest discomfort, cease activity and sit or lie down.
- Place one nitroglycerin tablet or spray under your tongue, allowing the tablet to dissolve.
- Wait 5 minutes for relief.
- If no relief results, repeat the nitroglycerin and wait 5 more minutes.
- If there is no relief, repeat and wait 5 more minutes.
- If there is still no relief, call for transportation to a health care facility.
- Carry a medical identification card or wear a bracelet or necklace that identifies a history of heart problems.

heavy as 15 pounds (such as 2 gallons of milk) but should avoid lifting or pulling heavier objects for the first 6 to 8 weeks. Chart 41-11 lists suggested instructions for exercise.

Clients may begin a simple walking program by walking 400 feet twice a day at the rate of 1 mile/hr the first week after discharge and increasing the distance and rate as tolerated, usually weekly, until they can walk 2 miles at 3 to 4 miles/hr. Instruct clients to take their pulse reading before, halfway through, and after exercise. The client should stop exercising if the target pulse rate is exceeded or if dyspnea or angina develops.

After a limited exercise tolerance test, the physical therapist or nurse encourages the client to join a formal exercise program, ideally one that assists the client in monitoring cardiovascular progress. The program should include 5- to 7-minute warm-up and cool-down periods, as well as 30 minutes of aerobic exercise. The client should engage in aerobic exercise a minimum of three (and preferably five) times a week.

The benefits of lowering BP following exercise were reported by Zanabria and Welch (2003). After 30 to 45 minutes, SBP was lowered by 10 to 20 mm Hg. This effect usually lasts for 9 hours. BP changes can be seen as soon as 3 weeks to 3 months after beginning an exercise program.

Complementary and Alternative Therapies. Additional therapies can aid in reducing the client's anxiety about progressive activity both in the immediate postoperative period and during the rehabilitation phase. The overall use of complementary and alternative medicine is about 75% in clients undergoing heart surgery procedures (*Heart Disease Weekly*, 2000). However, many clients do not share with their health care providers that they use complementary therapies. Techniques such as progressive muscle relaxation, guided imagery, music therapy, pet therapy, and therapeutic touch have been shown to decrease anxiety, reduce depression, and increase compliance with activity/exercise regimens after heart surgery. A recent study examined the use of therapeutic touch as a relaxation intervention to lessen perceived stress, heart rate variability, and BP following surgery (Sneed et al., 2001).

SEXUAL ACTIVITY. Sexual activity is often a subject of great concern to clients and their partners. Inform the client and partner that engaging in their usual sexual activity is unlikely to cause any damage to the heart. Clients can resume sexual intercourse on the advice of the health care provider, usually after an exercise tolerance assessment. In general, clients who can walk one block or climb two flights of stairs without symptoms can usually safely resume sexual activity.

Suggest that initially clients schedule intercourse after a period of rest. They might try having intercourse in the morning when they are well rested or wait $1\frac{1}{2}$ hours after exercise or a heavy meal. The position selected should be comfortable for both the client and his or her partner so that no undue stress is placed on the heart or suture line.

BLOOD PRESSURE CONTROL. Make arrangements for the client to have blood pressure (BP) measurements taken at regular intervals, and collaborate with the health care provider to establish parameters for reporting the BP. Lifestyle modifications such as weight reduction, physical activity, and reduced-sodium diets may assist in the management of hypertension. If the client is taking medication, assess compliance with the medication regimen.

BLOOD GLUCOSE CONTROL. Clients with diabetes mellitus are assessed for their participation in efforts to control hyperglycemia. Review the prescribed dosage of insulin or oral hypoglycemic agents with the client and family. The client should demonstrate accurate testing of blood for glucose levels.

CARDIAC MEDICATIONS. Assist the client in understanding the type of cardiac medications prescribed, the benefit of each drug, potential side effects, and the correct dosage and time of day to take each drug. Medication regimens vary considerably; however, many clients with angina are discharged while taking aspirin, a beta blocker, a calcium channel blocker, an anti-hyperlipidemic agent, and a nitrate. Clients who have experienced an MI may require aspirin, a beta blocker, an anti-hyperlipidemic agent, and an angiotensin-converting enzyme (ACE) inhibitor. The regimen can be complex. Determine whether the client can comply with the instructions.

Use of sublingual or spray nitroglycerin (NTG) deserves special attention. Instruct the client to carry NTG at all times. Keep the tablets in a glass, light-resistant container. NTG should be replaced every 3 to 5 months, before it loses its potency or stops producing a tingling sensation when placed under the tongue. Chart 41-12 gives instructions for clients for management of chest discomfort at home.

SEEKING MEDICAL ASSISTANCE. Clients are encouraged to notify their health care provider if they experience the following:

- Heart rate remaining less than 50 after arising
- Wheezing or difficulty breathing

- Weight gain of 3 pounds in 1 week or 1 to 2 pounds overnight
- Show persistent increase in NTG use
- Dizziness, faintness, or shortness of breath with activity

Clients are encouraged to call for transportation to the hospital if they experience the following:

- Chest discomfort that does not improve after 20 minutes or three NTG tablets
- Extremely severe chest or epigastric discomfort with weakness, nausea, or fainting
- Other symptoms that are particular to the client, such as fatigue and nausea

HEALTH CARE RESOURCES

The AHA is an excellent source for booklets, films, videocassettes, cookbooks, and professional service referrals for the client with CAD. Many local affiliates have their own cardiac rehabilitation programs.

Within the community, cardiac rehabilitation programs may be affiliated with local hospitals, community centers, or other facilities, such as clinics. Many shopping malls open before shopping hours to allow a measured walking program indoors; this is particularly popular with older clients because it provides a good support group and allows for an appropriate place to exercise in inclement weather.

Mended Hearts is a nationwide program with local chapters that provides education and support to CABG clients and their families. Smoking-cessation programs and clinics as well as weight-reduction programs are found within the community. Many hospitals also sponsor health fairs, BP screening, and risk factor modification programs.

Evaluation: Outcomes

Evaluate the client with CAD on the basis of the identified nursing diagnoses and collaborative problems. The expected outcomes are that the client will:

- State that discomfort or other symptoms are alleviated
- Have adequate blood flow through the coronary vasculature to ensure heart function
- Walk 200 feet four times a day without discomfort, shortness of breath, or other symptoms of CAD
- Take personal actions to manage stressors related to CAD

Specific indicators for these outcomes are listed for each nursing diagnosis and collaborative problem under the Planning and Implementation section (see earlier).

GET READY for the NCLEX Examination!

KEY POINTS

Safe Effective Care Environment

- Manage and use aseptic techniques when caring for all sternal and leg wound incisions, and any invasive lines.
- Refer clients who have had heart surgery for consultation with interdisciplinary health care team members (e.g., physical therapist, case manager, and home care providers).
- Evaluate the client's support options for meeting self-care needs.
- Interview the client and assess the client's home for environmental hazards and accessibility.
- Assist clients in securing personal medical identification alert devices that provide information regarding their heart conditions.

Health Promotion and Maintenance

- In collaboration with the dietitian, identify a healthy pattern of eating that helps reduce the incidence of CAD.
- In collaboration with the multidisciplinary health team, assess the client for activity tolerance and help design an appropriate exercise regimen.
- Teach the client about the signs and symptoms of cardiovascular disease and when to seek medical assistance.
- Assess the client for lifestyle risk factors of coronary artery disease (CAD), such as obesity, smoking, positive family history, cholesterol management, and the diagnosis and treatment of hypertension.
- Teach clients ways to decrease their risk for CAD.
- Teach clients about drug therapy, including therapeutic and adverse effects.
- Refer clients to appropriate community programs and support groups.

Psychosocial Integrity

- Allow clients to verbalize and express feelings of fear, anxiety, anger, denial, and grief regarding their CAD.
- Address the needs of the family and significant others and provide teaching and information regarding the disease process; clarify any misconceptions.
- Explain to the client the significance of reporting any pain or discomfort, and help identify barriers in seeking medical assistance.
- Identify and explain various diagnostic tests and procedures for clients experiencing cardiac compromise. Examples include electrocardiography, stress and exercise testing, nuclear scans, and cardiac catheterization.

Physiological Integrity

- Identify and interpret diagnostic values for cardiac enzymes and other indicators of CAD.
- Monitor clients receiving thrombolytics and anticoagulants, such as heparin, for bleeding.
- For clients undergoing invasive cardiac procedures, assess for signs and symptoms of active bleeding.
- Interpret and assess the client with CAD for dysrhythmias.
- Evaluate the client for pain characteristics (e.g., type, location, duration, cause, intensity, and measures taken to relieve symptoms).
- Identify and assess for complications for post–cardiac surgical clients, especially stroke, heart failure, bleeding, and pulmonary dysfunction.

ADDITIONAL STUDY RESOURCES

Go to your Student CD-ROM for Review Questions for the NCLEX Examination.

evolve Go to http://evolve.elsevier.com/Iggy/ for Integrated Management of Care Questions for the NCLEX Examination.

SELECTED BIBLIOGRAPHY

Asterisk indicates a classic or definitive work on this subject.

Allen, J.K. (2000). Cholesterol management: An opportunity for nurse case managers. *Journal of Cardiovascular Nursing, 14*(2), 50-58.

Angioplasty: Copper chelation holds promise for clogged arteries. (2003). *Heart Disease Weekly, June 28,* 3-4.

Angioplasty: Gene therapy during procedure improves blood flow. (2003). *Heart Disease Weekly, June 15,* 10-11.

Aronow, W.S. (2003). Silent MI: Prevalence and prognosis in older patients diagnosed by routine electrocardiogram. *Geriatrics, 59*(1), 24-40.

Becker, C. (2003). Bypassing the pump. *Modern Healthcare, 35*(10), 36-40.

Bialous, S.A., & Sarna, L. (2004). Sparing a few minutes for tobacco cessation. *American Journal of Nursing, 104*(12), 54-60.

Boersma, E., et al. (2003). Acute myocardial infarction. *Lancet, 361*(9630), 847-859.

Cadroy, Y., et al. (2003). Strenuous activity may pose a risk of plaque injury. *Journal of Applied Physiology, 93*(3), 829-835.

Cardiac medication: Study newer anticoagulation is as effective as gold standard. (2003). *Heart Disease Weekly, March 23,* 22-23.

Cheek, D., & Cesan, A. (2003). What's different about heart disease in women? *Nursing 2003, 33*(8), 36-42.

Chen-Scarabelli, C. (2002). Beating-heart coronary artery bypass surgery: Indications, advantages, and limitations. *Critical Care Nurse, 22*(5), 44-58.

Clinical trials: Enrollment completed for gamma in-stent restenosis study. (2002). *Heart Disease Weekly, March 3,* 7-8.

Coronary artery bypass surgery versus percutaneous coronary intervention with stent implantation in patients with multivessel coronary artery disease. (2002). *Lancet, 360*(9360), 965-971.

Coronary artery occlusion: Heart attack victims to benefit from drug-coated stents. (2003). *Heart Disease Weekly, June 8,* 25-26.

Coronary bypass: Procedure without general anesthesia studied. (2000). *Heart Disease Weekly, October 15,* 11-12.

Cronin, S.N., et al. (2000). Recovery after percutaneous transluminal coronary angioplasty: Assessment after discharge. *Critical Care Nurse, 20*(2), 70-84.

Crumlish, C.M., et al. (2000). When time is muscle. *American Journal of Nursing, 100*(1), 26-36.

Daly, J., et al. (2000). Health status, perceptions of coping, and social support immediately after discharge of survivors of acute myocardial infarction. *American Journal of Critical Care, 9*(1), 62-69.

Davis, S.L. (2002). How the heart failure picture has changed. *Nursing, 32*(11), 36-44.

Ditlea, S. (2000). Robosurgeons. *Technology Review, 103*(6), 74-82.

Estabrooks, P.A., Glasgow, R.E., & Dzewaltowski, D.A. (2003). Physical activity promotion. *JAMA, 289*(22), 2913-2917.

Furry, B., & House-Fancher, M.A. (2000). Reviewing the drug lineup against AMI. *Nursing 2000, 30*(7), 32hn1-32hn3.

Futterman, L.G., & Lemberg, L. (2000). Update on management of acute myocardial infarction: Facilitated percutaneous coronary intervention. *American Journal of Critical Care, 9*(1), 70-76.

Gentz, C.A. (2000). Perceived learning needs of the patient undergoing coronary angioplasty: An integrative review of the literature. *Heart and Lung, 29*(3), 161-172.

Gorman, C., et al. (2003). The no. 1 killer of women. *Time Canada, 161*(17), 42-49.

Gradman, J. H., & Schell, M. (2002). *Managing cardiac emergencies.* Eau Claire, WI: PESI HealthCare.

Graham, H. (2003). A conceptual map for studying long-term exercise adherence in a cardiac population. *Rehabilitation Nursing, 28*(3), 80-86.

Grech, E. (2003a). ABC of interventional cardiology: Pathophysiology and investigation of coronary artery disease. *British Medical Journal, 326*(7399), 1027-1030.

Grech, E. (2003b). Percutaneous coronary intervention. I: History and development. *British Medical Journal, 326*(7398), 1080-1083.

Grech, E. (2003c). Percutaneous coronary intervention. II: The procedure. *British Medical Journal, 326*(7359), 1135-1141.

Grech, E., & Ramsdale, D. (2003). ABC of interventional cardiology: Acute coronary syndrome, unstable angina and non-ST segment elevation myocardial infarction. *British Medical Journal, 326*(7359), 1259-1261.

Hamilton, A. (2001). Forceps! Scalpel! Robot! *Time, 157*(22), 64-66.

Heart disease and stroke statistics–2003 update. (2003). Dallas: American Heart Association.

Heart disease mortality: Gene for cellular receptors could be key for lower heart risk. (2003). *Genomics & Genetics Weekly, May 2,* 19-20.

Henke, K., & Eigsti, J. (2003). After cardiopulmonary bypass: Watching for complications. *Nursing, 35*(3), cc1-cc4.

Here's a pet therapy for stressed caregivers. (2001). *Work & Family Life, 2.*

High cholesterol: Gene therapy lowers cholesterol in a model of familial hypercholesterolemia. (2003). *Heart Disease Weekly, June 22,* 36-35.

Hooker, S., Holbrook, L. F., & Stewart, P. (2002). Pet therapy research: A historical review. *Holistic Nursing Practice, 17*(1), 17-23.

Hussey, L. C., Hynan, L., & Leeper, B. (2001). Risk factors for sternal wound infection in men versus women. *American Journal of Critical Care, 10*(2), 112-116.

Hyett, J.M. (2004). Caring for a patient after CABG surgery, *Nursing 2004, 34*(7), 48-49.

Intracoronary radiation: Intima may become so thin that stent struts are exposed, may lead to thrombosis. (2003). *Heart Disease Weekly, June 1,* 53-54.

Kohli, M., et al. (2003). A risk index for sternal surgical wound infection after cardiovascular surgery. *Infection Control and Hospital Epidemiology, 24*(1), 17-22.

Lapchak, P.A., et al. (2002). The nonpeptide glycoprotein IIb/IIIa platelet receptor antagonist SM-20302 reduces tissue plasminogen activator-induced intracerebral hemorrhage after thromboembolic stroke. *Stroke, 35*(1), 147-152.

Litton, K. (2002). Left vs. right ventricular MI: Which is it? *RN, 65*(5), 36ac5-36ac10.

Liu, E.H. (2000). Use of alternate medicine by patients undergoing cardiac surgery. *Journal Thoracic Cardiovascular Surgery, 120*(2), 355-361.

Low-cost intranasal antibiotic reduces sternal wound infections in open-heart surgery patients. (2001). *Formulary, 36*(7), 483-484.

Madias, J. E. (2000). Killip and Forrester classifications: Should they be abandoned, kept, reevaluated, or modified? *Chest, 117*(5), 1223-1226.

Manson, J.E., et al. (2001). Heart disease in older women. *Patient Care for the Nurse Practitioner, 4*(5), 28-40.

McAvoy, J.A. (2000). Cardiac pain: Discover the unexpected. *Nursing 2000, 30*(3), 36-40.

McCance, K., & Huether, S. (2002). *Pathophysiology: The biologic basis for disease in adults* (4th ed.). St. Louis: Mosby.

Meadows, M. (2002). Robots lend a helpful hand to surgeons. *FDA Consumer,36*(3), 10-16.

Nguyen, T., et al. (2000). Catheter based interventions in acute myocardial infarction. In T. Nguyen et al. (Eds.), *Management of complex cardiovascular problems* (pp. 35-56). Armonk, NY: Futura Publishing.

O'Toole, L., Grech, E., & Grech, E. (2003). ABC of interventional cardiology. Chronic stable angina: Treatment options. *British Medical Journal, 326*(7400), 1185-1189.

Pagana, K.D., & Pagana, T.J.(2002). *Mosby's manual of diagnostic and laboratory tests* (2nd ed.). St. Louis: Mosby.

Palatnik, A.M. (2001). Acute coronary syndrome: New advances and nursing strategies. *Nursing 2001, 31*(5), 32cc1-32cc6.

Peterson, D.A. (2000). Managing hypotension after cardiac surgery: An algorithm for treatment. *Critical Care Nurse, 20*(2), 36-49.

Quality assurance: Half of heart patients unable to recall details of informed consent. (2003). *Heart Disease Weekly, April 20,* 74-75.

Rademaker, F.E. (2003). Magnetic resonance imaging in cardiology. *Lancet, 361*(9355), 359-361.

Richards, S.B., Funk, M., & Milner, K.A. (2000). Differences between blacks and whites with coronary artery disease in initial symptoms and delay in seeking care. *American Journal of Critical Care, 9*(4), 235-244.

Riemsma, R.P., et al. (2003). Systematic review of the effectiveness of stage based interventions to promote smoking cessation. *British Medical Journal, 326*(74), 1175-1178.

Robinson, A.W. (2002). Older women's experiences if living alone after heart surgery. *Applied Nursing Research, 15*(3), 118-125.

Robotic heart surgery (2002). *Science News, 162*(23), 365.

Ryan, D. (2000). Is it an MI? A lab primer for myocardial infarction. *RN, 63*(1), 26-31.

Sadovsky, R. (2003a). Clopidogrel vs. aspirin in preventing acute MI. *American Family Physician, 67*(5), 1085.

Sadovsky, R. (2003b). Preventing plaque rupture: New clinical strategies. *American Family Physician, 67*(6), 1362-1365.

Sakallaris, et al. (2000). Same-day transfer of patients to the cardiac telemetry unit after surgery: The rapid after bypass back into telemetry (Rabbit) program. *Critical Care Nurse, 20*(2), 50-68.

Skidmore-Roth, L. (2002). *Mosby's nursing drug reference.* St. Louis: Mosby.

Sneed, N.V., et al. (2001). Influence of a relaxation intervention on perceived stress and power spectral analysis of heart rate variability. *Progress in Cardiovascular Nursing, 16*(2), 57-62.

Solomon, A.J., & Gersh, B.J. (2000). Unstable coronary artery disease. In T. Nguyen et al. (Eds.), *Management of complex cardiovascular problems* (pp. 1-14). Armonk, NY: Futura Publishing.

Verosky, D. (2003). Using pharmacologic stress testing to evaluate cardiac perfusion. *Nursing 2003, 33*(8), 68.

Watson, R.D., Chin, B.S.P., & Lip, G.Y.H. (2002). ABC of antithrombotic therapy. *British Medical Journal, 325*(7356), 1348-1352.

*Wenger, N.K., et al. (1995). *Cardiac rehabilitation as secondary prevention. Clinical practice guideline. Quick reference guide for clinicians, No. 17.* AHCPR Pub. No. 96-0673. Rockville, MD: Agency for Health Care Policy and Research and National Heart, Lung, and Blood Institute, Public Health Service, U.S. Department of Health and Human Services.

Wilson, J. (2000). Beating-heart surgery. *Popular Mechanics, 177*(4), 50-52.

Women and heart disease. (2003). *Harvard Heart Letter, 13*(9), 7.

Woods, A. (2004). Loosening the grip of hypertension. *Nursing 2004, 34*(12), 36-43.

Yates, B.C., Braklow-Whitton, J.L., & Agrawal, S. (2003). Outcomes of cardiac rehabilitation participants and nonparticipants in a rural area. *Rehabilitation Nursing, 28*(2), 57-64.

Yoshihiro, M. (2002). Coronary artery disease: Repeat stenting not always durable. *Heart Disease Weekly, June 16,* 12-13.

Zanabria, E., & Welch, G. (2003). Hypertension and exercise. *American Fitness, 21*(2), 56-60.

Zepf, B. (2003a). Walking vs. vigorous exercise for heart health in women. *American Family Physician, 67*(3), 599.

Zepf, B. (2003b). Choosing anticoagulation or aspirin after heart attack. *American Family Physician, 67*(6), 1399.

UNIT **NINE**

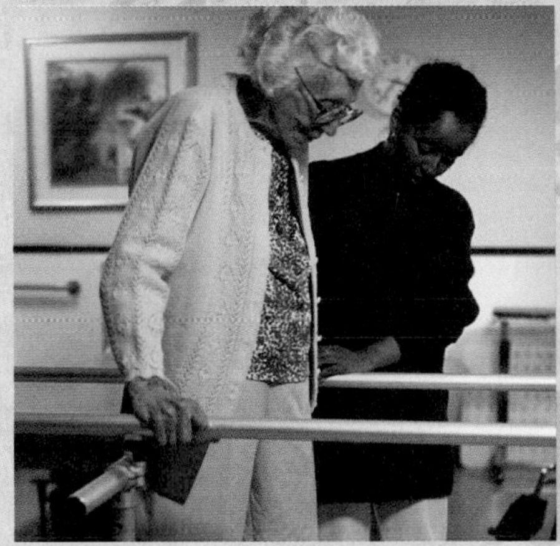

PROBLEMS of TISSUE PERFUSION

Management of Clients with Problems of the Hematologic System

CHAPTER

42 Assessment of the Hematologic System

M. LINDA WORKMAN

LEARNING OUTCOMES

After studying this chapter, you should be able to:

1. Describe the hematologic changes associated with aging.
2. Explain the process of erythrocyte maturation.
3. Describe the role of platelets in hemostasis.
4. Compare the structure and function of platelet plugs and fibrin clots.
5. Interpret blood cell counts and clotting tests to assess the client's hematologic status.
6. Compare the actions and uses of anticoagulants, fibrinolytics, and inhibitors of platelet activity.
7. Develop a community-based teaching plan for the client on anticoagulant therapy at home.
8. Prioritize nursing care for the client after bone marrow aspiration.

Go to your Student CD-ROM for Review Questions
for the NCLEX Examination keyed to these Learning Outcomes.

The hematologic system is the blood, blood cells, lymph, and organs involved with blood formation or blood storage. All systems depend on circulation; thus any problem of the hematologic system affects total body health and well-being. This chapter, together with Chapter 23, reviews the normal physiology of the hematologic system and assessment of hematologic status.

ANATOMY AND PHYSIOLOGY REVIEW

Bone Marrow

Bone marrow is the blood-forming **(hematopoietic)** organ. It produces most of the cells of the blood, including red blood cells **(RBCs, erythrocytes),** white blood cells (WBCs), and platelets. Bone marrow also is involved in the immune responses (see Chapter 23).

Each day the bone marrow in a healthy adult releases about 2.5 billion RBCs, 2.5 billion platelets, and one billion white blood cells **(leukocytes)** per kilogram of body weight.

In the fetus, blood components are formed in the liver and spleen and, by the last trimester, the bone marrow. At birth, blood-producing marrow is present in every bone. The flat bones (sternum, skull, pelvic and shoulder girdles) contain active blood-producing marrow throughout life. As a person ages, the amount of blood-producing marrow decreases in the long bones and in small, irregularly shaped bones. By the age of 18 years, blood production is limited to the ends of the long bones. During adulthood, fatty tissue replaces inactive bone marrow. In older adults the amount of fatty marrow increases and only a small portion of the remaining marrow continues with active blood production.

The bone marrow first produces stem cells. Stem cells are immature, undifferentiated cells that are capable of maturing into any one of several types of blood cells: RBCs, WBCs, or platelets, depending on the body's needs (Figure 42-1).

The next stage in blood cell development is the committed stem cell (also called the precursor cell or the unipotent stem cell). A committed stem cell enters one maturational pathway and can at that point differentiate into only one cell type. Committed stem cells actively divide but require the presence of a specific growth factor for maturation. For example, **erythropoietin** is a growth factor made in the kidneys that is specific for the RBC. Many different growth factors influence WBC and platelet maturation (see Chapters 23, 28, and 43).

Blood Components

Blood is composed of plasma and cells. Plasma is part of the body's extracellular fluid. It is similar to the interstitial fluid found between tissue cells, but plasma contains several times more protein than interstitial fluid contains. The three major types of plasma proteins are albumin, globulins, and fibrinogen.

Albumin increases the osmotic pressure of the blood, which prevents the plasma from leaking into the tissues (see

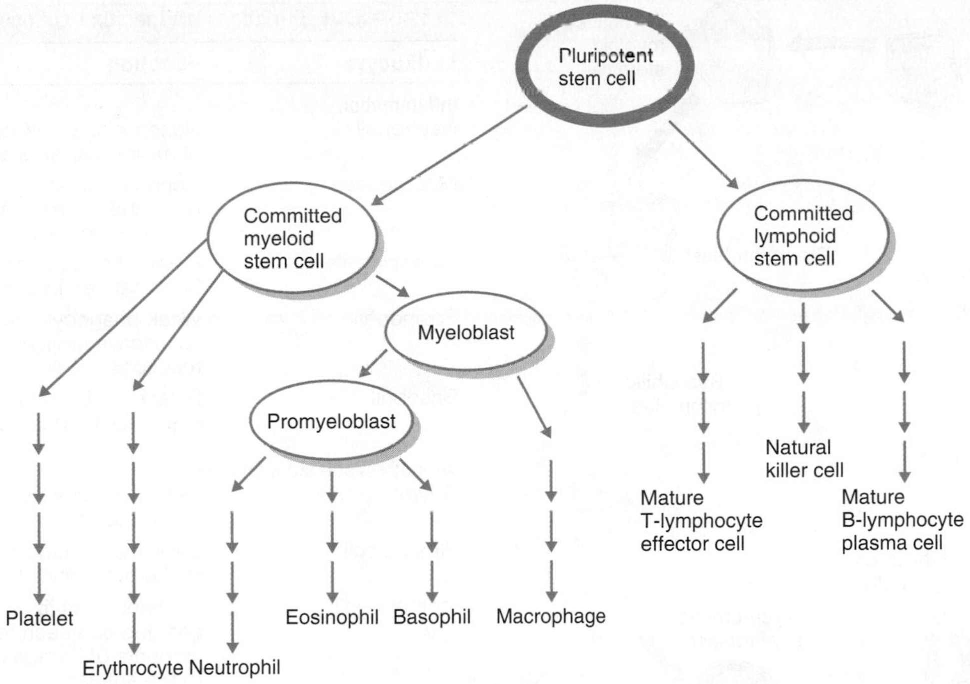

Figure 42-1 ■ Bone marrow cell differentiation and maturational pathways.

Chapter 14). Globulins have many functions, such as transporting other substances and protecting the body against infection. Globulins are also the main component of antibodies. **Fibrinogen** is a protein molecule that can be activated to form fibrin. Fibrin molecules assemble together to form structures important in the blood clotting process.

The blood cells include RBCs, WBCs, and platelets. These cells differ in structure, site of maturation, and function.

RED BLOOD CELLS (ERYTHROCYTES)

Red blood cells, or **erythrocytes,** are the largest proportion of blood cells. Mature RBCs have no nucleus and have a biconcave disk shape. Together with a flexible membrane, this feature allows RBCs to change their shape without breaking as they pass through narrow, winding capillaries. The number of RBCs a person has varies according to gender, age, and general health, but the normal range is from 4,200,000 to 6,100,000/mm^3.

As shown in Figures 42-1 and 42-2, RBCs start out as stem cells, enter the myeloid pathway, and progress in stages to the mature RBC (i.e., the erythrocyte). Healthy, mature RBCs have a life span of about 120 days after being released into the blood. As RBCs age, their membranes become more fragile. These old cells are trapped and destroyed in the tissues, spleen, and liver. Some parts of destroyed RBCs (e.g., iron), are recycled and used to make new RBCs.

The RBCs produce hemoglobin (Hgb). Each normal mature RBC contains thousands of hemoglobin molecules (Berne et al., 2004). The heme part of each hemoglobin molecule needs a molecule of iron. Only when the heme molecule is complete with iron can it transport up to four molecules of oxygen. *Therefore iron is a critical component of hemoglobin.* The globin portion of hemoglobin carries carbon dioxide. RBCs also are buffers and help maintain acid-base balance.

The most important feature of hemoglobin is its ability to combine loosely with oxygen. With only a small drop in oxygen level in the tissues, a greater increase in the transfer of oxygen from hemoglobin to tissues occurs. This transfer is also known as **oxygen dissociation.** Some problems change the speed and amount of oxygen released to the tissues.

The total number of RBCs a person has is carefully controlled through **erythropoiesis** (selective maturation of stem cells into mature erythrocytes). This process ensures that enough RBCs are present for good oxygenation without having too many cells that could "thicken" the blood and slow its flow. The trigger for control of erythropoiesis is tissue oxygenation. The kidney produces the RBC growth factor erythropoietin at the same rate as RBC destruction occurs to maintain a constant normal level of circulating RBCs. When tissue oxygenation is less than normal **(hypoxia),** the kidney increases the production of erythropoietin. This growth factor stimulates the bone marrow to increase RBC production. When tissue oxygenation is normal or high, the kidney reduces erythropoietin levels, slowing the production of RBCs. Synthetic erythropoietin (Procrit, Epogen, EPO) has the same effect on bone marrow as the naturally occurring erythropoietin.

Many substances are needed to form hemoglobin and RBCs, including iron, vitamin B_{12}, folic acid, copper, pyridoxine, cobalt, and nickel. A lack of any of these substances can lead to anemia. Anemia is the result of any problem that reduces the function or the number of erythrocytes to the point that tissue oxygen demands are not completely met (see Chapter 43).

WHITE BLOOD CELLS (LEUKOCYTES)

White blood cells (WBCs), or leukocytes, perform actions critical to inflammation or immunity (Table 42-1). The many types of WBCs all have specialized functions. Most

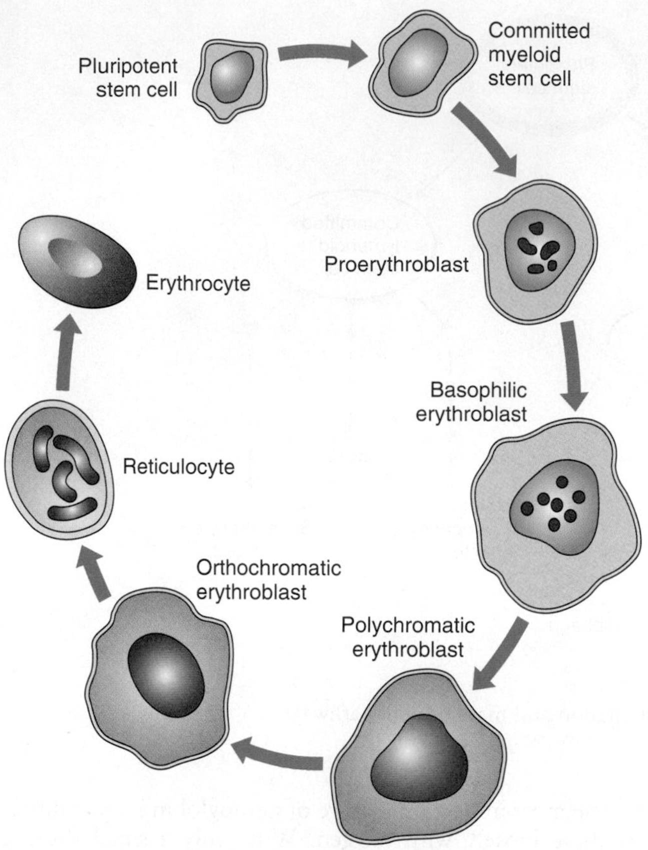

Figure 42-2 ■ Erythrocyte maturational pathway.

TABLE 42-1 Functions of Specific Leukocytes

Leukocyte	Function
Inflammation	
Neutrophil	Nonspecific ingestion and phagocytosis of microorganisms and foreign protein
Macrophage	Nonspecific recognition of foreign proteins and microorganisms; ingestion and phagocytosis
Monocyte	Destruction of bacteria and cellular debris; matures into macrophage
Eosinophil	Weak phagocytic action, releases vasoactive amines during allergic reactions
Basophil	Releases histamine and heparin in areas of tissue damage
Antibody-Mediated Immunity	
B-lymphocyte	Becomes sensitized to foreign cells and proteins
Plasma cell	Secretes immunoglobulins in response to the presence of a specific antigen
Memory cell	Remains sensitized to a specific antigen and can secrete increased amounts of immunoglobulins specific to the antigen
Cell-Mediated Immunity	
T-lymphocyte helper/ inducer T-cell	Enhances immune activity through the secretion of various factors, cytokines, and lymphokines
Cytotoxic-cytolytic T-cell	Selectively attacks and destroys non-self cells, including virally infected cells, grafts, and transplanted organs
Natural killer cell	Nonselectively attacks non-self cells, especially body cells that have undergone mutation and become malignant; also attacks grafts and transplanted organs

WBCs are formed in the bone marrow and are part of the hematopoietic system. WBC function is presented in Chapter 23 because these cells provide immunity and protect against invasion and infection.

PLATELETS

Platelets are the third type of blood cells. They are the smallest of the blood cells, formed as fragments of a giant precursor cell in the bone marrow, the **megakaryocyte.** Figure 42-1 shows the overall blood cell developmental pathway, and Figure 42-3 shows specific platelet development.

Platelets stick to injured blood vessel walls and form platelet plugs that can stop the flow of blood from the injured site. They also produce substances important to coagulation. Platelets help keep blood vessels intact by beginning the repair of damage to small blood vessels. They perform most of their functions by **aggregation** (clumping).

Bone marrow production of platelets also is precisely controlled by growth factors (thrombopoietin). After platelets leave the bone marrow, they are stored in the spleen and then released slowly to meet the body's needs. Normally 80% of platelets circulate and 20% are stored in the spleen. Each platelet has a life span of 1 to 2 weeks.

Accessory Organs of Hematopoiesis

The spleen and liver are important accessory organs of the hematopoietic system. They help to regulate the maturation of blood cells to help maintain hematologic homeostasis.

SPLEEN

The spleen is located under the diaphragm to the left of the stomach. It contains three types of tissue: white pulp, red pulp, and marginal pulp. These tissues all help to balance blood cell production with blood cell destruction and assist with immunity. White pulp is filled with white blood cells (WBCs), especially lymphocytes and macrophages. As whole blood filters through the white pulp, unwanted cells (such as bacteria and old RBCs) are removed. Red pulp contains vascular enlargements **(sinuses)** that store RBCs and platelets. Marginal pulp contains the ends of many arteries and other blood vessels.

The spleen destroys old or imperfect RBCs, breaks down the hemoglobin released from these destroyed cells, stores platelets, and filters antigens. A client who has had a splenectomy has reduced immune functions. Thus, after a splenectomy, clients are not as efficient at ridding the body of disease-causing organisms and are at greater risk for infection and sepsis.

LIVER

The liver is the main production site for prothrombin and most of the blood clotting factors. In addition, proper liver function and bile production are critical to the formation of vitamin K in the intestinal tract. (Vitamin K is essential for

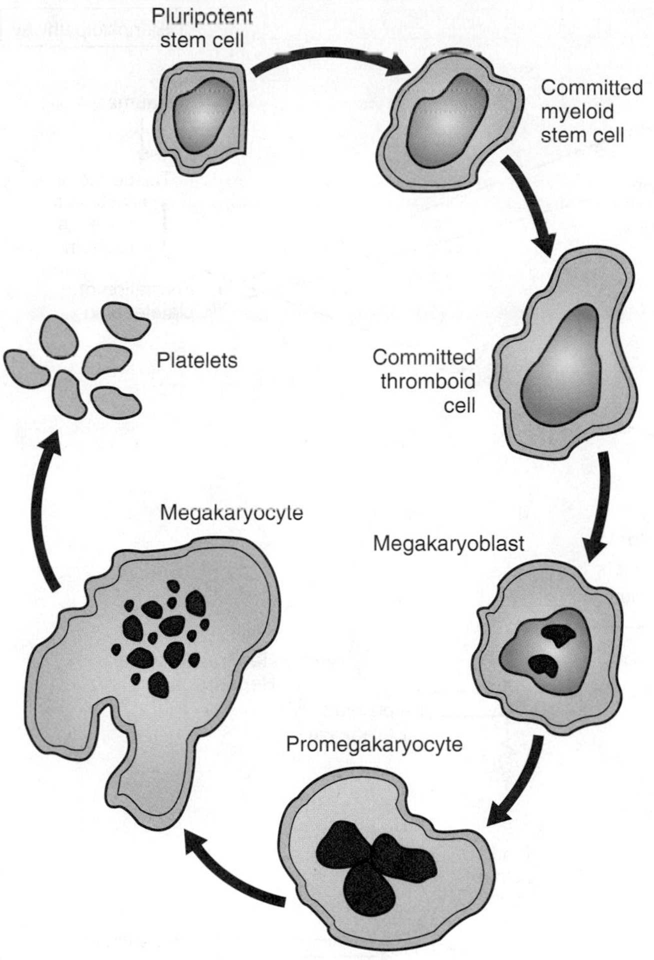

Figure 42-3 ■ Platelet maturational pathway.

producing blood clotting factors VII, IX, and X and prothrombin.) Large quantities of whole blood and blood cells can be stored in the liver. The liver also converts bilirubin (one end product of hemoglobin breakdown) to bile and stores extra iron within the protein ferritin. Small amounts of erythropoietin are produced in the liver.

Hemostasis/Blood Clotting

In hemostasis, localized blood clotting occurs in damaged blood vessels while blood continues to circulate to all other areas. Hemostasis is a complex process that balances the production of clotting and dissolving factors. It begins with the formation of a platelet plug and continues with a series of events that eventually cause the formation of a fibrin clot. Intrinsic and extrinsic factors are involved in blood clotting. Three sequential processes result in blood clotting: platelet aggregation with formation of a platelet plug, the blood clotting cascade, and the formation of a complete fibrin clot.

PLATELET AGGREGATION

Forming a platelet plug by causing platelets to clump together is essential for blood clotting. Platelets normally circulate as individual cell-like structures. They are not attracted to each other and do not clump together until activated. Usually activation causes platelet membranes to become sticky, allowing clumping to occur. When platelets become activated and clump, they form large, semisolid plugs within the lumens and walls of blood vessels and disrupt local blood flow. *These platelet plugs are not clots and cannot provide complete hemostasis.*

Some substances that cause platelets to clump include adenosine diphosphate (ADP), calcium, thromboxane A_2, and collagen. Platelets themselves can be stimulated to secrete some of these substances, whereas other substances that activate platelets are exogenous. Platelet plugs start the cascade reaction that leads to fibrin clot formation and blood coagulation.

THE BLOOD CLOTTING CASCADE

The blood clotting cascade is triggered by the formation of a platelet plug. Platelet plugs can occur from both intrinsic and extrinsic factors. The beginning of the blood clotting cascade is rapidly amplified or enhanced; that is, the final result is much larger than the triggering event. Cascades work like a landslide. A few small pebbles rolling down a steep hillside can dislodge large rocks and pieces of soil, causing a final enormous movement of earth. Just like landslides, cascade reactions are hard to stop once set into motion.

Intrinsic Factors

Intrinsic factors are problems or substances directly in the blood itself that first make platelets clump and then activate the blood clotting cascade (Figure 42-4). These factors or conditions include antigen-antibody reactions, circulating debris, prolonged venous stasis, and bacterial toxins. Continuing the cascade to the point of fibrin clot formation depends on the presence of sufficient amounts of all the various clotting factors and cofactors (Table 42-2).

Extrinsic Factors

Platelet plugs also can form as a result of changes in the blood vessels rather than in the blood. When platelet plugs form in response to blood vessel changes, the response is said to be caused by **extrinsic factors** (outside the blood). The most common extrinsic event is trauma that damages blood vessels and exposes the platelets to collagen. Collagen then activates platelets and causes clumping. The platelet plug is formed within seconds of the trauma. The blood clotting cascade is started sooner by the extrinsic pathway because some of the steps of the intrinsic pathway are bypassed.

Whether the platelet plugs were formed because of abnormal blood (intrinsic factors) or by exposure of substances from damaged blood vessels (extrinsic factors), the end result of the cascade is the same: *formation of a fibrin clot and coagulation.*

Many steps of the cascade that occur between the formation of a platelet plug and the formation of a fibrin clot are dependent on the presence of specific clotting factors as well as calcium and more platelets.

Clotting factors (see Table 42-2) are inactive enzymes that become activated in a sequence. The last part of the sequence is the activation fibrinogen into fibrin. At each step, the activated enzyme from the previous step activates the next enzyme. The last two steps in the cascade are the activation of thrombin from prothrombin and the conversion (by thrombin) of fibrinogen into fibrin. Only fibrin molecules can begin the formation of a true clot.

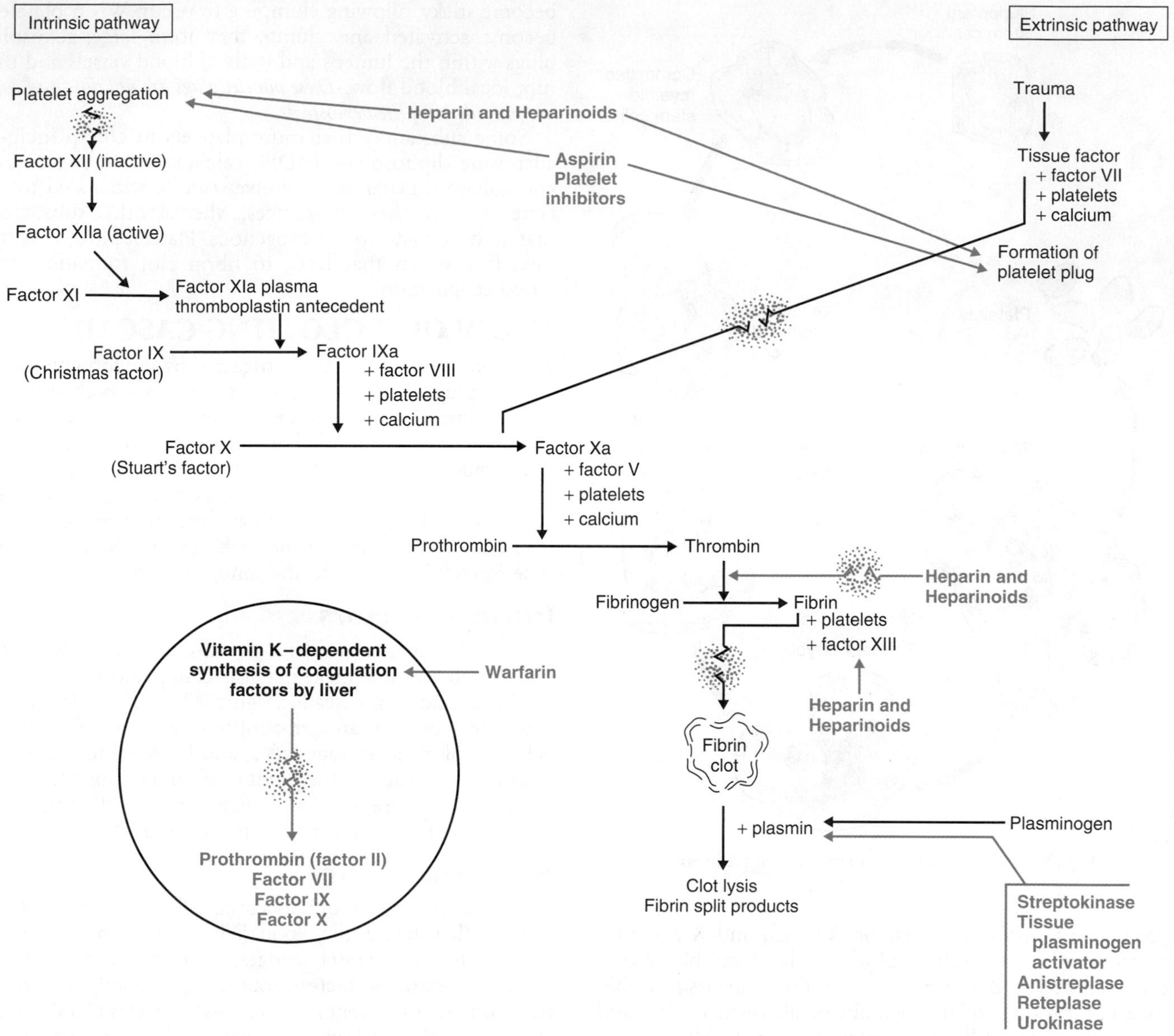

Figure 42-4 ■ Summary of blood clotting cascade.

FIBRIN CLOT FORMATION

Fibrinogen is a large, inactive protein made in the liver. The enzyme thrombin removes the end portions of fibrinogen, converting it to active fibrin. Individual fibrin molecules link together to form fibrin threads. The fibrin threads make a netlike meshwork that forms the base of a blood clot (Figure 42-5).

After the fibrin mesh is formed, clotting factor XIII tightens up the mesh, making it more dense and stable. More platelets stick to the threads of the mesh and attract other blood cells and proteins to form an actual blood clot. As this clot retracts, the **serum** (plasma without the clotting factors) is extruded, and clot formation is complete.

FIBRINOLYSIS

Because blood clotting occurs through a rapid cascade process, in theory it keeps forming fibrin clots whenever the cascade is set into motion until all blood throughout the entire body has coagulated. Such widespread clotting would lead to death. Therefore, whenever the blood clotting cascade is started, counterclotting or **anticoagulant** forces are also started. These forces limit clot formation to damaged areas only so that normal blood flow is maintained everywhere else. When blood clotting and anticlotting actions are normal and balanced, clotting occurs only where it is needed and normal blood flow elsewhere is maintained.

The fibrinolytic system dissolves the fibrin clot with special enzymes (Figure 42-6). The key to fibrinolysis is activating plasminogen to plasmin. Plasmin, an active enzyme, then digests fibrin, fibrinogen, and prothrombin, thus breaking down the fibrin clot.

Hematologic Changes Associated with Aging

Aging changes the cellular and plasma components of blood. Chart 42-1 lists assessment tips for older adults. Sev-

TABLE 42-2 The Clotting Factors

Factor	Action	Factor	Action
I: Fibrinogen	Factor I is converted to fibrin by the enzyme thrombin. Individual fibrin molecules form fibrin threads, which are the scaffold for clot formation and wound healing.	VIII: Antihemophilic factor	Factor VIII together with activated factor IX enzymatically activates factor X. In addition, factor VIII combines with another protein (von Willebrand's factor) to help platelets adhere to capillary walls in areas of tissue injury. A lack of factor VIII is the basis for classic hemophilia (hemophilia A).
II: Prothrombin	Factor II is the inactive precursor of thrombin. Prothrombin is activated to thrombin by coagulation factor X (Stuart-Prower factor). After it is activated, thrombin converts fibrinogen (coagulation factor I) into fibrin and activates factors V and VIII. Synthesis is vitamin K–dependent.	IX: Plasma thromboplastin component (Christmas factor)	Factor IX, when activated, activates factor X to convert prothrombin to thrombin. This factor is essential in the common pathway between the intrinsic and extrinsic clotting cascades. A lack of factor IX is the basis for hemophilia B. Synthesis is vitamin K–dependent.
III: Tissue thromboplastin	Factor III interacts with factor VII to initiate the extrinsic clotting cascade.	X: Stuart-Prower factor	Factor X, when activated, converts prothrombin into thrombin. Synthesis is vitamin K–dependent.
IV: Calcium	Calcium (Ca^{2+}), a divalent cation, is a cofactor for most of the enzyme-activated processes required in blood coagulation. Calcium also enhances platelet aggregation and makes red blood cells clump together.	XI: Plasma thromboplastin antecedent	Factor XI, when activated, assists in the activation of factor IX. However, a similar factor must exist in tissues. People who are deficient in factor XI have mild bleeding problems after surgery but do not bleed excessively as a result of trauma.
V: Proaccelerin	Factor V is a cofactor for activated factor X, which is essential for converting prothrombin to thrombin.	XII: Hageman factor	Factor XII is critically important in the intrinsic pathway for the activation of factor XI.
VI: Discovered to be an artifact	No factor VI is involved in blood coagulation.	XIII: Fibrin-stabilizing factor	Factor XIII assists in forming cross-links among the fibrin threads to form a strong fibrin clot.
VII: Proconvertin	Factor VII activates factors IX and X, which are essential in converting prothrombin to thrombin. Synthesis is vitamin K–dependent.		

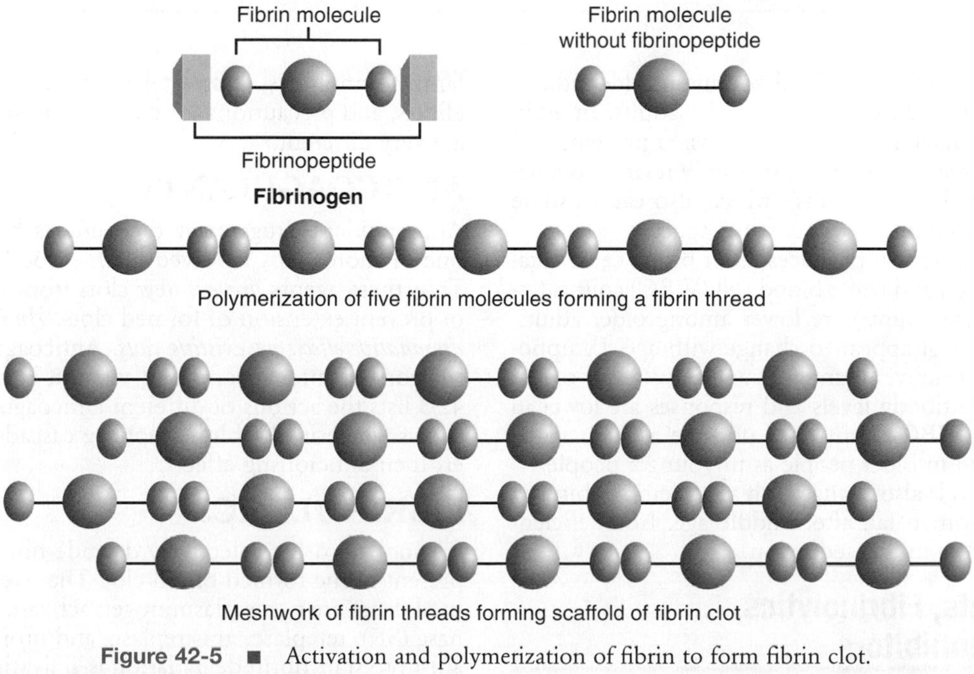

Figure 42-5 ■ Activation and polymerization of fibrin to form fibrin clot.

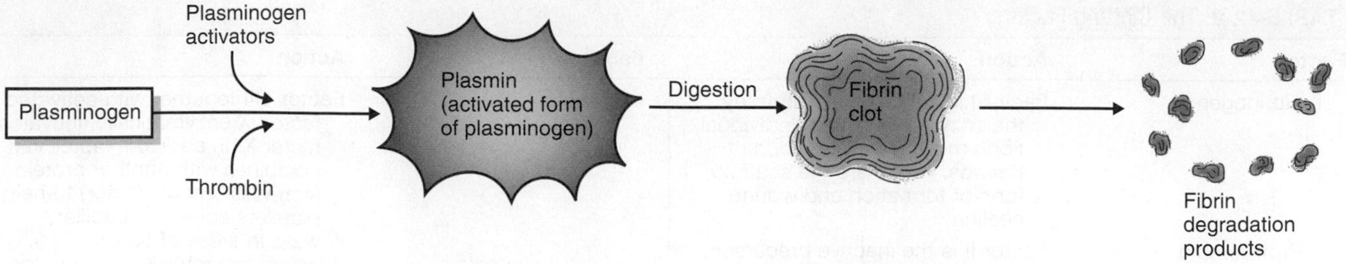

Figure 42-6 ■ The process of fibrinolysis.

CHART 42-1

NURSING FOCUS on the OLDER ADULT
Hematologic Assessment

Findings in Hematologic Disorders	Normal Changes in the Older Adult	Significance/Alternatives
Nail Beds (for Capillary Refill)		
Pallor or cyanosis may indicate a hematologic disorder.	Thickened or discolored nails make visualization of skin color beneath the nails impossible.	Use another body area, such as the lip, to assess central capillary refill.
Hair Distribution		
Thin or absent hair on the trunk or extremities may indicate poor circulation to a particular area.	Progressive loss of body hair is a normal facet of aging.	A relatively even pattern of hair loss that has occurred over an extended period is not significant.
Skin Moisture		
Skin dryness may indicate any of a number of hematologic disorders.	Skin dryness is a normal result of aging.	Skin moisture is not usually a reliable indicator of an underlying pathologic condition in the older adult.
Skin Color		
Skin color changes, especially pallor and jaundice, are associated with some hematologic disorders.	Pigment loss and skin yellowing are common changes associated with aging.	Pallor in an older adult may not be a reliable indicator of anemia; laboratory testing is required. Yellow-tinged skin in an older adult may not be a reliable indicator of increased serum bilirubin levels; laboratory testing is required.

eral factors cause a decreased blood volume in older adults. Total body water is decreased among older adults. In addition, they tend to have lower levels of plasma proteins and decreased plasma osmotic pressure (possibly related to a decreased dietary intake of proteins), which also causes some loss of blood volume into the interstitial space.

As bone marrow ages, it produces fewer blood cells. Total red blood cell (RBC) and white blood cell (WBC) counts (especially lymphocyte counts) are lower among older adults. Platelet counts do not appear to change with age. Lymphocytes become less reactive to antigens and have a loss of immune function. Antibody levels and responses are lower in older adults. The WBC count does not rise as high in response to infection in older people as in younger people.

Hemoglobin levels also change with age. Hemoglobin levels in men and women fall after middle age. Iron-deficient diets may play a role in this reduction.

Anticoagulants, Fibrinolytics, and Platelet Inhibitors

Drug therapy is used to reduce clotting ability or to destroy existing clots when circulation is at risk. The broad categories of drugs that perform these functions are anticoagulants, fibrinolytics, and platelet inhibitors. The actions, side effects, and precautions for drugs in each of these categories are very different.

ANTICOAGULANTS

Anticoagulant drugs exert their effects by interfering with one or more steps involved in the blood clotting cascade. Thus these agents *prevent* new clots from forming and limit or prevent extension of formed clots. *Anticoagulants have no degradative effects on existing clots.* Anticoagulants are further categorized into heparin and vitamin K antagonists. Table 42-3 lists the actions of different anticoagulants. Figure 42-4 shows where in the blood clotting cascade these agents exert their anticlotting effects.

FIBRINOLYTICS

Fibrinolytic drugs selectively degrade fibrin threads already present in the formed blood clot. The five most commonly used drugs are tissue plasminogen activator (t-PA), streptokinase (SK), reteplase, anistreplase, and urokinase. The mechanism to start fibrin degradation is activation of the inactive tissue protein **plasminogen** to its active form, **plasmin**. Plasmin directly attacks and degrades the fibrin molecule, having fewer effects on the fibrinogen molecule. Thus the ac-

TABLE 42-3 Anticoagulants, Fibrinolytics, and Platelet Inhibitors

Agent	Mechanism of Action	Side Effects/Precautions	Nursing Implications
Anticoagulants			
Heparin (Calciparin, Hepalean✱)	Potentiates the inhibiting actions of antithrombin III Interferes with thrombin formation Prevents conversion of fibrinogen to fibrin	Prevents clot formation	Check client for bleeding
		Has no effect on existing clots	Used for prevention of clot formation or extension
		Must be given parenterally	Teach client proper technique for home administration
		Antidote is protamine sulfate	Keep protamine sulfate on the unit when a client is receiving heparin
		Half-life is 1 to 6 hr	Client is most at risk for excessive bleeding in the first few hours after administration
		Derived from animal sources	Check client for possible allergic reactions
		Can induce thrombocytopenia	Monitor platelet count, monitor for blood in urine, stool, emesis; check skin for increasing bruises or petechiae
Low-Molecular-Weight Heparins			
Enoxaparin (Lovenox)	Same as heparin	Same as heparin, less allergenic, does not alter laboratory value	Does not require monitoring of drug levels or aPTT Same as for heparin
Dalteparin (Fragmin, Tedelparin)	Similar to heparin Also inhibits clotting factor Xa	Same as for enoxaparin	Same as for enoxaparin
Vitamin K Antagonists			
Warfarin (Coumadin, Warfilone✱)	Disrupts liver synthesis of vitamin K–dependent clotting factors (factors II, VII, IX, X)	Requires 48-96 hr to peak effect	May be started while the client is still receiving heparin
		Requires 1 wk to clear after drug is discontinued	Instruct client that bleeding precautions are still needed for at least a week after stopping the drug
		Anticoagulation is additive to that of platelet inhibitors	Warn clients not to take aspirin or other platelet inhibitors unless prescribed by the health care provider who also prescribed the warfarin
		Blood levels fluctuate with diet and other factors	Instruct clients to keep all appointments for drug level checks and not to self adjust drug dosages
Fibrinolytics			
Reteplase (Retavase)	Activates plasminogen into plasmin, which breaks degrades fibrin, disintegrating clots	Peak activity is immediate, lasting about an hour	Avoid venipunctures during and for one hour after administration
		May induce intracranial hemorrhage in older clients	Do not place clients in a position in which the head is dependent to the body; assess neurologic status every 30 minutes for the first 3 hours after administration
		Affects all existing clots <24 hr old	Assess any incisions, venipuncture sites, previous areas of trauma for bleeding
Anistreplase (Eminase)	Binds with plasminogen to form a complex that digests fibrin	Activity persists for 2-4 hr after administration	Avoid venipunctures during and for 4 hours after drug administration
		Others same as for reteplase	Same as for reteplase
Alteplase (Activase)	Same as for reteplase	Same as for reteplase	Same as for reteplase
Streptokinase (Streptase)	Same as for anistreplase	Made from exogenous substances and is allergenic	Check client for mild and severe allergic reactions during and after treatment (rash, hypotension, difficulty breathing, wheezing); keep emergency equipment and medications in client's room
		Not clot specific, also disrupts clotting cascade-greater risk for hemorrhage	Use bleeding precautions when handling the client; assess for excessive bleeding at least every 15 minutes during and for 2 hours after drug administration
		May not be effective in clients who have had multiple *Streptococcal* infections	Assess for drug effectiveness during administration

Data from Facts and Comparisons. (2004). *Drug facts and comparisons* (58th ed.). St. Louis: Author.

Continued

TABLE 42-3 Anticoagulants, Fibrinolytics, and Platelet Inhibitors—*cont'd*

Agent	Mechanism of Action	Side Effects/Precautions	Nursing Implications
Fibrinolytics—*cont'd*			
Urokinase (Abbokinase)	Same as for reteplase	Fibrinogen levels remain low for 12-24 hr	Use bleeding precautions for at least 24 hours after drug administration; assess for bleeding at least every 2 hours for the first 24 hours.
		Produced by cultured human cells, thus has the potential to transmit infectious disease	Assess client for manifestations of infection at least every shift during hospitalization; teach client to have regular monitoring for blood-borne diseases for at least 1 year after therapy.
Platelet Inhibitors			
Aspirin	Disrupts production of thromboxane A-2, preventing platelets aggregation	Can trigger asthma when taken frequently or in high doses	Instruct clients to stop aspirin if wheezing occurs
		Platelet aggregation is affected for up to 10 days after a single dose	Instruct clients to discontinue aspirin at least a week before scheduled dental work, surgery and other invasive procedures
		Irritates gastric lining and promotes gastrointestinal ulceration	Teach clients to take drug with food and to observe stools for evidence of bleeding (bright red blood, black tarry-looking stools)
Abciximab (ReoPro)	Is an antibody that binds to the receptors on the platelet surface that normally bind the sticky glycoproteins, preventing platelet adhesion	Contains human and mouse proteins that may induce an allergic reaction	Teach client to observe for any skin rashes, swelling, or difficulty breathing that may indicate an allergy to the drug
Clopidogrel (Plavix)	Prevents ADP from binding to platelet receptors, inhibiting platelet activation	Platelet function remains low for up to 5 days after the drug is discontinued	Instruct clients to avoid dental work and invasive procedures while taking this drug or to inform health care professionals that he or she is taking the drug
		Irritates gastric lining and promotes gastrointestinal ulceration	Teach clients to take drug with food and to observe stools for evidence of bleeding (bright red blood, black tarry-looking stools)
		Prolongs bleeding	Same as for aspirin
Dipyridamole (Persantine)	Increases levels of adenosine which then inhibits ADP formation and platelet activation	Produces peripheral vasodilation	Teach clients that their blood pressure could be lower than normal during position changes and that they should move slowly when changing from a sitting or lying position to a standing position
		Prolongs bleeding	Same as for aspirin

Data from Facts and Comparisons. (2004). *Drug facts and comparisons* (58th ed.). St. Louis: Author.

tion of fibrinolytic drugs is the selective breakdown of formed fibrin clots with less effect on clot formation.

The use of fibrinolytic drugs results in the best clot breakdown with less disruption of blood clotting. These drugs are the first-line therapy for problems caused by small, localized formed clots such as myocardial infarction (MI), limited arterial thrombosis, and thrombotic strokes. For some problems, such as MI, these drugs are only given within the first 6 hours after the onset of symptoms. This time limitation is not related to drug activity because fibrinolytic agents can break down clots older than 6 hours. Rather, the tissue that has been anoxic for more than 6 hours as a result of an acute event is not likely to benefit from this therapy, making the risks to the client greater than the advantages.

Fibrinolytic therapy has a limited role when clotting is extensive, such as in deep vein thrombophlebitis. With these problems, clots are very large compared with the size of the clots found in the coronary arteries. The amount of drug and the duration of therapy needed for breakdown of such large clots are cost prohibitive and risky. Many of these clots are not easily accessed for direct infusion of the fibrinolytic drug. In addition, these clots are large and the drug response creates many small clots that can enter circulation **(emboli).** These emboli could potentially occlude other blood vessels. The chance of emboli formation is much greater when degrading large venous clots than it is for degrading smaller arterial clots. In such cases, mechanical thrombolytic devices may be able to debulk the clot. These devices remove debris or break it into fragments small enough to pass through capillary beds without causing vessel occlusion.

One exception for using fibrinolytics in large clots is the newly approved use of urokinase for adults who have massive pulmonary emboli with obstruction of blood flow either to an entire lobe or to multiple segments (see Chapter 35 for further discussion of pulmonary emboli therapy).

PLATELET INHIBITORS

Platelet inhibitors are drugs that either prevent platelets from becoming active or prevent activated platelets from clumping together. The most widely used drug for this effect is aspirin, which inhibits the production of substances that can trigger platelet activation, such as thromboxane. Other drugs change the platelet membrane, reducing its "stickiness," or prevent activators from binding to platelet receptor sites. Table 42-3 lists the actions and nursing implications for specific platelet inhibitors.

ASSESSMENT TECHNIQUES

History

DEMOGRAPHIC DATA

Chart 42-2 lists questions based on Gordon's Functional Health Patterns to ask during assessment of hematologic function. Age and gender are important variables to obtain when assessing the client's hematologic status. Bone marrow and immune activity diminish with age.

WOMEN'S HEALTH CONSIDERATIONS

At all ages, women have lower blood cell counts than do men. This difference is greater during menstrual years. This gender difference may be related to a blood dilution caused by fluid retention from female hormones or to differences in bone marrow activity.

FAMILY HISTORY AND GENETIC RISK

Obtaining an accurate family history is important because many bleeding disorders are inherited. Ask whether anyone in the family has had hemophilia, frequent nosebleeds, postpartum hemorrhages, excessive bleeding after tooth extractions, or heavy bruising after relatively mild trauma. Obtain family information about sickle cell disease or sickle cell trait. Although sickle cell disease is seen most often among African Americans, anyone can have the trait.

PERSONAL HISTORY

Personal factors to be included in the hematologic assessment are liver function, the presence of known immunologic or hematologic disorders, and current drug use. Because the liver makes clotting factors, ask about manifestations that may indicate liver problems, such as jaundice, anemia, and gallstones.

Ask the client about use of blood "thinners" such as warfarin (Coumadin, Warfilone✱), aspirin, and other nonsteroidal anti-inflammatory drugs (NSAIDs). A person who takes aspirin daily may have bleeding problems, and many over-the-counter drugs contain aspirin or other drugs that disrupt platelet clumping. Check all drugs that the client is using or has used in the past 3 weeks. Ask about the use of antibiotics because prolonged antibiotic therapy can lead to clotting problems or bone marrow depression. Table 42-4 lists drugs known to change hematologic function. Previous radiation therapy may result in some permanent impairment of hematologic function if marrow-forming bones were in the radiation path.

CHART 42-2

Hematologic Assessment
USING GORDON'S FUNCTIONAL HEALTH PATTERNS

Activity-Exercise Pattern
- How does your energy level seem to you compared with last year at this time?
- Do you feel rested after a typical night's sleep?
- Have you experienced any dizziness or light-headedness?
- Does your heart ever seem to pound?
- How much exercise do you get? How often? What type?
- Do you feel you have enough energy to do what you want or need to do?

Nutrition-Metabolic Pattern
- Have you noticed any change in your skin lately?
- How easily do you bruise?
- Do your gums ever bleed? Under what conditions?
- How much meat do you eat in a week?
- How often do you eat salads or other green leafy vegetables?
- Are you taking any vitamin or mineral supplements?
- Do your feet and hands usually feel warm or cold?
- Has your weight changed by 5 pounds or more this year?
- How often do you take aspirin or any other nonsteroidal anti-inflammatory drug?
- What medications do you take daily?

Modified from Gordon, M. (2002). *Manual of nursing diagnosis* (10th ed.). St. Louis: Mosby.

It is also important to collect information about occupation, hobbies, and the location of housing. This information may indicate an exposure to agents or chemicals that affect bone marrow growth and hematologic function.

DIET HISTORY

Dietary pattern can alter cell quality and affect blood clotting. Ask clients to record everything eaten during the previous week. Use this information to determine the causes of anemias and of protein, mineral, or vitamin deficiencies. Diets high in fat and carbohydrates and low in protein, iron, and vitamins can cause many types of anemia and decrease the functions of all blood cells.

Ask the clients about alcohol consumption. Chronic alcoholism can cause nutritional deficiencies and liver impairment, both of which reduce blood clotting.

Certain dietary habits can enhance blood clotting. Diets high in vitamin K may increase the rate of blood clotting. Assess the amount of raw, leafy green vegetables that the client eats and whether he or she routinely takes supplemental vitamins. Also assess the amount of calcium in the diet or in supplements.

SOCIOECONOMIC STATUS

Assess the client's ability to understand and follow instructions related to diet, procedures and tests, and therapeutic regimens. Ask about personal resources, such as finances and social support. A person with a poor income may have a diet low in iron and protein.

CURRENT HEALTH PROBLEMS

Determine whether the client has had swelling of lymph nodes or excessive bruising or bleeding and whether the bleeding was spontaneous or induced by trauma. Ask about the amount and duration of bleeding after routine dental work.

TABLE 42-4 Drugs Impairing the Hematologic System

Generic Name	Common Trade Names
Drugs Causing Bone Marrow Suppression	
Altretamine	Hexalen, Hexastat✱
Amphotericin B	Fungizone
Azathioprine	Imuran
Chemotherapeutic agents*	
Chloramphenicol	Chloromycetin, Novochlorocap✱
Chromic phosphate	Phosphocol
Colchicine	(Generic only)
Didanosine	Videx
Eflornithine	Ornidyl
Foscarnet sodium	Foscavir
Ganciclovir	Cytovene
Interferon alfa	Actimmune, Alferon, Intron-A, Roferon-A, Wellferon
Pentamidine	Pentam 300, NebuPent, Pentacarinat✱
Sodium iodide	Iodopen
Zalcitabine	HIVID
Zidovudine	AZT, Retrovir, Novo-AZT✱
Drugs Causing Hemolysis	
Acetohydroxamic acid	Lithostat
Chlorpropamide	Diabinese, Glucamide, Novo-Propamide✱
Doxapram	Dopram
Glyburide	DiaBeta, Micronase, Euglucon✱
Mefenamic acid	Ponstel, Ponstan✱
Menadiol diphosphate	Synkayvite
Methyldopa	Aldomet, Dopamet✱
Nitrofurantoin	Macrodantin, Novo-Furantoin✱
Amoxicillin	Amoxil, Augmentin, Apo-Amoxi✱
Drugs Causing Hemolysis—*cont'd*	
Penicillin G benzathine	Bicillin, Crystapen
Penicillin V	Pen-Vee K, Pen Vee, Nu-Pen-VK✱
Primaquine	(Generic only)
Procainamide hydrochloride	Procan-SR, Promine, Pronestyl
Quinidine polygalacturonate	Cardioquin, Quinalan, Novoquinidin✱
Quinine	Legatrin, Quindan
Sulfonamides	Sulfamethoxazole (Gantanol), sulfisoxazole (Gantrisin, Novo-Soxazole✱)
Tolbutamide	Oramide, Orinase, Apo-Tolbutamide✱, Mobenol✱
Vitamin K	AquaMEPHYTON, Konakion
Drugs Disrupting Platelet Action	
Aspirin	Anacin, Ascriptin, Bufferin, Ecotrin, Entrophen✱, Riphen✱, Triaphen✱
Carbenicillin	Geopen, Pyopen✱
Carindacillin	Geocillin
Dipyridamole	Persantine, Apo-Dipyridamole✱, Novo-Dipiradol✱
Moxalactam	Moxam
Pentoxifylline	Trental
Sulfinpyrazone	Anturane, Antazone✱, Novopyrazone✱
Ticarcillin	Ticar
Ticlopidine	Ticlid
Valproic acid	Dalpro, Depakene, Epival✱

Data from United States Pharmacopeia Dispensing Information (USP DI): Vol. I. *Drug information for the health care professional* (20th ed.). Englewood, CO: Micromedix.
* General categories of chemotherapeutic agents include alkylating agents, antimitotics, antitumor antibiotics, and antimetabolites.

Determine whether a woman has **menorrhagia** (excessive menstrual flow). Ask her to estimate the number of pads or tampons used during the most recent menstrual cycle and whether this amount represents a change from her usual pattern of menstrual flow. Determine whether clots are present in menstrual blood. If the client has had menstrual clots, ask her to estimate clot size using coins or fruit for comparison ("clots are dime-sized" or "clots are the size of lemons").

Assess whether the client has dyspnea on exertion, palpitations, frequent infections, fevers, recent weight loss, headaches, or paresthesias. Any or all of these symptoms may occur with hematologic disease.

The single most common symptom of anemia is fatigue. Ask clients about feeling tired, needing more rest, or losing endurance during normal activities. Ask them to compare their activities during the past month with those of the same month a year ago. Determine whether they have other symptoms of anemia, such as vertigo, tinnitus, and a sore tongue.

Physical Assessment

Assess the whole body; hematologic dysfunction affects all systems. Certain problems are specific for hematologic assessment in older adults (see Chart 42-1).

SKIN ASSESSMENT

Inspect the color of the skin for pallor or jaundice and of the mucous membranes and nail beds for pallor or cyanosis. Pallor of the gums, conjunctivae, and palmar creases indicates decreased hemoglobin levels. Assess the gums for active bleeding in response to light pressure or brushing the teeth with a soft-bristled brush and any lesions or draining areas. Inspect for petechiae and large bruises **(ecchymoses). Petechiae** are pinpoint hemorrhagic lesions in the skin. Bruises may be confluent or clustered. For hospitalized clients, determine whether there is bleeding from sites such as nasogastric tubes, endotracheal tubes, central lines, peripheral intravenous (IV) sites, or Foley catheters. Check the skin turgor and ask about itching because dry skin or itching can indicate hematologic disease.

CULTURAL CONSIDERATIONS

Pallor and cyanosis are more easily detected in people with darker skin by examining the oral mucous membranes and the conjunctiva of the eye. Jaundice can be seen more easily on the roof of the mouth. Petechiae may be visible only on the palms of the hands or the soles of the feet. Bruises can be seen as darker areas of skin and palpated as slight swellings or irregular skin surfaces. Ask the client about pain when skin surfaces are touched lightly or palpated. (Chapter 69 provides tips for assessing darker skin.)

HEAD AND NECK ASSESSMENT

Check for pallor or ulceration of the oral mucosa. The tongue may be completely smooth in pernicious anemia and iron deficiency anemia or smooth and red in nutritional deficiencies. These manifestations may occur with fissures at the corners of the mouth. Assess for jaundice of the sclera.

Inspect and palpate all lymph node areas. Document any lymph node enlargement, including whether palpation of the enlarged node causes pain. It is important to determine whether the enlarged node moves or remains fixed with palpation.

RESPIRATORY ASSESSMENT

Assess the rate and depth of respiration while the client is at rest as well as during and after mild physical activity (e.g., walking 20 steps in 10 seconds). Note whether the client can complete a 10-word sentence without stopping for a breath. Assess whether the client is fatigued easily, has shortness of breath at rest or on exertion, or needs extra pillows to sleep comfortably at night. Many anemias cause these symptoms.

CARDIOVASCULAR ASSESSMENT

Observe for heaves, distended neck veins, edema, or signs of phlebitis. Auscultate for murmurs, gallops, irregular rhythms, and abnormal blood pressure (BP). Systolic BP tends to be lower than normal in clients with anemia. If hypercellularity is present, BP is higher than normal. Severe anemias can cause enlargement of the right ventricle and heart disease.

RENAL AND URINARY ASSESSMENT

The kidneys have many blood vessels, and bleeding problems may manifest as overt or occult **hematuria** (blood in the urine). Inspect a voided sample of urine for color. Hematuria may appear as grossly bloody red or dark brownish gold urine. Test the urine for proteins with a urine test dipstick because hematologic problems may increase the protein content of the urine. Also test the urine sample for occult blood (Hemoccult test).

MUSCULOSKELETAL ASSESSMENT

Rib or sternal tenderness is an important sign of hematologic malignancy. Examine the superficial surfaces of all bones, including the ribs and sternum, by applying intermittent firm pressure with the fingertips. Assess the range of joint motion and document any swelling or joint pain.

ABDOMINAL ASSESSMENT

The normal adult spleen is usually not palpable. An enlarged spleen, however, occurs with many hematologic problems. An enlarged spleen may be detected by percussion, although palpation is more reliable. The spleen lies just beneath the abdominal wall, under the ribs on the left side. When it is enlarged, the spleen can be identified by its movement during respiration. During palpation have the client lie in a relaxed, supine position while you stand on the client's right and palpate the left upper quadrant. *Palpate gently and cautiously because an enlarged spleen may be tender and easily ruptured.*

Palpating the edge of the liver in the right upper quadrant of the abdomen can detect hepatic enlargement, which is often associated with hematologic problems. The normal liver may be palpable as much as 4 to 5 cm below the right costal margin but is usually not palpable in the epigastrium.

A common cause of anemia among older adults is a chronically bleeding gastrointestinal lesion. If the lesion or open area is located in the stomach or the small intestine, obvious blood may not be visible in the stool, or such a small amount is passed each day that the client is not aware of it. Therefore obtain a stool specimen for occult blood testing.

CENTRAL NERVOUS SYSTEM ASSESSMENT

Examination of cranial nerves and neurologic function is important in hematologic assessment because some problems cause specific nervous system manifestations. Vitamin B_{12} deficiency impairs cerebral, olfactory, spinal cord, and peripheral nerve function, and severe chronic deficiency may cause permanent neurologic degeneration. Many neurologic problems can develop in clients who have hematologic malignancies as a consequence of bleeding, infection, or tumor spread. When the client with a known or suspected bleeding disorder has any head trauma, expand the assessment to include frequent neurologic checks and mental status examinations (see Chapter 44).

Other clinical manifestations that occur with impaired hematologic function include fever, chills, and night sweats.

Psychosocial Assessment

The client with hematologic problems may have a chronic illness (e.g., hemophilia or cancer) or an acute episode of a chronic disease (e.g., pernicious anemia). In either case, each person brings his or her own coping style to the illness. Develop a rapport with the client and learn what coping mechanisms he or she has used successfully during past illness or crises.

Ask the client and family members about social support networks, community resources, and financial health. A problem in any of these areas can interfere with the client's adherence to therapy and, ultimately, recovery.

Critical Thinking Challenge

The client is a 22-year-old woman who is in the emergency room for an ankle injury that occurred while she was playing volleyball at a family picnic. Her complete blood count indicates a total white blood count of 8000, erythrocyte count of 200,000, hematocrit of 22%, and hemoglobin level of 8.5 g. She says she is very tired and has palpitations on exertion. Her vital signs are P 94, R 26, BP 102/70. Her oxygen saturation measured by pulse oximetry is 98% on room air.

1. Are these counts considered normal or abnormal? If any are abnormal, are they high or low?
2. Do her vital signs indicate any type of hematologic problem? Explain why or why not.
3. What specific questions regarding family history, recent health history, diet history, and personal history should you ask?

evolve For suggested answer guidelines, go to http://evolve.elsevier.com/Iggy/.

Diagnostic Assessment

LABORATORY TESTS

In hematologic disease, the most definitive signs are often the laboratory test results. Chart 42-3 lists laboratory data associated with hematologic function.

CHART 42-3

LABORATORY PROFILE
Hematologic Assessment

Test	Reference	Range	International Reference Units	Significance of Abnormal Findings
Red blood cell (RBC) count	18-64 yr	*Females:* 4.2-5.4 million/μL	4.2-5.4 × 10^{12} cells/L	*Decreased levels* indicate possible anemia or hemorrhage.
		Males: 4.7-6.1 million/μL	4.7-6.1 × 10^{12} cells/L	*Increased levels* indicate possible chronic hypoxia or polycythemia vera.
	>64 yr	*Females:* 3.8-5.2 million/μL	3.8-5.2 × 10^{12} cells/L	
		Males: 3.8-5.8 million/μL	3.8-5.8 × 10^{12} cells/L	
Hemoglobin (Hgb)	18-64 yr	*Females:* 12-16 g/dL	112-160 g/L	Same as for RBC.
		Males: 14-18 g/dL	140-180 g/L	
	>64 yr	*Females:* 11.7-16.1 g/dL	117-161 g/L	
		Males: 12.6-17.4 g/dL	126-174 g/L	
Hematocrit (Hct)	18-64 yr	*Females:* 37-47%	0.37-0.47 fraction	Same as for RBC.
		Males: 42-52%	0.42-0.52 fraction	
	>64 yr	*Females:* 35%-47%	0.35-0.47 fraction	
		Males: 37%-51%	0.37-0.51 fraction	
Mean cell hemoglobin (MCV)		80-95 mm^3	Same as reference range	*Increased levels* indicate macrocytic cells, possible anemia. *Decreased levels* indicate microcytic cells, possible iron deficiency anemia.
Mean cell hemoglobin (MCH)		27-31 pg/cell	Same as reference range	Same as for MCV.
Mean cell hemoglobin concentration (MCHC)		32-36 g/dL cells	320-370 g/L	*Increased levels* may indicate spherocytosis or anemia. *Decreased levels* may indicate iron deficiency anemia or a hemoglobinopathy.
White blood cell (WBC) count		5000-10,000/μL	5.0-10.0 × 10^9 cells/L	*Increased levels* are associated with infection, inflammation, autoimmune disorders, and leukemia. *Decreased levels* may indicate prolonged infection or bone marrow suppression.
Reticulocyte count		0.5%-0.2% of RBCs	0.005-0.020 fraction	*Increased* levels may indicate chronic blood loss. *Decreased levels* indicate possible inadequate RBC production.
Total iron binding capacity (TIBC)		250-460 mcg/dL	45-82 μmol/L	*Increased levels* indicate iron deficiency. *Decreased levels* may indicate anemia, hemorrhage, hemolysis.
Iron (Fe)		*Females:* 60-160 mcg/dL	11-29 μmol/L	*Increased levels* indicate iron excess, hemochromocytosis, liver disorders, megaloblastic anemia.
		Males: 80-180 mcg/dL	14-32 μmol/L	*Decreased levels* indicate possible iron deficiency anemia, hemorrhage.
Serum ferritin		*Females:* 10-150 ng/mL	Same as reference range	Same as for iron.
		Males: 12-300 ng/mL		
Platelet count		150,000-400,000 mm^3	150-400 × 10^9/L	*Increased levels* may indicate polycythemia vera or malignancy. *Decreased levels* may indicate bone marrow suppression, autoimmune disease, hypersplenism.
Hemoglobin electrophoresis		Hgb A_1: 95%-98%	>0.95 fraction	*Variations* indicate hemoglobinopathies.
		Hgb A_2: 2%-3%	0.020-0.030 fraction	
		Hgb F: 0.8%-2%	<0.02 fraction	
		Hgb S: 0%	0.0 fraction	
		Hgb C: 0%	0.0 fraction	

Values for people over 64 years from Tietz, N. (1995). *Clinical guide to laboratory tests* (3rd ed.). Philadelphia: W.B. Saunders.
pg, picogram; *INR*, International Normalized Ratio.

CHART 42-3

LABORATORY PROFILE
Hematologic Assessment—*cont'd*

Test	Reference	Range	International Reference Units	Significance of Abnormal Findings
Direct Coombs' and indirect Coombs' test		Negative	Negative	*Positive findings* indicate antibodies to RBCs.
Prothrombin time (PT)		11-12.5 sec	Patient PT/normal PT (INR)	*Increased time* indicates possible deficiency of clotting factors V and VII. *Decreased time* may indicate vitamin K excess.
Bleeding time		1-9 min	Same as reference range	*Increased time* may indicate inadequate platelet function or number, clotting factor deficiencies.
Fibrin degradation products		<10 mcg/mL	<10 mg/L	*Increased levels* may indicate disseminated intravascular coagulation of fibrinolysis.

Tests of Cell Number and Function

COMPLETE BLOOD COUNT

A complete blood count (CBC) includes a number of studies: red blood cell (RBC) count, white blood cell (WBC) count, hematocrit, and hemoglobin level. The RBC count measures circulating RBCs in 1 mm^3 of blood. The WBC count measures all leukocytes present in 1 mm^3 of blood. To determine the percentages of different types of leukocytes circulating in the blood, a WBC count with differential leukocyte count is performed (Chapter 23). The hematocrit (Hct) is calculated as the percentage of red blood cells in the total blood volume. The hemoglobin level is the total amount of hemoglobin in blood.

The CBC can measure other variables of the RBCs, including mean corpuscular volume (MCV), mean corpuscular hemoglobin (MCH), and mean corpuscular hemoglobin concentration (MCHC). MCV measures the average volume or size of a single RBC and is useful for classifying anemias. When the MCV is elevated, the cell is abnormally large **(macrocytic)**, as seen in megaloblastic anemias. When the MCV is decreased, the cell is abnormally small **(microcytic)**, as seen in iron deficiency anemia. The MCH is the average amount of hemoglobin by weight in a single RBC. The MCHC measures the average amount of hemoglobin by percentage in a single RBC. When the MCHC is decreased, the cell has a hemoglobin deficiency and is hypochromic, as in iron deficiency anemia.

RETICULOCYTE COUNT

Another hematologic test helpful in determining bone marrow function is the reticulocyte count. A reticulocyte is an immature RBC that still has its nucleus. An elevated reticulocyte count indicates increased RBC production by the bone marrow. Normally about 2% of circulating RBCs are reticulocytes. An elevated reticulocyte count is desirable in an anemic client or after hemorrhage because this indicates that the bone marrow is responding appropriately to a decrease in the total RBC mass. An elevated reticulocyte count without a precipitating cause usually indicates health problems, such as polycythemia vera.

HEMOGLOBIN ELECTROPHORESIS

Hemoglobin electrophoresis detects abnormal forms of hemoglobin, such as hemoglobin S in sickle cell disease. Hemoglobin A is the major type of hemoglobin in the normal RBC from an adult. Decreased hemoglobin A levels with increasing levels of other types of hemoglobin indicate some hematologic problems, such as sickle cell disease.

LEUKOCYTE ALKALINE PHOSPHATASE

Leukocyte alkaline phosphatase (LAP) is an enzyme produced by normal mature neutrophils. Elevated LAP levels occur during episodes of infection or stress. An elevated neutrophil count without an elevation in LAP level occurs with chronic myelogenous leukemia

COOMBS' TEST

The two Coombs' tests (direct and indirect) are used for blood typing. The direct test detects the presence of antibodies (also called antiglobulins) against RBCs that may be attached to a person's RBCs. Although healthy people can make these antibodies, in certain diseases (e.g., systemic lupus erythematosus, mononucleosis, lymphomas) these antibodies are directed against the client's own RBCs. The presence of these antibodies usually causes a hemolytic anemia.

The indirect Coombs' test detects the presence of circulating antiglobulins. The test is used to determine whether the client has serum antibodies to the type of RBCs that he or she is about to receive by blood transfusion.

SERUM FERRITIN, TRANSFERRIN, AND TOTAL IRON-BINDING CAPACITY

Serum ferritin, transferrin, and the total iron-binding capacity (TIBC) tests measure iron levels. Abnormal levels of iron and TIBC occur with hematologic problems, including iron deficiency anemia.

The serum ferritin test measures the amount of iron present as free iron in the plasma. The amount of serum ferritin is related to the amount of intracellular iron and represents 1% of the total body iron stores. Therefore the serum ferritin level provides a means to assess total iron stores. People with serum ferritin levels within 10 g of the normal range for their gender have adequate iron stores; people with levels 10 g or more lower than the normal range have inadequate iron stores and have difficulty recovering from any hemorrhagic event.

Transferrin is a protein that transports iron from the intestines to cell storage sites. Transferrin is not easily measured, but by measuring the amount of iron that can be bound to serum transferrin indirectly one can determine whether an adequate amount of transferrin is present. This test is the total iron binding capacity (TIBC) test. In healthy people only about 30% of the transferrin is bound to iron in the blood. TIBC is measured by taking a sample of blood and adding measured amounts of iron to it. TIBC is calculated when the blood no longer binds the iron but allows it to precipitate. TIBC increases when a person is deficient in serum iron and stored iron levels. Such a value indicates that an adequate amount of transferrin is present but less than 30% of it is bound to serum iron.

Tests Measuring Bleeding and Coagulation

CAPILLARY FRAGILITY TEST

The capillary fragility test, or Rumpel-Leede test, measures vascular hemostatic function. The intracapillary pressure in the arm is increased by occluding venous outflow or by applying controlled negative pressure to a skin area. A blood pressure cuff is usually inflated to a pressure halfway between the systolic and diastolic pressures. This pressure is maintained for 5 minutes and the petechiae that appear distal to the cuff are counted. Normally 5 to 10 petechiae appear. When the number of petechiae that form increases, the cause of excessive bleeding or bruising is capillary fragility rather than poor platelet action.

BLEEDING TIME TEST

The bleeding time test evaluates vascular and platelet activity during hemostasis. A special spring-loaded lancet that makes a uniform wound depth is applied to the forearm while a blood pressure cuff remains inflated at 40 mm Hg. Blood is blotted from the site at 30-second intervals, and the time required for the bleeding to stop is recorded. Normal bleeding time ranges from 1 to 9 minutes.

PROTHROMBIN TIME

The prothrombin time (PT) measures how long blood takes to clot. This test reflects how much of the clotting factors II, V, VII, and X is present and how well they are functioning. When enough of these clotting factors are present and functioning, the PT shows blood clotting between 11 and 13 seconds or within 85% to 100% of the time needed for a control sample of blood to clot. PT is prolonged when one or more clotting factors is deficient, such as when liver disease is present. Sodium warfarin (Coumadin, Warfilone✱) therapy is also monitored using PT levels. Usually warfarin therapy is considered appropriate when the PT is prolonged by one and a half to two times the client's normal PT value.

Facilities are using the PT test less often to assess blood clotting because control blood is taken from different people and may not be the same even in one laboratory from one day to the next. To reduce PT errors as a result of control blood variation or in some of the chemicals used in the test, the **International Normalized Ratio (INR)** is used to assess clotting time.

INTERNATIONAL NORMALIZED RATIO

The INR measures the same process as the PT in a slightly different way: by establishing a normal mean or standard for PT. The INR is calculated by dividing the client's PT by the established standard PT. A normal INR ranges between 0.7 and 1.8. When using the INR to monitor warfarin therapy, the goal is usually to maintain the client's INR is between 2.0 and 3.0 regardless of the actual PT in seconds. It is important to remember, however, that the desired INR range for any client is individualized for specific client factors.

PARTIAL THROMBOPLASTIN TIME

The partial thromboplastin time (PTT) assesses the intrinsic clotting cascade and evaluates the action of factors II, V, VIII, IX, XI, and XII. PTT is prolonged whenever any of these factors is deficient, such as in hemophilia or disseminated intravascular coagulation (DIC). Because factors II, IX, and X are vitamin K–dependent and are produced in the liver, liver disease can decrease their levels and prolong the PTT. Heparin (Calciparin, Hepalean✱) therapy is monitored by PTT. Desired therapeutic ranges for anticoagulation are 1.5 to 2.0 times normal values.

Controversy exists as to whether this test is accurate when the blood sample is taken through a vascular access device (e.g., arterial line or a normal saline lock) instead of through a separate new venipuncture. With an appropriate discard, samples obtained through vascular access devices accurately reflect the client's aPTT.

PLATELET AGGLUTINATION/AGGREGATION

Platelet aggregation, or the ability to clump, is tested by mixing the client's plasma with a substance called ristocetin. The degree of clumping is noted. Aggregation can be impaired in von Willebrand's disease and during the use of drugs such as aspirin, anti-inflammatory agents, psychotropic agents, and platelet inhibitors.

RADIOGRAPHIC EXAMINATIONS

Assessment of the client with a suspected hematologic abnormality can include radioisotopic imaging. Isotopes are used to evaluate the bone marrow for sites of active blood cell formation and sites of iron storage. Radioactive colloids are used to determine organ size and liver and spleen function.

The client is given a radioactive isotope intravenously about 3 hours before the procedure. The client is then taken to the nuclear medicine department for the scan, where he or she must lie still for about an hour. No special client preparation or follow-up care is needed for these tests.

Standard x-rays may be used to diagnose some hematologic disorders. For example, multiple myeloma causes characteristic bone destruction, with a "Swiss cheese" appearance on x-ray.

BONE MARROW ASPIRATION AND BIOPSY

Bone marrow aspiration or biopsy is often performed to evaluate the client's hematologic status when other tests show persistent abnormal findings. Results can provide important information about bone marrow function, including the production of red blood cells (RBCs), white blood cells (WBCs), and platelets. Bone marrow aspiration and bone marrow biopsy are similar invasive procedures. In a bone marrow aspiration, cells and fluids are suctioned from the bone marrow. In a bone marrow biopsy, solid tissue and cells are obtained by coring out an area of bone marrow with a large-bore needle.

A physician's order and a signed informed consent are obtained from the client before a bone marrow aspiration or biopsy is performed. Bone marrow aspiration may be performed by a physician, a sanctioned clinical nurse specialist, a nurse practitioner, or a physician assistant, depending on the agency's policy and regional law. The procedure may be performed at the client's bedside, in an examination room, or in a laboratory.

After learning what specific tests will be performed on the marrow, check the facility's procedure manual and the hematology laboratory to determine how to handle the specimen. Some tests require that heparin or other solutions be added to the specimen.

CLIENT PREPARATION. Most clients have anxiety or fear before a bone marrow aspiration. Clients who have had a bone marrow aspiration in the past may have less anxiety or more anxiety, depending on their previous experience. You can help reduce anxiety and allay fears by providing accurate information and emotional support. Some clients like to have their hand held during the procedure; others may want you to hug or hold their entire upper body.

Explain the procedure to the client and tell him or her that you will stay during the entire procedure. Occasionally a friend or family member is permitted to be present to hold the client's hand and provide additional emotional support. If a local anesthetic is used, tell the client that the injection will feel like a stinging or burning sensation. Tell him or her to expect a heavy sensation of pressure and pushing while the needle is being inserted. Some clients also can hear a crunching sound or feel a scraping sensation as the needle punctures the bone. Explain that a brief sensation of painful pulling will be experienced as the marrow is being aspirated by mild suction in the syringe. If a biopsy is performed, the client may feel more pressure and discomfort as the needle is rotated into the bone.

The client is assisted onto an examining table, and the site (most commonly the iliac crest) is exposed. If this site is not available or if more marrow is needed, the sternum can be used. If the iliac crest is the site, the client is usually placed in the prone position or, occasionally, in the side-lying position. Depending on the tests to be performed on the specimen, a laboratory technician may also be present to ensure appropriate handling of the specimen.

PROCEDURE. The procedure usually lasts from 5 to 15 minutes. Clients may have pain. The type and the amount of anesthesia or sedation depend on the physician's preference, the client's preference and previous experience with bone marrow aspiration and biopsy, and the setting.

A local anesthetic agent is injected into the skin around the site. The client may also receive a mild tranquilizer or a rapid-acting sedative, such as midazolam (Versed) or lorazepam (Ativan, Apo-Lorazepam✱, Novo-Lorazem✱). Some clients do well with guided imagery or autohypnosis.

Aspiration or biopsy procedures are invasive, and sterile precautions are observed. The skin over the site is cleaned with a disinfectant solution. For an aspiration, the needle is inserted with a twisting motion and the marrow is aspirated by pulling back on the plunger of the syringe. When sufficient marrow has been aspirated to ensure accurate analysis, the needle is rapidly withdrawn while the tissues are supported at the site. For a biopsy, a small skin incision is made and the biopsy needle is inserted through the skin opening. Pressure and several twisting motions are needed to ensure coring and loosening of an adequate amount of marrow tissue. Apply external pressure to the site until hemostasis is ensured. A pressure dressing or sandbags may be applied to reduce bleeding at the site.

FOLLOW-UP CARE. Cover the site with a dressing after bleeding is controlled, and closely observe it for 24 hours for signs of bleeding and infection. A mild analgesic (aspirin free) may be given for discomfort, and ice packs can be placed over the site to limit bruising. Instruct the client to inspect the site every 2 hours for the first 24 hours and to note the presence of active bleeding or bruising. Advise him or her to avoid contact sports or any activity that might result in trauma to the site for 48 hours.

Information obtained from bone marrow aspiration or biopsy reflects the degree and quality of bone marrow activity present. The counts made on a marrow specimen can indicate whether stem cells, blast cells, committed cells, and more mature cell forms are present in the expected quantities and proportions. In addition, bone marrow aspiration or biopsy can confirm the spread of cancer cells from other tumor sites.

Critical Thinking Challenge

The client is a 70-year-old man who is scheduled to have a bone marrow aspiration in 1 week to determine the cause of abnormal white blood cell and red blood cell counts. He has been healthy otherwise, and his only drugs are a daily multiple vitamin and one aspirin per day (81 mg). He is very concerned about the pain of the procedure and the possible results. In addition, he wants to travel by air to attend his grandson's graduation in 10 days.

1. What is your care priority for this client?
2. What will you tell him regarding pain or pain management?
3. What should you tell him about air travel within 4 days after having the procedure?

evolve For suggested answer guidelines, go to http://evolve.elsevier.com/Iggy/.

GET READY for the NCLEX Examination!

KEY POINTS

Safe Effective Care Environment

- Use good handwashing techniques before providing any care to a client who is either immunocompromised or immunodeficient.
- Use bleeding precautions (see Chart 43-11) for any client with a bleeding problem or who is receiving anticoagulants, thrombolytics, or platelet inhibitors.

Health Promotion and Maintenance

- Teach people to avoid unnecessary contact with environmental chemicals or toxins. If contact cannot be avoided, teach people to use safety precautions.
- Instruct clients about the importance of eating a diet with adequate amounts of foods that are good sources of iron, folic acid, and vitamin B_{12}.
- Teach clients who are taking anticoagulants or platelet inhibitors on a daily basis to use a soft-bristled toothbrush and to avoid flossing.
- Encourage clients who are confined to bed for any reason or who are recovering from surgery to turn and perform leg exercises at least every 2 hours.
- Instruct clients to stop taking aspirin, aspirin-containing products, or most nonsteroidal anti-inflammatory drugs (NSAIDs) 10 days to 2 weeks before having surgery or dental work.

Psychosocial Integrity

- Explain all procedures, restrictions, medications, and follow-up care to the client and family.
- Ask clients about their activity level and whether they are satisfied with the energy they have for activities.

Physiological Integrity

- Teach the side effects of the drugs to clients who are taking anticoagulants or platelet inhibitors at home.
- Teach clients who are taking anticoagulants or platelet inhibitors to assess themselves daily for increased bleeding. They should check their gums and toothbrush for fresh bleeding, look at voided urine or evacuated stool for color changes indicating bleeding, and examine their skin for the presence of bruises or petechiae.
- Stress the importance of keeping all appointments for blood testing for clients who are receiving anticoagulation therapy.
- Instruct clients taking warfarin to keep a food diary to determine whether eating habits are influencing blood clotting (especially keeping track of the amount of leafy, green raw vegetables).
- Apply an ice pack to the needle site after a bone marrow aspiration or biopsy.
- Check the needle site at least every 2 hours after a bone marrow aspiration or biopsy. If the client is going home, teach the client and family how to assess the site for bleeding and when to seek assistance.
- Instruct clients to avoid activities that may traumatize the site after a bone marrow aspiration or biopsy.

ADDITIONAL STUDY RESOURCES

Go to your Student CD-ROM for Review Questions for the NCLEX Examination.

evolve Go to http://evolve.elsevier.com/Iggy/ for Integrated Management of Care Questions for the NCLEX Examination.

SELECTED BIBLIOGRAPHY

Beitz, J. (2004). Anticoagulant-induced skin necrosis. *American Journal of Nursing, 104*(4), 31-32.

Berne, R., et al. (2004). *Physiology* (5th ed.). St. Louis: Mosby.

Buchsel, P., Murphy, B., & Newton, S. (2002). Epoetin alfa: Current and future indications and nursing implications. *Clinical Journal of Oncology Nursing, 6*(5), 261-267.

Cagen, D., Franco, M., & Vasquez, D. (2002). The ABCs of low blood cell count. *Clinical Journal of Oncology Nursing, 6*(1), 34-36.

Cleveland, K. (2003). Argatroban: A new treatment option for heparin-induced thrombocytopenia. *Critical Care Nurse, 23*(6), 61-66.

Ebersole, P., Hess, P., & Luggen, A. (2004). *Toward healthy aging: Human needs and nursing response* (6th ed.). St. Louis: Mosby.

Facts and Comparisons. (2004). Drug facts and comparisons (58th ed.). St. Louis: Author.

Gibbar-Clements, T., et al. (2000). The challenge of warfarin therapy. *American Journal of Nursing, 100*(3), 38-40.

Gordon, M. (2002). *Manual of nursing diagnosis* (10th ed.). St. Louis: Mosby.

Hirsh, J., Dalen, J., & Guyatt, G. (2001). Oral anticoagulants: Mechanisms of action, clinical effectiveness, and optimal therapeutic range. *Chest, 119*(Suppl 1), 8S-21S.

Horner, B., & Myers, S. (2004). Don't miss HIT (heparin-induced thrombocytopenia). *Burns, 30*(1), 88-90.

Jarvis, C. (2004). *Physical examination and health assessment* (4th ed.). Philadelphia: W. B. Saunders.

McCance, K., & Huether, S. (2002). *Pathophysiology: The biologic basis for disease in adults and children* (4th ed.). St. Louis: Mosby.

Mullaney, S., Letizia, M., & Jennrich, J. (2001). Enoxaparin (Lovenox): An effective and convenient anticoagulant. *MEDSURG Nursing, 10*(6), 326-329.

Nussbaum, R., McInnes, R., & Willard, H. (2001). *Thompson & Thompson: Genetics in medicine* (6th ed.). Philadelphia: W.B. Saunders.

Ogedegbe, H. (2002). Your lab focus: An overview of hemostasis. *Laboratory Medicine, 948-953*, 955-956.

O'Malley, P. (2003). Clotting and bleeding: Anticoagulation update for the clinical nurse specialist. *Clinical Nurse Specialist, 17*(2), 83-85.

Pagana, K., & Pagana, T. (2002). *Mosby's manual of diagnostic and laboratory tests* (2nd ed.). St. Louis: Mosby.

Rempher, K., & Little, J. (2004). Assessment of red blood cell and coagulation laboratory data. *AACN Clinical Issues, 15*(4), 622-637.

Stevens, S. (2000). Heparin-induced thrombocytopenia. *Journal of Vascular Nursing, 18*(2), 54-58.

Trewhitt, K. (2001). Bone marrow aspiration and biopsy: Collection and interpretation. *Oncology Nursing Forum, 28*(9), 1409-1416.

Weitz, J., & Hirsh, J. (2001). New anticoagulant drugs. *Chest, 119*(Suppl 1), 95S-107S.

Wheatley, M., Cox, J., & Nemis-White, J. (2003). Optimizing anticoagulation therapy. *Canadian Nurse, 99*(6), 16-19.

Woodrow, P. (2003). Assessing blood results in older people: Haematology and liver function tests. *Nursing Older People, 15*(3), 29-31.

CHAPTER

43

Interventions for Clients with Hematologic Problems

CONSTANCE VISOVSKY

LEARNING OUTCOMES

After studying this chapter, you should be able to:

1. Identify three clinical manifestations common to clients who have any type of anemia.
2. Explain the pattern of inheritance for sickle cell disease.
3. Prioritize nursing care for the client who has sickle cell disease.
4. Plan a diet for a client who has iron deficiency anemia or vitamin B_{12} deficiency anemia.
5. Explain the mechanism of action and potential side effects of epoetin alpha therapy.
6. Compare the pathologic mechanisms of hemolytic anemia versus aplastic anemia.
7. Compare leukemia and lymphoma for etiology, pathophysiology, and clinical manifestations.
8. List four risk factors for the development of leukemia.
9. Analyze laboratory data and clinical manifestations to determine the presence of infection in a client who has neutropenia.
10. Compare the purposes and scheduling of induction therapy, consolidation therapy, and maintenance therapy for leukemia.
11. Prioritize nursing interventions for the client with neutropenia.
12. Prioritize nursing interventions for the client with thrombocytopenia.
13. Develop a community-based teaching plan for a client with thrombocytopenia.
14. Prioritize nursing responsibilities during transfusion therapy.
15. Identify clients at risk for complications of transfusion therapy.

Go to your Student CD-ROM for Review Questions for the NCLEX Examination keyed to these Learning Outcomes.

Hematologic disorders or diseases are the result of impaired production or function, or the abnormal destruction of any type of blood cell. The type and severity of the disorder determine the impact it has on the health of individuals. This chapter discusses mild hematologic disorders and those that are potentially life threatening, such as sickle cell disease and leukemia.

Red Blood Cell Disorders

Red blood cells (RBCs), also known as **erythrocytes**, are the major cell in the blood. Tissue oxygenation depends on keeping the circulating number of RBCs within the normal range for the person's age and gender. Tissue oxygenation also depends on the ability of RBCs to perform their normal functions. RBC disorders include problems in production, function, and destruction. Problems may result in a deficient number or poor function of RBCs **(anemia)** or an excess of RBCs **(polycythemia).**

ANEMIA

Anemia is a reduction in either the number of RBCs, the amount of hemoglobin, or the **hematocrit** (percentage of packed RBCs per deciliter of blood). Anemia is a clinical sign, not a specific disease, because it is a manifestation of several abnormal conditions. Anemia can result from dietary problems, genetic disorders, bone marrow disease, or excessive bleeding. Gastrointestinal bleeding is the most common reason for anemia in adults.

There are many types and causes of anemia. Some anemias are caused by a deficiency in one or more of the components needed to make fully functional RBCs. Such anemias can be caused by deficiencies of iron, vitamin B_{12}, folic acid, or intrinsic factor. Other causes include a decreased rate of RBC

TABLE 43-1 Common Causes of Anemia

Type of Anemia	Common Causes
Sickle cell disease	Autosomal recessive inheritance of two defective gene alleles for hemoglobin synthesis
Glucose-6-phosphate dehydrogenase (G6PD) deficiency anemia	X-linked recessive deficiency of the enzyme G6PD
Autoimmune hemolytic anemia	Abnormal immune function in which a person's immune reactive cells fail to recognize his or her own red blood cells as self cells
Iron deficiency anemia	Inadequate iron intake caused by ■ Iron-deficient diet ■ Chronic alcoholism ■ Malabsorption syndromes ■ Partial gastrectomy Rapid metabolic (anabolic) activity caused by ■ Pregnancy ■ Adolescence ■ Infection
Vitamin B_{12} deficiency anemia	Dietary deficiency Failure to absorb vitamin B_{12} from intestinal tract as a result of ■ Partial gastrectomy ■ Pernicious anemia
Folic acid deficiency anemia	Dietary deficiency Malabsorption syndromes Drugs ■ Oral contraceptives ■ Anticonvulsants ■ Methotrexate
Aplastic anemia	Exposure to myelotoxic agents ■ Radiation ■ Benzene ■ Chloramphenicol ■ Alkylating agents ■ Antimetabolites ■ Sulfonamides ■ Insecticides Viral infection (unproven) ■ Epstein-Barr virus ■ Hepatitis B ■ Cytomegalovirus

production and increased RBC destruction. Table 43-1 lists common causes of many anemias. Despite the many causes of anemia, the effects of anemia on the client (Chart 43-1) and the nursing care needed are similar for all types of anemia.

ANEMIAS RESULTING FROM INCREASED DESTRUCTION OF RED BLOOD CELLS

Sickle Cell Disease

PATHOPHYSIOLOGY

Sickle cell disease is a genetic disorder that results in chronic anemia, pain, disability, organ damage, increased risk for infection, and early death. There is a difference between sickle cell disease state and sickle cell trait. In addition, there is great variation among clients in how severe the disease is and when complications start.

CHART 43-1

KEY FEATURES of
Anemia

Integumentary Manifestations
- Pallor, especially of the ears, the nail beds, the palmar creases, the conjunctiva, and around the mouth
- Cool to the touch
- Intolerance of cold temperatures
- Nails become brittle and may lose the normal convex shape; over time, nails become concave and fingers assume clublike appearance

Cardiovascular Manifestations
- Tachycardia at basal activity levels, increasing with activity and during and immediately after meals
- Murmurs and gallops heard on auscultation when anemia is severe
- Orthostatic hypotension

Respiratory Manifestations
- Dyspnea on exertion
- Decreased oxygen saturation levels

Neurologic Manifestations
- Increased somnolence and fatigue
- Headache

The main problem in this disorder is the formation of abnormal hemoglobin chains. In adults, the normal hemoglobin molecule has two alpha chains and two beta chains of amino acids. This normal adult hemoglobin is called **hemoglobin A (HbA).** Normal adult hemoglobin usually contains 98% to 99% HbA, with a small percentage of a fetal form of hemoglobin (HbF).

In sickle cell disease, at least 40% of the total hemoglobin contains an abnormality of the beta chains, known as hemoglobin S (HbS). HbS is sensitive to changes in the oxygen content of the RBC. When RBCs having large amounts of HbS are exposed to decreased oxygen states, the abnormal beta chains contract and pile together within the cell, distorting the shape of the RBC. These cells assume a sickle shape, become rigid, clump together, and form masses of sickled RBCs that block blood flow (Figure 43-1). Thus blood vessel obstruction leads to further tissue **hypoxia** (reduced oxygen supply) and more sickling, with more blood vessel obstructions and ischemia in the affected tissues. Repeated episodes of ischemia lead to progressive organ damage from infarction (Larsen, Neverett, & Larsen, 2001). Conditions that cause sickling include hypoxia, dehydration, infections, venous stasis, low environmental or body temperatures, acidosis, strenuous exercise, and anesthesia.

Usually, sickled cells go back to normal shape when the low oxygen condition is removed and proper oxygenation occurs. Although the cells then appear normal, at least some of the hemoglobin remains twisted, decreasing cell flexibility. The cell membranes become damaged over time, and cells are permanently sickled. The membranes of cells with HbS are more fragile and more easily broken. The average life span of an RBC containing 40% or more of HbS is about 12 to 15 days, much less than the 120-day life span of normal RBCs. This reduced RBC life span causes **hemolytic** (blood cell–destroying) anemia in clients with sickle cell disease.

The client with sickle cell disease has periodic episodes of extensive cellular sickling, called **crises.** The crises have a

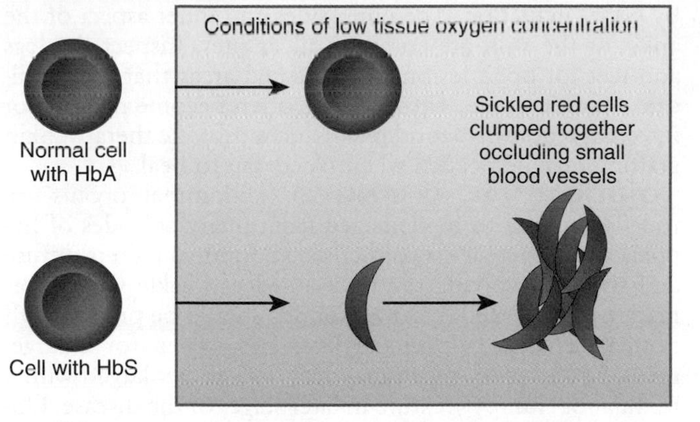

Figure 43-1 ■ Red blood cell actions under conditions of low tissue oxygenation. *HbA,* Hemoglobin A; *HbS,* hemoglobin S.

CHART 43-2

KEY FEATURES of Sickle Cell Disease

Hematologic Manifestations
- Fragile red blood cells that sickle and clump under conditions of low tissue oxygenation, venous stasis, lower environmental or body temperature
  - Anemia
- Tissue hypoxia and ischemia
  - Pain
  - Hardened, enlarged spleen

Respiratory Manifestations
- Pulmonary infarcts
  - Chest pain
  - Pneumonia

Genitourinary Manifestations
- Renal ischemia
  - Decreased urine concentration
- Priapism

Cardiovascular Manifestations
- Cardiac ischemia
  - Myocardial infarctions
  - Chest pain
  - Heart failure
- Strokes

Musculoskeletal Manifestations
- Necrosis of femur head
- Pain in extremities with moderate physical exercise
- Delayed growth—small stature

Integumentary Manifestations
- Leg ulcers
- Pale, cyanotic skin

sudden onset and can occur as often as weekly or as seldom as once a year. Many clients are in good health much of the time, with crises occurring only in response to conditions that cause local or systemic **hypoxemia** (deficient oxygen in the blood).

Repeated occlusions of larger blood vessels have long-term poor effects on tissues and organs (Chart 43-2). Most effects occur as a result of blood vessel occlusion leading to tissue hypoxia, anoxia, ischemia, and cell death. Tissues and organs begin to have small infarcted areas. Eventually,

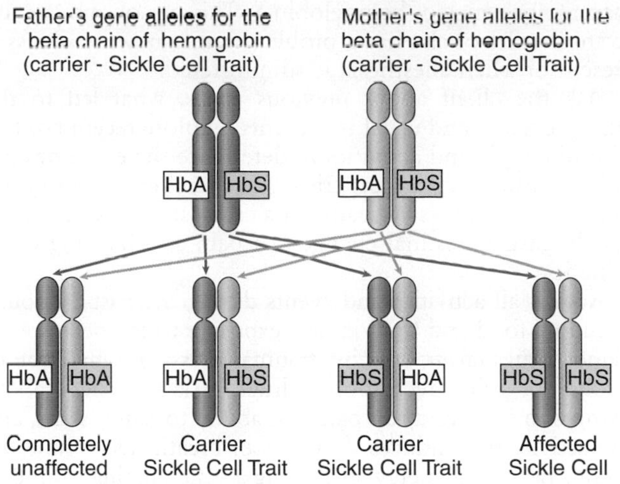

Figure 43-2 ■ Inheritance pattern for sickle cell disease.

enough healthy cells are destroyed that organ failure results. Organs most often affected in this way are the spleen, liver, heart, kidney, brain, bones, and retina.

Etiology and Genetic Risk

Sickle cell disease is a genetic disorder with an autosomal recessive pattern of inheritance (see Chapter 11). The formation of the beta chains of the hemoglobin molecule is dependent on a pair of gene alleles. A mutation in these alleles leads to the formation of hemoglobin S (HbS) instead of HbA. In sickle cell disease, the client has inherited one hemoglobin S gene allele from each parent, resulting in 80% to 100% of the total hemoglobin containing HbS. Clients with sickle cell disease have severe manifestations of the disease, even under mild precipitating conditions. If a client with sickle cell disease has children, each child will inherit one of the two abnormal gene alleles and at least have sickle cell trait.

In sickle cell trait, one normal gene allele and one abnormal gene allele are inherited, so that only half of the hemoglobin chains produced will be abnormal. The client is a carrier of the HbS gene allele (Figure 43-2). The client can pass the trait on to his or her children, but the client has only mild manifestations of the disease under severe precipitating conditions because less than 40% of the hemoglobin is abnormal.

Incidence/Prevalence

Sickle cell trait and different forms of sickle cell disease occur in people of all races and ethnicities but less often among white individuals. In the United States, about 70,000 people have sickle cell disease, most commonly in African Americans (Sickle Cell Information Center, 2003). Sickle cell disease occurs in 1 in 400 African Americans, and 8% to 10% of all African Americans are carriers of one sickle cell gene allele and have sickle cell trait (Platt et al., 2002).

◆COLLABORATIVE MANAGEMENT

◆Assessment

HISTORY

An adult with sickle cell disease usually has a long-standing diagnosis of the disorder. Adults with sickle cell trait usually have no symptoms or abnormal laboratory findings other than the presence of hemoglobin S. This person may be unaware that he or she has a problem until an acute illness is present or when anesthesia is administered.

Ask the client about previous crises, what led to the crises, severity, and usual treatments. Explore recent contact with ill people and activities to determine the event or condition causing the current crisis. Ask the client about symptoms of infection as the cause of a crisis, such as sore throat, cough, gastrointestinal changes, or pain and burning upon urination.

Review all activities and events during the past 24 hours, including food and fluid intake, exposure to temperature extremes, drugs taken, exercise, trauma, stress, and ingestion of alcohol or other recreational drugs. Ask the client about changes in sleep and rest patterns, ability to climb stairs, and any activity that induces shortness of breath. Determine the client's perceived energy level using a scale ranging from 0 to 10 (0 = not tired with plenty of energy; 10 = total exhaustion) to evaluate the degree of fatigue. This activity review provides important information about fatigue, activity tolerance, and participation in activities of daily living (ADLs).

PHYSICAL ASSESSMENT/CLINICAL MANIFESTATIONS

Pain is the most common symptom of sickle cell crisis. Jaundice may also be present as a result of RBC destruction and release of bilirubin. Other manifestations vary with the site of tissue damage.

CARDIOVASCULAR CHANGES. Clients with sickle cell disease are at risk for high output heart failure because of the anemia. Assess the client for shortness of breath, dyspnea upon exertion, and weakness. Other problems may include murmurs and the presence of an S_3 heart sound. Assess the client's cardiac and vascular status by comparing peripheral pulses, temperature, and capillary refill in all extremities. Extremities distal to blood vessel occlusion are cool to the touch with slow capillary refill and may have reduced or absent pulses. The heart rate may be rapid and the blood pressure low to average, with a decreased pulse pressure, because breakage of RBCs leads to anemia.

SKIN CHANGES. The skin may be pale or cyanotic because of decreased perfusion and anemia. Examine the lips, tongue, nail beds, conjunctivae, palms, and soles of the feet at least once per shift for subtle color changes. With cyanosis, the lips and tongue are gray, and the palms, soles, conjunctivae, and nail beds have a bluish tinge.

Another skin manifestation of sickle cell disease is jaundice. Bilirubin, present inside RBCs, is released when fragile cells are damaged, leading to jaundice. Assess for jaundice in clients with darker skin by inspecting the roof of the mouth for yellow discoloration. Yellow-tinged sclera may be misleading because of normal deposits of fat that appears yellowish in contrast to the dark skin around the eye. Examine the sclera closest to the cornea to assess jaundice more accurately. The palms and soles of dark-skinned clients may appear yellow if callused and should not be mistaken for jaundice. Jaundice often causes intense itching.

Despite the anemia, clients with sickle cell disease usually are not iron deficient. In fact, with increased RBC production and destruction, iron released from the cells may increase the pigmentation of the skin.

As many as 75% of adult clients with sickle cell disease have open sores or ulcers on the lower legs that are caused by poor circulation. The outer sides and inner aspect of the ankle or the shin are common ulcer sites. Inspect the legs and feet for open lesions or darkened areas that may indicate necrotic tissue. These lesions often become necrotic or infected, requiring debridement and antibiotic therapy. Skin grafting may be needed when ulcers fail to heal.

ABDOMINAL CHANGES. Abdominal organs are usually the first to be damaged from many episodes of hypoxia and ischemia. In pain crisis, abdominal pain is diffuse and steady, involving the back and legs (Sickle Cell Information Center, 2003). Bowel sounds should be present with normal activity. Palpate the liver and spleen for enlargement. The liver or spleen may feel firm and enlarged with a nodular or "lumpy" texture in later stages of the disease. Observe whether the client has guarding or rebound tenderness to palpation. A rapidly enlarging liver or spleen that occurs with increasing jaundice may indicate blood trapping in those organs.

MUSCULOSKELETAL CHANGES. Arms and legs are common sites of blood vessel occlusion in clients with sickle cell disease. Joints also may be damaged from many hypoxic episodes and have necrotic degeneration. Inspect the arms and legs for symmetry and record any areas of swelling or color difference. Ask clients to move all joints and record the range of motion and any pain with movement.

CENTRAL NERVOUS SYSTEM CHANGES. Changes in central nervous system (CNS) function may occur in sickle cell disease. During crises, clients may have a low-grade fever. If the CNS has infarcts or repeated episodes of hypoxia, clients may have seizures or manifestations of a stroke. Assess hand grasps on both sides. Also assess the client's gait and coordination.

PSYCHOSOCIAL ASSESSMENT

Psychosocial assessment is important because behavioral changes are early manifestations of cerebral hypoxia. Observe the client and document behavior. Ask family members whether the current behavior and mental status are usual for the client.

Sickle cell disease is a chronic, painful, life-limiting disorder that can be passed on to one's children. Assess the client's psychosocial needs in terms of new factors, established support systems, previous and current coping patterns, and disease progression. Ask the client about how he or she views the disease and what changes in lifestyle have been made as limitations increased.

LABORATORY ASSESSMENT

The diagnosis of sickle cell disease is based on the large percentage of hemoglobin S (HbS) seen on electrophoresis. A person who has sickle cell trait usually has less than 40% HbS, and the client with sickle cell disease may have 80% to 100% HbS. *This percentage does not change during crises.* Another indicator of sickle cell disease is the number of RBCs with permanent sickling. This value is less than 1% among people who do not have sickle cell disease, is 5% to 50% among people with sickle cell trait, and may exceed 90% among clients with sickle cell disease.

Other laboratory tests can indicate the problems or complications of the disease, especially during crises. The hematocrit of clients with sickle cell disease is low (between 20% and 30%). This value decreases even more during crises or when the bone marrow fails to produce cells during stress (aplastic crisis). The reticulocyte count is high, indicating anemia of long duration. Often the mean corpuscular hemoglobin concentration (MCHC) and total bilirubin levels are high in clients with sickle cell disease.

The total white blood cell (WBC) count is usually elevated in clients with sickle cell disease. This elevation is related to chronic inflammation caused by tissue hypoxia and ischemia.

RADIOGRAPHIC ASSESSMENT

Bone changes occur as a result of chronically stimulated marrow and hypoxic bone tissue. The skull may show changes on x-ray as a result of chronic bone surface cell destruction and new growth, giving the skull a "crew cut" appearance on x-ray. X-rays of joints may show necrosis and destruction.

OTHER DIAGNOSTIC ASSESSMENTS

Electrocardiographic (ECG) changes document cardiac infarcts and tissue damage. Specific ECG changes are related to the area of the heart that has been damaged. Ultrasonography, computed tomography (CT), positron emission tomography (PET), and magnetic resonance imaging (MRI) may show soft-tissue and organ changes from poor oxygenation and chronic inflammation.

Common Nursing Diagnoses and Collaborative Problems

Nursing diagnoses and collaborative problems that may apply to clients with sickle cell disease include the following:

- Acute Pain related to poor tissue oxygenation
- Chronic Pain related to joint destruction
- Potential for Sepsis
- Potential for Multiple Organ Dysfunction and Death

Interventions

PAIN. The most common problem of sickle cell disease is pain. The pain with sickle cell crisis is the result of ischemic tissue injury caused by obstructed blood flow. At times, clients have mild pain episodes that can be managed at home. However, pain is often severe enough to require hospitalization and large doses of opioid analgesics. Acute pain episodes have a sudden onset, usually involving the chest, back, abdomen, and extremities (Platt et al., 2002). Complications of sickle cell disease, such as bone necrosis, can cause severe, chronic pain, requiring large doses of opioid analgesics.

Ask the client if the pain is typical of past pain episodes. If not, other pain causes or disease complications must be explored. Use of a pain rating scale can help proper pain management. Ask the client to rate pain on a scale ranging from 0 to 10 and evaluate the effectiveness of interventions based on the ratings.

Concerns about substance abuse can lead to inadequate pain treatment in these clients. Opioid addiction is rare, occurring in only 2% to 5% of clients with sickle cell disease (Platt et al., 2002). Treatment of pain is based on past pain history, previous drug use, disease complications, and current pain assessment. Health care providers must be aware of their own attitudes when caring for this population. If substance abuse is suspected, the treatment of addiction is incorporated into the client's overall treatment plan. Treatment of substance abuse and sickle cell disease pose many challenges, because the client usually cannot be expected to be totally opioid-free. Addicted clients with acute pain crisis may need opioids for short periods. The use of individual contracts as plans for pain control can also be helpful.

Drug Therapy. Clients in acute sickle cell crisis often need at least 48 hours of intravenous (IV) analgesics. (Chart 43-3 lists best practices for nursing care of the client in sickle cell crisis.) Morphine and hydromorphone (Dilaudid) are given IV on a routine schedule, or by infusion pump using patient-controlled analgesia (PCA) (see Chapter 7). Once relief is obtained, the IV dose can be tapered and the drug given orally. Avoid "as needed" (PRN) schedules because they do not provide adequate relief. Avoid intramuscular (IM) injections because absorption is impaired by poor circulation and sclerosed skin. Moderate pain may be treated with oral doses of opioids or nonsteroidal anti-inflammatory drugs (NSAIDs). (See Chapter 7 for more information on pain management.)

Hydroxyurea (Droxia) has been successfully used to reduce the number of sickling and pain episodes. Hydroxyurea works by stimulating fetal hemoglobin (HbF) production. HbF is present during fetal development, but production of hemoglobin F is turned off before birth. Increasing the level of HbF reduces sickling of red blood cells in persons with sickle cell disease. However, this drug is associated with an increased incidence of leukemia (Weiner & Brugnara, 2003). Long-term complications should be discussed with the client before this therapy is started. Hydroxyurea also suppresses bone marrow function, and regular follow-up to monitor complete blood counts (CBCs) for drug toxicity is important. *Hydroxyurea also causes birth defects, thus female clients of childbearing age should use at least two methods of birth control while taking this drug.*

Oral Hydration. Oral or IV hydration helps reduce the duration of pain episodes. Urge the client to drink water or juices. Hydration with hypotonic fluids, such as dextrose 5% with water (D_5W) or with dextrose 5% in 0.45% sodium chloride, is infused at 250 mL/hr for 4 hours. The IV rate is then reduced to 125 mL/hr if more hydration is needed.

Complementary and Alternative Therapies. Complementary therapies and other measures, such as keeping the room warm, using distraction and relaxation tech-

CHART 43-3

BEST PRACTICE for Care of the Client in Sickle Cell Crisis

- Administer oxygen.
- Administer pain medication as prescribed.
- Hydrate the client with normal saline intravenously and with beverages of choice (without caffeine) orally.
- Remove any constrictive clothing.
- Encourage the client to keep extremities extended to promote venous return.
- Do not raise the knee gatch of the bed.
- Elevate the head of the bed no more than 30 degrees.
- Keep room temperature at or above 72° F (22.2° C).
- Avoid taking blood pressure with external cuff.
- Check circulation in extremities every hour:
  - Pulse oximetry of fingers and toes
  - Capillary refill
  - Peripheral pulses
  - Toe temperature

niques, positioning with support for painful areas, aromatherapy, therapeutic touch, and warm soaks or compresses all help reduce pain perception. *Do not assume that these methods alone will provide adequate pain relief. Analgesics are needed to treat sickle cell pain.*

POTENTIAL FOR SEPSIS. The client with sickle cell disease is at greater risk for infection by such organisms as *Streptococcus pneumoniae* and *Haemophilus influenzae,* because of decreased spleen function. Interventions aim at preventing infection, controlling infection, and initiating early treatment for specific infections. The client who develops a fever should have diagnostic testing for sepsis including CBC with differential, blood cultures, reticulocyte count, urine culture, and a chest x-ray. Usually, these clients are started on prophylactic antibiotics.

Prevention/Early Detection. A major objective is to protect the client in sickle cell crisis from infection. Frequent, thorough handwashing is of the utmost importance. Any person with an upper respiratory tract infection who must enter the client's room wears a mask. Use strict aseptic technique for all invasive procedures.

Continually assess the client for infection and monitor the daily complete blood count (CBC) with differential WBC count. Inspect the mouth during every shift for lesions indicating fungal or viral infection. Auscultate the lungs every 8 hours for crackles, wheezes, or reduced breath sounds. Each time the client voids, inspect the urine for odor and cloudiness, and ask about urgency, burning, or pain during urination. Take vital signs at least every 4 hours to assess for fever.

Drug Therapy. Drug therapy is a major defense against the infections that develop in the client with sickle cell disease. Prophylactic therapy with twice-daily oral penicillin reduces the number of pneumonia and other streptococcal infections. Encourage yearly influenza vaccination. Drug therapy for an actual infection can control infection and prevent sepsis. Agents used depend on the sensitivity of the specific organism causing the infection as well as on the extent of the infection.

POTENTIAL FOR MULTIPLE ORGAN DYSFUNCTION. Continued blood vessel occlusion by clumping of sickled cells increases the risk for multiple organ dysfunction. Management of sickle cell disease focuses on prevention of blood vessel occlusion and promotion of oxygenation.

The client in sickle cell crisis is admitted to the acute care hospital. Assess for adequacy of circulation to all body areas. Remove restrictive clothing and instruct the client to avoid flexing the knees and hips.

Hydration. Dehydration increases cell sickling and must be avoided. Assist the client in maintaining adequate hydration. The client in acute crisis needs an oral or IV intake of at least 200 mL/hr.

Oxygen Therapy. Oxygen is given during crises because deoxygenation is the main cause of sickling. Ensure that oxygen therapy is delivered with nebulization to prevent dehydration. Monitor oxygen saturation using pulse oximetry. Clients with low oxygen saturation should have an arterial blood gas (ABG) drawn and a chest x-ray obtained.

Transfusion Therapy. RBC transfusions can be helpful to increase HbA levels and dilute HbS levels. During transfusion, monitor the client for complications of the procedure (discussed under Transfusion Reactions, p. 916).

Transfusions are prescribed cautiously to prevent iron overload with repeated transfusions. Iron overload damages the heart, liver, and endocrine organs (Sickle Cell Information Center, 2003). Monitor the client's serum ferritin, serum iron (Fe), and total iron binding capacity (TIBC). Deferoxamine mesylate (Desferal, Desferrioxamine) may be prescribed to treat transfusion-induced iron overload.

In some treatment centers, bone marrow transplantation is performed to correct abnormal hemoglobin permanently. Because bone marrow transplantation is expensive and may result in chronic and life-threatening complications, its risks and benefits need to be considered for each client.

Critical Thinking Challenge

A 20-year-old African-American woman with sickle cell disease comes to the outpatient clinic with complaints of joint and back pain, cough, runny nose, and a temperature of 100° F (38° C). She states her pain level is 7/10.

1. What questions related to pain would you ask this client?
2. What drugs and by which route would you expect this client to receive?
3. What diagnostic tests would you expect to be ordered for this client?
4. What nursing assessments would be most important for you to make at this time?

evolve For suggested answer guidelines, go to http://evolve.elsevier.com/Iggy/.

Community-Based Care

Sickle cell disease is progressive with periods of disease exacerbation. Rarely is there a true remission, although the number of crisis episodes may be reduced. Care focuses on prevention of complications. The client with sickle cell disease may receive care in a variety of settings, including acute care, subacute care, extended or assistive care, and home care.

Teach the client to avoid specific activities that lead to hypoxia and hypoxemia. (See the Resource Management box on p. 893.) Emphasize the recognition of the early manifestations of crisis so that treatment can be started early to prevent undue pain, complications, and permanent tissue damage. The client is often given opioid analgesics for self-management of sickle cell crises at home. Teach the client and family about the correct use of these drugs. In addition, counsel clients about the hereditary aspects of sickle cell disease, and provide information about prenatal diagnosis, birth control methods, and pregnancy options.

WOMEN'S HEALTH CONSIDERATIONS

Pregnancy in women with sickle cell disease may be life threatening. Clients who have damage to vital organs are advised against becoming pregnant. Usually, barrier methods of contraception (cervical cap, diaphragm, or condoms with or without spermicides) are recommended for women with sickle cell disease. The use of oral contraceptives (OCs) among these women is controversial, however. OCs may increase clot formation, especially among smokers, predisposing them to crises. However, the use of oral contraceptives also can reduce menstrual blood loss and decrease the degree of anemia. The risks versus benefits of OCs must be examined for each client.

RESOURCE MANAGEMENT

SICKLE CELL DISEASE

Cost of Care

- Each year in the United States, an average of 75,000 hospitalizations are due to sickle cell disease, costing about $475 million.
- The National Institutes of Health report that about $47 million per year is spent on sickle cell research.
- In pharmacies, the average price of 100 capsules of hydroxyurea is between $121 and $164.
- Most clients take two to three capsules daily, which would cost about $100 per month.

Implications for Nursing

The costs related to the treatment of sickle cell disease are the direct result of the need for frequent health-related interventions and hospitalizations related to a lifelong chronic disease. Preventive educational interventions aimed at ways to prevent pain crisis may assist in reducing the costs related to hospitalizations.

Data from Sickle Cell Information Center. (2004). Emory University, Atlanta, GA. Available at http://www.scinfo.org.

Glucose-6-Phosphate Dehydrogenase Deficiency Anemia

PATHOPHYSIOLOGY

Many forms of **hemolytic** (blood cell–destroying) anemia are present from birth as a result of defects or deficiencies of one or more enzymes within the red blood cell (RBC). More than 200 such disorders have been identified. Most of these enzymes are needed to complete some critical step in RBC energy production. The most common type of congenital hemolytic anemia is the deficiency of the enzyme glucose-6-phosphate dehydrogenase (G6PD). This disease is inherited as an X-linked recessive disorder and affects about 10% of all African Americans (McCance & Huether, 2002).

G6PD stimulates reactions in glucose metabolism. RBCs contain no **mitochondria** (sites of production of adenosine triphosphate [ATP]), so active glycolysis is needed for energy metabolism. Newly produced RBCs from clients with G6PD deficiency have sufficient levels of G6PD; however, as the cells age, the level decreases rapidly. Cells with reduced amounts of G6PD break more easily during exposure to some drugs (e.g., phenacetin, sulfonamides, aspirin, quinine derivatives, and thiazide diuretics) and toxins.

The client is usually asymptomatic until exposed to these agents or when a severe infection develops. After exposure to any of these agents, clients have acute breakage of RBCs lasting from 7 to 12 days. During this acute phase, anemia and jaundice develop. The hemolytic reaction is limited because only older RBCs, containing less G6PD, are destroyed.

COLLABORATIVE MANAGEMENT

It is critical that the drug or toxin responsible for the hemolytic reaction be identified and totally removed. People should be screened for this deficiency before donating blood, because cells deficient in G6PD can be hazardous for the recipient.

Hydration is essential during an episode of hemolysis to prevent precipitation of debris and hemoglobin in the kidney tubules, which can lead to acute tubular necrosis. Osmotic diuretics, such as mannitol (Osmitrol), may help prevent this complication. Transfusion therapy is needed when anemia is present and kidney function is normal. Table 43-6 lists indications for transfusion with various types of blood components (see discussion under Transfusion Therapy, p. 913).

Immunohemolytic Anemia

PATHOPHYSIOLOGY

Increased RBC destruction through hemolysis occurs in response to many situations, including trauma, malarial infection, and autoimmune reactions. All increase the rate of RBC destruction by causing membrane **lysis** (breakage). The most common types of hemolytic anemias in North America are the immunohemolytic anemias, also referred to as autoimmune hemolytic anemias (McCance & Huether, 2002).

In immunohemolytic anemia, immune system products attack a person's own RBCs for unknown reasons. Some hemolytic anemias occur with other autoimmune disorders (e.g., systemic lupus erythematosus). Regardless of the cause, RBCs are viewed as non-self by the immune system and are destroyed.

There are two types of immunohemolytic anemia: warm antibody anemia and cold antibody anemia. **Warm antibody anemia** occurs with immunoglobulin G (IgG) antibody excess. These antibodies are most active at 98° F (37° C) and may be triggered by drugs, chemicals, or other autoimmune problems. **Cold antibody anemia** occurs with complement protein fixation on immunoglobulin M (IgM) and occurs most at 86° F (30° C). This problem often occurs with a Raynaud-like response in which the arteries in the hands and feet constrict profoundly in response to cold temperatures or stress.

COLLABORATIVE MANAGEMENT

Treatment depends on symptom severity. Steroid therapy to cause immunosuppression is the first line of treatment and is temporarily effective in most clients. Splenectomy and more intense immunosuppressive therapy with cyclophosphamide (Cytoxan, Procytox✱) and azathioprine (Imuran) may be used if steroid therapy fails. Plasma exchange therapy to remove attacking antibodies is effective for clients who do not respond to immunosuppressive therapy.

ANEMIAS RESULTING FROM DECREASED PRODUCTION OF RED BLOOD CELLS

Anemias caused by decreased red blood cell (RBC) production can occur in response to many problems. Some anemias are caused by failure or inability of the bone marrow to properly produce RBCs. Other anemias are caused by failure of the body to make or absorb a substance needed for RBC production.

CONSIDERATIONS FOR OLDER ADULTS

Older clients often have restricted diets and may be unable to eat meat because of tooth loss or economic reasons, and thus are at risk for iron deficiency anemia (McCance & Huether, 2002). Ask about a family history of anemia. B_{12} deficiency anemia often occurs in clients 50 to 80 years of age and may be genetically transmitted.

Iron Deficiency Anemia

PATHOPHYSIOLOGY

Adults usually have between 2 and 6 g of iron, depending on the size of the person and the amount of hemoglobin in the cells. About two thirds of this iron is contained in hemoglobin; the other one third is stored in the bone marrow, spleen, liver, and muscle (see Chapter 42). With iron deficiency, the iron stores are depleted first, followed by the hemoglobin stores. As a result, RBCs are small **(microcytic),** and the client has mild manifestations of anemia, including weakness and pallor. In iron deficiency anemia, serum ferritin values are less than 12 g/L.

Iron deficiency anemia is a common type of anemia and can result from blood loss, poor intestinal absorption, and an inadequate diet. The basic problem is a decreased iron supply for the developing RBC. Iron deficiency anemia can occur at any age but is more frequent in women, older adults, and people with poor diets.

COLLABORATIVE MANAGEMENT

Any adult with iron deficiency should be evaluated for abnormal bleeding, especially from the gastrointestinal tract. The treatment of iron deficiency anemia is to increase the oral intake of iron from common food sources (Table 43-2). An adequate diet supplies about 10 to 15 mg of iron per day. However, only 5% to 10% of dietary iron is absorbed. This amount is enough to meet the needs of men and women after childbearing age but is not sufficient to supply the greater needs of menstruating women. Fortunately, if iron intake is inadequate, or if bleeding or pregnancy occurs, the intestinal tract increases iron absorption to about 20% to 30% of the total daily intake (McCance & Huether, 2002).

If iron losses are mild, oral iron supplements, such as ferrous sulfate, are started. This treatment should cause the hemoglobin level to rise about 2 g/dL in 4 weeks. Treatment continues until the hemoglobin level returns to normal. When iron deficiency anemia is severe, iron solutions can be given IM. These solutions must be given using the Z-track best practice method outlined in Chart 43-4.

TABLE 43-2 Common Food Sources of Iron, Vitamin B_{12}, and Folic Acid

Iron	Vitamin B_{12}
▪ Liver (especially pork and lamb)	▪ Liver
▪ Red meat	▪ Organ meats
▪ Organ meats	▪ Dried beans
▪ Kidney beans	▪ Nuts
▪ Whole-wheat breads and cereals	▪ Green leafy vegetables
▪ Leafy green vegetables	▪ Citrus fruit
▪ Carrots	▪ Brewer's yeast
▪ Egg yolks	
▪ Raisins	**Folic Acid**
	▪ Liver
	▪ Organ meats
	▪ Eggs
	▪ Cabbage
	▪ Broccoli
	▪ Brussels sprouts

Data from Pennington, J. (1998). *Bowe's and Church's food values of portions commonly used* (17th ed.). Philadelphia: J. B. Lippincott.

CHART 43-4

BEST PRACTICE for
Administering Intramuscular Medications by the Z-Track Method

- Draw the medication up into the syringe using aseptic technique.
- Add 0.25 mL of air to the syringe.
- Discard the needle used to draw up the medication.
- Place a new needle (22-gauge, 2 to 3 inches long) on the syringe.
- Make certain that the injection site is in bright light.
- *Select the dorsal gluteal site only.*
- Identify appropriate landmarks for administration into the upper, outer quadrant.
- Once the site is selected, pull the skin and subcutaneous tissues sideways away from the muscle.
- Clean the site while holding the skin and subcutaneous tissues off to the side.
- Insert the needle deeply into the muscle tissue.
- Aspirate to determine needle placement.
- Iron dextran is black; look very closely to determine whether or not blood is being aspirated into the syringe.
- If blood is aspirated, withdraw the needle and begin the procedure again from the first step.
- If no blood is aspirated, inject the medication slowly, followed by injection of the air bubble.
- Quickly withdraw the needle.
- Release the skin and subcutaneous tissue.
- *Do not massage the injection site.*

Vitamin B_{12} Deficiency Anemia

PATHOPHYSIOLOGY

Proper production of RBCs depends on adequate **deoxyribonucleic acid (DNA)** synthesis in the precursor cells so that cell division and growth into functional RBCs can occur. All cell division requires adequate amounts of folic acid to make DNA. One function of vitamin B_{12} is to activate the enzymes that move folic acid into the cell, where DNA synthesis occurs. Vitamin B_{12} deficiency causes anemia by inhibiting folic acid transport and reducing DNA synthesis in precursor cells. These precursor cells then undergo improper DNA synthesis and increase in size. Only a few are released from the bone marrow. This type of anemia is called **megaloblastic (macrocytic)** because of the large size of these abnormal cells.

Vitamin B_{12} deficiency results result from poor intake of foods containing vitamin B_{12}. This can occur with vegetarian diets or diets lacking dairy products. Conditions such as small bowel resection, diverticula, tapeworm, or overgrowth of intestinal bacteria can lead to poor absorption of vitamin B_{12}. Anemia caused by failure to absorb vitamin B_{12} **(pernicious anemia)** is caused by a deficiency of **intrinsic factor** (a substance normally secreted by the gastric mucosa), which is needed for intestinal absorption of vitamin B_{12}.

Vitamin B_{12} deficiency anemia may be mild or severe, usually develops slowly, and produces few symptoms. Clients usually have pallor and jaundice, as well as **glossitis** (a smooth, beefy-red tongue), fatigue, and weight loss. Because vitamin B_{12} is needed for normal nerve function, clients with pernicious anemia may also have **paresthesias** (abnormal sensations) in the feet and hands and poor balance (Chart 43-5).

COLLABORATIVE MANAGEMENT

When anemia is caused by a dietary deficiency, the client must increase the intake of foods rich in vitamin B_{12} (animal proteins, eggs, dairy products). Vitamin supplements may

CHART 43-5

KEY FEATURES of
Vitamin B_{12} Deficiency Anemia

- Severe pallor
- Slight jaundice
- Smooth, beefy red tongue
- Fatigue
- Weight loss
- Paresthesias of the hands and feet
- Difficulty with gait

be prescribed when anemia is severe. Vitamin B_{12} and folic acid levels are monitored. Clients who may have pernicious anemia, are tested using the Shilling test of vitamin B_{12} absorption. Clients who have pernicious anemia are given vitamin B_{12} injections weekly at first, then monthly for maintenance.

Folic Acid Deficiency Anemia

PATHOPHYSIOLOGY

Folic acid deficiency can also cause megaloblastic anemia. Manifestations are similar to those of vitamin B_{12} deficiency but nervous system functions remain normal, because folic acid does not affect nerve function. The absence of neurologic problems helps distinguish folic acid deficiency from vitamin B_{12} deficiency. The disease develops slowly, and symptoms may be attributed to other problems or diseases.

The three common causes of folic acid deficiency are poor nutrition, malabsorption, and drugs. Poor nutrition, especially a diet lacking green leafy vegetables, liver, yeast, citrus fruits, dried beans, and nuts, is the most common cause. Malabsorption syndromes, such as Crohn's disease, are the second most common cause. Chronic alcohol abuse with malnutrition is another cause. Anticonvulsants and oral contraceptives slow or prevent the absorption and conversion of folic acid to its active form, leading to folic acid deficiency and anemia.

COLLABORATIVE MANAGEMENT

Prevention of folic acid deficiency anemia is aimed at identifying high-risk clients, such as older, debilitated clients with alcoholism; clients susceptible to malnutrition; and those with increased folic acid requirements. A diet high in folic acid and vitamin B_{12} prevents a deficiency (see Table 43-2). By assessing dietary habits for all clients, you can determine which clients are at risk for diet-induced anemias. This type of anemia is treated with scheduled folic acid replacement therapy.

Aplastic Anemia

PATHOPHYSIOLOGY

Aplastic anemia is a deficiency of circulating red blood cells (RBCs) because of failure of the bone marrow to produce these cells. It is caused by an injury to the hematopoietic precursor cell, the **pluripotent stem cell.** Although aplastic anemia sometimes occurs alone, it usually occurs with **leukopenia** (a reduction in white blood cells) and **thrombocytopenia** (a reduction in platelets). These three problems occur together because the damaged bone marrow loses the ability to produce any of these cells. **Pancytopenia** (a deficiency of all three cell types) is common in aplastic anemia. The onset of aplastic anemia may be slow or rapid.

Aplastic anemia may be caused by long-term exposure to toxic agents, ionizing radiation, or infection (see Table 42-4). In about 50% of cases, the cause of aplastic anemia is unknown. Aplastic anemia may follow viral infection (McCance & Huether, 2002), but the exact mechanism of bone marrow damage is unknown.

COLLABORATIVE MANAGEMENT

Assess for symptoms of bone marrow failure such as weakness, pallor, and petechiae or ecchymosis. A complete blood count (CBC) shows severe macrocytic anemia, leukopenia and thrombocytopenia. A bone marrow biopsy may show replacement of cells by fat.

Blood transfusions are the mainstay of treatment for clients with aplastic anemia. Transfusion is used only when the anemia causes disability or when bleeding is life threatening because of thrombocytopenia. Unnecessary transfusion, however, increases the chances of developing immune reactions to platelets and shortens the life span of the transfused cell. Transfusions are discontinued as soon as the bone marrow begins to produce RBCs.

Immunosuppressive therapy helps clients who have the types of aplastic anemia with a disease course similar to that of autoimmune problems. Agents that suppress lymphocyte activity, such as antilymphocyte globulin (ALG), antithymocyte globulin (ATG), and cyclosporine (Sandimmune), have brought about partial or complete remissions. In more severe cases, stronger immunosuppressive agents, such as prednisone and cyclophosphamide (Cytoxan, Procytox✱), have been effective.

Splenectomy (removal of the spleen) may be performed for clients with an enlarged spleen that is either destroying normal RBCs or suppressing their development. Bone marrow transplantation replaces defective stem cells and can cure the disorder. Cost, availability, and complications limit this treatment of aplastic anemia.

POLYCYTHEMIA

In polycythemia, the number of red blood cells (RBCs) in the blood is greater than normal. The blood of a client with polycythemia is **hyperviscous** (thicker than normal blood). The problem may be temporary (occurring as a result of other conditions) or chronic. One type of polycythemia, polycythemia vera (PV), is fatal if left untreated.

Polycythemia Vera

PATHOPHYSIOLOGY

Polycythemia vera (PV) is a disease with a sustained increase in blood hemoglobin levels to 18 g/dL, an RBC count of 6 million/mm^3, or a hematocrit of 55% or greater. PV is a cancer of the RBCs with three major hallmarks: massive production of RBCs, excessive leukocyte production, and excessive production of platelets. Extreme **hypercellularity** (cell excess) of the peripheral blood occurs in people with PV (Chart 43-6).

At the time of diagnosis, the client's facial skin and mucous membranes have a dark, flushed **(plethoric)** appearance. These

CHART 43-6

KEY FEATURES of
Polycythemia Vera

- Persistently elevated hematocrit value (>55%)
- Hypertension
- Dark, flushed appearance of the hands and face
- Distention of superficial veins
- Weight loss
- Fatigue
- Intense itching
- Enlarged hemorrhoids
- Swollen, painful joints
- Enlarged, firm spleen
- Infarctions of the heart
  - Chest pain
  - Heart failure
- Strokes
- Bleeding tendency

CHART 43-7

CLIENT EDUCATION GUIDE
Polycythemia Vera

- Drink at least 3 L of liquids each day.
- Avoid tight or constrictive clothing, especially garters or girdles.
- Wear gloves when outdoors in temperatures lower than 50° F (10° C).
- Keep all health care–related appointments.
- Contact your physician at the first sign of infection.
- Take anticoagulants as prescribed.
- Wear support hose or stockings while you are awake and up.
- Elevate your feet whenever you are seated.
- Exercise slowly and only on the advice of your physician.
- Stop activity at the first sign of chest pain.
- Use an electric shaver.
- Use a soft-bristled toothbrush to brush your teeth.
- Do not floss between your teeth.

areas appear purplish or cyanotic because the blood in these tissues is poorly oxygenated. Many clients have intense itching caused by dilated blood vessels and varied tissue oxygenation. Blood viscosity is increased, causing an increase in peripheral resistance. Superficial veins are visibly distended. The thick blood moves more slowly through all tissues and places increased demands on the heart, resulting in hypertension. In some highly vascular areas, blood flow may become so slow that stasis occurs. Vascular stasis causes **thrombosis** (clot formation) within the smaller vessels, occluding blood vessels. The blood vessel occlusion leads to tissue hypoxia, anoxia and, later, to infarction and necrosis. Tissues most at risk for this problem are the heart, spleen, and kidneys, although infarction and damage can occur in any organ or tissue.

Because the actual number of cells in the blood is greatly increased and the cells are not completely normal, cell life spans are shorter. The shorter life spans and increased cell production cause a rapid turnover of circulating blood cells. This rapid turnover increases the amount of cell debris (released when cells die) in the blood, adding to the general "sludging" of the blood. This debris includes uric acid and potassium, which cause the symptoms of gout and **hyperkalemia** (elevated serum potassium level).

Other manifestations of PV are related to abnormal RBCs. Even though the number of RBCs is greatly increased, their oxygen-carrying capacity is impaired, and clients have severe hypoxia. Clients with PV also have bleeding problems because of platelet impairment (McCance & Huether, 2002).

COLLABORATIVE MANAGEMENT

Polycythemia vera (PV) is a malignant disease that progresses in severity over time. If left untreated, few people with PV live longer than 2 years after diagnosis. Monitor the CBC to assess response to treatment. Conservative treatment of repeated phlebotomies (two to five times per week) can prolong life for 10 to 20 years. (**Phlebotomy** is the blood drawing with removal of the client's RBCs to decrease the number of RBCs and reduce blood viscosity.) Increasing hydration and promoting venous return help prevent clot formation. Therapy aims to prevent clot formation and includes the use of anticoagulants. Chart 43-7 lists health tips for clients with PV.

As the disease progresses, more intensive therapies are needed to suppress bone marrow activity. Therapy includes oral chemotherapy agents and radiation therapy with injections of radioactive phosphorus. Bone marrow transplantation is promising, but the results are too limited to determine its application to PV. A significant number of clients with PV go on to develop acute leukemia.

MYELODYSPLASTIC SYNDROME

PATHOPHYSIOLOGY

Myelodysplastic syndromes (MDS) are a group of disorders caused by the formation of abnormal cells in the bone marrow. These abnormal cells are usually destroyed shortly after they are released into the blood. As a result, clients with MDS have decreases in the type of blood cell lines affected. MDS occurs in about 5 per 100,000 people, with older adults being affected more frequently (National Comprehensive Cancer Network, 2004). Although not officially a type of cancer, MDS has cancer-like features and is considered to be a precursor to cancer. Like cancer, MDS arises from a single population of abnormal cells. About 30% of all clients with MDS do eventually have acute leukemia. There are many subtypes of MDS and problems can range from unresponsive anemia to cytopenia with increased numbers of blast cells.

Diagnosis is made by examination of the chromosomes and the genes within the chromosomes (cytogenetic testing) of the bone marrow cells. Peripheral blood smears are used to assess marrow cell maturation and the degree of abnormal cells present.

COLLABORATIVE MANAGEMENT

Supportive care of the client with MDS includes blood transfusions for anemia and platelet transfusions for severe thrombocytopenia. Erythropoietin may be given in addition to transfusions. Clients with neutropenia may receive granulocyte colony stimulating factor (G-CSF) or granulocyte-monocyte colony-stimulating factor (GM-CSF). Treatment can include low-dose chemotherapy. For clients with more advanced disease and a high risk for leukemia, bone marrow transplantation is considered.

TABLE 43-3 Differentiating Characteristics of the Four Types of Leukemia

Age at Onset (yr)	Gender Predilection	Racial Predilection	Cell of Origin	Specific Markers	Comments
Acute Lymphocytic (ALL)					
<15	Males	White	B-cell	CALLA+ Hyperdiploidy TDT+	Prognosis poorer for adults than for children Prognosis better than in AML Curable in children
Acute Myelogenous (AML)					
15-39	Equal incidence	None	Myelocyte Promyelocyte Myelomonocyte	TDT− t(9;22) t(15;17)	Prognosis generally poor Heterogeneous tumor cell populations Best prognosis with bone marrow transplant
Chronic Myelogenous (CML)					
>50	Males	None	Myeloid cell	Ph^1 chromosome	Prognosis generally poor; worse if no Ph^1 chromosome No blockage of maturation of nonmalignant leukocytes Blastic crisis indicative of more acute disease
Chronic Lymphocytic (CLL)					
>50	Males	White	B-cell	Trisomy 12	Prognosis poor Long (4-10 yr) course with rare conversion to acute form Only leukemia with a possible genetic predisposition

White Blood Cell Disorders

As discussed in Chapter 23, white blood cells (WBCs), or **leukocytes,** provide protection from infection and cancer development. These protective functions depend on maintaining normal numbers and ratios of the different mature, circulating WBCs. When any one type of WBC is present in either abnormally high or abnormally low amounts, immune function is altered to some degree, as are the functions of oxygen transport and blood clotting, placing clients at risk for many complications. This section covers the changes and nursing care for clients with disorders involving overgrowth of specific types of WBCs. (See Chapter 25 for the problems and care needs for clients with immunodeficiency.)

LEUKEMIA

PATHOPHYSIOLOGY

Leukemia is a type of cancer with uncontrolled production of immature WBCs (usually blast cells) in the bone marrow. As a result, the bone marrow becomes overcrowded with immature, nonfunctional cells and production of normal blood cells is greatly decreased. **Leukemia** may be **acute,** with a sudden onset and short duration, or **chronic,** with a slow onset and symptoms that persist for a period of years.

Leukemias are classified by cell type. Abnormal leukemic cells coming from the lymphoid pathways (see Figure 23-3) are **lymphocytic** or **lymphoblastic.** Leukemias in which the abnormal cells come from the myeloid pathways are **myelocytic** or **myelogenous.** Several subtypes exist for each of these diseases, which are classified according to the degree of maturity of the abnormal cell and the specific cell type involved (Table 43-3).

With leukemia, cancer occurs in the stem cells or early precursor leukocyte cells, causing excessive growth of a specific type of leukocyte. These cells are abnormal and their excessive production in the bone marrow stops normal bone marrow production of red blood cells, platelets, and mature leukocytes. Anemia, thrombocytopenia, and leukopenia result. The number of immature, abnormal WBCs in the blood is greatly elevated. Leukemic cells can also be found in the spleen, liver, lymph nodes and central nervous system. Without treatment, the client dies of infection or hemorrhage. For clients with acute leukemia, these changes occur rapidly and, without intervention, progress to death. Chronic leukemia may be present for years before changes appear.

Etiology and Genetic Risk

The exact cause of leukemia is unknown, although many genetic and environmental factors are involved in its development. The basic mechanism involves damage to genes controlling cell growth. This damage then changes cells from a normal to a **malignant** (cancer) state. Analysis of the bone marrow of a client with acute leukemia shows abnormal chromosomes about 50% of the time (McCance & Huether, 2002). Possible risk factors for the development of leukemia include ionizing radiation, exposure to chemicals and drugs, bone marrow **hypoplasia** (reduced production blood cells), genetic factors, immunologic factors, environmental factors, and the interaction of these factors.

Ionizing radiation exposures such as radiation therapy for cancer treatment or environmental irradiation (e.g., the atomic bomb at Hiroshima or the nuclear accident at Chernobyl) increase the risk for leukemia development, particularly acute myelogenous leukemia (AML) (Stone, 2002).

Certain chemicals and drugs have been linked to the development of leukemia because of their ability to damage DNA. Previous treatment for cancer that included melphalan, cyclophosphamide, doxorubicin, and etoposide poses risks for leukemia development about 5 to 8 years after treatment (Stone, 2002). Table 42-4 lists chemicals and drugs that increase the risk for leukemia.

Bone marrow hypoplasia can increase leukemia risk by reducing or changing bone marrow cell production. Disorders that have marrow hypoplasia and may lead to leukemia development include Fanconi's anemia, paroxysmal nocturnal hemoglobinuria, and myelodysplastic syndromes.

Genetic factors influence leukemia development. There is an increased incidence of the disease among clients with hereditary conditions such as Down syndrome, Bloom syndrome, Klinefelter syndrome, and Fanconi's anemia. Identical siblings of clients with leukemia have a higher incidence of leukemia than does the general population.

Immunologic factors, especially immune deficiencies, may promote the development of leukemia. Leukemia among immunodeficient people may be a result of immune surveillance failure, or the same mechanisms that cause the immune deficiency may also trigger cancer in the WBC population.

Interaction of many host and environmental factors may result in leukemia. Because each person tolerates the interaction of these factors differently, it is difficult to determine the origin of any specific leukemia.

Incidence/Prevalence

Leukemia accounts for 2% of all new cases of cancer and for 4% of all deaths from cancer (American Cancer Society, 2005). The incidence depends on many factors, including the type of WBC affected, age, gender, race, and geographic locale.

In the United States, about 28,800 new cases of leukemia occur each year (American Cancer Society, 2005), with most cases occurring among adults older than 60 years of age (Stone, 2002). Leukemia is classified into any one of four types based on the cell type affected and the rate of progression of the leukemia:

- *Acute myelogenous leukemia (AML)* is the most common form of adult leukemia. *Acute promyelocytic leukemia (APL)* is a subtype of AML that makes up about 10% of adult-onset AML.
- *Acute lymphocytic leukemia (ALL)* constitutes about 10% of adult leukemias but is most common in children.
- *Chronic myelogenous leukemia (CML)* constitutes about 20% of adult leukemias, occurring more often in people older than 50 years of age.
- *Chronic lymphocytic leukemia (CLL)* is the rarest type of leukemia and occurs most often in people older than 50 years of age.

Features of and risk factors for leukemia are listed in Table 43-3.

COLLABORATIVE MANAGEMENT

Assessment

HISTORY

Ask the client about exposure to risk factors and related genetic factors. Age is important because the risk for adult leukemia increases with age. Occupation and hobbies may also reveal exposure to agents that increase the risk for leukemia. Previous illnesses and the medical history may reveal exposure to ionizing radiation or drugs that increase risk.

Changes in immune function increase the risk for infection in the client with leukemia. Ask about the frequency and severity of infections, such as colds, influenza, pneumonia, bronchitis, or unexplained fevers, during the preceding 6 months.

Platelet function is reduced with leukemia. Ask the client about any excessive bleeding episodes, such as the following:

- A tendency to bruise easily
- Nosebleeds
- Increased menstrual flow
- Bleeding from the gums
- Rectal bleeding
- Hematuria (blood in the urine)
- Prolonged bleeding after minor abrasions or cuts

If the client has experienced such an episode, ask whether this type and extent of bleeding is his or her usual response to injury or represents a change.

The client with leukemia often has weakness and fatigue from anemia and increased metabolism of the leukemic cells. Ask whether the client has had any of the following:

- Headaches
- Behavior changes
- Increased somnolence
- Decreased alertness
- Decreased attention span
- Lethargy, muscle weakness
- Loss of appetite
- Weight loss
- Increased fatigue

Listing activities in the previous 24 hours may reveal information about activity intolerance, changes in behavior, and unexplained fatigue. Determine how long the client has had any of these debilitating symptoms.

PHYSICAL ASSESSMENT/CLINICAL MANIFESTATIONS

Leukemia affects all blood cells, and blood influences the health and function of all organs and systems, thus many body areas and systems cells may be affected (Chart 43-8). The following manifestations occur with the acute leukemias (McCance & Huether, 2002). Some of these findings may also be present in the client with chronic leukemia in the blast phase.

CARDIOVASCULAR CHANGES. Cardiovascular changes are usually related to anemia. The heart rate is increased and blood pressure is decreased. **Murmurs** (abnormal blood flow sounds through the heart) and **bruits** (abnormal blood flow sounds heard over arteries) may be present. Capillary filling time is increased.

RESPIRATORY CHANGES. Respiratory changes are related to anemia and infections. The respiratory rate increases as anemia becomes more severe. If respiratory infections are present, the client may have manifestations of pneumonia, including cough and shortness of breath. Abnormal breath sounds are present on auscultation.

SKIN CHANGES. The skin may be pale and cool to the touch as a result of anemia. Pallor is most evident on the face, around the mouth, and in the nail beds. The conjunctiva of the eye also is pale, as are the creases on the palm of the hand (most evident when the skin over the palm of the

CHART 43-8

KEY FEATURES of Acute Leukemia

Integumentary Manifestations
- Ecchymoses
- Petechiae
- Open infected lesions
- Pallor of the conjunctiva, nail beds, palmar creases, and around the mouth

Gastrointestinal Manifestations
- Bleeding gums
- Anorexia
- Weight loss
- Enlarged liver and spleen

Renal Manifestations
- Hematuria

Cardiovascular Manifestations
- Tachycardia at basal activity levels
- Orthostatic hypotension
- Palpitations

Respiratory Manifestations
- Dyspnea on exertion

Neurologic Manifestations
- Fatigue
- Headache
- Fever

Musculoskeletal Manifestations
- Bone pain
- Joint swelling and pain

hand is stretched). **Petechiae** (raised red spots) may be present on any area of skin surface, especially the legs and feet. The petechiae may be unrelated to any obvious trauma. Inspect for skin infections or injured areas that have failed to heal. Inspect the mouth for gum bleeding and any sore or lesion of the oral cavity indicating infection.

INTESTINAL CHANGES. Intestinal manifestations may be related to an increased bleeding tendency and to fatigue. Weight loss, nausea, and anorexia are common. Examine the rectal area for fissures and test the stool for occult blood. Many clients with leukemia have reduced bowel sounds and constipation. Enlargement of the liver and spleen and abdominal tenderness also may be present from leukemic infiltration of abdominal viscera.

CENTRAL NERVOUS SYSTEM CHANGES. Cranial nerve disturbances, headache, and papilledema may occur as a result of leukemic invasion of the central nervous system (CNS). In advanced cases, seizures and coma may occur. Clients often have fever, although this is more related to infection than to changes in the CNS.

MISCELLANEOUS CHANGES. Other problems include bone and joint tenderness as the marrow is damaged and the bone resorbs. Leukemic cells invade lymph nodes, causing enlargement or masses.

PSYCHOSOCIAL ASSESSMENT

The client with newly diagnosed leukemia is very anxious and fearful of the disease outcome. Current therapies have greatly improved the prognoses of leukemia. Spend time with the client and family to assess what the diagnosis means to them and what they expect in the future. Without knowing the client's expectations and feelings, you cannot educate and provide individualized support.

A diagnosis of leukemia has serious consequences for a person's lifestyle. Hospitalization for initial treatment often lasts weeks and may result in boredom, loneliness, isolation, and financial stress. Assess coping patterns, including activities that the client finds enjoyable and methods that help the client relax. After initial therapy, the client may be able to resume work, depending on his or her occupation. Often the client must make adjustments for changes in functional status. Repeated hospitalizations for complications are common.

LABORATORY ASSESSMENT

The client with acute leukemia usually has decreased hemoglobin and hematocrit levels, a low platelet count, and an abnormal white blood cell (WBC) count. The WBC count may be low, normal, or elevated but usually is quite high, with counts of 20,000 to 100,000. The client with a high WBC count at diagnosis has a poorer prognosis.

The definitive test for leukemia is an examination of cells obtained from bone marrow aspiration and biopsy. The bone marrow is full of leukemic **blast phase cells** (immature cells that are dividing). The proteins **(antigens)** on the surfaces of the leukemic cells help diagnose the type of leukemia. These proteins are "markers" of certain types of leukemia or may indicate prognosis. Such markers include the T11 protein, terminal deoxynucleotidyl transferase (TDT), the common acute lymphoblastic leukemia antigen (CALLA), and the CD33 antigen.

Blood-clotting times and factors are usually abnormal with acute leukemia. Reduced levels of fibrinogen and other clotting factors are common. Whole blood–clotting time (Lee-White clotting test) is increased, as is the activated partial thromboplastin time (aPTT).

Chromosome analysis (cytogenetic studies) of the leukemic cells may identify marker chromosomes to help diagnose the type of leukemia, predict the prognosis, and determine therapy effectiveness. An example is the Philadelphia chromosome, which is important in the diagnosis and treatment of chronic myelogenous leukemia (CML).

RADIOGRAPHIC ASSESSMENT

Specific manifestations determine the need for specific tests. For example, in a client with dyspnea, a chest x-ray is needed to determine whether leukemic infiltrates are present in the lung. Skeletal x-rays may help determine whether bone **resorption** (loss of bone minerals and density) is present.

Critical Thinking Challenge

The client is a 44-year-old man who has been recently diagnosed with acute myelogenous leukemia (AML). His past medical history includes Hodgkin's disease at 22 years of age, for which he was treated with chemotherapy and radiation. He also has hypertension, gout, and hypercholesterolemia. He is admitted to your unit to begin induction chemotherapy.

1. What risk factors would predispose this client to development of AML?
2. What are some of the physical findings you would expect to see when examining him?
3. What abnormalities would you expect when reviewing his laboratory tests and bone marrow biopsy?

evolve For suggested answer guidelines, go to http://evolve.elsevier.com/Iggy/.

◆Analysis

COMMON NURSING DIAGNOSIS AND COLLABORATIVE PROBLEMS

The following are priority nursing diagnoses for adult clients with acute myelogenous leukemia (AML), the most common type of adult leukemia:

1. Risk for Infection related to decreased immune response
2. Risk for Injury related to thrombocytopenia
3. Fatigue related to decreased tissue oxygenation and increased energy demands

The primary collaborative problem is Potential for Antineoplastic Therapy Adverse Effects.

ADDITIONAL NURSING DIAGNOSES AND COLLABORATIVE PROBLEMS

In addition to the common nursing diagnoses and collaborative problems, clients with AML may have one or more of the following:

- Impaired Skin Integrity related to prolonged immobility
- Impaired Oral Mucous Membrane related to effects of chemotherapy and pancytopenia
- Self-Care Deficit (Total) related to progressive debilitation and weakness
- Imbalanced Nutrition: Less Than Body Requirements related to anorexia, nausea, and vomiting
- Anxiety related to fear of death
- Powerlessness related to an inability to control disease progression
- Interrupted Family Processes related to acute, life-threatening illness of a family member
- Ineffective Role Performance related to perceived inability to fulfill parental and other family roles and prolonged hospitalization
- Deficient Diversional Activity related to prolonged hospitalization.

◆Planning and Implementation

RISK FOR INFECTION

NOC **PLANNING: EXPECTED OUTCOMES.** The client with leukemia is expected to remain free from infection. Indicators include the following:

- Absence of fever and foul-smelling or purulent drainage
- Absence of cough, chest pain, and dyspnea
- Absence of urinary frequency, urgency, or pain and burning

INTERVENTIONS. Infection is a major cause of death in the client with leukemia, and sepsis is a common complication. Infection occurs through both **autocontamination** (normal flora overgrows and penetrates the internal environment) and **cross-contamination** (organisms from another person or the environment are transmitted to the client). The three most common sites of infection are the skin, respiratory tract, and intestinal tract.

Gram-negative bacteria are the most common cause of infection, although other infections do occur. Interventions aim to halt infection and control specific infections early. Chart 43-9 lists areas to assess for the client at risk for infection.

Drug Therapy for Acute Leukemia. Drug therapy for clients with AML is divided into three distinctive phases: induction, consolidation, and maintenance.

CHART 43-9

FOCUSED ASSESSMENT of
Hospitalized or Home Care Clients with Potential or Actual Risk for Infection

General Condition
- Age, fatigue, malaise
- History of allergies
- History of chemotherapy, radiation therapy, or other immunosuppressive therapies, such as steroid use
- Chronic diseases
- History of febrile neutropenia and associated symptoms
- Nutritional status
- Functional status—problems with immobility
- Tobacco use—cigarettes, pipe, cigars, oral
- Recreational drug use
- Alcohol use
- Prescribed and over-the-counter medication use
- Baseline and ongoing vital signs—blood pressure, heart rate, respiratory rate, and temperature

Skin and Mucous Membranes
- Thorough inspection of all skin surfaces with special attention to axilla, perineum (particularly the anorectal area), and under breasts; inspection of skin for color, vascularity, bleeding, lesions, edema, moist areas, excoriation, irritation, erythema; general condition of hair and nails, pressure areas, swelling, pain, tenderness, biopsy or surgical sites, wounds, enlarged lymph nodes, catheters, or other devices
- Inspection of oral cavity, including lips, tongue, mucous membranes, gingiva, teeth, and throat—color, moisture, bleeding, ulcerations, lesions, exudate, mucositis, stomatitis, plaque, swelling, pain, tenderness, taste changes, amount and character of saliva, ability to swallow, changes in voice, dental caries, client's oral hygiene routine
- History of current skin disorders or problems with mucous membranes

Head, Eyes, Ears, Nose
- Pain, tenderness, exudate, crusting, enlarged lymph nodes

Cardiopulmonary
- Respiratory rate and pattern, breath sounds (presence/absence, adventitious sounds), quantity and characteristics of sputum, shortness of breath, use of accessory muscles, dysphagia, diminished gag reflex, tachycardia, blood pressure

Gastrointestinal
- Pain, diarrhea, bowel sounds, character and frequency of bowel movements, constipation, rectal bleeding, hemorrhoids, change in bowel habits, sexual practices, erythema, ulceration

Genitourinary
- Dysuria, frequency, urgency, hematuria, pruritus, pain, vaginal or penile discharge, vaginal bleeding, burning, lesions, ulcerations, characteristics of urine

Central Nervous System
- Cognition, level of consciousness, personality, behavior

Musculoskeletal
- Tenderness, pain, loss of function

Modified from Dean, G.E., Haeuber, D., & Rivera, L.M. (1996). Infection. In R. McCorkle, et al. (Eds.), *Cancer nursing: A comprehensive textbook* (2nd ed., p. 975). Philadelphia: W. B. Saunders.

Induction Therapy. Induction therapy is intensive and consists of combination chemotherapy started at the time of diagnosis. The goal of this therapy is to achieve a rapid, complete remission of all manifestations of disease. Agencies and physicians differ in drugs used and the treatment schedule. A commonly prescribed course of aggressive chemotherapy includes continuous IV cytosine arabinoside for 7 days together with a brief infusion of daunorubicin for the first 3 days. Fifty percent to 90% of clients receiving this therapy achieve a complete remission (Scigliano et al., 2001).

A major side effect of this therapy is severe bone marrow suppression. As a result, the client is at even more risk for infection than before the treatment started. Prolonged hospitalizations are common while the client is immunosuppressed. Recovery of bone marrow function requires at least 2 to 3 weeks, during which time the client must be protected from life-threatening infections. Other side effects include nausea, vomiting, diarrhea, **alopecia** (hair loss), **stomatitis** (mouth sores), kidney toxicity, liver toxicity, and cardiac toxicity. (See Chapter 28 for information on effects of anticancer agents.) Older clients have a greater infection-related death rate during this phase than do younger clients (Stone, 2002).

For clients with APL type of AML, induction therapy typically consists of all-trans retinoic acid (ATRA) plus combination chemotherapy. If a remission of APL is not achieved with induction, the client may be treated with arsenic trioxide (Trisenox), or referred for bone marrow transplantation.

Consolidation Therapy. Consolidation therapy often consists of another course of either the same drugs used for induction at a different dosage or a different combination of chemotherapeutic agents. This treatment occurs early in remission, and its intent is to cure. Consolidation therapy may be either a single course of chemotherapy or repeated courses of chemotherapy for 1 to 2 years.

Maintenance Therapy. Maintenance therapy may be prescribed for months to years after successful induction and consolidation therapies. It is indicated for clients with acute lymphocytic leukemia (ALL) and acute promyelocytic leukemia (APL). The purpose is to maintain the remission achieved through induction and consolidation. Maintenance agents for ALL are milder and are often given orally for 2 to 5 years. Not all types of leukemia respond to maintenance therapy.

Maintenance therapy for clients with APL may consist of additional chemotherapy with mercaptopurine plus methotrexate and/or ATRA (National Comprehensive Cancer Network, 2004). Older clients who have a relapse of previously treated AML may be treated with gemtuzumab ozogamicin (Mylotarg), a monoclonal antibody-based chemotherapy agent.

New Drug Therapies. Currently, clinical trials are underway exploring the use of such therapies as targeted therapy, radioimmunotherapy, and tumor vaccines in the treatment of leukemia. See Chapter 28 for further information on cancer therapies. Imatinib mesylate (Gleevec) is targeted therapy for chronic myelogenous leukemia (CML) that is Philadelphia chromosome positive. This drug prevents the activation of an enzyme (tyrosine kinase) needed for growth of CML cells.

Drug Therapy for Infection. Drug therapy is the main defense against infections that develop in clients undergoing therapy for AML. Agents used depend on the sensitivity of the organism causing the infection, as well as infection severity. Drugs for infection are classified as antibacterial, antiviral, or antifungal. Figure 43-3 outlines the drug therapy for management of the febrile neutropenic client.

Antibiotic and Antibacterial Agents. Antibiotic and antibacterial drugs used for prevention or treatment of infection in clients with AML usually include an aminoglycoside antibiotic (amikacin, gentamicin, and tobramycin) and a penicillin, or a third-generation cephalosporin (ceftazidime). Additional, powerful antibiotics used may include vancomycin in cases of methicillin-resistant *Staphylococcus aureus* or when indwelling venous catheter infection is suspected (Peterson, 2003; Moran & Camp-Sorrell, 2002).

Antifungal Agents. Systemic antifungal agents are used when a fungal infection has been diagnosed or is strongly suggested, or when a neutropenic client remains febrile 4 to 7 days after starting antibiotic therapy. Common antifungal drugs include amphotericin B, ketoconazole (Nizoral), voriconazole (Vfend), and nystatin (Mycostatin, Nadostine✱, Nilstat). In neutropenic clients, antifungal creams (e.g., miconazole nitrate) are given intravaginally to prevent yeast infections.

Antiviral Agents. Antiviral agents are used in clients with leukemia to prevent and treat viral infections. Acyclovir is given at the start of chemotherapy, especially for clients who are cytomegalovirus (CMV) positive. If a viral infection is suspected or diagnosed, drug treatments may include ganciclovir, foscarnet, or steroids. The antivirals, although helpful in combating severe infections, have serious adverse effects, especially **ototoxicity** (disruption of hearing and/or balance) and **nephrotoxicity** (disruption of kidney function). Carefully monitor the client treated with such drugs for signs of hearing impairment and renal insufficiency.

NIC **Infection Protection.** A major objective in caring for the client with leukemia is protection from infection. Chart 43-10 lists NIC interventions for the client with leukemia. All personnel must use extreme care during all nursing procedures. Frequent, thorough handwashing is of the utmost importance. Anyone with an upper respiratory tract infection who must enter the client's room must wear a mask. Observe strict procedures when performing dressing changes or accessing a central venous catheter. Maintain strict aseptic technique in the care of these catheters at all times.

If possible, ensure that the client is in a private room to reduce cross-contamination. Other environmental precautions are used, such as allowing no standing collections of water in vases, denture cups, or humidifiers in the client's room, because they are excellent breeding grounds for organisms.

Some treatment centers prescribe a "minimal bacteria diet" during the neutropenic period. Any uncooked foods, such as raw fruits and vegetables, and pepper are removed from the diet because they contain large numbers of organisms. Whether clients benefit from this diet is controversial.

The immunosuppressed client may be placed in a room with a high-efficiency particulate air (HEPA) filtration or laminar airflow system. These systems decrease the number of airborne pathogens. Again, whether these systems benefit clients is not known.

Continually assess the client for the presence of infection. This task is difficult because manifestations may not be obvious in the client with leukopenia. The development of fever and the formation of pus (both common indicators of infection) depend on the presence of white blood cells (WBCs). The client with leukopenia may have a severe infection without pus and with a relatively low fever.

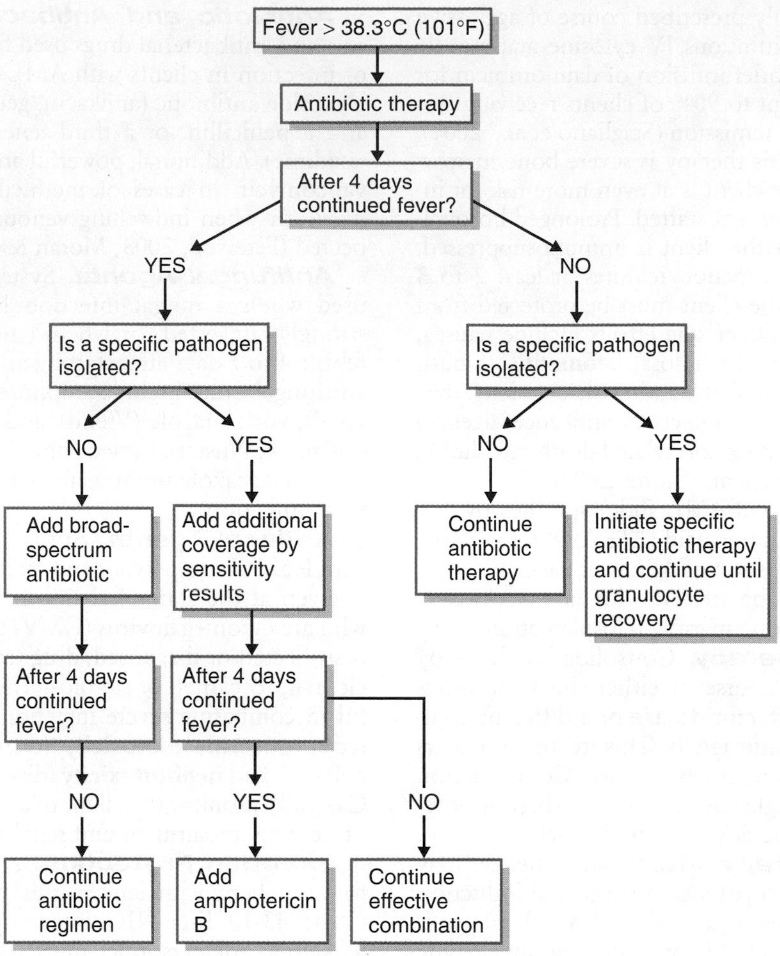

Figure 43-3 ■ Example of antibiotic management for fever in the neutropenic client.

Monitor the client's daily CBC with differential WBC count. Inspect the oral mucosa during every shift for lesions. Auscultate the lungs every 8 hours for crackles, wheezes, or reduced breath sounds. Each time the client voids, assess the urine for odor and cloudiness. Ask the client about any urgency, burning, or pain present on urination.

Take vital signs at least every 4 hours to assess for fever. A temperature elevation of even 0.5° F (or 0.5° C) above baseline is significant for a client with leukopenia and indicates infection until it has been proved otherwise.

Many hospital units that specialize in the care of clients with neutropenia have specific protocols for antibiotic therapy if infection is suspected. Usually, the health care provider is notified immediately, and specific specimens are obtained for culture. Obtain blood for bacterial and fungal cultures from peripheral sites and from the central venous catheter. Obtain urine specimens, sputum specimens, and specimens from open lesions for culture. Chest x-rays are taken. After the specimens are obtained, the client begins IV antibiotics.

Skin Care. Skin care is important for preventing infection in the client with leukemia. The skin may be the only intact defense. Teach the client about thorough hygiene care and encourage daily bathing. If the client is immobile, turn him or her every hour and apply skin lubricants.

Respiratory Care. Perform pulmonary hygiene every 2 to 4 hours. Auscultate the lungs for crackles, wheezes, or reduced breath sounds. Urge the client to cough and deep breathe or to perform sustained maximal inhalations every hour while awake.

Critical Thinking Challenge

The previously described client has completed induction therapy for 7 days. A few days later, he has a temperature of 38.4° C. He complains of having sores in his mouth and a burning sensation in his throat when he swallows.

1. What assessments should you make at this time?
2. What infection protection measures should be instituted for this client?
3. What is the most likely source of the client's infection?

evolve For suggested answer guidelines, go to http://evolve.elsevier.com/Iggy/.

Bone Marrow Transplantation. Bone marrow transplantation (BMT) is a standard treatment for leukemia. BMT is the treatment of choice for the client with leukemia who has a closely matched donor and who is in temporary remission after induction therapy. This therapy is also used for lymphoma, aplastic anemia, sickle cell disease, and many solid tumors.

The bone marrow is the actual site of production of leukemic cells. It can be difficult to ensure that all leukemic cells have been eradicated during induction therapy; therefore, before BMT, additional chemotherapy treatments and total body irradiation are given to purge (condition) the marrow

CHART 43-10

NIC INTERVENTION ACTIVITIES for
The Client with Leukemia or the Client Undergoing Bone Marrow/Stem Cell Transplantation

Infection Protection: *Prevention and early detection of infection in a client at risk*

- Monitor absolute granulocyte count, WBC count, and differential results.
- Screen all visitors for communicable disease.
- Maintain asepsis for client at risk.
- Inspect skin and mucous membranes for redness, extreme warmth, or drainage.
- Obtain cultures, as needed.
- Promote sufficient nutritional intake.
- Encourage fluid intake, as appropriate.
- Encourage deep breathing and coughing, as appropriate.
- Instruct client to take antibiotics as prescribed.
- Teach the client and family about signs and symptoms of infection and when to report them to health care provider.
- Remove fresh flowers and plants from client areas, as appropriate.
- Provide private room, as needed.

Bleeding Precautions: *Reduction of stimuli that may induce bleeding or hemorrhage in at-risk clients*

- Monitor the client closely for hemorrhage.
- Note hemoglobin/hematocrit levels before and after blood loss, as indicated.
- Monitor for signs and symptoms of persistent bleeding (e.g., check all secretions for frank or occult blood).
- Monitor coagulation studies, including prothrombin time (PT), partial thromboplastin time (PTT), fibrinogen, fibrin degradation/split products, and platelet counts, as appropriate.
- Administer blood products (e.g., platelets and fresh frozen plasma), as appropriate.
- Protect the client from trauma, which may cause bleeding.
- Avoid injections (IV, IM, or SC), as appropriate.
- Use soft toothbrush or toothettes for oral care.
- Use electric razor, instead of straight-edge, for shaving.
- Instruct client to avoid aspirin or other anticoagulants.
- Instruct client to increase intake of foods rich in vitamin K.
- Avoid constipation (e.g., encourage fluid intake and stool softeners), as appropriate.
- Instruct the client and/or family on signs of bleeding and appropriate actions (e.g., notify the nurse), should bleeding occur.

Energy Management: *Regulating energy use to treat or prevent fatigue and optimize function*

- Determine client's/significant other's perception of causes of fatigue.
- Encourage verbalization of feelings about limitations.
- Monitor nutritional intake to ensure adequate energy resources.
- Monitor/record client's sleep pattern and number of sleep hours.
- Limit number of visitors and interruptions by visitors, as appropriate.
- Provide calming diversionary activities to promote relaxation.
- Encourage an afternoon nap, if appropriate.
- Avoid care activities during scheduled rest periods.
- Plan activities for periods when the client has the most energy.
- Monitor client's oxygen response (e.g., pulse rate, cardiac rhythm, and respiratory rate) to self-care or nursing activities.
- Instruct client/significant other to recognize signs and symptoms of fatigue that require reduction in activity.

NIC intervention activities selected from Dochterman, J.M., & Bulechek, G.M. (2004). *Nursing interventions classification (NIC)* (4th ed.). St. Louis: Mosby. No part of this work is to be altered without prior written permission from the Publisher.
WBC, White blood cell.

of leukemic cells. These treatments are lethal to the bone marrow, and without replacement of bone marrow through transplantation, the client would die of infection or hemorrhage.

After conditioning, new, healthy marrow is given to the client. The new marrow then begins the process of hematopoiesis, which results in normal, properly functioning cells and, ideally, a permanent cure.

BMT units are commonplace, even in community hospital settings. With long-term survival after transplantation increasing, nurses can expect to be caring for these people, if not during the actual transplantation or recovery period, then during the post-transplantation period, in a variety of health care settings.

Sources of Stem Cells. BMT started with the use of **allogeneic bone marrow transplantation** (transplantation of bone marrow from a sibling) and has advanced to the use of human leukocyte antigen (HLA)-matched stem cells from the umbilical cords of unrelated donors. Transplants are classified by the source of stem cells. In **autologous transplants,** clients receive their own stem cells (which were collected before high-dose therapy). **Syngeneic transplants** are those with the stems cells taken from the client's own identical sibling. In **allogeneic transplants,** a closely HLA-matched sibling or an unrelated but matched donor provides the stem cells. Stem cells for transplantation may be obtained by bone marrow harvest, peripheral stem cell pheresis, or umbilical cord blood stem cell banking. Table 43-4 lists the types of transplants.

TABLE 43-4 Classification of Transplants

Type of Transplant	Sources of Stem Cells
Autologous	
Self-donation	Bone marrow harvest Peripheral stem cell pheresis Umbilical cord blood
Syngeneic	
Client's HLA identical twin	Bone marrow harvest Peripheral stem cell pheresis
Allogeneic	
HLA-matched relative, usually a sibling Unrelated HLA-matched donor Mismatched or partially HLA-matched family member or unrelated donor (donor registries)	Bone marrow harvest Peripheral stem cell pheresis Umbilical cord blood

HLA, Human leukocyte antigen.

Transplantation has five phases: stem cell obtainment, conditioning regimen, transplantation, engraftment, and post-transplantation recovery.

Obtaining the Stem Cells. Bone marrow is taken either from the client directly (autologous marrow) or from an HLA-matched person (allogeneic marrow). For allogeneic marrow, a donor is selected from family members tested for HLA type. The best results occur when the donor is an HLA-identical sibling, but BMT can also be successful between those with closely matched HLA types. The chance of matching with any given sibling is 25%.

Donor registries keep records of people willing to donate marrow to provide marrow for clients who do not have a family member HLA match. The chance of matching with an unrelated donor is one in 5000.

CULTURAL CONSIDERATIONS

About 70% of people on the bone marrow donor lists are white. It is estimated that the chance of finding an HLA-matched unrelated donor is 30% to 40% for white individuals, but for African Americans the chance is less than 20% because there are fewer African Americans among registered donors. Unlike blood types, which are present in all racial groups, tissue types can be very different among racial and ethnic groups. Nationally, efforts are made to publicize the need for donors from all cultural backgrounds.

After a suitable donor is identified by tissue typing, the donor is taken to the operating room, where sufficient marrow for transplant is removed through multiple aspirations from the iliac crests. About 500 to 1000 mL of marrow is aspirated; this amount is about 5% to 10% of the donor's marrow supply and regrows within a few weeks. The marrow is then filtered and, if autologous, is treated to rid the marrow of any remaining cancer cells. Allogeneic marrow is transfused into the recipient immediately; autologous marrow is frozen for later use.

Monitor the donor for manifestations of fluid loss, assess for complications of anesthesia, and manage postoperative pain. During surgery, donors may lose a large amount of fluid in addition to the volume of marrow donated. Donors are hydrated with saline infusions before and immediately after surgery. Occasionally the donor may need an RBC transfusion. Assess the harvest sites to ensure that the dressings are dry and intact and that the donor is not bleeding excessively.

Marrow donation is usually a same-day surgical procedure. Teach the donor to inspect the harvest sites for bleeding and to take analgesics for pain. Pain at the harvest sites (hip) is common and is managed with oral non–aspirin-containing analgesics. Some donors may require opioid analgesics for pain control.

There are three phases to obtaining **peripheral blood stem cells (PBSCs):** mobilization, collection, and reinfusion. During the mobilization phase, chemotherapy or hematopoietic growth factors are given to the client. These agents increase the numbers of stem cells and WBCs in the peripheral blood. The stem cells are then collected by **pheresis** (withdrawing whole blood, filtering out the cells, and returning the plasma to the client). One to five pheresis procedures, each lasting 2 to 4 hours, are usually needed to obtain enough stem cells for transplantation. The stem cells are then frozen and stored for reinfusion after the conditioning regimen.

Monitor the client closely during pheresis. Complications include catheter clotting and hypocalcemia (caused by anticoagulants). Hypocalcemia may cause chills, numbness, abdominal or muscle cramping, or chest pain. Oral calcium supplements may be used to manage these symptoms. Monitor vital signs at least every hour during pheresis. The client may become hypotensive from fluid volume changes during the procedure.

Stem cells may also be obtained from umbilical cord blood of newborns. This blood has a high concentration of stem cells. Umbilical stem cells are obtained via a simple phlebotomy procedure. After birth, before the placenta detaches, a syringe is used to withdraw 43 to 150 mL of blood from the umbilical vein from the placenta. The syringes are placed in a kit, which is returned to the Cord Blood Registry for processing and storage. The stem cells may be used later for an unrelated recipient or stored in case the infant develops a serious illness later in life and needs them. The cost of banking and processing umbilical cord stem cells is about $1500, with an additional charge of $100 per year for storage. Umbilical stem cells can last for years when stored properly in liquid nitrogen.

Conditioning Regimen. Figure 43-4 outlines the timing and steps involved in BMT. The day the client receives the bone marrow is day T-0. The pretransplantation conditioning days are counted in reverse order from T-0, just like a rocket countdown. Post-transplantation days are counted in order from the day of transplantation.

The client must first undergo a conditioning regimen, which varies with the diagnosis and type of transplant to be received. The conditioning regimen serves two purposes: (1) to "wipe out" the client's own bone marrow, thus preparing the client for optimal graft take and (2) to give higher than normal doses of chemotherapy and/or radiotherapy to rid the person of cancer cells (myeloablation). Usually a period of 5 to 10 days is required. The regimen usually includes high-dose chemotherapy and sometimes includes total-body irradiation (TBI). Each conditioning regimen is individually tailored, with the client's specific disease, overall health, and previous treat-

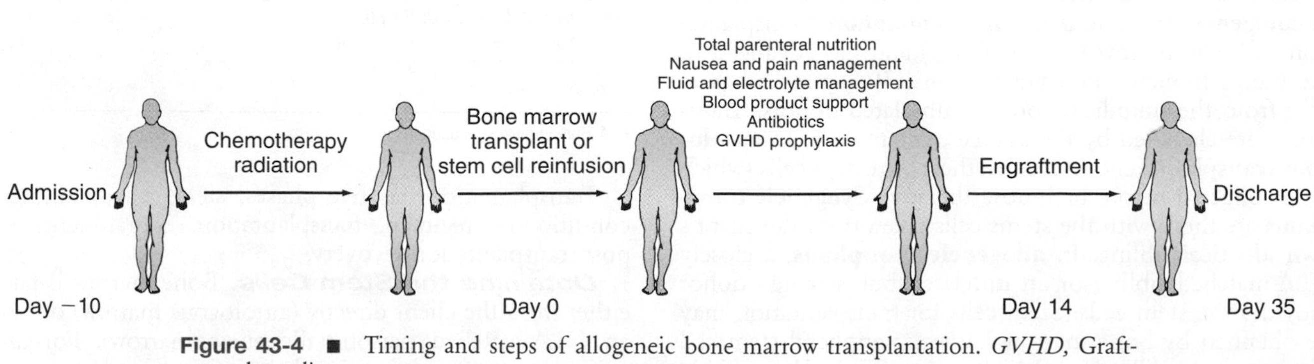

Figure 43-4 ■ Timing and steps of allogeneic bone marrow transplantation. *GVHD,* Graft-versus-host disease.

ment taken into account. A typical conditioning regimen for an adult with acute myelogenous leukemia (AML) receiving an allogenic BMT for treatment is as follows:

- *Days T-7 through T-5:* High-dose chemotherapy to obliterate the client's own bone marrow cells and to kill off any remaining leukemic cells. Specific agents include busulfan, carmustine, cyclophosphamide, cytosine arabinoside, etoposide, and melphalan. The dosages are much higher than those used for normal chemotherapy.
- *Days T-4 through T-2:* Delivery of TBI. The total radiation dose for TBI is 1200 rads given as 200 rads twice daily over 3 days.

Because of the morbidity and mortality associated with this conditioning regimen, a nonmyeloablative approach is being studied. There are many variations in nonmyeloablative conditioning regimens. This approach uses lower chemotherapy doses and low-dose TBI to reduce side effects (Kim, 2002).

During conditioning, bone marrow and normal tissues respond immediately to the chemotherapy and radiation. The client has all of the expected side effects associated with both therapies. When chemotherapy is given in high doses, these side effects are more intense than those seen with standard doses. Side effects include nausea and vomiting, mucositis, capillary leak syndrome, diarrhea, and bone marrow suppression.

Late effects from the conditioning regimen are also common, occurring as late as 3 to 10 years after transplantation. These problems include veno-occlusive disease (VOD), skin toxicities, cataracts, lung fibrosis, second cancers, cardiomyopathy, endocrine complications, and neurologic complications.

Transplantation. Day T-0, the day of transplantation, is separated from the conditioning by at least 2 days to ensure that the chemotherapy drugs have been cleared and will not kill off the transplanted stem cells. The client has few circulating WBCs, indicating successful conditioning.

The transplantation itself is very simple. Frozen marrow, PBSCs, or umbilical cord blood cells are thawed and then infused through the client's central catheter like an ordinary blood transfusion *(but not using blood administration tubing).* Usually the marrow is infused over a 30-minute period, although it can be given by IV push directly into the central catheter. In nonablative transplants, the new marrow plus stem cells from the umbilical cord are also infused.

Side effects of all types of stem cell transfusions are similar. The client may have fever and hypertension as a reaction to the preservative used in stem cell storage. To prevent these reactions, acetaminophen (Tylenol), hydrocortisone, and diphenhydramine (Benadryl) are given before the infusion. Antihypertensives or diuretics may be needed to treat fluid volume changes. The client may have red urine as a result of red blood cell hemolysis in the infused stem cells.

Engraftment. The transfused PBSCs and marrow cells circulate briefly in the peripheral blood. The stems cells find their way to the marrow-forming sites of the client's bones and establish residency there. How the donated marrow cells "home in" on the bone marrow sites is not yet understood.

Engraftment, successful "take" of the transplanted cells in the client's bone marrow, is key to the whole transplantation process. For the donated marrow or stem cells to "rescue" the client after large doses of chemotherapy or radiotherapy have wiped out his or her own bone marrow, the transfused stem cells must survive and grow in the client's bone marrow sites. Engraftment takes 8 to 12 days for peripheral blood stem cell transplantation and 12 to 28 days for bone marrow stem cell transplantation. To aid engraftment, growth factors, such as granulocyte colony-stimulating factor or granulocyte-macrophage colony-stimulating factor, may be given. When engraftment occurs, the client's WBC, RBC, and platelet counts begin to rise.

Prevention of Complications. The period after transplantation is difficult. Infection and bleeding are severe problems because the client remains without any natural immunity until the transfused stem cells grow and engraftment occurs. The nursing care for this client is the same as for the client during induction therapy for AML. Helping the client to maintain hope through this long recovery period is difficult. Complications are often severe and life threatening. Help the client to have a positive attitude and be involved in his or her own recovery.

In addition to the problems related to the period of **pancytopenia** (too few circulating blood cells), other complications of BMT include failure to engraft, development of graft-versus-host disease (GVHD), and VOD.

Failure to Engraft. Sometimes the donated marrow or stem cells fail to engraft. This possibility is discussed in advance with the client and the donor. Failure to engraft occurs more often with transplants using allogeneic stem cells than those using autologous stem cells. The causes include insufficient numbers of cells transplanted, attack or rejection of donor cells by the remaining immune system cells of the recipient, infection of transplanted cells, and unknown biologic factors. If the transplanted cells fail to engraft, the client will die unless another transplantation is successful.

Graft-Versus-Host Disease. Graft-versus-host disease (GVHD) occurs mostly in allogeneic transplants. The immunocompetent cells of the donated marrow recognize the client's (recipient) cells, tissues, and organs as foreign and start an immunologic attack against them. The graft is actually trying to attack the host tissues and cells.

Although all host tissues can be attacked and harmed, the tissues usually damaged are the skin, intestinal tract, and liver. About 25% to 50% of all allogeneic BMT recipients have some degree of GVHD, and more than 15% of the clients who develop GVHD die of its complications. The presence of some GVHD indicates successful engraftment.

Management of GVHD involves limiting the activity of donor T-cells by using immunosuppressive drugs such as cyclosporine, methotrexate, corticosteroids, and antithymocyte globulin (Kim, 2002). Care is taken to avoid suppressing the new immune system to the extent that either the client is at risk for infection or the transplanted cells stop engrafting.

Veno-occlusive Disease. Veno-occlusive disease (VOD) is the occlusion of liver blood vessels by clotting and inflammation (phlebitis). This problem occurs in up to 20% of clients who undergo BMT. Problems usually begin within the first 30 days after transplantation. Clients who received high doses of chemotherapy, especially alkylating agents, are at risk for life-threatening liver complications. Manifestations include jaundice, pain in the right upper quadrant, ascites, weight gain, and liver enlargement.

There is no known way of opening the liver vessels, thus treatment is supportive. Early detection improves the chance for survival. Fluid management is also crucial. Assess the client daily for weight gain, fluid retention, increases in abdominal girth, and hepatomegaly.

RISK FOR INJURY

Normal bone marrow production of platelets is severely limited with acute myelogenic leukemia (AML), leading to thrombocytopenia. The client is at great risk for excessive bleeding in response to minimal trauma. Thrombocytopenia can also be caused by induction therapy for AML or high-dose chemotherapy for transplantation.

NOC **PLANNING: EXPECTED OUTCOMES.** The client with leukemia is expected to remain free from bleeding. Indicators include the following:

- Maintenance of hematocrit and hemoglobin within normal limits
- Absence of frank bleeding, petechiae, or ecchymosis

INTERVENTIONS. The client's platelet count is decreased as a side effect of chemotherapy. During the period of greatest bone marrow suppression (the **nadir**), the platelet count may be very low (<10,000/mm³). The client is at extreme risk for bleeding once the platelet count falls below 50,000/mm³, and spontaneous bleeding often occurs when the platelet count is lower than 20,000/mm³.

NIC **Bleeding Precautions.** The goals are to protect the client from injury with bleeding and to closely monitor any bleeding that does occur (see Chart 43-10). Assess the client at least twice per shift for evidence of bleeding: oozing, enlarging bruises, petechiae, or purpura. Inspect all stool, urine, drainage, and vomitus for blood and test for occult blood. Measure any blood loss as accurately as possible and measure the client's abdominal girth daily. Increases in abdominal girth can indicate internal hemorrhage. Institute bleeding precautions (Chart 43-11).

CHART 43-11

BEST PRACTICE for
The Client with Thrombocytopenia

- Handle the client gently.
- Use a lift sheet when moving and positioning in bed.
- Avoid IM injections and venipunctures.
- When injections or venipunctures are necessary, use the smallest-gauge needle for the task.
- Apply firm pressure to the needle stick site for 10 minutes or until the site no longer oozes blood.
- Apply ice to areas of trauma.
- Test all urine and stool for the presence of occult blood.
- Observe IV sites every 2 hours for bleeding.
- Avoid trauma to rectal tissues:
  - Do not take temperatures rectally.
  - Do not give enemas.
  - Administer well-lubricated suppositories with caution.
  - Advise client not to have anal intercourse.
- Measure abdominal girth daily.
- Advise the client to use an electric shaver.
- Teach the client to avoid mouth trauma:
  - Use soft-bristled toothbrush or tooth sponges.
  - Do not floss between teeth.
  - Avoid dental work, especially extractions.
  - Avoid hard foods.
  - Make sure that dentures fit and do not rub.
- Encourage the client not to blow the nose or insert objects into the nose.
- Advise the client to avoid contact sports.
- Teach client to wear shoes with firm soles whenever ambulating.

Monitoring. Monitor laboratory values daily. Review CBC results daily to determine the risk for bleeding, as well as actual blood loss. The client with a platelet count below 20,000/mm³ may need a platelet transfusion. Oprelvekin (Neumega), a platelet (thrombopoietic) growth factor, may be prescribed to induce platelet growth after the completion of chemotherapy. For the client with severe blood loss, packed RBCs may be prescribed (see later discussion under Red Blood Cell Transfusions, p. 914).

FATIGUE

Normal production of red blood cells is limited in leukemia, causing anemia, which results in fatigue. Additionally, leukemic cells have high rates of metabolism, increasing fatigue in the anemic client with leukemia. Anemia may also occur as a side effect of chemotherapy treatment.

NOC **PLANNING: EXPECTED OUTCOMES.** The client with leukemia is expected to have no increase in fatigue. Indicators include that the client consistently demonstrates the following behaviors:

- Participation in self-care
- Recognition of symptoms of fatigue and alteration of activity before fatigue becomes excessive

NIC **INTERVENTIONS.** Interventions aim to reduce fatigue through energy management (see Chart 43-10) and improving red blood cell (RBC) counts.

Diet Therapy. The client must eat enough calories to meet at least basal energy requirements, but increasing dietary intake can be difficult when the client is fatigued. Provide small, frequent meals high in protein and carbohydrates. Food items that are liquid or semisolid require less effort to eat.

Blood Replacement Therapy. Blood transfusions are sometimes indicated for the client with fatigue. Transfusions increase the blood's oxygen-carrying capacity and replace missing RBCs. For the client with leukemia who has fatigue related to anemia, packed RBCs are the blood component choice. (See Table 43-6 under Transfusion Therapy, p. 913, for a discussion of nursing care during transfusions.)

Drug Therapy. Clients may receive colony-stimulating factors to reduce the severity and duration of anemia and/or neutropenia following intensive chemotherapy. For anemia, subcutaneous injections of epoetin alfa (Epogen or Procrit) 50 to 100 units/kg may be given three times per week, or darbepoetin alfa (Aranesp) 2 to 2.5 mcg/kg may be given subcutaneously weekly. This growth factor boosts the production of RBCs. This agent causes a stinging sensation when injected. Assess for side effects such as hypertension, headaches, fever, **myalgia** (muscle aches), and rashes. (See Chapter 28 for information on hematopoietic growth factors.)

Energy Conservation. Examine the client's schedule of prescribed and routine activities. Assess those activities that do not have a direct positive effect on the client's condition in terms of their usefulness. If the benefit of an activity is less than its worsening of fatigue, consult with other members of the health care team about eliminating or postponing it. Candidates for cancellation or postponement include physical therapy and any invasive diagnostic tests not needed for assessment or treatment of current problems.

Community-Based Care

The client with leukemia is discharged after induction chemotherapy and recovery of blood cell production. Follow-up care continues on an outpatient basis. Although many transplant centers discharge clients following engraftment, some centers give high-dose chemotherapy and stem cell infusion on an outpatient basis. This plan involves daily clinic visits and frequent follow-up by nurses in the home care setting.

HOME CARE MANAGEMENT

Planning for home care for the client with leukemia begins as soon as remission is achieved. The client will need help at home until the condition improves. Assess the available support mechanisms. Many clients need a visiting nurse to assist with dressing changes for central venous catheters, hyperalimentation infusions, platelet infusions, and to answer questions. Home transfusion therapy for blood components may be needed.

The home care team is critical for the client receiving stem cell transplantation in the home setting. Potential candidates are evaluated in advance. Criteria include a knowledgeable caregiver, a clean home environment, location near the hospital, telephone access, and emotional stability on the part of the client and caregiver.

Home care nurses give chemotherapy and monitor the client for complications. Nurses visit the client once or twice per day and spend between 4 and 8 hours per day in the home. The client receives the stem cell transplant infusion in the outpatient clinic. Nursing care is similar to that provided in the hospital. If complications such as sepsis or veno-occlusive disease (VOD) occur, the client is admitted to the inpatient facility.

HEALTH TEACHING

Instruct the client and family about the importance of continuing therapy and medical follow-up. Many clients go home with a central venous catheter in place and need instructions about its care. Chart 43-12 lists guidelines for central venous catheter care at home. These guidelines may be altered depending on the home setting, assistance available, and agency policy.

Protecting the client from infection at home is just as important as it was during hospitalization. (See Chart 43-9 for focused assessment for the client at risk for infection.) Urge the client to use proper hygiene and to avoid crowds or others with infections. Neither the client nor any household member should receive live virus immunization (poliomyelitis, measles, or rubella) for 2 years after transplantation. Instruct the client to continue mouth care regimens at home. Emphasize that the client should immediately notify the physician if he or she has a fever or any other sign of infection. Chart 43-13 lists guidelines for clients for infection prevention.

Many clients return home still at risk for bleeding because platelet recovery is slower than recovery of white blood cells (WBCs). Platelet levels may be low for 6 months after transplantation. Reinforce safety and bleeding precautions, and emphasize that the client must follow these precautions until the platelet count is above 50,000/mm^3. Instruct the client and family to assess for petechiae, avoid trauma and sharp objects, apply pressure to wounds for 10 minutes, and report blood in the stool or urine, or headache that does not respond to acetaminophen. Chart 43-14 lists guidelines for clients at risk for bleeding.

PSYCHOSOCIAL PREPARATION

A diagnosis of leukemia threatens self-esteem and the family role. The client faces the possibility of death, and treatment causes major changes in self-image. The client and family also experience changes in the client's body image,

CHART 43-12

CLIENT EDUCATION GUIDE
Home Care of the Central Venous Catheter

- To maintain patency, flush the catheter briskly with heparinized saline (10 units/mL) once a day and after completing infusions.
- Change the Luer-Lok cap on each catheter lumen weekly.
- Change the dressing every other day:
  - Use clean technique with thorough handwashing.
  - Clean the exit site with alcohol and povidone-iodine (Betadine).
  - Apply antibacterial ointment to the site.
  - Cover the site with dry sterile gauze dressing, taped securely, or with transparent adherent dressing.
- To prevent tension, always tape the catheter to yourself.
- Look for and report any signs of infection (redness, swelling, or drainage at the exit site).
- In case of a break or puncture in the catheter lumen, immediately clamp the catheter between yourself and the opening. *Notify your physician immediately*.

CHART 43-13

CLIENT EDUCATION GUIDE
Prevention of Infection

- Avoid crowds and other large gatherings of people who might be ill.
- Do not share personal toilet articles, such as toothbrushes, toothpaste, washcloths, or deodorant sticks, with others.
- If possible, bathe daily.
- Wash the armpits, groin, genitals, and anal area at least twice a day with an antimicrobial soap.
- Clean your toothbrush daily by either running it through the dishwasher or rinsing it in liquid laundry bleach and water.
- Wash your hands thoroughly with an antimicrobial soap before you eat or drink, after touching a pet, after shaking hands with anyone, as soon as you come home from any outing, and after using the toilet.
- Eat a low-bacteria diet, and avoid salads, raw fruits and vegetables, undercooked meat, pepper, and paprika.
- Wash dishes between uses with hot, sudsy water, or use a dishwasher.
- Do not drink water that has been standing for longer than 15 minutes.
- Do not reuse cups and glasses without washing.
- Avoid changing pet litter boxes. If unavoidable, use gloves or wash hands immediately.
- Avoid keeping turtles and reptiles as pets.
- Do not feed pets raw or undercooked meat.
- Take your temperature at least twice a day.
- Report any of the following manifestations of infection to your physician immediately:
  - Temperature greater than 100° F (38° C)
  - Persistent cough (with or without sputum)
  - Pus or foul-smelling drainage from any open skin area or normal body opening
  - Presence of a boil or abscess
  - Urine that is cloudy or foul smelling, or burning on urination
- Take all medications as prescribed.
- Do not dig in the garden or work with houseplants.
- Avoid travel to areas of the world with poor sanitation or less-than-adequate health care facilities.

CHART 43-14

CLIENT EDUCATION GUIDE
The Client at Risk for Bleeding

- Use an electric shaver.
- Use a soft-bristled toothbrush, and do not floss.
- Do not have dental work done without consulting your doctor.
- Do not take aspirin or any aspirin-containing products. Read the label to be sure that the product does not contain aspirin or salicylates.
- Do not participate in contact sports or any activity likely to result in your being bumped, scratched, or scraped.
- If you are bumped, apply ice to the site for at least 1 hour.
- Notify your doctor if you:
  - Experience an injury and persistent bleeding results
  - Have excessive menstrual bleeding
  - See blood in your urine or bowel movement
  - Have a headache that does not respond to acetaminophen.
- Avoid anal intercourse.
- Take a stool softener to prevent straining during a bowel movement.
- Do not use enemas or rectal suppositories.
- Avoid bending over at the waist.
- Do not wear clothing or shoes that are tight or that rub.
- Avoid blowing your nose or placing objects in your nose. If you must blow your nose, do so gently without blocking either nasal passage.

level of independence, and lifestyle. Some feel threatened by their environment, seeing everything as potentially infectious. Clients who are cared for in protective isolation may feel lonely and isolated. Help the client and family define priorities, understand the illness and its treatment, and find hope. Make referrals to support groups sponsored by organizations such as the American Cancer Society ("I Can Cope" and "Make Today Count"), which may benefit both the client and the family. (See the Evidence-Based Practice for Nursing box at right.)

HEALTH CARE RESOURCES

The client with limited social support may need help at home until strength and energy return. A home care aide may suffice for some clients, whereas for others a visiting nurse may be needed to reinforce teaching. The client may also need equipment for activities of daily living (ADLs) and ambulation. Assess financial resources. Cancer treatment is expensive, and you must work closely with the social services department to ensure that insurance is adequate. If the client is uninsured, explore other sources, such as drug company-sponsored compassionate aid programs. The Leukemia Society of America offers limited financial help for clients with leukemia, sponsors support groups, and provides information for clients and families.

Prolonged outpatient contact and follow-up is necessary and clients need transportation to the outpatient facility. Many local units of the American Cancer Society offer free transportation to clients with cancer, including leukemia.

Critical Thinking Challenge

The client has received a bone marrow transplant for treatment of leukemia.

1. For what complications from this procedure should you assess?
2. What discharge instructions should be given to this client?

evolve For suggested answer guidelines, go to http://evolve.elsevier.com/Iggy/.

EVIDENCE-BASED PRACTICE for Nursing

What is the best measure of quality of life for clients undergoing bone marrow or peripheral blood stem cell transplantation?

Danaher Hacker, E. (2003). Quantitative measurement of quality of life in adult patients undergoing bone marrow transplant or peripheral blood stem cell transplant: A decade in review. *Oncology Nursing Forum, 30*(4), 613-629.

The evaluation of quality of life (QOL) becomes important as cancer treatments impact all aspects of a person's life. The purpose of this review was to evaluate the quantitative means of measuring QOL in clients undergoing bone marrow transplantation (BMT) or peripheral blood stem cell transplantation (PBSCT) over the past 10 years. Thirty-two research studies were included in the review. In terms of sample size, 22 studies (69%) had more than 100 participants, whereas 10 studies (31%) had fewer than 100 participants. Eighty-eight percent of the studies evaluated QOL in clients who had undergone BMT, but only 9% (n = 3) focused on QOL following PBSCT. In 66% of the studies, QOL was measured only once, from 1 to 5 years after transplantation. Two studies measured QOL in long-term transplant survivors, and 34% measured QOL before transplantation, 100 days after transplantation, and 1 year after transplantation. Most studies used measurement tools that captured the multidimensional nature of QOL. The severe toxicities associated with transplant underscore the need to assess the client's QOL as well as overall survival and disease-free survival when looking at client outcomes. Controversy remains regarding whether to use one or more instruments to measure QOL, and no gold standard measure for QOL, either in research or practice, yet exists.

Level of Evidence: 1—Quantitative systematic review.

Critique. Few studies had actually defined QOL, and a lack of consensus remains as to what QOL represents. Study sample sizes were relatively small, limiting the generalizability of the study findings. The majority of the studies used a cross-sectional design, measuring QOL only once rather than over time. A review of a decade of research fails to resolve the controversy regarding the use of single or multiple instruments to measure QOL.

Implications for Nursing. The assessment of QOL as a client outcome of transplantation is receiving increased attention. Therefore the inclusion of a QOL measure that captures the multidimensional nature of QOL, but is not too burdensome for the client should be a consideration in clinical practice and research. The determination of research findings that are clinically relevant regarding QOL in transplant recipients will provide the basis for evidence-based nursing practice and ultimately improve care for transplant recipients.

Evaluation: Outcomes

Evaluate the care of the client with leukemia on the basis of the identified nursing diagnoses and collaborative problems. The expected outcomes include that the client will:

- Remain free of infection and sepsis
- Not experience episodes of bleeding
- Be able to balance activity and rest
- Use energy conservation techniques
- Adapt lifestyle to energy level

Specific indicators for these outcomes are listed for each nursing diagnosis and collaborative problem under the Planning and Implementation section (see earlier).

MALIGNANT LYMPHOMA

Malignant lymphomas are the abnormal overgrowth of one type of leukocyte, the lymphocyte. They differ from the leukemias in the degree of maturation of the affected cells and the location of cancer cell production. Lymphomas are cancers of committed lymphocytes rather than stem cell precursors (as in leukemia). This growth occurs in lymphoid tissues scattered throughout the body, especially the lymph nodes and spleen, rather than in the bone marrow. Lymphomas are solid tumors rather than cellular suspensions within the blood and bone marrow. There are two major categories of lymphoma among adults: Hodgkin's lymphoma (HL) and non-Hodgkin's lymphoma (NHL).

Hodgkin's Lymphoma

PATHOPHYSIOLOGY

Hodgkin's lymphoma (HL) is a cancer that can affect any age-group. It occurs most often in people in their mid to late 20s and in people older than 50 years of age (McCance & Huether, 2002). HL equally affects younger men and women, but the disease is more prevalent in men in the older group.

Possible causes of HL include viral infections and exposure to chemical agents. This cancer usually starts in a single lymph node or a single chain of nodes. The tissue in the node becomes cancerous. These nodes contain a specific cancer cell type, the **Reed-Sternberg cell,** a marker for Hodgkin's lymphoma. The disease first spreads in a predictable manner to nearby lymph tissues and eventually invades nonlymphoid tissues.

COLLABORATIVE MANAGEMENT

Assessment

The most common first assessment finding is a large but painless lymph node or nodes, usually in the neck. The client also often has fever, malaise, and night sweats (Table 43-5). Specific manifestations depend on the site and extent of disease.

Diagnosis and grade are established when biopsy of a node or mass reveals Reed-Sternberg cells (McCance & Huether, 2002). The client then undergoes staging procedures to determine the extent of disease. Staging is detailed and accurate because the treatment regimen is determined by the extent of disease. Staging procedures for HL include biopsies of distant lymph nodes, computed tomography (CT) of the chest and abdomen, laparotomy, a complete blood count (CBC), liver function studies, and bilateral bone marrow biopsies.

Interventions

Hodgkin's lymphoma (HL) is one of the most curable types of cancer. Generally, for stage I and stage II disease, the treatment of choice is external radiation of involved lymph node regions. With more extensive disease, radiation is used along with combination chemotherapy to achieve a cure. (See Chapter 28 on general care of clients receiving radiation and chemotherapy.)

Nursing management of the client undergoing treatment for HL focuses on the side effects of therapy, especially the following:

- Drug-induced pancytopenia, which increases the risk for infection, bleeding, and anemia
- Severe nausea and vomiting
- Skin problems at the site of radiation
- Impaired hepatic function either by metastasis to the liver or by multiagent chemotherapy

TABLE 43-5 Manifestations and Staging Criteria for Hodgkin's Lymphoma

Stage Ia
Disease is confined to a single lymph node region or only one extranodal site.

Stage Ib
Disease is confined to a single lymph node region or only one extranodal site. The client also experiences some or all of the following systemic symptoms: persistent fever, night sweats, and significant weight loss (>10%).

Stage IIa
Disease is confined to either two or more lymph node regions on the same side of the diaphragm or contiguous extranodal sites on the same side of the diaphragm.

Stage IIb
Disease is confined to either two or more lymph node regions on the same side of the diaphragm or contiguous extranodal sites on the same side of the diaphragm. Client also experiences some or all of the following systemic symptoms: persistent fever, night sweats, and significant weight loss (>10%).

Stage IIIa
Disease extends to lymph node regions on both sides of the diaphragm.

Stage IIIb
Disease extends to lymph node regions on both sides of the diaphragm. The client also experiences some or all of the following systemic symptoms: persistent fever, night sweats, and significant weight loss (>10%).

Stage IIIc
Disease extends to lymph node regions on both sides of the diaphragm. The client also experiences some or all of the following systemic symptoms: persistent fever, night sweats, and significant weight loss (>10%). The spleen is also involved in disease.

Stage IV
Disease has widely disseminated foci of involvement, including one or more extranodal tissues and organs.

- Permanent sterility for male clients receiving radiation to the abdominopelvic region in the pattern of an inverted Y in combination with specific chemotherapeutic agents (The client is informed of this side effect and given the option to store sperm in a sperm bank before treatment.)
- Secondary cancer development as a result of HL treatment (Long-term follow-up includes screening for recurrence, as well as the possible development of a secondary cancer.)

Non-Hodgkin's Lymphoma

PATHOPHYSIOLOGY

Non-Hodgkin's lymphoma (NHL) includes all lymphoid cancers that do not have the Reed-Sternberg cell. There are more than 12 subtypes of NHL, including low-grade, intermediate, and high-grade lymphomas. NHLs arise from altered B or T lymphocytes. The low-grade lymphomas usually arise from B-cell lymphocytes and progress slowly. Although clients with low-grade lymphomas have longer survival rates, the diseases are less responsive to treatment and cures are rare (Strauss, 2003).

High-grade lymphomas are aggressive tumors of mixed cell types with rapid growth. High-grade lymphomas are more responsive to chemotherapy, and the chances for a long-term cure are greater. A low-grade lymphoma can convert to a higher-grade lymphoma. When this occurs, the prognosis is poor.

NHL is the sixth most common cause of cancer-related death in the United States (American Cancer Society, 2005). The disease is more common in men, white individuals, and people older than 50 years of age. The long-term prognosis is better for women and clients younger than 65 years of age. Most NHLs start in lymph nodes, but they can originate in any tissue or organ. NHL may be related to inherited problems that result in gene damage. Gene damage may result in loss of tumor suppressor gene function, allowing cancer development to occur. Viral infection, autoimmune disease, and exposure to radiation or to toxic chemicals have all been implicated in the development of NHL.

◆COLLABORATIVE MANAGEMENT

Enlarged lymph nodes may be the only manifestation of lymphoma because these nodes can arise from lymphoid cells in any tissue and can spread to any organ. Painless swelling of the cervical, axillary, inguinal, and femoral nodes are most often seen. Diagnosis is made from the histologic features of cells obtained by biopsy of a node or mass. Classification of the lymphoma subtype is based on a complex grading of surface markers, chromosomes, cell size, and presence of viral antigens. Staging is similar to that for Hodgkin's lymphoma (HL) (see Table 43-5).

Treatment consists of radiation therapy and multiagent chemotherapy, or single-agent therapy with fludarabine. In relapsed disease, newer agents including monoclonal antibodies (e.g., rituximab and alemtuzumab) and radiolabeled antibodies (^{131}I tositumomab and ^{90}Y ibritumomab) are being used. Nursing care needs are similar to those for clients with HL, with additional organ-specific problems taken into account if the disease is widely spread.

Multiple Myeloma

PATHOPHYSIOLOGY

Multiple myeloma is a white blood cell (WBC) cancer that involves a more mature lymphocyte than either leukemia or lymphoma. There is overgrowth of B-lymphocyte plasma cells in the bone marrow. These cells normally make antibodies. When they become cancerous, these plasma cells overproduce both complete and incomplete antibodies or gamma globulins. Thus the disorder is called a "gammopathy." Similar to the leukemias, when the myeloma cells are overproduced, fewer functional red blood cells (RBCs), WBCs, and platelets are produced.

In addition to the excess antibodies, multiple myeloma cells also produce excess cytokines (see Chapter 23) that increase the cancer cell growth rates and destroy bone. The excess antibodies are released into the blood, increasing the serum protein levels and clogging blood vessels in the kidney and other organs. Without treatment, the disease causes progressive bone destruction, bleeding problems, kidney failure, immunosuppression, and death.

Multiple myeloma is an uncommon cancer, accounting for 1% of all cancers (Rice & Sheridan, 2001). This disorder occurs mostly in people older than 50 years of age and is about twice as common among African Americans as white individuals. It occurs equally in men and women. The cause of multiple myeloma is unknown, although radiation and chemical exposure may be risk factors.

◆COLLABORATIVE MANAGEMENT

The client with multiple myeloma usually first notices fatigue, easy bruising, and bone pain. Other manifestations, such as bone fractures, hypertension, increased infection, hypercalcemia, and fluid imbalance, occur as the disease progresses. Diagnosis is made by bone marrow biopsy, x-ray findings of bone thinning with areas of bone loss that resemble "Swiss cheese," electrophoresis of plasma proteins, and the presence of "Bence-Jones" protein in the urine.

Standard treatment for multiple myeloma is chemotherapy. Agents most commonly used are melphalan, prednisone, vincristine, cyclophosphamide, doxorubicin, and carmustine. Recently, thalidomide is showing promise in controlling the disease. Autologous bone marrow transplantation is being used with clients who have a good response to the chemotherapy. For client's whose disease progresses despite treatment, a recently approved proteasome inhibitor, bortezomib (Velcade), may be used. Bortezomib acts by blocking processes needed for the cancer cells' growth and survival. Side effects include fatigue, nausea, diarrhea, neuropathy, thrombocytopenia, and neutropenia.

Coagulation Disorders

Coagulation disorders are bleeding disorders with increased bleeding resulting from defects in one or more components regulating the blood clotting system. Bleeding disorders may be spontaneous or traumatic, localized or generalized, lifelong or acquired. They can arise from a defect in the clotting processes at the vascular, platelet, or clotting factor level. Figure 43-5 outlines the blood-clotting cascade and sites where specific defects and drugs disrupt the clotting processes.

PLATELET DISORDERS

Platelets have a vital role in blood clotting. Blood clotting always starts with platelets sticking together and forming a platelet plug. Any condition that either reduces the number of platelets or interferes with their ability to adhere (to one another, blood vessel walls, collagen, or fibrin threads) can result in increased bleeding. Platelet disorders can be inherited, acquired, or temporarily induced by drugs that limit platelet production or inhibit aggregation.

A decrease in the number of platelets below the level needed for normal coagulation is called **thrombocytopenia.** Thrombocytopenia may occur as a result of other conditions or treatments that suppress general bone marrow activity. It also can occur through processes that limit platelet formation or increase the rate of platelet destruction. The two thrombocytopenic conditions affecting adults are autoim-

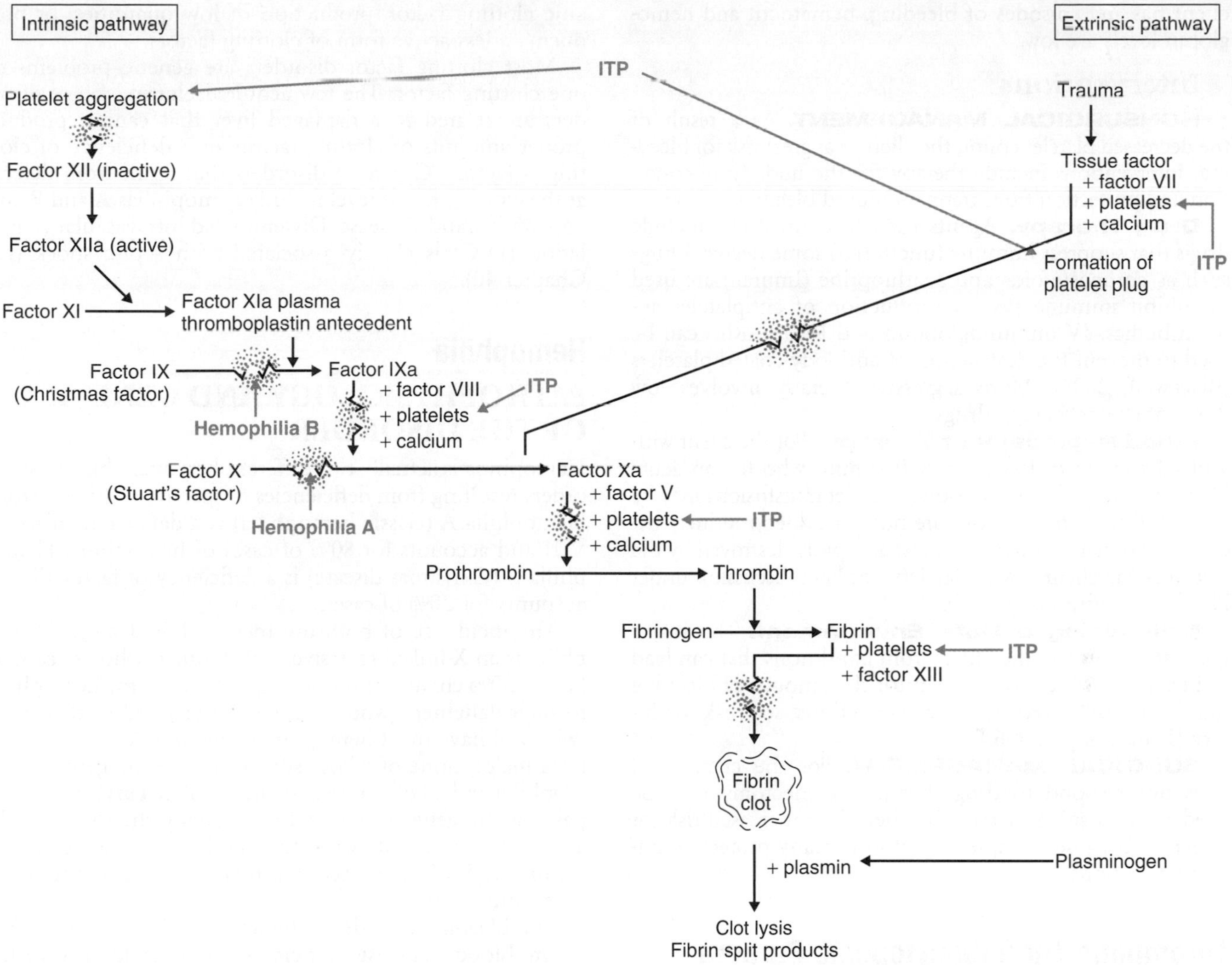

Figure 43-5 ■ Sites of disruption of the coagulation mechanisms by disease. *ITP,* Idiopathic thrombocytopenic purpura.

mune thrombocytopenic purpura and thrombotic thrombocytopenic purpura.

Autoimmune Thrombocytopenic Purpura

PATHOPHYSIOLOGY

Autoimmune thrombocytopenic purpura is also called idiopathic thrombocytopenic purpura (ITP). The total number of circulating platelets is greatly reduced in ITP, even though platelet production in the bone marrow is normal.

Clients with this disorder make an antibody directed against the surface of their own platelets (an antiplatelet-antibody). This antibody coats the surface of the platelets, making them more likely to be destroyed by macrophages (see Chapter 23). The spleen contains a large number of macrophages and the blood vessels of the spleen are long and twisted. Both of these conditions allow antibody-coated platelets to be destroyed in the spleen (Blackwell, 2003). When the rate of platelet destruction exceeds that of production, the number of circulating platelets decreases and blood clotting slows.

Although the cause of this disorder is autoimmune, the trigger for the production of autoantibodies is unknown. ITP is most common among women between the ages of 20 and 40 and among people who have other autoimmune disorders, such as systemic lupus erythematosus (McCance & Huether, 2002).

COLLABORATIVE MANAGEMENT

Assessment

Clinical manifestations of ITP are at first limited to the skin and mucous membranes: large **ecchymoses** (bruises) or a petechial rash on the arms, legs, upper chest, and neck. Mucosal bleeding occurs easily. If the client has had significant blood loss, anemia may also be present.

A rare complication is an intracranial bleed–induced stroke. Assess for neurologic function and mental status (see Chapter 44). Ask family members whether the client's behavior and responses to questions are typical or represent a change.

ITP is diagnosed by a decreased platelet count and large numbers of megakaryocytes in the bone marrow. Antiplatelet antibodies may be detected in the blood. If the client has any episodes of bleeding, hematocrit and hemoglobin levels are low.

Interventions

NONSURGICAL MANAGEMENT. As a result of the decreased platelet count, the client is at great risk for bleeding. Interventions include therapy for the underlying condition and protection from trauma-induced bleeding episodes.

Drug Therapy. Agents used to control ITP include drugs that suppress immune function to some degree. Drugs such as corticosteroids and azathioprine (Imuran) are used to inhibit immune system production of antiplatelet autoantibodies. IV immunoglobulin and IV anti-Rho can be used to prevent the destruction of antibody-coated platelets (Blackwell, 2003). More aggressive therapy involves low doses of chemotherapy drugs.

Blood Replacement Therapy. For the client with a platelet count of less than 20,000/mm^3 who has an acute life-threatening bleeding episode, platelet transfusions may be needed. Platelet transfusions are not performed routinely because the donated platelets are just as rapidly destroyed by the spleen as the client's own platelets (see later discussion under Platelet Transfusions, p. 915).

Maintaining a Safe Environment. The major goals are to protect the client from conditions that can lead to bleeding and to closely monitor the amount of bleeding that is occurring. (For nursing care actions, see Risk for Injury [Leukemia], p. 906.)

SURGICAL MANAGEMENT. For the client who does not respond to drug therapy, splenectomy may be needed. After splenectomy, the client is at increased risk for infection because the spleen performs many protective immune functions.

Thrombotic Thrombocytopenic Purpura

PATHOPHYSIOLOGY

Thrombotic thrombocytopenic purpura (TTP) is a rare disorder in which platelets clump together abnormally in the capillaries and too few platelets remain in circulation. The client has inappropriate clotting, yet the blood fails to clot properly when trauma occurs. The underlying cause of TTP appears to be an autoimmune reaction in blood vessel cells (endothelial cells) that makes platelets clump together in very small blood vessels. As a result, tissues become ischemic. Manifestations include renal failure, myocardial infarction, and stroke. If left untreated, this condition is often fatal within 3 months.

COLLABORATIVE MANAGEMENT

Treatment for the client with TTP focuses on preventing platelet clumping and stopping the underlying autoimmune process. Treatment consists of plasma pheresis and the infusion of fresh frozen plasma. This treatment provides platelet aggregation inhibitors. Drugs that inhibit platelet clumping, such as aspirin, alprostadil (Prostin), and plicamycin, also may be helpful. Immunosuppressive therapy reduces the intensity of this disorder.

CLOTTING FACTOR DISORDERS

Coagulation or bleeding disorders can result from a clotting factor defect. Defects include the inability to produce a specific clotting factor, production of low quantities, or producing a less active form of clotting factors.

Most clotting factor disorders are genetic problems of one clotting factor. The few acquired clotting factor disorders are related to a damaged liver that cannot produce proper amounts of clotting factors or a deficiency of clotting cofactors. Common disorders that result from defects at the clotting factor level include hemophilias A and B and von Willebrand's disease. Disseminated intravascular coagulation (DIC) is closely associated with septic shock (see Chapter 40).

Hemophilia

PATHOPHYSIOLOGY AND GENETICS OF THE DISORDER

Hemophilia is actually two different hereditary bleeding disorders resulting from deficiencies of specific clotting factors. Hemophilia A (classic hemophilia) is a deficiency of factor VIII and accounts for 80% of cases of hemophilia. Hemophilia B (Christmas disease) is a deficiency of factor IX and accounts for 20% of cases.

The incidence of both disorders is 1 in 10,000. Hemophilia is an X-linked recessive trait. Women who are carriers have a 50% chance of transmitting the gene for hemophilia to their daughters (who then are carriers) and to their sons (who will have overt hemophilia). Hemophilia A mostly affects males, none of whose sons will have the gene for hemophilia and all of whose daughters will be **carriers** (able to pass on the gene without actually having the disorder). In about 30% of clients with hemophilia, there is no family history, and it is presumed that their disease is the result of a new mutation.

The bleeding disorder of hemophilia A is so severe that before blood transfusions were available, children with hemophilia rarely survived past age 3 years. With blood transfusion and factor VIII therapy, survival time has increased so greatly that hemophilia now is often seen among adult clients.

The clinical pictures of hemophilia A and B are identical. The client has abnormal bleeding in response to any trauma because of a deficiency of the specific clotting factor. Clients with hemophilia do not bleed more frequently or even more rapidly than those without the disease, but they do bleed for a longer period. Hemophiliacs form platelet plugs at the bleeding site, but the clotting factor deficiency impairs the clotting response and stable fibrin clots do not form. This allows excessive bleeding, which may be mild, moderate, or severe, depending on the degree of factor deficiency.

COLLABORATIVE MANAGEMENT

Assessment

Assessment of the client with hemophilia shows the following:

- Excessive hemorrhage from minor cuts, bruises, or abrasions (as a result of abnormal platelet function)
- Joint and muscle hemorrhages that lead to disabling long-term problems
- A tendency to bruise easily
- Prolonged and potentially fatal postoperative hemorrhage

The laboratory test results for a client with hemophilia show a prolonged partial thromboplastin time (PTT), a normal bleeding time, and a normal prothrombin time (PT). The most common problem that occurs with hemophilia is degenerating joint function as a result of chronic bleeding into the joints, especially at the hip and knee.

Interventions

The bleeding problems of hemophilia A are managed by either regularly scheduled IV infusions of factor VIII cryoprecipitate (Bioclate, Helixate, ReFacto) or intermittent infusions as needed (see Cryoprecipitate Transfusions, p. 915). The cost of cryoprecipitate is prohibitive for many people with hemophilia. In addition, because the precipitated clotting factors are made from pooled human serum, a risk for viral contamination remains, even with the use of heat-inactivated serum. Infectious complications of hemophilia therapy include hepatitis B, hepatitis C, cytomegalovirus, and human immunodeficiency virus (HIV). Although newer serum processing techniques have reduced these risks, they have not yet been eliminated.

Transfusion Therapy

Any blood component may be removed from a donor and transfused to a recipient. Components may be transfused individually or collectively, with varying degrees of benefit to the recipient. Table 43-6 lists indications for transfusion therapy.

PRETRANSFUSION RESPONSIBILITIES

Nursing actions during transfusions aim at prevention or early recognition of adverse transfusion reactions. Preparation of the client for transfusion therapy is imperative, and institutional blood product administration procedures must be carefully followed. Before administering any blood product, review the agency's policies and procedures. Chart 43-15 lists best practices for transfusion therapy.

Legally, a physician's prescription is needed to administer blood or its components. The prescription specifies the type of component, the volume, and any special conditions the physician judges to be important. Verify the prescription for accuracy and completeness. In many hospitals a separate consent form must be obtained before a transfusion is performed.

A blood specimen is obtained for crossmatching (testing of the donor's blood and the recipient's blood for compatibility). The procedure and responsibility for obtaining this specimen are specified by hospital policy. The laboratory requires at least 45 minutes to complete the crossmatch testing. In most hospitals a new crossmatching specimen is required at least every 48 hours.

Blood components are viscous, requiring that a large needle (at least 20-gauge) be used, whenever possible, for venous access. Both Y-tubing and straight tubing sets are used for blood component infusion. A blood filter (about 170 μm) to remove sediment from the stored blood products is included with blood administration sets and must be used to transfuse most blood products. In massive transfusion, a microaggregate filter (20 to 43 μm) may be used.

Use normal saline as the solution to administer with blood products. Ringer's lactate and dextrose in water are not used for infusion with blood products because they cause clotting or hemolysis of blood cells. *Never add drugs to blood products.*

Before the transfusion is started, it is essential to determine that the blood component delivered is correct and that identification of the client is correct. Check the physician's prescription simultaneously with another registered nurse to determine the client's identity and whether the hospital identification band name and number are identical to those on the blood component tag. *Checking the client's room number is not an acceptable form of identification* (Joint Commission on Accreditation of Healthcare Organizations, 2004). Examine the blood bag label, the attached tag, and the requisition slip to ensure that the ABO and Rh types are compatible. Check the expiration date and inspect the product for discoloration, gas bubbles, or cloudiness, all indicators of bacterial growth or hemolysis.

TRANSFUSION RESPONSIBILITIES

Before starting the transfusion, explain the procedure to the client. Take the vital signs, including temperature, immediately before starting the transfusion. Begin the infusion slowly. Remain with the client for the first 15 to 30 minutes. Any severe reaction usually occurs with infusion of the first 50 mL of blood. Ask the client to report unusual

TABLE 43-6 Indications for Treatment with Blood Components

Component	Volume	Infusion Time	Indications
Packed red blood cells (PRBCs)	200-250 mL	2-4 hr	Anemia; hemoglobin <6 g/dL, 6-10 g/dL, depending on symptoms
Washed red blood cells (WBC-poor PRBCs)	200 mL	2-4 hr	History of allergic transfusion reactions Bone marrow transplant clients
Platelets			
Pooled	About 300 mL	15-30 min	Thrombocytopenia, platelet count <20,000 Clients who are actively bleeding with a platelet count <80,000
Single donor	200 mL	30 min	History of febrile or allergic reactions
Fresh frozen plasma	200 mL	15-30 min	Deficiency in plasma coagulation factors Prothrombin or partial thromboplastin time 1.5 times normal
Cryoprecipitate	10-20 mL/unit	15-30 min	Hemophilia VIII or von Willebrand's disease Fibrinogen levels <100 mg/dL
White blood cells (WBCs)	400 mL	1 hr	Sepsis, neutropenic infection not responding to antibiotic therapy

CHART 43-15

BEST PRACTICE for
Transfusion Therapy

Nursing Actions	Rationales
Before Infusion	
1. Assess laboratory values.	Many institutions have specific guidelines for blood product transfusions (i.e., platelet count <20,000 or hemoglobin <6 g/dL).
2. Verify the medical prescription.	Legally, a physician's prescription is required for transfusions. The order should state the type of product, dose, and transfusion time.
3. Assess the client's vital signs, urine output, skin color, and history of transfusion reactions.	Determine whether the client can tolerate infusion. Baseline information may be needed to help identify transfusion reactions.
4. Obtain venous access. Use a central catheter or 19-gauge needle if possible.	The larger-bore needle allows cells to flow more easily without occluding the lumen of the catheter.
5. Obtain blood products from a blood bank. Transfuse immediately.	Once a blood product has been released from the blood bank, the product should be transfused as soon as possible (e.g., red blood cell transfusions should be completed within 4 hours of removal from refrigeration).
6. With another registered nurse, verify the client by name and number, check blood compatibility, and note expiration time.	Human error is the most common cause of ABO incompatibility reactions.
During Infusion	
7. Administer the blood product using the appropriate filtered tubing.	Filters are needed to remove aggregates and possible contaminants.
8. If the blood product needs to be diluted, use only normal saline solution.	Hemolysis occurs if any other IV solution is used.
9. Remain with the client during the first 15 to 30 minutes of the infusion.	Hemolytic reactions occur most often within the first 50 mL of the infusion.
10. Infuse the blood product at the prescribed rate.	Fluid overload is a potential complication of rapid infusion.
11. Monitor vital signs.	Vital sign changes often indicate transfusion reactions.
After Infusion	
12. When the transfusion is completed, discontinue infusion and dispose of the bag and tubing properly.	Bloodborne pathogens may be spread inadvertently through improper disposal.
13. Document.	The client record should indicate the type of product infused, product number, volume infused, time of infusion, and any adverse reactions.

sensations such as chills, shortness of breath, hives, or itching. Assess vital signs 15 minutes after starting the transfusion to detect signs of a reaction. If there are none, the infusion rate can be increased to transfuse 1 unit in about 2 hours (depending on the client's cardiac status). Take vital signs every hour throughout the transfusion or as specified by agency policy.

Blood components without large amounts of red blood cells (RBCs) can be infused more quickly. The identification checks are the same as for RBC transfusions. It may be necessary to infuse blood products at a slower rate for older clients. Best practices related to the nursing care needs of older clients during transfusion therapy are listed in Chart 43-16.

TYPES OF TRANSFUSIONS

Red Blood Cell Transfusions

RBCs are given to replace cells lost as a result of trauma or surgery. Clients with problems that destroy RBCs or impair RBC maturation also may benefit from RBC transfusions. Packed RBCs, supplied in 250-mL bags, are a concentrated source of RBCs and are the most common component given to RBC-deficient clients. Packed RBCs are given to clients with a hemoglobin level less than 6 g/dL (or a hemoglobin value of 6 to 10 g/dL if manifestations are present).

Blood transfusions are actually transplantations of tissue from one person to another. The donor and recipient blood must thus be carefully checked for compatibility to prevent lethal reactions (Table 43-7). Compatibility is determined by two different types of antigen systems (cell surface proteins): the ABO system antigens and the Rh antigen, which is present on the membrane surface of RBCs.

RBC antigens are inherited. For the ABO antigen system, a person inherits one of the following:

- A antigen (type A blood)
- B antigen (type B blood)
- Both A and B antigens (type AB blood)
- No A or B antigens (type O blood)

Within the first few years of life, circulating antibodies develop against the blood type antigens that were not inherited. For example, a person with type A blood forms antigens against type B blood. A person with type O blood has not inherited either A or B antigens and will form antibodies against RBCs that have either A or B antigens. If RBCs that contain an antigen are infused into a recipient who does not share the antigen, the donated tissue is recognized by the immune system of the recipient as non-self, and the recipient has a reaction to the transfused products.

CHART 43-16

BEST PRACTICE for
The Older Adult Receiving a Transfusion

- Assess the client's circulatory, renal, and fluid status before initiating the transfusion.
- Use no larger than a 19-gauge needle.
- Try to use blood that is less than 1 week old. (Older blood cell membranes are more fragile, break easily, and release potassium into the circulation.)
- Take vital signs (especially pulse, blood pressure, and respiratory rate) every 15 minutes throughout the transfusion. Changes in these parameters can indicate fluid overload and may also be the only indicators of adverse transfusion reactions.

Overload
- Rapid bounding pulse
- Hypertension
- Swollen superficial veins

Transfusion Reaction
- Rapid thready pulse
- Hypotension
- Increased pallor, cyanosis
- Administer blood slowly, taking 2 to 4 hours for each unit of whole blood, packed red blood cells, or plasma.
- Avoid concurrent fluid administration into any other IV site.
- If possible, allow 2 full hours after the administration of 1 unit of blood before administering the next unit.

The Rh antigen system is slightly different. An Rh-negative person is born without the Rh-antigen on his or her RBCs and does not form antibodies unless he or she is specifically sensitized to it. Sensitization can occur with RBC transfusions from an Rh-positive person or from exposure during pregnancy and birth. Once an Rh-negative person has been sensitized and antibody development has occurred, any exposure to Rh-positive blood can cause a transfusion reaction. Antibody development can be prevented by giving Rh-immune globulin as soon as exposure to the Rh antigen is suspected. *People who have Rh-positive blood can receive an RBC transfusion from an Rh-negative donor, but Rh-negative people should not receive Rh-positive blood.*

Platelet Transfusions

Platelets are given to clients with platelet counts below 20,000 mm^3 and to clients with thrombocytopenia who are actively bleeding or are scheduled for an invasive procedure. Platelet transfusions are usually pooled from as many as 10 donors and do not have to be of the same blood type as the client. For clients who are going to receive a bone marrow transplant (BMT) or who need multiple platelet transfusions, single-donor platelets may be prescribed. Single-donor platelets are taken from just one donor and decrease the amount of antigen exposure to the recipient, helping to prevent the formation of platelet antibodies. The chances of allergic reactions to future platelet transfusions are thus reduced.

Platelet infusion bags usually contain 300 mL for pooled platelets and 200 mL for single-donor platelets. Platelets are fragile and must be infused immediately after being brought to the client's room, usually over a 15- to 30-minute period. A special transfusion set with a smaller filter and shorter tubing is used. *Standard transfusion sets are not used with platelets because the filter traps the platelets, and the longer tubing increases platelet adherence to the lumen.* Additional platelet filters help remove white blood cells (WBCs) from the platelet concentrate. These filters are connected directly to the platelet transfusion set and are used for clients who have a history of febrile reactions or who need multiple platelet transfusions.

TABLE 43-7 Compatibility Chart for Red Blood Cell Transfusions

	Recipient			
Donor	**A**	**B**	**AB**	**O**
A	X		X	
B		X	X	
AB			X	
O	X	X	X	X

Take the vital signs before the infusion, 15 minutes after the infusion is initiated, and at its completion. The client may be premedicated with meperidine (Demerol) or hydrocortisone to reduce the chances of a reaction. He or she can become febrile and have **rigors** (severe chills) during transfusion, but these symptoms are not considered a true transfusion reaction. IV infusion of amphotericin B (Amphotec, Fungizone), an antifungal agent given to many clients with leukemia, is discontinued during platelet transfusion and not resumed for at least 1 hour after transfusion. This drug can cause severe allergic reactions that are difficult to distinguish from transfusion reactions.

Plasma Transfusions

Plasma infusions may be given fresh to replace blood volume. More commonly, plasma is frozen immediately after donation, forming **fresh frozen plasma (FFP)**. Freezing preserves the clotting factors, and the plasma can then be used for clients with clotting disorders. Infuse FFP immediately after thawing while the clotting factors are still active. Clients who are actively bleeding with a prothrombin time (PT) or partial thromboplastin time (PTT) greater than 1.5 times normal are candidates for an FFP infusion.

ABO compatibility is required for transfusion of plasma products. The infusion bag contains about 200 mL. Infuse FFP as rapidly as the client can tolerate, generally over a 30- to 60-minute period, through a regular Y-set or straight-filtered tubing.

Cryoprecipitate Transfusions

Cryoprecipitate is a product derived from plasma. Clotting factors VIII and XIII, von Willebrand's factor, and fibrinogen are precipitated from pooled plasma to produce cryoprecipitate. Clients with a fibrinogen level of less than 100 mg/dL are candidates for a cryoprecipitate infusion. Give this highly concentrated blood product to clients with clotting factor disorders at a volume of 10 to 15 mL/unit. Although cryoprecipitate can be infused, it is usually given by IV push within 3 minutes. Dosages are individualized, and it is best if the cryoprecipitate is ABO compatible.

Granulocyte (White Cell) Transfusions

At some centers, neutropenic clients with infections receive white blood cell (WBC) replacement transfusions. This practice is controversial because the potential benefit to the client must be weighed against the potential severe reactions that often occur with WBC transfusions. The surfaces of WBCs contain many antigens that can cause severe reactions when infused into a client whose immune system recognizes these antigens as non-self. In addition, transfused WBCs have a short life span and provide minimal protection (see Chapter 23).

WBCs are suspended in 430 mL of plasma and should be infused over a 45- to 60-minute period. Agency policies often require more stringent monitoring of clients receiving WBCs. A physician may need to be present in the hospital unit, and vital signs may need to be taken every 15 minutes throughout the transfusion. Amphotericin B infusion and WBC transfusions should be separated by 4 to 6 hours.

CULTURAL CONSIDERATIONS

Although transfusion with blood products is common in acute care settings, you must remain sensitive to those clients who view receiving blood or blood products of others as repugnant, even sinful. More than 800,000 Jehovah's Witnesses live in the United States. A belief of Jehovah's Witnesses is that receiving autotransfusion or donated blood is the same as "consuming" blood, an act specifically prohibited in the Old Testament. Often Jehovah's Witnesses will accept the use of dialysis and heart-lung equipment, as well as intraoperative blood salvage if the blood outside the body remains intact with circulatory system. Whenever possible, transfusion therapy with human blood products is avoided for this group. If in an emergency situation, clients are transfused with blood products against their will, show respect for the client's distress and religious beliefs (Glendenning, 2002).

Newer therapies for clients with anemia or hypovolemia may reduce the need for transfusion of human blood products. One therapy is the use of hemoglobin substitutes, also known as "artificial blood," which increases the oxygen-carrying power of the client's own blood. In addition, pretreating or treating these clients with epoetin alfa (Procrit) or darbepoetin alfa (Aranesp) can reduce the recovery time from blood loss without transfusion.

TRANSFUSION REACTIONS

Clients can develop any of the following transfusion reactions: hemolytic, allergic, febrile, or bacterial reactions; circulatory overload; or transfusion-associated graft-versus-host disease (GVHD). Remain vigilant during transfusions to prevent complications through early detection and initiation of appropriate treatment.

Hemolytic Transfusion Reactions

Hemolytic transfusion reactions are caused by blood type or Rh incompatibility. When blood containing antigens different from the client's own antigens is infused, antigen-antibody complexes are formed in the client's blood. These complexes destroy the transfused cells and start inflammatory responses in the client's blood vessel walls and organs. The reaction may be mild, with fever and chills, or life threatening, with disseminated intravascular coagulation (DIC) and circulatory collapse. Other manifestations include the following:

- Apprehension
- Headache
- Chest pain
- Low back pain
- Tachycardia
- Tachypnea
- Hypotension
- Hemoglobinuria
- A sense of impending doom

The onset of a hemolytic reaction may be immediate or may not occur until subsequent units have been transfused (McConnell, 2000; Atterbury, 2001).

Allergic Transfusion Reactions

Allergic transfusion reactions are most often seen in clients with a history of allergy. They may have urticaria, itching, bronchospasm, or anaphylaxis. Onset of this type of reaction usually occurs during or up to 24 hours after the transfusion. Clients with a history of allergy can be given leukocyte-reduced or washed red blood cells (RBCs) in which the white blood cells (WBCs) and plasma have been removed. This procedure reduces the possibility of an allergic reaction.

Febrile Transfusion Reactions

Febrile transfusion reactions occur most often in the client with anti-WBC antibodies, a situation that can develop after multiple transfusions. The recipient develops the following:

- Chills
- Tachycardia
- Fever
- Hypotension
- Tachypnea

Giving leukocyte-reduced blood or single-donor HLA-matched platelets reduces the risk for this type of reaction. WBC filters may be used to trap WBCs and prevent their infusion into the client (Baldwin, 2002).

Bacterial Transfusion Reactions

Bacterial transfusion reactions occur as a result of infusion of contaminated blood products. Usually a gram-negative organism is the source because these bacteria grow rapidly in blood stored under refrigeration. Symptoms include the following:

- Tachycardia
- Hypotension
- Fever
- Chills
- Shock

The onset of a bacterial transfusion reaction is rapid. (See Chapter 40 for care of the client experiencing septic shock.)

Circulatory Overload

Circulatory overload can occur when a blood product is infused too quickly. This complication is most common with whole-blood transfusions or when the client requires multiple transfusions. Older adults are most at risk for this condition (see Chart 43-16). Symptoms include the following:

- Hypertension
- Bounding pulse
- Distended jugular veins
- Dyspnea

- Restlessness
- Confusion

You can both manage and prevent this complication by monitoring intake and output, infusing blood products more slowly, and giving diuretics. (See Chapter 15 for management of clients with fluid overload.)

Transfusion-Associated Graft-Versus-Host Disease

Transfusion-associated graft-versus-host disease (TA-GVHD) is a rare but life-threatening problem that can occur in both immunosuppressed and immunocompetent clients. Its cause in immunosuppressed clients is similar to that of GVHD that occurs with allogeneic bone marrow transplantation (BMT), discussed on p. 902, in which donor T-cell lymphocytes attack host tissues.

Manifestations usually occur within 1 to 2 weeks and include thrombocytopenia, anorexia, nausea, vomiting, chronic hepatitis, weight loss, and recurrent infection.

TA-GVHD has a 90% mortality rate but can be prevented by using irradiated blood products. Irradiation destroys T-cells and their cytokine products.

AUTOLOGOUS BLOOD TRANSFUSIONS

Autologous blood transfusions involve collection and infusion of the client's own blood. This type of transfusion eliminates compatibility problems and reduces the risk for transmitting bloodborne diseases. The four types of autologous blood transfusions are preoperative autologous blood donation, acute normovolemic hemodilution, intraoperative autologous transfusion, and postoperative blood salvage.

Preoperative autologous blood donation, the most common type of autologous blood transfusion, involves collection of whole blood from the client, division into components, and then storage for later use (e.g., after a scheduled surgical procedure). As long as hematocrit and hemoglobin levels are within a safe range, the client can donate blood on a weekly basis until the prescribed amount of blood is obtained. Fresh packed RBCs may be stored for 43 days. For clients with rare blood types, blood may be frozen for up to 10 years. Platelets and plasma may be collected by pheresis. Some cardiac problems and bacteremia are contraindications for autologous blood donation.

Acute normovolemic hemodilution involves withdrawal of a client's RBCs and volume replacement just before a surgical procedure. The goal is to decrease RBC loss during surgery. The blood is stored at room temperature for up to 6 hours and reinfused after surgery. This type of autologous transfusion is contraindicated for anemic clients or those with poor renal function.

Intraoperative autologous transfusion and postoperative blood salvage are the recovery and reinfusion of a client's own blood, collected either from an operative field or from a bleeding wound. Special devices collect, filter, and drain the blood into a transfusion bag. This autologous blood is often used for trauma or surgical clients with severe blood loss. The salvaged blood must be reinfused within 6 hours.

Transfuse autologous blood products using the guidelines previously described. Although the client receiving autologous blood is not at risk for most types of transfusion reactions, you must still assess for circulatory overload or bacterial transfusion reactions that occur as a result of contamination.

GET READY for the NCLEX Examination!

KEY POINTS

Safe Effective Care Environment

- Use aseptic technique during all central line dressing changes or any invasive procedure.
- Use standard precautions for all clients regardless of age, gender, race or ethnicity, sexual orientation, education level, and profession.
- Ask all clients about advance directives and document their status.
- Use good handwashing techniques before providing any care to a client who is either immunocompromised or immunodeficient.
- Use bleeding precautions for any client with thrombocytopenia pancytopenia (see Chart 43-10).
- Verify prescriptions for transfusion of blood products with another registered nurse.
- Use at least two forms of identification for the client who is to receive a blood product transfusion (name and identification number). *Do not use a room number to identify the client.*

Health Promotion and Maintenance

- Teach people to avoid unnecessary contact with environmental chemicals or toxins. If contact cannot be avoided, teach people to use safety precautions.
- Identify clients at high risk for infection because of disease or therapy.
- Teach the client and family about the manifestations of infection and when to seek medical advice.
- Instruct clients who have anemia as a result of dietary deficiency which foods are good sources of iron, folic acid, and vitamin B_{12}.
- Teach precautions to take to avoid injury (Chart 43-14) to clients at risk for bleeding.

Psychosocial Integrity

- Allow the client the opportunity to express fear or anxiety regarding the diagnosis of leukemia or lymphoma or the treatment regimen, including bone marrow transplantation.
- Explain all procedures, restrictions, medications, and follow-up care to the client and family.
- Offer alternative therapies for relaxation, pain reduction, and distraction, such as massage, music therapy, and guided imagery.
- Refer clients and family members to local cancer resources and support groups.
- Reassure clients having pain that using opioid analgesics for needed pain relief is not drug abuse.

Physiological Integrity

- Teach the client about any medications to be continued after discharge from the hospital.
- Instruct the client and family in the manifestations of complications and when to seek assistance.
- Pace nonurgent health care activities to reduce the risk for fatigue among clients with anemia or pancytopenia.

- Assess the client in the induction phase of chemotherapy and those after BMT every shift for manifestations of infection.
- Assess the skin integrity of the perianal region of a client with leukemia after every bowel movement.
- Administer analgesics on a schedule rather than PRN.
- Use normal saline as the solution infusing with blood products.
- Transfuse blood products more slowly to older clients or those who have a cardiac problem.
- Remain with the client during the first 15 minutes of infusion of any blood product.
- Do not administer any drugs with infusing blood products.

ADDITIONAL STUDY RESOURCES

Go to your Student CD-ROM for Review Questions for the NCLEX Examination.

evolve Go to http://evolve.elsevier.com/Iggy/ for Integrated Management of Care Questions for the NCLEX Examination.

SELECTED BIBLIOGRAPHY

Asterisk indicates a classic or definitive work on this subject.

American Cancer Society. (2005). *Cancer facts and figures 2005*. Report No. 01-300M-No. 5008.05. Atlanta: Author.

Anastasia, P. (2001). Nursing considerations for managing topotecan- related hematologic side effects. *Clinical Journal of Oncology Nursing, 5*(1), 9-13.

Applebaum, F. (2003). Update on treatment for acute myeloid leukemia. *Oncology (Special Edition),* 6, 45-49.

Atterbury, C. (2001). Blood transfusions. *Nursing Times, 97*(27), 45-46.

Baldwin, P. (2002). Febrile nonhemolytic transfusion reactions. *Clinical Journal of Oncology Nursing, 6*(3), 171-172.

Bedell, C. (2003). Pegfilgrastim for chemotherapy-induced neutropenia. *Clinical Journal of Oncology Nursing, 7*(1),55-64.

Bennett, C., & Schumock, G. (2003). Cost analyses of adjunct colony stimulating factors for older patients with acute myeloid leukemia: Can they improve clinical decision making? *Drugs & Aging,* 20(7), 479-483.

*Bilodeau, B.B., & Fessele, K.L. (1998). Non-Hodgkin's lymphoma. *Seminars in Oncology Nursing, 14*(4), 273-283.

Birner, A. (2003). Safe administration of oral chemotherapy. *Clinical Journal of Oncology Nursing, 7*(2), 158-162.

Blackwell, J. (2003). Diagnosis and treatment of idiopathic thrombocytopenia purpura. *Journal of the American Academy of Nurse Practitioners, 15*(6), 244-245.

Blash, J. (2002). Systemic candida infections in patients with leukemia: An overview of drug therapy. *Clinical Journal of Oncology Nursing, 6*(6), 323-331.

Brown, C., & Yoder, L. (2002). Stomatitis: An overview. *American Journal of Nursing, 102*(4), 20-23.

Buchsel, P., Murphy, B., & Newton, S. (2002). Epoetin Alfa: Current and future indications and nursing implications. *Clinical Journal of Oncology Nursing, 6*(5), 261-267.

Cagen, D., Franco, M., & Vasquez, D. (2002). The ABCs of low blood cell count. *Clinical Journal of Oncology Nursing, 6*(1), 34-36.

*Callaghan, M. (1998). Hodgkin's disease. *Seminars in Oncology Nursing 14*(4), 262-272.

*Chielens, D. (1999). Chronic myelogenous leukemia. In C. Miaskowski & P. Buchsel (Eds.), *Oncology nursing: Assessment and clinical care* (pp. 1239-1250). St. Louis: Mosby.

Clark, P., & Gomez, E. (2001). Details on demand: Consumers, cancer information, and the Internet. *Clinical Journal of Oncology Nursing, 5*(1), 19-26.

Cleveland, K. (2003). Argatroban: A new treatment option for heparin-induced thrombocytopenia. *Critical Care Nurse, 23*(6), 61-66.

Cook, L. (2000). A simple case of anemia: Pathophysiology of a common symptom. *Journal of Intravenous Nursing, 23*(5), 271-281.

Cope, D. (2002). Patients' and physicians' experiences with sperm banking and infertility issues related to cancer treatment. *Clinical Journal of Oncology Nursing, 6*(5), 293-295, 309.

D'Arcy, Y. (2004). Managing sickle-cell crisis. *Nursing2004, 34*(1), 24-25.

Davey, M. (2002). Imatinib mesylate. *Clinical Journal of Oncology Nursing, 6*(2), 118-120

Day, S., & Wynn, L. (2000). Sickle cell pain & hydroxyurea. *American Journal of Nursing, 100*(11), 34-39.

Decker, G. (2000). Pharmacologic and biologic therapies in cancer care. *Clinical Journal of Oncology Nursing, 4*(5), 242-244.

Dillman, R. (2001). Monoclonal antibody therapy for lymphoma. *Cancer Practice,* 9(2), 71-80.

Dochterman, J.M., & Bulechek, G.M. (2004). *Nursing interventions classification (NIC)* (4th ed.). St. Louis: Mosby.

Ebersole, P., Hess, P., & Luggen, A. (2004). *Toward healthy aging: Human needs and nursing response* (6th ed.). St. Louis: Mosby.

Facts and Comparisons. (2004). *Drug facts and comparisons* (58th ed.). St. Louis: Author.

Folloder, J. (2005). Effects of darbepoetin alfa administration every two weeks on hemoglobin and quality of life of patients receiving chemotherapy. *Oncology Nursing Forum, 32*(1), 81-89.

Franck, L., et al. (2002). Assessment of sickle cell pain in children and young adults using the Adolescent Pediatric Pain Tool. *Journal of Pain and Symptom Management, 23*(2), 114-120.

Garcia-Manero, G., & Kantarjian, H. (2003). Treatment innovations in chronic myelogenous leukemia. *Oncology (Special Edition), 6*, 25-30.

Giving Z-track injections. (2002). *Nursing2002, 32*(9), 81.

Glendenning, J. (2002). Refusal of blood because of religious beliefs: A patient's right to die. *Journal of Emergency Nursing, 28*(3), 196-198.

Golden, C. (2003). Polycythemia: A review. *Clinical Journal of Oncology Nursing, 7*(5), 553-556.

Goldman, D. (2000). Chronic lymphocytic leukemia and its impact on the immune system. *Clinical Journal of Oncology Nursing, 4*(5), 233-236.

Hacker, E.D. (2003). Quantitative measurement of quality of life in adult patients undergoing bone marrow transplant or peripheral blood stem cell transplant: A decade in review. *Oncology Nursing Forum, 30*(4). 613-629.

Hadaway, L. (2002). What you can do to decrease catheter-related infections. *Nursing2002, 32*(9), 46-48.

Hadaway, L. (2004). Preventing extravasation from a central line. *Nursing2004, 34*(6), 22-23.

Hendrix, C., deLeon, C., & Dillman, R. (2002). Radioimmunotherapy for non-Hodgkin's lymphoma with yttrium 90 ibritumomab tiuxetan. *Clinical Journal of Oncology Nursing, 6*(3), 144-148.

Hood, L. (2003). Chemotherapy in the elderly: Supportive therapy for chemotherapy-induced myelotoxicity. *Clinical Journal of Oncology Nursing, 7*(2), 185-190.

Horrell, C., & Rothman, J. (2000). Establishing the etiology of thrombocytopenia. *The Nurse Practitioner, 25*(6), 68-77.

Iovino, C. (2003). Acute myeloid leukemia: A classification and treatment update. *Clinical Journal of Oncology Nursing, 7*(5), 535-540.

Joint Commission on Accreditation of Healthcare Organizations (2004). National Patient Safety Goals. Patient Identification. Available at http://www.jcaho.com.

Kantarjian, H., et al. (2002). Hematologic and cytogenetic responses to imatinib mesylate in chronic myelogenous leukemia. *The New England Journal of Medicine, 346*(9), 645-652.

Kemp, J. (2002). Interdisciplinary modular teaching for patients undergoing progenitor cell transplantation. *Clinical Journal of Oncology Nursing, 6*(3), 157-160.

Kim, H. (2002). Mini-allogeneic stem cell transplantation. *Cancer Practice, 10*(3), 170-172.
Kirschman, A. (2004). Finding alternatives to blood transfusions. *Nursing2004, 34*(6), 58-62.
Kosits, C. (2000). Rituximab: A new monoclonal antibody therapy for non-Hodgkin's lymphoma. *Oncology Nursing Forum,* 27(1), 51-59.
Larsen, L., Neverett, S., & Larsen, R. (2001). Clinical nurse specialist as facilitator of interdisciplinary collaborative program for adult sickle cell population. *Clinical Nurse Specialist, 15*(1), 15-22.
Lynn, A., et al. (2003). Treatment of chronic lymphocytic leukemia with alemtuzumab: A review for nurses. *Oncology Nursing Forum, 30*(4), 689-696.
Maloy, B. (2000). Hematopoiesis, stem cells, and transplantation. *Journal of Intravenous Nursing, 23*(5), 298-303.
Mayorga, J., Richardson-Hardin, C., & Dicke, K. (2002). Arsenic trioxide as effective therapy for relapsed acute promyelocytic leukemia. *Clinical Journal of Oncology Nursing, 6*(6), 341-346.
McCance, K., & Huether, S. (2002). *Pathophysiology: The biologic basis for disease in adults and children* (4th ed.). St. Louis: Mosby.
McConnell, E. (2000). Infusion perfusion: IV pumps for every need. *Nursing Management, 31*(10), 49-50.
McGuire, D. (2002). Mucosal tissue injury in cancer therapy. *Cancer Practice, 10*(4), 179-191.
McSweeney, P., et al. (2001). Hematopoietic cell transplantation in older patients with hematologic malignancies: Replacing high-dose cytotoxic therapy with graft-versus-tumor effects. *Blood,* 97, 3390-3400.
Moorhead, S., Johnson, M., & Maas, M. (Eds.). (2004). *Nursing outcomes classification (NOC)* (3rd ed.). St. Louis: Mosby.
Moran, A., & Camp-Sorrell, D. (2002). Maintenance of venous access devices in patients with neutropenia. *Clinical Journal of Oncology Nursing, 6*(3), 126-130.
Mower-Wade, D., Bartley, M., & Chiari-Allwein, J. (2001). How to respond to shock. *Dimensions of Critical Care Nursing, 20*(2), 22-27.
National Comprehensive Cancer Network. (2004). Clinical practice guidelines in oncology nursing. Available at http://www.nccn.org.
Nussbaum, R., McInnes, R., & Willard, H. (2001). *Thompson & Thompson: Genetics in medicine* (6th ed.). Philadelphia: W. B. Saunders.
O'Malley, P. (2003). Clotting and bleeding. *Clinical Nurse Specialist, 17*(2), 83-85.
Ott, M. (2002). Complementary and alternative therapies in cancer symptom management. *Cancer Practice, 10*(3), 162-166.
Parker, D., Deel, P., & Arner, S. (2004). Iron out the details of therapeutic phlebotomy. *Nursing2004, 34*(2), 46-47.
Parmar, K., & King, R. (2001). Imatinib mesylate: A new pill for chronic myelogenous leukemia. *Cancer Practice, 9*(5), 263-265.
Pearl, R., & Pohlman, A. (2002). Understanding and managing anemia in critically ill patients. *Critical Care Nurse, Supp* (December), 1-14.
Penwarden, L., & Montgomery, P. (2002). Developing a protocol for obtaining blood cultures from central venous catheters and peripheral sites. *Clinical Journal of Oncology Nursing, 6*(5), 268-270.
Peterson, K. (2003). Central line sepsis. *Clinical Journal of Oncology Nursing, 7*(2), 218-221.
Plaisance, L., & Ellis, J. (2002). Opioid-induced constipation. *American Journal of Nursing, 102*(3), 72-73.
Platt, A., et al. (2002). Treating sickle cell pain: An update from the Georgia Comprehensive Sickle Cell Center. *Journal of Emergency Nursing, 28*(4), 297-303.
Pohlman, A., Carven, J., & Lindsay, K. (2001). Conserving blood in the intensive care unit. *Critical Care Nurse, Supp* (December), 1-6.
Rice, D., & Sheridan, C. (2001). Nursing care of patients with multiple myeloma: A paradigm for the needs of a special population. *Clinical Journal of Oncology Nursing, 5*(3), 89-93.
Rudnicke, C. (2003). Transfusion alternatives. *Journal of Infusion Nursing, 26*(1), 29-33.
Scigliano, E., et al. (2001). The leukemias. In Rubin & Williams (Eds.). *Clinical oncology: A multidisciplinary approach for physicians & students.* Philadelphia: W. B. Saunders.
Seeley, K., & DeMeyer, E. (2002). Nursing care of patients receiving Campath. *Clinical Journal of Oncology Nursing, 6*(3), 138-143.
Shannon-Dorcy, K. (2002). Nursing implications of Mylotarg: A novel antibody-targeted chemotherapy for CD 33+ acute myeloid leukemia in first relapse. *Oncology Nursing Forum, 29*(4), 52-57.
Sickle Cell Information Center. (2003). Emory University. Atlanta, GA. Available at http://www.scinfo.org.
Simmons, P. (2003). A primer for nurses who administer blood products. *MEDSURG Nursing, 12*(3), 184-192.
Sorokin, P. (2002). New agents and future directions in biotherapy. *Clinical Journal of Oncology Nursing, 6*(1), 19-26.
Stevens, S. (2000). Heparin-induced thrombocytopenia. *Journal of Vascular Nursing, 18*(2), 54-68.
Stone, R. (2002). The difficult problem of acute myeloid leukemia in the older adult. *CA: A Cancer Journal for Clinicians, 52*(6), 363-372.
Strauss, D. (2003). Therapeutic strategies for indolent B-cell non-Hodgkin's lymphoma: Toward a cure. *Oncology Special Edition,* 6, 33-37.
Tariman, J. (2003). Thalidomide: Current therapeutic uses and management of its toxicities. *Clinical Journal of Oncology Nursing, 7*(2), 143-147.
Tasota, F., & Tate, J. (2001). Interpreting the highs and lows of platelet counts. *Nursing2001, 31*(2), 25.
Tennant, L. (2001). Chronic myelogenous leukemia: An overview. *Clinical Journal of Oncology Nursing, 5*(5), 218-220.
Triesh, I. (2000). Targeting leukemia cells with gemtuzumab ozogamicin. *Cancer Practice,* 8(5), 254-256.
Tuinstra, N. (2003). Outpatient administration of radiolabeled monoclonal antibodies. *Clinical Journal of Oncology Nursing, 7*(1), 106-111.
Vernon, S., & Pfeifer, G. (2003). Blood management strategies for critical care patients. *Critical Care Nurse, 23*(6), 34-41.
Viele, C. (2002). Gentuzumab ozogamicin. *Clinical Journal of Oncology Nursing, 6*(5), 298-299, 304.
Wagner, H., et al. (2002). Administration guidelines for radioimmunotherapy of non-Hodgkin's lymphoma with ^{90}Y-labeled anti CD20 monoclonal antibody. *The Journal of Nuclear Medicine, 43*(2), 267-272.
Waldman, A. (2003). Understanding non-Hodgkin's lymphomas. *Clinical Journal of Oncology Nursing, 7*(1), 93-96.
Weiner, D., & Brugnara, C. (2003). Hydroxyurea and sickle cell disease: A chance for every patient. *Journal of the American Medical Association, 289*(13), 1692-1694.
White, C. (2002). Painful lesions in a pancytopenic patient. *Clinical Journal of Oncology Nursing, 6*(1), 47-49, 51.
Witt, J. (2002). Living with fatigue. *American Journal of Nursing, 102*(4), 28-31.
Witzig, T, et al. (2002). Randomized controlled trial of Yttrium-90-labeled ibritumomab immunotherapy for patients with relapsed or refractory low-grade, follicular, or transformed B-cell non-Hodgkin's lymphoma. *Journal of Clinical Oncology, 20*(10), 2453-2463.
Wolff, S., et al. (2000). Fluconazole vs low-dose amphotericin for the prevention of fungal infections in patients undergoing bone marrow transplantation: A study of the North American Marrow Transplant Group. *Bone Marrow Transplantation, 25,* 853-859.
Wu, H. (2002). Tretinoin for the treatment of acute promyelocytic leukemia. *Cancer Practice, 10*(2), 109-111.
Young, J. (2000). Transfusion reaction. *Nursing2000, 30*(12), 33.
Zitella, L. (2000). Tyrosine kinase inhibitors: A cure for chronic myeloid leukemia? *Clinical Journal of Oncology Nursing, 4*(5), 227-231.

UNIT **TEN**

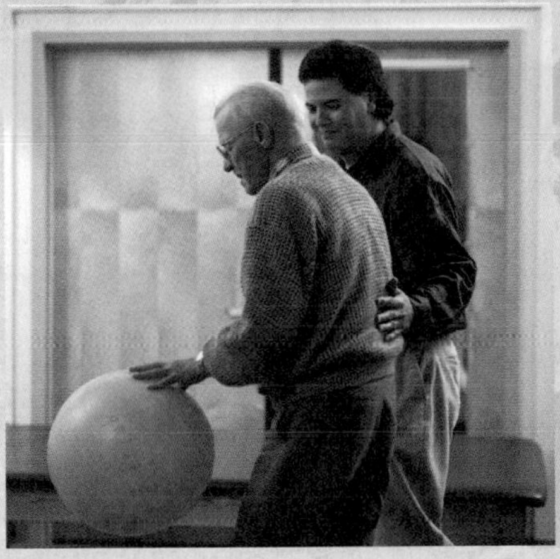

PROBLEMS of MOBILITY, SENSATION, and COGNITION

Management of Clients with Problems of the Nervous System

CHAPTER

44 Assessment of the Nervous System

KATHY A. HAUSMAN

LEARNING OUTCOMES

After studying this chapter, you should be able to:

1. Compare the functions of the major divisions of the nervous system.
2. Describe the mechanisms of nerve impulse transmission.
3. Identify the structure and function of different areas of the central and peripheral nervous system.
4. Identify common physiologic changes associated with aging that affect the nervous system.
5. Perform a neurologic history.
6. Perform a comprehensive neurologic physical assessment.
7. Perform a rapid neurologic assessment and interpret findings.
8. Interpret results of cerebrospinal fluid analysis.
9. Plan and implement pretest and follow-up care for clients undergoing common neurologic diagnostic tests.

Go to your Student CD-ROM for Review Questions for the NCLEX Examination keyed to these Learning Outcomes.

The nervous system is the center of thinking, memory, judgment, sensation, movement, cognition, communication, behavior, and personality. In addition to its direct control over many processes, the nervous system innervates many other body systems and thus indirectly influences their functions. For example, damage to the spinal nerves that innervate the diaphragm may result in respiratory arrest.

Refer to current anatomy, physiology, pathophysiology, and assessment books for complete information about the nervous system and neurologic assessment. A brief review is presented in this chapter.

ANATOMY AND PHYSIOLOGY REVIEW

The major divisions of the nervous system are the central nervous system (CNS) and the peripheral nervous system (PNS).

The brain and spinal cord are the major components of the CNS. The PNS is composed of 12 pairs of cranial nerves, 31 pairs of spinal nerves, and the autonomic nervous system. The autonomic nervous system is further subdivided into sympathetic and parasympathetic fibers.

The nervous system contains two types of cells: neurons, which transmit or conduct nerve impulses, and neuroglial cells, which have an interdependent role with the neuron.

Nervous System Cells

NEURONS

Structure

The basic unit of the nervous system, the neuron, transmits impulses. Some neurons are **motor** (facilitating movement), and some are **sensory** (facilitating sensation). Some process information, and some retain information. When a neuron receives an impulse from another neuron, the effect may be excitation or inhibition as well as conduction of the impulse. Each neuron has a cell body, or soma; short, branching processes called a dendrite; and a single axon (Figure 44-1).

Dendrites may have many branches or few. Each dendrite synapses with another cell body, axon, or dendrite and brings information to the cell body from other neurons. The dendritic process is described as an afferent pathway. The axonal process, called the efferent pathway, transmits impulses from its cell body to other neurons. Although only one axon extends from each neuron, it may extend long distances.

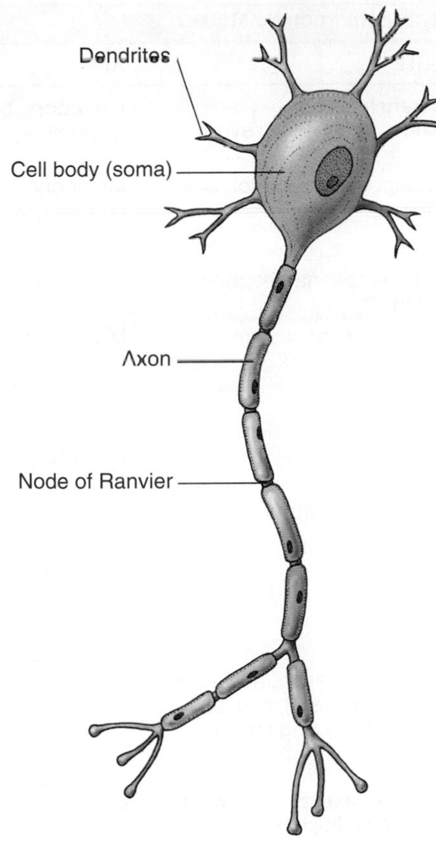

Figure 44-1 ■ The structure of a typical neuron.

Many (but not all) axons are covered by a myelin sheath, a white, lipid covering. Myelinated axons appear whitish and therefore are also called white matter. Nonmyelinated axons have a grayish cast and are called gray matter. Myelinated axons have gaps in the myelin called nodes of Ranvier. The nodes of Ranvier play a major role in impulse conduction (see Figure 44-1). The enlarged, distal end of each axon is called the synaptic, or terminal, knob. Within the synaptic knobs are the mechanisms for manufacturing, storing, and releasing a transmitter substance. Each neuron produces a specific transmitter substance (e.g., acetylcholine or serotonin) that is capable of either enhancing or inhibiting the impulse, but not both.

Mechanism for Nerve Impulse Conduction

Sodium (Na^+) and chloride (Cl^-) ions are heavily concentrated in the area outside of the cell (interstitial space). Potassium ions (K^+) and other organic material are present within the cell (intracellular space). The inside of the cell is negatively charged compared with the interstitial space. Because of the different concentration of Na^+ and K^+, a neuron is constantly charged, even at rest.

When a stimulus is strong enough, the permeability of the cell membrane to Na^+ and K^+ is changed, and **depolarization** (impulse conduction) begins. Certain proteins within the membrane function as gates, or channels, that open for either sodium or potassium. With depolarization, sodium diffuses through the membrane first. It is believed that calcium plays a part in controlling the amount of sodium that diffuses through the membrane by controlling the gates. After sodium has entered the cell, potassium begins to leave the cell. Sodium is actively pumped out of the cell, and **repolarization** (return to baseline) occurs in preparation for another impulse. As an action potential or impulse occurs at one point on the cell membrane, the impulse excites adjacent cells so the impulse is conducted all along the nerve fiber membrane. If the impulse is not of sufficient strength, there will be no action potential.

Synapses

Impulses are transmitted to their eventual destination through **synapses**. There are two distinct types of synapses: *neuron to neuron* and *neuron to muscle* (or gland). Between the terminal knob and the next cell is a small space called the synaptic cleft. The knob, the cleft, and the portion of the cell to which the impulse is being transmitted constitute the synapse.

Factors Affecting Transmission

Several factors affect the transmission of an impulse. Distance is one of the established factors. Synapses on or near the body of the cell have greater influence than those farther along the dendrite. The strength of the stimulus can also be influenced by other mechanisms, such as inhibition by another neuron, inadequate supply of transmitter substance, and extracellular fluid (ECF) changes. Lack of oxygen or the effects of hypnotics and anesthetics can quickly depress nerve cell activity.

Changes in the pH of ECF also affect neuron transmission. For example, acidosis depresses nerve cell activity. Alkalosis, on the other hand, excites nerve cells. Increased nerve cell activity occurs with the use of some drugs, such as caffeine (in coffee), theophylline (in tea and asthma drugs), and theobromine (in cocoa).

Neurotransmitters

Neurotransmitters are chemical substances that enhance or inhibit nerve impulses. Other substances, although not specifically identified as transmitters, are considered probable transmitters. Table 44-1 summarizes what is currently known about them.

NEUROGLIAL CELLS

Neuroglial cells, which vary in size and shape, provide protection, structure, and nutrition for the neurons. There are 5 to 10 times more neuroglial cells than neurons in the central nervous system (CNS), and they account for 40% of the CNS cell mass. Neuroglial cells are classified into four types: astroglial cells, ependymal cells, oligodendrocytes, and microglial cells. Microglial cells play a scavenger role by responding to infection in or trauma to the CNS. Astroglial (star-shaped) cells provide the physical support for the neurons, regulate the chemical environment, and nourish the neurons. Oligodendrocytes form myelin sheaths around the axons. Ependymal cells form the lining of ventricles and the central canal of the spinal cord. They are also part of the blood-brain barrier and help regulate the composition of cerebrospinal fluid (CSF).

Central Nervous System

The central nervous system (CNS) is composed of the brain, which directs the regulation and function of the nervous system and all other systems of the body, and the spinal

TABLE 44-1 Sites, Functions, and Actions of Transmitters, Probable Transmitters, and Neuromodulators

Transmitter Substance	Site	Function/Comments	Action
Acetylcholine	Brain, brainstem, basal ganglia, autonomic nervous system	Nerve and muscle transmission Parasympathetic and preganglionic sympathetic system	Excitatory, but some inhibitory
Serotonin	Medial brainstem, hypothalamus, dorsal horn of spinal cord	Possible onset of sleep, mood control; pain pathway inhibitor in spinal cord	Inhibitory
Catecholamines			
Dopamine	Substantia nigra to basal ganglia	Complex movements, emotional response regulation, attention	Usually inhibitory
Norepinephrine (epinephrine parallels)	Hypothalamus, brainstem, reticular formation, cerebellum, sympathetic nervous system	Maintenance of arousal, reward system, dreaming sleep, mood regulation	Mainly excitatory
Amino Acids			
Aspartate	Brain, spinal cord interneurons	Sensation	Excitatory
Gamma-aminobutyric acid (GABA)	Brain, brainstem, basal ganglia, autonomic nervous system	Nerve and muscle transmission Possibly one third of brain neurons	Inhibitory
Glutamate	Sensory pathways	Sensation	Excitatory
Glycine	Spinal cord interneurons	Muscle control	Inhibitory
Peptides*			
Substance P	Brain, neurons in spinal cord	Pain transmission	Excitatory
Endorphins, enkephalins	Thalamus, hypothalamus, spinal cord, pituitary	Pleasure sensation, reward system, analgesia, (inhibits release of substance P), released with ACTH (corticotropin) during stress	Probably excitatory
Gases			
Nitric acid	Neurons	Not stored in specific site; made by enzymes as needed; released by diffusion	Excitatory
Carbon monoxide	Neurons	Function not well understood	Questionable

*Other peptides under investigation as probable transmitters are vasopressin (ADH), gastrin, cholecystokinin, glucagon, insulin, somatostatin, angiotensin, melanocyte-stimulating hormone (MSH), luteinizing hormone–releasing hormone (LH-RH), and thyrotropin-releasing hormone (TRH). Prostaglandins, also under investigation, are thought to be modulators.

cord, which initiates reflex activity and transmits impulses to and from the brain.

BONE

The brain and spinal cord are encased in the cranium and vertebral column, respectively. For the most part, they are well protected. However, there are some areas of vulnerability, such as the nasal sinuses, the palate of the throat, the ears, and the cervical spine. The upright position of humans creates additional strain on the vertebrae and musculature. Although there are some differences in structure, all of the vertebrae protect the spinal cord and give structure to the body.

Animation: Functional Brain Areas

BRAIN

Meninges

The **meninges** form the immediate protective covering of the brain and the spinal cord:

Situated between the arachnoid and pia mater is the subarachnoid space, where CSF circulates. The subdural space is located between the inner dura and the arachnoid. A *potential* space, referred to as the epidural space, is located between the skull and the outer layer of the dura. This area also extends down the spinal cord and is important in the delivery of epidural analgesia.

Between the two layers of dura are the venous sinuses. The inner layer of dura dips down between the two hemispheres and is called the falx. The dura also lies between the cerebral hemispheres and the cerebellum and is called the tentorium. The falx and the tentorium decrease or prevent the transmission of force from one hemisphere to another and protect the lower brainstem. Clinical references may be made to a lesion (e.g., a tumor) as being **supratentorial** (above the tentorium) or **infratentorial** (below the tentorium).

Cerebrum

The right and left hemispheres of the cerebrum are joined by the corpus callosum. The *left* hemisphere is the dominant hemisphere in most people (even in many left-handed people). Within the deeper structures of the cerebrum are the right and left lateral ventricles. At the base of the cerebrum near the ventricles is a group of neurons called the basal ganglia that regulate movement and body tone.

The motor cortex, located anterior to the central fissure of Rolando of the cerebrum, controls voluntary movement. Corticospinal tracts, also called pyramidal tracts, begin in the motor cortex and travel through the internal capsule and diencephalons and cross at the decussation of the pyramids in the medulla. Nerve fibers continue to the target muscle to initiate movement on each side of the body. The crossing of the fibers in the medulla (decussation of the pyramids) is responsible for the contralateral control of motor movement. In the motor cortex, the motor homunculus is the spatial arrangement of motor nuclei controlling voluntary muscles of the body. The cerebrum is divided into

TABLE 44-2 Brain Lobe Functions

Frontal Lobe
- The primary motor area (also known as the motor "strip" or cortex)
- Broca's speech center on the dominant side
- Voluntary eye movement
- Access to current sensory data
- Access to past information or experience
- Affective response to a situation
- Regulates behavior based on judgment and foresight
- Judgment
- Ability to develop long-term goals
- Reasoning, concentration, abstraction

Parietal Lobe
- Understand sensation, texture, size, shape, and spatial relationships
- Three-dimensional (spatial) perception
- Important for singing, playing musical instruments, and processing nonverbal visual experiences
- Perception of body parts and body position awareness
- Taste impulses for interpretation

Temporal Lobe
- Auditory center for sound interpretation
- Complicated memory patterns
- Wernicke's area for speech

Occipital Lobe
- Primary visual center

Limbic Lobe
- Emotional and visceral patterns connected with survival
- Learning and memory

lobes by sulci (fissures). Except for the limbic lobes, these are given the same name as the overlying bone. The name and function of each lobe is listed in Table 44-2.

Two important speech areas of the cerebrum are Broca's area and Wernicke's area. **Broca's area**, located in the frontal lobe, is composed of neurons responsible for the formation of words, or speech. This requires respiratory activation of the vocal cords, which must occur at the same time as tongue and mouth movements. This association area, **Wernicke's area**, is located in the temporal lobe and plays a significant role in higher-level brain function. It enables processing of words into coherent thought and recognition of the idea behind written or printed words (language).

The general interpretive area, which is located where the temporal, parietal, and occipital lobes meet at the junction of the lateral fissure, enables a person to process complex thoughts, remember the notes of music, recite a speech heard or read long ago, recall childhood experiences, and so forth. Damage to this area on the dominant side after 5 years of age is catastrophic.

Diencephalon

The diencephalon, which lies below the cerebrum, includes the thalamus, hypothalamus, and epithalamus (Figure 44-2).

The **thalamus** is the major "relay station," or "central switchboard," for the CNS. The **hypothalamus** is an integral part of the autonomic nervous system control (controlling temperature and other functions), and plays an essential role in intellectual function. The epithalamus contains the roof of the third ventricle and the pineal gland. See Table 44-3 for additional information concerning the diencephalon.

TABLE 44-3 Diencephalon Functions

Thalamus
- All sensation except smell
- Sensation perceived at the thalamic level is crude and cannot be localized or quantified

Hypothalamus
- Regulates water metabolism, appetite, sleep-wake cycle, temperature control, and thirst
- Hormonal activity
- Posterior pituitary hormones, such as vasopressin and oxytocin
- Anterior pituitary hormone excretion
- Growth, thyrotropin, and follicle-stimulating hormones; prolactin and corticotropin
- Regulates emotions and controls basic drive for self-preservation

Epithalamus
- Often calcified by young adulthood and is radiopaque
- Used as a point of reference on an x-ray film or a computed tomography scan

Subthalamus
- Contains sensory tracts
- Connections to basal ganglia

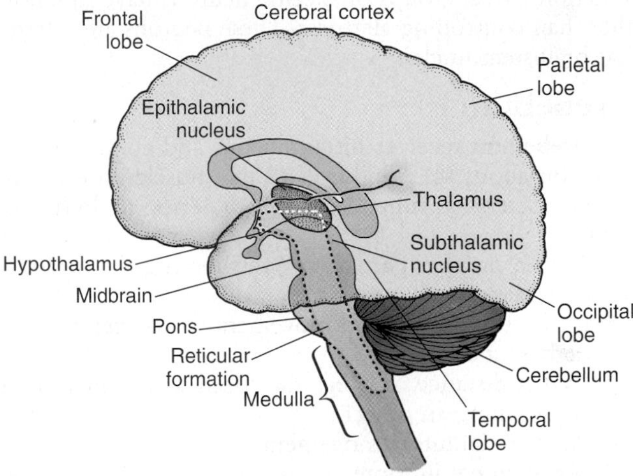

Figure 44-2 ■ The structures of the brainstem and diencephalons.

Hypophysis (Pituitary Gland)

The **hypophysis (pituitary gland)** is situated in the sella turcica of the ethmoid bone and is connected to the hypothalamus by tissue called the hypophyseal stalk. It has two lobes, each releasing specific hormones into the circulation under the regulation of the hypothalamus. The pituitary is often referred to as the "master gland" because of its control of numerous hormonal functions.

Brainstem

The brainstem (see Figure 44-2) includes the midbrain, pons, and medulla. The functions of these structures are presented in Table 44-4.

Throughout the brainstem are special cells that constitute the **reticular activating system (RAS),** which controls awareness and alertness. For example, this tissue awakens a person from sleep when presented with a noxious stimuli,

TABLE 44-4 Brainstem Structure Functions

Medulla
- Cardiac-slowing center
- Respiratory center
- Cranial nerves IX (glossopharyngeal), X (vagus), XI (accessory), and XII (hypoglossal) emerge from the medulla, as do portions of cranial nerves VII (facial) and VIII (acoustic)

Pons
- Cardiac acceleration and vasoconstriction centers
- Pneumotaxic center helps control respiratory pattern and rate
- Four cranial nerves originate from the pons: V (trigeminal), VI (abducens), VII (facial), and VIII (acoustic)

Midbrain
- Contains the cerebral aqueduct or aqueduct of Sylvius
- Location of periaqueductal gray, which may abolish pain when stimulated
- Cranial nerve nuclei III (oculomotor) and IV (trochlear) located here

when there is pain, or when it is time to rise. Many sensory fibers branch and terminate here. The reticular formation area has abundant connections with the cerebrum, the rest of the brainstem, and the cerebellum. Within the reticular formation tissue, groups of specific neurons have functions other than controlling alertness. These neurons are referred to as brainstem nuclei.

Cerebellum

The **cerebellum** receives instantaneous and continuous information about the condition of the muscles, joints, and tendons. Cerebellar function enables a person to do the following:

- Keep a moving part from overshooting the intended destination
- Move from one skilled movement to another in an orderly sequence
- Predict distance or gauge the speed with which one is approaching an object
- Control voluntary movement
- Maintain equilibrium

Cerebellar control of the body is **ipsilateral** (situated on the same side). The right side of the cerebellum controls the right side of the body, and the left cerebellum controls the left side of the body.

Cerebral Circulation

Circulation in the brain originates from the carotid and vertebral arteries (Figure 44-3). The internal carotid arteries branch into the anterior cerebral artery (ACA) and middle cerebral arteries (MCA). The two posterior vertebral arteries become the basilar artery, which then divides into two posterior cerebral arteries. The anterior, middle, and posterior cerebral arteries are joined together by small communicating arteries to form a ring at the base of the brain known as the **circle of Willis.**

The circle of Willis is located at about the level of the pons, or the general level of the upper nose and lower border of the eye. The middle cerebral artery supplies the lateral surface of the cerebrum from about the mid-temporal lobe upward (i.e., the area for hearing and upper body motor and sensory neurons). The anterior cerebral artery supplies the midline, or medial, aspect of the same area (i.e., the lower body motor and sensory neurons). The posterior cerebral arteries supply the area from the mid-temporal region down and posteriorly (occipital lobe), as well as much of the brainstem.

Venous drainage occurs through the cerebral veins into the dural sinuses, which are large venous reservoirs between the inner and outer dura mater. From the dural sinuses, the blood drains into the jugular vein and then into the superior vena cava. Because cerebral veins have no valves, intracranial pressure (ICP) can be affected by central venous pressure (CVP).

Two sinuses are of particular importance: the superior sagittal sinus (SSS) and the cavernous sinus. The superior sagittal sinus receives cerebrospinal fluid (CSF) after it circulates through the ventricular system. The cavernous sinus is located near the eye and receives venous blood from the eye. In addition, the carotid artery passes through the cavernous sinus (the only place in the body where an artery passes through a vein); thus the potential exists for development of a fistula between an artery and a vein (usually from trauma).

Blood-Brain Barrier

The **blood-brain barrier (BBB)** seems to exist because the endothelial cells of the cerebral capillaries (along with ependymal cells) are joined tightly together. This keeps some substances in the plasma out of the cerebrospinal circulation and out of brain tissue. Substances that can pass through the blood-brain barrier include oxygen, glucose, carbon dioxide, alcohol, anesthetics, and water. Large molecules such as albumin, any substance bound to albumin, and many antibiotics are prevented from crossing the blood-brain barrier.

Cerebrospinal Fluid Circulation

Cerebrospinal fluid (CSF) surrounds and cushions the brain and spinal cord. While circulating through the subarachnoid space, the fluid is continuously produced by the choroid plexus, reabsorbed by the arachnoid villi, and then channeled into the superior sagittal sinus (Figure 44-4). Expanded areas of subarachnoid space, where there are large amounts of CSF, are called *cisterns.* The largest cistern is the lumbar cistern, the site of lumbar puncture, from the level of the second lumbar vertebra to the second sacral vertebra (L2-S2).

SPINAL CORD

The spinal cord controls body movement; regulates visceral function; processes sensory information from the extremities, trunk, and many internal organs; and transmits information to and from the brain. It contains H-shaped **gray matter** (neuron cell bodies) that is surrounded by **white matter** (myelinated axons). The white matter is divided into posterior, lateral, and anterior columns. Groups of cells in the white matter (ascending and descending tracts) have been fairly well identified (Figure 44-5). The gray matter divisions are posterior, intermediolateral, and anterior.

Ascending Tracts

As a general rule, **ascending tracts** originate in the spinal cord and end in the brain. Three ascending tracts are important for understanding the client with neurologic problems: spinothalamic tracts, spinocerebellar tracts, and fasciculi gracilis and cuneatus (posterior white columns).

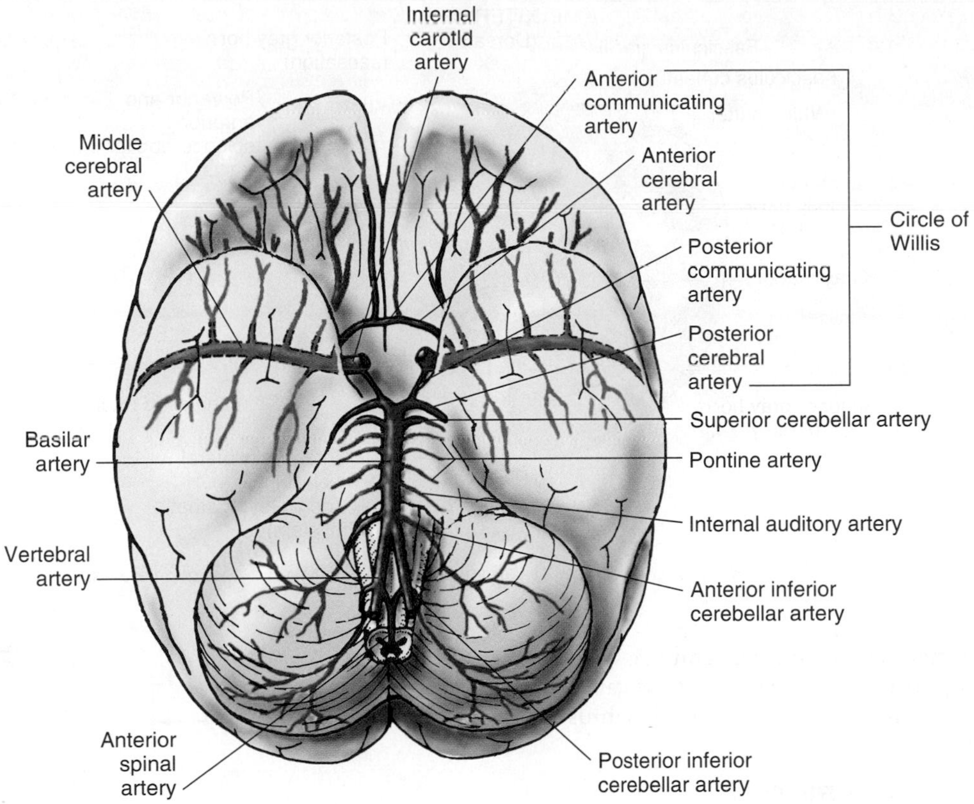

Figure 44-3 ■ Cerebral circulation and the circle of Willis at the base of the brain.

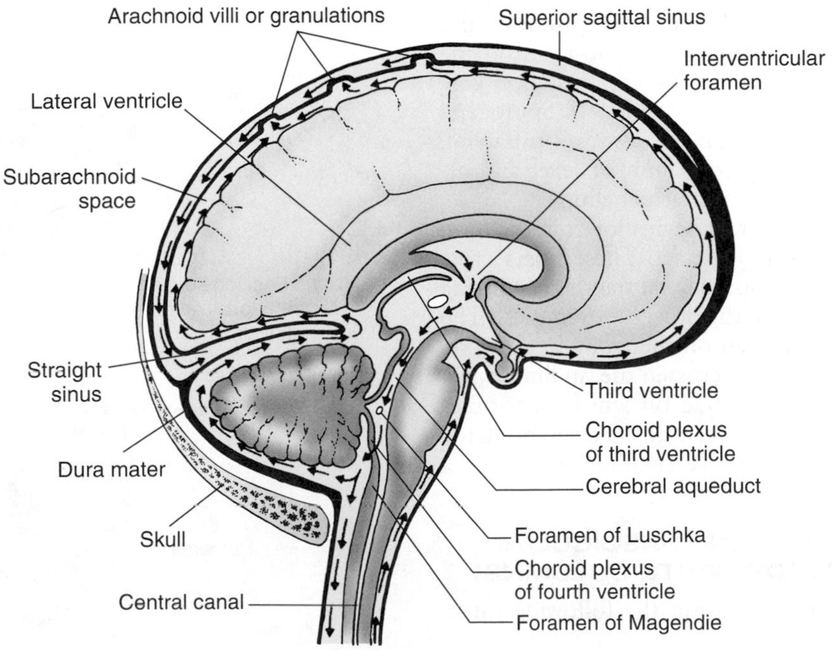

Figure 44-4 ■ Circulation of cerebrospinal fluid. Note that the fluid also extends down into the spinal column.

SPINOTHALAMIC TRACTS

As the name indicates, spinothalamic tracts begin in the spinal cord and end primarily in the thalamus. These tracts carry sensations of pain, temperature, light touch, and pressure. The axon fibers from the cells decussate (cross) the anterior white and gray commissures to the opposite side and become the contralateral (situated on the opposite side) spinothalamic tract. These fibers continue up to the thalamus. Some branches terminate in the reticular formation of the medulla and pons.

A pain or temperature impulse enters the posterior horn on the same side on which the sensation occurs. It

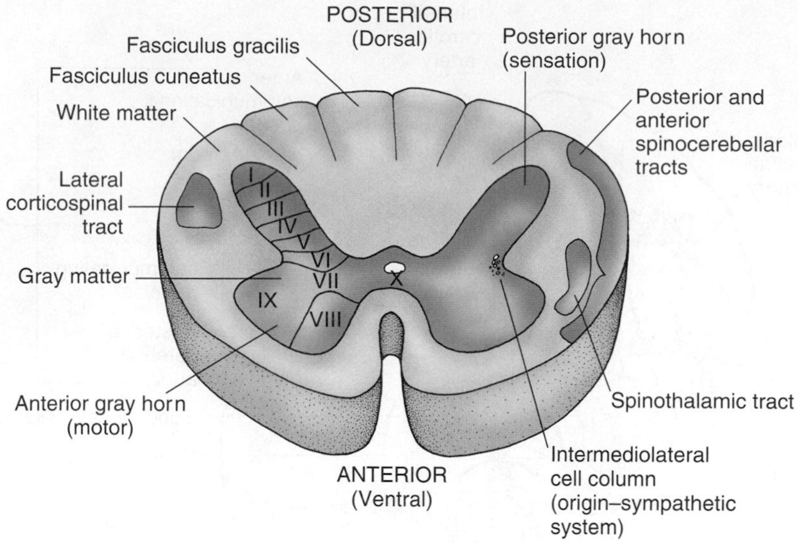

Figure 44-5 ■ A cross section of the spinal cord showing the common tracts.

is transmitted to other cells in several laminae, is further propelled to the opposite spinothalamic tract, and continues up to its ultimate destinations–the thalamus and the parietal lobe (Figure 44-6).

POSTERIOR AND ANTERIOR SPINOCEREBELLAR TRACTS

Spinocerebellar tracts begin in the spinal cord and end in the cerebellum. The *posterior* spinocerebellar tract transmits impulses of proprioception (awareness of position and movements of body parts) or kinesthesia, mostly from the lower extremities. The impulses enter the posterior gray horn and synapse with tract cells in lamina VII. Spinocerebellar axons then form the tract on the *same,* or ipsilateral, side. This tract begins at the second lumbar level and ascends to the medulla and then to the cerebellum.

The *anterior* spinocerebellar tract begins lower in the lumbar spine than does the posterior tract. These fibers cross immediately and ascend as a contralateral tract, transmitting proprioceptive impulses from the lower extremities. The fibers cross again in the midbrain on their way to the cerebellum. Because these fibers have crossed the midline twice, the sensations terminate on the side on which they originated. The *right* cerebellum receives information about the *right* side of the body, and the *left* cerebellum receives data about the *left* side.

FASCICULUS GRACILIS AND FASCICULUS CUNEATUS (POSTERIOR WHITE COLUMNS)

The posterior white columns transmit the following information to the thalamus:

- The sensation of proprioception from muscles, joints, and tendons
- Vibratory sense
- Light touch from the skin
- Discrete localization
- Two-point discrimination

Most of the fibers ascend on the *same* side as their origin to the medulla, where they cross and then synapse in the thalamus, with termination in the parietal lobe. This tract enables identification of the exact point of pressure on the skin. Recognition of pressure includes the shape of an object (with eyes closed), movement across the skin (a number being written), and acknowledgment of two points of touch close together.

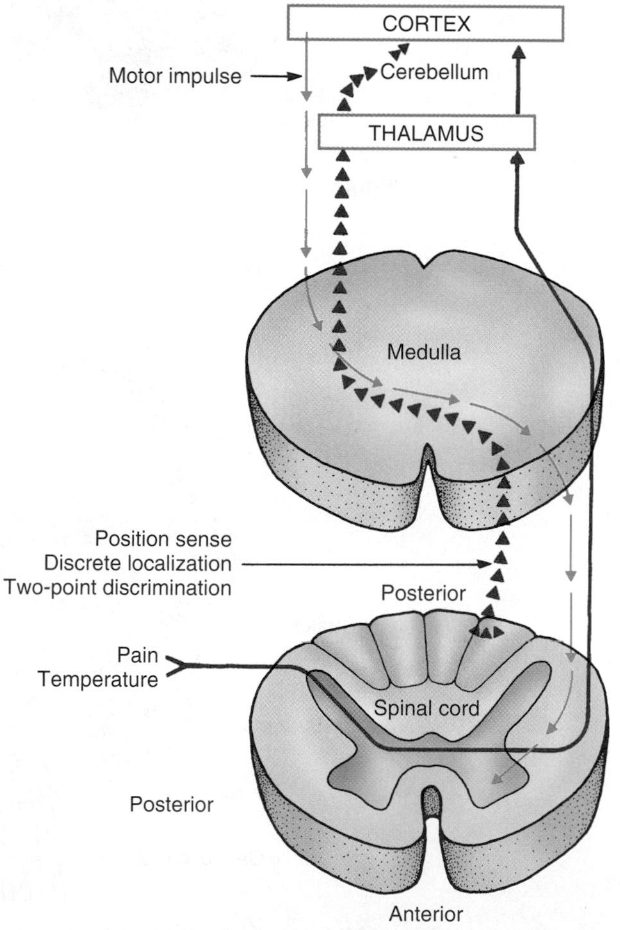

Figure 44-6 ■ Examples of common spinal tract pathways.

Descending Tracts

Descending tracts *begin* in the brain and *end* in the spinal cord. The major descending tract of importance for understanding neurologic problems is the lateral corticospinal, or pyramidal, tract. The corticospinal tract originates in the motor cortex of the frontal lobe and portions of the parietal lobe. The lateral tract fibers cross to the opposite side at the level of the medulla. After crossing, the fibers descend to a predetermined level and synapse with interneurons of the gray matter. A few fibers connect directly with lower motor neurons (LMNs). The cervical area has a high concentration of fibers synapsing with interneurons, which possibly reflects the complexity of hand and finger movements.

The motor neurons of the other descending tracts and the basal ganglia used to be referred to as an extrapyramidal system. It was thought that pyramidal neurons initiated voluntary muscle activity and that extrapyramidal neurons initiated automatic or nonvoluntary muscle action. The descending tracts and the basal ganglia are necessary for the smooth function of all motor activity. The term *extrapyramidal* is still often used clinically to connote the origin of abnormal spontaneous movement.

Spinal Cord Circulation

The blood supply for the spinal cord comes from three main arteries. The anterior spinal artery originates from a branch of the vertebral arteries. The two posterior spinal arteries originate from either the vertebral or posterior inferior cerebellar artery. Additional circulation is supplied by branches of the descending aorta.

Peripheral Nervous System

The peripheral nervous system (PNS) is composed of the spinal nerves, cranial nerves, and autonomic nervous system.

SPINAL NERVES

There are 31 pairs of spinal nerves (8 cervical, 12 thoracic, 5 lumbar, 5 sacral, and 1 coccygeal) exiting from the spinal cord. Each of the nerves has a posterior and an anterior branch. The posterior branch carries sensory information to the cord **(afferent pathway).** The anterior branch transmits motor impulses to the muscles of the body **(efferent pathway).**

Each spinal nerve is responsible for the muscle innervation and sensory reception of a given area of the body. The cervical and thoracic spinal nerves are relatively close to their areas of responsibility, whereas the lumbar and sacral spinal nerves are some distance from theirs. Because the spinal cord ends between L1 and L2, the axons of the lumbar and sacral cord extend downward before exiting the appropriate intervertebral foramen. The area controlled by each spinal nerve is roughly reflected in the dermatomes. **Dermatomes** represent sensory input from spinal nerves to specific areas of the skin (Figure 44-7). For example, the client with an injury to cervical spinal nerve root C6 and C7 exhibits sensory changes in the thumb, index finger, middle finger, middle of the palm, and back of the hand.

SENSORY RECEPTORS

Animation: Sensory Pathways ▶

Sensory receptors throughout the body monitor and transmit impulses of pain, temperature, touch, vibration, pressure, visceral sensation, and proprioception. Sensory receptors also monitor and transmit the sensations of the special senses—vision, taste, smell, and hearing.

LOWER MOTOR NEURONS AND PLEXUSES

Animation: Motor Pathways ◀

The cell bodies of the anterior spinal nerves are located in the anterior gray matter (anterior horn) of each level in the spinal cord. The anterior motor neurons are also referred to as lower motor neurons. As each nerve axon leaves the spinal cord, it joins other spinal nerves to form **plexuses** (clusters of nerves). Plexuses continue as trunks, divisions, and cords and finally branch into individual peripheral nerves.

The major plexuses are cervical, brachial, lumbar, and sacral. The latter two plexuses are also referred to as lumbosacral. An awareness of the location of the plexuses is helpful because a major concentration of nerves is present. In addition, the nerves of each plexus pass through or are surrounded by bone. Injury to the area or entrapment of a nerve by bone can cause multiple problems.

REFLEXES

Animation: Reflex Arc ◀

Reflexes consist of sensory input from the following (Figure 44-8):

- The muscles, tendons, skin, organs, and special senses
- Small cells in the spinal cord lying between the posterior and anterior gray matter (interneurons)
- The anterior motor neurons, along with the muscles they innervate

Sensory data from a specific peripheral location account for a change in the motor impulses going to that location. This closed circuit, which requires no mediation in the cerebral cortex, is called the reflex arc.

Muscle tone is achieved by special fibers in the middle of the muscle. These special fibers, called muscle spindles or intrafusal fibers, are attached to the surrounding muscle and are able to contract only at their ends. The contractible ends are innervated by special motor fibers from the anterior horn. The middle portion of the intrafusal fibers contains special receptors that measure the degree of stretch of the muscle.

CRANIAL NERVES

There are 12 cranial nerves. The name, number, origin, type, and function of the cranial nerves are summarized in Table 44-5.

Autonomic Nervous System

The **autonomic nervous system (ANS)** is composed of two parts: the sympathetic nervous system (SNS) and the parasympathetic nervous system (PNS). Through the use of biofeedback and other mechanisms, some ANS functions can be brought under conscious control.

SYMPATHETIC NERVOUS SYSTEM

The cells of origin for the SNS are located in the gray matter of the spinal cord from T1 and through L2 or L3. This part of the ANS is considered *thoracolumbar* because of its anatomic location.

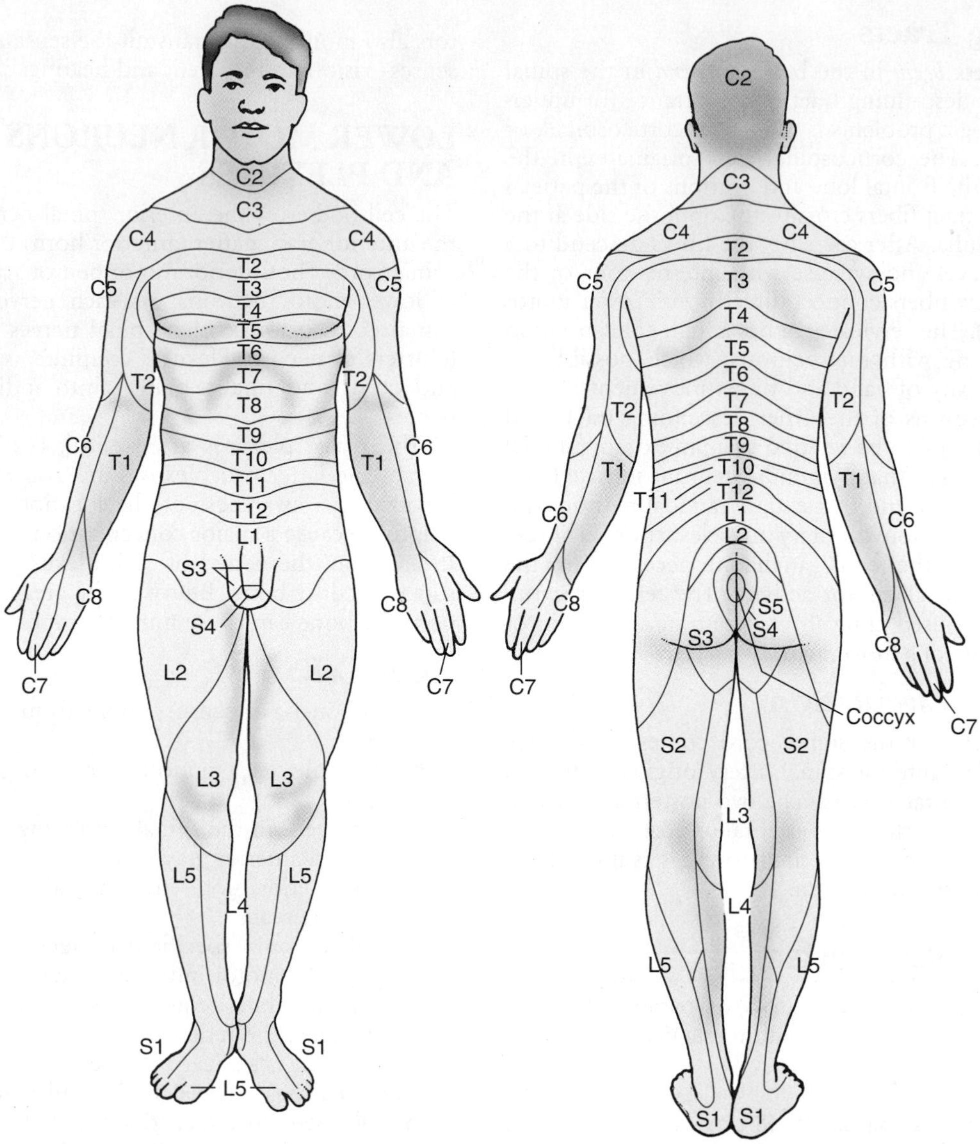

Figure 44-7 ■ Dermatomes (cutaneous innervation of spinal nerves)

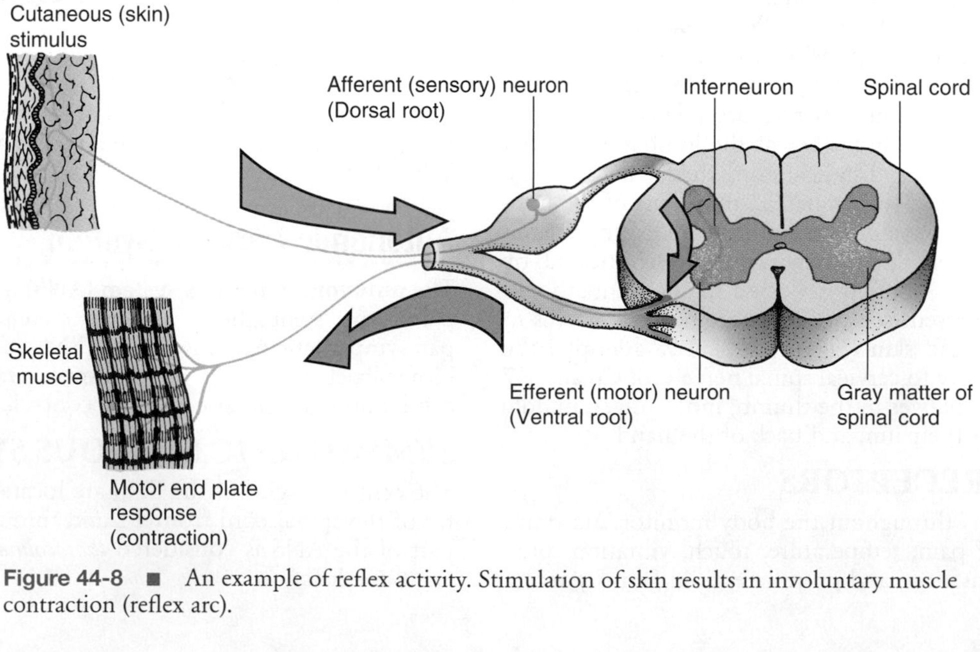

Figure 44-8 ■ An example of reflex activity. Stimulation of skin results in involuntary muscle contraction (reflex arc).

TABLE 44-5 Origins, Types, and Functions of the Cranial Nerves

Cranial Nerve	Origin	Type	Function
I: Olfactory	Olfactory bulb	Sensory	Smell
II: Optic	Midbrain	Sensory	Vision
III: Oculomotor	Midbrain	Motor to eye muscles	Eye movement via medial and lateral rectus and inferior oblique and superior rectus muscles; lid elevation via the levator muscle
		Parasympathetic-motor	Pupil constriction; ciliary muscles
IV: Trochlear	Lower midbrain	Motor	Eye movement via superior oblique muscles
V: Trigeminal	Pons	Sensory	Sensation from skin of face and scalp and mucous membranes of mouth and nose
		Motor	Muscles of mastication (chewing)
VI: Abducens	Inferior pons	Motor	Eye movement via lateral rectus muscles
VII: Facial	Inferior pons	Sensory	Pain and temperature from ear area; deep sensations from the face; taste from anterior two thirds of the tongue
		Motor	Muscles of the face and scalp
		Parasympathetic-motor	Lacrimal, submandibular, and sublingual salivary glands
VIII: Vestibulocochlear	Pons-medulla junction	Sensory	Hearing Equilibrium
IX: Glossopharyngeal	Medulla	Sensory	Pain and temperature from ear; taste and sensations from posterior one third of tongue and pharynx
		Motor	Skeletal muscles of the throat
		Parasympathetic-motor	Parotid glands
X: Vagus	Medulla	Sensory	Pain and temperature from ear; sensations from pharynx, larynx, thoracic and abdominal viscera
		Motor	Muscles of the soft palate, larynx, and pharynx
		Parasympathetic-motor	Thoracic and abdominal viscera; cells of secretory glands; cardiac and smooth muscle innervation to the level of the splenic flexure
XI: Accessory	Medulla (anterior gray horn of the cervical spine)	Motor	Skeletal muscles of the pharynx and larynx and sternocleidomastoid and trapezius muscles
XII: Hypoglossal	Medulla	Motor	Skeletal muscles of the tongue

PARASYMPATHETIC NERVOUS SYSTEM

The cells of origin for the PNS are located in the gray matter of the sacral area of the spinal cord (from S2 to S4) plus portions of cranial nerves III, VII, IX, and X (*craniosacral*). The PNS conserves the body's resources.

Parasympathetic fibers to the viscera have some sensory ability in addition to motor function. Sensations of irritation, stretching of an organ, or a decrease in tissue oxygen are transmitted to the thalamus through pathways not yet fully understood. Because pain from internal organs is often felt below the body wall innervated by the spinal nerve, it is presumed that there are connections between the viscera and body structure that relay pain sensations. Table 44-6 compares the action of sympathetic and parasympathetic systems in the body.

Neurologic Changes Associated with Aging

MOTOR/SENSORY ABILITY

Motor changes in late adulthood are interrelated with sensory function and musculoskeletal status (Chart 44-1). Any problems that affect the nerves, bones, muscles, or joints also affect motor ability. The older adult may have tremors without rigidity, and deep tendon reflexes may be hypoactive. Balance and coordination may be impaired as a result.

Sensory changes in older adults can affect their daily activities. Pupils decrease in size, which restricts the amount of light entering the eye. The pupils also adapt more slowly. Touch sensation decreases, which may precipitate falls because the older person may not feel pebbles or small objects underfoot. Vibration sense may be lost in the ankles and feet. (See also the discussion on fall prevention in Chapter 5.) Hearing also decreases, especially for high-pitched sounds **(presbycusis).**

MENTAL STATUS

Intellect does not decline as a result of aging; however, a person with certain pathologic conditions may experience a decrease in intellectual level caused by drug interactions or an insufficient oxygen supply to the brain. Some older adults may need more time than a younger person to process questions, learn new information, solve problems, or complete analogies.

Subtle memory changes are typical for many older people. Long-term memory seems better than recall (recent) or immediate (registration) memory. Older adults may need more time to retrieve information. These changes may be partly due to the loss of cerebral neurons, which is associated with the aging process.

Insomnia, anxiety, and depression in late adulthood may cause some changes in mental status. Circadian rhythm disorders may lead to wakefulness until later at night, with

TABLE 44-6 Effects of the Autonomic Nervous System on Various Organs of the Body

Organ	Effect of Sympathetic Stimulation	Effect of Parasympathetic Stimulation
Eye		
Pupil	Dilated	Constricted
Ciliary muscle	Slight relaxation	Constricted
Glands Nasal Lacrimal Parotid Submandibular Gastric Pancreatic	Vasoconstriction and slight secretion	Stimulation of copious (except pancreas) secretion (containing many enzymes for enzyme-secreting glands)
Sweat glands	Copious sweating (cholinergic)	Sweating of the palms of the hands
Apocrine glands	Thick, odoriferous secretion	None
Heart		
Muscle	Increased rate Increased force of contraction	Slowed rate Decreased force of contraction
Coronary arteries	Dilated ($beta_2$); constricted (alpha)	Dilated
Lungs		
Bronchi	Dilated	Constricted
Blood vessels	Mildly constricted	? Dilated
Gut		
Lumen	Decreased peristalsis and tone	Increased peristalsis and tone
Sphincter	Increased tone (most times)	Relaxed (most times)
Liver	Glucose released	Slight glycogen synthesis
Gallbladder and bile ducts	Relaxed	Contracted
Kidney	Decreased output and renin secretion	None
Bladder		
Detrusor	Relaxed (slight)	Excited
Trigone	Contracted	Relaxed
Penis	Ejaculation	Erection
Systemic arterioles		
Abdominal	Constricted	None
Muscle	Constricted (alpha-adrenergic) Dilated ($beta_2$-adrenergic) Dilated (cholinergic)	None
Skin	Constricted	None
Blood		
Coagulation	Increased	None
Glucose	Increased	None
Lipids	Increased	None
Basal metabolism	Increased up to 100%	None
Adrenal medullary secretion	Increased	None
Mental activity	Increased	None
Piloerector muscles	Contracted	None
Skeletal muscle	Increased glycogenolysis Increased strength	None
Fat cells	Lipolysis	None

From Guyton, A.C. (1991). *Textbook of medical physiology* (8th ed.). Philadelphia: W.B. Saunders.

extended sleeping in the morning (a pattern opposite that of most health care facility routines). Many older adults require less sleep than do their younger counterparts.

Mental status may also be compromised as the result of infection. Many times this change in mental status is a key early sign of an infectious process in the older client.

ASSESSMENT TECHNIQUES

History

The neurologic history and assessment begin the moment the nurse first meets the client. During the introduction, note the client's appearance and assess his or her speech, affect, and motor function. If the client appears to have cognitive deficits or has trouble speaking or hearing, ask a family member or significant other to stay during the history taking to help secure accurate information. Charts 44-2 and 44-3 elaborate on the information that should be obtained from the client or family.

FAMILY HISTORY AND GENETIC RISK

Ask the client questions about family history such as a history of stroke or heart attack. Ethnic and cultural background may influence the development of a neurologic disorder. For example, it has been long established that Huntington disease is

CHART 44-1

NURSING FOCUS on the OLDER ADULT
Changes in the Nervous System Related to Aging

Physiologic Changes	Nursing Implications	Rationales
Recent memory loss	Reinforce teaching by repetition and written teaching aids.	Intellect is not impaired, but the learning process is slowed. Repetition helps the client learn new information and recall it when needed.
Decreased touch sensation	Remind the client to look where his or her feet are placed when walking. Instruct the client to wear shoes that provide good support when walking. If the client is unable, change his or her position frequently (every hour) while he or she is in bed or the chair.	Decreased sensation may cause the client to fall.
Change in perception of pain	Ask the client to describe the nature and specific characteristics of pain. Monitor additional assessment variables to detect possible health problems.	Accurate and complete nursing assessment ensures that the interventions will be appropriate for the older adult (see Chapter 7).
Change in sleep patterns	Ascertain sleep patterns and preferences. Adjust the client's daily schedule to his or her sleep pattern and preference as much as possible (e.g., evening versus morning bath).	Most older adults require less sleep than do younger adults. However, frequent rest periods are needed.
Altered balance and/or decreased coordination	Instruct the client to move slowly when changing positions. If needed, advise the client to hold on to handrails when ambulating. Assess the need for an ambulatory aid, such as a cane.	The client may fall if moving too quickly. Assistive and adaptive aids provide support and prevent falls.

inherited. With the advent of the Human Genome Project and intensive research, several other neurologic diseases have been found to have a genetic basis, and the list is expanding. Neuromuscular disorders, movement disorders, migraine headaches, and epilepsy have been determined to be caused by inherited mutations of ion channels (Kullman & Hanna, 2002). Other disorders related to genetic factors include Alzheimer's disease and multiple sclerosis. Neurofilament mutations have now been associated with Parkinson disease and amyotropic lateral sclerosis (Al-Chalabi & Miller, 2003).

PERSONAL HISTORY

Questions about the client's medical history and dietary history are necessary for any bearing they might have on the present problem. Questions about the client's level of activities of daily living (ADLs) may highlight subtle changes in neurologic function. Knowing the level of daily activity also helps establish a baseline for later comparison with changes resulting from improving or worsening neurologic function. Ask whether the client is right-handed or left-handed. This information is important for several reasons:

- The client may be somewhat stronger on the dominant side, which is expected.
- The effects of cerebral injury or disease are more pronounced if the dominant hemisphere is involved.

CURRENT HEALTH PROBLEMS AND SOCIAL HISTORY

Obtain information from the client as outlined in Charts 44-2 and 44-3.

CHART 44-2

BEST PRACTICE for
Establishing a Nursing Database: History

Demographic Data

Age
Gender

Past Medical History

Client's medical history
Family's medical history
Previous injuries or congenital problems
Chronic diseases
- Hypertension
- Diabetes mellitus
- Lung disease

Previous neurologic problems
- Headaches
- Seizures
- Head or spine trauma
- Eye problems

Current History

Current symptoms
- Blurred vision
- Headache
- Speech or swallowing difficulty
- Numbness, tingling
- Weakness, clumsiness
- Bowel or bladder difficulties
- Nausea or vomiting
- Personality seizures

Allergies
- Food
- Medications
- Environment

Pain tolerance
- Medications taken for pain
- Behaviors to reduce pain

Medications
- Prescribed
- Illicit
- Over-the-counter

Activities of daily living

Social History

Usual recreational activities
Level of physical activity each day
Hobbies
Alcohol consumption and use of recreational drugs
Smoking, use of any tobacco products
Sleep habits
- Changes in pattern, duration, or intensity

Work history
- Exposure to toxic agents

Ethnic and cultural background
Handedness (right or left)
Educational background

CHART 44-3

Neurologic Assessment
USING GORDON'S FUNCTIONAL HEALTH PATTERNS

Health Perception–Health Management Pattern
- How would you describe your general health?
- Has your health changed significantly over the past few weeks or months?
- Have you had to miss any work because of changes in your health?

Cognitive-Perceptual Pattern
- Have you noticed any changes in your vision? Hearing? Memory?
- Do you feel you are having any difficulty in making decisions? In learning?
- Are you experiencing any discomfort? Pain? Weakness?

Activity-Exercise Pattern
- Do you have enough energy for your activities?
- What is your perceived ability for the following (code for level according to key below):

Feeding?	Level 0: Full self-care
Bathing?	Level I: Requires use of equipment or device
Toileting?	Level II: Requires assistance or supervision of another person
Bed mobility?	Level III: Requires assistance or supervision of another person and equipment or device
Dressing?	Level IV: Is dependent and does not participate
Grooming?	
General mobility?	
Cooking?	
Home maintenance?	
Shopping?	

Based on Gordon, M. (2002). *Manual of nursing diagnosis* (10th ed.). St. Louis: Mosby.

Physical Assessment

Perform a focused assessment based on the client's presenting symptoms or diagnosis. The establishment of baseline data is important. Make comparisons with each assessment (e.g., to findings 5 minutes or an hour earlier, to the client's baseline, between the right and left sides, between upper and lower extremities, and to the expected progression for the client). Much of the assessment can be performed with the client sitting or lying down. Two types of neurologic assessments may be performed–a complete assessment and a "rapid" assessment. The method chosen depends upon the information needed, the time available with your client, and your skill level. Advanced practice nurses (APNs) and other health care providers usually perform the complete assessment, although parts of it can be done by any health care professional. It is important that you understand each component of the assessment and what the results might indicate. The complete assessment is described first.

ASSESSMENT OF MENTAL STATUS

While collecting the history data, make observations about the client's mental status, speech, and behavior as noted in Chart 44-4. An organized head-to-toe physical assessment begins with the mental status. It is better to start with this part of the assessment, especially when neurologic problems have been noted. For example, if the client is confused, you need to differentiate the cause of the confusion. It may be related to hypoxia rather than the immediate neurologic problem. In older adults, acute confusion may be indicative of a urinary tract infection or other health problem.

CHART 44-4

BEST PRACTICE for
Assessment of Mental Status

- Are the client's answers appropriate?
- Is the client's behavior and facial expression appropriate?
- Is the speech pattern of normal tone, rate, rhythm, and volume?
- Are the answers complete?
- Is the client's appearance neat or untidy; appropriate for age and weather conditions?
- Is the client cooperative, euphoric, hostile, anxious, withdrawn, or guarded?
- Is the client experiencing hallucinations or delusions?
- Is the client's posture and hygiene appropriate for the situation?

Level of Consciousness and Orientation

Determine **level of consciousness (LOC)** by observing the client's level of responsiveness to the environment. *A change in LOC is the **first** indication that central neurologic function has declined!* The client who is **alert** is awake and responsive. Clients who are less than alert are labeled lethargic, stuporous, or comatose. To better identify the client's level of cognitive function or exact state of consciousness, describe behavior in response to stimulation. Ask the client questions that indicate **orientation** to *person, place,* and *time.* Varying the sequence of questioning on repeated assessments prevents the client from memorizing the answers. During the history taking, responses that indicate orientation to person, place, and time include the following:

- The client's ability to relate the onset of symptoms
- The name of his or her physician/nurse practitioner/nurse
- The year and month
- His or her address
- The name of the referring physician or health care agency

Advanced age, time of day, medications, and the need for sleep may affect client responses.

Memory

Memory is one of the most important criteria for neurologic assessment. If the client cannot remember, most of the verbal assessment tests are either not feasible or are at best unreliable. Loss of memory, especially recent memory, tends to be an *early* sign of neurologic problems. Three facets of memory are tested: long-term (remote) memory, recall (recent) memory, and immediate memory.

Remote, or long-term, **memory** can be tested by asking clients about their birth date, schools attended, the city of birth, or anything from the past that can be verified. Nurses often ask the maiden name of the client's mother; this is sometimes listed on the admission form and can be checked.

Recall (recent) **memory** can be tested fairly well during the history taking by assessing the following:

- The accuracy of the medical history
- Dates of clinic or physician appointments
- The time of admission
- Health care providers seen within the past few days
- Mode of transportation to the hospital or clinic

Immediate (new) **memory** is tested by giving the client two or three unrelated words, such as "apple," "street," and "chair," and asking him or her to repeat the words to make sure they were heard. After about 5 minutes, while continuing with the examination, ask the client to repeat the words. A person normally should be able to do this correctly. An alternative to this method is to give a three-step command and observe whether it is carried out correctly.

Attention

To assess attention, ask the client to repeat a series of three numbers, such as 4, 7, and 3. The series is increased by one number with each successful repetition until seven or eight digits are achieved. If the client has difficulty at any level (cannot repeat the series), repeat the numbers. If the client cannot repeat, stop the procedure. Next, ask the client to repeat the numbers backward, starting again with three digits and increasing by one each time. Normally, a person should be able to repeat five to eight digits forward and four to six backward. Education, occupation, interest, culture, anxiety, and depression affect mental status, and what is considered normal may not be so for a particular client.

The serial seven test to determine attention may also be used. The client is asked to count backward from 100 by 7 (the examiner stops when the client reaches 65 successfully). Depending on education and other factors, it may be better to ask the person to subtract by three or to add forward by five. Use judgment and assessment skills in deciding which of these tests to use.

Language and Copying

If desired, most language and copying skills can be assessed during the initial interview. The client demonstrates language comprehension by following directions on admission (e.g., getting undressed and providing a urine specimen). If there is hesitancy in speech, indicating that the client groped for words, point to items and ask the client to name them, such as a drinking glass, the door, or the bed.

The advanced practice nurse or speech-language pathologist tests reading comprehension by writing a simple command and giving it to the client (e.g., "close your eyes"). Writing can be tested by asking the client to write a sentence. The practitioner must remember that some clients are not able to read or write and modify the examination accordingly. The practitioner usually tests copying ability by having the client copy something the nurse has drawn, such as a cross, circle, diamond, or square.

Cognition

Higher intellectual functions are assessed by asking about favorite hobbies, current events, the names of the last few presidents, or the meaning of a statement. Abstract reasoning can be evaluated by asking the meaning of proverbs (e.g., "A stitch in time saves nine" or "A rolling stone gathers no moss"). The client's judgment can be assessed, at least partially, during the interview. Did he or she make rational decisions in dealing with his or her symptoms? Ask questions such as, "What would you do if stopped for speeding?" and "What would you do if there was a fire in the wastepaper basket?" Remember that testing of cognition (general knowledge, abstraction, and judgment) is influenced by culture.

Video Clips: Smell and Central Vision

ASSESSMENT OF CRANIAL NERVES

Cranial nerves are typically tested to establish a baseline from which to compare progress or deterioration. However, they are not routinely tested unless the client has a suspected problem affecting one or more of the cranial nerves (see Table 44-5). The testing of cranial nerve III is usually a part of the rapid neurologic assessment described on p. 938. Adding the specific cranial nerves to be tested on the flowsheet of a client with a problem affecting the cranial nerves helps ensure continued comparison and evaluation.

ASSESSMENT OF SENSORY FUNCTION

Video Clip: Sensory Evaluation

For the most part, the assessment of sensory function is reserved for clients with problems affecting the spinal cord or spinal nerves, such as trauma, intervertebral disk disease, Guillain Barré syndrome (GBS), neoplasm, infection, stenosis, or transverse myelitis. Components of the sensory assessment include pain, superficial and deep sensation, light touch, and proprioception. Pain and light touch are the most commonly assessed component of sensory function. Sensory assessment of the face may be completed with testing of the trigeminal nerve.

The acuity level of the client will determine the frequency of the sensory assessment and the targeted sensory parameter. Clients with acute spinal cord trauma or GBS should be assessed every hour until stable, then every 4 hours. As the condition improves, sensory assessment may be needed only once each shift. Findings of the sensory assessment are documented according to agency protocol. A special spinal cord assessment flowsheet may be used to document sensory and/or motor findings for the client with a spinal cord injury.

Pain and Temperature

Pain and temperature sensations are transmitted by the same nerve endings. Therefore if one sensation is tested and found to be intact, it can safely be assumed that the other is intact. Testing temperature sensation can usually be accomplished using a cold reflex hammer and the warm touch of the hand for clients with known or suspected spinal problems. Testing pain sensation is relatively easy and more reliable.

Assess for pain sensation with any object perceived as being sharp or dull. A cotton-tipped applicator or paper clip has a sharp end and a dull end. Instruct the client to keep eyes closed and to indicate whether the touch is sharp or dull. It is necessary to demonstrate what will be done while the client's eyes are open. The sharp and dull stimuli should be interchanged at random so the client does not anticipate the type of the next stimulus. Not all areas need to be tested unless he or she has suffered a spinal cord injury. If testing begins on the hands and feet, there is no need to test the more proximal parts of the extremities because the tracts transmitting pain and temperature sensations are intact. Compare reactions on each side. A sensation reported as dull when the stimulus was actually sharp necessitates more finite testing. A client with sensory loss as a result of diabetes mellitus or peripheral vascular disease may or may not be aware of the loss until tested. Some clients may in fact point out their sensory losses to the nurse.

Video Clip: Light Touch

Touch

Light touch discrimination is likely to be normal if pain and temperature sensations are intact. Touch discrimination and two-point discrimination are performed as part of a complete neurologic examination by the health care provider.

For testing **touch discrimination,** the client closes his or her eyes. The practitioner touches him or her with a finger and asks that he or she point to the area touched. This procedure is repeated on each extremity at random rather than at sequential points. Next, the practitioner touches the client on each side of the body on corresponding sites at the same time. The client should be able to point to both sites. An inability to sense touch on one side is called the extinction phenomenon and is a subtle test for sensory loss.

The practitioner then touches the client in two places on the same extremity with two objects, such as cotton-tipped applicators. A person can normally identify two points fairly close together depending on the location of the stimuli. The more nerve innervation in an area, the closer the two-point discrimination.

Abnormal Sensory Findings

Abnormal sensory findings may have a peripheral nervous system (PNS) or a central nervous system (CNS) cause. The neuropathies of diabetes, malnutrition, and vascular problems are due to a PNS cause and generally involve the entire extremity or both extremities. Damage to a specific spinal nerve may not result in significant sensory loss because the spinal nerves overlap. Injury to several adjacent spinal nerves is manifested as decreased or absent sensation in the dermatomes of those nerves.

CNS problems can occur within the spinal cord, the brainstem, the cerebellum, and the cerebral cortex. Sensory deficits from spinal cord damage vary with the location of the damage. Involvement of only the posterior column leads to lost **proprioception** (position sense) below the level of the damage on the same side or on both sides (if both the right and left posterior columns are involved). A lesion involving only the right spinothalamic tract results in a loss of pain and temperature sensation below the lesion on the *left* side. Problems in the brainstem, thalamus, and cortex generally result in loss of sensation on the **contralateral** (opposite) side of the body. Cerebellar lesions affect sensation on the *same* side of the body.

ASSESSMENT OF MOTOR FUNCTION

Throughout the physical assessment, observe the client for involuntary tremors or movements. Such movements need to be characterized as accurately as possible, such as "pill rolling with the thumbs and fingers at rest" or "intention tremors of both hands" (tremors that occur when the client tries to do something).

Muscle Strength

Measure hand strength by asking the client to grasp and squeeze two fingers of each of your hands. Then compare the grasps for equality of strength. As another means of evaluating strength, try to withdraw the fingers from the client's grasp and compare the ease or difficulty. He or she should release the grasps on command–another assessment of consciousness and the ability to follow commands.

To test the client's strength against resistance, ask him or her to resist your bending or straightening of the arm, hand, leg, or foot being tested (Figure 44-9). A five-point rating scale is commonly used (see Chapter 53, Table 53-1). Test results are sometimes recorded as 5/5, 3/5, and so forth, indicating the criteria that were used and the status of the client at that testing. Always evaluate and compare strength on each side. Later testing results are compared with previous results to indicate progress or regression.

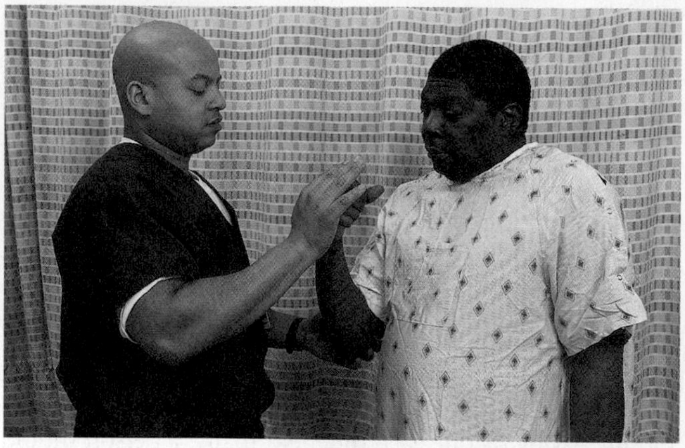

Figure 44-9 ■ Testing for strength against resistance.

Cerebral/Brainstem Integrity

Cerebral motor or brainstem integrity may also be assessed. Ask the client to close his or her eyes and hold the arms perpendicular to the body with the palms up for 15 to 30 seconds. If there is a cerebral or brainstem reason for muscle weakness, the arm on the weak side will start to fall, or "drift," with the palm pronating (turning inward). This is called a **pronator drift**. The same can be done for the lower extremities, with the client lying on his or her stomach with the legs bent upward at the knees. However, it is easier for most clients to sit on the side of the bed and extend the legs outward.

Abnormal Motor Findings

Peripheral motor problems are caused by injury, neuropathies, vascular problems, or a localized lesion in the opposite motor cortex. Tremors, unintentional movements, and changes in gait or posture represent problems in the basal ganglia or specialized nuclei of the brainstem or cerebellum. Motor cortex lesions, such as strokes, cause weakness or paralysis on the contralateral side of the body.

Video Clips: Fine Motor Coordination

ASSESSMENT OF CEREBELLAR FUNCTION

Coordination

Most of the assessment of cerebellar function can be performed with the client sitting on the side of the bed or examining table. Fine coordination of muscle activity is tested. Ask the client to perform the following with his or her eyes closed:

- Run the heel of one foot down the shin of the other leg, and repeat with the other leg (the client should be able to do this smoothly and keep the heel on the shin).
- Place the hands palm-up and then palm-down on each thigh, repeating as fast as possible (this can normally be done rapidly).
- With arms out at the side, touch the finger to the nose two or three times, with eyes open and then with eyes closed (this can be done with alternating arms or with each arm individually).

Gait and Equilibrium

For the last part of the cerebellar assessment, the ambulatory client stands for testing of gait and equilibrium. Gait and equilibrium are usually tested at the end of the entire neurologic assessment. Ask the client to walk across the room, turn, and return. Observe for inequality in steps, difficulty maneuvering, and so forth. To evaluate balance, the client is asked to stand on one foot and then on the other. Tiptoe walking and heel-to-toe walking can also demonstrate gait problems.

To test equilibrium, ask the client to stand with arms at the sides, feet and knees close together, and eyes open. Check for swaying and then ask the client to close his or her eyes and maintain position. The examiner should be close enough to prevent falling if the client cannot stay erect. If he or she sways with the eyes closed but not when the eyes are open (the **Romberg sign**), the problem is probably **proprioceptive** (awareness of body position). If the client sways with the eyes both open and closed, the neurologic disturbance is probably *cerebellar* in origin.

If the client is not able to perform any of these activities smoothly, the problem is manifested on the same side as the cerebellar lesion. If both lobes of the cerebellum are involved, the incoordination is bilateral.

ASSESSMENT OF REFLEX ACTIVITY

Procedure

Video Clip: Deep Tendon Reflex

The health care provider assesses deep tendon reflexes (DTRs) and superficial (cutaneous) reflexes. The **deep tendon reflexes** of the biceps, triceps, brachioradialis, and quadriceps muscles and of the Achilles tendon can be tested as part of the routine neurologic assessment. Striking the tendon with the hammer should cause contraction of the muscle (Figure 44-10). The appropriate muscle contraction indicates an intact reflex arc. The tendon is tapped quickly but not with too much force. If the client is tensing the muscle, the reflexes cannot be elicited. Having the client interlock his or her hands and pull outward will help to decrease muscle tensing so the reflex can be tested.

The **cutaneous (superficial) reflexes** usually tested are the plantar reflexes and sometimes the abdominal reflexes. The plantar reflex is tested with a pointed (but not sharp) object, such as the handle end of the reflex hammer or the rounded end of bandage scissors. The normal response is plantar flexion of all toes. Dorsiflexion of the great toe and fanning of the other toes **(Babinski's sign)** is abnormal in anyone older than 2 years and represents the presence of central nervous system (CNS) disease. The term "positive Babinski's sign" (abnormal response) and "negative Babinski's sign" (normal response) are clinically used terms but are not correct. **Babinski's sign** is a pathologic, or abnormal, reflex. Health care providers may also use the terms "upgoing" or "downgoing" to refer to the toes of the stimulated foot. "Upgoing" toes is an abnormal response that indicates the presence of pathology in the CNS. Babinski's sign can occur with drug and alcohol intoxication or after a seizure.

To test the abdominal reflex, stroke the client's abdomen in all four quadrants diagonally toward the umbilicus. The umbilicus should deviate toward the stimulus, but obesity may mask the reflex. The abdominal reflex can be absent in both upper and lower motor neuron disease.

Abnormal Reflex Findings

Hyperactive reflexes indicate possible upper motor neuron disease, tetanus, or hypocalcemia. Hypoactive reflexes may result from lower motor neuron disease (damage to the spinal cord), disease of the neuromuscular junction, muscle disease, or metabolic diseases such as diabetes mellitus, hypothyroidism, or hypokalemia.

Although people can display hyperactive, hypoactive, or even absent reflexes, *asymmetry* is an important finding because it probably indicates a disease process. The results of reflex testing are recorded by the use of a stick figure and a scale of 0 to 4 (Figure 44-11). A score of 2 is considered normal, although scores of 1 (hypoactive) or 3 (stronger than normal) may be normal for a particular client. **Clonus** is the sudden, brief, jerking contraction of a muscle or muscle group often seen in seizures.

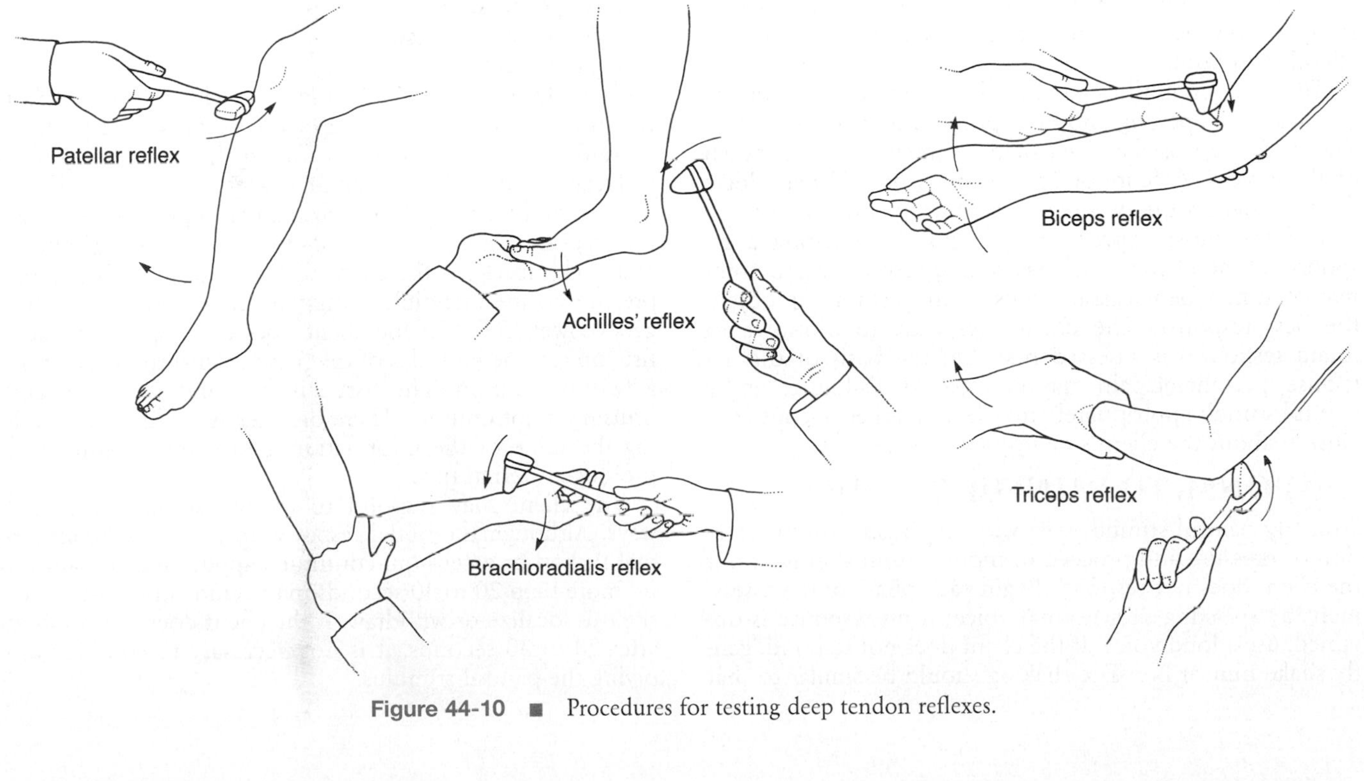

Figure 44-10 ■ Procedures for testing deep tendon reflexes.

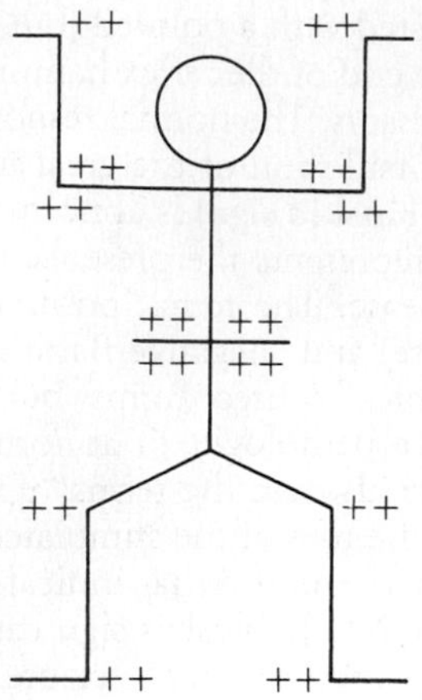

0	Absent, no response
1 (+)	Weaker than normal, hypoactive
2 (+ +)	Normal
3 (+ + +)	Stronger or more brisk than normal
4 (+ + + +)	Hyperactive
	(Note: 1 and 3 may be normal for some individuals)

Figure 44-11 ■ A stick figure and scale for recording reflex activity.

Rapid Neurologic Assessment

A rapid neurologic assessment is completed when the client is admitted to a health care facility on an emergent basis, or as part of the client's routine or ongoing assessment or in the event of a sudden change in neurologic status. This is the most common type of neurologic assessment you will perform when caring for adult clients.

GLASGOW COMA SCALE

A form of the **Glasgow Coma Scale** (GCS) (Figure 44-12) is used in many health care agencies. This tool has been shown to be reliable as one measure of neurologic assessment. Some agencies may use the GCS along with other assessment findings for a more comprehensive picture of the client's condition.

The GCS establishes baseline data in each of the following areas: eye opening, motor response, and verbal response. The client is assessed and assigned a numerical score for each of these areas. A score of 15 represents normal neurologic functioning; a score of 3 represents a deep coma state.

Use the most appropriate stimulus for eliciting a response. If the client is not awake and responding to commands, it may be necessary to use painful stimuli to obtain the best response. The client's response to central pain (brain response) is assessed first. On the basis of this response, peripheral pain may be assessed. Failure to apply painful stimuli appropriately may lead to an erroneous conclusion about the client's neurologic status.

RESPONSE TO PAINFUL STIMULI

To apply painful stimuli, start with the least noxious irritation or pressure and proceed to more painful stimulation if the client does not respond. Begin each phase of the assessment by speaking in a normal voice; if no response is obtained, use a loud voice. If the client does not respond, gently shake him or her. The shaking should be similar to that used in attempting to wake up a child. If that is unsuccessful, painful stimuli are applied using one of the following methods:

- Supraorbital pressure
- Trapezius squeeze
- Mandibular pressure
- Sternal rub

First, apply supraorbital pressure by placing a thumb under the orbital rim in the middle of the eyebrow and pushing upward. This technique is not used if the client has orbital or facial fractures (Lower, 2003).

A second technique to elicit pain is to pinch or squeeze the trapezius muscle located at the angle of the shoulder and neck muscle. If the client remains unresponsive, apply pressure to the mandible using your index and middle fingers (Lower, 2003). If the client does not respond, make a fist and rub the knuckles of the hand against the sternum in a twisting motion. The tissue in this area is tender, and bruising is not unusual. Therefore exercise judgment regarding the value of the information gained from frequent or prolonged sternal rubs.

The client may respond to painful stimuli in several ways. Although the initial response to pain may be abnormal flexion or extension, continued application of pain for no more than 20 to 30 seconds may demonstrate that he or she can localize or withdraw. If the client does not respond after 20 to 30 seconds, it is not necessary to continue applying the painful stimulus.

GLASGOW COMA SCALE*	
Eye Opening	
Spontaneous	4
To sound	3
To pain	2
Never	1
Motor Response	
Obeys commands	6
Localizes pain	5
Normal flexion (withdrawal)	4
Abnormal flexion	3
Extension	2
None	1
Verbal Response	
Oriented	5
Confused conversation	4
Inappropriate words	3
Incomprehensible sounds	2
None	1

* The highest possible score is 15

Figure 44-12 ■ The Glasgow Coma Scale. The highest possible score is 15.

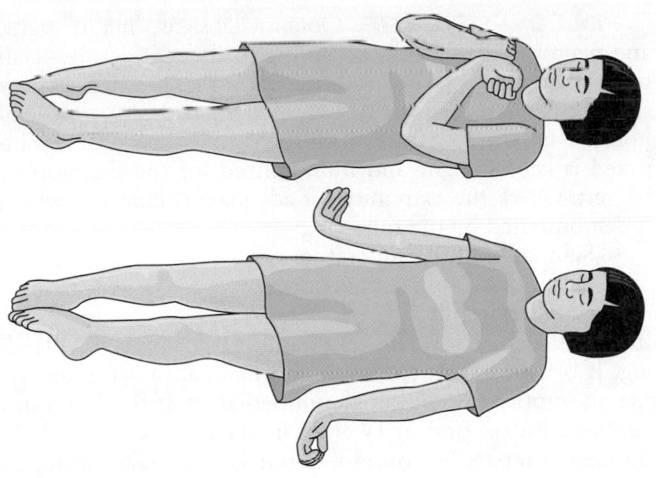

Figure 44-13 ■ Posturing. **A,** Decorticate posturing. **B,** Decerebrate posturing.

If the client responds by moving, but not all extremities move, assess the peripheral response to pain. Place a pen or pencil on top of the client's nail bed at the base of the cuticle and apply pressure. This maneuver is performed only on the extremity that did not move.

LEVEL OF CONSCIOUSNESS

In addition to using the Glasgow Coma Scale, assess the client's level of consciousness (LOC). This area of the assessment must be meticulously recorded and described as a change in LOC. *Even a subtle change is the **first** indicator of a decline in neurologic status!* These changes include complaints of headache; restlessness, irritability, or being unusually quiet; slurred speech; and a change in the level of orientation.

Decerebrate or decorticate posturing, as well as pinpoint or dilated and nonreactive pupils, is a late sign of deterioration. The physician should be notified immediately of any change in the client's status. **Decortication** is abnormal posturing seen in the client with lesions that interrupt the corticospinal pathways (Figure 44-13, *A*). The client's arms, wrists, and fingers are flexed with internal rotation and plantar flexion of the legs. **Decerebration** is abnormal posturing and rigidity characterized by extension of the arms and legs, pronation of the arms, plantar flexion, and opisthotonos (Figure 44-13, *B*). Decerebration is usually associated with dysfunction in the brainstem area.

PUPIL ASSESSMENT

▶ Video Clip: Pupil Responses

The pupils are assessed as part of ongoing "neuro" checks. Pupil constriction is a function of cranial nerve III. *P*upils should be *e*qual in size, *r*ound and *r*egular in shape, and react to *l*ight and *a*ccommodation **(PERRLA).** Estimate the size of both pupils using a millimeter ruler. Clients who have had eye surgery for cataracts or glaucoma often have irregularly shaped pupils. Clients using eyedrops for either cataracts or glaucoma may have unequal pupils if only one eye is being treated, and the pupillary response may be altered.

To test for pupil constriction, the client should be asked to close his or her eyes. Bring a penlight in from the side of the client's head and shine the light in the eye being tested as soon as the client opens his or her eyes. The pupil should constrict **(direct response);** the other eye should also constrict slightly **(consensual response).** To test accommodation, the client focuses on a distant object and then immediately focuses on an object 4 to 5 inches from the nose. The eyes should converge, and the pupils should constrict.

Diagnostic Assessment

LABORATORY TESTS

For clients with a neurologic problem resulting from or concomitant with systemic infection, blood cultures are necessary to identify the causative agent of the infection. Although the cause of infection must be determined for any client, this is especially true for those with central nervous system (CNS) disease. The blood-brain barrier is often not intact in neurologic disease, and the client is more susceptible to infection of the nervous system, such as meningitis or encephalitis.

RADIOGRAPHIC EXAMINATIONS

X-ray Examinations of the Skull and Spine

Plain x-rays of the skull and spine are used to determine bony fractures, curvatures, bone erosion, bone dislocation, and possible calcification of soft tissue, which can damage the nervous system.

Several views are taken–anteroposterior, lateral, oblique, and, when necessary, special views of the facial bones. In head trauma and multiple injuries, one of the first priorities is to rule out cervical fracture by radiography.

Explain that the x-ray procedure for the skull and spine is similar to that for a chest x-ray procedure, that he or she will need to remain still during the procedure, and that the exposure to radiation is minimal. If the client is in traction and a portable x-ray unit is not available, the nurse may need to accompany him or her to assist with positioning. Any client who cannot walk from a wheelchair to the x-ray table should go to the radiology department on a stretcher. The client is positioned for each of the desired views and is asked not to move just before each x-ray. Follow-up care is not required.

Cerebral Angiography

Cerebral angiography (arteriography) is done to visualize the cerebral circulation (carotid and vertebral arteries). A contrast medium is injected into an artery (usually the femoral) to identify aneurysms, traumatic injuries, strictures/occlusions, tumors, and arteriovenous malformations.

CLIENT PREPARATION. Determine whether the client is allergic to iodinated contrast agents (Chart 44-5). The procedure is initially explained to the client by the person obtaining the written consent, usually the radiologist. Clarify the explanation by answering questions and reinforcing the following important points:

- The necessity for not moving during the procedure
- The necessity for immobilization of the head

The client is allowed nothing by mouth for 4 to 6 hours before the test. Most hospitals require that the nurse complete a preoperative checklist. Be sure to:

- Remove the client's hairpins and jewelry.
- Record neurologic and vital signs.
- Ask the client to empty his or her bladder before the procedure.

CHART 44-5

BEST PRACTICE for Studies Involving the Injection of Contrast Agent

Special precautions are taken for clients who will receive a contrast agent as part of their diagnostic test. These measures include the following:

- Following institutional guidelines regarding informed consent
- Determining whether the client has any food or fluid restriction before the test
- Asking the client about allergies to contrast agents, shellfish, or iodine.
- Determining risk factors for contrast-induced nephropathy (renal damage)
  - Pre-existing renal disease
  - Diabetic nephropathy
  - Heart failure
  - Dehydration
  - Medications that interfere with renal perfusion, such as metformin (Diabetic clients on the metformin require preprocedure and postprocedure changes in their medication regimen.)
- Notifying the health care provider if the client has reported a risk factor
- Checking the client's creatinine level (Clients with a level greater than 1.5 mg/dL are more at risk for contrast-induced nephropathy.)

PROCEDURE. The client is placed on an examining table and made as comfortable as possible. At this time, dentures and hearing aids must be removed. The client's head is placed in a positioning headrest or sponge. He or she is then connected to cardiac monitoring throughout the procedure. Many institutions avoid sedating these clients because sedation may mask neurologic changes.

The radiologist numbs an area at the groin and inserts a needle into the femoral artery. A soft-tip guiding wire goes through the needle and into the aorta. A thin catheter is inserted into the artery over the wire. Under fluoroscopic guidance, the catheter is advanced into a carotid or vertebral artery. Then, the physician injects 6-8 mL of iodinated contrast material into each vessel several times while recording images from different angles over the head and neck. The newest radiographic systems come with software to create three-dimensional images that can be rotated to reveal overlapping anatomic structures.

After all the vessels have been imaged, the radiologist reviews all the images and consults with the referring physician to decide whether the client could benefit from any therapeutic radiologic procedure to treat the problem. It is common to use an arterial closure device to seal the artery and prevent bleeding.

Prior to the mid-1980s, images were taken by film. Imaging now is done almost exclusively by digital means (without film). The new equipment couples x-ray machines with a digital camera and computer. The x-ray images are stored on a computer. These systems could display the so-called "subtracted image," made from two images–one just before the contrast was injected and one with the contrast in the artery. Technologic improvements allow high-resolution images and three-dimensional rotational imaging, especially useful in cerebral studies.

The risks for the procedure are contrast reaction, thrombosis (clotting), vasospasm, and bleeding from the entry site. Clients with known contrast sensitivity are pre-treated with steroids. The overall risk for complications is less than 1%.

FOLLOW-UP CARE. Obtain vital signs, "neuro" signs, and neurovascular checks according to the written physician orders. Compare these findings with the pre-angiography signs. The client is usually restricted to bedrest for several hours. The extremity into which the contrast medium was injected is kept straight and immobilized for the duration of bedrest. Check the extremity for adequate circulation, which is demonstrated by the following:

- Skin color and temperature
- Pulses distal to the injection site
- Capillary refill

Inspect the injection site frequently for evidence of bleeding. If bleeding is noted, maintain manual pressure on the site and notify the radiologic immediately. If fluids are not contraindicated, oral or IV fluid intake is increased to help the client excrete the contrast material, which takes about 24 hours.

Computed Tomography

Computed tomography (CT) scanning is relatively accurate and is the quickest, easiest, and least expensive method of diagnosing neurologic problems. With the aid of a computer, pictures are taken at many horizontal levels, or slices, of the brain or spinal cord. The cross-sectional slices build up three-dimensional pictures of the brain or spinal cord. A contrast medium may be used to enhance the image. CT scans distinguish bone, soft tissue (e.g., the brain, vascular system, and ventricular system), and fluids such as cerebrospinal fluid (CSF) or blood. Tumors, infarctions, hemorrhage, hydrocephalus, and bone malformations can be identified. A CT scan may also be performed after a myelogram (see Chapter 53 for brief discussion of this test).

CLIENT PREPARATION. Follow the guidelines listed in Chart 44-5 if a contrast agent is to be given. If a contrast medium is used, food is withheld for 4 to 6 hours before the test. Fluids are generally not withheld. Instruct the client to remove hairpins, hairpieces, or wigs.

PROCEDURE. The client is placed on a movable table. His or her head is positioned in a head-holding device. The client must remain completely still during the test, which may be difficult. The table is positioned in the machine, a large donut-shaped structure. Some clients are fearful of the machine or of being confined in a small space. A noncontrast series of pictures is taken first. Then, if needed, the client is withdrawn from the scanner and given an injection of the iodinated contrast medium. The scan is then repeated. Each set of head scans takes less than 5 minutes in newer scanners. Spine studies take about 10 minutes per body section (cervical, thoracic, lumbar) and are less likely to require contrast injection.

Most clients with new neurologic symptoms get both the precontrast and postcontrast study of the head. Contrast-enhanced CT is especially useful in locating and identifying tumor types and abscesses. For situations in which bleeding is the only concern (e.g., in trauma clients), contrast scans are not usually required.

New CT scanners can provide CT-angiography (CTA) images. Computer software can assemble three-dimensional reconstruction of the blood vessels of the neck or brain. These images are not yet as detailed as angiographic images, but are faster, cheaper, and less invasive than angiography.

FOLLOW-UP CARE. Check for a delayed allergic response to the contrast medium if it was used. If a contrast medium was used, the resultant diuresis may require the administration of replacement fluids.

Positron Emission Tomography

Positron emission tomography (PET) is a diagnostic tool that is becoming available to more medical centers. Its benefit over a computed tomography (CT) scan or magnetic resonance imaging (MRI) is that it provides information about the *function* of the brain, specifically glucose and oxygen metabolism and cerebral blood flow. Current CT scanners provide information about the *structure* of the central nervous system (CNS). Some research centers have functional magnetic resonance imaging (fMRI).

The physician or nuclear medicine technologist injects the client with the molecule deoxyglucose, which is tagged to an isotope. The isotope emits activity in the form of positrons, which are scanned and converted into a color image by computer. The more active a given part of the brain, the greater the glucose uptake. This test is used to evaluate drug metabolism and detect areas of metabolic alteration that occur in dementia, epilepsy, psychiatric and degenerative disorders, neoplasms, and Alzheimer's disease. The level of radiation is equivalent to that of five or six x-rays but much less than exposure during CT. Recently, the half-life of these isotopes has increased and more centers are able to offer this test. Regional cyclotrons can now provide isotopes for medical centers within two hours of the generator.

CLIENT PREPARATION. Explain the test and instruct the client to withhold caffeine, alcohol, and tobacco for 24 hours before the test, according to agency policy. The client is on NPO status (nothing by mouth) for 6 to 12 hours before the procedure (if the client is diabetic, no insulin is given before the test). Do not give any glucose solutions and any other drugs that alter glucose metabolism.

PROCEDURE. The client is placed on a stretcher. An IV line is started to inject the isotope. An arterial line may be used to obtain blood samples. The client may be blindfolded and have earplugs inserted for all or part of the test. The total procedure takes 2 to 3 hours. The client is asked to perform certain mental functions to activate different areas of the brain.

FOLLOW-UP CARE. The radioisotope is eliminated in the urine and requires no special precautions. However, encourage the client to increase fluid intake. Follow-up care is not required.

Single-Photon Emission Computed Tomography

The limitation of PET may be overcome through the use of **single-photon emission computed tomography (SPECT).** With SPECT, a radiopharmaceutical, an agent that enables radioisotopes to cross the blood-brain barrier is administered by IV injection. Gamma-emitting radionuclides have longer half-lives, therefore eliminating the need for a cyclotron near the scanner. Although SPECT is less expensive than PET, the resolution of the images is limited. SPECT is particularly useful in studying the following:

- Cerebral blood flow
- Stroke
- Dementia
- Acquired immunodeficiency syndrome (AIDS)
- Amnesia
- Neoplasms
- Head trauma
- Seizures
- Persistent vegetative state
- Brain death
- Psychiatric disorders

SPECT is contraindicated in pregnant women or women who are breastfeeding.

CLIENT PREPARATION. Client preparation is similar to that for PET. Determine whether the client has recently had other nuclear medicine screenings which may leave traces of the radiopharmaceutical agent in the client. Recent scanning may interfere with test results. As with other tests that involve the injection of contrast material, determine whether the client has renal disease or has had a reaction to dye in the past.

PROCEDURE. The client is injected with the material about 1 hour before the actual scan by the radiologist, certified nuclear medicine technologist, or specially trained RN.

He or she is positioned on an x-ray table in a quiet dark room for the actual scans. Several gamma cameras scan the client's head. When completed, the images are downloaded to a computer.

FOLLOW UP CARE. The client can return to his or her previous activity level. There are no food or fluid restrictions as a result of the test.

OTHER DIAGNOSTIC TESTS

Magnetic Resonance Imaging

Magnetic resonance imaging (MRI) produces images considered superior to the CT scan. It does not use ionizing radiation but instead relies on magnetic fields. Special precautions must be taken when entering the MRI procedure room. Images may be enhanced with the use of gadolinium, a non-iodine-based contrast. MRIs of the spine have replaced CT scans and myelography in most instances (see Chapter 53).

Two newer uses for MRI are **magnetic resonance angiography (MRA)** and **magnetic resonance spectroscopy (MRS).** MRA is used to identify arterial blockages, intracranial aneurysms, and arteriovenous malformations. MRS is used to detect abnormalities in the brain's biochemical processes, such as that which occurs in Alzheimer's disease and brain attack (Pagana & Pagana, 2002).

CLIENT PREPARATION. A signed consent form is obtained; no food or fluid restrictions are necessary. Tell the client that the procedure is noisy and that earplugs are available. In addition, the client should know that he or she will lie on a hard surface inside a hollow tube. If the client is claustrophobic, a mild sedative may be prescribed before the procedure.

Newer, open-sided units ("open MRI") now produce adequate images for those clients who do not wish to be sedated for standard long-bore MRI scanners. MRI is contraindicated for clients with cardiac pacemakers, other implanted pumps or devices, and ferromagnetic aneurysm clips. Other implanted devices, such as vascular stents, intravascular catheter (IVC) filters, and metal vascular embolic devices may be scanned immediately or after a certain period of time, depending on manufacturers' recommendations. MRI may also be contraindicated in clients who are confused, pregnant, or agitated; have unstable vital signs; are on continuous life support; or have tattoos. New physiologic monitoring systems made specifically for MRI allow some clients who are unstable to be scanned. A comprehensive online list of medical devices tested for MRI safety and compatibility can be found at http://www.mrisafety.com (Carr, 2002). Medical personnel must remove any medical devices they are carrying or wearing, and ensure that only approved devices are allowed in the MRI room.

PROCEDURE. MRI uses a powerful magnet to align hydrogen nuclei (usually) in the plane of the magnetic field. The scanner emits a radio frequency (RF) pulse, which is transmitted to change the hydrogen alignment. Between RF pulses, the hydrogen realigns with the magnet and nuclei transmit an RF signal back to the scanner. This signal is then converted to an image that locates hydrogen on the body. Multiple sets of images are taken that are used to determine normal and abnormal anatomy.

FOLLOW-UP CARE. No special post-procedure or follow-up care is required.

Statscan Critical Imaging System

The Statscan was first used in the United States in the Shock Trauma Center at the University of Maryland in Baltimore. This low-dose digital imaging system, small enough to fit into an average-sized trauma room, can take full-body images. In just 13 seconds, the trauma team has information about fractures and other injuries that may not be readily apparent on the initial trauma survey. No special preparation or care is needed.

Lumbar Puncture

Lumbar puncture (spinal tap) is the insertion of a spinal needle into the subarachnoid space between the third and fourth (sometimes the fourth and fifth) lumbar vertebrae. A lumbar puncture is used to do the following:

- Obtain pressure readings with a manometer
- Obtain cerebrospinal fluid (CSF) for analysis
- Check for spinal blockage attributable to a spinal cord lesion
- Inject contrast medium or air for diagnostic study
- Inject spinal anesthetics
- Inject certain medications
- Reduce mild to moderate increased intracranial pressure (ICP) in certain conditions

Because of the danger of sudden release of CSF pressure, a lumbar puncture is contraindicated in clients with symptoms suggestive of increased ICP. The procedure is also contraindicated in clients with skin infections at or near the puncture site because of the danger of introducing infective organisms into the CSF.

CLIENT PREPARATION. A consent form is signed by the client. Explain the procedure, noting that some discomfort may be felt when the local anesthetic is injected. Some clients experience pain in the leg when the spinal needle is inserted. Ask the client to empty his or her bladder as a comfort measure. Position the client on whichever side he or she is most comfortable, with his or her back close to the edge of the bed or examining table. When the health care provider is ready, ask the client to bring the knees up as close as possible to the trunk and to assume a "fetal" position (using the arms to hold the knees in place) with the head bent forward. Some clients need help in achieving and maintaining this position. To help maintain the position, grasp the client behind the knees and the back of the lower neck. A pillow under the head and between the knees aids body alignment.

PROCEDURE. The health care provider cleans the skin site thoroughly. The injection site is determined, and the local anesthetic is injected. In a few minutes, the health care provider inserts a spinal needle between the third and fourth lumbar vertebrae. Instruct the client to inform the provider if there is shooting pain or a tingling sensation. After determining proper placement in the subarachnoid space by removing the stylet and seeing CSF, the client is asked to relax a little so the pressure reading will be more accurate. Opening and closing pressure readings are taken and recorded. Three to five test tubes of CSF are usually collected and numbered sequentially. After specimen collection, the needle is withdrawn, slight pressure is applied, and an adhesive bandage strip is placed over the insertion site. The nurse may or may not be able to help with the collection and numbering of the specimens, depending on the client's ability to remain quiet. If the client is restless or unable to cooperate, two people may need to assist instead of one. Consider this possibility before beginning the procedure.

Examination of CSF has been a useful diagnostic tool for some time, and recent technical advances are increasing the number of analyses that can be done on CSF. The normal characteristics of CSF and some of the more common abnormalities are given in Table 44-7. Gram stain smears can test for particular types of meningitis, such as tubercular meningitis. CSF can be cultured, and sensitivity studies determine the best choice of antibiotic if an infection is diagnosed. A specific test for neurosyphilis is the fluorescent treponemal antibody absorption (FTA-ABS) test. Cytologic studies of CSF can identify tumor cells.

FOLLOW-UP CARE. After a lumbar puncture (LP), the client is generally restricted to bedrest in a flat position for 4 to 8 hours as prescribed by the physician or as determined by hospital policy. This prevents CSF leakage from the puncture site. However, a report by the Therapeutics and Assessment Subcommittee of the American Academy of Neurology found that the duration of bedrest does not influence the occurrence of post-LP headache (Evans et al., 2000). Instruct the client to increase fluid intake (to 3000 mL unless contraindicated) for 24 to 48 hours to facilitate CSF production, although research has not supported or refuted this practice.

A decrease in CSF may cause a severe, throbbing headache (also called a **spinal headache**). Administer analgesics as prescribed for headache if it occurs. If the lumbar puncture was done to reduce intracranial pressure, perform a rapid neurologic assessment (especially level of consciousness) more frequently until stability is ensured. Complications of lumbar puncture, although uncommon, include infection, CSF leakage, and hematoma formation.

Electroencephalography

Electroencephalography (EEG) records the electrical activity of the cerebral hemispheres. Each graphic recording represents the voltage changes in various areas of the brain (determined by recording the difference between two electrodes). The EEG may be normal even when a pathologic condition is present. The test is performed to:

- Determine the general activity of the cerebral hemispheres
- Determine the origin of seizure activity (epilepsy)

TABLE 44-7 Significance of Cerebrospinal Fluid Findings

Findings	Significance
Pressure	
Less than 20 cm H_2O	Normal range
Color/Appearance	
Clear, colorless	Normal
Pink-red to orange	Red blood cells present
Yellow	Bilirubin present owing to hemolysis of red blood cells; possible causes include subarachnoid hemorrhage, jaundice, increased cerebrospinal fluid (CSF) protein, hypercarotenemia, or hemoglobinemia
Brown	Methemoglobin present, indicating previous meningeal hemorrhage
Unclear or hazy	Cell count is elevated
Cells	
0-5 small lymphocytes/mm^3	Normal
More than 5 lymphocytes/mm^3	Reaction to infection, tumor, chemical substance, or blood
Proteins	
Total	
15-45 mg/dL	Normal
45-100 mg/dL	Paraventricular tumor
50-200 mg/dL	Viral infection
More than 500 mg/dL	Bacterial infection, Guillain-Barré syndrome
Less than 15 mg/dL	Meningismus, pseudotumor cerebri, hyperthyroidism, normal finding after lumbar puncture
Immune Gamma Globulin (IgG, the most important protein)	
3%-12% of total protein	Normal
More than 3%-12% of total protein	Multiple sclerosis, neurosyphilis, or viral infection
Albumin/Globulin Ratio	
8:1	Normal
Glucose	
50-75 mg/dL or 60%-70% of blood glucose level	Normal
Less than 50 mg/dL (usually accompanied by the presence of pathologic organisms)	Bacterial, fungal, or viral meningitis; central nervous system (CNS) leukemia; or cancer
Other Characteristics	
Lactic Acid	
10-25 mg/dL	Normal
More than 10-25 mg/dL	Systemic acidosis or increased CSF glucose metabolism
Glutamine	
Less than 20 mg/dL	Normal
More than 20 mg/dL	Hepatic coma or cirrhosis of liver
Lactate Dehydrogenase	
10% of serum level or 2.0-7.2 units/mL	Normal
More than 10% of serum level	Bacterial meningitis, inflammatory diseases of CNS

- Determine cerebral function in pathologic conditions other than epilepsy, such as tumors, abscesses, cerebrovascular disease, hematomas, injury, metabolic diseases, degenerative brain disease, and drug intoxication
- Differentiate between organic and hysterical or feigned blindness or deafness
- Monitor cerebral activity during surgical anesthesia
- Diagnose sleep disorders (all-night EEG)
- Determine brain death

CLIENT PREPARATION. This test is done on an ambulatory care basis. Chart 44-6 lists instructions for the client preparing to have an EEG.

Explain the purpose of and procedure for the test. If the EEG is ordered with the client "sleep deprived," he or she should be kept awake from about 2 to 3 AM through the rest of the night. CNS depressants and stimulants are usually not given for 24 hours before the test. The health care provider indicates whether anticonvulsants are to be withheld. If anticonvulsants are withheld, monitor the client for signs of seizure activity. Remind the client to avoid coffee, tea, and other stimulants. Food and other fluids may be consumed because hypoglycemia (low blood glucose) affects brain activity. The client's hair should be shampooed, clean, and free from hairpins, sprays, or oils.

CHART 44-6

BEST PRACTICE for
The Client Having an Electroencephalogram

- Thoroughly explain the procedure to the client.
- If the order is for the client to be "sleep deprived," tell the client to awaken about 2 to 3 AM and to stay awake for the rest of the night.
- Instruct the client to avoid central nervous system depressants or stimulants; withhold anticonvulsants only if instructed by the physician.
- Tell the client not to drink caffeine-containing fluids, such as coffee or tea, on the day of the test.
- Reassure the client that the test is not dangerous or uncomfortable.
- Ask the client to wash his or her hair on the morning of the test and to remove all hairpins, sprays, or oils.
- Inform the client that the hair will need to be washed again after the test to remove the electrode glue.

PROCEDURE. The client is placed on a reclining chair or bed. According to an internationally accepted procedure, 16 to 24 electrodes are usually attached to the scalp with a jelly-like substance and connected to the machine. The physician or EEG technician places glue over the electrodes to prevent slippage. The client must lie still with his or her eyes closed during the initial recording. The rest of the test engages the client in certain activities: hyperventilation, photic stimulation, and sleep. A portable EEG may be performed at the bedside if necessary, but the preference is for the EEG to be done in a room devoid of stimuli.

Hyperventilation produces cerebral vasoconstriction and alkalosis, which increases the likelihood of seizure activity. The client is asked to breathe deeply 20 to 30 times for 3 minutes.

In *photic stimulation,* a strobe light (bright light) is placed in front of the client. Frequencies of 1 to 20 flashes per second are used with the client's eyes open and then closed. If the client's seizures are photosensitive in origin, the EEG will show waves corresponding to each flash of light or waves indicating seizure activity.

Sleep is either natural or induced by an oral or IV sedative. EEG waves indicative of temporal lobe epilepsy can be demonstrated best during sleep.

Throughout the test, which takes 40 to 60 minutes, the technician watches the client closely and records any movement. These movements alter the record and must be labeled as artifacts. Examples of artifacts are tongue movement, eye blinking, muscle tenseness, and nervousness.

FOLLOW-UP CARE. If not removed in the EEG laboratory, the client removes the jelly-like substance and glue from the scalp and hair with acetone and then with shampoo. Any medications that were withheld are reinstituted. The client may need a nap if he or she was deprived of sleep before the test.

Electromyography

Electromyography (EMG) records the electrical activity of peripheral nerves by testing muscle activity (see Chapter 53 for a description of client preparation, procedure, and follow-up care). Electromyography and **electroneurography** or nerve conduction velocity studies (NCVS) are usually used together and are referred to as **electromyoneurography.**

Cerebral Blood Flow Evaluation

Cerebral blood flow (CBF) can be measured in many areas of the brain with the use of radioactive substances. It is particularly useful in evaluating cerebral vasospasm. Explain the test and, if drugs have previously been prescribed, withhold central nervous system (CNS) depressants and stimulants for 24 hours before the test.

Because xenon readily diffuses into brain tissue, it is the most common choice as an inhaled or injected tracer. The xenon travels through the vasculature to the brain, where it is detected by external scintillation counters placed on the skull. Normal CBF is 50 to 55 mm/min/100 g of cerebral tissue. The client receives various stimuli during the test. Increases in local blood flow can be seen with any neuronal activity, such as reading, hand movement, seizures, and temperature elevation (up to 107.6° F [42° C]). Local blood flow decreases with degenerative disease, comas of metabolic origin, increased intracranial pressure (ICP), or subarachnoid hemorrhage. Follow-up care for this test is not required.

Brain Scan

The **brain scan** is a radionuclide imaging study. A radioactive substance is injected to detect certain pathologic conditions. The test is especially useful in evaluating vascular abnormalities such as aneurysms and in locating tumors, hematomas, and abscesses. As technologic advances in diagnostic testing continue, this test is being performed less frequently.

Explain the test and ask the client to empty the bladder as a comfort measure immediately before the test is done. A signed consent form may be necessary, depending on agency policy.

During the procedure, the physician injects the client with a radioactive isotope, usually technetium (Tc 99m). There is a delay in the test of up to 2 hours while the brain absorbs the isotope. The client is placed on a table and must remain still with the hands at his or her side for the duration of the test. The test takes 1 to 2 hours, depending on the number of scannings used.

For follow-up care, teach the client to increase fluids to promote elimination of the isotope (urine does not need special handling).

Transcranial Doppler

Intracranial hemodynamics can be evaluated through the use of the **transcranial Doppler (TCD).** TCD does not measure cerebral blood flow or visualize the vessels, but it does measure the time needed for pulse waves to travel a specific depth and return to the skull's surface. It is particularly valuable in evaluating cerebral vasospasm. TCD is safe and repeatable and is an inexpensive alternative to angiography.

GET READY for the NCLEX Examination!

KEY POINTS

Safe Effective Care Environment

- When caring for older adults, remind them to move slowly and use caution when ambulating; older adults have an altered balance and decreased coordination.

- For tests that use contrast media, use precautions as listed in Chart 44-5.
- Check for bleeding after clients have an angiography; if bleeding is observed, call the radiologist immediately.
- Before MRI, check for ferromagnetic devices, such as pacemakers, vascular stents, and implanted pumps.

Health Promotion and Maintenance

- Reinforce teaching and use teaching aids for older adults who typically have recent memory loss.
- Explain what clients should expect before diagnostic testing for neurologic structure and function.
- Encourage clients who receive contrast media or isotopes to push fluids to increase elimination of the material.
- Teach clients having an EEG to follow the precautions listed in Chart 44-6.

Psychosocial Integrity

- Assess the mental status of clients as part of the neurologic assessment, including orientation.
- Remember that a change in level of consciousness (LOC) is the first indicator of neurologic decline.
- Assess the client's memory because loss of memory, especially recent memory, tends to be an early sign of neurologic problems.

Physiological Integrity

- Evaluate the client's sensory and motor abilities, as well as gait, balance, and coordination.
- Use the Glasgow Coma Scale as one measure of neurologic functioning; the lower the score, the poorer the function.
- Check pupils for size, shape, and reaction; pupils should be equal in size, round and regular in shape, and reactive to light and accommodation.
- Be aware that decerebrate or decorticate posturing, and pinpoint or dilated nonreactive pupils are late signs of neurologic deterioration.
- Assist with client positioning during a lumbar puncture (fetal position preferred).
- Recall that normal cerebrospinal fluid (CSF) is clear and colorless with few cells.

ADDITIONAL STUDY RESOURCES

Go to your Student CD-ROM for Review Questions for the NCLEX Examination.

evolve Go to http://evolve.elsevier.com/Iggy/ for Integrated Management of Care Questions for the NCLEX Examination.

SELECTED BIBLIOGRAPHY

Al-Chalabi, A., & Miller, C.C. (2003). Neurofilaments and neurological disease. *Bioessays, 25*(4), 346-355.

Altizer, L. (2002). Orthopaedic essentials. Neurovascular assessment. *Orthopaedic Nursing, 21*(4), 48-50.

Barker, E. (2003). *Neuroscience nursing: A spectrum of care* (2nd ed.). St. Louis: Mosby.

Brenner, Z.R., & Myers, S.A. (2003). Acetylcysteine and nephropathy. *American Journal of Nursing, 103*(3), 64AA-64EE.

Carr, M.W., & Grey, M.L. (2002). Magnetic resonance imaging. *American Journal of Nursing, 102*(12), 26-32.

Chaudhuri, A. (2002). The role of neurodiagnostics in functional disorders. *Physical Medicine & Rehabilitation: State of the Art Reviews, 16*(1), 63-75.

Evans, R.W. (2003). *Saunders manual of neurological practice.* Philadelphia: W.B. Saunders.

Evans, R.W., et al. (2000). Assessment: Prevention of post-lumbar puncture headaches: Report of the Therapeutics and Technology Assessment Subcommittee of the American Academy of Neurology. *Neurology, 55*(7), 909-911.

Gambrell, M., & Flynn, N. (2004). Seizures 101. *Nursing 2004, 34*(8), 36-41.

Goetz, C.G. (2003). *Textbook of Clinical Neurology* (2nd ed.). Philadelphia: W.B. Saunders.

Hickey, J. (2002). The clinical practice of neurological and neurosurgical nursing. Philadelphia: J.B. Lippincott.

Hinkle, J. (2002). SPECT: A powerful imaging tool. *American Journal of Nursing* (March), *102*(3), 24A-24G.

Huether, S.E., & McCance, K.L. (2004). *Understanding pathophysiology* (3rd ed.). St. Louis: Mosby.

Jarvis, C. (2003). *Physical examination and health assessment* (4th ed.). Philadelphia: W.B. Saunders.

Kullman, D.M., & Hanna, M.G. (2002). Neurological disorders caused by inherited ion-channel mutations. *Lancet: Neurology, 1*(3), 157-166.

Lower, J. (2002). Facing neuro assessment fearlessly. *Nursing, 32*(2), 58-65.

Lower, J. (2003). Using pain to assess neurologic response. *Nursing 2003, 33*(6), 56-57.

Pagana, K.D., & Pagana, T.J. (2002). *Mosby's manual of diagnostic and laboratory tests* (2nd ed.). St. Louis: Mosby.

Solomon, E.P. (2003). *Introduction to human anatomy and physiology* (2nd ed.). Philadelphia: W.B. Saunders.

CHAPTER 45

Interventions for Clients with Problems of the Central Nervous System

The Brain

KATHY A. HAUSMAN

LEARNING OUTCOMES

After studying this chapter, you should be able to:

1. Compare the assessment findings of migraine, cluster and tension headaches.
2. Develop a teaching plan for a client diagnosed with migraine headaches.
3. Differentiate the common types of seizures, including presenting clinical manifestations.
4. Identify collaborative management options for treating clients diagnosed with epilepsy.
5. Explain the nursing interventions required when providing care for a client having a seizure.
6. Outline the priorities for care of clients with meningitis and encephalitis.
7. Describe the pathophysiology of Parkinson disease.
8. Develop a community-based plan of care for a client with Parkinson disease.
9. Identify nursing implications related to giving medications for Parkinson disease.
10. Identify the roles of the interdisciplinary health care team and family in developing a comprehensive individualized treatment plan for the client with Alzheimer's disease.
11. Explain the use of drug therapy for clients with Alzheimer's disease.
12. Prioritize care for clients with Alzheimer's disease.
13. Develop a teaching plan for caregivers of clients with Alzheimer's disease.
14. Analyze legal/ethical concerns related to genetic counseling of clients with Huntington disease.

Go to your Student CD-ROM for Review Questions for the NCLEX Examination keyed to these Learning Outcomes.

Dysfunction of the brain may be a mild disorder that a person can learn to live with or a devastating disorder that drastically affects the client and the family. With newer diagnostic tools and treatment methods, the rate and the quality of recovery and rehabilitation are improving steadily. Neurologic impairment tends to involve many aspects of the person's life:

- The neurologic problem itself
- Family life alteration or disruption
- Occupational changes
- Body image
- Self-worth conflicts
- The realization of a continuous need for numerous resources

HEADACHES

Headaches are a common symptom of a variety of neurologic and non-neurologic disorders. The challenge to the health care provider is to determine the cause of the headache so appropriate treatment may begin. To assist the health care provider in this endeavor, the International Headache Society developed a classification and diagnostic criteria of all headache disorders. This system, which identifies common terminology, has gained acceptance as a common standard throughout the world (Evans & Olesen, 2003). Three of the most common types of headaches are migraine headaches, cluster headaches, and tension headaches. Clients are managed in the ambulatory care setting by the primary health care provider.

Clients with headaches are encouraged to keep a headache diary, which may help identify the type of headache they are experiencing. They need to understand the importance of notifying their health care provider if the severity, intensity, or nature of the headache increases or changes. Clients also need to report whether the headache is associated with unusual visual changes and whether the prescribed medication is no longer effective.

Migraine Headache

PATHOPHYSIOLOGY

A **migraine headache** is an episodic familial disorder manifested by unilateral, frontotemporal, throbbing pain in the head, which is often worse behind one eye or ear. It is often accompanied by a sensitive scalp, anorexia, **photophobia** (sensitivity to light), and nausea with or without vomiting. Clients tend to have the same clinical manifestations each time they have a migraine headache. Some may have to refrain from regular activities for several days if they cannot control or relieve the pain in its early stage.

Several theories have emerged regarding the causes of migraines, which involve vascular, genetic, neurologic (central neuronal hyperexcitability) and chemical factors. It is generally agreed that migraine headaches are mediated via the trigeminal vascular system and its central projections (Welch, Cutrer, & Peter, 2003). Blood vessels in the brain overreact to a triggering event, causing spasm in the arteries at the base of the brain. This response is followed by arterial constriction and a decrease in cerebral blood flow; cerebral hypoxia may occur. Platelets clump together and serotonin, a vasoconstrictor, is released. Other arteries dilate, which triggers the release of **prostaglandins,** chemicals that cause inflammation and swelling, and substances that increase sensitivity to pain. This theory is supported by the success of medications that affect 5-HT (serotonin) in the brain.

COLLABORATIVE MANAGEMENT

Assessment

Migraines fall into three categories: migraines with aura, migraines without aura, and atypical migraines. An **aura** is a sensation that signals the onset of a headache or seizure. In a migraine, the aura occurs immediately before the migraine episode. Most headaches are migraines without aura. The signs and symptoms of both migraines with aura and those without are listed in Chart 45-1. **Atypical migraines** are less common and include menstrual and cluster migraines. Kolb-Lucas describes the stages of migraine as:

- Prodrome phase, in which the client has specific symptoms such as food cravings or mood changes
- Aura phase (if present), which generally involves visual changes, flashing lights, or **diplopia** (double vision)
- Headache phase, which may last a few hours to a few days
- Termination phase, in which the intensity of the headache decreases
- Postprodrome phase, in which the client is often fatigued, may be irritable, and has muscle pain

The diagnosis of migraine headache is based on the client's history, and physical and neurologic assessment. Neuroimaging, such as magnetic resonance imaging (MRI), may be indicated if the client has other neurologic findings, a history of seizures, findings not consistent with a migraine, or a change in the severity of symptoms or frequency of the attacks. Neuroimaging is recommended in clients older than 50 years of age with a new onset of headaches.

CHART 45-1

KEY FEATURES of Migraine Headaches

Phases of Migraine with Aura (Classic Migraine)

First, or Prodromal, Phase

- Aura develops over a period of several minutes and lasts no more than 1 hour.
- Well-defined transient focal neurologic dysfunction exists.
- Pain may be preceded by:
  - Visual disturbances
  - Flashing lights
  - Lines or spots
  - Shimmering or zigzag lights
- Pain may be preceded by a variety of neurologic changes, including the following:
  - Numbness, tingling of the lips or tongue
  - Acute confusional state
  - Aphasia
  - Vertigo
  - Unilateral weakness
  - Drowsiness

Second Phase

- Headache is accompanied by nausea and vomiting.
- Pain usually begins in the temple; it increases in intensity and becomes throbbing within 1 hour.

Third Phase

- Pain changes from throbbing to dull.
- Headache, nausea, and vomiting usually last from 4 to 72 hours. (Older clients may have aura without pain, known as a visual migraine.)

Migraine without Aura (Common Migraine)

- Migraine begins without an aura before the onset of the headache.
- Pain is aggravated by performing routine physical activities.
- Pain is unilateral and pulsating.
- One of the following symptoms is present:
  - Nausea and/or vomiting
  - **Photophobia** (light sensitivity)
  - **Phonophobia** (sound sensitivity)
- Headache lasts for 4 to 72 hours.
- Migraine often occurs in the early morning, during periods of stress, or in those with premenstrual tension or fluid retention.

Atypical Migraine

- Status migrainous
  - Headache lasts longer than 72 hours.
- Migrainous infarction
  - Neurologic symptoms are not completely reversible within 7 days.
  - Ischemic infarct is noted on neuroimaging.
- Unclassified
  - Headache does not fulfill all of the criteria to be classified a migraine.

Common Nursing Diagnoses and Collaborative Problems

Nursing diagnoses that may apply to clients with migraine headaches include the following:

- Chronic Pain related to chronic physical disability

- Acute Pain related to biologic and chemical factors
- Anxiety related to change in or threat to health status
- Hopelessness related to deteriorating physiologic condition

Interventions

The priority for interdisciplinary care of the client experiencing a migraine is pain management, which may be achieved by abortive and preventive drug therapy, as well as nondrug measures. Many of the medications have significant side effects, contraindications, and nursing implications.

Drug Therapy. Drug therapy is prescribed to manage migraine headaches. Headaches that occur more frequently than two to three times a month require preventive therapy. Mild migraine headaches may be relieved with aspirin or acetaminophen (Tylenol, Abenol✱). The health care provider must take into consideration any comorbid medical conditions when prescribing medications. In general, the client is started on a low dose of medication that is adjusted upward until the desired clinical effect is obtained.

Abortive Therapy. Abortive drug therapy is aimed at alleviating pain during the aura phase (if present) or soon after the headache has started. These medications include ergotamine derivatives, nonsteroidal anti-inflammatory drugs (NSAIDs), triptans, and isometheptene combinations. A potential side effect of these medications is rebound headache, in which another headache occurs after the medication seems effective.

Acetaminophen and NSAIDs, such as naproxen (Naprosyn, Novo-Naprox✱), are usually effective for mild migraine headaches. The health care provider may prescribe antiemetics, such as prochlorperazine (Compazine), to help control nausea and vomiting. Often, metoclopramide (Reglan, Clopra) is administered with the NSAID to promote gastric emptying and decrease vomiting.

Ergotamine tartrate (Cafergot) is given at the start of the headache; the client may take up to six tablets in 24 hours. Dihydroergotamine (DHE) may be given intravenously (IV) or intramuscularly (IM), along with an antiemetic, if satisfactory pain control and relief of nausea are not achieved with other medications. DHE should not be given within 24 hours of a triptan medication.

The triptan preparations activate the 5-HT (serotonin) receptors on the cranial arteries, the basilar artery, and the vasculature of the dura mater to produce a vasoconstrictive effect. Sumatriptan succinate (Imitrex) is given or self-administered for acute migraine relief. It is available in tablets, as a subcutaneous injection, or as a nasal spray. Examples of other drugs in this category include rizatriptan (Maxalt), naratriptan (Naramig✱), zolmitriptan (Zomig), eletriptan (Relpax), almotriptan (Axert), and frovatriptan (Frova)–all available as tablets. For many clients, these drugs are highly effective for pain, nausea, vomiting, and light and sound sensitivity, with few side effects. Most are contraindicated in clients with actual or suspected ischemic heart disease, hypertension, and peripheral vascular disease or in those with Prinzmetal's angina because of the potential of coronary vasospasm.

Teach clients taking the triptan drugs to report chest pain or tightness to their health care providers immediately. Remind them to use contraception (birth control) while taking the drug because it may not be safe for women who are pregnant. Common expected side effects include flushing, tingling, and a hot sensation. Triptan medications should not be taken with selective serotonin reuptake inhibitor (SSRI) antidepressants or St. John's wort, an herb used commonly for depression.

Preventive Therapy. Unless otherwise contraindicated, the health care provider may initially prescribe an NSAID, a beta-adrenergic blocker, or a calcium channel blocker. Propranolol (Inderal, Apo-Propranolol✱, Novopranol✱) and timolol (Blocadren, Apo-Timol✱) are the only beta blockers approved for migraine prophylaxis, but others such as atenolol are also effective. These medications lower blood pressure and decrease pulse rate. Teach the client, especially older adults, how to assess vital signs and observe for beginning clinical manifestations of heart failure.

Calcium channel blockers may be used if beta blockers are contraindicated. Although they have fewer side effects than beta blockers, they are not as effective. Other effective medications to prevent migraine headaches include tricyclic or SSRI antidepressants, antiepileptic drugs, or riboflavin (vitamin B_2). The tricyclic drugs should not be used in older adults because they have a long half-life.

Studies are ongoing concerning the use of sustained-release niacin. Low plasma levels of serotonin have been implicated in migraine pathogenesis, and niacin may act as a negative feedback regulator on the kynurenine pathway to shunt tryptophan into the serotonin pathway, thus increasing plasma serotonin levels (Velling, Dodick, & Muir, 2003).

Table 45-1 lists commonly used medications for migraine headaches. This table is not inclusive; new medications are introduced on the market regularly.

Complementary and Alternative Therapies. Many clients seek complementary and alternative therapies as an adjunct to their medications because medications are

TABLE 45-1 Commonly Used Drugs for Migraine Headache

Nonsteroidal Anti-inflammatory Drugs (NSAIDs)
- Diclofenac
- Ibuprofen
- Naproxen
- Flurbiprofen

Beta Blockers
- Propranolol
- Timolol
- Metoprolol
- Nadolol
- Atenolol

Calcium Channel Blockers
- Verapamil
- Nifedipine
- Divalproex

Antidepressants
- Amitriptyline
- Doxepin
- Fluoxetine
- Imipramine
- Nortriptyline

Abortive Drugs

Analgesics
- Aspirin
- Acetaminophen

Ergotamine Preparations
- Ergotamine with caffeine (oral or suppository)
- Ergotamine metered dose inhaler (MDI) or sublingual (SL)
- Dihydroergotamine (DHE)

Triptan Preparations
- Almotriptan
- Eletriptan
- Frovatriptan
- Naratriptan
- Rizatriptan
- Zolmitriptan
- Sumatriptan tablets, injection, or nasal spray

Opioid Analgesic
- Butorphanol
- Hydromorphone

Investigational
- Cyproheptadine
- Droperidol

not completely effective. Some drugs do not offer any pain relief or are associated with unpleasant side effects. Yoga, meditation, message, exercise, biofeedback, and relaxation techniques are helpful for some clients. For example, at the beginning of a migraine attack, the client may be able to alleviate pain by lying down and darkening the room. The client may want both eyes covered and a cool cloth on the forehead. If the client falls asleep, he or she should remain undisturbed until awakening.

Several small studies have found acupuncture to be effective for migraine management for some participants (Melchart et al., 2003). The studies provide suggestive, but not convincing, evidence of the efficacy of acupuncture. Further research is needed to determine the role of acupuncture in migraine treatment

There is even less scientific evidence on the efficacy of herbs and other nutritional therapies in the treatment of headaches. However, a number of herbs are also used for headaches, both for prevention and pain management. Table 45-2 describes commonly used herbs for migraines. Some clients have found that eliminating tyramine-containing products, such as pickled products, caffeine, beer, wine, preservatives, and artificial sweeteners, reduce their headaches. All herbs and nutritional remedies should be approved by the client's health care provider before they are used.

Other clients have identified specific factors that trigger an attack (Chart 45-2). Remind clients to avoid these triggers to prevent migraine episodes.

Cluster Headache

PATHOPHYSIOLOGY

The **cluster headache,** also referred to as histamine cephalalgia, is less common than the migraine headache. It occurs six times more frequently in young adult men between 20 and 50 years of age than in women. The cause and mechanism of cluster headaches are not known, but have been attributed to vasoreactivity and oxyhemoglobin desaturation. Neuroimaging studies suggest that cluster headaches are related to hypothalamic hyperactivity. In a recent study, positron emission tomography (PET) scans and magnetic resonance imaging (MRI) demonstrated an increase in neuronal hypothalamic density and hypothalamic size in clients with cluster headaches (Franzini et al., 2003). There is no genetic or family link, diet has no effect, and the disorder is unrelated to personality type.

The pain of these unilateral (one-sided), oculotemporal, or oculofrontal headaches is often described as excruciating, boring, and nonthrobbing. The intense pain is felt deep in and around the eye. The headaches occur every 8 to 12 hours and up to 24 hours daily at the same time for about 6 to 8 weeks (hence the term *cluster*), followed by a period of remission for 9 months to a year. This episodic form is the most common, although there is a chronic form in which there may not be a remission for more than a year. The average duration of each headache is 10 to 45 minutes.

The pain may radiate to the forehead, temple, or cheek. It may also radiate, but to a lesser extent, to the ear, occiput, and neck. The temporal artery may be prominent and tender. Physical activity during the attack consists of pacing, walking, or sitting and rocking. A cluster is the only headache type in which this behavior occurs. During periods of remission, alcohol does not induce a headache (as it does during the headache period). The onset of the headache is associated with relaxation, napping, or rapid eye movement (REM) sleep.

The headache is usually accompanied by **ipsilateral** (same side) tearing of the eye, **rhinorrhea** ("runny nose") or congestion, **ptosis** (drooping eyelid), eyelid edema, facial sweating, and **miosis** (abnormal constriction of pupils). The ptosis may become permanent. There may be bradycardia, flushing or pallor of the face, increased intraocular pressure, and increased skin temperature.

◆COLLABORATIVE MANAGEMENT

Question the client about prescribed and nonprescribed drugs for both the prevention and the alleviation of the headache, as well as over-the-counter (OTC) drugs he or she may be taking. Interventions used by the client may include relaxation techniques, meditation, acupuncture, or massage therapies. Ask the client to recall a typical week's activities and any recent changes in lifestyle, and specifically to identify

TABLE 45-2 Commonly Used Herbs to Prevent Migraine Headaches

- Feverfew *(Tanacetum parthenium)*
- Bay *(Laurus nobilis)*
- Willow *(Salix)*
- Ginger *(Zingiber officinale)*
- Red pepper *(Capsicum)*
- Lemon balm *(Melissa officinalis)*
- Purslane *(Portulaca oleracea)*

CHART 45-2

CLIENT EDUCATION GUIDE

Factors That May Trigger a Migraine Attack

Teach clients to avoid the foods, medications, and other factors that may trigger a migraine attack.

Food and beverages (tyramine-containing):
- Alcoholic drinks: beer, wine, and hard liquor
- Aged cheese
- Caffeine found in beverages such as coffee, tea, cola
- Chocolate
- Foods with yeast such as pastry and fresh breads
- Monosodium glutamate (MSG)
- Nitrates (food preservatives), pickled or fermented foods
- Nuts
- Artificial sweeteners
- Smoked fish

Medications:
- Cimetidine (Tagamet)
- Estrogens
- Nitroglycerin
- Nifedipine (Procardia, Nifed✱)

Other factors:
- Anger, conflict
- Fatigue
- Hormonal fluctuations, such as menstruation, pregnancy, and menopause
- Light glare
- Missed meals
- Psychological stress
- Sleep problems
- Smells, such as tobacco smoke
- Travel to different altitudes

bedtimes and waking times, which helps assess changes in activity or lack of continuity in the sleep-wake cycle.

NONSURGICAL MANAGEMENT

Drug Therapy. The health care provider typically prescribes the same types of drugs used for migraines. Because an informed person is better able to comply with the therapeutic plan, instruct the client in all aspects of the drugs being taken.

Other Pain Relief Measures. During the periods of attack, teach the client to wear sunglasses and to sit facing away from the window, which helps decrease exposure to light and glare. If the health care provider prescribes oxygen, 100% oxygen via mask at 5 L/min is typically administered with the client in a sitting position. The oxygen is administered for no longer than 15 minutes and is discontinued when the headache is relieved. Oxygen reduces cerebral blood flow and inhibits activity of the carotid bodies, which are sensitive to oxygen levels in the body. To prevent future attacks brought on by precipitating factors (bursts of anger, prolonged anticipation, excessive physical activity, and excitement), discuss their relationship to the onset of cluster headaches. The necessity and importance of a consistent sleep-wake cycle should also be explained.

SURGICAL MANAGEMENT. Surgical intervention may be recommended for clients with chronic drug-resistant cluster headaches. Invasive procedures, such as radiofrequency rhizotomy and glycerol rhizolysis, have been performed with varying success rates. Findings from a small clinical trial found that long-term high frequency electrical stimulation of the posterior hypothalamus reduced or eliminated pain (Franzini et al., 2003).

Tension Headache

Tension headaches are characterized by neck and shoulder muscle tenderness and bilateral pain at the base of the skull and in the forehead. They share many of the characteristics, precipitating factors, and epidemiologic factors as migraine headaches, and distinguishing between the two is very difficult. The International Headache Society criteria define tension headaches as head pain without associated symptoms. However, the classic signs of nausea, vomiting and photophobia, phonophobia, and aggravation of the headache with activity that are part of the diagnostic criteria for migraine may also occur with a tension headache.

Treatment of tension headaches includes non-opioid analgesics, such as acetaminophen, aspirin, and nonsteroidal anti-inflammatory drugs [NSAIDs]). Muscle relaxants may be included in the treatment plan and occasionally opioids may be needed. A study by Sparano (2001) found that the combination of ibuprofen plus caffeine was more effective in relieving pain than NSAIDs alone. Prophylactic treatment is similar for migraine headaches.

SEIZURES AND EPILEPSY

PATHOPHYSIOLOGY

A **seizure** is an abnormal, sudden, excessive, uncontrolled electrical discharge of neurons within the brain that may result in alteration in consciousness, motor or sensory ability, and/or behavior. A single seizure may occur for no known reason. Seizures may be due to a pathologic condition of the brain, such as a tumor. In this case, once the underlying problem is treated, the client is often asymptomatic.

Epilepsy is a chronic disorder characterized by recurrent, unprovoked seizure activity. It may be caused by an abnormality in electrical neuronal activity, an imbalance of neurotransmitters, especially gamma aminobutyric acid (GABA), or a combination of both.

Types of Seizures

The International Classification of Epileptic Seizures recognizes three broad categories of seizure disorders: generalized seizures, partial seizures, and unclassified seizures (Table 45-3).

GENERALIZED SEIZURES

Six types of **generalized seizures** may occur and involve both cerebral hemispheres. The **tonic-clonic seizure** lasting 2 to 5 minutes begins with a tonic phase that is characterized by stiffening or rigidity of the muscles, particularly of the arms and legs, and immediate loss of consciousness. **Clonic** or rhythmic jerking of all extremities follows it. The client may bite his or her tongue and may become incontinent of urine or feces. Fatigue, confusion, and lethargy may last up to an hour after the seizure.

Occasionally, only tonic or clonic movement may occur. **Tonic seizures** are characterized by an abrupt increase in muscle tone, loss of consciousness, and loss of autonomic signs lasting from 30 seconds to several minutes. The **clonic seizure** lasts several minutes and is characterized by muscle contraction and relaxation.

The **absence seizure** is more common in children and tends to run in families. It consists of brief (often just seconds) periods of loss of consciousness and blank staring, as though the person is daydreaming. The client returns to baseline immediately after the seizure. Left undiagnosed or untreated, the seizures may occur frequently throughout the day, interfering with work or school.

The **myoclonic seizure** is characterized by a brief jerking or stiffening of the extremities, which may occur singly or in groups. Lasting for just a few seconds, the contractions may be symmetric or asymmetric.

The **atonic (akinetic) seizure** is characterized by a sudden loss of muscle tone, lasting for seconds, followed by **postictal** (after the seizure) confusion. In most cases, these seizures cause the client to fall, which may result in injury.

PARTIAL SEIZURES

Partial seizures, also called *focal* or *local* seizures, begin in a part of one cerebral hemisphere. They are further subdivided

TABLE 45-3 Classification of Epileptic Seizures

Generalized Seizures
- Absence (formerly petit mal)
- Generalized tonic-clonic (formerly grand mal)
- Myoclonic
- Atonic
- Clonic
- Tonic

Partial Seizures (Focal/Local Seizures)
- Simple partial
- Complex partial

Unclassified Seizures

into two main classes: complex partial seizures and simple partial seizures. In addition, some partial seizures can evolve into generalized tonic-clonic, tonic, or clonic seizures (also called "secondary generalization") (Pena, 2003). Partial seizures are most often seen in adults and generally are less responsive to medical treatment.

Complex partial seizures cause the client to lose consciousness, or "black out," for 1 to 3 minutes. Characteristic behavior known as **automatisms** (the client is not aware of the behavior) may occur, such as lip smacking, patting, picking at clothes, and so forth. In the period after the seizure, the client may experience amnesia. Because the area of the brain most often involved in this type of epilepsy is the temporal lobe, complex partial seizures are often called *psychomotor* seizures or *temporal lobe* seizures.

The client with a **simple partial seizure** remains conscious throughout the episode. He or she often reports an **aura** (unusual sensation) before the seizure takes place. This may consist of a "déjà vu" (already seen) phenomenon, perception of an offensive smell, or sudden onset of pain. During the seizure, the client may have unilateral movement of an extremity, experience unusual sensations, or have autonomic or psychic symptoms. Autonomic changes include a change in heart rate, skin flushing, and epigastric discomfort.

UNCLASSIFIED SEIZURES

Unclassified, or **idiopathic,** seizures account for about half of all seizure activity. They occur for no known reason and do not fit into the generalized or partial classifications.

Etiology and Genetic Risk

Primary or **idiopathic epilepsy** is not associated with any identifiable brain lesion. Secondary epilepsy results from an underlying brain lesion, most commonly a tumor or trauma. Seizures may also be caused by:

- Metabolic disorders
- Acute alcohol withdrawal
- Electrolyte disturbances (e.g., hyperkalemia, water intoxication, hypoglycemia)
- Heart disease.

Seizures resulting from these problems are not considered epilepsy. Certain risk factors can trigger a seizure, such as increased physical activity, emotional stress, excessive fatigue, alcohol or caffeine consumption, or certain foods or chemicals.

Several alterations in gene function that lead to seizures have been identified (Hickey, 2003):

- Defective genes for channels regulate neuronal signals or the flow of ions in and out of the cells.
- Clients with progressive myoclonus are missing the cystatin B protein.
- An abnormally active version of a gene that increases resistance to antiepileptic drugs has been identified in clients who are unable to obtain seizure control with varied and multiple drugs.
- An abnormal gene that controls neuronal migration can lead to areas of misplaced or abnormally formed neurons or dysplasia.

Incidence/Prevalence

It is estimated that 2 million people in the United States have epilepsy, 80% of whom are able to control their seizures with medications. Prevalence of epilepsy in the United States is 0.5% to 1% (Hickey, 2003).

HEALTH PROMOTION/ILLNESS PREVENTION

It is important for clients with epilepsy to take their medication as prescribed and to notify their health care provider if they are unable to take their medications. A balanced diet, proper rest, and stress reduction techniques usually minimize the risk of breakthrough seizures. Encourage the client to keep a seizure diary to determine whether there are factors that tend to be associated with seizure activity. Clients should follow state law concerning driving a motor vehicle. The client's employment may need to be modified within applicable state and federal regulations.

COLLABORATIVE MANAGEMENT

Assessment

A complete description of the type of seizure activity that occurs and events surrounding the seizure assists in determining the best treatment plan. Obtain information from the client and family or significant others regarding the presence of an aura before the seizure (**preictal phase**). Diagnosis is based on the history and physical examination. A variety of diagnostic tests are performed to rule out other causes of seizure activity and to confirm the diagnosis of epilepsy. Typical diagnostic tests include an electroencephalogram (EEG), computed tomography (CT) scan, MRI, or positron emission tomography (PET) scan. Laboratory studies are performed to identify metabolic or genetic disorders that may cause or contribute to seizure activity.

Common Nursing Diagnoses and Collaborative Problems

Nursing diagnoses that may apply to clients with epilepsy include the following:

- Risk for Falls related to impaired balance
- Ineffective Coping related to uncertainty and inadequate level of perception of control
- Risk for Ineffective Breathing Pattern related to neuromuscular dysfunction
- Potential for Status Epilepticus

Interventions

Removing or treating the underlying condition or cause of the seizure manages secondary epilepsy and seizures that are not considered epileptic. In most cases, primary epilepsy is managed through drug therapy.

NONSURGICAL MANAGEMENT. Most seizures can be completely or almost completely controlled through the administration of **antiepileptic drugs (AEDs),** sometimes referred to as anticonvulsants, for specific types of seizures.

Drug Therapy. Drug therapy is the major component of management (Chart 45-3). The health care provider introduces one drug at a time to achieve seizure control. If the chosen drug is not effective, the dosage may be increased or another drug introduced. At times, seizure control is achieved only through a combination of medications. The dosage of medications is adjusted to achieve therapeutic blood levels without causing major side effects.

Before administering an AED, the client's laboratory values are evaluated for the most current blood level of the medication, if appropriate. Be aware of drug-drug and drug-food

CHART 45-3

DRUG THERAPY for Commonly Used Antiepileptic Drugs

Drug	Indication for Use	Nursing Interventions
Carbamazepine (Tegretol, Tegretol-XR, Carbatrol)	Partial, generalized tonic-clonic seizures	Monitor for headache, dizziness, diplopia or blurred vision, N/V, and leukopenia. Monitor CBC. Do not crush or chew sustained-release capsules.
Clonazepam (Klonopin)	Absence, myoclonic, and akinetic seizures	Monitor results of liver function tests.
Clorazepate dipotassium	Adjunctive management of partial seizures	Give with food; monitor blood pressure.
Diazepam (Valium, Apo-Diazepam ✱), lorazepam (Ativan), Diastat (Valium rectal gel delivery system)	Status epilepticus	Monitor airway, breathing, circulation (ABCs).
Divalproex (Depakote), valproic acid (Depakene)	All types of seizures	Monitor for hair loss, tremor, increased liver enzymes, bruising, and N/V. Monitor CBC, PT, PTT, and AST.
Ethosuximide (Zarontin)	Absence seizures	Watch for N/V, skin rash, lethargy, and anorexia. Monitor CBC and liver function tests. (Drug used infrequently.)
Felbamate (Felbatol)	Adjunctive therapy for intractable complex partial seizures	Note that aplastic anemia and liver failure are major sequelae of treatment. Client must sign consent for use, acknowledging risk for aplastic anemia and liver failure. Monitor CBC. Monitor liver function tests. Watch for anorexia and weight loss.
Gabapentin (Neurontin)	Partial seizures	Watch for increased appetite and weight gain. Monitor for ataxia, irritability, dizziness, and fatigue.
Lamotrigine (Lamictal)	Partial seizures	Watch for diplopia, headaches, dizziness, drowsiness, ataxia, N/V, and life-threatening rash when given with valproic acid.
Levetiracetam (Keppra)	Adjunct management of partial seizures	Monitor renal function carefully. Notify health care provider for gait or coordination problems.
Oxcarbazepine (Trileptal)	Partial seizures	Monitor for hyponatremia.
Phenobarbital (Barbita, Luminal)	Generalized tonic-clonic seizures, partial seizures	Note that this is less desirable than other antiepileptic drugs (AEDs) because of sedation. Be aware that overdose can be fatal. Monitor for drowsiness, sleep disturbances, cognitive impairment, and depression.
Phenytoin (Dilantin), fosphenytoin (Cerebyx)	All types, except absence, myoclonic, and atonic seizures; for status epilepticus	Monitor for gastric distress, gingival hyperplasia, anemia, ataxia, and nystagmus. Check CBC and calcium levels. For IV phenytoin, flush catheter with saline before and after administration. For fosphenytoin, use phenytoin equivalent for dosing.
Primidone (Mysoline, Sertan ✱)	Partial seizures, generalized tonic-clonic seizures	Monitor for vertigo and lethargy. Watch for drug interactions with phenobarbital and isoniazid.
Tiagabine (Gabitril)	Partial seizures	Monitor for dizziness, weakness, nervousness, psychomotor slowing, nystagmus, and paresthesias. Administer with food.
Topiramate (Topamax)	Adjunctive therapy for intractable partial seizures	Monitor for ataxia, confusion, dizziness, and fatigue. Be aware of increased risk for renal calculi.
Valproate (Depakote), valproate sodium injection (Depacon)	Simple and complex absence seizures Adjunct therapy for partial complex and generalized tonic-clonic seizures	Monitor for hair loss, tremor, increased liver enzymes, bruising, and N/V. Monitor CBC, PT, PTT, AST.
Zonisamide (Zonegran)	Adjunctive therapy for partial seizures	Monitor CBC, platelets, and renal function. Assess mental status, especially memory.

***Med Error Alert!** Do not confuse Keppra with Kaletra, an antiretroviral drug used to treat HIV.*

N/V, Nausea and vomiting; *CBC*, complete blood count; *PT*, prothrombin time; *PTT*, partial thromboplastin time; *AST*, aspartate aminotransferase.

CHART 45-4

CLIENT EDUCATION GUIDE
Instructions for the Client with Epilepsy

- Avoid alcohol consumption and excessive fatigue.
- Do not take any medication, including over-the-counter drugs, without asking your health care provider.
- Wear a medical alert bracelet or necklace or carry ID indicating epilepsy.
- Contact the Epilepsy Foundation of America or other organized epilepsy group.
- Investigate your local state laws covering driving and operating machinery.
- Medication information:
  - Name, dosage, time of administration
  - Actions to take if side effects occur
  - Importance of taking as prescribed and not missing a dose
  - What to do if a medication is missed or cannot be taken
  - Importance of having blood drawn for therapeutic levels
- Instruct family member or significant other on care of client during and after a seizure, including when to call health care provider or emergency medical services (911).

CHART 45-5

BEST PRACTICE for
Care of the Client During a Tonic-Clonic or Complete Partial Seizure

- Protect the client from injury.
- Do not force anything into the client's mouth.
- Turn the client to the side.
- Loosen any restrictive clothing the client is wearing.
- Maintain the client's airway and suction as needed.
- Do not restrain the client; guide the client's movements if necessary.
- At the completion of the seizure:
  - Take the client's vital signs.
  - Perform neurologic checks.
  - Keep the client on his or her side.
  - Allow the client to rest.
  - Document the seizure (see Chart 45-6).

interactions. Medications need to be taken on time to maintain therapeutic blood levels and maximal effectiveness. Instruct the client to avoid drugs and foods that might interfere with the absorption or metabolism of the AED. For instance, warfarin (Coumadin, Warfilone✱) should not be given with phenytoin (Dilantin). Document side and adverse effects of the prescribed medications and report to the health care provider.

Client and Family Education. An educational program must be provided for the client and family (Chart 45-4). Ask them what they understand about the disorder and correct any misinformation. As new information is presented, be sure that the client and family are able to understand it.

Emphasize that antiepileptic drugs (AEDs) must not be stopped even if the seizures have stopped. Discontinuing AEDs can lead to the recurrence of seizures or the life-threatening complication of status epilepticus (discussed later). Some clients may stop taking their medications simply because they do not have the money to purchase them. Refer limited-income clients to the social services department for financial assistance or to a case manager to locate other resources.

All states prohibit discrimination against people who have epilepsy. Clients who work in occupations in which a seizure might cause serious harm to themselves or others (e.g., construction workers, operators of dangerous equipment, pilots, railroad engineers) may need to find alternative employment. They may need to curtail or modify strenuous or potentially dangerous physical activity to avoid harm, although this varies with the individual. Various local state and federal agencies can help with finances, living arrangements, and vocational rehabilitation.

Seizure Precautions. Precautions are taken to prevent the client from injury if a seizure occurs. **Seizure precautions** vary, depending on health care agency policy. In most agencies it is recommended that oxygen and suctioning equipment with an airway be readily available. It is also appropriate to insert a saline lock in hospitalized clients who do not have an IV access and are at significant risk for generalized tonic-clonic seizures. The saline lock provides ready access if IV medication must be given to stop the seizure.

Although side rails are rarely the source of significant injury, they should be in the "up" position at all times. The use of padded side rails is controversial as to whether they maintain safety. Padded side rails may embarrass the client and the family. Keep the bed in the lowest position in case the client falls out of bed.

Padded tongue blades do not belong at the bedside and should never be inserted into the client's mouth after a seizure begins, because the jaw may clench down as soon as the seizure begins! Forcing a tongue blade or airway into the mouth is more likely to chip the teeth and increase the risk of aspiration of tooth fragments than it is to prevent the client from biting the tongue. Furthermore, improper placement of a padded tongue blade can obstruct the airway.

Seizure Management. The actions taken during a seizure should be appropriate for the type of seizure (Chart 45-5). For example, for a simple partial seizure, observe the client and document the time that the seizure lasted. Direct the client engaged in activities away from the activity to prevent injury. Turn the client on the side during a generalized tonic-clonic or complex partial seizure because he or she may lose consciousness. If possible, turn the client's head to the side to prevent aspiration and allow secretions to drain. Remove any objects that might injure the client.

It is not unusual for the client to become cyanotic during a generalized tonic-clonic seizure. The cyanosis is generally self-limiting, and no treatment is needed. Some health care providers prefer to give the high-risk client (e.g., older adult; critically ill or debilitated client) oxygen by nasal cannula or face mask during the postictal phase. He or she is not restrained, because this may cause injury and may exacerbate the situation, causing more seizure activity. However, the client with atonic seizures may benefit from wearing a protective vest to keep from falling when sitting in a chair. Follow institutional policy and procedures for use of a protective vest. For any type of seizure, careful observation of the seizure and documentation of assessment findings must be done (Chart 45-6).

Emergency Care: Acute Seizure and Status Epilepticus Management. Seizures occurring in greater intensity, number, or length than the client's usual seizures are considered **acute.** They may also appear in clusters that are different from the client's typical seizure pattern. Treatment with lorazepam (Ativan, Apo-Lorazepam✱) or diazepam (Valium, Meval✱, Vivol✱, Diastat [rectal diazepam

CHART 45-6

FOCUSED ASSESSMENT of
Seizures: Nursing Observations and Documentation

How often the seizures occur
- Date, time, and duration of the seizure

Description of each seizure
- Tonic, clonic
- Staring spells, blinking
- Automatism

Whether more than one type of seizure occurs
Sequence of seizure progression
- Where the seizure began
- Body part first involved

Observations during the seizure
- Changes in pupil size and any eye deviation
- Level of consciousness
- Presence of apnea, cyanosis, and salivation
- Incontinence of bowel or bladder during the seizure
- Eye fluttering
- Movement and progression of motor activity
- Lip smacking or other automatism
- Tongue or lip biting

How long the seizures last
When the last seizure took place
Whether the seizures are preceded by an aura
- Dizziness, numbness, or visual disturbances
- Gustatory (taste) or auditory disturbances

What the client does after the seizure
- Feels drowsy or weak
- May resume normal behavior
- May be unaware that the seizure took place

How long it takes for the client to return to preseizure status

gel]) may be given to stop the clusters to prevent the development of status epilepticus. Phenytoin or fosphenytoin may be added (Gambrell & Flynn, 2004).

Status epilepticus is characterized by prolonged seizures lasting more than 5 minutes or repeated seizures over the course of 30 minutes. It is a potential complication of all types of seizures. The usual causes of status epilepticus include the following:

- Sudden withdrawal from antiepileptic drugs
- Infections
- Acute alcohol withdrawal
- Head trauma
- Cerebral edema
- Metabolic disturbances

Convulsive status epilepticus is a neurologic emergency and must be treated promptly and aggressively! Notify the health care provider immediately if this problem occurs, and establish an airway. (Intubation by an anesthesiologist, nurse anesthetist, or respiratory therapist may be necessary.) Administer oxygen as indicated by the client's condition. If not already in place, establish IV access with a large-bore catheter, and start 0.9% sodium chloride (Chart 45-7). The client is usually placed in the intensive care unit for continuous monitoring and management for several days.

Blood is drawn to determine arterial blood gases and to identify metabolic, toxic and other causes of the uncontrolled seizure. Brain damage and death may occur in the client with tonic-clonic status epilepticus. Left untreated, metabolic changes occur, leading to hypoxia, hypotension, hypoglycemia, cardiac dysrhythmias, or lactic acidosis. Further harm to the client occurs when muscle breaks down and myoglobin accumulates in the kidneys, which can lead to renal failure and electrolyte imbalance.

CHART 45-7

BEST PRACTICE for
Emergency Care for the Client in Status Epilepticus

EMERGENCY CARE

- Support the ABCs (*a*irway, *b*reathing, and *c*irculation).
- Prepare for possible intubation.
- Protect the client from injury.
- Do not force an airway into the client's mouth; provide oxygen via nasal cannula or face mask.
- Establish IV access if not already available, and begin infusion of 0.9% saline.
- Administer drugs as prescribed, and observe the client for side effects or signs of toxicity from the medications.
- Monitor vital signs and cardiac rhythm.

Medications used to treat status epilepticus include IV diazepam (Valium, Meval✱, Vivol✱), IV lorazepam (Ativan, Apo-Lorazepam✱), or diazepam rectal gel (Diastat), to stop motor movement. Lorazepam is typically the drug of choice and is given 2 to 4 mg over a 2-minute period. This procedure may be repeated, if necessary, until a total of 8 mg is reached. To prevent recurrence or arrest tonic-clonic seizures, a loading dose of phenytoin (Dilantin) or fosphenytoin (Cerebyx) is prescribed.

Initially, phenytoin is administered at no more than 50 mg/min using an infusion pump. Additional doses of 100 mg/min may be necessary. An alternative to phenytoin is fosphenytoin, a water-soluble phenytoin prodrug. Fosphenytoin can be administered IM as well as IV, and is compatible with most IV solutions. It also causes less cardiovascular complications than phenytoin and can be given in an IV dextrose solution (Pena, 2003). After administration, fosphenytoin converts to phenytoin in the body. Therefore the Food and Drug Administration (FDA) requires the dosage to be written as a phenytoin equivalent (PE); 150 mg of fosphenytoin equals 100 mg of phenytoin. Fosphenytoin may be administered at a rate of 100 to 150 mg/min IV piggyback (Pena, 2003).

Serum drug levels should be checked every 6 to 12 hours after the loading dose and then 2 weeks after oral phenytoin has started. Fosphenytoin is not available in an oral form. Teach the client about the side and adverse effects of any AED that is prescribed (see Chart 45-3).

General anesthesia may be used as a treatment of last resort to stop the seizure activity. The nurse, physician, or clinical pharmacist monitors serum drug levels closely for the first 3 days after the start of the AED and thereafter as indicated.

SURGICAL MANAGEMENT. Clients whose case cannot be managed effectively with medication may be candidates for surgery, including vagal nerve stimulation (VNS) and conventional surgical procedures. VNS is a fairly new procedure that has been very successful for many clients with epilepsy.

Vagal Nerve Stimulation. Vagal nerve stimulation (VNS) is performed for control of medically intractable simple or complex partial seizures with or without secondary generalization. Clients with multifocal or bihemisphere seizure foci, who are not candidates for surgical excision (because this may result in severe neurologic deficits), and those in whom other, less invasive treatment options are not effective may also qualify for the use of VNS. The stimulating device is surgically implanted in the left chest wall. An electrode lead is attached to the left vagus nerve, tunneled under the skin, and connected to a generator. The procedure usually takes 2 hours with the client under general anesthesia. The stimulator is activated by the physician to deliver intermittent VNS. Programming is adjusted gradually over a period of time. The pattern of stimulation is individualized to the client's tolerance. A typical amount of stimulation is 30 seconds on and five minutes off, although these time frames vary among clients.

The client can activate the VNS with a handheld magnet when experiencing an aura, thus aborting the seizure. Clients experience a change in voice quality, which signifies that the vagus nerve has been stimulated. They report a relief in intensity and duration of seizures and an improved quality of life. However, the exact mechanism for how VNS works continues to be studied.

Conventional Surgical Procedures. A small percentage of clients with epilepsy cannot be fully controlled with medications or VNS. When all other medication and treatment options are exhausted, conventional surgery may be indicated to improve the quality of life.

The largest group of surgical candidates includes clients with complex partial seizures of temporal lobe origin. Partial seizures of frontal origin and from other extratemporal sites may also be treated surgically when the clinical manifestations and diagnostic studies indicate an epileptic region in a resectable area.

Preoperative care is similar to that described for clients undergoing a craniotomy (see Chapter 48). Preoperative diagnostic tests include magnetic resonance imaging (MRI) and single-photon emission computed tomography (SPECT)/positron emission tomography (PET) scans as described in Chapter 44. An intracarotid amobarbital test (Wada test) and neuropsychological testing are also done. The Wada test assesses hemispheric lateralization of language and memory after intracarotid injection of amobarbital, a short-acting anesthetic. This procedure establishes the safety of surgery in terms of language preservation and memory. Neuropsychological testing evaluates memory, visuospatial function, language function, and intelligence quotient to identify deficiencies in a restricted brain region that might correspond to areas believed to be the epileptogenic region. It is also used to compare preoperative and postoperative cognitive functioning.

Clients with seizures that do not respond to medication may benefit from surgical excision of the seizure area of the brain. The procedure involves continuous electroencephalogram (EEG) recording, close observation, and in many hospitals, video monitoring of the client at all times except during personal care activities. After the seizure area is identified, electrodes are surgically implanted into the brain tissue to identify the extent of the focal area. This step is followed by additional continuous EEG and video monitoring at all times (except during personal care), as well as close observation by the nursing staff. The area is excised if it can be safely removed without affecting vital areas of brain function.

Anterior temporal lobe resection is the safest and most effective procedure for complex partial seizures of temporal origin. Multiple suboccipital transections done over all areas of seizure foci, as well as over other stereotactic volumetric radiofrequency lesions of the intracranial structures, may be performed.

The more traditional surgical approach, the **corpuscallostomy,** is used to treat tonic-clonic or atonic seizures in clients who are not candidates for other surgical procedures. The surgeon sections the anterior two thirds of the corpus callosum, preventing neuronal discharges from passing between the two hemispheres of the brain. This surgery usually reduces the number and severity of the seizures, making them more amenable to more conventional drug therapy.

INFECTIONS

Meningitis

PATHOPHYSIOLOGY

Meningitis is an inflammation of the arachnoid and pia mater of the brain and spinal cord and the cerebrospinal fluid (CSF). Bacterial and viral organisms are most often responsible for meningitis, although fungal meningitis and protozoal meningitis also occur. Bacterial meningitis occurs most frequently; early detection and treatment are associated with a more favorable outcome. Viral meningitis is usually self-limiting, and the client has a complete recovery. It is not considered as serious or potentially life threatening. Regardless of the causative organism, symptoms are the same.

The organisms responsible for meningitis enter the central nervous system (CNS) via the bloodstream at the blood-brain barrier. Direct routes of entry occur as a result of penetrating trauma, surgical procedures, or a ruptured cerebral abscess. **Otorrhea** (ear discharge) or **rhinorrhea** (nasal discharge, or "runny nose"), which may be caused by a basilar skull fracture, may lead to meningitis as a result of the direct communication of CSF with the environment. The invading organisms migrate throughout the CNS via the subarachnoid space. The presence of the organism in the subarachnoid space produces an inflammatory response in the pia mater, the arachnoid, the CSF, and the ventricles. The exudate formed may spread to both cranial and spinal nerves, causing further neurologic deterioration.

Viral Meningitis

Viral meningitis, the most common type, is sometimes referred to as **aseptic meningitis**. It often occurs as a sequela to a variety of viral illnesses, including measles, mumps, herpes simplex, and herpes zoster. The formation of exudate that is common in bacterial meningitis does not occur, and no organisms are obtained from the CSF. Inflammation occurs over the cerebral cortex, the white matter, and the meninges. The susceptibility of the brain tissue to the virus varies, depending on which type of cell is involved. The herpes simplex virus alters cellular metabolism, which quickly results in necrosis of the cells. The coxsackievirus and echovirus families also may cause viral meningitis. Other viruses cause an alteration in the production of enzymes or neurotransmitters, which results in dysfunction of the cells and possible neurologic defects.

Clinical manifestations of viral meningitis include fever, photophobia, headache, myalgias, and nausea. Herpes simplex type 2 may cause genital lesions. A maculopapular rash is seen when the causative organism is an enterovirus.

Treatment is symptomatic. If genital lesions are also present, acyclovir may be prescribed.

Fungal Meningitis

Cryptococcus neoformans meningitis is the most commonly seen fungal infection that affects the CNS of clients with acquired immunodeficiency syndrome (AIDS). Fulminant invasive

TABLE 45-4 Common Bacteria That Cause Meningitis

- *Neisseria meningitidis* (meningococcal)
- *Diplococcus pneumoniae* (pneumococcal)
- Streptococci, group A
- *Staphylococcus aureus*
- *Escherichia coli*
- *Klebsiella*
- *Proteus*
- *Pseudomonas*
- *Listeria monocytogenes*
- *Haemophilus influenzae* (not as common due to immunization)

fungal sinusitis is also a recognized cause of fungal meningitis. The clinical manifestations vary because the compromised immune system affects the inflammatory response. For example, some clients have fever and others do not. Almost all clients have headache, nausea, and vomiting and show a decline in mental status. Treatment is symptomatic and includes IV antifungal agents.

Bacterial Meningitis

Bacterial meningitis is a *medical emergency* with a mortality rate of about 25%. It is seen most often in fall and winter when upper respiratory tract infections commonly occur. The most frequently involved organisms responsible for bacterial meningitis include *Streptococcus pneumoniae* (pneumococcal disease), and *Neisseria meningitidis* (Table 45-4). An estimated 17,500 cases of acute bacterial meningitis occur in the United States each year.

Meningococcal meningitis is the only type of bacterial meningitis that occurs in outbreaks, and it is most likely to occur in areas of high population density, such as college dormitories, military barracks, crowded living areas, and prisons. The number of outbreaks on college campuses has been decreasing over the past few years because many states require students to be vaccinated against meningitis. A meningitis polysaccharide vaccine (Menomune) is available to prevent infection by certain groups of meningococcal bacteria.

Most often, the client has a predisposing condition, such as otitis media, pneumonia, acute sinusitis, or sickle cell anemia that increases the likelihood of meningitis. A fractured skull or brain, or spinal surgery may also contribute to the development of meningitis. Vulnerable populations include clients who are immunosuppressed, have immunocompromised disorders, or have infections elsewhere in the body, and older adults, especially those with chronic debilitating diseases

◆COLLABORATIVE MANAGEMENT

◆Assessment

A complete neurologic and neurovascular assessment is done to detect clinical manifestations associated with a diagnosis of meningitis or suspected meningitis as outlined in Chart 45-8.

PHYSICAL ASSESSMENT/CLINICAL MANIFESTATIONS

Presenting signs and symptoms of meningitis result from meningeal irritation and include headache, nausea, vomiting, and fever. The client may also complain of photophobia and have indications of increased intracranial pressure.

CHART 45-8

KEY FEATURES of Meningitis

Decreased (or change in) level of consciousness
Disoriented to person, place, and year
Pupil reaction and eye movements
- Photophobia
- Nystagmus
- Abnormal eye movements

Motor response
- Normal early in disease process
- Hemiparesis, hemiplegia, and decreased muscle tone possible later
- Cranial nerve dysfunction, especially CN III, IV, VI, VII, VIII

Memory changes
- Attention span (usually short)
- Personality and behavior changes
- Bewilderment

Severe, unrelenting headaches
Generalized muscle aches and pain
Nausea and vomiting
Fever and chills
Tachycardia
Red macular rash (meningococcal meningitis)

Although nuchal rigidity (stiff neck) and positive Kernig's and Brudzinski's signs may be positive, newer research indicates that these sign are present in only 9% of client's with a definitive diagnosis of meningitis. Seizure, decreased mental status, or focal neurologic deficits may also occur, particularly in bacterial meningitis.

Assess the client for complications that may occur, including increased intracranial pressure (ICP) resulting from the presence of exudate, which can lead to hydrocephalus and cerebral edema. Left untreated, increased ICP can lead to herniation of the brain and death (see Chapter 48).

Seizure activity may be caused by irritation of the cerebral cortex. Because of abnormal stimulation of the hypothalamic area, excessive amounts of antidiuretic hormone (ADH) (vasopressin) are produced. This results in water retention and dilution of serum sodium attributable to increased excretion of sodium by the kidneys. This syndrome of inappropriate antidiuretic hormone (SIADH) production may lead to further increases in ICP (see Chapter 48).

The client's vascular status is assessed by:
- Observing the color and temperature of the extremities
- Determining the presence of peripheral pulses
- Identifying any indicators of abnormal bleeding

Septic emboli in the blood may block circulation in the small vessels of the hands and feet, leading to gangrene. Excessive fibrinolysis that occurs in bacteremia and infections from viruses, fungi, or protozoa may lead to disseminated intravascular coagulation (DIC). Vascular involvement of the cerebral arteries, veins, and venous sinuses may lead to seizures and hemiparesis.

LABORATORY ASSESSMENT

The most significant laboratory test used in the diagnosis of meningitis is the analysis of the cerebrospinal fluid (CSF). Clients older than 60 years of age, those who are immunocompromised, or those who have signs of increased ICP usually have a CT scan preformed before the lumbar puncture. If there will be a delay in obtaining the CSF, blood is drawn for culture and sensitivity and a broad-spectrum an-

TABLE 45-5 Cerebrospinal Fluid Findings in Bacterial and Viral Meningitis

Finding	Bacterial Meningitis	Viral Meningitis
Appearance	Cloudy, turbid	Clear
White blood cells	Increased	Increased
Protein	Increased	Increased, slightly elevated
Glucose	Decreased	Normal
CSF pressure	Elevated	Varies

tibiotic should be given before the lumbar puncture. The CSF is analyzed for cell count, differential count, and protein. Glucose concentrations are determined, and culture, sensitivity, and Gram stain studies are performed.

Counterimmunoelectrophoresis (CIE) may be performed to determine the presence of viruses or protozoa in the CSF. CIE is also indicated if the client has received antibiotics before the CSF was obtained. To identify a possible bacterial source of infection, specimens for culture are obtained and Gram stains of the blood, urine, throat, and nose are performed. Table 45-5 compares CSF findings in bacterial meningitis and in viral meningitis.

Polymerase chain reaction (PCR) may be used to detect viral deoxyribonucleic acid (DNA) or ribonucleic acid (RNA) in the CSF. Specificity and sensitivity in diagnosing encephalitis are excellent, especially with herpes simplex virus (HSV). The test is rapid and noninvasive, replacing the brain biopsy for diagnosis.

A complete blood count (CBC) is performed, with attention to the white blood cell (WBC) count, which is generally elevated well above the normal value. Serum electrolyte values are also assessed with attention to the sodium value. Dilutional hyponatremia may occur secondary to syndrome of inappropriate antidiuretic hormone (SIADH), a complication of bacterial meningitis. A blood culture is always performed.

OTHER DIAGNOSTIC ASSESSMENTS

X-rays of the chest, air sinuses, and mastoids are obtained to determine the presence of infection. A computed tomography (CT) or magnetic resonance imaging (MRI) scan may be performed to identify increased ICP, the presence of a brain abscess, or developing hydrocephalus.

Interventions

The most important nursing intervention for clients with meningitis is the accurate monitoring and recording of their neurologic status, vital signs, and vascular assessment. Other areas of nursing care are found in Chart 45-9.

Monitoring Neurologic Status. The client's neurologic status and vital signs are assessed at least every 4 hours or more often if clinically indicated. Assess for neurologic changes indicative of cerebral complications, especially increased ICP. The health care team provides interventions for the client with increased ICP as discussed in Chapter 48. The client is at risk for seizure activity, and care should be provided as discussed under Interventions (Seizures and Epilepsy), p. 951.

Complete cranial nerve testing is included as part of the routine neurologic assessment because of possible cranial

CHART 45-9

BEST PRACTICE for
Care of the Client with Meningitis

- Follow ABCs (airway, breathing, circulation).
- Take vital signs and perform neurologic checks every 2 to 4 hours, as required.
- Perform cranial nerve assessment, with particular attention to cranial nerves III, IV, VI, VII, and VIII, and monitor for changes.
- Manage pain through drug and nondrug methods.
- Perform vascular assessment and monitor for changes.
- Give medications and IV fluids as prescribed, and document the client's response.
- Record intake and output.
- Decrease environmental stimuli.
  - Provide a quiet environment.
  - Minimize exposure to bright lights from windows and overhead lights.
  - Maintain bedrest with head of bed elevated 30 degrees.
- Maintain isolation precautions per hospital policy (for meningococcal meningitis).
- Monitor for and prevent complications.
  - Increased intracranial pressure
  - Vascular dysfunction
  - Fluid and electrolyte imbalance
  - Seizures
  - Shock

TABLE 45-6 Anti-Infective Therapy for Meningitis

Causative Organism	Anti-Infective Agent
Staphylococcus	Vancomycin Ceftazidime
Haemophilus influenzae	Cefotaxime Ceftriaxone
Streptococcus	Third-generation cephalosporins (ceftriaxone) Rifampin Vancomycin
Neisseria meningitidis	Third-generation cephalosporins (ceftriaxone) Other cephalosporins
Fungus	Amphotericin B Flucytosine Fluconazole

nerve involvement. Particular attention is given to cranial nerves III, IV, VI, VII, and VIII (see Chapter 44). A sixth cranial nerve defect (inability to move the eyes laterally) may indicate the development of hydrocephalus. Other indicators of hydrocephalus include the usual signs of increased ICP and the presence of urinary incontinence in the previously continent client. Urinary incontinence occurs secondary to the decreasing level of consciousness (LOC).

Drug Therapy. To avoid life-threatening complications, the health care provider prescribes a broad-spectrum antibiotic until the results of the culture and Gram stain are available. After this information is available, the appropriate medication to treat the specific type of meningitis is given. Table 45-6 lists some of anti-infective medications commonly used. The medication should begin within 1 to 2 hours after it is prescribed. The client's response to the medication is monitored and documented.

The client with bacterial meningitis may experience increased ICP, and seizure activity may occur. Medications used by the physician to treat these complications include hyperosmolar agents and anticonvulsants. Controversy exists as to whether steroids have any place in the treatment of adults with meningitis. It is, however, recommended for clients with S. pneumoniae (de Gans & van de Beek, 2002). People who have been in close contact with a client with *N. meningitides* have prophylaxis treatment with rifampin, ciprofloxacin, or ceftriaxone. Prophylaxis treatment with rifampin may be prescribed for those in close contact with a client with *H. influenzae* meningitis.

Monitoring for Complications. A complete vascular assessment during each nursing shift or more often, if indicated, is performed to prevent and detect early vascular compromise from septic emboli. This severe complication is most often seen in circulation to the hand. Assess the client's temperature, color, pulses, and capillary refill. If vascular compromise is left unrecognized and untreated, gangrene can develop quickly, possibly leading to loss of the involved extremity. The health care team monitors the client for other complications, including shock, coagulation disorders, septic complications (bacterial endocarditis), and prolonged fever.

Encephalitis

PATHOPHYSIOLOGY

Encephalitis is an inflammation of the brain parenchyma (brain tissue) and often the meninges. It affects the cerebrum, the brainstem, and the cerebellum. The incidence of encephalitis is 1 in 200,000 people (Hickey, 2003). A viral agent most often causes it, although bacteria, fungi, or parasites may also be involved (e.g., malaria). Viral encephalitis is almost always preceded by a viral infection. The virus gains access to the central nervous system (CNS) via the bloodstream, along peripheral or cranial nerves, or in the meninges (e.g., varicella zoster).

After the virus invades the brain tissue, it begins to reproduce, causing an inflammatory response. Unlike in meningitis, this response does not cause exudate formation. Inflammation extends over the cerebral cortex, the white matter, and the meninges, causing degeneration of the neurons of the cortex. Demyelination of axons occurs in the involved area because the white matter is destroyed. This leads to hemorrhage, edema, necrosis, and the development of small lacunae (hollow cavities) within the cerebral hemispheres. Widespread edema can cause compression of blood vessels, leading to a further increase in intracranial pressure (ICP). Death may occur from herniation and increased ICP.

Arboviruses

Arboviruses can be transmitted to humans through the bite of an infected mosquito or tick. The most common types of encephalitis caused by arboviruses are eastern or western equine encephalitis, St. Louis encephalitis, California encephalitis, and West Nile virus.

West Nile virus has gained attention in the United States because it has spread rapidly throughout the country. This infection is generally mild and usually the client is asymptomatic. The incubation period is 3 to 12 days after being bitten by an infected mosquito. Other sources of transmission include blood products, breast milk, or an organ transplant. In most cases the client is asymptomatic or has flu-like symptoms. Diagnostic tests to determine the presence of West Nile virus include enzyme-linked immunosorbent assay and West Nile virus–specific IgM antibody in serum or cerebrospinal fluid (CSF).

CONSIDERATIONS FOR OLDER ADULTS

Older adults are more likely to have severe infections that can result in long-term residual fatigue and weakness, as well as death. Teach older adults to avoid areas where mosquitoes or ticks are likely to be, such as near rivers and lakes. When they are near these areas, instruct the older adults to wear long-sleeved shirts and long pants and to use insect repellent.

Enteroviruses

Echovirus, coxsackievirus, poliovirus, herpes zoster, and viruses that cause mumps and chickenpox are the common enteroviruses associated with encephalitis.

Herpes Simplex Virus Type 1

Herpes simplex virus type 1 (HSV1) encephalitis is the most common nonepidemic type of encephalitis in North America. Clients with herpes encephalitis often have a history of cold sores. Mortality rates for HSV1 encephalitis can be as high as 80%, whereas mortality for the other types is much lower (Hickey, 2003).

Amebae

Amebic meningoencephalitis is caused by the amebae *Naegleria* and *Acanthamoeba.* Both are found in warm freshwater areas and can enter the nasal mucosa of people swimming in ponds or lakes. The amebae may also be found in soil and decaying vegetation. Although this infection has not often been seen in the past, the incidence in North America is increasing, perhaps because the ponds and lakes are becoming more polluted.

COLLABORATIVE MANAGEMENT

Assessment

The typical client with encephalitis has a fever and complains of nausea, vomiting, and a stiff neck. Other signs and symptoms include the following:

- Changes in the level of consciousness (LOC) and mental status
- Motor dysfunction
- Focal neurologic deficits
- Fatigue
- Symptoms of increased intracranial pressure (ICP)

Assess the client's LOC using the Glasgow Coma Scale (see Chapter 44). The client may be lethargic, stuporous, or comatose. Mental status changes include acute confusion, irritability, and personality and behavior changes (especially noted in the presence of herpes simplex). Signs of meningeal irritation include the presence of nuchal rigidity, and motor changes may vary from a mild weakness to hemiplegia. The client may have muscle tremors, spasticity, an ataxic gait (postencephalitic parkinsonism), myoclonic jerks, and increased deep tendon reflexes. Seizure activity is not uncommon. Fever, nausea, vomiting, headache, and vertigo may also occur.

Cranial nerve involvement is exhibited by ocular palsies, facial weakness, and nystagmus. The herpes zoster lesion affects cranial and spinal nerve root ganglia, which is clinically manifested by a rash, severe pain, itching, burning, or tingling in the areas innervated by these nerves.

In severe cases of encephalitis, the client may exhibit increased ICP resulting from cerebral edema, hemorrhage, and necrosis of brain tissue. Monitor vital signs for indications of a widened pulse pressure, bradycardia, and irregular respirations. The pupils become increasingly dilated and less responsive to light. Left untreated, increased ICP leads to herniation of the brain tissue and possibly death.

Interventions

Nursing interventions for encephalitis are similar to those for meningitis, with the exception of drug therapy. Supportive nursing care and prompt recognition and treatment of increased ICP are essential components of management. A patent airway is maintained to prevent the development of atelectasis or pneumonia, which can lead to further brain hypoxia from inadequate amounts of oxygen in the circulating blood.

Unlicensed assistive personnel help and encourage the client to turn, cough, and deep breathe at least every 2 hours. Deep tracheal suctioning may be performed, even in the presence of increased ICP, if the findings of the respiratory assessment indicate that respiratory status is compromised, possibly causing cerebral hypoxia.

Assess vital signs and neurologic signs every 2 hours or more frequently if clinically indicated. Elevate the head of the bed 30 to 45 degrees unless contraindicated (e.g., after lumbar puncture or in the client with severe hypotension).

Acyclovir (Zovirax) is the drug of choice for the treatment of herpes encephalitis and is associated with a significantly lower mortality rate than vidarabine (Vira-A). Drug therapy is most effective if begun early, before the client becomes stuporous or comatose. This usually occurs within 4 to 6 days after the appearance of the initial neurologic symptoms. No specific drug therapy is available for infection by arboviruses or enteroviruses.

If there are permanent neurologic disabilities, the client with encephalitis is usually discharged to a rehabilitation setting or a long-term care facility. The client with minimal neurologic problems is discharged to the home setting.

PARKINSON DISEASE

PATHOPHYSIOLOGY

Parkinson disease (PD), also referred to as paralysis agitans, is the third most common neurologic disorder of older adults. PD has a large economic impact in the form of direct medical costs, as well as indirect costs, such as lost wages and decreased productivity. It is a debilitating disease affecting motor ability and is characterized by four cardinal symptoms: tremor, rigidity, **akinesia** (slow movement), and postural instability.

Motor activity occurs as a result of integration of the actions of the cerebral cortex, basal ganglia, and cerebellum. The basal ganglia are a group of neurons located deep within the cerebrum at the base of the brain near the lateral ventricles. When the basal ganglia are stimulated, muscle tone in the body is inhibited and voluntary movements are refined. The secretion of two neurotransmitters accomplishes this process: dopamine and acetylcholine (ACh).

Dopamine is produced in the substantia nigra, as well as in the adrenal glands, and is transmitted to the basal ganglia along a connecting neural pathway for secretion when needed. ACh is produced and secreted by the basal ganglia, as well as in the nerve endings in the periphery of the body. ACh-producing neurons transmit excitatory messages throughout the basal ganglia. Dopamine inhibits the function of these neurons, allowing control over voluntary movement. This system of checks and balances allows for refined, coordinated movement, such as picking up a pencil and writing.

Widespread degeneration of the substantia nigra leads to a decrease in the amount of dopamine. Dopamine produced in the adrenal glands is not available, because it is quickly metabolized in the body. When dopamine levels are decreased, a person loses the ability to refine voluntary movement. The large number of excitatory ACh-secreting neurons remains active, creating an imbalance between excitatory and inhibitory neuronal activity. The resulting excessive excitation of neurons prevents a person from controlling or initiating voluntary movement.

New evidence has found that because PD involves postganglionic sympathetic noradrenergic lesions, the disease seems to be not only a movement disorder with dopamine loss in the nigrostriatal system of the brain but also a dysautonomia, with norepinephrine loss in the sympathetic nervous system of the heart. This loss results in the orthostatic hypotension frequently seen in the client with PD.

PD is separated into stages according to the symptoms and degree of disability (Table 45-7). Stage 1 is mild disease with unilateral limb involvement. Bilateral limb involvement occurs in stage 2. In stage 3, the client exhibits significant gait disturbances and moderate generalized disability. Stage 4 is characterized by severe disability, akinesia (no initiation of movement), and muscle rigidity. The client with stage 5 disease is completely dependent in all activities of daily living (ADLs). Other classifications refer simply to mild, moderate, and severe disease.

Etiology and Genetic Risk

Although the exact cause of PD is not known, evidence suggests it is due to environmental and genetic factors. Endotoxin (lipopolysaccharide [LPS]), a common airborne environmental and occupational contaminate in agriculture and other industries, may be an environmental factor in the development of PD. Other factors that increase the risk of PD include rural living, well water consumption, and living near wood pulp mills.

There is evidence of a number of inherited forms of the disease associated with gene mutation. Recently, it has been

TABLE 45-7 Stages of Parkinson Disease

Stage 1: Initial Stage ▪ Unilateral limb involvement ▪ Minimal weakness ▪ Hand and arm trembling	**Stage 3: Moderate Disease** ▪ Increased gait disturbances
Stage 2: Mild Stage ▪ Bilateral limb involvement ▪ Masklike facies ▪ Slow, shuffling gait	**Stage 4: Severe Disability** ▪ Akinesia ▪ Rigidity **Stage 5: Complete Dependence**

found that some clients with PD have an extra copy of a normal gene (alpha-synuclein [SNCA]) that causes too much protein to build up in their brains (Guttman, Kish, & Furukawa, 2003).

Incidence/Prevalence

According to data from the National Institutes of Health, 500,000 people in the United States currently suffer from PD with some 50,000 new cases identified each year. As the population ages, the number of those affected is expected to dramatically increase. It is estimated that males are affected more often than females. Symptoms typically begin between 40 and 70 years of age with a peak onset in the 60s. However, Michael Fox, a popular actor, was diagnosed with PD in his 30s.

HEALTH PROMOTION/ILLNESS PREVENTION

There is no known way to prevent or cure PD. However, researchers from the Harvard School of Public Health have found that regular users of nonsteroidal anti-inflammatory drugs (NSAIDs) had a 45% lower risk for Parkinson disease than nonusers (Chen et al., 2003). A similar decrease in risk was observed among participants who took two or more tablets of aspirin per day compared with nonusers, but not among those taking smaller amounts of aspirin. However, because of the gastrointestinal side effects of these medications and the need for additional studies, people with PD should not take these drugs unless under the care of their health care provider.

COLLABORATIVE MANAGEMENT

Assessment

Collect data related to the time and progression of symptoms noticed by the client or the family. The older adult, who may assume that these behaviors are normal changes associated with aging, may ignore early signs and symptoms, such as fatigue, slight tremor, and problems with manual dexterity. Other signs and symptoms are listed in Chart 45-10, which summarizes the clinical manifestations of Parkinson disease. The client assessment consists of checking for evidence of **rigidity,** or resistance to passive movement of the extremities. Rigidity is classified as follows:

- Cogwheel, manifested by a rhythmic interruption of the muscle movement
- Plastic, defined as mildly restrictive movement
- Lead pipe, or total resistance to movement

Rigidity is present early in the disease process and progresses over time. Observe the client's ability to relax a muscle or move a selected muscle group.

Changes in facial expression or a masklike facies with wide-open, fixed, staring eyes are caused by rigidity of the facial muscles (Figure 45-1). This rigidity can lead to difficulties in chewing and swallowing, particularly if the pharyngeal muscles are involved. As a result, the client may have inadequate nutrition. Uncontrolled drooling may occur. Some clients develop dementia later as the disease progresses. In addition to changes in voluntary movement, many clients experience autonomic nervous system symptoms, such as excessive perspiration and orthostatic hypotension. Orthostatic hypotension was originally thought to be a side effect of levodopa therapy. Evidence suggests that it is related to baroreflex failure and loss of sympathetic innervation, most noticeably in the heart.

CHART 45-10

KEY FEATURES of Parkinson Disease

Posture
- Stooped posture
- Flexed trunk
- Fingers abducted and flexed at the metacarpophalangeal joint
- Wrist slightly dorsiflexed

Gait
- Slow and shuffling
- Short, hesitant steps
- Propulsive gait
- Difficulty stopping quickly

Motor
- Bradykinesia
- Akinesia
- Tremors
- "Pill-rolling" movement
- Masklike facies
- Difficulty chewing and swallowing
- Uncontrolled drooling, especially at night
- Fatigue
- Difficulty getting in and out of bed
- Little arm swinging when walking
- Change in handwriting (micrographia, or gets smaller)

Speech
- Soft, low-pitched voice
- **Dysarthria** (slurred speech)
- **Echolalia** (automatic repetition of what another person says) and repetition of sentences
- Change in voice volume, phonation, or articulation

Autonomic dysfunction
- Orthostatic hypotension
- Excessive perspiration
- Oily skin
- Seborrhea
- Flushing
- Changes in skin texture
- Blepharospasm (eyelid spasm)

Psychosocial assessment
- Emotionally labile
- Depression
- Paranoia
- Easily upset
- Rapid mood swings
- Cognitive impairments (i.e., dementia)
- Delayed reaction time
- Sleep disturbances

The diagnosis of PD is made on the basis of the clinical findings and after other neurologic diseases are eliminated as possibilities. There are no specific diagnostic tests. Analysis of cerebrospinal fluid (CSF) may show a decrease in dopamine levels, although the results of other studies are usually normal.

Common Nursing Diagnoses and Collaborative Problems

Nursing diagnoses that may apply to clients with Parkinson disease include the following:

- Impaired Physical Mobility related to neuromuscular impairment
- Risk for Falls related to decreased lower extremity strength and orthostatic hypotension
- Risk for Self-Care Deficit related to neuromuscular impairment

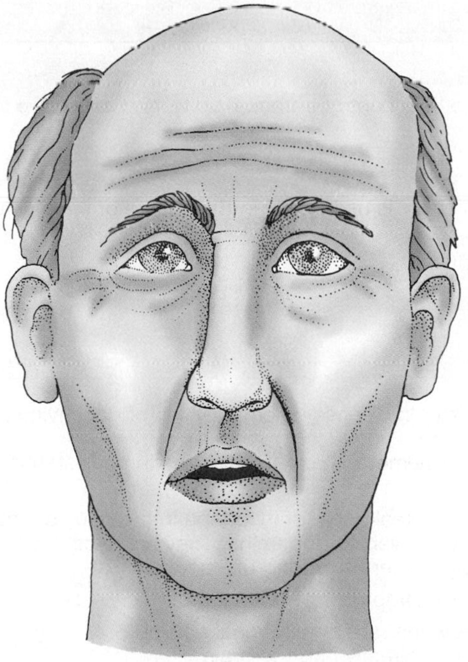

Figure 45-1 ■ The masklike facial expression typical of clients with Parkinson disease.

CHART 45-11

BEST PRACTICE for
Care of the Client with Parkinson Disease

- Administer medications promptly on schedule to maintain continuous therapeutic drug levels.
- Monitor for side effects of medications, especially orthostatic hypotension, hallucinations, and acute confusional state (delirium).
- Collaborate with physical and occupational therapists to keep the client as mobile and as independent as possible in activities of daily living (ADLs).
- Allow the client time to perform ADLs and mobility skills.
- Implement interventions to prevent complications of immobility, such as constipation, pressure ulcers, and contractures.
- Schedule appointments and activities late in the morning to prevent rushing the client, or schedule them at the time of the client's optimal level of functioning.
- Teach the client to speak slowly and clearly; use alternative communication methods, such as a communication board; refer to speech-language pathologist.
- Monitor the client's ability to eat and swallow; monitor actual food and fluid intake; collaborate with dietitian.
- Provide high-protein, high-calorie foods or supplements to maintain weight.
- Recognize that Parkinson disease affects the client's body image; focus on the client's strengths.
- Assess for depression and anxiety.

- Risk for Impaired Verbal Communication related to physiologic conditions
- Chronic Confusion related to dementia
- Risk for Imbalanced Nutrition: Less Than Body Requirements related to inability to ingest food due to biologic factors

Interventions

In addition to the physician and nurse practitioner, the registered nurse, physical or occupational therapist, speech-language pathologist, and social worker collaborate with the client and family to develop an interdisciplinary treatment plan. In some cases, palliative surgery may be performed to assist the client in remaining mobile for as long as possible. Chart 45-11 summarizes best practices for nursing management of the client with PD.

NONSURGICAL MANAGEMENT. Drug therapy is an essential part of management, which decreases signs and symptoms and allows the client to provide self-care and have a reasonable quality of life.

Drug Therapy. Medications are prescribed to treat the symptoms of PD with the goal of maximizing the client's functional abilities. An equally important goal is to prescribe medications with minimal long-term side effects. Many questions and controversies remain about which drugs to use, when to start therapy, and how to prevent complications. Medication administration is closely monitored, and the health care provider adjusts the dosage or changes the medication as the client's condition warrants. Teach the client and family how to monitor for and report side effects of medications. See Table 45-8 for more information on drug therapy.

Older Drugs. **Anticholinergic** drugs benefit the client whose primary symptom is tremor. The health care provider prescribes anticholinergic drugs less frequently to the older adult because they often cause confusion or other cognitive deficits. Amantadine (Symmetrel) may be prescribed as the first line of treatment to younger clients when tremor is the main problem (Guttman, Kish, & Furukawa, 2003). Selegiline (Carbex, Eldepryl, Novo-Selegiline✱) may be prescribed to confer mild, symptomatic benefit before initiating dopaminergics in the treatment of PD.

Dopamine agonists stimulate dopamine receptors and are typically the most effective during the first 3 to 5 years of use. The benefit of these agents is the less frequent incidents of **dyskinesias** (problems with movement) and **"wearing off" phenomenon** (loss of response to the medication), which is characterized by periods of good mobility ("on") alternating with periods of poor mobility ("off"). However, dopamine agonists are associated with side effects such as nausea, postural hypotension, hallucinations, and drowsiness.

Levodopa (Dopar, L-dopa) and its combination with carbidopa (Sinemet) is the most efficacious treatment for PD, and all clients are on it at some point in the disease process. It may be the initial drug of choice if the client's presenting symptoms are severe or interfere with work or school. Both an immediate-release (IR) and controlled-release (CR) form of Sinemet are available, although there is no difference in reducing response fluctuations. The levodopa agents are less expensive than the dopamine agonists and are better at improving motor function. Long-term use leads to dyskinesia.

When the classic dopaminergics and anticholinergics fail or are no longer effective, bromocriptine mesylate (Parlodel) or pergolide may be prescribed to activate the release of dopamine. They may be used alone or in combination with carbidopa/levodopa (Sinemet). Some providers may prescribe bromocriptine mesylate early in the course of treatment. It is especially useful in the client who has experienced side effects such as dyskinesias or orthostatic hypotension while receiving Sinemet.

Amantadine (Symmetrel) is an antiviral drug that has anti-Parkinson benefits. It may be used early in disease to

TABLE 45-8 Medications Used for Parkinson Disease

Medication	Use
Anticholinergics Benztropine (Cogentin) Procyclidine (Kemadrin) Trihexyphenidyl (Artane)	Older drugs are used to help control tremor, rigidity, and excessive sweating.
Selegiline (Eldepryl)	Monoamine oxidase inhibitor is used early in the course of the disease.
Dopamine agonists (given more often to younger clients) Bromocriptine mesylate (Parlodel) Cabergoline Pergolide (Permax) Pramipexole (Mirapex) Ropinirole (Requip)	These drugs mimic dopamine. Do not give to older adults.
Levodopa combinations Carbidopa/levodopa (Sinemet IR) Carbidopa/levodopa (Sinemet CR) Carbidopa/levodopa/entacapone (Stalevo)	These drugs are used later in disease when activities of daily living (ADLs) are impaired. Some clients take both Sinemet CR and IR to maintain consistent therapeutic blood levels.
Catechol *O*-methyltransferase (COMT) inhibitors Tolcapone (Tasmar) Entacapone (Comtan)	These inhibitors block the breakdown of levodopa in the body so more can travel to the brain and convert to dopamine. They are used in conjunction with Sinemet and help prevent "wearing off" periods.
Amantadine (Symmetrel)	This drug is given to treat symptoms of "wearing off."
Investigational Coenzyme Q10 Dextromethorphan glial-derived neurotrophic factor	Coenzyme Q10 may slow the rate of functional decline. This factor is administered directly into the brain.

reduce symptoms. It is also prescribed with Sinemet to reduce dyskinesias.

Newer Drugs. **Catechol *O*-methyltransferase (COMT) inhibitors** are enzymes that inactivate dopamine. Therefore COMT inhibitors block this activity, thus increasing the effectiveness of levodopa. For example, entacapone (Comtan) is used in combination with levodopa and carbidopa. Stalevo is a combination of levodopa, carbidopa, and entacapone. The benefit of these medications is that the client only needs to take one medication. However, it is not beneficial for those clients who need more specific dosages of the individual medication. Additional therapeutic strategies used for PD include the administration of monoamine oxidase (MAO) inhibitors, such as selegiline (Eldepryl), to reduce the metabolic breakdown of dopamine.

Studies are ongoing to search for more effective ways of delivering the best medications. For example, topical patches rather than pills may be available to treat PD. Neuroprotective drugs, such as coenzyme Q10, are currently in clinical trials and may replace traditional drug therapy for some clients.

Drug Toxicity. For the client on long-term drug therapy regimens, drug tolerance or drug toxicity often develops. Drug toxicity is evidenced by delirium (acute confusion), cognitive impairment, decreased effectiveness of the drug, or hallucinations. Delirium may be difficult to assess in the client who is already suffering from chronic dementia as a result of PD or another disease. If possible, compare the client's current cognitive and behavioral status with his or her baseline before drug therapy began.

When drug tolerance is reached, the drug's effects do not last as long as previously. The treatment of drug toxicity or tolerance includes the following:

- A reduction in medication dosage
- A change of medications or in the frequency of administration
- A drug holiday (particularly with levodopa therapy)

During a drug holiday, which typically lasts up to 10 days, the client receives no medications. He or she must be carefully monitored during this time.

Exercise and Ambulation. Nontraditional exercise programs, such as yoga and tai chi, may help elevate mood as well as improve mobility in the early stage of the disease. Early in the disease process, physical and occupational therapists should be consulted to plan and implement a program to keep the client mobile and flexible by incorporating active and passive range-of-motion (ROM) exercises, muscle stretching, and activity. The client is instructed to avoid watching his or her feet when walking to prevent falls.

Self-Care. The nurse and rehabilitation team encourage the client to participate as much as possible in the performance of self-care or activities of daily living (ADLs). The team makes the environment conducive to independence in activity and as stress-free and safe as possible. Occupational and physical therapists provide training in ADLs and the use of adaptive devices, if needed, to facilitate independence. The occupational therapist (OT) evaluates the client in all aspects of ADLs and determines the need for adaptive devices, for example, special utensils for eating.

Injury Prevention. Clients with PD tend to not sleep well at night. Some clients nap for short periods during the day and may not be aware that they have done so. This sleep misperception may put the client at risk for injury. For example, the client may fall asleep while driving an automobile. Therefore teach the client and family to monitor the client's sleeping pattern and discuss whether or not the client is safe to operate machinery or perform other potentially dangerous tasks.

Nutrition. A registered dietitian (RD) should see the client to evaluate his or her food intake. The client's intake of calcium, vitamin K, and other key elements is evaluated, especially in the client who is susceptible to falling or has difficulty swallowing. The RD takes into consideration the client's bowel habits and adjusts the diet if constipation occurs. If the client has trouble swallowing, a speech-language pathology consultation is made and an extensive swallowing evaluation is conducted. Based on these findings and the client interview, an individualized dietary plan is developed. Usually a soft diet or thick, cold fluids, such as milk shakes, are more easily tolerated.

Smaller, more frequent meals or a commercial powder, such as Thick-It, added to liquids may assist the client who has difficulty swallowing. The client is positioned with the head elevated to facilitate swallowing and prevent aspiration. The speech-language pathologist can be very helpful in evaluating swallowing ability and recommending specific strategies. Food intake is recorded daily or as needed. The client may experience weight loss as a result of altered food intake and the increased number of calories burned secondary to muscle rigidity. The client should be weighed once a week and adjustments made to the diet as indicated. As the disease progresses and swallowing becomes more of a problem, supplemental feedings become the main source of nutrition to maintain weight, with meals and other foods taken as the client is able to tolerate. (See Chapter 64 for additional interventions for clients with undernutrition.)

Communication. Collaborate with the speech-language pathologist if the client has speech difficulties. Together with the health care team, client, and family, a communication plan is developed. The client is taught exercises to strengthen muscles used for breathing, speech, and swallowing. The client is instructed to speak slowly and clearly and to pause and take deep breaths at appropriate intervals during each sentence. Unnecessary environmental noise should be eliminated to maximize the listener's ability to hear and understand the client. The client is asked to repeat words that the listener does not understand, and the listener watches the client's lips and nonverbal expressions for cues as to the meaning of conversation. The client is instructed to organize his or her thoughts before speaking and is encouraged to use facial expression and gestures, if possible, to assist with communication. In addition, the client should exaggerate words to increase the listener's ability to understand. If the client cannot communicate verbally, he or she must use alternative methods of communication, such as a communication board, mechanical voice synthesizer, or computer. The speech-language pathologist assesses the client's ability to use these devices before a decision is made about which method to use.

Psychosocial Support. Although not all clients with PD have dementia, impaired cognitive function and memory deficits are common. Clients may also experience changes in gait and tremors that are uncontrollable. In the late stages of the disease, they cannot move without assistance, have difficulty with articulation, have minimal facial expression, and may drool. Clients often state that they are embarrassed, and they tend to avoid social events or groups of people. They should not be forced into situations in which they feel ashamed of their appearance. They should be encouraged to undertake activities that do not require small-muscle dexterity, such as light, modified aerobic exercises.

A social worker may be able to help the family with financial and health insurance issues. The client and family may be referred to social and state agencies as well as support groups. The case manager and social workers collaborate on discharge planning issues as well as respite issues when they become necessary.

The client's abilities or strengths are emphasized and positive reinforcement is provided when he or she meets the daily goals. The client, the family or significant others, and the rehabilitation team mutually set realistic goals that can be achieved. Assisting the client with grooming and hygiene is also important in maintaining a positive body image.

The long-term management of PD presents a special challenge in the home care setting. A case manager may be required to coordinate interdisciplinary care and provide support for the client and family. Impaired mobility affects the daily lifestyle, including sexuality. The case manager or home care nurse uses a holistic approach to ensure that psychosocial, as well as physical, needs are addressed.

SURGICAL MANAGEMENT. Several options are available if surgery for the client with Parkinson disease (PD) is needed. Surgery is a last resort when drugs are ineffective in symptom management. The most common surgeries are stereotactic pallidotomy and thalamotomy, although newer surgical procedures are being tried.

Stereotactic Pallidotomy/Thalamotomy. **Stereotactic pallidotomy** can be a very effective treatment for controlling the symptoms associated with PD. First, the target area within the pallidum is identified via a computed tomography (CT) or magnetic resonance imaging (MRI) scan. Next, the stereotactic head frame is placed on the client. IV sedation is given, and a burr hole is made into the cranium; an electrode or cylindric rod is inserted into the target area. The target area receives a mild electrical stimulation, and the client's reaction is assessed for reduction of tremor and rigidity. If this result does not occur, or if unexpected visual, motor, or sensory symptoms appear, the probe is repositioned. When the probe is in the ideal location, a temporary lesion is made. If this is successful, the permanent lesion is made. The client is monitored in the postanesthesia care unit (PACU) for about 1 hour and is then returned to the inpatient unit for continuing postoperative care.

As an alternative to stereotactic pallidotomy, the surgeon may perform a **thalamotomy** for treatment of tremor through thermocoagulation of brain cells. This procedure is effective for a limited number of clients. Because bilateral procedures have increased surgical complication rates, only unilateral surgery is done to benefit the side of the body that is most affected by the disease.

Deep Brain Stimulation. Deep brain stimulation (DBS) is used when medications are no longer effective in controlling the client's symptoms. A thin electrode is implanted in the thalamus or subthalamus and then connected to a "pacemaker" that delivers electrical current to interfere with "tremor" cells. The electrodes are connected to an implantable pulse generator (IPG) that is placed underneath the skin in the client's chest, similar to a cardiac pacemaker. The client uses a magnet placed over the IPG to adjust the settings and to check the battery status.

Fetal Tissue Transplantation. Fetal tissue transplantation is an experimental and highly controversial procedure. Fetal substantia nigra tissue, either human or pig, is transplanted into the caudate nucleus of the brain. Preliminary reports suggest that clients show substantial clinical improvement in motor symptoms without dyskinesias after receiving the transplanted tissue. Long-term results are yet to be seen.

New therapies currently in clinical trials include the following:

- Gene therapy to replace lost gamma aminobutyric acid (GABA) inputs to the subthalamic nucleus and globus pallidus interna/substantia nigra pars reticulata
- Infusion of recombinant glial-derived neurotrophic factor directly into the brain to support at-risk nigrostriatal neurons
- Other stem cell research methods

ALZHEIMER'S DISEASE

PATHOPHYSIOLOGY

Alzheimer's disease (AD), also known as dementia, Alzheimer type (DAT), is a chronic, progressive, degenerative disease that accounts for 60% of the dementias occurring in people older than 65 years of age. It may also be seen less commonly in people in their 40s and 50s, which is referred to as early dementia, Alzheimer type, or presenile dementia, Alzheimer type. It is characterized by loss of memory, judgment, and visuospatial perception, and by a change in personality. Over time, the client becomes increasingly cognitively impaired; severe physical deterioration takes place and death occurs as a result of complications of immobility.

Structural Changes in the Brain

The brain of the older adult weighs less and occupies less space in the cranial vault than does the brain of a younger person. Other changes in the brain that occur with aging include widening of the cerebral sulci, narrowing of the gyri, and enlargement of the ventricles. In the presence of AD, these normal changes are greatly accelerated. Brain weight is reduced further, and there is marked cerebral atrophy. The cerebral sulci and fissures, as well as the ventricles, are enlarged more than those of persons of the same age without AD. The following areas of the brain are particularly affected:

- Precentral gyrus of the frontal lobe
- Superior temporal gyrus
- Hippocampus
- Substantia nigra

Microscopic changes of the brain found in people with AD include **neurofibrillary tangles,** senile or **neuritic plaques,** and granulovascular degeneration. Neurofibrillary tangles are a classic finding at autopsy in the brains of clients with AD. They consist of tangled masses of fibrous elements throughout the neurons. The same tangles and chemical changes are found in people with Down syndrome.

Senile plaques are composed of degenerating nerve terminals and are found particularly in the hippocampus, an important part of the limbic system. Deposited within the plaques are increased amounts of an abnormal protein called **beta amyloid.** Increased amounts of beta amyloid are being studied carefully for their role in the development of AD. Research is focusing on the following:

- Does beta amyloid disrupt the normal sodium, potassium, and calcium channels that are responsible for nerve function and signal transmission from one nerve cell to another?
- How does the overproduction of oxidants as a result of beta amyloid breakdown affect genetic material in the DNA of cells?
- What is the role of overproduction of immune factors in response to oxidation in the development of AD?

Although vascular degeneration occurs in the normally aging brain, its presence is significantly increased in clients with AD. Vascular degeneration accounts for at least partial loss of the ability of nerve cells to function properly. This pathologic change contributes to the mortality associated with this disorder.

Chemical Changes in the Brain

In addition to the structural changes in the brain associated with AD, abnormalities in the neurotransmitters (acetylcholine [ACh], norepinephrine, dopamine, serotonin) may occur. High levels of beta amyloid are associated with reduced ACh by as much as 75%, which leads to a decrease in the amount of acetyltransferase in the hippocampus. This loss is significant because the decrease in acetyltransferase interferes with cholinergic innervation to the cerebral cortex. This results in dysfunction of cognition, recent memory, and the ability to acquire new memories. The exact role of the reduction of neurotransmitters in the development of AD is not well understood.

Etiology and Genetic Risk

The exact cause of AD is unknown. Several theories and risk factors have been proposed: genetics, chemical imbalances, environmental agents, and immunologic changes. It is well established that age is the most important risk factor. Older adults tend to get sporadic AD rather than the familial genetic type.

There is little doubt that for many clients with AD there is a genetic predisposition to the development of the disease. The clients who seem to have this predisposition have familial AD (FAD). Studies of families are ongoing to determine the exact genetic pathway that is responsible. Most cases of early onset of AD are associated with mutations in genes (Table 45-9).

Early onset FAD seems to be related to an acceleration of beta amyloid plaque formation and apoptosis, which are caused by defective genes. Late stage AD research focuses on

TABLE 45-9 Alzheimer's Disease and Genetic Disposition

Generalized Seizures

Most cases of early onset of AD are associated with mutations in genes:

- Presenilin I gene on chromosome 14
- Presenilin I gene on chromosome 1
- Amyloid precursor protein on chromosome 21

Research shows an acceleration of beta amyloid plaque formation and apoptosis, a process by which cells self-destruct.

Late stage AD research focuses on the role of apolipoprotein, specifically:

- Apolipoprotein E (Apo E)-4 on chromosome 19 is a major risk factor.
  - The presence of two copies of Apo E-4 is associated with even higher risk of developing AD.
  - Some clients with Apo E-4 may not develop AD.
  - Conversely, some clients without Apo E-4 may develop AD.
- Apolipoprotein E (Apo E)-2 lowers risk of AD.

Other genetic research is focusing on the following:

- Chromosome 10 as a location for genetic factors, mutations in the proteins amyloid precursor protein (APP)
- Ubiquitin-B

the role of apolipoprotein E on chromosome 19. People with Down syndrome often develop dementia with characteristic features of AD. The importance of alpha-2 macroglobulin on chromosome 12 continues to be studied as another factor in the development of Alzheimer's disease.

Environmental agents, especially certain viruses such as herpes zoster and herpes simplex, and metal ions such as zinc and copper, have also been suggested as causes. Clients who have experienced a head injury may be more at risk for AD, and at an earlier age, than others.

Incidence/Prevalence

AD may affect anyone older than 40 years of age, although it occurs more often in those older than 65 years of age. The cost of care for clients with AD is tremendous, making it the third most expensive disease in the United States (see the Resource Management box below). Loss of wages and productivity in society adds to the increasing costs of health care.

HEALTH PROMOTION/ILLNESS PREVENTION

There are no proven ways to prevent AD. Current research activities are focusing on eating a balanced diet, eating dark-colored fruits and vegetables, using soy products and sufficient amounts of folate and vitamins B_{12}, C, and E. These substances have been associated with less risk of developing AD. Walking, swimming, and other exercise not only increase tone and muscle strength but also have been shown to decrease mental decline in AD as well as other dementias.

The use of ibuprofen and other nonsteroidal anti-inflammatory drugs (NSAIDs) has been demonstrated to reduce the risk of developing AD if taken in the years before symptoms develop (Zandi, Breitner, & Anthony, 2002). The exact mechanism of action is not fully understood. Unfortunately the long-term use of these agents, especially in the older adult, may result in significant complications such as a high risk of bleeding and gastrointestinal (GI) ulcerations. Therefore these agents should not be taken to prevent AD unless under careful health care provider supervision.

RESOURCE MANAGEMENT

THE CLIENT WITH ALZHEIMER'S DISEASE

Cost of Care

- Most clients live at home where care is provided by family and friends. The average out-of-pocket expenses for home care is $12,500.
- Average annual cost per client is $18,400 for clients with mild disease, $30,100 for moderate disease, and $36,100 for advanced disease, not including indirect costs such as productivity or wages.
- Overall cost of a lifetime of care for a client with Alzheimer's disease (AD) is staggering; average lifetime cost per client is more than $200,000.
- AD is the third most expensive disease in the United States, after heart disease and cancer.
- U.S. society spends at least $100 billion per year on AD.
- Lost productivity of caregivers (due to absenteeism, productivity, cost of replacement workers) averages $33 billion.
- Seven billion dollars is spent annually on health care and long-term care.
- Half of all nursing home clients suffer from AD; average cost per client for nursing home care is $42,000 per year, but cost can exceed $70,000 in some areas.
- In 1999 the federal government spent about $400 million for AD research.

Implications for Nursing

It is important for all health care providers to understand the staggering costs of caring for clients with AD, not only the monetary cost but also the psychological and emotional costs to the family and caregivers. Even with increased research funds, no cure for AD has been found. Care continues to be symptomatic; thus costs of providing care for clients increases as clients progress through the stages of the disease. Clients often require nursing home care and specialized equipment as the disease progresses.

Data from http://www.alzheimers.org.

◆COLLABORATIVE MANAGEMENT

PHARM REVIEW

◆Assessment

The client with Alzheimer's disease (AD) often presents with cognitive impairment, although many other disorders, drugs, and environmental factors can cause changes in cognition as well. A thorough history and physical examination are necessary to differentiate AD from other, possibly reversible causes (Table 45-10). Obtain information from family members or significant others, as well as from the client, because the client may be unaware of the problems, denying their existence or covering them up.

The most important information to be obtained concerns the onset, duration, progression, and course of the symptoms obtained. Question the client and the family about changes in memory or increasing forgetfulness and about the ability to perform activities of daily living (ADLs). Further information obtained includes current employment status, work history, and ability to fulfill household responsibilities,

TABLE 45-10 Causes of Cognitive Impairment in the Older Adult

Neurologic Causes ▪ Vascular insufficiency ▪ Infections ▪ Trauma ▪ Tumors ▪ Normal-pressure hydrocephalus	**Drug Intoxication** ▪ Misuse of prescribed medications ▪ Side effects of medications ▪ Incorrect use of over-the-counter medications ▪ Ingestion of heavy metals
Cardiovascular Causes ▪ Myocardial infarction ▪ Dysrhythmias ▪ Heart failure ▪ Cardiogenic shock ▪ Endocarditis	**Nutritional Deficiencies** ▪ B vitamins ▪ Vitamin C ▪ Hypoproteinemia
Pulmonary Causes ▪ Infection ▪ Pneumonia ▪ Hypoventilation	**Environmental Causes** ▪ Hypothermia/hyperthermia ▪ Unfamiliar environment ▪ Sensory deprivation/overload
Metabolic Causes ▪ Electrolyte imbalance ▪ Acidosis/alkalosis ▪ Hypoglycemia/hyperglycemia ▪ Acute and chronic renal failure ▪ Fluid volume deficit ▪ Hepatic failure	**Psychological Causes** ▪ Depression ▪ Anxiety ▪ Pain ▪ Fatigue ▪ Grief ▪ Paranoia

CHART 45-12

KEY FEATURES of
Alzheimer's Disease

Early (Mild), or Stage I
- Forgets names; misplaces household items
- Mild memory loss
- Short attention span
- Subtle changes in personality and behavior
- No social or employment problems
- Cognitive impairment, problems with judgment
- Decreased performance, especially when stressed
- Unable to travel alone to new destinations
- Decreased knowledge of current events
- Loss of judgment
- Wandering
- Decreased sense of smell

Middle (Moderate), or Stage II
- Severe impairment of all cognitive functions
- Gross intellectual impairments
- Complete disorientation to time, place, and event
- Possible depression, agitated
- Physical impairment
- Loss of ability to care for self
- Visuospatial deficits
- Speech and language deficits
- Incontinent
- Wandering

Late (Severe), or Stage III
- Completely incapacitated
- Totally dependent in activities of daily living
- Motor and verbal skills lost
- General and focal neurologic deficits

including cleaning, grocery shopping, and preparing meals. Elicit a history concerning changes in driving ability, ability to handle routine financial transactions, and language and communication skills. In addition, document any changes in personality and behavior.

There is increasing evidence that olfactory dysfunction is associated with the development of AD (Peters et al., 2003). Therefore ask about changes in the ability to smell or changes in the sense of smell. The history taking concludes with a review of the client's medical history. Of importance is a history of head trauma, viral illness, or exposure to metal or toxic waste, as well as any family history of AD or Down syndrome.

PHYSICAL ASSESSMENT/CLINICAL MANIFESTATIONS

STAGES OF ALZHEIMER'S DISEASE. The clinical manifestations associated with AD can be grouped into three broad stages on the basis of the progress of the disease (Chart 45-12). The client does not necessarily progress from one stage to the next in an orderly fashion. A stage may be bypassed, or he or she may exhibit symptoms of one or several stages. Each client exhibits different disease stages and clinical manifestations. Consequently, some authorities now use broader terms, such as early (mild), middle (moderate), and late (severe) stages.

The primary focus of the neurologic assessment of clients with AD is to identify abnormalities in cognition, including language, personality, and behavior. Physical manifestations of neurologic impairment (seizures, tremors, or ataxia) tend to occur late in the disease process.

CHANGES IN COGNITION. Cognition refers to the ability of the brain to process, store, retrieve, and manipulate information. Therefore the client is assessed for deficits in the following abilities:

- Attention and concentration
- Judgment and perception
- Learning and memory
- Communication and language
- Speed of information processing

Typical symptoms experienced by the client include memory impairment, as well as new memory, and defects in information retrieval resulting from dysfunction in the hippocampal, frontal, or parietal region. Alterations in communication abilities, such as **apraxia** (inability to use objects appropriately), **aphasia** (inability to speak or understand), **anomia** (inability to find words), and **agnosia** (loss of sensory comprehension), are due to dysfunction of the temporal and parietal lobes. Frontal lobe impairment produces difficulties with judgment, inability to make decisions, decreased attention span, and diminished ability to concentrate. As the disease progresses, the client loses all cognitive abilities, is totally unable to communicate, and becomes less aware of the environment.

To assess the presence of cognitive impairment, the nurse or other health care provider can use one of several assessment tools. One of the most popular tools is Folstein's Mini-Mental State Examination (MMSE), also known as the "mini-mental." The MMSE assesses five major areas—orientation, registration, attention and calculation, recall, and speech-language (including reading). Figure 45-2 lists examples of the questions asked on this test. The client performs certain cognitive tasks that are scored and added together for a total score of 0 to 30. The lower the score, the greater the severity of the dementia. It is not unusual for a client with advanced AD to score below 5.

Although the MMSE is used frequently, the client must be able to read. For the client who cannot read, or for a quicker screening test, the SET test can be used, which is especially useful for the older adult. The client is asked to name 10 items in each of four categories: fruits, animals, colors, and towns (FACT). Other categories can be used, if necessary. The client receives 1 point for each item, for a possible maximum score of 40. Clients who score above 25 do not have dementia. Although this assessment is more comprehensive and easy to administer, it should not be used for clients with hearing impairments or aphasia. References describing other available tests to measure cognitive impairment may be found in the Selected Bibliography.

CHANGES IN BEHAVIOR AND PERSONALITY. One of the most difficult aspects of AD that families, significant others, and health care professionals cope with are the behavioral changes that can occur in advanced disease. The client is assessed for the following:

- Aggressiveness, especially verbal and physical abusive tendencies
- Rapid mood swings
- Increased confusion at night **(sundowning)** or in excessively fatigued clients

The client may wander and become lost or may go into other rooms to rummage through another's belongings. Hoarding objects such as washcloths is also common.

For some clients with dementia, emotional and behavioral problems accompany the primary disease. They may experience paranoia, delusions, hallucinations, and depression. These behaviors are documented, care is taken to en-

Orientation to Time
"What is the date?"

Registration
"Listen carefully, I am going to say three words. You say them back after I stop. Ready? Here they are...
HOUSE (pause), CAR (pause), LAKE (pause). Now repeat those words back to me." [Repeat up to 5 times, but score only the first trial.]

Naming
"What is this?" [Point to a pencil or pen.]

Reading
"Please read this and do what it says." [Show examinee the words on the stimulus form.]
CLOSE YOUR EYES

A

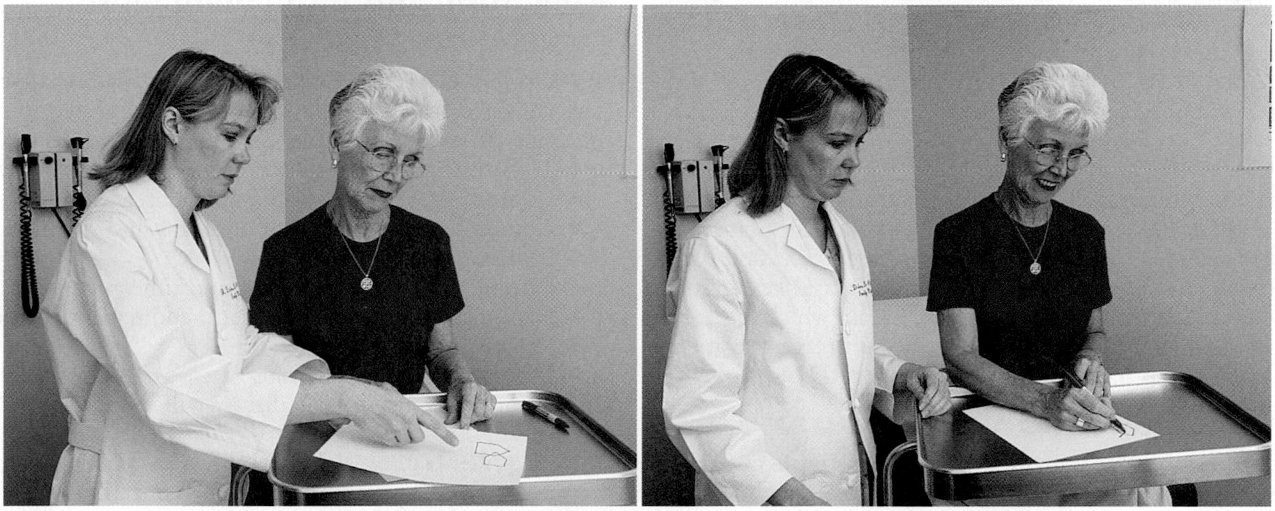

B

Figure 45-2 ■ **A,** Examples of questions that are asked on the Mini-Mental State Examination. **B,** Copying is one of the tasks on the MMSE. (**A** from Mini-Mental State Examination © 1975, 1998, 2001 by MiniMental, LLC. All rights reserved. Published 2001 by Psychological Assessment Resources, Inc. May not be reproduced in whole or in part in any form or by any means without written permission of Psychological Assessment Resources, Inc., P.O. Box 998, Odessa, FL 33556; (800) 331-8378 or (813) 968-3003. **B** from Seidel, H.M., et al. (1999). *Mosby's guide to physical examination* (4th ed.). St. Louis: Mosby.)

sure the client's safety, and the health care provider is notified. (Refer to a mental health/behavior health nursing textbook for a complete discussion of these disorders.)

Although drug therapy is not effective in treating dementia, certain drugs may help control the emotional and psychiatric manifestations, such as depression, anxiety, paranoia, and aggression associated with the primary disease.

CHANGES IN SELF-CARE SKILLS. Changes in the client's self-care skills that may be observed by the family, significant others, or nurse include the following:

- Decreased interest in personal appearance
- Selection of clothing that is inappropriate for the weather or event
- Loss of bowel and bladder control
- Decreased appetite or ability to eat

Over time, the client becomes less mobile and muscle contractures develop. He or she eventually becomes totally immobile and requires total physical care.

PSYCHOSOCIAL ASSESSMENT

In people with AD, the cognitive changes, as well as biochemical and structural dysfunctions, affect personality and behavior. In the early stage, clients often recognize that they are experiencing memory or cognitive changes and may attempt to hide the problems, deny them, or become depressed over the changes. Older clients typically attribute the changes to "old age."

As the disease progresses, clients begin to display major changes in emotional and behavioral affect. Of particular importance is the need for an assessment of the clients' reactions to changes in routine or environment. For example, a hospital admission is very traumatic for most clients with dementia. It is not unusual for them to exhibit a catastrophic response or overreact to any change by becoming excessively aggressive or abusive.

As clients become unaware of their behavior, the focus of the psychosocial assessment shifts to the family or significant others. The health care team assesses their ability to cope with the chronicity and progression of the disease and identifies possible support systems.

LABORATORY ASSESSMENT

No laboratory tests exist to confirm the diagnosis of AD. Diagnosis is made on the basis of brain tissue examination at autopsy, which confirms the presence of neurofibrillary tangles and neuritic plaques.

Genetic testing, specifically for apolipoprotein E (Apo E), may be helpful as an ancillary test (not a predictive test) for the differential diagnosis of AD. Testing for other genes that have been shown to predispose a person to AD has not become routine. A variety of laboratory tests may be performed to rule out other treatable causes of dementia or delirium, including the following:

- A complete blood count (CBC)
- Determination of serum electrolyte levels, blood urea nitrogen, and glucose
- Determination of vitamin B_{12} levels
- Determination of folate levels
- Thyroid and liver function tests
- A serologic test for syphilis
- Drug toxicity screening tests (over-the-counter and illegal drugs)
- Alcohol screening tests

RADIOGRAPHIC ASSESSMENT

Computed tomography (CT) and positron emission tomography (PET) may be performed to rule out other causes of disease. The CT scan typically shows cerebral atrophy and ventricular enlargement, wide sulci, and shrunken gyri in the later stages of the disease. The PET scan, which measures glucose in living cells, shows a significant decrease in metabolic activity in the brains of people with AD.

OTHER DIAGNOSTIC ASSESSMENTS

Magnetic resonance imaging (MRI) can also rule out other causes of neurologic disease. The electroencephalogram (EEG) shows slow-wave delta activity indicative of dementia in the second and third stages of AD.

To identify clearly the nature and extent of the client's cognitive dysfunction, the physician, usually a neurologist, administers several neuropsychological tests. The tests used depend on physician preference and the ability of the client to participate in testing. All of the tests focus on cognitive ability and may be repeated over time to measure changes.

◆Analysis

COMMON NURSING DIAGNOSES AND COLLABORATIVE PROBLEMS

The following are priority nursing diagnoses for clients with Alzheimer's disease (AD):

1. Chronic Confusion related to Alzheimer's disease
2. Risk for Injury related to problems with orientation
3. Compromised Family Coping and Caregiver Role Strain related to the client's prolonged progression of disability and client's increasing care needs
4. Disturbed Sleep Pattern related to changes in sleep phases, anxiety, and/or depression

ADDITIONAL NURSING DIAGNOSES AND COLLABORATIVE PROBLEMS

In addition to the common nursing diagnoses, clients with AD may have one or more of the following:

- Impaired Verbal Communication related to aphasia, anomia, agnosia, and/or apraxia
- Imbalanced Nutrition: Less Than Body Requirements related to self-care deficit and/or anorexia
- Total Urinary Incontinence and Bowel Incontinence related to cognitive and self-care deficits
- Social Isolation related to personality and behavior changes
- Risk for Impaired Physical Mobility related to progression of disability
- Risk for Impaired Skin Integrity related to immobility and/or impaired nutritional status
- Self-Care Deficit (Total) related to cognitive deficit
- Risk for Other-Directed Violence and Risk for Self-Directed Violence related to behavior changes
- Hopelessness related to inability to control the progression of disease

◆Planning and Implementation

CHRONIC CONFUSION

NOC **PLANNING: EXPECTED OUTCOMES.** In early stages of the disease, the client with AD is expected to have the ability to execute complex mental processes. Indicators include that the client will have noncompromised ability to:

- Communicate clearly and appropriately
- Comprehend the meaning of events and situations
- Be attentive and concentrate
- Be oriented to person, place, and time
- Demonstrate immediate, recent, and remote memory
- Process information
- Make appropriate decisions

Clients with late stages of the disease will cannot meet these criteria.

INTERVENTIONS. The health care provider should answer the client's questions truthfully concerning the diagnosis of AD. In this manner the client can more fully participate in the interdisciplinary treatment plan. Interventions are the same whether the client is cared for at home, in an adult day care center, in an assisted living center, or in a long-term care facility. The client with memory problems benefits from a structured and consistent environment. Many variables, including physical illness and environmental factors, can worsen or exacerbate the clinical manifestations of AD (Table 45-11). The client with AD frequently has other medical problems such as cardiovascular disease, arthritis, renal insufficiency, and pulmonary disease. Changes in vision and hearing may also be present. Treating and controlling these conditions optimize the client's functional abilities.

NIC **Cognitive Stimulation/ Memory Training.** The purpose of cognitive stimulation and memory training is to

TABLE 45-11 Factors That Can Worsen Alzheimer's Disease

- Stroke
- Subdural hematoma
- Space-occupying lesion
- Decrease in blood supply to the brain
- Myocardial infarction
- Dysrhythmias
- Hypoglycemia
- Impaired renal function
- Impaired hepatic function
- Infection
- Impaired vision and hearing
- Sudden changes in surroundings
- Pain and discomfort
- Drugs
- Physical restraint

reinforce or promote desirable cognitive function and facilitate memory (Chart 45-13). An individualized cognitive therapy program may provide some benefit to the client; however, reported clinical studies have not demonstrated its efficacy for early-stage AD (Clare et al., 2003).

Structuring the Environment. The health care team collaborates to identify conditions in the environment that can be modified to increase the client's ability to function. The two most important actions that are necessary for the client with AD are preventing overstimulation and providing a structured and orderly environment.

Preventing Overstimulation. Environmental distractions and noise should be kept to a minimum. The client's home (hospital or institution room) should not have pictures on the wall or other decorations that could be misinterpreted as people or animals that could harm the client. An abstract painting or wallpaper might look like a fire or an explosion and might scare the client. The room should have adequate, nonglare lighting and no potentially frightening shadows.

In addition to disturbed sleep, other negative effects of high noise levels include decreased nutritional intake, changes in blood pressure and pulse rates, and feelings of increased stress and anxiety. The client with AD is especially susceptible to these changes and needs to have as much undisturbed sleep at night as possible. Fatigue increases confusion and behavioral manifestations such as agitation and aggressiveness.

When a client is in a new setting or environment (hospital, assisted-living, or long-term care facility), the staff works with the admitting department to select a room that is in the quietest area of the unit and away from obvious exits, if possible. A private room may be needed if the client has a history of agitation or wandering. The television should remain off unless the client turns it on or requests that it be turned on.

Providing Consistency. Objects such as furniture, a hairbrush, and eyeglasses should be kept in the same place. A daily routine is established and followed as much as possible. The client's bedroom could have a communication board on which scheduled activities and other data to promote orientation are listed, such as the day of the week, the month, and the year. Pictures of people familiar to the client can be placed on this board.

Orientation and Validation Therapy. Changes in routine need to be explained to the client before the occurrence, repeating the explanation immediately before the changes take place. Clocks and single-date calendars also help the client maintain day-to-day orientation to the environment in the early stages of the disease process. For the client with early disease, **reality orientation** is usually appropriate. Family members and health care professionals should frequently reorient the client to the environment.

For the client in the later stages of AD, reality orientation is ineffective and often increases agitation. The health care team uses validation therapy for the client with moderate or severe AD. In **validation therapy,** the staff member recognizes and acknowledges the client's feelings and concerns. For example, if the client is looking for a deceased mother, ask the client to talk about what the mother looks like and what she might be wearing. This response does not refute the client, but also does not reinforce the client's belief that the mother is still living.

Promoting Independence in Activities of Daily Living. As the disease progresses, altered thought processes affect the ability to perform activities of daily living (ADLs). Encourage the client to perform as much self-care as possible and to maintain independence in daily living skills as long as possible. For example, in the home setting, complete clothing outfits that can be easily removed and put on (e.g., shirt, slacks, underwear, and socks) can be placed on a single hanger; the client selects from these groupings. When possible, the client should participate in meal preparation, grocery shopping, and other household routines.

The occupational and physical therapists provide a complete evaluation and assistance in helping the client become more independent. Adaptive devices, such as grab bars in the bathtub or shower area, an elevated commode, and adapted eating utensils, may enable the client to maintain independence in grooming, toileting, and feeding. The physical therapist prescribes an exercise program for the client to improve physical health and functionality.

Promoting Bowel and Bladder Continence. The client may remain continent of bowel and bladder for long periods if taken to the bathroom or given a bedpan or urinal every 2 hours or more often during the day, and possibly less frequently at night. The caregiver encourages the client to drink adequate fluids to promote optimal voiding. A client may refuse to drink enough fluids because of a fear of incontinence. Assure the client that he or she will be toileted on a regular schedule to prevent incontinent episodes.

When clients with AD are in the hospital or other unfamiliar place, they may get out of bed unassisted during the

CHART 45-13

NIC INTERVENTION ACTIVITIES for The Client with Alzheimer's Disease

Cognitive Stimulation: *Promotion of awareness and comprehension of surroundings by utilization of planned stimuli*

- Offer environmental stimulation through contact with varied personnel.
- Present change gradually.
- Provide a calendar.
- Allow for rest periods.
- Use repetition to present new material.
- Present information in small, concrete portions.
- Use touch therapeutically.

Memory Training: *Facilitation of memory*

- Discuss with client/family any practical memory problems experienced.
- Stimulate memory by repeating client's last expressed thought, as appropriate.
- Reminisce about past experiences with client, as appropriate.
- Implement appropriate memory techniques such as visual imagery, mnemonic devices, memory games, memory cues, association techniques, making lists, using computers, using name tags, or rehearsing information.
- Provide for orientation training, such as client rehearsing personal information and dates, as appropriate.
- Provide for picture recognition memory, as appropriate.
- Encourage client to participate in group memory training programs, as appropriate.
- Monitor client's behavior during therapy.

night and fall while trying to locate the bathroom. In some hospitals, the side rails on beds are required to be up for all clients older than 60 or 65 years of age. However, if the client climbs over the side rail and falls, the injury is likely to be worse than if the bed had been left in the lowest position and the side rail left down (preferably the lower rail in a split rail system). Maintain an unobstructed path between the bed and bathroom at all times. For clients who are too weak to walk to the bathroom, a bedside commode may be used. (See Chapter 5 for further discussion on fall prevention.) Some clients may void in inappropriate places, such as the sink or a wastebasket. As a reminder of where they should toilet, place a picture of the commode on the bathroom door. Depending on written signs for identification is useless because most clients lose their ability to read as the disease progresses.

Assisting with Facial Recognition. As the disease progresses, the client may experience **prosopagnosia,** an inability to recognize oneself and other familiar faces. Encourage the family to provide pictures of family members and close friends that are labeled with the person's name on the picture. In addition, advise the family to reminisce with the client about pleasant experiences from the past. The nurse may also conduct reminiscence therapy while assisting the client with ADLs or performing a treatment or assessment. Referring to a personal item in the room may help the client begin to talk about its meaning in the present and in the past.

It is not unusual for the client to talk to his or her image in the mirror. This behavior should be allowed as long as it is not harmful. If the client becomes frightened by the mirror image, remove or cover the mirror. In some health care settings, a picture of the client is placed on the room door to help with facial recognition and to help the client locate his or her room. This picture also helps the staff locate the client in case of elopement (running away).

Promoting Communication. With the intervention known as **redirection,** attracting the client's attention before conversing helps with communication problems and nonlistening behaviors. The environment should be as free of distractions as possible. The caregiver speaks directly to the client in a distinct manner. Sentences should be clear and short. The client is asked to perform one task at a time, and sufficient time must be allowed for completion. It may be necessary to break each task down into many small steps.

As the disease progresses, the client is unable to perform tasks when asked. Show the client what needs to be done or provide cues to remind the client how to perform the task. When possible, explain and demonstrate the task that the client is asked to perform.

Drug Therapy. Cholinesterase inhibitors are drugs approved for symptomatic treatment of AD. These drugs improve cholinergic neurotransmission in the central nervous system (CNS) by delaying the destruction of acetylcholine (ACh) by acetylcholinesterase, thus delaying the onset of cognitive decline. None of these drugs affects the course of the disease. Examples include donepezil (Aricept), galantamine (Reminyl), and rivastigmine (Exelon).

Memantine (Namenda) is the first of a new class of medications that is a low to moderate affinity NMDA (N-methyl-D-aspartate) receptor antagonist. Overexcitation of NMDA receptors by the neurotransmitter glutamate may play a role in AD. This drug therefore blocks excess amounts of glutamate that can damage nerve cells. It is indicated for advanced AD and has been shown to slow the pace of deterioration, and it maintains functionality for a few months longer. Some clients show improved memory and thinking skills. This drug may also be given with donepezil (Aricept), a cholinesterase inhibitor.

Some clients with AD experience depression and may be treated with antidepressants. Selective serotonin reuptake inhibitors (SSRIs), such as paroxetine (Paxil) and sertraline (Zoloft), are usually prescribed. Tricyclic antidepressants, such as amitriptyline (Elavil, Levate✱), should not be used because of their anticholinergic effect.

Psychotropic drugs, also called antipsychotic and neuroleptic drugs, should be reserved for clients with emotional and behavioral health problems that sometimes accompany dementia, such as hallucinations and delusions. In clinical practice, however, these drugs are sometimes inappropriately used for agitation, combativeness, or restlessness. Psychotropic drugs are considered chemical restraints because they decrease mobility and clients' ability to care for themselves. Therefore most geriatricians recommend that these medications be used as a last resort and with caution in low doses for a specific emotional or behavioral health problem, because most clients with dementia are in late adulthood (see Chapter 5). The specific drug prescribed depends on side effects, the condition of the client, and anticipated outcomes. Institutional policy should be followed concerning the use of chemical restraints.

Complementary and Alternative Therapies. A number of complementary and alternative therapies are being researched that may prevent AD, slow its occurrence, or slow its progression in older adults. Examples of these therapies include vitamin E (antioxidants), ibuprofen, estrogen, melatonin, and nicotine patches. Art, massage, dance, and music therapy are often used in long-term care settings to minimize agitation.

RISK FOR INJURY

NOC **PLANNING: EXPECTED OUTCOMES.** The client with Alzheimer's disease (AD) is expected to remain free from physical harm and not injure anyone else. A safe home environment is also expected for those clients at home or in a homelike environment, such as assisted-living. Indicators include that there will be totally adequate:

- Provision of lighting
- Placement of handrails
- Safe storage of medications
- Provision of assistive devices in accessible locations
- Arrangement of furniture to reduce risks

INTERVENTIONS. Many clients with AD tend to wander and may easily become lost. In later stages of the disease, some clients may become severely agitated and physically or verbally abusive to others.

Coping with Restlessness and Wandering. The Alzheimer's Disease Association estimates that almost two thirds of clients will wander and become temporarily lost in the community. The client should always wear an identification badge or bracelet when at home. The badge should include how to contact the primary caregiver. In an inpatient setting, the client is checked frequently and placed in a room that can be monitored easily. The room may need to be close to the nurses' station (if the noise level in the nurses' station can be managed) and away from exits and stairs. Some health care agencies place large stop signs or red tape on the floor in front of exits. Others have installed alarm systems to indicate when a client is opening the door.

The client's family may choose to enroll in the Safe Return Program, a national, government-funded program of the Alzheimer's Association that assists in the identification and safe, timely return of individuals with Alzheimer's disease and related dementias who wander off and become lost. The program includes registration of the client and a 24-hour hotline to be called to assist in finding a lost client. If a client wanders and becomes lost, the family (or health care institutions) should immediately notify the police department. An up-to-date picture of the client makes it easier for local authorities, the public, and neighbors to identify the missing client.

Restlessness may be decreased if the client is taken for frequent walks. If the client begins to wander, he or she is redirected. For example, if the client insists on going shopping for clothes, the client is redirected to his or her closet to select clothing that will not be recognized as his or her own. This type of activity can be repeated a number of times because the client has lost short-term memory.

In any setting, clients should be kept busy with structured activities. In a health care agency, an activity therapist or volunteer may work with clients as a group or individually to determine the type of activity that is appropriate for the stage of the disease. Puzzles, board games, and art activities are often appropriate. Music and art therapy are becoming very popular in acute and long-term care for clients with dementia.

Physical restraints, such as waist belts and geri-chairs with lapboards, should be applied only as a last resort because they often increase the restlessness and cause agitation. Federal regulations in long-term care facilities in the United States mandate that all residents have the right to be free of both physical and chemical restraints. In addition, agencies accredited by the Joint Commission on Accreditation of Healthcare Agencies (JCAHO) are required to minimize the use of restraints and use alternatives (see Chapter 5).

Ensuring Safety. Clients with AD may become injured because they cannot recognize objects or situations as harmful. All potentially dangerous objects (e.g., knives, needles, and cleaning solutions) are removed or secured. Clients are often unaware that their driving ability is impaired and usually want to continue this activity even if their driver's license has been suspended secondary to the disease. Automobile keys must be secured and the client appropriately informed.

Late in the disease process, the client may experience seizure activity. If the client is cared for at home, teach caregivers what action to take when a seizure occurs (see earlier discussion under Interventions [Seizures and Epilepsy], p. 951).

Minimizing Agitation. Talking calmly and softly and attempting to redirect the client to a more positive behavior or activity is an effective strategy when he or she is agitated. Use calm, positive statements and reassure the client that he or she is safe. Statements such as "I'm sorry that you are upset. I know it's hard. I will stay until you feel better" may help.

Actions to avoid when the client is agitated include raising the voice, confrontation, arguing, reasoning, taking offense, or explaining. The caregiver should not show alarm or make sudden movements out of the person's view. If the client remains agitated, ensure the client's safety and leave the room after explaining that you will return later. Frequent visual checks must be done during this time. If the client is connected to any type of tubing or other device, he or she may try to disconnect it or pull it out. These devices should be used sparingly in the client with dementia. If IV access, for example, is needed, the catheter or cannula is placed in an area that the client cannot easily see.

Another way to manage this problem is to provide a diversion. For example, if the client is doing an activity or holding an item such as a stuffed animal or doll, he or she might be less likely to pay attention to medical devices. Additional strategies to minimize behavioral problems are listed in Table 45-12.

TABLE 45-12 Minimizing Behavioral Problems at Home

Carefully evaluate the client's environment.
- Ensure environment is safe:
  - Remove throw rugs.
  - Consider replacing tile floors with nonslippery floors.
  - Arrange furniture and room decorations to maximize the client's safety when walking.
  - Minimize clutter in all rooms in and outside of the house.
  - Install night lights in client's room, bathroom, and hallway.
  - Install and maintain smoke alarms, fire alarms, and natural gas detectors.
- Install safety devices for the bathroom.
- Install alarm system or bells on outside doors; place safety locks on doors and gates.
- Ensure that door locks cannot be easily opened by the client.

Assist the client to remain oriented as long as possible.
- Place single-date calendars in client's room and in kitchen.
- Use large-faced clocks with a neutral background.

Communicate with the client based on his or her ability to understand.
- As the disease progresses, use simple language and explain activities before the client needs to carry it out.
- Break complex tasks down to simple steps.

Encourage the client to be as independent as possible in activities of daily living.
- Place complete outfits for the day on hangers; have the client select one to wear.
- Develop and maintain a predictable routine (e.g., meals, bedtime, morning routine)

When a problem behavior occurs, use distraction to divert client to another activity.

Minimize excessive stimulation.
- Take the client on outings when crowds are small.
- If crowds cannot be avoided, minimize the amount of time the client is present in a crowd, for example, at family gatherings, provide a quiet room for the client to rest throughout the visit.

Arrange for a day care program if possible.

Register the client with the Alzheimer's Association Safe Return Program.

COMPROMISED FAMILY COPING/CAREGIVER ROLE STRAIN

NOC **PLANNING: EXPECTED OUTCOMES.** The family or other caregivers of the client with Alzheimer's disease (AD) are expected to have a positive perception of their health status and life circumstances. Indicators include that they will be completely satisfied with their:
- Physical health
- Psychological health

- Lifestyle
- Performance of usual roles
- Social support
- Availability of respite

INTERVENTIONS. The client with AD requires continual, 24-hour supervision and caregiving. Severe cognitive changes leave the client unable to manage finances, property, or personal care. The family needs to seek legal counsel regarding the client's competency and the need to obtain guardianship or a durable medical power of attorney when necessary. The family can be referred to the local AD support group for literature and information concerning the disease and related problems.

Family members and other caregivers must be aware of their own health and stress levels. Signs of stress include anger, social withdrawal, anxiety, depression, lack of concentration, sleepiness, irritability, and health problems. When signs of stress occur, the caregiver should be referred to their health care provider or should seek one on his or her own.

DISTURBED SLEEP PATTERN

PLANNING: EXPECTED OUTCOMES. The client with AD is expected to sleep through the night and be awake at appropriate times.

INTERVENTIONS. The client with AD often has difficulty sleeping at night but tends to nap frequently during the day. Suggest ways to enhance sleep to the family or other caregiver. One way to establish the usual day-night pattern is to keep the client very active during the day. A daily routine that consists of a balance between passive activities and those requiring more strenuous exercise, such as walking or stretching activities, usually facilitates sleep at night. The client may want to take a nap in the late afternoon, but this should be discouraged if possible. In the last stage of the disease, the client may sleep during much of the day and night.

To facilitate sleep, instruct the family to establish a before-bedtime ritual. The routine usually consists of personal hygiene activities (e.g., bathing, toileting, brushing teeth) and environmental control measures to reduce noise and eliminate distractions. A back rub or small snack may help the client prepare for sleep.

The client's treatment and medication schedule is adjusted to provide for uninterrupted sleep. If more conventional measures fail to induce sleep, the health care provider may prescribe a mild antianxiety agent or hypnotic.

Community-Based Care

HOME CARE MANAGEMENT

Alzheimer's disease (AD) is a chronic, progressive condition that eventually leaves the client completely disoriented and totally dependent on others for all aspects of care. In the early stages, clients may be cared for at home with little need for outside intervention. Whenever possible, the client and family should be assigned a case manager who can assess their needs for health care resources and facilitate appropriate placement throughout the continuum of care.

The client usually begins to withdraw from friends and social events as memory impairment and personality and behavior changes become more apparent. This increases the family's responsibilities to minimize the impact of social isolation and decreased activity. The family may begin to decrease their own social activities as the demands of the client's care take more of their time. Emphasize to the family the importance of maintaining their own social contacts and leisure activities. Many family members experience caregiver stress, which affects their physical, mental, and emotional health. Chart 45-14 lists strategies for reducing caregiver stress. (See Chapter 5 for further discussion on caregiver role strain and interventions.)

CHART 45-14

BEST PRACTICE for Reducing Caregiver Stress

- Maintain realistic expectations for the person with Alzheimer's disease (AD).
- Take each day one at a time.
- Try to find the positive aspects of each incident or situation.
- Use humor with the person who has AD.
- Use the resources of the Alzheimer's Association, including attending local support group meetings.
- Explore alternative care settings early in the disease process for possible use later.
- Establish advance directives with the AD client early in the disease process.
- Set aside time each day for rest or recreation away from the client, if possible.
- Seek respite care periodically for longer periods of time.
- Take care of yourself by watching your diet, exercising, and getting plenty of rest.
- Be realistic about what you or they can do, and accept help from family, friends, and community resources.
- Use relaxation techniques.

It is now possible in most areas of the United States for the family to arrange respite care. The client may be placed in a respite facility or nursing home for the weekend or for several weeks to give the family a rest from the constant care demands. The family may also be able to obtain respite care in the home through a home care agency or the Alzheimer's Disease and Related Disorders Association (often called the Alzheimer's Association). Stress that respite care is for a short period of time; it is not a permanent placement. Some health care agencies have opened adult day care centers or specialty units for clients with AD. In the day care center, clients spend all or part of the day at the facility and participate in activities as their condition permits. Although these centers are usually open only on weekdays, this arrangement allows the caregiver to work or participate in other activities.

Teach the family how to be prepared in case the client becomes restless, agitated, abusive, or combative. In addition, the family can learn how to use reality orientation or validation therapy, depending on the stage of the disease.

HEALTH TEACHING

Usually the client with AD is cared for in the home until late in the disease process. Because health insurance coverage in the United States and family finances are usually insufficient to cover the services of a private duty nurse or home care aide, family members typically provide the care. The client care plan developed by the nurse or case manager, in conjunction with the family, must be reasonable and realistic for the family to implement.

Review how to assist with bathing, dressing, toileting, and other self-care activities. The occupational therapist teaches the family and the client how to use adaptive equipment, such as a brace, a sling, a cane, or modified eating utensils.

The client may have difficulty chewing, swallowing, or tasting foods and may not be able to eat without assistance.

The family and the dietitian should develop a diet plan to maximize the client's nutritional intake. In the late stage of AD, the client's intake often decreases, and he or she loses weight.

Provide information to the family on what to do in the event of a seizure and how to protect the client from injury. Instruct the family to notify the health care provider if the seizure is prolonged or if the client's seizure pattern changes.

DRUG THERAPY. The name, time, and route of administration; the dosage; and the side effects of all medications are explained to the family or other caregiver. Remind the family to check with the health care provider before using any over-the-counter medications because they may interact with prescribed medication.

EXERCISE. Emphasis is placed on the need for the client to have an established exercise program to maintain mobility as long as possible, as well as to prevent complications of immobility. In collaboration with the family, the physical therapist develops an individualized exercise program. The physical therapist may continue to work with the client at home until goals are achieved, depending on the payer source.

SAFETY. Remind the family or other caregiver to take special precautions to maintain the client safely at home. The environment must be uncluttered, consistent, and structured. All hazardous items (e.g., cleaning fluids, power tools, insect spray) are removed or secured. All electrical sockets not in use should be covered with safety plugs. Handrails and grab bars should be installed in the bathroom; handrails should be along all stairways, and a guardrail should be placed around porches or open stairwells. Because the client may have a tendency to wander, especially at night, the family may want to install alarms to all outside doors, the basement, and the client's bedroom. All outside and basement doors should have deadbolt locks to prevent the client from going outside unsupervised. The temperature of the water heater should be adjusted to prevent accidental burns. Night lights should be used in the client's bedroom, hallway, and bathroom.

When the client can no longer be cared for at home, referral to an assisted-living or long-term care facility may be needed. Early in the course of the disease, advise the family that placement might be needed in the late stages of the disease. This allows the family to begin the search process for an appropriate facility before a crisis develops and immediate placement is needed. A number of facilities specialize in the care of clients with AD and other dementias. These units generally have a high staff-to-client ratio and are architecturally designed to meet the special needs of this type of client. The national office of the Alzheimer's Association publishes an outline of criteria for a dementia unit.

All families should be referred to their local chapter of the Alzheimer's Association. This organization provides information and support services to clients and their families, including seminars, audiovisual aids, and publications.

◆Evaluation: Outcomes

Evaluate the care of the client with Alzheimer's disease (AD) on the basis of the identified nursing diagnoses. The expected outcomes include that the client will:

- Have the ability to execute complex mental processes (early AD)
- Remain free from injury and have a safe home environment
- Sleep through the night and be awake at appropriate times

The caregiver will have a positive perception of his or her health status and life circumstances. Specific indicators for these outcomes are listed for each nursing diagnosis under the Planning and Implementation section (see earlier).

HUNTINGTON DISEASE

OVERVIEW

Huntington disease (HD), formerly called Huntington chorea, is a hereditary disorder transmitted as an autosomal dominant trait at the time of conception.

Genetic Considerations

Huntington disease is a single gene disorder caused by a mutation in the HD gene located on chromosome 4. The mutation is a multiple repeat of the specific base triplet CAG, increasing the length of the gene. An autosomal dominant trait with high penetrance means that a person who inherits just one mutated allele has nearly a 100% chance of developing the disease. This gene mutation has different expressions depending on whether it is inherited from the mother or father. People who inherit the mutation from their fathers have an earlier onset and a shorter life expectancy than do those who inherit from their mothers. In addition, there is some variation in the disease depending on the size (length) of the mutation. The longer the mutation, the more severe the disease is at an earlier age.

It is estimated that 25,000 people in the United States have HD, and another 20,000 to 50,000 are thought to carry the gene. Men and women are equally affected, and symptoms begin between 35 and 50 years of age, striking at a highly productive time in life. The clinical onset of HD is gradual. The two main symptoms of the disease are progressive mental status changes, leading to dementia, and **choreiform movements** (rapid, jerky movements) in the limbs, trunk, and facial muscles. Dementia is related to the destruction of neurons within the cerebral cortex; it may also be associated with excessive amounts of dopamine found within the cerebral cortex and limbic systems of those affected. Two structures within the basal ganglia are involved in the development of HD: the caudate nucleus and the putamen. Both structures have close connections to the cerebral cortex and are closely associated with neurotransmitters. Neurotransmitters are secreted at the synapse, or junction, of one neuron with another, and it is through their specific excitation or inhibition of neurons that fine, controlled, integrated motor activity occurs.

In the presence of HD, there is a decrease in the amount of gamma-aminobutyric acid (GABA) and acetylcholine (ACh), both excitatory neurotransmitters. Dopamine is not affected. This shift in balance between dopamine (an inhibitory neurotransmitter) and GABA at the synapse leads to uninhibited motor activity. The result is brisk, jerky, purposeless movements, particularly of the hands, face, tongue, and legs, which the client is unable to stop.

There are three stages of HD, each lasting roughly 5 years, corresponding to the average 15-year course of the disease. Stage 1 is the onset of neurologic or psychological symptoms; stage 2 is characterized by an increasing dependence on others for care; stage 3 results in loss of independent function.

The diagnosis of HD is made on the basis of a family history of the disease and clinical assessment. The triad of dominant inheritance, choreoathetosis (neuromuscular symptoms), and dementia are hallmarks of the disease. The symptoms exhibited by the client vary in range and severity, age of onset, and rate of progression. Clinical manifestations include chorea, poor balance, hesitant or explosive speech, dysphagia, impaired respiration, and bowel and bladder incontinence. Mental status changes include decreased attention span, poor judgment, memory loss, personality changes, and dementia (later in the disease process).

COLLABORATIVE MANAGEMENT

There is no known cure or treatment for HD. The only way to prevent transmission of the gene is for those affected to refrain from having children. Genetic counseling is important for children of clients with the disease. People at risk for the disease can be tested to determine whether or not the gene is present on chromosome 4. Before the testing procedure is undertaken, counseling is necessary to ensure that the client has voluntarily decided in favor of testing and is not being pressured by family or friends. In addition, counseling helps determine whether the benefits of knowing the results outweigh the risks of a positive result (e.g., depression or suicide).

Antipsychotic agents or monoamine-depleting agents may be used to manage movement abnormalities that interfere with ADLs or are functionally disabling. They are also used to help control agitation, hallucinations, or psychotic delusions. Medications may be use to treat other symptoms such as depression, anxiety, or obsessive-compulsive behaviors. Many of the medications used to treat HD may cause side effects that may be difficult to differentiate from signs of HD.

The care of the client with HD is managed by the collaborative efforts of the family and health care team:

- Speech-language pathologist helps with communication and swallowing.
- Registered dietitian plans meals.
- Physical and occupational therapists determine exercise conditioning and assistive devices
- Home care nurse and home health care aide give direct care and assessment of the client and assistance to the care provider.
- Case manager and social worker coordinate care and referrals to community agencies.

GET READY for the NCLEX Examination!

KEY POINTS

Safe Effective Care Environment

- For a client having a tonic-clonic or complete partial seizure, protect the client from injury. Other interventions are listed in Chart 45-5.
- For clients who have had one or more seizures, place on "seizure precautions," which includes having oxygen and suctioning emergency equipment available, starting an IV access, and putting the side rails up at all times.
- Implement interventions as summarized in Chart 45-7 for clients having status epilepticus, a life-threatening emergency.
- For clients with meningitis, carefully monitor neurologic status, including vital signs; observe for signs and symptoms of increased intracranial pressure (ICP).
- Assess level of consciousness (LOC) as a priority in clients with encephalitis.
- Monitor for drug toxicity when clients are taking medications for Parkinson disease, especially levodopa combinations, such as Sinemet. Delirium and decreased drug effectiveness are the most common indicators of toxicity.
- Observe clients with Alzheimer's disease closely because they tend to wander and make inappropriate decisions; safety is a priority for these clients.

Health Promotion and Maintenance

- Teach clients with an aura before migraine headaches the importance of taking abortive drugs to prevent a migraine episode.
- Teach clients with cluster headaches about precipitating factors, such as anger episodes, excitement, and excessive physical activity.
- In addition to prescribed drug therapy, encourage clients with headaches to use complementary and alternative therapies to help relieve pain, such as ice, darkened room, and relaxation techniques. Dietary changes help some clients by avoiding certain trigger foods (e.g., caffeine, beer, wine, pickled products).
- Teach the client with epilepsy the importance of continuing prescribed antiepileptic drugs (AEDs), even if he or she is seizure-free; additional instructions for the client and family are listed in Chart 45-4.
- If not contraindicated by other condition or age, encourage people who are in areas of high population density, such as college dormitories and crowded living areas, to become immunized against meningococcal meningitis.
- Teach people who enjoy outdoor activities to avoid areas where mosquitoes and ticks are likely to populate, especially near lakes and wooded areas. If in contact with these areas, remind them (especially older adults) to use insect repellent and keep skin exposure at a minimum.
- Teach clients and caregivers how to provide a safe home environment for clients with Parkinson or Alzheimer's disease.

Psychosocial Integrity

- Remind caregivers of clients with chronic neurologic diseases, such as Alzheimer's disease, to find ways to cope with their stress to remain physically and psychologically healthy, as suggested in Chart 45-14.
- Teach caregivers of clients with dementia to use validation therapy, rather than reality orientation; acknowledge the client's feelings and concerns.
- Be aware that clients with Parkinson disease may develop dementia as the disease progresses.

Physiological Integrity

- Assess for characteristic clinical manifestations in clients with classic migraine headaches as listed in Chart 45-1.

- Recall that the pain of cluster headaches is usually accompanied by ipsilateral (same side) eye tearing, rhinorrhea, congestion, ptosis, facial sweating, eyelid edema, and/or miosis.
- Recognize that generalized seizures, such as the tonic-clonic seizure, involve both cerebral hemispheres; partial seizures, also called focal or local seizures, usually involve only one hemisphere.
- During a seizure, document client's body movements and other assessments as described in Chart 45-6.
- Monitor for side and adverse effects of antiepileptic drugs (AEDs) as listed in Chart 45-3.
- Assess for clinical manifestations of meningitis as listed in Chart 45-8.
- Assess for key features of Parkinson disease as described in Chart 45-10.
- Collaborate with physical and occupational therapists, dietitian, and speech-language pathologist in planning and providing care for clients with Parkinson or Alzheimer's disease.
- Keep in mind that newer surgical procedures, such as deep brain stimulation, and experimental stem cell therapies are becoming available as options to control symptoms of Parkinson disease.
- Assess cognitive and functional abilities of the client with Alzheimer's disease, recognizing that it is a progressive dementia with several stages as listed in Chart 45-12.
- Recall that both familial (early onset) and late onset (advanced age) Alzheimer's disease has a genetic predisposition that continues to be researched.
- For clients with Alzheimer's disease, recall that the newer drugs seem to improve function and cognition (cholinesterase inhibitors; e.g., donepezil [Aricept]) or slow the disease process (Memantine), but they do not cure the disease.
- Administer psychotropic medications to clients with Alzheimer's disease who also have mental/behavioral health problems, such as depression and severe agitation.
- Remember that Huntington disease is a chronic, hereditary illness that is transmitted as an autosomal dominant trait at the time of conception; refer clients with the disease for genetic counseling.

ADDITIONAL STUDY RESOURCES

Go to your Student CD-ROM for Review Questions for the NCLEX Examination.

evolve Go to http://evolve.elsevier.com/Iggy/ for Integrated Management of Care Questions for the NCLEX Examination.

SELECTED BIBLIOGRAPHY

Armstrong, T., Kanusky, J.T., & Gilbert, M.R. (2003). Seize the moment to learn about epilepsy in people with cancer. *Clinical Journal of Oncology Nursing, 7*(2), 163-171.

Bender, K., & Thompson, F.E. (2003). West Nile virus: A growing challenge. *American Journal of Nursing, 103*(6), 32-40.

Berg, A. (2003). How long does it take for epilepsy to become intractable? *Neurology, 60*(2), 186.

Betchen, S.A., & Kaplitt, M. (2003). Future and current surgical therapies in Parkinson's disease. *Current Opinion in Neurology, 16*(4), 487-493.

Bridy MA. (2001).The importance of quickly initiating antibiotic therapy in a 20-year-old man with bacterial meningitis. *Journal of Emergency Nursing, 27*(5), 437-439.

Burdick, W.P. (2003). Computed tomography of the head before lumbar puncture in adults with suspected meningitis. *Annals of Emergency Medicine, 41*(1), 161-162.

Chen, H., et al. (2003). Nonsteroidal anti-inflammatory drugs and the risk of Parkinson disease. *Archives of Neurology, 60*(8), 1059-1064.

Clare, L., et al. (2003). A. Cognitive rehabilitation and cognitive training for early-stage Alzheimer's disease and vascular dementia. In *The Cochrane Library,* Issue 4. Chichester, UK, John Wiley & Sons.

Clark, C.M., & Karlawish, J.H.T. (2003). Alzheimer disease: Current concepts and emerging diagnostic and therapeutic strategies. *Annals of Internal Medicine, 138*(5):400-410.

Cohen, J. (2003). Management of bacterial meningitis in adults: Algorithm from the British Infection Society represents current standard of care. *British Journal of Medicine, 326*(7397), 996-997.

Cummings, J.L., et al. (2002a). Guidelines for managing Alzheimer's disease, Part 1. *American Family Physician, 65*(11), 263-272.

Cummings, J.L., et al. (2002b). Guidelines for managing Alzheimer's disease, Part 2. *American Family Physician, 65*(12), 525-534.

de Gans, J., & van de Beek, D. (2002). Dexamethasone in adults with bacterial meningitis. *New England Journal of Medicine, 347*(20), 1549-1556, 1639-1640.

Edwards, N.E., & Scheetz, P.S. (2002). Predictors of burden for caregivers of patients with Parkinson's disease. *Journal of Neuroscience Nursing, 34*(4), 184-190.

Evans, R.W., & Olesen, J. (2003). Migraine classification, diagnostic criteria, and testing. *American Academy of Neurology, 60*(7) Supplement 2, S24-S30.

Franzini, A., et al. (2003). Stimulation of the posterior hypothalamus for treatment of chronic intractable cluster headaches. *Neurosurgery, 52*(5), 1095-1101.

Gambrell, M., & Flynn, N. (2004). Seizures 101. *Nursing 2004, 34*(8), 36-41.

Gilliam, F. (2002). Optimizing health outcomes in epilepsy. *Neurology, 8*(Supplement 5), S9-S20.

Guttman, M., Kish, S.J., & Furukawa, Y. (2003). Current concepts in the diagnosis and management of Parkinson's disease. *Canadian Medical Association Journal, 168*(3), 293-301.

Hickey, J.V. (2003). *The clinical practice of neurological and neurosurgical nursing* (5th ed.). Philadelphia: Lippincott-Raven.

Holroyd, K.A., & Mauskop, A. (2003). Complementary and alternative treatments. *Neurology, 60*(7) (Supplement 2), S58-S62.

Kolb-Lucas, K. (2003). Strategies for treating migraine. *Nursing, 33*(5), 32cc4-32cc6.

Lipton, R.B., et al. (2003). A self-administered screener for migraine in primary care. *Neurology, 61*(3), 375-382.

Lockey, A.S. (2002). Emergency department drug therapy for status epilepticus in adults. *Emergency Medicine Journal, 19*(2):96-100.

Lopez, O.L., et al. (2002). Cholinesterase inhibitor treatment alters the natural history of Alzheimer's disease. *Journal of Neurology, Neurosurgery & Psychiatry, 72*(3):310-314.

Matchar, D.B. (2003). Acute management of migraine. Highlights of the U.S. Headache Consortium. *Neurology, 60*(7) (Supplement 2), S21-S23.

McNamara, P., et al. (2003). Counterfactual cognitive deficit in persons with Parkinson's disease. *Journal of Neurology, Neurosurgery & Psychiatry, 74*(8):1065-1070.

Meador, K.J. (2002). Cognitive outcomes and predictive factors in epilepsy. Optimizing epilepsy management: Seizure control, medication tolerability, and co-morbidities. *American Academy of Neurology, 58* (Supplement 5), S21-S26.

Melchart, D., et al. (2003). Acupuncture versus placebo versus sumatriptan for early treatment of migraine attacks: A randomized controlled trial. *Journal of Internal Medicine, 253*(2), 181-188.

Miller, J.L. (2002). Parkinson's disease primer. *Geriatric Nursing, 23*(2), 69-74.

Miyasaki, J.M., et al. (2002). Practice parameter: Initiation of treatment for Parkinson's disease: An evidenced based review. *Neurology, 58*(1), 11-17.

Nussbaum, R.L., & Ellis, C.E. (2003). Alzheimer's disease and Parkinson's disease. *New England Journal of Medicine, 348*(14), 1356-1364.

Pena, C.G. (2003). Emergency: Seizure. *American Journal of Nursing, 103*(11), 73-81.

Peters, J.M., et al. (2003). Olfactory function in mild cognitive impairment and Alzheimer's disease: An investigation using psychophysical and electrophysiological techniques. *American Journal of Psychiatry, 160,* 1995-2002.

Ravina, B.M., et al. (2003). Neuroprotective agents for clinical trials in Parkinson's disease: A systematic assessment. *Neurology, 60*(8):1234-1240.

Redington, J.J., & Tyler, K.L. (2002). Viral infections of the nervous system, 2002: Update on diagnosis and treatment. *Archives of Neurology, 59,* 712-718.

Rowe, M.A. (2003). People with dementia who become lost. *American Journal of Nursing, 103*(5), 32-40.

Sheth, R. (2002). Epilepsy surgery: Presurgical evaluation. *Neurology Clinics, 20*(4), 1195.

Smith, L.P. (2003). Steady the course of Parkinson's disease. *Nursing Management, 34*(4), 35-39.

Smolowitz, J., & Waters, C. (2001). Clinical management of the adult with Parkinson's disease. *The American Journal for Nurse Practitioners, 5*(7), 9-34.

Souder, E., & Beck, C. (2004). Overview of Alzheimer's disease. *Nursing Clinics of North America, 39*(3), 545-559.

Sparano, N.I. (2001). Is the combination of ibuprofen and caffeine effective for the treatment of a tension-type headache? *Journal of Family Practice, 50*(1), 10.

Tammelleo, A.D. (2003). Was there a duty to warn nurse of meningitis risk? *Nursing Law's Regan Report, 43*(12), 1.

Thomas, E., et al. (2003). The diagnostic accuracy of Kernig's sign, Brudzinski's sign, and nuchal rigidity in adults with suspected meningitis. *Annals of Emergency Medicine, 42*(2), 311-312.

Tolosa, E. (2003). Advances in the pharmacological management of Parkinson disease. *Journal of Neural Transmission, Supplementum* (64), 65-78.

Tunkel, A.R., & Scheld, W.M. (2003). Corticosteroids for everyone with meningitis? *New England Journal of Medicine, 347*(20), 1613-1615.

United Health Care. (2002). *Clinical evidence concise.* London: BMJ Publishing Group.

Van Den Eeden, S.K, et al. (2003). Incidence of Parkinson's disease: Variation by age, gender, and race/ethnicity. *American Journal of Epidemiology, 157*(11), 1015-1022.

Vaughan, J., & Hardie, R.J. (2002). The differential diagnosis of Parkinson's disease. *Reviews in Clinical Gerontology, 12*(1):40-51.

Velling, D.A., Dodick, D.W., & Muir, J.J. (2003). Sustained-release niacin for prevention of migraine headache. *Mayo Clinic Proceedings, 78*(6), 770-771.

Welch, K.M, Cutrer, F.M., & Peter, J. (2003). Migraine pathogenesis: Neural and vascular mechanisms. *Neurology, 60*(7) (Supplement 2), S9-S14.

Zandi, P.P., Breitner, J.C., & Anthony, J.C. (2002). Is pharmacological prevention of Alzheimer's a realistic goal? *Expert Opinion on Pharmacotherapy, 3*(4), 365-380.

Zingmark, K., Sandman, P.O., & Norberg, A. (2002). Promoting a good life among people with Alzheimer's disease. *Journal of Advanced Nursing, 38*(1), 50-58.

CHAPTER 46

Interventions for Clients with Problems of the Central Nervous System
The Spinal Cord

KATHY A. HAUSMAN

LEARNING OUTCOMES

After studying this chapter, you should be able to:

1. Identify risk factors that contribute to back pain.
2. Explain health promotion measures to prevent back pain.
3. Plan care for the client having a diskectomy, laminectomy, or spinal fusion.
4. Analyze the common nursing diagnoses and collaborative problems for the client with an acute spinal cord injury (SCI).
5. Describe the role of the health care team in the recognition and treatment of typical medical complications that are experienced by clients with an SCI.
6. Prioritize the nursing care of the client with an SCI.
7. Evaluate the expected outcomes for the client with an SCI.
8. Identify the clinical manifestations and treatment options associated with spinal cord tumors.
9. Explain the pathophysiology of multiple sclerosis (MS), including the six basic types.
10. Discuss the role of medications in managing clients with MS.
11. Develop a community-based teaching plan for the client with MS.
12. Compare and contrast the clinical manifestations of MS and amyotrophic lateral sclerosis.

Go to your Student CD-ROM for Review Questions for the NCLEX Examination keyed to these Learning Outcomes.

Problems of the spinal cord may be either acute or chronic and either short term or long term. Some problems require surgery, whereas others require extensive rehabilitation. Spinal cord neurons do not regenerate, and damage to nerve fibers is permanent.

BACK PAIN

Lumbosacral Back Pain (Low Back Pain)

OVERVIEW

Back pain is one of the most common reasons for visiting a health care provider. Back problems are very costly in terms of time lost from work and medical treatment, and they are the most common cause of disability for persons younger than 43 years of age. Disabling low back pain is the single greatest cause of compensable injury in the working population. The lumbosacral (lower back) vertebrae and cervical (neck) vertebrae are most commonly affected.

PATHOPHYSIOLOGY

Lumbosacral back pain, referred to as **low back pain (LBP),** is more common than cervical pain. Acute pain is caused by muscle strain or spasm, ligament sprain, disk degeneration, or herniation of the nucleus pulposus from the center of the disk. Herniated disks occur most often between the fourth and fifth lumbar vertebrae (L4-5) but may occur at other levels. A **herniated nucleus pulposus (HNP)** in the lumbosacral area can press on the adjacent spinal nerve (usually the sciatic nerve), causing severe burning or stabbing pain down into the leg or foot. The HNP may press on the spinal cord itself, causing leg weakness and bowel and bladder dysfunction. The specific area of pain depends on the level of herniation.

Muscle spasms of the affected leg may also occur. The pain is usually aggravated by sneezing, coughing, or straining. If LBP continues for 3 months or if repeated episodes of pain occur, the client has chronic back pain.

Etiology and Genetic Risk

Acute back pain usually results from trauma. The client typically hyperflexes or twists the back during a vehicular accident, or the injury occurs when the client lifts a heavy object. Obesity places increased stress on the back muscles and typically contributes to the occurrence or severity of back pain. Smoking has been linked to disk degeneration. Congenital spinal conditions and scoliosis can also lead to back discomfort.

CONSIDERATIONS FOR OLDER ADULTS

For older adults the cause of low back pain is usually osteoarthritis (OA), a type of arthritis seen primarily in this population. OA may be related to genetic factors, especially when the disease affects the hands and knees (Birchfield, 2001). Other factors contributing to low back pain in older adults are presented in Chart 46-1.

WOMEN'S HEALTH CONSIDERATIONS

Chronic low back pain in women often results from having poor posture or from wearing high-heeled shoes. Excessive high heels cause the body to compensate to maintain balance. The back becomes more **lordotic** (anteriorly curved), which strains back muscles.

Incidence/Prevalence

Eighty percent of the U.S. population has LBP at some time. About 85% to 90% of adults over 50 years of age have degenerative disk disease.

HEALTH PROMOTION/ILLNESS PREVENTION

Many of the problems related to acute back pain can be prevented by recognizing the cause of back pain and taking appropriate preventive measures. For example, good posture, proper lifting techniques, and exercise can significantly decrease the incidence of low back pain. Chart 46-2 summarizes ways to prevent LBP.

CHART 46-1

NURSING FOCUS on the OLDER ADULT
Factors Contributing to Low Back Pain

- Changes in support structures
  - Spinal stenosis
  - Hypertrophy of the intraspinal ligaments
  - Arthritis
- Changes in vertebral support and malalignment
  - Scoliosis
  - Lordosis
- Vascular changes
  - Diminished blood supply to the spinal cord or cauda equina caused by arteriosclerosis
  - Blood dyscrasias
- Intervertebral disk degeneration

COLLABORATIVE MANAGEMENT

Assessment

PHYSICAL ASSESSMENT/CLINICAL MANIFESTATIONS

The client's *primary* complaint is continuous acute pain. Some clients have so much pain that they walk in a stiff, flexed state, or they may be unable to bend at all. The client who has low back pain (LBP) may walk with a limp, indicating possible sciatic nerve impairment. Walking on the heels or toes often causes severe pain in the affected leg, the back, or both.

Inspect the client's back for vertebral alignment and for tenderness and swelling caused by muscle spasm. Local muscle spasm in the back and affected leg is common. It is thought that a compressed nerve becomes inflamed and irritates adjacent muscle tissue. Clients complain of stabbing, continuous pain in the muscle close to the affected disk. In clients with lumbosacral involvement, pain radiates down the posterior leg. The pain usually does not extend the entire length of the limb. Clients with LBP report sharp, burning posterior thigh or calf pain that may radiate to the ankle or toes. They may also report the same type of pain in the middle of one buttock.

Ask the client whether **paresthesia** (tingling sensation) or numbness is present in the involved limb. Both extremities may be checked for sensation by using a pin or paper clip and a cotton ball for comparison of light and deep touch. The client may feel sensation in both limbs but may experience a stronger sensation on the unaffected side. The client with a severe problem may lose both bowel and bladder control from spinal nerve involvement.

If the sciatic nerve is compressed, the client reports severe pain when raising a straight leg. Foot, ankle, and leg weakness may accompany the pain. To complete the neurologic assessment, evaluate the client's muscle tone and strength. Muscles in the extremity or in the back atrophy in severe, chronic conditions. The client has difficulty with movement, and certain movements elicit more pain than others.

DIAGNOSTIC ASSESSMENT

The health care provider often orders magnetic resonance imaging (MRI) or a computed tomography (CT) scan, performed with or without contrast media enhancement, to vi-

CHART 46-2

CLIENT EDUCATION GUIDE
Prevention of Low Back Pain and Injury

- Use proper body mechanics, with specific attention to bending, lifting, and sitting.
- Assess the need for assistance with your household chores or other activities.
- Participate in a regular exercise program, especially one that promotes back strengthening, such as swimming and walking.
- Do not wear high-heeled shoes.
- Use good posture when sitting, standing, or walking.
- Avoid prolonged sitting or standing. Use a foot stool and ergonomic chairs and tables to lessen back strain.
- Keep weight within 10% of ideal body weight. Ensure adequate calcium intake.
- Stop smoking. If you are not able to stop, cut down on the number of cigarettes or decrease the use of other forms of tobacco.

sualize the herniated disk and pressure on the nerve root or spinal cord.

Electrodiagnostic testing, such as electromyography (EMG) and nerve-conduction studies, may help to differentiate motor neuron diseases, peripheral neuropathies, peripheral nerve entrapment, and radiculopathies. These are especially useful in chronic diseases because it takes at least 3 weeks for pathologic changes to produce symptoms. Chapter 44 describes these tests in more detail.

Interventions

Management of clients with back pain varies with the severity and chronicity of the problem. Most clients with acute low back pain (LBP) need only a short-term treatment regimen. The health care provider initially implements conservative measures; if these are unsuccessful, surgery may be indicated. Some clients experience chronic pain that must be managed for an extended period.

NONSURGICAL MANAGEMENT. Nonsurgical management of back pain may include proper positioning, exercise, anti-inflammatory analgesics, heat or ice therapy, and other pain-relief measures and preventive measures in the work setting.

Positioning. The **Williams position** is typically more comfortable and therapeutic for the client with LBP. In this position, the client lies in the semi-Fowler's position and flexes the knees to relax the muscles of the lower back and relieve pressure on the spinal nerve root.

A firm mattress or a backboard placed under a soft mattress provides back support. A flat position is particularly helpful for the client with a muscle injury. For a herniated disk causing spinal nerve root compression in the lumbar spine, a flat position may aggravate the pain. The client usually gains pain relief from reclining or sleeping in the Williams position.

Exercise. Exercises are used to strengthen the back, relieve pressure on compressed nerves, and protect the back from reinjury. A variety of exercise programs are available to treat LBP. Isometric exercises are generally the most effective.

The physical therapist (PT) works with the client to develop an individualized exercise program. The type of exercises prescribed depends on the location and nature of the injury and the type of pain. The client does not begin exercises until acute pain is reduced by other means. Several specific exercises for LBP are provided in Chart 46-3.

Drug Therapy. The health care provider often prescribes muscle relaxants, such as cyclobenzaprine hydrochloride (Flexeril) and tizanidine (Zanaflex), and nonsteroidal anti-inflammatory drugs (NSAIDs), such as naproxen (Naprosyn, Naxen✱) and ibuprofen (Motrin, Novoprofen✱). Opioid analgesics are no more effective than nonsteroidal analgesics and should be avoided if at all possible. If they must be used, the course of therapy should be short to prevent adverse side effects. An epidural or local steroid injection may also be helpful. Short-term oral steroids may be prescribed for some clients. Clients experiencing chronic back pain may require an antiepileptic drug (AED), such as gabapentin (Neurontin) and oxcarbazepine (Trileptal). For clients with chronic back problems, these drugs are used to treat neuropathic pain. Most of the drugs in this class can cause hyponatremia (low serum sodium). Older clients should be monitored very carefully for this adverse effect. Chapter 7 describes in detail the drug therapy and nursing implications for the care of clients in acute or chronic pain.

Heat and Ice Therapy. Some clients with back pain experience temporary relief from the application of heat. Heat increases blood flow to the affected area and promotes the healing of injured nerves. Moist heat in the form of heat packs or hot towels applied for 20 to 30 minutes at least four times per day may be recommended. Hot showers or baths are also often beneficial. The physical therapist (PT) may administer deep heat therapy, such as ultrasound treatments and diathermy. The PT and nurse monitor the effects of heat treatment by assessing the client's skin condition and the relief of pain.

Some clients prefer ice instead of heat to relieve pain and inflammation. Ice therapy using ice packs or ice massage may be applied over the affected area for 10 to 15 minutes every 1 to 2 hours. For some clients, a course of alternating ice and heat applications may be effective.

Diet Therapy. Weight control often helps to reduce chronic back pain by decreasing the work on the vertebrae caused by excess weight. If the client's weight exceeds the ideal by more than 10%, caloric restriction is necessary.

Health care providers must be sensitive when reinforcing the need for clients to lose weight to prevent or to lessen chronic back pain. Collaborate with the dietitian to plan and implement an appropriate calorie-restricted diet plan. Positive reinforcement and self-esteem building are integral to the diet plan.

Other Pain Relief Measures. Physical therapy with manipulation of the lower back during the first month of symptoms may be beneficial. Shoe insoles may also help to decrease pain when standing for prolonged periods. Preventive measures for the occupational setting may include a corset, supportive back belt, and ergonomic office furniture. A structured educational program about low back problems in the work setting has also been helpful in decreasing both injuries and time lost from work.

Complementary and Alternative Therapies. The client may find that other nontraditional and complementary therapies provide short-term pain relief. Distraction,

CHART 46-3

CLIENT EDUCATION GUIDE

Typical Exercises for Chronic or Postoperative Low Back Pain

Extension Exercises

- **Stomach lying:** Lie face down with a pillow under your chest; lift legs straight up (alternate legs).
- **Upper trunk extension:** Lie face down with your arms at your sides, and lift your head and neck.
- **Prone pushups:** Lie face down on a mat and, keeping your body stiff, and push up to extend your arms.

Flexion Exercises

- **Pelvic tilt:** Lying on your back with your knees bent, tighten your abdominal muscles to push your lower back against the mat.
- **Semi-sit-ups:** Lying on your back with your knees bent, raise your upper body at a 45-degree angle, and hold this position for 5 to 10 seconds.
- **Knee to chest:** Lying on your back with your knees bent, tighten your abdominal muscles to push your lower back against the mat. Now bring one or both knees to your chest and hold this position for 5 to 10 seconds.

imagery, magnetic-field therapy, and music therapy are examples of pain-relief therapies. Chapters 4 and 7 describe these techniques in detail.

Percutaneous Laser Disk Decompression. A nonsurgical procedure known as **percutaneous laser disk decompression (PLDD)** may relieve the pain of a herniated disk by drawing the herniated portion away from the nerve root. This treatment is performed in special spinal centers around the United States and throughout the world.

Using advanced laser technology and a local anesthetic, a thin needle is inserted under fluoroscopy. An optical fiber is placed through the needle to enable laser energy to travel and vaporize the disk nucleus. Most clients walk away from this half-hour procedure pain free and with just a small bandage. Physicians typically prescribe 24 hours of bedrest after the procedure before beginning progressive ambulation. Depending on the type of work, most clients can resume work within a week.

SURGICAL MANAGEMENT. Surgery is usually performed when conservative measures fail to relieve back pain after a month or so or if neurologic deficits progress.

Conventional Operative Procedures. The most common conventional operative procedures are diskectomy, laminectomy, and spinal fusion. These procedures involve extensive muscle and soft-tissue dissection to expose the anatomic landmarks. Major complications include nerve injuries, diskitis, and dural tears.

In a conventional **diskectomy,** the spinal nerve is usually lifted to remove the offending portion of the disk. A **laminectomy** is the removal of one or more vertebral laminae plus osteophytes, if present, and the herniated nucleus pulposus. Both procedures are performed through a 3- to 4-inch (7.5- to 10-cm) longitudinal incision. The standard hospital stay is 1 to 2 days but may be shorter or longer, depending on the client's condition and the reimbursement source.

When repeated laminectomies are performed or the spine is unstable, the surgeon may perform a **spinal fusion (arthrodesis)** to stabilize the affected area. Chips of bone are removed, typically from the iliac crest or obtained from donor bone, and are grafted between the vertebrae for support and to strengthen the back. Before closing, the surgeon may give an **intrathecal** (spinal) dose of morphine to decrease postoperative pain and respiratory complications.

An adjunct for clients for whom fusion may be difficult is the placement of an implantable **direct current stimulation (DCS)** to promote bone fusion. External bone stimulators may also be effective for healing bone fusions.

Alternative Operative Procedures. Minimally invasive lumbar procedures have the advantage of being associated with less muscle injury, decreased blood loss, and decreased postoperative pain. Three alternatives to a laminectomy that have varying degrees of popularity are percutaneous lumbar diskectomy, microdiskectomy, and laser-assisted laparoscopic lumbar diskectomy. The primary advantage of these surgical procedures is a shortened hospital stay and the possibility of an ambulatory procedure. Spinal cord complications are also less likely. New procedures for spinal fusions include laparoscopic lumbar fusion and intervertebral body fusion devices (e.g., titanium-threaded and mesh interbody cages). When possible, these procedures are preferred over conventional ones.

For a **percutaneous lumbar diskectomy,** a local anesthetic is given. The surgeon uses fluoroscopy to insert a metal cannula, or endoscope, adjacent to the affected disk. A special cutting tool is threaded through the cannula for removal of disk pieces that are compressing the nerve root. Inpatient hospitalization is not necessary.

A **microdiskectomy** involves microscopic surgery through a 1-inch incision. This procedure allows easier identification of anatomic structures, improved precision in removing small fragments, and decreased tissue trauma and pain.

Laser-assisted laparoscopic lumbar diskectomy combines a laser with modified standard disk instruments inserted periumbilically through the laparoscopic cannula. It may be used to treat herniated disks that, although bulging, have not encroached on the vertebral canal. The primary risks of this surgery are infection and nerve-root injury. The client is typically discharged in 24 to 48 hours but may be discharged the same day.

Another new treatment for herniated disks involves a hard plastic prosthesis that replaces the client's natural disk. The disk is shaped to allow full spinal movement. Recently approved for widespread use, this device could revolutionize care for clients with herniated disks.

Preoperative Care. Preoperative care of the client preparing for a lumbar laminectomy is similar to that for any client undergoing surgery (see Chapter 20). The nurse and physical therapist teach the client what to expect postoperatively and how to move in bed. The client should be warned that various sensations, such as numbness and tingling, may be experienced in the affected leg or in both legs because of the manipulation of nerves and muscles during surgery.

The client who has undergone a spinal fusion typically wears a back brace postoperatively. This brace is fitted before surgery. The nurse in the surgeon's office or clinic teaches about the importance of wearing the brace as instructed during the healing process.

The surgeon explains where the bone for grafting will be obtained. The client's own bone is used whenever possible, but supplemental bone from a bone bank may be needed. The surgeon provides verbal and written information about the type and the source of bone for surgery. The client signs an informed consent form before surgery.

Postoperative Care. Early postoperative nursing care focuses on preventing and assessing complications that might occur in the first 24 to 48 hours (Chart 46-4). As for any client undergoing surgery, take vital signs at least every 4 hours during the first 24 hours to assess for fever and for hypotension, which could indicate bleeding or severe pain. Perform a neurologic assessment every 4 hours. Of particular importance is the client's ability to move and feel sensation in the extremities.

Carefully check the client's ability to void. Pain and a flat position in bed make voiding difficult, especially for men. An inability to void may indicate damage to the sacral spinal nerves, which control the detrusor muscle in the bladder. Opioid analgesics have been associated with difficulty voiding. The client with a diskectomy or laminectomy typically gets out of bed with assistance on the evening of surgery, which may facilitate voiding.

Pain control may be achieved with patient-controlled analgesia (PCA) or intravenous (IV) medications such as

CHART 46-4

BEST PRACTICE for
Assessing and Managing the Client with Major Complications of Lumbar Spinal Surgery

Complication	Assessment/Interventions
Cerebrospinal fluid (CSF) leakage	Observe for clear fluid on or around the dressing. If CSF is present, test for glucose. (The test result is positive if glucose is present.) Report CSF leakage immediately to the surgeon. (The client is usually kept on flat bedrest for several days while the dural tear heals.)
Fluid volume deficit	Monitor intake and output; monitor drain output, which should not be more than 250 mL in 8 hr during the first 24 hr. Monitor vital signs carefully for hypotension and tachycardia.
Acute urinary retention	Assist the client to the bathroom or a bedside commode as soon as possible postoperatively. Assist male clients to stand at the bedside as soon as possible postoperatively. Give bethanechol (Urecholine) chloride as prescribed to stimulate the detrusor muscle of the bladder.
Paralytic ileus	Monitor for the return of bowel sounds. Assess for abdominal distention, nausea, and vomiting.
Fat embolism syndrome (FES) (more common in people with spinal fusion)	Observe for and report chest pain, dyspnea, anxiety, and mental status changes (particularly common in older adults). Note petechiae around the neck, upper chest, buccal membrane, and conjunctiva. Monitor arterial blood gas values for decreased Pao_2.
Persistent or progressive lumbar radiculopathy (nerve root pain)	Report pain not responsive to opioids. Document the location and nature of pain. Administer analgesics as ordered.
Infection (e.g., wound diskitis, hematoma)	Monitor the client's temperature carefully (a slight elevation is normal). Increased temperature elevation or a spike after the second postoperative day is possibly indicative of infection. Report increased pain at the wound site or in the legs. Give antibiotics as prescribed. Use sterile technique for dressing changes.

morphine. Pain medication is changed to oral administration when the client is able to take fluids. Hospital policy should be followed regarding pain management.

Inspect the surgical dressing for blood or any other type of drainage. Clear drainage may mean cerebrospinal fluid (CSF) leakage. Report such a finding to the surgeon immediately. Bulging at the incision site may be due to a CSF leak or a hematoma, both of which are reported to the surgeon.

Empty the surgical drain, usually a Jackson-Pratt or Hemovac, and record the amount of drainage every 8 hours. The surgeon usually removes the drain in 24 to 36 hours.

Correct turning of the client in bed is especially important. Teach the client to log roll every 2 hours from side to back and vice versa. In log rolling, the client turns all at once while his or her back is kept as straight as possible. A turning sheet may be used for large clients. Either turning method may require additional assistance, depending on how much the client can assist. Instruct the client to keep his or her back straight when getting out of bed. The client should sit in a straight-backed chair with the feet resting comfortably on the floor.

Teach the client to deep breathe every 2 hours to prevent atelectasis and pneumonia. Until the client can ambulate independently, he or she wears graduated compression stockings, sequential compression devices (SCDs), or pneumatic compression boots (PCBs) to prevent deep vein thrombosis (DVT) and possible pulmonary emboli. Older adults are especially susceptible to these complications of immobility.

When a spinal fusion is performed in addition to a laminectomy, more care is taken with mobility and positioning. The client usually stays in bed for 24 hours, with the nurse or assistive nursing personnel log rolling him or her every 2 hours. For the conventional fusion, inspect both the iliac and spinal incision areas for problems, as described earlier in this section. A brace or other type of thoracolumbar support is worn when the client is out of bed. Remind the client to avoid prolonged sitting or standing.

Community-Based Care

The client with back pain who does not undergo surgery is typically managed at home. If back surgery is performed, the client is usually discharged to home with support from family or significant others. For older adults without a community support system, a short-term stay in a nursing home or subacute unit may be needed. The case manager or discharge planner collaborates with the health care team, client, and family to determine the most appropriate placement.

HOME CARE MANAGEMENT

Inform the client and family members or significant other that the client should have a firm mattress to provide support for the entire vertebral column. A bed board or large piece of plywood placed under a soft mattress may suffice. After back surgery, the client may be limited in the number of times he or she is allowed to climb stairs each day. However, daily walking is encouraged. The client can usually return to work in 4 to 6 weeks, depending on the nature of the job and the extent and type of surgery. Weight that may be lifted is initially limited to 5 pounds. The amount is gradually increased as healing occurs. Driving is not permitted for several weeks until the surgeon re-evaluates the client.

HEALTH TEACHING

In collaboration with the dietitian and physical therapist, instruct the client to do the following:

- Continue with a weight-reduction diet, if needed.
- Stop smoking, if applicable.
- Use moist heat as needed.
- Perform strengthening exercises as initiated preoperatively and in the hospital setting.

The physical therapist reviews and demonstrates the principles of body mechanics and muscle-strengthening exercises. The client is then asked to demonstrate these principles (Chart 46-5).

The health care provider may want the client to continue taking medications such as anti-inflammatory drugs and muscle relaxants. The nurse reminds the client and family about the possible side effects of drugs and what to do if they occur. If the client has a conventional spinal fusion, he or she may need to wear a brace or thoracolumbar support for 3 to 6 months while the fusion heals completely. The client may not be able to return to full functioning for 6 to 12 months after a spinal fusion, depending on the type of work that is done.

The client with an acute episode of back pain typically returns to his or her usual activities but may fear a recurrence. Remind the client that he or she may never have another episode if caution is used. However, continuous or repeated pain can be frustrating and tiring. If pain is unremitting, surgery is indicated. Encourage the client and family members to set short-term goals and to take steps toward recovering slowly.

In a few clients, back surgery is not successful. This situation, referred to as **failed back surgery syndrome (FBSS),** is a complex combination of organic, psychological, and socioeconomic factors. Repeated surgical procedures often discourage these clients, who must continue nonsurgical management of pain after multiple operations. Nerve blocks and other chronic pain-management modalities may be needed on a long-term basis (see Chapter 7).

A new drug for severe chronic pain, ziconotide (Prialt), has recently been approved for intrathecal infusion with a surgically implanted pump. Ziconotide is the first available drug in a new class called N-type calcium channel blockers (NCCBs). NCCBs seem to selectively block calcium channels on those nerves that usually transmit pain signals to the brain. Ziconotide is also used for clients with cancer, AIDS, and unremitting pain for other nervous system disorders. It can be given with opioid analgesics but should not be given to clients with severe mental health/behavioral health problems (http://www.prialt.com).

HEALTH CARE RESOURCES

Assist the client in identifying support systems (e.g., family, church groups, and clubs) after back surgery or FBSS. For example, a spouse may help the client with exercises or perform the exercises with the client. Members of a church group may help run errands and do household chores.

The client with back pain may continue physical therapy on an ambulatory basis after discharge. For unresolved pain, the client may be referred to pain specialists or clinics, which are usually found in large metropolitan hospitals. A case manager may be assigned to the client to help with resource management and utilization.

CHART 46-5

CLIENT EDUCATION GUIDE
Use of Proper Body Mechanics to Prevent Back Injury

- Size up the load to determine the number of persons needed to perform the task.
- When lifting an object, keep your back straight and do not bend at the waist; lift with your large thigh muscles.
- Push objects rather than pull them.
- Do not twist your back.
- Avoid prolonged sitting or standing. Use a footstool to lessen back strain.
- Sit in chairs with good support; sleep on a firm mattress.
- Avoid shoulder stooping; use proper posture.
- Do not walk or stand in high-heeled shoes for prolonged periods (for women).

Cervical Neck Pain

PATHOPHYSIOLOGY

Cervical neck pain usually results from a herniation of the nucleus pulposus in an intervertebral disk. As seen in Figure 46-1, the herniation usually occurs laterally where the annulus fibrosus is weakest and the posterior longitudinal lig-

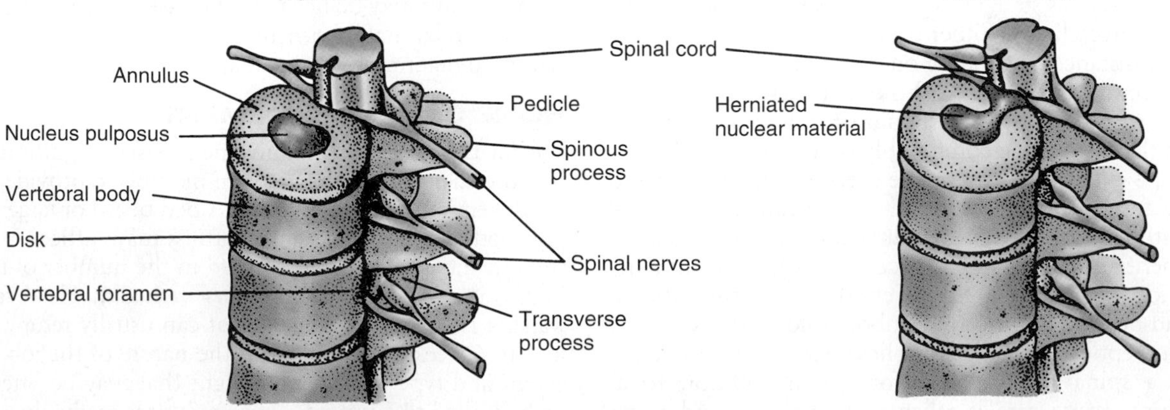

Figure 46-1 ■ Herniation of the nucleus pulposus.

ament is thinned. The result is spinal nerve root compression, with subsequent motor and sensory manifestations, typically in the neck and down the affected arm. The disk between the fifth and sixth cervical vertebrae (C5-6) is affected most often.

If the disk does not rupture, nerve compression may be caused by osteophyte (bony outgrowth) formation from osteoarthritis. The osteophyte presses on the intervertebral foramen, which results in a narrowing of the disk and pressure on the nerve root. A client with nerve compression may experience either continuous or intermittent chronic pain. When the disk herniates centrally, pressure on the spinal cord occurs.

Cervical pain–acute or chronic–may also occur from muscle strain, ligament sprain resulting from aging or poor posture, lifting incorrectly, tumor, or infection. The typical history of the client includes complaints of pain when moving the neck, which radiates to the scapula and down the arm. The pain may interrupt sleep and may be accompanied by a headache or numbness and tingling in the affected arm. To determine the exact cause of the pain, the health care provider orders diagnostic tests, such as computed tomography (CT) or magnetic resonance imaging (MRI), x-rays of the neck, electromyography (EMG), or a combination of these.

COLLABORATIVE MANAGEMENT

Conservative treatment for neck pain is the same as described for back pain except the exercises focus on the shoulders and neck. The physical therapist teaches the client the correct techniques for performing "shoulder shrug," "shoulder squeeze," and "seated rowing." If these treatments do not work, the health care provider may prescribe a soft collar, especially at night. The collar is used no longer than 10 days, or it can lead to increased pain and decreased muscle strength and range of motion.

If conservative treatment is ineffective, surgery may be required. Depending on the causative factor, either an anterior or posterior approach is used. An anterior cervical diskectomy and fusion (ACDF) is commonly performed. The client requires routine preoperative and postoperative care as described in Chapters 20 and 22. Chart 46-6 summarizes best practices for postoperative care and discharge planning. Potential complications of the anterior surgical approach can be found in Chart 46-7.

CHART 46-6

BEST PRACTICE for
Care of the Client Following an Anterior Cervical Diskectomy and Fusion

Postoperative Interventions
- Assess airway, breathing, and circulation (ABCs).
- Check for bleeding and drainage at the incision site.
- Monitor vital signs and neurologic status frequently.
- Check for swallowing ability.
- Monitor intake and output.
- Assess the client's ability to void (may be a problem secondary to opiates).
- Manage pain adequately.
- Assist the client with ambulation within a few hours of surgery, if he or she is able.

Discharge Teaching
- Review drug therapy.
- Teach care of the incision.
- Review activity restrictions:
  - No lifting
  - No driving until physician permission
  - No strenuous activities
- Walk every day.
- Call the surgeon if symptoms of pain, numbness, and tingling worsen or if difficulty in swallowing occurs.
- Wear collar per surgeon's orders.

Critical Thinking Challenge

You have been assigned to a woman admitted to the medical-surgical unit following an anterior cervical diskectomy and fusion (ACDF). She is wearing a soft collar. Her diet order is clear liquids and advance as tolerated. She may ambulate with assistance. The client tells you that her pain score is 7/10; she is having difficulty swallowing, and you notice that her voice is hoarse. According to the client, no one told her she "would feel like this."

1. What is your best nursing action in response to these symptoms?
2. What would you tell the client about her symptoms?
3. What are the possible complications of an ACDF, and why might they occur?

evolve For suggested answer guidelines, go to http://evolve.elsevier.com/Iggy/.

SPINAL CORD INJURY

Despite increased awareness and the sophistication of treatment for spinal cord injury (SCI), the effects of the initial injury cannot be reversed. However, research with clients with SCI has increased, led by actor Christopher Reeve, who experienced a complete cervical spinal injury. The cost of care for clients with an SCI varies with the neurologic deficit. Clients experiencing **tetraplegia** (also called quadriplegia)–paralysis from the neck down–are the most expensive for society in terms of both health care and living expenses (see the Resource Management box on p. 984).

Loss of motor function, sensation, reflex activity, and bowel and bladder control often result from an SCI. In addition, the client may experience significant behavior and emotional problems as a result of changes in body image, role performance, and self-concept.

The SCIs are classified as complete or incomplete. A **complete** injury is one in which the spinal cord has been severed or damaged in a way that eliminates all innervation below the level of the injury. Injuries that allow some function or movement below the level of the injury are described as **incomplete.**

CHART 46-7

KEY FEATURES of
Postoperative Complications of Cervical Diskectomy and Fusion

- Hoarseness due to laryngeal injury; may be temporary or permanent
- Temporary dysphagia; may last few days to several months; usually not severe
- Esophageal, tracheal, or vertebral artery injury
- Wound infection
- Injury to the spinal cord or nerve roots
- Dura mater tears with associated cerebrospinal fluid leaks
- Pseudoarthrosis caused by nonunion of fusion
- Graft extrusion and screw loosening if a fusion was performed.

RESOURCE MANAGEMENT

SPINAL CORD INJURIES

Cost of Care

- The average annual cost (health care and living expenses) and the estimated lifetime costs for a client with a spinal cord injury (SCI) varies greatly with the severity of injury.
- The cost of care for a C1-4 quadriplegic is $626,588 for the first year; each subsequent year the cost is $112,237.
- The cost of care for a paraplegic is more than $200,000 for the first year and more than $20,000 for each subsequent year.
- Estimated lifetime costs for a C1-4 quadriplegic, 25 years old, is $2,393,507; 50 years old, $1,409,070.
- Cost-of-care estimates do not include loss of income, fringe benefits, and productivity, which could average $46,000, depending on the client's education, occupation, and work history.
- The average length of stay in the acute setting in 1974 was 26 days; in 1998 it was 15 days. The average length of stay in the rehabilitation setting has decreased from 115 to 44 days. Clients with more neurologically complete injuries require longer acute and rehabilitation stays.
- Only 4% of clients with an SCI are discharged to nursing homes; 91.3% are sent to noninstitutional residences, usually their home. The remaining SCI clients are discharged to hospitals, group living situations, or other places.

Implications for Nursing

The high cost of care for quadriplegic clients requires nurses to be more vigilant in the prevention of complications of immobility that would extend the average length of stay, increase morbidity, and increase the cost of care. Inherent in this preventive strategy is the need to educate the client and family thoroughly on potential complications that would lengthen recovery and delay discharge to rehabilitation. The use of rehabilitation principles from the time of admission would facilitate earlier discharge and a smoother transition back into society.

PATHOPHYSIOLOGY

Mechanisms of Injury

When sufficient force is applied to the spinal cord, damage results in neurologic deficits. Sources of force include injury to the vertebral column (fracture, dislocation, and subluxation) or penetrating trauma (gunshot or knife wounds). Although in some cases the cord itself may remain intact, at other times the cord undergoes a destructive process caused by a contusion, compression, or concussion.

The causes of SCI can be divided into primary and secondary mechanisms of injury (Okonkwo, 2003). Four primary mechanisms may result in an SCI: hyperflexion; hyperextension; axial loading, or vertical compression; and excessive rotation. Penetrating injuries to the cord may also occur.

A **hyperflexion** injury occurs when the head is suddenly and forcefully accelerated forward, causing extreme flexion of the neck (Figure 46-2). This type of injury often occurs in head-on collisions and diving accidents. Flexion injury to the lower thoracic and lumbar spine may occur when the trunk is suddenly flexed on itself, such as occurs in a fall on the buttocks. The posterior ligaments can be stretched or torn, or the vertebrae may fracture or dislocate. Either process may disrupt the integrity of the spinal cord, causing hemorrhage, edema, and necrosis.

Hyperextension injuries occur most often in automobile accidents in which the client's vehicle is struck from behind or during falls when the client's chin is struck (Figure 46-3).

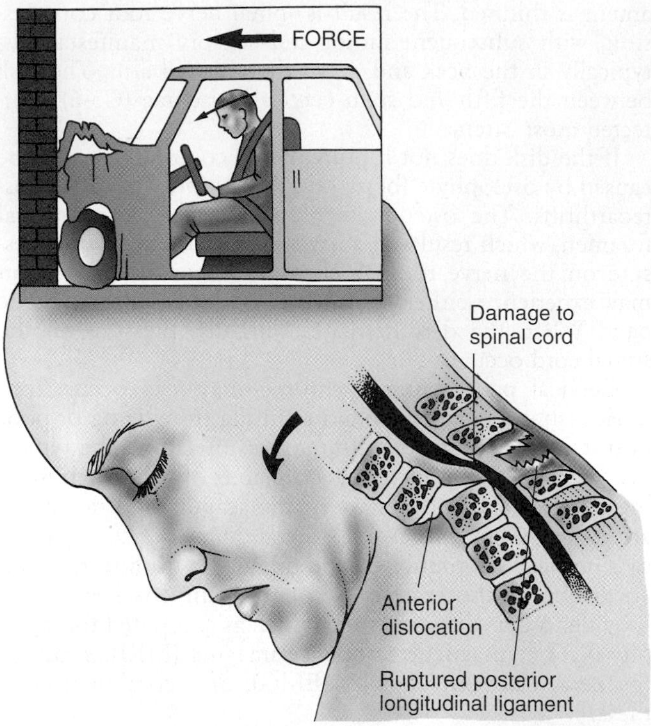

Figure 46-2 ■ Hyperflexion injury of the cervical spine.

The head is suddenly accelerated and then decelerated. This stretches or tears the anterior longitudinal ligament, fractures or subluxates the vertebrae, and perhaps ruptures an intervertebral disk. As with flexion injuries, the spinal cord may easily be damaged.

Diving accidents, falls on the buttocks, or a jump in which a person lands on the feet can cause many of the injuries attributable to **axial loading** (vertical compression) (Figure 46-4). The blow to the top of the head causes the vertebrae to shatter. Pieces of bone enter the spinal canal and damage the cord.

Rotation injuries are caused by turning the head beyond the normal range.

Penetrating injuries to the spinal cord are classified by the velocity of the vehicle (e.g., knife or bullet) causing the injury. Low-velocity or low-impact injuries cause damage directly at the site or localized damage to the spinal cord or spinal nerves. In contrast, high-velocity injuries that occur from gunshot wounds cause both direct and indirect damage.

Secondary injury exacerbates the primary injury and worsens morbidity. Secondary injuries include the following:

- Neurogenic shock
- Vascular insult
- Hemorrhage
- Ischemia
- Fluid and electrolyte imbalance

The spinal cord may be contused, lacerated, or compressed as a result of injury. Petechial hemorrhage into the central gray matter, and later into the white matter, can be caused by a contusion and laceration of the spinal cord. Spinal cord edema occurs as a result of cord compression by hemorrhage, bony fragments, or laceration. Necrosis of the spinal cord occurs from compromised capillary circulation and venous return.

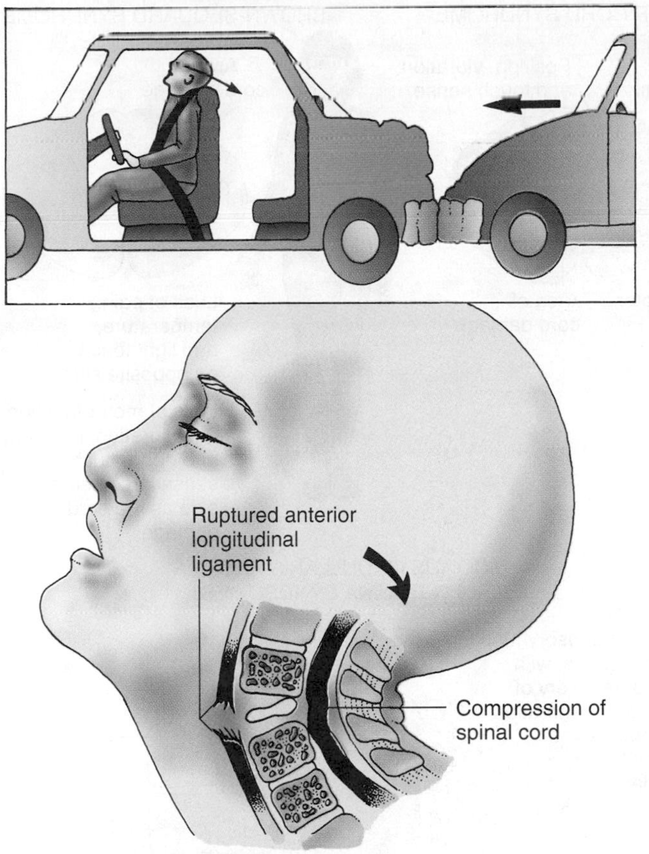

Figure 46-3 ■ Hyperextension injury of the cervical spine.

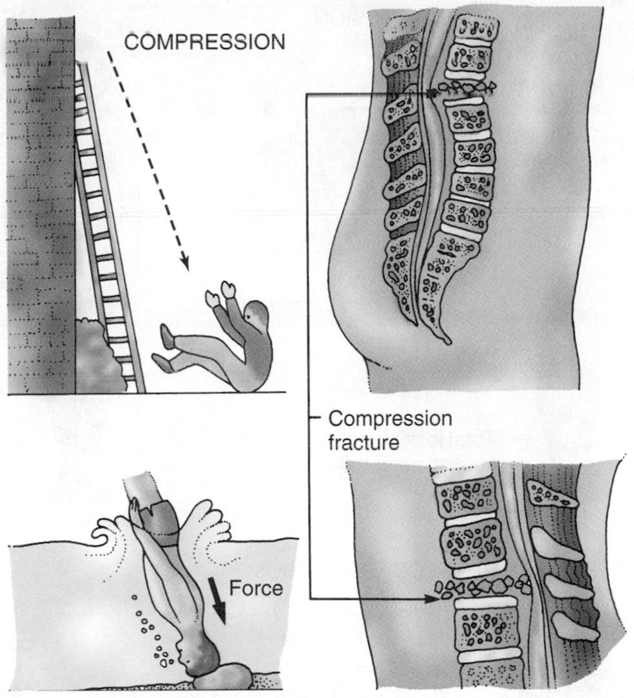

Figure 46-4 ■ Axial loading (vertical compression) injury of the cervical spine and the lumbar spine.

Extent of Injury

Incomplete SCIs are more common than complete lesions. A client experiencing an incomplete lesion typically has preservation of a mixed pattern of motor, sensory, and reflex function. Specific syndromes result from incomplete lesions (Figure 46-5). A "pure" syndrome may not be seen. Cervical injuries may produce the following:

- Anterior cord syndrome
- Posterior cord syndrome
- Brown-Séquard syndrome
- Central cord syndrome

Conus medullaris and cauda equina syndromes are associated with injuries to the lumbar and sacral cord.

CERVICAL INJURIES

Anterior cord syndrome results from damage to the anterior portion of both gray and white matter of the spinal cord, usually as a result of decreased blood supply. Although motor function and pain and temperature sensation are lost below the level of injury, the sensations of touch, position, and vibration remain intact. More than 50% of clients with this syndrome are older than 40 years, with most between 50 and 70 years. Functional motor control is recovered in 10% to 20% of clients with cervical spine injuries.

Just the opposite transpires in a rarely encountered **posterior cord lesion**, which also occurs from damage to the posterior gray and white matter of the spinal cord. Motor function remains intact, but the client experiences a loss of vibratory sense, crude touch, and position sensation.

Brown-Séquard syndrome generally results from penetrating injuries that cause hemisection of the spinal cord or injuries that affect half of the spinal cord. Motor function, proprioception, vibration, and deep touch sensations are lost on the same side of the body as the lesion (ipsilateral). On the opposite side of the body (contralateral) from the injury, the sensations of pain, temperature, and light touch are affected.

Lesions of the central portion of the spinal cord produce a **central cord syndrome.** Loss of motor function is more pronounced in the upper extremities than in the lower extremities. Varying degrees and patterns of sensation remain intact.

LUMBOSACRAL INJURIES

Damage to the cauda equina or conus medullaris produces a variable pattern of motor or sensory loss because the peripheral nerves have the potential for recovery and regrowth. In addition, this injury usually results in a neurogenic bowel and bladder.

Etiology

Trauma is the leading cause of spinal cord injuries (SCIs); almost 45% result from motor vehicle accidents. The second leading cause is acts of violence (24%), followed by falls (22%) and sports accidents (8%) (National Spinal Cord Injury Data Base [NSCIDB], 2001). Spinal cord damage can also result from diseases such as polio, spina bifida, and tumors.

Incidence/Prevalence

Between 250,000 and 400,000 persons in the United States have SCIs, and about 14,000 new injuries occur each year (Gibson, 2003). The client may be hospitalized for 3 months or longer, including acute care and rehabilitation. Life expectancy has increased, but it is still below that of individuals without an SCI. Clients usually die from complications of immobility or infection.

A typical client with an SCI is an unmarried man between 16 and 30 years of age. Peak incidence of injury occurs in the

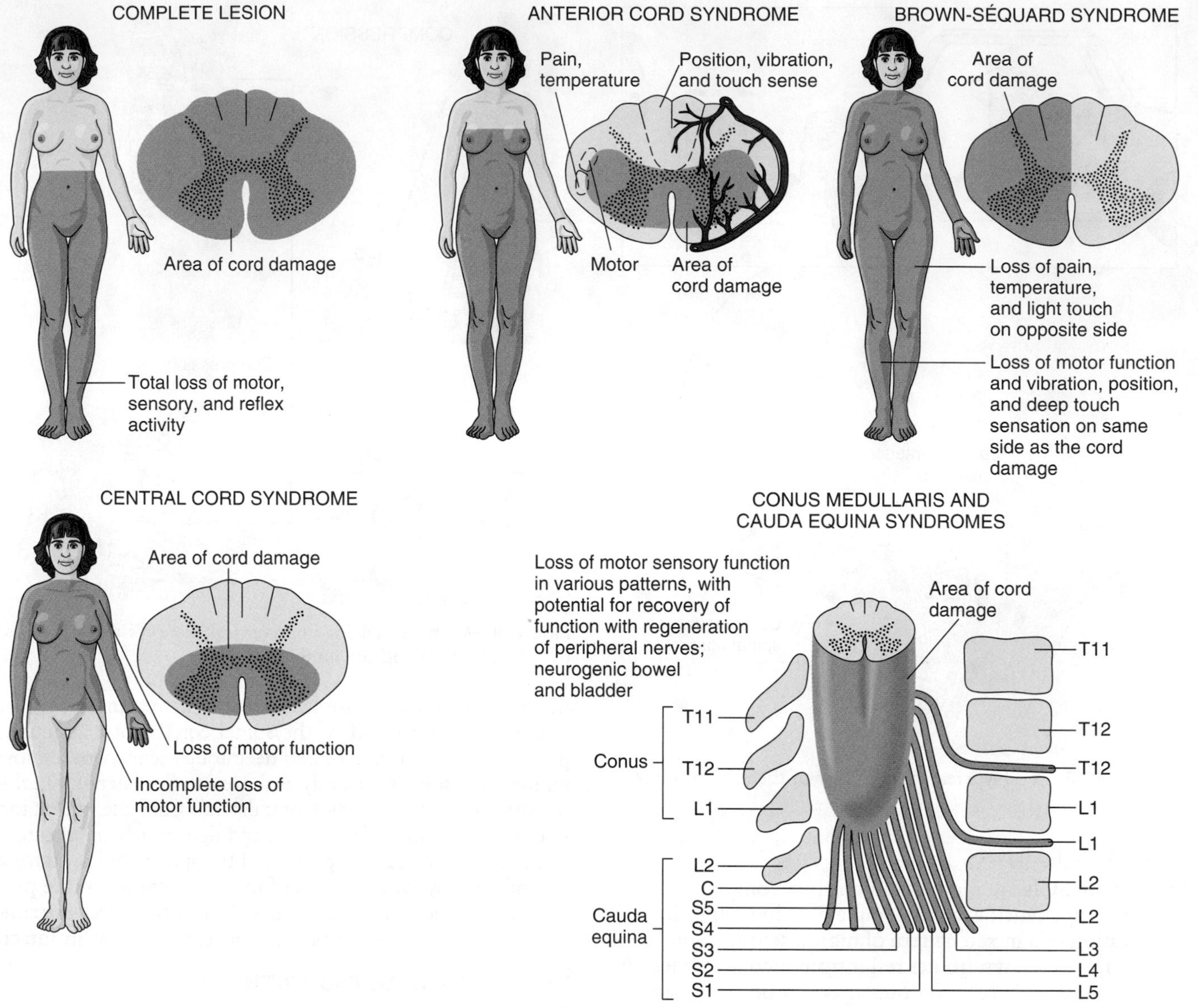

Figure 46-5 ■ Common spinal cord syndromes.

summer or warmer months. Men constitute 82% of SCI clients, and most are white. Most injuries are cervical. The percentage of persons over the age of 60 is 10% (NSCIDB, 2001).

COLLABORATIVE MANAGEMENT

PHARM e REVIEW

Assessment

HISTORY

When obtaining a history from a client with a spinal cord injury (SCI), the nurse gathers as much data as possible about how the accident occurred and the probable mechanism of injury. Questions include the position of the client immediately after the injury, the symptoms that occurred after the injury, and the changes that have occurred since the initial appearance of signs and symptoms. If possible, prehospital rescue personnel are questioned about the type of immobilization devices used and whether any problems occurred during stabilization and transport to the hospital. Information is obtained about the medical treatment given at the scene of injury or in the emergency department (e.g., medications and IV fluids).

Obtain the client's medical history, including a history of arthritis of the spine, congenital deformities, osteoporosis or osteomyelitis, cancer, and previous injury or surgery of the neck or back. These health problems may cause or contribute to an SCI. A detailed history of any respiratory problems is particularly important if the client has experienced a cervical SCI.

PHYSICAL ASSESSMENT/CLINICAL MANIFESTATIONS

INITIAL ASSESSMENT. The *first priority* for the client with an SCI is assessing the respiratory pattern and ensuring an adequate airway. The client with a cervical SCI is at high risk for respiratory compromise because the cervical spinal nerves (C3-5) innervate the phrenic nerve, which controls the diaphragm. Endotracheal intubation may be necessary to prevent respiratory arrest.

The client is assessed for indications of intra-abdominal hemorrhage or hemorrhage or bleeding around fracture sites. Other indicators of hemorrhage include hypotension and tachycardia with a weak and thready pulse.

Use the Glasgow Coma Scale (see Chapter 44) to assess the client's level of consciousness (LOC). Cognitive impairment as a result of an associated traumatic brain injury (TBI) or substance abuse is seen in about half of all traumatic SCIs. A detailed assessment of the client's motor and sensory status is performed to assist in determining the level of injury and to serve as baseline data for future comparison. The level of injury is the lowest neurologic segment with intact or normal motor and sensory function. **Tetraplegia,** also called **quadriplegia** (paralysis), and **quadriparesis** (weakness) involve all four extremities, as seen with cervical cord injury. **Paraplegia** (paralysis) and **paraparesis** (weakness) involve only the lower extremities, as seen in lower thoracic and lumbosacral injuries or lesions.

Spinal shock occurs immediately after injury as a result of disruption in the communication pathways between upper motor neurons and lower motor neurons. This condition is characterized by the following:

- Flaccid paralysis
- Loss of reflex activity below the level of the lesion
- Bradycardia
- Paralytic ileus (occasionally)
- Hypotension

Spinal shock may last from a few days to several months; its reversal is indicated by the return of reflex activity.

ASSESSMENT OF SENSATION. Sensation is carried from the peripheral nerves to the spinal cord and up to the cerebral cortex via a variety of sensation-specific tracts. Injury to the spinal cord may prohibit sensory impulses from reaching the brain. To test sensory abilities, the client is asked to close his or her eyes. Touch the skin with a clean safety pin or cotton-tipped applicator and ask the client whether he or she can feel the pinprick or light touch. Bilateral responses are compared. Follow the sensory distribution of the skin dermatomes (see Figure 44-7), with the examination beginning in the area of reported loss of sensation and ending where sensation becomes normal. For example, sensation of the top of the foot and calf of the leg is spinal skin segment (dermatome) levels L3, L4, and L5. The area at the level of the umbilicus is T10, the clavicle is C3 or C4, and finger sensation is C7 and C8. The client may report a complete sensory loss, **hypoesthesia** (decreased sensation), or **hyperesthesia** (increased sensation).

The client's proprioceptive function may be assessed. Ask the client again to close his or her eyes. Next move one of his or her fingers or toes up or down. Ask the client to identify the position of the digits.

ASSESSMENT OF MOTOR ABILITY. In addition to performing a routine motor evaluation of the client, selected muscles are tested in a more systematic fashion (Chart 46-8). Many scales are available to measure motor function. The American Spinal Injury Association (ASIA) recommends a five-point grading scale, with 0 being no movement and 5 being normal strength. Ask the client to flex and extend the elbows, elevate both arms off the bed, flex and extend the wrists and fingers, and touch each finger to the thumb. Clients with spinal injuries at the fifth or sixth cervical vertebra are often able to flex but not extend

CHART 46-8

BEST PRACTICE for
Assessing Motor Function in the Client with a Spinal Cord Injury

- To assess C4-5, apply downward pressure while the client shrugs his or her shoulders upward.
- To assess C5-6, apply resistance while the client pulls up his or her arms.
- To assess C7, apply resistance while the client straightens his or her flexed arms.
- To assess C8, make sure the client is able to grasp an object and form a fist.
- To assess L2-4, apply resistance while the client lifts his or her legs from the bed.
- To assess L5, apply resistance while the client dorsiflexes his or her feet.
- To assess S1, apply resistance while the client plantar flexes his or her feet.

their arms. Observe the client's ability to move the lower extremities. Ask him or her to wiggle the toes, flex and extend the feet and knees, and move one or both hips.

The advanced practice nurse or health care provider may also test deep tendon reflexes (DTRs), including the biceps (C5), triceps (C7), patella (L3), and ankle (S1). It is not unusual for these reflexes, as well as all motor function or sensation, to be absent immediately after the injury because of spinal shock. After spinal shock has resolved, the reflexes may return if the lesion is incomplete or involves upper motor neurons.

CARDIOVASCULAR ASSESSMENT. Cardiovascular dysfunction is usually the result of disruption of the autonomic nervous system, especially if the injury is above the sixth thoracic vertebra. Bradycardia, hypotension, and hypothermia result from a loss of sympathetic input and may lead to cardiac dysrhythmias. A systolic blood pressure below 90 mm Hg requires treatment because lack of perfusion to the spinal cord would worsen the client's condition. In addition, the lack of sympathetic or hypothalamic control causes the client to lose thermoregulatory functions. As a result, the body tends to assume the temperature of the environment and attempts to compensate by increasing extracellular fluid.

EMERGENCY CARE. The client with an upper SCI must be observed for signs of **autonomic dysreflexia** (hyperreflexia). Dysreflexia is characterized by severe hypertension, bradycardia, severe headache, nasal stuffiness, and flushing (Chart 46-9). The cause of this syndrome is a noxious stimulus, most often a distended bladder or constipation. *This is a neurologic emergency and must be promptly treated to prevent a hypertensive stroke*! Chart 46-10 lists emergency care for autonomic dysreflexia.

RESPIRATORY ASSESSMENT. A client with a cervical SCI is at risk for respiratory problems resulting from immobility or from an interruption of spinal innervation to the respiratory muscles. Some clients require intubation and mechanical ventilation. A complete respiratory assessment is done in collaboration with the respiratory therapist, if available. The respiratory therapist should evaluate vital capacity and minute volume as part of the assessment. Periodic repetition of these tests should be performed as the client's clinical status indicates.

Closely monitor the client for life-threatening respiratory complications, such as an impaired gas exchange resulting

CHART 46-9

KEY FEATURES of
Autonomic Dysreflexia

- Sudden onset of severe, throbbing headache
- Severe, rapidly occurring hypertension
- Bradycardia
- Flushing above level of lesion (face and chest)
- Pale extremities below level of lesion
- Nasal stuffiness
- Sweating
- Nausea
- Blurred vision
- Piloerection
- Feeling of apprehension

CHART 46-10

BEST PRACTICE for
Emergency Care of the Client Experiencing Autonomic Dysreflexia: Immediate Interventions

EMERGENCY CARE

- Place client in sitting position.
- Page/notify health care provider.
- Loosen tight clothing on the client.
- Assess for and treat the cause.
- Check the Foley catheter tubing (if present) for kinks or obstruction.
- If a Foley catheter is not present, check for bladder distention and catheterize immediately.
- Place anesthetic ointment on tip of catheter before insertion.
- Check the client for fecal impaction; if present, disimpact immediately using anesthetic ointment.
- Check the room temperature to ensure that it is not too cool or drafty.
- Monitor blood pressures every 10 to 15 minutes.
- Give nitrates or hydralazine (Apresoline, Novo-Hylazin ✱) as prescribed.

from pneumonia, pulmonary emboli, and atelectasis. Pneumonia and pulmonary emboli decrease the life expectancy of SCI clients and have replaced renal failure as the leading cause of death.

GASTROINTESTINAL AND GENITOURINARY ASSESSMENT. Assess the client's abdomen for indications of hemorrhage, distention, or paralytic ileus. Hemorrhage may result from the trauma, or it may occur later from a stress ulcer or the administration of steroids. Paralytic ileus may develop within 72 hours of hospital admission. During the period of spinal shock, peristalsis decreases, leading to a loss of bowel sounds and gastric distention. This lack of or interference with autonomic innervation may lead to a reflex or hypotonic bowel.

Autonomic dysfunction initially causes an areflexic bladder, which later leads to urinary retention and a neurogenic bladder. The client is at risk for urinary tract infection from an indwelling urinary catheter, from intermittent catheterizations, or from bladder distention, stasis, and overflow.

MUSCULOSKELETAL ASSESSMENT. Assess the client's muscle tone and size. Muscle wasting results from the long-term flaccid paralysis seen in clients with **lower motor neuron** (LMN) lesions. Incomplete lesions or **upper motor neuron** (UMN) lesions may cause muscle spasticity, which can lead to contractures after spinal shock has resolved.

Observe the condition of the client's skin, especially over pressure points, at least twice daily. Any reddened area is carefully assessed and monitored for change. A pressure-reducing mattress or special bed is used to prevent skin breakdown.

Another complication of prolonged immobility is **heterotopic ossification** (bony overgrowth, often into muscle), which occurs in 15% to 20% of all clients with spinal cord injury (SCI). It is evidenced by swelling, redness, warmth, and decreased range of motion (ROM) of the involved extremity. Changes in the bony structure are not visible until several weeks after initial symptoms appear.

PSYCHOSOCIAL ASSESSMENT

If possible, obtain information about the client's preinjury psychosocial status, usual methods of coping with illness, difficult situations, and disappointments. Determine the client's level of independence or dependence and his or her comfort level in discussing feelings and emotions with family members or close friends. Clients who are emotionally secure and have a positive self-image, supportive family, and financial and job security often adapt to their injury. Information about the client's religious beliefs or cultural background also assists the nurse in developing the plan of care. The client with an SCI must cope with changes in body image, self-esteem, independence, role relationships, and sexuality.

In addition, assess family members or significant others to determine how well they are coping with the client's injury and their role changes. The client and significant others must be prepared for extensive rehabilitation and changes in lifestyle. Financial constraints may pose additional stress.

LABORATORY ASSESSMENT

The health care provider orders routine laboratory studies for the client with an SCI to establish baseline data or to prepare for surgery. A urinalysis is used to check for the presence of blood in the urine after trauma. Arterial blood gas analysis is used to monitor the respiratory status of a client at risk for respiratory insufficiency. The findings should be within normal limits unless the client has a history of heavy smoking or preinjury pulmonary disease or is experiencing respiratory failure. Failure is indicated by decreased oxygen levels, increased carbon dioxide levels, and respiratory acidosis.

RADIOGRAPHIC AND OTHER DIAGNOSTIC ASSESSMENTS

The health care provider orders a complete radiographic series of the spine to identify vertebral fractures, subluxation, or dislocation. Computed tomography (CT) or magnetic resonance imaging (MRI) may be performed to determine the degree and extent of damage to the spinal cord and to detect the presence of blood and bone within the spinal column.

◆Analysis

COMMON NURSING DIAGNOSES AND COLLABORATIVE PROBLEMS

The following are the most common nursing diagnoses for clients with a spinal cord injury (SCI):

1. Ineffective Tissue Perfusion (Spinal Cord) related to interruption of arterial flow
2. Ineffective Airway Clearance, Ineffective Breathing Pattern, and Impaired Gas Exchange related to spinal cord injury

3. Impaired Physical Mobility or Self-Care Deficit (the level depends on the extent and level of the injury) related to decreased or absent muscle control
4. Impaired Urinary Elimination and Constipation related to sensory/motor impairment
5. Impaired Adjustment related to disability or health status change requiring change in lifestyle

ADDITIONAL NURSING DIAGNOSES AND COLLABORATIVE PROBLEMS

In addition to the common nursing diagnoses, clients with an SCI may have one or more of the following:

- Risk for Impaired Skin Integrity related to physical immobilization
- Sexual Dysfunction related to altered body function
- Acute Pain related to physical injury
- Risk for Injury related to altered mobility
- Imbalanced Nutrition: Less Than Body Requirements related to hypermetabolism or inability to absorb nutrients

Collaborative problems include the following:

- Potential for Deep Vein Thrombosis (DVT)
- Potential for Sepsis
- Potential for Hypoxemia
- Potential for Atelectasis, Pneumonia

Planning and Implementation

INEFFECTIVE TISSUE PERFUSION (SPINAL CORD)

PLANNING: EXPECTED OUTCOMES. The client with an SCI is expected to demonstrate adequate spinal cord tissue perfusion as evidenced by no further deterioration in neurologic status.

INTERVENTIONS. If the client has a fractured vertebra, the primary concern of the health care team is to reduce and immobilize the fracture to prevent further damage to the spinal cord from bone fragments. The health care provider typically uses nonsurgical techniques with traction or external fixation, but surgery may be necessary to stabilize the spine and prevent further spinal cord damage.

NONSURGICAL MANAGEMENT. Assess the client's vital signs and neurologic status, especially respiratory function and motor and sensory changes in the extremities every 4 hours or more often if clinically indicated. In the first 24 hours after injury, the client is at risk for **neurogenic shock** as manifested by hypotension and bradycardia. Neurogenic shock is most often associated with cervical spinal injuries and is caused by a loss of autonomic function.

NIC **Positioning: Neurologic.** Regardless of the level of SCI, keep the client in optimal body alignment to prevent further cord injury or irritability (Chart 46-11). Devices such as traction, orthoses, or collars may be used to keep the spine immobilized during healing and rehabilitation.

Immobilization for Cervical Injuries. The client with a cervical spine injury is usually placed in fixed skeletal traction to realign the vertebrae, facilitate bone healing, and prevent further injury. The most commonly used devices for immobilization are the halo fixation device and cervical tongs (Gardner-Wells, Barton, or Crutchfield tongs) (Figure 46-6). These devices may be used in conjunction with a Stryker frame, rotational bed, or kinetic treatment table to allow frequent turning. Either device is inserted by the physician into the outer aspect of the skull. The addition of traction to the cervical tongs assists in reducing the fracture. Traction may or may not be used with the halo fixator. Traction weights may be prescribed by the physician.

The halo fixator is a static traction device (see Figure 46-6). Four pins (or screws) are inserted into the skull. The metal halo ring may be attached to a plastic vest or cast when the spine is stable, allowing increased client mobility. Never move or turn the client by holding or pulling on the halo device. Check the client's skin frequently to ensure that the jacket or cast is not causing pressure. The nurse should be able to insert one finger easily under the jacket or cast.

Monitor the client's neurologic status for changes in movement or decreased strength. The weights of the traction should hang freely at all times. Releasing the traction could cause further neurologic damage. Maintain the client in alignment, and ensure that the ropes for the traction remain within the pulley and hang freely. The insertion sites of the tongs or halo device are monitored for signs of infection. Hospital policy is followed for pin site care, which may specify the use of solutions such as hydrogen peroxide and saline.

CHART 46-11

NIC **INTERVENTION ACTIVITIES for The Client with a Spinal Cord Injury**

Positioning: Neurologic: *Achievement of optimal, appropriate body alignment for the client experiencing or at risk for spinal cord injury or vertebral irritability.*

- Immobilize or support the affected body part, as appropriate.
- Place in the designated therapeutic position.
- Maintain proper body alignment.
- Position with head and neck in alignment.
- Turn using the log roll technique.
- Apply an orthosis collar.
- Instruct on orthosis collar care, as needed.
- Apply and maintain a splinting or bracing device.
- Monitor skin integrity under bracing device/orthosis collar.
- Instruct on pin site care, as needed.
- Monitor traction pin insertion site.
- Perform traction/orthosis device pin insertion site care.
- Monitor traction device setup.

Airway Management: *Facilitation of patency of air passages*

- Position client to maximize ventilation potential.
- Identify client requiring actual/potential airway insertion.
- Insert oral or nasopharyngeal airway, as appropriate.
- Perform chest physical therapy, as appropriate.
- Remove secretions by encouraging coughing or by suctioning.
- Encourage slow, deep breathing; turning; and coughing.
- Instruct how to cough effectively.
- Assist with incentive spirometer, as appropriate.
- Auscultate breath sounds, noting areas of decreased or absent ventilation and presence of adventitious sounds.
- Perform endotracheal or nasotracheal suctioning, as appropriate.
- Administer humidified air or oxygen, as appropriate.
- Regulate fluid intake to optimize fluid balance.
- Position to alleviate dyspnea.
- Monitor respiratory and oxygenation status, as appropriate.

NIC intervention activities selected from Dochterman, J.M., & Bulechek, G.M. (Eds.). (2004). *Nursing interventions classification (NIC)* (4th ed.). St. Louis: Mosby.

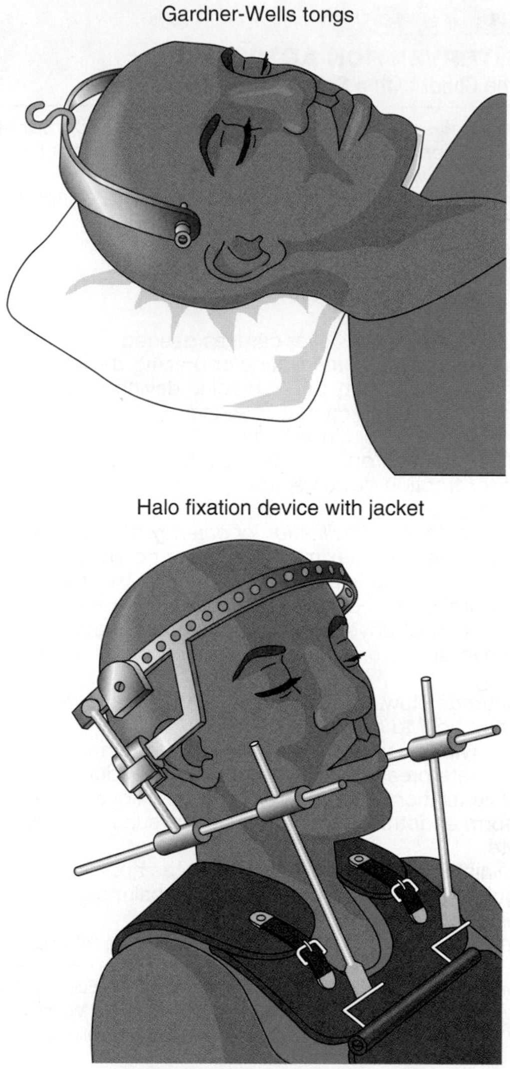

Figure 46-6 ■ Types of cervical spine traction.

Immobilization of Thoracic and Lumbar/Sacral Injuries. The client with a thoracic injury is placed on bedrest; immobilization with a fiberglass or plastic body cast may be done (see also Chapter 55). For lumbar and sacral injuries, immobilization of the spine is typically accomplished with a brace or a corset worn when the client is out of bed. Newer lightweight, custom-fit thoracic lumbar sacral orthoses (TLSOs) are preferred over heavier braces or splints, such as the Taylor splint.

Drug Therapy. The administration of methylprednisolone (Solu-Medrol) is controversial. Previously it was thought that when given within 8 hours of injury the client showed improvement in motor and sensory function. Recent clinical trials do not support this as an evidenced-based standard of care for SCI because the adverse effects of the drug outweigh the benefits (Gibson, 2003). Dextran, a plasma expander, may be used to increase capillary blood flow within the spinal cord and to prevent or treat hypotension. Atropine sulfate is used to treat bradycardia if the pulse rate falls below 50 to 60 beats/min. Hypotension, if severe, is treated with inotropic and sympathomimetic agents such as dopamine hydrochloride (Intropin) and isoproterenol.

Research continues to explore interventions in pharmacologic and surgical management of SCIs. Naloxone (Narcan) and thyrotropin-releasing hormone (TRH) have shown promise in improving spinal cord blood flow. Sygen is being researched for use in acute SCI but may also be studied for its use for chronic SCI. Another drug, 4-AP, a potassium channel blocker, is thought to improve spinal cord conduction and remains in clinical trials for clients whose SCI is older than 18 months. Research in the areas of muscle stimulation and neural regeneration also shows promise.

Dantrolene (Dantrium) and baclofen (Lioresal) may help to control severe muscle spasticity (usually upper motor neuron [UMN] injuries). Severe spasticity may also be managed with intrathecal baclofen (ITB) therapy. The drug is administered through a programmable infusion pump and intrathecal catheter directly into the cerebrospinal fluid.

Other drugs to prevent or treat complications of immobility may be needed later during the rehabilitative phase. For example, etidronate disodium (Didronel) may be prescribed for the client with **heterotopic ossification** (bony overgrowth).

Critical Thinking Challenge

A 19-year-old college student is admitted to your neurosurgical/orthopedic unit from the neuroscience intensive care unit. He has a Halo fixator in place for an incomplete spinal cord injury following a car accident. His best friend was killed in the accident. The client has an indwelling urinary catheter and is sitting in a semi-Fowler's position when you enter his room. You notice that his face is flushed and he complains of being very hot.

1. What additional assessment data should you obtain at this time? Why?
2. Could you delegate part of the assessment to unlicensed assistive personnel? Why or why not?
3. What should you do *first* if you suspect an emergency situation? Why?

evolve For suggested answer guidelines, go to http://evolve.elsevier.com/Iggy/.

SURGICAL MANAGEMENT. Emergency surgery may be indicated if there is evidence of spinal cord compression. The procedure is usually necessary to remove bone fragments from a vertebral fracture, evacuate a hematoma, or remove penetrating objects such as a bullet. A **decompressive laminectomy** (removal of one or more laminae) allows for cord expansion from edema if more conventional measures fail to prevent neurologic deterioration. Postoperative care of clients having back surgery is discussed earlier in this chapter on p. 980.

Additional surgical procedures to stabilize and support the spine may be performed at the discretion of the physician, depending on the client's condition and the extent of the injury. Typical procedures include a spinal fusion and the insertion of metal or steel rods, such as Harrington rods, to stabilize thoracic spinal injuries. After surgery, the client usually wears a brace, a corset, or lumbosacral support (TLSO) to keep the operative area immobilized during recovery. (See also Chapter 55, Collaborative Management of Scoliosis.)

Postoperatively, assess the client's neurologic status and vital signs at least every hour for the first 4 to 6 hours after surgery and then, if the client is stable, every 4 hours. Complications of surgery, such as hematoma and edema, are manifested by a deterioration in neurologic status.

The client is also at risk for cardiovascular instability because of a loss of sympathetic innervation. In some cases the client may require a pacemaker. Log roll the client when he or she is being moved to maintain skeletal alignment or placed on a special bed such as a kinetic treatment table. Monitor the client's cardiovascular status carefully, especially with position changes. A complete discussion of postoperative nursing care is found in Chapter 22.

INEFFECTIVE AIRWAY CLEARANCE; INEFFECTIVE BREATHING PATTERN; IMPAIRED GAS EXCHANGE

NOC **PLANNING: EXPECTED OUTCOMES.** The client with an SCI is expected to have airway patency, alveolar exchange to maintain arterial blood gas (ABG) concentrations, and adequate ventilation. Indicators include that the following will not be compromised:

- Ease of breathing
- Respiratory rate and rhythm
- ABGs
- Oxygen saturation
- Auscultated breath sounds

INTERVENTIONS. Airway management is the priority for a client with spinal cord injury. Clients with injuries at or above the sixth thoracic vertebra are especially at risk for respiratory complications (e.g., pneumonia) and pulmonary embolus as a result of impaired functioning of the intercostal muscles. Depending on the level of injury, intubation or tracheotomy with mechanical ventilation may be needed.

Turn the client at least every 2 hours, and instruct him or her to breathe as deeply as possible. Assist the client who is tetraplegic to cough by placing his or her hands on either side of the rib cage or upper abdomen below the diaphragm. This technique is sometimes called "assisted coughing," "quad cough," or "**cough assist**." As the client inhales, push upward to help expand the lungs and cough.

Encourage the client to use an incentive spirometer. The nurse or respiratory therapist performs a respiratory assessment every 8 hours to determine the effectiveness of these strategies. In some cases it may be necessary to perform oral or nasal suctioning if the client cannot clear the airway of secretions effectively (see Chart 46-11).

IMPAIRED PHYSICAL MOBILITY; SELF-CARE DEFICIT

NOC **PLANNING: EXPECTED OUTCOMES.** The client with an SCI is expected to be free from complications of immobility and perform the most basic physical tasks and personal care activities as independently as possible with or without assistive/adaptive devices. Indicators include that the client will have no consequences of immobility, including the following:

- Pressure ulcers
- Venous thrombosis
- Contracted joints
- Bone fracture

Additional indicators include that the following will not be compromised:

- Transfer performance
- Wheelchair mobility
- Eating
- Dressing
- Bathing and grooming
- Oral hygiene

INTERVENTIONS. The client with an SCI is especially at risk for pressure ulcers, contractures, and deep vein thrombosis (DVT) or pulmonary emboli. Proper positioning not only helps to prevent complications but also provides alignment to prevent further spinal cord injury or irritability, as described under Positioning: Neurologic, p. 989.

Preventing Complications of Immobility. To decrease the high risk of pressure ulcers, the nurse or assistive nursing personnel turns and repositions the client in bed at least every 2 hours. When sitting in a chair, the client is repositioned or taught to reposition himself or herself more often than every 2 hours because in the sitting position most of the weight is placed on one area, the ischial tuberosities. Special pressure-relief devices, such as gel pads, may be used in the wheelchair or the bed, but these do not eliminate the need for regular turning and repositioning.

Inspect (and teach the client to inspect) the skin frequently to determine the client's tolerance for sitting and to detect reddened areas. Press on any reddened areas over the ischial tuberosities and look for blanching. If blanching does not occur, the area is vulnerable to skin breakdown.

To decrease the risk of contractures as a result of immobility, range-of-motion (ROM) exercises are performed at least once every 8 hours. The physical therapist and the occupational therapist will do the following:

- Determine the most appropriate positioning and exercise techniques
- Assess the need for hand and wrist splints
- Develop a plan to prevent footdrop (usually clients wear high-topped tennis shoes for prevention)

Assess the client's lower extremities for indications of DVT. Signs and symptoms include leg or calf pain, localized tenderness, swelling, and redness. Some clients may be totally asymptomatic. Recent guidelines for acute spinal cord injury (SCI) recommend a combination of low-molecular-weight heparin (LMWH) (e.g., enoxaparin [Lovenox]) and rotational bed, or adjusted-dose unfractionated heparin (Guides for Management of Acute Cervical Spinal Injury, 2002). Lovenox provides the same level of antithrombotic activity as heparin but may decrease the risk for hemorrhage. Graduated compression stockings (GCSs), also called sequential compression devices (SCDs), or pneumatic compression boots (PCBs) may be used with this regimen or in addition to these measures. Lovenox provides the same level of antithrombotic activity as heparin but may decrease the risk for hemorrhage (see Chapter 39 for a complete discussion of DVT prevention).

Preventing Orthostatic Hypotension. Clients with cervical cord injuries are especially at high risk for orthostatic (postural) hypotension, but any client who is immobilized may have this problem. If the client moves from a lying position to a sitting or standing position too quickly, he or she may experience hypotension, which could result in dizziness and falls. Because of interrupted autonomic innervation, the blood vessels do not constrict quickly enough to

CHART 46-12

BEST PRACTICE for
Care of the Client with a Spinal Cord Injury

- Assess the client's respiratory status; monitor for atelectasis, pneumonia, and pulmonary embolus.
- Take vital signs every 4 hours or more often if clinically indicated; monitor for orthostatic hypotension.
- Perform neurologic status checks every 4 hours or more often if clinically indicated.
- Notify the physician immediately of deterioration in motor status.
- Watch for and immediately treat autonomic dysreflexia.
- Give pain medication as prescribed; document the client's response.
- Prevent immobility complications.
  - Have the client turn, cough, and deep breathe (TCDB) every 2 hours.
  - Use pneumatic compression boots or gradated compression stockings.
  - Check the skin and bony prominences for redness and breakdown.
- Assess bladder function.
  - Palpate the abdomen for distention.
  - Begin a bladder retraining program as appropriate.
  - Assess intake and output.
- Assess bowel function.
  - Auscultate bowel sounds.
  - Palpate for distention.
  - Chart stool frequency.
  - Begin a bowel program as appropriate.
- Monitor nutritional status, including a calorie count, and collaborate with the dietitian to identify an appropriate diet.
- Assess psychological status.
  - Communicate with the client.
  - Answer questions honestly; refer questions that you cannot answer to someone who can.
  - Assess for signs of depression or anger.

push blood up into the brain; this causes the dizziness or light-headedness often experienced by these clients.

Observe the client carefully for indications of orthostatic hypotension when the head of the bed is raised and when the client is permitted to dangle the legs over the side of the bed or to be up in a chair. Blood pressure is measured in each position.

To help prevent orthostatic hypotension, teach the client to change positions slowly. Some clients wear elastic corsets around the trunk to help facilitate blood flow. Thigh-high antiembolism stockings or elastic (Ace) wraps around both legs may also be used. A tilt table may be used to help the client get used to postural changes. Chart 46-12 summarizes the most important aspects of care for clients with an SCI.

Promoting Self-Care. The most important part of promoting self-care is setting realistic outcomes on the basis of the client's potential mobility and functional level. Even clients with a cervical SCI may be able to learn how to perform most activities of daily living (ADLs) independently. Collaborate with the physical therapist (PT) and occupational therapist to evaluate how the client can best transfer from a bed to the wheelchair and feed, dress, and bathe. Various assistive/adaptive devices are available to help clients regain their independence. Chapter 10 discusses self-care promotion in more detail.

Many clients with an SCI can no longer walk. They become wheelchair dependent and must learn new skills. The PT carefully measures the client and orders a custom-made wheelchair. If the client is unable to self-propel the chair manually, electronic devices are available so he or she can use the mouth, neck, or upper arm to ambulate in the chair.

IMPAIRED URINARY ELIMINATION AND/OR CONSTIPATION

NOC **PLANNING: EXPECTED OUTCOMES.** The client with an SCI is expected to achieve control of elimination of urine and stool. Indicators include that the client will consistently demonstrate the following:

- Predictable pattern of voiding
- Voiding more than 150 mL each time
- Emptying the bladder completely
- Managing clothing independently
- No urinary incontinence
- No urinary infection
- Control of bowel movements
- Ease of stool passage

INTERVENTIONS. Clients with SCIs have reflex or neurogenic loss of bowel and bladder control. Many can become continent if they rigorously adhere to an established program. The type of program depends on the usual elimination pattern and whether the injury involved upper motor neurons (UMNs) or lower motor neurons (LMNs). A urologic evaluation may be needed to identify bladder type.

Establishing a Bladder Retraining Program. As soon as the client is medically stable, the indwelling Foley catheter is removed. Initially the physician may prescribe an intermittent catheterization program. The nurse typically catheterizes the client every 4 hours as ordered and more frequently if the urine output is greater than 500 mL. Over time the intervals between catheterizations are increased and adjusted to the client's fluid intake and sleep times. A bedside **bladder ultrasound** device is often used to measure bladder residual.

After the acute care phase has passed, the client may be able to initiate voiding by using specific techniques. Clients with UMN, or **spastic, bladder** problems (injury above the sacrum) may be able to stimulate voiding by doing the following:

- Stroking the inner thigh
- Pulling on pubic hair and hair of the upper thigh
- Pouring warm water over the perineum
- Tapping the bladder area to stimulate the detrusor muscle

Some health care providers prescribe a drug to stimulate voiding, such as bethanechol chloride (Urecholine). Bethanechol is a cholinergic agent that facilitates contraction of the detrusor muscle and is usually given two to four times daily about 1 hour before attempts to void.

Clients with injuries to the lumbosacral area usually have an LMN (flaccid) bladder. Clients with **flaccid bladders** may achieve emptying of the bladder by performing a Valsalva maneuver or tightening the abdominal muscles. These techniques are not successful for all LMN injuries. To ascertain the effectiveness of these maneuvers, catheterize the client for residual urine after voiding. Some clients rely solely on intermittent catheterization two or three times daily to empty the bladder. Obese clients and those with very high-level SCIs may need an indwelling urinary catheter (Gibson, 2003).

All clients are encouraged to drink 2000 to 2500 mL of fluid each day to prevent urinary tract infection (UTI) and calculus formation. Clients with an LMN injury may decrease fluid intake after 6 or 7 PM each evening to prevent the need for catheterization in the middle of the night.

The client with any SCI is at risk for long-term renal complications, such as hydronephrosis, renal failure, and kidney stones. UTIs are common because organisms are introduced into the urinary tract by urinary catheters. Clients with SCI may not be aware of the infection because he or she cannot perceive dysuria, urgency, or back pain. They must rely on other signs and symptoms, such as foul-smelling urine or fever.

Establishing a Bowel Retraining Program. The following are essential elements of a bowel program:

- A consistent time for bowel elimination
- A high fluid intake (at least 2000 mL/day) unless fluid intake is restricted
- A high-fiber diet
- Rectal stimulation with or without suppositories
- If needed, stool softener medications such as docusate sodium (Colace) and docusate sodium and casanthranol (Peri-Colace)

If the client has sustained an LMN injury, the resulting flaccid large bowel may require the client to perform or undergo manual disimpaction. Additional stimuli to facilitate a bowel movement include scheduling toileting 30 minutes to 1 hour after meals to optimize the gastrocolic reflex and teaching the client to perform a Valsalva maneuver. Massaging the abdomen from right to left along the outline of the large intestine may also be helpful. Additional information about bladder and bowel retraining is provided in Chapter 10.

IMPAIRED ADJUSTMENT

NOC **PLANNING: EXPECTED OUTCOMES.** The client with an SCI is expected to develop an adaptive psychosocial response to a significant life change. Indicators include that the client will consistently demonstrate the following:

- Setting realistic goals
- Maintaining self-esteem
- Reporting feeling useful
- Verbalizing optimism about the present and future
- Identifying effective coping strategies

INTERVENTIONS. Information obtained from the psychosocial assessment is used by the interdisciplinary team to identify strategies to help the client adjust to the disability. Invite the client to ask questions, and answer them openly and honestly. Questions about prognosis and potential for complete recovery are referred to the health care provider because the timing and extent of recovery are different for each client.

Encourage the client to discuss his or her perceptions of the situation and the coping strategies that can be used. He or she should feel free to express personal feelings and emotions in an acceptable manner. The client may behave in a socially unacceptable manner (e.g., excessive anger, verbal abuse, use of illegal drugs); attempt to redirect this behavior. Begin a client education program to clarify misconceptions and provide health teaching. Referrals to clergy, rabbis, other spiritual leaders, or a psychologist or psychiatric liaison nurse may be needed to help clients adjust to their unexpected life change. Support groups are available for clients and their families.

Clients with SCIs should be referred to a social worker or financial counselor for a review of their insurance and financial status and also should be referred to the appropriate social service agencies as necessary. Many insurance policies do not provide coverage for extended rehabilitation services.

Community-Based Care

Case managers are ideal care coordinators to act as SCI client advocates. In some settings, case managers begin working with clients in the emergency department to establish a positive image of SCI rehabilitation. Rehabilitation begins in the critical care unit when clients are hemodynamically stable and spinal shock has subsided. They are usually transferred from the acute care setting to a rehabilitation setting, where they learn more about self-care, mobility skills, and bladder and bowel retraining. The length of stay in the rehabilitation hospital or unit is typically 1 to 3 months, depending on the medical complications that may occur, such as infections.

Psychosocial adaptation is one of the critical factors in determining the success of rehabilitation. The case manager or acute care nurse can help the client prepare for discharge or transfer to a rehabilitation hospital. Assist in verbalizing feelings and fears about body image, self-concept, role performance, and self-esteem. The client should be told about the expected reactions of those outside the security of the hospital environment. In the acute care setting, the nurse, family members, or friends can take the client to the hospital lobby or, if permitted, to the cafeteria or outside on the hospital grounds. Let the client know, in a tactful and nonjudgmental manner, when his or her behavior is unacceptable for the time and place in which it occurs, and encourage more positive behaviors. Role-playing or anticipating responses to potential problems is helpful. For example, the client can practice answering questions from children about why he or she is in a wheelchair or cannot move certain parts of the body.

HOME CARE MANAGEMENT

If the client is discharged home or returns home for a weekend visit from the rehabilitation setting, the environment must be assessed to ensure that it is free from hazards and can accommodate the client's special needs (e.g., a wheelchair). The occupational or physical therapist, in collaboration with rehabilitation and the home care nurse, usually assesses the client's temporary or permanent home environment. Ease of accessibility is particularly important at the entrance of the home as well as the bathroom, kitchen, and bedroom. The height of the client's bed may need to be adjusted to facilitate a smooth transfer into or out of the bed.

All adaptive devices that the client will use at home should be ordered and delivered to the rehabilitation facility. This enables the nurse and other therapists to ensure that the items fit correctly and that the client and family know how to use them correctly.

HEALTH TEACHING

The teaching plan for the client with an SCI includes the following:

- Physical mobility and activity skills (including skin care)
- Activities of daily living (ADLs) skills

CHART 46-13

CLIENT EDUCATION GUIDE

Use of a Halo Device*

- Be aware that the weight of the halo device alters balance. Be careful when leaning forward or backward.
- Wear loose clothing, preferably with hook and loop (Velcro) fasteners or large openings for head and arms.
- Bathe in the bathtub or sponge bath. (Some physicians allow showers.)
- Wash under the lamb's wool liner of the vest to prevent rashes or sores; use powders or lotions sparingly under the vest.
- Have someone change the liner if it becomes odorous.
- Support the head with a small pillow when sleeping to prevent unnecessary pressure and discomfort.
- Try to resume usual activities to the extent possible; keep as active as possible. (The weight of the device may cause fatigue or weakness.) Avoid contact sports or swimming, however.
- Do not drive because vision is impaired with the device.
- Keep straws available for drinking fluids.
- Cut meats and other food into small pieces to facilitate chewing and swallowing.
- Before going outside in cold temperatures, wrap the pins with cloth to prevent the metal from getting cold.
- Have someone clean the pin sites as recommended by physician or hospital protocol.
- Observe the pin sites daily for redness, drainage, or loosening; report changes to the physician.
- Increase fluids and fiber in the diet to prevent constipation.
- Use a position of comfort during sexual activity.

*Home care instructions may vary depending on hospital or physician preference.

- Bowel and bladder retraining program
- Medication regimen
- Sexuality education

This information should be reinforced with written handouts or other client education material that the client, family members, or significant others can use after discharge to the home.

MOBILITY AND ACTIVITIES OF DAILY LIVING. It is important that the client learn mobility skills so that he or she can negotiate movement on sidewalks, carpeting, and other flooring surfaces. The client must also be able to negotiate sidewalk curbs while walking independently with crutches or a cane or while in a wheelchair.

Some clients are discharged home or to a rehabilitation setting with a halo vest. A halo vest has a significant physical and psychological impact on clients. Physically, clients find it difficult to perform mobility skills and ADLs independently, especially dressing, bathing, and feeding. From a psychological perspective, clients perceive an altered body image. Teach the client or other caregiver going home or to a rehabilitation setting how to care for and adjust to the halo device (Chart 46-13).

The ADL training for the client with an SCI includes a structured exercise program to promote strength and endurance. The occupational therapist instructs the client in the correct use of all adaptive equipment. In collaboration with the therapists, instruct family members or the caregiver in transfer skills, feeding, bathing, dressing, positioning, and skin care as discussed previously in this chapter and in Chapter 10.

BOWEL AND BLADDER TRAINING. Collaborate with the dietitian to help the client maintain an ideal body weight and to promote bowel and bladder elimination. Reinforce the need to follow the client's individualized bowel and bladder program, and teach the client in the procedures to follow if problems develop.

CHART 46-14

NURSING FOCUS on the OLDER ADULT

What Clients Need to Know About Aging with Spinal Cord Injury

Nursing Intervention	Rationales
Get flu shots annually, tetanus shots every 10 years, and the pneumonia vaccine as required.	Respiratory complications are the most common cause of death following spinal cord injury (SCI).
For women, have annual Papanicolaou (Pap) smears and mammograms.	Limitations in movement may make breast self-examination difficult. All older women should have an annual Pap smear.
Take measures to prevent osteoporosis, such as increasing calcium intake, exercising, and avoiding caffeine and smoking.	Women over 50 years of age often lose bone density, which can result in fractures.
Practice meticulous skin care, including moisturizing and drinking plenty of water.	As a person ages, skin becomes dry and less elastic, predisposing the client to pressure ulcers.
Take measures to prevent constipation, such as drinking adequate fluids, eating a healthy diet with fiber, and exercising.	Constipation is a problem for most clients with SCI, and they are more likely to develop the problem later in life.
Modify activities if joint pain occurs; use a powered rather than a manual wheelchair. Ask the health care provider about treatment options.	Arthritis occurs in more than half of people over 65 years of age. Clients with SCI are more likely to develop arthritis as a result of added stress on the upper extremities when using a wheelchair.

MEDICATION REGIMEN. Teach the client and his or her family or other caregiver about the name, purpose, dosage, timing of administration, and side effects of all medications. They should also understand the possible interaction of prescribed medications with over-the-counter medications or alcohol and illegal drugs.

SEXUALITY EDUCATION. The goal of sexuality education is to answer questions and correct any misinformation. Women with SCI are able to have sexual intercourse and conception, although menses may be temporarily interrupted initially. For men, SCIs often affect fertility and sexual function. Erection and ejaculation are impaired for many clients. Unless the nurse has specific training or experience in sexuality counseling of people with SCIs, detailed questions should be directed to a sexuality counselor or urologist.

CONSIDERATIONS FOR OLDER ADULTS

Many clients with SCI are living into middle and older adulthood. Thinking and planning about preventive health care for the future are important parts of health teaching. Chart 46-14 outlines important interventions for maintaining health in older adults with SCI.

HEALTH CARE RESOURCES

The nurse or case manager refers the client and family or significant others to the local, state or province, and national organizations for those with SCIs. These organizations include the National Spinal Cord Injury Association and the Spinal Cord Injury Hotline. Many consumer-oriented books, journals, and films are also available. Support groups may help the client and family adjust to a changed lifestyle and provide solutions to commonly encountered problems.

A full-time caretaker or personal assistant is usually required if the quadriplegic client returns home. The caretaker may be a family member or a nursing assistant employed to help provide care and companionship. A paraplegic client is often able to function without assistance after an appropriate rehabilitation program.

Critical Thinking Challenge

The college student with an incomplete cervical spinal cord injury will soon be discharged to home with his parents. He continues to have a Halo device but is able to void using bladder stimulation techniques rather than catheterization. The client has been reluctant to discuss the death of his friend in the car accident in which he was injured.

1. What are the priorities for discharge planning in this situation?
2. What health care resources will the client require?
3. What health teaching will he require and why?

evolve For suggested answer guidelines, go to http://evolve.elsevier.com/Iggy/.

Evaluation: Outcomes

Evaluate the care of the client with an SCI on the basis of the identified nursing diagnoses and collaborative problems. The expected outcomes are that the client:

- Exhibits no deterioration in neurologic status
- Maintains a patent airway, an alveolar exchange to maintain arterial blood gas concentration, and adequate ventilation
- Is free from complications of immobility
- Performs basic activities of living as independently as possible with or without the use of assistive/adaptive devices
- Achieves control of elimination of stool and urine
- Develops an adaptive psychosocial response to a significant life change

Specific indicators for these outcomes are listed for each nursing diagnosis under the Planning and Implementation section (see earlier).

SPINAL CORD TUMORS

Spinal cord tumors occur most often in the thoracic area, followed by an almost equal distribution in the lumbar and cervical region. Signs and symptoms depend on the location of the tumor and its speed of growth.

PATHOPHYSIOLOGY

The pathologic effects of a spinal cord tumor are more often related to compression of the cord than to invasion of the spinal cord itself. As the tumor expands within the vertebral column, it compresses the cord or the spinal nerve roots. Further growth leads to displacement of the cord. In addition, a large tumor may disrupt the vascular supply to the cord by compression or obstruct the normal flow of cerebrospinal fluid (CSF). Venous occlusion by the tumor may lead to spinal cord congestion and infarction.

The appearance of neurologic signs and symptoms is related to the rate of tumor growth. The spinal cord can often accommodate a slowly growing lesion. With time, the cord may become significantly misshapen and displaced, but the client has surprisingly few symptoms. On the other hand, a rapidly growing tumor quickly leads to spinal cord compression and edema and the development of neurologic symptoms, such as numbness and paralysis.

Primary spinal cord tumors arise from the epidural vessels, spinal meninges, or glial cells of the cord. Their cause is unknown. About 20% to 30% of spinal cord tumors (called secondary tumors) develop as a consequence of metastatic tumors from the lungs, breasts, prostate, colon, and uterus.

Anatomically, spinal cord tumors may be extramedullary or intramedullary. **Intramedullary tumors** account for 10% of spinal cord tumors and are usually malignant. They originate within the spinal cord itself, in the central gray matter and the anterior commissure. **Extramedullary tumors,** representing 90% of spinal cord tumors, are found within the spinal dura but outside the cord. They are further defined anatomically as extradural and intradural tumors. Extradural or epidural tumors occur between the vertebrae and the spinal dura. They develop in the surrounding bone and cause destruction of the vertebral bodies. Intradural tumors are located within the dura and originate from the pia-arachnoid, spinal roots, or denticulate ligaments.

Spinal cord tumors account for only about 0.5% of all tumors in adults and 10% to 15% of primary central nervous system (CNS) tumors. Thoracic tumors account for 50% of all spinal cord tumors. Cervical tumors occur 30% of the time, followed by lumbosacral tumors (20%). Most of these tumors are benign. They occur equally in both men and women between 20 and 60 years of age.

COLLABORATIVE MANAGEMENT

Assessment

PHYSICAL ASSESSMENT/CLINICAL MANIFESTATIONS

The clinical manifestations of a spinal cord tumor depend on its location (Chart 46-15) and rate of growth. The most common complaint of the client with a spinal cord tumor is pain. Pain results from spinal cord compression, infiltration of the spinal tracts, or irritation of the spinal roots. Assess the quality, severity, and intensity of the pain. In addition, ask the client to describe factors that exacerbate and relieve the pain. **Radicular** (nerve root) pain is described as stabbing or dull, with intermittent episodes of sharp, piercing pain. The term **radiculopathy** is commonly used to refer to radicular pain. The pain may be increased during coughing, straining, or sneezing. Lying flat may increase the pain as a consequence of stretching the involved spinal nerve roots.

Involvement of the corticospinal tract may lead to motor deficits. The nurse assesses for weakness, clumsiness, spasticity, and hyperactive reflexes and compares the responses on both sides of the body. Other presenting signs include ataxia, hypotonia, and a positive Babinski's reflex. Spastic

CHART 46-15

KEY FEATURES of Spinal Cord Tumors

General Manifestations
- Pain
- Sensory loss or impairment
- Motor loss or impairment
- Sphincter disturbance (bladder before bowel)

Cervical Manifestations

High Cervical
- Respiratory distress
- Diaphragm paralysis
- Occipital headache
- Quadriparesis
- Stiff neck
- Nystagmus
- Cranial nerve dysfunction

Low Cervical
- Pain in the arms and the shoulders
- Weakness
- Paresthesia
- Motor loss
- Horner's syndrome
- Increased reflexes

Thoracic Manifestations
- Sensory loss
- Spastic paralysis
- Positive Babinski's sign
- Bladder and bowel dysfunction
- Pain in the chest and the back
- Muscle atrophy
- Muscle weakness in the legs
- Foot drop

Lumbosacral Manifestations
- Low back pain
- Paresis
- Spastic paralysis
- Sensory loss
- Bladder and bowel dysfunction
- Sexual dysfunction
- Decreased-to-absent ankle and knee reflexes

paralysis is seen most often, although a flaccid paralysis may be seen in a tumor that affects the spinal roots, in an intramedullary tumor in the enlargements of the cervical or lumbar area, or in an extramedullary tumor complicated by spinal shock. A flaccid paralysis may also be noted in the presence of a cauda equina lesion.

Determine sensory loss on each side of the body and compare the responses. Early symptoms of sensory loss include a slowly progressive numbness or tingling, pain, and temperature loss. The sensory deficit is further marked by a decreased appreciation of touch, an inability to sense vibration, and a loss of position sense. The client often reports a tight, bandlike feeling around the trunk. Brown-Séquard syndrome or central cord syndrome may be manifested (see Extent of Injury [Spinal Cord Injury], pp. 984 and 985).

Loss of bladder control often occurs before a loss of bowel control in the client with a spinal cord tumor. Typically, bladder dysfunction is manifested by hesitancy, dribbling, incontinence, urgency, or acute retention. Bowel dysfunction is manifested by constipation. Keep in mind that the client is often embarrassed to admit to bladder or bowel dysfunction.

A lesion in the sacral area may cause a decrease in genital sensation and thus impair the client's sexual function and enjoyment. Men may be unable to have an erection or to ejaculate.

DIAGNOSTIC ASSESSMENT

Routine x-ray examinations or tomographic scans of the spine are obtained to detect a narrowing of the spinal canal, destruction of the vertebrae, or the presence of calcification. A myelogram may be useful when a block is incomplete; it indicates the level, extent, and boundaries of a tumor. This test is being performed less today due to newer imaging techniques.

A magnetic resonance imaging (MRI) scan with and without enhancement provides more detail of the pathologic condition of the spinal cord than either a computed tomography (CT) scan or myelography. EMG may help make a differential diagnosis to rule out multiple sclerosis (MS) or amyotrophic lateral sclerosis (ALS).

◆Interventions

Nursing care of the client with a spinal cord tumor includes obtaining the vital signs and checking neurologic status at least every 4 hours and more often as clinically indicated. As for any client with a spinal cord problem, report any change in motor and sensory status immediately to the physician.

SURGICAL MANAGEMENT. The primary management of a spinal cord tumor is surgery. The goal of surgical intervention is to remove as much of the tumor as possible. Often this is not feasible, and other treatment is indicated (e.g., radiation therapy). Emergency surgery is indicated if the client experiences a rapid loss of motor and sensory function or a loss of bladder and bowel control. Surgical decompression may be performed to maintain bladder, bowel, or motor function and to preserve quality of life—even with a poor prognosis.

The neurosurgeon performs a laminectomy and surgical decompression and total or partial resection of the tumor. Depending on the extent of the tumor, a spinal fusion may be necessary. Rarely, a cordotomy or a palliative sectioning of sensory roots is done to control intractable pain. Laminectomies are discussed under Surgical Management (Back Pain), p. 980.

After surgery, assess the client's vital signs and neurologic status every 1 to 2 hours until they are stable and then every 4 hours. The client is log rolled (turned as a unit) and repositioned every 2 hours. Inspect the incision site for drainage, especially of cerebrospinal fluid (CSF), and signs of infection. The client with a cervical cord tumor must also be carefully monitored for respiratory compromise. Postoperative nursing care for a client undergoing a laminectomy is discussed under Postoperative Care (Back Pain), pp. 980 and 981.

NONSURGICAL MANAGEMENT

Radiation Therapy. Radiation therapy may be necessary, depending on the tumor type. It is usually used with low-grade malignant tumors that are not completely resected, with metastatic tumors, or with recurrent tumors when there is no other treatment option. The spinal cord cannot tolerate high doses of radiation. Overexposure to radiation may lead to radiation myelopathy, which develops over 6 to 12 months. It is manifested by progressive spinal cord degeneration and neurologic deficits such as Brown-Séquard syndrome. With time, the client experiences spastic paralysis, loss of sensation, and bowel and bladder dysfunction; death may occur. Care of the client undergoing radiation therapy is described in detail in Chapter 28.

Chemotherapy. The use of chemotherapy in the treatment of spinal cord tumors is very limited. There are no reports of clinical trials with chemotherapy for primary spinal cord tumors. However, chemotherapy may be used as an adjunctive therapy for tumors metastasized to the spinal cord from other primary sites, such as the breast. Leptomeningeal involvement may benefit from intrathecal (spinal) chemotherapy.

Pain Control. Pain control may be accomplished by pharmacologic and nonpharmacologic measures. Patient-controlled analgesia (PCA) with morphine is often used to provide immediate postoperative pain relief. The client is gradually switched to oral analgesics before discharge. As per the standard of care, assess the client's level of pain, provide appropriate pain relief medication, and document the response to the medication. If drug therapy does not provide pain relief, collaborate with the health care provider to identify a more effective medication.

Turning and proper positioning of the client often enhances pain relief. The nurse or assistive nursing personnel provides range-of-motion (ROM) exercises to prevent atrophy and contractures, which can increase pain. Hypnosis, music therapy, and imagery techniques are other methods of pain relief (see Chapters 4 and 7).

Preventing Complications of Immobility. The client who is immobilized from a spinal cord tumor or spinal surgery is especially at risk for pressure sores and deep vein thrombosis (DVT) or pulmonary emboli. The nurse or assistive nursing personnel turns the client in bed at least every 2 hours. When the client is sitting in a chair, he or she is repositioned every 30 to 60 minutes.

Inspect the client's skin frequently to determine tolerance for sitting and to detect the presence of reddened areas. Press on the reddened areas over the ischial tuberosities and look for blanching. If blanching does not occur, the area is vulnerable to skin breakdown. The physical and occupational therapists determine the most appropriate positioning and exercise techniques and assess the need for assistive devices. It may be necessary for the client to be placed on a waterbed or an air mattress to prevent or treat pressure ulcers.

Monitor the client's lower extremities for indications of DVT. Sequential compression devices may be used in place of or as an adjunct to graduated compression stockings. The health care provider may prescribe sodium heparin 5000 units subcutaneously every 12 hours, low-molecular-weight heparin (enoxaparin [Lovenox]), or sodium warfarin (Coumadin, Warfilone✱) in therapeutic dosages to help prevent DVT or embolus formation.

Bowel and Bladder Program. Ask the client about his or her normal defecation pattern. On the basis of this information, establish a bowel program. The following are the essential elements of this program:

- A consistent time for bowel elimination
- A high fluid intake (2000 mL/day) unless fluid intake is restricted
- A high-fiber diet
- Rectal stimulation with or without suppositories
- If needed, stool softener medications, such as docusate sodium (Colace) and docusate sodium and casanthranol (Peri-Colace)

Manual disimpaction may be necessary if the client has lower motor neuron (LMN) symptoms.

The client's bladder program is determined by the specific dysfunction, usually urinary retention. The nurse or assistive nursing personnel monitors the voiding pattern and strictly measures and records intake and output. Assess for suprapubic distention and other indications of retention, such as overflow and dribbling. Encourage the client to empty the bladder every 2 hours.

Community-Based Care

HOME CARE MANAGEMENT

Collaborate with the client and his or her family members or significant others to identify and suggest corrections for potential hazards in the home. If needed, make a referral to a home care nurse, social worker, or case manager to assess the need for structural alterations to the home. Structural alterations may be needed to accommodate ambulatory aids (e.g., a walker) and to enable the client to perform activities of daily living (ADLs).

Some clients may be discharged from the acute care hospital to a rehabilitation setting, where they can learn to function as independently as possible. Chapter 10 describes rehabilitation in detail.

HEALTH TEACHING

The teaching plan for the client with a spinal cord tumor depends on his or her level of dysfunction. With decompression of the tumor, the severity of the client's symptoms often lessens. Deficits that may remain include mobility and sensory loss. Learning mobility skills can enable the client to negotiate movement on sidewalks, carpeting, and other flooring surfaces. The client must also be able to negotiate sidewalk curbs independently. The physical or occupational therapist instructs the client in the correct use of all adaptive equipment. Review the individualized bowel and bladder program with the client, family member, or other caregiver.

The goal of sexuality education in the acute care setting is to answer questions and correct any misinformation. Unless the nurse has had specific training or experience in sexuality counseling of people with spinal cord tumors or injuries, more detailed questions should be directed to a sexuality counselor.

HEALTH CARE RESOURCES

The prognosis for the client with malignant tumors or secondary tumors is poor. Determine what the physician and family members have told the client about diagnosis and prognosis. Encourage the client to verbalize feelings and fears about prognosis, body image, self-concept, role performance, and self-esteem.

Clients and family members or significant others should be referred to local, state or province, and national organizations for people with spinal cord injuries, which are applicable to spinal cord tumors. These groups often have information for clients with spinal cord tumors. Refer clients with a malignancy to the American Cancer Society. Referral to support groups may also assist clients and family with adapting to lifestyle changes.

MULTIPLE SCLEROSIS

Multiple sclerosis (MS) is a chronic autoimmune disease that affects the myelin sheath and conduction pathway of the central nervous system (CNS). It is one of the leading causes of neurologic disability in persons 20 to 40 years of age.

PATHOPHYSIOLOGY

This chronic disease is characterized by periods of remission and **exacerbation** (flare). As the severity and duration of the disease progress, the periods of exacerbation become more frequent. MS has received increased public attention since actress Annette Funicello and talk show host Montel Williams were diagnosed with the disease.

Multiple sclerosis is characterized by an inflammatory response that results in random or patchy areas of plaque in the white matter of the central nervous system (CNS). When this occurs, the myelin sheath is damaged and its thickness is reduced. Myelin is responsible for the electrochemical transmission of impulses between the brain and spinal cord and the rest of the body. Impulses are still transmitted but are not as effective as before; over time they may be completely blocked. The white fiber tracts (especially the axons) that connect the neurons in the brain and spinal cord are generally involved in MS. The areas particularly affected include optic nerves, pyramidal tracts, posterior columns, brainstem nuclei, and the periventricular region of the brain. Eventually, with repeated exacerbations of the disease, damage to the axons becomes permanent.

Major types of MS include the following:

- Relapsing-remitting
- Progressive-relapsing
- Primary progressive
- Secondary progressive

The classic picture of the **relapsing-remitting** type of MS (RRMS) occurs in 85% of cases. The course of the disease may be mild or moderate, depending on the degree of disability. Relapses develop over 1 to 2 weeks and resolve over 4 to 8 months, after which the client returns to baseline. Of the 85% who start with relapsing-remitting disease, more than 50% will develop secondary progressive MS (SPMS) within 10 years; 90% develop it within 25 years (Costello & Harris, 2003).

Progressive-relapsing MS (PRMS) occurs less often, that is, in only 5% of clients with MS. It is characterized by the absence of periods of remission, and the client's condition does not return to baseline. Progressive, cumulative symptoms and deterioration occur over several years.

Primary progressive MS (PPMS) involves a steady and gradual neurologic deterioration without remission of symptoms. The client has progressive disability with no acute attacks. Clients with this type of MS tend to be between 40 and 60 years of age at onset of the disease.

Secondary progressive MS (SPMS) begins with a relapsing-remitting course that later becomes steadily progressive. Attacks and partial recoveries may continue to occur.

Etiology and Genetic Risk

The exact cause of MS remains unknown. Research continues on viral, immunologic, and genetic and environmental etiologic factors. Viruses are well recognized as causes of demyelination and inflammation; so it may be possible that a virus or other infectious agent is the triggering factor in MS. Although a number of viruses have been studied, no single virus has been identified as causing MS.

The immune theory suggests that an unidentified factor triggers an autoimmune response in the brain, spinal cord, and visual system. Both humoral and cell-mediated immune system dysfunction have been implicated. This theory is supported by research data that show elevated immunoglobulin G (IgG) and oligoclonal bands in the CSF of clients with MS (Costello & Harris, 2003).

According to the National Multiple Sclerosis Society:

- Having a first-degree relative such as a parent or sibling with MS increases an individual's risk of developing the disease.
- There is a higher prevalence of certain genes in populations with higher rates of MS.
- Common genetic factors have been found in some families in which there is more than one person with MS.
- The environment may also contribute to the development of MS. The disease is seen more often in the colder climates of the northeastern, Great Lakes, and Pacific northwestern states as well as in Canada.

Incidence/Prevalence

Multiple sclerosis (MS) usually occurs in people between the ages of 20 and 40 years, but cases may occur in those younger than 15 years and older than 50 years. It is known as the disease of young adults. Only 20% of clients with MS report that the first symptom occurred in their 40s or 50s. About 500,000 people in the United States are currently affected. Women are affected slightly more often than men (1.5:1). The incidence in first-degree relatives of persons with MS is 15 times greater than in the general population The life expectancy for those with MS is about 85% of that of the general population, or about 35 years after the onset of symptoms (Finesilver, 2003).

◆COLLABORATIVE MANAGEMENT

◆Assessment

HISTORY

Multiple sclerosis (MS) often mimics other neurologic diseases, which often makes the diagnosis difficult and prolonged. Therefore obtaining a thorough history is essential for accurate diagnosis. The client is queried for a history of vision changes, motor skills, and sensations, all of which are early indicators of MS. The symptoms are often vague and nonspecific in the early stages of the disease. Of significance is the client's report that symptoms were first noticed several years earlier but that medical attention was not sought because the symptoms disappeared. Other information to be obtained includes questions about the progression of symptoms, with particular attention given to determining whether the symptoms are intermittent or are becoming progressively worse. Document the date (month and year) when the client first noticed the clinical manifestations.

Next question about factors that aggravate the symptoms, such as fatigue, stress, overexertion, temperature extremes, or a hot shower or bath. Ask the client and the family about any personality or behavioral changes that have occurred (e.g., euphoria, poor judgment, inattentiveness). In addition, determine whether there is a family history of MS.

PHYSICAL ASSESSMENT/CLINICAL MANIFESTATIONS

Multiple sclerosis produces a wide variety of manifestations. Any myelinated fibers of the brain and spinal cord may be affected. To determine a client's specific manifestations, the nurse performs a complete neurologic assessment.

MOTOR ASSESSMENT. First assess the client's motor status. The client often reports increased fatigue and stiffness of the extremities, particularly the legs. Fatigue is one of the most disabling manifestations, affecting 70% to 90% of clients with MS. Unlike fatigue in others, MS fatigue is characterized by persistent sensitivity to temperature (Costello & Harris, 2003).

Flexor spasms at night may awaken the client from sleep. Further examination reveals increased, or hyperactive, deep tendon reflexes; clonus; positive Babinski's reflex; and absent abdominal reflexes. Gait may be unsteady because of leg weakness and spasticity.

Significant cerebellar findings include **intention tremor** (tremor when performing an activity), **dysmetria** (inability to direct or limit movement), and dysdiadochokinesia (inability to stop one motor impulse and substitute another). Motor movements are often clumsy; the client may lose balance easily and may exhibit signs of poor coordination.

During examination of the cranial nerves and brainstem function, the client may report tinnitus (ringing in the ears), vertigo (dizziness), and hearing loss. The client may show indications of facial weakness and have dysphagia. Speech problems include dysarthria (slurred speech), ataxia, and slow, scanning speech.

Typical clinical findings from assessment of the client's visual acuity, visual fields, and pupils include the following:

- Blurred vision
- **Diplopia** (double vision)
- Decreased visual acuity
- **Scotomas** (changes in peripheral vision)
- **Nystagmus** (involuntary, rapid eye movements)

SENSORY ASSESSMENT. Sensory findings include hypalgesia (diminished sensitivity to pain), paresthesia, facial pain, and decreased temperature perception. The client may report numbness, tingling, burning, or crawling sensations.

If demyelination of the spinal cord has occurred, the client may experience bowel and bladder dysfunctions as well as alterations in sexuality. The client may have an areflexic bladder or may experience frequency, urgency, or nocturia. Bowel problems include altered rectal tone, constipation, and incontinence. Problems with sexuality include impotence, difficulty sustaining an erection, and decreased vaginal secretion.

COGNITIVE ASSESSMENT. Finally, the client for is examined for mental status changes. Cognitive changes are usually seen late in the course of the disease and include decreased short-term memory, concentration, and ability to perform calculations; inattentiveness, and impaired judgment. Chart 46-16 summarizes the common clinical manifestations of MS.

PSYCHOSOCIAL ASSESSMENT

After the initial diagnosis of MS, the client is often anxious. Apathy, emotional lability, and depression are fairly common. The client may be euphoric or giddy, either as a result of the disease itself or because of the medications used to treat the disease. The nurse assesses the client's previously used coping and stress management skills in preparing him or her for a chronic, usually debilitating disease.

CHART 46-16

KEY FEATURES of Multiple Sclerosis

- Muscle weakness and spasticity
- Fatigue
- Intention tremors
- Dysmetria (inability to direct or limit movement)
- Numbness or tingling sensations (paresthesia)
- Hypalgesia
- Ataxia (decreased motor coordination)
- Dysarthria (slurred speech)
- Dysphagia (difficulty swallowing)
- Diplopia (double vision)
- Nystagmus (involuntary eye movements)
- Scotomas (changes in peripheral vision)
- Decreased visual and hearing acuity
- Tinnitus, vertigo (ringing in the ears, dizziness)
- Bowel and bladder dysfunction
- Alterations in sexual function, such as impotence
- Cognitive changes, such as memory loss, impaired judgment, and decreased ability to solve problems or perform calculations

LABORATORY ASSESSMENT

No single specific procedure is definitively diagnostic for multiple sclerosis (MS). However, the collective results of a variety of tests are usually conclusive. Changes may be evident during an acute attack. Abnormal cerebrospinal fluid (CSF) findings include an elevated protein level and a slight increase in the white blood cell count. CSF electrophoresis reveals an increase in the myelin basic protein and the presence of oligoclonal (IgG) bands. IgG bands are seen in most clients with MS.

OTHER DIAGNOSTIC ASSESSMENTS

The health care provider usually orders a computed tomography (CT) scan, which may show an increased density in the white matter and MS plaques. Magnetic resonance imaging (MRI) demonstrates the presence of plaques and is considered diagnostic for MS. A complete diagnostic evaluation is necessary to exclude other disease.

Results of visual, auditory, and brainstem-evoked potential studies are often abnormal. EMG findings may be grossly abnormal in people with advanced disease.

The diagnosis of MS is made by the exclusion of other neurologic diseases, laboratory and neuroimaging assessment, and on specific diagnostic criteria, including the presence of neurologic dysfunction that occurs over time and in more than one area of the central nervous system (CNS).

Common Nursing Diagnoses and Collaborative Problems

Nursing diagnoses that may apply to clients with MS include the following:

- Fatigue related to disease state
- Activity Intolerance related to generalized weakness
- Disturbed Sensory Perception (Visual) related to altered sensory reception
- Impaired Physical Mobility related to neuromuscular impairment

- Impaired Urinary Elimination related to sensory-motor impairment
- Chronic Pain related to chronic physical disability
- Self-Care Deficit related to neuromuscular impairment
- Disturbed Thought Processes related to disease state
- Imbalanced Nutrition: Less Than Body Requirements related to difficulty swallowing
- Sexual Dysfunction related to altered body function

Interventions

The client with MS is often weak and easily fatigued. The Concept Map below illustrates the common problems and interventions for the client with MS. Teach the client the importance of planning activities and allowing sufficient time to complete activities. For example, the client should check that all items needed for work are gathered before leaving the house. Items used on a daily basis should be easily accessible.

Drug Therapy. A variety of medications are used to treat and control the disease, decrease specific symptoms, and attempt to slow its progression (Table 46-1).

Biological Response Modifiers. The National Multiple Sclerosis Society recommends early and continuous treatment of relapsing-remitting MS with *one* of three drugs, all classified as **biological response modifiers (BRMs)** or immunomodulators–Avonex, Betaseron, or Copaxone–the ABCs of MS therapy. As the name implies, these drugs attempt to modify the course of the disease. Interferon beta-1a

CONCEPT MAP Multiple Sclerosis

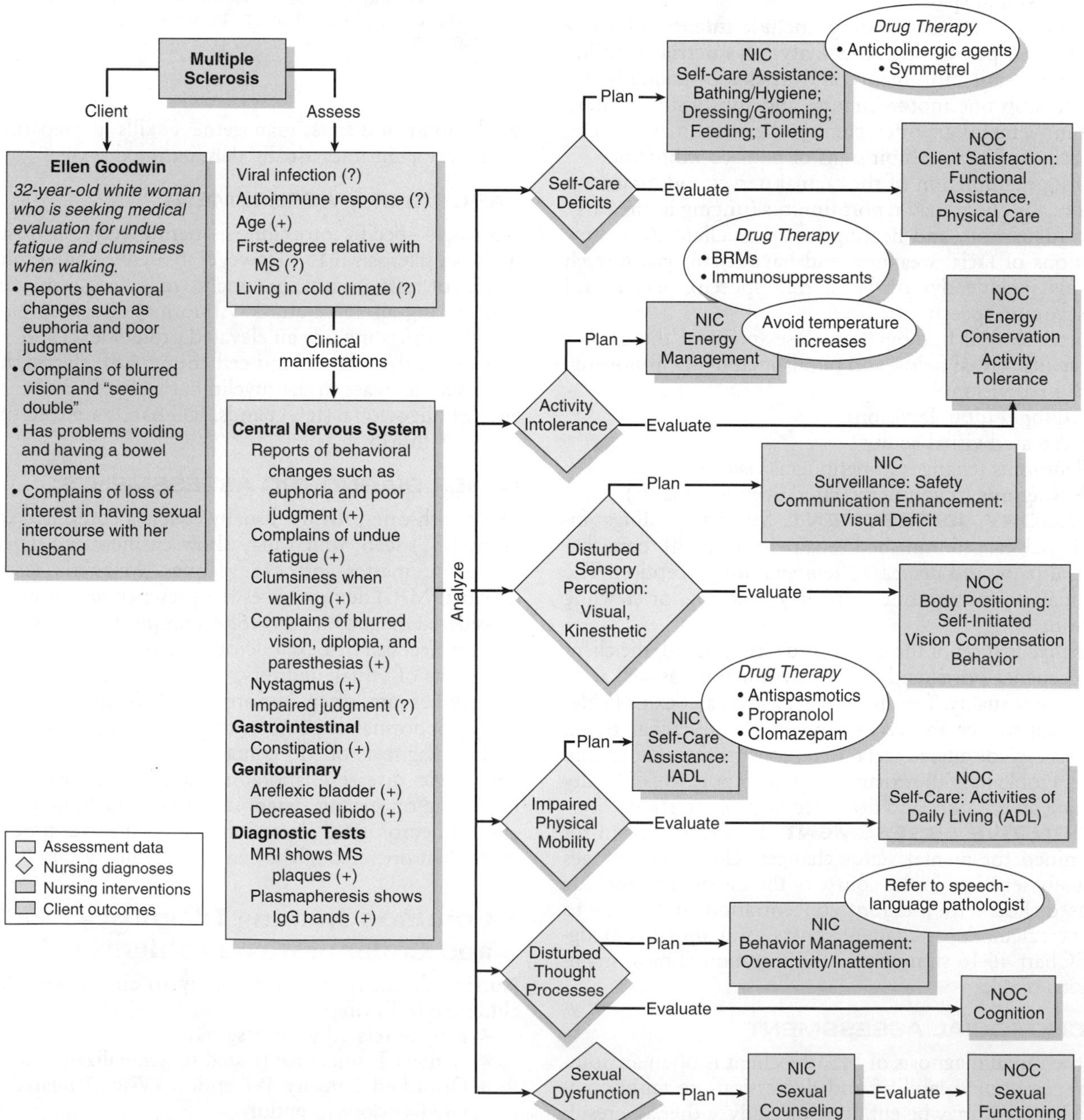

Concept Map by Elaine Bishop Kennedy, EdD, RN

(Avonex) has been approved by the Food and Drug Administration (FDA) for clients who have experienced their first episode of relapsing MS and have a magnetic resonance imaging (MRI) scan that demonstrates MS. This medication, given intramuscularly (IM) once a week, delays disability and decreases the number and severity of exacerbations. An alternative interferon beta-1a is Rebif, which is given subcutaneously three times a week (often self-administered). Interferon beta-1b (Betaseron) is administered subcutaneously every other day to reduce the frequency of exacerbations. Glatiramer acetate (Copaxone), given subcutaneously every day, decreases the clinical relapse rate and disease progression. Adherence to the self-administered daily Copaxone therapy is often difficult. Some clients feel that it is too challenging, and stop the therapy (Fraser, Hadjimichael, & Vollmer, 2001).

The interferons can cause depression, suicidal ideation, thrombocytopenia (low platelet count), leukopenia (low white blood cell count), and injection site reactions. Ice applied to the site before and after injection can help prevent redness, tenderness, or swelling. More than 20% of clients who take Copaxone experience transient chest pain.

TABLE 46-1 Commonly Used Medications for Clients with Multiple Sclerosis

Biological Response Modifiers
- Interferon beta-1a (Avonex or Rebif)
- Interferon beta-1b (Betaseron)
- Glatiramer acetate (Copaxone)

Immunosuppressive/Antineoplastic
- Cyclophosphamide (Cytoxan) and methylprednisolone combination
- Azathioprine (Imuran)
- Methotrexate
- Mitoxantrone (Novantrone)

Steroids
- Methylprednisolone (Solu-Medrol)
- IV immunoglobulin

Symptomatic Treatment of Fatigue
- Amantadine HCl (Symmetrel)
- Pemoline (Cylert)
- Methylphenidate HCl (Ritalin, Concerta, others)
- Modafinil (Provigil)

Symptomatic Treatment of Depression
- Fluoxetine HCl (Prozac)
- Sertraline HCl (Zoloft)

Symptomatic Treatment of Spasticity
- Baclofen (Lioresal)
- Tizanidine HCl (Zanaflex)
- Dantrolene sodium (Dantrium)
- Diazepam (Valium)
- Clonazepam (Klonopin)

Symptomatic Treatment of Bladder Dysfunction
- Oxybutynin chloride (Ditropan)
- Propantheline bromide (Pro-Banthine)
- Hyoscyamine sulfate (Anaspaz, Cystospaz-M)
- Desmopressin (DDA VP nasal spray)

Symptomatic Treatment of Chronic Pain
- Amitriptyline (Elavil)
- Carbamazepine (Tegretol)
- Clonazepam (Klonopin)
- Gabapentin (Neurontin)
- Nortriptyline (Pamelor)

Immunosuppressive Therapy. Mitoxantrone (Novantrone), an antineoplastic agent, has also been shown to be effective in reducing neurologic disability and the frequency of clinical relapses in clients with secondary-progressive, progressive-relapsing, or worsening relapsing-remitting MS. It is well tolerated, but its use over a long period causes cardiac problems, such as heart failure and life-threatening dysrhythmias.

Immunosuppressive therapy with a combination of cyclophosphamide (Cytoxan) and methylprednisolone (Solu-Medrol) may be used for treatment to stabilize the disease process. Methotrexate (MTX) may also have a modest benefit. Long-term side effects include sterility, mutations, and the increased risk of cancer.

Steroid Therapy. The health care provider may use methylprednisolone (Solu-Medrol) to reduce edema and the inflammatory response in acute exacerbations. One gram is administered IV daily for 3 to 14 days, depending on the provider and the extent of the client's symptoms. A course of oral prednisone 60 mg daily for 5 to 7 days may be used following the methylprednisolone. Adrenocorticotropic hormone (ACTH), 25 to 60 international units IV or IM, may be given instead of methylprednisolone and tapered gradually over 2 to 4 weeks.

Common nursing interventions while the client is receiving these medications include the following:

- Carefully monitoring fluid and electrolyte levels
- Testing the client's serum glucose concentration
- Providing dietary or supplemental potassium
- Observing for indications of gastrointestinal (GI) bleeding, such as gastric pain or blood in the stool
- Documenting any changes in personality (e.g., euphoria and insomnia)
- Minimizing the client's exposure to people with communicable or infectious diseases

Antispasmodic Therapy. The health care provider may prescribe baclofen (Lioresal), diazepam (Valium, Apo-Diazepam✱), or dantrolene sodium (Dantrium) to lessen muscle spasticity. Severe spasticity may be treated with intrathecal baclofen administered through a surgically implanted pump. A surgical tendon release may also be performed by the physician if spasms prevent the client from learning mobility and ADL skills.

Adjunctive Therapy. Paresthesia may be treated with carbamazepine (Tegretol) or tricyclic antidepressants (amitriptyline). Propranolol hydrochloride (Inderal) and clonazepam (Klonopin) have been used to treat cerebellar ataxia. If fatigue cannot be controlled through the use of nonpharmacologic measures, amantadine hydrochloride (Symmetrel) may be prescribed.

Bladder dysfunction (detrusor hyperreflexia) is treated with anticholinergic agents, including oxybutynin chloride (Ditropan) and hyoscyamine sulfate (Anaspaz, Cystospaz-M).

Pain and paresthesia are often problems for the MS client. Antispasmodics such as tizanidine (Zanaflex), antiepileptic drugs (AEDs) such as carbamazepine (Tegretol), analgesics, NSAIDs, tranquilizers, or antidepressants may be used, depending on the cause of the pain and the client's response.

Promoting Mobility and Self-Care. In collaboration with physical and occupational therapists, an exercise program is developed and includes range-of-motion (ROM) exercises and stretching and strengthening exercises. The client is encouraged to ambulate as tolerated and to use assistive ambulation devices as needed, including a cane, walker, wheelchair, or electric cart (Amigo). Additional assistive/adaptive devices may be needed to enable the client with tremor, spasticity, and weakness to remain independent in activities of daily living (ADLs). Chapter 10 describes additional interventions to increase physical mobility and promote ADL independence.

The importance of avoiding rigorous activities that increase body temperature is emphasized. Increased body temperature may lead to increased fatigue, diminished motor ability, and decreased visual acuity resulting from changes in the conduction abilities of the injured axons.

Managing Cognitive Problems. Cognitive impairment may occur early in the disease process. It is estimated that up to 65% of clients exhibit some neuropsychological dysfunction during the course of their disease (Halper et al., 2003). Areas affected include attention, memory, problem solving, visual perception, and use of speech. To assist the client with orientation, place a single date calendar in the client's room; give or encourage the client to use written lists or recorded messages. To maintain an organized environment, the client is encouraged to keep frequently used items in familiar places.

If the client experiences dysarthria, refer to the speech-language pathologist (SLP) for evaluation and treatment. It is not unusual for the client with dysarthria also to have dysphagia (difficulty swallowing). The SLP will do a swallowing evaluation. Further diagnostic testing may be indicated.

Adapting to Changes in Sexual Functioning. More than 70% of all women with MS and 90% of all men with MS report some change in their sexual life after onset of the disease (Gagliardi, 2003). Women report impaired genital sensation, diminished orgasm, and loss of sexual interest. Men most often complain of difficulty in achieving and maintaining an erection and delayed ejaculation. Many clients may be embarrassed to discuss their concerns about sexuality. Therefore, ask the client whether he or she has any concerns. The nurse with appropriate education and experience should answer the client's questions or refer the client to a therapist or urologist with experience in the field of sexuality and disability.

Managing Bladder and Bowel Problems. The client may experience a variety of bladder problems. In addition to drug therapy, other modalities include an intermittent self-catheterization program, indwelling urinary catheter, placement of a suprapubic catheter, or insertion of a bladder pacemaker. When the client activates the control on the pacemaker, the bladder is stimulated and voiding is initiated (Finesilver, 2003).

Clients with MS are at increased risk for urinary tract infections. Antibiotics may be prescribed by the health care provider. Remind the client to drink plenty of fluids unless contraindicated by other medical conditions. Teach the client procedures that stimulate bladder emptying, such as stroking the genitals and **Credé method** (applying manual pressure on the lower abdomen over the bladder to express urine). **Kegel exercises** (contracting and holding the pubococcygeal muscle) may also be helpful.

To prevent or control constipation, remind the client to increase fluid and fiber intake. If dietary control is not effective, medications such as bulk-forming agents, stool softeners, oral stimulants, mild laxatives, and suppositories or enemas may be prescribed. It is important for the client to develop a bowel program to maximize the effectiveness of dietary and medication interventions.

Treating Visual Disturbances. An eye patch that is alternated from eye to eye every few hours usually relieves **diplopia** (double vision). For peripheral visual deficits, teach scanning techniques by having the client move his or her head from side to side. Changes in visual acuity may be assisted by corrective lenses.

Complementary and Alternative Therapies. A number of complementary and alternative therapies have been reported by clients with MS to be successful in minimizing their symptoms, including beestings and nutritional supplements. These modalities continue to be researched for their efficacy.

The client may use moist, moderate heat; massage correction of posture abnormalities; exercises to increase muscle strength; and electrical stimulation of the affected area to increase their comfort level. Among other alternative treatments for pain are guided imagery, aromatherapy, and acupuncture (see Chapters 4 and 7).

Critical Thinking Challenge

You are a nurse in a family practice office in a small rural town. A young woman has requested a physical examination because she has "been feeling very tired lately." She has also been dropping things and has fallen twice when climbing stairs. After examination, the nurse practitioner tells her that he suspects multiple sclerosis or other neurodegenerative disease. The client begins to cry because she is planning to be married next month.

1. How should you respond to her at this time?
2. What diagnostic testing will most likely be prescribed for her?
3. What treatment options does she have?

evolve For suggested answer guidelines, go to http://evolve.elsevier.com/Iggy/.

Community-Based Care

HOME CARE MANAGEMENT

To help the client maintain maximum strength, function, and independence, continuity of care through an interdisciplinary team in both the rehabilitation and home setting is necessary. Admission to a rehabilitation center is brief but usually provides a program to improve functional ability. In collaboration with the discharge planner and the occupational therapist, the nurse or case manager assesses the client's home for any hazards before discharge. Any items that might interfere with mobility (e.g., scatter rugs) are removed. In addition, care must be taken to prevent injury resulting from visual problems. The home environment should remain as structured and as free from clutter as possible. As the disease progresses, the home may need to be adapted for wheelchair accessibility. Any necessary assistive/adaptive device should be readily available before discharge from the hospital.

HEALTH TEACHING

The health care provider explains to the client and family the development of MS and the factors that may exacerbate the symptoms. The importance of avoiding overexertion, stress, extremes of temperatures (fever, hot baths, overheating, excessive chilling), humidity, and people with upper respiratory tract infections is emphasized. Explain all medications to be taken on discharge, including the time and route of administration, dosage, purpose, and side effects. Teach the client how to differentiate expected side effects from adverse or allergic reactions, and provide the name of a resource person to call if questions arise. Written instructions are provided as a resource to the client and caregivers at home.

The physical therapist develops an exercise program appropriate for the client's tolerance level. The client is instructed in techniques for self-care, daily living skills, and the use of required adaptive equipment, such as walkers and electric carts. The nurse should also include information on the following programs: bowel and bladder management, skin care, nutrition, and positioning techniques. Chapter 10 describes these aspects of chronic illness and rehabilitation in detail.

Instruct clients about the importance of obtaining adequate rest and avoiding undue stress. It is equally important for them to engage in regular social activities. Often clients are anxious about discharge from the hospital and worry about how long the remission will last or when the disease will progress.

Because personality changes are not unusual, teach the family or significant others strategies to enable them to cope with these changes. For example, the family may develop a nonverbal signal to alert the client to potentially inappropriate behavior (e.g., a talkative person may be reminded to be quiet if a family member displays a prearranged signal). This action avoids embarrassment for the client.

HEALTH CARE RESOURCES

The client with MS is able to live independently in the early stages of the disease. As the condition deteriorates, the assistance of a home care nurse or a family member may be required.

Stuifbergen et al. (2003) found that setting incremental health goals was a useful strategy for women with MS. Assist clients in establishing realistic short-term goals.

In severe or late disease, placement in a long-term care facility is an appropriate alternative. The population of young and middle-aged residents in nursing homes is increasing as people with chronic, disabling diseases live longer.

The nurse or case manager refers the client and family members or significant others to the local and national MS societies. Other community resources include meal delivery services (e.g., Meals on Wheels), transportation services for the disabled, and homemaker services.

AMYOTROPHIC LATERAL SCLEROSIS

PATHOPHYSIOLOGY

Amyotrophic lateral sclerosis (ALS), also known as **Lou Gehrig's disease,** is a progressive and degenerative disease that involves the motor system. It is characterized by atrophy of the hands, forearms, and legs. ALS results in paralysis and death. There is no known cause, no cure, no specific treatment, no standard pattern of progression, and no method of prevention. Unlike with many other neural degenerative diseases, the sensory and autonomic nervous systems are not involved. Mental status changes do not result from the disease.

Amyotrophic lateral sclerosis may occur at any age. The incidence in the United States is 4.6 per 100,000. The usual age of onset is between 40 and 70 years; the incidence increases with each decade of life. ALS is more prevalent in men than in women. Death typically occurs within 2 to 5 years after the onset of symptoms and is attributable to respiratory failure.

The cause of the disease is unknown. Researchers are exploring genetic, viral, and environmental factors as potential causes.

COLLABORATIVE MANAGEMENT

Assessment

The clinical manifestations of ALS include fatigue, muscle atrophy, and weakness. Early symptoms include the following:

- Fatigue while talking
- Tongue atrophy
- **Dysphagia** (difficulty swallowing)
- Weakness of the hands and arms
- **Fasciculations** (twitching) of the face
- Nasal quality of speech
- **Dysarthria** (slurred speech)

As the disease progresses, muscle atrophy, particularly of the trapezius and sternocleidomastoid muscles, develops. Muscle weakness and atrophy extend until a flaccid quadriplegia develops. Eventually the respiratory muscles become involved, leading to respiratory compromise, pneumonia, and death.

Diagnosis is based on clinical and diagnostic test findings and by ruling out other causes of the motor changes. There is no specific test to diagnose ALS, but creatine kinase (CK) is increased. The electromyogram (EMG) demonstrates fibrillations and fasciculations of the muscles. A muscle biopsy specimen typically demonstrates small, angulated, atrophic fibers. Other diagnostic studies reveal motor strength deficits in serial muscle testing; abnormal pulmonary function test results, such as a decreased vital capacity (less than 2 L); and dysphagia.

Interventions

There is no known cure for ALS, but an interdisciplinary approach is needed for maintaining optimum functioning. Riluzole (Rilutek) is the only drug approved by the Food and Drug Administration for use with ALS clients. It is not a cure, but it does extend survival time. The usual dose is 50 mg twice daily on an empty stomach. The client is monitored for liver toxicity from the drug by frequent measures of liver enzymes, such as alanine aminotransferase (ALT) and aspartate aminotransferase (AST). The health care provider also prescribes medication for pain, fatigue, spasticity, excessive secretions, sleep disturbances, and other complications as they occur.

The interdisciplinary health care team collaborates with the client and family to develop an individualized treatment plan. The physical therapist and occupational therapist evaluate the client's home and make recommendations for modifications as the disease progresses. An exercise and mobility program is developed and special equipment is obtained as needed to help with activities of daily living and mobility. Other interventions are directed toward preventing complications of immobility and promoting comfort.

The speech-language pathologist (SLP) evaluates the client for speech and swallowing problems, and makes recommendations as needed. The SLP teaches clients various adaptive strategies, such as techniques to help them speak louder and more clearly. He or she works with the client and family to develop a communication system to be used when the client can no longer verbally communicate.

A dietary consult is made to help with planning meals that the client can swallow. The family is taught how to ensure that the client obtains sufficient nutrients, fiber, and fluids. When the client can no longer swallow, a feeding tube is placed. The dietician can recommend the appropriate enteral feedings.

At some point the client will require respiratory support. An intermittent positive pressure ventilation [IPPV] or bilevel positive airway pressure [BIPAP]) may be used to aid breathing during sleep or full time. Mechanical ventilation enables the client to breathe and prolongs survival; it will not alter progression of the disease. For this reason, many clients elect not to be placed on a mechanical ventilator.

Refer the client to a hospice program. The hospice team works closely with the family to ensure the client's comfort. They collaborate with the health care provider to ensure that the client has the needed medication and pain control as well as quality of life for the client and family.

The hospice nurse also provides ongoing support and counseling to the client and the family as they begin to cope with the impact of this terminal disease. The client should be informed about the need for advance directives, such as a living will. Community resources include clinics and other support services run by the ALS Association or the Muscular Dystrophy Association.

GET READY for the NCLEX Examination!

KEY POINTS

Safe Effective Care Environment

- To help prevent back injury, use proper body mechanics as described in Chart 46-5.
- For clients who have back surgery, observe the incision site for bleeding and cerebrospinal leakage (clear fluid).
- Log roll clients having spinal surgery, especially those who have fusions.
- Monitor clients with cervical spinal injuries for manifestations of autonomic dysreflexia (see Chart 46-9).
- Provide emergency care for clients who experience autonomic dysreflexia as listed in Chart 46-10.
- Observe clients with spinal injuries and diseases for complications of immobility.
- Monitor respiratory status carefully in clients with amyotrophic lateral sclerosis; clients experience respiratory failure in terminal stages of the disease.

Health Promotion and Maintenance

- Teach clients who have had spinal surgery to avoid lifting and driving and to use proper body mechanics.
- Teach overweight and obese clients the importance of losing weight to reduce back pain and strain.
- Teach young adults (especially young men) to avoid potentially dangerous activities that could result in a spinal cord injury (SCI).
- Instruct clients with SCI and disease how to prevent complications of immobility (e.g., inspect skin, drink adequate fluids).
- Assess clients with spinal cord injury and disease for the need for adaptive/assistive devices to become independent in ADLs.
- Implement bowel and bladder retraining programs for clients with SCI and spinal diseases.
- Teach clients with multiple sclerosis (MS) the importance of adhering to their medication regimen.

Psychosocial Integrity

- Recognize that spinal cord injury and progressive neurologic diseases, such as MS, require the client to adjust to major life changes.
- Determine client and family coping strategies to help clients adjust to spinal trauma or disease.
- Refer clients to appropriate resources, such as a sexuality counselor or urologist for sexual dysfunction resulting from illness or disease.
- Encourage clients to share their feelings about life-altering SCI or neurodegenerative disease.
- Refer clients with spinal cord cancer to appropriate resources, such as the American Cancer Society and its support groups.

Physiological Integrity

- Assess pain level in clients with back injury, including the nature of the pain and location.
- Implement drug and nondrug interventions for back pain, including analgesics, NSAIDs, and muscle relaxants; suggest heat and ice as adjuncts to medication.
- Provide postoperative care and discharge teaching for clients having cervical neck surgery as listed in Chart 46-6.
- For clients with an SCI, assess airway *first!*
- Provide care of clients with SCI as summarized in Chart 46-12.
- Assess clients with multiple sclerosis for clinical manifestations listed in Chart 46-16; fatigue is the most common symptom.
- Assess for adverse effects of drug therapy for multiple sclerosis; drugs that are commonly used are listed in Table 46-1.
- Provide supportive care for the client with amyotrophic lateral sclerosis; refer to hospice in the terminal stage of the disease.

ADDITIONAL STUDY RESOURCES

Go to your Student CD-ROM for Review Questions for the NCLEX Examination.

evolve Go to http://evolve.elsevier.com/Iggy/ for Integrated Management of Care Questions for the NCLEX Examination.

SELECTED BIBLIOGRAPHY

Arce, D., Sass, P., & Abul-Khoudoud, H. (2001). Recognizing spinal cord emergencies. *American Family Physician, 64*(4), 631-638, 561-563.

Barker, E., & Saulino, M.F. (2002). First-ever guidelines for spinal cord injuries. *RN, 65*(10), 32-37.

Birchfield, P.C. (2001). Osteoarthritis overview. *Geriatric Nursing, 22*(3), 124-131.

Borasio, G.D., Voltz, R., & Miller, R.G. (2001) Palliative care in amyotrophic lateral sclerosis. *Neurologic Clinics, 19*(4), 829-847.

Charles, T., & Swash, M. (2001). Amyotrophic lateral sclerosis: current understanding. *Journal of Neuroscience Nursing, 33*(5), 245-255.
Cherry, C. (2002). Home study program. Anterior cervical discectomy and fusion for cervical disc disease. *AORN Journal, 76*(6), 996, 998-1004, 1007-1012.
Costello, K., & Harris, C. (2003). Differential diagnosis and management of fatigue in multiple sclerosis: Considerations for the nurse. *Journal of Neuroscience Nursing, 35*(3), 139-148.
Costello, K., Hill, C.A., & Tranter, M.C. (2000) Multiple sclerosis in the primary care setting: Key issues for diagnosis and management. *The American Journal for Nurse Practitioners, 4,* 9-26.
Filippi, M., et al. (2003). Evidence for widespread axonal damage at the earliest clinical stage of multiple sclerosis. *Brain, 126*(2), 433-437.
Finesilver, C. (2003). Multiple sclerosis: defenses gone awry. *RN, 66*(4):36.
Finlayson, M., VanDenend, T., & Hudson, E. (2004). Aging with multiple sclerosis. *Journal of Neuroscience Nursing, 36*(5), 245-251.
Fraser, C., Hadjimichael, O., & Vollmer, T. (2001). Predictors of adherence to Copaxone therapy in individuals with relapsing-remitting multiple sclerosis. *Journal of Neuroscience Nursing, 33*(5), 231-239.
Gagliardi, B.A. (2003) The experience of sexuality for individuals living with multiple sclerosis. *Journal of Clinical Nursing, 12*(4), 571-578.
Gibson, K.L. (2003). Caring for a patient who lives with a spinal cord injury. *Nursng 2003, 33*(7), 36-41.
Goodin, D.S., et al. (2002) Disease modifying therapies in multiple sclerosis: report of the Therapeutics and Technology Assessment Subcommittee of the American Academy of Neurology and the MS Council for Clinical Practice Guidelines. *Neurology, 58*(2): 169-178.
Guides for management of acute cervical spinal injury. (2002), *Neurosurgery, 50*(3), Suppl, S1-S84.
Grudinskas, L.V., & Nee, M.A. (2002). As assessment tool for the older person with a spinal cord injury. *SCI Nursing, 19*(2), 61-66.
Halper, J., et al. (2003) Rethinking cognitive function in multiple sclerosis: a nursing perspective. *Journal of Neuroscience Nursing, 35*(2):70-81.
Hassounch-Phillips, D.S., & McNeff, E. (2004). Understanding care-related abuse and neglect in the lives of women with SCI. *SCI Nursing, 21*(2), 75-81.
Hedger, A. (2002a). Clinical corner. Clearance of cervical spines in adult trauma patients. *Journal of Neuroscience Nursing, 34*(6), 331-335, 337.
Hedger, A. (2002b). Spinal cord injury. *Nursing 2002, 32*(12), 96.
Higo, R., et al. (2002). Videomanofluorometric study in amyotrophic lateral sclerosis. *Laryngoscope, 112*(5), 911-917.
Holland, N., et al. (2001). Adherence to disease-modifying therapy in multiple sclerosis. *Rehabilitation Nursing, 26*(5), 172-176.
Kim, J. (2003). How do I respond to autonomic dysreflexia? *Nursing 2003, 33*(2), 18.
Lassmann, H. (2003). Axonal injury in multiple sclerosis. *Journal of Neurology, Neurosurgery & Psychiatry, 74*(6), 695-697.
Linovitz, R.J., et al. (2002) Combined magnetic fields accelerate and increase spine fusion: a double-blind, randomized, placebo controlled study. *Spine, 27*(13), 1383-1389.
Lyall, R.A., et al. (2001) A prospective study of quality of life in ALS patients treated with noninvasive ventilation. *Neurology, 57*(1), 153-156.
Lysberg, K., & Seversinsson, E. (2003). Spinal cord injured women's views of sexuality: A Norwegian survey. *Rehabilitation Nursing, 28*(1), 23-26.
Massey, R., & Jedlicka, D. (2002). The Massey Bedside Swallowing Screen. *Journal of Neuroscience Nursing, 34*(5):252-253, 257-260.
Okonkwo, D.O., & Stone, J.R. (2003). Basic science of closed head injury and spinal cord injuries. *Clinics in Sports Medicine, 22*(3).
Patel, S.A., & Maragakis, N.J. (2002). Amyotrophic lateral sclerosis: pathogenesis, differential diagnoses, and potential interventions. *Journal of Spinal Cord Medicine, 25*(4), 262-273.
Rammohan, K.W. (2003). Axonal injury in multiple sclerosis. *Current Neurology & Neuroscience Reports, 3(3),* 231-237.
Richmond, T.S., & Thompson, H.J. (2002). Quality care in challenging circumstances: a patient with a spinal cord injury. *Journal of Neuroscience Nursing, 34*(1), 44-48.
Rowland, L.P., & Shneider, N.A. (2001). Medical progress: Amyotrophic lateral sclerosis. *New England Journal of Medicine, 344*(22):1688-1700.
Saal, J.S. (2002) General principles of diagnostic testing as related to painful lumbar spine disorders: a critical appraisal of current diagnostic techniques. *Spine,* 27(22), 2538-2546.
Schoeggl, A., Reddy, M., & Matula, C. (2002) Neurological outcome following laminectomy in spinal metastases. *Spinal Cord, 40*(7):363-366.
Schwendimann, R.N. (2002). A conservative approach to acute low back pain. *RN, 34*(5), 22-26, 28.
Smeltzer, S.C. (2002). Reproductive decision making in women with multiple sclerosis. *Journal of Neuroscience Nursing, 34*(3), 145-157.
Stuifbergen, A.K.,et al. (2003). The use of individualized goal setting to facilitate behavior change in women with multiple sclerosis. *Journal of Neuroscience Nursing, 35*(2), 94-99, 106.
Urban, M.K., et al. (2002). Reduction in postoperative pain after spinal fusion with instrumentation using intrathecal morphine. *Spine, 27*(5), 535-537.
Vollmer TL, et al. (2002). Disability and treatment patterns of multiple sclerosis patients in United States: a comparison of veterans and nonveterans. *Journal of Rehabilitation Research & Development, 39*(2), 163-174.
Wassem, R., & Dudley, W. (2003). Symptom management and adjustment of patients with multiple sclerosis: A 4-year longitudinal intervention study. *Clinical Nursing Research, 12*(1), 102-117.
Wilson, T.C., Morgan, P., & Blumhardt, L. (2003). Pyramidal tract mapping by diffusion tensor magnetic resonance imaging in multiple sclerosis: improving correlations with disability. *Journal of Neurology, Neurosurgery, & Psychiatry, 74*(2), 203-207.

CHAPTER

47 Interventions for Clients with Problems of the Peripheral Nervous System

KATHY A. HAUSMAN

LEARNING OUTCOMES

After studying this chapter, you should be able to:

1. Compare and contrast the pathophysiology and etiology of Guillain-Barré syndrome (GBS) and myasthenia gravis (MG).
2. Analyze assessment data for a client with GBS or MG to determine common nursing diagnoses.
3. Prioritize nursing care for the client with GBS or MG.
4. Evaluate nursing care for the client with GBS or MG based on expected outcomes.
5. Differentiate between a myasthenic crisis and a cholinergic crisis.
6. Identify specific nursing actions regarding medication administration for the client with MG.
7. Develop a teaching plan for the client with peripheral neuropathy.
8. Prioritize postoperative care for the client undergoing peripheral nerve repair.
9. Compare and contrast trigeminal neuralgia and facial paralysis.
10. Discuss the role of drug therapy in managing the client with trigeminal neuralgia and facial paralysis.
11. Explain the purpose of surgery for clients with trigeminal neuralgia.

Go to your Student CD-ROM for Review Questions for the NCLEX Examination keyed to these Learning Outcomes.

Peripheral nervous system (PNS) disorders range in severity from potentially life-threatening conditions, such as Guillain-Barré syndrome, to relatively benign (but often painful) conditions, such as polyneuritis. Although hospitalization is rarely required for these less serious dysfunctions, you may encounter them as secondary disorders in hospitalized clients as well as in clients in ambulatory care, long-term care, or community settings.

GUILLAIN-BARRÉ SYNDROME

PATHOPHYSIOLOGY

Guillain-Barré syndrome (GBS) is an acute autoimmune disorder characterized by varying degrees of motor weakness and paralysis. It may be referred to by a variety of other names, such as *acute idiopathic polyneuritis* and *polyradiculoneuropathy.*

The client's life and ultimate potential for rehabilitation depend on appropriate interventions and the effectiveness of nursing care. Your expertise in providing care, monitoring for and preventing complications, and offering emotional support to the client and significant others is essential. With skilled care, the mortality rate can be very low. Mortality generally results from complications of respiratory compromise, such as pulmonary emboli or respiratory arrest.

In GBS, the immune system starts to destroy the myelin sheath that surrounds the axons. Segmental demyelination (the destruction of myelin between the nodes of Ranvier) is the major pathologic finding in GBS. This destruction affects saltatory conduction, or the leaping of impulses from node to node. The result is dispersion of impulses and slow conduction velocities or conduction block in the late stages of the disease. Although the heavily myelinated cranial and motor nerves are affected more often than are the thinly myelinated pain, touch, and temperature nerve fibers, sensory function is often affected. In addition, the brain may receive inappropriate sensory signals, resulting in tingling, "crawling skin," or pain.

On microscopic examination, aggregates of lymphocytes are seen at the points of myelin breakdown, yet the axons usually remain intact. In some instances there may be secondary damage to the cell body, the neurilemma, or the axon; this can delay recovery or result in permanent deficits.

Three stages make up the *acute* course of GBS:

- The *initial period* (1 to 4 weeks), which begins with the onset of the first definitive symptoms and ends when no further deterioration is noted
- The *plateau period* (several days to 2 weeks)
- The *recovery phase* (4 to 6 months, maybe up to 2 years), which is thought to coincide with remyelination and axonal regeneration

Chronic inflammatory demyelinating polyneuropathy (CIDP) is an unusual type of GBS that progresses over a longer period; complete recovery rarely occurs. The uncommon condition in which relapsing attacks of GBS occur is called chronic relapsing polyneuropathy.

Etiology and Genetic Risk

The cause of GBS remains obscure. Most of the evidence implicates a cell-mediated immunologic reaction. Research suggests that the humoral immune system is also involved. Defects of T-lymphocytes (T-cells) and B-lymphocytes (B-cells) of the lymphatic system may be the basis of the syndrome. T-cells are responsible for cell-mediated immunity and the phagocytosis of bacteria. B-lymphocytes produce and secrete immunoglobulin, which form the humoral part of the immune system. Normally these antibodies combine with antigens, such as viruses, and prevent the organisms from having a harmful effect. This antigen-antibody combination also induces an inflammatory reaction by attracting T-cells (Sulton, 2002).

The client with GBS often relates a history of acute illness, trauma, surgery, or immunization 1 to 3 weeks before the onset of neurologic manifestations. Other risk factors identified in epidemiologic studies include an upper respiratory tract infection or gastrointestinal (GI) illness (50% of cases) and positive antibodies to cytomegalovirus or Epstein-Barr virus (EBV). It is believed that the prodromal (earlier) event causes a limited malfunction of the immune system, which sensitizes the T-cells to the client's myelin. In response to several antigens, some clients apparently form a demyelinating antibody that has a direct toxic effect on nerves or attracts a cellular immune response; this ultimately destroys the myelin. Other factors associated with the development of Guillain-Barré syndrome (GBS) are listed in Table 47-1.

Incidence/Prevalence

The annual incidence of GBS throughout the world is about 1 to 4 cases per 100,000 population. It generally affects people between 15 and 36 and between 50 and 75 years of age.

TABLE 47-1 Factors Associated with Development of Guillain-Barré Syndrome

■ Acute illness	■ Vaccination
■ Gastrointestinal illness	Flu
■ *Campylobacter jejuni*	Group A *Streptococcus*
■ Human immunodeficiency virus infection	Rabies
■ *Mycoplasma pneumoniae*	■ Swine flu
■ Surgery	■ Medications
■ Upper respiratory infection	Captopril
■ Virus	Danazol
Cytomegalovirus	Penicillamine
Epstein-Barr virus	Streptokinase
Varicella-zoster virus	

GBS is seen more often in clients with Hodgkin's disease, systemic lupus erythematosus, and human immunodeficiency virus (HIV) infection. In 2% to 5% of cases, a chronic or recurrent GBS develops. Mortality is estimated at 4% to 15%; generally due to autonomic instability and complications of immobility (Hughes, 2003). The mortality rate in older adults is 5% higher than in the general population secondary to dysrhythmias.

CULTURAL CONSIDERATIONS

GBS has worldwide distribution, is not seasonal, and affects people of all races and ages. Higher rates have been noted in people 45 years of age or older. The incidence of the disease is 50% higher in white individuals than in black individuals, but the cause is not known (Hughes, 2003).

HEALTH PROMOTION/ILLNESS PREVENTION

There is no way to prevent GB. Once the illness develops about 25% of those affected require mechanical ventilation for a period of time. Fatigue is a major lingering symptom in more than two thirds of those affected. The cost to treat a typical client with GB in the United States is $110,000 for acute care and results in $360,000 in lost productivity per client. Complications of GB can be minimized through meticulous nursing care.

◆COLLABORATIVE MANAGEMENT

◆Assessment

HISTORY

In addition to biographic data (e.g., age, gender, cultural background), obtain a complete medical and surgical history. Any illness (infection or other illness) 1 to 8 weeks before the onset of Guillain-Barré syndrome (GBS) should be explored. Ask the client to describe the symptoms in chronologic order, if possible.

PHYSICAL ASSESSMENT/CLINICAL MANIFESTATIONS

Manifestations of GBS depend on the degree of weakness and the progression of symptoms. Although features may vary (Chart 47-1), most people with GBS relate an abrupt onset of muscle weakness and pain. Typically, GBS does not affect level of consciousness, cerebral function, or pupillary signs.

The clinical variations of GBS reflect the areas of earliest or most severe involvement. **Ascending GBS** is the most common clinical pattern. Weakness and paresthesias begin in the lower extremities and progress upward to include the trunk and arms or affect the cranial nerves. The client may exhibit symptoms of an ascending flaccidity or weakness that evolves over hours to several days (1 to 10 days). The extent of the motor deficit ranges from mild paresis to total quadriplegia. About half of the clients with GBS experience some degree of respiratory compromise. Although they may be diminished during the initial assessment, deep tendon reflexes are absent in limbs that become paralyzed. *Pure motor* GBS is identical to the ascending variant, except sensory manifestations are absent.

The client with **descending GBS** initially experiences weakness of the face or **bulbar** muscles of the jaw, the sternocleidomastoid muscles (head rotators), and the muscles of the tongue, pharynx, and larynx. Weakness progresses downward to involve the limbs. This type of GBS may quickly affect the respiratory function. The client is monitored for breathlessness during speech, shallow respirations, dyspnea, and decreased tidal volume.

Descending GBS often includes **ophthalmoplegia** (paralysis or weakness of the eye muscles), causing diplopia. If the pupillary response to light is affected, functional blindness may result. Thus the client's visual function is assessed. Clients who experience visual problems are provided with information, explanation, and support. In this variation, numbness is more common in the hands than in the feet. Deep tendon reflexes are decreased or absent.

The **Miller Fisher variant**, a rare polyneuropathy, consists of a triad of ophthalmoplegia (paralysis of ocular [eye] muscles), areflexia (absence of reflexes), and severe ataxia (defective muscle coordination). Motor strength and sensory function are normal. The pupillary response to light is occasionally affected by the ophthalmoplegia, which results in functional blindness. Although respiratory complications are rare in clients with this variant, respiratory function is monitored frequently.

With any of the variants, *cranial nerve* involvement most often affects the facial nerve (cranial nerve VII). Involvement of the facial nerve results in the inability to smile, frown, whistle, or drink from a straw. In addition to monitoring the functions of cranial nerve VII, assess the client for dysphagia and paralysis of the larynx. Less frequently affected cranial nerves include the glossopharyngeal (IX), vagus (X), accessory (XI), and hypoglossal (XII) nerves. The client's inability to cough, gag, or swallow results from the involvement of cranial nerves IX and X. Monitor the client closely for varying blood pressure (hypertensive and hypotensive episodes or orthostatic hypotension), bradycardia, heart block, and asystole. These symptoms are characteristic of *autonomic dysfunction,* which is linked to vagus nerve (X) deficit. Cranial nerve XI (accessory) is assessed by asking the client to perform shoulder shrugs. Hypoglossal nerve (XII) deficit is evidenced by deviation or paralysis of the tongue.

Pain related to paresthesias is a commonly encountered symptom that requires aggressive management.

CHART 47-1

KEY FEATURES of Guillain-Barré Syndrome

Motor Manifestations
- Ascending symmetric muscle weakness → flaccid paralysis without muscle atrophy
- Decreased or absent deep tendon reflexes (DTRs)
- Respiratory compromise (dyspnea, diminished breath sounds, decreased tidal volume and vital capacity) and respiratory failure
- Loss of bowel and bladder control (less common)

Sensory Manifestations
- Paresthesias
- Pain (cramping)

Cranial Nerve Manifestations
- Facial weakness
- Dysphagia
- Diplopia
- Difficulty speaking

Autonomic Manifestations
- Labile blood pressure
- Cardiac dysrhythmias
- Tachycardia

PSYCHOSOCIAL ASSESSMENT

In addition to determining the usual roles and responsibilities, occupation, motivation, and available support systems, the client's ability to cope with this devastating illness and the accompanying fear and anxiety is assessed. In general, GBS is self-limiting and the paralysis temporary (Gregory, 2003). It is not unusual for the client to experience depression throughout the recovery period due to a feeling of powerlessness.

LABORATORY ASSESSMENT

Although no single clinical or laboratory finding confirms the diagnosis of Guillain-Barré syndrome (GBS), the health care provider may perform a lumbar puncture (LP) to evaluate cerebrospinal fluid (CSF). An increase in CSF protein level without an increase (or only a slight to moderate increase) in cell count is a distinguishing feature of GBS. However, high protein levels may not be noted until after 1 to 2 weeks of illness, reaching a peak in 4 to 6 weeks. The CSF lymphocyte count is normal.

Peripheral blood tests may show a moderate leukocytosis early in the illness. The number of leukocytes rapidly returns to normal in the absence of complications or concurrent illness. Elevated liver function tests were found in one third of the clients in one reported study (Sharshar et al., 2003).

OTHER DIAGNOSTIC ASSESSMENTS

Electrophysiologic studies demonstrate demyelinating neuropathy. The degree of abnormality found on testing does not always correlate with clinical severity. Within 3 weeks of symptoms, nerve conduction velocities are depressed. In some cases, denervated potentials (fibrillations) develop later in the illness. Electromyographic (EMG) findings, which reflect peripheral nerve function, are normal early in the illness. Electrophysiologic changes appear only after denervation of muscle has been present for 4 weeks or longer. Nerve conduction velocity (NCV) testing is performed in conjunction with the EMG. An electrical impulse is applied to one end of a nerve in the client's arm or leg. The time it takes to reach the other end is measured. Nerve damage or disease may still exist despite normal NCV results. These tests are described in Chapter 44.

A magnetic resonance imaging (MRI) or computed tomography (CT) scan may be ordered to rule out other causes of motor weakness. Respiratory function is often compromised in clients with GBS. Vital capacity may be decreased, and arterial blood gas (ABG) values may be abnormal (decreased partial pressure of arterial oxygen [Pa_{O_2}], increased partial pressure of arterial carbon dioxide [Pa_{CO_2}], or increased pH).

Critical Thinking Challenge

An older adult client presents to the neurologist's office with complaints of lower extremity weakness, difficulty swallowing, and dizziness. She states that she has had these symptoms for almost a week and seems to be getting worse each day. As the office nurse interviewing this client, you suspect that her clinical manifestations are possibly due to GBS.

1. What important history questions should you ask her and why?
2. When you perform an initial physical assessment, what should your priority be?
3. What actions might the neurologist take to confirm a medical diagnosis of GBS?

evolve For suggested answer guidelines, go to http://evolve.elsevier.com/Iggy/.

Analysis

COMMON NURSING DIAGNOSES AND COLLABORATIVE PROBLEMS

The following are priority nursing diagnoses for clients with GBS:

1. Ineffective Breathing Pattern, Ineffective Airway Clearance, and Impaired Gas Exchange related to respiratory muscle weakness or paralysis, inability to cough and deep breathe effectively, and immobility
2. Acute Pain related to paresthesias
3. Impaired Physical Mobility and Self-Care Deficit related to weakness, paralysis, and ataxia
4. Impaired Verbal Communication related to intubation or paralysis of the muscles required for speech
5. Powerlessness related to the inability to perform activities of daily living (ADLs) and usual role responsibilities

ADDITIONAL NURSING DIAGNOSES AND COLLABORATIVE PROBLEMS

In addition to the common nursing diagnoses, clients with GBS may have one or more of the following:

- Risk for Impaired Skin Integrity related to altered sensation, altered nutrition, and/or immobility
- Impaired Home Maintenance related to lack of knowledge or inadequate support systems
- Disturbed Sensory Perception (Tactile, Kinesthetic, and Visual) related to paresthesias and diplopia
- Disturbed Body Image and Situational Low Self-Esteem related to loss of body function, physical changes, and dependency
- Imbalanced Nutrition: Less Than Body Requirements related to difficulty chewing, dysphagia, paralysis of the extremities, anxiety, or depression
- Risk for Aspiration related to dysphagia from motor weakness
- Risk for Deficient Fluid Volume related to cranial nerve paralysis, dysphagia, and paralysis of the extremities
- Constipation, Diarrhea, or Bowel Incontinence related to inadequate oral intake, immobility, and impaired communication
- Decreased Cardiac Output related to autonomic dysfunction
- Deficient Knowledge related to understanding the disease process and expectations

Planning and Implementation

INEFFECTIVE BREATHING PATTERN; INEFFECTIVE AIRWAY CLEARANCE; IMPAIRED GAS EXCHANGE

NOC **PLANNING: EXPECTED OUTCOMES.** The client with Guillain-Barré syndrome (GBS) is expected to have adequate ventilation, airway patency, and sufficient gas exchange in the lungs as indicated by:

- Noncompromised respiratory rate and rhythm
- Normal breath sounds
- Tidal volume and vital capacity within normal limits
- No dyspnea or cyanosis
- Arterial blood gases (ABGs) within normal limits
- Noncompromised cognitive status

INTERVENTIONS. The *priority* intervention for the client is to maintain adequate respiratory function and implement interdisciplinary actions, if necessary, to assist him or her in meeting the expected outcomes (Chart 47-2).

NIC **Respiratory Monitoring.** In the initial phase, the client is monitored closely (usually in a critical care unit) for signs of respiratory distress, such as dyspnea, air hunger, adventitious breath sounds, and cyanosis. In addition, the client's respiratory rate, rhythm, and depth are monitored every 1 to 4 hours; vital capacity is checked every 2 to 4 hours; and the lungs are auscultated at 4-hour intervals. The client's ability to cough and swallow should also be monitored for change. Assess cognitive status, especially in older adults; a decline often indicates hypoxia.

NIC **Airway Management.** The purpose of airway management is to promote airway patency and gas exchange. Elevate the head of the bed to at least 45 degrees or higher as determined by the client's response and level of dyspnea. Suctioning of the client is based on assessment data. During suctioning, the client is at risk for vagal nerve stimulation that could lead to bradycardia and cardiac arrest. Monitor the color, consistency, and amount of secretions obtained. Chest physiotherapy, performed by the respiratory therapist or nurse, and frequent position changes are combined with breathing exercises (coughing and deep breathing) to prevent pneumonia and atelectasis. Encourage the client to use the incentive spirometer to expand the lungs every few hours. Oxygen may be administered by nasal cannula at a flow rate prescribed by the health care provider.

Arterial blood gas (ABG) values are frequently monitored for acid-base abnormalities and decreasing oxygen saturation. A decrease in vital capacity to less than 15 to 20 mL/kg (or less than two thirds of the client's normal) and the inability to clear secretions may be indications for elective intubation. Keep equipment for performing an endotracheal intubation at the bedside, and keep a ventilator readily available in case of respiratory emergency. Sharshar and colleagues (2003) found the following characteristics were predictive of those clients who required intubation and mechanical ventilation:

- Rapidly progressing symptoms
- Inability to lift elbows off bed

CHART 47-2

NIC **INTERVENTION ACTIVITIES for The Client with Guillain-Barré Syndrome**

Respiratory Monitoring: *Collection and analysis of client data to ensure airway patency and adequate gas exchange*
- Monitor rate, rhythm, depth, and effort of respirations.
- Monitor breathing patterns: bradypnea, tachypnea, hyperventilation, Kussmaul respirations, Cheyne-Stokes respirations, apneustic breathing, Biot's respiration, and ataxic patterns.
- Auscultate breath sounds, noting areas of decreased/absent ventilation and presence of adventitious sounds.
- Monitor PFT values, particularly vital capacity, maximal inspiratory force, forced expiratory volume in 1 second (FEV_1), and FEV_1/FVC, as available.
- Monitor mechanical ventilator readings, noting increases in inspiratory pressures and decreases in tidal volume, as appropriate.
- Monitor for increased restlessness, anxiety, and air hunger.
- Note changes in Sao_2, Svo_2, end tidal CO_2, and changes in ABG values, as appropriate.
- Monitor client's ability to cough effectively.
- Monitor for dyspnea and events that decrease and worsen it.
- Monitor chest x-ray reports.
- Place the client on side, as indicated, to prevent aspiration; log roll if cervical aspiration suspected.
- Institute respiratory therapy treatments (e.g., nebulizer), as needed.

Airway Management: *Facilitation of patency of air passages*
- Position client to maximize ventilation potential.
- Identify client requiring actual/potential airway insertion.
- Perform chest physical therapy, as appropriate.
- Remove secretions by encouraging coughing or by suctioning.
- Instruct how to cough effectively.
- Auscultate breath sounds, noting areas of decreased or absent ventilation and presence of adventitious sounds.
- Perform endotracheal or nasotracheal suctioning, as appropriate.
- Administer humidified air or oxygen, as appropriate.
- Administer aerosol treatments, as appropriate.
- Administer ultrasonic nebulizer treatments, as appropriate.
- Position to alleviate dyspnea.
- Monitor respiratory and oxygenation status, as appropriate.

NIC intervention activities selected from Dochterman, J.M., & Bulechek, G.M. (Eds.). (2004). *Nursing interventions classification (NIC)* (4th ed.). St. Louis: Mosby. No part of this work is to be altered without prior written permission from the Publisher.

PFT, Pulmonary function test; *FEV_1*, forced expiratory volume in 1 second; *FVC*, forced vital capacity; *Svo_2*, venous oxygen saturation; *Sao_2*, arterial oxygen saturation; *CO_2*, carbon dioxide; *ABG*, arterial blood gas.

- Inability to stand
- Ineffective cough
- Elevated liver enzymes
- Vital capacity less than 60% of predicted value

Interventions for Cardiac Dysfunction. Both the sympathetic and parasympathetic systems may be affected. The client is placed on a cardiac monitor because of the risk for dysrhythmias. Monitor vital signs closely. Hypertension is treated with a beta blocker or nitroprusside. Hypotension is treated with intravenous (IV) fluids and placing the client in a supine position, unless he or she is in extreme respiratory distress. Atropine may be prescribed to treat bradycardia.

Some clients experience urinary retention; maintain strict intake and output. If the client is unable to void, an indwelling urinary catheter (Foley) may be needed or an intermittent catheterization program started.

Drug Therapy/Plasmapheresis. The health care provider should follow the best practice guidelines from the American Academy of Neurology for the treatment of GBS (Hughes, 2003). These include the following recommendations:
- Treat with either plasma exchange (plasmapheresis) *or* immunoglobulin; there is no benefit to combine these treatments.
- Implement plasma exchange (PE) for nonambulatory adult clients who seek treatment within 4 weeks of the development of symptoms. It is also recommended for ambulatory clients seen within 2 weeks of onset of symptoms.
- Use IV immunoglobulin (IVIg) for ambulatory clients who seek treatment within 2 weeks of onset of symptoms.
- Do not use corticosteroids.

IV Immunoglobulin. IVIg has been shown to be as effective as plasmapheresis. It is safer and immediately available. Side effects of immunoglobulin therapy range from minor annoyances (e.g., chills, mild fever, myalgia, and headache) to major complications (e.g., anaphylaxis, aseptic meningitis, retinal necrosis, and acute renal failure). A serum IgA is drawn before administration of the medication. Infuse IVIg slowly when it is started. Observe for side and adverse effects, and report their occurrence to the health care provider. The rate of administration can be increased based on the client's tolerance.

Plasmapheresis. **Plasmapheresis** removes the circulating antibodies thought to be responsible for the disease. In this procedure, plasma is selectively separated from whole blood. The blood cells are returned to the client without the plasma. Plasma usually replaces itself, or the client is transfused with colloidal substitute such as albumin. Fresh frozen plasma is generally not used because of the associated risk of infection and allergic pulmonary edema (Sulton, 2002). This procedure should be started 7 to 14 days after the onset of the illness. The client usually receives three to four treatments, 1 to 2 days apart. Some clients may require a second round of treatment if they deteriorate after the first plasmapheresis.

Nursing responsibilities for the client undergoing plasmapheresis include providing information and reassurance, weighing the client before and after the procedure, and administering proper care to the shunt. Proper shunt care includes maintaining shunt patency, checking for bruits every 2 to 4 hours, keeping double bulldog clamps at the bedside, and observing the puncture site for bleeding or ecchymosis (bruising). Observe for signs of complications throughout the procedure (Chart 47-3). Atropine is prescribed in the event of bradycardia.

ACUTE PAIN

PLANNING: EXPECTED OUTCOMES. The client with Guillain-Barré syndrome (GBS) is expected to experience adequate pain control as indicated by client report and consistent demonstration of ways to manage pain.

INTERVENTIONS. Assess the severity and nature of the client's pain, which is often worse at night. The typical pain experienced is often not relieved by medication other than opiates, which can be administered via a patient-controlled analgesia (PCA) pump or continuous IV drip.

CHART 47-3

BEST PRACTICE for
Preventing and Managing Complications of Plasmapheresis

Complication	Nursing Interventions
Trauma or infection at vascular access site	Keep the site clean and dry. Monitor the site for redness, swelling, drainage, or other signs of infection.
Hypovolemia with resultant hypotension, tachycardia, dizziness, and diaphoresis	Monitor fluid and electrolyte status and vital signs. Administer fluids as prescribed. Provide an explanation of side effects, and reassure the client.
Hypokalemia and hypocalcemia	Monitor fluid and electrolyte balance. Administer replacement electrolytes, as prescribed Observe for cardiac dysrhythmias.
Temporary circumoral and distal extremity paresthesias, muscle twitching, nausea, and vomiting related to administration of citrated plasma	Add calcium gluconate or calcium chloride to exchange fluids, as prescribed. Provide explanations, comfort measures, and reassurance.

Document the client's response to pain medication, and notify the health care provider if pain relief is not sufficient. Other pain control measures include frequent repositioning, massage, ice, heat, relaxation techniques, guided imagery, and distractions (e.g., music or visitors). Chapter 7 discusses these and other pain relief measures in detail.

IMPAIRED PHYSICAL MOBILITY AND SELF-CARE DEFICIT

NOC **PLANNING: EXPECTED OUTCOMES.** The client with GBS is expected to be free of physiologic immobility consequences as indicated by *no:*

- Pressure ulcers
- Constipation, paralytic ileus, or stool impaction
- Urinary retention, calculi, or infection
- Fracture or contractures
- Venous thrombosis
- Lung congestion or pneumonia
- Orthostatic hypotension

The client is also expected to perform basic activities of daily living (ADLs) as indicated by noncompromised:

- Eating
- Toileting
- Hygiene, dressing, and grooming
- Walking or wheelchair mobility
- Self-transfer and positioning

INTERVENTIONS. The client's emotional and mental status and his or her level of acceptance of the disability is determined. The client, family, nurse, physical and occupational therapist, speech-language pathologist, and dietitian collaborate to develop interventions to prevent complications of immobility and to address deficits in self-care. Assess the client's motor (muscle) function every 2 to 4 hours as part of the neurologic assessment. The interventions prescribed for mobility and self-care and to prevent complications depend on the degree of motor deficit experienced by the client. Assistive devices and instructions for their use are provided for the client. To ensure safety, assist the client with ambulation, transfers from bed to chair, position changes, and maintenance of proper body alignment until he or she is able to perform these activities independently. Maximal independence is always encouraged. Range-of-motion (ROM) exercises are performed actively or passively every 2 to 4 hours by the nurse or unlicensed assistive personnel (UAP). Family members may be instructed in these techniques. (See Chapter 10 for detailed discussion of ways to improve physical mobility and self-care, as well as ways to prevent immobility consequences.) Monitor the client's responses to or tolerance of activity. Provide adequate rest periods between activities and therapy sessions.

Decreased gastric motility, dysphagia, and depression can cause malnutrition. The dietitian develops an individualized nutrition plan. The client may require little assistance with feeding or may be totally dependent. If the client is unable to safely swallow food or liquids, enteral nutrition via feeding tube is prescribed. Weigh the client three times a week, and monitor serum albumin and prealbumin each week.

Malnutrition places clients at risk for pressure ulcers. Therefore special attention is paid to skin care, including interventions to prevent skin breakdown. Instruct the UAP to turn the client a minimum of every 2 hours. Assess the skin for any areas of redness that may lead to pressure ulcers. If the client's bed does not have a pressure-reducing mattress, use a mattress overlay to help prevent skin breakdown. Document changes in the client's skin condition every shift while in the acute care setting and at least daily in a subacute or rehabilitation setting. If an ulcer occurs, implement aggressive interventions to manage the wound. Chapters 10 and 70 discuss pressure ulcer care in detail.

Because pulmonary emboli and deep vein thrombosis are common complications of immobility, the health care provider may prescribe prophylactic anticoagulant therapy, such as subcutaneous heparin or Lovenox. Antiembolism stockings and sequential compression stockings may be used to promote venous return. Be sure that stockings are removed at least once every 24 hours for 15 to 30 minutes. Other prevention measures are determined by agency policy or health care provider preference. Chapter 10 describes additional interventions to prevent complications of immobility and promote self-care.

IMPAIRED VERBAL COMMUNICATION

PLANNING: EXPECTED OUTCOMES. The client with Guillain-Barré syndrome (GBS) is expected to communicate as indicated by the ability to receive, interpret, and express written and nonverbal messages to and from the staff, family, and/or significant others.

INTERVENTIONS. The client may have difficulty communicating because the muscles required for the production of speech are weak, or the client may be on a mechanical ventilator because the respiratory muscles are paralyzed. In either case, the nurse collaborates with the speech-language pathologist to develop a communication system. A simple technique involves eye blinking or moving a finger to indicate "yes" and "no." A communication board can be developed with the letters of the alphabet or a list of common requests, such as the need to be repositioned or the need for pain medication. Both the staff and the visitors must know how the client's communication system operates.

POWERLESSNESS

NOC **PLANNING: EXPECTED OUTCOMES.** The client with GBS is expected to maintain hope as indicated by consistently expressing:

- Expectation of a positive future
- Faith
- Meaning in life
- Sense of self-control
- Optimism

INTERVENTIONS. Assess the client and family or significant others for verbal and nonverbal behaviors that indicate powerlessness, anxiety, fear, and grieving. Encourage the client to verbalize feelings about the illness and its effects, if possible, while fostering hope. Previous decision-making patterns, roles, and responsibilities are examined. Ask the client and family to describe their usual lifestyles and the situations in which they coped both effectively and ineffectively to help identify factors that influence coping ability.

Refer clients who need further psychosocial support to the social worker, hospital chaplain or appropriate spiritual resource, and local support groups. If necessary, obtain a psychological consultation for further evaluation and intervention.

Community-Based Care

The severity and course of Guillain-Barré syndrome (GBS) are extremely variable, which makes it difficult to predict the prognosis. The most likely residual effects at discharge are related to motor status and mobility, self-care, and perhaps sensory alteration and disturbed self-concept. For clients who experience total quadriparesis or respiratory paralysis, the course of the rehabilitation phase is even more variable and may require weeks to years. The goal of the recovery phase is to move from dependence to independence, if possible. Cooke and Orb (2003) found that clients go through several phases during their recovery to meet that goal (see the Evidence-Based Practice for Nursing box above).

Planning for discharge begins on admission. The client may be discharged to home or to a rehabilitation unit. The nurse, discharge planner, or case manager (CM) makes appropriate referrals to a home care agency and community agencies for assistance in the home setting after discharge. Chapter 10 discusses various aspects of rehabilitation in detail.

A family member or significant other is included in the education process throughout the client's hospitalization. The client and family are given both oral and written instructions in techniques to facilitate mobility, use of adaptive-assistive devices, and prevent skin breakdown. If mobility remains markedly impaired, the physical therapist emphasizes the need for ROM exercises, positioning and frequent turning techniques, and prevention of skin breakdown.

If the client is discharged to home while still dependent on assistive devices, the interdisciplinary health care team makes certain that the necessary equipment has been delivered after evaluating the home setting. Home care management for clients with GBS is similar to that for those who have had a stroke or spinal cord injury, depending on the nature of the neurologic deficit (see Chapter 48).

EVIDENCE-BASED PRACTICE for Nursing

How do clients with Guillain-Barré syndrome gain independence during the recovery period?

Cooke, J.F., & Orb, A. (2003). The recovery phase in Guillain-Barré syndrome: Moving from dependency to independence. *Rehabilitation Nursing, 28*(4), 105-108, 130.

This small qualitative study followed five clients with Guillain-Barré syndrome (GBS) discharged from a major teaching hospital during their recovery period. Each participant was interviewed using a semistructured questionnaire to obtain data that were analyzed through a constant comparative method. Five phases were identified as these subjects progressed from dependency to independence:

- Experiencing dependency
- Encountering helplessness
- Wanting to know more about GBS
- Discovering inner strength
- Regaining independence

A central theme identified was that all clients discovered inner strengths that they did not realize they had. They also stated that when they were discharged, they had very little knowledge about their illness or prognosis.

Level of Evidence: 8—This was a very small number for subjects used for a qualitative study.

Critique. Although the sample size was very small, this study provides the groundwork for future nursing research. Qualitative research was an appropriate research method to answer the study question. This research needs to be replicated before any generalization can occur, especially focusing on themes that may emerge in varying cultural groups.

Implications for Nursing. Of particular interest are the findings related to lack of knowledge upon discharge and discovery of inner strengths. Nurses need to ensure that clients are well-informed about their health problems before hospital discharge. In collaboration with social workers, nurses should talk with clients to help them identify coping strategies and other strengths that have helped clients in other critical or stressful situations.

Self-help groups for clients with chronic illness are common. Consult with the client and the health care provider about referrals to these groups, if indicated. The Guillain-Barré Foundation provides information about local resources and information for clients and their families. The psychosocial adjustment needed may be minimal or dramatic depending on the client's residual deficit, age, gender, usual roles and responsibilities, usual coping strategies, available support systems, and occupation. Help the client identify other support systems, such as church members, social club members, or spiritual resources.

Evaluation: Outcomes

Evaluate the care of the client with GBS on the basis of the identified nursing diagnoses. The expected outcomes include that the client should:

- Have adequate ventilation, airway patency, and sufficient gas exchange in the lungs
- Experience adequate pain control
- Be free of physiologic immobility consequences
- Perform basic ADLs
- Communicate with staff, family, and significant others
- Maintain hope

Specific indicators for these outcomes are listed for each nursing diagnosis under the Planning and Implementation section (see earlier).

MYASTHENIA GRAVIS

PATHOPHYSIOLOGY

Myasthenia gravis (MG) is a chronic disease characterized by fatigue and weakness primarily in muscles innervated by the cranial nerves, as well as in skeletal and respiratory muscles (Chitnis & Khoury, 2003). This autoimmune disease of the neuromuscular junction may take many forms–from mild disturbances of the ocular muscles to a rapidly developing, generalized weakness that may lead to death from respiratory failure. It is characterized by remissions and exacerbations (worsening or "flare-ups").

MG is caused by an autoantibody attack on the acetylcholine receptors (AChR) in the muscle end plate membranes (Richman & Agius, 2003). As a result, nerve impulses are not transmitted to the skeletal muscle at the neuromuscular junction.

Etiology and Genetic Risk

Although the precipitating event remains unclear, research strongly suggests that MG is caused by antibodies to the ACh receptors. Although the disease is not hereditary, there is a 5% familial incidence. Evidence also suggests a relationship between MG and hyperplasia (overgrowth) of the thymus gland. The thymus gland is often abnormal. **Thymoma** (encapsulated thymus gland tumor) occurs in about 15% of cases, and 70% of the remaining cases show hyperplasia of the thymus. There is also a very strong association between MG and hyperthyroidism. D-penicillamine, interferon-alpha, and bone marrow transplantation have been associated with drug-induced (iatrogenic) autoimmune MG (Pascuzzi, 2003).

Incidence/Prevalence

The incidence of MG in the United States is estimated to be 0.5 per 100,000 people. Although it may begin at any age, the onset of MG before 10 years of age or after 60 years of age is rare. The peak age at onset is between 20 and 30 years of age. Women are affected three times more often than are men.

COLLABORATIVE MANAGEMENT

Assessment

Although the onset of MG is usually insidious, some instances of fairly rapid development have been preceded by infection, emotional upset, pregnancy, or anesthesia. Thus the nurse inquires about any history of these events. A temporary increase in weakness may be noted after vaccination, menstruation, and exposure to extremes in environmental temperature.

In addition to the biographic data and history, ask the client if he or she experienced the rapid onset of fatigue. Note complaints of muscle weakness that increases on exertion or as the day wears on and improves with rest. Ask the client to describe his or her symptoms, specifically noting the affected muscle groups and any limitation or inability in performing activities of daily living (ADLs).

Additional areas of inquiry include any history of **ptosis** (drooping eyelids) or **diplopia** (double vision), difficulty chewing or swallowing **(dysphagia),** and the type of diet best tolerated. Assess the client for previous manifestations of respiratory difficulty, choking, or voice weakness. Other areas of assessment include asking about any difficulty holding up the head, brushing teeth, combing hair, or shaving. Inquiry is made about the presence of paresthesias or aching in weakened muscles. Finally, assess for a history of thymus gland tumor.

CHART 47-4

KEY FEATURES of Myasthenia Gravis

Motor Manifestations
- Progressive muscle weakness (proximal) that usually improves with rest
- Poor posture
- Ocular palsies
- Ptosis
- Weak or incomplete eye closure
- Diplopia
- Respiratory compromise
- Loss of bowel and bladder control
- Fatigue

Sensory Manifestations
- Muscle achiness
- Paresthesias
- Decreased smell and taste

PHYSICAL ASSESSMENT/CLINICAL MANIFESTATIONS

MG may be diagnosed after the demonstration of *progressive* paresis of affected muscle groups that is resolved, at least in part, by rest (Chart 47-4). The most common symptoms (exhibited by more than 90% of clients) are related to involvement of the levator palpebrae or extraocular muscles. Assess for ocular palsies, ptosis, diplopia, and weak or incomplete eye closure. These symptoms may last only a few days at the onset and then resolve, only to return weeks or months later. Normal pupillary responses to light and accommodation are present.

For most clients, the muscles of facial expression, chewing, and speech are affected (**bulbar** involvement). Note the client's smile, which may be transformed into a snarl; the jaw may hang so that the client must prop it up with the hand. Chewing and swallowing difficulties, choking, and regurgitation of fluids through the nose may lead to considerable weight loss. Inquire about the client's nutritional status and any recent weight loss. It may be more difficult for the client to eat after talking. After extended conversations, the voice may become weaker or exhibit a nasal twang. In some clients, the tongue has one central and two lateral longitudinal fissures (sores or ulcers).

Less often involved are the muscles of the shoulders, the flexors of the neck, and the hip flexors. Because limb weakness is more often *proximal,* the client may have difficulty climbing stairs, lifting heavy objects, or raising the arms overhead. Neck weakness may be mild or severe enough to cause difficulty in holding the head erect. Among the trunk muscles, the erector spinae are most commonly affected. This results in difficulty sustaining a sitting or walking posture.

In the most advanced cases of MG, all muscles are weakened, including those associated with respiratory function and the control of bladder and bowel function. In these severe cases, inquire about bowel and bladder function. Assess respiratory function frequently.

Muscle atrophy, although rarely marked in degree, occurs in a small percentage of clients with myasthenia gravis (MG). The client's tendon reflexes should be assessed, but they are not often affected. Assess for pain, although this is seldom a major complaint. Some clients report aching of the weakened muscles. If present, paresthesias (painful tingling sensation) affecting the muscles of the face, hands, and thighs is not associated with any loss of sensation. Lost or decreased sensations of smell and taste have been reported. There is no alteration of consciousness.

In **Eaton-Lambert syndrome**, a form of myasthenia often observed in combination with small cell carcinoma of the lung, the muscles of the trunk and the pelvic and shoulder girdles are most commonly affected. Although weakness increases after exertion, there may be a temporary increase in muscle strength during the first few contractions, followed by rapid decline. Diagnosis is confirmed by electromyography (EMG). Management differs somewhat from other types of MG. Treatment includes removing the tumor, managing the cancer, and administering medications to release acetylcholine (ACh). Additional therapies may include plasmapheresis and immunosuppressive therapy (discussed later).

LABORATORY ASSESSMENT

In virtually all cases of MG, the diagnosis is obvious from the history and physical examination findings. MG may be immediately confirmed by the client's response to cholinergic drugs. A standard series of laboratory studies is usually performed for clients with known or suspected MG. Thyroid function should be tested because **thyrotoxicosis** (excessive thyroid hormone) is present in about 5% of myasthenic clients. Serum protein electrophoresis evaluates the client for immunologic disorders. Immunologic-based diseases, such as rheumatoid arthritis, systemic lupus erythematosus, and polymyositis, are associated with the disease.

Testing for acetylcholine receptor antibodies (AChR) has become an important diagnostic criterion, because 80% to 90% of clients with MG have elevated AChR. A positive antibody test result confirms the diagnosis, but a negative finding does not exclude the disease (Pagana & Pagana, 2002).

RADIOGRAPHIC ASSESSMENT

Some clients with MG have a thymoma, and therefore clients are assessed for this condition. The thymus, an H-shaped gland located in the upper mediastinum beneath the sternum, is one organ in which ACh receptor antibodies are formed. Although a thymoma can often be seen on routine frontal and lateral chest x-rays, special studies should be performed for any area suggestive of thymoma in the anterior mediastinum. The nurse prepares the client for these tests or for a computed tomography (CT) scan by explaining the equipment and what to expect during the tests.

OTHER DIAGNOSTIC ASSESSMENTS

TENSILON TESTING. Pharmacologic tests with the cholinesterase inhibitors edrophonium chloride (Tensilon) and neostigmine bromide (Prostigmin) have been in use since the 1950s. Tensilon is used more often because of its rapid onset and brief duration of action. This drug inhibits the breakdown of ACh at the postsynaptic membrane, which increases the availability of ACh for excitation of postsynaptic receptors. To perform the test, the physician first estimates the strength of cranial muscles. Initially, 2 mg (0.2 mL) is injected IV; if this is tolerated, an additional 8 mg (0.8 mL) is injected after 30 seconds. Within 30 to 60 seconds of the first dose, most myasthenic clients show a marked improvement in muscle tone that lasts 4 to 5 minutes. False-positive test results may be caused by increased muscle effort by the client. False-negative findings may be seen if the tested muscle is extremely weak or refractory to the drug (Pascuzzi, 2003).

Tensilon testing may also be used to help determine whether increasing weakness in the previously diagnosed myasthenic client is due to a **cholinergic crisis** (overmedication with cholinesterase inhibitors) or a **myasthenic crisis** (undermedication with cholinesterase inhibitors). In a cholinergic crisis, muscle tone does not improve after the administration of Tensilon. Instead, weakness may actually increase, and **fasciculations** (muscle twitching) may be noted around the eyes and face. The Tensilon test poses a danger of ventricular fibrillation and cardiac arrest, but these reactions rarely occur. Atropine sulfate is the antidote for Tensilon and must be available in case these complications occur.

ELECTROMYOGRAPHY. A common diagnostic test performed by the physician or technician is electromyography (EMG). Although electrical testing of the normal neuromuscular junction produces no change in the amplitude (force) of muscle contraction, the amplitude of the muscle's response diminishes with progressive stimulation. A decrease in amplitude of more than 10% between the first and fifth responses generally indicates the defective neuromuscular transmission characteristic of, but not unique to, MG. Several muscles may be tested to increase the likelihood of detecting an abnormality. Testing may be performed after exercise or exposure of the muscle to curare or to ischemia.

Single-fiber EMG is even more sensitive in detecting defects of neuromuscular transmission. This test compares the stability of the firing of one muscle fiber with that of another fiber innervated by the same motor neuron. The time interval between the two firings normally shows a minor degree of variability, called jitter. Defective transmission increases jitter or actually blocks successive discharges.

Critical Thinking Challenge

A young woman presents in the emergency department (ED) with new onset of muscle weakness in her shoulders, "droopy" eyelids, "double-vision," and extreme fatigue. During assessment, she tells you that she also has a "tingling" sensation in her hands at times. She came to the ED because her physician is out of town and she doesn't know the physician who is covering for him.

1. As her admitting ED nurse, what questions should you ask her?
2. What is the priority for care for the client at this time?
3. After physician evaluation, the probable diagnosis is myasthenia gravis. What diagnostic testing will the physician most likely prescribe and why?
4. What are the differences between Guillain-Barré syndrome and myasthenia gravis?

evolve For suggested answer guidelines, go to http://evolve.elsevier.com/Iggy/.

Common Nursing Diagnoses and Collaborative Problems

Nursing diagnoses that typically apply to clients with myasthenia gravis include the following:

- Risk for Ineffective Breathing pattern and Ineffective Airway Clearance related to intercostal muscle weakness
- Self-Care Deficit related to fatigue and muscle weakness
- Activity Intolerance related to fatigue
- Impaired Verbal Communication related to muscle weakness

Interventions

The classic presentation of MG is muscle weakness that increases when the client is fatigued and limits his or her mobility and ability to participate in activities. Management for this disease fall into two categories:

- Treatment that affects the symptoms of MG without influencing the actual course of the disease (anticholinesterases or cholinergic drugs)
- Therapeutic efforts for inducing remission, such as the administration of immunosuppressive drugs or corticosteroids, plasmapheresis, and thymectomy (removal of the thymus gland)

NONSURGICAL MANAGEMENT. Assess the client's motor strength before and after periods of activity. Provide assistance as necessary to prevent the client from becoming fatigued. He or she is scheduled for tests, treatments and other activities early in the day or during the energy peaks that follow the administration of medications. Assist the client in planning the periods of rest necessary for avoiding excess fatigue.

Providing Assistance with Activities. During periods of maximal weakness, assistance is provided for ambulation, transfers from bed to chair or toilet/commode, position changes, and maintenance of body alignment. Active or passive range-of-motion (ROM) exercises are performed every 2 to 4 hours with assistance of the nurse, unlicensed assistive personnel (UAP), or family. Assess the client's skin integrity and teach family members how to perform this skill. The client is repositioned, and bony prominences are assessed at least every 2 hours for skin breakdown and contractures. Pressure-reducing devices or mattresses are used to prevent pressure ulcers. Consult with the physical and occupational therapist to develop a program for the client to assist with mobility, self-care, and energy conservation techniques.

Drug Therapy. Two groups of drugs are typically prescribed for the treatment of myasthenia gravis (MG): anticholinesterases and immunosuppressants. These medications must be administered *on time* to maintain blood levels and thus facilitate increased muscle strength. The client's response to medications are monitored and documented. Provide information for the client and the family about the indications for, effectiveness of, and side effects of the drugs used in the treatment of MG.

Cholinesterase Inhibitor Drugs. Cholinesterase (ChE) inhibitor drugs are the *first-line* management of MG. These drugs are also referred to as anticholinesterase drugs or antimyasthenics. They enhance neuromuscular impulse transmission by preventing the decrease of ACh by the enzyme ChE, thus increasing the response of the muscles to nerve impulses and improving muscle strength. The ChE drug of choice is pyridostigmine (Mestinon, Regonol). Expect day-to-day variations in dosage depending on the client's fluctuating symptoms.

Administer ChE medications with a small amount of food to help alleviate gastrointestinal side effects. Instruct the client to eat meals 45 minutes to 1 hour after taking these medications to avoid aspiration. This is very important if the client has bulbar involvement. Drugs containing magnesium, morphine or its derivatives, curare, quinine, quinidine, procainamide, or hypnotics or sedatives should be avoided because they may increase the client's weakness. Antibiotics such as neomycin, kanamycin, polymyxin B, and certain tetracyclines impair transmitter release and also increase myasthenic symptoms.

A potential adverse effect of these drugs is cholinergic crisis. Sudden increases in weakness and the inability to clear secretions, swallow, or breathe adequately indicate that the client is experiencing crisis. There are two types of crises:

- Myasthenic crisis–an exacerbation of the myasthenic symptoms caused by undermedication with anticholinesterase drugs
- Cholinergic crisis–an acute exacerbation of muscle weakness caused by overmedication with cholinergic (anticholinesterase) drugs

Because myasthenic and cholinergic crises have many common characteristics, the type of crisis the client is experiencing must be identified for effective treatment to be provided (Table 47-2). Monitor carefully for early detection of these emergencies.

Emergency Care: Myasthenic Crisis. Myasthenic crisis is often preceded by some type of infection. For other clients, increasing muscle weakness leads to an overdose of anticholinesterase drugs. As a result, the client may experience a *mixed* crisis. The Tensilon test (described on p. 1014), although not always conclusive, is an important procedure for differentiation. Tensilon produces a temporary improvement in myasthenic crisis, but no improvement or worsening of symptoms in cholinergic crisis.

The *priority* for nursing management of the client in myasthenic crisis is maintaining adequate respiratory function. The acutely ill client may need intensive nursing care for monitoring and maintenance of body functions. He or she may require mechanical ventilation. Cholinesterase-inhibiting drugs are withheld because they increase respiratory secretions and are usually ineffective for the first few

TABLE 47-2 Characteristics of Myasthenic and Cholinergic Crises

Myasthenic Crisis	Cholinergic Crisis	Mixed Crisis
Increased pulse and respiration	Nausea	Apprehension
Rise in blood pressure	Vomiting	Restlessness
Anoxia	Diarrhea	Dyspnea
Cyanosis	Abdominal cramps	Dysphagia (difficult swallowing)
Bowel and bladder incontinence	Blurred vision	Dysarthria (painful joints)
Decreased urine output	Pallor	Increased lacrimation (tearing)
Absence of cough and swallow reflex	Facial muscle twitching	Increased salivation
	Pupillary miosis	Diaphoresis
	Hypotension	Generalized weakness

days after the crisis begins. Medications are restarted gradually and at lower dosages.

Emergency Care: Cholinergic Crisis. In *cholinergic* crisis, anticholinergic drugs are withheld while the client is maintained on a ventilator. Atropine 1 mg IV may be given and repeated, if necessary. When atropine is prescribed, the nurse must observe the client carefully; secretions are thickened by the drug, which causes more difficulty with airway clearance and possibly the development of mucous plugs. Unless complications such as pneumonia or aspiration develop, the client in crisis improves rapidly after the appropriate drugs have been given. Continue to provide assistance as necessary, because the client tires easily after minimal exertion.

Immunosuppression. Immunosuppression may be accomplished with the use of corticosteroids, such as prednisone (Deltasone, Winpred✱), or with chemotherapeutic agents, such as azathioprine (Imuran), or cyclophosphamide (Cytoxan, Procytox✱). Prednisone is used initially to reduce remission and to control and improve symptoms. The drug is tapered over a period of weeks to months. Some clients may need continuous low-dose therapy because of exacerbations of symptoms. For ocular MG, corticosteroid treatment that does not cause significant systemic complications may significantly reduce the prevalence of generalized myasthenia gravis after 2 years on the medication (Kupersmith, Latkany, & Homel, 2003).

Azathioprine and cyclophosphamide are used for long-term management. Cyclophosphamide is reserved for clients who are refractory to other treatments. IV immunoglobulins (IVIg) may also be used for acute disease management or as a long-term option for disease refractory to other treatment.

Plasmapheresis. Plasmapheresis is a method by which antibodies are removed from the plasma. It may be used to decrease symptoms. Six exchanges occur over a 2-week period, with follow-up exchanges weekly or monthly as needed. This is usually done on an ambulatory care basis. Nursing management of the client undergoing plasmapheresis is presented in the earlier discussion of Guillain-Barré syndrome, p. 1010.

Respiratory Support. Although not all clients with MG experience respiratory compromise, ongoing assessment and maintenance of respiratory function must be done. Both myasthenic crisis (undermedication) and cholinergic crisis (overmedication) increase muscle weakness and the client's risk for respiratory compromise. The diaphragm and the respiratory and intercostal muscles may be affected, which inhibits the client's ability to maintain adequate ventilation, breathe deeply, and cough effectively. In addition, dysphagia may result in the aspiration of foods, fluids, or saliva, which compounds the respiratory problems. Because of their respiratory muscle involvement, many of these clients have an increased risk of pulmonary infections.

The client who cannot cough effectively may require oropharyngeal or nasopharyngeal suctioning. The nurse may need to teach the assisted cough technique, similar to that used by clients who are quadriplegic (see Chapter 48). Chest physiotherapy consisting of postural drainage, percussion, and vibration mobilizes secretions and helps prevent pneumonia and atelectasis. A breathing bag (e.g., Ambu), equipment for oxygen administration, and endotracheal intubation equipment are kept at the bedside in case of respiratory distress.

Because breathing difficulty or the inability to breathe easily is frightening, the nurse should be aware of the client's mental and emotional status during periods of respiratory compromise. His or her response to medications prescribed for muscle weakness, bronchodilation, and pulmonary congestion are monitored and documented.

As an alternative to mechanical ventilation, BiPAP (continuous positive airway pressure) should be tried first in clients with acute respiratory failure from MG crisis while awaiting improvement from IV immunoglobulin (IVIg) therapy or plasma exchange. Repeat arterial blood gas (ABG) measurements and clinical assessment after using the device for a few hours are used to determine its effects (Evoli et al., 2002).

Promoting Self-Care. Generalized weakness and fatigue affect the client's ability to participate in activities of daily living (ADLs). Impaired fine motor control and shoulder weakness, which result in difficulty raising the arms, often compound the problem. Self-care deficits may be complete or partial depending on the severity of the illness, the client's response to drugs, and his or her ability to tolerate activity without excessive fatigue.

To establish abilities and limitations, assess the client's ability to perform ADLs. Although the client is encouraged to perform activities as independently as possible, assistance is provided as necessary to avoid undue frustration and fatigue. For maximizing independence and making attempts at self-care successful, activities are planned to follow the administration of medication. Monitor and document the client's response to or tolerance of activity, providing alternating periods of activity and rest. Rest is critical because increased fatigue can precipitate a crisis. In addition, occupational and physical therapists evaluate the client for assistive-adaptive devices. In collaboration with the nurse, they teach the client and family energy conservation techniques and ideas for making work and self-care easier after discharge from the hospital.

Assisting with Communication. Weakness of the speech and facial muscles often results in dysarthric and nasal speech. Thus it may be difficult for myasthenic clients to make their speech understood by others.

The speech-language pathologist and nurse determine the client's ability to communicate. The client is instructed to speak slowly while the nurse attempts to lip-read. The information is repeated back to the client to verify that it is correct. Questions that can be answered with "yes" or "no" or by gestures may be used along with alternative communication systems such as eye blinking, flash cards, magic slates, notebook and pencil, and picture, letter, or word boards.

Nutritional Support. The client with myasthenia gravis (MG) may have difficulty maintaining an adequate intake of food and fluid because the muscles needed for chewing and swallowing become weakened and tire easily. In collaboration with the dietitian, occupational therapist, and speech-language pathologist, the client's nutritional status and his or her ability to receive adequate oral nutrition are evaluated. Small, frequent meals and high-calorie snacks are often well tolerated. The effectiveness of the nutrition program is monitored by recording the client's calorie counts, intake and output, serum albumin levels, and daily weights (Chart 47-5). If the client is not able to swallow, a feeding tube may be used.

Eye Protection. The client's inability to completely close the eyes may lead to corneal abrasions and further compromise vision and comfort. During the day, artificial tears are applied to keep the corneas moist and free from

CHART 47-5

BEST PRACTICE for
Improving Nutrition in Clients with Myasthenia Gravis

- Assess the client's gag reflex and ability to chew and swallow.
- Provide frequent oral hygiene as needed.
- Collaborate with the dietitian, speech-language pathologist, and occupational therapist to plan and implement meals that the client can eat and enjoy.
- Offer small, frequent meals.
- Cut food into small bites, and encourage the client to eat slowly.
- Observe client for choking, nasal regurgitation, and aspiration.
- Provide high-calorie snacks or supplements (e.g., puddings).
- Keep the head of the bed elevated during meals and for 30 to 60 minutes after the client eats.
- Avoid liquids because they can easily cause choking and aspiration; provide a soft diet.
- Monitor food intake carefully.
- Weigh the client daily.
- Monitor serum prealbumin and albumin levels.
- Administer anticholinesterase drugs, as prescribed: 45 to 60 minutes before meals.

abrasion. A lubricant gel and shield may be applied to the eye at bedtime to provide more extensive coverage. To help relieve diplopia, the eyes should be alternately covered with a patch for 2 to 3 hours at a time.

SURGICAL MANAGEMENT. For clients with MG, **thymectomy** (removal of the thymus gland) is usually performed early in the disease. The procedure is not always immediately effective, and it may take several years for remission to occur–if it occurs at all. Clients who have surgery within 2 years of the onset of myasthenic symptoms show the most improvement.

Preoperative Care. Routine preoperative care is provided as discussed in Chapter 20. Because there is no way to predict whether remission or improvement will occur, it is important to avoid making promises, although optimism is warranted. Immediately before surgery, pyridostigmine (Mestinon) may be given with a small amount of water to keep the client stable during and after surgery. If steroids have been used, they are also given before surgery and are tapered during the postoperative period. Antibiotics are administered immediately before and for several days after surgery. Plasmapheresis may be used preoperatively and postoperatively to decrease circulative antibodies more quickly.

Operative Procedures. One of two surgical approaches may be used: the transcervical incision or the sternal split. Advocates of the transcervical approach claim a lower morbidity rate and more rapid recovery with less postoperative discomfort. The client often requires only a small dressing and an IV line. However, the sternal split allows the surgeon to directly visualize the mediastinum. Because more precise and complete removal of all thymic tissue is ensured, this may be the approach of choice.

When thymoma is present, all contiguous involved structures (e.g., the pericardium, the innominate vein, a portion of the superior vena cava, and a portion of the lung) are removed. A single chest tube is placed in the anterior mediastinum. The client may be admitted to the critical care unit postoperatively. Thymoma should be considered as a potentially malignant tumor requiring prolonged follow-up. The presence of myasthenic weakness can still complicate its management. Thymoma-related deaths are bound to outnumber those due to MG in the future.

Postoperative Care. Although clients with adequate respiratory function may be extubated immediately after the procedure, most require a gradual weaning from the ventilator. Prolonged ventilatory assistance is rare. After the client is extubated, conscientious attention is paid to pulmonary hygiene. Suctioning is performed as necessary, and the client is encouraged to turn, cough, and breathe deeply and to use incentive spirometry every 2 hours. In addition to monitoring respiratory function and providing bronchial hygiene, observe for signs of pneumothorax or hemothorax, such as the following:

- Chest pain
- Sudden shortness of breath
- Diminished or delayed chest wall expansion
- Diminished or absent breath sounds
- Restlessness or a change in vital signs (decreasing blood pressure or a weak, rapid pulse)

For the sternal surgical technique, perform chest tube care (see Chapter 35). Both surgical approaches require special wound care. Observe the client for signs of infection, such as increasing or purulent drainage; redness, warmth, or swelling around the wound; and elevated temperature. Appropriate client and family teaching is needed before discharge from the hospital.

Community-Based Care

The client with myasthenia gravis (MG) may be cared for in a variety of settings, including the home, subacute unit, rehabilitation setting, or long-term care facility. The client discharged from the hospital may be weak and may require the assistance of a family member, home care nurse, physical therapist, occupational therapist, or home care aide.

HEALTH TEACHING

The more the client and family know about the disease and the drugs used for treatment, the less likely it is that complications will develop.

Encourage the client and the family to ask questions. Discuss the episodic nature (exacerbations and remissions) of the disease, including factors that predispose the client to exacerbation, such as infection, stress, surgery, hard physical exercise, sedatives, and enemas or strong cathartics (Table 47-3). Instruct the client to collaborate with the health care team to monitor muscle strength, ability to perform activities of daily living (ADLs), and the need to adjust medications.

The importance of lifestyle adaptations such as avoiding heat (e.g., sauna, hot tubs, and sunbathing), crowds, overeating, erratic changes in sleep habits, or emotional extremes is stressed. Teach the signs of exacerbation, such as increased weakness, increased diplopia, ptosis, and problems with chewing or swallowing. Instruct the client to plan activities to allow for rest periods and to conserve energy.

Provide the medication regimen in a written format that includes the names, purposes, dosages, scheduled administration times, administrative routes, and side effects of the drugs. Explain that the drugs are normally taken before activities such as eating, participating in sports, or engaging in work. The importance of maintaining therapeutic blood levels by taking the medications on time and as prescribed and not missing or postponing doses is also stressed. In addition, inform the client of the side effects of anticholinesterase

TABLE 47-3 Factors Precipitating or Worsening Myasthenia Gravis

Various medications, including the following:
- Strong cathartics
- Antidysrhythmics
- Beta-blocking agents
- Antibiotics
- Antirheumatic drugs
- Antispasmodics
- Antihistamines
- Opioids
- Phenytoin (Dilantin)
- Antidepressants (tricyclics)

Rheumatoid arthritis
Alcohol
Hormonal changes
Stress
Infection
Seasonal temperature changes
Heat
Surgery
Enemas

drugs. Advise him or her to avoid medications such as morphine, curare, quinine, quinidine, procainamide, mycin-type antibiotics, and drugs containing magnesium. These agents markedly increase muscle weakness. Additional health teachings regarding medications are listed in Chart 47-6.

In preparing the client for discharge, explain the signs and symptoms of myasthenic and cholinergic crises and the need to contact the physician or other health care professional whenever either type of crisis is suspected. Because respiratory compromise often occurs in myasthenic clients, family members are encouraged to gain skills in resuscitation procedures. A manual resuscitation bag, suctioning equipment, and oxygen should be available in the home for clients susceptible to crisis. Family members should be instructed in the proper use of equipment.

The episodic nature of MG, the potential or actual loss of independence, and body image changes (e.g., the inability to smile) affect the client's adjustment. Kittiwatanapaisan and colleagues (2003) found that fatigue was moderately correlated with depression. During discharge planning, the case manager (CM) considers factors such as age, gender, usual roles and responsibilities, available support systems, occupation, and financial status. Because the client's and family's need for psychosocial adjustment may range from minimal to dramatic, the CM remains sensitive to their needs and provides information and support. The CM encourages family members or significant others to discuss their feelings with one another.

HOME CARE MANAGEMENT

Clients with MG are usually managed at home. Hospitalization is restricted to the diagnostic and evaluation processes, myasthenic or cholinergic crisis resulting in respiratory failure, or periods of exacerbation when respiratory function is threatened.

Unless the client requires assistive devices, little preparation of the home setting is required. In consultation with physical and occupational therapists, the CM makes certain that the necessary equipment has been delivered and properly installed. In addition, the CM makes sure that the client and family members can use the equipment safely. If the client becomes wheelchair dependent, the discharge planner or CM ensures that any necessary modifications to the home (e.g., the installation of ramps or widening of doorways) have been completed before discharge from the hospital.

CHART 47-6

CLIENT EDUCATION GUIDE
Helpful Hints for Medication Teaching of Clients with Myasthenia Gravis

- Keep medications and a glass of water at your bedside if you are weak in the morning.
- Wear a watch with an alarm function (or beeper) to remind you to take your medications.
- Post your medication schedule so others know it.
- Plan strenuous activities, when possible, when the medication peaks.
- Keep an extra supply of medications in your car or at work. Be sure they are secured.
- Do not take any over-the-counter medications without checking with your health care provider.

HEALTH CARE RESOURCES

In consultation with the health care provider, client, and family, the staff nurse or CM may initiate referrals to home care agencies and to local self-help groups for people who have chronic illnesses and for their families. The Myasthenia Gravis Foundation, headquartered in New York City, has education and research programs and provides assistance with financial aid and community resources. The CM encourages the client to obtain and wear a medical alert (MedicAlert) bracelet or necklace and to carry identification at all times.

POLYNEURITIS AND POLYNEUROPATHY

PATHOPHYSIOLOGY

Systemic diseases, vitamin B_{12} deficiency, drug toxicity, infections, trauma, vascular or metabolic disturbances, and exogenous substances such as alcohol, medications, industrial agents, and heavy metals may damage cranial and peripheral nerves. Although the term polyneuritis implies an inflammatory process, it may also denote noninflammatory lesions. Thus the terms **polyneuritis, polyneuropathy,** and **peripheral neuropathy** may describe syndromes whose clinical hallmarks are muscle weakness with or without atrophy, pain that is described as stabbing, cutting or searing, and paresthesias or loss of sensation, impaired reflexes, autonomic manifestations, or combinations of these symptoms.

The most common type of neuropathy is a symmetric polyneuropathy in which the client experiences decreased sensation along with the feeling that an extremity is asleep. Tingling, burning, tightness, or aching sensations generally start in the feet and progress to the level of the knee before being noted in the hands **("glove and stocking" neuropathy).** Other clients may complain of unsteadiness, clumsiness, an inability to recognize objects by feel, and injury without pain. Diabetic neuropathy is a common example, as are the neuropathies resulting from renal or hepatic failure, alcoholism, acquired immunodeficiency syndrome (AIDS),

TABLE 47-4 Factors Associated with Polyneuropathy

Diseases ■ Amyloidosis ■ Alcoholism ■ Carcinomas ■ Diabetes mellitus ■ Diphtheria ■ Hepatic failure ■ Malabsorption or malnutrition ■ Porphyria ■ Renal failure (uremia) ■ Vascular disease	**Drug Use** ■ Vincristine ■ Isoniazid ■ Phenytoin ■ Amitriptyline ■ Hydralazine **Environmental Exposures** ■ Heavy metals ■ Industrial solvents
Trauma	
Vitamin Deficiencies ■ Vitamin B_1 (thiamine) ■ Vitamin B_6 (pyridoxine) ■ Vitamin B_2 (riboflavin) ■ Vitamin B_c (folic acid) ■ Vitamin B_{12} ■ Niacin	

and drug or toxic exposures. Common factors associated with polyneuropathy are presented in Table 47-4.

Peripheral neuropathy is a condition that can be caused or exacerbated by the administration of certain chemotherapeutic agents. The effects of **chemotherapy-induced peripheral neuropathy (CIPN)** are dose limiting and could lead to permanent, debilitating disabilities. Oncology nurses should know the pathophysiology, pre-existing conditions contributing to an increased risk of CIPN, causative agents, and interventions used in managing CIPN. Be aware that the peripheral nervous system is divided into small fibers, large fibers, and the autonomic nervous system, which is important in the assessment, detection, and treatment of this neuropathy. Presenting symptoms are related to the specific fibers that are damaged. Because of the different mechanisms of action, symptoms vary depending on the chemotherapeutic agents used (Marrs & Newton, 2003). Early intervention and client education can have a positive effect on the quality of life for clients with this disorder.

COLLABORATIVE MANAGEMENT

Assessment

Although peripheral neuropathy rarely necessitates hospitalization, you are likely to encounter clients with this condition in a variety of settings, particularly among older adults or in clients with a related illness. Nursing assessment includes an examination of the client's sensory and motor abilities. The client can often outline a specific area of sensory deficit. Because the client may be unaware of decreased sensation, his or her distal extremities may be assessed for light touch using cotton balls or cotton-tipped applicators and for pain using a safety pin. Assess position sense, or kinesthetic sensation by gently grasping the involved digit or extremity on its sides. With the client's eyes closed, change the position of the digit or extremity, and ask the client to describe how the position was changed. The client should be able to acknowledge even slight movements. Advanced practice nurses may use a tuning fork placed on bone prominences to test for sensitivity to vibration. The examination is started at the distal sites. More proximal areas are tested only if the client fails to perceive the duration of vibration at the distal site.

The client's extremities are examined for any signs of injury of which the he or she may be unaware. Also assess the client for the following:

- Orthostatic hypotension
- Abnormal sweating
- **Miosis** (abnormal constriction of the pupil)
- Sphincter disturbances, such as loss of bowel and bladder control
- Other autonomic dysfunctions that may accompany the neuropathy

All abnormal findings are documented and brought to the health care provider's attention.

Interventions

Medical management of clients with peripheral neuropathy consists of the removal or treatment of the underlying cause and symptomatic therapy, including supportive care and physiotherapy. The diet is generally supplemented with vitamins, especially if vitamin deficiency is an underlying cause. However, there is no evidence that vitamins in excess of those contained in a well-balanced diet have any effect on the forms of polyneuropathy unrelated to vitamin deficiency.

With removal of the toxic agent or correction of the metabolic defects, recovery may be rapid if the continuity of the nerves has not been interrupted. If there has been axonal destruction, recovery may require several months. After severe degeneration, there may be permanent weakness, atrophy, decreased reflexes, and sensory deficits.

Extensive client teaching is essential. For clients with decreased sensation in their feet and legs, explain the importance of proper foot care (Chart 47-7). In addition, teach the client who has decreased sensation to recognize potential hazards, such as:

- Exposure to extremes of environmental temperature (e.g., frostbite)
- Bath water or dishwater that may be too hot
- Contact of the feet with heat sources (e.g., heating pads, radiators) while sleeping
- Burns associated with cooking

Smoking is discouraged because the resulting vasoconstriction may worsen the neuropathy. If needed, refer the client to a smoking cessation program. Clients with postural hypotension are taught to arise slowly and wear support or elastic stockings to minimize the pooling of blood in the legs.

Many clients, especially those with the acute forms of polyneuropathy associated with drugs or exposure to toxic substances, experience anxiety, impaired coping, and changes in family processes such as role responsibilities and sexual functioning. Thus it is vital for the health care team to establish a trusting nurse/client relationship and to provide psychosocial support. The physician, social worker, chaplain or religious leader, physical and occupational therapists, and nurse focus on the client's abilities and strengths and help identify new ways of coping, meeting needs, and restructuring activities.

Adjuvant analgesics prescribed for neuropathic pain include desipramine, nortriptyline, gabapentin, and valproic acid (Davis & Srivastava, 2003). High doses of the opioid levorphanol are more effective than low doses in reducing the intensity of chronic neuropathic pain originating in the central or peripheral nervous system. However, in many clients, pain relief is not achieved or there are intolerable side effects (Rowbotham et al., 2003).

CONSIDERATIONS FOR OLDER ADULTS

Pain management for the older adult presents unique challenges due to physiologic changes that alter the pharmacokinetics and pharmacodynamics of analgesics. The results of these changes are decreased drug effectiveness, and increased drug toxicity and drug-drug interactions.

CHART 47-7

CLIENT EDUCATION GUIDE

Peripheral Neuropathy of the Lower Extremities

- Wash your feet and legs with mild soap each day; rinse and dry them well.
- Apply lanolin or lubricating lotion to your feet and legs once or twice daily.
- Inspect your feet and legs daily; report skin changes or open areas to your physician or other health care provider.
- Wear white or colorfast stockings or socks, and change them daily.
- Check the temperature of your bath water with a thermometer before putting your feet into the water.
- Do not use heating pads or other heat sources on your feet.
- Do not use sharp devices to remove corns or calluses (use a pumice stone) or to cut nails. Seek professional podiatry care on a regular basis.
- Wear support or elastic stockings if you have orthostatic hypotension or dependent edema.
- Wear well-fitted shoes; avoid going barefoot.

PERIPHERAL NERVE TRAUMA

PATHOPHYSIOLOGY

The peripheral nerves are subject to injuries associated with mechanical or vehicular accidents, certain sports, the injection of particular drugs, military conflicts or wars, and acts of violence (e.g., knife or gunshot wounds). Specific mechanisms of injury include the following:

- Partial or complete severance of a nerve or nerves
- Contusion, stretching, constriction, or compression of a nerve or nerves
- Ischemia
- Electrical, thermal, or radiation injury

Most commonly affected are the median, ulnar, and radial nerves of the arms and the peroneal, femoral, and sciatic nerves of the legs (Figure 47-1).

After a nerve is transected, the nerve distal to the injury degenerates and retracts within 24 hours. Motor and sensory dysfunction distal to the lesion coincide with the loss of electrical excitability as the nerve fibers degenerate. Recovery occurs as Schwann cells of the neurilemma proliferate from both the proximal and distal stumps. Dividing mitotically, these cells form neurilemmal cords, which act as guidelines for the regenerating axon. Tiny unmyelinated sprouts are generated at the proximal axon and grow 1 to 4 mm each day. Some can

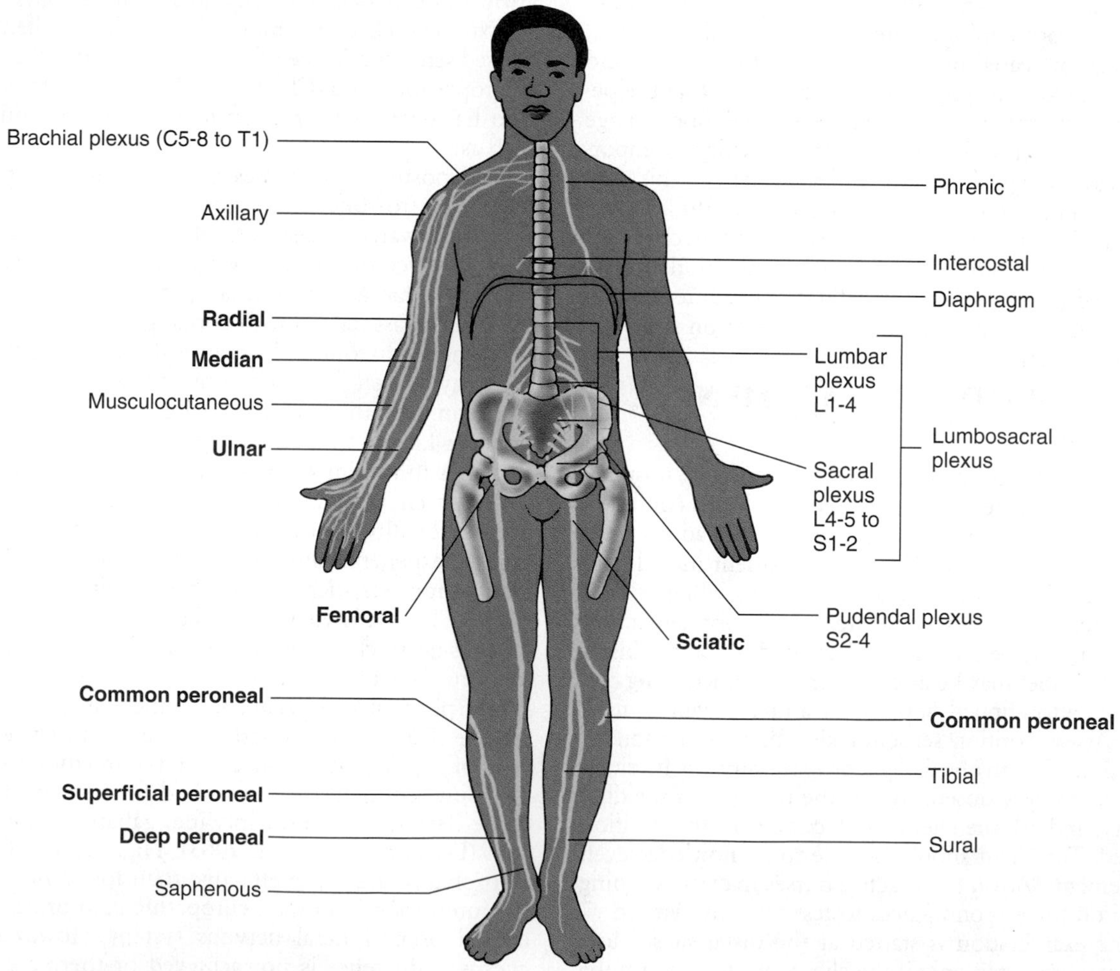

Figure 47-1 ■ Distribution of selected peripheral nerves in the body. The nerves most commonly affected by trauma are highlighted in bold type.

cross the transected gap through guidance by the neurilemma to find their way to the distal stump. The better aligned the union, the more normal the functional return (Figure 47-2).

Successfully realigned nerves remyelinate, grow to their former size, and eventually claim conduction velocities of 80% of their former capacity (Hickey, 2002). Successful reinnervation is adversely affected by the loss of anatomic continuity of the nerve, infection, and increasing age. Disorganization of the nerve or mismatched realignments may result in functional weakness, unintentional muscle movements, and poor sensory discrimination and localization of stimuli.

Some sensory function may return before the regeneration process can occur. This is because nerves proximal to the injured neurons are stimulated to produce collateral innervation to the affected areas. These collaterals provide some innervation before the axon itself has regenerated sufficiently.

COLLABORATIVE MANAGEMENT

Assessment

The client may relate a history of extremity or pelvic trauma, penetrating injury, recent surgery, the use of crutches, or pain after medication injections. Peripheral nerve trauma is especially common in wartime combat or other injury. In addition to weakness or flaccid paralysis, the client may complain of burning sensations distal to the trauma or pain that increases with tactile or environmental stimulation. Skin and nail changes of the affected extremities may also be noted by the client.

A physical assessment is performed to determine which neurologic functions are intact. In acute trauma, the injury should first be evaluated by the physician to determine whether movement is contraindicated. If movement is not contraindicated, the client's motor function is assessed by putting the limb through the normal range of motion. Any abnormal movements, tremor, atrophy, contractions, paresis or paralysis, and weak or absent deep tendon reflexes are documented. The client is questioned about abnormal sensations.

After complete denervation, the extent of vasomotor function is reflected in skin temperature, skin color, and edema. A warm phase and a cold phase have been identified. During the **warm phase**, the extremity is warm, and the skin appears flushed or rosy. Over 2 to 3 weeks, this phase is gradually superseded by a **cold phase**, during which the skin appears cyanotic, mottled, or reddish blue and feels cool compared with the contralateral, unaffected extremity. The dorsal surface of the hand of the examiner is used to compare skin temperatures because the abundance of temperature receptors in this area facilitates more accurate assessments. Edema may be noted immediately after injury or later as a result of surgical procedures. Any evidence of trophic changes (e.g., scaling of skin, brittleness of nails, or loss of body hair) is recorded. This initial assessment serves as the baseline for comparison during subsequent examinations, which are performed every 2 to 4 hours or less frequently as the client's condition indicates.

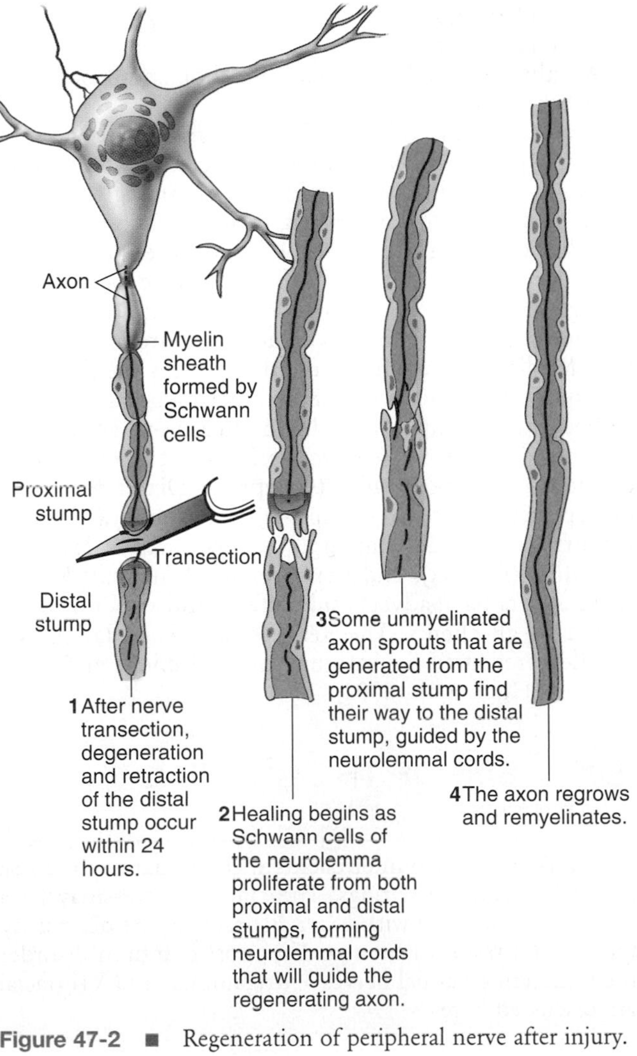

Figure 47-2 ■ Regeneration of peripheral nerve after injury.

Interventions

Interventions for the client with peripheral nerve trauma depend on the location as well as the type and degree of injury. If the nerve trauma results from a primary lesion, such as a tumor, the underlying problem is addressed first.

The health care provider may prescribe immobilization of the involved area by splint, cast, or traction to provide the rest needed to limit and resolve any inflammation. The purpose of surgical management is to restore the function of the damaged nerve.

Preoperative Care. There are usually no special preoperative interventions for the client undergoing peripheral nerve repair. Chapter 20 describes the general care of the client before surgery.

Operative Procedures. If the nerve is lacerated or transected, surgery may be indicated. Restorative procedures include resecting and suturing to reapproximate the severed nerve ends, nerve grafts, and nerve and tendon transplants.

Since surgeons first began to repair injured nerves, the timing of these procedures has been controversial. In the past, a repair delay of 3 to 8 weeks after injury allowed associated injuries to heal, after which the surgeon could better assess the extent of nerve damage. Although microsurgery and the use of lasers now allow primary nerve repair at the time of injury, the physician's judgment in selecting the optimal time and surgical procedure remains crucial.

After an injury, the two severed nerve segments contract and may form scar tissue. Before surgical anastomosis, the surgeon dissects these stumps to remove any damaged nerve tissue. This further decreases the lengths of the ends to be joined. To compensate for this shortening and to avoid excessive tension on the sutured nerve, the involved extremity is positioned in exaggerated flexion. The surgeon aligns the segments under magnification, bringing proximal motor and sensory fibers to distal motor and sensory fibers, and then sutures the nerve tissue.

Postoperative Care. After suturing, the extremity is placed in a cast to maintain the flexed position and to avoid tension on the suture line. Ten to 14 days after nerve repair, the entire dressing is removed, the joint flexion is eased, and a new splint may be applied for an additional 2 weeks. At that time, a removable splint may be applied and physiotherapy begun. Protection of the nerve sutures is continued for a minimum of 6 weeks.

If a large segment of nerve has been damaged and direct anastomosis would be impossible without stretching the nerve more than 10% to 15% of its total length, the surgeon may interpose a nerve graft. Motor and sensory axons may regenerate through the graft, joining proximal and distal segments through the two sites of anastomosis. The amount of sensory and motor regeneration depends on the length of the graft, the type of nerve involved, the condition of the end plates, and the number of axons able to traverse the graft and suture sites. Thus the results are not usually as favorable as with direct reanastomosis. In the case of grafted nerve repairs, maintenance of the flexed position is less essential, although immobilization by splints or casts to facilitate healing of the surgical sites remains imperative.

Splints are usually held in place with elastic wrapping or hook-and-loop (Velcro) closures, which can become too tight if edema develops. Check the skin around the splints and casts frequently (hourly, initially) for tightness, warmth, and color. If the client complains of discomfort, tingling, or coolness or if the color is blanched, the cast or splint may be too tight, inform the physician. Immediately report any indication of drainage under a splint or cast.

Skin care is essential. Atrophy of the epidermis and underlying tissue causes the skin to become more fragile and more susceptible to injury and breakdown. The decreased skin nutrition and decreased vascularity associated with denervation cause delayed healing, which further compounds the problem. Thoroughly examine the skin for evidence of irritation or injury and assist or instruct the client to wash and dry the involved areas carefully. If the skin is dry, lanolin or cocoa butter may be used as a lubricant. Because sensation may be absent or inhibited, instruct the client to protect the involved areas from temperature extremes or other sources of potential trauma.

Rehabilitation. Physiotherapy is the major approach for rehabilitation after surgical repair. The nurse reinforces and helps the client perform the exercises learned in these sessions. Because the regeneration of nerves and subsequent return of sensory and motor function may be extremely slow and produce pain, the client may become discouraged and depressed. If the disability is permanent, he or she needs encouragement and assistance to cope with the changes in body image, self-esteem, and lifestyle.

RESTLESS LEGS SYNDROME

PATHOPHYSIOLOGY

Restless legs syndrome (RLS) is characterized by leg paresthesias associated with an irresistible urge to move. It affects 20 million Americans, but few health care providers know that it exists (Cuellar, 2003). The more common type is associated with peripheral and central nerve damage in the legs and spinal cord (Kapur & Friedman, 2002). Many of those affected have a positive family history, indicating a genetic basis (Hogl et al., 2002). The incidence may be higher in nursing home and home care clients, who often have diabetes and renal failure—two very common conditions correlated with RLS. The incidence is equal in men and women. The client complains of intense burning or "crawling-type" sensations in the limbs and subsequently feels the need to move the limbs repeatedly. These symptoms are worse in the evening and at night and when the client is still for a period of time. Clients feel they need to move to relieve the symptoms. For that reason, clients with RLS often refer to themselves as "night walkers."

COLLABORATIVE MANAGEMENT

Diagnosis is made on the history; there is no known etiology. Potential contributing factors include the following:

- Vitamin and mineral deficiencies
- Anemias
- Polyneuropathies
- Diabetes mellitus (type II)
- Pregnancy
- Peripheral nerve disease
- Pinched nerves
- Lumbar surgical procedures
- Renal failure
- Substances such as caffeine, alcohol, and beta blockers
- Parkinson disease

The management of RLS is symptomatic and involves treating the underlying cause or contributing factor, if known. The client is provided with strategies to minimize insomnia such as limiting caffeine, nicotine, and alcohol and setting a routine bedtime. Strenuous activity should not be done 2 to 3 hours before bedtime. Although there are few research studies that support their use, massage, biofeedback, and acupuncture may be effective. Medications are not prescribed unless the severity of the symptoms and functional impairment are not controlled with nonpharmacologic measures. Medications that have proven to be effective for some clients include clonidine hydrochloride (Catapres, Dixarit✱), carbamazepine (Tegretol, Mazepine✱), clonazepam (Klonopin, Rivotril✱), and dopaminergic agents such as levodopa, pergolide (Permax), and pramipexole (Mirapex). Most of these agents have adverse side effects and may not be tolerated by all clients. The Restless Legs Foundation is an excellent resource for information and client and family support (Hogl et al., 2002).

DISEASES OF THE CRANIAL NERVES

The nurse may encounter clients with cranial nerve disease in various practice settings. The cranial nerves may be affected in association with other disorders of the nervous system or as a result of trauma. The most common disorders, those affecting cranial nerves V (trigeminal) and VII (facial), are discussed here.

Trigeminal Neuralgia

PATHOPHYSIOLOGY

Trigeminal neuralgia also known as tic douloureux:

- Is a disease that affects the trigeminal or fifth cranial nerve
- Entails a specific type of unilateral facial pain, which occurs in abrupt, intense paroxysms (spasms)
- Is usually provoked by minimal stimulation of a trigger zone
- Is unilateral and confined to the area innervated by the trigeminal nerve, most often the second and third branches (Figure 47-3)

Clients younger than 30 years of age with pain in more than one branch of the trigeminal nerve may be further evaluated to rule out the possibility of a tumor or multiple sclerosis.

CONSIDERATIONS FOR OLDER ADULTS

Trigeminal neuralgia usually appears in people older than 50 years of age. The female-to-male ratio is 2:1.

When describing the pain, clients use terms such as "excruciating," "sharp," "shooting," "piercing," "burning," and "jabbing." Between bursts of pain, which last from seconds to minutes, there is usually no pain. Often no sensory or motor deficits are found on examination, but the condition can be agonizing for the client. The fear of precipitating attacks often causes clients to avoid talking, smiling, eating, or attending to hygienic needs such as shaving, washing the face, and brushing the teeth.

The cause of trigeminal neuralgia is thought to be related to impaired inhibitory mechanisms in the brainstem caused by excessive firing of irritated fibers in the trigeminal nerve. In addition, trauma and infection of the teeth, jaw, or ear may be contributing factors.

The course of trigeminal neuralgia is characterized by bouts of pain for several weeks or months followed by spontaneous remissions. The length of these remissions may vary from days to years, but attack-free periods tend to become shorter as the client grows older. Symptoms rarely disappear permanently.

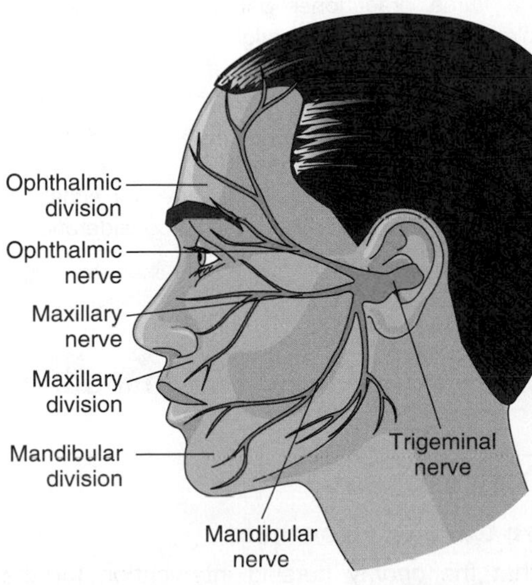

Figure 47-3 ■ Distribution of the trigeminal nerve and its three divisions: ophthalmic, maxillary, and mandibular.

COLLABORATIVE MANAGEMENT

Management of the client with trigeminal neuralgia is determined by the amount of pain he or she is experiencing. Conservative measures are usually tried first.

NONSURGICAL MANAGEMENT. Medical management is accomplished with the use of drugs such as carbamazepine (Tegretol, Apo-Carbamazepine✱, Mazepine✱), phenytoin (Dilantin), baclofen (Lioresal), and occasionally amitriptyline (Elavil, Meravil✱) or diazepam (Valium, E-Pam✱). Initial therapy should always be nonsurgical, and drugs may be used singly or in combination. Surgical management may be considered if the client and the physician agree that the pain or the toxic effects of drug therapy are worse than the risk of surgery.

About 70% of clients respond to carbamazepine, 20 to 1200 mg daily, alone or in combination with phenytoin in average daily doses of 200 to 400 mg. Fosphenytoin (Cerebyx) may also be given IV to abort an acute attack. Phenytoin and fosphenytoin are anticonvulsants believed to decrease the paroxysmal afferent impulses in much the same way as when they are used to treat seizure disorders.

Injection of alcohol or phenol into the affected branch of the trigeminal nerve may relieve pain for up to 16 months. Injection into the gasserian ganglion, where sensory root fibers arise, may provide permanent pain control but carries with it a greater risk of extraocular palsies, keratitis, blindness, or masticatory paralysis. In both blocking procedures, there is complete anesthesia to the portion of the face innervated by the injected branch.

SURGICAL MANAGEMENT. Surgery is performed if the client is unable to tolerate the side effects of medications or they are ineffective in controlling pain. Surgical procedures include microvascular decompression, percutaneous balloon compression, and radiofrequency thermocoagulation.

Preoperative Care. In addition to the general preoperative care provided to all clients (see Chapter 20), the surgeon thoroughly explains the surgical benefits and any expected neurologic deficits.

Operative Procedures. In some clients, a small artery compresses the trigeminal nerve as it enters the pons. Surgical relocation of this artery **(microvascular decompression)** may relieve the pain of trigeminal neuralgia without compromising facial sensation. The surgeon carefully lifts the loop of artery off the nerve and places a small silicone (Silastic) sponge between the vessel and the nerve. Complications include aseptic meningitis, cerebrospinal fluid leak, ataxia, **ipsilateral** (same side) hearing loss, and seventh and eighth nerve defects (Filipchuk, 2003). Older adults and clients with other medical problems may not be a candidate for this procedure.

Radiofrequency thermalcoagulation may provide lasting relief of pain without compromising touch or motor function. During this procedure, the client is sedated with small doses of diazepam (Valium), midazolam hydrochloride (Versed), or fentanyl (Sublimaze) but is alert and able to follow commands in response to sensory and motor testing. The physician inserts a needle electrode and, under radiographic control, advances it to the appropriate area, where a heat lesion is made. The advantages of this procedure include long-term pain relief, tolerance by older adults, absence of facial paralysis and preservation of the sensation of touch. The possibility of puncturing the internal carotid artery and the occurrence of anesthesia dolorosa are disadvantages (Hickey, 2002). The affected side is permanently insensitive to pain.

A **percutaneous balloon microcompression** is performed under general anesthesia. Under guided fluoroscopy, a balloon catheter is threaded through a large-bore needle and inflated, compressing the gasserian ganglion and nerve root (Filipchuk, 2003). Complications that may occur during this procedure include bradycardia and hypotension.

Unlike the other procedures, the **injection of glycerol** to destroy the myelinated fibers of the trigeminal nerve may take up to 3 weeks for pain relief to occur.

Postoperative Care. In addition to general post-craniotomy care (see Chapter 48), monitor the client for complications associated with these procedures, including headache, permanent cranial nerve dysfunction, and hemorrhage. The client's corneal reflex, extraocular muscles, and facial nerve are assessed and abnormal findings are documented and reported to the surgeon.

Apply an ice pack to the operative site on the jaw for 3 to 4 hours. A soft diet is prescribed, and the client is discouraged from chewing on the affected side until the paresthesias is abated. Instruct the client to avoid rubbing the eye on the affected side because the protective mechanism of pain will no longer warn of injury. He or she should inspect the eye daily for redness or irritation and report any change or blurred vision to the physician. Regular dental examinations are encouraged because the absence of pain may not warn the client of potential problems.

Psychosocial considerations for the client with trigeminal neuralgia include disappointment with ineffective drug protocols or surgical procedures, as well as the fear that the pain may recur with any activity. The client may fail to move the face in an attempt to prevent pain. This behavior may be misinterpreted by others as withdrawal, antisociability, or depression.

Facial Paralysis

PATHOPHYSIOLOGY

Facial paralysis, or **Bell's palsy** (acute paralysis of cranial nerve VII), was first described by Sir Charles Bell of England in 1821. The incidence is 23 persons per 100,000 population; men and women are equally affected (Hickey, 2002). Although the incidence may be slightly higher among people with diabetes, the condition occurs in all ages and at all times of the year.

The onset of Bell's palsy is acute. Maximal paralysis is attained within 48 hours in about half the clients and within 5 days in almost all clients. Pain behind the ear or on the face may precede paralysis by a few hours or days. The disorder is characterized by a drawing sensation and paralysis of all facial muscles on the affected side. The client cannot close the eye, wrinkle the forehead, smile, whistle, or grimace. The face appears masklike and sags. Taste is usually impaired to some degree, but this symptom seldom persists beyond the second week of paralysis.

Although the cause of Bell's palsy remains obscure, it may be the result of an inflammatory process. Clients with Bell's palsy are rarely hospitalized, but the nurse may encounter them in community-based settings such as clinics, physicians' offices, or emergency departments.

◆COLLABORATIVE MANAGEMENT

Medical management consists of the administration of prednisone (Deltasone, Winpred✱), 30 to 60 mg daily, during the first week after the onset of symptoms. Analgesics may help relieve the pain. Nursing care is directed toward managing the major neurologic deficits and providing psychosocial support. Because the eye does not close, the cornea must be protected from drying and subsequent ulceration or abrasion. Instruct the client to manually close the eyelid at intervals and to instill artificial tears four times daily. The eye may be patched or taped closed at bedtime.

The client may be unable to chew, sip fluids through a straw, or control drooling on the affected side. Thus mealtime may become a problem. Encourage the client to eat and drink using the unaffected side of the mouth. Frequent, small meals may be better tolerated, and clients may require a soft diet. Simple techniques of massage; the application of warm, moist heat; and facial exercises are explained to the client.

A facial sling may prevent drooping of the affected side. As muscle tone improves, instruct the client to grimace, wrinkle the brow, force the eyes closed, whistle, and blow air out of the cheeks three or four times daily for 5 minutes in front of a mirror.

Although most clients recover fully within a few weeks or months, about 15% to 20% experience some residual weakness; a few have permanent neurologic deficits. These clients require a great deal of support because body image and self-esteem are drastically affected. The nurse is a valuable source of both information and psychosocial support.

Critical Thinking Challenge

An older adult in a long-term care setting complains to you that the left side of her face is very painful. She has had this problem before, but does not recall what her health care provider told her about the cause of her problem. After a thorough pain assessment, you decide to call the nurse practitioner to inform her of the client's complaint and your findings.

1. How will the nurse practitioner determine whether the client's problem is trigeminal neuralgia or facial paralysis (Bell's palsy)?
2. What is the difference between the nerve involvement and subsequent clinical manifestations of trigeminal neuralgia and Bell's palsy?
3. What options for treatment will the client have for either of these diseases, taking her advanced age into consideration?

evolve For suggested answer guidelines, go to http://evolve.elsevier.com/Iggy/.

GET READY for the NCLEX Examination!

KEY POINTS

Safe Effective Care Environment

- Remember that the *priority* nursing intervention for the client with Guillain-Barré syndrome (GBS) is to assess for and maintain his or her respiratory function.

- Observe for and report side and adverse effects of IV immunoglobulin (IVIg), such as chills, fever, headache, and anaphylaxis; infuse the drug slowly when it is started.
- Observe for, prevent, and/or manage complications of plasmapheresis as outlined in Chart 47-3.
- Monitor clients on cholinesterase (ChE) inhibitor drugs for early manifestations of cholinergic or myasthenic crisis as listed in Table 47-2.
- Use caution when feeding clients with dysphagia to prevent aspiration, a common potential problem in clients with GBS and myasthenia gravis (MG).

Health Promotion and Maintenance

- In collaboration with the physical and occupational therapists, plan interventions to promote self-care for clients with GBS.
- Demonstrate to clients and family members basic measures to prevent complications of immobility, such as turning and repositioning, and range-of-motion exercises.
- For clients with MG, reinforce the importance of taking medications at appropriate times as listed in Chart 47-6.
- For clients with MG, teach them to rest frequently and avoid stressors that may exacerbate their illness (see Table 47-3).
- Teach care of lower extremities for clients with peripheral neuropathy, as detailed in Chart 47-7.
- Refer clients with chronic peripheral nervous system (PNS) diseases to appropriate community resources and support groups, such as the Restless Legs Foundation and Myasthenia Gravis Foundation.

Psychosocial Integrity

- Encourage clients with GBS and MG to verbalize feelings about their illness and its effects, while fostering hope and optimism.
- Assist clients with PNS diseases to identify coping strategies they have used in the past as they adapt to their health problems.
- Assess clients with PNS disease for depression; teach clients and families to notify the health care provider if changes in mental status or outlook occur.

Physiological Integrity

- Ask clients with suspected GBS about recent history of acute illness, trauma, surgery, or immunization.
- For clients with GBS, implement interventions and associated activities as listed in Chart 47-2.
- Be aware that edrophonium (Tensilon) testing is commonly used for diagnosing MG and for differentiating myasthenic (undermedication) crisis and cholinergic (overmedication) crisis.
- Evaluate clients with GBS or MG to determine whether outcomes related to adequate ventilation and airway patency were met.
- For clients having a thymectomy, maintain adequate respiratory function and observe for signs of pneumothorax or hemothorax, such as chest pain and sudden shortness of breath.
- Assess clients who have peripheral nerve injury for a warm phase (extremity is warm and skin is flushed initially) or a cold phase (extremity later becomes cold and skin is cyanotic, mottled, or reddish blue).
- Recognize that restless legs syndrome is a common, underdiagnosed disorder in which the client has leg paresthesias with urges to move the legs frequently, especially at night; pain is described as an intense burning.
- Assess clients with severe facial pain for associated clinical manifestations of trigeminal neuralgia or facial paralysis; evaluate effect of pain control measures.
- Recognize that trigeminal neuralgia is unilateral (one-sided) and usually provoked by minimal stimulation, such as talking or eating.

ADDITIONAL STUDY RESOURCES

Go to your Student CD-ROM for Review Questions for the NCLEX Examination.

evolve Go to http://evolve.elsevier.com/Iggy/ for Integrated Management of Care Questions for the NCLEX Examination.

SELECTED BIBLIOGRAPHY

Chitnis, T., & Khoury, S.J. (2003). Immunological neuromuscular disorders. *Journal of Allergy and Clinical Immunology, 111,* 231-246.

Cooke, J.F., & Orb, A. (2003). The recovery phase in Guillain-Barré syndrome: Moving from dependency to independence. *Rehabilitation Nursing, 28*(4), 105-108, 130.

Cuellar, N. (2003). Restless legs syndrome: A case study. *Journal of Neuroscience Nursing, 35*(4), 193-201.

Cunning, S. (2000). When the Dx is myasthenia gravis. *RN, 63*(4), 26-30.

Davis, M.P., & Srivastava, M. (2003). Demographics, assessment and management of pain in the elderly. *Drugs & Aging, 20*(1):23-57.

Dochterman, J.M., & Bulechek, G.M. (2004). *Nursing interventions classification (NIC).* St. Louis: Mosby.

Evoli, A., et al. (2002). Thymoma in patients with MG: Characteristics and long-term outcome. *Neurology, 59*(12), 1844-1850.

Filipchuk, D. (2003), Classic trigeminal neuralgia: A surgical perspective. *Journal of Neuroscience Nursing, 35*(2), 82-86.

Gregory, R.J. (2003). Recovery from depression associated with Guillain Barré syndrome. *Issues in Mental Health Nursing, 24*(2), 129-135.

Hickey, J.V. (2002). *The clinical practice of neurological and neurosurgical nursing* (5th ed.). Philadelphia: Lippincott-Raven.

Hogl, B., et al. (2002). Transient restless legs syndrome after spinal anesthesia: A prospective study. *Neurology, 59,* 1705-1707.

Hughes, R.C., et al. (2003). Practice parameter: Immunotherapy for Guillain-Barré syndrome: Report of the Quality Standards Subcommittee of the American Academy of Neurology. *Neurology, 61,* 736-740.

Kapur, N., & Friedman, R. (2002). Oral ketamine: A promising treatment for restless legs syndrome. *Anesthesia and Analgesia, 94,*1558-1559.

Kittiwatanapaisan, W., et al. (2003). Fatigue in myasthenia gravis patients. *Journal of Neuroscience Nursing, 35*(2), 87-93, 106.

Kupersmith, M.J., Latkany, R., & Homel, P. (2003). Development of generalized disease at 2 years in patients with ocular myasthenia gravis. Neurology, *60*(2), 243-248.

Marrs, J, & Newton, S. (2003). Updating your peripheral neuropathy "know-how." *Clinical Journal of Oncology Nursing, 7*(3), 299-303.

Moorhead, S., Johnson, M., & Maas, M. (2004). *Nursing outcomes classification (NOC).* St. Louis: Mosby.

Pagana, K.D., & Pagana, T.J. (2002). *Mosby's manual of diagnostic and laboratory tests.* St. Louis: Mosby.

Parker, J.N., & Parker, P.M. (2002). *The official patient's source book for Guillain-Barré syndrome.* San Diego: Icon Health Publications.

Pascuzzi, R.M. (2003). The edrophonium test. *Seminars in Neurology, 23*(1), 83-88.

Rabinstein, A., & Wijdicks, E.F. (2002). BiPAP in acute respiratory failure due to myasthenic crisis may prevent intubation. *Neurology,* 59(10), 1647-1649.

Richman, D., & Agius, M. (2003). Treatment of autoimmune myasthenia gravis. *Neurology, 61*(12), 1652-1661.

Rowbotham, M.C., et al. (2003). Oral opioid therapy for chronic peripheral and central neuropathic pain. *New England Journal of Medicine, 348*(13), 1223-1232.

Sharshar, T., et al. (2003). Early predictors of mechanical ventilation in Guillain-Barré syndrome. *Critical Care Medicine, 31*(1), 278-283.

Sulton, L.L. (2002). Meeting the challenges of Guillain-Barré syndrome. *Nursing Management, 33*(7), 25-30.

Sweeney, C.W. (2002). Understanding peripheral neuropathy in patients with cancer: Background and patient assessment. *Clinical Journal of Oncology Nursing,* 6(3), 163-166.

Worsham, T.L. (2000). Easing the course of Guillain-Barré syndrome. *RN, 63*(3), 46-50.

Zimmermann, P.G. (2003). Lessons learned: On watching for zebras. *Journal of Emergency Nursing, 29(*1), 85-86.

CHAPTER 48

Interventions for Critically Ill Clients with Neurologic Problems

RICHARD B. ARBOUR

LEARNING OUTCOMES

After studying this chapter, you should be able to:

1. Identify the common types of strokes.
2. Discuss risk factors that increase the likelihood of strokes.
3. Describe typical clinical manifestations associated with stroke.
4. Analyze assessment data to determine common nursing diagnoses that are pertinent to clients with strokes.
5. Identify the purpose of intracranial pressure (ICP) monitoring and signs of increasing ICP.
6. Explain the role of drug therapy in managing clients with strokes.
7. Prioritize nursing care for a client who has experienced a stroke.
8. Discuss the purpose of rehabilitation for the client who has had a stroke.
9. Develop a teaching plan for the client who has experienced a stroke.
10. Differentiate the common types of traumatic brain injury (TBI).
11. Explain the pathophysiologic changes that can result from moderate or severe TBI.
12. Describe the psychosocial and behavioral manifestations associated with TBI.
13. Prioritize nursing care for the client with TBI.
14. Explain the role of sedation and analgesia in managing the client with intracranial hypertension.
15. Describe common complications of brain tumors.
16. Develop a postoperative plan of care for a client having a craniotomy.

Go to your Student CD-ROM for Review Questions for the NCLEX Examination keyed to these Learning Outcomes.

Certain neurologic problems can cause clients to become critically ill or die. Stroke, head injury, brain tumor, and brain abscess can cause increased intracranial pressure (ICP), a life-threatening complication that may easily compound disability and risk of death from the initial brain insult. Permanent neurologic dysfunction or death may be prevented by prompt recognition and aggressive management of this complication by the interdisciplinary health care team.

STROKE

A **stroke** is caused by a disruption in the normal blood supply to the brain. This disruption in blood supply may be in the form of an interruption in blood flow to the brain, in which case the stroke is ischemic in origin. The blood supply disruption may also take the form of bleeding within or around the brain. This is called a hemorrhagic stroke. Formerly called *cerebrovascular accident* (CVA), the National Stroke Association now uses the term *brain attack* to describe a stroke. A stroke is a *medical emergency* that strikes suddenly, and it should be treated immediately to prevent neurologic deficit and permanent disability.

Stroke is the second most common cause of death and major disability worldwide. Although the number of stroke deaths has decreased during the past several years in the United States, stroke remains the third most common cause of death and the primary cause of adult disability (Goldszmidt

RESOURCE MANAGEMENT

STROKE

Cost of Care

- The direct and indirect cost of stroke is $53 billion annually, including medical care, lost wages, and lost productivity.
- The cost of rehabilitation is $30,000 to $50,000 per client.
- Hospitalization costs are higher for clients receiving thrombolytic therapy, but rehabilitation costs are significantly lower than for those not receiving thrombolytics.
- Clinical pathways for clients with strokes decrease the length of stay and costs.
- The use of specialized stroke teams to enhance the rapid diagnosis and treatment of stroke improves outcomes and decreases morbidity and mortality.

Implications for Nursing

The institution of specialized stroke teams has had a significant impact on clients with ischemic stroke. A decreased length of stay and improved outcomes have significantly affected the cost of care. Nurses must be aware of the revised focus of stroke as an emergency (much like a myocardial infarction) and the valuable contributions of the stroke team to improve client outcomes.

Data from http://www.strokeassociation.org (Stroke Facts 2004: All Americans).

& Caplan, 2003). The direct and indirect costs of stroke are more than $41 billion annually (see the Resource Management box above).

PATHOPHYSIOLOGY

Pathophysiologic Changes in the Brain

The brain is unable to store oxygen or glucose and therefore must receive a constant flow of blood to provide these substances to function normally. In addition, blood flow is important for the removal of metabolic waste, carbon dioxide, and lactic acid. If blood supply to any part of the brain is interrupted for more than a few minutes, this may lead to death of cerebral tissue. This in turn can cause death as well as varying degrees of disability, depending on the location and amount of brain tissue affected.

Through the processes of cerebral **autoregulation,** blood flow is maintained at a fairly constant rate of 1000 mL/min. Put another way, the brain receives at least 20% of the available cardiac output. To maintain stability of cerebral blood flow, the cerebral arteries dilate or constrict in response to changes in blood pressure, carbon dioxide tension, and oxygen tension. For example, with normal, intact autoregulation, low blood pressure, high arterial carbon dioxide, or low arterial oxygen tension will cause a dilation of cerebral arteries to maintain cerebral blood flow.

In an **occlusive stroke,** ischemia occurs in the brain tissue supplied by the affected artery, and brain dysfunction results. **Ischemia** leads to hypoxia or anoxia and hypoglycemia within the affected brain tissue. These processes set in motion a series of events that ultimately lead to **infarction** or death of neurons, glia, and the involved area of the brain. In addition, brain metabolism and blood flow after a stroke is affected in stroke "watershed" area as well as in the **contralateral** (opposite side) hemisphere. Effects of a stroke on the contralateral side may be due to brain swelling as well as to further changes in blood flow throughout the brain.

Small lacunar infarctions may also occur. Lacunae are small, deep cavities within the brain that result first from occlusion of a small vessel. This occlusion leads to infarct and necrosis of the area of the brain supplied by the affected vessel. Lacunar infarcts occur almost exclusively in the internal capsule, basal ganglia, and thalamus. They produce either a pure motor deficit (internal capsule) or a pure sensory deficit (thalamus). A lacunar infarct is generally regarded as a type of ischemic stroke.

Types of Strokes

Strokes are generally classified as ischemic (occlusive) or hemorrhagic. Most ischemic strokes are either thrombotic strokes or embolic strokes (Table 48-1).

ISCHEMIC STROKE

An **ischemic stroke** is caused by the occlusion of a cerebral artery by either a thrombus or an embolus. A stroke that is caused by a thrombus is referred to as a thrombotic stroke, whereas a stroke caused by an embolus is referred to as an embolic stroke. About 80% of all strokes are ischemic.

THROMBOTIC STROKE. Thrombotic strokes account for more than half of all strokes and are commonly associated with the development of atherosclerosis of the blood vessel wall. Atherosclerosis is a complex process that includes altered function of the inner lining of arterial vessels, inflammation, and increased growth of vascular smooth muscle cells. It is the process by which plaques develop on the inner wall of the affected arterial vessel.

The first step in plaque development is accumulation of low-density lipoprotein (LDL) particles within the arterial vessel wall. These may undergo chemical changes and then stimulate endothelial cells to adhere to **monocytes** (inflammatory cells) and **T-cells** (immune system cells). The endothelium produces chemical messengers, which signal the monocytes and T-cells to incorporate within the intimal layer.

The second step is maturation of monocytes into macrophages. The macrophages, in turn, ingest LDL particles.

The third step occurs when the macrophages ingest a "critical mass" of LDL particles; they are then called foam cells. These cells constitute the fatty streak on the inner arterial wall, the earliest manifestation of arterial plaque.

The fourth step is additional growth of the lesion through influence of inflammatory molecules, which also help form a fibrous cover or cap over the lipid core. This covering makes the plaque larger but also separates it from blood flow through the vessel.

The fifth step occurs with plaque rupture. Rupture of the plaque exposes foam cells to clot-promoting elements in the blood. The end result is clot formation. If the clot is of sufficient size, it may interrupt blood flow to the brain tissue supplies by the vessel, causing an occlusive stroke. This process may occur over many years because collateral circulation to the involved area develops to compensate for the occlusion.

As the artery becomes completely occluded, blood flow to the area is markedly diminished. Decreased blood flow causes transient ischemia, which progresses to complete ischemia and infarction of the brain tissue. Within 72 hours, the area is edematous and necrotic, and cavities develop. The **bifurcation** (point of division) of the common carotid artery and the vertebral arteries at their junction with the

TABLE 48-1 Differential Features of the Types of Stroke

	Ischemic		
Feature	**Thrombotic**	**Embolic**	**Hemorrhagic**
Evolution	Intermittent or stepwise improvement between episodes of worsening Completed stroke	Abrupt development of completed stroke Steady progression	Usually abrupt onset
Onset	Daytime (10 AM to 12 PM) Gradual (minutes to hours)	Daytime Sudden	Daytime Sudden, may be gradual if caused by hypertension
Level of consciousness	Preserved (client is awake)	Preserved (client is awake)	Deepening stupor or coma
Contributing associated factors	Hypertension Atherosclerosis	Cardiac disease	Hypertension Vessel disorders
Prodromal symptoms	Transient ischemic attack		
Neurologic deficits	Deficits during the first few weeks Slight headache Speech deficits Visual problems Confusion	Maximal deficit at onset Paralysis Expressive aphasia	Focal deficits Severe, frequent
Cerebrospinal fluid	Normal; possible presence of protein	Normal	Bloody
Seizures	No	No	Usually
Duration	Improvements over weeks to months Permanent deficits possible	Rapid improvements	Variable Permanent neurologic deficits possible

basilar artery are the most common sites involved. Because of the gradual occlusion of the arteries, thrombotic strokes tend to have a *slow* onset.

A **lacunar stroke** is another type of thrombotic stroke. A lacunar stroke causes a soft area or cavity to develop in the white matter or deep gray matter of the brain. This type of stroke may result in significant neurologic dysfunction if it damages a critical area in the brain.

EMBOLIC STROKE. An **embolic stroke** is caused by an **embolus** or a group of emboli (clots) that break off from one area of the body and travel to the cerebral arteries via the carotid artery or vertebrobasilar system. The usual sources of emboli are cardiac. Emboli can occur in clients with nonvalvular atrial fibrillation, ischemic heart disease, rheumatic heart disease, and mural thrombi following a myocardial infarction (MI) or insertion of a prosthetic heart valve. Another source of emboli may be plaque that breaks off from the carotid sinus or internal carotid artery. Emboli tend to become lodged in the smaller cerebral blood vessels at their point of bifurcation or where the lumen narrows. Embolic strokes account for almost half of all strokes.

The middle cerebral artery (MCA) is most commonly involved in an embolic stroke. As the emboli occlude the vessel, ischemia develops, and the client experiences the clinical manifestations of the stroke. However, the occlusion may be temporary if the embolus breaks into smaller fragments, enters smaller blood vessels, and is absorbed. For these reasons, embolic strokes are characterized by the *sudden* development and rapid occurrence of focal neurologic deficits. The symptoms may resolve over several hours or a few days. A cerebral hemorrhage may result if significant damage to the wall of the involved vessel has occurred. Conversion of an occlusive stroke to a hemorrhagic stroke may occur because the arterial vessel wall is also vulnerable to ischemic damage from blood supply interruption. Sudden hemodynamic stress may result in vessel rupture, causing bleeding directly within the brain tissue.

CHART 48-1

KEY FEATURES of Transient Ischemic Attack

Visual Deficits
- Blurred vision
- Diplopia (double vision)
- Blindness in one eye
- Tunnel vision

Motor Deficits
- Transient weakness (arm, hand, or leg)
- Gait disturbance (ataxic)

Sensory Deficits
- Transient numbness (face, arm, or hand)
- Vertigo

Speech Deficits
- Aphasia
- Dysarthria (slurred speech)

TRANSIENT ISCHEMIC ATTACK AND REVERSIBLE ISCHEMIC NEUROLOGIC DEFICIT. Ischemic strokes are often preceded by warning signs, such as a **transient ischemic attack (TIA),** also called a "silent" stroke (Chart 48-1) or a **reversible ischemic neurologic deficit (RIND).** Both warning signs cause transient focal neurologic dysfunction resulting from a brief interruption in cerebral blood flow, possibly resulting from cerebral vasospasm or transient systemic arterial hypertension. The difference between a TIA and an RIND is the length of time the client is symptomatic. A TIA lasts a few minutes to fewer than 24 hours,

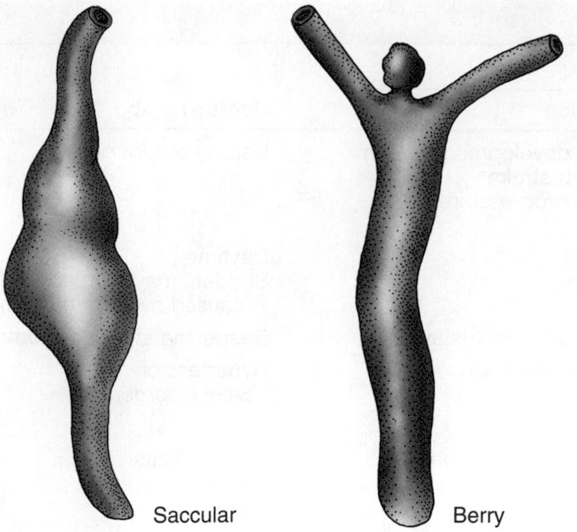

Figure 48-1 ■ Two common types of cerebral aneurysms.

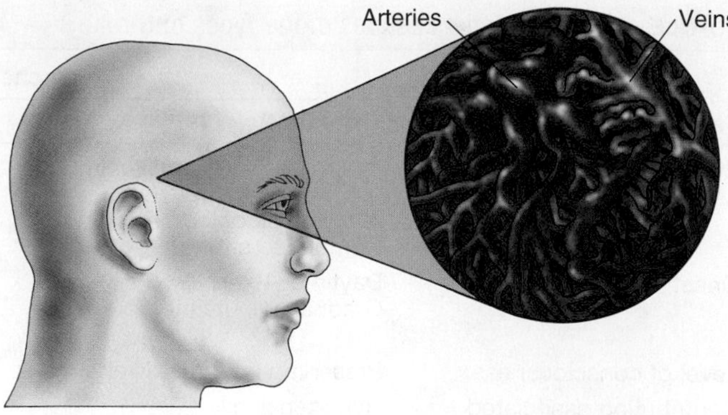

Figure 48-2 ■ Appearance of an arteriovenous malformation. Note the dilated, entangled blood vessels.

whereas RIND symptoms last longer than 24 hours but less than a week. Both TIAs and RINDs may damage the brain tissue with repeated insults, as evidenced by magnetic resonance imaging (MRI) or computed tomography (CT). Multiple TIAs indicate significant increased stroke risk.

HEMORRHAGIC STROKE

The second major classification of stroke is **hemorrhagic stroke.** In this type of stroke, vessel integrity is interrupted, and bleeding occurs into the brain tissue or into the spaces surrounding the brain (ventricular, subdural, subarachnoid). Hemorrhage into the brain tissue generally results from a ruptured aneurysm (localized weakening and distortion of vessel wall); rupture of an arteriovenous malformation; or, more commonly, severe hypertension.

ANEURYSM. A ruptured cerebral aneurysm results in hemorrhagic stroke. An **aneurysm** is an abnormal ballooning or blister on the involved artery (Figure 48-1). Aneurysms may be congenital or traumatic. A congenital aneurysm is a developmental defect in the media and elastica (adventitia or outer layer) of the vessel wall. Both etiologies weaken the vessel wall. Continued force on the weakened vessel wall from elevated blood pressure stretches and thins the vessel wall, causing the intimal or innermost vessel layer to protrude. This is the point most vulnerable to rupture. Although the rupture may occur at any time, it usually happens during activity. Aneurysms are often found at the bifurcations (branching) of major cerebral arteries.

Aneurysm rupture causes the development of an intracerebral hematoma, bleeding into the subarachnoid space, or bleeding directly into the ventricles. **Vasospasm,** a sudden and transient constriction of a cerebral artery, often occurs after a cerebral hemorrhage from aneurysm rupture. This occurs because blood is also an irritant to arterial vessels. Blood flow to distal areas of the brain supplied by the artery is markedly diminished, which leads to cerebral ischemia and infarction and further neurologic dysfunction.

ARTERIOVENOUS MALFORMATION. An **arteriovenous malformation (AVM)** is a developmental abnormality that occurs during embryonic development. It is a tangled or spaghetti-like mass of malformed, thin-walled, dilated vessels (Figure 48-2). The congenital absence of a capillary network in these vessels forms an abnormal communication between the arterial and venous systems. The vessels may eventually rupture, causing bleeding into the subarachnoid space or into the intracerebral tissue. The risk of rupture and cerebral hemorrhage exists because normally the capillary network intervenes between the arterial and venous systems. In the absence of the capillary network, the thin-walled veins are subjected to arterial pressure.

HYPERTENSION. Although the exact mechanisms involved are unknown, it is hypothesized that elevated systolic and diastolic blood pressures cause changes within the arterial wall that leave it susceptible to rupture. An intracerebral hemorrhage occurs when the vessel ruptures. Damage to the brain occurs from bleeding, causing distortion or displacement. Brain tissue edema acts as a direct irritant to brain tissue. Hemorrhagic strokes may be more likely with sudden, dramatic blood pressure elevations, such as those seen with cocaine intoxication.

Etiology and Genetic Risk

Certain major risk factors increase the likelihood of strokes, especially the following:

- Hypertension
- Diabetes mellitus
- Heart disease
- Hypercholesteremia
- **Hypercoagulable** (increased clotting) state
- Illicit drug use (especially cocaine)
- Obesity
- Nonvalvular atrial fibrillation

Most of these disorders have a familial or genetic predisposition and are discussed elsewhere in this text. For example, relative stroke risk increases with a strong family history of hypertension or atherosclerotic disease. Close blood relatives of a client with an aneurysm may be at higher risk for intracranial aneurysms and are potential candidates for diagnostic testing and follow-up.

CULTURAL CONSIDERATIONS

Black individuals tend to have one of the highest rates of strokes compared with other groups, possibly because they have a high rate of hypertension and diabetes mellitus. The cause for the higher occurrence is unknown, but it might be due to dietary habits or problems with access to health care, especially in rural areas.

CHART 48-2

CLIENT EDUCATION GUIDE

Common Risk Factors for Developing a Stroke

- Atrial fibrillation or heart murmur
- Myocardial infarction
- Previous stroke or transient ischemic attack (TIA)
- Heart surgery
- Valvular heart disease
- Diabetes mellitus
- Smoking
- Substance abuse (particularly cocaine)
- Obesity
- Sedentary lifestyle
- Oral contraceptive use
- Elevated serum cholesterol, lipoprotein, triglyceride, low-density lipoprotein (LDL) and high-density lipoprotein (HDL) levels
- Previous stroke or TIA
- Heavy alcohol use
- Sudden discontinuation of antihypertensive medications (causes hemorrhagic stroke)
- Heredity/familial tendency
- Migraines
- Older age
- Male
- Black heritage
- Sickle cell anemia
- Use of phenylpropanolamine (PPA), which is found in antihistamine drugs (causes catastrophic strokes, primarily in young and middle-aged women)
- Hypercoagulable states

Incidence/Prevalence

It is estimated that there are more than 4.7 million stroke survivors in the United States. About 730,000 strokes occur each year, and more than 150,000 deaths result. About 25% of strokes occur in people under 65 years of age. The number of strokes occurring in the younger population is increasing as a result of chronic intravenous (IV) drug abuse. Those using crack cocaine experience an increased incidence of stroke resulting from changes in the clotting mechanism caused by the drugs, spasm of cerebral vessels or hemodynamic stress from the sudden increase in systolic blood pressure.

Between 5% and 15% of all clients who have had strokes have a recurrence within 1 year. By 5 years, about 40% have recurrence, and half of those die from stroke complications (Goldszmidt & Caplan, 2003). Strokes tend to occur more often in the southern United States ("stroke belt"), which is probably related to the geographic distribution of the older population, an increased use of tobacco, obesity, and a diet higher in fats.

HEALTH PROMOTION/ILLNESS PREVENTION

Individuals with predisposing health conditions should be aware that they could have a stroke unless they change their lifestyle. Teach them the importance of seeking professional health care and being compliant with the recommended treatment plan. Also remind them that other risk factors contribute to stroke, some of which can be avoided, such as smoking, a sedentary lifestyle, and high-fat diet (Chart 48-2). Recommend a diet high in fruits and vegetables and low in saturated and trans fats. Light to moderate alcohol consumption may reduce the risk of stroke, but a higher consumption may increase it. Additional information about diet, weight control, and smoking cessation can be found in the Cardiac Unit and in the discussion on obesity in Chapter 64.

Nurses or other health care providers can assess a client's risk for stroke by completing a Stroke Risk Screening tool (Figure 48-3).

◆COLLABORATIVE MANAGEMENT

PHARM REVIEW

◆Assessment

HISTORY

An accurate history is important in the diagnosis of a stroke. The information obtained assists in identifying the area of the brain involved as well as the cause. Obtain a history of the client's activity when the stroke began. Ischemic strokes often occur during sleep, whereas hemorrhagic strokes tend to occur during activity. Next ask the client or a family member how the symptoms progressed. Be sure to elicit a history of the onset of the stroke. Symptoms of an embolic or hemorrhagic stroke tend to occur abruptly, whereas thrombotic strokes generally have a more gradual progression. Determine the severity of the symptoms, such as whether they worsened after the initial onset (hemorrhagic stroke) or began to improve (embolic stroke). It is important to determine whether the symptoms come and go, possibly indicating a transient ischemic attack (TIA) or a reversible ischemic neurologic deficit (RIND).

During the interview, observe the client's level of consciousness (LOC), and assess for indications of intellectual or memory impairments or difficulties with speech or hearing. Question the client or family member about the presence of any sensory or motor changes, visual problems, problems with balance or gait, and changes in reading or writing abilities.

In addition, ask about the client's medical history, with specific attention directed toward a history of head trauma, diabetes, hypertension, heart disease, anemia, obesity, and headache. Obtain a list of current medications, including prescribed, over-the-counter (OTC), and recreational (illicit) drugs. Always ask about herbal supplements. Medications that could contribute to stroke include anticoagulants, aspirin, vasodilators, and illegal drugs as well as OTC products containing ephedra or herbal products that affect blood clotting. To complete the history, obtain data about the client's social history, including education, employment, travel, leisure activities, and personal habits (e.g., smoking, diet, exercise pattern, drug and alcohol use).

PHYSICAL ASSESSMENT/CLINICAL MANIFESTATIONS

NEUROLOGIC ASSESSMENT. Perform a neurologic assessment of the client. Specific neurologic signs and other manifestations depend on the extent and location of the ischemia and the arteries involved (Chart 48-3).

COGNITIVE CHANGES. The client may exhibit a variety of cognitive problems in addition to changes in level of consciousness (LOC). LOC may vary, depending on the extent of increased intracranial pressure (ICP) caused by the stroke and on the location of the stroke. LOC changes may also vary according to concurrent conditions, such as drug or alcohol intoxication as well as hypoxemia or metabolic disturbances. Always assess for indications of the following:

- Denial of the illness
- Spatial and **proprioceptive** (awareness of body position in space) dysfunction

STROKE RISK SCREENING

Site and address of Screening ______________________________ Date:____/____/____

PART I - DEMOGRAPHICS, AGE AND ETHNICITY

Name: (last)______________________ (first) ______________________ (middle initial)____

Gender: __ Male __Female Highest Level of Education: ___ High School or less __ College __ Graduate School

Address:______________________ (city)__________ (state)____ (zip)______ (county)______

Phone: Home (__)______________ Work (__)______________ Date of Birth:___/___/___ Age today____

Do you have a primary health care provider? ______Yes______No

Have you seen a health care provider in the past year? ______Yes______No

Do you have medical insurance? ______Yes______No

Ethnicity/Race: _____ African American _____Caucasian _____Hispanic White _____ Hispanic Non-White

_____ Asian/Pacific Islander _____ American Indian or Alaskan Native _____ Other or Unknown

PART II - HISTORY FOR KNOWN AND ESTABLISHED HIGH RISK FACTORS FOR STROKE

1. Have you ever been told that you have high blood pressure? ______Yes______No
2. Do you take medication for high blood pressure? ______Yes______No
3. Do you have a history of abnormal heart rate or rhythm called atrial fibrillation? ______Yes______No
4. Have you ever been checked for or been told that you have narrowing of the arteries to the brain? ______Yes______No
5. Have you had a heart attack, heart bypass surgery, angioplasty or another disease of the heart? ______Yes______No
6. Have you had a previous stroke, mini-stroke or TIA? ______Yes______No
7. Do you have diabetes mellitus (DM) or are you on insulin or medication for high blood sugar? ______Yes______No
8. Have you ever smoked cigarettes? ______Yes______No
9. Do you currently smoke cigarettes? ______Yes______No

PART III - HISTORY FOR SIGNIFICANT BUT SLIGHTLY LOWER RISK FACTORS FOR STROKE

10. Has a family member had a stroke or heart attack when they were less than 45 years of age? ______Yes______No
11. Do you consume more than two ounces of alcohol per day on a daily basis? ______Yes______No
12. Do you have a cholesterol level greater than 200? ______Yes______No

PART IV - HISTORY OF OTHER/UNCOMMON IMPORTANT RISK FACTORS FOR STROKE

13. Do you smoke cigarettes and take birth control pills? ______Yes______No
14. Do you have Sickle Cell Anemia? ______Yes______No
15. Do you use one or more of the following drugs: Cocaine, Crack, Heroin, Amphetamines? ______Yes______No
16. Are you overweight or obese? ______Yes______No
17. Do you consider your activity level as generally inactive? ______Yes______No

Figure 48-3 ■ Stroke Risk Screening Tool.

PART V - BLOOD PRESSURE AND PULSE

Blood Pressure (BP) recorded sitting ________(Systolic) ________(Diastolic) ______ Right Arm ______ Left Arm

Radial Pulse rate for 60 seconds (beats/minute) ________________ Irregular pulse rate? ______ Yes ______ No

PART VI - IDENTIFICATION OF RISK FOR STROKE AND RECOMMENDATION

1. ______ **Low Risk for Stroke:**

Under the age of 55, responded "**NO**" to questions 1-17 (self-reported risk factors) and was not identified to have an irregular pulse rate or a measured Systolic BP equal to or greater than or equal to 140 or Diastolic equal to or greater than 90.

RECOMMENDATION: Take this completed screening form to your health care provider at your next appointment.

2. ______ **Moderate Risk for Stroke:**

Age equal to or greater than 55 with no self-reported risk factors and no risk factors identified on screening

OR - Age up to 64 with one self-reported risk factor, or an irregular pulse rate or a measured Systolic BP equal to or greater than 140 or a Diastolic equal to or greater than 90.

RECOMMENDATION: Notify your health care provider within a week with the results of your screening and request an appointment for an evaluation and care to prevent a stroke.

3. ______ **High Risk for Stroke:**

Age equal to or greater than 65 with one self-reported risk factor, or irregular pulse, or a measured Systolic BP equal to or greater than 140 or a Diastolic BP equal to or greater than 90.

OR - Any age with **two or more risk factors**, either self-reported and/or identified on measurement of an irregular pulse or Systolic BP equal to or greater than 140 or a Diastolic equal to or greater than 90.

RECOMMENDATION: Notify your health care provider TODAY with the results of your screening and request an appointment for an evaluation of your risks for stroke and care to prevent a stroke.

4. ______ **PRESENTS WITH WARNING SIGNS OF STROKE, OR TIA (MINI-STROKE)**
RECOMMENDATION: CALL OR HAVE SOMEONE CALL 9-1-1 IMMEDIATELY!

PART VII - THE EARLY WARNING SIGNS OF STROKE

*** SUDDEN WEAKNESS, NUMBNESS, OR PARALYSIS OF THE FACE, ARM OR LEG, ON ONE OR BOTH SIDES OF THE BODY**

*** SUDDEN BLURRED VISION OR BLINDNESS IN ONE OR BOTH EYES**

*** SUDDEN DIFFICULTY SPEAKING, SLURRING OF SPEECH OR DIFFICULTY UNDERSTANDING**

*** SUDDEN SEVERE HEADACHE WITH SUDDEN ONSET THAT OCCURS WITHOUT APPARENT REASON**

*** SUDDEN LOSS OF BALANCE, DIZZINESS, OR FALLING WITHOUT ANY APPARENT REASON**

CALL 9-1-1 IMMEDIATELY IF YOU EXPERIENCE ANY OF THESE SYMPTOMS

I have received a screening for the risk of stroke and agree to follow up with the recommendations. I understand this is only a screening. I agree that this data can be entered into a database for research without identifying me by name.

(Signature of Participant) ________________ **Signature of Health care provider** ________________

The **Stroke Risk Screening** was developed in 1999 jointly by the Division on Research, Delaware Nurses Association and Ellen Barker, MSN, RN, CNRN, Neuroscience Nursing Consultants, Wilmington, Delaware. Marian P. LaMonte, M.D., M.S.N., Assistant Professor of Neurology and Co-Director of the Maryland Brain Attack Center, University of Maryland Medical Center, Baltimore, Maryland, served as Nurse/Neurologist advisor. There is no Copyright and permission is not needed to duplicate this form.

Figure 48-3 ■ *cont'd.*

CHART 48-3

KEY FEATURES of
Stroke Syndromes

Middle Cerebral Artery Strokes
- Contralateral hemiparesis: arm > leg
- Contralateral sensory deficit
- Homonymous hemianopsia
- Unilateral neglect or inattention
- Aphasia, anomia, alexia, agraphia, and acalculia
- Impaired vertical sensation
- Spatial deficit
- Perceptual deficit
- Visual field deficit
- Altered level of consciousness: drowsy to comatose

Posterior Cerebral Artery Strokes
- Perseveration
- Aphasia, amnesia, alexia, agraphia, visual agnosia, and ataxia
- Loss of deep sensation
- Decreased touch sensation
- Possible choreoathetoid movements
- Stupor; coma

Internal Carotid Artery Strokes
- Contralateral hemiparesis
- Sensory deficit
- Hemianopsia, blurred vision, blindness
- Aphasia (dominant side)

Internal Carotid Artery Strokes
- Headache
- Bruit

Anterior Cerebral Artery Strokes
- Contralateral hemiparesis: leg > arm
- Bladder incontinence
- Personality and behavior changes
- Aphasia, gait apraxia, and amnesia
- Positive grasp and sucking reflex
- Perseveration
- Sensory deficit (lower extremity)
- Memory impairment
- Apraxic gait

Vertebrobasilar Artery Strokes
- Headache and vertigo
- Coma
- Memory loss and confusion
- Flaccid paralysis
- Areflexia, ataxia, and vertigo
- Cranial nerve dysfunction
- Dysconjugate gaze
- Visual deficits (uniorbital) and homonymous hemianopsia
- Sensory loss: numbness

- Impairment of memory, judgment, or problem-solving and decision-making abilities
- Decreased ability to concentrate and attend to tasks

Dysfunction in one or more of these areas may be more pronounced, depending on the hemisphere involved (Chart 48-4).

The right cerebral hemisphere is more involved with visual and spatial awareness and proprioception. A person who has a stroke involving the right cerebral hemisphere is often unaware of any deficits and may be disoriented to time and place. Personality changes include impulsivity (poor impulse control) and poor judgment. The left cerebral hemisphere, the dominant hemisphere in all but about 15% to 20% of the population, is the center for language, mathematic skills, and analytic thinking. Therefore a left hemisphere stroke results in **aphasia** (inability to use or comprehend language), **alexia** (reading problems), and **agraphia** (difficulty with writing). Persons with left-hemisphere strokes tend to be slow and cautious.

CHART 48-4

KEY FEATURES of
Left and Right Hemisphere Strokes

Feature	Left Hemisphere*	Right Hemisphere
Language	Aphasia Agraphia Alexia (word blindness)	Impaired sense of humor
Memory	Possible deficit	Disorientation to time, place, and person Inability to recognize faces
Vision	Inability to discriminate words and letters Reading problems Deficits in the right visual field	Visual spatial deficits Neglect of the left visual field Loss of depth perception
Behavior	Slowness Cautiousness Anxiety when attempting a new task Depression or a catastrophic response to illness Sense of guilt Feeling of worthlessness Worries over future Quick anger and frustration Intellectual impairment	Impulsiveness Lack of awareness of neurologic deficits Confabulation Euphoria Constant smiling Denial of illness Poor judgment Overestimation of abilities (risk for injury)
Hearing	No deficit	Loss of ability to hear tonal variations

*Location for speech in all but 15% to 20% of people.

MOTOR CHANGES. The motor examination provides information about which part of the brain is involved. A right **hemiplegia** (paralysis on one side of the body) or **hemiparesis** (weakness on one side of the body) indicates a stroke involving the left cerebral hemisphere because the motor nerve fibers cross in the medulla before entering the spinal cord and periphery. Conversely, a left hemiplegia or hemiparesis indicates a stroke in the right cerebral hemisphere. If the brainstem or cerebellum is affected, the client may experience hemiparesis or quadriparesis and ataxia.

In collaboration with the physical and occupational therapist, gauge the client's muscle tone. The client with **hypotonia,** or **flaccid paralysis**, is unable to overcome the forces of gravity, and the extremities tend to fall to the side. The extremities feel heavy, and muscle tone is inadequate for balance, equilibrium, or protective mechanisms. **Hypertonia (spastic paralysis)** tends to cause fixed positions or contractures of the involved extremities. Range of motion (ROM) of the joints is restricted, and shoulder subluxation may easily occur from either spasticity or flaccidity. Also assess proprioception, head and trunk control, balance, coordination, and gait.

Loss of inhibitory nervous control from the cerebral cortex results in a spastic (upper motor neuron), uninhibited bladder. Bowel function may also be affected.

SENSORY CHANGES. The sensory examination evaluates the client's response to touch and painful stimuli. In addition to diminished motor function, decreased sensation typically occurs on the affected side of the body. The client who has had a stroke may also be unable to write, comprehend reading material, use an object correctly **(agnosia),** or carry out a purposeful motor activity **(apraxia).**

Evaluate for indications of **neglect syndrome,** which is particularly evident with strokes in the right cerebral hemisphere. In this syndrome, the client is unaware of the existence of his or her left or paralyzed side. The typical picture is that of the client sitting in a wheelchair, leaning to the left with the arm caught in the wheelchair wheel. When questioned, the client often states that everything is fine and believes that he or she is sitting up straight in the chair. Another typical example of neglect syndrome is the client who washes or dresses only one side of the body.

Another important part of the nursing assessment focuses on visual ability. Infarction or ischemia involving the carotid artery may cause pupillary abnormalities, **ptosis** (eyelid drooping), visual field deficits, or pallor and petechiae of the conjunctiva. **Amaurosis fugax,** a brief episode of blindness in one eye, results from retinal ischemia caused by ophthalmic or carotid artery insufficiency. **Hemianopsia,** or blindness in half of the visual field, results from damage to the optic tract or occipital lobe. Most often this deficit occurs as homonymous hemianopsia, in which there is blindness in the same side of both eyes (Figure 48-4). The client with this condition must turn his or her head to scan the complete range of vision. Otherwise, he or she does not see half of the visual field. For example, the client eats only half of a meal because that is the only portion seen. Clients with brainstem or cerebellar damage may experience abnormal eye movements.

CRANIAL NERVE FUNCTION. Assessment of the client's ability to chew reflects cranial nerve (CN) V. Assessment of the client's ability to swallow reflects CNs IX and X. In addition, note any facial paralysis or paresis (CN VII), absent gag reflex (CN IX), or impaired tongue movement (CN XII). The client who has difficulty chewing or swallowing foods and liquids is at risk for aspiration pneumonia and may become constipated from inadequate fluid intake.

CARDIOVASCULAR ASSESSMENT. Clients with embolic strokes may have a heart murmur, dysrhythmias, or hypertension. It is not unusual for the client to be admitted to the hospital with a blood pressure greater than 180-200/110-120 mm Hg. Although a somewhat higher blood pressure (150/100 mm Hg) is needed to maintain cerebral perfusion after a stroke, pressures above this limit may lead to another stroke.

PSYCHOSOCIAL ASSESSMENT

A typical client with a stroke is older than 60 years of age, is hypertensive, and has varying degrees of motor weakness and level of consciousness. Language and cognitive deficits, as well as behavior and memory problems, may also occur. It is possible for stroke to occur at much younger ages.

Determine the client's reaction to the illness, especially in relation to changes in body image, self-concept, and ability to perform activities of daily living (ADLs). In collaboration with the client's family and friends, identify any difficulties in coping mechanisms or personality changes.

Determine the client's financial status and occupation because these aspects may be altered by the residual neurologic deficits of the stroke. Clients who do not have disability or health insurance may worry about how their family will cope financially with the disruption in their lives. Early involvement of social services or psychological counseling may enhance coping skills.

Assess for **emotional lability,** especially if the frontal lobe of the brain has been affected. In such cases, the client laughs and then cries unexpectedly for no apparent reason. It is important that the nurse explain these uncontrollable emotions to the family or significant others so they do not feel responsible for these reactions.

LABORATORY ASSESSMENT

Clinical history and presentation are usually sufficient to identify a stroke. No definitive laboratory tests confirm its diagnosis. Elevated hematocrit and hemoglobin levels are often associated with a severe or major stroke as the body attempts to compensate for lack of oxygen to the brain. An elevated white blood cell count may indicate the presence of an infection, possibly subacute bacterial endocarditis or a response to physiologic stress as well as inflammation. The health care provider typically orders a prothrombin time (PT) or International Normalized Ratio (INR) as well as a partial thromboplastin time (PTT) to establish baseline coagulation information in case anticoagulation therapy is initiated. These diagnostic tests may also provide supportive evidence that a hemorrhagic stroke has occurred. If there is no indication of increased intracranial pressure (ICP), a lumbar puncture may be performed to obtain cerebrospinal fluid (CSF) for analysis. Blood in the spinal fluid or a high red blood cell count in the CSF in all samples obtained is indicative of a subarachnoid hemorrhage.

RADIOGRAPHIC ASSESSMENT

Computed tomography (CT) and CT angiography (CTA) assist in the differential diagnosis of a stroke. The primary purpose of the initial scan is to identify the presence of cerebral hemorrhage. Cerebral aneurysms, if large enough, may be identified. For a client with an ischemic or occlusive stroke, the head CT is usually initially negative. After the first 24 hours, CT shows progressive changes of ischemia, infarction, and associated cerebral edema. This test is invaluable in establishing baseline information for future comparison in case the client's condition deteriorates. In addition, the scans enable the physician to identify pathologic changes that may mimic a stroke, such as a brain tumor or cerebral hematoma, both of which may be unrelated to cerebrovascular disease.

OTHER DIAGNOSTIC ASSESSMENTS

Magnetic resonance imaging (MRI) may show the presence of edema, ischemia, and tissue necrosis earlier than a CT scan. Information about the status of the cerebral vessels is

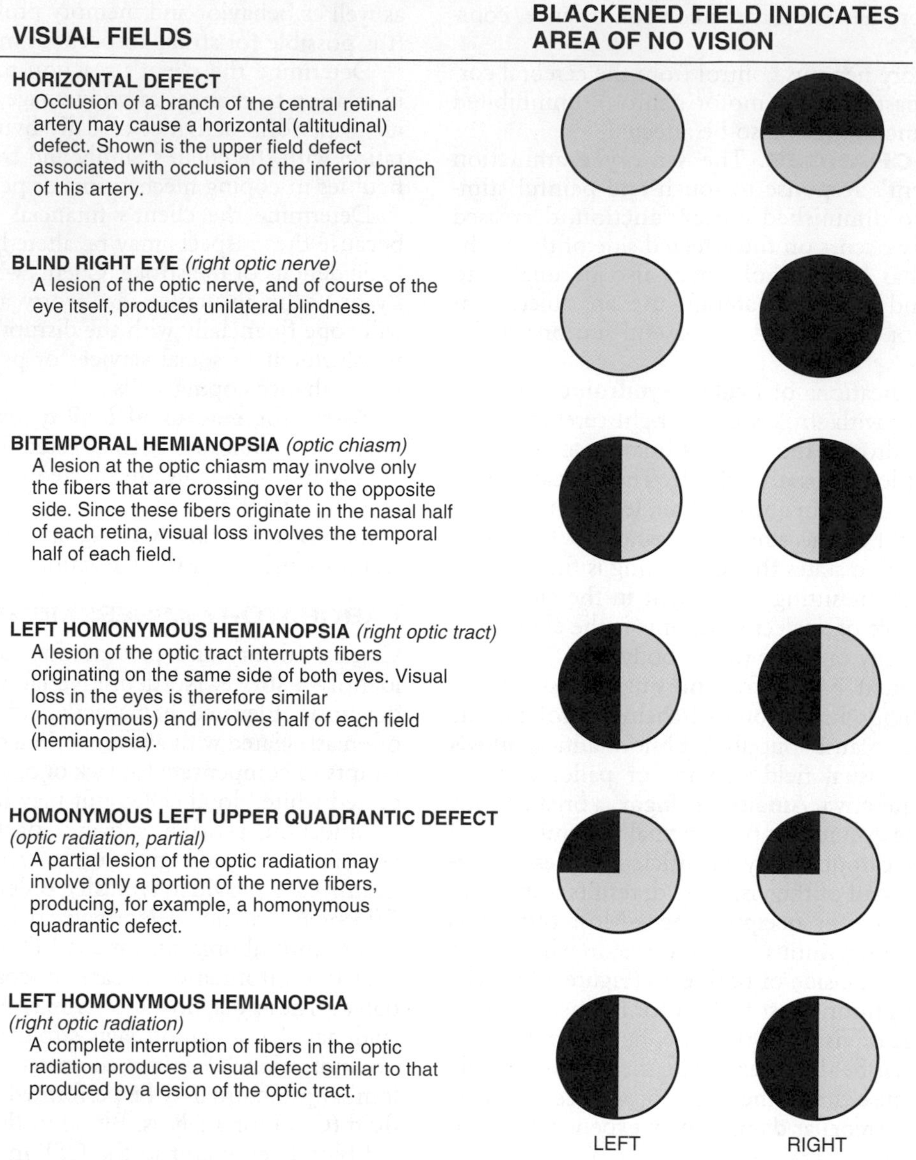

Figure 48-4 ■ Visual field defects produced by selected lesions in the visual pathways. (Modified from Bates, B. [2000]. Bates' guide to physical examination and history taking [7th ed.]. Philadelphia: J.B. Lippincott.)

obtained by angiography, digital subtraction angiography, diffusion/perfusion-weighted MRI, or magnetic resonance angiography (MRA). These studies reveal abnormal vessel structures (aneurysm location) or identify the area of vessel wall rupture and vasospasm. Following angiography, a narrowed vessel can be treated by catheter injection of papaverine or by using angioplasty techniques. Diffusion/perfusion MRI or MRA helps to locate areas that are underperfused but not yet infarcted. Single-photon emission computed tomography (SPECT) studies can also provide information on regional perfusion of blood flow in the brain.

To assist in the determination of a cardiac cause of a stroke, the health care provider may request an electrocardiogram (ECG), a Holter monitor test, cardiac enzymes evaluation, and an echocardiogram. As with other neurovascular diseases, it is not unusual to find the following changes on the ECG: inverted T wave, ST depression, and prolongation of the Q-T interval in the cardiac cycle.

Critical Thinking Challenge

You have been floated from a medical unit to the emergency department (ED) for the night shift. Two clients present with possible stroke—a middle-aged black man and an older white woman. The man's history reveals that he is a construction worker who collapsed on the job. His wife states that he has been noncompliant with his antihypertensive medications and he "drinks too much." The female client has a history of diabetes mellitus type 2 and mild hypertension, but she has been very diligent in following her physician's treatment plan.

1. What other information would you want to obtain from these clients or their families or significant others?
2. What factors do you already know put these clients at risk for stroke?
3. What physical assessment should you perform at this time?
4. What diagnostic testing would you anticipate for these clients?

evolve For suggested answer guidelines, go to http://evolve.elsevier.com/Iggy/.

Analysis

COMMON NURSING DIAGNOSES AND COLLABORATIVE PROBLEMS

The following are the most common nursing diagnoses for clients with a stroke:

1. Ineffective Tissue Perfusion (Cerebral) related to interruption of arterial blood flow and a possible increase in ICP
2. Impaired Physical Mobility and Self-Care Deficit related to neuromuscular impairment or cognitive impairment
3. Disturbed Sensory Perception related to altered sensory reception, transmission, and integration
4. Unilateral Neglect related to effects of disturbed perceptual abilities or hemianopsia
5. Impaired Verbal Communication related to decreased circulation in the brain
6. Impaired Swallowing related to neuromuscular impairment
7. Total Urinary Incontinence and Bowel Incontinence related to neurologic dysfunction

ADDITIONAL NURSING DIAGNOSES AND COLLABORATIVE PROBLEMS

In addition to the common nursing diagnoses, clients with stroke may have one or more of the following:

- Risk for Aspiration related to impaired swallowing
- Disturbed Body Image related to biophysical or cognitive disability
- Ineffective Role Performance related to health alterations
- Risk for Falls related to visual difficulties, urgency or incontinence, decreased lower extremity strength, impaired balance, difficulty with gait, or proprioceptive deficits
- Sexual Dysfunction related to altered body function
- Constipation related to lack of adequate fluid intake or insufficient physical activity
- Imbalanced Nutrition: Less Than Body Requirements related to impaired swallowing

Additional collaborative problems include the following:

- Potential for Deep Vein Thrombosis or Pulmonary Embolism
- Potential for Increased Intracranial Pressure
- Potential for Seizures
- Potential for Hypoxemia
- Potential for Atelectasis and Pneumonia
- Potential for Hypercarbia

Planning and Implementation

INEFFECTIVE TISSUE PERFUSION (CEREBRAL)

NOC **PLANNING: EXPECTED OUTCOMES.** The client with a stroke is expected to have an adequate blood flow through the cerebral vasculature to maintain brain function. Indicators include that the following will be noncompromised in this client:

- Neurologic function
- Intracranial pressure
- Systolic blood pressure
- Diastolic blood pressure

CHART 48-5

KEY FEATURES of
Increased Intracranial Pressure

- Decreased level of consciousness (lethargy to coma)
- Behavior changes: restlessness, irritability, and confusion
- Headache
- Nausea and vomiting
- Change in speech pattern
- Aphasia
- Slurred speech
- Change in sensorimotor status
- Pupillary changes: dilated and nonreactive pupils ("blown pupils") or constricted and nonreactive pupils
- Cranial nerve dysfunction
- Ataxia
- Seizures
- Cushing's triad
- Abnormal posturing (see Chapter 44)
    - Decerebrate (extensor)
    - Decorticate (flexion)

INTERVENTIONS. Interventions are determined primarily by the type and extent of the stroke. For selected clients with ischemic strokes, early intervention with systemic thrombolytic therapy to dissolve the clot is indicated to address neurologic deficits if implemented within 3 hours of the onset of stroke.

Unless major medical complications occur, the health care provider manages the client conservatively with drug therapy and aggressive rehabilitation to promote an optimal level of well-being and function. In some cases, as with cerebral hemorrhage causing progressive damage, the physician may need to intervene surgically to prevent further neurologic dysfunction.

NONSURGICAL MANAGEMENT. Nursing interventions are initially aimed at monitoring for neurologic changes or complications associated with stroke. The client is at risk for continued progression of the stroke or increased intracranial pressure (ICP) (Chart 48-5). Perform a neurologic assessment when the client is admitted to the hospital and at intervals as indicated thereafter, including the beginning of each nursing shift. Periodic neurologic checks using the Glasgow Coma Scale (GCS) (see Chapter 44) or other neurologic assessment tools are indicated at least every 2 to 4 hours or more frequently, depending on the client's condition.

NIC **Intracranial Pressure Monitoring.** The client is most at risk for increased ICP resulting from edema during the first 72 hours after onset of the stroke (Chart 48-6). Be alert for symptoms of increased ICP, and report any deterioration in the client's neurologic status to the health care provider *immediately. The first sign of increased ICP is a declining level of consciousness (LOC).*

Current nursing practice for the care of clients with ischemic strokes is to elevate the head of the bed (HOB) to 30 degrees. However, evidence to support this practice is lacking. Wojner, El-Mitwalli, and Alexandrov (2002) found that lowering the HOB increases blood flow to the ischemic brain, which decreases further infarction (see the Evidence-Based Practice for Nursing box on p. 1038). The physician or clinical pathway may designate the desired HOB position. Maintain the head in a midline, neutral position to facilitate venous drainage from the brain.

In collaboration with other team members, plan care to avoid activities and procedures that may increase ICP,

CHART 48-6

NIC INTERVENTION ACTIVITIES for The Client with a Stroke

Intracranial Pressure Monitoring: *Measurement and interpretation of client data to regulate intracranial pressure*
- Assist with ICP monitoring device insertion.
- Provide information to family/significant others.
- Calibrate and level the transducer.
- Set alarms.
- Record ICP pressure readings and analyze waveforms.
- Note client's change in response to stimuli.
- Monitor cerebral perfusion pressure.
- Monitor client's ICP and neurologic response to care activities.
- Monitor intake and output.
- Monitor insertion site for infection.
- Monitor temperature and WBC count.
- Administer pharmacologic agents to maintain ICP within specified range.
- Space nursing care to minimize ICP elevation.
- Notify health care provider of elevated ICP that does not respond to treatment protocols.

NIC intervention activities selected from Dochterman, J.M., & Bulechek, G.M. (Eds.). (2004). *Nursing interventions classification (NIC)* (4th ed.). St. Louis: Mosby. No part of this work is to be altered without prior written permission from the Publisher.
ICP, Intracranial pressure; *WBC*, white blood cell.

particularly if the client has focal neurologic deficits and indications of cerebral edema. Extreme hip and neck flexion should be avoided. Extreme hip flexion may increase intrathoracic pressure, which may make ICP more difficult to control. Extreme neck flexion interferes with venous drainage from the brain, also making ICP more difficult to control.

Additional nursing considerations include avoiding the clustering of nursing procedures (e.g., giving a bath followed immediately by changing the bed linen) within a short time. This is because the effect on ICP elevation is more dramatic when multiple activities are clustered within a narrow time interval. Hyperoxygenating the client before suctioning may also be appropriate to avoid even transient hypoxemia and resultant ICP elevation from dilation of cerebral arteries. Fully assess the need for suctioning because it may increase ICP. A quiet environment is particularly important for the client experiencing a headache, which is common with an aneurysm or increased ICP. The client may have **photophobia** (sensitivity to light); therefore the room lights should be kept low.

Monitor vital signs closely, at least every 4 hours. Notify the health care provider if the blood pressure exceeds acceptable levels. Generally, the health care provider allows the client to be slightly hypertensive (150/100 mm Hg) to facilitate adequate cerebral tissue perfusion. A higher blood pressure could lead to a hemorrhagic stroke or rebleeding of an aneurysm (if present).

Clients admitted to a critical care unit are connected to a cardiac monitor and observed for dysrhythmias. The critical care nurse performs a cardiac assessment, with particular attention directed toward auscultation of heart sounds to identify the presence of cardiac murmurs or atrial fibrillation (AF). Murmurs or AF may place the client at increased risk for emboli. Close physical assessment for indications of hemodynamic stability is indicated. Invasive hemodynamic monitoring may be needed to monitor and evaluate physiologic stability and response to therapy. (See also Chapter 37 for a discussion of AF.)

EVIDENCE-BASED PRACTICE for Nursing

Head elevation: A critical new look at traditional practice

Wojner, A.W., El-Mitwalli, A., & Alexandrov, A.V. Effect of head positioning on intracranial blood flow velocities in acute ischemic stroke: A pilot study. *Critical Care Nurse Quarterly*, 25(4), 57-66.

Evidence has been lacking regarding the current nursing practice of elevating the head of the bed (HOB) to 30 degrees following an acute ischemic stroke. The practice might be taken from studies of clients with traumatic brain injury. This small pilot study of 11 clients examined cerebral artery mean flow velocities (MCA-MFV) when the HOB was placed in various positions. On average, a 9.2% increase in MCA-MFV occurred when the HOB was lowered to 15 degrees from a 30-degree elevation. An additional increase of 3.9% resulted when the bed was lowered from 15 degrees to a flat position. The researchers concluded that the clients in the sample benefited from lowering the HOB because the total increase was 13.1% ($p = 0.054$).

Level of Evidence: 6—The study sample is small and not randomized, but it illustrates the need for further study and has questioned a traditional practice that has not been research based in the past.

Critique. No substantial research has been conducted that examined HOB positioning in clients immediately following an ischemic stroke. This study clearly demonstrated that in this small convenience sample whose average age was 60 years, there was an increase in cerebral blood flow that could possibly reduce additional infarction. The authors did not state the race or ethnic origin of the sample, so it is assumed that the sample population was white. Additional studies using larger numbers, varying ages, and an ethnically diverse group might help to validate these early findings.

Implications for Nursing. This study begins to provide an evidence base for changing practice in the positioning of clients after an acute ischemic stroke. Further study needs to be conducted to ensure that clients have optimal clinical outcomes.

Drug Therapy. The medications prescribed by the health care provider for a stroke depend on the type of stroke and the resulting neurologic dysfunction. In general, the goals of drug therapy are to prevent further thrombotic episodes (anticoagulation), increase blood flow, and protect the neurons (cytoprotection).

Thrombolytic Therapy. **Intravenous (systemic) thrombolytic therapy** for an acute ischemic stroke (AIS) dissolves the cerebral artery occlusion to re-establish blood flow and prevent cerebral infarction. Recombinant tissue plasminogen activator (rt-PA [Retavase]) was the first definitive drug with Food and Drug Administration (FDA) approval for the treatment of acute ischemic stroke. Thrombolytics activate plasminogen, which degrades the thrombus by breaking down fibrin. Fibrin breakdown results in the release of fibrin degradation products, such as D-dimers and other D-polymers (Goldszmidt & Caplan, 2003).

Clients must meet strict eligibility criteria for rt-PA administration. Contraindications to thrombolytic therapy include, but are not limited to, stroke or serious head injury in the past 3 months, hemorrhagic stroke, recent myocardial infarction (MI), increased partial thromboplastin time (PTT), anticoagulant therapy, or pregnancy. When considering thrombolytic therapy, the client should be quickly evaluated for any concurrent clinical state that might increase bleeding risk. Some health care facilities refer to an admission of a client having a stroke as a **Code Gray**

(Nolan, Naylor, & Burns, 2003). This label alerts the health care team of the importance of treating the client quickly.

For treatment of ischemic or occlusive stroke, the initial head CT should be negative. The presence of changes on head CT indicating progression of ischemia or infarction rules out systemic thrombolytic therapy because the time interval from symptom onset to medical evaluation exceeds 3 hours. The rt-PA should be given within 3 hours of the onset of symptoms. However, when the occlusion affects the basilar artery, thrombolysis may be effective even after 12 to 18 hours of ischemia (Goldszmidt & Caplan, 2003).

Catheter-directed thrombolytic therapy may be attempted if systemic therapy is not effective in improving the client's condition. As an option, catheter-directed therapy into an obstructed vessel may be initiated without attempting the systemic method based on agency protocols. This type of therapy should be prescribed within 6 hours of the ischemic event. Current lytic agents for this purpose include urokinase (Abbokinase), t-PA (alteplase), and rt-PA (Retavase). These agents may also be used with heparin and a platelet inhibitor such as abciximab (ReoPro).

Anticoagulants. The use of **anticoagulants** and **antiplatelet agents** to treat stroke is controversial and depends on the health care provider's preference. The principal drugs used are aspirin, heparin, low-molecular weight heparin (enoxaparin [Lovenox]), and warfarin (Coumadin). If the client received thrombolytic therapy, an IV anticoagulant is usually prescribed as a follow-up treatment.

The provider typically prescribes sodium heparin (Hepalean✱) subcutaneously or via a continuous IV infusion to prevent the progression of transient ischemic attacks (TIAs) or evolving strokes. This drug is also effective in prevention of deep vein thrombosis (DVT), a hazard of immobility. Baseline prothrombin time (PT) and partial thromboplastin time (PTT) values are usually obtained before initiating of heparin therapy, 6 to 8 hours after the start of the infusion, and every morning while the client is receiving heparin therapy. The therapeutic goal is to achieve 1.5 to 2 times the client's normal baseline PT and PTT values. PT is used to monitor oral anticoagulant therapy, whereas PTT is used to monitor heparin therapy. The World Health Organization advocates use of the International Normalized Ratio (INR) to monitor warfarin therapy. The target INR value for most clients with strokes is 2.0 to 3.0; for strokes of cardiac origin, the goal is usually 3.0 to 4.5.

Sodium heparin and other anticoagulants, such as warfarin (Coumadin, Warfilone✱), can cause bleeding. Observe for signs of blood in the urine or stool, epistaxis, bleeding gums, and easy bruising. Anticoagulant therapy is contraindicated in clients who have ulcers, uremia, or hepatic failure.

Enteric-coated or other forms of aspirin (Ecotrin, Ancasal✱) have proved useful primarily in the prevention of recurrent stroke or embolic stroke. These drugs prevent blood clotting by reducing platelet adhesiveness. Other commonly used **antiplatelet medications** include ticlopidine hydrochloride (Ticlid), clopidogrel (Plavix), and dipyridamole (Persantine, Apo-Dipyridamole✱). These agents can cause bruising, hemorrhage, and liver disease. Always teach the client to report any unusual bruising or bleeding to the health care provider. Liver function and coagulation studies are carefully monitored during the course of drug therapy. Clopidogrel should be taken with food to prevent gastric distress.

Other Drugs. To treat seizures, lorazepam (Ativan), a benzodiazepine, is administered with close neurologic and cardiorespiratory monitoring. For long-term anticonvulsant therapy, the health care provider may also prescribe antiepileptic drugs (AEDs), such as phenytoin (Dilantin), gabapentin (Neurontin), or topiramate (Topamax). Calcium channel blockers (e.g., nimodipine [Nimotop]) are used to treat or prevent cerebral vasospasm following a subarachnoid hemorrhage, which usually occurs between 4 and 14 days after the stroke, inhibits blood flow to the area, and worsens ischemia. These drugs work by relaxing the smooth muscles of the vessel wall and reducing the incidence and severity of the spasm. Neurologic functioning is improved and further deterioration from ischemia is prevented. In addition, calcium channel blockers possibly dilate collateral vessels to ischemic areas of the brain. Stool softeners, analgesics for pain, and antianxiety drugs may also be prescribed.

Monitoring for Other Complications. The client with an aneurysm or arteriovenous malformation (AVM) must be monitored for the presence of hydrocephalus and vasospasm. **Hydrocephalus** (increased CSF within the ventricular and subarachnoid spaces) may occur as a consequence of blood in the CSF, which prevents it from being reabsorbed properly by the arachnoid villi. It may also occur resulting from cerebral edema, interfering with flow of CSF out from the ventricular system. Eventually the ventricles become enlarged and, if hydrocephalus is left untreated, increased intracranial pressure (ICP) occurs. Observe for clinical manifestations of hydrocephalus, which mirror those of ICP elevation, including a change in the level of consciousness (LOC). Clinical findings may also include headache, alterations in pupils, seizures, poor coordination, gait disturbances (if ambulatory), and behavior changes.

Vasospasm, or a narrowing of the cerebral vessels in response to stimulus such as bleeding or irritation, leads to cerebral ischemia and infarction. Clinical manifestations may include decreased LOC, motor and reflex changes, and increased neurologic deficits (e.g., CN dysfunction, motor weakness and aphasia). The symptoms may fluctuate with the occurrence and degree of vasospasm present.

Rebleeding or rupture is a common complication for the client with an aneurysm or AVM. It may occur within 24 hours of the initial bleed or rupture and up to 7 to 10 days later. It is manifested by severe headache, nausea and vomiting, a decreased LOC, and additional neurologic deficits. Potential consequences of aneurysm rebleed may be catastrophic.

Carotid Artery Angioplasty. Although angioplasty was introduced in the mid-1980s, it was rarely used on the carotid arteries. However, with the development and refinement of vascular stents, carotid artery angioplasty has become more common. A device called a **distal protection device (DSP)** can make carotid angioplasty safer than endarterectomy. The DSP is placed beyond the stenosis, which catches any debris that breaks off during the angioplasty/stenting procedure. This interventional radiology procedure is done under moderate sedation and may eventually be performed as an outpatient procedure.

Other Nonsurgical Techniques. New early techniques are being tried for clients who are not candidates for thrombolytic therapy. For example, hypothermia treatment started during the first few hours after onset of a stroke may result in preservation of neurologic function in select clients. Techniques for cooling need further evaluation with well-structured research to identify optimal client selection criteria, target temperature, and duration of therapy. Cytoprotective drugs such as sodium channel blockers, opioid antagonists, free radical scavengers, magnesium, estrogens, gamma-aminobutyric acid (GABA) antagonists, glutamate receptor antagonists, calcium channel blockers, and membrane stabilizers are being tested as a therapy for stroke. A clot-dissolving substance in vampire bat saliva is also being tested and may be used to develop a new drug to treat occlusive strokes. No conclusive results have been demonstrated, and research is ongoing. Cell and tissue transplants are also being investigated for their potential benefit in replacing dead or damaged neurons and restoring otherwise lost brain function.

SURGICAL MANAGEMENT. Some clients are candidates for surgery to prevent or treat strokes. The surgical procedure depends on the cause of the stroke.

Endarterectomy. Carotid endarterectomy is the most widely used surgical procedure to prevent progressing stroke in symptomatic clients with recurrent TIAs or carotid stenosis. The purpose of a **carotid endarterectomy** is to remove atherosclerotic plaque from the inner lining of the carotid artery. The goal is to open the artery enough to re-establish blood flow and decrease stroke risk.

Extracranial-Intracranial Bypass. In an **extracranial-intracranial bypass**, the surgeon performs a craniotomy and bypasses the blocked artery by making a graft or a bypass from the first artery to the second artery. This procedure establishes blood flow around the blocked artery and re-establishes blood flow to the involved areas. The two most common techniques are the superficial middle temporal artery-to-middle cerebral artery (STA-MCA) graft and the occipital-to-posterior inferior cerebellar artery (PICA) bypass. Clinical trials have shown little or no differences in the effectiveness and benefit of this procedure in preventing stroke. Despite this finding, this procedure continues to be performed.

Management of Arteriovenous Malformations. The usual treatment of an arteriovenous malformation (AVM) is interventional therapy to occlude abnormal arteries or veins and prevent bleeding from the vascular lesion. The same procedure may be performed to occlude the vessels surrounding an aneurysm. Under fluoroscopic guidance, the physician inserts a microcatheter into the carotid artery, typically using a femoral artery approach, and threads it to the vessel to be embolized. The physician then injects an embolic agent, such as platinum coils, detachable silicone balloons, liquid acrylic, or polyvinyl alcohol, to embolize the involved arteries (Figure 48-5). If the AVM is large, the physician may elect to occlude the artery gradually to allow a gradual change in the blood supply to the surrounding brain. In this case, the embolization procedure is carried out over 1 to 2 weeks. Whenever possible, the involved vessels are totally removed surgically. The surgeon ligates the vessels and removes the defect. Gamma radiation delivered through the Gamma Knife produces fibrous thickening of the endothelial lining of the vessels to prevent further vessel enlargement and ultimately eliminated the lesion from the cerebral circulation. Improved microsurgical techniques have significantly reduced morbidity and mortality rates, and these procedures are becoming the treatment of choice in many medical centers.

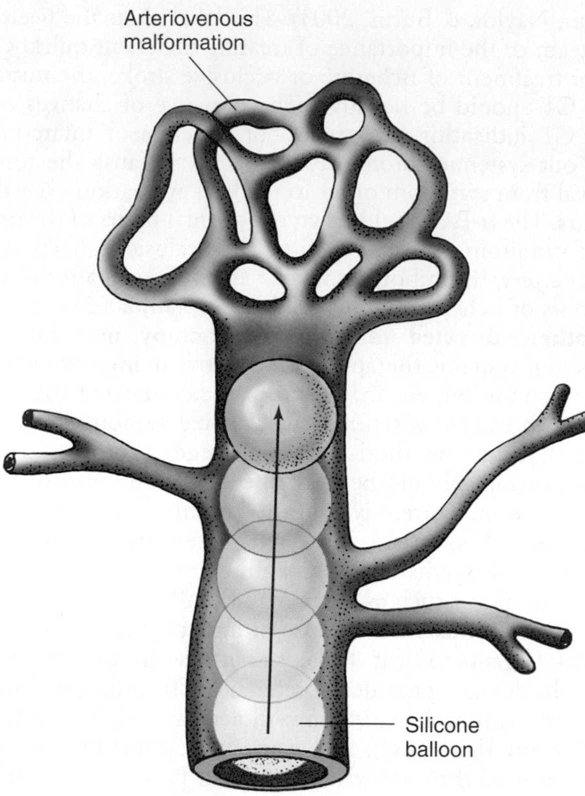

Figure 48-5 ■ Embolization procedure to treat an arteriovenous malformation. The embolic agent travels to the area to cause vessel thrombosis.

Management of Cerebral Aneurysms. Cerebral aneurysms may be repaired via a craniotomy as soon as the client's condition is stabilized. Surgery may be postponed for clients with ruptured aneurysms that caused stupor or coma because their condition makes them high-risk surgical candidates. During surgery, the aneurysm is clipped or a clamp is placed at the base, or neck, of the aneurysm to prevent blood from entering the area. If the aneurysm does not have a neck, it may be wrapped with muscle, muslin, or a plastic coating to reinforce the wall and prevent rebleeding. Timing of the surgery and specific interventions are usually determined by individual physician preferences. Visitors may be limited, and measures to decrease the client's stress and increase comfort are usually initiated.

A less invasive method for treating cerebral aneurysms is interventional radiology. An interventional neuroradiologist directs a small catheter into the femoral artery and advances the catheter into the aneurysm. Specially designed, detachable platinum wire coils are advanced into the aneurysm, which helps to seal the area with a clot. It is predicted that this method will soon treat most intracranial aneurysms, thus avoiding craniotomies and their complications.

Management of Intracranial Bleeding. For some clients who have hemorrhagic strokes, blood clots may be removed via a craniotomy to relieve intracranial pressure (ICP). Particular indications for clot removal would be a progressively worsening neurologic examination and extension of the intracranial lesion with significant ICP elevation. Craniotomies are discussed on p. 1053.

Critical Thinking Challenge

The two clients who presented in the ED with possible strokes have been diagnosed through history, physical examination, and diagnostic testing. The middle-aged man has a small intracerebral bleed and a current blood pressure of 210/120. The woman has a resolving transient ischemic attack (TIA) and a current blood pressure of 160/92. Both clients are being admitted to the hospital as soon as beds are available.

1. What do you suspect is the cause of the male client's intracerebral bleed?
2. The ED techs can take vital signs as part of their responsibility. Would you delegate that activity to a tech when caring for these clients? Why or why not?
3. Which client will be your priority for nursing care? Why?
4. The female client is placed on clopidogrel (Plavix) and is given her first dose while in the ED. Why did the physician prescribe this medication for her?

evolve For suggested answer guidelines, go to http://evolve.elsevier.com/Iggy/.

IMPAIRED PHYSICAL MOBILITY; SELF-CARE DEFICIT

NOC **PLANNING: EXPECTED OUTCOMES.** The client with a stroke is expected to be able to move purposefully in his or her own environment independently, with or without assistive device. Indicators include that the following will be noncompromised in this client:

- Balance and coordination
- Gait
- Transfer performance

The client is also expected to perform basic personal care activities and household tasks. Indicators include that the client will not be compromised in the following:

- Bathing self
- Dressing self
- Feeding self
- Maintaining personal cleanliness
- Toileting
- Performing household tasks

INTERVENTIONS. Clients who have experienced a stroke may exhibit flaccid or spastic paralysis. It is not unusual for the client to have a spastic arm and flaccid leg on the affected side. The affected leg often regains function more quickly than the arm. The nurse or family member performs passive range-of-motion (ROM) exercises at least every 2 to 3 hours for the involved extremities. The client is taught how to do active ROM exercises for the unaffected side. When able, he or she may perform passive exercises on the affected side. Physical therapy consultation should be initiated on admission, and intervention should continue through discharge.

Careful positioning is necessary to maintain proper body alignment and decrease spasticity or increase muscle tone in flaccid extremities. The affected hand or lower leg may need splinting to prevent contractures. Collaborate with the physical and occupational therapists (PT/OT) to determine the most appropriate splinting technique and client positions when lying, sitting, and transferring from the bed to a chair.

A major complication of impaired physical mobility is the development of deep vein thrombosis (DVT). Provide care to prevent this complication by applying sequential compression stockings or pneumatic compression boots, changing the client's position frequently, and mobilizing the client. Always report any indications of DVT to the health care provider, and document your assessment in the client's chart.

The rehabilitation therapists also evaluate the client in the ability to perform basic activities of daily living (ADLs) and household tasks that will be performed on discharge to home. After a thorough evaluation, the PT and OT develop a treatment plan to promote client independence, with or without assistive or adaptive devices. Therapy begins in the hospital setting and continues after discharge in most cases.

DISTURBED SENSORY PERCEPTION

PLANNING: EXPECTED OUTCOMES. The major concern of clients with sensory or perceptual changes is adapting to the deficits. Therefore the client with stroke is expected to adapt to sensory or perceptual changes in vision, proprioception (position sense), and sensation and to be free from injury.

INTERVENTIONS. Clients with right hemisphere brain damage typically have difficulty with visual-perceptual or spatial-perceptual tasks. They have problems with depth and distance perception and with discrimination of right from left or up from down. Because of these problems, they have difficulty performing routine activities of daily living (ADLs). Caregivers help the client adapt to these disabilities by using frequent verbal and tactile cues and by breaking down tasks into discrete steps. Always approach the client from the unaffected side, which should face the door of the room.

The client who has experienced a stroke may have difficulties with ambulating, lack depth perception, and proprioception. Objects should be placed within the client's field of vision; a mirror may help in visualizing more of the environment. If the client has diplopia (double vision), a patch may be placed over the affected eye. Ensure a safe environment by removing clutter from the room.

The client with a left hemisphere lesion generally experiences memory deficits and may show significant changes in the ability to carry out simple tasks. To assist with memory problems, reorient the client to the month, year, day of the week, and circumstances surrounding hospital admission. Establish a routine or schedule that is as structured, repetitious, and consistent as possible. Information is presented in a simple, concise manner. A step-by-step approach is often most effective because the client can master one step before moving to the next. When possible, the family or significant other should bring in pictures and other familiar objects.

The client may be unable to plan and execute tasks in an organized manner. Apraxia, or the inability to perform previously learned motor skills or commands, may be present. Typically, the client with apraxia exhibits a slow, cautious, and hesitant behavior style. Physical therapy involvement will assist the client in compensating for loss of position sense.

UNILATERAL NEGLECT

PLANNING: EXPECTED OUTCOMES. The client with stroke is expected to adjust and use techniques to compensate for one-sided neglect.

INTERVENTIONS. Unilateral neglect, or neglect syndrome, occurs most commonly in clients who have had a right cerebral stroke. However, it can occur in any client who experiences hemianopsia, in which the vision of one or both eyes is affected. This problem places the client at additional risk for injury because of an inability to recognize his or her physical impairment or because of a lack of proprioception.

Teach the client to touch and use both sides of the body. For example, encourage the client to wash both the affected and unaffected sides of the body. When dressing, remind the client to dress the affected side first. If hemianopsia is present, teach the client to turn his or her head from side to side to expand the visual field. This scanning technique is also useful when the client is eating or ambulating.

IMPAIRED VERBAL COMMUNICATION

NOC **PLANNING: EXPECTED OUTCOMES.** Ideally, the client with a stroke is expected to receive, interpret, and express spoken, written, and nonverbal messages. However, some clients may need to develop strategies for alternative methods of communication, such as pictures or nonverbal language.

INTERVENTIONS. Language or speech problems are usually the result of a stroke involving the dominant hemisphere. The left cerebral hemisphere is the speech center in all but 15% to 20% of the population. Speech and language problems may be the result of aphasia or dysarthria. Although aphasia is caused by cerebral hemisphere damage, **dysarthria** is due to a loss of motor function to the tongue or to the muscles of speech, causing slurred speech. Involvement of the speech-language pathologist as early as possible in the hospitalization will maximize the client's chances for optimal recovery.

Aphasia can be classified in a number of ways. Most commonly, aphasia is classified as expressive, receptive, or global (mixed) (Table 48-2). **Expressive (Broca's, or motor) aphasia** is the result of damage in Broca's area of the frontal lobe. It is a motor speech problem in which the client generally understands what is said but is unable to communicate verbally. He or she also has difficulty writing. Rote speech and automatic speech, such as responses to a greeting, are often intact. The client is aware of the deficit and may become frustrated and angry.

Receptive (Wernicke's, or sensory) aphasia is due to injury involving Wernicke's area in the temporoparietal area. The client is unable to understand the spoken and often the written word. Although he or she may be able to talk, the language is often meaningless. Neologisms (made-up words) are common parts of speech.

More often, the client exhibits dysfunction in both the areas of expression and reception; this is known as a global, or mixed, aphasia. Reading and writing ability are equally affected. Few clients exhibit either expressive *or* receptive aphasia. In most cases, one type is dominant but two or more types are present.

Collaborate with the speech-language pathologist (SLP) in working with the client who has aphasia or dysarthria. The aphasic client requires repetitive directions to understand or complete a task. Each task should be broken down into component parts and given one step at a time. Face the client and speak slowly and clearly. The client should be given sufficient time to understand and process the information and to respond. Encourage the client to communicate and reinforce this behavior positively.

Family members or significant others and staff repeat the names of objects used on a routine basis. For example, state, "This is the toothbrush" when assisting the client to brush his or her teeth. If necessary, a picture board or communication board should be developed by the SLP for the client with Broca's aphasia. This board consists of a picture of an activity (e.g., someone eating) and the printed description below. The client can point to the activity or object desired.

It is difficult to understand a client with dysarthria. The same techniques used for the client with aphasia can be used for dysarthria. Facial muscle exercises may be performed to strengthen the muscles used for speech. Many clients who are dysarthric are also aphasic.

TABLE 48-2 Types of Aphasia

Expressive
- Referred to as Broca's, or motor, aphasia
- Difficulty speaking
- Difficulty writing

Receptive
- Referred to as Wernicke's, or sensory, aphasia
- Difficulty understanding spoken words
- Difficulty understanding written words
- Speech often meaningless
- Neologisms

Global (Mixed)
- Combination of difficulty understanding words and speech
- Difficulty with reading and writing

IMPAIRED SWALLOWING

NOC **PLANNING: EXPECTED OUTCOMES.** The client with a stroke is expected to have safe passage of fluids and solids from the mouth to the stomach. Indicators include that the client will have noncompromised ability to do the following:
- Maintain food in the mouth
- Handle oral secretions
- Chew
- Deliver bolus to hypopharynx in time with swallow reflex
- Clear oral cavity

INTERVENTIONS. Before feeding, assess the client's ability to swallow. Observe for facial drooping, drooling, and a weak, hoarse voice. To assess the swallowing reflex, place the thumb and the index finger on either side of the client's Adam's apple, or laryngeal protuberance, and ask him or her to swallow. You should be able to feel the larynx elevate. Next check the gag and cough reflex. Collaborate with the SLP, who specializes in swallowing evaluation, to determine the extent of the swallowing problem. In some cases, the health care provider may order a barium swallow to detect the specific cause of the swallowing problem.

Positioning the client to facilitate the swallowing process is extremely important. He or she should eat all meals sitting in a chair or sitting straight up in bed. The head and neck are positioned slightly forward and flexed. In general, clients with swallowing problems are able to tolerate or swallow soft or semisoft foods and fluids (mechanically soft or dental diet, junior baby foods, custards, scrambled eggs) better than thin liquids (water, juice, or milk) or a regular meal. Powdered thickener (Thick-It) may be added to thicken foods to a more manageable consistency.

Collaborate with the dietitian to find an appropriate diet for the client with dysphagia. Monitor the client's weight at least twice a week to ensure that he or she is receiving adequate nutrition. Supplements such as milkshakes and Ensure may be needed to meet caloric and protein requirements. Calorie counts may be necessary to evaluate nutritional intake fully.

Foods that stimulate saliva production and thus facilitate swallowing include beef broth and sweet, sour, or salty foods. Instruct the client to place food in the back of the mouth on the unaffected side to prevent trapping food in the affected cheek.

Some clients are able to swallow without difficulty but are at risk for aspiration because they are easily distracted and impulsive. These clients require a distraction-free environment with minimal disruption from television, visitors, or environmental noise. Observe for indications of fatigue because this can significantly interfere with the desire and ability to eat.

TOTAL URINARY INCONTINENCE; BOWEL INCONTINENCE

NOC **PLANNING: EXPECTED OUTCOMES.** The client with a stroke is expected to control elimination of urine and stool. Indicators include that the client will consistently demonstrate the ability to do the following:

- Recognize the urge to void and defecate
- Maintain predictable pattern of urinary and bowel elimination
- Respond to urge in timely manner
- Get to toilet between urge and passage of urine or stool
- Empty bladder and bowel completely

INTERVENTIONS. The client may be incontinent of urine and stool because of an altered level of consciousness, impaired innervation, or an inability to communicate the need to urinate or defecate. Before beginning an education program to correct these problems, the cause must first be established. Typically, the client who has had a stroke can relearn both bowel and bladder control. To begin a bladder training program, place the client on the bedpan or the commode or offer the urinal every 2 hours. Encourage a total fluid intake of at least 2000 mL daily unless contraindicated. Catheterizations to check for residual urine after voiding (postvoiding residuals) may be done in the early part of the bladder retraining program to ensure that the client is emptying the bladder. A bedside ultrasound can also be used for this purpose and is less invasive. Retained urine can lead to a urinary tract infection.

Before establishing a bowel training program, determine the client's normal time for bowel elimination and any routine that helps to ensure an acceptable evacuation. This routine is followed, if possible, and the client is placed on the bedpan or commode at the same time as the previous schedule at home. Collaborate with the dietitian to provide a diet high in bulk and fiber. Encourage the client to drink apple or prune juice to help promote bowel elimination. A stool softener (Colace) may be prescribed. Suppositories or digital stimulation may also assist in re-establishing a bowel routine. Chapter 10 provides a complete discussion of bowel and bladder training programs.

Community-Based Care

The client with a stroke without complications may be discharged within 2 to 3 days to home, a rehabilitation center, or a long-term care facility, depending on the extent of the disability and the availability of family or caregiver support. Some clients experience no significant neurologic dysfunction and are able to return home and live independently or with minimal support. Other clients are able to return home but require ongoing assistance with activities of daily living as well as supervision to prevent accidents or injury. Speech, physical, or occupational therapy may continue in the home or on an ambulatory care basis. Clients admitted to a rehabilitation or long-term care facility require continued or more complex nursing care as well as extensive physical, occupational, recreational, speech-language, or cognitive therapy, which is coordinated by a case manager. The goal of rehabilitation is to maximize the client's abilities in all aspects of life.

HOME CARE MANAGEMENT

Collaboration with the case manager is needed if the client is discharged to the home setting. Needs for assistive or adaptive and safety equipment must be identified. The extent of this assessment depends on the disabilities experienced by the client. The home of the client with hemiparesis should be free from scatter rugs or other obstacles in the walking pathways. The bathtub and toilet should be equipped with grab bars. Anti-skid patches or strips should be placed in the bathtub to prevent slipping. The PT or OT works with the client and the family or significant others to obtain all needed assistive devices *before* the client is discharged from the hospital, rehabilitation setting, or long-term care facility. Appointments for outpatient speech, physical, and occupational therapy must also be arranged before discharge. Involvement of the case manager and utilization of critical pathways have been shown to be very effective in facilitating optimal timing of diagnostic testing, consultations with SLT and physical therapy, as well as facilitating discharge to home or rehabilitation.

HEALTH TEACHING

The teaching plan for the client with a stroke includes the medication schedule, ambulation/transfer skills, communication skills, safety precautions, dietary management, activity levels, and self-care skills. Health teaching should focus on tasks that must be performed by the client and the family after hospital discharge. Provide both written and verbal instruction in all these areas. Return demonstrations assist in evaluating the family members' competency in tasks required for the client's care.

The client must take the prescribed medication to prevent another stroke and to keep hypertension under control. Teach the client and the family the name of the drug, the dosage, the timing of administration and how to take it, and possible side effects. In collaboration with the PT and OT, teach the client how to climb stairs safely, if he or she is able; transfer from the bed to a chair; get into and out of a car; and use any aids for mobility. The client and family members are also taught how to use any equipment needed to increase independence in self-care skills. The most important information provided is what to do in an emergency and whom to call for nonemergency questions.

It is not unusual for clients, particularly older white men, to become depressed within 6 months after discharge. In general, this depression is self-limiting, but the client may require antidepressants for a short time. Emotional lability is also common. The family is advised to avoid being overprotective and is assisted in establishing realistic and achievable goals.

Families may feel overwhelmed by the continuing demands placed on them. Depending on the location of the lesion, the client may be anxious, slow, cautious, hesitant, and lack initiative (left hemisphere lesions), or he or she may be impulsive and seemingly unaware of any deficit. Family members and other caregivers need to spend time away from the client on a routine basis to continue to provide full-time care without sacrificing their own physical and emotional health. Refer the family to social services for further support and counseling.

HEALTH CARE RESOURCES

Available resources include a variety of publications from the American Heart Association, including *Stroke: A Guide for Families* and *Stroke: Why Do They Behave That Way?* The National Stroke Association also provides publications and videotapes for caregivers and clients. *Recovering After a Stroke: A Patient and Family Guide* is available from the Agency for Healthcare Research and Quality (http://www.ahrq.gov), formerly the Agency for Health Care Policy and Research. Refer the client and family members or significant others to local stroke support groups.

Evaluation: Outcomes

Evaluate the care of the client with stroke on the basis of the identified nursing diagnoses and collaborative problems. The expected outcomes are that the client:

- Has an adequate blood flow through the cerebral vasculature to maintain brain function
- Moves purposefully in his or her own environment with or without assistive devices
- Learns to adapt to sensory and perceptual changes
- Adjusts and uses techniques to compensate for one-sided neglect
- Receives, interprets, and expresses messages or develops strategies for alternative communication methods
- Has safe passage of fluids and solids from the mouth to the stomach
- Controls elimination of urine and stool

Specific indicators for these outcomes are listed for each nursing diagnosis under the Planning and Implementation section (see earlier).

TRAUMATIC BRAIN INJURY

Traumatic brain injury (TBI) occurs as a result of an external force applied to the head and brain causing disruption of physiologic stability locally, at the point of injury, as well as globally with elevations in ICP and potentially dramatic changes in blood flow within and to the brain. These changes may produce a diminished or altered state of consciousness. TBI may result in the impairment of cognitive abilities or physical functioning as well as a disturbance of behavior or emotional functioning. These impairments may be either temporary or permanent and may cause partial or total functional disability or psychosocial maladjustment. In the United States, TBI has taken more lives of people 18 to 34 years of age than all other causes combined for that age group. The annual cost of care for TBI survivors in the United States is higher than that for stroke survivors.

PATHOPHYSIOLOGY

Various terms are used to describe the brain injuries that occur when a mechanical force is applied either directly or indirectly to the brain. A force produced by a blow to the head is a direct injury, whereas a force applied to another body part with a rebound effect to the brain is an indirect injury. The brain responds to these forces by movement within the rigid cranial vault. The brain may also rebound or rotate on the brainstem, causing diffuse axonal injury (shearing injuries). The moving brain may be contused or lacerated as it moves over the inner surfaces of the cranium, which is irregularly shaped and sharp. Damage most commonly occurs to the frontal and temporal lobes of the brain, especially the raised surfaces of the gyri. Movement or distortion of the brain within the cranial cavity is possible due to multiple factors. The first factor is how the brain is supported. The brain is supported by cerebrospinal fluid (CSF) within the cranial cavity. As such, when external force is applied to the head, the brain can be injured by the internal surfaces of the skull and meninges. The second factor is the consistency of brain tissue. It is exceedingly fragile and prone to injury.

Primary Brain Injury

Primary brain damage results from the physical stress (force) within the brain tissue caused by open or closed trauma. An **open head injury** occurs when there is a skull fracture or when the skull is pierced by a penetrating object. The integrity of the brain and the dura is violated, and there is exposure to outside, or environmental, contaminants. Damage may occur to the underlying vessels, dural sinus, brain, and cranial nerves. A **closed head injury** is the result of blunt trauma; the integrity of the skull is not violated. It is the more serious of the two types of injury, and the damage to brain tissue depends on the degree and mechanisms of injury.

Brain injury may also be described as mild, moderate, or severe. A Glasgow Coma Scale (GCS) score of 13 to 15 and a loss of consciousness for 0 to 15 minutes characterize a mild TBI (MTBI). A moderate TBI often includes a period of loss of consciousness (LOC) up to 6 hours and may be accompanied by other systemic injury and a GCS score of 9 to 12. A short critical care stay maybe needed for close monitoring. After injury, these clients may have difficulty with work, learning, and role function. Severe head injury (GCS score of 3 to 8 and LOC greater than 6 hours) is more serious and requires management in critical care with ongoing monitoring of multiple physiologic parameters, including hemodynamic stability and intracranial pressure (ICP).

OPEN HEAD INJURY

The types of fractures associated with an open head injury are linear, depressed, open, and comminuted. A **linear fracture** is a simple, clean break in which the impacted area of bone bends inward and the area around it bends outward; linear fractures account for about 80% of all skull fractures. In a **depressed fracture,** the bone is pressed inward into the brain tissue to at least the thickness of the skull. In an **open fracture,** the scalp is lacerated, creating a direct opening to the brain tissue. A **comminuted fracture** involves fragmentation of the bone with depression of bone into the brain tissue.

A unique fracture is a basilar skull fracture. It occurs at the base of the skull, usually extending into the anterior, middle, or posterior fossa and results in cerebrospinal fluid (CSF) leakage from the nose or ears. Of significance with this fracture is the potential development of hemorrhage caused by damage to the internal carotid artery; damage to cranial nerves (CN) I, II, VII, and VIII; and infection.

Most penetrating injuries to the skull are caused by gunshot wounds (GSWs) and knife injuries. The degree of injury to brain tissue depends on the velocity, mass, shape, and direction of impact. High-velocity injuries produce the greatest damage to brain tissue. As with any open head injury, the client with a penetrating injury is at high risk for infection from the object that pierced the skull and from other environmental contaminants.

CLOSED HEAD INJURY

Closed head injuries are caused by blunt trauma and lead to concussions, contusions, and lacerations of the brain. The damage to the brain may be mild, as occurs in a concussive injury, or it may be more severe, causing diffuse axonal injury or widespread injury to the white matter of the brain.

A **mild concussion** is characterized by a brief LOC. Possibly as many as 30% of these clients experience "post-concussion" syndrome (PCS). The mechanism of injury is typically acceleration/deceleration with shearing stress on the reticular formation. PCS symptoms may include headache, irritability, memory deficits, fatigue and sleep disturbances, and depression (Mateo, 2003). Severity of concussion is measured by duration of unconsciousness.

Diffuse axonal injury (DAI) is usually related to high-speed acceleration/deceleration as with automobile accidents. In DAI significant damage occurs to axons in the white matter. Lesions may also be found in the corpus callosum, midbrain, cerebellum, and upper brainstem. Depending on severity, small areas of hemorrhage may be found on computed tomography (CT) scanning followed by possible enlargement of the lateral ventricles. Severe DAI may present with immediate coma, and most survivors require long-term care.

A **contusion** is a bruising of the brain tissue and is most commonly found at the site of impact (coup injury) or in a line opposite the site of impact **(contrecoup injury)** (Figure 48-6). The base of the frontal and temporal lobes is most often involved.

A **laceration** causes actual tearing of the cortical surface vessels, which may lead to secondary hemorrhage and significant cerebral edema and inflammation. This condition is more serious than a contusion.

Types of Force

Other factors that must be considered in the dynamics of head injury are the type of force and the mechanisms of injury involved (Figure 48-7). An **acceleration injury** is caused by an external force contacting the head, suddenly placing the head in motion. A **deceleration injury** occurs when the moving head is suddenly stopped or hits a stationary object. These forces may be sufficient to cause the cerebrum to rotate about the brainstem, resulting in shearing, straining, and distortion of the brain tissue, particularly of the axons in the brainstem and cerebellum. Small areas of hemorrhage may develop around the blood vessels that sustain the impact of these forces (stress), with destruction of adjacent brain tissue. Particularly affected are the basal nuclei and the hypothalamus.

Secondary Responses and Insults

Secondary responses to brain injury include any neurologic damage that occurs after the initial injury. Secondary injuries or responses increase the morbidity and mortality after head trauma. The most common response is the development of increased intracranial pressure (ICP) attributable to edema, hemorrhage, hematoma development, impaired cerebral autoregulation, or hydrocephalus. Hypoxemia, hypercapnia (increased carbon dioxide), or systemic hypotension may precipitate increased ICP. Damage to the brain tissue occurs primarily because the delivery of oxygen and glucose to the brain is interrupted.

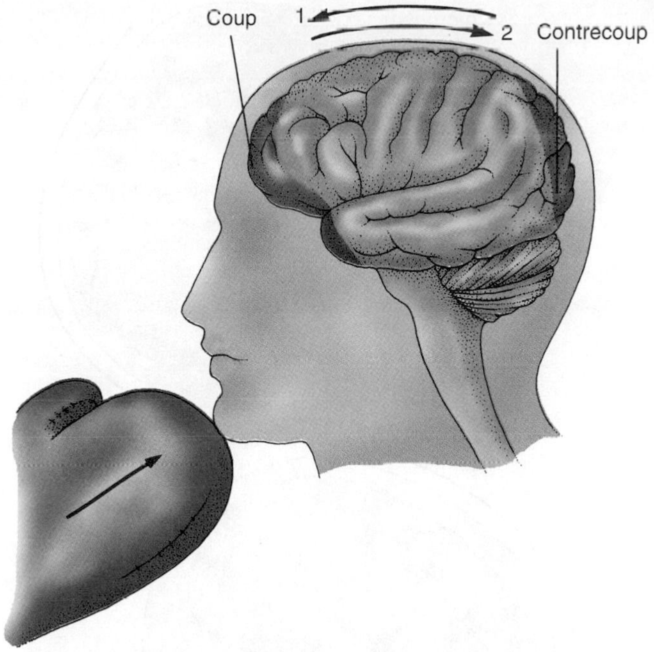

Figure 48-6 ■ Coup (site of impact) injury to frontal area of brain, and contrecoup injury to frontal and temporal areas of the brain.

INCREASED INTRACRANIAL PRESSURE

The cranial contents include brain tissue, blood, and cerebrospinal fluid (CSF). These components are encased in the relatively rigid skull. Within this space, there is little room for any of the components to expand or increase in volume. Through the processes of accommodation and compliance, ICP is maintained at its normal level of 10 to 15 mm Hg despite transient increases in pressure that occur with straining during defecation, coughing, or sneezing. According to the Monro-Kellie hypothesis, any increase in the volume of one component must be compensated for by a decrease in the volume of one of the other components.

As a first response to an increase in the volume of any of these components, the CSF is shunted or displaced from the cranial compartment to the spinal subarachnoid space or the rate of CSF absorption is increased. An additional response, if needed, is a decrease in cerebral blood volume by displacement of cerebral venous blood into the sinuses. As long as the brain is able to compensate for the increase in volume and remain compliant, increases in ICP are minimal.

Increased ICP is the leading cause of death from head trauma in clients who reach the hospital alive. It occurs when compliance no longer takes place and the brain cannot accommodate further volume changes. As ICP increases, cerebral perfusion decreases, leading to tissue hypoxia, a decrease in serum pH level, and an increase in the level of carbon dioxide. This process causes cerebral vasodilation, edema, and a

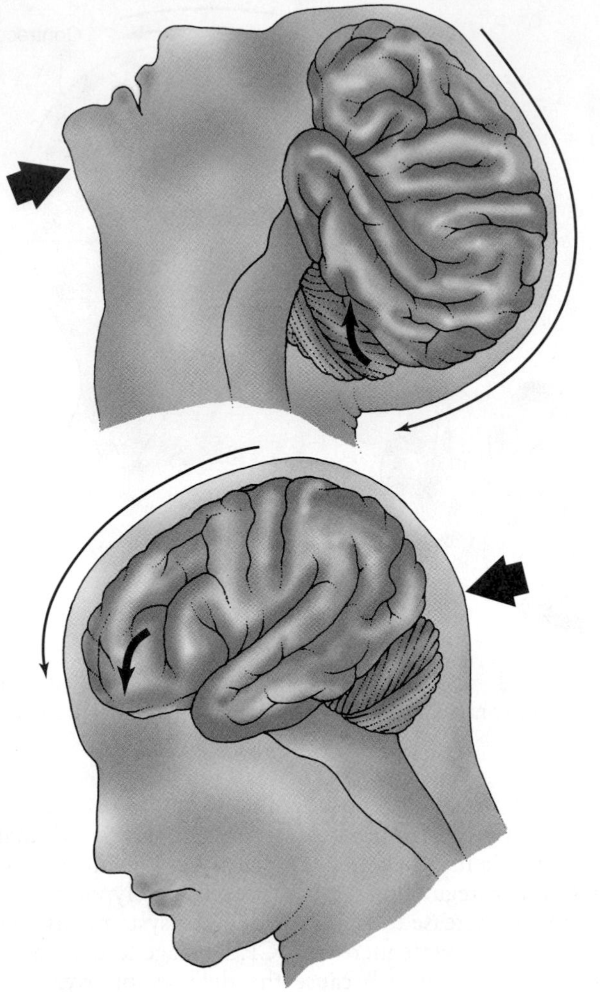

Figure 48-7 ■ Head movement during acceleration-deceleration injury, which is typically seen in motor vehicle accidents.

further increase in ICP, and the cycle continues. If the condition remains untreated, the brain may herniate downward toward the brainstem or laterally from a unilateral lesion within one cerebral hemisphere, causing irreversible brain damage and possibly death **(brain herniation syndromes).**

Two types of edema may cause increased ICP: vasogenic edema and cytotoxic edema. A third type (interstitial edema) occurs in the presence of acute brain swelling. Vasogenic edema is seen most often as a cause of increased ICP in the adult. It is characterized by an increase in the volume of brain tissue. This increase is caused by an abnormal permeability of the walls of the cerebral vessels, which allows protein-rich plasma infiltrate to leak into the extracellular space of the brain. The fluid collects primarily in the white matter.

Cytotoxic, or cellular, edema may occur as a result of a hypoxic insult, which causes a disturbance in cellular metabolism, the sodium pump, and active ion transport. The brain is quickly depleted of available oxygen, glucose, and glycogen and converts to anaerobic metabolism. The sodium pump fails, and sodium enters the cells and pulls water from the extracellular space. A concomitant decrease occurs in the serum sodium level to less than 120 mEq/L. As a result, an abnormal accumulation of fluid in the brain cells and a decrease in the extracellular fluid space occur. Cytotoxic edema may lead to vasogenic edema and a further increase in ICP.

Interstitial edema occurs in the presence of acute brain swelling and is associated with elevated blood pressure or increased CSF pressure. Edema develops rapidly in the perivascular and periventricular white space and can be controlled through measures to reduce blood pressure, decrease CSF pressures, or increase the **cerebral perfusion pressure (CPP).** The CPP is the pressure gradient over which the brain is perfused. It is influenced by oxygenation, cerebral blood volume, blood pressure, cerebral edema, and ICP and is determined by subtracting the mean ICP from the mean arterial pressure. Maintenance of a CPP above 70 mm Hg is generally accepted as an appropriate goal of therapy.

HEMORRHAGE

Hemorrhages, which cause brain hematoma or clot formation, may occur as part of the primary injury and begin at the moment of impact. They may also be a secondary event arising from vessel damage and occur somewhat later or worsen later in the client's clinical course. Classically they are caused by vascular damage from the shearing force of the trauma or direct physical damage from skull fractures or penetrating injury. All hematomas are potentially life threatening because they act as space-occupying lesions and are surrounded by edema. Three types of hemorrhages include **epidural, subdural, and intracerebral hemorrhage**. Subarachnoid hemorrhage may also occur following head trauma. The pathophysiology of subarachnoid hemorrhage is discussed under Stroke earlier in this chapter.

EPIDURAL HEMATOMA. An **epidural hematoma** results from arterial bleeding into the space between the dura and the inner table of the skull (Figure 48-8). It is often caused by a fracture of the temporal bone, which houses the middle meningeal artery. Epidural hematomas may be characterized by the presence of a "lucid interval" that lasts for minutes, during which time the client is awake and talking. This follows a momentary unconsciousness that occurred within minutes of the injury. Following the initial lucid interval, symptoms progress very quickly with potentially catastrophic ICP elevation and structural changes. The client becomes increasingly symptomatic, loses consciousness, and may become increasingly unstable. An epidural hematoma is a neurosurgical emergency.

SUBDURAL HEMATOMA. A **subdural hematoma (SDH)** results typically from venous bleeding into the space beneath the dura and above the arachnoid (see Figure 48-8). It results most often from a tearing of the bridging veins within the cerebral hemispheres or from a laceration of brain tissue. Bleeding from this injury occurs more slowly than from an epidural hematoma and mirrors the slower development of symptoms. SDHs are subdivided into acute, subacute, and chronic. An acute SDH presents within 48 hours after impact; the subacute SDH, between 48 hours and 2 weeks; and the chronic SDH, from 2 weeks to several months following injury. SDHs have the highest mortality rate.

INTRACEREBRAL HEMORRHAGE. An intracerebral hemorrhage (ICH) is the accumulation of blood within the brain tissue caused by the tearing of small arteries and veins in the subcortical white matter (see Figure 48-8). ICH may act as a space-occupying lesion and may be potentially devastating, depending on its location. ICH may also produce significant brain edema and ICP elevations. A brainstem hemorrhage occurs as a result of direct trauma, fractures, or torsion injuries to the brainstem.

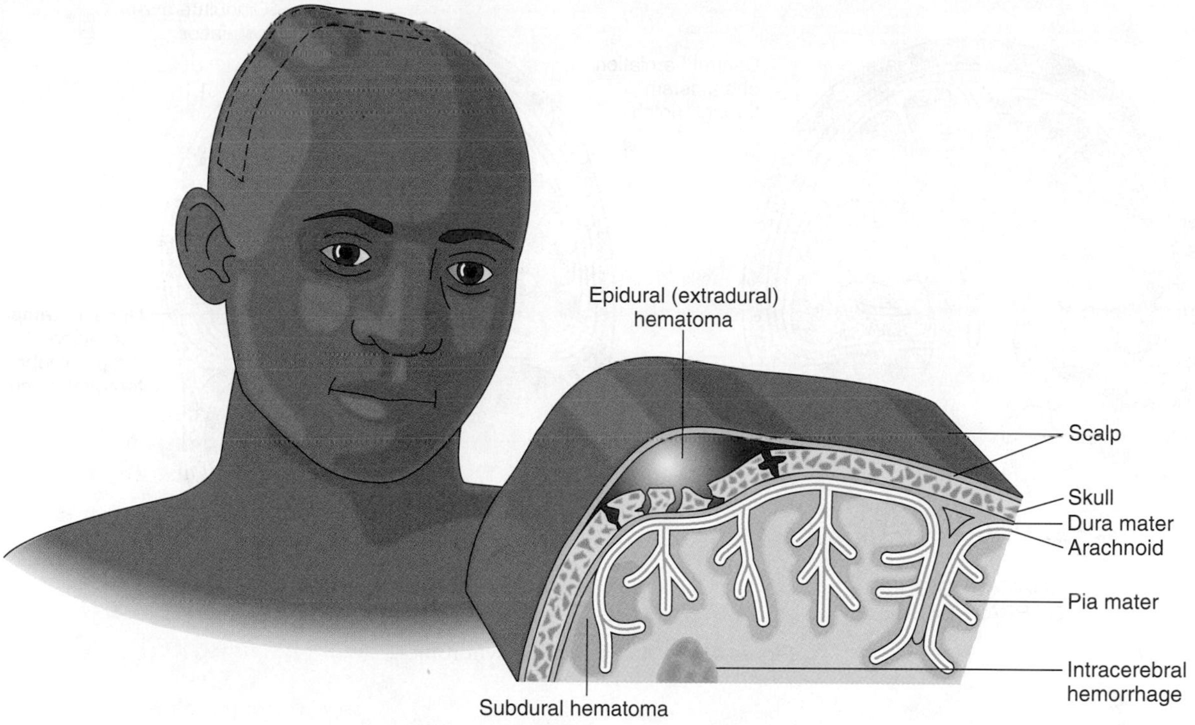

Figure 48-8 ■ Epidural hematoma (outside the dura mater of the brain), subdural hematoma (under the dura mater), and intracerebral hemorrhage (within the brain tissue).

LOSS OF AUTOREGULATION

Through the process of cerebral autoregulation, blood flow to the brain remains relatively constant despite variations in systemic blood pressure. A loss of autoregulation causes the cerebral blood flow to fluctuate passively with the systemic blood pressure. Systemic hypertension may cause an increase in ICP (from an increase in cerebral blood flow) and the potential for vasogenic edema. Hypoxemia and hypercapnia cause marked cerebral vasodilation and therefore an increase in cerebral blood flow, which contributes to increased ICP.

HYDROCEPHALUS

Hydrocephalus is an abnormal increase in CSF volume. It may caused by impaired reabsorption of CSF at the arachnoid villi (from subarachnoid hemorrhage or meningitis). This is called a communicating hydrocephalus. It may also be caused by interference or blockage with CSF outflow from the ventricular system (from cerebral edema, tumor or debris). The ventricles may dilate from the relative increase in CSF volume. Ultimately, if not treated, this increase in CSF volume may lead to increased ICP.

BRAIN HERNIATION

In the presence of increased ICP, the brain tissue may shift and herniate downward. Of the several types of herniation syndromes (Figure 48-9), uncal (transtentorial) herniation is one of the most clinically significant because it is life threatening. It is caused by a shift of one or both areas of the temporal lobe, known as the uncus. This shift creates pressure on the third cranial nerve. Late findings include dilated and nonreactive pupils, ptosis, and a rapidly deteriorating level of consciousness. Central herniation is caused by a downward shift of the brainstem and the diencephalon from a supratentorial lesion. It is clinically manifested by Cheyne-Stokes respirations, pinpoint and nonreactive pupils, and potential hemodynamic instability.

A shift of the cingulate gyrus below the falx cerebri is known as cingulate herniation. Cingulate herniation is diagnosed most frequently on head computed tomography (CT). It is a sign of brain decompensation and poor intracranial compliance. A type of infratentorial herniation, cerebellar tonsillar herniation, occurs when the cerebellar tonsils shift and compress the medulla. This may lead to respiratory and cardiovascular compromise or arrest. All herniation syndromes are potentially life threatening, and the physician must be notified immediately when they are suspected.

Etiology

The most common causes of traumatic brain injury (TBI) in the United States are accidents involving motor vehicles, including both automobiles and motorcycles. All too often, alcohol and drugs are contributing factors to the accident. Falls, acts of violence, and sports-related injuries are the next most common causes.

Incidence/Prevalence

Each year seven million people in the United States sustain some type of TBI. Of these, 500,000 require hospitalization and 100,000 are permanently disabled, with 2000 remaining in a persistent vegetative state (Hickey, 2003). Summer and spring months, evenings, nights, and weekends are associated with the greatest number of injuries.

HEALTH PROMOTION/ILLNESS PREVENTION

Head injuries occur three times more often in males than in females. Males tend to play more sports, take more risks when

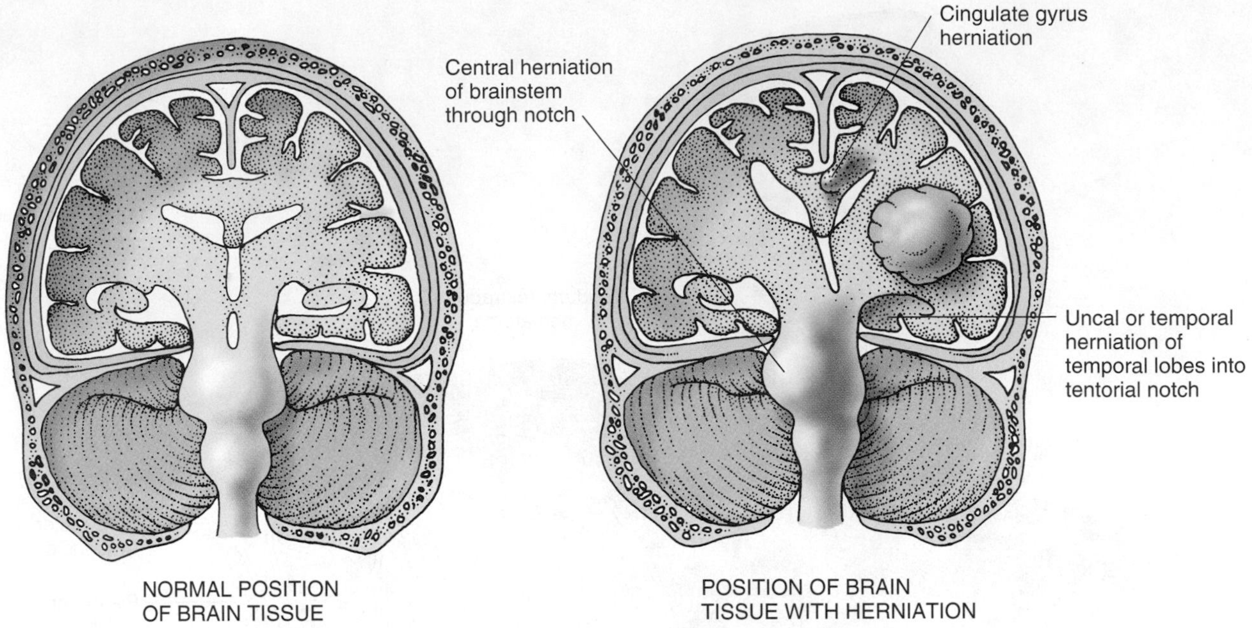

Figure 48-9 ■ Herniation syndromes.

driving, and consume large amounts of alcohol. More than 70% of these injuries occur in people between 10 and 39 years of age. Therefore, teach adolescents and young adults to do the following:

- Avoid driving when drinking.
- Follow the game rules for sports.
- Be cautious when engaging in sports (e.g., do not try to "show off" on ski slopes).
- Avoid vehicular speeding.
- Wear helmet and other protective gear when engaging in contact sports or driving motorcycles/all-terrain vehicles (ATVs).
- Avoid dangerous risk-taking activities unless trained to participate in them.

COLLABORATIVE MANAGEMENT

Assessment

HISTORY

Obtaining an accurate history from a client who has sustained craniocerebral trauma may be difficult because of either the seriousness of the injury or the presence of amnesia. It is not unusual for the client to experience **amnesia** (loss of memory) for the events before or after the injury. The client with a serious head injury is often admitted to the hospital unconscious or in a confused and combative state. If the client is unable to provide information, the history can be obtained from rescue workers or witnesses to the injury. Always ask when, where, and how the injury occurred. Did the client lose consciousness? If so, for how long? Has there been a change in the level of consciousness (LOC)? If trauma is related to drug or alcohol intoxication, it may be difficult to differentiate neurologic changes from head trauma from those produced by intoxication.

Obtain as much information about the events as possible immediately after the injury. Clients with a severe injury may have several different presentations. The client may be completely unresponsive after the injury; alternatively, the client may initially be responsive and deteriorate rapidly within a few minutes to several hours. In another typical presentation, the client is initially unconscious for a few minutes as a result of the primary brain injury, returns to a normal level of consciousness, and then rapidly deteriorates as a consequence of secondary insult to the brain.

Determine whether the client experienced any seizure activity before or after the injury and whether there is a history of a seizure disorder. It is important to obtain precise information about the circumstances of falls, particularly in the older client (Chart 48-7). Other pertinent information includes hand dominance, any diseases of or injuries to the eyes, and any allergies to medications or food, particularly seafood. People allergic to seafood are often allergic to the intravenous (IV) contrast media used in diagnostic tests. Inquire about a history of alcohol or drug use and abuse because drugs or alcohol may mask the symptoms of increased ICP.

PHYSICAL ASSESSMENT/CLINICAL MANIFESTATIONS

No two injuries are alike. The client with a TBI may have a variety of manifestations depending on the severity of injury and the resulting increase in intracranial pressure (ICP) (see Chart 48-5). The goals of the nursing assessment are the establishment of baseline data and the early detection of and prevention of increased ICP, systemic hypotension, hypoxia, or hypercapnia (increased blood levels of carbon dioxide). The early detection of subtle changes in the client's neurologic status enables the health care team to prevent or treat potentially life-threatening complications.

Because it is estimated that 5% to 20% of clients with TBI have associated cervical spinal cord injuries, all clients with head trauma are treated as though they have spinal cord injury until radiographic studies prove otherwise. Assess for indicators of spinal cord injury, such as loss of motor and sensory function, tenderness along the spine, and abnormal head tilt. The client may experience respiratory problems and diaphragmatic breathing, and his or her re-

CHART 48-7

NURSING FOCUS on the OLDER ADULT
Head Injury

- Head injury is the fifth leading cause of death in older adults.
- The 65- to 75-year age-group has second highest incidence of head injury of all age-groups.
- Falls and motor vehicle accidents are the most common cause of head injury.
- The following factors contribute to high mortality:
  - Falls causing subdural hematomas (closed head injuries), especially chronic subdural hematomas
  - Poorly tolerated systemic stress, which is increased by admission to a high-stimuli environment
  - Medical complications, such as hypotension, hypertension, and cardiac problems
  - Decreased protective mechanisms, which make clients susceptible to infections (especially pneumonia)
  - Decreased immunologic competence, which is further diminished by head injury

flexes may be diminished or absent. The client may also experience severe hemodynamic instability from an existing spinal cord injury.

AIRWAY AND BREATHING PATTERN ASSESSMENT. The *first priority* is the assessment of the client's airway and breathing pattern. Hypoxia and hypercapnia are best detected through arterial blood gas analysis, but the nursing assessment is vital to identify the client at risk for respiratory-related complications. Direct observation of chest wall movement and lung auscultation are paramount. Any suspicion of respiratory inadequacy should be reported immediately to the physician. The client's lung ventilation should be supported as appropriate, and they may need controlled ventilation through an endotracheal tube. Injuries to the brainstem may cause a change in the client's breathing pattern, such as Cheyne-Stokes respirations, central neurogenic hyperventilation, and/or apnea.

VITAL SIGNS ASSESSMENT. The mechanisms of autoregulation are often impaired as the result of craniocerebral trauma. The more serious the injury, the more severe the impact on autoregulation. Depending on the severity of the injury, the nurse or assistive nursing personnel monitors the client's blood pressure and pulse to detect possible changes in cerebral blood flow caused by impaired autoregulation as a result of hypotension or hypertension. The **Cushing reflex,** a classic yet late sign of increased ICP, is manifested by severe hypertension with a widened pulse pressure and bradycardia. As ICP increases, the pulse becomes thready, irregular, and rapid. Cerebral blood flow increases in response to hypertension, and vasogenic edema may occur, further increasing ICP. In contrast, hypotension and tachycardia are symptomatic of hypovolemic shock. This decrease in blood volume may lead to decreased cerebral perfusion pressure and eventually to ischemia and infarct of the brain tissue.

Hypovolemic shock is usually due to intra-abdominal bleeding or bleeding into the soft tissue around major fractures–not to intracranial bleeding. Cardiac dysrhythmias may result from chest trauma, bruising of the heart, or interference with the autonomic nervous system. Cardiac dysrhythmias may also result from severe ICP elevations and brainstem pressure.

NEUROLOGIC ASSESSMENT. Many hospitals use the Glasgow Coma Scale to assess neurologic status (see Chapter 44). The *most important* variable to assess is level of consciousness. A decrease or change in level of consciousness is typically the *first sign* of deterioration in neurologic status. Changes in consciousness or orientation are due to injury to the cerebral cortex and may also involve damage to the reticular formation. A decrease in arousal or increased sleepiness and coma are caused by pressure on the reticular activating system within the brainstem. Early indicators of a change in level of consciousness include behavior changes (e.g., restlessness or irritability), which are often subtle in nature.

EYE ASSESSMENT. Elicit a history of previous eye injury or medications that affect pupillary dilation and constriction, such as anticholinergics and adrenergics. Check pupils for size and reaction to light. Any changes in pupil size, shape, and reactivity must be reported to the health care provider immediately because such changes indicate an increase in ICP. Pupillary changes or eye signs differ depending on which areas of the brain are damaged. Pinpoint and nonresponsive pupils are indicative of brainstem dysfunction at the level of the pons. Of particular importance is the **ovoid pupil,** which is regarded as the midstage between a normal-sized pupil and a dilated pupil. This finding indicates the development of increased ICP. Pupils that are fixed (nonreactive) and dilated are a poor prognostic sign, resulting from a marked increase in ICP. Clients with this problem are sometimes referred to as having "blown" pupils.

Check gross vision if the client's condition permits. Have the client read any printed material (e.g., the nurse's name tag) or count the number of fingers that you hold within the client's visual field. Loss of vision is usually caused by injury to the occipital lobe, which produces temporary cortical blindness.

If the client is able to cooperate, the health care provider or neurosurgical nurse tests CN III, IV, and VI. Extraocular movements may be diminished because of the presence of increased ICP and hydrocephalus. Damage to the optic chiasm, optic tract, or optic radii may cause visual-field deficits or diplopia. In the unconscious client, additional oculocephalic and oculovestibular tests are performed to test the integrity of the brainstem and of CN III, VI, and VII.

MOTOR ASSESSMENT. Assess for bilateral motor responses to avoid missing lateralizing signs. The client's motor loss or dysfunction usually appears contralateral to the site of the lesion. For example, a left-sided hemiparesis is indicative of an injury to the right cerebral hemisphere. A deterioration in motor function or the development of abnormal posturing **(decerebrate** or **decorticate posturing)** or flaccidity is another indicator of increased ICP. These changes are attributable to dysfunction within the pyramidal system or cerebral peduncles. Brainstem or cerebellar injury may cause ataxia, decreased or increased muscle tone, and weakness.

ADDITIONAL NEUROLOGIC ASSESSMENT. If the client is able to cooperate, a full neurologic assessment is completed as outlined in Chapter 44. Particular attention is given to cranial nerves I, V, VII, IX, and X. The first cranial nerve is often damaged where the frontal lobe passes over the irregularly shaped bones of the anterior and middle fossa; this results in the loss of smell (anosmia). CN V, VII, IX, and X are important for chewing and swallowing abilities and phonation. The client's ability to speak must be assessed, with particular attention directed toward differentiating aphasias (caused by injury to the cerebral cortex) from communication impairments (caused by damage to the cranial nerves and cerebellum). Damage to the cranial nerves occurs from disruption of the nerve trunk, either intracranially or along its extracranial course in the skull or face. Cranial nerve damage may result from direct trauma or compression associated with pressure or hemorrhage.

Assess for additional signs of increased ICP (see Chart 48-5). These include severe headache, nausea, vomiting, seizures, and papilledema (seen by ophthalmoscopic examination). **Papilledema,** also known as a **choked disc,** is edema and hyperemia of the optic disc. It is always a sign of increased ICP. Headache and seizures are a response to the injury and may or may not be associated with increased ICP. Findings on the neurologic examination should be interpreted over time, in response to interventions, and may also indicate progression of injury. Always remember that the client with a head injury is at risk for potentially devastating ICP elevations.

Carefully observe the client's ears and nose for any signs of cerebrospinal fluid (CSF) leaks that result from a basilar skull fracture. CSF placed on a white absorbent background can be distinguished from other fluids by the "halo" sign, a yellowish stain surrounded by bloody drainage. CSF tests positively for glucose when a strip testing method (Dipstix) is used, but this method of determining a CSF leak is not always reliable. If there is a CSF leak, the client should be assessed for any signs of **nuchal rigidity** (stiff neck), which may indicate infection or blood in the CSF. Nuchal rigidity is not checked until a spinal cord injury has been ruled out.

The client's head is palpated carefully to detect the presence of fractures or hematomas. The nurse looks for areas of ecchymosis (bruising), tender areas of the scalp, and lacerations.

Clients with a *minor* head injury should be assessed for manifestations of post-concussion syndrome. Symptoms include a wide array of physical and cognitive problems that range from persistent headache, weakness, and dizziness to personality and behavior changes, loss of memory, and problems with perception, reasoning abilities, and concept formation. The symptoms may persist for a few days or weeks to several months after the injury. For some clients, severe physical and cognitive problems remain despite a relatively benign initial clinical presentation and normal diagnostic test findings.

PSYCHOSOCIAL ASSESSMENT

The person who has had a moderate or severe head injury is never the same as before the injury. Most often, the client with a major head injury has personality changes manifested by temper outbursts, depression, risk-taking behavior, and denial of disability. The client may become talkative and develop a very outgoing personality. Memory, especially recent or short-term memory, is affected and should not be confused with problems of aphasia. The ability to learn new information and concentration may be affected. Finally, the client may exhibit problems with insight and planning. All these problems may lead to difficulties within the family structure and with social and work-related interactions. Coping strategies that have been used in the past must be assessed to determine the client's ability to adapt to the changes in physical and cognitive abilities. Although they have no focal signs, clients with a mild head injury may still have symptoms of disability 1 year after injury.

Assess family dynamics, particularly if the client is discharged to the family's care directly from the acute care hospital. The family or significant others must also cope with changes in the client's physical appearance and cognitive abilities. Many families are angry with the client for being injured, especially when his or her behavior or their own behavior resulted in an injury that could have been prevented. They may feel guilty that they did not or were not able to prevent the injury. The family or significant others may feel overwhelmed by the complexity of care required and the long recovery period. Both the family and the client need to develop coping strategies to deal with the potential role reversals and role changes caused by the injury. Consultation with social services or utilization of available counseling services may assist the family in developing appropriate coping strategies.

Critical Thinking Challenge

A female college student who had been treated for clinical depression attempted suicide by jumping from her fourth-floor dormitory room. Although she has multiple orthopedic injuries, she sustained only a mild traumatic brain injury (MTBI). You are assigned to care for her in the step-down surgical unit. When you enter her room, you find that her family is visiting and she is crying.

1. What should you do at this time? Give a rationale for your answer.
2. What are some reasons she is so upset? (Think of all the possibilities.)
3. The neurologist explained to the client's mother that she could have long-lasting neurologic problems as a result of the MTBI. What problems might she have, and how might they compound her existing health problems?

evolve For suggested answer guidelines, go to http://evolve.elsevier.com/Iggy/.

LABORATORY ASSESSMENT

There are no laboratory tests to diagnose a primary brain injury; however, several laboratory tests are used to diagnose or indicate measures to prevent secondary brain insult. Arterial blood gases (ABGs) are analyzed, with particular attention given to oxygen and carbon dioxide levels. The health care provider also orders a complete blood count (CBC) and determination of serum glucose and electrolyte levels and osmolarity. These tests are performed to monitor hemodynamic status or to identify electrolyte imbalance or the presence of infection. Severe electrolyte imbalances can also contribute to secondary injury as well as increase the risk of seizures.

RADIOGRAPHIC ASSESSMENT

The health care provider immediately orders computed tomography (CT) scanning to identify the extent and scope of injury to the brain. This diagnostic test can identify the presence of a lesion that requires surgical intervention, such as epidural or subdural hematoma. Radiography and CT scanning of the cervical spine and the skull are done to rule out fractures and dislocations. A chest x-ray is done to identify fractured ribs or other chest injuries. A flat plate of the abdomen, abdominal ultrasound, or abdominal CT may be obtained to assist in the diagnosis of abdominal bleeding or bowel laceration.

OTHER DIAGNOSTIC ASSESSMENTS

Magnetic resonance imaging (MRI) is particularly useful in the diagnosis of diffuse axonal injury, but it is not recommended for clients with ICP monitoring devices or other invasive monitoring devices. As the client's condition stabilizes, the physician may order other diagnostic tests to identify the extent of injury to the brain. For example, the integrity of the cerebral vessels is measured through the use of Doppler flow studies or an arteriogram; cerebral perfusion is measured by cerebral blood flow studies. Evoked potentials provide information on the functioning sensory pathways and may be useful in predicting outcome.

Interventions

The client with a *severe* head injury is admitted to the critical care unit or a trauma center. Clients with moderate head injuries are admitted to either the general nursing unit or the critical care unit, where they are closely observed for at least 24 hours. Clients with mild TBI may possibly be sent home from the emergency department with instructions (Chart 48-8).

NONSURGICAL MANAGEMENT. Nursing interventions for all clients with a head injury are directed toward preventing or detecting increased ICP, promoting fluid and electrolyte balance, and monitoring the effects of treatments and medications.

Assessment of Vital Signs. Take and record the client's vital signs at least every 1 to 2 hours and as indicated based on client acuity. The health care provider may prescribe medications to prevent severe hypertension or hypotension. The client in the critical care unit is connected to a cardiac monitor to detect any cardiac dysrhythmias. Nonspecific ST-segment or T-wave changes may occur, possibly in response to stimulation of the autonomic nervous system or an increase in the level of circulating catecholamines. Documents and report cardiac irregularities to the health care provider.

The client with a head injury is often admitted with a fever—a defense mechanism in the presence of trauma or an indication of inflammatory response. Fever as a consequence of infection may develop later in the course of the disease. A third cause of fever is a central fever caused by hypothalamic damage. It is manifested by an absence of sweating and no diurnal (daily) variation; this type of fever is high and lasts several days to weeks. In addition, this type of fever responds better to cooling (hypothermia blanket, sponge bath) than to the administration of antipyretic drugs such as acetaminophen (Tylenol, Ace-Tabs✱).

Positioning. Position the client to avoid extreme flexion or extension of the neck and to maintain the head in the midline, neutral position. Log roll the client during turning to avoid extreme hip flexion, and keep the head of the bed elevated at least 30 degrees or as recommended by the health care provider. Head positioning should be based on both intracranial pressure (ICP) and systemic blood pressure. If increasing head elevation lowers ICP but also significantly lowers systemic blood pressure, the client does not benefit and may actually be harmed. Base head elevation on cerebral perfusion pressure when possible. All these measures enhance venous drainage, which helps prevent increased ICP.

Pulmonary Ventilation and Management. Prophylactic hyperventilation during the first 20 hours after injury is usually avoided because it may produce ischemia by causing cerebral vasoconstriction with a resulting decrease in cerebral blood volume and ICP. In acute neurologic deterioration, however, hyperventilation may be used for brief periods of central ICP elevations pending use of other therapies.

The client who requires mechanical ventilation is ventilated to maintain a partial pressure of arterial carbon dioxide ($Paco_2$) of about 35 mm Hg. One major goal is to prevent hypercarbia. Carbon dioxide is a very potent vasodilator that can contribute to increases in ICP. The $Paco_2$ must not be allowed to fall significantly, which may result in tissue hypoxia caused by *severe* vasoconstriction. Arterial oxygen levels (Pao_2) are maintained between 80 and 100 mm Hg to prevent cerebral vasodilation resulting from hypoxemia. Arterial blood gas values are monitored at least twice daily and after each change in the ventilator setting.

Pulmonary secretions tend to pool as the result of a decreased level of consciousness, an ineffective cough, or an altered breathing pattern. The secretions may be thick because of the diuretics or fluid intake restriction that may be used to prevent cerebral edema. Chest physiotherapy and frequent turning may be needed as indicated by the results of the respiratory assessment, with close attention given to the ICP response.

The client with increased ICP should be carefully observed when suctioned. If the client is intubated, he or she should be manually hyperventilated carefully with 100% oxygen before each pass of the catheter. Overly aggressive hyperventilation with endotracheal suctioning may be dangerous because of the cerebral vasoconstriction caused by even transient hypocapnia (low arterial carbon dioxide levels). This may increase the risk of cerebral ischemia as a secondary event. The

CHART 48-8

CLIENT EDUCATION GUIDE
Minor Head Injury

- If the person is sleeping, wake him or her every 3 to 4 hours for the first 2 days, asking his or her name, where he or she is, and the name of the caregiver.
- Expect the person to complain of headache, nausea, or dizziness for at least 24 hours. If these symptoms are severe or do not improve, contact the physician immediately or take the person back to the emergency department.
- For a headache, give acetaminophen (Tylenol) every 4 hours as needed.
- Avoid giving the person sedatives, sleeping pills, or alcoholic beverages for at least 24 hours unless the physician instructs otherwise.
- Do not allow the person to engage in strenuous activity for at least 48 hours.
- Do not allow nose blowing or ear cleaning for 48 hours.
- If any of the following symptoms occur, take the person back to the emergency department immediately:
  - Blurred vision
  - Drainage from the ear or nose
  - Weakness
  - Slurred speech
  - Progressive sleepiness
  - Vomiting
  - Worsening headache
  - Unequal pupil size
- Keep follow-up appointments with the health care provider.

client should be allowed a rest period of a few minutes after suctioning to prevent increased ICP. Lidocaine given IV or endotracheally may be used to suppress the cough reflex, which would increase ICP.

Drug Therapy. Glucocorticoids (dexamethasone [Decadron, Dexasone]) and methylprednisolone sodium succinate [Solu-Medrol, Medrol]) have no demonstrated benefit in the management of increased ICP as a result of head injury or cerebral infarction. Mannitol (Osmitrol), an **osmotic diuretic,** is used to treat cerebral edema by pulling water out of the extracellular space of the edematous brain tissue, but it does not cross the blood-brain barrier. It is most effective when given in boluses rather than as a continuous infusion. Furosemide (Lasix), a loop diuretic, is often used as adjunctive therapy to reduce the incidence of rebound from mannitol and also enhances its therapeutic action. Furosemide also reduces edema and blood volume, decreases sodium uptake by the brain, and decreases the production of CSF at the choroid plexus.

Administer mannitol through a filter in the IV tubing or, if given by IV push, draw it up through a filtered needle to eliminate microscopic crystals. Monitor the client receiving either osmotic or loop diuretics for intake and output and severe dehydration as well as for indications of acute renal failure, weakness, edema, and changes in urine output. Serum electrolyte and osmolarity levels are measured every 6 hours. Mannitol is used to obtain a serum osmolarity of 310 to 320 mOsm/L, depending on physician preference and the goals of therapy. A Foley catheter must be inserted to maintain strict measurement of output. The client's serum and urine osmolarity are checked daily.

Opioids, such as morphine sulfate or fentanyl citrate, may be used with ventilated clients to decrease agitation and control restlessness if the agitation is caused by pain. Fentanyl has fewer hemodynamic consequences than morphine and may therefore be a safer agent to manage pain. These agents may be reversed with naloxone (Narcan), but opioid reversal should be avoided if at all possible to reduce risk of withdrawal and rebound pain and agitation. Sedatives such as lorazepam (Ativan) and midazolam (Versed) may be used for anxiety to promote comfort and treat agitation. Sedatives and opioids may mask the neurologic assessment and potentially lower blood pressure. As such, they should be administered in small incremental doses to a predetermined endpoint with close assessment of hemodynamic stability and neurologic status.

Neuromuscular blocking agents (NMBAs), such as vecuronium bromide or cisatracurium (Nimbex), may be used for the client following head trauma if the client is experiencing dangerous agitation or if the increased activity is causing ICP elevations (Arbour, 2000). NMBAs have no analgesic and sedative effects and *must never be used without aggressive sedation/analgesia.* NMBAs are associated with an increased risk of pneumonia and other complications. Therefore they are not used routinely.

Antiepileptic drugs, such as phenytoin (Dilantin), to prevent seizures that occur initially more than 7 days **(late-onset seizures)** following injury are not recommended. However, they may be recommended as an option to prevent seizure activity that may occur within 7 days following injury **(early-onset seizures).** Acetaminophen (Tylenol, Ace-Tabs✱) and aspirin (acetylsalicylic acid [ASA], Ancasal✱) are given to clients who are febrile (temperature greater than 101° F [39° C]) to reduce fever.

Induction of Barbiturate Coma. Clinical trials in the use of **barbiturate coma** have been disappointing yet remain an option for clients whose ICP cannot be controlled by other means. Pentobarbital sodium (Nembutal, Novopentobarb✱) or sodium thiopental are the drugs of choice (Censullo & Sebastian, 2003). These drugs decrease the metabolic demands of the brain and cerebral blood flow, stabilize cell membranes, decrease the formation of vasogenic edema, and produce a more uniform blood supply. The provider adjusts the dosage to maintain complete unresponsiveness. Barbiturate coma is optimally managed using hemodynamic assessment, ICP monitoring, and electroencephalographic (EEG) monitoring to document endpoints. As a consequence, it is difficult to recognize subtle or unsubtle neurologic changes. The client requires mechanical ventilation, sophisticated hemodynamic monitoring, and ICP monitoring. Complications of barbiturate coma include decreased gastrointestinal motility, cardiac dysrhythmias, hypotension, and fluctuations in body temperature. **Therapeutic hypothermia** is being widely researched as a better option for lowering elevated ICP (Bayir, Clark, & Kochanek, 2003).

Fluid and Electrolyte Management. The client with craniocerebral trauma is at risk for diabetes insipidus (DI) and the syndrome of inappropriate antidiuretic hormone (SIADH) because the pituitary gland may be injured or compressed from cerebral edema (see Chapter 14). Fluid overload can occur and cerebral edema can be worsened in the client with multiple trauma from the rapid administration of IV fluids, plasma expanders, or corticosteroids. Fluids management may be titrated to optimize volume resuscitation but minimize brain swelling and ICP elevation. Fluid management is also influenced by the response to diuretic therapy and an evaluation of laboratory values. Serum osmolarity should be maintained below 310 to 320 mOsm as ordered by the physician. Check urine specific gravity every 1 to 4 hours. Monitor serum and urine osmolarity and electrolytes frequently.

Strategies for Sensory/Perceptual Alterations. The client with a *major* head injury following the acute phase of management may exhibit changes in the following areas: sense of smell; ability to taste, swallow, or feel the presence of food within the oral cavity; and vision, pain, and temperature sensation. As a result, the client is at risk for nutritional deficits, which may interfere with the healing process. The client may be injured from falling over objects outside the field of vision, or burn injuries could occur because of the inability to perceive variations in water temperatures.

Ensure that mealtime and the surrounding environment are a pleasant experience, and position the client to maximize swallowing ability. The speech-language pathologist identifies strategies to prevent food from accumulating in the cheek of the affected side. In general, clients who have swallowing problems are able to tolerate or swallow soft or semisoft foods and liquids (mechanical soft or dental diet, junior baby foods, custards, scrambled eggs) better than thin liquids (water, juice, or milk). Powdered thickener (Thick-It) may be added to thicken foods to a more manageable consistency. Collaborate with the dietitian to find a diet appropriate for the client with dysphagia.

If a large lesion of the parietal lobe is present, the client may experience a loss of sensation for pain, temperature, touch, and proprioception, which prevents the client from responding appropriately to environmental stimuli. A hazard-free environment is necessary to prevent injury (e.g., from burns if the client's coffee is too hot or from falls if the siderails on the bed are not kept up). A sensory stimulation program should be integrated into the comatose or stuporous client's routine care activities. Sensory stimulation is done to facilitate a meaningful response to the environment. Present visual, auditory, or tactile stimuli one at a time and explain the purpose and the type of stimulus presented. For example, show a picture of the client's mother and say, "This is a picture of your mother." The picture is shown several times, and the same words are used to describe the picture. If auditory tapes are used, they should not be longer than 10 to 15 minutes. If the stimulus is presented for a longer period, it simply becomes "white" noise, or meaningless background noise.

The client may be disoriented and experience a short-term memory loss. Always introduce yourself to the client before any interaction. Explanations of procedures and activities should be short and simple and given immediately before and throughout the procedure. A sleep-wake cycle must be maintained, with scheduled rest periods. Orient the client to time (day, month, and year), and place and explain the reason for the hospitalization. Reassure the client that he or she is safe and that family members know where he or she is. Ask the family to bring in familiar objects, such as pictures. Orientation cues within the environment, such as a large clock with numbers or a single-date calendar, should be provided.

Behavioral Management. The client is at risk for seizure activity, and actions are taken as outlined in the discussion of epilepsy (see Chapter 45). Keep the bed in low position with the side rails up. Hand mittens may be applied if the client attempts to pull out the IV line or nasogastric tube. Restraining any extremity increases agitation and fear. The client's behavior is observed and documented at least every hour. Alternatives to restraints should be attempted according to hospital policy. For example, covering the client's IV site with the I.V. House or other device may prevent dislodgment. Keeping the client's hands busy with activity pillows or puzzles accomplishes the same goal.

Orient the client to the surroundings as needed, and provide a quiet environment. Closely monitor the client's response to television programs or the radio. Often he or she is unable to differentiate these situations or programs from what is happening within his or her own environment.

Strategies for Preventing Complications of Immobility. Chapter 10 discusses mobility and activities of daily living (ADLs) skills in detail as well as ways to prevent complications of immobility.

Nutrition Management. The client who is moderately to severely injured usually has a decreased level of consciousness, at least temporarily. As a result, the client is unable to chew or swallow and must receive nutrition and fluids by an alternative method. The client initially receives IV fluids until he or she has stabilized. If there is no improvement in level of consciousness, long-term nutritional support via enteral feeding is usually instituted. A small-lumen nasogastric or nasoduodenal tube or a percutaneous endoscopic gastrostomy (PEG) tube is used for continuous or intermittent feeding. Small-bore tubes decrease the risk for aspiration in a client who is at high risk. Care of the client receiving enteral feeding is described in Chapter 64.

With the use of either type of tube, the client should be weighed daily. Collaborate with the dietitian to determine whether caloric needs are being met, and monitor serum albumin and prealbumin levels to assess adequacy of protein intake. Assess the client daily for signs of dehydration, such as dry mucous membranes and poor skin turgor. Supplements such as milkshakes and Ensure may be needed to meet the client's caloric and protein requirements if he or she is not receiving total enteral nutrition.

SURGICAL MANAGEMENT. The physician may elect to insert an intracranial pressure (ICP) monitoring device to evaluate the client's ICP more closely. All devices are inserted through a burr hole that is placed in the skull using a twist drill. Each device is connected to an electronic transducer that converts ICP to electronic impulses and provides information that can be viewed real-time using a monitor at the client's bedside. The monitor is able to record the pressure waves and provide a digital readout of the pressure.

Intracranial Pressure Monitoring. Various types of devices for monitoring ICP are used. An **intraventricular catheter (IVC)** is a small tube that is inserted into the anterior horn of the lateral ventricle of the nondominant cerebral hemisphere. The advantage of this system is that cerebrospinal fluid (CSF) can be drained to decrease ICP, and specimens can be obtained for laboratory analysis. The **subarachnoid screw or bolt** is a hollow device placed into the subarachnoid space for direct pressure measurement. A disadvantage of the system is that CSF cannot be drained to treat increased ICP; however, it is less invasive, which lowers the risk of infection (Table 48-3).

An **epidural catheter** or sensor is a transducer that is placed between the skull and the dura, leaving the dura intact. A similar device is the **subdural catheter**, which is placed under the dura mater. Its major advantage is the decreased risk of infection from an open dural space. The **fiberoptic transducer-tipped pressure sensor** is a commonly used device for ICP monitoring. It is easily transported and can be placed in the subdural or subarachnoid space, in the ventricle, or directly into brain tissue. The critical care nurse follows the agency's protocols for the management of these devices.

Craniotomy. In extreme cases in which the client's ICP cannot be controlled, the physician may elect to perform a craniotomy to remove ischemic tissue or the tips of the temporal lobes. The removal of nonvital brain tissue allows expansion of brain tissue without further compromise of ICP. A craniotomy may also be performed to remove epidural or subdural hematomas. Care of the client with a craniotomy is discussed under Postoperative Care (Brain Tumor), p. 1058.

Community-Based Care

The client with a *major* head injury requires case management and ongoing rehabilitation following the acute phase of hospitalization. Information on the selection of a head injury rehabilitation facility can be obtained from the National Head Injury Foundation (NHIF). Other preparation includes the development of a detailed client care plan to be

TABLE 48-3 Advantages and Disadvantages of Intracranial Pressure Monitoring Devices

Monitoring Device	Advantages	Disadvantages
Intraventricular catheter (IVC)	Allows accurate measurement of intracranial pressure (ICP) Allows drainage or sampling of cerebrospinal fluid (CSF) Allows instillation of contrast media Provides reliable evaluation of cerebral compliance	Provides additional site for potential infection Most invasive method for monitoring ICP Must be balanced and recalibrated frequently Catheter can become occluded by blood or tissue Insertion can be difficult with small or collapsed ventricles CSF leakage can occur around insertion site Associated with increased infection rate
Subarachnoid bolt or screw	Lower infection rates than with IVC Quickly and easily placed Can be used with small or collapsed ventricles Does not penetrate brain parenchyma	Tendency for dampened waveform Less accurate at high ICP May become occluded by blood or tissue Must be balanced and recalibrated frequently (i.e., every 4 hr and whenever client is repositioned) Baseline drift and tendency for dampened waveform Does not provide for CSF sampling
Subdural/epidural catheter or sensor	Least invasive Decreased risk for infection Easily and quickly placed	Increasing baseline drift over time; therefore accuracy and reliability are questionable Does not provide for CSF sampling or drainage
Fiberoptic transducer tipped catheter	Can be placed in subdural or subarachnoid space, in ventricle, or into brain tissue Easily transported Requires zeroing only once (during insertion) Baseline drift to 1 mm Hg/day Decreased risk of infection Less waveform artifact No need to adjust transducer to client's position Easy to insert	Does not provide for CSF sampling or drainage Cannot be recalibrated after placement Probe needs periodic replacement Fragile fiberoptic cable easily damaged and broken

given to the rehabilitation facility. This enables the provision of consistent care and decreases the initial anxiety related to the changes the client may experience. The discharge summary states medications, including dosage, possible reactions, and special preparation; the current client care plan; techniques used to motivate or calm the client; and strategies to assist the family to adapt to the situation.

The goal of rehabilitation after head injury is to maximize the client's ability to return to his or her highest level of functioning. Rehabilitation activities such as occupational therapy (OT), physical therapy (PT), and speech therapy may continue in the home after discharge from the rehabilitation facility. Adaptation of the home environment to accommodate the client safely may be needed. The family may require assistance in obtaining adaptive devices needed for ADLs and ambulation.

HOME CARE MANAGEMENT

Little home care preparation is needed for the client with a concussion unless he or she is experiencing post-traumatic symptoms. The client's home should be assessed for potential hazards before discharge from the hospital. Functioning smoke and fire alarms must be present because the client with a head injury often loses the sense of smell. This information can be obtained from the admission data or by a home visit. Home adaptations and referrals to outside agencies should be completed before discharge. Case management and use of critical pathways can facilitate optimal timing of diagnostic testing, clinical consults, and involvement of other health care providers, such as physical/occupational therapy.

HEALTH TEACHING

The staff nurse or case manager provides the client and family with both written and verbal instructions. The teaching plan for the client with craniocerebral trauma includes a review of seizure precautions and strategies to adapt to sensory dysfunction and to cope with the personality or behavior problems that may arise. Explain the purpose, dosage, schedule, and route of administration of any medications. The client is encouraged to participate in activities as tolerated. Demonstrations and return demonstrations of care activities may facilitate the competence of family members in skill performance. Stress the importance of regular follow-up visits with therapists and health care providers.

With the family and the client, reinforce the same strategies used in the hospital to treat sensory or perceptual changes. In addition, the family or significant others are taught about the importance of not moving furniture or other objects in the home to a different place because this can lead to an injury in the client with visual problems or might confuse the client with cognitive impairments.

Clients with personality and behavior problems respond best to a structured and consistent environment. Instruct the family to develop a home routine that provides structure, repetition, and consistency. The family must also be reminded about the importance of reinforcing positive behaviors and not reinforcing negative behaviors.

Teach the client who has sustained a *minor* head injury (e.g., a concussion) that post-concussion syndrome may occur. As stated earlier, this syndrome is a group of clinical manifestations including, but not limited to, the following:

- Personality changes
- Irritability
- Headaches
- Dizziness
- Restlessness
- Nervousness
- Insomnia

- Memory loss
- Depression

Many clients with head injuries experience some of these manifestations during recovery. However, some clients have these problems for weeks, months, or even years to the extent that they interfere with daily activities such as employment. The prolonged pattern is classified as post-trauma syndrome. The exact cause of the phenomenon is not known, but physiologic and psychological theories have been espoused. Support groups and professional counseling are the most effective interventions.

Most clients with moderate to severe craniocerebral trauma are discharged with physical and cognitive disabilities. Changes in personality and behavior are not unusual. The family must learn to cope with the client's increased fatigue, irritability, temper outbursts, depression, and memory problems. These clients often require constant supervision at home, and eventually the families feel socially isolated. Instruct the family to plan for regular respite care, either in a structured day-care respite program or through relief provided by a friend or neighbor. Family members, particularly the primary caretaker, may become depressed and experience feelings of loneliness. They may also experience isolation, increased responsibilities, and role reversals. In addition, the family may feel angry with the client because of the additional responsibilities (financial or emotional) that his or her care has placed on them. To help the family cope with these problems, suggest that they join and actively participate in a local head injury support group.

The client needs assistance in identifying realistic expectations for discharge. Because of cognitive deficits, it may not be possible for the client to return to his or her previous employment or educational pursuits. The client may experience a sense of isolation and loneliness because personality and behavior changes make it difficult to resume or maintain the social contacts he or she had before the injury.

HEALTH CARE RESOURCES

The nurse or case manager refers families and significant others and clients to the National Head Injury Foundation (NHIF) as well as to the local or state group for information and support. The NHIF and its state chapters maintain lists of rehabilitation facilities for clients with head injuries. The NHIF will send family members and other interested persons guidelines for selecting a rehabilitation facility. Families should inquire about the facility's experience in caring for the person with a head injury, how many admissions the facility has had in the previous 2 to 3 years, and the results or outcome statistics on those clients (e.g., how many went home and at what functional recovery level–poor, fair, or good). Other helpful groups include the National Easter Seal Society and the National Institute of Handicapped Research.

BRAIN TUMORS

Brain tumors can arise anywhere within the brain structures and are named according to the cell or tissue from which they originate. *Primary* tumors originate within the central nervous system (CNS) and rarely metastasize outside this area. *Secondary* brain tumors result from metastasis from other areas of the body, such as the lungs, breast, kidney, and gastrointestinal tract.

PATHOPHYSIOLOGY

Regardless of origin, the tumor expands and invades, infiltrates, compresses, and displaces normal brain tissue. This leads to the following problems:

- Cerebral edema/brain tissue inflammation
- Increased intracranial pressure (ICP)
- Focal neurologic deficits
- Obstruction of the flow of cerebrospinal fluid (CSF)
- Pituitary dysfunction

Complications of Cerebral Tumors

Cerebral edema, or more specifically vasogenic edema, results from changes in capillary endothelial tissue permeability, which allows plasma to seep into the extracellular spaces. This leads to increased ICP and, depending on the location of the primary lesion, brain herniation syndromes may occur. A variety of focal neurologic deficits result from edema, infiltration, distortion, and compression of surrounding brain tissue. The cerebral blood vessels may become compressed because of edema and increased ICP. This compression leads to ischemia of the area supplied by the vessel. In addition, the tumor may infiltrate the walls of the vessel, causing it to rupture and hemorrhage into the tumor bed or adjacent brain tissue. About 33% of clients who have brain tumors experience seizure activity attributable to interference with the brain's normal electrical activity.

Increased ICP may also result from hydrocephalus related to obstruction of the flow of CSF or displacement of the lateral ventricles by the expanding lesion. Typically, a tumor obstructs the aqueduct of Sylvius or one of the ventricles or encroaches on the subarachnoid space. Posterior fossa tumors may obstruct the flow of CSF from the fourth ventricle to the foramen of Luschka or Magendie. With any brain tumor, the obstruction of normal CSF flow causes hydrocephalus and eventually leads to increased ICP.

Pituitary dysfunction may occur as the tumor compresses the pituitary gland and causes the syndrome of inappropriate antidiuretic hormone (SIADH) or diabetes insipidus (DI). These disorders result in severe fluid and electrolyte imbalances and can be life threatening (see Chapter 66 for a complete description).

Classification of Tumors

Brain tumors are usually classified as either malignant or benign (Table 48-4). Benign tumors are generally associated with a favorable outcome, which is often not the case with malignant tumors. However, benign tumors may be malignant by virtue of their location. If the tumor cannot be completely removed or treated, it continues to grow. As it invades other brain tissue, cerebral edema, focal neurologic deficits, and increased ICP occur. Herniation of brain tissue may eventually lead to death. Benign tumors also may undergo histologic changes and become malignant.

A second classification system is based on location. **Supratentorial** tumors, which occur most often in adults, are located in the area above the tentorium cerebelli, the tentlike fold of dura that surrounds the cerebellar hemisphere and supports the occipital lobe. In other words, supratentorial tumors are located within the cerebral hemispheres. Located beneath the tentorium is the **infratentorial** area, the area of the brainstem structures and cerebellum.

TABLE 48-4 Classification of Brain Tumors

Benign	Malignant
▪ Acoustic neuroma ▪ Meningioma ▪ Pituitary adenoma ▪ Astrocytoma Grade 1 (may undergo changes and become malignant) ▪ Chondroma ▪ Craniopharyngioma ▪ Hemangioblastoma	▪ Astrocytoma Grade 2 Grade 3 Grade 4 (also known as glioblastoma multiforme) ▪ Oligodendroglioma ▪ Ependymoma ▪ Medulloblastoma ▪ Chondrosarcoma ▪ Glioma ▪ Lymphoma

A third classification system depends on the cellular, histologic, or anatomic origins of the tumor. The nervous system is composed of two types of cells: (1) neurons, which are responsible for nerve impulse conduction; and (2) neuroglial cells, which provide support, nourishment, and protection for neurons. Four specific types of cells are neuroglial cells: astrocytes, oligodendroglia, ependymal cells, and microglia. When classifying tumors according to this system, tumors are named by their cell type. For example, an astrocytoma is a tumor of astrocytes.

GLIOMAS

Gliomas are malignant tumors. They account for 60% of all brain tumors in adults and arise from the neuroglial cells of the brain and brainstem. Malignant gliomas have a peak incidence in people 40 to 60 years of age. They infiltrate and invade surrounding brain tissue. The most common type of glioma is the astrocytoma, which may be found anywhere within the cerebral hemispheres. It is usually treated by surgery to remove as much tumor bulk as possible, followed by radiation and chemotherapy. Oligodendrogliomas, another type of glioma, are generally located within the frontal lobes of the brain. These tumors are slow-growing and are usually calcified. Surgical removal is possible, and the long-term prognosis is good. A glioblastoma is a highly malignant, grade 3 or higher, rapidly growing, invasive astrocytoma. Although improved surgical techniques and advanced treatment have improved the outlook and quality of life for a client with this type of tumor, fewer than 15% of affected clients survive 18 months after diagnosis.

Ependymomas arise from the lining of the ventricles and are difficult to treat surgically because of their location. The treatment of choice involves radiation and shunting procedures to control the hydrocephalus caused by the blocking of normal CSF flow by the tumor. Chemotherapy may also be used to treat these tumors.

Gliomas are graded according to their cellular differentiation or how closely the tumor cells resemble normal cells. Grade 1 tumors are well differentiated, grade 2 tumors are moderately differentiated, and grade 3 tumors are poorly differentiated. Grade 3 tumors can rapidly change to grade 4 tumors, which are also very poorly differentiated. A grade 3 or 4 astrocytoma is referred to as glioblastoma multiforme and is associated with a poor outcome. Grade 1 and 2 tumors may undergo cellular changes and become grade 3 or 4 tumors.

MENINGIOMAS

Meningiomas arise from the coverings of the brain (the meninges). They are the most common benign tumor, with a peak incidence at age 50 years. Females are affected more than males by a 2:1 ratio. This tumor is encapsulated, globular, and well demarcated and causes compression and displacement of adjacent brain tissue. Although complete removal of the tumor is possible, it tends to recur. It tends to occur in areas where the meninges predominate.

PITUITARY TUMORS

Pituitary tumors that occur in the anterior lobe account for 10% to 25% of brain tumors and may cause endocrine dysfunction. The most common type of pituitary tumor is the adenoma, which is subdivided into chromophobe, secretory, and nonsecretory adenomas. These tumors are benign and often occur in young and middle-aged adults. The presenting symptoms are often visual disturbances. These tumors also produce hypopituitary signs, such as loss of body hair, diabetes DI, sterility, visual field defects, and headaches.

ACOUSTIC NEUROMAS

Acoustic neuromas arise from the sheath of Schwann cells in the peripheral portion of cranial nerve VIII. They are also referred to as cerebellar pontine angle (CPA) tumors to describe their anatomic location. Acoustic neuromas compress brain tissue and tend to surround adjacent cranial nerves (VII, V, IX, X), making surgical removal difficult without causing permanent cranial nerve dysfunction. Females are twice as likely as males to have acoustic neuromas. Common symptoms include hearing loss, **tinnitus** (ringing in the ears), and dizziness or vertigo.

METASTATIC TUMORS

Metastatic, or secondary, tumors account for nearly 30% of brain tumors. Metastatic cells from the lungs, breast, colon, pancreas, and kidney can travel to the brain via the blood and the lymphatic system. Multiple metastatic lesions are not uncommon.

Etiology

The exact cause of brain tumors is unknown. Several areas under investigation include genetic changes, heredity, errors in fetal development, ionizing radiation, electromagnetic fields, environmental hazards, diet, viruses, and injury. Recently, the use of cellular phones has been investigated in the development of brain tumors, but findings are inconclusive.

Incidence/Prevalence

Brain tumors account for less than 2% of all cancer deaths. About 18,000 people per year are diagnosed with a primary brain tumor in the United States. Another 150,000 have metastatic brain tumors. Brain tumors in the adult population are seen primarily in clients 40 to 60 years of age, and the survival rate is low compared with other cancers.

◆COLLABORATIVE MANAGEMENT

◆Assessment

The clinical manifestations of brain tumors vary with the site of the tumor (Chart 48-9). In general, symptoms of a brain tumor include the following:

- Headaches that are usually more severe on awakening in the morning
- Nausea and vomiting
- Visual symptoms
- Seizures

CHART 48-9

KEY FEATURES of
Common Brain Tumors

Cerebral Tumors
- Headache (most common feature)
- Vomiting unrelated to food intake
- Changes in visual acuity and visual fields; diplopia (visual changes caused by papilledema)
- Hemiparesis or hemiplegia
- Hypokinesia
- Hyperesthesia, paresthesia, decreased tactile discrimination
- Seizures
- Aphasia
- Changes in personality or behavior

Brainstem Tumors
- Hearing loss (acoustic neuroma)
- Facial pain and weakness
- Dysphagia, decreased gag reflex
- Nystagmus
- Hoarseness
- Ataxia and dysarthria (cerebellar tumors)

- Changes in mentation or personality
- **Papilledema** (swelling of the optic disc)

Neurologic deficits result from the destruction, distortion, or compression of brain tissue. *Supratentorial* tumors usually result in paralysis, seizures, memory loss, cognitive impairment, language impairment, or vision problems. *Infratentorial* tumors produce ataxia, autonomic nervous system dysfunction, vomiting, drooling, hearing loss, and vision impairment. As the tumor grows, ICP increases, and the symptoms become progressively more severe.

Diagnosis is based on the history, neurologic assessment, clinical examination, and results of neurodiagnostic testing. Noninvasive diagnostic studies such as computed tomography (CT), magnetic resonance imaging (MRI), and skull films are conducted first. The CT and MRI identify the size, location, and extent of the tumor. The MRI may be used for initial diagnostic evaluation and is a more sensitive diagnostic study, whereas the CT is often used for follow-up during the hospital course.

Cerebral angiography is usually not indicated to diagnose a brain tumor but may be used to provide additional information about vascular supply to the tumor. Electroencephalography (EEG), lumbar puncture (LP), myelography, brain scan, and positron emission tomography (PET) may be indicated to provide further information about the size, location, and characteristics of the tumor. LP should not be performed if the client is exhibiting signs of ICP elevation to prevent brain herniation. Laboratory tests may also be ordered to evaluate endocrine function, renal status, and electrolyte balance.

Interventions

When possible, obtain a history from both the client and the family, including current signs and symptoms. A complete neurologic assessment is needed to establish baseline data and to determine the nature and extent of neurologic deficits.

NONSURGICAL MANAGEMENT. The goal of treatment of brain tumors is to decrease tumor size, improve quality of life, and improve survival time. The type of treatment selected depends on the tumor size and location, client symptoms and general condition, and whether the tumor is recurrent. The treatment of brain tumors may include radiation, chemotherapy, and surgery. A number of experimental treatment modalities are being investigated, including blood-brain barrier disruption, recombinant deoxyribonucleic acid (DNA), monoclonal antibodies, new antineoplastic drugs, immunotherapy, and hyperthermia.

Radiation Therapy. Radiation therapy may be used alone, after surgery, or in combination with chemotherapy and surgery. Chapter 28 discusses radiation treatment for cancer in detail. An anti-tenascin radioactive monoclonal antibody treatment (81C6) that is directly injected into the cavity where the tumor was removed is being investigated. The antibodies deliver radiation directly into the brain but are less potent than traditional radiation (Wood, 2004).

Drug Therapy. The health care provider may prescribe a variety of medications to treat the tumor as well as manage the client's symptoms and prevent complications.

Chemotherapy. Chemotherapy may be given alone, in combination with radiation and surgery, and with tumor progression. Although these drugs may control tumor growth or decrease tumor burden, the benefit usually is very short-lived. Chemotherapy usually involves more than one agent and may be given IV, intra-arterially, or intrathecally through an Ommaya reservoir placed in a cranial ventricle.

The most commonly used drugs are alkylating agents, especially nitrosoureas such as carmustine (BCNU) and lomustine (CCNU). A combination of procarbazine, lomustine, and vincristine (PCV) may be given for selected clients. Tamoxifen may also be used for selected types of tumors. A newer drug, temozolomide (Temodar), crosses the blood-brain barrier and is widely used today. It is administered orally, unlike most other agents. Side effects of these drugs are similar to those of any chemotherapeutic medication. Chapter 28 describes nursing implications for care of a client receiving chemotherapy.

Most chemotherapeutic agents have difficulty crossing the blood-brain barrier. Therefore direct drug delivery to the tumor is an emerging practice. Disk-shaped drug wafers called Gliadel wafers may be placed directly into the cavity created during surgical tumor removal. The major drug in the wafer is carmustine. This therapy is usually used for newly diagnosed high-grade malignant gliomas, but recurrent tumors may also be treated with this method. Other drugs that are awaiting approval from the Food and Drug Administration (FDA or have been recently approved include erlotinib (Tarceva) for malignant glioma, gefitinib (Iressa), and tipifarnib (Zarnestra) (Wood, 2004). New drugs are continuously emerging for all types of cancers.

Other Drugs. Analgesics, such as codeine and acetaminophen (Tylenol, Ace-Tabs✱), are given for headache. Dexamethasone (Decadron) is usually given to control cerebral edema. Research supports the efficacy of administering glucocorticoids for the treatment of edema resulting from brain tumors. Phenytoin (Dilantin) may be used to prevent or treat seizure activity. Histamine blockers such as ranitidine hydrochloride (Zantac, Apo-Ranitidine✱) or proton pump inhibitors such as pantoprazole (Protonix) are given to decrease gastric acid secretion and prevent the development of stress ulcers. Metoclopramide (Reglan) and other antiemetics are used to treat nausea and vomiting.

Radiosurgery. Radiosurgical procedures are an alternative to surgery. These techniques include the modified linear accelerator using accelerated x-rays (LINAC), a particle accelerator using beams of protons (cyclotron), and isotope seeds implanted in the tumor (brachytherapy). The Gamma Knife and CyberKnife are newer treatments.

Gamma Knife. The Gamma Knife is a type of stereotactic radiosurgical procedure that uses a single high dose of ionized radiation to focus 201 beams of gamma radiation produced by the radioisotope cobalt 60 to destroy intracranial lesions selectively without damaging surrounding healthy tissue (Figure 48-10). Combining neurodiagnostic imaging tools–including magnetic resonance imaging (MRI), computed tomography (CT), magnetic resonance angiography (MRA), and angiography–with the Gamma Knife allows for precise localization of deep-seated or anatomically difficult lesions. Treatment usually takes less than an hour, and clients require only overnight hospitalization. Advantages of this technique include its noninvasive nature; a lower risk than the traditional craniotomy; surgical precision; and decreased cost, morbidity, length of hospital stay, and recovery time.

The Gamma Knife is used primarily for brain tumors or arteriovenous malformations (AVMs) that are in an inaccessible location and therefore unresectable by craniotomy. Tumors typically treated in this manner are acoustic neuromas, meningiomas, and metastatic tumors. The procedure may also be used with clients who refuse conventional surgery, for clients whose age and physical condition preclude general anesthesia, as an adjunct to radiation therapy, and for recurrent or residual AVM or tumors after embolization or craniotomy. Additional potential applications of Gamma Knife radiosurgery are being evaluated.

Other Radiosurgical Procedures. The LINAC has an advantage over the Gamma Knife in that the Gamma Knife uses a rigid head frame that is difficult to position. The LINAC employs a skull-conforming mask. In another system called the CyberKnife, no frame is needed.

SURGICAL MANAGEMENT. The most important modality in the treatment of brain tumors is a biopsy to determine the specific pathology. A craniotomy is the most common surgical treatment and may be done to improve symptoms related to the lesion or to decrease pressure effects. The challenge for the surgeon is to remove the tumor as completely as possible without damaging normal tissue. Complete removal is possible with some benign tumors,

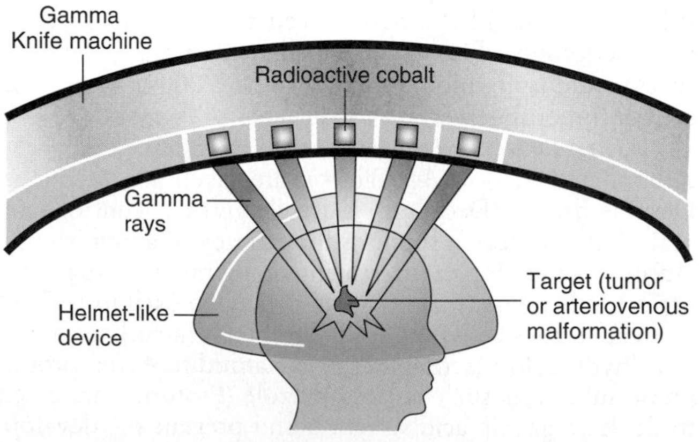

Figure 46-10 ■ A Gamma Knife treatment. The treatment beams are widely dispersed over the surface of the head to prevent damage to healthy brain tissue. The beams are intense only at the point of target.

which results in a "surgical cure." Postoperatively, the client is usually admitted to the critical care unit.

Postoperative Care. The Plan of Care on pp. 1059 to 1063 highlights the major aspects of postoperative nursing care following a craniotomy. The focus of postoperative care is to monitor the client to detect changes in status and to prevent or minimize complications, especially increased intracranial pressure (ICP). Assess neurologic and vital signs every 30 minutes for the first 4 to 6 hours after surgery and then every hour. If the client is stable for 24 hours, the frequency of these checks may be decreased to every 2 to 4 hours, depending on the agency's policy. Potential neurologic deficits include a decreased level of consciousness, motor weakness or paralysis, aphasia, visual changes, and personality changes. Periorbital edema and ecchymosis of one or both eyes is not unusual and is treated with cold compresses to decrease swelling. Irrigate the affected eye with warm saline solution or artificial tears to improve client comfort. If the client is still recovering from anesthesia, has a decreased level of consciousness, or may not be able to protect the airway, he or she may remain intubated and receive controlled ventilation.

The client in the critical care unit is routinely connected to the cardiac monitor. Dysrhythmias may occur after posterior fossa surgery, or they may result from fluid and electrolyte imbalance. Other nursing interventions include strict recording of the client's intake and output and possibly fluid restriction to 1500 mL daily as clinically indicated. Range-of-motion exercises to all extremities are performed at least every 2 to 3 hours. Assist the client to turn, cough, and breathe deeply every 2 hours. To prevent the development of deep vein thrombosis, sequential compression stockings or pneumatic compression boots are kept in place until the client is ambulating.

Positioning. Clients who have undergone supratentorial surgery should have the head of the bed elevated 30 degrees or as tolerated to promote venous drainage from the head. Position the client to avoid extreme hip or neck flexion and maintain the head in a midline, neutral position. The client may be turned side-to-side or remain supine. If a large tumor has been removed, it is recommended that the client be placed on the nonoperative side to prevent displacement of the cranial contents by gravity. The client with an infratentorial craniotomy should be kept flat and positioned on either side for 24 to 48 hours. This prevents pressure on the neck-area incision site. It also prevents pressure on the internal tumor excision site from higher cerebral structures. The client should receive nothing by mouth (NPO status) for 24 hours because edema around the medulla and lower cranial nerves may place the client at risk for vomiting and aspiration.

Monitoring the Dressing. Check the head dressing every 1 to 2 hours for signs of drainage. Mark the area of drainage once during each shift for baseline comparison. A small or moderate amount of drainage is expected. Some clients may have a Hemovac, Jackson-Pratt, or other surgical drain in place for 24 hours after surgery. Measure the drainage every 8 hours and record the amount and color; a typical amount of drainage is 30 to 50 mL per shift (8 hours). Follow the manufacturer's and surgeon's instructions to maintain suction within the drain. Excessive amounts of drainage (a saturated head dressing or drainage greater than 50 mL/8 hr should be reported immediately to the physician.

Text continued on p. 1064.

PLAN of CARE MEDICAL DIAGNOSIS: CRANIOTOMY

NURSING DIAGNOSIS NO. 1 ■ Decreased Intracranial Adaptive Capacity

	Expected Outcomes	Nursing Interventions	Rationales
RELATED FACTORS Decreased cerebral perfusion <60-70 mm Hg Sustained increase in intracranial pressure (ICP) = >15-20 mm Hg Systemic hypotension with intracranial hypertension Brain injuries **DEFINING CHARACTERISTICS** Baseline ICP ≥10-15 mm Hg Disproportionate increase in ICP following a single environmental or nursing maneuver stimulus	Baseline ICP remains ≤15-20 mm Hg Has an ICP that remains stable following nursing activities or environmental stimuli Remains oriented to time, place, person, and situation Has a level of consciousness (LOC) that remains stable	NIC **Cerebral Perfusion Promotion** Monitor neurologic status.	A decrease or change in LOC is typically the first sign of a deterioration in neurologic status.
		Calculate and monitor cerebral perfusion pressure (CPP).	A CPP ≥60-70 mm Hg is needed to provide adequate oxygenation and nutrition to brain tissue.
		Monitor client's ICP and neurologic response to care activities.	ICP may elevate in response to stimulation from care activities. An elevation in ICP decreases CPP.
		Monitor central venous pressure (CVP) if central venous access is present. Also perform regular physical examinations to assess fluid balance (edema, rales/crackles on lung auscultation), as well as jugular venous distension.	CVP measures fluid status. ICP elevates with fluid overload.
		Monitor pulmonary artery wedge pressure (PAWP) and pulmonary artery pressure (PAP).	Elevated PAWP and PAP indicates ineffective pumping force of the heart and increased fluid pressure in the lungs, upper extremities, head, and neck.
		Monitor respiratory status (e.g., rate, rhythm, and depth of respirations; Po_2, Pco_2, pH, and bicarbonate levels).	Adequate gas exchange is required for tissue oxygenation.
		Maintain Pco_2 level at 35 mm Hg to avoid hypercarbia.	CO_2 is a powerful vasodilator, which causes cerebral vasodilation and increases ICP.
		Monitor $Paco_2$, Sao_2, and hemoglobin levels and cardiac output, if available.	$Paco_2$, Sao_2, and hemoglobin levels and cardiac output are determinants of tissue oxygen delivery.
		Administer colloid, blood products, and crystalloid, as appropriate.	Volume expanders maintain hemodynamic parameters.
		Administer and titrate vasoactive drugs, as ordered.	Vasoactive drugs maintain hemodynamic parameters.
		Maintain serum glucose level within normal range.	The brain does not store glucose and needs a constant supply for cellular energy. Hypoglycemia can cause brain damage. Hyperglycemia is associated with increased morbidity and mortality.
		Consult with physician to determine optimal head of bed (HOB) placement (e.g., 0, 15, or 30 degrees), and monitor the client's responses to head positioning.	The client's head should be positioned to best facilitate drainage of blood and cerebrospinal fluid.
		Avoid neck flexion or extreme hip/knee flexion.	Absence of neck or hip flexion enhances venous drainage, which prevents increased ICP.

Continued

PLAN of CARE   MEDICAL DIAGNOSIS: CRANIOTOMY—*cont'd*

NURSING DIAGNOSIS NO. 1 ■ Decreased Intracranial Adaptive Capacity—*cont'd*

	Expected Outcomes	Nursing Interventions	Rationales
		Administer and monitor the effects of osmotic and loop-active diuretics and corticosteroids.	Osmotic diuretics are used to treat cerebral edema by pulling fluid out of edematous brain tissue. A loop-active diuretic may be used to counteract rebound from the osmotic diuretic.
		Administer pain medication, as appropriate.	Pain may increase ICP and other stress-related complications.
		Test stool and nasogastric (NG) drainage for blood.	Clients receiving anticoagulant medication should be observed for signs of bleeding.
		NIC **Intracranial Pressure Monitoring**	
		Check client for nuchal rigidity or other meningeal signs.	Nuchal rigidity indicates irritation of the meninges and may indicate inflammation or infection, such as meningitis.
		Administer antibiotics.	Antibiotics will treat an infectious process and lower the risk of systemic or intracranial infection.
		Record ICP pressure readings and analyze waveforms.	ICP pressure readings and the characteristics of the waveforms provide indicators of changes in CPP, ICP, and intracranial compliance.
		Other Interventions	
		Give simple, clear explanations.	Increased ICP may affect cognition and make information processing difficult.
		Keep surroundings as quiet and calm as possible.	Stimulation may cause ICP to increase.
		Continuing Care Considerations	
		Provide the client and family with written explanations and instructions.	Brain injury and/or anxiety may affect cognition.
		Refer the family to the National Head Injury Foundation (NHIF), as appropriate.	The foundation provides information and support for clients and their families who are dealing with head injury.

NURSING DIAGNOSIS NO. 2 ■ Impaired Memory

	Expected Outcomes	Nursing Interventions	Rationales
RELATED FACTORS Neurologic impairment Hypoxia, acute **DEFINING CHARACTERISTICS** Inability to recall factual information Inability to recall recent events Inability to learn or retain new skills or information Observed or reported experience of forgetting	Able to recall factual information Able to recall recent or past events Able to learn or retain new skills or information No verbal report or observation of forgetting Able to perform previously learned skill (specify) Has cognitive functions that remain stable No verbal report or observation of impaired memory No verbal report or observation of diminished ability to learn	NIC **Memory Training** Discuss with the client and family any practical memory problems experienced. Reminisce about past experiences with the client, as appropriate. Implement visual imagery, mnemonic devices, memory games, memory cues, association techniques, list making, computers, name tags, or rehearsing of information.	 Determine the extent of memory problems and the client's and family's response to those difficulties. Reminiscing about past experiences may assist the client to remember problem-solving skills and techniques previously used. Appropriate memory techniques can assist the client with storage and retrieval of information.

NURSING DIAGNOSIS NO. 2 ■ Impaired Memory—*cont'd*

	Expected Outcomes	Nursing Interventions	Rationales
		D Assist in associated learning tasks, as appropriate.	Practice in learning and recalling verbal and pictorial information as presented helps the client to exercise memory and information retrieval.
		Provide for orientation training, as appropriate.	The client can rehearse personal information and dates to improve retention of key information.
		D Have the client engage in games such as matching pairs of cards, as appropriate.	Matching games provide an opportunity for concentration.
		Question the client about a recent outing or other recent notable event.	Questioning the client about a recent event provides an opportunity to use memory for recent events.
		Provide for picture recognition memory, as appropriate.	Pictures trigger memories from storage areas of the brain that are different from those used for speech.
		Structure the teaching methods according to the client's organization of information.	The client's organization of information will determine the logical sequence of learning for the individual.
		Encourage the client to participate in group memory training programs, as appropriate.	Group support and understanding of memory difficulties makes memory problems less threatening.
		Monitor the client's behavior during therapy.	The client may get agitated and frustrated during therapy, which signals the need to stop the session.
		Other Interventions	
		D Encourage the client to use previously learned skills.	Distant memory may remain intact and provide a sense of control to the client.
		Assist the family to understand that assaultive behavior may be the result of poor memory.	Aggressive or combative behavior by the client may signal a threat to self-esteem from memory loss.
		Continuing Care Considerations	
		Collaborate with the client and family to manage tasks that may be difficult for the client (e.g., paying bills).	The client may need to have financial or other protection.

NURSING DIAGNOSIS NO. 3 ■ Impaired Physical Mobility

	Expected Outcomes	Nursing Interventions	Rationales
RELATED FACTORS Discomfort Sensoriperceptual impairments Musculoskeletal impairment Neuromuscular impairment Intolerance to activity **DEFINING CHARACTERISTICS** Limited ability to perform gross motor skills Limited ability to perform fine motor skills Uncoordinated or jerky movement Limited range of motion Difficulty turning	Has full or improved range of motion in all joints Has smooth, coordinated movements Able to turn without assistance Has stable posture during performance of activities of daily living Has no movement-induced tremor Has skin that remains intact with no bruising or rashes Able to perform fine motor skills Able to perform gross motor skills	NIC **Exercise Therapy: Joint Mobility** Collaborate with physical therapy in developing and executing an exercise program.	The physical therapist is the primary health care professional responsible for developing and executing an exercise program.
		Initiate pain control measures before beginning joint exercise.	Initiating pain control measures before joint exercise increases the likelihood of client comfort and willingness to engage in the exercise.
		D Dress the client in nonrestrictive clothing.	Nonrestrictive clothing permits full range of joint motion.

Continued

D Indicates tasks that can be delegated to unlicensed assistive nursing personnel at the discretion of the nurse.

PLAN of CARE MEDICAL DIAGNOSIS: CRANIOTOMY—*cont'd*

NURSING DIAGNOSIS NO. 3 ■ Impaired Physical Mobility—*cont'd*

Expected Outcomes	Nursing Interventions	Rationales
	D Encourage active range-of-motion exercises according to regular, planned schedule.	Regular periods of active range-of-motion exercise maximize the exercise benefit to joints.
	Assist the client to develop a schedule for active range-of-motion exercises.	Regular exercise maximizes the benefit of the exercise.
	D Encourage ambulation, if appropriate.	Ambulation is a form of active joint exercise and also improves cardiovascular tone.
	NIC **Positioning**	
	Premedicate the client before turning, as appropriate.	Premedicating the client before turning will increase client comfort and decrease resistance to repositioning from fear of pain.
	D Place the client in the designated therapeutic position.	The designated therapeutic position should cause no undue stress on muscles or joints.
	D Position the client in proper body alignment.	Proper body alignment preserves the functionality of muscles and bony skeleton.
	D Minimize friction and shearing forces when positioning and turning the client.	Friction and shearing forces will cause damage to the skin and underlying tissues.
	D Turn using the log roll technique.	The log roll technique keeps the spinal column in alignment during the turn, which prevents injury to the spinal nerves.
	Apply a foot board to the bed.	A foot board will prevent foot drop.
	D Elevate the head of the bed, as appropriate.	The head of the bed may be elevated to provide countertraction or for comfort if permitted.
	D Turn the client as indicated by skin condition.	Clients should be turned at least every 2 hours and have small position shifts more frequently to prevent pressure injury.
	D Place frequently used objects within reach.	Placing frequently used objects within reach permits the client safe and convenient access.
	Other Interventions	
	Instruct the client in the use of assistive devices.	The client will need instruction to properly use canes, crutches, walkers, splints, or other assistive devices.
	Continuing Care Considerations	
	Refer the client to rehabilitative services, as appropriate.	Ongoing support from physical therapists, occupational therapists, and others may be needed to help the client resume activities of daily living.
	Refer the client to a vocational counselor, as appropriate.	Long-term physical impairment may require the client to change employment.
	Collaborate with community organizations to inform the public about injury prevention.	Injury prevention saves the individual and society as a whole an enormous economic burden.

D Indicates tasks that can be delegated to unlicensed assistive nursing personnel at the discretion of the nurse.

PLAN of CARE MEDICAL DIAGNOSIS: CRANIOTOMY—*cont'd*

NURSING DIAGNOSIS NO. 4 ■ Risk for Infection

	Expected Outcomes	Nursing Interventions	Rationales
RELATED FACTORS Invasive procedures Insufficient knowledge to avoid exposure to pathogens Trauma or injury Tissue destruction and increased environmental exposure Increased environmental exposure to pathogens Immunosuppression (steroids)	Denies fatigue Denies weakness Denies nausea Has a blood pressure that remains ±10 mm Hg of baseline Has no observable alterations in personality No verbal report or observation of urgency Has skin with warm undertones Has a heart rate that remains regular, strong, and between 60 and 100 beats/min No verbal report or observation of altered eating habits No verbal report or observation of vomiting Denies headache No verbal report or observation of diarrhea Has a body temperature that remains between 97° and 99.6° F (36.1° and 37.5° C)	NIC **Infection Protection** Monitor for systemic and localized signs and symptoms of infection.	Elevated temperature, pulse, respirations, and fever indicate systemic infection. Redness, heat, swelling, and pain indicate local infection.
		Monitor absolute granulocyte count, white blood cell (WBC) count, and differential results.	Elevations in these laboratory tests demonstrate the body's response to infection.
		Obtain cultures, as needed.	Purulent wound drainage indicates infection. A culture will identify the causative agent and indicate the appropriate antibiotic therapy.
		Inspect the condition of any surgical incision/wound.	A surgical incision may be slightly reddened and swollen from tissue damage but remain free of the purulent drainage, excess swelling, or excess local pain that indicates infection.
		Maintain asepsis for the client at risk.	Asepsis will minimize client exposure to pathogenic agents and thus minimize the incidence of infection.
		D Encourage deep breathing and coughing, as appropriate.	Coughing and deep breathing clears the lungs of secretions that may encourage the growth of pathogenic microbes.
		D Promote sufficient nutritional intake.	Adequate nutrition is essential for immune system cell formation and for the repair of damaged body tissues to provide protection against external pathogens.
		D Encourage fluid intake, as appropriate.	Adequate fluid intake provides for renal clearance of toxins produced by pathogens.
		D Encourage rest.	Mending tissues requires energy. A fatigued client is stressed and requires greater expenditure of energy to accomplish tasks.
		NIC **Infection Control** Administer antibiotic therapy, as appropriate.	Antibiotic therapy should assist the body to destroy pathogens.
		Continuing Care Considerations Teach the client and family about the signs and symptoms of infection and when to report them to the health care provider.	Early intervention to treat infection prevents untoward complications from the infection and its therapy.

Monitoring Laboratory Values. The laboratory studies monitored postoperatively include complete blood count (CBC), serum electrolyte levels and osmolarity, coagulation studies, and arterial blood gas (ABG) measurements.

The client's hematocrit and hemoglobin concentration may be abnormally low from blood loss during surgery or elevated if the blood was replaced. Hyponatremia (low serum sodium) may occur as a result of fluid volume overload, syndrome of inappropriate antidiuretic hormone (SIADH), or steroid administration. Hypokalemia (low serum potassium) may cause cardiac irritability. Weakness, a change in level of consciousness, and confusion are symptoms of hyponatremia and hypokalemia. Hypernatremia may be caused by meningitis, dehydration, or diabetes insipidus (DI). It is manifested by muscle weakness, restlessness, extreme thirst, and dry mouth. Additional signs of dehydration such as poor skin turgor, thickened lung secretions, and hypotension may be present. Untreated hypernatremia may lead to seizure activity. ABG values are monitored to ensure adequate cerebral oxygenation. DI should be considered if the client voids large amounts of very dilute urine with an increasing serum osmolarity and electrolyte concentration.

Ventilating the Client. Often the client is electively mechanically ventilated and hyperventilated for the first 24 to 48 hours after surgery to prevent increased intracranial pressure (ICP). The goal of controlled ventilation is to keep the partial pressure of arterial carbon dioxide ($PaCO_2$) at about 35 mm Hg, with normal arterial oxygen levels. This is designed to avoid cerebral vasodilation from hypercarbia (increased carbon dioxide) with the resulting rise in ICP. If the client is awake or attempting to breathe at a rate other than that set on the ventilator, medications such as fentanyl citrate or midazolam (Versed) are given to treat pain and anxiety as well as to promote rest and comfort. The client who is intubated is suctioned if indicated by the findings of frequent respiratory assessments. Remember to hyperoxygenate the client carefully before suctioning.

Drug Therapy. Medications routinely given postoperatively include antiepileptic drugs, histamine blockers, proton pump inhibitors, and corticosteroids, such as dexamethasone (Decadron). Analgesics such as codeine are given for pain, and acetaminophen is given for fever or mild pain. Some physicians may elect to administer prophylactic antibiotics to prevent infection.

Preventing Postoperative Complications. Postoperative complications are listed in Table 48-5.

Increased Intracranial Pressure. The major postoperative complication of supratentorial surgery is increased ICP from cerebral edema, hemorrhage, or obstruction of the normal flow of cerebrospinal fluid (CSF). Symptoms of increased ICP include severe headache, deteriorating level of consciousness, restlessness, irritability, and dilated or pinpoint pupils that are slow to react or nonreactive to light. Treatment of increased ICP is the same as that described in the Interventions section of Traumatic Brain Injury on p. 1051.

Hematomas. Subdural and epidural hematomas and intracranial hemorrhage are manifested by severe headache, a change in level of consciousness, progressive neurologic deficits, and herniation syndromes. Bleeding into the posterior fossa may lead to sudden cardiovascular and respiratory arrest. Treatment of a hematoma necessitates surgical removal, whereas an intracranial hemorrhage is treated with aggressive medical management (e.g., osmotic diuretics and ICP monitoring).

TABLE 48-5 Postoperative Complications of Craniotomy

Increased intracranial pressure (ICP)
Hematomas
- Subdural hematoma
- Epidural hematoma
- Subarachnoid hemorrhage

Hypovolemic shock
Hydrocephalus
Respiratory complications
- Atelectasis
- Hypoxia
- Pneumonia
- Neurogenic pulmonary edema

Wound infection
Meningitis
Fluid and electrolyte imbalances
- Dehydration
- Hyponatremia
- Hypernatremia

Seizures
Cerebrospinal fluid (CSF) leak
Cerebral edema

Hydrocephalus. Hydrocephalus is caused by obstruction of the normal CSF pathway from edema, an expanding lesion such as a hematoma, or blood in the subarachnoid space. Rapidly progressive hydrocephalus produces the classic symptoms of increased ICP. Slowly progressive hydrocephalus is manifested by headache, decreased level of consciousness, irritability, blurred vision, and urinary incontinence. Emergently, an intraventricular catheter **(ventriculostomy)** may be placed to drain CSF for rapidly deteriorating neurologic function. If long-term treatment is required for chronic hydrocephalus, a surgical shunt is inserted to drain CSF to another area of the body. A ventriculoperitoneal or, less often, a ventriculoatrial or lumbar peritoneal shunt procedure is usually performed. A major complication of the shunting procedure is a subdural hematoma from the tearing of bridging veins. An external lumbar drain may also be used temporarily. Additional information about shunts may be found in neuroscience nursing textbooks.

Respiratory Problems. Respiratory complications include atelectasis, pneumonia, and neurogenic pulmonary edema. Atelectasis and pneumonia can be prevented by providing appropriate pulmonary hygiene, turning the client frequently, and encouraging the client to take frequent deep breaths to expand the lungs each hour. The provision of humidified air and incentive spirometry are useful techniques to prevent these complications. Other treatment modalities include endotracheal or oral tracheal suctioning and chest physiotherapy. These measures may cause an increase in ICP. However, close monitoring of the client's status and ICP waveforms allows him or her to receive the benefits of aggressive pulmonary hygiene despite the potential risk.

Neurogenic pulmonary edema is an infrequent but life-threatening complication of neurologic insult such as traumatic brain injury (TBI), brain tumors, or surgery. Its symptoms are the same as those of acute pulmonary edema, but there are no associated cardiac problems. In spite of aggressive treatment, most clients with neurogenic pulmonary edema do not survive the insult.

Wound Infection. Wound infections occur more often in older and debilitated clients and in clients with a history of diabetes, long-term steroid use, obesity, and previous infections. The client may contribute to the problem by rubbing or scratching the wound. If infection is present, the wound appears reddened and puffy. It may begin to separate, is sensitive to touch, and feels warm. The client may or may not be febrile. Treatment is based on the degree and extent of the infection. The nurse may treat a localized infection by simply cleaning it with alcohol or by applying local antibiotics. For more severe infections, systemic antibiotic administration may be required. If the underlying bone is involved, it may need to be removed.

Meningitis. Meningitis is an inflammation of the meninges and may occur as a result of surgery or wound infection, a cerebrospinal fluid (CSF) leak, or contamination during surgery. (See the discussion of meningitis in Chapter 45 for a more complete explanation of this complication.)

Fluid and Electrolyte Imbalances. Complications related to fluid and electrolyte imbalance include DI, syndrome of inappropriate antidiuretic hormone (SIADH), and cerebral salt wasting (CSW). DI is seen most often after supratentorial surgery, especially procedures involving the pituitary gland or hypothalamus. Failure of the posterior pituitary gland to secrete antidiuretic hormone (ADH) leads to failure of the renal tubules to reabsorb water. The client's urine output increases dramatically (it may be up to 10 L/day), and the urine specific gravity drops to below 1.005. Urine osmolarity decreases, whereas serum osmolarity increases. The client may become dehydrated, and hypovolemic shock may develop if this condition is left untreated. Fluid replacement to replace urinary losses and prevent dehydration may be accomplished by having the client increase oral intake or use IV fluids if he or she can do so. Hormonal replacement may also be necessary, especially if fluid loss is greater than 6 L/24 hr. Aqueous vasopressin is short-acting, lasting only 6 to 8 hours. Desmopressin acetate (DDAVP) may be administered for long-term replacement therapy.

Syndrome of inappropriate antidiuretic hormone (SIADH) occurs when the posterior pituitary gland secretes too much ADH, causing water retention. The urine output decreases dramatically, with a urine output of less than 20 mL/hr. Sodium concentration in the urine is normal or elevated, whereas the serum sodium level falls. Other indications of SIADH are loss of thirst, irritability, muscle weakness, and decreased level of consciousness. SIADH is treated by fluid restriction, which is usually sufficient to correct the hyponatremia. Slow, controlled IV infusion of 3% hypertonic sodium may be needed for severe hyponatremia (<118 mEq/L).

Cerebral salt-wasting (CSW) is thought to result from the extrarenal influence of atrial natriuretic factor (ANF). ANF cells are located in the hypothalamus and the right atrium and regulate fluid volume. CSW is believed to be the primary cause of hyponatremia in the neurosurgical population. It is characterized by hyponatremia, decreased serum osmolarity, and decreased blood volume. Serum vasopressin and ANF levels can differentiate CSW and SIADH. CSW is treated with the replacement of sodium and isotonic fluid volume.

Clients with complications related to fluid and electrolyte imbalance undergo strict measurement of their intake and output. An accurate daily weight measurement is an essential aspect of nursing care. The nurse assesses carefully for indications of fluid overload or dehydration during treatment. Serum electrolyte levels and osmolarity are measured daily (or more often if clinically indicated). Chapters 15 and 16 provide additional information on fluid and electrolyte imbalances, and Chapter 66 provides further discussion of SIADH and DI.

Critical Thinking Challenge

A young woman was employed as an accountant for a well-known firm. She was planning to be married in 6 months but began to have frequent headaches with occasional nausea and vomiting. After a thorough medical evaluation, she was diagnosed as having a grade 3 astrocytoma. She is scheduled for a craniotomy before radiation via a Gamma Knife and chemotherapy with PCV.

1. What preoperative teaching would you provide for this client?
2. What postoperative complications should you look for? How will you know if she develops any of these problems, and what should you do if she does?
3. What can you tell her to expect during the Gamma Knife procedure?
4. What health teaching does she need regarding her PCV treatments? (Hint: You might need to refer to Chapter 28 to help answer this question.)
5. How can you help her meet her psychosocial needs while her tumor is being treated?

evolve For suggested answer guidelines, go to http://evolve.elsevier.com/Iggy/.

Community-Based Care

The client with a brain tumor is managed at home if possible. The nurse or case manager mobilizes health resources to support the client and family at home. Maintaining a reasonable quality of life is an important goal for recovery and rehabilitation.

HOME CARE MANAGEMENT

Unless the client has a significant degree of disability, no special preparation for home care is needed. Clients with hemiparesis need assistance to ensure that their home is accessible according to their method of mobility (e.g., cane, walker, wheelchair). The environment should be made safe to prevent falls. For example, scatter rugs should be removed and grab bars placed in the bathroom.

Information about the selection of rehabilitation or chronic care facility, if needed, can be obtained from the social worker or discharge planner. The selected facility should have experience in providing care for neurologically impaired clients. A psychologist should be available to provide input in the evaluation of the cognitive disabilities often exhibited by the client.

HEALTH TEACHING

It is important that the client and family fully understand the importance of any recommended follow-up health care appointments. The discharge summary should state the name of the person who has given the follow-up information.

Information given to the client and the family or significant others includes the name of the medications, the dosage, the timing of administration, the number of days to take the medication, and any side effects. Explain what to do or whom to call if any adverse reactions occur. Remind the client to refrain from taking any over-the-counter medications unless authorized by the health care provider.

Instruct the client to maintain a program of regular physical exercise within the limits of any disabilities. Referral to the dietitian may be necessary to ensure adequate caloric intake for the client receiving radiation or chemotherapy.

Seizures are a potential complication that can occur at any time for as long as 1 year or more postoperatively. Provide the client and the family with information about seizure precautions and what to do if a seizure occurs.

If long-term changes or disability is expected, the client needs to be prepared for major lifestyle changes. Chapter 10 discusses coping with disability in more detail.

HEALTH CARE RESOURCES

Refer the client and the family or significant others to the American Brain Tumor Association or the National Brain Tumor Foundation. The American Cancer Society is also an appropriate community resource for clients with malignant tumors. Home care agencies are available to provide both the physical and rehabilitative care that the client may need at home. Hospice services and palliative care may be needed for the terminally ill client. Brain tumor support groups may also be a valuable asset to the client and family.

BRAIN ABSCESS

A **brain abscess** is a purulent infection of the brain in which pus forms in the extradural, subdural, or intracerebral area of the brain. The causative organisms are most often bacteria, which invade the brain directly or indirectly. Cerebral abscesses may be a complication of meningitis infection.

PATHOPHYSIOLOGY

In general, organisms from the ear, sinus, or mastoid area enter the brain by traveling along the wall of the cerebral veins, and therefore they may spread to any area of the brain. At times, the organisms (especially those from the ear) erode the bone, form a tract, and enter the brain directly. Septic emboli from the heart, the lungs, or a dental or peritonsillar abscess may break off and enter the systemic circulation. These organisms may become lodged in a cerebral vessel and produce a localized infection. Penetrating trauma, open head injuries, and neurosurgical procedures provide a potential means for the direct entry of an organism into the brain. In the past 15 years, the number of clients with a brain abscess as a consequence of immunosuppression, organ transplantation, and acquired immunodeficiency syndrome (AIDS) has increased rapidly.

The organisms cause a local infection, and acute inflammation surrounds the involved area. Within a few days, necrosis of the tissue takes place, and pus formation and liquefaction of the tissue occur. This is followed by the development of cerebral edema resulting from localized vascular congestion and tissue swelling in response to inflammation. During the subsequent 2 weeks, the area becomes encapsulated, first by fibrous granulation tissue and later by collagenous connective tissue. The abscess usually occurs deep within the cerebral hemisphere and involves the white matter of the brain. Occasionally the abscess does not become encapsulated but instead spreads through the brain tissue to the subarachnoid space and ventricular system.

The organism varies with the source of the abscess. *Streptococci* are the most common organisms and are often found with other anaerobes such as *Bacteroides. Enterobacteriaceae* such as *Escherichia coli* and *Proteus* organisms may also be combined with *Streptococcus.* Yeast and fungi are now implicated in 9% to 17% of cases of cerebral abscess formation, particularly in clients who are immunosuppressed. *Toxoplasma gondii* is the most commonly seen central nervous system (CNS) opportunistic infection in the AIDS population.

Most brain abscesses occur in the frontal and temporal lobes. It is estimated that 5% to 20% of affected clients have more than one abscess. Mortality rates vary from 30% to 60%; abscesses that occur in immunosuppressed clients are associated with a higher mortality rate.

COLLABORATIVE MANAGEMENT

Assessment

PHYSICAL ASSESSMENT/CLINICAL MANIFESTATIONS

The clinical manifestations of a brain abscess are insidious and are similar to some of the manifestations of meningitis. The client may present with headache, fever, and focal neurologic deficits or nonspecific signs and symptoms. Perform a complete neurologic assessment. The client may be mildly lethargic or somewhat confused. The pupillary response to light is normal in the early stages. As increased intracranial pressure (ICP) progresses, the pupils may become sluggish, unequal, dilated, and nonresponsive to light. The client's level of consciousness declines to a state in which he or she loses the ability to interact with the environment. Airway and respiratory function may also be altered.

Examination of the client's visual fields often reveals a **temporal field blindness** (decrease in peripheral vision laterally). If the abscess affects the cerebral hemispheres, nystagmus and a dysconjugate gaze may be noted. Motor examination reveals a generalized weakness. More significant motor problems, such as hemiplegia, may be apparent in the presence of a frontal lobe abscess. An ataxic gait is seen with a cerebellar abscess. Sensory impairment varies, although the client often exhibits no sensory deficits. The client may have varying degrees of aphasia in the presence of a frontal or temporal lobe abscess. Seizure activity may occur because of irritation of the cortical tissue. Late in the disease process, more severe symptoms of increased ICP occur and include severe headache, coma, a widened pulse pressure, bradycardia, and irregular respirations. The client with AIDS often presents with systemic infection, CNS involvement, and lymphoma.

Some clients may have atypical presentations. Clients with atypical presentations include age extremes, such as older adults (age-related compromise in immune function) and pediatric populations (immature immune system), those receiving steroid therapy, immune-modulating drugs, and clients with later stages of human immunodeficiency virus (HIV) infection (immune system compromise). Particularly in the earlier stages, the inflammatory response (arising from immune system function) is responsible for much of the clinical presentation, particularly if cerebral abscess formation is a consequence of meningitis infection. Any clinical state that affects immune system function or the inflammatory response can lead to an atypical clinical presentation. The risk is that the client may progress to severe abscess formation before the onset of "classic" manifestations.

DIAGNOSTIC TESTS

A complete blood count (CBC) and erythrocyte sedimentation rate (ESR) are typically performed. The white blood cell count (WBC) and ESR are usually elevated, indicating the presence of infection. If the abscess is encapsulated, the WBC may be normal. Obtain specimens for aerobic and, when possible, and anaerobic cultures of the blood, ear, nose, and throat to determine the primary source of infection.

The health care provider orders a computed tomography (CT) scan to determine the presence of cerebritis, hydrocephalus, or a midline shift. Magnetic resonance imaging (MRI) is also useful in detecting the presence of an abscess early in the course of the disease. An EEG can localize the lesion in most cases and shows high-voltage, slow-wave activity; electra-cerebral silence may be noted in the area of the abscess. Radiography of the sinuses and the mastoid is often indicated. A lumbar puncture may be performed if meningitis is also suspected and the client does not exhibit indications of ICP elevation.

◆Interventions

Medications are prescribed by the physician to treat the abscess. Typically used antibiotics include penicillin G benzathine (Bicillin) and nafcillin sodium (Nafcil, Unipen). Metronidazole (Flagyl, Novonidazol✱) or vancomycin may be used if an anaerobic organism is the causative agent. Antibiotic dosing may be adjusted upward to ensure adequate CNS penetration. These agents are particularly useful in the early stages (cerebritis) of abscess formation. A combination of antibiotics is used, particularly if the abscess resulted from septic emboli. Antiepileptic drugs, such as phenytoin (Dilantin), may be used prophylactically to prevent seizures. The medication schedule is strictly followed to maintain therapeutic blood levels. Analgesics may be prescribed to treat headache.

The physician may surgically drain an encapsulated abscess via a burr hole to reduce the mass effect of the lesion. In certain cases a craniotomy may be performed to remove the abscess. The decision to perform surgery is based on the client's general condition, the stage of abscess development, and the site of the abscess. Provide routine preoperative and postoperative care for the client undergoing a craniotomy, as discussed earlier under Postoperative Care (Brain Tumor), p. 1058.

The client with a brain abscess is discharged to home if few or no neurologic deficits are present. Clients with severe dysfunction are usually transferred to long-term care or a rehabilitation facility. Thirty percent of surviving clients have neurologic deficits.

GET READY for the NCLEX Examination!

KEY POINTS

Safe Effective Care Environment

- When caring for a client experiencing a stroke ("brain attack"), assess airway, breathing, and circulation status first.
- Monitor clients with stroke, brain tumor, traumatic brain injury (TBI), and brain abscess for signs and symptoms of increased intracranial pressure (ICP).
- Be aware that the *first* sign of increasing ICP is a decreased level of consciousness (LOC); notify the health care provider immediately if this occurs.
- Monitor for other signs and symptoms of increased ICP as described in Chart 48-5.
- Keep the head of the bed at 30 degrees or as otherwise ordered and the head in a neutral position to prevent increasing ICP and promote venous drainage.
- Collaborate with the case manager to plan care for clients being discharged from the hospital with stroke, brain tumor, TBI, or brain abscess.
- Collaborate with other members of the health care team, especially physical and occupational therapists, and speech-language pathology (SLP), following the acute phase of a stroke.
- Be aware that clients having strokes and traumatic brain injuries are at risk for falls.
- For clients receiving thrombolytics and anticoagulants, monitor carefully for bleeding.

Health Promotion and Maintenance

- Teach clients with risk factors for strokes to avoid or manage them to prevent the chance of having a stroke; risk factors are listed in Chart 48-2.
- Teach the client with hemianopsia to turn his or her head to scan from side to side.
- Remind clients, their families, and significant others to employ home safety measures for clients who have had a stroke.
- Teach young adults, especially men, to avoid risk-taking behaviors, such as driving a motorcycle without a helmet.
- Teach clients with critically ill neurologic problems about their medications, including adverse effects (e.g., antiplatelet drugs for clients who had a stroke).

Psychosocial Integrity

- Recognize that clients with strokes, especially men, may become depressed; monitor for signs of depression, and teach families about what to observe and report to the health care provider.
- Teach the family and significant others of clients with TBI that mood disorders, including depression, are very common, even in mild injury.
- Refer clients with brain tumors and their families to health care resources, such as the American Brain Tumor Association and American Cancer Society, and suggest a brain tumor support group.
- Refer clients who have had a stroke to a local stroke support group.

Physiological Integrity

- Recall that the two major classifications of strokes are ischemic and hemorrhagic; thrombotic and embolic strokes are common types of ischemic strokes.
- Remember that hemorrhagic strokes result most often from severe hypertension, ruptured aneurysms, and arteriovenous malformations (AVMs).
- Assess common clinical manifestations of stroke as listed in Charts 48-3 and 48-4.

- Determine the specific speech and language problems manifested by stroke clients; expressive and receptive aphasia are common.
- In collaboration with the speech-language pathologist (SLP), determine whether the client experiencing a stroke has impaired swallowing; if so, modify the diet and implement swallowing precautions.
- Be aware that traumatic brain injury TBI can be either open head injury or closed head injury and can range in severity from mild to severe.
- Recognize that the priority concern for a client with TBI is prevention and management of increased ICP; interventions are described in Chart 48-6.
- Recall that brain tumors may be benign or malignant, as listed in Table 48-4.
- Note that a brain abscess is an infection within the brain that produces localized inflammation and pus; assess for signs and symptoms similar to those for meningitis (e.g., fever and headache).
- Observe for postoperative complications of craniotomy as listed in Table 48-5.

ADDITIONAL STUDY RESOURCES

Go to your Student CD-ROM for Review Questions for the NCLEX Examination.

evolve Go to http://evolve.elsevier.com/Iggy/ for Integrated Management of Care Questions for the NCLEX Examination.

SELECTED BIBLIOGRAPHY

Asterisk indicates a classic or definitive work on this subject.

*American Brain Tumor Association. (1996). *A primer of brain tumors.* Des Plaines, IL: American Brain Tumor Association.

Arbour, R. (2000). "Mastering neuromuscular blockade". *Dimensions of Critical Care Nursing,_19*(5), 4-18.

Arbour, R. (2004). Intracranial hypertension: Monitoring and nursing assessment. *Critical Care Nurse, 24*(5), 19-34.

Armstrong, T., & Gilbert, M.R. (2000). Metastatic brain tumors: Diagnosis, treatment and nursing interventions. *Clinical Journal of Oncology Nursing, 4*(5), 217-225.

Bader, M.K., & Palmer, S. (2000). Keeping the brain in the zone: Applying the severe head trauma guidelines to practice. *Critical Care Nursing Clinics of North America, 12*(4), 413-427.

Bayir, H., Clark, R.S.B., & Kochanek, P.M.. (2003). Promising strategies to minimize secondary brain injury after head trauma. *Critical Care Medicine, 31*(1 suppl), S-112- S-117.

Becskee, T., & Jallo, G. (2002). Subarachnoid hemorrhage. eMedicine Journal. Accessed February 7, 2002, from http://www.emedicine.com.

*Blank-Reid, C. (1996). How to have a stroke at an early age: The effects of crack, cocaine, and other illicit drugs. *Journal of Neuroscience Nursing, 28*(1), 19-27.

*Bohan, E.M., & Weingart, J. (1998). Neurosurgical management of primary brain tumors: Diagnosis, treatment and future trends. *Journal of Neuroscience Nursing, 30*(6), 361-362.

Bonnono, C., et al. (2000). Emergi-paths and stroke teams: An emergency department approach to acute ischemic stroke. *Journal of Neuroscience Nursing, 32*(6), 298-305.

Brown, D.M., & and Levine, S.R. (2003). Highlights from the 28th international stroke conference. Accessed April 20, 2003, from http://www.medscape.com/viewarticle/451138_print.

Censullo, J.L., & Sebastian, S. (2003). Pentobarbital sodium coma for refractory intracranial hypertension. *Journal of Neuroscience Nursing, 35*(5), 252-262.

Davis, A. (2000). Mechanisms of traumatic brain injury: Biomechanical, structural and cellular considerations. *Critical Care Nurse Quarterly, 23*(3), 1-13.

Del Castillo, M.A. (2001). Monitoring neurologic patients in intensive care. *Curr Opin in Crit_Care, 7,* 49-60.

Felberg, R.A., and Naidech, A.M. (2003). The 5 Ps of acute ischemic stroke treatment: Parenchyma, pipes, penumbra and prevention of complications. *Southern Medical Journal, 96*(4), 336-342.

Fernandes H.M., et al. (2000) Continuous monitoring of ICP and CPP following ICH and its relationship to clinical, radiological and surgical parameters. *Acta Neurochir (Suppl), 76,* 463-466.

Georgiadis, D., et al. (2001). Influence of positive end-expiratory pressure in intracranial pressure and cerebral perfusion pressure in patients with acute stroke. *Stroke 32,* 2088-2092.

Goldszmidt, A.J., & Caplan, L.R. (2003). *Stroke essentials.* Royal Oak, MI: Physicians' Press.

Guidelines for cerebral perfusion pressure. (2000). *Journal of Neurotrauma, 17*(6/7), 507-512.

Harvey, J. (2004). Countering "brain attacks." *Nursing Management, 35*(8), 27-32.

Hickey, J.V. (2003). *The clinical practice of neurological and neurosurgical nursing* (5th ed.). Philadelphia: J.B. Lippincott.

Hilton, G. (2000) Cerebral oxygenation in the traumatically brain-injured patient: Are ICP and CPP enough? *Journal of Neuroscience Nursing,* 32, 278-282.

Hinkle, J.L., & Bowman, L. (2003). Pharmacology update: Neuroprotection for ischemic stroke. *Journal of Neuroscience Nursing, 35*(2), 114-118.

Hlatky, R., et al. (2003). Intracranial hypertension and cerebral ischemia after severe traumatic brain injury. Retrieved May 14, 2003, from http://www.medscape.com/viewarticle/452766_print.

Hung, O.R., et al. (2000). Head elevation reduces head-rotation associated increased ICP in patients with intracranial tumors. *Canadian Journal of Anesthesia, 47*(5), 415-420.

*Indications for intracranial pressure monitoring. (2000). *Journal of Neurotrauma, 17,* 479-491.

Intracranial pressure treatment threshold. (2000). *Journal of Neurotrauma, 17*(6/7), 493-495.

Jacobi, J., et al. (2002). Clinical practice guidelines for the sustained use of sedatives and analgesics in the critically ill adult. *Critical Care Medicine, 30*(1), 119-141.

*Jauch, E.C., & Elias, B. (1999). Intracerebral hemorrhage: Pathophysiology and management. *Air Medical Journal, 18*(2), 62-67.

Kelley, R.E., & Minagar, A. (2003). Cardioembolic stroke: An update. *Southern Medical Journal,* 96(4), 343-349.

Kondziolka, D., et al. (2002). The role of cell therapy in stroke. Accessed January 26, 2003, from http://www.medscape.com/viewarticle/446194_print.

Libby, P. (2002). Atherosclerosis: The new view. *Scientific American, May,* 47-55.

Littlejohns, L.R., & Bader, M.K. (2001). Guidelines for the management of severe head injury: Clinical application and changes in practice. *Critical Care Nurse, 21*(6), 48-65.

Liu, J.K., et al. (2003). Conduits for cerebrovascular bypass and lessons learned from the cardiovascular experience. Accessed April 24, 2003, from http://www.medscape.com/viewarticle/451256_print.

Lutz, B.J. (2004). Determinants of discharge destination for stroke patients. *Rehabilitation Nursing, 29*(5), 154-163.

March, K. (2000a). Intracranial pressure monitoring and assessing intracranial compliance in brain injury. *Critical Care Nursing Clinics of North America, 12,* 429-436.

March, K. (2000b). Application of technology in the treatment of traumatic brain injury. *Critical Care Nursing Quarterly, 23*(3), 26-37.

Mateo, M.A. (2003). Evaluation of patients with mild traumatic brain injury. *Lippincott's Case Management, 8*(5), 203-207.

NIH Consensus Development Panel on rehabilitation of Persons with Traumatic Brain Injury. (2000). Rehabilitation of persons with traumatic brain injury. *Journal of the American Medical Association, 282*(10), 974-986.

Nolan, S., Naylor, G., & Burns, M. (2003). Code Gray–An organized approach to inpatient stroke. *Critical Care Nurse Quarterly, 26*(4), 296-302.

Recommendations for intracranial pressure monitoring technology. (2000). *Journal of Neurotrauma,* 17 (6/7), 497-506.

Resuscitation of blood pressure and oxygenation. (2000). *Journal of Neurotrauma, 17*(6/7), 471-478.

Rhoney, D.H., & Parker, D. (2001). Use of sedative and analgesic agents in neurotrauma patients: Effects on cerebral physiology. *Neurological Research, 23,* 237-259.

Robertson, C.S. (2001) Management of cerebral perfusion pressure after traumatic brain injury. Anesthesiology, *95,* 1513-1517.

Roth, P., & Farls, K. (2000). Pathophysiology of traumatic brain injury. *Critical Care Nursing Quarterly, 23*(3), 14-25.

Shepard, S. (2001). Head trauma. Accessed February 7, 2002, from http://www.medscape.com.

Smillova, A., & Walker, E. (2000). Meningococcemia: A critical care emergency. *Critical Care Nurse, 20*(5), 28-38.

Stubgen, J.-P., & Caronna, J.J. (2002). Coma. In J. E. Parillo & R.P. Dellinger (Eds.), *Critical care medicine: Principles of diagnosis and management in the adult.* St. Louis: Mosby.

Thompson, H.J. (2000). Managing patients with lumbar drainage devices. *Critical Care Nurse, 20*(5), 59-68.

Tolias, C., & Sgouros, S. (2001). Initial evaluation and management of CNS injury. *eMedicine Journal, 2*(10). Accessed November 29, 2001 from http://www.emedicine.com/med/topic3216.htm.

Torbey, M.T., & Bhardwaj, A. (2001). How to manage blood pressure in critically ill neurologic patients. *The Journal of Critical Illness, 16*(4), 179-192.

Tummala, R.P., et al. (2003). Extracranial-intracranial bypass for symptomatic occlusive cerebrovascular disease not amenable to carotid endarterectomy. Accessed April 24, 2003, from http://www.medscape.com/viewarticle/451261_print.

Vinas, F.C. (2001). Bedside invasive monitoring techniques in severe brain-injured patients. *Neurological. Research, 23,* 157-166.

Winkleman, C. (2000). Effect of backrest position on intracranial and cerebral perfusion pressures in traumatically brain-injured adults. *American Journal of Critical Care, 9,* 373-382.

Wojner, A.W., El-Mitwalli, A., & Alexandrov, A.V. (2002). Effect of head positioning on intracranial blood flow velocities in acute ischemic stroke: A pilot study. *Critical Care Nurse Quarterly, 25*(4), 57-66.

Wong, F.W.H. (2000). Prevention of secondary brain injury. *Critical Care Nurse, 20*(5), 18-27.

Wood, D. (2004). Into the brain: Unlocking new brain cancer treatments. *Cure: Cancer Updates, Research, and Education, 3*(1), 22-30.

Xavier, A.R., et al. (2003). Neuroimaging of stroke: A review. *Southern Medical Journal, 96*(4), 367-379.

Zuccarelli, L.A. (2000). Altered cellular anatomy and physiology of acute brain injury and spinal cord injury. *Critical Care Nursing Clinics of North America, 12*(4), 403-412.

Zweifler, R.M. (2003). Management of acute stroke. *Southern Medical Journal, 96*(4), 380-385.

UNIT **ELEVEN**

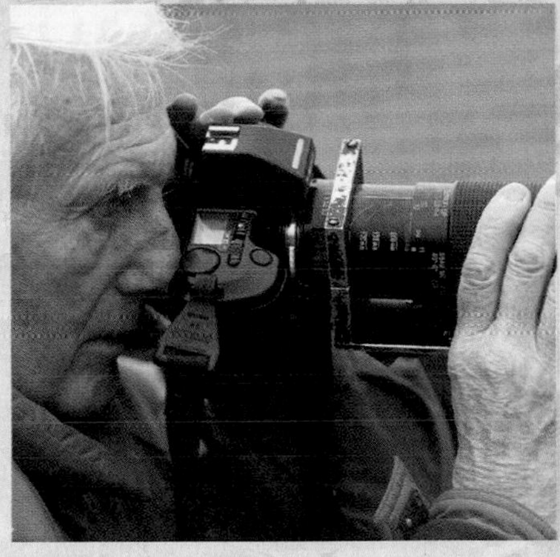

PROBLEMS of SENSATION

Management of Clients with Problems of the Sensory System

CHAPTER

49 Assessment of the Eye and Vision

M. LINDA WORKMAN

LEARNING OUTCOMES

After studying this chapter, you should be able to:

1. Explain the concept of refraction in relation to how the cornea, lens, aqueous humor, and vitreous humor contribute to vision.
2. Describe age-related changes in the eye, eyelids, and vision.
3. List five systemic disorders that have an impact on the eye and vision.
4. Discuss which elements of a client's history might predict visual impairment later in life.
5. Interpret the findings of visual acuity by the Snellen chart.
6. Describe two methods of assessing extraocular muscle function.
7. Describe the proper technique for examining the client's eyes with an ophthalmoscope.
8. Discuss the educational needs of a client undergoing fluorescein angiography.
9. Explain the relationship between intraocular pressure and eye health.
10. Use proper technique to instill eyedrops.

Go to your Student CD-ROM for Review Questions for the NCLEX Examination keyed to these Learning Outcomes.

Vision is considered by many people to be their most important sense. Vision begins with the eye and is fully perceived in the brain. Many conditions can affect the eye and change vision temporarily or permanently. Changes in the eye and vision can provide information about the client's general health status and problems that might occur in self-care.

ANATOMY AND PHYSIOLOGY REVIEW

Structure

The eyeball, a round, ball-shaped organ about 2.5 cm long and 2.3 cm in diameter, is located in the front part of the eye orbit. The **orbit** is the bony socket of the skull that surrounds and protects the eye along with the attached muscles, nerves, vessels, and tear-producing glands.

LAYERS OF THE EYEBALL

The eye has three layers, or coats (Figure 49-1). The external layer is the **sclera** (the opaque tissue making up the "whites" of the eye) and the transparent cornea on the front of the eye.

The middle layer, or **uvea,** is heavily pigmented. This layer consists of the choroid, the ciliary body, and the iris. The choroid, a dark brown membrane between the sclera and the retina, lines most of the sclera. The choroid has many blood vessels that supply nutrients to the retina.

The ciliary body connects the choroid with the iris and secretes aqueous humor. The **iris** is the colored portion of the external eye; its center opening is the **pupil.** The muscles of the iris contract and relax to control pupil size and the amount of light entering the eye.

The innermost layer is the **retina,** a thin, delicate structure made up of sensory receptors that transmit impulses to the optic nerve. The retina contains blood vessels and two types of photoreceptors called rods and cones. The rods work at low light levels and provide peripheral vision. The cones are active at bright light levels and provide color and central vision.

The **optic fundus** is the area at the inside back of the eye that can be seen with an ophthalmoscope. This area contains the **optic disc,** a creamy pink to white depressed area in the retina (Figure 49-2). The optic nerve enters the eyeball at this point. The optic disc is sometimes called the "blind spot" because it contains only nerve fibers and no photoreceptor cells. To one side of the optic disc is a small, yellow-

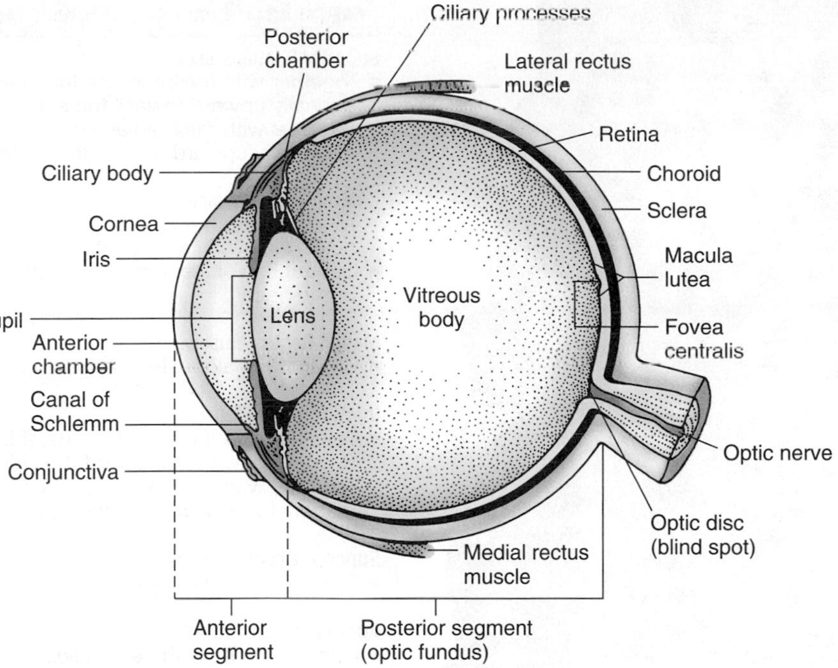

Figure 49-1 ■ Anatomic features of the eye.

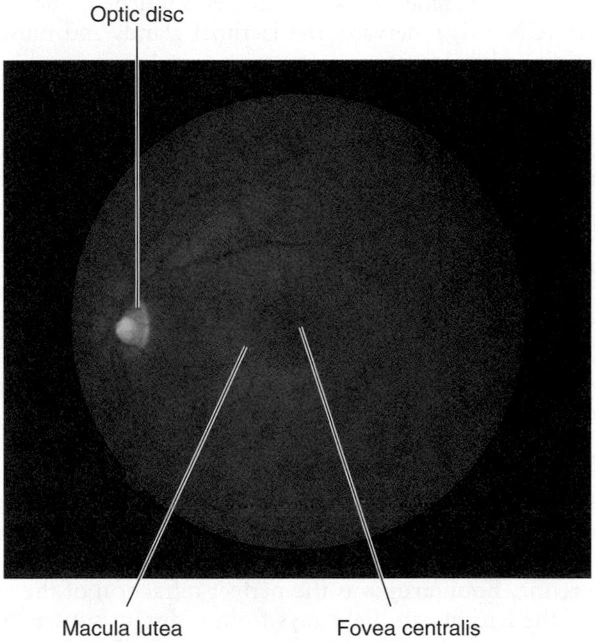

Figure 49-2 ■ A normal optic fundus.

ish pink area called the macula lutea. The center of the macula is the *fovea centralis*, where vision is the most acute.

REFRACTIVE STRUCTURES AND MEDIA

Light waves pass through the following structures on the way to the retina: cornea, aqueous humor, lens, and vitreous humor. Each of these structures has a different density, which causes the light waves to bend **(refract)** to some degree and focus images on the retina. These structures are the eye's refracting media.

The **cornea** is the clear layer that forms the external coat on the front of the eye (see Figure 49-1). The **aqueous humor** is a clear, watery fluid that fills the anterior and posterior chambers of the eye. Aqueous humor is continually produced by the ciliary processes and passes from the posterior chamber, through the pupil, and into the anterior chamber. This fluid drains through the canal of Schlemm into the blood to maintain a balanced intraocular pressure (IOP), the pressure within the eye.

The **lens** is a circular, convex structure that lies behind the iris and in front of the vitreous body. It is normally transparent. The lens bends the rays of light entering through the pupil so that they focus properly on the retina. The curve of the lens changes to focus on near or distant objects.

The **vitreous body** is a clear, thick gel that fills the vitreous chamber (the space between the lens and the retina). This gel transmits light and shapes the eye.

EXTERNAL STRUCTURES

The eyelids are thin, movable folds of skin that protect the eyes, shut out light during sleep, and keep the cornea moist. The upper eyelid is larger than the lower one. The **canthus** is the place where the two eyelids meet at the corner of the eye.

The **conjunctivae** are the mucous membranes of the eye. The palpebral conjunctiva is a thick membrane with many blood vessels that lines the under surface of each eyelid. Located over the sclera is the thin, transparent bulbar conjunctiva.

Tears are produced by a small **lacrimal gland,** which is located in the upper outer part of each orbit (Figure 49-3). Tears flow across the front of the eye, toward the nose, and into the inner canthus. They drain through the **punctum** (an opening at the nasal side of the lid edges), into the lacrimal duct and sac, and then into the nose through the nasolacrimal duct.

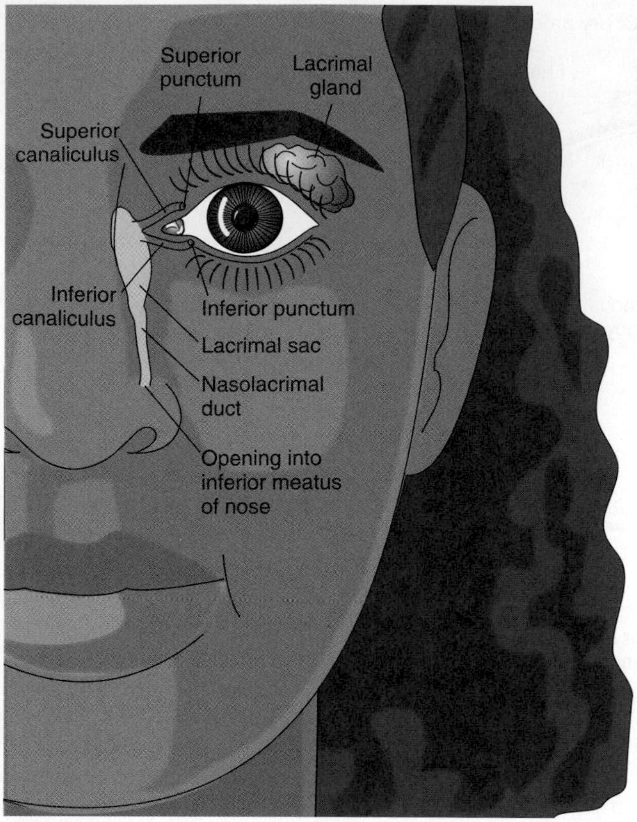

Figure 49-3 ■ Anterior view of the eye and adjacent structures.

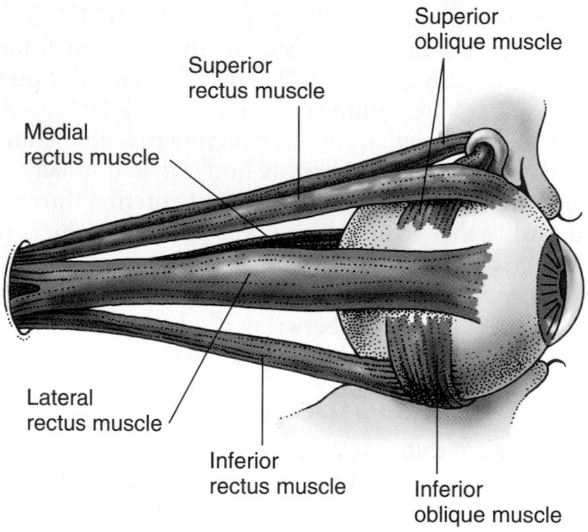

Figure 49-4 ■ The extraocular muscles.

MUSCLES

Six voluntary muscles rotate the eye and coordinate eye movements (Figure 49-4). Table 49-1 lists the functions of these muscles. Coordinated eye movements ensure that the retina of each eye receives an image at the same time so only a single image is seen.

NERVES

The muscles around the eye are innervated by cranial nerves (CN) III (oculomotor), IV (trochlear), and VI (abducens). The **optic nerve** (CN II) is the nerve of sight, connecting the optic disc to the brain. Part of the trigeminal nerve (CN V) stimulates the blink reflex when the cornea is touched. The facial nerve (CN VII) innervates the lacrimal glands and muscles controlling lid closure.

TABLE 49-1 Functions of Ocular Muscles

Superior Rectus Muscle
- Together with the lateral rectus, this muscle moves the eye diagonally upward toward the side of the head.
- Together with the medial rectus, this muscle moves the eye diagonally upward toward the middle of the head.

Lateral Rectus Muscle
- Together with the medial rectus, contraction of this muscle holds the eye in a straight position.
- Contracting alone, this muscle turns the eye toward the side of the head.

Medial Rectus Muscle
- Contracting alone, this muscle turns the eye toward the nose.

Inferior Rectus Muscle
- Together with the lateral rectus, this muscle moves the eye diagonally downward toward the side of the head.
- Together with the medial rectus, this muscle moves the eye diagonally downward toward the middle of the head.

Superior Oblique Muscle
- Contraction pulls the eye downward.

Inferior Oblique Muscle
- Contraction pulls the eye upward.

BLOOD VESSELS

The ophthalmic artery brings oxygenated blood to the eye and structures in the orbit. This artery branches to supply blood to the retina. The ciliary arteries supply the sclera, choroid, ciliary body, and iris. Venous drainage occurs through the two ophthalmic veins.

Function

The four eye functions that provide clear images of near and far objects are refraction, pupillary constriction, accommodation, and convergence.

REFRACTION

The different curved surfaces and refractive media of the eye allow light to pass through to the retina. Each surface and media bends (refracts) light differently to focus an image on the retina. **Emmetropia** is the perfect refraction of the eye: With the lens at rest, light rays from a distant source (6 m or more) are focused into a sharp image on the retina. Figure 49-5 shows the normal refraction of light within the eye. Images fall on the retina inverted and reversed left to right. For example, an object in the lower nasal visual field strikes the upper outer area of the retina.

Errors of refraction are common. **Hyperopia** (also called hypermetropia or farsightedness) occurs when the eye does not refract light enough. As a result, images actually fall (converge) behind the retina (see Figure 49-5). Vision beyond 20 feet is normal, but near vision is poor. Hyperopia is corrected with a convex lens in eyeglasses or contact lenses.

Myopia (nearsightedness) occurs when the eye overrefracts or overbends the light. As a result, images are focused in front of the retina (see Figure 49-5). Near vision is normal, but dis-

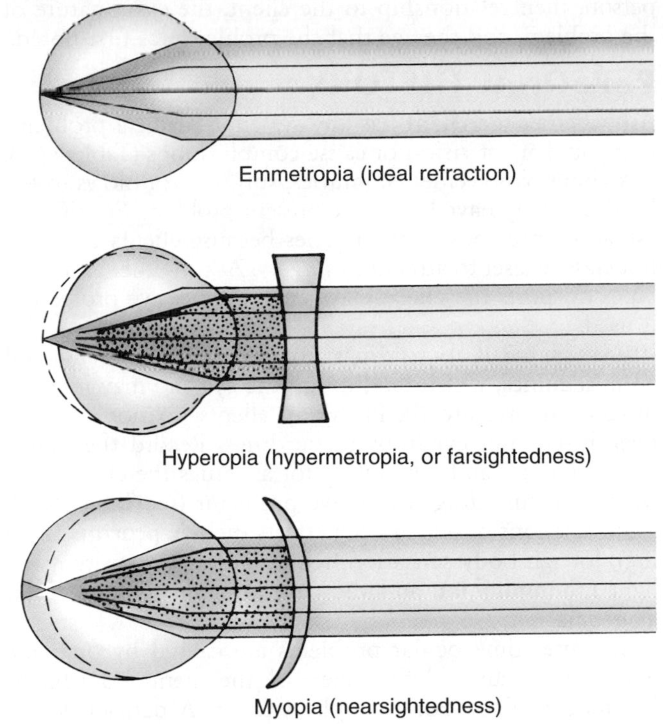

Figure 49-5 ■ Refraction and correction in emmetropia, hyperopia, and myopia.

tance vision is poor. Myopia is corrected with a biconcave lens in eyeglasses or contact lenses.

Astigmatism is a refractive error caused by unevenly curved surfaces on or in the eye, especially of the cornea. These uneven surfaces distort vision.

PUPILLARY CONSTRICTION

The pupil controls the amount of light that enters the eye. If the level of light to one or both eyes is increased, both pupils constrict (become smaller). The amount of constriction depends on how much light is available and how well the retina can adapt to light changes. Pupillary constriction is called **miosis,** and pupillary dilation is called **mydriasis.** Drugs can alter pupillary constriction.

ACCOMMODATION

The healthy eye can focus images sharply on the retina whether the image is close to the eye or distant. The process of maintaining a clear visual image when the gaze is shifted from a distant to a near object is known as **accommodation.** The eye is able to adjust its focus by changing the curve of the lens.

Eye Changes Associated with Aging

Changes inside the eye cause visual acuity to decrease with age. Age-related changes of the nervous system and in the eye support structures also reduce visual function (Chart 49-1).

Age-Related Structural Changes

In the older adult, decreased eye muscle tone reduces the ability to keep gaze focused on a single object. The lower eyelid may relax and fall away from the eye (ectropion), exposing more of the eye and leading to dry-eye symptoms.

Arcus senilis, an opaque, bluish white ring within the outer edge of the cornea, is caused by fat deposits (Figure 49-6). Although it is very common, not all older people have arcus senilis. Its presence does not affect vision.

The clarity and shape of the cornea change with age. After age 65, the cornea flattens and the curve of its surface becomes irregular. This change causes or worsens astigmatism and distorts or blurs vision.

Fatty deposits cause the sclera to develop a yellowish tinge. A bluish color may be seen as the sclera thins. With increasing age, the iris has less ability to dilate, which leads to difficulty in adapting to dark environments. Older adults may need additional light for reading.

CHART 49-1

NURSING FOCUS on the OLDER ADULT

Changes in the Eye Related to Aging

Structure/Function	Change
Appearance	Eyes appear to be sunken. Arcus senilis forms. Sclera yellows or appears blue.
Cornea	Cornea flattens, which causes blurring of vision.
Ocular muscles	Muscle strength is reduced, which results in a diminished capacity to maintain an upward gaze and to maintain a single image.
Lens	Elasticity is lost, which increases the near point of vision. Lens hardens and becomes compact. Cataracts form.
Iris	Decrease in ability to dilate results in small pupil size and poor adaptation to darkness.
Pupil	Pupil size is smaller. Aperture size takes longer to change, which reduces the ability to see in dim light.
Color vision	Discrimination among colors of short wavelength (green, blue, violet) decreases.
Tears	Diminished tear production results in dry eyes, increasing discomfort and risk for infection.

Age-Related Functional Changes

The lens yellows with aging, reducing the ability of the eye to transmit and focus light. The aging lens hardens, shrinks, and loses elasticity. As the lens loses elasticity, the ability of the eye to accommodate is gradually lost. The **near point of vision** (the closest distance at which the eye can see an object clearly) increases. Near objects (especially reading material) must be placed farther from the eye to be seen clearly. This age-related change is called **presbyopia.** In addition, the **far point** (farthest point at which an object can be distinguished) decreases. Thus the older person has a narrower visual field.

As a person ages, general color perception decreases, especially among the colors of green, blue, and violet. More light is needed to stimulate the visual receptors. Intraocular pressure (IOP) is slightly higher in older adults.

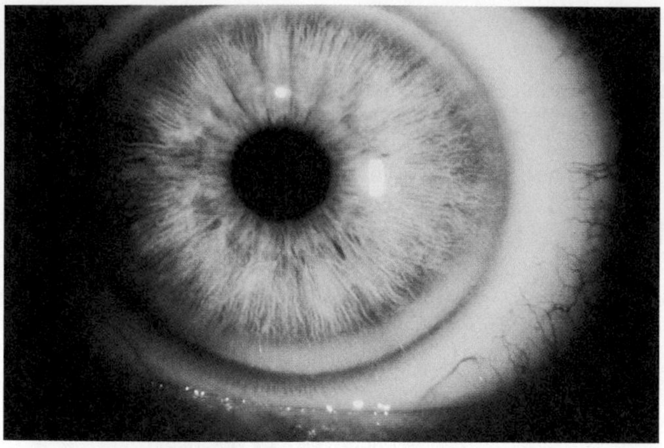

Figure 49-6 ■ Arcus senilis of the iris.

CHART 49-2

Eye and Vision Assessment
USING GORDON'S FUNCTIONAL HEALTH PATTERNS

Cognition Perceptual Pattern
- Do you have any difficulty seeing objects at a distance?
- Do you have any difficulty reading fine print or doing close work?
- Do you wear eyeglasses or contact lenses?
- What type of light do you use for reading?
- Do you wear sunglasses or a hat when outdoors?
- Do you have frequent headaches?
- Have you noticed any change in your ability to see things at night?
- When did you last have your eyes examined?
- Do you go to an ophthalmologist or an optometrist?
- When were you last tested for glaucoma?

Based on Gordon, M. (2002). *Manual of nursing diagnosis* (10th ed.). St. Louis: Mosby.

ASSESSMENT TECHNIQUES

History

Collect subjective information from the client to determine whether problems with the eye or vision have an impact on daily functioning. Chart 49-2 lists some questions to ask when assessing eye and vision history.

DEMOGRAPHIC DATA

Age is an important factor to consider when assessing the visual processes and eye structure. The incidence of glaucoma and cataract formation increases with aging. Presbyopia commonly begins in the 40s.

Gender also may be important. For example, retinal detachments are more common in men, and dry-eye symptoms are more common in women.

FAMILY HISTORY AND GENETIC RISK

Ask the client about a family history of eye problems. Some conditions, such as a refractive error, show a familial tendency. In addition, some genetic problems lead to visual impairment in adulthood. Table 49-2 lists some eye and vision problems that may have a genetic basis. When a client tells you that other relatives, especially first-degree relatives, have eye problems, be sure to record the gender of the affected person, their relationship to the client, the exact nature of the problem, and the age that the problem was first noted.

PERSONAL HISTORY

Ask whether the client has any systemic medical problems that could affect vision or cause complications (Table 49-3). Ask about past accidents, injuries, surgeries, or blows to the head that may have led to the present problem. Specifically ask about previous laser surgeries because clients often do not classify laser treatment as surgery. Ask whether and what types of sports the client plays and whether eye protection is used.

Ask the client about drugs, especially decongestants and antihistamines, which tend to dry the eye and may increase intraocular pressure (IOP). Many clients do not consider over-the-counter eyedrops to be drugs. Record the name, strength, dose, and scheduling for all drugs the client uses. Many systemic drugs cause eye problems (see Table 49-3). Manifestations of ocular drug effects include **pruritus** (itching), foreign body sensation, redness, tearing, sensitivity to light **(photophobia)**, and the development of cataracts or glaucoma.

Because some ocular problems are caused by or made worse with vitamin deficiencies, ask the client about his or her food choices. For example, vitamin A deficiency can cause eye dryness, keratomalacia, and blindness.

Ask the client about his or her work and specifically how the eyes are used. In some occupations, such as computer programming, constant exposure to monitor screens may lead to eyestrain and the need for eyeglasses. Machine operators are at risk for eye injury because of the high speeds at which particles can be thrown at the eye. Ask the client who works in industrial settings about the use of protective eyewear, such as goggles. Chronic exposure to infrared or ultraviolet light may cause photophobia and cataract formation.

CURRENT HEALTH PROBLEMS

Ask the client about the onset of visual changes. Did the change occur rapidly or slowly? *A client with a sudden or persistent loss of vision within the past 48 hours should be seen immediately by an ophthalmologist, as should the client experiencing trauma, a foreign body in the eye, sudden ocular pain, or sudden redness.* Determine whether the same symptoms are present to the same degree in both eyes.

Ask the following questions if ocular injury or eye trauma is involved:
- How long ago did the injury occur?
- What was the client doing when it happened?
- If a foreign body was involved, what was its source?
- Was any first aid administered at the scene? If so, what actions were taken?

Physical Assessment

INSPECTION

Look for head tilting, squinting, or other noticeable actions that offer clues to compensatory stances for attaining clear vision. For example, clients with double vision may cock the head to the side in an attempt to focus the two images into one, or they may close one eye to see more clearly.

TABLE 49-2 Genetic Disorders Affecting the Eye and Vision in Adults

Disorder	Eye and Vision Problems	Related Health Problems	Inheritance Pattern
Retinitis pigmentosa	Increased pigmentation leading to night blindness and reduced visual fields, eventually progressing to total blindness	None consistently present	AR (85%-90% AD (10%) XL (<1%)
Cone-rod retinal dystrophy	Colorblindness, night blindness, reduced peripheral vision, eventually progressing to total blindness	None consistently present	AR
Bothnia retinal dystrophy	Atrophy of rods, night blindness, eventually progressing to total blindness	None consistently present	AD
Ocular albinism	Decreased visual acuity, myopia, colorblindness	None consistently present	XL
Pericentral pigmentary retinopathy	Progressive retinal degeneration and atrophy in young adults, progressing to total blindness by 6th and 7th decades of life	None consistently present	AD
Alström syndrome	Retinal atrophy and progressive blindness	Diabetes mellitus, obesity	AR
Usher syndrome	Progressive retinal pigmentation and total blindness	Progressive hearing loss	AR
Amyloidosis	Corneal dystrophy, reduced acuity	Cutaneous amyloidosis	XL
Choroidal sclerosis	Progressive degeneration of choroidal capillaries and retinal epithelial atrophy, blindness	None consistently present	XL
Rieger syndrome	Early onset glaucoma	None consistently present	AD

AD, Autosomal dominant; *AR*, autosomal recessive; *XL*, X-linked.

TABLE 49-3 Extraocular Conditions Affecting the Eye and Vision

Systemic Disorders	Drugs
■ Diabetes mellitus	■ Antihistamines
■ Hypertension	■ Decongestants
■ Lupus erythematosus	■ Antibiotics
■ Sarcoidosis	■ Opioids
■ Thyroid dysfunction	■ Anticholinergics
■ Acquired immunodeficiency syndrome	■ Cholinergic agonists
■ Cardiac disease	■ Sympathomimetics
■ Multiple sclerosis	■ Oral contraceptives
■ Pregnancy	■ Antineoplastic agents
	■ Corticosteroids
	■ Carbonic anhydrase inhibitors
	■ Beta blockers

Video Clip: External Eye ▶

Assess for symmetry in the appearance of the eyes. Check the eyes to determine whether they are equal distance from the nose, the same size, and of the same degree of prominence. Assess the eyes for their placement in the orbits and for symmetry of movement. **Exophthalmos** (proptosis) is protrusion of the eye. **Enophthalmos** is the sunken appearance of the eye.

Assess the eyebrows and eyelashes for hair distribution, and determine the direction of the eyelashes. Eyelashes normally point outward and away from the eyelid. Assess the eyelids for **ptosis** (drooping), redness, lesions, or swelling. The lids normally close completely, with the upper and lower lid edges touching. When the eyes are open, the upper lid covers a small portion of the iris. The edge of the lower lid lies below the line between the cornea and sclera. No sclera should be visible between the eyelid and the iris.

Scleral and Corneal Assessment

Examine the sclera for color; it is usually white. A yellow color may indicate jaundice or systemic problems. In dark-skinned people the normal sclera may appear yellow, and small, pigmented dots may be visible (Jarvis, 2004).

The cornea is best observed by directing a light at it from the side using several angles. The cornea should be transparent, smooth, shiny, and bright. Any cloudy areas or specks may be the result of accidents or injuries.

Assess the blink reflex by bringing a fist quickly toward the client's face; clients with vision will blink. This reflex can also be assessed by expelling a syringe full of air toward the eyes. The client blinks if the reflex is intact.

Pupillary Assessment

Video Clip: Pupil Responses ◀

The pupils are usually round and of equal size. About 5% of people normally have a noticeable difference in the size of their pupils **(anisocoria).** Pupil size varies in people exposed to the same amount of light. Pupils are smaller in older adults. People with myopia have larger pupils; people with hyperopia have smaller pupils. The normal pupil diameter is between 3 and 5 mm.

Observe the pupils for their response to light. Increasing light causes constriction, whereas decreasing light causes dilation. Constriction of both pupils is the normal response to direct light and to accommodation. Assess pupillary reaction to light by asking the client to look straight ahead while quickly bringing the beam of a penlight in from the side and directing it at the right pupil. Constriction of the right pupil is a direct response to shining the penlight into that eye. Constriction of the left pupil when light is shined at the right pupil is known as a **consensual response.** Assess the direct and consensual responses for each eye.

Evaluate each pupil for speed of reaction. The pupil should immediately constrict when a light is directed at it. This rapid response is termed **brisk.** If the pupil takes more than 1 second to constrict, the response is termed **sluggish.** Pupils that fail to react are termed **nonreactive** or **fixed.** Compare the reactivity speed of right and left pupils and document any difference.

In assessing for accommodation, hold the index finger about 18 cm from the client's nose and move it toward the nose. The client's eyes normally converge during this movement, and the pupils constrict equally. When accommodation stops, the pupils begin to enlarge and return to their normal size.

MEASUREMENT OF VISION

Vision is measured by various tests. First test each eye separately, and then test both eyes together. Clients who wear corrective lenses are tested both without and with their lenses.

Acuity

Video Clip: Central Vision

Visual acuity tests measure both distance and near vision. The Snellen chart, or "eye chart," is a simple tool to measure distance vision. This chart has letters, numbers, pictures, or a single letter presented in various positions (Figure 49-7). Have the client stand 20 feet from the chart, cover one eye, and use the other eye to read the line that appears most clear. If the client can do this accurately, ask him or her to read the next lower line. Repeat this sequence to the last line on which the client can correctly identify most characters. Repeat the procedure with the other eye. Record findings as a comparison between what the client can read at 20 feet and the distance at which a person with normal vision can read the same line. For example, 20/50 means that the client is able to see at 20 feet from the chart what a "healthy eye" can see at 50 feet.

For clients who are in a confined space that does not permit a 20-foot distance to the eye chart or who cannot see the 20/400 character, visual acuity is assessed by holding fingers in front of their eyes and asking them to count (Figure 49-8). This procedure is repeated five times. Acuity is recorded as "count fingers vision at 5 feet," or the farthest distance at which the client can count the fingers correctly.

Clients who cannot count fingers are tested for hand motion (HM) acuity. Stand about 2 to 3 feet in front of the client. Ask the client to cover the eye not being tested. Direct a light onto your hand from behind the client. Demonstrate the three possible directions in which the hand can move during the test (stationary, left-right, or up-down). Move your hand slowly (1 second per motion) and ask the client, "What is my hand doing now?" Repeat this procedure at least five times. Visual acuity is recorded as HM at the farthest distance at which the client correctly identifies most of the hand motions.

If the client cannot detect hand movement, test acuity by measuring light perception (LP). Ask the client first to cover the left eye. In a darkened room, direct the beam of a penlight at the client's right eye from a distance of 2 to 3 feet for 1 to 2 seconds. Instruct the client to say "on" when the beam of light is perceived and "off" when it is no longer detected. Repeat this procedure five times. If the client identifies the presence or absence of light three times correctly, acuity is recorded as LP.

Near-Vision Testing

Near vision is tested for clients who have difficulty reading and in clients over 40 years of age. Use a small, handheld Snellen chart called a Rosenbaum Pocket Vision Screener (Figure 49-9) or a Jaeger card. Ask the client to hold the card 14 inches away from his or her eyes and read the characters. Test each eye separately and then together. Record the value of the lowest line on which the client can identify more than half the characters.

Assessment of Visual Fields

A **confrontation test** is used to examine the client's visual fields, or peripheral vision. During the test, sit facing the client and ask him or her to look directly into your eyes while you look into the client's eyes. Cover your right eye, and have the client cover his or her left eye so that you both have the same

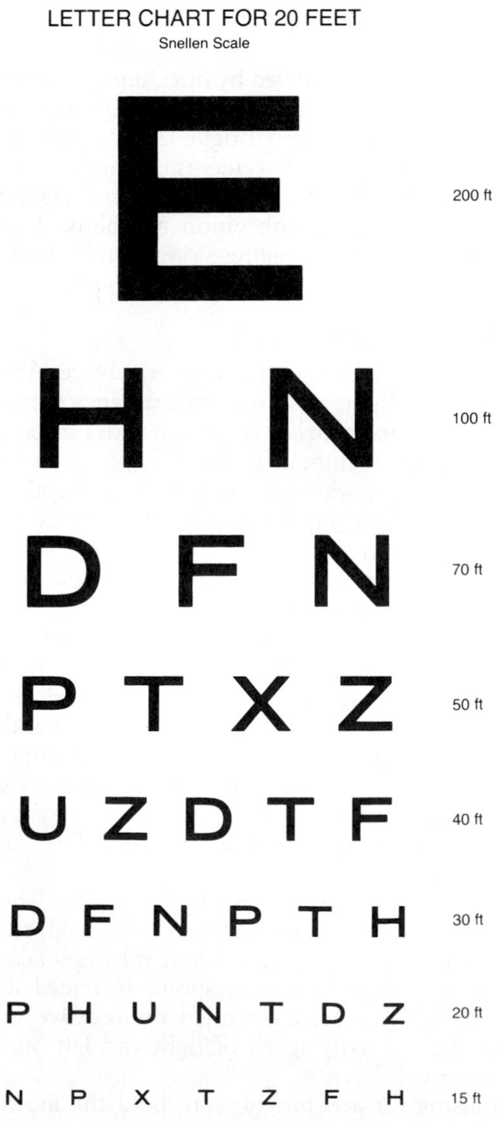

Figure 49-7 ■ A typical Snellen chart. (Courtesy of the National Society to Prevent Blindness, Schaumburg, IL.)

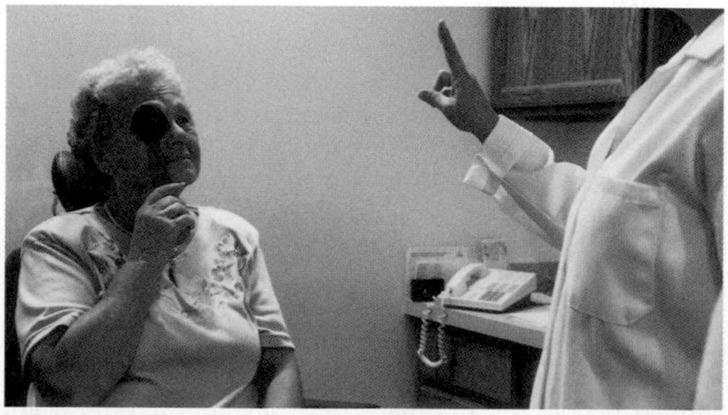

Figure 49-8 ■ Client counting fingers during determination of visual acuity.

visual field. Then move a finger or an object from a nonvisible area into the client's line of vision. The client with normal peripheral vision should notice the object at about the same time you do. Repeat this examination by covering your left eye and the client covering his or her right eye.

This test provides only a crude estimate of the client's visual fields but can reveal large-field defects such as **hemianopia** (blindness in one half the field of vision), **quadrantanopia** (blindness in one fourth of the field of vision), or large **scotomas** (blind spots in the visual field).

Assessment of Extraocular Muscle Function

Assessment of extraocular muscle function uses three tests: the corneal light reflex, the six cardinal positions of gaze, and the cover-uncover test. Also observe for parallelism of the eyes and smoothness of ocular movements.

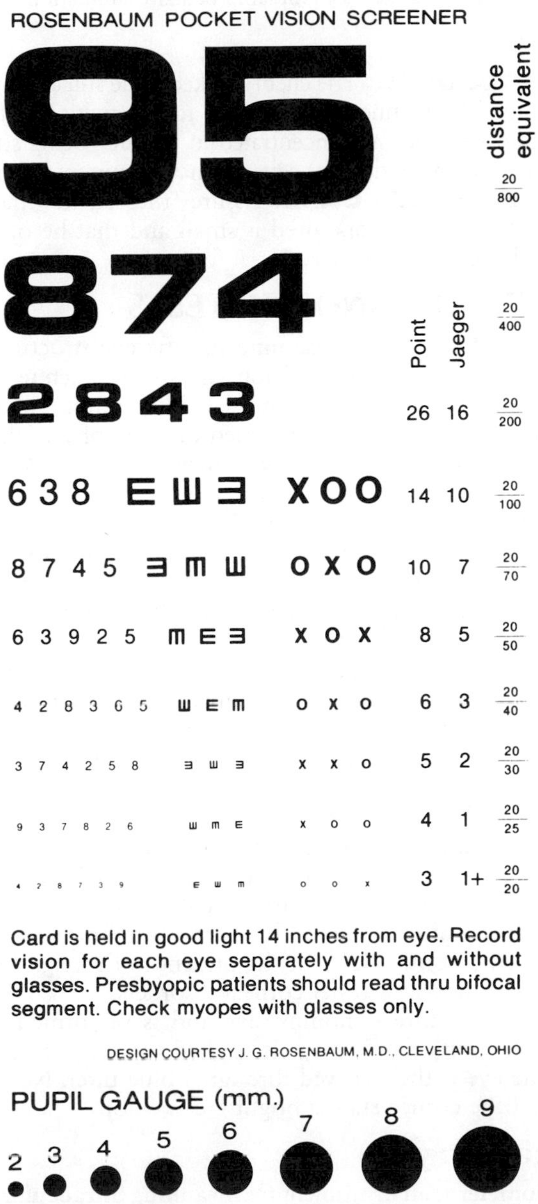

Figure 49-9 ■ A Rosenbaum Pocket Vision Screener. (Courtesy J.G. Rosenbaum, M.D., Cleveland, OH).

The corneal light reflex determines alignment of the eyes. After asking the client to stare straight ahead, shine a penlight at both corneas from a distance of 12 to 15 inches. The bright dot of light reflected from the shiny surface of the cornea should be in a symmetric position (e.g., at the 1 o'clock position in the right eye and at the 11 o'clock position in the left eye). An asymmetric reflex indicates a deviating eye and possible muscle imbalance.

Use the six cardinal positions of gaze to assess muscle function (Figure 49-10). The eye will not turn to a particular position if the muscle is weak or if the controlling nerve is affected. Ask the client to hold his or her head still and to move the eyes to follow a small object such as a pen. Move the object to the client's right (lateral), upward and right (temporal), down and right, left (lateral), upward and left (temporal), and down and left (see Figure 49-10). While the client moves the eyes to these positions, observe for parallel eye movements and any deviation of movement. **Nystagmus,** an involuntary and rapid twitching of the eyeball, is a normal finding for the far lateral gaze. It may also be caused by abnormal nerve function or prolonged reduced vision.

Another method of assessing muscle function is the cover-uncover test. Ask the client to use both eyes to look at a specific fixed point, such as your nose. Then place a card over one of the client's eyes, and observe the uncovered eye to see if it moves to fix on the object. If muscle function is normal, the eye does not move. If the eye moves, it was not focused on the fixed point before the other eye was covered. Then remove the cover and observe for any movement in the eye just uncovered. Record the presence and direction of any eye movement deviation.

Assessment of Color Vision

Several methods are used to test color vision. The most commonly used tool is the **Ishihara chart,** which shows numbers composed of dots of one color within a circle of dots of a different color (Figure 49-11). Test each eye separately by asking the client what numbers he or she sees on the chart. Reading the numbers correctly indicates normal color vision.

Psychosocial Assessment

A client with changes in visual perception may be anxious or fearful about a possible loss of vision. Clients with severe visual defects may be unable to perform normal activities of daily living and may need to change their leisure activities. The sense of dependency resulting from reduced vision can affect self-esteem. Ask the client how he or she feels about the vision changes and assess the effectiveness of coping techniques. Discuss his or her concerns with family members to determine whether support is available. Also assess the client's knowledge and use of services for the visually impaired.

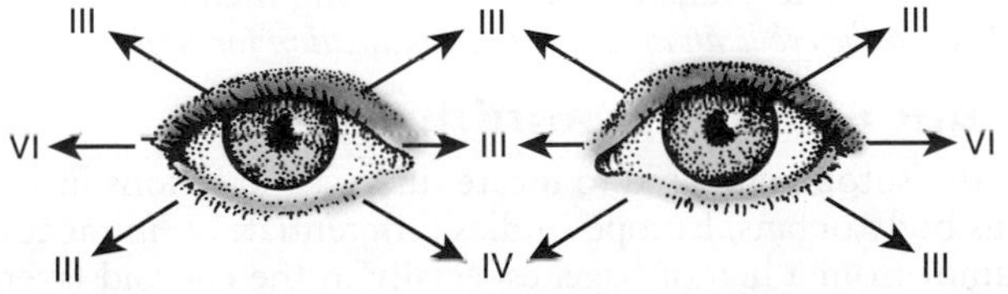

Figure 49-10 ■ Checking extraocular movements in the six cardinal positions indicates the functioning of cranial nerves III, IV, and VI.

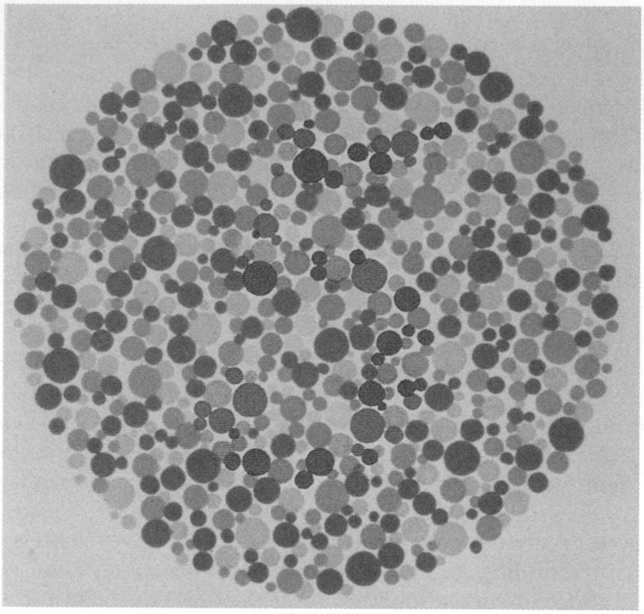

Figure 49-11 ■ An Ishihara chart for testing color vision.

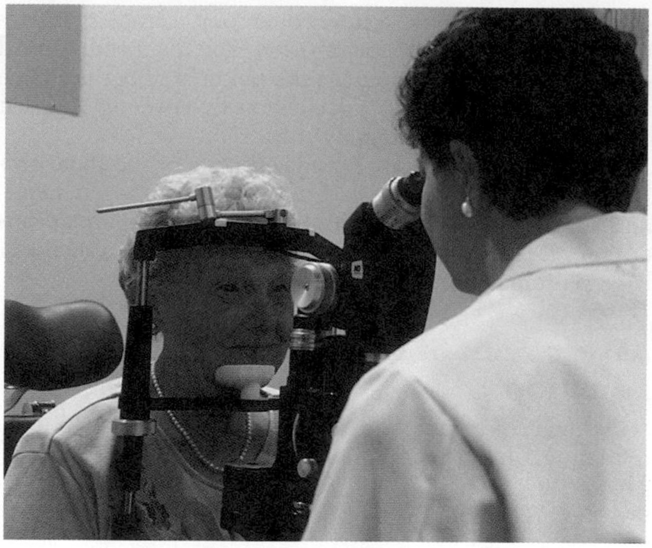

Figure 49-12 ■ Slit-lamp ocular examination.

Diagnostic Assessment

LABORATORY TESTS

Cultures and smears of corneal or conjunctival swabs and scrapings help to diagnose infections. Obtain a sample of the exudate for culture before antibiotics or topical anesthetics are instilled. Take swabs from the conjunctivae and any ulcerated or inflamed areas.

RADIOGRAPHIC EXAMINATIONS

Computed Tomography

Computed tomography (CT) is a useful diagnostic tool for looking at the eyes, bony structures around the eye, and the extraocular muscles. CT is also used for detecting tumors in the orbital space. The use of contrast dye is common unless trauma is suspected. Usually two sets of CT scans are performed, one set taken in the supine position (called axial images) and one set taken with the head tipped back as far as possible (called coronal images). The coronal images provide the "front view" needed to determine the extent of many eye problems. Inform the client that this test is not painful but does require that he or she be positioned in a confined space and keep the head still during the procedure.

Magnetic Resonance Imaging

Magnetic resonance imaging (MRI) has replaced CT in many settings for looking at the orbits and the optic nerves. MRI is also useful for evaluating ocular tumors. MRI cannot be used to evaluate injuries involving metal in the eyes. *Metal in the eye is an absolute contraindication for MRI.*

Radioisotopic Scanning

Radioisotopes are used to locate tumors and lesions in various body organs. Isotope studies differentiate an intraocular tumor from a hemorrhage, especially in the choroid layer.

CLIENT PREPARATION. After the informed consent process, the client receives a tracer dose of the radioactive isotope, either orally or by injection.

PROCEDURE. The client is asked to lie still and breathe normally. The scanner measures the radioactivity emitted by the radioactive atoms concentrated in the area being studied. Clients who are anxious or agitated may require sedation.

FOLLOW-UP CARE. Assure the client that the amount of radioisotope used is small and that he or she is not radioactive. No other special follow-up care is required.

OTHER DIAGNOSTIC TESTS

Many tests are used to examine specific eye structures but are not needed for routine vision assessment. Such tests may be indicated for those with special risks, symptoms, or exposures. These tests are performed only by physicians, optometrists, or advanced practice nurses.

Slit-Lamp Examination

The slit lamp permits the examination of anterior ocular structures under microscopic magnification (Figure 49-12). The client leans on a chin rest to stabilize the head. A narrow beam (slit) of light is aimed so that only a narrow segment of the eye is brightly lighted. The examiner can then locate the position of any abnormality in the cornea, lens, or anterior vitreous humor. The slit beam also may help identify the presence of cells in the aqueous humor.

Corneal Staining

Corneal staining consists of placing fluorescein or other topical dye into the conjunctival sac. The dye outlines irregularities of the corneal surface that are not easily visible. Corneal staining is used for corneal trauma, problems caused by a contact lens, or the presence of foreign bodies, abrasions, ulcers, or other corneal disorders.

This procedure is noninvasive and is performed under aseptic conditions. The dye is applied topically to the eye, and the eye is then viewed through a blue filter. Nonintact areas of the cornea stain a bright green color.

Tonometry

A **tonometer** is an instrument for measuring **intraocular pressure (IOP).** Normal IOP readings are 10 to 21 mm Hg. About 5% of clients with healthy eyes have a slightly higher pressure.

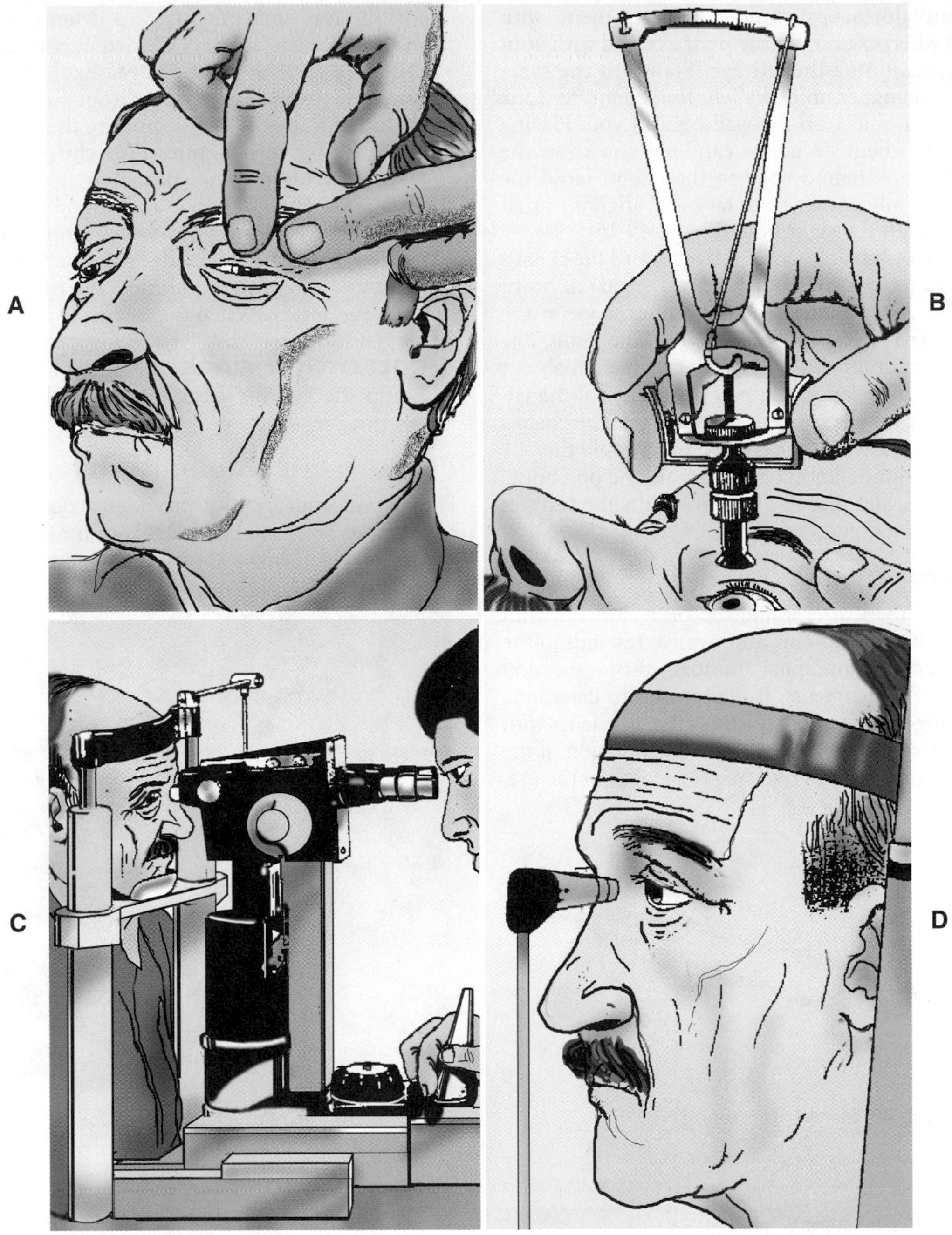

Figure 49-13 ■ Methods of intraocular pressure estimation. **A,** Finger palpation is useful only when a large difference exists between the intraocular pressure of the two eyes, as in unilateral angle-closure glaucoma. **B,** Schiötz tonometry can be learned readily. Because the tonometer is relatively inexpensive, it can be used in every physician's office to screen for chronic simple glaucoma. **C,** The air-puff tonometer can be used for screening large numbers of clients but is far more expensive than Schiötz's tonometer. **D,** Goldman's applanation tonometer, used with a slit-lamp, is the standard instrument for glaucoma diagnosis and management for most ophthalmologists. It is expensive and requires considerable skill.

Tonometer readings are indicated for all clients older than 40 years of age. Adults with a family history of glaucoma should have their IOP measured once or twice a year.

Intraocular pressure varies throughout the day. It is often higher in the morning but may peak at any time of the day. Therefore always document the time of IOP measurement.

Several methods and instruments are available to measure IOP (Figures 49-13 and 49-14). Some involve direct contact with the eye, whereas others use a noncontact technique. Table 49-4 compares the advantages and disadvantages of each method.

Ophthalmoscopy

The ophthalmoscope allows viewing of the eye's external and interior structures. It is easiest to examine the fundus when the room is dark because the pupil will dilate. When performing ophthalmoscopy, hold the instrument with your right hand when examining the right eye and with your left hand when examining the left eye. Stand on the same side as the eye being examined. Tell the client to look straight ahead at an object on the wall behind you. Placing your thumb on the client's eyebrow can help you know the distance from the ophthalmoscope to the client. Hold the ophthalmoscope firmly against your face and align it so that your eye sees through the sight hole (Figure 49-15).

When using the ophthalmoscope, move toward the client's eye from about 12 to 15 inches away and to the side of his or her line of vision. As you direct the ophthalmoscope at the pupil, a red glare **(red reflex)** should be seen in the pupil. The red reflex is a reflection of the light on the retina. An absent red reflex may indicate a lens opacity or cloudiness of the vitreous. With both of your eyes open, move toward the client's pupil while following the red reflex. The retina should then be visible through the ophthalmoscope. Examine the optic disc, optic vessels, fundus, and macula. Table 49-5 lists the features that should be observed in each structure.

Ultrasonography

Ultrasonography is used to examine the orbit and eye with high-frequency sound waves. This noninvasive test aids in the diagnosis of trauma, intraorbital tumors, proptosis, and choroidal or retinal detachments. It is also used to determine gross outline changes in the eye and the orbit in clients with cloudy corneas or lenses that reduce direct examination of the fundus. Ultrasonography helps calculate the length of the eye, one of the measurements used to determine the strength of the intraocular lens implant needed after cataract removal.

CLIENT PREPARATION. Explain the test to the client and instill anesthetic drops into the lower lid. Caution the client to avoid rubbing the eye. Seat the client upright with his or her chin in the chin rest.

PROCEDURE. The probe is touched against the client's anesthetized cornea and sound waves are bounced through the eye. The sound waves return to the transducer when they strike a non–fluid-filled structure. Structures that reflect sound waves are the cornea, anterior and posterior lens capsule, and retina. When these reflected sound waves return to the transducer, a "spike" pattern appears on the screen.

FOLLOW-UP CARE. Remind the client not to rub or bump the eye until the effects of the anesthetic drops have worn off.

Fluorescein Angiography

Fluorescein angiography provides a detailed image of eye circulation. Photographs are taken in rapid succession after the dye is given intravenously. This test is useful for assess-

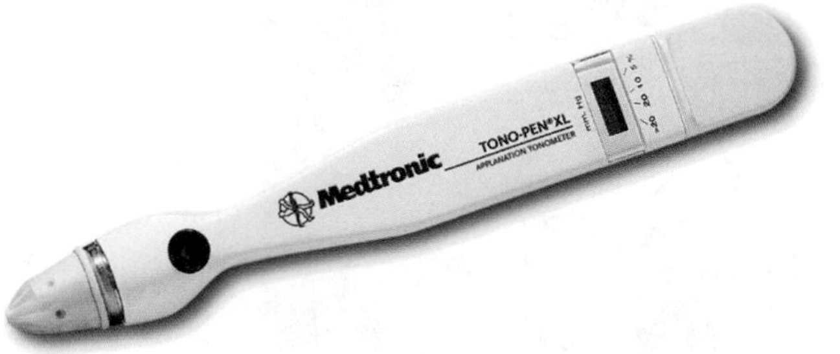

Figure 49-14 ■ The Tono-Pen.

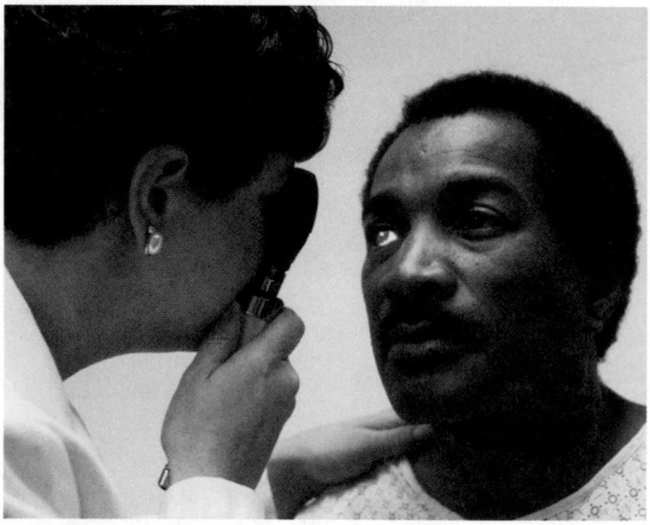

Figure 49-15 ■ Proper technique for direct ophthalmoscopic visualization of the retina.

TABLE 49-4 Types of Tonometry

Type of Tonometry	Advantages	Disadvantages
Noncontact (air-puff) tonometer A puff of air indents the cornea	No direct contact with the client's cornea No anesthesia needed Very rapid	Less accurate than direct contact methods The puff of air is unpleasant and may startle the client
Schiötz tonometer A small pressure gauge is placed on the cornea, and a weighted plunger is depressed	Reliable readings Portable Low cost	Touches the client's cornea Requires topical anesthetic May abrade or infect the cornea
Goldman's applanation tonometer The machine exerts a force against the cornea	Highly accurate Rapid	Touches the client's cornea Requires topical anesthetic Danger of infection Machine is expensive
Tono-Pen XL A penlight-sized appliance is placed against the cornea and exerts a force against the cornea	Rapid Portable Accurate Uses a sleeve to prevent infection	Touches the client's cornea Requires topical anesthetic

ing problems of retinal circulation (e.g., diabetic retinopathy, retinal hemorrhage, and macular degeneration) or for the diagnosis of intraocular tumors.

CLIENT PREPARATION. Explain the procedure to the client, and instill mydriatic eyedrops (cause pupil dilation) 1 hour before the test. Chart 49-3 lists the best practice for correct eyedrop instillation. Check that the informed consent has been signed by the client or responsible person. Warn that the dye may cause the skin to appear yellow for several hours after the test. The stain is eliminated through the urine, which also changes color.

PROCEDURE. Intravenous access must be obtained. After the needle is in the vein, 5 mL of a 10% solution of fluorescein is injected. A digital camera is set up with equipment to photograph retinal and choroidal blood vessels as the dye passes through them. The results can be viewed immediately on a computer screen. The procedure takes only minutes because the vessels fill quickly.

FOLLOW-UP CARE. After the test, encourage clients to drink fluids to help eliminate the dye. Emphasize that any yellow or green staining of the skin will disappear in a few hours. After the test, the urine will be bright green until the dye is excreted. Instruct the client to avoid direct sunlight until pupil dilation returns to normal.

TABLE 49-5 Structures to Assess by Direct Ophthalmoscopy

Red Reflex ▪ Presence or absence **Optic Disc** ▪ Color ▪ Margins (sharp or blurred) ▪ Cup size ▪ Presence of rings or crescents **Optic Blood Vessels** ▪ Size ▪ Color ▪ Kinks or tangles ▪ Light reflection ▪ Narrowing ▪ Nicking at arteriovenous crossings	**Fundus** ▪ Color ▪ Tears or holes ▪ Lesions ▪ Bleeding **Macula** ▪ Presence of blood vessels ▪ Color ▪ Lesions ▪ Bleeding

CHART 49-3

BEST PRACTICE for Instillation of Ophthalmic Drops

- Wash your hands.
- Don gloves if secretions are present.
- Explain the procedure to the client.
- Check the name, strength, and expiration date of the solution.
- Stand behind the client.
- Instruct the client to tilt the head backward, open the eyes, and look up.
- Have the client's head rest against your body.
- Pull the lower lid downward against the cheekbone.
- Hold the medication bottle like a pencil, with the tip down.
- Rest the wrist holding the bottle on the client's cheek.
- Without touching the tip of the bottle to the client's conjunctiva, squeeze the bottle gently and release the correct number of drops into the conjunctival pocket.
- Gently release the lower eyelid.
- Instruct the client to close the eyes gently, without squeezing the lids together.

Electroretinography

Electroretinography is the process of graphing the retina's response to light stimulation. This test is helpful in detecting and evaluating blood vessel changes from disease or drugs. The graph is obtained by placing a contact lens electrode on an anesthetized cornea. Lights at varying speeds and intensities are flashed, and the neural response is graphed. The measurement from the cornea is identical to the response that would be obtained if electrodes were placed directly on the retina.

Preparation includes instilling an anesthetic into the eye. Afterward, remind the client to avoid rubbing the eye until the effects of the anesthetic have disappeared.

Critical Thinking Challenge

The client is a 90-year-old woman who has experienced many vision changes within the last year. She has bilateral cataracts, macular degeneration, and has had retinal bleeding. Her other health problems include hypertension and chronic heart failure. She is being evaluated today with fluorescein angiography to determine whether surgical intervention is needed. She lives alone, no longer drives, and is accompanied today by her 60-year-old son. She is extremely anxious and repeats over and over again, "I want you to fix my eyes so I can do everything that I used to do."

1. How would you address this client's expectations of having her eyes "fixed?"
2. What could you do to reduce her anxiety over the angiography?
3. Should you include her son during any explanations or procedures? Why or why not?

evolve For suggested answer guidelines, go to http://evolve.elsevier.com/Iggy/.

GET READY for the NCLEX Examination!

KEY POINTS

Safe Effective Care Environment

- Wash your hands before moving a client's eyelids.
- If a client has discharge from one eye, examine the eye without the discharge first.
- Use contact precautions with any client who has drainage from the eyes.
- Avoid performing an examination using an ophthalmoscope on a confused or uncooperative client.

Health Promotion and Maintenance

- Teach clients not to rub their eyes.
- Teach clients who have discharge from one eye to use a tissue to wipe the drainage and discard the tissue. Use a clean tissue on the second eye.
- Identify clients at risk for eye injury as a result of work environment or leisure activities.
- Encourage all clients to wear eye protection when performing yard work, working in a woodshop or metal shop, using chemicals, or are in any environment where drops or particulate matter are airborne.

Psychosocial Integrity

- Pace your interview to match the learning needs and style of the individual client.
- Allow the client the opportunity to express fear or anxiety regarding a possible change in vision status.
- Refer clients newly diagnosed with permanent vision impairment to local resources and support groups.
- Explain all diagnostic procedures, restrictions, and follow-up care to the client scheduled for tests.
- Offer large print or auditory educational materials for the client with decreased visual acuity.

Physiological Integrity

- Ask the client about vision problems in any other members of the family because some vision problems have a genetic component.
- Test the visual acuity of both eyes immediately of any person who experiences an eye injury.

ADDITIONAL STUDY RESOURCES

Go to your Student CD-ROM for Review Questions for the NCLEX Examination.

evolve Go to http://evolve.elsevier.com/Iggy/ for Integrated Management of Care Questions for the NCLEX Examination.

SELECTED BIBLIOGRAPHY

Berne, R., et al. (2004). *Physiology* (5th ed.). St. Louis: Mosby.

Bron, A. (2001). The architecture of the corneal stroma. *British Journal of Ophthalmology, 85*(4), 379-381.

Bron, A. (2002). Danger: Ultraviolet light! *Insight (American Society of Ophthalmic Registered Nurses), 27*(3), 80-81.

Ebersole, P., Hess, P., & Luggen, A. (2004). *Toward healthy aging: Human needs and nursing response* (6th ed.). St. Louis: Mosby.

Garber, N. (2000a). A guide to performing basic manifest refractometry. *Journal of Ophthalmic Nursing and Technology, 19*(2), 84-95.

Garber, N. (2000b). Performing direct ophthalmoscopy. *Journal of Ophthalmic Nursing and Technology, 19*(3), 120-133.

Gordon, M. (2002). *Manual of nursing diagnosis* (10th ed.). St. Louis: Mosby.

Jarvis, C. (2004). *Physical examination and health assessment* (4th ed.). Philadelphia: W. B. Saunders.

Nussbaum, R., McInnes, R., & Willard, H. (2001). *Thompson & Thompson: Genetics in medicine* (6th ed.). Philadelphia: W.B. Saunders.

Pagana, K., & Pagana, T. (2002). *Mosby's manual of diagnostic and laboratory tests* (2nd ed.). St. Louis: Mosby.

Sackett, C., & Schenning, S. (2002). The age-related eye disease study: The results of the clinical trial. *Insight (American Society of Ophthalmic Registered Nurses), 27*(1), 5-7.

Sackett, C., & Schenning, S. (2003). Eye safety in the workplace. *Insight (American Society of Ophthalmic Registered Nurses), 27*(4), 101-102.

Segal, W., et al. (2001). Disinfection of Goldman tonometers after contamination with hepatitis C virus. *American Journal of Ophthalmology, 131*(2), 184-187.

Smith, S. (2003). Reducing ophthalmic drug-related injuries in older patients. *Insight (American Society of Ophthalmic Registered Nurses), 28*(2), 33-34.

Vaughan, D., Asbury, T., & Riordan-Eva, P. (Eds.). (2004). *General ophthalmology* (16th ed.). New York: McGraw-Hill.

CHAPTER 50

Interventions for Clients with Eye and Vision Problems

M. LINDA WORKMAN

LEARNING OUTCOMES

After studying this chapter, you should be able to:

1. Describe how to correctly instill ophthalmic drops and ointment into the eye.
2. Explain the consequences of increased intraocular pressure (IOP).
3. Identify common actions, conditions, and positions that increase IOP.
4. Prioritize educational needs for the client after cataract surgery with and without lens replacement.
5. Compare myopia with hyperopia for pathophysiology and the correction needed for each.
6. Describe the pathologic bases, manifestations, and nursing care priorities for primary open-angle glaucoma and acute angle-closure glaucoma.
7. Describe the mechanism of action, side effects, and nursing implications of drug therapy for glaucoma.
8. Identify the nursing care priorities for the donor when corneal donation is planned.
9. Explain how diabetes mellitus and hypertension affect vision.
10. Develop a community-based teaching plan for the client after corneal transplantation.
11. Describe the common visual deficits for the client with dry macular degeneration.
12. Identify nursing interventions to promote home safety for the client with reduced vision.

Go to your Student CD-ROM for Review Questions for the NCLEX Examination keyed to these Learning Outcomes.

Many conditions affect vision. Some conditions occur gradually, such as cataracts, and others can result from an acute insult or illness. Even when reduced vision is temporary, the client must make some changes in function or lifestyle.

EYELID DISORDERS

The eyelid is composed of thin skin attached to small muscles. It protects the eye surface and spreads tears. Eyelid problems can be related to changes in the structure, function, or position of the eyelid. Lid structure may also be altered by age (Figures 50-1 and 50-2).

Blepharitis

PATHOPHYSIOLOGY

Blepharitis, an inflammation of the eyelid edges, occurs most often in the older adult and those with dry-eye syndrome (see Keratoconjunctivitis Sicca, p. 1090). Reduced tear production often leads to bacterial infection of the eye structures, because tears inhibit bacterial growth.

COLLABORATIVE MANAGEMENT

Clients usually have itchy, red, and burning eyes. **Seborrhea** (greasy, itchy scaling) of the eyebrows and eyelids is often present. On close inspection, greasy scales and mattering may be seen where the eyelashes exit the eyelid.

Blepharitis is controlled with eyelid care using warm, moist compresses followed by gentle scrubbing with dilute baby shampoo. Instruct the client to avoid rubbing the eyes, because this action can spread the infection to other eye structures.

Entropion

PATHOPHYSIOLOGY

An **entropion** is the turning inward of the eyelid causing the lashes to rub against the eye. Entropion can be caused by eyelid muscle spasms or by scarring and deformity of the

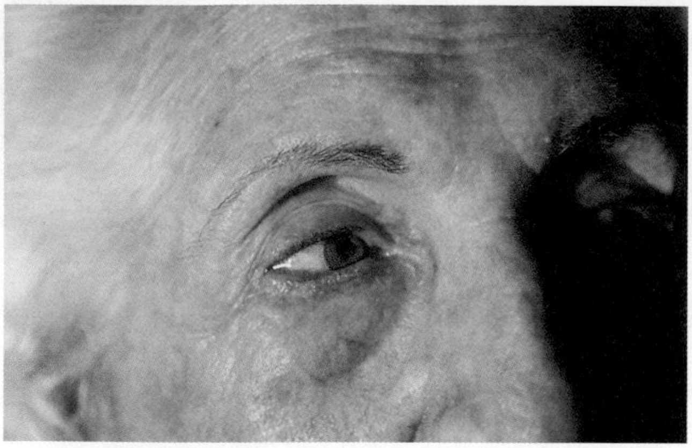

Figure 50-1 ■ Eyelid eversion (ectropion).

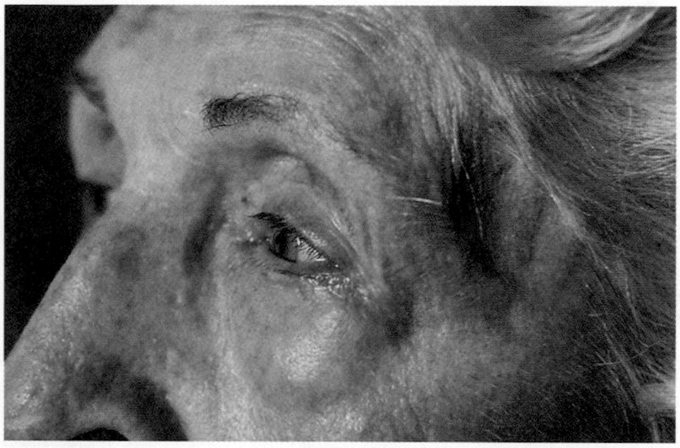

Figure 50-2 ■ "Bags" under the eyes.

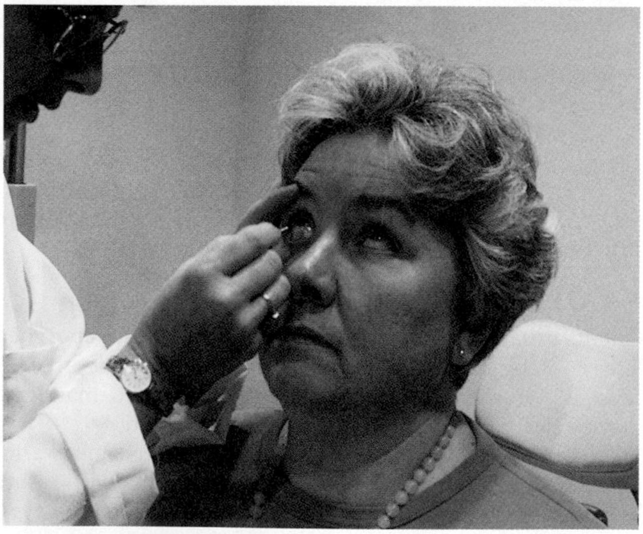

Figure 50-3 ■ Application of ophthalmic ointment.

eyelid as a result of trauma. Entropion occurs often among older adults because of age-related loss of tissue support.

COLLABORATIVE MANAGEMENT

The client usually reports "feeling something in my eye." Pain and tears may also be present. The eyelid is turned inward, and the conjunctiva is red. Corneal abrasion may result from constant irritation.

CHART 50-1

BEST PRACTICE for
Instillation of Ophthalmic Ointments

- Wash your hands.
- Wear gloves.
- Explain the procedure to the client.
- Check the name, strength, and expiration date of the medication.
- Instruct the client to tilt the head backward, open the eyes, and look up.
- Pull the client's lower lid downward, toward the cheekbone, creating a "pocket" in the lower lid.
- Hold the tube like a pencil, with the tip downward.
- Rest the wrist holding the tube on the client's cheek.
- Do not touch the tip of the tube to the conjunctiva.
- Squeeze the tube gently until a small amount of ointment is in the pocket.
- Release the lower eyelid.
- Instruct the client to close the eye gently.
- Tell the client that vision may be blurred by the ointment.
- Instruct the client to remove the ointment before driving or operating equipment.
- Remove ointment by closing the eye and wiping the closed lid from the inner canthus outward with a clean tissue.

Surgery corrects eyelid position by either tightening the orbicular muscles and moving the eyelid to a normal position or by preventing inward rotation of the eyelid. After surgery, the eye is covered with a patch, and the client is discharged a few hours later.

Demonstrate instillation of eyedrops and evaluate the client's ability to instill the drops. Instruct the client to leave the patch in place until he or she is seen by the ophthalmologist and to report any pain or drainage under the patch. Teach the client or family member how to clean the suture line with a cotton swab and the prescribed solution. A small amount of antibiotic ointment may be applied (Figure 50-3). Chart 50-1 describes how to apply ophthalmic ointment; Chart 50-2 lists important information on ophthalmic drugs.

Ectropion

PATHOPHYSIOLOGY

An **ectropion** is the turning outward and sagging of the eyelid (see Figure 50-1), which often occurs with aging. It is caused by relaxation of the orbicular muscle. This lid position reduces the washing action of tears, leading to corneal drying and ulceration.

COLLABORATIVE MANAGEMENT

Clients often have constant tears and a sagging lower eyelid. Surgery can restore proper lid alignment. After surgery, the eye is covered with a patch and the client is discharged. Nursing care is the same as for an entropion.

Hordeolum

PATHOPHYSIOLOGY

A hordeolum, or stye, can be external or internal. An external hordeolum is an infection of the sweat glands in the eyelid at the place where the eyelashes exit from the eyelid. A red, swollen, tender area is found on the skin surface side of

CHART 50-2

DRUG THERAPY for Eye Problems

Drug ❗	Nursing Interventions*,†	Rationales
Topical Anesthetics		
Proparacaine HCl, or proxymetacaine (AK-Taine, Alcaine, Ocu-Caine, Ophthetic) Tetracaine HCl, cocaine HCl (Pontocaine)	Remind the client not to rub or touch the eye while it is anesthetized.	Touching may injure the eye.
	Patch the eye if the client leaves the facility before the anesthetic wears off.	The use of a patch prevents injury, such as corneal abrasion.
	Do not use discolored solution.	Discoloration is a sign of altered drug composition.
	Store the bottle tightly closed.	Air may cause drug contamination and oxidation.
Topical Steroids		
Prednisolone acetate (Ocu-Pred, Ophtho-Tate♣) Prednisolone phosphate (Inflamase) Dexamethasone (Dexair, Dexotic, Maxidex) Betamethasone (Betnesol) Fluorometholone (Fluor-Op, Liquifilm)	Shake vigorously before use.	Medication is a suspension; shaking is required to distribute the medication evenly in the solution.
	Monitor the client for signs of corneal ulceration.	Steroid use predisposes the client to local infection.
	Advise the client not to share eyedrops with others.	Disease transmission is possible when sharing eyedrops.
Anti-Infective Agents		
Gentamicin (Alcomicin♣, Garamycin, Genoptic) Tobramycin (Tobrex) Ciprofloxacin (Ciloxan) Erythromycin (Ilotycin) Chlortetracycline (Aureomycin) Sulfisoxazole (Gantrisin) Ofloxacin (Ocuflox)	Be sure to obtain a specimen for culture before use.	Use of an antibiotic before a culture specimen is obtained may alter culture results.
	Clean exudate from the eyes before administering drops.	Cleansing decreases the risk of contaminating the medication and increases contact of the conjunctiva with the medication.
	Reinforce the importance of completing the prescribed medication regimen.	Compliance is critical to maintain a therapeutic level of medication.
Antibiotic-Steroid Combinations		
Tobramycin with dexamethasone (TobraDex) Neomycin sulfate with polymyxin B sulfate and dexamethasone (Maxitrol)	This is the same as for each component alone.	This is the same as for each component alone.
Topical Antiviral Agents		
Idoxuridine (Herplex, Stoxil) Trifluridine (Viroptic) Vidarabine (Vira-A)	Refrigerate and protect from light.	Cool temperatures and absence of light ensures medication stability.
	Monitor the client for itching lids and burning eyes.	Sensitivity to this drug is common.
Nonsteroidal Anti-Inflammatory Agents		
Flurbiprofen (Ocufen) Diclofenac (Voltaren) Ketorolac (Acular)	Monitor the client for bleeding in the eye.	These drugs disrupt platelet aggregation.
	Instruct the client not to wear soft contact lenses during therapy with these drugs.	These drugs interact with contact lens materials and increase the risk for infection.
Agents for Glaucoma		
Alpha-2 Adrenergic Agonist		
Brimonidine tartrate (Alphagan)	Do not give to clients who take an MAOI (monoamine oxidase inhibitor).	Drug can precipitate hypertensive crisis.
	Teach clients not to insert soft contact lenses for at least 15 minutes after instilling the drug.	Soft contact lenses absorb the preservative.
Sympathomimetics		
Epinephrine (Epifrin, Glaucon) Dipivefrin HCl (Propine)	Do not use with soft contact lenses.	Drug discolors soft contact lenses.
	Clients taking epinephrine eyedrops for glaucoma need to discontinue epinephrine therapy before starting dipivefrin.	Taking the two drugs together increases the side effects and can cause an acute angle-closure glaucoma.
Apraclonidine (Iopidine)	Do not give this drug to clients who have a hypersensitivity to the drug clonidine.	This drug contains the same active ingredient as clonidine.

❗ ***Med Error Alert!*** *All of these drugs are administered by the eye instillation route, not the oral route. Oral administration of these agents can cause systemic side effects in addition to not having the correct effect on the eyes.*

*When instilling eyedrops, teach clients to use nasal punctal occlusion to reduce the risk for systemic absorption and side effects.

†When more than one topical ophthalmic drug is prescribed, teach clients to separate the instillation of each drug by at least 5 minutes.

Continued

CHART 50-2

DRUG THERAPY for Eye Problems—*cont'd*

Drug	Nursing Interventions*,†	Rationales
Agents for Glaucoma—*cont'd*		
Beta-Adrenergic Blockers		
Levobunolol HCl (Betagan Liquifilm) Betaxolol HCl (Betoptic) Metipranolol HCl (Metipranolol, OptiPranolol) Carteolol HCl (Ocupress) Timolol (Betimol, Timoptic) Levobetaxolol (Betaxon)	Use of any beta-adrenergic blocker is contraindicated in clients with severe asthma or chronic obstructive pulmonary disease.	These drugs, if absorbed systemically, constrict bronchiolar smooth muscle and narrow the airways.
	Caution diabetic clients using beta-adrenergic blockers to check blood glucose levels frequently.	These drugs mask the hypoglycemic symptoms.
	Teach clients who are taking these drugs along with systemic beta-adrenergic blockers to take their pulse at least twice per day.	These drugs can potentiate the effects of systemic beta-adrenergic drugs on heart rate and blood pressure.
Mitotics, Direct-Acting		
Acetylcholine chloride Carbachol (Carboptic, Carbastat, Isopto Carbachol, Miostat) Pilocarpine (Isopto Carpine, Pilocar, Akarpine, Pilopine)	Do not use this class of drugs in clients with corneal abrasion.	Drug increases penetration of drug and the risk for side effects.
	Caution clients to not exceed the dose or scheduling of this drug class.	Drug excess can lead to systemic side effects.
Mitotics, Cholinesterase Inhibitors		
Demecarium bromide (Humorsol)	Tell clients that pupil changes may not be present for the first 24 hours.	Drug has a slow onset of action and a long duration of action.
Echothiophate iodide (Phospholine Iodide)	Teach clients to have their intraocular pressure measured more frequently when using this drug.	Tolerance develops quickly with this drug; a rest period of several days restores response.
Carbonic Anhydrase Inhibitors		
Dorzolamide (TruSopt) Brinzolamide (Azopt)	Do not give this class of drugs to clients who have a known hypersensitivity to sulfonamides.	Drug contains similar proteins, and allergic reactions are possible.
	Teach clients to not wear contact lenses during or within 15 minutes of instilling these drugs.	Contact lenses absorb the drug and may cloud or discolor.
Prostaglandin Agonist		
Latanoprost (Xalatan)	Inform clients that a change in the color of the iris does not interfere with vision.	Many clients have increased iris pigmentation that may be permanent.
Travoprost (Travatan)	Drug should not be used in pregnant clients or those who may become pregnant.	Drug has been associated with increased pregnancy loss.
Bimatoprost (Lumigan)	Pigment changes are the same as for latanoprost.	
Unoprostone isopropyl (Rescula)	Same pigment changes as with latanoprost.	

*When instilling eyedrops, teach clients to use nasal punctal occlusion to reduce the risk for systemic absorption and side effects.
†When more than one topical ophthalmic drug is prescribed, teach clients to separate the instillation of each drug by at least 5 minutes.

the eyelid. An internal hordeolum is caused by an infection of the eyelid sebaceous glands. The most common causative organisms are *Staphylococcus aureus*, *Staphylococcus epidermidis*, and *Streptococcus*. The hordeolum usually affects only one eyelid at a time. Vision is not affected.

COLLABORATIVE MANAGEMENT

Small, beady, swollen areas may be seen on the skin side of the eyelid or on the conjunctival side of the eyelid. As the hordeolum forms, it fills with purulent material, causing pain.

Treatment includes the use of warm compresses four times a day and an antibacterial ointment. When the lesion opens, the purulent material drains and the pain subsides.

Nursing interventions include applying compresses and instructing the client in this application. Chart 50-3 lists the proper technique for application of an eye compress.

After compresses have been applied, instill antibiotic ointment. Advise the client that ointments may cause blurred vision, and tell him or her to remove the ointment from the eyes before driving or operating machinery. To remove the ointment, tell the client to close the eye and then gently wipe the closed eyelid from the nasal side of the eye outward.

Chalazion

PATHOPHYSIOLOGY

A **chalazion** is an inflammation of a sebaceous gland in the eyelid. It begins with redness and tenderness (similar to the hordeolum), followed by a gradual painless swelling at the gland. In its fully developed state, no inflammatory signs are present.

CHART 50-3

CLIENT EDUCATION GUIDE
Application of an Ocular Compress

1. Wash your hands.
2. Fold a clean washcloth into fourths.
3. Soak the washcloth with running tap water that is warm to your inner wrist. (If cool compresses are needed, follow the same steps using cold running tap water.)
4. Place the cloth over your closed eye.
5. Keep the cloth in place with minimal pressure until the cloth cools.
6. Refold the washcloth so that a different "fourth" will be held against the eye.
7. Resoak the cloth with running tap water.
8. Repeat applications three times for as many times each day as prescribed by your physician.

COLLABORATIVE MANAGEMENT

Most chalazia protrude on the inside of the eyelid. The client has eye fatigue, light sensitivity, and excessive tears.

Treatment includes the use of warm compresses for 15 minutes four times a day, followed by instillation of ophthalmic ointment. If the chalazion is large enough to affect vision, is cosmetically displeasing to the client, or recurs frequently, it may be removed surgically.

After surgery, antibiotic ointment is instilled and the eye is covered with a patch. Best practices for application of a nonpressure eye patch are listed in Chart 50-4.

Instruct the client to leave the eye patch in place for about 6 hours, then remove the patch and apply warm, wet compresses. Instill antibiotic eyedrops after use of the compresses.

CHART 50-4

BEST PRACTICE for
Application of an Eye Patch

Nonpressure Eye Patch

1. Assemble the equipment:
   - Eye patch
   - Skin preparation
   - Nonallergenic paper tape
2. Explain the procedure to the client.
3. Wash your hands.
4. Apply a skin preparation to the client's forehead and cheek.
5. Instruct the client to close both eyes gently.
6. Place a patch over the closed eyelid.

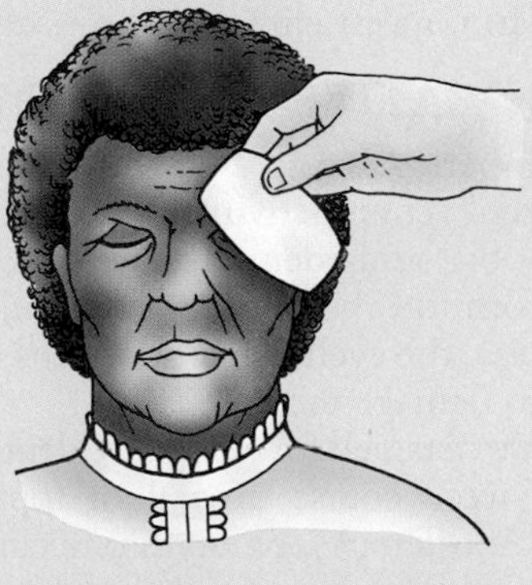

7. Apply tape from the cheek to the middle of the forehead in a diagonal line.

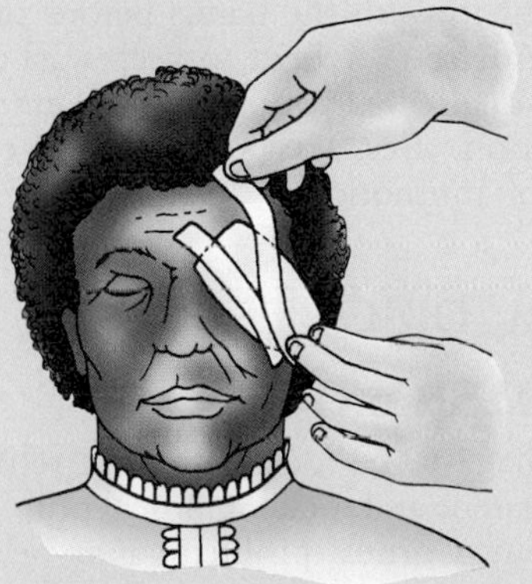

8. Cover the patch with overlapping pieces of tape.

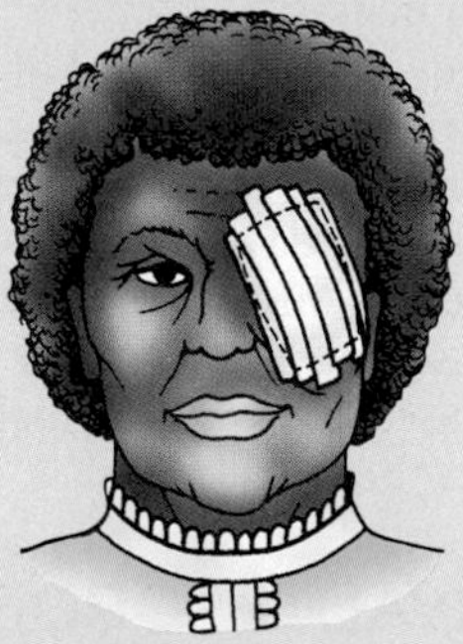

Pressure Eye Patch

1. Assemble the equipment:
   - Two eye patches for each eye requiring treatment
   - Skin preparation pad
   - Nonallergenic paper tape

2-5. Follow corresponding steps under Nonpressure Eye Patch.

6. Fold one eye patch in half, place it over the closed eyelid, and apply a second eye patch (unfolded) over the folded one.

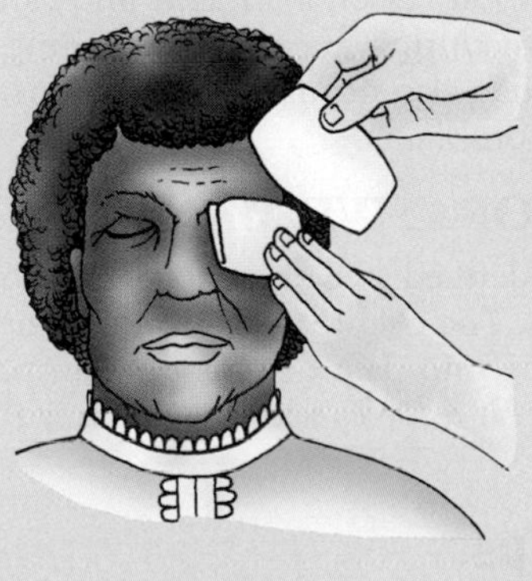

7, 8. Follow corresponding steps under Nonpressure Eye Patch.

Tell the client to immediately report increasing redness, purulent drainage, or reduced vision to the ophthalmologist.

KERATOCONJUNCTIVITIS SICCA

PATHOPHYSIOLOGY

The lacrimal system moistens the eye surface with tears and removes tears from the eye. Problems arise from reduced tear production, infection, or inflammation in the lacrimal system.

Keratoconjunctivitis sicca, or dry-eye syndrome, results from changes in tear composition, lacrimal gland malfunction, or altered tear distribution. Decreased tear production can also occur with the use of some drugs, such as antihistamines, beta-adrenergic blocking agents, or anticholinergic drugs. Diseases associated with decreased tear production include rheumatoid arthritis, leukemia, sarcoidosis, and multiple sclerosis. Radiation or chemical burns to the eye also decrease tear production. Injury to the facial nerve (cranial nerve VII) inhibits tears. Eye dryness may follow vision-enhancing surgery.

COLLABORATIVE MANAGEMENT

The client may feel as if a foreign body is in the eye, burning and itching eyes, and photophobia (sensitivity to light). The corneal light reflex is dulled or distorted. Tears may contain strands of mucus.

Treatment depends on the severity of the manifestations. Restasis, a cyclosporine ophthalmic emulsion, may be prescribed to increase tear production. Artificial tears (HypoTears, Refresh) are prescribed for daytime use to reduce dryness and can be used as often as necessary. A lubricating ointment (Lacri-Lube S.O.P., Refresh P.M.) is used at night. If the dry-eye syndrome is caused by an abnormal eyelid position or function, surgery may be needed.

CONJUNCTIVAL DISORDERS

The conjunctiva is a thin mucous membrane that covers and protects the eye. Because of its location, the conjunctiva is subject to trauma and infection.

Hemorrhage

PATHOPHYSIOLOGY

Conjunctival blood vessels are fragile and can break with increased pressure during sneezing, coughing, or vomiting. Hemorrhages may also occur with hypertension, trauma, or blood clotting problems.

COLLABORATIVE MANAGEMENT

The small, well-defined area of hemorrhage is bright red under the conjunctiva. The client is usually concerned about its appearance although no pain or visual impairment occurs with the hemorrhage. It resolves within 14 days without treatment.

Conjunctivitis

PATHOPHYSIOLOGY

Conjunctivitis is an inflammation or infection of the conjunctiva. Inflammation occurs from exposure to allergens or irritants and is not contagious. Infectious conjunctivitis occurs with bacterial or viral infection and is readily transmitted from person to person.

COLLABORATIVE MANAGEMENT

Manifestations of allergic conjunctivitis include edema, a sensation of burning, engorgement of blood vessels ("bloodshot" appearance), excessive tears, and itching.

Treatment includes the instillation of vasoconstrictors and corticosteroid eyedrops. Instruct the client to avoid using makeup until all symptoms have subsided.

Bacterial conjunctivitis, or "pink eye," is usually caused by *Staphylococcus aureus, Haemophilus influenzae,* or *Pseudomonas aeruginosa.* Manifestations include blood vessel dilation, mild conjunctival edema, tears, and discharge. The discharge is watery at first and then becomes thicker, with shreds of mucus.

Cultures of the drainage are obtained to identify the organism. Treatment is aimed at controlling the infection. Appropriate topical antibiotics are given.

Nursing interventions focus on preventing the spread of the disease to the other eye or to other people. Document the amount, color, and type of drainage. Review hygiene with the client, including handwashing after touching the eye and before instilling eyedrops. Warn the client not to touch the unaffected eye without first washing the hands and to avoid sharing washcloths and towels with others.

Trachoma

PATHOPHYSIOLOGY

Trachoma is a chronic, bilateral scarring form of conjunctivitis caused by *Chlamydia trachomatis.* Trachoma is the chief cause of preventable blindness in the world. The incidence is highest in warm, moist climates where sanitation is poor.

COLLABORATIVE MANAGEMENT

The incubation period is 5 to 14 days. At first, trachoma resembles bacterial conjunctivitis. Manifestations include tears, photophobia, and edema of the eyelids and conjunctiva. Follicles form on the upper eyelid conjunctiva. As the disease progresses, the eyelid scars and turns inward, causing the eyelashes to damage the cornea.

Specimens are obtained for culture to identify the causative organism. A 4-week course of oral or topical tetracycline (Achromycin, Apo-Tetra✱) or erythromycin (Apo-Erythro-EC✱, E-Mycin, E.E.S.) is given. Azithromycin (Zithromax) can be used once per week for 1 to 3 weeks.

Nursing interventions focus on infection control. Instruct the client to wash the hands before and after touching the eyes. Advise the client to keep washcloths separate from those of unaffected people and to launder them separately. In addition, stress the importance of completing the entire course of antibiotics.

CORNEAL DISORDERS

PATHOPHYSIOLOGY

For a sharp image to be focused on the retina, the cornea must be transparent and intact. Corneal problems lead to visual impairment. Corneal problems may be caused by degeneration of the cornea (keratoconus) (Figure 50-4); deposits in the cornea, reducing the refracting power (dystrophies); irritation or infection (keratitis); or ulceration of the corneal surface. Table 50-1 lists common causes of corneal disorders.

COLLABORATIVE MANAGEMENT

Assessment

The client with a corneal disorder usually has pain, reduced vision, photophobia, and eye secretions. Cloudy or purulent (pus-filled) fluid may be present on the eyelids or eyelashes. Wear gloves during the examination when drainage is present.

The cornea may look hazy or cloudy. An altered corneal light reflex may occur. The cornea may no longer be intact, and patchy areas may be visible on examination. When fluorescein stain is used, these areas appear green.

No definitive tests confirm corneal disease, although microbial culture and corneal scrapings can help determine which organism is causing a corneal ulcer. For culture, obtain swabs from the ulcer and its edges. For corneal scrapings, the cornea is anesthetized with a topical agent, and a sterile spatula is used to remove samples from the center and edge of the ulcer.

Interventions

NONSURGICAL MANAGEMENT. Treatment for a corneal disorder is aimed at reducing symptoms, restoring corneal clarity, and enhancing the client's ability to use the remaining vision.

TABLE 50-1 Common Causes of Corneal Disorders

Keratoconus ■ Autosomal recessive trait ■ Down syndrome ■ Aniridia ■ Marfan syndrome ■ Atopic allergy ■ Retinitis pigmentosa	**Keratitis (Acanthamoeba)** ■ Protozoal infection
Keratitis (Exposure) ■ Ectropion/entropion ■ Exophthalmos ■ Neurologic deficits	**Corneal Ulcers** ■ Mechanical injury ■ Chemical injury ■ Drying ■ Infection

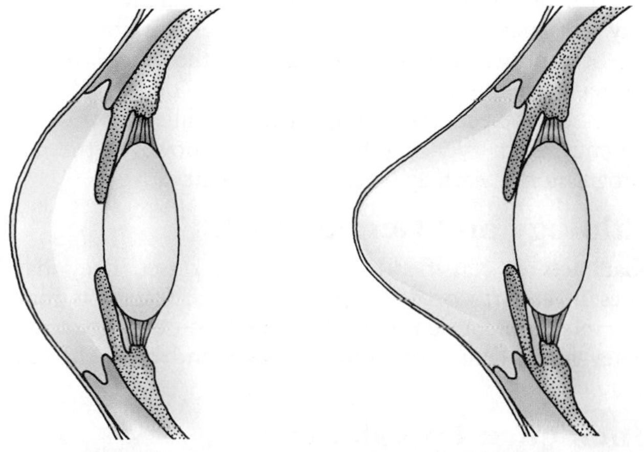

Figure 50-4 ■ Profiles of a normal eyeball and one with keratoconus.

Drug Therapy. Antibiotics, antifungals, and antivirals are prescribed to reduce or eliminate microorganisms. Usually, a broad-spectrum antibiotic is prescribed first and may be changed when culture results are known. Steroids may be used with antibiotics to reduce the inflammatory response in the eye. Drugs can be given topically as eyedrops, injected subconjunctivally, or injected intravenously (IV). Chart 50-5 lists best practices for instilling eyedrops.

Vision Enhancement. Assist clients in using their functional vision, suggesting sunglasses and indirect lighting if glare creates difficulties. Inform clients about magnifiers and special light fixtures.

SURGICAL MANAGEMENT. **Keratoplasty** (corneal transplant) is the surgical removal of diseased corneal tissue and replacement with tissue from a human donor cornea. This process restores vision by removing corneal deformities and replacing them with healthy corneal tissue.

Preoperative Care. Corneal transplantation is performed when the donor tissue becomes available. Usually the client is quite anxious. Use a calm approach to assess the client's knowledge of the surgery and of expected care before and after surgery.

Examine the client's eyes for signs of infection and report any redness, drainage, or edema to the ophthalmologist. Instill antibiotic drops into the eye to reduce the risk for infection. IV access is placed before surgery.

Operative Procedures. Usually regional anesthesia is used. The nerves around and behind the eye are numbed so that the client cannot move or see out of the eye. The surgeon removes the center 7 to 8 mm of the diseased cornea (Figure 50-5) with a **trephine,** an instrument that works like a cookie cutter. The same trephine is used to cut the tissue graft from the donor cornea. The donor corneal graft is sutured into place on the eye. Figure 50-6 shows the eye after transplantation.

Postoperative Care. After the procedure is completed, a subconjunctival antibiotic injection is given and an antibiotic ointment instilled. The eye is covered with a pressure patch and a protective shield. This dressing is left in place until the next day. Usually, the surgeon removes this dressing.

Notify the ophthalmologist of changes in vital signs or of drainage on the dressing. Instruct the client to lie on the nonoperative side to reduce intraocular pressure (IOP).

CHART 50-5

BEST PRACTICE for Eyedrop Administration

- Administer drugs at frequent, precise intervals. *The timing of administration is critical.* Clients with eye problems are often given several broad-spectrum antibiotics. If each drug is administered every hour, create separate dosage schedules. For example, give antibiotic A at 7:00, 8:00, 9:00, and 10:00. Then give antibiotic B at 7:30, 8:30, 9:30, and 10:30.
- If two medications must be administered *at the same time, separate the instillation by 5 minutes.* For example, a client with glaucoma and a bacterial ulcer receives timolol (Apo-Timop✱, Timoptic) at 7:00 and tobramycin (Tobrex) at 7:05.
- If the same medication is required for both eyes and one eye is infected, use *separate* bottles of medication.
- Clearly label each bottle with "left" or "right" for the appropriate eye.
- Wear gloves when ocular drainage is present.
- Wash your hands before and after administering eyedrops.

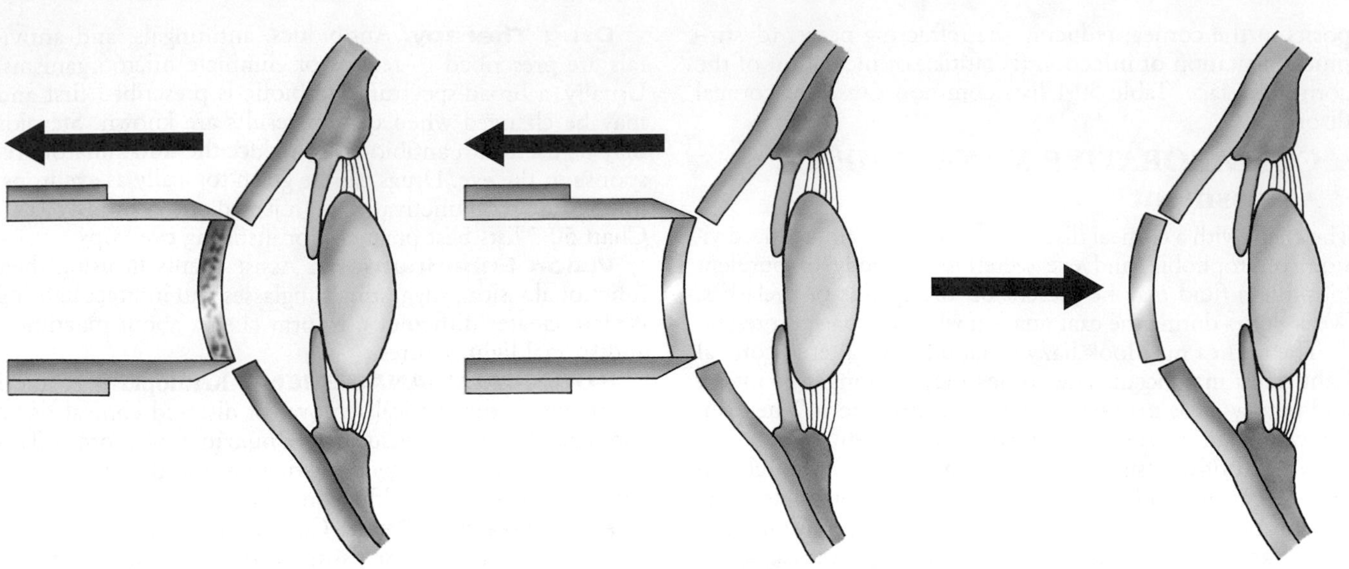

Figure 50-5 ■ The steps involved in corneal transplantation (penetrating keratoplasty).

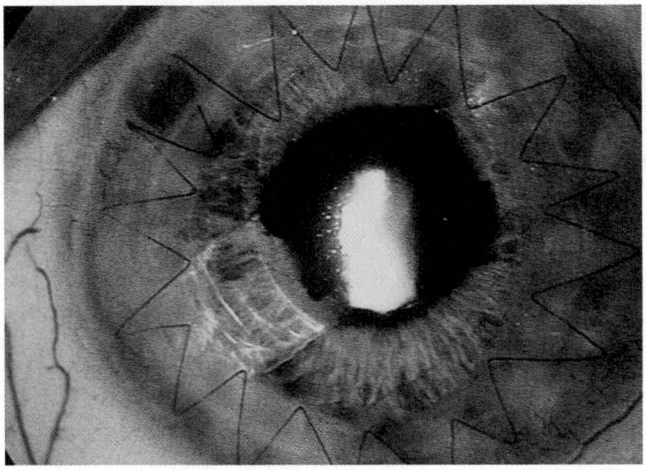

Figure 50-6 ■ The appearance of the eye with sutures in place after corneal transplantation. (Courtesy of John A. Costin, MD.)

During the early period after surgery, the client cannot see out of the affected eye because of the eye patch and shield.

If the patches are to remain in place after discharge, show the client how to apply a patch and obtain a return demonstration. Instruct the client to wear the shield at night for the first month after surgery and whenever he or she is around small children or pets. Complications after surgery include bleeding, wound leakage, infection, and graft rejection.

Although the cornea has no blood supply, graft rejection is possible. Inflammation starts in the donor cornea near the graft edge and moves toward the center. Vision is reduced and the cornea becomes cloudy. Frequent applications of topical corticosteroids are used. If rejection continues, the graft becomes opaque and blood vessels branch into the opaque tissue.

Eye Donation. Corneal tissue is obtained from a local eye or tissue bank. An eye bank obtains its supply of corneal tissue from volunteer donors. These donors must be free of infectious disease or cancer at the time of death. If a deceased client is a potential eye donor, follow the steps listed below:

- Raise the head of the bed 30 degrees.
- Instill antibiotic eyedrops, such as Neosporin or tobramycin.
- Close the eyes and apply a *small* ice pack to the closed eyes.
- Contact the family and physician to discuss eye donation.

CATARACT

PATHOPHYSIOLOGY

The lens is a biconvex, transparent, refractive elastic structure suspended behind the iris. A cataract is an opacity of the lens that distorts the image projected onto the retina (Figure 50-7). With aging, the lens gradually loses water and increases in density. This increased density occurs as older lens fibers are compressed and new fibers are produced in the outer layers. Lens proteins dry out and form crystals. As the density of the lens increases, it becomes opaque with a painless loss of transparency. Both eyes may have cataracts; however, the rate of progression in each eye is usually different.

Etiology and Genetic Risk

Cataracts are classified by nature or by onset. They may be present at birth or develop at any time. Cataracts may be age related or caused by trauma or exposure to toxic agents. They also occur with other diseases and ocular disorders (Table 50-2).

Incidence/Prevalence

Cataracts develop in 5 to 10 million people worldwide every year. The age-related cataract is the most common type. Some

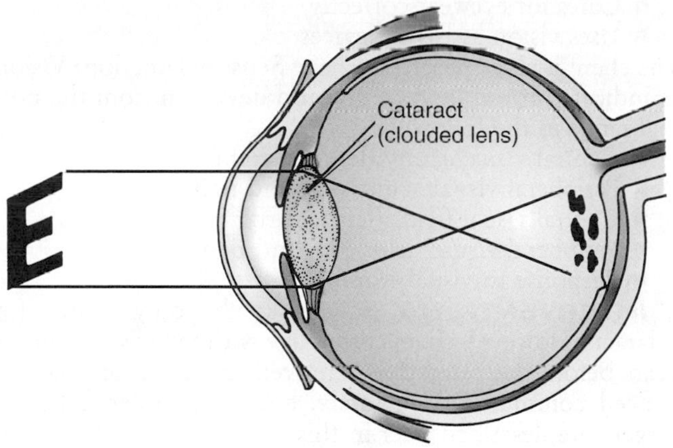

Figure 50-7 ■ The visual impairment produced by the presence of a cataract.

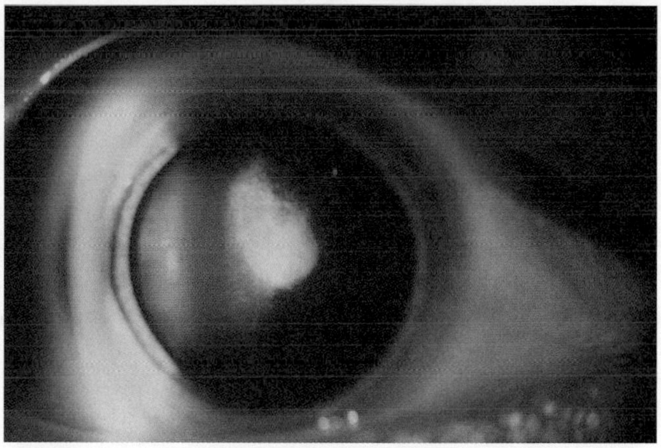

Figure 50-8 ■ The appearance of an eye with a mature cataract. (Courtesy of John A. Costin, MD.)

TABLE 50-2 Common Causes of Cataracts

Age-Related Cataracts
- Lens water loss and fiber compaction

Traumatic Cataracts
- Blunt injury to eye or head
- Penetrating eye injury
- Intraocular foreign bodies
- Radiation exposure, therapy

Toxic Cataracts
- Corticosteroids
- Phenothiazine derivatives
- Miotic agents

Associated Cataract
- Diabetes mellitus
- Hypoparathyroidism
- Down syndrome
- Chronic sunlight exposure

Complicated Cataracts
- Retinitis pigmentosa
- Glaucoma
- Retinal detachment

CHART 50-6

KEY FEATURES of Cataracts

Early
- Blurred vision
- Decreased color perception

Late
- Diplopia
- Reduced visual acuity progressing to blindness
- Absence of red reflex
- Presence of white pupil

degree of cataract formation is expected in all people older than 70 years of age (Vaughan, Asbury, & Riordan-Eva, 2004).

HEALTH PROMOTION/ILLNESS PREVENTION

Although most cases of cataracts in North America are age related, the onset of cataract formation occurs earlier with heavy sun exposure or exposure to other sources of ultraviolet light. Wearing sun glasses that limit penetration of ultraviolet light is a major way to reduce cataract formation. Additionally, cataracts are caused by direct eye injury. Urging all people to wear eye and head protection during sports, such as baseball, or any activity that increases the risk for the eye being hit by objects in motion, can help reduce the incidence of cataracts.

◆COLLABORATIVE MANAGEMENT

PHARM e REVIEW

◆Assessment

HISTORY

Age is important because cataracts are most prevalent in the older adult. Ask about the following predisposing factors:

- Recent or past trauma to the eye
- Exposure to radioactive materials or x-rays
- Systemic disease (such as diabetes mellitus, hypoparathyroidism, Down syndrome, or atopic dermatitis)
- Use of corticosteroids, chlorpromazine, or miotic drugs
- Intraocular disease (such as recurrent uveitis)

Ask the client to describe his or her vision. For example, you might say, "Tell me what you can see well and what you have difficulty seeing." This technique helps determine the impact of visual deficits on the client.

PHYSICAL ASSESSMENT/CLINICAL MANIFESTATIONS

Early manifestations of cataracts include slightly blurred vision and decreased color perception (Chart 50-6). As lens cloudiness continues, the client may have vision reduced to such an extent that daily activities are adversely affected. Blurred and double vision may occur. Without surgical intervention, visual impairment can progress to blindness. *No pain or eye redness is associated with age-related cataract formation.*

Visual acuity is very reduced. Vision is tested using a Snellen chart and brightness acuity testing (see Chapter 49). Evaluate the client's acuity under various lighting conditions, which can help determine the degree of visual disability.

Examine the lens with the direct ophthalmoscope and describe any observed densities by size, shape, and location. As the cataract matures, the opacity makes it difficult to see the retina and the red reflex may be absent. When this occurs, the pupil is white (Figure 50-8).

PSYCHOSOCIAL ASSESSMENT

Loss of vision is gradual, and the client may not be aware of the change until reading or driving is affected. Fear of losing one's eyesight can be overwhelming, and the client may have great anxiety during an eye evaluation.

Analysis

COMMON NURSING DIAGNOSES AND COLLABORATIVE PROBLEMS

The most common nursing diagnosis for clients with cataracts is Disturbed Sensory Perception: Visual related to altered sensory reception.

ADDITIONAL NURSING DIAGNOSES AND COLLABORATIVE PROBLEMS

In addition to the most common nursing diagnosis, clients with cataracts may have one or more of the following:

- Fear related to sensory impairment, loss of eyesight, scheduled surgery, or inability to regain eyesight
- Risk for Injury related to decreased vision
- Social Isolation related to reduced visual acuity, fear of injury, or fear of embarrassment
- Self-Care Deficit (dressing/grooming) related to perceptual impairment
- Deficient Knowledge (Cataract Pathophysiology and Treatment) related to lack of information or misconceptions
- Impaired Home Maintenance related to age, limited vision, or activity restrictions imposed by surgery

Critical Thinking Challenge

The client is a 62-year-old woman who works as a stockbroker. She has recently been diagnosed with bilateral cataracts. She lives in the Denver area and her hobbies include long-distance biking and downhill skiing. She has a glass or two of wine with dinner every night. She smoked when she was in college but has not smoked for more than 30 years. She is surprised by her diagnosis because she is a vegetarian and keeps herself physically fit. She also tells you that neither her parents nor any of her four brothers and sisters have cataracts.

1. How should you explain the influence of genetics on the development of cataracts?
2. What factors may have influenced the development of her cataracts?
3. What additional personal and family information should you obtain from this client?

evolve For suggested answer guidelines, go to http://evolve.elsevier.com/Iggy/.

Planning and Implementation

DISTURBED SENSORY PERCEPTION: VISUAL

NOC **PLANNING: EXPECTED OUTCOMES.** The client with cataracts is expected to have Vision Compensation Behavior as indicated by consistent demonstration of the following behaviors:

- Monitors symptoms of vision deterioration
- Positions self to advantage vision
- Uses adequate lighting for activity being performed
- Wears eyeglasses or contact lenses correctly
- Cares for eyewear correctly
- Uses vision assistive devices

The client is also expected to have Sensory Function: Vision as indicated by an increase to mild deviation from the normal range in the following:

- Central visual acuity (left and right)
- Peripheral visual acuity (left and right)
- Central visual fields (left and right)
- Peripheral visual fields (left and right)
- Response to visual stimuli

INTERVENTIONS. Surgery is the only "cure" for cataracts. However, clients often live with reduced vision for years before the cataract is removed. Interventions for enhanced communication, safety, and independence before surgery are described later in this chapter in the Collaborative Management section for Reduced Vision (see p. 1108).

Preoperative Care. The health care provider gives the client accurate information so that he or she can make informed decisions about treatment. Teach about the nature of cataracts, their progression, and their treatment.

Because cataract surgery is usually an outpatient procedure and most clients are older, adequate preoperative teaching is problematic. Assess how the client's vision affects the activities of daily living, especially dressing, eating, and ambulating.

Stress to the client that care after surgery requires the instillation of different types of eyedrops several times a day for 2 to 4 weeks. Careful assessment of eye appearance is also needed. If the client is unable to perform these tasks, help him or her make arrangements for this care.

An IV infusion may be started in the operating room. A sedative is given before surgery, and oral acetazolamide (Acetazolam✱, Diamox) may be given on the morning of surgery to reduce intraocular pressure (IOP). A series of ophthalmic drugs are instilled just before surgery to dilate the pupils and cause vasoconstriction. Other eyedrops are instilled to induce paralysis to prevent lens movement. When the client is in the surgical area, a local anesthetic is injected into the muscle cone behind the eye for anesthesia and eye paralysis.

Operative Procedures. Extraction of the lens can be intracapsular or, more commonly, extracapsular (Figure 50-9). The front portion of the capsule is opened and removed. Usually the surgeon then uses sound waves to break the cataractous lens into small pieces, a process known as **phacoemulsion.** The small pieces are then sucked out. The posterior lens capsule is left inside the eye to anchor the replacement lens.

In intracapsular surgery, the surgeon removes the lens and capsule completely. A disadvantage of this approach is that the protective posterior capsule is removed, placing the eye at greater risk for retinal detachment and resulting in the loss of a supportive structure for the intraocular lens (IOL) implant.

After the lens with the cataract is removed, the eye has no accommodative power and has lost most of its refractive ability **(aphakia).** A replacement lens is needed to focus light rays in the retina. Most often, a small, clear, plastic lens is implanted at the time of cataract removal. Replacement lenses can be selected to allow correction of a specific refractive error. Some clients have distant vision restored to 20/20 and may need glasses only for reading or close work. Some replacement lenses have multiple focal planes and may correct all vision for a client to the extent that glasses or contact lenses are not needed at all or are only minimally needed.

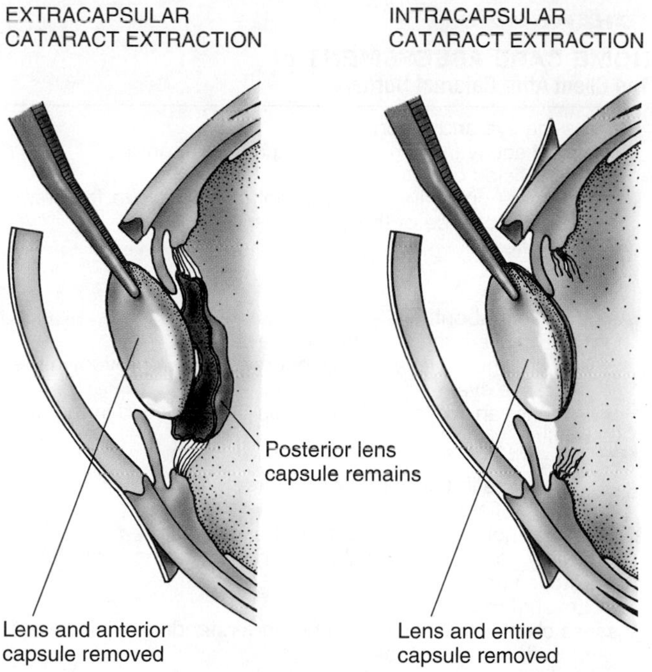

Figure 50-9 ■ Surgical approaches to lens removal for cataracts.

Postoperative Care. Immediately after surgery, antibiotics are given subconjunctivally. Usually an antibiotic plus steroid ointment also is instilled. The eye is usually left unpatched and often the client is discharged within an hour after surgery. Instruct the client to wear dark glasses outdoors or in brightly lit environments until the pupil responds to light.

The ophthalmologist examines the eye with a slit-lamp microscope the next day. Antibiotic-steroid eyedrops, such as tobramycin combined with dexamethasone (TobraDex), are instilled.

Mild itching is normal, as is a "bloodshot appearance." The eyelid may be slightly swollen; however, significant swelling or bruising is abnormal. Cool compresses may be beneficial. Discomfort at the site is controlled by a mild analgesic such as acetaminophen (Abenol✱, Tylenol) or acetaminophen with oxycodone (Endocet✱, Percocet, Tylox). Instruct the client to avoid aspirin because of its effects on blood clotting.

Pain early after surgery may indicate a complication, such as increased IOP or hemorrhage. Instruct the client to contact the ophthalmologist if pain occurs with nausea or vomiting.

To reduce increases in IOP (the major complication after surgery), teach the client and family about activity restrictions. Activities that can cause a sudden rise in IOP are listed in Table 50-3.

Another major complication is infection. Instruct the client to observe for increasing redness of the eye, a change in visual acuity, tears, and photophobia. Creamy white, dry, crusty drainage on the eyelids and lashes is normal. Yellow or green drainage indicates infection and must be reported.

Bleeding into the anterior chamber of the eye also may occur, usually several days after surgery. Blood may come from the incision, iris, or ciliary body. Instruct the client to report any change in vision immediately to the ophthalmologist.

TABLE 50-3 Activities That Increase Intraocular Pressure

- Bending from the waist
- Sneezing, coughing
- Blowing the nose
- Straining to have a bowel movement
- Vomiting
- Sexual intercourse
- Keeping the head in a dependent position
- Wearing tight shirt collars

Most clients experience a dramatic improvement in vision as early as the day of surgery. Caution the client that final best vision will not be present until 4 to 6 weeks after surgery.

Critical Thinking Challenge

Your 62-year-old client with bilateral cataracts is scheduled to have an extracapsular cataract removal with immediate intraocular lens implantation for her left eye (the one with the worse vision). She asks why both eyes can't be done at the same time so that she will not have to go "through all of this rigmarole twice." She also is concerned about her facial appearance after surgery and whether any bruising will be present.

1. Should both eyes be done at the same time? Why or why not?
2. How will her appearance be changed during the first week after surgery?

evolve For suggested answer guidelines, go to http://evolve.elsevier.com/Iggy/.

Community-Based Care

The client is usually discharged within 2 hours after cataract surgery. Nursing interventions focus on helping the client and family with plans for return to the home, assisted living, or extended care setting.

HOME CARE MANAGEMENT

If the client has difficulty instilling eyedrops, a supportive neighbor, friend, or family member can be taught the procedure. Adaptive equipment that positions the bottle of eyedrops directly over the eye can also be purchased.

HEALTH TEACHING

Review the following indications of complications after cataract surgery with the client and family before discharge:

- Sharp, sudden pain in the eye
- Bleeding or increased discharge
- Lid swelling
- Decreased vision
- Flashes of light or floating shapes

Tell the client to avoid activities that might increase IOP (see Table 50-3). The client may wash his or her hair a day or two after surgery, but only with the head tilted back, such as in a beauty salon or barber shop, to avoid getting water in the eye. For the first week after surgery, advise the client to stand in the shower with the face held away from the showerhead.

Cooking and light housekeeping are permitted, but vacuuming should be avoided for several weeks because of the forward flexion involved and the rapid, jerky movements required. Advise the client to refrain from driving, operating machinery, and participating in certain sports, such as golf, until given specific permission from the ophthalmologist.

CHART 50-7

NIC **INTERVENTION ACTIVITIES for**
The Client Requiring Topical Eye Medication

Medication Administration: *Eye: Preparing and instilling ophthalmic medications*

- Follow the five rights of medication administration.
- Note client's medical history and history of allergies.
- Determine client's knowledge of medication and understanding of method of administration.
- Position client supine or sitting in a chair with neck slightly hyperextended; ask client to look at ceiling.
- Instill medication onto the conjunctival sac using aseptic technique.
- Apply gentle pressure to nasolacrimal duct if medication has systemic effects.
- Instruct client to close eye gently to help distribute medication.
- Monitor for local, systemic, and adverse effects of medication.

Review the procedure for instilling eyedrops with the client or caretaker. If the client is concerned that the drops may not be correctly instilled, advise him or her to refrigerate the eyedrops. Then, when the eyedrop falls into the conjunctival sac, the client will notice a cool feeling. Eyedrops are often prescribed for 4 to 6 weeks after cataract surgery (Chart 50-7). Chart 50-8 lists items to cover in the focused assessment of a client in the home environment after cataract surgery.

HEALTH CARE RESOURCES

If the client lives alone and has no family or significant others, arrange for a home care nurse to assess the client and the home situation. If the client is unable to instill eyedrops independently, a friend, neighbor, or family member can be taught this technique.

Critical Thinking Challenge

Your 62-year-old client had the cataract removed from her left eye and a multifocal lens implanted on Friday afternoon. She plans to go back to work on Monday and does not want her co-workers to know about the surgery. (She worries that people will think she is "old" and not on the cutting edge of her profession.)

1. Should she go back to work on Monday? Why or why not?
2. What accommodations will she have to make at her work place?
3. What specific activities will you tell her to avoid?

evolve For suggested answer guidelines, go to http://evolve.elsevier.com/Iggy/.

Evaluation: Outcomes

Evaluate the care of the client with cataracts on the basis of the identified nursing diagnoses. The expected outcomes include that the client having cataracts will:

- Demonstrate Vision Compensation Behavior
- Remain free from injury

The client having cataract surgery will:

- Have improved Sensory Function: Vision
- Recognize manifestations of complications

CHART 50-8

HOME CARE ASSESSMENT of
The Client After Cataract Surgery

Assess the eye and vision:
- Visual acuity in both eyes using a Jaeger card
- Visual fields of both eyes
- Compare operative eye with nonoperative eye for presence or absence of the following:
  - Redness
  - Tearing
  - Drainage

Ask the client about:
- Pain in or around the operative eye
- Any change in visual acuity (decreased or improved) in the operative eye
- Whether any of the following has been noticed in the operative eye:
  - Dark spots
  - Increase in the number of floaters
  - Bright flashes of light

Assess the home environment for the following:
- Safety hazards (especially tripping and falling hazards)
- Kitchen hazards
- Level of room lighting

Assess client adherence with and understanding of treatment and limitations, such as:
- Signs and symptoms to report
- Medication regimen
- Activity restrictions

Assess functional ability:
- Activities of daily living
- Compliance with medication regimen

Specific indicators for these outcomes are listed for each nursing diagnosis under the Planning and Implementation section (see earlier).

GLAUCOMA

PATHOPHYSIOLOGY

Glaucoma is a group of ocular diseases resulting in increased IOP. Intraocular pressure (IOP) is the fluid (aqueous humor) pressure within the eye. A normal IOP of 10 to 21 mm Hg is maintained when there is a balance between production and outflow of aqueous humor. IOP can be raised by decreasing the outflow of aqueous fluid or by overproducing aqueous humor. In people with glaucoma, aqueous humor builds up inside the eye, and the increased pressure reduces blood flow to the optic nerve and retina. The sensitive nerve tissue becomes ischemic and dies. Tissue damage usually starts in the periphery and moves inward toward the fovea centralis. Left untreated, glaucoma can result in blindness. Glaucoma is commonly painless and the client may be unaware of a gradual reduction in vision.

Etiology

There are several causes and types of glaucoma (Table 50-4). Glaucoma is classified as primary, secondary, or associated. In primary glaucoma, the most common form, the structures involved in circulation and reabsorption of the aqueous humor undergo direct pathologic change.

Primary open-angle glaucoma (POAG), the most common form of primary glaucoma, is usually bilateral and asymptomatic in the early stages. There is reduced outflow

TABLE 50-4 Common Causes of Glaucoma

Primary Glaucoma
- Aging
- Heredity
- Central retinal vein occlusion

Secondary Glaucoma
- Uveitis
- Iritis
- Neovascular disorders
- Trauma
- Ocular tumors
- Degenerative disease
- Eye surgery

Associated Glaucoma
- Diabetes mellitus
- Hypertension
- Severe myopia
- Retinal detachment

CHART 50-9

KEY FEATURES of Glaucoma

Early
- Increased intraocular pressure
- Diminished accommodation

Late
- Diminished visual fields (loss of peripheral vision)
- Decreased visual acuity not correctable with glasses
- Halos around lights
- Headache or eye pain (acute closed-angle glaucoma)
- Increased cup-disc ratio
- Pale optic disc

of aqueous humor through the chamber angle. Because the fluid cannot leave the eye at the same rate it is produced, IOP gradually increases.

Angle-closure glaucoma (also called closed-angle glaucoma, narrow-angle glaucoma, or acute glaucoma) is less common, has a sudden onset, and is an emergency. The basic problems are a narrowed angle and forward displacement of the iris. Movement of the iris against the cornea narrows or closes the chamber angle, obstructing the outflow of aqueous humor. This can happen suddenly and without warning.

Secondary glaucoma results from ocular diseases that cause a narrowed angle or an increased volume of fluid within the eye. This can happen suddenly and without warning.

Incidence/Prevalence

Glaucoma is a common cause of blindness in affluent countries. It is age related, occurring in about 10% of people older than 80 years of age (McCance & Huether, 2002).

COLLABORATIVE MANAGEMENT

Primary open-angle glaucoma develops slowly, usually without symptoms. The gradual loss of visual fields may go unnoticed because central vision is unaffected. At times, the client may have foggy vision, reduced accommodation, mild aching in the eyes, or headaches and may require frequent changes in eyeglass prescriptions. Late manifestations occur after irreversible damage to optic nerve function and include visual field losses along with decreased visual acuity not correctable with eyeglasses. Chart 50-9 lists other manifestations of glaucoma. The Concept Map on p. 1098 addresses assessment and nursing care issues for clients who have glaucoma.

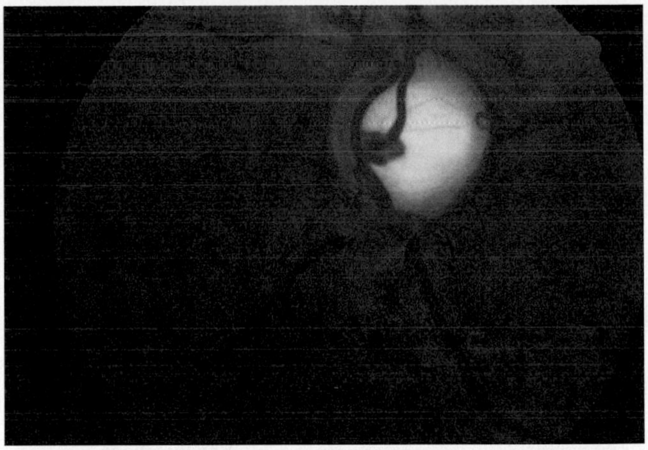

Figure 50-10 ■ The optic fundus of a client with glaucoma.

Assessment

PHYSICAL ASSESSMENT/CLINICAL MANIFESTATIONS

Ophthalmoscopic examination of the client with glaucoma shows cupping and atrophy of the optic disc. The disc becomes wider and deeper and turns white or gray (Figure 50-10).

To determine the extent of peripheral field losses, visual fields are measured. In chronic open-angle glaucoma, the visual fields first show a small crescent-shaped defect that gradually progresses to a larger field defect. In acute angle-closure glaucoma, the visual fields can quickly decrease.

The manifestations of acute angle-closure glaucoma differ from those of open-angle glaucoma. The onset of symptoms is acute, and the client has sudden, severe pain around the eyes that radiates over the face. Headache or brow pain, nausea, and vomiting also may occur. Other manifestations include seeing colored halos around lights and sudden blurred vision with decreased light perception.

On examination, the sclera may appear reddened and the cornea foggy. Ophthalmoscopic examination reveals a shallow anterior chamber, cloudy aqueous humor, and a moderately dilated, nonreactive pupil.

OTHER DIAGNOSTIC ASSESSMENTS

TONOMETRY. Intraocular pressure (IOP), as measured by tonometry, is elevated in glaucoma. If an elevated reading is found during routine screening examination, take several readings over a period of time at various times of the day to determine a pattern, because IOP varies during the day. In open-angle glaucoma, the tonometry reading is between 22 and 32 mm Hg (normal is 10 to 21 mm Hg). In angle-closure glaucoma, the tonometry reading may be 30 mm Hg or higher.

TONOGRAPHY. Tonography combines the use of an electronic indentation tonometer with a recording device. The outflow of aqueous humor from the eye is measured while a weight rests on the globe. The slope of the graph indicates IOP changes. A steep downhill tracing (normal) indicates adequate drainage. A flat tracing indicates reduced outflow, as in glaucoma.

GONIOSCOPY. A special lens that eliminates the corneal curve helps view the drainage angle in the anterior chamber. The entire 360-degree circumference of the angle

CONCEPT MAP Glaucoma

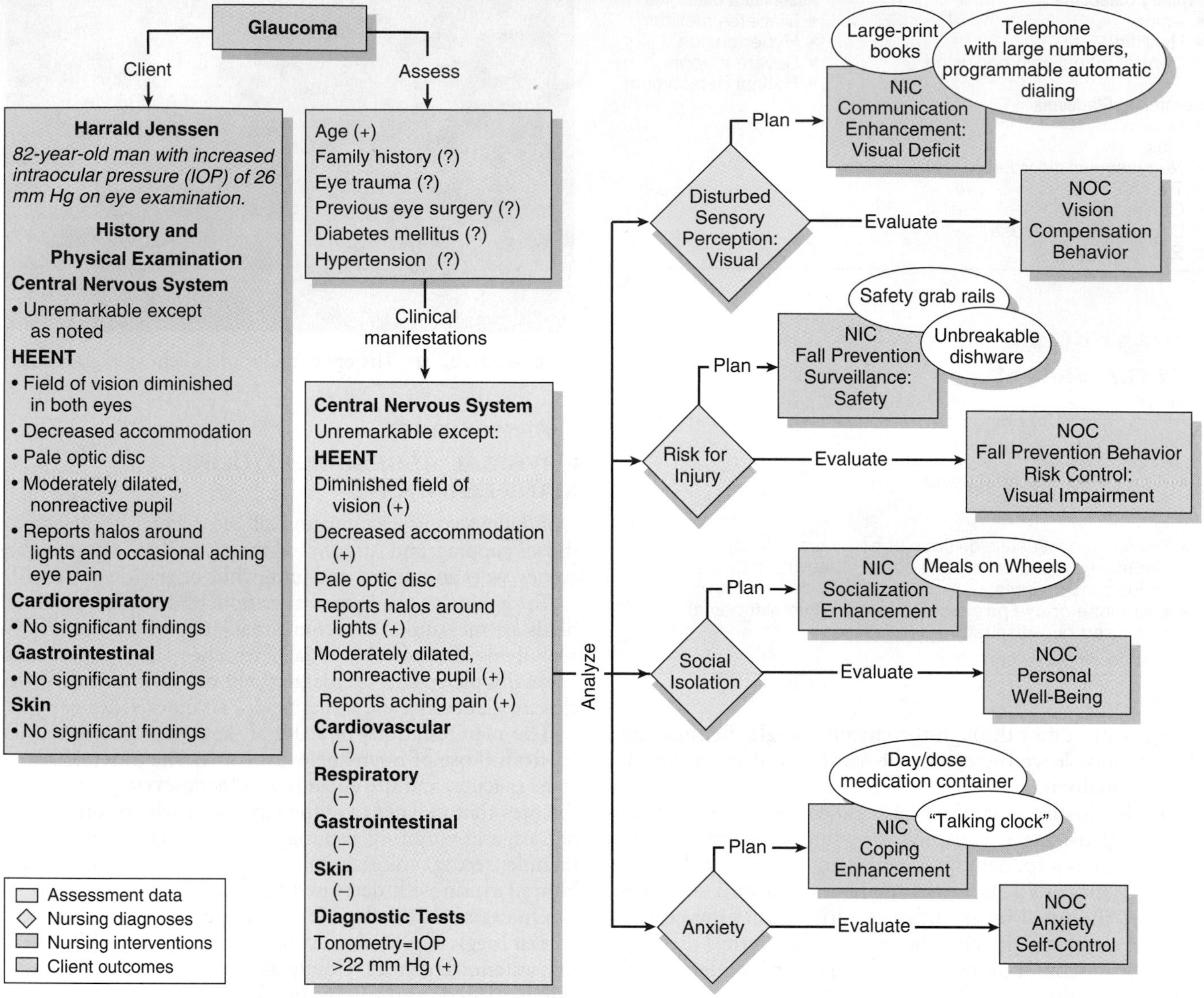

Concept Map by Elaine Bishop Kennedy, EdD, RN

between the iris and the cornea is examined. Adhesions, abnormal blood vessels, sites of trauma, and other changes as possible causes of secondary glaucoma can be seen.

Interventions

NONSURGICAL MANAGEMENT. Blindness from glaucoma can be prevented by early detection, lifelong treatment, and a regimen of close monitoring and follow-up care. Some degree of vision loss occurs, although use of topical agents that reduce ocular hypertension have been found to delay or prevent damage from glaucoma. (See the Evidence-Based Practice for Nursing box on p. 1099.) Chart 50-10 lists ways to assist the older client with impaired vision to remain as independent as possible.

Drug Therapy. Drug therapy for glaucoma focuses on reducing IOP through the following mechanisms:

- Constricting the pupil so that the ciliary muscle is contracted, allowing better circulation of the aqueous humor to the site of absorption
- Reducing the production of aqueous humor

Pupillary Constriction. Drugs that constrict the pupil and contract the ciliary muscle **(miotics),** such as pilocarpine hydrochloride (Isopto Carpine, Pilocar, Spersacarpine✱), are commonly used to treat glaucoma. In acute angle-closure glaucoma, pupil constriction is helpful because it enhances aqueous outflow. Carbachol (Isopto Carbachol, Miostat) may be used with or in place of pilocarpine. Echothiophate iodide (Phospholine Iodide) produces miosis and increases outflow. Remind the client that miotics may cause blurred vision for 1 to 2 hours after use and that vision in low light environments is difficult because of the pupillary constriction. Another group of drugs that improve outflow of aqueous humor are the prostaglandin agonists. Drugs from this class include latanoprost (Xalatan), travoprost (Travatan), bimatoprost (Lumigan), and unoprostone (Rescula). Nursing interventions for these drugs are listed in Chart 50-2.

Inhibition of Aqueous Humor. Beta blockers such as timolol (Apo-Timop✱, Timoptic) and levobunolol (Betagan) are used to decrease IOP. When used as eyedrops,

EVIDENCE-BASED PRACTICE for Nursing

Encourage clients to adhere to their ocular hypotensive drug therapy

Kass, M., et al. (2002). The ocular hypertension treatment study: Medication delays or prevents the onset of primary open-angle glaucoma. *Archives of Ophthalmology, 120*(6), 701-713.

The purpose of this multicenter, randomized, controlled clinical trial was to determine whether topical ocular hypotensive agents could delay or prevent the onset of primary open-angle glaucoma (POAG). The study subjects were 1500 individuals between 40 and 80 years of age who were identified as having mild to moderate elevations of intraocular pressure (IOP of 24 to 32 mm Hg) in at least one eye and who had no evidence of damage from glaucoma (as determined by visual field examination). The subjects were randomized to one of two groups, an observation-only control group or a treatment group receiving daily ocular hypotensive drugs with a goal of lowering IOP by at least 20%. Subjects in both groups were followed at 6-month intervals for 5 years. Purposive sampling of 400 African-American subjects was performed to ensure adequate representation of this population who are at high risk for glaucoma. The two groups were statistically homogeneous for baseline measures, ages, education, socioeconomic factors, gender, and study completion.

Measures performed at follow-up visits included IOP, slit-lamp examination, direct ophthalmoscopy, optic disc photographs, refraction, visual acuity, and full threshold visual field tests performed by clinicians who were masked to the participant category and to the previous examination findings for each subject.

At the conclusion of the study, subjects receiving the ocular hypotensive drugs had an average reduction in IOP of 22.5% and those in the observational group had an average reduction in IOP of 4.0%. A total of 36 subjects in the treatment group developed glaucoma compared to 89 subjects in the observation group. The researchers concluded that intervention with ocular hypotensive agents could delay or prevent glaucoma in clients with an elevated IOP.

Level of Evidence: 1—Well-designed, randomized, controlled clinical trial at multiple sites of adequate quality.

Critique. The study was well designed and well controlled to answer the questions posed. The multicentered nature of the study contributes to its validity but has the potential to reduce the reliability. The researchers used appropriate methods to ensure reliability. The large sample size also increases the generalizability of the findings.

Implications for Nursing. Many clients are not aware that they have ocular hypertension until glaucoma is present and vision is affected. In addition, many people are poorly adherent to drug regimens involving eyedrops. The results of this study can be used as an inducement for nurses to strongly encourage all clients to have yearly eye examinations that include measurement of intraocular pressure. Explaining the findings of this study to clients under treatment for ocular hypertension could improve client adherence to the treatment regimen and delay vision loss.

beta blockers reduce aqueous humor production without causing pupillary constriction.

Carbonic anhydrase inhibitors, such as acetazolamide (Acetazolam✱, Diamox) and methazolamide (Neptazane), reduce aqueous humor production to help maintain a lowered IOP. Epinephrine 0.5% to 2% and dipivefrin hydrochloride (Propine) also reduce aqueous humor production. *Epinephrine-containing agents are not used in angle-closure glaucoma because they dilate the pupil.*

Osmotic drugs may be given angle-closure glaucoma as part of emergency treatment to rapidly reduce IOP. Such agents include oral glycerin (Osmoglyn) and IV mannitol (Osmitrol).

SURGICAL MANAGEMENT

Laser Surgery. When drugs for the client with open-angle glaucoma are not effective at controlling IOP, laser surgery is indicated.

Preoperative Care. Nursing interventions include informing the client about laser technology, expected sights and sounds often heard during this procedure, and expected outcomes.

Operative Procedures. A laser trabeculoplasty burns the trabecular meshwork, scarring it and causing the meshwork fibers to tighten. Fiber tightening increases the size of the spaces between the fibers, improving outflow of aqueous humor and a reduction in IOP. Topical or local anesthesia is used. Clients may have a temporary increase in IOP immediately after this procedure.

Laser surgery is also indicated for clients with angle-closure glaucoma. The laser makes a hole near the edge of the iris, allowing aqueous humor to flow from the posterior chamber to the anterior chamber and then into the drainage meshwork.

Postoperative Care. Instruct the client to arrange for transportation home because driving is prohibited right after the surgery. Because laser procedures can sometimes increase IOP, the pressure should be re-evaluated 1 hour after surgery and before discharge. An ocular steroid, such as prednisolone acetate (Ocu-Pred, Ophtho-Tate✱), may be prescribed.

Standard Surgical Therapy. For open-angle glaucoma that fails to respond to drug and laser therapy and for some cases of angle-closure glaucoma, surgery is needed. This surgery either creates a new drainage channel for aqueous humor or destroys the structures that produce it.

Glaucoma surgery is performed either in a hospital or on an outpatient basis. The usual length of stay is several hours to several days.

After surgery, the ophthalmologist injects an antibiotic under the conjunctiva. The eye is then covered with a patch and a protective shield is applied over it. Instruct the client to avoid taking aspirin, to avoid lying on the operative side, and to report any brow pain, severe eye pain, or nausea.

The most serious complication after glaucoma surgery is choroidal hemorrhage. If IOP is too low, fluid may enter the suprachoroid space and cause a choroidal detachment. Extra fluid in this space may break blood vessels located there. Manifestations of choroidal hemorrhage include the following:

- Acute pain deep in the eye
- Decreased vision
- Vital sign changes

VITREOUS HEMORRHAGE

PATHOPHYSIOLOGY

The vitreous is the gel that fills the posterior two thirds of the eye and maintains the eye's shape. Vitreous hemorrhage (bleeding into the vitreous cavity) may result from aging, systemic diseases, or trauma, or it may occur spontaneously. With aging, the vitreous may spontaneously detach from the retina. Torn blood vessels allow bleeding into the vitreous. Diseases that disrupt the retinal blood vessels, such as

CHART 50-10

NURSING FOCUS on the OLDER ADULT
Promote Independent Living in Clients with Impaired Vision

Medications
- Having a neighbor, relative, friend, or visiting nurse visit once a week to measure the proper medications for each day may be helpful.
  If the client is to take medications more than once each day, it is helpful to use a container of a different shape (with a lid) each time. For example, if the client is to take medications at 9 AM, 1 PM, and 9 PM, the 9 AM medications would be placed in a round container, the 1 PM medications in a square container, and the 9 PM medications in a triangular container.
  It is helpful to place each day's medication containers in a separate box with raised letters on the side of the box spelling out the day.
- "Talking clocks" are available for the client with low vision.

Communication
- Telephones with large, raised block numbers may be helpful. The best models are those with black numbers on a white phone or white numbers on a black phone.
- Telephones that have a programmable, automatic dialing feature are very helpful. Programmed numbers should include those for the fire department, police, relatives, friends, neighbors, and 911.

Safety
- It is best to leave furniture the way the client wants it and not move it.
- Throw rugs are best eliminated.
- Appliance cords should be short and kept out of walkways.
- Lounge-style chairs with built-in footrests are preferable to footstools.
- Nonbreakable dishes, cups, and glasses are preferable to breakable ones.
- Cleansers and other toxic agents should be labeled with large, raised letters.
- Hook-and-loop (Velcro) strips at hand level may help to mark the locations of switches and electrical outlets.

Food Preparation
- Meals on Wheels is a service that many older adults find helpful. This service brings meals at mealtime, cooked and ready to eat. The cost of this service varies, depending on the client's ability to pay.
- Many grocery stores offer a "shop by telephone" service. The client can either complete a computer booklet indicating types, amounts, and brands of items desired, or the store will complete this booklet over the telephone by asking the client specific information. The store then delivers groceries to the client's door (many stores also offer a "put away" service) and charges the client's bank card.
- A microwave oven is a safer means of cooking than a standard stove, although many older clients are afraid of microwave ovens. If the client has and will use a microwave oven, others can prepare meals ahead of time, label them, and freeze them for later use. Also, many complete, microwavable frozen dinners that comply with a variety of dietary restrictions are available.
- Friends or relatives may be able to help with food preparation. Often relatives do not know what to give an older person for birthdays or other gift-giving occasions. One suggestion is a homemade prepackaged frozen dinner that the client enjoys.

Personal Care
- Handgrips should be installed in bathrooms.
- The tub floor should have a nonskid surface.
- Male clients should use an electric shaver rather than a razor.
- Choosing a hairstyle that is becoming but easy to care for (avoiding parts) helps in independent living.
- Home hair care services may be available.

Diversional Activity
- Some clients are able to use large-print books, newspapers, and magazines (available through local libraries and vision services).
- Books, magazines, and some newspapers are available on audiotape.
- Clients experienced in knitting or crocheting may be able to create items fashioned from straight pieces, such as afghans.
- Card games, dominoes, and some board games that are available in large, high-contrast print may be helpful for clients with low vision.

hypertension and diabetes mellitus, also cause blood leakage into the vitreous.

COLLABORATIVE MANAGEMENT

The main manifestation of vitreous hemorrhage is reduced visual acuity. The degree of reduced vision varies with the severity of the hemorrhage. A mild hemorrhage may cause the client to see a red haze or "floaters." A moderate hemorrhage may cause the client to see "black streaks" or "tiny black dots." Severe hemorrhage may reduce visual acuity to hand motion. Eye examination shows a reduced red reflex because light rays are blocked from reaching the retina. Ultrasonography is used to determine the location and extent of the hemorrhage.

A vitreous hemorrhage may absorb slowly with no treatment. Leaking blood vessels can be sealed with laser therapy. If the hemorrhage is still present several weeks to months later, a **vitrectomy** (surgical removal of the vitreous) is indicated.

UVEITIS

PATHOPHYSIOLOGY

The uveal tract has three related parts: the iris, the ciliary body, and the choroid. A common problem within these structures is inflammation, or **uveitis.** Uveitis may occur in the anterior or posterior portion of the eye.

Anterior uveitis is inflammation of the iris, inflammation of the ciliary body, or both. The cause of anterior uveitis is unknown, but often follows exposure to allergens, infectious agents, trauma, or systemic disease (rheumatoid arthritis, herpes simplex, herpes zoster). It can follow any local or systemic bacterial infection. Manifestations include aching around the eye; tearing; blurred vision; photophobia; a small, irregular, nonreactive pupil; and a "bloodshot" appearance of the sclera.

Posterior uveitis is the common term for **retinitis** (inflammation of the retina) and **chorioretinitis** (inflammation of both the choroid and the retina). Posterior uveitis occurs with tuberculosis, syphilis, and toxoplasmosis.

The onset of symptoms is slow and painless. Visual impairment in the affected eye results from fluid, fibrin, and cells leaking into the vitreous cavity. The pupil is small, nonreactive, and irregularly shaped. Black dots are visible against the red background of the fundus. Lesions appear as grayish yellow patches on the retinal surface.

COLLABORATIVE MANAGEMENT

Treatment of uveitis includes resting the ciliary body with a cycloplegic agent. The pupil is dilated to prevent adhesions between the iris and the lens. Steroid drops are given hourly to reduce the inflammation and to prevent adhesion of the iris to the cornea and lens. Ocular injections of steroids are used in posterior uveitis or when topical steroids have been ineffective. Analgesics that contain neither aspirin nor opioids are prescribed for pain. Systemic antibiotic therapy may be started for posterior uveitis or when infection is present with anterior uveitis.

Cool or warm compresses are applied for ocular pain. Darkening the room and wearing sunglasses reduce the discomfort of photophobia. Because of blurred vision from the cycloplegic drops, instruct the client not to drive or operate machinery. Review the manifestations of bacterial and fungal ulcers and those of increased intraocular pressure (IOP).

RETINAL DISORDERS

Hypertensive Retinopathy

PATHOPHYSIOLOGY

Many Americans have hypertension. Hypertension causes blood vessel changes in the eyes that damage the retina and reduce vision. Hypertensive retinopathy is classified by grades. With each increasing grade, progressive changes occur in the retina.

COLLABORATIVE MANAGEMENT

As blood pressure increases, retinal arterioles narrow and take on a classic "copper wire" appearance (Figure 50-11). Nicking, or narrowing, of the vessel at arteriovenous crossings is present. If blood pressure remains elevated, areas of ischemia, known as soft exudates or "cotton wool" spots, develop from blood vessel occlusion. Small hemorrhages may be seen. The client may also have headaches and vertigo. Left untreated, hypertensive retinopathy can cause retinal detachment.

Treatment focuses primarily on management of the systemic hypertension (see Chapter 39) and controlling IOP.

Diabetic Retinopathy

PATHOPHYSIOLOGY

Diabetic retinopathy is a retinal blood vessel complication. The longer the person has diabetes, the greater the incidence and severity of retinopathy (McCance & Huether, 2002). Poor glucose control worsens the retinopathy. Good control lessens the disease severity. The two types of diabetic retinopathy are background retinopathy and proliferative retinopathy.

In **background diabetic retinopathy,** the cells of the retinal vessels die and fluid leaks into the eye. As this fluid is absorbed, thick yellow-white hard exudates, are formed. The capillaries lose their ability to transport needed oxygen and nutrients. Small outpouches **(microaneurysms)** form in the walls of capillaries. These fragile capillaries bleed easily and cause hemorrhages in the nerve layer of the retina (Figure 50-12). Visual acuity is reduced by retinal ischemia or by macular edema.

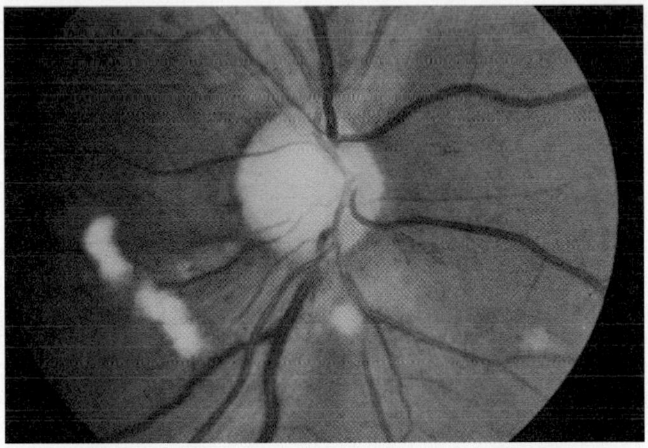

Figure 50-11 ■ The optic fundus of a client with hypertension.

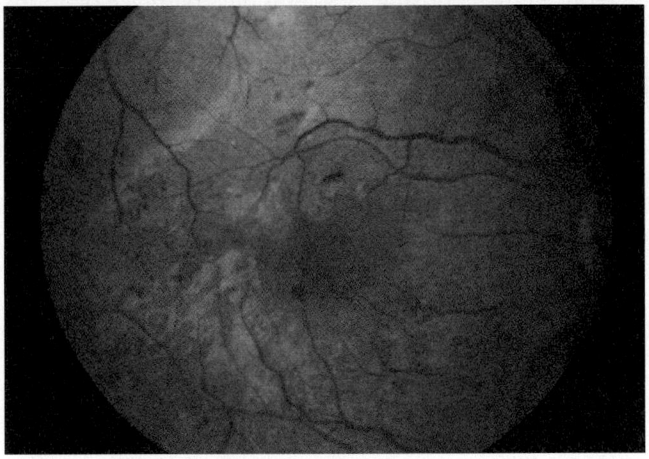

Figure 50-12 ■ The optic fundus of a client with diabetes.

In clients with **proliferative diabetic retinopathy,** a network of fragile new blood vessels develops, leaking blood and protein into the surrounding tissue. These new blood vessels are stimulated by retinal hypoxia that results from poor capillary perfusion of retinal tissues. New blood vessels grow in the retina, onto the iris, and into the back of the vitreous. The vitreous contracts and pulls away from the retina, causing blood vessels to break and bleed into the vitreous.

COLLABORATIVE MANAGEMENT

Treatment of diabetic retinopathy depends on the severity of retinal damage. Laser therapy can seal microaneurysms and decrease bleeding. Scattering of laser burns across the retina can decrease the retina's need for oxygen and control the growth of new blood vessels.

A vitrectomy is performed if frequent bleeding into the vitreous occurs and fibrin bands threaten to detach the retina. Fibrin bands within the vitreous are severed and removed. A laser may be used in the eye during surgery to seal leaking or bleeding blood vessels.

Macular Degeneration

PATHOPHYSIOLOGY

Macular degeneration (deterioration of the macula, the area of central vision) can be atrophic (age related, or *dry*) or exudative *(wet)*. Age-related degeneration is caused by gradual blockage of retinal capillaries, allowing retinal cells in the macula to become ischemic and necrotic. Rod and cone photoreceptors die. Central vision declines, and clients describe "mild blurring and distortion." This type of degeneration is more common and progresses at a faster rate among smokers than among nonsmokers. Current research findings suggest that the risk for atrophic macular degeneration can be reduced by increasing long-term dietary intake of antioxidants and the carotenoids lutein and zeaxanthin. The same dietary treatments appear to slow the progression of macular degeneration.

Clients with exudative ("wet") degeneration have a sudden decrease in vision after a serous detachment of pigment epithelium in the macula. Newly formed blood vessels invade this injured area and cause fluid and blood to collect under the macula (like a blister), resulting in scar formation and visual distortion.

Critical Thinking Challenge

The client is a 75-year-old man who was diagnosed with age-related "dry" macular degeneration after he was involved in a car accident in which he failed to stop at an intersection and hit another car at a low rate of speed. No injuries resulted from the car accident although the client received a citation for a moving violation. The client is very upset with the diagnosis. His wife has never driven nor has she managed the household accounts. He is concerned about "going blind" and wants to know if the LASIK procedure would restore his vision.

1. Can the client continue to drive? Why or why not?
2. Will a LASIK procedure be helpful for this problem? Why or why not?
3. How will you address the issue of "going blind?"

evolve For suggested answer guidelines, go to http://evolve.elsevier.com/Iggy/.

COLLABORATIVE MANAGEMENT

Treatment of age-related macular degeneration aims to help the client maximize remaining vision. The loss of central vision reduces the ability to read, write, recognize safety hazards, and drive. Suggest alternative strategies (such as large-print books and public transportation) and referrals to community organizations that provide a wide range of adaptive equipment.

Management of clients with exudative or "wet" macular degeneration is geared toward slowing the process and identifying further changes in visual perception. Fluid and blood may resorb in some clients with exudative degeneration. Laser therapy to seal the leaking blood vessels in or near the macula can limit the extent of the damage. Another method used with some success at sealing or destroying the leaking retinal blood vessels is photodynamic therapy (Gottlieb, 2002; Rechtman et al., 2002). In this treatment, the client is given an IV agent to increase photosensitivity (Verteporfin). After the agent is absorbed, a special nonheating light is applied in the specific area to activate the agent. Activation causes local formation of oxygen radicals that occlude the leaking vessels and prevent excessive formation of new vessels.

Critical Thinking Challenge

Your client with macular degeneration (dry) wants to know if continuing to use his limited vision will increase the progression of the macular degeneration. He also worries that he will "lose his mind" if he has to give up all his usual activities.

1. How will you address his concerns?
2. How will you proceed to assist the client and his wife in maintaining independence and quality of life?

evolve For suggested answer guidelines, go to http://evolve.elsevier.com/Iggy/.

Retinal Holes, Tears, and Detachments

PATHOPHYSIOLOGY

A retinal hole is a break in the retina. Retinal holes can be caused by trauma or can occur with aging. A retinal tear is a more jagged and irregularly shaped break in the retina. It can result from traction on the retina. A retinal detachment is the separation of the retina from the epithelium. Detachments are classified by the nature of their development.

Rhegmatogenous detachments occur following a hole or tear in the retina caused by mechanical force, creating an opening for the vitreous to move under the retina. When sufficient fluid collects in this space, the retina detaches. *Traction* detachments occur when the retina is pulled away from the support tissue by bands of fibrous tissue in the vitreous. *Exudative* detachments are caused by fluid collecting under the retina. These often occur with a systemic disease or with ocular tumors. No retinal break occurs.

COLLABORATIVE MANAGEMENT

The onset of a retinal detachment is usually sudden and painless because no pain fibers are located in the retina. Clients may suddenly see bright flashes of light **(photopsia)** or floating dark spots in the affected eye. During the initial phase of the detachment or if the detachment is partial, the client may describe the sensation of a curtain being pulled over part of the visual field. The visual field loss corresponds to the area of detachment.

Assessment

On ophthalmoscopic examination, detachments are seen as gray bulges or folds in the retina that quiver. Depending on the cause of the detachment, a hole or tear also may be seen at the edge of the detachment.

Interventions

If a retinal hole or tear is discovered before it causes a detachment, the defect may be closed or sealed. Closure prevents fluid from collecting under the retina and reduces the risk for a detachment. Treatment involves creating an inflammatory response that will bind the retina and choroid together around the break. The inflammatory response can be created with the application of **cryotherapy** (a freezing probe), **photocoagulation** (laser), or **diathermy** (high-frequency current).

Spontaneous reattachment of the retina is rare. Surgical repair is usually needed to place the retina in contact with the underlying structures. A common repair procedure is scleral buckling.

Preoperative Care. The client is usually anxious and fearful about a possible permanent loss of vision. Provide information and reassurance to allay fears.

Activity is often restricted before surgery to prevent further tearing or detachment and to promote drainage of any fluid under the retina. An eye patch is placed over the client's affected eye to reduce eye movement. Topical drugs are given before surgery to inhibit pupil constriction and accommodation.

Operative Procedures. The surgery is performed with the client under general anesthesia. In scleral buckling, the ophthalmologist repairs wrinkles or folds in the retina so that the retina can assume its normal smooth position. To promote reattachment, a small piece of silicone is placed against the sclera and held in place by an encircling band (Figure 50-13). This device keeps the retina in contact with the choroid and sclera to promote attachment. Any fluid under the retina is drained.

A gas or silicone oil placed inside the eye can be used to promote retinal reattachment. These agents float up against the retina to hold it in place until healing occurs.

Postoperative Care. After surgery, an eye patch and shield are applied. Monitor the client's vital signs and check the eye patch and shield for any drainage.

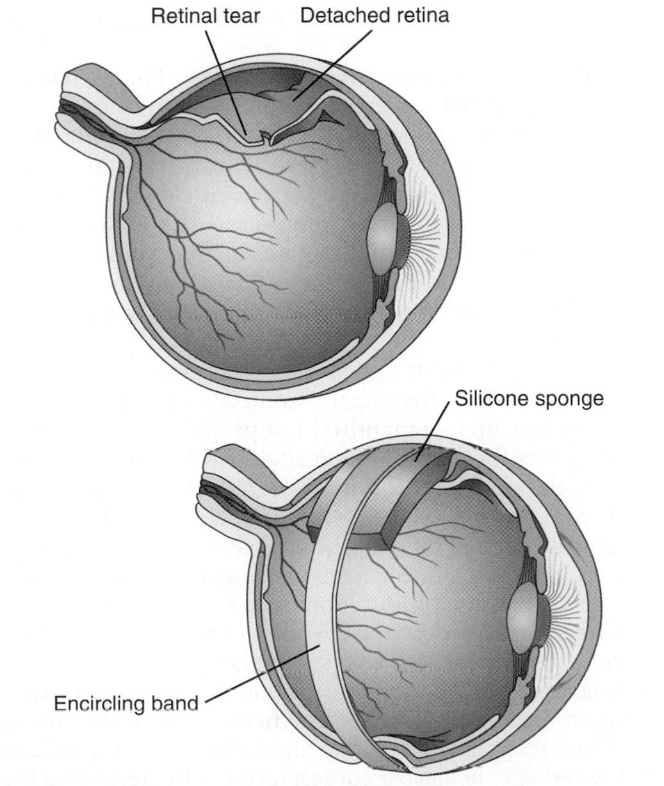

Figure 50-13 ■ The scleral buckling procedure for repair of retinal detachment.

Activity after surgery varies. If gas or oil has been used, position the client on his or her abdomen to allow the gas to float against the retina. Instruct the client to lie with the head turned so that the affected eye is facing up, for several days or until the gas has been absorbed. As an alternative, he or she can sit on the side of the bed and place the head on an over-the-bed table. Bathroom privileges are allowed once the client is fully awake.

The client may have nausea and pain after surgery. Give analgesics and antiemetics as prescribed. Report any sudden increase in pain or pain occurring with nausea to the surgeon because these symptoms may indicate the development of complications. Instruct the client to avoid activities that increase intraocular pressure (IOP) (see Table 50-3).

In the first week after retinal detachment surgery, the client must avoid reading, writing, and close work, such as sewing, because these activities cause rapid eye movements and promote detachment. Teach the client the manifestations of infection and detachment. Instruct the client to notify the nurse or physician if any signs or symptoms occur.

Retinitis Pigmentosa

PATHOPHYSIOLOGY

Several types of retinal disorders can cause progressive degeneration of the retina and lead to blindness. Retinitis pigmentosa (RP) is a condition in which retinal nerve cells degenerate and the pigmented cells of the retina grow and move into the sensory areas of the retina, causing further degeneration.

Genetic Considerations

Different forms of this disorder can be inherited as an autosomal dominant trait, an autosomal recessive trait, or an X-linked recessive trait (Nussbaum, McInnes, & Willard, 2001). Mutations in several genes have been identified as being responsible for retinitis pigmentosa and screening of people who are at high risk is available in some medical centers (Majewski, et al., 2003).

COLLABORATIVE MANAGEMENT

The most common early manifestation of retinitis pigmentosa is night blindness, often occurring in childhood. Over time, decreased visual acuity progresses to total blindness. Examination of the retina shows heavy pigmentation in a lacy pattern. Cataracts may accompany this disorder.

No current therapy has proved effective in preventing or slowing the degenerative process. Because some retinal destruction resembles that seen with vitamin A deficiency, a regimen of vitamin A, along with decreased exposure of the retina to bright light, is being tried. An experimental treatment of a retinal microchip implant (artificial retina) is under investigation (Smith, 2002).

REFRACTIVE ERRORS

PATHOPHYSIOLOGY

The ability of the eye to focus images on the retina depends on the length of the eye from front to back and the refractive power of the lens system. **Refraction** is the bending of light rays. Problems in either eye length or refraction can result in refractive errors.

Myopia

In **myopia** (nearsightedness), the refractive ability of the eye is too strong for the eye length. Images are bent and fall in front of, not on, the retina.

Hyperopia

In **hyperopia,** or **hypermetropia** (farsightedness), the refractive ability of the eye is too weak, causing images to be focused behind the retina. A short eye length may contribute to the development of hyperopia.

Presbyopia

As people age, the lens loses its elasticity and is less able to alter its shape to focus the eye for close work **(presbyopia).** As a result, images fall behind the retina. Presbyopia usually occurs in people in their 30s and 40s.

Astigmatism

Astigmatism occurs when the curve of the cornea is uneven. Because light rays are not refracted equally in all directions, the image does not focus on the retina.

◆COLLABORATIVE MANAGEMENT

◆Assessment

Refractive errors are diagnosed through a process known as **refraction.** The client is asked to view an eye chart while lenses of different strengths are systematically placed in front of the eye. With each lens strength, the client is asked whether the lenses sharpen or worsen vision. The strength of the lens needed to focus the image on the retina is expressed in measurements called diopters.

◆Interventions

NONSURGICAL MANAGEMENT. Errors of refraction can be corrected with a lens that focuses light rays on the retina (see Figure 49-5). Hyperopic vision is corrected to bring the image forward onto the retina with a concave lens. Myopic vision is corrected with a convex lens to move the focused image back to the retina.

Eyeglasses. Eyeglasses are used to correct refractive errors. Advantages of eyeglasses are ease of use, durability, availability, and low cost. Disadvantages include a change in appearance, the weight of the frame on the nose, and reduced peripheral vision (vision is corrected only when the client looks through the center of the lens).

Contact Lenses. Contact lenses also correct refractive errors. Round plastic disks rest against the cornea and fit under the eyelid.

Hard Lenses. Hard contact lenses correct errors in two ways, by changing the shape of the cornea and by providing direct refraction. Changing corneal shape increases its refracting ability. Direct refraction from the contact lens places the specific refractive power and shape needed in front of the eye so that light rays are correctly focused onto the retina.

Complications of hard contact lens wear include corneal edema, which occurs when the lenses are worn for an extended period. Corneal abrasions can result from overwear, which dries the cornea and causes minute breaks, or from the irritation of the contact lens against the cornea.

Soft Lenses. Soft contact lenses are larger but better tolerated than hard contact lenses. They resemble the thickness of plastic wrap and can be worn for longer periods because this type of lens allows greater corneal access to moisture and oxygen. Most problems with wearing soft lenses are related to lens deterioration, deposits in the lens, and failure to follow correct lens care practices.

There are two types of soft contact lenses: daily-wear lenses (worn during waking hours) and extended-wear lenses. Extended-wear contact lenses can be worn continuously for several days to several weeks, depending on the client's environment, activities, and tolerance of the lenses.

SURGICAL MANAGEMENT. Surgery is a popular alternative for the treatment of refractive errors. Vision-enhancing surgeries include radial keratotomy, photorefractive keratectomy, laser in-situ keratomileusis (LASIK), and placement of Intacs corneal ring segments. All surgical procedures are much more expensive than eyeglasses or any type of contact lens. These procedures, performed as outpatient surgery, are rarely covered by insurance.

Radial Keratotomy. Radial keratotomy (RK) is an outpatient surgical procedure for the treatment of mild to moderate myopia. Eight to 16 diagonal incisions are made through 90% of the peripheral cornea. Because the central cornea is not incised, vision is not reduced. These incisions flatten the cornea, which allows the image to be focused closer to the retina.

Most clients have several days of moderate discomfort after surgery. Slight overcorrection or undercorrection of the refractive error is possible, in which case the client still must wear some form of visual correction after the surgery. Other complications include corneal scarring and chronic dry eyes. This procedure is less popular now in North America as a result of increased availability of laser surgeries to correct myopia.

Photorefractive Keratotomy. Photorefractive keratectomy (PRK) is used for people with mild to moderate stable myopia and low astigmatism. It is also used to correct corneal complications following other types of surgery for myopia. PRK is not a laser version of radial keratotomy but a completely different procedure. An excimer laser pulses a brief but powerful beam on the outer surface of the central cornea. This beam removes small portions of the tissue surface, reshaping the cornea to properly focus an image on the retina.

One eye is treated at a time, usually at least 3 months apart. The eye is patched after surgery. Complete healing to best vision may take up to 6 months. Most people do not need corrective lenses for distance vision after PRK but may still need reading glasses. Expected side effects of PRK after surgery include pain, hazy vision, light sensitivity, tearing, and pupil enlargement. Complications include reduced night vision, corneal clouding, undercorrection, far-sightedness, increased intraocular pressure (IOP), chronic dry eyes, and glare.

Laser In-Situ Keratomileusis. Laser-in-situ keratomileusis (LASIK) is a very popular procedure for correcting near-sightedness, far-sightedness, and astigmatism using the excimer laser. The superficial layers of the cornea are lifted temporarily as a flap and brief but powerful laser pulses reshape the deeper corneal layers. After reshaping the deeper layers, the corneal flap is placed back into its original position.

Usually both eyes are treated at the same time. Most clients have improved vision within an hour after surgery; complete healing to best vision may take up to 4 weeks.

This procedure is thought to be superior to PRK because the outer corneal layer is not damaged. Pain is less than for PRK, and the time to best vision is reduced. A wider variety of refractive errors can be treated with LASIK than with PRK.

After LASIK correction of refractive errors, many clients no longer require eyeglasses or contact lenses. Overcorrection or undercorrection is possible, however, and some clients may need a mild prescription for a continued refractive error.

The risk for complications is reported to be less than for other types of vision-enhancing surgery, although clients must be informed that serious complications are possible. Complications include corneal clouding, chronic dry eyes, and refractive errors. Some clients have developed blurred vision and other refractive errors months to years after this surgery as a result of keratectasia (Kymionis et al, 2003; Rojas & Manche, 2002). This problem is related to the formation of the corneal flap during surgery and laser-thinning of the cornea. The cornea then becomes unstable and does not refract appropriately.

Intacs Corneal Ring. Intacs corneal ring placement enhances vision for near-sightedness. This surgery does not involve the use of a laser and has the advantage of being reversible. With this procedure, the shape of the cornea is changed by placing a flexible ring in the outer edges of the cornea (outside of the optical zone).

Intacs ring placement is performed on both eyes during one surgery under local anesthesia. Healing to best vision is immediate. Overcorrection or undercorrection of refraction is possible; however, removal, replacement, or adjustment of ring tightness can enhance satisfaction. In addition, replacements can be made if the client's vision changes further as a result of aging. Because the ring is applied to the cornea outside of the optical zone, the risk for corneal clouding or scarring is lower than with other surgical procedures.

TRAUMA

Trauma to the eye or orbital area can result from almost any activity. Care varies depending on the area of the eye affected and whether the globe of the eye has been penetrated.

Hyphema

PATHOPHYSIOLOGY

A **hyphema** is a hemorrhage in the anterior chamber. It occurs when a force is applied to the eye and breaks the blood vessels.

COLLABORATIVE MANAGEMENT

If the hyphema is large, it may block the pupil and reduce vision, possibly causing pain and photophobia. Hemolysis of the blood occurs, and the blood is filtered out of the eye through the trabecular meshwork. If the blood particles obstruct the meshwork, increased intraocular pressure (IOP) results.

The client with a hyphema is treated by bedrest in semi-Fowler's position to use gravity as an aid in keeping the hyphema away from the optical center of the cornea. Minimal or no sudden eye movements are permitted for 3 to 5 days to decrease the risk for rebleeding. Cycloplegic eyedrops may be prescribed to place the eye at rest, and the eye is protected by a patch and shield. Television and reading are restricted. A hyphema usually resolves in 5 to 7 days.

Contusion

PATHOPHYSIOLOGY

A contusion of the eyeball and surrounding tissue is caused by traumatic contact with a blunt object. The force of the blow pushes the eye back in the socket. The globe is compressed, and stretching of the ocular soft tissues occurs, which can produce damage and possibly rupture the globe.

Results of the injury may not be seen immediately. These results include edema of the eyelids, subconjunctival hemorrhage, corneal edema, and hyphema.

COLLABORATIVE MANAGEMENT

Periorbital ecchymosis, or "black eye," a common contusion injury, is usually caused by blunt trauma. Bleeding into the soft tissue occurs, creating the bruise. The color fades gradually and disappears in 10 to 14 days. Visual acuity is usually not affected, although orbital pain, photophobia, eyelid edema, and diplopia may be present.

Treatment begins at the time of injury. Ice is applied immediately. The client should have a thorough eye examination to rule out any other eye injuries.

Foreign Bodies

PATHOPHYSIOLOGY

Eyelashes, dust, fingernails, dirt, and airborne particles can come in contact with the conjunctiva or cornea and irritate or abrade the surface. If nothing is seen on the cornea or conjunctiva, the eyelids are everted to examine the conjunctivae.

COLLABORATIVE MANAGEMENT

The client usually has a feeling of something being in the eye and may have blurry vision. Pain occurs if the corneal surface is injured. Tearing and photophobia may be present.

Evaluation of vision is done before treatment. The eye of any client with a suspected corneal abrasion is examined with fluorescein, followed by irrigation with normal saline (0.9%) to gently remove the particles. Best practices for ocular irrigation are listed in Chart 50-11.

After the foreign body is removed and if an eye patch is applied, tell the client how long the patch must be left in place (patching over corneal abrasions is controversial). Follow-up with the ophthalmologist is needed.

Lacerations

PATHOPHYSIOLOGY

Lacerations are wounds caused by sharp objects and projectiles. Lacerations can occur to any part of the eye, but the most commonly injured areas are the eyelids and the cornea.

COLLABORATIVE MANAGEMENT

Initially, close the eye and apply a small ice pack to decrease bleeding. The client should receive medical attention as soon as possible.

CHART 50-11

BEST PRACTICE for
Ocular Irrigation

1. Assemble equipment:
   - Normal saline IV (1000-mL bag)
   - Macrodrip IV tubing
   - IV pole
   - Eyelid speculum
   - Topical anesthetic (proparacaine hydrochloride)
   - Gloves
   - Collection receptacle (emesis basin works well)
   - Towels
   - pH paper
2. Quickly obtain a history from the client while flushing the tubing with normal saline:
   - Nature and time of the injury
   - Type of irritant or chemical (if known)
   - Type of first aid administered at the scene
   - Any allergies to the "caine" family of medications
3. Evaluate the client's visual acuity *before* treatment:
   - Ask the client to read your name tag with the affected eye while covering the good eye.
   - Ask the client to "count fingers" with the affected eye while covering the good eye.
4. Put on gloves.
5. Place a strip of pH paper in the cul-de-sac of the client's affected eye.
6. Instill proparacaine hydrochloride eyedrops as prescribed.
7. Place the client in a supine position with the head turned slightly toward the affected eye.
8. Have the client hold the affected eye open, or position an eyelid speculum.
9. Direct the flow of normal saline across the affected eye from the nasal corner of the eye toward the outer corner of the eye.
10. Assess the client's comfort during the procedure.
11. If both eyes are affected, irrigate them simultaneously using separate personnel and equipment.

If the client can open the eye, check visual acuity and clean the eyelids. Minor lacerations of the eyelid can be sutured in an emergency department, an urgent care center, or an ophthalmologist's office. A microscope is needed in the operating room if the client has a laceration that involves the eyelid margin, affects the lacrimal system, involves a large area, or has jagged edges.

Corneal lacerations are an emergency because eye contents may prolapse through the laceration. Manifestations include severe eye pain, photophobia, tearing, decreased visual acuity, and inability to open the eyelid. If the laceration is the result of a penetrating injury, an object may be seen protruding from the eye. *The object is removed only by the ophthalmologist, because it may be holding eye structures in place.*

Antibiotics are given to reduce the risk for infection. Depending on the depth of the laceration, scarring may develop. If the scar alters vision, a corneal transplant may be needed later. If the eye contents have prolapsed through the laceration or if the injury is severe, enucleation (surgical eye removal) may be indicated.

Penetrating Injuries

PATHOPHYSIOLOGY

Clients with penetrating eye injuries have the poorest chance of retaining vision in the injured eye. Glass, high-speed metal or wood particles, BB pellets, and bullets are common causes of penetrating injuries. The particles can enter the eye and lodge in or behind the eyeball.

COLLABORATIVE MANAGEMENT

The client usually has some eye pain and says he or she "suddenly felt something hit my eye." An entrance wound may be visible. Depending on the location of the entrance and the resting place of the projectile, vision may be affected.

X-rays and computed tomography (CT) scans of the orbit are usually performed. Computer-generated reconstructions of the CT images are created to study this complex area to ensure the orbit is intact and to look for fractures that might entrap orbital muscles. *Magnetic resonance imaging (MRI) is contraindicated because the procedure may move any metal-containing projectile and cause more injury.*

Surgery is usually needed to remove the foreign object. In some cases, foreign bodies need to be removed by a vitrectomy. IV antibiotics are started before surgery to reduce the risk for infection. A tetanus booster is given if necessary.

Assess and document visual acuity. If the client cannot see print, determine whether he or she can count fingers or see hand motions. If the client cannot see movement, assess his or her ability to see light.

OCULAR MELANOMA

PATHOPHYSIOLOGY

Melanoma is the most common malignant eye tumor in adults. This tumor occurs most often in the uveal tract among people in their 30s and 40s.

Because of its rich blood supply, a melanoma can spread easily. Spread occurs by extension through the sclera or invasion of other eye structures into nearby tissue and the brain.

COLLABORATIVE MANAGEMENT

Assessment

Manifestations of melanoma may not be readily apparent; the tumor may be discovered during a routine examination. Blurring of vision may occur if the macular area is invaded. Visual acuity is reduced if the tumor grows inward toward the center of the eye from the choroid and alters the visual pathway. Increased intraocular pressure (IOP) can result if the tumor invades the canal of Schlemm and obstructs flow of aqueous humor. A change in iris color may occur if the tumor infiltrates the iris. Sudden loss of a portion of the visual field may result from tumor invasion of the space under the retina, producing retinal detachment.

Diagnostic tests for a melanoma depend on the size and tumor growth rate. Ultrasonography is performed to determine the tumor's location and size.

Interventions

Treatment also depends on the tumor's size and growth rate, as well as the condition of the other eye. Small lesions of the iris not affecting the iris root are monitored until growth is observed. Tumors of the choroid are treated by surgical enucleation or by radiation therapy with a radioactive plaque.

SURGERY. Enucleation (surgical removal of the entire eyeball) is performed under general anesthesia. After the eye is removed, a ball implant is inserted to provide a base for the socket prosthesis and to ensure the best cosmetic result.

CHART 50-12

BEST PRACTICE for
Insertion and Removal of an Ocular Prosthesis

Insertion

1. Assemble equipment:
   - Prosthesis
   - Gloves
   - Towel
2. Explain the procedure to the client.
3. Wash your hands.
4. Cover the work area with a cloth or towel.
5. Don gloves.
6. Remove the prosthesis from its container and rinse it with tepid water.
7. Lift the client's upper lid using your nondominant hand.

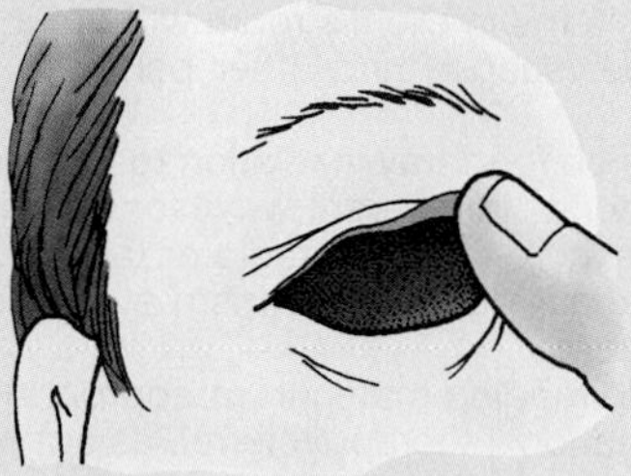

8. Place the prosthesis between the thumb and forefinger of your dominant hand. The notched end of the prosthesis should be closest to the client's nose.

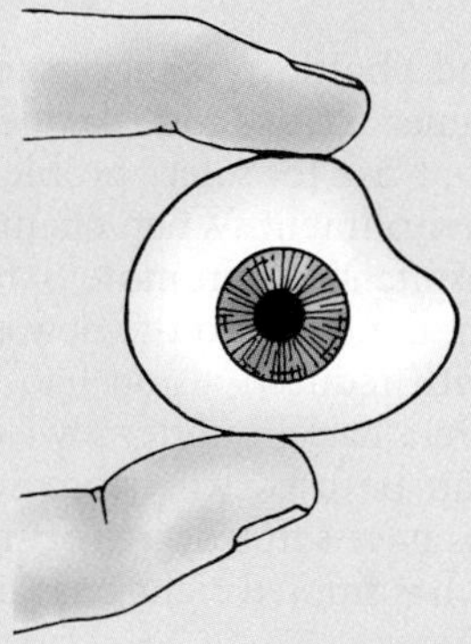

9. Insert the prosthesis with the top edge slipping under the upper lid. Continue until most of the iris is covered by the upper lid.

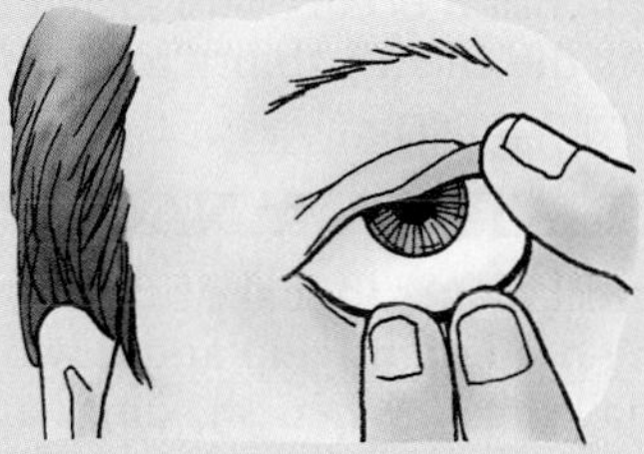

10. Gently release the upper eyelid.
11. Retract the lower lid slightly until the bottom edge of the prosthesis slips behind it.

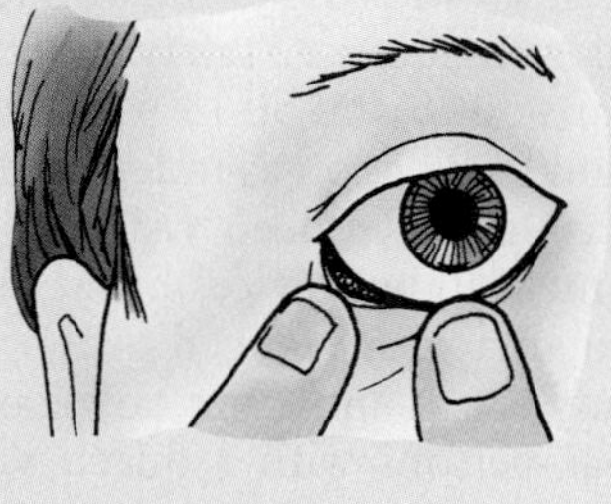

12. Release your hands slowly.

Removal

1. Assemble equipment:
   - Normal saline-filled labeled container
   - Gloves
2. Explain the procedure to the client.
3. Wash your hands.
4. Don gloves.
5. Instruct the client to sit up and tilt the head slightly downward.
6. Place your hand against the client's cheek, palm side up.
7. Pull the lower lid slightly down and laterally.
8. Allow the prosthesis to slide out onto your hand, or pull gently if necessary.
9. Place the prosthesis in a container filled with normal saline labeled with the client's name. Cover the container.

The implant is covered with surrounding tissue, muscles, and conjunctiva. A plastic conformer is placed over the conjunctiva to maintain the shape of the eyelids until a prosthesis can be fitted. After the dressing is removed, a pressure patch is placed over the eye for 24 hours.

Until the prosthesis is fitted (about 1 month after surgery), an antibiotic-steroid ointment is inserted into the cul-de-sac once a day. Best practices for the insertion and removal of the prosthesis are listed in Chart 50-12.

RADIATION. Radiation therapy can reduce the size and thickness of melanomas. The radioactive plaque, a round, flat disk about the size of a dime and containing a radioactive material, is sutured to the sclera overlying the tumor site. The length of time the plaque remains sutured to the sclera depends on the size of the tumor and the dose of radiation to be delivered.

Complications of radiation therapy include vascular changes, retinopathy, glaucoma, necrosis of the sclera, and cataract formation. Vitreous hemorrhage may develop as the tumor becomes smaller and pulls or breaks blood vessels.

While the plaque is in place, the eye may or may not be covered with a patch. Cycloplegic eyedrops and an antibiotic-steroid combination are given. Teach the client how to instill eyedrops.

REDUCED VISION

PATHOPHYSIOLOGY

Different forms of reduced vision may affect any or all aspects of vision, including color, light, image, movement, and acuity. Some periods of reduced vision may be temporary, such as when cataracts obscure vision but surgery has not yet been planned or performed. Clients are legally blind if their best visual acuity with corrective lenses is 20/200 or less in the better eye or if the widest diameter of the visual field in that eye is no greater than 20 degrees.

Blindness can occur in one or both eyes. When one eye is affected, the field of vision is narrowed and depth perception is impaired.

Central vision can be impaired by diseases involving the macula, such as macular edema or macular degeneration. Loss of peripheral vision occurs with glaucoma. The loss of side vision affects the client's ability to drive and awareness of hazards in the periphery.

COLLABORATIVE MANAGEMENT

Teach the client techniques to make better use of existing vision. Moving the head slightly up and down can enhance a three-dimensional effect. When shaking hands or pouring water, the client can line up the object and move toward it. He or she should choose a position that favors the good eye; for example, people with vision in the right eye should position people and items on their right.

Nursing interventions for the client with reduced sight fall into the areas of communication, safety, ambulation, self-care, and support. Charts 50-10 and 50-13 list ways to help clients with reduced vision to function as independently as possible.

Communication. Reduced vision is a common occurrence and many adaptive devices have been developed to help the person living with reduced vision to maintain independence. Many towns and cities now have auditory traffic signals so that persons with reduced vision can know when it is safe to cross a street. Curbs in these areas may have high contrast color paint to let the person know when to step up or down. Libraries have large-print books and books on tape. "Talking" clocks, watches, and timers are available. Playing cards, games, restaurant menus, calendars, and instruction booklets are available in large print sizes. Computer keyboards with high contrast and larger letters in the keys are available as are large screens. Direct the client with reduced vision to the local resources to obtain adaptive items and to learn how best to use them.

Safety. For clients at home with reduced vision, the home is the place where the client feels most safe. He or she is familiar with room and item location. For example, they may have counted the number of footsteps needed to move from one area to another within the home. It is important to stress to family and friends that changes in item location should not be made without input from the person with reduced vision.

Even people who have experienced gradually reduced vision over time and who use Vision Compensation Behaviors in the home may benefit from having a person with vision assist in making adaptations in the home. Such adaptations may include the following:

- Using tape and a heavy black marker, mark
  - the 350-degree temperature setting on the oven
  - the 70-degree temperature setting on the heating or cooling thermostat
- Paint or mark light switches in a deep color that contrasts with the surrounding wall.
- Label canned goods with large, bold, black letters on white tape.
- Teach the client to feel for the crease in paper milk cartons that indicates the place to open the spout.
- Help the client differentiate different drugs by altering the shape or contours of a bottle. Rubber bands can be wound around a bottle to change its texture. Raised symbols can be glued to caps to make identification easier.

CHART 50-13

NIC INTERVENTION ACTIVITIES for The Client with Reduced Vision

Communication Enhancement: Visual Deficit: *Assistance in accepting and learning alternate methods for living with diminished vision*

- Identify yourself when you enter the client's space.
- Note client's reaction to diminished vision (e.g., depression, withdrawal, or denial).
- Accept client's reaction to diminished vision.
- Assist client in setting new goals to learn how to "see" with other senses.
- Build on client's remaining vision, as appropriate.
- Walk one or two steps ahead of the client, with client's hand on your elbow.
- Describe environment to client.
- Do not move items in client's room without informing client.
- Read mail, newspaper, and other pertinent information to client.
- Identify items on food tray in relation to numbers on a clock.
- Fold paper money in different ways for easy identification.
- Inform client where to locate radio or talking books.
- Provide a magnifying glass or prism eyeglasses, as appropriate, for reading.
- Provide braille reading material, as appropriate.
- Initiate occupational therapy referral, as appropriate.
- Refer client with visual problems to appropriate agency.

NIC intervention activities selected from Dochterman, J.M., & Bulechek, G.M. (Eds.). (2004). *Nursing interventions classification (NIC)* (4th ed.). St. Louis: Mosby. No part of this work is to be altered without prior written permission from the Publisher.

The client is most at risk for safety problems in an unfamiliar or changing environment. When clients with reduced vision must be hospitalized, promote safety and independence by orienting the client to the new environment.

Most clients with reduced vision had full sight at some time and thus have a background knowledge regarding size and shape that can be used when providing information. Many blind clients have some degree of sight. When talking with a client who has limited sight or is blind, always use a normal tone of voice.

First orient the client to the immediate environment, including the size of the room. Use one object in the room, such as a chair or hospital bed, as the focal point during your description. Guide the client to the focal point and orient him or her to the environment from that point. For example, you might say, "To the left of the bed is a chair." Then describe all other objects in relation to the focal point. Go with the client to other important areas, such as the bathroom, so that the client can learn their locations. Highlight the location of the toilet, sink, and toilet paper holder. *Never leave the client with reduced vision in the center of an unfamiliar room.*

Clients with reduced vision prefer to establish the location of important objects, such as the call bell, water pitcher, and clock. Once their location has been fixed, do not move these items without the client's consent. Do not move the location of chairs, stools, and wastebaskets without consulting the client.

At mealtime, set up food on the tray using clock placement. For example, "There is sliced ham at 6 o'clock; peas are located at 3 o'clock; to the right of the plate is coffee; salt and pepper are next to the coffee."

Ambulation. When helping a client with reduced vision to ambulate, allow him or her to grasp your arm at the elbow. Keep the arm close to your body so that the client can detect your direction of movement. Alert the client when obstacles are in the path ahead.

Clients may use a cane to detect obstacles, such as furniture, walls, or curbs. The cane is held in the dominant hand several inches off the floor and sweeps the ground where the client's foot will be placed next. The laser cane sends out signals to help detect obstacles.

Self-Care. The ability to control the environment is important to the client with reduced vision. Knock on the door before entering the hospital room or any other environment of a client with reduced vision. State your name and the reason for visiting when entering the room.

Support. Clients' reaction to the loss of sight is similar to the reaction to loss of a body part. Newly blind clients may need a period of grieving for the "dead" (nonseeing) eye. Clients often feel hopeless and angry. With time, anger usually gives way to acceptance. The ability to cope may begin within days, but some clients mourn for months or years.

Clients benefit from the honest support that you can provide. They need to hear that it is normal to mourn, to cry, and to feel the loss. Help clients move toward acceptance by encouraging the mastery of one task at a time and by providing positive reinforcement for each success.

GET READY for the NCLEX Examination!

KEY POINTS

Safe Effective Care Environment

- Use contact precautions with any client who has drainage from the eye or lacrimal apparatus.
- Avoid performing an ophthalmoscopic examination on a confused or uncooperative client.
- Orient the client with reduced vision to his or her immediate surroundings, including how to call for help and where the bathroom is located.
- Identify the room of a client with reduced vision.

Health Promotion and Maintenance

- Identify clients at risk for visual impairment as a result of work environment or leisure activities.
- Encourage all clients to wear eye protection when performing yard work, working in a woodshop or metal shop, using chemicals, or are in any environment where drops or particulate matter are airborne.
- Encourage all adult clients older than 40 years of age to have an eye examination with measurement of intraocular pressure every year.
- Encourage all clients to use polarizing sunglasses whenever outdoors in bright sunlight.
- Teach all clients to wash their hands before and after touching the eyes.

Psychosocial Integrity

- Use a normal tone of voice to talk with a client who has a vision problem and normal hearing.
- Pace your interview to match the learning needs and style of the individual client.
- Knock on the door before entering the room of a client with reduced vision and introduce yourself.
- Allow the client the opportunity to express fear or anxiety regarding a change in vision.
- Refer clients newly diagnosed with visual impairment to appropriate local resources and support groups.
- Explain all diagnostic procedures, restrictions, and follow-up care to the client scheduled for tests.

Physiological Integrity

- Ask the client about vision problems in any other members of the family, because many vision problems have a genetic component.
- Teach clients the proper technique to use for self instillation of eyedrops and eye ointment.
- Stress the importance of completing an antibiotic regimen when an infection is present in the eye.
- Teach clients who are at risk for increased intraocular pressure what activities to avoid (see Table 50-3).
- Teach clients with an infection of the eye or eyelid not to rub the eye (to avoid infecting the other eye).
- Never attempt to remove any object protruding from the eye.

ADDITIONAL STUDY RESOURCES

Go to your Student CD-ROM for Review Questions for the NCLEX Examination.

evolve Go to http://evolve.elsevier.com/Iggy/ for Integrated Management of Care Questions for the NCLEX Examination.

SELECTED BIBLIOGRAPHY

Ackley, B., & Ladwig, G. (2002). *Nursing diagnosis handbook: A guide to planning care* (5th ed.). St. Louis: Mosby.

American Cancer Society. (2005). *Cancer facts and figures 2005.* Report No. 00-300M-No. 5008.05. Atlanta: Author.

Barnie, D. (2002). Restoring vision in older patients. *RN, 65*(1), 30-36.

Bickerton, R. (2000). Identifying and treating ocular emergencies. *Journal of Ophthalmic Nursing and Technology, 19*(5), 224-229.

Collins, M., et al. (2001). Effect of laser in situ keratomileusis (LASIK) on the corneal endothelium three years postoperatively. *American Journal of Ophthalmology, 131*(1), 1-6.

Craffey, A. (2000). Look on the bright side: A case study of uveitis. *Insight (American Society of Ophthalmic Registered Nurses), 25*(4), 119-124.

Dochterman, J., & Bulechek, G. (Eds.). (2004). *Nursing interventions classification (NIC)* (4th ed.). St. Louis: Mosby.

Ebersole, P., Hess, P., & Luggen, A. (2004). *Toward healthy aging: Human needs and nursing response* (6th ed.). St. Louis: Mosby.

Facts and Comparisons. (2004). *Drug facts and comparisons* (58th ed.). St. Louis: Author.

Gordon, M., et al. (2002). The ocular hypertension treatment study: Baseline factors that predict the onset of primary open-angle glaucoma. *Archives of Ophthalmology, 120*(6), 714-720.

Jarvis, C. (2004). *Physical examination and health assessment* (4th ed.). Philadelphia: W. B. Saunders.

Kass, M., et al. (2002). The Ocular Hypertension Treatment Study: Medication delays or prevents the onset of primary open-angle glaucoma. *Archives of Ophthalmology, 120*(6), 701-713.

Kushner, B., & Kowal, L. (2003). Diplopia after refractive surgery: Occurrence and prevention. *Archives of Ophthalmology, 121*(3), 315-321.

Kymionis, G., et al. (2003). Management of post-LASIK corneal ectasia with Intacs inserts: One-year results. *Archives of Ophthalmology, 121*(3), 322-326.
Majewski, J., et al. (2003). Age-related macular degeneration–A genome scan in extended families. *American Journal of Human Genetics, 73*(3), 540-550.
McCance, K., & Huether, S. (2002). *Pathophysiology: The biologic basis for disease in adults and children* (4th ed.). St. Louis: Mosby.
Milder, L., & Smith, S. (2002). Refractive surgery: An overview. *Insight (American Society of Ophthalmic Registered Nurses), 27*(2), 46-49.
Moore, L. (2000). Severe visual impairment in older women. *Western Journal of Nursing Research, 22*(5), 571-595.
Moore, L., & Miller, M. (2003). Older men's experiences of living with severe visual impairment. *Journal of Advanced Nursing, 43*(1), 10-18.
Moorhead, S., Johnson, M., & Maas, M. (Eds.). (2004). *Nursing outcomes classification (NOC)* (3rd ed.). St. Louis: Mosby.
Nicholls, P. (2004). Consult stat: Traumatic glaucoma can arise years after an injury. *RN, 67*(10), 65.
Nussbaum, R., McInnes, R., & Willard, H. (2001). *Thompson & Thompson: Genetics in medicine* (6th ed.). Philadelphia: W. B. Saunders.
Pagana, K., & Pagana, T. (2002). *Mosby's manual of diagnostic and laboratory tests* (2nd ed.). St. Louis: Mosby.
Ramponi, D. (2000). Go with the flow during an eye emergency. *Nursing2000, 30*(8), 54-56.
Rapaport, M. (2000). Eyelid dermatitis. *Dermatology Nursing, 12*(5), 352-354.
Rechtman, E., et al. (2002). An update on photodynamic therapy in age-related macular degeneration. *Expert Opinion on Pharmacotherapy, 3*(7), 931-938.
Rojas, M., & Manche, E. (2002). Phototherapeutic keratectomy for anterior basement membrane dystrophy after laser in situ keratomileusis. *Archives of Ophthalmology, 120*(6), 722-727.
Sackett, C., & Schenning, S. (2002). The age-related eye disease study: The results of the clinical trial. *Insight (American Society of Ophthalmic Registered Nurses), 27*(1), 5-7.
Shelswell, N. (2002). Perioperative patient education for retinal surgery. *AORN Journal, 75*(4), 801-807.
Smith, S. (2002). Eye on research: Retinal microchip implants. *Journal of the American Society of Ophthalmic Registered Nurses, 27*(3), 88.
Smith, S. (2003). Reducing ophthalmic drug-related injuries in older patients. *Insight (American Society of Ophthalmic Registered Nurses), 28*(2), 33-34.
Vaughan, D., Asbury, T., & Riordan-Eva, P. (Eds.) (2004). *General ophthalmology* (16th ed.). New York: McGraw-Hill.

CHAPTER

51

Assessment of the Ear and Hearing

JUDY MALKIEWICZ

LEARNING OUTCOMES

After studying this chapter, you should be able to:

1. Describe the key elements to inspect when performing assessment of the external ear.
2. Describe age-related changes in the structure of the ear and hearing.
3. Identify 10 common drugs that affect hearing.
4. Demonstrate the correct use of an otoscope.
5. Describe the landmarks of the tympanic membrane (eardrum).
6. Compare air conduction of sound with bone conduction of sound.
7. Demonstrate the correct use of a tuning fork in performing the Weber and Rinne tests for hearing.
8. Prioritize educational needs for the client about to undergo pure-tone audiometry and electronystagmography.

Go to your Student CD-ROM for Review Questions for the NCLEX Examination keyed to these Learning Outcomes.

Ear and hearing problems are common among adults of all ages. Assessment of the ear and hearing is an important skill for nurses in any care environment. Many problems with the ear and hearing develop over a long period, and hearing may also be affected by many drugs. An understanding of the anatomy and physiology of the ear is essential. Table 51-1 defines terms commonly used in assessing the ear and hearing.

ANATOMY AND PHYSIOLOGY REVIEW

Structure

The ear has three divisions or parts: the external ear, the middle ear, and the inner ear. Each part is important to the hearing process.

EXTERNAL EAR

The external ear develops in the embryo at the same time as the kidneys and urinary tract. Any person with a defect of the external ear should also be examined for possible problems or defects of the renal and urinary systems.

The external ear **(pinna),** which is composed of cartilage covered by skin, is embedded in the temporal bone on both sides of the head at the level of the eyes. The ear is attached to the head by skin and cartilage at about a 10-degree angle. The external ear extends from the pinna through the external canal to the **tympanic membrane** (eardrum) (Figure 51-1). The external ear canal is slightly S-shaped and lined with **cerumen** (wax)-producing glands (which help protect and lubricate the ear canal), sebaceous glands, and hair follicles. The hair follicles and cerumen protect the eardrum and the middle ear. In the adult, the distance from the opening of the external canal to the eardrum is about 1 to 1½ inches (2.5 to 3.75 cm). The external ear includes the **mastoid process,** the bony ridge located over the temporal bone behind the pinna.

MIDDLE EAR

The middle ear begins at the medial side of the eardrum. It consists of the **epitympanum,** a compartment containing the three bony **ossicles** (Figure 51-2): the malleus, the incus, and the stapes. The beginning of the eustachian tube also opens in the middle ear.

The eardrum **(tympanic membrane)** is a thick, transparent sheet of tissue providing a barrier between the external ear and the middle ear. The landmarks on the eardrum include the annulus, the pars flaccida, and the pars tensa. The eardrum is attached to the first bony ossicle, the **malleus** (hammer), at the **umbo** (Figure 51-3). The bony ossicles behind the eardrum are joined loosely, moving with vibrations from the eardrum.

The pars flaccida and pars tensa are parts of the eardrum. The pars flaccida is that portion of the eardrum above the short process of the malleus; the pars tensa is that portion surrounding the long process of the malleus. The eardrum is usually transparent, opaque, or pearly gray, and it moves when air is injected into the external canal. The umbo is seen through the eardrum membrane as a white dot at the end of the long process of the malleus. The short process of the malleus, the long process of the malleus, and the umbo are structures that can be seen through the transparent eardrum.

The middle ear is separated from the inner ear by the round window and the oval window. The eustachian tube begins at the floor of the middle ear at the proximal end and opens at the distal end in the throat. The distal opening in the throat is surrounded by adenoid lymphatic tissue (Figure 51-4). The eustachian tube allows the pressure on both sides of the eardrum to equalize. Secretions from the middle ear drain through it.

INNER EAR

The inner ear, which lies on the other side of the oval window, contains the semicircular canals, the cochlea, the vestibule, and the distal end of the eighth cranial nerve (see Figure 51-2). The **semicircular canals** are tubes made of cartilage that contain fluid and hair cells. These canals are connected to the sensory nerve fibers of the vestibular portion of the eighth cranial nerve. The fluid and hair cells within the canals help to maintain the sense of balance.

The **cochlea,** the spiral organ of hearing, is divided into the scala tympani and the scala vestibuli. Reissner's membrane stretches across the scala vestibuli and forms the duct of the cochlea, or the scala media. The scala media is filled with **endolymph,** a fluid similar to intracellular fluid. The scala tympani and scala vestibuli are filled with **perilymph.** Endolymph and perilymph protect the cochlea and the semicircular canals by allowing these structures to "float" in the fluids and be cushioned against abrupt head movements.

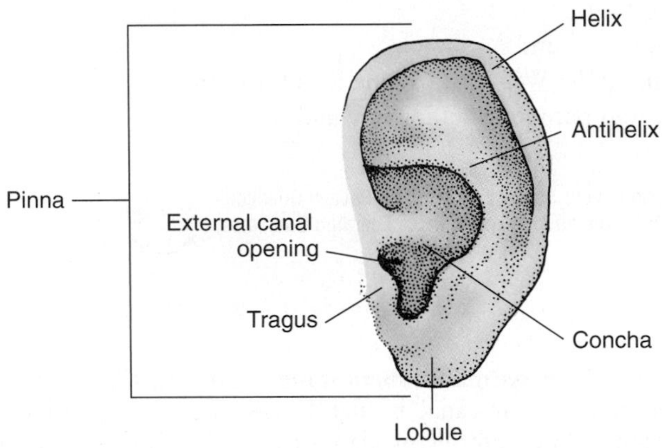

Figure 51-1 ■ Anatomic features of the external ear.

TABLE 51-1 Terminology Commonly Used in Ear and Hearing Assessment

cerumen Waxlike secretion of the external ear canal
conductive hearing loss Hearing loss resulting from a physical disruption in the transmission of sound waves
decibel A unit of sound for expressing loudness
masking The process of hiding a specific sound from one ear while the other ear is tested for its ability to hear that sound
Ménière's disease An intermittent but progressive deterioration of hearing and balance
otitis media Inflammation/infection of the middle ear
otosclerosis Formation of spongy bone around structures of the middle and inner ear, leading to low-tone hearing impairment
ototoxic Damaging to the structures important for hearing
presbycusis Age-related degenerative changes in the ear, leading to decreased hearing acuity
sensorineural Hearing loss resulting from neural defects
spondee Words of two syllables on which equal stress is placed during pronunciation
tympanic membrane The eardrum; a thin membrane that separates the middle ear from the external ear canal. This membrane vibrates when sound waves strike it
vestibular Relating to the functions of the ear for the sense of balance and position

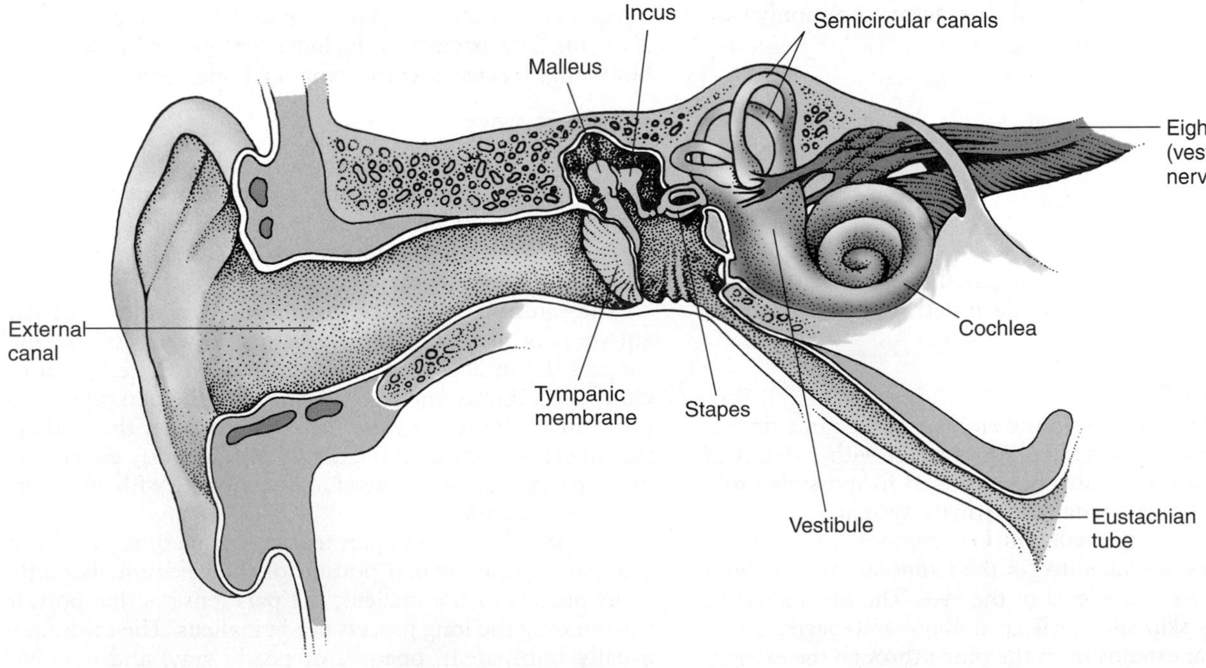

Figure 51-2 ■ Anatomic features of the internal ear.

The **organ of Corti** is the receptor end-organ of hearing located on the basilar membrane of the cochlea. The cochlea contains hair cells that detect vibration from sound and stimulate the eighth cranial nerve.

Function

The ear's main function is hearing, which occurs when sound is delivered through the air to the external ear canal and the temporal bone covering the mastoid air cells. The sound waves strike the mastoid and the movable eardrum, which is connected to the first bony ossicle. The sound wave vibrations are transferred from the eardrum to the malleus, the incus, and the stapes. From the stapes the vibrations are transmitted to the cochlea. Receptors there **transduce** (change) the vibrations into action potentials, conducted to the brain as nerve impulses by the cochlear portion of the eighth cranial (or auditory) nerve. Sound is processed and interpreted by the brain.

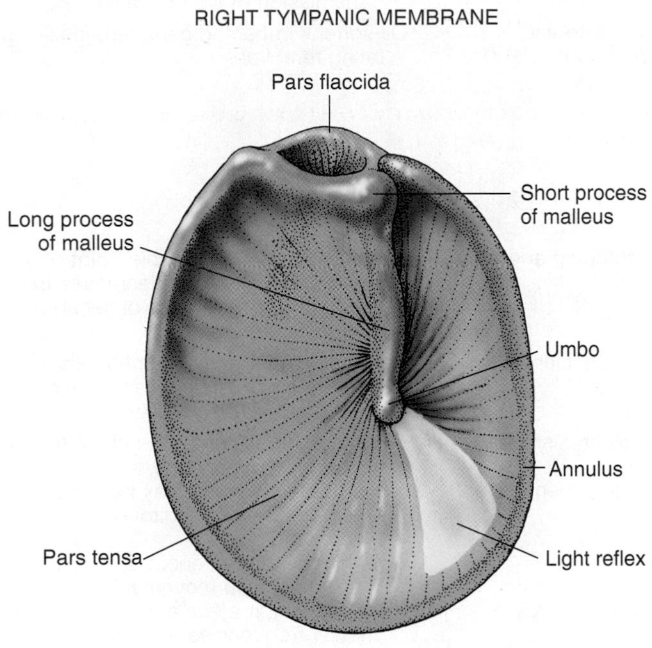

Figure 51-3 ■ Landmarks on the tympanic membrane.

Ear and Hearing Changes Associated with Aging

Ear and hearing changes related to aging are listed in Chart 51-1. Some of these changes are harmless; others pose serious threats to the hearing ability of older clients and call for nursing interventions.

All older adults should be screened for hearing acuity. Many scales or tools can be used to obtain the client's perception of hearing loss. These scales may not be any more helpful than just asking, "Do you have a hearing problem now?" (see the Evidence-Based Practice for Nursing box on p. 1114).

ASSESSMENT TECHNIQUES

History

First obtain a thorough history from the client. Informal hearing assessment begins as you observe the client listening to and answering questions. The client's posture and appropriateness of responses provide additional information about his or her hearing acuity.

During the interview, sit in adequate light, facing the client, which allows him or her to see you speaking. Be careful to use ordinary language. Also assess demographic data, personal and family history, socioeconomic status, current health problems, and the use of any remedies for

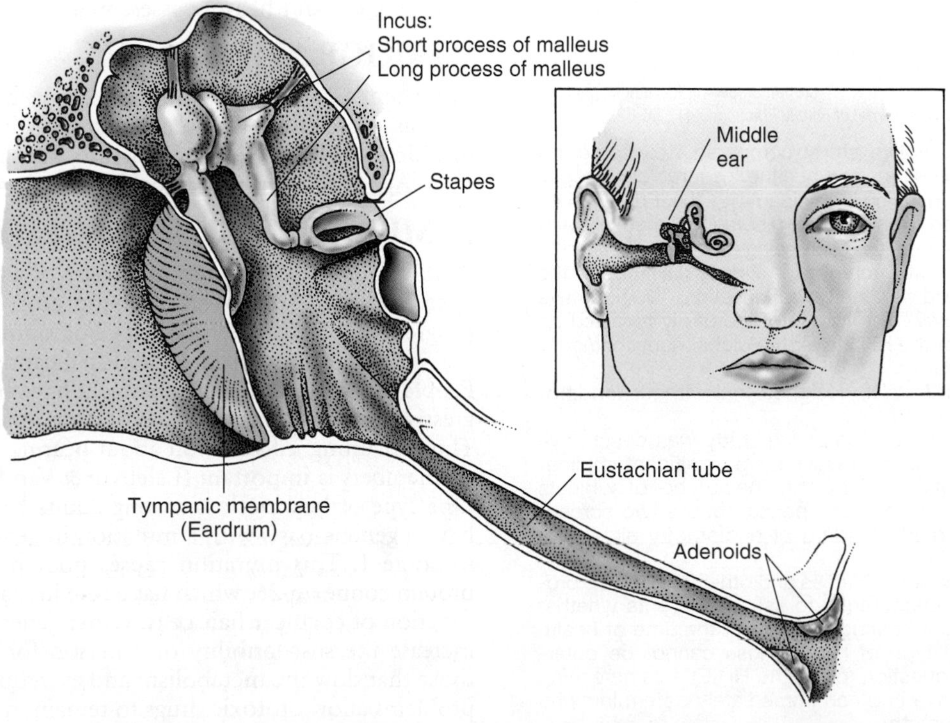

Figure 51-4 ■ Anatomic features and attached structures of the middle ear.

CHART 51-1

NURSING FOCUS on the OLDER ADULT
The Ear and Hearing

Physiologic Change	Nursing Interventions	Rationales
The pinna becomes elongated because of normal loss of subcutaneous tissue and decreased tissue elasticity.	When asked, explain that larger-appearing ears are associated with the normal aging process.	Explanation allays anxiety about the change in ear size.
Hair becomes coarser and longer, especially in men.		
Cerumen-producing glands decrease in number and function.	Irrigate ear canal weekly.	Irrigation removes excess cerumen, preventing impaction and enhancing transmission of sound waves.
Cerumen tends to be drier in older clients; it becomes impacted, which causes hearing loss.	Place 1 or 2 drops of oil into ear canal 8 hr before irrigation.	Oil softens impacted cerumen, facilitating removal.
The tympanic membrane loses elasticity; it may normally appear dull and retracted.		
Bony ossicles have decreased movement.		
The cochlea undergoes degenerative changes.		
Disturbed vestibular function results in occasional dizziness, vertigo, and sensations of unsteadiness in 50%-60% of older adults.	Assist the client with standing and initial ambulation.	The nurse provides a stable point of reference. Assistance decreases the risk of falling as a result of vestibular disorientation.
Hearing acuity diminishes with advancing age.	Establish that a hearing deficiency exists.	Determine whether interventions are needed. Not all older clients have diminished hearing acuity.
The ability to hear high-frequency sounds is nearly gone by age 60 years, which affects speech reception and increases auditory reaction time greatly. Clients have particular difficulty with the *f, s, sh,* and *pa* sounds. Some older clients hear a persistent noise (tinnitus). Presbycusis (a sensorineural type of hearing loss) is common in older adults.	When speaking to an older client with a hearing deficiency: ▪ Provide a quiet environment. ▪ Face the client. ▪ Speak slowly in a deeper voice.	This makes it easier for the client to hear and communicate. ▪ Extraneous noise may interfere with the client's auditory perception. ▪ The client can benefit by being able to see lip movement. ▪ The client may be able to discern lower frequencies more easily.

EVIDENCE-BASED PRACTICE for Nursing

Sometimes clients know best

Gates, G., Murphy, M., Rees, T., & Fraher, A. (2003). Screening for handicapping hearing loss in the elderly. *The Journal of Family Practice,* 52(1), 56-62.

This prospective descriptive study compared two screening methods to identify unrecognized hearing loss in older people. The 546 subjects, continuing participants in the Framingham Heart Study, consented to using the two screening methods and had audiometry performed. One screening method consisted of the Hearing Handicap Inventory for the Elderly (HHIE), and the other screening method was the global question, "Do you have a hearing problem now?" The results of the study revealed no improved specificity of the HHIE over the global questioning related to a hearing problem.

Level of Evidence: 3—Well-designed trial without randomization, with a large cohort.

Critique. Although the design of the study was descriptive rather than experimental, the results have significant implications for health care of the older adult. The number of subjects involved in the study and the comparison of the two screening methods to the gold standard of audiometry allows for generalization of the findings.

Implications for Nursing. Nurses and other health care professionals should be encouraged to ask their clients whether they are experiencing a hearing problem at the time of health history. Although the type of hearing loss cannot be determined by the global question (or by the HHIE), this screening method is cost-effective and can immediately determine who should undergo audiometry.

ear problems. Chart 51-2 lists important questions to ask regarding ear and hearing assessment.

DEMOGRAPHIC DATA

The client's gender is important. Some hearing disorders, such as otosclerosis, are more common in women. Other disorders, such as Ménière's disease, are more common in men. Age is also an important factor in hearing loss.

FAMILY HISTORY AND GENETIC RISK

Although most hearing loss as a result of a genetic mutation is seen in childhood, some genetic problems can lead to progressive hearing loss in adults. For example, 70% of people with Down syndrome develop hearing loss as adults. People with osteogenesis imperfecta have bilateral and progressive hearing loss in the second or third decade of life. Thus obtaining information about hearing loss among family members is important (Lefebvre & Van De Water, 2000). One type of hearing loss among adults has been found to have a genetic basis with a mutation in gene *GJB2* on chromosome 1. This mutation causes poor production of the protein connexin-26, which has a role in maintaining proper function of cochlear hair cells. Other genetic problems that increase the susceptibility of a person for hearing loss are those that slow the metabolism and excretion of drugs. Such problems allow ototoxic drugs to remain in a client's system longer and do more damage to the hearing system.

CHART 51-2

Ear and Hearing Assessment
USING GORDON'S FUNCTIONAL HEALTH PATTERNS

Cognitive-Perceptual Pattern
- Do you have any hearing difficulty?
- Do you use any type of hearing aid?
- Do you notice that you have the volume of the television or radio set at an increased level?
- Are you sitting closer to the television or radio in order to hear more clearly?
- Do you have difficulty in your ability to hear or follow conversations in a noisy environment, such as a restaurant?
- Do you have difficulty hearing high-pitched sounds like the doorbell?

Health Perception/Health Management Pattern
- Have you had your hearing checked?
- If you are or were exposed to environmental noise, have you consistently used appropriate hearing protection?
- Do you avoid cleaning your ear canals with foreign objects such as toothpicks or paper clips?
- Have you discussed with your health care provider the side effects of any drugs you may be taking that might affect your ear and hearing?

Based on Gordon, M. (2002). *Manual of nursing diagnosis* (10th ed.). St. Louis: Mosby.

Specific questions to ask the client include the following:
- Who in your family has hearing problems?
- In those who have hearing problems, are the problems present in men and women equally, or are they present more in one gender?
- At what age was hearing loss diagnosed in your relative(s)?
- Are both ears affected?

PERSONAL HISTORY

Personal history includes information on past or current manifestations of ear pain, ear discharge, vertigo, tinnitus, decreased hearing, and difficulty understanding people when they talk or difficulty hearing environmental noises. Ask the client about the following:
- Ear trauma
- Ear surgery
- Past infections
- Excessive cerumen
- Ear itch
- Any invasive instruments routinely used to clean the ear
- Type and pattern of ear hygiene
- Exposure to loud noise or music
- Air travel (especially in unpressurized aircraft)
- Swimming habits and the use ear protection when swimming
- History of hereditary factors and health problems causing changes in the blood supply to the ear (heart disease, hypertension, diabetes)
- History of vitiligo (a pigment disorder in which there may be a loss of melanin-containing cells [and their protective function] in the inner ear, resulting in hearing loss)
- History of smoking (nicotine increases the carboxyhemoglobin in the blood, reducing the oxygen supply to the cochlea, and possibly increasing sensory cell damage)
- History of vitamin B_{12} and folate deficiency (associated with age-related hearing loss)

TABLE 51-2 Ototoxic Drugs

Drug Type	Drug
Antibiotics	Amikacin Capreomycin Chloramphenicol Dihydrostreptomycin Erythromycin Gentamicin (Garamycin, Cidomycin) Kanamycin Metronidazole (vestibulotoxicity rarely) Neomycin Netilmicin Streptomycin Tobramycin
Diuretics	Acetazolamide (Apo-Acetazolamide, Diamox) Ethacrynic acid (Edecrin) Bumetanide Furosemide (Apo-Furosemide✱, Lasix, Furoside✱)
Nonsteroidal anti-inflammatory agents	Ibuprofen (Advil, Nuprin, Motrin) Indomethacin (Indocin) Naproxen (Aleve, Naprosyn, Anaprox) Feldene, Dolobid, Lodine, Relafen, Toradol, Voltaren Salicylates (aspirin, Disalcid, Bufferin, Ecotrin, Trilisate, Ascriptin, Empirin, Excedrin, Fiorinal)
Chemotherapy agents	Actinomycin Bleomycin Cisplatin (Abiplatin, Platinol) Carboplatin Nitrogen mustard (Mustargen) Vincristine
Miscellaneous	Carbamazepine Hydroxychloroquine (Plaquenil) Quinine (Legatrin, NovoQuinine✱, Quinamm) Quinidine (Apo-Quinidine✱, Cardioquin, Quinidex)

If the client uses a hearing aid, determine how well it works, the date of the last hearing test, the type of test given, and the results. Ask the client about other problems that may impair hearing, such as allergies; upper respiratory infections; hypothyroidism; arteriosclerosis; head trauma; and recent head, facial, or dental surgery. A thorough drug history is crucial because many drugs are ototoxic (Table 51-2).

Ask the client about his or her occupation and any hobbies that involve exposure to loud environmental noise or music. Also determine whether the client uses protective ear devices or any devices inserted into the ear, such as a telephone headset or a stethoscope.

SOCIOECONOMIC STATUS

Assess the client's socioeconomic status to determine the availability of health care. Clients of lower socioeconomic status often do not seek health care for ear-related problems until hearing damage is extensive. Clients at any socioeconomic level, however, might hesitate to have their hearing loss diagnosed because of the fear of needing to wear a hearing aid.

CURRENT HEALTH PROBLEMS

Assess current ear-related health problems by asking whether the client has noticed any "trouble with" his or her ears, ear pain, or discharge, including any earwax. Ask about any change in hearing, such as intolerance for sound levels that do not bother other people (hyperacusis), or other problems, such as ringing in the ears. If a change in hearing is reported, ask whether one or both ears are involved and whether the change was sudden or gradual. Also ask the client about any problems with dizziness, sensations of being "off balance" or **vertigo** (sense of spinning movement).

Physical Assessment

Inspection and palpation are the only examination techniques used to assess the ear. Begin the examination by placing the client in either a sitting or a supine position. Do not attempt to examine an uncooperative or confused client. Remove any hearing aids during the examination. After the otoscopic examination, inspect the hearing aid for cracks, debris, and a proper fit. Ear examination is divided into external ear and mastoid assessment, otoscopic assessment, and auditory assessment.

Video Clip: External Ear

EXTERNAL EAR AND MASTOID ASSESSMENT

Inspect the mastoid process for redness and swelling, which indicate inflammation. To assess for tenderness, gently tap with one finger over the mastoid process, compress the tragus with one finger, and gently manipulate the pinna forward and backward. Any tenderness suggests an inflammatory process in either the external ear or the mastoid.

Inspect the entire external ear for shape, location of attachment to the head, and condition of the visible external canal. The normal pinna is uniformly shaped without skin tags or deformity. The pinna should be attached vertically to the side of the head at a posterior angle of no greater than 10 degrees. It should fall within or touch the eye-occiput line, an imaginary line drawn from the greatest protuberance on the occiput to the lateral canthus of the eye. Record any variation from the normal ear shape and attachment.

Abnormalities of the pinna include swelling, nodules, and lesions. In chronic gout, collection of uric acid crystals results in hard, irregular, painless nodules called **tophi** on the helix and antihelix portions of the pinna. Other painless nodules on the pinna might be due to basal cell carcinoma or rheumatoid arthritis. Small, crusted, ulcerated, or indurated lesions on the pinna that fail to heal could be squamous cell carcinoma.

The normal external canal is free from lesions, dry, clean, and not reddened. Assess for the following problems:

- Furuncles
- Large amounts of cerumen
- Scaliness
- Redness
- Swelling of or drainage from the ear associated with a foreign object (insects or other substances), trauma, or infection

Also record any other drainage (blood, cerebrospinal fluid, pus, or serous fluid) and its character.

OTOSCOPIC ASSESSMENT

An instrument called an otoscope is used to examine the ear. Many types are available. An **otoscope** (Figure 51-5) consists of a light, a handle, a magnifying lens, and a pneumatic bulb for injecting air into the external canal to test mobility of the eardrum.

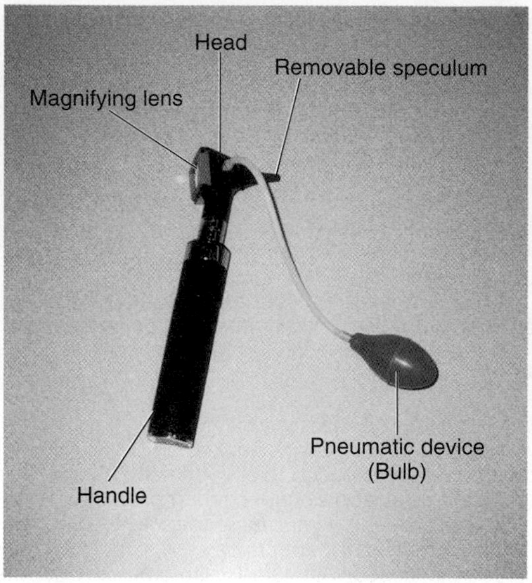

Figure 51-5 ■ Functional components of an otoscope.

Specula of various diameters attach to the head of the otoscope. Select the largest that most comfortably fits the client's external canal. *Never blindly insert the speculum into the external canal because of the risk of perforating the eardrum.*

If the client has any pain during external ear examination, cautiously attempt an otoscopic examination. (The speculum will cause extreme pain if it comes in contact with inflamed tissue in the external canal.) Become familiar with and memorize all the structures of the eardrum and middle ear before attempting to visualize them with an otoscope.

When performing an otoscopic examination, tilt the client's head slightly away and hold the otoscope upside down, like a large pen (Figure 51-6). This position permits your hand to lie against the client's head for support. If the client moves, both your hand and the otoscope also move, preventing damage to the external canal or eardrum. Hold the otoscope in the dominant hand and gently pull the pinna up and back with the nondominant hand. Visualize the external canal while you slowly insert the speculum. Use caution and avoid jamming the speculum into the walls of the external canal, which causes pain.

Video Clip: Ear Canal

After the pinna is correctly displaced and the otoscope is comfortably introduced in the external canal, observe the eardrum for color, intactness, and shape. Assess for lesions and the amount and consistency of cerumen and hair. The normal external canal is skin colored, intact, and without lesions. It contains various amounts of soft cerumen and has small, fine hairs.

Next assess the eardrums for intactness; normal structures seen through the eardrum (the long and short processes of the malleus and the umbo); portions of the eardrum itself (light reflex, pars flaccida, and pars tensa); and the color, shape, and mobility of the membrane as well as any lesions. Figure 51-7 shows an otoscopic view of a normal eardrum. *The normal eardrum is always intact.* The long process of the malleus is seen through the eardrum as a whitish streak extending from the short process of the malleus to the umbo.

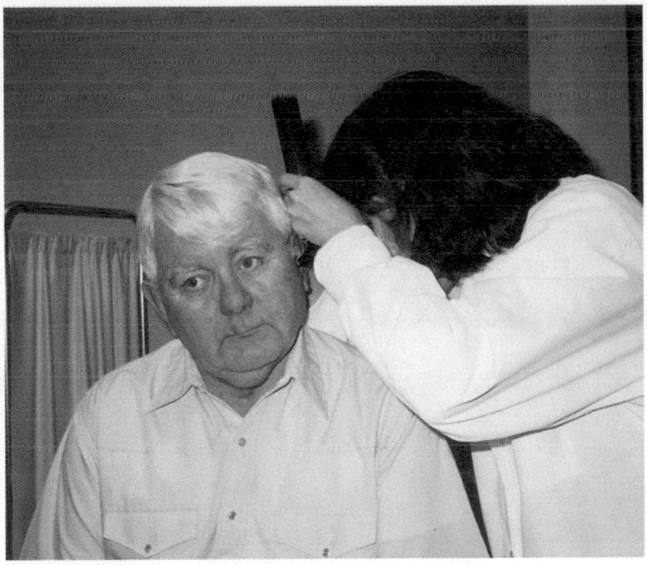

Figure 51-6 ■ Proper technique for an otoscopic examination.

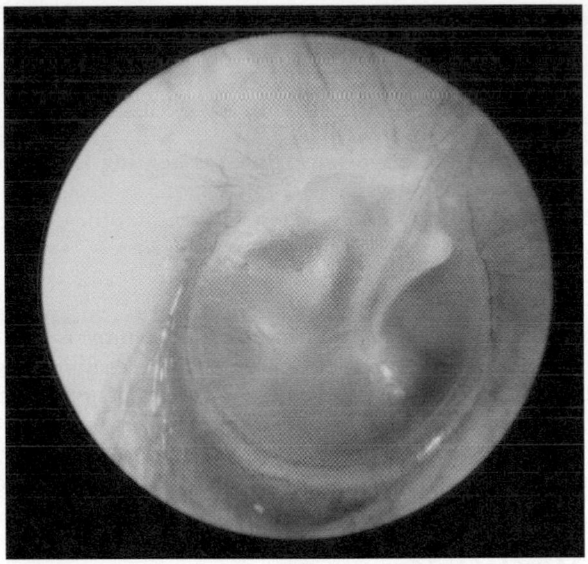

Figure 51-7 ■ Otoscopic view of a normal tympanic membrane.

In some people with allergies, visible blood vessels may be present on the long process, although this finding also occurs as an early indication of otitis media.

The short process of the malleus is seen through the eardrum as a white structure that seems more three-dimensional (projecting out toward the otoscope) than the other structures on the eardrum. The umbo appears as a round, white dot.

The long and short processes of the malleus, in addition to the umbo, are always easily identified in the normal ear. Abnormal variations are caused by serous otitis and otitis media, among other disorders.

Reflection of the otoscope's light off of the eardrum is the **light reflex,** a clearly demarcated triangle of light in the normal ear. The base of the triangle is on the annulus, and the point of the triangle is on the umbo. When the light reflex is spotty or multiple because of a changed eardrum shape from either retraction or bulging, the light reflex is termed **diffuse.**

The eardrum is normally shiny, transparent, and opaque or pearly gray. Abnormal variations include redness (as seen in otitis media) and dullness or retraction (as seen in serous otitis).

The normal eardrum is slightly concave, allowing the pars tensa portion to move gently on testing with a puff of air from the pneumatic bulb on the otoscope.

The normal eardrum is free of lesions. The most common lesion is scarring caused by previous ear infection and perforation. A scar thickens the eardrum, which makes it difficult or impossible to see through the membrane at the point of the scar and reduces the mobility of the eardrum.

Test the mobility of the eardrum by gently injecting a small puff of air through the pneumatic bulb into the external canal and watching the pars tensa portion for movement. The normal eardrum moves gently. Decreased or absent mobility results from scarring, retraction, bulging, the presence of fluid in the middle ear, and decreased mobility of the ossicles associated with aging.

CULTURAL CONSIDERATIONS

Cerumen is generally moist and tan or brown in black clients and white clients. It is dry and light brown to gray in Asians and Native Americans/American Indians. The color of the lining of the external ear canal varies with the client's skin tone. Clients with more moist earwax may form cerumen impactions more easily than do clients with drier, flaky earwax.

Critical Thinking Challenge

The client is an older woman who lives with her son's family. The family immigrated from Mexico 3 years ago. She speaks limited English and is fluent in Spanish. She arrives at the clinic with her 15-year-old granddaughter, who is bilingual in English and Spanish. They tell you that Abuela's (Grandmother's) left ear has been painful for some time. She seems reluctant to tell you how she has tried to treat her ear at home. You are about to perform an external and otoscopic examination on her.

1. How will you explain these procedures to the client?
2. Describe variations in home treatments for ear pain.
3. Describe the otoscopic examination results you would expect if her eardrum is infected.

evolve For suggested answer guidelines, go to http://evolve.elsevier.com/Iggy/.

Auditory Assessment

After completing bilateral external ear and otoscopic examinations, assess the client's hearing acuity. Sound is transmitted by air conduction and bone conduction. Air conduction of sound is normally more sensitive than bone conduction. If hearing acuity is decreased, the hearing loss is categorized as follows:

- **Conductive hearing loss,** which results from any physical obstruction of sound wave transmission (such as a foreign body in the external canal, a retracted or bulging tympanic membrane, or fused bony ossicles)

- **Sensorineural hearing loss,** which results from a defect in the cochlea, the eighth cranial nerve, or the brain itself. Exposure to loud noises and music may cause this type of hearing loss resulting from damage of the cochlear hair cells.
- **Mixed conductive-sensorineural hearing loss,** a profound hearing loss.

Each of the auditory function tests determines the degree of hearing loss and differentiates the type of loss.

VOICE TEST

A simple hearing acuity test can be conducted by asking the client to block one external ear canal while standing 1 to 2 feet (30 to 60 cm) away. Quietly whisper a statement and then ask the client to repeat it. Test each ear separately. If the client does not respond correctly, use a louder whisper. If you suspect the client is lip-reading, use your hand to block the view of your mouth.

WATCH TEST

A ticking watch is used to test hearing acuity for high-frequency sounds. Hold a ticking watch about 5 inches (12.7 cm) from each of the ears and ask whether the ticking is heard. The client with normal hearing should be able to hear it.

AUDIOSCOPY

The lightweight audioscope allows you to visualize the external ear and eardrum. Hearing can be measured at a 40-decibel (dB) intensity at frequencies of 510, 1000, 2000, and 4000 cycles per second (cps), or hertz (Hz). The audioscope is larger than a standard otoscope, and you can easily use it to assess hearing.

TUNING FORK TESTS

Hearing acuity can be tested by the Weber and Rinne tuning fork tests. Tuning fork tests are useful, although limited, in distinguishing between conductive and sensorineural hearing losses. The frequency range of the tuning fork used for these tests corresponds to that of normal speech: 512 or 1024 Hz. To perform this assessment, stand in front of the sitting client.

Animation: Weber Test

Weber Tuning Fork Test

To perform the Weber tuning fork test, strike the tuning fork to make it vibrate. Place the vibrating tuning fork on the middle of the client's head, at the midline of the forehead, or above the upper lip over the teeth. Many clients object to the vibration over the upper lip; so the preferred site is the midline of the skull (Figure 51-8). Take care to hold the vibrating tuning fork by the stem only, not by the vibrating fork. Ask the client in which ear the sound is louder. The normal test result is sound heard equally in both ears. If the client hears the sound louder in one ear, the term *lateralization* describes the side on which the sound is the loudest.

Rinne Tuning Fork Test

The Rinne tuning fork test compares hearing by air conduction with hearing by bone conduction. Sound is normally heard two to three times longer by air conduction than by bone conduction. Perform the Rinne tuning fork test by placing the vibrating tuning fork stem on the client's mastoid process. When the client indicates that he or she no longer hears the sound, quickly bring the tuning fork in front of the pinna without touching the client, and ask whether he or she still hears the sound (Figure 51-9). Record the duration of both phases, bone conduction followed by air conduction, and compare the times. The client normally continues to hear the sound two times longer in front of the pinna after not hearing it with the tuning fork touching the mastoid process.

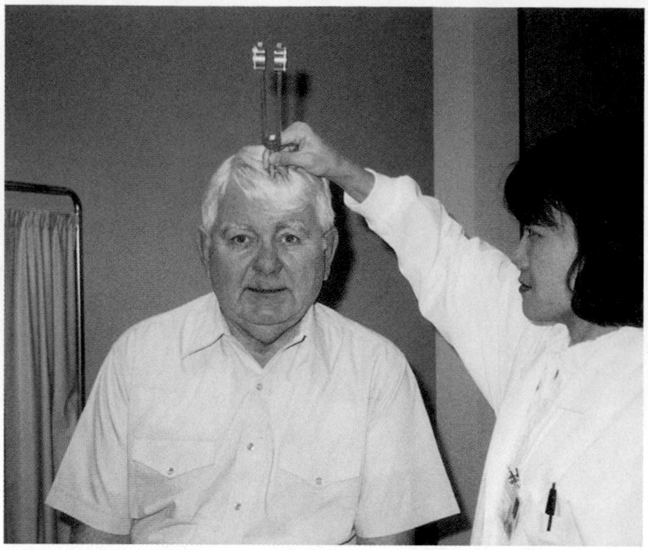

Figure 51-8 ■ Correct placement of the tuning fork for the Weber test.

Psychosocial Assessment

The client may become irritable, frustrated, and depressed by an inability to hear and respond appropriately. The inability to hear often isolates the client from the world. Depression may result from the sensory isolation of hearing loss. You must be sensitive to the client and conduct the interview at a pace appropriate for that person.

Ask about social and work relationships to determine whether the client is isolated because of hearing problems. In addition, encourage the client to express feelings related to hearing loss and discuss changes in daily living activities for coping. Also obtain information from family members, especially if the client does not acknowledge having a hearing problem. Throughout the assessment, remain patient and empathetic.

Diagnostic Assessment

LABORATORY TESTS

Laboratory tests generally are not of value in determining hearing acuity. For an external ear infection, microbial culture and antibiotic sensitivity tests can determine the causative organism and the most appropriate antibiotic.

RADIOGRAPHIC EXAMINATIONS

Computed Tomography

Computed tomography (CT), with or without contrast enhancement, reveals the structures of the ear in great detail by multiple x-ray scans of the head. These scans are then av-

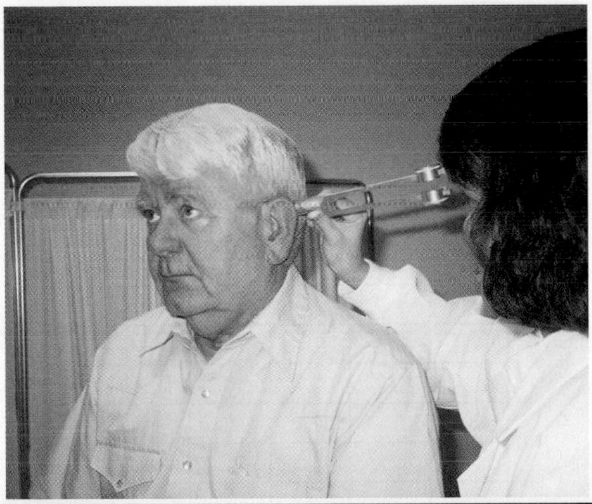

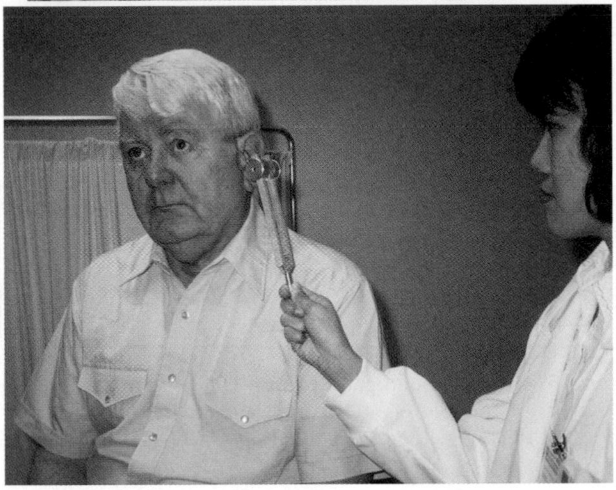

Figure 51-9 ■ Correct placement of the tuning fork for the Rinne test.

eraged by a computer. CT is especially helpful in diagnosing acoustic tumors.

OTHER DIAGNOSTIC ASSESSMENTS

Magnetic Resonance Imaging

Magnetic resonance imaging (MRI) is a noninvasive, nonradioactive diagnostic tool that uses a computer to generate images. Because of its superior contrast resolution, no bony artifacts can obscure tissue. Therefore MRI has great sensitivity to soft-tissue changes. Clients with internal metal vascular clips cannot have MRI.

Auditory Brainstem-Evoked Response

Auditory brainstem-evoked response (ABR) assesses hearing in clients who are unable to indicate or unreliable in indicating their recognition of sound stimuli during hearing testing. This test helps to diagnose both conductive and sensorineural hearing losses. Electrodes are placed on the scalp during the test. After the test, the client's hair should be cleansed to remove the electrode gel.

To prepare the client for ABR testing, you must do the following:

- Tell the client that no fasting or sedation is needed
- Carefully explain the procedure and its purpose
- Inform the client that the procedure usually takes about 30 minutes

Elcctronystagmography

Electronystagmography (ENG) is a cost-effective test that is sensitive in detecting both central and peripheral disease of the vestibular system in the ear. The ENG detects **nystagmus** (involuntary eye movements) that can be recorded. (The eyes and ears depend on each other for good balance.) Electrodes are taped to the skin near the eyes, and one or more procedures (caloric testing, changing gaze position, or changing head position) are performed to stimulate nystagmus. Failure of nystagmus to occur with cerebral stimulation suggests an abnormality in the vestibulocochlear apparatus, the cerebral cortex, the auditory nerve, or the brainstem. To prepare the client for ENG, you must do the following:

- Carefully explain the procedure and its purpose. The examiners will be asking the client to name names or do simple math problems during the test to ensure the client stays alert.
- Tell the client to fast for several hours before the test and to avoid caffeine-containing beverages for 24 to 48 hours before the test.
- Tell clients with pacemakers that they should not have the test.
- Carefully introduce fluids after the test to prevent nausea and vomiting.

Caloric Testing

Caloric testing is performed to evaluate the vestibular (inner-ear) portion of the auditory nerve. Water warmer or cooler than body temperature is infused into the ear. A normal response is the onset of **vertigo** (spinning sensation) and nystagmus (involuntary eye movements) within 20 to 30 seconds. To prepare the client for caloric testing, you must do the following:

Carefully explain the procedure and its purpose.

- Tell the client to fast for several hours before the test.
- Tell the client that the affected side will be tested first.
- Explain that the client will be maintained on bedrest after the procedure with careful introduction of fluids to prevent nausea and vomiting.

Dix-Hallpike Test for Vertigo

The Dix-Hallpike test for vertigo is performed by assisting the client to a sitting position on an examination table. Stand to the side of the client, and quickly reposition him or her from sitting to supine with the head extending beyond the end of the table. This change of position is done first to one side and then to the other side. A client with benign positional vertigo will have a burst of nystagmus after a delay of 5 to 10 seconds.

To prepare the client for the Dix-Hallpike test, you must do the following:

- Carefully explain the procedure and its purpose.
- Tell the client that he or she should keep the eyes open and try not to blink.
- Explain that double vision may occur during the test.

Audiometry

Audiometry is the measurement of hearing acuity. **Frequency** is the highness or lowness of tones (expressed in

TABLE 51-3 Decibel Intensity and Safe Exposure Time for Common Sounds

Sound	Decibel Intensity (dB)	Safe Exposure Time*
Threshold of hearing	0	
Whispering	20	
Average residence or office	40	
Conversational speech	60	
Car traffic	70	>8 hr
Motorcycle	90	8 hr
Chain saw	100	2 hr
Rock concert, front row	120	3 min
Jet engine	140	Immediate danger
Rocket launching pad	180	Immediate danger

*For every 5-dB increase in intensity, the safe exposure time is cut in half.

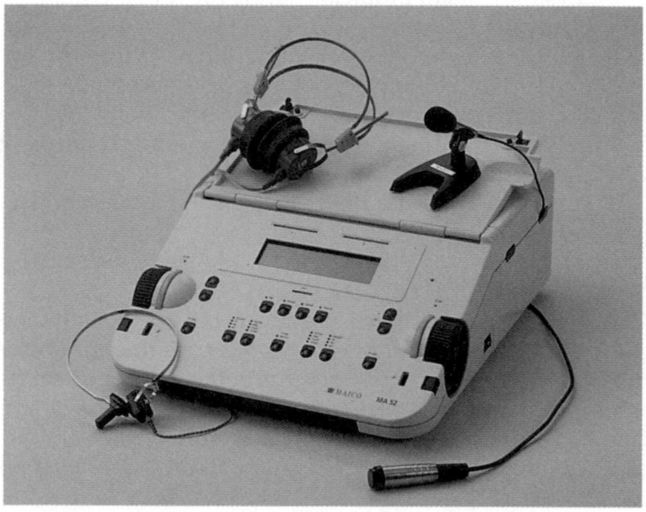

Figure 51-10 ■ A pure-tone audiometer. (Courtesy of Maico, Inc., Minneapolis, MN.)

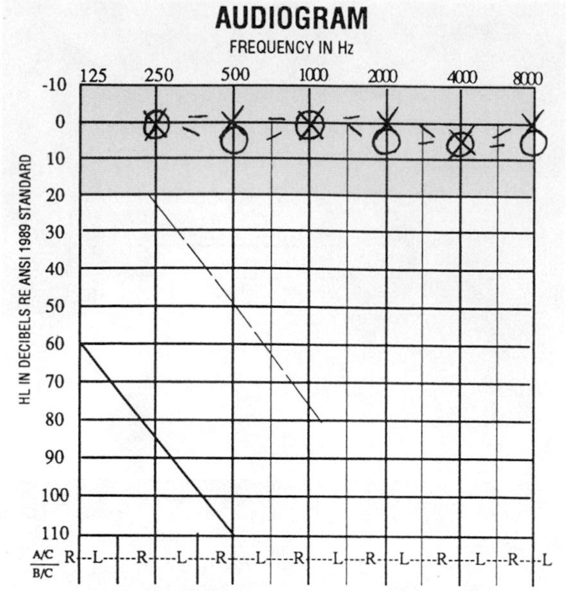

Audiogram Key	Left	Right		Left	Right
AC Unmasked	x	o	AC Masked	□	Δ
BC Unmasked	>	<	BC Masked	]	[
No Response	↘	↙	SF		S

Figure 51-11 ■ Audiogram pattern depicting normal hearing. (Courtesy of the Cleveland Hearing and Speech Center, Cleveland, OH.)

hertz). The greater the number of vibrations per second, the higher the frequency (pitch) of the sound; the fewer the number of vibrations per second, the lower the pitch.

Intensity of sound is expressed in decibels. The lowest intensity at which a young, normal ear can detect sound (about 51% of the time) is 0 dB. Sound at 110 dB is so intense (loud) that it is painful for most people with normal hearing. Conversational speech is around 60 dB, and a soft whisper is around 20 dB (Table 51-3). A hearing loss of 45 to 51 dB renders the person unable to hear speech without a hearing aid. A person with a hearing loss of 90 dB may not be able to hear speech even with a hearing aid.

Threshold is the lowest level of intensity at which pure tones and speech are heard by a client (about 50% of the time).

Pure tones are generated by an **audiometer** (Figure 51-10) to determine hearing acuity. The two types of audiometry are pure-tone audiometry and speech audiometry.

Pure-Tone Audiometry

Tones generated by an audiometer are presented to the client at frequencies for hearing speech, music, and other common sounds. Pure-tone audiometry is performed by air-conduction testing or bone-conduction testing. The results of pure-tone audiometry are plotted on an **audiogram** (Figure 51-11). For some clients, the hearing of one ear is "masked" while the hearing of the other ear is tested.

AIR-CONDUCTION TEST

Pure-tone air-conduction testing determines whether a client hears normally or has a hearing loss. It is designed to test air-conduction hearing sensitivity (through earphones) at frequencies of 125, 251, 510, 751, 1000, 1510, 2000, 3000, 4000, 6000, and 8000 Hz, but thresholds are usually confined to the frequencies of 251, 510, 1000, 2000, 4000, and 8000 Hz. The intensities for the pure tones generally range from 10 to 110 dB.

CLIENT PREPARATION. Place the client in a sound-isolated room in which background noise does not exceed American National Standards Institute noise standards. Sit facing the client because his or her facial expressions are often helpful in evaluating responses. Hearing-impaired clients may benefit from lip-reading your instructions. Instruct the client as follows:

"I am going to test your hearing. The object of the test is to find the point at which you can just barely hear the tones. The tones will sound like soft bells or tuning forks. Every time you hear one, no matter how soft, signal by raising your hand (or pushing the button) on the side you hear the tone." (If the client cannot raise a hand or push a button because of physical or motor disabilities, a yes-no verbal response can be used.)

"When you no longer hear the tone, lower your hand (or release the button). This lets me know when you hear the tone and when it goes away."

PROCEDURE. Test the ear with the better hearing first. Before beginning the test, adjust the audiometric equipment by doing the following:

1. Setting the frequency control at 1000 Hz and the hearing level control at 40 dB.
2. Putting on the earphones and listening to the tone while switching from one ear to the other.
3. In each earphone, listening to the tone while gradually turning the hearing level control toward 0 dB.
4. Testing the signal cord and light to make sure they are working.

Best practices for conduction audiometry to obtain a profile of the client's hearing for pure tones from low to high frequencies are listed in Chart 51-3. No special follow-up care is needed.

BONE-CONDUCTION TEST

Pure-tone bone-conduction testing determines whether the hearing loss detected by air-conduction testing is due to conductive or sensorineural factors or to a combination of the two. It is used only when the results of air-conduction testing are abnormal. There are restrictions on both the frequency and the intensity of the sound produced by the device. The frequencies are usually restricted to those between 251 and 4000 Hz. Because a bone-conduction oscillator requires great power to vibrate the skull, maximal outputs for bone conduction are also lower.

CLIENT PREPARATION. Explain that hearing sensitivity for bone conduction is going to be checked. The sounds and how the client should respond are the same as those for the air-conduction test.

PROCEDURE. The ear with greater acuity is tested first. If neither ear is "better," it makes no difference which is tested first.

The bone-conduction vibrator is placed behind the pinna, firmly on the mastoid process. Then follow steps 4 through 9 of Chart 51-3. Remember that restrictions are placed on both the intensity and the frequency used in bone-conduction testing. Restrictions are usually described on the face of the audiometer. No special follow-up care is needed.

INTERPRETATION OF RESULTS

Audiometric evaluation determines whether the client's hearing is within normal limits or, with a hearing impairment, whether the hearing loss is conductive, sensorineural, or mixed. The type of loss can be determined by the shape of the audiogram after completion of pure-tone air- and bone-conduction audiometry.

For an experienced clinician, the audiometer is a useful tool for evaluating the extent and type of hearing loss. For interpreting the results of a hearing test, the expertise of the person who performed the test and the reliability of the client's responses must be considered. In reality the audiogram is the diagnostician's best estimate of hearing, based on observations of the client's hearing behavior in the testing situation.

Figure 51-11 is an audiogram showing normal results of air- and bone-conduction tests. Hearing is considered normal when the pure-tone thresholds are at 10 dB or better. The line at 0 dB on the audiogram represents the hearing thresholds of a young person with normal hearing. Figure 51-12 shows audiogram graphs of various types of hearing loss.

CHART 51-3

BEST PRACTICE for
Pure-Tone Air-Conduction Audiometry

1. After explaining the procedure to the client, place the earphones on the client. Make sure that the side marked *left* is on the left ear and the side marked *right* is on the right ear. The earphones must cover the ears.
2. If the client reports a hearing difference between the two ears, test the ear with better hearing first.
3. Begin the testing at 1000 Hz. This frequency is near the middle of the ear's sensitivity spectrum, and it has been demonstrated to have good test-retest reliability.
4. Adjust the audiometer so that the tone is inaudible unless the interrupter switch is depressed. Start with the hearing level control at its lowest setting, either 0 or −10 dB. Depress the interrupter switch, and gradually increase the intensity of the tone until the client signals that the tone is heard. Increase the intensity of the tone beyond this point by about 20 dB to give the client an opportunity to hear it well.
5. Now reduce the intensity of the tone in 5-dB steps until the client indicates that the tone is no longer heard. Note the last intensity level, in 5-dB decrement steps, at which the client signaled. The last point at which the client indicated that the tone was still heard should be his or her threshold for hearing for that frequency. The threshold can be tested for reliability by increasing the tone by 20 dB once again and then descending in 5-dB steps until once again the lowest point in intensity is reached.
6. If you have succeeded in obtaining a consistent threshold at 1000 Hz, change the frequency control to 500 Hz and start again. The preferred method is to test the lower frequencies first (500 and 250 Hz) and then move higher, usually to 2000, 4000, and 8000 Hz. At each frequency, the procedure is the same as for 1000 Hz.
7. After you have completed the threshold measurements on the first ear, switch the output selector to the opposite earphone. Proceed in the same manner to obtain thresholds for the other ear, also beginning at 1000 Hz.
8. If the thresholds of the second ear seem to differ by 40 dB or more from those of the first ear, masking of the better-hearing ear is indicated to rule out its participation in the test.
9. In operating the interrupter switch, make sure that you do not fall into rhythmic patterns that the client can follow. The pattern of tonal presentations should be irregular so that the client cannot predict when the tone will be presented.

Speech Audiometry

In speech audiometry, the client's ability to hear spoken words is measured through a microphone connected to an audiometer. The two components of speech audiometry are the speech reception threshold and speech discrimination.

SPEECH RECEPTION THRESHOLD

The **speech reception threshold** is the minimum loudness at which a client can repeat simple words. In testing this threshold, try to determine how intense (or loud) a simple speech stimulus must be before the client can hear it well enough to repeat it correctly. In one common test, lists of two-syllable words called **spondee** are used (i.e., words in which there is generally equal stress on each syllable, such as *airplane, railroad,* and *cowboy*).

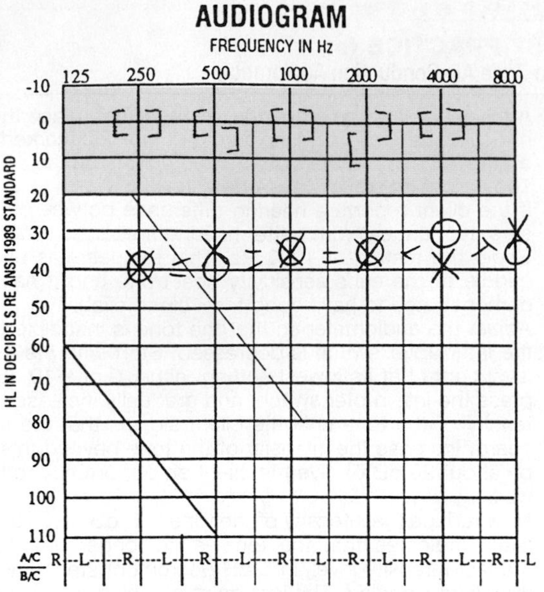

Pattern Depicting Conductive Hearing Loss

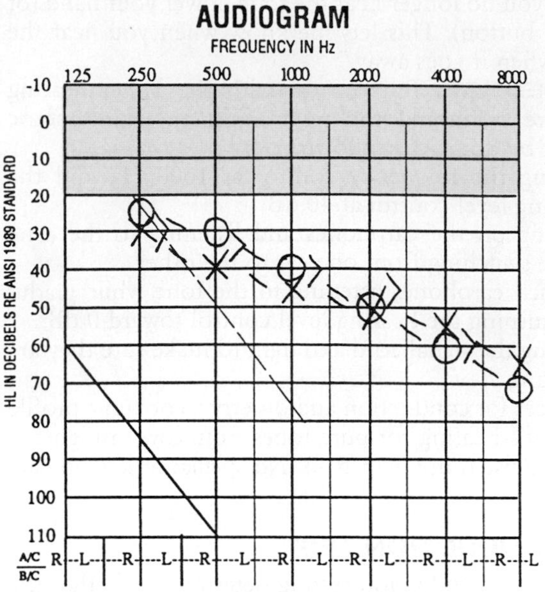

Pattern Depicting Sensorineural Hearing Loss

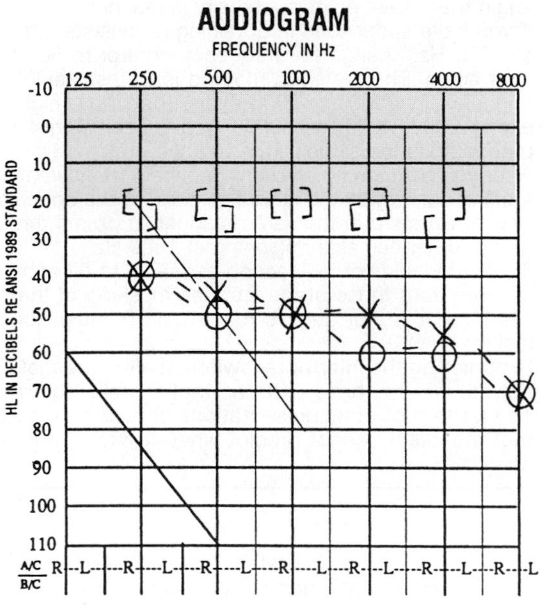

Pattern Depicting Conductive and Sensorineural Hearing Loss

Audiogram Key	Left	Right		Left	Right
AC Unmasked	x	o	AC Masked	□	Δ
BC Unmasked	>	<	BC Masked	]	[
No Response	↘	↙	SF		S

Figure 51-12 ■ Audiogram patterns depicting various types of hearing loss. (Courtesy of the Cleveland Hearing and Speech Center, Cleveland, OH.)

The speech reception threshold measured by the audiometer is the hearing level at which the client can repeat simple words correctly 50% of the time. The test is conducted in a manner similar to the pure-tone tests, but the microphone is activated through the audiometer. The intensity dial on the audiometer regulates word level intensity.

SPEECH DISCRIMINATION

Speech discrimination testing determines the client's ability to discriminate among similar sounds or among words that contain similar sounds. The ability to understand speech is the most important measurable aspect of human hearing. Speech discrimination testing assesses understanding of speech. A hearing loss may decrease sensitivity to sound and impair understanding of what is being said.

A standard format contains lists of 25 to 50 **monosyllabic** (one-syllable) words, such as *carve, day, toe,* and *ran,* phonemically balanced (designed to include the phonemes of American English in the proper proportion) and with equal word difficulty between lists. The lists are presented to the client through earphones at a selected loudness level, generally about 30 to 40 dB above the speech reception threshold, or at the client's most comfortable listening level. A percentage score is derived from the number of words repeated correctly.

Tympanometry

Tympanometry assesses mobility of the eardrum and structures of the middle ear by systematically varying air pressure in the external auditory canal. The progression or resolution of serous otitis and otitis media can be accurately monitored with this procedure.

Tympanometry is helpful in distinguishing middle-ear pathologic conditions, such as otosclerosis, ossicular disarticulation, otitis media, and perforation of the eardrum. It is also useful for assessing patency of the eustachian tube and for check recovery of middle-ear function after surgery.

Critical Thinking Challenge

Your client is a 24-year-old man who arrives at the clinic on his motorcycle from his construction job. He is wearing a headset with a compact disc (CD) player hooked to his belt. You are to perform a hearing assessment on him.

1. What should you tell him regarding the preparation and actual audiometry procedures?
2. What recommendations would you make to him regarding the protection of his hearing in the future?

evolve For suggested answer guidelines, go to http://evolve.elsevier.com/Iggy/.

GET READY for the NCLEX Examination!

KEY POINTS

Safe Effective Care Environment

- Use a separate speculum cover for each ear when conducting an otoscopic examination.
- Slowly and gently introduce the otoscopic speculum into the external ear canal during assessment.
- Use contact precautions with any client who has drainage from the ear canal.
- Do not perform an otoscopic examination on a confused or uncooperative client.
- Use the suggestions presented under the History section to enhance communication with a client who has a hearing impairment.

Health Promotion and Maintenance

- Teach clients the proper way to clean the pinna and external ear canal.
- Identify clients at risk for hearing impairment as a result of work environment or leisure activities.
- Encourage all clients, even if they already have a hearing impairment, to use ear protection in loud environment.
- Inform all clients who smoke that smoking increases the risk for development of hearing problems.
- Assist clients interested in smoking cessation to find an appropriate smoking cessation program.

Psychosocial Integrity

- Pace your interview to match the learning needs and style of the individual client.
- Allow the client the opportunity to express fear or anxiety regarding a change in hearing status.
- Refer clients newly diagnosed with hearing impairment to local resources and support groups.
- Explain all diagnostic procedures, restrictions, and follow-up care to the client scheduled for tests.

Physiological Integrity

- Ask the client about hearing problems in any other members of the family because many hearing problems have a genetic component, such as osteogenesis imperfecta, retinitis pigmentosa, Usher's syndrome, Waardenburg's syndrome, Alport's syndrome, and Treacher Collins syndrome.
- Ask the client whether any ototoxic drugs have ever been used (Table 51-2).

ADDITIONAL STUDY RESOURCES

Go to your Student CD-ROM for Review Questions for the NCLEX Examination.

evolve Go to http://evolve.elsevier.com/Iggy/ for Integrated Management of Care Questions for the NCLEX Examination.

SELECTED BIBLIOGRAPHY

Asterisk indicates a classic or definitive work on this subject.

Baker, C. (2002). Caring for patients with hearing impairments. *Dermatology Nursing, 14*(1), 49, 52.

*Benjamin, B., et al. (1994). *A color atlas of otorhinolarynogology.* Philadelphia: Lippincott-Raven.

Bess, F.H., & Humes, L.E. (2003). *Audiology: The fundamentals* (3rd ed.). Baltimore: Williams & Wilkins.

Borg-Stein, J., Rauch, S., & Krabak, B. (2001). Evaluation and management of cervicogenic dizziness. *Critical Reviews in Physical and Rehabilitation Medicine, 13*(4), 255-264.

Boys Town National Research Hospital. Retrieved April 2003 from http://www.boystownhospital.org/services/AudioVest/basic.asp#Basic.

Dean, W.A., & Davidson, M. (2002). Hearing loss in adults: Physical limitation, psychosocial barrier. *Clinician Reviews, 12*(6), 62-67.

Demers, K. (2002). Try this: Hearing screening. *Home Health Care Nurse, 20*(2), 132-133.

Diagnostic tests (February 22, 2003). Retrieved April 2003 from http://www.vestibular.org/tests.html.

Dowden, C. (2002). What is the best treatment for impacted cerumen? *The Journal of Family Practice, 51*(2), 117-119.

Ebersole, P., Hess, P., & Luggen, A. (2004). *Toward healthy aging: Human needs and nursing response* (6th ed.). St. Louis: Mosby.

Fields, R. Borderlands: An El Paso Community College local history project: Food, spices double as folk cures. Retrieved June 2003 from http://www.epcc.edu/ftp/Homes/monicaw/borderlands/09_food.htm.

Finesilver, C. (2002). A new age for childhood diseases: Down syndrome. *RN, 64*(11), 43-49.

Gates, G., et al. (2003). Screening for handicapping hearing loss in the elderly. *The Journal of Family Practice, 52*(1), 56-62.

Gill-Body, K. (2001). Current concepts in the management of patients with vestibular dysfunction. *PT: Magazine of Physical Therapy, 9*(12), 40-58.

Gordon, M. (2002). *Manual of nursing diagnosis* (10th ed.). St. Louis: Mosby.

Hain, T. Ototoxic mezdication. Retrieved April 2003 from http://www.tchain.com/otoneurology/disorders/bilat/ototoxins.html.

Jarvis, C. (2004). *Physical examination and health assessment* (4th ed.). Philadelphia: W.B. Saunders.

Kuurila, K., et al. (2002). Hearing loss in Finnish adults with osteogenesis inperfecti: A nationwide study. *Annals of Otology, Rhinology & Laryngology, 111*(10), 939-946.

Lefebvre, P., & Van De Water, T. (2000). Connexins, hearing and deafness: Clinical aspects of mutations in the connexin 26 gene. *Brain Research Reviews, 32*, 159-162.

Lucas, L., & Matthews-Flint, L. (2001). Sound advice about hearing aids. *Nursing 2001, 31*(2), 59-61.

Lucas, L., & Matthews-Flint, L. (2003). Heed the word about hearing impairment. *Nursing 2003, 33*(10), 32hn1-32hn3.

*Lusk, S.L. (1997). Noise exposures: Effects of hearing and prevention of noise induced hearing loss. *AAORN Journal, 45*(8), 397-405, 409-410.

Martin, F.N. (2000). *Introduction to audiology* (7th ed.). Boston: Allyn & Bacon.

McCance, K., & Huether, S. (2002). *Pathophysiology: The biologic basis for disease in adults and children* (4th ed.). St. Louis: Mosby.

McConnell, E. (2002). How to converse with a hearing-impaired patient. *Nursing 2002, 32*(8), 20.

National Council on Aging. (2000). The consequences of untreated hearing loss in older persons. *ORL-Head and Neck Nursing, 18*(1), 12-16.

Nussbaum, R., McInnes, R., & Willard, H. (2001). *Thompson & Thompson: Genetics in medicine* (6th ed.). Philadelphia: W.B. Saunders.

Pagana, K., & Pagana, T. (2002). *Mosby's manual of diagnostic and laboratory tests* (2nd ed.). St. Louis: Mosby.

Phillips, M. (2003). Genetics of hearing loss. *MEDSURG Nursing, 12*(6), 386-390, 411.

Sheehan, J. (2000). Caring for the deaf: Do you do enough? *RN, 63*(3), 69-72.

Sommer, S., & Sommer, N. (2002). When your patient is hearing impaired. *RN, 65*(12), 28-32.

*Ventry, I., & Selsnick, S. (1983). Identification of elderly people with hearing problems. *American Speech-Language Hearing Association, July*, 37-42.

Zadeh, M., & Selesnick, S. (2001). Evaluation of hearing impairment. *Comprehensive Therapy, 27*(4), 302-310.

CHAPTER 52

Interventions for Clients with Ear and Hearing Problems

JANICE HOOT MARTIN

LEARNING OUTCOMES

After studying this chapter, you should be able to:

1. Compare the clinical manifestations and interventions for external otitis with those of otitis media.
1. Describe how to correctly instill medications into the ear.
3. Describe the mechanisms of action, side effects, and nursing interventions of drug therapy for ear infections.
4. Explain the procedures to safely remove impacted cerumen from the ear canal of an older client.
5. Prioritize educational needs for the client with Ménière's disease.
6. Describe the mechanisms of action, side effects, and nursing implications of drug therapy for Ménière's disease.
7. Compare the causes and interventions for conductive hearing loss with those for sensorineural hearing loss.
8. Prioritize nursing care needs for the client after tympanoplasty.
9. Prioritize educational needs for the client after stapedectomy.
10. Identify an appropriate method for communicating with a client who has recently become hearing impaired.
11. Develop a community-based teaching plan for a client who is learning to use a hearing aid.

Go to your Student CD-ROM for Review Questions for the NCLEX Examination keyed to these Learning Outcomes.

The ears play an important role in daily functioning. Ear disorders can cause many problems ranging from hearing difficulty to problems of balance and functional ability. Hearing problems can lead to confusion, mistrust, social isolation, and the inability to give and receive accurate information. Disorders of the ear and of hearing are often easily treated with proper diagnosis; however, early recognition and intervention are necessary to prevent additional damage and to promote a maximal level of wellness.

CONDITIONS AFFECTING THE EXTERNAL EAR

The external ear is the outermost part of the ear structures and is subject to outside factors that can cause problems. Disorders of the external ear include congenital malformation (birth defects), trauma, and infectious or noninfectious lesions of the pinna, auricle, or auditory canal. Ear structures (external, middle, and inner ear) develop at different times during fetal life; thus the presence of birth defects in one area does not necessarily mean that other areas also will be affected. Abnormalities of the external ear range from crumpling or falling forward of the pinna to complete absence **(atresia)** of the auditory canal. In addition, trauma can damage or destroy the auricle and external canal. Surgical reconstruction can re-form the pinna with skin grafts and plastic prostheses. Trauma to the auricle resulting in a hematoma requires the removal of blood via needle aspiration to prevent calcification and hardening, which is often referred to as a **cauliflower** or **boxer's ear.**

Benign cysts or polyps of the auricle or external canal are surgically removed if they block the canal and affect hearing. Cancer cells, most often basal cell carcinoma, can also be found on the pinna. In general, treatment consists of simple excision. As the lesion becomes larger, its location near the skull and facial nerve makes treatment more difficult.

TABLE 52-1 Comparison of Features Between External Otitis and Otitis Media

Etiology	Clinical Manifestations	Treatment
External Otitis		
Allergic reactions Bacterial or fungal infection Swimming Local trauma	Pain Itching Hearing loss Plugged feeling in ear Redness and edema	Topical antibiotics Corticosteroids Oral analgesics Local heat
Otitis Media		
Bacterial or viral infection Fluid accumulation	Exudate Pain Pressure in ear Hearing loss Tinnitus Fever Malaise Nausea or vomiting Bulging tympanic membrane Fluid behind tympanic membrane	Systemic antibiotics Analgesics Local heat Antipyretics Antihistamines Decongestants Myringotomy

External Otitis

PATHOPHYSIOLOGY

External otitis is a painful condition caused when irritating or infective agents come into contact with the skin of the external ear. The result to the external ear canal or the auricle is either an allergic response or inflammation with or without infection. Affected skin becomes red, swollen, and tender to touch or movement. Swelling of the ear canal can lead to hearing loss due to canal obstruction. Allergic external otitis is commonly caused by contact with cosmetics, hair sprays, earphones, earrings, or hearing aids. The most common infectious organisms, usually bacterial or fungal, are *Pseudomonas aeruginosa, Streptococcus, Staphylococcus,* and *Aspergillus.* Table 52-1 compares external otitis and otitis media.

External otitis occurs more often in hot, humid environments, especially in the summer, and is commonly referred to as **swimmer's ear** because of the high incidence in people involved in water sports. In addition, clients who have traumatized their external ear canal with sharp or small objects (such as hairpins or cotton-tipped applicators) or through headphones are more susceptible to external otitis.

Necrotizing or *malignant otitis* is the most virulent form of external otitis. Organisms spread beyond the external ear canal into the ear and skull. The high mortality rate seen with malignant external otitis results from complications such as meningitis, brain abscess, and destruction of cranial nerve VII.

COLLABORATIVE MANAGEMENT

Assessment

Manifestations of external otitis include many problems, ranging from mild itching to pain with movement of the pinna or tragus. Clients have pain with movement of the pinna and tragus or when upward pressure is applied to the external canal. They report feeling as if the ear is plugged and hearing is reduced.

Use caution during otoscopic examination to avoid pressing on the walls of the external canal, which causes pain. Drainage from the ear is often greenish white. To prevent cross-contamination, dispose of the otoscope tip and wash your hands before examining the opposite ear. Hearing loss in the affected ear can be severe when inflammation obstructs the ear canal and prevents sounds from reaching the eardrum **(tympanic membrane).**

CHART 52-1

BEST PRACTICE for Instillation of Eardrops

1. Gather the solutions to be administered.
2. Check the labels to ensure correct dosage and time.
3. Remove and discard any ear packing.
4. Irrigate the ear if the eardrum is intact.
5. Place the bottle of eardrops (with the top on tightly) in a bowl of warm water for 5 minutes.
6. Tilt the client's head in the opposite direction of the affected ear and place the drops in the ear.
7. With the head tilted, gently move the head back and forth five times.
8. Insert a cotton ball into the opening of the ear canal to act as packing.

Interventions

Treatment focuses on reducing inflammation, edema, and pain. Heat is applied locally for 20 minutes three times a day, using towels warmed with water and then wrapped in a plastic bag, or heating pads placed on a low setting. Bedrest limits head movements, thereby reducing pain.

Topical antibiotic and steroid therapies are most effective in decreasing inflammation and pain. Review best practices for instilling eardrops with the client, as shown in Chart 52-1. Observe the client to make sure that he or she uses proper technique. If edema obstructs the external canal, an earwick is inserted past the blockage, with medicated drops applied to the outside end (Figure 52-1). A long piece of gauze dressing serves as an earwick, which the health care provider inserts using forceps to push carefully through the blocked external auditory canal to the eardrum. The earwick may be removed when medication can flow freely into the canal. Thorough handwashing is strictly enforced. Systemic oral or intravenous antibiotics are used in severe cases, especially when cellulitis is present or the auricular lymph nodes are enlarged.

Analgesics, including opioids, may be needed for pain relief during the initial days of therapy. Acetylsalicylic acid (aspirin, Entrophen✱), ibuprofen (Advil), or acetaminophen (Tylenol, Abenol✱) may relieve less severe pain.

After the inflammation has subsided, diluted alcohol may be dropped into the ear to keep it clean and dry and to prevent recurrence. Teach the client not to use cotton-tipped applicators to dry the ears, because this use could damage the canal and increase the risk for infection or inflammation. Recommend that clients with recurrent episodes of external otitis use ear plugs when engaging in water sports.

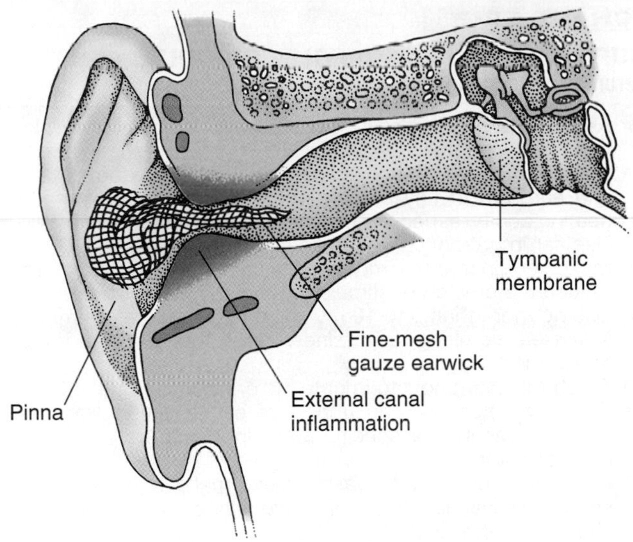

Figure 52-1 ■ Earwick for instillation of antibiotics into the external canal. When edema occludes the external auditory canal, it is difficult for antibiotic solutions to enter the canal adequately. An earwick is placed through the meatus. Solutions placed on the external portion of the earwick are absorbed through the canal.

Furuncle

PATHOPHYSIOLOGY

A **furuncle** is a localized external otitis caused by bacterial infection, usually *Staphylococcus,* of a hair follicle. Most furuncles occur on the outer half of the external canal.

COLLABORATIVE MANAGEMENT

The manifestations of a furuncle include intense local pain to light touch. The area is swollen and red, with tight skin covering the area, possibly with a purulent head. No drainage is seen unless the furuncle has ruptured. Hearing is impaired if the lesion blocks the canal.

Treatment consists of local and systemic antibiotics and local heat application. An earwick may be used with one-half strength Burow's solution to relieve pain. The furuncle may need to be incised and drained if it does not resolve with the use of antibiotics.

Cerumen or Foreign Bodies

PATHOPHYSIOLOGY

Many objects can enter or be placed in the external ear canal. **Cerumen** (wax) is the most common cause of an impacted canal. Vegetables, beads, pencil erasers, and insects are other common items that may also enter the ear, with or without the client's help. Although uncomfortable, cerumen or foreign bodies are rarely true emergencies, and can be carefully removed by a health care professional. Remember, cerumen impaction in the older adult is common and research has shown that removal of cerumen from residents of a long-term care facility not only improves hearing but also improves mental status (see the Evidence-Based Practice for Nursing box above).

EVIDENCE-BASED PRACTICE for Nursing

Effect of cerumen impaction on cognition in older adults

Moore, A., et al. (2002). Cerumen, hearing, and cognition in the elderly. Journal of the American Medical Directors Association, 3(3), 136-139.

The purpose of this study was to confirm the high incidence of cerumen impaction among older adult residents admitted to skilled nursing facilities and to evaluate the impact of hearing loss caused by cerumen impaction on cognition in these residents. The design was a prospective pretest-posttest design conducted in a 160-bed long-term care facility. Subjects included 29 newly admitted residents who were older than 65 years of age. All residents were tested using the Folstein Mini-Mental Status Exam (MMSE) [mental status measure] and electronic audiometry [hearing measure]. The residents were divided into two groups, those without 50% cerumen occlusion and those with 50% cerumen occlusion. The intervention included removal of cerumen in those residents with 50% or more occlusion. Residents were tested for mental status and hearing both before and after cerumen removal. Residents with less than 50% cerumen occlusion were used as a control.

As suspected, a large percentage of the residents (65.5%) had cerumen occlusions of more than 50%. A statistically significant hearing improvement was found for 80% of the residents who had cerumen removed. Additionally, mental status was significantly improved for residents after removal of cerumen.

Level of Evidence: 3—Well-designed trial without randomization; single pretest and post-test.

Critique. This was a well-designed study with reliable and valid measurement tools. Statistical significance was found even though there was small variability in the measurement score for the hearing (improvement, no change, loss of frequency). The sample size was ample although it may not be representative of other long-term care facilities. Further study is needed to determine whether the mental status changes again as cerumen impaction develops again or whether these findings are similar for clients hospitalized with acute illnesses.

Implications for Nursing. Nurses are responsible for assessing the mental status of clients and making judgments based on these findings. This study suggests that hearing loss has a direct effect on mental status and that the simple task of cerumen removal to improve hearing will also improve mental status in a significant number of clients. Nursing care aimed at improving sensory hearing that leads to improved mental status might also lead to improved client outcomes and adherence to health care needs.

COLLABORATIVE MANAGEMENT

Assessment

Clients have a sensation of fullness in the ear, with or without hearing loss, and may have ear pain, itching, or bleeding from the ear. The object may be visible with direct inspection.

Interventions

When the occluding material is cerumen, irrigate the canal with a mixture of water and hydrogen peroxide at body temperature (Figure 52-2), following best practices for proper irrigation (Chart 52-2). Wax removal by irrigation is a slow process and may take more than one sitting. When cerumen obstruction is the cause of hearing loss, its removal improves hearing. Between 50 and 70 mL of solution is the maximum amount that the client can tolerate at one sitting. *Do not irrigate an ear that has an eardrum perforation or otitis media.*

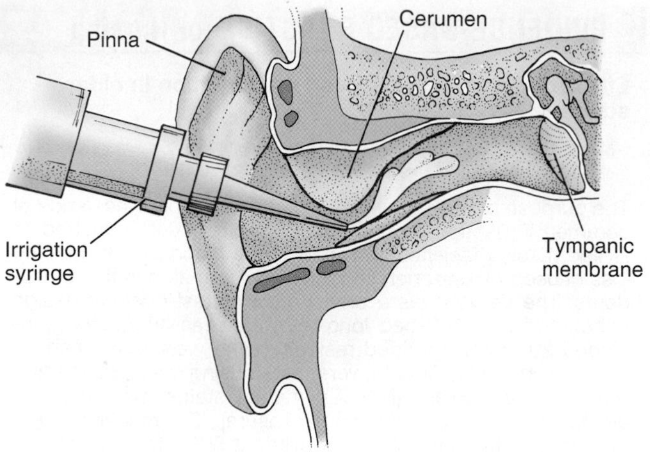

Figure 52-2 ■ Irrigation of the external canal. Cerumen and debris can be removed from the ear by irrigation with warm water. The stream of water is aimed above or below the impaction to allow back pressure to push it out rather than further down the canal.

CHART 52-2

BEST PRACTICE for Ear Irrigation

1. Gather the proper equipment: basin, syringe, otoscope, towel.
2. Warm tap water to body temperature.
3. Fill a syringe with warm water.
4. Place a towel around the client's neck.
5. Place a basin under the ear to be irrigated.
6. Use an otoscope to check the location of the impacted cerumen; ascertain that the eardrum is intact and that the client does not have otitis media.
7. Place the tip of the syringe at an angle so that the fluid pushes on one side and not directly on the impaction (this helps to loosen the impaction instead of forcing it further into the canal).
8. Watch the fluid return for signs of cerumen plug removal.
9. Continue to irrigate the ear with about 70 mL of fluid.
10. If the cerumen does not drain out, wait 10 minutes and repeat the irrigation procedure.
11. Monitor the client for signs of nausea.
12. If the client becomes nauseated, stop the procedure.
13. If the cerumen cannot be removed by irrigation, the client may place mineral oil into the ear three times a day for 2 days to soften dry, impacted cerumen, after which irrigation may be repeated.

If the cerumen is thick and dry or cannot be removed easily, the health care provider may prescribe a ceruminolytic product such as Cerumenex to soften the wax before trying to remove it. Another way to soften cerumen is to add 3 drops of glycerin or mineral oil to the ear at bedtime and 3 drops of hydrogen peroxide twice a day. After several days of this treatment, the cerumen is more easily removed by irrigation. In some cases, a small curette or cerumen spoon may be used to scoop out the wax. Only trained health care providers should use this method, because damage to the canal or the eardrum is likely with improper technique. Refer to Chart 52-3 for nursing care considerations of older adult clients with cerumen impaction.

Irrigation is *not* used when the foreign object is vegetable matter, because this material expands when wet, making the impaction worse. The object needs to be physically removed by an experienced health care provider.

CHART 52-3

NURSING FOCUS on the OLDER ADULT Cerumen Impaction

- Assess the hearing of all older clients using simple voice tests (see Chapter 51).
- Perform a gentle otoscopic inspection of the external canal and eardrum of any older client who has a problem with hearing acuity, especially the client who wears a hearing aid.
- Use ear irrigation to remove any impacted cerumen.
- Make certain that the irrigating fluid is about 98° F (37° C) to reduce the chance of stimulating the vestibular sense.
- Use no more than 5 to 10 mL of irrigating fluid at a time.
- If nausea, vomiting, or dizziness develops, stop the irrigation immediately.
- Teach the client how to irrigate his or her own ears.
- Obtain a return demonstration of ear irrigation from the client, observing for specific areas in which the client may need assistance.
- Encourage the client to wash the external ears daily using a soapy, wet washcloth over the index finger (best done in the shower or while washing the hair).

Insects are killed before removal unless they can be coaxed out by a flashlight or a humming noise. Mineral oil or diluted alcohol is instilled into the ear to suffocate the insect, which is then removed with ear forceps.

If the client has local irritation, an antibiotic or steroid ointment may be applied to prevent infection and reduce local irritation. Hearing acuity is tested if hearing loss is not resolved by removal of the object.

In rare cases, surgical removal of the foreign object is required. The object is removed through the transcanal route using a wire bent at a 90-degree angle. The wire is looped around the object, and the object is pulled out. Because this procedure is painful, general anesthesia is necessary.

CONDITIONS AFFECTING THE MIDDLE EAR

Otitis Media

PATHOPHYSIOLOGY

The three most common forms of otitis media are acute otitis media, chronic otitis media, and serous otitis media. Each type affects the middle ear but has slightly different causes, incidences, and pathologic changes. If otitis progresses or remains untreated, permanent conductive hearing loss may occur. Otitis media is less common in adults than in children.

Acute otitis media and chronic otitis media, also known as suppurant or purulent otitis media, are similar. An infecting agent introduced into the middle ear causes inflammation of the mucosa, leading to swelling and irritation of the ossicles within the middle ear. A purulent inflammatory exudate follows. Acute disease has a sudden onset and a duration of 3 weeks or less. Chronic otitis media often follows repeated acute episodes, has a longer duration, and causes greater middle-ear injury.

The eustachian tube and mastoid, connected to the middle ear by a sheet of cells, are also affected by the infection. If the eardrum membrane perforates and infective materials

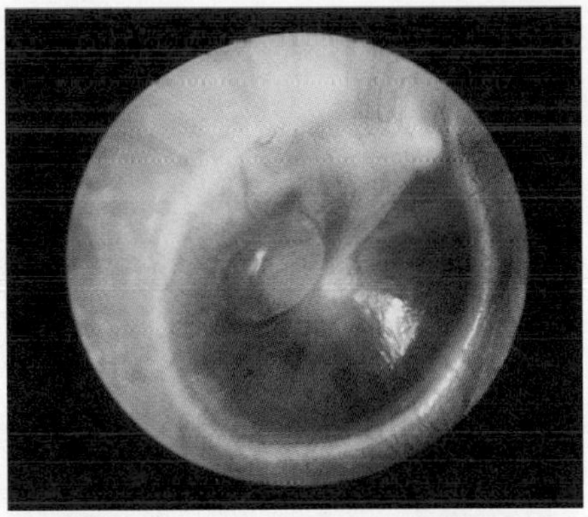

Figure 52-3 ■ Otoscopic view of otitis media.

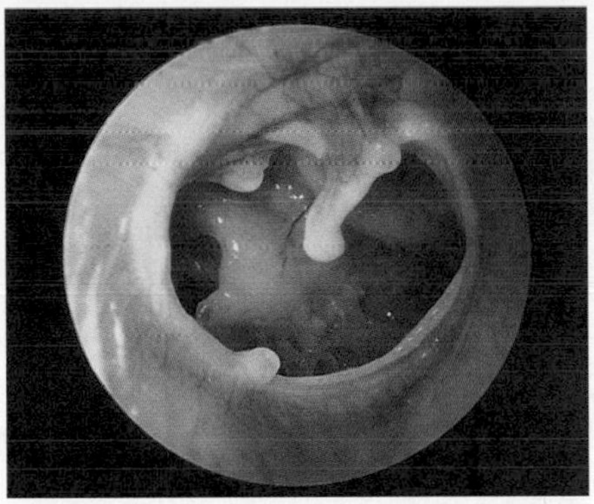

Figure 52-4 ■ Otoscopic view of a perforated tympanic membrane.

spill into the external ear, external otitis also develops, which thickens and scars the middle ear if left untreated. Necrosis of the ossicles destroys middle-ear structures.

COLLABORATIVE MANAGEMENT

Assessment

The chief complaint of the client with acute or chronic otitis media is ear pain with or without movement of the external ear. Pain with chronic otitis media is much less severe than that occurring with acute otitis media. As the pressure in the middle ear increases, there is a sensation of fullness in the ear. Hearing is reduced and distorted. The client may notice a sticking or cracking sound in the ear on yawning or swallowing or may have tinnitus in the form of a low hum or a low-pitched sound. Conductive hearing loss may occur as sound wave transmission is obstructed. Headaches are common, and systemic symptoms such as malaise, fever, nausea, and vomiting can occur. As the pressure on the middle ear pushes against the inner ear, the client may have dizziness or vertigo.

Otoscopic examination findings vary, depending on the stage of the disease. The eardrum is initially retracted, which allows landmarks of the ear to be seen clearly. At this early stage, the client has only vague ear discomfort. As the disease progresses, the eardrum's blood vessels dilate and appear red (Figure 52-3). In the third stage, the eardrum becomes red, thickened, and bulging, with loss of landmarks. Decreased eardrum mobility is evident on inspection with a pneumatic otoscope. Pus may be seen behind the membrane.

If the disease progresses, the eardrum spontaneously **perforates** (breaks open) and pus or blood drains from the ear (Figure 52-4). This discharge may be pulsating when viewed through the otoscope. When the membrane ruptures, the client notices a marked decrease in pain as the pressure on middle-ear structures is relieved (Figure 52-5). Tympanic perforations from any cause may heal if the underlying problem is controlled. The membrane covering initially appears thinner over the healed perforation. A simple central perforation does not interfere with hearing unless the ossicles of the middle ear are damaged or the perforation is large. However, repeated perforations with extensive scarring can cause hearing loss.

Cultures of drainage after a perforation from uncontrolled otitis media may reveal the infecting agent. Cultures are taken only when previous treatment has been ineffective. When the eardrum is not perforated, a needle aspiration or myringotomy draws fluid for culture.

Interventions

NONSURGICAL MANAGEMENT. Treatment can be as simple as putting the client in a quiet environment. Bedrest limits head movements that intensify the pain. Heat may be applied by using a heating pad adjusted to a low setting. Application of cold may occasionally relieve pain.

Systemic antibiotic therapy decreases pain by reducing inflammation. Topical antibiotics are not used to treat otitis media. Analgesics such as aspirin and acetaminophen (Tylenol, Abenol✱) or nonsteroidal anti-inflammatory drugs (NSAIDs) such as ibuprofen (Advil) relieve pain and reduce fever. When the client has severe pain, opioid analgesics such as codeine and meperidine hydrochloride (Demerol) also may be used.

Antihistamines and decongestants are prescribed to decrease mucus production and to decrease fluid in the middle ear. The body can then reabsorb the fluid, reducing pressure and pain.

SURGICAL MANAGEMENT. If the pain persists after antibiotic therapy and the eardrum continues to bulge, a **myringotomy** (surgical opening of the pars tensa of the eardrum) is performed. A myringotomy drains middle-ear fluids and immediately relieves pain.

Preoperative Care. Reassure the client that the myringotomy will relieve pain and is usually performed without anesthesia. Many people are concerned about a perforation and its effect on hearing. To relieve some of this anxiety, discuss the reasons for the procedure and encourage the client to use techniques such as deep breathing before and during the procedure. Systemic antibiotic therapy continues before and after this procedure. Clean the external canal with a bacteriostatic solution such as povidone-iodine (Betadine) before the myringotomy.

Operative Procedures. The small surgical incision is performed in an office or clinic setting and heals rapidly. Another approach is the removal of fluid from the middle ear with a needle. For relief of pressure caused by serous otitis media, a small **grommet** (polyethylene tube) may be surgically placed through the tympanic membrane to allow continuous drainage of middle-ear fluids (Figure 52-6).

Postoperative Care. Take care to keep the external ear and canal free of other substances while the incision is healing. Instruct the client to keep his or her head dry by not washing the hair or showering for several days. Other instructions after surgery are listed in Chart 52-4.

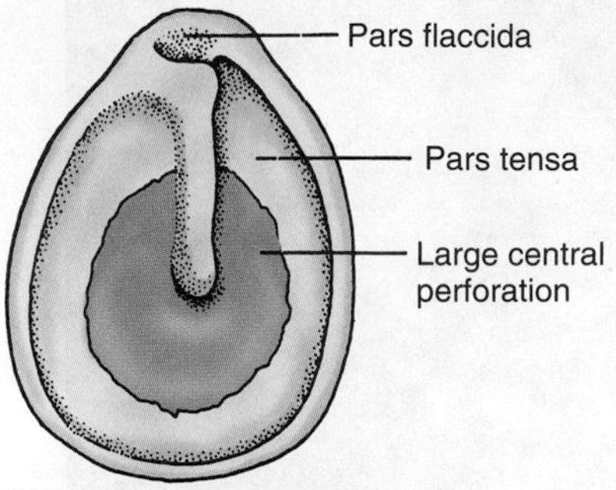

With a **large central perforation,** clients complain of significant hearing loss.

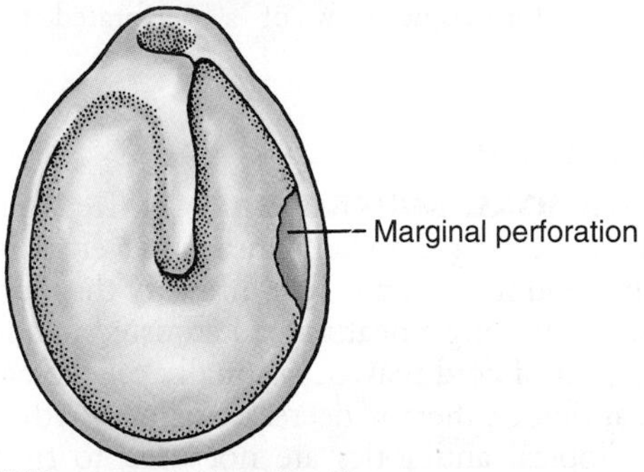

With a **marginal perforation,** clients might complain of significant hearing loss.

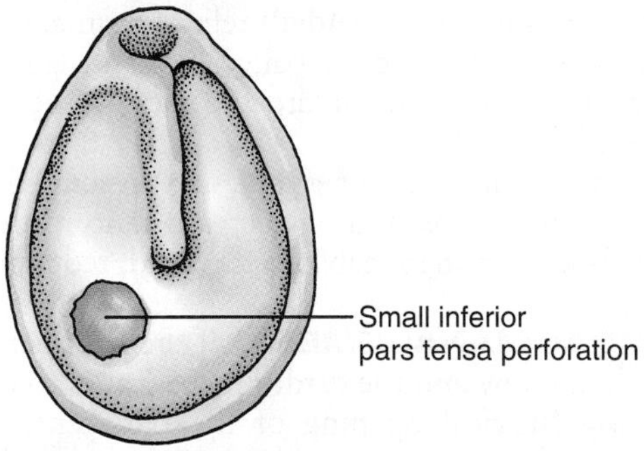

With a **small inferior pars tensa perforation,** clients do not complain of much interference with hearing.

Figure 52-5 ■ Perforations of the tympanic membrane. Central perforations heal more quickly than marginal perforations. Marginal perforations that do not heal allow cholesteatoma formation.

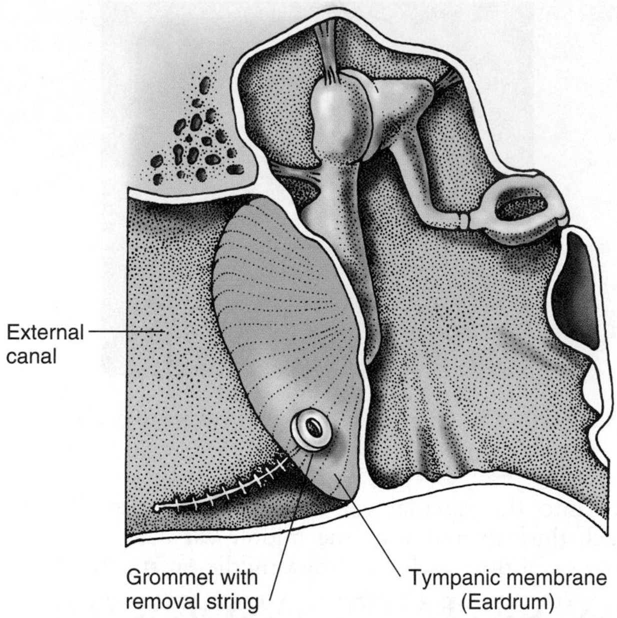

Figure 52-6 ■ Grommet through the tympanic membrane. A small grommet is placed through the tympanic membrane away from the margins, which allows prolonged drainage of fluids from the middle ear. The grommet can be removed later and the tympanic membrane allowed to heal naturally or patched with a small piece of homogenous tissue.

CHART 52-4

CLIENT EDUCATION GUIDE
Recovery from Ear Surgery

- Avoid straining when you have a bowel movement.
- Do not drink through a straw for 2 to 3 weeks.
- Avoid air travel for 2 to 3 weeks.
- Avoid excessive coughing for 2 to 3 weeks.
- Stay away from people with colds.
- If you need to blow your nose, blow gently, one side at a time, with your mouth open.
- Avoid getting your head wet, washing your hair, and showering for 1 week.
- Keep your ear dry for 6 weeks by placing a ball of cotton coated with petroleum jelly (such as Vaseline) in your ear. Change the cotton ball daily.
- Avoid rapidly moving the head, bouncing, and bending over for 3 weeks.
- Change your ear dressing every 24 hours as directed.
- Report excessive drainage immediately to your physician.

Mastoiditis

PATHOPHYSIOLOGY

The lining of the middle ear is continuous with the lining of the mastoid air cells, which are embedded in the temporal bone. **Mastoiditis** is an infection of the mastoid air cells caused by untreated or inadequately treated otitis media. This infection can be acute or chronic. Antibiotic therapy is aimed at treating the middle-ear infection before it progresses to mastoiditis.

COLLABORATIVE MANAGEMENT

Assessment

The manifestations of mastoiditis include swelling behind the ear and pain with minimal movement of the tragus, the pinna, or the head. Pain is not relieved by myringotomy. **Cellulitis** (infection spreading laterally through the tissues of the skin) develops on the skin or external scalp over the mastoid process. Otoscopic examination shows a red, dull, thick, immobile eardrum with or without perforation. Lymph nodes behind the ear are tender and enlarged. Clients may have low-grade fever, malaise, ear drainage, and anorexia.

Interventions

NONSURGICAL MANAGEMENT. Intravenous antibiotics are prescribed to prevent the spread of infection. These drugs have limited use in actual mastoiditis treatment because they do not easily penetrate the infected bony structure of the mastoid. Cultures of the ear drainage determine which antibiotics should be most effective.

SURGICAL MANAGEMENT. Surgical removal of the infected tissue is needed if the infection does not respond to antibiotic therapy within a few days. A simple or modified radical mastoidectomy with tympanoplasty is the most common treatment. All infected tissue must be removed so that the infection does not spread to other structures. A tympanoplasty is then performed to reconstruct the ossicles and the eardrum to restore hearing. Client preparation, the operative procedure, and follow-up care for tympanoplasty are discussed on pp. 1137 and 1138.

Complications occur when infective material is not removed completely or when other structures are contaminated. Such complications include damage to cranial nerves VI and VII, decreasing the client's ability to look laterally (cranial nerve VI) and causing a drooping of the mouth on the affected side (cranial nerve VII). Other complications include vertigo, meningitis, brain abscess, chronic purulent otitis media, and wound infection.

Trauma

PATHOPHYSIOLOGY

Trauma and damage may occur to the eardrum and ossicles by infection, by direct damage, or through rapid changes in the middle-ear cavity pressure. Foreign objects placed in the external canal exert pressure on the eardrum and cause perforation. If the objects continue through the canal, the bones of the stapes, incus, and malleus may be damaged. Blunt injury to the skull and ears can also damage middle-ear structures through fractures extending to the middle ear. Slapping of the external ear increases the pressure in the ear canal, tearing the eardrum when the pressure is great enough. The eardrum has a limited stretching ability and gives way under high pressure. Excessive nose blowing and rapid changes of pressure that occur with nonpressurized air flight **(barotrauma)** can cause an increase in pressure within the middle ear. High pressure damages the ossicles and can perforate the eardrum.

◆COLLABORATIVE MANAGEMENT

Most eardrum perforations heal within 1 or 2 weeks. Repeated perforations, especially from chronic otitis media, heal more slowly, with scarring. Depending on the amount of damage to the ossicles, hearing may or may not return. Hearing aids can improve hearing in this type of hearing loss. Surgical reconstruction of the ossicles and eardrum through a tympanoplasty or a myringoplasty may also improve hearing (see later discussion of nursing care under Tympanoplasty, pp. 1137 and 1138).

Preventive measures should be taken to avoid trauma. Instruct clients to avoid inserting objects into the external canal. Ear protectors should be used when blunt trauma is likely, especially in sports such as boxing.

Neoplasms

PATHOPHYSIOLOGY

Tumors of the middle ear are rare. The most common type of tumor is the *glomus jugulare*, a highly vascular benign lesion arising from the jugular vein. Malignant ear tumors include adenocarcinoma, adenoid cystic carcinoma, and mucoepidermoid carcinoma. The growth of any lesion within the middle-ear fossa disrupts conductive hearing, erodes the ossicles, and may spread to the inner ear and adjacent cranial nerves.

◆COLLABORATIVE MANAGEMENT

Clients have progressive hearing loss and tinnitus. Infection and pain rarely occur with *glomus jugulare* tumors. Otoscopic examination reveals bulging of the eardrum or a mass extending to the external ear canal. The many blood vessels of the *glomus jugulare* tumor give it a reddish color and a visible pulsation when seen through the eardrum.

Diagnosis is made by physical examination, tomography, and angiography. Tumors are removed by surgery, which often destroys hearing in the affected ear. If all of the edges of the tumor can be seen clearly through the eardrum, a transcanal approach is used to remove the lesion. When the tumor edges extend past the eardrum, more testing is needed to determine the extent of involvement. Radiation therapy is used to decrease the vascularity of the *glomus jugulare* tumor but is not the preferred method of treatment.

Benign lesions are removed because, with continued growth of the neoplasm, other structures can be affected, further damaging the facial or trigeminal nerve. When possible, reconstruction of the middle-ear structures is performed later to restore conductive hearing.

CONDITIONS AFFECTING THE INNER EAR

Tinnitus

PATHOPHYSIOLOGY

Tinnitus (continuous ringing or noise perception in the ear) is a common ear or hearing disorder. Diagnostic testing cannot confirm tinnitus. However, some tests are performed to assess for hearing loss and to rule out other ear problems. Tinnitus can have disturbing emotional consequences for the person afflicted with this disorder.

◆COLLABORATIVE MANAGEMENT

Symptoms of tinnitus range from mild ringing, which can go unnoticed during the day, to a loud roaring in the ear, which can interfere with thinking and attention span. When clients report tinnitus, you must be alert to the many factors that cause tinnitus: presbycusis, **otosclerosis** (irregular bone growth around ossicles), Ménière's disease, certain drugs, exposure to loud noise, and other inner-ear problems.

The exact pathophysiology and treatment of tinnitus vary with the underlying cause. When no cause can be found or the disorder is untreatable, therapy focuses on ways to mask the tinnitus with background sound, noisemakers, and music during sleeping hours. Ear mold hearing aids can amplify sounds to drown out the tinnitus during the day. The American Tinnitus Association assists clients in coping with tinnitus when other therapy is unsuccessful.

Vertigo and Dizziness

PATHOPHYSIOLOGY

Vertigo and dizziness are common manifestations of many ear disorders. Dizziness is a disturbed sense of a person's proper relationship to space. Clients vary greatly in defining dizziness. Vertigo is often used interchangeably with dizziness, but the definition, as well as the cause, is somewhat different. True **vertigo** is a real sense of whirling or turning in space.

The visual system, the vestibular system (cochlea, semicircular canals), and the proprioceptive system (muscles and nerve endings) combine to give input to the brain about balance. Problems in any of these areas leads to a disturbed sense of balance or motion. Factors affecting the ear that cause vertigo include Ménière's disease, labyrinthitis, acoustic neuromas, motion sickness, and drug or alcohol ingestion.

COLLABORATIVE MANAGEMENT

Manifestations of vertigo include nausea, vomiting, falling, nystagmus, hearing loss, and tinnitus. Until the cause of the vertigo can be treated, each manifestation is treated. Advise clients to:

- Restrict head motions and move more slowly.
- Maintain adequate hydration, especially after vomiting.
- Take drugs with antivertiginous effects, such as dimenhydrinate (Dramamine, Gravol✱), diazepam (Valium, Apo-Diazepam✱), and scopolamine (Transderm Scop, Transderm-V✱).

Many clients are dissatisfied with treatment because side effects of the drugs, especially drowsiness, can be worse than the vertigo. Caution clients to maintain a safe, uncluttered environment to prevent accidents during periods of vertigo and to use a cane or walker to maintain balance. Also instruct them not to drive or operate machinery when taking these drugs.

Labyrinthitis

PATHOPHYSIOLOGY

Labyrinthitis is an infection of the labyrinth, which may occur as a complication of acute or chronic otitis media. Infection results from an erosion of the bony capsule, allowing organisms to invade the inner ear. Labyrinthitis often results from the growth of a **cholesteatoma** (benign overgrowth of squamous cell epithelium) from the middle ear into the semicircular canal. Labyrinthitis may follow middle-ear or inner-ear surgery when infection is present. Labyrinthitis may be part of a systemic viral infection such as an upper respiratory infection or infectious mononucleosis.

COLLABORATIVE MANAGEMENT

Manifestations include hearing loss, tinnitus, spontaneous nystagmus to the affected side, and vertigo with nausea and vomiting. **Meningitis** (infection of the brain covering) is a common complication of labyrinthitis.

Treatment of labyrinthitis includes the use of systemic antibiotics such as ampicillin (Omnipen, Apo-Ampi✱). Advise clients to stay in bed in a darkened room until manifestations are reduced. Antiemetics, such as chlorpromazine hydrochloride (Thorazine, Novo-Chlorpromazine✱), and antivertiginous medications, such as dimenhydrinate (Dramamine, Gravol✱), relieve symptoms.

The client also needs psychosocial support. Hearing loss on the affected side may be permanent, although vertigo subsides as the inflammation resolves. Persistent balance problems may improve with gait training and physical therapy.

Ménière's Disease

PATHOPHYSIOLOGY

Ménière's disease has three features: tinnitus, one-sided sensorineural hearing loss, and vertigo, occurring in attacks that can last for several days. Clients are almost totally incapacitated during an attack, and several days are needed for full recovery. The pathology of Ménière's disease is either overproduction or decreased reabsorption of endolymphatic fluid, causing a distortion of the entire inner-canal system. This distortion decreases hearing from dilation of the cochlear duct, vertigo because of damage to the vestibular system, and tinnitus from unknown cause. The initial hearing loss is reversible, but repeated damage to the cochlea from increased fluid pressure, leads to permanent hearing loss.

The cause of Ménière's disease is unknown but it often occurs with infections, allergic reactions, and fluid imbalances. Long-term stress may have a role in Ménière's disease.

COLLABORATIVE MANAGEMENT

Assessment

Ménière's disease usually first occurs in people between the ages of 20 and 50 years. The prevalence is greater in men and in white individuals. Times of severe, debilitating attacks alternate with symptom-free periods. Clients often have certain manifestations before an attack of vertigo, such as headaches, increasing tinnitus, and a feeling of fullness in the affected ear. Manifestations are usually unilateral.

Clients describe the tinnitus as a continuous, low-pitched roar or a humming sound, which worsens just before and during a severe attack. Hearing loss is initially of the low-frequency tones but worsens to include all levels after repeated episodes. In the early stages of Ménière's disease, periods of remission are marked by normal or nearly normal hearing, but permanent hearing loss develops as the attacks increase.

Clients describe the vertigo as periods of whirling, which might even cause them to fall. The vertigo is so intense that even while lying down, clients hold the bed or ground to prevent the whirling sensation. Severe vertigo usually lasts 3 to 4 hours, but clients may feel dizzy long after the attack. Nausea and vomiting are common. Other manifestations include rapid eye movements **(nystagmus)** and severe headaches.

Common Nursing Diagnoses and Collaborative Problems

Nursing diagnoses that may apply to clients with Ménière's disease include the following:

- Anxiety related to loss of control
- Risk for Injury related to loss of balance
- Powerlessness related to loss of control
- Activity Intolerance related to perception of dizziness
- Risk for Deficient Fluid Volume related to nausea and vomiting
- Fear related to potential of hearing loss

Interventions

NONSURGICAL MANAGEMENT. Instruct clients to make slow head movements to prevent worsening of the vertigo. Dietary and lifestyle changes, such as salt and fluid restrictions that reduce the amount of endolymphatic fluid, are helpful. Advise clients to stop smoking because of the blood vessel constricting effects.

Drug therapy aims to control the vertigo and vomiting and restore normal balance. Mild diuretics are prescribed to decrease endolymph volume. Nicotinic acid has been found to be useful because of its vasodilatory effect. Antihistamines such as diphenhydramine hydrochloride (Benadryl, Allerdryl✱) and dimenhydrinate (Dramamine, Gravol✱) help reduce the severity of or stop an acute attack. Antiemetics such as chlorpromazine hydrochloride (Thorazine, Novo-Chlorpromazine✱), droperidol (Inapsine), and trimethobenzamide hydrochloride (Arrestin, Tigan) help control the nausea and vomiting. Diazepam (Valium, Apo-Diazepam✱) calms the client; controls vertigo, nausea, and vomiting; and allows the client to rest quietly during an attack.

SURGICAL MANAGEMENT. Surgical treatment of Ménière's disease is a last resort because the hearing in the affected ear is often sacrificed. When medical therapy is ineffective and the client's hearing level has decreased significantly, surgery is performed. The most radical procedure involves resection of the vestibular nerve or total removal of the labyrinth **(labyrinthectomy),** performed via the transcanal route. The footplate of the stapes is moved aside, and the labyrinth is removed through the oval window.

Another procedure performed early in the course of the disease is endolymphatic decompression with drainage and a shunt. The endolymphatic sac is drained, and a small tube is inserted to improve fluid drainage. Some clients report relief of vertigo with retention of their hearing.

If endolymphatic decompression has been performed, movement of the vestibular structures of the inner ear causes postoperative vertigo. Reassure the client that the vertigo is temporary as a result of the surgical procedure, not the disease.

Critical Thinking Challenge

The client is a 52-year-old man who is the conductor of a symphony in a large city. He is admitted to the emergency department with severe dizziness and vomiting. He tells you he was eating dinner in a restaurant when his symptoms began suddenly. He has had such episodes in the past and has been diagnosed with Ménière's disease. He tells you he would rather die than lose his hearing because music is his life.

1. What vital signs should you take first for this client? Why?
2. What nursing diagnoses are appropriate at this time for this client?
3. What interventions can you initiate for the symptoms he has before he is seen by a physician?
4. What lifestyle changes can you suggest for his chronic problem?

evolve For suggested answer guidelines, go to http://evolve.elsevier.com/Iggy/.

Acoustic Neuroma

PATHOPHYSIOLOGY

An **acoustic neuroma** is a benign tumor of cranial nerve VIII. The tumor is destructive as it grows, often damaging structures in the cerebellum. Depending on the size and exact location of the tumor, damage to hearing, facial movements, and sensation can occur. The presence of an acoustic neuroma can cause many neurologic manifestations as the tumor enlarges in the brain.

COLLABORATIVE MANAGEMENT

Manifestations begin with tinnitus and progress to gradual sensorineural hearing loss in most clients. Later, clients have constant mild vertigo. As the tumor enlarges, nearby cranial nerves are damaged.

Acoustic neuromas are diagnosed with computed tomography (CT) scanning and magnetic resonance imaging (MRI). Audiograms detect sensorineural hearing loss. Cerebrospinal fluid assays show increased pressure and the presence of protein.

Surgical removal via a craniotomy is performed, and the remaining hearing is sacrificed. Extreme care is taken to preserve the function of the facial nerve (cranial nerve VII). Routine postcraniotomy care is discussed in Chapter 48. Acoustic neuromas rarely recur after surgical removal.

HEARING LOSS

PATHOPHYSIOLOGY

Hearing loss is one of the most common physical handicaps in North America. Hearing loss may be conductive, sensorineural, or a combination of the two (Figure 52-7). Conductive hearing loss occurs when sound waves are blocked from contact with inner-ear nerve fibers because of external-ear or middle-ear disorders. If the inner-ear nerve, or sensory, fibers that lead to the cerebral cortex are damaged, the hearing loss is termed sensorineural. Combined hearing loss is known as mixed conductive-sensorineural.

The differences in conductive and sensorineural hearing loss are listed in Table 52-2. Disorders that cause conductive hearing loss are often corrected with no or minimal permanent damage. Sensorineural hearing loss is often permanent, and measures must be taken to prevent further damage or to amplify sounds as a means to improve hearing.

Etiology and Genetic Risk

COMMON CAUSES OF CONDUCTIVE HEARING LOSS

Any inflammatory process or obstruction of the external or middle ear by cerumen or foreign objects leads to conductive hearing loss. Changes in the eardrum such as bulging, retraction, and perforations may indicate damage to middle-ear structures, which leads to conductive hearing loss. Tumors, scar tissue buildup, and overgrowth of soft bony tissue **(otosclerosis)** on the ossicles from previous middle-ear surgery also lead to conductive hearing loss.

COMMON CAUSES OF SENSORINEURAL HEARING LOSS

When the inner ear or auditory nerve (cranial nerve VIII) is damaged, sensorineural hearing loss develops. Prolonged exposure to loud noise can damage the hair cells of the cochlea. Many drugs are toxic **(ototoxic)** to the inner ear structures, and their effects on hearing can be transient or permanent, dose related or non–dose related, and affect one or both ears. When ototoxic drugs (such as those listed in Table 51-2) are given to clients with reduced renal function, increased ototoxicity can result because drug elimination is slower. Older clients are especially at risk for ototoxicity because of reduced kidney function.

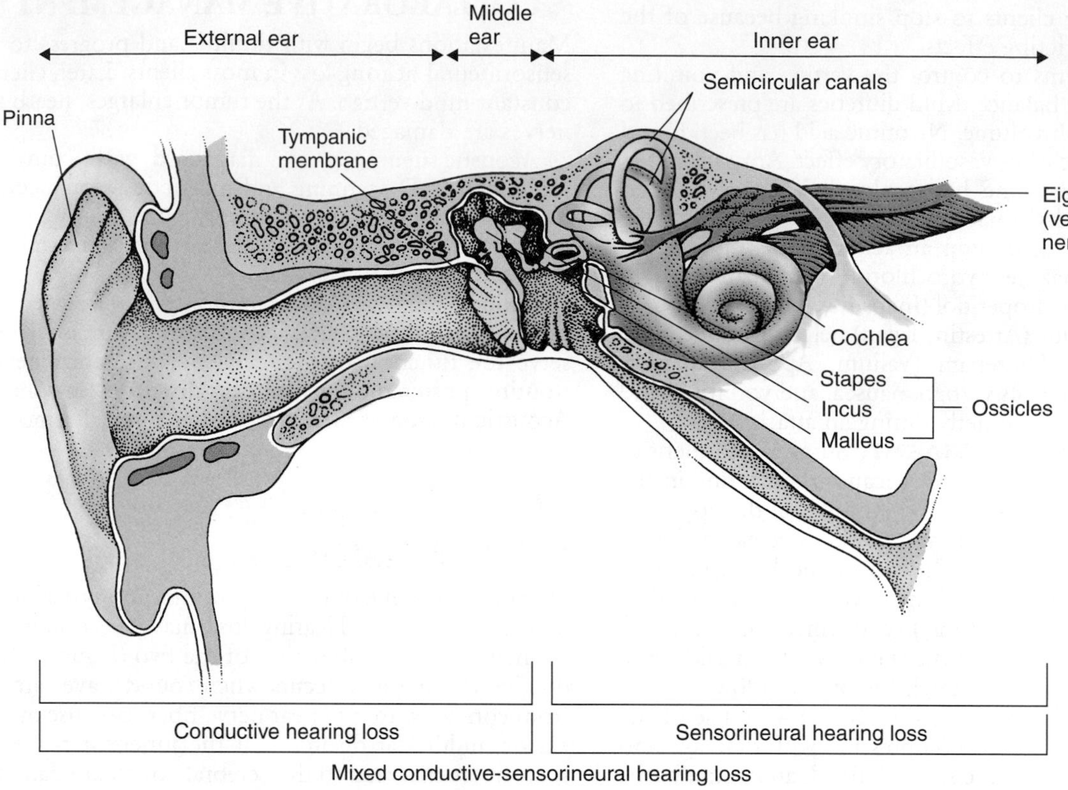

Figure 52-7 ■ Anatomy of hearing loss. Hearing loss can be divided into three types: (1) conductive (difficulty in the external or the middle ear), (2) sensorineural (difficulty in the inner ear or the acoustic nerve), and (3) mixed conductive-sensorineural (a combination of the two).

TABLE 52-2 Differential Features of Conductive and Sensorineural Hearing Loss

Conductive Hearing Loss	Sensorineural Hearing Loss
Causes	
Cerumen	Prolonged exposure to noise
Foreign body	Presbycusis
Perforation of the tympanic membrane	Ototoxic substances
Edema	Ménière's disease
Infection of the external ear or middle ear	Acoustic neuroma
Tumors	Diabetes mellitus
Otosclerosis	Labyrinthitis
	Infection
	Myxedema
Assessment Findings	
Evidence of obstruction with otoscope	Normal appearance of external canal and tympanic membrane
Abnormality in tympanic membrane	Tinnitus common
Speaking softly	Occasional dizziness
Hearing best in a noisy environment	Speaking loudly
Rinne test: air conduction greater than bone conduction	Hearing poorly in loud environment
Weber test: lateralization to affected ear	Rinne test: air conduction less than bone conduction
	Weber test: lateralization to unaffected ear

Presbycusis is a sensorineural hearing loss that occurs as a result of aging. This hearing loss is caused by degeneration or atrophy of the ganglion cells in the cochlea, loss of elasticity of the basilar membrane, or a decreased blood supply to the inner ear. Research findings suggest that deficiencies of vitamin B_{12} and folic acid may play a role in presbycusis. Other causes include atherosclerosis, hypertension, infections, prolonged fever, Ménière's disease, diabetes mellitus, and ear surgery. Each disorder appears to accelerate degenerative changes of the cochlea. Trauma to the ear or the head also contributes to sensorineural hearing loss.

Genetic Considerations

In some cases, hearing loss in adults can have a genetic origin. Some syndromes in which a single gene mutation results in many abnormal manifestations also increase the risk for progressive hearing loss in adults. Two such syndromes are Usher's syndrome and Alport's syndrome. Usher's syndrome, in addition to hearing loss, occurs with blindness as a result of retinitis pigmentosa. This syndrome has an autosomal recessive pattern of inheritance. Alport's syndrome, which causes abnormal renal function in addition to progressive hearing loss, has many forms and patterns of inheritance, including autosomal dominant, autosomal recessive, and X-linked recessive (Online Mendelian Inheritance in Man, 2000). One type of adult-onset progressive hearing loss that does not have any other physical problems is associated with a mutation in the GJB2 gene on chromosome 1. This problem has an autosomal dominant pattern of inheritance.

Incidence/Prevalence

Because hearing loss may be gradual and affect only some aspects of hearing, many adults are unaware that their hearing is impaired. The actual incidence of hearing loss is not known, although about 30% to 35% of people ages 65 to 75

CHART 52-5

NIC INTERVENTION ACTIVITIES for Care of the Ears

Ear Care: *Prevention or minimization of threats to ear or hearing*
- Monitor for drainage from ears, as appropriate.
- Irrigate the ear, as appropriate.
- Avoid placing sharp objects in the ear.
- Administer eardrops, as appropriate.
- Explain the relationship between balance and the inner ear, as appropriate.
- Monitor for episodes of dizziness associated with ear problems, as appropriate.
- Determine if cerumen in the ear canal is causing pain or hearing loss.
- Instill mineral oil in the ear to soften impacted cerumen before irrigation.
- Irrigate the ear canal with a WaterPik (or similar device) on a low setting using warm water (80° to 90°F), as appropriate.
- Demonstrate proper technique for ear irrigation to caregiver, as appropriate.
- Monitor frequency of ear infections.
- Instruct clients how to administer eardrops, as appropriate.
- Instruct how to monitor and regulate high-volume noise exposure.
- Instruct client to wear hearing protection for exposure to high-intensity noise.
- Instruct client with pierced ears how to avoid infection at the insertion site.
- Encourage use of ear plugs for swimming, if client is susceptible to ear infections.

years have a hearing loss. As many as half of the people older than 85 years of age have some degree of hearing loss (National Institute on Deafness and Other Communications Disorders, 1999).

HEALTH PROMOTION/ILLNESS PREVENTION

For most people, hearing is as an important factor in social interactions and to gain knowledge. With special care to the ears, hearing can be preserved at maximal levels (Chart 52-5).

◆COLLABORATIVE MANAGEMENT

PHARM e REVIEW

◆Assessment

HISTORY

Ask clients how long they have noticed a difference in their hearing and whether the changes occurred suddenly or gradually. Age is an important factor, because some ear and hearing changes occur with advanced age. Chronic otitis media occurs more often in the older adult. Ask about occupational exposure to loud or continuous noises, as well as current or previous use of ototoxic drugs. Also ask about any history of external-ear or middle-ear infection and whether eardrum perforation occurred with the infection. Ask clients about any direct trauma to the ears. Because some types of hearing loss have a genetic predisposition, ask whether any family members are hearing impaired.

When pain occurs with acute-onset hearing loss, ask about recent upper respiratory infection and allergies affecting the nose and sinuses.

CHART 52-6

FOCUSED ASSESSMENT of The Client with Suspected Hearing Loss

Assess whether the client has any of the following ear complaints:
- Pain
- Feeling of fullness or congestion
- Dizziness or vertigo
- Tinnitus
- Difficulty understanding conversations, especially in a noisy room
- Difficulty hearing sounds
- The need to strain to hear
- The need to turn the head to favor one ear or the need to lean forward to hear

Assess visible ear structures, particularly the external canal and tympanic membrane:
- Position and size of the pinna
- Patency of the external canal; presence of cerumen or foreign bodies, edema, or inflammation
- Condition of the tympanic membrane: intact, edema, fluid, inflammation

Assess functional ability, including:
- Frequency of asking people to repeat statements
- Withdrawal from social interactions or large groups
- Shouting in conversation
- Failing to respond when not looking in the direction of the sound
- Answering questions incorrectly

PHYSICAL ASSESSMENT/CLINICAL MANIFESTATIONS

Chart 52-6 lists focused assessment techniques for clients with suspected hearing loss. Hearing loss may be sudden or gradual and often affects both ears. The ability to hear high-frequency soft, consonants, especially *s, sh, f, th,* and *ch* sounds, is lost first. Clients often state that they have no problem with hearing but cannot understand specific words. They might think that the speaker is mumbling. They often experience high-pitched, continuous bilateral tinnitus. Vertigo may be present, depending on the extent of inner-ear involvement.

TUNING FORK TESTS. Tuning fork tests help diagnose hearing loss (see Chapter 51). With the Weber test, the client can usually hear sounds well in the ear with a conductive hearing loss because of bone conduction. With the Rinne test, the client reports that sound transmitted by bone conduction is louder and more sustained than that transmitted by air conduction.

OTOSCOPIC EXAMINATION. An otoscopic examination is performed to assess the external ear canal, the eardrum, and structures of the middle ear visible through the eardrum (see Chapter 51). Findings from examination vary, depending on the cause of the hearing loss.

Obstruction of the external ear canal can result in hearing loss. Inspect the canal, looking for the following:
- Whether the canal is open
- The amount and character of cerumen present
- The integrity of the skin lining the canal
- The presence of redness, exudates, lesions, or foreign objects

Middle-ear infections can also reduce hearing. In infection or inflammation, the eardrum appears red, thickened, and bulging, with a loss of landmarks. Loss of eardrum mobility is seen with inspection through a pneumatic otoscope. Document the presence of any scars or perforations on the eardrum. With close observation, you may be able to see exudate behind the membrane.

PSYCHOSOCIAL ASSESSMENT

For persons with a hearing loss, communication can become a struggle, and they may isolate themselves because of the difficulty in talking and listening. Social isolation can lead to depression, fear, and despair. You must be sensitive to emotional changes that may be related to reduced hearing and a decline in conversational skills.

LABORATORY ASSESSMENT

No laboratory test diagnoses hearing loss. However, some laboratory findings can indicate problems that affect hearing.

White blood cell counts are elevated in the client with acute or chronic otitis media. Microbial culture and antibiotic sensitivity tests can determine the causative organism and the most appropriate drug therapy when infection causes hearing loss.

The client with hearing loss from peripheral neuropathy may have other systemic diseases, including poorly controlled diabetes mellitus. The blood glucose level may be elevated, and the blood may be positive for serum acetone.

RADIOGRAPHIC ASSESSMENT

Radiographic assessment can determine nonauditory problems affecting hearing ability. Some hearing problems can be diagnosed using radiographic techniques. Skull x-rays are used to determine bony involvement in otitis media and the location of otosclerotic lesions, and computed tomography (CT) and magnetic resonance imaging (MRI) are used to determine soft-tissue involvement and the presence and location of tumors.

OTHER DIAGNOSTIC ASSESSMENTS

Audiometry can help to determine the extent and type of hearing loss. An audiogram shows whether hearing loss is only conductive or whether it has a sensorineural component. This is important in determining possible causes of the hearing loss and in planning interventions.

Critical Thinking Challenge

You are the home care nurse for a 74-year-old woman with diabetes, stasis ulcers, and rheumatoid arthritis who lives alone at home. She has had a conductive hearing loss for 10 years and has been using a hearing aid successfully for that time. She has had a kidney infection for the past 2 weeks and was seen by her internist for this problem. At first she was taking Septra orally (prescribed by her internist) for the infection but when her symptoms didn't subside, she went to an urgent care center and was started on streptomycin 8 days ago. The other drugs she takes routinely are insulin, bumetanide, and ibuprofen. She says her hearing has decreased during the last 4 days.

1. What questions should you ask this client?
2. Exactly how will you test her hearing in this setting?
3. What interventions could you perform immediately for her change in hearing?
4. Can you determine whether she has any sensorineural hearing loss? Why or why not?
5. What drugs or health factors could be contributing to her difficulty hearing?

evolve For suggested answer guidelines, go to http://evolve.elsevier.com/Iggy/.

Analysis

COMMON NURSING DIAGNOSES AND COLLABORATIVE PROBLEMS

The following are priority nursing diagnoses for clients with any degree of hearing impairment:

1. Disturbed Sensory Perception (Auditory) related to obstruction, infection, damage to the middle ear, or damage to the auditory nerve
2. Impaired Verbal Communication related to reduced sensory perception (auditory)

ADDITIONAL NURSING DIAGNOSES AND COLLABORATIVE PROBLEMS

In addition to the common nursing diagnoses, clients with hearing loss or impairment may have one or more of the following:

- Deficient Knowledge related to treatment and prevention
- Activity Intolerance related to pain
- Social Isolation related to pain and decreased hearing
- Risk for Injury related to altered auditory perception and infection
- Acute Pain related to an inflammatory process and fluid in the middle ear
- Impaired Physical Mobility related to vertigo

Planning and Implementation

DISTURBED SENSORY PERCEPTION (AUDITORY)

NOC **PLANNING: EXPECTED OUTCOMES.** The client with hearing loss or impairment is expected to either experience an increase in auditory sensory perception to a functional level or maintain existing levels of hearing. Indicators include the following:

- Mild to no loss of high pitch tones
- Mild to no loss of ability to distinguish conversation from background environmental noise
- Turning to sound
- Maintaining auditory discrimination of discrete sounds

INTERVENTIONS. Interventions aim at identifying the problem, halting the pathologic processes, and improving auditory sensory perception.

NONSURGICAL MANAGEMENT. Interventions include early detection of hearing impairment, use of drug therapy and comfort measures, and use of assistive devices to amplify or augment the client's auditory perception.

Early Detection. Early detection helps correct the problem causing the hearing loss. When hearing loss is gradual, the client can compensate. Assess for indications of hearing loss, as listed in Chart 52-6.

Drug Therapy. Drug therapy is aimed at either correcting the underlying pathologic change or reducing the side effects of disorders occurring with hearing loss. Local (topical) antibiotics are given to clients with external otitis. Systemic antibiotics are needed when clients have other auditory infections. By treating the infection, antibiotics reduce local edema and improve hearing. When pain occurs with hearing disorders, analgesics are used, depending on the location and type of pain. Many ear disorders disturb equilibrium, causing vertigo and dizziness with nausea and vomiting. Antiemetic, antihistamine, antivertiginous, and benzodiazepine drugs can help correct nausea, vertigo, and dizziness.

Assistive Devices. Many devices are useful for clients with permanent, progressive hearing loss. Telephone amplifiers increase telephone volume, allowing the caller to speak in a normal voice. Flashing lights activated by the ringing telephone or a doorbell alert clients visually. In some cases, clients may have a specially trained dog to help them be aware of sounds (ringing telephones or doorbells, cries of other people, and potential dangers), in much the same way that a seeing eye dog assists a blind person.

Small, portable audio amplifiers can assist you in communicating with clients with hearing loss but who have chosen not to use a hearing aid. The use of audio amplifiers or allowing clients to use a stethoscope helps you to communicate with anyone who requires additional volume to hear speech.

Hearing Aids. A hearing aid is a miniature electronic amplifier that is usually used for clients with conductive hearing loss. Hearing aids are less effective for sensorineural hearing loss and may make hearing worse by amplifying background noise. The amplifier can be worn in one or both ears. Local agencies offer special classes for the hearing impaired that help the user benefit from this device.

Offer some special tips to help the client adjust to the hearing aid. Hearing with a hearing aid can be different from natural hearing. Encourage the client to start using the hearing aid slowly, at first wearing it only at home and only during part of the day. Listening to television and the radio and reading aloud can help the client get used to new sounds. The tone or volume of the hearing aid can be adjusted. The most important and difficult aspect of a hearing aid is the amplification of background noise, as well as voices. The client must learn to concentrate and filter out background noises.

The client must also learn to care for the hearing aid (Chart 52-7). Hearing aids are delicate devices that should be handled only by people who know how to care for them properly. The cost of the aids varies greatly but is a significant investment.

Cochlear Implants. Cochlear implantation may help clients with sensorineural hearing loss. A small computer converts sound waves into electronic impulses. Electrodes are placed by the internal ear, with the computer attached to the external ear. The electronic impulses then directly stimulate nerve fibers. Some clients have a 50% return of their hearing with this method.

SURGICAL MANAGEMENT. Many surgical interventions are available for clients with specific disorders leading to hearing loss.

Tympanoplasty. Tympanoplasty reconstructs the middle ear to improve hearing caused by conductive hearing loss. The procedures vary from simple reconstruction of the eardrum **(myringoplasty)** to replacement of the ossicles within the middle ear. A type I tympanoplasty is used for a myringoplasty; a type II tympanoplasty is used in cases of greater damage and to provide more extensive reconstruction (Figure 52-8).

CHART 52-7

CLIENT EDUCATION GUIDE
Hearing Aid Care

- Keep the hearing aid dry.
- Clean the ear mold with mild soap and water while avoiding excessive wetting.
- Clean debris from the hole in the middle of the part that goes into your ear with a toothpick or a pipe cleaner.
- Turn off the hearing aid and remove the battery when not in use.
- Check and replace the battery frequently.
- Keep extra batteries on hand.
- Keep the hearing aid in a safe place.
- Avoid dropping the hearing aid or exposing it to temperature extremes.
- Adjust the volume to the lowest setting that allows you to hear, to prevent feedback squeaking.
- Avoid using hair spray, cosmetics, oils, or other hair and face products that might come into contact with the receiver.
- If the hearing aid does not work:
  - Change the battery.
  - Check the connection between the ear mold and the receiver.
  - Check the on/off switch.
  - Clean the sound hole.
  - Adjust the volume.
  - Take the hearing aid to an authorized service center for repair.

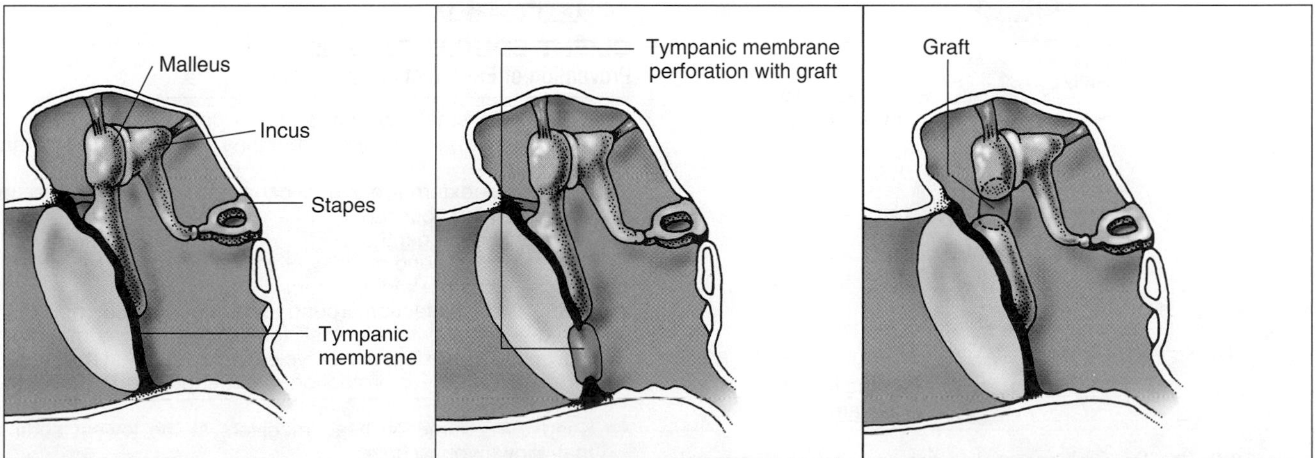

Normal tympanic membrane and ossicles.

In **type I tympanoplasty (myringoplasty)**, a graft is placed over a perforation in the tympanic membrane; other middle ear structures are normal.

In **type II tympanoplasty (ossiculoplasty)**, the malleus, which has become disconnected from the tympanic membrane, is grafted to reconnect the structures.

Figure 52-8 ■ A normal tympanic membrane and two types of tympanoplasties.

Preoperative Care. The client requires specific instructions before surgery. Systemic antibiotics reduce the risk for infection. Before surgery, irrigate the ear with a solution of equal parts of vinegar and sterile water to restore normal ear pH. Teach the client to follow other measures to decrease the risks for infection, such as avoiding people with upper respiratory infections, getting adequate rest, eating a balanced diet, and maintaining an adequate fluid intake.

Assure the client that hearing loss immediately after surgery is normal because of canal packing, and that hearing will improve on packing removal. Explain the importance of deep breathing and coughing after surgery but emphasize that forceful coughing increases middle-ear pressure and must be avoided.

Operative Procedures. Surgery is performed only when the middle ear is free of infection and if the condition of the eustachian tube does not promote continued infection. If an infection is present, the graft is more likely to become infected and not heal properly. Surgery of the eardrum and ossicles requires the use of a microscope and is a delicate procedure. Local anesthesia can be used, although general anesthesia is often used to prevent the client from moving.

The surgeon can repair the eardrum with many materials, including muscle fascia, a skin graft, and venous tissue. If the ossicles are damaged, more extensive surgery is needed for repair or replacement. The ossicles are reached via a transcanal approach, an endaural incision, or the postauricular route with a mastoidectomy (Figure 52-9).

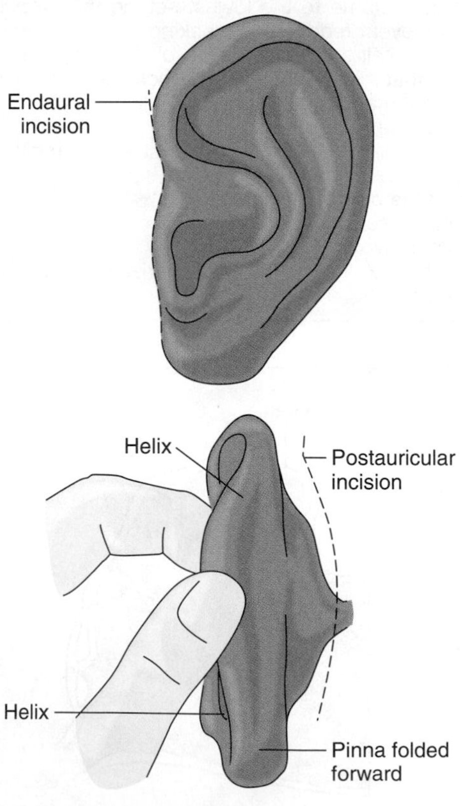

Figure 52-9 ■ Surgical approaches for the ear. The endaural approach is used when the external canal is too small to use for a transcanal approach (not shown because no external incision is used). The postauricular approach is used for more extensive repair of the middle-ear and inner-ear structures.

The surgeon removes diseased tissue and cleans the middle-ear cavity. The ossicles are assessed for damage and the extent of needed repair or replacement. The surgeon uses the client's cartilage or bone, cadaver ossicles, stainless steel wire, or special polymers (Teflon) to repair or replace the ossicles.

Postoperative Care. An antiseptic-soaked gauze, such as iodoform gauze (Nu Gauze), is packed in the ear canal. If a postauricular or endaural incision is used, a dressing is placed over the incision. Keep the dressing clean and dry, using sterile technique for changes. Keep the client flat, with the head turned to the side and the operative ear facing up for at least 12 hours after surgery. Give prescribed antibiotics to prevent infection.

Clients often report hearing improvement after removal of the canal packing. Until that time, communicate as with a hearing-impaired client, directing conversation to the unaffected ear. Instruct the client in care and activity restrictions (see Chart 52-4).

Stapedectomy. A partial or complete stapedectomy with a prosthesis corrects hearing loss. This procedure is most effective for clients with hearing loss related to otosclerosis.

Preoperative Care. To prevent infection, the client must be free from external otitis at surgery. Instruct the client to follow measures that prevent middle-ear or external-ear infections (Chart 52-8).

Review with the client the expected outcomes and possible complications of the surgery. Hearing is initially worse after a stapedectomy. The success rate of this procedure is high; however, there is always a risk of failure that might lead to total deafness on the affected side. Possible complications include prolonged vertigo, infection, and facial nerve damage. A decision to proceed with surgery should be made with the client's full knowledge and understanding of these complications.

Operative Procedures. A stapedectomy is usually performed through the external ear canal with the client under local anesthesia. The head and neck of the stapes and, less often, the footplate are removed. After removal of the bone, a small hole is drilled in the footplate and a prosthesis in the shape of a piston is connected between the incus

CHART 52-8

CLIENT EDUCATION GUIDE
Prevention of Ear Infection or Trauma

- Do not use small objects, such as cotton-tipped applicators, matches, toothpicks, or hairpins, to clean your external ear canal.
- Wash your external ear and canal daily in the shower or while washing your hair.
- Blow your nose gently.
- Do not occlude one nostril while blowing your nose.
- Sneeze with your mouth open.
- Wear sound protection around loud or continuous noises.
- Avoid activities with high risk for head or ear trauma, such as wrestling, boxing, motorcycle riding, and skateboarding; wear head and ear protection when engaging in these activities.
- Keep the volume on head receivers at the lowest setting that allows you to hear.
- Frequently clean objects that come into contact with your ear (e.g., headphones, telephone receivers).
- Avoid environmental conditions with rapid changes in air pressure.

and the footplate (Figure 52-10). Sounds cause the prosthesis to vibrate as the stapes did. After stapedectomy, up to 90% of clients have restoration of practical hearing.

Postoperative Care. Inform the client that improvement in hearing may not occur until 6 weeks after surgery. Initially, the ear packing interferes with hearing. Swelling in the ear after surgery reduces hearing until the edema has resolved. Drugs for pain help reduce discomfort, and antibiotics are given to reduce the risk for infection. Instruct the client to follow the procedures in Chart 52-4.

The surgical procedure is performed in an area where cranial nerves VII, VIII, and X can be damaged by trauma or by swelling after surgery. Assess for facial nerve damage or muscle weakness and changes in tactile sensation or taste. Vertigo, nausea, and vomiting are common after surgery because of the nearness to inner-ear structures.

Antivertiginous drugs, such as meclizine hydrochloride (Antivert, Bonamine✱), and antiemetic drugs, such as droperidol (Inapsine), are given. Take care to prevent injury, especially during times of increased vertigo. Assist the client with ambulating during the first 1 to 2 days after surgery. Keep bed siderails up and remind the client to move his or her head slowly when changing position to avoid vertigo.

IMPAIRED VERBAL COMMUNICATION

NOC **PLANNING: EXPECTED OUTCOMES.** The client with hearing loss or impairment is expected to become proficient in hearing compensation behaviors to maintain or improve expressive and receptive communication. Indicators include that the client consistently demonstrates the following behaviors:

- Uses hearing assistive devices
- Cares for external hearing assistive devices
- Uses sign language, lip reading, or closed captioning (for television viewing)
- Accurately interprets messages received
- Uses nonverbal language
- Exchanges messages accurately with others

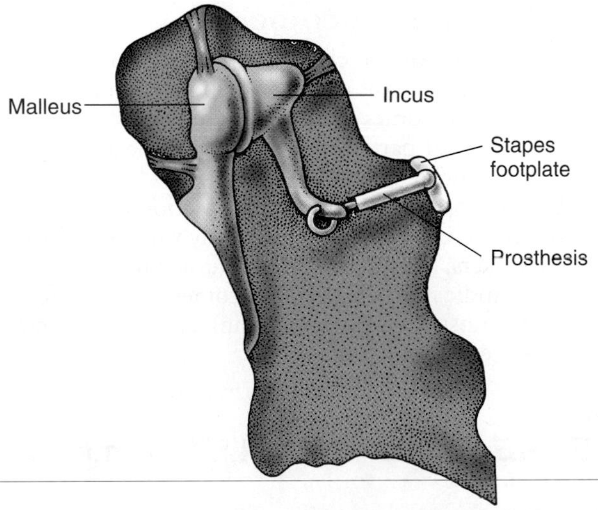

Figure 52-10 ■ Prosthesis used with stapedectomy. The stapes is removed, leaving the footplate. After a hole is drilled in the footplate, a metal or plastic prosthesis is connected to the incus and inserted through the hole to act as a vibration device, much as the stapes worked before the development of otosclerosis.

INTERVENTIONS. Interventions focus on facilitating communication and reducing anxiety.

Use best practices for communicating with a hearing-impaired client that are listed in Chart 52-9. Shouting to the client is of little benefit, because the sound may be projected at a higher frequency, making him or her less able to understand. The most obvious means of communicating with such a client is by the written word (if he or she is able to see, read, and write) or with pictures of familiar phrases and objects. Many television programs are now closed captioned (subtitled).

Assistive Devices. Assistive devices, described on p. 1137, can greatly increase communication for the client with a hearing impairment.

Lip-Reading. Lip-reading and sign language can also enhance communication. In lip-reading classes, clients are taught the special cues to look for when lip-reading and how to understand body language. However, the best lip-reader still misses more than 50% of what is being said. Because hearing is assisted by even minimal lip-reading, urge clients to wear their eyeglasses when talking with someone to see lip movement.

Sign Language. For clients with more severe hearing loss, special languages have been developed, including American Sign Language (ASL). Such languages combine speech with hand movements that signify letters, words, and phrases. These languages take time and effort to learn, and many people are unable to learn them, just as many people cannot learn foreign languages. However, as the hearing-impaired person becomes less able to function, motivation to learn may increase.

Managing Anxiety. A major source of anxiety is the possibility of permanent hearing loss. Provide honest and accurate information about the likelihood of hearing returning. When the hearing impairment is likely to be permanent or become more profound, reassure clients that communication and social interaction can be maintained.

To reduce anxiety and prevent social isolation, clients use remaining resources to make social contact satisfying. The most obvious way to decrease social isolation is by improving communication (as previously described). Ask about past or present diversional activities to identify the

CHART 52-9

BEST PRACTICE for
Communicating with a Hearing-Impaired Client

- Position yourself directly in front of the client.
- Make sure that the room is well lighted.
- Get the client's attention before you begin to speak.
- Move closer to the better-hearing ear.
- Speak clearly and slowly.
- Do not shout (shouting raises the frequency of the sound and often makes understanding more difficult).
- Keep hands and other objects away from your mouth when talking to the client.
- Attempt to have conversations in a quiet room with minimal distractions.
- Have the client repeat your statements rather than just indicating assent.
- Rephrase sentences and repeat information to aid in understanding.
- Use appropriate hand motions.
- Write messages on paper if the client is able to read.

client's most satisfying activities and social interactions and determine the amount of effort necessary to continue them. Activities can be altered to maximize client satisfaction. Someone accustomed to large gatherings might choose smaller groups instead. A quiet evening meal at home with friends might substitute for dinner in a noisy restaurant.

Community-Based Care

Lengthy hospitalization is rare for most clients with ear and hearing disorders. If surgical repair is necessary and the procedure is completed without complications, the procedure may be completed as an outpatient, or the hospital stay is usually only 1 day.

HOME CARE MANAGEMENT

Clients who have persistent vertigo, either with the disorder or as a side effect of surgery, remain in danger of falling. Assess the home for potential hazards and to determine whether family members or significant others are available to assist with meal preparation and other activities of daily living. A nurse case manager can, in collaboration with the home care nurse, assist clients and their families in determining the best ways to maintain adequate self-care abilities, maintain a safe environment, decide about assistance needs, and provide needed care.

HEALTH TEACHING

Give clients written instructions about how to take drugs and when to return for follow-up care. If the client cannot read, give these instructions to a family member who may assist with care. Teach clients how to instill eardrops (see Chart 52-1) and irrigate the ears (see Chart 52-2), and ask for a return demonstration.

To promote health and prevent infections after surgery, clients are instructed to follow the suggestions in Chart 52-8. For clients who use a hearing aid, teach them how to use it effectively.

HEALTH CARE RESOURCES

If clients do not have family or friends to help during the time before surgery, a referral to a home care agency is needed. Help with meal preparation, cleaning, and personal hygiene can be arranged by the hospital discharge planners.

Follow-up hearing tests are scheduled for clients when the lesions are well healed, in about 6 to 8 weeks. Audiograms done before and after treatment are compared, and evaluation for further intervention to improve hearing begins. A complication of an unsuccessful surgery is continued disability or complete loss of hearing in the affected ear. Surgery is performed on the ear with the greatest hearing loss. If the surgery does not improve hearing, clients must decide to either attempt surgical correction of the other ear or continue to use an amplification device. When the underlying disorder causing the hearing impairment is progressive, this decision is difficult. Support clients by listening to their concerns and giving additional information when needed.

Costs to the person with a hearing impairment can be extensive. Information and support can come from several organizations that publish informative articles to help clients reduce hearing loss (Table 52-3). Many public and private agencies offer hearing evaluations as well as supply information and counseling for clients with hearing disorders.

TABLE 52-3 Agencies Offering Services for Ear and Hearing Disorders

House Ear Institute
2100 West Third Street, Fifth Floor
Los Angeles, CA 90057
Voice: (800) 352-8888
TTY: (213) 484-2642
Internet: http://www.hei.org

National Information Center on Deafness
Gallaudet University
800 Florida Avenue NE
Washington, DC 20002
Voice: (202) 651-5051
TTY: (202) 651-5000
E-mail: nidc@gallux.gallaudet.edu
Internet: http://www.gallaudet.edu

American Academy of Otolaryngology/Head and Neck Surgery
One Prince Street
Alexandria, VA 22314
Voice: (703) 519-1589
TTY: (703) 836-4444
Internet: http://www.entnet.org

American Speech-Language-Hearing Association
10801 Rockville Pike
Rockville, MD 20852
Voice/TTY: (301) 897-5700
Voice: (800) 638-8255
Internet: http://www.asha.org

Self-Help for Hard of Hearing People, Inc. (SHHH)
7910 Woodmont Avenue, Suite 1200
Bethesda, MD 20814
Voice: (301) 657-2248
TTY: (301) 657-2249
Fax: (301) 913-9413
E-mail: info@hearingloss.org
Internet: http://www.hearingloss.org

Evaluation: Outcomes

Evaluate the care of the client with hearing loss or hearing impairment on the basis of the identified nursing diagnoses. The expected outcomes include that the client will:

- Have at least partial improvement of hearing
- Have reduced anxiety
- Use appropriate hearing compensation behaviors
- Be able to communicate effectively with family, friends, co-workers, and health care professionals

Specific indicators for these outcomes are listed for each nursing diagnosis under the Planning and Implementation section (see earlier).

GET READY for the NCLEX Examination!

KEY POINTS

Safe Effective Care Environment

- Use a separate speculum cover for each ear when conducting an otoscopic examination.

- Slowly and gently introduce the otoscopic speculum into the external ear canal during assessment.
- Use contact precautions with any client who has drainage from the ear canal.
- Avoid performing an otoscopic examination on a confused or uncooperative client.
- Use the suggestions presented under "History" to enhance communication with a client who has a hearing impairment.
- Initiate fall precautions with clients with vertigo or dizziness and assist with ambulation.

Health Promotion and Maintenance

- Teach clients the proper way to clean the pinna and external ear canal.
- Identify clients at risk for hearing impairment as a result of work environment or leisure activities.
- Encourage all clients, even if they already have a hearing impairment, to use ear protection in loud environment.
- Teach clients how to properly care for their hearing aids.
- Instruct clients to avoid closing off one nares when blowing the nose.
- Tell clients who engage in water sports and who are at risk for external otitis either to wear earplugs when in the water or to rinse the ear canal with drops of dilute alcohol after any immersion of the head in water.
- Teach proper ear hygiene for cleaning cerumen from external canal.
- Urge everyone to avoid exposure to loud noises for extended periods of time without proper OSHA-approved ear protection.

Psychosocial Integrity

- Pace your interview to match the learning needs and style of the individual client.
- Allow the client the opportunity to express fear or anxiety regarding a change in hearing status.
- Refer clients newly diagnosed with hearing impairment or any chronic ear problem to appropriate local resources and support groups.
- Explain all diagnostic procedures, restrictions, and follow-up care to the client scheduled for tests.
- Teach family members ways to communicate with a hearing impaired client with and without a hearing aid.

Physiological Integrity

- Ask the client about hearing problems in any other members of the family, because many hearing problems have a genetic component.
- Check the hearing of any client receiving an ototoxic medication (Table 51-2) for more than 5 days.
- Teach clients the proper technique to use for self-instillation of eardrops and ear irrigation.
- Stress the importance of completing an antibiotic regimen when an infection is present in the ear.
- Follow the guidelines in Chart 52-2 when irrigating the ear canal.
- Avoid ear canal irrigation if the eardrum is perforated or if the canal contains vegetative matter.

ADDITIONAL STUDY RESOURCES

Go to your Student CD-ROM for Review Questions for the NCLEX Examination.

evolve Go to http://evolve.elsevier.com/Iggy/ for Integrated Management of Care Questions for the NCLEX Examination.

SELECTED BIBLIOGRAPHY

Asterisk indicates a classic or definitive work on this subject.

Ackley, B., & Ladwig, G. (2002). *Nursing diagnosis handbook: A guide to planning care* (5th ed.). St. Louis: Mosby.

Alper, C., Myers, E., & Eibling, D. (2001). Decision making in ear, nose, and throat disorders, Philadelphia: W. B. Saunders.

Baker, C. (2002). Caring for patients with hearing impairments. *Dermatology Nursing, 14*(1), 49, 52.

Ball, A. (2002). Caring for older people who have a hearing disability. *Nursing Older People, 14*(4), 39.

Battaglia, S., Sabri, A., & Jackson, C. (2002). Management of chronic otitis media in the only hearing ear. *Laryngoscope, 112*(4), 681-685.

Berry, J., et al. (2002). Patient-based outcomes in patients with primary tinnitus undergoing tinnitus retraining therapy. *Archives of Otolaryngology: Head and Neck Surgery, 128*(10), 1153-1157.

Burton, M. (2000). Hall and Colman's diseases of the ear, nose, and throat *(15th ed.). New York: Churchill Livingstone.*

Canalis, R., & Lambert, P. (2000). *The ear comprehensive otology.* Philadelphia: Lippincott Williams & Wilkins.

Carmen, R., & Uram, S. (2002). Hearing loss and anxiety in adults. *Hearing Journal,* 55(4), 48, 50, 52-54.

Cattel, C., Manna, R., & Carbonin, P. (2003). Case report: a swollen and red ear. *Journal of the American Geriatrics Society,* 51(1),138-139.

Chasin, M. (2000). Middle ear implants: what are surgically-implanted hearing aids and who are they for? *Hearing Loss,* 21(3), 13-15.

Dean, W. A., & Davidson, M. (2002). Hearing loss in adults: Physical limitation, psychosocial barrier. *Clinician Reviews,* 12(6), 62-67.

Demers, K. (2001). Try this: best practices in nursing care to older adults. Hearing screening. *Journal of Gerontological Nursing,* 27(11), 8-9.

Devaiah, A. (2000). Clinical indicators useful in predicting response to the medical management of Meniere's disease. *Laryngoscope,* 110(11), 1884-1889.

*Dhillon, R., & East, C. (1999). *Ear, nose, and throat, and head and neck surgery: An illustrated colour text.* New York: Churchill Livingstone.

Dochterman, J., & Bulechek, G. (Eds.). (2004). *Nursing interventions classification (NIC)* (4th ed.). St. Louis: Mosby.

Dowden, C. (2002). What is the best treatment for impacted cerumen? *The Journal of Family Practice,* 51(2), 117-119.

Ebersole, P., Hess, P., & Luggen, A. (2004). *Toward healthy aging: Human needs and nursing response* (6th ed.). St. Louis: Mosby.

Erber, S., & Garstecki, D. (2002). Hearing loss and hearing aid related stigma: Perceptions of women with age-normal hearing. *American Journal of Audiology,* 11(2), 83-91.

Facts and Comparisons. (2004). *Drug facts and comparisons* (58th ed.). St. Louis: Author.

Garber, S., et al. (2002). Payment under public and private insurance and access to cochlear implants. *Archives of Otolaryngology B Head & Neck Surgery,* 128(10), 1145-1152.

Gates, G., et al. (2003). Screening for handicapping hearing loss in the elderly. *The Journal of Family Practice,* 52(1), 56-62.

Green, C., & Pope, C. (2001). Effects of hearing impairment on use of health services among the elderly, *Journal of Aging & Health,* 13(3), 315-328.

Grossan, M. (2000). Safe, effective techniques for cerumen removal. *Geriatrics,* 55(1), 80-86.

Humes, L., et al. (2002). Longitudinal changes in hearing aid satisfaction and usage in the elderly over a period of one or two years after hearing aid delivery. *Ear & Hearing,* 23(5), 428-438.

Jafek, B., & Murrow, B. (2001). *ENT secrets.* Philadelphia: Hanley & Belfus

Larrabee, T. (2002). Prescribing practices that promote antibiotic resistance: Strategies for change. *Journal of Pediatric Nursing,* 17(2), 126-132.

Lucas, L., & Matthews-Flint, L. (2001). Sound advice about hearing aids. *Nursing2001, 31*(2), 59-61.

Lucas, L., & Matthews-Flint, L. (2003). Heed the word about hearing impairment. *Nursing 2003,* 33(10), 32hn1-32hn3.

McCance, K., & Huether, S. (2002). *Pathophysiology: The biologic basis for disease in adults and children* (4th ed.). St. Louis: Mosby.

McConnell, E. (2002). How to converse with a hearing-impaired patient. *Nursing 2002,* 32(8), 20.

Meyer, S., & Megerian, C. (2000). Patients' perceived outcomes after stapedectomy for otosclerosis. *ENT-Ear, Nose & Throat Journal,* 79(11), 846-856.

Moore, A., et al. (2002). Cerumen, hearing, and cognition in the elderly. *Journal of the American Medical Directors Association,* 3(3), 136-139.

Moorhead, S., Johnson, M., & Maas, M. (Eds.). (2004). *Nursing outcomes classification (NOC)* (3rd ed.). St. Louis: Mosby.

National Council on the Aging. (2000). The consequences of untreated hearing loss in older persons. *ORL-Head and Neck Nursing,* 18(1), 12-16.

*National Institute on Deafness and Other Communication Disorders. (1999). What is presbycusis? NIH Publication No. 97-4233. Available at http://www. nidcd.nih.gov/.

Ng, M., & Nipako, J. (2000). Otosclerosis: Causes, surgical and medical treatment. *Hearing Loss, 21(2), 26-28.*

*Nusbaum, N. (1999). Aging and sensory senescence. Southern Medical Journal, 92(3), 267-275. Also available at http://www.medscape.com/SMA/SMJ/1999/v92.n03/smj9203.02.nusb/smj9203.02.nusb-01.html.

Nussbaum, R., McInnes, R., & Willard, H. (2001). *Thompson & Thompson: Genetics in medicine* (6th ed.). Philadelphia: W. B. Saunders.

Online Mendelian Inheritance in Man, OMIM (TM). McKusick-Nathans Institute for Genetic Medicine, Johns Hopkins University (Baltimore, MD) and National Center for Biotechnology Information, National Library of Medicine (Bethesda, MD), 2000. Available at http://www.ncbi.nlm.nih.gov/omim/.

Pagana, K., & Pagana, T. (2002). *Mosby's manual of diagnostic and laboratory tests* (2nd ed.). St. Louis: Mosby.

Phillips, M. (2003). Genetics of hearing loss. *MEDSURG* Nursing, 12(6), 386-390, 411.

Pichichero, M. (2000). Acute otitis media: Part I. Improving diagnostic accuracy, *American Family Physician,* 61 (7), 2052-2056.

Ruholl, L. (2003). Tips for teaching the elderly. *RN,* 66(5), 48-52.

*Sanna, M. (1999). *Color atlas of otoscopy: From diagnosis to surgery.* New York: Thieme.

Sheehan, J. (2000). Caring for the deaf: Do you do enough? *RN,* 63(3), 69-72.

Sommer. S., & Sommer, N. (2002). When your patient is hearing impaired. *RN,* 65(12), 28-32.

Summerfield, A.Q., Marshall, D., Barton, G., & Bloor, K. (2002). A cost-utility scenario analysis of bilateral cochlear implantation. *Archives of Otolaryngology-Head and Neck Surgery, 128*(11), 1255-1262.

Wilson, S., & Lopez, R. (2002). What is the best treatment for impacted cerumen? *The Journal of Family Practice,* 51(2), 117.

Woodson, G. (2001). Ear, nose, and throat disorders in primary care. Philadelphia: W. B. Saunders.

UNIT **TWELVE**

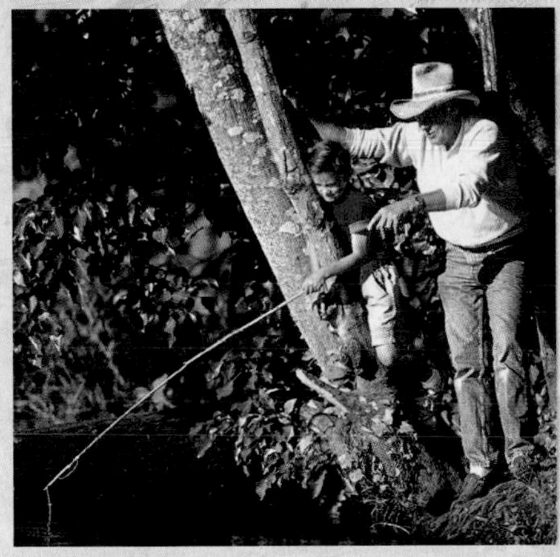

PROBLEMS of MOBILITY

Management of Clients with Problems of the Musculoskeletal System

CHAPTER 53

Assessment of the Musculoskeletal System

CATHY A. MURRAY

LEARNING OUTCOMES

After studying this chapter, you should be able to:

1. Recall the anatomy and physiology of the musculoskeletal system.
2. Explain how physiologic aging changes of the musculoskeletal system affect care of older adults.
3. Conduct a musculoskeletal history using Gordon's Functional Health Patterns.
4. Evaluate important assessment findings in a client with a musculoskeletal health problem.
5. Explain the use of laboratory testing for a client with a musculoskeletal health problem.
6. Identify the use of radiography in diagnosing musculoskeletal health problems.
7. Plan follow-up care for clients undergoing musculoskeletal diagnostic testing.
8. Develop a teaching plan for clients undergoing arthroscopic procedures.

Go to your Student CD-ROM for Review Questions
for the NCLEX Examination keyed to these Learning Outcomes.

The musculoskeletal system is the second largest body system; it includes the bones, joints, and skeletal muscles, as well as their supporting structures. Disease, surgery, and trauma often affect one or more parts of this system, yet nurses often overlook assessment of this system. This chapter does not include diagnostic testing related to arthritis or specific tests for osteoporosis. Descriptions of those tests are found in Chapters 24 and 54 under discussions of those diseases.

ANATOMY AND PHYSIOLOGY REVIEW

Skeletal System

The skeletal system consists of 206 bones and multiple joints. The growth and development of these structures occur during childhood and adolescence and are not discussed in this text.

BONES

Types

Bone can be classified in two ways, by shape and by structure. In regard to shape, *long bones,* such as the femur, are cylindrical with rounded ends and often bear weight. *Short bones,* such as the phalanges, are small and bear little or no weight. *Flat bones,* such as the scapula, protect vital organs and often contain blood-forming cells. Bones that have unique shapes are known as *irregular bones.* The carpal bones in the wrist and the small bones in the inner ear are examples of irregular bones. The *sesamoid bone* is the least common type and develops within a tendon; the patella is a typical example.

Structure

The second way bone is classified is by structure or composition. As shown in Figure 53-1, the outer layer of bone, or **cortex**, is composed of dense, compact bone tissue. The inner layer, in the medulla, contains spongy, cancellous tissue. Almost every bone has both tissue types but in varying quantities. The long bone typically has a shaft, or **diaphysis,** and two knoblike ends, or **epiphyses.**

The structural unit of the cortical, compact bone is the haversian system, which is detailed in Figure 53-1. The haversian system is a complex canal network containing microscopic blood vessels, which supply nutrients and oxygen to bone, and lacunae, which are small cavities that house osteocytes (bone cells). The canals run longitudinally within the hard, cortical bone tissue.

The softer, **cancellous** tissue contains large spaces, or trabeculae, which are filled with red and yellow marrow. **Hematopoiesis** (production of blood cells) occurs in the red marrow. The yellow marrow contains fat cells, which can be dislodged and enter the bloodstream to cause fat embolism

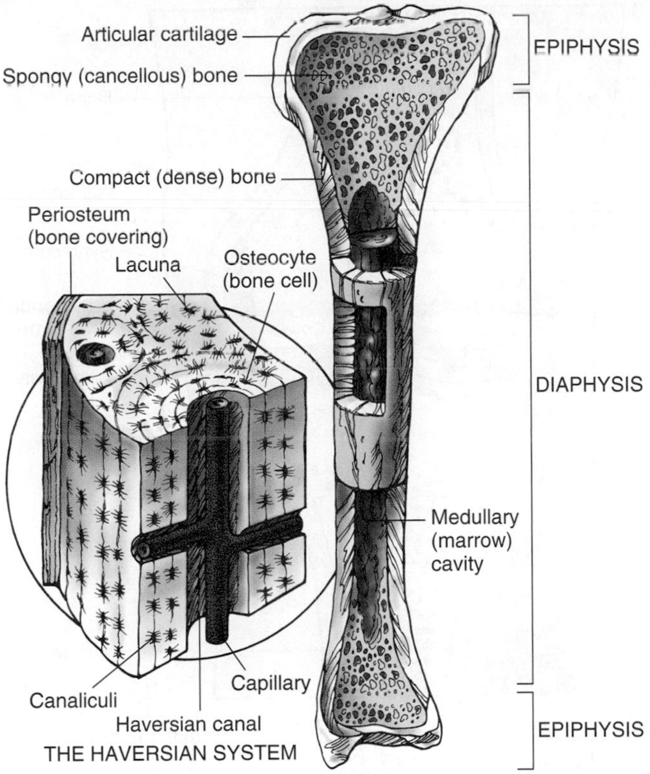

Figure 53-1 ■ The structure of a typical long bone. The cortex, or outer layer, is composed of dense, compact tissue. The microscopic structure of this compact cortical tissue is the haversian system.

syndrome (FES), a life-threatening complication. Volkmann's canals connect bone marrow vessels with the haversian system and periosteum, the outermost covering of the bone. Osteogenic cells, which later differentiate into **osteoblasts** (bone-forming cells) and **osteoclasts** (bone-destroying cells), are found in the deepest layer of the periosteum.

Bone also contains a **matrix** (also called *osteoid*) consisting chiefly of collagen, mucopolysaccharides, and lipids. Deposits of inorganic calcium salts (carbonate and phosphate) in the matrix provide the hardness of bone.

Bone is a very vascular tissue; its estimated total blood flow is between 200 and 400 mL/min. Each bone has a principal nutrient artery, which enters near the middle of the shaft and branches into ascending and descending vessels. These vessels supply the cortex, the marrow, and the haversian system. Sympathetic and afferent (sensory) fibers constitute the sparse nerve supply to bone. Sympathetic nerve fibers control dilation of blood vessels. Afferent nerve fibers transmit pain signals experienced by clients who have primary lesions of the bone.

Function

The skeletal system:

- Provides a framework for the body and allows the body to be weight bearing, or upright
- Supports the surrounding tissues (e.g., muscle and tendons)
- Assists in movement through muscle attachment and joint formation
- Protects vital organs, such as the heart and lungs
- Manufactures blood cells in red bone marrow
- Provides storage for mineral salts (e.g., calcium and phosphorus)

Growth and Metabolism

After puberty, bone reaches its maturity and maximal growth. Bone is a dynamic tissue, however, that undergoes a continuous process of formation and resorption, or destruction, at equal rates until the age of 35 years. In later years, bone resorption accelerates, decreasing bone mass and predisposing clients to injury. (See Chapter 54 for a discussion of the effects of aging on bone metabolism.)

Numerous minerals and hormones, including the following, affect bone growth and metabolism:

- Calcium
- Phosphorus
- Calcitonin
- Vitamin D
- Parathyroid hormone (PTH)
- Growth hormone
- Glucocorticoids
- Estrogens and androgens
- Thyroxine
- Insulin

CALCIUM AND PHOSPHORUS

Bone accounts for about 99% of the calcium in the body and 90% of the phosphorus. The serum concentrations of calcium and phosphorus maintain an inverse relationship; for example, as calcium levels rise, phosphorus levels decrease. When serum levels of calcium and phosphorus are altered, calcitonin and PTH work to maintain equilibrium. If the calcium level of the blood is decreased, the bone, which stores calcium, releases calcium into the vascular system in response to PTH stimulation.

CALCITONIN

Calcitonin is produced by the thyroid gland and *decreases* the serum calcium concentration if it is increased above its normal level. Calcitonin inhibits bone resorption and increases renal excretion of calcium and phosphorus as needed to maintain equilibrium.

VITAMIN D

Vitamin D and its metabolites are produced in the body and transported in the blood to promote the absorption of calcium and phosphorus from the small intestine. They also seem to enhance PTH activity in the release of calcium from the bone. A decrease in the body's vitamin D level can result in osteomalacia in the adult. An external source of vitamin D may be given to clients at risk for or diagnosed with osteomalacia. Vitamin D metabolism and osteomalacia are detailed in Chapter 54.

PARATHYROID HORMONE

When serum calcium levels are lowered, parathyroid hormone (PTH, or parathormone) secretion increases and stimulates bone to promote osteoclastic activity and *release* calcium to the blood. PTH reduces the renal excretion of calcium and facilitates its absorption from the intestine. Conversely, when serum calcium levels increase, PTH secretion diminishes to preserve the bone calcium supply; this is an example of the feedback loop system of the endocrine system.

GROWTH HORMONE

Growth hormone secreted by the anterior lobe of the pituitary gland is responsible for increasing bone length and determining the amount of bone matrix formed before puberty. During childhood, an increased secretion results in gigantism, and a decreased secretion results in dwarfism. In the adult, an increase causes acromegaly, which is characterized by bone and soft-tissue deformities (see Chapter 66).

GLUCOCORTICOIDS

Adrenal glucocorticoids regulate protein metabolism, either increasing or decreasing catabolism to reduce or intensify the organic matrix of bone. They also aid in regulating intestinal calcium and phosphorus absorption.

ESTROGENS AND ANDROGENS

Estrogens stimulate osteoblastic activity and inhibit PTH. When estrogen levels decline at menopause, women are susceptible to low serum calcium levels with subsequent bone loss (osteoporosis). Androgens, such as testosterone, promote anabolism and increase bone mass. External sources of estrogen and testosterone may be prescribed for clients at risk for or diagnosed with osteoporosis.

THYROXINE AND INSULIN

Thyroxine is one of the principal hormones secreted by the thyroid gland. Its primary function is to increase the rate of protein synthesis in all types of tissue, including bone. Insulin works together with growth hormone to build and maintain healthy bone tissue.

JOINTS

A **joint** is a space in which two or more bones come together. This is also referred to as *articulation* of the joint. The primary function of a joint is to provide movement and flexibility in the body.

Types

There are three types of joints in the body:

- Synarthrodial, or completely immovable, joints (e.g., in the cranium)
- Amphiarthrodial, or slightly movable, joints (e.g., in the pelvis)
- Diarthrodial (synovial), or freely movable, joints (e.g., the elbow and knee)

Although any of these joints can be affected by disease or injury, the diarthrodial joints are most commonly involved.

Structure and Function

The **diarthrodial,** or **synovial, joint** is the most common type of joint in the body. Synovial joints are so named because they are the only type lined with synovium, a membrane that secretes synovial fluid for lubrication and shock absorption. As illustrated in Figure 53-2, the synovium lines the internal portion of the joint capsule but does not normally extend onto the surface of the cartilage at the spongy bone ends. Articular cartilage consists of a collagen fiber matrix impregnated with a complex ground substance. Clients with inflammatory types of arthritis often have synovitis (synovial inflammation) and breakdown of the cartilage. **Bursae,** small sacs lined with synovial membrane, are located at joints and bony prominences to prevent friction between bone and structures adjacent to bone. These structures can also become inflamed, causing bursitis.

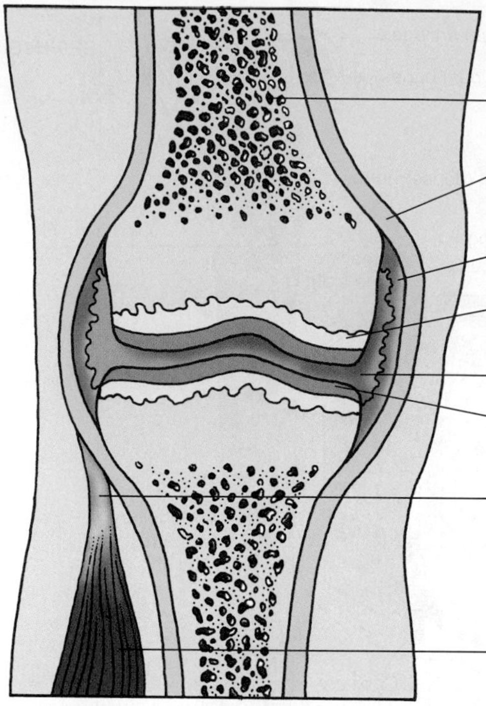

Figure 53-2 ■ The structure of a diarthrodial joint. Synovium lines the joint capsule but does not extend into the articular cartilage.

Animations: Joints

Synovial joints are subtyped by their anatomic structures. *Ball-and-socket* joints (shoulder, hip) permit movement in any direction. *Hinge* joints (elbow) allow motion in one plane, flexion, and extension. The knee is often classified as a hinge joint, but it rotates slightly, as well as flexes and extends. It is best described as a *condylar* type of synovial joint. The gliding movement of the wrist is characteristic of the *biaxial* joint. *Pivot* joints permit rotation only, as in the radioulnar area.

Muscular System

There are three types of muscle in the body: smooth muscle, cardiac muscle, and skeletal muscle. Smooth, or nonstriated, involuntary muscle is responsible for contractions of organs and blood vessels and is controlled by the autonomic nervous system. Cardiac muscle, or striated, involuntary muscle is also controlled by the autonomic nervous system. The smooth and cardiac muscles are discussed with the body systems to which they belong in the assessment chapters.

Structure

In contrast to smooth and cardiac muscle, skeletal muscle is **striated**, voluntary muscle controlled by the central and peripheral nervous systems. The junction of a peripheral motor nerve and the muscle cells that it supplies is sometimes referred to as a motor end plate. Muscle fibers are held in place by connective tissue in bundles, or fasciculi. The entire mus-

CHART 53-1

NURSING FOCUS on the OLDER ADULT

Changes in the Musculoskeletal System Related to Aging

Physiologic Change	Nursing Interventions	Rationales
Decreased bone density	Teach safety tips to prevent falls. Reinforce need to exercise, especially weight-bearing exercise.	Porous bones are more likely to fracture. Exercise slows bone loss.
Increased bone prominence	Prevent pressure on bone prominences.	There is less soft tissue to prevent skin breakdown.
Kyphotic posture: widened gait, shift in the center of gravity	Teach proper body mechanics; instruct the client to sit in supportive chairs with arms.	Correction of posture problems prevents further deformity; the client should have support for bony structures.
Cartilage degeneration	Provide moist heat, such as a shower or warm, moist compresses.	Moist heat increases blood flow to the area.
Decreased ROM	Assess the client's ability to perform ADLs and mobility.	The client may need assistance with self-care skills.
Muscle atrophy, decreased strength	Teach isometric exercises.	Exercises increase muscle strength.
Slowed movement	Do not rush the client; be patient.	The client may become frustrated if hurried.

ROM, Range of motion; *ADLs*, activities of daily living.

cle is surrounded by dense, fibrous tissue, or fascia, which contains the muscle's blood, lymph, and nerve supply.

Function

The primary function of skeletal muscle is movement of the body and its parts. When bones, joints, and supporting structures are adversely affected by injury or disease, the adjacent muscle tissue is often involved, limiting mobility. During the aging process, muscle fibers decrease in size and number, even in well-conditioned people. Atrophy results when muscles are not regularly exercised, and they deteriorate from disuse.

Supporting Structures

In addition to the articular cartilage of joints, several types of cartilage occur in other areas. *Costal* cartilage connects the sternum to the rib cage. *Hyaline* cartilage is in the septum of the nose, larynx, and trachea. The external ear and epiglottis contain *yellow* cartilage. In all areas, the tissue is flexible and elastic and can withstand enormous tension.

Other important supporting structures that are susceptible to injury include **tendons** (bands of tough, fibrous tissue that attach muscles to bones) and **ligaments,** which attach bones to other bones at joints.

Musculoskeletal Changes Associated with Aging

As one ages, bone density often decreases, causing postural changes and predisposing a person to fractures (osteoporosis). Synovial joint cartilage can become less elastic and compressible as a person ages. As a result of these cartilage changes and continued use of joints, trauma to the joint cartilage can occur. The result is sometimes described as osteoarthritis (OA); however, genetic defects in cartilage may contribute to joint disease. The most common joints affected are the weight-bearing joints of the hip, knee, and cervical and lumbar spine, but joints in the shoulder and upper extremity, feet and hands can be affected. Refer to Chapter 24 for a complete discussion of OA. Muscle tissue atrophy occurs, but increased activity and exercise can slow the progression of atrophy and restore muscle strength. Collectively, these changes cause decreased coordination, muscle strength loss, gait changes, and predisposition to falls with injury. Chart 53-1 lists the major anatomic and physiologic changes and suggested nursing interventions.

CULTURAL CONSIDERATIONS

The body proportions of African Americans differ from those of white individuals, Asian Americans, and Native Americans/American Indians. African-American men typically have denser bones than African American women. White women have the least amount of bone density of any group, which makes them more likely to have osteoporosis and fractures (Jarvis, 2004).

Many African Americans and some white individuals have a **lactose intolerance** (inability to convert lactose to glucose and galactose). Milk and dairy products are high in lactose, but are also rich in calcium, a bone-building mineral. Therefore, lactose-intolerant individuals need to obtain their calcium from other food sources, such as dark, green leafy vegetables.

ASSESSMENT TECHNIQUES

History

In the assessment of a client with an actual or potential musculoskeletal problem, a detailed history aids the nurse in identifying diagnoses and subsequent interventions (Chart 53-2).

DEMOGRAPHIC DATA

Young men are at the greatest risk for trauma related to motor vehicle crashes. Older adults are at the greatest risk for falls that result in fractures and soft-tissue injury (see Chapter 5).

FAMILY HISTORY AND GENETIC RISK

Certain disorders have a familial or genetic tendency. Osteoporosis (age-related bone loss), for instance, often occurs in several generations of a family, and bone cancer tends to

CHART 53-2

Musculoskeletal Assessment
USING GORDON'S FUNCTIONAL HEALTH PATTERNS

Activity-Exercise Pattern
- Do you have sufficient energy for desired/required activities?
- What is your exercise pattern? Type of exercise? Regularity?
- What spare time (leisure) activities do you engage in?
- What is your perceived ability for (code for level according to key below):

Feeding?	Level 0: Full self-care
Bathing?	Level I: Requires use of equipment or device
Toileting?	
Bed mobility?	Level II: Requires assistance or supervision of another person
Dressing?	
Grooming?	Level III: Requires assistance or supervision of another person and equipment or device
General mobility?	
Cooking?	
Home maintenance?	Level IV: Is dependent and does not participate
Shopping?	

Cognitive-Perceptual Pattern
- Do you experience any discomfort?
- Do you have pain? If so, how do you manage it?
- What is the easiest way for you to learn things?
- Do you have any difficulty learning?

Based on Gordon, M. (2002). *Manual of nursing diagnosis* (10th ed.). St. Louis: Mosby.

be genetically linked. The risk for osteoarthritis may also be strongly linked to genetic factors. Chapters 24 and 54 provide a more complete description of musculoskeletal disease processes that have strong genetic links.

PERSONAL HISTORY

Accidents, illnesses, lifestyle and medications may relate to a client's current problem. When taking a personal health history, question the client about current level of physical activity, all traumatic injuries, participation in sports and sports injuries, regardless of the date of occurrence. An injury to the lumbar spine 30 years previously may contribute to a client's current complaint of low back pain. A motor vehicle accident or sports injury can be the cause of osteoarthritis years after the event.

Previous or concurrent diseases may affect musculoskeletal status. For example, a client with diabetes who is treated for a foot ulcer is at high risk for acute or chronic osteomyelitis (bone infection). In addition, diabetes slows the healing process. It is also important to determine a history of previous hospitalizations and illnesses or complications.

Ask about previous and current use of medications. Some drugs, such as steroids, can affect calcium metabolism and promote bone loss. Other drugs may be taken to relieve musculoskeletal pain. Inquire about herbal, vitamin and mineral supplements, or biologic compounds that may be used for arthritis and other musculoskeletal problems, such as glucosamine and chondroitin. Complementary and alternative therapies are commonly employed by clients with various types of arthritis and arthralgias (joint aching) (see Chapter 24).

DIET HISTORY

An evaluation of the client's diet history will help determine any risks of inadequate nutrition. For example, most people, especially women, do not consume adequate amounts of calcium. Asking a client for a recall of a typical day of food intake helps identify deficiencies and excesses in the diet. Lactose intolerance is a common problem and can affect adequate calcium intake. People who cannot afford to buy food are especially at risk for undernutrition.

Inadequate protein or insufficient vitamin C or D in the diet inhibits healing of bone and tissue. Obesity places excess stress and strain on bones and joints, with resultant fractures and trauma to joint cartilage. In addition, obesity inhibits mobility in clients with musculoskeletal problems, which predisposes them to complications such as respiratory and circulatory problems.

SOCIOECONOMIC STATUS

When assessing a client with a possible musculoskeletal alteration, inquire about lifestyle. A person's occupation can cause or contribute to an injury. For instance, fractures are not uncommon in clients whose jobs require manual labor, such as housekeepers and mechanics. Certain occupations, such as computer-related jobs, may predispose a person to carpal tunnel syndrome (entrapment of the median nerve in the wrist). Construction workers and health care workers may experience back injury from prolonged standing and excessive lifting. Amateur and professional athletes often experience acute musculoskeletal injuries, such as joint dislocations and fractures, or chronic disorders, such as joint cartilage trauma, which can lead to osteoarthritis.

Socioeconomic status may be related to the client's occupation and therefore affect the likelihood of musculoskeletal problems. For example, an executive working in an office is less likely to sustain a musculoskeletal injury than is a painter or roofer engaged in manual labor and activities such as climbing ladders.

CURRENT HEALTH PROBLEMS

Collect data pertinent to the client's presenting complaint as follows:

- Date and time of onset
- Factors that cause or exacerbate (worsen) the problem
- Course of the problem (e.g., intermittent or continuous)
- Clinical manifestations (as expressed by the client) and the pattern of their occurrence
- Measures that improve clinical manifestations (e.g., heat)

The most common complaint of people with musculoskeletal problems is pain. The pain may be acute or chronic, depending on its onset and duration. Use the PQRST model or other tool to elicit a complete assessment of the client's pain:

P Provoking incident? (Was there a certain incident or event that precipitated the pain or caused an exacerbation of the pain?)

Q Quality of pain? (What does the pain feel like in descriptive terms? For example, is it burning, throbbing, stabbing?)

R Region, radiation, and relief? (Exactly where is the pain located? Does the pain travel or radiate? Does anything help relieve the pain?)

S Severity of the pain? (How severe is the pain? The client may use a pain scale [see Chapter 7] or describe how the pain has interfered with his or her ability to function.)

T Time? (How long does the pain last? When does it occur? Is it worse at night or during the day? If the pain awakens a person at night, the source of the pain is most likely inflammatory, not degenerative.)

With any pain assessment, it is always best if the client describes the pain in his or her own words and points to its location, if possible.

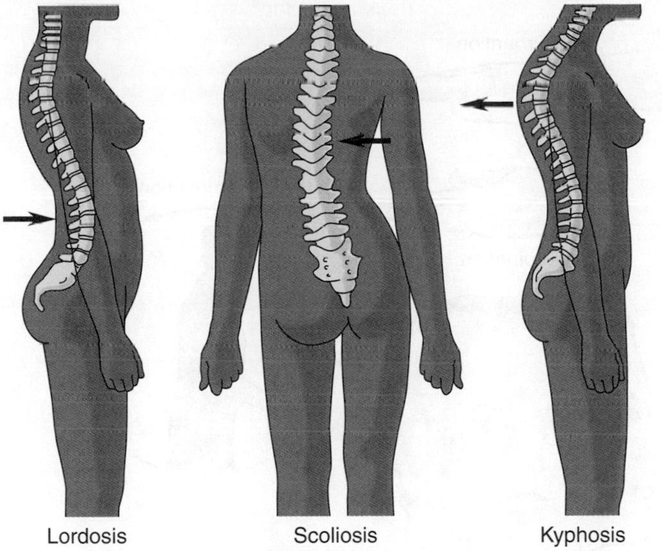

Figure 53-3 ■ Common spinal deformities.

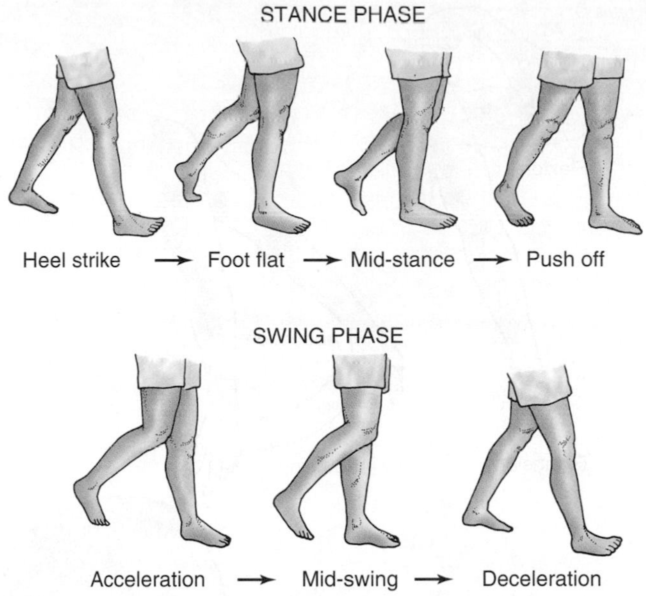

Figure 53-4 ■ The phases of gait.

Physical Assessment

Although bones, joints, and muscles are usually assessed simultaneously in a head-to-toe approach, each subsystem is described separately for emphasis and understanding. For physical assessment of the musculoskeletal system, the nurse incorporates inspection, palpation, range of motion (ROM), which may be active (AROM) or passive (PROM), and special techniques for specific problems. A general assessment is described in this chapter. More specific assessment techniques are discussed in the interventions chapters that follow for each musculoskeletal problem.

ASSESSMENT OF THE SKELETAL SYSTEM

General Inspection

Observe the client's posture, gait, and general mobility for gross deformities and impairment. Note unusual findings and collaborate with the physical or occupational therapist for an in-depth physical assessment.

POSTURE

Posture includes the person's body build and alignment when standing and walking. Assess the curvature of the spine and the length, shape, and symmetry of extremities. Figure 53-3 illustrates some common spinal deformities. Muscle mass is also inspected for size and symmetry.

GAIT

Video Clip: Gait

Most clients with musculoskeletal problems eventually have a problem with gait. The two phases of normal, automatic gait are the stance phase and the swing phase (Figure 53-4).

The nurse or therapist evaluates the client's balance, steadiness, and ease and length of stride; any limp or other asymmetric leg movement or deformity is noted. An abnormality in the stance phase of gait is called an **antalgic** gait. When part of one leg is painful, the person shortens the stance phase on the affected side. An abnormality in the swing phase is called a **lurch**. This abnormal gait occurs when the muscles in the buttocks and/or legs are too weak to allow the person to change weight from one foot to the other. In this case, the shoulders are moved either side-to-side or front-to-back for help in shifting the weight from one leg to the other. Some clients, such as those with chronic hip pain and muscle atrophy from arthritic disorders, have a combination of an antalgic gait and lurch.

MOBILITY

In collaboration with the physical or occupational therapist, monitor the client's need for or use of ambulatory devices, such as canes and walkers, during transfer from bed to chair and while walking and climbing stairs. Assess mobility by asking the client to perform activities of daily living (ADLs) such as dressing and bathing. Pain and deformity may limit physical mobility and function. A complete discussion of functional assessment is found in Chapter 10.

After performing a functional assessment, assess major bones, joints, and muscles by inspection, palpation, and determination of ROM. Pay special attention to areas that are affected or may be affected, according to the client's history or current complaint.

A **goniometer** is a tool that may be used by physical therapists or nurses to provide an exact measurement of ROM. Active range of motion (AROM) can be evaluated by asking the client to move each joint through the ROM himself or herself. If a client is unable to actively move a joint through range of motion, ask the client to relax the muscles in the extremity. Hold the part with one hand above and one hand below the joint to be evaluated and allow passive range of motion to evaluate joint mobility. Movements shown in Figure 53-5 may be used to evaluate active and passive ROM. Circumduction is a movement that can also be evaluated in the shoulder by having the client move the arm in circles from the shoulder joint. As long as the client can function to meet personal needs, a limitation in ROM may not be significant. For each anatomic location, the skin is observed for color, elasticity, and lesions that may relate to musculoskeletal dysfunction. This also includes inspection of skin over bony prominences.

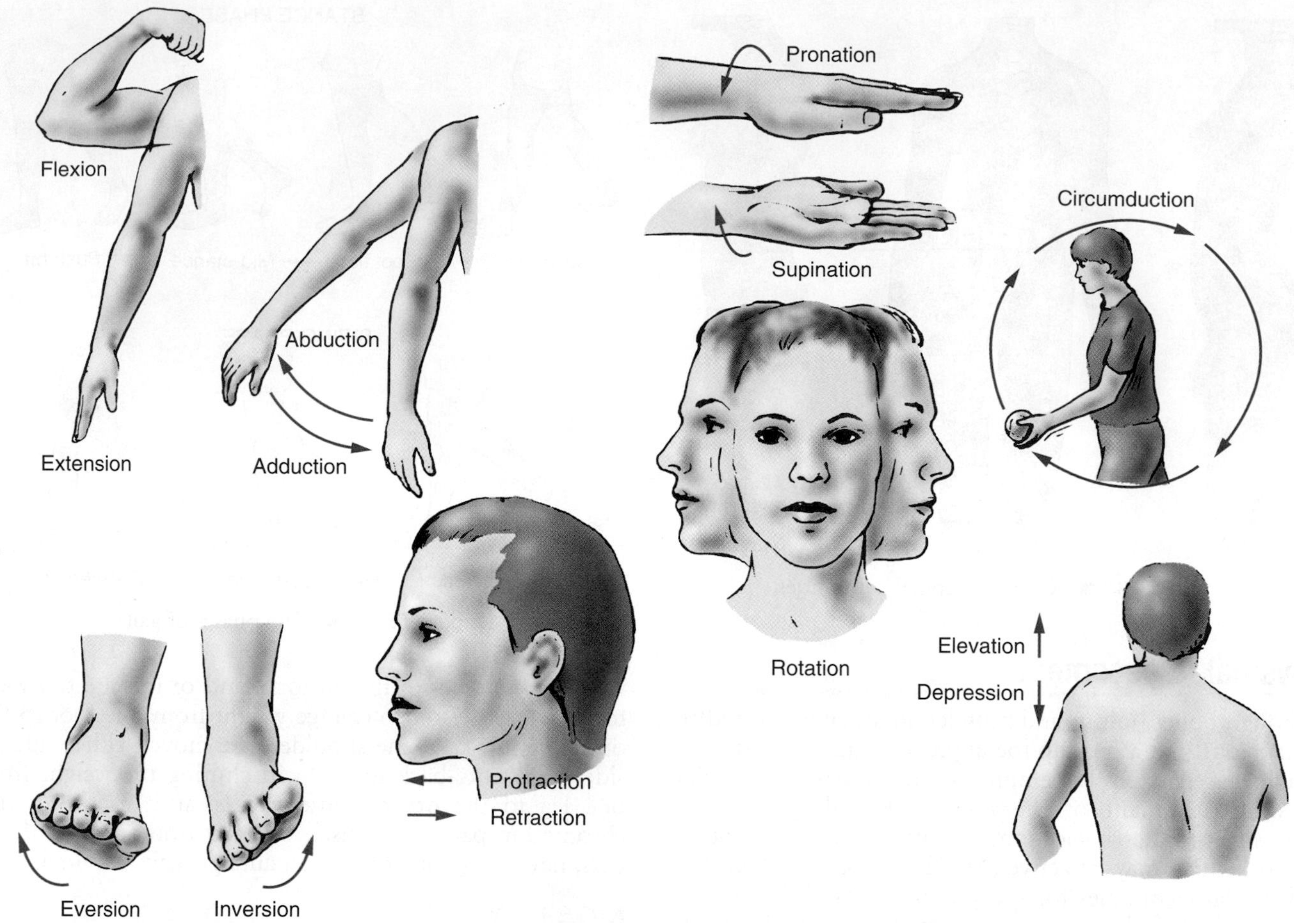

Figure 53-5 ■ Movements of the skeletal muscles. (Modified from Jarvis, C. [2000]. Physical examination and health assessment [3rd ed.]. Philadelphia: W. B. Saunders.)

Assessment of the Head and Neck

Inspect and palpate the skull for shape, symmetry, tenderness, and masses. The temporomandibular joints (TMJs) are best evaluated by palpation. Ask the client to open his or her mouth while palpating the TMJs. Common abnormal findings are tenderness or pain, **crepitus** (a grating sound), and a spongy swelling caused by excess synovium and fluid.

Then inspect and palpate each vertebra of the spine in the neck. Clinical findings may include malalignment; tenderness; or inability to flex, extend, and rotate the neck as expected.

Assessment of the Spine

The thoracic spine, lumbar spine, and sacral spine are evaluated in the same manner as the neck. Spinal alignment problems are common (see Figure 53-3). Place both hands over the lumbosacral area and apply pressure with the thumbs along the spine to elicit tenderness. Many clients do not complain of discomfort until the area is palpated. **Lordosis** is a common finding in pregnancy and in abdominal obesity. During screening for **scoliosis**, ask the client to flex forward from the hips and inspect for a lateral curve in the spine.

Assessment of the Upper Extremities

Assess both extremities at the same time. For example, both shoulders are inspected and palpated for size, swelling, deformity, malalignment, tenderness or pain, and mobility. A shoulder injury may prevent the client from combing his or her hair with the affected arm, but severe arthritis may inhibit movement in both arms. Assess the elbows and wrists in a similar way.

Because the hand has multiple joints in a single digit, assessment of hand function is perhaps the most critical part of the examination. Inspect and palpate the metacarpophalangeal (MCP), proximal interphalangeal (PIP), and distal interphalangeal (DIP) joints. The same digits are compared on the right and left hands (Figure 53-6). Determine the range of motion (ROM) for each joint by observing active movement. If movement is not possible, evaluate passive motion. For a quick and easy assessment of ROM, the client is asked to make a fist and then appose each finger to the thumb. If he or she can perform these maneuvers, ROM of the hand is not seriously restricted.

Assessment of the Lower Extremities

Evaluation of the hip joint relies primarily on determination of its degree of mobility, because the joint is deep and difficult to inspect or palpate. The client with hip pain usually experiences pain in the *groin* area, or the pain may radiate to the knee. The knee is readily accessible for nursing assessment, particularly when the client is sitting and the knee is flexed. Fluid accumulation, or **effusion**, is easily detected in the knee joint; limitations in movement with accompanying pain are common findings. The knees may be maligned, as

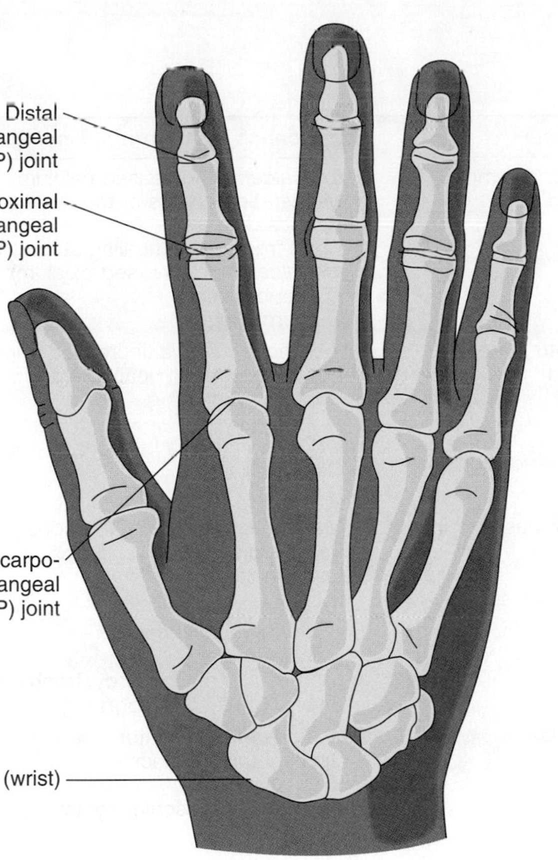

Figure 53-6 ■ The small joints of the hand.

in **genu valgum** ("knock-knee") or **genu varum** ("bow-legged") deformities.

The ankles and feet are often neglected in the physical examination; however, they contain multiple bones and joints that can be affected by disease and injury. Observe and palpate each joint and test for ROM.

Neurovascular Assessment

While completing a physical assessment of the musculoskeletal system, it is important to include assessment of peripheral vascular and peripheral nerve integrity. As with other physical assessment, always compare one extremity to the other, beginning with the injured side. Neurovascular assessment includes inspection of skin color, temperature, and capillary refill distal to an injury or cast. Palpation of pulses in the extremities below level of injury and assessment of sensation, movement, and pain in the injured part give a complete neurovascular assessment. If pulses are not palpable, a Doppler should be used to evaluate pulses in the extremities. See Chart 55-3 for more detail of neurovascular assessment.

▶ Video Clips: Muscular Development and Strength

ASSESSMENT OF THE MUSCULAR SYSTEM

During the skeletal assessment, evaluate the size, shape, tone, and strength of major skeletal muscles. The circumference of each muscle may be measured and compared symmetrically for an estimation of muscle mass.

In addition to inspecting and palpating the skeletal muscles, ask the client to demonstrate muscle strength. For instance, to determine grip strength, ask the client to squeeze a sphygmomanometer (blood pressure cuff) bulb to record the level of pressure achieved. This method provides a precise measurement that can be used to observe improvement or deterioration of muscle ability. In another method, apply resistance by holding the extremity and asking the client to move against resistance. For example, place your hands on the client's upper arms and ask the client to try to raise the arms. Although movement against resistance is not easily quantified, several scales are available for grading the client's strength. A commonly used scale is delineated in Table 53-1.

TABLE 53-1 Lovett's Scale for Grading Muscle Strength

Rating	Description
5	Normal: ROM unimpaired against gravity with full resistance
4	Good: can complete ROM against gravity with some resistance
3	Fair: can complete ROM against gravity
2	Poor: can complete ROM with gravity eliminated
1	Trace: no joint motion and slight evidence of music contractility
0	Zero: no evidence of muscle contractility

ROM, Range of motion.

Psychosocial Assessment

The data from the history and physical examination provide clues for the nurse in anticipating psychosocial problems. For instance, the client with multiple fractures who requires extensive immobilization and therapy is at high risk for sensory deprivation. Prolonged absence from employment or permanent disability may cause the client to lose his or her job or occupation. Further stress may be experienced if chronic pain ensues and he or she cannot cope with numerous stressors simultaneously. Deformities resulting from musculoskeletal disease or injury can affect a person's body image and self-concept. Assessment of a client's support systems and coping mechanisms from previous stressful situations will assist in planning for possible stressors that may occur with a current injury or illness.

Diagnostic Assessment

LABORATORY TESTS

Chart 53-3 lists the common laboratory tests used in assessing clients with musculoskeletal disorders. There is no special client preparation or follow-up care for any of these tests. Teach the client the purpose of the test and the procedure that can be expected. Additional tests performed for clients with connective tissue diseases, such as rheumatoid arthritis, are described in Chapter 24.

Serum Calcium and Phosphorus

The concentrations of calcium and phosphorus, or phosphate (inorganic phosphorus), have an inverse relationship. In a healthy state, when the calcium level decreases, the phosphorus level increases, and vice versa. Disorders of bone and the parathyroid gland are often reflected in an alteration of the serum calcium or phosphorus level.

CHART 53-3

LABORATORY PROFILE
Musculoskeletal Assessment

Test	Normal Range for Adults	Significance of Abnormal Findings
Serum calcium	9.0-10.5 mg/dL (2.25-2.75 mmol/L) *Older adults:* decreased	*Hypercalcemia* (increased calcium) ■ Metastatic cancers of the bone ■ Paget's disease ■ Bone fractures in healing stage *Hypocalcemia* (decreased calcium) ■ Osteoporosis ■ Osteomalacia
Serum phosphorus	3.0-4.5 mg/dL (0.97-1.45 mmol/L) *Older adults:* decreased	*Hyperphosphatemia* (increased phosphorus) ■ Bone fractures in healing stage ■ Bone tumors ■ Acromegaly *Hypophosphatemia* (decreased phosphorus) ■ Osteomalacia
Alkaline phosphatase (ALP)	30-120 units/L *Older adults:* slightly increased	*Elevations* may indicate: ■ Metastatic cancers of the bone ■ Paget's disease ■ Osteomalacia
Serum muscle enzymes		
Creatine kinase (CK)	Total CK: *Men:* 55-170 units/L *Women:* 30-135 units/L	*Elevations* may indicate: ■ Muscle trauma ■ Progressive muscular dystrophy ■ Effects of electromyography
Lactate dehydrogenase (LDH)	Total LDH: 100-190 units/L *LDH_1:* 17%-27% *LDH_2:* 27%-37% *LDH_3:* 18%-25% *LDH_4:* 3%-8% *LDH_5:* 0% to 5%	*Elevations* may indicate: ■ Skeletal muscle necrosis ■ Extensive cancer ■ Progressive muscular dystrophy
Aspartate aminotransferase (AST)	0-35 units/L *Older adults:* increased	*Elevations* may indicate: ■ Skeletal muscle trauma ■ Progressive muscular dystrophy
Aldolase (ALD)	3.0-8.2 units/dL	*Elevations* may indicate: ■ Polymyositis and dermatomyositis ■ Muscular dystrophy

Alkaline Phosphatase

Alkaline phosphatase (ALP) is an enzyme normally present in blood. The concentration of ALP increases with bone or liver damage. In metabolic bone disease and bone cancer, the enzyme concentration rises in proportion to the osteoblastic activity, which indicates bone formation. The level of ALP is normally slightly increased in older adults.

Serum Muscle Enzymes

The major muscle enzymes affected in skeletal muscle disease or injuries are as follows:

- Creatine kinase (CK-MM)
- Aspartate aminotransferase (AST)
- Aldolase (ALD)
- Lactic dehydrogenase (LDH)

As a result of damage, the muscle tissue releases additional amounts of these enzymes, which increases serum levels.

The serum CK level begins to rise 2 to 4 hours after muscle injury and is elevated early in muscle disease, such as muscular dystrophy. The CK molecule has two subunits: M (muscle) and B (brain). Three isoenzymes have been identified. Skeletal muscle CK (CK-MM, or CK_3) is the only isoenzyme that rises in concentration with damage to skeletal muscle.

AST is moderately elevated (three to five times normal) in certain muscle diseases, such as muscular dystrophy and dermatomyositis. The levels of the isoenzymes aldolase A (ALD-A) and LDH_5 also increase in clients with these disorders.

RADIOGRAPHIC EXAMINATIONS

Standard Radiography

The skeleton is readily visible on standard x-rays. Anteroposterior and lateral projections are the initial screening views. Other approaches, such as oblique or stress views, depend on the part of the skeleton to be evaluated and the necessity of the x-ray.

Observations of bone density, alignment, swelling, and intactness are made. The conditions of joints can be determined, including the size of the joint space, the smoothness of articular cartilage, and synovial swelling. Soft-tissue involvement may be evident but not clearly differentiated.

Inform the client that the x-ray table is hard and cold and instruct him or her to remain still during the filming process.

Tomography and Xeroradiography

Whereas standard x-rays superimpose one structure on another, **tomography** produces planes, or slices, for focus and blurs the images of other structures. This procedure is helpful in detailing the musculoskeletal system, because the many close structures make visualization difficult.

Xeroradiography highlights the contrast between structures. Margins and edges can be clearly seen (edge enhancement). Disadvantages of xeroradiography are the higher radiation dose to the client and inability of xeroradiography to determine tissue densities.

Myelography

Myelography involves the injection of contrast medium, or dye, into the subarachnoid space of the spine, usually by spinal puncture. The vertebral column, intervertebral disks, spinal nerve roots, and blood vessels can be visualized. Although this test is still performed, it is far less popular; computed tomography (CT) and magnetic resonance imaging (MRI) have often replaced such invasive, and potentially painful, diagnostic techniques. The post-test care is similar to that for lumbar puncture, except that the client is usually placed in a sitting position to prevent the contrast medium from getting into the brain. (See Chapter 44.)

Arthrography

An **arthrogram** is an x-ray study of a joint after contrast medium (air or solution) has been injected to enhance its visualization. Double-contrast arthrography, which uses both air and contrast, may be performed when a traumatic injury is suspected. The physician can often determine bone chips, torn ligaments, or other loose bodies within the joint.

The most common joints studied are the knee and the shoulder. The client is questioned about allergy to contrast media. Most joints are now studies by magnetic resonance imaging.

Computed Tomography

Computed tomography (CT) has gained wide acceptance for the detection of musculoskeletal problems, particularly those of the vertebral column. The scanned images can be used to create additional images from other angles or to create three-dimensional images, and therefore view complex structures from any position. CT scans may be requested with intravenous (IV) contrast if tumor or postsurgical changes are suspected. The nurse or radiology technologist should ask the client about iodine-based contrast allergies. The current class of CT scans takes less than 20 minutes per body part. Because scanners are faster, claustrophobia (fear of small spaces) is rarely an issue.

Critical Thinking Challenge

An older adult comes to the oncology clinic for follow-up of her treatment for breast cancer. She has been experiencing severe lower back pain for the past 2 weeks. The physician suspects metastatic cancer to her bone.

1. What assessment should you perform at this time? Consider a complete assessment, including interview, physical assessment, and psychosocial assessment.
2. For the following laboratory values, what changes might you expect in this client and why?
   Alkaline phosphatase
   Calcium
   Phosphorus
3. What other diagnostic assessment would you anticipate the physician to request?

evolve For suggested answer guidelines, go to http://evolve.elsevier.com/Iggy/.

OTHER DIAGNOSTIC TESTS

Bone and Muscle Biopsy

In a **bone biopsy**, the physician extracts a specimen of bone for microscopic examination. This invasive test may confirm the presence of infection or neoplasm, but it is not commonly done today. One of two techniques may be used to retrieve the specimen: needle (closed) biopsy or incisional (open) biopsy.

Muscle biopsy is done for the diagnosis of atrophy (as in muscular dystrophy) and inflammation (as in polymyositis). The procedure and care for clients undergoing muscle biopsy are the same as those for clients undergoing bone biopsy.

Electromyography

Electromyography (EMG) is usually accompanied by nerve conduction studies for determining the electrical potential generated in an individual muscle. EMG helps in the diagnosis of neuromuscular, lower motor neuron, and peripheral nerve disorders.

CLIENT PREPARATION. Inform the client that EMG may cause temporary discomfort, especially when the client is subjected to episodes of electrical current. For selected clients, mild sedation is prescribed. The physician may also prescribe a temporary discontinuation of skeletal muscle relaxants several days before the procedure to prevent medication from having effects on the test results.

PROCEDURE. The test may be performed at the bedside or in an EMG laboratory. When both EMG and nerve conduction studies are done, nerve conduction is usually tested first. Flat electrodes are placed along the nerve to be evaluated, and low electrical currents are passed through the electrodes to the nerve and muscle innervated. If nerve conduction is accomplished, the muscle contracts.

For testing muscle potential, multiple needle electrodes varying from ½ to 3 inches (1.3 to 7.5 cm) are inserted. The client may be asked to perform activities for measurement of muscle potential during minimal and maximal contraction. The degree of nerve and muscle activity is recorded on an oscilloscope, which provides a graphic readout for later interpretation.

FOLLOW-UP CARE. A few medical complications are associated with EMG. The nurse provides comfort measures and inspects the needle sites for hematoma formation. The application of ice can prevent this complication. The client may also complain of increased pain and anxiety after the test.

Arthroscopy

The **arthroscopy** may be used as a diagnostic test or a surgical procedure. An arthroscope is a fiberoptic tube inserted into a joint for direct visualization; the knee and shoulder are most commonly evaluated. In addition, synovial biopsy and surgical procedures to repair traumatic injury can be accomplished through the arthroscope.

CLIENT PREPARATION. Because the knee is most commonly "scoped," the care described for the client undergoing arthroscopy relates to that joint. Arthroscopy is performed on an ambulatory basis or as same-day surgery. Clients who cannot flex their knees at least 40 degrees or who have infected knees are not candidates for the procedure. The client must be able to flex the knee. Joint infection may worsen from the mechanical trauma of arthroscope insertion.

If the procedure is surgical, the client may have a physical therapy consultation before arthroscopy to learn the leg exercises that are necessary after the test. Straight-leg raises (SLRs) and quadriceps setting exercises (isometrics with the leg extended) are practiced in sets of 10 each. Range-of-motion (ROM) exercises are also taught but may not be allowed immediately after arthroscopic surgery. The nurse in the surgeon's office or at the surgical center can teach these exercises or reinforce the information provided by the physical therapist. The nurse also explains the procedure and post-test care.

PROCEDURE. The client is usually given local, light general, or epidural anesthesia, depending on the purpose of the procedure. In some settings, a large pneumatic tourniquet is used around the thigh to minimize bleeding during the procedure. Medications promoting vasoconstriction for control of bleeding may be used alone or in conjunction with the tourniquet.

The knee is flexed to at least 40 degrees, and the knee is irrigated. As shown in Figure 53-7, the arthroscope is inserted through a small incision less than ¼ inch (0.6 cm) long. Multiple incisions may be required to allow inspection at a variety of angles. After the procedure, a dressing may be applied, depending on the amount of manipulation during the test or surgery.

FOLLOW-UP CARE. Evaluate the neurovascular status of the client's affected limb frequently, in accordance with the nursing standard of care. Monitor distal pulses, warmth, color, capillary refill, pain, movement, and sensation of the affected extremity.

Encourage the client to perform exercises as taught before the examination, if appropriate. For the mild discomfort experienced after the diagnostic arthroscopy, the physician prescribes a mild analgesic, such as acetaminophen (Tylenol, Ace-Tabs✱). If postoperative, the client has short-term activity restrictions, depending on the musculoskeletal problem. Ice is often used for 24 hours, and the extremity should be elevated for 24 to 48 hours. When arthroscopic surgery is performed, the health care provider usually prescribes an opioid-analgesic combination, such as oxycodone and acetaminophen (Percocet, Tylox).

Although complications are not common, monitor and teach the client to observe for the following:

- Swelling
- Hypothermia (decreased body temperature) resulting from the use of the tourniquet during the procedure
- Increased joint pain attributable to mechanical injury
- Thrombophlebitis
- Infection

Severe joint or limb pain after discharge may indicate a possible complication and warrants that the client contacts the physician immediately. The health care provider may see the client about 1 week after the test to check for complications.

Bone Scan

The **bone scan** is a radionuclide test in which radioactive material is injected for visualization of the entire skeleton. It is used primarily to detect tumors, arthritis, osteomyelitis, osteoporosis, vertebral compression fractures, and unexplained bone pain. Bone scans are used less commonly today as magnetic resonance imaging (MRI) becomes more available. However, it is very useful for detecting hairline fractures in clients with unexplained bone pain and diffuse metastatic bone disease.

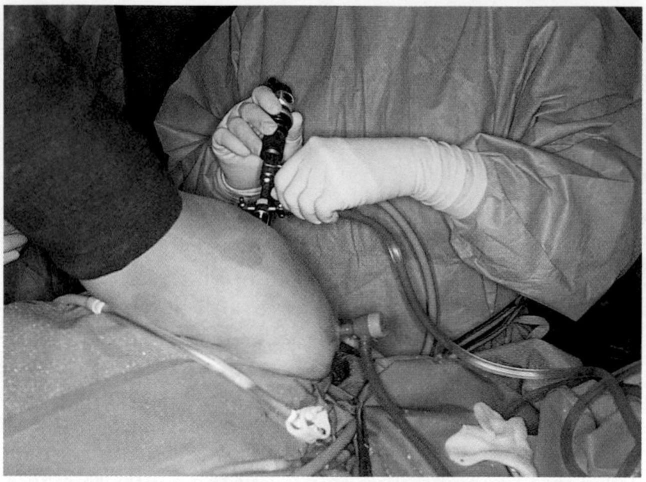

Figure 53-7 ■ An arthroscope is used in the diagnosis of pathologic changes in the joints. This client is undergoing arthroscopy of the shoulder.

Gallium/Thallium Scans

The **gallium** or **thallium scan** is similar to the bone scan but is more specific and sensitive in detecting bone problems. Gallium citrate (^{67}Ga) is the radioisotope most commonly used. This substance also migrates to brain, liver, and breast tissue and therefore is used in examination of these structures when disease is suspected.

For clients with osteosarcoma, thallium (^{201}Tl) is better than gallium or technetium for diagnosing the extent of the disease. Thallium has traditionally been used for the diagnosis of myocardial infarctions, but can be used for additional evaluation of cancers of the bone.

CLIENT PREPARATION. Because bone takes up gallium slowly, the nuclear medicine physician or technician administers the isotope 1 to 2 days before scanning. Other tests that require contrast media or other isotopes cannot be given during this time.

Instruct the client that the radioactive material poses no threat because it readily deteriorates in the body. Because gallium is excreted through the intestinal tract, it tends to collect in feces before the scanning procedure.

PROCEDURE. Depending on the tissue to be examined, the client is taken to the nuclear medicine department 1 to 2 days after injection. The procedure takes 30 to 60 minutes, during which time the client must lie still for accurate test results to be achieved. Mild sedation may be necessary to facilitate relaxation and cooperation during the procedure for confused older clients or those in severe pain.

FOLLOW-UP CARE. No special care is required after the test. The radioisotope is excreted in stool and urine, but no precautions are taken in handling the excreta. Encourage the client to push fluids to facilitate urinary excretion.

Magnetic Resonance Imaging

Magnetic resonance imaging (MRI), with or without the use of contrast media, can be used to diagnose musculoskeletal disorders. It is more accurate than computed tomography (CT) and myelography for many spinal and knee problems. MRI is most appropriate for joints, soft tissue, and bony tumors that involve soft tissue. CT is still the test of choice for injuries or pathology that involve only bone.

CHART 53-4
BEST PRACTICE for
The Client Preparing for Magnetic Resonance Imaging

- Is the client pregnant?
- Does the client have ferromagnetic fragments or implants, such as an older style aneurysm clip?
- Does the client have a pacemaker or electronic implant?
- Can the client lie still in the supine position for 45 to 60 minutes (may require sedation)?
- Does the client need life support equipment available?
- Can the client communicate clearly and understand verbal communication?

The image is produced through the interaction of magnetic fields, radio waves, and atomic nuclei showing hydrogen density. Simply put, the radio waves "bounce" off the body tissues being examined. Because each tissue has its own density, the computer image clearly distinguishes normal and abnormal tissues. For some tissues, the cross-sectional image is better than that produced by radiography or CT. The lack of hydrogen ions in cortical bone makes it easily distinguishable from soft tissues. The test is particularly useful in identifying problems with muscles, tendons, and ligaments.

Ensure that the client removes all metal objects and checks for clothing zippers and metal fasteners. Although joint implants made of titanium or stainless steel are safe, pacemakers and surgical clips are not. Chart 53-4 lists questions that the nurse or technician should consider in preparing the client for MRI. Open MRIs prevent the claustrophobia that occurs with the older, encased machines.

Gadolinium-DTPA (diethylenetriamine-pentaacetic acid) is the contrast agent approved for MRI. It is most commonly used to diagnose degenerative vertebral disease and recurrent disk herniation–sometimes referred to as the failed back surgery syndrome (Patel & Lauerman, 1997).

Ultrasonography

Sound waves produce an image of the tissue in ultrasonography. An ultrasound procedure may be used to visualize the following:

- Soft-tissue disorders, such as masses and fluid accumulation
- Traumatic joint injuries
- Osteomyelitis
- Surgical hardware placement

A jelly-like substance applied to the skin over the site to be examined promotes the movement of a metal probe. No special preparation or post-test care is necessary. A quantitative ultrasound (QUS) may be done for determining fractures or bone density.

Critical Thinking Challenge

A young male client complains of severe left knee pain following a ski trip last weekend. The orthopedic surgeon suspects damage to the meniscus and schedules the client for an arthroscopy.

1. As his office nurse, what health teaching will you need to provide to prepare the client for this procedure?
2. What immediate post-test care will the client require?
3. What discharge instructions will the postanesthesia care unit (PACU) nurse need to review?

evolve For suggested answer guidelines, go to http://evolve.elsevier.com/Iggy/.

GET READY for the NCLEX Examination!

KEY POINTS

Safe Effective Care Environment

- Be aware that older adults are at high risk for falls due to decreased bone density.
- Ask the client about allergy to iodine-based contrast media prior to diagnostic testing, such as computerized tomography (CT).
- Monitor the client for bleeding following an open bone biopsy.
- Assess the client to ensure that he or she is an appropriate candidate for magnetic resonance imaging; use the guidelines in Chart 53-4.

Health Promotion and Maintenance

- Teach clients to eat a diet sufficient in vitamin D, calcium, and protein to promote bone healing.
- Teach the client that mild discomfort can be expected during electromyography, a test to assess the electrical potential of muscles and their innervation.
- Instruct the client to report swelling, infection, and increased pain following an arthroscopy.

Psychosocial Integrity

- Assess the client's support systems and coping mechanisms when musculoskeletal trauma or disease affects his or her body image.
- Ask about the client's occupation because heavy, manual labor may cause back injury and other musculoskeletal trauma.

Physiological Integrity

- Assess the client's pain using the P-Q-R-S-T model.
- Assess the client's mobility, including gait, posture, and muscle strength.
- Interpret the client's laboratory values that are related to musculoskeletal disease (see Chart 53-3).
- Evaluate the neurovascular status of the client's affected extremity after an arthroscopic procedure.
- Encourage clients to drink additional fluids after tests that require contrast media or radioisotopes to help eliminate these substances.

ADDITIONAL STUDY RESOURCES

Go to your Student CD-ROM for Review Questions for the NCLEX Examination.

evolve Go to http://evolve.elsevier.com/Iggy/ for Integrated Management of Care Questions for the NCLEX Examination.

SELECTED BIBLIOGRAPHY

Asterisk indicates a classic or definitive work on this subject.

Gordon, M. (2002). *Manual of nursing diagnosis* (10th ed.). St. Louis: Mosby.

Jarvis, C. (2004). *Physical examination and health assessment* (3rd ed.). Philadelphia: W. B. Saunders.

Maher, A. B. (2002). Assessment of the musculoskeletal system. In A.B. Maher, S.W. Salmond, & T.A. Pellino (Eds.). *Orthopaedic nursing* (3rd ed.) Philadelphia: W. B. Saunders.

*Mangini, M. (1998). Physical assessment of the musculoskeletal system. *Nursing Clinics of North America, 33*(4), 643-652.
*Martsolf, D.S. (1999). Cultural aspects of orthopaedic nursing. *Orthopaedic Nursing, 18*(2), 65-71.
*Neal, L. (1997). Basic musculoskeletal assessment: Tips for the home health nurse. *Home Healthcare Nurse, 15*(4), 227-235.
*O'Hanlon-Nichols, T. (1998). Basic assessment series: A review of the adult musculoskeletal system. *American Journal of Nursing, 98*(6), 48-52.
Pagana, K.D., & Pagana, T.J. (2002). *Mosby's diagnostic and laboratory test reference* (2nd ed.). St. Louis: Mosby.
*Patel, P.R., & Lauerman, W.C. (1997). The use of magnetic resonance imaging in the diagnosis of lumbar disc disease. *Orthopaedic Nursing, 16*(1), 59-65.

CHAPTER 54

Interventions for Clients with Musculoskeletal Problems

CATHY A. MURRAY

LEARNING OUTCOMES

After studying this chapter, you should be able to:

1. Explain the risk factors for primary and secondary osteoporosis.
2. Implement interventions to decrease the risk for developing osteoporosis.
3. Develop a teaching plan for all age-groups concerning osteoporosis.
4. Describe the role of drug therapy in the prevention and management of osteoporosis.
5. Compare and contrast osteoporosis and osteomalacia.
6. Identify common assessment findings in clients with Paget's disease of the bone.
7. Differentiate acute and chronic osteomyelitis.
8. Prioritize care for clients with osteomyelitis.
9. Analyze assessment data to determine common nursing diagnoses and collaborative problems for the client with a malignant bone tumor.
10. Discuss the psychosocial aspects associated with a diagnosis of bone cancer.
11. Evaluate the nursing care of a client with a bone tumor using expected outcome criteria.
12. Explain the pathophysiology and risk factors for carpal tunnel syndrome.
13. Identify treatment options for the client diagnosed with carpal tunnel syndrome.
14. Describe common disorders of the foot, including hallux valgus and plantar fasciitis.
15. Explain the role of the nurse when caring for an adult client with muscular dystrophy.

Go to your Student CD-ROM for Review Questions for the NCLEX Examination keyed to these Learning Outcomes.

Musculoskeletal disorders include metabolic bone diseases, such as osteoporosis and Paget's disease, bone tumors and lesions, and a variety of deformities and syndromes. Whereas the older adult is at the greatest risk for the development of most of these health problems, young persons and adults can experience these musculoskeletal disorders. The incidence of bone cancer is increasing in both the younger and the older population. As technologic advances occur and clients survive longer with primary cancers, metastatic lesions become more prevalent. This chapter focuses on selected disorders not covered in Chapter 24 on arthritis and other connective tissue diseases.

METABOLIC BONE DISEASES

Osteoporosis

PATHOPHYSIOLOGY

Osteoporosis is a metabolic disease in which bone demineralization results in decreased density and subsequent fractures. Osteoporosis is often referred to as a "silent disease" because the first indication of osteoporosis in most persons follows some kind of a fracture. The wrist, hip, and vertebral column are most often affected (National Osteoporosis Foundation, 2003a).

TABLE 54-1 Causes of Secondary Osteoporosis

Diseases/Conditions
- Diabetes mellitus
- Hyperthyroidism
- Hyperparathyroidism
- Cushing's syndrome
- Growth hormone deficiency
- Metabolic acidosis
- Female hypogonadism
- Paget's disease
- Osteogenesis imperfecta
- Rheumatoid arthritis
- Prolonged immobilization
- Marfan syndrome
- Bone cancer
- Cirrhosis
- Chronic airway limitation

Drugs (Chronic Use)
- Corticosteroids
- Heparin
- Anticonvulsants
- Ethanol (alcohol)
- Drugs that induce hypogonadism (decreased levels of sex hormones)
- High levels of exogenous (external) thyroid hormone

Bone is a dynamic tissue that is constantly undergoing changes in a process referred to as bone remodeling. Osteoporosis and **osteopenia** (low bone mass) occur when there is a disruption in the bone remodeling process. This disruption can be described when **osteoclastic** (bone resorption) activity is greater than **osteoblastic** (bone building) activity. The result is a decreased **bone mineral density (BMD).** BMD determines bone strength and peaks between 30 and 35 years of age. Before and during the peak years, osteoclastic activity is followed by osteoblastic activity at a constant rate. After the peak years, bone resorption activity exceeds bone-building activity, and bone density decreases. BMD decreases rapidly in postmenopausal women as serum estrogen levels diminish. About 40% to 45% of a woman's bone mass is lost during her life span. **Trabecular**, or **cancellous** (spongy), bone is lost first, followed by loss of **cortical** (compact) bone. This results in thin, fragile bone tissue that is susceptible to fracture.

The World Health Organization (WHO) has developed a standard for osteoporosis diagnosis based on BMD values using T-scores. A T-score is obtained during dual-energy x-ray absorptiometry. A T-score is the number of standard deviations above or below the average BMD for young, healthy white women. **Osteopenia** is present when the T-score is between 1 and 2.5. **Osteoporosis** in postmenopausal women is defined as a BMD T-score more than 2.5 standard deviations below normal (or −2.5 or below) (National Institutes of Health, 2000).

The exact pathophysiology of osteoporosis is unclear, but two theories of disease development have been advocated. First, osteoporosis may result from decreased osteoblastic activity. The osteoblasts, or bone-forming cells, may have a shortened life span or may be less efficient in the client with osteoporosis. The second and more popular theory suggests an increase in osteoclastic (bone resorption) activity. The latter theory has gained increased recognition over the past decade and has resulted in treatment directed toward measures to prevent rapid bone resorption.

CHART 54-1

BEST PRACTICE for
Assessing Risk Factors for Primary Osteoporosis

Assess for the following:
- Client's age older than 60 years of age
- Family history of osteoporosis
- White or Asian race
- Thin, lean body build
- Low lifetime calcium intake
- Estrogen deficiency
- Androgen deficiency
- Smoking history
- High alcohol intake
- Lack of physical exercise or prolonged immobility

Classification of Osteoporosis

Osteoporosis can be classified as generalized or regional. **Generalized osteoporosis** involves many structures in the skeleton and is further divided into two categories, primary and secondary. *Primary* osteoporosis is more common and occurs in postmenopausal women and in men in their sixth or seventh decade of life. Estrogen presumably prevents or decreases the rate of bone resorption in women and is unavailable in sufficient quantities after menopause. Even though men do not experience the rapid bone loss that women experience after menopause, they do experience decreasing levels of testosterone and altered ability to absorb calcium. This results in a slower loss of bone mass in men, especially those over 75 years of age. *Secondary* osteoporosis results from an associated medical condition, such as hyperparathyroidism; long-term drug therapy, such as with corticosteroids; or prolonged immobility, such as that seen with spinal cord injury (Table 54-1). Treatment of the secondary type is directed toward the cause of the osteoporosis when possible.

Regional osteoporosis occurs when a limb is immobilized related to a fracture, injury, paralysis, or joint inflammation. Immobilization for periods of time greater than 8 to 12 weeks can result in this type of osteoporosis. Bone loss also occurs when persons spend prolonged time in a gravity-free or weightless environment.

Etiology and Genetic Risk

The exact cause of primary osteoporosis is unknown; however, numerous risk factors have been identified (Chart 54-1). About 98% of peak bone mass is achieved by around 20 years of age in most women. The rate of bone loss accelerates after menopause. These two factors together determine bone density. Building strong bone as a young person may be the best defense against osteoporosis in later adulthood (National Osteoporosis Foundation, 2003a). Young women need to be aware of appropriate health and lifestyle practices that can prevent this potentially disabling disease (see the Meeting Healthy People 2010 Objectives box on p. 1159). A nursing study by Berarducci et al. (2000) found that most health care providers focus on the risk of osteoporosis in women older than 50 years of age and do not assess risk as often in women 49 years of age and younger (see the Evidence-Based Practice for Nursing box on p. 1159).

Primary osteoporosis most often occurs in women after menopause as a result of decreased estrogen levels. Women

Meeting HEALTHY PEOPLE 2010 Objectives

OSTEOPOROSIS

Objective 2.10: Reduce the proportion of adults who are hospitalized for vertebral fractures associated with osteoporosis.

- Teach women of all ages about osteoporosis as a disease and cause of potentially life-threatening fractures.
- Teach young and middle-aged women the need to practice a lifestyle that reduces the risk factors for osteoporosis (e.g., no smoking, increased exercise, increased calcium intake).
- Teach middle-aged and older adults to have bone mineral density screening tests to determine their bone loss percentage (often available at no or minimal cost at local health fairs or pharmacies).
- Remind clients to use proper body mechanics, such as using large leg muscles rather than back muscles for lifting.
- If clients are at high risk for osteoporosis, tell them to avoid jarring activities such as jogging or horseback riding.
- If clients are at high risk for osteoporosis, tell them to consult with a health care provider and comply with preventive treatment.

EVIDENCE-BASED PRACTICE for Nursing

Do health care providers assess knowledge of osteoporosis in young women?

Berarducci, A., et al. (2000). Health-promoting educational practices related to osteoporosis. *Applied Nursing Research, 13*(4), 173-180.

This descriptive study was designed to determine whether health care providers educate women of all ages about osteoporosis, including assessing risk factors for the disease. The researchers surveyed 90 health care providers in southwest Florida. Forty-nine surveys were returned, and 47 were usable. The responses of the providers showed significant differences between women 49 years of age and younger and women older than 50 years of age. Health care providers routinely assessed risk factors in older women and educated these women, but they did not identify risk factors or provide education for younger women.

Level of Evidence: 6—Study sample is small and not randomized.

Critique. Although the sample size was small and the subjects constituted a convenience sample, this research is one of the few studies that address the issue of health promotion to prevent osteoporosis in young women. The study cannot be generalized and needs to be repeated using a larger sample in a larger geographic area.

Implications for Nursing. Nurses and other health care professionals in any setting have a responsibility to educate all women, regardless of age, about the risk factors for osteoporosis and how to reduce them. Other studies have supported the belief that lifestyle changes in young adulthood can prevent or minimize the risk for osteoporosis as women age.

lose about 2% of their bone mass every year in the first 5 years after menopause. For women of any age who cannot take estrogen replacement, such as breast cancer survivors, the risk of osteoporosis increases.

In addition, body build seems to predict the occurrence of the disease. Osteoporosis occurs more often in thin, lean-built white and Asian women, particularly those who do not exercise regularly. Obese women can store estrogen in their tissues for use as necessary to maintain a normal level of serum calcium. Exercise decreases bone resorption and stimulates bone formation. Immobilization, such as prolonged bedrest, produces rapid bone loss.

The relationship of osteoporosis to dietary factors is becoming more well-established. A diet deficient in calcium and vitamin D stimulates the parathyroid gland to produce parathyroid hormone (PTH). PTH triggers the release of calcium from the bony matrix. Malabsorption, caused by disease or drugs, also contributes to low serum calcium levels. Institutionalized or homebound people who are not exposed to sunlight may be at a higher risk because they do not receive adequate vitamin D for the metabolism of calcium.

Protein deficiency may contribute to the incidence of bone demineralization, although this theory is controversial. Because 50% of serum calcium is protein bound, protein is needed for calcium utilization; however, excessive protein intake may increase calcium loss in the urine. Protein is needed for bone healing when a fracture occurs.

Alcohol consumption and cigarette smoking are other possible risk factors. Although the exact mechanisms are not known, these substances may promote acidosis, which in turn increases bone loss. Alcohol also has a direct toxic effect on bone tissue, resulting in decreased bone formation and increased bone resorption (Leslie, 2000). Excessive caffeine intake can increase calcium loss in the urine.

Osteoporosis is also reported in persons who participate in excessive exercise or experience eating disorders, such as anorexia nervosa or bulimia. Excessive exercise and eating disorders can result in a low body mass index with resulting amenorrhea and estrogen deficiency in adolescents and young women.

Genetic factors may play a role for both men and women, but this hypothesis has not been confirmed (Orwell, 2000). Several of the suspected risk factors, such as body build, are determined in part by heredity. History of fracture in a first-degree relative may be a risk factor; however, heredity or a genetic influence alone probably is not predictive for osteoporosis.

Incidence/Prevalence

Osteoporosis is a major health problem in the United States and many countries. A World Congress on Osteoporosis was convened in 2000 to explore how to best prevent and treat this costly health problem. The estimated cost for osteoporosis-related health care in the United States alone was more than $17 billion in 2001 with continual cost increases each year (National Osteoporosis Foundation, 2003a).

Osteoporosis is a potential health problem for more than 44 million Americans. About 10 million persons have the disease and about 34 million persons 50 years of age and older experience osteopenia and are at risk for development of osteoporosis. Women remain the largest group affected by osteoporosis at about 80%, and 20% of men experience osteoporosis. Persons of all ethnic backgrounds are at risk (National Osteoporosis Foundation, 2003a).

Osteoporosis results in more than 1.5 million fractures each year, 300,000 of which are hip fractures. In people older than 90 years of age, one third of women and one fifth of men experience at least one hip fracture. The mortality rate for older clients with hip fractures is very high, especially within the first 6 months, and the debilitating effects can be devastating (McClung, 2000).

HEALTH PROMOTION/ILLNESS PREVENTION

The focus of osteoporosis prevention is to minimize risk factors, as described earlier under the Assessment section (see Chart 54-1). For example, for clients who ingest inadequate amounts of calcium, teach them which foods should be included. Clients who have sedentary lifestyles should be taught about the importance of exercise and what types of exercise they should do. Weight-bearing exercises are preferred; activities that cause jarring, such as horseback riding, should be avoided to prevent further damage.

Rather than wait until adulthood, osteoporosis education should begin in childhood to prevent possible pain and disability later in life. Lypaczewski, Lappe, and Stubby (2002) published the short-term results of an educational intervention on bone health for 50 prepubertal Girl Scouts and their mothers. The program stressed the importance of exercise and increased dietary calcium intake for both children and women to prevent osteoporosis. The authors suggested that nurses must take opportunities to teach bone health to school-age children as one way to improve health of future adults.

◆COLLABORATIVE MANAGEMENT

◆Assessment

A complete health history with assessment of risk factors is important in the prevention, early detection, and treatment of osteoporosis. Clients who have risk factors for osteoporosis are at increased risk for fractures when falls occur. A fall risk assessment may be included in the health history. Assess for fall risk factors, including the following:

- Delirium
- Dementia
- Immobility
- Muscular weakness
- History of falls
- Visual or hearing deficits
- Current medications

Chapter 5 discusses falls in older adults in more detail.

PHYSICAL ASSESSMENT/CLINICAL MANIFESTATIONS

When performing a musculoskeletal assessment, inspect and palpate the vertebral column. The classic "dowager's hump," or kyphosis of the dorsal spine, is usually present (Figure 54-1). The client often states that height has been shortened, perhaps as much as 2 to 3 inches (5 to 7 cm) within the previous 20 years. Height and weight should be measured and compared with previous measurements if they are available.

Accompanying the spinal deformity is the complaint of back pain, which often occurs after lifting, bending, or stooping. The pain may be sharp and acute in onset. Pain is worse with activity and is relieved by rest. Palpation of the vertebrae, particularly the lower thoracic and lumbar vertebrae, usually increases the client's discomfort. Therefore palpation should be gentle.

Back pain accompanied by tenderness and voluntary restriction of spinal movement suggests one or more compression vertebral fractures, the most common type of osteoporotic fracture. Movement restriction and spinal deformity may result in constipation, abdominal distention, reflux esophagitis, and respiratory compromise in severe cases. The most likely area for fracture occurrence is between T8 and L3.

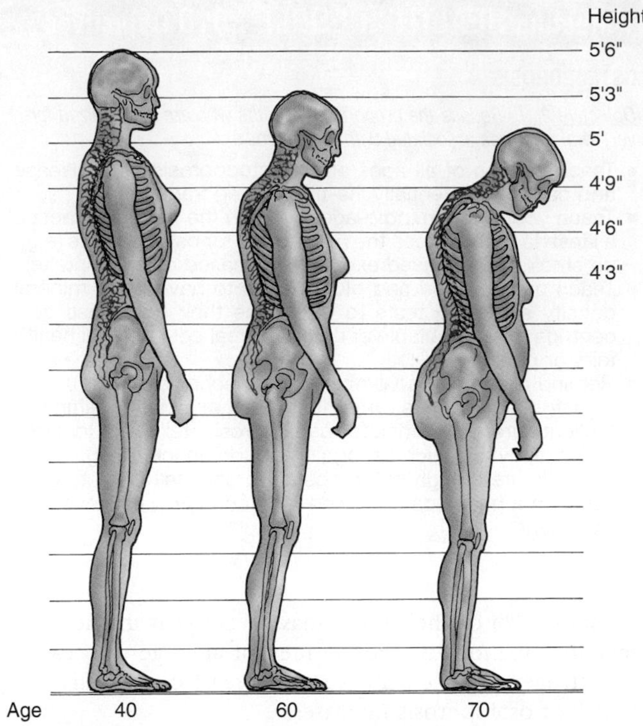

Figure 54-1 ■ A normal spine at age 40 years of age and osteoporotic changes at ages 60 and 70 years of age. These changes can cause a loss of as much as 6 inches in height and can result in the so-called dowager's hump (far right) in the upper thoracic vertebrae.

Fractures are also common in the distal end of the radius and the upper third of the femur (hip). The nurse directs special attention to these areas as part of the physical assessment.

PSYCHOSOCIAL ASSESSMENT

Women often associate osteoporosis with menopause, getting older, and becoming less independent. The disease can result in suffering, deformity, and disability that can affect the client's well-being and life satisfaction. The quality of life may be further impacted by pain, insomnia, depression, and **fallophobia** (fear of falling).

Assess the client's concept of body image, especially if the client is severely kyphotic. For example, the client may have difficulty finding clothes that fit properly. Social interactions may be curtailed because of a change in appearance or the physical limitations of being unable to sit in chairs in restaurants, movie theaters, and other places. Alterations in sexuality may occur as a result of poor self-esteem or the discomfort imposed by positioning during intercourse.

Because osteoporosis readily predisposes a client to fractures, the client must be extremely cautious about activities. As a result, the threat of fracture can create anxiety and fear and result in further limitation of social or physical activities. Assessment for the presence of these feelings assists in individualization of treatment and client teaching. For example, the client may not exercise as prescribed for fear that a fracture will occur.

LABORATORY ASSESSMENT

There are no definitive laboratory tests that confirm a diagnosis of primary osteoporosis, although a number of biochemical markers can provide information about bone modeling. A battery of tests can be performed to rule out secondary osteoporosis or other metabolic bone diseases, such as osteomalacia and Paget's disease. These include determination of serum calcium, vitamin D, phosphorus, and alkaline phosphatase levels.

Urinary calcium levels may also be assessed. Serum protein measurements and thyroid function tests are performed to exclude hyperthyroidism.

A simple, specific, and sensitive test to evaluate bone resorption is being used with clients with spinal cord injury and others at risk. The uPYR Crosslinks assay measures urinary concentrations of pyridinium, a collagen substance found in bone and cartilage. An increase in urinary levels indicates increased bone resorption (loss). The advantage of this test is its ability to detect bone loss early. In addition, no special client preparation is required. The disadvantage of the test is its cost, which is high because the test is relatively new. However, pyridinium and other biochemical markers of bone modeling may be used in the future as a routine screening test.

RADIOGRAPHIC ASSESSMENT

X-rays of the spine and long bones show loss of bone density and the presence of fractures. However, radiographic findings of bone density changes are evident only after a 25% to 40% bone loss has occurred.

In the past decade, technologic advances have enabled the detection of early changes in bone density. A popular screening and diagnostic tool is **dual-energy x-ray absorptiometry (DEXA).** Many physicians recommend that women in their 40s have a baseline DEXA scan so that later bone changes can be detected and compared. DEXA is a painless scan that measures bone mineral density (BMD) in the hip, wrist, or vertebral column. It is the best tool currently available for diagnosis and follow-up evaluation of treatment of osteoporosis. No special client preparation or follow-up care is required.

Qualitative ultrasound (QUS) of the heel or calcaneus is an effective and low-cost screening tool that can detect osteoporosis and predict risk for hip fracture. The test requires no special preparation, is quick, and has no radiation exposure or specific follow-up care.

Common Nursing Diagnoses and Collaborative Problems

The most common nursing diagnoses and collaborative problems that apply to clients with diagnosed osteoporosis include the following:

- Risk for Falls related to being female 65 years of age or older and environmental hazards
- Impaired Physical Mobility related to decreased muscle strength, pain, and musculoskeletal impairment
- Acute Pain and/or Chronic Pain related to effects of acute physical illness (fracture) or chronic disability

The primary collaborative problem for clients with the disease is Potential for Fractures. (See the Plan of Care box below and on pp. 1162 to 1165.)

Interventions

Because the client is predisposed to fractures, medications, nutritional therapy, and exercise are used to retard bone resorption and form new bony tissue. Client education can help prevent osteoporosis or slow the progress. These measures help reduce the chance of fracture and subsequent

Text continued on p. 1165.

PLAN of CARE MEDICAL DIAGNOSIS: OSTEOPOROSIS

NURSING DIAGNOSIS NO. 1 ■ Imbalanced Nutrition: Less Than Body Requirements

	Expected Outcomes	Nursing Interventions	Rationales
RELATED FACTORS Inability to ingest or digest food or absorb nutrients due to biologic, psychological, or economic factors **DEFINING CHARACTERISTICS** Reported or evidence of lack of food Misconceptions Lack of information or misinformation	Has muscle tone ≥4+ Has skin with warm undertones No verbal report or observation of altered eating habits	NIC **Nutrition Management** Determine, in collaboration with the dietitian as appropriate, the number of calories and type of nutrients needed to meet nutrition requirements.	Individual client needs for nutrients and calories should be the basis of a sound dietary plan.
		Provide appropriate information about nutritional needs and how to meet them.	Clients need accurate and timely information to make informed decisions about nutritional needs and how to meet them.
		Other Interventions Teach the client and family about nutritional supplements, as appropriate.	Additional vitamins and minerals, calories, dietary fiber, or other nutritional components may need to be added to the diet of a client who is unable to eat a nutritionally adequate diet.
		Teach the client and family about the prevention of constipation.	Clients on diets low in fiber may need additional fluids and supplemental fiber to maintain bowel regularity.

Continued

PLAN of CARE MEDICAL DIAGNOSIS: OSTEOPOROSIS—*cont'd*

NURSING DIAGNOSIS NO. 1 ■ Imbalanced Nutrition: Less Than Body Requirements—*cont'd*

	Expected Outcomes		Nursing Interventions	Rationales
			Continuing Care Considerations	
			Refer the client to appropriate community nutritional programs, as needed.	Resources such as Weight Watchers, Overeaters Anonymous, and Take Off Pounds Sensibly provide support for the client attempting to maintain appropriate body weight.
			Refer the client to community support groups and encourage attendance, as appropriate.	Clients may need support to maintain healthy eating patterns. In addition, support groups can offer advice on how to overcome common problems.
			Encourage the client and family to use the home nutritional therapy team.	The home nutritional therapy team is able to monitor and adjust the nutritional plan of care to maximize client nutritional status.

NURSING DIAGNOSIS NO. 2 ■ Impaired Physical Mobility

	Expected Outcomes		Nursing Interventions	Rationales
RELATED FACTORS Discomfort Pain Lack of knowledge regarding value of physical activity Musculoskeletal impairment Intolerance to activity Decreased strength and endurance **DEFINING CHARACTERISTICS** Postural instability during performance of routine activities of daily living Gait changes Reaction time: Decreased	Has full or improved range of motion in all joints Has smooth, coordinated movements Has stable posture during performance of activities of daily living Has no movement-induced tremor Has skin that remains intact with no bruising or rashes Able to perform fine motor skills Able to perform gross motor skills	NIC	**Exercise Therapy: Joint Mobility**	
			Collaborate with physical therapy in developing and executing an exercise program.	Physical therapists are the primary health care professionals responsible for developing and executing an exercise program.
			Initiate pain control measures before beginning joint exercise.	Initiating pain control measures before joint exercise increases the likelihood of client comfort and willingness to engage in the exercise.
		D	Dress the client in nonrestrictive clothing.	Nonrestrictive clothing permits full range of joint motion.
		D	Protect the client from trauma during exercise.	Stretching exercises may cause the client to be off balance.
		D	Encourage ambulation, if appropriate.	Ambulation is a form of active joint exercise and also improves cardiovascular tone.
			Continuing Care Considerations	
			Refer the client to a vocational counselor, as appropriate.	Long-term physical impairment may require the client to change his or her employment.

NURSING DIAGNOSIS NO. 3 ■ Ineffective Health Maintenance

	Expected Outcomes		Nursing Interventions	Rationales
RELATED FACTORS Lack of material resources Ineffective individual coping **DEFINING CHARACTERISTICS** Demonstrated lack of knowledge regarding basic health practices	Able to accurately perform needed health care tasks No verbal report or observation of lack of equipment, financial, and/or other resources	NIC	**Health System Guidance**	
			Identify and facilitate communication among health care providers, client, or family, as appropriate.	Faulty communication may increase the time delays for service or foster distrust among the health care providers, client, and family.

D Indicates tasks that can be delegated to unlicensed assistive nursing personnel at the discretion of the nurse.

NURSING DIAGNOSIS NO. 3 ■ Ineffective Health Maintenance—*cont'd*

	Expected Outcomes	Nursing Interventions	Rationales
Expressed interest in improving health behaviors Reported or observed lack of equipment, financial, and/or other resources	Able to ask for or seek out assistance Practices basic health maintenance activities	Give written instructions for the purpose and location of posthospitalization and outpatient activities, as appropriate.	Written instructions provide clear information that can be referred to for memory assistance.
		Identify and facilitate transportation needs for obtaining health care services.	Ensuring that the client/family has suitable, timely transportation increases the likelihood that appointments will be kept as scheduled.
		NIC **Support System Enhancement**	
		Determine the adequacy of existing social networks.	The client's/family's perception of the adequacy of social networks provides the basis of planning.
		Identify degree of family support.	Family support is not guaranteed, even with proximity.
		Determine barriers to using support systems.	The client/family needs to plan ways to overcome barriers as needed, because they may impair health maintenance.
		Encourage the client to participate in social and community activities.	Participation in social and community activities provides the client with the opportunity to form friendships that may provide emotional support.
		Assess community resource adequacy to identify strengths and weaknesses.	Understanding the strengths and weaknesses of available community resources permits realistic expectations of assistance from those sources.
		Refer to a community-based promotion, prevention, treatment, and/or rehabilitation program, as appropriate.	A community-based promotion, prevention, treatment, and/or rehabilitation program may provide the client/family with essential services and emotional support.
		Other Interventions	
		Teach the client and family about the care necessary to manage their health state.	Lack of knowledge will render efforts at health maintenance less effective.
		Continuing Care	
		Refer the family to appropriate counseling services.	Families in distress may be unable to provide essential support to a family member with a health maintenance problem.

NURSING DIAGNOSIS NO. 4 ■ Risk for Falls

	Expected Outcomes	Nursing Interventions	Rationales
RELATED FACTORS		NIC **Fall Prevention**	
Age 65 or older History of falls Use of assistive devices (e.g., walker, cane) Impaired physical mobility Impaired balance Difficulty with gait Cluttered environment Throw or scatter rugs	No falls No injuries	Identify characteristics of the environment that may increase potential for falls (e.g., slippery floors and open stairways).	Removal or modification of the environment to prevent falls decreases the risk for injury.
		Monitor gait, balance, and fatigue level with ambulation.	Tired, unsteady clients are more likely to fall and suffer injury.

Continued

NURSING DIAGNOSIS NO. 4 ■ Risk for Falls—*cont'd*

Expected Outcomes	Nursing Interventions	Rationales
	D Assist the unsteady client with ambulation and provide assistive devices (e.g., cane and walker).	Assistance with mobility and assistive devices serves to steady gait and diminish fall risk.
	D Provide adequate lighting.	Increased visibility assists the client to locate hazards and avoid them.
	D Place a mechanical bed in the lowest position or provide a sleeping surface close to the floor, as needed.	For clients who are at high risk for falling out of bed, placing the bed in a low position or providing a sleeping surface close to the floor diminishes the distance that the client may fall, thereby lowering the force of the fall.
	D Assist with toileting at frequent, scheduled intervals.	Frequent toileting assists the client to remain continent and decreases the necessity for unassisted attempts to toilet himself or herself.
	D Ensure that the client wears shoes that fit properly, fasten securely, and have nonskid soles, and ensure that the client wears prescription glasses, as appropriate, when out of bed.	Nonskid, properly fitting shoes and corrected vision increase the client's ability to remain stable and to see hazards.
	D Instruct the client to call for assistance with movement, as appropriate.	Giving assistance to unsteady clients prevents falls.
	Other Interventions	
	Collaborate with other health care team members to minimize the side effects of medications that contribute to falling (e.g., orthostatic hypotension and unsteady gait).	Clients should be evaluated carefully for adverse effects that create an injury hazard. Medications should be reviewed and dosages altered to minimize the adverse effects whenever possible.
	Provide safety equipment (e.g., nonslip, nontrip floor surfaces, grab bars in the bathroom, nonslip surfaces in tubs, and nonglare lighting).	Environmental safety equipment permits the unsteady client to ambulate safely.
	Continuing Care Considerations	
	Encourage the client to develop a routine physical exercise program that includes walking.	Exercise helps strengthen muscles and improves coordination.
	Have the client's doors, thresholds, and steps clearly marked.	Having clearly identified geographic markers will help the client maneuver over and through uneven spots with fewer bumps or falls.
	Instruct the client to remain indoors during inclement weather to avoid ice and other slippery outdoor surfaces.	Outdoor surfaces made slippery with water or ice increase the risk of falls.

D Indicates tasks that can be delegated to unlicensed assistive nursing personnel at the discretion of the nurse.

PLAN of CARE MEDICAL DIAGNOSIS: OSTEOPOROSIS—*cont'd*

NURSING DIAGNOSIS NO. 5 ■ Disturbed Body Image

	Expected Outcomes	Nursing Interventions	Rationales
RELATED FACTORS Biophysical Developmental changes Trauma or injury **DEFINING CHARACTERISTICS** Verbal report of feelings that reflect an altered view of one's body in appearance, structure, or function Actual change in structure and/or function	Acknowledges changes in body that reflect a realistic appraisal of altered appearance or function	NIC **Body Image Enhancement** Use anticipatory guidance.	Anticipatory guidance prepares the client for predictable changes in body image.
		Assist the client to discuss changes caused by aging, as appropriate.	The client may be unaware of the normal body changes caused by aging and may associate negative feelings about those changes.
		Assist the client to discuss stressors affecting body image.	Stressors affecting body image may be due to congenital condition, injury, disease, or surgery.
		Identify the significance of the client's culture, religion, race, gender, and age on body image.	Culture, religion, race, gender, and age influence the client's perception of a positive or negative body image.
		Determine the client's and family's perceptions of the alteration in body image versus reality.	The client's and family's perceptions of the alteration in body image may vary significantly from the reality of the change.
		Assist the client to identify actions that will enhance appearance.	Assisting the client to enhance his or her appearance will improve his or her self-concept.
		Other Interventions D Provide an atmosphere of caring and acceptance.	A client with traumatic changes in body parts or functioning may be especially sensitive to cues that indicate an aversive reaction.

complications. The role of drug therapy has increased over the past decade and helps to prevent fractures related to osteoporosis.

Drug Therapy. The health care provider may prescribe hormone replacements, calcium supplements, vitamin D, bisphosphonates (BPs), selective estrogen receptor modulators (SERMs), calcitonin, or a combination of several drugs to treat, as well as prevent, osteoporosis (Chart 54-2). Other agents have been given, but with limited success. Estrogen and combination hormone therapy are the least expensive of the drugs used for osteoporosis, but they do increase other health risks for women.

Hormone Replacement Therapy. Hormone replacement therapy (HRT) has been used as a primary *prevention* strategy for reducing bone loss in the postmenopausal woman. However, recent studies by the Women's Health Initiative demonstrated that long-term effects of HRT may increase a woman's risk of breast cancer, cardiovascular disease, and stroke. Warnings for drugs such as conjugated estrogens/medroxyprogesterone (Prempro, Premphase) state that the use of these drugs for prevention of osteoporosis must be carefully evaluated by the health care provider and the client. If taken, the benefit of the medication should outweigh the risks to the client (U.S. Food and Drug Administration, 2003).

Parathyroid Hormone. The use of parathyroid hormone is approved for *treatment* of osteoporosis in men and women. Clients must be instructed to self-administer teriparatide (Forteo) as a daily subcutaneous injection. Teriparatide stimulates new bone formation, thus increasing BMD. Reduced risk of fracture in hip, spine, and wrist is reported in women and reduced risk of hip fracture is reported in men (National Osteoporosis Foundation, 2003b). For clients taking this medication, teach them the signs and symptoms of hypercalcemia, including the following:

- Fatigue
- Anorexia
- Nausea/vomiting
- Constipation
- Polyuria

Calcium. Intake of calcium alone is not a treatment for osteoporosis, but calcium is an important part of a prevention program to promote bone health. Most persons cannot ingest sufficient quantities of calcium in the diet, and therefore calcium supplements may be used. Calcium carbonate, found in over-the-counter (OTC) drugs such as Tums or Os-Cal, is one of the most cost-effective supplement formulas. Calcium citrate, available OTC as Citracal, is often recommended for those persons who experience gastric upset when

CHART 54-2

DRUG THERAPY for Osteoporosis

Drug	Usual Dosage	Nursing Interventions	Rationales
Calcium (e.g., Os-Cal, Tums, Caltrate-600, Citracal)	1-1.5 g in divided doses PO	Give a third of daily dose at bedtime. Push fluids.	Calcium is most readily utilized by the body when the client is fasting and immobile. Increased fluid intake aids in preventing the formation of calcium-based urinary stones.
		Assess for a history of urinary stones.	Calcium supplements are not given to clients who are susceptible to urinary stone formation.
		Monitor serum calcium level.	Hypercalcemia, or calcium excess, is a side effect of calcium supplementation.
		Monitor urinary calcium level (no more than 4 mg/kg in 24 hr).	The kidneys attempt to excrete excess calcium.
		Observe for signs of hypercalcemia.	Hypercalcemia can result in urinary stones, cardiac dysrhythmias, and an increase or decrease in skeletal muscle tone.
Estrogen or estrogen/progesterone (e.g., Premarin, Prempro)	0.425-1.25 mg PO for 25 days/mo 0.625 mg conjugatedl estrogens/2.5 mg medroxyprogesterone acetate (Prempro) (dose may be lower)	Assess for history of tumors, hypertension, thromboembolytic disease, or liver or gallbladder disease.	Estrogen therapy is withheld from clients with susceptibility to an exacerbation of one or more of these problems.
		Teach the importance of gynecologic examinations every 6 months.	Endometrial and breast cancer can result from estrogen therapy.
		Teach breast self-examination.	Clients can detect potentially malignant lesions early so that treatment can begin immediately.
		Observe for vaginal bleeding.	Vaginal bleeding is a side effect of estrogen therapy and a sign of possible endometrial cancer.
		Monitor blood pressure.	Hypertension and other cardiovascular complications may result from combined estrogen-progesterone therapy.
		Observe for thrombus formation.	Deep vein thrombosis is a complication of combined estrogen-progesterone therapy.
		Monitor serum liver enzyme and cholesterol levels.	An elevation of liver enzyme levels may be indicative of liver involvement resulting from estrogen. An elevated cholesterol level can result in hypertension and thrombus formation.
! Alendronate (Fosamax)	5 mg PO daily	Take early in AM with 8 oz water; do not lie down until after breakfast.	Although not common, esophagitis or esophageal ulcers may result from alendronate therapy.
Risedronate (Actonel)	5 mg daily	Give ≥30 min before a meal (preferably breakfast); follow interventions for alendronate	Same as for alendronate.
		Observe for CNS side/adverse effects, such as drowsiness, anxiety, agitation	Drug can cause CNS effects that may not be tolerated.
Ibandronate (Boniva)	2.5 mg daily	Same as for alendronate.	Same as for alendronate.
Raloxifene (Evista)	60 mg daily	Teach client to monitor weight and BP frequently.	Drug causes increased water and sodium retention.
		Monitor liver function tests (LFTs) in collaboration with health care provider.	Raloxifene can cause increased LFTs or worsen hepatic disease (should not be given to client who has liver disease).
Calcitonin (e.g., Calcimar [salmon], Cibacalcin [human], Miacalcin [salmon; nasal spray])	100 International Units SC or IM daily 200 International Units intranasally daily, alternating nostrils	Rotate injection sites for parenteral administration.	Injection sites become irritated and reddened.
		Monitor for flushing, headache, nausea, and vomiting.	These are common side effects of calcitonin.
		Monitor renal function, calcium, and vitamin D levels.	Toxicity from calcitonin can cause renal problems.

! ***Med Error Alert!** Do not confuse Fosamax with Flomax, a selective alpha-adrenergic blocker used for benign prostatic hyperplasia (BPH).*

SC, Subcutaneous.

taking a calcium supplement. Teach clients to take calcium supplements with food and 6 to 8 ounces of water. It is best to divide the daily dose, with one third of the daily dose being taken in the evening. Supplements should be started in high-risk persons in young adulthood to assist in building peak bone mass (Sedlak & Doheny, 2002).

Clients should take calcium supplements under the supervision of a health care provider. **Hypercalcemia** (excess serum calcium) can cause serious damage to the urinary system. The amount of calcium prescribed is affected by the addition of HRT and the presence of risk factors for osteoporosis. Chart 16-13 lists the clinical manifestations associated with hypercalcemia.

In the United States the typical daily intake of dietary calcium is between 450 and 550 mg. The recommended daily allowance (RDA) of calcium is 1200 mg. Many clinicians and researchers believe that the RDA is insufficient to meet the calcium requirements of postmenopausal women, who may require as much as 1500 mg or more daily to prevent osteoporosis. An increased calcium intake may prevent bone loss in men as well. The nurse teaches the client to consume foods rich in calcium, such as milk and dairy products and dark green, leafy vegetables (see Chapter 14 for a list of foods high in calcium).

Vitamin D. Vitamin D supplementation may be necessary for the institutionalized or homebound client or for those who do not meet daily requirements. An adequate level of vitamin D is needed for optimal calcium absorption in the intestines. The prescribed dosage is usually 400 to 800 International Units/day. Higher doses can produce toxic effects, such as hypercalcemia and hyperphosphatemia.

Bisphosphonates. Bisphosphonates (BPs) inhibit bone resorption by binding with crystal elements in bone, especially spongy, trabecular bone tissue. Three BPs, alendronate (Fosamax), ibandronate (Boniva), and risedronate (Actonel), are commonly used for the *prevention and management* of osteoporosis and hypercalcemia associated with cancer. They are also approved for use in the prevention and treatment of osteoporosis in men and postmenopausal women. New bisphosphonates are being approved every year.

Although side effects are not common, when they do occur, they tend to be serious. **Esophagitis** (inflammation of the esophagus) and esophageal ulcers have been reported with the use of BPs, especially when the tablet is not completely swallowed. Teach clients taking this drug to take it early in the morning with 8 ounces of water and wait 30 minutes before eating. They should remain upright during the 30 minutes before eating. If chest pain occurs, a symptom of esophageal irritation, instruct them to discontinue the drug and contact their health care provider. Clients with poor renal function, hypocalcemia, or gastrointestinal reflux disease (GERD) should not take BPs.

Selective Estrogen Receptor Modulators. Selective estrogen receptor modulators (SERMs), a newer class of drugs, are designed to mimic estrogen in some parts of the body while blocking its effect elsewhere. Raloxifene (Evista) is used for *prevention and management* of osteoporosis in postmenopausal women. It increases BMD, reduces bone resorption, and lowers serum cholesterol. The drug should not be given to women who have a history of venous thromboembolism (VTE) (Leslie, 2000). Research continues to evaluate the effect of raloxifene as a cardiovascular protective agent.

Calcitonin. Calcitonin is a thyroid hormone that inhibits osteoclastic activity, thus decreasing bone loss. It is used for the *treatment* of osteoporosis, Paget's disease, and hypercalcemia associated with cancer. The drug also has an analgesic effect after vertebral fracture, thereby promoting early recovery.

Calcitonin (salmon) can be given intramuscularly, subcutaneously, or intranasally (Miacalcin). Nasal administration is preferred because it improves compliance, minimizes side effects, and is convenient. However, the effect of salmon calcitonin may decrease after use for two or more years. Clients may require a holiday from this treatment to maintain effectiveness. The nurse teaches the client to alternate nostrils to prevent nasal mucosal irritation, a common side effect. Salmon calcitonin must be refrigerated.

Other Agents. Androgens, such as testosterone propionate (Testex, Malogen✱), have been successful in decreasing bone resorption and increasing bone growth. Androgens may decrease bone resorption in men, particularly in older men. When given to postmenopausal women, however, androgens cause masculine traits and may lead to liver disease.

Diet Therapy. The dietary considerations for the treatment of a client with a diagnosis of osteoporosis are the same as those for preventing the disease. Adequate amounts of protein, magnesium, vitamin K, and trace minerals are needed for bone formation. Calcium and vitamin D intake needs to be increased, and alcohol and caffeine consumption should be discouraged. For the client who has sustained a fracture, intake of protein, vitamin C, and iron is increased to promote bone healing. Education for persons of all ages must focus on the importance of adequate intake of calcium to build strong bones (Lypaczewski, Lappe, Stubby, 2002).

Fall Prevention. The client must be careful to prevent falls and other activities that can cause a fracture. A hazard-free environment is necessary to meet this goal, and the nurse must teach the client about its importance.

Many hospitals and long-term care facilities have risk management programs in which clients are assessed for their risk for falls. For those at high risk, programs such as the Falling Star protocol have reduced falls by making the staff aware of the client's high risk. In this program, a star is placed at the head of the bed to designate a person at high risk. Chapter 5 discusses fall prevention in health care agencies and at home in more detail.

Hip protectors are inexpensive devices that can prevent hip fracture if the client experiences a fall. A **hip protector** is a pad that is worn while ambulating. If the client falls onto his or her trochanter, the probability of hip fracture is lessened.

Exercise. Exercise is important in the prevention and management of osteoporosis. It also plays a vital role in pain management, cardiovascular function, and an improved sense of well-being.

In collaboration with the health care provider, the physical therapist prescribes exercises for strengthening the abdominal and back muscles. These exercises improve posture and provide an improved support for the spine. Abdominal isometrics, deep breathing, and pectoral stretching are stressed in order to increase pulmonary capacity. Exercises for the extremity muscles include isometric, resistive, and range-of-motion (ROM) exercises. The nurse encourages active ROM exercises, which improve joint mobility and increase muscle tone.

In addition to exercises for muscle strengthening, a general weight-bearing exercise program is implemented. Walking for 30 minutes three times a week, swimming, or bicycling are recommended activities. Teach the client that certain high-impact recreational activities, such as bowling and horseback riding, may cause vertebral compression and should be avoided.

Pain Management. The pain management program depends on the intensity and duration of the pain. With treatment, pain from spinal fractures often resolves 6 to 8 weeks after injury; treatment usually includes drug therapy and orthotic devices. The health care provider prescribes analgesics (opioid and non-opioid) during the acute phase of the pain (i.e., from the time of injury to as long as several weeks afterward). Muscle relaxants, which ease the discomfort associated with muscle spasms, are often used for spinal fractures. Nonsteroidal anti-inflammatory drugs (NSAIDs) are beneficial for pain relief and for decreasing spinal nerve root inflammation from crushed vertebrae. However, monitor for problems associated with NSAIDs, such as gastrointestinal bleeding and heart failure, particularly in older adults.

Orthotic Devices. Known as dorsolumbar orthoses, orthotic devices immobilize the spine during the acute pain phase and provide spinal column support (Figure 54-2). The physical therapist or orthotist custom fits the client for this lightweight device. Teach the client to inspect the skin for irritation and report tolerance to the device.

Community-Based Care

Clients with osteoporosis are usually managed at home. However, some experience fractures that may require hospitalization. In any setting, assess for risk factors of osteoporosis and provide health teaching as appropriate, and described under the Interventions section above.

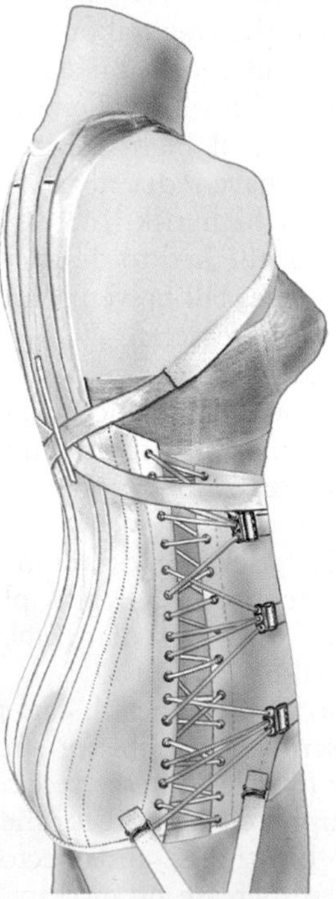

Figure 54-2 ■ A dorsolumbar orthosis. (Courtesy Truform Orthotics and Prosthetics, Cincinnati, OH.)

The client with osteoporosis who has one or more fractures can be discharged to the home setting. In some instances, the client is discharged to a long-term care facility for rehabilitation or permanent residence when support systems are not available. Case managers, social workers, and discharge planners assist in preparing clients and their families for placement in long-term care facilities. Chapter 55 discusses continuing care for clients who experience fractures.

The National Osteoporosis Foundation provides information to clients and health care professionals regarding the disease and its treatment. Large metropolitan hospitals often have osteoporosis specialty clinics and support groups for clients with osteoporosis.

Osteomalacia

PATHOPHYSIOLOGY

Osteomalacia is described as softening of the bone tissue and is characterized by inadequate mineralization of osteoid. Mineralized osteoid results in mature compact and cancellous (spongy) bone. In osteomalacia, normal remodeling of the bone is disrupted and mineralization or calcification does not occur. Osteomalacia is the adult equivalent of rickets, or vitamin D deficiency, in children.

Vitamin D deficiency is the most important factor in development of osteomalacia. In its natural form, vitamin D is obtained from the ultraviolet radiation of the sun, from certain foods, and as a nutritional supplement. In combination with calcium and phosphorus, the vitamin is necessary for bone formation.

Osteomalacia is frequently confused with osteoporosis because of similar characteristics shared by the two disease processes. Table 54-2 shows a comparison and contrast of osteoporosis and osteomalacia.

CONSIDERATIONS FOR OLDER ADULTS

Osteomalacia is not thought to be common, but researchers and clinicians are exploring its incidence in older adults. Although there are no accurate statistical data to indicate the incidence of osteomalacia in the United States, health care professionals are continuing to study its occurrence in nursing homes and other residences for older adults.

TABLE 54-2 Differential Features of Osteoporosis and Osteomalacia

Characteristic	Osteoporosis	Osteomalacia
Definition	Decreased bone mass	Demineralized bone
Pathophysiology	Lack of calcium	Lack of vitamin D
Radiographic findings	Osteopenia, fractures	Pseudofractures, Looser's zones, fractures
Calcium level	Normal	Low or normal
Phosphate level	Normal	Low or normal
Parathyroid hormone	Normal	High or normal
Alkaline phosphatase	Normal	High

Etiology and Genetic Risk

In addition to primary vitamin D deficiency related to lack of sunlight exposure or dietary intake, vitamin D deficiency attributable to various pathologic conditions may result in osteomalacia (Table 54-3). Malabsorption of the vitamin from the small bowel is a common postsurgical complication of partial or total gastrectomy and bypass or resection surgery of the small intestine. Disease of the small bowel, such as Crohn's disease, may cause decreased vitamin absorption.

Liver and pancreatic disorders interrupt vitamin D metabolism and decrease the production of usable substance. Chronic renal insufficiency interferes with the synthesis of calcitriol, the most active vitamin metabolite. Osteomalacia can also be caused by malignant bone tumors (**oncogenic** or **tumor-induced osteomalacia**).

Conditions that contribute to phosphate depletion (hypophosphatemia) lead to osteomalacia. Osteomalacia is also a complication of the intake of certain drugs, particularly anticonvulsants, barbiturates, and fluoride. The exact mechanism for the drug effects is not known. Genetic deviations in vitamin D or phosphate metabolism may commonly cause bone changes seen in osteomalacia.

Incidence/Prevalence

Osteomalacia is rarely seen in the United States and Western Europe, however, it is more common in nonindustrialized nations or in countries where famine is common. In the United States, older adults are most at risk. This group may have inadequate exposure to sunlight or intake of vitamin D–fortified foods. Persons who adhere to very restrictive vegetarian diets without adequate supplement of vitamin D can also be at risk. The risk for osteomalacia should be assessed in any person who has poor nutritional intake related to homelessness or severe drug or alcohol abuse or who is very poor.

HEALTH PROMOTION/ILLNESS PREVENTION

Because the nursing diagnoses for osteomalacia are the same as those for osteoporosis, client outcomes are also similar. An increase in vitamin D through dietary intake, sun exposure, and drug supplementation is promoted. Teach the at-risk client about foods high in vitamin D and the importance of frequent sun exposure for the manufacture of the vitamin.

Some persons are lactose intolerant or choose not to use dairy products related to strict vegetarian diets. Many products are available for persons who need to make dietary choices other than dairy products. Soy and rice milk, tofu, and other soy products are readily available. Instruct clients to choose those products that are fortified with vitamin D. Other foods rich in vitamin D are eggs, swordfish, chicken, liver, as well as cereals and bread products enriched with vitamin D.

TABLE 54-3 Causes of Osteomalacia

Vitamin D Disturbance	**Kidney Disease**
Inadequate production	Chronic renal failure
Lack of sunlight exposure	Renal tubular disorders
Dietary deficiency	▪ Acidosis
Abnormal metabolism	▪ Hypophosphatemia
Drug therapy	
▪ Phenytoin (Dilantin)	**Familial Metabolic Error**
▪ Fluoride	Hypophosphatemia
▪ Barbiturates	
Liver disease	
Renal disease	
Inadequate absorption	
▪ Postgastrectomy	
▪ Malabsorption syndrome	
Inflammatory bowel disease	

◆COLLABORATIVE MANAGEMENT

◆Assessment

Important data to collect for a client with osteomalacia or suspected osteomalacia include age, exposure to sunlight, and skin pigmentation. The older adult who has been homebound or chronically institutionalized is at the greatest risk. People who have dark skin and consume minimal protein are more at risk than light-skinned people with the same dietary habits. Take a thorough diet history to determine the intake of foods containing vitamin D and calcium.

Assessment will also include any history of chronic disease processes of the gastrointestinal tract including inflammatory bowel disease, gastric or intestinal bypass surgery, or any syndrome that interferes with absorption from the gastrointestinal tract. A history of renal or liver dysfunction may lead to ineffective metabolism of vitamin D. Drugs such as phenytoin (Dilantin) or fluoride preparations may interfere with metabolism of vitamin D.

PHYSICAL ASSESSMENT/CLINICAL MANIFESTATIONS

Osteomalacia is easily confused with osteoporosis. Many of the clinical manifestations are similar, and both disorders may occur at the same time.

In the early stages of osteomalacia, the manifestations are nonspecific. Muscle weakness and bone pain are often misdiagnosed as arthritis or other connective tissue disorder. In some cases, proximal muscle weakness in the shoulder and pelvic girdle areas is the only complaint.

Muscle weakness in the lower extremities may cause a waddling and unsteady gait, which contributes to falls and subsequent fractures. Hypophosphatemia leads to an inadequate production of muscle cell adenosine triphosphate, thus resulting in a decrease in muscle cell energy. If hypocalcemia is present, muscle cramping may accompany the weakness.

Assessment of muscle strength and observation of the client's gait will be made. Document complaints of muscle cramps and bone pain. Skeletal discomfort is often vague and generalized. The spine, ribs, pelvis, and lower extremities are most often affected. The client usually describes the pain as aggravated by activity and worse at night.

In addition to the client's subjective complaint of pain, palpate the affected bones for tenderness. Bone tenderness can be elicited by pressure on the tibia or rib cage. Observation of skeletal malalignment as in long-bone bowing or spinal deformity may be similar to that seen in osteoporosis. In extreme cases, the pelvis narrows, so that vaginal childbirth is difficult.

If osteomalacia is untreated, vertebral, rib, and long-bone fractures may occur. The client may be misdiagnosed as having bone cancer or osteoporosis.

DIAGNOSTIC ASSESSMENT

Table 54-2 shows the changes in laboratory values that help support the diagnosis of osteomalacia. X-rays of bone tissue with osteomalacia reveal a decrease in the trabeculae of cancellous bone and lack of osteoid sharpness. The classic diagnostic finding specific to the disease, however, is the presence of radiolucent bands (Looser's lines or zones). Looser's zones are pseudofractures; they represent stress fractures that have not mineralized. They often appear symmetrically in the medial area of the femoral neck, ribs, and inferior pubic rami and may progress to complete fractures with minimal trauma. Bone biopsy of these areas may be necessary for complete diagnosis. DEXA scan may assist in diagnosis of osteomalacia.

Interventions

The major treatment for osteomalacia is vitamin D. The recommended daily allowance (RDA) of vitamin D is 400 International Units. Because older adults are at risk for bone demineralization from aging, as well as for osteomalacia, a safe and adequate daily requirement may be as high as 600 to 800 International Units. Chart 54-3 lists interventions for helping older clients meet the daily requirement of vitamin D. Other interventions for clients with osteomalacia are discussed under Health Promotion/Illness Prevention.

Critical Thinking Challenge

An older woman who lives in an assisted-living complex tells you that she had a recent DEXA scan that revealed beginning osteoporosis. She is very upset because she has always had a "normal" scan, and thought she was not a high risk for the disease. Her mother suffered a fractured hip and died of complications in a nursing home. The client is worried that this complication could happen to her and wants to know how she can "slow this disease down."

1. What further information do you need to complete her history?
2. What physical assessment should you perform?
3. What health teaching is appropriate at this time?
4. What options does she have for treatment?
5. Is this client also at risk for osteomalacia? Why or why not?

evolve For suggested answer guidelines, go to http://evolve.elsevier.com/Iggy/.

Paget's Disease of the Bone

PATHOPHYSIOLOGY

Paget's disease, or **osteitis deformans**, is a metabolic disorder of bone remodeling, or turnover, in which increased resorption or loss results in bone deposits that are weak, enlarged, and disorganized.

CHART 54-3

NURSING FOCUS on the OLDER ADULT
Meeting the Daily Requirement for Vitamin D

- Advise clients to get sun exposure for at least 5 minutes weekly, even in the summer and winter.
- Recommend that clients eat food high in calcium to promote vitamin D absorption and utilization in the small intestines.
- Suggest that clients eat natural and fortified foods containing vitamin D, including milk and dairy products, such as ice cream (or ice milk), yogurt, and cheese.
- Recommend that clients exercise on a regular basis (at least three times a week for 20 to 30 minutes) to prevent bone loss.

Three pathophysiologic phases of the disorder have been described: active, mixed, and inactive. In the first phase (the active phase), a prolific increase in osteoclasts (cells that break down bone) causes massive bone destruction and deformity. The osteoclasts of pagetic bone are large and multinuclear, unlike the osteoclasts of normal bone tissue.

In the mixed phase, the osteoblasts (bone-forming cells) react to compensate in forming new bone. The result is bone that is vascular, structurally weak, and deformed. Paget's disease occurs in one bone or in multiple sites. The most common areas of involvement are the vertebrae, the femur, the skull, the sternum, and the pelvis.

When the osteoblastic activity exceeds the osteoclastic activity, the inactive phase occurs. The newly formed bone becomes sclerotic and very hard. The number of osteoclasts begins to return toward normal.

Bone biopsy specimens have revealed an antigen from a respiratory virus and measles. Because the disorder is present in monozygotic twins, a familial autosomal dominant pattern has been suggested. The disease has been noted in up to 30% of people with a positive family history for Paget's disease.

Paget's disease is the second most common bone disease, after osteoporosis, in the older population. The exact cause of Paget's disease is unknown but it may be the result of a latent viral infection contracted in young adulthood and manifesting as a disease 20 to 40 years later. The risk for developing Paget's disease increases as a person ages, particularly in those 80 years old and older.

CONSIDERATIONS FOR OLDER ADULTS

About 1 to 3 million people in the United States suffer from Paget's disease. It is primarily a disease of older adults and occurs in a very small percentage of those younger than 40 years of age.

CULTURAL CONSIDERATIONS

Because Paget's disease occurs more often in Europe and less often in Asia, there may be a link between the disease and ethnic origin. This linkage has not been well researched.

COLLABORATIVE MANAGEMENT

Assessment

Of clients with Paget's disease, 80% are asymptomatic. The disease may be confined to one bone. The disease is often accidentally discovered during a routine laboratory or radiographic examination. In more severe disease, the manifestations are diverse and potentially fatal (Chart 54-4).

Assessment should include history of fracture and a thorough pain assessment. Bone pain causes the client to seek medical attention. The pain is aching, poorly described, deep, and worsened by pressure and weight bearing. It is most noticeable at night or when the client is resting, and the pain is typically mild to moderate. Back pain and headache are common complaints.

The pain associated with the disorder may result from metabolic bone activity, secondary arthritis, impending fracture, or nerve impingement. Arthritis occurs at the joints of the affected bones, but its relationship to Paget's disease is unclear. Nerve impingement is particularly common in the lumbosacral area of the vertebral column, presenting as back pain that radiates along one or both lower extremities.

In addition to these assessments, inquire about any changes in hearing, vision, swallowing, balance, or speech. As bony changes progress in the skull and temporal regions, deficits in these areas may appear.

PHYSICAL ASSESSMENT/CLINICAL MANIFESTATIONS

MUSCULOSKELETAL AND NEUROLOGIC ASSESSMENT. Posture, stance, and gait are observed to identify gross bony deformities. Because of the enlargement of the vertebrae, loss of normal spinal curvature, and lower extremity malalignment, the client is usually short. Long-bone bowing in the arms and legs with subsequent varus deformity of the elbows and knees may be asymmetric. Flexion contracture in the hip joint is often present.

When performing a musculoskeletal assessment in a client with Paget's disease, pay particular attention to the size and shape of the skull, which is typically soft, thick, and enlarged. Involvement of the temporal bone may lead to deafness and vertigo, whereas basilar complications can compress any of the cranial nerves and result in neurologic compromise. Assess the client for impairments in vision, swallowing, and speech. **Platybasia**, or basilar invagination, causes brainstem manifestations that threaten life. In some cases, the bony enlargement of the skull blocks cerebrospinal fluid (CSF), resulting in hydrocephalus.

Pathologic fractures may be the presenting clinical manifestation of the disorder. Up to 30% of clients with Paget's disease can sustain at least one incomplete or complete fracture. The femur and the tibia are most often affected, and fracture of these bones can result from minimal trauma. The fracture line is usually perpendicular to the long axis of the bone, and healing is unpredictable because of abnormal metabolic activity within the bone.

The most dreaded complication of Paget's disease is neoplasm, most commonly osteogenic sarcoma (see the discussion later under Malignant Bone Tumors, p. 1176). Sarcomas occur in about 1% of clients with pagetic bone. They appear primarily in the pelvis, the femur, and the humerus and carry a grave prognosis because of early metastasis to the lung or extensive local invasion. They are often multifocal, and they occur more often in men. When severe bone pain is present in a client with Paget's disease, neoplasm is suspected.

SKIN ASSESSMENT. Assess the skin for its color and temperature. In people with Paget's disease, the skin is typically flushed and warm because of increased vascularity. In addition, the nurse assesses the client's energy level. The client usually complains of apathy, lethargy, and fatigue.

OTHER MANIFESTATIONS. Other, less common manifestations of Paget's disease include hyperparathyroidism and gout. Secondary hyperparathyroidism leads to an increase in serum and urinary calcium levels. In severe cases, calcium excess results from prolonged immobilization. Calcium deposits occur in joint spaces or as stones in the urinary tract. **Hyperuricemia** (serum uric acid excess) and gout occur because the increased metabolic activity of bone creates an increase in nucleic acid catabolism.

In a few cases, increased vascularity causes an increase in cardiac output, resulting in heart failure. Cardiac complications tend to occur only when more than a third of the skeleton is involved.

CHART 54-4

KEY FEATURES of Paget's Disease of the Bone

Musculoskeletal Manifestations
- Bone and joint pain (may be in a single bone) that is aching, poorly described, and aggravated by walking
- Low back and sciatic nerve pain
- Bowing of long bones
- Loss of normal spinal curvature
- Enlarged, thick skull
- Pathologic fractures
- Osteogenic sarcoma

Skin Manifestations
- Flushed, warm skin

Other Manifestations
- Apathy, lethargy, fatigue
- Hyperparathyroidism
- Gout
- Urinary or renal stones
- Heart failure from fluid overload

LABORATORY ASSESSMENT

Increases in serum alkaline phosphatase (ALP) and urinary hydroxyproline levels are the primary laboratory findings indicating the probability of Paget's disease. Overactive osteoblasts cause the alteration in ALP level. Clients who are receiving medications to manage Paget's disease should have an assessment of ALP three or four times a year to assess treatment effectiveness.

The 24-hour urinary hydroxyproline level reflects bone collagen turnover and indicates the degree of disease severity. The higher the hydroxyproline, the more severe the disease.

The calcium levels in blood and urine are normal or elevated. The immobilized client is more likely to have an increase in calcium levels as a result of calcium moving from bone into the blood.

Paget's disease often causes an elevation of uric acid because nucleic acid from overactive bone metabolism increases. This finding may be misinterpreted as primary gout.

RADIOGRAPHIC ASSESSMENT

Radiologic studies are the primary means of diagnosis of Paget's disease. X-rays of pagetic bone reveal radiolucent, or punched-out, areas indicative of increased bone resorption. Depending on the phase of the disease, the overall bone mass is enlarged and the cortices are thickened. Malalignment deformities, fractures, and secondary arthritic changes may be present.

Computed tomography (CT) is useful in the detection of sarcomas, changes in the skull, and spinal cord or nerve compression.

OTHER DIAGNOSTIC ASSESSMENTS

Magnetic resonance imaging (MRI) may also be used for the same purpose as the CT scan. Bone biopsy may also be used to rule out suspicion of malignancy.

Interventions

Nonsurgical or surgical management may be necessary to reduce pain. Nonsurgical interventions are used initially.

NONSURGICAL MANAGEMENT. Drug therapy is the primary intervention used for treatment and pain relief. Not only can drugs relieve pain, but they also may cause the disease to go into remission for a period of time by reducing pagetic bone resorption. Other pain relief measures are also used.

Drug Therapy. The purpose of drug therapy in Paget's disease is to relieve pain and to decrease bone resorption. Management of mild to moderate pain may include the use of aspirin or nonsteroidal anti-inflammatory drugs (NSAIDs), such as ibuprofen (Motrin, Apo-Ibuprofen ✱). When the calcium level is more than twice the normal value and the disease is widespread, the physician usually prescribes more potent drugs, such as calcitonin, selected bisphosphonates, alendronate (Fosamax), or mithramycin.

Calcitonin. Calcitonin is a thyroid hormone and is one of the treatments of choice for Paget's disease. It seems to retard bone resorption and, subsequently, relieve pain. The drug often causes a dramatic decrease in the alkaline phosphatase level in a few weeks. Calcitonin is approved for parenteral administration in treating Paget's disease. Side effects include nausea, flushing, and skin rash. Skin testing should be done before administration of the first dose.

Bisphosphonates. Etidronate (Didronel), an older bisphosphates (BP), may be prescribed orally in a dose of 5 mg/kg/day. Etidronate must be given in a 6-month on and 6-months off schedule. The dosage is kept to a minimum because high dosages may increase the risk of pathologic fracture. The major disadvantage is that the drug is poorly absorbed from the small intestine. Etidronate should be taken on an empty stomach 1 to 2 hours after breakfast or at bedtime with water or juice. Milk or milk products inhibit the drug's absorption. Diarrhea may occur in a few clients, but this problem can be treated with an antidiarrheal medication.

Calcitonin and etidronate are often the first drugs prescribed and are often used in combination. If repeated courses of these drugs are not effective, mithramycin or other BPs may be added to the drug regimen. Alendronate (Fosamax) and tiludronate (Skelid) are BPs that are also approved for treatment of Paget's disease.

Mithramycin. Mithramycin (Mithracin) is a potent antineoplastic and antibiotic with many side effects and is rarely used. It is reserved for clients with marked hypercalcemia or severe disease with neurologic compromise. Observe for signs of toxicity to the liver, gastrointestinal tract, and kidneys. Liver and kidney function studies and intake and output are monitored daily. Because mithramycin also suppresses platelets, daily platelet counts and bleeding precautions are taken. When liver enzyme levels become extremely high, drug therapy is interrupted temporarily.

The nurse and health care provider monitor the client's alanine phosphatase levels periodically to determine drug effectiveness. Periodic x-rays may also be ordered to assess bone changes during and after drug therapy.

Other Interventions. In addition to administering medication, implement physical measures to reduce pain. These measures may include application of heat and gentle massage. An exercise program may be started with the help of a physical therapist. Exercise may be difficult because of pain and danger of fracture. Nonimpact exercise should be used, but the client may benefit from strengthening and weight-bearing exercises. ROM and gentle stretching should be taught to the client. The client may be fitted for an orthotic device to immobilize and provide support for the vertebrae or long bones. Additional interventions for pain relief, such as relaxation techniques, are discussed in Chapter 7.

Measures to promote bone health are also important and include a diet rich in calcium. Diet therapy for bone health is described earlier under the interventions for Osteoporosis.

Provide the client with information to contact the local chapter of the Paget's Disease Foundation and the Arthritis Foundation. These resources provide information and support for the client and family or significant others. Dietary instruction should be similar to information given to the person with osteoporosis.

SURGICAL MANAGEMENT. When a client with Paget's disease has secondary arthritis and pain relief is not achieved, he or she may undergo a tibial osteotomy, or partial or total joint replacement (see Chapter 24). Surgical decompression and stabilization of the spine may be used to retain function, decrease pain, and reduce potential cardiac and respiratory complications.

OSTEOMYELITIS

PATHOPHYSIOLOGY

Invasion by one or more pathogenic microorganisms stimulates the inflammatory response in bone tissue, a condition known as **osteomyelitis.** The inflammation produces an increased vascularity and edema often involving the surrounding soft tissues. Once inflammation is established, the vessels in the area become thrombosed and release exudate into bony tissue. Ischemia of bone tissue follows and necrotic bone results. This area of necrotic bone separates from surrounding bone tissue and **sequestrum** is formed. The presence of sequestrum retards bone healing and causes superimposed infection, often in the form of bone abscess. As shown in Figure 54-3, the cycle repeats itself as the superimposed infection leads to further inflammation, vessel thromboses, and necrosis.

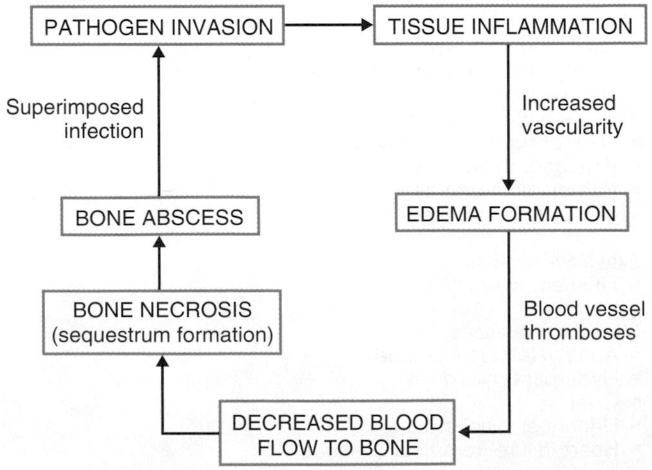

Figure 54-3 ■ Infection cycle of osteomyelitis.

Osteomyelitis is categorized as **exogenous,** in which infectious organisms enter from outside the body as in an open fracture, or **endogenous,** in which organisms are carried by the bloodstream from other areas of infection in the body. Endogenous osteomyelitis may also be referred to as **hematogenous** osteomyelitis. A third category is **contiguous,** in which bone infection results from skin infection of adjacent tissues. Osteomyelitis can be further divided into two major types: acute osteomyelitis and chronic osteomyelitis.

Etiology

Each type of bone infection has its own causative factors. Pathogenic microbes favor bone that has a rich vascular supply and a marrow cavity. **Acute hematogenous** infection results from bacteremia, underlying disease, or nonpenetrating trauma. Urinary tract infections, particularly in older men, tend to spread to the lower vertebrae. Long-term intravenous (IV) catheters, such as Hickman catheters, are primary sources of infection. Clients undergoing long-term hemodialysis and IV drug abusers are also at risk for osteomyelitis. *Salmonella* infections of the gastrointestinal tract may spread to bone. Clients with sickle cell anemia and other hemoglobinopathies often experience multiple episodes of salmonellosis, which can cause bone infection.

Poor dental hygiene and gum infection can be a causative factor in **contiguous** osteomyelitis in facial bones. Minimal trauma of the nonpenetrating type can cause hemorrhages or small-vessel occlusions, leading to bone necrosis. Regardless of the source of infection, many infections are caused by *Staphylococcus aureus.* Treatment of infection may be complicated further by the presence of methicillin-resistant *Staphylococcus aureus,* which is becoming more common in institutionalized persons.

CONSIDERATIONS FOR OLDER ADULTS

Malignant external otitis media involving the base of the skull is sometimes seen in older adults with diabetes. The most common cause of contiguous spread in older adults, however, is found in clients with diabetes or peripheral vascular disease who have slow-healing foot ulcers. Multiple organisms tend to be responsible for the resulting osteomyelitis.

In contrast, penetrating trauma leads to acute osteomyelitis by direct inoculation. A concurrent soft-tissue infection may be present as well. Animal bites, puncture wounds, and bone surgery can result in bone infection. The most common offending organism is *Pseudomonas aeruginosa,* but other gram-negative bacteria may be found.

If bone infection is misdiagnosed or inadequately treated, **subchronic** or **chronic osteomyelitis** occurs. Inadequate treatment results when the treatment period is too short or when the treatment is delayed or inappropriate. About 50% of cases of chronic osteomyelitis are caused by gram-negative bacteria. Remaining infections may be the result of a mixture of gram-negative and gram-positive organisms. Although bacteria are the most common causes of osteomyelitis, fungal organisms and virus also may cause infection.

Incidence/Prevalence

Hematogenous osteomyelitis is the most common type of osteomyelitis. Osteomyelitis occurs more often in children but is becoming increasingly common in adults, particularly older adults. Acute infection is more common in children; subchronic and chronic infection is more common in adults. Men experience osteomyelitis more frequently than women related to a higher incidence of blunt or penetrating trauma. Accompanying conditions such as malnutrition, alcoholism, renal or liver disease, and immunosuppressive disorders increase the risk and complicate effective treatment. Bone tissue in the vertebrae and long bones are common sites of infection. The adult with a compromised vascular supply is at greatest risk for chronic infection. Advanced age and concurrent disease may prolong the course of the infection for as long as a year or more.

COLLABORATIVE MANAGEMENT

Assessment

Bone pain, with or without other manifestations, is a common complaint of clients with bone infection. The pain is described as a constant, localized, pulsating sensation that intensifies with movement.

The client with *acute* osteomyelitis manifests fever, usually with temperature greater than 101° F (38° C). The area around the infected bone swells and is tender when palpated. Erythema (redness) and heat may also be present. When there is severe vascular compromise, clients may not feel discomfort because of nerve damage from lack of blood supply.

When vascular insufficiency is suspected, assess circulation in the distal extremities. Draining ulcers may be present on the feet or hands, indicating inadequate healing ability as a result of poor circulation.

Fever, swelling, and erythema are less common in those with *chronic* osteomyelitis. Ulceration resulting in sinus tract formation, localized pain, and drainage are more characteristic of chronic infection (Chart 54-5).

The client with osteomyelitis usually has an elevated white blood cell (leukocyte) count, which may be double the normal value. In chronic infection, normal values or slight elevations may be seen.

The erythrocyte sedimentation rate (ESR) may be normal early in the course of the disease but rises as the condition progresses. The rate may remain elevated for as long as 3 months after drug therapy is discontinued.

If bacteremia is present, a potentially life-threatening complication that could lead to septic shock, a blood culture identifies the offending organisms to determine which an-

CHART 54-5

KEY FEATURES of
Acute and Chronic Osteomyelitis

Acute Osteomyelitis
- Fever; temperature usually above 101° F (38° C)
- Swelling around the affected area
- Erythema of the affected area
- Tenderness of the affected area
- Bone pain that is constant, localized, and pulsating; intensifies with movement

Chronic Osteomyelitis
- Ulceration of the skin
- Sinus tract formation
- Localized pain
- Drainage from the affected area

tibiotics should be used in treatment. Both aerobic and anaerobic blood cultures should be collected at the initiation of therapy. About 50% of clients with acute hematogenous infection have positive blood cultures.

Although bone changes cannot be detected early with standard x-rays, changes in blood flow can be seen early in the course of the disease by radionuclide scanning. A bone scan, using technetium or gallium, is extremely helpful in the diagnosis of osteomyelitis and identifies most cases. In some cases, magnetic resonance imaging (MRI) may be more sensitive than traditional bone scanning in the diagnosis of osteomyelitis.

The definitive diagnosis of osteomyelitis may be made by bone biopsy. A culture of soft tissue or of the sinus tract may not identify the offending microbes invading the bone. Often the organisms affecting soft tissue and bone are different, and each must be treated.

Common Nursing Diagnoses and Collaborative Problems

Nursing diagnoses and collaborative problems that may apply to clients with osteomyelitis include the following:

- Acute Pain or Chronic Pain related to inflammation
- Hyperthermia related to pathogenic invasion of the bone
- Ineffective Tissue Perfusion (peripheral) related to tissue swelling
- Potential for Sepsis and Septic Shock

Interventions

The specific treatment protocol depends on the type and number of microbes present in the infected tissue. If other measures fail to resolve the infectious process, surgical management may be needed.

NONSURGICAL MANAGEMENT. To reverse osteomyelitis, the health care provider initiates antibiotic therapy as soon as possible. Contact precautions prevent the spread of the offending organism to other clients and health care personnel (see Chapter 29 for a discussion of contact precautions).

Drug Therapy. IV antibiotic therapy is usually prescribed for several weeks for acute osteomyelitis. More than one antibiotic may be needed to combat the presence of multiple types of organisms. The hospital or home care nurse gives the drugs at specifically prescribed times so that therapeutic serum levels are achieved. The nurse must become familiar with the actions, side effects, toxicity, interactions, and precautions for administration of the drugs. Family members in the home setting may be taught how to administer the antibiotics.

The optimal drug regimen for clients with chronic osteomyelitis is not well established. Prolonged therapy for more than 3 months may be needed to eliminate the infection. Because of the cost of lengthy hospital stays, clients are typically discharged to the home setting with long-term vascular access catheters, such as the peripherally inserted central catheter (PICC), for medication administration. After discontinuation of IV drugs, oral antibiotic therapy may be needed for weeks or months. Clients and families must understand the complications of inadequate treatment or failure to follow-up with health care providers. Teach the client and family that antibiotic therapy must be continued over a long period of time to be effective. Even when symptoms of the disease appear to be improved, the full course of IV and oral antibiotics must be completed.

In addition to parenteral or oral drug administration, the wound may be irrigated, either continuously or intermittently, with one or more antibiotic solutions. Use sterile technique at all times. A technique in which beads are impregnated with an antibiotic and packed into the wound can provide direct contact of the antibiotic with the offending organism.

Medications are also needed to control pain. Clients experience acute and chronic pain, and must receive regimen drug therapy for control. Chapter 7 describes pharmacologic and nonpharmacologic interventions for both acute and chronic pain.

Infection Control. If an open wound or ulcer is present in the hospital or long-term care setting, the client's treatment usually includes standard precautions for limited infections in which the wound is covered. This practice may vary according to health care agency policy. Contact precautions are reserved for more severe infections, particularly when the purulent material cannot be adequately contained by a dressing. The open area is covered, and strict aseptic technique is used when dressings are changed to prevent further contamination. Wounds may be managed through the window of a cast, which must remain dry during dressing or irrigation procedures.

Hyperbaric Oxygen Therapy. A treatment to increase tissue perfusion for clients with chronic, unremitting osteomyelitis is the use of a hyperbaric chamber or portable device to administer hyperbaric oxygen (HBO) therapy. These devices are usually available in large teaching hospitals and may not be accessible to all clients who might benefit from them. With HBO therapy, the affected area is exposed to a high concentration of oxygen that diffuses into the tissues to promote healing. In conjunction with high-dose antibiotic therapy and surgical debridement, HBO has proved very useful in treating a number of anaerobic infections.

SURGICAL MANAGEMENT. Antibiotic therapy alone may not be sufficient to meet the goals of treatment. Surgical techniques are used to minimize the disfigurement that heretofore has been a devastating result of severe osteomyelitis. Most often, surgery is reserved for clients with chronic osteomyelitis.

Sequestrectomy. Because bone cannot heal in the presence of necrotic tissue, a sequestrectomy is performed to debride the infected bone and allow revascularization of tissue.

Bone Grafts. The excision of devitalized and infected bone often results in a sizable cavity, or bone defect. The use of cancellous bone grafts to obliterate bone defects began in the 1940s and is still widely used. One of the most popular surgical techniques is the Papineau procedure, or open cancellous bone graft, which is used primarily with large bone and soft-tissue defects.

The surgeon excises necrotic bone, grafts the bone, and covers the skin, if necessary. The donor bone is most often taken from the client's posterior ileum, but can be taken from other sites. If needed, the surgeon performs a skin graft, usually a simple split-thickness graft, often between 8 and 16 weeks after the bone graft.

Bone Segment Transfers. When infected bone is extensively resected, reconstruction with microvascular bone transfers may be useful. In general, a bone transfer is reserved for larger skeletal defects.

The most common donor sites are the client's fibula and iliac crest. The bone graft may have an attached muscle or skin flap, if necessary. The steps of the procedure are similar to those of cancellous grafting in that debridement precedes bone transfer.

Nursing care of the client after surgery is similar to that for any postoperative client (see Chapter 22). However, the important difference is that neurovascular (NV) assessments must be done frequently because the client experiences swelling after the surgical procedure. Elevate the affected extremity to increase venous return, and thus control swelling. Assess the client's NV status, including the following:

- Pain
- Movement
- Sensation
- Warmth
- Temperature
- Distal pulses
- Capillary refill (not as reliable as the above indicators)

Muscle Flaps. If the bony defect is relatively small, a muscle flap may be the only surgery required. Local muscle flaps are used in the treatment of chronic osteomyelitis when soft tissue does not obliterate the dead space, or cavity, resulting from bone debridement. The flap provides wound coverage and enhances blood flow to promote healing. A split-thickness skin graft is often applied several days after the muscle flap.

Amputation. When the previously described surgical procedures are not appropriate or successful, the affected limb may need to be amputated. The physical and psychological care for a client who has undergone an amputation is discussed in Chapter 55.

For all of the surgical procedures and their recovery phases, long-term antibiotic treatment is necessary. The preoperative and postoperative nursing care is similar to that for repair of musculoskeletal trauma.

Critical Thinking Challenge

An older adult has a history of type II diabetes and peripheral vascular disease. He was recently admitted to your medical unit with a draining foot ulcer. A blood culture reveals septicemia, and an MRI scan shows osteomyelitis. The client is placed on IV antibiotic therapy and analgesics for pain control. Today, his wife tells you that the doctor told her that her husband will be going home on IV antibiotics. She is angry that he has not taken better care of himself, and she doesn't know if she can take care of him at home because she is not well herself.

1. What is your best response to the client's wife at this time?
2. Who should you collaborate with when planning the client's discharge to home?
3. If the wife refuses to care for him at home, what options for care might he have?
4. What health teaching is needed for both the client and his wife after he is discharged?
5. What infection control measures will you use while he is hospitalized, and what measures will be necessary at home?

evolve For suggested answer guidelines, go to http://evolve.elsevier.com/Iggy/.

BONE TUMORS

Benign Bone Tumors

Benign (noncancerous) bone tumors are often asymptomatic and may be discovered on routine x-ray examination or as the cause of pathologic fractures. The cause of benign bone tumors is not known. Tumors may arise from several types of tissue. The major classifications include **chondrogenic** tumors (from cartilage), **osteogenic** tumors (from bone), and **fibrogenic** tumors (from fibrous tissue and found most often in children) (Table 54-4). As with other neoplasms, the cause of bone tumors is unknown. Although many specific benign tumors have been identified, only the common ones are described in the following sections.

CHONDROGENIC TUMORS

Osteochondroma

The most common benign bone tumor is the **osteochondroma**. Although its onset is usually in childhood, the tumor grows until skeletal maturity and may not be diagnosed until adulthood. The tumor may be a single growth or multiple growths and can occur in any bone. The femur and the tibia are most often involved.

On gross appearance, the tumor has a large cartilaginous cap with a bony stalk protruding from the bone. As the cap grows, the tumor ossifies (calcified) and may become malignant (cancerous). About 10% of osteochondromas change into sarcomas. Osteochondromas account for about 40% of all benign bone tumors and typically affect males more often than females.

Chondroma

The **chondroma,** or endochondroma, is closely related to the osteochondroma in histologic (cellular) presentation. Unlike the osteochondroma, however, the chondroma is a lesion of mature hyaline cartilage affecting primarily the hands and the feet. The ribs, the sternum, the spine, and the long bones may also be involved. Chondromas are slow growing and often cause pathologic fractures after minor injury.

Chondromas are found in people of all ages, occur in both males and females, and can affect any bone.

OSTEOGENIC TUMORS

Osteoid Osteoma

The **osteoid osteoma** is distinguished by its pinkish, granular appearance, resulting from the proliferation of osteoblasts. Unlike other tumors, a single lesion is usually less than 0.4

TABLE 54-4 Classification of Primary Bone Tumors

Benign	Malignant
Chondrogenic	***Chondrogenic***
Osteochondroma	Chondrosarcoma
Chondroma	
Osteogenic	***Osteogenic***
Osteoid osteoma	Osteosarcoma
Osteoblastoma	***Fibrogenic***
Giant cell tumor	Fibrosarcoma
	Unknown Origin
	Ewing's sarcoma

inch (1 cm) in diameter. Any bone can be affected, but the femur and the tibia are most often involved. When the osteoid osteoma occurs in the spinal column and sacrum, the clinical manifestations resemble those of the lumbar disk syndrome. The client complains of unremitting bone pain, probably attributable to the increase in prostaglandin levels associated with the tumor.

About 10% of all benign bone tumors are osteoid osteomas. The lesion occurs in children and young adults, with predominance among males.

Osteoblastoma

Often called *giant osteoid osteoma,* the **osteoblastoma** affects the vertebrae and long bones. The tumor is larger than the osteoid osteoma and lies in cancellous bone. Its reddish, granular appearance facilitates diagnosis.

The lesion accounts for less than 1% of primary bone tumors and affects adolescent boys and young adults of both genders.

Giant Cell Tumor

The origin of the **giant cell tumor** remains uncertain. This lesion is aggressive and can be extensive. On gross examination, the lesions are gray to reddish brown and may involve surrounding soft tissue. Although classified as benign, giant cell tumors can metastasize (spread) to the lung.

Unlike most other benign bone tumors, giant cell tumors affect women older than 20 years of age; the peak incidence occurs in clients in their 30s.

COLLABORATIVE MANAGEMENT

Assessment

PHYSICAL ASSESSMENT/CLINICAL MANIFESTATIONS

If a client experiences clinical manifestations of a benign bone tumor, pain is the most frequent complaint. The pain can range from mild to moderate, as seen with chondromas, to unremitting and intense, as is typical with osteoid osteomas. Pain can be caused by direct tumor invasion into soft tissue, compressing peripheral nerves, or by a resulting pathologic fracture.

In addition to collecting information regarding the nature of the client's pain, observe and palpate the suspected involved area. When the tumor affects the lower extremities or the small bones of the hands and feet, local swelling may be detected as the neoplasm enlarges. In some cases, muscle atrophy or muscle spasm may be present. Palpate the bone and muscle to detect these changes and elicit tenderness.

DIAGNOSTIC ASSESSMENT

Routine radiography and conventional tomography are extremely beneficial in localizing and visualizing neoplasms of the bone. Benign tumors are characterized by sharp margins, intact cortices, and smooth, uniform periosteal bone.

Computed tomography (CT) is less useful, except in complex anatomic areas, such as the spinal column and sacrum. The test is helpful in evaluating the extent of soft-tissue involvement.

When the diagnosis of a benign tumor is uncertain, an open or needle biopsy of the bone is performed. The open surgical method is preferred to obtain a sufficient amount of tissue.

Magnetic resonance imaging (MRI) may be especially helpful in viewing problems of the spinal column.

Interventions

The physician uses drug therapy and surgery in combination when possible. Nondrug pain relief measures are also used. Depending on the client's preference and tolerance, measures such as application of heat or cold may be helpful to relieve pain.

In addition to prescribing analgesics to reduce pain, the health care provider usually prescribes one or more nonsteroidal anti-inflammatory drugs (NSAIDs) to inhibit prostaglandin synthesis and thus relieve pain in the client with an osteoid osteoma. Observe for drug actions and side effects, administering the drug after meals or with milk and crackers.

The most common surgical procedure used for clients with benign bone tumors is curettage, or simple excision of the tumor tissue. If the tumor is small, surgery may not be indicated. When the lesion is extremely extensive, as in a giant cell tumor, the neoplasm is removed with care to restore or maintain the function of the adjacent joint, most often the knee. In some cases, the knee is replaced with a prosthetic device, and less often, is fused **(arthrodesis).** Bone grafting may be needed. The nursing care for clients undergoing these surgical procedures is discussed in Chapter 24.

Malignant Bone Tumors

Malignant bone tumors may be **primary** (those that originate in bone; see Table 54-4) or **secondary** (those that originate in other tissues and metastasize to bone). Primary tumors occur most often in people between 10 and 30 years of age and make up a small percentage of bone cancers. As for other forms of cancer, the exact cause of bone cancer is unknown. Metastatic lesions most often occur in the older age-group and account for most bone cancers.

Primary Tumors

OSTEOSARCOMA

Osteosarcoma, or osteogenic sarcoma, is the most common type of primary malignant bone tumor. More than 50% occur in the distal femur, followed in decreasing order of occurrence by the proximal tibia and humerus. Flat-bone and long-bone incidence is about equal in people older than 25 years of age.

The lesion is relatively large, causing pain and swelling of short duration. The involved area is usually warm, because the vascularity to the site increases. The central portion of the mass is sclerotic from increased osteoblastic activity; the periphery is soft, extending through the bone cortex in the classic sunburst appearance associated with the neoplasm. An inward expansion into the medullary canal is also common.

Osteosarcoma may be osteoblastic, chondroblastic, or fibroblastic, depending on the tissue of origin. Regardless of its source, the lesion typically metastasizes to the periphery of the lung within 2 years of treatment; metastasis usually results in death.

Osteosarcoma occurs more often in males than in females (2:1), between ages 10 and 30 years, and in older clients with Paget's disease. Clients who have received radiation for other forms of cancer or who have benign lesions are also at high risk.

EWING'S SARCOMA

Although **Ewing's sarcoma** is not as common as other tumors, it is the most malignant. Like other primary tumors, it causes pain and swelling. In addition, systemic manifestations, particularly low-grade fever, leukocytosis, and anemia, characterize the lesions. The pelvis and the lower extremity are most often affected. Pelvic involvement is a poor prognostic sign.

On a cellular level, the tumor is similar to bone lymphoma. On x-ray examination the characteristic mottled destructive pattern and "onion skin" appearance of the bone surface distinguish the neoplasm as Ewing's sarcoma. Like other malignant tumors, it is not encapsulated and often extends into soft tissue. Death results from metastasis to the lungs and other bones.

Five percent of all malignant bone tumors are Ewing's sarcoma. Although the tumor can be seen in clients of any age, it usually occurs in children and young adults in their 20s. Men are affected more often than women.

CHONDROSARCOMA

In contrast to the client with osteosarcoma, the client with **chondrosarcoma** experiences dull pain and swelling for a long period. The tumor typically affects the pelvis and proximal femur near the diaphysis. Arising from cartilaginous tissue, the lesion destroys bone and often calcifies. The client with chondrosarcoma usually has a better prognosis than the client with osteogenic sarcoma.

Chondrosarcoma occurs in middle-aged and older people, with a slight predominance in men, and accounts for fewer than 10% of all malignant bone tumors.

FIBROSARCOMA

Arising from fibrous tissue, **fibrosarcomas** can be divided into subtypes, of which malignant fibrous histiocytoma (MFH) is the most malignant. Most often, the clinical presentation of MFH is gradual, without specific symptoms. Local tenderness, with or without a palpable mass, occurs in the long bones of the lower extremity. As with other bone cancers, the lesion can metastasize to the lungs.

Although MFH affects people of all ages, it typically occurs in middle-aged men. Fortunately, the lesion is not common.

Metastatic Bone Disease

PATHOPHYSIOLOGY

Primary tumors of the prostate, breast, kidney, thyroid, and lung are called *bone-seeking* cancers; they metastasize to the bone more often than other primary tumors. The vertebrae, pelvis, femur, and ribs are the bone sites commonly affected. Simply stated, primary tumor cells, or seeds, are carried to bone through the bloodstream. Almost all metastatic lesions are of epithelial origin and begin in the bone marrow. **Pathologic fractures** are a major concern in management. The most commonly affected areas for fracture are the acetabulum and the proximal femur.

Metastatic bone tumors greatly outnumber primary malignant neoplasms. Metastatic bone disease primarily affects people older than 40 years of age. In clients with a history of cancer and local pain, metastasis is suspected. The incidence of bone metastasis ranges from 20% to 70%, depending on the statistical reporting source. It is suspected that the reported incidence of metastasis is grossly understated.

COLLABORATIVE MANAGEMENT

Assessment

HISTORY

The data collected for the client suspected of having a malignant tumor are similar to the data required for the client with a benign growth. In addition, ask whether the client has had previous radiation therapy for cancer and elicit information about the client's general health.

PHYSICAL ASSESSMENT/CLINICAL MANIFESTATIONS

The clinical manifestations seen in the client with a primary malignant tumor or metastatic disease vary, depending on the specific type of lesion. Most often, the client has a group of nonspecific complaints, including pain, local swelling, and a tender, palpable mass. Marked disability may be present in advanced metastatic bone disease.

In a client with Ewing's sarcoma, a low-grade fever may occur because of the systemic features of the neoplasm. For this reason, Ewing's sarcoma is often confused with osteomyelitis. Fatigue and pallor resulting from anemia are also common.

In performing a musculoskeletal assessment, inspect the involved area and palpate the mass for size characteristics and tenderness. The client's ability to perform mobility tasks and activities of daily living (ADLs) is also determined. If possible, observe the client performing mobility tasks and record the results on a functional assessment tool (see Chapter 10). The degree of disability can then be determined for comparison with later measurements after medical and nursing intervention.

PSYCHOSOCIAL ASSESSMENT

Often, clients with malignant bone tumors are young adults whose socially productive lives are just beginning. They need support systems to help cope with the diagnosis and its treatment. Family, significant others, and health care professionals are major components of the needed support. Determine what systems are available to clients.

Clients often experience a loss of control over their lives when a diagnosis of malignancy is made. As a result, they become anxious and fearful about the outcome of their illness. Coping with the diagnosis becomes a challenge. All clients go through the grieving process; initially, there is denial. Identify the anxiety level and assess the stage or stages of the grieving process. Explore any maladaptive behavior, indicating ineffective coping mechanisms. Chapter 28 further elaborates on the psychosocial assessment for clients with malignancy.

LABORATORY ASSESSMENT

The client with a primary malignant or metastatic bone tumor typically shows elevated serum alkaline phosphatase (ALP) levels, indicating the body's attempt to form new bone by increasing osteoblastic activity. The client with Ewing's sarcoma or metastatic bone lesions often has normocytic anemia. In addition, leukocytosis is common with Ewing's sarcoma. The progression of Ewing's sarcoma may be evaluated by elevated serum lactate dehydrogenase (LDH) levels.

In some clients with bone metastasis from the breast, kidney, or lung, the serum calcium level is elevated. Massive bone destruction stimulates release of the mineral into the bloodstream.

In clients with Ewing's sarcoma and bone metastasis, often the erythrocyte sedimentation rate (ESR) is elevated, which is probably attributable to secondary tissue inflammation.

RADIOGRAPHIC ASSESSMENT

As with benign bone tumors, routine x-rays and computed tomography (CT) allow for adequate visualization of malignant lesions. Although each tumor type has its own characteristic radiographic pattern, certain findings are common to all. Malignant tumors typically show poor margination, bone destruction, irregular periosteal new bone, and cortical breakthrough.

Metastatic lesions may increase or decrease bone density, depending on the amount of osteoblastic and osteoclastic activity. CT is helpful in determining the extent of soft-tissue damage.

OTHER DIAGNOSTIC ASSESSMENTS

The client may have magnetic resonance imaging and a bone scan. In some cases, a bone biopsy may be performed. After biopsy, the cancer is staged according to the grade of the tumor. One popular method is the TNM staging system, which uses determinations of *t*umor size, *n*odal involvement, and evidence of *m*etastasis.

Another surgical staging method is to correlate the tumor grade (high or low), tumor site (intracompartmental or extracompartmental), and presence of metastatic disease (positive or negative). Staging guides the health care team in their decision regarding treatment.

Analysis

COMMON NURSING DIAGNOSES AND COLLABORATIVE PROBLEMS

The following are priority nursing diagnoses for clients with malignant bone tumors:

1. Acute Pain and Chronic Pain related to physical injury (direct tumor invasion into soft tissue)
2. Anticipatory Grieving related to a change in body image or impending death
3. Disturbed Body Image related to the effects of illness treatment, including surgery

A primary collaborative problem is Potential for Fractures.

ADDITIONAL NURSING DIAGNOSES AND COLLABORATIVE PROBLEMS

In addition to the common nursing diagnoses and collaborative problems, clients with malignant bone tumors may have one or more of the following:

- Fear and Anxiety related to the medical diagnosis, possible disfiguring surgery, or impending death
- Ineffective Coping related to inadequate level of confidence in ability to cope
- Compromised Family Coping related to prolonged disease
- Dysfunctional Grieving related to actual loss
- Impaired Physical Mobility related to pain and musculoskeletal impairment
- Imbalanced Nutrition: Less Than Body Requirements related to an increased metabolic process
- Disturbed Sleep Pattern related to pain
- Self-Care Deficit (Total) related to impaired physical mobility and weakness
- Ineffective Role Performance related to a temporary or permanent inability to maintain the family or community role
- Spiritual Distress related to fear of death

Planning and Implementation

ACUTE PAIN; CHRONIC PAIN

NOC **PLANNING: EXPECTED OUTCOMES.** The client with a malignant bone tumor is expected to take personal actions to control pain. Indicators include that the client will consistently demonstrate the ability to:

- Recognize pain onset
- Use preventive measures
- Use analgesics appropriately
- Use nonanalgesic relief measures
- Report pain control

INTERVENTIONS. Because the pain is often due to direct tumor invasion, treatment is aimed at reducing the size of or removing the tumor. A combination of nonsurgical and surgical management is often used to promote client comfort and eliminate the complications of bone cancer.

NONSURGICAL MANAGEMENT. In addition to analgesics for local pain relief, chemotherapeutic agents and radiation therapy are often administered to cause tumor regression. In clients with vertebral metastatic disease, bracing and immobilization with cervical traction reduce back pain.

Drug Therapy. The physician may prescribe chemotherapy to be given alone or in combination with radiation or surgery. Certain proliferating tumors, such as Ewing's sarcoma, are sensitive to cytotoxic medications. Others, such as chondrosarcomas, are often totally drug resistant. Chemotherapy seems to work best for small, metastatic lesions and may be administered before or after surgery. For most tumors, the physician prescribes a combination of agents. At present, there is no universally accepted protocol of chemotherapeutic agents. The drugs selected are determined in part by the primary source of the cancer in metastatic disease. For example, when metastasis occurs from breast cancer, estrogens and progesterone may be used.

Observe the client carefully for side and toxic effects and monitors laboratory tests diligently. Chapter 28 discusses the nursing care associated with the administration of cytotoxic agents.

Radiation Therapy. Radiation is used for selected types of malignant tumors. For clients with Ewing's sarcoma and early osteosarcoma, radiation may be the treatment of choice in reducing tumor size and thus pain.

For clients with metastatic disease, radiation is given primarily for palliation. The therapy is directed toward the painful sites to provide a more comfortable life span. One or more treatments are given, depending on the extent of disease. With precise planning, radiation therapy can be used with minimal complications. The nursing care for clients receiving radiation therapy is described in Chapter 28.

SURGICAL MANAGEMENT. The treatment of primary bone tumors is surgery, often combined with radiation or chemotherapy.

Preoperative Care. Preoperatively, thoroughly evaluate the client to assist the physician in the selection of the surgical procedure to be performed. In addition to the nature, progression, and extent of the tumor, the client's age and general health state are taken into consideration. Chemotherapy may be administered preoperatively.

As for any client preparing for cancer surgery, the client with bone cancer needs psychological support from the nurse and other members of the health care team. Assess the level of understanding of the client and the family or significant others. As a client advocate, encourage the expression of concerns and questions and provide information regarding hospital routines and procedures. Spiritual support is important to some clients, who may prefer to contact their own clergy, rabbi, or spiritual leader or talk with the clergy affiliated with the hospital. Assist in arranging for spiritual assistance if needed.

Postoperative needs are anticipated and planned for as much as possible before the client undergoes surgery. Remind the client what to expect postoperatively and how to help ensure adequate recovery.

Operative Procedures. Wide or radical resection procedures are commonly performed for clients with bone sarcomas. Wide excision is removal of the lesion surrounded by an intact cuff of normal tissue and leads to cure of low-grade tumors only. A radical resection includes removal of the lesion, the entire muscle, bone, and other tissues directly involved. It is the only procedure adequate for high-grade tumors.

Bone defects that result from tumor removal include the following:

- Total joint replacements with prosthetic implants, either whole or partial
- Custom metallic implants
- Allografts from the iliac crest, rib, or fibula

As an alternative to total replacement, an allograft may be implanted with internal fixation for those clients who do not have metastases. This is a common procedure for sarcomas of the proximal femur. Allograft procedures for the knee are also performed, particularly in young adults. Preoperative chemotherapy is given to enhance the likelihood of success. **Allografts** with adjacent tendons and ligaments are harvested from cadavers and can be frozen or freeze-dried for a prolonged period. The graft is fixed with a series of bolts, screws, or plates. Observe for signs of hemorrhage, infection, or fracture.

For clients with metastatic disease, intractable pain is surgically treated with percutaneous **cordotomy** (cutting of the spinal nerve roots). **Cryosurgery** (cold application) may reduce pain and tumor size.

Postoperative Care. The surgical incision for a limb salvage procedure is often extensive. A pressure dressing with wound suction is typically maintained for several days.

The client who has undergone a limb salvage procedure has resulting impaired physical mobility and a self-care deficit. The nature and extent of the alterations depend on the location and extent of the surgery.

Promotion of Physical Mobility. Usually, muscle strengthening and range-of-motion (ROM) exercises begin immediately postoperatively and continue for at least a year. After upper extremity surgery, the client can engage in active-assistive exercises by using the opposite hand to help achieve motions such as forward flexion and abduction of the shoulder. Continuous passive motion (CPM) using a CPM machine may be initiated as early as the first postoperative day for either upper extremity or lower extremity procedures.

After lower extremity surgery, the emphasis is on strengthening the quadriceps muscles by using passive and active motion when possible. Maintaining muscle tone is an important prerequisite to weight bearing, which progresses from toe touch or partial weight bearing to full weight bearing by 3 months postoperatively.

The client who has had a bone graft has a plaster cast that remains in place for several months. Weight bearing is prohibited until there is evidence that the graft is incorporated into the adjacent bone tissue.

During the recovery phase, the client also needs assistance with activities of daily living (ADLs), particularly if the surgery involves the upper extremity. Assist if needed, but at the same time try to encourage the client to do as much as possible unaided.

Neurovascular Assessment. Surrounding tissues, including nerves and blood vessels, may be sacrificed during surgery. Vascular grafting is common, but the lost nerve is usually not replaced. Assess the neurovascular status of the affected extremity and its digits thoroughly and frequently. Splinting or casting of the limb may also cause neurovascular compromise and needs to be checked for proper placement.

Pelvic lesions, although not commonly seen, are also excised. Reconstruction generally entails bone fusion with muscle and nerve preservation. A hip spica cast or brace may be necessary until graft incorporation has occurred. The client may need a cane for ambulation.

The major complications peculiar to reconstructive surgery for which you should observe are superficial and deep wound infection, dislocation or loosening of the implants, and rapid neurovascular compromise. Report an increase in pain or temperature, or a rapid deterioration in circulatory status to the physician promptly.

Psychological Support. In addition to needing psychological help in coping with physical disabilities, the client may need help coping with the surgery and its effects postoperatively. Having identified the available support systems preoperatively, you can help mobilize them for use after surgery.

As a result of most of the surgical procedures, the client experiences an alteration in body image. Suggest ways to minimize cosmetic changes. For example, a lowered shoulder can be covered by a custom-made pad worn under clothing. The client can cover lower extremity defects with pants.

ANTICIPATORY GRIEVING

NOC **PLANNING: EXPECTED OUTCOMES.** The client with a malignant bone tumor is expected to adjust to actual or impending loss. Indicators include that the client will have the ability to:

- Resolve feelings about loss
- Verbalize reality of loss

- Discuss unresolved conflicts
- Seek social support
- Progress through stages of grief

INTERVENTIONS. The nurse's most important role is to be an active listener and to encourage the client and family or significant others to verbalize their feelings. Counselors and members of the clergy or spiritual leaders may provide additional assistance in promoting acceptance of the diagnosis, treatment, or, possibly, impending death. Chapter 9 provides information about death and dying.

Regardless of the prognosis, a diagnosis of bone cancer is a major stressor that causes the client and family or significant others to grieve. Help the client and others to cope with the loss and resolve the grief (Chart 54-6).

The nurse also acts as an advocate for the client and the family and often promotes the physician-client relationship. For instance, the client may not completely understand the medical or surgical treatment plan but may be hesitant to question the physician. The nurse's intervention increases communication, which is essential in successful management of the client with cancer.

DISTURBED BODY IMAGE

NOC **PLANNING: EXPECTED OUTCOMES.** The client with a malignant bone tumor is expected to experience a positive perception of his or her own appearance and body functions. Indicators include that the client will have a consistently positive:

- Internal picture of self
- Satisfaction with body appearance
- Adjustment to changes in health status
- Adjustments to body changes due to surgery

INTERVENTIONS. The client's self-perception of body image is closely associated with his or her ability to accept the illness. Recognize and accept the client's view about the body image alteration. A trusting nurse-client relationship allows the client freedom to verbalize negative feelings. Emphasize the client's strengths and remaining capabilities. Establish realistic mutual goals regarding lifestyle (see Chart 54-6).

POTENTIAL FOR FRACTURES

PLANNING: EXPECTED OUTCOMES. As with other bone diseases in which pathologic fracture is a possible complication (e.g., osteoporosis), the client with a malignant bone tumor is expected to avoid falls and minimize trauma to prevent fractures. In people with metastatic bone disease, fractures occur more readily and are not as preventable because of resulting destructive bone resorption. A more realistic outcome for people with metastatic disease, then, may be that the client's pain will be minimized through treatment of the fracture.

INTERVENTIONS. Radiation or surgery may be required to reinforce or replace the diseased bone to prevent fracture. In recent years, surgical techniques have also been improved for fracture fixation.

NONSURGICAL MANAGEMENT. Newer techniques in radiation therapy have improved the incidence of bone healing for actual and impending pathologic fractures. To improve muscle tone and, consequently, to reduce the risk for fracture, the client performs strengthening exercises. Physical therapy on an ambulatory basis is commonly prescribed.

One of two bisphosphonates, zoledronic acid (Zometa) and pamidronate (Aredia), may be used to inhibit bone resorption and subsequent hypercalcemia. Both medications are given by IV infusion and place clients at risk for flulike symptoms, hypokalemia, hypomagnesemia, and hypophosphatemia. Inform clients that osteonecrosis of the jaw may also occur, especially in those who have dental procedures (Aschenbrenner, 2005).

SURGICAL MANAGEMENT. The principles of surgery for metastatic fractures include the following:

- Replacing as much defective bone as possible
- Being thorough in technique to avoid a second procedure
- Aiming to return the client to a functional state with a minimum of hospitalization and immobilization

Fractures of the proximal femur are very common. Prosthetic replacement reinforced with polymethylmethacrylate ("bone glue") is preferred over open reduction with internal fixation (ORIF) when feasible. The surgeon uses intramedullary rods and compression screws for more distal fractures. Prophylactic fixation may be indicated for microscopic fractures that cause chronic pain. Chapter 55 discusses the nursing management for clients undergoing repair of a fractured hip.

Community-Based Care

After medical treatment for a primary malignant tumor, the client is usually managed at home with follow-up care. The client with metastatic disease may remain in the home or,

CHART 54-6

NIC INTERVENTION ACTIVITIES for The Client with Bone Cancer (Psychosocial Care)

Grief Work Facilitation: *Assistance with the resolution of a significant loss*

- Identify the loss.
- Assist the client to identify the nature of the attachment to the lost object or person.
- Assist the client to identify the initial reaction to the loss.
- Encourage expression of feelings about the loss.
- Instruct in phases of the grieving process, as appropriate.
- Support progression through personal grieving stages.
- Include significant others in discussion and decisions, as appropriate.
- Assist client to identify personal coping strategies.
- Communicate acceptance of discussing loss.
- Identify sources of community support.
- Reinforce progress made in the grieving process.
- Assist in identifying modifications needed in lifestyle.

Body Image Enhancement: *Improving a client's conscious and unconscious perceptions and attitudes toward his/her body*

- Assist client to discuss changes caused by illness or surgery, as appropriate.
- Help client determine the extent of actual changes in the body or its level of functioning.
- Assist client to determine the influence of a peer group on the client's perception of present body image.
- Identify the effects of the client's culture, religion, race, sex, and age in terms of body image.
- Monitor whether client can look at the changed body part.
- Determine if a change in body image has contributed to increased social isolation.
- Assist client to identify actions that will enhance appearance.
- Identify support groups available to client.

NIC intervention activities selected from Dochterman, J.M., & Bulechek, G.M. (Eds.). (2004). *Nursing interventions classification (NIC)* (4th ed.). St. Louis: Mosby.

when home support is not available, may be admitted to a long-term care facility for extended or hospice care. A case manager may assist with management of the client's care.

HOME CARE MANAGEMENT

In collaboration with the occupational therapist, evaluate the client's home environment for structural barriers that may hinder mobility. The client may be discharged with a cast, crutches, or a wheelchair.

Accessibility to eating and toileting facilities is essential to promote independence. Because the client with metastatic disease is susceptible to pathologic fractures, potential hazards that may contribute to falls or injury should be removed.

HEALTH TEACHING

For the client receiving intermittent chemotherapy on an ambulatory basis, emphasize the importance of keeping appointments. Review the expected, side, and toxic effects of the medications with the client. Teach the client how to treat minor side effects and when to alert the health care provider. If the drugs are administered at home via long-term IV catheter, explain the care involved with daily dressing changes and potential catheter complications. Chapter 17 describes the health teaching required for a client receiving infusion therapy at home.

The client receiving radiation therapy is also taught the importance of keeping appointments and recognizing the complications of treatment. Review interventions that can be used at home for minor complications.

If the client has undergone surgery, he or she has a wound and limited mobility. Teach the client, family, and/or significant others how to care for the wound. Help the client learn how to perform activities of daily living (ADLs) and mobility activities independently. Physical and occupational therapists assist in ADL teaching and provide or recommend assistive and adaptive devices if necessary. The physical therapist also teaches the proper use of ambulatory aids, such as crutches, and exercises.

Pain management can be a major problem, particularly in the client with metastatic bone disease. Discuss the various options for pain relief, including relaxation and music therapy. Emphasize the importance of those techniques that worked during hospitalization.

The client with bone cancer typically fears that the malignancy will return. Acknowledge this fear, but reinforces confidence in the health care team and medical treatment chosen.

Realistic goals regarding return to work, recreational activities, and so forth are mutually established. Encourage the client to resume a functional lifestyle, but caution that it should be gradual. Certain activities, such as participating in sports, may be prohibited.

The client with advanced metastatic bone disease needs to prepare for death. The nurse and other support personnel assist the client through the stages of death and dying (see Chapter 9). Identify resources that can help the client write a will, visit with distant family members, or do whatever he or she thinks is needed to die in peace. In the later stages of the disease, hospice care may be an option. Nurses working in this area of care can be most helpful in managing end-of-life care.

HEALTH CARE RESOURCES

In addition to family and significant others, cancer support groups are helpful to the client with bone cancer. Some organizations, such as I Can Cope, provide information and emotional support; others, such as CanSurmount, are geared more toward client and family education.

The hospital staff nurse, discharge planner, or case manager also ensures that follow-up care, including nursing care and physical or occupational therapy, is available in the home. The client with terminal cancer may choose to become part of a hospice program (see Chapter 9).

◆Evaluation: Outcomes

Evaluate the care of the client with a malignant bone tumor on the basis of the identified nursing diagnoses and collaborative problems. The expected outcomes may include that the client will:

- Demonstrate ability to control pain
- Adjust to actual or impending loss
- Experience positive perception of own appearance and body function

Specific indicators for these outcomes are listed for each nursing diagnosis and collaborative problem under the Planning and Implementation section (see earlier).

DISORDERS OF THE HAND

Carpal Tunnel Syndrome

PATHOPHYSIOLOGY

Carpal tunnel syndrome (CTS) is a common condition in which the median nerve in the wrist becomes compressed, causing pain and numbness. The carpal tunnel is a rigid canal lying between the carpal bones and a fibrous tissue sheet called the flexor retinaculum. As seen in Figure 54-4, a group of nine tendons enveloped by synovium share space with the median nerve in the carpal tunnel. When the synovium becomes swollen or thickened, the nerve is compressed.

The median nerve supplies the motor, sensory, and autonomic function for the first three digits of the hand and the palmar aspect of the fourth digit. Because of the median nerve's proximity to other structures, wrist flexion causes nerve impingement against the flexor retinaculum; extension causes increased pressure in the distal portion of the carpal tunnel.

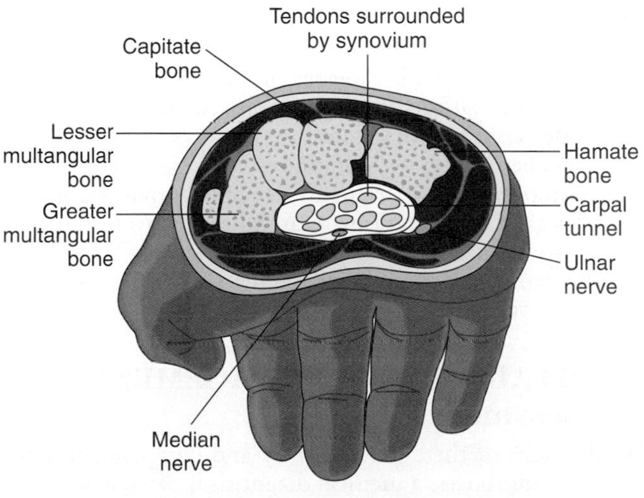

Figure 54-4 ■ Anatomy of the carpal tunnel.

Etiology and Genetic Risk

CTS usually presents as a chronic problem; acute cases are rare. Excessive hand exercise, edema or hemorrhage into the carpal tunnel, or thrombosis of the median artery can lead to acute CTS. Clients with a Colles' fracture of the wrist or hand burns are particularly at risk for rapid CTS development.

In most cases, however, the causative factors may not result in neurologic deficit for years. CTS is a common complication of certain metabolic and connective tissue diseases. For example, **synovitis** (inflammation of the synovium) occurs in clients with rheumatoid arthritis. The hypertrophied synovium compresses the median nerve. In other chronic disorders such as diabetes mellitus, inadequate blood supply can cause median nerve neuropathy, or dysfunction, resulting in CTS.

CTS is the most **common repetitive strain injury (RSI)**—the fastest growing type of occupational injury. People whose jobs require repetitive hand activities involving pinch or grasp during wrist flexion, such as factory workers, computer operators, and jackhammer operators, are predisposed to CTS. CTS can also result from overuse in sports activities such as golf, tennis, or racquetball.

In a few cases, CTS may be a familial or congenital problem, manifesting in adulthood. Space-occupying lesions, such as ganglia, tophi, and lipomas, can also result in nerve compression.

Incidence/Prevalence

CTS occurs in adults of all ages but peaks between ages 30 and 60 years of age. Women are five times more likely to experience the problem than men. Most often, CTS affects the dominant hand, but it can occur in both hands simultaneously. Children and adolescents are also beginning to experience CTS as a result of the increased use of computers in everyday life.

HEALTH PROMOTION/ILLNESS PREVENTION

Many businesses have recognized the hazards of repetitive motion as a primary cause of occupational injury and disability. Both men and women in the labor force are experiencing increasing numbers of repetitive strain injuries (RSIs). Occupational health nurses have played an important role in the development of ergonomically appropriate furniture and other aids to decrease CTS and other musculoskeletal injuries. Federal and state legislation has been passed to ensure that businesses provide ergonomically appropriate workstations for their employees, but furniture for the home cannot be mandated.

Teach clients who use computers frequently or have jobs that require repetitive strain to use appropriate ergonomically designed work stations. Remind clients to take regular breaks from activities that predispose them to CTS. If beginning symptoms occur, tell them to seek medical attention for prompt, early treatment.

COLLABORATIVE MANAGEMENT

Assessment

On the basis of the client's history and complaint of hand pain and numbness, a medical diagnosis is often made without further assessment. Question clients regarding the nature, intensity, and location of the pain. Clients often state that the pain is worse at night as a result of flexion or direct pressure during sleep. The pain may radiate to the arm, the shoulder and neck, or the chest.

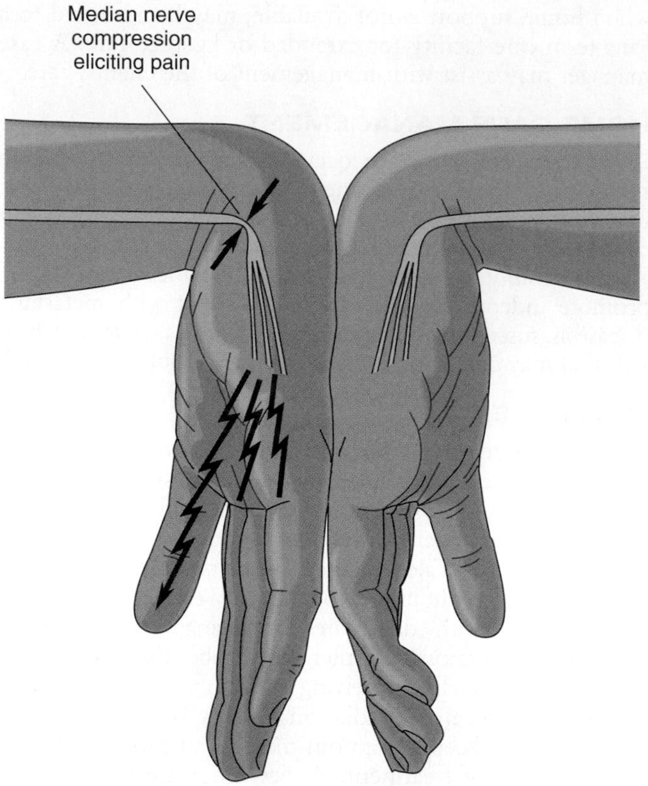

Figure 54-5 ■ Phalen's maneuver for detection of carpal tunnel syndrome.

In addition to the complaint of numbness, clients with carpal tunnel syndrome (CTS) may also experience **paresthesia** (painful tingling). Sensory changes usually precede motor manifestations by weeks or months.

PHYSICAL ASSESSMENT/CLINICAL MANIFESTATIONS

The health care provider performs several tests to elicit abnormal sensory findings. Phalen's wrist test, sometimes called **Phalen's maneuver,** produces paresthesia in the median nerve distribution (palmar side of the thumb, index, and middle finger, and radial half of the ring finger) within 60 seconds. The client is asked to relax the wrist into flexion or place the back of the hands together and flex both wrists simultaneously (Figure 54-5). Most clients with CTS have a positive Phalen's test result.

The same sensation can be elicited by tapping lightly over the area of the median nerve in the wrist **(Tinel's sign).** If the test is unsuccessful, a blood pressure cuff can be placed on the upper arm and inflated to the client's systolic pressure. The result is often pain and tingling.

Motor changes begin with a weak pinch, clumsiness, and difficulty with fine movements and then progress to muscle weakness and wasting. The nurse may test for pinching ability and ask the client to perform a fine-movement task, such as threading a needle. Strenuous hand activity worsens the subjective complaints.

In addition to inspecting for muscle atrophy and task performance, observe the wrist for swelling. Palpate the area and note unusual findings. Autonomic changes may be evidenced by skin discoloration, nail changes (e.g., brittleness), and increased or decreased palmar sweating.

DIAGNOSTIC ASSESSMENT

Routine x-rays are ordered to visualize bone changes, space-occupying lesions, and synovitis. If these causative factors are not suspected, a client with CTS may not have x-rays done.

The health care provider may order electromyography (EMG), magnetic resonance imaging (MRI), or ultrasonography when a definitive diagnosis is uncertain. Problems of the cervical spine and spinal nerves can mimic the clinical manifestations of CTS. EMG testing reveals nerve dysfunction before muscle atrophy is observed. MRI is very useful for helping to diagnose CTS. The most common finding is an enlarged median nerve within the carpal tunnel. The newest technique for diagnosis is the use of ultrasound.

Interventions

The health care provider uses conservative measures before surgical intervention. With either type of treatment, however, CTS can recur.

NONSURGICAL MANAGEMENT. Drug therapy and immobilization of the wrist are the major components of nonsurgical management. Teach the client the importance of these modalities in the hope of preventing surgical intervention.

The most commonly prescribed drugs for the relief of pain and inflammation, if present, are nonsteroidal anti-inflammatory drugs (NSAIDs). In addition to or instead of systemic medications, the physician may inject corticosteroids directly into the carpal tunnel. If the client responds to the medication, several additional weekly or monthly injections are given. As with any medication, monitor the effects of drug therapy. NSAIDs are given with or after meals to reduce gastric irritation.

A splint may be used to immobilize the wrist during the day, during the night, or both. Many clients experience temporary relief with splinting. The occupational therapist places the wrist in the neutral position or in slight extension. Even when a splint is not used, instruct the client to minimize hand activities, at least temporarily.

SURGICAL MANAGEMENT. Surgery is necessary in about half of clients with CTS. Surgery can relieve the pressure on the median nerve by providing nerve decompression.

Preoperative Care. The nurse in the physician's office or same-day surgical center reinforces the teaching provided by the surgeon regarding the nature of the surgery. Postoperative care is reviewed so that the client knows what to expect.

Operative Procedures. The two most common surgeries are the open carpal tunnel release (OCTR) and the newer endoscopic carpal tunnel release (ECTR). When CTS is a complication of rheumatoid arthritis, a **synovectomy** (removal of excess synovium) through a small inner-wrist incision may resolve the problem. Removal of a space-occupying lesion, if present, also decompresses the nerve. Whatever the cause of nerve compression, the physician removes it either by cutting or by the newer laser technique. In some cases, CTS recurs months to years after surgery.

An alternative to OCTR is the endoscopic release. The surgeon makes a very small incision (less than ½ inch [1.2 cm]) through which the endoscope is inserted. The surgeon then uses special instruments, which may include a laser, to free the trapped median nerve.

Postoperative Care. Although ECTR is less invasive and costs less than the open procedure, the client may experience pain and numbness for a longer time postoperatively as compared with recovery from OCTR. Major surgical complications are rare following CTS surgery.

After surgery, monitor vital signs and check the dressing carefully for drainage and tightness. If the endoscopic procedure has been performed, the dressing is very small. The surgeon may require that the client's hand and arm be elevated above heart level for several days to reduce swelling from surgery. Check the neurovascular status of the digits every hour during the immediate postoperative period, encouraging the client to move all fingers of the affected hand frequently. Offer pain medication and assure the client that he or she will be given a prescription for analgesics for use at home during recovery.

Hand movements, including lifting heavy objects, may be restricted for 4 to 6 weeks after surgery. The client can expect weakness and discomfort for weeks or perhaps months. Teach the client to report any changes in neurovascular status.

The client must realize that the surgical procedure might not be a cure. For instance, synovitis may recur in the client with rheumatoid arthritis and may recompress the median nerve. Multiple operations and other treatments are not uncommon with CTS.

The client may need assistance with routine daily tasks or even self-care activities during recovery. Ensure the client that assistance in the home should be available; this is usually provided by the family or significant others.

Critical Thinking Challenge

You are a nurse working for a large factory in an urban area. One of the employees comes to you complaining of pain and tingling in his right hand, and he is right-handed. He has been working at the factory for 37 years and has worked every piece of equipment there during that period. He is upset that "this place" doesn't care about its workers and makes them work too long in one station without adequate breaks. He plans to file a complaint for worker's compensation and notify the local Occupational Safety and Health board to report this problem.

1. What history questions should you ask him at this time?
2. What physical assessment findings would you expect and why?
3. What options does he have for management of his health problem?
4. How should you respond to his perception regarding the employer's lack of caring for its employees?

EVOLVE For suggested answer guidelines, go to http://evolve.elsevier.com/Iggy/.

Dupuytren's Contracture

Dupuytren's contracture, or deformity, is a slowly progressive contracture of the palmar fascia, resulting in flexion of the fourth or fifth digit of the hand. The third digit is occasionally affected. Although Dupuytren's contracture is a fairly common problem, the cause is unknown. It usually occurs in older men, tends to occur in families, and can be bilateral.

When function becomes impaired, surgical release is required. A partial or selective fasciectomy (removal of fascia) is performed. After removal of the dressing and drain, a splint may be used. Nursing care is similar to that for the client with carpal tunnel repair.

Ganglion

A **ganglion** is a round, cystlike lesion, often overlying a wrist joint or tendon. The synovium surrounding the tendon degenerates, allowing the tendon sheath tissue to become weak and distended. Ganglia are painless on palpation, but they can cause joint discomfort after prolonged joint use or minor trauma, such as a strain. The lesion can disappear and then recur. Ganglia are most likely to develop in people between 15 and 50 years of age.

Although the fluid within the lesion can be aspirated, total excision is preferred. The postoperative care is the same as that for the client undergoing other hand surgery.

DISORDERS OF THE FOOT

Hallux Valgus

The **hallux valgus** deformity, sometimes referred to as a bunion, is a common foot problem. The great toe deviates laterally at the metatarsophalangeal (MTP) joint (Figure 54-6). Although hallux valgus is often congenital, it can occur as a result of arthritis or poorly fitted shoes. As the deviation worsens, the bony prominence enlarges and causes pain, particularly when shoes are worn. Women are affected more often than men.

The surgical procedure, a simple **bunionectomy,** involves removal of the bony overgrowth and bursa. When other toe deformities accompany the condition or if the bony overgrowth is large, several osteotomies, or bone resections, may be performed. Fusions may also be performed. Screws or wires are often inserted to stabilize the bones during the healing process. If both feet are affected, one foot is usually treated at a time. Most clients are allowed partial weight bearing while wearing an orthopedic boot or shoe.

Hammertoe

Often clients have hammertoes and hallux valgus deformities simultaneously. As shown in Figure 54-7, a **hammertoe** is the dorsiflexion of any MTP joint with plantar flexion of the adjacent proximal interphalangeal (PIP) joint. The second toe is most often affected. As the deformity worsens, corns may develop on the dorsal side of the toe and calluses may appear on the plantar surface. Clients are uncomfortable when wearing shoes and walking.

Hammertoe is often treated by surgical correction of the deformity with **osteotomies** (bone resections) and the insertion of wires or screws for fixation. The postoperative course is similar to that for the client with hallux valgus repair. The client uses crutches until full weight bearing is allowed several weeks postoperatively.

Morton's Neuroma

In the client with **Morton's neuroma,** or plantar digital neuritis, a small tumor grows in a digital nerve of the foot. The client usually describes the pain as an acute, burning sensa-

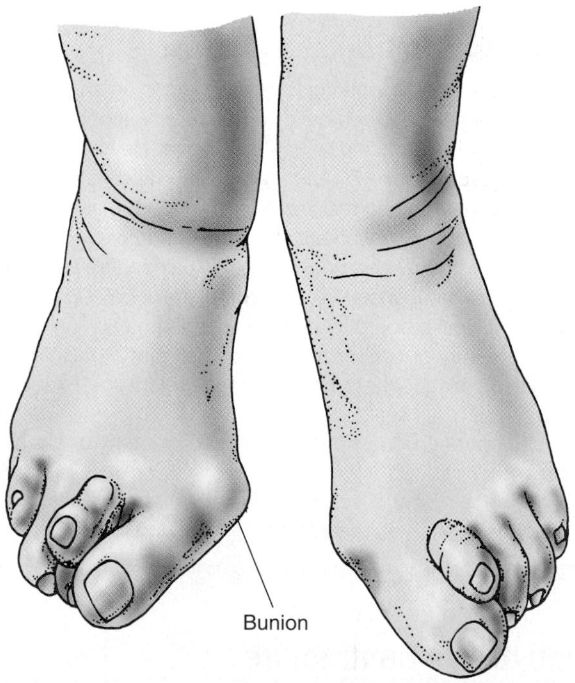

Figure 54-6 ■ Appearance of hallux valgus with a bunion.

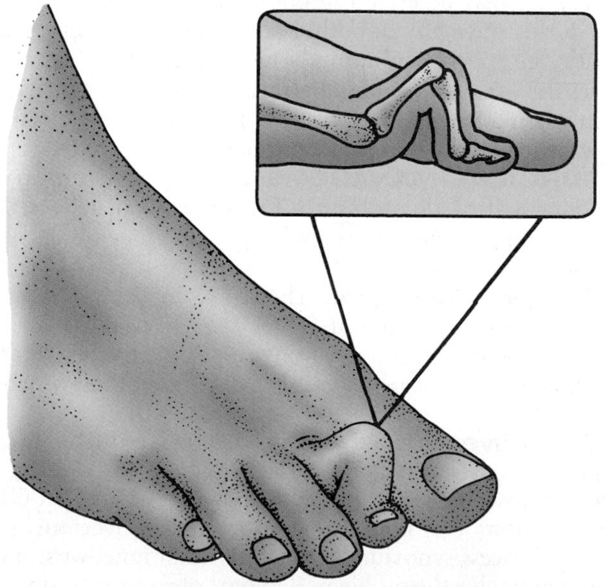

Figure 54-7 ■ Hammertoe of the second metatarsophalangeal joint.

tion in the web space. The pain involves the entire surface of the third and fourth toes.

Treatment involves surgical removal of the neuroma and application of a pressure dressing. Ambulation is usually permitted immediately after surgery.

Tarsal Tunnel Syndrome

Tarsal tunnel syndrome is the ankle version of carpal tunnel syndrome (CTS). The posterior tibial nerve in the ankle becomes compressed, resulting in loss of sensation and pain in a portion of the foot. Typically, the median and lateral plantar branches, which supply the sole of the foot and the distal phalanges, are affected by the nerve compression. Diagnosis and treatment are similar to those for CTS.

Plantar Fasciitis

Plantar fasciitis is an inflammation of the plantar fascia, which is located in the area of the arch of the foot. It is often seen in middle-aged and older adults, as well as in athletes, especially runners. In ambulatory care settings, plantar fasciitis accounts for 10% of running injuries. Obesity is also a contributing factor.

Clients complain of pain in the arch of the foot, especially when getting out of bed. The pain is worsened with weight bearing. Although most clients experience unilateral plantar fasciitis, the problem can affect both feet.

More than 90% of clients respond to conservative management, which includes rest, ice, stretching exercises, strapping of the foot to maintain the arch, shoes with good support, and orthotics. Nonsteroidal anti-inflammatory drugs (NSAIDs) or steroids may be needed to control pain and inflammation. If conservative measures are unsuccessful, endoscopic surgery to remove the inflamed tissue may be required.

Nursing care involves teaching the client about the importance of complying with the treatment plan and coordinating care with the physical therapist for instruction in exercise.

Other Problems of the Foot

Table 54-5 cites other common foot problems. Although clients are usually not hospitalized for these conditions, the nurse may recognize a foot disorder and alert the physician.

OTHER DISORDERS OF THE SKELETON

Scoliosis

PATHOPHYSIOLOGY

In early scoliosis, changes in muscles and ligaments on the concave side of the spinal column occur. These structures shorten and over time progressive deformity of the vertebra result. The vertebra rotate, begin to compress, and the spinal column begins to move into a lateral curve, a condition known as **scoliosis** (see Figure 53-3). As the degree of curvature increases, damage to the vertebral bodies occurs. The degree of the curvature increases during periods of growth, such as in adolescence. Curvature of greater than 50 degrees results in an unstable spine and curvature of greater than 60 degrees in the thoracic spine results in compromise of cardiopulmonary function.

The exact cause of scoliosis is not well understood. The process may result from some deviation in the balance mechanism located in the central nervous system. Females are affected more often than males and onset is often in adolescence. Children are screened for scoliosis during the middle school years. Information about caring for children with scoliosis is presented in most pediatric nursing textbooks.

Three types of scoliosis can be described: congenital, neuromuscular, and idiopathic. Congenital scoliosis occurs during embryonic development. Neuromuscular scoliosis can result from a neuromuscular condition in childhood or adulthood, such as cerebral palsy or spinal cord tumors. Idiopathic scoliosis is the most common form of scoliosis and results from no known cause.

Scoliosis can be further classified as structural or nonstructural. Nonstructural scoliosis results from a cause outside the spine itself, such as a leg length discrepancy. Structural scoliosis follows some deviation of the spinal column.

◆COLLABORATIVE MANAGEMENT

◆Assessment

Complete history of the client with spinal deformity should include onset of problem, in adolescence or adulthood and what treatments may be been used in the past. Clients who experienced surgery for scoliosis during adolescence are returning with progressive, debilitating back pain from degenerative disk disease below the fusion. A loss of lumbar curvature, or **lordosis**, described as "flat back" syndrome, may be present. A thorough pain assessment must be completed for those clients presenting with complaint of back pain.

The client is observed from the front and back, while standing and during forward flexion from the hips. Physical examination reveals asymmetry of hip and shoulder height, prominence of the thoracic ribs and scapula on one side, and visible curve in the spinal column. Observation from the side may reveal kyphosis of the thoracic spine. Leg length discrepancy must be ruled out.

TABLE 54-5 Treatment of Common Foot Problems

Description/Cause	Treatment
Corn	
Induration and thickening of the skin caused by friction and pressure, painful conical mass	Surgical removal by podiatrist
Callus	
Flat, poorly defined mass on the sole over a bony prominence caused by pressure	Padding and lanolin creams; overall good skin hygiene
Ingrown Nail	
Nail sliver penetration of the skin, causing inflammation	Removal of sliver by podiatrist; warm soaks; antibiotic ointment
Hypertrophic Ungual Labium	
Chronic hypertrophy of nail lip caused by improper nail trimming; results from untreated ingrown nail	Surgical removal of necrotic nail and skin; treatment of secondary infection

Interventions

Methods of treating adult scoliosis differ from those used for children. The adult spinal column is less flexible and therefore less likely to respond to exercises, weight reduction, bracing, and casting for correction of the deformity. In the adult, the disorder is progressive and can result in an additional one degree of deviation each year.

Adults with less than 50 degrees of curvature of the spine may be treated conservatively but those with greater than 50 degrees of curvature may require surgical intervention. The procedure consists of surgical fusion and insertion of instrumentation or rods to stabilize the spine. The surgeon performs spinal fusion by packing cancellous bone chips, usually from the iliac crest, between the affected vertebrae for support and stabilization. Both an anterior and a posterior approach may be needed. If so, the surgeon may perform both procedures during the same operative day or may stage them 7 to 10 days apart. The metal instrumentation supports the spine and immobilizes the fused area during healing.

The nursing care of the client undergoing corrective surgery for scoliosis is similar to that for the client undergoing a laminectomy or spinal fusion (see Chapter 46). Some procedures may require several days of immobilization postoperatively while other procedures allow the client to begin mobility the next day after surgery. A thoracolumbosacral orthosis (TLSO) is typically used to support the vertebral column (see Figure 54-2).

The client usually returns to work in about 3 weeks and can resume activities such as swimming and bicycling. Recreational sports, such as tennis, are usually resumed in 6 weeks. Other surgical procedures may prevent the client from performing these activities until 3 to 6 months postoperatively.

Osteogenesis Imperfecta

Osteogenesis imperfecta (OI) is a rare genetic disorder in which the bones are fragile and fracture easily resulting in bone deformity. The pathophysiology of the disease involves errors in synthesis of collagen, a connective tissue. OI is described by the Sillence classification system. The Sillence system describes four types of OI based on inheritance as autosomal dominant or autosomal recessive and clinical findings of each type. Types I and IV are more mild manifestations of the disease and can persist into adulthood. Types II and III are more severe and can result in fractures in utero, during the birth process, or in early childhood. Types II and III are associated with a high mortality rate.

Clinical manifestations include osteoporosis, history of multiple fractures, bony deformity, and poor skeletal development. Blue sclerae; soft, brownish teeth; and hearing loss may also be found upon assessment. Serum alkaline phosphatase will be elevated. In children with milder types of OI, child abuse is often considered until the diagnosis of OI can be made.

The treatment is palliative, and the client's life span is often shortened. The physician prescribes steroids, calcium, vitamin C, and, possibly, sodium fluoride. Physical therapy, casting or bracing, and telescoping intramedullary rods are used to maintain mobility and promote ambulation if possible. Research is ongoing in the use of bisphosphonates for treatment of OI. The nurse refers the client to the Osteogenesis Imperfecta Foundation in the United States or to the Brittle Bones Society in other countries for information and support.

MUSCULAR DISEASES

Progressive Muscular Dystrophies

PATHOPHYSIOLOGY

At least nine types of **muscular dystrophy (MD)** have been clinically identified. They can be broadly categorized as slowly progressive or rapidly progressive. The slowly progressive types are most commonly seen in adults. Most pediatric nursing books describe the care for clients with MD in detail. Five forms of MD are often seen in adults. Each type has its own distinct characteristics and causes, but all are progressive (Table 54-6).

The exact pathophysiologic mechanisms are unknown, but three theories have been advocated. The vascular theory suggests that a lack of blood flow causes the typical degeneration of muscle tissue seen in MD. Microscopic necrotic areas in atrophied muscle tissue support this hypothesis, although this finding does not explain the marked degree of degeneration often seen in the disease.

The neurogenic theory proposes a disturbance in nerve-muscle interaction. Research has failed, however, to locate the nature of the disturbance.

The most popular belief is the membrane theory. This theory suggests that cell membranes are genetically altered, causing a compromise in cell integrity. An increase in the activity of muscle proteolytic enzymes may accompany the membrane alteration, leaving the muscle cell vulnerable to degeneration. Increased enzyme activity has been documented in the client with atrophied muscles.

The cause of MD is unknown, but there may be a genetic influence for most of the major types. Some forms of MD are transmitted as autosomal dominant or recessive traits, whereas others are sex linked.

The most commonly occurring type of MD is the severe X-linked recessive variety initially described by Guillaume Duchenne in 1868. Each year, 20 to 33 cases are reported per 100,000 live male births. In an X-linked recessive disorder, one half of the male children of an unaffected mother, or carrier, manifest the disease. Becker's dystrophy is also inherited in an X-linked recessive manner, but it is less common than Duchenne's dystrophy. The other types of MD seen in adults can occur in either gender.

COLLABORATIVE MANAGEMENT

Diagnosis of MD is often difficult because the clinical manifestations are similar to those of other muscular disorders. Muscle biopsy often confirms the diagnosis. Muscle weakness and trophic changes are characteristic of all types of MD. Serum muscle enzyme values may be elevated, and electromyographic (EMG) findings are often abnormal.

Management of the client with MD is supportive and involves the entire health care team. Physical and occupational therapy helps the client maintain as much function and independence as possible. Major organ or body system involvement is medically managed, but the life span is often short-

TABLE 54-6 Differential Features of Common Muscular Dystrophies

Onset	Genetics	Clinical Manifestations	Progression
Duchenne (Severe X-Linked) Dystrophy			
18 mo-4 yr	Sex-linked recessive; expression in males	Symmetric pelvic and shoulder girdle muscle weakness; waddling gait; cardiac involvement common; mental retardation in one third of clients	Severely progressive, leading to inability to walk between 7 and 11 yr of age; death from cardiac or respiratory failure in 20s or 30s
Becker (Benign X-Linked) Dystrophy			
5-25 yr	Sex-linked recessive; expression in males	Wasting of pelvic and shoulder muscles; normal cardiac and mental function	Gradual progression; inability to walk 25 yr after onset; usually normal life span
Limb-Girdle Dystrophy			
Usually 20s or 30s	Usually autosomal dominant; expression in either gender	Upper extremity and neck muscles and lower extremity and hip muscle weakness	Extremely variable; severe disability within 10-20 yr after onset; life span shortened by 10-20 yr
Facioscapulohumeral (Landouzy-Dejerine) Dystrophy			
Usually in 20s	Autosomal dominant; expression in either gender	Facial and shoulder girdle muscle involvement	Usually benign; normal life span
Myotonic (Steinert) Dystrophy			
Birth to 40s	Autosomal dominant; expression in either gender	Muscle atrophy with multiple organ involvement (e.g., heart, lungs, smooth muscle, and endocrine system)	Usually gradual if onset in adulthood

ened from these manifestations of the disease. With the exception of prednisone, no drug has been found to slow the progression of the disorder, although immunosuppressive agents, anabolic steroids, and growth factors have been tried.

An experimental treatment, myoblast transfer therapy (MTT), has been supported by the Food and Drug Administration (FDA). MTT involves injections of healthy muscle cells (myoblasts) taken from a donor and multiplied in a laboratory. The cells are then given to the client with MD, where they theoretically fuse with each other and the recipient's unhealthy muscle cells. Effective gene therapy may also be an option for curing MD in the future.

Nursing interventions focus on making the client as comfortable as possible and reinforcing techniques and exercises taught in the physical therapy program. The nurse's role in caring for a client with cardiac or other organ involvement is the same as for any client with dysfunction of these areas.

Other Muscular Disorders

Most muscular disorders are classified as neuromuscular disorders, such as myasthenia gravis, or as connective tissue diseases, such as polymyositis. Therefore these disorders are discussed in Chapters 47 and 24, respectively.

GET READY for the NCLEX Examination!

KEY POINTS

Safe Effective Care Environment

- Assess clients with osteoporosis for risk for falls; fractures are common in these clients.
- Use strict aseptic technique when caring for clients with an open wound associated with osteomyelitis.
- Differentiate key features of acute and chronic osteomyelitis as listed in Chart 54-5; acute osteomyelitis can lead to bacteremia, a potentially life-threatening complication.
- For clients who have surgery for bone cancer, report postoperative manifestations of infection, dislocation, or neurovascular compromise to the surgeon promptly.

Health Promotion and Maintenance

- Teach clients at risk for osteoporosis to minimize risk factors, such as stopping smoking, decreasing alcohol intake, exercising regularly, and increasing dietary calcium.
- Remind clients at risk for osteoporosis to have screening tests, such as the DEXA scan.
- Remind clients taking bisphosphonates (BPs) to take them early in the morning, at least 30 minutes before breakfast with a full glass of water, and to remain sitting upright during that time to prevent esophagitis, a common complication of BP therapy.
- Instruct older adults to have at least 5 minutes of sun per week and to eat vitamin D–fortified foods to prevent osteomalacia.
- Teach clients who have repetitive hand activities to be alert to clinical manifestations of carpal tunnel syndrome, the fastest growing occupational injury; use techniques to avoid repetitive strain.

Psychosocial Integrity

- Assist clients with osteoporosis to overcome fear of falling, or fallophobia, which prevents them from socializing or going outside their homes; collaborate with the physical therapist to determine whether ambulatory devices such as canes are indicated.

- Help clients with bone cancer cope with their illness as described in Chart 54-6.
- Refer clients with musculoskeletal problems to appropriate community resources, such as the Paget's Disease Foundation and the National Osteoporosis Foundation.

Physiological Integrity

- Most clients are unaware that they have osteoporosis until they experience a fracture, the most common complication of the disease.
- Secondary generalized or regional osteoporosis can be caused by any of the risk factors listed in Table 54-1.
- Osteomalacia, caused by a deficiency in vitamin D, can be caused by the factors listed in Table 54-3.
- Assess for key features of Paget's disease as summarized in Chart 54-4.
- Remember that bone tumors can be benign or malignant, as summarized in Table 54-4.
- Be aware that carpal tunnel syndrome (CTS) can be treated conservatively with medications and splinting; the goal of surgery is to release the pressure from the median nerve in the wrist.
- Assess clients having CTS surgery for changes in neurovascular status.
- Be aware that even minor hand and foot problems can be very painful; common foot problems are described in Table 54-5.
- Recognize that most major types of muscular dystrophy are genetic and manifest usually in childhood; care is supportive.

ADDITIONAL STUDY RESOURCES

Go to your Student CD-ROM for Review Questions for the NCLEX Examination.

evolve Go to http://evolve.elsevier.com/Iggy/ for Integrated Management of Care Questions for the NCLEX Examination.

SELECTED BIBLIOGRAPHY

Asterisk indicates a classic or definitive work on this subject.

Aschenbrenner, D.S. (2005). Drug watch: new warnings and safety concerns: medications and adverse effects. *American Journal of Nursing, 105*(1), 29.

Bayles, C.M., Cochran, K., & Anderson, C. (2000). The psychosocial aspects of osteoporosis in women. *Nursing Clinics of North America, 35*(1), 279-286.

Berarducci, A., et al. (2000). Health-promoting educational practices related to osteoporosis. *Applied Nursing Research, 13*(4), 173-180.

Carroll, K.L. (2002). Alterations in musculoskeletal function in children. In K.L. McCance & S.E. Huether (Eds.), *Pathophysiology: The biologic basis for disease in adults and children* (pp. 1409-1433). St. Louis: Mosby.

Crowther, C.L., & Mourad, L.A. (2002). Alterations in musculoskeletal function. In K.L. McCance & S.E. Huether (Eds.), *Pathophysiology: The biologic basis for disease in adults and children* (pp. 1364-1408). St. Louis: Mosby.

*Dowd, R., & Cavalieri, R.J. (1999). Help your patient live with osteoporosis. *American Journal of Nursing, 99*(4), 55, 57-60.

Geier, K.A. (2001). Osteoporosis in men. *Orthopaedic Nursing, 20*(6), 49-56.

*Hall, J., & Riley, R.E. (1999). Nutritional strategies to reduce the risk of osteoporosis. *MEDSURG Nursing, 8*(5), 281-293.

*Hunt, A.H. (1996). The relationship between height change and bone mineral density. *Orthopaedic Nursing, 15*(3), 57-71.

Lehne, R.A. (2001). *Pharmacology for nursing care.* Philadelphia: W. B. Saunders.

Leslie, M. (2000). Issues in the nursing management of osteoporosis. *Nursing Clinics of North America, 35*(1), 189-197.

*Lewis, T., et al. (1999). Caring for the patient with Paget's disease of the bone. *Nurse Practitioner, 24*(7), 53, 57-58.

Lypaczewski, G., Lappe, J., & Stubby, J. (2002). "Mom & me" and healthy bones: An innovative approach to teaching bone health. *Orthopaedic Nursing, 21*(2), 35-43.

*Mahon, S.M. (1998). Osteoporosis: A concern for cancer survivors. *Oncology Nursing Forum, 25*(5), 843-851.

McClung, B.L. (2000). *Nursing practice guideline: Clinical management of patients at risk for or diagnosed with osteoporosis.* New York: Medical Information Services.

National Institutes of Health. (2000). *Consensus statements: Osteoporosis prevention, diagnosis, and therapy.* Accessed July 27, 2003, from http://www.consensus.nih.gov/cons/111/111_statement.htm.

*National Osteoporosis Foundation. (1995). *Position paper: Current perspective on diagnosis, prevention, and treatment of osteoporosis.* Washington, DC: Author.

National Osteoporosis Foundation. (2003a). *Disease statistics.* Accessed July 26, 2003, from http://www.nof.org/osteoporosis/stats.htm.

National Osteoporosis Foundation. (2003b). *Medications to prevent and treat osteoporosis.* Accessed July 26, 2003, from http://www.nof.org/patientinfo/medications.htm.

Orwell, E. (2000). Men with osteoporosis. Presented at the World Congress on Osteoporosis 2000, June 17, 2000, Chicago.

Peterson, J.A. (2001). Osteoporosis overview. *Geriatric Nursing, 22*(1), 17-23.

*Piasecki, P.A. (1996). Nursing care of the patient with metastatic bone disease. *Orthopaedic Nursing, 15*(4), 25-33.

*Quaschnick, M.S. (1996). The diagnosis and management of plantar fasciitis. *Nurse Practitioner, 21*(4), 50-63.

Rodts, M.F. (2002). Disorders of the spine. In A.B. Maher, S.W. Salmond, & T.A. Pellino (Eds.), *Orthopaedic nursing* (pp. 515-550). Philadelphia: W. B. Saunders.

Sedlak, C.A. & Doheny, M.O. (2002). Metabolic conditions. In A.B. Maher, S.W. Salmond, & T.A. Pellino (Eds.), *Orthopaedic nursing* (pp. 423-467). Philadelphia: W. B. Saunders.

Sedlak, C.A., Doheny, M.O., & Estok, P.J. (2000). Osteoporosis in older men: Knowledge and health beliefs. *Orthopaedic Nursing, 19*(3), 38-46.

Sedlak, C.A., et al. (1998). Osteoporosis prevention in young women. *Orthopaedic Nursing, 17*(3), 53-60.

Taft, L.B., Looker, P.A., & Cella, D. (2000). Osteoporosis: A disease management opportunity. *Orthopaedic Nursing, 19*(2), 67-76.

*Tawil, R. (1999). Outlook for therapy in the muscular dystrophies. *Seminars in Neurology, 19*(1), 81-86.

U.S. Food and Drug Administration. (2003). *FDA approves new labeling and provides new advice to postmenopausal women who use or who are considering using estrogen and estrogen with progestin.* Accessed July 26, 2003, from http://www.fds.gov/bbs/topics/factsheets/2003/fsl.htm.

CHAPTER 55

Interventions for Clients with Musculoskeletal Trauma

MARY R. HERON EVANS

LEARNING OUTCOMES

After studying this chapter, you should be able to:

1. Compare and contrast common types of fractures.
2. Discuss the usual healing process for bone.
3. Identify common complications of fractures.
4. Explain the typical clinical manifestations that are seen in clients with fractures.
5. Analyze common nursing diagnoses for the client with a fracture.
6. Describe the nursing care of the client with a cast, including client education.
7. Describe the nursing care of the client in traction.
8. Discuss pain management for the client with a fracture.
9. Prioritize nursing care for the postoperative client who has undergone open reduction with internal fixation of the hip.
10. Evaluate the nursing care of a client with a fracture.
11. Identify common types of amputations.
12. Explain the psychosocial aspects related to amputations.
13. Develop a community-based teaching plan for a client who has undergone an elective amputation.
14. Describe the collaborative management for the client with complex regional pain syndrome.
15. Identify the common types of sports-related injuries and their management.

Go to your Student CD-ROM for Review Questions for the NCLEX Examination keyed to these Learning Outcomes.

Musculoskeletal injury accounts for about 66% of all injuries and is one of the primary causes of disability in the United States. Trauma to the musculoskeletal system ranges from simple muscle strain to multiple bone fractures with severe soft-tissue damage. With advancing age, a person is more likely to develop decreased bone mass (osteoporosis), which causes fractures. Hip, wrist, vertebral, and pelvic fractures are common in late adulthood.

FRACTURES

PATHOPHYSIOLOGY

A **fracture** is a break or disruption in the continuity of a bone. Fractures can occur anywhere in the body and at any age. All fractures have the same basic pathophysiologic mechanism and nursing management, regardless of fracture type or location.

Classification of Fractures

A fracture is classified by the extent of the break as follows:

- *Complete fracture.* The break is across the entire width of the bone in such a way that the bone is divided into two distinct sections.
- *Incomplete fracture.* The fracture does not divide the bone into two portions because the break is through only part of the bone.

A fracture is described by the extent of associated soft-tissue damage as **open** (or **compound**) or **closed** (or **simple**). The skin surface over the broken bone is disrupted in a compound fracture, which causes an external wound. These fractures are often graded to define the extent of tissue damage. Grade I is the least severe injury, and skin damage is minimal. In grade II an open fracture is accompanied by skin and muscle contusions. The most severe injury is grade III, in which there is damage to skin, muscle, nerve tissue, and blood vessels; the wound is more than

2.4 to 3.2 inches (6 to 8 cm) in diameter. A closed (simple) fracture does not extend through the skin and therefore has no visible wound.

Figure 55-1 illustrates common types of fractures. The nurse needs to be familiar with the differences in these types because they often dictate the specific nursing care required for the client. In addition to being identified by type, fractures are characterized by their cause. A **pathologic (spontaneous) fracture** occurs after minimal trauma to a bone that has been weakened by disease. For example, a client with bone cancer or osteoporosis can easily sustain a pathologic fracture. A **fatigue or stress fracture** results from excessive strain and stress on the bone. **Compression fractures** are produced by a loading force applied to the long axis of cancellous bone. They commonly occur in the vertebrae of clients with osteoporosis.

Stages of Bone Healing

When a bone is broken, the body immediately begins the healing process to repair the injury and restore the body's equilibrium. Within 48 to 72 hours after the injury, a hematoma forms at the site of the fracture because bone is extremely vascular. Blood supply to and within the bone usually diminishes because of the injury, which causes an area of bone necrosis. The dead cells prompt the migration of fibroblasts and osteoblasts to the fracture site as part of the inflammatory process. This then prompts the formation of fibrocartilage, providing the foundation for bone healing (within 3 days to 2 weeks).

As a result of vascular and cellular proliferation, the fracture site is surrounded by new vascular tissue known as a callus (within 2 to 6 weeks). **Callus** formation is the beginning of a nonbony union. As healing continues, it is transformed

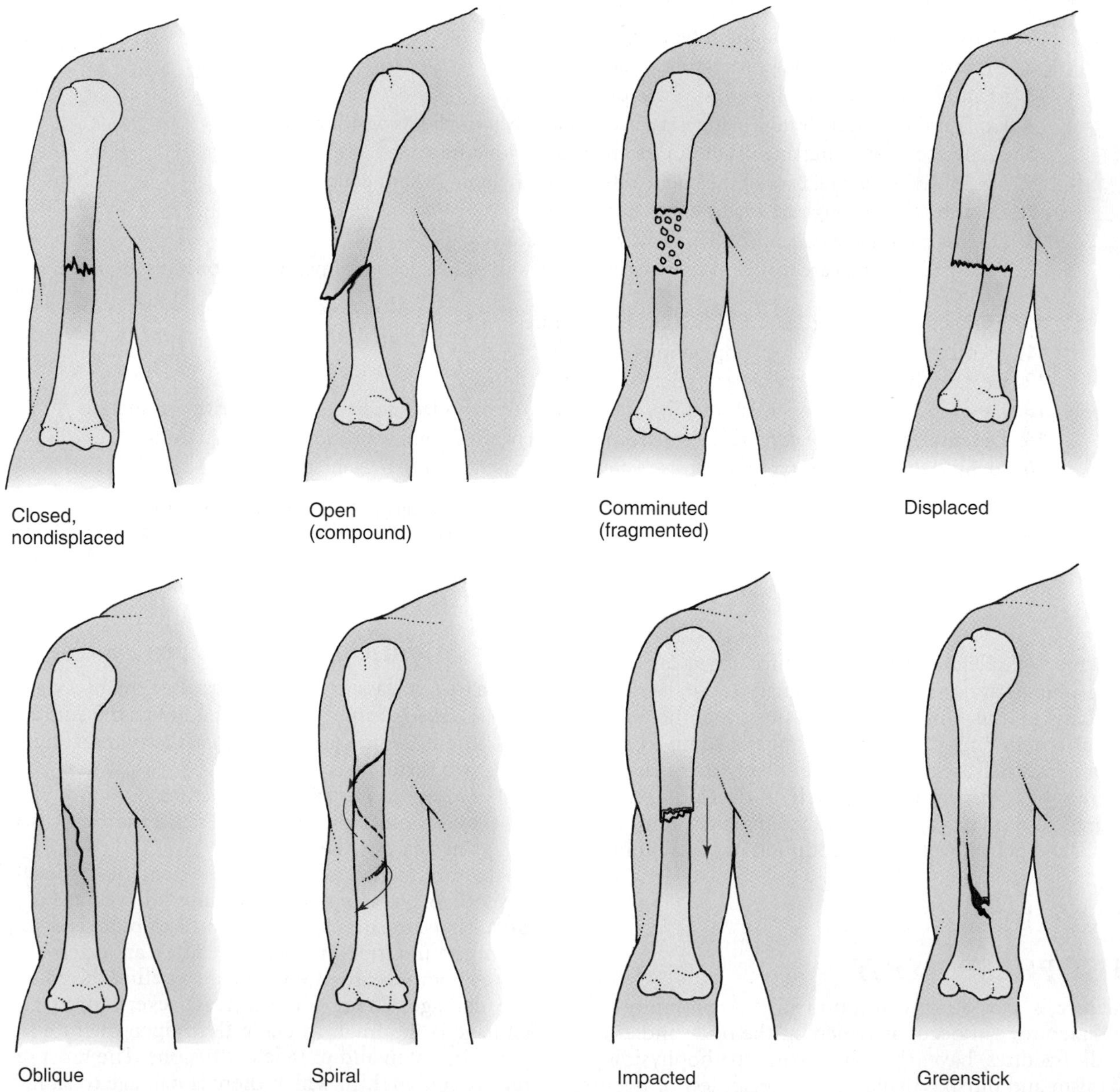

Figure 55-1 ■ Common types of fractures.

from a loose, fibrous tissue into bone (within 3 weeks to 6 months). Excess callus is resorbed. During the final phase of healing, consolidation, and remodeling, bone continues to be resorbed and deposited in response to stress, reshaping to meet mechanical demands. This process may start as early as 6 weeks after fracture and can continue for up to 1 year. Figure 55-2 summarizes the stages of bone healing.

In young, healthy adult bone, healing takes about 6 weeks. In the older person who has reduced bone mass, healing time is lengthened; complete healing often takes 3 to 6 months. Other factors that affect healing include the severity of the trauma, the type of bone injured, inadequate immobilization, infections at the fracture site, and ischemic or avascular necrosis (AVN).

CONSIDERATIONS FOR OLDER ADULTS

Healing can be affected by a number of factors in addition to the aging process. Bone formation and strength rely on adequate nutrition. Calcium, phosphorus, vitamin D, and protein are necessary for the production of new bone (see Chapter 54). For women the loss of estrogen after menopause is detrimental to the body's ability to form new bone tissue. Concurrent diseases can also affect the rate at which bone heals. For instance, peripheral vascular diseases, such as arteriosclerosis, reduce arterial circulation to bone; thus the bone receives less oxygen and lesser amounts of nutrients, both of which are needed for repair.

Complications of Fractures

Regardless of the type or location of the fracture, several limb- and life-threatening complications can result from the injury. The nurse must be able to recognize the clinical manifestations of impending complications so that treatment can be started immediately. In some cases, careful monitoring and assessment can prevent these complications.

ACUTE COMPARTMENT SYNDROME

Compartments are sheaths of inelastic fascia that support and partition muscles, blood vessels, and nerves in the body. **Acute compartment syndrome (ACS)** is a serious condition in which increased pressure within one or more compartments causes massive compromise of circulation to the area. The most common sites for ACS in clients experiencing musculoskeletal trauma are the compartments in the lower leg and the dorsal and volar compartments of the forearm.

PREVENTION. The pressure to the compartment can be from an external or internal source. Tight, bulky dressings and casts are examples of external pressure. Blood or fluid accumulation is a common source of internal pressure. ACS is not limited to clients with musculoskeletal problems; clients with severe burns, extensive insect bites, or massive infiltration of intravenous (IV) fluids are also susceptible to compartment syndrome. In these situations, edema increases pressure in one or more compartments.

Identify clients who may be at risk for ACS and monitor them closely. If ACS is suspected, notify the health care provider immediately and, if possible, implement interventions to relieve the pressure. For example, for the client with constricting bulky dressings, loosen the bandage or tape. If the client has a cast, request an order to cut the cast. In some agencies, protocols permit this procedure without a physician's order.

PATHOPHYSIOLOGIC CHANGES. The primary pathophysiologic changes of increased compartment pressure are sometimes referred to as the ischemia-edema cycle. Capillaries within the viable muscle dilate, which raises capillary pressure. Capillaries then become more permeable because of the release of histamine by the ischemic muscle tissue. As a result, plasma proteins leak into the interstitial fluid space, and edema occurs. Edema causes pressure on nerve endings and subsequent pain. Blood flow to the area is reduced, and further ischemia results. Sensory deficits

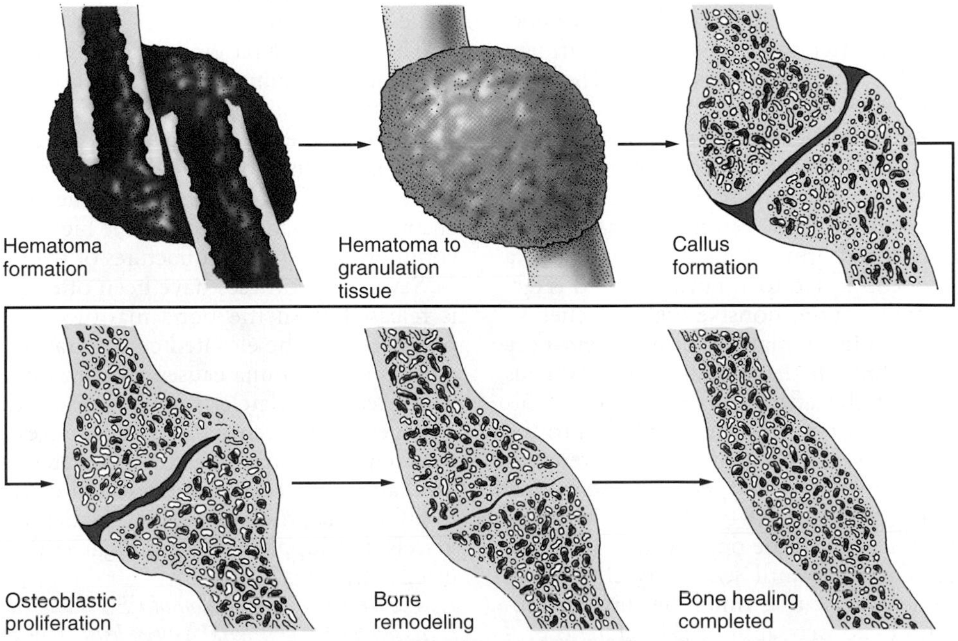

Figure 55-2 ■ The stages of bone healing.

CHART 55-1

KEY FEATURES of Compartment Syndrome

Physiologic Change	Clinical Findings
Increased compartment pressure	No change
Increased capillary permeability	Edema
Release of histamine	Increased edema
Increased blood flow to area	Pulses present Pink tissue
Pressure on nerve endings	Pain
Increased tissue pressure	Referred pain to compartment
Decreased tissue perfusion	Increased edema
Decreased oxygen to tissues	Pallor
Increased production of lactic acid	Unequal pulses Flexed posture
Anaerobic metabolism	Cyanosis
Vasodilation	Increased edema
Increased blood flow	Tense muscle swelling
Increased tissue pressure	Tingling Numbness
Increased edema	Paresthesia
Muscle ischemia	Severe pain unrelieved by medication
Tissue necrosis	Paresis/paralysis

(e.g., paresthesia) generally appear before changes in vascular or motor signs. The color of the tissue pales, and pulses begin to weaken but rarely disappear; the affected area is usually palpably tense, and pain can be elicited with passive motion of the extremity. If the condition is not treated, cyanosis, tingling, numbness, paresis, and severe pain occur. Chart 55-1 summarizes the sequence of pathophysiologic events in compartment syndrome and the associated clinical assessment findings.

EMERGENCY CARE. Fortunately, ACS is not common, but it creates an emergency situation when it does occur. Within 4 to 6 hours after the onset of compartment syndrome, neuromuscular damage is irreversible. The limb can become useless in 24 to 48 hours.

In a few cases, clients at especially high risk for ACS are monitored by an invasive procedure. Compartment pressures can be monitored on a one-time basis with a handheld device with a digital display, or they can be monitored continuously. Continuous monitoring requires placement of a wick or slit-tip catheter connected to a transducer and is recommended for comatose or unresponsive high-risk clients.

If ACS is verified, the surgeon may perform a **fasciotomy** by making an incision through the skin and subcutaneous tissues into the fascia of the affected compartment. This procedure relieves the pressure to restore circulation to the affected area. No consensus exists on what pressure requires fasciotomy (normal is 0 to 8 mm Hg); compartment pressures must be considered in relation to the client's hemodynamic status. After fasciotomy, the open wound is packed and dressed on a regular basis until secondary closure occurs, usually in 4 to 5 days. At that time, the surgeon usually debrides the wound and may apply a skin graft to promote healing.

POSSIBLE RESULTS. Although uncommon, specific problems resulting from compartment syndrome include infection, persistent motor weakness in the affected extremity, contracture, and myoglobinuric renal failure. In extreme cases, amputation becomes necessary.

Infection from the necrotic tissue may become severe enough that amputation of the limb is warranted. *Motor weakness* from injured nerves is not reversible, and the client may require braces or other orthotic devices for assistance in movement. Volkmann's *contractures* of the forearm, which can begin within 12 hours of the pressure increase, result from shortening of the ischemic muscle and from nerve involvement.

Myoglobinuric renal failure, from muscle tissue breakdown **(rhabdomyolysis),** is a potentially fatal complication of compartment syndrome. It commonly occurs when large or multiple compartments are involved. Injured muscle tissues release myoglobulin (muscle protein) into the circulation, where it can occlude the distal convoluted tubule and precipitate acute renal failure. Although the exact pathophysiologic mechanisms are unknown, it is suspected that myoglobulin has a direct toxic effect on the kidney. Damaged muscle cells also release potassium, which cannot be excreted because of the renal failure. The resulting hyperkaliemia may cause cardiac dysrhythmias and cardiac arrest.

SHOCK

Bone is quite vascular; therefore there is a risk of bleeding with bone injury. In addition, trauma can sever adjacent arteries and cause hemorrhage; consequently, hypovolemic shock can develop rapidly. (The pathophysiology of hypovolemic shock is described in Chapter 40.)

FAT EMBOLISM SYNDROME

Fat embolism syndrome (FES) is a serious complication, usually resulting from a fracture, in which fat globules are released from the yellow bone marrow into the bloodstream. FES may also occur, although less often, with pancreatitis, diabetic coma, osteomyelitis, blunt trauma, or sickle cell anemia.

The release of fat emboli is most likely with fractures of long bones or multiple fractures, although a break in any bone with sufficient bone marrow content can cause the complication. The problem can occur at any age or in either gender, but young men between ages 20 and 40 years and older adults between ages 70 and 80 years are at the greatest risk. The older client with a fractured hip has the highest risk, but FES is also common in clients with fractures of the pelvis.

Several hypotheses have been offered to explain how fat is released from the bone marrow. The metabolic theory proposes that the elevated concentration of catecholamines as a result of trauma causes mobilization of free fatty acids, which leads to platelet aggregation and the formation of fat globules. The mechanical theory suggests that the pressure within yellow bone marrow is greater than capillary pressure, and therefore fats are released directly from the bone. In either case, the fat globules are deposited in small blood vessels that supply the major organs of the body, most commonly the lungs.

The earliest manifestation of FES is altered mental status, which is caused by a low arterial oxygen level. The client then typically experiences respiratory distress, tachycardia, tachypnea, fever,

CHART 55-2

KEY FEATURES of
Pulmonary Emboli: Fat Embolism Versus Blood Clot Embolism

Fat Embolism	Blood Clot Embolism
Definition	
Obstruction of the pulmonary vascular bed by fat globules	Obstruction of the pulmonary artery by a blood clot or clots
Origin	
95% from fractures of the long bones; occurs usually within 48 hr	85% from deep vein thrombosis in the legs or pelvis; can occur anytime
Assessment Findings	
Altered mental status (earliest sign) Increased respirations, pulse, temperature Chest pain Dyspnea Crackles Decreased SaO_2 Petechiae (50%-60%) Retinal hemorrhage (not common) Mild thrombocytopenia	Same as for fat embolism, except no petechiae
Treatment	
Bedrest Gentle handling Oxygen Hydration (IV fluids) Possibly steroid therapy Fracture immobilization	Preventive measures (e.g., leg exercises, antiembolism stockings, SCDs) Bedrest Oxygen Possibly mechanical ventilation Anticoagulants Thrombolytics Possible surgery: pulmonary embolectomy, vena cava umbrella

SaO_2, Arterial oxygen saturation; SCD, sequential compression device.

and **petechiae** (a macular, measles-like rash over the neck, upper arms, or chest and abdomen). Petechiae are characteristic of fat emboli, but the physiologic basis for their development is not known.

Laboratory findings in FES include the following:

- Increased erythrocyte sedimentation rate (ESR)
- Decreased serum calcium levels
- Decreased red blood cell and platelet counts
- Increased serum lipase level

These changes in blood values are poorly understood, but they aid in diagnosis of the condition.

Fat embolism usually occurs within 48 hours of the fracture and can result in respiratory failure or death, often from pulmonary edema. When the lungs are affected, the complication may be misdiagnosed as a pulmonary embolism from a blood clot (Chart 55-2). Care of the client is similar to that for those with pulmonary emboli, with the primary exception that FES is not treated with anticoagulant agents.

VENOUS THROMBOEMBOLISM

Venous thromboembolism (VTE) includes deep vein thrombosis (DVT) and its complication, pulmonary embolism (PE). DVT often develops in people who are immobile because of trauma, surgery, or disability. It is the *most common* complication of lower extremity surgery or trauma and the most often fatal complication of musculoskeletal surgery. A person who smokes, is obese, has heart disease, is taking oral contraceptives or hormones, or has a history of thromboembolitic complications is at increased risk for DVT. The incidence of life-threatening embolic conditions is highest in older adults, particularly during the first 2 to 3 days after musculoskeletal surgery, usually hip repair.

Certain fracture sites are more often associated with life-threatening thrombi. For example, DVT that leads to PE is more likely to develop in clients with fractures of the lower extremities and pelvis. Local venous stasis secondary to trauma or surgical procedures (e.g., use of tourniquets in lower extremity injuries) increases the chance of VTE in clients with musculoskeletal trauma. A further discussion of VTE is found in Chapter 39.

INFECTION

Anytime there is trauma to tissues, the body's defense system is disrupted. Wound infections are the most common type of infection resulting from orthopedic trauma; they range from superficial skin infections to deep wound abscesses. Infection can also be caused by implanted hardware used to repair a fracture surgically, such as pins, plates, or rods. Clostridial infections can result in gas gangrene or tetanus and can prevent the bone from healing properly.

Bone infection, or **osteomyelitis,** is most common with open fractures in which skin integrity is lost and after surgical repair of a fracture (see Chapter 54). For clients experiencing this type of trauma, the risk of hospital-acquired **(nosocomial)** infections is increased.

ISCHEMIC NECROSIS

Ischemic necrosis is sometimes referred to as aseptic or avascular necrosis or **osteonecrosis.** Blood supply to the bone is disrupted, which results in the death of bone tissue. This problem is most often a complication of hip fractures or any fracture in which there is displacement of bone. Surgical repair of fractures also can lead to necrosis because the hardware can interfere with circulation.

FRACTURE BLISTERS

Fracture blisters are associated most commonly with high-energy fractures and twisting injuries in the lower extremities. Extensive tissue edema allows fluid to move into the weakened space between the epidermis and the dermis. The increased colloidal osmotic pressure then pulls more fluid into the space. Fracture blisters can lead to wound infection and delayed fracture treatment, which may then contribute to potential nonunion. Nursing measures that can assist in preventing or minimizing fracture blisters include maintaining proper immobilization before definitive treatment and elevation to limit edema.

DELAYED UNION, NONUNION, AND MALUNION

Delayed union describes a fracture that has not healed within 6 months of injury. Some fractures never achieve union; that is, they never completely heal (nonunion); others heal incorrectly (malunion). These problems are most common in clients with tibial fractures, fractures for which a number of different treatment techniques have been used (e.g., cast, traction), and pathologic fractures. Union may also be delayed or not achieved in the older client. If bone does not heal, the client typically experiences pain and immobility from deformity.

Etiology and Genetic Risk

The primary cause of a fracture is trauma from a motor vehicle accident or fall and is spread over all socioeconomic groups. The trauma experienced may be a direct blow to the bone or an indirect force from muscle contractions or pulling forces on the bone. Sports, vigorous exercise, and malnutrition are contributing factors. Bone diseases, such as osteoporosis, increase the risk of a fracture in older adults. Genetic factors that increase risk of fracture will be discussed with the specific problems throughout the text.

Incidence/Prevalence

The incidence of fractures depends on the location of the injury. Rib fractures are the most common type in the adult population. Femoral shaft fractures occur most often in young and middle-aged adults. The incidence of proximal femur (hip) fractures is highest in older adults. Humeral fractures are common in adults; the older the person, usually the more proximal the fracture. Wrist (Colles') fractures are typically seen in middle and late adulthood.

WOMEN'S HEALTH CONSIDERATIONS

It is estimated that more than 1.5 million fractures occur annually in the United States as a result of osteoporosis, and most occur in middle-aged and older women. By age 80, one in five women has suffered a hip fracture.

HEALTH PROMOTION/ILLNESS PREVENTION

The introduction of airbags and seatbelts has decreased the number of severe injuries and deaths, but it has increased the number of lower extremity and ankle fractures, especially in older adults. Nurses need to encourage the use of seatbelts and support legislation for improved vehicle design and reevaluation of the federal standards for motor vehicle safety. Health promotion and illness prevention activities should focus on decreasing falls and motor vehicle crashes. Such activities might include programs regarding the following:

- Osteoporosis screening and education
- Fall prevention
- Home assessment and modification
- Drinking and driving
- Medication safety
- Older adults and driving

COLLABORATIVE MANAGEMENT

PHARM e REVIEW

Assessment

HISTORY

Collect data to determine the cause of the fracture, which helps in developing an individualized plan of care for the client.

PRECEDING EVENTS. Ask the client to recall the specific events up to the time of the injury. Some type of force, such as incisional, crush, acceleration or deceleration, shearing, or friction, leads to most musculoskeletal injuries. As a result, several body systems are often affected.

Incisional (as from a knife wound) and crush injuries cause hemorrhage and disrupt blood flow to major organs. Acceleration or deceleration injuries cause direct trauma to the spleen, brain, and kidneys when these organs are moved from their fixed locations in the body. Shearing and friction damage the skin and cause a high level of wound contamination.

By asking about the events leading to the injury, you can determine which forces have been experienced and therefore which body systems or parts of the body to assess. For example, a forward fall often results in Colles' fracture of the wrist because the person tries to catch himself or herself with an outstretched hand. Knowing the mechanism of injury also helps the nurse to determine whether other types of injury, such as head and spinal cord injury, might be present.

OTHER HISTORY. A medication history, including substance abuse (recreational drug use), is important regardless of the client's age. For example, a young adult may have had an excessive amount of alcohol, which contributed to a motor vehicle accident or to a fall at the work site. Many older adults also consume alcohol and an assortment of prescribed and over-the-counter drugs, which can cause dizziness and loss of balance.

A medical history elicits possible causes of the fracture and gives clues as to how long it will take for the bone to heal. Certain diseases, such as bone cancer and Paget's disease, cause pathologic fractures that often do not achieve union.

Ask about the client's occupation and recreational activities. Some occupations are more hazardous than others; for instance, construction work is potentially more physically dangerous than office work. Certain hobbies and recreational activities are also extremely hazardous (e.g., skiing, in-line skating). Contact sports, such as football and ice hockey, often result in musculoskeletal injuries, including fractures. Other activities do not have such an obvious potential for injury but can cause fractures nonetheless. For instance, daily jogging and frequent marching in a band can lead to fatigue fractures.

Because inadequate nutrition contributes to fractures and can inhibit bone healing, take a complete diet history. Health-promotion counseling is a major focus for comprehensive health care today.

PHYSICAL ASSESSMENT/CLINICAL MANIFESTATIONS

BODY SYSTEM ASSESSMENT. The client with a fracture often sustains trauma to other body systems. Consequently, assess all major body systems *first* for life-threatening complications, including head, thoracic, and abdominal injuries. The assessment of these areas is described elsewhere in this text.

MUSCULOSKELETAL ASSESSMENT. When inspecting the site of a possible fracture, look for a change in bone alignment. The bone may appear deformed, or a limb may be internally or externally rotated. Accompanying these deviations may be an alteration in the length of the extremity (usually a shortening) or a change in bone shape. Ask the client to move the involved body part, but if pain is elicited, stop the movement immediately. Range of motion (ROM) is

CHART 55-3

BEST PRACTICE for
Assessment of Neurovascular Status in Clients with Musculoskeletal Injury

Assessment Technique	Normal Findings
Skin Color	
Inspect the area distal to the injury.	No change in pigmentation compared with other parts of the body.
Skin Temperature	
Palpate the area distal to the injury (the dorsum of the hands is most sensitive to temperature).	The skin is warm.
Movement	
Ask the client to move the affected area or the area distal to the injury (active motion).	The client can move without discomfort.
Move the area distal to the injury (passive motion).	No difference in comfort compared with active movement.
Sensation	
Ask the client if numbness or tingling is present (paresthesia).	No numbness or tingling.
Palpate with a paper clip (especially the web space between the first and second toes or the web space between the thumb and forefinger).	No difference in sensation in the affected and unaffected extremities. (Loss of sensation in these areas indicates perineal nerve or median nerve damage.)
Pulses	
Palpate the pulses distal to the injury.	Pulses are strong and easily palpated; no difference in the affected and unaffected extremities.
Capillary Refill (least reliable)	
Press the nail beds distal to the injury until blanching occurs (or the skin near the nail if nails are thick and brittle).	Blood returns (return to usual color) within 3 sec (5 sec for older clients).
Pain	
Ask the client about the location, nature, and frequency of the pain.	Pain is usually localized and is often described as stabbing or throbbing. (Pain out of proportion to the injury and unrelieved by analgesics might indicate compartment syndrome.)

typically decreased. When the affected part is moved, the nurse may hear **crepitation,** a grating sound created by bone fragments.

Observe the skin for integrity. If the skin is intact (closed fracture), the area over the fracture may be **ecchymotic** (bruised) from bleeding into the underlying soft tissues. **Subcutaneous emphysema,** the appearance of bubbles under the skin because of air trapping, is not uncommon but is seen later.

Swelling at the fracture site is rapid and can result in marked neurovascular compromise. Perform a thorough neurovascular assessment and compare the injured area with its symmetric counterpart. Skin color and temperature, sensation, mobility, pain, and pulses are assessed distal to the fracture site. If the fracture involves an extremity, check the nails for capillary refill by applying pressure to the nail and observing for the speed of blood return. If nails are brittle or thick, the skin adjacent to the nail is assessed. *Checking for capillary refill is not as reliable as other indicators of perfusion.* Chart 55-3 describes the procedure for a neurovascular assessment, which evaluates circulation, movement, and sensation.

For an open fracture, determine the degree of soft-tissue damage and the amount of overt bleeding. The area may be lightly palpated for tenderness, but a sterile glove is worn if the skin is disrupted.

Clients often complain of moderate to severe pain at the site of the fracture or in an adjacent or distal area. For example, clients with a fractured hip may have groin pain or pain referred to the back of the knee. Pain is usually due to muscle spasm and edema, which result from the fracture. In clients with one or more fractured ribs, severe pain occurs when deep breaths are taken. Assess respiratory status, which may be severely compromised from pain or pneumothorax (air in the pleural cavity).

SPECIAL ASSESSMENT CONSIDERATIONS. For fractures of the shoulder and upper arm, the physical assessment is best done with the client in a sitting or standing position, if possible, so that shoulder drooping or other abnormal positioning can be seen. Support the affected arm and flex the elbow to promote comfort during the assessment. For more distal areas of the arm, the assessment is done with the client in a supine position so that the extremity can be elevated to reduce swelling.

Place the client in a supine position for assessment of the lower extremities and pelvis. A client with an impacted hip fracture may be able to walk for a short time after injury, although this is not recommended. The client with any type of hip fracture has pain in addition to decreased ROM in the hip.

Some fractures can cause internal organ damage, resulting in hemorrhage. When a pelvic fracture is suspected, assess vital signs, skin color, and the level of consciousness for indications of possible hypovolemic shock. The urine is checked for blood, which indicates damage to the urinary system, often the bladder. If the client is unable to void, the nurse suspects damage to the urethra.

PSYCHOSOCIAL ASSESSMENT

The psychosocial status of a client with a fracture depends on the extent of the injury and other complications. Hospitalization is usually not required for a single, uncomplicated fracture, and the client may return to usual daily activities within a few days. Healing is usually complete in a young adult in 4 to 6 weeks.

In contrast, a client suffering multiple trauma can be hospitalized for weeks and may undergo many surgical procedures, treatments, and prolonged rehabilitation. For these clients, disruptions in lifestyle can create a high level of stress.

The stresses that result from a chronic condition affect relationships between the client and family members or significant others. Assess the client's feelings about himself or herself as a person, and ask about how he or she coped with previously experienced stressful events. Body image and sexuality may be altered by deformity, treatment modalities for fracture repair, or long-term immobilization.

Critical Thinking Challenge

A 30-year-old man arrives at the emergency department via ambulance. He was the driver of a motorcycle involved in a collision with an SUV. Paramedics report that the client was hit from the side; the bike fell on him, and he was trapped underneath the SUV. Initial reports from the ambulance en route describe an individual in shock with a mangled left leg below the knee and a left wrist fracture. The client was wearing a helmet at the time of the crash.

1. What information given above is helpful in predicting other injuries this client may have sustained?
2. What are the priority assessments you should perform when he arrives at the hospital?
3. What assessments of the leg injury will determine the type and grade of the fracture?
4. What initial assessments of the injured leg should you perform?

evolve For suggested answer guidelines, go to http://evolve.elsevier.com/Iggy/.

LABORATORY ASSESSMENT

No special laboratory tests are available for assessment of fractures. The client's hemoglobin and hematocrit levels are often low because of bleeding caused by the injury. If extensive soft-tissue damage accompanies the fracture, the erythrocyte sedimentation rate (ESR) may be elevated, which indicates the expected inflammatory response. If the ESR increases during fracture healing, the client may have a bone infection. During the healing stages, serum calcium and phosphorus levels are often increased as the bone releases these elements into the blood.

RADIOGRAPHIC ASSESSMENT

The health care provider orders standard x-rays and tomograms to confirm a diagnosis of fracture. These reveal the bone disruption, malalignment, or deformity. If the x-ray film does not show a fracture but the client is symptomatic, the x-ray is usually repeated with additional views.

The computed tomography (CT) scan is useful in detecting fractures of complex structures, such as the hip and pelvis. It also identifies compression fractures of the spine.

OTHER DIAGNOSTIC ASSESSMENTS

Although not commonly used, the health care provider may order a bone scan (with technetium or gallium) for help in detecting certain types of fractures, particularly pathologic fractures. It is impossible for fractures of small bones or occult fractures to be visualized by conventional x-rays as early as by a bone scan. In addition, the bone scan can better determine fracture complications, such as delayed bone healing, nonunion, infection, and ischemic necrosis.

Magnetic resonance imaging (MRI) is useful in determining the amount of soft-tissue damage that may have occurred with the fracture. It is also very helpful in visualizing vertebral and skull fractures.

Analysis

COMMON NURSING DIAGNOSES AND COLLABORATIVE PROBLEMS

The following are priority nursing diagnoses for clients with fractures:

1. Risk for Peripheral Neurovascular Dysfunction related to fractures (bone and soft-tissue trauma)
2. Acute Pain related to biologic injury (bone disruption, soft-tissue damage, muscle spasm, and edema)
3. Risk for Infection related to trauma
4. Impaired Physical Mobility related to pain
5. Imbalanced Nutrition: Less Than Body Requirements related to additional metabolic need for healing of bone and soft tissues

ADDITIONAL NURSING DIAGNOSES AND COLLABORATIVE PROBLEMS

In addition to the common nursing diagnoses, clients with fractures may have one or more of the following:

- Activity Intolerance related to pain and impaired mobility
- Constipation related to opioids and prolonged immobility (particularly in older adults)
- Ineffective Coping related to prolonged immobility, hospitalization, or lifestyle changes
- Compromised Family Coping related to prolonged hospitalization or lifestyle changes
- Self-Care Deficit related to pain and immobility
- Disturbed Body Image related to deformity and/or treatment modality
- Sexual Dysfunction related to pain and immobility
- Disturbed Sleep Pattern related to chronic pain or prolonged hospitalization
- Fear related to possible nursing home placement or death (particularly in older adults)
- Impaired Skin Integrity and Impaired Tissue Integrity related to bone injury and immobility

The following collaborative problems may be appropriate for clients with *severe* fractures:

- Potential for Acute Compartment Syndrome
- Potential for Hypovolemic Shock
- Potential for Fat Embolism Syndrome
- Potential for Venous Thromboembolism
- Potential for Ischemic Necrosis
- Potential for Delayed Healing, Malunion, or Nonunion

Planning and Implementation

RISK FOR PERIPHERAL NEUROVASCULAR DYSFUNCTION

NOC **PLANNING: EXPECTED OUTCOMES.** The client with a fracture is expected to have adequate blood flow through the small vessels of the extremities to maintain tissue function. Indicators include that the client will have noncompromised:

- Capillary refill
- Sensation
- Skin color
- Muscle function
- Extremity skin color
- Pedal pulses

CHART 67-4

BEST PRACTICE for
Emergency Care of the Client with an Extremity Fracture

EMERGENCY CARE

1. Remove the client's clothing (cut it necessary) to inspect the affected area while supporting the injured area above and below the injury. Do not remove shoes because this can cause increased trauma.
2. Apply direct pressure on the area if there is bleeding and pressure over the proximal artery nearest the fracture.
3. Keep the client warm and in a supine position.
4. Check the neurovascular status of the area distal to the extremity: temperature, color, sensation, movement, and capillary refill. Compare affected and unaffected limbs.
5. Immobilize the extremity by splinting; include joints above and below the fracture site. Recheck circulation after splinting.
6. Cover the affected area with a dressing (preferably sterile).

INTERVENTIONS. A fracture can happen anywhere, and it may be accompanied by multiple injuries to vital organs. In some cases, one or more fractures occur in the community setting, often as a result of an accident (e.g., fall, vehicle).

EMERGENCY CARE: FRACTURE. For any client who experiences trauma, first assess for respiratory distress, bleeding, and head injury. If any of these is present, provide lifesaving care before being concerned about the fracture. In the community setting, provide emergency interventions until medical treatment in a hospital is available, or call 911 for the emergency team.

The fracture injury is then assessed (Chart 55-4). If the person is clothed, the emergency team member (first responder) cuts away clothing from the fracture site for best visualization. Bleeding is controlled by direct pressure on the area and digital pressure over the proximal artery nearest the fracture. At the same time, to prevent shock, check vital signs, place the client in a supine position, and keep him or her warm.

The emergency team also does the following:

- Inspects the fracture site for intactness of skin, swelling, and deformity (e.g., shortening and rotation)
- Palpates the area *lightly* to determine temperature (coolness), decreased sensation, and blanching
- Assesses distal pulses by comparing affected and unaffected extremities, if applicable
- Assesses for motor function by asking the client to move an area distal to the fracture (e.g., if a femoral fracture is suspected, he or she is asked to move the ankle and foot on the affected side; the upper portion of the leg remains immobilized)

To prevent further damage, reduce pain, and increase circulation, the emergency team immobilizes the area of the fracture by splinting. Any object or device that extends to the joints above and below the fracture can be used as a splint. At the scene of an accident, the emergency team may need to improvise by using available materials, such as a board. If the skin is broken, loosely apply a clean (preferably sterile) cloth to prevent further contamination of the wound. Neurovascular assessment is rechecked after splinting.

In the emergency department, physician's office, or clinic, fracture management begins with reduction and immobilization of the fracture:

- Reduction, or realignment of the bone ends for proper healing, is accomplished by a closed method (e.g., traction) or an open (surgical) procedure.

CHART 55-5

NIC **INTERVENTION ACTIVITIES for**
The Client at Risk for Peripheral Neurovascular Dysfunction

Circulatory Care (Arterial Insufficiency/Venous Insufficiency): *Promotion of arterial and venous circulation*

- Perform a comprehensive appraisal of peripheral circulations (e.g., check peripheral pulses, edema, capillary refill, color, and temperature).
- Monitor degree of discomfort or pain.
- Protect the extremity from injury.
- Place extremity in a dependent position, as appropriate.

Peripheral Sensation Management: *Prevention or minimization of injury or discomfort in the client with altered sensation*

- Monitor for paresthesia: numbness, tingling, hyperesthesia, and hypoesthesia.
- Monitor fit of bracing devices, prostheses, shoes, and clothing.
- Administer analgesics, as necessary.
- Discuss or identify causes of abnormal sensations or sensation changes.

NIC intervention activities selected from Dochterman, J.M., & Bulechek, G.M. (Eds.) (2004). *Nursing interventions classification (NIC)* (4th ed.). St. Louis: Mosby. No part of this work is to be altered without prior written permission from the Publisher.

- Immobilization is achieved by the use of bandages, casts, traction, internal fixation, or external fixation.

The health care provider selects the treatment method on the basis of the type, location, and extent of the fracture. These interventions prevent further injury and reduce discomfort.

NONSURGICAL MANAGEMENT. Nonsurgical management typically involves closed reduction and immobilization with a bandage, splint, cast, or traction. For each modality, the nurse's *primary* concern is assessment and prevention of neurovascular dysfunction or compromise (Chart 55-5). Assess the neurovascular status of the client who has sustained a fracture every hour for the first 24 hours and every 4 to 8 hours thereafter (see Chart 55-3). Elevate the fractured extremity higher than the heart, and apply ice for the first 24 to 48 hours, as appropriate, to reduce edema. Assess dressings, splints, casts, and traction for neurovascular compromise. The client will usually complain of discomfort that is unrelieved by analgesics if the bandage, splint, or cast is too tight.

Pay particular attention to *early* signs and symptoms of acute compartment syndrome (ACS) by doing a thorough pain assessment. The client with early ACS typically complains of severe, diffuse pain that is not relieved by analgesics; pain during passive motion is greater than pain during active motion. If the client presents with this complaint, notify the health care provider *immediately*. Additional preventive measures and interventions for ACS are described earlier in this chapter under Complications of Fractures.

Closed Reduction. Closed reduction is the most common nonsurgical method for managing a simple fracture. While applying a manual pull, or traction, on the bone, the health care provider manipulates the bone ends so that they realign. Anesthesia or analgesia is typically used during this procedure to minimize pain. An x-ray verifies that the bone ends are approximated before the bone is immobilized.

Bandages and Splints. For certain areas of the body, such as the scapula and clavicle, an elastic bandage or commercial mobilizer may be used to immobilize the bone during healing. Because upper extremity bones do not bear

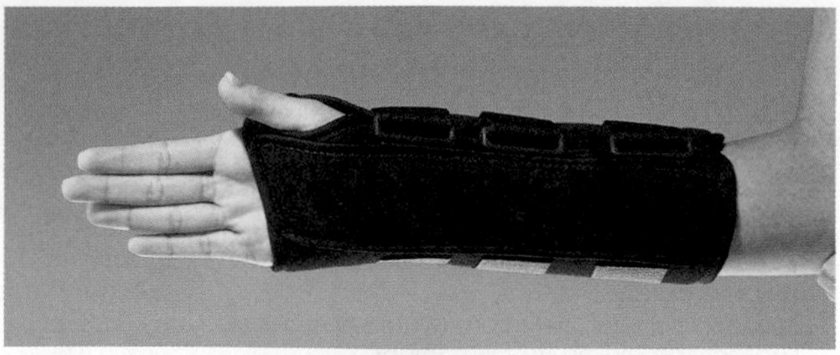

Figure 55-3 ■ A universal wrist and forearm splint used for immobilization. (Courtesy Smith & Nephew, Inc., Orthopaedics Divisions, Memphis, TN.)

weight, splints may be sufficient to keep bone fragments in place. Figure 55-3 illustrates the use of a wrist splint for fracture immobilization. Thermoplast, a durable, flexible material for splinting, allows custom fitting to the client's body part.

The nurse's primary responsibility is to assess the area distal to the bandage or splint for neurovascular compromise. The client usually complains of increased discomfort that is not relieved by analgesics if the splint or bandage is too tight. Reinforce the need for elevation as appropriate and teach how to assess for circulatory changes. The client is reminded to keep the device as dry and clean as possible to prevent skin breakdown and infection.

Casts. For more complex fractures or fractures of the lower extremity, the physician or orthopedic technician applies a cast to hold bone fragments in place after reduction. A **cast** is a rigid device that immobilizes the affected body part while allowing other body parts to move. It also allows early mobility and reduces pain. Although its most common use is for fractures, a cast may be applied for correction of deformities (such as clubfoot) or for prevention of deformities (such as those seen in some clients with rheumatoid arthritis).

Cast Materials. Several types of materials are used to make casts. The traditional plaster-of-Paris (anhydrous calcium sulfate) cast requires application of a well-fitted stockinette under the material. If the stockinette is too tight, it may impair circulation; if it is too loose, wrinkles can lead to the development of pressure ulcers and subsequent skin breakdown. Padding is applied over the stockinette, followed by wet plaster rolls wrapped around the extremity or other body part. The cast feels hot because an immediate chemical reaction occurs, but it soon becomes damp and cool. This type of cast takes 24 to 72 hours to dry, depending on the size and location of the cast. A wet cast feels cold, smells musty, and is grayish. The cast is dry when it feels hard and firm, is odorless, and has a shiny white appearance.

On occasion, the plaster cast may have rough edges, which can crumble and cause skin irritation. Petaling the cast will resolve this problem, if the underlying stockinette does not cover the edges of the cast. Small strips of tape are placed over the rough edges to protect the skin. If the skin under the cast was disrupted, the health care provider, orthopedic technician, or specially trained nurse cuts a window into the cast so that the wound can be observed and cared for. A window is also an access for taking pulses, removing wound drains, or relieving abdominal distention when the client is in a body or spica cast.

If the cast is too tight, it may be cut with a cast cutter to relieve pressure or allow tissue swelling. The health care provider may choose to bivalve the cast (i.e., cut it lengthwise into two equal pieces) if bone healing is almost complete. Either half of the cast can be removed for inspection or for provision of care. The two halves are then reunited by an elastic bandage wrap.

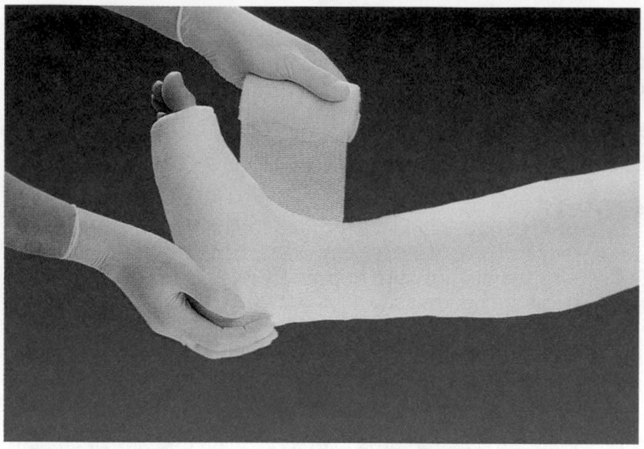

Figure 55-4 ■ Application of fiberglass synthetic cast. (Courtesy Smith & Nephew, Inc., Orthopaedics Divisions, Memphis, TN.)

Synthetic materials for casts include fiberglass and polyester-cotton knit (Figure 55-4). These materials are lighter than plaster and require minimal drying time. Fiberglass casts are dry in 10 to 15 minutes and can bear weight 30 minutes after application. Polyester-cotton knit casts take 7 minutes to dry and can withstand weight bearing in about 20 minutes. Some health care providers use synthetic casts for upper extremities and plaster-of-Paris casts for lower extremities because plaster casts can bear more weight for a longer time. However, synthetic casts are used much more commonly overall.

Types of Casts. Casts can be generally divided into four main groups: arm casts, leg casts, cast braces, and body or spica casts. Table 55-1 describes specific casts that are used for various parts of the body.

When a client is in bed with an *arm cast,* the arm is elevated above the heart to reduce swelling. The hand should be higher than the elbow. Ice may be prescribed for the first 24 to 48 hours. When the client is out of bed, the arm is supported with a sling placed around the neck to alleviate fatigue caused by the weight of the cast. The sling should distribute the weight over a large area of the shoulders and trunk, not just the neck. Some health care providers prefer that after the first few days in an arm cast, particularly a short-arm cast, the client not use a sling; this encourages normal movement of the mobile joints and enhance bone healing.

A *leg cast* permits mobility and requires the client to use ambulatory aids, such as crutches. A cast shoe, sandal, or boot that attaches to the foot or a rubber walking pad attached to the sole of the cast assists in ambulation (if weight bearing is allowed) and helps prevent damage to the cast. The affected leg is elevated on several pillows to reduce swelling, and ice is applied for the first 24 hours or as prescribed.

A *cast brace* enables the client to bend unaffected joints while the fracture is healing. The fracture must show signs of healing and minimal tissue edema before application of

TABLE 55-1 Types of Casts Used for Musculoskeletal Trauma

Type and Characteristics of Cast	Use
Upper Extremity Casts	
Short-arm cast (SAC) (extends from below the elbow to and including part of the hand)	Stable fractures of the wrist (metacarpals, carpals, or distal radius)
Long-arm cast (LAC) (includes the upper arm to and including part of the hand)	Unstable fractures of the wrist, distal humerus, radius, or ulna
Hanging-arm cast (same as LAC but heavier, with added loop at the mid-forearm)	Fractures of the humerus that cannot be aligned by LAC (light traction is possible while the client is in bed or by an attached strap that extends around the neck).
Thumb spica (gauntlet) cast (similar to SAC with the thumb casted in abduction)	Fractures of the thumb
Shoulder spica cast (the shoulder is casted in abduction with the elbow flexed)	Unstable fractures of the shoulder girdle or humerus; dislocations of the shoulder
Lower Extremity Casts	
Short-leg cast (SLC) (from below the knee to the base of the toes)	Fractures of the ankle, metatarsals, or foot
Long-leg cast (LLC) (from the mid-upper thigh to the base of the toes)	Unstable fractures of the tibia, fibula, or ankle
Walking cast (a walking device on the bottom of SLC or LLC)	Same as for SLC or LLC
Leg cylinder (similar to SLC, but the ankle and foot are not casted)	Stable fractures of the tibia, fibula, or knee
Long-leg cylinder (similar to LLC, but the ankle and foot are not casted)	Stable fractures of the distal femur, proximal tibia, or knee
Cast Braces (or Brace Casts)	
Patellar weight-bearing cast (similar to SLC or leg cylinder)	Midshaft or distal shaft fractures of the femur
External polycentric knee hinge cast (a hinge connects the lower and upper leg and allows 90 degrees of knee flexion)	Same as for the patellar weight-bearing cast
Body Casts	
Hip spica (extends from below the nipple line down the affected leg [single], down the leg and half of the unaffected leg [1½], or down both legs [double])	Dislocation of the hip; pelvic or hip injuries
Risser's cast (the body jacket extends from the shoulders to beyond the iliac crests and hips, with a large opening over the anterior chest)	Scoliosis; thoracic spinal fractures
Halo cast (the body jacket contains a halo brace)	Fractures of the cervical spine

this cast. Two cylindrical casts are made and connected by a hinge to allow joint movement. As healing occurs, the casts may be removed and replaced with a soft brace. Commercial immobilizers, which serve the same function as a cast brace, are available and may be used in some cases.

A *body cast* encircles the trunk of the body; a **spica cast** encases a portion of the trunk and one or two extremities. A client with either of these casts presents a special challenge for nursing care. Potential complications related to severe impairment in mobility include the following:

- Skin breakdown
- Respiratory dysfunction, such as pneumonia and atelectasis
- Constipation
- Joint contractures

Cast syndrome (superior mesenteric artery syndrome), an uncommon but serious complication, is most often seen in orthopedic clients who have been placed in a hip spica or body cast. Partial or complete upper intestinal obstruction results in classic symptoms: abdominal distention, epigastric pain, nausea, and vomiting. The vomiting often occurs after meals, and clients may have normal bowel sounds. Partial obstruction occurs initially from compression of the third portion of the duodenum between the superior mesenteric artery and the aorta. This progresses to complete obstruction from duodenal edema caused by continued vomiting and distention. Placing a window in the abdominal portion of the cast or bivalving the cast may be sufficient to relieve pressure on the duodenum. Management of intestinal obstruction is the same as for any client with this complication.

Cast Care. Before the cast is applied, explain the purpose of the cast and the procedure for its application. With a plaster cast, it is particularly important to warn the client about the heat that will be felt immediately after the wet cast is applied. The new cast is not covered; this facilitates air-drying.

When a client with a wet plaster cast is moved and turned, the cast is handled with the palms of the hands to prevent indentations and resultant areas of pressure on the skin. The client is turned every 1 to 2 hours to allow air to circulate and dry all parts of the cast. If the client is hospitalized, a sign is placed at the head of the bed as a reminder that the cast is wet and requires special handling. If the health care provider requests that the cast be elevated to reduce swelling, a cloth-covered pillow is used instead of one encased in plastic, which could cause the cast to retain heat and prevent drying. Elevation of the casted extremity reduces edema but may impair arterial circulation to the affected limb. Uniform support is needed while the cast is drying to prevent development of pressure points.

For preventing contamination by urine or feces, the perineal area of a dry long leg or body cast is encased in a plastic protective covering. Fracture pans are preferred over traditional bedpans because they are smaller and more comfortable for the client. Care is taken to prevent spillage onto the cast.

Check to ensure that the cast is not too tight and frequently monitor the client's neurovascular status, usually every hour for the first 24 hours after application. You should be able to insert a finger between the cast and the skin. Ice may be applied for the first 24 to 36 hours to reduce swelling and inflammation.

Once the plaster cast is dry, it is inspected at least once every 8 hours for drainage, cracking, crumbling, alignment, and fit. Plaster casts act like sponges and absorb drainage, whereas synthetic casts act like a wick, pulling drainage away from the drainage site. Padding can also absorb wound drainage. Drainage on any cast should always be measured and documented in the client record; however, sources disagree on whether drainage should be circled on the cast because it may increase anxiety. Immediately report to the health care provider any sudden increases in the amount of drainage or change in the integrity of the cast. After swelling decreases, it is not uncommon for the cast to become too loose and need replacement. If the client is not admitted to the hospital, he or she is given instructions regarding cast care, as discussed later under Community-Based Care, p. 1205.

Cast Complications. During hospitalization, assess for other complications resulting from casting that can be serious and life threatening, such as infection, circulation impairment, and peripheral nerve damage. If the client returns home after cast application, the client and family are taught how to monitor for these complications and when to notify the health care provider.

Infection most often results from the breakdown of skin under the cast (pressure necrosis). If pressure necrosis occurs, the client typically complains of a very painful "hot spot" under the cast, and the cast may feel warmer in the affected area. Smell the area for mustiness or an unpleasant odor that would indicate infected material. If the infection progresses, a fever may develop.

Circulation impairment and peripheral nerve damage can result from constriction of the cast. Perform frequent neurovascular assessments as described in Chart 55-3. A client with a new cast may require hourly assessments. A client with a cast that is 3 or 4 days old usually requires assessments every 4 to 8 hours.

The client with a cast may be immobilized for a prolonged period, depending on the extent of the fracture and the type of cast. Assess for complications of immobility, such as skin breakdown, pneumonia, atelectasis, thromboembolism, and constipation. Before the cast is removed, inform the client that the cast cutter will not injure the skin but that heat may be felt during the procedure.

Because of prolonged immobilization, a joint may become contracted, usually in a fixed state of flexion, or degenerative arthritis may develop from lack of weight bearing, which is necessary for cartilage viability. Muscle can also atrophy from lack of exercise during prolonged immobilization of the affected body part, usually an extremity.

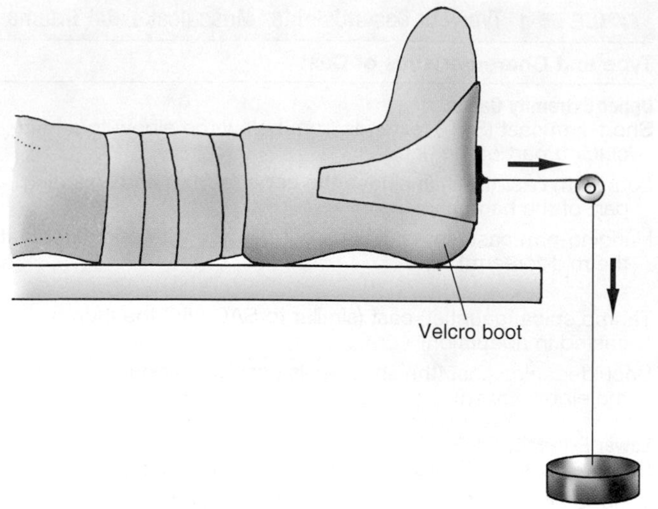

Figure 55-5 ■ Buck's traction with a hook-and-loop fastener (Velcro) boot, commonly used for hip fractures.

Traction. **Traction** is the application of a pulling force to a part of the body to provide reduction, alignment, and rest. Traction can also decrease muscle spasm (thus relieving pain) and prevent or correct deformity and tissue damage. A client in traction is usually hospitalized longer, but in some cases home care is possible even for skeletal traction.

Mechanical traction can be either of the following:

- Continuous, as in fracture treatment
- Intermittent, for relief of muscle spasm in other types of musculoskeletal/neurologic trauma, such as cervical nerve root compression

Traction may also be classified as running traction or balanced suspension. In running traction, the pulling force is in one direction and the client's body acts as countertraction. Moving the body or bed position can alter the countertraction force. Balanced suspension provides the countertraction so that the pulling force of the traction is not altered when the bed or client is moved. This allows for increased client movement and facilitates care.

Types of Traction. Traction is typically one of five types: skin traction, skeletal traction, plaster traction, brace traction, or circumferential traction. Skin traction involves the use of a Velcro boot (Buck's traction) (Figure 55-5), belt, or halter, which is secured around a body part. The primary purpose of skin traction is to decrease painful muscle spasms that accompany fractures. The weight is used as a pulling force is limited (5 to 10 pounds [2.3 to 4.5 kg]) to prevent injury to the skin.

In skeletal traction, pins, wires, tongs (e.g., Crutchfield), or screws are surgically inserted directly into bone. These allow the use of longer traction time and heavier weights (usually 15 to 30 pounds [6.8 to 13.6 kg]). Skeletal traction aids in bone realignment.

Plaster traction combines skeletal traction and a plaster cast. A brace traction device exerts a pull for correction of alignment deformities. Circumferential traction uses a belt around the body, such as pelvic traction for low back problems. Table 55-2 describes commonly used types of traction for various parts of the body.

Traction Care. The nurse may set up or assist in the setup of traction. In larger or specialty hospitals or units, or-

TABLE 55-2 Types of Traction Used for Musculoskeletal Trauma

Type and Characteristics of Traction	Use
Upper Extremity Traction	
Sidearm skin or skeletal traction (the forearm is flexed and extended 90 degrees from the upper part of the body)	Fractures of the humerus with or without involvement of the shoulder and clavicle
Overhead or 90-90 traction, skin or skeletal (the elbow is flexed and the arm is at a right angle to the body over the upper chest)	Same as above (depends on the physician's preference)
Plaster traction (pins inserted through the bone are fixed in the cast)	Fractures of the wrist
Lower Extremity Traction	
Buck's extension traction (skin) (the affected leg is in extension)	Fractures of the hip or femur preoperatively Prevention of hip flexion contractures Hip dislocation
Russell's traction (similar to Buck's traction, but a sling under the knee suspends the leg)	Fractures of the hip or end of the femur
Balanced skin or skeletal traction (the limb is usually elevated in a Thomas splint with Pearson's attachment, or a Böhler-Braun splint is used)	Fractures of the femur or pelvis (acetabulum)
Spinal Column and Pelvic Traction	
Cervical halter (a strap under the chin)	Cervical muscle spasms, strain/sprain, or arthritis
Cervical skeletal (e.g., halo brace, Crutchfield tongs)	Cervical fractures of the spine Muscle spasms
Pelvic belt (a strap around the hips at the iliac crests is attached to weights at the foot of the bed)	Pain, strain, sprain, or muscle spasms, in the lower back
Pelvic sling (a wide strap around the hips is attached to an overhead bar to keep the pelvis off the bed)	Pelvic fractures; other pelvic injuries

thopedic technicians may set up traction. Once traction is applied, maintain the correct balance between traction pull and countertraction force. Weights are not usually removed without an order; they are not usually lifted manually or allowed to set on the floor. Weights should be freely hanging at all times. Teach this important point to staff members on the unit and to other personnel, such as those in the radiology department.

Inspect the skin at least every 8 hours for signs of irritation or inflammation. When possible, remove the belt or boot that is used for skin traction every 8 hours to inspect under the device.

When skeletal traction is used, pay particular attention to the points of entry of pins, wires, or screws for signs of inflammation or infection. A small amount of clear fluid drainage ("weeping") is expected. Most health care providers prefer that pin care is preformed every day. No standardized method or protocol for pin care has been established throughout the United States. Some health care providers and nurse specialists believe that cleaning the pins disrupts the skin's natural barrier to infection and advise against this practice. In any case, observe pin sites at least every 8 hours for drainage, color, odor, and severe redness, which indicate inflammation and possible infection. Infection of the pin tract may result in osteomyelitis.

The nurse is responsible for checking traction equipment to ensure its proper functioning. All ropes, knots, and pulleys are inspected at least every 8 hours for loosening, fraying, and positioning. Check the weight for consistency with the health care provider's order. At times the health care provider or qualified technician changes the weight without notifying the nurse or modifying the written order; contact the person responsible to confirm the change. Sometimes one of the weights is accidentally displaced by a staff member or visitor who bumps into it. Replace the weights if they are not correct, and notify the health care provider or orthopedic technician.

If the client complains of severe pain from muscle spasm, the weights may be too heavy or the client may need realignment. Report the pain to the health care provider if body realignment fails to reduce the discomfort. Also assess the neurovascular status of the affected body part to detect circulatory compromise and subsequent tissue damage. The circulation is usually monitored every hour for the first 24 hours after traction is applied and every 4 hours thereafter.

SURGICAL MANAGEMENT. For some types of fractures, casts and traction are not appropriate or sufficient treatment techniques. Surgical intervention may be needed to realign the bone for the healing process.

Preoperative Care. For stabilizing the fracture, the client may be placed in traction before surgery. This procedure is typical for managing a fractured hip when Buck's traction may be used preoperatively (see Figure 55-5). Teach the client and family or significant others what to expect during and after the surgery. The preoperative care for a client undergoing musculoskeletal surgery is similar to that for any client preparing for surgery with general or epidural anesthesia. (See Chapter 20 for a thorough discussion of preoperative nursing care.)

Operative Procedures. Open reduction with internal fixation (ORIF) is a common method of reducing and immobilizing a fracture. When this method is not feasible, external fixation with closed reduction is used. Although nurses do not decide which surgical technique is used, understanding the procedures enhances client teaching and care.

Open Reduction with Internal Fixation. Because ORIF permits early mobilization, it is often the preferred surgical method for an older adult who is susceptible to the complications of immobility.

Open reduction allows the surgeon direct visualization of the fracture site. **Internal fixation** uses metal pins, screws, rods, plates, or prostheses to immobilize the fracture during healing. The surgeon makes an incision to gain access to the broken bone and implants one or more devices. A newer bioabsorbable plate was recently introduced for internal fixation. This device is strong enough to fix the fracture but is reabsorbed by the body in about 3 months.

After the bone achieves union, the metal hardware may be removed, depending on the location and type of fracture (e.g., fractured ankle). Specific types of internal fixation devices are discussed later under Fractures of Specific Sites, p. 1206.

External Fixation. An alternative modality for the initial management of fractures is the external fixation apparatus, as shown in Figure 55-6. After fracture reduction, the physician makes small percutaneous incisions so that pins may be implanted into the bone. All pins are self-drilling. The pins are held in place by an external metal frame to prevent bone movement.

ADVANTAGES AND DISADVANTAGES. External fixation has several advantages over other immobilization techniques:

- There is minimal blood loss in comparison with internal fixation.
- The device allows early ambulation and exercise of the affected body part while relieving pain.
- The device maintains alignment in closed fractures that will not maintain position in a cast and stabilizes comminuted fractures that require bone grafting.
- In open fractures, in which skin and tissue trauma accompanies the fracture, the device permits easy access to the wound and promotes healing. This method is often preferred over the use of a window in a cast for wound care.

A disadvantage of external fixation is pin-tract infection. Pin-tract infections can lead to osteomyelitis, which is serious and difficult to treat (see Chapter 54). For prevention of these infections, some agencies have a pin-care procedure that is performed several times a day. The procedure is similar to that described earlier for skeletal traction pins (see Traction Care, pp. 1200 and 1201). As with skeletal traction, the need for special cleaning of the pins and the area around the pins is controversial. Regardless of whether pin care is done, inspect the pin sites at least daily for severe redness, swelling, and purulent drainage.

CARE OF THE CLIENT WITH AN EXTERNAL FIXATOR. As with any fracture treatment, assess the neurovascular status of the extremity distal to the fracture. External fixators may be used for an extremity or for fractures of the pelvis. External fixation is not definitive treatment for fractures. After a fixator is removed, the client may be placed in a cast until healing is complete.

The client with an external fixator may experience a disturbed body image. The frame may be large and bulky, and the affected area may have massive tissue damage with dressings. Be sensitive to this possibility in planning care.

CIRCULAR EXTERNAL FIXATION. The Ilizarov technique of circular external fixation is sometimes used to treat new fractures (closed, comminuted fractures and open fractures with bone loss) as well as malunion or nonunion of fractures. It may also be used to treat congenital bone deformities, especially in children. This procedure originated in Russia about 50 years ago and was introduced in the United States in 1986.

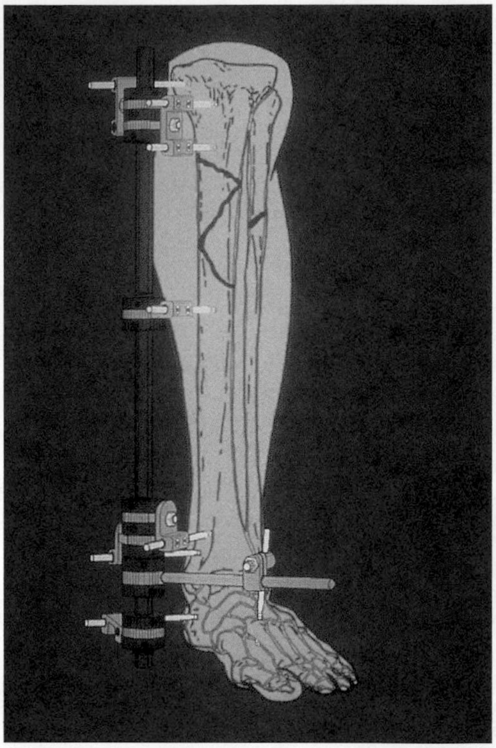

Figure 55-6 ■ The Hex-Fix external fixations system for tibial fractures. (Courtesy of Smith & Nephew, Inc., Orthopaedics Divisions, Memphis, TN.)

A circular external fixation device stimulates bone growth. Unlike the traditional fixator, the Ilizarov external fixator promotes rotation, angulation, shortening, lengthening, or widening of bone while allowing healing of the soft-tissue defect. The nursing care of the client with this device is similar to the care of the client with other external fixation systems except in one major exception: if the device is being used for filling bone gaps, using bone transport or distraction, the client must be taught how to manually turn the four-sided nuts (clickers), usually four times a day, unless he or she has an automated device. Daily distraction rates vary among clients, but 1 mm daily is common. Screening and teaching are particularly important because the client adjusts and cares for the apparatus for a prolonged time.

Postoperative Care. The postoperative care for a client undergoing ORIF or external fixation is similar to that provided for any client undergoing surgery (see Chapter 22). Because bone is a vascular, dynamic body tissue, the client is at risk for certain complications specific to fractures and musculoskeletal surgery. These problems (e.g., fat embolism and venous thromboembolism) were discussed earlier under Complications of Fractures, p. 1191.

Procedures for Nonunion. Some surgical repairs are not successful because the bone does not heal. Several additional options are available to the surgeon to promote bone union, such as electrical bone stimulation, bone grafting, and the newest therapy, ultrasound fracture treatment.

For selected clients, **electrical bone stimulation** may be successful. This procedure is based on research showing that bone has inherent electrical properties that are used in healing. The exact mechanism of action is unknown. Several types of devices have been developed. A noninvasive system uses magnetic coils applied on the skin or over a cast to deliver a pulsed magnetic field. There are no known risks with this system, although clients with pacemakers cannot use this device on an upper extremity. Implanted direct-current stimulators are placed directly in the fracture site and have no external apparatus. Both systems require about 6 months of treatment, and weight bearing is at the discretion of the health care provider.

Another method of treating nonunion is **bone grafting.** A bone graft may also replace diseased bone or increase bone tissue for joint replacement. In most cases, chips of bone are taken from the client's iliac crest or other site and are packed or wired between the bone ends to facilitate union. Allografts from cadavers may also be used. These grafts are frozen or freeze-dried and stored under sterile conditions in a bone bank.

Bone banking from living donors is becoming increasingly popular. If qualified, clients undergoing total hip replacement may donate their femoral heads to the bank for later use as bone grafts for other clients. Careful screening ensures that the bone is healthy and that the donor has no communicable disease. The bone cannot be donated without the client's written consent.

One of the newest modalities for fracture healing is **low-intensity pulsed ultrasound** (Exogen therapy). Used for slow-healing fractures or for new fractures as an alternative to surgery, ultrasound treatment has yielded excellent results. The client applies the treatment for about 20 minutes each day. It has no contraindications or adverse effects.

ACUTE PAIN

NOC **PLANNING: EXPECTED OUTCOMES.** The client with a fracture is expected to take personal actions to control pain. Indicators include that the client will consistently demonstrate the ability to:

- Use preventive measures
- Use nonanalgesic relief measures
- Use analgesic relief measures appropriately
- Report changes in pain symptoms or sites to health care professional
- Report uncontrollable pain symptoms to health care professional
- Report that pain is controlled

INTERVENTIONS. The nonsurgical or surgical management of fractures through reduction and immobilization helps reduce pain and prevents neurovascular injury. However, the client often requires drug therapy and other pain relief measures.

Drug Therapy. Musculoskeletal pain related to soft-tissue damage, bone disruption, and muscle spasm is one of the most severe types of pain that can be experienced. The client often has the pain for a prolonged time, which makes pain management difficult. The health care provider commonly prescribes opioid analgesics, anti-inflammatory drugs, and muscle relaxants.

For clients with chronic, severe pain, opioid and nonopioid drugs are alternated or given together to manage pain both centrally and peripherally. The nurse and client mutually decide on the best times for the strong pain relievers to be administered (e.g., before a complex dressing change, physical therapy, and at bedtime). Observe the client carefully for the effectiveness of the medication and its side effects. An early sign of acute compartment syndrome (ACS) is often the sudden inability of pain medication to relieve pain. Chapter 7 discusses the various methods of pain management, including epidural analgesia and patient-controlled analgesia.

Complementary and Alternative Therapies. With chronic, severe pain, the client cannot depend solely on drugs for relief. The client uses temporary pain relief measures, such as ice or heat, depending on the cause of the pain. If swelling causes pressure on the affected area, ice and elevation of the affected body part may be appropriate. Muscle spasms are best relieved by application of heat and massage. Other physical measures include a warm, soothing bath, a back rub, and the use of therapeutic touch.

If these measures are not effective in reducing pain, distraction, imagery, or music therapy may be used as alternatives. Teach the client relaxation techniques, such as deep breathing, for use during periods of severe pain. Chapters 4 and 7 discuss these techniques in detail.

RISK FOR INFECTION

NOC **PLANNING: EXPECTED OUTCOMES.** The client with a fracture is expected to be free of a wound or bone infection. Indicators include that the client will have none of the following:

- Foul-smelling discharge
- Purulent drainage
- Fever
- Lethargy
- Wound-site culture colonization (if wound present)
- White blood cell (WBC) elevation

INTERVENTIONS. When caring for a client with a fracture, particularly an open fracture, use strict aseptic technique for dressing changes and wound irrigations. Manifestations of local inflammation with purulent drainage are reported immediately to the health care provider. Other infections, such as pneumonia and urinary tract infection, may occur days after the fracture. The client's vital signs are monitored every 4 to 8 hours because increases in temperature and pulse often indicate systemic infection.

For most clients with an open fracture, the health care provider prescribes one or more broad-spectrum antibiotics prophylactically. This treatment is especially important for fractures requiring surgical repair.

IMPAIRED PHYSICAL MOBILITY

NOC **PLANNING: EXPECTED OUTCOMES.** The client with a fracture is expected to be free of physiologic consequences of impaired mobility. Indicators include that the client will have none of the following:

- Pressure ulcers
- Constipation
- Urinary retention
- Contracted joints
- Pneumonia
- Venous thrombosis

The client is also expected to move purposefully in his or her own environment independently with or without an assistive device. Indicators include that the following will not be compromised for the client:

- Balance
- Coordination
- Muscle movement
- Transfer performance
- Ambulation

INTERVENTIONS. The interventions necessary for this diagnosis can be grouped into two types: those that help to prevent complications of impaired mobility and those that help to increase mobility.

Prevention of Complications. The nurse plays a vital role in preventing and assessing for complications in immobilized clients with fractures. Additional information about nursing care for preventing problems associated with immobility is found in Chapter 10 and earlier in this chapter in the discussion of specific complications under Complications of Fractures, p. 1191.

Promotion of Mobility. The use of crutches or a walker increases mobility and assists in ambulation. The client may progress to use of a cane.

Crutches. Crutches are the most commonly used ambulatory aid for many types of musculoskeletal trauma (e.g., fractures, sprains, amputations). In most agencies, the physical therapist fits the client for crutches and teaches him or her how to ambulate with them on flat surfaces and stairs. The nurse's role may be to reinforce the instructions and evaluate whether the client is using the crutches correctly. However, in emergency department and ambulatory settings, nurses routinely teach clients how to use crutches.

Walking with crutches requires strong upper extremities, balance, and coordination. For this reason, crutches are not used as often for older adults. The therapist pads the tips and axillary bars of the crutches; padding prevents the tips

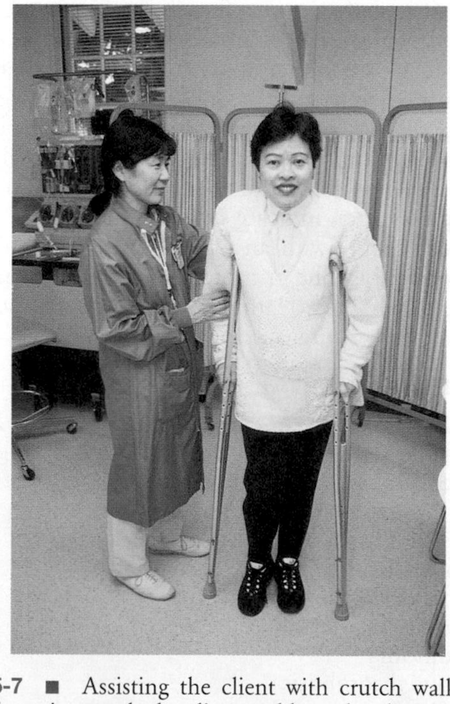

Figure 55-7 ■ Assisting the client with crutch walking. Note how the therapist guards the client and how the client's elbows are at no more than 30 degrees of flexion.

from slipping and the bars from damaging the axillae. To prevent pressure on the axillary nerve, there should be two to three finger breadths between the axilla and the top of the crutch when the crutch tip is at least 6 inches (15 cm) diagonally in front of the foot. The crutch is adjusted so that the elbow is flexed no more than 30 degrees when the palm is on the handle (Figure 55-7).

There are several types of gaits for walking with crutches. The most common one for musculoskeletal injury is the three-point gait, which allows minimal weight bearing on the affected leg.

Walkers and Canes. A walker is most often used by the older client who needs additional support for balance. The physical therapist assesses the strength of the upper extremities and the unaffected leg. Strength is improved with exercise as needed.

A cane is sometimes used if the client needs only minimal support for an affected leg. The straight cane offers the least support. A hemi-cane or quad-cane provides a broader base for the cane and therefore more support. The cane is placed on the *unaffected* side and should create no more than 30 degrees of flexion of the elbow. The top of the cane should be parallel to the greater trochanter of the femur.

IMBALANCED NUTRITION: LESS THAN BODY REQUIREMENTS

NOC **PLANNING: EXPECTED OUTCOMES.** The client with a fracture is expected to maintain an adequate dietary intake to meet metabolic needs. Indicators include that the client will have no deviation from normal range in the following:

- Nutrient intake
- Food intake
- Fluid intake
- Hematocrit

INTERVENTIONS. Nursing interventions focus on meeting the client's nutritional needs. The dietitian assesses the client's food likes and dislikes and collaborates with him or her to plan meals that are both appealing and nutritional. For promotion of bone and tissue healing, the client needs a high-protein, high-calorie diet. Supplements of vitamins B and C are also required for tissue nutrition. Clients with fractures may be immobilized for extended periods; thus they are predisposed to hypocalcemia, which results in loss of calcium from bone and in subsequent bone fragility. Teach the client to increase the intake of foods high in calcium, particularly milk and milk products if the client can tolerate them.

A negative nitrogen balance can develop 7 to 10 days after injury in an immobilized client because of an increase in catabolism without compensatory protein intake. Suggest frequent small feedings and supplements of high-protein liquids, such as Boost or Carnation Instant Breakfast preparations. Milk shakes are an excellent protein and calorie supplement as well as a source of calcium.

Because of less weight bearing on long bones, the immobilized client with a fracture often becomes anemic. Blood loss from the injury or reparative surgery contributes to the anemic state. Encourage intake of foods high in iron content. The health care provider may prescribe a daily multivitamin with iron supplement.

Critical Thinking Challenge

Following initial assessment in the emergency department, your client, who was injured in a motorcycle accident, has a closed reduction of the wrist fracture and application of a long-arm cast. He is alert and oriented when he arrives on the orthopedic unit.

1. What assessments should you perform to evaluate the client's injured arm?
2. What is a potential cause of compartment syndrome in this client's fractured arm?
3. What symptoms would raise suspicion of compartment syndrome?

evolve For suggested answer guidelines, go to http://evolve.elsevier.com/Iggy/.

Community-Based Care

The client with an uncomplicated fracture is usually discharged to home from the emergency department. Older adults with hip or other fractures or clients with multiple trauma are hospitalized and then transferred to home, a rehabilitation setting, or a long-term care facility for rehabilitation. To ensure continuity of care, the case manager or the discharge planner in the hospital communicates the plan of care to the health care agency receiving the client (see the Evidence-Based Practice for Nursing box below).

HOME CARE MANAGEMENT

If the client is discharged to home, the nurse, therapist, or case manager assesses the home environment for structural barriers to mobility, such as stairs. Most clients are taught how to use stairs, but older adults may not be able to perform this difficult task.

HEALTH TEACHING

The client with a fracture may be discharged from the hospital, emergency department, office, or clinic with a bandage, splint, cast, or external fixator. Provide verbal and written instructions on the care of these devices. Chart 55-6 describes care of the affected extremity after removal of the cast.

The client may also need to continue wound care at home. Instruct the client and caregiver about how to assess and dress the wound to promote healing and prevent infection. Teach the client also how to recognize complications (see Complications of Fractures, p. 1191) and when and where to seek professional health care if complications occur.

Additional educational needs depend on the type of fracture and fracture repair. Care of external fixators and casts is discussed earlier in this chapter under Cast Care (p. 1199) and External Fixation (p. 1202).

HEALTH CARE RESOURCES

Identify potential or actual problems in the hospital and arrange for follow-up care at home. For example, professional counseling for depression may need to continue after discharge from the hospital. A social worker may need to help the client apply for funds to pay medical bills. If there is severe bone and tissue damage, be realistic and help the client understand the long-term nature of the recovery period, particularly if he or she experiences a major complication, such as infection, while in the hospital. Multiple treatment techniques and surgical procedures required for complications can be mentally and emotionally draining for the client and family. A vocational counselor may be needed to help the client seek a different type of job, depending on the nature of the fracture.

The client with a severe injury and multiple treatment modalities may need follow-up care in the home by a home care nurse. An older or incapacitated client may need assistance with activities of daily living (ADLs), which is provided by home care aides. The nurse in the hospital anticipates the client's needs and arranges for these services, usually with the assistance of the case worker or discharge planner.

It is extremely important for the hospital nurse to communicate the client's needs to the nurse or aide who will care for the client at home. A physical therapist may come to the home, or the client may go to a clinic, hospital, or private office for follow-up physical therapy after discharge

EVIDENCE-BASED PRACTICE for Nursing

Improving client outcomes through trauma case management

Curtis, K., et al. (2002). The impact of trauma case management on patient outcomes. *The Journal of Trauma Injury, Infection, and Critical Care, 53*(3), 477-482.

This study examined the use of nurse case managers for trauma clients with injury severity scores (ISS) of 8-15, length of stay, length of stay for age over and under age 50, missed injury detection, complication rated overall, over/under age 50, and utilization and days/client of allied health intervention (physical, occupational, or other therapies).

Results demonstrated a trend toward reduced length of stay overall, more so in the older and more severely injured. The trauma case management greatly improved the missed injury detection rates and coordinated allied health use more efficiently. Staff surveys exhibited dramatic improvement in the effectiveness of client care. There was an overall reduction in complication rates, especially in the older group of clients; however, it was not statistically significant.

Level of Evidence: 6—This study serves as a pilot study for future research regarding the utilization of nurse case managers, a growing trend.

Critique. The sample sizes of both the control (327) and study (149) groups were relatively small, which makes generalization more difficult. Also, the use of age 50 to divide the older and younger populations is an unusual age and makes interpretation of data more difficult to relate to other studies.

Implications for Nursing. Nurses play an important role in improving client care and follow-up. Nurses should (1) coordinate care between various health care providers, (2) listen to all the client's complaints and concerns, and (3) be alert for early signs and symptoms of complications.

CHART 55-6

CLIENT EDUCATION GUIDE
Care of the Extremity After Cast Removal

- Remove scaly, dead skin carefully by soaking; do not scrub.
- Move the extremity carefully. Expect discomfort, weakness, and decreased range of motion.
- Support the extremity with pillows or your orthotic device until strength and movement return.
- Exercise slowly as instructed by your physical therapist.
- Wear support stockings or elastic bandages to prevent swelling (for lower extremity).

from the hospital. An occupational therapist assists with retraining in the home environment for ADLs; adaptations in the home enable the client to be independent.

The cost to individuals and society at large is enormous (see the Resource Management box at right). The cost for direct medical care, rehabilitation, lost wages, and lost productivity is more than $224 billion each year (http://www.cdc.gov). Each year about 90,000 people sustain injuries serious enough to cause long-term disability. Injury is a definable, correctable event with specific identifiable risks. It is imperative that nurses be active in educating the public on prevention of injury through programs that highlight the major risk factors, including alcohol, illicit drugs, and firearms among the young and falls in older adults.

Evaluation: Outcomes

Evaluate the care of the client with a fracture on the basis of the identified nursing diagnoses and collaborative problems. The expected outcomes include that the client:

- Has adequate blood flow through the small vessels to maintain tissue perfusion
- Takes personal actions to control pain
- Is free of infection
- Is free of physiologic consequences of impaired mobility
- Moves purposefully independently in his or her own environment with or without an assistive device
- Meets metabolic needs

Specific indicators for these outcomes are listed for each nursing diagnosis under the Planning and Implementation (see earlier).

RESOURCE MANAGEMENT

MUSCULOSKELETAL TRAUMA

Cost of Care

- The cost of fractures attributable to osteoporosis could escalate to about $62 billion by the year 2020.
- The cost of hip fracture includes not only the cost of the fracture during hospitalization but also the cost of associated morbidities and post-hospital care. Annual costs in the year following hip fracture have been estimated at $37,250 per person.
- The cost for musculoskeletal injury is estimated at over $224 billion each year. Most of this sum is related to the indirect cost of productivity: loss from death or disability. The direct cost of medical services accounts for about 30%.

Implications for Nursing

Injuries are the primary cause of musculoskeletal trauma. Injuries are not accidents; they have identifiable risk factors and patterns. Nurses can play a major role in injury prevention by educating the community about these risks. Prevention is a key factor in reducing costs related to musculoskeletal trauma.

Data from National Osteoporosis Foundation (2003). Physician's guide to prevention and treatment of osteoporosis. National Osteoporosis Foundation, Washington, DC. Available at http://www.cdc.gov.

FRACTURES OF SPECIFIC SITES

Upper Extremity Fractures

Fractures of the Clavicle

Fractures of the clavicle typically result from a fall on an outstretched hand, a fall on the shoulder, or a direct injury. Most clavicular fractures are self-healing; a splint or bandage is used for immobilization. Complicated fractures, although uncommon, may require open reduction with internal fixation (ORIF) by pins, wires, or screws.

Fractures of the Scapula

Scapular fractures are not common and are usually caused by direct impact to the area. Serious internal trauma, including pneumothorax, pulmonary contusion, and fractured ribs, can accompany these fractures.

The shoulder is immobilized with a sling and swathe or a shoulder immobilizer until the fracture heals, usually in 2 to 4 weeks. Intra-articular neck and glenoid fractures may require surgical intervention with plate and screw fixation.

Fractures of the Humerus

Fractures of the proximal humerus, particularly impacted or displaced fractures, are common in the older adult. An impacted injury is usually treated conservatively with a sling for immobilization. A displaced fracture often requires ORIF with pins or a prosthetic device.

Humeral shaft fractures are generally corrected by closed reduction and application of a hanging-arm cast or splint. If necessary, the fracture is repaired surgically (with an intramedullary rod or metal plate and screws) or with external fixation. Nonunion of the bone and radial nerve palsy are frequent complications of this fracture. Bone grafting facilitates union; prolonged splinting is necessary while the radial nerve regenerates.

A direct blow to the condyles of the distal humerus can cause either or both condyles to fracture, usually in a T- or Y-shaped configuration. The most serious complication is damage to the brachial or median nerve. Condylar fracture is usually treated by ORIF with a series of screws, although skeletal traction and casting can be used.

Fractures of the Olecranon

Fractures of the olecranon are relatively common in adults and typically result from a fall on the elbow. Many are successfully treated by closed reduction and application of a cast. The healing process usually takes more than 2 months, and several additional months may be needed before full use of the elbow is achieved. ORIF is performed for displaced fractures, and a splint is worn during the healing phase.

Fractures of the Radius and Ulna

Forearm fractures of the ulna without accompanying injury to the radius are rare. As with other fractures of long bones, closed reduction with casting may be the appropriate treatment. If the fracture is displaced, ORIF with intramedullary rods or plates and screws is required.

Fractures of the Wrist and Hand

One or more of the bones in the wrist and hand can break, but the most common fracture is of the carpal scaphoid bone in young adult men. This is also one of the most misdiagnosed fractures because it is poorly visualized on an x-

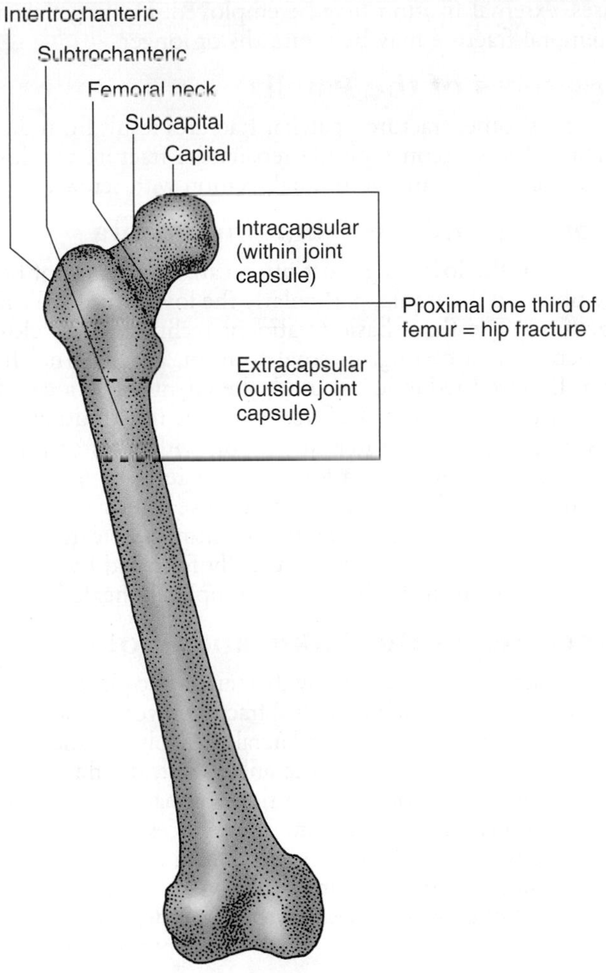

Figure 55-8 ■ Types of hip fractures.

ray film. Closed reduction and casting for 6 to 12 weeks is the treatment of choice. If the bone does not heal, open reduction and bone grafting are performed.

Fractures of the metacarpals and phalanges are usually not displaced, which makes their treatment less difficult than that of other fractures. Metacarpal fractures are immobilized for 3 to 4 weeks. Phalangeal fractures are immobilized in finger splints for 10 to 14 days.

Lower Extremity Fractures

Fractures of the Hip

Hip fractures include those involving the upper third of the femur and are classified as **intracapsular** (within the joint capsule) or **extracapsular** (outside the joint capsule). These types are further divided according to fracture location (Figure 55-8).

Falls cause most hip fractures; impaction or displacement, especially of the femoral neck, often results. If the degree of osteoporosis is so severe that it prevents surgical intervention, the client may be incapacitated for the remainder of his or her life. The cost of hip fractures is increasing as baby boomers age and increased Medicare funds are needed (see the Evidence-Based Practice for Nursing box above).

EVIDENCE-BASED PRACTICE for Nursing

Evaluating costs for older adults with musculoskeletal injury

Bishop, C.E., et al. (2002). Medicare spending for injured elders: Are there opportunities for savings? *Health Affairs, 21*(6), 215-223.

This study examined Medicare spending for injuries in 1999 on all paid claims from a randomly selected 5% sample. The study found that fractures were the most common and costly injury (67% / $5.5 billion), followed by open wounds (11% / $873 million), then internal injuries (6% / $503 million). Sprains and strains accounted for 4% of the injuries and resulted in an additional $323 million expenditure. More than 70% of these unintentional injuries are musculoskeletal.

Level of Evidence: 2—The study used a large sample and randomized the sample.

Critique. The 5% randomly selected sample and calculation of costs for the HMO portion of Medicare may or may not be accurate. Because the study reviewed paid claims, it did identify expenses that would be missed by more traditional studies, which review only hospitalization or emergency department records. The findings related to cost for fractures generally confirm other studies related to the cost of fractures and incidence of fractures in this age group.

Implications for Nursing. Results of this study and prior research can be used to develop guidelines reduce the incidence and related cost of musculoskeletal injuries in older adults. Nurses should (1) continue osteoporosis screening and education to increase bone mineral density for both women and men; (2) provide fall prevention education; (3) support special programs for older drivers to reduce injuries to pedestrians, passengers, and drivers; (4) teach about medication safety; and (5) encourage exercise programs to increase gait, strength, and coordination.

CONSIDERATIONS FOR OLDER ADULTS

Hip fractures occur most often in older persons, particularly women who have osteoporosis. Repair of hip fracture is rapidly becoming the most common surgical procedure for people older than 85 years of age. As many as one third of older clients who sustain a hip fracture die within 1 year of injury from medical complications caused by the fracture or by the immobility that occurs after the fracture. About 50% cannot return home or live independently after the fracture (Schmitt, 2000). Because of the poor prognosis of clients experiencing hip fractures, public education on osteoporosis and fracture prevention is crucial. Studies suggest that older, thin, white women are at the greatest risk for hip fracture.

The treatment of choice is surgical repair, when possible, to allow the older client to get out of bed. Buck's traction may be applied before surgery, which should be scheduled within 24 hours of injury if at all possible. Depending on the exact location of the fracture, open reduction with internal fixation (ORIF) may include an intramedullary rod, pins, a prosthesis, or a fixed sliding plate (such as a compression screw). The client with a compression screw can usually ambulate a few days after surgery and has a decreased chance of infection and nonunion in comparison with clients for whom other procedures are used. If the femoral neck or head is fractured, a prosthetic device is implanted. Depending on the age of the client and prior mobility status, the surgeon replaces the femoral head only or performs a total hip replacement. Figures 55-9 and 55-10 illustrate examples of these devices used for ORIF of the hip. Nonsurgical options are Buck's traction and skeletal traction, followed by use of a cast brace (Taggart, 1999).

CONSIDERATIONS FOR OLDER ADULTS

Older clients often have peripheral vascular disease, connective tissue disease, or diabetes. Therefore they are at high risk for problems caused by skin or skeletal traction because of inadequate circulation and sensation. Traction of any type is not the ideal treatment for the older client because it necessitates a prolonged period of immobilization; serious complications can result, such as pneumonia and pulmonary emboli. Abrasions, ulcers, and other skin problems should be reported to the health care provider. Care must be taken to avoid pressure on the bony prominences and superficial nerves. Pressure on the peroneal nerve at the point where it passes around the neck of the fibula must also be avoided, or footdrop could occur.

Hip fractures are very common. Nurses in all health care settings need to know how to care for the special needs of the older adult with a hip fracture (see the Plan of Care on pp. 1209 to 1217). Some of the postoperative care is similar to that needed by older clients undergoing total hip replacement (see Chapter 22).

Fractures of the Femur

Fractures of the lower two thirds of the femur usually result from trauma (often from a motor vehicle accident). A femoral fracture is seldom immobilized by casting because the powerful muscles of the thigh become spastic, which causes displacement of bone ends. Extensive hemorrhage is associated with femoral fracture.

Skeletal traction, followed by a cast brace or hip spica cast, is the typical nonsurgical treatment. Surgical treatment is ORIF with nails, rods, or a compression screw. In a few cases, external fixation may be employed. Healing time for a femoral fracture may be 6 months or longer.

Fractures of the Patella

Like most other fractures, patellar fractures result from direct impact. The surgeon typically repairs the fracture by closed reduction and casting or internal fixation with screws.

Fractures of the Tibia and Fibula

Trauma to the lower leg most often causes fractures of both the tibia and the fibula, particularly the lower third ("tib-fib" fractures). The three basic treatment techniques are closed reduction with casting, internal fixation, and external fixation. If closed reduction is used, the client wears a cast for at least 8 to 10 weeks. Delayed union is not unusual with this type of fracture. Internal fixation with nails or a plate and screws, followed by a long leg cast for 4 to 6 weeks, is another option. When the fractures cause extensive skin and soft-tissue damage, the initial treatment may be external fixation, often for 6 to 10 weeks, usually followed by application of a cast until the fracture is completely healed.

Fractures of the Ankle and Foot

Ankle fractures are described by their anatomic place of injury. For example, a bimalleolar (Pott's) fracture involves the medial malleolus of the tibia and the lateral malleolus of the fibula. Because of the instability of the ankle joint, the fracture can result from supination and eversion, pronation and abduction, or pronation and eversion. These forces generally create spiral, transverse, or oblique breaks, which are often difficult to treat and present problems in healing. A combination of closed and open techniques may be used, depending on the

Text continued on p. 1217.

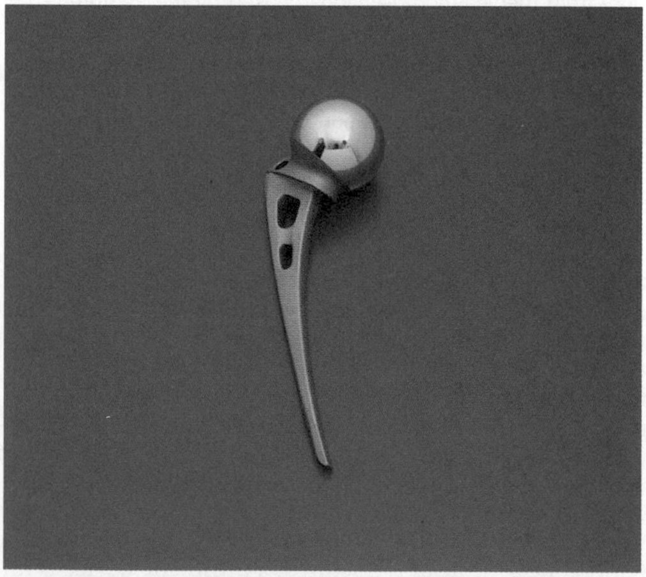

Figure 55-9 ■ The Moore prosthesis, which is used for hip fractures. (Courtesy of Smith & Nephew, Inc., Orthopaedics Divisions, Memphis, TN.)

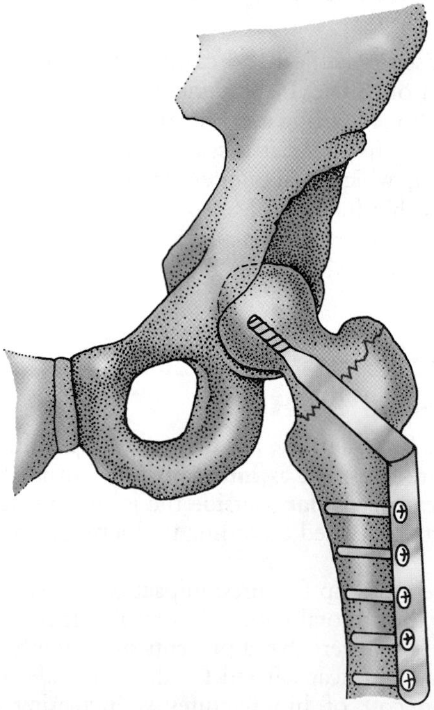

Figure 55-10 ■ A compression hip screw used for open reduction with internal fixation (ORIF) of the hip.

PLAN of CARE MEDICAL DIAGNOSIS: FRACTURES

NURSING DIAGNOSIS NO. 1 ■ Risk for Peripheral Neurovascular Dysfunction

	Expected Outcomes	Nursing Interventions	Rationales
RELATED FACTORS Trauma or injury Vascular obstruction Orthopedic surgery Fracture Mechanical compression (e.g., tourniquet, cane, cast, brace, dressing, restraint)	No verbal report or observation of altered interpretation or response to stimuli No verbal report or observation of guarding or protective gestures Has skin with warm undertones Has a pulse that remains strong and equal at all pulse points No verbal report or observation of delayed healing Denies paresthesias or numbness	NIC **Peripheral Sensation Management** Monitor for paresthesia: numbness, tingling, hyperesthesia, and hypoesthesia.	Changes in sensation are clinical indicators of changes in circulation or nerve functioning.
		Monitor for thrombophlebitis and deep vein thrombosis.	Pooling of blood from impaired circulation or impaired mobility may facilitate the formation of thrombophlebitis and deep vein thrombosis.
		Instruct the client or family to examine the skin daily for alterations in skin integrity.	Frequent skin inspection may prevent breaks in skin integrity.
		Other Interventions Assist the client to develop a plan to manage the stress in his or her life.	Emotional stress may cause vasoconstriction.
		Administer hemorheologic and antiplatelet agents as prescribed.	Hemorheologic agents increase the flexibility of red blood cells, and antiplatelet agents inhibit the platelet aggregation that could impede blood flow in the extremities.
		Prepare the client for surgical intervention as ordered by the physician.	Procedures such as percutaneous transluminal angioplasty, laser-assisted angioplasty, atherectomy, or arterial revascularization may be needed to restore peripheral tissue perfusion.
		D Instruct the client to avoid crossing his or her legs.	Crossing the legs will interfere with blood flow.
		D Instruct the client to completely abstain from tobacco products.	Nicotine causes vasoconstriction.
		D Instruct the client to abstain from caffeine.	Caffeine causes vasoconstriction.
		Continuing Care Considerations Teach the client and family how to assess tissue perfusion to the affected extremity.	Pain, pallor, paresthesias, pulselessness, paralysis, and poikilothermia are indicators of poor tissue perfusion.
		Instruct the client about the therapeutic regimen.	The client needs to follow foot care instructions, cease smoking, and avoid exposure of the affected extremity to heat/cold to prevent further injury to the extremity.
		D Remove safety hazards in the home.	Fall prevention and prevention of injury to the lower extremities is essential if the client has circulatory or nervous system impairments.

D Indicates tasks that can be delegated to unlicensed assistive nursing personnel at the discretion of the nurse.

Continued

PLAN of CARE MEDICAL DIAGNOSIS: FRACTURES—*cont'd*

NURSING DIAGNOSIS NO. 2 ■ Acute Pain

	Expected Outcomes	Nursing Interventions	Rationales
RELATED FACTORS Injury agents: Biologic, chemical, physical, psychological **DEFINING CHARACTERISTICS** Verbal or coded report of pain Observed evidence of pain Protective gestures Facial mask Self-focus	Denies experiencing pain greater than 5 on a 0 to 10 pain scale No verbal report or observation of guarding or protective gestures No verbal report or observation of self-focusing behavior No verbal report or observation of facial mask of pain	NIC **Pain Management** Perform a comprehensive pain assessment that includes location, characteristics, onset/duration, frequency, quality, intensity or severity of pain, and precipitating factors.	A plan for pain management must be based on the client's unique responses to pain.
		D Observe for nonverbal cues of discomfort, especially in those who are unable to communicate effectively.	Nonverbal cues provide support for the existence of pain.
		Consider cultural influences on the pain response.	Cultural stereotypes may lead to an inaccurate assessment of pain.
		Determine the needed frequency of making an assessment of client comfort, and implement a monitoring plan.	Initial pain management strategies may require frequent evaluation to adjust dosing to maintain adequate comfort.
		D Reduce or eliminate factors that precipitate or increase the pain experience.	Preventing a pain experience is preferred to trying to control or eliminate pain.
		Encourage the client to monitor his or her own pain and to intervene appropriately.	The client is the best person to manage his or her own pain.
		Use pain control measures before pain becomes severe.	Medicating the client in a timely manner prevents pain from reaching acutely unpleasant levels.
		Provide information about the pain, such as causes, how long it will last, and anticipated discomforts from procedures.	The client is better able to monitor his or her own discomfort and to intervene appropriately when informed.
		Teach the use of nonpharmacologic techniques before, after and, if possible, during painful activities; before pain occurs or increases; and along with other pain relief measures.	Nonpharmacologic techniques help the client to establish a sense of control over his or her pain experience.
		NIC **Analgesic Administration** D Monitor vital signs before and after administering opioid analgesics with a first-time dose or if unusual signs are noted.	Opioid analgesics may depress respirations or cause other adverse effects.
		Choose the IV rather than the IM route for frequent pain medication injections, when possible.	The IV route avoids tissue trauma and the unpredictable absorption of medication.
		Administer analgesics around-the-clock.	Administration around-the-clock prevents the peaks and troughs of analgesia, especially with severe pain.
		Set positive expectations regarding the effectiveness of analgesics.	Positive expectations will optimize the client's response to the analgesics.

D Indicates tasks that can be delegated to unlicensed assistive nursing personnel at the discretion of the nurse.

PLAN of CARE MEDICAL DIAGNOSIS: FRACTURES—*cont'd*

NURSING DIAGNOSIS NO. 2 ■ Acute Pain—*cont'd*

Expected Outcomes	Nursing Interventions	Rationales
	Institute safety precautions for a client who is receiving opioid analgesics, as appropriate.	Opioid analgesics may impair the client's judgment and/or coordination.
	After each administration of the analgesic, evaluate the effectiveness at regular and frequent intervals, especially after the initial dose; in addition, observe for any signs or symptoms of untoward effects.	Frequent evaluation of analgesic effectiveness permits the nurse to adjust the dose and timing interval to the client's need and provides an early warning of adverse responses.
	Instruct the client to request a PRN pain medication before the pain becomes severe.	Pain may be managed with lower doses of analgesics and fewer untoward effects if PRN pain medications are used before pain becomes severe.
	Inform the client that drowsiness sometimes occurs during the first 2 to 3 days of opioid administration and then subsides.	Drowsiness poses a hazard to the client, making accidents more likely to occur.
	Correct any misconceptions or myths that the client or family members may hold regarding analgesics, particularly opioids.	A client's misconceptions may prevent him or her from using opioid analgesics.
	Teach about the use of analgesics, strategies to decrease side effects, and expectations for involvement in decisions about pain relief.	Information about analgesics and the expectations for client involvement increase the client's sense of control over his or her pain.
	NIC **Environmental Management: Comfort**	
	Determine sources of discomfort, such as damp dressings, tubing position, constrictive dressings, wrinkled bed linens, and environmental irritants.	Control of environmental discomforts may decrease the need for pharmacologic intervention.
	Monitor skin, especially over bony prominences, for signs of pressure or irritation.	Skin irritation or tissue damage add a source of discomfort.
	D Prevent unnecessary interruptions and allow for rest periods.	Rest may improve the client's pain tolerance.
	D Provide a clean, comfortable bed.	Clean bed linens decrease exposure to infectious agents and increase the client's sense of well-being.
	D Facilitate hygiene measures to keep the client comfortable.	Hygiene measures may improve the client's overall sense of well-being.
	D Position the client to facilitate comfort.	The nurse may decrease sources of discomfort by using principles of body alignment, supporting with pillows, supporting joints during movement, splinting over incisions, and immobilizing painful body parts.

Continued

PLAN of CARE MEDICAL DIAGNOSIS: FRACTURES—*cont'd*

NURSING DIAGNOSIS NO. 2 ■ Acute Pain—*cont'd*

	Expected Outcomes	Nursing Interventions	Rationales
		Other Interventions	
		Refer the client to the Pain Advisory Committee.	The Pain Advisory Committee is a multidisciplinary committee with wide expertise in pain relief interventions.
		Consider the use of alternative therapies such as yoga, meditation, spirituality, and/or religion.	The experience of meditation and prayer and the reflection on meaning may help the client to relax, thereby easing the muscle tension that contributes to pain sensation.
		Consider the use of alternative therapies such as imagery, aromatherapy, music, touch, and laughter/humor.	Cognitive and behavioral strategies may be used as adjuncts to or in place of pharmacologic or surgical interventions for chronic pain. Each therapy has a different mode of action, which may or may not benefit the client.
		Consider using other cutaneous skin stimulation techniques such as massage and/or vibration to complement pain management strategies.	Massage may cause muscle relaxation, which decreases pain signals; vibration interrupts pain signal transmission to decrease pain perception.
		Continuing Care Considerations	
		Refer the client to an advanced practice nurse pain specialist, social worker, home care nurse, and/or psychologist, as appropriate.	The health care team members are able to provide continuing support for the client facing chronic pain.

NURSING DIAGNOSIS NO. 3 ■ Risk for Infection

	Expected Outcomes	Nursing Interventions	Rationales
RELATED FACTORS		NIC **Infection Protection**	
Invasive procedures Trauma or injury Inadequate secondary defenses (decreased hemoglobin, leukopenia, suppressed inflammatory response) Inadequate primary defenses (broken skin, traumatized tissue, decrease in ciliary action, stasis of body fluids, changes in pH secretions, altered peristalsis)	Denies fatigue Denies weakness Denies nausea Has no observable alterations in personality Has skin with warm undertones Has a heart rate that remains regular, strong, and between 60 and 100 beats/min Has a body temperature that remains between 97° and 99.6° F (36.1° and 37.5° C)	Monitor for systemic and localized signs and symptoms of infection.	An elevated temperature, pulse, and respirations indicate systemic infection; redness, heat, swelling, and pain indicate local infection.
		Monitor absolute granulocyte count, white blood cell (WBC) count, and differential results.	Elevations in these laboratory tests demonstrate the body's response to infection.
		Inspect the condition of any surgical incision/wound.	A surgical incision may be slightly reddened and swollen from tissue damage but remain free of the purulent drainage, excess swelling, or excess local pain that indicate infection.
		D Provide appropriate skin care to edematous areas.	Edematous skin is particularly susceptible to injury, and edematous tissue may encourage the growth of pathogenic agents.
		D Maintain asepsis for the client at risk.	Asepsis will minimize the client's exposure to pathogenic agents and thus minimize the incidence of infection.

D Indicates tasks that can be delegated to unlicensed assistive nursing personnel at the discretion of the nurse.

PLAN of CARE MEDICAL DIAGNOSIS: FRACTURES—*cont'd*

NURSING DIAGNOSIS NO. 3 ■ Risk for Infection—*cont'd*

	Expected Outcomes	Nursing Interventions	Rationales
		D Encourage coughing and deep breathing, as appropriate.	Coughing and deep breathing clears the lungs of secretions that may encourage the growth of pathogenic microbes.
		D Promote sufficient nutritional intake.	Adequate nutrition is essential for the formation of immune system cells and for the repair of damaged body tissues to provide protection against external pathogens.
		D Encourage fluid intake, as appropriate.	Adequate fluid intake provides for renal clearance of the toxins produced by pathogens.
		Report positive cultures to infection control personnel.	Early intervention to treat infection improves the client's response to therapy.
		NIC **Infection Control**	
		Administer antibiotic therapy, as appropriate.	Antibiotic therapy should assist the body to destroy pathogens.
		Continuing Care Considerations	
		Numerous visitors should be limited, and visits from individuals with known infections should be discouraged.	Visitors may provide a needed diversion for the client, but too many visitors may cause fatigue and bring unwanted exposure to pathogens.
		Teach the client and family about the signs and symptoms of infection and when to report them to the health care provider.	Early intervention to treat infection prevents untoward complications from the infection and its therapy.

NURSING DIAGNOSIS NO. 4 ■ Impaired Physical Mobility

	Expected Outcomes	Nursing Interventions	Rationales
RELATED FACTORS Medications Prescribed movement restrictions Pain Musculoskeletal impairment	Has full or improved range of motion in all joints Has smooth, coordinated movements Able to turn without assistance	NIC **Exercise Therapy: Joint Mobility** Collaborate with physical therapy in developing and executing an exercise program.	Physical therapists are the primary health care professionals responsible for developing and executing an exercise program.
DEFINING CHARACTERISTICS Limited ability to perform gross motor skills Limited range of motion Difficulty turning	Has skin that remains intact with no bruising or rashes Able to perform gross motor skills	Explain to the client and family the purpose of and plan for joint exercises.	An informed client and family is more likely to comply with a joint exercise regimen.
		Initiate pain control measures before beginning joint exercise.	Initiating pain control measures before joint exercise increases the likelihood of client comfort and his or her willingness to engage in the exercise.
		D Dress the client in nonrestrictive clothing.	Nonrestrictive clothing permits full range of joint motion.
		D Protect the client from trauma during exercise.	Stretching exercises may cause the client to be off balance.
		D Assist the client to an optimal body position for passive/active joint movement.	Neutral alignment is the optimal positioning for joint movement.

Continued

PLAN of CARE MEDICAL DIAGNOSIS: FRACTURES—*cont'd*

NURSING DIAGNOSIS NO. 4 ■ Impaired Physical Mobility—*cont'd*

Expected Outcomes	Nursing Interventions	Rationales
	D Encourage active range-of-motion exercises, according to a regular, planned schedule.	Periods of regular active range-of-motion exercise maximize the exercise benefit to the joints.
	D Perform passive range-of-motion (PROM) or assisted range-of-motion (AROM) exercises, as indicated.	The use of PROM or AROM exercises depends on the client's ability to initiate muscle and joint movement, the restrictions imposed by medical therapies, and the client's endurance.
	Assist the client to develop a schedule for active range-of-motion exercises.	Regular exercise maximizes the benefit of the exercise.
	D Encourage the client to sit in bed, on the side of the bed ("dangle"), or in a chair, as tolerated.	Sitting in bed, on the edge of the bed, or in a chair exercises the joints by the shift in position.
	D Encourage ambulation, if appropriate.	Ambulation is a form of active joint exercise and also improves cardiovascular tone.
	NIC **Positioning**	
	D Provide a firm mattress.	A firm mattress offers support.
	D Encourage the client to get involved in positioning changes, as appropriate.	Involving the client in positioning changes actively exercises the muscles and joints and permits the client a measure of control in the positioning process.
	Premedicate the client before turning, as appropriate.	Premedicating the client before turning will increase comfort and decrease resistance to repositioning from fear of pain.
	D Position in proper body alignment.	Proper body alignment preserves the functionality of the muscles and bony skeleton.
	D Immobilize or support the affected body part, as appropriate.	Immobilization or support of the affected body part permits healing and decreases further injury.
	D Provide support to edematous areas (e.g., pillow under the arms, scrotal support), as appropriate.	Support to edematous areas is necessary because edematous tissue is more susceptible to pressure injury.
	D Provide appropriate support for the neck.	The neck should be kept in neutral alignment, neither hyperflexed nor hyperextended.
	D Avoid placing the client in a position that increases pain.	Repositioning should provide the client with a measure of comfort. Pain may indicate improper body positioning.
	D Minimize friction and shearing forces when positioning and turning the client.	Friction and shearing forces will cause damage to the skin and underlying tissues.
	D Turn the client using the log roll technique.	The log roll technique keeps the spinal column in alignment during the turn, thereby preventing injury to the spinal nerves.

D Indicates tasks that can be delegated to unlicensed assistive nursing personnel at the discretion of the nurse.

PLAN of CARE MEDICAL DIAGNOSIS: FRACTURES—*cont'd*

NURSING DIAGNOSIS NO. 4 ■ Impaired Physical Mobility—*cont'd*

Expected Outcomes	Nursing Interventions	Rationales
	D Position the client to avoid placing tension on the wound, as appropriate.	Tension on a wound will cause pain and impede healing.
	Apply a foot board to the bed.	A foot board will prevent foot drop.
	D Elevate the affected limb 20 degrees or more, above the level of the heart.	Elevating the affected limb 20 degrees or more, above the level of the heart, improves venous return.
	Monitor traction devices.	Traction devices need to be monitored for proper setup.
	Maintain the position and integrity of the traction.	The traction must be intact and in the prescribed position to provide the desired therapeutic effect.
	D Elevate the head of the bed, as appropriate.	The head of the bed may be elevated to provide countertraction or comfort if permitted.
	Develop a written schedule for repositioning, as appropriate.	A written schedule for repositioning permits all health care workers to participate in repositioning.
	D Use a hand roll or trochanter roll, as appropriate.	Hand rolls and trochanter rolls support the limbs.
	D Place frequently used objects within reach.	Placing frequently used objects within reach permits the client safe and convenient access.
	D Place the bed-positioning switch within easy reach.	Placing the bed-positioning switch within easy reach permits the client to change positions safely and conveniently.
	Place the call light within reach.	Placing the call light within reach allows the client to summon assistance conveniently.
	Other Interventions	
	Instruct the client in the use of assistive devices.	The client will need instruction to properly use canes, crutches, walkers, splints, or other assistive devices.
	Continuing Care Considerations	
	Refer the client to rehabilitative services, as appropriate.	Ongoing support from physical therapists, occupational therapists, and others may be needed to help the client resume his or her activities of daily living.
	Refer the client to a vocational counselor, as appropriate.	Long-term physical impairment may require a change in employment.
	Collaborate with community organizations to inform the public about injury prevention.	Injury prevention saves the individual—and society as a whole—an enormous economic burden.

Continued

PLAN of CARE MEDICAL DIAGNOSIS: FRACTURES—*cont'd*

NURSING DIAGNOSIS NO. 5 ■ Imbalanced Nutrition: Less Than Body Requirements

	Expected Outcomes	Nursing Interventions	Rationales
RELATED FACTORS Inability to ingest or digest food or absorb nutrients due to biologic, psychological, or economic factors **DEFINING CHARACTERISTICS** Poor muscle tone Lack of interest in food Capillary fragility Information: Lack of or misinformation	Has muscle tone ≥4+ Denies changes in taste sensation Has bowel sounds that remain at 3 to 5 per quadrant per minute Has skin with warm undertones No verbal report or observation of altered eating habits No verbal report or observation of alteration in appetite Weight remains within ±5 pounds of desired weight	NIC **Nutrition Management** Determine, in collaboration with a dietitian as appropriate, the number of calories and type of nutrients needed to meet nutrition requirements.	Individual client needs for nutrients and calories should be the basis for a sound dietary plan.
		Provide appropriate information about nutritional needs and how to meet them.	Clients need accurate and timely information to make informed decisions about nutritional needs and how to meet them.
		NIC **Weight Gain Assistance** Monitor the daily calories consumed.	Calorie consumption that is inadequate for individual need causes weight loss.
		Monitor levels of serum albumin, lymphocytes, and electrolytes.	Serum albumin and lymphocyte production and electrolyte levels reflect nutritional intake.
		Provide oral care before meals, as needed.	A clean mouth improves taste sensation.
		Ensure that the client is in a sitting position before eating or feeding.	The sitting position minimizes the risk of aspiration and prevents an increasingly full stomach from pressing on the diaphragm.
		Assist clients with eating or feed them, as appropriate.	Clients who are unable to feed themselves should be fed to maintain adequate nutrition.
		Administer medications to reduce nausea and pain before eating, as appropriate.	Medicating for nausea and pain before a meal improves the client's willingness to expend the energy to eat.
		Encourage increased calorie intake.	Clients with a diminished appetite need reminders and encouragement to consume adequate nutrition.
		Provide the client with a variety of high-calorie and nutritious foods from which to select.	Monotony in food choices may lead to disinterest in the foods offered.
		Consider the client's food preferences as governed by personal choices and cultural and religious preferences.	Selecting appropriate foods according to personal, cultural, and religious preferences increases the likelihood that the client will eat the food.
		Other Interventions Teach the client and family about high-calorie, high-protein meal planning, as appropriate.	Meal planning that considers the client's and family's budget and other resources increases the likelihood that appropriate meals will be prepared.
		Teach the client and family about nutritional supplements, as appropriate.	Additional vitamins and minerals, calories, dietary fiber, or other nutritional components may need to be added to the diet of a client who is unable to eat a nutritionally adequate diet.
		Teach the client and family about preventing constipation.	Clients on low-fiber diets may need additional fluids and supplemental fiber to maintain bowel regularity.

PLAN of CARE MEDICAL DIAGNOSIS: FRACTURES—*cont'd*

NURSING DIAGNOSIS NO. 5 ■ Imbalanced Nutrition: Less Than Body Requirements—*cont'd*

Expected Outcomes	Nursing Interventions	Rationales
	Continuing Care Considerations	
	Refer the client to appropriate community nutritional programs, as needed.	Resources such as Weight Watchers, Overeaters Anonymous, and Take Off Pounds Sensibly provide support to the client who is attempting to maintain appropriate body weight.
	Refer the client to community support groups and encourage attendance, as appropriate.	Clients may need support to maintain healthy eating patterns. In addition, support groups can offer advice on how to overcome common problems.
	Encourage the client and family to use the home nutritional therapy team.	The home nutritional therapy team is able to monitor and adjust the nutritional plan of care to maximize the client's nutritional status.

severity and extent of the fracture. An arthrodesis (fusion) may be needed if the bone does not heal.

Treatment of fractures of the foot or phalanges is similar to that of other fractures, with either closed or open reduction. Phalangeal fractures are more painful than, but not as serious as, most other types of fractures.

Fractures of the Ribs and Sternum

Chest trauma may cause fractures of the ribs or sternum; the most commonly fractured ribs are numbers 4 through 8. The major concern with rib and sternal fractures is the potential for puncture of the lungs, heart, or arteries by bone fragments or ends. Fractures of the lower ribs may damage underlying organs, such as the liver, spleen, or kidneys. These fractures tend to heal spontaneously without surgical intervention. The client is often uncomfortable during the healing process and requires analgesia.

Fractures of the Pelvis

Because the pelvis is very vascular and is close to major organs and blood vessels, associated internal damage is the chief concern in fracture management. After head injuries, pelvic fractures are the second most common cause of death from trauma. In young adults, pelvic fractures typically result from motor vehicle accidents or falls from buildings; falls are the most common cause in older adults. The major concern related to pelvic injury is venous oozing or arterial bleeding. Loss of blood volume leads to hypovolemic shock.

Internal abdominal trauma is assessed by checking for the presence of blood in the urine and stool and by watching the abdomen for the development of rigidity or swelling. The trauma team may use peritoneal lavage, computed tomography (CT) scanning, or ultrasound (the newest diagnostic modality) for assessment of hemorrhage. Ultrasound is noninvasive, rapid, reliable, and cost effective, and it can be done at the bedside.

There are many classification systems for pelvic fractures. A system that is particularly useful divides fractures of the pelvis into two broad categories: non–weight-bearing fractures and weight-bearing fractures.

When a non–weight-bearing part of the pelvis is fractured, such as one of the pubic rami or the iliac crest, treatment can be as minimal as bedrest on a firm mattress or bed board. This type of fracture can be quite painful, and the client may need stool softeners to facilitate defecation because of hesitancy to move. Well-stabilized fractures usually heal in 2 months.

A weight-bearing fracture, such as multiple fractures of the pelvic ring creating instability or a fractured acetabulum, necessitate external fixation or open reduction with internal fixation (ORIF) or both. Progression to weight bearing depends on the stability of the fracture after fixation. Some clients can fully bear weight within days of surgery, whereas others managed with traction may not be able to bear weight for as long as 12 weeks.

Compression Fractures of the Spine

Most vertebral fractures are associated with osteoporosis rather than acute spinal injury. Multiple hairline fractures, called **compression fractures,** result when bone mass diminishes. The client experiences pain, deformity, and occasional neurologic compromise. As discussed in the Osteoporosis section of Chapter 54, the client's quality of life is reduced by the negative emotional impact of this problem.

Nonsurgical management with bedrest, analgesics, and physical therapy has been the traditional treatment. However, two new procedures have been successful in managing vertebral fractures in clients with osteoporosis. **Vertebroplasty** and **kyphoplasty** are both minimally invasive surgeries in which bone cement is injected directly into the fracture site to provide immediate pain relief. Kyphoplasty includes the additional step of using an inflated balloon to restore height to the vertebra. For most clients, these procedures are very successful in controlling pain (http://www.spine-health.com).

Fractures at Other Sites

Because the skull and vertebral column protect the brain and spinal cord, these acute fractures are described in Chapters 46 and 48. The nurse must be aware of the special care required for these clients because of possible neurologic damage resulting from these fractures. Fractures of the mandible or nose and other facial trauma are discussed elsewhere in the text.

AMPUTATIONS

PATHOPHYSIOLOGY

An **amputation** is the removal of a part of the body. The nurse recognizes that the psychosocial ramifications of the procedure are often more devastating than the physical impairment that results. The loss experienced is complete and permanent and causes a change in body image and often in self-esteem. As with other types of loss, the client can be expected to progress through phases of the grieving process.

Surgical Amputation

Amputations range from removal of part of a digit to removal of nearly half the entire body. The surgeon performs an amputation by one of two methods: open (guillotine) method or closed (flap) method. Surgical amputations are often referred to as "elective" surgeries.

The open method is used for clients who have, or are likely to develop, an infection. The wound remains open, and drains allow exudate to escape from the site until the infection clears. The surgeon may suture the skin flaps over the wound at a later time. In the closed technique, the surgeon pulls the skin flaps over the bone end and sutures them in place as part of the amputation procedure. One or more drains are typically inserted.

In either the closed or open method, the surgeon attempts to preserve as much of the part as possible and to keep major joints intact for maximal postoperative mobility.

Traumatic Amputation

Not all amputations are surgically planned. Some, classified as traumatic amputations, occur when a body part is severed unexpectedly (e.g., by a chain saw). Because the amputated part in these clients is usually healthy, attempts to replant it may be made.

One of the most likely replantations involves one or more digits. The current recommendation for prehospital care is that the severed digit be wrapped in a cool, dry cloth and moistened with normal saline, if possible, or bottled water. The digit should then be placed in a sealed plastic bag. The bag is placed in ice water, never directly on ice. Contact between the digit and the water is avoided to prevent tissue damage. Any semidetached parts of the digit should not be removed.

Levels of Amputation

LOWER EXTREMITY

Lower extremity amputations are performed much more frequently than upper extremity amputations. Five types of lower extremity amputations may be performed (Figure 55-11).

The loss of any or all of the small toes presents a minor disability. Loss of the great toe is significant because it affects balance, gait, and "push off" ability during walking. Midfoot amputations (e.g., the Lisfranc amputation and the Chopart amputation) and the Syme amputation are common procedures for peripheral vascular disease. In the Syme amputation, most of the foot is removed but the ankle remains. The advantage of this surgery over traditional amputations below the knee is that weight bearing can be accomplished without use of a prosthesis and without pain.

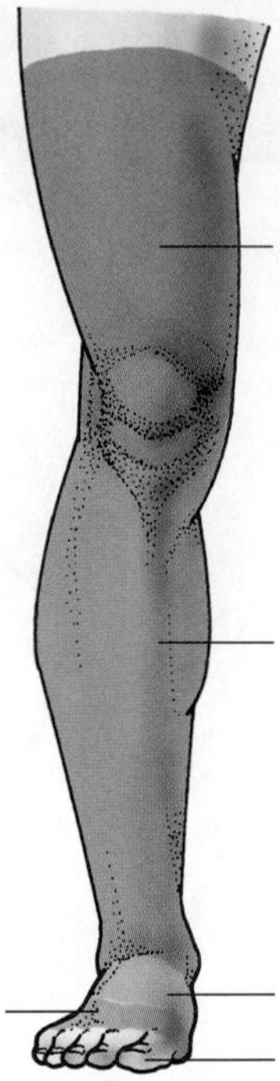

Figure 55-11 ■ Common levels of lower extremity amputation.

An intense effort is made to preserve knee joints with below-knee amputation (BKA) rather than above-knee amputation (AKA). When the cause for the amputation extends beyond the knee, however, above-knee or higher amputations are performed. Hip disarticulation, or removal of the hip joint, and hemipelvectomy procedures are more common in younger clients than in older clients, who cannot easily handle the cumbersome prostheses required for ambulation. The higher the level of amputation, the more energy is required for ambulation. These higher-level procedures are typically done for cancer of the bone, osteomyelitis, or trauma.

UPPER EXTREMITY

Fewer than 10% of all amputations are upper extremity amputations. An amputation of any part of the upper extremity is generally more incapacitating than one of the leg. The arms and hands are necessary for activities of daily living (ADLs), such as feeding, bathing, dressing, and driving a car. As much length as possible is saved to maintain function. Early replacement with a prosthetic device is vital for the client with this type of amputation.

Complications of Amputations

The following are common complications of elective or traumatic amputations:

- Hemorrhage
- Infection
- Phantom limb pain

- Problems associated with immobility
- Neuroma
- Flexion contractures

HEMORRHAGE

When a person loses part or all of an extremity either by surgery or by trauma, major blood vessels are severed, which causes bleeding. If the bleeding is uncontrolled, the client is at risk for hypovolemic shock and possibly death.

INFECTION

As with any surgical procedure or trauma, infection can occur in the wound or the bone (osteomyelitis). The older adult who is debilitated and confused is at the greatest risk because excreta may soil the wound, or the client may remove the dressing and pick at the incision.

PHANTOM LIMB PAIN

Phantom limb pain (PLP) is a frequent complication of amputation. Most clients experience phantom limb sensation in the early postoperative period, most often after an AKA. Sensation is perceived in the phantom foot or hand and diminishes over time. When phantom limb sensation persists and is unpleasant or painful, it is referred to as PLP. PLP is more common in clients who have experienced chronic limb pain before surgery and rare in those who experience traumatic amputations.

No one theory explains or predicts PLP. Three theories continue to be researched:

- Peripheral nervous system theory
- Central nervous system theory
- Psychological theory

The peripheral nervous system theory implies that sensations remain as a result of severing peripheral nerves during the amputation. The central nervous system theory states that PLP results from a loss of inhibitory signals that are usually generated through afferent impulses from the amputated limb. When many sensory fibers are destroyed by amputation, the loss of inhibitory influences allows repetitive neural activity, which results in pain. Neither of these physiologic theories completely explains PLP. Most likely, a psychological component helps to predict and explain this phenomenon. Stress, anxiety, and depression often worsen or trigger an episode of PLP but are not likely to be the causative factors.

When experiencing PLP, the client complains of pain in the removed body part, most often shortly after surgery. The pain is often described either as an intense burning or crushing sensation or as cramping. Some clients say they feel as if the removed part is in a distorted, uncomfortable position; they experience numbness and tingling (sometimes called phantom limb sensation) as well as pain.

Some clients report that the most distal area of the removed part feels as if it is retracted into the residual limb end. For most clients, the pain is triggered by touching the residual limb, by temperature or barometric pressure changes, by concurrent illness, by fatigue, or by emotional stress. Routine activities, such as urination, can trigger the pain in other clients. If pain is long-standing, especially if it existed before the amputation, any stimulus can cause it, including touching any part of the body.

Pain does interfere with the amputee's activities of daily living. Some clients report that residual limb pain (RLP) accounted for more pain-related impairment than PLP or back pain (Marshall et al., 2002).

PROBLEMS ASSOCIATED WITH IMMOBILITY

Because the client experiences reduced mobility as a result of surgery, the complications of immobility can readily occur. These problems are discussed earlier under Complications of Fractures, p. 1191.

NEUROMA

Neuroma–a sensitive tumor consisting of nerve cells found at severed nerve endings–forms most often in amputations of the upper extremity but can occur anywhere.

FLEXION CONTRACTURES

Flexion contractures of the hip or knee are seen in clients with amputations of the lower extremity. This complication must be avoided so that the client can ambulate with a prosthesis.

Etiology

Most knowledge about amputations was obtained during World War II, when trauma often necessitated a loss of one or more body parts. Today, with highly sophisticated microsurgery for revascularization of tissues, amputations related to trauma are less likely to be needed. Limb salvage procedures, such as those described in Chapter 54 (under Surgical Management in the section on malignant bone tumors), have reduced the need for amputation.

Traumatic amputations most often result from accidents. A person may be cleaning lawn mower blades or a snow blower without disconnecting the machine. A motor vehicle or industrial machine accident may also cause an amputation. Individuals with a family history of peripheral vascular disease and diabetes have a higher risk for amputation.

Incidence/Prevalence

Surgical amputations are not as common as they were in the past because the success rates of revascularization and limb salvage techniques have improved over the last 30 years. However, more than 100,000 amputations are performed yearly in the United States, about half of these in clients with coexisting diabetes.

CONSIDERATIONS FOR OLDER ADULTS

The primary indication for surgical amputation is *ischemia* from peripheral vascular disease in the older client. The rate of lower extremity amputation, for example, is much greater among clients with diabetes than among other clients because of peripheral neuropathy and peripheral vascular disease (Collins et al., 2002). In addition, these older diabetic clients have visual, cardiac, and kidney problems. A client with an amputation of one leg because of poor circulation will often have an amputation of the other leg within 5 years. Older adults of advanced age may not be candidates for prostheses because of the energy required for ambulation. The more proximal (higher) the amputation in the lower extremity, the more energy required for ambulation.

CULTURAL CONSIDERATIONS

The incidence of lower extremity amputations is greater in the black and Hispanic populations because the incidence of

Continued

major diseases leading to amputation, such as diabetes and arteriosclerosis, is greater in this population. Limited access to health care for these minority groups may also play a major role in limb loss (Collins et al., 2002).

HEALTH PROMOTION/ILLNESS PREVENTION

The typical client undergoing the procedure is a middle-aged or older man with diabetes and a lengthy history of smoking. The client most likely has failed to care for his feet properly, which has resulted in a nonhealing, infected foot ulcer and possibly gangrene. Therefore compliance with the disease management plan may help prevent the need for later amputation.

The second largest group with amputations consists of young men who experience motorcycle or other vehicular accidents or who are injured at work by industrial equipment. These men may either experience a traumatic amputation or undergo a surgical amputation because of a severe crushing injury and massive soft-tissue damage. Teach young male adults the importance of taking safety precautions to prevent injury at work and to avoid speeding or driving while drinking alcohol.

◆COLLABORATIVE MANAGEMENT

◆Assessment

PHYSICAL ASSESSMENT/CLINICAL MANIFESTATIONS

When the client has peripheral vascular disease, the nurse's primary concern preoperatively is to assess circulation in other parts of the body. Assess skin color, temperature, sensation, and pulses in both affected and unaffected extremities. Capillary refill is evaluated by applying pressure to the nail bed and waiting for the brisk return of normal color. In the older adult, however, this test may be difficult to do because the nails may be thick and opaque. In this situation, the skin near the nail bed can be assessed (see Chart 55-3). Capillary refill may not be as reliable as other indicators.

PSYCHOSOCIAL ASSESSMENT

People react differently to the loss of a body part. Be aware that an amputation of a portion of one finger can be traumatic to the client; therefore the loss must not be underestimated. The client undergoing an amputation faces a complete, permanent loss. Evaluate the client's psychological preparation for a planned amputation, and expect him or her to experience the grieving process. Adjustment to a traumatic, unexpected amputation is often more difficult than accepting a planned one. The young client may be bitter, hostile, and uncooperative. In addition to loss of a body part, the client may lose a job, the ability to participate in favorite recreational activities, or a social relationship if the other person cannot accept the body change.

The client is faced with an altered self-concept. The physical alteration that results from an amputation affects body image and self-esteem. For example, a client may think that an intimate relationship with a mate is no longer possible. An older adult may feel a loss of independence. Assess the client's feelings about himself or herself to identify areas in which he or she needs emotional support.

Attempt to determine the client's willingness and motivation to withstand prolonged rehabilitation after the amputation. Asking questions about how the client has dealt with previous life crises can provide clues. The client's willingness to change careers or other activities is also determined. Adjustment to the amputation and rehabilitation is less difficult if the client is willing to make necessary changes.

In addition to assessing the client's psychosocial status, assess the family's or significant others' reaction to the surgery. The family's response usually correlates directly with the client's progress during recovery and rehabilitation. The family can be expected to grieve for the loss and must be allowed to adjust to the change in the client.

Also assess the client's coping abilities, and help him or her to identify personal strengths and weaknesses. Ascertain that the client's religious or spiritual beliefs have been determined because certain groups require that the amputated body part be stored for later burial with the rest of the body or be buried immediately.

DIAGNOSTIC ASSESSMENT

Routine preoperative x-rays, such as a chest x-ray, are done as appropriate for any client undergoing surgery. The surgeon determines which tests are performed to assess for viability of the limb. A large number of noninvasive techniques are available to assist the physician in this evaluation. For complete accuracy, the health care provider does not rely on any single test.

One procedure is measurement of segmental limb blood pressures, which can also be used by the nurse at the bedside. In this test, an ankle-brachial index (ABI) is calculated by dividing ankle systolic pressure by brachial systolic pressure. A normal ABI is greater than or equal to 1.

Blood flow in an extremity can also be assessed by many other noninvasive tests, including Doppler ultrasonography, laser Doppler flowmetry, and transcutaneous oxygen pressure ($TcPO_2$). The ultrasonography measures the velocity of blood flow in the limb. The $TcPO_2$ measures oxygen pressure to indicate blood flow in the limb. Angiography is the most commonly used invasive method; however, it is not helpful in predicting healing of amputations. Transcutaneous oxygen pressure has proved reliable for predicting healing.

◆Interventions

Clients undergoing amputation today are not confined to a wheelchair. Advancements in the design of prosthetics have enabled clients to become independent in ambulation. Therefore complications from extended bedrest are not common, even for older adults.

Assessment of Tissue Perfusion. *The nurse's primary focus is to monitor for signs indicating that there is sufficient tissue perfusion but no hemorrhage.* The skin flap at the end of the residual limb should be pink in a light-skinned person and not discolored (lighter or darker than other skin pigmentation) in a dark-skinned client. The area should be warm but not hot. Assess the closest proximal pulse for strength and compare it with that in the other extremity. If the client has bilateral vascular disease, however, comparison of limbs is not an accurate way of measuring blood flow.

Management of Pain. Phantom limb pain (PLP) must be distinguished from stump pain because they are managed differently. Pain management related to stump pain is not unlike that for any client in pain (see Chapter 7). If the client complains of PLP, recognize that the pain is real. It is not therapeutic to remind the client that the limb cannot be hurting because it is missing. To prevent increased pain, handle the residual limb carefully when assessing the site or changing the dressing.

Drug Therapy. Some studies have shown that opioids are not as effective for PLP as they are for residual limb pain. For unknown reasons, IV infusions of calcitonin (Miacalcin, Calcimar) during the week after amputation can reduce phantom limb pain. The health care provider prescribes other medications on the basis of the type of PLP the client experiences. For instance, beta-blocking agents such as propranolol (Inderal, Apo-Propranolol✱, Detensol✱) are used for constant, dull burning. Anticonvulsants, such as carbamazepine (Tegretol) and gabapentin (Neurontin), may be used for knifelike pain; antispasmodics such as baclofen may be prescribed for muscle spasms or cramping.

Complementary and Alternative Therapies. More than 50 treatments for PLP have been used worldwide. Transcutaneous electrical nerve stimulation (TENS) has had the most consistent pain relief rates. Other treatment measures include the following:

- Ultrasound therapy
- Massage
- Exercises
- Biofeedback
- Distraction therapy
- Hypnosis
- Psychotherapy

These modalities are described in Chapters 4 and 7.

Prevention of Infection. The surgeon typically prescribes broad-spectrum prophylactic antibiotics for several days postoperatively. The initial pressure dressing and drains are usually removed by the surgeon 48 to 72 hours after surgery. The nurse does the following:

- Inspects the wound site for signs of inflammation (e.g., redness and swelling)
- Monitors the healing process
- Records the characteristics of drainage, if present
- Changes the soft dressing every day until the sutures are removed

The below-the-knee limb may be casted in the operating room for protection, prevention of edema, and prevention of knee contractures. On the third postoperative day, a window is opened in the distal end of the cast to inspect the suture line.

Promotion of Ambulation. The nurse or health care provider consults with a physical therapist to initiate exercises as soon as possible after surgery. If the amputation is a planned one, the therapist often works with the client before surgery to start muscle-strengthening exercises and to evaluate the need for aids, such as crutches. If the client can be instructed preoperatively in the use of these devices, learning how to ambulate after surgery is facilitated.

Exercise. For clients with above-knee amputations (AKAs) or below-knee amputations (BKAs), teach range-of-motion (ROM) exercises for prevention of flexion contractures, particularly of the hip and knee. A trapeze and an overhead frame, as shown in Figure 55-12, aid in strengthening the upper extremities and allow the client to move independently in bed.

A firm mattress is essential for preventing contractures with a lower extremity amputation. Assist the client into a prone position every 3 to 4 hours for 20- to 30-minute periods. This position may be uncomfortable initially, but it is necessary to prevent hip flexion contractures. Instruct the prone client to pull the residual limb close to the other leg and contract the gluteal muscles of the buttocks. For BKAs, also teach the client to push the residual limb down toward the bed while supporting it on a pillow. After the sutures are removed, the physical therapist may begin resistive exercises with a "sling-and-spring" apparatus, which can also be used at home.

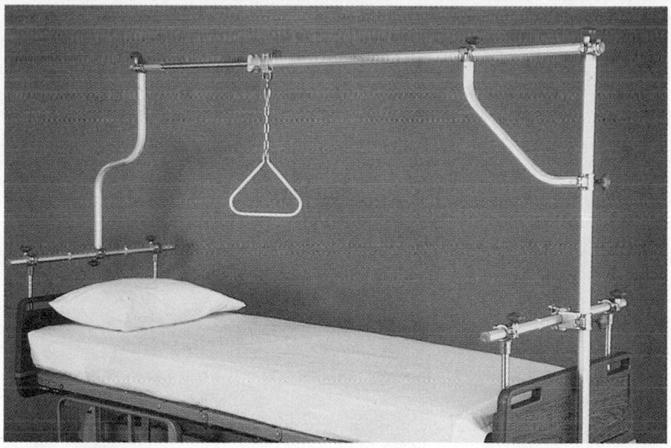

Figure 55-12 ■ The placement of an overhead frame and trapeze on a bed.

Elevation of a lower-leg residual limb on a pillow while the client is in a supine position is controversial. Some practitioners advocate avoiding this procedure at all times because it promotes hip or knee flexion contracture. Others allow elevation for the first 24 hours to reduce swelling and subsequent discomfort. Inspect the residual limb daily to ensure that it lies completely flat on the bed.

Prostheses. Following an amputation, arrange for the client to see a certified prosthetist-orthotist (CPO) so that planning can begin for the client's postoperative needs. Arrangements for replacing an upper extremity are especially important so that the client can provide self-care. Some clients are fitted with a temporary prosthesis at the time of surgery. Other clients, particularly older clients with vascular disease, are fitted after the residual limb has healed.

The client being fitted with a lower extremity prosthesis should bring a sturdy pair of shoes to the fitting. The prosthesis will be adjusted to that heel height.

Several devices help to shape and shrink the residual limb in preparation for the prosthesis. Rigid, removable dressings are preferred because they decrease edema, protect and shape the limb, and allow easy access to the wound for inspection. The Jobst air splint, a plastic inflatable device, is sometimes used for this purpose. This device is usually inflated to 20 mm Hg for 22 of every 24 hours. One of its disadvantages is air leakage.

Wrapping with elastic bandages can be effective in reducing edema, shrinking the limb, and holding the wound dressing in place. Most surgeons prefer elastic bandages over a shrinker sock, although it is easier for the client to apply a sock than to wrap elastic bandages.

For wrapping to be effective, reapply the bandages every 4 to 6 hours or more often if they become loose. Figure-eight wrapping prevents restriction of blood flow. Decrease

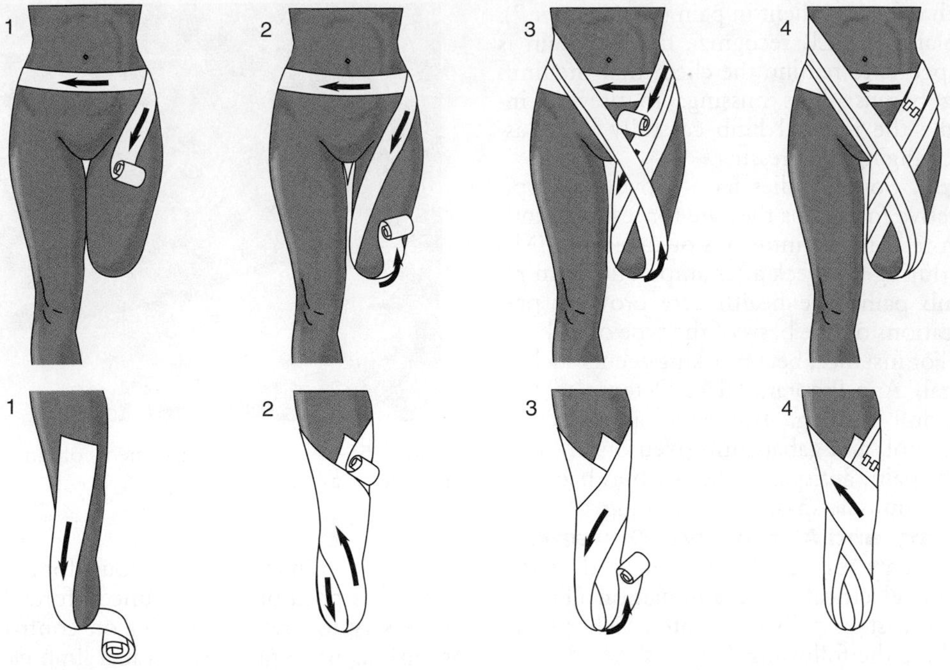

Figure 55-13 ■ A common method of wrapping an amputation stump. *Top,* Wrapping for above-knee amputation. *Bottom,* Wrapping for below-knee amputation.

the tightness of the bandages while wrapping in a distal-to-proximal direction. After wrapping, anchor the bandages to the most proximal joint, such as above the knee for BKAs (Figure 55-13).

The design of and materials for prostheses have improved dramatically over the years. Computer-assisted design and manufacturing (CAD-CAM) is now available for a custom fit. One of the most important developments in lower extremity prosthetics is the ankle-foot prosthesis. The Flex-Foot is used by more active amputees.

Promotion of Body Image. The client often experiences feelings of inadequacy as a result of losing a body part, especially the older adult who was in poor health before surgery. If possible, arrange for the client to meet with a rehabilitated amputee. If the client is older, an older amputee is the ideal person with whom the client should interact.

Use of the word *stump* for referring to the remaining portion of the limb (residual limb) is controversial. Clients have reported feeling as if they were part of a tree when the term was used. However, some rehabilitation specialists who routinely work with amputees believe the term is appropriate because it forces the client to realize what has happened and enhances adjustment to the amputation.

Assess the client's verbal and nonverbal references to the affected area. Some clients behave euphorically and seem to have accepted the loss. Do not jump to the conclusion that acceptance has occurred. Ask the client to describe his or her feelings about changes in body image and self-esteem. The client may verbalize acceptance but refuse to look at the area during a dressing change. This inconsistent behavior is not unusual and should be noted.

Promotion of Lifestyle Adaptations. The client may believe that it will be impossible to return to a previous lifestyle, including intimate relationships, his or her job, and recreational activities. With advancements in prostheses, many clients can return to their jobs and other activities. Professional athletes who use prostheses are quite successful in sports. Clients with amputations ski, hike, bowl, and participate in other physically demanding activities. More than 20,000 amputees in the United States currently participate actively in sports; about a fourth of these individuals are engaged in organized competition.

If a job or career change is necessary, consult with a social worker for evaluation of the client's other skills that could be used in another capacity. A supportive family or significant other is important for the client's adjustment to this change. The client may also think that an intimate relationship is no longer possible because of physical changes. Work with the sexual partner to help in the client's adjustment to the amputation. Professional assistance from a sex counselor or psychologist may be needed.

Help the client to set realistic goals and to take one day at a time. Help him or her to recognize personal strengths, which are emphasized and taken into account in setting goals. If the goals are not realistic, frustration and disappointment may dampen the client's motivation during rehabilitation. Basic principles of rehabilitation are discussed in Chapter 10.

Community-Based Care

The client is discharged directly to home or to a rehabilitation facility, depending on the extent of the amputation. In the few cases in which rehabilitation is not feasible (e.g., for a debilitated, confused older client), he or she may be discharged to a long-term care facility. The case manager or discharge planner coordinates this transfer.

HOME CARE MANAGEMENT

The client with a lower extremity amputation needs to have enough room at home to maneuver a wheelchair if the leg prosthesis is not yet available. He or she must be able to use

CHART 55-7

HOME CARE ASSESSMENT of
The Client with a Lower Extremity Amputation in the Home

Assess the residual limb for the following:
- Adequate circulation
- Infection
- Healing
- Flexion contracture
- Dressing/elastic wrap

Assess the client's ability to perform activities of daily living (ADLs) in the home.
Evaluate the client's ability to use ambulatory aids and care for the prosthetic device (if available).
Assess the client's nutritional status.
Assess the client's ability to cope with body image change.

toileting facilities and have access to areas necessary for self-care, such as the kitchen. Structural changes may be required before the client goes home.

HEALTH TEACHING

After the sutures are removed (several weeks after surgery), the client begins residual limb care. The home care nurse teaches the client how to care for the residual limb and how to care for the prosthesis if it is available. The limb should be rewrapped three times a day with an elastic bandage applied in a figure-eight manner (see Figure 55-13) by the client or family member. After the residual limb is healed, it is cleaned each day with the rest of the body during bathing with soap and water, and it is inspected for signs of inflammation or skin breakdown.

Prostheses require special care for ensuring their reliability and proper function, and the prosthetist plays an important role in the rehabilitation team effort. Prostheses are custom made, taking into account the client's level of amputation, lifestyle, and occupation. Proper teaching regarding correct cleansing of the socket and inserts, wearing the correct liners, assessing shoe wear, and a schedule of follow-up care is essential before discharge.

A client who seems to adjust to the amputation during hospitalization may realize that it is difficult to cope with the loss after discharge from the hospital. The nurse in the hospital setting should tell the client that this can happen. During the hospital stay, help the client to identify strong support systems on which he or she can rely after discharge. The home care or rehabilitation nurse reinforces this supporting information.

HEALTH CARE RESOURCES

For the older adult or for the client with an extensive amputation, such as a hemipelvectomy, the case manager or discharge planner arranges for follow-up care in the home by a home care nurse (Chart 55-7). Physical therapy may continue in the home or on an ambulatory care basis.

The client with an upper extremity amputation may need occupational therapy to relearn activities of daily living (ADLs). The nurse or case manager also makes arrangements for vocational or family counseling as needed. Some clients are discharged to a rehabilitation facility for 2 to 3 weeks for these services. Chapter 10 describes the rehabilitation phase of health care in detail. Teach the client to explore support groups for amputees that may be available in the client's community.

Critical Thinking Challenge

Four days ago, an adolescent client had closed reduction and external fixation for a severely comminuted left tibia and fibula. Today he becomes febrile, has an elevated white blood cell count, and a decreased hematocrit level. He returns to the operating suite for debridement and exploration, where his surgeon finds extensive tissue loss and damage. After this surgery, he recommends a BKA for the client.

1. What teaching will the client and family require in preparation for surgery?
2. What psychosocial assessment and interventions will this client need?
3. What can you tell him about changes in his lifestyle after the BKA?

evolve For suggested answer guidelines, go to http://evolve.elsevier.com/Iggy/.

CRUSH SYNDROME

When multiple compartments in the leg or arm are injured, crush syndrome (CS) can occur. CS is a potentially life-threatening, systemic complication after a severe crush injury. Its pathophysiologic mechanism is similar to that of acute compartment syndrome (see p. 1191).

Specific causes of CS include the following:
- Wringer-type injuries
- Natural disasters, such as earthquakes
- Work-related injuries, such as being trapped under heavy equipment or material
- Drug or alcohol overdose, when one or more limbs may be compressed by body weight for a prolonged time

Regardless of the cause, CS is characterized by the following:
- Acute compartment syndrome
- Hypovolemia
- Hyperkalemia
- **Rhabdomyolysis** (myoglobulin release from skeletal muscle into the bloodstream)
- Acute tubular necrosis (ATN) resulting from hypovolemia and rhabdomyolysis

Nursing assessments include signs and symptoms of hypovolemia, hyperkalemia, and compartment syndrome. Treatments focus on preventing acute tubular necrosis secondary to myoglobin release and cardiac dysrhythmias related to hyperkalemia. Adequate IV fluids, diuretics, and low-dose dopamine to enhance renal perfusion may be prescribed. An output of 100 to 200 mL/hr is the goal. Sodium bicarbonate is given to treat acidosis. Kayexalate may reduce serum potassium adequately, but hemodialysis may be required if potassium levels remain high or renal failure occurs.

COMPLEX REGIONAL PAIN SYNDROME

PATHOPHYSIOLOGY

Complex regional pain syndrome (CRPS), formerly called **reflex sympathetic dystrophy (RSD),** is a poorly understood complex disorder that includes debilitating pain, atrophy, autonomic dysfunction (excessive sweating, vascular changes), and motor impairment (most notably muscle paresis). It is probably caused by an abnormally hyperactive sympathetic nervous system. CRPS most often results from traumatic injury and commonly occurs in the feet and hands. In some cases, specific nerve injuries are present, but in others no definable injury can be identified.

The syndrome tends to progress through three classic stages. In stage 1, which lasts 1 to 3 months, the client complains of locally severe, burning pain; edema; vasospasm; and muscle spasm. Over the next 3 months, clients in stage 2 have more severe, diffuse pain and edema, muscle atrophy, and spotty osteoporosis, as shown on x-ray examination. In stage 3, the final stage, the client presents with marked muscle atrophy, intractable (unrelenting) pain, severely limited mobility of the affected area, contractures, and marked, diffuse osteoporosis. Timing of diagnosis is important because the syndrome is more difficult to treat when diagnosed in the later stages.

COLLABORATIVE MANAGEMENT

The first priority of management is pain relief. Nurses play an important role in pain management, which includes drug therapy and an array of nonpharmacologic modalities. Chapter 7 discusses pain management in detail.

In collaboration with the physical and occupational therapist, the nurse also assists in maintaining adequate range of motion (ROM). The skin of a client with CRPS tends to alternate between warm, swollen, and red to cool, clammy, and bluish. Skin care needs to be gentle, with minimal stimulation.

A new procedure to control hyperhidrosis (excessive sweating), the **endoscopic thoracic sympathectomy (ETS)**, has also been successful for some clients with CRPS. Only one extremely small incision is made in the axilla, through which an endoscope is inserted. The surgeon identifies and cuts the sympathetic nerve branches involved. Topical skin adhesive is used to close the microincision. The client is discharged to home a few hours later with a follow-up examination the next day. Usual activities can resume a few days later.

Assist the client in coping with CRPS, realizing that psychotherapy may be indicated. The Reflex Sympathetic Dystrophy Syndrome Association (RSDSA) is available to help clients organize or locate support groups and other resources for clients with this syndrome.

SPORTS-RELATED INJURIES

In addition to the bone and muscle problems already discussed, trauma can cause cartilage, ligament, and tendon injury. Many musculoskeletal injuries are the result of participation in sports (professional and amateur) or other strenuous physical activities. The popularity of all-terrain vehicles (ATVs) and skateboarding has increased injuries in younger clients. Sports injuries have become so common that large metropolitan hospitals have sports medicine clinics and physicians who specialize in this field.

Although the specific types of injury are numerous, this chapter includes only the most common ones seen in a hospital or ambulatory care setting. The principles of injury to one part of the body are analogous to those of similar injuries in other parts. For example, a tendon rupture in a knee is cared for in the same manner as a tendon rupture in the wrist. Chart 55-8 lists general emergency measures for sports-related injuries.

CHART 55-8

BEST PRACTICE for Emergency Care of Sports-Related Injuries

EMERGENCY CARE

- Do not move the victim until spinal cord injury is ascertained (see Chapter 46 for assessment of spinal cord injury).
- Immobilize the injured part, and immobilize the joint above and below the injury by applying a splint.
- Apply ice intermittently for the first 24 to 48 hours (heat may be used thereafter).
- Elevate the affected limb to decrease swelling.
- Always assume the area is fractured until x-ray studies are done.
- Assess neurovascular status in the area distal to the injury.

Because the knee is most often injured, it is discussed as a typical example of other areas of the body. Trauma to the knee results in **internal derangement,** a broad term for disturbances of an injured knee joint. When surgery is required to resolve the problem, most surgeons prefer to perform the procedure through an arthroscope when possible. A general description of arthroscopy is presented in Chapter 53.

Knee Injuries: Meniscus

PATHOPHYSIOLOGY

There are two semilunar cartilaginous structures, or menisci, in the knee joint: the medial meniscus and the lateral meniscus. These pads act as shock absorbers, but they can tear. Tearing is usually a result of twisting the leg when the knee is flexed and the foot is placed firmly on the ground. The medial meniscus is much more likely to tear than the lateral meniscus because it is less mobile. Internal rotation causes a tear in the medial meniscus; external rotation causes a tear in the lateral meniscus.

Tears can be anterior or posterior, longitudinal or transverse. In the medial meniscus, a longitudinal tear, or "bucket handle" injury, often causes the knee to lock; that is, the torn cartilage jams between the femur and the tibia and prevents extension of the knee. Surgery is often required for this type of injury. In transverse tears, the knee does not lock, and surgery may not be required.

COLLABORATIVE MANAGEMENT

The client with a torn meniscus typically has pain, swelling, and tenderness in the knee. A clicking or snapping sound can often be heard when the knee is moved.

A common diagnostic technique is the **McMurray test.** The examiner flexes and rotates the knee and then presses on the medial aspect while slowly extending the leg. The test result is positive if clicking is palpated or heard. A negative finding, however, does not rule out a tear.

For a locked knee, the treatment may be manipulation followed by casting for 3 to 6 weeks. If the problem recurs, a partial or total **meniscectomy** is performed. An open meniscectomy requires a surgical incision for removal of all or part of the meniscus and is rarely performed. Most surgeons prefer to remove only the affected portion, during a closed meniscectomy, which can be accomplished through an arthroscope as a same-day surgical procedure. As described in Chapter 53, an arthroscope is a metal tubular instrument used for examination or surgery of joints. One or more small incisions (less than ¼ inch [0.6 cm] long) are made in the knee for insertion of the arthroscope. The surgeon threads a cutting device through the arthroscope for removal of the torn cartilage while the knee is irrigated. The surgeon may use a laser during the procedure, depending on the type and severity of the injury. A bulky pressure dressing is applied after the procedure, and the affected leg is wrapped in elastic bandages.

As for any postoperative client, check the surgical dressing for bleeding and monitor vital signs after the client is readmitted to the unit. Perform circulation checks, as outlined in Chart 55-3, usually every hour for the first few hours and then every 4 hours.

The client begins leg exercises immediately after surgery to strengthen the leg, prevent thrombophlebitis, and reduce swelling. Quadriceps setting, in which the client straightens the leg while pushing the knee against the bed, is done in sets of 10 or more. Straight-leg raises are also performed as soon as the client awakens from anesthesia. Range-of-motion (ROM) exercises are usually not started for several days.

To prevent the client from bending the affected knee, the physician may order a knee immobilizer, such as the one shown in Figure 55-14. Elevate the leg on one or two pillows according to the physician's preference, and apply ice to reduce postoperative swelling. Full weight bearing is restricted for several weeks, depending on the amount of cartilage removed. The client is usually discharged from the hospital with crutches in less than 23 hours.

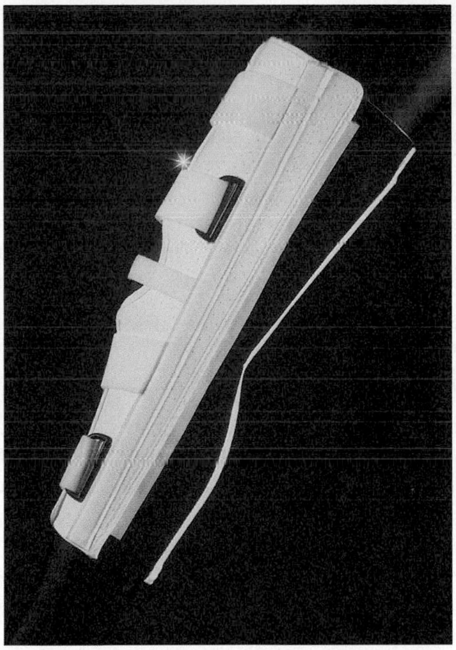

Figure 55-14 ■ A knee immobilizer. (Courtesy Zimmer, Inc., Warsaw, IN.)

Knee Injuries: Ligaments

PATHOPHYSIOLOGY

The cruciate and collateral ligaments in the knee are predisposed to injury, often from sports or vehicular accidents. The anterior cruciate ligament (ACL) is the most commonly torn ligament in the knee. Athletes often experience ACL injuries during skiing or gymnastics.

When the ACL is torn, the person feels a snap; the knee gives way because of ACL laxity. Within hours, the knee is swollen, stiff, and painful.

COLLABORATIVE MANAGEMENT

Physical examination by the health care provider shows positive ligamentous laxity. The diagnosis of ACL deficiency is confirmed by x-rays, magnetic resonance imaging (MRI), or assessment with an arthrometer (an instrument for measuring the amount of tibial displacement).

Treatment may be nonsurgical or surgical, depending on the severity of the injury and the anticipated activity of the client. Exercises, bracing, and limits on activities while the ligament heals may be sufficient. If medical management is not effective, surgery may be needed.

The surgeon repairs the tear by reattaching the torn portions of the ligament, and the leg is placed in a cast. If the ligament cannot be repaired, reconstructive surgery may be performed with the use of autologous grafts. Since the early 1980s, the Food and Drug Administration (FDA) has approved several artificial knee ligaments. The Gore-Tex ligament is a permanent implant. A ligament augmentation device is used temporarily while the autograft heals. Both of these materials can be implanted through an arthroscope.

Complete healing of knee ligaments after surgery can take 6 to 9 months or longer. Nursing management is similar to the care of any client in a cast, which is described earlier in this chapter under Cast Care, p. 1199. These clients may have postoperative orders for a continuous passive motion machine (CPM). CPM use is discussed with the postoperative care of the total knee client in Chapter 24.

Tendon Ruptures

Rupture of the Achilles tendon is common in adults who participate in strenuous sports. In the older adult, quadriceps tendon rupture may occur from a fall down several steps. For severe damage, the tendon is surgically repaired and the leg is immobilized in a cast for 6 to 8 weeks. If the tendon is beyond repair, a **tendon transplant** (also known as tendon reconstruction) is performed. A tendon is removed from one part of the body and transplanted to the affected area. The nursing care for these clients is similar to that discussed earlier for a client with a cast (see Cast Care, p. 1199).

Dislocations and Subluxations

Dislocation of a joint occurs when the articulating surfaces are no longer in proximity. If the dislocation is not complete, the joint is partially dislocated, or subluxed. Dislocation can occur in any diarthrodial (synovial) joint but is common in the shoulder, hip, knee, and fingers. This injury is most often the result of trauma but can be congenital or pathologic (resulting from joint disease, such as arthritis).

The following are the typical manifestations of dislocation:

- Pain
- Immobility
- Alteration in contour of the joint

- Deviation in length of the extremity
- Rotation of the extremity

The health care provider performs a closed manipulation, or reduction, of the joint and forces it back into its original position while the client is anesthetized or under conscious sedation. The joint is immobilized by a cast or immobilizer until healing occurs.

Recurrent dislocations are common in the knee and shoulder. For this problem, the joint is fixed with wires to prevent further displacement; a cast, splint, or traction is applied for 3 to 6 weeks.

Strains

A strain is excessive stretching of a muscle or tendon when it is weak or unstable. Strains are sometimes referred to as muscle pulls. Falls, lifting of heavy items, and exercise often cause this injury.

Strains are classified according to their severity:

- A first-degree (mild) strain causes mild inflammation but little bleeding. Swelling, ecchymosis, and tenderness are usually present.
- A second-degree (moderate) strain involves tearing of the muscle or tendon fibers without complete disruption. Muscle function may be impaired.
- A third-degree (severe) strain involves a ruptured muscle or tendon with separation of muscle from muscle, tendon from muscle, or tendon from bone. Severe pain and disability result from severe strains.

Management usually involves cold and heat applications, exercise, and activity limitations. The health care provider may prescribe anti-inflammatory drugs to decrease inflammation and pain. Muscle relaxants may also be used. In third-degree strains, surgical repair of the ruptured muscle or tendon may be necessary.

Sprains

A sprain is excessive stretching of a ligament. Twisting motions from a fall or sports activity typically precipitate the injury. Sprains are classified according to severity:

- A first-degree (mild) sprain involves tearing of a few fibers of a ligament. Function of the joint is not impaired.
- In a second-degree (moderate) sprain, more fibers are torn, but stability of the joint remains intact.
- A third-degree (severe) sprain causes marked instability of the joint.
- Pain and swelling characterize ligament injuries. The treatment for mild (first-degree) sprains is minimal:
- Rest
- Use of ice for the first 24 to 48 hours
- Application of a compression bandage for a few days to reduce swelling and provide joint support
- Elevation

Second-degree sprains require immobilization (elastic bandage and Air Stirrup ankle brace, splint, or cast) and partial weight bearing while the tear heals. For severe ligament damage (third-degree sprain), immobilization for 4 to 6 weeks is necessary. Surgery may be recommended, particularly for chronic instability, as discussed earlier under Knee Injuries: Ligaments, p. 1225.

For more specific client education, refer to the Clinical Pathway on the Evolve website.

Rotator Cuff Injuries

The musculotendinous, or rotator, cuff of the shoulder functions to stabilize the head of the humerus in the glenoid cavity during shoulder abduction. The rotator cuff typically undergoes degenerative changes as one ages. Young adults usually sustain a tear of the cuff by substantial trauma, such as may occur during a fall, while throwing a ball, or with heavy lifting. Older adults tend to have small tears related to aging, repetitive motions, or falls.

Clients with a torn rotator cuff have shoulder pain and cannot initiate or maintain abduction of the arm at the shoulder. When the arm is abducted, the client usually drops the arm because abduction cannot be maintained (drop arm test).

The health care provider usually treats the client conservatively with nonsteroidal anti-inflammatory drugs (NSAIDs), physical therapy, sling support, and ice/heat applications while the tear heals.

For clients who do not respond to conservative treatment or for those who have a complete tear, the surgeon repairs the cuff. After surgery, the affected arm is usually immobilized in a sling for several weeks. Pendulum exercises are started on the third or fourth postoperative day and progress to active exercises in about 2 weeks. If the surgery is extensive, the client's arm may be immobilized for a longer time before exercises begin.

GET READY for the NCLEX Examination!

KEY POINTS

Safe Effective Care Environment

- Identify the client at risk for acute compartment syndrome; loosen bandages or request that the client's cast be cut if neurovascular compromise.
- As a priority, assess neurovascular status frequently in clients with musculoskeletal injury, traction, or cast as described in Chart 55-3.
- Identify clients at risk for venous thromboembolism (VTE), and monitor for early signs of this potentially fatal complication.
- Implement interventions to prevent complications of immobility in clients having musculoskeletal injury or surgery.
- Observe for hemorrhage in the client having an amputation.

Health Promotion and Maintenance

- Encourage the use of seat belts in motor vehicles and helmets for skateboarding to help prevent serious injury.
- Educate individuals in the community about the importance of osteoporosis screening, medication safety, fall prevention, and programs for older drivers.
- Teach clients and their family members and significant others how to care for casts or traction at home.
- Reinforce teaching for ambulating with crutches, walkers, or canes.
- Teach exercises to clients with leg amputation to prevent hip flexion contractures.

- Provide health care resource information for clients with musculoskeletal trauma, such as RSDS Association for clients with complex regional pain syndrome.
- Teach clients to take precautions when operating machinery to avoid traumatic amputations or other severe injury.

Psychosocial Integrity

- Be aware that clients with severe musculoskeletal trauma may have a prolonged hospitalization and recovery period.
- For clients with severe trauma or amputation, assess the client's coping skills and encourage verbalization.
- Recognize that the client having an amputation may need to adjust to an altered lifestyle; however, new custom prosthetics improve mobility.
- Help the client with an amputation or other musculoskeletal trauma to set realistic goals and take one day at a time.
- Be aware that clients with complex regional pain syndrome may require psychotherapy.

Physiological Integrity

- Be aware that open fractures cause a higher risk for infection than do closed fractures.
- Assess clients with fractures for complications, such as VTE, infection, and acute compartment syndrome.
- Differentiate fat embolism syndrome from pulmonary (blood clot) embolism as outlined in Chart 55-2.
- Provide emergency care of the client experiencing a fracture as described in Chart 55-4.
- Provide appropriate cast care, depending on the type of cast (plaster or synthetic); check for pressure necrosis under the cast by feeling for heat, assessing the client's pain level, and smelling the cast for an unpleasant odor.
- Provide pin care for clients with skeletal traction or external fixator; assess for manifestations of infection at the pin sites.
- Provide postoperative care for the client having a hip repair as described in the Client Care Plan.
- Postoperatively, assess for and manage phantom limb pain in the client who has an amputation.
- Provide emergency care for clients experiencing a sports-related injury as outlined in Chart 55-8.

ADDITIONAL STUDY RESOURCES

Go to your Student CD-ROM for Review Questions for the NCLEX Examination.

evolve Go to http://evolve.elsevier.com/Iggy/ for Integrated Management of Care Questions for the NCLEX Examination.

SELECTED BIBLIOGRAPHY

Asterisk indicates a classic or definitive work on this subject.

Altizer, L. (2002). Fractures. *Orthopaedic Nursing, 21*(6), 51-58.

Altizer, L. (2003). Hand and wrist fractures. *Orthopaedic Nursing, 22*(2), 131-138.

Bartley, M.K., & Telford, G. (2004). The latest in trauma care. *Critical Care Choices 2004,* 26-29.

Bishop, C.E., et al. (2002). Medicare spending for injured elders: Are there opportunities for savings? *Health Affairs, 21*(6), 215-223.

Collins, T.C., et al. (2002). Lower extremity nontraumatic amputation among veterans with peripheral arterial disease: Is race an independent factor? *Medical Care, 40*(1), Suppl I106-I116.

Curtis, K., et al. (2002). The impact of trauma cast management on patient outcomes. *The Journal of TRAUMA Injury, Infection, and Critical Care, 53*(3), 477-482.

Fletcher, D.D., et al. (2002). Trends in rehabilitation after amputation for geriatric patients with vascular disease: Implications for future health resource allocation. *Archives of Physical Medicine and Rehabilitation, 83*(10), 1389-1393.

Geier, K. (2001). Osteoporosis in men. *Orthopaedic Nursing, 20*(6), 49-56.

Harvey, C. (2001). Compartment syndrome: When it is least expected. *Orthopaedic Nursing, 20*(3), 15-25.

Injury fact book 2001-2002. Available at http://www.cdc.gov.

Jacobs, D.J., et al. (2003). Practice management guideline for geriatric trauma: The EAST practice management guidelines work group. *The Journal of TRAUMA Injury, Infection, and Critical Care, 54*(2), 391-416.

Kyphoplasty–A new treatment for osteoporotic fractures. Available at http://www.spine-health.com.

Maher, A.B. (2001). Trauma. In D.C. Schoen (Ed.), *Core curriculum for orthopaedic nursing* (4th ed.) Pitman, NJ: National Association of Orthopaedic Nurses.

Maher, A.B., Salmond, S.W., & Pellino, T.A. (Eds.). (2002). *Orthopaedic nursing* (3rd ed.) Philadelphia: W.B. Saunders.

Marshall, H.M., et al. (2002). Pain site and impairment in individuals with amputation pain. *Archives of Physical Medicine & Rehabilitation, 83*(8), 1116-1119.

Michaels, A., et al. (2001). Traditional injury scoring underestimates the relative consequences of orthopedic injury. *The Journal of TRAUMA Injury, Infection, and Critical Care, 50*(3), 389-396.

Miller, R.L.S. (2003). Reflex sympathetic dystrophy. *Orthopaedic Nursing, 22*(2), 91-101.

Moran, S.G., et al. (2003). Relationship between age and lower extremity fractures in frontal motor vehicle collisions. *The Journal of TRAUMA Injury, Infection, and Critical Care, 54*(2), 261-265.

National Osteoporosis Foundation. (2003). *Physician's guide to prevention and treatment of osteoporosis.* Washington D.C.: National Osteoporosis Foundation.

Pudelek, B. (2002). Geriatric trauma: Special needs for a special population. *AACN Clinical Issues, 13*(1), 61-72.

*Roberts, D. (1999). Introduction to bone: Structure and function, fractures, and osteoporosis. In C.M. Ceccio, J.A. Deuschle, & D.R. Eckhouse-Ekeberg (Eds.), *An introduction to orthopaedic nursing* (2nd ed., pp. 3-16). Pitman, NJ: National Association of Orthopaedic Nurses.

Rudman, N., & McIlmail, D. (2000). Emergency department evaluation and treatment of hip and thigh injuries. *Emergency Medicine Clinics of North America, 18*(1), 29-66.

Schmitt, M. (2000) Osteoporosis: Focus on fractures. *Patient Care for the Nurse Practitioner, 3*(2), 61-71.

Swiontkowski, M.F., et al. (2002). Factors influencing the decision to amputate or reconstruct after high-energy lower extremity trauma. *The Journal of TRUAMA Injury, Infection, and Critical Care, 52*(4), 641-649.

*Taggart, H. (1999). Caring for the elderly hip fracture patient. In C.M. Ceccio, J.A. Deuschle, & D.R. Eckhouse-Ekeberg (Eds.), *An introduction to orthopaedic nursing* (2nd ed., pp. 113-122). Pitman, NJ: National Association of Orthopaedic Nurses.

UNIT **THIRTEEN**

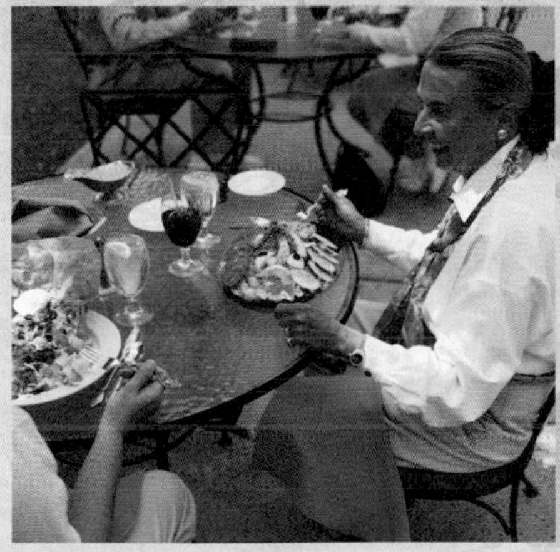

PROBLEMS of DIGESTION, NUTRITION, and ELIMINATION

Management of Clients with Problems of the Gastrointestinal System

CHAPTER

56 Assessment of the Gastrointestinal System

KARRIE K. DIETZEN

LEARNING OUTCOMES

After studying this chapter, you should be able to:

1. Recall the anatomy and physiology of the gastrointestinal (GI) system.
2. Identify GI system changes associated with aging.
3. Perform a GI history using Gordon's Functional Health Patterns.
4. Evaluate important physical assessment findings in a client with digestion, nutrition, and elimination (GI) health problems.
5. Explain the use of laboratory testing for a client with a GI health problem.
6. Describe the use of radiography in diagnosing GI health problems.
7. Explain follow-up care for clients who have invasive radiographic examinations.
8. Plan preprocedure and follow-up care for clients having endoscopic procedures.

Go to your Student CD-ROM for Review Questions for the NCLEX Examination keyed to these Learning Outcomes.

The gastrointestinal (GI) system includes the GI tract (alimentary canal), consisting of the mouth, esophagus, stomach, small and large intestines, and rectum. The salivary glands, liver, gallbladder, and pancreas secrete substances into the GI tract by connecting ducts (Figure 56-1). The adult GI tract is about 25 feet long (mouth to anus). The main function of the GI tract, with the aid of organs such as the pancreas and the liver, is the digestion of food and the elimination of waste. The GI tract is susceptible to many pathologic conditions, including structural problems, impaired motility, infection, and cancer.

ANATOMY AND PHYSIOLOGY REVIEW

Overview of the Gastrointestinal System

Structure

The GI tract consists of a hollow muscular tube surrounded by four tissue layers. The **lumen**, inner wall, of the GI tract consists of four layers: mucosa, submucosa, muscularis, and serosa. The **mucosa**, the innermost layer, includes a thin layer of smooth muscle and specialized exocrine gland cells. The mucosa is surrounded by the submucosa, which is made up of connective tissue. Submucosa layer is surrounded by the muscularis. The muscularis is composed of both circular and longitudinal smooth muscles, which work to keep contents moving through the tract. The outermost layer, serosa, is composed of connective tissue. Although the GI tract is continuous from the mouth to the anus, it is divided into specialized regions. The mouth, pharynx, esophagus, stomach, and small and large intestines each perform a specific function. In addition, the secretions of the salivary, gastric, and intestinal glands; liver; and pancreas empty into the GI tract to aid digestion.

Function

The functions of the GI tract include secretion, digestion, absorption, motility, and elimination. Food and fluids are ingested, swallowed, and propelled along the lumen of the GI tract to the anus for elimination. The smooth muscles contract to move food from the mouth to the anus. Before food can be absorbed, it must be broken down to a liquid, called **chyme.** Digestion is the mechanical and chemical process whereby complex foodstuffs are broken down into simpler forms that can be used by the body. During digestion, the stomach secretes hydrochloric acid, the liver se-

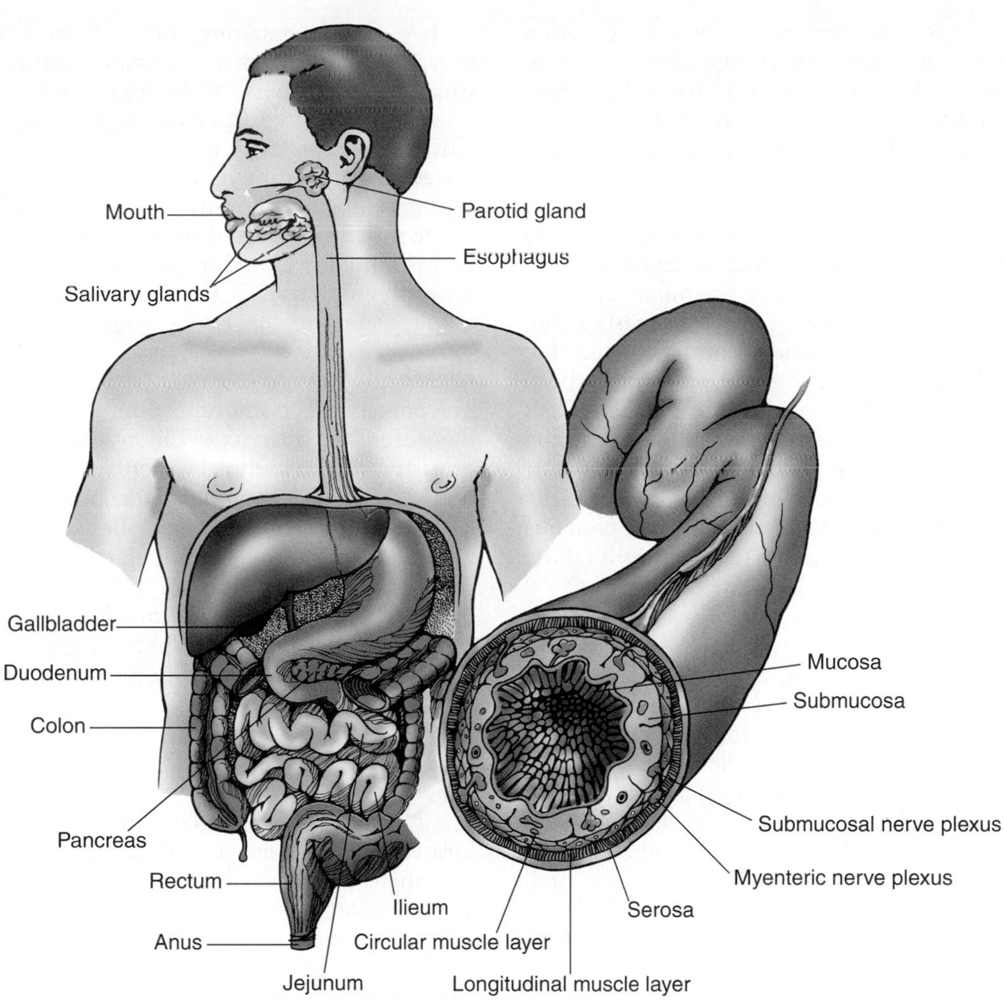

Figure 56-1 ■ The gastrointestinal system (GI tract) can be thought of as a tube (with necessary structures) extending from the mouth to the anus for a 25-foot length. The structure of this tube (shown enlarged) is basically the same throughout its length.

cretes bile, and digestive enzymes are released from accessory organs, aiding in food breakdown. After the digestive process is complete, absorption takes place. **Absorption** is carried out as the nutrients produced by digestion move from the lumen of the GI tract into the body's circulatory system for uptake by individual cells.

Nerve Supply

Innervation of the GI tract occurs in two ways. First, intrinsic contractile stimulation is provided by two internal nerve plexuses: the *myenteric* plexus (an outer plexus found in the longitudinal and circular smooth muscle) and the *submucosal* plexus (an inner nerve plexus in the submucosa). These nerve plexuses connect with each other along the entire length of the GI tract to maintain the tone of the smooth muscle and to stimulate movements.

The second type of innervation is provided by the autonomic nervous system, which connects with nerve fibers from the intrinsic nerve plexuses. Parasympathetic stimulation is provided primarily by the vagus nerve (cranial nerve X). The vagus nerve innervates the esophagus, the stomach, and to a lesser extent, the small intestine, the gallbladder, and part of the large intestine. This stimulation causes increased motor and secretory activity and relaxation of sphincters. Sympathetic stimulation via the thoracic and lumbar splanchnic nerves is provided to all parts of the GI tract. It slows movement, inhibits secretions, and contracts sphincters.

Blood Supply

The blood supply to the GI tract originates from the aorta and branches to the many arteries throughout the length of the tract. The venous system that carries absorbed nutrients away from the lumen of the GI tract consists of the gastric vein, the splenic vein, and other veins that drain into the portal vein of the liver. This blood circulates through the liver to the hepatic vein and returns to the heart via the inferior vena cava.

ORAL CAVITY

Structure

The oral cavity (mouth) includes the buccal mucosa, lips, tongue, hard palate, soft palate, teeth, and salivary glands. The buccal mucosa is the mucous membrane lining the inside of the mouth. The lips are external to the mouth and are pink-red. The tongue is involved in speech, taste, and

mastication (chewing). The mucous membrane covering the tongue consists of small projections, called papillae, which accommodates the taste buds and provides a roughened surface, permitting the movement of food in the mouth during chewing. The hard palate and the soft palate together form the roof of the mouth.

Adults have 32 permanent teeth: 16 each in upper and lower arches. The teeth are composed of a hard, calcified substance called dentin, and are covered by enamel. There are four types of teeth: incisors, canines, premolars, and molars. The teeth are important for speech and mastication. The oral cavity contains three major salivary glands: the parotid glands, the submandibular glands, and the sublingual glands. These glands produce about 1 L of saliva per day to assist in digestion by moistening food, thus enabling it to be formed into a bolus for swallowing.

The **pharynx** (throat) extends from the soft palate to the esophagus. It is lined with mucous membrane and contains three pairs of organs: the adenoids, the lingual tonsils (at the base of the tongue), and the tonsils.

Function

The different types of teeth function to prepare food for digestion by cutting, tearing, crushing, or grinding the food. Swallowing begins after food is taken into the mouth and chewed. Saliva is secreted in response to the presence of food in the mouth and begins to soften the food. Saliva contains mucin and an enzyme called salivary amylase (also known as ptyalin), which begins the breakdown of carbohydrates.

The four phases of swallowing are oral preparatory, oral, pharyngeal, and esophageal. The *oral preparatory* phase begins with the intake of food into the mouth. The mandible (jaw), teeth, and tongue work to soften the food and form a bolus. The tongue acts to move the bolus toward the back of the mouth. The *oral* phase begins with the movement of the bolus toward the back of the mouth. The tongue presses the bolus against the hard palate, toward the glossopalatine arch, elevating the larynx, which forces the food bolus to pass into the pharynx, triggering the swallowing reflex. The oral phase is under voluntary control of the individual.

The *pharyngeal* phase begins as the swallowing reflex is triggered. As the bolus is forced into the pharynx, the soft palate elevates, which seals the nasal cavity. At this time, the swallowing reflex also inhibits respiration and allows the opening of the esophagus so that the food can enter. The oral and pharyngeal phases are extremely rapid, usually taking less than 1 second. The pharyngeal phase is under both voluntary and involuntary control of the individual.

The *esophageal* phase begins when the bolus enters the esophagus at the cricopharyngeal juncture. A peristaltic wave passes the food to the stomach, which takes about 9 seconds. The esophageal phase is completely under involuntary control.

ESOPHAGUS

Structure

The esophagus is a muscular canal about 10 inches (24 cm) long; it extends from the pharynx to the stomach and passes through the hiatus in the center of the diaphragm. The wall of the esophagus consists of mucosa, submucosa, and muscularis propria. The mucosal layer is composed of squamous epithelial cells. The submucosa is composed of loose connective tissue containing blood vessels, lymphatics, and nerve fibers. The muscularis propria consists of smooth and striated muscle fibers. At the upper end of the esophagus is a sphincter referred to as the **upper esophageal sphincter (UES).** When at rest, the UES is closed to prevent air into the esophagus during respiration. The portion of the esophagus proximal to the gastroesophageal junction is referred to as the **lower esophageal sphincter (LES).** When at rest, the LES is normally closed to prevent reflux of gastric contents into the esophagus. If this is not done adequately, gastroesophageal reflux disease (GERD) can develop.

Function

The primary function of the esophagus is to propel food and fluids from the pharynx to the stomach and to prevent reflux of gastric contents into the esophagus. The propulsive function is the result of coordinated contractions of the muscular layers of the esophagus. The esophageal walls secrete mucus to lubricate the food and aid in the transport of the bolus to the stomach. As peristalsis pushes the bolus along the esophagus, the cardiac sphincter relaxes to allow the bolus to enter the stomach. The activity of the LES is regulated by smooth muscle, as well as by neural and hormonal influences.

STOMACH

Structure

The stomach is a glandular digestive and endocrine organ located in the midline and left upper quadrant (LUQ) of the abdomen. The stomach has four anatomic regions. The *cardia* is the narrow portion of the stomach that is distal to the gastroesophageal junction. The *fundus* is the area to the left above the gastroesophageal junction. The main area of the stomach is referred to as the *body* or *corpus.* The *antrum* (pylorus) is the distal portion of the stomach and is separated from the duodenum by the pyloric sphincter. Both ends of the stomach are guarded by sphincters (cardiac and pyloric), which aid in the transport of food through the gastrointestinal (GI) tract and prevent backflow (Figure 56-2).

The surface of the stomach is covered with *rugae,* or folds of mucosa and submucosa that extend longitudinally.

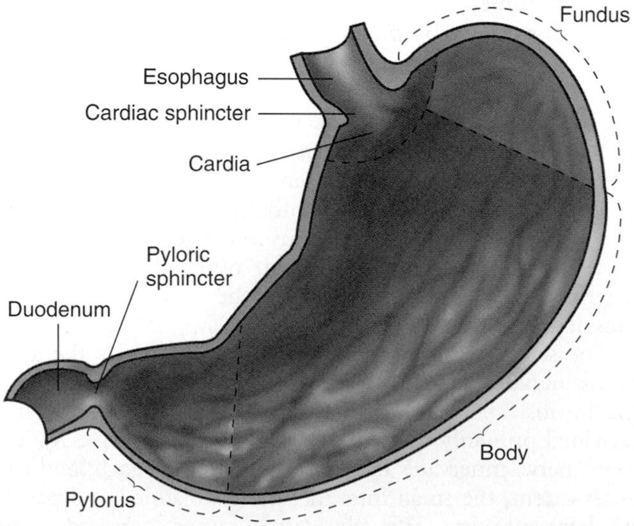

Figure 56-2 ■ The anatomy of the stomach.

Smooth muscle cells that line the stomach are responsible for gastric motility. The stomach is also richly innervated with intrinsic and extrinsic nerves. Parietal cells lining the wall of the stomach secrete hydrochloric acid, whereas chief cells secrete pepsinogen (a precursor to pepsin, a digestive enzyme). Parietal cells also produce intrinsic factor, which works to facilitate the absorption of vitamin B_{12}. Absence of the intrinsic factor causes pernicious anemia.

Function

The stomach performs several functions. Following ingestion of food, the stomach functions as a food reservoir. The primary function of the stomach is to begin the digestive process by using both mechanical movements and chemical secretions. Gastric secretion can be divided into three phases: cephalic, gastric, and intestinal.

The *cephalic phase* begins with the sight, smell, and taste of food and is regulated by the vagus nerve. Sympathetic nerve fibers activate neurons in the GI nerve plexus, which then initiate secretory and contractile activity. The *gastric phase* begins with the presence of food in the stomach. The G-cells in the antrum secrete the hormone gastrin, which promotes the secretion of hydrochloric acid and pepsinogen. Hydrochloric acid transforms inactive pepsinogen into active pepsins, which aid in the digestion of proteins. The secretion of mucus and bicarbonate protect the stomach from mechanical and chemical damage. The fluids secreted into the stomach are collectively referred to as gastric juice (Table 56-1).

The stomach also mixes or churns the food, breaking apart the large food molecules and mixing them with gastric secretions to form chyme, which then empties into the duodenum. The *intestinal phase* begins as the chyme passes from the stomach into the duodenum, causing distention. The intestinal phase is mediated by secretin, a hormone that inhibits further acid production and decreases gastric motility.

TABLE 56-1 Gastrointestinal Hormones

Hormone	Source	Effect
Gastrin	Secreted by the gastric mucosa in the presence of peptides	Stimulates gastric motility and secretion of hydrochloric acid
Secretin	Secreted by the duodenum in the presence of hydrochloric acid	Stimulates the secretion of pancreatic juice and bile from the liver
Pancreozymin	Secreted by the duodenum in the presence of hydrochloric acid and peptides	Stimulates the secretion of pancreatic juice
Cholecystokinin	Secreted by the duodenum in the presence of amino acids and fatty acids	Stimulates the secretion of pancreatic enzymes and bile from the gallbladder

PANCREAS

Structure

The pancreas is a fish shaped gland that lies retroperitoneally in the upper abdominal cavity behind the stomach and extends horizontally from the duodenal C-loop to the spleen. The pancreas is divided into portions known as the head, the body, and the tail (Figure 56-3).

Function

Two major cellular bodies within the pancreas have separate functions: exocrine and endocrine. The *exocrine* part of the pancreas constitutes about 80% of the organ and consists of acinar cells, which secrete the enzymes that are necessary for the digestion of carbohydrates, fats, and proteins (trypsin, chymotrypsin, amylase, and lipase) (Table 56-2). The *endocrine* part of the pancreas is made up of the islets of Langerhans, with alpha cells producing glucagon and beta cells producing insulin. Although the islet cells account for less than 2% of the volume of the pancreas, the hormones produced

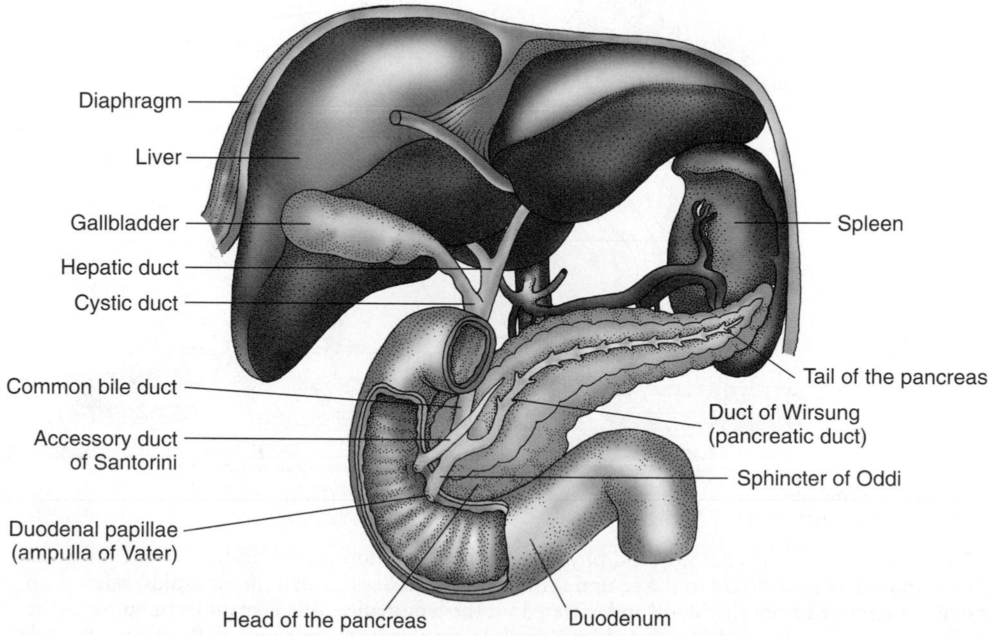

Figure 56-3 ■ The anatomy of the pancreas, the liver, and the gallbladder.

are essential in the regulation of metabolism. Chapter 65 describes the endocrine function of the pancreas.

LIVER AND GALLBLADDER

Structure

The liver is the largest organ in the body and is mainly located in the right upper quadrant (RUQ) of the abdomen. The liver is divided into two major regions: a larger right lobe and a smaller left lobe. It is made up of functioning units called lobules (Figure 56-4). The right and left hepatic ducts transport bile from the liver. The liver receives its blood supply from the hepatic artery and the hepatic portal vein. About 1500 mL of blood flows through the liver every minute.

The gallbladder is a pear-shaped bulbous sac that is located in a depression on the inferior surface of the liver. The gallbladder has three portions: the neck, which is continu-

TABLE 56-2 Major Digestive Enzymes and Bile

Substance	Source	Substrate	End Product
Salivary amylase (ptyalin)	Salivary glands	Starch	Dextrins, maltose
Gastric pepsin (protease)	Stomach	Proteins	Polypeptides
Gastric lipase	Stomach	Emulsified fats	Fatty acids* and glycerol*
Bile (contains no enzymes)	Liver; stored and released from the gallbladder	Unemulsified fats	Emulsified fats
Trypsin	Pancreas	Proteins and polypeptides	Polypeptides and amino acids*
Chymotrypsin	Pancreas	Proteins and polypeptides	Polypeptides and amino acids*
Carboxypeptidase	Pancreas	Polypeptides	Smaller polypeptides
Amylase	Pancreas	Starch	Maltose, lactose, and sucrose
Lipase	Pancreas	Bile and emulsified fats	Glycerol* and fatty acids*
Enterokinase	Duodenal mucosa	Trypsinogen	Trypsin
Peptidases	Intestine	Peptides	Amino acids*
Lactase	Intestine	Lactose (milk sugar)	Glucose* and galactose*
Maltase	Intestine	Maltose (malt sugar)	Glucose*
Sucrase	Intestine	Sucrose (cane sugar)	Glucose* and fructose*

*End product ready for digestion.

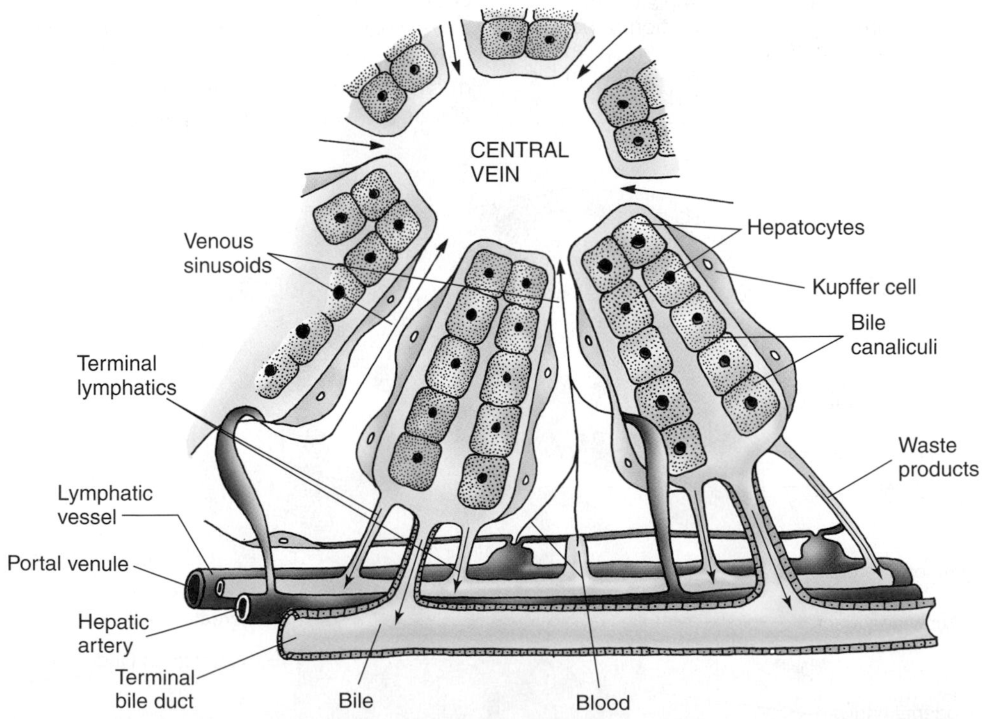

Figure 56-4 ■ The anatomy and physiology of the liver lobule. Blood flows from the portal vein and the hepatic artery to the central vein. As blood passes through the sinusoids, waste products are removed from the blood and excreted via the lymphatics. Bile is manufactured by the hepatocytes (liver cells) and is secreted into the bile canaliculi. From there, it flows into the bile ducts and then to the gallbladder.

ous with the cystic duct; the body, or main portion; and the fundus, the lower bulbous section. The gallbladder is drained by the cystic duct, which joins with the hepatic duct from the liver to form the common bile duct.

Function

The liver performs more than 400 functions in three major categories: storage, protection, and metabolism. The liver stores several minerals and vitamins, such as the following:

- Copper
- Iron
- Magnesium
- Vitamin B_2
- Vitamin B_{12}
- Folic acid
- Vitamin B_6
- Fat-soluble vitamins A, D, E, and K

The protective function of the liver involves phagocytic **Kupffer cells**, which are part of the body's reticuloendothelial system. They engulf harmful bacteria and anemic red blood cells. The liver also detoxifies potentially harmful compounds (such as drugs, chemicals, and alcohol) that are ingested.

The liver functions in the metabolism of proteins considered vital for human survival. It breaks down amino acids to remove ammonia, which is then converted to urea and is excreted via the kidneys. In addition, the liver synthesizes several plasma proteins, including albumin, prothrombin, and fibrinogen. The liver's role in carbohydrate metabolism involves storing and releasing glycogen as the body's energy requirements change. The liver synthesizes, breaks down, and temporarily stores fatty acids and triglycerides.

The liver forms and continually secretes bile. **Bile** is essential for the emulsification of fat. The secretion of bile increases in response to gastrin, secretin, and cholecystokinin. Bile is secreted into small ducts that empty into the common bile duct and into the duodenum at the sphincter of Oddi. However, if the sphincter is closed, the bile goes to the gallbladder for storage.

The gallbladder collects, concentrates, and stores the bile that has come from the liver. It releases the bile into the duodenum via the common bile duct when fat is present.

SMALL INTESTINE

Structure

The small intestine is the longest and most convoluted portion of the digestive tract, measuring 16 to 19 feet (5 to 6 m) in length in an adult. It is composed of three different regions: duodenum, jejunum, and ileum. The *duodenum* is the first 12 inches (30 cm) of the small intestine and is attached to the distal end of the pylorus. It is C-shaped, curving left around the head of the pancreas and bending behind the transverse portion of the large intestine. The common bile duct and pancreatic duct join to form the ampulla of Vater, emptying into the duodenum at the duodenal papilla. This papillary opening is surrounded by muscle known as the **sphincter of Oddi**. The 8-foot (2.5 m) portion of the small intestine that follows the sphincter of Oddi is the *jejunum*. The last 8 to 12 feet (2.5 to 4 m) of the small intestine is called the *ileum*. The ileocecal valve separates the entrance of the ileum from the cecum of the large intestine.

The inner surface of the small intestine has a velvety appearance because of numerous mucous membrane finger-like projections. These projections are called intestinal villi. In addition to the intestinal villi, the small intestine has circular folds of mucosa and submucosa, which increase the surface area for digestion and absorption.

Function

The small intestine has three main functions: movement (mixing and peristalsis), digestion, and absorption. Because the intestinal villi increase the surface area of the small intestine, the small intestine is the major organ of absorption of the digestive system. The small intestine mixes and transports the chyme by movements called segmental contractions. The contents are moved back and forth over short distances, thereby allowing the chyme to mix with many digestive enzymes. The ileocecal valve opens only to allow the passage of chyme. It takes an average of 3 to 10 hours for the contents to be propelled by peristalsis through the small intestine. The intestinal glands secrete intestinal juice containing epithelial cells that are used to replace surface epithelial cells of the villi as they are lost. The intestinal cells also produce cells that contain enzymes aiding in the digestion of proteins, carbohydrates, and lipids (see Tables 56-1 and 56-2).

LARGE INTESTINE

Structure

The large intestine extends about 5 to 6 feet in length from the ileocecal valve to the anus and is lined with columnar epithelium that has absorptive and mucous cells. It begins with the *cecum*, a dilated pouchlike structure that is inferior to the ileocecal opening. At the base of the cecum is the vermiform appendix, which has no known digestive function. The large intestine then extends upward from the cecum as the colon. The colon consists of four divisions: ascending colon, transverse colon, descending colon, and sigmoid colon. The sigmoid colon empties into the rectum.

Following the sigmoid colon, the large intestine bends downward to form the rectum. The last 6 to 8 inches (3 to 4 cm) of the large intestine is called the anal canal, which opens to the exterior of the body through the anus. The anal canal is surrounded by sphincter muscles.

Function

The large intestine's functions are movement, absorption, and elimination. Movement in the large intestine consists mainly of segmental contractions, like those in the small intestine, to allow enough time for the absorption of water and electrolytes. In addition, three or four strong peristaltic contractions per day are triggered by colonic distention in the proximal large intestine to propel the contents toward the rectum, where the material is stored until the urge to defecate occurs.

Absorption of water and some electrolytes occurs in the large intestine to reduce the fluid volume of the chyme, which creates a more solid material, the feces, for elimination.

Gastrointestinal Changes Associated with Aging

Like other systems, physiologic changes occur as individuals age, especially when they become 65 years of age or older. Changes in digestion, nutrition, and elimination are common, and affect nursing care as outlined in Chart 56-1.

CHART 56-1

NURSING FOCUS on the OLDER ADULT

Changes in the Gastrointestinal System Related to Aging

Physiologic Change	Disorders Related to Change	Nursing Interventions	Rationales
Stomach			
Atrophy of the gastric mucosa is characterized by a decrease in the ratio of gastrin-secreting cells to somatostatin-secreting cells. This change leads to decreased hydrochloric acid levels (hypochlorhydria).	Decreased hydrochloric acid levels lead to decreased absorption of iron and vitamin B_{12} and to proliferation of bacteria. Atrophic gastritis occurs as a consequence of bacterial overgrowth.	Encourage bland foods high in vitamins and iron. Assess for epigastric pain.	Bland foods help prevent gastritis. Assessment helps detect gastritis.
Large Intestine			
Peristalsis decreases, and nerve impulses are dulled.	Decreased sensation to defecate can result in postponement of bowel movements, which leads to constipation and impaction.	Encourage a high-fiber diet and 1500 mL of fluid intake daily (if not contraindicated). Encourage as much activity as tolerated.	These interventions increase the sensation of needing to defecate.
Pancreas			
Distention and dilation of pancreatic ducts change. Calcification of pancreatic vessels occurs with a decrease in lipase production.	Decreased lipase level results in decreased fat absorption and digestion. Steatorrhea, or excess fat in the feces, occurs because of decreased fat digestion.	Encourage small, frequent feedings. Assess for diarrhea.	Small, frequent feedings help prevent steatorrhea. Diarrhea may be steatorrhea.
Liver			
A decrease in the number and size of hepatic cells leads to decreased liver weight and mass. This change and an increase in fibrous tissue lead to decreased protein synthesis and changes in liver enzymes. Enzyme activity and cholesterol synthesis are diminished.	Decreased enzyme activity depresses drug metabolism, which leads to accumulation of drugs—possibly to toxic levels.	Assess all clients for adverse effects of all drugs, even those administered in normal doses.	Assessment detects drug toxicity.

ASSESSMENT TECHNIQUES

History

One method of assessing gastrointestinal (GI) functioning is to use the nutritional-metabolic and elimination patterns found in Gordon's Functional Health Patterns (Chart 56-2). The goal of the health history is to determine the events related to the current health problem.

DEMOGRAPHIC DATA

Collect demographic data about the client, such as age, gender, culture, and occupation. This information can provide information regarding predispositions to particular GI system disorders.

FAMILY HISTORY AND GENETIC RISK

Inquire about a family history of gastrointestinal (GI) disorders. Some GI health problems have a genetic predisposition. For example, familial adenomatous polyposis (FAP) is an inherited autosomal dominant disorder that predisposes the client to colon cancer.

PERSONAL HISTORY

A thorough review of the client's overall health status is an important part of every nursing history. Question the client regarding previous GI disorders or abdominal surgeries. Ask about prescription medications being taken, including how much, when the drugs are administered, and why they have been prescribed. It is also important to explore whether the client takes over-the-counter medications, which he or she may use independently. In particular, you should ask whether aspirin, nonsteroidal anti-inflammatory drugs (NSAIDs) (such as ibuprofen), laxatives, herbal preparations, or enemas are routinely taken. Large amounts of aspirin or NSAIDs can predispose the client to peptic ulcer disease and GI bleeding. Long-term use of laxatives or enemas can cause dependence on such stimulation and result in constipation. Some herbal preparations can affect absorption and elimination, or enhance the action of certain medications.

Finally, investigate the client's travel history. Ask the client whether he or she has traveled outside of the country recently. This information may provide clues as to the origin of symptoms such as diarrhea.

CHART 56-2

Gastrointestinal Assessment
USING GORDON'S FUNCTIONAL HEALTH PATTERNS

Nutritional-Metabolic Pattern
- What is your typical daily food intake? Describe a day's meals, snacks, and vitamins.
- How much salt do you typically add to your food? Do you use salt substitutes?
- How is your appetite? Any recent change?
- Do you have any difficulty chewing or swallowing?
- Do you wear dentures? How well do they fit?
- Do you ever experience indigestion or "heartburn"? How often? What seems to cause it? What helps it?
- Do you have pain, diarrhea, gas, or any other problems? Do any specific foods cause this for you?
- What is your typical daily fluid intake? What types of fluids (water, juices, soft drinks, coffee, tea)? How much?
- Have you had any recent change in your weight? Weight gain? Weight loss? How much?
- Have you noticed a change in the tightness of your rings or shoes? Tighter? Looser?
- Have you noticed any difference in the size of your abdomen?

Elimination Pattern
- What is your usual bowel elimination pattern? Frequency? Character? Discomfort? Laxatives?
- Do you have any pain or bleeding associated with bowel movements?
- Have you experienced any changes in your usual bowel pattern?
- When was your last rectal examination?
- Have you ever had an endoscopy or a colonoscopy?
- What is your usual urinary elimination pattern? Frequency? Amount? Color? Odor? Control?
- Have you noticed a change in the amount of urine?

Based on Gordon, M. (2002). *Manual of nursing diagnosis* (10th ed.). St. Louis: Mosby.

DIET HISTORY

A diet history is important when assessing GI system function. Many conditions manifest themselves as a result of alterations in dietary intake and absorption of nutrients. The goal of a nutritional assessment is to gather information about how well the client's nutritional needs are being met. You should inquire about any special diet and whether there are any known food allergies. Ask the client to describe the usual foods that are eaten daily and the times that meals are taken.

Illness changes dietary intake, so explore with the client any changes that have occurred in eating habits as a result of illness. **Anorexia** (loss of appetite for food) can occur with GI disease. Assess changes in taste and any difficulty or pain with swallowing (dysphagia) that could be associated with esophageal disorders. Also ascertain whether abdominal pain or discomfort accompanies eating, and whether the client has experienced any nausea, vomiting, or **dyspepsia** (indigestion or heartburn). Unknown food allergies often cause these symptoms. Inquire about any unintentional weight loss, because some cancers of the GI tract may present in this manner. It is also important to assess alcohol and caffeine consumption, because both substances are associated with many GI disorders, such as gastritis and peptic ulcer disease.

CULTURAL CONSIDERATIONS

Cultural and religious patterns are important in obtaining a complete diet history. The nurse determines whether culturally based foods pose a problem for the client. For example, the spices or hot pepper used in cooking in many cultures can aggravate or precipitate GI tract complaints, such as indigestion. Note religious patterns such as fasting or abstinence.

About 80% to 90% of black individuals are lactose intolerant. A much smaller percentage of white individuals also have this problem. Lactose intolerance causes bloating, cramping, and diarrhea as a result of lack of the enzyme lactase. Lactase is needed to convert lactose in milk and other dairy products to glucose and galactose.

SOCIOECONOMIC STATUS

The client's socioeconomic status may have a profound impact on his or her nutritional status. Knowledge of the client's socioeconomic status can provide valuable clues for determining his or her ability to obtain food, medications, and medical care. People who have limited budgets, such as some older adults or the unemployed, may not be able to purchase foods required for a balanced diet. In addition, they may substitute less expensive, and perhaps less effective, over-the-counter medications for prescription medications. Necessary medical care may be delayed, and clients may not seek health care until conditions are well advanced. Clients who are financially restricted may benefit from suggestions for managing nutrition while on a budget.

CURRENT HEALTH PROBLEMS

Because GI clinical manifestations are often vague and difficult for the client to describe, it is important to obtain a chronologic account of the current problem, symptoms, and any treatments taken. Furthermore, explore the characteristics associated with each symptom, including the location, quality, quantity, timing (onset, duration), and factors that may aggravate or alleviate the symptom (see Chart 56-2).

For example, a change in bowel habits is a significant complaint. Obtain the following information from the client:
- Pattern of bowel movements
- Color and consistency of the feces
- Occurrence of diarrhea or constipation
- Effective action taken to relieve diarrhea or constipation
- Presence of frank blood or tarry stools
- Presence of abdominal distention or gas

An unintentional weight gain or loss is another symptom that warrants further investigation. Assess the following:
- Normal weight
- Weight gain or loss
- Period of time for weight change
- Changes in appetite or oral intake

Smoking predisposes the client to several types of cancer, especially oral cancer, because nicotine and other chemicals found in tobacco are GI irritants. Obtain the client's smoking history, including the number of packs of cigarettes smoked per day times the number of years smoked. For example, if the client smoked two packs of cigarettes per day for 20 years, then he or she would have a 40-year cigarette smoking history. Also ask about any history or current use of cigars, pipe tobacco, or chewing tobacco.

Pain is a common complaint in clients with GI tract disorders. The mnemonic **PQRST** may be helpful in assisting you to organize the current problem assessment (Jarvis, 2004):

P: Precipitating or palliative. What brings it on? What makes it better? Worse? When did you first notice it?
Q: Quality or quantity. How does it look, feel, or sound? How intense/severe is it?
R: Region or radiation. Where is it? Does it spread anywhere?
S: Severity scale. How bad is it (on a scale of 1 to 10)? Is it getting better, worse, or staying the same?
T: Timing. Onset–Exactly when did it first occur? Duration–How long did it last? Frequency–How often does it occur?

Abdominal pain is often vague and difficult to evaluate. Asking the client to apply descriptors to the type of pain, such as burning, gnawing, or stabbing, is often helpful. The location of the pain can be determined by asking the client to point to the involved site. Ask about the relationship of food intake to the onset or worsening of pain. For example, a high-fat meal often triggers gallbladder pain.

Changes in the skin can result from several GI tract disorders, such as liver and biliary system obstruction. Ask the client about whether these clinical manifestations have occurred, or assess whether they are present:

- Skin discolorations or rashes
- Itching
- Jaundice
- Increased susceptibility to bruising
- Increased tendency to bleed

Physical Assessment

Physical assessment of the gastrointestinal (GI) system involves a comprehensive examination of the client's nutritional status, the mouth and pharynx, the abdomen, and the extremities. Nutritional assessment is discussed in detail in Chapter 64.

MOUTH AND PHARYNX

Assessment of the mouth involves inspection and palpation. To begin the examination of the mouth, put on gloves, face the client, and inspect the lips for color, moisture, cracking, or lesions. You will need a penlight and a tongue depressor to continue inspecting the inner surfaces of the lips and the oral mucosa, starting on the client's left side and moving in a clockwise fashion. Carefully palpate the U-shaped area under the tongue for nodules, because oral malignancies are most likely to develop in this area. The tongue is inspected for color, coating, ulcers, and variations in size and shape.

It is important to examine the teeth for evidence of dental caries and note the absence of teeth. Tooth discoloration may be the result of excessive tobacco use. Refer the client to a dentist if you detect abnormalities or decay.

The gums should be pink, moist, and smooth. Dark-skinned clients may have a dark line on the margins of the gingiva. If the client wears dentures, they are removed to facilitate a thorough examination of the mouth. Throughout this examination, be alert to any significant mouth odors that suggest disease. For instance, a fruity smell may indicate uncontrolled diabetes mellitus.

Oral lesions or nodules are noted. For example, lesions from Kaposi's sarcoma may be seen in clients with acquired immunodeficiency syndrome (AIDS).

ABDOMEN

In preparation for examination of the abdomen, the client is instructed to empty his or her bladder and then to lie in a supine position with knees bent, keeping the arms at the sides to prevent inadvertent tensing of the abdominal muscles.

The abdominal examination usually begins at the client's right side and proceeds in a systematic fashion (Figure 56-5):

- Right upper quadrant (RUQ)
- Left upper quadrant (LUQ)
- Left lower quadrant (LLQ)
- Right lower quadrant (RLQ)

Table 56-3 lists the organs that lie in each of these areas.

If areas of pain or discomfort are noted from the history, this area is examined last in the examination sequence. This sequence should prevent the client from tensing abdominal muscles because of the pain, which would make the examination difficult. Examine any area of tenderness cautiously and instruct the client to state whether it is too painful. Observe the client's face for signs of distress or pain.

Assess the abdomen by using the four techniques of examination, but in a sequence different from that used for other body systems: inspection, auscultation, percussion, and then palpation. This sequence is preferred so that palpation and percussion do not increase intestinal activity and hence increase bowel sounds. Palpation is not performed if appendicitis or an abdominal aneurysm is suspected.

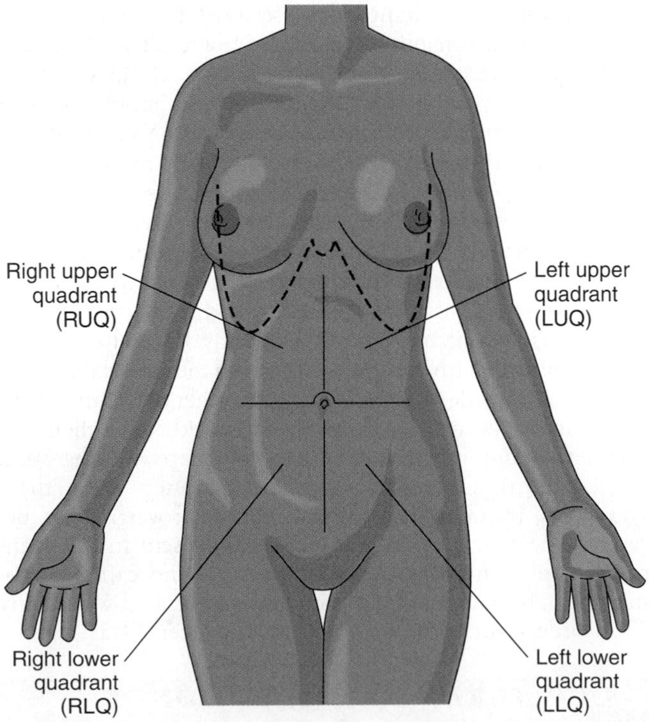

Figure 56-5 ■ A topographic division of the abdomen into quadrants.

Inspection

Inspect the skin and note the following:

- Overall symmetry of the abdomen
- Presence of discolorations (rashes, lesions, striae, petechiae, scars, distended superficial veins, jaundice, and any other pigmentation changes)
- Abdominal distention
- Bulging flanks
- Taut, glistening skin

Assess the shape of the abdomen by observing its contour and symmetry. The contour of the abdomen can be rounded, flat, concave, or distended. It is best determined when standing at the side of the bed or treatment table and looking down on the abdomen. View the abdomen at eye level from the side. Note whether the contour is symmetric or asymmetric. Asymmetry of the abdomen can indicate problems affecting the underlying body structures (see Table 56-3). Note the shape and position of the umbilicus for any deviations. The presence of ecchymosis around the umbilicus **(Cullen's sign)** is an indication of intra-abdominal bleeding.

Finally, observe the client's abdominal movements, including the normal rising and falling with inspiration and expiration, and note any distress during movement. Occasionally, pulsations may be visible, particularly in the area of the abdominal aorta. Peristaltic movements are rarely seen on inspection unless the client is thin and has markedly increased peristalsis. If these movements are observed, note the quadrant of origin and the direction of peristaltic flow. This finding is reported to the health care provider, because it may indicate an intestinal obstruction.

Auscultation

Video Clip: Abdomen, Bowel Sounds

Auscultation of the abdomen is performed with the diaphragm of the stethoscope because bowel sounds are usually high pitched. The stethoscope is placed lightly on the abdominal wall while listening for bowel sounds in all four quadrants, beginning in the RLQ at the ileocecal valve area.

Bowel sounds are created as air and fluid move through the GI tract. They are normally heard as relatively high-pitched gurgles every 5 to 15 seconds, with a normal frequency range of 5 to 30 per minute. Bowel sounds are characterized as normal, hypoactive, or hyperactive. Listen for the character and frequency of the sounds. Bowel sounds may be irregular, so you must listen for *at least* 1 full minute in each quadrant to confirm the absence of bowel sounds. Bowel sounds are diminished or absent after abdominal surgery or in the client with peritonitis or paralytic ileus. Increased bowel sounds, especially loud gurgling sounds, result from hypermotility of the bowel **(borborygmus).** These sounds are usually heard in the client with diarrhea or gastroenteritis or above a complete intestinal obstruction.

When auscultating the abdomen, also listen for vascular sounds or **bruits** ("swooshing" sounds) over the abdominal aorta, the renal arteries, and the iliac arteries. A bruit heard over the aorta usually indicates the presence of an aneurysm. *If this sound is heard, do not percuss or palpate the abdomen. Notify the health care provider of your findings!*

TABLE 56-3 Location of Body Structures in Each Abdominal Quadrant

Right Upper Quadrant (RUQ) ▪ Most of the liver ▪ Gallbladder ▪ Duodenum ▪ Head of the pancreas ▪ Hepatic flexure of the colon ▪ Part of the ascending and transverse colon	**Left Lower Quadrant (LLQ)** ▪ Part of the descending colon ▪ Sigmoid colon ▪ Left ureter ▪ Left ovary and fallopian tube ▪ Left spermatic cord
Left Upper Quadrant (LUQ) ▪ Left lobe of the liver ▪ Stomach ▪ Spleen ▪ Body and tail of the pancreas ▪ Splenic flexure of the colon ▪ Part of the transverse and descending colon	**Right Lower Quadrant (RLQ)** ▪ Cecum ▪ Appendix ▪ Right ureter ▪ Right ovary and fallopian tube ▪ Right spermatic cord **Midline** ▪ Abdominal aorta ▪ Uterus (if enlarged) ▪ Bladder (if distended)

Percussion

Video Clip: Percussion, Abdomen

Percussion may be used during the abdominal assessment to determine the size of solid organs; to detect the presence of masses, fluid, and air; and to estimate the size of the liver and spleen. This part of the physical assessment is usually performed by a physician or advanced practice nurse (APN). The examiner elicits percussion notes by placing the middle finger of the nondominant hand over the abdominal area to be percussed, striking his or her finger lightly with the tip of the middle finger of the dominant hand several times. Each quadrant is systematically assessed by comparing sounds over different areas. The **percussion notes** normally heard in the abdomen are termed **tympanic** (the high-pitched, loud, musical sound of an air-filled intestine) or **dull** (the medium-pitched, softer, thudlike sound over a solid organ, such as the liver).

Video Clip: Percussion, Liver

To percuss the size of the liver span, the physician or APN begins from below the right nipple in the midclavicular line and is careful to percuss between ribs. The percussion note should change from resonance of the lung tissue to dullness of the liver when the upper liver border is reached. The examiner marks the area where percussion tones change, then percusses up from the iliac crest in the midclavicular line until the percussion note changes from tympany of the bowel to dullness of the liver at the lower border. Again, this area is marked. The distance between the two marks is the approximate liver span, which is normally 2.4 to 5 inches (6 to 12 cm). An enlarged liver span indicates **hepatomegaly** (liver enlargement).

Video Clip: Percussion, Spleen

The examiner may also use percussion techniques to determine the size and position of the spleen at the tenth intercostal space in the left midaxillary line. Dullness heard forward of the midaxillary line or in the left anterior axillary line indicates enlargement of the spleen **(splenomegaly).** Mild to moderate splenomegaly can be detected before the spleen becomes palpable. Percussion can also be used to detect a distended bladder. Dullness is heard over a distended bladder.

Palpation

The purpose of palpation is to determine the size and location of abdominal organs and to assess for the presence of masses or tenderness. Palpation of the abdomen consists of two types: light palpation and deep palpation. Only physicians and APNs, such as clinical nurse specialists and nurse practitioners, should perform deep palpation. Deep palpation is used to further determine the size and shape of abdominal organs and masses.

Video Clip: Palpation of Abdomen

The technique of *light palpation* is used to detect large masses and areas of tenderness and to help the client achieve muscular relaxation. Place the first four fingers of the palpating hand close together and then place them lightly on the abdomen and proceed smoothly and systematically from quadrant to quadrant. The abdomen is depressed to a depth of 0.5 to 1 inch (1.25 to 2.5 cm), and the assessment proceeds with a rotational movement of the palpating hand. Any areas of tenderness or guarding are noted, because these areas are examined last and cautiously during deep palpation. While performing light palpation, be alert to signs of rigidity which, unlike voluntary guarding, is a sign of peritoneal inflammation. Areas of pain should be evaluated for rebound tenderness **(Blumberg's sign).** With fingers placed at a 90-degree angle in relation to the abdomen, the examiner pushes slowly and deeply, releasing quickly. Pain felt on release is a positive sign for rebound tenderness and should be reported to the health care provider.

Psychosocial Assessment

Psychosocial assessment focuses on how the current complaint affects the client's lifestyle. Remember that clients are often reluctant to discuss elimination problems, which are very personal. The interview focus is whether there has been any interruption of, or disturbance to, usual activities, including employment. Question the client about recent stressful events. Emotional stress has been associated with the development or exacerbation of irritable bowel syndrome (IBS) and other GI disorders.

Critical Thinking Challenge

A middle-aged female client is seen in the emergency department where you work complaining of RUQ abdominal pain and cramping for the last 2 days. Because she travels extensively for her job, her usual dietary pattern consists of eating at restaurants several times weekly. The symptoms began 1 to 2 hours after eating a dinner of fried or spicy foods.

1. About which specific areas of the history should you seek further information or clarification?
2. What physical assessment findings would you be most likely to find during the abdominal examination?

evolve For suggested answer guidelines, go to http://evolve.elsevier.com/Iggy/.

Diagnostic Assessment

LABORATORY TESTS

To make an accurate assessment of the many possible causes of gastrointestinal (GI) system abnormalities, laboratory testing of blood, urine, and stool specimens may be performed.

Blood Tests

A *complete blood count (CBC)* aids in the diagnosis of anemia and infection; it also detects changes in the blood's formed elements. In adults, GI bleeding is the most frequent cause of anemia.

Because the liver is the main site of all proteins involved in coagulation, the prothrombin time is useful in evaluating the levels of these clotting factors. *Prothrombin time (PT)* measures the rate at which prothrombin is converted to thrombin, a process that is dependent on most of the vitamin K–associated clotting factors. Severe acute or chronic liver damage leads to a prolonged PT secondary to impaired synthesis of clotting proteins.

Many *electrolytes* are altered in GI tract dysfunction. For example, calcium is absorbed in the GI tract and may be measured to detect malabsorption. Excessive vomiting or diarrhea causes electrolyte depletion, thus requiring replacement.

Assays of serum enzymes are important in the evaluation of liver damage. **Aspartate aminotransferase (AST)** and **alanine aminotransferase (ALT)** are two enzymes found in the liver and other organs. These enzymes are elevated in most liver disorders, but they are highest in conditions that cause necrosis, such as severe viral hepatitis.

Elevations in serum **amylase** and **lipase** are indicative of acute pancreatitis. In acute pancreatitis, serum amylase levels begin to elevate within 24 hours of onset and remain elevated for up to 5 days. Serum amylase and lipase are not elevated when extensive pancreatic necrosis is present because there are few pancreatic cells manufacturing the enzymes. Serum amylase and lipase measurements are the best indicators of the presence of acute pancreatitis, with elevations in 80% to 85% of pancreatitis cases (Avunduk, 2002).

Bilirubin is the primary pigment in bile, which is normally conjugated and excreted by the liver and biliary system. It is measured as total serum bilirubin, conjugated (direct) bilirubin, and unconjugated (indirect) bilirubin. These measurements are important in the evaluation of jaundice and in the evaluation of liver and biliary tract functioning. Elevations in direct and indirect bilirubin levels can indicate impaired secretion or conjugation.

The serum level of ammonia is also measured to evaluate hepatic function. Ammonia is normally used to rebuild amino acids or is converted to urea for excretion. Elevated ammonia levels are seen in conditions that cause severe hepatocellular injury, such as cirrhosis of the liver or fulminant hepatitis (Pagana & Pagana, 2002).

Two primary **oncofetal antigens**–CA19-9 and CEA–are evaluated to diagnose, monitor the success of cancer therapy, and assess for the recurrence of cancer in the GI tract. These antigens may also be increased in benign GI conditions. Chart 56-3 lists blood tests commonly used by the health care provider in the diagnosis of GI disorders.

Urine Tests

The presence of amylase can be detected in the urine. In acute pancreatitis, there is increased renal clearance of amylase. Amylase levels in the urine remain high even after serum levels return to normal. This becomes an important finding in clients who are symptomatic for 3 days or longer (Pagana & Pagana, 2002).

Urine urobilinogen is a form of bilirubin that is converted by the intestinal flora and excreted in the urine. Its measurement is useful in the evaluation of hepatic and biliary obstruction, because the presence of bilirubin in the urine often precedes the development of jaundice (Chart 56-4).

CHART 56-3

LABORATORY PROFILE
Gastrointestinal Assessment

Test	Normal Range for Adults	Significance of Abnormal Findings
Calcium (total)	9.0-10.5 mg/dL (Values decrease in older adults)	*Decreased* values indicate possible: Malabsorption Renal failure Acute pancreatitis
Potassium	3.5-5.0 mEq/L or 3.5-5.0 mmol/L	*Decreased* values indicate possible: Vomiting Gastric suctioning Diarrhea Drainage from intestinal fistulas
Albumin	3.5-5.0 g/dL	*Decreased* values indicate possible: Hepatic disease
Alanine aminotransferase (ALT)	3-35 International Units/L or 8-20 units/L (SI units)	*Increased* values indicate possible: Liver disease Hepatitis Cirrhosis
Aspartate aminotransferase (AST)	5-40 units/L	*Increased* values indicate possible: Liver disease Hepatitis Cirrhosis
Lactate dehydrogenase (LDH)	115-225 International Units/L	*Increased* values indicate possible: Damaged liver caused by hepatitis and other hepatocellular disorders
Alkaline phosphatase	30-85 International Units/L or 42-128 units/L (SI units)	*Increased* values indicate possible: Hepatic disease Biliary obstruction
Bilirubin Total serum	0.1-1.0 mg/dL	*Increased* values indicate possible: Hemolysis Biliary obstruction Hepatic damage
Conjugated (direct)	0.1-0.3 mg/dL	*Increased* values indicate possible: Biliary obstruction
Unconjugated (indirect)	0.2-0.8 mg/dL	*Increased* values indicate possible: Hemolysis Hepatic damage
Ammonia	15-110 mg/dL	*Increased* values indicate possible: Hepatic disease such as cirrhosis
Xylose absorption	*5-g dose in 2 hr:* >20 mg/dL or >1.3 mmol/L *25-g dose in 2 hr:* >25 mg/dL or >1.7 mmol/L	*Decreased* values in blood and urine indicate possible: Malabsorption in the small intestine
Serum amylase	56-90 International Units/L or 25-125 units/L (SI units)	*Increased* values indicate possible: Acute pancreatitis
Serum lipase	0-110 units/L	*Increased* values indicate possible: Acute pancreatitis
Cholesterol	<200 mg/dL	*Increased* values indicate possible: Pancreatitis Biliary obstruction *Decreased* values indicate possible: Liver cell damage
Carbohydrate antigen 19-9 (CA19-9)	<37 units/mL	*Increased* values indicate possible: Cancer of the pancreas, stomach, colon Acute pancreatitis Inflammatory bowel disease
Carcinoembryonic antigen (CEA)	*Nonsmoker:* <2.5 ng/mL *Smoker:* up to 5 ng/mL	*Increased* values indicate possible: Colorectal, stomach, pancreatic cancer Ulcerative colitis Crohn's disease Hepatitis Cirrhosis

CHART 56-4

LABORATORY PROFILE

Common Urine and Stool Tests Used in Gastrointestinal Assessment

Test	Normal Range for Adults	Significance of Abnormal Findings
Urine bilirubin	Negative	*Increased* values indicate possible: Biliary obstruction Cirrhosis Hepatitis
Urobilinogen	Urine 0.1-1.0 Ehrlich unit/mL	*Increased* values indicate possible: Hepatitis Cirrhosis *Absence* indicates possible obstructive jaundice
Urine amylase	Various levels, depending on unit of measure	*Increased* values indicate possible: Acute pancreatitis Pancreatic obstruction
Stool for occult blood (FOBT)	Negative	*Presence* indicates possible: Carcinoma Peptic ulcer Ulcerative colitis
Ova and parasites	Negative	*Presence* is diagnostic of infection.
Fecal fat	<5 g/24 hr with normal diet	*Increased* values indicate possible: Crohn's disease Malabsorption syndrome Pancreatic disease

Stool Tests

Several stool examinations are used in the evaluation of GI tract dysfunction (see Chart 56-4). Stool studies are conducted to evaluate the function and integrity of the GI tract. Stool testing for occult blood is called the **fecal occult blood test (FOBT).** The FOBT measures the presence of blood in the stool from GI bleeding, a common finding associated with colorectal cancer.

Stool samples are collected to test for ova and parasites to aid in the diagnosis of parasitic infection. Stool samples tested for fecal fats are evaluated for steatorrhea and malabsorption. Fat is normally absorbed in the small intestine in the presence of biliary and pancreatic secretions. In malabsorption, fat is abnormally excreted in the stool.

Another common stool examination is for the presence of a bacterial infection called *Clostridium difficile.* This test is indicated on clients who have been on antibiotic therapy. The antibiotic therapy depresses the natural intestinal flora causing an overgrowth of *C. difficile.* The bacterium releases a toxin, which causes colonic epithelium necrosis resulting in severe diarrhea (Pagana & Pagana, 2002).

WOMEN'S HEALTH CONSIDERATIONS

Compared with women of lower socioeconomic status, women of higher socioeconomic status are more likely to have regular physical examinations that include an annual FOBT and a proctosigmoidoscopy every 3 to 5 years after the age of 50. An annual FOBT may reduce mortality from colorectal cancer in women. Most physicians include an FOBT as part of the gynecologic examination.

RADIOGRAPHIC EXAMINATIONS

Radiographic examinations and similar diagnostic procedures are useful in detecting structural and functional disorders of the gastrointestinal (GI) system. Your role is to properly prepare the client for the examination, to provide an explanation of the procedure, and to provide the necessary postprocedure care. As with most invasive procedures, many of the diagnostic tests outlined here require a witnessed and signed informed consent.

Plain Films of the Abdomen

A plain film of the abdomen is generally the first x-ray study that the health care provider requests when diagnosing a GI problem. This film, taken in the supine position, has the ability to reveal abnormalities such as masses, tumors, and strictures or obstructions to normal movement. Patterns of bowel gas appear light on the abdominal film and can be useful in detecting an obstruction (ileus). There is no required client preparation except to wear a hospital gown and remove any jewelry or belts, which may interfere with the film.

When abdominal pain is severe or when there is a suspicion of bowel perforation, a set of films called an *acute abdomen series* is requested. This procedure consists of a chest x-ray, supine abdomen film, and an upright abdomen film. The chest x-ray may reveal a hiatal hernia and an upright abdomen film may show air in the peritoneum for a bowel perforation.

Upper Gastrointestinal Series and Small Bowel Series

An **upper GI radiographic series** is an x-ray visualization from the oral part of the pharynx to the duodenojejunal junction. The upper GI series is used to detect disorders of structure or function of the esophagus (barium swallow), stomach, or duodenum. An extension of the upper GI series, the small bowel follow-through (SBFT), continues tracing the barium through the small intestine–up to and including the ileocecal junction–to detect disorders of the jejunum or ileum.

CLIENT PREPARATION. Remind the client to withhold foods or liquids for 8 hours before the test. If possible, opioid analgesics and anticholinergic medications are withheld for 24 hours before the test, because they decrease intestinal tract motility.

Instruct the client about the barium preparation and the need to drink about 16 ounces of the barium. The radiology nurse or technician explains that a rotating examination table will be used to assist the client in assuming the vertical, supine, prone, and lateral positions required for this test.

PROCEDURE. The procedure takes about 30 minutes for the radiologist to perform. Fluoroscopy is used to trace the barium through the esophagus and stomach. The client stands against the x-ray table for this part of the test. The table then moves the client to a lying position for more views of the stomach and duodenum. Lying in a prone position, the client drinks more barium as quickly as possible while x-rays are taken. To attempt to make the client as comfortable as possible, a pillow for the head and a sheet to prevent chilling are supplied whenever possible. The position changes help to coat the mucosa and identify gastroesophageal reflux and hiatal hernia.

If a small bowel radiographic series is included, the client drinks additional barium, and more x-rays are taken at specific intervals. This series can take several hours, depending on how long it takes the barium to reach the cecum.

FOLLOW-UP CARE. After either of these series, teach the client to drink plenty of fluids to help eliminate the barium. The client may be given a mild laxative or stool softener to assist in its elimination. The radiology nurse or technician instructs the client that stools may be chalky white for 24 to 72 hours as barium is excreted. The client is informed that when all barium is passed, brown stools return. If the client is at home, he or she is instructed to report abdominal fullness, pain, or a delay in return to brown stools.

Barium Enema

A **barium enema** examination, also known as a **lower GI series**, is a radiographic visualization of the large intestine. This test is usually ordered for a client with a complaint of blood or mucus in the stool or a change in bowel pattern, such as diarrhea or constipation. A barium enema can also detect bowel obstruction from the twisting of the colon upon itself **(volvulus).** This test is usually contraindicated in clients when colon perforation or fistula is suspected because there is the potential for barium to enter the venous circulation, causing cardiac arrest.

CLIENT PREPARATION. Adequate client preparation for a barium enema study is very important. The client consumes only clear liquids 12 to 24 hours before the examination to reduce the amount of fecal matter in the bowel. The client is allowed nothing by mouth (NPO) after midnight on the night before the test. In addition, the health care provider prescribes a potent laxative. Oral liquid preparations, such as magnesium citrate or GoLYTELY, are used for cleaning the bowel the evening before the examination. In some cases, a cleansing enema is needed or required according to the agency's procedure.

PROCEDURE. To begin the barium enema examination, a rectal catheter with an inflatable balloon is inserted. About 500 to 1500 mL of barium is instilled slowly by gravity, and the client is instructed to hold the barium. Films are taken with the client in supine, prone, and lateral positions. He or she may experience abdominal cramps and the urge to defecate as the barium enema is given. This procedure can be extremely uncomfortable, especially for older adults. The client is instructed to take slow, deep breaths and to hold the anal sphincter as tightly closed as possible. The test takes about 45 minutes to 1 hour. In some cases, a double-contrast study (ACBE) is requested. In this study, air is instilled to enhance the contrast and outline small lesions.

FOLLOW-UP CARE. After the study is completed, the client is allowed to expel the barium. The radiology nurse or technician teaches the client to drink plenty of fluids to assist in eliminating the barium. A laxative is given to help remove the barium from the intestinal tract. The client is informed that the stools will be chalky white for about 24 to 72 hours, until all barium is expelled.

Percutaneous Transhepatic Cholangiography

Percutaneous transhepatic cholangiography (PTC) is an x-ray study of the biliary duct system using an iodinated dye instilled via a percutaneous needle inserted through the liver into the intrahepatic ducts. This procedure may be performed when a client has jaundice or persistent upper abdominal pain, even after cholecystectomy, but is rarely done as a diagnostic procedure any more. Information about dilated biliary ducts can be obtained using ultrasound and ERCP (discussed later).

CLIENT PREPARATION. A laxative is usually given to the client the evening before the procedure. The client is NPO for 12 hours before the test. It is important to ask about allergies to iodine or seafood. Steroids are administered if the client has one of these allergies. Coagulation tests are monitored, because impaired clotting is a contraindication to this procedure. Before the procedure begins, an intravenous (IV) infusion is started for the administration of sedatives.

PROCEDURE. The client is placed in a supine position on the fluoroscopy table. The site is prepared and draped, and a local anesthetic is injected into the skin. During the test, the client is instructed to hold his or her breath on expiration while a needle is inserted into the liver under x-ray visualization. The dye is injected slowly until the biliary tree is filled. X-ray images are taken as the dye reaches the biliary duct system. A tilt table may be used to place the client in various positions to visualize the entire biliary tree. At the end of the test, the biliary ducts are aspirated of the contrast medium. The procedure usually takes 30 minutes to 1 hour.

FOLLOW-UP CARE. After a PTC, the client is confined to bed for several hours. The client's vital signs are checked frequently, because there is a risk of hemorrhage and sepsis. The client is placed on the right side with a firm pillow or sandbag placed against the lower ribs and abdomen. Observe the lower right rib cage area for signs of bleeding, hematoma, ecchymosis (bruising), or bile leakage with each postprocedure vital sign assessment.

Computed Tomography of the Gastrointestinal System

Computed tomography (CT), also referred to as a CT scan, is a noninvasive cross-sectional x-ray visualization that can detect tissue densities and abnormalities in the abdomen, liver, pancreas, spleen, and biliary tract. CT may be performed with or without contrast media.

The client is instructed that he or she will need to lie still in a rather enclosed space of the machine. The client is instructed to remove jewelry or metal. If the use of a contrast medium is scheduled, ask about allergies to seafood and iodine. The client is NPO for at least 4 hours before the test if a contrast medium is to be used. IV access will be required for injection of the contrast medium. The client is advised that a warm, flushing feeling may be felt on injection. The client who is mildly claustrophobic may require a mild sedative to tolerate the study.

The radiologic technician instructs the client to lie still and to hold his or her breath when asked. The client is placed on the examining table, and a series of x-ray images are taken. The contrast medium may be given by IV injection for a second set of images. The test takes about 1 to 2 hours to complete.

No particular follow-up care is needed after a CT scan unless sedatives were administered. If the client was sedated, monitor vital signs until the client is alert and fully awake.

OTHER DIAGNOSTIC TESTS

Endoscopy

Endoscopy is direct visualization of the gastrointestinal (GI) tract by means of a flexible fiberoptic endoscope. Endoscopes of various sizes are used for different areas of the GI tract. Visualization of the esophagus, stomach, biliary system, and bowel is possible. Endoscopy is usually ordered to evaluate bleeding, ulceration, inflammation, masses, tumors, and cancerous lesions. Obtaining specimens for biopsy and cytologic studies is also possible through the endoscope. There are several types of endoscopic examinations.

Esophagogastroduodenoscopy

Esophagogastroduodenoscopy (EGD), a visual examination of the esophagus, stomach, and duodenum, is accomplished using a fiberoptic endoscope. The distal end of the endoscope is flexible, allowing visualization of the entire area. This procedure has significantly reduced the number of upper GI series that are done.

The client preparing for an upper GI endoscopic examination is usually placed on NPO status 6 to 8 hours before the procedure. Instruct the client that a flexible tube will be passed down the esophagus while he or she is under conscious sedation. Midazolam hydrochloride (Versed), meperidine (Demerol), and fentanyl (Fentanyl, Sublimaze) are commonly used medications to sedate the client. Atropine may be administered to dry secretions. In addition, a local anesthetic is sprayed to inactivate the gag reflex and facilitate passage of the tube. Explain that this anesthetic will depress the gag reflex and that swallowing will be difficult. If the client has dentures, they are removed. Evaluate the strength of the gag reflex before giving the anesthetic spray, so that you can adequately assess the return of the client's gag reflex following the procedure.

After the medications are administered, the client is usually placed in the left lateral decubitus (Sims', or side-lying) position with a towel or basin at the mouth for secretions. A bite block is inserted to prevent the client from biting down on the endoscope and to protect the client's teeth. The physician passes the tube through the mouth and into the esophagus (Figure 56-6). The procedure takes about 20 to 30 minutes.

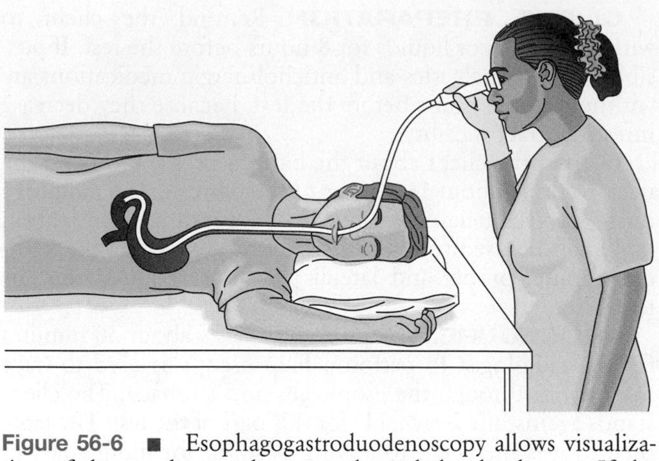

Figure 56-6 ■ Esophagogastroduodenoscopy allows visualization of the esophagus, the stomach, and the duodenum. If the esophagus is the focus of the examination, the procedure is called esophagoscopy. If the stomach is the focus, the procedure is called gastroscopy.

After the test, vital signs are checked frequently (usually every 30 minutes) until the sedation wears off. The siderails of the bed are raised during this time. The client remains NPO until the gag reflex returns (usually in 1 to 2 hours). *Do not offer fluids or food by mouth until the gag reflex is intact to prevent aspiration!* Monitor for signs of perforation, such as pain, bleeding, or fever. The client is instructed not to drive for 12 hours following the procedure. He or she is informed that a hoarse voice or sore throat may persist for several days following the test. Throat lozenges can be used to relieve throat discomfort.

Endoscopic Retrograde Cholangiopancreatography

Endoscopic retrograde cholangiopancreatography (ERCP) includes visual and radiographic examination of the liver, gallbladder, bile ducts, and pancreas to identify the cause and location of obstruction. After the cannula is inserted into the common bile duct, a radiopaque dye is inserted, followed by several x-ray images. The physician may perform a **papillotomy**, a small incision in the sphincter around the ampulla of Vater, to remove gallstones.

The client is prepared in the same manner as for an EGD, including being NPO for 6 to 8 hours before the test. The client will require IV access for the administration of sedation. Ask about prior exposure to x-ray dye and any sensitivities or allergies. If the client has dentures, they are removed. It is important to evaluate the strength of the gag reflex before giving the anesthetic spray, so that you can adequately assess the return of the client's gag reflex following the procedure.

The endoscopic portion of an ERCP is similar to that of an EGD, except that the endoscope is advanced farther, to the duodenum and into the biliary tract. Once the cannula is in the common duct, contrast medium is injected, and x-rays are taken to evaluate the biliary tract. A tilt table assists in distributing the contrast medium to all branches of the biliary tree. The client is placed in a left lateral position for the cannulization of the common bile duct; once the cannula is placed, the client is placed in a prone position. Following examination of the biliary tree, the cannula is directed into the pancreatic duct for examination. The ERCP lasts from 30 minutes to 2 hours.

After the test, assess vital signs frequently, usually every 15 minutes, until the client is stable. Check to ensure that the gag reflex has returned before offering fluids or food. Monitor the client for several postprocedure complications, including cholangitis, perforation, sepsis, and pancreatitis. The client will complain of pain if any of these complications occur. These problems do not occur immediately after the procedure but may take several hours to 2 days to develop. Colicky abdominal pain can occur secondary to the air instilled during the procedure. The client is instructed to report abdominal pain, fever, nausea, or vomiting that fails to resolve. He or she remains on NPO status until the gag reflex returns.

Small Bowel Capsule Enteroscopy

Enteroscopy is the visualization of the small intestine. Capsule endoscopy (M2A) is a small bowel enteroscopy that visualizes the entire small bowel, including the distal ileum. It is used to evaluate and locate the source of GI bleeding. Before the development of the M2A Capsule Endoscope, visualization of the small intestine was inadequate, and physicians relied primarily on barium x-rays for diagnosing disorders of the small intestine (Yu, 2002).

Prepare the client by explaining the procedure, the purpose, and what to expect during the testing. The client must fast (water only) for 8 to 10 hours before the test and be NPO for the first 2 hours of the testing.

At the time of the procedure the client's abdomen is marked for the location of the sensors, and the eight-lead sensors (Sensor Array) are applied. The client wears an abdominal belt that houses a recorder (DataRecorder) to capture the transmitted images. After the capsule is taken with a glass of water, the client may return to normal activity for the remainder of the study. The client can resume a normal diet 4 hours after capsule ingestion. At the conclusion of the procedure, the client returns to the facility with the capsule equipment for downloading to a central computer. The procedure lasts about 8 hours (Yu, 2002).

Because the M2A Capsule Endoscope is a single-use device that is propelled through the GI tract by peristalsis and excreted naturally, explain to the client the capsule will be excreted in the stool. No other follow-up is necessary.

Colonoscopy

Colonoscopy is an endoscopic examination of the entire large bowel. The physician may also obtain tissue biopsy specimens or remove polyps through the colonoscope. A colonoscopy is also used to evaluate the cause of chronic diarrhea or locate the source of GI bleeding. An alternative to this invasive procedure is the **virtual colonoscopy**, which is not invasive and uses a scanner to view the colon.

CLIENT PREPARATION. The client should have a liquid diet for 12 to 24 hours before a colonoscopy and is usually NPO 6 to 8 hours before the procedure.

An oral liquid preparation for cleaning the bowel (e.g., polyethylene glycol electrolyte solution [GoLYTELY] or sodium phosphate [Phospho-Soda]) is given to the client the evening before the examination and may be repeated the morning of the study. The solutions should be chilled to make them more palatable. Instruct the client to drink the preparation quickly. These solutions produce a watery diarrhea that begins in about 1 hour. The bowel clears in 4 to 5 hours. In some cases, the client may require laxatives, suppositories (e.g., bisacodyl [Dulcolax]), or one or more cleansing enemas. IV access is necessary for the administration of conscious sedation. A bowel preparation is needed for both the endoscopic procedure and the virtual colonoscopy.

PROCEDURE. The physician prescribes medication to aid in relaxation, usually midazolam hydrochloride (Versed) and/or an opiate. Initially, the client is placed on the left side with the knees drawn up while the endoscope is passed into the rectum to the cecum. Air may be instilled for better visualization. The entire procedure lasts about 30 to 60 minutes. Atropine sulfate is kept available in case of bradycardia resulting from vasovagal response.

FOLLOW-UP CARE. Check vital signs every 15 minutes until the client is stable. Siderails are kept up until the client is fully alert. Observe for signs of perforation (causes severe pain) and hemorrhage. Instruct the client that a feeling of fullness, cramping, and passage of flatus are expected for several hours after the test. If a polypectomy or tissue biopsy was performed, there may be a small amount of blood in the first stool after the colonoscopy. However, excessive bleeding should be reported immediately to the health care provider (Chart 56-5). If the procedure was performed in an ambulatory care setting, the client will need another person to provide transportation home. The client should avoid driving for 8 to 12 hours after the procedure because of the effects of sedation.

If a polyp is detected during a virtual colonoscopy, the client must have an endoscopic procedure at a later time to have it removed. Therefore the advantage of the invasive method is that both diagnostic testing and minor surgical procedures can be done at the same time.

CHART 56-5

BEST PRACTICE for
Care of the Client After a Colonoscopy

- Do not allow the client to take anything by mouth until sedation wears off and the client is alert.
- Take vital signs every 15 to 30 minutes until the client is alert.
- Keep the siderails up until the client is alert.
- Assess for rectal bleeding or blood clots.
- Remind the client that fullness and mild abdominal cramping are expected for several hours.
- Assess for manifestations of bowel perforation, including *severe* abdominal pain and guarding. Fever may occur later.
- Assess for manifestations of hypovolemic shock, including dizziness, light-headedness, decreased blood pressure, tachycardia, pallor, and altered mental status (may be the first sign).
- If the procedure is performed in an ambulatory care setting, arrange for another person to drive the client home.

Proctosigmoidoscopy

Proctosigmoidoscopy is an endoscopic examination of the rectum and sigmoid colon using a flexible or rigid scope. The purpose of this test is to screen for colon cancer, investigate the source of GI bleeding, or diagnose or monitor inflammatory bowel disease. If proctosigmoidoscopy is used as an alternative to colonoscopy for colorectal cancer screening, it is recommended that screening begin at 50 years of age.

The client should have a liquid diet for at least 24 hours before a sigmoidoscopy; a cleansing enema or sodium biphosphate (Fleet's) enema is usually given the morning of the procedure. A laxative may also be prescribed the evening before the test.

For a proctosigmoidoscopy, the client is placed on the left side in the knee-chest position or on a special table in the proctoscopic position. No sedation is required. The endoscope is lubricated and inserted into the anus to the required depth for visualization. Tissue biopsy may be performed during this procedure. The examination usually lasts about 30 minutes.

The client is informed that mild gas pain and flatulence may be experienced from air instilled into the rectum during the examination. If a biopsy was obtained, a small amount of bleeding may be observed. Instruct the client that excessive bleeding should be reported immediately to the health care provider.

Critical Thinking Challenge

In the endoscopy clinic today, you are assigned to a middle-aged man who is having his first colonoscopy. He tells you that his aunt died of colon cancer 5 years ago and he is very worried about the procedure. The client also mentions that he's not sure his wife will be able to leave work to pick him up after the test.

1. How should you respond to his comments about his worries and his aunt's death?
2. What would you tell him about what he can expect during the procedure?
3. What discharge instructions will he need after the procedure is finished? When can you discharge him? Will he be able to drive home alone? Why or why not?

evolve For suggested answer guidelines, go to http://evolve.elsevier.com/Iggy/.

Gastric Analysis

Gastric analysis measures the hydrochloric acid and pepsin content for evaluation of aggressive gastric and duodenal disorders (e.g., Zollinger-Ellison syndrome). There are two tests in gastric analysis: basal gastric secretion and gastric acid stimulation. Basal gastric secretion measures the secretion of hydrochloric acid between meals. If only small amounts of secretion are collected, a follow-up gastric stimulation test is given.

The client is NPO for at least 12 hours before the test. Alcohol, tobacco, and medications that may affect gastric secretion are avoided for 24 hours before the study. A nasogastric (NG) tube is inserted and gastric residual contents are aspirated and discarded.

The NG tube is attached to suctioning equipment for collecting the contents at 15-minute intervals for 1 hour. Samples are collected and labeled with basal acid output (BAO), time, and volume of each specimen.

For the gastric acid stimulation test, the NG tube is left in place, and a drug that stimulates gastric acid secretion (e.g., pentagastrin or betazole dihydrochloride [Histalog]) is given subcutaneously. Fifteen minutes after injection of the drug, specimens are again collected at 15-minute intervals for 1 hour. Samples are collected and labeled with maximal acid output (MAO), time, and volume of each specimen.

Depressed levels of gastric secretion suggest the presence of gastric carcinoma. Increased levels of gastric secretion indicate Zollinger-Ellison syndrome and duodenal ulcers (see Chapter 59).

After the test is completed, the NG tube is removed and the client can resume normal eating patterns. No other follow-up is necessary.

Ultrasonography

Ultrasonography is a technique in which high-frequency, inaudible vibratory sound waves are passed through the body via a transducer; the echoes of the sound waves created are then recorded. The echoes are converted into images and photographed for analysis. Ultrasound testing is commonly used to image soft tissues, such as the liver, the spleen, the pancreas, the gallbladder, and the biliary system. The advantages of ultrasonography are that it is painless, noninvasive, and requires no radiation.

The client may be fasting depending on the abdominal organs to be examined. Inform the client that it will be necessary to lie still during the study. He or she is instructed to drink 1 to 2 L of fluid just before the test, because a full bladder is necessary for accurate visualization.

The client is placed in a prone or supine position. The technician applies insulating gel to the end of the transducer and on the area of the abdomen under study. This gel allows airtight contact of the transducer with the skin. The technician moves the transducer back and forth over the skin until the desired images are obtained. The study takes about 15 to 30 minutes. No follow-up care is necessary after ultrasonography.

Endoscopic Ultrasonography

Endoscopic ultrasonography (EUS) provides images of the gastrointestinal (GI) wall and high-resolution images of the digestive organs. The ultrasonography is performed through the endoscope. This procedure is useful in diagnosing the presence of lymph node tumors, mucosal tumors, and tumors of the pancreas, stomach, and rectum. The client preparation and follow-up care are similar to the preparation and follow-up care for both endoscopy and ultrasonography.

Liver-Spleen Scan

A liver-spleen scan uses IV injection of a radioactive material that is taken up primarily by the liver and secondarily by the spleen. The scan evaluates the liver and the spleen for tumors or abscesses, organ size and location, and vascularity. This scan is useful in evaluating hepatocellular disease.

Instruct the client about the need to lie still during the scanning. The client is assured that the colloid injection has only small amounts of radioactivity and is not dangerous. Ask female clients of childbearing age if they may be pregnant or are currently breastfeeding. The radionuclide can be found in breast milk, and radiation from x-rays should be avoided in pregnancy.

The technician or the physician gives the radioactive injection through an IV line, and a wait of about 15 minutes is necessary for uptake. The client is placed in many different positions while the scanning takes place. No follow-up care is necessary after a liver scan.

The client should be instructed that the radionuclide is eliminated from the body through the urine in 24 hours. Careful handwashing following toileting will decrease the exposure to any radiation present in the urine.

GET READY for the NCLEX Examination!

KEY POINTS

Safe Effective Care Environment

- Check for the return of the gag reflex after an upper endoscopic procedure before offering fluids or food; aspiration may occur if the gag reflex is not intact.
- Monitor vital signs carefully for the client having any endoscopic procedure and conscious sedation.
- Monitor clients having a percutaneous transhepatic cholangiogram (PTC) for bleeding, the most common and life-threatening complication.

Health Promotion and Maintenance

- Teach clients to limit caffeine and alcohol in their diets to reduce risk of gastrointestinal health problems.
- If the client is having an endoscopic procedure on an ambulatory basis, remind him or her to have someone available to drive him or her home due to the effects of conscious sedation.
- Teach clients having invasive colon diagnostic procedures to follow instructions carefully for the bowel preparation before testing; the bowel must be clear to allow visualization of the colon.
- Instruct the client to drink plenty of fluids and take a laxative as prescribed to eliminate barium if used during diagnostic testing.
- Teach clients having a PTC to report pain following the procedure, which could indicate bleeding.

Psychosocial Integrity

- Because most clients do not openly express their elimination patterns and complaints, provide support and education.
- Remember that problems of digestion, nutrition, and elimination can markedly affect lifestyle.

Physiological Integrity

- Assess and report any complications of GI testing to the health care provider.
- Review laboratory results, report abnormal findings to the health care provider.

ADDITIONAL STUDY RESOURCES

Go to your Student CD ROM for Review Questions for the NCLEX Examination.

evolve Go to http://evolve.elsevier.com/Iggy/ for Integrated Management of Care Questions for the NCLEX Examination.

SELECTED BIBLIOGRAPHY

Avunduk, C. (2002). *Manual of gastroenterology: Diagnosis and therapy* (3rd ed.). Philadelphia: Lippincott Williams & Wilkins.

Carpenito, L.J. (2001). *Nursing diagnosis: Application to clinical practice* (9th ed.). Philadelphia: Lippincott Williams & Wilkins.

Donley, K.M. (2003). Surfing an acidic wave: pH monitoring technologies swim in sea of innovation. *EndoNurse, 3*(1), 22-24.

Dykes, C.M. (2001). Virtual colonoscopy: A new approach for colorectal cancer screening. *Gastroenterology Nursing, 24*(1), 5-11.

Given Imaging. (2002). M2A Capsule Endoscopy: Given diagnostic system. (Available from Given Imaging, Inc., Oakbrook Technology Center, 5555 Oakbrook Parkway, # 355, Norcross, GA 30093.

Gordon, M. (2002). *Manual of nursing diagnosis* (10th ed.). St. Louis: Mosby.

Huether, S.E. (2002). Structure and function of the digestive system. In K.L. McCance & S.E. Huether (Eds.), *Pathophysiology: The biologic basis for disease in adults & children* (4th ed., pp. 1231-1260). St. Louis: Mosby.

Jarvis, C. (2004). *Physical examination and health assessment* (4th ed.). Philadelphia: W. B. Saunders.

National Institutes of Health. (2000). National digestive disease information clearinghouse publications. Available at http://www.nih.gov.

Pagana, K.D. & Pagana, T.J. (2002). *Mosby's manual of diagnostic and laboratory tests* (2nd ed.). St. Louis: Mosby.

Price, A.S. (2003). Primary and secondary prevention of colorectal cancer. *Gastroenterology Nursing, 26*(2), 73-81.

Shier, D., Butler, J., & Lewis, R. (2003). Digestive system. In *Hole's human anatomy and physiology* (10th ed., pp. 655-702). Boston: McGraw-Hill.

Skidmore-Roth, L. (2004). *Mosby's nursing drug reference.* St. Louis: Mosby.

Society of Gastroenterology Nurses and Associates. (2004). *Gastroenterology nursing: A core curriculum* (3rd ed.). St. Louis: Mosby.

Whitney, E.N., et al. (2000). Nutrition assessment: History, drug history, and physical examination. In *Nutrition for health and health care* (2nd ed., pp. 299-319). St. Paul, MN: West.

Yu, M. (2002). M2A Capsule Endoscopy: A breakthrough diagnostic toll for small intestine imaging. *Gastroenterology Nursing, 25*(1), 24-27.

CHAPTER 57

Interventions for Clients with Oral Cavity Problems

KARRIE K. DIETZEN

LEARNING OUTCOMES

After studying this chapter, you should be able to:

1. Develop a teaching plan for clients who have stomatitis.
2. Explain the common causes of malignant oral tumors.
3. Describe health promotion strategies to prevent oral cancer.
4. Identify common nursing diagnoses for clients with oral cancer.
5. Prioritize postoperative care for clients undergoing surgery for oral cancer.
6. Develop a teaching plan for community-based care of clients with oral cancer.
7. Plan care for clients who have disorders of the salivary glands.

Go to your Student CD-ROM for Review Questions for the NCLEX Examination keyed to these Learning Outcomes.

Oral cavity disorders can severely impact speech, nutrition, body image, and overall quality of life. Although there are numerous oral health problems, this chapter discusses the most common disorders. Nurses play an important role in maintaining and restoring oral cavity health in their clients through nursing interventions and client education. Chart 57-1 lists ways for clients to maintain a healthy oral cavity.

STOMATITIS

PATHOPHYSIOLOGY

Stomatitis is characterized by painful single or multiple ulcerations of the oral mucosa that appear as inflammation and denudation of the oral mucosa, impairing the protective lining of the mouth. These ulcerations are commonly referred to as canker sores. The ulceration causes pain, and open areas predispose the individual to bleeding and infection. Mild erythema (redness) may respond to topical treatments, whereas extensive stomatitis may require treatment with opioid analgesics. Stomatitis is classified according to the cause of the inflammation. *Primary stomatitis* includes aphthous (noninfectious) stomatitis, herpes simplex stomatitis, and traumatic ulcers. *Secondary stomatitis* generally results from infection by opportunistic viruses, fungi, or bacteria in clients who are immunocompromised.

A common type of secondary stomatitis is caused by *Candida albicans.* **Candidiasis,** also called moniliasis, is a fungal infection resulting from an overgrowth of normal flora. In most cases, antibiotic therapy destroys the normal flora that usually prevents fungal infections; thus candidiasis can occur in clients receiving long-term antibiotic therapy. Candidiasis of the oral cavity is also common in clients undergoing immunosuppressive therapy (chemotherapy, radiation, steroid therapy, or antirejection medication). In addition, the mouth is susceptible to the effects of human immunodeficiency virus (HIV) disease; therefore HIV-positive individuals commonly present with candidiasis.

CONSIDERATIONS FOR OLDER ADULTS

Older adults are especially at high risk for candidiasis because aging causes a decrease in immune function. The risk increases for clients who are diabetic, malnourished, or under emotional stress. Older adults who wear dentures may use soft denture liners that provide comfort but can also be colonized by *C. albicans,* contributing to denture stomatitis.

CHART 57-1

CLIENT EDUCATION GUIDE
Maintaining a Healthy Oral Cavity

- Perform a self-examination of your mouth every month; report any unusual finding.
- Be sure to eat a balanced diet.
- Brush and floss your teeth every day. Set a routine and keep to it.
- Manage your stress as much as possible; learn how to maintain your emotional health.
- Avoid contact with agents that may cause inflammation of the mouth, such as mouthwashes that contain alcohol.
- If possible, avoid medications that may cause inflammation of the mouth or reduce the flow of saliva.
- Be aware of any changes in the occlusion of your teeth, mouth pain, or swelling; seek medical attention promptly.
- See your dentist regularly: have problems attended to promptly.
- If you wear dentures, make sure they are in good repair and fit properly.

Etiology and Genetic Risk

Stomatitis can result from infection, allergy, vitamin deficiency, systemic disease, irritants (e.g., tobacco and alcohol), chemotherapy, or radiation. Infectious agents, such as bacteria and viruses, may have a role in the development of recurrent stomatitis. Although viruses have not been successfully cultured from aphthous lesions, recurrent lesions have been associated with latent zoster or cytomegalovirus (CMV).

Certain foods may trigger allergic responses that result in the formation of aphthous ulcers, although this remains controversial. Foods such as coffee, potatoes, cheese, nuts, citrus fruits, and gluten may be precipitating factors. In some cases, strict elimination diets have resulted in the improvement of ulcers. Deficiencies in complex B vitamins, folate, zinc, and iron associated with malnutrition can contribute to the formation of recurrent stomatitis. Recurrent aphthous ulcers (RAU) are reported to run in families, but may be environmental rather than genetic (Rini & Bloom, 2002).

Systemic diseases such as HIV infection, chronic renal failure, and inflammatory bowel disease can also predispose a person to stomatitis. Treatment of cancer with antineoplastic agents or radiation can predispose an individual to the development of painful stomatitis or mucositis. The severity of stomatitis is related to the type and dose of therapy as well as to client-related factors, such as pretreatment oral health. (See Chapter 28 for nursing care of the client undergoing radiation and chemotherapy.)

Incidence/Prevalence

Aphthous stomatitis is the most common oral lesion. Recurrent aphthous lesions have been found to affect at least 30% of the population (Scully & Shotts, 2001). Data for other types of stomatitis are not readily available.

WOMEN'S HEALTH CONSIDERATIONS

A hormonal influence has been suggested in relation to women and aphthous stomatitis. Women generally have a higher prevalence of the disorder, with an increased incidence of oral ulceration during the luteal phase of the menstrual cycle. A moderation or absence of lesions during pregnancy has been attributed to increased steroid levels.

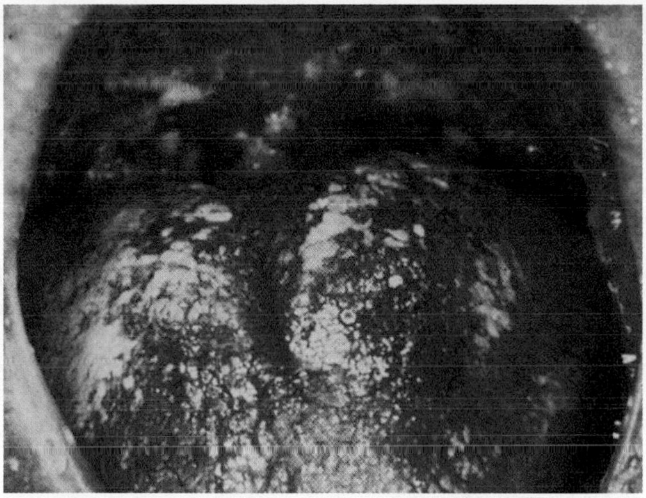

Figure 57-1 ■ Oral candidiasis. (From Radford, J., & Thatcher, N. [1988]. The toxicity of cancer chemotherapy in adults. Cancer Care, 5, 4-7.)

COLLABORATIVE MANAGEMENT

Assessment

HISTORY

When performing an oral assessment, collect information concerning possible etiologic factors, such as recent infections, a history of stomatitis, nutritional compromise, oral hygiene habits, oral trauma, stress, or immunocompromise. A medication history should also be collected, including over-the-counter (OTC) agents and herbals. Document the course of the current outbreak, and ascertain whether episodes of stomatitis are recurrent. Ask the client if the lesions interfere with swallowing or eating.

PHYSICAL ASSESSMENT/CLINICAL MANIFESTATIONS

The symptoms of stomatitis range in severity from a dry, painful mouth to open ulcerations, predisposing the client to infection. Mouth ulcerations can alter nutritional status as a result of difficulty with food ingestion or swallowing. When they are severe, stomatitis and the accompanying edema have the potential to compromise the airway.

Stomatitis lesions appear most commonly on the buccal mucosa, soft palate, oropharyngeal mucosa, and lateral and ventral areas of the tongue. The painful lesions appear as shallow ulcerations covered by a whitish gray pseudomembrane and outer erythematous ring (Jarvis, 2004).

In oral candidiasis, a type of yeast infection, white plaque-like lesions appear on the tongue, palate, pharynx, and buccal mucosa (Figure 57-1). When these patches are wiped away, the underlying surface appears red and sore (Walton, Miller, & Tordecilla, 2001). Clients rarely complain of actual pain but describe the lesions as dry or hot.

While examining the oral cavity, wear nonsterile gloves for protection against infection. Adequate lighting, including a flashlight or penlight, and a tongue blade facilitate the examination. Assess the oral cavity for lesions, coating, cracking, and fissures. Characteristics of the lesions are described in terms of location, size, shape, color, and drainage. Any odors are noted and described.

If lesions are noted along the pharynx, and the client reports dysphagia or pain on swallowing, you should suspect that the lesions might extend down the esophagus. Additional diagnostic testing may be required.

The physical examination should also include examination of the cervical and submandibular lymph nodes for swelling. Any elevation in temperature is noted.

LABORATORY ASSESSMENT

Laboratory tests are usually not needed. However, serum albumin, vitamin B_{12}, folate, and iron levels may be obtained if nutritional status appears to be compromised. A complete blood count may reveal the presence of infection, neutropenia, or anemia. Cytologic; routine, viral, or bacterial cultures; and Gram stain testing can assist in distinguishing organisms causing the stomatitis ulcerations.

Interventions

Interventions for stomatitis are aimed toward the promotion of oral health through meticulous oral hygiene and careful food selection.

Oral Hygiene. When providing oral care for your client, use a soft-bristled toothbrush or disposable foam swabs to stimulate gums and clean the oral cavity. Encourage frequent rinsing of the mouth with any of the following: sodium bicarbonate solution, warm saline, or hydrogen peroxide solution. The client should avoid commercial mouthwashes because they have high alcohol content, causing a burning sensation in irritated or ulcerated oral mucosa.

Instruct the client or provide mouth care every 2 hours and twice at night if the stomatitis is not controlled. Frequent gentle mouth care enhances debridement of ulcerated lesions and can prevent superinfections. Frequent oral care also promotes a general feeling of well-being. Chart 57-2 lists measures for special oral care.

Drug Therapy. Medications used include antimicrobials, immune modulators, symptomatic topicals, and complementary and alternative therapies.

Antimicrobial Agents. Antimicrobials, including antibiotics and antifungals, may be necessary for control of infection in the client with stomatitis. Tetracycline syrup (swish/swallow) 250 mg/10 mL four times daily for 10 days may be prescribed, especially for RAU. The client rinses for 2 minutes and swallows the syrup, thus obtaining both topical and systemic therapy. Minocycline swish/swallow and chlorhexidine mouthwashes may also be used.

A regimen of intravenous (IV) acyclovir (Zovirax) is typically prescribed for immunocompromised clients who contract herpes simplex stomatitis. Acyclovir is typically administered to clients with normal renal function at a dose of 5 mg/kg, infused at a constant rate over a 1-hour period, every 8 hours for 7 days. Clients with competent immune systems may be given acyclovir in oral or topical form.

For fungal infections, nystatin (Mycostatin) oral suspension 600,000 units four times daily for 7 to 10 days is the agent most often used. The client swishes and swallows the topical preparation. Ice pop troches (lozenges) of the antifungal preparation allow the medication to slowly dissolve, and the cold provides an analgesic effect.

Anti-Inflammatory Agents and Immune Modulators. Topical triamcinolone in benzocaine (Kenalog in Orabase) and oral dexamethasone elixir used as a swish/expectorate preparation are commonly used for stomatitis, especially recurrent aphthous ulcers (RAU).

CHART 57-2

BEST PRACTICE for
Care of Clients with Problems of the Oral Cavity

- Remove dentures if the client has severe stomatitis or oral pain.
- Encourage the client to perform oral hygiene, or provide it after each meal and as often as needed.
- Increase mouth care to every 2 hours or more often if stomatitis is not controlled.
- Use a soft toothbrush, toothette, or gauze for oral care.
- Encourage frequent rinsing of the mouth with hydrogen peroxide, warm saline, sodium bicarbonate (baking soda) solution, or a combination of these solutions.
- Teach the client to avoid commercial mouthwashes and lemon-glycerin swabs.
- Assist the client in selecting soft, bland, and nonacidic foods.
- Apply topical analgesics or anesthetics as prescribed by the physician and monitor their effectiveness.

Immune modulating agents that may be prescribed include the following:

- Oral levamisole
- Topical amlexanox (Aphthasol)
- Topical granulocyte-macrophage colony-stimulating factor (GM-CSF)
- Thalidomide

The exact mechanism for how these drugs work is not clear. However, they may inhibit release of mediators that contribute to the inflammation seen in clients with RAU (Rini & Bloom, 2002).

Symptomatic Topical Agents. Other agents can be used to minimize pain, such as over-the-counter (OTC) benzocaine anesthetics (e.g., Orabase, Anbesol) and camphor phenol (Campho-Phenique).

Fifteen mL of 2% viscous lidocaine every 3 hours (maximum of 8 doses per day) can be used as a gargle or mouthwash.

Critical Thinking Challenge

You are a nurse on a busy medical-surgical nursing unit where you are caring for an older adult with cellulites and type 2 diabetes mellitus. She was on oral antibiotics at home before admission yesterday and is now receiving IV antibiotics. The client's daughter states that her mother is not eating well and complains that her mouth is burning and sore. When you check her oral cavity, you note white patches that can be partially scraped away.

1. What problem do you think this client has and why?
2. What risk factors does she have for her oral cavity problem?
3. What treatment will she most likely receive as a result of her problem?
4. How will you describe the special oral care this client needs to your nursing assistant?

evolve For suggested answer guidelines, go to http://evolve.elsevier.com/Iggy/.

ORAL TUMORS

Oral cavity tumors can be benign, premalignant, or malignant. Whether benign or malignant, tumors of the oral cavity impact many daily functions. Activities such as swallowing, chewing, and speaking can be affected. Pain accompanying the tumor can also impose limitations on daily activities and self-care. Oral cavity tumors affect body image, especially if treatment involves removal of the tongue or part of the mandible, or requires a tracheostomy.

Premalignant Lesions

Leukoplakia

PATHOPHYSIOLOGY

Leukoplakia presents as slowly developing changes in the oral mucous membranes that are characterized by thickened, white, firmly attached patches. These patches appear slightly raised and sharply circumscribed. Ninety percent of leukoplakial lesions are benign; however, about 7% of lesions become malignant after a mean of 8 years (Palkhivala, 2003). Although leukoplakia can be found anywhere on the oral mucosa, lesions on the lips or tongue are more likely to progress to malignancy.

Etiology

Leukoplakia results from mechanical factors that cause long-term oral mucous membrane irritation, such as poorly fitting dentures, chronic cheek nibbling, or broken or poorly repaired teeth. In addition, oral hairy leukoplakia can be found in clients with HIV infection. The use of tobacco products has also been implicated in the development of leukoplakia, which is sometimes referred to as "smoker's patch." Oral leukoplakia can be confused with oral candidal infection. However, unlike candidal infection, leukoplakia cannot be removed by scraping.

Incidence/Prevalence

Leukoplakia is the most common oral lesion among adults. Oral hairy leukoplakia is an early manifestation of HIV infection and is highly correlated with progression from HIV infection to acquired immunodeficiency syndrome (AIDS). Leukoplakia not associated with HIV infection is more often seen in people over 40 years of age. Men have twice the incidence of leukoplakia that women have, but this ratio is changing because increasing numbers of women are smoking.

Erythroplakia

Erythroplakia presents as a red, velvety mucosal lesion on the surface of the oral mucosa. There is a higher degree of malignant transformation in erythroplakia than in leukoplakia. As such, these lesions should be regarded with suspicion and analyzed by biopsy. Erythroplakia is most commonly found on the floor of the mouth, tongue, palate, and mandibular mucosa, and it can be difficult to distinguish from inflammatory or immune reactions.

Malignant Tumors

Squamous Cell Carcinoma

PATHOPHYSIOLOGY

More than 90% of oral cancers are squamous cell carcinomas that begin on the surface of the epithelium. Over a period of many years, premalignant (or dysplastic) changes begin. Cells begin to vary in size and shape; alterations in the thickness of the lining of the epithelium develop, resulting in atrophy. These tumors usually grow slowly, and the lesions may be large before the onset of symptoms unless ulceration is present. Mucosal erythroplasia is the earliest sign of oral carcinoma. Oral lesions that appear as red, raised, eroded areas are suspicious for carcinoma.

The American Joint Committee on Cancer has devised the TNM (tumor, node, metastasis) classification system for tumors of the lip and oral cavity. Each lesion is defined by the following:

T–the size of the tumor or degree of penetration
N–the presence, size, number, and location of cervical lymph nodes involved
M–the presence of distant metastasis (spread)

Etiology

Squamous cell carcinoma is the most common oral malignancy. It can be found on the lips, tongue, buccal mucosa, and oropharynx. The major risk factors in the development of oral cancers are increasing age, tobacco use, and alcohol ingestion. Ninety-five percent of all oral cancers occur in people over 40 years of age. Tobacco use in any form (e.g., smoking or chewing tobacco) can increase the risk of cancer. Alcohol ingestion can potentiate the carcinogenic effects of tobacco products.

An increased rate of oral carcinoma is found in individuals with certain occupations, such as textile workers, plumbers, and coal and metal workers. Additional factors, such as sun exposure, poor dietary habits, poor oral hygiene, and infection with the human papillomavirus (HPV) may also contribute to oral cancer (Neville & Day, 2002).

Incidence/Prevalence

Carcinomas of the oral cavity account for about 3% of all cancers in men and 2% of all cancers in women in the United States. Nearly 30,000 new cases are diagnosed each year, with almost 8000 deaths, or 2% of all cancer deaths (American Cancer Society, 2004; Weinberg & Estefan, 2002). Most cancers occur in middle-aged and older individuals, although in recent years more younger adults have been affected, most likely as a result of sun exposure. Oral and oropharyngeal cancers are more common in black individuals than in white individuals, but the reason for this disparity is not known.

Basal Cell Carcinoma

Basal cell carcinoma of the oral cavity occurs primarily on the lips. The lesion is asymptomatic and resembles a raised scab. With time, the lesion evolves into a characteristic ulcer with a raised pearly border. Basal cell carcinomas do not metastasize but can aggressively involve the skin of the face. The major etiologic factor in basal cell carcinoma is exposure to sunlight.

Basal cell carcinoma occurs as a result of the failure of basal cells to mature into keratinocytes. It is the second most common type of oral cancer, but it is much less common than squamous cell carcinoma.

Kaposi's Sarcoma

Kaposi's sarcoma is a malignant lesion that arises in blood vessels. Kaposi's sarcoma is usually painless and appears as a raised purple nodule or plaque. In the mouth the hard palate is the most common site of Kaposi's sarcoma, but it can also be found on the gums, tongue, or tonsils. It is most often associated with AIDS. (See Chapter 25 for a complete discussion of Kaposi's sarcoma.)

Health Promotion/Illness Prevention

In the past decade, dentists and other physicians have begun systematically screening their clients for oral cancer. Oral examination has become a part of the routine dental examination. Individuals should visit a dentist at least once per year for professional dental hygiene and oral examination.

In addition to medical screening, prevention strategies for oral cancer include minimizing sun exposure, including tanning beds, tobacco cessation, and decreasing alcohol intake. Teach clients to follow the guidelines in Chart 57-1 to maintain oral health.

COLLABORATIVE MANAGEMENT

Assessment

HISTORY

A priority for nurses in the prevention and detection of oral cancers is the identification of high-risk groups. Individuals at high risk for developing oral cancer tend to use large amounts of alcohol and tobacco and are over 40 years of age. It is important to conduct a functional assessment. Ask about occupation and exposure to known oral carcinogens or irritants, such as sunlight or other source of ultraviolet radiation. A family history of cancer and a history of previous oral cancer alert health care providers to be especially observant for signs of cancer.

Begin by assessing the client's routine oral hygiene regimen and use of dentures or oral appliances, which might add to discomfort or mechanically irritate the mucosa. Ask the client about oral bleeding, which might indicate an ulcerative lesion. Determine the status of the client's past and current appetite and nutritional state, including difficulty with chewing or swallowing. A continuing trend of weight loss may be related to metastasis, heavy alcohol intake, difficulty in eating or chewing, or an underlying disorder.

PHYSICAL ASSESSMENT/CLINICAL MANIFESTATIONS

Common signs and symptoms of oral carcinoma include unusual lumps or thickening of the buccal mucosa or red or white patches appearing on the gums, tongue, or oral mucous membranes. Cancers of the lip are strongly associated with chronic exposure to the sun and often present as a sore that fails to heal. Soreness, pain, or a burning sensation may also be present. In later stages, the client may experience difficulty chewing or swallowing. Advanced cancers of the tongue can cause pain that radiates to the ear. Cervical lymph nodes may become enlarged, hardened, and fixed secondary to metastatic invasion.

An examination of the oral cavity requires adequate lighting for proper visualization. Thoroughly inspect the oral cavity for any lesions, evidence of pain, or restriction of movement. Using a tongue blade, visually examine all areas of the oral cavity. Carefully note any alteration in speech attributable to tongue restriction. Following inspection, the advanced practice nurse uses bimanual palpation of any visible nodules to determine size and fixation. The cervical lymph nodes should also be palpated (Figure 57-2).

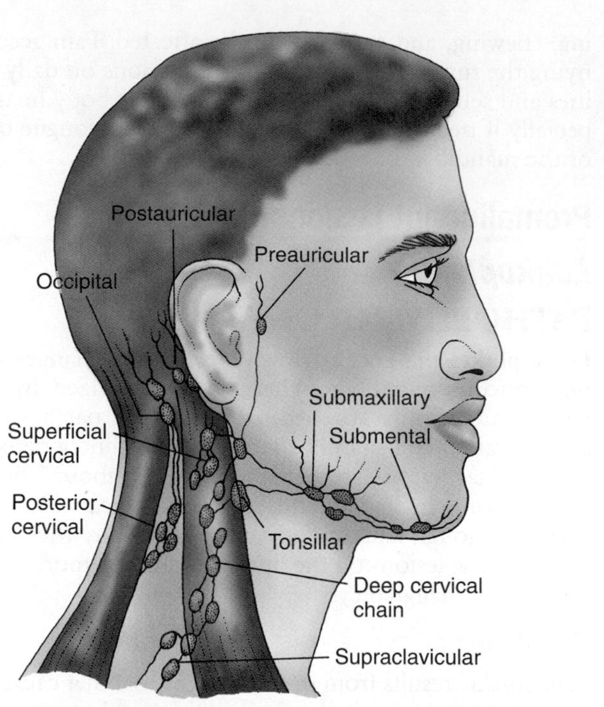

Figure 57-2 ■ The lymph nodes of the cervical region.

PSYCHOSOCIAL ASSESSMENT

The functioning and appearance of the oral cavity are strongly linked with body image and quality of life. Therefore, it is important to assess the impact of oral lesions on the client's self-concept. In addition, assess the client for any educational or cultural needs regarding instruction or therapy. Evaluate the client's support system and past mechanisms of coping.

RADIOGRAPHIC ASSESSMENT

The purpose of radiologic diagnostic tests for cancer of the oral cavity is to assess the extent and spread of the tumor. Computed tomography (CT) scans are helpful in determining the extent of the tumor and lymphatic or bone involvement.

OTHER DIAGNOSTIC ASSESSMENTS

Biopsy is the definitive method for diagnosis of oral cancer. Therefore the physician obtains a needle biopsy specimen of the oral tissue to assess for malignant or premalignant changes. Incisional biopsies may also be performed. An intraoral biopsy can be done with the client under local anesthesia. In very small lesions, an excisional biopsy can permit complete tumor removal. Magnetic resonance imaging (MRI) is useful in detecting perineural involvement and in evaluating thickness in cancers of the tongue. Both CT and MRI can be used to determine metastatic spread to the liver or lungs if further staging of the disease is warranted.

An aqueous solution of toluidine blue 1% can be applied to oral lesions to determine if they are malignant. This preparation stains malignant lesions, leaving normal tissue unaffected. However, a lesion that is the result of an inflammatory process may also pick up the stain, leading to a false-positive result. Although a biopsy is still needed to confirm a cancer diagnosis, toluidine blue may be useful for screening high-risk individuals.

◆Analysis

COMMON NURSING DIAGNOSES AND COLLABORATIVE PROBLEMS

The following are priority nursing diagnoses for clients with malignant tumors of the oral cavity:

1. Risk for Ineffective Airway Clearance related to obstructed airway by the tumor, edema, or secretions
2. Impaired Oral Mucous Membrane related to pathologic conditions from the tumor

ADDITIONAL NURSING DIAGNOSES AND COLLABORATIVE PROBLEMS

In addition to the common nursing diagnoses, clients with tumors of the oral cavity may have one or more of the following:

- Impaired Verbal Communication related to physical barrier or anatomic defect
- Disturbed Body Image related to surgery
- Acute Pain related to physical injury
- Risk for Infection related to invasive procedures
- Impaired Swallowing related to oral cavity or oropharnygeal abnormalities
- Imbalanced Nutrition: Less Than Body Requirements related to inability to ingest food
- Potential for Metastasis

◆Planning and Implementation

RISK FOR INEFFECTIVE AIRWAY CLEARANCE

NOC **PLANNING: EXPECTED OUTCOMES.** The client with a malignant tumor of the oral cavity is expected to have open, clear tracheobronchial passages for air exchange. Indicators include that the client will have noncompromised:

- Ease of breathing
- Respiratory rate
- Respiratory rhythm
- Ability to move sputum out of airway

INTERVENTIONS. Extensive tumor involvement and tenacious secretions can inhibit airway patency. Nursing measures for maintaining airway patency is a primary focus. Assessment should be centered on the client's dyspnea, inability to cough effectively, or inability to swallow.

NONSURGICAL MANAGEMENT. Assess for difficulty breathing and decreased air exchange and dysphagia. Institute measures to increase air exchange, remove secretions, and prevent aspiration (Chart 57-3).

NIC **Airway Management.** Assess for dyspnea resulting from the obstructive presence of the tumor or from excessive secretions. Assess the quality, rate, and depth of respirations, and auscultate the lungs for decreased or absent ventilation or for the presence of adventitious sounds. If oral secretions are excessive or thick, aid the client in expectorating secretions. To increase air exchange, place the client in a semi-Fowler's or high Fowler's position to maximize ventilation potential. Secretions can be mobilized by encouraging fluids to help liquefy secretions, by chest physiotherapy, and by measures to encourage effective coughing.

CHART 57-3

NIC INTERVENTION ACTIVITIES for The Client with Oral Cancer

Airway Management: *Facilitation of patency of air passages*

- Position client to maximize ventilation potential.
- Remove secretions by encouraging coughing or by suctioning.
- Instruct how to cough effectively.
- Auscultate breath sounds, noting areas of decreased or absent ventilation and presence of adventitious sounds.
- Administer humidified air or oxygen, as appropriate.
- Position to alleviate dyspnea.
- Monitor respiratory and oxygenation status, as appropriate.

Cough Enhancement: *Promotion of deep inhalation by the client with subsequent generation of high intrathoracic pressures and compression of underlying lung parenchyma for the forceful expulsion of air*

- Assist client to a sitting position with the head slightly flexed, shoulders relaxed, and knees flexed.
- Encourage client to take several deep breaths.
- Encourage client to take a deep breath, hold it for 2 seconds, and cough two or three times in succession.
- Instruct client to inhale deeply, bend forward slightly, and perform three or four huffs (against an open glottis).
- Instruct client to inhale deeply several times, to exhale slowly, and to cough at the end of exhalation.
- Instruct client to follow coughing with several maximal inhalation breaths.
- Promote systemic fluid hydration, as appropriate.

Aspiration Precautions: *Prevention or minimization of risk factors in the client at risk for aspiration*

- Monitor level of consciousness, cough reflex, gag reflex, and swallowing ability.
- Monitor pulmonary status.
- Maintain an airway.
- Position upright 90 degrees or as far as possible.
- Feed in small amounts.
- Avoid liquids or use thickening agent.
- Offer foods or liquids that can be formed into a bolus before swallowing.
- Cut food into small pieces.
- Request medication in elixir form.
- Break or crush pills before administration.
- Keep head of bed elevated 30 to 45 minutes after eating.

NIC intervention activities selected from Dochterman, J.M., & Bulechek, G.M. (Eds.) (2004). *Nursing interventions classification (NIC)* (4th ed.). St. Louis: Mosby. No part of this work is to be altered without prior written permission from the Publisher.

If oral secretions remain problematic, oral suction equipment with a dental tip or a tonsil tip (Yankauer catheter) can be used.

If edema is associated with oral cavity lesions, the client may receive steroids for reducing inflammation. Antibiotics may be prescribed if infection is present because infection can increase inflammation and edema. A cool mist supplied by a face tent may assist with oxygen transport and control of edema.

NIC **Cough Enhancement.** Measures that promote deep inhalation generate high intrathoracic pressure, which assists the client in producing an effective cough to mobilize secretions. Assist the client to a sitting position with the head slightly flexed and the knees flexed. Then instruct the client to take several deep breaths, hold the breath for 2 seconds, and then cough two to three times in succession. He or she is instructed to follow coughing with several maximal inhalation breaths. The client can also be instructed to enhance coughing by inhaling deeply several times and coughing at the end of exhalation.

NIC **Aspiration Precautions.** Aspiration precautions prevent or minimize the risk factors associated with aspiration. The client's level of consciousness, gag reflex, and ability to swallow are assessed. To prevent aspiration, place the client sitting upright at 90 degrees (high Fowler's position). As a precaution, suction equipment should be kept nearby. Clients at risk of aspiration should be fed in small amounts. Thickened liquids can be used as an aid to prevent aspiration.

SURGICAL MANAGEMENT. The client with an oral lesion may require a tracheostomy. This may be due to the extent of surgical excision required to remove the tumor, or it may be due to excessive edema. A tracheostomy re-establishes a patent airway and can be performed by the physician with the client under local or general anesthesia. The tracheostomy tube is usually left in place until edema resolves and the airway is patent. If the tumor is the major cause of the oral airway blockage, however, the tracheostomy may be maintained through the perioperative period until oral healing begins. In some cases, it may be permanent. After postoperative edema resolves, the client is **decannulated** (i.e., the tracheostomy tube is removed). (Refer to Chapter 31 for nursing care of the client with a tracheostomy.)

IMPAIRED ORAL MUCOUS MEMBRANE

NOC **PLANNING: EXPECTED OUTCOMES.** The client with a malignant tumor of the oral cavity is expected to maintain or re-establish structural intactness and normal physiologic function of mucous membranes. Indicators include that the client will not have the following:

- Mucous membrane lesions
- Induration
- Erythema

INTERVENTIONS. Both the presence of tumors of the oral cavity and the effects of treatment of oral tumors pose threats to the integrity of the oral mucosa. Oral cavity lesions can be treated by surgical excision, by nonsurgical treatments such as radiation or chemotherapy, or by a combination of treatments (referred to as multimodal therapy). Multimodal therapy is the treatment option that incurs the most cost. Nursing interventions focus primarily on the restoration and maintenance oral health.

NONSURGICAL MANAGEMENT. The purpose of nonsurgical management is to promote tissue healing and to maintain and promote oral hygiene for the client with oral lesions.

Oral Care. It is important to work with the client to establish an oral hygiene routine. Ideally, oral hygiene is performed every 2 hours for ulcerated lesions, infection, or in the immediate postoperative period. Modifications might be needed because of oral discomfort, bleeding, or edema. Oral care with a soft-bristled toothbrush is preferred. In the event of a fall in the platelet count below 40,000/mm^3, the client should be switched to an ultrasoft "chemobrush." The use of "toothettes" or a disposable foam brush is discouraged because these products may not adequately control bacteremia-promoting plaque. Lubricant can be applied to moisten the lips and oral mucosa as needed.

Clients with ulcerative or bleeding lesions should avoid using commercial mouthwashes and lemon-glycerin swabs. Commercial mouthwashes contain alcohol, and lemon-glycerin swabs are acidic. These substances can cause a burning sensation and contribute to drying of the oral mucous membranes. Encourage frequent rinsing of the mouth with sodium bicarbonate solution, warm saline, or hydrogen peroxide solution (see also Chart 57-2).

Radiation Therapy. Radiation therapy has been used alone as well as in conjunction with surgery and chemotherapy in the treatment of cancer of the oral cavity. The goal of radiation therapy is tumor eradication while preserving function and appearance. There are several ways to apply radiotherapy. In collaboration with the client, the physician chooses the best mode on the basis of the tumor site and staging.

Radiation therapy for oral cancers can be given by external beam or interstitial implantation. External-beam radiation passes through the skin or mucous membrane to the tumor site. Typically, treatments are given as five daily treatments per week over a 6- to 9-week period. Special precautions are taken to minimize the dose of radiation to the brain or spinal cord. Another option is the implantation of radioactive substances (interstitial radiation therapy) either to boost the dosage or to deliver a radiation dose close to the tumor bed. This form of implant therapy can be curative in early stage lesions in the floor of the mouth or anterior tongue or to add an additional boost of radiation to a tumor that received external-beam radiation.

Interstitial radiation is used for smaller lesions that do not infiltrate surrounding tissues. The following can be radioactive materials:

- Seeds, which are permanently implanted into the tissue (usually for tumors unable to be completely excised or in neck nodes)
- Needles or wires, which are removed at the end of therapy
- Radiation catheters or holders, which are loaded with radioactive materials
- A "mold" of radioactive material placed directly over the lesion for a specific time

With the exception of radioactive seeds, which have a low level of activity, clients receiving interstitial radiation are usually hospitalized for the duration of treatment. Radiation isolation precautions must be instituted while the materials are active or in place. A tracheostomy may be required with interstitial implants because of edema and increased oral secretions. (See Chapter 28 for nursing care of clients undergoing radiation therapy.)

Chemotherapy. The client may receive one or more chemotherapeutic agents. The advantages of chemotherapy instead of, or as an adjunct to, surgery or radiation for cancer of the oral cavity continue to be evaluated.

It is important to instruct the client undergoing chemotherapy about the anticipated side effects of the medication, which vary with each antineoplastic agent. Administer antiemetic medications as prescribed and provide other comfort measures as needed (see Chapter 28 for care of clients receiving chemotherapy).

SURGICAL MANAGEMENT. The physician can often excise small, noninvasive lesions of the oral cavity in an ambulatory setting with local anesthesia. The surgical defect is usually small enough to be closed by sutures. These smaller lesions are also responsive to carbon dioxide laser therapy or *cryotherapy* (extreme cold application), which can be performed as an ambulatory care procedure in a surgical center (but may require general anesthesia).

Small oral cancers are equally responsive to radiation therapy and to surgery. More invasive lesions (stage III and IV) require more extensive surgical excision and result in a greater loss of function and disfigurement. Not all lesions can be excised by the peroral approach (through the mouth). The goal of surgical resection is removal of the tumor with a surgical margin that is free of tumor involvement.

Preoperative Care. Before excision of a lesion in the oral cavity, it is important to assess and document the client's level of understanding of the disease process, the rationale for the surgery, and the planned intervention. Problems associated with cancer therapy can be minimized or optimally managed with client preparation and instruction (Robins-Sadler et al., 2003). Information is reinforced as needed. Family members or other caregivers are included in the health teaching.

For small, local excisions, postoperative restrictions include a liquid diet for a day and then advancing as tolerated. There are no activity limitations, and postoperative analgesics are prescribed.

Instructions for the client undergoing large surgical resections may include, but are not limited to, the following postoperative expectations:

- Placement of a temporary tracheostomy and the concomitant nursing care (oxygen therapy and suctioning)
- Temporary loss of speech due to the tracheostomy
- Frequent monitoring of postoperative vital signs
- Nothing by mouth (remain on NPO status) until intraoral suture lines are healed
- Need to have IV lines in place for medication delivery and hydration
- Postoperative medications and activity (out of bed on the first postoperative day)
- Possibility of surgical drains

Because communication is interrupted, you need to assess the client's ability to read and write. In collaboration with the client, select the method of communication to use postoperatively with staff and family members (e.g., Magic Slate, computer, picture board, or pad and pencil).

Operative Procedures. Three factors influence the extent of surgery performed for oral cancers: the size and location of the tumor, tumor invasion into the bone, and the presence of metastasis to neck lymph nodes. Small, noninvasive tumors located near the mouth opening can be excised perriorally (inside the mouth). Otherwise, an external approach may be used. The most extensive oral operations are composite resections, which combine partial or total **glossectomy** (tongue removal) and partial mandibulectomy. In the *commando* (co-mandible) *procedure,* the surgeon excises a segment of the mandible with the oral lesion, usually in conjunction with a radical neck dissection (see Chapter 32).

Metastasis to cervical lymph nodes usually indicates a poor prognosis for clients with cancer of the oral cavity. In clients with cervical node metastasis, a neck dissection may also be performed. A radical neck dissection involves the removal of submental; submandibular; upper, mid, and lower jugular; and posterior triangular levels of the cervical lymph nodes, along with cranial nerve XI, the internal jugular vein, and the sternocleidomastoid muscle. Modified and selective neck dissections may be done in individuals with minimal lymph node involvement.

CHART 57-4

FOCUSED ASSESSMENT of
The Postoperative Older Adult with Oral Cancer

- Assess the mouth and surrounding tissues for candidiasis, mucositis, pain, and loss of appetite and taste.
- Monitor the client's weight.
- Monitor nutritional and fluid intake.
- Assess for difficulty in eating or speech.
- Assess pain status and measures used to control pain.
- Monitor the client's response to medications.
- Identify psychosocial problems, such as depression, anxiety, and fear.

Postoperative Care. Airway management is a priority postoperatively for the client with cancer of the oral cavity. The client will have a temporary or permanent tracheostomy, requiring intensive nursing care to promote airway clearance. In addition, care must be taken to protect the surgical incision site from mechanical damage and infection. Nursing interventions to relieve pain or discomfort and promote nutrition are also important. Older adults are a special risk for surgery and need to be monitored very carefully (Chart 57-4).

Maintaining Airway Patency. After extensive excision or resection, the most important nursing intervention is maintaining airway patency. The client may not recall on awakening from anesthesia that a tracheostomy tube is in place and may initially panic because of the inability to speak. Remind the client why he or she cannot speak, and provide reassurance that the vocal cords are intact (unless a total laryngectomy has been performed, then the loss of voice is permanent). Ensure that the predetermined method of communication is available for the client, family members, and staff.

Nursing interventions are aimed at keeping the temporary tracheostomy patent. Frequent suctioning, using sterile technique, may be required for excessive secretions. Humidified oxygen may be prescribed to help liquefy secretions in the early postoperative phase. After the immediate postoperative phase, the client may be able to cough effectively enough to decrease the need for suctioning. After oral edema has decreased and the tracheostomy tube has been changed to a noncuffed type, the client can speak by plugging the stoma with the fingertip. Collaboration between the nurse and physician determine the appropriateness of instructing the client in this technique. (See Chapter 31 for care of the client with a tracheostomy.)

When the client has been determined to have an adequate airway through the aerodigestive tract and can effectively clear secretions by coughing, the tracheostomy tube may be removed. When the tracheostomy tube is removed, an airtight dressing is placed over the site, and the tracheostomy incision heals without the need for sutures.

Clients who have undergone extensive resection may have slurred speech or difficulty in speaking. A consultation with a speech-language pathologist may be indicated.

Protecting the Operative Area. The surgical incision site requires careful attention to avoid infection. It is important to provide gentle mouth care for cleaning away thick secretions and stimulating the flow of saliva. The delivery of oral care depends on the nature and extent of the surgical procedure. Oral care should be provided every 4 hours in the early postoperative phase. The presence of unusual odors from the mouth can indicate infection. In the early postoperative phase, care must be taken to avoid disruption of the suture line during oral hygiene.

Elevate the head of the bed to at least 30 degrees to assist in decreasing edema by gravity. If skin grafting was done, the nurse inspects the donor site (generally on the anterior thigh) during every nursing shift for bleeding or signs of infection. (See Chapter 32 for specific nursing care of the client with a radical neck dissection.)

Relieving Pain. To provide optimal pain relief in the postoperative period, rely on subjective and objective data to assess the need for analgesics and the effectiveness of the medications given. The goal of pain medication during this period is relief of pain while allowing the client to function at an optimal level. Clients who have undergone surgery for oral carcinomas describe their pain as throbbing or pounding. IV morphine is usually the initial postoperative pain medication given. Tylox or Percocet (Percodan plus acetaminophen) may be used for systemic relief of moderate pain.

Promoting Nutrition. Clients who have undergone extensive resections of the oral cavity remain on NPO status for several days. This allows healing in the oral cavity before food contacts the incision. Nasogastric feeding or total parenteral nutrition may be needed during this time (see Chapter 64).

When oral fluid intake is begun, it is important to assess for and document difficulty in swallowing, aspiration, or leakage of saliva or fluids from the suture line. Nursing care should also include the monitoring of weight and hydration. Nutritional supplementation may be used to improve the client's quality of life (see the Legal/Ethical Issues box above). Clients who experience weight loss or who are having difficulty maintaining hydration may be candidates for the surgical placement of a gastrostomy tube.

Encourage the client to perform swallowing exercises. A speech-language pathologist is often consulted to assist with swallowing techniques. A swallowing impairment may be temporary or permanent.

Community-Based Care

Continuing care for the client with an oral tumor depends on the severity of the tumor, the treatment for the tumor, and available support systems. Most clients are maintained at home during follow-up care. Ongoing nutritional management remains a vital part of the treatment plan. In addition, the client and family may benefit from a community-based support group for cancer victims.

HOME CARE MANAGEMENT

If radiation therapy is part of the client's treatment plan, home care considerations include preparatory information and management strategies. Complications due to radiation to the head or neck can be acute or delayed. Acute effects include treatment-related mucositis, stomatitis, and alterations in taste. Long-term effects such as xerostomia (excessive mouth dryness) and dental decay require ongoing oral care, the use of saliva substitutes, and follow-up dental visits. Although ongoing dental care is important, the possible adverse effects that radiation has on the cellular elements of the bone make elective oral surgical procedures, such as tooth extraction, impossible in the area of the radiation. Fatigue is a common side effect of radiation and chemotherapy.

LEGAL/ETHICAL ISSUES

NUTRITIONAL SUPPLEMENTATION IN CLIENTS UNDERGOING RADIATION TREATMENTS

Maintaining optimal nutritional status for individuals with oral carcinoma is a difficult task, considering the many aspects of digestion impacted by the disease and treatment. Radiation therapy can pose additional challenges to nutrition because of the decreased saliva flow and alterations in taste that can result. Not only does increasing evidence point to nutritional status as a predictor of overall survival, but the ability to eat and enjoy food is an important component of quality of life.

The purpose of the study by McCarthy and Weihofen (1999) was to describe the effect of nutritional supplements on the food intake of clients undergoing radiotherapy. Forty clients beginning external-beam radiation therapy were given weekly dietary counseling. The daily food intake was recorded 3 days per week for 4 weeks. One half of the subjects were assigned to ingest a nutritional supplement between meals and at bedtime. Findings suggested that those who ingested the nutritional supplements significantly increased their total caloric and protein intake while not reducing their food-derived caloric and protein intake. Based on this study, the addition of nutritional supplements to the normal food intake for clients undergoing radiotherapy for the treatment of oral cancer may be a viable option in helping to maintain adequate nutrition.

From McCarthy, D., & Weihofen, D. (1999). The effect of nutritional supplements on food intake in patients undergoing radiotherapy. *Oncology Nursing Forum, 26*(5), 897-900.

The client whose tracheostomy has been removed is often taking a soft diet by mouth before discharge. Occasionally, however, clients are discharged from the hospital while still requiring tracheostomy suction, oral suction, and nasogastric feedings. Suction equipment, nutritional supplies, and nursing care can be provided by home care companies. (See Chapter 64 for home care preparation for the client receiving home parenteral nutrition and Chapter 31 for home care preparation for the client with a tracheostomy.)

HEALTH TEACHING

It is vitally important to instruct the client and family about medications, diet or feedings, any treatments (such as tracheostomy care, suture line care, and dressing changes), and early symptoms of infection before hospital discharge.

Alterations in taste and dysphagia make maintaining adequate nutrition a challenge for the oral cancer client. Alterations in taste occur when the taste buds are included in the radiation treatment field. Taste sensation begins to return several weeks after the completion of treatment.

Changes in taste include aversions for meat, such as beef or pork, and metallic tastes in the mouth. Teach clients to add seasonings to foods, to use gravies or sauces to make foods more palatable, and to use high-protein foods such as cheeses, milk, eggs, puddings, and legumes in place of meat. Instruct clients with dysphagia in swallowing exercises. Recommend thickened liquids because thin liquids, such as water, are difficult to control during swallowing. In collaboration with the dietitian, instruct the client and family on how to assess the nutritional intake of the client who is just beginning to eat. Liquid dietary supplements are usually recommended at this time. If bleeding or stomatitis is present, a diet of soft foods is recommended so as to not cause further injury to the mucous membranes.

Instruct the client or family members to inspect the oral cavity daily for areas of redness, indicating the onset of stomatitis. Meticulous oral hygiene should be continued in the postoperative phase, especially with adjuvant chemotherapy or radiation. When instructing the client, reinforce the oral hygiene routine, emphasizing the need for frequent rinsing of the oral cavity to reduce the number of microorganisms and to maintain adequate hydration. The client should use a chemobrush, rinse the chemobrush with hydrogen peroxide and water after each use, and change chemobrushes weekly.

Saliva production is greatly reduced as a consequence of radiation. The resulting xerostomia results in the inability to eat dry foods. Instruct the client regarding the use of saliva substitutes.

Skin reactions are also a common side effect of radiation. Instruct the client to avoid sun exposure, to avoid perfumed lotions or powders, and to cleanse the face or neck area with a gentle nondeodorant soap.

Assess and document the client and family's understanding of health teaching. The client and family should provide a return demonstration of learned skills. This activity increases retention of the health information provided.

HEALTH CARE RESOURCES

Clients who have undergone composite resection often require community services because they have both physical and psychosocial needs. Depression related to a change in body image is common. Excision of a portion of the mandible can leave a facial defect that may be difficult to hide. A social worker or other health care professional may be needed for client and family counseling. Clients who have undergone a total glossectomy may be able to speak with special training and the use of an intraoral prosthesis fashioned by a maxillofacial prosthodontist. The prosthesis is similar to dentures, with augmentation to approximate the oral articulating surfaces.

A social worker or case manager provides assistance in obtaining special equipment or nutritional resources required by the client at home. The case manager assesses the financial needs of the client and makes referrals to government, community, and religious organizations as needed. Refer the client to the American Cancer Society for local support groups.

Critical Thinking Challenge

A middle-aged man with a long history of smoking is admitted to your surgical unit for surgery for oral cancer. His cancer involves the epiglottis and tongue on the left side. The surgeon performs a commando procedure in which part of his mandible and tongue are removed as well as lymph nodes and muscle tissue from his neck (radical neck dissection). Postoperatively he has a tracheostomy and is receiving oxygen via a tracheostomy mask.

1. What is your priority for care for this client? Why?
2. How will you meet his communication needs?
3. How will you meet his nutritional needs at this time?
4. What health teaching will he and his wife need before discharge to home?

evolve For suggested answer guidelines, go to http://evolve.elsevier.com/Iggy/.

Evaluation: Outcomes

Evaluate the care of the client with a malignant tumor of the oral cavity on the basis of the identified nursing diagnoses and collaborative problems. The expected outcomes include that the client will:

- Maintain open, clear tracheobronchial passages for air exchange
- Maintain the structural intactness and physiologic integrity of the oral mucous membrane

Specific indicators for each of these outcomes are listed for each nursing diagnosis under the Planning and Implementation section (see earlier).

DISORDERS OF THE SALIVARY GLANDS

Acute Sialadenitis

PATHOPHYSIOLOGY

Acute sialadenitis, the inflammation of a salivary gland, can be caused by infectious agents, irradiation, or immunologic disorders. Salivary gland inflammation can have a bacterial or viral etiology. Acute sialadenitis can be caused by infection with cytomegalovirus (CMV). The most common bacterial organisms are *Staphylococcus aureus, Staphylococcus pyogenes, Streptococcus pneumoniae,* and *Escherichia coli.* This disorder most commonly affects the parotid or submandibular gland in adults.

A decrease in the production of saliva (as in dehydrated or debilitated clients or in those who are on NPO status postoperatively for an extended time) usually precipitates acute sialadenitis. The bacteria or viruses enter the gland through the ductal opening in the oral cavity. Systemic medications, such as phenothiazines and the tetracyclines, can also precipitate an episode of acute sialadenitis. Untreated infections of the salivary glands can evolve into abscesses, which can rupture and spread infection into the tissues of the neck and the mediastinum.

Clients who receive radiation for the treatment of cancers of the head and neck or thyroid may develop decreased salivary flow, predisposing them to acute or persistent sialadenitis. The effect of radiation on the salivary glands is rapid and dose related. Immunologic disorders such as HIV infection can cause enlargement of the parotid gland that result from secondary infection. Sjögren's syndrome, an autoimmune disorder, is characterized by chronic salivary gland enlargement and inflammation (see Chapter 24).

COLLABORATIVE MANAGEMENT

Assessment

During the initial interview, assess for any predisposing factors for sialadenitis, such as ionizing radiation to the head or neck area. Collect a thorough medication history and ask about systemic illnesses, such as HIV infection.

The presence of dehydration can be noted by assessing the oral cavity and the skin for turgor. Other assessment findings include pain and swelling of the face over the affected gland. Cranial nerve function is tested because the branches of the facial nerve lie close to the salivary glands. Fever and general malaise also occur, and purulent drainage can often be massaged from the affected duct in the oral cavity (Chart 57-5).

CHART 57-5

KEY FEATURES of
Sialadenitis

- Swelling on the sides of the face or under the tongue, which increases when the client eats
- Alteration in the quantity or appearance of saliva
- Pain, especially during eating
- Purulent drainage from the affected duct

Interventions

Collaborative management includes the administration of IV fluids and measures such as the following to treat the underlying cause and increase the flow of saliva:

- Hydration
- Application of warm compresses
- Massage of the gland
- Use of a saliva substitute
- Use of **sialagogues** (substances that stimulate the flow of saliva)

Sialagogues include lemon slices and fruit- or citrus-flavored candy. Massage is accomplished by milking the edematous gland with the fingertips toward the ductal opening. Elevation of the head of the bed promotes gravity drainage of the edematous gland.

Acute sialadenitis is best prevented by adherence to routine oral hygiene. This practice prohibits infections from ascending to the salivary glands from the oral cavity.

Postirradiation Sialadenitis

The salivary glands are sensitive to ionizing radiation, such as from radiation therapy or radioactive iodine treatment of thyroid cancers. Exposure of the glands to radiation produces **xerostomia** (very dry mouth caused by a severe reduction in the flow of saliva) within 24 hours. Radiation to the salivary glands can also produce pain and edema, which generally abate after several days.

Xerostomia may be temporary or permanent, depending on the dose of radiation and the percentage of total salivary gland tissue irradiated. Little can be done to relieve the client's dry mouth during the course of radiation therapy. Frequent sips of water and frequent mouth care, especially before meals, are the most effective interventions. After the course of radiation therapy has been completed, saliva substitutes may provide moisture for 2 to 4 hours at a time. Over-the-counter solutions are available, or solutions may be mixed with methylcellulose (Cologel), glycerin, and saline.

Salivary Gland Tumors

PATHOPHYSIOLOGY

Of all oral tumors, those of the salivary glands are relatively rare. Initially, malignant tumors present as slow-growing, painless masses. Involvement of the facial nerve, more common with malignant tumors, results in facial weakness or paralysis (partial or total) on the affected side. Needle aspiration biopsy and open biopsy are useful procedures in establishing a diagnosis.

COLLABORATIVE MANAGEMENT

Assessment

It is important to collect information about any prior radiation exposure because radiation to the head and neck areas is associated with the occurrence of salivary gland tumors. Salivary gland malignancies present as localized, firm masses. In advanced stages of salivary gland tumors, you may note a large preauricular mass accompanied by facial nerve paralysis. Submandibular and minor salivary gland tumors may be tender or painful. Tumor invasion of the hypoglossal nerve causes impaired movement of the tongue, and a loss of sensation can follow. Pay particular attention to assessment of the facial nerve because of its close proximity to the salivary glands. Assess the client's ability to do the following:

- Wrinkle the brow
- Raise the eyebrows
- Squeeze the eyes shut
- Wrinkle the nose
- Pucker the lips
- Puff out the cheeks
- Grimace or smile

Interventions

The treatment of choice for both benign and malignant tumors of the salivary glands is surgical excision. However, radiation therapy is often used for salivary gland cancers that are large, have recurred, show evidence of residual disease after excision, or are highly malignant.

Clients who have undergone **parotidectomy** (surgical removal of the parotid glands) or submandibular gland surgery are at risk for weakness or loss of function of the facial nerve because the nerve courses directly through the gland. Facial nerve repair with autogenous nerve grafting can be done at the time of surgery. A combination of surgery with postoperative radiation is common for advanced disease. Care for clients following parotidectomy is similar to that required for clients having oral cancer surgery, described on pp. 1254 and 1255.

GET READY for the NCLEX Examination!

KEY POINTS

Safe Effective Care Environment

- Be aware that airway management is the priority for care for clients having surgery for oral cancer.
- Place clients having oral cancer surgery in a high-Fowler's, sitting position to facilitate breathing and prevent aspiration.
- Be sure to assess for swallowing ability before offering liquids or food to the client who has had oral cancer surgery to prevent aspiration.

Health Promotion and Maintenance

- Teach clients to seek medical attention for oral lesions that do not heal; these lesions could be oral carcinomas.
- Remind clients to visit their dentist regularly for dental hygiene and oral examination.
- Instruct clients to avoid harsh commercial mouthwashes if they have oral lesions.

- Teach clients to avoid tobacco, alcohol, and sun exposure to decrease their chance of having oral cancer.
- Instruct clients with acute sialadenitis to use sialagogues to stimulate saliva, such as citrus foods or candies.

Psychosocial Integrity

- Recognize that clients with stomatitis are often unable to eat or swallow without discomfort.
- Be aware that those who have had surgery for oral cancer may have difficulty coping with the disease.
- Remember that clients having oral cancer may have an impaired body image because of their reconstructive surgery.
- Refer clients with oral cancer to support groups, such as those available through the American Cancer Society.

Physiological Integrity

- Remember that stomatitis usually manifests as painful single or multiple ulcerations within the mouth.
- Recognize that stomatitis can be caused by a variety of organisms; candida infections are very common in clients who receive antibiotic therapy and in those who are immunocompromised.
- Provide gentle oral care for clients with oral lesions, including the need for chemobrushes and warm saline, hydrogen peroxide, or sodium bicarbonate.
- Be aware that clients with stomatitis receive antimicrobials, anti-inflammatory agents, immune modulators, and topical agents for relief of symptoms, including pain.
- Differentiate leukoplakia and erythroplakia: leukoplakia presents as thin, white patches, and erythroplakia presents as red, velvety lesions.
- Provide care for clients having cancer surgery as summarized in Chart 54-3.
- Be aware that sialadenitis can occur as result of radiation therapy.
- For clients with salivary gland tumors, assess for facial nerve involvement.
- Remember that a parotidectomy involves the removal of the salivary glands; postoperative are is similar to that for clients who have oral cancer surgery.

ADDITIONAL STUDY RESOURCES

Go to your Student CD-ROM for Review Questions for the NCLEX Examination.

evolve Go to http://evolve.elsevier.com/Iggy/ for Integrated Management of Care Questions for the NCLEX Examination.

SELECTED BIBLIOGRAPHY

Asterisk indicates a classic or definitive work on this subject.

Anonymous. (2001). Oral care update. *Nursing Management, 34*(5), S1.

Capenito-Moyet, L.J. (2003). *Nursing care plans & documentation: Nursing diagnosis and collaborative problems* (10th ed.). Philadelphia: Lippincott, Williams, & Wilkins.

Chia-Hui Chen, C. (2003). The Geriatric Oral Health Assessment Index (GOHAI). *Try This: Best Practices in Nursing for Older Adults, 14*(6), 5-6.

Fitzpatrick, J. (2000). Oral health needs of dependent older people: Responsibilities of nurses and care staff. *Journal of Advanced Nursing, 32*, 1325-1332.

Freer, S.K. (2000). Use of an oral assessment tool to improve practice. *Professional Nurse, 15*(10), 635-639.

Greenlee, R., et al. (2000). Cancer statistics, 2000. *Ca: A Cancer Journal for Clinicians, 50*(1), 7-33.

Jarvis, C. (2004). *Physical examination and health assessment* (4th ed.). Philadelphia: W.B. Saunders.

*Mandel, S., & Mandel, R. (1999). Persistent sialadenitis after radioactive iodine therapy: Report of two cases. *Journal of Oral Maxillofacial Surgery, 57*(7), 738-741.

McCance, K.L., & Huether, S.E. (2002). *Pathophysiology: The biologic basis for disease in adults & children* (4th ed.). St. Louis: Mosby.

*McCarthy, D., & Weihofen, D. (1999). The effect of nutritional supplements on food intake in patients undergoing radiotherapy. *Oncology Nursing Forum, 26*(5), 897-900.

Miller, M., & Kearney, N. (2001). Oral care for patients with cancer: A review of the literature. *Cancer Nursing, 24*(4), 241-254.

Neville, B.W., & Day, T.A. (2002). Oral cancer and precancerous lesions. *CA: A Cancer Journal for Clinicians, 52*(4), 195-215.

Palkhivala, A. (2003). Leukoplakia. *Dermatology Times, 24*(5), 36-39.

*Pearson, L. (1996). A comparison of the ability of foam swabs and toothbrushes to remove dental plaque: Implications for nursing practice. *Journal of Advanced Nursing, 23*, 62-69.

*Peterson, M.J., & Baughman, R. (1996). Recurrent aphthous stomatitis: Primary care management. *Nurse Practitioner, 21*(5), 36-47.

*Ransier, A., et al. (1995). A combined analysis of a toothbrush, foam brush, and a chlorhexidine-soaked foam brush in maintaining oral hygiene. *Cancer Nursing, 18*(5), 393-396.

Rini, A., & Bloom, K.C. (2002). Down in the mouth: Update on treatment of oral aphthous ulcers. *The Clinical Advisor, February*, 67-72.

Robins-Sadler, G., et al. (2003). Managing the oral sequelae of cancer therapy. *MedSurg Nursing, 12*(1), 28+.

Scully, C., & Shotts, R. (2001). Mouth ulcers and other causes of orofacial soreness and pain. *Western Journal of Medicine, 174*(6), 421+.

Walton, J.C., Miller, J., & Tordecilla, L. (2001). Elder oral assessment and care. *MEDSURG Nursing, 10*(1), 37-44.

Weinberg, M.A., & Estefan, D.J. (2002). Assessing oral malignancies. *American Family Physician, 65*(7), 1379-1384.

CHAPTER

58 Interventions for Clients with Esophageal Problems

CONSTANCE VISOVSKY

LEARNING OUTCOMES

After studying this chapter, you should be able to:

1. Explain the pathophysiology of gastroesophageal reflux disease (GERD).
2. Assess the client who is experiencing GERD.
3. Plan the nursing care for clients with GERD.
4. Identify medications that are used for GERD and nursing implications for each classification.
5. Develop a postoperative teaching plan for the client having a hiatal hernia repair.
6. Identify the differences in the incidence of esophageal cancer among cultural groups.
7. Describe the risk factors for esophageal cancer.
8. Analyze assessment data to determine common nursing diagnoses for the client with esophageal cancer.
9. Discuss the priorities for postoperative care of the client undergoing surgery for esophageal cancer.
10. Plan community-based care for clients diagnosed with esophageal cancer.

Go to your Student CD-ROM for Review Questions for the NCLEX Examination keyed to these Learning Outcomes.

The esophagus is a hollow tube located behind the trachea, passing through the diaphragm at the esophageal hiatus and extending to the gastroesophageal junction. The function of the esophagus is to allow the passage of food from the mouth to the stomach. Disorders of the esophagus can be of inflammatory, structural, motor, and neoplastic origin. Collaborative management involves dietary and lifestyle modifications in conjunction with medical and surgical therapies. Gastroesophageal reflux and related esophageal disorders affect as much as 20% of the population in the United States (Hubbard, 2002). Approximately two million ambulatory care visits yearly can be attributed to GERD. Impaired gastroesophageal motility resulting from achalasia or diverticula is responsible for 400,000 visits to health care providers annually.

GASTROESOPHAGEAL REFLUX DISEASE

Gastroesophageal reflux disease (GERD) is the most common upper gastrointestinal disorder in the United States. It occurs as a result of the backward flow **(reflux)** of gastrointestinal contents into the esophagus. Reflux produces symptoms by exposing the esophageal mucosa to the irritating effects of gastric or duodenal contents, resulting in inflammatory changes of the esophageal mucosa. A person with acute symptoms of inflammation is often described as having **reflux esophagitis,** a hallmark of GERD. Reflux esophagitis is graded according the extent and severity of the lesions.

PATHOPHYSIOLOGY

Several physiologic factors are implicated in the development of GERD (Hubbard, 2002):

- Inappropriate relaxation of the lower esophageal sphincter
- Irritation from the refluxed material
- Delayed gastric emptying
- Abnormal esophageal clearance

The reflux of gastric contents into the esophagus is normally prevented by the presence of two high-pressure areas that remain relatively contracted in the resting phase. A 3-cm (1.2-inch) segment at the proximal end of the esophagus is called the upper esophageal sphincter (UES). Another 2- to 4-cm (0.8- to 1.6-inch) portion just proximal to the gastroesophageal junction is called the **lower esophageal sphincter (LES).** The function of the LES is supported by its anatomic placement in the abdomen, where the surrounding pressure is significantly higher than in the low-pressure thorax. Sphincter function is also supported by the acute angle (angle of His) that is formed as the esophagus enters the stomach. Esophageal reflux can occur when the following occur:

- Gastric volume or intra-abdominal pressure is elevated
- The sphincter tone of the LES is decreased
- The LES undergoes inappropriate relaxation

An individual experiencing reflux may be asymptomatic and relatively unaware that reflux is occurring. However, the esophagus has only limited resistance to the damaging effects of the acidic gastrointestinal (GI) contents. The pH of acid secreted by the stomach ranges from 1.5 to 2.0, whereas the pH of the distal esophagus is normally neutral (6.0 to 7.0). Repeated exposure of the esophageal mucosa to highly acid gastric secretions is associated with the development of erosive esophagitis.

Refluxed material is returned to the stomach by a combination of gravity, saliva, and peristalsis. The effectiveness of the clearance mechanism is very important. An inflamed esophagus cannot eliminate the refluxed material as quickly or efficiently as a healthy one, and therefore the duration of exposure increases with each reflux episode. Hyperemia (increased blood flow) and erosion occur in the esophagus in response to the chronic inflammation. Gastric acid and pepsin are responsible for the tissue injury. Minor capillary bleeding often accompanies the erosion, but frank hemorrhage is rare.

During the process of healing, the body may substitute a columnar epithelium **(Barrett's epithelium)** for the normal squamous cell epithelium of the lower esophagus. Although this new tissue is more resistant to acid and therefore supports esophageal healing, it is considered premalignant and is associated with an increased risk of cancer in clients with prolonged GERD (Field, 2003). The fibrosis and scarring that accompany the healing process can produce esophageal stricture, resulting in a narrowing of the esophageal lumen. The stricture leads to progressive difficulty in swallowing. Uncontrolled esophageal reflux also creates a risk for other serious complications, such as esophageal ulceration, hemorrhage, and aspiration pneumonia. GERD has been implicated as one of the causes of adult-onset asthma, laryngitis, and dental deterioration.

Etiology

The most common cause of GERD is inappropriate relaxation of the LES, which allows the reflux of gastric contents into the esophagus and exposure of the esophageal mucosa to gastric contents from impaired esophageal clearance. Nighttime reflux tends to result in prolonged exposure of the esophagus to acid because recumbency tends to impair peristalsis and gravity clearance mechanisms.

Gastric distention caused by the ingestion of large meals or by conditions associated with delayed gastric emptying predispose the client to reflux. A number of individual factors, including certain foods and medications, have been identified as influencing the tone and contractility of the LES (Table 58-1). Clients who have a nasogastric tube often experience compromised esophageal sphincter function. The tube keeps the cardiac sphincter open and allows acidic contents from the stomach to enter the esophagus. Other factors that increase intra-abdominal and intragastric pressure (e.g., pregnancy, wearing tight belts, obesity, bending over, and ascites) overcome the gastroesophageal pressure gradient maintained by the LES and allow reflux to occur.

TABLE 58-1 Factors Contributing to Decreased Lower Esophageal Sphincter Pressure

■ Fatty foods	■ Calcium channel blockers
■ Caffeinated beverages, such as coffee, tea, and cola	■ Nitrates
■ Chocolate	■ Peppermint, spearmint
■ Citrus fruits	■ Alcohol
■ Tomatoes and tomato products	■ Anticholinergic drugs
■ Nicotine in cigarette smoke	■ High levels of estrogen and progesterone
	■ Nasogastric tube placement

Incidence/Prevalence

Gastroesophageal reflux disease (GERD) affects about 5% to 7% of the world population and 20% of the U.S. population (Hubbard, 2002). Forty percent of the population reports experiencing symptoms of heartburn once monthly, and 20% report experiencing symptoms weekly (Fennerty et al., 2002). GERD can occur at any age, but it is more common in people over 45 years of age. The incidence of GERD may be underestimated because many people with mild disease relate the symptoms to episodes of stress or dietary indiscretion.

COLLABORATIVE MANAGEMENT

Assessment

HISTORY

Ask the client about a history of heartburn or atypical chest pain associated with the reflux of gastrointestinal contents. Assess the client for dysphagia (difficulty swallowing) or odynophagia (painful swallowing), either of which can indicate the development of a stricture. Ask the client whether he or she has been newly diagnosed asthma or has experienced morning hoarseness or pneumonia. These symptoms are suggestive of severe reflux reaching the pharynx or mouth or pulmonary aspiration.

PHYSICAL ASSESSMENT/CLINICAL MANIFESTATIONS

The clinical manifestations of reflux may vary substantially in severity (Chart 58-1).

DYSPEPSIA. Heartburn, also known as **dyspepsia,** is the characteristic symptom of GERD. Clients often describe this pain as a substernal or retrosternal burning sensation that tends to move up and down the chest in a wavelike fashion. Because heartburn might not be viewed as a serious concern, clients may delay seeking treatment for GERD. If the heartburn is severe, the pain may radiate to the neck or jaw or may be referred to the back. The pain typically worsens when the client bends over, strains, or is in a recumbent position.

With severe GERD, the pain occurs after each meal and persists for 20 minutes to 2 hours. Clients usually experience prompt relief by ingesting fluids or antacids or by maintaining an upright posture.

REGURGITATION. Regurgitation of food particles or fluids is common. The client reports the occurrence of warm fluid traveling up the throat, unaccompanied by nausea. If the fluid reaches the level of the pharynx, he or she notes a

CHART 58-1

KEY FEATURES of
Gastroesophageal Reflux Disease

- Dyspepsia (heartburn)
- Regurgitation (may lead to aspiration or bronchitis)
- Coughing, hoarseness, or wheezing at night
- Water brash (hypersalivation)
- Dysphagia
- Odynophagia (painful swallowing)
- Epigastric pain
- Belching
- Flatulence
- Nausea
- Pyrosis (retrosternal burning)
- Globus (feeling of something in back of throat)
- Pharyngitis
- Dental caries (severe cases)

sour or bitter taste in the mouth. This effortless regurgitation can even occur when the client is in an upright position. The danger of aspiration is increased if regurgitation occurs when the client is in a recumbent (lying down) position.

The client experiencing regurgitation should be carefully monitored for crackles in the lung, which is an indication of associated aspiration. Assess the client for coughing, hoarseness, or wheezing at night, which may be related to recumbent regurgitation. Assessment for bronchitis may be necessary in clients experiencing long-term regurgitation.

HYPERSALIVATION. A reflex salivary hypersecretion known as **water brash** occurs in response to reflux. Water brash must be carefully distinguished from regurgitation. The client reports a sensation of fluid in the throat, but unlike with regurgitation, there is no bitter or sour taste.

DYSPHAGIA AND ODYNOPHAGIA. Chronic GERD can involve **dysphagia** (difficulty swallowing). Dysphagia usually indicates a narrowing of the esophagus because of stricture or inflammation. Careful assessment is required if a client reports progressive or persistent dysphagia because it usually indicates the development of a stricture or cancer. Assessment of the client should include the following:

- The degree of dysphagia
- Whether dysphagia occurs with the ingestion of solids, liquids, or both
- Whether dysphagia is intermittent or occurs with each swallowing effort

Odynophagia (painful swallowing) is a possible symptom of GERD, but it is relatively rare in people with uncomplicated reflux disease. Severe and long-lasting chest pain may be present if spasms occurring in the esophagus cause the muscle to contract with excess force. The resulting pain can be agonizing and may last for hours.

OTHER MANIFESTATIONS. Other symptoms include chronic cough that occurs mostly at night or when the client is in a recumbent position, asthma, and atypical chest pain. Cough and symptoms of asthma occur when refluxed acid is spilled over into the tracheobronchial tree (Field, 2003). *Atypical chest pain* is thought to be caused by stimulation of pain receptors in the esophageal wall and by esophageal spasm. This type of chest pain can mimic angina and needs to be carefully differentiated from cardiac disease.

Eructation (belching), flatulence (gas), or bloating after eating are other common complaints. Nausea and vomiting occur infrequently, and unplanned weight loss is rare.

DIAGNOSTIC ASSESSMENT

The most accurate method of diagnosing gastroesophageal reflux disease (GERD) is **24-hour ambulatory pH monitoring** (McCormick, 2004). This test involves placing a small catheter through the nose into the distal esophagus. The client is asked to keep a diary of activities and symptoms, and the pH is continuously monitored and recorded. Ambulatory pH monitoring is very useful in establishing a diagnosis in clients with atypical symptoms.

Endoscopy, in particular esophagogastroduodenoscopy (EGD), is useful in diagnosing or evaluating reflux esophagitis or in monitoring complications such as Barrett's esophagus. Endoscopy requires the use of conscious sedation during the procedure and the clients must have someone accompany them home after recovery. During the procedure, tissue samples can be obtained for biopsy, and strictures can be dilated (see Chapter 56).

Esophageal manometry, or motility testing, can be performed when the diagnosis is uncertain. Water-filled catheters are inserted via the client's nose or mouth and slowly withdrawn while measurements of LES pressure and peristalsis are recorded. When used alone, manometry is not sensitive or specific enough to establish a diagnosis of GERD.

◆Common Nursing Diagnoses and Collaborative Problems

Nursing diagnoses that may apply to clients with GERD include the following:

- Acute Pain and Chronic Pain related to physical (esophageal irritation) injury
- Risk for Aspiration related to incompetent LES
- Impaired Swallowing related to stricture or inflammation

◆Interventions

Inform the client that GERD is a chronic disorder that requires ongoing management. Clients will need to make lifestyle modifications and adhere to medication regimens for the successful treatment of GERD.

NONSURGICAL MANAGEMENT. The goals of treatment for GERD are the relief of symptoms, treatment of esophagitis, and prevention of complications such as strictures or Barrett's esophagus. Although GERD can be controlled by diet therapy, education, lifestyle changes, and drug therapy, it is important to note that, even after esophagitis is healed, 40% to 80% of clients relapse in 6 months after their medication is discontinued.

Diet Therapy. Diet therapy is used to relieve symptoms in clients with relatively mild GERD. In collaboration with the dietitian, explore the client's basic meal patterns and food preferences. Collaborate with the dietitian, client, and family to plan modifications that may decrease reflux symptoms. For adherence at home to be successful, it is essential that family members who do the shopping and cooking be included in this discussion.

Advise the client to limit or eliminate foods that decrease LES pressure, such as chocolate, fat, and mints. The client should also restrict spicy and acidic foods (e.g., orange juice, tomatoes) until esophageal healing can occur because these foods irritate the inflamed tissue and cause heartburn.

Large meals increase the volume of and pressure in the stomach and delay gastric emptying. Therefore, teach the client to eat four to six small meals each day rather than three large ones. Carbonated beverages should also be avoided because they increase pressure in the stomach. Encourage clients to avoid evening snacks and to eat no food for at least 3 hours before going to bed. Reflux episodes are most damaging at night. Clients may have the most difficulty adhering to the restriction of evening snacks. Advise the client to eat slowly and chew thoroughly to facilitate digestion and prevent eructation (belching).

Client Education. Teach the client about the risk factors for the development of reflux, including contributing lifestyle factors. Lifestyle factors that can exacerbate the disease need to be reviewed, and the client should be given instructions on ways to avoid recurrence. Educate the client regarding the need for ongoing monitoring, particularly if the client has developed strictures, ulcerations, or Barrett's esophagus.

Lifestyle Changes. The control of GERD involves lifestyle adjustments to promote health and control reflux (Chart 58-2). Instruct the client to elevate the head of the bed by 6 inches for sleep to prevent nighttime reflux. This can be done by placing blocks under the head of the bed or by using a large, wedge-style pillow instead of a standard pillow (Hubbard, 2002). Emphasize the importance of this intervention, and investigate all possible approaches for achieving compliance.

Instruct the client to sleep in the left lateral decubitus (side-lying) position to minimize the effects of nighttime episodes of reflux. Nighttime reflux is extremely common, and infrequent swallowing in combination with a recumbent position significantly impairs esophageal clearance. Smoking and alcohol cause decreased LES pressure. Explore the possibility and means of smoking cessation, and make appropriate referrals for the client. Ask the client about the normal pattern and amount of alcoholic beverages. If appropriate, assist the client in finding appropriate alcohol cessation programs.

For the obese client, collaborate with the dietitian to examine approaches to weight reduction. Decreasing intra-abdominal pressure often reduces reflux symptoms. Wearing constrictive clothing, lifting heavy objects or straining, and working in a bent-over or stooped position should be avoided. Emphasize that these general adaptations are an essential and effective component of disease management and can produce prompt results in uncomplicated cases.

Drug Therapy. Some medications lower LES pressure and cause reflux, such as oral contraceptives, anticholinergic agents, sedatives, tranquilizers, beta-adrenergic agonists, nitrates, and calcium channel blockers (Hubbard, 2002). The possibility of eliminating those medications in reflux should be explored with the health care provider.

Three principles guide drug therapy for gastroesophageal reflux:

- Inhibit gastric acid secretion
- Accelerate gastric emptying
- Protect the gastric mucosa (Chart 58-3)

Antacids. In uncomplicated cases of GERD, antacids may be effective for occasional episodes of heartburn. Antacids act by elevating the pH level of the gastric contents, thereby deactivating pepsin. They are inadequate for the control of frequent symptoms because their duration of action is too short and their nighttime effectiveness is minimal.

Antacids containing aluminum hydroxide or magnesium hydroxide may be used. Maalox and Mylanta consist of a combination of these two agents. Clients often tolerate them better because they produce fewer side effects, such as constipation and diarrhea. Instruct the client to take the antacid 1 hour before and 2 to 3 hours after each meal. Some antacids are prepared as double-strength (DS) suspensions or tablets. The advantage of DS preparations is that the client can take a smaller amount of the drug. For example, 30 mL of regular Mylanta equals 15 mL of Mylanta-II (DS preparation).

Gaviscon, a combination of aluminum hydroxide and magnesium carbonate, is a commonly used and very effective medication for GERD. It forms a viscous foam that floats on top of the gastric contents and theoretically decreases the incidence of reflux. If reflux occurs, the foam enters the esophagus first and buffers the acid in the refluxed material. Remind the client to take this drug when food is in the stomach.

Histamine Receptor Antagonists. Histamine blockers, such as famotidine (Pepcid), ranitidine (Zantac), cimetidine (Tagamet), and nizatidine (Axid) decrease acid. With histamine receptor antagonists available over the counter (OTC) and widely advertised for heartburn, many clients self-medicate before seeking professional assistance from their health care provider. When clients who have self-medicated with OTC preparations experience uncontrolled symptoms, the health care provider usually prescribes a *higher* dose of a histamine receptor antagonist.

Cimetidine (Tagamet) is not used as often as the longer-acting preparations. It has an inhibitory effect on the elimination of certain other medications, and therefore significant drug interactions can occur in clients taking warfarin (Coumadin), theophylline (Theo-Dur), phenytoin (Dilantin), nifedipine (Procardia), or propranolol (Inderal). Ranitidine and the other preparations are longer acting, and less frequent dosing is necessary. They also appear to produce fewer side effects and are safe for long-term administration. Although these drugs do not affect the occurrence of reflux directly, they do reduce gastric acid secretion, improve symptoms, and promote healing of inflamed esophageal tissue.

Proton Pump Inhibitors. The proton pump inhibitors (PPIs), such as omeprazole (Prilosec), lansoprazole (Prevacid), rabeprazole (Aciphex), pantoprazole (Protonix), and esomeprazole (Nexium), are the *main* treatment for

CHART 58-2

CLIENT EDUCATION GUIDE

Health Promotion Modifications to Control Reflux

- Eat four to six small meals a day.
- Limit or eliminate fatty foods, coffee, tea, cola, and chocolate.
- Reduce or eliminate from your diet any food or spice that increases gastric acid and causes pain.
- Limit or eliminate alcohol and tobacco.
- Do not snack in the evening, and take no food for 2 to 3 hours before you go to bed.
- Eat slowly, and chew your food thoroughly to reduce belching.
- Remain upright for 1 to 2 hours after meals, if possible.
- Elevate the head of your bed 8 to 12 inches using wooden blocks or a foam wedge. Never sleep flat in bed.
- If you are overweight, lose weight.
- Do not wear constrictive clothing.
- Avoid heavy lifting, straining, and working in a bent-over position.
- Chew "chewable" antacids thoroughly and follow with a glass of water.

CHART 58-3

DRUG THERAPY for Gastroesophageal Reflux Disease (GERD)

Drug	Usual Dosage	Nursing Interventions	Rationales
Antacids			
Aluminum or magnesium salts (Mylanta, Maalox)	30 mL PO between meals and as needed (PRN) throughout the day and at bedtime	Give 1 hr before meals, 2-3 hr after meals and at bedtime. Give PRN as instructed by physician.	
		Observe the client for constipation or diarrhea.	Aluminum products produce constipation, and magnesium products induce diarrhea.
		Suggest the use of combination mixtures or alternating use of aluminum and magnesium products.	Balancing their effects is important for client adherence.
Gaviscon, antacid plus alginic acid	1 tablet or 10-20 mL PO throughout the day and at bedtime	Give after meals and at bedtime.	Alginic acid forms a viscous foam that floats on top of the gastric contents, impeding reflux or buffering its effects when it occurs.
Histamine receptor antagonists			
Cimetidine (Tagamet) (Peptol)	300 mg PO four times daily or 900-1200 mg PO at bedtime	Observe the client for side effects; fatigue, headache, and diarrhea are common. Instruct client about potential toxicity with some medications.	Tagamet causes interactions with common medications and is not used as often.
Ranitidine (Zantac)	150 mg PO twice daily	Administer with meals and at bedtime.	Ranitidine and famotidine are more potent, longer-acting drugs but produce fewer side effects.
Famotidine (Pepcid)	40 mg PO daily or 20 mg PO twice daily		
Nizatidine (Axid)	150 mg PO twice daily	Use cautiously and in reduced dosages in clients with renal disease.	Clients need an adequate creatinine clearance to prevent drug toxicity.
		Observe for dysrhythmias.	Dysrhythmias are common adverse effects of the drug.
		Do not mix with tomato-based, mixed-vegetable juices; apple juice is the preferred choice.	Nizatidine may be less potent when mixed with tomato-based, mixed-vegetable juices.
Metoclopramide (Reglan)	10 mg PO three or four times daily	Instruct the client to take the drug before meals.	This drug increases the rate of gastric emptying.
		Teach the client to report any neurologic or psychotropic side effects, such as restlessness, anxiety, ataxia, or hallucinations.	Long-term drug use produces adverse effects in up to one third of clients.
Proton Pump Inhibitors			
Omeprazole (Prilosec, Losec 🍁)	20-30 mg PO daily	Instruct the client to take the drug before meals. Observe the client for typical side effects: abdominal cramping, diarrhea, headache.	Gastric acid suppression is greater than 90%. Action is prolonged, but gastrointestinal effects are severe in some clients.
Lansoprazole (Prevacid)	15 mg PO daily for gastroesophageal reflux disease (GERD)	Instruct the client to take the drug before meals.	Same as omeprazole.
	Up to 60 mg PO for gastrointestinal ulcers or Zollinger-Ellison syndrome	For the client who has difficulty swallowing or has a nasogastric tube, open the capsule and mix granules in apple juice (or applesauce if not tube fed).	The drug is safe to administer by opening (not crushing) the capsule.
Rabeprazole (Aciphex)	60 mg PO daily (may increase to 120 mg in two divided doses)	Do not crush, break, or chew delayed release tablets.	This form of the drug is released into the body slowly throughout the day
		Teach client to wear sunscreen.	The drug predisposes the client to burns.
Pantoprazole (Protonix, Protonix IV)	40 mg daily or 40 mg IV daily for 7-10 days	Do not crush, break, or chew delayed release tablets.	This form of the drug is released slowly into the body throughout the day.
Esomeprazole (Nexium)	20-40 mg PO daily	Do not administer with digoxin, rabeprazole, or iron salts.	This drug may alter the effect and absorption of these agents.

GERD. These agents provide effective, long-acting inhibition of gastric acid secretion through inhibition of the proton pump of the gastric parietal cell. PPIs reduce gastric acid secretion by about 90% over a 24-hour period and can be given in a single daily dose. If once-a-day dosing fails to control symptoms, twice-daily dosing is appropriate. PPIs promote rapid tissue healing, but recurrence is common when the drug is stopped.

Other Drugs. Prokinetic drugs may used to increase gastric emptying and improve lower esophageal sphincter (LES) pressure and esophageal peristalsis. Metoclopramide (Reglan) is a prokinetic agent that acts to increase the rate of gastric emptying. It does not affect gastric acid secretion or directly heal esophageal tissue. Its use is also associated with a high incidence of neurologic and psychotropic side effects such as fatigue, anxiety, ataxia, and hallucinations. Long term use is not recommended.

Endoscopic Therapies. In the past decade, several noninvasive endoscopic procedures have been approved for GERD. Three of these newer techniques are the Stretta procedure, the Enteryx procedure, and the Bard EndoCinch Suturing System (BESS). Although not as common as other treatment measures, these methods are becoming more popular.

In the Stretta procedure, the physician applies radiofrequency (RF) energy through needles placed near the gastroesophageal junction. The RF energy inhibits the activity of the vagus nerve, thus reducing discomfort for the client (McCormick, 2004).

The Enteryx procedure also requires an endoscopy and needles. The physician injects a soft, spongy permanent implant made of liquid polymeric material into the LES muscle. This technique tightens the LES and prevents reflux. Similarly, the BESS procedure tightens the LES, but the physician sutures near the sphincter. Chart 58-4 outlines discharge instructions for endoscopic therapies.

The advantage of these therapies compared with surgery include the following:

- Moderate sedation (rather than general anesthesia)
- Ambulatory procedure (rather than an inpatient stay)
- Shorter procedure (45 minutes versus several hours)
- 1 to 2 days absence from work (rather than 2 to 3 weeks)
- No antibiotics and lower complication rate

CHART 58-4

CLIENT EDUCATION GUIDE

Postoperative Instructions for Clients Having Endoscopic Therapies for Gastroesophageal Reflux Disease (e.g., Stretta Procedure)

- Remain on clear liquids for 24 hours after the procedure.
- After the first day, consume a soft diet, such as custard, pureed vegetables, mashed potatoes, and applesauce.
- Avoid nonsteroidal anti-inflammatory drugs and aspirin for 10 days.
- Continue medications as prescribed, usually proton pump inhibitors.
- Ingest liquid medications whenever possible.
- Do not allow nasogastric tubes for at least 1 month because esophageal perforation could occur.
- Contact the health care provider if the following problems occur:
  - Chest or abdominal pain
  - Bleeding
  - Dysphagia
  - Shortness of breath
  - Nausea or vomiting

Critcal Thinking Challenge

You are a nurse in an internist's office and take the history of a middle-aged man with complaint of heartburn. He tells you that he especially has problems when he eats tomatoes, onions, and citrus fruits or juice. For the past month he has been taking over-the-counter Tagamet or Prilosec, and finds that Prilosec is best.

1. What other data should you collect from this client and why?
2. What diagnostic testing might he have to confirm a diagnosis of GERD?
3. Why does he get more relief from the Prilosec compared with Tagamet?
4. If the client is diagnosed with GERD, what health teaching does this client need?

evolve For suggested answer guidelines, go to http://evolve.elsevier.com/Iggy/.

SURGICAL MANAGEMENT. A very small percentage of clients with GERD require antireflux surgery. It is usually indicated for otherwise healthy clients who have failed to respond to medical treatment or have developed complications related to GERD. Various surgical procedures may be used through conventional open techniques or laparoscope.

Laparoscopic Nissen fundoplication (LNF) is the gold standard for surgical management. A discussion of this procedure can be found in the next section under Surgical Management (Hiatal Hernia). Clients who have surgery are encouraged to continue following the basic antireflux regimen of antacids and diet therapy because the rate of recurrence is significant.

Placement of the synthetic Angelchik esophageal antireflux prosthesis may be used for clients with severe reflux. The surgeon performs a laparotomy (abdominal approach) and ties a C-shaped silicone prosthesis filled with gel around the distal esophagus. The prosthesis anchors the LES in the abdomen and reinforces sphincter pressure. This device is not used as often as in previous years because of complications, such as long-term dysphagia and migration of the prosthesis. About 25% of clients with Angelchik devices have them removed.

HIATAL HERNIA

Hiatal hernias, also called diaphragmatic hernias, involve the protrusion of the stomach through the esophageal hiatus of the diaphragm into the thorax. The esophageal hiatus is the opening in the diaphragm through which the esophagus passes from the thorax to the abdomen. Clients with hiatal hernias may be completely asymptomatic or may experience daily symptoms similar to those of clients with GERD.

PATHOPHYSIOLOGY

The two major types of hiatal hernias are sliding hernias and paraesophageal (rolling) hernias.

Sliding Hernia

Sliding hernias are the most common type of hernia and account for 90% of the total number of hiatal hernias. The esophagogastric junction and a portion of the fundus of the

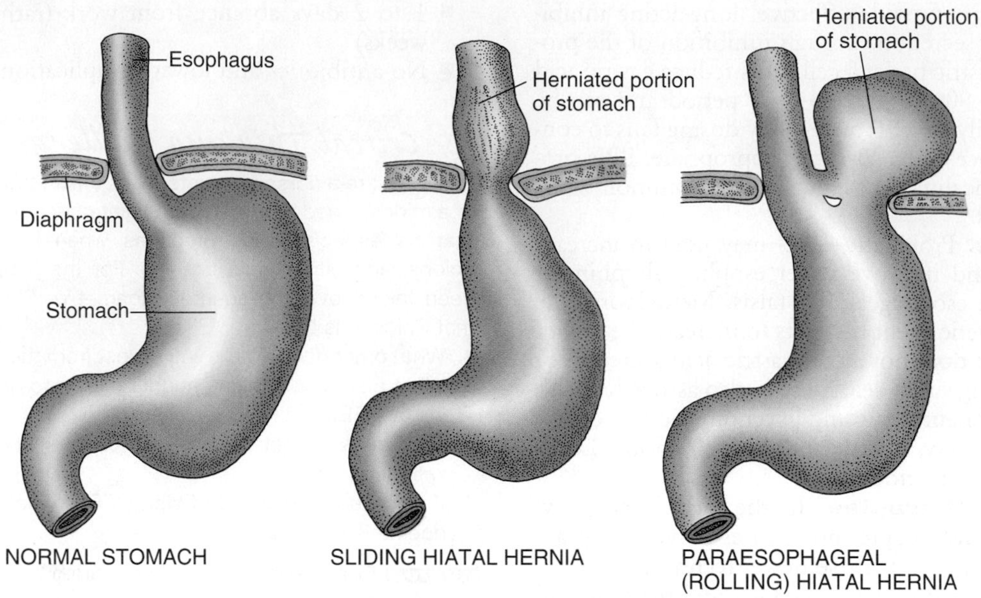

Figure 58-1 ■ A comparison of the normal stomach and sliding and paresophageal (rolling) hiatal hernias.

stomach slide upward through the esophageal hiatus into the thorax (Figure 58-1). The hernia generally moves freely and slides into and out of the thorax during changes in position or intra-abdominal pressure. Although **volvulus** (bowel twisting) and obstruction do occur rarely, the major concern in a client with a sliding hernia is the development of esophageal reflux and its complications. The development of reflux appears to be related to chronic exposure of the lower esophageal sphincter (LES) to the low pressure of the thorax, which significantly reduces the effectiveness of the LES. Symptoms associated with LES pressure are worsened by positions that favor reflux, such as bending or lying supine.

Rolling Hernia

With paraesophageal hernias, the gastroesophageal junction remains in its normal intra-abdominal location, but the fundus (and possibly portions of the stomach's greater curvature) rolls through the esophageal hiatus and into the thorax beside the esophagus (see Figure 58-1). The herniated portion of the stomach may be small or quite large; in rare cases, the stomach completely inverts into the thorax. Reflux is rarely a concern because the LES remains anchored below the diaphragm, but the risks of volvulus, obstruction, and strangulation are high. The development of iron deficiency anemia is common because slow bleeding secondary to venous obstruction causes the gastric mucosa to become engorged and ooze. Significant bleeding or hemorrhage is rare.

Etiology

Sliding hiatal hernias develop from muscle weakening in the esophageal hiatus, which loosens the esophageal supports and permits the lower portion of the esophagus to rise into the thorax. Congenital weaknesses, trauma, obesity, or surgery may also play a significant role. The development of the hernia is the result of the combined effects of weakened support structures and prolonged increases in abdominal pressure.

Paraesophageal hernias are thought to develop from an anatomic defect occurring when the stomach is not properly anchored below the diaphragm rather than from muscle weakness. Paraesophageal hernias can also be caused by previous esophageal surgeries, including sliding hernia repair.

Incidence/Prevalence

Hiatal hernia is one of the most common disorders affecting the upper gastrointestinal tract, and it affects women more often than men. Hiatal hernias have been reported in up to 20% of adults.

COLLABORATIVE MANAGEMENT

Assessment

Assess the client for heartburn, regurgitation, pain, dysphagia, and belching. An assessment of general physical appearance and nutritional status is also included. Note the location, onset, duration, quality, and aggravating and alleviating factors associated with the presence of pain. The primary symptoms of sliding hiatal hernias are associated with reflux. Auscultate the thorax and lungs because pulmonary symptoms similar to asthma may be triggered by episodes of aspiration, particularly at night. A detailed history is crucial in attempting to differentiate angina from noncardiac chest pain caused by gastroesophageal reflux. Symptoms resulting from hiatal hernia typically worsen after a meal or when the client is in a recumbent position (Chart 58-5).

In clients with paraesophageal (rolling) hernias, assess for symptoms related to the stretching or displacement of thoracic contents by the hernia. Clients may report a feeling of fullness after eating and may even experience breathlessness or a feeling of suffocation if the hernia interferes with

CHART 58-5

KEY FEATURES of Hernias

Sliding Hiatal Hernias	Paraesophageal Hernias
■ Heartburn	■ Feeling of fullness after eating
■ Regurgitation	■ Breathlessness after eating
■ Chest pain	■ Feeling of suffocation
■ Dysphagia	■ Chest pain that mimics angina
■ Belching	■ Worsening of manifestations in a recumbent position

breathing. Some clients experience chest pain associated with reflux that mimics angina.

The barium swallow study with fluoroscopy is the most specific diagnostic test for identifying hiatal hernia. Paraesophageal hernias are usually clearly visible, and sliding hernias can often be observed as the client is moved through a series of positions that increase intra-abdominal pressure.

Clients with sliding hernias usually experience symptoms of reflux. Therefore any or all of the diagnostic tests used for gastroesophageal reflux disease (GERD) may be used to evaluate the extent of reflux and the degree of esophageal damage (see Diagnostic Assessment [GERD], p. 1262).

Interventions

Clients with hiatal hernias may be managed either medically or surgically. The health care provider's choice of management is based on the severity of the client's symptoms and the risk of serious complications. Sliding hiatal hernias are most commonly treated medically. Large paraesophageal hernias can become strangulated or obstructed; therefore early surgical repair is encouraged.

NONSURGICAL MANAGEMENT. The interventions for clients with hiatal hernia closely follow those outlined for clients with GERD and include drug therapy, diet therapy, lifestyle modifications, and client education. The health care provider typically prescribes antacids and histamine receptor antagonists, such as ranitidine (Zantac), in an attempt to control reflux and its symptoms.

Diet therapy is also an integral part of the conservative management of hiatal hernia and follows the guidelines discussed earlier for GERD, p. 1262.

Encourage the client to avoid eating in the late evening and to avoid foods associated with reflux. In collaboration with the dietitian, teach the client to modify the diet to reduce body weight (if appropriate). Obesity increases intra-abdominal pressure and worsens both the hernia and the symptoms of reflux. Explain the underlying condition to increase the client's understanding of the disorder and increase adherence to the treatment regimen. Teaching about positioning, as described earlier for GERD (p. 1263) is also extremely important. It is essential that clients do the following:

- Sleep at night with the head of the bed elevated 6 inches.
- Remain upright for several hours after eating.
- Avoid straining or excessive vigorous exercise.
- Refrain from wearing clothing that is tight or constrictive around the abdomen.

SURGICAL MANAGEMENT. Surgery may be required when the risk of complications is high or when damage from chronic reflux becomes severe.

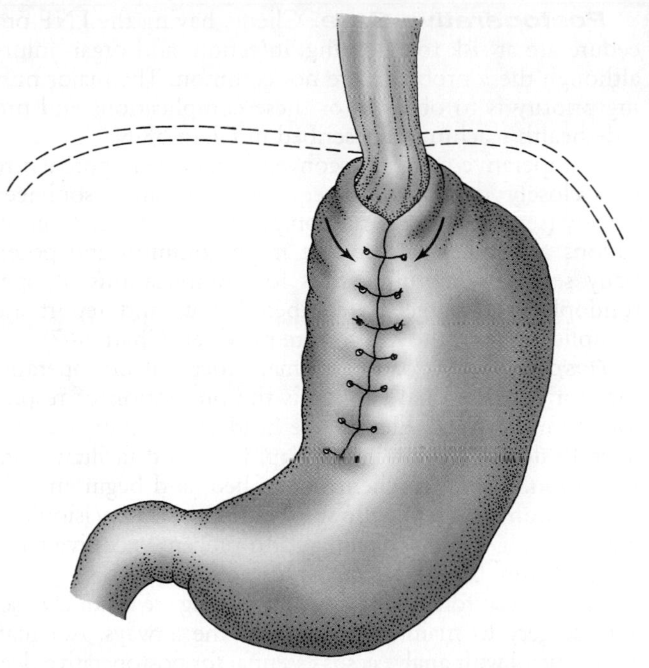

Figure 58-2 ■ Open surgical approach for Nissen fundoplication for gastroesophageal reflux disease or hiatal hernia repair.

Preoperative Care. If the surgery is not urgent, the surgeon encourages clients who are overweight to lose weight before surgery. They are advised to quit or significantly reduce smoking. As part of preoperative teaching, you should reinforce the surgeon's instructions and prepare the client for the postoperative course.

You must know which surgical approach is chosen to develop an appropriate teaching plan. For example, for the trans-thoracic surgical approach, teach the client about chest tubes. Inform the client that a nasogastric tube will be inserted during surgery and will remain in place for several days. Oral intake is started gradually with clear liquids after peristalsis is re-established or to stimulate peristalsis. Instruct the client about techniques for effective deep breathing and use of the incentive spirometer. These measures are essential to prevent postoperative respiratory complications. The high incision makes deep breathing extremely painful for the client. Educate the client concerning the aspects of postoperative pain, and assure the client that adequate postoperative analgesia will be administered.

Operative Procedures. Although several hiatal hernia repair procedures are in use, each involves reinforcement of the lower esophageal sphincter (LES) through some degree of fundoplication. The surgeon wraps a portion of the stomach fundus around the distal esophagus to anchor it and reinforce the LES. The eventual recurrence for either type of hernia following surgical repair is 10% to 15% over 5 years.

Laparoscopic Nissen fundoplication (LNF) is the most common surgical technique for hiatal hernia repair. However, a small percentage of clients are not candidates for laparoscopic procedures and require a conventional open fundoplication (Figure 58-2). In laparoscopic surgery, the repair is performed through several (usually five) ½-inch incisions in the abdomen.

Postoperative Care. Clients having the LNF procedure are at risk for bleeding, infection, and organ injury, although these problems are not common. The major nursing priority is to observe for these complications and provide health teaching as described in Chart 58-6.

Postoperative care after conventional open approach repair closely follows that required after any esophageal surgery (see the Plan of Care on pp. 1269 to 1272). Complications after open surgery are more common and potentially serious. Carefully assess for complications of open fundoplication surgery, described below, and report any complications to the health care provider (Chart 58-7).

Respiratory Care. The primary focus of postoperative care for conventional surgery is the prevention of respiratory complications. Elevate the head of the client's bed at least 30 degrees to lower the diaphragm and facilitate lung expansion. Assist the client out of bed, and begin ambulation as soon as possible. Be sure to support the incision during coughing to reduce pain and to prevent excessive strain on the suture line, especially with obese clients.

Incentive spirometry and deep breathing are routinely used after surgery to maintain patency of the airways. Adequate pain control with analgesics is essential for postoperative deep breathing and coughing, and it should be administered as needed. Clients with a smoking history or chronic airway limitation (e.g., chronic obstructive pulmonary disease, asthma) require more aggressive respiratory management by the respiratory therapist to prevent atelectasis and pneumonia. Clients with large hiatal hernias are at high risk for developing respiratory complications.

Nasogastric Tube Management. Postoperative management for open surgery also involves the care of the nasogastric (NG) tube. Inserting a large-diameter NG tube during surgery prevents the fundoplication wrap from becoming too tight around the esophagus. The NG drainage is initially dark brown with old blood but should become normal yellowish green within the first 8 hours after surgery. Check the NG tube every 4 to 8 hours for proper placement in the stomach. The NG tube should be properly anchored so it cannot be displaced because it cannot be safely reinserted without risking perforation of the incision. Follow the surgeon's requests for care of the client with an NG tube.

Frequent assessment of the patency of the tube is essential to keep the stomach decompressed; this prevents retching or vomiting, which can strain or rupture the stomach sutures. The NG tube is irritating; therefore provide frequent oral hygiene to increase comfort. Assess the client's hydration status regularly, including accurate measures of intake and output. Adequate fluid replacement helps to thin respiratory secretions.

Nutritional Care. The client may begin oral intake with clear fluids after peristalsis is re-established or in an effort to stimulate peristalsis. Some surgeons create a temporary gastrostomy for feeding to allow for undisturbed healing of the repair. The client gradually progresses to a near-normal diet during the first 6 weeks. A few foods, such as caffeinated or carbonated beverages and alcohol, are either restricted or eliminated. The food storage area of the stomach is reduced by the surgery, and meals need to be both smaller and more frequent.

The first oral feedings should be carefully supervised because temporary dysphagia is common. Persistent dysphagia usually indicates that the fundoplication is too tight, and dilation may be required.

Another common complication of fundoplication surgery is the **gas bloat syndrome,** in which clients are unable to voluntarily eructate (belch). The syndrome is usually temporary but may persist, even in clients who have the lap-aroscopic approach. Teach the client to avoid drinking carbonated beverages and to avoid eating gas-producing foods (especially high-fat foods), chewing gum, and drinking with a straw.

Many clients acquire the habit of **aerophagia** (air swallowing) from attempting to reverse or clear acid reflux. Teach these clients to relax consciously before and after meals, to eat and drink slowly, and to chew all food thoroughly. Air in the stomach that cannot be removed by belching can be extremely uncomfortable. Frequent position changes and ambulation are often effective interventions for eliminating air from the gastrointestinal tract. If gas pain is still present, clients are encouraged to take simethicone, 80 mg four times daily as needed. Be sure to remind the client to crush and dissolve the medication in water before taking.

Community-Based Care

Clients undergoing one of the open surgical repairs require activity restrictions during the 3- to 6-week postoperative recovery period. For laparoscopic surgery, activity is typically restricted for a shorter time, and the client can return to his or her usual lifestyle more quickly, usually in a few days to

Text continued on p. 1272.

CHART 58-6

CLIENT EDUCATION GUIDE
Postoperative Instructions for Clients Having Laparoscopic Nissen Fundoplication (LNF)

- Stay on a soft diet for about a week, including mashed potatoes, puddings, custard, and milkshakes; avoid carbonated beverages, tough foods, and raw vegetables that are difficult to swallow.
- Remain on antireflux medications as prescribed for at least a month.
- Do not drive for a week after surgery; do not drive if taking opioid pain medication.
- Walk every day, but do not do any heavy lifting.
- Remove gauze dressings 2 days after surgery and shower; do not remove Steri-strips until 10 days after surgery.
- Wash incisions with soap and water, rinse well, and pat dry; report any redness or drainage from the incisions to your surgeon.
- Report fever above 101° F, nausea, vomiting, or uncontrollable bloating or pain.
- Schedule an appointment for follow-up with your surgeon in 3 to 4 weeks.

CHART 58-7

BEST PRACTICE for
Assessment of Postoperative Complications Related to Fundoplication Procedures

Complication	Assessment Findings
Temporary dysphagia	The client has difficulty swallowing when oral feeding begins.
Gas bloat syndrome	The client has difficulty belching to relieve distention.
Atelectasis, pneumonia	The client experiences dyspnea, chest pain, or fever.
Obstructed nasogastric tube	The client experiences nausea, vomiting, or abdominal distention. The nasogastric tube does not drain.

PLAN of CARE MEDICAL DIAGNOSIS: ESOPHAGEAL SURGERY

NURSING DIAGNOSIS NO. 1 ■ Ineffective Breathing Pattern

	Expected Outcomes	Nursing Interventions	Rationales
RELATED FACTORS Pain Musculoskeletal impairment **DEFINING CHARACTERISTICS** Altered chest excursion	No verbal report or observation of dyspnea Respiratory rate remains between 11 and 22 breaths/min Has respirations that remain regular and deep	NIC **Airway Management** Place the client in semi-Fowler's position, if possible.	Semi-Fowler's position ensures that abdominal contents do not press against the diaphragm and restrict chest expansion.
		Encourage the client to cough frequently, or suction the client as necessary.	Coughing or suction will rid the airway of secretions.
		D Encourage the client to take slow, deep breaths; to turn; and to cough.	Effective aeration and coughing will help rid the body of secretions. Frequent position changes will prevent secretions from pooling in one area.
		D Assist the client with an incentive spirometer, as appropriate.	Incentive spirometry encourages the client to deep breathe.
		D Regulate fluid intake to optimize fluid balance.	Fluids will help keep lung secretions thin and easier to cough out of the airways.
		NIC **Respiratory Monitoring** D Monitor the rate, rhythm, depth, and effort of respirations.	Changes in respiratory rate, rhythm, depth, or effort may signal a descent into respiratory failure.
		Note chest movement, watching for symmetry, the use of accessory muscles, and supraclavicular and intercostal muscle retractions.	The use of accessory muscles indicates an increased respiratory effort.
		Auscultate breath sounds, noting areas of decreased/absent ventilation and the presence of adventitious sounds.	Absent breath sounds or adventitious breath sounds indicate poor gas exchange or poor movement of air through the airways.
		Note changes in Sao_2, Svo_2, end tidal CO_2, and arterial blood gas (ABG) values, as appropriate.	These tests indicate the effectiveness of gas exchange or gas transport.
		D Monitor the client's respiratory secretions.	Changes in the color, consistency, or odor of the secretions may indicate infection.
		Other Interventions Provide pain relief.	Deep breathing and coughing causes diaphragmatic movement and may increase pain.
		Continuing Care Considerations Teach the client relaxation techniques.	Stress management and relaxation techniques help to control the anxiety resulting from hypoxia.
		D Encourage the client to engage in regular physical exercise.	Cardiopulmonary efficiency and endurance improve with exercise.
		Encourage the client to enroll in a smoking cessation program, as indicated.	Smoking damages the airways and alveoli.

D Indicates tasks that can be delegated to unlicensed assistive personnel at the discretion of the nurse.

Continued

PLAN of CARE MEDICAL DIAGNOSIS: ESOPHAGEAL SURGERY—*cont'd*

NURSING DIAGNOSIS NO. 2 ■ Imbalanced Nutrition: Less Than Body Requirements

	Expected Outcomes	Nursing Interventions	Rationales
RELATED FACTORS Inability to ingest or digest food or absorb nutrients due to biologic factors: Surgery **DEFINING CHARACTERISTICS** Pain: Abdominal with or without pathology Perceived inability to ingest food	Has bowel sounds that remain at 3 to 5 per quadrant per minute Denies abdominal pain No verbal report or observation of diarrhea Weight remains within ±5 pounds of desired weight	Determine, in collaboration with a dietitian as appropriate, the number of calories and type of nutrients needed to meet nutrition requirements.	Individual client needs for nutrients and calories should be the basis for a sound dietary plan.
		D Provide foods appropriate for the client—blenderized or commercial formula via nasogastric or gastrostomy tube, or total parenteral nutrition—as ordered by physician.	Diet therapy and type of surgery dictate the type and form of foods that may be offered to the client.
		D Create a pleasant and relaxing environment at mealtime.	A pleasant and relaxing environment at mealtime improves digestion.
		Other Interventions Teach the client and family about high-calorie, high-protein meal planning, as appropriate.	Meal planning that considers the client's and family's budget and other resources increases the likelihood that appropriate meals will be prepared.
		Administer medication such as simethicone (crushed and dissolved in water) as ordered.	Simethicone may alleviate or eliminate painful gastrointestinal gas.
		Teach the client to consciously relax before and after meals.	Clients may have the habit of aerophagia to clear acid reflux. The excess air may be extremely uncomfortable.
		Teach the client and family about nutritional supplements, as appropriate.	Additional vitamins and minerals, calories, dietary fiber, or other nutritional components may need to be added to the diet of clients who are unable to eat a nutritionally adequate diet.
		Teach the client and family about preventing constipation.	Clients on low-fiber diets may need additional fluids and supplemental fiber to maintain bowel regularity.
		Continuing Care Consideration Encourage the client and family to use the home nutritional therapy team.	The home nutritional therapy team is able to monitor and adjust the nutritional plan of care to maximize the client's nutritional status.

NURSING DIAGNOSIS NO. 3 ■ Acute Pain

	Expected Outcomes	Nursing Interventions	Rationales
RELATED FACTORS Injury agents (biologic, chemical, physical, psychological): Surgery **DEFINING CHARACTERISTICS** Verbal or coded report of pain Observed evidence of pain	Denies experiencing pain greater than a 5 on a 0 to 10 pain scale No verbal report or observation of guarding or protective gestures No verbal report or observation of an alteration in sleep patterns No verbal report or observation of self-focusing behavior	NIC **Pain Management** Perform a comprehensive pain assessment that includes location, characteristics, onset/duration, frequency, quality, intensity or severity of pain, and precipitating factors.	A plan for pain management must be based on the client's unique responses to pain.
		Consider the cultural influences on the pain response.	Cultural stereotypes may lead to an inaccurate assessment of pain.

D Indicates tasks that can be delegated to unlicensed assistive personnel at the discretion of the nurse.

PLAN of CARE MEDICAL DIAGNOSIS: ESOPHAGEAL SURGERY—*cont'd*

NURSING DIAGNOSIS NO. 3 ■ Acute Pain—*cont'd*

Expected Outcomes	Nursing Interventions	Rationales
No verbal report or observation of facial mask of pain No verbal report or observation of an alteration in activity level	Select and implement a variety of measures to facilitate pain relief, as appropriate.	Pharmacologic, nonpharmacologic, and interpersonal strategies may provide pain relief depending on the client's unique responses to the therapeutic interventions.
	Use pain control measures before pain becomes severe.	Medicating the client in a timely manner prevents pain from reaching acutely unpleasant levels.
	Teach the use of nonpharmacologic techniques before, after and, if possible, during painful activities; before pain occurs or increases; and along with other pain relief measures.	Nonpharmacologic techniques help the client establish a sense of control over his or her pain experience.
	NIC **Analgesic Administration**	
	Choose the IV rather than the IM route for frequent pain medication injections, when possible.	The IV route avoids tissue trauma and the unpredictable absorption of medication.
	D Institute safety precautions for clients who are receiving opioid analgesics, as appropriate.	Opioid analgesics may impair the client's judgment and/or coordination.
	Document the client's response to the analgesic and any untoward effects.	Documentation provides the health care team with the information needed to accurately evaluate the client's response to the analgesic regimen.
	Implement actions to decrease the untoward effects of analgesics.	Actions taken to prevent the predictable but unwanted effects of narcotic analgesics (e.g., constipation) increase client comfort.
	Instruct the client to request PRN pain medication before the pain is severe.	Pain may be managed with lower doses of analgesics and fewer untoward effects if PRN drugs are used before pain becomes severe.
	NIC **Patient-Controlled Analgesia (PCA) Administration**	
	Consult with the client, family members, and physician to adjust lockout interval, basal rate, and demand dosage.	The client's response to the analgesic will determine the PCA settings.
	Teach the client and family to monitor pain intensity, quality, and duration.	This information will help the client and family determine when to administer a bolus dose of analgesic, if appropriate, or when to request an increase in basal rate of the analgesic.
	Teach the client and family members to monitor respiratory rate and blood pressure.	This information will help the health care team to adjust the analgesic doses to the client's responses and decrease the untoward effects.

Continued

PLAN of CARE MEDICAL DIAGNOSIS: ESOPHAGEAL SURGERY—*cont'd*

NURSING DIAGNOSIS NO. 3 ■ Acute Pain—*cont'd*

Expected Outcomes	Nursing Interventions	Rationales
	Teach the client and family how to use the PCA device.	The PCA device will not be used if the client and/or family do not know how to use or are afraid of the device.
	NIC **Environmental Management: Comfort**	
	D Facilitate hygiene measures to keep the client comfortable.	Hygiene measures may improve the client's overall sense of well-being.
	D Position the client to facilitate comfort.	The nurse may decrease sources of discomfort by using principles of body alignment, supporting with pillows, supporting joints during movement, splinting over incisions, and immobilizing painful body parts.
	Other Interventions	
	Refer the client to the Pain Advisory Committee.	The Pain Advisory Committee is a multidisciplinary committee with wide expertise in pain relief interventions.
	Consider the use of alternative therapies such as yoga, meditation, spirituality, and/or religion.	The experience of meditation and prayer and the reflection on meaning may help the client to relax, thereby easing the muscle tension that contributes to pain sensation.
	Consider the use of alternative therapies such as imagery, aromatherapy, music, touch, and laughter/humor.	Cognitive and behavioral strategies may be used as adjuncts to or in place of pharmacologic or surgical interventions for chronic pain. Each therapy has a different mode of action that may or may not benefit the client.
	Consider using other cutaneous skin stimulation techniques such as massage and/or vibration to complement pain management strategies.	Massage may cause muscle relaxation, which decreases pain signals; vibration interrupts pain signal transmission to decrease pain perception.
	Continuing Care Considerations	
	Refer the client to an advanced practice nurse pain specialist, social worker, home care nurse, and/or psychologist, as appropriate.	Health care team members are able to provide continuing support to the client who is facing chronic pain.

D Indicates tasks that can be delegated to unlicensed assistive personnel at the discretion of the nurse.

a week. For long-term management, teach the client and family about appropriate diet modifications. The use of stool softeners or bulk laxatives is recommended for the first postoperative weeks until healing is complete. Instruct the client to avoid straining and to prevent constipation. Teach the client to inspect the healing incision daily and to notify the health care provider if swelling, redness, tenderness, discharge, or fever occurs. Advise the client to avoid contact with people with respiratory infections and to contact the health care provider if symptoms of a cold or influenza develop. Persistent coughing can cause the incision or the fundoplication to dehisce. The client is also advised to avoid smoking.

Consult with the dietician to educate the family and significant others about dietary changes. Full support is essential for the client to modify the size and timing of meals successfully. Relatively few ongoing diet restrictions are needed, but overeating or eating the wrong types of foods can produce discomfort if the client cannot belch. Instruct the client to report the recurrence of reflux symptoms to the health care provider.

Although severe surgical complications are relatively rare, conditions such as gas bloat syndrome and dysphagia are common and may persist. Prepare the client for these problems and for the potential that reflux may not be completely controlled or may occur again. Although surgery controls the condition, a cure is rare, and lifestyle modifications need to be ongoing.

ACHALASIA

PATHOPHYSIOLOGY

Achalasia is an esophageal motility disorder believed to result from esophageal **denervation** (loss of nerve impulse passage). Its exact cause is unknown. A genetic basis to the disorder has been proposed as suggested by occasional familial clustering and phenotype (observable characteristics) association. As a result, the lower esophageal sphincter (LES) fails to relax properly with swallowing and in which the normal peristalsis of the esophagus is replaced with abnormal contractions. Achalasia is characterized by chronic and progressive dysphagia. Over time, peristaltic failure plus spasm can produce a massively dilated esophagus, which further slows food passage (Strader, 2001). Epigastric pain, a sensation of food sticking in the lower esophagus, and regurgitation of ingested food may also occur (Goroll & Mulley, 2000). Nighttime regurgitation of food occurs in 33% of people and can be the cause of cough, aspiration, or pneumonia (Strader, 2001). If left untreated, progressive dysphagia can result in weight loss.

Achalasia is an uncommon disorder that usually occurs between 20 and 40 years of age. Both genders appear to be equally affected. About 5% to 10% of individuals with this disorder develop esophageal squamous cell carcinoma. Complications of achalasia also include esophageal candidiasis, lower esophageal diverticula, airway obstruction, and aspiration pneumonia.

COLLABORATIVE MANAGEMENT

Assessment

Assess for the primary symptoms of achalasia, such as dysphagia and regurgitation of solids, liquids, or both. Ask the client about the presence of chest pain associated with these symptoms. Inquire about factors that aggravate the symptoms (e.g., body position or diet changes) as well as medications or home treatments that relieve the symptoms. Ask the client about a history of previous esophageal surgery or trauma, which can compound the progressive dysphagia. A respiratory history and current respiratory-associated symptoms are particularly important with regard to their direct relationship to reflux, regurgitation, and aspiration.

Take a nutritional history to determine the effect of the esophageal symptoms. Collect information about dietary habits, food tolerances, and weight loss. Note the presence of **halitosis** (foul mouth odor), which can be caused by the regurgitation of previously ingested food. Auscultate the lungs for adventitious sounds secondary to pulmonary aspiration of retained saliva and food. The client's current and usual weight should be noted and compared for weight loss resulting from dysphagia.

A barium swallow is the most sensitive test for visualizing the esophagus and is likely to show esophageal dilation with a persistent beaklike narrowing at the terminal esophagus, the hallmark of a nonrelaxing LES. A chest x-ray can show a distorted and dilated tubular esophagus, the absence of a gastric air bubble, and occasionally a tubular mediastinal mass next to the aorta. Esophageal manometry typically reveals an increased LES pressure and incomplete sphincter relaxation when the client swallows. Endoscopy is used to evaluate the appearance of the esophageal mucosa, especially for changes associated with cancer or the presence of candida.

Interventions

The symptoms associated with achalasia can be treated with a variety of approaches. A combination of dietary measures, pharmacologic agents, esophageal dilation, and surgery is used.

Drug and Diet Therapy. Mild cases of achalasia can be managed with calcium channel blockers (nifedipine [Procardia]) or nitrates (sublingual nitroglycerin) to reduce LES pressure. Drug therapy is given for symptom relief and is not recommended as an alternative to more definitive therapy. Achalasia can also be treated with the direct injection of botulinum toxin (Botox) into the LES muscle via endoscopy. Botulinum toxin acts to denervate cholinergic nerves in the distal esophagus by suppression of acetylcholine release. Ninety percent of clients have improvement after this procedure; however, repeated regular dosing is required, and the long-term effects are unknown.

Advise the client to experiment with changes in diet because they can often ease the pressure and reflux associated with achalasia. Discuss any food habits he or she has noted that aggravate or relieve the symptoms. Semisoft foods are often better tolerated, as are warm foods and liquids. Eating four to six smaller meals rather than three large meals during the day facilitates the passage of food. Collaborate with the dietitian for additional suggestions about diet changes and nutritional balance. Nocturnal reflux of foods and liquids from the dilated esophagus into the hypopharynx and oral cavity often can be prevented if the client sleeps with the head of the bed elevated or in a semi-sitting position. Advise the client to experiment with various changes in position while eating because such changes can reduce pressure sensations during meals. Some clients benefit from arching the back while swallowing. Caution the client to avoid wearing restrictive clothing, which can increase esophageal pressure and regurgitation.

Esophageal Dilation. More severe cases of achalasia require dilation of the LES. The traditional treatment involves the passage of progressively larger sizes of esophageal bougies (dilators) using polyurethane balloons on a catheter. The procedure is performed on an ambulatory care basis. Large-diameter metal **stents** may be used to keep the esophagus open for longer durations.

After the procedure, monitor the client for complications of bleeding and signs of perforation, such as chest and shoulder pain, elevated temperature, **subcutaneous emphysema** (air under the skin), or **hemoptysis** (coughing up blood). Teach the client to expectorate rather than swallow any secretions that are be produced. Instruct the client to take nothing by mouth (NPO) for 1 hour and to limit dietary intake to liquids for 24 hours. The procedure may be repeated in 2 to 3 months if needed. Most clients report improvement in swallowing.

Esophagomyotomy. Surgical procedures for the client with achalasia are aimed at facilitating the passage of food. **Esophagomyotomy,** in which the LES is incised, has been used successfully for decades. Open thoracic and abdominal approaches can be used, but laparoscopic surgery has become more common. An antireflux wrap **(fundoplication)** may or may not be part of the procedure.

Conventional esophagomyotomy is a more complex surgical treatment for achalasia. Using an open approach, general anesthesia is required, and the client is hospitalized for several days. A thoracotomy approach permits exposure of the esophagus. The surgeon cuts muscle fibers around the LES to open the sphincter and thereby provide less obstruction to food passage.

For long-term refractory achalasia, the surgeon may attempt excision of the affected portion of the esophagus, with or without replacement by a segment of colon or jejunum (partial esophagectomy).

Postoperative care for clients undergoing trans-thoracic esophagomyotomy includes managing chest tubes and drains, assessing healing of the thoracotomy or abdominal incision, pain control, and managing NG feedings. (See Chapter 22 for general postoperative care and Chapter 33 for care of the client with a thoracotomy.)

Laparoscopic surgery permits a shorter length of stay and fewer complications compared with either open surgical approach. Clients receive conscious sedation rather than general anesthesia. Teach clients having laparoscopic surgery to report complications, such as bleeding and fever. Instruct the client as described in Chart 58-6.

ESOPHAGEAL TUMORS

PATHOPHYSIOLOGY

Esophageal tumors can be benign or malignant. However, benign esophageal tumors, known as leiomyomas, are extremely uncommon. These tumors are removed if they cause discomfort but otherwise require no specific treatment. Most malignant esophageal tumors arise from the epithelium. Squamous cell carcinomas of the esophagus are located in the upper two thirds of the esophagus. Adenocarcinomas are more commonly found in the distal third and at the gastroesophageal junction, and these tumors account for 50% of all esophageal cancers (Brooks-Brunn, 2000). The local and regional lymphatic spread of the disease differs according to the site of the original tumor. Esophageal tumors exhibit rapid local growth because there is no serosal layer to limit their extension. Because the esophageal mucosa is richly supplied with lymphatics, there is early spread of tumors to lymph nodes. Esophageal tumors can protrude into the esophageal lumen and can cause thickening of the lumen or invade deeply into surrounding tissue. In rare cases the lesion may be confined to the epithelial layer (in situ). In the most cases, the tumor is relatively large and well established on diagnosis. More than 50% of esophageal cancers **metastasize** (spread throughout the body).

Etiology and Genetic Risk

In Western societies, the two primary risk factors associated with the development of squamous cell carcinoma of the esophagus are tobacco use and heavy alcohol intake. The compounds in tobacco smoke may be responsible for the genetic mutations seen in one half of esophageal tumors. A smoker has two to six times the risk of eventually developing esophageal cancer than does a nonsmoker. Some alcoholic beverages contain potent carcinogens that may be responsible for the development of esophageal tumors. Smoking and alcohol ingestion act together in the development of esophageal cancer.

Long-term, untreated gastroesophageal reflux disease (GERD) can play a role in esophageal cancer development. For individuals with Barrett's esophagus, the risk of developing esophageal cancer is increased 30 to 150 times as compared with the general population. Exposure to acid and pepsin leads to the replacement of normal distal squamous mucosa with columnar epithelium as a response to tissue injury, known as **Barrett's esophagus.** This tissue undergoes dysplasia and, ultimately, malignant transformation. In other parts of the world where esophageal cancer is common, the incidence of squamous cell carcinoma appears to be linked to high levels of nitrosamines (which are found in pickled and fermented foods) and foods high in nitrate. Diets that are chronically deficient in fresh fruits and vegetables have also been implicated in the development of squamous cell carcinoma.

Certain genetic factors may have a role in the development of esophageal cancer. It has been proposed that esophageal cancers result from mutations in suppressor genes and proto-oncogenes (see Chapter 11 for a more complete discussion). Overexpression and mutations of the *p53* tumor suppressor gene have been found in persons with esophageal cancer. In addition, the presence of the *p53* gene may be an indication of advanced disease. Tumor cells with a mutated *p53* gene have demonstrated resistance to chemotherapy.

Incidence/Prevalence

Esophageal cancer, the second most common cancer of the thoracic cavity, accounts for 6% of all cancers of the GI tract, and mortality from the disease remains very high (American Cancer Society, 2003). In 2003 about 14,000 new cases of esophageal cancer were diagnosed and as many related deaths in the United States (American Cancer Society, 2003). The incidence of squamous cell carcinoma of the esophagus has remained stable, but the rate of adenocarcinoma has continued to rise 4% to 5% per year. This increased rate seems to be directly related to the increase in cases of GERD.

CULTURAL CONSIDERATIONS

Squamous cell carcinoma is more commonly found in African-American men, whereas adenocarcinoma is more prevalent in white men. Squamous cell carcinoma of the esophagus is the seventh leading cause of cancer deaths in African Americans. By contrast, white men have a higher prevalence of adenocarcinoma of the esophagus (Brooks-Brunn, 2000).

COLLABORATIVE MANAGEMENT

PHARM REVIEW

Assessment

HISTORY

Assess for risk factors related to the development or symptoms of esophageal cancer, such as the client's racial and cultural background, age, gender, history of alcohol consumption, tobacco use, dietary habits, and other esophageal problems (e.g., dysphagia, stricture, reflux). Ask the client about the ingestion of pickled foods, changes in appetite, changes in taste, or a decline in weight. Cancer of the esophagus is a silent tumor in its early stages, with few signs to identify on assessment. By the time the tumor causes symptoms, it usually has spread rather extensively.

PHYSICAL ASSESSMENT/CLINICAL MANIFESTATIONS

Dysphagia (difficulty swallowing) is the most common symptom of esophageal cancer, but it may not be present until the lumen of the esophagus is significantly narrowed. Dysphagia is both persistent and progressive. It is initially associated with swallowing solids, particularly meat, and then progresses rapidly over a period of weeks or months to difficulty in swallowing soft foods and liquids. Late in the disease, even saliva can induce choking. Clients usually report a sensation that food is sticking in the throat or in the substernal area. Careful assessment of the dysphagia is an important part of the diagnosis because dysphagia associated with other esophageal disorders is not usually continuous. Weight loss often accompanies dysphagia and can exceed 20 pounds.

Odynophagia (painful swallowing) is present in most clients and is reported as a steady, dull, substernal pain that may radiate. The presence of severe or persistent pain often indicates tumor invasion of the mediastinal structures. Assess for the occurrence of regurgitation, vomiting, foul breath, and chronic hiccups, which often accompany advanced disease. In most clients, pulmonary complications develop at some point. Assess for the presence of chronic cough, increased secretions, and a history of recent infections. Tumors in the upper esophagus may involve the larynx and thus cause hoarseness. Chart 58-8 summarizes the clinical manifestations of esophageal tumors.

PSYCHOSOCIAL ASSESSMENT

The diagnosis of esophageal cancer is a great source of anxiety to the client. The disease is accompanied by distressing symptoms and is often terminal. The fear of choking can place unusual stress on normal mealtimes. Assess the client's response to the diagnosis and prognosis, and explore his or her coping strengths and resources. The impact of the disease on the usual pattern of activities is also assessed. Determine the availability of support systems and the potential financial impact of the disease and its treatment. Refer the client and family members to psychological counseling, pastoral care, and the social worker as needed.

RADIOGRAPHIC ASSESSMENT

A barium swallow study with fluoroscopy is usually the first diagnostic test ordered to evaluate dysphagia. In a barium swallow, the margins of a tumor may be seen. However, to make a definitive diagnosis of cancer, a tissue biopsy via endoscopy is needed.

CHART 58-8

KEY FEATURES of Esophageal Tumors

- Persistent and progressive dysphagia (most common feature)
- Feeling of food sticking in the throat
- Odynophagia (painful swallowing)
- Severe, persistent chest or abdominal pain or discomfort
- Regurgitation
- Chronic cough with increasing secretions
- Hoarseness
- Anorexia
- Nausea and vomiting
- Weight loss (often more than 20 pounds)
- Changes in bowel habits (diarrhea, constipation, bleeding)

OTHER DIAGNOSTIC ASSESSMENTS

The definitive diagnosis of esophageal cancer is made by esophagogastroduodenoscopy (EGD) with biopsies of the esophagus and tumor. During an EGD, the esophagus is inspected and tissue specimens are obtained for cytologic studies and disease staging. Multiple tissue samples may be required when the suspected tumor is in the distal esophagus, because clear tissue samples are difficult to obtain. A complete staging workup is performed to determine the extent of the disease.

A computed tomography (CT) scan assists in identifying metastatic disease, which might be present in the chest or abdomen. Positron emission tomography (PET) is a newer technology that may identify metastatic disease with more accuracy than a CT scan. An endoscopic ultrasound (EUS) is a staging technique that can help determine the size and depth of tumor invasion. (These tests are described elsewhere in Chapter 56.)

Critical Thinking Challenge

You are caring for an older adult recently diagnosed with esophageal cancer. He states he smoked two packs of cigarettes per day for 30 years but quit 5 years ago. He also states that he drinks alcohol occasionally but tends to eat late at night and as a result often has heartburn. He also complains of food "sticking" in his throat.

1. What lifestyle factors in this client's history would predispose him to esophageal cancer?
2. What questions would you ask him regarding symptoms he might be experiencing as a result of his diagnosis?
3. What complications will he experience if his dysphagia worsens?

evolve For suggested answer guidelines, go to http://evolve.elsevier.com/Iggy/.

Analysis

COMMON NURSING DIAGNOSES AND COLLABORATIVE PROBLEMS

The following is a priority nursing diagnosis for adult clients with esophageal cancer:

- Imbalanced Nutrition: Less Than Body Requirements related to impaired swallowing

ADDITIONAL NURSING DIAGNOSES AND COLLABORATIVE PROBLEMS

In addition to the common nursing diagnosis, the client with esophageal cancer may develop any of the following resulting from the impact of the disease and its treatment:

- Risk for Aspiration related to impaired swallowing secondary to esophageal strictures
- Impaired Swallowing related to obstruction by the tumor or the effects of radiotherapy
- Acute Pain or Chronic Pain related to the physical injury (pressure of the tumor mass in the esophagus or mediastinum)
- Ineffective Coping and Compromised Family Coping related to the effects of the disease and to the terminal prognosis
- Anticipatory Grieving related to declining physical status and terminal prognosis
- Spiritual Distress related to impending death

The additional collaborative problem is Potential for Metastasis resulting from the close proximity of the esophagus to other body structures.

◆Planning and Implementation

IMBALANCED NUTRITION: LESS THAN BODY REQUIREMENTS

NOC **PLANNING: EXPECTED OUTCOMES.** The major concern for a client with esophageal cancer is weight loss secondary to dysphagia. Therefore the client is expected to maintain adequacy of his or her usual pattern of nutrient intake. Indicators include that the client will have totally adequate:

- Caloric intake
- Protein and fat intake
- Carbohydrate intake
- Vitamin and mineral intake

INTERVENTIONS. Interventions to maintain or improve the nutritional status of the client must focus on treatments that remove or shrink the obstructive tumor. Methods to reduce the effects of treatment that can impact nutritional status are also a priority.

NONSURGICAL MANAGEMENT. Treatment options for cancer of the esophagus that can assist in both disease and nutrition management include the following:

- Nutrition therapy
- Swallowing therapy
- Chemotherapy
- Radiation therapy
- Photodynamic therapy
- Esophageal dilation
- Endoscopic therapies
- Surgical removal of the tumor

The treatment of esophageal cancer often involves a combination of the above therapies **(multimodal therapies).** Clients with cancer of the esophagus can experience many problems, and relieving symptoms becomes an essential consideration.

NIC **Nutrition Therapy.** The purpose of nutrition therapy is the administration of food and fluids to support the client who is malnourished or at high risk of becoming malnourished. A thorough nutritional assessment provides members of the health care team with baseline information concerning the client's nutritional status. The dietitian determines the caloric needs of the client to meet nutritional requirements. Weigh the client daily. Careful positioning is essential for a client who is experiencing frequent regurgitation or who has prosthetic tubes to keep the esophagus patent. Teach the client to remain upright for several hours after meals and to avoid lying completely flat. The head of the bed should remain elevated to a 30-degree angle or more to prevent reflux.

Semisoft foods and thickened liquids are preferred because they are easier to swallow. The total number of calories taken in daily and the amount of fluids ingested are monitored daily to monitor progress toward nutritional goals. Liquid nutritional supplements (e.g., Boost, Ensure) are used between feedings to increase caloric intake. Ongoing efforts are made to preserve the ability to swallow, but feeding tubes may be needed temporarily when dysphagia is severe. In clients with complete obstruction or life-threatening fistula formation, it may be necessary to create a gastrostomy or jejunostomy. Laboratory and clinical indicators of nutritional status are also monitored on a regular basis. The client and family are encouraged to meet with the dietician for diet teaching and planning.

NIC **Swallowing Therapy.** Consult with the speech-language pathologist to assist the client with oral exercises to improve swallowing. A lollipop given to the client to suck on can enhance tongue strength. The client is instructed to reach for food particles on the lips or chin using the tongue. In preparation for swallowing, you should assist the client to position the head in forward flexion (chin tuck). The client is then instructed to place food at the back of the mouth. Monitor the client for the sealing of lips and for tongue movements while eating and also check for pocketing of food after swallowing. It is important to monitor for signs of aspiration. Family members and caregivers are taught how to feed the client, monitor for aspiration, and institute appropriate measures if choking occurs. Chart 58-9 provides a summary of NIC interventions.

Chemotherapy. The use of chemotherapy in the treatment of esophageal cancer has been only moderately effective. It can be given as a primary treatment if the client is not a candidate for surgery. However, chemotherapy is most often given in combination with radiation therapy. This treatment is thought to provide the client with the best chance of cure. The rationale behind this approach is to shrink the tumor and eliminate any tumor that may be in the local lymph nodes, improving the odds for a complete surgical resection. The two most commonly used chemotherapeutic agents are 5-fluorouracil (5-FU) and cisplatin. Cisplatin and 5-FU make the tumor cells more sensitive to the effects of radiation.

Radiation Therapy. Radiation therapy to manage esophageal cancer is only moderately effective and can be used alone or in combination with other modalities. Radiation given alone can provide palliation of symptoms by shrinking the tumor. It is contraindicated for clients with tracheoesophageal fistula, mediastinitis, mediastinal hemorrhage, or infiltration of the cancer to the trachea or bronchus. Normal esophageal tissue is very sensitive to the effects of radiation, and although higher doses of radiation demonstrate better results, esophageal stricture or stenosis can result in 30% to 50% of clients requiring esophageal dilation.

Radiation therapy is typically administered in 20 episodes over 4 weeks. In the first weeks of treatment, it produces edema and epithelial desquamation, which often create

CHART 58-9

NIC INTERVENTION ACTIVITIES for The Client with Esophageal Problems

Nutrition Therapy: *Administration of food and fluids to support metabolic processes of a client who is malnourished or at high risk for becoming malnourished*

- Determine—in collaboration with the dietitian, as appropriate—the number of calories and type of nutrients needed to meet nutrition requirements.
- Assist client to a sitting position before eating or feeding.
- Encourage client to select semisoft food, if lack of saliva hinders swallowing.
- Monitor food/fluid ingested and calculate daily caloric intake, as appropriate.
- Determine need for enteral tube feedings.

Swallowing Therapy: *Facilitating swallowing and preventing complications of impaired swallowing*

- Collaborate with speech therapist to instruct client/family about swallowing exercise regimen.
- Explain rationale of the swallowing regimen to client/family.
- Provide a lollipop for client to suck on to enhance tongue strength, if appropriate.
- Assist client to position head in forward flexion in preparation for swallowing ("chin tuck").
- Assist client to place food at back of mouth and on unaffected side.
- Monitor for signs and symptoms of aspiration.
- Instruct family/caregiver how to position, feed, and monitor client.
- Instruct client/caregiver on emergency measures for choking.

NIC intervention activities selected from Dochterman, J.M., & Bulechek, G.M. (Eds.). (2004). *Nursing interventions classification (NIC)* (4th ed.). St. Louis: Mosby. No part of this work is to be altered without prior written permission from the Publisher.

acute esophagitis and odynophagia (painful swallowing). Profound anorexia, nausea, and vomiting may also result. Symptoms persist until treatment is completed. Assess the client frequently to determine the incidence and severity of symptoms. Systemic analgesics are often required to control discomfort, and topical lidocaine (Viscous Xylocaine) can be administered before each attempt at oral feeding.

Assist the client to modify the diet to meet nutritional needs and maintain comfort. Small, frequent, soft or semiliquid meals are offered. Sweet, light foods are often tolerated best, and protein powder may be used to supplement the nutritional content of the diet. An accurate record of calorie counts, intake and output, and daily weights should be maintained. Assess skin turgor and mucous membranes regularly. In collaboration with the health care provider and dietitian, assess the need for enteral nutrition if oral intake is insufficient. Frequent, gentle mouth care is important for clients receiving radiation therapy because clients are at risk for monilial esophagitis. Chapter 28 describes additional nursing interventions for the client undergoing radiation therapy.

Photodynamic Therapy. Photodynamic therapy (PDT) was originally used for the treatment of skin cancer. In 1995 it was approved for use as a palliative treatment for individuals with advanced esophageal cancer, who are not candidates for surgery. The client is injected with porfimer sodium (Photofrin), a light-sensitive drug that acts to amass cancer cells. Two days after the injection, a fiberoptic probe with a light at the tip is threaded into the esophagus. The light activates the Photofrin, destroying only cancer cells. PDT is far less invasive than surgery and is performed on an ambulatory care basis under conscious sedation.

The side effects of Photofrin are rare but include nausea, fever, and constipation. After the procedure, the client is given written guidelines concerning photosensitivity measures. Instruct the client to avoid exposure to sunlight for 1 month. Sunglasses and protective clothing that covers all exposed body areas are essential. The client may experience chest pain secondary to tissue damage and will require pain relief with opioid analgesics for a short time. Remind the client to follow a clear liquid diet for 3 to 5 days after the procedure and advance to full liquids as tolerated.

Esophageal Dilation. Esophageal dilation may be performed as necessary throughout the course of the disease to achieve temporary but immediate relief of dysphagia. Esophageal dilation can be performed on an ambulatory care basis. Dilators are used to tear soft tissue, thereby widening the esophageal lumen. In most cases, malignant tumors can be dilated safely, but perforation remains a significant risk. Large metal stents may be used to keep the esophagus open for longer durations. A stent covered with graft material can be used to seal a perforation. Bacteremia can also occur. To reduce the risk of endocarditis, the American Heart Association recommends prophylaxis with antibiotics. The treatment is repeated as often as needed to preserve the client's ability to swallow.

Endoscopic Therapies. When clients are not candidates for surgery or the tumor is too large to remove surgically, laser therapy or electrocoagulation may be performed as a palliative measure. Both of these methods destroy cancer cells to improve swallowing.

SURGICAL MANAGEMENT. The goals of surgical resection vary from palliation to cure. **Esophagectomy** is the removal of all or part of the esophagus. An **esophagogastrostomy** involves the removal of part of the esophagus and proximal stomach. The remaining stomach may be "pulled up" to take the place of the esophagus, or the jejunum or colon may be used as a conduit. Conventional open surgical techniques can take 6 to 8 hours and are associated with significant morbidity and mortality. Mortality as a result of open surgery ranges from 10% to 20%. Complications (e.g., fistula formation, abscess, respiratory complications) occur in 20% to 50% of individuals.

For clients with early stage cancer, a **minimally invasive esophagectomy (MIE)** via laparoscopy may be performed. However, most clients require the conventional open surgery because of tumor size and metastasis.

Preoperative Care. Preoperative preparation for clients undergoing esophagectomy or esophagogastrostomy can be quite extensive, especially before conventional techniques. Clients are advised to stop smoking 2 to 4 weeks before surgery to enhance their pulmonary functioning. Client preparation may include 5 days to 2 to 3 weeks of nutritional support in an effort to improve nutritional status and decrease postoperative morbidity. Ideally this supplementation is given orally, but many clients require tube feeding or parenteral nutrition. The role of parenteral nutritional support in these clients remains controversial. Monitor the client's weight, intake and output, and fluid and electrolyte balance. A preoperative dental evaluation may be required to remove pre-existing dental caries. Provide meticulous oral care four times daily to decrease the risk of postoperative infection.

Preoperative nursing care also focuses on teaching and on psychological support regarding the surgical procedure and preoperative and postoperative instructions. Educate the client about the following:

- The number and sites of all incisions and drains
- The placement of a jejunostomy tube for initial enteral feedings
- The need for chest tubes if the pleural space is entered
- The purpose of the nasogastric tube
- The need for intravenous (IV) infusion

Instruct the client about routines for turning, coughing, deep breathing, and chest physiotherapy. Emphasize the crucial nature of postoperative respiratory care. If colon interposition (resecting a piece of colon and creating an esophagus) is planned, the client also undergoes a complete bowel preparation with laxatives and enemas before surgery.

The client facing a serious illness and extensive surgery can be expected to display feelings of grief and anxiety. Encourage the client to talk about personal feelings and fears, and involve the family or significant others in all preoperative teaching and discussions. A primary nurse or case manager can be extremely helpful in providing continuity of care and support to the entire family.

Operative Procedures. In the MIE procedure, the surgeon makes four or five small incisions in the chest and abdomen. The lower esophagus and gastric fundus are removed. The remaining portion of the esophagus is then anastomosed (reconnected) to the stomach.

For most clients, an open subtotal or total esophagectomy is required because tumors are often quite large and involve distant lymph nodes. The diseased portion of the esophagus is removed, and the cervical portion is anastomosed (connected) to the stomach. The cervical portion of the stomach is then brought up into the thorax through the esophageal hiatus (Figure 58-3). A **pyloromyotomy** is created to prevent gastric motility disturbances. Finally, a jejunostomy tube may be placed for postoperative enteral feeding.

For clients with early stage tumors of the lower third of the esophagus, a transhiatal esophagectomy is the preferred surgical approach. The surgery is performed through an upper midline cervical incision. With this approach there is no entry into the pleural space, reducing respiratory complications. For clients with tumors in the upper esophagus, a radical neck dissection and laryngectomy may also be needed if the disease has spread to the larynx. The surgeon may perform a **colon interposition** when the tumor involves the stomach or the stomach is otherwise unsuitable for anastomosis. A section of right or left colon is removed and brought up into the thorax to substitute for the esophagus (see Figure 58-3).

Postoperative Care. These surgical procedures pose cardiovascular risks for the client. Intraoperative hypotension can result from pressure on the posterior heart. Pulmonary edema can occur when mediastinal lymph nodes and lymphatics are resected due to decreased pulmonary clearance and lymphatic congestion. The stress placed on the heart by extensive surgery can increase the risk of myocardial ischemia and dysrhythmias, especially if the client has underlying coronary disease.

The client with compromised nutritional status or prior radiation or chemotherapy is predisposed to an increased risk of infection. For clients who undergo more radical surgical procedures, there is a serious risk of leakage at the anastomosis site. This situation is especially true with colon interpositions because several anastomosis sites are vulnerable to the effects of tension, poor blood supply, and delayed healing. Mediastinitis resulting from an anastomotic leak can lead to fatal sepsis.

The client requires meticulous postoperative care and is at risk for multiple serious complications. The Plan of Care on pp. 1269 to 1272 outlines client interventions for esophageal surgery.

Respiratory Care. Respiratory care is the highest postoperative priority. For the client having traditional surgery, intubation with mechanical ventilation is needed for at least the

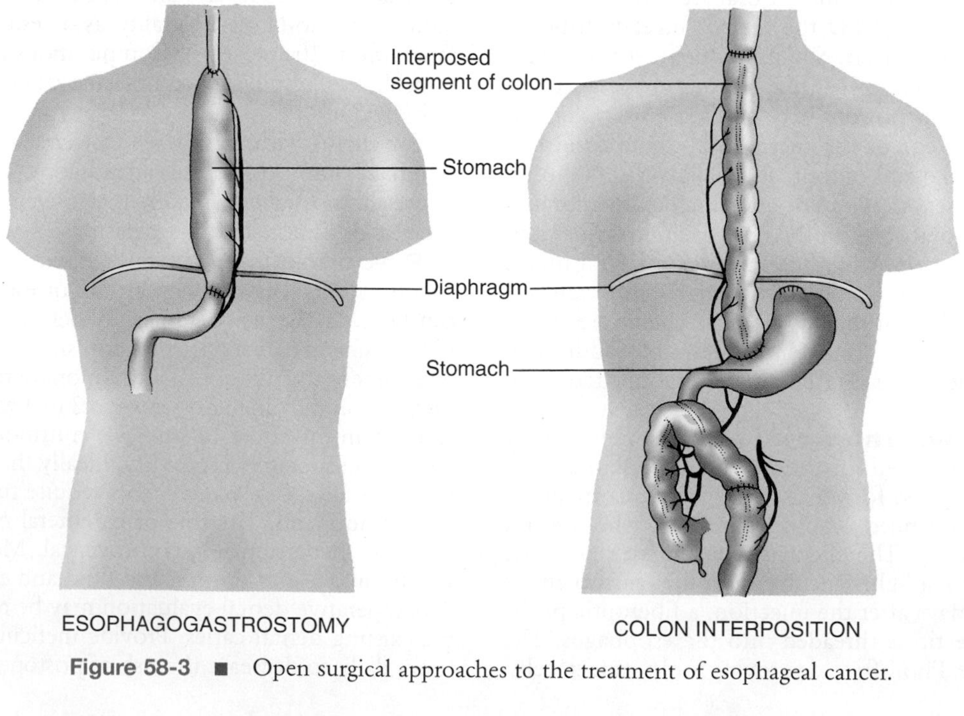

Figure 58-3 ■ Open surgical approaches to the treatment of esophageal cancer.

first 24 hours. Postoperative pulmonary complications include atelectasis and pneumonia. The risk of postoperative pulmonary complications is increased in the client who has received preoperative radiation. Once the client is extubated, deep breathing, turning, and coughing routines should begin. Chest physiotherapy is initiated as ordered, usually every 2 to 4 hours. Assess the client for decreased breath sounds and shortness of breath every 1 to 2 hours. Incisional support and adequate analgesia are essential for effective coughing and should be administered regularly if the client's vital signs remain stable. Keep the client in a semi-Fowler's or high Fowler's position to support ventilation and prevent reflux. The health care provider prescribes prophylactic antibiotics and supplemental oxygen; blood gases are ordered regularly. Ensure the patency of the chest tube drainage system, and monitor for changes in the volume or color of the drainage.

Cardiovascular Care. Cardiovascular complications, particularly hypotension, can occur secondary to pressure placed on the posterior heart, and usually respond well to IV fluid administration. Monitor for manifestations of fluid volume overload, particularly in older clients and in those who have undergone lymph node dissection. Assess for edema, crackles in the lungs, and increased jugular venous pressure. In the immediate postoperative phase, the client may be admitted to the intensive care unit. Critical care nurses assess hemodynamic parameters such as cardiac output, cardiac index, and systemic vascular resistance every 2 hours to monitor for myocardial ischemia. Atrial fibrillation is a dysrhythmia that results from irritation of the vagus nerve during surgery and must be managed.

Wound Management. Wound management is another significant postoperative concern for conventional surgery because the client typically has multiple incisions and drains. Provide incisional support during turning and coughing to prevent dehiscence. Wound infection usually occurs 4 to 5 days after surgery. Postoperative leakage from the site of anastomosis is a dreaded complication that can appear 2 to 10 days after surgery. If an anastomotic leak occurs, all oral intake is discontinued and is not resumed until the leak has healed. Nutrition may be given through the jejunostomy tube during the healing process. Carefully assess for fever, fluid accumulation, general signs of inflammation, and symptoms of early shock (e.g., tachycardia, tachypnea), and report these findings to the health care provider immediately.

Nasogastric Tube Management. A nasogastric (NG) tube is placed intraoperatively to decompress the suture line. Monitor the NG tube for patency and carefully secure the tube to prevent dislodgment, which can disrupt the sutures at the anastomosis. *Do not independently irrigate or reposition the NG tube in clients who have undergone esophageal surgery!* The initial nasogastric drainage is bloody but should change to a greenish yellow color by the end of the first postoperative day. The continued presence of blood may indicate bleeding at the suture line. Oral hygiene should be provided to the client every 2 to 4 hours while the tube is in place (Chart 58-10).

Nutritional Care. The nutritional management of the client who has undergone an esophageal surgery is an early postoperative concern. After conventional surgery, on the second postoperative day, initial feedings begin through the jejunostomy tube. The feedings are slowly increased over the next several days. Feeding by this method can be discontinued once the client is taking adequate oral nutrition. However, some clients may require jejunostomy feedings for about 1 month if small amounts of aspiration are detected.

Before beginning oral feedings, a cine-esophagram study is performed to detect the presence of anastomotic leaks, strictures, or signs of aspiration. If no leaks are detected, an esophageal diet is begun, starting with liquids. If liquids are well tolerated, the client's diet is advanced to include semisolid foods and then solid foods. The client should be placed in an upright position and supervised during all initial swallowing efforts. The food storage area of the stomach has been radically decreased, and gravity is the client's only real defense against reflux. The client is instructed to consume six to eight meals per day and to ingest fluids between, rather than with, meals to prevent diarrhea. Diarrhea can occur 20 minutes to 2 hours after eating and can be symptomatically managed with loperamide (Imodium) before meals. The diarrhea is thought to be the result of **vagotomy syndrome,** which develops as a result of the interruption of vagal fibers to the abdominal viscera during surgery. This syndrome is diminished by pyloroplasty. Assessment for signs of anastomotic leakage should be continued throughout hospitalization.

Critical Thinking Challenge

Your client has been told he is not a candidate for curative surgery for his esophageal cancer and will be receiving combination chemoradiation as a palliative treatment.

1. What should you teach the client about these treatments?
2. What other types of services should you anticipate this client will require?
3. What psychological issues is this client facing?

evolve For suggested answer guidelines, go to http://evolve.elsevier.com/Iggy/.

Community-Based Care

Clients with esophageal cancer have many challenges to face once they are discharged home. The combination treatment regimens cause long-lasting side effects, such as fatigue and

CHART 58-10

BEST PRACTICE for
Managing the Client with a Nasogastric Tube After Esophageal Surgery

- Check for tube placement every 4 to 8 hours.
- Ensure that the tube is patent (open) and draining; drainage should turn from bloody to yellowish green by the end of the first postoperative day.
- Secure the tube well to prevent dislodgment.
- Do not irrigate or reposition the tube without a physician's order.
- Provide meticulous oral and nasal hygiene every 2 to 4 hours.
- Keep the head of the bed elevated to at least 30 degrees.
- When the client is permitted to have a small amount of water, place the client in an upright position and observe for dysphagia (difficulty swallowing).
- Observe for leakage from the anastomosis site, as indicated by fever, fluid accumulation, and manifestations of early shock (tachycardia, tachypnea, altered mental status).

weakness. These complex treatments also require the client to be knowledgeable about symptom management and to know when to report issues of concern to the health care provider. (See Chapter 28 for care of the client undergoing radiation therapy and chemotherapy.)

HOME CARE MANAGEMENT

The client having minimally invasive surgery has a shorter hospital stay and fewer complications compared with conventional surgical clients. Clients with MIE usually stay several days in the hospital and return to usual activities sooner than those having traditional surgical procedures. Many clients have chemotherapy and radiation after surgery.

Once the client is discharged home, ongoing respiratory care is a priority. Give the client and family members instructions about ambulation and incentive spirometer use. Encourage the client to be as active as possible and to avoid excessive bedrest because this can lead to complications. Teach the family to protect the client from infection and to contact the health care provider immediately if signs of respiratory infection develop.

HEALTH TEACHING

Teach the client and family to inspect the incisions daily for redness, tenderness, swelling, odor, and discharge because proper wound healing is still a concern at the time of discharge. Instruct the client and family to report a temperature greater than 101° F (38.3° C). Prepare written instructions about the signs of anastomosis leakage and the importance of reporting them to the health care provider immediately. Instruct the client and family members to report the presence of fever and a swollen, painful neck incision, which indicate a cervical anastomotic leak.

Nutritional support also remains a concern. Encourage the client to continue increasing oral feedings as tolerated. Instruct the client to eat small, frequent meals containing high-calorie, high-protein foods that are soft and easily swallowed. Instruct the client to use supplemental eggnogs and milkshakes between meals, and instruct the client to eat slowly. Individuals who have undergone esophageal resection can lose up to 10% of their body weight. Teach the client to monitor his or her weight at home and to report a weight loss of 5 pounds or more. If sufficient oral intake is not possible, the family may need instruction about tube feedings or parenteral nutrition at home.

Emphasize the importance of remaining upright after meals. Dysphagia or odynophagia may recur because of stricture, reflux, or cancer recurrence. These symptoms should be promptly reported to the health care provider. Despite radical surgery, the client with cancer of the esophagus still has a terminal illness and a relatively short life expectancy. Emphasis is placed on maximizing quality of life. (See Evidence-Based Practice for Nursing box above). Realistic planning is important as the client's condition eventually worsens, and the client and family are assisted to plan for the future together. Assist family members in exploring formal and informal sources of support. Help the family or significant others arrange for hospice care when it is needed.

HEALTH CARE RESOURCES

Referrals to community or home care organizations should be initiated to assist the family in providing care in the home. The client may need transportation to the radiation treatment center five times per week for up to 6 weeks. Oncology nursing care may be needed to monitor and evaluate the client who is receiving chemotherapy at home through venous access devices or portable infusion pumps. Inform the client and family about the services available through the American Cancer Society. Familiarize the family with area hospice services for future planning.

EVIDENCE-BASED PRACTICE for Nursing

What is the quality of life for a client who has undergone esophagectomy for cancer?

Sweed, M.R., et al. (2002). Quality of life after esophagectomy for cancer. *Oncology Nursing Forum, 29*(7), 1127-1131.

The purpose of this longitudinal, descriptive pilot study was to evaluate the quality of life (QOL) in 23 clients who had undergone esophagectomy for esophageal cancer. The European Organization for Research and Treatment of Cancer (EORTC) questionnaire was used to measure QOL at four time points. This tool contains five subscales that measure function, three symptom subscales, a global health status, a QOL scale, and six single items scored from 0 to 100, with higher scores equaling a higher response level. Measures were taken at baseline (before chemoradiation), 2 weeks following esophagectomy, 3 months after surgery and 6 months after surgery.

The study supported previous findings of weight loss, diarrhea, and acid reflux occurring post-esophagectomy. Increased hoarseness was also found, but it could not be attributed to the surgery itself. The study concluded that overall QOL remains stable after esophagectomy, but severity of symptoms can affect QOL.

Level of Evidence: 6—This research was a descriptive pilot that serves as a basis for future study.

Critique. Although the study is limited by the small sample size and some findings that were not statistically significant, it provides important beginning data on symptoms that affect QOL after curative esophagectomy for esophageal cancer. This study should be replicated with a larger sample to confirm findings to assist in helping nurses to develop interventions to improve QOL in this population.

Implications for Nursing. Nurses need to be supportive and yet realistic when caring for clients with esophageal cancer and surgery. Expected changes in QOL tend to occur when symptoms become more severe.

◆Evaluation: Outcomes

Evaluate the care of the client with esophageal cancer on the basis of the identified nursing diagnoses. The major expected outcome is that the client will be able to consume adequate nutrition and maintain a stable weight. Other outcomes for postoperative esophageal surgical clients are outlined in the Plan of Care on pp. 1269 to 1272. Specific indicators for this outcome are listed for the nursing diagnosis under the Planning and Implementation section (see earlier).

DIVERTICULA

PATHOPHYSIOLOGY

Diverticula are sacs resulting from the herniation of esophageal mucosa and submucosa into surrounding tissue. Diverticula may develop anywhere along the length of the esophagus. No environmental risk factors are known to be involved in the development of esophageal diverticula. The incomplete or late opening of the cricopharyngeal muscle during swallowing leads to high pressures in the hypopharynx and leads to *Zenker's diverticulum,* the most common form. Zenker's diverticulum occurs most often in older adults. Clients complain of dysphagia, regurgitation, nocturnal cough, and halitosis (bad breath). Clients with esophageal diverticula can be at risk for esophageal perforation because the mucosa is without the protection of the normal esophageal muscle layer.

COLLABORATIVE MANAGEMENT

Esophageal diverticula are diagnosed by barium swallow and esophagogastroduodenoscopy (EGD). If endoscopy is done, it must be performed with strict care because of the risk of perforation. Diet therapy and positioning are the major interventions for controlling symptoms related to diverticula. The dietitian assists the client in exploring variations in the size and frequency of meals and in food texture and consistency. Semisoft foods and smaller meals are often best tolerated and may reduce or relieve the symptoms of pressure and reflux. Nocturnal reflux associated with diverticula is managed by instructing the client to sleep with the head of the bed elevated and to avoid the recumbent position for at least 2 hours after eating. Counsel the client to avoid vigorous exercise after meals. Advise the client to avoid restrictive clothing and frequent stooping or bending.

Surgical management is aimed at excising the diverticula and reapproximating the mucosa. Postoperatively the client takes nothing by mouth for several days to promote healing. During that period, the client receives IV fluids for hydration, tube feedings, and then oral fluid and food. Provide pain relief measures, and monitor for complications such as bleeding or perforation. A nasogastric (NG) tube is placed during surgery for decompression and is *not* irrigated or repositioned unless specifically ordered by the surgeon.

Community-based care includes teaching the client and family about the following:

- Tube feeding and resuming an oral diet
- Positioning guidelines to prevent reflux
- Warning signs of complications

Community resources are usually not needed for uncomplicated cases.

ESOPHAGEAL TRAUMA

PATHOPHYSIOLOGY

Trauma to the esophagus can result from blunt injuries, chemical burns, surgery or endoscopy, or the stress of protracted severe vomiting (Table 58-2). Trauma may affect the esophagus directly, impairing swallowing and nutrition, or it may create problems and complications in related structures such as the lungs or mediastinum. The incidence of most forms of esophageal trauma is low in adults. When excessive force is exerted on the esophageal mucosa, it may perforate or rupture, allowing the caustic acid secretions to enter the mediastinal cavity. These tears are associated with a high mortality rate related to shock, respiratory impairment, or sepsis.

Chemical injury is usually a result of the accidental or intentional ingestion of caustic substances. The oral cavity is also usually damaged, and the damage is rapid and severe. Acid burns tend to affect the superficial layers of the esophagus, whereas alkaline substances cause deeper penetrating injuries. Strong alkalis can cause full perforation of the esophagus within 1 minute. Additional problems may include aspiration pneumonia and hemorrhage. Strictures may develop as scar tissue forms.

TABLE 58-2 Common Causes of Esophageal Perforation

- Straining
- Seizures
- Trauma
- Foreign objects
- Instrument or tubes
- Chemical injury
- Complications of esophageal surgery
- Ulcers

COLLABORATIVE MANAGEMENT

Clients with esophageal trauma are initially evaluated and treated in the emergency department. Assessment focuses on the nature of the injury and the circumstances surrounding it. Assess for the presence of an airway, chest pain, dysphagia, vomiting, or bleeding. If the risk of extending the damage is not excessive, an x-ray or endoscopic study may be ordered to evaluate tears or perforation. A computed tomography (CT) scan of the chest can be done to assess for the presence of mediastinal air.

After the injury, keep the client NPO (nothing by mouth) to prevent further leakage of esophageal secretions. Esophageal and gastric suction can be used for drainage and to rest the esophagus. Esophageal rest is maintained for at least 10 days after injury to allow for initial healing of the mucosa. Total parenteral nutrition (TPN) is prescribed to provide calories and protein for wound healing while the client is not eating.

To prevent sepsis, broad-spectrum antibiotics are prescribed. High-dose corticosteroids may be administered to suppress inflammation and prevent strictures. In addition, opioid and nonopioid analgesics are prescribed for pain management. When caustic burns involve the oral cavity, topical agents, such as 50/50 diphenhydramine hydrochloride (Benadryl) and kaolin with pectin (Kapectolin) or topical lidocaine (Viscous Xylocaine), may be used for topical analgesia and local anti-inflammatory action.

If nonsurgical management is not effective in healing traumatized esophageal tissue, the client may need surgery to remove the damaged tissue. The client with severe injuries may require resection of part of the esophagus with a gastric pull-through and repositioning or replacement by a bowel segment. (See Surgical Management [Esophageal Tumors], p. 1277.)

GET READY for the NCLEX Examination!

KEY POINTS

Safe Effective Care Environment

- Teach client and family to recognize the symptoms of dysphagia.
- Remain with the dysphasic client during meals to prevent or assist with choking episodes.
- Teach the client oral exercises aimed at improving swallowing.

Health Promotion and Maintenance

- Consult with dietitian, client, and family regarding dietary restrictions for clients with GERD.
- Stress the importance of recognizing and controlling reflux through dietary and medications to avoid further esophageal damage that could lead to Barrett's esophagus.
- Teach the client to elevate the head of the bed by 6 inches for sleep to prevent nighttime reflux.
- Instruct the client to sleep in the left lateral decubitus position to minimize the effects of nighttime episodes of reflux.
- Teach the client with esophageal cancer to monitor his or her body weight and to notify the health care provider for a loss of 5 pounds or greater.
- Teach the client to avoid alcoholic beverages, smoking, and other substances as listed in Chart 58-2 because they lead to increased gastroesophageal reflux.
- Teach the client to prevent gas bloat syndrome by avoiding drinking carbonated beverages, eating gas-producing foods, chewing gum, and drinking with a straw.
- Review post-procedure instructions for clients having endoscopic therapies for GERD as outlined in Chart 58-4.

Psychosocial Integrity

- Allow the client the opportunity to express fear or anxiety regarding the diagnosis of esophageal cancer and related treatment regimen of surgery, chemotherapy, and radiation.
- Explain all procedures, restrictions, medications, and follow-up care to the client and family.
- Refer the client or family members to psychological counseling, hospice, pastoral care, and the social worker as needed.

Physiological Integrity

- For clients with GERD, teach the importance of strict adherence to antifeflux agents in preventing esophageal damage (see Chart 58-3).
- Be aware that laparoscopic Nissen fundoplication (LNF) is the most common surgical procedure for clients with GERD and hiatal hernia; LNF may also be performed for clients with achalasia.
- Recall that achalasia is an esophageal motility disorder caused by esophageal denervation, which can lead to severe complications, such as carcinoma and aspiration pneumonia.
- Assess for complications and provide postoperative care for clients having the LNF procedure as described in Charts 58-6 and 58-7.
- Teach the client having open esophageal surgery about incisions, drains, and jejunostomy tube placement before he or she undergoes surgery for esophageal cancer.
- For the client with a nasogastric (NG) tube, check the NG tube every 4 to 8 hours for proper placement and anchorage; follow guidelines as outlines in Chart 58-10.
- Assess the postoperative esophageal surgical client for pulmonary and cardiac complications of surgery, and report changes to the health care provider.
- Assess clients for key features of esophageal tumors as listed in Chart 58-8.
- Provide care for clients with esophageal surgery as discussed in the Plan of Care.

ADDITIONAL STUDY RESOURCES

Go to your Student CD-ROM for Review Questions for the NCLEX Examination.

evolve Go to http://evolve.elsevier.com/Iggy/ for Integrated Management of Care Questions for the NCLEX Examination.

SELECTED BIBLIOGRAPHY

American Cancer Society. (2003). *Cancer facts and figures 2003.* Report No. 01-300M-No. 5008.03. Atlanta: Author.

Arbogast, D. (2002). Enteral feedings with comfort and safety. *Clinical Journal of Oncology Nursing, 6*(5), 275-282.

Brooks-Brunn, J.A. (2000). Esophageal cancer: An overview. *MEDSURG Nursing, 9*(5), 248-254.

Bruce, S. (2001). Photodynamic therapy: Another option in cancer treatment. *Clinical Journal of Oncology Nursing, 5*(3), 95-100.

Daly, B. (2000). The special challenges of withholding artificial nutrition and hydration. *Journal of Gerontological Nursing, 26*(9), 25-31.

Fackler, W.K., & Richter, J.E., (2000). Refractory GERD: What next? *Consultant,* May, pp. 973-983.

Fennerty, B., et al. (2002). New paradigms for the treatment of acid-related reflux disorders. *Patient Care for the Nurse Practitioner, Special Edition*, Fall, 3-12.

Field, S. (2003). Detecting patients with hidden GERD. *Clinical Advisor*, 23-34.

Goroll, A., & Mulley, A. (2000). Evaluation of dysphagia and suspected esophageal chest pain. *Primary Care Medicine* (4th ed., pp. 389-394). Philadelphia: Lippincott Williams & Wilkins.

Hemminger, L.L., & Wolfsen, H.C. (2002). Photodynamic therapy for Barrett's esophagus and high-grade dysplasia: results of a patient satisfaction survey. *Gastrointestinal Nursing, 25*(4), 139-141.

Hubbard, P.M. (2002). Update on gastroesophageal reflux disease. *The American Journal for Nurse Practitioners, 2,* 9-18.

Maguire, M. (2000). Nutritional care of surgical oncology patients. *Seminars in Oncology Nursing, 16*(2), 128-134.

McCormick, D.G. (2004). Stretta procedure for the treatment of gastroesophageal reflux disease. *Gastroenterology Nursing, 27*(1), 22-28.

Nilsson, G., et al. (2002). Patient's experience of illness, operation and outcome with reference to gastroesophageal reflux disease. *Journal of Advanced Nursing, 40*(3), 307-315.

Parkman, H., MacMillan Rooney, W., & Rogers, H. (2000). Empiric therapy for nonulcer dyspepsia. *Patient Care for the Nurse Practitioner, 3*(1), 23-34.

Rayhorn, N., Argel, N., & Demchak, K. (2003). Understanding gastroesophageal reflux disease. *Nursing 2003, 33*(10), 36-41.

Rockney, A.D. (2002). What you need to know about Barrett's esophagus. *Gastroenterology Nursing, 25*(6), 237-240.

Strader, S.L. (2001). Esophageal motor disorders: Achalasia and esophageal spasm. *Journal of the American Academy of Nurse Practitioners, 13*(11), 502-507.

Sweed, M., et al. (2002). Quality of life after esophagectomy for cancer. *Oncology Nursing Forum, 29*(7), 1127-1131.

Terrado, M., Russell, C., & Bowman, J. (2001). Dysphagia: An overview. *MEDSURG Nursing, 10*(5), 233-248.

CHAPTER 59

Interventions for Clients with Stomach Disorders

JACQUELYN R. GIBBS

LEARNING OUTCOMES

After studying this chapter, you should be able to:

1. Compare etiologies and assessment findings of acute and chronic gastritis.
2. Describe the key components of collaborative management for clients with gastritis.
3. Compare and contrast assessment findings associated with gastric and duodenal ulcers.
4. Identify the most common medical complications that can result from peptic ulcer disease (PUD).
5. Analyze assessment data to determine common nursing diagnoses associated with PUD.
6. Discuss drug therapy for gastritis and PUD.
7. Develop a teaching plan related to drug therapy for clients experiencing PUD.
8. Prioritize interventions for clients with upper gastrointestinal bleeding.
9. Plan preoperative and postoperative care for the client undergoing gastric surgery.
10. Develop a community-based plan of care for clients who have undergone gastric surgery.
11. Evaluate outcomes for clients with PUD.
12. Explain Zollinger-Ellison syndrome and its associated clinical manifestations.
13. Analyze risk factors for gastric carcinoma, including cultural considerations.
14. Plan postoperative care for clients who have undergone surgery for gastric cancer.
15. Discuss the psychological and emotional concerns of clients with gastric cancer.

Go to your Student CD-ROM for Review Questions for the NCLEX Examination keyed to these Learning Outcomes.

Although only a few diseases affect the stomach, they can be very serious and in some cases life threatening. The most common disorders include gastritis, peptic ulcer disease, Zollinger-Ellison syndrome, and gastric carcinoma (cancer).

GASTRITIS

Gastritis is defined as inflammation of the gastric mucosa (stomach lining). It can be scattered or localized and can be classified according to cause, cellular changes, or distribution of the lesions. Gastritis can be designated as erosive (acute gastritis, stress ulcers) or nonerosive (chronic gastritis). Although the mucosal changes accompanying acute gastritis typically resolve after several months, this is not true for chronic gastritis.

PATHOPHYSIOLOGY

Prostaglandins provide a protective mucosal barrier that prevents the stomach from digesting itself by a process called acid **autodigestion.** If there is a break in the protective barrier, mucosal injury occurs. The resulting injury is compounded by histamine release and vagal nerve stimulation. Hydrochloric acid can then diffuse back into the mucosa and injure small vessels. This back-diffusion results in edema, hemorrhage, and erosion of the stomach's lining. The pathologic changes of gastritis include vascular congestion, edema, acute inflammatory cell infiltration, and degenerative changes in the superficial epithelium of the stomach lining.

The early pathologic manifestation of gastritis is a thickened, reddened mucous membrane with prominent **rugae**, or folds. As the disease progresses, the walls and lining of the stomach thin and atrophy. With progressive gastric atrophy from chronic mucosal injury, the function of the parietal (acid-secreting) cells decreases and the source of intrinsic factor is lost. The intrinsic factor is critical for absorption of vitamin B_{12}. When body stores of vitamin B_{12} are eventually depleted, **pernicious anemia** results. The amount and concentration of acid in stomach secretions gradually decrease until the secretions consist of only mucus and water.

Chronic gastritis is associated with an increased risk of gastric cancer as the persistent inflammation extends deep into the mucosa, causing destruction of the gastric glands and cellular changes. Hemorrhage may occur after an episode of acute gastritis or with ulceration caused by chronic gastritis.

Acute Gastritis

Inflammation of the gastric mucosa or submucosa after exposure to local irritants can result in **acute gastritis**. Various degrees of mucosal necrosis and inflammatory reaction occur in acute disease. The diagnosis cannot be based solely on clinical symptoms. Complete regeneration and healing usually occur within a few days. If the stomach muscle is not involved, complete recovery usually occurs with no residual evidence of gastric inflammatory reaction.

Chronic Gastritis

Chronic gastritis appears as a patchy, diffuse (spread out) inflammation of the mucosal lining of the stomach. Chronic gastritis usually heals without scarring, but it can progress to hemorrhage and the formation of an ulcer.

Chronic gastritis may be categorized as type A, type B, or atrophic. Type A (nonerosive) chronic gastritis refers to an inflammation of the glands, as well as the fundus and body of the stomach. Type B chronic gastritis usually affects the glands of the antrum but may involve the entire stomach. In atrophic chronic gastritis, diffuse inflammation and destruction of deeply located glands accompany the condition. Chronic atrophic gastritis affects all layers of the stomach, thus decreasing the number of cells. The muscle becomes thickened, and inflammation is present. Chronic atrophic gastritis is characterized by total loss of fundal glands, minimal inflammation, thinning of the gastric mucosa, and intestinal metaplasia (abnormal tissue development).

Etiology and Genetic Risk

ACUTE GASTRITIS

The onset of infection with *Helicobacter pylori* can result in acute gastritis. *H. pylori* is a gram-negative, spiral-shaped bacterium that penetrates the mucosal gel layer of the gastric epithelium. Although it is uncommon, other forms of bacterial gastritis from organisms such as staphylococci, streptococci, *Escherichia coli,* or salmonella can cause life-threatening consequences such as sepsis and extensive tissue necrosis (death). Other infectious causes of acute gastritis can be found in clients with immunosuppressive disorders. In clients with acquired immunodeficiency syndrome (AIDS), for example, gastric erosions can be found with herpes simplex viral infection and disseminated cytomegalovirus (CMV) infection.

Nonsteroidal anti-inflammatory drug (NSAID) use poses a risk for the development of acute gastritis. Gastritis occurs in 5% to 25% of NSAID users, but the exact mechanism of the role of NSAIDs in the development of gastritis is not well understood. Other drugs, including alcohol, cytotoxic agents, caffeine, and corticosteroids, have also been implicated; however, scientific evidence is lacking. Acute gastritis is also caused by local irritation from radiation therapy and accidental or intentional ingestion of corrosive substances, including acids or alkalis (e.g., lye and drain cleaners). In the client who is allowed nothing by mouth (NPO), gastritis may result from lack of stimulation of normal secretions. Acute stress-induced gastritis, characterized by multiple shallow erosions of the proximal stomach, may be present in 80% to 100% of critically ill clients.

CHRONIC GASTRITIS

Type A gastritis has been associated with the presence of antibodies to parietal cells and intrinsic factor; therefore an autoimmune pathogenesis for this type of gastritis has been proposed. Parietal cell antibodies have been found in 90% of clients with pernicious anemia and in more than one half of individuals with type A gastritis. A genetic link to this disease, with an autosomal dominant pattern of inheritance, has been noted in the relatives of clients with pernicious anemia.

The most common form of the disease is **type B gastritis**, caused by *H. pylori* infection. There is a direct correlation between the number of organisms and the degree of cellular abnormality present. Although serum antibodies have been isolated in some clients, it is believed that these antibodies are not representative of an autoimmune process but are the result of prolonged inflammation. Fifty percent of clients who have gastric ulcers have associated chronic gastritis.

Chronic local irritation and toxic effects caused by alcohol ingestion, radiation therapy, and smoking have been implicated in the development of chronic gastritis. Surgical procedures that involve the pyloric sphincter, such as the Billroth II procedure, can lead to gastritis by causing reflux of alkaline secretions into the stomach. Other systemic disorders such as Crohn's disease, graft-versus-host disease, and uremia can also precipitate the development of chronic gastritis.

Atrophic gastritis is a type of chronic gastritis that is seen most often in older adults. It can occur after exposure to toxic substances in the workplace (e.g., benzene, lead, and nickel) or *H. pylori* infection, or it can be related to autoimmune factors.

Although atrophic gastritis is often present in people with gastric cancer, it is not always considered a precancerous lesion. Gastric carcinoma develops in fewer than 10% of clients who have atrophic gastritis. Chart 59-1 lists guidelines for preventing gastritis.

Incidence/Prevalence

About 2.7 million people in the United States have gastritis. The incidence of gastritis is higher in men than in women; although it has been suggested that more women have chronic

CHART 59-1

CLIENT EDUCATION GUIDE
Gastritis Prevention

- Avoid drinking excessive amounts of alcoholic beverages.
- Use caution in taking large doses of aspirin, nonsteroidal anti-inflammatory drugs (e.g., ibuprofen), and corticosteroids. Prolonged use of small doses of corticosteroids may also cause gastritis.
- Avoid excessive intake of caffeine-containing beverages.
- Avoid eating contaminated foods or drinking contaminated water.
- Stop smoking.
- Protect yourself against exposure to toxic substances in the workplace, such as lead and nickel.
- Seek medical treatment if you are experiencing symptoms of esophageal reflux (see Chapter 58).

atrophic gastritis. Acute and chronic forms of the disease are more prevalent in heavy smokers and persons who abuse alcohol. The incidence of chronic gastritis increases with age.

HEALTH PROMOTION/ILLNESS PREVENTION

Balanced diet, regular exercise, and stress reduction techniques help prevent gastritis. A balanced diet includes following the recommendations of the U.S. Department of Agriculture (USDA) food pyramid and limiting intake of foods and spices that can cause gastric distress such as tea, coffee, cola, chocolate, mustard, paprika, cloves, pepper, and hot spices. Alcohol and tobacco consumption should be avoided. Regular exercise maintains peristalsis, which helps prevent gastric contents from irritating the gastric mucosa. Stress reduction techniques can include cardiovascular exercise, meditation, reading, and/or yoga depending on individual preferences. Psychotherapy may also be considered.

Excessive use of aspirin and other NSAIDs should also be avoided. Clients with problems such as back pain that find themselves needing to take NSAIDs frequently need to see their health care provider promptly so the pain can be managed under medical supervision. If a family member or significant other has *H. pylori* infection or has had it in the past, then testing should be considered. This test could diagnose, treat, and eradicate the bacteria before it causes gastritis.

COLLABORATIVE MANAGEMENT

Assessment

PHYSICAL ASSESSMENT/CLINICAL MANIFESTATIONS

Physical assessment findings may include abdominal tenderness and bloating, **hematemesis** (vomiting blood), or **melena** (traces of blood in the stool). In stress-induced gastritis, symptoms of intravascular volume depletion and shock may be present.

ACUTE GASTRITIS. Symptoms of acute gastritis can range from mild to severe. Epigastric discomfort, anorexia, cramping, nausea, and vomiting may be present. In some cases, gastric hemorrhage is the presenting symptom (Chart 59-2). The symptoms last only a few hours or days and vary with the cause. Aspirin-related gastritis may result in dyspepsia (heartburn). Gastritis from alcohol abuse may cause vomiting and hematemesis. Gastritis or food poisoning caused by endotoxins, such as staphylococcal endotoxin, has an abrupt onset; severe nausea and vomiting often occur within 5 hours of ingestion of the contaminated food.

CHRONIC GASTRITIS. Chronic gastritis causes few symptoms. Clients may complain of nausea, vomiting, or upper abdominal discomfort. Periodic epigastric pain may simulate ulcer-like distress, which is relieved on ingestion of food. Some clients may have anorexia, and pain may be exacerbated by eating fatty or spicy foods (see Chart 59-2).

CHART 59-2

KEY FEATURES of Gastritis

Acute Gastritis
- Rapid onset of epigastric pain or discomfort
- Nausea and vomiting
- Hematemesis (vomiting blood)
- Gastric hemorrhage
- Dyspepsia (heartburn)
- Anorexia

Chronic Gastritis
- Vague complaint of epigastric pain that is relieved by food
- Anorexia
- Nausea or vomiting
- Intolerance of fatty and spicy foods
- Pernicious anemia

DIAGNOSTIC ASSESSMENT

Esophagogastroduodenoscopy (EGD) via an endoscope with biopsy is the gold standard for diagnosing gastritis, as well as detecting the presence of *H. pylori.* The health care provider uses biopsy to establish a definitive diagnosis of the type of gastritis. If lesions are patchy and diffuse, biopsy of several suspicious areas may be necessary to avoid misdiagnosis. A cytologic examination of the biopsy specimen is performed to confirm or rule out gastric cancer.

Common Nursing Diagnoses and Collaborative Problems

Nursing diagnoses and collaborative problems that may apply to clients with gastritis include the following:

1. Acute Pain or Chronic Pain related to physical injury (inflammation)
2. Nausea related to gastric irritation
3. Deficient Knowledge related to unfamiliarity with information resources
4. Potential for Hemorrhage

Interventions

Clients with gastritis are not often seen in the acute care setting unless they have an exacerbation ("flare up") of acute or chronic gastritis that results in fluid and electrolyte imbalance or bleeding. Management is directed toward supportive care for relieving the symptoms and removing the cause of discomfort.

Acute gastritis is treated symptomatically and supportively because the healing process is spontaneous, usually occurring within a few days. When the cause is removed, pain and discomfort usually subside. If hemorrhage is severe, a blood transfusion may be necessary. Fluid replacement is indicated in clients with severe fluid loss. Surgery, such as partial gastrectomy, pyloroplasty, and/or vagotomy, may be indicated for clients with major bleeding or ulceration. Treatment of chronic gastritis varies with the cause. General treatment goals include the elimination of causative agents, treatment of any underlying disease (e.g., uremia, Crohn's disease), and avoidance of toxic substances (e.g., alcohol, tobacco, nonsteroidal anti-inflammatory drugs [NSAIDs]).

NONSURGICAL MANAGEMENT. The identification and elimination of the causative factors, such as *H. pylori* infection, is the primary treatment modality. Drugs and diet therapy are also used in the treatment of gastritis.

Drug Therapy. In the acute phase, the health care team directs actions toward relief of pain and discomfort. The health care provider may prescribe medications that block and buffer gastric acid secretions to relieve pain.

CHART 59-3

DRUG THERAPY for Peptic Ulcer Disease

Drug	Usual Dosage	Nursing Interventions	Rationales
Antacids			
Magnesium hydroxide with aluminum hydroxide (Maalox, Mylanta)	50-80 mEq 1 hr and 3 hr after meals and at bedtime	Give 2 hr after meals and at bedtime.	Hydrogen ion load is high after ingestion of foods.
		Use liquid rather than tablets.	Suspensions are more effective than chewable tablets.
		Do not give other drugs within 1-2 hr of antacids.	Antacids interfere with absorption of other drugs.
		Assess the client for a history of renal disease.	Hypermagnesemia may result. These antacids have a high sodium content. These antacids contain magnesium, which cannot be excreted by poorly functioning kidneys, thus causing toxicity.
		Assess the client for a history of heart failure.	Inadequate renal perfusion from heart failure decreases the ability of the kidneys to excrete magnesium, thus causing toxicity.
		Observe the client for the side effect of diarrhea.	Magnesium often causes diarrhea.
Aluminum hydroxide (Amphojel)	50-80 mEq 1 hr and 3 hr after meals and at bedtime	Give 1 hr after meals and at bedtime.	Hydrogen ion load is high after ingestion of food.
		Use liquid rather than tablets if palatable.	Suspensions are more effective than chewable tablets.
		Do not give other drugs within 1-2 hr of antacids.	Antacids interfere with absorption of other drugs.
		Observe the client for the side effect of constipation. If constipation occurs, consider alternating with magnesium antacid.	Aluminum causes constipation, and magnesium has a laxative effect. Aluminum binds with phosphates in the gastrointestinal (GI) tract.
		Use for clients with renal failure.	This antacid does not contain magnesium.
H_2 Antagonists			
Ranitidine (Zantac)	150 mg PO twice daily or 300 mg PO at bedtime; 50 mg IV q6h or 8 mg/hr IV (continuous)	Give single dose at bedtime for treatment of GI ulcers. **NOTE:** IV ranitidine may also be given to prevent surgical stress ulcers.	Bedtime administration suppresses nocturnal acid production.
Famotidine (Pepcid)	40 mg PO once daily or in two divided doses; 20 mg IV q12h	Give single dose at bedtime.	Bedtime administration suppresses nocturnal acid production. Compliance may improve with less frequent administration.
Nizatidine (Axid)	150 mg PO twice daily or 300 mg at bedtime	Give single dose at bedtime.	Bedtime administration suppresses nocturnal acid production. Compliance may improve with less frequent administration.

H_2-receptor antagonists are typically used to block gastric secretions. The most common agents include ranitidine (Zantac), famotidine (Pepcid), and nizatidine (Axid). Sucralfate (Carafate, Sulcrate✱), a mucosal barrier fortifier, may also be prescribed. Antacids used as buffering agents include aluminum hydroxide combined with magnesium hydroxide (Maalox) and aluminum hydroxide combined with simethicone and magnesium hydroxide (Mylanta). Antisecretory agents (proton-pump inhibitors) such as omeprazole (Prilosec) or esomeprazole magnesium (Nexium) may also be used to suppress gastric acid secretion (Chart 59-3). Monitor for symptom relief and side effects of these medications and notify the health care provider of any untoward effects or worsening of gastric distress.

Clients with chronic gastritis may require vitamin B_{12} for prevention or treatment of pernicious anemia. If *H. pylori* is found in biopsy specimens, the health care provider may treat the infection and reverse or prevent impairment of mucosal defenses. A common drug regimen for *H. pylori* infection includes triple therapy, which may include bismuth subsalicylates (Pepto-Bismol) or a proton-pump inhibitor such as omeprazole (Prilosec), and a combination of two antibiotics such as metronidazole (Flagyl, Novonidazol✱) and tetracycline or clarithromycin and amoxicillin.

The nurse, health care provider, or pharmacist instructs clients about the medications associated with gastric irritation. These medications include chemotherapeutic agents, corticosteroids, erythromycin (E-Mycin, Erythromid✱), and

CHART 59-3

DRUG THERAPY for Peptic Ulcer Disease—*cont'd*

Drug	Usual Dosage	Nursing Interventions	Rationales
Mucosal Barrier Fortifiers			
Sucralfate (Carafate, Sulcrate✱)	1 g PO four times daily or 2 g twice daily	Give 1 hr before and 2 hr after meals, and at bedtime.	Food may interfere with drug's adherence to mucosa.
		Do not give within 30 min of giving antacids or other drugs.	Antacids may interfere with effect.
Antisecretory Agents			
Omeprazole (Prilosec, Losec✱)	20 mg PO twice daily or 40 mg at bedtime	Have the client take capsule whole; do not crush.	Delayed-release capsules allow absorption after granules leave the stomach.
		Give single dose at bedtime for ulcer disease.	Bedtime administration suppresses nocturnal acid production.
Lansoprazole (Prevacid)	15 or 30 mg PO at bedtime	Give single dose at bedtime for ulcer disease; do not crush.	Bedtime administration suppresses nocturnal acid production.
Rabeprazole (AcipHex)	20 mg PO once daily	Take following the morning meal.	Drug promotes healing and symptom relief of duodenal ulcers.
		Do not crush capsule.	Drug is a sustained-release capsule.
Pantoprazole (Protonix)	40 mg PO or IV daily	Do not crush.	Drug is enteric-coated.
		IV form must be given with filter and in a separate line.	Given IV, drug precipitates easily.
Esomeprazole (Nexium)	20 or 40 mg PO daily	Give 1 hr before meals.	Food decreases absorption.
		Assess for hepatic impairment.	Clients with severe hepatic problems need a low dose.
Prostaglandin Analogues			
Misoprostol (Cytotec)	200 mcg PO four times daily	Take with food.	Drug protects against nonsteroidal anti-inflammatory drug (NSAID)–induced ulcers.
		Avoid magnesium-containing antacids.	Both misoprostol and magnesium-containing antacids can cause diarrhea.
Antimicrobials			
Clarithromycin (Biaxin)	500 mg PO three times daily	Antimicrobials should be given as part of therapy to eradicate *Helicobacter pylori* infection.	*H. pylori* is a gram-negative bacterium implicated in the development of peptic ulcer disease (PUD).
Amoxicillin (Amoxil)	1 g PO twice daily		
Tetracycline	500 mg PO four times daily	The selection of the specific drug depends on its effectiveness, side effects, and drug interactions.	
Metronidazole (Flagyl)	250 mg PO three times daily and at bedtime		

NSAIDs, such as aspirin, naproxen (Naprosyn), and ibuprofen (Motrin, Advil, Amersol✱, Novo-Profen✱).

The health care provider may change the dose, frequency, or type of medication if symptoms of gastric irritation appear or persist. Instruct clients to avoid stomach-irritating over-the-counter (OTC) medications, such as aspirin and ibuprofen.

Diet Therapy. Instruct the client with gastric disease to limit intake of any foods and spices that cause distress. Tea, coffee, cola, chocolate, mustard, paprika, cloves, pepper, and hot spices may increase discomfort. Alcohol and tobacco should also be avoided.

After the client has an acute episode of gastritis, help him or her identify foods that cause discomfort. New foods should be introduced one at a time. Avoidance of substances that cause symptoms is important. Most clients seem to progress better with a soft, bland diet and smaller, more frequent meals.

Stress Reduction. Assist the client with various techniques that reduce stress and discomfort, such as progressive relaxation, cutaneous stimulation, guided imagery, and distraction. (See Chapter 4 for a discussion of these therapies.)

SURGICAL MANAGEMENT. Partial gastrectomy, pyloroplasty, vagotomy, or even total gastrectomy may be indicated for clients who have major bleeding caused by severe erosive gastritis. Such surgery is necessary only if more conservative measures have not controlled the bleeding. Surgical interventions are discussed under Surgical Management (Peptic Ulcer Disease), p. 1296.

PEPTIC ULCER DISEASE

A **peptic ulcer** is a mucosal lesion of the stomach or duodenum. The term *peptic ulcer* is used to describe both gastric and duodenal ulcers. **Peptic ulcer disease (PUD)** results when gastric mucosal defenses become impaired and no longer protect the epithelium from the effects of acid and pepsin (Figure 59-1).

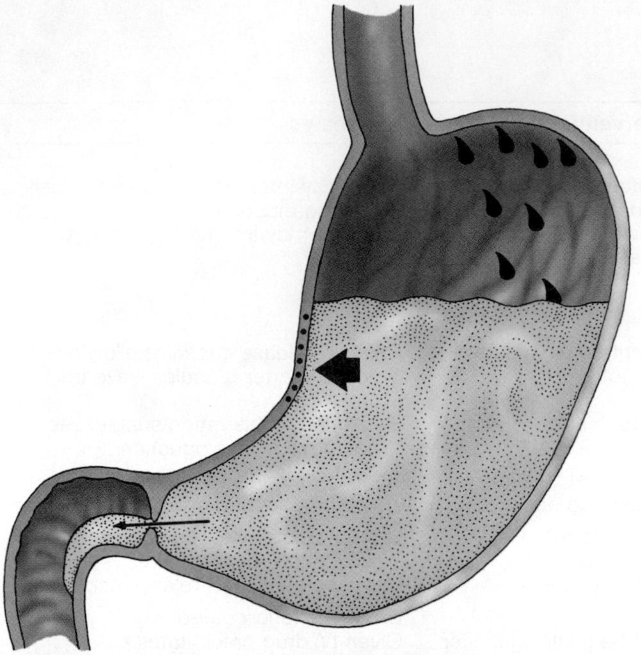

Conditions favoring the development of **gastric ulcers** are normal gastric acid secretion and delayed stomach emptying with *increased diffusion of gastric acid back into the stomach tissues.*

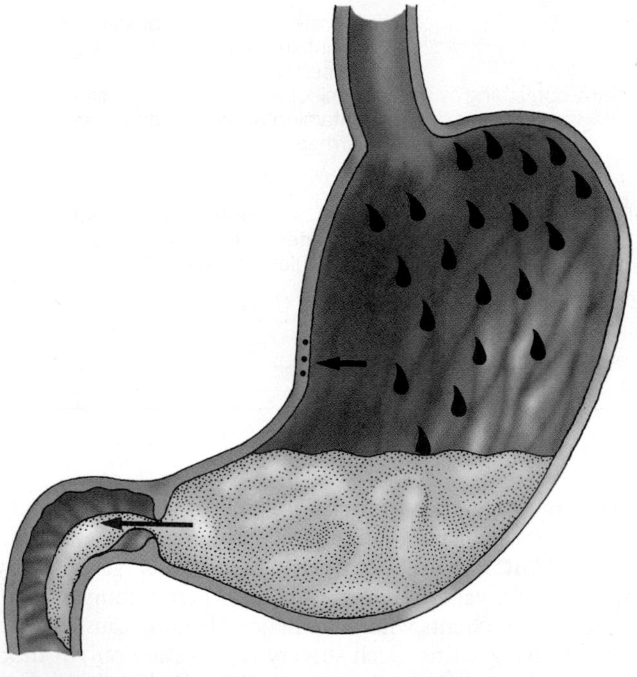

Conditions favoring the development of **duodenal ulcers** are normal diffusion of acid back into stomach tissues with *increased secretion of gastric acid* and *increased stomach emptying.*

Figure 59-1 ■ The pathophysiology of peptic ulcer.

PATHOPHYSIOLOGY

Gastric Ulcers

Acid, pepsin, and *H. pylori* infection play an important role in the development of gastric ulcers. The gastric mucosal barrier overlies the epithelium. The secretion of mucus and

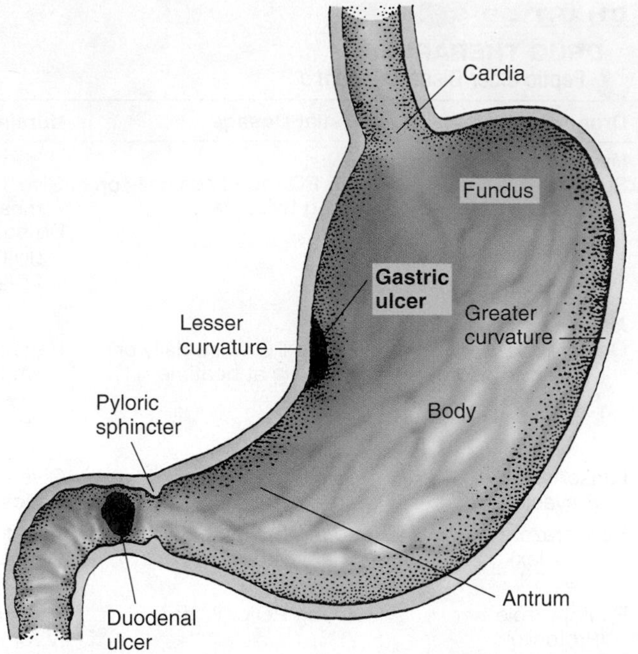

Figure 59-2 ■ The most common sites for peptic ulcers.

bicarbonate provides a first line of defense in maintaining a near-normal pH on the gastric epithelium and protects the mucosal barrier against acid. Gastromucosal prostaglandins increase the barrier's resistance to ulceration. The integrity of the barrier is enhanced by the rich blood supply of the mucosa of the stomach and duodenum.

When a break in the mucosal barrier occurs, hydrochloric acid injures the epithelium. Gastric ulcers may then result from back-diffusion of acid or dysfunction of the pyloric sphincter (see Figure 59-1). Without normal functioning of the pyloric sphincter, bile refluxes (backs up) into the stomach. This reflux of bile acids may break the integrity of the mucosal barrier and produce hydrogen ion back-diffusion, which leads to mucosal inflammation. Toxic agents and bile then destroy the lipid plasma membrane of the gastric mucosa.

Gastric emptying is often delayed in clients with gastric ulceration. This causes regurgitation of duodenal contents, which compounds the gastric mucosal injury. A decreased blood flow to the gastric mucosa may also alter the defense barrier and thereby allow ulceration to occur. Characteristically, gastric ulcers are deep and penetrating, and they usually occur on the lesser curvature of the stomach, near the pylorus (Figure 59-2).

Duodenal Ulcers

Most duodenal ulcers occur in the first portion of the duodenum. Duodenal ulcers present as deep, sharply demarcated lesions that penetrate through the mucosa and submucosa into the muscularis propria (muscle layer). The floor of the ulcer consists of a necrotic area residing on granulation tissue and surrounded by areas of fibrosis.

The characteristic feature of a duodenal ulcer is high gastric acid secretion, although a wide range of secretory levels is found. In clients with duodenal ulcers, pH levels are low in the duodenum for long periods. Protein-rich meals, calcium, and vagal excitation stimulate acid secretion. Combined with hypersecretion, a rapid emptying of food from the stomach reduces the buffering effect of food and delivers a large acid bolus to the duodenum (see Figure 59-1). Inhibitory secretory mechanisms and pancreatic secretion may be insufficient to control the acid load.

Many clients with duodenal ulcer disease have confirmed *H. pylori* infection. *H. pylori* produces substances that damage the gastric mucosa. Urease produced by *H. pylori* catalyzes the hydrolysis of urea to ammonia. Hydrogen ions are then released in response to the presence of ammonia and contribute further to gastric mucosal damage.

Stress Ulcers

Stress ulcers are acute gastric mucosal lesions occurring after an acute medical crisis or trauma. Stress ulcers have been associated with head injury, major surgery, burns, respiratory failure, shock, and sepsis. Bleeding caused by gastric erosion is the principal manifestation of acute stress ulcers. Multifocal lesions associated with stress ulcers occur in the proximal portion of the stomach and duodenum. These lesions begin as focal areas of ischemia and evolve into erosions and ulcerations that may progress to massive hemorrhage. Little is known of the exact etiology of stress ulcers; however, in the presence of elevated levels of hydrochloric acid, ischemic areas can progress to erosive gastritis and subsequent ulcerations. Stress ulcers are associated with lengthened hospital stay by as much as 11 days and mortality rates greater than 50% (Rotello, 2003).

Complications of Ulcers

The most common complications of PUD are hemorrhage, perforation, pyloric obstruction, and intractable disease.

HEMORRHAGE

Hemorrhage occurs in about 15% to 25% of clients with PUD and is the most serious complication (Figure 59-3). It tends to occur more often in clients with gastric ulcers and in older adults. Of those with an initial bleed, 40% experience a recurrence of bleeding if underlying infection with *H. pylori* remains untreated or if therapy does not include an H_2 antagonist. With massive bleeding, the client vomits bright red or coffee-ground blood (**hematemesis**). Hematemesis usually indicates bleeding at or above the duodenojejunal junction (**upper gastrointestinal [GI] bleeding**).

Minimal bleeding from ulcers is manifested by occult blood in a tarry stool (melena). Melena may occur in clients with gastric ulcers but is more common in those with duodenal ulcers. Gastric acid digestion of blood typically results in a granular dark vomitus (coffee-ground appearance); the digestion of blood within the duodenum and small intestine may result in a black stool.

PERFORATION

Gastric and duodenal ulcers can perforate or bleed. Perforation occurs when the ulcer becomes so deep that the entire thickness of the stomach or duodenum is worn away. The stomach or duodenal contents can then leak into the surrounding abdomen. In clients with perforation, the gastroduodenal contents (acid peptic juice, bile, and pancreatic juice) empty through the anterior wall of the stomach or duodenum into the peritoneal cavity. Sudden, sharp pain begins in the midepigastric region and spreads over the entire abdomen. The amount of pain correlates with the amount and type of GI contents spilled. The characteristic pain causes the client to be apprehensive. The abdomen is tender, rigid, and boardlike. The client assumes the knee-chest ("fetal") position to decrease the tension on the abdominal muscles. The client may become desperately ill within hours. Chemical peritonitis soon occurs; bacterial septicemia and hypovolemic shock follow. Peristalsis diminishes, and paralytic ileus develops. Peptic ulcer perforation is considered a surgical emergency and can be life threatening.

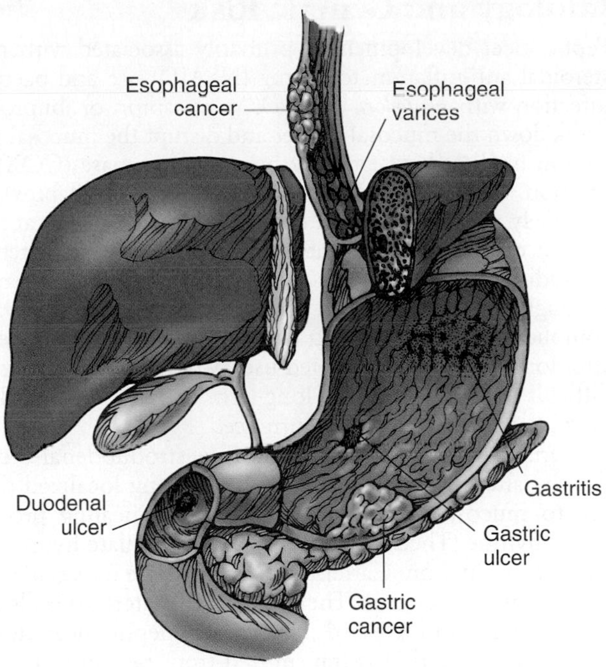

Figure 59-3 ■ Common causes of upper gastrointestinal bleeding.

PYLORIC OBSTRUCTION

Pyloric obstruction (blockage) occurs in a small percentage of clients and is manifested by vomiting caused by stasis and gastric dilation. Obstruction occurs at the pylorus (the gastric outlet) and is caused by scarring, edema, inflammation, or a combination of these factors.

Symptoms of gastric outlet obstruction include abdominal bloating, nausea, and vomiting. When vomiting persists, the client may experience hypochloremic (metabolic) alkalosis from loss of large quantities of acid gastric juice (hydrogen and chloride ions) in the vomitus. Hypokalemia may also result from the vomiting or metabolic alkalosis. The health care provider typically hospitalizes the client so he or she may receive intravenous (IV) fluid and electrolyte replacement.

INTRACTABLE DISEASE

One third of all clients with ulcers have a single episode with no recurrence. However, intractability may develop from complications of ulcers, excessive stressors in the client's life, or an inability to adhere to long-term therapy. The client no longer responds to conservative management, or recurrences of symptoms interfere with activities of daily living (ADLs). In general, the client continues to have recurrent pain and discomfort despite treatment. Clients who fail to respond to traditional treatments or who have a relapse following discontinuation of therapy should be referred to a gastroenterologist.

Etiology and Genetic Risk

Peptic ulcer development is primarily associated with nonsteroidal anti-inflammatory drug (NSAID) use and bacterial infection with *H. pylori*. NSAIDs (e.g., aspirin or ibuprofen) break down the mucosal barrier and disrupt the mucosal protection mediated systemically by cyclooxygenase (COX) inhibition. COX-2 inhibitors, such as celecoxib (Celebrex), are less likely to cause mucosal damage but place clients at high risk for cardiovascular events, such as myocardial infarction. In addition, NSAIDs cause the depletion of endogenous prostaglandins, resulting in local gastric mucosal injury. GI complications from NSAID use can occur at any time, even after long-term uncomplicated use. NSAID-related ulcers are difficult to treat, even with long-term therapy, because these ulcers have a high rate of recurrence.

Certain drugs may contribute to gastroduodenal ulceration by altering gastric secretion, producing localized damage to mucosa and interfering with the healing process. Theophylline (Theo-Dur) and caffeine stimulate hydrochloric acid production. Caffeine may contribute to vascular stasis and mucosal anoxia. The use of corticosteroids is also associated with an increased incidence of peptic ulceration.

H. pylori infection is transmitted from person to person, but the exact mode of transmission remains uncertain. Studies have suggested that it is spread either fecally–orally or by mouth-to-mouth contact, such as by kissing or perhaps by ingesting contaminated food or water (Perry, 2002).

Genetic factors may be important. Some studies found that 50% of children with PUD have a first- or second-degree relative with PUD. First-degree relatives of clients with duodenal ulcers have a threefold increase in the prevalence of duodenal (but not gastric) ulcers, and relatives of clients with gastric ulcers have a threefold increase in the prevalence of gastric (but not duodenal) ulcers (Soll, 2002).

Incidence/Prevalence

In the United States, PUD affects about 4.5 million people annually. One in 10 Americans develops an ulcer at some time in his or her life (see the Resource Management box above). Physician office visits and hospitalizations for PUD have decreased in the last few decades. The mortality rate has also decreased in the last few decades and is about 1 death per 100,000 cases. The hospitalization rate is about 30 clients per 100,000 cases. Duodenal ulcers are increasing in older women, which may be the result of increased NSAID use for arthritic pain (Fantry, 2003).

HEALTH PROMOTION/ILLNESS PREVENTION

Health promotion and illness prevention practices are the same as for gastritis. For critically ill clients, health care providers may consider prophylactic therapy to prevent stress ulcers from occurring. This includes focusing on optimal oxygenation and circulation, which may involve finding and treating the underlying cause of bleeding aggressively. In addition health care providers may consider starting a client on enteral nutrition. Enteral nutrition is suggested to have a beneficial effect on the stomach mucosa because the artificial enteral products are alkaline. Finally, health care providers may consider drug therapy with H_2 antagonists, antacids, sucralfate, or antisecretory agents to prevent stress ulcers from occurring (McCarthy, 2003).

RESOURCE MANAGEMENT

PEPTIC ULCER DISEASE

Cost of Care

- In the early 1990s, health care costs attributed to management of acute or chronic ulcer disease totaled over $13.9 billion per year.
- The most extreme treatment, vagotomy or ulcer surgery, costs about $17,000 and requires an average of 307 days of treatment over a 15-year period. Maintenance therapy with antisecretory agents costs about $11,000 and requires 187 days of treatment over 15 years.
- In comparison, antibiotic therapy for *H. pylori* takes about 17 days and costs less than $1,000, over the same 15 year period.

Treatment of *H. pylori*–associated PUD decreases the need for hospitalization secondary to bleeding episodes. This reduces the economic burden to the health care system.

Treatment of *H. pylori*–related PUD provides substantial savings in terms of direct costs (e.g., medications, office visits) and indirect costs (lost workdays due to the illness).

Implications for Nursing

Nurses need to encourage clients to see their health care provider for continual symptoms of abdominal tenderness, dyspepsia, melena, and/or abdominal fullness to determine whether they possibly have *H. pylori*. *H. pylori* can be eradicated if clients follow the proper medication regimen for a relatively low cost compared to the high cost of chronic ulcer treatment. In addition, nurses need to educate clients regarding the role of *H. pylori* and ulcer disease and the importance of complying with the medication regimen to completely eradicate *H. pylori*.

Data from Gold, B.D. (2001). *Helicobacter pylori* and peptic ulcer disease: The key to cure for most patients. *Center for Disease Control.* Retrieved June 10, 2003, from http://www.cdc.gov/ulcer/keytocure.htm.

◆COLLABORATIVE MANAGEMENT

PHARM E REVIEW

◆Assessment

HISTORY

Collect data related to the causes and risk factors for peptic ulcer disease (PUD). Question the client about dietary factors that can influence the development of PUD, such as alcohol intake and tobacco use. Note if certain foods, such as tomatoes, or caffeinated beverages precipitate or worsen symptoms. Information regarding actual or perceived daily stressors is also elicited.

A history of current or past medical conditions focuses on gastrointestinal (GI) tract problems, particularly any history of diagnosis or treatment for *H. pylori* infection. A complete evaluation of all prescription and OTC medications is obtained. Specifically inquire whether the client is taking corticosteroids, aspirin, or other nonsteroidal anti-inflammatory drugs (NSAIDs). Also ask whether the client has ever undergone radiation treatments.

A history of GI upset, pain and its relationship to eating and sleep patterns, and actions taken to relieve pain is also important. Inquire about any changes in the character of the pain, because this may signal the development of complications. For example, if pain that was once intermittent and relieved by food and antacids becomes constant and radiates to the back or upper quadrant, this may indicate impending ulcer perforation. It is important to note that many individuals with active duodenal or gastric ulcers report having no ulcer symptoms.

TABLE 59-1 Differential Features of Gastric and Duodenal Ulcers

Feature	Gastric Ulcer	Duodenal Ulcer
Age	Usually 50 yr or older	Usually 50 yr or older
Gender	Male/female ratio of 1.1:1	Male/female ratio of 1:1
Blood group	No differentiation	Most often type O
General nourishment	May be malnourished	Usually well nourished
Stomach acid production	Normal secretion or hyposecretion	Hypersecretion
Occurrence	Mucosa exposed to acid-pepsin secretion	Mucosa exposed to acid-pepsin secretion
Clinical course	Healing and recurrence	Healing and recurrence
Pain	Occurs 30-60 min after a meal; at night: rarely	Occurs 1½ -3 hr after a meal; at night: often awakens client between 1 and 2 AM
	Accentuated by ingestion of food	Relieved by ingestion of food
Response to treatment	Healing with appropriate therapy	Healing with appropriate therapy
Hemorrhage	Hematemesis more common than melena	Melena more common than hematemesis
Malignant change	Perhaps in less than 10%	Rare
Recurrence	Tends to heal and recurs often in the same location	60% recur within 1 yr; 90% recur within 2 yr
Surrounding mucosa	Atrophic gastritis	No gastritis

PHYSICAL ASSESSMENT/CLINICAL MANIFESTATIONS

Physical assessment findings may reveal epigastric tenderness, usually located at the midline between the umbilicus and the xiphoid process. If perforation into the peritoneal cavity is present, the client exhibits a rigid, boardlike abdomen accompanied by rebound tenderness. Initially, auscultation of the abdomen may reveal hyperactive bowel sounds, but these may diminish with progression of the disorder.

Dyspepsia (indigestion), which is defined as discomfort centered around the epigastrium or upper abdomen, is the most commonly reported symptom associated with PUD. It is typically described as sharp, burning, or gnawing. Some clients may perceive discomfort as a sensation of abdominal pressure or of fullness or hunger.

CONSIDERATIONS FOR OLDER ADULTS

Both duodenal and gastric ulcers occur more often following the sixth decade of life. Pain is less often the initial complaint in the older client. In this age group, **melena** (occult blood) is often the presenting sign. Acute confusion and dizziness may also occur as a result of the lack of oxygen to the brain.

Gastric ulcer pain often occurs in the upper epigastrium with localization to the left of the midline and may be relieved by food. *Duodenal* ulcer pain is usually located to the right of the epigastrium (Table 59-1). The pain associated with a duodenal ulcer occurs 90 minutes to 3 hours after eating and often awakens the client at night. Pain may also be exacerbated by certain foods (e.g., tomatoes, hot spices, fried foods, onions, alcohol, or caffeine drinks) and certain medications (e.g., aspirin, NSAIDs, or corticosteroids).

Vomiting may be a symptom accompanying ulcer disease, most commonly with pyloric sphincter dysfunction. It results from gastric stasis associated with pyloric obstruction. Appetite is generally maintained in clients with a peptic ulcer unless pyloric obstruction is present.

To assess for fluid volume deficit, which can occur secondary to bleeding, take orthostatic vital signs of all clients suspected of having PUD. Orthostatic changes are characterized by a decrease of more than 20 mm Hg in systolic blood pressure, a decrease of 10 mm Hg in diastolic blood pressure, and/or an increase in pulse when the client rises from a lying to an erect (sitting or, if possible, standing) position. Also assess for dizziness, especially when the client is upright, because this is another symptom of fluid volume deficit.

PSYCHOSOCIAL ASSESSMENT

Assess the impact of ulcer disease on the client's lifestyle, occupation, family, and social and leisure activities. Questions about lifestyle, occupation, and leisure can yield important information. Evaluate the impact that lifestyle changes will have on the client. This assessment determines the client's ability to comply with the prescribed treatment regimen and to obtain the needed social support to alter his or her lifestyle.

LABORATORY ASSESSMENT

Hemoglobin and hematocrit values may be low, indicating bleeding. The stool specimen may be positive for occult (not apparent on visual inspection) blood if bleeding is present.

RADIOGRAPHIC ASSESSMENT

A barium examination of the GI tract can be used to establish a duodenal ulcer. A duodenal ulcer appears as a discrete crater in the duodenal bulb. This is often the initial test for a client who does not have severe symptoms. If perforation is suspected, the health care provider usually requests an upright abdomen series to demonstrate free air in the peritoneum. In any instance where free air is a possibility, barium should not be used.

OTHER DIAGNOSTIC ASSESSMENTS

The major diagnostic test for PUD is esophagogastroduodenoscopy (EGD), which is the most accurate means of establishing a diagnosis. Visualization of the ulcer crater by EGD allows the health care provider to take specimens for *H. pylori* testing and for biopsy and cytologic studies for ruling out gastric cancer (see the Legal/Ethical Issues box on p. 1292). EGD may be repeated at 4- to 6-week intervals while the health care provider evaluates the progress of healing in response to therapy.

LEGAL/ETHICAL ISSUES

QUALITY OF CARE FOR MEDICARE CLIENTS WITH PEPTIC ULCER DISEASE

Economic constraints on the health care system have resulted in efforts to provide cost-effective, high-quality care. To improve the quality of care delivered to Medicare beneficiaries with peptic ulcer disease (PUD), a chart review of 2644 Medicare beneficiaries was conducted to measure compliance with National Institutes of Health (NIH) guidelines for the detection and treatment of *Helicobacter pylori* in PUD.

In this particular study, only 57% of hospitalized Medicare recipients with PUD were tested for *H. pylori.* In addition, only 74% of clients with known *H. pylori* infection were treated with appropriate antimicrobial therapy. Medical record review also noted that 74% of clients were screened for nonsteroidal anti-inflammatory drug (NSAID) use. Only 24% had documented counseling regarding the risks associated with NSAID use, and only 2% had documented education of the ulcer-associated risks of NSAID use.

Although limited documented education may be in part to blame for the poor quality of care regarding *H. pylori*–related ulcers, NIH clinical practice guidelines for the diagnosis and treatment of peptic ulcer disease are clearly underutilized. Quality improvement initiatives are needed to improve the care delivered to Medicare beneficiaries with PUD. *H. pylori* screening and treatment guidelines need to be enforced to ensure that appropriate treatment is received, especially by older adults.

Data from Offman, J., et al. (2000). The quality of care for Medicare patients with peptic ulcer disease. *American Journal of Gastroenterology 95*(1), 106-113.

A common noninvasive test for *H. pylori* involves IgG serologic testing. Infection with *H. pylori* causes immunoglobulin antibodies to form. Although antibody assays have a high sensitivity and specificity (>95%) for detecting *H. pylori,* antibody assays cannot be used to document elimination of the organism, because antibody levels can remain elevated despite successful treatment.

Urea breath testing has been employed to detect *H. pylori* when endoscopy is not clinically indicated. To perform this test, the client must be on NPO status after midnight on the night before the test. The client drinks a carbon-enriched urea solution. The presence of *H. pylori* causes the bacteria to break down the solution and release carbon dioxide, which the client exhales in a collection container for analysis. The carbon dioxide excreted in the breath is then measured and compared with a baseline measurement to determine the presence of *H. pylori.* In addition to its noninvasive nature, this test assesses the entire stomach and may prove especially helpful in determining whether treatment was successful. The breath test is 96% to 98% accurate.

Stool tests may also be used to detect *H. pylori.* The test detects *H. pylori* antigen in the stool (National Digestive Diseases Information Clearinghouse, 2002).

A complete medication history needs to be obtained before diagnostic testing is done for *H. pylori.* False-negative results could be obtained if the client has received antibiotic treatment, used a bismuth preparation (Pepto-Bismol), or used a proton-pump inhibitor within the 4-week period before testing for *H. pylori.* Other medications, such as misoprostol, sucralfate, or an H_2-blocker administered within the week before the test may also yield a false-negative result. Use of over-the-counter medications (OTC), such as Pepcid AC, Tagamet, and Zantac, can also affect test results.

◆Analysis

COMMON NURSING DIAGNOSES AND COLLABORATIVE PROBLEMS

The priority nursing diagnosis for clients with peptic ulcer disease (PUD) is Acute Pain or Chronic Pain related to physical (gastric and/or duodenal mucosal) injury.

The collaborative problem that is of most concern is Potential for Gastrointestinal (GI) Bleeding.

ADDITIONAL NURSING DIAGNOSES AND COLLABORATIVE PROBLEMS

In addition to the common nursing diagnosis and collaborative problem, clients with PUD may have one or more of the following:

- Deficient Knowledge related to management of PUD
- Imbalanced Nutrition: Less Than Body Requirements related to anorexia, nausea, or diet constraints
- Disturbed Sleep Pattern related to discomfort
- Risk for Falls related to orthostatic hypotension
- Fatigue related to loss of blood and chronic illness
- Nausea related to gastrointestinal irritation
- Ineffective Health Maintenance related to lack of knowledge regarding health practices to prevent ulcer formation
- Fear related threat to well-being or potential death

Possible collaborative problems include the following:

- Potential for Shock
- Potential for Metabolic Alkalosis

◆Planning and Implementation

ACUTE PAIN; CHRONIC PAIN

NOC **PLANNING: EXPECTED OUTCOMES.** PUD causes significant discomfort that impacts many aspects of daily living. The client with PUD is expected to take personal actions to control pain. Indicators include that the client will:

- Report that pain is controlled.
- Use available resources.
- Use previous measures.
- Report uncontrolled symptoms to health care professionals.

INTERVENTIONS. Interventions to manage pain related to PUD are accomplished with specific ulcer therapy and dietary modifications. One of the primary purposes for employing drug therapy in the management of PUD is to reduce or eliminate pain. Analgesics are not the mainstay of pain relief for PUD. Instead, the ulcer drug regimen itself promotes relief of pain by eradicating *H. pylori* infection and promoting healing of gastric mucosa.

CONSIDERATIONS FOR OLDER ADULTS

Older adults tend to use over-the-counter (OTC) remedies, often delaying appropriate treatment for symptoms of PUD. In addition, they often suffer from one or more chronic illnesses that require the use of medications that can precipitate or worsen PUD. Older adults may also be at increased risk for complications and death following acute peptic ulcer bleeding.

Perform a comprehensive pain assessment that includes the following aspects of pain:

- Location
- Characteristics
- Onset/duration
- Frequency
- Quality
- Severity
- Precipitating and alleviating factors

Any changes in the characteristics or location of peptic ulcer pain are carefully assessed, because such changes often accompany the development of complications. Teach the client to eliminate irritants (e.g., spicy foods) that can precipitate or increase pain from ulcer disease.

Measures to promote adequate rest and sleep may be necessary, because ulcer pain can cause the client to awaken. Assist the client in achieving compliance with the medication regimen, because adherence to the drug regimen promotes relief of pain and discomfort. Monitor the client's satisfaction with the level of pain relief.

Drug Therapy. The primary goals of drug therapy in the treatment of PUD are (1) to provide pain relief, (2) to eradicate *H. pylori* infection, (3) to heal ulcerations, and (4) to prevent recurrence (see Chart 59-3). Several different regimens can be used to achieve these goals. In selecting a therapeutic drug regimen, the health care provider must consider the efficacy of the treatment, the anticipated side effects, the ability of the client to comply with the regimen, and the cost of the treatment.

Although numerous drugs have been evaluated for the treatment of *H. pylori* infection, no single agent has been used successfully against the organism. Current practice involves using a combination of agents to achieve treatment goals. The most successful regimen used is a triple therapy consisting of a bismuth compound or a proton-pump inhibitor such as omeprazole (Prilosec), and a combination of two antibiotics such as metronidazole (Flagyl, Novonidazol✱) and tetracycline or clarithromycin and amoxicillin. Although this regimen is the most effective and least expensive, adherence to the regimen is difficult for most clients. A client must consume medications four times daily for up to 14 days, and adverse effects occur in 20% to 30% of individuals, especially in older adults. Some strains of *H. pylori* have begun to demonstrate metronidazole resistance, raising concerns about long-term treatment with this regimen.

Hyposecretory Drugs. Hyposecretory drugs produce a reduction in gastric acid secretions. These drugs include antisecretory agents, H_2-receptor antagonists, and prostaglandin analogues (see Chart 59-3).

Antisecretory Agents. These medications are also called proton pump inhibitors and have emerged as the drug class of choice for treating clients with acid-related disorders (Horn, 2000). Omeprazole (Prilosec), lansoprazole (Prevacid), rabeprazole (Aciphex), pantoprazole (Protonix), and esomeprazole magnesium (Nexium) suppress the H, K-ATPase enzyme system of gastric acid production. Omeprazole, lansoprazole, and esomeprazole magnesium are each available as delayed-release capsules designed to release their contents outside of the stomach. Omeprazole and lansoprazole may be dissolved in a solution of sodium bicarbonate and given through any feeding tube. Bicarbonate protects the dissolved omeprazole and lansoprazole granules in gastric acid. Therefore the drugs are still absorbed correctly. These capsules can also be opened. The enteric-coated capsules can be put in apple juice or orange juice and given through a large-bore feeding tube (McCarthy, 2003). Rabeprazole (Aciphex) and pantoprazole (Protonix) are enteric-coated tablets that quickly dissolve after the tablet has moved through the stomach and cannot be crushed before administration. Pantoprazole (Protonix) is also available in an IV form, which may be helpful for clients who are NPO.

H_2-Receptor Antagonists. Drugs that block histamine-stimulated gastric secretions are effective in the management of ulcer disease. These medications may be used for indigestion and heartburn. Lower-dose forms are available in over-the-counter (OTC) products. H_2-receptor antagonists block the action of the H_2 receptors of the parietal cells, thus inhibiting gastric acid secretion. The most common drugs are ranitidine (Zantac), famotidine (Pepcid), and nizatidine (Axid). These drugs are typically administered in a single dose at bedtime and are used for 4 to 6 weeks in combination with other therapy.

Prostaglandin Analogues. Prostaglandins are naturally abundant in the gastrointestinal (GI) tract. Prostaglandin analogues have been shown to be effective in clinical trials in the treatment of duodenal ulcers. They reduce gastric acid secretion and enhance gastric mucosal resistance to tissue injury. Misoprostol (Cytotec), the most commonly used drug in this category, *helps prevent* NSAID-induced ulcers. Some NSAIDs are being manufactured in combination with misoprostol. A significant adverse effect of this drug is uterine contraction; therefore its use is contraindicated in pregnant women.

Antacids. Antacids buffer gastric acid and prevent the formation of pepsin. Antacids have demonstrated effectiveness in accelerating the healing of duodenal ulcers. Liquid suspensions are the most therapeutic form, but tablets may be more convenient and enhance compliance. The most widely used preparations are mixtures of aluminum hydroxide and magnesium hydroxide. This combination overcomes the unpleasant GI side effects of either of these preparations when used alone. Mylanta and Maalox are examples of this type of combination antacid formulation. The aluminum and magnesium hydroxide combination products neutralize well at small doses. These products must be administered cautiously to those with renal impairment. These substances cannot be eliminated adequately by the kidneys and are consequently retained in excessive amounts in the body.

Instruct the client that to achieve a therapeutic effect, sufficient antacid must be ingested to neutralize the hourly production of acid. For optimal effect, teach the client to take antacids about 2 hours after meals to reduce the hydrogen ion load in the duodenum. Antacids may be effective from 30 minutes to 3 hours after ingestion. Antacids taken with an empty stomach are quickly evacuated; thus the neutralizing effect is reduced. Calcium carbonate (Tums) is a potent antacid, but it triggers gastrin release, causing a rebound acid secretion. Therefore its use in acid inhibition is not recommended.

Antacids can interact with certain drugs, such as phenytoin (Dilantin), tetracycline, and ketoconazole, and interfere with their effectiveness. Determine what other drugs the client is using before a specific antacid is prescribed. Medications are administered 1 to 2 hours before or after the antacid. Inform the client that flavored antacids, especially wintergreen, should be avoided. The flavoring increases the emptying time of the stomach; thus the desired effect of the antacid is negated.

Teach the client with past or present heart failure to avoid antacids containing a high sodium content, such as aluminum hydroxide, magnesium hydroxide, sodium bicarbonate, and simethicone combination products (Gelusil and Mylanta). Magaldrate (Riopan) has the lowest sodium concentration.

Mucosal Barrier Fortifiers. Sucralfate (Carafate) is sulfonated disaccharide that forms complexes with proteins at the base of a peptic ulcer. This protective coat prevents further digestive action of both acid and pepsin.

Sucralfate does not inhibit acid secretion. Rather, it binds bile acids and pepsins, reducing injury from these substances. Sucralfate may be used in conjunction with H_2-receptor antagonists and antacids but should not be administered within 1 hour of the antacid. Sucralfate is given on an empty stomach 1 hour before each meal and at bedtime. The main side effect of this drug is constipation.

Diet Therapy. The value of diet in the management of ulcer disease is highly controversial. There is no evidence that dietary restriction reduces gastric acid secretion or promotes tissue healing, although a bland diet may assist in relieving symptoms. Food itself acts as an antacid by neutralizing gastric acid for 30 to 60 minutes. An increased rate of gastric acid secretion, called rebound, may follow. If diet therapy is used, it may be directed toward neutralizing acid and reducing hypermotility, which may alleviate symptoms.

Instruct the client to avoid substances that increase gastric acid secretion. This includes caffeine-containing beverages (coffee, tea, and cola). Both caffeinated and decaffeinated coffees should be avoided, because coffee contains peptides that stimulate gastrin release.

In collaboration with the dietitian, teach the client to exclude any foods that cause discomfort. A bland, nonirritating diet is recommended during the acute symptomatic phase. Bedtime snacks are avoided because they may stimulate gastric acid secretion. Eating six smaller daily meals may help, but this regimen is no longer a regular part of therapy. There is no evidence to support the theory that eating six daily meals promotes healing of the ulcer. This practice actually stimulates gastric acid secretion. Clients should avoid alcohol and tobacco because of their stimulatory effects on gastric acid secretion.

Complementary and Alternative Therapies. The use of Kundalini yoga meditation techniques is currently being studied to see how they can help manage gastrointestinal disorders such as peptic ulcer disease. Kundalini yoga techniques have been demonstrated to have a dramatically beneficial effect on obsessive-compulsive disorders and anxiety disorders. Many have suggested that GI disorders result from the dysfunction of both the GI tract itself and the brain. This means that stress is thought to make GI disorders such as peptic ulcer disease worse. Yoga is thought to alter the activities of the central and autonomic nervous system (Shannahoff-Khalsa, 2002).

Other modalities include herbs, such as powders of slippery elm and marshmallow root, quercetin, and licorice. These herbs are thought to heal inflamed tissue and increase blood flow to the gastric mucosa. Other substances include zinc, vitamin C, essential fatty acids, acidophilus, vitamins E and A, and glutamine. All of these substances enhance healing.

POTENTIAL FOR GASTROINTESTINAL BLEEDING

PLANNING: EXPECTED OUTCOMES. Fluid volume loss secondary to the development of complications is a risk associated with PUD. Blood loss due to hemorrhage can carry significant morbidity and mortality. Fluid volume loss secondary to vomiting can lead to dehydration and electrolyte imbalances. The client with peptic ulcer disease (PUD) is expected to maintain vascular, cellular, and intracellular perfusion. Indicators include that the client will:

- Have intact mental status
- Have stable blood pressure
- Have warm, dry skin
- Excrete at least 30 mL/hr of urine

INTERVENTIONS. Monitoring and early recognition of complications are critical to the successful management of PUD. Interventions aimed at managing complications associated with PUD include prevention and/or management of bleeding, perforation, and gastric outlet obstruction. In some cases, surgical treatment of complications becomes necessary.

NIC **HYPOVOLEMIA MANAGEMENT.** The purpose of managing hypovolemia is to expand intravascular fluid in a client who is volume depleted. Monitor vital signs and observe for fluid loss from bleeding and vomiting. Carefully monitor the client's fluid status, including intake and output. Fluid replacement in older adults should be closely monitored to prevent fluid overload. An infusion pump is used to ensure accurate delivery of the desired volume. Serum electrolytes are also monitored, because depletions from vomiting or nasogastric suctioning must be replaced. Ensure that two large-bore peripheral IV catheters are inserted so that both fluids and blood lost to vomiting and/or hemorrhage can be replaced. Volume replacement with isotonic crystalloid solutions (0.9 normal saline solution, or lactated Ringer's solution) should be started immediately, because adequate fluid volume replacement is essential. The health care provider may order blood products, such as packed red blood cells, to expand volume and correct abnormalities in the complete blood count (CBC). For clients with active bleeding, fresh frozen plasma may be given if the prothrombin time is 1.5 times higher than the midrange control value. To prevent injury from falls secondary to orthostatic hypotension, the client is assisted with ambulation. Orthostatic hypotension is common in clients with decreased fluid volume.

NIC **BLEEDING REDUCTION: GASTROINTESTINAL.** The purpose of activities to reduce bleeding is to limit the amount of blood loss from the upper and lower gastrointestinal (GI) tract resulting from complications related to PUD. Monitor the client for manifestations indicating GI bleeding. All excretions are observed for the presence of frank (obvious) or occult (not apparent on visual inspection) bleeding. With GI bleeding, the presence of frank blood or coffee-ground vomitus may be observed. Stools can contain frank blood or appear black and tarry.

CHART 59-4

KEY FEATURES of
Gastrointestinal Bleeding

- Coffee-ground vomitus
- Tarry stools or frank (obvious) blood in stools
- Melena (occult blood)
- Decreased blood pressure
- Increased weak and thready pulse
- Decreased hemoglobin and hematocrit
- Vertigo
- Acute confusion (in older adults)
- Dizziness
- Syncope

Occult blood loss may be detected by stool examination and may be accompanied by progressive iron deficiency anemia (Chart 59-4).

Monitor the client's hematocrit, hemoglobin, and coagulation studies for changes from the baseline measurements. Monitor vital signs frequently. With mild bleeding (less than 500 mL), slight feelings of weakness and mild perspiration may be present. When blood loss exceeds 1 L/24 hr, manifestations of shock may be manifested, such as hypotension, chills, palpitations, diaphoresis, and a weak, thready pulse. (See Chapter 40 for the treatment of shock.)

Immediately notify the health care provider of major bleeding. Transfusion therapy may be required to replace blood loss. (See Chapter 43 for nursing interventions for clients undergoing blood transfusion.) The health care provider may prescribe H_2 blockers to avoid extremes in gastric pH levels. If appropriate and as prescribed, insert a nasogastric (NG) tube, monitor secretions, and perform nasogastric lavage to decompress the stomach and alleviate bleeding. In addition, instruct the client and family to avoid the use of anti-inflammatory medications that can precipitate or worsen GI bleeding. NIC interventions and activities are summarized in Chart 59-5.

NONSURGICAL MANAGEMENT. Because prevention or early detection of complications is critical in obtaining a satisfactory outcome, monitor the client carefully and immediately report changes to the health care provider. The type of nonsurgical intervention selected will depend on the type and severity of the complication.

The goals of therapeutic interventions for bleeding secondary to PUD are as follows:

- Stop the acute bleeding episode
- Prevent rebleeding

A combination of several different therapeutic interventions, including endoscopic therapy, acid suppression, NG tube placement, and saline lavage, can be used to control acute bleeding and prevent rebleeding. Therapeutic trials have been conducted to determine the optimal treatment for bleeding due to peptic ulcers. Endoscopic therapy and suppression of gastric acid are the primary therapies used to control active bleeding caused by PUD. H_2-receptor antagonists, proton pump inhibitors, and antacids are the primary medications used to treat this bleeding.

Endoscopic Therapy. Endoscopic therapy via an esophagogastroduodenoscopy (EGD) can assist in achieving homeostasis during an acute bleeding episode. The primary methods of endoscopic therapy are (1) thermal contact using a heater probe or multielectrocoagulation, (2) injection of the bleeding site with diluted epinephrine, (3) laser therapy, and (4) clipping the bleeding vessel with a mechanical clip. All methods are effective in achieving blood clot formation. Thermal contact and injection with epinephrine are most commonly used. Laser therapy is costly and therefore is used less often. Clipping is used mostly when a bleeding vessel is visible. Generally, endoscopic therapy is beneficial for clients with active bleeding; however, ulcers that continue to bleed or continue to rebleed despite endoscopic therapy may require surgical repair. Sometimes endoscopists (physicians) may scope a client daily during an acute bleed of a peptic ulcer to assess and possibly re-treat the ulcer if it continues to bleed or begins bleeding again. Sometimes this regimen will prevent the client from having to have surgery.

Pre-EGD nursing care involves inserting a large-bore IV catheter. A large catheter allows the client to receive IV conscious sedation (e.g., midazolam [Versed] and meperidine [Demerol]) to remain comfortable during the procedure. In addition, ensure that the client remains NPO six hours before the procedure. This prevents the risk of aspiration and allows the endoscopist (physician) to visualize and treat the ulcer. A client must sign a consent before the EGD after the physician informs the client about the procedure. During the EGD, a trained endoscopy nurse and technician assist the physician with the procedure. Post-EGD care involves

CHART 59-5

NIC **INTERVENTION ACTIVITIES for**
The Client with Peptic Ulcer Disease

Hypovolemia Management: *Expansion of intravascular fluid volume in a client who is volume depleted*

- Monitor vital signs, as appropriate.
- Monitor fluid status, including intake and output, as appropriate.
- Monitor for fluid loss (e.g., bleeding, vomiting, diarrhea, perspiration, and tachypnea).
- Arrange availability of blood products for transfusion, if necessary.
- Administer blood products (e.g., platelets and fresh frozen plasma), as appropriate.
- Monitor for blood reaction, if appropriate.

Bleeding Reduction: *Gastrointestinal: Limitation of the amount of blood loss from the upper and lower gastrointestinal tract and related complications*

- Monitor for signs and symptoms of persistent bleeding (e.g., check all secretions for frank or occult blood).
- Hematest all excretions and observe for blood loss in emesis, sputum, feces, urine, NG tube drainage, and wound drainage, as appropriate.
- Document color, amount, and character of stools.
- Monitor coagulation studies and complete blood count (CBC) with WBC differential.
- Insert nasogastric tube to suction and monitor secretions, if appropriate.
- Perform nasogastric lavage, as appropriate.
- Avoid extremes in gastric pH level by administration of appropriate medication (e.g., antacids or histamine-blocking agent).
- Instruct the client and/or family on the need for blood replacement, as appropriate.
- Instruct the client and/or family to avoid the use of antiinflammatory medications (e.g., aspirin and ibuprofen).

NIC intervention activities selected from Dochterman, J.M., & Bulechek, G.M. (Eds.). (2004). *Nursing interventions classification (NIC)* (4th ed.). St. Louis: Mosby. No part of this work is to be altered without prior written permission from the Publisher.
WBC, White blood cell.

checking the vital signs, heart rhythm, and oxygen saturation frequently until they return to baseline. In addition, assess the client's ability to swallow saliva frequently. The client's gag reflex may initially be absent after an EGD due to the anesthetizing (numbing) the throat with a spray before the procedure. The client will not be able to resume a pre-procedure diet until the gag reflex is intact.

Acid Suppression. Aggressive acid suppression is used to prevent rebleeding. When acute bleeding is stopped and clot formation has taken place within the ulcer crater, the clot remains in contact with gastric contents. Acid-suppressive agents are used to stabilize the clot by raising the pH level of gastric contents. Several drugs are used to achieve acid suppression in clients with a bleeding episode. H_2-receptor antagonists prevent acid from being produced by parietal cells. Proton pump inhibitors prevent the transport of acid across the parietal cell membrane, whereas antacids buffer acid produced in the stomach.

Somatostatin analogue may also be used and has shown excellent hemostatic results. Somatostatin analogue is actually a synthetic gastrointestinal (GI) hormone that suppresses gastric acid secretion by a direct action on parietal and chief cells. Somatostatin analogue vasoconstricts splanchnic arteries, which reduces hemorrhage (Yabuki et al., 2002).

Nasogastric Tube Placement. Upper GI bleeding may require the health care provider or nurse to insert a nasogastric (NG) tube to:

- Ascertain the presence or absence of blood in the stomach
- Assess the rate of bleeding
- Prevent gastric dilation
- Administer saline lavage

Nasogastric aspiration is an important part of diagnostic and prognostic evaluation of the client. The presence of red blood in emesis, nasogastric aspirate, or stools is correlated with a poor outcome.

Once the NG tube is placed, confirmation of proper positioning of the tube is determined by x-ray examination. Irrigate the NG tube to maintain its patency and prevent obstruction with clotted blood.

Saline Lavage. Saline lavage requires the insertion of a large-bore NG tube with instillation of saline in volumes of 50 to 200 mL. The saline and blood are repeatedly withdrawn until returns are clear or light pink and without clots. For protection against exposure to blood, practitioners may use the following procedure with a closed system for irrigation and suction. A Y-connector is attached to the NG tube, and an IV bag of normal saline is attached to tubing at one end of the Y-connector. The opposite connector is attached to tubing connected to wall suction. After the stomach is initially drained by suctioning, the tubing attached to the wall suction is clamped, and up to 200 mL of normal saline is allowed to drain into the client through the NG tube. After the saline is instilled, the tube connecting the saline to the NG tube is clamped, and the clamp to suction is released. Instruct the client to lie on the left side during this procedure to limit the flow of saline out of the stomach and prevent aspiration.

NONSURGICAL MANAGEMENT OF PERFORATION. To prevent peritonitis from GI contents that have entered the peritoneum, perforation is managed by immediately replacing fluid, blood, and electrolytes, administering antibiotics, and keeping the client NPO. Maintain nasogastric suction to drain gastric secretions and thus prevent further peritoneal spillage. Carefully monitor intake and output and check vital signs at least hourly and monitor the client for clinical manifestations of septic shock, such as fever, pain, tachycardia, lethargy, or anxiety.

NONSURGICAL MANAGEMENT OF PYLORIC OBSTRUCTION. Pyloric obstruction is caused by edema, spasm, or scar tissue. Symptoms of obstruction related to difficulty in emptying the stomach include feelings of fullness, distention, or nausea after eating, as well as vomiting of copious amounts of undigested food.

Treatment of obstruction is directed toward restoration of fluid and electrolyte balance and decompression of the dilated stomach. Obstruction related to edema and spasm generally responds to medical therapy. First, the stomach must be decompressed with nasogastric suction; next, interventions are directed at correcting metabolic alkalosis and dehydration. The NG tube is clamped after about 72 hours, and the client is checked for retention of gastric contents. If the amount retained is not more than 350 mL in 30 minutes, the health care provider may allow oral fluids. In some cases, surgical intervention may be required.

SURGICAL MANAGEMENT. New guidelines for the treatment of PUD that include *H. pylori* eradication and the development of nonsurgical means of controlling bleeding have led to a decline in the need for surgical intervention. In PUD, surgical intervention is used to:

- Reduce the acid-secreting ability of the stomach
- Treat clients who do not respond to medical therapy
- Treat a surgical emergency that develops as a complication of PUD

Two general surgical approaches are available for PUD—minimally invasive partial gastrectomy and conventional open surgery.

Minimally invasive gastrectomy (MIG) via laparoscopy (a type of endoscope) may be performed to remove a chronic gastric ulcer or treat hemorrhage from perforation. Several small incisions allow access to the stomach and duodenum. The client may have partial gastric removal and/or a vagotomy (vagus nerve cutting) to control acid secretion. The advantages of laparoscopic surgery over traditional procedures include a shorter hospital stay, less postoperative complications, less pain, and better, quicker recovery.

Preoperative Care. Before conventional open-approach surgery, an NG tube is inserted and connected to suction to remove secretions and empty the stomach. This allows surgery to take place without contamination of the peritoneal cavity by gastric secretions. Chart 59-6 describes the procedure for inserting the NG tube and nursing care associated with NG tube maintenance. The NG tube remains in place postoperatively to prevent the accumulation of secretions, which may lead to vomiting or gastrointestinal (GI) distention and pressure on the suture line.

Other preoperative nursing measures for the client undergoing open gastric surgery are the same as those for any client undergoing abdominal surgery and general anesthesia (see Chapter 20).

Operative Procedures. There is no definitive single procedure for PUD. The most commonly performed conventional surgical procedures are gastroenterostomy, vagotomy, and pyloroplasty.

CHART 59-6

BEST PRACTICE for
Nasogastric Tubes

1. Inform the client about the procedure and its potential discomfort.
2. Seat the client with pillows behind the shoulders.
3. Lubricate the tube with a water-soluble lubricant.
4. Measure the length of the tube to be passed.
   a. Measure from the bridge of the nose to the earlobe to the xiphoid process.
   b. Indicate this length with a piece of tape on the tube.

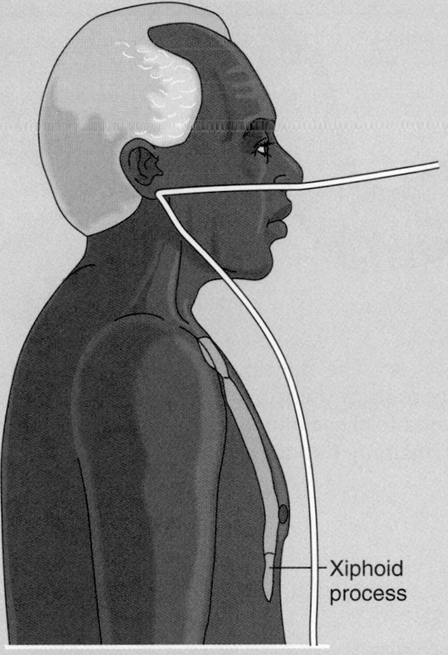

5. Determine which nostril is more patent.
6. Encourage the client to swallow or drink water if the level of consciousness and treatment plan permit.
7. Insert the tube.
   a. Pass the tube gently into the nasopharynx. Ask the client to swallow repeatedly while the tube is advanced.
   b. If resistance is met, rotate the tube slowly, aiming downward and toward the closer ear.
   c. In the intubated or semiconscious client, flex the client's head toward the chest while passing the tube.
8. Withdraw the tube immediately if any change is noted in the client's respiratory status.
9. Test for tube placement by using the following techniques:
   a. Obtain a sample of the gastric contents by aspirating with a 50-mL catheter-tipped syringe.
   b. Test the pH of the gastric contents (should be between 1 and 3.5).
   c. Obtain an order for an x-ray study to confirm placement.
10. Connect the tube to suction at low pressure.
    a. The Levin tube is connected to intermittent low suction.
    b. The Salem sump or Anderson tube is connected to continuous low suction.
11. Secure the tube to the client's nose with tape and to the client's gown.
    a. Tie a slipknot around the tube with a rubber band.
    b. Pin a rubber band to the client's gown.
12. Check the client's intake and output every 4 hr or more often, as indicated.
13. Observe the client for nausea, vomiting, abdominal fullness, or distention.
14. If irrigation is indicated, use only a normal saline solution.
15. Observe the client for alterations in fluid and electrolyte balance.
16. If indicated, instruct the client about movement that will not dislodge the tube and cause nasal irritation.
17. Remove the tape securing the tube to the nose daily and PRN to clean skin; reapply tape.

Gastroenterostomy. A simple **gastroenterostomy** permits neutralization of gastric acid by regurgitation of alkaline duodenal contents into the stomach. The surgeon creates a passage between the body of the stomach and the small bowel, often the jejunum (Figure 59-4). The benefit may be offset by interference with acid inhibition of gastrin release, which results in a net increase in acid secretion.

If the gastroenterostomy drains the stomach, it reduces motor activity in the pyloroduodenal area. Drainage of the gastric contents diverts acid from the ulcerated area and facilitates healing. However, the secretory capacity of the parietal cell mass of the stomach has not been reduced, and the gastrin mechanism continues to function. For this reason, a vagotomy is usually combined with gastroenterostomy for reduction of the vagal influences.

Vagotomy. Three types of **vagotomy** have been used in the treatment of duodenal ulcers: truncal vagotomy, selective vagotomy, and proximal gastric vagotomy (Figure 59-5). Vagotomy eliminates the acid-secreting stimulus to gastric cells and decreases the responsiveness of parietal cells. In a truncal vagotomy, the vagal trunks are transected and the antrum is removed. The remaining stomach is anastomosed to the proximal duodenum (Billroth I) or to a loop of jejunum (Billroth II) (Figures 59-6 and 59-7).

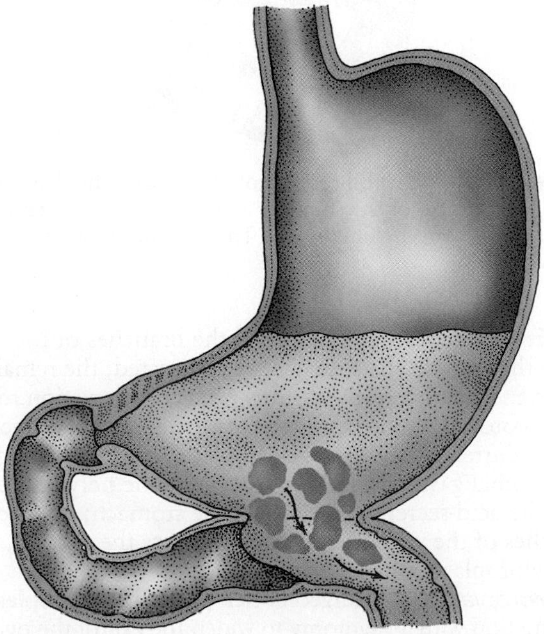

Figure 59-4 ■ Gastroenterostomy (the creation of a passage between the body of the stomach and the jejunum).

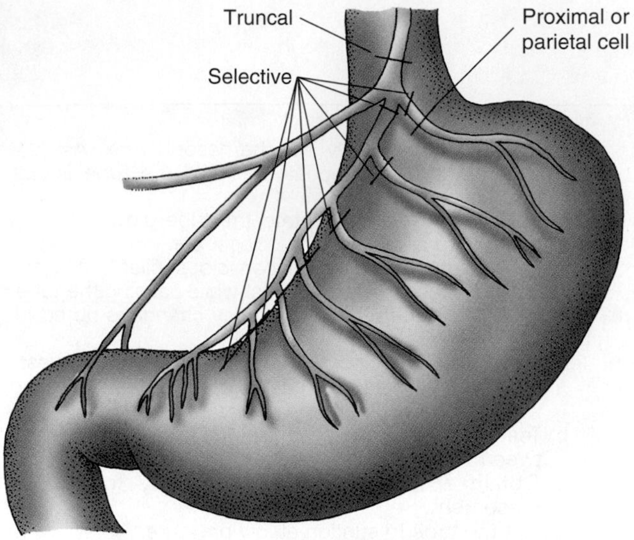

Figure 59-5 ■ Various types of vagotomies.

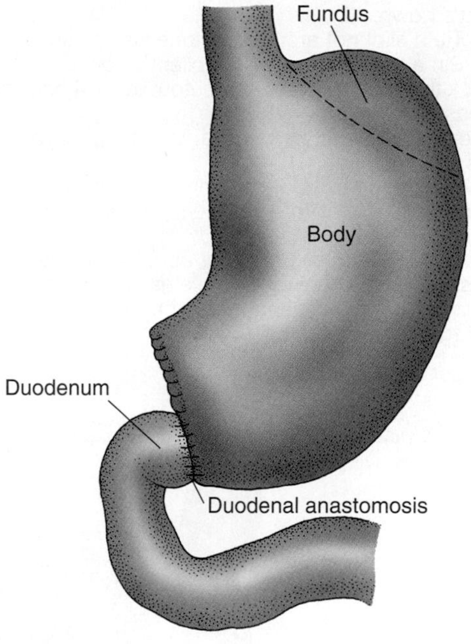

Figure 59-6 ■ The Billroth I procedure (gastroduodenostomy). The distal portion of the stomach is removed, and the remainder is anastomosed to the duodenum. The shading shows the portion removed.

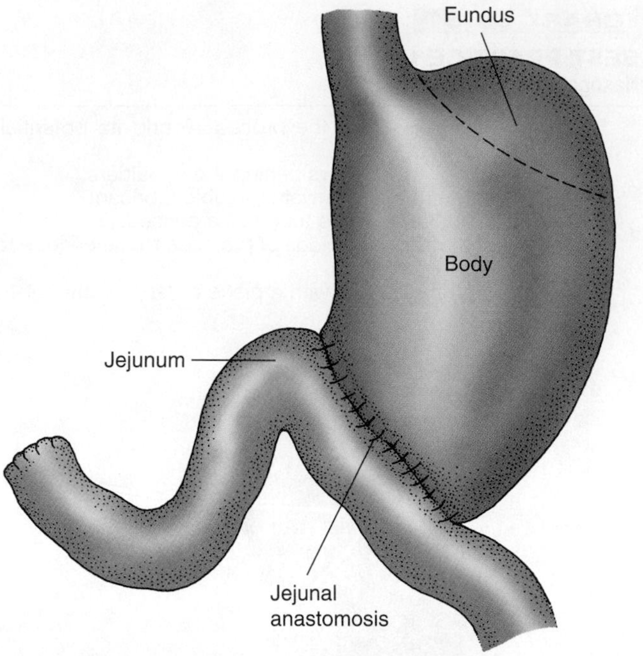

Figure 59-7 ■ The Billroth II procedure (gastrojejunostomy). The lower portion of the stomach is removed, and the remainder is anastomosed to the jejunum. The shading shows the portion removed. A remaining duodenal stump is closed.

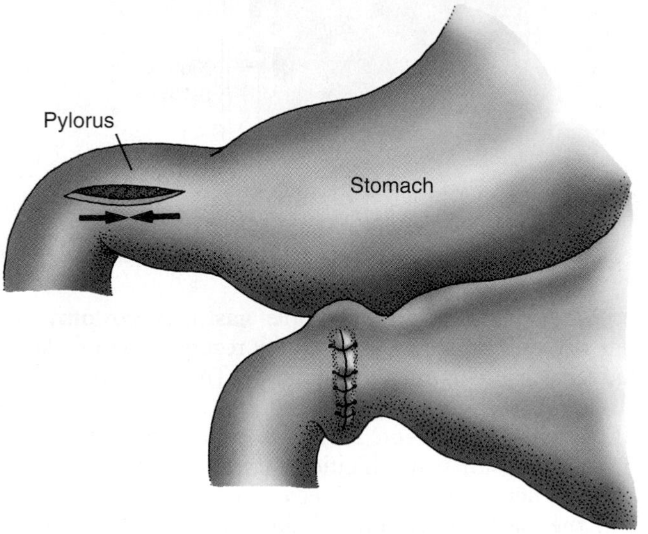

Figure 59-8 ■ The Heineke-Mikulicz pyloroplasty.

With selective vagotomy, only the branches of the vagus nerve that supply the stomach are transected; the remaining abdominal viscera still has intact vagal innervation. Selective vagotomy results in a more complete response, reduced ulcer recurrence, and fewer postoperative complications.

Proximal gastric vagotomy interrupts the nerve supply to only the acid-secreting portion of the stomach; it spares the branches of the vagus nerve that innervate the antrum, making pyloroplasty unnecessary.

Pyloroplasty. The surgeon often performs **pyloroplasty** in conjunction with a vagotomy to widen the exit of the pylorus. This facilitates emptying of stomach contents. The most common procedure is the Heineke-Mikulicz pyloroplasty (Figure 59-8). In this procedure the surgeon enlarges the pyloric stricture by incising the pylorus longitudinally and sutures the incision transversely.

Postoperative Care. The postoperative care is similar for all of the surgical procedures (see the Plan of Care on pp. 1299 to 1302). Provide the usual postoperative care for clients who have had general anesthesia (see Chapter 22). In addition, monitor the client for the development of postoperative complications.

Nasogastric Tube Management. Monitor the nasogastric (NG) tube for patency and carefully secure the tube to prevent dislodgment; this is critical for preventing the retention of gastric secretions. Monitor the client to make sure that no

PLAN of CARE MEDICAL DIAGNOSIS: GASTRECTOMY

NURSING DIAGNOSIS NO. 1 ■ Acute Pain

	Expected Outcomes	Nursing Interventions	Rationales
RELATED FACTORS Injury agents: Surgery **DEFINING CHARACTERISTICS** Verbal or coded report of pain Observed evidence of pain	Denies experiencing pain greater than 5 on a 0 to 10 pain scale No verbal report or observation of guarding or protective gestures No verbal report or observation of an alteration in sleep patterns No verbal report or observation of self-focusing behavior No verbal report or observation of facial mask of pain No verbal report or observation of an alteration in activity level	NIC **Pain Management** Perform a comprehensive pain assessment that includes location, characteristics, onset/duration, frequency, quality, intensity or severity of pain, and precipitating factors.	A plan for pain management must be based on the client's unique responses to pain.
		D Reduce or eliminate factors that precipitate or increase the pain experience.	Preventing a pain experience is preferred to trying to control or eliminate pain.
		Provide information about the pain, such as causes, how long it will last, and anticipated discomforts from procedures.	The client is better able to monitor his or her own discomfort and to intervene appropriately when informed.
		NIC **Analgesic Administration** Choose the IV rather than the IM route for frequent pain medication injections, when possible.	The IV route avoids tissue trauma and the unpredictable absorption of medication.
		Administer analgesics around-the-clock.	Administration around-the-clock prevents the peaks and troughs of analgesia, especially with severe pain.
		D Institute safety precautions for a client who is receiving opioid analgesics, as appropriate.	Opioid analgesics may impair the client's judgment and/or coordination.
		Document the client's response to the analgesic and any untoward effects.	Documentation provides the health care team with the information needed to accurately evaluate the client's response to the analgesic regimen.
		Implement actions to decrease the untoward effects of analgesics.	Actions taken to prevent the predictable but unwanted effects of opioid analgesics (e.g., constipation) increase client comfort.
		Teach about the use of analgesics, strategies to decrease side effects, and expectations for involvement in decisions about pain relief.	Information about analgesics and the expectation for involvement increase the client's sense of control over his or her pain.
		NIC **Patient-Controlled Analgesia (PCA) Administration** Validate that the client can use a PCA device.	To use a PCA, the client must be able to communicate, comprehend explanations, and follow directions.
		Document the client's pain, amount and frequency of drug dosing, and response to pain treatment on a pain flow sheet.	Information on the pain flow sheet assists the health care team to adjust the analgesic regimen to the client's needs.
		Teach the client and family how to use the PCA device.	The device will not be used if the client and/or family do not know how to use or are afraid of the device.

D Indicates tasks that can be delegated to unlicensed assistive nursing personnel at the discretion of the nurse.

Continued

PLAN of CARE MEDICAL DIAGNOSIS: GASTRECTOMY—*cont'd*

NURSING DIAGNOSIS NO. 1 ■ Acute Pain—*cont'd*

	Expected Outcomes	Nursing Interventions	Rationales
		NIC **Environmental Management: Comfort**	
		D Position the client to facilitate comfort.	The nurse may decrease sources of discomfort by using principles of body alignment, supporting with pillows, supporting joints during movement, splinting over incisions, and immobilizing painful body parts.
		Other Interventions	
		Consider the use of alternative therapies such as imagery, aromatherapy, music, touch, and laughter/humor.	Cognitive and behavioral strategies may be used as adjuncts to or in place of pharmacologic or surgical interventions for chronic pain. Each therapy has a different mode of action, which may or may not benefit the client.

NURSING DIAGNOSIS NO. 2 ■ Ineffective Breathing Pattern

	Expected Outcomes	Nursing Interventions	Rationales
RELATED FACTORS		NIC **Airway Management**	
Pain	No verbal report or observation of dyspnea	D Place the client in semi-Fowler's position, if possible.	Semi-Fowler's position ensures that the abdominal contents do not press against the diaphragm and restrict chest expansion.
DEFINING CHARACTERISTICS	Respiratory rate remains between 11 and 22 breaths/min		
Altered chest excursion			
Depth of breathing: Adult tidal volume 500 mL at rest	Has respirations that remain regular and deep	D Encourage the client to take slow, deep breaths; to turn; and to cough.	Effective aeration and coughing will help rid the body of secretions. Frequent position changes will prevent secretions from pooling in one area.
		D Assist the client with an incentive spirometer, as appropriate.	Incentive spirometry encourages the client to deep breathe.
		NIC **Respiratory Monitoring**	
		D Monitor the rate, rhythm, depth, and effort of respirations.	Changes in respiratory rate, rhythm, depth, or effort may signal a descent into respiratory failure.
		Note chest movement, watching for symmetry, the use of accessory muscles, and supraclavicular and intercostal muscle retractions.	The use of accessory muscles indicates increased respiratory effort.
		Auscultate breath sounds, noting areas of decreased/absent ventilation and the presence of adventitious sounds.	Absent or adventitious breath sounds indicate poor gas exchange or poor movement of air through the airways.
		Continuing Care Considerations	
		D Encourage the client to engage in regular physical exercise.	Cardiopulmonary efficiency and endurance improve with exercise.
		D Encourage the client to enroll in a smoking cessation program, as indicated.	Smoking damages the airways and alveoli.

D Indicates tasks that can be delegated to unlicensed assistive nursing personnel at the discretion of the nurse.

PLAN of CARE MEDICAL DIAGNOSIS: GASTRECTOMY—*cont'd*

NURSING DIAGNOSIS NO. 3 ■ Imbalanced Nutrition: Less Than Body Requirements

	Expected Outcomes	Nursing Interventions	Rationales
RELATED FACTORS Inability to ingest or digest food or absorb nutrients due to biologic, psychological, or economic factors **DEFINING CHARACTERISTICS** Satiety immediately after ingesting food Perceived inability to ingest food Abdomen: Cramping Pain: Abdominal with or without pathology Diarrhea	Has bowel sounds that remain at 3 to 5 per quadrant per minute Denies abdominal pain No verbal report or observation of diarrhea Weight remains within ±5 pounds of desired weight	NIC **Nutrition Management** Determine, in collaboration with a dietitian as appropriate, the number of calories and type of nutrients needed to meet nutrition requirements.	Individual client needs for nutrients and calories should be the basis for a sound dietary plan.
		Adjust the diet to the client's lifestyle, as appropriate.	The dietary division of nutrients, calories, and meals should be adjusted to the client's lifestyle to increase compliance.
		D Provide foods appropriate for the client—general diet; mechanical soft, blenderized or commercial formula via a nasogastric or gastrostomy tube; or total parental nutrition—as ordered by the health care provider.	Diet therapy dictates the types and form of foods that may be offered to the client.
		D Create a pleasant, relaxing environment at mealtime.	A pleasant, relaxing environment at mealtime improves digestion.
		Other Interventions	
		Teach the client and family about high-calorie, high-protein meal planning as appropriate, as well as refraining from drinking liquids with meals.	Meals must be nutritionally adequate to promote healing and to avoid events such as reflux and dumping syndrome.
		Monitor for early signs and symptoms of dumping syndrome—vertigo, tachycardia, syncope, sweating, pallor, palpitations, and the desire to lie down.	Dumping syndrome poses a threat to client safety.
		Teach the client and family about nutritional supplements, as appropriate.	Additional vitamins and minerals, calories, dietary fiber, or other nutritional components may need to be added to the diet of a client who is unable to eat a nutritionally adequate diet.
		Continuing Care Considerations	
		Refer the client to appropriate community nutritional programs, as needed.	Resources such as Weight Watchers, Overeaters Anonymous, and Take Off Pounds Sensibly provide support to the client who is attempting to maintain appropriate body weight.

Continued

PLAN of CARE MEDICAL DIAGNOSIS: GASTRECTOMY—*cont'd*

NURSING DIAGNOSIS NO. 4 ■ Risk for Infection

	Expected Outcomes	Nursing Interventions	Rationales
RELATED FACTORS Invasive procedures Malnutrition Increased environmental exposure to pathogens Inadequate primary defenses (broken skin, traumatized tissue, decrease in ciliary action, stasis of body fluids, changes in pH secretions, altered peristalsis)	Denies fatigue Denies weakness Denies nausea Has a blood pressure that remains ±10 mm Hg of baseline Has a heart rate that remains regular, strong, and between 60 and 100 beats/min No verbal report or observation of vomiting Has a body temperature that remains between 97° and 99.6° F (36.1° and 37.5° C)	NIC **Infection Protection** Monitor for systemic and localized signs and symptoms of infection.	An elevated temperature, pulse, and respirations indicate systemic infection; redness, heat, swelling, and pain indicate local infection.
		Monitor absolute granulocyte count, white blood cell (WBC) count, and differential results.	Elevations in these laboratory tests demonstrate the body's response to infection.
		Inspect the condition of any surgical incision/wound.	A surgical incision may be slightly reddened and swollen from tissue damage but remain free of the purulent drainage, excess swelling, or excess local pain that indicate infection.
		D Maintain asepsis for the client at risk.	Asepsis will minimize the client's exposure to pathogenic agents and thus minimize the incidence of infection.
		D Encourage coughing and deep breathing, as appropriate.	Coughing and deep breathing clears the lungs of secretions that may encourage the growth of pathogenic microbes.
		D Promote sufficient nutritional intake.	Adequate nutrition is essential for the formation of immune system cells and for the repair of damaged body tissues to provide protection against external pathogens.
		D Encourage fluid intake, as appropriate.	Adequate fluid intake provides for renal clearance of the toxins produced by pathogens.
		D Encourage rest.	Mending tissues require energy. A fatigued client is stressed and requires greater expenditure of energy to accomplish tasks.
		NIC **Infection Control** Administer antibiotic therapy, as appropriate.	Antibiotic therapy should assist the body to destroy pathogens.
		Continuing Care Considerations Numerous visitors should be limited, and visits from individuals with known infections should be discouraged.	Visitors may provide a needed diversion for the client, but too many visitors may cause fatigue and bring unwanted exposure to pathogens.
		Teach the client and family about the signs and symptoms of infection and when to report them to the health care provider.	Early intervention to treat infection prevents untoward complications from the infection and its therapy.

D Indicates tasks that can be delegated to unlicensed assistive nursing personnel at the discretion of the nurse.

TABLE 59-2 Diet for Dumping Syndrome

Food Group	Foods Allowed or Encouraged	Foods to Use with Caution	Foods That Must Be Excluded
Soups		Fluids 1 hr before and after meals	Spicy soups
Meat and meat substitutes	8 oz or more per day: fish, poultry, beef, pork, veal, lamb, eggs, cheese, and peanut butter		Spicy meats or meat substitutes
Potato and substitutes	Potato, rice, pasta, starchy vegetables (small amount)		Highly spiced potatoes or substitutes
Bread and cereal	White bread, rolls, muffins, crackers, and cereals (small amount)	Whole-grain bread, rolls, crackers, and cereals	Breads with frosting or jelly, sweet rolls, and coffee cake
Vegetables	Two or more cooked vegetables	Gas-producing vegetables, such as cabbage, onions, broccoli, or raw vegetables	
Fruits	Limit three per day: unsweetened cooked or canned fruits	Unsweetened juice or fruit drinks 30-45 min after meals; fresh fruit	Sweetened fruit or juice
Beverages	Dietetic drinks	Limit to 1 hr after meals; caffeine-containing beverages, such as coffee, tea, and cola; if tolerated, diet carbonated beverages	Milk shakes, malts, and other sweet drinks; regular carbonated beverages and alcohol
Fats	Margarine, oils, shortening, butter, bacon, and salad dressings	Mayonnaise	Any fats with milk products
Desserts	Fruit (see Fruits)	Sugar-free gelatin, pudding, and custard	All sweets, cakes, pies, cookies, candy, ice cream, and sherbet
Seasonings and miscellaneous	Diet jelly, diet syrups, sugar substitutes	Excessive amounts of salt	Excessive amounts of spices, sugar, jelly, honey, syrup, or molasses

General Principles

- Several small meals daily
- Relatively high fat and protein content
- Low roughage
- Relatively low carbohydrate content
- No milk, sweets, or sugars
- Liquid between meals *only*

more than a scant amount of blood drains from the tube and that abdominal distention does not develop. If these problems occur, report them immediately to the surgeon. Irrigation or repositioning of the NG tube is not done after gastric surgery unless specifically prescribed by the surgeon.

Monitoring for Postoperative Complications. Observe the client carefully for possible complications and report them immediately to the health care provider. In the immediate postoperative period, many complications may occur.

A disruption in the patency of the NG tube can result in *acute gastric dilation* postoperatively; this is manifested by epigastric pain and a feeling of fullness, hiccups, tachycardia, and hypotension. Irrigation or replacement of the NG tube by order of the surgeon can relieve these symptoms.

Dumping syndrome is a term that refers to a constellation of vasomotor symptoms after eating, especially following a Billroth II procedure. This syndrome is believed to occur as a result of the rapid emptying of gastric contents into the small intestine, which shifts fluid into the gut, causing abdominal distention. Observe for *early* manifestations of this syndrome, which typically occurs within 30 minutes of eating. Symptoms include vertigo, tachycardia, syncope, sweating, pallor, palpitations, and the desire to lie down.

Late dumping syndrome, which occurs 90 minutes to 3 hours after eating, is caused by a release of an excessive amount of insulin. The insulin release follows a rapid rise in the blood glucose level that results from the rapid entry of high-carbohydrate food into the jejunum. Observe for intestinal manifestations, including dizziness, light-headedness, palpitations, diaphoresis, and confusion.

Dumping syndrome is managed by dietary measures that include decreasing the amount of food taken at one time and eliminating liquids ingested with meals. In collaboration with the dietitian, instruct the client to consume a high-protein, high-fat, low- to moderate-carbohydrate diet (Table 59-2). Pectin administered in the form of a dry powder may *prevent* the syndrome. A somatostatin analogue, octreotide (Sandostatin), 50 to 150 mcg subcutaneously daily, may be prescribed in severe cases. Octreotide is a synthetic form of the hormone, somatostatin, which is found in the gastrointestinal tract. It is thought to inhibit the gastric and pancreatic hormones that probably cause the signs and symptoms of dumping syndrome.

Alkaline **reflux gastropathy,** also known as *bile reflux gastropathy,* is a complication of gastric surgery in which the pylorus is bypassed or removed (e.g., pyloroplasty, gastric resection with gastroduodenostomy [Billroth I procedure], and gastrojejunostomy [Billroth II procedure]). Endoscopic examination reveals regurgitated bile in the stomach and mucosal hyperemia. Symptoms include early satiety, abdominal discomfort, and vomiting.

Delayed gastric emptying is often present after gastric surgery and usually resolves within 1 week. Edema at the anastomosis or adhesions obstructing the distal loop may have mechanical causes. Metabolic causes (e.g., hypokalemia, hypoproteinemia, or hyponatremia) should be considered. The edema is resolved with nasogastric suction, maintenance of fluid and electrolyte balance, and proper nutrition.

Afferent loop syndrome may occur when the duodenal loop is partially obstructed after a Billroth II resection. Pancreatic and biliary secretions fill the intestinal loop, which becomes distended. Painful contractions attempt to propel these secretions from the loop. Monitor for clients reporting abdominal bloating and pain 20 to 60 minutes after eating, often followed by nausea and vomiting. Treatment consists of surgical correction of the incomplete loop obstruction.

Recurrent ulceration occurs in about 5% of clients who have undergone gastric surgery for PUD. Recurrent ulcers can be due to incomplete vagotomy or persistent *H. pylori* infection. Recurrence is most common following vagotomy with antrectomy, and ulcerations tend to occur at the site of anastomosis (stomal or marginal ulcer) or immediately distal in the small intestine. Abdominal pain, usually located in the epigastrium, is the most commonly reported symptom of recurrent peptic ulcer. The health care provider may prescribe H_2-receptor antagonists and proton pump inhibitors to assist with the healing process. The eradication of *H. pylori* in the case of recurrent ulcerations is controversial.

NUTRITIONAL MANAGEMENT. Several problems related to nutrition develop as a result of partial removal of the stomach, including deficiencies of vitamin B_{12}, folic acid, and iron; impaired calcium metabolism; and reduced absorption of calcium and vitamin D. These problems are caused by a shortage of intrinsic factor. The shortage results from the resection and from inadequate absorption because of rapid entry of food into the bowel. In the absence of intrinsic factor, clinical manifestations of pernicious anemia occur. Assess for the development of atrophic glossitis secondary to vitamin B_{12} deficiency. In atrophic glossitis, the tongue takes on a shiny and "beefy" appearance. The client may also have signs of anemia secondary to folic acid and iron deficiency. Monitor the complete blood count (CBC) for signs of megaloblastic anemia and leukopenia. These manifestations are corrected by the administration of vitamin B_{12}. The health care provider may also prescribe folic acid or iron preparations.

Critical Thinking Challenge

A 40-year-old Hispanic client has been experiencing stomach pain for many years "off and on." Recently, the pain has been getting worse and she is fatigued, short of breath, and dizzy with exertion. She notices that the pain hurts most in her right upper quadrant 2 to 3 hours after she eats. The primary health care provider admits the client to the hospital because she is pale and has a blood pressure of 90/50 (normal for her is 130/82) and a pulse of 120 (normal for her is 86).

1. As the nurse admitting this client, what other data should you gather?
2. What are some explanations for why this client did not seek medical attention for this problem sooner?
3. What do you anticipate her complete blood count (CBC) to be?
4. What diagnostic and therapeutic procedures do you anticipate for this client?
5. Would you delegate taking her vital signs to an unlicensed person? Why or why not?
6. What is the priority for her care at this time?

evolve For suggested answer guidelines, go to http://evolve.elsevier.com/Iggy/.

Community-Based Care

Clients may be discharged from the hospital as long as there is no evidence of ongoing bleeding, orthostatic changes, or cardiopulmonary distress or compromise. Clients discharged following treatment for peptic ulcer disease (PUD) and/or complications secondary to the disease must face several challenges in order to manage the disease successfully. Long-term adherence to medication regimens requires the client to take several oral medications on a daily basis. Permanent lifestyle alterations in dietary habits must also be made. Clients must be knowledgeable about complications related to PUD and know when to report symptoms to the health care provider.

HOME CARE MANAGEMENT

Clients are discharged to the home, subacute unit, or skilled nursing facility to continue recuperation. Clients who have undergone surgery or have had complications, such as hemorrhage, may require visits from a home care nurse to assess clinical progress (Chart 59-7).

CHART 59-7

HOME CARE ASSESSMENT of The Client with Ulcer Disease

Assess gastrointestinal and cardiovascular status, including:
- Vital signs, including orthostatic vital signs
- Skin color
- Presence of abdominal pain (location, severity, character, duration, precipitating factors, and relief measures)
- Character, color, and consistency of stools
- Changes in bowel elimination pattern
- Hemoglobin and hematocrit
- Bowel sounds; palpate for areas of tenderness

Assess nutritional status, including:
- Dietary patterns and habits
- Intake of caffeine and alcohol
- Relationship of food to symptoms

Assess medication history.
- Use of steroids
- Use of nonsteroidal anti-inflammatory drugs (NSAIDs)
- Use of over-the-counter medications

Assess client's coping style.
- Recent stressors
- Past coping style

Assess client's understanding of illness and ability to comply with therapeutic regimen.
- Symptoms to report to health care provider
- Expected and side effects of medications
- Food and drug interactions
- Need for smoking cessation

HEALTH TEACHING

The primary focus of home care preparation is client teaching regarding risk factors for the recurrence of PUD; clients are also taught to recognize and report the development of complications related to the disease process or surgical intervention.

Instruct the client and family or significant others about factors related to the development of an ulcer. A risk assessment assists in identifying gastric irritants and lifestyle stressors that may be contributory to ulcer formation. Strategies for lifestyle changes are developed together with the client. Teach about symptoms that should be brought to the attention of the health care provider after discharge from the hospital, such as abdominal pain; nausea and vomiting; black, tarry stools; and weakness or dizziness. To demonstrate understanding, have the client describe the symptoms.

Also teach the client about diets to be used for avoiding postprandial distention or dumping syndrome. For postsurgical clients, especially those who have undergone partial stomach removal, a smaller meal may be required. In collaboration with the dietitian, instruct the client to:

- Eat small, frequent meals
- Avoid drinking liquids with meals
- Abstain from foods that contribute to discomfort
- Eliminate caffeine and alcohol consumption
- Begin a smoking cessation program
- Receive B_{12} injections, as appropriate
- Lie flat after eating for a short time

The client is also taught to avoid any over-the-counter (OTC) product containing aspirin or other NSAID. Emphasize the importance of adhering to the treatment regimen. Long-term medication compliance is critical for eradicating *H. pylori* infection and achieving healing of the ulcer. The importance of keeping all follow-up appointments is also emphasized, because early detection of recurrence or the development of complications is desirable.

Help the client identify situations that cause stress, describe feelings during stressful situations, and develop a plan for coping with stressors. Encourage the client to learn and use relaxation techniques, such as exercise, biofeedback, humor, and imagery (see Chapter 4). Psychotherapy may be indicated to help some clients cope with excessive anxiety or stress. Ulcer disease is difficult to eradicate, so it is essential for the client and family to understand how modifying living, working, and eating habits minimizes the risk of ulcer recurrence.

HEALTH CARE RESOURCES

Following discharge, home care nursing visits may be indicated if clients and family members or significant others require instruction or assistance with follow-up care, such as dressing changes, monitoring of potential complications, and continued nutritional problems.

◆Evaluation: Outcomes

Evaluate the care of the client with peptic ulcer disease (PUD) on the basis of the identified nursing diagnoses and collaborative problems. The expected outcomes are that the client:

- Maintains hemodynamic stability, free of disease or surgical complications
- Takes personal actions to control pain

Specific indicators for these outcomes are listed for each nursing diagnosis and collaborative problem under the Planning and Implementation section (see earlier).

ZOLLINGER-ELLISON SYNDROME

Zollinger-Ellison syndrome (ZES) is manifested by upper gastrointestinal (GI) tract ulceration, increased gastric acid secretion, and the presence of a non–beta cell islet tumor of the pancreas, called a **gastrinoma**. Affected individuals may have more than one gastrinoma. About two thirds of gastrinomas are malignant. Although most gastrinomas grow slowly, a small portion of them develop rapidly and metastasize widely. Metastasis occurs mainly in the liver and regional lymph nodes. Gastrinoma remains a relatively uncommon disease, with an incidence of one to three new cases per year per million people.

PATHOPHYSIOLOGY

ZES is caused by a non–beta islet cell, gastrin-secreting tumor of the pancreas that stimulates the acid-secreting cells of the stomach to maximal activity. This large quantity of acid causes gastrointestinal ulceration.

In the early course of the disease, symptoms are similar to those of peptic ulcer disease (PUD). However, these symptoms tend to progress, and they respond poorly to traditional ulcer therapy. Diarrhea may be a manifestation of this disorder, occurring in almost half of clients. The diarrhea may be associated with large amounts of hydrochloric acid secreted into the proximal duodenum. **Steatorrhea** (an excessive amount of fat in the feces) results from the inactivation of pancreatic lipase secondary to the large concentrations of acid and decreased amounts of bile acids.

Etiology and Genetic Risk

In 20% to 60% of clients with ZES, the gastrinoma results from an autosomal dominant disorder called multiple endocrine neoplasia type 1 (MEN-1) syndrome. Gastrinomas contain multiple hormones, but adrenocorticotropic hormone (ACTH) is most commonly found. As a result, Cushing's syndrome with increased ACTH levels is reported in about 8% of clients with ZES (Praveen, 2002).

Incidence/Prevalence

ZES occurs in about 1% of clients with duodenal ulcers. Currently, the morbidity and mortality of ZES is low because of better medical and surgical management of the disease. Fewer than 5% of clients develop a complication, such as abdominal perforation or gastric outlet obstruction. All races can be affected (Praveen, 2002).

HEALTH PROMOTION/ILLNESS PREVENTION

Again, health promotion and illness prevention practices are the same as for gastritis and peptic ulcer disease (PUD). In addition, clients with a known family history of Zollinger-Ellison syndrome (ZES) may consider genetic counseling and possible surgery to prevent the syndrome from developing.

◆COLLABORATIVE MANAGEMENT

◆Assessment

Clients may complain of PUD symptoms and may have diarrhea and/or steatorrhea. Inquire whether any relatives have had ZES. Radiographic and endoscopic findings for

ZES are similar to those for PUD. However, infection with *H. pylori* is usually absent. The diagnosis is usually made by radioimmunoassay studies that reveal increased serum gastrin levels in conjunction with the clinical features of the disease.

◆Interventions

The aim of therapy is to suppress acid secretion in order to control the client's symptoms. The H,K-ATPase inhibitors, such as lansoprazole (Prevacid) and omeprazole (Prilosec, Losec✱) (given as 60 mg daily in a single dose) are the drugs of choice to reduce gastric acid secretion and heal ulcers in clients with ZES. High doses of H_2-receptor antagonists, such as ranitidine (Zantac), are also effective in reducing gastric acid and providing symptom relief.

If medical therapy fails, the health care provider may choose to perform a vagotomy and pyloroplasty to supplement pharmacologic means of controlling hypersecretion. A total gastrectomy is the surgical approach of choice for this disorder when vagotomy, pyloroplasty, and medical therapy are inadequate. Laparoscopic or open gastrectomy may be performed. (See the earlier discussion of these surgeries under Surgical Management [Peptic Ulcer Disease], p. 1296.)

The consequences of the malignant properties of the tumor are now being more widely recognized, and complete surgical resection of the tumor appears to be the optimal treatment. Clients with aggressive disease can also be treated with chemotherapeutic agents such as 5-fluorouracil and doxorubicin to reduce the tumor and control symptoms.

GASTRIC CARCINOMA

Gastric carcinoma refers to malignant neoplasms in the stomach. Most cancers of the stomach are adenocarcinomas. This is a type of cancer that develops in the mucosal cells that form the innermost lining of any portion or all of the stomach. Other types of cancers include lymphomas and sarcomas (Antigenics, 2003). The remaining cases of gastric carcinoma involve the entire stomach. Often there are no symptoms in the early stages and the disease is often advanced when detected.

PATHOPHYSIOLOGY

Gastric adenocarcinoma can be characterized as *intestinal* or *diffuse* (scattered). Intestinal adenocarcinomas result from atrophic gastritis or intestinal metaplasia, both of which are considered precancerous conditions. The diffuse form of the disease is found primarily in areas where gastric cancer is endemic. Early, superficial gastric cancers produce no notable symptoms. On microscopic examination, the cells resemble intestinal metaplasia (abnormal tissue development).

Gastric cancers spread by direct extension through the gastric wall and into regional lymphatics. The intramural lymphatics readily allow horizontal spread within the gastric wall. Extramural lymphatics carry tumor deposits to lymph nodes in more than 50% of operable cases. Direct invasion of and adherence to adjacent organs (e.g., the liver, pancreas, and transverse colon) may also result. Hematogenous spread via the portal vein to the liver and via the systemic circulation to the lungs and bones is the most common mode of metastasis. Peritoneal seeding of cancer cells from the involved gastric serosa to the omentum, peritoneum, ovary, and pelvic cul-de-sac can also occur.

In people with advanced gastric cancer, there is invasion of the muscularis (stomach muscle) or beyond. These lesions are not amenable to curative resection. The overall 5-year survival rate of people with stomach cancer in the United States is about 21%. The 5-year survival rate for early stage cancers of the upper part of the stomach is about 10% to 15%. For early stage cancer of the lower portion of the stomach, the 5-year survival rate is 50% (Antigenics, 2003).

Etiology and Genetic Risk

Recent evidence has provided a strong link between infection with *H. pylori* and the subsequent development of gastric cancer. Metabolic products produced by the organism transform the gastric mucosa while producing a state of chronic inflammation. Such chronic inflammatory states can induce cancer by increasing cell proliferation and free radical formation.

Clients with pernicious anemia, gastric polyps, chronic atrophic gastritis, and **achlorhydria** (absence of secretion of hydrochloric acid) are two to three times more likely to develop gastric cancer.

Gastric cancer seems to be positively correlated with the ingestion of pickled foods, salted fish, salted meat, and nitrates from processed foods, as well as a high consumption of salt. The ingestion of these foods over a long period of time can lead to atrophic gastritis, a precancerous condition.

The role of cigarette smoking and alcohol consumption in the development of gastric carcinoma is controversial, although some studies support the conclusion that smokers are more likely to develop gastric cancer than are nonsmokers.

Genetic factors play a role in the development of gastric cancer. Familial diffuse gastric cancer is a disease with autosomal dominant inheritance in which gastric cancer develops at a young age. Mutations in the E-cadherin gene (CDH1) have been found in many families with hereditary diffuse gastric cancer (Huntsman et al., 2001). Gastric cancer can also be related to mutations in repair genes MLH1 and MSH2. These genes are generally related to an increased risk of colorectal cancer, specifically hereditary nonpolyposis colon cancer (HNPCC), but they also have been related to an increased risk for gastric, ovarian, biliary tract, urinary, and endometrial cancers. This is also inherited in an autosomal dominant fashion.

Gastric surgery, especially a Billroth II procedure, seems to increase the risk for gastric cancer because of the eventual development of atrophic gastritis, which results in changes to the mucosa. Clients with Barrett's esophagus have an increased risk of adenocarcinoma of the gastric cardia (where the stomach connects to the esophagus).

Incidence/Prevalence

Gastric cancer is the second leading cause of cancer death in the world and 5-year survival rates are low (National Cancer Institute, 2000). The American Cancer Society estimated that in 2003, about 22,400 new cases would be diagnosed in the United States and 12,100 people would die of the disease. Men appear to have a slightly greater risk for developing stomach cancer than women. Most people with diagnosed stomach cancer are in their 60s and 70s.

CULTURAL CONSIDERATIONS

In the United States, *H. pylori* is more common in Hispanics (62%) and black individuals (53%) than among non-Hispanic whites (26%). *H. pylori* infection increases the risk of stomach cancer. In the United States, the incidence of stomach cancer is about twice as high among black individuals as it is among non-Hispanic whites. Native Americans/American Indians and Hispanic Americans are also at an increased risk for stomach cancer. The U.S. National Institute of Diabetes and Digestive and Kidney Diseases (NIDDK) is currently focusing research efforts on *H. pylori* and minority populations. The goal of this research is to determine how *H. pylori* is transmitted in these populations so strategies can be developed to decrease *H. pylori* infection in these populations (NIDDK, 2003).

HEALTH PROMOTION/ILLNESS PREVENTION

Clients with gastritis and/or *H. pylori* infection must follow the recommended guidelines from their health care providers to ensure that the gastritis heals correctly and *H. pylori* is eradicated. This helps prevent gastric cancer. In addition, eating a well-balanced diet following the recommendations of the USDA food pyramid and limiting intake of foods that have been attributed to possibly causing gastric cancer such as pickled foods, salted foods, and processed foods can help prevent gastric cancer. Alcohol and tobacco consumption should be avoided. Clients with a family history of gastric cancer or colon, endometrial, biliary tract, ovarian, or urinary tract cancers should consider genetic counseling to determine whether they are more at risk genetically. Proper genetic counseling can help determine whether a client has a high risk for developing cancer and may prevent cancer if prophylactic treatment such as surgery is performed.

COLLABORATIVE MANAGEMENT

Assessment

HISTORY

Question the client regarding the known risk factors for the development of gastric cancer. Elicit information regarding preferred foods, especially pickled, salted, or smoked foods. Information regarding tobacco use and alcohol ingestion is also gathered. Inquire whether the client has ever been diagnosed with or treated for *H. pylori* infection, gastritis, or pernicious anemia. Note whether the client has a history of gastric surgery or polyps. Also inquire whether any of the client's immediate relatives have gastric cancer.

PHYSICAL ASSESSMENT/CLINICAL MANIFESTATIONS

Although clients with *early* gastric cancer may be asymptomatic, indigestion (heartburn) and abdominal discomfort are the *most* common symptoms (Chart 59-8). These symptoms are often ignored, however, or a change in diet or use of antacids relieves them. As the tumor grows, these symptoms become more severe and do not respond to diet changes or antacids. Epigastric or back pain is also an early symptom that may go unrecognized.

CHART 59-8

KEY FEATURES of
Early Versus Advanced Gastric Cancer

Early Gastric Cancer
- Indigestion
- Abdominal discomfort initially relieved with antacids
- Feeling of fullness
- Epigastric, back, or retrosternal pain

(NOTE: Many clients with early gastric cancer have no clinical manifestations.)

Advanced Gastric Cancer
- Nausea and vomiting
- Obstructive symptoms
- Iron deficiency anemia
- Palpable epigastric mass
- Enlarged lymph nodes
- Weakness and fatigue
- Progressive weight loss
- Signs of distant metastasis
  - Virchow's nodes
  - Blumer's shelf
  - "Sister Mary Joseph nodes"
  - Krukenberg's tumor

In *advanced* gastric carcinoma, progressive weight loss, nausea, and vomiting can occur. Vomiting represents pronounced dilation, thickening of the stomach wall, or pyloric obstruction. Obstructive symptoms appear earlier with tumors located near the pylorus than with fundic lesions. Clients with advanced disease may have weakness, fatigue, and anemia.

Physical assessment findings in advanced disease may be absent, or a palpable epigastric mass may suggest hepatomegaly (liver enlargement) from metastatic disease. Hard, enlarged lymph nodes in the left supraclavicular chain, left axilla, or umbilicus may be the result of metastasis from gastric cancer. Masses on the right suggest metastasis in the perigastric lymph nodes or liver. Signs of distant metastasis include the following:

- Virchow's (sentinel or signal) nodes (enlarged supraclavicular lymph nodes, especially on the left)
- Blumer's shelf, resulting from peritoneal seeding that produces a firm mass palpable on rectal or vaginal examination
- "Sister Mary Joseph nodes" (subcutaneous periumbilical deposits)
- Krukenberg's tumor (metastatic ovarian nodules)

LABORATORY ASSESSMENT

In clients with advanced disease, anemia is evidenced by low hematocrit and hemoglobin values. Clients may have macrocytic or microcytic anemia associated with decreased iron or vitamin B_{12} absorption. The stool may be positive for occult blood.

Hypoalbuminemia and abnormal results of liver tests (e.g., bilirubin and alkaline phosphatase) occur with advanced disease and with hepatic metastasis. The level of carcinoembryonic antigen (CEA) is elevated in *advanced* cancer of the stomach.

RADIOGRAPHIC ASSESSMENT

A double-contrast upper gastrointestinal (GI) series is usually the first diagnostic test. The use of a double-contrast medium assists in the detection of small lesions. A polypoid mass, ulcer crater, or thickened fibrotic gastric wall may suggest gastric cancer.

A computed tomography (CT) scan is used to evaluate gastric malignancies. CT scans of the chest, abdomen, and pelvis are used in determining the extent of the disease.

OTHER DIAGNOSTIC ASSESSMENTS

The health care provider uses esophagogastroduodenoscopy (EGD) for definitive diagnosis of gastric cancer. The lesion can be visualized directly, and biopsies of all visible lesions can be obtained to determine the presence of cancer cells. During the endoscopy, an endoscopic ultrasound (EUS) of the gastric mucosa can also be performed. This technology allows the health care provider to evaluate the depth of the tumor and the presence of lymph node involvement that permits more accurate staging of the disease.

Interventions

Management of gastric cancer includes drug therapy, radiation, and/or surgery.

NONSURGICAL MANAGEMENT. The treatment of gastric cancer is highly dependent on the stage of the disease. Surgical resection of the tumor is usually combined with chemotherapy and/or radiation. Radiation and chemotherapy commonly prolong survival of clients with advanced gastric disease.

Drug Therapy. The role of chemotherapy in gastric cancer remains uncertain. No specific chemotherapeutic protocol has had a positive effect on survival. Chemotherapy with single agents such as fluorouracil (5-FU), doxorubicin, mitomycin-C, cisplatin, and etoposide have been used, but the use of a combination of agents appears to have superior results. Bone marrow suppression, nausea, and vomiting are common side effects. Chapter 28 discusses chemotherapy in detail.

Radiation Therapy. Although gastric cancers are somewhat sensitive to the effects of radiation, the use of this treatment is limited, because the disease is often widely disseminated to other abdominal organs on diagnosis. Organs such as the liver and kidneys, as well as the spinal cord, have limits as to the amount of radiation they can endure. Postoperative radiation has not significantly increased survival. Intraoperative radiotherapy (IORT) is available at only a few institutions in the United States, because special operative suites, equipment, and personnel are required.

The most common side effects experienced by clients undergoing radiation include impaired skin integrity, fatigue, and anorexia. Nausea, vomiting, and diarrhea may occur about 1 week after treatment is initiated and diminish a month or more after treatment ends. (See Chapter 28 for more information on radiation therapy.) The most common potential problems of IORT are hemorrhage and fistula development.

SURGICAL MANAGEMENT. Surgical resection is the preferred method for treating gastric cancer. The primary surgical procedures for the treatment of gastric cancer are total gastrectomy and subtotal gastrectomy. In early stages, laparoscopic surgery plus adjuvant chemotherapy or radiation may be curative. Clients having laparoscopic surgery have less pain, shorter hospital stays, rare postoperative complications, and quicker recovery.

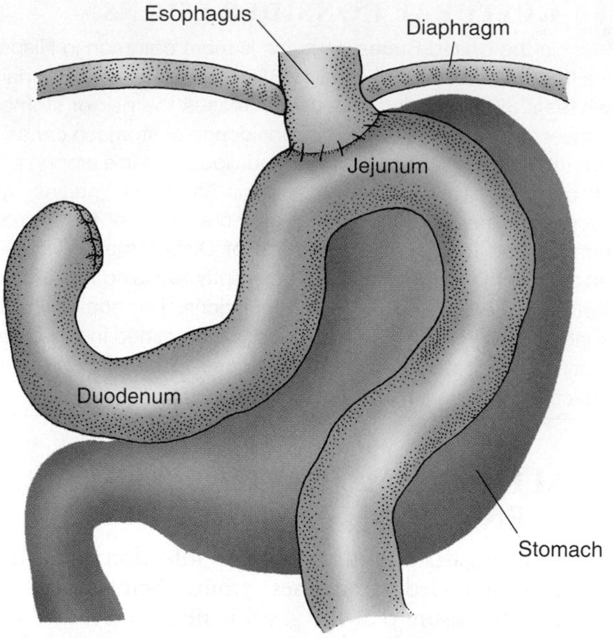

Figure 59-9 ■ Total gastrectomy, with anastomosis of the esophagus to the jejunum (esophagojejunostomy), is the principal medical intervention for extensive gastric cancer.

Most clients with advanced disease are candidates for palliative surgical treatment. Metastasis in the supraclavicular lymph nodes (Virchow's nodes), inguinal lymph nodes, liver, umbilicus, or perirectal wall indicates that the opportunity for cure by resection has been lost. Palliative resection may significantly improve the quality of life for a client suffering from obstruction, hemorrhage, or pain.

Preoperative Care. The health care provider gives the client and family an explanation of the disease and the available treatment options (potentially curative or palliative). Reinforce and clarify the information given. Preoperative care is similar to that provided for the client undergoing general anesthesia and abdominal surgery (see Chapter 20).

Operative Procedures. When the tumor is located in the mid or distal (lower) portions of the stomach, a subtotal gastrectomy is typically performed. The surgeon may use a Billroth I or Billroth II procedure (discussed earlier under Operative Procedures [Peptic Ulcer Disease], pp. 1296 to 1298). The omentum, spleen, and relevant nodes are also removed.

For the client with a resectable growth in the proximal (upper) third of the stomach, a total gastrectomy is performed (Figure 59-9). In this procedure the surgeon removes the entire stomach along with en bloc removal of the lymph nodes and omentum. The surgeon sutures the esophagus to the duodenum or jejunum to reestablish continuity of the GI tract. More radical surgery involving removal of the spleen and distal pancreas is controversial. The overall mortality rate for clients undergoing total gastrectomy surgery is 10% to 15%. For clients with advanced disease, total gastrectomy is performed only when gastric bleeding or obstruction is present.

Clients with tumors at the gastric outlet who are not candidates for subtotal or total gastrectomy may undergo gastroenterostomy for palliation. The surgeon creates a passage between the body of the stomach and the small bowel, often the duodenum (see Figure 59-4).

Postoperative Care. Clients require the standard postoperative care that is given to those who have had general anesthesia (see Chapter 22). Complications after *conventional* gastric surgery may include the following:

- Pneumonia
- Anastomotic leak
- Hemorrhage
- Reflux aspiration
- Sepsis
- Reflux (acute) gastritis (discussed earlier under Acute Gastritis, p. 1284)
- Paralytic ileus
- Bowel obstruction
- Wound infection
- Dumping syndrome (discussed earlier under Monitoring for Postoperative Complications [Peptic Ulcer Disease], p. 1303).

Monitor the client for the development of postoperative complications. Auscultate the lungs for adventitious sounds and monitor for the return of bowel sounds. Monitor vital signs as appropriate to detect signs of infection or bleeding. Aggressive pulmonary exercises and early ambulation can help prevent respiratory complications and deep vein thrombosis. Also inspect the operative site every 8 hours for the presence of redness, swelling, or drainage, which indicates wound infection. Also ensure proper positioning of the client to prevent aspiration from reflux.

Because weight loss is problematic for clients with gastric cancer, nutrition therapy is a vital aspect of preoperative and postoperative management. Preoperatively, compression by the tumor can impede adequate nutritional intake. To correct malnutrition before surgery, the health care provider may prescribe supplements to the diet and/or total parenteral nutrition (TPN). Vitamin, mineral, iron, and protein supplements are essential for correction of nutritional deficits.

Postoperatively, the client's inability to ingest normal-size meals, along with poor nutrient absorption due to decreased stomach size, can prevent the client from taking in adequate nutrition. Therefore the surgeon may place an enteral feeding tube during surgery for continued nutritional support. When feasible, oral intake should begin with fluids and progress to solids as tolerated. For clients who have undergone gastric surgery, regurgitation may result from overeating or from eating too quickly. Experiences with food and fluid are often unsatisfactory for many clients (see the Evidence-Based Practice for Nursing box above).

After oral feedings are restarted, observe the client for signs and symptoms of dumping syndrome and teach the manifestations and management of this syndrome. Advise the client to eat six small meals per day and to consume a diet high in protein and fat but low in carbohydrate-rich foods (see Table 59-2). Liquids should not be taken with meals. Milk and dairy products are usually eliminated because many clients are lactose-intolerant and have symptoms after the ingestion of milk-containing products.

In collaboration with the dietitian, guide the client and family in providing the most nutrients and calories. Counseling about methods of preparation and types of foods that increase caloric and protein intake is essential. Maintain intake, output, and calorie counts on a daily basis and record weights at least weekly. Anemia, as well as vitamin B_{12} and folate deficiency, can result following gastrectomy. Oral folate and iron replacement and vitamin B_{12} injections can help correct these deficiencies.

EVIDENCE-BASED PRACTICE for Nursing

What are clients' experiences with food and fluid intake following gastrectomy due to tumor?

Olsson, V., Bergbom, I., & Bosaeus, I. (2002). Patients' experiences of their intake of food and fluid following gastrectomy due to tumor. *Gastroenterology Nursing, 25*(4), 146-153.

The purpose of this qualitative study was to describe clients' experiences of their appetite, hunger, changes in weight, and intake of food and fluid 3 months after gastrointestinal surgery due to tumor. This study was conducted due to the lack of knowledge regarding clients' experiences of intake of food and fluid following gastrointestinal surgery.

Fifteen clients were interviewed regarding their experiences following gastrointestinal surgery. The interviews were tape recorded and transcribed. The interviews were then read several times and repeated phrases and words were identified. Finally, content analysis was performed to identify themes, which included the struggle to eat and drink, bodily estrangement, and nutritional treatment regimens. These three themes consisted of subthemes, such as having no appetite, having difficulty drinking and eating, feeling nauseous, and stress and adaptation.

Some clients felt unhappy because they did not feel hunger, a sensation that made them want to eat and eating was joyful. Eating made many of the clients feel full quickly, which then caused them to dread eating. The full feeling also made them feel nauseous. Many clients felt they were being forced to eat by family members and that food was a medical treatment and not enjoyable. Clients also felt isolated because their eating regimen had to be altered to adhere to medical guidelines.

Level of Evidence: 6—This qualitative research is very small, but serves as a pilot study.

Critique. Although the convenience sample was small, it does give nurses some insight on how to help clients manage nutritional intake after gastrectomy. Qualitative research is an appropriate method for studying this topic. Additional larger studies with diverse subjects are needed to generalize findings.

Implications for Nursing. Nurses need to encourage clients and families to enjoy food after a gastrectomy. They should not view oral nutrition as a medical treatment but as a source of enjoyment. Clients need to be encouraged to eat what they feel like as much as possible. If new eating and drinking habits must be adopted, they should be integrated into the family's existing mealtimes and patterns.

Community-Based Care

Clients who have undergone total gastrectomy and those who are debilitated with advanced gastric cancer are discharged to home with maximal assistance or to a subacute unit or skilled nursing facility. Clients who have undergone subtotal gastrectomy and are not debilitated may be discharged to home with partial assistance for activities of daily living (ADLs). Recurrence of cancer is common, and clients need regular follow-up examinations and radiographic assessments. A case manager may be assigned to ensure continuity of care and thorough follow-up with diagnostic testing.

HOME CARE MANAGEMENT

Gastric cancer is considered a life-threatening illness; therefore the client and family members require physical and emotional care from the health care team. The side effects of gastric cancer treatment can be debilitating, and clients need to learn symptom management strategies. Hospice programs can help both the client and the family cope with these physical and emotional needs.

Clients may fear returning home because of their inability to care for themselves adequately. Enlisting family and health care resources for the client may ease some of this anxiety. The family needs adequate information and support systems to make the transition to home care easier for the client. If the prognosis is poor, the client and family need continued professional support from case managers, social workers and/or nurses to cope with death and dying. (See Chapter 9 for a discussion of end-of-life care.)

HEALTH TEACHING

Instruct the client and family members about any continuing postoperative needs, adjuvant (assistive) treatment, and nutrition therapy. If clients are discharged to home with surgical dressings, teach the client and family to perform dressing changes. Identify the manifestations of incisional infection (e.g., fever, redness, and drainage) that are to be reported.

Clients who will be receiving radiation therapy or chemotherapy require instructions related to the side effects of these treatments. Nausea and vomiting are common side effects of chemotherapy, and instruction in the use of prescribed antiemetics may be needed. (See Chapter 28 for education for clients receiving chemotherapy or radiation therapy.)

In collaboration with the dietitian, educate the client and family concerning the type and quantity of foods that will provide optimal nutritional value. Interventions to minimize dumping syndrome are also emphasized (see Table 59-2).

HEALTH CARE RESOURCES

A home care referral provides ongoing assessment, assistance, and encouragement to the client and family or significant others at home. A home care nurse can help with physical care procedures and can also provide valuable psychological support. Additional referrals to a dietitian, professional counselor, or clergy may be necessary. Referral to a hospice agency can be of great assistance. Hospice care may be delivered in the home or in an institutional setting. Appropriate support groups (e.g., I Can Cope, provided by the American Cancer Society) can be a major resource.

Critical Thinking Challenge

One of your clients has just been diagnosed with gastric cancer. The client lives alone and is scheduled for surgery tomorrow. He has just completed a prescribed 2-week series of antibiotics but does not know what it was for. The client lives alone.

1. Why might the client have taken antibiotics?
2. What are some possible postoperative complications that you should anticipate?
3. What teaching should you provide to this client if these complications arise?
4. What resources might you consider for the client upon discharge?

evolve For suggested answer guidelines, go to http://evolve.elsevier.com/Iggy/.

GET READY for the NCLEX Examination!

KEY POINTS

Safe Effective Care Environment

- For clients with gastric cancer, initiate a consultation or referral to a social worker, grief counselor, and/or community support group.
- For clients undergoing surgical procedures such as esophagogastroduodenoscopy (EGD), make sure that the client has been informed by the physician regarding what the procedure entails, including the benefits and risks and that the client signs a consent form.
- For clients with terminal gastric cancer, encourage them to talk with an attorney or family members regarding their advanced directives.
- Teach clients the importance to of complying with *H. pylori* treatment regimens to eradicate the bacteria, thus preventing its spread.

Health Promotion and Maintenance

- Identify clients at risk for PUD, especially older clients who take large amounts of NSAIDs and clients with *H. pylori.*
- Teach clients behaviors to prevent PUD, such as avoiding large consumption of caffeine, alcohol, coffee, ASA (acetylsalicylic acid), and NSAIDs. Also teach them to avoid contaminated foods and water and smoking.
- Teach clients the importance of complying with *H. pylori* treatment to prevent the risk of gastric cancer.
- Encourage families that have a high incidence of gastric cancer to see a genetic counselor to determine whether specific family members have a high risk for cancer. This action may possibly prevent cancer if prophylactic measures such as surgery are taken.

Psychosocial Integrity

- Allow clients with *H. pylori* to express feelings of anxiety.
- Allow clients with gastric carcinoma to express feelings of grief, fear, and anxiety.
- Address the reactions of family and significant others to the diagnosis of cancer; provide support and education.
- For clients with advanced metastatic gastric cancer, provide end-of-life care, including referral to hospice care.

Physiological Integrity

- For clients who have undergone a gastrectomy, collaborate with the dietitian and instruct the client regarding diet changes to avoid abdominal distention and dumping syndrome.
- Teach clients with abnormal symptoms, such as abdominal tenderness, abdominal pain that is relieved by food or pain or that becomes worse 3 hours after eating, dyspepsia, melena, and/or distention to consult with their physician immediately for a prompt diagnosis and treatment.
- Teach clients that hematemesis is a medical emergency and that they should go to the emergency department for prompt treatment.
- Teach the proper administration of antacids (one to two after meals). Tell clients that antacids can interfere with the effectiveness of certain drugs, such as phenytoin (Dilantin), so other medications must be taken 1 to 2 hours before or after the antacid.

- Teach the client with past or present heart failure to avoid antacids containing a high sodium content. Magaldrate (Riopan) has the lowest sodium concentration.
- Teach the proper administration of H_2 antagonists. Explain that ranitidine, famotidine, and nizatidine are all given at bedtime and sucralfate must be given on an empty stomach.
- Teach the proper administration of antisecretory agents, noting that most cannot be crushed because they are sustained-release or enteric-coated tablets.
- Monitor clients with ulcers for any of the signs and symptoms of GI bleeding that are listed in Chart 59-4. Report any of these symptoms if noted to a physician immediately.
- Post-EGD, monitor the client's vitals signs, heart rhythm, and oxygen saturation frequently until they return to baseline. Assess the gag reflex and ensure that it is intact before giving the client food to prevent aspiration.
- Observe the client for signs and symptoms of dumping syndrome after vagotomy; teach the manifestations and management of this syndrome. Advise the client to eat six small meals per day and to consume a diet high in protein and fat but low in carbohydrate-rich foods. Liquids should not be taken with meals.

ADDITIONAL STUDY RESOURCES

Go to your Student CD-ROM for Review Questions for the NCLEX Examination.

evolve Go to http://evolve.elsevier.com/Iggy/ for Integrated Management of Care Questions for the NCLEX Examination.

SELECTED BIBLIOGRAPHY

Ackley, B.J., & Ladwig, G. B. (2002). *Nursing diagnosis handbook.* St. Louis: Mosby.

Antigenics. (2003). *Gastric cancer.* Retrieved June 19, 2003, from http://www.antigenics.com/diseases/gastriccancer.html.

Barham Solutions. (2003). *Endoscopy Clinic web page.* Retrieved July 9, 2003, from http://www.endo-world.com/peptic.html.

Braunwald, E., et al. (Eds.). *Harrison's manual of medicine* (15th ed., pp. 691). New York: McGraw-Hill.

Carroll, M. (2002). Peptic ulcer disease. *Emedicine.* Retrieved June 16, 2003, from http://www.emedicine.com/PED/topic2341.htm.

Deglin, J.L., & Vallerand, A.J. (2002). *Davis's drug guide for nurses* (8th ed.). Philadelphia: F. A. Davis.

Fantry, G. (2003). Peptic ulcer disease. *Emedicine.* Retrieved June 16, 2003, from http://www.emedicine.com/MED/topic1776.htm.

Giuli, R. (2002). Breast and gastric cancer. *Journal of Surgical Oncology, 2*(8), 1. Retrieved June 19, 2003, from http://www.geocities.com/surgoncnet/roukos.htm.

Horn, J. (2000). The proton-pump inhibitors: Similarities and differences. *Clinical Therapeutics, 22*(3), 266-280.

Huntsman, D.G., et al. (2001). Early gastric cancer in young, asymptomatic carriers of germ-line E-cadherin mutations. *The New England Journal of Medicine, 344*(25), 1904-1909.

Kuremu, R.T. (2002). Surgical management of peptic ulcer disease. *East African Medical Journal, 79*(9), 454-456.

Marshall, J., Collins, S., & Gafni, A. (2000). Prediction of resource utilization and case cost for acute nonvariceal upper gastrointestinal hemorrhage at a Canadian community hospital. *American Journal of Gastroenterology, 94*(7), 1841-1846.

Matheson, A.J. & Jarvis, B. (2001). Lansoprazole: An update of its place in the management of acid-related disorders. *Drugs, 61*(12), 1801-1833.

McCarthy, M.S. (2003). Changing perspectives of stress ulcer prophylaxis. *CME-Today 1*(1), 15-22.

Medical Letter. (2002). Pantoprazole IV (Protonix IV). *Medical Letter on Drugs and Therapeutics, 44*(1129), 41.

National Cancer Institute. (2000). Vitamins, anti-bacterials may prevent stomach cancer. *Stomach Cancer Home Page.* Retrieved June 16, 2003, from http://www.cancer.gov/clinicaltrials/results/vitamins-and-antibacterials1200.

National Cancer Institute. (2001). Radiation and chemotherapy after surgery improves survival in stomach cancer. *Stomach Cancer Home Page.* Retrieved June 16, 2003, from http://www.cancer.gov/clinicaltrials/results/survival-in-stomach-cancer0901.

National Digestive Disease Information Clearinghouse. (2002). *H. pylori* and peptic ulcer. *National Institute of Diabetes and Digestive and Kidney Diseases Home Page.* Retrieved June 27, 2003, from http://www.niddk.nih.gov./health/digest/pubs/hpylori/hypylori.htm.

National Institute of Diabetes and Digestive and Kidney Diseases. (2003). Area of focus #7. Peptic ulcer disease and *Helicobacter pylori.* Retrieved June 27, 2003, from http://www.niddk.nih.gov/federal/planning/Area7.pdf.

Offman, J., et al. (2000). The quality of care for Medicare patients with peptic ulcer disease. *American Journal of Gastroenterology 95*(1), 106-113.

Parkman, H., MacMillan Rodney, W., & Rogers, H. (2001). Empiric therapy for nonulcer dyspepsia. *Patient Care for the Nurse Practitioner, 3*(1), 23-24.

Perry, M. (2002). Peptic ulceration. *Practice Nurse, 24*(8), 39-41.

Praveen, R. (2002). Zollinger-Ellison syndrome. *Emedicine.* Retrieved June 19, 2003, from http://www.emedicine.com/med/byname/zollinger-ellison-syndrome.htm.

Rotello, L.C. (2003). Managing critically ill patients at risk for stress ulcers. *CME-Today, 1*(1), 27-30.

Shannahoff-Khalsa, D. (2002). Stress management for gastrointestinal disorders: The use of Kundalini yoga meditation techniques. *Gastroenterology Nursing, 25*(3), 126-129.

Soll, A.H. (2002). Epidemiology of and risk factors for peptic ulcer disease. *University of California Los Angeles Center for Health Sciences.* Retrieved June 16, 2003, from http://www.uptodate.com/patient_info/topicpages/topics/AcidPep/6089.asp?usd=987106559&r=/patie.

Sukhdeep, P. (2002). Dumping syndrome. *Emedicine.* Retrieved June 30, 2003, from http://www.emedicine.com/medhopic589.htm.

Yabuki, K., et al. (2002). Extensive hemorrhagic erosive gastritis associated with acute pancreatitis successfully treated with a somatostatin analog. *Journal of Gastroenterology, 37*(9), 737-741.

CHAPTER

60 Interventions for Clients with Noninflammatory Intestinal Disorders

MARCIA M. BOEHMKE

LEARNING OUTCOMES

After studying this chapter, you should be able to:

1. Develop a teaching-learning plan for clients with irritable bowel syndrome (IBS).
2. Differentiate the most common types of hernias.
3. Develop a plan of care for a client undergoing a minimally invasive inguinal hernia repair.
4. Interpret assessment findings for clients with colorectal cancer (CRC).
5. Identify health promotion practices to prevent CRC.
6. Discuss the psychosocial aspects associated with CRC and related surgeries.
7. Explain the role of the nurse in managing the client with CRC.
8. Develop a perioperative plan of care for a client undergoing a colon resection and colostomy.
9. Construct a community-based teaching-learning plan for clients requiring colostomy care.
10. Identify community-based resources for clients with CRC.
11. Analyze the differences between small-bowel and large-bowel obstructions.
12. Explain the role of the nurse when caring for clients with nasogastric tubes.
13. Develop a plan of care for a client experiencing intestinal obstruction.
14. Prioritize nursing care for the client with abdominal trauma.
15. Develop a teaching-learning plan for clients having hemorrhoid surgical procedures.
16. Explain the pathophysiology of malabsorption syndrome.

Go to your Student CD-ROM for Review Questions for the NCLEX Examination keyed to these Learning Outcomes.

Intestinal disorders commonly present with symptoms of rectal bleeding, changing bowel patterns and abdominal pain. Thorough investigation is imperative to differentiate those caused by a serious condition from those caused by benign processes. Figure 60-1 depicts locations and common causes of gastrointestinal bleeding.

IRRITABLE BOWEL SYNDROME

PATHOPHYSIOLOGY

Irritable bowel syndrome (IBS) is a chronic gastrointestinal (GI) disorder, characterized by the presence of chronic or recurrent diarrhea, constipation, and/or abdominal pain and bloating. It is sometimes referred to as spastic colon, mucous colon, or nervous colon. The disease exacerbates whenever the client is exposed to causative agents.

IBS is believed to be due to impairment in the motor or sensory function of the GI tract. Motility changes, often associated with meals, result in changes in the normal bowel elimination pattern to a pattern of diarrhea, constipation, or alternating diarrhea and constipation. Even with these symptoms, the mucosal lining of the bowel remains essentially unchanged. Symptoms of IBS typically begin to appear in young adulthood. The disease is characterized by remissions and exacerbations ("flare-ups").

Etiology

No structural or infectious etiology has been identified, so the exact cause is unknown. Physical factors, such as diverticular disease, ingestion of coffee or other gastric stimulants, or lactose intolerance may contribute to IBS. There is also considerable evidence to implicate the roles of stress and mental or behavioral illness. Clients who seek medical

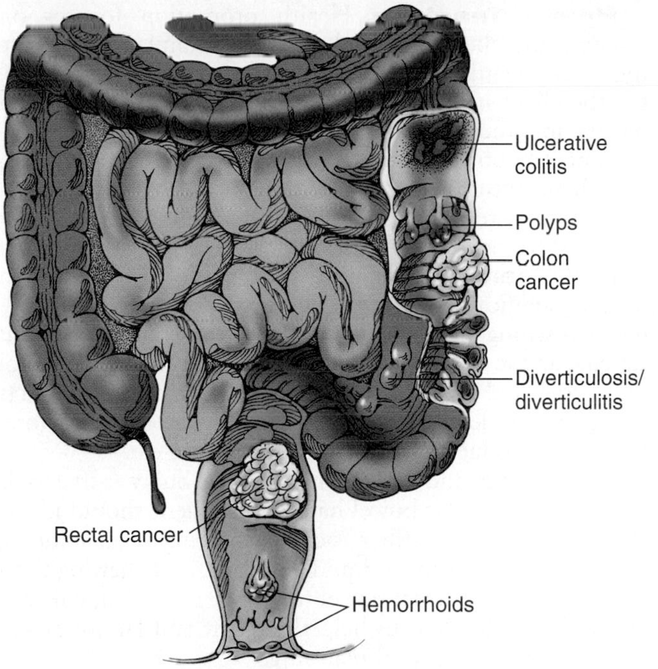

Figure 60-1 ■ Common causes of lower gastrointestinal bleeding.

care for IBS have a higher incidence of panic disorder, anxiety disorder, and major depression than control populations (Lehrer & Lichtenstein, 2004). A familial predisposition has also been noted for some clients.

Incidence/Prevalence

IBS is the most common digestive disorder seen in clinical practice and is estimated to occur in 10% to 22% of the U.S. population. Women are two to three times more likely to have the disease than men. IBS causes 34,000 hospitalizations in the United States each year, and more than 2 million prescriptions are issued for treatment (Lehrer & Lichtenstein, 2004).

COLLABORATIVE MANAGEMENT

Assessment

HISTORY

Ask the client about a history of abdominal pain, changes in the bowel pattern or consistency of stools, and the passage of mucus. Collect information on all medications the client is taking, because many medications cause GI symptoms similar to those of IBS. A careful dietary history, including the use of caffeinated beverages or beverages sweetened with sorbitol or fructose, which can cause bloating or diarrhea, should be elicited.

The course of the illness is generally specific to the client, and most clients can identify factors that precipitate exacerbations, such as diet, stress, or anxiety. There are no changes in the bowel mucosa and therefore no serious health consequences. Food intolerance may be associated with IBS. Dairy products and grains can contribute to bloating, flatulence, and distention. In one study, individuals who reported intolerances to multiple foods were more likely to report IBS (Locke et al., 2000). Finally, IBS symptoms have also been associated with analgesic use (see the Evidence-Based Practice for Nursing box above).

EVIDENCE-BASED PRACTICE for Nursing

What are the possible risk factors for irritable bowel syndrome?

Locke, G.R., et al. (2000). Risk factors for irritable bowel syndrome: Role of analgesics and food sensitivities. *American Journal of Gastroenterology, 95*(1), 157-164.

The purpose of this study was to identify additional risk factors for the development of irritable bowel syndrome (IBS), because previous evaluations of traditional risk factors have not led to insight into the pathogenesis of this disorder. Questionnaires were mailed to a sample of 892 individuals residing in Olmsted County, Minnesota, who were stratified by age (30 to 64 years) and gender. Six hundred forty-three individuals returned the surveys. A self-report questionnaire listed gastrointestinal symptoms required for a diagnosis of IBS, measures of potential risk factors, and psychosomatic symptoms. Logistic regression was used in the analysis. The survey controlled for age, gender, and psychosomatic symptoms.

Results showed that 12% of respondents reported IBS symptoms. IBS was significantly associated with the use of analgesics, particularly aspirin. IBS was also correlated with reports of food allergies and ratings of somatic symptoms. The incidence of IBS was higher among subjects taking analgesics and among those reporting multiple food sensitivities.

Level of Evidence: 5—Case control study with adequate sample size.

Critique. Although this study provides early insight into possible risk factors not before associated with IBS, the results must be interpreted with caution. Although the sample size is adequate, the self-selection, cross-sectional design, and limited geographic area lend bias and an inability to generalize the results to the study. Moreover, the self-report method and the fact that the subjects were not necessarily medically evaluated for their symptoms limits the interpretation of the findings.

Implications for Nursing. Although the study results cannot be generalized to the population, nurses collecting history information can include questions concerning analgesic use and food allergies in individuals suspected of having IBS. Individuals who identify themselves as having food sensitivities may also have symptoms of IBS that require investigation. Although analgesics in themselves may not be causative, it is possible that clients with IBS present with other forms of pain induced by the disorder. Careful questioning during the intake history can provide more information into the pathogenesis of IBS.

PHYSICAL ASSESSMENT/CLINICAL MANIFESTATIONS

There are no specific biomarkers for IBS, but the following characteristic symptoms known collectively as the **Manning criteria** are typically present:

- Abdominal pain relieved by defecation or associated with changes in stool frequency or consistency
- Abdominal distention
- The sensation of incomplete evacuation of stool
- The presence of mucus with stool passage

Bowel function changes progressively and eventually forms the characteristic pattern.

A flare-up consisting of worsening cramps, abdominal pain, and diarrhea or constipation usually brings the client to the health care provider. The most common symptom of IBS is pain in the left lower quadrant of the abdomen. The client typically reports increased pain after eating and relief after a bowel movement. Nausea may be associated with

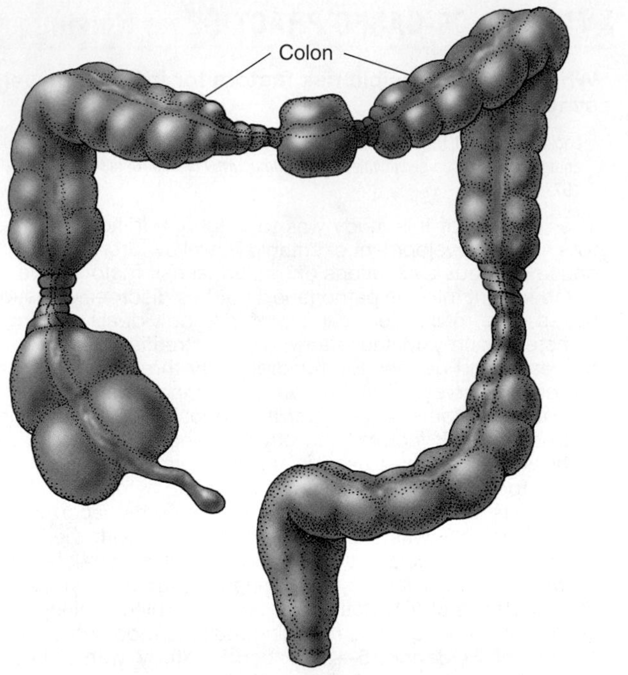

Figure 60-2 ■ Spastic contractions of the colon as they occur with irritable bowel syndrome.

mealtime and defecation. The crampy abdominal patterns are accompanied by constipation or diarrhea. The constipated stools are small and hard and are generally followed by several softer stools. The diarrheal stools are soft and watery, and mucus is often present in the stools. Clients with IBS often complain of belching, gas, anorexia, and bloating.

The client generally appears well, with a stable weight, and nutritional and fluid levels are within normal ranges. Inspect and auscultate the abdomen. Bowel sounds are generally within normal range and may be somewhat quiet with constipation. On percussion of the abdomen, tympanic sounds may be heard over loops of filled bowel. On palpation, there may be diffuse (widespread) tenderness, which is generally worse if the sigmoid colon is palpable.

DIAGNOSTIC ASSESSMENT

Routine laboratory work (including a complete blood count [CBC], serologic tests, serum albumin, erythrocyte sedimentation rate, and stools for occult blood) is normal in IBS. The health care provider typically orders a barium enema examination for clients suspected of having IBS. Colonic spasm is often noted during the procedure; however, this finding is not diagnostic. In the absence of other diagnostic findings, colonic spasm supports the diagnosis (Figure 60-2).

The evaluation of IBS is not complete without flexible sigmoidoscopy in adults younger than 40 years of age or colonoscopy in adults older than 40 years of age. A colonoscopy often demonstrates intense spastic contractions, which often stimulate painful sensations. Otherwise, the bowel mucosa appears continuous, smooth, and pink.

Interventions

The client with IBS is most often cared for on an ambulatory basis. Interventions are directed at education, dietary modification, drug therapy, and stress management. Some clients use complementary and alternative therapies as well.

Health Teaching. Health promotion focuses on teaching the client to avoid problem stimulants. Educate the client regarding the chronic nature of the disorder. Assist the client in identifying food intolerances and needed dietary modifications. Information regarding what constitutes normal bowel function and laxative abuse is provided. The client must be alert to the urge to defecate and evacuate promptly to avoid straining and should plan to allow time and privacy in the bathroom.

Diet Therapy. The initial treatment of IBS focuses on dietary modifications. Instruct the client to eliminate offending or upsetting foods. They should be further advised to limit caffeine and to avoid alcohol, beverages that contain sorbitol or fructose, and other gastric irritants. Milk and milk products should be avoided if lactose intolerance is suspected. Lactose-free or soy products can be used as a substitute.

Dietary fiber and bulk help produce bulky, soft stools and establish regular bowel habits. The client should ingest about 30 to 40 g of fiber each day. Eating regular meals, drinking 8 to 10 cups of liquid each day, and chewing food slowly promote normal bowel function. If needed, collaborate with the dietitian to help the client and family or significant others with meal planning.

Drug Therapy. Drug therapy is directed at the major symptom. The health care provider may prescribe bulk-forming laxatives, antidiarrheal agents, anticholinergic agents, tricyclic antidepressants, and 5-HT_4 agonists.

For the treatment of constipation-predominant IBS, bulk-forming laxatives, such as psyllium hydrophilic mucilloid (Metamucil) or calcium polycarbophil (Mitrolan), are generally taken at mealtimes with a glass of water. The hydrophilic properties of these medications help prevent dry, hard, or liquid stools.

Diarrhea-predominant IBS is typically treated with antidiarrheal agents, such as diphenoxylate hydrochloride with atropine sulfate (Lomotil) or loperamide (Imodium) (Chart 60-1). A newer group of drugs called muscarinic (M3)-receptor antagonists also inhibit intestinal motility. Examples of medications in this group currently undergoing clinical trials are darifenacin and zamifenacin.

For IBS in which pain is the predominant symptom, anticholinergics or antispasmodics, such as dicyclomine hydrochloride (Bentyl), help relieve abdominal cramping and intestinal spasm. Tricyclic antidepressants, such as amitriptyline (Elavil), have also been successfully used in this form of IBS. It is unclear whether their effectiveness is due to the antidepressant or anticholinergic effects of the drugs. If clients experience postprandial discomfort (discomfort after eating), they should take these medications 30 to 45 minutes before mealtime.

Recently approved 5-HT_4 medications, such as the selective partial agonist tegaserod (Zelnorm) and more potent prucalopride, possess GI prokinetic activity. These drugs are given only to women who have constipation as their primary symptom. Zelnorm imitates the action of serotonin to stimulate peristalsis in the GI tract. The usual dosage is 6 mg twice daily before meals for 4 to 6 weeks. The course may be repeated if needed. Teach clients that the medication should be taken at least 30 minutes before meals because food decreases the drug's absorption. Zelnorm decreases the effects of oral contraceptives, and therefore an additional form of birth control should be used to prevent pregnancy. Prucalopride appears to be a very promising

CHART 60-1

DRUG THERAPY for
Treatment of Irritable Bowel Syndrome (IBS)

Drug	Usual Dosage	Nursing Interventions	Rationales
For Diarrhea-Predominant IBS			
Diphenoxylate hydrochloride and atropine sulfate (Lomotil)	1 tablet 6 times daily; no more than 6 tablets in 24 hr	Teach client to report abdominal distention, pain, and fever.	These symptoms may indicate a bacterial organism in the gastrointestinal (GI) tract. Diarrhea should not be suppressed in the presence of GI infection.
		Teach client to report sedation, dry mouth, urinary retention, and rash.	These are common side effects.
Loperamide (Imodium)	2 mg after each loose stool; maximum of 16 mg daily	Teach client to report abdominal distention, pain, and fever.	These symptoms may indicate a bacterial organism in the GI tract. Diarrhea should not be suppressed if GI infection is present.
For Constipation-Predominant IBS			
Tegaserod (Zelnorm)	6 mg PO twice daily 30 min before meals for 4 to 6 wk (women; dose for men not established)	Teach client to take extra birth control precautions, if appropriate.	The drug decreases effect of oral contraceptives.
		Teach client to report dizziness, irregular pulse, angina.	The drug can cause cardiovascular side effects/adverse effects.
Psyllium (Metamucil, Karacil✱)	1-2 tsp. in 8 oz. H_2O two to three times daily	Teach client to report excessive cramping, rectal bleeding, nausea, or vomiting.	The drug should be discontinued if these problems occur.

drug that is being tested as another choice for clients with IBS who have chronic constipation.

Stress Management. Stress management is based on the client's current and ongoing stressors and available resources. After completing a detailed psychosocial assessment, set expected outcomes and plan appropriate interventions with the client. Relaxation techniques can help the client learn skills for managing the illness. Understanding the illness empowers the client to take certain actions (e.g., diet modification and exercise) that can significantly affect the course of the illness.

If the client is in a stressful work or family situation, personal counseling may be helpful. Make appropriate referrals or assist in making appointments, if necessary. The opportunity to discuss problems and attempt creative problem solving is often helpful. Instruct the client that regular exercise is important for managing stress and promoting regular bowel elimination.

Complementary and Alternative Therapies. Some clients use other modalities as supplements to their medical treatment regimen. The following are examples of therapies that are used to reduce symptoms and reduce discomfort:

- Peppermint and caraway oil combination
- Evening primrose oil
- Chamomile
- Yoga and other relaxation techniques
- Hypnosis
- Acupuncture

Critical Thinking Challenge

A 45-year-old woman is admitted to your hospital unit with acute IBS, severe dehydration, and hyponatremia. On history you find that she is a middle-school teacher who is currently under psychiatric care for acute depression and anxiety disorder. She states that she has a poor memory and has problems with concentration. She is married with no children and states that she is very religious. The client did not want to be admitted because she misses her husband, her primary support system.

1. Why do you think she is dehydrated and has hyponatremia? What other historical data do you need right now?
2. What risk factors does this client have for IBS?
3. What are her primary nursing diagnoses and expected outcomes?
4. What actions should you take at this time?

evolve For suggested answer guidelines, go to http://evolve.elsevier.com/Iggy/.

HERNIATION

PATHOPHYSIOLOGY

A **hernia** is a weakness in the abdominal muscle wall through which a segment of the bowel or other abdominal structure protrudes. Hernias can also penetrate through any other defect in the abdominal wall, through the diaphragm, or through other structures in the abdominal cavity.

The most common types of abdominal hernias (Figure 60-3) are indirect, direct, femoral, umbilical, and incisional.

- An **indirect inguinal hernia** is a sac formed from the peritoneum that contains a portion of the intestine or omentum. The hernia pushes downward at an angle into the inguinal canal. In males, indirect inguinal hernias can become large and often descend into the scrotum.
- **Direct inguinal hernias**, in contrast, pass through a weak point in the abdominal wall.
- **Femoral hernias** protrude through the femoral ring. A plug of fat in the femoral canal enlarges and eventually

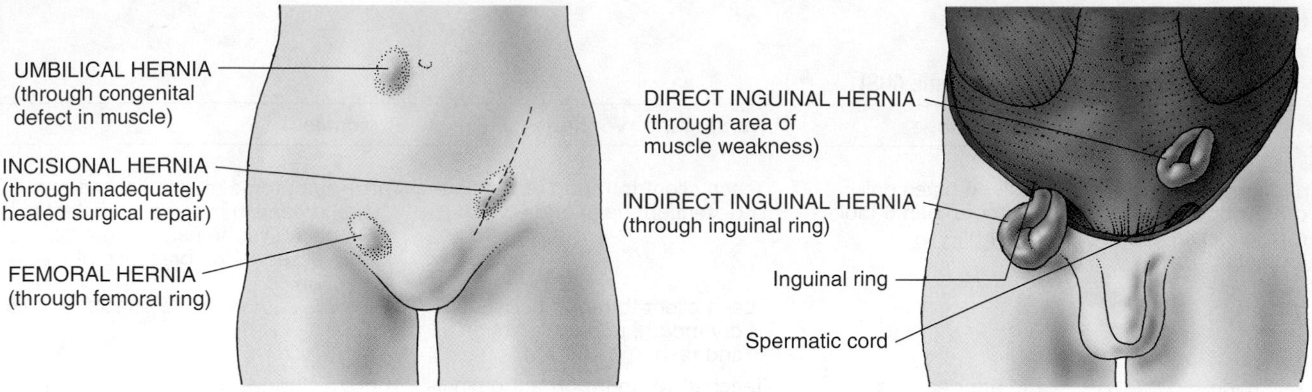

Figure 60-3 ■ Types of abdominal hernia.

pulls the peritoneum and often the urinary bladder into the sac.

- **Umbilical hernias** are congenital or acquired. Congenital umbilical hernias appear in infancy. Acquired umbilical hernias directly result from increased intra-abdominal pressure. They are most commonly seen in obese individuals.
- **Incisional, or ventral, hernias** occur at the site of a previous surgical incision. These hernias result from inadequate healing of the incision, which is most often caused by postoperative wound infections, inadequate nutrition, and obesity.

Hernias may also be classified as **reducible,** irreducible (incarcerated), or strangulated. A hernia is reducible when the contents of the hernial sac can be placed back into the abdominal cavity by gentle pressure. An **irreducible** (incarcerated) hernia cannot be reduced or placed back into the abdominal cavity. Any hernia that is not reducible requires immediate surgical evaluation.

A hernia is **strangulated** when the blood supply to the herniated segment of the bowel is cut off by pressure from the hernial ring (the band of muscle around the hernia). If a hernia is strangulated, there is ischemia and obstruction of the bowel loop. This can lead to necrosis of the bowel and possibly bowel perforation. Signs of strangulation are abdominal distention, nausea, vomiting, pain, fever, and tachycardia.

The most important elements in the development of a hernia are congenital or acquired muscle weakness and increased intra-abdominal pressure. The most significant factors contributing to increased intra-abdominal pressure are obesity, pregnancy, and lifting of heavy objects.

Indirect inguinal hernias, the most common type, are most frequent in men because they follow the tract that develops when the testes descend into the scrotum before birth. Direct hernias occur more often in older adults. Femoral and adult umbilical hernias are most common in obese or pregnant women. Incisional hernias can occur in people who have undergone abdominal surgery.

Defects in the muscle wall result from weakened collagen or widened spaces at the inguinal ligament. These muscle weaknesses can be inherited or acquired as part of the aging process. Increases in intra-abdominal pressure as a result of pregnancy, obesity, abdominal distention, ascites, heavy lifting, or coughing can contribute to their occurrence.

HEALTH PROMOTION/ILLNESS PREVENTION

Even though the muscle weakness cannot be prevented, exercises can be performed to strengthen muscles. Obesity is considered a contributing factor because it causes increased intra-abdominal pressure. Weight control helps to decrease the likelihood of hernias by decreasing pressure on the abdominal muscles. Heavy lifting and straining also increases intra-abdominal pressure and should be avoided.

COLLABORATIVE MANAGEMENT

Assessment

The client with a hernia typically comes to the health care provider's office or the emergency department with a complaint of a "lump" or protrusion felt at the involved site. The development of the hernia may be associated with straining or lifting.

Perform an abdominal assessment inspecting the abdomen when the client is lying and again when he or she is standing. If the hernia is reducible, it may disappear when the client is lying flat. The advanced practice nurse or other health care provider asks the client to strain or perform the Valsalva maneuver and observes for bulging. The abdomen is auscultated for active bowel sounds. Absent bowel sounds may indicate obstruction and strangulation.

To palpate an inguinal hernia, the health care provider gently examines the ring and its contents by inserting a finger in the ring and noting any changes when the client coughs. The hernia is never forcibly reduced; that maneuver could cause strangulated intestine to rupture.

If a male client suspects a hernia in his groin, the health care provider has him stand for the examination. Using the right hand for the client's right side and the left hand for the client's left side, the examiner invaginates the loose scrotal skin with the index finger, following the spermatic cord upward to the external inguinal cord. At this point, the client is asked to cough, and any palpable herniation is noted.

Interventions

The type of treatment selected depends on client factors, as well as the type of hernia.

NONSURGICAL MANAGEMENT. If the client is not a surgical candidate, often an older adult with multiple health problems, the health care provider may prescribe a truss for an inguinal hernia. A **truss** is a pad made with firm material; it is held in place over the hernia with a belt to help keep the abdominal contents from protruding into the hernial sac. If a truss is used, it is applied only after the physician has reduced the hernia if incarcerated. The client usually applies the truss before arising. Teach the client to assess the skin under the truss daily and to protect it with a light layer of powder.

SURGICAL MANAGEMENT. Most hernias are inguinal. Surgical repair of a hernia is the treatment of choice. Surgery is usually performed on an ambulatory care basis for adult clients who have no pre-existing health conditions that would complicate the operative course. In same-day surgery centers, anesthesia may be local, regional, or general, and the surgery is typically laparoscopic. More extensive surgery, such as a bowel resection or temporary colostomy, may be necessary if strangulation results in a gangrenous section of bowel. Clients undergoing extensive surgery are hospitalized for a longer period of time.

A **minimally invasive inguinal hernia repair (MIIHR)** through a laparoscope, also called **herniorrhaphy,** is the surgery of choice. An open, conventional herniorrhaphy may be performed when laparoscopy is not appropriate.

Preoperative Care. In addition to client education about the procedure, the most important preoperative preparation is to teach the client to remain NPO (given nothing by mouth) from midnight the day of surgery. If same day surgery is planned, assist the client in making appropriate arrangements for travel to home and for home care. For clients having an open surgical approach, provide preoperative care as described in Chapter 20.

Operative Procedures. During an MIIHR, the surgeon makes several small incisions, identifies the defect, and covers the weakened area with a mesh patch on the *inside* of the abdominal wall. During a traditional herniorrhaphy, the surgeon makes an abdominal incision and places the contents of the hernial sac back into the abdominal cavity before closing the opening. When a **hernioplasty** is also performed, the surgeon reinforces the weakened *outside* muscle wall with a mesh patch. MIIHR procedures tend to be more successful because the surgeon can reinforce the weakened area inside the abdominal wall and the client has a shorter recovery time. Therefore recurring hernias are not common after laparoscopic herniorrhaphy.

Postoperative Care. The client who has had MIIHR is discharged from the surgical center in 3 to 5 hours. Teach the client to rest for several days before returning to work and a normal routine. Remind the client to observe the small incisions for redness, induration, heat, drainage, and increased pain, and promptly report their occurrence to the surgeon. The client should complain of soreness and discomfort rather than severe, acute pain following laparoscopy.

Postoperative care of the client having an open surgical approach is the same as that described in Chapter 22, except that clients who have undergone surgery for hernias are told to avoid coughing. To promote lung expansion, encourage deep breathing and ambulation. With repair of an indirect inguinal hernia, the physician may suggest a scrotal support and ice bags to be applied to the scrotum to prevent swelling, which often contributes to pain. Elevation of the scrotum with a soft pillow helps prevent and control swelling.

In the immediate postoperative period, the client may experience difficulty voiding. Encourage male clients to stand to allow a more natural position for gravity to facilitate voiding and bladder emptying. Techniques to stimulate voiding, such as allowing water to run, may also be used. A fluid intake of at least 1500 to 2500 mL daily prevents dehydration and maintains urinary function. A "straight" catheterization is required if the client cannot void. Clients usually remain the hospital less than 24 hours.

Most clients have uneventful recoveries after an open hernia repair. Surgeons generally allow clients to return to their usual activities after surgery, with avoidance of straining and lifting for 1 to 2 weeks. Depending on the site and the extent of repair, as well as the client's general physical condition, this period may be extended to 4 to 6 weeks.

Provide oral instructions and a written list of symptoms to be reported, including fever, chills, wound drainage, redness or separation of the incision, and increasing incisional pain. Instruct the client to keep the wound dry and clean with antibacterial soap and water. Showering is usually permitted in a few days.

COLORECTAL CANCER

PATHOPHYSIOLOGY

"Colorectal" refers to the colon and rectum, which together make up the large intestine, also known as the large bowel. Colorectal cancer (CRC) is cancer of the colon or rectum, and is a major health problem worldwide. In the United States, it is one of the most prevalent malignancies, utilizing a significant proportion of health care dollars.

Ninety-five percent of CRCs are adenocarcinomas. **Adenocarcinomas** are tumors that arise from the glandular epithelial tissue of the colon. CRC develops as a multistep process, resulting in a number of molecular changes, such as loss of key tumor suppressor genes and activation of certain oncogenes that alter colonic mucosa cell division. The increased proliferation of the colonic mucosa forms polyps that can be transformed into malignant tumors. Most CRCs are believed to arise from adenomatous polyps that present as a visible protrusion from the mucosal surface of the bowel.

Tumors occur in different areas of the colon, with about two thirds occurring within the rectosigmoidal region. The percentages in Figure 60-4 indicate an increased incidence of cancer in the proximal sections of the large intestine over the past 25 years.

Colorectal cancer (CRC) can metastasize by means of direct extension or by spreading through the blood or lymph. The tumor may spread locally into the four layers of the bowel wall and into neighboring organs. It may enlarge into the lumen of the bowel or spread through the lymphatics or the circulatory system. The circulatory system is entered directly from the primary tumor through blood vessels in the bowel or via the lymphatics. The liver is the most frequent site of metastasis from circulatory spread. Of clients with colorectal cancer, metastasis to the liver develops in 15% to 30% even with surgical resection of the tumor. Metastasis to the lungs, brain, bones, and adrenal glands may also occur. Colon tumors can also spread by peritoneal seeding during surgical resection of the tumor. Seeding occurs when a tumor

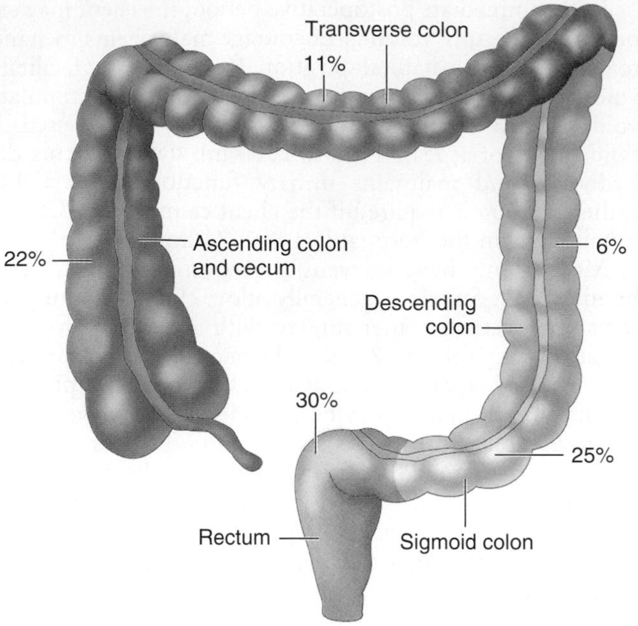

Figure 60-4 ■ The incidence of cancer in relation to colorectal anatomy.

is excised and cancer cells break off from the tumor into the peritoneal cavity.

Complications related to the increasing growth of the tumor locally or through metastatic spread include bowel obstruction or perforation with resultant peritonitis, abscess formation, and fistula formation to the urinary bladder or the vagina. The tumor may invade neighboring blood vessels and cause frank bleeding. A tumor growing into the bowel lumen can gradually obstruct the intestine and eventually block it completely. Tumor extending beyond the bowel wall may place pressure on neighboring organs (uterus, urinary bladder, and ureters) and cause symptoms that mask those of the cancer. Chapter 27 discusses cancer pathophysiology in more detail.

Etiology

Risk factors for the development of colorectal cancer (CRC) include genetic predisposition, personal and dietary factors, and inflammatory bowel disease.

GENETIC CONSIDERATIONS

Individuals with a first-degree relative (sister, sibling, or child) diagnosed with colorectal cancer (CRC) have a threefold to fourfold risk of developing the disease. An autosomal dominant inherited genetic disorder known as **familial adenomatous polyposis (FAP)** accounts for 1% of CRCs. FAP is the result of one or more mutations in the adenomatous polyposis coli gene (APC) (Zangwill, 2004). In these clients, thousands of adenomatous polyps develop over the course of 10 to 15 years and have nearly a 100% chance of becoming malignant. By 20 years of age, most individuals require surgical intervention, usually a colectomy with colostomy, to prevent cancer. New treatment approaches, such as COX-2 drug therapy, are being researched as an alternative to invasive surgical procedures for these clients (Zangwill, 2004). However, COX-2 inhibitors have recently been associated with cardiovascular events, such as myocardial infarction and stroke.

TABLE 60-1 Foods That Affect a Person's Risk for Colorectal Cancer

Foods To Avoid
- Red meat
- Animal fat
- Fatty foods
- Fried meats and fish
- Refined carbohydrates (e.g., concentrated sweets)

Foods To Consume
- Fruits and vegetables, especially cruciferous vegetables from the cabbage family (e.g., broccoli, cabbage, cauliflower, brussels sprouts)
- Whole-grain products
- Adequate fluids, especially water
- Baked or poached fish and poultry

Hereditary nonpolyposis colorectal cancer (HNPCC) is another autosomal dominant disorder and accounts for 10% of all colorectal cancers (CRCs). HNPCC is also caused by gene mutations. Individuals with these mutations have an 80% chance of developing CRC at an average of 45 years of age. They also tend to have a higher incidence of endometrial, ovarian, stomach, and ureteral cancers. Genetic testing is available for these familial CRC syndromes (Zangwill, 2004).

PERSONAL FACTORS

About 75% of all colorectal cancers (CRCs) have no known predisposing cause. Age is considered a risk factor in the development of colorectal cancer, in that 95% of cases are diagnosed in persons over 50 years of age. Clients who have been diagnosed with and treated for CRC have an increased risk of developing a second primary CRC, often at the site of the surgical anastomosis. Those with adenomatous polyps are at an increased risk of developing colorectal cancer. Such individuals need regular follow-up with colonoscopy to visualize and remove polyps.

DIETARY FACTORS

Decreased bowel transit time and certain foods containing chemical mutagens may place individuals at risk for colorectal cancer (Table 60-1). These foods also aid in decreasing bowel transit time, which would increase the time that the bowel is exposed to **carcinogens** (cancer-causing substances). A high-fat diet, particularly animal fat from red meats, increases bile acid secretion and anaerobic bacteria, which are thought to be carcinogenic within the bowel. Fried and broiled meats and fish are also thought to contain chemical mutagens that are carcinogenic. Diets with large amounts of refined carbohydrates that lack fiber decrease bowel transit time as well.

INFLAMMATORY BOWEL DISEASE

Inflammatory bowel diseases (IBDs), such as ulcerative colitis and Crohn's disease, pose an increased risk of colorectal cancer, especially if the disease has had a long, severe course.

Incidence/Prevalence

Colorectal cancer (CRC) is the third most common malignancy (after prostate and lung cancer in men and after breast and lung cancer in women), with an estimated 150,000 new cases each year (Jemal et al., 2002). Americans have a 6% lifetime risk for development of CRC. It is rare before 30 years of age, but incidence increases with age. The median age at diagnosis is 67 years (Ellenhorn, Coia, & Hoff, 2002). The overall incidence is equivalent in men and women, with cancer of the rectum being more common in men. Anal cancers account for about 4% of colorectal cancers.

CULTURAL CONSIDERATIONS

Both black men and black women have an increased frequency of colorectal cancer (CRC) in advanced stages at the time of diagnosis compared with both white men and women; consequently, they also have a greater death rate from CRC. The cause for this difference is not known.

HEALTH PROMOTION/ILLNESS PREVENTION

Individuals at risk can take action to decrease their chance of having CRC. For example, clients whose family members have had hereditary CRC should be genetically tested for FAP and HNPCC. If gene mutations are present, the individual can collaborate with the health care team to decide what treatment plan to implement.

All people, regardless of risk, should modify their diets to decrease fat, refined carbohydrates, and low-fiber foods. Encourage broiled or baked foods, especially those high in fiber and low in animal fat.

Nonsteroidal anti-inflammatory drugs (NSAIDs), including aspirin, decrease the incidence of colon cancer (McCance & Huether, 2002). Regular exercise, daily multivitamins, and female hormonal therapy (e.g., oral contraceptives) also contribute to cancer prevention.

Regular CRC screening, including fecal occult blood testing (FOBT), should be a part of health promotion practices for men and women older than 50 years of age. Individuals who have a personal or family history of the disease should begin screening earlier and more frequently. Teach individuals to follow the American Cancer Society Recommendations for CRC screening listed in Chart 60-2.

CHART 60-2

BEST PRACTICE for
Screening Recommendations for Men and Women Age 50 and Older at Average Risk for Colorectal Cancer

Procedure: Choice of One of the Following	Interval after Screening Initiated at Age 50 Years	Comments
Fecal occult blood test (FOBT)	Every year	Procedure: two samples from three consecutive bowel movements obtained at home; tested by physician or nurse
OR		
Flexible sigmoidoscopy	Every 5 yr	
OR		
FOBT plus flexible sigmoidoscopy	FOBT every year; flexible sigmoidoscopy every 5 yr	Procedure for FOBT as above. This combination is preferred over either test alone
OR		
Double-contrast barium enema	Every 5 yr	
OR		
Colonoscopy	Every 10 yr	

Data from American Cancer Society. (2003). Colorectal cancer. *CA: A Cancer Journal for Clinicians, 53*(1), 44-51.

COLLABORATIVE MANAGEMENT

Assessment

HISTORY

In taking a history from a client with colorectal cancer, obtain the client's diet history and ask about major risk factors, such as a personal history of breast, ovarian, or endometrial cancer; ulcerative colitis; Crohn's disease; familial polyposis or adenomas; or a family history of colorectal cancer (CRC). Also assess the client's participation in age-specific screening guidelines for CRC (see Chart 60-2).

Ask whether the client has had changes in bowel habits, such as diarrhea or constipation, with or without blood in the stool. The client may also report fatigue (related to anemias), abdominal fullness, pain, or weight loss, which are signs of advanced disease.

PHYSICAL ASSESSMENT/CLINICAL MANIFESTATIONS

The signs of CRC depend on the location of the tumor. However, the most common signs are rectal bleeding, anemia, and a change in the stool. Stools may contain microscopic amounts of blood that are not noticeably visible, or the client may have mahogany-colored or bright red stools. Gross blood is not usually detected with tumors of the right side of the colon, but is common (but not massive) with tumors of the left side of the colon and the rectum.

Tumors arising in the transverse and descending colon result in symptoms of obstruction as growth of the tumor impedes the passage of stool. The client may complain of "gas pains," cramping, or incomplete evacuation. Tumors arising in the rectosigmoid colon are associated with **hematochezia** (the passage of red blood via the rectum), straining to pass stools, and narrowing of stools. Clients may complain of dull pain. Right-sided tumors can grow quite large without disrupting bowel patterns or appearance, because the stool consistency is more liquid in this part of the colon. These tumors ulcerate and bleed intermittently, so stools can contain dark or mahogany-colored blood. A mass may be palpated in the lower right quadrant, and the client often has anemia secondary to blood loss.

Examination of the abdomen begins with assessment for obvious distention or masses. Visible peristaltic waves accompanied by high-pitched or "tingling" bowel sounds may indicate a partial bowel obstruction from the tumor. Total absence of bowel sounds after listening for 5 full minutes indicates a complete bowel obstruction. Palpation and percussion are performed by the advanced practice nurse or other health care provider to determine whether there is liver or spleen enlargement, or whether there are masses along the colon. The examiner may also perform a digital rectal examination to palpate the rectum and lower sigmoid colon for masses.

PSYCHOSOCIAL ASSESSMENT

The psychological consequences associated with a diagnosis of colorectal cancer (CRC) are many. Clients must cope with a diagnosis that inspires fear and anxiety about treatment, pain, possible disfigurement, and death. In addition, if the cancer is believed to have a genetic origin, there is anxiety concerning implications for the client's immediate family members. Possible loss of health insurance and excessive costs of genetic testing are also sources of fear and anxiety.

LABORATORY ASSESSMENT

Hemoglobin and hematocrit values are usually decreased as a result of the intermittent bleeding associated with the tumor. Colorectal cancer (CRC) that has metastasized to the liver causes liver function tests to be elevated.

A positive test result for occult blood in the stool **(fecal occult blood test [FOBT])** indicates bleeding in the gastrointestinal (GI) tract. These tests can yield false-positive results if certain foods, vitamins, or drugs are ingested before taking the test (Levin et al., 2003). The client should avoid foods such as meat, peroxidase-containing foods (horseradish and beets), and medications, such as aspirin and vitamin C, for 48 hours before giving a stool specimen. Also assess whether the client is taking anti-inflammatory drugs (e.g., ibuprofen, corticosteroids, or salicylates). These medications may be discontinued in consultation with the primary care provider for a designated period before the test. Two separate stool samples should be tested on 3 consecutive days. Negative results do not completely rule out the possibility of CRC.

Carcinoembryonic antigen (CEA), an oncofetal antigen, may be elevated in 70% of people with CRC. There is no relationship between the CEA level and the cancer stage. This antigen is not specifically associated with the colorectal cancer, and it may be elevated in the presence of other benign or malignant diseases and in smokers. CEA is often used to monitor the effectiveness of treatment and identify disease recurrence.

RADIOGRAPHIC ASSESSMENT

A double-contrast barium enema (air and barium are instilled into the colon) provides better visualization of polyps and small lesions than a barium enema alone. This test may demonstrate an occlusion in the bowel, where the tumor is decreasing the size of the lumen.

Computed tomography (CT) of the abdomen, pelvis, lungs, or liver helps confirm the existence of a mass and the extent of disease.

A chest x-ray and liver scan may locate distant sites of metastasis.

OTHER DIAGNOSTIC ASSESSMENTS

A sigmoidoscopy provides visualization of the lower colon using a fiberoptic scope. Polyps can be visualized, and samples can be taken for biopsy. A colonoscopy provides visualization of the entire large bowel from the rectum to the ileocecal valve. As with sigmoidoscopy, polyps can be visualized and removed, and tissue samples can be taken for biopsy. Colonoscopy is the definitive test for the diagnosis of colorectal cancer. A liver scan may locate distant sites of metastasis.

◆Analysis

COMMON NURSING DIAGNOSES AND COLLABORATIVE PROBLEMS

The priority nursing diagnosis for clients with colorectal cancer (CRC) is Anticipatory Grieving related to the diagnosis of a potentially terminal illness, a disturbance in body image, and the possible loss of fecal continence. The priority collaborative problem is Potential for Metastasis.

ADDITIONAL NURSING DIAGNOSES AND COLLABORATIVE PROBLEMS

In addition to the common nursing diagnoses and collaborative problems, clients with colorectal cancer may develop one or more of the following:

- Acute Pain or Chronic Pain related to physical injury agents (e.g., tumor obstruction of the intestine with possible pressure on other organs or chronic physical disability)
- Fatigue related to disease state, anemia, and stress
- Disturbed Body Image related to biophysical factors, illness treatment, and/or surgery
- Ineffective Coping related to uncertainty and high degree of threat
- Imbalanced Nutrition: Less Than Body Requirements related to inability to digest or absorb food due to biologic factors
- Powerlessness related to illness-related regimen

◆Planning and Implementation

ANTICIPATORY GRIEVING

NOC **PLANNING: EXPECTED OUTCOMES.** A client faced with a diagnosis of colorectal cancer is expected to adjust to actual or impending loss. Indicators include that the client will consistently demonstrate the ability to:

- Resolve feelings about loss
- Express spiritual beliefs about death
- Verbalize acceptance of loss
- Report decreased preoccupation with loss
- Report absence of sleep disturbance
- Seek social support
- Progress through stages of grief

INTERVENTIONS. The client and family are faced with a possible loss of or alteration in body functions. Medical and surgical interventions for the treatment of colorectal cancer may result in cure, disease control, or palliation. Interventions are designed to assist the client in formulating effective strategies for expressing feelings of grief and developing coping skills.

Observe and identify the following:

- The client and family's current methods of coping
- Effective sources of support used in past crises
- The client's and family's present perceptions of the health problem
- Signs of anticipatory grief, such as crying, anger, and withdrawal from usual relationships

Encourage the client to verbalize feelings about the diagnosis, treatment, and anticipated alteration in body functions if a colostomy is planned (see later discussion of the operative procedure under Surgical Management, p. 1322). Sadness, anger, feelings of loss, and depression are normal responses to this change in body functions.

If a colostomy is planned, instruct the client what to expect about the appearance and care of the colostomy. Postoperatively, encourage the client to look at and touch the stoma. When the client is physically able, ask him or her to participate in colostomy care. Participation helps to restore the client's sense of control over his or her lifestyle and thus facilitates improved self-esteem.

NIC **Grief Work Facilitation.** The purpose of grief work is to assist the client with the resolution of a significant loss. Assist in identifying the nature of and reaction to the loss. Encourage the client to verbalize feelings and identify fears to help move him or her through the appropriate phases of the grief process. Establish a trusting, ongoing relationship with the client and provide support through the personal grieving stages.

In collaboration with the psychologist or psychiatric clinical nurse specialist and when appropriate, assist the client in identifying personal coping strategies. Encourage the client to implement cultural, religious, and social customs associated with the loss, and identify sources of community support available to the client and family. Modifications in lifestyle can be anticipated in clients with a diagnosis of CRC. Help the client and family to identify the necessary modifications in lifestyle. The chaplain, social worker, or family assists in discussions and decisions concerning treatment, the prognosis, and end-of-life decisions, as appropriate.

NIC **Genetic Counseling.** Genetic counseling entails the use of an interactive helping process focusing on the prevention of a genetic disorder or on the ability to cope with a family member who has a genetically based disorder. Referral to a genetics center for clients with familial CRCs may be needed. Specially trained nurses can discuss the purposes and goals of genetic testing. Privacy and confidentiality need to be ensured. A review of the family history may provide important information concerning the pattern of colorectal cancer inheritance. To make an informed decision, the client and family need information about the advantages, risks, and costs of appropriate genetic tests. Monitor the client's response regarding genetic risk factors. NIC interventions are summarized in Chart 60-3.

CHART 60-3

NIC INTERVENTION ACTIVITIES for The Client with Noninflammatory Intestinal Disorders

Grief Work Facilitation: *Assistance with the resolution of a significant loss*

- Assist the client to identify the nature of the attachment to the lost object or person.
- Assist the client to identify the initial reaction to the loss.
- Encourage expression of feelings about the loss.
- Instruct in phases of the grieving process, as appropriate.
- Support progression through personal grieving stages.
- Include significant others in discussions and decisions, as appropriate.
- Assist client to identify personal coping strategies.
- Encourage client to implement cultural, religious, and social customs associated with the loss.
- Identify sources to community support.
- Assist in identifying modifications needed in lifestyle.

Genetic Counseling: *Use of an interactive helping process focusing on assisting an individual, family, or group, manifesting or at risk for developing or transmitting a birth defect or genetic condition, to cope*

- Provide privacy and ensure confidentiality.
- Determine the client's purpose, goals, and agenda for the genetic counseling session.
- Monitor response when client learns about own genetic risk factors.
- Provide referral to genetic health care specialists, as necessary.

NIC intervention activities selected from Dochterman, J.M., & Bulechek, G.M. (Eds.) (2004). *Nursing interventions classifications (NIC)* (4th ed.). St. Louis: Mosby.

POTENTIAL FOR METASTASIS

PLANNING: EXPECTED OUTCOMES. The client with colorectal cancer (CRC) is expected to not have the cancer spread to vital organs; thus the client's life expectancy will be increased and the quality of life will be improved.

INTERVENTIONS. Although surgical resection is the primary means used to control the disease, several adjuvant therapies are employed as well. Adjuvant therapies are administered before or after surgery to affect a cure and to prevent recurrence.

NONSURGICAL MANAGEMENT. The type of therapy used is based on the pathologic staging of the disease. **Dukes' staging classification** may be used to classify colorectal tumors by designating them as A, B, C, or D, according to the depth of invasion into the mucosa and distant spread.

- Dukes' stage A indicates that the tumor has penetrated into, but not through, the bowel wall.
- Stage B indicates that the tumor has penetrated through the bowel wall.
- Stage C indicates that the tumor has penetrated through the bowel wall and that there is lymph node involvement.
- Stage D indicates that the tumor has metastasized to any of a number of distant sites.

Radiation Therapy. The administration of preoperative radiation therapy has not improved overall survival rates for colon cancer but it has been effective in providing local or regional control of the disease. Postoperative radiation has not demonstrated any consistent improvement in survival or recurrence. As a palliative measure, radiation therapy may be used to control pain, hemorrhage, bowel obstruction, or metastasis to the lung in advanced disease. For rectal cancer, unlike the for colon cancer, radiation therapy is almost always a part of the treatment plan. Reinforce information about the radiation therapy procedure to the client and family and monitor for possible side effects (e.g., diarrhea and fatigue). (See Chapter 28 for care of clients undergoing radiation therapy.)

Drug Therapy. Adjuvant *chemotherapy* after primary surgery is recommended for clients with stage II (Dukes' stage B_2) or stage III (Dukes' stage C) disease to interrupt the DNA production of cells and improve survival. The drug of choice is intravenous (IV) 5-fluorouracil (5-FU) with or without leucovorin (folinic acid). These medications cannot discriminate between cancer and healthy cells. Therefore the side effects are diarrhea, mucositis, leucopenia, mouth ulcers, and skin effects.

Oxaliplatin (Eloxatin) is a relatively new platinum analogue chemotherapeutic agent used in combination with 5-FU and leucovorin for clients with treatment-resistant CRC (FOLFOX regimen). The dose-limiting toxicity for this agent is peripheral sensory neuropathy. It may also be used for the initial treatment of advanced colorectal cancer (CRC).

In 1997, irinotecan (Camptosar) was approved as second-line treatment for *metastatic (stage IV or Dukes' D)* disease if it has recurred or progressed after treatment with 5-FU. With this drug, **myelosuppression** (bone marrow suppression, causing **pancytopenia** [decreased blood cells]) and diarrhea are the most frequent dose-limiting toxicities. Camptosar is now given commonly with 5-FU (Saltz regimen). More recently, Camptosar is administered with 48-hour infusions of 5-FU/leucovorin.

In 2004, two new drugs were approved for CRC. Bevacizumab (Avastin) is the first antiangiogenesis medication to be approved for advanced CRC. This type of drug reduces blood flow to the growing tumor cells, thereby depriving them of necessary nutrients needed to grow. Avastin is usually given in combination with other chemotherapeutic agents. Cetuximab (Erbitux), a monoclonal antibody, was also approved for advanced disease. This drug works by binding to a protein (epidural growth factor receptor) to slow cell growth. Erbitux is usually given in combination with another drug.

Current clinical trials using other monoclonal antibodies and a colorectal tumor vaccine are in progress. In addition, new oral agents consisting of a fluorinated pyrimidine and leucovorin are being tested. Additional antiangiogenesis drugs are also being tested. Intrahepatic arterial chemotherapy, often with 5-FU, may be administered to clients with liver metastasis.

Clients with advanced CRC and metastasis also receive drugs for relief of symptoms, such as analgesics and antiemetics. These medications are discussed in Chapter 9.

SURGICAL MANAGEMENT. Surgical removal of the tumor with margins free of disease is the best method of ensuring removal of CRC. The size of the tumor, its location, the extent of metastasis, the integrity of the bowel, and the condition of the client determine which surgical procedure is performed for colorectal cancer (Table 60-2). The most common surgeries performed are **colon resection** (removal of the tumor and regional lymph nodes) with reanastomosis, **colectomy** (colon removal) with *colostomy (temporary or permanent),* and **abdominoperineal (AP) resection.** A **colostomy** is the surgical creation of an opening of the colon onto the surface of the abdomen. An AP resection is performed when rectal tumors are present. The surgeon removes the sigmoid colon, rectum, and anus through combined abdominal and perineal incisions. Most surgeries are done using an open approach, requiring 6 to 7 inch incisions. An alternative is laparoscopic surgery.

Small tumors indicate an early stage of cancer and are well differentiated without evidence of vascular or lymphatic invasion. They can be removed with clean margins and may be treated with local excision and close follow-up. A **transanal approach** without an abdominal incision is the technique most commonly used; this approach decreases the risk for postoperative complications and shortens the hospital stay. Only 5% of clients with colorectal cancer (CRC), however, meet the criteria of early-stage cancer.

Preoperative Care. Reinforce the physician's explanation of the planned surgical procedure. The client is told as accurately as possible what anatomic and physiologic changes will occur with surgery. The location and number of incision sites and drains are also discussed.

Before evaluating the tumor and colon during surgery, the surgeon may not be able to determine whether a colostomy will be necessary. In this case, the client is informed that a colostomy is a possibility. If a colostomy is inevitable, consult an enterostomal therapist (ET) to advise on optimal placement of the ostomy and instruct the client about the rationale and general principles of ostomy care. An ET is a registered nurse who has completed specialized training and is certified in ostomy nursing care. Some are also certified in wound and incontinence care.

The client who requires low rectal surgery (AP resection) is faced with the risk of postoperative sexual dysfunction and urinary incontinence as a result of nerve damage during surgery. The surgeon discusses the risk for these problems with the client before surgery and allows him or her to verbalize concerns and questions related to this risk. Reinforce teaching about abdominal surgery performed with the client under general anesthesia and review the routines for turning and deep breathing (see Chapter 20).

If the bowel is not obstructed or perforated, elective surgery is planned. The client is instructed to thoroughly clean the bowel, or "bowel prep," to minimize bacterial growth and prevent complications. In preparation for the bowel prep, the client is usually instructed to restrict the diet to clear liquids for 1 to 2 days before surgery. Mechanical cleaning is accomplished with laxatives and enemas or with "whole-gut lavage." For whole-gut lavage, the client usually ingests large quantities of a sodium sulfate and polyethylene glycol solution (e.g., GoLYTELY). This solution overwhelms the absorptive capacity of the small bowel and clears feces from the colon.

To reduce the risk of infection, the surgeon may prescribe oral or IV antibiotics to be given the day before surgery. A nasogastric (NG) tube may be placed for decompression of the stomach following surgery. A peripheral IV line is also placed for fluid and electrolyte replacement while the client is taking nothing by mouth (NPO) postoperatively.

The client with colorectal cancer faces a serious illness with long-term consequences of the disease and treatment. A case manager can be very helpful in identifying client and family needs, as well as continuity of care and support.

Operative Procedures. For the conventional open surgical approach, the surgeon makes an incision in the abdomen and explores the abdominal cavity to determine whether the tumor can be removed. For a colon resection, the portion of the colon with the tumor is excised, and the two open ends of the bowel are irrigated before **anastomosis** (reattachment) of the colon. If an anastomosis is not feasible because of the location of the tumor or the bowel is inflamed, a colostomy is created.

TABLE 60-2 Surgical Procedures for Colorectal Cancers in Various Locations

Right-Sided Colon Tumors
- Right hemicolectomy for smaller lesions
- Right ascending colostomy or ileostomy for large, widespread lesions
- Cecostomy (opening into the cecum with intubation to decompress the bowel)

Left-Sided Colon Tumors
- Left hemicolectomy for smaller lesions
- Left descending colostomy for larger lesions

Sigmoid Colon Tumors
- Sigmoid colectomy for smaller lesions
- Sigmoid colostomy for larger lesions
- Abdominoperineal resection for large, low sigmoid tumors (near the anus) with colostomy (the rectum and the anus are completely removed, leaving a perineal wound)

Rectal Tumors
- Resection with anastomosis or pull-through procedure (preserves anal sphincter and normal elimination pattern)
- Colon resection with permanent colostomy
- Abdominoperineal resection with colostomy

A colostomy may be created in the ascending, transverse, descending, or sigmoid colon (Figure 60-5). One of several techniques is used to construct a colostomy. A loop **stoma** (surgical opening) is made by bringing a loop of colon to the skin surface, severing and everting the anterior wall, and suturing it to the abdominal wall. Loop colostomies are usually performed in the transverse colon and are usually temporary. An external rod may be used to support the loop until the intestinal tissue adheres to the abdominal wall. Care must be taken to avoid displacing the rod, especially during appliance changes.

An end stoma is often constructed, most often in the descending or sigmoid colon, when a colostomy is intended to be permanent. It may also be done when the surgeon oversews the distal stump of the colon and places it in the abdominal cavity, preserving it for future reattachment. An end stoma is constructed by severing the end of the proximal portion of the bowel and bringing it out through the abdominal wall.

The least common colostomy is the **double-barrel stoma,** which is created by dividing the bowel and bringing both the proximal and distal portions to the abdominal surface to create two stomas. The proximal stoma (closest to the client's head) is the functioning stoma and eliminates stool; the distal stoma (farthest from the head) is considered nonfunctioning, although it may secrete some mucus. The distal stoma is sometimes referred to as a mucous fistula.

Some surgeons use minimally invasive techniques for colon resection via laparoscopy. Laparoscopic colon resection or total colectomy allows complete tumor removal with an adequate surgical margin and removal of associated lymph nodes. This technique is as safe and effective as the conventional surgical method, but it requires more surgical time.

Postoperative Care. Clients who have undergone an open colon resection without a colostomy receive care similar to that of clients undergoing any abdominal surgery (see Chapter 22). In addition, clients require colostomy and wound management. The client typically has a nasogastric (NG) tube after surgery and receives PCA for the first 24 to 36 hours. After NG tube removal, the diet is slowly progressed from liquids to solid foods as the client can tolerate. The care of clients with an NG tube is discussed under Interventions (Intestinal Obstruction) on p. 1329.

By contrast, clients who have laparoscopic surgery do not have an NG tube and can progress from liquids to solids more quickly. They usually have less pain and are able to ambulate earlier than those who have the conventional approach. The hospital stay is usually shorter for the client with minimally invasive surgery–usually 4 to 5 days.

Colostomy Management. The client who has a colostomy created may return from surgery with an ostomy pouch system in place. If there is no pouch system in place, a petrolatum gauze dressing is usually placed over the

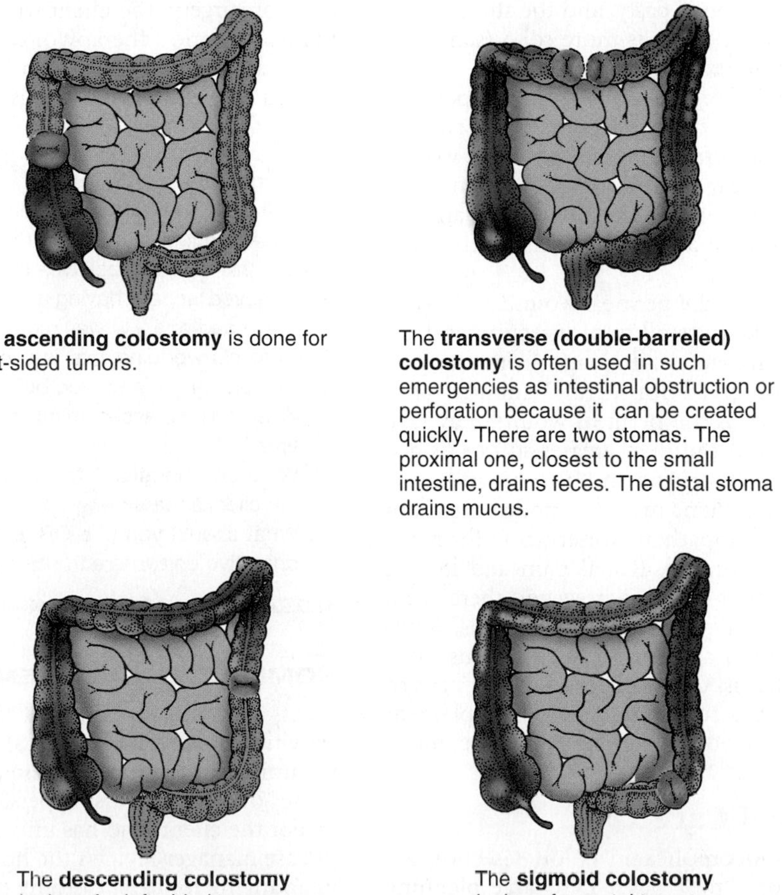

The **ascending colostomy** is done for right-sided tumors.

The **transverse (double-barreled) colostomy** is often used in such emergencies as intestinal obstruction or perforation because it can be created quickly. There are two stomas. The proximal one, closest to the small intestine, drains feces. The distal stoma drains mucus.

The **descending colostomy** is done for left-sided tumors.

The **sigmoid colostomy** is done for rectal tumors.

Figure 60-5 ■ Different locations of colostomies in the colon.

stoma to keep it moist, and this is covered with a dry, sterile dressing. In collaboration with the enterostomal therapist (ET), place a pouch system as soon as possible. The colostomy pouch system, also called an appliance, allows more convenient and acceptable collection of stool than a dressing does.

Assess the color and integrity of the stoma. A healthy stoma should be reddish pink and moist and will protrude about ¾ inch (2 cm) from the abdominal wall. A small amount of bleeding at the stoma is common.

Report any of the following problems related to the colostomy to the surgeon:

- Signs of ischemia and necrosis (dark red, purplish, or black color; dry, firm, or flaccid)
- Unusual bleeding
- Mucocutaneous separation (breakdown of the suture line securing the stoma to the abdominal wall)

Also assess the condition of the peristomal skin (skin around the stoma) and frequently check the pouch system for proper fit and signs of leakage. The peristomal skin should be intact, smooth, and without redness or excoriation.

The colostomy should start functioning 2 to 4 days postoperatively. When the colostomy begins to function, the pouch may need to be emptied frequently because of excess gas collection. It should be emptied when it is one-third to one-half full of stool. Stool is liquid immediately postoperatively but becomes more solid, depending on where in the colon the stoma was placed. For example, the stool from a colostomy in the ascending colon is liquid, the stool from a colostomy in the transverse colon is pasty, and the stool from a colostomy in the descending colon is more solid (similar to usual stool expelled from the rectum).

Wound Management. For an AP resection, the perineal wound is generally surgically closed, and two bulb suction drains, such as Jackson-Pratt drains, are placed in the wound or through stab wounds near the wound. The drains help prevent drainage from collecting within the wound and are usually left in place for several days, depending on the character and amount of drainage.

Monitoring drainage from the perineal wound and cavity is important because of the possibility of infection and abscess formation. Serosanguineous drainage from the perineal wound may be observed for 1 to 2 months after surgery. Complete healing of the perineal wound may take 6 to 8 months. This wound can be a greater source of discomfort than the abdominal incision and ostomy, and more care may be required. The client may experience phantom rectal sensations because sympathetic innervation for rectal control has not been interrupted. Rectal pain and itching may occasionally occur after healing; however, there is no known physiologic explanation for these sensations. Interventions may include use of antipruritic medications, such as benzocaine, and sitz baths. Continually assess for signs of infection, abscess, or other complications and implement methods for promoting wound drainage and comfort (Chart 60-4).

CHART 60-4

BEST PRACTICE for Perineal Wound Care

Wound Care

- Place an absorbent dressing (Kerlix or abdominal pad) over the wound.
- Instruct the client that he or she may:
  - Use a feminine napkin as a dressing.
  - Wear jockey-type shorts rather than boxers.

Comfort Measures

- If prescribed, soak the wound area in a sitz bath for 10 to 20 minutes three or four times per day.
- Administer pain medication as prescribed and assess its effectiveness.
- Instruct the client about permissible activities. The client should:
  - Assume a side-lying position in bed; avoid sitting for long periods.
  - Use foam pads or a soft pillow to sit on whenever in a sitting position.
  - Avoid the use of air rings or rubber doughnut devices.

Prevention of Complications

- Maintain fluid and electrolyte balance by monitoring intake and output and by monitoring output from the perineal wound.
- Observe incision integrity and monitor wound drains; watch for erythema, edema, bleeding, drainage, unusual odor, and excessive or constant pain.

Community-Based Care

Clients undergoing an uncomplicated colon resection are typically hospitalized for 5 to 7 days. Discharge planning with the assistance of a discharge planner or case manager assists clients and their families in coping with the immediate postoperative phase of recovery. Following hospitalization for surgery, the client with CRC is usually managed at home. Radiation therapy or chemotherapy is typically done on an ambulatory (outpatient) basis. For the client with advanced cancer, hospice care is an option (see Chapter 9).

Critical Thinking Challenge

A 55-year-old client is admitted to the surgical suite for a colon resection secondary to colorectal cancer (CRC). Although his surgeon believes the cancer is contained and can be removed without having a colostomy, the client is afraid that he may need one. He was recently engaged and is looking forward to his wedding that is scheduled in 6 weeks. His father had colon cancer and died before he was 60 years of age.

1. What further assessment data should you obtain at this time?
2. What collaborative interventions would be useful in view of the client's fears?
3. What should you (the OR nurse) communicate to the postoperative unit where the client will be discharged?

evolve For suggested answer guidelines, go to http://evolve.elsevier.com/Iggy/.

HOME CARE MANAGEMENT

Assess all clients for their ability to perform incision care and activities of daily living (ADLs) within limitations. For clients requiring assistance with these activities, home care visits by nurses or assistive nursing personnel can be provided.

For the client who has undergone a colostomy, the nurse or case manager reviews the home situation to aid the client in arranging for care. Ostomy products should be kept in an area (preferably the bathroom) where the temperature is neither hot nor cold (skin barriers may become stiff or melt in extreme temperatures) to ensure proper functioning. The enterostomal therapist (ET) may serve as a consultant after the client is discharged home to ensure continuity of care.

No changes are needed in sleeping accommodations. A rubber covering may initially be placed over the bed mattress if clients feel insecure about the pouch system. The client may consume his or her usual diet on discharge.

HEALTH TEACHING

Before discharge, clients are instructed to avoid lifting heavy objects or straining on defecation to prevent tension on the anastomosis site. If the client had the open surgical approach, driving should be avoided for 4 to 6 weeks while the incision heals. Clients who had laparoscopy can usually return to all usual activities in 1 to 2 weeks.

A stool softener may be prescribed to keep stools at a soft consistency for ease of passage. Clients are instructed to note the frequency, amount, and character of the stools. In addition to this information, teach all clients with colon resections to watch for and report clinical manifestations of intestinal obstruction and perforation (e.g., cramping, abdominal pain, nausea, and vomiting). A normal diet may be resumed; however, the client is advised to avoid gas-producing foods and carbonated beverages. Four to six weeks may be required to establish the effects of certain foods on bowel patterns.

COLOSTOMY CARE. Rehabilitation after ostomy surgery requires that clients and family members learn the principles of colostomy care and the psychomotor skills needed to facilitate this care. Providing information is important, but the nurse must also allow adequate opportunity for clients to learn the psychomotor skills involved in ostomy care before discharge. Sufficient practice time is planned for clients and family or significant others so that they can handle, assemble, and apply all ostomy equipment. Teach clients and families or other caregivers about the following:

- The normal appearance of the stoma
- Signs and symptoms of complications
- Measurement of the stoma
- The choice, use, care, and application of the appropriate appliance to cover the stoma
- Measures to protect the skin adjacent to the stoma
- Dietary measures to control gas and odor
- Resumption of normal activities, including work, travel, and sexual intercourse

The appropriate pouch system must be selected and fitted to the stoma. Clients with flat, firm abdomens may use either flexible (bordered with paper tape) or nonflexible (full skin barrier wafer) pouch systems. A firm abdomen with lateral creases or folds requires a flexible system. Clients with deep creases, flabby abdomens, a retracted stoma, or a stoma that is flush or concave to the abdominal surface benefit from a convex appliance with a stoma belt. This type of system presses into the skin around the stoma, causing the stoma to protrude. This protrusion helps tighten the skin and prevents leaks around the stoma opening onto the peristomal skin.

Measurement of the stoma is necessary to determine the correct size of the stomal opening on the appliance. The opening should be large enough not only to cover the peristomal skin but also to avoid stomal trauma. The stoma will shrink within 6 to 8 weeks of surgery; therefore it needs to be measured at least once weekly during this time and as needed if the client gains or loses weight. The client and family caregiver should be taught to trace the pattern of the stomal area on the wafer portion of the appliance and to cut an opening about $\frac{1}{8}$- to $\frac{1}{16}$-inch larger than the stomal pattern to ensure that stomal tissue will not be constricted.

Skin preparation may include clipping peristomal hair or shaving the area to achieve a smooth surface, prevent unnecessary discomfort when the wafer is removed, and minimize the risk of infected hair follicles. The client is advised to avoid using moisturizing soaps to clean the area because the lubricants can interfere with adhesion of the appliance. The client and family caregiver are taught to apply a skin sealant and allow it to dry before application of the appliance (colostomy bag) to facilitate less painful removal of the tape or adhesive. If peristomal skin becomes raw, the client or caregiver checks to see whether the sealant contains alcohol and, if so, reconsiders using it to avoid causing a burning sensation to the skin. Stoma powder or paste, or a combination, may also be used for erythematous peristomal skin. The paste is also used to fill in crevices and creases to create a flat surface for the faceplate of the colostomy bag. If the client develops a fungal rash, an antifungal cream or powder is used, as prescribed.

Control of gas and odor from the colostomy is often a significant goal for clients with new ostomies. Although a leaking or inadequately closed pouch is the usual cause of odor, flatus can also contribute to the odor. Remind the client and family caregiver that although there are generally no forbidden foods for ostomates, certain foods and habits can cause flatus or contribute to odor when the pouch is open. Broccoli, brussels sprouts, cabbage, cauliflower, cucumbers, mushrooms, and peas often cause flatus, as does chewing gum, smoking, drinking beer, and skipping meals. Crackers, toast, and yogurt can help prevent gas. Asparagus, broccoli, cabbage, turnips, eggs, fish, and garlic contribute to odor when the pouch is open. Buttermilk, cranberry juice, parsley, and yogurt will help prevent odor; charcoal filters, pouch deodorizers, or placement of a breath mint in the pouch will eliminate odors. The client should be cautioned not to put aspirin tablets in the pouch because they may cause ulceration of the stoma.

The client with a sigmoid colostomy may benefit from colostomy irrigation to regulate elimination. However, most clients with a sigmoid colostomy can become regulated through diet. An irrigation is similar to an enema, but is administered through the stoma rather than the rectum.

In addition to instructing the client about the clinical manifestations of obstruction and perforation, advise the client with a colostomy to report any fever or sudden onset of pain or swelling around the stoma. Other home care assessment is listed in Chart 60-5.

PSYCHOSOCIAL PREPARATION. The diagnosis of cancer can be emotionally immobilizing for the client and family or significant others, but treatment may be welcomed because it may provide hope for control of the disease. Explore the client's reactions to the illness and perceptions of planned interventions.

The client's reaction to ostomy surgery, which may include disfigurement, may involve the following:

- Fear of not being accepted by others
- Feelings of grief related to disturbance in body image
- Concerns about sexuality

CHART 60-5

HOME CARE ASSESSMENT of
The Client with a Colostomy

Assess gastrointestinal status, including:
- Dietary and fluid intake and habits
- Presence or absence of nausea and vomiting
- Weight gain or loss
- Bowel elimination pattern and characteristics and amount of effluent (stool)
- Bowel sounds

Assess condition of stoma, including:
- Location, size, protrusion, color, and integrity
- Signs of ischemia, such as dull coloring or dark or purplish bruising

Assess peristomal skin for:
- Presence or absence of excoriated skin, leakage underneath drainage system
- Fit of appliance and effectiveness of skin barrier and appliance

Assess client's and family's coping skills, including:
- Self-care abilities in the home
- Acknowledgment of changes in body image and function
- Sense of loss

Allow the client to verbalize his or her feelings. By teaching how to physically manage the ostomy, help the client begin to restore self-esteem and improve body image. Inclusion of family and significant others in the rehabilitation process may help maintain relationships and raise the client's self-esteem. Anticipatory instruction includes information on leakage accidents, odor control measures, and adjustments to resuming sexual relationships.

HEALTH CARE RESOURCES

Several resources are available to complement nursing care, maintain continuity of care in the home environment, and provide for client needs that the nurse is not able to meet. Make referrals to case managers or social workers, who can provide further emotional counseling to the client and family or significant others, aid in managing the financial concerns that the client and family may have, or arrange home care or extended care (e.g., in a nursing home, group home, or hospice) as needed.

If needed, make a referral to the enterostomal therapist (ET) to aid in preoperative stoma teaching, evaluate the stoma site, and provide consultation for problems in care. The enterostomal therapist (ET) may also conduct an ambulatory care clinic for ongoing client needs.

Information about the United Ostomy Association, a self-help group of people who have ostomies, is provided. Literature, such as the organization's publication *(Ostomy Quarterly)*, and information about a local chapter are given to the client. This organization conducts a visitor program that sends specially trained visitors (who have an ostomy) to talk with clients. After obtaining the client's consent, you can also make a referral to the visitor program so that the visitor can see the client both preoperatively and postoperatively. A physician's consent for visitation is generally necessary.

The local division or unit of the American Cancer Society (ACS) can help provide necessary medical equipment and supplies, home care services, travel accommodations, and other resources for the client who is undergoing cancer treatment or ostomy surgery. Inform the client and family of the programs available through the local division or unit.

Because of short hospital stays, clients with new ostomies receive most of their instruction on colostomy care from nurses working for home care agencies. This resource also facilitates provision for physical care needs, medication management, and emotional support for clients with or without colostomies. If the client has advanced colorectal cancer, a referral for hospice services in the home, nursing home, or other long-term care setting may be appropriate. The home care nurse informs the client and family about what ostomy supplies are needed and where they can be purchased. Price and location are considered before recommendations are made.

Evaluation: Outcomes

Evaluate the care of the client with colorectal cancer on the basis of the identified nursing diagnoses and collaborative problems. The expected outcomes are that the client:
- Adjusts to actual or impending loss
- Is free of complications or metastasis associated with CRC

Specific indicators for these outcomes are listed for each nursing diagnosis and collaborative problem under the Planning and Implementation section (see earlier).

INTESTINAL OBSTRUCTION

PATHOPHYSIOLOGY

Intestinal obstructions can be partial or complete and are classified as mechanical or nonmechanical. In **mechanical obstruction,** the bowel is physically obstructed by disorders outside the intestine (e.g., adhesions or hernias) or by blockages in the lumen of the intestine (e.g., tumors, inflammation, strictures, or fecal impactions). **Nonmechanical obstruction** (also known as paralytic ileus or adynamic ileus because it is a result of neuromuscular disturbance) does not involve a physical obstruction in or outside the intestine. Instead, peristalsis is decreased or absent, resulting in a slowing of the movement or a backup of intestinal contents.

Intestinal contents are composed of ingested fluid and saliva; gastric, pancreatic, and biliary secretions; and swallowed air. In both mechanical and nonmechanical obstructions, the intestinal contents accumulate at and above the area of obstruction. Intestinal distention results from the intestine's inability to absorb the contents and mobilize them down the intestinal tract. To compensate for the lag, peristalsis increases in an effort to move the intestinal contents forward. The increase in peristalsis stimulates more secretions, which leads to additional distention. This causes edema of the bowel with increased capillary permeability. Plasma leaking into the peritoneal cavity and fluid trapped in the intestinal lumen markedly decrease the absorption of fluid and electrolytes into the vascular space. Reduced circulatory blood volume and electrolyte imbalances typically occur. Hypovolemia ranges from mild to extreme (hypovolemic shock).

Specific fluid and electrolyte problems result, depending on the part of the intestine that is blocked. An obstruction high in the small intestine causes a loss of gastric hydrochloride, which can lead to *metabolic alkalosis.* Obstruction below the duodenum but above the large bowel results in loss of both acids and bases, so that acid-base imbalance is usually not compromised. Obstruction at the end of the small intestine and lower in the intestinal tract causes loss of alkaline fluids, which can lead to *metabolic acidosis*.

If the resultant hypovolemia is severe, renal insufficiency or even death can occur. Bacterial peritonitis with or without actual perforation can also result. Bacteria in the intestinal contents lie stagnant in the obstructed intestine. This is not a problem unless the blood flow to the intestine is compromised. However, with so-called closed-loop obstruction (blockage in two different areas) or a **strangulated obstruction** (obstruction with compromised blood flow), the risk for peritonitis is greatly increased. Bacteria without blood supply can form an endotoxin, and release of the endotoxin into the peritoneal or systemic circulation results in septic shock. With a strangulated obstruction, major blood loss into the intestine and the peritoneum can result. Current mortality rates for bowel obstruction range from 3.5% to 6% but may be as high as 14% in older adults.

Etiology

Intestinal obstruction is a common and serious disorder caused by a variety of conditions and is associated with significant morbidity. It can occur anywhere in the intestinal tract, although the ileum in the small intestine (the narrowest part of the intestinal tract) is the most common site.

Mechanical obstruction can result from the following:

- Adhesions
- Tumors
- Hernias
- Fecal impactions (especially in older adults)
- Strictures due to Crohn's disease or radiation
- **Intussusception** (telescoping of a segment of the intestine within itself)
- **Volvulus** (twisting of the intestine)
- Fibrosis due to disorders such as endometriosis
- Vascular disorders (e.g., emboli and arteriosclerotic narrowing of mesenteric vessels) (Figure 60-6).

In individuals age 65 or older, diverticulitis and tumors are the most common causes of obstruction.

Regardless of age, adhesions are the most common cause of mechanical obstruction, accounting for 45% to 60% of cases. Adhesions are bands of granulation and scar tissue that develop as a result of an inflammatory response, encircling the intestine and constricting its lumen.

Paralytic, or **adynamic, ileus** is a nonmechanical obstruction caused by physiologic, neurogenic, or chemical imbalances associated with decreased peristalsis from trauma or the effect of a toxin on autonomic intestinal control. Adynamic ileus occurs to some degree following abdominal surgery or trauma. Paralytic ileus can be caused by handling of the intestines during abdominal surgery; intestinal function is lost for a few hours to several days.

Thoracic diseases such as myocardial infarction, rib fracture, and pneumonia can also cause paralytic ileus. Electrolyte disturbances, especially hypokalemia, predispose the client to ileus. Paralytic ileus can be a consequence of peritonitis, because leakage of colonic contents causes severe irritation and triggers an inflammatory response. Vascular insufficiency to the bowel, also referred to as intestinal ischemia, is a potential cause of adynamic ileus. Vascular insufficiency results when arterial or venous thrombosis or an embolus decreases blood flow to the mesenteric blood vessels surrounding the intestines, as in heart failure or severe shock. Severe insufficiency of blood supply can result in infarction of surrounding organs (e.g., bowel infarction).

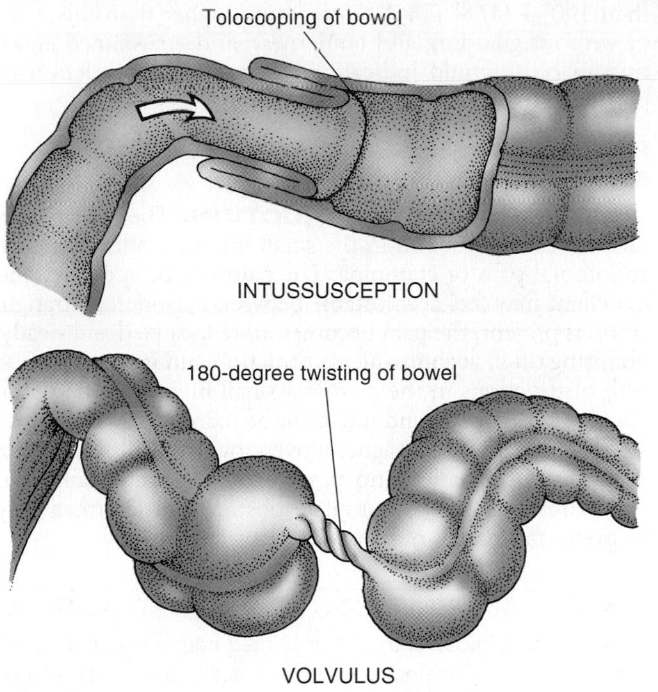

Figure 60-6 ■ Two types of mechanical obstruction.

Incidence/Prevalence

Obstruction of the intestines occurs in about 20% of all clients who are seen for acute abdominal pain. It is the most common reason for surgery of the small intestine. Because bowel obstruction is a result of other disorders, statistics on the incidence of bowel obstruction are not readily available.

Obstruction of the intestines occurs in all age groups, but the incidence differs with age. In adults, 75% of all obstructions occur in the small intestine and 15% occur in the large intestine.

COLLABORATIVE MANAGEMENT

Assessment

HISTORY

Collect information concerning the following:

- Past or recent abdominal surgery
- Radiation therapy
- History of inflammatory bowel disease
- Gallstones
- Hernias
- Trauma
- Peritonitis
- Cancer

Question the client about recent nausea or vomiting. Ask about the passage of flatus and the time, character, and consistency of the last bowel movement. Singultus (hiccups) is common with all types of intestinal obstruction.

Assess for a family history of colorectal cancer (CRC) and ask about blood in the stool or a change in bowel pattern. The body temperature with obstruction is rarely higher than 100° F (37.8° C). A temperature higher than this, with or without guarding and tenderness, and a sustained elevation in pulse could indicate a strangulated obstruction or peritonitis.

PHYSICAL ASSESSMENT/CLINICAL MANIFESTATIONS

MECHANICAL OBSTRUCTION. The client with mechanical obstruction in the small intestine often has mid-abdominal pain or cramping. The pain can be sporadic, and the client may feel comfortable between episodes. If strangulation is present, the pain becomes more localized and steady. Vomiting often accompanies obstruction and is more profuse with obstructions in the proximal small intestine. The vomitus may contain bile and mucus or be orange-brown and foul smelling as a result of bacterial overgrowth with low ileal obstruction. **Obstipation** (no passage of stool) and failure to pass flatus accompany complete obstruction. Diarrhea may be present in partial obstruction.

CONSIDERATIONS FOR OLDER ADULTS

The older adult with a strangulated hernia may not complain of pain but instead may only present with nausea and vomiting. Evaluate the client complaining of any of these symptoms, because they may require immediate medical and eventually surgical intervention.

Mechanical colonic obstruction causes a milder, more intermittent colicky abdominal pain than is seen with small-bowel obstruction. Lower abdominal distention may be present, as well as obstipation, or ribbon-like stools if obstruction is partial. Alterations in bowel patterns and blood in the stools accompany the obstruction if colorectal cancer or diverticulitis is the cause.

On examination of the abdomen, observe for abdominal distention, which is common in all forms of intestinal obstruction. Peristaltic waves may also be visible. Auscultate for proximal high-pitched bowel sounds **(borborygmi),** which are associated with cramping early in the obstructive process as the intestine tries to push the mechanical obstruction forward. In later stages of mechanical obstruction, bowel sounds are absent, especially distal to the obstruction. Abdominal tenderness and rigidity are usually minimal. The presence of a tense, fluid-filled bowel loop mimicking a palpable abdominal mass may signal a closed-loop, strangulating small-bowel obstruction.

NONMECHANICAL OBSTRUCTION. In most types of nonmechanical obstruction (paralytic, or adynamic, ileus), the pain is described as a constant, diffuse discomfort. Colicky cramping is not characteristic of this type of obstruction. Pain associated with obstruction attributable to vascular insufficiency or infarction is usually severe and constant. On inspection, abdominal distention is typically present. On auscultation of the abdomen, note decreased bowel sounds in early obstruction and absent bowel sounds in later stages. Vomiting of gastric contents and bile is frequent, but the vomitus rarely has a foul odor and is rarely profuse. Obstipation may or may not be present. Chart 60-6 compares small-bowel and large-bowel obstructions.

CHART 60-6

KEY FEATURES of Small-Bowel and Large-Bowel Obstructions

Small-Bowel Obstructions	Large-Bowel Obstructions
Abdominal discomfort or pain possibly accompanied by visible peristaltic waves in upper and middle abdomen	Intermittent lower abdominal cramping
Upper or epigastric abdominal distention	Lower abdominal distention
Nausea and early, profuse vomiting	Minimal or no vomiting (may contain fecal material)
Obstipation	Obstipation or ribbon-like stools
Severe fluid and electrolyte imbalances	No major fluid and electrolyte imbalances
Metabolic alkalosis	Metabolic acidosis

LABORATORY ASSESSMENT

There is no definitive laboratory test to confirm a diagnosis of mechanical or nonmechanical obstruction. White blood cell (WBC) counts may be normal unless there is a strangulated obstruction, in which case there may be leukocytosis (increased WBCs). Hemoglobin, hematocrit, creatinine, and blood urea nitrogen (BUN) values are often elevated, indicating dehydration. Serum sodium, chloride, and potassium concentrations are reduced because of loss of fluid and electrolytes. Elevations in serum amylase levels may be found with strangulating obstructions, which can damage the pancreas.

High obstruction in the small intestine is likely to show an elevated serum venous carbon dioxide concentration and other values indicative of metabolic alkalosis. Obstruction in the large intestine is likely to show a low serum venous carbon dioxide concentration and other values suggestive of metabolic acidosis.

RADIOGRAPHIC ASSESSMENT

The health care provider obtains flat-plate and upright abdominal x-rays as soon as an obstruction is suspected. Distention of loops of intestine with fluid and gas in the small intestine, in conjunction with the absence of gas in the colon, indicates an obstruction in the small intestine. However, x-ray findings are often normal when a strangulated obstruction actually exists in the small intestine. Therefore obstruction cannot be ruled out on the basis of x-ray findings.

Obstruction of the large intestine often shows gas distention of the colon on abdominal x-rays. A finding of free air under the diaphragm on abdominal x-ray examination indicates a perforated intestine.

OTHER DIAGNOSTIC ASSESSMENTS

The diagnostic examination chosen depends on the suspected location of the obstruction. The physician may perform endoscopy (sigmoidoscopy or colonoscopy) or a barium enema study to determine the cause of the obstruction, except when perforation is suspected. A computed tomography (CT) scan is useful in uncovering the cause and location of the obstruction and may be the diagnostic tool of choice when symptoms are severe.

Interventions

Interventions are aimed at uncovering the cause and relieving the obstruction. Intestinal obstructions can be relieved by nonsurgical or surgical means. If the obstruction is partial and there is no evidence of strangulation, nonsurgical management is the treatment of choice. Decompression of the intestinal tract is initiated along with fluid and electrolyte replacement.

NONSURGICAL MANAGEMENT. Paralytic ileus responds well to nonsurgical methods of relieving obstruction. Nonsurgical approaches are also preferred in the treatment of clients with terminal disease associated with bowel obstruction. In addition to being on NPO status, clients with intestinal obstruction typically have a nasogastric or, more rarely, nasointestinal tube inserted. These tubes provide decompression of the bowel by draining fluid and air and are attached to suction; the type of suction depends on the type of tube inserted.

Nasogastric Tubes. Most clients with an obstruction have at least a **nasogastric (NG) tube** in place unless the obstruction is mild. Salem sump and Anderson tubes are examples of NG tubes that sit distally in the stomach and are attached to *low continuous* suction. Levin tubes are connected to *low intermittent* suction.

At least every 4 hours, assess for proper placement of the tube, tube patency, and output (quality and quantity). The nasal skin is also monitored daily for integrity. Assess for peristalsis by auscultating for bowel sounds with the suction disconnected (suction masks peristaltic sounds).

Question the client regarding the passage of flatus and record the passage, amount, and character of bowel movements daily. Abdominal girth is measured at the same point each day. The client is also assessed for nausea and asked to report this manifestation.

NG tubes must be monitored for proper functioning. Occasionally, NG tubes move out of optimal drainage position or become plugged. In this case, note a decrease in gastric output or stasis of the tube's contents. Assess the client for nausea, vomiting, increased abdominal distention, and placement of the tube. If the NG tube is repositioned or replaced, confirmation of proper placement is obtained by x-ray examination before use. After appropriate placement is established, the contents are aspirated and the tube is irrigated with 30 mL of normal saline every 4 hours or as needed to maintain patency.

Nasointestinal Tubes. The physician *occasionally* inserts nasointestinal (NI) tubes (such as the Miller-Abbott, Cantor, and Harris tubes) for obstruction of the small intestine. These longer tubes extend into the small intestine. Mercury-filled balloons at the end of a lumen act as a bolus of food, stimulating peristalsis and advancing down the intestinal tract. The Cantor and Harris tubes are single-lumen tubes with mercury-filled balloons at the tips and suction ports within the same lumen, proximal to the tip. The Miller-Abbott tube has two separate lumens for mercury and drainage.

Assist with progression of the tube by helping the client change position every 2 hours and, if ordered, by advancing the tube 3 to 4 inches at specified times. These tubes are *never* taped to the nose until they reach a specified position in the intestine. As the tube is being inserted and advanced, it drains by gravity. Monitor the drainage; if drainage stops, obtain a physician's order to inject 10 mL of air. *Do not irrigate the NI tube with fluid without an order by the health care provider!* If ordered, attach low intermittent suction to the suction lumen when the tube has stopped advancing.

Most health care providers avoid the use of NI tubes because insertion of the mercury-filled lumen is often difficult; the time it takes to insert the tube also delays treatment. Insertion of this tube can be uncomfortable for clients.

Other Nonsurgical Techniques. Most types of nonmechanical obstruction respond to nasogastric decompression in conjunction with medical treatment of the primary disorder. Incomplete mechanical obstruction can sometimes be successfully treated without surgery. Obstruction caused by fecal impaction usually resolves after disimpaction and enema administration. Intussusception may respond to hydrostatic pressure changes during a barium enema.

Fluid and Electrolyte Replacement. IV fluid replacement and maintenance are indicated for all clients with intestinal obstruction, because the client is on NPO status and fluid and electrolyte loss (particularly potassium) through vomiting and nasogastric suction is great. On the basis of serum electrolytes and blood urea nitrogen (BUN) levels, the health care provider orders aggressive fluid replacement with 2 to 4 L of normal saline or lactated Ringer's solution with potassium added. Care must be taken with clients who are susceptible to fluid overload (e.g., the client with a history of heart failure). Monitor lung sounds, weight, and intake and output. Blood replacement may be indicated in strangulated obstruction because of blood loss into the bowel or peritoneal cavity.

Monitor the client's vital signs and other measures of fluid status (e.g., urine output, skin turgor, and mucous membranes). Edema from third spacing is assessed because fluid is lost, mostly from the vascular space, into surrounding spaces (e.g., the peritoneal cavity). In collaboration with the dietitian, the physician may prescribe total parenteral nutrition (TPN) to improve the nutritional status of the client, especially if he or she has had chronic nutritional problems and has been on NPO status for an extended period. Chapter 64 discusses the nursing care of clients receiving TPN.

The client with intestinal obstruction is characteristically thirsty. Provide or delegate frequent mouth care to help maintain moist mucous membranes. A small amount of ice chips may be allowed if the client is not having surgery; however, the health care provider should be consulted first. Ice chips can provide more free water than electrolytes; thus potassium and hydrochloric acid are washed out of the NG tube.

Pain Management. The abdominal distention commonly noted with intestinal obstruction can cause a great deal of discomfort, especially when distention is severe. The colicky, crampy pain that comes and goes with mechanical obstruction and the nausea, vomiting, dry mucous membranes, and thirst contribute to the client's discomfort. Continually assess the character and location of the pain and immediately report any pain that significantly increases or changes from a colicky, intermittent type to a constant discomfort. Such changes can indicate perforation of the intestine or peritonitis.

Opioid analgesics are normally withheld in the diagnostic period so that clinical manifestations of perforation or peritonitis are not masked. Explain to the client and family the rationale for not giving analgesics. In addition, if analgesics such as morphine or meperidine are given, they slow intestinal motility and can cause vomiting. Be alert to this side effect because nausea and vomiting are also signs of NG tube obstruction or worsening bowel obstruction.

Help the client obtain a position of comfort with frequent position changes to promote increased peristalsis. A semi-Fowler's position helps alleviate the pressure of abdominal distention on the chest. Not only is this a good comfort technique, but it also facilitates adequate thoracic excursion and normal breathing patterns.

Discomfort is generally less with nonmechanical obstruction than with mechanical obstruction. With both types of obstruction, discomfort is aggravated by ingestion of food or fluids.

Drug Therapy. If strangulation is thought to be likely, the health care provider prescribes IV broad-spectrum antibiotics. In addition, in cases of partial obstruction or paralytic ileus, medications that enhance gastric motility, such as octreotide acetate (Sandostatin), may be used.

SURGICAL MANAGEMENT. In all cases of complete mechanical obstruction and in many cases of incomplete mechanical obstruction, surgical intervention is necessary to relieve the obstruction. A strangulated obstruction is inevitably complete, and surgical intervention is always required. An **exploratory laparotomy** (a surgical opening of the abdominal cavity to investigate the cause of the obstruction) is initially performed for most clients with obstruction. More specific surgical procedures depend on the cause of the obstruction.

Preoperative Care. Provide preoperative teaching as discussed in Chapter 20. If time permits, all clients who require surgery for obstruction undergo nasogastric intubation and suction before surgery. However, in cases of complete obstruction, surgery should proceed without delay.

Operative Procedures. The surgeon enters the abdominal cavity and explores for obstruction. If adhesions are found to be the cause of the obstruction, the adhesions are lysed (cut and released). Obstruction caused by a tumor or diverticulitis requires a colon resection with primary anastomosis or a temporary or permanent colostomy. If obstruction is caused by intestinal infarction, an embolectomy, thrombectomy, or resection of the gangrenous bowel may be necessary.

Postoperative Care. Postoperative care for the client undergoing an exploratory laparotomy with lysis of adhesions, colon resection, thrombectomy, or embolectomy is similar to that described in Chapter 22. In addition, all clients have an NG tube in place until peristalsis (as characterized by the return of bowel sounds) resumes. The NG tube is removed slowly by first discontinuing suction and then clamping the tube for a scheduled amount of time. Residual drainage is checked at each stage to assess peristalsis without decompression before removing the NG tube entirely.

Critical Thinking Challenge

An older adult from a nursing home is admitted to your medical-surgical unit with severe vomiting and abdominal pain from possible bowel obstruction. She is very "confused" and unable to communicate when you ask her questions. The transfer form from the nursing home states that she is usually alert and oriented but that she began to become confused last night after dinner. She has a long history of diverticulitis and had surgery for colorectal cancer 10 years ago.

1. How will you assess this client's pain level?
2. What fluid, electrolyte, and acid-base imbalances is she likely to have or develop?
3. How will the health care provider determine if she has an obstruction?
4. What do you expect when you listen for bowel sounds?
5. What part of her care would you delegate to the nursing assistant?

evolve For suggested answer guidelines, go to http://evolve.elsevier.com/Iggy/.

Community-Based Care

All clients with intestinal obstruction are hospitalized for monitoring and treatment. The length of stay varies according to the type of obstruction, the treatment, and the presence of complications. Clients who have complicated obstruction, such as strangulation or incarceration, are at greater risk for peritonitis, sepsis, and shock. The hospital stay may be longer than a week, depending on the severity of complications.

Clients with nonmechanical (adynamic) intestinal obstruction are less likely to require a lengthy hospitalization because of the obstruction alone. Adynamic obstruction generally responds to NG intubation and suction within a few days.

HOME CARE MANAGEMENT

For the client who has had an intestinal obstruction, preparation for home care depends on the cause of the obstruction and the treatment required. Clients who have resolution of obstruction without surgical intervention are assessed for their knowledge of strategies to avoid recurrent obstruction. For example, if fecal impaction was the cause of the obstruction, assess the client's ability to carry out a bowel regimen independently. For clients who have undergone surgery, evaluate their ability to function at home with the added tasks of incision care and possibly colostomy care.

HEALTH TEACHING

Instruct the client to report any abdominal pain or distention, nausea, or vomiting, with or without constipation, because these symptoms might indicate recurrent obstruction. The client should be reassured, however, that recurrent paralytic ileus is not usually a problem. The client who has had mechanical obstruction as a result of fecal impaction (often the older adult) needs to have a structured bowel regimen to prevent recurrence (Chart 60-7). Instruct this client to adhere to high-fiber diets, to exercise, and to drink adequate amounts of water daily, unless contraindicated. The physician may also prescribe bulk-forming laxatives to help maintain a consistent elimination pattern.

Instruct the client who has had surgery about incision care, drug therapy, and activity limitations. Drug therapy consists of an oral opioid analgesic, such as oxycodone hydrochloride with acetaminophen (Tylox, Percocet, Endocet✱), to be taken as needed for incisional discomfort. As with any opioid therapy, a stool softener is added to the medication regimen to prevent constipation and possible recurrent obstruction.

CHART 60-7

NURSING FOCUS on the OLDER ADULT
Fecal Impaction

- Teach the client to eat high-fiber foods, including plenty of raw fruits and vegetables and whole-grain products.
- Encourage the client to drink adequate amounts of fluids, especially water.
- Do not routinely administer a laxative; teach the client that laxative abuse decreases abdominal muscle tone and contributes to an atonic colon.
- Encourage the client to exercise regularly, if possible. Walking every day is an excellent exercise for promoting intestinal motility.
- Use natural foods to stimulate peristalsis, such as warm beverages and prune juice.
- Take bulk-forming products, such as Metamucil, to provide fiber.
- Check the client's stool for amount and frequency; oozing of soft or diarrheal stool often indicates a fecal impaction.
- Have the client sit on a toilet or bedside commode, rather than on a bedpan, for elimination.

With resolution of obstruction, educational efforts by the nurse are aimed at prevention of obstruction by examining the cause of the obstruction and how to prevent recurrence. The nurse also reinforces important signs and symptoms to report to the health care provider. The client who had curative treatment of the underlying cause most likely requires less support than the client who underwent treatment of obstruction related to a serious disease that will require further treatment. Encourage the client to express fears and concerns about the future. Assess the client's understanding and needs with regard to treatment plans.

HEALTH CARE RESOURCES

The need for follow-up appointments depends on the cause of the obstruction and the treatment required. If the client is at risk for fecal impaction, arrange for a home care nurse to assess the gastrointestinal (GI) function and dietary habits of the client on an ongoing basis. Arrangements should also be made for the services of a home care nurse if the client needs help with incision or colostomy care. Medicare guidelines or insurance precertification requirements must be met before approval is given for home care visits. The discharge planner or case manager assists in setting up home care follow-up.

ABDOMINAL TRAUMA

PATHOPHYSIOLOGY

Abdominal trauma is defined as injury to the structures located between the diaphragm and the pelvis, which occurs when the abdomen is subjected to blunt or penetrating forces. Organs injured may include the large or small bowel, liver, spleen, duodenum, pancreas, kidneys, and urinary bladder.

At least one half of all blunt abdominal trauma occurs from motor vehicle accidents (MVAs). Other causes of blunt trauma include falls, aggravated assaults, and contact sports. *Penetrating abdominal trauma* is caused by gunshot wounds, stabbing, or impalement with an object. The liver is the most commonly injured organ in blunt and penetrating trauma. The spleen is the most commonly injured organ in blunt abdominal trauma. The small intestine is the third most commonly injured organ in abdominal trauma; 80% of injuries are caused by gunshot wounds (GSWs). Trauma is the leading cause of death in young adults (under 40 years of age) and the fifth leading cause of death in adults in the United States.

Because most abdominal or blunt trauma cases are the result of automobile accidents, encourage health promotion and illness prevention through the wearing of seat belts, which decreases abdominal trauma during accidents.

◆COLLABORATIVE MANAGEMENT

◆Assessment

First, assess any client experiencing trauma for airway, breathing, and circulation (ABC). Once these parameters are stabilized, focus on the risks of hemorrhage, shock, and peritonitis. Mental status, vital signs, and skin perfusion are *priority* nursing assessments, with skin perfusion being the most reliable clinical guide in assessing hypovolemic shock:

- In a person with mild shock, the skin is pale, cool, and moist.
- With moderate shock, diaphoresis is more marked and urine output ceases.
- With severe shock, changes in mental status are manifested by agitation, disorientation, and recent memory loss.

Assess for abdominal trauma by asking the client about the presence, location, and quality of pain. The abdomen, flanks, back, genitalia, and rectum are inspected for contusions, abrasions, lacerations, ecchymosis, penetrating injuries, and symmetry. All of the client's clothes must be removed.

Inspection of the abdomen may reveal distention. To perform an adequate inspection, turn the client while maintaining spinal immobilization. Ecchymosis may signify internal bleeding. Ecchymosis present in the distribution of a lap seat belt should be reported to the health care provider immediately, because investigation for occult injury to the bowel is necessary. Ecchymosis around the umbilicus is known as **Cullen's sign,** and ecchymosis on either flank (known as **Turner's sign**) may indicate retroperitoneal bleeding into the abdominal wall.

Auscultate the abdomen for bowel sounds. Absent or diminished bowel sounds may be caused by the presence of blood, bacteria, or a chemical irritant in the abdominal cavity. Also auscultate for bruits in the abdomen, which could indicate renal artery injury.

During percussion, an abnormal sign associated with abdominal trauma is resonance over the right flank with the client lying on the left side. This is known as **Ballance's sign** and is found with a ruptured spleen. Resonance over the normally dull liver is due to free air, which is pathologic. Palpation for lower rib fractures should increase suspicion of liver or spleen injuries. Injury to the spleen is present in 20% of individuals with left lower rib fractures. Liver injury is present in 10% of individuals with right lower rib fractures. The presence of **Kehr's sign,** left shoulder pain resulting from diaphragmatic irritation, may be present in splenic injury.

Dullness over hollow organs that normally contain gas, such as the stomach and the large and small intestines, may indicate the presence of blood or fluid. Light abdominal palpation identifies areas of tenderness, rebound tenderness, guarding, rigidity, and spasm. If you palpate a mass, it may be blood or a fluid collection.

The client without obvious significant bleeding or definite signs of peritoneal irritation undergoes abdominal radiography, diagnostic peritoneal lavage (DPL), and computed tomography (CT). For peritoneal lavage, the physician inserts a large-bore catheter into the abdomen and allows fluid to enter the abdominal cavity. If the return drainage from the abdomen is pink or grossly bloody, the health care team prepares the client for surgery. Abdominal ultrasound is used to diagnose blunt abdominal trauma and may replace CT and DPL for diagnosis (Levins, 2000). Clients with hemodynamic instability or peritonitis are candidates for immediate laparotomy.

Interventions

Nonsurgical and surgical interventions are aimed at preserving or restoring hemodynamic stability, preventing or decreasing blood loss, and preventing complications.

EMERGENCY CARE: ABDOMINAL TRAUMA. Nursing interventions include placement of at least two large-bore IV catheters in the upper extremities. IV catheters are not used in the lower extremities; if the vasculature has been injured, fluid can pool in the abdomen. The health care provider may insert a central venous catheter to assist with rapid fluid volume infusion. IV fluid consists of a balanced saline solution, crystalloids, and possibly blood.

The following physiologic parameters are monitored:

- Arterial blood gases
- Complete blood count (CBC)
- Serum electrolyte, glucose and amylase, and blood urea nitrogen (BUN) determinations
- Liver function tests
- Clotting studies

Measuring arterial blood gases may be of assistance in determining the severity of shock. Hemoglobin and hematocrit values do not initially reflect true blood loss; values can be skewed because of hemoconcentration from volume loss or the dilutional effects of IV fluids. Serial hemoglobin and hematocrit measurements may be more accurate in determining true blood loss. An elevated white blood cell (WBC) count may indicate a ruptured spleen or intestinal injury. Elevated levels of serum transaminases may indicate liver injury. Elevation of serum amylase activity may signal injury to the pancreas or the bowel. All laboratory work is compiled so that values can be compared and subtle changes noted.

Continuous hemodynamic monitoring is begun in the emergency department. Insert an indwelling urinary (Foley) catheter unless there is blood at the urinary meatus. Initially and hourly thereafter, evaluate urine output for bleeding and specific gravity. Laboratory tests indicate the amount of blood and protein in the urine. If there is an open abdominal wound or evisceration, cover it with a sterile dry dressing unless the physician orders otherwise. Unless it is contraindicated, as in the case of a concomitant skull fracture, the physician or nurse inserts a nasogastric (NG) tube, which is kept in place to identify bleeding and to minimize the risk of vomiting and aspiration. Antibiotics are administered as prescribed to reduce the risk of peritonitis.

If the client with known abdominal trauma has no definite clinical manifestations of active bleeding or abdominal injury, he or she is admitted to the hospital for observation. Blunt trauma can cause active, but often not obvious, damage. Assess for abdominal or referred pain and nausea. Every 15 to 30 minutes in the early postinjury period and then hourly, evaluate the following:

- Mental status
- Vital signs
- Clinical findings, such as vomiting, guarding, rigidity, or rebound tenderness
- Skin temperature
- Bowel sounds
- Urine output

Report any change immediately to the health care provider. It is more important to recognize the high risk of an active abdominal injury and assess for general signs of abdominal injury (e.g., hemorrhage and peritonitis) than to identify the exact nature of the abdominal injury. Analgesics for pain are not prescribed at this time so that clinical manifestations are not masked or overlooked. Explain the rationale for withholding analgesics to the client and family or significant others.

SURGICAL MANAGEMENT. For the client with severe abdominal trauma, the surgeon performs an exploratory laparotomy and repairs abdominal injuries immediately if there are definite signs of peritoneal irritation. These signs include rebound tenderness, significant blood loss, evisceration, or a gunshot wound (GSW) with possible peritoneal involvement.

Most stab wounds require exploratory laparotomy, but as many as 25% are superficial and do not involve the peritoneum. Using local anesthesia, the surgeon explores and cleans superficial stab wounds; the client does not require an exploratory laparotomy.

Before discharge from the hospital, the client who has experienced abdominal trauma is taught the signs and symptoms of abdominal bleeding whether or not surgery has been performed. Instruct the client to report abdominal pain, nausea, vomiting, bloody or black stools, fever, weakness, and dizziness.

Hemorrhage can occasionally occur weeks after blunt abdominal trauma, despite medical evaluation. For the client who undergoes surgery or exploration of wounds, provide instructions on wound care before discharge from the hospital.

POLYPS

PATHOPHYSIOLOGY

Polyps in the intestinal tract are small growths covered with mucosa and attached to the surface of the intestine. Although most are benign, polyps are significant in that some have the potential to become malignant.

Polyps are identified by their tissue type. The presence of adenomas always necessitates medical consultation because of their malignant potential. Although only 2% to 5% of adenomas progress to cancer, almost all colorectal cancers develop from an adenoma. Adenomas are further classified as villous or tubular. Of these, villous adenomas pose a greater cancer risk.

Familial adenomatous polyposis (FAP) and hereditary nonpolyposis colorectal cancer (HNPCC) are inherited syndromes characterized by progressive development of colorectal adenomas. Unless these syndromes are treated, colorectal cancer (CRC) inevitably occurs by the fourth to fifth decade of life. These conditions were discussed earlier under Genetic Considerations in the Colorectal Cancer section of this chapter.

Other types of polyps include hyperplastic and hamartomatous polyps. Hyperplastic polyps, which include mucosal and inflammatory varieties, are entirely benign with no malignant potential. Hamartomatous polyps include juvenile and Peutz-Jeghers syndrome polyps. Although both types are generally benign, rare reports of malignant changes have been reported in juvenile polyps.

In addition to being classified by their tissue type, polyps are described according to their appearance (Figure 60-7). Pedunculated polyps are stalklike; a thin stem attaches them to the intestinal wall. They become elongated as peristalsis pulls them into the lumen of the intestine. Polyps attached to the intestinal walls by a broad base are described as sessile. A malignant polyp may be pedunculated or sessile.

COLLABORATIVE MANAGEMENT

Polyps are usually asymptomatic and are discovered during routine diagnostic testing, including tests for blood in the stool. However, they can cause gross rectal bleeding, intestinal obstruction, or intussusception (telescoping of the bowel). Diagnostic studies involve a barium enema examination and proctosigmoidoscopy or colonoscopy for ruling out cancer. Biopsy specimens of polyps can be obtained, or the entire polyp can be removed (polypectomy) with the use of an electrocautery snare that fits through the sigmoidoscope or colonoscope. This often eliminates the need for abdominal surgery to remove a suspicious or definitely malignant polyp. The client with FAP often requires a total colectomy (colon removal) to prevent the development of cancer.

Nursing care focuses on client education. Instruct the client about the following:

- The nature of the polyp
- Clinical manifestations to report to the health care provider
- The need for regular, routine monitoring

If the client has undergone a polypectomy, follow-up sigmoidoscopic or colonoscopic examinations are needed, because there is an increased risk of multiple polyps in the client who has had at least one polyp.

Nursing care of the client who has undergone a polypectomy of the colorectal area includes monitoring for abdominal distention and pain, rectal bleeding, mucopurulent rectal drainage, and fever. A small amount of blood might appear in the stool after a polypectomy, but this should be temporary.

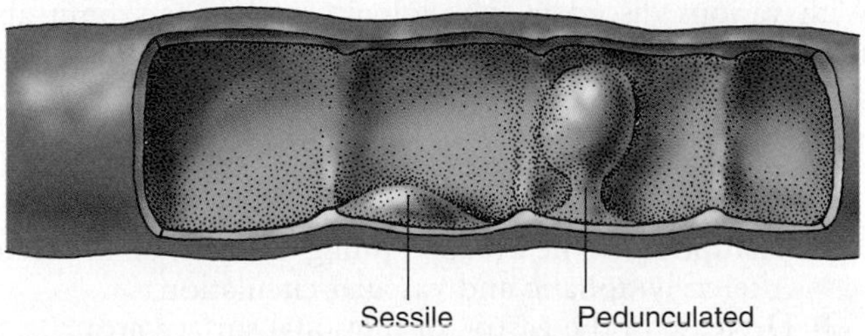

Figure 60-7 ■ Pedunculated and sessile polyps. Pedunculated polyps, such as tubular adenomas, are stalklike. Sessile polyps, such as villous adenomas, are broad based.

HEMORRHOIDS

PATHOPHYSIOLOGY

Hemorrhoids are unnaturally swollen or distended veins in the anorectal region. The veins involved in the development of hemorrhoids are part of the normal structure in the anal region. With limited distention, the veins function as a valve overlying the anal sphincter that assists in continence. Increased intra-abdominal pressure causes elevated systemic and portal venous pressure, which is transmitted to the anorectal veins. Arterioles in the anorectal region shunt blood directly to the distended anorectal veins, which increases the pressure. With repeated elevations in pressure from increased intra-abdominal pressure and engorgement from arteriolar shunting of blood, the distended veins eventually separate from the smooth muscle surrounding them. The result is prolapse of the hemorrhoidal vessels.

Hemorrhoids can be internal or external (Figure 60-8). **Internal hemorrhoids**, which cannot be seen on inspection of the perineal area, lie above the anal sphincter. **External hemorrhoids** lie below the anal sphincter and can be seen on inspection of the anal region. Prolapsed hemorrhoids can become thrombosed or inflamed, or they can bleed.

Etiology

Hemorrhoids are common and not significant unless they cause pain or bleeding. Caused by increased abdominal pressure, the condition exacerbates during pregnancy, constipation with straining, obesity, heart failure, prolonged sitting or standing, and strenuous exercise and weight lifting. Decreased fluid intake can also cause hemorrhoids due to the development of hard stool and subsequent constipation. Straining while evacuating stool causes them to enlarge.

Incidence/Prevalence

One in three individuals, or more than one third of the population of the United States will have hemorrhoids sometime in their lives. For adults over 50 years of age, the numbers

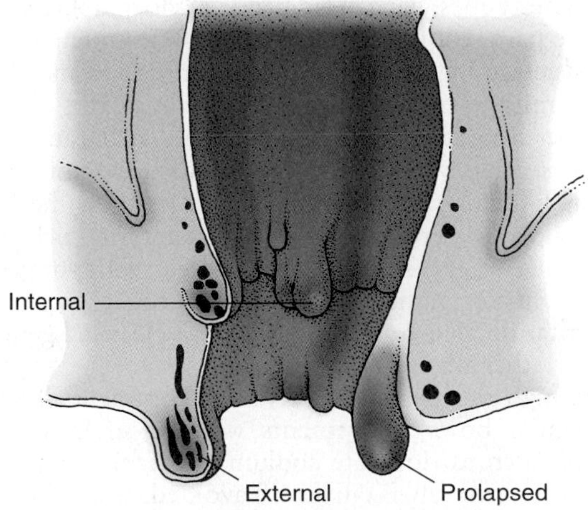

Figure 60-8 ■ Internal, external, and prolapsed hemorrhoids. Internal hemorrhoids lie above the anal sphincter and cannot be seen on inspection of the anal area. External hemorrhoids lie below the anal sphincter and can be seen on inspection of the anal region. Hemorrhoids that enlarge, fall down, and protrude through the anus are called prolapsed hemorrhoids.

increase to 50%, or 1 in every 2. However, only a small percentage of affected individuals actually become symptomatic. Men tend to be affected more often than women. The prevalence of hemorrhoids is highest in affluent countries of the Western World.

HEALTH PROMOTION/ILLNESS PREVENTION

Prevention of constipation is key, and is accomplished by increasing fiber in the diet, such as eating more whole grains, nuts, and raw vegetables and fruits. Encourage individuals to drink plenty of water. Remind the client to avoid straining at stool. Exercise, while encouraged, should be done in moderation with a gradual buildup in intensity. Maintaining a healthy weight also helps prevent hemorrhoids.

COLLABORATIVE MANAGEMENT

Assessment

The most common symptoms of hemorrhoids are bleeding, swelling, and prolapse. Blood is characteristically bright red and is present on toilet tissue or outside the stool. Pain is a common symptom and is often associated with thrombosis, especially if thrombosis occurs suddenly. Other symptoms include itching and a mucous discharge. Diagnosis is made by inspection, digital examination, proctoscopy, or proctoscopic ultrasonography.

Interventions

Interventions are typically conservative and are aimed at reducing symptoms with a minimum of discomfort, cost, and time lost from usual activities.

NONSURGICAL MANAGEMENT. Local treatment and diet therapy are initiated when symptoms begin. Cold packs applied to the anorectal region for a few minutes at a time beginning with the onset of pain and tepid sitz baths three or four times per day are often enough to relieve discomfort, even if the hemorrhoids are thrombosed.

Witch hazel soaks (e.g., Tucks) are also effective for pain. Topical anesthetics, such as lidocaine (Xylocaine), are useful for severe pain. Dibucaine (Nupercainal) ointment and similar products are available over-the-counter and may be applied for mild to moderate pain and itching. This ointment should be used only temporarily, however, because it can mask worsening symptoms and delay diagnosis of a severe disorder. If itching or inflammation is present, the health care provider prescribes a steroid preparation, such as hydrocortisone. Cleansing the anal area with moistened cleansing tissues rather than standard toilet tissue helps avoid irritation. The anal area should be cleansed gently by dabbing, rather than by wiping.

Diets high in fiber and fluids are recommended to promote regular bowel movements without straining. Stool softeners, such as docusate sodium (Colace), can be used temporarily. Irritating laxatives are avoided, as are foods and beverages that can make hemorrhoids worse. Spicy foods, nuts, coffee, and alcohol can be irritating. Remind clients to avoid sitting for long periods of time. The health care provider may prescribe oral analgesics for pain if the hemorrhoids are thrombosed.

Conservative treatment should alleviate symptoms in 3 to 5 days. If symptoms continue or recur frequently, the client may require surgical intervention.

SURGICAL MANAGEMENT. The surgeon can perform several procedures for symptomatic internal hemorrhoids on an ambulatory basis. Ultrasound, sclerotherapy, circular stapling, or simple resection of the hemorrhoids are examples of techniques that can be performed. The type of surgery depends on the degree of prolapse, whether there is thrombosis, and the overall condition of the client.

The harmonic scalpel is an ultrasonically activated instrument that vibrates to coagulate small and medium-size vessels. In sclerotherapy, the surgeon injects a sclerosing agent into the tissues around the hemorrhoids to obliterate the vessels. However, it can be done only for low-grade hemorrhoids. If the hemorrhoid is prolapsed, a circular stapling device is used to excise a band of mucosa above the prolapse and restore the hemorrhoidal tissue back into the anal canal.

Hemorrhoidectomy, or simple resection of the hemorrhoid, tends to cause more pain than the other procedures. Urinary retention can also occur because of rectal spasms and anorectal tenderness. Hemorrhage, which may be internal and not visible or external, is a rare but potential complication.

Teach clients with hemorrhoids about the need to consume high-fiber, high-fluid diets to promote regular bowel patterns before and after surgery. Advise clients to avoid stimulant laxatives, which are habit forming.

For clients who undergo any type of surgical intervention, monitor for bleeding and pain postoperatively and teach clients to report these problems to their health care provider.

Use of moist heat (e.g., sitz baths) three or four times per day can help promote comfort.

The first postoperative bowel movement may be very painful. The physician usually prescribes stool softeners, such as docusate sodium (Colace) to begin preoperatively and continue after surgery. Analgesics and anti-inflammatory medications are administered postoperatively. A mild laxative should be administered if the client has not had a bowel movement by the third postoperative day.

MALABSORPTION SYNDROME

PATHOPHYSIOLOGY

Malabsorption is a syndrome associated with a variety of disorders and intestinal surgical procedures. It interferes with the ability to absorb nutrients and is a result of a generalized flattening of the mucosa of the small intestine. With various disorders, physiologic mechanisms limit absorption of nutrients because of one or more of the following abnormalities:

- Bile salt deficiencies
- Enzyme deficiencies
- Presence of bacteria
- Disruption of the mucosal lining of the small intestine
- Altered lymphatic and vascular circulation
- Decrease in the gastric or intestinal surface area

The nutrient involved in malabsorption depends on the type and location of the abnormality in the intestinal tract.

Deficiencies of bile salts can lead to malabsorption of fats and fat-soluble vitamins. Bile salt deficiencies can result from decreased synthesis of bile in the liver, bile obstruction, or alteration of bile salt absorption in the small intestine.

Enzymes normally found in the intestine split disaccharides (complex sugars) to monosaccharides (simple sugars). Examples of these enzymes are lactase, sucrase, maltase, and isomaltase. Lactase deficiency is the most common disaccharide enzyme deficiency. Without sufficient amounts of this enzyme, the body is not able to break down lactose. Lactase deficiency can be due to genetic transmission, injury to intestinal mucosa from viral hepatitis, bacterial proliferation in the intestine, or sprue. Deficiencies of the other disaccharide enzymes are rare.

Pancreatic enzymes are also necessary for absorption of vitamin B_{12}. With destruction or obstruction of the pancreas or insufficient pancreatic stimulation, these nutrients are malabsorbed. Chronic pancreatitis, pancreatic carcinoma, resection of the pancreas, and cystic fibrosis can cause these malabsorption problems.

Loops of bowel can accumulate intestinal contents, resulting in bacterial overgrowth, when there is a decrease in peristalsis. Bacteria at these sites break down bile salts, and fewer salts are available for fat absorption. These bacteria can also ingest vitamin B_{12}, which contributes to vitamin B_{12} deficiency. This phenomenon can occur after a gastrectomy or with progressive systemic sclerosis and diabetic enteropathy.

Disruption of the mucosal lining of the intestine is responsible for the malabsorption that occurs with celiac (nontropical) sprue, tropical sprue, Crohn's disease, and ulcerative colitis.

In celiac (nontropical) sprue, the absorptive surface area in the small intestine is lost; there is malabsorption of most nutrients. Celiac sprue is thought to be due to a genetic immune hypersensitivity response to gluten or its breakdown products or to result from the accumulation of gluten in the diet with peptidase deficiency.

Tropical sprue is caused by an infectious agent that has not been identified but is thought to be bacterial. Mucosal changes occur in a more widespread manner than in celiac sprue. However, the changes are not as severe as in celiac sprue. Tropical sprue results in malabsorption of fat, folic acid, and vitamin B_{12} in later stages of the disease.

The inflammation in Crohn's disease interferes with the surface of cells absorbing bile salts and therefore leads to fat malabsorption. In ulcerative colitis, protein loss may occur.

Obstruction to lymphatic flow in the intestine can lead to loss of plasma proteins along with loss of minerals (such as iron, copper, and calcium), vitamin B_{12}, folic acid, and lipids. Lymphatic obstruction can be caused by many conditions. Certain cancers, such as lymphoma, inflammatory states, radiation enteritis, Crohn's disease, Whipple's disease, heart failure, and constrictive pericarditis, are causes of lymphatic obstruction.

Interference with blood flow to the intestinal mucosa, which occurs in celiac and superior mesenteric artery disease, results in malabsorption. With intestinal surgery, there is loss of the surface area needed to facilitate absorption. Resection of the ileum results in vitamin B_{12}, bile salt, and other nutrient deficiencies. Gastric surgery is one of the most common causes of malabsorption and maldigestion. Other conditions associated with maldigestion and malabsorption include small-bowel ischemia and radiation enteritis.

◆ COLLABORATIVE MANAGEMENT

◆ Assessment

Diarrhea is the classic symptom of malabsorption. It occurs secondary to unabsorbed nutrients, which add to the bulk of the stool, and unabsorbed fat. **Steatorrhea** (greater than normal amounts of fat in the feces) is a common sign. Steatorrhea is a result of bile salt deconjugation, nonabsorbed fats, or bacteria in the intestine. Not all clients with malabsorption will have diarrhea; instead, many clients manifest an increased stool mass. Other clinical manifestations include the following:

- Weight loss
- Bloating and flatus (carbohydrate malabsorption)
- Decreased libido
- Easy bruising (purpura)
- Anemia (with iron and folic acid or vitamin B_{12} deficiencies)
- Bone pain (with calcium and vitamin D deficiencies)
- Edema (caused by hypoproteinemia)

Laboratory studies reveal a decrease in mean corpuscular volume (MCV), mean corpuscular hemoglobin (MCH), and mean corpuscular hemoglobin concentration (MCHC). These decreases indicate hypochromic microcytic anemia resulting from iron deficiency. Increased MCV and variable MCH and MCHC values indicate macrocytic anemia resulting from vitamin B_{12} and folic acid deficiencies. Serum iron levels are low in protein malabsorption because of insufficient gastric acid for use of iron. Serum cholesterol levels may be low from decreased absorption and digestion of fat. Low serum calcium levels may indicate malabsorption of vitamin D and amino acids. Low levels of serum vitamin A (retinol) and carotene, its precursor, indicate a bile salt deficiency and malabsorption of fat. Serum albumin and total protein levels are low if protein loss occurs. A quantitative fecal fat analysis is elevated in either malabsorption or maldigestion.

A lactose tolerance test result that shows less than a 20% rise in the blood glucose level over the fasting blood glucose level indicates lactose intolerance. A monosaccharide test validates or rules out lactase deficiency. The xylose absorption test can reveal low urine and serum D-xylose levels if malabsorption in the small intestine is present, a common finding in celiac sprue. An abnormal D-xylose test can indicate bacterial overgrowth in the small intestine.

The Schilling test measures urinary excretion of vitamin B_{12} for diagnosis of pernicious anemia and a variety of other malabsorption syndromes. The bile acid breath test assesses the absorption of bile salt. If the client has bacterial overgrowth, the bile salts will become deconjugated, and the carbon dioxide level in the breath will peak earlier than expected.

Biopsy of the small intestine is performed via an oral endoscopic procedure for diagnosis of tropical sprue or celiac sprue. Ultrasonography is used to diagnose pancreatic tumors and tumors in the small intestine that are causing malabsorption. X-rays of the gastrointestinal (GI) tract reveal pancreatic calcifications, tumors, or other abnormalities that cause malabsorption. Barium enema examination shows mucosal changes representative of celiac sprue or other abnormalities.

Interventions

Interventions for most malabsorption syndromes focus on avoidance of dietary substances that aggravate malabsorption and supplementation of nutrients. Surgical or nonsurgical management of the primary disease may be indicated. Drug therapy may also improve or resolve malabsorption.

Dietary management includes a low-fat diet for clients who have gallbladder disease, severe steatorrhea, cystic fibrosis, and progressive systemic sclerosis. A low-fat diet may or may not be indicated for pancreatic insufficiency, because this disorder improves with enzyme replacement. Some clinicians believe that limitation of fat intake is not necessary with enzyme replacement. Dietary intake of fat is actually beneficial to the client because it has a high number of calories. After a total gastrectomy, a high-protein, high-calorie diet and small, frequent meals are recommended. Lactose-free or lactose-restricted diets are available for clients with lactase deficiency, and gluten-free diets are available for clients with celiac sprue.

The physician prescribes nutritional supplements according to the specific deficiency. Common supplements include the following:

- Water-soluble vitamins, such as folic acid and vitamin B complex
- Fat-soluble vitamins, such as vitamin A, vitamin D, and vitamin K
- Minerals, such as calcium, iron, and magnesium
- Pancreatic enzymes, such as pancrelipase (Pancrease, Viokase)

Antibiotics are used to treat tropical sprue, Whipple's disease, and other disorders involving bacterial overgrowth. Tropical sprue is treated with trimethoprim/sulfamethoxazole (Bactrim, Septra). Bacterial overgrowth can be caused by a variety of disorders but is often treated with tetracycline and metronidazole (Flagyl, Novonidazol✱). Steroids are sometimes given in celiac disease to decrease inflammation.

Drug therapy is used to control the clinical manifestations of malabsorption. Antidiarrheal agents, such as diphenoxylate hydrochloride and atropine sulfate (Lomotil), are often used to control diarrhea and steatorrhea (see Chart 60-1). Anticholinergics, such as dicyclomine hydrochloride (Bentyl, Bentylol✱), are often given before meals to inhibit gastric motility. IV fluids may be necessary to replenish fluid losses associated with diarrhea.

CHART 60-8

BEST PRACTICE for
Special Skin Care for Clients with Chronic Diarrhea

- Use medicated wipes or premoistened disposable wipes rather than toilet tissue to clean the perineal area.
- Clean the perineal area well with mild soap and warm water after each stool; rinse soap from the area well.
- If the physician allows, provide a sitz bath several times per day.
- Apply a thin coat of vitamin A & D ointment or other medicated protective barrier, such as aloe products, after each stool.
- Keep the client off the affected buttock area.
- For open areas, cover with thin DuoDerm or Tegaderm occlusive dressing to promote rapid healing.
- Observe for fungal or yeast infections, which appear as dark red rashes. Obtain prescription for medication if this problem occurs.

Provide special measures to protect the skin when diarrhea occurs (Chart 60-8). Conduct an ongoing assessment for clinical manifestations of malabsorption and relate these to activities and dietary intake. For example, clients with steatorrhea are monitored for fluid and electrolyte imbalances and are encouraged to ingest electrolyte-rich liquids liberally. Teach clients the rationale for dietary, drug, and surgical management of nutritional deficiencies and evaluate interventions on the basis of changes in or resolution of clinical manifestations.

GET READY for the NCLEX Examination!

KEY POINTS

Safe Effective Care Environment

- Be aware that a strangulated hernia can cause ischemia and bowel obstruction, requiring immediate intervention.
- Assess the characteristics of the colostomy stoma, which should be reddish pink and moist; report abnormalities such as ischemia and necrosis (purplish or black) or unusual bleeding to the surgeon.
- Prioritize care for clients experiencing abdominal trauma: First assess airway, breathing, and circulation (ABC), then monitor mental status, vital signs, and skin perfusion to assess for hypovolemic shock.

Health Promotion and Maintenance

- Teach clients with irritable bowel syndrome (IBS) to avoid GI stimulants, such as caffeine, alcohol, and milk and milk products.
- Instruct client on dietary modifications to decrease the occurrence of colorectal cancer (CRC) as listed in Table 60-1.
- Refer clients with familial CRC syndromes for genetic counseling and testing.
- Teach adults over 50 years of age to have routine screening for CRC as listed in Chart 60-2; individuals with genetic predispositions should have earlier and more frequent screening.
- Teach clients and caregivers how to provide colostomy care, including dietary measures, skin care, and ostomy products.
- Refer ostomy clients to the United Ostomy Association and the American Cancer Society for additional information and support groups.
- Teach individuals measures for preventing constipation to minimize hemorrhoid occurrence.
- Teach clients having hemorrhoid surgery to take mild laxatives before and after surgery to decrease discomfort during defecation.

Psychosocial Integrity

- Assess effects of IBS on client lifestyle; recommend stress management techniques.
- Assist the client with CRC with grief work, as listed in Chart 60-3.
- Be aware that having a colostomy is a life-altering event that severely impacts one's body image; issues related to sexuality and fear of acceptance should be discussed.

Physiological Integrity

- Assess clients with IBS for elimination pattern, abdominal pain, and nausea.

- Be aware that minimally invasive inguinal hernia repair is an ambulatory procedure done via laparoscopy; postoperative management requires health teaching regarding rest for a few days and inspection of incisions for signs of infection.
- Monitor clients who have conventional, open herniorrhaphy for ability to void.
- Recognize that surgical procedures for CRC vary depending on tumor location as specified in Table 60-2.
- Consult with the enterostomal therapist (ET) when a client is scheduled for or has a new colostomy.
- Keep the peristomal skin clean and dry; observe for leakage around the pouch seal.
- Provide meticulous perineal wound care for clients having an abdominoperineal (AP) resection, as described in Chart 60-4.
- Recall that bowel sounds are altered in clients with obstruction; absent bowel sounds imply total obstruction.
- Assess the client's nasogastric tube for proper placement, patency, and output at least every 4 hours.
- Monitor clients with bowel obstruction for signs and symptoms of fluid, electrolyte, and acid-base imbalances.
- Be aware that intestinal polyps are usually benign, but can become malignant if not removed.

ADDITIONAL STUDY RESOURCES

Go to your Student CD-ROM for Review Questions for the NCLEX Examination.

evolve Go to http://evolve.elsevier.com/Iggy/ for Integrated Management of Care Questions for the NCLEX Examination.

SELECTED BIBLIOGRAPHY

Asterisk indicates a classic or definitive work on this subject.

*Alderman, J. (1999). Managing irritable bowel syndrome. *ADVANCE for Nurse Practitioners, 7*(1), 40-46.

American Cancer Society. (2003). Colorectal cancer. *CA: A Cancer Journal for Clinicians, 53*(1), 44-51.

American Cancer Society. (2004). *Cancer facts and figures 2004.* Atlanta: Author.

Beackington, E. (2000). Irritable bowel syndrome: An update on treatment options. *Advance for Nurse Practitioners,* October, pp. 32-36.

*Bradley, M., & Pupiales, M. (1997). Essential elements of ostomy care. *American Journal of Nursing, 97*(7), 38-46.

Chung-Park, M. (2002). A look at colorectal cancer screening in women. *Nurse Practitioner, 27*(6), 43-48.

Ellenhorn, J.D.L., Coia, L.R., & Hoff, P.M. (2002). Colorectal and anal cancers. In R. Pazdur, et al. (Eds.). *Cancer management: A multidisciplinary approach* (6th ed., pp. 295-318). Melville, NY: PRR, Inc.

Jacobs, L.A. (2002). Health beliefs of first-degree relatives of individuals with colorectal cancer and participation in health maintenance visits: A population-based survey. *Cancer Nursing, 25*(4), 251-265.

Jarrett, M., Visser, R., Heitkemper, M. (2001). Diet triggers symptoms in women with irritable bowel syndrome: The patient's perspective. *Gastroenterology Nursing, 24*(5), 246-252.

Jemal, A., et al. Cancer statistics, 2002. *A Cancer Journal for Clinicians, 2002, 52*(1), 23-47.

Koloski, N., Talley, N., & Boyce, P. (2000). The impact of functional gastrointestinal disorders on quality of life. *American Journal of Gastroenterology, 95*(1), 67-71.

Lehrer, J.K., & Lichtenstein, G.R. (accessed June 8, 2004). Irritable bowel syndrome. Available at http://www.emedicine.com/med/topic1190.htm.

*Lerman, C., et al. (1999). Genetic testing in families with hereditary nonpolyposis colon cancer. *Journal of the American Medical Association, 281*(17), 1618-1622.

Levin, B., et al. (2003). Emerging technologies in screening for colorectal cancer: CT colonography, immunochemical fecal occult blood tests, and stool screening using molecular markers. *CA: A Cancer Journal for Clinicians, 53*(1), 44-51.

Levins, T.T. (2000). Using ultrasound to assess blunt abdominal trauma. *Nursing2000, 30*(5), 32cc14-32cc15.

Locke, G.R., et al. (2000). Risk factors for irritable bowel syndrome: Role of analgesics and food sensitivities. *American Journal of Gastroenterology, 95*(1), 157-164.

Lustyk, M.K., et al. (2001). Does a physically active lifestyle improve symptoms in women with irritable bowel syndrome? *Gastroenterology Nursing, 24*(3), 129-137.

McCance, K.L., & Huether, S.E. (2002). *Pathophysiology: The biologic basis for disease in adults and children (4th ed.).* St. Louis: Mosby.

Motzer, S.A., et al. (2003). Sense of coherence and quality of life in women with and without irritable bowel syndrome. *Nursing Research, 52*(2), 329-337.

*O'Brien, B. (1999). Coming of age with an ostomy. *American Journal of Nursing, 99*(8), 71-74.

Pontieri-Lewis, V. (2000). Colorectal cancer: Prevention and screening. *MEDSURG Nursing, 9*(1), 9-13.

Schmulson, M., et al. (2000). Correlation of symptom criteria with perception thresholds during rectosigmoid distension in irritable bowel syndrome patients. *American Journal of Gastroenterology, 95*(1), 152-155.

*Shelton, B. (1999). Intestinal obstruction. *AACN Clinical Issues: Advanced Practice in Acute and Critical Care, 10*(4), 478-491.

Shelton, B.K. (2002). Introduction to colorectal cancer. *Seminars in Oncology Nursing, 18*(2), Suppl 2, 2-12.

Toner, B., & Akman, D. (2000). Gender role and irritable bowel syndrome: Literature review and hypothesis. *American Journal of Gastroenterology, 95*(1), 11-16.

Weber, T., et al. (1999). Novel hMLH1 and hMLH2 germline mutations in African-Americans with colorectal cancer. *Journal of the American Medical Association, 281*(24), 2316-2320.

Zangwill, M. (2004). Closing in on colon cancer. *CURE: Cancer updates, research, and education, (3),*1, 46-49.

CHAPTER

61 Interventions for Clients with Inflammatory Intestinal Disorders

MARCIA M. BOEHMKE

LEARNING OUTCOMES

After studying this chapter, you should be able to:

1. Differentiate common types of acute inflammatory bowel disease.
2. Prioritize nursing care for the client who has peritonitis.
3. Discuss the common causes of gastroenteritis.
4. Compare and contrast the pathophysiology and clinical manifestations of ulcerative colitis and Crohn's disease.
5. Analyze priority nursing diagnoses and collaborative problems for clients with chronic inflammatory bowel disease (IBD).
6. Explain the purpose of and nursing implications related to drug therapy for clients with IBD.
7. Formulate a postoperative plan of care for a client undergoing a colon resection/colectomy and colostomy or ileostomy.
8. Identify expected outcomes for clients with chronic IBD.
9. Explain the role of diet therapy in managing the client with diverticular disease.
10. Describe the comfort measures that the nurse can use for the client with an anal abscess, fissure, or fistula.
11. Discuss ways that helminthic infestation, parasitic infection, and food poisoning can be prevented.

Go to your Student CD-ROM for Review Questions for the NCLEX Examination keyed to these Learning Outcomes.

Nonspecific **inflammatory bowel disease (IBD)** is used to describe two conditions of unknown etiology: ulcerative colitis and Crohn's disease. However, IBD is a condition of the small or large intestine or both involving inflammation that can be acute or chronic in duration. Acute conditions are treated and resolved. Chronic forms of IBD are characterized by periods of exacerbation and remission. Inflammatory and infectious intestinal disorders are often difficult to differentiate because many of the characteristics of infectious processes mimic those of more chronic conditions.

ACUTE INFLAMMATORY BOWEL DISORDERS

Appendicitis, peritonitis, and gastroenteritis are the most common acute inflammatory bowel problems. These disorders are potentially life threatening and can have major systemic complications if not treated promptly.

Appendicitis

PATHOPHYSIOLOGY

Appendicitis is acute inflammation of the vermiform appendix–the blind pouch attached to the cecum of the colon that is usually located in the right iliac region, just below the ileocecal valve. The appendix has no known function in adults. Inflammation of the appendix can occur when the lumen (opening) of the appendix is obstructed. Inflammation leads to infection as bacteria invade the wall of the appendix.

When the lumen is blocked, the mucosa continues to secrete fluid until the pressure within the lumen exceeds venous pressure. Blood flow to the appendix is restricted, and infection causes more swelling, which further impedes blood flow. Gangrene from hypoxia or perforation can occur within 24 to 36 hours. If this process occurs slowly, adjacent organs may wall off the area, and a localized abscess develops. If the infectious process occurs rapidly, peritonitis (inflammation of the peritoneum) may result. All complications of peritonitis are serious. Acute appendicitis is the most common cause of acute inflammation in the right lower quadrant. Consequently, it is one of the most common indications for emergency abdominal surgery.

When obstruction is present, calculi composed of fecal material (fecaliths), calcium phosphate–rich mucus, and inorganic salts may be the most common cause of the initial obstruction. Other causes of obstruction include tumors, viral infections, and worms. However, ulceration of the mucosa may be the primary cause of appendicitis. Infection by viral or fungal pathogens has been suggested as the cause of ulceration. Although appendicitis affects a person at any age, the peak incidence is between the ages of 20 and 30 years. Appendicitis affects men and women equally, except before 25 years of age, when males are affected more often than females at a 3:2 ratio.

CONSIDERATIONS FOR OLDER ADULTS

Appendicitis is relatively rare at extremes in age; however, perforation is more common in older people, causing a higher mortality rate. The diagnosis of appendicitis is difficult to establish in older adults because symptoms of pain and tenderness are not as pronounced in this age-group. As a result, a significant number of older clients with appendicitis develop perforation due to a delay in diagnosis.

It is thought that chronic infection of the appendix can occur, but this is not usually the cause of abdominal pain that lasts for weeks or months. Recurrent acute appendicitis does sometimes occur, often with complete remission of inflammation between acute attacks. In rare instances, acute appendicitis may be the first manifestation of Crohn's disease.

COLLABORATIVE MANAGEMENT

Assessment

Early history taking and the identification of risk factors such as adolescent males, familial tendency, and intra-abdominal tumors should be obtained from the client. The most common symptom is abdominal pain, which results from contractions of the appendix or distention of its lumen. With *classic* appendicitis, abdominal pain in the epigastric or periumbilical area is the initial symptom. Pain may not be localized, however, and can exist anywhere in the abdomen or flanks. The pain at this time is described as mild or cramping. Nausea and vomiting follow in 50% to 60% of cases. As the inflammation spreads to the peritoneal surface, the pain becomes more steady and severe and the location shifts to the right lower quadrant. Abdominal pain that increases with cough or movement and is relieved by flexion of the right hip or the knees suggests a perforated appendix with peritonitis. Anorexia is a frequent finding associated with acute appendicitis.

Abdominal tenderness on palpation is the most common, important, and reliable symptom. In later stages of inflammation, tenderness becomes more localized and is noted with palpation of the right lower quadrant. This area is referred to as **McBurney's point;** it is located midway between the anterior iliac crest and the umbilicus in the right lower quadrant (Figure 61-1). The nurse may feel tenseness of the muscles (muscle rigidity) over the tender area. Rigidity over the whole

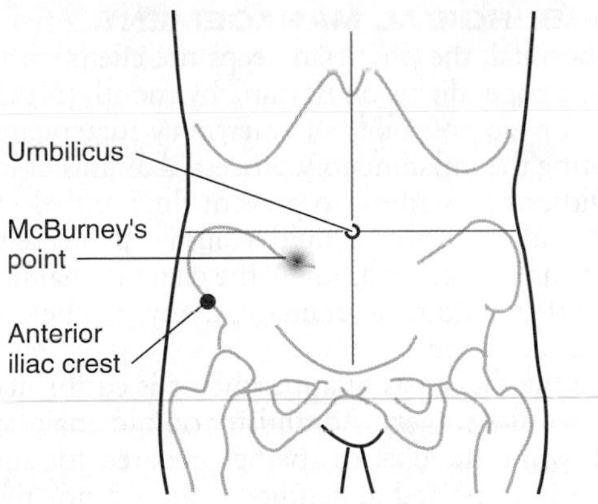

Figure 61-1 ■ McBurney's point is located midway between the anterior iliac crest and the umbilicus in the right lower quadrant. This is the classic area for localized tenderness during the later stages of appendicitis.

abdomen, accompanied by tense positioning and guarding, indicates a perforated appendix with peritonitis.

Perforation (rupture) rarely occurs within 24 hours of the onset of symptoms, but the incidence of peritonitis rises to as high as 80% after 48 hours. **Rebound tenderness** is a term used to describe a sensation of severe pain that occurs after deep pressure is applied and released. This maneuver involves pressing a finger into the abdomen at a point away from the pain and is performed by the physician or advanced-practice nurse.

The client's temperature is usually normal or slightly elevated at 99° to 100.5° F (37.2° to 38° C). A temperature of 101° F (38.2° C) or higher suggests the presence of peritonitis. As the temperature rises, a corresponding rise in pulse rate will be noted.

Because the clinical manifestations associated with many other medical conditions are similar to those of acute appendicitis, arriving at a diagnosis is often difficult. It is important to determine the sequence of symptoms. For example, nausea and vomiting that precede abdominal pain often indicate gastroenteritis.

Clinical manifestations that do not follow the classic pattern can occur as a result of variations in the anatomic location of the appendix. The appendix can be located deep in the pelvis, in the right upper quadrant, or even in the left lower quadrant.

Laboratory findings do not establish the diagnosis, but there is often a moderate elevation of the white blood cell (WBC) count (leukocytosis) to 10,000 to 18,000/mm^3 with a "shift to the left" (an increased number of immature WBCs). A WBC elevation greater than 20,000/mm^3 may indicate a perforated appendix. An ultrasound study may show the presence of an enlarged appendix. If symptoms are recurrent or prolonged, a barium enema or computed tomography (CT) scan can be diagnostic and may reveal the presence of a fecalith.

Interventions

All clients with suspected or confirmed appendicitis are hospitalized and examined by a surgeon. If the diagnosis is questionable, the health care team observes the client before surgical exploration.

NONSURGICAL MANAGEMENT. After admission to the hospital, the physician keeps the client with suspected or known appendicitis on nothing by mouth (NPO) status to prepare for the possibility of emergency surgery and to avoid aggravating the inflammatory process. Administer intravenous (IV) fluids, as prescribed, to prevent fluid and electrolyte imbalance and to replenish fluid volume. If the semi-Fowler's position can be tolerated, advise the client to maintain this position so that abdominal drainage, if any, can be contained in the lower abdomen.

Once the diagnosis of appendicitis is confirmed, the surgeon schedules surgery. Administer opioid analgesics, as prescribed, while the client is being prepared for surgery. The client with suspected appendicitis should not receive laxatives or enemas, which can cause perforation of the appendix. Heat should never be applied to the abdomen because this may increase circulation to the appendix and result in increased inflammation and perforation.

SURGICAL MANAGEMENT. Surgery is required as soon as possible. If the diagnosis is not definitive but the client is at high risk for complications from suspected appendicitis, the surgeon may perform an exploratory laparoscopy or laparotomy to rule out appendicitis. A **laparoscopy** is a minimally invasive procedure in which the surgeon makes several small incisions near the umbilicus, through which a small endoscope is placed. Various instruments are put through the laparoscope to perform the needed procedure. A **laparotomy** is an open approach in which a large abdominal incision is made.

Preoperative Care. Preoperative teaching is often limited because the client is in pain or may be transferred to the operating suite for emergency surgery. The client is prepared for general anesthesia and surgery (see Chapter 20).

Operative Procedures. An **appendectomy** is the removal of the inflamed appendix. In an open, conventional, and uncomplicated appendectomy, the surgeon removes the appendix through an incision approximately 3 inches (7.5 cm) long in the right lower quadrant. The incision is larger if the appendix is in an atypical position or if peritonitis is present. Most uncomplicated appendectomies today are done via **laparoscopy**.

Postoperative Care. Postoperative care of the client who has undergone an appendectomy includes the care required for any client who has received general anesthesia (see Chapter 22). For clients who have undergone a conventional appendectomy, the incision is located over McBurney's point if the appendix was in the typical location. The incision may be as long as the length of the abdomen, depending on the area explored in surgery and the location of the appendix. Drains may have been inserted during the procedure if an abscess was present or if the appendix perforated.

If peritonitis was present, a nasogastric (NG) tube is placed to decompress the stomach and prevent abdominal distention. IV antibiotics are typically prescribed if peritonitis or abscess is present. Opioid analgesics are administered for pain as needed. The client is typically out of bed on the evening of surgery or the first postoperative day. The client who has had an uncomplicated appendectomy via laparoscopy may stay overnight or may be discharged on the day of surgery. In this case, no NG tubes or drains are needed. The client experiences less pain and recovers much more quickly with this surgical approach. Most clients can return to usual activities in 1 to 2 weeks.

The client who has undergone an open, uncomplicated appendectomy usually recovers rapidly and can resume normal activity in 2 to 4 weeks. If surgery has been complicated by perforation or peritonitis, the client may be hospitalized for as long as 5 to 7 days.

Peritonitis

Peritonitis is an acute inflammation of the visceral/parietal peritoneum and endothelial lining of the abdominal cavity, or peritoneum. Peritonitis can be classified as primary or secondary, localized or generalized. Peritonitis is a life-threatening illness and is associated with several abdominal disorders.

PATHOPHYSIOLOGY

Normally the peritoneal cavity contains approximately 50 mL of sterile fluid (transudate), which serves to prevent friction in the abdominal cavity during peristalsis. When the peritoneal cavity is contaminated by bacteria, the body initially produces an inflammatory reaction that walls off a localized area to fight the infection. This local reaction involves vascular dilation and increased capillary permeability, allowing transport of leukocytes and subsequent phagocytosis of the offending organisms. If this walling off process fails, the inflammation spreads and contamination becomes massive, resulting in diffuse peritonitis.

Complications of Peritonitis

Vascular dilation continues, along with hyperemia (increased blood flow) and a fluid shift. The body responds to the infectious process by shunting extra blood to the area of inflammation. Fluid is shifted from the extracellular fluid (ECF) compartment into the peritoneal cavity, connective tissues, and gastrointestinal (GI) tract ("third spacing"). This shift of fluid out of the vascular space can result in a significant decrease in circulatory volume. The rate of decreasing circulatory volume is proportional to the degree of peritoneal involvement. Severely decreased circulatory volume can result in insufficient perfusion of the kidneys, leading to renal failure with electrolyte imbalance.

Peristalsis slows or stops in response to severe peritoneal infection, and the lumen of the bowel becomes distended with gas and fluid. Fluid that normally flows to the small bowel and the colon for reabsorption accumulates in the intestine in volumes of 7 to 8 L daily. The toxins or bacteria responsible for the peritonitis can also enter the bloodstream from the peritoneal area, leading to bacteremia or **septicemia** (bacterial invasion of the blood).

Respiratory problems can occur as a result of increased abdominal pressure against the diaphragm from intestinal distention and fluid shifts to the peritoneal cavity. Pain can interfere with ventilatory efforts when the client has an increased oxygen demand because of the infectious process.

Types of Peritonitis

Primary peritonitis is an acute bacterial infection that develops as a result of contamination of the peritoneum through the vascular system. Tuberculous peritonitis that arises from a tuberculin infection originating elsewhere in the body is a type of primary peritonitis. Clients with alcoholic cirrhosis and ascites, in the absence of a perforated organ, often manifest peritonitis, which may be due to leakage of bacteria through the wall of the intestine.

Secondary peritonitis is usually caused by bacterial invasion as a result of an acute abdominal disorder. Secondary peritonitis can develop as a result of a gangrenous bowel, perforation of the viscera by blunt or penetrating trauma, or bile leakage.

Etiology

Peritonitis is caused by contamination of the peritoneal cavity by bacteria or chemicals. Bacteria gain entry into the peritoneum by perforation or from an external penetrating wound. The most common causes of bacterial peritonitis are appendicitis and perforations associated with peptic ulcer disease, diverticulitis, a gangrenous gallbladder, or bowel obstruction. Bacterial invasion can also occur from an ascending infection through the reproductive tract, as in salpingitis (fallopian tube inflammation) or a septic abortion. Other causes of peritonitis include perforating tumors, ulcerative colitis, foreign bodies (from trauma), leakage or contamination during a surgical procedure, and infection by skin pathogens in clients undergoing continuous ambulatory peritoneal dialysis (CAPD). Bacteria responsible for peritonitis include *Escherichia coli, Streptococcus, Staphylococcus, Pneumococcus,* and *Gonococcus.* Chemical peritonitis arises from leakage of bile, pancreatic enzymes, and gastric acid.

COLLABORATIVE MANAGEMENT

Assessment

HISTORY

Question the client regarding a history of abdominal pain and determine whether the pain is localized or generalized. Ask about a history of a low-grade fever or recent spikes in temperature.

PHYSICAL ASSESSMENT/CLINICAL MANIFESTATIONS

Physical findings of peritonitis (Chart 61-1) depend on several factors: the stage of the disease, the ability of the body to localize the process by walling off the infection, and whether the inflammation has progressed to generalized peritonitis. The client typically appears acutely ill, lying still, possibly with the knees flexed. Movement is guarded, and the client may report and show signs of pain (e.g., facial grimacing) with coughing or movement of any type. During inspection, observe for progressive abdominal distention if the inflammation markedly reduces intestinal motility. Auscultate for bowel sounds, but these usually disappear with progression of the inflammation.

The cardinal signs of peritonitis are abdominal pain and tenderness. In the client with localized peritonitis, the abdomen is tender on palpation in a well-defined area of the abdomen with rebound tenderness in this area. With generalized peritonitis, tenderness is widespread. *Abdominal wall rigidity is a classic finding, sometimes referred to as a "board-like" abdomen.* The client may have a high fever because of the infectious process, with tachycardia occurring in response to the fever. Assess whether the client has dry mucous membranes and a low urine output. The latter occurs because fluid accumulates in the peritoneal cavity, the GI tract, and connective tissues, resulting in a fluid deficit in the vascular space (dehydration). Nausea and vomiting may also be present. Hiccups may occur as a result of diaphragmatic irritation. Depending on the severity of the peritonitis, the nurse may find that the client has a compromised respiratory status.

CHART 61-1

KEY FEATURES of Peritonitis

- Rigid, boardlike abdomen (classic)
- Abdominal pain (localized, poorly localized, or referred to the shoulder or thorax)
- Distended abdomen
- Nausea, anorexia, vomiting
- Diminishing bowel sounds
- Inability to pass flatus or feces
- Rebound tenderness in the abdomen
- High fever
- Tachycardia
- Dehydration from high fever (poor skin turgor)
- Decreased urine output
- Hiccups
- Possible compromise in respiratory status

DIAGNOSTIC ASSESSMENT

White blood cell (WBC) counts are commonly elevated to $20{,}000/mm^3$ with a high neutrophil count. A series of blood culture studies may be done to determine whether septicemia has occurred and to identify the causative organism to enable appropriate therapy. The health care provider orders laboratory tests to assess fluid and electrolyte balance and renal status, including the following:

- Electrolytes
- Blood urea nitrogen (BUN)
- Creatinine
- Hemoglobin
- Hematocrit

Arterial blood gas values are obtained to assess respiratory function and acid-base balance.

Abdominal x-rays may be obtained to assess for free air or fluid in the abdominal cavity, which indicates perforation. The x-rays may also show dilation, edema, and inflammation of the small and large intestines. An abdominal sonogram is also useful in locating the problem.

The physician may perform a diagnostic peritoneal lavage by instilling 1 L of fluid through a peritoneal dialysis catheter. Lavage fluid positive for peritonitis is characterized by the following: more than 500 WBCs/mL of fluid, more than 50,000 red blood cells (RBCs)/mL, or the presence of bacteria on a Gram stain. Bile-stained green fluid may indicate a ruptured gallbladder or perforated intestine, which can lead to chemical peritonitis.

Interventions

All clients with peritonitis are hospitalized because of the severe nature of the illness. If complications are extensive, the client may be admitted to a critical care unit. Nursing interventions focus on the early identification of complications.

NONSURGICAL MANAGEMENT. The physician prescribes IV fluids and broad-spectrum antibiotics immediately after establishing the diagnosis of peritonitis. IV fluids are necessary to replace fluids collected in the peritoneum and bowel. Monitor daily weight and intake and output carefully to assess fluid status. A nasogastric (NG) tube is inserted to decompress the stomach and the intestine, and the client is on NPO status. Administer oxygen, as prescribed, according to the client's respiratory status. The health care provider will most likely institute pain management with IV analgesics, such as morphine sulfate administered via a patient-controlled analgesia (PCA) pump. Expect the health care provider to request a surgical consultation in the event that surgery becomes necessary.

SURGICAL MANAGEMENT. Abdominal surgery is the optimal treatment for identifying and repairing the cause of the peritonitis. If the client is so critically ill that surgery would be life threatening, it may be delayed. Surgery focuses on controlling the contamination, removing foreign material from the peritoneal cavity, and draining collected fluid.

The surgeon typically performs an **exploratory laparotomy** to remove or repair the inflamed or perforated organ. The abdominal cavity is opened surgically and explored for inflamed and perforated organs or other abnormalities. For example, an appendectomy is performed for an inflamed appendix; a colon resection, with or without a colostomy, is indicated for a perforated diverticulum or perforated colon secondary to a tumor. Before the abdominal cavity is closed, the surgeon irrigates the peritoneum with antibiotic solutions. Several catheters may also be inserted to drain the cavity and provide a route for irrigation postoperatively.

The preoperative care is similar to that described in Chapter 20 for clients having general anesthesia. Postoperative care is also similar to that for other clients undergoing surgery (see Chapter 22). Clients with peritonitis may have actual or potential multisystem complications. Therefore monitor the level of consciousness, vital signs, respiratory status (respiratory rate and breath sounds), and fluid and electrolyte status (intake and output and laboratory values) at least hourly immediately after surgery.

Positioning. Maintain the client in a semi-Fowler's position to promote drainage of peritoneal contents in the inferior region of the abdominal cavity. This position also facilitates adequate respiratory excursion because the diaphragm and abdominal contents are impinging on respiratory muscles.

Wound Care. The client is likely to have multiple incisions and drains. Because contamination at the time of surgery impedes healing of an incision with edges well approximated (by first intention), incisions are allowed to heal by second or third intention. These incisions necessitate meticulous care involving manual irrigation or packing as ordered by the surgeon. If the surgeon requests peritoneal irrigation through a drain, maintain strict sterile technique during manual irrigation, usually by using a catheter-tipped syringe. Determine that the client is not retaining irrigant by ensuring the absence of abdominal distention or pain and by monitoring irrigant intake and output.

As a result of the loss of fluids from the extracellular space to the peritoneal cavity, IV fluid replacement and maintenance are indicated for all clients with peritonitis. Fluid volume deficit also occurs as a result of NG suctioning and NPO status. Normal saline or a balanced saline solution with potassium is administered IV according to electrolyte, BUN, and serum creatinine values. To assess fluid volume, monitors vital signs, urine output, skin turgor, integrity of mucous membranes, and most importantly weight. Also assess for edema from third spacing.

Community-Based Care

The length of hospitalization depends on the extent and severity of the infectious process. Clients who have a localized abscess drained and who respond to antibiotics and IV fluids without multisystem complications are discharged in less than a week. Those who experience complications of peritonitis, along with sepsis or shock, may require mechanical ventilation or hemodialysis, with hospital stays lasting longer. Discharge planning varies with the degree of involvement of all body systems. Some clients may be transferred to a transitional care unit to complete their antibiotic therapy and recovery.

If the client is being discharged to home, assess his or her ability to function at home with the added task of incision care and a diminished activity tolerance. Provide the client and family or significant other with written and oral instructions to report the following:

- Unusual or foul-smelling drainage
- Swelling, redness, or warmth or bleeding from the incision site
- A temperature higher than 101° F (38.2° C)
- The presence of abdominal pain

Also instruct the client in proper handwashing and dressing change techniques, which include directions to dress wounds separately to avoid cross-contamination.

The physician typically prescribes an oral opioid analgesic and possibly an antibiotic. Review information about these medications with the client and caregiver. For clients taking opioid analgesics for any length of time, a stool softener should be prescribed.

Explain diet and activity limitations. Diet depends on the type of surgery performed and the client's specific food tolerances at discharge. All clients are told to refrain from any lifting for *at least* 6 weeks. Other activity limitations are made on an individual basis with the physician's recommendation.

Peritonitis is a life-threatening and consequently frightening illness. Incisional care can be demanding, and activity intolerance can be overwhelming. If complications have resolved, the nurse reassures clients that they can realistically expect to resume their previous lifestyle. Convalescence is often longer than that required for other types of surgery, however, because of the multisystem involvement.

Clients with an incision healing by second or third intention may require dressings, solution, and catheter-tipped syringes to irrigate the wound. A home care nurse may be needed to assess, irrigate, or pack the wound and change the dressing as needed. If a client needs assistance with activities of daily living, a home care aide or temporary placement in a skilled care facility may be indicated. The case manager collaborates with the health care team to determine the most appropriate setting for community-based care.

Gastroenteritis

PATHOPHYSIOLOGY

Acute diarrheal illnesses cause significant morbidity among young children and older adults, especially in less-industrialized nations of the world. **Gastroenteritis** is an increase in the frequency and water content of stools or vomiting as a result of inflammation of the mucous membranes of the stomach and intestinal tract. It primarily affects the small bowel and can be of either viral or bacterial origin. Both forms have similar manifestations and are considered self-limiting in their course unless complications occur. All organisms that are implicated in gastroenteritis cause diarrhea; however, the organisms discussed in this section have distinguishing characteristics.

Authors disagree on classification of the infectious diseases described as gastroenteritis. Some include shigellosis when discussing gastroenteritis; others consider shigellosis separately as a dysentery type of illness. Dysenteries affect the *large* bowel; gastroenteritis affects the *small* bowel. Other authors classify infectious disease of the intestine as bacterial, viral, or parasitic, without using the term *gastroenteritis.*

Food poisoning is sometimes described in conjunction with gastroenteritis, with specific reference to the organism causing the food poisoning. Gastroenteritis, however, differs from food poisoning with regard to transmission in the body, incubation time, and effect on immunity.

The following discussion of gastroenteritis includes the epidemic viral form and the bacterial forms (*Campylobacter, Escherichia coli,* and shigellosis) (Table 61-1). Organisms associated with food poisoning and parasitic infections are discussed under Food Poisoning, p. 1365.

Infection with viral and bacterial organisms can produce gastrointestinal (GI) illnesses in which watery diarrhea is the primary feature. These disorders can be caused by noninflammatory, inflammatory, or penetrating mechanisms. The infecting organism (e.g., enterotoxigenic *E. coli*) can release enterotoxin (a noninflammatory toxic substance specific to the intestinal mucosa), which results in diarrhea. The organism (e.g., *Shigella* or *Campylobacter*) can also attach itself to mucosal epithelium without penetrating it. Cells of the intestinal villi are then destroyed, and malabsorption results. Infections that are mediated by bacterial toxins cause the absorptive capacity of the distal small bowel and proximal colon to be overcome, resulting in diarrhea. Finally, the organism can penetrate the intestine, causing cellular destruction, necrosis, and a potential for ulceration. Diarrhea occurs often with white blood cells (WBCs) or red blood cells (RBCs) present in the stool.

All these situations result in *increased* GI motility, with fluids and electrolytes being secreted into the intestine at rapid rates. Invading organisms have increased capabilities of attaching to the intestinal mucosa if the normal intestinal flora is altered. This can occur in clients who are receiving antibiotics, are malnourished, or are debilitated. Two groups of viruses, the rotaviruses (which affect young children) and Norwalk virus, as well as bacterial pathogens, are primary etiologic agents involved in the development of gastroenteritis.

TABLE 61-1 Common Types of Gastroenteritis and Their Characteristics

Type	Characteristics
Viral Gastroenteritis	
Epidemic viral	Caused by many parvovirus-type organisms Transmitted by the fecal-oral route in food and water Incubation period 10-51 hr Communicable during acute illness
Rotarvirus and Norwalk virus	Transmitted by the fecal-oral route and possibly the respiratory route Incubation in 48 hr Rotavirus is most common in infants and young children Norwalk virus affects young children and adults
Bacterial Gastroenteritis	
Campylobacter enteritis	Transmitted by the fecal-oral route or by contact with infected animals or infants Incubation period 1-10 days Communicable for 2-7 weeks
Escherichia coli diarrhea	Transmitted by fecally contaminated food, water, or fomites
Shigellosis	Transmitted by direct and indirect fecal-oral routes Incubation period 1-7 days Communicable during the acute illness to 4 wk after the illness Humans possibly carriers for months

Types of Gastroenteritis

VIRAL GASTROENTERITIS

Norwalk virus infection can occur year-round and affects adults and children alike. This virus is spread by the oral-fecal route and is responsible for one third of all epidemics of viral gastroenteritis in developed countries. The virus is also a common cause of waterborne epidemics of gastroenteritis.

BACTERIAL GASTROENTERITIS

The following are the three common types of bacterial gastroenteritis:

- *E. coli* diarrhea ("traveler's diarrhea")
- *Campylobacter enteritis* (another "traveler's diarrhea")
- *Shigellosis* (bacillary dysentery)

E. coli is the most common organism implicated in traveler's diarrhea. The reservoirs of *E. coli* are humans, who are often asymptomatic. The organism is transmitted through fecally contaminated food, water, or fomites (any other substance that transmits infection).

The etiologic feature of *Campylobacter* enteritis is the bacterium *Campylobacter jejuni;* reservoirs are domestic or wild animals and birds. *C. jejuni* is transmitted through the fecal-oral route by ingestion of water or food contaminated with feces or by direct contact with infected animals or infants. Incubation ranges from 1 to 10 days. The organism is communicable for several days to weeks throughout the course of the infection (usually 2 to 7 weeks).

Shigellosis is caused by infection with *Shigella* bacteria. Direct or indirect fecal-oral transmission can occur from an infected person or carrier. The incubation period before the illness is 1 to 7 days. The illness can be communicated during the acute phase and for up to 4 weeks after the onset of illness. A person can be a carrier of this illness for months after the acute illness.

Incidence/Prevalence

As a group, acute GI illnesses are the second most common disease worldwide. Acute diarrheal illnesses are the most common cause of morbidity and mortality among children and older adults in Asia, Africa, and Latin America. Gastroenteritis often occurs in epidemic outbreaks.

Campylobacter enteritis occurs worldwide, commonly in epidemic outbreaks. Its incidence is highest during warm months. Diarrhea caused by *E. coli* also occurs worldwide, commonly in epidemics. The highest incidence is in areas of poor sanitation during warm months. Shigellosis occurs worldwide in every age-group but most frequently in children under the age of 10 years. Children and older adults are more susceptible to *Shigella* because of their immature or depressed immune systems. Outbreaks of shigellosis are common in areas with crowded living conditions.

COLLABORATIVE MANAGEMENT

Assessment

The history elicited from the client can provide information related to the potential cause of the illness. Question the client regarding a recent history of travel, especially to tropical regions of Asia, Africa, or Central or South America. Traveler's diarrhea can begin 3 days to 2 weeks after the client's arrival.

The client who has gastroenteritis usually appears ill. Nausea and vomiting can occur with all types of gastroenteritis but are usually limited to the first 1 or 2 days of the illness. All clients with gastroenteritis classically have diarrhea, which varies in consistency and amount with the causative organism.

In clients with epidemic viral gastroenteritis, myalgia (muscle aches), headache, and malaise are often reported. Note any slight abdominal distention, auscultate for hyperactive bowel sounds, and be mindful of any diffuse tenderness on palpation. However, there should be *no* rebound tenderness, which might indicate peritonitis. Depending on the amount of fluids lost through diarrhea and vomiting, the client may have varying degrees of dehydration manifested by the following:

- Poor skin turgor
- Dry mucous membranes
- Orthostatic blood pressure changes
- Hypotension
- Oliguria

In some cases, dehydration may be severe, and shock may occur if diarrhea is prolonged. Dehydration occurs rapidly in older adults and may require hospitalization.

Diarrhea associated with epidemic viral gastroenteritis is typically limited to 24 to 48 hours. Infection with the Norwalk virus is characterized by the rapid onset of nausea, abdominal cramps, vomiting, and diarrhea. The illness is usually mild, lasting 24 to 48 hours. *Campylobacter* enteritis is a more severe disease with foul-smelling stools that contain blood and that can number 20 to 30 per day for up to 7 days. *E. coli* gastroenteritis may or may not involve blood or mucus in the stool; diarrhea can last for up to 10 days. *Shigella* causes stools containing blood and mucus, which can continue for up to 5 days.

As part of the laboratory assessment, Gram stain of stool is usually done before culture. Many white blood cells (WBCs) on Gram stain suggest shigellosis. The presence of WBCs and red blood cells (RBCs) in the stool indicates *Campylobacter* gastroenteritis.

A stool culture that is positive for enterotoxigenic *E. coli* is diagnostic of *E. coli* diarrhea. Culture of stool that is positive for *Shigella* when pus cells or WBCs are present in the stool is diagnostic of shigellosis.

Interventions

For clients with most types of gastroenteritis, supportive treatment is instituted. Therapy is focused on fluid replacement, and the amount and route of fluid administration are determined by fluid status.

Fluid Replacement. For mild cases of gastroenteritis, the client is treated on an ambulatory care basis or in the nursing home if he or she is a resident there. If the fluid volume is severely depleted, the client is admitted to the hospital for administration of IV fluids. For older clients at home or in a long-term care setting, oral rehydration therapy (ORT) with commercially prepared rehydration products, such as Resol, may prevent hospitalization.

Obtain a weight, orthostatic blood pressure, and other vital sign measurements at admission. Hypotonic IV fluids, such as half-strength normal saline (0.45% sodium chloride), are infused as prescribed. Monitor the client's vital signs, intake and output, and weight. A rapid gain or loss of 1 kg (2.2 pounds) of body weight is equivalent to the gain or loss of 1 L of fluid. Standard precautions are consistently observed when handling vomitus and stool.

The health care provider may prescribe a potassium supplement to be added to IV fluids if the serum potassium level is low. To help assess renal function and prevent hyperkalemia, verify that the client is voiding before and during potassium replacement. The client is advised to rest in bed, especially during periods of nausea or vomiting.

Depending on the type of gastroenteritis, the local health department may need to be notified. It is mandatory that every case of shigellosis be reported. In some endemic areas, *Campylobacter* enteritis needs to be reported on a case-by-case basis. Other types of gastroenteritis must be reported only if they occur in epidemic proportions.

Diet Therapy. Diet therapy is the same for the client who remains at home as for the client in the hospital. If the client is not actively vomiting, recommend small volumes of clear liquids with electrolytes (e.g., Pedialyte) for 24 hours. The frequency and amount of oral intake can be increased if nausea and vomiting are *not* present. If nausea and vomiting continue, suggest that food and fluids be withheld until these symptoms subside. Advise the client *not* to drink water because it does not contain any electrolytes to replace those lost. After 24 hours, the diet for most clients can be advanced to include saltine crackers, toast, and jelly. When the client can tolerate this diet, bland foods (e.g., nonfat soup, custard, yogurt, cottage cheese, mashed or baked potatoes, cooked vegetables) can be added. Caffeine is avoided because it can increase intestinal motility. The client may progress to a regular diet as tolerated.

Drug Therapy. Drugs that suppress intestinal motility, such as anticholinergics and antiemetics, are *not* routinely given for bacterial or viral gastroenteritis. Use of these drugs can prevent the infecting organisms from being eliminated from the body. If the health care provider determines that antiperistaltic agents are necessary, an initial dose of loperamide (Imodium) 4 mg can be administered orally, followed by 2 mg after each loose stool, up to 16 mg daily. Bismuth subsalicylate (Pepto-Bismol) 30 mL or two tablets every 30 minutes for a maximum of eight doses can be given to reduce the watery volume of the stool.

Treatment with antibiotics may be warranted if the gastroenteritis is due to bacterial infection with fever and severe diarrhea. The health care provider may prescribe norfloxacin (Chibroxin, Noroxin) 400 mg twice daily PO or ciprofloxacin (Cipro) 500 mg twice daily PO for 3 days. If the gastroenteritis is due to shigellosis, anti-infective agents, such as trimethoprim/sulfamethoxazole (Septra DS, Bactrim DS, Roubac*), are administered.

For relatively short-term diarrhea of 24 to 48 hours' duration, the diagnosis is based primarily on the client's history and clinical manifestations without validation by a stool examination. When diarrhea is severe or persists for long periods, the stool is examined in an effort to determine the causative organism and to begin specific treatment. It should be determined whether the diarrhea is caused by *Salmonella* or by parasites because these organisms respond to specific medications (see Parasitic Infection, p. 1362). Diarrhea that continues longer than 10 days is probably *not* due to gastroenteritis, and a thorough investigation for the cause is warranted.

Skin Care. Frequent stools that are rich in electrolytes and enzymes, as well as frequent wiping and washing of the anal region, can irritate the skin. Teach the client to avoid toilet paper and harsh soaps. Ideally, the client can gently clean the area with warm water or absorbent cotton, followed by thorough drying with absorbent cotton. Cream, oil, or gel can be applied to a damp, warm washcloth to remove excrement adhering to excoriated skin. Hydrocortisone cream or protective barrier cream should be applied to the skin between stools. Witch hazel compresses (e.g., Tucks) and sitz baths for 10 minutes, two to three times daily, can also relieve discomfort.

If leakage of stool is a problem, the client can put absorbent cotton next to the anal orifice and keep it in place with snug underwear. For clients who are incontinent, remind assistive nursing personnel to keep the perineal and buttock areas clean and dry. The use of incontinent pads instead of briefs allows air to circulate to the skin and prevents irritation.

Health Teaching. During the acute phase of the illness, teach the client about the importance of fluid replacement. The client should follow the diet, described earlier under Diet Therapy, p. 1344. Instruction of the client and family about the importance of minimizing the risk of transmission of gastroenteritis is also important. Furthermore, clients are advised to do the following:

- Wash hands meticulously with an antibacterial soap, especially after bowel movements, and maintain good personal hygiene.
- Restrict the use of glasses, dishes, eating utensils, and tubes of toothpaste to themselves only.
- Maintain clean bathroom facilities to avoid exposure to stool.
- Inform the health care provider if symptoms persist beyond 3 days.

Clients adhere to these precautions for up to 7 weeks after the illness or up to several months if *Shigella* was the offending organism. If the client is employed as a food handler, the public health department should be consulted for recommendations about the return to work (Chart 61-2).

CHART 61-2

CLIENT EDUCATION GUIDE

Measures to Prevent the Transmission of Gastroenteritis

- Wash your hands meticulously with an antibacterial soap, especially after having a bowel movement.
- Do not share your dishes, glasses, or toothpaste.
- Keep the commode clean to prevent exposure to your stool.
- Do not prepare or handle food that will be consumed by others.

CHRONIC INFLAMMATORY BOWEL DISEASE

Chronic inflammatory bowel disease (chronic IBD, also sometimes just called IBD) refers to several inflammatory disorders of the gastrointestinal (GI) tract with no known etiology. Chronic IBDs may be divided into two major groups: ulcerative colitis and Crohn's disease (Table 61-2).

Ulcerative Colitis

PATHOPHYSIOLOGY

Ulcerative colitis (UC) is one of a group of bowel diseases of unknown etiology, characterized by remissions and exacerbations ("flare-ups"). This chronic inflammatory process affects the mucosal lining of the colon or rectum. It can result in loose stools containing blood and mucus, poor absorption of vital nutrients, and thickening of the colon wall. Over time, the client experiences episodes of abdominal discomfort and extraintestinal (other than intestinal) manifestations of the disease that cause disruption of lifestyle. The affected client may have only minor periodic health problems, necessitating only ambulatory care, or the client may have serious problems, such as malnutrition and physical debilitation, requiring multiple hospitalizations.

Ulcerative colitis is characterized by diffuse inflammation of the intestinal mucosa; the result is a loss of surface epithelium with ulceration and possibly abscess formation. Generally the disease begins in the rectum and proceeds in a uni-

TABLE 61-2 Differential Features of Ulcerative Colitis and Crohn's Disease

Feature	Ulcerative Colitis	Crohn's Disease
Location	Begins in the rectum and proceeds in a continuous manner toward the cecum	Most often in the terminal ileum, with patchy involvement through all layers of the bowel
Etiology	Unknown	Unknown
Peak incidence at age	15-25 yr and 55-65 yr	15-40 yr
Stools	10-20 liquid, bloody stools per day	5-6 soft, loose stools per day, rarely bloody
Common complications	Hemorrhage Perforation Fistulas Nutritional deficiencies	Fistulas Nutritional deficiencies

TABLE 61-3 Complications of Ulcerative Colitis and Crohn's Disease

Complication	Description
Hemorrhage/perforation	Lower gastrointestinal bleeding results from erosion of the bowel wall.
Abscess formation	Localized pockets of infection develop in the ulcerated bowel lining.
Toxic megacolon	Paralysis of the colon causes dilation and subsequent bowel obstruction.
Malabsorption	Essential nutrients cannot be absorbed through the diseased intestinal wall, causing anemia and malnutrition (most common in Crohn's disease).
Bowel obstruction	Obstruction results from toxic megacolon or cancer.
Fistulas	Fistulas can occur anywhere but usually track between the bowel and bladder. Pyuria and fecaluria result.
Colorectal cancer	Clients with ulcerative colitis for 7-10 yr or longer have a high risk for colorectal cancer. This complication accounts for about one third of all deaths related to ulcerative colitis.
Extraintestinal complications	Complications include arthritis, hepatic and biliary disease (especially cholelithiasis), oral and skin lesions, and ocular disorders, such as iritis. The cause is unknown.

form, continuous manner proximally toward the cecum. The process progresses to epithelial cell damage and loss, leaving areas of ulceration, redness, and bleeding in the *acute* stage.

As the disease course progresses, *chronic* changes in the colon occur. Fibrosis and retraction of the bowel result in muscle hypertrophy, deposition of fat and fibrous tissue, and a narrower and shorter colon. With long-term disease, dysplastic changes to the surface epithelium occur. These changes are associated with an increased risk of colon cancer.

Complications of UC include the following:

- Intestinal perforation with resultant peritonitis and fistula formation
- Toxic megacolon
- Hemorrhage
- Increased risk of colon cancer
- Abscess formation
- Malabsorption
- Bowel obstruction
- Extraintestinal clinical manifestations, such as arthritis

Table 61-3 describes these common complications.

Etiology and Genetic Risk

The exact cause of UC is unknown. A genetic basis of the disease has been proposed because of the increased incidence seen in families, certain ethnic groups, and twins. Immunologic hypotheses, including autoimmune dysfunction, have been explored because of the extraintestinal manifestations of the disease. One hypothesis suggests that IBD results from an abnormal response to normal flora present in the intestines; another possibility is that there may be a defect in intestinal permeability that permits antigens to leak through the mucosa, stimulating an inflammatory response. Psychological factors have also been implicated because stress often results in a flare-up of the disease. However, little evidence has been found to relate psychological factors to the cause of the disease.

Incidence/Prevalence

There is a higher geographic distribution of the disease in northern Europe and North America. The annual incidence of ulcerative colitis is about 2 to 10 new cases per 100,000 persons. The prevalence is 40 to 100 cases per 100,000 people in the United States. There is a 10-fold risk of the disease if an individual has a first-degree relative with the disease.

CULTURAL CONSIDERATIONS

Ulcerative colitis is four to five times more common among people of Jewish origin and commonly affects white individuals in developed Western society. It is seen more often in individuals of Jewish European or Ashkenazi origin but not in those of Sephardic origin. Although the disease is more common in white individuals, the incidence in black individuals is increasing.

Peak incidence is between the ages of 15 and 25 years, with another peak occurring between ages of 55 and 65 years. Females are more often affected than men.

COLLABORATIVE MANAGEMENT

Assessment

HISTORY

Collect data on any family history of inflammatory bowel disease (IBD) and previous and current therapy for the illness, as well as dates and types of surgery. Obtaining a diet history is essential. It should include the client's usual dietary patterns and the relationship of elimination patterns to intolerance of milk and milk products and greasy, fried, spicy, or hot foods. A history of weight loss may be seen in clients with severe disease.

Ask about the symptoms of acute ulcerative colitis, which often include abdominal pain, cramping, urgency, and diarrhea with up to 10 to 20 liquid, bloody stools per day, as well as anorexia and fatigue. Furthermore, question the client regarding his or her usual bowel elimination pattern; the color, consistency, and character of stools; and the presence or absence of blood in all stools. Note any relationship between the occurrence of diarrhea and the timing of meals, pain, emotional distress, and activity. Question the client regarding extraintestinal symptoms such as arthritis, mouth sores, vision problems, and skin disorders.

PHYSICAL ASSESSMENT/CLINICAL MANIFESTATIONS

The client with ulcerative colitis may have symptoms that vary with the acuteness of onset and with complications of the disease process. They may complain of abdominal pain, bloody diarrhea, and **tenesmus** (uncontrollable straining).

Vital signs are usually within normal limits in mild disease. In more severe cases, the client may have a low-grade fever (99° to 100° F [37.2° to 37.8° C]). The physical assessment findings are typically nonspecific, and in milder cases the physical examination may be normal.

Note any mild abdominal distention along the colon. Palpation may reveal areas of increased or localized tenderness. Rebound tenderness may suggest peritonitis. You should further note any localized areas of abdominal pain or cramping over areas of diseased bowel. The client may be febrile and tachycardic, indicating possible complications, such as peritonitis, dehydration, and bowel perforation.

PSYCHOSOCIAL ASSESSMENT

The intestinal and extraintestinal symptoms associated with ulcerative colitis can be taxing. Evaluate the client's understanding of the illness and its impact on his or her lifestyle. Encourage and support the client while simultaneously exploring the following:

- The relationship of life events to disease exacerbations
- Stress factors that produce symptoms
- Family and social support systems
- Concerns regarding the possible genetic basis and associated cancer risks of the disease

Many clients are very apprehensive regarding the frequency of stools and the presence of blood. The uncontrollability of the disease symptoms, particularly diarrhea, can be disruptive and stress producing. More severe illness may limit the client's activities outside the home. As a result of the excessive diarrhea, the client may become dependent on the proximity of a bathroom. Eating may be associated with pain and cramping as well as an increased frequency of stools. Mealtimes may become unpleasant experiences. Frequent visits to health care providers and vigilant monitoring of the colonic mucosa for dysplastic (irregular) changes can be anxiety provoking.

LABORATORY ASSESSMENT

As a result of chronic blood loss, hematocrit and hemoglobin levels may be low, reflecting anemia and a chronic disease state. An increased white blood cell (WBC) count and elevated erythrocyte sedimentation rate (ESR) are consistent with inflammatory disease. Sodium, potassium, and chloride concentrations may be depleted secondary to frequent diarrheal stools and malabsorption resulting from the diseased bowel. Hypoalbuminemia (decreased serum albumin) is found in clients with extensive disease.

Viral and bacterial dysenteries can cause symptoms similar to those of ulcerative colitis. Before an invasive diagnostic workup, the stools are examined for occult blood, ova (eggs), and parasites, and specimens for culture are obtained. Other problems must be ruled out before a definitive diagnosis of ulcerative colitis is made.

RADIOGRAPHIC ASSESSMENT

Barium enemas with air contrast demonstrate differences between Crohn's disease and ulcerative colitis and identify complications, mucosal patterns, and the distribution and depth of disease involvement. In early disease, the barium enema will show incomplete filling as a result of inflammation and fine ulcerations along the bowel contour. These ulcerations appear deeper in more advanced disease.

> **Critical Thinking Challenge**
>
> A 42-year-old client visits the physician's office where you work. She complains of abdominal pain and numerous diarrheal stools each day. She also states that she has abdominal cramping and often feels "bloated." Her activity level has decreased because of her fatigue and the need to stay near a bathroom most of the day.
>
> 1. What questions should you ask her to elicit a thorough history?
> 2. What physical assessment findings would you expect and why?
> 3. What psychosocial assessment questions would be appropriate?

evolve For suggested answer guidelines, go to http://evolve.elsevier.com/Iggy/.

Analysis

COMMON NURSING DIAGNOSES AND COLLABORATIVE PROBLEMS

The following are priority nursing diagnoses for clients with ulcerative colitis:

1. Diarrhea related to inflammation of the bowel mucosa
2. Acute and Chronic Pain related to inflammation and ulceration of the bowel mucosa and accompanying skin irritation

The primary collaborative problem is Potential for Gastrointestinal Bleeding.

ADDITIONAL NURSING DIAGNOSES AND COLLABORATIVE PROBLEMS

In addition to the common nursing diagnoses and collaborative problems, clients with ulcerative colitis may have one or more of the following:

- Imbalanced Nutrition: Less Than Body Requirements related to inability to absorb food due to biologic factors
- Disturbed Body Image related to biophysical factors and possible surgery
- Activity Intolerance related to generalized weakness
- Ineffective Coping related to high degree of threat and uncertainty
- Risk for Deficient Fluid Volume related to diarrhea

Planning and Implementation

DIARRHEA

NOC **PLANNING: EXPECTED OUTCOMES.** A major concern for a client with ulcerative colitis is the occurrence of frequent, bloody diarrhea. Therefore the client is expected to have formed stools. Indicators include that the client will have noncompromised:

- Elimination pattern
- Control of bowel movements
- Stool color
- Stool amount for diet

INTERVENTIONS. Many measures are used to relieve symptoms and to reduce intestinal motility, decrease inflammation, and promote intestinal healing. Medical management is the preferred and initial treatment option.

The purpose of diarrhea management (Chart 61-3) is the prevention and alleviation of diarrhea. It is important to instruct the client with exacerbations of diarrhea to record the

CHART 61-3

NIC INTERVENTION ACTIVITIES for The Client with Inflammatory Bowel Disease

Diarrhea Management: *Management and alleviation of diarrhea*

- Instruct client/family members to record color, volume, frequency, and consistency of stools.
- Identify factors (e.g., medications, bacteria, tube feedings) that may cause or contribute to diarrhea.
- Teach the client to eliminate gas-forming and spicy foods from diet.
- Suggest trial elimination of foods containing lactose.
- Instruct in low-fiber, high-protein, high-calorie diet, as appropriate.
- Teach client appropriate use of antidiarrheal medications.
- Monitor skin in perianal area for irritation and ulceration.
- Weigh client regularly.
- Perform actions to rest the bowel (NPO, liquid diet).

Pain Management: *Alleviation of pain or a reduction in pain to a level of comfort that is acceptable to the client*

- Perform a comprehensive assessment of pain to include location, characteristics, onset/duration, frequency, quality, intensity or severity of pain, and precipitating factors.
- Evaluate, with the client and the health care team, the effectiveness of past pain control measures that have been used.
- Reduce or eliminate factors that can precipitate or increase the pain experience (e.g., fear, fatigue, monotony, and lack of knowledge).
- Teach the use of nonpharmacologic techniques (e.g., biofeedback, TENS, hypnosis, relaxation, guided imagery, music therapy, distraction, activity therapy, acupressure, hot/cold application, and massage) before, after and, if possible, during painful activities; before pain occurs or increases; and along with other pain relief measures.

NIC intervention activities selected from Dochterman, J.M., & Bulechek, G.M. (Eds.) (2004). *Nursing interventions classification (NIC)* (4th ed.). St. Louis: Mosby. No part of this work is to be altered without prior written permission from the Publisher.
TENS, Transcutaneous electrical nerve stimulation.

color, volume, frequency, and consistency of stools to determine the severity of the problem. In collaboration with the dietitian, assist in identifying factors that may cause or contribute to diarrhea.

Monitor the skin in the perianal area for irritation and ulceration resulting from loose, frequent stools. Stool cultures may be sent for analysis if diarrhea continues. Instruct the client and family members about the appropriate use of antidiarrheal medications. If the client is hospitalized, have the assistive nursing personnel weigh the client daily. Clients at home should weigh themselves one to two times each week.

NONSURGICAL MANAGEMENT. Nonsurgical management includes drug and diet therapy. The provision of physical and emotional rest is also important considerations.

Drug Therapy. The health care provider prescribes a combination of drugs, including salicylate compounds, corticosteroids, immunosuppressants, and antidiarrheals.

Salicylate Compounds. Sulfasalazine (Azulfidine, PMS-Sulfasalazine✱) is one of the primary treatments for ulcerative colitis. It is thought to act by inhibiting prostaglandin synthesis to reduce inflammation. Sulfasalazine is used to prevent recurrences of the disease as well as to treat acute exacerbations of mild to moderate severity. The usual dose of sulfasalazine is 2 to 4 g daily. Remind the client to take the drug with a full glass of water and to increase fluids throughout the day. The drug should be taken after meals to prevent GI discomfort. Because severe hypersensitivity reactions, blood dyscrasias such as leukopenia, and anemia may occur, newer drugs that are less likely to cause these adverse effects are often given as alternatives.

Other 5-aminosalicylic acid agents, such as mesalamine (Asacol, Pentasa, Salofalk✱), olsalazine (Dipentum), and balsalazide (Colazal), are also used for their anti-inflammatory effect. The recommended dose of Asacol is 800 mg three times daily or Pentasa 4 g daily in divided doses for acute illness. Tablets should not be crushed, broken, or chewed. Clients with mild to moderate colitis of the distal bowel may be treated with mesalamine suppositories given two or three times daily or with retention enemas (Rowasa enema) given once daily at bedtime.

Dipentum 1 g daily in divided doses may be used for maintenance therapy. Colazal is used for acute illness at the usual dose of 2.25 g three times daily for 8 to 12 weeks.

Corticosteroids. Oral or IV corticosteroid therapy may be prescribed during exacerbations of the disease. Prednisone (Deltasone, Winpred) 40 to 65 mg daily is usually given orally. For a severely ill client, prednisolone (Delta-Cortef) 45 to 60 mg daily may be given IV. Once clinical improvement has been established, the corticosteroids are tapered over a 2- to 3-month period after discharge because of the long-term adverse effects that commonly occur with steroid therapy. Examples include hyperglycemia (increased blood glucose), osteoporosis, peptic ulcer disease, and increased risk for infection. For clients with rectal symptoms, topical steroids in the form of small-retention enemas may be prescribed. Hydrocortisone rectal foam (Cortifoam) is prescribed as one to two times daily for 2 to 3 weeks and then every other day. Hydrocortisone enemas (Cortenema) are given at bedtime for 21 days, tapered, and discontinued.

Immunosuppressive Drugs. As single agents, immunosuppressive drugs (also known as immunomodulators) are not effective in the treatment of ulcerative colitis. However, when given in combination with steroids, they may help to reduce the amount of steroids necessary to obtain a response. For example, cyclosporine (Gengraf) given at 4 mg/kg/day can be beneficial in severely ill clients who might otherwise require a colectomy. Oral 6-mercaptopurine (Purinethol) may be given at a dose of 1.5 to 2.5 mg/kg/day. Observe for side effects of this medication, which include thrombocytopenia (decreased platelets), leukopenia (decreased white blood cells [WBCs]), anemia, renal failure, infection, headache, GI ulceration, stomatitis (oral cavity inflammation), and hepatotoxicity. Therefore it is important to monitor blood counts and note signs of infection. Other drugs in the same class, such as tacrolimus (Prograf), are being used experimentally for ulcerative colitis when other medications are not effective.

Antidiarrheal Drugs. To provide symptomatic management of diarrhea, antidiarrheal drugs may be prescribed. These drugs are given very cautiously, however, because they can precipitate colonic dilation and toxic megacolon. Common antidiarrheal drugs include diphenoxylate hydrochloride and atropine sulfate (Lomotil) and loperamide (Imodium).

Other Drugs. Although not approved as a first-line medication for ulcerative colitis, infliximab (Remicade) may be used for **refractory disease** (disease that does not respond to any other type of therapy) or for severe complications,

TABLE 61-4 Guidelines for a Low-Fiber Diet

Foods Allowed	Foods Not Allowed
Beverages	
Only 2 glasses of milk, if allowed, boiled or evaporated; strained fruit juices, coffee, tea, and carbonated beverages	Alcohol
Eggs	
Prepared in any manner, except fried	Fried
Cheese	
Cottage, cream, milk, American, and Tillamook (use in small amounts)	Highly flavored
Meats or Poultry	
Roasted, baked, or broiled tender beef, lamb, liver, veal, fish, chicken, or turkey	Tough meats, pork; fried or highly spiced meats
Soups	
Bouillon, broth, and strained cream soups from foods allowed	Any others
Fats	
Butter, margarine, oils, 30 mL (1 oz) of cream daily	None
Vegetables	
Canned or cooked vegetables, such as asparagus, beets, carrots, peas, potatoes, pumpkin, squash, spinach, and young string beans; tomato juice	Raw or whole cooked vegetables (e.g., potato with skin)
Fruits	
Strained fruit juices; cooked or canned apples, apricots, Royal Ann cherries, peaches, pears, dried fruit purée, and ripe banana and avocado; all of the above without skins or seeds	All other raw or cooked fruits
Bread and Crackers	
Refined bread, toast, rolls, and crackers	Pancakes, waffles, and whole-grain bread or rolls
Cereals	
Cooked cereal, such as Cream of Wheat, Malt-O Meal, strained oatmeal, cornmeal, cornflakes, puffed rice, Rice Krispies, and puffed wheat	Whole-grain cereals; other prepared cereals
Potatoes/Rice/Pasta	
White rice, macaroni, noodles, and spaghetti	Fried potato, potato chips, and brown rice
Desserts	
Gelatin desserts, tapioca, angel food or sponge cake, plain custards, water ice or ice cream without fruit or nuts, and rennet or simple puddings	Rich pastries, pies, and anything with nuts or dried fruit
Sweets	
Sugar, jelly, honey, syrups, gumdrops, hard candy, plain creams, milk chocolate	Other candy; jam, marmalade
Miscellaneous Foods	
Cream sauce and plain gravy	Nuts, olives, popcorn, rich gravies, pepper, spices and vinegar

Modified from Williams, S.R. (2001). *Basic nutrition and diet therapy* (11th ed.). St. Louis: Mosby.

such as toxic megacolon. This drug is an immunoglobulin G (IgG) monoclonal antibody that neutralizes the activity of tumor necrosis factor (TNF) to decrease inflammation. It is used more commonly for managing Crohn's disease.

Diet Therapy. The severity of the client's ulcerative colitis determines the type of diet required. Clients may begin with one form of diet therapy and progress to a more advanced diet as symptoms diminish, with the goal of preventing hyperactive bowel activity.

Clients with severe symptoms are kept on NPO status to ensure bowel rest. The physician often prescribes total parenteral nutrition (TPN) for these clients (see Chapter 64). Clients with slightly less severe symptoms may be given elemental formulas, such as Vivonex, which are absorbed in the upper bowel, thus minimizing bowel stimulation. Clients with significant but less severe symptoms may be restricted to a low-fiber (low-residue) diet. Clients following a low-fiber diet should avoid foods such as whole-wheat grains, nuts, and fresh fruits or fresh vegetables (Table 61-4). Whether fiber needs to be restricted during the chronic phase of the illness remains controversial. If fiber intake does not induce symptoms, the intake of fiber need not be limited. However, because the role of diet in inflammatory bowel disease (IBD) is not well defined, and because individual tolerance to foods vary, clients with controlled symptoms may only need to limit or omit those foods that cause them discomfort or diarrhea.

Typically, lactose-containing foods are poorly tolerated and should be reduced or eliminated. All clients should be cautioned that caffeinated beverages, pepper, alcohol, and smoking are common GI stimulants that could cause discomfort.

Rest. At the onset of treatment, activity is generally restricted because rest can reduce intestinal activity, provide comfort, and promote healing. Ensure that the client has easy access to a bedpan, commode, or bathroom in case of urgency or tenesmus.

Complementary and Alternative Therapies. In addition to dietary changes, complementary and alternative therapies have become very popular to supplement traditional management of ulcerative colitis. Examples include the following:

- Herbs, such as flaxseed
- Selenium
- Vitamin C
- Biofeedback
- Hypnosis
- Yoga
- Acupuncture
- Ayurveda (a combination of diet, yoga, herbs, breathing exercises)

SURGICAL MANAGEMENT. About a fourth of individuals with ulcerative colitis will require a colectomy. Indications for surgery include bowel perforation, toxic megacolon, hemorrhage, colon cancer, and failure of conventional treatment. The surgeon may choose one of several surgical procedures to alleviate these problems.

Total Proctocolectomy with a Permanent Ileostomy. Total proctocolectomy (or colectomy) with a permanent ileostomy has traditionally been the standard surgical procedure for clients undergoing a colectomy.

Preoperative Care. When an ileostomy is indicated, provide an extensive explanation to the client and family or significant other. Preoperative teaching includes aspects that relate to abdominal surgery (see Chapter 20) and those that relate to ileostomy. The surgeon consults with the enterostomal therapist (ET) preoperatively for recommendations on the location of the ostomy (stoma). (An ET is a nurse specializing and certified in skin and ostomy care.) A visit from an **ostomate** (a client with an ostomy) may be appropriate before surgery if the client agrees to this. The surgeon prescribes oral or parenteral antibiotics, such as neomycin sulfate (Mycifradin), as a bowel antiseptic. Mechanical cleansing of the bowel with enemas or laxatives may also be required.

Operative Procedures. During a total proctocolectomy with a traditional permanent **ileostomy,** the colon, rectum, and anus are removed, followed by closure of the anus. The surgeon brings the end of the terminal ileum out through the abdominal wall and forms a stoma, or ostomy. The stoma is usually placed in the right lower quadrant of the abdomen, below the belt line (Figure 61-2). The surgeon makes a perineal incision to remove the rectum and supporting tissues.

Postoperative Care. Initially after surgery the output from the ileostomy is a loose, dark green liquid that may contain some blood. Over time, a process called ileostomy adaptation occurs. The small intestine begins to absorb increased amounts of sodium and water (a former function of the large intestine, which was removed by surgery). Stool volume decreases, becomes thicker (pastelike), and turns yellow-green or yellow-brown. The effluent (fluid material) usually has little odor or a sweet odor. Any foul or unpleasant odor may be a symptom of some underlying problem (e.g., blockage or infection).

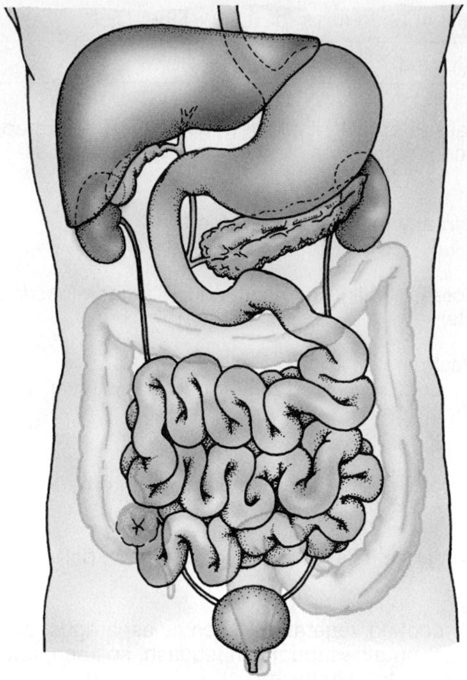

Figure 61-2 ■ Total proctocolectomy with a permanent ileostomy. This involved removal of the colon, the rectum, and the anus with closure of the anus. Note the missing colon, rectum, and anus with the resultant stoma in the right lower quadrant.

Depending on the frequency and irritation of stool drainage, the client must wear a pouch system at all times. Prevention of skin problems (irritation, excoriation, ulceration) is *a priority* for the client with an ileostomy. The output from the small intestine is rich in proteolytic enzymes and bile salts, which can quickly irritate and injure the skin. A pouch system that has some type of skin barrier (gelatin or pectin) provides sufficient protection for most clients. Other products are also available.

Most clients undergoing surgical intervention for ulcerative colitis have lived with chronic illness for some time. They may view surgery positively as a relief from the multiple problems caused by the disease. Initially, however, they may not perceive life with an ileostomy as a positive alternative.

Total proctocolectomy with a permanent ileostomy results in an alteration in appearance and body function. The goals for a client undergoing this procedure are to become proficient in self-care, to adapt his or her lifestyle to include care of an ostomy, and to resume presurgery activities successfully.

Total Colectomy with a Continent Ileostomy. As an alternative to the traditional ileostomy with an external pouch, the surgeon may create an internal system: a Kock's ileostomy or ileal reservoir. This procedure is sometimes referred to as a continent ileostomy. The surgeon constructs an intra-abdominal pouch or reservoir from the ter-

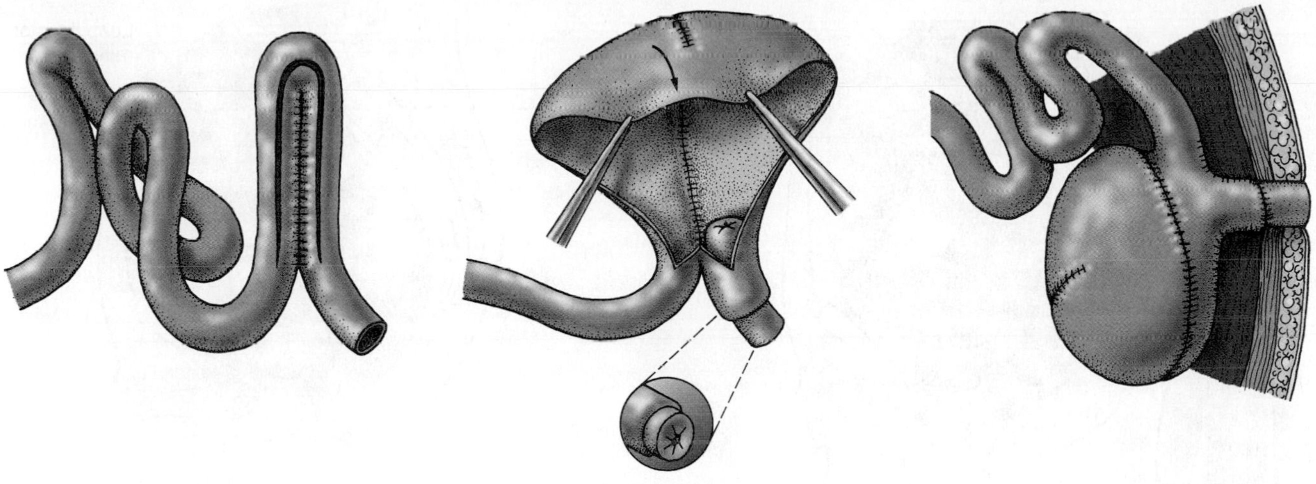

1. A reservoir, in which the client will retain stool until draining it, is constructed from a loop of ileum folded and sutured together, then cut.

2. A portion of the ileum is intussuscepted to form a nipple valve, and the upper part of the stitched and cut ileum is pulled down and sutured to form a pouch.

3. The nipple valve, which shuts tight against pressure from a filled pouch, is pulled through the stoma and sutured flush with the abdomen.

Figure 61-3 ■ The creation of a Kock's (continent) ileostomy.

minal ileum (Figure 61-3), where stool is stored in the pouch until the client drains it by using a catheter. The care of a Kock's ileostomy involves the connection of the pouch to the stoma, which is constructed with a nipple-like valve made from an intussuscepted portion of the ileum. The stoma is flush with the skin.

The nursing care of the client undergoing this procedure is similar to the care of the client undergoing a procto-colectomy with a permanent ileostomy (see the previous section). Immediately postoperatively, an indwelling Foley catheter is placed in the pouch, which is connected to low intermittent suction and irrigated as ordered.

Monitor the character and quality of **effluent** (drainage). Teach the client to drain the stoma. Initially the pouch holds only 50 to 75 mL; over time, the pouch capacity reaches 500 to 700 mL. When the pouch needs to be emptied, the client experiences a sensation of fullness. The client drains the pouch several times a day and wears a small dressing over the stoma to keep it moist and to protect clothing from the moist stoma. This procedure has several advantages. The client does not need to wear an external pouch for collection of stool and experiences minimal skin problems. Unfortunately, the need for frequent revisions and problems with leakage have made this procedure less desirable.

Total Colectomy with Ileoanal Anastomosis; Ileoanal Reservoir. During a total colectomy with ileoanal anastomosis, the surgeon removes the colon and the rectum and sutures the ileum into the anal canal. Usually continence is excellent after this procedure, but up to 20% of clients will have some nocturnal leakage of stool. Care of the client undergoing this procedure is similar to the care of clients undergoing a colectomy. With an ileoanal anastomosis, perineal irritation is a common occurrence as a result of frequent, loose stools. The nurse or assistive nursing personnel should provide careful perineal care.

The creation of an **ileoanal reservoir,** also known as a **J pouch**, has become popular for clients with ulcerative colitis, especially young adults, because it spares the rectal sphincter and eliminates the need for an ostomy. During this procedure, the surgeon removes the colon and sutures the ileum into the rectal stump to form a reservoir. If residual rectal mucosa remains after either an ileoanal anastomosis or a reservoir procedure, proctoscopy is done at predetermined intervals to monitor for dysplasia.

Preoperative Care. The preoperative care for a client undergoing an ileoanal anastomosis is similar to that for a client undergoing an ileostomy. However, clients will not have an ostomy and therefore do not require consultation with an enterostomal therapist (ET).

Operative Procedures. Ileoanal anastomosis occurs in two stages (Figure 61-4). In the first stage the surgeon excises the rectal mucosa, performs an abdominal colectomy, constructs the reservoir or pouch to the anal canal, and creates a temporary loop ileostomy. The loop ileostomy is necessary to allow adequate healing of the internal pouch and all anastomosis sites and to allow for an increase in the capacity of the internal reservoir through fluid instillations. After 3 to 4 months the client returns to have the loop ileostomy closed. Stool formation resembles that in clients who have undergone a traditional ileostomy.

Postoperative Care. Provide the usual postoperative interventions for clients who have undergone abdominal surgery. All clients requiring surgical intervention for ulcerative colitis have an abdominal incision. Initially most clients are maintained on NPO status and a nasogastric (NG) tube is used for suction.

ACUTE PAIN; CHRONIC PAIN

NOC **PLANNING: EXPECTED OUTCOMES.** The client with ulcerative colitis is expected to take personal action to control pain. Indicators include that the client will be able to demonstrate consistently the ability to:

- Use preventive measures
- Use non-analgesic relief measures

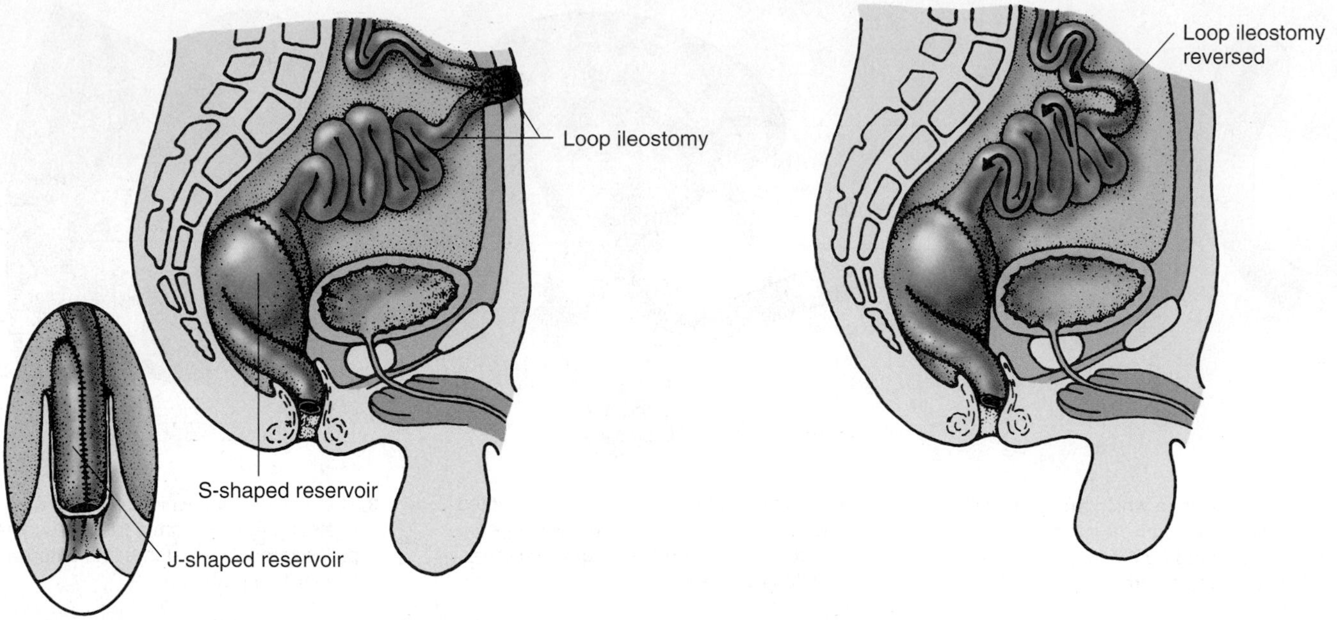

Stage 1.
After removal of the colon, a temporary loop ileostomy is created and an ileoanal reservoir is formed. The reservoir is created in an S-shaped reservoir (using three loops of ileum) or a J-shaped reservoir (suturing a portion of ileum to the rectal cuff, with an upward loop).

Stage 2.
After the reservoir has had time to heal–usually several months–the temporary loop ileostomy is reversed, and stool is allowed to drain into the reservoir.

Figure 61-4 ■ The creation of an ileoanal reservoir.

- Report changes in pain symptoms to health care professional
- Use available resources
- Recognize associated symptoms of pain
- Report that pain is controlled

INTERVENTIONS. Pain control may be accomplished through pharmacologic and nonpharmacologic measures. The client's symptoms can cause physical discomfort, which can also contribute to emotional discomfort. The use of a variety of symptom-reducing interventions and supportive measures can provide increased comfort.

NIC **Pain Management.** The purpose of pain management is alleviation of pain or a reduction in pain to a level of comfort that is acceptable to the client (see Chart 61-3). The client with ulcerative colitis experiences abdominal pain and cramping, particularly with exacerbations of the disease. Increases in pain may also signal the development of complications such as peritonitis. Frequent bowel movements can cause skin irritation and increase the client's discomfort. The nurse performs a comprehensive pain assessment. With the client and the health care team, the nurse evaluates the effectiveness of past pain control measures that were used.

Assist the client in reducing or eliminating factors that can precipitate or increase the pain experience. Antidiarrheal medications may be prescribed to control diarrhea but must be used cautiously because they can precipitate toxic megacolon. The client may benefit from diet teaching and meal planning as a means of decreasing abdominal discomfort related to cramping and bloating. Excoriated skin can contribute to pain and discomfort. Scrupulous skin care prevents painful excoriation of the skin. Also teach the client to use nonpharmacologic measures (e.g., biofeedback, music therapy, guided imagery) as a means of pain modification (see Chapter 7).

Drug Therapy. Antidiarrheal medications are used to control diarrhea and thereby reduce the resulting discomfort. These must be used with caution because toxic megacolon can develop. **Toxic megacolon** is characterized by an enlarged colon, along with fever, leukocytosis, and tachycardia. The abdomen is often distended and tender; bowel elimination patterns differ from one person to another. The physician may prescribe anticholinergics, such as dicyclomine (Bentyl, Bentylol✱), before meals to provide relief from the pain and cramping that may occur with diarrhea. Opioids are used sparingly and cautiously because they can mask symptoms of life-threatening complications.

Diet Therapy. Dietary measures help to control symptoms and thereby promote relief from discomfort. Assess the client's needs for diet teaching, and evaluate the effects of implemented dietary measures on an ongoing basis.

Perineal Skin Care. Perineal skin can be irritated by frequent contact with loose stools and frequent cleaning, and it can cause discomfort. Explain special measures for skin care. For example, cleaning the perineal area with mild soap and warm water after each bowel movement keeps the skin free of any stool. Frequent sitz baths may be helpful, particularly after a bowel movement. The application of a thin coat of barrier creams, vitamin A and D ointment, aloe creams, or medicated foam applications may provide relief. Use of medicated wipes with witch hazel (e.g., Tucks) is soothing if the rectal area is tender or sensitive from the use of toilet tissue.

Various manufacturers of ostomies (e.g., Hollister and ConvaTec) produce a three-product system for skin care that may help prevent and heal perineal skin irritation, thus relieving discomfort. Such systems include a skin-cleaning solution, a moisturizing and healing cream, and a petroleum jelly–like barrier that prevents contact of moisture and stool with the skin.

POTENTIAL FOR GASTROINTESTINAL BLEEDING

PLANNING: EXPECTED OUTCOMES. The client with ulcerative colitis is expected to experience a reduction in or cessation of the gastrointestinal (GI) bleeding that accompanies chronic ulcerative colitis. The client is also expected to remain free of complications of the disease that can cause bleeding, such as perforation.

INTERVENTIONS. Primary responsibility is to monitor the client closely for signs and symptoms of GI bleeding resulting from acute disease or complications. All stools are monitored for blood, using both gross and occult examination. Monitor the client's hematocrit, hemoglobin, and electrolyte values for abnormalities as well as the client's vital signs. Observe the client for the development of fever, tachycardia, fluid volume depletion, electrolyte imbalances, and severe abdominal pain. Changes in mental status may be noted, especially among older adults.

If symptoms of GI bleeding are present, notify the health care provider immediately because surgical intervention may be necessary. Blood products may be necessary for clients with severe anemia. Prepare the client for transfusion by inserting a large-bore IV catheter for the administration of blood. Chapter 59 describes the management of GI bleeding in detail.

Community-Based Care

HOME CARE MANAGEMENT

The client with ulcerative colitis is managed at home but may require hospitalization during exacerbations. In addition, clients experiencing extraintestinal manifestations of the disease will require ongoing management of joint or skin problems. Clients with moderate to severe ulcerative colitis have more acute exacerbations than those with milder forms of the disease. Such clients may benefit from case manager services to coordinate and facilitate quality care in a cost-effective way.

For clients with ulcerative colitis, home care management focuses on managing symptoms and monitoring for complications. Instruct the client in measures to reduce or control abdominal pain, cramping, and diarrhea. Also teach the client and family members regarding symptoms that should be reported immediately to the health care provider. For clients returning home or transferring to nursing home or subacute care after surgery, ongoing respiratory care, incision care, ostomy care, and pain management are additional concerns.

HEALTH TEACHING

Educate the client about the nature of ulcerative colitis with regard to its acute episodes, remissions, and symptom management. Furthermore, emphasize that even though the cause is unknown, relapses can be resolved with proper health care.

CHART 61-4

CLIENT EDUCATION GUIDE
Ileostomy Care

Skin Protection
- Use a pectin-based skin barrier to protect your skin from contact with contents from the ostomy.
- Use skin care products, such as skin sealants and ostomy skin creams. If your skin continues to come into contact with ostomy contents.
- Watch your skin for any irritation or redness.

Pouch Care
- Empty your pouch when it is one third to one half full.
- Change the pouch during inactive times, such as before meals, before retiring at night, on waking in the morning, and 2 to 4 hours after eating.
- Change the entire pouch system every 3 to 7 days.

Diet
- Chew food thoroughly.
- Be cautious of high-fiber and high-cellulose foods. You may need to eliminate these from the diet if they cause severe problems (diarrhea, constipation, or blockage). Examples include popcorn, peanuts, coconut, Chinese vegetables, string beans, tough-fiber meats, shrimp and lobster, rice, bran, and skinned vegetables (tomatoes, corn, and peas).

Medications
- Avoid taking enteric-coated and capsule medications.
- Inform any health care provider who is prescribing medications for you that you have an ostomy. Before having prescriptions filled, inform your pharmacist that you have an ostomy.
- Do not take any laxative or enemas. You should usually have loose stool and should contact a physician if no stool has passed in 6 to 12 hours.

Symptoms to Watch for
- Report any drastic increase or decrease in drainage to your health care provider.
- If stomal swelling, abdominal cramping, or distention occurs or if ileostomy contents stop draining, do the following:
  - Remove the pouch with faceplate.
  - Lie down, assuming a knee-chest position.
  - Begin abdominal massage.
  - Apply moist towels to the abdomen.
  - Drink hot tea.
  - If none of these maneuvers is effective in resuming ileostomy flow or if abdominal pain is severe, call your health care provider right away.

Instruct the client about dietary measures to reduce bloating and cramping. The client needs to learn what foods are best tolerated, and adjust his or her diet accordingly. Teach about prescribed medications and medication side effects for which the client should remain alert. Clients taking immunosuppressive drugs should be taught to report signs of infection, such as sore throat, to the health care provider. Prepare written instructions for the client and family members about the signs of colonic dilation and perforation, and reiterate the importance of notifying the health care provider if these signs occur.

If the client has undergone a surgical diversion to manage colon effluent, you or the enterostomal therapist (ET) explains and demonstrates the required care. The client is encouraged to demonstrate self-care of the ileostomy. Also teach clients with an ileostomy to include adequate amounts of salt and water in their diets because the ileostomy promotes the loss of these elements. They will also be taught to be cautious in situations that promote profuse sweating or fluid loss, such as during strenuous physical activities, when environmental heat is excessive, and during episodes of diarrhea and vomiting. Chart 61-4 describes ileostomy care in detail.

A client with an ileostomy may have multiple concerns about management at home and about sexual and social adjustments. Considering possible sexual issues helps the client to identify and discuss these concerns with the sexual partner. Social situations may precipitate some anxieties related to decreased self-esteem and a disturbance in body image. Help the client explore possible concerns in addressing and resolving these potentially stressful events.

HEALTH CARE RESOURCES

If the client requires assistance with activities of daily living, the case manager or social worker may help to arrange the services of a home care aide. If the client is discharged from the hospital with an ileostomy, the case manager makes a referral to a home care agency. A home care nurse can provide assessment and guidance in integrating ostomy care into the client's lifestyle and possibly provide wound care, including the monitoring of wound healing (Chart 61-5). The client needs to know where to purchase ostomy supplies, along with the name, size, and manufacturer's order number. The ET or case manager contacts local and regional supply companies for prices and availability of supplies.

Identify the local ostomy support group by contacting the United Ostomy Association. A support group or the Crohn's and Colitis Foundation of America may be of assistance in obtaining supplies as well as providing education for ostomates. Inform the client and family or significant others of available ostomy outpatient clinics and ETs. If the client agrees, a visit from an ostomate can be initiated or continued on an ambulatory care basis.

CHART 61-5

HOME CARE ASSESSMENT of The Client with Inflammatory Bowel Disease

Assess gastrointestinal function and nutritional status, including the following:
- Abdominal cramping or pain
- Bowel elimination pattern, specifically frequency, characteristics and amount of stools, presence or absence of blood in stools
- Dietary and fluid intake and habits (include relationship of specific foods to cramping and stools)
- Weight gain or loss
- Signs and symptoms of dehydration
- Presence or absence of fever, rectal tenesmus, or urgency
- Bowel sounds
- Condition of perianal skin, including presence or absence of perianal fistula or abscess

Assess client's and family's coping skills, including the following:
- Current and ongoing stress level and coping style
- Availability of support system

Assess home environment, including the following:
- Adequacy and availability of bathroom facilities
- Opportunity for rest and relaxation

Assess ability to manage therapeutic regimen, including the following:
- Knowledge of medications
- Signs and symptoms to report
- Dietary management
- Availability of community resources
- Importance of follow-up care

Evaluation: Outcomes

Evaluate the care of the client with ulcerative colitis on the basis of the identified nursing diagnoses and collaborative problems. Expected outcomes may include that the client will:
- Have formed stools
- Take personal action to control pain

In addition, the client with an ileostomy can be expected to:
- Engage in self-care of the ileostomy
- Maintain peristomal skin integrity
- Demonstrate behaviors that integrate ostomy care into his or her lifestyle
- Verbalize signs and symptoms of stoma complications

Critical Thinking Challenge

A 42-year-old woman with ulcerative colitis is placed on several drugs to manage her disease. Unfortunately, the medications are not successful and she requires a colectomy and ileostomy. Her husband recently left her, and she has no children. She also lost her job because she missed a lot of time from work because of her illness.

1. What discharge teaching will she require?
2. What support systems can you suggest for her after discharge from the hospital?
3. In your hospital, patient care technicians (PCTs) are allowed to provide ostomy care. Would you delegate health teaching about the client's ostomy to the PCT? Why or why not?

evolve For suggested answer guidelines, go to http://evolve.elsevier.com/Iggy/.

Crohn's Disease

PATHOPHYSIOLOGY

Crohn's disease is an idiopathic inflammatory disease of the small intestine (60%), the colon (20%), or both. It involves all layers of the bowel but most commonly involves the terminal ileum. It is a slowly progressive and recurrent disease with predominant involvement of multiple regions of the intestine with normal sections between.

Chronic, nonspecific inflammation of the entire intestinal tract characterizes the disease, with the terminal ileum the site most often affected. Eventually deep fissures and ulcerations develop and often extend through all bowel layers, predisposing the individual to the development of bowel fistulas. The result is severe diarrhea and malabsorption of vital nutrients. Chronic pathologic changes include thickening of the bowel wall, resulting in narrowing of the bowel lumen and strictures. In advanced disease, the bowel mucosa demonstrates nodular swelling (granulomas) intermingled with deep ulcerations.

The complications associated with Crohn's disease are similar to those of ulcerative colitis. As shown in Table 61-3, hemorrhage is more common in ulcerative colitis, but it can occur in Crohn's disease as well. Severe malabsorption by the small intestine is more common in clients with Crohn's disease. Rarely, cancer of the small bowel and colon develop but usually occurs after the disease has been present for 15 to 20 years. Fistula formation is a common complication of Crohn's disease. Fistulas can occur between segments of the intestine or manifest as cutaneous fistulas or perirectal abscesses. Fistulas can also extend from the bowel to other organs and body cavities, such as the bladder or vagina (Figure 61-5). Twenty to thirty percent of individuals with the disease will develop intestinal obstruction. Initially obstruction results from inflammation and edema. Over time, fibrosis develops and obstruction results secondary to a narrowing of the bowel.

Etiology and Genetic Risk

Mycobacterium paratuberculosis has been proposed as an environmental stimulus that could be implicated in the development of Crohn's disease because granulomas similar to those seen in individuals with pulmonary tuberculosis have been found on biopsy of the intestines of people with the disease. A genetic predisposition to the disease has also been found because the disease tends to cluster in families and appears equally in identical twins (Dooley et al., 2004). Fifteen percent of clients have first-degree relatives with inflammatory bowel disease (IBD). Family members develop the disease with similar patterns and similar age of onset. The most widely accepted cause of Crohn's disease is a combination of reasons–a defect in the immunoregulation of inflammation in the intestinal tract along with a genetic predisposition for the disease.

Incidence/Prevalence

More than one million people in the United States have the disease; peak incidence is between 15 and 40 years of age (Goldstein et al., 2004).

COLLABORATIVE MANAGEMENT

Assessment

HISTORY

Although the exact cause is not clear, Crohn's disease is aggravated by bacterial infection, inflammation, and smoking cessation. Therefore a detailed history assists in uncovering manifestations specific to the disease. A history of fever, abdominal pain, and loose stools is commonly seen in a client with Crohn's disease. Ask about recent unintentional loss of weight and the frequency, consistency, and presence of blood in the stool.

PHYSICAL ASSESSMENT/CLINICAL MANIFESTATIONS

Perform a thorough abdominal examination, assess for clinical manifestations of the disease, and evaluate the client's nutritional and hydration status. When performing an abdominal assessment, note findings that are consistent with those in acute appendicitis (e.g., tenderness, guarded movement, a palpable mass in the right lower quadrant).

On inspection of the abdomen, assess for distention, masses, or visible peristalsis. Inspection of the perianal area may reveal ulcerations or fissures. During auscultation, bowel sounds may be decreased or absent in the client with severe inflammation or obstruction. An increase in high-pitched or rushing sounds may be present over areas of narrowed bowel loops. Muscle guarding, masses, rigidity, or tenderness may be noted on palpation.

The clinical presentation of Crohn's disease can vary greatly from client to client. Most clients report diarrhea, abdominal pain, and low-grade fever. Fever is also commonly present with complications such as fistulas and severe inflammation. If the disease occurs in only the ileum, diarrhea occurs five or six times per day, often with a soft, loose stool. **Steatorrhea** (fatty diarrheal stools) is common. The stool may contain bright red blood, but this is a rare finding.

Abdominal pain from the inflammatory process is usually constant and is located in the right lower quadrant. Clients also experience periumbilical pain before and after bowel movements. If the lower colon is diseased, pain is often experienced in both lower abdominal quadrants.

Weight loss is experienced by about 80% of individuals with Crohn's disease. Clients often experience nutritional problems as a result of increased catabolism secondary to chronic inflammation, anorexia, malabsorption, or self-imposed dietary restrictions. The result is fluid and electrolyte imbalances and protein, iron, vitamin, and mineral deficiencies.

The marked inflammatory bowel changes decrease the small bowel's ability to absorb nutrients, which may be worsened by surgery and fistulas. Be acutely aware of the importance of detecting the clinical manifestations of peritonitis, bowel obstruction, and nutritional and fluid imbalances. Early detection of a change in the client's status helps to minimize these life-threatening complications.

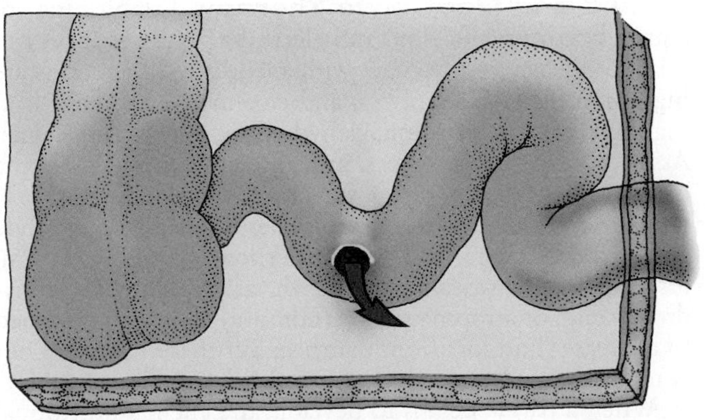

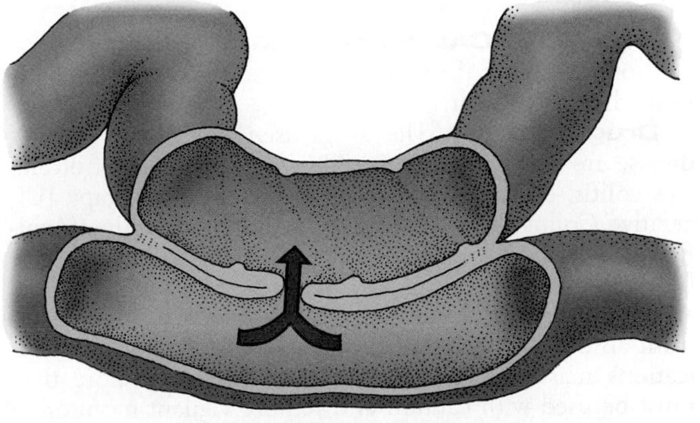

Figure 61-5 ■ The types of fistulas that are complications of Crohn's disease.

PSYCHOSOCIAL ASSESSMENT

The client experiencing Crohn's disease needs a complete psychosocial assessment. The chronicity of the problem and the troublesome complications can greatly affect clients and their families. The assessment should be ongoing and should continuously reflect the client's status as well as the family's. Lifestyle changes are necessary to cope with such a disruptive and painful chronic illness. Assess the client's coping skill and identify support systems.

DIAGNOSTIC ASSESSMENT

The health care provider may order a number of laboratory studies for clients with Crohn's disease; however, no disease-specific tests are available to confirm the diagnosis. The results of laboratory tests often indicate the extent and severity of inflammation associated with the disease.

If bleeding is present, decreased hemoglobin and hematocrit values are likely. Serum levels of folic acid and cobalamin (vitamin B_{12} group) are generally low because of malabsorption, further contributing to anemia. Amino acid malabsorption may result in decreased albumin levels. An elevated erythrocyte sedimentation rate (ESR) is consistent with the presence of inflammation. White blood cells (WBCs) in the urine may indicate infection (pyuria), which may be caused by ureteral obstruction or an **enterovesical** (bowel to bladder) **fistula.** If significant diarrhea is present, the client will experience electrolyte losses, particularly potassium and magnesium.

The results of the contrast barium enema and upper gastrointestinal (GI) series often provide more specific diagnostic information. X-rays show narrowing, ulcerations, strictures, and fistulas consistent with Crohn's disease. In acute illness these tests are often deferred until the risk of perforation lessens.

Depending on which areas of the bowel are diseased, the sigmoidoscopic examination may not be diagnostic. If the rectosigmoid colon is involved, the physician may see ulcerations and inflamed mucosa, areas of fissure, fistula, and abscess formation of the perianal and perirectal areas.

Colonoscopy is used when other tests, especially the barium enema examination, have not led to a specific diagnosis.

◆Interventions

Treatment of Crohn's disease is similar to that described earlier under Nonsurgical Management (Ulcerative Colitis), p. 1348.

NONSURGICAL MANAGEMENT. Specific interventions vary with the severity of disease and the complications that are present.

Drug Therapy. The drugs used to manage Crohn's disease are similar to those used in the treatment of ulcerative colitis, except for mesalamine (see Drug Therapy [Ulcerative Colitis], p. 1348). For example, sulfasalazine (Azulfidine, PMS-Sulfasalazine✱) 1.5 to 2 g twice daily PO has been effective in treating exacerbations of Crohn's disease. Although glucocorticoids can be effective, sepsis can result from abscesses or fistulas that may be present. These medications mask the symptoms of infection; therefore they must be used with caution and require vigilant monitoring by the nurse for signs of infection.

Metronidazole (Flagyl, Novonidazole✱) 250 to 500 mg three times daily PO has been helpful in clients with fistulas. Immunosuppressive therapy has been effective in clients with refractory disease or fistulas. Azathioprine (Imuran), an immunosuppressive agent, 50 mg daily for 12 months, may be instituted. After that time the health care provider may attempt to withdraw the drug, but long-term therapy may be needed in some cases. Methotrexate (Rheumatrex) may also be given to suppress immune activity.

Because a defect in the immunoregulation of inflammation may be implicated in the development of Crohn's disease, neutralization of a cytokine (specifically, tumor necrosis factor) may prove useful in decreasing bowel inflammation. Infliximab (Remicade), a monoclonal antibody form of antitumor necrosis factor alpha, has been approved for IV use at monthly intervals. The usual dose of 5 mg/kg has demonstrated efficacy in the treatment of active Crohn's disease and fistulas. Clients who have infections or those with hypersensitivity to murine proteins should not take this medication.

Nutritional Management. Long-standing nutritional deficits can have severe consequences for the client with Crohn's disease. Malnutrition can result in poor fistula and wound healing, loss of lean muscle mass, decreased immune system response, and increased morbidity and mortality. With severe exacerbations of the disease, the health care provider may recommend hospitalization to provide bowel rest and nutritional enhancement with total parenteral nutrition (TPN). For less severe exacerbations, the health care provider may prescribe an elemental diet using products such as Vivonex to induce remission. Elemental diets are absorbed in the jejunum and therefore permit the distal small intestine and colon to rest. Once remission is achieved, the health care provider usually prescribes a low-residue diet. Nutritional supplements, such as Ensure or Sustacal, can be added to provide nutrients and added calories. GI stimulants, such as caffeinated beverages and alcohol, should be avoided.

Complication Management. Fistulas (abnormal tract from intestine to skin or intestine to intestine) are common occurrences with acute exacerbations of Crohn's disease. Clients with fistulas often experience complications such as systemic infections, skin problems, malnutrition, and fluid and electrolyte imbalances. Treatment of the client with a fistula is multidimensional and includes nutrition and electrolyte therapy, skin care, and prevention of infection.

Fluid and Electrolyte Therapy. Establishing adequate nutrition and fluid and electrolyte balance takes priority in the care of the client with a fistula. GI secretions are high in volume, electrolytes, and enzymes. The client is at high risk for malnutrition, dehydration, and hypokalemia. Assess for these complications, and collaborate with the health care team to manage them.

The health care provider prescribes fluids and electrolyte replacement by oral liquids and nutrients as well as IV fluids. An antidiarrheal agent, such as diphenoxylate hydrochloride or atropine sulfate (Lomotil), may be prescribed to decrease fluid loss from diarrhea, but these drugs are not commonly used and must be given with caution.

When a fistula begins to develop, the client's nutritional status is usually compromised. After the fistula has developed, nutritional status worsens. The client requires at least 3000 calories daily to promote healing of the fistula. If the client cannot take adequate oral fluids and nutrients, the physician may prescribe TPN. In collaboration with the dietitian, do the following:

- Carefully monitor the client's tolerance to diet
- Assist the client in selecting high-calorie, high-protein, high-vitamin, low-fiber meals
- Offer enteral supplements, such as Ensure and Vivonex
- Record food intake for accurate calorie counts

Skin Care. Proteolytic enzymes and bile contribute to the problem of skin irritation and excoriation. Skin irritation needs to be prevented; this is usually accomplished through the use of skin barriers, application of pouches, and insertion of drains (Figure 61-6). By applying a pouch to the draining fistula, the risk of skin irritation is minimized and **effluent** (drainage) can be measured.

One approach to drainage management is to cover the area surrounding the fistula with barriers, such as Stomahesive or DuoDerm, and subsequently apply a wound drainage system over the fistula, securing it to the protective dressing. The skin adjacent to the fistula is cleaned with normal saline solution and gently patted dry.

Collaborate with the enterostomal therapist (ET) to provide wound management. Wound drainage must *never* be allowed to be in direct contact with skin without prompt cleaning because intestinal fluid enzymes are caustic.

Prevention of Infection. Clients with fistulas are at extremely high risk for intra-abdominal abscesses and sepsis. Intra-abdominal fistulas are treated with careful nursing interventions, containment of wound drainage, and antibiotic therapy. Observe for subtle signs of infection or sepsis, such as fever, abdominal pain, or a change in mental status.

Complementary and Alternative Therapies. Other options for disease management that are used to relax the client and soothe the GI tract include the following modalities:

- Naturopathy
- Herbs (e.g., ginger and peppermint oil)
- Acupuncture
- Hypnotherapy
- Ayurveda (a combination of diet, herbs, yoga, breathing exercises)

SURGICAL MANAGEMENT. Surgery for Crohn's disease is confined to those who have demonstrated failure on medical management or those who exhibit complications from the disease. Those who continue to have symptoms after long-term medical treatment and those with complications such as fistulas may undergo resection of the diseased area. Other indications include the following:

- Perforation
- Massive hemorrhage
- Intestinal obstruction (often caused by stricture)
- Abscesses
- Adenocarcinoma (rare)

In some cases the resection can be performed as minimally invasive surgery via laparoscopy. Both small bowel resection (usually the ileum) and ileocecal resections can be done using this procedure. The advantages of laparoscopic surgery over conventional open techniques include the following:

- Smaller incisions
- Less postoperative pain
- Quicker surgical recovery and return to usual lifestyle

Stricturoplasty may be performed for bowel strictures related to Crohn's disease. This procedure, which involves incising along the length of the stricture and suturing the incised area on the horizontal plane, allows for an increase in the bowel diameter. Preoperative and postoperative care for each of these surgical procedures is similar to care for clients undergoing other types of abdominal surgery. (See Surgical Management [Ulcerative Colitis], p. 1350.)

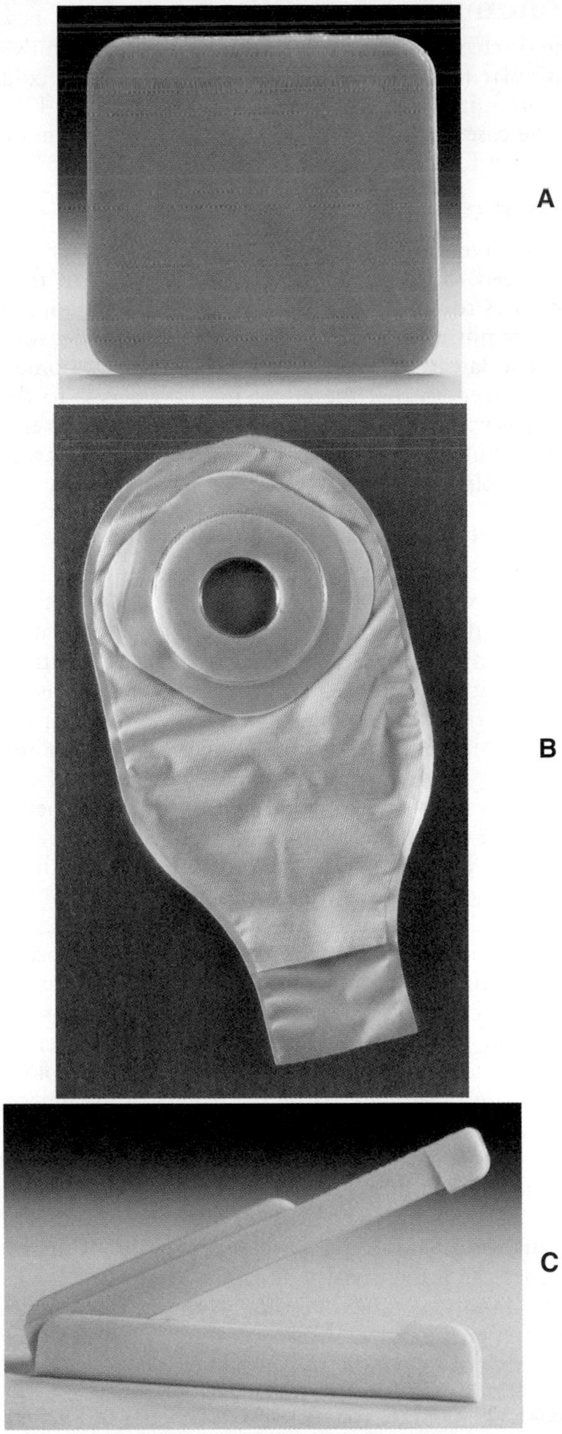

Figure 61-6 ■ Skin barriers, such as wafers **(A),** are cut to fit $\frac{1}{8}$ inch around the fistula. A drainable pouch **(B)** is applied over the wafer and clamped **(C)** until the pouch is to be emptied. Effluent should drain into the bag and not contact the skin. (Courtesy ConvaTec, A Bristol-Myers Squibb Company, Skillman, NJ.)

Community-Based Care

The discharge care plan for the client with Crohn's disease is similar to that for the client with ulcerative colitis (see Community-Based Care [Ulcerative Colitis], p. 1353). You or the case manager will help the client with a draining fistula plan for care of the fistula at home.

HOME CARE MANAGEMENT

The interventions begun in the hospital to manage the disease need to be carried out to some extent in the home. Measures to control the disease and related symptoms and manage nutrition need to be reinforced. Supplies for wound and fistula care may be required. The client's home should be arranged so that the client has easy access to the bathroom as well as privacy to perform fistula care. To ensure adequate nutrition, the client should have easy access to a well-supplied kitchen of readily prepared foods.

HEALTH TEACHING

The teaching plan for Crohn's disease is similar to that for the client with ulcerative colitis. Inform the client about the usual course of the disease, symptoms of complications, and when to notify the health care provider. Medication teaching, including purpose, dose, and side effects, is incorporated into the teaching plan. In addition to other drugs, vitamin supplements, including monthly vitamin B_{12} injections may be needed due to the inability of the ileum to absorb nutrients. In collaboration with the dietitian, instruct the client to follow a low-residue, high-calorie diet and to avoid foods that cause discomfort, such as milk, gluten, and other GI stimulants.

Remind the client to provide for rest periods, especially during exacerbations of the disease. If stress appears to increase symptoms of the disease, stress management techniques or counseling should be recommended. For long-term follow-up, the client is educated regarding the increased risk of bowel cancer and the advisability of having a colonoscopy as a means of early detection of changes in the mucosa.

If a client has developed a fistula, explain and demonstrate fistula care. The client needs opportunities to practice the care in the hospital. Ideally the client should be independent in fistula care before leaving the hospital. However, because of the perirectal or vaginal location of the fistula or an obese abdomen, assistance may be needed. If this is the case, a family member or a caregiver must learn and practice the care, or the nurse or case manager can arrange for home care services.

HEALTH CARE RESOURCES

The client discharged to home after undergoing resection and anastomosis may require visits from a home care nurse to assess the surgical wound and monitor for complications. Assess the client's and his or her family's ability to monitor the progress of fistula healing and to watch for signs and symptoms of infection and sepsis. Home care nursing visits may also be appropriate for this purpose. A home care aide might be considered for clients who cannot meet their nutritional needs, who need help with meal preparation, and who need help in purchasing groceries.

If the client needs equipment for fistula care, such as skin barriers and wound drainage bags, the nurse or case manager contacts medical supply companies or local pharmacies to ascertain their availability and price. A support group sponsored by the United Ostomy Association or a local hospital in the community may also be available to assist the client and family with physical as well as psychosocial needs.

Diverticular Disease

Diverticula are congenital or acquired pouchlike herniations of the mucosa through the muscular wall of the small intestine or colon. **Diverticulosis** is the presence of many abnormal pouchlike herniations (diverticula) in the wall of the intestine. **Diverticulitis** is the term used to describe an inflammation of one or more diverticula.

PATHOPHYSIOLOGY

Diverticula can occur in any part of the small or large intestine, but they occur most commonly in the sigmoid colon (Figure 61-7). The musculature of the colon hypertrophies, thickens, and becomes rigid, and herniation of the mucosa and submucosa through the colon wall is seen. Diverticula seem to occur at points of weakness in the intestinal wall, often at areas where blood vessels interrupt muscular continuity. The muscle weakness develops as part of the aging process.

In and of themselves, diverticula cause few problems. If undigested food or bacteria become trapped in a diverticulum, however, blood supply to that area diminishes and bacteria invade the diverticulum. Diverticulitis results when the diverticulum perforates and a local abscess forms. The perforated diverticulum can also progress to an intra-abdominal perforation with generalized peritonitis.

Bleeding from diverticula can range from minor, localized bleeding to massive hemorrhage. Minor bleeding is often due to localized inflammation in areas of vascular granulation tissue at the base of the diverticulum. Hemorrhage can result when a blood vessel is eroded within a diverticulum. Inflammation secondary to recurrent diverticulitis can lead to narrowing of the bowel lumen, which may result in obstruction. Inflammation can also result in fistulas to other organs, such as the bladder and the vagina.

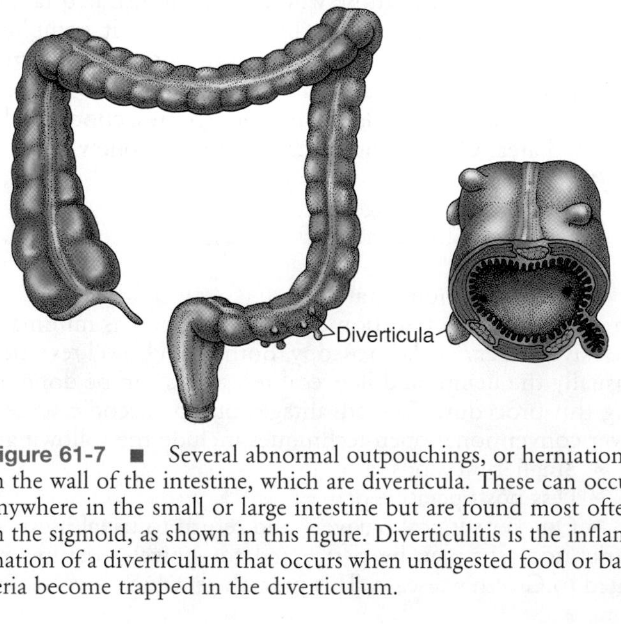

Figure 61-7 ■ Several abnormal outpouchings, or herniations, in the wall of the intestine, which are diverticula. These can occur anywhere in the small or large intestine but are found most often in the sigmoid, as shown in this figure. Diverticulitis is the inflammation of a diverticulum that occurs when undigested food or bacteria become trapped in the diverticulum.

Etiology

Diets with small amounts of fiber have been implicated in the development of diverticula in that they cause less bulky stool and possibly constipation. For diverticulosis and diverticulitis to occur, there must be an increase in intraluminal pressure and muscle contractions to move fecal material through the colon.

The etiologic factor in diverticulitis might be retained undigested food in diverticula, which compromises the blood supply to that area and facilitates bacterial invasion of the sac.

Incidence/Prevalence

The incidence of diverticulosis is difficult to determine, but it is estimated that millions of people are affected. Diverticulitis affects one third of adults over age 60 years, with more men than women affected. Although diverticulosis is common, only one of five people with this disease displays symptoms.

COLLABORATIVE MANAGEMENT

Assessment

HISTORY

Clients with diverticulosis are usually asymptomatic, and unless pain or bleeding develops, the condition may go undiagnosed or found incidentally on routine colonoscopy. Occasionally diverticulosis causes symptoms. For clients with uncomplicated diverticulosis, the nurse asks about a history of intermittent pain in the left lower quadrant and a history of constipation. If diverticulitis is suspected, the client is asked about a history of fever and abdominal pain. Inquire about recent bowel elimination patterns because constipation may develop as a result of intestinal inflammation. The client is also questioned about the presence of bleeding from the rectum.

PHYSICAL ASSESSMENT/CLINICAL MANIFESTATIONS

On physical examination of the client with uncomplicated diverticulosis, no clinical manifestations of the disorder may be present. Occasionally tenderness is elicited on abdominal palpation.

The client with diverticulitis has abdominal pain, most often localized to the left lower quadrant. The pain may be intermittent at first but becomes progressively steady. Occasionally pain may be suprapubic, or it may occur on one side. Abdominal pain is generalized if peritonitis has occurred. The client's temperature is elevated, ranging from a low-grade fever to 101° F (38.2° C), and may be accompanied by chills. Note any tachycardia secondary to fever. Nausea and vomiting are also commonly present.

On examination of the abdomen, observe for distention. Tenderness on palpation may be noted over the area involved (usually the left lower quadrant). The colon may be palpable. If localized peritoneal irritation is present, localized muscle spasm, guarded movement, and rebound tenderness are usually present. If generalized peritonitis is present, abdominal muscle spasm, guarding, and rebound tenderness are more diffuse.

If the perforated diverticulum is close to the rectum, the health care provider may palpate a tender mass during the rectal examination. Blood pressure checks may show orthostatic changes. If bleeding is massive, the client may have hypotension and dehydration that result in shock. If generalized peritonitis has occurred, sepsis and manifestations of hypotension and septic or hypovolemic shock can occur.

DIAGNOSTIC ASSESSMENT

For the client with uncomplicated diverticulosis, laboratory studies are not indicated. The client with diverticulitis, however, has an elevated white blood cell (WBC) count. Decreased hematocrit and hemoglobin values are noted if chronic or severe bleeding is present. In stool tests for occult blood, results are positive in 20% of clients (also called a fecal occult blood test [FOBT]). Urinalysis may show a few red blood cells (RBCs) if the left ureter is in proximity to a perforated diverticulum.

X-rays of the intestinal tract with barium contrast show diverticula. An upper gastrointestinal (GI) series shows diverticula of the small intestine, and barium enema examination shows diverticula of the large intestine. X-rays are not indicated for clients with uncomplicated diverticulosis because symptoms are usually minimal or nonexistent.

The client with diverticulitis usually does *not* undergo a barium enema examination in the acute phase of the illness because of the risk of rupture of the inflamed diverticulum. A barium enema examination may be completed after the client has been treated with antibiotics and the inflammation has resolved. A flat-plate film of the abdomen may reveal free air and fluid in the left lower quadrant, suggesting an abscess or free air under the diaphragm, indicating perforation. The health care provider may also order a computed tomography (CT) scan to diagnose an abscess or thickening of the bowel related to diverticulitis.

Ultrasonography, a noninvasive test, may reveal bowel thickening or an abscess. The physician may perform a sigmoidoscopy or colonoscopy *after the acute phase* of the illness, usually to rule out the presence of a tumor in the large intestine, particularly if the client has rectal bleeding. If the sigmoidoscope or colonoscope enters a diverticulum, however, the chances of perforating the diverticulum are high.

Interventions

Clients may be treated on an ambulatory care basis when symptoms are mild, with a temperature lower than 101° F (38.2° C) and a WBC count ranging from 13,000 to 15,000/mm^3. The client who is an outpatient should be monitored for any prolonged or increased fever, abdominal pain, or blood in the stool.

Clients with moderate to severe diverticulitis usually require hospitalization. Clinical manifestations that suggest the need for admission are a temperature higher than 101° F (38.2° C), persistent abdominal pain for more than 3 days, or evidence of lower GI bleeding.

NONSURGICAL MANAGEMENT. For the client with diverticulitis, a combination of drug and diet therapy with rest to decrease inflammation and improve tissue perfusion is indicated. This plan is preferred for older adults and others with mild to moderate disease (Chart 61-6).

For clients with mild diverticulitis, the health care provider prescribes broad-spectrum antibiotics, such as metronidazole (Flagyl) plus trimethoprim/sulfamethoxazole (Bactrim, Septra) or ciprofloxacin (Cipro). A mild analgesic may be given for pain.

CHART 61-6

NURSING FOCUS on the OLDER ADULT
Diverticulitis

- Provide antibiotics, analgesics, and anticholinergics as prescribed. Observe older clients carefully for side effects of these drugs, especially confusion (or increased confusion), urinary retention or failure, and orthostatic hypotension.
- Do not give laxatives or enemas. Teach the client and the family about the importance of avoiding these measures.
- Encourage the client to rest and to avoid activities that may increase intra-abdominal pressure, such as straining and bending.
- While diverticulitis is active, provide a *low*-fiber diet (see Table 61-4). When the inflammation resolves, provide a *high*-fiber diet. Teach the client and family about these diets and when they are appropriate.
- Because older clients do not always experience the typical pain or fever expected, observe carefully for signs of active disease.
- Perform frequent abdominal assessments to determine distention and tenderness on palpation.
- Check stools for occult or frank bleeding.

The health care provider admits clients with more severe pain to the hospital and prescribes IV fluids to correct dehydration as well as IV antibiotics such as cefoxitin plus metronidazole. Anticholinergics may reduce intestinal hypermotility. For clients with moderate to severe diverticulitis, an opioid analgesic, such as meperidine hydrochloride (Demerol) or morphine sulfate, can alleviate pain.

Laxatives are avoided because they increase intestinal motility. Enemas are avoided because they increase intraluminal pressure. The nurse assesses the client for clinical manifestations of fluid and electrolyte imbalance on an ongoing basis.

Instruct the client to remain in bed during the acute phase of illness. He or she is advised to refrain from lifting, straining, coughing, or bending to avoid an increase in intra-abdominal pressure, which can result in perforation of the diverticulum.

During the acute phase of the illness, the client's diet is restricted to clear liquids. Clients who have more severe symptoms are admitted to the hospital and are kept on NPO status. A nasogastric (NG) tube is inserted if nausea, vomiting, or abdominal distention is severe. Administer IV fluids, as prescribed, for hydration. In collaboration with the dietitian, the client increases dietary intake slowly as symptoms subside. When inflammation has resolved and bowel function returns to normal, a fiber-containing diet is introduced gradually. If active diverticulitis recurs, fiber intake is stopped for the acute phase of the illness.

SURGICAL MANAGEMENT. The client with diverticulitis may need to undergo surgery for any of the following complications:

- Rupture of the diverticulum with subsequent peritonitis
- Pelvic abscess
- Bowel obstruction
- Fistula
- Persistent fever or pain after 4 days of medical treatment
- Uncontrolled bleeding

The surgeon performs emergency surgery if peritonitis, bowel obstruction, or pelvic abscess is present. Colon resection, with or without a colostomy, is the most common surgical procedure for clients with diverticular disease.

Preoperative Care. Preparation of the client for surgery depends on the severity of the condition. The surgery might be performed on an emergency basis, or it might be done with a few weeks' notice. The surgeon informs the client whether a temporary or permanent colostomy might be required.

If the client is *not* in the acute stage of diverticulitis, a thorough bowel preparation *may* be given, consisting of enemas and laxatives daily for 1 to 2 days before surgery. Because of the risk of perforation, however, the surgeon may forgo an aggressive bowel preparation. If the client has an acutely inflamed diverticulum or persistent fever and abdominal pain, the bowel preparation is most likely withheld.

For clients without acute inflammation, a well-structured preoperative diet is ordered. The client usually has a low-fiber diet for 4 to 5 days, followed by a full-liquid diet for 2 days, then a clear-liquid diet the evening before surgery.

Preoperative teaching may include information about the possible need for a colostomy. If a colostomy is a possible outcome, the enterostomal therapist (ET) or office nurse describes its function and purpose. The nurse need not discuss colostomy care in detail unless the client wishes this information at this time.

Operative Procedures. In a resection of the colon, the surgeon excises the portion that is inflamed or diseased and, if possible, creates an anastomosis of the colon to restore patency. Inflammation and infection, however, may preclude the feasibility of an anastomosis. If this is the case, the surgeon may perform a colostomy. Select clients may be candidates for colostomy closure and anastomosis after the bowel has been allowed to rest for 3 to 6 months.

Postoperative Care. The immediate physical care for clients undergoing a colon resection for diverticulitis is the same as that for clients undergoing abdominal surgery (see Chapter 22).

The client has a drain in place at the abdominal incision site for 2 to 3 days. If a colostomy has been performed, the stoma may be covered with petroleum gauze dressing because the colostomy does not drain for approximately 2 days, or a colostomy bag may be placed over the stoma. If the stoma is visible, monitor for color and integrity. The stoma should be pinkish to cherry red without retraction or prolapse into the abdomen.

The client is maintained on NPO status with a possible NG tube in place for 2 to 3 days after a colon resection, with or without a colostomy. When peristalsis returns, remove the NG tube, according to the health care provider's order, and introduce clear liquids *slowly*. *Gradually*, the diet is advanced to solids, depending on the return of peristalsis and bowel function.

If the client has had a colostomy created, it should begin functioning in 2 to 4 days. Most clients who undergo surgery and colostomy formation for diverticulitis have a sigmoid colostomy because the sigmoid colon is the most common site of diverticulitis. Drainage from a sigmoid colostomy initially consists of loose stool, but eventually the stool becomes formed. A tight seal around the stoma is essential to avoid contact of feces with the skin. Colostomy care is detailed in Chapter 60.

If a colostomy has been performed, give the client an opportunity to express feelings about the ostomy. Discuss these feelings with the client, acknowledging that anger and depression are normal responses. When the client is physically able, encourage him or her to look at the stoma and touch the apparatus.

Community-Based Care

The length of hospitalization for clients with diverticulitis ranges from 3 days to longer than a week, depending on the response to medical treatment and the need for surgery. Discharge plans vary according to the treatment.

HOME CARE MANAGEMENT

For the client with diverticulitis who has responded to medical treatment, home care focuses on proper diet. Assess the client's ability to obtain and prepare the recommended high-fiber foods. The client who has required surgical intervention has the added responsibilities of incision care and possibly colostomy care, with some temporary limitations placed on activities.

HEALTH TEACHING

All clients with diverticular disease require education regarding a high-fiber diet. For clients with diverticulosis, an increase in dietary fiber can regulate bowel function and bring about partial relief of symptoms. The nurse and dietitian encourage the client with diverticulosis to eat a diet high in cellulose and hemicellulose types of fiber. These substances can be found in wheat bran, whole-grain breads, and cereals. The client should ingest at least 25 to 35 g of fiber per day. This requirement can be derived from four slices of 100% whole-wheat bread and a 3-ounce serving of all-bran cereal. Teach the client to eat fresh fruits and vegetables with high-fiber content to add bulk to stools.

The client who is not accustomed to eating high-fiber foods should add them to the diet gradually to avoid flatulence and abdominal cramping. If the client cannot tolerate the recommended fiber requirement, a bulk-forming laxative, such as psyllium hydrophilic mucilloid (Metamucil), can be taken to increase fecal size and consistency. An adequate intake of fluids will help to prevent the bloating that may accompany a high-fiber diet. The client should also avoid alcohol because it irritates the bowel. Clients are instructed to avoid foods containing seeds or indigestible material that may block a diverticulum, such as nuts, corn, popcorn, cucumbers, tomatoes, figs, strawberries, and caraway seeds. In collaboration with the dietitian, the nurse teaches the client that dietary fat intake should not exceed 30% of the total daily caloric intake.

Clients should *avoid all fiber* when they have symptoms of *diverticulitis* because high-fiber foods are irritating. As diverticulitis resolves, fiber can gradually be added until progression to a high-fiber diet is once again obtained. The client who has undergone surgery is usually taking solid food by the time of discharge from the hospital.

Explain the usual disease course and factors that can exacerbate the disease to the client. Follow-up with the health care provider approximately 1 month after resolution of symptoms is recommended, and a repeat flexible sigmoidoscopy or barium enema may be preformed at that time.

Clients who have had abdominal surgery need oral and written instructions on incision care and the signs and symptoms to report to the health care provider. These are similar to the instructions given to clients after other types of abdominal surgery. Provide instructions on colostomy care for clients who have a temporary or permanent colostomy.

Instruct clients *with any type of diverticular disease,* orally and in writing, about the manifestations of acute diverticulitis, including fever, abdominal pain, and bloody, mahogany, or tarry stools. The client should be advised to avoid the use of laxatives (other than bulk-forming types) and enemas. All clients can also benefit from avoiding the activities that increase intra-abdominal pressure, such as straining at stool, bending, or lifting heavy objects.

Reassure clients with diverticulosis that this disorder need not cause problems if a proper diet is followed. The client is informed that this illness does not commonly recur and that with proper diet and elimination patterns, recurring episodes and potential complications can be avoided.

The client with a colostomy has special needs with regard to the alteration in body image and loss of body function. Encourage the client to verbalize concerns about body image.

HEALTH CARE RESOURCES

Clients who have undergone surgery may need assistance with incision and colostomy care. The nurse or case manager arranges for a home care nurse to assess wound healing and proper functioning of the ostomy and the appliance. If the client is interested, the nurse can arrange for a visit from an ostomy volunteer or an enterostomal therapist (ET). For information about other ostomy resources, instruct the client to contact the United Ostomy Association.

Critical Thinking Challenge

A middle-aged man is informed that his colonoscopy revealed moderate diverticulosis and several polyps, which were removed. His mother died of colon cancer last year, and he is very nervous about his chances for cancer. He has had gastroesophageal reflux disease (GERD) and irritable bowel syndrome (IBS) for longer than 10 years and currently takes Metamucil daily.

1. Is this client a candidate for drug therapy? Why or why not?
2. What dietary modifications and restrictions should he follow and why? (Keep his GERD and IBS in mind also.)
3. What other health teaching does he need?

evolve For suggested answer guidelines, go to http://evolve.elsevier.com/Iggy/.

ANORECTAL ABSCESS

PATHOPHYSIOLOGY

Anorectal abscess is a localized induration and fluctuance caused by inflammation of the soft tissue near the rectum or anus. It is most often the result of obstruction of the ducts of glands in the anorectal region by feces, foreign bodies, or trauma. Stasis of obstructing contents occurs and causes infection that spreads into adjacent tissue. Most abscesses begin as cryptitis (a pocket of infection in an anal crypt).

The client may experience rectal pain as the first symptom. There may be no clinical manifestations at the time of the first physical assessment, but local swelling, erythema, and tenderness on palpation are apparent within a few days after the onset of pain. If the abscess becomes chronic, discharge, bleeding, and pruritus (itching) may exist. Fever occurs if larger abscesses are present.

CHART 61-7

BEST PRACTICE for Promoting Perineal Comfort

- Keep the perineal area clean with mild soap.
- Pat the perineal area dry instead of rubbing it.
- Provide warm sitz baths, or apply warm compresses to the area.
- If the area is acutely inflamed, apply cold packs.
- Provide a chair cushion or a soft, inflatable ring for the seated client. For the older or debilitated client, monitor the skin carefully to prevent pressure sores.
- Use absorbent pads for drainage, if any, and change them often.
- Use premoistened wipes for cleaning the perineal area after a bowel movement.
- Use witch hazel wipes (e.g., Tucks) to relieve pain.
- Give bulk-forming agents, such as psyllium mucilloid (Metamucil), as prescribed, to reduce pain associated with defecation.
- Apply a topical anesthetic cream to the perineal area, as prescribed.
- Give oral analgesics, as prescribed, for pain relief.
- Do not administer enemas or give potent laxatives.

COLLABORATIVE MANAGEMENT

Anorectal abscesses are managed by surgical incision and drainage. The physician can often incise simple perianal and ischiorectal abscesses using a local anesthetic. For clients with more extensive abscesses, a regional or general anesthetic may be needed. Systemic antibiotics are given only for clients who are immunocompromised, are diabetic, have valvular disease or a prosthetic valve, or have extensive subcutaneous fat. Incision and drainage in these clients are performed after antibiotic therapy.

Nursing interventions are focused on helping the client to maintain comfort and optimal perineal hygiene (Chart 61-7). Encourage the use of warm sitz baths, analgesics, bulk-producing agents, and stool softeners during the perioperative period until healing occurs. Emphasize the importance of ongoing perineal hygiene after all bowel movements and the maintenance of a regular bowel pattern with a high-fiber diet.

ANAL FISSURE

PATHOPHYSIOLOGY

An **anal fissure** is a common anorectal condition of particular concern because of the degree (if acute) of discomfort and disability. First-degree fissures are associated with diarrhea or constipation; second-degree fissures are associated with another disorder (e.g., Crohn's disease, tuberculosis, leukemia, or neoplasm) or with trauma (e.g., from a foreign body, childbirth, or perirectal surgery).

COLLABORATIVE MANAGEMENT

An acute anal fissure is superficial and resolves spontaneously or heals quickly with conservative treatment. Chronic fissures recur, and surgical treatment may be needed. Pain during and after defecation and bleeding noted outside the stool are the most common symptoms. Other clinical manifestations associated with chronic fissures are pruritus, urinary frequency or retention, dysuria, and **dyspareunia** (painful intercourse).

The health care provider makes the diagnosis by inspecting and stretching the perianal skin. If the client is having pain at the time of the examination, diagnostic testing is usually limited to inspection. If the client is not in severe pain, a digital examination and possibly a sigmoidoscopy are performed. When painless or multiple fissures are present, the physician may perform a barium enema and sigmoidoscopy to rule out an associated inflammatory bowel disorder.

Management of an acute fissure is typically nonsurgical, with interventions aimed at local, symptomatic pain relief and softening of stools to reduce trauma to the area. Warm sitz baths and analgesia are recommended along with the use of bulk-producing agents, such as psyllium hydrophilic mucilloid (Metamucil), which help to minimize pain associated with defecation. Topical anti-inflammatories (Hydrocortisone creams and suppositories) or opiate suppositories (opium and belladonna suppositories) are helpful if spasms are severe.

Explain the appropriate pain control measures to the client. When nonsurgical management is initiated, instruct the client to notify the health care provider if pain is not relieved within a few days. If fissures do not respond to medical management within several days to weeks, surgical excision of the fissure with a local anesthetic may be necessary. Teach the client who undergoes surgery to continue with the same pain management and bowel regimen, including sitz baths, analgesics, and bulk-forming agents. He or she is reminded to report any drainage or bleeding from the rectum to the health care provider.

ANAL FISTULA

An anal fistula, or *fistula in ano,* is an abnormal tract leading from the anal canal to the perianal skin. Most anal fistulas result from anorectal abscesses, which are caused by obstruction of anal glands (see Anorectal Abscess, p. 1361). Fistulas can also be associated with tuberculosis, Crohn's disease, or cancer.

The client with an anal fistula has pruritus (itching), purulent discharge, and tenderness or pain that is worsened by bowel movements. The physician uses a proctoscope to identify the source of symptoms and to locate the fistula. Because fistulas do not heal spontaneously, surgery is necessary. To perform a **fistulotomy,** the surgeon incises the tissue overlying the tract and performs curettage (scraping) of the base. The incision site heals by secondary intention. In a client with a high fistula, a special surgical technique is necessary because important sphincters are often affected. Postoperatively the nurse instructs the client about sitz baths, analgesics, and the use of bulk-producing agents or stool softeners to minimize pain.

PARASITIC INFECTION

PATHOPHYSIOLOGY

Parasites can enter and invade the gastrointestinal (GI) tract and cause infections leading to varying degrees of illness. Parasites commonly enter through the mouth by means of fecal-oral transmission from the following:

- Contaminated food or water
- Oral-anal sexual practices
- Contact with feces from a contaminated person

Common **parasites** that cause infection in humans are *Entamoeba histolytica*, which causes amebiasis (amebic dysentery); *Giardia lamblia*, which causes giardiasis; and *Cryptosporidium*.

Infection with *Entamoeba histolytica*

Humans are the only known hosts for *E. histolytica* (also known as amebiasis). This organism occurs in cysts and trophozoites (sporozoan parasites). Trophozoites die rapidly after they leave the body in stool. Cysts, however, can remain viable in the right type of environment for weeks or months. Humans who eliminate cysts are infectious. Flies have been found to be vectors for transmission of the cysts, and transmission is increased in areas that use human excrement for fertilizer. Transmission occurs by the fecal-oral route.

Amebiasis occurs worldwide, but it is most prevalent and most severe in tropical areas. Prevalence rates are as high as 40% in areas with poor sanitation, crowding, and poor nutrition. Amebiasis causes 40,000 to 100,000 deaths annually worldwide. The disease causes less severe symptoms and often goes undiagnosed in temperate climates. The organism may occur in 5% of some populations in the United States.

E. histolytica either feeds on bacteria in the intestine or invades and ulcerates the mucosa of the large intestine. The parasite can be limited to the GI tract (intestinal amebiasis), or it can extend outside the intestines (extraintestinal amebiasis). People can have intestinal amebiasis without having any symptoms, or symptoms can range from mild to severe.

Infection with *Giardia lamblia*

G. lamblia is a protozoal parasite that causes superficial invasion, destruction, and inflammation of the mucosa in the small intestine. Like *E. histolytica*, *G. lamblia* has a trophozoite and cysts form, and cysts can transmit the organism. Humans are hosts to this organism, but beavers and dogs may be reservoirs for infection. *G. lamblia* is transmitted by the fecal-oral route. Giardiasis is a well-recognized problem in travelers, campers, male homosexuals, and immunosuppressed people.

Modes of transmission are similar to those for amebiasis; in the United States, however, giardiasis is much more prevalent and is the most common parasitic infection. Giardiasis affects only the intestinal system, causing acute diarrhea, chronic diarrhea, or malabsorption syndrome. The acute phase usually is self-limiting, lasting days or weeks. The chronic phase can last for years. Diarrhea is usually mild in both forms, but it can be severe. As stools increase in frequency, they become more watery, greasy, frothy, and malodorous with mucus. Weight loss and weakness are also common. Malabsorption can occur with diarrhea that continues for longer than 3 weeks. Manifestations result from malabsorption of fat, protein, vitamin B_{12}, and lactase deficiency.

Infection with *Cryptosporidium*

Cryptosporidium is another parasitic infestation transmitted by the fecal-oral route that is manifested by diarrhea. This infection commonly occurs in immunosuppressed clients, particularly those with human immunodeficiency virus (HIV). (See Chapter 25 for a discussion of HIV infection.)

COLLABORATIVE MANAGEMENT

Assessment

A thorough history can provide information about potential sources of exposure to parasitic infection. A history of travel to parts of the world where such infections are prevalent increases suspicion for infection with parasites. GI symptoms related to travel may be delayed as long as 1 to 2 weeks after the return home. A diet history is especially helpful if several people become ill. Common water supplies may be infected with *Giardia* or *Cryptosporidium*. Trichinosis should be considered if the client has ingested pork products.

Mild to moderate *E. histolytica* infestation causes clinical manifestations, including the daily passage of several strongly odoriferous stools, possibly with mucus but without blood, accompanied by abdominal cramping, flatulence, fatigue, and weight loss.

Clients experience characteristic remissions and recurrences. Severe amebic dysentery is manifested by frequent, more liquid, and odoriferous stools with mucus *and* blood. Fever up to 105° F (40° C), **tenesmus** (painful straining to defecate), generalized abdominal tenderness, and vomiting can also occur. The ulcerations characteristic of invading amebiasis that occur in the colon can cause pain, bleeding, and obstruction. Ulcerations can also be localized in the rectum, resulting in formed stool with blood. Complications are rare but include appendicitis and bowel perforation.

Extraintestinal amebiasis can occur without symptoms of intestinal infection. The most common form is amebic liver abscess, which causes symptoms of fever, pain, and an enlarged liver. The abscess can rupture, and death can result if the infection is not treated and complications occur.

The diagnosis of *amebiasis* is made by examination of stool for parasites. Because *E. histolytica* is difficult to detect, serial stool examinations are needed if the disease is suspected. The use of sigmoidoscopy may detect ulcerations in the rectum or colon. Exudate obtained during sigmoidoscopic examination is studied for the parasite. The white blood cell (WBC) count can be as high as 20,000/mm^3 when severe dysentery is present.

The diagnosis of *giardiasis* is also confirmed by stool examination for parasites. Because organisms may not be detected for at least 1 week after symptoms appear, multiple stool samples should be examined. Duodenal aspirate can also be examined for the parasite.

Infection with *Cryptosporidium* is usually self-limiting in individuals who are not immunocompromised. Drug therapy for clients with immunosuppression may consist of paromomycin 500 to 750 mg four times daily.

Interventions

Interventions for Amebiasis. Treatment for all types of amebiasis mandate the use of amebicide drugs. The physician commonly prescribes metronidazole (Flagyl, Novonidazole✱) and diloxanide furoate (Entamide) or diloxanide furoate and tetracycline hydrochloride (Sumycin) followed by chloroquine. Clients with severe dysentery require IV fluids for replacement and maintenance of fluid volume and possibly opiates, such as diphenoxylate hydrochloride and atropine sulfate (Lomotil), to control bowel motility. Clients with extraintestinal amebiasis or severe dehydration are hospitalized. Clients with asymptomatic, mild, or moderate disease are treated as outpatients with drug therapy. For all clients, at least three stools are examined for parasites at 2- to 3-day intervals, starting 2 to 4 weeks after drug therapy has been completed.

Interventions for Giardiasis. Treatment for giardiasis is drug therapy. Metronidazole is the drug of choice, and the usual dose, is 250 mg three times daily PO for 5 days. Tinidazole (Fasigyn) can be used as an alternative. Stools are examined 2 weeks after treatment is begun to assess for eradication.

Explain modes of transmission and means to avoid the spread of infection and recurrent contact with parasitic organisms. Clients are taught that they can transmit the infection to others until amebicides effectively kill the parasites. The nurse instructs clients to do the following:

- Avoid contact with stool
- Keep toilet areas clean
- Wash their hands meticulously with an antimicrobial soap after bowel movements
- Maintain personal hygiene
- Avoid stool from dogs and beavers

The client is also advised to avoid sexual practices who allow rectal contact until drug therapy is completed. Inform the client that all household and sexual contacts should undergo stool examinations for parasites. If the water supply is suspected as the source, a sample is obtained and sent for analysis. Multiple infections are common in households, often as a result of contaminated water supplies. Well water and water from areas with inadequate or no filtration equipment can be sources of contamination.

HELMINTHIC INFESTATION

Helminths are wormlike animals; they are often parasitic and capable of causing infectious disease in humans. There are many species of helminths, which for purposes of classification are divided into three general categories:

- Roundworms (nematodes)
- Flukes (trematodes)
- Tapeworms (cestodes)

Helminths can cause various degrees of gastrointestinal (GI) symptoms in humans. Most often they enter the human body through the skin or via the oral route with ingestion of food, water, or other substances contaminated with worms. Some helminths gain access to the human body via insects, such as flies and mosquitoes. Helminths that are typically transmitted via insects are limited to tropical areas, however, and are not discussed here. Flukes (trematodes), which are passed to humans via snail-contaminated water, are also limited to tropical and subtropical areas outside the United States and are not discussed here.

Roundworms

Roundworms are commonly the cause of helminthic infections in the United States and worldwide. These infections include enterobiasis, trichinosis, and hookworm.

Enterobiasis

Enterobiasis ("pinworm infection") is caused by *Enterobius vermicularis* and is the most common helminthic infection in the United States. It is transmitted by oral ingestion of contaminated food, drink, or fomites. The most common clinical manifestations of infection include nocturnal perianal pruritus, vaginitis, insomnia, and restlessness.

The client may have vague GI symptoms, such as abdominal pain, nausea, vomiting, and diarrhea. However, many infected clients have no symptoms. Diagnosis is made when eggs of the helminth are found on the perianal skin or on cellulose tape that has been applied to the perianal skin.

Treatment of enterobiasis includes meticulous handwashing techniques after defecation and before meals to prevent spread of the worms to others. Drug therapy is indicated for all clients with symptoms and in some clients who are infected but are not symptomatic. Household cohabitants of an infected client may be treated with drug therapy even if they are asymptomatic. Pyrantel pamoate (Antiminth, Combantrin✱) or mebendazole (Vermox, Nemasol✱) is given orally in one dose, repeated at 2 and 4 weeks.

Infection with pinworms is curable and is not usually associated with complications; however, recurrences are common.

Trichinosis

Trichinosis is another helminthic disease caused by roundworms. The incidence in the United States is 50 to 100 cases annually, but many mild or asymptomatic cases are not diagnosed because the person is usually asymptomatic. *Trichinella spiralis,* which lives in the intestine of humans, pigs, bears, and rats, causes trichinosis. The organism is usually transmitted to people who ingest undercooked pork or pork products. Ingestion of other meats, such as ground beef, can also promote transmission if a meat grinder has been used for both beef and pork. Following ingestion, the larvae, encased in cysts, are released by the digestive action of acid and pepsin. Incubation is 12 hours to 28 days after ingestion. Clinical manifestations range from none to severe; death rarely results.

During the first week after infection, diarrhea results from the invasion of the gut by large numbers of the parasite. Abdominal pain, nausea, and vomiting may follow. During the second week, the larvae begin to invade the muscle, instigating a hypersensitivity reaction characterized by fever, periorbital and facial edema, and subconjunctival hemorrhage. Occasionally a rash or dyspnea develops. Two to three weeks after infection, symptoms of myositis, myalgia, and muscle weakness develop, particularly in the lower back, neck, jaw, biceps, and extraocular muscles. Vague muscle pain and malaise characterize the convalescence phase, which can last several months.

A diagnosis of trichinosis is confirmed by a history of ingestion of raw or undercooked meat. White blood cell (WBC) and eosinophil counts are elevated for 2 weeks after meat is ingested. Biopsy of skeletal muscle shows larvae of the *Trichinella* organism. Worms are rarely seen in feces.

During the first week after infection, the client is treated with oral mebendazole. During the stage of muscle invasion, he or she must be hospitalized to receive high doses of corticosteroids.

Hookworms

Hookworms are also roundworms. They differ from pinworms and *Trichinella* in that they initially enter the human body through the skin. Hookworm disease is caused by either *Ancylostoma duodenale* or *Necator americanus.*

Hookworms infect a quarter of the world's population, but the disease is rare in areas outside the tropics or in areas with little rain. Worms are infective outside the body in warm, moist soil for up to 1 week. Transmission occurs when larvae penetrate through the skin. The organism can migrate to pulmonary capillaries via the bloodstream and enter alveoli. Cilia carry the organisms up the respiratory tree to the pharynx and the mouth, where they are swallowed and enter the GI tract. Hookworms probably also enter the GI tract when a person ingests contaminated food.

Early symptoms of hookworm disease include a pruritic, erythematous, raised vesicular inflammation of the skin. Infection in the GI tract may produce no symptoms, or it may cause anorexia, diarrhea, or mild abdominal and epigastric discomfort. Bleeding and anemia may occur when worms suck blood at sites of attachment in the GI tract. If blood loss is severe, the client may have symptoms of iron deficiency anemia, such as pallor, hair thinning, deformed nails, pica, and shortness of breath.

Diagnosis of hookworm infection is based on the presence of ova (eggs) in the feces. Occult blood is often present in the stool. There may be a low hemoglobin concentration and hematocrit value or a low serum iron level and high iron-binding capacity, indicating hypochromic microcytic anemia. The WBC counts and eosinophil counts are elevated.

All clients with symptoms receive iron therapy and a diet high in protein and vitamins for at least 3 months after anemia is corrected. Pyrantel pamoate (Antiminth) or mebendazole (Vermox) is given for a complete recovery. Severe hookworm disease can cause malabsorption and protein loss, necessitating nutritional support in addition to other treatments.

Tapeworms

Five types of tapeworms (cestodes) may infect humans: tapeworms found in cattle, fish, dogs, pigs, and rodents. Tapeworm infections generally cause either no symptoms or only occasional GI upset, such as nausea, diarrhea, or abdominal pain.

Transmission of tapeworms occurs when a person ingests undercooked beef, raw fish, or other contaminated food or water or accidentally swallows infected lice or fleas from dogs. People can also accidentally ingest arthropods, such as cockroaches, in stored foods or cereals.

The diagnosis of tapeworm infestation is made by laboratory examination of eggs found in the stool (test of stool for ova and parasites). Clients are treated with medications for this type of infection.

When caring for clients with helminths, follow standard precautions or body substance precautions when in contact with any stool. All clients are taught to wash their hands after defecating and before eating. They should avoid ingesting undercooked beef, fish, or pork and drinking water that might be contaminated. After petting dogs, clients should take care to keep their mouth closed and wash their hands. All stored foods should be kept tightly closed to avoid contamination by cockroaches and other insects.

FOOD POISONING

Foodborne illnesses are a common problem, with 6.5 cases occurring in the United States every year (Van Benden et al., 1999). Food poisoning has been linked to as many as 9000 deaths per year in the United States. Food poisoning results when a person ingests infectious organisms in food. Unlike gastroenteritis, food poisoning is not directly communicable from person to person, and incubation periods are shorter. Like gastroenteritis, it causes diarrhea, nausea, and vomiting. You can differentiate food poisoning from gastroenteritis by obtaining a thorough history of common food intake in clients who have common symptoms of acute diarrhea, nausea, and vomiting.

The common types of food poisoning are caused by pathogens and include the following (Table 61-5):

- Gram-negative *Salmonella*
- *Staphylococcal aureus*
- *Escherichia coli*
- Botulism

All cases of botulism and salmonellosis need to be reported to the local health department. Cases of staphylococcal and *E. coli* food poisoning are reported if epidemic outbreaks occur.

Salmonellosis

Salmonellosis is a bacterial infection caused by the *Salmonella* organism. It can be transmitted by the "five Fs": flies, fingers, food, feces, and fomites.

Incubation is 8 to 48 hours after the person has ingested the contaminated food or liquid. Symptoms usually last for 3 to 5 days and include fever with or without chills, nausea, vomiting, cramping abdominal pain, and diarrhea, which may be bloody.

Salmonellosis is usually self-limiting, but bacteremia with localization in joints or bone may occur. The definitive diagnosis is made by stool culture. Treatment is symptomatic, and drug therapy is not usually indicated unless bacteremia occurs; in that case, the physician prescribes antibiotics.

Clients may be carriers of the bacterium for up to 1 year. The nurse instructs all clients with *Salmonella* gastroenteritis and their contacts to wash their hands before meals and after defecating to avoid transmission of the organism. The treatment for *Salmonella* infection is controversial because antibiotics tend not to shorten the illness. In some studies,

TABLE 61-5 Common Types of Food Poisoning

Staphylococcal Infection
- Caused by contaminated meats and dairy products
- Can be transmitted by human carriers
- Causes abrupt onset of vomiting and diarrhea without fever

***Escherichia coli* Infection**
- Caused by meat contaminated with animal feces
- Causes abrupt vomiting, diarrhea, abdominal cramping, and fever

Botulism
- Commonly associated with improperly canned foods, especially fruits and vegetables
- Nausea, vomiting, diarrhea, and weakness progressing to paralysis
- Diplopia, dysphagia, and dysarthria

Salmonellosis
- Caused by contaminated food or drink but can be transmitted by the fecal-oral route
- Fever, nausea, vomiting, abdominal cramping, and diarrhea lasting for 3 to 5 days

quinolones have been effective, but these are usually reserved for individuals with severe manifestations of the illness.

Staphylococcal Infection

Staphylococcus is associated with 25% of reported food poisoning outbreaks. *Staphylococcus* is found in meats and dairy products and can be transmitted by carriers of the organism. For staphylococcal food poisoning to occur, there must be contamination of food and a period of time (hours) during which the organisms multiply. This can take place during the slow cooling of food after it is cooked.

Symptoms of staphylococcal food poisoning include an abrupt onset of vomiting, abdominal cramping, and diarrhea. The person usually has symptoms 2 to 4 hours after ingesting the contaminated food. There is no fever, but the client is weak.

A diagnosis can be made when stool culture yields 100,000 enterotoxin-producing staphylococci; however, symptoms rarely last more than 24 hours, and people do not always seek medical attention. Antimicrobial drug therapy is not usually indicated unless an agent produces progressive systemic involvement. Parenteral fluids may be necessary if fluid volume is grossly depleted.

Escherichia coli Infection

E. coli is not usually associated with food poisoning. Since 1992, however, there have been several outbreaks of *E. coli* food poisoning in the United States. Enterohemorrhagic strains of *E. coli* produce cytotoxins that cause outbreaks of hemorrhagic colitis and hemolytic-uremic syndrome. Treatment of the client with *E. coli* food poisoning includes IV fluids and antibiotic therapy.

Botulism

Botulism is a paralytic disease resulting from ingestion of a toxin in food contaminated with *Clostridium botulinum*. Botulism is most commonly associated with home-canned foods, particularly vegetables, fruits, condiments and, less commonly, meat and fish. It can be associated with commercially prepared products and with products not adequately heated to destroy toxins before they are eaten.

Incubation is usually 18 to 36 hours. After this time, symptoms occur; illness may be mild or severe, with paralysis, respiratory failure, and death. Initial symptoms include diplopia, dysphagia, and dysarthria.

Weakness can progress rapidly from the neck to the arms, thorax, and legs. Paralytic ileus, severe constipation, and urinary retention can also occur. Nausea, vomiting, and abdominal pain may occur before or after the onset of paralysis.

The diagnosis is made on the basis of the client's history and a stool culture of *C. botulinum*. The serum may be positive for toxins.

Treatment with trivalent botulism antitoxin (ABE) is given as soon as the diagnosis is made if the client is not hypersensitive to it. The physician may lavage the stomach to stop absorption of toxin. All clients are hospitalized to observe for and treat respiratory paralysis. Nothing is given orally until swallowing and respiratory difficulties pass. The physician prescribes IV fluids as needed. If respiratory paralysis occurs, tracheostomy and mechanical ventilation are implemented. If ventilation can be maintained, the client can survive with no neurologic deficits after the illness.

To prevent botulism, teach clients the importance of discarding cans of food that are punctured or swollen or that have defective seals. Containers for home-canned foods must be sterilized by boiling for 20 minutes to destroy *C. botulinum* spores before canning.

GET READY for the NCLEX Examination!

KEY POINTS

Safe Effective Care Environment

- Recognize that perforation (rupture) of the appendix requires prompt intervention and can result in peritonitis.
- Be alert for GI bleeding in the client with chronic inflammatory bowel disease (IBD).
- Prioritize care for clients with IBD according to their major nursing diagnoses: diarrhea and acute or chronic pain or both.
- Be aware that clients with Crohn's disease are at high risk for malnutrition as a result of an inability to absorb nutrients via the small intestine.

Health Promotion and Maintenance

- Teach individuals ways to prevent transmission of gastroenteritis as stated in Chart 61-2.
- Teach clients with chronic IBD to avoid gastrointestinal stimulants, such as alcohol and caffeine; each client's response to foods differs.
- Teach clients taking immunosuppressive agents, such as 6-mercaptopurine, that these medications can cause decreased blood cell count, infection, and other adverse effects typical of this class of medications.
- Teach clients how to provide ileostomy care, paying particular attention to skin care; the effluent has a high enzyme content that can easily cause severe skin excoriation (see Chart 61-4).
- Consult with an ET nurse for ileostomy teaching and care.
- Instruct clients with diverticulosis about diet modifications, such as avoiding nuts, foods with seeds, and GI stimulants.
- Teach clients with diverticulosis to eat a high-fiber diet; diverticulitis requires a low-fiber diet.
- Instruct clients with anorectal disorders to use sitz baths, bulk-forming agents (such as Metamucil), and stool softeners to decrease pain.

Psychosocial Integrity

- Be aware that all inflammatory bowel diseases (acute and chronic) are very disruptive to one's daily routine; chronic IBD requires a lifetime of modifications.
- Recognize that having an ileostomy impacts the client's body image and self-esteem; assess for coping strategies that the client has previously used and identify personal support systems to assist in coping and acceptance of loss.

Physiological Integrity

- Assess for the classic clinical manifestations of appendicitis, which include abdominal pain, nausea and vomiting, and abdominal tenderness upon palpation (McBurney's point); some clients also have leukocytosis.

- Assess for the key features of peritonitis as listed in Chart 61-1.
- Assess for signs and symptoms of dehydration in clients who have inflammatory bowel disease.
- Administer antidiarrheal medications, as prescribed, to decrease stools and therefore prevent dehydration in clients with inflammatory bowel diseases.
- Be aware that there are two types of chronic inflammatory bowel disease (IBD): ulcerative colitis (UC) and Crohn's disease; both have similarities but also have differences (see Table 61-2).
- Monitor for complications of UC as listed in Table 61-3.
- Provide nursing interventions for clients with IBD as listed in Chart 61-3.
- Administer 5-aminosalicylic acid drugs, as prescribed (e.g., Pentasa and Dipentum), to decrease inflammation in clients with UC; most of these same drugs are also used for Crohn's disease management.
- Administer corticosteroids and 6-mercaptopurine, as prescribed, for both UC and Crohn's disease; infliximab (Remicade) is used primarily for Crohn's but may be useful for those with UC in selected cases.
- Observe for gastrointestinal bleeding in clients with diverticular disease.
- Be aware that gastrointestinal problems, including diarrhea, may also be caused by parasites and helminths.

ADDITIONAL STUDY RESOURCES

Go to your Student CD-ROM for Review Questions for the NCLEX Examination.

evolve Go to http://evolve.elsevier.com/Iggy/ for Integrated Management of Care Questions for the NCLEX Examination.

SELECTED BIBLIOGRAPHY

Asterisk indicates a classic or definitive work on this subject.

Bernstein, C., et al. (2000). Direct hospital costs for patients with inflammatory bowel disease in a Canadian tertiary care university hospital. *American Journal of Gastroenterology, 95*(3), 677-683.

Casellas, F., et al. (2000). Impact of surgery for Crohn's disease on health-related quality of life. *American Journal of Gastroenterology, 95*(1), 177-181.

Cohen, R., et al. (2000). The cost of hospitalization for Crohn's disease. *American Journal of Gastroenterology, 95*(2), 524-530.

*Delco, F., & Sonnenberg, A. (1999). Commonalities in the time trends of Crohn's disease and ulcerative colitis. *American Journal of Gastroenterology, 94*(8), 2172-2176.

Dooley, T.P., et al. (2004). Regulation of gene expression in inflammatory bowel disease and correlation with IBD drugs: Screening by DNA microassays. *Inflammatory Bowel Disease, 10*(1), 1-14.

Goldstein, E.S., Marion, J.F., & Present, D.H. (2004). 6-mercaptopurine is effective in Crohn's disease without concomitant steroids. *Inflammatory Bowel Disease, 10*(2), 79-84.

Joachim, G. (2002). An assessment of social support in people with inflammatory bowel disease. *Gastroenterology Nursing, 25*(6), 246-252.

*Klonowski, E., & Masoodi, J. (1999). The patient with Crohn's disease. *RN, 62*(3), 32-37.

*Martin, F. (1997). Ulcerative colitis. *American Journal of Nursing 97*(8), 38-39.

*Mikula, C. (1999). Anti-TNF alpha: New therapy for Crohn's disease. *Gastroenterology Nursing, 22*(6), 245-248.

*Mishkin, S. (1997). Dairy sensitivity, lactose malabsorption, and elimination diets in inflammatory bowel disease. *American Journal of Clinical Nutrition, 65*(2), 564-567.

*Northouse, L.L., et al. (1999). The concerns of patients and spouses after the diagnosis of colon cancer: A qualitative analysis. *Journal of Wound, Ostomy, and Incontinence Nursing, 26*(1), 8-17.

*Norton, B. (1998). Crohn's disease: A review of medical, surgical and nutritional management. *ADVANCE for Nurse Practitioners, 6*(9), 42-50.

*Olmstead, J. (1998). Evaluation and management of the patient with ulcerative colitis. *Gastroenterology Nursing, 21*(4), 176-180.

Pearson, C. (2004). Inflammatory bowel disease. *Nursing Times, 100*(9), 86-90.

*Rayhorn, N. (1999). Understanding inflammatory bowel disease. *Nursing 99, 29*(12), 57-61.

Tanaka, M., Miyawaki, I., & Kazuma. K. (2003). A study of relationships between self-evaluation of physical condition and perception of life in ulcerative colitis patients. *Gastroenterology Nursing,* 26(3), 115-124.

*Van Benden, C., et al. (1999). Multiple outbreak of *Salmonella enterica* serotype Newport infections due to contaminated alfalfa sprouts. *Journal of the American Medical Association, 281*(2), 158-162.

*Worley, J. (1999). Diagnosis and management of inflammatory bowel disease. *Journal of the American Academy of Nurse Practitioners, 11*(1), 23-31.

CHAPTER

62 Interventions for Clients with Liver Problems

MADELEINE B. MURPHY

LEARNING OUTCOMES

After studying this chapter, you should be able to:

1. Describe the pathophysiology and complications associated with cirrhosis of the liver.
2. Interpret laboratory test findings commonly seen in clients with cirrhosis.
3. Analyze assessment data from clients with cirrhosis to determine priority nursing diagnoses and collaborative problems.
4. Formulate a collaborative plan of care for the client with severe late-stage cirrhosis.
5. Identify emergency interventions for the client with bleeding esophageal varices.
6. Evaluate care for clients with cirrhosis.
7. Develop a community-based teaching plan for the client with cirrhosis of the liver.
8. Compare and contrast the transmission of hepatitis A, B, and C viral infections.
9. Explain ways in which each type of hepatitis can be prevented.
10. Discuss the primary concerns about the increasing incidence of hepatitis C in the United States.
11. Identify treatment options for clients with cancer of the liver.
12. Describe the typical complications that result from liver transplantation.

Go to your Student CD-ROM for Review Questions for the NCLEX Examination keyed to these Learning Outcomes.

The liver is the largest and one of the most vital internal organs, performing more than 400 functions and affecting every system in the body. When the liver cannot perform its complex activities, hepatic failure results. Liver diseases range in severity from mild hepatic inflammation to chronic end-stage cirrhosis.

CIRRHOSIS

Cirrhosis is extensive scarring of the liver, usually caused by a chronic irreversible reaction to hepatic inflammation and necrosis. The disease typically develops insidiously and has a prolonged, destructive course.

The most common causes for cirrhosis in the United States are alcoholic liver disease and hepatitis C. Worldwide, hepatitis B is the leading cause.

PATHOPHYSIOLOGY

Cirrhosis is characterized by diffuse fibrotic bands of connective tissue that distort the liver's normal architecture. Inflammation caused by either toxins or disease results in extensive degeneration and destruction of **hepatocytes** (liver cells). As cirrhosis develops, the tissue becomes nodular. These nodules can block bile ducts and normal blood flow throughout the liver. Flow alterations in the vascular system and lymphatic bile duct channels result from compression caused by the proliferation of fibrous tissue. In early disease, the liver is usually enlarged, firm and hard. As the pathologic process continues, the liver shrinks in size.

Complications of Cirrhosis

Common problems and complications associated with hepatic cirrhosis depend on the amount of damage sustained by the liver. In **compensated cirrhosis**, the liver has significant scarring but is still able to perform essential functions without causing significant symptoms.

In **decompensated cirrhosis**, liver function is significantly impaired with obvious manifestations of liver failure.

The loss of hepatic function contributes to the development of metabolic abnormalities. Hepatic cell degeneration may lead to the following:

- Portal hypertension
- Ascites
- Bleeding esophageal varices
- Coagulation defects
- Jaundice
- Portal-systemic encephalopathy (PSE) with hepatic coma
- Hepatorenal syndrome
- Spontaneous bacterial peritonitis

PORTAL HYPERTENSION

Portal hypertension, a persistent increase in pressure within the portal vein, is a major complication of cirrhosis. It results from increased resistance to or obstruction of the flow of blood through the portal vein and its tributaries. The blood meets resistance to flow and seeks collateral venous channels around the high-pressure area.

Blood flow backs into the spleen, causing splenomegaly. Veins in the esophagus, stomach, intestines, abdomen, and rectum become dilated. Portal hypertension can result in ascites, esophageal varices, prominent abdominal veins (caput medusae), and hemorrhoids.

ASCITES

Ascites is the accumulation of free fluid within the peritoneal cavity. Increased hydrostatic pressure from portal hypertension causes this fluid to leak into the peritoneal cavity. The accumulation of plasma protein, primarily albumin, in the peritoneal fluid reduces the amount of circulating plasma protein in the blood. When this decrease is combined with the inability of the liver to synthesize albumin because of impaired hepatocyte functioning, the effective serum colloid osmotic pressure is decreased in the circulatory system.

The decrease of effective intravascular circulation from massive ascites may cause renal vasoconstriction, triggering the renin-angiotensin system. This results in sodium and water retention, which increases hydrostatic pressure and the intravascular volume, which perpetuates the cycle of ascites.

BLEEDING ESOPHAGEAL VARICES

As a result of portal hypertension, the blood backs up from the liver and enters the esophageal and gastric vessels that carry it into the systemic circulation. **Esophageal varices** occur when fragile, thin-walled esophageal veins become distended from increased pressure. The potential for varices to bleed depend upon their size; size is determined by direct endoscopic observation. Varices occur most often in the distal esophagus but can also be present in the stomach.

Bleeding esophageal varices represent a life-threatening medical emergency. There can be significant blood loss, resulting in shock from hypovolemia. The bleeding may be manifested by **hematemesis** (vomiting blood) or **melena** (black, tarry stools). Loss of consciousness may precede any observed bleeding. Variceal bleeding can occur spontaneously with no precipitating factors. However, any activity that increases abdominal pressure may increase the likelihood of a variceal bleed. Clients with this problem should be advised against heavy lifting and vigorous physical exercise. There is no clear evidence that poorly chewed food, medications, or refluxed gastric acid cause variceal bleeding.

Clients with portal hypertension may also have **portal hypertensive gastropathy**. This complication can occur with or without the presence of esophageal varices. Slow gastric mucosal bleeding occurs, which may result in chronic slow blood loss, occult positive stools, and anemia.

COAGULATION DEFECTS

With cirrhosis, there is a decrease in the synthesis of bile in the liver; this prevents the absorption of fat-soluble vitamins (e.g., vitamin K). Without vitamin K, clotting factors II, VII, IX, and X are not produced in sufficient quantities, and the client is susceptible to bleeding and easy bruising. These abnormalities are manifested in abnormal prothrombin times (prolonged or elevated).

Splenomegaly (enlarged spleen) results from the backup of blood into the spleen. The enlarged spleen destroys platelets, causing thrombocytopenia (low serum platelet count). Thrombocytopenia is often the first clinical sign that a client has liver dysfunction.

JAUNDICE

Jaundice in clients with hepatic cirrhosis is caused by one of two mechanisms: hepatocellular disease or intrahepatic obstruction (Table 62-1). Hepatocellular jaundice develops because the liver cells cannot effectively excrete bilirubin. This decreased excretion results in excessive circulating bilirubin levels. Intrahepatic obstructive jaundice results from edema, fibrosis, or scarring of the hepatic bile channels and bile ducts, which interferes with normal bile and bilirubin excretion.

PORTAL-SYSTEMIC ENCEPHALOPATHY

Portal-systemic encephalopathy (PSE) is also known as **hepatic encephalopathy** and **hepatic coma** in the later stages. It is a clinical disorder seen in hepatic failure and cirrhosis. PSE is manifested by neurologic symptoms and is characterized by an altered level of consciousness, impaired thinking processes, and neuromuscular disturbances. Encephalopathy may be acute and reversible with early intervention.

The exact mechanisms causing hepatic encephalopathy are not clearly understood but most likely are the result of the shunting of portal venous blood into the central circulation so that the liver is bypassed. As a result, toxic substances absorbed by the intestine are not broken down or detoxified and may lead to metabolic abnormalities, most significantly elevated serum ammonia. Elevated ammonia levels are usually cited as the cause of hepatic encephalopathy. However, ammonia levels are not a clear indicator of the presence of encephalopathy. Some clients may have significant impairment without dramatic elevations of serum ammonia, and elevations of ammonia can occur without evidence of encephalopathy.

TABLE 62-1 Laboratory Diagnostic Differentiation of Jaundice

Test	Hepatocellular Jaundice	Obstructive Jaundice	Hemolytic Jaundice
Serum bilirubin			
Indirect (unconjugated)	Increased	Slightly increased	Increased
Direct (conjugated)	Increased	Moderately increased	Normal
Urine bilirubin	Increased	Increased	None
Urobilinogen			
Stool	Normal to decreased	None	Increased
Urine	Normal to increased	None	Increased

TABLE 62-2 Stages of Portal-Systemic Encephalopathy

Stage I Prodromal
- Subtle manifestations that may not be recognized immediately
- Personality changes
- Behavior changes (agitation, belligerence)
- Emotional lability (euphoria, depression)
- Impaired thinking
- Inability to concentrate
- Fatigue, drowsiness
- Slurred or slowed speech
- Sleep pattern disturbances

Stage II Impending
- Continuing mental changes
- Mental confusion
- Disorientation to time, place, or person
- Asterixis (see Figure 62-3)

Stage III Stuporous
- Progressive deterioration
- Marked mental confusion
- Stuporous, drowsy but arousable
- Abnormal electroencephalogram tracing
- Muscle twitching
- Hyperreflexia
- Asterixis

Stage IV Comatose
- Unresponsiveness, leading to death in 85% of clients progressing to this stage
- Unarousable, obtunded
- Response to painful stimulus
- No asterixis
- Positive Babinski's sign
- Muscle rigidity
- Fetor hepaticus (characteristic liver breath—musty, sweet odor)
- Seizures

PSE may develop insidiously in clients with chronic liver disease and go undetected until the late stages. Symptoms develop rapidly in acute liver dysfunction. Four stages of development have been identified: prodromal, impending, stuporous, and comatose (Table 62-2). The client's symptoms may gradually progress to coma or fluctuate among the four stages.

Factors that may precipitate PSE include the following:
- High-protein diet
- Infections
- Hypovolemia (deficient fluid volume)
- Hypokalemia (deficient serum potassium)
- Constipation
- Gastrointestinal (GI) bleeding (causes a large protein load in the intestines)
- Drugs (e.g., hypnotics, opioids, sedatives, analgesics, diuretics)

PSE may also occur after paracentesis or shunting procedures. The prognosis depends on the severity of the underlying cause, the precipitating factors, and the degree of liver dysfunction.

HEPATORENAL SYNDROME

The development of **hepatorenal syndrome** indicates a poor prognosis for the client with hepatic failure. It is often the cause of death in clients with cirrhosis. Progressive oliguric renal failure associated with hepatic failure results in functional impairment of kidneys with normal anatomic and morphologic features. This syndrome is manifested by the following:
- A sudden decrease in urinary flow
- Elevated blood urea nitrogen and creatinine levels, with abnormally decreased urine sodium excretion
- Increased urine osmolarity

Hepatorenal syndrome often occurs after clinical deterioration from GI bleeding or the onset of PSE. It may also complicate other liver diseases, including acute hepatitis and fulminant liver failure.

TABLE 62-3 Common Causes of Cirrhosis

Alcoholic liver disease	Drugs and toxins
Viral hepatitis	Biliary disease
Autoimmune hepatitis	Metabolic/genetic causes
Steatohepatitis	Cardiovascular disease

SPONTANEOUS BACTERIAL PERITONITIS

Clients with cirrhosis and ascites may develop acute spontaneous bacterial peritonitis (SBP). Those who are particularly susceptible are clients with very advanced liver disease. This may be the result of low concentrations of proteins; proteins normally provide some protection against bacteria.

The bacteria responsible for SBP are typically from the bowel and reach the ascitic fluid after transmigrating through the bowel wall and transversing the lymphatics. Clinical manifestations vary, but may include fever, chills, and abdominal pain and tenderness. However, symptoms can also be minimal with only mild or vague complaints in the absence of fever. Worsening encephalopathy and increased jaundice may also be present without abdominal complaint.

The diagnosis of SBP is made when a sample of ascitic fluid is obtained by paracentesis for cell counts and culture. An ascitic fluid leukocyte count of more than 250 polymorphonuclear (PMN) leukocytes can be the basis for treatment.

Etiology

Cirrhosis can occur as a result of many factors and diseases. Table 62-3 lists the most common etiologies, which are described in the following sections.

ALCOHOL

Alcohol has a direct toxic effect on the hepatocytes and causes liver inflammation (**alcoholic hepatitis**). The liver becomes enlarged, with cellular degeneration and infiltration by fat, leukocytes, and lymphocytes. Over time, the inflammatory process decreases and the destructive phase increases. Early scar formation is caused by fibroblast infiltration and collagen formation. Damage to liver tissue progresses as a result of malnutrition and repeated exposure to the alcohol. If alcohol is withheld, the fatty infiltration and inflammation is reversible. If alcohol abuse continues, widespread scar tissue formation and fibrosis infiltrate the liver as a result of cellular necrosis.

The amount of alcohol necessary to cause cirrhosis varies widely from person to person and there are gender differences. In women, it may take as few as two to three drinks per day over a minimum of 10 years. In men, perhaps six drinks per day over the same time period may be needed to cause disease. However, there are other individuals, both male and female, who consume far more alcohol per day over a period of several years without ever developing cirrhosis.

VIRAL HEPATITIS

Hepatitis C is an infectious bloodborne illness that usually causes chronic disease. Inflammation caused by infection over time leads to progressive scarring of the liver. It usually takes decades for cirrhosis to develop, although alcohol use in combination with hepatitis C may accelerate the process.

Hepatitis B is the most common cause of cirrhosis worldwide. Hepatitis B also causes inflammation and low-grade damage over decades that can ultimately lead to cirrhosis. The role that concomitant use of alcohol plays in hepatitis B cirrhosis is not as clear as that of hepatitis C cirrhosis.

Hepatitis D is another virus that infects the liver, but only in people who already have hepatitis B (see later discussion on hepatitis in this chapter).

AUTOIMMUNE HEPATITIS

Unlike viral hepatitis, this is not an infectious disease. For reasons not clearly understood, the host's immune system produces a high level of circulating autoantibodies, causing inflammation of the liver. This chronic inflammation can lead to fibrosis and eventual cirrhosis.

STEATOHEPATITIS

Frequently referred to as "fatty liver," **steatohepatitis** occurs when fat and cholesterol deposits in the liver cause chronic inflammation. Over time, this inflammation may cause liver damage, or fibrosis and eventual cirrhosis. Obesity and elevated lipid profile are risk factors for steatohepatitis. This complication is discussed as a separate health problem later in this chapter.

DRUGS AND TOXINS

Medications, herbal supplements, and environmental exposure to toxins may damage the liver so significantly that cirrhosis occurs. Sometimes the development of cirrhosis occurs decades after the initial exposure.

BILIARY DISEASE

Biliary cirrhosis develops as a result of chronic biliary obstruction, bile stasis, inflammation, or diffuse hepatic fibrosis. The most common causes of biliary cirrhosis are primary biliary cirrhosis and primary sclerosing cholangitis. Both of these forms of biliary cirrhosis may also present as secondary to either stones or strictures affecting the common bile duct.

Primary biliary cirrhosis (PBC) is a disease, probably with an immunologic basis, that involves the slow progressive destruction of small intrahepatic ducts, resulting in cholestasis. The disease usually affects middle-aged women. One of the most common presenting features is an asymptomatic elevation of the alkaline phosphatase.

Primary sclerosing cholangitis (PSC) is an illness that is characterized by diffuse inflammation and fibrosis that involves the biliary system. It has the potential to cause cirrhosis because this process leads to a narrowing and eventual obliteration of the intrahepatic bile ducts. There is a strong association between PSC and inflammatory bowel disease. This disease predominantly affects men.

METABOLIC/GENETIC CAUSES

There are many metabolic and genetic disorders that can cause cirrhosis of the liver:

- **Hemachromatosis**, which is characterized by excessive iron storage
- **Wilson's disease**, a disorder of copper metabolism
- **Alpha$_1$ antitrypsin deficiency**, which may cause an abnormal accumulation of antitrypsin and produce inflammatory activity
- **Cystic fibrosis,** which can cause cirrhosis from intrahepatic bile duct plugging

CARDIOVASCULAR DISEASE

Vascular (cardiac) cirrhosis is associated with severe right-sided heart failure. The liver becomes enlarged, is congested with venous blood, and appears edematous and dark in color. The liver serves as a reservoir for large amounts of venous blood that the failing heart cannot pump back into the systemic circulation. The increase in hepatic volume and pressure causes severe venous congestion. The decrease in nourishing blood flow to the liver results in hepatic cell necrosis and fibrosis.

UNKNOWN CAUSES

Cryptogenic cirrhosis is a diagnosis given when no known etiology for liver disease can be demonstrated by serologic testing, liver biopsy, or diagnostic scanning. Cryptogenic cirrhosis occurs in about 10% of clients with cirrhosis.

Incidence/Prevalence

The incidence of cirrhosis is not well known, although the number of deaths from all liver diseases is about 43,000 per year in the United States.

> **CULTURAL CONSIDERATIONS**
>
> Deaths from chronic liver disease and cirrhosis are about four times more prevalent among Native Americans/American Indians and Alaskan Natives than among the general U.S. population. The cause of increased death rates is not known but may be related to a lack of health care access.

COLLABORATIVE MANAGEMENT

Assessment

HISTORY

It is important to obtain historical data from clients with suspected cirrhosis, including age, gender, race, and employment history, especially history of exposure to harmful chemical toxins. Keep in mind that all exposures are important regardless of how long ago they occurred. Determine whether there has ever been a needle stick injury. Sexual history may be important in determining an infectious cause for liver disease.

Elicit whether there is a family history of alcoholism and/or liver disease in the family. Ask the client to describe his or her alcohol intake, including the amount consumed during a given period of time. Is there a history of drug use? Oral? Intravenous (IV)? Intranasal? For clients previously or currently in an alcohol or drug recovery program, how long have they been in sobriety? What does their participation consist of in the treatment program? This information is sensitive and many times difficult for the client to answer.

Be sure to establish with the client why you are asking these questions and accept them in a nonjudgmental manner. For many people, the behaviors causing the liver disease occurred years before the onset of their current illness and they are regretful and often embarrassed.

Ask the client about previous medical conditions, such as an episode of jaundice or acute viral hepatitis, biliary tract disorders, viral infections, blood transfusions, autoimmune disorders, obesity, altered lipid profile and a history of heart failure or respiratory disorders.

PHYSICAL ASSESSMENT/CLINICAL MANIFESTATIONS

Because cirrhosis has an insidious onset, many of the early manifestations are vague and nonspecific. The client may report the following:

- Fatigue
- Significant change in weight
- Gastrointestinal (GI) symptoms
- Abdominal pain and liver tenderness (both of which may be ignored by the client)
- Pruritus

Hepatic function abnormalities are often detected when a physical examination or laboratory tests are completed for an unrelated illness or problem. It is not uncommon for a client with *compensated cirrhosis* to be completely unaware that there is a liver problem. The first sign of cirrhosis may present before the onset of symptoms when routine laboratory tests, presurgical evaluations, or life and health insurance assessments show abnormalities. These tests could indicate abnormal hepatic function or thrombocytopenia, prompting a more thorough diagnostic workup.

The development of late signs of advanced cirrhosis may cause the client to seek medical treatment. GI bleeding, jaundice, ascites, and spontaneous bruising indicate deteriorating hepatic function and represent complications of cirrhosis.

Thoroughly assess the client with liver dysfunction or hepatic failure, because it affects every body system (Figure 62-1). The clinical picture and course vary from client to client depending on the severity of hepatic failure. An inspection may reveal the following:

- Obvious yellowing of the skin (jaundice) and the sclerae (icterus)
- Dry skin

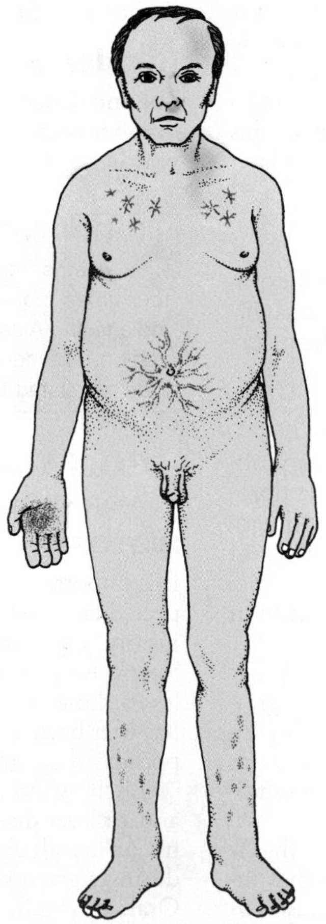

Figure 62-1 ■ The clinical picture of a client with liver dysfunction. Manifestations vary according to the progression of the disease. Early manifestations are noted in color.

- Rashes
- Purpuric lesions, such as **petechiae** (round, pinpoint, red-purple lesions) or **ecchymosis** (large purple, blue, or yellow bruises)
- Warm and bright red palms of the hands (palmar erythema)
- Vascular lesions with a red center and radiating branches, known as "**spider angiomas**" (telangiectasias, spider nevi, or vascular spiders), on the nose, cheeks, upper thorax, and shoulders
- Peripheral dependent edema of the extremities and sacrum

ABDOMINAL ASSESSMENT. Usually *massive* ascites can be detected as a distended abdomen with bulging flanks. The umbilicus may protrude, and dilated abdominal veins (caput medusae) may radiate from the umbilicus. Ascites can cause physical problems; for example, orthopnea and dyspnea from increased abdominal distention can interfere with lung expansion. The client may have difficulty maintaining an erect body posture, and problems with balance may affect walking. Inspect and palpate for the presence of inguinal or umbilical hernias, which are likely to develop in clients with ascites because of increased intra-abdominal pressure.

Minimal ascites is often more difficult to detect. Advanced assessment techniques, such as the percussion test for shifting dullness and the presence of a fluid wave, may be performed by the health care provider.

When performing an assessment of the abdomen, keep in mind that **hepatomegaly** (liver enlargement) occurs in 60% of all cases of early cirrhosis. As the liver deteriorates it may become hard and small. The advanced practice nurse or other health care provider palpates the right upper quadrant for hepatomegaly below the costal (rib cage) border. The presence of hepatomegaly may be determined by percussing for dullness over the enlarged liver.

Measure the client's abdominal girth to evaluate the progression of ascites (Figure 62-2). To measure abdominal girth, the client lies flat while the nurse pulls a tape measure around the largest diameter of the abdomen. The girth is measured at the end of exhalation. Mark the abdominal skin and flanks to ensure the same tape measure placement on subsequent readings.

OTHER PHYSICAL ASSESSMENTS. Assess nasogastric (NG) tube drainage (if present), vomitus, and stool for the presence of blood. This may be indicated by frank blood in the excrement or by a positive result of an *o*-toluidine test for occult blood content (Hema-Check, Hematest). Gastritis, stomach ulceration, or oozing esophageal varices may be responsible for the presence of blood **(melena).**

Note the presence of **fetor hepaticus**, which is the distinctive breath odor of chronic liver disease and portal-systemic encephalopathy (PSE) and is characterized by a fruity or musty odor. Fetor hepaticus results from the inability of the damaged liver to metabolize and detoxify mercaptan, which is produced by bacterial degradation of methionine, a sulfurous amino acid.

Amenorrhea may occur in women, and men may exhibit testicular atrophy, **gynecomastia** (enlarged breasts), and impotence as a result of inactive hormones and certain diuretics. Clients with problems of the hematologic system caused by hepatic failure may have bruising, petechiae (small, purplish hemorrhagic spots on the skin), and an enlarged spleen.

Continually assess the client's neurologic functioning. Subtle changes in mentation and personality often progress to coma, a late complication of PSE. Monitor for **asterixis** (liver flap or flapping tremor), a coarse tremor characterized by rapid, nonrhythmic extensions and flexions in the wrists and fingers. Figure 62-3 illustrates the technique used to elicit asterixis during physical assessment.

PSYCHOSOCIAL ASSESSMENT

The client with hepatic cirrhosis may undergo subtle or obvious personality, cognitive, and behavior changes, such as agitation and belligerence. He or she may experience sleep pattern disturbances or may exhibit signs of emotional lability, euphoria, or depression. A psychosocial assessment identifies needs and helps guide client care.

Repeated hospitalizations are common for clients with cirrhosis. It is a life-altering chronic disease, impacting not only the client, but immediate and extended family members as well. There are significant emotional, physical, and

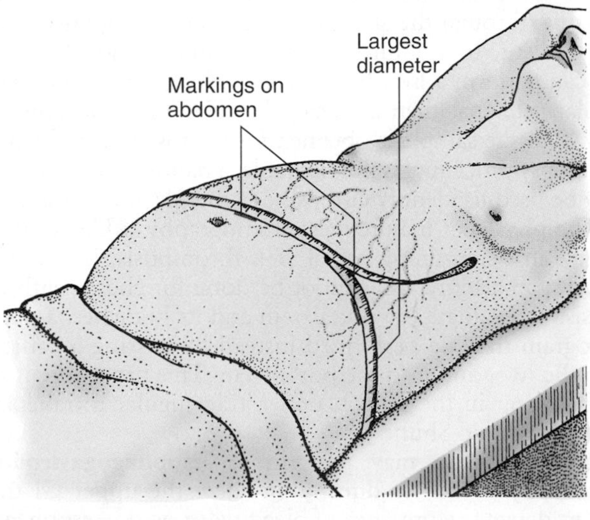

Figure 62-2 ■ How to measure abdominal girth. With the client supine, bring the tape measure around the client and take a measurement at the level of the umbilicus. Before removing the tape, mark the client's abdomen along the sides of the tape on the client's flanks (sides) and midline to ensure that later measurements are taken in the same place.

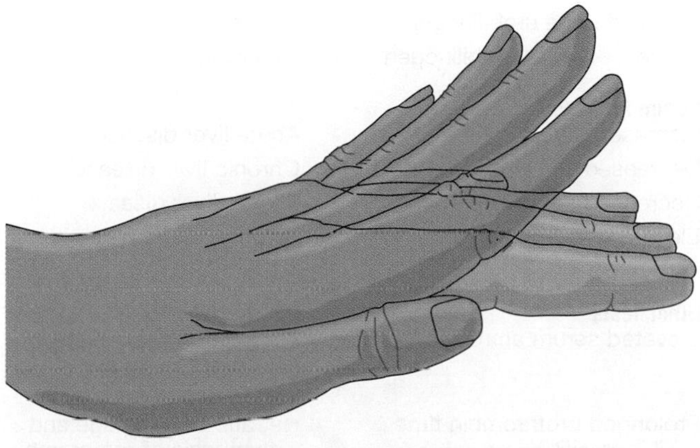

Figure 62-3 ■ To elicit asterixis (flapping tremor), have the client extend the arm, dorsiflex the wrist, and extend the fingers. Observe for rapid, nonrhythmic extensions and flexions.

financial changes. Substance abuse may continue in the face of deteriorating health. It is important, whenever possible, to use resources available to these individuals and their families. Social workers, substance abuse counselors, and mental health/behavioral health professionals should be involved in client management.

LABORATORY ASSESSMENT

Characteristic abnormalities are common in laboratory studies of clients with liver disease (Table 62-4). Serum levels of aspartate aminotransferase (AST), alanine aminotransferase (ALT), and lactate dehydrogenase (LDH) may be elevated because these enzymes are released into the blood during hepatic inflammation. However, as the liver deteriorates, the hepatocytes may be unable to create an inflammatory response and the AST and ALT may be normal.

Alkaline phosphatase levels are sensitive to mild extrahepatic or intrahepatic biliary obstruction and therefore may increase in clients with cirrhosis. Total serum bilirubin levels also rise. Indirect bilirubin levels increase in clients with cirrhosis because of the inability of the failing liver to excrete bilirubin. Therefore bilirubin is present in the urine (urobilinogen) in increased amounts. Fecal urobilinogen concentration is decreased in clients with biliary tract obstruction. These clients exhibit light- or clay-colored stools.

Total serum protein and albumin levels are decreased in clients with severe or chronic liver disease as a result of decreased synthesis by the liver. Prothrombin time (PT/INR) is prolonged because the liver decreases the synthesis of prothrombin. The platelet count is low, resulting in a characteristic thrombocytopenia of cirrhosis. Anemia may be reflected by an altered complete blood count (CBC), with decreased hemoglobin and hematocrit values. The white blood cell (WBC) count may also be decreased. Ammonia levels may be elevated in clients with advanced liver disease. Serum creatinine may be elevated as well due to deteriorating kidney function.

TABLE 62-4 Assessment of Abnormal Laboratory Findings in Liver Disease

Abnormal Finding	Significance
Serum Enzymes	
Elevated serum aspartate aminotransferase (AST)	Hepatic cell destruction, hepatitis (most specific indicator)
Elevated serum alanine aminotransferase (ALT)	Hepatic cell destruction, hepatitis
Elevated lactate dehydrogenase (LDH)	Hepatic cell destruction
Elevated serum alkaline phosphatase	Obstructive jaundice, hepatic metastasis
Bilirubin	
Elevated serum total bilirubin	Hepatic cell disease
Elevated serum direct conjugated bilirubin	Hepatitis, liver metastasis
Elevated serum indirect unconjugated bilirubin	Cirrhosis
Elevated urine bilirubin	Hepatocellular obstruction, viral or toxic liver disease
Elevated urine urobilinogen	Hepatic dysfunction
Decreased fecal urobilinogen	Obstructive liver disease
Serum Proteins	
Increased serum total protein	Acute liver disease
Decreased serum total protein	Chronic liver disease
Decreased serum albumin	Severe liver disease
Elevated serum globulin	Immune response to liver disease
Other Tests	
Elevated serum ammonia	Advanced liver disease or portal-systemic encephalopathy (PSE)
Prolonged prothrombin time (PT) or INR	Hepatic cell damage and synthesis of prothrombin

INR, International Normalized Ratio.

RADIOGRAPHIC ASSESSMENT

Plain x-rays of the abdomen may show hepatomegaly, splenomegaly, or massive ascites. A computed tomography (CT) scan may be requested if the diagnosis is more complex and ultrasound is not definitive.

OTHER DIAGNOSTIC ASSESSMENTS

Ultrasound (US) of the liver is often the first assessment for an individual with suspected liver disease to detect ascites, hepatomegaly, and splenomegaly. It can also determine the presence of biliary stones or biliary duct obstruction. Liver US is useful in detecting portal vein thrombosis and evaluating whether portal blood flow is from the portal vein into liver (normal flow) or vice versa.

Magnetic resonance imaging is another test used to diagnose and treat the client with liver disease. It can reveal mass lesions, giving additional specific information about their character. This information is helpful in determining whether the condition is malignant or benign.

Most clients being assessed for liver disease require biopsies to determine the exact pathology and the extent of disease progression. This procedure can be problematic because a large number of clients are at risk for bleeding. Even a **percutaneous** (through the skin) biopsy can pose a significant risk to the client. To minimize this risk, an interventional radiologist can perform a liver biopsy using a long sheath through a jugular vein that then is threaded into the hepatic vein and liver. A tissue sample is obtained for microscopic evaluation. If a biopsy procedure is not desirable, a radioisotope liver scan may be used to identify cirrhosis or other diffuse disease.

The physician may request arteriography if US is inconclusive in determining portal vein thrombosis. In most instances, an arteriogram cannot be done for clients with cirrhosis. To evaluate the portal vein and its branches, a portal venogram may be performed instead by passing a catheter into the liver and into the portal vein. This procedure is described later in the section under Transjugular Intrahepatic Portal-Systemic Shunt.

The physician may perform an **esophagogastroduodenoscopy** (EGD) to directly visualize the upper GI tract and to detect the presence of bleeding or oozing esophageal varices, stomach irritation and ulceration, or duodenal ulceration and bleeding. EGD is performed by introducing a flexible tube into the mouth, esophagus, and stomach while the client is under conscious sedation. A camera attached to the scope permits direct visualization of the mucosal lining of the upper gastrointestinal tract. This test is discussed in detail in Chapter 56.

Analysis

COMMON NURSING DIAGNOSES AND COLLABORATIVE PROBLEMS

The most common nursing diagnosis for clients with cirrhosis is Excess Fluid Volume related to edema (portal hypertension).

The following are the primary collaborative problems for clients with cirrhosis:

1. Potential for Hemorrhage
2. Potential for Portal-Systemic Encephalopathy (PSE)

ADDITIONAL NURSING DIAGNOSES AND COLLABORATIVE PROBLEMS

In addition to the common nursing diagnoses and collaborative problems, clients with cirrhosis may have one or more of the following:

- Risk for Imbalanced Nutrition: Less Than Body Requirements related to inability to ingest or digest food due to biologic factors
- Ineffective Breathing Pattern related to decreased diaphragmatic excursion and pressure on the diaphragm from ascites
- Chronic Pain related to abdominal pressure
- Risk for Infection related to inadequate secondary defenses (leukopenia)
- Risk for Impaired Skin Integrity related to pruritus and altered nutritional state
- Ineffective Coping related to a high degree of threat (chronic and potentially fatal disease)
- Sexual Dysfunction related to altered hormonal function and decreased libido
- Disturbed Body Image related to biophysical changes (distended abdomen and skin lesions)

Additional collaborative problems include the following:

- Potential for Drug Toxicity
- Potential for Hypokalemia

Planning and Implementation

EXCESS FLUID VOLUME

NOC **PLANNING: EXPECTED OUTCOMES.** The client with cirrhosis is expected to have water balance in the intracellular and extracellular compartments of the body. Indicators include that the client will have:

- Noncompromised blood pressure
- Noncompromised peripheral pulses
- Noncompromised mean arterial pressure
- 24-hour intake and output balance
- Stable body weight
- Moist mucous membranes
- Noncompromised serum electrolytes
- Noncompromised hematocrit
- Noncompromised urine specific gravity

INTERVENTIONS. Fluid accumulations are minimal during the early stages of ascites, and therefore interventions are aimed at preventing the accumulation of additional fluid and mobilizing the existing fluid collection. Nonsurgical treatment measures usually control ascites. If respiratory or abdominal functioning is compromised, surgical measures may be necessary. (See the Concept Map for chronic liver failure on p. 1376.)

NONSURGICAL MANAGEMENT. Supportive measures to control abdominal ascites include diet therapy, drugs, paracentesis, and comfort measures. The client's fluid and electrolyte status is also carefully monitored.

Diet Therapy. The health care provider usually places the client with abdominal ascites on a low sodium diet as an initial means of controlling fluid accumulation in the abdominal cavity. The amount of daily sodium intake restriction typically varies from 500 mg to 2 g. In collaboration with the dietitian, explain the purpose of the diet and advise the client and family to read the sodium content labels on all food and beverages. Table salt should be completely excluded. The absence of salt in low-sodium diets is distasteful to most people, so the dietitian suggests alternative flavoring additives such as lemon, vinegar, parsley, oregano, and pepper. Remind the client that seasoned and salty food is an acquired taste; in time he or she will become used to the decrease in dietary sodium.

The health care provider may limit the client's fluid intake if serum sodium levels fall. The kidneys retain sodium, and dilutional hyponatremia results, primarily from excessive fluid volume. IV and oral fluids are restricted to 1000 to 1500 mL/day in an effort to reverse the fluid overload and raise the serum sodium level. Calculate the permitted amount of oral fluids on the basis of the ordered IV intake. However, *it is not necessary for a client with ascites and a normal serum sodium to have fluid restriction.*

In general, clients with cirrhosis are malnourished and have multiple dietary deficiencies. Vitamin supplements, such as thiamine, folate, and multivitamin preparations, are typically added to the IV fluids because of the inability of the liver to store vitamins. Oral vitamins are given when IV fluid administration is discontinued.

Drug Therapy. The health care provider usually prescribes a diuretic to reduce fluid accumulation and to prevent cardiac and respiratory impairment. Monitor the effect of diuretic therapy by assessing intake and output, weighing the client daily, measuring abdominal girth, documenting peripheral edema, and assessing electrolyte levels. Serious electrolyte imbalances, such as hypokalemia (decreased potassium) and hyponatremia (decreased sodium), may accompany diuretic therapy. (See Chapter 16 for a discussion of electrolyte imbalances.) Depending on the diuretic selected, the provider may prescribe an oral or IV potassium supplement. Many clinicians prescribe a combination of furosemide (Lasix) and spironolactone (Aldactone) as a combination diuretic therapy for the treatment of ascites. Because of their different mechanisms of action, they are utilized for maintenance of sodium and potassium balance.

Keep in mind that all clients with ascites have the potential to develop SBP (spontaneous bacterial peritonitis). In some individuals, the presentation can be with very mild symptoms of low-grade fever and loss of appetite. In others, there may be abdominal pain, fever, rigors, and change in mental status.

Paracentesis. Abdominal **paracentesis** may be indicated if dietary restrictions and drug administration fail to control ascites (Chart 62-1). The procedure is performed at the bedside. The physician inserts a trocar catheter into the abdomen to remove and drain ascitic fluid from the peri-

CONCEPT MAP Cirrhosis

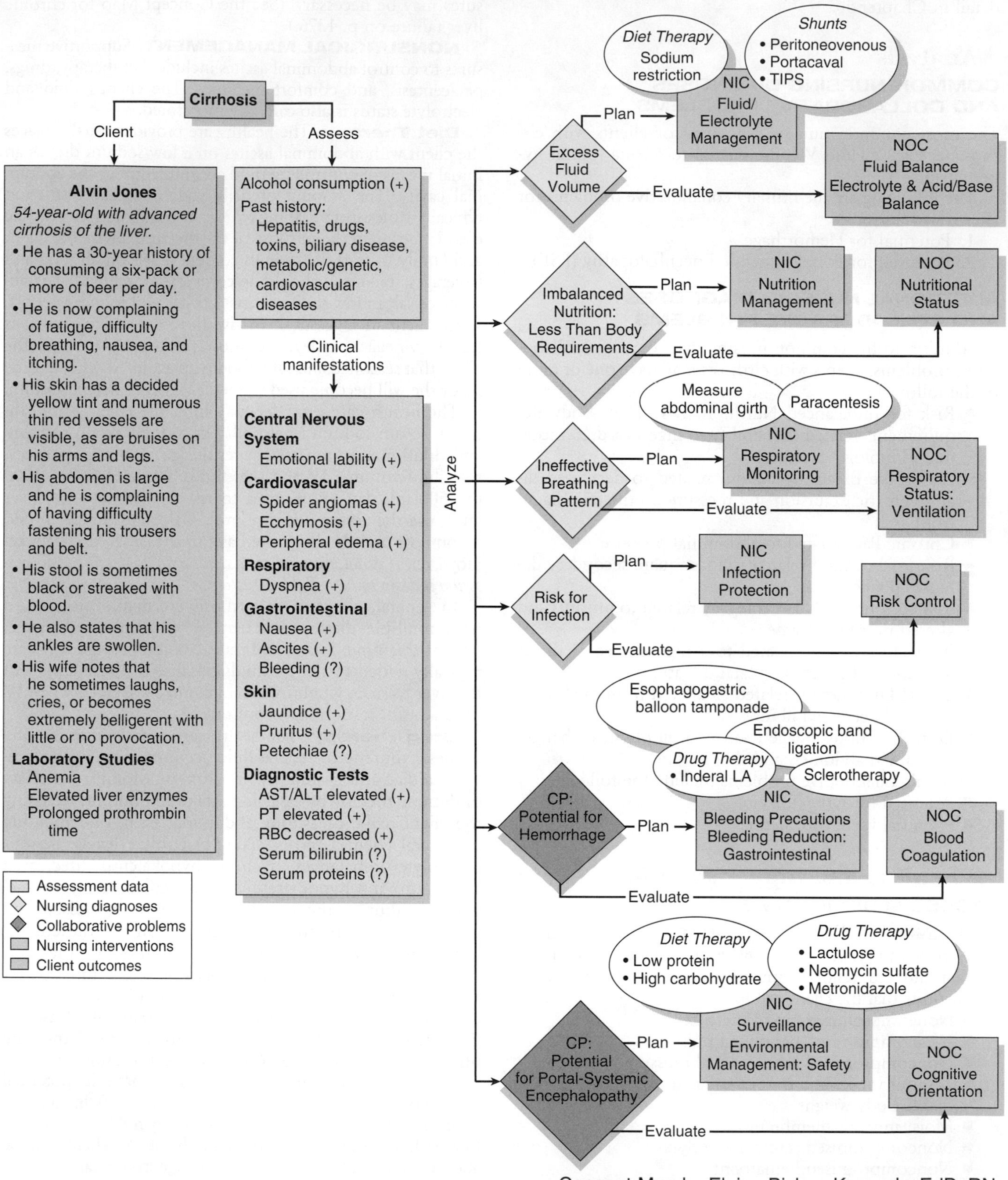

Concept Map by Elaine Bishop Kennedy, EdD, RN

CHART 62-1

BEST PRACTICE for
The Client with Paracentesis

- Explain the procedure and answer client questions.
- Obtain vital signs, including weight.
- Ask the client to void.
- Position the client in bed with the head of the bed elevated.
- Monitor vital signs per protocol or physician's orders.
- Measure the drainage and record accurately.
- Describe the collected fluid.
- Label and send the fluid for laboratory analysis; document in the client record that specimens were sent.
- After the physician removes the catheter, apply a dressing to the site; assess for leakage.
- Maintain bedrest per protocol.
- Weigh the client after the paracentesis; document in the client record weight both before and after paracentesis.

toneal cavity. This procedure is also done using ultrasound for added safety. In some situations, a short-term ascites drain catheter may be placed while the client is awaiting surgical intervention.

Once a primary treatment modality for ascites, paracentesis is more commonly used as a diagnostic tool to examine ascitic fluid. If SBP is suspected, ascitic fluid is withdrawn (10 to 20 mL) and sent for cell count and culture. If the client is symptomatic for infection, the physician may prescribe antibiotics while awaiting the culture results.

Paracentesis is also used as a palliative measure to relieve abdominal pressure because ascites may cause severe respiratory and abdominal distress. To relieve acute symptoms, the physician slowly drains the ascitic fluid (usually 1 to 3 L). Hypovolemia with a fluid volume deficit may occur with rapid fluid removal because these clients have adjusted to the excessive fluid volume in the abdomen. *Rapid, drastic removal of ascitic fluid leads to decreased abdominal pressure, which may contribute to vasodilation and shock.* Observe for impending signs of shock, such as hypotension and tachycardia, from fluid shifts during and immediately after the procedure.

Some physicians prescribe an albumin or other volume replacer infusion during paracentesis to avoid depleting the intravascular space and to avoid hypotension.

Repeated paracentesis procedures are discouraged because of the increased incidence of protein depletion, hypovolemia, and electrolyte imbalances. A low-sodium diet and diuretics are preferred as ways to control ascites.

Comfort Measures. Excessive ascitic fluid volume in the abdomen may cause the client to experience respiratory difficulty. Dyspnea may develop as a result of increased intra-abdominal pressure, which limits thoracic expansion and diaphragmatic excursion. The nurse or assistive nursing personnel elevates the head of the bed to at least 30 degrees or as high as the client wishes in an effort to minimize shortness of breath. The client is encouraged to sit in a chair. This upright position, with his or her feet elevated to discourage dependent ankle edema, often relieves dyspnea.

To weigh the client, the nurse or assistive nursing personnel uses a standard upright bedside scale if the client can stand. Weighing on a bed scale necessitates that the client lie flat; this supine position can cause the client to feel increasingly short of breath and can increase anxiety.

NIC **Fluid/Electrolyte Management.** Fluid and electrolyte imbalances are common as a result of the disease or

CHART 62-2

NIC **INTERVENTION ACTIVITIES for**
The Client with Cirrhosis

Fluid/Electrolyte Management: *Regulation and prevention of complications from altered fluid and/or electrolyte levels*
- Obtain laboratory specimens for monitoring of altered fluid and electrolyte levels (e.g., hematocrit, BUN, protein, sodium, and potassium levels), as appropriate.
- Keep an accurate record of intake and output.
- Weigh client daily and monitor trends.
- Monitor for signs and symptoms of fluid retention.
- Monitor vital signs, as appropriate.
- Administer prescribed supplemental electrolytes, as appropriate.

Bleeding Precautions: *Reduction of stimuli that may induce bleeding or hemorrhage in at-risk clients*
- Monitor the client closely for hemorrhage.
- Monitor for signs and symptoms of persistent bleeding (e.g., check all secretions for frank or occult blood)
- Monitor coagulation studies, including prothrombin time (PT), partial thromboplastin time (PTT), fibrinogen, fibrin degradation/split products, and platelet counts, as appropriate.
- Monitor orthostatic vital signs, including blood pressure.
- Use electric razor, instead of straight-edge, for shaving.
- Use soft toothbrush or toothettes for oral care.
- Avoid injections (IV, IM, or SC), as appropriate.
- Protect the client from trauma, which may cause bleeding.

Neurologic Monitoring: *Collection and analysis of client data to prevent or minimize neurologic complications*
- Monitor level of consciousness.
- Monitor level of orientation.
- Monitor recent memory, attention span, past memory, mood, affect, and behaviors.
- Monitor vital signs: temperature, blood pressure, pulse, and respirations.

NIC intervention activities selected from Dochterman, J.M., & Bulechek, G.M. (Eds.). (2004). *Nursing interventions classification (NIC)* (4th ed.). St. Louis: Mosby. No part of this work is to be altered without prior written permission from the Publisher.
BUN, Blood urea nitrogen; *SC*, subcutaneous.

treatment. Laboratory tests, such as blood urea nitrogen (BUN), serum protein, hematocrit, and electrolytes help determine fluid and electrolyte status. Nursing intervention activities are listed in Chart 62-2.

SURGICAL MANAGEMENT. When medical management fails to control ascites, the physician may choose surgical intervention to divert ascites into the venous system by creating a shunt. Clients with ascites are poor surgical risks. The **peritoneovenous shunt** has a pressure-sensitive one-way valve allowing ascitic fluid to flow from the abdominal cavity to the superior vena cava. Complications associated with this procedure include infection and thrombosis of the shunt. The **portacaval shunt** may also result in improvement in ascites (Figure 62-4). If symptoms return after placement of a shunt, a nuclear medicine examination called a peritoneal shunt evaluation may be requested. A radiologist injects a radioisotope tracer into the ascitic fluid in the abdomen or directly into the valve of the shunt. If functioning normally, the tracer should be seen in the shunt within about 10 minutes.

More recently, the **TIPS (transjugular intrahepatic portal-systemic shunt)** nonsurgical procedure has been the used to control refractory ascites and to reduce variceal bleeding. This procedure is described under the Interventions section for Potential for Hemorrhage on p. 1379.

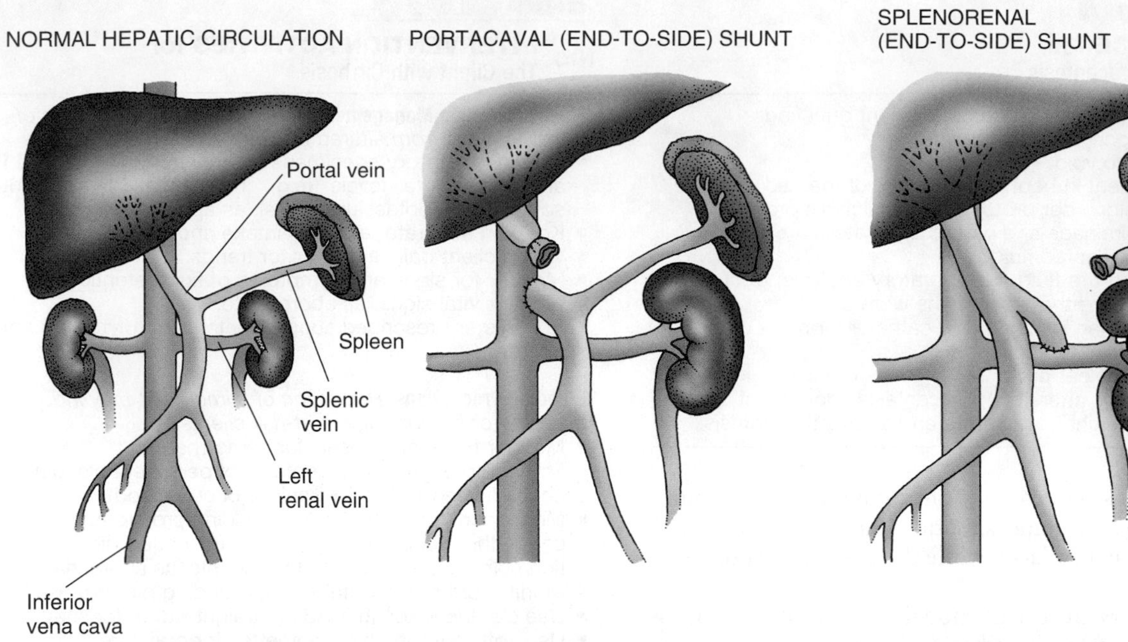

Figure 62-4 ■ Surgical shunting diverts portal venous blood flow from the liver to decrease portal and esophageal pressure.

The client with cirrhosis has many underlying medical problems; an optimal physical state is desired before surgery is performed. Electrolyte imbalances are corrected, and abnormal coagulation is treated with the administration of fresh frozen plasma and vitamin K. Packed red blood cells are made available for transfusion, because these clients have bleeding tendencies.

Provide the usual postoperative care for a client undergoing abdominal surgery (see Chapter 22). Remain aware that the ascitic fluid is routed into the venous system, resulting in vascular volume expansion and hemodilution. Vital signs are monitored carefully; an increase in blood pressure reflects an increase in vascular volume. If the client has a central venous or pulmonary artery catheter in place, determine whether pressure is elevated. Breath sounds are auscultated for the presence of crackles, which indicates excessive lung fluid. A diuretic, such as furosemide (Lasix), is usually prescribed to rid the body of excessive fluid. Note any abnormal results of coagulation studies (prothrombin time [PT] and partial thromboplastin time [PTT]). The nurse or assistive nursing personnel measures the client's weight, abdominal girth, and urine output each shift to determine the effectiveness of the shunting procedure.

POTENTIAL FOR HEMORRHAGE

PLANNING: EXPECTED OUTCOMES. The client is expected to not have bleeding episodes. However, if the client experiences hemorrhage, it is expected to be controlled through medical and nursing interventions.

INTERVENTIONS. During the acute phase of bleeding, early interventions are based on identifying the source of bleeding and initiating treatment to halt it. Because massive esophageal bleeding can cause rapid blood loss, emergency interventions are initiated. If the client is a known alcoholic with a history of variceal bleeding, measures to treat the esophageal varices are initiated and therefore valuable time is not wasted looking for another source of bleeding.

NONSURGICAL MANAGEMENT. The role of drug therapy is to *prevent* bleeding in clients where varices are present. If bleeding occurs, the health care team intervenes quickly to control it by providing interventions, such as gastric intubation, balloon tamponade, blood products, endoscopic band ligation, or endoscopic injection sclerotherapy. After the acute bleeding episode has been controlled, the client may require a transjugular intrahepatic portal-systemic shunt (TIPS) to decrease portal hypertension, thereby decreasing the risk of further variceal bleeding. The client is managed in the critical care unit.

Drug Therapy. To *prevent* the incidence of esophageal hemorrhage, the client with esophageal varices may be placed on a nonselective beta-blocking agent such as the long-acting form of propranolol (Inderal LA). The client is started on a low dose that is increased every 3 to 5 days until the heart rate is about 55 beats/min. By decreasing heart rate and the hepatic venous pressure gradient, the chance of bleeding may be reduced.

Gastric Intubation. The client's reports of hematemesis or melena should be rapidly investigated. A nasogastric tube is placed when GI bleeding is known or suspected and gastric lavage is performed until the fluid returned is clear. **Lavage** is the introduction of saline or water into the nasogastric tube to achieve vasoconstriction of the bleeding gastric ulceration or varices. When lavage is unsuccessful, more aggressive therapy is indicated.

Esophagogastric Balloon Tamponade. If hematemesis has occurred because of bleeding esophageal varices, gastric lavage has been unsuccessful, and emergent endoscopy is not available, the physician usually inserts an esophagogastric tamponade tube. This is a temporary measure to avoid the complications of hemorrhage.

The classic method of treating bleeding esophageal varices is by compressing the bleeding vessels with an esophagogastric tube, such as the Sengstaken-Blakemore tube (Blakemore tube), which has two balloons. This type of tube is also referred to as a **tamponade tube.** When inflated, the large esophageal balloon compresses the esophagus. The smaller gastric balloon helps anchor the tube and exerts pressure against bleeding varices in the distal esophagus and the cardia of the stomach. A third lumen terminates in the stomach and is connected to suction, allowing the aspiration of gastric contents and blood. A Salem sump tube is used in conjunction with the Sengstaken-Blakemore tube and is placed in the proximal esophagus to enable clearing of collected esophageal secretions, saliva, and blood.

Before the physician inserts the tube, the nurse should inspect it and inflate and deflate the balloons to check for integrity and leaks. Each lumen is identified and labeled to prevent errors in adding or removing pressure and air volume.

The physician typically anesthetizes the client's nose and oropharynx, introduces the tube, and gently inserts it into the stomach. Alert clients who can follow directions to take sips of water through a straw. Often, though, these clients are encephalopathic and unable to cooperate, requiring soft restraints or sedation. After tube placement is verified, the stomach is aspirated and irrigated. The balloon is inflated with the recommended volume of air. The correct lumens are clamped, and the tube is then pulled back gently until the correct resistance is felt. Assist the physician in securing the tube and applying traction, which provides additional tamponading pressure. This is accomplished through various traction devices. One method is to secure it to an overbed traction apparatus and applying a 1-pound (0.45-kg) traction weight. Inflation of the balloon should be monitored using a manometry device at the bedside.

The most serious complications of esophageal tamponade are aspiration and airway occlusion. Aspiration of blood and gastric contents may lead to pneumonia. Airway occlusion and asphyxia can occur from tube displacement. It is imperative to monitor the client's respiratory status. Asphyxia can be prevented by tube deflation and extraction. It is standard practice to have surgical scissors at the bedside of these clients so that in an emergency, all tube lumens can be quickly cut distally to the bifurcation points to allow for removal.

Placement of the tamponade tube should halt variceal bleeding. After bleeding is controlled, the traction is released, and esophageal pressure is gradually decreased. The gastric balloon is deflated, and the tube is removed. Another tube should be kept at the bedside for potential reinsertion if bleeding recurs.

Blood Transfusions. Massive hemorrhage necessitates replacement by blood products. Blood is drawn to identify the client's blood type. Until the blood is available, administer IV fluids or colloid (plasma) volumes, as prescribed, into large-bore IV access routes to maintain blood pressure.

Give packed red blood cells and fresh frozen plasma (per physician order and agency policy) to replace blood volume and clotting factors. The physician and the nurse monitor trends in hemoglobin and hematocrit levels, and additional blood products are transfused as indicated.

Endoscopic Procedures. Esophageal varices may be treated with **endoscopic band ligation**. This involves the application of small "O" bands around the base of the varices to cut off blood supply. The client is unaware of the bands and they cause no discomfort. An IV infusion of the drug octreotide may be given to the client with bleeding esophageal varices before the procedure to reduce blood flow.

Injection **sclerotherapy** may also be employed to stop variceal bleeding. This is also done through an endoscopic procedure. The varices are injected with a sclerosing agent via a catheter. There is potential for this procedure to cause mucosal ulceration, which could result in further bleeding. Because of the lower potential for treatment-related side effects, band ligation is typically used for long-term obliteration.

Transjugular Intrahepatic Portal-Systemic Shunt. Insertion of a transjugular intrahepatic portal-systemic shunt (TIPS) is a nonsurgical procedure performed in larger interventional radiology departments. This procedure is done for clients who have not responded to other modalities for hemorrhage or intractable ascites. If time permits, clients have an ultrasound to assess vein anatomy and patency. The client receives moderate IV sedation or heavy general anesthesia for this procedure. The radiologist places a large sheath into the jugular vein and places it into a hepatic vein. A needle is guided through the sheath and pushed through the liver into the portal vein. A balloon enlarges this tract and a metal stent keeps it open. Most clients have an ultrasound Doppler study of the liver after the TIPS procedure to record the blood flow through the shunt.

Serious complications of a TIPS are not common. Clients are discharged in 2 to 4 days and are followed up with ultrasounds for the first year after the shunt is placed. About one third of clients with a TIPS need to be re-ballooned once during the first year as an ambulatory care procedure.

SURGICAL MANAGEMENT. Traditional portal-systemic shunts are considered a last resort intervention for clients with portal hypertension and bleeding esophageal varices. Surgical bypass shunting procedures decrease portal hypertension by diverting a portion of the portal vein blood flow from the liver.

Recurrent esophageal variceal bleeding after a portal-systemic shunt is not uncommon and may indicate the return of elevated portal pressures caused by a thrombosed (clotted) shunt. A rapid reaccumulation of abdominal fluid may also suggest a failed shunt. Continue to measure the client's abdominal girth and report sudden girth increases to the physician. Be alert for the development of post-shunt encephalopathy, because it is common in clients receiving either a shunt or TIPS procedure (see care measures for portal-systemic encephalopathy [PSE] in the next section).

Monitor the client closely for hemorrhage. Coagulation studies, including prothrombin time (PT), partial thromboplastin time (PTT), platelet count, and International Normalized Ratio (INR), are also monitored carefully. Chart 62-2 lists additional interventions for clients at risk for bleeding.

Other techniques that are being used are electrocautery, cryoablation, and laser procedures via laparoscopic surgery.

Critical Thinking Challenge

You are the nurse for a middle-aged client with cirrhosis caused by alcoholic liver disease. You go into the client's room and find the client in the bathroom vomiting what appears to be hematemesis (blood in the vomitus).

1. What actions will you take immediately?
2. In what order of priority should you implement these interventions?
3. How can you differentiate between a gastrointestinal bleed and an esophageal bleed?

evolve For suggested answer guidelines, go to http://evolve.elsevier.com/Iggy/.

POTENTIAL FOR PORTAL-SYSTEMIC ENCEPHALOPATHY

PLANNING: EXPECTED OUTCOMES. It is expected that the nurse report and document findings for clients who exhibit early signs of portal-systemic encephalopathy (PSE).

INTERVENTIONS. The mechanisms that produce portal systemic encephalopathy are not completely clear, but ammonia probably plays a significant role. The poorly functioning liver cannot convert ammonia and other byproducts of metabolism to a less toxic form. They are carried by the circulatory system to the brain where there is interference with normal cerebral function. The aim of PSE management is to halt this process.

Because ammonia is formed in the gastrointestinal (GI) tract by the action of bacteria on protein, nonsurgical treatment measures to decrease ammonia production include dietary limitations and drug therapy to reduce bacterial breakdown. Collaborate with the dietitian and physician to plan and implement these treatment measures.

Diet Therapy. The client with cirrhosis has increased nutritional requirements. In general, the client needs high-carbohydrate, moderate-fat, and high-protein foods. However, the diet is often modified for clients who have elevated serum ammonia levels and exhibit the signs of PSE.

The diet for a client with PSE or elevated ammonia levels usually includes low-protein foods and simple carbohydrates. There have been suggestions that vegetable protein is preferred over animal protein for this population. It is important to include family members or significant others in nutritional counseling. The client is often weak and unable to remember complicated guidelines. Brief, simple directions regarding dietary do's and don'ts are recommended. Keep in mind any financial or cultural limitations when discussing food choices.

When a client with cirrhosis experiences GI bleeding, it can result in the formation of increased amounts of ammonia as intestinal bacteria attempt to metabolize the blood cells. GI bleeding may precipitate hepatic coma (stage IV of PSE). These clients are maintained on nothing by mouth (NPO) status with a nasogastric (NG) tube or an esophageal tamponade tube, depending on the source of the bleeding.

Drug Therapy. Medications are used sparingly because they are difficult for the failing liver to metabolize. In particular, opioid analgesics, sedatives, and barbiturates should be restricted, especially for the client with a history of encephalopathy.

Several types of drugs, however, can eliminate or reduce ammonia levels in the body. These include lactulose, neomycin sulfate, and metronidazole.

Lactulose. The health care provider prescribes lactulose to promote the excretion of ammonia in the stool. Lactulose, a disaccharide with high molecular weight, is a viscous, sticky, sweet-tasting liquid that is administered either orally or by NG tube. The purpose is to obtain a laxative effect; cleansing the bowels rids the intestinal tract of the toxins that contribute to encephalopathy. The drug is prescribed to the client who has manifested signs of PSE, regardless of the stage.

Lactulose retention enemas may be necessary when the client cannot tolerate oral administration or when liquids are contraindicated in the upper GI tract.

Lactulose creates an acidic environment in the bowel by keeping ammonia in its ionized state; this decreases the pH of the colon from 7 to 5. A decreased pH causes ammonia to leave the circulatory system and move into the colon, which reverses the normal passage of ammonia from the colon to the bloodstream.

The desired effect of the drug is production of two to five soft stools per day and a decrease in client confusion caused by PSE. During the acute phase of PSE, 20 to 30 g of lactulose is administered at 4-hour intervals until stools are achieved; the dosage is then decreased to three or four times daily.

Observe for response to lactulose. The client may complain of intestinal bloating and cramping. Serum ammonia levels may be monitored but do not always correlate with symptoms. Hypokalemia and dehydration may result from excessive stools.

Neomycin Sulfate. Neomycin sulfate (Mycifradin), a broad-spectrum antibiotic, is given to act as an intestinal antiseptic. It destroys the normal flora in the bowel, diminishing protein breakdown and decreasing the rate of ammonia production. Maintenance doses of neomycin are given orally, but may also be administered as a retention enema. Long-term use has the potential for renal toxicity and, therefore, it is used with caution.

Metronidazole. Metronidazole (Flagyl, Novonidazole✱) is a broad-spectrum antibiotic with similar action to neomycin, but it has less potential for renal toxicity. It is used both as a single agent or in combination with lactulose for treatment and prophylaxis of PSE.

NIC **Neurologic Monitoring.** The nurse or assistive nursing personnel continually assesses for changes in level of consciousness and orientation (see Chart 62-2). An individualized neurologic assessment is developed for each client and includes the assessment of simple tasks such as name writing, bilateral hand grasping, and serial subtractions and additions. Continually assess for the presence of asterixis (liver flap) and fetor hepaticus (liver breath). These signs suggest worsening encephalopathy.

> ***Critical Thinking Challenge***
>
> You are caring for a client in the prodromal stage of portal systemic encephalopathy (PSE).
>
> 1. In planning care, which common medications are hepatotoxic and should be avoided?
> 2. What type of dietary restrictions might be ordered?
> 3. How will you maintain the client's safety?
> 4. For what signs and symptoms indicating worsening PSE will you be observing?

evolve For suggested answer guidelines, go to http://evolve.elsevier.com/Iggy/.

Community-Based Care

If the client with hepatic cirrhosis survives life-threatening complications, he or she is usually discharged to the home or to a long-term care facility after treatment measures have combated the acute medical problems. A home care referral may be needed if the client is discharged to the home. These chronically ill clients are often readmitted, and community-based care is aimed at preventing rehospitalization. The client may benefit from hospice care. A case manager is often needed to coordinate interdisciplinary care.

CHART 62-3

CLIENT EDUCATION GUIDE
Cirrhosis

Diet Therapy
- Consume a diet that adheres to the guidelines set by your physician, nurse, or dietitian.
- If you have excessive fluid in your abdomen, follow the low-sodium diet prescribed for you.
- Eat small, frequent meals that are nutritionally well balanced.
- Include in your diet daily supplemental liquids (e.g., Ensure or Ensure Plus) and a multivitamin; low-protein supplements are available if needed.

Drug Therapy
- Take the diuretics or preventive beta blocker prescribed for you. If you experience muscle weakness, irregular heartbeat, or light-headedness, contact your health care provider right away.
- Take the medication prescribed for you that helps prevent gastrointestinal bleeding.
- Take the lactulose syrup as prescribed to maintain three to five bowel movements every day.
- Do *not* take any other medication unless specifically prescribed by your health care provider.

Alcohol Abstinence
- Do not consume any alcohol.
- Seek support services for help if needed.

HOME CARE MANAGEMENT

The nurse, case manager, client, and family or significant other should identify any physical adaptations needed to prepare the client's home for convalescence. The client's rest area needs to be close to a bathroom, because diuretic therapy increases the frequency of urination. If the client has difficulty reaching the toilet, additional equipment (e.g., urinals, bedpans, and bedside commodes) is necessary. Special, adult-sized incontinence pads or briefs may be helpful if the client has an altered mental status and has urinary incontinence.

Initial home activity may be limited for the client who has undergone surgical intervention. If the client experiences shortness of breath from massive ascites, elevating the head of the bed and maintaining the client in a semi-Fowler's to high Fowler's position may help alleviate respiratory distress. Alternatively, a reclining chair with a foot elevator may be used.

HEALTH TEACHING

The client is discharged to the home setting with an individualized teaching plan (Chart 62-3) that covers diet therapy, drug therapy, and alcohol abstinence.

DIET THERAPY. In collaboration with the dietitian, and in keeping with the client's financial and cultural status, provide dietary instructions. The client with portal-systemic encephalopathy (PSE) must avoid high-protein foods at home to decrease the incidence of progressive neurologic dysfunction. If the client's nutritional intake is decreased after discharge, multivitamin supplements and supplemental liquid feedings (e.g., Ensure, Boost) are usually needed.

DRUG THERAPY. The client is often discharged while receiving diuretics. Provide instructions regarding the health care provider's prescription for the diuretic. Teach the client about side effects of therapy, such as hypokalemia. The client may need to take a potassium supplement.

If the client has had problems with bleeding from gastric ulcers, the provider may prescribe an H_2-receptor antagonist agent or proton pump inhibitor. Clients who have had episodes of SBP (spontaneous bacterial peritonitis) may be on a daily maintenance antibiotic. Because many of these individuals have alienated relatives over the years because of substance abuse, it may be necessary to help the client identify a friend, neighbor, or person in their recovery group to assist with medications.

Families and significant others should be informed about how to recognize signs of PSE and be instructed that it is necessary and safe to increase the daily lactulose at the first sign of encephalopathy. The health care provider should also be contacted. Clients and family members are reminded that constipation, bleeding, and infections may lead to PSE. They should also understand that PSE is usually reversible.

Advise the client to avoid all over-the-counter medications and to consult the physician for follow-up medical care. Remind the client and family to notify the physician immediately if any gastrointestinal (GI) bleeding is noted so that re-evaluation can be initiated quickly.

ALCOHOL ABSTINENCE. One of the most important aspects of ongoing care for the nurse to stress is the need to avoid alcohol and illicit drugs (see Chapter 8). By avoiding alcohol and drugs, the client:
- Prevents further fibrosis of the liver from scarring
- Allows the liver to heal and regenerate
- Prevents gastric and esophageal irritation
- Reduces the incidence of bleeding
- Prevents other life-threatening complications

HEALTH CARE RESOURCES

The client with chronic cirrhosis may require a home care nurse. The home care nurse can also monitor the effectiveness of drug therapy or the surgical shunt in controlling ascites. The encephalopathic client may need to be monitored for compliance with medications. For the individual recovering from bacterial peritonitis, home infusion of antibiotics may be needed. Individual and group therapy sessions may be arranged to assist clients in dealing with alcohol abstinence if they are too ill to attend a formal treatment program. The nurse may refer the client and family to self-help groups, such as Alcoholics Anonymous and Al-Anon. The client may also desire spiritual support. Finances are frequently a problem for the chronically ill client and family; social support and community services need to be identified. The American Liver Foundation is an excellent source for more information about liver disease.

◆Evaluation: Outcomes

Evaluate the care of the client with cirrhosis on the basis of the identified nursing diagnoses and collaborative problems. The expected outcomes include that the client will:
- Experience a decrease in or no ascites
- Have electrolytes within normal limits (WNL)
- Have blood pressure WNL
- Not experience hemorrhage or will be managed immediately if bleeding occurs
- Not experience PSE or will be managed immediately if PSE occurs

- Avoid the development of SBP (spontaneous bacterial peritonitis)
- Have the optimal quality of life possible

Specific indicators for these outcomes are listed for each nursing diagnosis and collaborative problem under the Planning and Implementation section (see earlier).

HEPATITIS

PATHOPHYSIOLOGY

Hepatitis is the widespread inflammation of liver cells. *Viral* hepatitis is the most prevalent type and can be either acute or chronic. **Viral hepatitis** results from an infection caused by one of five major categories of viruses:

- Hepatitis A virus (HAV)
- Hepatitis B virus (HBV)
- Hepatitis C virus (HCV)
- Hepatitis D virus (HDV)
- Hepatitis E virus (HEV)

Hepatitis F and G have also been identified but are uncommon.

Liver injury with inflammation can also develop after exposure to a number of pharmacologic and chemical agents by inhalation, ingestion, or parenteral (IV) administration. **Toxic and drug-induced hepatitis** can result from exposure to hepatotoxins (e.g., industrial toxins, alcohol, and medications).

Hepatitis may also occur as a secondary infection during the course of infections with other viruses, such as Epstein-Barr, herpes simplex, varicella-zoster, and cytomegalovirus.

After the liver has been exposed to causative agents (e.g., a virus), it becomes enlarged and congested with inflammatory cells, lymphocytes, and fluid, resulting in right upper quadrant pain and discomfort. As the disease progresses, the liver's normal lobular pattern becomes distorted as a result of widespread inflammation, necrosis, and hepatocellular regeneration. This distortion increases pressure within the portal circulation, interfering with the blood flow into the hepatic lobules. Edema of the liver's bile channels results in intrahepatic obstructive **jaundice** (yellowing of the skin).

Classification of Hepatitis and Etiologies

VIRAL HEPATITIS

The five types of acute viral hepatitis vary by mode of transmission, manner of onset, and incubation periods (Table 62-5).

HEPATITIS A. The causative agent of **hepatitis A**, hepatitis A virus (HAV), is a ribonucleic acid (RNA) virus of the enterovirus family. HAV is characterized by a mild course similar to that of a typical viral syndrome and often goes unrecognized. It is spread via the fecal-oral route by the oral ingestion of fecal contaminants. Sources of infection include contaminated water, shellfish caught in contaminated water, and food contaminated by food handlers infected with HAV. The virus may also be spread by oral-anal sexual activity. The incubation period of hepatitis A is usually 15 to 50 days. The disease is usually not life threatening, but its course may be more severe in individuals older than 40 years of age. Hepatitis A can also complicate pre-existing liver disease.

Many people have had hepatitis A and do not know it. The course is similar to that of a gastrointestinal illness and the disease and recovery are usually uneventful.

HEPATITIS B. The **hepatitis B** virus (HBV) is not transmitted like HAV. It is a double-shelled particle containing deoxyribonucleic acid (DNA) composed of a core antigen (HBcAg), a surface antigen (HBsAg), and another antigen found within the core (HBeAg) that circulates in the blood. HBV may be spread through the following modes of transmission:

- Unprotected sexual intercourse with an infected partner (heterosexual and homosexual)
- Sharing needles
- Accidental needle sticks or injuries from sharp instruments (primarily in health care workers)
- Blood transfusions (that have not been screened for the virus)
- Hemodialysis
- Maternal-fetal route

The clinical course of hepatitis B may be varied. Symptoms usually occur within 25 to 180 days of exposure and include the following:

- Anorexia, nausea, and vomiting
- Fever
- Fatigue
- Right upper quadrant pain
- Dark urine with light stool
- Joint pain
- Jaundice

Blood tests confirm the disease, although about 40% of people with hepatitis B have no symptoms.

Most adults who get hepatitis B recover, clear the virus from their body, and develop immunity. However, up to 10% of clients with the disease do not develop immunity become carriers. **Hepatitis carriers** can infect others even though they are not sick and demonstrate no obvious signs of hepatitis B. Chronic carriers are at high risk for cirrhosis and liver cancer.

HEPATITIS C. The causative virus of **hepatitis C (HCV)** is an enveloped, single-stranded RNA virus. Transmission is blood to blood. The rate of sexual transmission is very low, and it is rarely transmitted from mother to fetus.

HCV is most commonly spread by:

- Illicit IV drug needle sharing (highest incidence)
- Blood, blood products, or organ transplants received before 1992
- Needle stick injury with HCV-contaminated blood (health care workers at high risk)
- Tattoos (unsanitary tattoo equipment)
- Intranasal cocaine use (sharing of intranasal cocaine)

The disease is **not** transmitted by casual contact or by intimate household contact. However, those infected are advised not to share razors, toothbrushes or pierced earrings, because there may be microscopic blood on these items.

The incubation period for HCV is 21 to 140 days, with an average incubation period of 7 weeks. Acute infection and illness is not common. Most individuals are completely unaware that they have been infected. They are asymptomatic and not diagnosed until many months or years after the initial exposure when an abnormality is detected during a routine laboratory evaluation or when symptoms of liver impairment appear. Unlike with hepatitis B, most people infected with hepatitis C do not clear the virus and a chronic infection develops.

HCV usually does its damage over decades by causing a chronic inflammation in the liver that eventually causes the

TABLE 62-5 Differential Features of the Five Types of Viral Hepatitis

Hepatitis A	Hepatitis B	Hepatitis C	Hepatitis D	Hepatitis E
Synonyms				
Infectious hepatitis	Serum hepatitis	Non-A, non-B hepatitis		Epidemic non-A, non-B hepatitis or enterically transmitted hepatitis
Diagnosis of Acute Disease				
Anti-HAV IgM in serum	HBsAg in serum	Anti-HCV in serum	Anti-HDV in serum	Anti-HEV in serum
Incubation Period				
15-50 days	48-180 days	14-180 days	14-56 days	15-64 days
High-Risk Groups				
More common in young children and institutional settings	All age-groups affected, especially drug addicts and health care workers	All ages of drug users Persons with hemophilia	Drug addicts Persons with hepatitis B	Persons living in underdeveloped countries
Season				
Fall and early winter	All year	All year	All year	All year
Transmission				
Usually by oral-fecal route among persons living in close contact; ingestion of contaminated water or contaminated shellfish	Primarily blood; drug abuse, sexual contact, mother to child at birth	Primarily blood; drug abuse, sexual contact (rarely), mother to child at birth	Co-infects with hepatitis B; nonpercutaneous; close personal contact	Oral-fecal route; transmitted principally by contaminated water
Clinical Findings				
Majority of type A infections (mild and anicteric); symptoms similar to those of influenza	Changes similar to those of hepatitis A Fatigue, anorexia, low-grade fever, abdominal discomfort, arthralgias, rashes, enlarged and tender liver, light stools, dark urine, jaundice Elevated serum AST and ALT levels (early), hyperbilirubinemia, abnormal liver function test results	Changes similar to those of hepatitis A Tends to have more severe symptoms; sometimes necessitates hospitalization for extended periods	Changes similar to those of hepatitis A, but symptoms often more severe than those in hepatitis A and hepatitis B Often asymptomatic	Resembles hepatitis A
Virus in Feces?				
Yes	Not infectious	Not identified	Not identified	Possible
Virus in Serum?				
Anti-HAV in serum during acute phase and incubation period is rare	HBsAg is in serum throughout the clinical course	Anti-HVC test is about 95% reliable; often takes up to 8 weeks to show antibody	Anti-HDV in serum	
Nosocomial Problem?				
No	Yes	Yes	Yes	No
Mortality				
Less frequent	More frequent, chronic form can be fatal	More frequent, chronic form can be fatal	Increased	Unknown

Anti-HAV, Antibody to HAV; *IgM*, immunoglobulin M; *HBsAg*, hepatitis B surface antigen; *anti-HCV*, antibodies to HCV; *anti-HDV*, antibodies to HDV; *anti-HEV*, antibodies to HEV; *AST*, aspartate aminotransferase; *ALT*, alanine aminotransferase.

hepatocytes (liver cells) to scar. This scarring may progress to cirrhosis. Concomitant use of alcohol hastens the progression to cirrhosis. Those infected with hepatitis C and in whom cirrhosis has developed are at risk for development of liver cancer.

Hepatitis C–induced cirrhosis is the leading indication for liver transplantation in the United States (National Institutes of Health Consensus Development Conference Statement, 2002). Unfortunately, the newly transplanted liver often becomes reinfected with the virus.

HEPATITIS D. Hepatitis D (delta hepatitis, or HDV) is caused by a defective RNA virus that needs the helper function of HBV. HDV co-infects with HBV and needs its presence for viral replication. Hepatitis D can co-infect a client with HBV or can occur as a superinfection in a client with chronic HBV. Superinfection usually develops into chronic

HDV. The incubation period is about 14 to 56 days. As with HBV, the disease is transmitted primarily by parenteral routes.

HEPATITIS E. The **hepatitis E** virus (HEV) was originally identified by its association with waterborne epidemics of hepatitis in the Indian subcontinent. Since then, it has occurred in epidemics in Asia, Africa, the Middle East, Mexico, and Central and South America. Many large outbreaks have occurred after heavy rains and flooding.

In the United States, hepatitis E has been found only in travelers returning from these endemic areas. The nonenveloped, single-stranded RNA virus is transmitted via the fecal-oral route, and the clinical course resembles that of hepatitis A. HEV has an incubation period of 15 to 64 days. There is no evidence at this time of a chronic form of HEV.

TOXIC AND DRUG-INDUCED HEPATITIS

Chemicals that are inhaled or swallowed can damage the liver. Prescription medications, over-the-counter (OTC) medications, herbals supplements, industrial solvents, pollutants, and even mushrooms have all been implicated as causes of hepatitis.

Complications of Hepatitis

Failure of the liver cells to regenerate, with progression of the necrotic process, results in a severe acute and often fatal form of hepatitis known as **fulminant hepatitis.** Hepatitis is considered to be chronic when liver inflammation lasts longer than several months (usually defined as 6 months). **Chronic hepatitis** usually occurs as a result of hepatitis B or C. Superimposed infection with hepatitis D (HDV) in clients with chronic HBV may also result in chronic hepatitis. As mentioned earlier, chronic hepatitis can lead to cirrhosis and liver cancer.

Incidence/Prevalence

Each year about 250,000 people in the United States become infected with hepatitis A. However, only a small portion of these cases is reported. Hepatitis B and C are much more of a concern, though, because of their connection to cirrhosis and liver cancer. Although exact numbers are not known, it is estimated that about 200 million people worldwide have the hepatitis C virus (HCV), making this type of hepatitis the most common type. In the United States, the rate of HCV is increasing among young adults, Hispanics, and war veterans who used IV drugs, experienced needle sticks, or had tattoos. About 3.9 million people in the United States have been exposed to HCV and about 3 million have chronic liver disease, making HCV very costly in dollars and quality of life (Centers for Disease Control and Prevention, 2002) (see the Resource Management box above).

Deaths from liver disease have been estimated at 43,000 per year, but that number is predicted to increase by 60% or more in the next decade. This increase will require a major increase in transplantations and lead to many more deaths.

HEALTH PROMOTION/ILLNESS PREVENTION

Measures for preventing hepatitis A (HAV) include the following:

- Proper handwashing
- Avoiding contaminated food or water

> **RESOURCE MANAGEMENT**
>
> **HEPATITIS C**
>
> **Cost of Care**
>
> - An estimated 3.9 million Americans, nearly 2% of the population, are chronically infected with hepatitis C.
> - The cost of hepatitis C infections and related diseases is more than $600 million per year.
> - More than half of the liver transplants performed in the United States are for hepatitis C. The average first-year cost for a liver transplant exceeds $200,000.
> - From the year 2010 through 2019, the projected cost in direct medical expenses is $10.7 billion, with 165,900 deaths due to chronic liver disease and 27,200 deaths due to hepatocellular carcinoma.
>
> **Implications for Nursing**
>
> Nurses are at high risk for getting hepatitis C and becoming part of these statistics. As these costs rise, health care will be impacted further from this disease. Nurses must strive to disseminate information about this disease to prevent others from obtaining it and to help reduce costs.

Data from Wong, J.B., et al. (2000). Estimating future hepatitis C morbidity, mortality, and costs in the United States. *American Journal of Public Health, 90*(10), 1562-1569.

- Receiving the HAV vaccine before traveling to areas where the disease is common (e.g., Mexico, Caribbean)
- Receiving immune globulin within 14 days if exposed to the virus

For hepatitis B (HBV) prevention, a vaccine can provide protection against the disease. There is no vaccine yet available for the other types of viral hepatitis. HBV vaccine is now recommended as part of the routine schedule of childhood vaccinations in the United States. It is also recommended for the following:

- Infants born to HBV-infected mothers
- People who have unprotected sexual intercourse with more than one partner
- People with any chronic liver disease
- People who are exposed to blood or body fluids in the workplace, including health care workers, firefighters, and police
- People who live in close living accommodations, such as college dormitories, correctional institutions, and long-term care facilities

Case reporting to local health departments for all types of *viral* hepatitis is mandatory (reporting is usually the responsibility of the laboratory). Additional measures to prevent viral hepatitis for health care workers and others in contact with infected clients are listed in Charts 62-4 and 62-5.

COLLABORATIVE MANAGEMENT

Assessment

HISTORY

In any client who presents with the manifestations of acute hepatitis, it is important to obtain a focused history. First, ask the client whether he or she has had known exposure to a person with hepatitis. The client should also be asked about the following:

- Exposure to either inhaled or ingested chemical
- Use of herbal supplement
- Use of any new prescribed medication
- Recent ingestion of shellfish

CHART 62-4

BEST PRACTICE for
Prevention of Viral Hepatitis in Health Care Workers

- Use standard precautions to prevent the transmission of disease between clients or between clients and health care staff (see Chapter 29).
- Eliminate needles and other sharp instruments by substituting needleless systems. (Needle sticks are the major source of hepatitis B transmission in health care workers.)
- Take the hepatitis B vaccine (Heptavax-B, Recombivax HB), which is given in a series of three injections. This vaccine also prevents hepatitis D.
- For postexposure prevention of hepatitis A or B, seek medical attention immediately for immunoglobulin (Ig) administration.
- Report all cases of hepatitis to the local health department.

CHART 62-5

CLIENT EDUCATION GUIDE
Health Promotion/Illness Prevention of Viral Hepatitis

- Maintain adequate sanitation and personal hygiene. Wash your hands before eating and after using the toilet.
- Drink water treated by a water purification system.
- If traveling in underdeveloped or nonindustrialized countries, drink only bottled water. Avoid food washed or prepared with tap water, such as raw vegetables, fruits, and soups.
- Use adequate sanitation practices to prevent the spread of the disease between family members.
- Do not share bed linens, towels, eating utensils, or drinking glasses.
- Do not share needles for injection, body piercing, or tattooing.
- Do not share razors, nail clippers, toothbrushes, or WaterPiks.
- Use a condom during sexual intercourse or abstain from this activity.
- Cover cuts or sores with bandages.
- If ever infected with hepatitis, never donate blood, body organs, or other body tissue.

- Exposure to a possibly contaminated water source
- Employment
- Recent foreign travel
- Sexual activities with men, women, or both, and whether it was protected or unprotected
- Injectable drug use
- For health care workers, recent needle stick exposure
- Recent body piercing or tattooing
- Close living accommodations, such as military barracks, correctional institutions, and overcrowded dormitories, long-term facilities, or employment in any such setting

For the client who presents with few or no symptoms of liver disease but who has had an abnormality detected by a laboratory evaluation (e.g., an elevated ALT or AST level), the history may need to include additional questions regarding the following:

- Blood or blood products received before 1992
- Military service or other travel to a foreign country
- Place of birth (United States or other country) and parents' place of birth
- Sharing of needles or cocaine straw at any time in the past
- Sexual history
- History of alcohol use (how many drinks each day or week)

PHYSICAL ASSESSMENT/CLINICAL MANIFESTATIONS

Assess whether the client is experiencing the following:

- Abdominal pain
- Changes in skin or eye color
- **Arthralgia** (joint pain)
- **Myalgia** (muscle pain)
- Diarrhea/constipation
- Changes in color of urine or stool
- Fever
- Lethargy
- Malaise
- Nausea/vomiting
- Pruritus

Lightly palpate the right upper abdominal quadrant to assess for liver tenderness. The client may report right upper quadrant pain with jarring movements. Inspect the skin, sclerae, and mucous membranes for the presence of jaundice. The client may present for medical treatment only after jaundice appears, believing that other vague symptoms are related to an influenza-like syndrome.

Jaundice in hepatitis results from intrahepatic obstruction and is caused by edema of the liver's bile channels. Dark urine and clay-colored stools are often reported by the client. If possible, obtain a urine and stool specimen for visual inspection and laboratory analysis. The client may also report pruritus (itching) and may have skin abrasions from scratching.

PSYCHOSOCIAL ASSESSMENT

Viral hepatitis has various presentations, but for most infected individuals, the initial course is mild with few symptoms. It is the long-term complications of fibrosis and cirrhosis that cause the more serious problem. This is especially true for clients who have HBV and HCV infection.

When the presentation is dramatic with jaundice and significant impairment of liver function, the client is acutely ill and needs supportive care.

Emotional problems for affected clients often center on their feeling sick and fatigued. General malaise, inactivity, and vague complaints contribute to depression and despondency. These clients worry about the long-term effects and complications. They often feel guilty and are remorseful about decisions made that caused the disease. These feelings are most likely to occur when the source of infection is from drug abuse.

Infectious diseases such as hepatitis continue to have a social stigma. The client may feel embarrassed by the isolation and hygiene precautions that are imposed in the hospital and continue to be necessary at home. This embarrassment may cause the client to limit social interactions. Self-imposed visitor restrictions may be instituted by the client out of fear of spreading the virus to family and friends.

Family members are sometimes afraid of contracting the disease and may distance themselves from the client. Allow the client and family to verbalize these feelings and explore the reasons for these fears. The nurse also plays an important role in educating client and family members about modes of transmission. It is essential to dispel any misconceptions that would contribute to the client's isolation.

Clients may be unable to return to work for several weeks during the acute phases of illness. The loss of wages and the cost of hospitalization for a client without insurance coverage may produce great anxiety and financial burden for the client and the family.

LABORATORY ASSESSMENT

The presence of hepatitis A, B, and C is usually indicated by acute elevations in levels of liver enzymes, indicating liver cellular damage, and by specific serologic markers.

SERUM LIVER ENZYMES. Levels of alanine aminotransferase (ALT) and aspartate aminotransferase (AST) levels may rise into the thousands in acute or fulminant cases of hepatitis. Alkaline phosphatase levels may be normal or elevated. Serum total bilirubin levels are elevated and are consistent with the clinical appearance of jaundice. Elevated levels of bilirubin are also present in the urine.

SEROLOGIC MARKERS/ENZYME ASSAYS. The presence of *hepatitis A* is established when hepatitis A virus (HAV) antibodies (anti-HAV) are identified in the blood. Ongoing inflammation of the liver by HAV is evidenced by the presence of immunoglobulin M (IgM) antibodies, which persist in the blood for 4 to 6 weeks. Previous infection is indicated by the presence of immunoglobulin G (IgG) antibodies. These antibodies persist in the serum and provide permanent immunity to HAV.

The presence of the *hepatitis B* virus (HBV) is established when serologic testing confirms the presence of hepatitis B antigen-antibody systems in the blood. HBV is a double-shelled DNA virus consisting of an inner core and an outer shell. Antigens located on the surface (shell) of the virus (HBsAg) and IgM antibodies to hepatitis B core antigen (anti-HBc IgM) are the most significant serologic markers. The presence of these markers establishes the diagnosis of hepatitis B. The client is considered infectious as long as HBsAg (hepatitis B surface antigen) is present in the blood. Persistence of this serologic marker after 6 months or longer indicates a carrier state or chronic hepatitis. HBsAg levels normally decline and disappear after the acute hepatitis B episode. The presence of antibodies to HBsAb (hepatitis B surface antibody) in the blood indicates recovery and immunity to hepatitis B. Keep in mind that people who have been vaccinated against HBV have a positive HBsAb because they also have immunity to the disease.

Enzyme-linked immunosorbent assay (ELISA) is the initial screening test for clients suspected of being infected with *hepatitis C* virus (HCV). It is also the most commonly used enzyme test for HCV antibodies (anti-HCV). The antibodies can be detected within 4 weeks of the infection (Pagana & Pagana, 2002). A more specific assay called the recombinant immunoblot assay (RIBA) has been used as a confirmatory test. These tests confirm that the client has been exposed to HCV and has developed the antibody. To confirm the presence of actual circulating virus, the HCV polymerase chain reaction (PCR) RNA test is used. This confirms active virus and can quantify the viral load.

The presence of *hepatitis D* virus (HDV) can be confirmed by the identification of intrahepatic delta antigen or, more often, by a rise in the hepatitis D virus antibodies (anti-HDV) titer. This increase can be seen within a few days of infection (Pagana & Pagana, 2002).

Hepatitis E virus (HEV) testing is usually reserved for travelers in whom hepatitis is present but the virus cannot be detected. The presence of the hepatitis E antibodies (anti-HEV) is found in individuals infected with the virus.

OTHER DIAGNOSTIC ASSESSMENTS

Liver biopsy is also used to confirm the diagnosis of hepatitis. Characteristic changes help the pathologist distinguish among a virus, drug, toxin, fatty liver, and other disease. It is usually performed on in an ambulatory care setting and performed percutaneously (through the skin) after a local anesthetic is given. If coagulation is abnormal, however, it may be done using either a CT guided or transjugular route.

◆Interventions

The client with viral hepatitis can be mildly or acutely ill depending on the severity of the inflammation. Most clients are not hospitalized, although older adults and those with dehydration may be admitted for a short-term stay. Some clients are hospitalized during administration of potent medications to treat hepatitis B or C. The plan of care for all clients with viral hepatitis is based on measures to rest the liver, promote cellular regeneration, and prevent complications (see the Plan of Care on pp. 1387 to 1390).

NONSURGICAL MANAGEMENT. During the acute stage of viral hepatitis, interventions are aimed at resting the inflamed liver to promote hepatic cell regeneration. Rest is an essential intervention to reduce the liver's metabolic demands and increase its blood supply. Treatment is generally supportive.

Physical Rest. Assess the client's response to activity and rest periods. Strict bedrest may be indicated during the early icteric phase of hepatitis. The client is usually tired and expresses feelings of general malaise. Complete bedrest is usually not required, but rest periods alternating with periods of activity are indicated and are often sufficient to promote hepatic healing. Individualize the client's plan of care and change it as needed to reflect the severity of symptoms, fatigue, and the results of liver function tests and enzyme determinations. Teach the client to adhere to scheduled rest periods. Activities such as self-care and ambulating are gradually added to the activity schedule as tolerated.

Psychological Rest. Emotional and psychological rest is essential for the client. Because bedrest and inactivity can produce anxiety, the client should include diversional activities.

Diet Therapy. A special diet is usually not required. The diet should be high in carbohydrates and calories with moderate amounts of fat and protein. Small, frequent meals are often preferable to three standard meals. Ask the client about food preferences, because favorite foods are tolerated better than randomly selected foods. Encourage the client to select foods that are appealing. High-calorie snacks may be needed.

The health care provider typically prescribes supplemental vitamins. If caloric intake is low, the client may need supplemental commercial feedings, such as Ensure or Boost.

PLAN of CARE MEDICAL DIAGNOSIS: HEPATITIS

NURSING DIAGNOSIS NO. 1 ■ Fatigue

	Expected Outcomes	Nursing Interventions	Rationales
RELATED FACTORS Disease states Malnutrition **DEFINING CHARACTERISTICS** Energy: Lack of Rest requirements: Increased Inability to maintain usual routines Increase in physical complaints	Denies fatigue No verbal report or observation of being lethargic or listless Denies feeling tired Denies an increase in rest requirements No verbal report or observation of lack of energy	NIC **Energy Management** D Monitor the client for evidence of excess physical and emotional fatigue.	Extended periods of inactivity may place the client at risk for excessive fatigue when carrying out desired activities.
		D Monitor nutritional intake.	Monitoring nutritional intake ensures that the client has adequate energy resources.
		D Reduce physical discomforts.	Physical discomforts could interfere with cognitive function and self-monitoring/regulation of activity.
		D Arrange physical activities (e.g., avoid activity immediately after meals).	Arranging physical activities reduces competition for oxygen supply to vital body functions.
		Encourage alternate rest and activity periods.	This avoids extended periods of either activity or exercise.
		Assist the client to schedule rest periods and avoid care activities during scheduled rest periods.	Rest periods should help restore client energy levels.
		Teach activity organization and time management techniques (e.g., assigning priority to activities to accommodate energy levels, establishing realistic activity goals).	Activity organization and time management techniques are used to prevent fatigue.
		Instruct the client/significant other to recognize the signs and symptoms of fatigue.	Symptoms of undue fatigue require a reduction in activity.
		Other Interventions Consider the use of complementary and alternative therapies.	Complementary and alternative therapies may be used to cope with chronic disease and disability, especially if chronic pain is a problem.
		Continuing Care Considerations Collaborate with the client/family and the rehabilitation team.	Effective interdisciplinary interventions facilitate the client's ability to manage his or her life.

NURSING DIAGNOSIS NO. 2 ■ Nausea

	Expected Outcomes	Nursing Interventions	Rationales
RELATED FACTORS Irritation to the gastrointestinal system Stimulation of neuropharmacologic mechanisms **DEFINING CHARACTERISTICS** Verbal reports of "nausea" or being "sick to stomach"	Denies nausea No verbal report or observation of vomiting	NIC **Nausea Management** Assess nausea, including frequency, duration, severity, and precipitating factors. If possible, use an established nausea assessment tool.	Performing a complete assessment of nausea using tools such as Self-Care Journal, Visual Analog Scales, Duke Descriptive Scales, and Rhodes Index of Nausea and Vomiting (INV) Form 2 can better monitor the client's nausea patterns.

D Indicates tasks that can be delegated to unlicensed assistive nursing personnel at the discretion of the nurse.

Continued

PLAN of CARE MEDICAL DIAGNOSIS: HEPATITIS—*cont'd*

NURSING DIAGNOSIS NO. 2 ■ Nausea—*cont'd*

Expected Outcomes	Nursing Interventions	Rationales
	Identify factors (e.g., medication and procedures) that may cause or contribute to nausea.	Identifying the source of nausea permits using strategies to prevent or diminish nausea.
	Ensure that effective antiemetic drugs are given, when possible.	Antiemetics are given to prevent nausea.
	D Control environmental factors such as aversive smells, sound, and unpleasant visual stimulation.	Environmental factors may evoke nausea.
	Encourage the use of nonpharmacologic techniques, as well as other nausea control measures, before nausea occurs or increases.	The use of nonpharmacologic techniques helps the client to control nausea and may amplify the relief obtained by other control measures.
	Inform other health care professionals and family members of any nonpharmacologic strategies being used by the client with nausea.	Health care professionals and family members can support the use of nonpharmacologic strategies and encourage their use.
	D Use frequent oral hygiene unless it stimulates nausea.	Frequent oral hygiene may promote comfort by removing unpleasant tastes from the mouth.
	D Encourage the client with nausea to eat small amounts of food that are appealing to him or her.	Foods that are appealing to the client with nausea are less likely to trigger nausea.
	Instruct in high-carbohydrate and low-fat food, as appropriate.	High-carbohydrate and low-fat food is absorbed more quickly in the intestinal tract and is less likely to add bulk, which might trigger nausea.
	D Give cold and clear liquid and odorless and colorless food, as appropriate.	Cold beverages are less likely to have an odor that may trigger nausea.
	Provide information about the causes of the nausea and how long it will last.	The client may believe that the nausea is not going to improve and may not understand why the nausea is occurring.
	Other Interventions	
	D Encourage supplemental commercial feedings, such as Ensure or Boost.	Commercial food supplements increase calories and are easy to ingest.
	Continuing Care Considerations	
	Collaborate with the client/family to monitor the client's weight and amount of nausea.	Continuing nausea is debilitating and significantly decreases the client's quality of life. Continuing therapy is essential to maintain nutrition.

D Indicates tasks that can be delegated to unlicensed assistive nursing personnel at the discretion of the nurse.

PLAN of CARE MEDICAL DIAGNOSIS: HEPATITIS—*cont'd*

NURSING DIAGNOSIS NO. 3 ■ Ineffective Health Maintenance

	Expected Outcomes	Nursing Interventions	Rationales
RELATED FACTORS Ineffective family coping Lack of material resources Lack of ability to make deliberate and thoughtful judgments Ineffective individual coping	Able to accurately perform needed health care tasks No verbal report or observation of lack of equipment, financial, and/or other resources	NIC **Health System Guidance** Inform the client of appropriate community resources and contact persons.	Clients and their families may not know what resources are available or how to contact the appropriate agencies or services.
DEFINING CHARACTERISTICS Knowledge: Demonstrated lack regarding basic health practices Reported or demonstrated inability to take responsibility for meeting basic health practices in any or all functional pattern areas History of lack of health-seeking behaviors	No verbal report or observation of failure to adhere to treatment plan Keeps medical appointments Practices basic health maintenance activities	Identify and facilitate communication among health care providers and the client/family, as appropriate.	Faulty communication may increase the time delays for service or foster distrust among the health care providers, client, and family.
		Give written instructions for the purpose and location of posthospitalization/outpatient activities, as appropriate.	Written instructions provide clear information to which the client can refer for memory assistance.
		Provide a report to posthospital caregivers, as appropriate.	Posthospital caregivers need information about the client's current condition and changes in status in order to provide appropriate care.
		NIC **Support System Enhancement**	
		Identify the degree of family support.	Family support is not guaranteed, even with proximity.
		Determine the support systems currently used.	Identify what the client is currently doing for support and the client's satisfaction with the amount of support.
		Determine barriers to using support systems.	This intervention assists the client and family in identifying methods to overcome barriers as needed.
		Monitor the current family situation.	The strain of providing emotional and financial support may stress family bonds.
		Assess community resource adequacy to identify strengths and weaknesses.	Understanding the strengths and weaknesses of available community resources permits realistic expectations of assistance from those sources.
		Refer to a community-based promotion/prevention/treatment program, as appropriate.	A community-based promotion/prevention/treatment program may provide the client/family with essential services and emotional support.
		Provide services in a caring and supportive manner.	Clients and their families deal with health status changes in individual ways; these ways need to be recognized in a caring manner.
		Involve the family/significant others/friends in the care and planning.	The involvement of family, significant others, and friends in the care and planning for the client shares the burden and builds bonds from shared experiences.
		Explain to concerned others how they can help.	Giving concerned others concrete suggestions for assistance provides them with guidance and provides the client with necessary aid.

Continued

PLAN of CARE MEDICAL DIAGNOSIS: HEPATITIS—*cont'd*

NURSING DIAGNOSIS NO. 3 ■ Ineffective Health Maintenance—*cont'd*

Expected Outcomes	Nursing Interventions	Rationales
	NIC **Other Interventions**	
	Teach the client and family about the care necessary to manage the health state.	Lack of knowledge will render efforts at health maintenance less effective.
	Assist the client/family to identify areas in which they need help and to whom or where they might go to get the help they need.	Clients/families are not always able to ask for help when aid is needed, either because they do not recognize the need or do not know how to secure aid.
	Continuing Care Considerations	
	Refer the family to appropriate counseling services.	Families in distress may be unable to provide essential support to a family member with a health maintenance problem.

Drug Therapy. Medications are used sparingly for clients with acute hepatitis to allow the liver to rest. An antiemetic to relieve nausea may be prescribed.

For clients with chronic hepatitis B and C, a number of drugs are being used, including antiviral medications and immunomodulators. Lamivudine (Epivir-HBV) and adefovir dipivoxil (Hepsera) are oral antiviral drugs given to destroy the hepatitis B virus in clients with chronic disease. Both of these medications can cause renal toxicity and granulocytopenia. A number of types of interferon, immunomodulating drugs, are being administered to treat both hepatitis B and C. Research on other possible drugs for hepatitis B is ongoing.

The most common treatment for hepatitis C is a combination of subcutaneous interferon (peginterferon alfa-2a [Pegasys]) and oral ribavirin. The length of treatment is dependent upon genotype, or strain of hepatitis. There are several different genotypes; most Americans who have hepatitis C are genotype 1. This genotype usually requires 48 weeks of treatment. Genotypes 2 and 3 have a better response rate and usually only need 24 weeks of treatment. The goal of treatment is to have a negative HCV PCR RNA level and to sustain a negative level after treatment has ended. Response rates vary, but in general, clients who are young, have a low viral load, and have minimal scarring on liver biopsy have a better chance of clearing the virus and remaining free of hepatitis C after treatment has ended.

Critical Thinking Challenge

You are the nurse caring for a 52-year-old man recently diagnosed with chronic hepatitis C. He denies any high-risk behavior but admits to getting a tattoo in Vietnam. How will you reply to his following questions?

1. "Could I have gotten this by a tattoo?"
2. "Could my wife and children have hepatitis?"
3. "How could I not have known I had hepatitis?"
4. "What is the treatment for hepatitis C?"

evolve For suggested answer guidelines, go to http://evolve.elsevier.com/Iggy/.

Community-Based Care

Home care management varies according to the type of hepatitis and whether the disease is acute or chronic. A primary focus in any case is preventing the spread of the infection. For hepatitis transmitted by the fecal-oral route, careful handwashing and sanitary disposal of feces are important. Standard precautions are used for hepatitis transmitted percutaneously and permucosally. Education is therefore very important. If the nurse and or assistive personnel are not sure about modes of transmission or precautions that need to be taken once the client is home and in the community, then the advice of hospital-based infection control personnel or infectious disease specialist should be sought. These experts can also suggest resources for the client and family.

Teach the client and the family to observe measures to prevent infection transmission (see Chart 62-5). In addition, instruct the client with viral hepatitis to avoid alcohol and check with the health care provider before taking any medication or vitamin, supplement, or herbal preparation.

The client must determine patterns for rest on the basis of physical tolerance of increased activity. Encourage the client to increase activity gradually to prevent fatigue. The client should eat small, frequent meals of high-carbohydrate and low-fat foods (Chart 62-6).

FATTY LIVER (STEATOHEPATITIS)

A **fatty liver** is caused by the accumulation of fats in and around the hepatic cells. Causes include the following:

- Diabetes mellitus
- Obesity
- Elevated lipid profile

Fatty infiltration of the liver may result from faulty fat metabolism in the liver and the mobilization of fatty acids from adipose tissue. Many clients with a fatty liver are asymptomatic. The most common and typical finding is asymptomatic elevation of alanine aminotransferase (ALT) and aspartate aminotransferase (AST).

CHART 62-6

CLIENT EDUCATION GUIDE
Viral Hepatitis

- Avoid all medications, including over-the-counter drugs, such as acetaminophen (Tylenol, Exdol✱), unless prescribed by your physician.
- Avoid all alcohol.
- Rest frequently throughout the day, and get adequate sleep at night.
- Eat small, frequent meals with a high-carbohydrate, low-fat content.
- Avoid sexual intercourse until antibody testing results are negative.
- Follow the guidelines for preventing transmission of the disease (see Chart 62-5).

Magnetic resonance imaging, ultrasound, and nuclear medicine examinations can be used to confirm excessive fat in the liver. A percutaneous biopsy can provide the same information. Interventions are aimed at removing the underlying cause of the infiltration. Weight loss, glucose control, and improving cholesterol and triglyceride levels may help.

HEPATIC ABSCESS

PATHOPHYSIOLOGY

Although hepatic abscesses are uncommon, they carry a high mortality rate. **Liver abscesses** occur when the liver is invaded by bacteria or protozoa. These organisms destroy the liver tissue, producing a necrotic cavity filled with infective agents, liquefied liver cells and tissue, and leukocytes. The infectious necrotic tissue walls off the abscess from the healthy liver.

A **pyogenic liver abscess** occurs when bacteria invade the liver. Infecting organisms include *Escherichia coli* and *Klebsiella, Enterobacter, Salmonella, Staphylococcus,* and *Enterococcus* species. A pyogenic abscess is generally solitary and confined to the right lobe, but occasionally abscesses are multiple. The usual cause is acute cholangitis, which occurs as a complication of cholelithiasis. Pyogenic liver abscesses may also result from liver trauma, abdominal peritonitis, and sepsis, or an abscess can extend to the liver after pneumonia or bacterial endocarditis.

The protozoan *Entamoeba histolytica* causes an **amebic hepatic abscess**, which may occur after amebic dysentery. These abscesses usually occur in the form of a single abscess in the right hepatic lobe.

◆COLLABORATIVE MANAGEMENT

Clients with hepatic abscesses are generally quite ill. On occasion, an abscess is not diagnosed until autopsy. In clients with a pyogenic liver abscess, the onset of symptoms is usually sudden. Amebic abscesses cause a more insidious onset of symptoms. Common complaints include the following:

- Right upper abdominal pain with a palpable, tender liver
- Anorexia
- Weight loss
- Nausea and vomiting
- Fever and chills
- Shoulder pain
- Dyspnea
- Pleural pain if the diaphragm is involved

A hepatic abscess is usually diagnosed by contrast-enhanced computed tomography (CT) scan or ultrasound. These abscesses are usually drained under CT or ultrasound guidance. Specimens may be sent for laboratory analysis so that the optimal antibiotic can be selected.

CHART 62-7

KEY FEATURES of
Liver Trauma

- Right upper quadrant pain with abdominal tenderness
- Abdominal distention and rigidity
- Guarding of the abdomen
- Increased abdominal pain exaggerated by deep breathing and referred to the right shoulder (Kehr's sign)
- Indicators of hemorrhage and hypovolemic shock:
  - Hypotension
  - Tachycardia
  - Tachypnea
  - Pallor
  - Diaphoresis
  - Cool, clammy skin
  - Confusion or other change in mental state

LIVER TRAUMA

PATHOPHYSIOLOGY

The liver is the most common organ to be injured in clients with penetrating trauma of the abdomen (e.g., gunshot wounds, stab wounds, and rib fractures) and is the second most commonly injured organ in clients who have blunt abdominal trauma. Liver damage or injury should be suspected whenever any upper abdominal or lower chest trauma is sustained. The liver is often injured by steering wheels in vehicular accidents. Common injuries to the liver include simple lacerations, multiple lacerations, avulsions (tears), and crush injuries.

◆COLLABORATIVE MANAGEMENT

◆Assessment

The liver is a highly vascular organ and receives about 29% of the body's cardiac output. When hepatic trauma occurs, blood loss can be massive. The client may exhibit signs of hemorrhagic shock (Chart 62-7).

An ultrasound or CT scan of the abdomen is often done to determine the presence of a hematoma. A decreased hematocrit may confirm suspected blood loss. Clinical manifestations include right upper quadrant pain with abdominal tenderness, distention, guarding, and rigidity. Abdominal pain exaggerated by deep breathing and referred to the right shoulder may indicate diaphragmatic irritation.

◆Interventions

When hepatic and other abdominal organ trauma is confirmed, a surgeon performs an exploratory laparotomy to identify and control the source and type of bleeding. Minor surgical interventions, such as suture placement, wound packing, decompression, or a combination of these procedures, are often performed to halt bleeding. Liver lobe resection is required in some extensive liver injuries. This procedure may be done using laparoscopy.

Clients with hepatic trauma require the administration of multiple blood products, packed red blood cells, and fresh frozen plasma, as well as massive volume infusion to maintain adequate hydration. Postoperatively, the client with hepatic trauma is admitted to a critical care unit. The nurse monitors the client for persistent bleeding. Complete blood count and coagulation studies must be closely monitored for trends in changes.

CANCER OF THE LIVER

PATHOPHYSIOLOGY

Primary hepatic cancer, or hepatocellular carcinoma (HCC), is one of the most common tumors in the world. It is more prevalent in regions of Asia and Africa where the annual incidence is up to 500 cases per 100,000 people.

In the United States, the incidence of HCC is increasing. In 1975 to 1977, age-adjusted incidence rates were 1.4 cases of HCC per 100,000 people. The age-adjusted incidence rates of HCC for 1999-2000 was 3.1 persons per 100,000 population. The fastest rising rates have been observed in men between 45 and 55 years of age, especially African-American men (Velazquez et al., 2003).

Chronic infection with HBV and HCV frequently lead to cirrhosis, which is a risk factor for developing hepatocellular carcinoma. It is important to remember that cirrhosis from any cause, including alcoholic liver disease, increases the risk for HCC.

COLLABORATIVE MANAGEMENT

The most common complaint is abdominal discomfort. Elevated serum alpha-fetoprotein and alkaline phosphatase are also common. Ultrasound and contrast-enhanced computed tomography (CT) are both useful in detecting metastasis. If the primary tumor site is not known, a CT- or ultrasound-guided liver biopsy can confirm the diagnosis.

Surgical management may be indicated for clients with a lesion confined to one liver lobe and may be performed through a laparoscope. Liver lobe resection has been successful in achieving survival rates of up to 5 years.

Unfortunately, 75% of clients are not candidates for surgical excision because their tumors are unresectable. The liver cannot tolerate high doses of radiation, so radiation treatments are not an option. Other approaches include hepatic artery embolization and chemotherapy (chemoembolization), alcohol ablation, and ultrasound-guided cryoablation. A newer device uses a radiofrequency (RF) generator as a heat source to "burn" a tumor in a percutaneous procedure. This procedure, called RF ablation, is done using CT or ultrasound guidance.

Chemotherapy may be administered by a surgically implanted infusion pump, which enables controlled infusion. It may also be given in a catheter-directed method. The interventional radiologist places a catheter into the hepatic tumor that supplies the tumor and injects a mixture of chemotherapy and contrast agent into the tumor. This procedure has the unique effect of depositing chemotherapeutic drugs directly into the tumor and blocking further blood flow into the tumor for weeks. Liver transplantation may also be used to treat liver cancer.

LIVER TRANSPLANTATION

Liver transplantation has become a common operation worldwide. The client with end-stage liver disease or acute liver failure who has not responded to conventional medical or surgical intervention is a potential candidate for liver transplantation. Liver transplantation may also be considered for the client with a primary malignant neoplasm of the liver.

The client for potential transplantation undergoes extensive physiologic and psychological assessment and evaluation by physicians and transplant coordinators to identify contraindications to the procedure. Clients who are not considered candidates for transplantation are those with the following:

- Severe cardiovascular instability with advanced cardiac disease
- Severe respiratory disease
- Active alcohol and/or substance abuse
- Metastatic malignant disease
- Inability to follow instructions regarding medications and self-care

Liver transplantation has become the most effective treatment for clients with an increasing number of acute and chronic liver diseases. Inclusion and exclusion criteria may vary among transplantation centers and are continually revised as treatment options change and surgical techniques improve.

Donor livers are obtained primarily from trauma victims who have not had liver damage. They are distributed through a nationwide program, the United Network of Organ Sharing (UNOS). This system distributes donor livers on the basis of regional considerations and recipient acuity. Candidates with the highest level of acuity receive highest priority.

The donor liver is transported to the surgery center in a cooled saline solution that preserves the organ for up to 8 hours. The diseased liver is removed through an incision made in the upper abdomen. The new liver is carefully put in its place and is attached to the client's blood vessels and bile ducts. The procedure can take up to 12 hours to complete and requires a highly specialized team and large volumes of fluid and blood replacement.

Living donors have also been used. This is done on a voluntary basis after careful psychological and physiologic preparation and testing. The donor's liver is resected (usually removal of one lobe) and implanted into the recipient after removal of the diseased liver. In both the donor and the recipient, the liver regenerates and grows in size to meet the demands of the body.

PATHOPHYSIOLOGY

Although liver transplantations are commonly done, complications can occur. Some problems can be medically managed, whereas others require removal of the transplant. The two most common complications are acute graft rejection and infection.

Acute Graft Rejection

The success of all transplantations has greatly improved since the introduction in 1980 of cyclosporine (cyclosporin A), an immunosuppressant drug. Now there are several other antirejection medications used, such as FK-506, CellCept, Prograf, Imuran, sirolimus, and prednisone.

Clinical manifestations of rejection may include tachycardia, fever, right upper quadrant or flank pain, decreased bile pigment and volume, and increasing jaundice. Laboratory findings include elevated serum bilirubin, rising ALT and AST levels, elevated alkaline phosphatase levels, and increased prothrombin time/International Normalized Ratio (INR).

Transplant rejection is treated aggressively with immunosuppressive medication. As with all rejection treatments, the client is at a greater risk for infection. If therapy is not effective, a rapid deterioration of liver function occurs. Multisystem organ failure, including respiratory and renal involvement, develops along with diffuse coagulopathies and portal-systemic encephalopathy (PSE). The only alternative for treatment is emergency retransplantation.

Infection

Infection is another potential threat to the transplanted graft and the client's survival. Immunosuppressant therapy, which must be used to prevent and treat organ rejection, significantly increases the client's susceptibility to and risk for infection. Other risk factors include the presence of multiple tubes and intravascular lines, immobility, and prolonged anesthesia.

In the early post-transplantation period, common infections include pneumonia, wound infections, and urinary tract infections. Opportunistic infections usually develop after the first postoperative month and include cytomegalovirus, mycobacterial infections, and parasitic infections. Latent infections such as tuberculosis and herpes simplex may be reactivated.

The physician prescribes broad-spectrum antibiotics for prophylaxis during and after surgery. Obtain culture specimens from all lines and tubes and collect specimens for culture at predetermined time intervals as dictated by the agency's policy. If an infection is detected, the physician prescribes organism-specific anti-infective agents.

Other Complications

The biliary anastomosis is susceptible to breakdown, obstruction, and infection. If leakage occurs or if the site becomes necrotic or obstructed, an abscess can form or peritonitis, bacteremia, and cirrhosis may develop. Other potential complications include the following:

- Hemorrhage
- Hepatic artery thrombosis
- Fluid and electrolyte imbalances
- Pulmonary atelectasis
- Acute renal failure
- Chronic graft rejection
- Psychological maladjustment

Transplant complications cause clients to be very anxious. The nurse and other members of the health care team assure the client that these problems are common and usually successfully treated.

EVIDENCE-BASED PRACTICE for Nursing

What is the psychosocial experience of clients who receive a liver transplant?

Forsberg, A., Backman, L., & Moller, A. (2002). Experiencing liver transplantation: A phenomenological approach. *Journal of Advanced Nursing, 32*(2), 327.

The aim of this study was to investigate the subjective experience of the meaning of having a liver transplant. Seven categories emerged from interviews of 12 clients who volunteered for the study:

- Facing the inevitable
- Recapturing the body
- Emotional chaos
- Leaving the experts
- Family and friends
- Threat of graft rejection
- Honoring the donor

Social support was found to be essential for recovery. Meeting other transplant survivors helped to deal with the identity crisis of suddenly feeling totally unique.

Level of Evidence: 6—The research serves as a small pilot study that should be replicated to better understand the needs of the client undergoing transplantation.

Critique. The study population consisted of nine women and three men. A more balanced gender number may have changed the selected categories. The race/ethnic origin of the subjects is assumed to be white. It is difficult to generalize study findings, and additional study is needed using more diverse and larger groups.

Implications for Nursing. The authors believe that the clinical implications from this study are that interventions such as client education and social and mental support are important tools to optimize both self-care capacity and the ability to maintain a healthy perception of identity after liver transplantation. Nurses should also keep in mind how stressful it may be for the client to leave the hospital after receiving a transplant. "Leaving the experts" was identified as a significant milestone.

COLLABORATIVE MANAGEMENT

Care of the client undergoing liver transplantation requires an interdisciplinary team approach. Receiving a transplant has a major psychosocial impact on the client. Forsberg and colleagues found seven themes that emerged from their research on clients who received liver transplants (see the Evidence-Based Practice for Nursing box above).

After the client is identified as a candidate and a donor organ is procured, the actual liver transplantation surgical procedure usually takes 8 hours. The length of the procedure can vary greatly.

In the immediate postoperative period, the client who has undergone liver transplantation is managed in the critical care unit and requires aggressive monitoring and care. The nurse assesses for signs and symptoms of complications of surgery and immediately reports their occurrence to the physician (Table 62-6).

Monitor the client's temperature and report elevations, increased abdominal pain, distention, and rigidity, which are indicators of peritonitis. Nursing assessment also includes monitoring for a change in neurologic status that could indicate encephalopathy from a nonfunctioning liver. Signs of coagulopathy (e.g., continuous bloody oozing from a catheter, drain, and incision sites; petechiae; or ecchymosis) are reported to the physician immediately because they can indicate impaired function of the transplanted liver.

TABLE 62-6 Assessment and Prevention of Common Postoperative Complications Associated with Liver Transplantation

Assessment	Prevention
Acute Graft Rejection	
Occurs from the 4th to 10th postoperative day Manifested by tachycardia, fever, right upper quadrant (RUQ) or flank pain, diminished bile drainage or change in bile color, or increased jaundice Laboratory changes: (1) increased levels of serum bilirubin, transaminases, and alkaline phosphatase: (2) prolonged prothrombin time	Prophylaxis with immunosuppressant agents, such as cyclosporine Early diagnosis to treat with more potent antirejection drugs, such as muromonab-CD3 (OKT3)
Infection	
Can occur at any time during recovery Frequent cultures of tubes, lines, and drainage Manifested by fever or excessive, foul-smelling drainage (urine, wound, or bile); other indicators depend on location and type of infection Early removal of invasive lines Good handwashing	Antibiotic prophylaxis Early diagnosis and treatment with organism-specific anti-infective agents
Hepatic Complications (Bile Leakage, Abscess Formation, Hepatic Thrombosis)	
Manifested by decreased bile drainage, increased RUQ abdominal pain with distention and guarding, nausea or vomiting, increased jaundice, and clay-colored stools Laboratory changes: increased levels of serum bilirubin and transaminases	Keep T-tube in dependent position and secure to client; empty frequently, recording quality and quantity of drainage. Report manifestations to physician immediately. May necessitate surgical intervention.
Acute Renal Failure	
Caused by hypotension, antibiotics, cyclosporine, acute liver failure, or hypothermia Indicators of hypothermia: shivering, hyperventilation, increased cardiac output, vasoconstriction, and alkalemia Early indicators of renal failure: changes in urine output, increased BUN and creatinine levels, and electrolyte imbalance	Monitor all drug levels with nephrotoxic side effects. Prevent hypotension. Observe for early signs of renal failure and report them immediately to the physician.

BUN, Blood urea nitrogen.

GET READY for the NCLEX Examination!

KEY POINTS

Safe Effective Care Environment

- Monitor the client with cirrhosis for bleeding and neurologic changes as described in Chart 62-2.
- For the client who has an esophagogastric tube, ensure airway patency because the tube may become displaced.
- Use standard precautions for all clients, especially for clients with hepatitis.
- Take precautions to prevent needle sticks or injury from other sharp instruments.
- Observe for hypovolemic shock from hemorrhage in the client with liver trauma.

Health Promotion and Maintenance

- Follow the guidelines listed in Chart 62-4 to prevent viral hepatitis in the workplace.
- Teach clients to take precautions to prevent viral hepatitis in the community as described in Chart 62-5.
- For clients with viral hepatitis, instruct them to follow the guidelines listed in Chart 62-6.

Psychosocial Integrity

- Recognize that clients with cirrhosis have mental and emotional changes due to portal systemic-encephalopathy (PSE).
- Be aware that clients with cirrhosis and/or chronic hepatitis may feel guilty about their disease because of past habits such as drug and alcohol abuse.
- Be aware that family members and friends may fear getting the disease from the client, causing client isolation.
- Encourage clients with cirrhosis and/or chronic hepatitis to verbalize their feelings.
- Be aware that clients having liver transplantation have major concerns about the possibility of complications, such as organ rejection.

Physiological Integrity

- Be aware that there are many causes of cirrhosis in addition to alcohol abuse (see Table 62-3).
- Monitor laboratory values of clients suspected of or diagnosed with cirrhosis of the liver as listed in Tables 62-1 and 62-4.
- Observe for clinical manifestations of portal-systemic encephalopathy (PSE) as listed in Table 62-2.
- Assess for manifestations of cirrhosis as shown in Figure 62-1.
- Provide care for the client having a paracentesis as described in Chart 62-1.
- Administer medications to decrease ammonia levels (which cause PSE) in clients with cirrhosis, such as lactulose, neomycin sulfate, and metronidazole.
- Differentiate the five major types of hepatitis as outlined in Table 62-5.

- Be aware that clients with chronic viral hepatitis often acquire cirrhosis and cancer of the liver.
- Recognize that potent immunomodulators, such as the interferons, and antivirals are being used to treat hepatitis B and C.
- Observe the client having a liver transplantation for complications, such as those described in Table 62-6.

ADDITIONAL STUDY RESOURCES

Go to your Student CD-ROM for Review Questions for the NCLEX Examination.

evolve Go to http://evolve.elsevier.com/Iggy/ for Integrated Management of Care Questions for the NCLEX Examination.

SELECTED BIBLIOGRAPHY

Asterisk indicates a classic or definitive work on this subject.

Banasik, J. (2001). Diagnosing alpha 1 antitrypsin deficiency. *The Nurse Practitioner, 26*(1), 58-67.

Bockhold, K.M. (2000). Who's afraid of hepatitis C? *American Journal of Nursing, 100*(5), 26-31.

Centers for Disease Control and Prevention. (2002). *Hepatitis fact sheet.* Available at http://www.cdc.gov/ncidod/diseases/hepatitis.htm.

Compton, P. (2002). Caring for the alcohol dependent patient. *Nursing2002, 32*(12), 58-63.

DeCarlis, L., et al. (2003). Surgical treatment of hepatocellular cancer in the era of hepatic transplantation. *Journal of American College of Surgeons, 196*(6), 887-897.

Dougherty, A.S., & Dreher, H.M. (2001). Hepatitis C: Current treatment strategies for an emerging epidemic. *MEDSURG Nursing, 10*(1), 9-13.

Freeman, A.J., et al. (2003). Predicting progression to cirrhosis in chronic hepatitis C virus infection. *Journal of Viral Hepatitis, 10*(4), 285-293.

Hepatitis Liver Cirrhosis/HCC. Available at http://www.extremehealthusa.com/hepatitis.html.

Hilsabeck, R., et al. (2002). Neuropsychological impairment in patients with chronic hepatitis C. *Hepatology, 35*(2), 440-446.

Iosue, K. (2002). Chronic hepatitis C: Latest treatment options. *The Nurse Practitioner, 27*(4), 32-49.

Ma, Y., et al. (2002). Antibodies to conformational epitopes of soluble liver antigen define a severe form of autoimmune liver disease. *Hepatology, 35*(3), 658-664.

National Institutes of Health Consensus Development Conference Statement. *Management of hepatitis C: 2002.* June 10-12, 2002, Washington, DC: National Institutes of Health.

Ohata, K., et al. (2003). Hepatic steatosis is a risk factor for hepatocellular carcinoma in patients with chronic hepatitis C virus infection. *Cancer, 97*(12), 3036-3043.

Pagana, K., & Pagana, T. (2002). *Mosby's manual of diagnostic and laboratory tests* (2nd ed.). St. Louis: Mosby.

Portal hypertension-New treatments. (March 2, 2004). Available at http://www.ccspublishing.com/journals5a/portal_hypertension.htm.

*Starzl, T., et al. (1997). Liver transplantation. *Gastroenterology, 112*(1), 288-291.

Velazquez, R., et al. (2003). Prospective analysis of risk factors for hepatocellular carcinoma in patients with liver cirrhosis. *Hepatology, 37*(3), 520-527.

Wong, J.B., et al. (2000). Estimating future hepatitis C morbidity, mortality, and costs in the United States. *American Journal of Public Health, 90*(10), 1562-1569.

Yeung, E., Wong, F.S. (2002). The management of cirrhotic ascites. *Medscape General Medicine, 4*(4), 8. Review. No abstract available.

CHAPTER 63

Interventions for Clients with Problems of the Biliary System and Pancreas

DONNA D. IGNATAVICIUS

LEARNING OUTCOMES

After studying this chapter, you should be able to:

1. Identify the common causes of cholecystitis and cholelithiasis (gallbladder disease).
2. Interpret diagnostic test results associated with gallbladder disease.
3. Compare postoperative care of clients undergoing a traditional cholecystectomy with that of clients undergoing a laparoscopic cholecystectomy.
4. Develop a community-based teaching plan for clients with gallbladder disease, including care of a T-tube.
5. Compare and contrast the pathophysiology of acute and chronic pancreatitis.
6. Interpret common assessment findings associated with acute pancreatitis and those associated with chronic pancreatitis.
7. Prioritize nursing care for clients with acute pancreatitis and clients with chronic pancreatitis.
8. Explain the use and precautions associated with enzyme replacement for chronic pancreatitis.
9. Develop a postoperative plan of care for clients undergoing a Whipple procedure.
10. Construct a discharge plan for care of clients with pancreatic cancer in the community.
11. Discuss the psychosocial needs of the client with pancreatic cancer and associated nursing interventions.

Go to your Student CD-ROM for Review Questions for the NCLEX Examination keyed to these Learning Outcomes.

Disorders of the biliary system and pancreas begin as single-organ processes, but the inflammatory response may extend to other organs if the primary disorder is not treated. This occurs because of the anatomic proximity of the liver, gallbladder, and pancreas and because the flow of bile from the liver through the biliary (gallbladder) ductal system may be impeded. Inflammation of the gallbladder, liver, or pancreas is caused by obstruction in the biliary system from gallstones, edema, stricture, or tumors. For example, gallstones impacted in the cystic duct cause cholecystitis; gallstones lodged in the ampulla of Vater impede the flow of bile and pancreatic secretions, which can result in pancreatitis.

BILIARY DISORDERS

Cholecystitis

PATHOPHYSIOLOGY

The two most common problems that occur within the biliary tree are stone formation (cholelithiasis) and associated chronic inflammation (cholecystitis). Cholecystitis may be either acute or chronic.

Acute Cholecystitis

Acute **cholecystitis** (inflammation of the gallbladder) usually develops in association with **cholelithiasis** (gallstones).

Either condition may occur singly, but most often they occur together.

Acalculous cholecystitis (inflammation occurring in the absence of gallstones) is typically associated with biliary stasis caused by any condition that affects the regular filling or emptying of the gallbladder. For example, a decrease in blood flow to the gallbladder or anatomic problems such as twisting or kinking of the gallbladder neck or cystic duct can result in pancreatic enzyme reflux into the gallbladder, causing inflammation.

Acute **calculous cholecystitis** usually follows obstruction of the cystic duct by a stone (calculus), which creates the inflammatory response. This response may be the result of a mechanical, chemical, or bacterial process. When the gallbladder is inflamed, trapped bile is reabsorbed and acts as a chemical irritant to the gallbladder wall; that is, the bile has a toxic effect. The presence of bile, in combination with impaired circulation, edema, and distention of the gallbladder, causes ischemia of the gallbladder wall. The result is tissue sloughing with necrosis and gangrene. Perforation (rupture) of the gallbladder wall may eventually occur. If the perforation is small and localized, an abscess may form. **Peritonitis**, infection of the peritoneum, may result if the perforation is large.

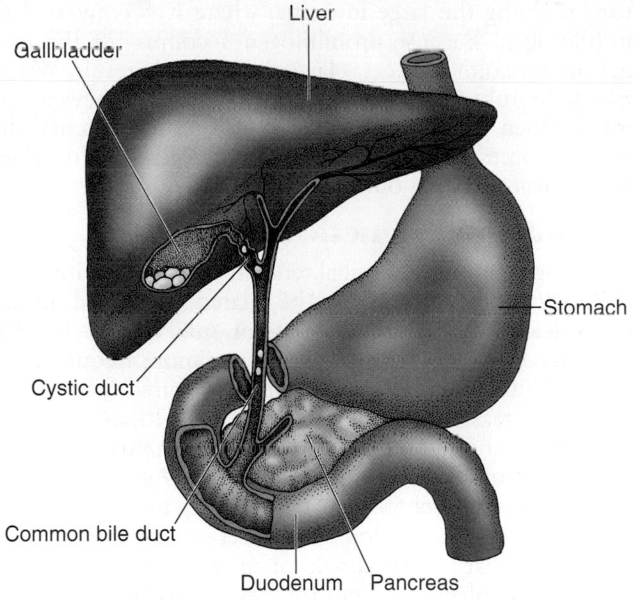

Figure 63-1 ■ Gallstones within the gallbladder and obstructing the common bile and cystic ducts.

PATHOLOGIC CHANGES

The exact pathophysiology of gallstone formation is not clearly understood, but abnormal metabolism of cholesterol and bile salts plays an important role in their formation. Contributing factors may include the following:

- Supersaturation of bile with cholesterol
- Excessive bile salt losses
- Decreased gallbladder-emptying rates
- Changes in bile concentration or bile stasis within the gallbladder

Gallstones may lie dormant within the gallbladder or may move to other areas of the biliary tree as the gallbladder empties and refills with bile. They may migrate and lodge within the gallbladder neck, cystic duct, or common bile duct, causing obstruction (Figure 63-1). Gallstones interfere with or totally obstruct normal bile flow from the gallbladder to the duodenum, causing vascular congestion as a result of impeded venous return. Edema and congestion occur and contribute to the initial inflammatory process. When bile cannot flow from the gallbladder, the stasis of bile and local irritation from the gallstones lead to cholecystitis.

Cholangitis, usually associated with **choledocholithiasis** (common bile duct stones), involves infection of the bile ducts. *Ascending* **cholangitis** (inflammation of the biliary tree) occurs after bacterial invasion of the ducts. Bacterial invasion can lead to life-threatening *suppurative* cholangitis when symptoms are not recognized quickly and pus accumulates in the ductal system.

TYPES OF GALLSTONES

The gallbladder provides an excellent environment for the production of gallstones. In particular, the gallbladder only occasionally mixes its normally abundant mucus with its highly viscous, concentrated bile. The constant temperature within the gallbladder also contributes to stone formation by delaying bile emptying, causing biliary stasis.

Gallstones are composed of substances normally found in bile, such as cholesterol, bilirubin, bile salts, calcium, and various proteins. They are classified as either cholesterol stones or pigment stones. Cholesterol calculi form as a result of metabolic imbalances of cholesterol and bile salts. They are the most common type found in people in the United States, accounting for 90% of all gallstones, and generally originate from the gallbladder.

Chronic Cholecystitis

Chronic cholecystitis results when repeated episodes of cystic duct obstruction result in chronic inflammation. Calculi are almost always present. In chronic cholecystitis, the gallbladder becomes fibrotic and contracted, which results in decreased motility and deficient absorption.

Pancreatitis and cholangitis can occur as complications of cholecystitis. These problems result from the backup of bile throughout the biliary tract. Bile obstruction leads to jaundice.

Jaundice (yellow discoloration of the skin and mucous membranes) and **icterus** (yellow discoloration of the sclerae) can occur in clients with acute cholecystitis but is most commonly seen in clients with the chronic form of the disease. Impeded or obstructed bile flow caused by edema of the ducts or gallstones contributes to *extrahepatic* **obstructive jaundice**. Jaundice in cholecystitis may also be caused by direct liver involvement. Inflammation of the liver's bile channels or bile ducts may cause *intrahepatic* obstructive jaundice, resulting in an increase in circulating levels of bilirubin, the principal pigment of bile.

When the concentration of bilirubin in the blood increases to greater than 2.5 mg/dL, jaundice occurs (Pagana & Pagana, 2002). In a person with obstructive jaundice, the normal flow of bile into the duodenum is blocked, allowing excessive bile salts to accumulate in the skin. This accumulation of bile salts leads to **pruritus** (itching) or a burning sensation. The bile flow blockage also prevents bilirubin from reaching the large intestine, where it is converted to urobilinogen. Because urobilinogen accounts for the normal brown color of feces, clay-colored stools result. Water-soluble bilirubin is normally excreted by the kidneys in the urine. When an excess of circulating bilirubin occurs, the urine becomes dark and foamy because of the kidneys' effort to clear the bilirubin.

Etiology and Genetic Risk

There appears to be a familial tendency in the development of cholelithiasis, but this may be related to familial dietary habits (excessive dietary cholesterol intake) and familial sedentary lifestyles. Gallstones are seen more frequently in obese clients, probably as a result of impaired fat metabolism or increased cholesterol. Cholesterol-lowering drugs, which lower cholesterol levels in the blood, actually increase the amount of cholesterol secreted in bile. Age is also a factor, with people over 60 years of age being more likely than younger people to develop stones. Persons with type I diabetes are also at increased risk for the development of gallstones and cholecystitis because they generally have higher levels of fatty acids (triglycerides).

Cholesterol is increased following rapid weight loss, when the liver excretes extra cholesterol into bile. The ingestion of low-calorie or liquid protein diets also increases the susceptibility to gallstone development. These diets cause the liberation of cholesterol from tissues; the cholesterol is excreted as crystals in bile. Alcohol abuse may contribute to the formation of pigment stones, but alcohol in moderate amounts appears to reduce the formation of cholesterol stones. Cholelithiasis is seen with hemolytic blood disorders, with bowel disease such as Crohn's disease, and after gastric bypass surgery as a treatment of morbid obesity.

Cholecystitis is triggered by a number of other processes and health problems. In addition to the formation of gallbladder calculi, causes of acute cholecystitis include the following:

- Trauma
- Inadequate blood supply
- Prolonged anesthesia and surgery
- Adhesions
- Edema
- Neoplasms (tumors)
- Diabetes mellitus
- Cardiac events
- Long-term fasting
- Prolonged dehydration
- Gallbladder trauma
- Prolonged immobility
- Excessive opioid use
- Hormone replacement therapy

Incidence/Prevalence

More than 20 million persons in the United States have gallbladder disease, resulting in over 500,000 surgeries each year. Gallstones are very common, with about 20% of the U.S. population being affected. Native Americans/American Indians, particularly the Pima Indians of Arizona, have an unusually high incidence of gallstones, with Mexican Americans and white individuals following (Everhart et al., 1999). A high incidence of biliary tract disease and cholecystitis occurs in people with a sedentary lifestyle, a familial tendency to biliary disease, obesity, or diabetes mellitus. Middle-aged white women have a high incidence of gallbladder disease, but the exact cause is unknown.

WOMEN'S HEALTH CONSIDERATIONS

Women who are between 20 and 60 years of age are twice as likely to develop gallstones as men. Obesity is a major risk factor for gallstone formation, especially in women. Pregnancy tends to worsen gallstone formation. Pregnancy, as well as drugs such as estrogen and birth control pills, especially the older oral contraceptives, alter hormone levels and delay muscular contraction of the gallbladder, causing a decreased rate of bile emptying. The incidence of gallstones is higher in women who have had multiple pregnancies. Combinations of causative factors increase the incidence of stone formation, especially in women. For example, an obese pregnant woman or an obese woman taking birth control pills may be at higher risk.

COLLABORATIVE MANAGEMENT

Assessment

PHYSICAL ASSESSMENT/CLINICAL MANIFESTATIONS

Clients with acute cholecystitis frequently present with pain, although clinical manifestations vary in intensity and frequency (Chart 63-1).

Ask assistive nursing personnel to obtain the client's height, weight, and vital signs, and assess gender, age, race, and ethnic group. Ask about food preferences and determine whether excessive fat and cholesterol are included in the diet. The client is asked whether any foods are not tolerated. Question whether any of the following gastrointestinal (GI) symptoms occur in relation to the intake of fatty food: **flatulence** (gas), **dyspepsia** (indigestion), **eructation** (belching), anorexia, nausea, vomiting, and abdominal pain or discomfort.

Ask the client to describe the pain, including its intensity and duration, precipitating factors, and any measures that relieve it. The pain may be described as indigestion of varying intensity, ranging from a mild, persistent ache to a steady, constant pain in the right upper abdominal quadrant. The pain may radiate to the right shoulder or scapula.

CHART 63-1

KEY FEATURES of Cholecystitis

- Episodic or vague upper abdominal pain or discomfort that can radiate to the right shoulder
- Pain triggered by a high-fat or high-volume meal
- Anorexia
- Nausea or vomiting
- Dyspepsia
- Eructation
- Flatulence
- Feeling of abdominal fullness
- Rebound tenderness (Blumberg's sign)
- Fever
- Jaundice, clay-colored stools, dark urine, steatorrhea (most common with chronic cholecystitis)

The abdominal pain of chronic cholecystitis may be vague and nonspecific. The usual pattern of more acute pain is episodic. Clients often refer to these episodes as "gallbladder attacks."

The severe pain of **biliary colic** is produced by obstruction of the cystic duct of the gallbladder. When a stone is moving through or is lodged within the duct, tissue spasm occurs in an effort to mobilize the stone through the small duct. This intense pain may be so severe that it is accompanied by tachycardia, pallor, diaphoresis, and **prostration** (extreme exhaustion).

Ask the client to describe his or her daily activity or exercise routines to determine whether his or her lifestyle is sedentary. Question whether there is a family history of gallbladder disease, because there is a familial tendency for biliary tract diseases. If the client is female, determine whether hormone replacement therapy (HRT) is being taken, because this therapy may contribute to biliary disorders.

Because of gallbladder tenderness, it is difficult to use abdominal palpation and percussion in assessment of the client with acute cholecystitis. With right subcostal palpation, pain increases with deep inspiration **(Murphy's sign).** Guarding and rigidity, as well as rebound tenderness **(Blumberg's sign),** are reliable indicators of peritoneal irritation.

Assessment for rebound tenderness and deep palpation are reserved for physicians and advanced practice nurses. To elicit rebound tenderness, the health care provider pushes his or her fingers deeply and steadily into the client's abdomen, then quickly releases the pressure. Pain that results from the rebound of the palpated tissue may indicate peritoneal inflammation. Deep palpation below the liver border in the right upper quadrant may reveal a sausage-shaped mass, representing the distended, inflamed gallbladder. Percussion over the posterior rib cage intensifies localized abdominal pain.

CONSIDERATIONS FOR OLDER ADULTS

Older adults and clients with diabetes mellitus have atypical manifestations, including the absence of pain and fever. Localized tenderness may be the only presenting sign. The older client may become acutely confused (delirium).

In *chronic* cholecystitis, clients may have insidious symptoms and may not seek medical treatment until late symptoms such as jaundice, clay-colored stools, and dark urine result from an obstructive process. Jaundice may also be seen as yellowing of the skin, sclerae, and oral mucous membranes. **Steatorrhea** (fatty stools) occurs because fat absorption is decreased owing to the lack of bile. Bile is needed for the absorption of fats and fat-soluble vitamins in the intestine. As with any inflammatory process, the client may have an elevated temperature of 99° to 102° F (37° to 39° C), tachycardia, and dehydration from fever and vomiting.

DIAGNOSTIC ASSESSMENT

There are no laboratory tests specific for gallbladder disease. A differential diagnosis must rule out other diseases that may cause similar symptoms, such as peptic ulcer disease, gastroesophageal reflux disorder, and pancreatitis. Serum levels of alkaline phosphatase, aspartate aminotransferase (AST), and lactate dehydrogenase (LDH) may be elevated, indicating abnormalities in liver function. The direct (conjugated) and indirect (unconjugated) serum bilirubin levels are elevated if an obstructive process is present. An increased white blood cell (WBC) count with a left shift on the differential count indicates inflammation. If there is pancreatic involvement, serum amylase and lipase levels are elevated.

Calcified gallstones are easily visualized on abdominal x-ray. Stones that are not calcified cannot be seen.

Ultrasonography of the right upper quadrant is the best diagnostic test for cholecystitis and has largely replaced the older cholecystogram. It is safe, accurate, and painless. Acute cholecystitis is evidenced by edema of the gallbladder wall and pericholecystic fluid, both of which are determined by the ultrasound. The health care provider may also order an upper GI radiographic series to rule out other causes of abdominal pain, such as gastritis and peptic ulcer disease.

A hepatobiliary scan can be performed to visualize the gallbladder and determine patency of the biliary system. The pretest fasting period for this scan can be as short as 4 hours, making it preferable to a diagnostic study that would require a longer fasting time. Visualization of the gallbladder excludes the diagnosis of acute cholecystitis with a high degree of certainty (Fischbach, 2004).

Interventions

Nonsurgical treatment measures prescribed during the acute phase of cholecystitis are directed at resting the inflamed gallbladder to reduce the inflammatory process and relieve pain. Because of the risk for sepsis and perforation, however, acute cholecystitis is generally managed surgically.

NONSURGICAL MANAGEMENT. Two thirds of gallstones are asymptomatic, or silent (Howard & Fromm, 1999). Asymptomatic stones are usually managed conservatively with no medical or surgical intervention. Acute pain occurs when the gallstones partially or totally obstruct the cystic or common bile duct.

Diet Therapy. In general, the client must adhere to a low-fat diet to prevent further pain of biliary colic. If gallstones are causing an obstruction of bile flow, the health care provider may prescribe replacement of fat-soluble vitamins (such as vitamins A, D, E, and K) and the administration of bile salts to facilitate digestion and vitamin absorption. Food and fluids are withheld if nausea and vomiting occur.

Drug Therapy. Pain caused by acute obstruction with gallstones necessitates opioid analgesia with meperidine hydrochloride (Demerol). Older clients should not be given Demerol, because it can cause acute confusion, seizures, or nausea (see Chapter 7). Morphine is usually not used, because it is thought to cause biliary spasm and constrict the sphincter of Oddi. Antispasmodic or anticholinergic drugs, such as atropine and dicyclomine (Bentyl, Lomine✱), may be given to relax smooth muscles and decrease ductal tone and spasm. The health care provider prescribes antiemetics to control nausea and vomiting.

Percutaneous Transhepatic Biliary Catheter Insertion. The physician may insert a **percutaneous transhepatic biliary catheter** under fluoroscopic guidance. This procedure decompresses obstructed extrahepatic ducts so that bile can flow. It is primarily used for inoperable hepatic, pancreatic, or bile duct carcinoma. It may be a nonsurgical alternative for the treatment of biliary obstruction caused by gallstones and hepatic dysfunction associated with obstructive jaundice and biliary sepsis in high-risk candidates. Nursing care associated with this treatment is outlined in Chart 63-4.

SURGICAL MANAGEMENT. The usual surgical treatment of clients with acute and chronic cholecystitis is **cholecystectomy**, the removal of the gallbladder. Two operative procedures are available to the surgeon for performing a cholecystectomy: the laparoscopic cholecystectomy and, less often, the traditional open approach cholecystectomy.

Laparoscopic Cholecystectomy. **Laparoscopic cholecystectomy,** a minimally invasive surgery (MIS), is considered the "gold standard," and is performed much more often than the traditional open cholecystectomy. The advantages of MIS versus the open technique include the following:

- Complications are not common.
- The death rate is very low (i.e., <0.1%).
- Bile duct injuries are rare.
- Client recovery is faster.
- Postoperative pain is less severe.

Preoperative Care. The laparoscopic procedure is commonly done on an ambulatory care basis in a same-day surgery suite. The surgeon explains the procedure; the nurse answers questions and reinforces the physician's instructions. There is no special preoperative preparation for the client. However, the physician typically orders the usual preoperative laboratory tests and requires the client to be on NPO (nothing by mouth) status before the surgery. Chapter 20 describes general preoperative care for the client undergoing anesthesia.

Operative Procedures. The surgeon makes a very small midline puncture at the umbilicus. The abdominal cavity is insufflated with 3 to 4 L of carbon dioxide. Gasless laparoscopic cholecystectomy using abdominal wall lifting devices is a more recent innovation. This technique results in improved pulmonary and cardiac function. A trocar catheter is inserted, through which a laparoscope is introduced. The laparoscope is attached to a video camera, and the abdominal organs are viewed on a monitor. The surgeon makes several small punctures through which to introduce laparoscopic forceps to manipulate the gallbladder. The gallbladder is dissected from the liver bed and the cystic artery and duct are closed. The surgeon mobilizes the gallbladder, aspirates the bile and crushes any large stones, and then extracts the gallbladder through the umbilical port.

Postoperative Care. Removing the gallbladder with the laparoscopic technique reduces the risk of wound complications. Some clients have a problem with "free air pain" from carbon dioxide retention in the abdomen. Teach about the importance of early ambulation to promote absorption of the carbon dioxide. Far less opioid analgesia is necessary after the laparoscopic procedure than following the open procedure.

The client is usually discharged from the hospital or surgery center within 1 day. Following laparoscopic surgery, the client can return to usual activities, including work, much sooner than if an open cholecystectomy had been done. Most clients are able to resume usual activities within 1 to 3 weeks.

Traditional Cholecystectomy. Use of the traditional surgical approach has markedly declined during the past decade. The client undergoing this surgery is usually hospitalized for several days following the procedure.

Preoperative Care. The surgical nurse provides the usual preoperative care and teaching in the operating suite on the day of surgery (see Chapter 20).

Operative Procedures. The surgeon not only removes the gallbladder through a right subcostal incision but also often explores the biliary ducts for the presence of stones. If the common bile duct is explored, the surgeon typically inserts a T-tube drain to ensure patency of the duct. Trauma to the common bile duct stimulates inflammation, which can impede bile flow and contribute to bile stasis. In addition, the surgeon usually inserts a drainage tube, such as a Jackson-Pratt (JP) drain. This drainage tube is positioned in the gallbladder bed to prevent fluid accumulation. The drainage is usually serosanguinous (serous fluid mixed with blood) and is stained with bile in the first 24 hours postoperatively.

Postoperative Care. Postoperative incisional pain relief after a traditional cholecystectomy is usually achieved with meperidine hydrochloride (Demerol) using a patient-controlled analgesia (PCA) pump. Older adults should not receive this medication because its toxic metabolite can cause seizures and other mental status changes. The client participates in coughing and deep breathing exercises more readily when pain is minimized.

Antiemetics may be necessary for clients with episodes of postoperative nausea and vomiting. Administer the antiemetic early, as prescribed, to prevent retching associated with vomiting and thus decrease the incidence of pain related to muscle straining.

Provide care for the incision, the surgical drain, and the T-tube. The surgeon typically removes the surgical dressing and drain within 24 to 48 hours after surgery. The T-tube, however, may remain in place for 6 weeks or longer. Chart 63-2 highlights the important nursing care activities associated with the T-tube system.

The client usually receives nothing by mouth (NPO) until the client is fully awake postoperatively. Gradually advance the diet from clear liquids to solid foods as tolerated. Within a day or two, the client resumes the ingestion of solid foods and is discharged to home.

The amount of fat allowed in the client's diet after a cholecystectomy depends on his or her tolerance of fat. In the early postoperative period, if bile flow is reduced, a low-fat diet may reduce discomfort and prevent nausea. For most clients, a special diet is not required. Advise the client to eat nutritious meals and avoid excessive intake of fat. If the client is obese, recommend a weight reduction program. Collaborate with the physician and the dietitian in planning the appropriate diet.

Community-Based Care

HOME CARE MANAGEMENT

After a traditional cholecystectomy, clients may need short-term assistance with procuring foods, preparing meals, performing dressing changes, and caring for the T-tube. Clients who have undergone traditional gallbladder surgery may also need transportation to follow-up appointments with the health care provider. The surgeon typically allows these clients to return to their usual activities 4 to 6 weeks after surgery.

HEALTH TEACHING

Following a cholecystectomy, discharge teaching for the client and the family may include the following:

- Pain management
- Diet therapy
- Wound, drain, and incision care
- Activity restrictions

CHART 63-2

BEST PRACTICE for
Care of the Client with a T-Tube

- Keep the drainage system below the level of the gallbladder. Maintain the client in the semi-Fowler's position.
- Assess the amount, color, consistency, and odor of drainage initially every 2 to 4 hours, then every 8 hours after the first 24 hours. In the immediate postoperative period, expect bloody drainage, which changes to green-brown bile. Bile output is about 400+ mL/day with a gradual decrease in amount. Report bile drainage amounts in excess of 1000 mL/day to the physician.
- Collect and administer excess bile output to the client by the nasogastric tube (uncommon), or give synthetic bile salts, such as dehydrocholic acid (Decholin).
- Report sudden increases in bile output after a normally decreasing output pattern is established. (The hospital-based nurse does not normally observe this, because it occurs 9 to 10 days postoperatively, but this information should be included in client discharge teaching.)
- Assess for foul odor and purulent drainage, which indicate infection or extensive inflammation. Report changes in drainage to the physician.
- Inspect the skin around the T-tube insertion site for signs of inflammation, including redness, swelling, and erythema, and observe for frank bile leakage. Keep the dressing dry. (Use the hospital's procedure and provide drain care and dressing change per protocol. The site is usually cleaned and the dressing changed daily.)
- *Never* irrigate, aspirate, or clamp a T-tube without a physician's order.
- Assess the drainage system for pulling, kinking, or tangling of tubing, especially when the client is positioned toward the right side. Assist the client with early turning and ambulation. Drape and secure the section of the T-tube emerging from the stab wound over a small roll of gauze taped to the client's skin to help prevent its lumen from occluding as a result of pressure.
- When the client is allowed to eat, clamp the T-tube for 1 to 2 hours (per physician's orders) before and after meals. Assess the client's response to determine tolerance of food.
- Teach client to observe stools for return of brown color 7 to 10 days postoperatively.

- Complication recognition
- Health care follow-up

During postoperative teaching and discharge planning, include a supportive spouse, family member, or significant other to provide reinforcement of information and to assist the client in adhering to the treatment plan.

Diet therapy for the client who has undergone a cholecystectomy is based on his or her tolerance of fats. The nurse or dietitian consults with the client to develop a nutrition program that includes nutritious, well-balanced meals that include the client's preferences, when possible. If the client has a poor tolerance of fats, a low-fat diet is developed and a list of foods to avoid is provided (Table 63-1). The dietitian may provide printed menu-planning guidelines. Some clients need to maintain a low-fat diet for 6 months or longer. They are advised to add fatty foods to the diet slowly and as tolerated.

If the client has problems tolerating three large meals a day, suggest trying smaller, more frequent meals. If the client is obese, a weight reduction diet is recommended and teaching is tailored to provide appropriate dietary guidelines.

Clients are leaving the hospital sooner after traditional open gallbladder surgery than they did in the past. Because a T-tube is usually left in place for several weeks, clients are sent home with the drainage systems intact. Instruct the client and one or more family members to inspect the incision wound and the T-tube drainage site for inflammation. Signs and symptoms include redness, swelling, warmth, extreme tenderness, excessive drainage, and increased incisional pain. Any of these findings should be reported to the health care provider. The nurse provides oral and written instructions for drainage tube care (Chart 63-3).

Provide information to the client and family about the potential for **postcholecystectomy syndrome,** in which the clinical manifestations of biliary tract disease occur following cholecystectomy in a small percentage of clients. Postcholecystectomy syndrome is caused by residual or recurring calculi, inflammation, or stricture of the common bile duct.

Remind the client to report symptoms of biliary tract disease, including jaundice of the skin or sclera, darkened urine,

TABLE 63-1 Foods for Clients with Cholecystitis or Cholelithiasis to Avoid

Foods High in Cholesterol/Fat	Gas-Forming Vegetables
Dairy Products	Cabbage
Whole milk	Onions
Ice cream	Broccoli
Butter	Cauliflower
Cream	Sauerkraut
Cheese	Radishes
	Cucumbers
Other Foods	Beans
Fried, fatty foods	
Rich pastries	
Gravies	
Nuts	
Chocolate	
Egg yolks	
Avocado	

CHART 63-3

CLIENT EDUCATION GUIDE
Home Care for the Client with a T-Tube

- Coil the drainage tubing and secure it to your abdomen by taping or using a belt with Velcro fasteners. Keep the drainage bag below the level of the T-tube.
- Wear loose-fitting clothes.
- Wear older clothes to prevent ruining good-quality clothes.
- If staining occurs, soak the garment in a solution of detergent, baking soda, and bleach.
- Take showers instead of baths.
- Avoid heavy lifting and strenuous activity.
- Remove the dressing around the T-tube every day. Hold the tube in place and clean the skin around the tube. Apply a precut dressing around the catheter and tape it in place.
- Empty the drainage bag at the same time each day. Allow the bile to flow from the bag's spout; do not disconnect the system.
- The physician may advise you to clamp the T-tube for 1 to 2 hours before and after meals. Otherwise, keep the T-tube unclamped.
- Observe the amount, color, and odor of the drainage. Report any change in drainage, abdominal pain, nausea, or vomiting to your physician.
- Inspect the wound for signs of infection, including redness, swelling, warmth, abdominal firmness, pain, and purulent drainage at the tube site. Take your temperature, and report a temperature of 100° F (37° C) or greater to your physician.
- Return to the health care provider as scheduled for follow-up.

light-colored stools, pain, fever, or chills, to the physician or nurse practitioner.

The client with cholecystitis who either refuses or postpones surgery must be instructed on the signs of potential complications of chronic cholecystitis, including fever, recurrent abdominal pain, and jaundice. If these signs occur, the client should notify the health care provider for prompt medical care.

HEALTH CARE RESOURCES

For clients at home with a T-tube or for those older adults who cannot manage self-care, a home care nurse may be needed to provide support and follow-up nursing care and teaching. The nurse assesses the client's adaptation to the treatment plan and evaluates wound healing and the integrity of the T-tube drainage system. The need for further wound and skin care interventions is also determined.

Critical Thinking Challenge

An older morbidly obese woman is admitted to the same-day surgical department where you work for a laparoscopic cholecystectomy. She has had severe episodic pain for several months following ingestion of fatty and spicy foods. Her history states that she has type 2 diabetes and has multiple lower extremity varicosities for which she has undergone two surgical procedures. The client stands all day for 6 days a week because she runs and cooks for a small, but busy restaurant in the local community.

1. The client is especially at risk for what postoperative complications?
2. What interventions should you implement to decrease these problems when she returns from the operating suite?
3. What discharge teaching will she need?

evolve For suggested answer guidelines, go to http://evolve.elsevier.com/Iggy/.

Cancer of the Gallbladder

PATHOPHYSIOLOGY

Primary cancer of the gallbladder is rare and is more common in women than in men. Adenocarcinoma and squamous cell carcinoma of the gallbladder account for the majority of gallbladder cancers, and may be hereditary in a small percentage of clients. They typically infiltrate the liver and ducts, as well as the gallbladder. These rare gallbladder carcinomas appear more frequently in clients with pre-existing chronic cholecystitis and cholelithiasis.

The diagnosis of gallbladder cancer is difficult. Early symptoms, when present, are insidious in onset and similar to those of chronic cholecystitis and cholelithiasis. Characteristic manifestations include the following:

- Anorexia
- Weight loss
- Nausea
- Vomiting
- General malaise
- Jaundice
- Hepatosplenomegaly
- Chronic, progressively severe epigastric or right upper quadrant pain

A moderately tender, irregularly shaped mass may be palpated. Gallbladder carcinoma is typically discovered during other procedures for diagnosis of suspected cholecystitis or during cholecystectomy.

CHART 63-4

BEST PRACTICE for
The Client with a Transhepatic Biliary Catheter

- Change the catheter dressing twice a week or more often if it is wet. Be extremely careful not to allow the catheter to pull out during the dressing change. Apply hydrogen peroxide and antibiotic ointment to the site.
- Check the chart for radiology orders on drainage bag instructions. Be very careful regarding sterile technique when emptying and changing the bag. Do not raise the bag above the insertion site and teach this precaution to the client.
- Do not irrigate or flush the catheter without specific orders to do so.
- Assess the client for decreasing jaundice. Stools should change from clay color to normal brown, and urine should change from dark to straw color. Monitor serum bilirubin test results for decreasing levels.
- Assess the client for fever, chills, and hypotension; report these findings to the physician.
- Inspect the catheter for the presence of blood, and notify the physician immediately if any is present.
- Inspect the catheter for patency.
- Affix the bag to the client's gown (not to the bed).
- Provide discharge instructions to the client or a family member, including:
  - Dressing care
  - Signs of catheter malfunction, infection, and dislodgment
  - Outpatient and diagnostic testing appointments

COLLABORATIVE MANAGEMENT

The prognosis for the client with cancer of the gallbladder is poor. Three treatments are used: surgery, radiation therapy, and chemotherapy. Surgical intervention, when performed, is usually extensive. Nursing care is similar to that for clients who have a cholecystectomy or Whipple procedure, depending on the extent of disease. (These procedures are described elsewhere in this chapter.) A bile drainage tube (transhepatic biliary catheter) may be inserted to relieve symptoms such as jaundice and itching (Chart 63-4).

PANCREATIC DISORDERS

Acute Pancreatitis

PATHOPHYSIOLOGY

Acute pancreatitis is a serious and, at times, life-threatening inflammatory process of the pancreas. This process is caused by a premature activation of pancreatic enzymes that destroy ductal tissue and pancreatic cells, resulting in autodigestion and fibrosis of the pancreas. The pathologic changes occur in variable degrees. The severity of pancreatitis depends on the extent of inflammation and tissue destruction. Pancreatitis can range from mild involvement evidenced by edema and inflammation to **necrotizing hemorrhagic pancreatitis (NHP).** NHP affects about 20% of clients with pancreatitis and is characterized by diffusely bleeding pancreatic tissue with fibrosis and tissue death.

The pancreas is unusual in that it functions as both an exocrine gland and an endocrine gland. The primary endocrine disorder is diabetes and is discussed in Chapter 68. The exocrine function of the pancreas is responsible for secreting enzymes that assist in the breakdown of starches,

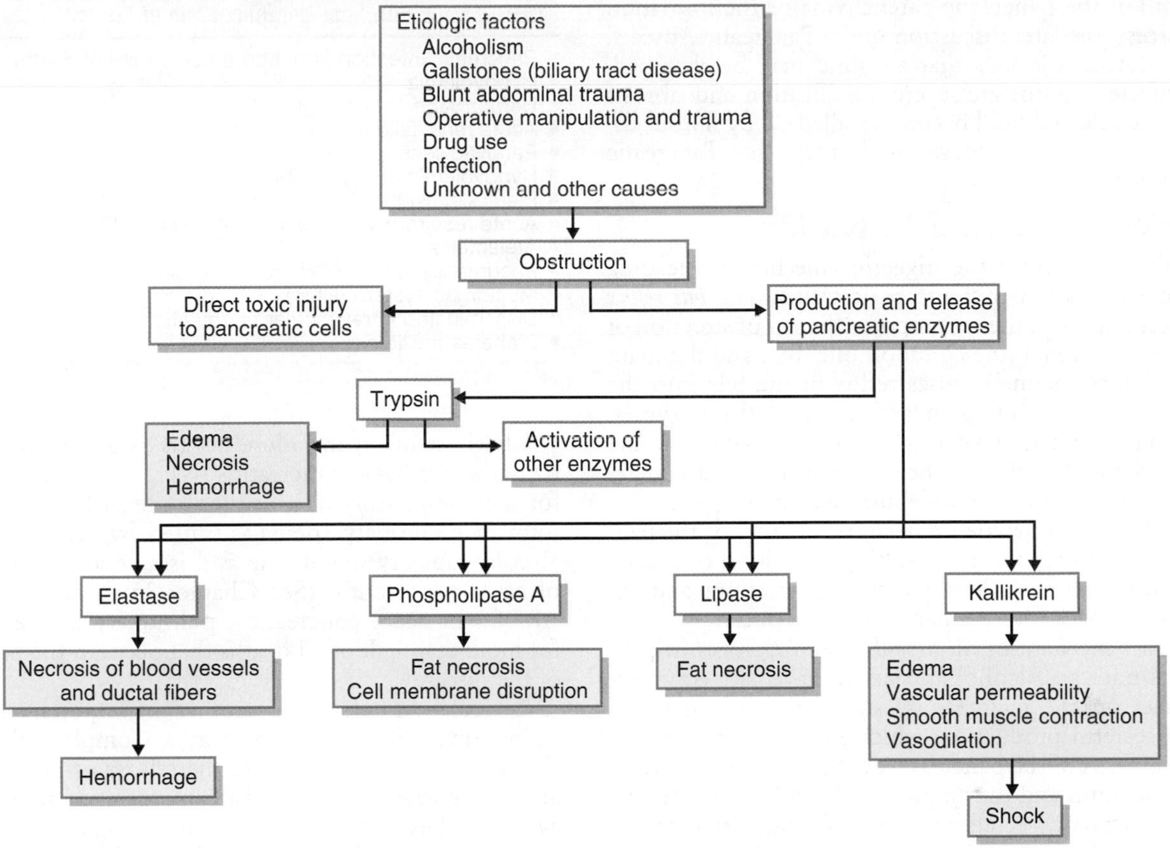

Figure 63-2 ■ The process of autodigestion in acute pancreatitis.

proteins, and fats. These enzymes are normally secreted in the inactive form and become activated once they enter the intestine. Early activation (i.e., activation within the pancreas rather than the intestinal lumen) results in the inflammatory process of pancreatitis. Direct toxic injury to the pancreatic cells and the production and release of pancreatic enzymes (trypsin, elastase, phospholipase A, lipase, and kallikrein) result from the obstructive damage. Following pancreatic duct obstruction, increased pressure within the pancreas and the pancreatic ducts may contribute to ductal rupture, allowing spillage of trypsin and other enzymes into the pancreatic parenchymal tissue. In acute pancreatitis, four major pathophysiologic processes occur: lipolysis, proteolysis, necrosis of blood vessels, and inflammation.

Lipolysis

The hallmark of pancreatic necrosis is enzymatic fat necrosis of the endocrine and exocrine cells of the pancreas caused by the enzyme lipase. Fatty acids are released during this lipolytic process and combine with ionized calcium to form a soaplike product. The initial rapid lowering of serum calcium levels is not readily compensated for by the parathyroid gland. Because the body needs ionized calcium and cannot use bound calcium, hypocalcemia occurs.

Proteolysis

The pathogenesis of pancreatitis involves **autodigestion** of the pancreatic parenchyma by the enzymes normally produced by the pancreas (Figure 63-2). **Trypsin** is the key element that activates all other proteolytic enzymes involved in autodigestion. The agent that triggers the premature activation of trypsin to trypsinogen has not been identified and is being investigated. Proteolysis involves the splitting of proteins by hydrolysis of the peptide bonds, resulting in the formation of smaller polypeptides. Proteolytic activity may lead to thrombosis and gangrene of the pancreas. Pancreatic destruction may be localized and confined to one area or may involve the entire organ.

Necrosis of the Blood Vessels

Elastase is activated by trypsin and causes elastic fibers of the blood vessels and ducts to dissolve. The necrosis of blood vessels results in bleeding, ranging from minor bleeding to massive hemorrhage of pancreatic tissue. Another pancreatic enzyme, kallikrein, causes the release of vasoactive peptides, bradykinin, and a plasma kinin known as kallidin. These substances contribute to vasodilation and increased vascular permeability, further compounding the hemorrhagic process. This massive destruction of blood vessels by necrosis may lead to generalized hemorrhage with blood escaping into the retroperitoneal tissues. The client with hemorrhagic pancreatitis is critically ill, and extensive pancreatic destruction and shock may lead to death. The majority of deaths in clients with acute pancreatitis result from irreversible shock.

Inflammation

The inflammatory stage occurs when leukocytes cluster around the hemorrhagic and necrotic areas of the pancreas. A secondary bacterial process may lead to suppuration (pus formation) of the pancreatic parenchyma or the formation of an abscess (see later discussion under Pancreatic Abscess, p. 1412). Infected lesions that are mild may be absorbed. When infected lesions are severe, calcification and fibrosis occur. If the infected fluid becomes walled off by fibrous tissue, a pancreatic pseudocyst is formed (see Pancreatic Pseudocyst, p. 1412).

Theories of Enzyme Activation

Several theories explain the triggering mechanisms leading to enzyme activation in acute pancreatitis. The *bile reflux* ("common channel") theory proposes that an obstruction of the common channel (the common bile duct and the main pancreatic duct channel) causes reflux of the bile into the pancreatic tissue, resulting in activation of the enzymes. Not all biliary tracts have this common channel. If the common channel is absent, the common bile and pancreatic ducts merge into the duodenum separately.

According to the *hypersecretion-obstruction* theory, the pancreatic duct ruptures and the resulting disruption or tearing of the cell membrane allows pancreatic secretions and enzymes to leak back into the parenchymal tissue.

The exact mechanism of *alcohol-induced* changes in pancreatitis is unclear. Alcohol appears to have a direct metabolic effect on the pancreas by stimulating hydrochloric acid and secretin production, which in turn stimulates exocrine functions of the pancreas. Alcohol also causes edema of the duodenum and the ampulla of Vater, obstructing the flow of pancreatic secretions. Alcohol may decrease the tone of the sphincter of Oddi and cause sphincter spasm and duodenal reflux.

According to the fourth theory, reflux of duodenal contents can occur from biliary tract disease, gallstones in the bile duct (causing the sphincter of Oddi to dilate), or a generalized loss of tone caused by alcohol ingestion. Duodenal contents can enter the pancreatic duct through the weakened sphincter, activating the pancreatic enzymes.

The generalized abdominal pain of acute pancreatitis is related to peritoneal irritation. Ductal release of digested proteins and lipids into the peripancreatic tissues, along with stretching of the pancreatic tissue, causes the seepage of these substances into the mesentery. The resultant peritonitis stimulates the sensory nerves, contributing to intense pain in the back and flanks.

Complications of Acute Pancreatitis

Acute pancreatitis may result in severe, life-threatening complications (Table 63-2). Jaundice occurs from swelling of the head of the pancreas, which impedes bile flow through the common bile duct. The bile duct may also be compressed by calculi or a pancreatic pseudocyst. The resulting total bile flow obstruction causes severe jaundice. Transient hyperglycemia occurs as a result of the release of glucagon, as well as the decreased release of insulin due to damage to the pancreatic islet cells. Total destruction of the pancreas may occur, leading to type 1 diabetes.

Left lung pleural effusions frequently develop in the client with acute pancreatitis. Amylase effusions probably occur when exudate containing pancreatic enzymes passes from the peritoneal cavity into the pleural cavity via the transdiaphragmatic lymph channels. Atelectasis and pneumonia may also occur, especially in older clients.

TABLE 63-2 Potential Complications of Acute Pancreatitis

- Pancreatic infection (most common cause of death)
- Hypovolemia
- Hemorrhage
- Acute renal failure
- Paralytic ileus
- Hypovolemic or septic shock
- Pleural effusion
- Acute respiratory distress syndrome (ARDS)
- Atelectasis
- Pneumonia
- Multiorgan system failure
- Disseminated intravascular coagulation (DIC)
- Diabetes mellitus

Multisystem organ failure occurs as a sequela to necrotizing hemorrhagic pancreatitis (NHP). The client is at risk for acute respiratory distress syndrome (ARDS). This severe form of pulmonary edema is caused by disruption of the alveolar-capillary membrane and is a serious complication of acute pancreatitis. (See Chapter 35 for a discussion of ARDS.) In acute pancreatitis, pulmonary failure accounts for more than half of all deaths that occur in the first 7 days of the disease.

Coagulation defects are another major potential complication and may result in death. Complex physiologic changes in the pancreas cause the release of necrotic tissue and enzymes into the bloodstream, resulting in altered coagulation. Disseminated intravascular coagulation (DIC) involves hypercoagulation of the blood, with consumption of clotting factors and the development of microthrombi.

Shock in acute pancreatitis results from peripheral vasodilation from the released vasoactive substances and the retroperitoneal loss of protein-rich fluid from proteolytic digestion. Hypovolemia may result in decreased renal perfusion and acute renal failure. Paralytic (adynamic) ileus results from peritoneal irritation and seepage of pancreatic enzymes into the abdominal cavity.

Etiology and Genetic Risk

In many cases, the cause of pancreatitis is not known. Many factors can produce injury to the pancreas. The most commonly cited factors are excessive alcohol ingestion and biliary tract disease, with gallstones accounting for almost half of the cases of obstructive pancreatitis. Older adults with pancreatitis typically have biliary obstruction. Iatrogenic acute pancreatitis may occur as a result of trauma from surgical manipulation after biliary tract, pancreatic, gastric, and duodenal procedures, such as cholecystectomy, the Whipple procedure, and partial gastrectomy. The trauma may also originate as a complication of the diagnostic procedure endoscopic retrograde cholangiopancreatography (ERCP).

Other etiologic factors include the following:

- Trauma: external (blunt trauma) or operative
- Pancreatic obstruction: tumors, cysts, or abscesses; abnormal organ structure
- Metabolic disturbances: hyperlipidemia, hyperparathyroidism, or hypercalcemia
- Renal disturbances: failure or transplantation
- Familial, inherited pancreatitis
- Penetrating gastric or duodenal ulcers, resulting in peritonitis

- Viral infections, such as coxsackievirus B infection
- Toxicities of drugs, including opiates, sulfonamides, thiazides, steroids, and oral contraceptives (The exact mechanism by which these and other drugs cause pancreatitis is unknown.)

Incidence/Prevalence

Pancreatic attacks are especially common during holidays and vacations when alcohol ingestion is usually high, especially in men. Women are affected most often after cholelithiasis and biliary tract disturbances. In addition, acute pancreatitis is the most common complication of endoscopic retrograde cholangiopancreatography (ERCP).

Death occurs in about 10% of clients with acute pancreatitis, but with early diagnosis and treatment, mortality can be reduced. Death occurs at a higher rate in older adults and in clients with postoperative pancreatitis. The prognosis for recovery is usually favorable for pancreatitis associated with biliary tract disease and poor if pancreatitis accompanies alcoholism. Mortality rises as high as 60% when necrosis and hemorrhage occur.

HEALTH PROMOTION/ILLNESS PREVENTION

In view of the causes of pancreatitis, individuals who drink alcohol should do so in moderation to prevent alcohol-related health problems, such as pancreatitis. Gallbladder disease, especially when triggered by gallstones, should be treated promptly to avoid complications.

To help reduce the incidence of acute pancreatitis in ERCP, several antisecretory agents may be given. The most widely investigated drugs used for this purpose are somatostatin and its analogue octreotide. These drugs appear to have anti-inflammatory and cytoprotective properties. SecreFlo (injectable secretin) and diclofenac have also been used with success. They are most useful during ERCP when measuring pressures of the sphincter of Oddi.

◆COLLABORATIVE MANAGEMENT

PHARM REVIEW

◆Assessment

HISTORY

Most often, the client indicates that he or she needs relief from abdominal pain. Ask whether the abdominal pain occurs when ingesting alcohol or eating a high-fat meal. Information about alcohol usage should be obtained, including the amount of alcohol consumed during what period of time (i.e., years of consumption, how much usually consumed over a particular period). Because of the familial connection, the client is questioned about a family or personal history of alcoholism, pancreatitis, or biliary tract disease. Determine whether any abdominal surgical interventions, such as cholecystectomy, or diagnostic procedures, such as ERCP, have been performed recently.

Assess for the presence of other medical problems known to cause pancreatitis, including peptic ulcer disease, renal failure, vascular disorders, hyperparathyroidism, and hyperlipidemia. Inquire about recent viral infections. Ask the client or family member/significant other to list all prescription and over-the-counter (OTC) drugs taken recently.

PHYSICAL ASSESSMENT/CLINICAL MANIFESTATIONS

The diagnosis of pancreatitis is made on the basis of the clinical presentation combined with the results of diagnostic studies–both laboratory and radiologic. Clinical manifestations of acute pancreatitis vary widely and depend on the severity of the inflammation. Typically, a client is diagnosed after presenting with abdominal pain that localizes in the epigastrium; this is the most frequent symptom. Assess the intensity and quality of pain. The client often states that the pain had a sudden onset, is located in the mid-epigastric area or the left upper quadrant, and radiates to the back, left flank, or left shoulder. The pain is described as intense, **boring** (feeling that it is going through the body), and continuous, and is worsened by lying in the supine position. Often the client finds relief by assuming the fetal position (with the knees drawn up to the chest and the spine flexed) or when sitting upright and bending forward. The client may report weight loss resulting from nausea and vomiting.

When performing an abdominal assessment, you may find the following on inspection:

- Generalized jaundice
- Gray-blue discoloration of the abdomen and periumbilical area **(Cullen's sign)**
- Gray-blue discoloration of the flanks **(Turner's sign),** caused by pancreatic enzyme leakage to cutaneous tissue from the peritoneal cavity

Listen for bowel sounds; absent or decreased bowel sounds usually indicate paralytic (adynamic) ileus. On light palpation, note abdominal tenderness, rigidity, and guarding as a result of peritonitis. A palpable mass may be found if a pancreatic pseudocyst is present. Pancreatic ascites creates a dull sound on percussion.

Assistive nursing personnel take and record vital signs frequently to assess for elevated temperature, tachycardia, and decreased blood pressure. Use these data to determine whether complications are occurring. Respiratory complications, such as left lung pleural effusions, atelectasis, and pneumonia, are common in clients with acute pancreatitis. Auscultate the lung fields for adventitious sounds or decreased aeration and observe respirations for dyspnea or orthopnea.

Significant changes in vital signs may indicate the life-threatening complication of shock. Hypotension and tachycardia may result from pancreatic hemorrhage, excessive fluid volume shifting, or the toxic effects of abdominal sepsis from enzyme damage. Observe the client for changes in behavior and sensorium that may be related to alcohol withdrawal, hypoxia, or impending sepsis with shock (see Chapter 8).

PSYCHOSOCIAL ASSESSMENT

Excessive alcohol intake, particularly in men, is the most frequent cause of acute pancreatitis. Therefore tactfully explore the client's alcohol intake history. You and the client should discuss the intake of alcohol and the reasons for overindulging. Ask him or her when increased drinking episodes occur, in particular, whether binges occur during holidays, vacations, or weekends or revolve around particular activities, such as television viewing. The client is also questioned about any recent traumatic event that may have contributed to increased alcohol consumption, such as the death of a family member or a job loss.

TABLE 63-3 Causes of Laboratory Diagnostic Abnormalities in Acute Pancreatitis

Abnormal Finding	Cause
Cardinal Diagnostic Tests	
Increased *serum* amylase	Pancreatic cell injury
Elevated *serum* lipase	Pancreatic cell injury
Elevated *serum* trypsin	Pancreatic cell injury
Elevated *serum* elastase	Pancreatic cell injury
Other Diagnostic Tests	
Elevated serum glucose	Pancreatic cell injury, resulting in impaired carbohydrate metabolism; decreased insulin release
Decreased serum calcium and magnesium	Fatty acids combined with calcium; seen in fat necrosis
Elevated bilirubin	Hepatobiliary obstructive process
Elevated alanine aminotransferase	Hepatobiliary involvement
Elevated leukocyte count	Inflammatory response

LABORATORY ASSESSMENT

Diagnostic laboratory abnormalities are found in clients with acute pancreatitis (Table 63-3). Amylase testing is quickly obtained and inexpensive. However, a variety of pancreatic and nonpancreatic disorders can cause increased serum levels. In clients with pancreatitis, amylase levels usually increase within 12 to 24 hours and remain elevated for 3 to 4 days. Persistent elevations may be an indicator of pancreatic abscess or pseudocyst. Lipase is considered more *specific* in the diagnosis of acute pancreatitis, and serum levels remain elevated for up to 2 weeks. Because serum lipase levels stay elevated for such a long time, the health care provider may find this test useful in diagnosing clients who are not examined until several days after the initial onset of symptoms. Trypsin testing is probably the most accurate serum indicator for acute pain, but is not widely available. Elastase has not proven to be better than lipase or trypsin in assisting the diagnosis of acute pancreatitis.

If pancreatitis is accompanied by biliary dysfunction (biliary pancreatitis), serum bilirubin and alkaline phosphatase levels are usually elevated. A sensitive indicator of biliary obstruction in acute pancreatitis is serum alanine aminotransferase (ALT). A threefold or greater rise in concentration offers a 95% probability that the diagnosis of acute biliary pancreatitis is correct. Elevated white blood cell (WBC) count and serum glucose levels are also common in acute pancreatitis.

Decreased serum calcium and magnesium levels are seen with fat necrosis. Calcium levels may fall and remain decreased for 7 to 10 days. Calcium levels that consistently remain below 8 mg/dL are associated with a poor prognosis.

RADIOGRAPHIC ASSESSMENT

A gas-filled duodenum (secondary to obstruction) on abdominal x-ray may support a diagnosis of pancreatitis. A chest x-ray may reveal elevation of the left side of the diaphragm or pleural effusion. Contrast-induced computed tomography (CT) provides a reliable diagnosis of acute pancreatitis. This noninvasive technique may be used to rule out pancreatic pseudocyst or ductal calculi.

OTHER DIAGNOSTIC ASSESSMENTS

In the client with severe pancreatitis, ultrasonography (US) and magnetic resonance imaging (MRI) of the pancreas help confirm an initial clinical impression, assess for the degree of inflammatory resolution, and reveal common bile duct dilation from obstruction or gallstones. US may be performed at the bedside.

◆Analysis

COMMON NURSING DIAGNOSES AND COLLABORATIVE PROBLEMS

The following are priority nursing diagnoses for clients with acute pancreatitis:

1. Acute Pain related to biologic and injury agents (pancreatic inflammation and enzyme leakage)
2. Imbalanced Nutrition: Less Than Body Requirements related to the inability to ingest food and absorb nutrients

ADDITIONAL NURSING DIAGNOSES AND COLLABORATIVE PROBLEMS

In addition to the common nursing diagnoses, clients with acute pancreatitis may have one or more of the following:

- Nausea related to pancreatic disease
- Risk for Deficient Fluid Volume related to abnormal and normal routines
- Risk for Infection related to necrotic pancreatic tissue
- Ineffective Breathing Pattern related to the complications of pleural effusion or acute respiratory distress syndrome (ARDS)
- Risk for Activity Intolerance related to generalized weakness
- Disturbed Sleep Pattern related to pain

The client with pancreatitis may also have the following collaborative problems:

- Potential for Hyperglycemia
- Potential for Hemorrhage
- Potential for Hypovolemic or Septic Shock
- Potential for ARDS
- Potential for Paralytic Ileus
- Potential for Multisystem Organ Failure

◆Planning and Implementation

ACUTE PAIN

PLANNING: EXPECTED OUTCOMES. The client with acute pancreatitis is expected to verbalize a decrease in or absence of abdominal pain, as evidenced by a pain scale measurement.

INTERVENTIONS. Abdominal pain is the prominent symptom of pancreatitis. The main focus of nursing care is aimed at reducing discomfort and pain by the use of interventions that decrease gastrointestinal (GI) tract activity, thus decreasing pancreatic stimulation. Pain assessment to measure the effectiveness of these interventions is a vital nursing activity (see Chapter 7).

NONSURGICAL MANAGEMENT. The health care team initially attempts to achieve pain relief with nonsurgical interventions, which include fasting, drug therapy, and comfort measures. If the client has a life-threatening complication or requires frequent monitoring, he or she is admitted to an intensive care unit.

CHART 63-5

NIC **INTERVENTION ACTIVITIES for The Client with Acute Pancreatitis**

Analgesic Administration: *Use of pharmacologic agents to reduce or eliminate pain*

- Determine pain location, characteristics, quality, and severity before medicating client.
- Check medical order for drug, dose, and frequency of analgesic prescribed.
- Choose the appropriate analgesic or combination of analgesics when more than one is prescribed.
- Choose the IV route, rather than IM, for frequent pain medication injections, when possible.
- Attend to comfort needs and other activities that assist relaxation to facilitate response to analgesia.
- Administer analgesics around-the-clock to prevent peaks and troughs of analgesia, especially with severe pain.
- Administer adjuvant analgesics and/or medications when needed to potentiate analgesia.
- Consider use of continuous infusion, either alone or in conjunction with bolus opioids, to maintain serum levels.
- Institute safety precautions for those receiving narcotic analgesics, as appropriate.
- Correct misconceptions/myths client or family members may hold regarding analgesics, particularly opioids (e.g., addiction and risks of overdose).
- Evaluate the effectiveness of analgesic at regular frequent intervals after each administration, but especially after the initial doses, also observing for any signs and symptoms of untoward effects (e.g., respiratory depression, nausea and vomiting, dry mouth, and constipation).
- Document response to analgesic and any untoward effects.
- Implement actions to decrease untoward effects of analgesics (e.g., constipation and gastric irritation).
- Collaborate with the health care provider if drug, dose, route of administration, or interval changes are indicated, making specific recommendations based on equianalgesic principles.

Pain Management: *Alleviation of pain or a reduction in pain to a level of comfort that is acceptable to the client*

- Perform a comprehensive assessment of pain to include location, characteristics, onset/duration, frequency, quality, intensity or severity of pain, and precipitating factors.
- Observe for nonverbal cues of discomfort, especially in those unable to communicate effectively.
- Ensure that client receives attentive analgesic care.
- Consider cultural influences on pain response.
- Determine the impact of the pain experience on quality of life (e.g., sleep, appetite, activity, cognition, mood, relationships, performance of job, and role responsibilities).
- Evaluate, with the client and the health care team, the effectiveness of past pain control measures that have been used.
- Control environmental factors that may influence the client's response to discomfort (e.g., room temperature, lighting, noise).
- Reduce or eliminate factors that precipitate or increase the pain experience (e.g., fear, fatigue, monotony, and lack of knowledge).
- Consider the client's willingness to participate, ability to participate, preference, support of significant others for method, and contraindications when selecting a pain relief strategy.
- Select and implement a variety of measures (e.g., pharmacologic, nonpharmacologic, interpersonal) to facilitate pain relief, as appropriate.
- Provide the person optimal pain relief with prescribed analgesics.
- Implement the use of patient-controlled analgesia (PCA), if appropriate.
- Use pain control measures before pain becomes severe.
- Verify level of discomfort with client, note changes in the medical record, inform other health professionals working with the client.
- Evaluate the effectiveness of the pain control measures used through ongoing assessment of the pain experience.
- Institute and modify pain control measures on the basis of the client's response.
- Promote adequate rest/sleep to facilitate pain relief.
- Notify the health care provider if measures are unsuccessful or if current complaint is a significant change from client's past experience of pain.
- Inform other health care professionals/family members of nonpharmacologic strategies being used by the client to encourage preventive approaches to pain management.
- Use a multidisciplinary approach to pain management, when appropriate.
- Consider referrals for client, family, and significant others to support groups, and other resources, as appropriate.
- Provide accurate information to promote family's knowledge of and response to the pain experience.
- Incorporate the family in the pain relief modality, if possible.
- Monitor client satisfaction with pain management at specified intervals.

Patient-Controlled Analgesia (PCA) Assistance: *Facilitating client control of analgesic administration and regulation*

- Collaborate with health care providers, client, and family members in selecting the type of narcotic to be used.
- Ensure that client is not allergic to analgesic to be administered.
- Teach client and family to monitor pain intensity, quality, and duration.
- Teach client and family to monitor respiratory rate and blood pressure.
- Teach client and family members how to use the PCA device.
- Teach client and family members the action and side effects of pain-relieving agents.
- Document client's pain, amount and frequency of drug dosing, and response to pain treatment in a pain flow sheet.
- Recommend a bowel regimen to avoid constipation.
- Consult with clinical pain experts for a client who is having difficulty achieving pain control.

NIC intervention activities selected from Dochterman, J.M., & Bulechek, G.M. (Eds.). (2004). *Nursing interventions classification (NIC)* (4th ed.). St. Louis: Mosby.

Fasting. To rest the pancreas and reduce pancreatic enzyme secretion, food and fluids are withheld in the acute period. The health care provider prescribes intravenous (IV) fluid administration to maintain hydration. IV replacement of calcium and magnesium may also be needed.

Nasogastric drainage and suction is reserved for clients who have continuous vomiting or biliary obstruction. Gastric decompression prevents gastric digestive juices from flowing into the duodenum. Because paralytic (adynamic) ileus is a common complication of acute pancreatitis, prolonged nasogastric intubation may be necessary. Assess frequently for the presence of bowel sounds, including before the nasogastric (NG) tube is removed.

Drug Therapy. To decrease pain, the primary drug class used is the opioid class of drugs. Other drugs may also be prescribed.

NIC ***Analgesic Administration.*** Pain management for acute pancreatitis typically begins with the administration of opioids by means of patient-controlled analgesia (PCA) or the intermittent intramuscular method (Chart 63-5). Meperidine

(Demerol) is the traditional drug of choice for relieving abdominal pain associated with acute pancreatitis. It has been thought that meperidine causes less incidence of spasm of the smooth musculature of the pancreatic ducts and the sphincter of Oddi than do other analgesics such as morphine.

However, the limitations and adverse drug reactions related to meperidine are well known (Waitman & McCaffery, 2001). Other options that have been used successfully to manage acute pain in clients with pancreatitis include transdermal fentanyl and epidural morphine with bupivacaine (Stevens, Esler, & Asher, 2002).

In mild pancreatitis, the pain usually subsides in 2 to 4 days; however, with severe acute pancreatitis, the abdominal pain and tenderness may persist for up to 2 weeks. The dosages and intervals of medication administration are individualized according to the severity of the disease and the symptoms.

Other Drugs. Anticholinergics, such as atropine (Urised), glucagons, calcitonin (Calcimar), histamine receptor antagonists (e.g., ranitidine [Zantac]), and protease inhibitors are indicated to decrease vagal stimulation, decrease GI motility, and inhibit pancreatic secretions. However, these drugs can cause unwanted side effects for older adults and have not been proven to alter clinical outcomes. Antibiotics may be used, but they are primarily indicated for clients with acute necrotizing pancreatitis. Common drugs used include cefuroxime (Zinacef), ceftazidime (Ceptaz), and imipenem cilastin (Primaxin).

Comfort Measures. Helping the client to assume the fetal position (with the legs drawn up to the chest) may decrease the abdominal pain of pancreatitis.

If the client has an NG tube in place, remind assistive nursing personnel to implement frequent oral hygiene measures to keep mucous membranes moist and free of inflammation or crusting. Because of the drying effect of medication and the absence of oral fluids, the mouth and oral cavity may be extremely dry, resulting in considerable discomfort.

Lowering the client's anxiety level may also substantially reduce pain. Provide thorough explanations of procedures. The client is encouraged to express the emotions and responses he or she is experiencing. Provide reassurance and offer diversional activities, such as television, music, and reading material, and encourage visitors to direct attention away from the pain.

Endoscopic Retrograde Cholangiopancreatography (ERCP). If pancreatitis was caused by gallstones, an ERCP with a **sphincterotomy** (opening of the sphincter of Oddi) may be performed on an urgent or emergent basis. If this procedure is not successful, surgery is required.

SURGICAL MANAGEMENT. Surgical intervention for acute pancreatitis is usually not indicated. However, if an ERCP is not successful in removing gallstones, a laparoscopic cholecystectomy is performed, as described under Surgical Management (Cholecystitis) on p. 1400.

Complications of pancreatitis, such as pancreatic pseudocyst and abscess, may also require surgical intervention. Laparoscopy (minimally invasive surgery [MIS]) may be performed for drainage of an abscess or pseudocyst. For clients who are high surgical risks, pseudocysts or abscesses can be treated by percutaneous drainage under computed tomography (CT) guidance.

Preoperative Care. In addition to general preoperative care measures, an NG tube may be inserted. The client is frequently in pain, a factor that inhibits the learning process. Provide preoperative teaching in a manner that takes the client's comfort level into account. Postoperative reminders may be needed to reinforce the preoperative learning. Teach the client having external drainage of the pseudocyst to expect a pancreatic drainage tube and explain its care during the postoperative period. Internal drainage via laparoscopy does not require an external tube and allows the client a faster recovery. Be certain that the client knows how to promote respiratory function by turning, coughing, deep breathing, and splinting the incision.

Operative Procedures. A laparoscopic **pseudocystojejunostomy** or **pseudocystogastrostomy** may be performed to drain a pseudocyst into the jejunum or stomach. Less often, an abscess or pseudocyst is incised and drained externally, drainage tubes are inserted, sutured in place, and connected to low suction to prevent further tissue erosion. An open approach, or laparotomy, may be used for this procedure.

Postoperative Care. The client having MIS typically spends less time in the hospital, requires less intense care, and recovers more quickly than those having open surgeries. If present, monitor drainage tubes for patency by assessing for kinks in the tubes and maintaining the ordered drain suction pressure and system integrity. Record the output amount from the drain and describe the character of the drainage. A sump type of drain is usually inserted. Ascertain that the drain is functioning, as indicated by the presence of a hissing noise from the sump lumen.

Provide meticulous skin care and dressing changes. Monitor for the first signs of redness or skin irritation because pancreatic enzyme drainage is particularly excoriating to the skin. Skin barriers, such as a Stomahesive wafer around the drainage tube, are applied to repel drainage from the skin. Collaborate with an enterostomal therapist (ET) for measures to promote skin integrity, such as the use of individualized ostomy appliances and the application of topical agents.

IMBALANCED NUTRITION: LESS THAN BODY REQUIREMENTS

NOC **PLANNING: EXPECTED OUTCOMES.** The client with acute pancreatitis is expected to have nutrients that are available to meet metabolic needs. Indicators include that the client will have normal:

- Nutrient intake
- Fluid intake
- Weight-height ratio
- Hematocrit
- Hydration

INTERVENTIONS. The client is maintained on NPO status in the early stages of pancreatitis. Antiemetics for nausea and vomiting are prescribed as needed. Clients who have severe pancreatitis and are unable to eat for 7 to 10 days should receive nutritional support in the form of total parenteral nutrition (TPN) (see Chapter 64) or total enteral nutrition (TEN). TEN has been shown to produce fewer episodes of glucose elevation and other complications associated with TPN, and to be as effective in maintaining nutritional status (Scolapio et al., 1999).

When food is tolerated during the recovery phase, the health care provider generally orders small, frequent, moderate- to high-carbohydrate, high-protein, low-fat meals. Foods should be bland with little spice; GI stimulants such as caffeine-containing foods (tea, coffee, cola, and chocolate), as well as alcohol, should be avoided.

To boost caloric intake, commercial liquid nutritional preparations, such as Ensure, supplement the diet. If caloric intake is less than desired, an NG tube may be required for additional nutrition via enteral feedings. The health care provider may also prescribe fat-soluble and other vitamin and mineral replacement supplements.

Critical Thinking Challenge

A middle-aged man is admitted to your medical unit with a diagnosis of acute pancreatitis. He has been admitted three other times for hepatic cirrhosis and has been treated for alcoholism for 15 years. Today he is complaining of excruciating abdominal pain that is "boring right through him." He has been nauseated and anorexic for over a week. His wife states that he just won't listen to her and she's very frustrated about his continued drinking; she is considering a divorce after he leaves the hospital.

1. What is his priority nursing diagnosis at this time?
2. What interventions will he need first?
3. How will you assess his nutritional status at this time?
4. What should you say to his wife who is so distraught about her husband's continued drinking despite his health problems?

evolve For suggested answer guidelines, go to http://evolve.elsevier.com/Iggy/.

Community-Based Care

HOME CARE MANAGEMENT

Home care preparation should be individualized for each client's circumstances. Some clients with acute pancreatitis may be severely weakened from their acute illness and need to confine activity to one floor, limiting stair climbing and other strenuous activities until they regain their strength.

HEALTH TEACHING

Education needs to be started early in the hospitalization period–as soon as the acute episodes of pain have subsided. Assess the client's and family members' or significant others' knowledge of the disease.

The goals of discharge planning and education are to avoid further episodes of pancreatitis and prevent progression to a chronic disease. Instruct the client to abstain from drinking alcohol to prevent further pain attacks and extension of inflammation and pancreatic insufficiency. The client is told that if alcohol is consumed, pain will be experienced, and further autodigestion of the pancreas will lead to chronic pancreatitis and chronic pain.

Teach the client to notify the health care provider after discharge to home if acute abdominal pain or biliary tract disease (as evidenced by jaundice, clay-colored stools, or darkened urine) occurs. These signs and symptoms are possible indicators of complications or disease progression.

HEALTH CARE RESOURCES

Clients with acute pancreatitis require visits by a home care nurse if the hospital course was complicated. In these cases, home care may be needed for wound care and assistance with activities of daily living (ADLs). The client requires medical follow-up with the primary care physician or nurse practitioner for monitoring of the disease process. For clients with alcoholism, provide information about groups such as Alcoholics Anonymous (AA). Family members may attend support groups such as Al-Anon and Alateen.

Evaluation: Outcomes

Evaluate the care of the client with acute pancreatitis on the basis of the identified nursing diagnoses and collaborative problems. The expected outcomes include that the client will:

- Experience an alleviation of or reduction in abdominal pain, as indicated by self-report
- Have adequate nutrients available to meet metabolic demand

Specific indicators for these outcomes are listed for each nursing diagnosis under the Planning and Implementation section (see earlier).

Chronic Pancreatitis

PATHOPHYSIOLOGY

Chronic pancreatitis is a progressive, destructive disease of the pancreas, characterized by remissions and exacerbations (recurrence). Inflammation and fibrosis of the tissue contribute to pancreatic insufficiency and diminished function of the organ. Chronic pancreatitis usually develops after repeated episodes of alcohol-induced acute pancreatitis. It may also be associated with chronic obstruction of the common bile duct. The disease may develop in the absence of a known acute disorder. Relief of pain, prevention of recurrence of attacks, prevention of complications, and nutritional support are the principal interventions.

Types of Chronic Pancreatitis

Alcohol-induced chronic pancreatitis is also known as **chronic calcifying pancreatitis (CCP).** Protein precipitates that plug the ducts and lead to ductal obstruction, atrophy, and dilation characterize CCP. As the protein plugging becomes diffuse, the epithelium of the ducts undergoes histologic changes, resulting in metaplasia (cell replacement) and ulceration. This inflammatory process causes fibrosis of the pancreatic tissue. Intraductal calcification and marked pancreatic parenchymal destruction develop in the late stages. Cystic sacs containing pancreatic secretions and enzymes form on the pancreas. The organ becomes hard and firm as a result of acinar cell atrophy and pancreatic insufficiency.

Chronic obstructive pancreatitis develops from inflammation, spasm, and obstruction of the sphincter of Oddi. Inflammatory and sclerotic lesions occur in the head of the pancreas and around the ducts, causing an obstruction and backflow of pancreatic secretions (see Complications of Acute Pancreatitis, p. 1404).

Pathologic Changes

Pancreatic insufficiency in chronic pancreatitis is characterized by the loss of exocrine function. Pancreatic exocrine secretion is divided into two components: aqueous bicarbonate and enzymes.

The aqueous component neutralizes the duodenal contents and pancreatic enzymes that are essential to normal digestion and absorption. Most clients with chronic pancreatitis have a decreased output of pancreatic secretion and bicarbonate. Pancreatic enzyme secretion must be reduced by more than 80% to produce steatorrhea resulting from severe malabsorption of fats. These characteristic stools are pale, bulky, and frothy and have an offensive odor. The action of colonic bacteria on unabsorbed lipids and proteins is responsible for the foul odor. On inspection of the stools, the fat content is visible. In severe chronic pancreatitis, stool fat output may exceed 40 g/day.

Fat malabsorption also contributes to weight loss and muscle wasting (a decrease in muscle mass) and leads to general debilitation of the client. Protein malabsorption results in a "starvation" edema of the feet, legs, and hands caused by decreased levels of circulating albumin.

The loss of pancreatic endocrine function is responsible for the development of frank diabetes mellitus in clients with chronic pancreatic insufficiency. (See Chapter 68 for a complete discussion of diabetes mellitus.)

The client with chronic pancreatitis may have pulmonary complications, such as pleuritic pain, pleural effusions, and pulmonary infiltrates. Pancreatic ascites may impede diaphragmatic excursion and decrease lung expansion, resulting in impaired ventilation. In the ill client with chronic pancreatitis, acute respiratory distress syndrome (ARDS) may develop.

Etiology

The cause of chronic calcifying pancreatitis is persistent excessive alcohol intake that results in repeated episodes of acute pancreatitis. The most common cause of chronic obstructive pancreatitis is cholelithiasis and biliary tract disease, which results in persistent inflammation. Other etiologic factors include pancreatic pseudocyst, postoperative ductal scarring, and cancer of the pancreas or duodenum. All of these factors can produce obstruction of the pancreatic duct. Interestingly, chronic pancreatitis is a risk factor for pancreatic cancer (McCance & Huether, 2002). Prolonged starvation and prolonged use of parenteral feedings for nutritional support can result in pancreatic atrophy, causing pancreatic insufficiency as well.

Incidence/Prevalence

Most clients with chronic pancreatitis are alcoholics (McCance & Huether, 2002). Alcohol-induced pancreatitis is predominantly found in men, but the incidence in women is increasing. In women, chronic pancreatitis occurs more commonly among those with biliary tract disease (cholecystitis and cholelithiasis). The age at occurrence of chronic pancreatitis is variable but is usually between 45 and 60 years.

COLLABORATIVE MANAGEMENT

Assessment

Clinical manifestations of chronic pancreatitis differ from those of an acute inflammation, although, as with acute pancreatitis, abdominal pain is the major clinical manifestation (Chart 63-6). The client with chronic pancreatitis typically describes the pain as a continuous burning or gnawing dullness with periods of acute exacerbation. The pain is intense and relentless. The frequency of acute exacerbations may increase as the pancreatic fibrosis develops.

CHART 63-6

KEY FEATURES of Chronic Pancreatitis

- Intense abdominal pain (major clinical manifestation) that is continuous and burning or gnawing
- Abdominal tenderness
- Ascites
- Possible left upper quadrant mass (if pseudocyst or abscess is present)
- Respiratory compromise manifested by adventitious or diminished breath sounds, dyspnea, or orthopnea
- Steatorrhea; clay-colored stools
- Weight loss
- Jaundice
- Dark urine
- Polyuria, polydipsia, polyphagia (diabetes mellitus)

Perform the same abdominal assessment as for clients with acute pancreatitis, but the findings may not be as significant. Abdominal tenderness is less intense. A mass may be palpated in the left upper quadrant, which is indicative of a pancreatic pseudocyst or abscess. Massive pancreatic ascites may be present, producing dullness on abdominal percussion. Because respiratory complications can accompany the condition, the nurse auscultates the lung fields for adventitious sounds or decreased aeration and observes for dyspnea or orthopnea.

Ask the client to collect a random stool specimen, if able, or ask him or her to describe the stools. The specimen may show the presence of steatorrhea (foul-smelling fatty stools that may increase in volume as pancreatic insufficiency progresses and lipase production decreases). The client may also experience weight loss, muscle wasting, jaundice, dark urine, and the manifestations of diabetes mellitus, such as polyuria, polydipsia, and polyphagia.

In chronic pancreatitis, significant laboratory findings include normal or moderately elevated serum amylase and lipase levels. Obstruction of the intrahepatic bile duct can cause elevated serum bilirubin and alkaline phosphatase levels. Transient elevations in serum glucose levels are common and can be detected by blood glucose monitoring, both fasting and nonfasting.

The only definitive diagnostic test for chronic pancreatitis is the identification of calcification of pancreatic tissue in a biopsy specimen. Pancreas ultrasonography is also a helpful diagnostic tool, especially to reveal pseudocysts. Endoscopic retrograde cholangiopancreatography (ERCP) may reveal ductal system abnormalities, such as calcification and strictures, or it may delineate the presence of pancreatic pseudocyst.

Interventions

The focus of caring for the client with chronic pancreatitis is to manage pain, assist in maintaining a sufficient nutritional intake, and prevent recurrence.

NONSURGICAL MANAGEMENT. Nonsurgical interventions primarily include drug and diet therapy.

Drug Therapy. The major intervention for the pain of chronic pancreatitis is drug therapy. In addition, teach the client to avoid ingesting irritating substances that can precipitate pain.

NIC ***Analgesic Administration.*** Medicate the client as prescribed according to the assessment of the level and intensity of pain and evaluate the effectiveness of the drug intervention (see Chart 63-5). Opioid analgesia with meperidine hydrochloride (Demerol) is most frequently used, but opioid dependency may become a problem. Non-opioid analgesics may be tried to relieve pain. (See Chapter 7 for other interventions for chronic pain.)

If drug dependency becomes a problem, behavior modification programs and drug and alcohol counseling will be necessary. The health care provider may need to admit these clients to drug and alcohol dependency programs.

Enzyme Replacement. Pancreatic enzymes are essential dietary supplements (Chart 63-7). These are given with meals or snacks to aid in digestion and absorption of fat and protein. Drugs such as pancreatin (Donnazyme, Creon) and pancrelipase (Cotazym, Cotazym-65B✱, Viokase, or Pancrease) are prescribed in capsule, tablet, or powder form and contain amylase, lipase, and protease. Teach the client to take these medications immediately before or during meals with a glass of water. Donnazyme should not be broken, crushed, or chewed because it has an enteric coating. At the client's request, mix the powder form in applesauce or fruit juice to make it more palatable. Enzyme preparations should not be mixed with foods containing proteins, because the enzymatic action dissolves the food into a watery substance. Advise the client to wipe his or her lips with a wet towel to prevent the skin irritation and breakdown that residual enzymes can cause. Remind the client not to inhale the enzymatic powder while preparing to take it.

The dosage of pancreatic enzymes depends on the severity of the malabsorption and maldigestion. Record the number and consistency of stools per day to monitor the effectiveness of enzyme therapy. If pancreatic enzyme treatment is effective, the stools should become less frequent and less fatty.

Insulin Therapy. If the client has diabetes, the health care provider prescribes insulin or oral hypoglycemic agents for glucose control. Clients maintained on total parenteral nutrition (TPN) are particularly susceptible to labile glucose levels and may require regular insulin additives to the solution. Closely monitor blood glucose levels so that hyperglycemia is controlled and insulin or diabetic shock is prevented. Check finger stick blood glucose or sugar (FSBG or FSBS) levels every 2 to 4 hours.

Other Drugs. The health care provider may also prescribe histamine receptor antagonists, such as ranitidine hydrochloride (Zantac), to decrease gastric acid. Gastric acid destroys the lipase needed to break down fats. Controlling the acidity of the stomach with H_2 blockers or proton pump inhibitors, or neutralizing stomach acid with oral sodium bicarbonate may enhance the effectiveness of the non-enteric-coated enzyme therapy. Subcutaneous octreotide (Sandostatin), a growth hormone similar to somatostatin, is used by some physicians if pain and diarrhea persist.

Diet Therapy. Protein and fat malabsorption results in significant weight loss and decreased muscle mass in the client with chronic pancreatitis. Therefore the nutritional interventions for acute pancreatitis are also relevant for the chronic phase of pancreatitis. The client often limits food intake to avoid the recurrent pain, which is exacerbated by eating. For this reason, nutrition maintenance is often difficult to achieve, and clients are provided with TPN or total enteral nutrition (TEN), including vitamin and mineral replacement.

CHART 63-7

CLIENT EDUCATION GUIDE

Enzyme Replacement for the Client with Chronic Pancreatitis

- Take pancreatic enzymes before or with meals and snacks.
- Administer pancreatin after antacid or H_2 blockers; decreased pH inactivates drug.
- Tell the client to swallow the tablets without chewing to minimize oral irritation.
- Mix the powder form in applesauce or fruit juice at client's request.
- Do not mix enzyme preparations in protein-containing foods.
- Have the client wipe his or her lips after taking enzymes to avoid skin irritation.
- Do not crush enteric-coated preparations.
- Follow up on all scheduled laboratory testing. (Pancrelipase can cause an increase in uric acid levels.)

For long-term dietary management, the client needs an increased number of calories, up to 4000 to 6000 calories/day, to maintain weight. Foods high in carbohydrates and protein also assist in the healing process. Foods high in fat are avoided because they cause or increase diarrhea.

SURGICAL MANAGEMENT. Surgery is not a primary intervention for the treatment of chronic pancreatitis. However, it may be indicated for intractable abdominal pain, incapacitating relapses of pain, or complications such as abscesses and pseudocysts.

The underlying pathologic changes determine the procedure indicated. Using laparoscopy, the surgeon incises and drains an abscess or pseudocyst. Laparoscopic cholecystectomy or choledochotomy (incision of the common bile duct) may be indicated if biliary tract disease is an underlying cause of pancreatitis. If the pancreatic duct sphincter is fibrotic, the surgeon performs a sphincterotomy (incision of the sphincter) to enlarge it. Endoscopic sphincterotomy may be used for clients who are poor surgical candidates.

In some cases, laparoscopic distal pancreatectomy may be appropriate for resection of the distal pancreas. This procedure is discussed later under Surgical Management (Pancreatic Carcinoma), p. 1415.

In a few cases, pancreas transplantation may be done. However, this procedure is performed most often for clients with severe, uncontrolled diabetes. Chapter 68 discusses pancreas transplantation.

Community-Based Care

HOME CARE MANAGEMENT

The care of the client with pancreatitis usually involves a case manager or discharge planner. A community-based case manager may continue to follow the client while he or she requires health care in the home or other community-based setting.

Clients with chronic pancreatitis are usually discharged to home, but some may require care in a long-term care setting. If the client is discharged to home, the activity area should be limited to one floor until he or she regains strength and can increase activity. Toilet facilities must be easily accessible because of chronic steatorrhea and frequent defecation. If toilet facilities are not available in the immediate rest area, a bedpan or bedside commode is obtained for the home.

HEALTH TEACHING

Because there is no known cure for chronic pancreatitis, client and family education is aimed at preventing further acute exacerbations of this chronic disease, providing long-term care, and promoting health maintenance (Chart 63-8).

DIET THERAPY. Instruct the client to avoid known precipitating factors, such as the ingestion of caffeinated beverages and alcohol. The dietitian elicits the participation of the family or significant other in diet planning and food preparation. Diet teaching focuses on eating bland, low-fat, frequent meals and avoiding rich, fatty foods. The nurse and dietitian stress the importance of dietary compliance and the need for increased nutritional intake to prevent acute exacerbations of this chronic illness. Written instructions on diet and pancreatic enzyme replacement therapy are essential.

Remind the client and family members or significant others on the importance of adhering to the pancreatic enzyme replacement treatment. The client must take the prescribed enzymes with meals and snacks to aid in the digestion of food and promote the absorption of fats and proteins. Teach the client to take the enzymes before or at the beginning of the meal and to report to the health care provider any increase in the occurrence of foul-smelling, frothy, fatty stools; abdominal distention; and cramping so that pancreatic enzyme replacement may be increased as needed. The client should report any skin excoriation or breakdown so that therapeutic interventions to promote skin integrity can be instituted.

SKIN CARE. The frequency of defecation (whether continent or incontinent) poses challenging skin care problems. Instruct the client to keep his or her skin dry and free of the abrasive fatty stools, which are excoriating to the skin. The skin should be cleaned thoroughly after each stool and a soothing emollient, such as Sween, applied. To prevent breakdown and maintain skin integrity, a skin barrier may be needed. Many products on the market, such as zinc oxide cream, actively repel stool from the skin.

DRUG THERAPY. The client and family members must be able to state the desired effect of the prescribed drugs, the schedule for drug administration, and potential side effects. Provide written guidelines as reinforcement.

If the client develops diabetes mellitus as a result of chronic pancreatitis from endocrine dysfunction, management of elevated glucose levels after discharge from the hospital may necessitate oral hypoglycemic agents or insulin injections. If this is the case, the client and the family require in-depth teaching concerning diabetes, its signs and symptoms, medical management, insulin administration, dietary management, urine and blood glucose monitoring, and general care information. (See Chapter 68 for a discussion of diabetes.)

CHART 63-8

CLIENT EDUCATION GUIDE
Prevention of Exacerbations of Chronic Pancreatitis

- Avoid things that make your symptoms worse, such as drinking caffeinated beverages.
- Avoid alcohol ingestion; refer to self-help group for assistance.
- Avoid nicotine.
- Eat bland, low-fat, high-protein, moderate-carbohydrate meals; avoid gastric stimulants, such as spices.
- Eat small meals and snacks high in calories.
- Take the pancreatic enzymes that have been prescribed for you with meals.
- Rest frequently; restrict your activity to one floor until you regain your strength.

HEALTH CARE RESOURCES

Chronic illnesses are devastating for families. The high costs of medical insurance, medical treatment, and drug therapy cause serious financial problems. Often the client with chronic pancreatitis is unable or unwilling to work. Case management to coordinate care and manage resources should be instituted during hospitalization and continue throughout the course of the illness.

The client may require home visits by nurses and a dietitian, depending on the severity of the chronic health problems and home maintenance and support needs. The home care nurse assesses the client for pain management, compliance with dietary guidelines and alcohol abstinence, the effectiveness of pancreatic enzyme therapy, and psychosocial adaptation to a chronic illness.

Refer the client to a counselor or a self-help group, such as Alcoholics Anonymous, if appropriate.

Pancreatic Abscess

PATHOPHYSIOLOGY

Pancreatic abscesses are the most serious complication of pancreatitis. If untreated, they are always fatal. After surgery, the recurrence rate is higher than 30%. The abscesses form from collections of purulent liquefaction of the necrotic pancreas.

Pancreatic abscesses occur after severe acute pancreatitis, exacerbations of chronic pancreatitis, or biliary tract surgery. The development of either a single abscess or multiple abscesses results from extensive inflammatory necrosis of the pancreas that is readily invaded by infectious organisms such as *Escherichia coli, Klebsiella, Bacteroides, Staphylococcus,* and *Proteus.* They can erode through the retroperitoneum into the bowel mesentery, the mediastinum, the pleural space, or the pelvis.

◆COLLABORATIVE MANAGEMENT

Clients with pancreatic abscesses often appear more seriously ill than clients with pseudocysts. Clinical manifestations are similar; however, the temperature in clients with abscesses may spike to as high as 104° F (40° C). Blood cultures are helpful in revealing the infective organism. Pleural effusions commonly accompany these abscesses. Ultrasonography and computed tomography (CT) cannot differentiate between pancreatic pseudocysts and abscesses.

Drainage via the percutaneous method or laparoscopy should be performed as soon as possible to prevent sepsis. Antibiotic treatment alone does not resolve the abscess. Mortality remains as high as 60%, even after surgical drainage. Many clients require multiple drainage procedures for recurrent abscesses.

Pancreatic Pseudocyst

PATHOPHYSIOLOGY

Pancreatic pseudocysts develop as a complication of acute or chronic pancreatitis and are caused by alcoholism, biliary tract disease, or abdominal or surgical trauma. They develop in 10% to 20% of all people with pancreatitis, and mortality is reported at about 10%.

Pancreatic pseudocysts, or false cysts, are so named because, unlike true cysts, they do not have an epithelial lining. They are encapsulated saclike structures that form on or surround the pancreas. The pseudocyst wall is inflamed, vascular, and fibrotic. It may contain up to several liters of straw-colored or dark-brown viscous fluid, the enzymatic exudate of the pancreas.

◆COLLABORATIVE MANAGEMENT

A pseudocyst can be palpated as an epigastric mass in about 50% of cases. The primary presenting symptom is epigastric pain radiating to the back. Other common clinical manifestations include abdominal fullness, nausea, vomiting, and jaundice.

Pseudocysts are diagnosed, and their growth and resolution monitored, by serial pancreatic ultrasonographic examination or CT.

Complications of pseudocyst formation include the following:

- Hemorrhage
- Infection
- Obstruction of the bowel, biliary tract, or splenic vein
- Abscess
- Fistula formation
- Pancreatic ascites

Pseudocysts may spontaneously resolve, or they may rupture and produce hemorrhage. Surgical intervention is necessary if the pseudocyst does not resolve within 6 weeks or if complications develop. To accomplish internal drainage, via laparoscopy, the surgeon creates an opening (ostomy) between the pseudocyst and the stomach **(pseudocystogastrostomy)** or the jejunum **(pseudocystojejunostomy).** To provide external drainage, the surgeon inserts a sump drainage tube to remove pancreatic secretions and exudate. Pancreatic fistulas are common after surgery, and skin breakdown from corrosive pancreatic enzymes in clients who have external drainage presents a major nursing care challenge (see earlier discussion under Postoperative Care [Acute Pancreatitis], p. 1408).

Insulinoma

Insulinoma is the most common type of neuroendocrine pancreatic tumor, even though it is rare. As the name implies, these tumors are typically benign tumors of the islets of Langerhans that cause excessive insulin secretion and subsequent hypoglycemia (low serum glucose). Endoscopic ultrasonography is usually done to locate the tumor.

Management includes removal of the tumor, usually via laparoscopic distal pancreatectomy. Nursing care associated with this surgery is described later under Pancreatic Carcinoma on pp. 1415 to 1417.

Pancreatic Carcinoma

PATHOPHYSIOLOGY

Cancer of the pancreas is one of the leading causes of cancer-related mortality, accounting for 2% to 3% of the new cancer cases each year. It is difficult to diagnose early because the pancreas is hidden and surrounded by other organs. The cost of care is almost $3 billion annually in the United States. Treatment has limited results, and 5-year survival rates are extremely low (American Cancer Society, 2004).

Pancreatic tumors usually originate from epithelial cells of the pancreatic ductal system. If the tumor is discovered in the early stages, the tumor cells may be localized within the glandular organ; however, this is highly unlikely. Most often, the tumor is discovered in the late stages of development and may be a well-defined mass or it is diffusely spread throughout the pancreas.

The tumor may be a primary cancer, or it may result from metastasis from cancers of the lung, breast, thyroid, kidney, or skin. Primary tumors are generally adenocarcinomas and grow in well-differentiated glandular patterns. They grow rapidly and spread to surrounding organs (stomach, duodenum, gallbladder, and intestine) by direct extension and invasion of lymphatic and vascular systems. This highly metastatic lesion may eventually invade the lung, peritoneum, liver, spleen, and lymph nodes.

Clinical manifestations depend on the site of origin or metastasis. The head of the pancreas is the most common site of pancreatic carcinoma. The tumors are usually small lesions with poorly defined margins. Jaundice results from tumor compression and obstruction of the common bile duct and from gallbladder dilation, causing the organ to enlarge.

Carcinomas of the body and tail of the pancreas are usually large and invade the entire tail and body. These tumors may be palpable abdominal masses, especially in the thin client. Through metastatic spread via the splenic vein, metastasis to the liver may cause **hepatomegaly** (enlargement of the liver up to two to three times its normal size). Carcinomas of the body and tail spread more extensively than do pancreatic head carcinomas, with invasion of the retroperitoneum, vertebral column, spleen, adrenal glands, colon, or stomach. Regardless of where it originates, pancreatic cancer spreads rapidly through the lymphatic and venous systems to other organs.

Venous thromboembolism is a common complication of pancreatic carcinoma. Necrotic products of the pancreatic tumor are believed to have thromboplastic properties, resulting in the blood's hypercoagulable state. Additionally, the client is at high risk due to decreased mobility and extensive surgical manipulation.

Etiology and Genetic Risk

The exact cause of pancreatic carcinoma is unknown. High-risk populations are those in their sixth to eighth decades of life and those with a personal history of smoking. About 10% of those with pancreatic cancer have an inherited risk. Mutations in certain oncogenes have been identified. Mutations have also been revealed in tumor suppressor genes, such as p16, p53, and BRCA2–the same mutation that makes some women susceptible to breast and ovarian cancer (Hahn et al., 2003).

A newly identified human pancreatic carcinoma cell line, FAMPAC, has a complex molecular pattern of mutations (Eisold et al., 2004). Clients with diabetes mellitus or chronic pancreatitis are slightly more at risk for pancreatic cancer, which may represent another genetic link. Research continues to explore the genetic origins of familial pancreatic cancer.

Incidence/Prevalence

About 30,000 people develop pancreatic cancer each year, and an equal number of people die of the disease each year (American Cancer Society, 2004). Fewer than 20% of persons diagnosed with pancreatic cancer survive longer than 1 year after diagnosis and less than 5% survive for 5 years (Konner & O'Reilly, 2002).

COLLABORATIVE MANAGEMENT

Assessment

PHYSICAL ASSESSMENT/CLINICAL MANIFESTATIONS

Pancreatic cancer often presents in an insidious, vague manner. The presenting symptoms depend somewhat on the location of the tumor. The first clue to the presence of pancreatic carcinoma may be the appearance of jaundice, which is actually a late sign (Chart 63-9). Jaundice appears as the initial sign in most cases because the gallbladder and liver are commonly involved. As the tumor spreads, the green-gold skin color associated with obstructive jaundice progressively worsens. On noting the jaundice, ask the client whether the color of the stool and urine has changed. As a result of the obstructive process, the stool is clay colored and the urine is dark and frothy. Inspect the skin for dryness and scratch marks, indicating pruritus from jaundice. Assess the sclerae for icterus and the mucous membranes for signs of jaundice.

By the time jaundice appears, the pancreatic carcinoma is usually in an advanced stage. The enlarged gallbladder and liver may be palpable. In advanced cases of pancreatic carcinoma, the tumor may be felt as a firm, fixed mass in the left upper abdominal quadrant or epigastric region.

The most common complaint, often misinterpreted by even the client, is fatigue. This fatigue is described as a diminished energy level and an increased need for rest disproportionate to the level of activity. The client notices an inability to perform usual physical or intellectual activities.

Question the client about abdominal pain, which may be described as a vague, constant dullness in the upper abdomen and nonspecific in nature. Pain, a common early complaint in clients with pancreatic carcinoma, is also present in the advanced stages of the disease. Pain may be related to eating or activity.

CHART 63-9

KEY FEATURES of Pancreatic Carcinoma

- Jaundice
- Clay (light) colored stools
- Dark urine
- Abdominal pain: usually vague, dull, or nonspecific that radiates into the back
- Weight loss
- Anorexia
- Nausea or vomiting
- Glucose intolerance
- Splenomegaly (enlarged spleen)
- Flatulence
- Gastrointestinal bleeding
- Ascites (abdominal fluid)
- Leg or calf pain (from thrombophlebitis)
- Weakness and fatigue

In addition, question whether the client is experiencing pain in other areas of the body. Referred back pain may be caused by pressure on the nerve plexus. Some clients have leg or calf pain with swelling and redness as a result of deep vein thrombosis or thrombophlebitis, a complication of pancreatic carcinoma.

Obtain the client's weight to determine the extent of weight loss and whether it has occurred rapidly. The client is questioned about food intake and intolerances. Anorexia accompanied by early satiety, nausea, flatulence, and vomiting is common. Gastrointestinal (GI) bleeding may develop from esophageal or gastric varices caused by the tumor pressing on the portal vein. A new diagnosis of diabetes is found in some clients.

In addition to the focused history, perform a general abdominal assessment. In particular, observe for distention and swelling, which may indicate **ascites** (abdominal fluid). Percussion over the ascitic abdomen elicits dullness. Pancreatic ascites occurs in the advanced stages of the disease process.

DIAGNOSTIC ASSESSMENT

There are no specific blood tests to diagnose pancreatic carcinoma. Serum amylase and lipase levels, as well as alkaline phosphatase and bilirubin levels, are elevated. The degree of elevation depends on the acuteness or chronicity of the pancreatic and biliary damage. Elevated carcinoembryonic antigen (CEA) levels occur in 80% to 90% of clients with pancreatic carcinoma. This test may provide early information about the presence of tumor cells. Other tumor markers, such as CA 19-9 and CA 242, have been found to be useful serologic tests for monitoring a proven diagnosis and for continuing surveillance for potential spread or recurrence. A recent study by Louhimo and colleagues (2004) found that serum HCG beta and CA 72-4 are the strongest independent prognostic indicators for pancreatic cancer.

Computed tomography (CT) can confirm the presence of a tumor and can differentiate the tumor from a cyst. Pancreatic ultrasonography (US) does not distinguish pancreatic carcinoma from other pancreatic disorders; however, it is an excellent test for identifying recurrence of the disease (Tanaka et al., 2004). Endoscopic retrograde cholangiopancreatography (ERCP) visualization and cytologic study of aspirate provide the most definitive diagnostic data. An alternative to ERCP is a percutaneous transhepatic biliary cholangiogram with placement of a percutaneous transhepatic biliary drain (PTBD). This drain decompresses the blocked biliary system by draining bile, either internally or externally. Aspiration of pancreatic ascitic fluid by abdominal paracentesis may reveal malignant cells and elevated amylase levels.

Interventions

Management of the client with pancreatic carcinoma is geared toward preventing tumor spread and decreasing pain. These measures are not curative, only palliative. The cancers are often metastatic and recur despite treatment.

NONSURGICAL MANAGEMENT. As in other types of cancer, chemotherapy or radiation is used to relieve pain. (See Chapter 28 for general nursing interventions associated with these treatment modalities.)

Drug Therapy. To keep the pain under control, the client takes high doses of opioid analgesics (usually morphine) as prescribed and uses other comfort measures before the pain escalates and reaches a peak. Because of the poor prognosis, drug dependency is not a consideration. Chapter 7 describes the care of the client with chronic cancer pain in detail.

Chemotherapeutic interventions for pancreatic carcinoma have had limited success. Combining agents has been more successful than single-agent chemotherapy. 5-fluorouracil (5-FU), a typically used drug, is an antimetabolite that interferes with deoxyribonucleic acid (DNA) synthesis in rapidly dividing cells. The following are other drugs that are commonly used:

- Mitomycin (Mutamycin)
- Gemcitabine (Gemzar)
- Docetaxel (Taxotere)
- Cisplatin (Platinol)

The major benefit of these drugs to the client is pain management, with shrinkage of tumor size and prolonged survival being of secondary benefit.

Radiation Therapy. Intensive external beam radiation therapy to the pancreas may offer pain relief by shrinking tumor cells, alleviating obstruction, and improving food absorption; it does not improve survival rates. Implantation of radioactive iodine (^{125}I) seeds, in combination with systemic or intra-arterial administration of floxuridine (FUDR), has also been used. The client may experience discomfort during and after the radiation treatments. Supportive nursing interventions for the relief of symptoms are indicated.

Biliary Stent Insertion. For clients experiencing biliary obstruction who are high surgical risks, **biliary stents** placed percutaneously (through the skin) can ensure patency to relieve pain. Stents are devices made of plastic or metal materials that keep the ducts of the biliary system open. Using another approach, self-expandable stents may be inserted endoscopically to relieve obstruction.

SURGICAL MANAGEMENT. Complete surgical resection of the pancreatic tumor offers the individual with pancreatic cancer the only effective treatment, but the surgery is only possible in a small percentage of cases. Recent technologic advances have expanded the role of **minimally invasive surgery (MIS)** via laparoscopy in the staging, palliation, and resection of pancreatic malignancies. The surgery selected depends on the purpose of the surgery and stage of the disease. For example, if the client experiences biliary obstruction, a laparoscopic procedure to relieve the obstruction, such as a cholecystojejunostomy, is performed. This procedure diverts bile drainage into the jejunum. Less often, a **distal pancreatectomy** to remove tumors in the tail of the pancreas is done. The spleen may also be removed as part of this surgery.

For extensive metastasis, the surgeon may perform either a total pancreatectomy or the Whipple procedure (pancreaticoduodenectomy). These procedures have traditionally been done using an open surgical approach, but new advances in laparoscopic technology using a hand-assist device is beginning to replace the conventional method. At this time, this new technology is not available for some surgeons because they are not yet trained in how to perform this exciting new technique. Therefore the traditional, open surgical approach remains the most common method of performing the Whipple procedure.

Preoperative Care. The client with pancreatic carcinoma is a poor surgical risk because of malnutrition and debilitation. Specific care depends on the type of surgical approach being used. A nasogastric (NG) tube for decompression may be inserted, and the administration of IV fluids or total parenteral nutrition (TPN) is typically started before surgery.

Tube Feedings. As long as intestinal function is adequate, the client may be maintained nutritionally with enteral tube feedings. When tube feedings are tolerated, a small-lumen silicone feeding tube, such as a Dobbhoff tube, is inserted to avoid the complications of larger-lumen tubes, such as sinusitis and nasal irritation. Commercially prepared products chosen by the health care provider or dietitian provide specific nutrients. Feedings are given by bolus or continuous infusion, depending on the client's tolerance and residual volumes.

Often, in the late stages of pancreatic carcinoma or during the Whipple procedure, the physician inserts a small catheter into the jejunum **(jejunostomy)** so that enteral feedings may be given. This feeding method is preferred to prevent reflux and to facilitate absorption. Feedings are initiated in low concentrations and volumes and are gradually increased as tolerated. Provide feedings by means of a pump to maintain a constant volume and assess for diarrhea frequency as a means of measuring tolerance (see Chapter 64).

Total Parenteral Nutrition. For optimal nutrition, hyperalimentation by TPN may be necessary in addition to tube feedings or as a single measure to provide nutrition. When central venous access is required, a Hickman catheter or other type of catheter may be necessary. Meticulous IV line care is an important nursing measure to prevent catheter sepsis. Sterile dressing changes and site observation are extremely important (see Chapter 17). Additional nursing care measures for the client receiving TPN are given in Chapter 64. Monitor nutrition indicators such as serum prealbumin and albumin.

For the laparoscopic procedure, no bowel preparation is needed. However, either approach requires that the client have nothing by mouth (NPO) at least 6 to 8 hours before surgery. Surgeon preference and agency policy dictates the preferred protocol for preoperative preparation.

Operative Procedures. The **Whipple procedure (radical pancreaticoduodenectomy)** involves extensive surgical manipulation and is used to treat cancer of the head of the pancreas. The procedure entails removal of the proximal head of the pancreas, the duodenum, a portion of the jejunum, the stomach (partial or total **gastrectomy**), and the gallbladder, with anastomosis of the pancreatic duct **(pancreaticojejunostomy),** the common bile duct **(choledochojejunostomy),** and the stomach **(gastrojejunostomy)** to the jejunum (Figure 63-3). In addition, the surgeon may remove the spleen **(splenectomy).**

Postoperative Care. In addition to routine postoperative care measures, the client who has undergone an open radical pancreaticoduodenectomy requires intensive nursing care and is usually admitted to a surgical critical care unit. Assess for multiple potential complications of the open Whipple procedure as listed in Table 63-4.

The primary benefit of MIS is the client's fast postoperative recovery and less pain when compared to traditional open procedures. The client having the laparoscopic Whipple surgery or distal pancreatectomy is also less at risk for severe complications, but some problems have occurred. For clients

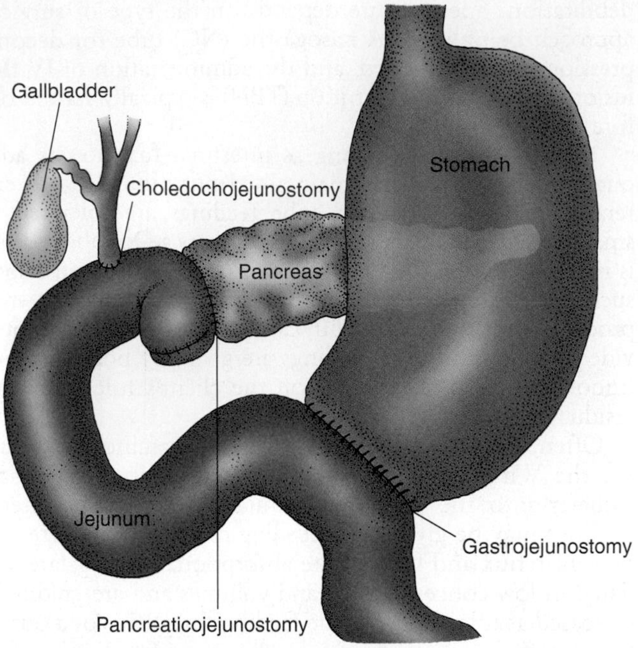

Figure 63-3 ■ The three anastomoses that constitute the Whipple procedure: choledochojejunostomy, pancreaticojejunostomy, and gastrojejunostomy.

TABLE 63-4 Potential Complications of the Whipple Procedure

Cardiovascular Complications
- Hemorrhage at anastomosis sites with hypovolemia
- Myocardial infarction
- Heart failure
- Thrombophlebitis

Pulmonary Complications
- Atelectasis
- Pneumonia
- Pulmonary embolism
- Acute respiratory distress syndrome
- Pulmonary edema

Gastrointestinal Complications
- Adynamic (paralytic) ileus
- Gastric retention
- Gastric ulceration
- Bowel obstruction from peritonitis
- Pancreatitis
- Hepatic failure
- Thrombosis to mesentery

Wound Complications
- Infection
- Dehiscence
- Fistulas: pancreatic, gastric, and biliary

Metabolic Complications
- Unstable diabetes mellitus
- Renal failure

having this procedure, observe for and implement preventive measures for the following surgical complications:

- Diabetes (Check blood glucose often.)
- Hemorrhage (Monitor pulse, blood pressure, skin color, and mental status.)
- Wound infection (Monitor temperature and wounds for redness and induration [hardness].)
- Bowel obstruction (Check bowel sounds and stools.)
- Intra-abdominal abscess (Monitor temperature and client's complaint of severe pain.)

Gastrointestinal Drainage Monitoring. If an NG tube is present, the monitoring of gastrointestinal (GI) drainage and tube patency is an important aspect of postoperative nursing care. In open approaches, drainage tubes are strategically placed during surgery to remove drainage and secretions from the area and to prevent stress on the anastomosis sites. Assess the tubes and drainage devices for stress or kinking and maintain the tubes in a dependent position. Check the suction pressure gauge frequently to maintain the desired suction level. Most often, Salem sump tubes are used and connected to low continuous suction (80 mm Hg or less) to maintain drain patency.

Monitor the drainage for color, consistency, and amount. The drainage should be serosanguineous; the appearance of clear, colorless, bile-tinged drainage or frank blood with an increase in output may indicate disruption or leakage of an anastomosis site. Most of the disruptions of the anastomosis site occur within 7 to 10 days after surgery. Hemorrhage can occur as an early or late complication.

If the NG tube is obstructed, instill air first. If this method does not keep the drainage lumen open, irrigation with 10 to 20 mL of normal saline is gently performed. If the problem continues, notify the physician for additional interventions.

The development of a fistula (an abnormal passageway) is the *most common and most serious* postoperative complication. Biliary, pancreatic, or gastric fistulas result from partial or total breakdown of an anastomosis site. The secretions that drain from the fistula contain bile, pancreatic enzymes, or gastric secretions, depending on which anastomosis site is ruptured. These secretions, particularly pancreatic fluid, are corrosive and irritating to the skin, and internal leakage causes a chemical peritonitis. Peritonitis (inflammation and infection of the peritoneum) necessitates treatment with multiple antibiotics. *If you suspect any postoperative complications resulting from MIS or open surgical approaches, call the physician immediately and provide assessment findings that support your concerns.*

Positioning. Place the client in the semi-Fowler's position to reduce stress on the suture line and anastomosis site as well as to optimize lung expansion. Stress on the gastric suture line of an open surgical procedure can be minimized by maintaining NG tube drainage at a low suction level to keep the remaining stomach (if a partial gastrectomy is done) or the jejunum (if a total gastrectomy is done) free of excessive fluid buildup and pressure. The NG tube also reduces stimulation of the remaining pancreatic tissue.

Assessment of Fluids and Electrolytes. Because the *open* Whipple procedure is extensive and can take 6 to 10 hours to complete, maintaining fluid and electrolyte balance can be difficult. Clients tend to experience significant intraoperative blood loss and postoperative bleeding. The intestine is exposed to air for long periods, and evaporation of fluid occurs. Significant losses of fluid and electrolytes occur from NG and other drainage tubes. In addition, these clients are usually malnourished and have low serum levels of protein and albumin, which maintain colloid osmotic pressure within the circulating system. Reduction in the serum osmotic pressure makes the client susceptible to third spacing of body fluids, with fluid moving from the intravascular to the interstitial space, resulting in shock. These problems are less likely to occur when MIS is used. Therefore, when possible, the trained surgeon prefers to perform laparoscopic Whipple procedures to shorten operating time and prevent the many complications that can occur.

Closely monitor vital signs for decreased blood pressure and increased heart rate, decreased vascular pressures with a pulmonary artery catheter (Swan-Ganz catheter), and decreased urine output to detect early signs of hypovolemia and prevent shock. Be alert for pitting edema of the extremities, dependent edema in the sacrum and back, and an intake that far exceeds output. Nutritional repletion via TPN helps promote the shift of fluid from the interstitial space back into the intravascular space.

Maintenance of ordered IV fluid volume replacement is important. Monitor hemoglobin and hematocrit values to assess for blood loss and the need for blood transfusions. Electrolyte values are reviewed for decreased serum levels of sodium, potassium, chloride, and calcium. IV fluid concentrations must be altered to correct these electrolyte imbalances. The physician orders replacement of electrolytes as needed.

Glucose Monitoring. Immediately after the Whipple procedure, the client may have transient hyperglycemia or hypoglycemia as a result of stress and surgical manipulation of the pancreas. Most of the endocrine cells (islets of Langerhans, responsible for insulin and glucose secretion) are located in the body and tail of the pancreas. In most clients, up to half of the gland remains, and diabetes does not develop; however, a large number of clients are diabetic before surgery. Monitor glucose levels frequently during the early postoperative period and administer insulin injections, as prescribed.

Critical Thinking Challenge

An older adult with a family history of pancreatic cancer is admitted to the intensive care unit where you work following a Whipple procedure for metastatic disease. He is alert but has acute delirium; he is unable to answer your questions. A head-to-toe assessment reveals that his breathing is very shallow. His color is normal, but his oxygen saturation is only 88%.

1. What are your priorities for his care at this time?
2. Why do you think he is acutely confused?
3. What complications is this client at risk for, in view of his age? How will you try to prevent them?
4. With what other members of the health care team might you collaborate?
5. Would you delegate his care to a licensed practical nurse at this time? Why or why not?

evolve For suggested answer guidelines, go to http://evolve.elsevier.com/Iggy/.

Community-Based Care

The client with pancreatic cancer is usually followed by a case manager, both in the hospital and in the home or other community-based setting. The role of the case manager is to ensure that the client receives cost-effective treatment and that his or her biopsychosocial needs are met.

HOME CARE MANAGEMENT

The stage of progression of pancreatic carcinoma and available home care resources dictate whether the client can be discharged to home or whether additional care is needed in a skilled nursing facility or with a hospice provider. Home care preparations depend on the client's physical and activity limitations and should be tailored to his or her needs. Coordinate care with the client and whoever will be providing care after discharge from the hospital–home care provider, hospice care provider, or extended care provider.

The client and family need emotional support to deal with issues related to this illness. Assist family members in ascertaining realistically and objectively the amount of physical care required for the client. The family members must be told that their own physical and emotional health is at risk during this stressful period and that supportive counseling is indicated. If the family does not have a religious affiliation or a spiritual leader (e.g., a minister or a rabbi) to provide support, suggest alternative counseling options. It is appropriate for the nurse to make the initial contact or appointment according to the client's or family's wishes.

HEALTH TEACHING

When the client is discharged to home, many of the care measures are palliative and aimed at providing relief of symptoms such as pain. Care measures and teaching information are similar to those for clients with chronic pancreatitis.

In many cases, the diagnosis of pancreatic cancer is made a few months before death occurs. The client needs time to adjust to the diagnosis, which is usually made too late for cure or prolonged survival. The nurse helps the client identify what needs to be done to prepare for death. For example, the client may want to write a will or see family members and friends whom he or she has not seen recently. The client needs to make specific requests for the funeral or memorial service known to family members or significant others. These actions help the client prepare for death in a dignified manner. Chapter 9 discusses anticipatory grieving and preparation for death in detail.

HEALTH CARE RESOURCES

Regular home care nursing and assistive nursing personnel visits are scheduled to assist the client and family by providing physical, psychological, and supportive care. Supply information about local hospice care (see Chapter 9) and cancer support groups.

GET READY for the NCLEX Examination!

KEY POINTS

Safe Effective Care Environment

- When caring for a client with a T-tube, do not place the drainage bag higher than the tube insertion site.
- Recognize that acute pain relief is the first priority for clients with acute pancreatitis.
- Be aware that clients with biliary and pancreatic disorders are at high risk for biliary obstruction, a serious and painful complication.
- Observe for and implement interventions to prevent life-threatening complications of the Whipple procedure as outlined in Table 63-4.

Health Promotion and Maintenance

- Teach clients having a cholecystectomy to avoid high-fat, high-cholesterol foods for several months following surgery; long-term food tolerances vary for each client.
- Provide health teaching for discharge with a T-tube as delineated in Charts 63-2 and 63-3.
- Teach clients about enzyme replacement therapy as described in Chart 63-7.
- Instruct clients about ways to prevent exacerbations of chronic pancreatitis as outlined in Chart 63-8.

Psychosocial Integrity

- Provide pain relief measures for clients with acute pancreatitis to reduce anxiety.
- Explore ways to decrease alcohol consumption in clients with pancreatitis who use excessive alcohol.
- Refer clients with pancreatic cancer for support services such as spiritual leaders and counselors.
- Help prepare the pancreatic cancer client and family for the death and dying process.

Physiological Integrity

- Be aware that autodigestion of the pancreas causes severe pain in clients with acute pancreatitis (see Figure 63-2).
- Monitor serum laboratory values, especially amylase and lipase, in clients with pancreatitis (see Table 63-3).
- Assess for common clinical manifestations of cholecystitis as listed in Chart 63-1.
- For clients with acute pancreatitis, provide interventions as specified in Chart 63-5; do not administer meperidine (Demerol).
- Assess for common clinical manifestations of chronic pancreatitis as listed in Chart 63-6.
- Recognize that obese, middle-aged white women are most likely to have gallbladder disease.
- Assess clients with presenting clinical manifestations of pancreatic carcinoma as described in Chart 63-9.

ADDITIONAL STUDY RESOURCES

Go to your Student CD-ROM for Review Questions for the NCLEX Examination.

evolve Go to http://evolve.elsevier.com/Iggy/ for Integrated Management of Care Questions for the NCLEX Examination.

SELECTED BIBLIOGRAPHY

Asterisk indicates a classic or definitive work on this subject.

American Cancer Society. (2004). *Cancer facts and figures–2004.* Atlanta: Author.

*Barton-Burke, M. (1999). Gemcitabine: A pharmacologic and clinical overview. *Cancer Nursing, 22*(2), 176-183.

Cole, L. (2001). Unraveling the mystery of acute pancreatitis. *Nursing2001, 31*(12), 58-63.

*Cooper, A.D. (1999). Bile salts: Metabolic, pathologic, and therapeutic considerations. *Gastroenterology Clinics of North America, 28*(1), xi, 1-245.

Eisold, S., et al. (2004). Characterization of FAMPAC, a newly identified human pancreatic carcinoma cell line with a hereditary background. *Cancer, 100*(1), 1978-1986.

Enzinger, P.C., & Mayer, R.J. (2004). Gastrointestinal cancer in older patients. *Seminars in Oncology, 31*(2), 206-219.

*Everhart, J.E., et al. (1999). Prevalence and ethnic differences in gallbladder disease in the United States. *Gastroenterology, 177*(3), 632-639.

Fischbach, F. (2004). *A manual of laboratory and diagnostic tests* (7th ed.). Philadelphia: J. B. Lippincott.

Gavaghan, M. (2002). The pancreas–Hermit of the abdomen. *AORN Journal, 75*(6), 1110-1114, 1117, 1119.

Hahn, S.A., et al. (2003). BRCA2 germline mutations in familial pancreatic carcinoma. *Journal of the National Cancer Institute, 95*(3), 214-221.

Hale, A.S., Moseley, M.J., & Warner, S.C. (2000). Treating pancreatitis in the acute care setting. *Dimensions of Critical Care Nursing, 19*(4), 15-21.

*Howard, D.E., & Fromm, H. (1999). Nonsurgical management of gallstone disease. *Gastroenterology Clinics of North America, 28*(1), 133-144.

*Izbicki, J.R., et al. (1999). Surgical treatment of chronic pancreatitis and quality of life after operation. *Surgical Clinics of North America, 79*(4), 913-944.

Klein, A.P., et al. (2004). Prospective risk of pancreatic cancer in familial pancreatic cancer kindreds. *Cancer Research, 64*(7), 2634-2638.

Konner, J., & O'Reilly, E. (2002). Pancreatic cancer: Epidemiology, genetics, and approaches to screening. *Oncology (Huntington), 16*(12), 1615-22, 1631-1632.

*Levin, B. (1999). Gallbladder carcinoma. *Annals of Oncology, 10*(Suppl. 4), 129-130.

Lightner, A.M., et al. (2004). Pancreatic resection in the elderly. *Journal of the American College of Surgery, 198*(5), 697-706.

Louhimo, J., et al. (2004). Serum HCG beta and CA 72-4 are stronger prognostic factors than CEA, CA-19 and CA 242 in pancreatic cancer. *Oncology, 66*(2), 126-131.

McCance, K.L., & Huether, S.E. (2002). *Pathophysiology: The biologic basis for disease in adults and children* (4th ed.). Philadelphia: W. B. Saunders.

*McCormick, M.E. (1999). Endoscopic retrograde cholangiopancreatography. *American Journal of Nursing, 99*(2), 24HH-JJ.

*Norton, I.D., & Petersen, B.T. (1999). Interventional treatment of acute and chronic pancreatitis: Endoscopic procedures. *Surgical Clinics of North America, 79*(4), 895-911, xii.

Pagana, K.D., & Pagana, T.J. (2002). *Mosby's manual of diagnostic and laboratory tests.* St. Louis: Mosby.

Quillen, S.M. (2001). Identification of pancreatitis in the ambulatory setting. *Gastroenterology Nursing, 24*(1), 20-22.

*Runzi, M., & Layer, P. (1999). Nonsurgical management of acute pancreatitis: Use of antibiotics. *Surgical Clinics of North America, 79*(4), 759-765, xii.

*Sauter, P.K., & Coleman, J. (1999). Pancreatic cancer: A continuum of care. *Seminars in Oncology Nursing, 15*(1), 36-47.

Sawabu, N., et al. (2004). Serum tumor markers and molecular diagnosis in pancreatic cancer. *Pancreas, 28*(3), 262-267.

*Scolapio, J.S., Mahli-Chowla, N., & Ukleja, A. (1999). Nutrition supplementation in patients with acute and chronic pancreatitis. *Gastroenterology Clinics of North America, 28*(3), 695-707.

Stevens, M., Esler, R., & Asher, G. (2002). Transdermal fentanyl for the management of acute pancreatitis pain. *Applied Nursing Research, 15*(2), 102-110.

*Strasberg, S. (1999). Laparoscopic biliary surgery. *Gastroenterology Clinics of North America, 28*(1), 117-130.

Tanaka, S., et al. (2004). Periodic ultrasonography checkup for the early detection of pancreatic cancer: A preliminary report. *Pancreas, 28*(3), 268-272.

*Understanding gallstone formation. (1999). *Nursing, 29*(4), 14.

Waitman, J., & McCaffery, M. (2001). Meperidine: A liability. *American Journal of Nursing, 101*(1), 57-58.

CHAPTER 64

Interventions for Clients with Malnutrition and Obesity

DONNA D. IGNATAVICIUS

LEARNING OUTCOMES

After studying this chapter, you should be able to:

1. Interpret findings of a nutritional assessment.
2. Explain the potential consequences and complications associated with malnutrition.
3. Describe the risk factors for malnutrition, especially for older adults.
4. Discuss the role of laboratory testing in the diagnosis of malnutrition.
5. Analyze assessment data to determine common nursing diagnoses for the client with malnutrition.
6. Identify expected outcomes for clients who are malnourished.
7. Describe the nursing care of clients receiving total enteral nutrition (TEN).
8. Prioritize nursing care for clients receiving total parenteral nutrition (TPN).
9. Identify complications associated with TEN and TPN.
10. Explain the potential consequences and complications associated with obesity.
11. Discuss the multiple causes of obesity.
12. Identify the role of drug therapy in the management of obesity.
13. Develop a postoperative teaching plan for clients having bariatric surgery.

Go to your Student CD-ROM for Review Questions for the NCLEX Examination keyed to these Learning Outcomes.

Nutrition plays a major role in promoting and maintaining health. Nutritional health not only contributes to positive care outcomes but also saves health care dollars. As part of a comprehensive health assessment, include nutritional screening to identify clients who have nutritional deficits or are at risk for developing nutritional deficits.

NUTRITION STANDARDS TO PROMOTE HEALTH

Dietary Recommendations

Several national standards are available for planning and evaluating nutrition. The standard most widely accepted in the United States is the Recommended Dietary Allowance (RDA). The RDA establishes recommendations for energy intake, protein, vitamins, and minerals for a healthy population. Healthy adults require about 1800 calories/day and 0.8 g of protein/kg of body weight to meet basal energy needs.

The RDA can be used to estimate the adequacy of nutrient intake over time. If a client does not meet 100% of the RDA, it is incorrect to assume that he or she is nutritionally deficient. The risk of inadequate intake for any nutrient is not presumed to be increased until less than 70% of the RDA is consumed. It is also incorrect to assume that all clients in a specific population who meet 100% of the RDA are not at risk for malnutrition.

The Food and Nutrition Board (FNB), with the involvement of Health Canada, has recommended that Dietary Reference Intakes (DRI) replace the RDA. The first DRI released recommended the intake of nutrients related to bone health (Food and Nutrition Board, 1997). The established standard of Canada, the Recommended Nutrient Intake (RNI), is similar to that of the United States.

The role of diet and nutrition in disease has been a subject of interest for many years. The current focus is on

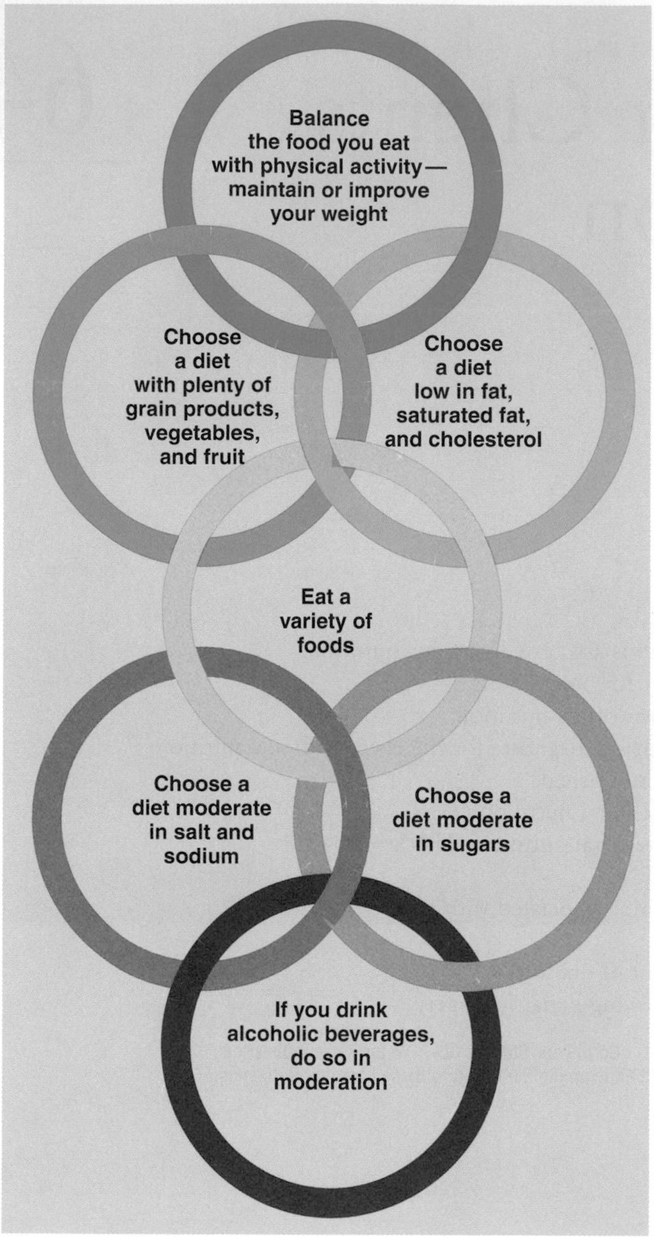

Figure 64-1 ■ Dietary guidelines developed by the U.S. Department of Agriculture and the U.S. Department of Health and Human Services.

health promotion and the prevention of disease. In 1995 the Dietary Guidelines for Americans were revised by the U.S. Department of Agriculture (USDA) and the U.S. Department of Health and Human Services (DHHS). These seven guidelines emphasize the importance of selecting foods to maintain a healthful diet with balance, moderation, and variety (Figure 64-1). One of the most noticeable changes from previous editions occurs in the weight guideline. For the first time, diet and physical activity were emphasized in the second guideline with the goal of maintaining or improving body weight.

The Nutrition Recommendations for Canadians (Table 64-1) are similar to the Dietary Guidelines for Americans. In addition, they recommend limiting the caffeine content of the diet to no more than the equivalent of four cups of coffee per day as well as adding fluoride to community water supplies to a level of 1 mg/L.

TABLE 64-1 Nutrition Recommendations for Canadians

- The sodium content of the Canadian diet should be reduced.
- The Canadian diet should include no more than 5% of total energy as alcohol, or two drinks daily, whichever is less.
- The Canadian diet should contain no more caffeine than the equivalent of four cups of regular coffee per day.
- Community water supplies containing less than 1 mg/L of fluoride should be fluoridated to that level.
- The Canadian diet should provide energy consistent with the maintenance of body weight within the recommended range.
- The Canadian diet should include essential nutrients in amounts specified in the Recommended Nutrient Intake.
- The Canadian diet should include no more than 30% of energy as fat (33 g/1000 kcal or 39 g/5000 kJ) and no more than 10% as saturated fat (11 g/1000 kcal or 13 g/5000 kJ).
- The Canadian diet should provide 55% of energy as carbohydrates (138 g/1000 kcal or 165 g/5000 kJ) from a variety of sources.

From Communications/Implementation Committee, Minister of National Health and Welfare. (1990). *Action towards healthy eating: Canada's guidelines for healthy eating and recommended strategies for implementation.* Cat. No. H39-166/1990E. Ottawa: Branch Publications Unit.

Food Pyramids

The USDA developed the **Food Guide Pyramid** in 1992 to translate food recommendations into a practical graphic format (Figure 64-2). A pyramid format was chosen to communicate three key dietary principles: variety, moderation, and proportionality. The pyramid design emphasizes building the diet on a base of grains, fruits, and vegetables. Moderate quantities of lean meats, protein sources, and dairy products are added, and the intake of fats and sweets is limited. Table 64-2 suggests the daily servings of each food group and clarifies the size of a serving. Adhering to this pattern results in a nutritionally adequate intake if a variety of foods is chosen.

A variety of vegetarian diet patterns is being adopted by increasing numbers of people for health, environmental, and moral reasons. In general, vegetarians are leaner than those who consume meat. The **lacto-vegetarian** eats milk, cheese, and dairy foods but avoids meat, fish, poultry, and eggs. The **lacto-ovo-vegetarian** also includes eggs. The **vegan** eats only foods of plant origin. Vegans can develop megaloblastic anemia as a result of vitamin B_{12} deficiency. Vegans should include a daily source of vitamin B_{12} in their diets, such as a fortified breakfast cereal, fortified soy beverage, or meat analogue. All vegetarians should ensure that they get adequate amounts of calcium, iron, zinc, and vitamins D and B_{12}. Well-planned vegetarian diets can provide adequate nutrition. The **Vegetarian Food Pyramid,** endorsed by the Vegetarian Resource Group, can assist vegetarians with daily food choices (Figure 64-3).

A third pyramid has recently been developed to reflect the current trend toward low-carbohydrate ("low-carb") diets, such as the Atkins and South Beach diets. The **Atkins pyramid** emphasizes building the diet on protein sources and vegetables rather than on grains, fruits, and vegetables as in the USDA-approved pyramid. Moderate quantities of fruits, dairy products, and nuts are added, and whole grain foods are limited. Refined carbohydrates are the least desirable foods, such as pasta, cakes, and white bread.

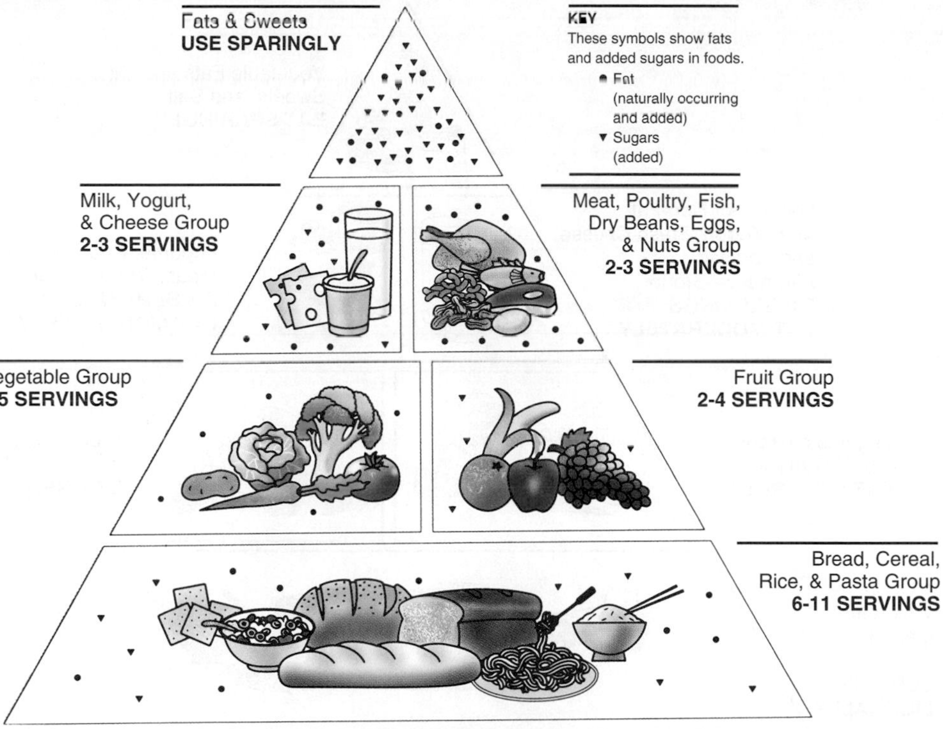

Figure 64-2 ■ The U.S. Department of Agriculture Food Guide Pyramid.

TABLE 64-2 Serving Sizes for Each Food Group

With the Food Guide Pyramid, what counts as a "serving" may not always be a typical "helping" of what you eat. The following are some examples of servings.

Bread, Cereal, Rice, and Pasta
6 to 11 servings recommended
Examples of one serving:
- 1 slice of bread
- 1 oz ready-to-eat cereal
- ½ c cooked cereal, rice, or pasta

Vegetables
3 to 5 servings recommended
Examples of one serving:
- 1 c raw leafy vegetables
- ½ c other vegetables, cooked or chopped raw
- ¾ c vegetable juice

Fruits
2 to 4 servings recommended
Examples of one serving:
- 1 medium apple, banana, or orange
- ½ c chopped, cooked, or canned fruit
- ¾ c fruit juice

Milk, Yogurt, and Cheese
2 to 3 servings recommended
Examples of one serving:
- 1 c milk or yogurt
- 1½ oz natural cheese
- 2 oz processed cheese

Meat, Poultry, Fish, Dry Beans, Eggs, and Nuts
2 to 3 servings recommended
Examples of one serving:
- 2 to 3 oz cooked lean meat, poultry, or fish
- ½ c cooked dry beans or 1 egg = 1 oz of lean meat
- 2 tbsp peanut butter or ⅓ c nuts = 1 oz of meat

How Much Is an Ounce of Meat?
Here is a handy guide for determining the weight of meat, chicken, fish, or cheese:
- 1 oz = the size of a matchbox
- 3 oz = the size of a deck of cards
- 8 oz = the size of a paperback book

Modified from Nutrition and your health: Dietary guidelines for Americans. (1995). *Home and Garden Bulletin No. 232* (4th ed.). Washington, D.C.: U.S. Department of Agriculture, U.S. Department of Health and Human Services.

CULTURAL CONSIDERATIONS

None of the food pyramids takes into account dietary preferences of diverse ethnic groups. For example, for individuals of Hispanic descent, tortillas, beans, and rice may be preferred over pasta, risotto, and potatoes. Therefore health teaching about diet should incorporate these variations (also see Chapter 6).

Some individuals have food allergies or intolerances. For instance, lactose intolerance (lactose is found in milk and milk products) is a relatively common condition that occurs in a number of ethnic groups. It is found more often in Mexican Americans and black individuals as well as in some Native American/American Indian tribes, Asian Americans, and Ashkenazic Jews. A small percentage of white individuals are also lactose intolerant. The cause of **lactose intolerance** is an insufficient amount of the lactase enzyme, which converts lactose into absorbable glucose.

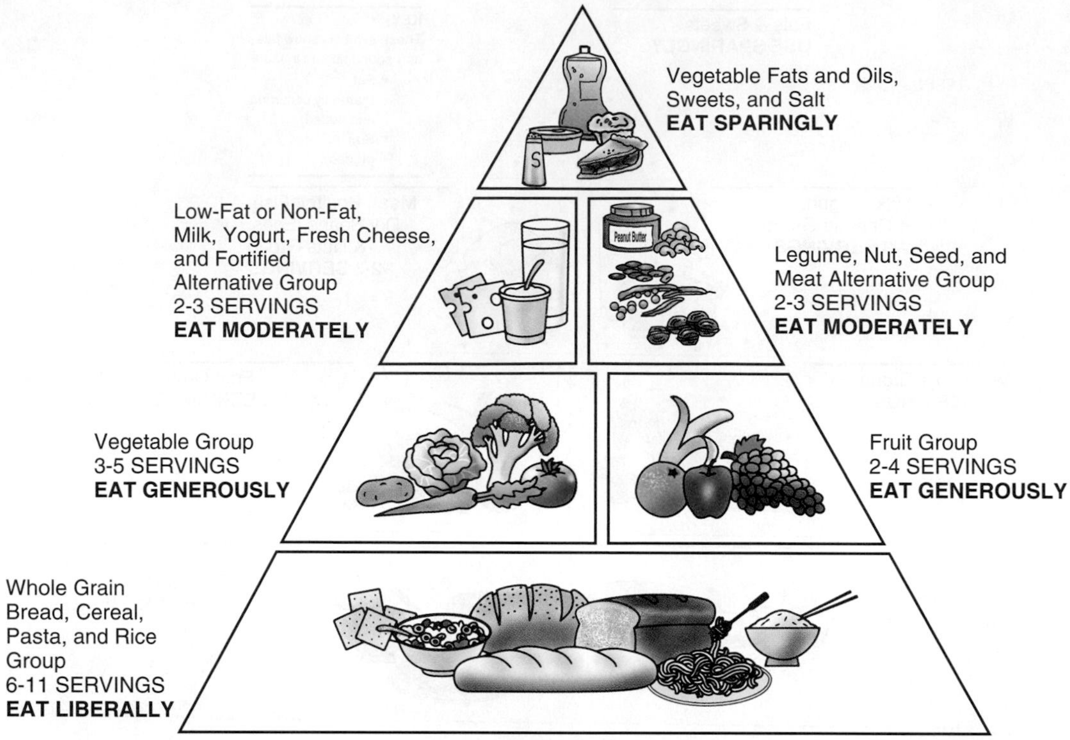

Figure 64-3 ■ Food pyramid for a vegetarian diet. (Courtesy The Health Connection, Hagerstown, MD.)

NUTRITIONAL ASSESSMENT

Malnutrition and obesity are common nutrition problems that occur as progressive changes within the client. When nutritional deficiencies or excesses develop, the body adapts through the use of homeostatic mechanisms. As the intake moves farther from the accepted range, however, the body accommodates by reducing functional levels or changing the status or size of the affected body compartments. The nutritional status of a client can be determined by the presence or absence of these adaptations.

Nutritional status reflects the balance between nutrient requirements and nutrient intake. Factors that affect nutrient requirements include disease, infection, and psychological stress. Nutrient intake is influenced by disease, eating behavior, economic factors, emotional stability, medication, and cultural factors.

Optimal nutritional care is a major interdisciplinary outcome for clients with malnutrition and obesity. Evaluation of nutritional status is an important part of total client assessment. A thorough assessment of nutritional status includes the following:

- Review of the diet history
- Food and fluid intake record
- Laboratory data
- Food-medication interactions
- Physical examination and health history
- Anthropometric measurements
- Psychosocial assessment

Monitoring the nutritional care of a client is as important as the initial assessment. The health care provider, nurse, and dietitian collaborate to identify clients at risk for nutritional problems.

Initial Nutritional Screening

Not every client needs a complete nutritional assessment, but it is important to identify clients at risk for nutritional problems through screening. An **initial nutritional screening** provides an inexpensive, quick way of determining which clients need more extensive nutritional assessment by the health care provider and dietitian.

The initial nutritional screening includes visual inspection, measured height and weight, weight history, usual eating habits, ability to chew and swallow, and any recent changes in appetite or food intake. Questions that may identify clients at risk for nutritional problems can be incorporated into the history and physical assessment (Chart 64-1).

The Mini Nutritional Assessment (MNA), which has been tested worldwide, provides a reliable, rapid assessment for clients in the community as well as in any health care setting (Stechmiller, 2003). The tool consists of six screening questions and, if needed, a follow-up set of more in-depth questions and arm and calf measurements. It can be completed in about 10 minutes; a low score indicates malnutrition or a risk for malnutrition (Figure 64-4).

Anthropometric Measurements

Anthropometric measurements are noninvasive methods of evaluating nutritional status. These measurements include height and weight and assessment of body fat.

CHART 64-1

BEST PRACTICE for
Initial Nutrition Screening Assessment

General
- Does the client have any conditions that cause nutrient loss, such as malabsorption syndromes, draining abscesses, wounds, fistulas, or protracted diarrhea?
- Does the client have any conditions that increase the need for nutrients, such as fever, burn, injury, sepsis, or antineoplastic therapies?
- Has the client been on NPO status for 3 days or more?
- Is the client receiving a modified diet or a diet restricted in one or more nutrients?
- Is the client being enterally or parenterally fed?
- Does the client describe food allergies, lactose intolerance, or limited food preferences?
- Has the client experienced a recent, unexplained weight loss?
- Is the client taking medications, either prescription, over-the-counter, or herbal/natural products?

Gastrointestinal
- Does the client complain of nausea, indigestion, vomiting, diarrhea, or constipation?
- Does the client exhibit glossitis, stomatitis, or esophagitis?
- Does the client have difficulty chewing or swallowing?
- Does the client have a partial or total gastrointestinal obstruction?
- What is the client's state of dentition?

Cardiovascular
- Does the client have ascites or edema?
- Is the client able to perform activities of daily living?
- Does the client have heart failure?

Genitourinary
- Does fluid input approximately equal fluid output?
- Does the client have an ostomy?
- Is the client hemodialyzed or peritoneally dialyzed?

Respiratory
- Is the client receiving mechanical ventilatory support?
- Is the client receiving oxygen via nasal prongs?
- Does the client have chronic obstructive pulmonary disease (COPD) or asthma?

Integumentary
- Does the client have nail or hair changes?
- Does the client have rashes or dermatitis?
- Does the client have dry or pale mucous membranes or decreased skin turgor?
- Does the client have pressure areas on the sacrum, hips, or ankles?

Extremities
- Does the client have pedal edema?
- Does the client exhibit cachexia?

Modified with permission of Ross Products Division, Abbott Laboratories, Columbus, OH.
NPO, Nothing by mouth.

MEASUREMENT OF HEIGHT AND WEIGHT

Height and weight provide a baseline determination of nutritional status. Be sure to obtain accurate measurements because clients who report their own measurements tend to overestimate height and underestimate weight. For clients who cannot stand, use a wheelchair or bed scales. Subsequent measurements may indicate an early change in nutritional status. Assistive nursing personnel often perform this activity.

Height

Clients should be measured and weighed while wearing minimal clothing and no shoes. Determine the client's height in inches or centimeters using the measuring stick of a weight scale if the client can stand. The client should stand erect and look straight ahead, with the heels together and the arms at the sides.

CONSIDERATIONS FOR OLDER ADULTS

Some older adults may have difficulty standing erect, and their actual height may be less than their height on recall. If height cannot be measured directly, it should be estimated by arm span or with use of a knee-height caliper, which provides a more precise height estimate.

Weight

The nurse or assistive nursing personnel weighs ambulatory clients with an upright balance-beam scale. Nonambulatory clients can be weighed with a movable wheelchair balance-beam scale or a bed scale. The manufacturer should calibrate weight scales twice yearly to ensure accurate readings. For daily or sequential weights, obtain the weight at the same time each day, if possible. Conditions such as congestive heart failure and renal disease cause weight gain; dehydration causes weight loss. *Weight is the most reliable indicator of fluid gain or loss.*

Normal weights for adult men and women are shown in the Metropolitan Life tables (Table 64-3). The latest U.S. Department of Agriculture (USDA) and U.S. Department of Health and Human Services (DHHS) Dietary Guidelines contain weight guidelines that emphasize both weight maintenance and weight loss. The same healthy weight guideline applies to all adults. Older adults are no longer permitted a higher weight standard. The weight range appears in the guidelines as a chart with three categories: healthy weight, moderate overweight, and severe overweight (Figure 64-5). Either the Metropolitan Life tables or the New Weight Guidelines from the USDA and the DHHS may be used for comparison with a client's height and weight. Some health care professionals prefer the Metropolitan Life tables because they consider body-build differences by gender.

Changes in body weight can be expressed by three different formulas:

1. Weight as a percentage of ideal body weight (IBW):

$$\%\text{IBW} = \frac{\text{Current weight} \times 100}{\text{Ideal weight}}$$

2. Current weight as a percentage of usual body weight (UBW):

$$\%\text{UBW} = \frac{\text{Current weight} \times 100}{\text{Usual weight}}$$

3. Change in weight:

$$\text{Weight change} = \frac{\text{Usual weight} - \text{Current weight}}{\text{Usual weight}} \times 100$$

NESTLÉ NUTRITION SERVICES

Nestlé

Mini Nutritional Assessment (MNA)

Last name: First name: Sex: Date:

Age: Weight, kg: Height, cm: I.D. Number:

Complete the screen by filling in the boxes with the appropriate numbers.
Add the numbers for the screen. If score is 11 or less, continue with the assessment to gain a Malnutrition Indicator Score.

Screening

A Has food intake declined over the past 3 months due to loss of appetite, digestive problems, chewing or swallowing difficulties?
0 = severe loss of appetite
1 = moderate loss of appetite
2 = no loss of appetite ☐

B Weight loss during last 3 months
0 = weight loss greater than 3 kg (6.6 lbs)
1 = does not know
2 = weight loss between 1 and 3 kg (2.2 and 6.6 lbs)
3 = no weight loss ☐

C Mobility
0 = bed or chair bound
1 = able to get out of bed/chair but does not go out
2 = goes out ☐

D Has suffered psychological stress or acute disease in the past 3 months
0 = yes 2 = no ☐

E Neuropsychological problems
0 = severe dementia or depression
1 = mild dementia
2 = no psychological problems ☐

F Body Mass Index (BMI) (weight in kg) / (height in m)^2
0 = BMI less than 19
1 = BMI 19 to less than 21
2 = BMI 21 to less than 23
3 = BMI 23 or greater ☐

Screening score (subtotal max. 14 points) ☐ ☐
12 points or greater Normal – not at risk – no need to complete assessment
11 points or below Possible malnutrition – continue assessment

Assessment

G Lives independently (not in a nursing home or hospital)
0 = no 1 = yes ☐

H Takes more than 3 prescription drugs per day
0 = yes 1 = no ☐

I Pressure sores or skin ulcers
0 = yes 1 = no ☐

J How many full meals does the patient eat daily?
0 = 1 meal
1 = 2 meals
2 = 3 meals ☐

K Selected consumption markers for protein intake
- At least one serving of dairy products (milk, cheese, yogurt) per day? yes ☐ no ☐
- Two or more servings of legumes or eggs per week? yes ☐ no ☐
- Meat, fish or poultry every day yes ☐ no ☐

0.0 = if 0 or 1 yes
0.5 = if 2 yes
1.0 = if 3 yes ☐.☐

L Consumes two or more servings of fruits or vegetables per day?
0 = no 1 = yes ☐

M How much fluid (water, juice, coffee, tea, milk...) is consumed per day?
0.0 = less than 3 cups
0.5 = 3 to 5 cups
1.0 = more than 5 cups ☐.☐

N Mode of feeding
0 = unable to eat without assistance
1 = self-fed with some difficulty
2 = self-fed without any problem ☐

O Self view of nutritional status
0 = views self as being malnourished
1 = is uncertain of nutritional state
2 = views self as having no nutritional problem ☐

P In comparison with other people of the same age, how does the patient consider his/her health status?
0.0 = not as good
0.5 = does not know
1.0 = as good
2.0 = better ☐.☐

Q Mid-arm circumference (MAC) in cm
0.0 = MAC less than 21
0.5 = MAC 21 to 22
1.0 = MAC 22 or greater ☐.☐

R Calf circumference (CC) in cm
0 = CC less than 31 1 = CC 31 or greater ☐

Assessment (max. 16 points) ☐ ☐.☐

Screening score ☐ ☐

Total Assessment (max. 30 points) ☐ ☐.☐

Malnutrition Indicator Score
17 to 23.5 points at risk of malnutrition ☐
Less than 17 points malnourished ☐

Ref.: Guigoz Y, Vellas B and Garry PJ. 1994. Mini Nutritional Assessment: A practical assessment tool for grading the nutritional state of elderly patients. *Facts and Research in Gerontology.* Supplement #2:15-59.
Rubenstein LZ, Harker J, Guigoz Y and Vellas B. Comprehensive Geriatric Assessment (CGA) and the MNA: An Overview of CGA, Nutritional Assessment, and Development of a Shortened Version of the MNA. In: "Mini Nutritional Assessment (MNA): Research and Practice in the Elderly". Vellas B, Garry PJ and Guigoz Y , editors. Nestlé Nutrition Workshop Series. Clinical & Performance Programme, vol. 1. Karger, Bâle, in press.

Figure 64-4 ■ The Mini Nutritional Assessment (MNA).

TABLE 64-3 Metropolitan Life Height and Weight Tables

Height*		Weight†			Height*		Weight†		
Feet	Inches	Small Frame	Medium Frame	Large Frame	Feet	Inches	Small Frame	Medium Frame	Large Frame
Men					**Women**				
5	2	128-134	131-134	138-150	4	10	102-111	109-121	118-131
5	3	130-136	133-143	140-153	4	11	103-113	111-123	120-134
5	4	132-138	135-145	142-156	5	0	104-115	113-126	122-137
5	5	134-140	137-148	144-160	5	1	106-118	115-129	125-140
5	6	136-142	139-151	146-164	5	2	108-121	118-132	128-143
5	7	138-145	142-154	149-168	5	3	111-124	121-135	131-147
5	8	140-148	145-157	152-172	5	4	114-127	124-138	134-151
5	9	142-151	148-160	155-176	5	5	117-130	127-141	137-155
5	10	144-154	151-163	158-180	5	6	120-133	130-144	140-159
5	11	146-157	154-166	161-184	5	7	123-136	133-147	143-163
6	0	149-160	157-170	164-188	5	8	126-139	136-150	146-167
6	1	152-164	160-174	168-192	5	9	129-142	139-153	149-170
6	2	155-168	164-178	172-197	5	10	132-145	142-156	152-173
6	3	158-172	167-182	176-202	5	11	135-148	145-159	155-176
6	4	162-176	171-187	181-207	6	0	138-151	148-162	158-179

Reprinted courtesy of Metropolitan Life Insurance Company, 1983.
*Shoes with 1-inch heels.
†Weight in pounds. Men: allow 5 pounds of clothing. Women: allow 3 pounds of clothing

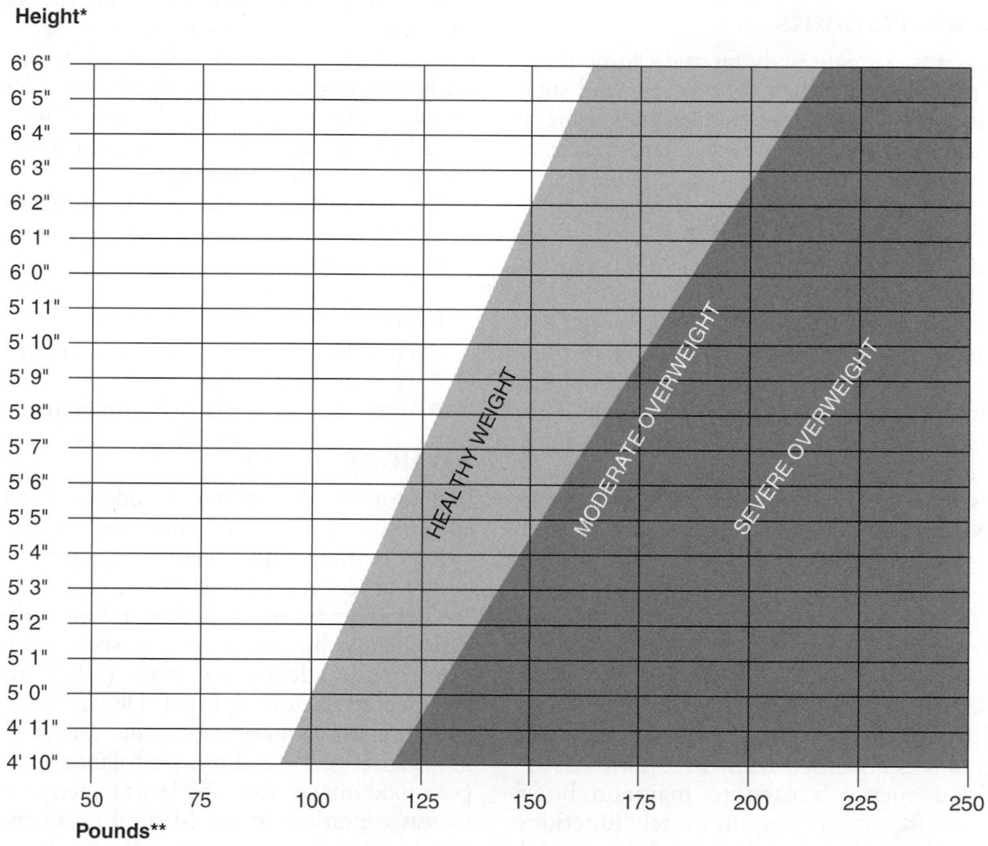

* Without shoes.
** Without clothes. The higher weights apply to people with more muscle and bone, such as many men.

Figure 64-5 ■ The U.S. Department of Agriculture and the U.S. Department of Health and Human Services guidelines for determining proper weight or degree of obesity. (Redrawn from http://www.nalusda.gov/fnic/Dietry/9dietgui.htm.)

An involuntary weight loss of 10% at any time significantly affects nutritional status. Weights may need to be taken daily, several times a week, or weekly for monitoring status and the effectiveness of nutritional support.

ASSESSMENT OF BODY FAT

Body Mass Index

The **body mass index (BMI)** is a measure of nutritional status that does not depend on frame size. The BMI indirectly estimates total fat stores within the body by the relationship of weight to height. Therefore an accurate height is as important as an accurate weight.

A simple calculation for estimating BMI can be programmed into handheld computers or calculators:

$$\text{BMI} = \frac{\text{Weight (lb)}}{\text{Height (inches)}^2} \times 703$$

BMI can also be determined using a nomogram. The least risk of malnutrition is associated with scores between 20 and 25. BMIs above and below these values are associated with increased health risks. Older adults should have a BMI between 24 and 27.

Skin Fold Measurements

Skin fold measurements estimate body fat and can be measured by either the nurse or dietitian. The triceps and subscapular skin folds are most commonly measured using a special caliper. Both are compared with standard measurements and recorded as percentiles.

Arm and Calf Circumferences

The midarm (MAC) and calf circumferences (CC) can be obtained to measure muscle mass and subcutaneous fat. These measurements are needed if the Mini Nutritional Assessment tool is used. To measure MAC, place a flexible tape around the arm at the midpoint, taking care to hold the tape firmly but gently to avoid compressing the tissue. This measurement is usually recorded in centimeters. The midarm muscle mass (MAMM) measures the amount of muscle in the body and is a sensitive indicator of protein reserves. It can be computed from the MAC and the triceps skin fold measure. The CC is obtained using a similar procedure on the calf.

MALNUTRITION

Carbohydrates, protein, and fat supply the body with energy. Under healthy conditions, most of this energy undergoes digestion and is absorbed from the gastrointestinal (GI) tract. Food energy is used to maintain body temperature, respiration, cardiac output, muscle function, protein synthesis, and the storage and metabolism of food sources.

Energy balance refers to the relationship between energy expended and energy stored. When energy expended exceeds energy intake, energy stores are used to supply the deficit; this results in weight loss. Body proteins are used for energy when calorie intake is insufficient. The body attempts to meet its calorie requirements even if it is at the expense of protein needs.

PATHOPHYSIOLOGY

Many severely ill or hospitalized clients experiencing trauma are at risk for **protein-calorie malnutrition (PCM),** also known as protein-energy malnutrition (PEM). PCM may present in three forms: marasmus, kwashiorkor, and marasmic-kwashiorkor. **Marasmus** is generally a calorie malnutrition in which body fat and protein are wasted. Serum proteins are often preserved. **Kwashiorkor** is a lack of protein quantity and quality in the presence of adequate calories. Body weight is more normal, and serum proteins are low. **Marasmic-kwashiorkor** is a combined protein and energy malnutrition. This problem often presents clinically when metabolic stress is imposed on a chronically starved client. The outcome of unrecognized or untreated PCM is often dysfunction or disability and increased morbidity and mortality.

Malnutrition is a multinutrient problem because foods that are good sources of calories and protein are also good sources of other nutrients. In the malnourished client, protein catabolism exceeds protein intake and synthesis, resulting in negative nitrogen balance, weight loss, decreased muscle mass, and weakness.

The functional ability of the liver, heart, lungs, GI tract, and immune system diminishes in the client with malnutrition. A decrease in serum proteins **(hypoproteinemia)** occurs as protein synthesis in the liver decreases. Vital capacity is also reduced as a result of respiratory muscle atrophy; cardiac output diminishes. Malabsorption occurs because of atrophy of GI mucosa and the loss of intestinal villi.

Other common complications of severe malnutrition in adults include the following:

- Leanness and **cachexia** (muscle wasting)
- Decreased activity tolerance
- Lethargy
- Intolerance to cold
- Edema
- Dry, flaking skin and various types of dermatitis
- Poor wound healing
- Infection, particularly postoperative infection

Etiology

Malnutrition, also known as undernutrition, results from inadequate nutrient intake, increased nutrient losses, and increased nutrient requirements. Inadequate nutrient intake can be linked to poverty, lack of education, substance abuse, decreased appetite, and a decline in functional ability to eat independently. Infectious diseases, such as tuberculosis and human immunodeficiency virus (HIV) infection, are also precipitating factors in PCM. Diseases that produce diarrhea and respiratory and other infections leading to anorexia result in negative calorie and protein balance; anorexia then leads to poor food intake. Vomiting leads to decreased absorption with increased nutrient losses. Medical treatments such as chemotherapy can also cause malnutrition. In addition, catabolic processes increase nutrient requirements and metabolic losses.

Inadequate nutrient intake can also result when a person is admitted to the hospital or nursing home (Cowan et al., 2004; Dudek, 2000). Many clients increase their nutritional risk during their hospitalization and therefore need to be frequently reassessed. For example, decreased staffing may not allow time for clients who need to be fed, especially older adults, who may eat slowly (Anderson, 2000). Many diagnostic tests, surgery, and unexpected medical complications require a period of having nothing by mouth (NPO) or anorexia.

CONSIDERATIONS FOR OLDER ADULTS

Unrecognized dysphagia is a common problem in nursing homes and can cause malnutrition, dehydration, and aspiration pneumonia. A nursing study by Kayser-Jones and Pengilly (1999) found that 45 of 82 residents in one nursing home had some degree of dysphagia (difficulty swallowing) ranging from mild to profound. Only 10 of the 45 residents had been referred for dysphagia evaluation by a speech-language pathologist.

Acute PCM may develop in clients who were adequately nourished before hospitalization if they experience starvation while in a catabolic state from infection, stress, or injury. *Chronic* PCM can occur in clients who have cancer, end-stage renal or hepatic disease, or chronic neurologic disease.

Eating disorders, such as anorexia nervosa and bulimia nervosa, also lead to malnutrition. **Anorexia nervosa** is a self-induced starvation resulting from a fear of fatness, even though the client is underweight. **Bulimia nervosa** is characterized by episodes of binge eating in which the client ingests a large amount of food in a short time. The binge eating is followed by some form of purging behavior, such as self-induced vomiting or excessive use of laxatives and diuretics. If not treated, death can result from starvation, infection, or suicide. Information about eating disorders can be found in textbooks on mental/behavioral health nursing.

Incidence/Prevalence

In a review of eight studies with more than 1347 hospitalized adults, 40% to 55% were determined to be malnourished or at risk for malnutrition, and up to 12% were severely malnourished (Dudek, 2000). Malnourished clients heal more slowly, suffer more complications, and have a higher mortality rate. Surgical clients with a likelihood of malnutrition were two to three times more likely to experience minor and major complications and excess mortality. Length of hospitalization in malnourished medical-surgical clients can be extended, which clearly increases health care costs.

COLLABORATIVE MANAGEMENT

PHARM REVIEW

Assessment

HISTORY

Review the medical history to determine the diagnosis, the possibility of increased metabolic needs or nutritional losses, chronic disease, recent surgery of the GI tract, drug and alcohol abuse, and recent significant weight loss. Each of these conditions can contribute to malnutrition. For older adults, explore mental status deterioration and note poor eyesight or hearing, diseases affecting major organs, constipation or incontinence, and slowed reactions. Review prescription and over-the-counter medications (including herbal and natural supplements) and physical disabilities (Chart 64-2).

For clients who live independently, the nurse or occupational therapist may assess the performance of instrumental activities of daily living (IADLs). Functional status can best be evaluated for institutionalized clients by assessing their performance of activities of daily living (ADLs). When functional status is evaluated with nutritional status, there appears to be a strong predictability of infections and complications among institutionalized adults. Chapter 10 describes functional assessment in detail.

CHART 64-2

NURSING FOCUS on the OLDER ADULT
Risk Assessment for Malnutrition

- Recognize that clinical manifestations of malnutrition may not be apparent because they are similar to physiologic changes associated with aging (e.g., dry skin, decreased muscle tone, dry hair).
- Assess body weight and compare it with the usual body weight or ideal body weight.
- Be aware that multiple chronic diseases, especially gastrointestinal disorders such as malabsorption syndromes, predispose the client to malnutrition.
- Assess the client's financial ability to buy healthy food.
- Assess the client's physical and mental ability to prepare food.
- Inspect the client's oral cavity for the presence of teeth or dentures, gum disease, or oral lesions that could affect food intake.
- Review the client's medications, including prescription and over-the-counter (OTC) drugs. Many drugs interact with food or cause anorexia or nausea.
- Use the Mini Nutritional Assessment.

Interview the client to obtain information about his or her usual daily food intake, eating behaviors, change in appetite, and recent weight changes. Ask the client to describe the usual foods eaten daily and the times of meals and snacks. The dietitian can more thoroughly analyze the diet, if necessary, based on the initial nutritional screening.

Explore changes in eating habits as a result of illness, and record any change in appetite, taste, and weight loss. A weight loss of 5% or more in 30 days, a weight loss of 10% in 6 months, or a weight that is below ideal body weight is significant for malnutrition.

Difficulty or pain in chewing or swallowing is also assessed. Ask the client whether any foods are avoided and why. The occurrence of nausea, vomiting, heartburn, or any other symptoms of discomfort with eating is also recorded. Finally, the client is asked about dental health problems, including the presence of dentures. Dentures or partial plates that do not fit well interfere with food intake.

PHYSICAL ASSESSMENT/CLINICAL MANIFESTATIONS

Assess for manifestations of various nutrient deficiencies (Table 64-4). Inspect the client's hair, eyes, oral cavity, nails, and musculoskeletal and neurologic systems. The condition of the skin, including any reddened or open areas, is observed. The previously described anthropometric measurements may also be obtained. The nurse or assistive nursing personnel monitors all food and fluid intake, observes the client at mealtime, and notes any mouth pain or difficulty in chewing or swallowing. A 3-day caloric intake may be collected and then calculated by the dietitian.

PSYCHOSOCIAL ASSESSMENT

The psychosocial history provides information about the client's economic status, occupation, educational level, living and cooking arrangements, and mental status. Determine

TABLE 64-4 Manifestations of Nutrient Deficiencies

Sign/Symptom	Potential Nutrient Deficiency
Hair	
Alopecia	Zinc, essential fatty acids
Easy pluckability	Protein, essential fatty acids
Lackluster hair	Protein, zinc
"Corkscrew" hair	Vitamin C, vitamin A
Decreased pigmentation	Protein, copper
Eyes	
Xerosis of conjunctiva	Vitamin A
Corneal vascularization	Riboflavin
Keratomalacia	Vitamin A
Bitot's spots	Vitamin A
Gastrointestinal Tract	
Nausea, vomiting	Pyridoxine
Diarrhea	Zinc, niacin
Stomatitis	Pyridoxine, riboflavin, iron
Cheilosis	Pyridoxine, iron
Glossitis	Pyridoxine, zinc, niacin, folic acid, vitamin B_{12}
Magenta tongue	Riboflavin
Swollen, bleeding gums	Vitamin C
Fissured tongue	Niacin
Hepatomegaly	Protein
Skin	
Dry and scaling	Vitamin A, essential fatty acids, zinc
Petechiae/ecchymoses	Vitamin C, vitamin K
Follicular hyperkeratosis	Vitamin A, essential fatty acids
Nasolabial seborrhea	Niacin, pyridoxine, riboflavin
Bilateral dermatitis	Niacin, zinc
Extremities	
Subcutaneous fat loss	Calories
Muscle wastage	Calories, protein
Edema	Protein
Osteomalacia, bone pain, rickets	Vitamin D
Arthralgia	Vitamin C
Hematologic	
Anemia	Vitamin B_{12}, iron, folic acid, copper, vitamin E
Leukopenia, neutropenia	Copper
Low prothrombin time, prolonged clotting time	Vitamin K, manganese
Neurologic	
Disorientation	Niacin, thiamine
Confabulation	Thiamine
Neuropathy	Thiamine, pyridoxine, chromium
Paresthesia	Thiamine, pyridoxine, vitamin B_{12}
Cardiovascular	
Congestive heart failure, cardiomegaly, tachycardia	Thiamine
Cardiomyopathy	Selenium

Used with permission of Ross Products Division, Abbott Laboratories, Columbus, OH.

whether financial resources are adequate for providing the necessary food. If resources are inadequate, the social worker may refer the client to available community services. Chapter 5 discusses nutrition in older adults in more detail.

LABORATORY ASSESSMENT

Laboratory tests supply objective data that can support subjective data and identify preclinical deficiencies. However, they must be carefully interpreted with regard to the total client; an isolated value may yield an inaccurate conclusion.

HEMATOLOGY. A low hemoglobin level may indicate anemia, recent hemorrhage, or hemodilution caused by fluid retention. Hemoglobin may also be low secondary to conditions such as low serum albumin, infection, catabolism, or chronic disease. High hemoglobin levels may indicate hemoconcentration or dehydration, or they may be secondary to liver disease.

Low hematocrit levels may reflect anemia, hemorrhage, excessive fluid, renal disease, or cirrhosis. High hematocrit levels may indicate dehydration or hemoconcentration.

PROTEIN STUDIES. Serum albumin, thyroxine-binding prealbumin, and transferrin can be measured in the laboratory. Serum albumin indicates the body's protein status but is not sensitive enough to detect early changes in nutritional status. The normal serum albumin level for men and women is greater than 3.5 g/dL.

Thyroxine-binding **prealbumin (PAB)** provides a more sensitive indicator of protein deficiency because of its short half-life of 2 days. Depending on the laboratory test used, the normal PAB range is 17 to 40 mg/dL. PAB can also assess improvement in nutritional status with refeeding; levels can increase by 1 mg/dL daily with adequate nutritional support.

Although not used as commonly, serum **transferrin,** an iron-transport protein, can be measured directly or calculated as an indirect measurement of total iron-binding capacity (TIBC). It has a short half-life of 8 to 10 days and therefore is also a more sensitive indicator of protein status than is albumin.

SERUM CHOLESTEROL. Cholesterol levels normally range between 160 and 200 mg/dL in adult men and women. Values are typically low with malabsorption, liver disease, pernicious anemia, terminal stages of cancer, or sepsis. A cholesterol level below 160 mg/dL has been identified as a possible indicator of malnutrition.

OTHER LABORATORY TESTS. Total lymphocyte count (TLC) can be used to assess immune function. Malnutrition suppresses the immune system and leaves the client more vulnerable to infection. When a client is malnourished, the TLC is usually decreased to below 1500 mm^3 (Bender et al., 2000).

Critical Thinking Challenge

An older adult was admitted to your unit following a colon resection secondary to cancer. He is a type 2 diabetic and had a coronary artery bypass graft 5 years ago. On admission he was 10 pounds less than ideal body weight. His primary language is German, and he speaks very few English words. Since surgery 2 days ago, his blood glucose levels have been very high and unstable, and he has experienced several episodes of atrial fibrillation. He has refused to eat since surgery because, his wife says, he does not like the food.

1. What risk factors does this client have for malnutrition?
2. What further nutritional assessment should you perform?
3. What laboratory tests would be appropriate for him at this time?
4. What could you suggest at this time to increase his food intake?

evolve For suggested answer guidelines, go to http://evolve.elsevier.com/Iggy/.

Analysis

COMMON NURSING DIAGNOSES AND COLLABORATIVE PROBLEMS

The most common diagnosis for the client with malnutrition is Imbalanced Nutrition: Less Than Body Requirements related to inability to ingest or digest food or absorb nutrients due to biologic, psychological, or economic factors.

ADDITIONAL NURSING DIAGNOSES AND COLLABORATIVE PROBLEMS

In addition to the common nursing diagnosis, clients with malnutrition may have one or more of the following:

- Risk for Impaired Skin Integrity related to alterations in nutritional state
- Risk for Infection related to malnutrition
- Risk for Disturbed Body Image related to biophysical changes from weight loss

Some clients with malnutrition are at risk for collaborative problems such as the following:

- Anemia
- Immunocompromised State
- Multisystem Failure

Planning and Implementation

IMBALANCED NUTRITION: LESS THAN BODY REQUIREMENTS

NOC **PLANNING: EXPECTED OUTCOMES.** The client with malnutrition is expected to have nutrients available to meet metabolic needs. Indicators include that the client will have no deviation from normal range in the following:

- Nutrient intake
- Fluid intake
- Energy
- Weight-height ratio
- Hematocrit
- Muscle tone
- Hydration

INTERVENTIONS. The preferred route for feeding is through the GI tract because it enhances the immune system and is safer, easier, less expensive, and more physiologically sound (Chart 64-3).

NIC **Nutrition Management.** In collaboration with the health care provider and dietitian, provide high-calorie, high-protein foods (e.g., milkshakes, cheese and crackers). A feeding schedule of six small meals benefits many clients. If the client has difficulty chewing or is **edentulous** (toothless), a pureed or dental soft diet may facilitate food intake.

Malnourished ill clients often need to be encouraged to eat. The nurse or assistive nursing personnel provides a quiet environment, which is conducive to eating. Some clients, especially older adults, may take a long time to eat even small quantities of food.

Restorative feeding programs help nursing home residents who need special assistance. These residents eat in a separate dining area so that time and attention can be given to them. Chart 64-4 offers additional interventions to increase nutritional intake for older adults in any setting.

Drug Therapy. Medications may be given to some clients to stimulate appetite. For example, cyproheptadine (Periactin), an antihistamine, may be prescribed for clients who are underweight, especially those with eating disorders. Megestrol acetate (Megace), an antineoplastic drug, may be used to increase appetite in clients who have cachexia, acquired immunodeficiency syndrome (AIDS), or unexplained weight loss. The mechanism for how these drugs work to increase appetite is unknown.

Partial Enteral Nutrition. The dietitian calculates the nutrients required daily and translates these requirements into meals for the client. If the client cannot ingest sufficient nutrients as food, **partial enteral nutrition (PEN)** with fortified medical nutritional supplements (MNSs) (e.g., Boost, Ensure, or Carnation Instant Breakfast) may be given, especially for older adults. Many commercial enteral products are available. For clients with medical diagnoses such as liver and renal disease or diabetes, special products that meet their needs are also available. The client must en-

CHART 64-3

NIC INTERVENTION ACTIVITIES for The Client with Malnutrition

Nutrition Management: *Assisting with or providing a balanced dietary intake of foods and fluids*

- Ascertain client's food preferences.
- Determine, in collaboration with dietitian as appropriate, number of calories and type of nutrients needed to meet nutrition requirements.
- Encourage increased intake of protein, iron, and vitamin C, as appropriate.
- Offer snacks (e.g., frequent drinks, fresh fruits/fruit juice), as appropriate.
- Adjust diet to client's lifestyle, as appropriate.
- Weigh client at appropriate intervals.
- Encourage client to wear properly fitted dentures and/or obtain dental care.
- Assist client in receiving help from appropriate community nutritional programs, as needed.

NIC intervention activities selected from Dochterman J.M., & Bulechek, G.M. (Eds.). (2004). *Nursing intervention classification (NIC)* (4th ed.). St Louis: Mosby. No part of this work is to be altered without prior written permission from the Publisher.

CHART 64-4

NURSING FOCUS on the OLDER ADULT
Promoting Nutritional Intake

- Observe the client during meals for food intake.
- Ask the client about food likes and dislikes.
- Encourage self-feeding, or feed the client slowly.
- Create an environment that is conducive to eating and socialization and relaxation, if possible.
- Decrease distractions, such as environmental noise from television, music, or other people.
- Provide adequate, nonglaring lighting.
- Keep away from offensive or medicinal odors.
- Keep eye contact with the client during the meal.
- Serve snacks with activities, especially in long-term care settings.
- Document the percentage of food eaten at each meal and snack.
- Ensure that meals are visually appealing, appetizing, and properly prepared.
- Review the client's medication profile, and discuss with the health care provider the use of drugs that might be suppressing appetite.
- If the client is depressed, be sure that the depression is treated by the health care provider.

joy the taste of the product for acceptability and optimal intake.

Nutritional supplements are supplied as liquid formulas, powders, bars, and puddings in a variety of flavors. They come in different degrees of sweetness and are also available as modular supplements that provide single nutrients. Examples of modular supplements are Polycose for carbohydrates and ProPac for protein. Carbohydrate modulars are useful only if additional calories are needed. Protein modulars are indicated when metabolic stress causes a need for higher protein intake.

CONSIDERATIONS FOR OLDER ADULTS

Supplements used in acute care, long-term care, and home care are costly. In addition, older adults may refuse them, and the supplements are then wasted. Bender at al. (2000) found that a more successful alternative to having the MNS distributed by food service or nursing assistant staff in the nursing home was to have the supplements delivered by nurses during their usual medication passes. In this study, the nurses gave 60 mL or more of the MNS at least four times a day with the clients' medications. The subjects increased weight and had fewer pressure ulcers, thus making the program very cost-effective.

LEGAL/ETHICAL ISSUES

TOTAL ENTERAL NUTRITION FOR OLDER ADULTS

Total enteral nutrition provides a client's total daily nutrient and fluid requirements. In some cases, this artificial nutrition and hydration may not be desired by the older adult. For example, some clients have advance directives stating that they do not want to be kept alive by artificial nutrition and hydration if certain conditions exist. However, questions arise when clients are not able to make their wishes known.

For many years it was believed that withholding food and fluids would cause discomfort. Recent cancer research indicates that clients who do not eat and drink do not suffer and in fact may be more comfortable if food and fluids are withheld. The decision to feed is complex, and there is no clear right or wrong answer. To compound this dilemma, medical complications (e.g., aspiration, pressure ulcers) are common in older adults who are tube fed.

When clinicians are making decisions about the desirability of tube feedings in these cases, the focus should be on achieving consensus by doing the following:

- Reviewing what is known about tube feedings, especially their risks and benefits
- Reviewing the medical facts about the client
- Investigating any available evidence that would help understand the client's wishes
- Obtaining the opinions of all stakeholders in the situation
- Delaying any action until consensus is achieved

The nurse or assistive nursing personnel maintains a daily calorie count and fluid intake to assess whether the client can meet the goals of nutritional therapy. The dietitian usually asks the nursing staff to keep the food intake record for at least three consecutive days. Accurate daily or weekly weights are also essential, depending on the amount of depletion.

Total Enteral Nutrition. Clients often cannot meet the goals of nutritional therapy through their usual oral intake because of increased metabolic demands or a decreased ability to eat. Therefore enteral tube feeding may be necessary to supplement oral intake or to provide total nutritional support.

Candidates for Total Enteral Nutrition. Clients likely to receive **total enteral nutrition (TEN)** can be divided into three groups:

- Clients who can eat but cannot maintain adequate nutrition by oral intake of food alone
- Clients who have permanent neuromuscular impairment and cannot swallow
- Clients who do not have permanent neuromuscular impairment but are critically ill and cannot eat because of their condition

Clients in the first group are often older adults or clients receiving cancer treatment who cannot meet their calorie and protein needs (see the Legal/Ethical Issues box above). Clients in the second group usually have permanent swallowing problems and require some type of feeding tube for delivery of the enteral product on a long-term basis. Examples of conditions that can cause permanent swallowing problems are strokes, severe head trauma, and advanced multiple sclerosis. Clients in the third group receive enteral nutrition for as long as their illness lasts. The feeding is discontinued when the client's condition improves and he or she can eat again. TEN is contraindicated for clients with diffuse peritonitis, severe pancreatitis, intestinal obstruction, intractable vomiting or diarrhea, and paralytic ileus.

Types of Enteral Products. Many commercially prepared enteral products are available. An appropriate combination of carbohydrates, fat, vitamins, minerals, and trace elements is available in liquid form. Differences among products allow the dietitian to select the right formula for each client. An order from the health care provider is required for enteral nutrition, but the dietitian usually makes the recommendation and computes the amount and type of product needed for each client.

Methods of Administration of Total Enteral Nutrition. Total enteral nutrition is administered as "tube feedings" through one of the available GI tubes, either via a **nasoenteric tube (NET)** or an **enterostomal tube.** It can be used in the client's home or any health care setting.

Types of Tubes. A NET is any feeding tube inserted nasally and then advanced into the GI tract. Commonly used NETs include the **nasogastric (NG) tube** and the **nasoduodenal tube (NDT).** A nasojejunal tube (NJT) is also available but is used less often than the other NETs. The NDTs and NJTs are usually indicated for critically ill clients at risk for aspiration or delayed stomach emptying.

The NETs are used for delivering short-term enteral feedings because they are easy to use and are safer for the client at risk for aspiration *if* the tip of the tube is placed below the pyloric sphincter of the stomach. Small-bore polyurethane or silicone tubes from 8 to 12 Fr external diameter are preferred over large-bore plastic or latex tubes. The smaller tubes are more comfortable and are less likely to cause complications such as nasal irritation, sinusitis, tissue erosion, and pulmonary compromise.

Enterostomal feeding tubes are used for clients who need long-term enteral feeding. The most common types are gastrostomies and jejunostomies. The physician directly accesses the GI tract using various surgical, endoscopic, and laparoscopic techniques.

A **gastrostomy** is a stoma created from the abdominal wall into the stomach, through which a short feeding tube

CHART 64-5

BEST PRACTICE for
Tube Feeding Care and Maintenance

- If nasogastric or nasoduodenal feeding is ordered, use a soft, flexible, small-bore feeding tube (smaller than 12 Fr). The initial placement of the tube should be confirmed by x-ray study. Secure the tube with tape or a commercial attachment device after applying a skin protectant; change the tape regularly.
- Check tube placement by x-ray study when the correct position of the tube is in question; an x-ray study is the only reliable method. Checking the pH of the aspirant is the preferred method for rechecking placement after an x-ray.
- If a gastrostomy or jejunostomy tube is used, assess the insertion site for signs of infection or excoriation (e.g., excessive redness, drainage). Rotate the tube 360 degrees each day, and check for in-and-out play of about ¼ inch (0.5 cm). If the tube cannot be moved, notify the health care provider immediately because the retention disk may be embedded in the tissue. Cover the site with a dry sterile dressing, and change the dressing at least once a day.
- Check and record the residual volume every 4 hours by aspirating stomach contents into a syringe. If residual feeding is obtained, check the health care provider's order for the appropriate intervention (usually to slow or stop the feeding for a time).
- Check the feeding pump to ensure proper mechanical operation.
- Ensure that the prescribed enteral product is infused at the prescribed rate (mL/hr).
- Change the feeding bag and tubing every 24 hours; label the bag with the date and time of the change. Use an irrigation set for no more than 24 hours.
- For continuous or cyclic feeding, add only 4 hours of product to the bag at a time to prevent bacterial growth; a closed system may be used for 24 hours.
- Wear clean gloves when changing or opening the feeding system or adding product; wear sterile gloves for critically ill or immunocompromised clients.
- Do not use blue (or any color) food dye in formula because it does not prevent aspiration and can cause serious complications (Maloney et al., 2002).
- To prevent aspiration, keep the head of the bed elevated at least 30 degrees during the feeding and at least 1 hour after the feeding for bolus feeding; maintain semi-Fowler's position for clients receiving cyclic or continuous feeding.
- Monitor laboratory values, especially blood urea nitrogen (BUN), serum electrolytes, hematocrit, prealbumin, and glucose.
- Monitor for complications of tube feeding, especially diarrhea.
- Monitor and carefully record the client's weight and intake and output.

is inserted by the physician. The gastrostomy may require a small abdominal incision, or it may be placed endoscopically; these tubes are called **percutaneous endoscopic gastrostomy (PEG)** or dual-access gastrostomy-jejunostomy (PEG/J) tubes. The PEG does not require general anesthesia and is more secure and more durable than traditional gastrostomies. An alternative to either device is the **low-profile gastrostomy device (LPGD).** The LPGD is available with a firm or balloon-style internal bumper or retention disk. An antireflux valve keeps GI contents from leaking onto the skin. This device is less irritating to the skin, longer lasting, and more cosmetically pleasing, and it allows greater client independence. However, skin-level devices do not allow easy access for checking residuals.

Jejunostomies are used less often than gastrostomies. A **jejunostomy** is used for long-term feedings when it is desirable to bypass the stomach, such as with gastric disease,

CHART 64-6

BEST PRACTICE for
Maintaining a Patent Feeding Tube

- Flush the tube with 30 to 60 mL of water (amount usually prescribed by the health care provider or dietitian):
  At least every 4 hours during a continuous tube feeding
  Before and after each intermittent tube feeding
  Before and after medication administration (use warm water)
  After checking residual volume
- If the tube becomes clogged, use 30 mL of water for flushing, applying gentle pressure with a 50-mL piston syringe.
- Avoid the use of carbonated beverage, except for existing clogs *when water is not effective*. Do not use cranberry juice.
- Whenever possible, use liquid medications instead of crushed tablets unless liquid forms cause diarrhea.
- Do not mix medications with the feeding product. Crush tablets as finely as possible and dissolve in warm water. *(Check to see which tablets are safe to crush. For example, do not crush slow-acting [SA] or slow-release [SR] medications.)*
- Consider use of automatic flush feeding pump such as Flexiflo, Quantum, or Kangaroo.

upper GI obstruction, and abnormal gastric or duodenal emptying.

Types of Feedings. Tube feedings are administered by bolus feeding, continuous feeding, and cyclic feeding. **Bolus feeding** is an intermittent feeding of a specified amount of enteral product at specified times during a 24-hour period, typically every 4 hours. This method can be accomplished manually or by infusion through a mechanical pump or controller device. A more popular method of tube feeding is continuous enteral feeding. **Continuous feeding** is similar to IV therapy in that small amounts are continuously infused (by gravity drip or by a pump or controller device) over a specified time. The most commonly seen type, **cyclic feeding,** is the same as continuous feeding except the infusion is stopped for a specified time in each 24-hour period, usually 6 to 10 or more hours ("down time"). Down time typically occurs in the morning to allow bathing, treatments, and other activities.

Infusion rates for cyclic feedings (and to some extent for intermittent bolus feeding) vary with the total amount of solution to be infused, the specific composition of the product, and the response of the client to the procedure. The health care provider and dietitian usually decide the type, rate, and method of tube feeding as well as the amount of additional water needed. If the client can swallow small amounts of food, he or she may also eat orally while the tube is in place.

The nurse is responsible for the care and maintenance of the feeding tube and the enteral feeding. Chart 64-5 lists best practices for the client receiving enteral nutrition (Padula et al., 2004).

Complications of Total Enteral Nutrition. The nurse is responsible for the prevention, assessment, and management of complications associated with tube feeding. Some complications of therapy result from the type of tube used to administer the feeding, and other complications result from the enteral product itself. The most common problem associated with feeding tubes is the development of a clogged tube. Chart 64-6 lists best practices for maintaining a patent tube.

Aspiration. A less common but more serious complication is dislodgment of the tube, which can cause aspiration.

Several techniques should be used to confirm proper placement. *An x-ray is the most accurate confirmation method and should always be done on initial tube insertion.* After the initial placement is confirmed, check the placement before each intermittent feeding or at least every 4 to 8 hours during continuous or cyclic feeding.

The traditional auscultatory method is *not* reliable, especially for clients with small-bore tubes. In this method, the nurse instills 20 to 30 mL of air into the tube while listening over the stomach with a stethoscope. *The resulting whooshing sound that results does not guarantee correct tube placement!* Instead, aspirate a sample of the GI content, observe its color, and test its pH. When aspirating fluid, wait at least 1 hour after medication administration, and then flush the tube with 20 mL of air to clear it. Collect the aspirate and test with pH paper. The pH of gastric fluid ranges from 0 to 4.0. If the tube has migrated down into the intestines, the pH will be between 7.0 and 8.0. If the tube is in the lungs, the pH will be greater than 6.0 (Metheny et al., 1998). The pH may also be as high as 6 if the client takes certain medications, such as H_2 blockers (e.g., ranitidine [Zantac] and famotidine [Pepcid]). Because these drugs affect pH, research using bilirubin testing is ongoing as perhaps a more reliable and valid method for predicting tube location (Metheny, Smith, & Stewart, 2000; Metheny & Stewart, 2002).

Fluid Excess. Clients receiving enteral nutrition therapy are at an increased risk for fluid imbalances. Clients who receive this therapy are often older or debilitated and may also have cardiac or renal problems. Fluid imbalances associated with enteral nutrition are usually related to the body's response to increased serum osmolarity, but fluid overload can also occur.

Increased Osmolarity. Osmolarity is the amount or concentration of particles dissolved in solution. This concentration exerts a specific osmotic pressure within the solution. Normal osmolarity of extracellular fluid (ECF) ranges between 270 and 300 mOsm. Enteral feeding products range in osmolarity from isotonic (about 300 mOsm) to extremely hypertonic (600 mOsm). Electrolytes (including sodium) contribute to this hypertonicity, but more of the osmolarity is determined by the concentration of proteins and sugar molecules in the enteral product. Even when the product is isotonic, the ECF can become hyperosmolar unless some hypotonic fluids are also administered to the client. This situation is most likely to develop in clients who are unconscious, unable to respond to the thirst reflex, on fluid restrictions, or receiving hyperosmotic enteral preparations.

An increase in the osmolarity of the plasma increases the osmotic pressure of the plasma. Because this increased osmolarity is largely a result of extra glucose and proteins (which tend to remain in the plasma rather than move to interstitial spaces), the plasma osmotic pressure (water-pulling pressure) is increased. In this situation, intracellular and interstitial water moves into and expands the plasma volume. This volume expansion results in an increased renal excretion of water (among clients with normal renal function) and leads to osmotic dehydration. If clients do not have normal renal and cardiac function, expansion of the plasma volume can lead to circulatory overload and the formation of pulmonary edema, especially in older adults. Assess for signs and symptoms of circulatory overload, and collaborate with the dietitian and physician in planning the correct amount of fluid to be provided to the client.

Dehydration. Excessive diarrhea may develop when hyperosmolar enteral preparations are delivered quickly. This situation can also lead to dehydration through excessive water loss. Consult with the health care provider and dietitian for recommendations to prevent diarrhea.

First the dietitian usually changes the feeding to a more iso-osmolar formula. Most of these formulas can be started full strength but slowly at 15 to 20 mL/hr. The rate is gradually increased as the client tolerates and as the expected nutritional outcome is achieved.

If diarrhea continues, the client should be evaluated for *Clostridium difficile* or other infectious organisms. Contamination can occur because of repeated and often faulty handling of the feeding solution and system. Some researchers recommend that clean gloves be used when changing systems and adding product. Sterile gloves may help to prevent infection in critically ill or immunocompromised clients. Tubes with medication ports also minimize contamination by preventing opening the feeding system to administer medications (Padula et al., 2004).

In some cases, diarrhea may be the result of liquid medications, such as elixirs and suspensions that have a very high osmolarity. Examples include acetaminophen, digoxin, furosemide, phenytoin, and potassium chloride. Clients receiving multiple liquid medications need to be evaluated to determine whether their drug regimen can be changed to prevent diarrhea. Diluting these liquids may also be an option.

Electrolyte Imbalances. Depending on the client's state of health, certain electrolyte imbalances can be avoided. This is achieved by the use of enteral preparations containing lower concentrations of the electrolytes that the client cannot handle well.

In addition to the client's specific electrolyte imbalances, the two most common electrolyte imbalances associated with enteral nutrition therapy are hyperkalemia and hypernatremia. Both of these conditions may be related to hyperglycemia-induced hyperosmolarity of the plasma and the resultant osmotic diuresis. Electrolyte imbalances are discussed in detail in Chapter 16.

Parenteral Nutrition. When a client cannot effectively use the GI tract for nutrition, parenteral nutrition therapy may maintain or improve his or her nutritional status. This form of IV therapy differs from standard IV therapy in that *all* nutrients (carbohydrates, proteins, fats, vitamins, minerals, and trace elements) can be delivered to the client. One liter of fluid containing 5% dextrose, which is often used as standard IV therapy, provides only 170 kcal. A hospitalized client typically receives 3 or 4 L a day, for a total number of calories ranging between 500 and 700 a day. This calorie intake is not sufficient when the client requires IV therapy for a prolonged period and cannot eat an adequate diet or has increased calorie needs for tissue repair and building.

Parenteral nutrition (**hyperalimentation,** or "hyperal") is subdivided into two categories:

- Partial parenteral nutrition, or peripheral parenteral nutrition
- Total parenteral nutrition, or central parenteral nutrition

As suggested by the names, these categories differ by the site of administration and the content of the solutions.

Partial Parenteral Nutrition. **Partial parenteral nutrition (PPN)** provides nutritional support to clients who are unable or unwilling to take a feeding via the GI tract. It is typically used when a client has a prolonged postoperative ileus or when placement of a central IV line is not advised. It is used when nutritional support is needed for less than 14 days. The client should be able to tolerate large fluid volumes and have readily accessible peripheral veins.

Usually PPN is delivered through a cannula or catheter in a large distal vein of the arm. Two types of solutions are commonly used in various combinations for PPN: lipid (fat) emulsions and amino acid dextrose solutions.

Most lipid emulsions (20%) are isotonic, but the tonicity of commercially prepared amino acid dextrose solutions ranges from 300 mOsm to nearly 1200 mOsm. Amino acid dextrose solutions are considered more stable than the lipid emulsions, and therefore additives (e.g., vitamins, minerals, electrolytes, and trace elements) tend to be mixed with the amino acid dextrose solutions. The amino acid dextrose solution must be delivered through an in-line filter. Lipids and amino acid dextrose solutions are administered by a pump or controller device for accuracy and constancy in delivery rate.

Most PPN products are a *mixture* of lipids (10% or 20% fat emulsion) and an amino acid dextrose (usually 10%) solution. This mixture of three types of nutrients is referred to as a 3:1, total nutrient admixture (TNA), or triple-mix solution.

Total Parenteral Nutrition. When the client requires intensive nutritional support for an extended time, the health care provider prescribes centrally administered **total parenteral nutrition (TPN).** TPN is delivered through access to central veins, usually the subclavian or internal jugular veins. Central venous catheters and associated nursing care are described in detail in Chapter 17.

Total parenteral nutrition solutions contain higher concentrations of dextrose and proteins, usually in the form of synthetic amino acids or protein hydrolysates (3% to 5%). These solutions are hyperosmotic (three to six times the osmolarity of normal blood). The base solutions are available as commercially prepared solutions. The hospital or community pharmacist adds components (specific electrolytes, minerals, trace elements, and insulin) according to the client's nutritional needs. This therapy provides needed calories and spares body proteins from catabolism for energy requirements.

The TPN solutions should be administered with an infusion pump. The osmolarity of the fluid and the concentrations of the specific components make controlled delivery essential.

Complications of Parenteral Nutrition. Clients receiving PPN or TPN are at risk for a wide variety of serious and potentially life-threatening complications. Complications may result from the PPN and TPN solutions or from the central venous catheter. The following discussion is limited to the complications of PPN and TPN that involve fluid or electrolyte balance. Complications of IV cannulas and central venous catheters are discussed in Chapter 17.

Fluid Imbalances. Clients receiving PPN or TPN are at increased risk for fluid imbalance. Not only is fluid delivered directly into the venous system, but the extreme hyperosmolarity of the solutions stimulates fluid shifts between body fluid compartments.

The hyperosmolarity of parenteral nutrition solutions is caused by their amino acid and dextrose concentrations. Increased dextrose causes hyperglycemia. As a result, some of the dextrose moves into the interstitial and intracellular spaces, where it is metabolized. However, dextrose remains in the plasma volume when the solutions are administered too rapidly, without enough insulin coverage, or in the presence of hyponatremia and hypokalemia. The result is a shift of water from the interstitial and intracellular spaces into the plasma. Expansion of the plasma volume together with hyperglycemia can cause osmotic diuresis and lead to serious dehydration and hypovolemic shock. If the client has an accompanying cardiac or renal dysfunction, the situation can lead to overhydration, congestive heart failure, and pulmonary edema.

Monitor for these complications by taking daily weights and by recording accurate intake and output while the client is receiving parenteral nutrition. Serum glucose and electrolyte values are also monitored (Chart 64-7). Any major changes or abnormalities are reported to the health care provider.

Electrolyte Imbalances. Clients receiving either PPN or TPN are at an increased risk for many different electrolyte imbalances, depending on the electrolyte composition of the solution and whether a fluid imbalance occurs. The health care provider usually orders daily determinations of serum electrolyte levels to detect these imbalances. The risk of metabolic and electrolyte complications is reduced when the rate of administration is carefully controlled and clients are closely monitored for response to treatment. Potassium and sodium imbalances are common among clients receiving PPN and TPN, especially when insulin is also administered as part of the therapy. Calcium imbalances, especially hypercalcemia, are associated with PPN and TPN, although immobility may play more of a role than the actual parenteral therapy in the development of this imbalance.

Effects of Medication. No specific drug therapy for malnutrition has been established, although multivita-

CHART 64-7

BEST PRACTICE for
Care and Maintenance of Total Parenteral Nutrition

- Check each bag of total parenteral nutrition (TPN) solution for accuracy by comparing it with the physician's order.
- Monitor the IV pump for accuracy in delivering the prescribed hourly rate.
- If the TPN solution is temporarily unavailable, give 10% dextrose/water (D/W) or 20% D/W until the TPN solution can be obtained.
- If the TPN administration is not on time ("behind"), do not attempt to "catch up" by increasing the rate.
- Monitor the client's weight daily or according to agency protocol.
- Monitor serum electrolytes and glucose daily or per agency protocol. (Some agencies require finger stick blood sugars [FSBSs] every 4 hours, especially if the client is receiving insulin. Urine testing for ketones may also be ordered.)
- Monitor and carefully record the client's intake and output.
- Assess the client's IV site for signs of infection or infiltration (see Chapter 17).
- Change the IV tubing every 24 hours or per agency protocol.
- Change the dressing around the IV site every 48 to 72 hours or per agency protocol.

mins and an iron preparation may be prescribed to treat or prevent anemia. Carefully review the client's medications because of food-medication interactions. Medications can affect nutritional status, and the foods ingested can affect the efficacy of medications.

Community-Based Care

Malnourished clients can be cared for in a variety of settings, including the acute care hospital, transitional care unit, nursing home, or their own home. Malnutrition is often diagnosed when the client is admitted to the acute care hospital or as a consequence of events that occur after hospitalization, such as poor wound healing or sepsis. If the client is severely compromised, he or she may require admission to a traditional nursing home for either transitional or long-term care and be followed by a case manager. If adequate home support is available, the client may be discharged to home in the care of a family member, significant other, or other caregiver. Home care nurses may be needed to monitor and direct the care.

HEALTH TEACHING

The dietitian instructs the malnourished client and the family about high-calorie, high-protein diet and nutritional supplements. The pharmacist reviews any parenteral solutions with the client and family or significant others.

Reinforce the importance of adhering to the diet, and review any medications the client may be taking. If the client takes an iron preparation, teach the importance of taking the medication immediately before or during meals. Caution the client that iron tends to cause constipation. For the older adult already susceptible to constipation, emphasize the importance of measures for prevention, including adequate fiber intake, adequate fluids, and exercise.

Some clients are discharged to home with enteral or parenteral nutrition. Teach the family or other caregiver how to continue these therapies. Remind caregivers to consider also the psychosocial aspects of these alternative methods for nutrition. For example, the caregiver can bring the enteral product, napkin, and funnel to the client on a decorative tray to make the feeding experience more elegant and "normal." Moving the feeding equipment out of view of the client when it is not in use is another consideration (Nickel, 2004).

HOME CARE MANAGEMENT

The malnourished client needs a variety of resources at home to continue aggressive nutrition support. If the client can consume food by the oral route, the case manager or other discharge planner determines whether his or her financial resources are adequate for providing the necessary food and nutrition supplements. If the hospital provides ambulatory nutrition counseling services, the client is scheduled for follow-up after discharge for assessment of weight gain.

HEALTH CARE RESOURCES

The malnourished client discharged to home on enteral or parenteral nutrition support needs the specialized services of a home nutrition therapy team. This team generally consists of the physician, nurse, dietitian, pharmacist, and social worker. Several commercial companies supply these services to clients in addition to the feeding supplies and formulas.

◆ Evaluation: Outcomes

Evaluate the care of the malnourished client on the basis of the identified nursing diagnoses and collaborative problems. The primary expected outcome is that the client has available nutrients to meet metabolic demands. Specific indicators for this outcome are listed for the nursing diagnosis under the Planning: Expected Outcomes section (see earlier).

OBESITY

PATHOPHYSIOLOGY

Obesity, like cancer, is not just one disease but rather many conditions with varying causes. The terms **obesity** and **overweight** are often used interchangeably, but they refer to different health problems. Overweight is an increase in body weight for height compared with a reference standard, such as the Metropolitan Life height and weight tables (see Table 64-3) or 10% greater than ideal body weight (IBW). However, this weight may not reflect excess body fat. It is possible for well-developed athletes to appear overweight because of increased muscle mass; in such cases the proportion of muscle to fat is greater than average.

An obese person weighs at least 20% above the upper limit of the normal range for ideal body weight. **Morbid obesity** refers to a weight that has a severely negative effect on health–usually more than 100% above IBW or a body mass index (BMI) greater than 40.

Obesity refers to an excess amount of body fat. It is possible to be obese at a weight that is within normal range according to a reference standard. The normal amount of body fat in *men* is between 15% and 20% of body weight. For *women,* the normal amount is 18% to 32%.

A number of chemicals in the body affect appetite and fat metabolism. Some of the most common ones that are thought to play a role in obesity include the following:

- **Leptin,** a hormone that is released by fat cells and possibly by gastric cells; it also acts on the hypothalamus to control appetite
- **Insulin,** a hormone that controls the metabolism of glucose, fat, and protein
- **Resistin,** a hormone produced by fat cells that creates resistance to insulin activity
- **Agouti-related protein,** a protein controlled by leptin that regulates calorie consumption
- **Wnt-10b,** a protein that inhibits fat cell formation
- **Cholecystokinin,** a hormone that stimulates digestive juices and may work with leptin to increase or decrease appetite
- **PYY,** a hormone that indicates stomach fullness and helps to limit food intake

Additional research is needed to determine the exact mechanisms by which these substances work together to cause weight gain.

Obesity Indexes

To establish the percentage of IBW, the height and weight of the client are compared with the midpoint of the desirable weight for a medium frame of the client's height and gender in the Metropolitan Life height and weight tables (see Table 64-3). The body mass index (BMI), as described previously on p. 1426, is a measure of heaviness and is only an indirect indicator of body fat. It reflects the combined effects of body build, proportions, lean body mass, and body fat. However, BMI has exhibited substantial correlations with fat mass for adult men and women and has been validated as a risk factor for cardiovascular disease. As a general rule, a BMI of 30 or more indicates obesity and an increased risk for health problems. A BMI of 27 to 30 indicates overweight. Arm and calf circumference and skin-fold measurements more completely define body composition and adiposity (described earlier).

The distribution of excess body fat rather than the degree of obesity has been used to predict increased health risks. For example, in premenopausal women, the waist circumference (WC) is a stronger predictor of coronary artery disease (CAD) than is the BMI. Lofgren et al. (2004) found that women with a WC greater than 88 cm had the highest risk for biomarkers of CAD.

The waist-to-hip ratio (WHR) is also a predictor of CAD. This measure differentiates a predominantly peripheral lower body obesity from a central upper body obesity. A WHR of 0.95 or greater in men (0.8 or greater in women) indicates android obesity with excess fat at the waist and abdomen; this pattern carries the greatest health risk. Excessive abdominal fat may also enhance the risk for gallbladder disease.

Complications of Obesity

The major complications of obesity include the following:

- Diabetes mellitus
- Hypertension
- **Hyperlipidemia** (increased serum lipids)
- CAD
- Obstructive sleep apnea
- Obesity hypoventilation syndrome
- Depression and other mental health/behavioral health problems
- Urinary incontinence
- **Cholelithiasis** (gallbladder stones)
- Chronic back pain
- Early osteoarthritis
- Decreased wound healing

Obese people are also more susceptible to infections and infectious diseases than are thinner people.

Etiology and Genetic Risk

The causes of obesity involve complex interrelationships of many environmental, genetic, and behavioral factors. A number of causes of both human and animal obesity have been identified.

The first cause is dietary obesity associated with *high-fat and high-cholesterol diets.* Data repeatedly suggest that obesity is associated with diet when it contains a significant amount of saturated fat, which increases low-density lipoproteins (LDL-C). Trans-fat (trans-fatty acids) and cholesterol also contribute significantly. By contrast, monosaturated and polysaturated fats are healthy fats.

Trans-fat is made when food manufacturers add hydrogen to vegetable oil, a process known as hydrogenation. This process increases the food's shelf life and flavor. Large amounts of trans-fat can be found in vegetable shortening, commercial cookies, snack foods, and French fries. For many years, food labels have included amounts of total fat, saturated fat, and cholesterol content per serving. However, the amount of trans-fat has not been revealed. Manufacturers will be required to publish the amount of trans-fat in their foods starting in 2006.

Physical inactivity has been identified as another cause. The major identified barriers to increasing physical activity include a lack of time or decreased mobility associated with prolonged illness. Regular exercise is associated with lower death rates for adults of any age. It also increases lean muscle, decreases body fat, aids in weight control, and enhances psychological well-being. Regular exercise can also decrease the risk of falling in older adults (see Chapter 5).

The third major cause of obesity is *drug treatment.* Some prescribed medications contribute to weight gain when they are taken on a long-term basis. Drugs that promote obesity include the following:

- Corticosteroids
- Estrogens and certain progestins
- Nonsteroidal anti-inflammatory drugs
- Antihypertensives
- Antidepressants and other psychoactive drugs
- Antiepileptic drugs
- Certain oral hypoglycemics

Familial and genetic factors play a very important role in obesity. When both parents are overweight, about 80% of their children will be overweight. If neither parent is overweight, fewer than 10% of the children will be overweight. In studies of identical twins, nonidentical twins, and parent-sibling relationships, about 50% of the difference in body fatness is transmitted to children and about 50% of this amount is genetically controlled.

Genetic composition may predispose some people, but not others, to obesity. Researchers have identified the ***ob* gene** in mice, which helps to regulate energy balance. Leptin, the hormone encoded by the *ob* gene, appears to send a message to the brain that the body has stored enough fat; this message serves as a signal to stop eating. In some obese individuals, other gene mutations have been identified, including an abnormality of the melano-cortin-4 receptor that inhibits appetite in families with a history of obesity. Other genetic factors have been associated with uncommon diseases, such as the Prader-Willi syndrome.

A small number of obese individuals have disorders of the neuroendocrine system. Examples include injury to the hypothalamus, Cushing's disease, polycystic ovary failure, hypogonadism, growth hormone deficiency, and insulinoma.

Incidence/Prevalence

More than one third of the U.S. population is obese, and another third is overweight. About 6% to 10% of adults are morbidly obese (Gallagher, 2004). The total cost (medical cost and lost productivity) of obesity is more than $100 billion each year. In 2000, more than 100 million adults in the United States were overweight or obese.

HEALTH PROMOTION/ILLNESS PREVENTION

Obesity is a major public health problem and is associated with many complications, including death. As a result of this increasing problem, the Healthy People 2010 agenda addresses the need to reduce the proportion of children,

Meeting HEALTHY PEOPLE 2010 Objectives

NUTRITION AND OVERWEIGHT

Objective 19.2: Reduce the proportion of adults who are obese.

- Teach the client the potential consequences and complications of obesity.
- Teach the client the importance of eating a healthy diet, including a variety of foods, especially grain products, vegetables, and fruits. The diet should be moderate in salt and sugar and low in fats and cholesterol.
- Remind the client that foods eaten away from home tend to be higher in fat, cholesterol, and salt and are lower in calcium than foods prepared at home.
- Reinforce the need to engage regularly in moderate physical activity for at least 30 minutes each day.
- Begin education regarding diet and physical activity for children and adolescents, and continue throughout adulthood. (Once an adolescent becomes overweight, he or she is likely to remain overweight.)

adolescents, and adults who are obese. Nurses can help meet this goal through education and role modeling (see the Meeting Healthy People 2010 Objectives box above).

COLLABORATIVE MANAGEMENT

Assessment

HISTORY

In collaboration with the dietitian, collect the following information about the client:

- Economic status
- Usual food intake
- Eating behavior
- Cultural background
- Attitude toward food
- Appetite
- Chronic diseases
- Medications
- Physical activity
- Family history of obesity

A diet history usually incorporates a 24-hour recall of food intake and the frequency with which foods are consumed. The adequacy of the diet can be rapidly evaluated by comparing the amount and types of foods consumed daily with the Dietary Guidelines for Americans (see Figure 64-1). Gross inadequacies for specific nutrients can be identified using this approach. The dietitian can provide a more detailed analysis of dietary intake.

PHYSICAL ASSESSMENT/CLINICAL MANIFESTATIONS

Obtain an accurate height and weight. The dietitian then calculates the percentage of ideal body weight (% IBW) and the body mass index (BMI). The dietitian may also do the following:

- Measure the waist circumference
- Calculate the waist-hip ratio
- Determine arm and calf circumferences

Examine the skin of the obese client for reddened or open areas. Lift skin-fold areas, such as pendulous breasts and abdominal apron (also called a **panniculus**), to observe for *Candida* (yeast) or other infections and excoriations. Infection of the panniculus is referred to as **panniculitis.**

PSYCHOSOCIAL ASSESSMENT

Obtain a psychosocial history to determine the client's circumstances and emotional factors that might prevent successful therapy or that might be worsened by therapy. Interview the client to determine his or her perception of current weight. Some clients do not view weight as a problem, which affects treatment and outcome. Others experience low self-esteem and have a disturbed body image.

Explore the client's past history to assess the following:

- Cause and duration of weight gain
- Family history of obesity
- Past attempts at weight reduction and outcomes
- Effects of obesity on lifestyle
- Effects of obesity on social interactions
- History of mental health/behavioral health problems, such as depression
- Effects of obesity on intimate relationships, especially sexuality

Obese men often experience erectile dysfunction, which can cause or worsen depression (Esposito et al., 2004).

Ask about the following:

- Current reasons for wanting to lose weight
- Stressors (e.g., home, employment, personal, financial, or community) that might prevent success
- Exercise patterns
- Current medications
- Perceptions of self-worth

The diet history provides a detailed analysis of the client's eating habits. As a member of the health care team, evaluate the data to coordinate an interdisciplinary approach that incorporates diet, exercise, behavior modification, and psychological support.

Interventions

Weight is lost only when energy expended is greater than intake. Weight loss may be accomplished by dietary modification with or without the aid of drugs and in combination with a regular exercise program. Clients who are candidates for surgical treatment include those with the following:

- Repeated failure of nonsurgical interventions
- A BMI equal to or greater than 40
- Weight more than 100% above IBW (i.e., morbidly obese)

NONSURGICAL MANAGEMENT. Various diet approaches and medications have attempted to help obese clients achieve permanent weight loss.

Diet Programs. Modalities for helping people lose weight include fasting, very-low-calorie diets, balanced and unbalanced low-energy diets, and novelty diets.

Fasting. Short-term fasting programs have not been successful in treating morbidly obese clients, and prolonged fasting does not produce permanent benefits. Most clients regain the weight that was lost by this method. In addition, the risks associated with fasting (e.g., severe ketosis) require close medical supervision.

Very-Low-Calorie Diets. Very-low-calorie diets generally provide 200 to 800 calories/day. Two types of these diets include the *protein-sparing modified fast* and the *liquid formula diet.*

The protein-sparing modified fast provides protein of high biologic value (1.5 g/kg of desirable body weight daily) within a limited number of calories. The diet produces rapid weight loss while preserving lean body mass. The liquid-formula diet provides between 33 and 70 g of protein daily.

Both diets require an initial cardiac evaluation, supervision by an interdisciplinary health team with monitoring by a physician, nutrition counseling by a registered dietitian, and supplementation with vitamins and minerals. These diets are only one part of a weight reduction program. Clients who are following these diets should receive nutrition education, psychological counseling, exercise, and behavior therapy. Comparable weight losses have been achieved with both diets, but most clients do not sustain the weight loss and regain the weight.

Balanced and Unbalanced Low-Energy Diets. Nutritionally balanced diets generally provide 1200 calories/day with a conventional distribution of carbohydrate, protein, and fat. Vitamin and mineral supplements may be necessary if energy intakes fall below 1200 calories for women and 1800 calories for men. This diet provides conventional foods that are economical and easy to obtain; thus the goal of weight loss is facilitated, and that loss is hopefully maintained. For example, Weight Watchers is an organization that provides education about nutritionally balanced diets based on a point system and weekly group support meetings

Unbalanced low-energy diets, such as the low-carbohydrate diet (e.g., Atkins or South Beach diet), restrict one or more nutrients. As described earlier, protein and vegetables are encouraged, but carbohydrates and fat foods are not. Although they remain controversial in the medical community, these diets are extremely popular. Scientific outcome data have been conflicting. However, a study by Yancy et al. (2004) found that compared with a low-fat diet, a low-carbohydrate diet had better participant retention and greater weight loss. Serum triglyceride levels decreased more and HDL-C levels increased more with the low-carb diet versus the low-fat diet.

Novelty Diets. Novelty diets, such as the grapefruit and Hollywood diet, are often nutritionally *inadequate.* This type of diet implies that a certain food or liquid increases metabolic rate or accelerates the oxidation of body fat. Weight loss is achieved because energy is restricted by food choice, but clients do not sustain weight loss after terminating the diet.

Diet Therapy. Diet recommendations for each client should be developed through close interaction between the client, physician, and dietitian. The diet should meet the client's needs and habits and should be realistic.

The dietitian develops a diet plan and instructs the client. At a minimum, the diet should do the following:

- Have a scientific rationale
- Be nutritionally adequate for all nutrients except energy
- Have a low risk-benefit ratio
- Be practical and conducive to long-term success

Calorie estimates are easily calculated. Resting metabolic rate is determined using a gender-specific formula that incorporates the appropriate activity factor. This figure reflects the total calories needed daily for maintaining current weight. To encourage a weight loss of 1 pound (2.2 kg) a week, the dietitian subtracts 500 calories each day. To encourage a weight loss of 2 pounds (4.4 kg) a week, the dietitian subtracts 1000 calories each day. The amount of weight lost varies with the client's food intake, level of physical activity, and water losses. A reasonable goal of 5% to 10% loss of body weight has been shown to improve glycemic control and reduce cholesterol and blood pressure, and these benefits continue if the weight loss is sustained.

Exercise Program. A major intervention for obesity is to increase the type and amount of daily exercise to create a calorie deficit along with modification of eating habits. For most people, adding exercise to a diet intervention produces more weight loss than just dieting alone. More of the weight lost is fat, which preserves lean body mass. An increase in exercise can produce a reduction in the waist-hip ratio.

Increasing and maintaining physical activity levels are important in maintaining weight loss. Many overweight or obese clients are so unfit that it may take several months of conditioning before they can exercise sufficiently to achieve weight loss.

The physical therapist or exercise physiologist or assistant first obtains a clinical exercise and health history. It is important to determine the client's current exercise pattern and exercise habits over a lifetime. The client should understand the importance of an exercise component in a weight loss program. The client's desire to participate in an exercise program and his or her preferred types of exercise is also ascertained.

The health care provider may evaluate the client by an exercise stress test. Not all clients need a stress test, but those with chronic disease may need the results to assist with individual exercise recommendations. Clients are counseled about unusual signs and symptoms during exercise (e.g., chest pain) and what to do if they occur. The physical therapist or exercise physiologist first emphasizes the importance of exercising consistently and then stresses the duration, intensity, and frequency.

A minimal-level workout should be developed for the client so that consistency can be achieved. The goal for the client is to maintain a lifetime of increased physical activity. The client is apt to be less fatigued and discouraged with a low-intensity, short-duration program. Sedentary clients are encouraged to increase their activity by walking 30 to 40 minutes daily (15 to 20 minutes per mile) or the equivalent. The activity may be performed all at once or divided over the course of the day. Remind the client to exercise only under the supervision of the physician. All members of the interdisciplinary team should provide encouragement and support for any increase in physical activity. Structured national programs with support staff, such as Curves, may be helpful for some clients. They typically offer diet counseling as well as cardiovascular and muscle-toning activities.

Drug Therapy. A BMI of 30 or a BMI of 27 with comorbidities is one indicator for the use of drug therapy. **Anorectic drugs** suppress appetite, which reduces food intake and over time may result in weight loss. These drugs play a valuable role in a comprehensive weight reduction program but should be used only as part of such a program. Currently available drugs to treat obesity act on either the noradrenergic or serotonergic systems in the central nervous system. The most commonly used anorectic drug for the treatment of obesity is sibutramine (Meridia). Sibutramine is an anorectic drug that inhibits the reuptake of serotonin (which enhances satiety [feeling full when eating]) and norepinephrine (which raises the metabolic rate). The usual dosage is 10 mg every day, which may be increased to 15 mg daily after 4 weeks or decreased to 5 mg daily, depending on the client's response. Adverse effects include dry mouth, constipation, and insomnia.

Orlistat (Xenical) is a different type of drug that inhibits lipase and leads to partial hydrolysis of triglycerides. Because fats are only partially digested and absorbed, calorie intake is decreased. The usual dosage is 120 mg three times daily with each main meal containing fat. Most clients taking orlistat experience GI symptoms that include loose stools, abdominal cramps, and nausea. Therefore this drug should be used with caution and limited to adults between 18 and 75 years of age. Treatment is usually not extended beyond 12 months.

A new drug is in the final stages of testing. Rimonabant (Acomplia) is the first of a new class of medications that reduces cravings for both food and smoking. It works by inhibiting a receptor found in a newly described physiologic system called the endocannabinoid system. Minor GI side effects may occur when the drug is first used, but these annoyances resolve after the first few weeks.

Behavioral Treatment. Behavioral treatment of obesity consists of various strategies to change daily eating habits to achieve weight loss. This ongoing process should produce a change in behavior. Self-monitoring techniques include keeping a record of foods eaten (food diary), exercise patterns, and emotional and situational factors. Stimulus control involves controlling the external cues that promote overeating. Reinforcement techniques are used to self-reward the behavior change. Cognitive restructuring involves modifying negative beliefs by learning positive coping self-statements.

Complementary and Alternative Therapies. Many other complementary and alternative therapies have been tested and used for obesity in both adults and children. These modalities aim to suppress appetite and therefore limit food intake to lose weight:

- Acupuncture
- Acupressure
- Ayurvedic (a combination of holistic approaches)
- Hypnosis

Descriptions of most of these methods can be found in Chapter 4.

SURGICAL MANAGEMENT. At any weight, some clients opt to improve their appearance by having a variety of cosmetic procedures to reduce the amount of adipose tissue in selected areas of the body. A typical example of this type of surgery is **liposuction,** which can be done in a physician's office. Whereas the client's appearance is improved, if weight gain continues, the fatty tissue will return. This procedure is not a solution for individuals who are morbidly obese.

Clients who do not respond to traditional dietary intervention may be considered for a major surgical procedure aimed at producing permanent weight loss. Clients with a body mass index (BMI) of 40 or greater or a BMI of 35 or greater along with additional risk factors should be considered for surgery.

Two major types of procedures may be performed for obesity:

- **Panniculectomy,** which is removal of any panniculus, most often the abdominal apron
- **Bariatric surgery,** which is surgical reduction of gastric capacity

For most clients, a panniculectomy is a safe, complication-free procedure that is usually done as a follow-up to bariatric surgery. Meticulous wound care is the priority for postoperative nursing care (Gallagher & Gates, 2003).

Most bariatric procedures today are of two types: gastric restrictive surgery and gastric restriction combined with malabsorption surgery, which offers the best results (Barrow, 2002). Every year, more than 100,000 individuals in the United States have these procedures, and that number is increasing. Many clients have minimally invasive surgery via laparoscopy. The decision of whether the client is a candidate for the laparoscopic procedure is based on weight, body build, history of abdominal surgery, and co-existing medical complications. With either approach, clients must agree to modify their lifestyle and follow stringent protocols to lose weight and keep the weight off. Following bariatric surgery, many clients no longer experience complications of obesity, such as diabetes mellitus, hypertension, depression, or sleep apnea.

Preoperative Care. Preoperative care is similar to that for any client undergoing abdominal surgery (see Chapter 20). However, obese clients are at increased surgical risks of pulmonary and thromboembolitic complications, as well as death. The primary role of the nurse is to reinforce health teaching in preparation for surgery.

Operative Procedures. **Gastric restriction** surgeries allow for normal digestion without the risk of nutritional deficiencies. As seen in Figure 64-6, for the **vertical banded gastroplasty,** the surgeon places a vertical line of staples to create a small stomach pouch to which a band is connected to provide an outlet to the small intestine. **Circumgastric banding** limits stomach size by placing an inflatable band around the fundus of the stomach. The band can be inflated or deflated through a subcutaneous port to change the size of the stomach as the client loses weight.

When gastric resection is combined with malabsorption surgery, the client's stomach, duodenum, and part of the jejunum is bypassed so that fewer calories can be absorbed. This procedure is commonly called a **gastric bypass** or **Roux-en-Y gastric bypass.**

Postoperative Care. Postoperative care depends on the type of surgical approach–the open conventional approach or minimally invasive technique (laparoscopy). Although many clients have laparoscopic surgery, they are considered as having major abdominal surgery along with all its risks. However, these clients usually require less than 24 hours in the hospital; some may need 1 to 2 days. Clients with open procedures may need 4 to 5 days to recover. All clients experience some degree of pain, but it is usually less severe when laparoscopy is used. Clients may use patient-controlled analgesia for the first day. All clients receive oral opioid analgesia as prescribed.

Care of the bariatric surgical client is similar to that for any client having abdominal or laparoscopic surgery. However, special bariatric equipment and accommodations, including an extra-wide bed and additional personnel for moving the client, are needed for both the surgical suite and postoperative care units. Beds must be wide enough to allow the client to turn. Bed rails should not be touching the body because they can cause pressure areas. Pressure be-

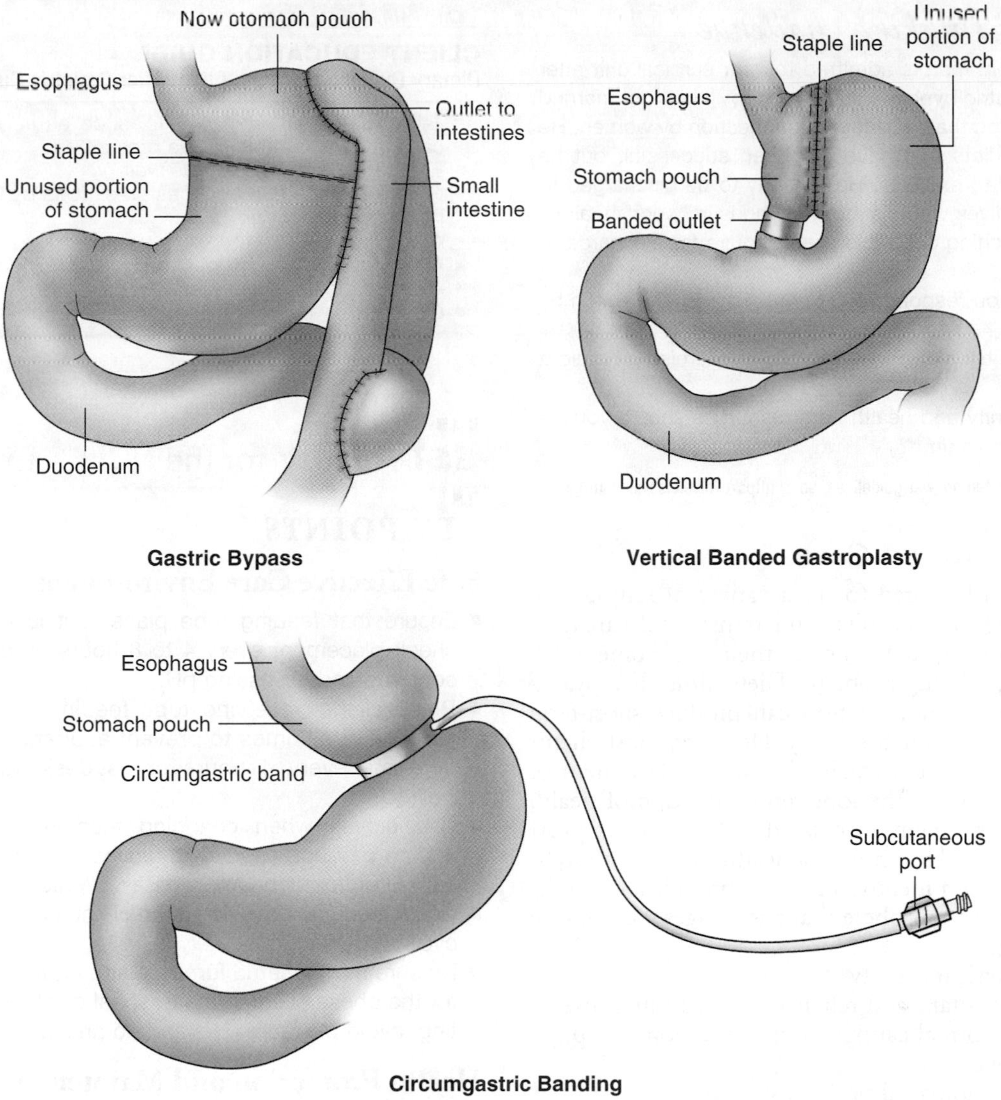

Figure 64-6 ■ Bariatric surgical procedures.

tween skin folds, as well as tubes and catheters, can also cause skin breakdown. Monitor the skin in these areas, and keep it clean and dry.

Some clients have a nasogastric (NG) tube put in place, especially after open surgical procedures. In gastroplasty procedures, the NG tube drains both the proximal pouch and the distal stomach. Closely monitor the tube for patency. *Never reposition the tube, because its movement can disrupt the suture line!* The NG tube is removed on the second or third day if the client has bowel sounds and is passing flatus. Clear liquids are introduced slowly if the client can tolerate water, and 1-ounce cups are used for each serving. Pureed foods, juice, and soups thinned with broth, water, or milk are added to the diet 24 to 48 hours after clear liquids are tolerated. Typically, the client can increase the volume to 1 ounce over 5 minutes or until satisfied, but the diet is limited to liquids or pureed foods for 6 weeks. The client then progresses to regular food, with an emphasis on nutrient-dense foods. Nausea, vomiting, or discomfort occurs if too much liquid is ingested.

In addition to the postoperative complications typically associated with abdominal surgery, bariatric clients have special needs and risks. Implement measures to prevent these complications:

- Apply an abdominal binder to prevent wound dehiscence.
- Place the client in semi-Fowler's position, or use continuous positive airway pressure (CPAP) ventilation at night to improve ventilation and decrease risk of sleep apnea.
- Observe skin areas and folds for redness, excoriation, or breakdown to treat these problems early.
- Use absorbent padding between folds to prevent pressure areas, particularly from tubes and catheters.
- In collaboration with the dietitian, provide six small feedings to prevent dehydration.
- Observe for signs and symptoms of **dumping syndrome** (caused by food entering the small intestine instead of the stomach) after gastric bypass, such as tachycardia, nausea, diarrhea, and abdominal cramping.

Critical Thinking Challenge

A 35-year-old man is admitted to your surgical unit after undergoing a gastric bypass via laparoscopy. He is not married and confides in you that he is fearful of rejection by women. He has tried many diets that have not been successful, but he never really liked to exercise. He is ready to be discharged to home, where he lives with his mother who is in "poor" health.

1. What diet teaching does this client require for discharge to home?
2. How should you respond to his concern about rejection by women?
3. What will you tell him about the role of exercise for weight loss?
4. What community and health care resources should you direct him to at this time?

evolve For suggested answer guidelines, go to http://evolve.elsevier.com/Iggy/.

Community-Based Care

Obese clients can be cared for in a variety of settings, including the acute care hospital and transitional care unit (particularly following surgery) or in their own home. Obesity is a chronic, lifelong problem. Diets, drug therapy, exercise, and behavior modification can produce short-term weight losses with reasonable safety. However, most clients who do lose weight often regain the weight. Treatment of obesity should focus on the long-term reduction of health risks and medical problems associated with obesity, improving quality of life, and promoting a health-oriented lifestyle. Interdisciplinary team members need to provide a nonjudgmental, supportive atmosphere that encourages the client to do the following:

- Increase physical activity
- Decrease fat intake and reliance on medication use
- Establish a normal eating pattern in response to physiologic hunger
- Address psychological problems

Frequent, long-term ambulatory care follow-up coordinated by a case manager is essential for successful treatment.

The most important features of client education for any obese client focus on health-related behavior patterns. In collaboration with the dietitian, counsel the client on a healthful eating pattern. The physical therapist or exercise physiologist recommends an appropriate exercise program. A psychologist may recommend cognitive restructuring approaches that help alter dysfunctional eating patterns. For clients who have surgery, additional modifications are needed (Chart 64-8).

Bariatric surgery results in a major lifestyle change as well as a variety of emotions. During weight loss, the client may become depressed or anxious. Some clients experience a "hibernation phase" for about a month after surgery because of physical and emotional adjustments (Gallagher, 2004). Plastic surgery, such as panniculectomy, may be performed after weight is stabilized, usually in about 12 to 15 months.

The chances for success in a weight control program are enhanced if additional support is available. Provide the client with a list of available community resources, such as Overeaters Anonymous and the American Obesity Association. For surgical clients, the American Society of Bariatric Surgery may be helpful.

CHART 64-8

CLIENT EDUCATION GUIDE
Dietary Guidelines for the Client After Bariatric Surgery

- Take nutritional supplements, such as iron, multivitamins, calcium, and vitamin B_{12} as prescribed.
- Eat slowly and chew foods well.
- Progress dietary amounts as prescribed by the dietitian and health care provider.
- Avoid high-protein foods.
- Avoid foods high in sugar (especially refined sugar) and fat.
- Avoid alcoholic beverages.
- Observe for and report signs and symptoms of dehydration.

GET READY for the NCLEX Examination!

KEY POINTS

Safe Effective Care Environment

- Ensure that feeding tube placement is verified by x-ray; check placement every 4 to 8 hours by aspirating gastric contents and assessing pH.
- Place clients receiving tube feeding in a semi-Fowler's position at all times to prevent aspiration; check residual contents every 4 hours or as designated per agency policy.
- Use gloves when changing feeding system tubing or adding product; use sterile gloves when working with critically ill or immunocompromised clients.
- Use a feeding pump when the client receives continuous or cyclic tube feeding.
- Be sure that bariatric furniture and equipment are available for the obese client in the hospital or other health care setting; avoid pressure on skin-fold areas.

Health Promotion and Maintenance

- For clients receiving enteral or parenteral nutrition at home, teach family members or other caregivers how to provide nutrition while avoiding complications.
- Teach clients who are undernourished to eat high-protein, high-calories foods and nutritional supplements.
- Instruct obese clients about the importance of health care provider–approved exercise for weight reduction.
- Provide health teaching about dietary guidelines after bariatric surgery as outlined in Chart 64-8.

Psychosocial Integrity

- Be aware that some obese clients may not view their weight as a problem and are therefore unlikely to be part of a weight reduction plan.
- Recognize that obesity can cause depression or anxiety, low self-esteem, and a disturbed body image.
- Be aware of legal and ethical issues related to tube feeding older adults with chronic or terminal illness.

Physiological Integrity

- Provide a nutritional screening for all inpatient clients (Charts 64-1 and 64-2); review serum prealbumin, hemoglobin, and hematocrit levels. Identify clients at nutritional risk, and refer to a dietitian.

- Assess clients with severe malnutrition for common complications, such as edema; cachexia; lethargy; and dry, flaking skin.
- Implement interventions to promote nutritional intake in older adults as specified in Chart 64-4.
- Provide nursing interventions for managing nutrition as listed in Chart 64-3.
- Provide care for clients receiving total enteral nutrition as described in Charts 64-5 and 64-6.
- Provide care for clients receiving total parenteral nutrition as specified in Chart 64-7.
- Recognize that many individuals are following low-carbohydrate rather than low-fat diets to lose weight.
- Recall that normal body mass index (BMI) for adults should be between 20 and 25; older adults should have a BMI between 24 and 27. A BMI of 27 to 30 indicates overweight, over 30 indicates obesity, and 40 and greater indicates morbid obesity.
- Recall that obesity causes early onset of many chronic illnesses, such as osteoarthritis, diabetes mellitus, hypertension, and coronary artery disease. Pulmonary problems, such as obstructive sleep apnea, delayed wound healing, and infections are also common.
- Remember that bariatric surgery includes gastric restriction procedures or gastric bypass; a panniculectomy may be performed to remove skin folds, especially the abdomen, once weight is stabilized.
- Provide postoperative care for clients having bariatric surgery including applying an abdominal binder, placing the client in semi-Fowler's position and using CPAP to increase ventilation, monitoring for skin breakdown and pressure, and observing for complications, such as dumping syndrome in clients who have a gastric bypass. Tachycardia, nausea, diarrhea, and abdominal cramping are common manifestations of dumping syndrome.

ADDITIONAL STUDY RESOURCES

Go to your Student CD-ROM for Review Questions for the NCLEX Examination.

evolve Go to http://evolve.elsevier.com/Iggy/ for Integrated Management of Care Questions for the NCLEX Examination.

SELECTED BIBLIOGRAPHY

Asterisk indicates a classic or definitive work on this subject.

*Ammon, P.K. (1999). Individualizing the approach to treating obesity. *Nurse Practitioner, 24*(2), 27-31, 36-38, 41-43.

Anderson, E.B. (2000). Facilitating quality of life through nutrition. *Advance for Nurses (DC/Baltimore), 2*(11), 17-18, 30.

Barrow, C.J. (2002). Roux-en-Y gastric bypass for morbid obesity. *AORN Journal, 76*(4), 595-604.

Bender, S., et al. (2000). Malnutrition: Role of the TwoCal® HN Med Pass Program. *MEDSURG Nursing, 9*(6), 284-296.

*Bowers, S. (1999). Nutrition support for malnourished, acutely ill adults. *MEDSURG Nursing, 8*(3), 145-166.

Bowers, S. (2000). All about tubes: Your guide to enteral feeding devices. *Nursing 2000, 30*(12), 41-48.

Cammon, S.A., & Hackshaw, H.S. (2000). Are we starving our patients? *American Journal of Nursing, 100*(5), 43-47.

Cowan, D.T., et al. (2004). Nutritional status of older people in long term care settings: Current status and future directions. *International Journal of Nursing Studies, 41*(3), 225-237.

Dudek, S.G. (2000). Malnutrition in hospitals: Who's assessing what patients eat? *American Journal of Nursing, 100*(4), 36-43.

Edwards, S.J., & Metheny, N.A. (2000). Measurement of gastric residual volume: State of the science. *MEDSURG Nursing, 9*(3), 125-128.

*Epley, D. (1999). Nutritional assessment in home care patients. *Home Care Provider, 4*(3), 102-105.

Esposito, K., et al. (2004). Effect of lifestyle changes on erectile dysfunction in obese men: A randomized controlled trial. *Journal of the American Medical Association, 291*(24), 2978-2984.

*Fairburn, C.G., & Cooper, Z. (1996). New perspectives on dieting and behavioural treatments for obesity. *International Journal of Obesity, 20* (suppl 1), S9-S13.

Fellows, L.S., et al. (2000). Evidence-based practice for enteral feedings: Aspiration prevention strategies, bedside detection, and practice change. *MEDSURG Nursing, 9*(1), 27-32.

*Food and Nutrition Board, Institute of Medicine, National Academy of Sciences. (1997). *Dietary reference intakes: Calcium, phosphorus, magnesium, vitamin D, and fluoride.* Washington, D.C.: National Academy Press.

*Food and Nutrition Board, National Research Council/National Academy of Sciences. (1989). *Recommended dietary allowances* (10th ed.). Washington, D.C.: National Academy Press.

Gallagher, S. (2004). Taking the weight off with bariatric surgery. *Nursing 2004, 34*(3), 58-63.

Gallagher, S., & Gates, J.L. (2003). Obesity, panniculitis, panniculectomy, and wound care: Understanding the challenges. *Journal of Wound, Ostomy, and Continence Nursing, 30*(6), 334-341.

*Grindel, C.G., & Costello, M.C. (1996). Nutrition screening: An essential assessment parameter. *MEDSURG Nursing, 5*(3), 145-156.

Holland, D.E., et al. (2001). How to creatively meet care needs of the morbidly obese. *Nursing Management, 32*(6), 39-41.

Kohn-Keeth, C. (2000). How to keep feeding tubes flowing freely. *Nursing 2000, 30*(3), 58-59.

Lofgren, I., et al. (2004). Waist circumference is a better predictor than body mass index of coronary heart disease risk in overweight premenopausal women. *Journal of Nutrition, 134*(5), 1071-1076.

Mackie, S.B. (2001). PEGs and ethics. *Gastroenterology Nursing, 24*(3), 138-142.

Maloney, J., et al. (2002). Food dye use in enteral feedings: A review and a call for a moratorium. *Nutrition and Clinical Practice, 17*, 169-181.

McGinnis, C. (2002). Parenteral nutrition focus: Nutrition assessment and formula composition. *Journal of Infusion Nursing, 25*(1), 54-64.

Metheny, N.A. & Titler, M.G. (2001). Assessing placement of feeding tubes. *American Journal of Nursing, 101*(5), 36-45.

Metheny, N.A. & Stewart, B.J. (2002). Testing feeding tube placement during continuous tube feedings. *Applied Nursing Research, 15*(4), 254-258.

Metheny, N.A., Smith, L., & Stewart, B.J. (2000). Development of a reliable and valid bedside test for bilirubin and utility for improving prediction of feeding tube location. *Nursing Research, 49*(6), 302-309.

Metheny, N.A., Schallom, M.E., & Edwards, S.J. (2004). Effect of gastrointestinal motility and feeding tube site on aspiration risk in critically ill patients: A review. *Heart and Lung, 33*(3), 131-145.

*Metheny, N.A., et al. (1998). Testing feeding tube placement: Auscultation vs. pH method. *American Journal of Nursing, 98*(5), 37-43.

Metheny, N.A., et al. (2002). Efficacy of dye-stained enteral formula in detecting pulmonary aspiration. *Chest, 122*(1), 276-281.

Mion, L.C., & O'Connell, A. (2003). Parenteral hydration and nutrition in the geriatric patient: Clinical and ethical issues. *Journal of Infusion Nursing, 26*(3), 144-152.

Nickel, K. (2004). Comparing voices. Tube feeding: Literature versus the textbook. *American Journal of Nursing, 104*(7), 65.

*Nutrition and your health: Dietary guidelines for Americans. (1995). *Home and Garden Bulletin No. 232* (4th ed.). Washington,

D.C.: U.S. Department of Agriculture and U.S. Department of Health and Human Services.

Padula, C.A., et al. (2004). Enteral feedings: What the evidence says. *American Journal of Nursing, 104*(7), 62-64, 66-69.

Payer, M., Ypungberg, B., & Pfister, S. (2003). Panniculectomy–An option for people who are morbidly obese. *AORN Journal, 77*(4), 782-794.

*Rotkoff, N. (1999). Care of the morbidly obese patient in a long-term care facility. *Geriatric Nursing, 20*(6), 309-313.

Schwarte, A. (2001). Ethical decisions regarding nutrition and the terminally ill. *Gastroenterology Nursing, 24*(1), 29-33.

Stechmiller, J.K. (2003). Early nutritional screening of older adults: A review of nutritional support. *Journal of Infusion Nursing, 26*(3), 170-177.

*Vegetarian food pyramid. (1994). *Vegetarian Journal, 13,* 21.

Voelker, M. (2004). Assessing quality of life in gastric bypass clients. *Journal of Perianesthesia Nursing, 19*(2), 89-101.

Wilson, J.A., & Clark, J.J. (2003). Obesity: Impediment to wound healing. *Critical Care Nursing Quarterly, 26*(2), 119-132.

Woodward, B. (2003). Bariatric surgery options. *Critical Care Nursing Quarterly, 26*(2), 89-100.

Yancy, W.S., et al. (2004). A low-carbohydrate, ketogenic diet versus a low-fat diet to treat obesity and hyperlipidemia: A randomized, controlled trial. *Annals of Internal Medicine, 140*(10), 769-777.

UNIT **FOURTEEN**

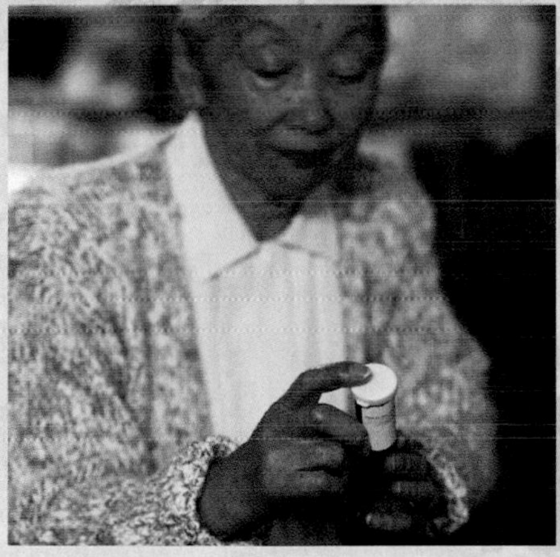

PROBLEMS of REGULATION and METABOLISM

Management of Clients with Problems of the Endocrine System

CHAPTER

65 Assessment of the Endocrine System

M. LINDA WORKMAN

LEARNING OUTCOMES

After studying this chapter, you should be able to:

1. Describe the relationship between hormones and receptor sites.
2. Explain negative feedback as a control mechanism for hormone secretion.
3. Discuss the structure and function of the hypothalamus.
4. Discuss the structure and function of the anterior and posterior pituitary glands.
5. Discuss the structure and function of the adrenal glands.
6. Discuss the structure and function of the thyroid and parathyroid glands.
7. Discuss the structure and function of the pancreas.
8. Describe changes in the endocrine system associated with aging.
9. Identify laboratory tests that aid in determining endocrine function and dysfunction.

Go to your Student CD-ROM for Review Questions for the NCLEX Examination keyed to these Learning Outcomes.

The endocrine system is made up of glands in many tissues and organs in a variety of body areas (Figure 65-1). A key feature of all endocrine glands is the secretion of hormones. **Hormones** are natural chemicals that exert their effects on specific tissues known as **target tissues.** Target tissues are usually located some distance from the endocrine gland, with no direct physical connection between the endocrine gland and its target tissue. For this reason endocrine glands are called "ductless" glands and must use the blood to transport secreted hormones to the target tissues. Endocrine glands include the following:

- Pituitary gland
- Adrenal glands
- Thyroid gland
- Islet cells of the pancreas
- Parathyroid glands
- Gonads

The endocrine system works with the nervous system to regulate overall body function, known as **neuroendocrine regulation.** Many interactions must occur between the endocrine system and all other body systems to ensure that each system maintains a constant normal balance **(homeostasis)** in response to environmental changes. For example, neuroendocrine control of other body systems keeps the internal body temperature at or near 98.6° F (37° C), even when environmental temperatures are lower or higher. Other neuroendocrine actions help keep the serum sodium level between 136 and 145 mEq/L (mmol/L), regardless of whether a person eats 2 g or 12 g of sodium per day.

Table 65-1 lists the specific hormones secreted by various endocrine glands. Hormones travel through the blood to all body areas but exert their actions only on target tissues. Hormones recognize their target tissues and exert their actions by binding to receptor sites on or within the target tissue cells. In general, each receptor site type is specific for only one hormone. Hormone-receptor actions work in a "lock and key" manner in that only the correct hormone (key) can bind to and activate the receptor site (lock) (Figure 65-2). Binding a hormone to its receptor causes the target tissue to change its activity. In this way, hormones produce specific responses even though they circulate throughout the body. Table 65-2 lists the key features of hormones.

Disorders of the endocrine system are related to either an excess or a deficiency of a specific hormone or to a defect at its receptor site. The onset of these disorders can be either slow and insidious or abrupt and life threatening.

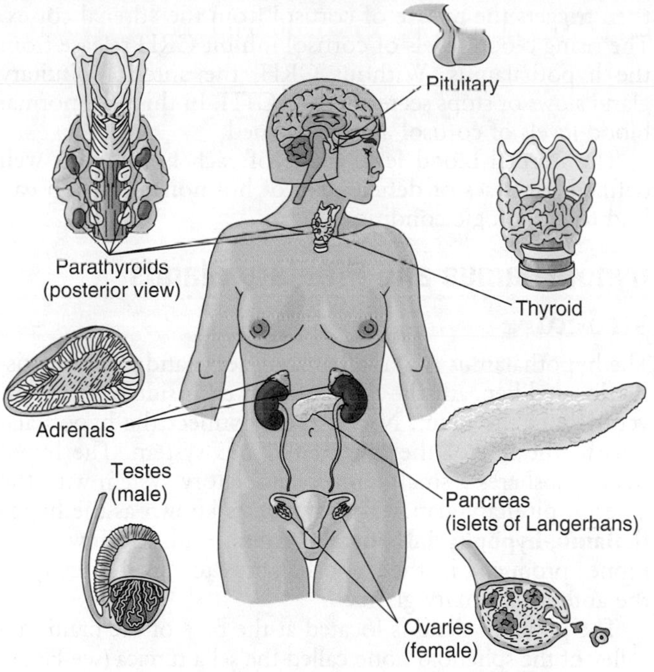

Figure 65-1 ■ The endocrine system.

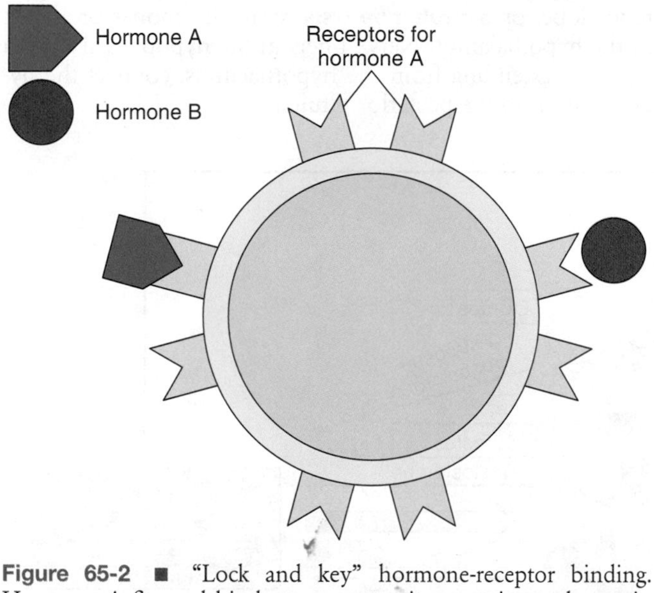

Figure 65-2 ■ "Lock and key" hormone-receptor binding. Hormone A fits and binds to receptor sites, causing a change in cell action. Hormone B does not fit or bind to receptor sites; no change in cell action results.

TABLE 65-1 Principal Hormones of the Endocrine Glands

Gland	Hormones
Hypothalamus	Corticotropin-releasing hormone (CRH) Thyrotropin-releasing hormone (TRH) Gonadotropin-releasing hormone (GnRH) Growth hormone–releasing hormone (GHRH) Growth hormone–inhibiting hormone (somatostatin GHIH) Prolactin-inhibiting hormone (PIH) Melanocyte-inhibiting hormone (MIH)
Anterior pituitary	Thyroid-stimulating hormone (TSH) Adrenocorticotropic hormone (ACTH, corticotropin) Luteinizing hormone (LH) Follicle-stimulating hormone (FSH) Prolactin (PRL) Growth hormone (GH) Melanocyte-stimulating hormone (MSH)
Posterior pituitary	Vasopressin (antidiuretic hormone [ADH]) Oxytocin
Thyroid	Triiodothyronine (T_3) Thyroxine (T_4) Calcitonin
Parathyroid	Parathyroid hormone
Adrenal cortex	Glucocorticoids (cortisol) Mineralocorticoids (aldosterone)
Ovary	Estrogen Progesterone
Testes	Testosterone
Pancreas	Insulin Glucagon Somatostatin

TABLE 65-2 Common Key Features of Hormones

- All hormones exert their effects at low blood concentrations.
- Receptors on or within target tissues are needed for *all* hormones to exert an effect.
- Most hormones (except for thyroid and adrenal medullary hormones) are not stored to any great extent and must be produced as needed.
- Hormones in the blood are bound to plasma proteins.
- Only free hormones (those not bound to plasma proteins) can bind to their receptor sites.
- Most hormones cause target tissues to increase or decrease their activity by changing gene activity either directly or indirectly. Exceptions are hormones that alter membrane permeability.
- The activity of most hormones is of short duration.
- Continued hormone activity requires continued production and secretion.
- The clearance of secreted hormones occurs through cellular uptake, enzymatic breakdown, gastrointestinal excretion, or urinary excretion.

ANATOMY AND PHYSIOLOGY REVIEW

The control of cellular function by any hormone depends on a series of reactions working through **negative feedback control mechanisms.** Hormone secretion is dependent on the need of the body for the final action of that hormone. When a body condition starts to move away from the normal range and a specific action or response is needed to correct this change, secretion of the hormone capable of causing the correcting action or response is stimulated until the need (demand) is met. As the correction occurs, hormone secretion decreases (and may halt). This type of control for hormone synthesis is "negative feedback" because the hormone causes the opposite action of the initial condition change.

An example of a simple negative feedback hormone response is the control of insulin secretion. When blood glucose levels start to rise above normal, the hormone insulin is secreted. Insulin increases glucose uptake by the cells, causing a decrease in blood glucose levels. Thus the action of insulin (decreasing blood glucose levels) is the opposite of the condition that stimulated insulin secretion (elevated blood glucose levels).

Some hormones that use negative feedback mechanisms have more complex interactions. These interactions involve a series of reactions in which more than one endocrine gland, as well as the final target tissues, is stimulated. In such a situation, the first hormone in the series may have another endocrine gland as its target tissue. For this type of mechanism to maintain homeostasis, the following series of interactions must occur:

- The central nervous system receives and reacts to various stimuli transmitted to the hypothalamus.
- The hypothalamus responds to the stimuli with the production and release of either releasing or inhibiting factors, which are transported to the pituitary.
- In the pituitary gland, the releasing or inhibiting factors either stimulate or inhibit the release of specific hormones.
- The anterior pituitary hormones then control the secretion of hormones in target organs or tissue (Figure 65-3).

One example of this complex control is the interaction of the hypothalamus and the anterior pituitary with the adrenal cortex. Low blood levels of cortisol stimulate the secretion of corticotropic-releasing hormone (CRH) in the hypothalamus. CRH stimulates the anterior pituitary gland to secrete adrenocorticotropic hormone (ACTH). ACTH then triggers the release of cortisol from the adrenal cortex. The rising blood levels of cortisol inhibit CRH release from the hypothalamus. Without CRH, the anterior pituitary gland slows or stops secretion of ACTH. In this way, normal blood levels of cortisol are maintained.

The normal blood level range of each hormone is well defined. Excesses or deficiencies of hormone secretion can lead to pathologic conditions.

Hypothalamus and Pituitary Glands

Structure

The hypothalamus is a small area of nerve and glandular tissue located beneath the thalamus on each side of the third ventricle in the brain. Nerve fibers connect the hypothalamus to the rest of the central nervous system. The hypothalamus shares a small, closed circulatory system with the anterior pituitary gland. This system is known as the **hypothalamic-hypophysial portal system,** and it allows hormones produced in the hypothalamus to travel directly to the anterior pituitary gland.

The pituitary gland is located at the base of the brain in a valley of the sphenoid bone called the sella turcica (see Figure 65-1). The oval pituitary gland is about 1 cm in diameter and is divided into two lobes (Figure 65-4). The anterior lobe, or **adenohypophysis,** makes up about 70% of the gland. The posterior lobe, or **neurohypophysis,** stores hormones produced in the hypothalamus. Nerve fibers in the hypophysial stalk, a structure extending from the hypothalamus, connect the hypothalamus to the posterior pituitary.

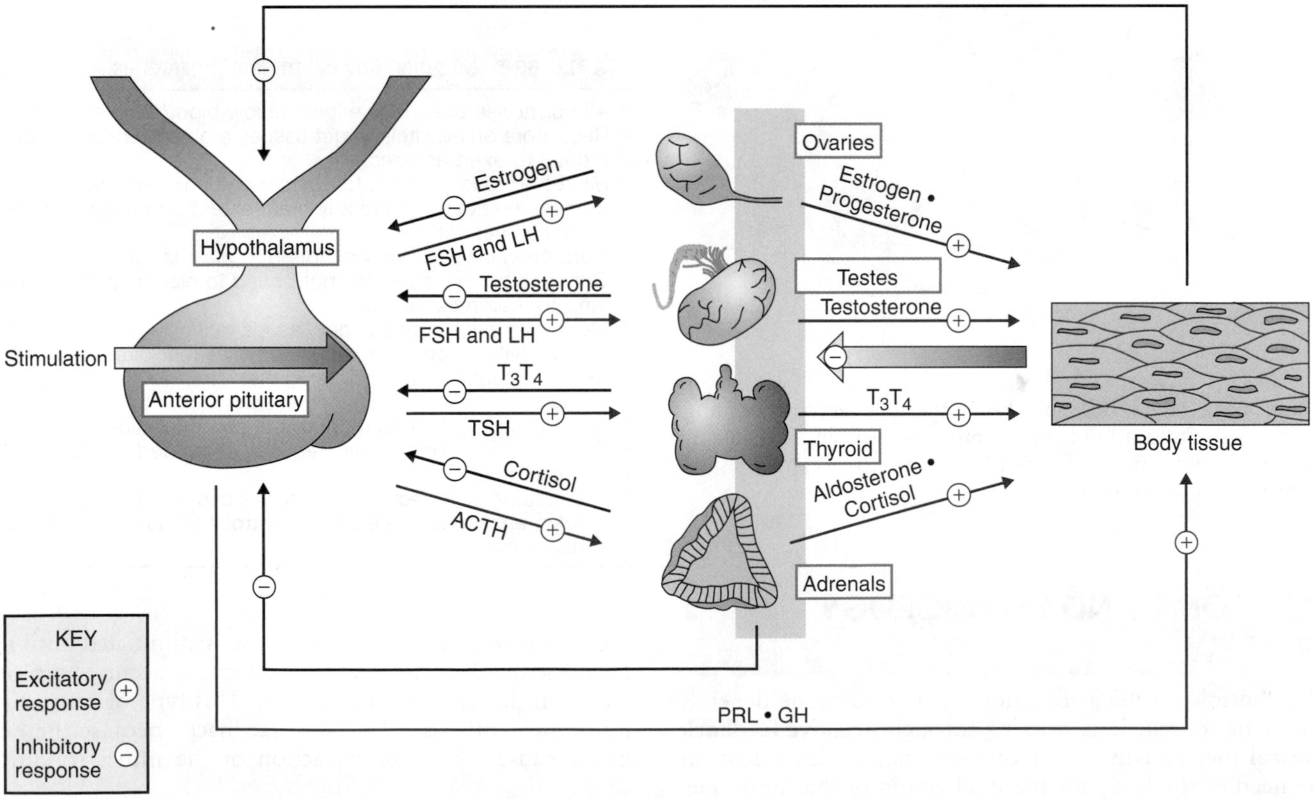

Figure 65-3 ■ The feedback system of the hypothalamic-pituitary-target gland axis. *ACTH,* Adrenocorticotropic hormone; *TSH,* thyroid-stimulating hormone; *T_3,* triiodothyronine; *T_4,* thyroxine; *FSH,* follicle-stimulating hormone; *LH,* luteinizing hormone; *PRL,* prolactin; *GH,* growth hormone.

Function

The hypothalamus has both endocrine and nonendocrine functions. The endocrine function is to produce regulatory hormones (see Table 65-1). Some of these hormones are released into the blood and travel to the anterior pituitary, where they either stimulate or inhibit the release of anterior pituitary hormones.

In response to the releasing hormones of the hypothalamus, the anterior pituitary secretes **tropic hormones**, which stimulate other endocrine glands. Other anterior pituitary hormones, such as prolactin, produce their effect directly on final target tissues (Table 65-3).

The hormones of the posterior pituitary, vasopressin (antidiuretic hormone [ADH]) and oxytocin, are produced in the hypothalamus and sent through the nerve tracts that connect the hypothalamus with the posterior pituitary. These hormones are stored in the nerve endings of the posterior pituitary and are released into the blood when needed.

Other conditions or substances can affect the release of hormones from the pituitary gland (Table 65-4). Drugs, diet, lifestyle, and pathologic conditions can increase or decrease pituitary hormone secretion.

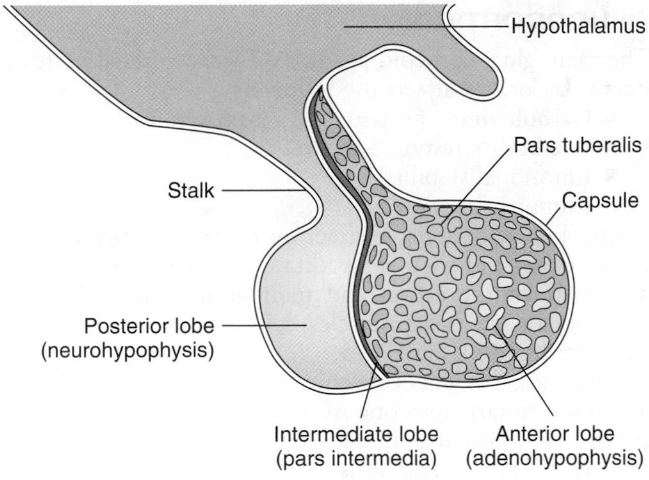

Figure 65-4 ■ The pituitary gland.

Gonads

The **gonads** are the male and female reproductive endocrine glands. Male gonads are the testes, and female gonads are the ovaries. Although these glands are formed before birth and are present at birth, their function does not begin until puberty.

During puberty in the male, the increased secretion of gonadotropins (luteinizing hormone [LH] and follicle-stimulating hormone [FSH]) from the anterior pituitary gland stimulates maturation of the testes, production of testosterone, and maturation of the external genitalia. During puberty in the female, increased secretion of the same gonadotropins stimulates ovarian maturation, estrogen production, ovulation, and maturation of the external genitalia. The function of the testes and ovaries is detailed in Chapter 76.

Adrenal Glands

The adrenal glands are vascular, tent-shaped organs on the top of each kidney (see Figure 65-1). The adrenal gland has an outer portion **(cortex)** and an inner portion **(medulla)**; each area has independent functions. The hormones of the adrenal glands have effects throughout the body.

ADRENAL CORTEX

Structure

The adrenal cortex makes up about 90% of the adrenal gland and has cells divided into three zones or layers (Figure 65-5). **Mineralocorticoids** are produced in the zona glomerulosa and help control the body's sodium and potassium content. Glucocorticoids, androgens, and estrogens are produced in the zona fasciculata and zona reticularis. The hormones produced and secreted by the cortex are often called **adrenal steroids** or **corticosteroids.**

TABLE 65-3 Pituitary Hormones: Target Tissues and Subsequent Actions

Hormone	Target Tissue	Actions
Anterior Pituitary		
TSH (thyroid-stimulating hormone)	Thyroid	Stimulates synthesis and release of thyroid hormone
ACTH (adrenocorticotropic hormone, corticotropin)	Adrenal cortex	Stimulates synthesis and release of corticosteroids and adrenocortical growth
LH (luteinizing hormone)	Ovary Testes	Stimulates ovulation and progesterone secretion Stimulates testosterone secretion
FSH (follicle-stimulating hormone)	Ovary Testes	Stimulates estrogen secretion and follicle maturation Stimulates spermatogenesis
PRL (prolactin)	Mammary glands	Stimulates breast milk production
GH (growth hormone)	Bone and soft tissue	Promotes growth through lipolysis, protein anabolism, and insulin antagonism
MSH (melanocyte-stimulating hormone)	Melanocytes	Promotes pigmentation
Posterior Pituitary*		
Vasopressin (antidiuretic hormone [ADH])	Kidney	Promotes water reabsorption
Oxytocin	Uterus and mammary glands	Stimulates uterine contractions and ejection of breast milk

*These hormones are synthesized in the hypothalamus and are stored in the posterior pituitary gland. They are transported from the hypothalamus to the posterior pituitary while bound to neurophysins.

Function

MINERALOCORTICOIDS

The adrenal cortex maintains life-sustaining physiologic activities. **Aldosterone,** the chief mineralocorticoid produced by the adrenal cortex, maintains extracellular fluid volume. It promotes sodium and water reabsorption and potassium excretion in the kidney tubules. Aldosterone secretion is regulated by the renin-angiotensin system, serum potassium ion concentration, and adrenocorticotropic hormone (ACTH).

Renin is produced by the juxtaglomerular cells of the renal afferent arterioles. Its release is triggered by a decrease in extracellular fluid volume, which can occur from blood loss, sodium loss, or posture changes. Renin converts renin substrate (formerly called angiotensinogen), a plasma protein made in the liver, to angiotensin I. Angiotensin I is converted by a converting enzyme to form angiotensin II, the active form of angiotensin. In turn, angiotensin II stimulates the secretion of aldosterone. Chapters 14 (Figure 14-8), 15 (Figure 15-2), and 72 further describe the renin-angiotensin system. Aldosterone causes the kidney to reabsorb sodium and water to bring the plasma volume and osmolarity back to normal.

Serum potassium level also controls aldosterone secretion. The adrenal cortex secretes aldosterone when the serum potassium level increases above normal by as little as 0.1 mEq/L.

TABLE 65-4 Factors Affecting Secretion/Release of Selected Pituitary Hormones

Vasopressin

Potential Causes of Increased Secretion
- Congestive heart failure
- Hemorrhage
- Diuretics
- Opioids
- Chlorpropamide
  - Diabinese
  - Novo-Propamide ✱
- Cyclophosphamide
- Vincristine
- Nicotine
- Stress
- Hypoxia

Potential Causes of Decreased Secretion
- Alcohol consumption
- Phenytoin

Growth Hormone

Potential Causes of Increased Secretion
- High-protein diet
- Deep sleep
- Hypoglycemia
- Fasting
- Estrogen
- Glucagon
- Dopamine

Potential Causes of Decreased Secretion
- REM (rapid eye movement) sleep
- Hyperglycemia
- Obesity
- Hypothyroidism

Prolactin

Potential Causes of Increased Secretion
- Stress
- Nipple manipulation
- Estrogen
- Dopamine antagonists
- Chlorpromazine
  - Thorazine
  - Chlorpromanyl ✱

Potential Causes of Decreased Secretion
- Dopamine
- Hyperthyroidism

Oxytocin

Potential Causes of Increased Secretion
- Nipple manipulation
- Orgasm
- Extracellular fluid hypertonicity

Potential Causes of Decreased Secretion
- Stress
- Opioids

Data from Wilson, J., et al. (Eds.). (1998). *William's textbook of endocrinology* (9th ed.). Philadelphia: W.B. Saunders.

GLUCOCORTICOIDS

The main glucocorticoid produced by the adrenal cortex is **cortisol.** Cortisol affects the following:
- Carbohydrate, protein, and fat metabolism
- The body's response to stress
- Emotional stability
- Immune function

Cortisol has a permissive effect on other body processes. It must be present for other important processes to occur, such as catecholamine action and maintaining the normal excitability of the heart muscles cells. Glucocorticoid functions are listed in Table 65-5.

The release of glucocorticoids is regulated directly by the anterior pituitary hormone ACTH and indirectly by the hypothalamic corticotropin-releasing hormone (CRH). The release of CRH and ACTH is affected by the serum level of free cortisol, the normal sleep-wake cycle, and stress.

As described earlier, when blood cortisol levels are low, the hypothalamus secretes CRH, which triggers the pituitary to release ACTH. Then ACTH triggers the adrenal cortex to se-

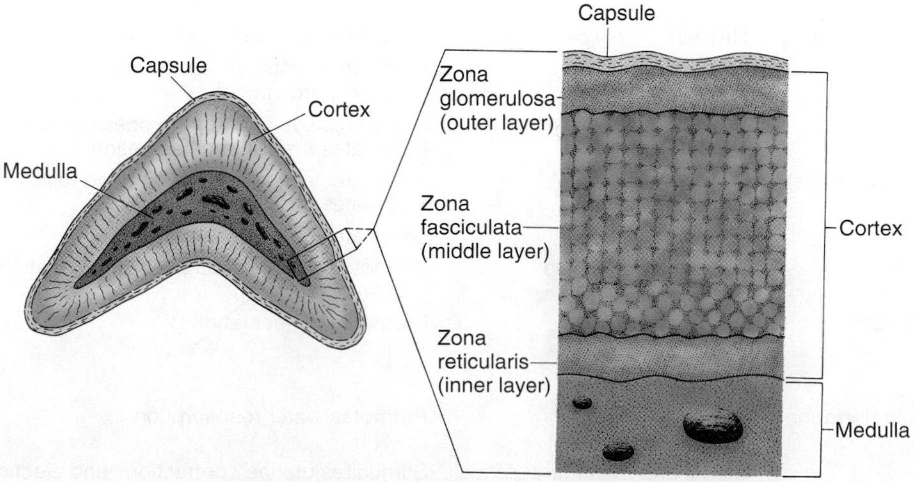

Figure 65-5 ■ The structural detail of the adrenal gland.

crete cortisol. Conversely, adequate or elevated blood levels of cortisol *inhibit* the release of CRH and ACTH. This inhibitory effect is an example of a negative feedback system.

Glucocorticoid release peaks in the morning and reaches its lowest level 12 hours after each peak. Emotional, chemical, or physical stress increases the release of glucocorticoids.

SEX HORMONES

Small amounts of androgens and estrogens are secreted by the adrenal cortex in both genders. Adrenal secretion of these hormones is usually not significant because the **gonads** (ovaries and testes) secrete much larger amounts of estrogens and androgens. In women, however, the adrenal gland is the major source of androgens. Women who have adrenal insufficiency or who have had surgical removal of the adrenals may need a small amount of testosterone replacement.

ADRENAL MEDULLA

Structure

The adrenal medulla is actually a sympathetic nerve ganglion that has secretory cells. Stimulation of the sympathetic nervous system results in the release of adrenal medullary hormones, the **catecholamines** (which includes epinephrine and norepinephrine). These hormones travel to all areas of the body through the blood and exert their effects on target cells. The adrenal medullary hormones are not essential for life but play a role in the physiologic stress response.

Function

The adrenal medulla secretes norepinephrine (NE) and epinephrine, in proportions of 15% and 85%, respectively. The effects of these hormones vary according to the specific receptor in the cell membranes of the target tissue.

These receptors are of two types: alpha adrenergic and beta adrenergic. Both types of receptors are further classified as $alpha_1$- and $alpha_2$-receptors and $beta_1$-, $beta_2$-, and $beta_3$-receptors. NE acts mainly on alpha-adrenergic receptors, and epinephrine most often stimulates beta-adrenergic receptors.

Catecholamines exert their actions on many target organs. Table 65-6 lists the effects of these hormones on body tissues and organs.

Activation of the sympathetic nervous system, which then releases adrenal medullary catecholamines, is an important part of the body's response to stress. Catecholamines are secreted in small amounts at all times to maintain homeostasis. Severe stress triggers increased secretion of catecholamines. This sympathetic activation results in the "fight-or-flight" response, a state of heightened physical and emotional awareness.

TABLE 65-5 Functions of Glucocorticoid Hormones

- Maintain blood glucose level by increasing hepatic gluconeogenesis and inhibiting peripheral glucose use
- Increase lipolysis, releasing glycerol and free fatty acids
- Increase protein catabolism
- Degrade collagen and connective tissue
- Increase the number of polymorphonuclear leukocytes released from bone marrow
- Exert anti-inflammatory effects that decrease the migration of inflammatory cells to sites of injury
- Maintain behavior and cognitive functions

Thyroid Gland

Structure

The thyroid gland is in the anterior neck, directly below the cricoid cartilage (Figure 65-6). It has two lobes joined by a thin strip of tissue (isthmus) in front of the trachea.

The thyroid gland has a rich blood supply, and the right lobe is slightly larger than the left lobe. It is composed of follicular and parafollicular cells. Follicular cells produce the thyroid hormones **thyroxine (T_4)** and **triiodothyronine (T_3).**

TABLE 65-6 Catecholamine Receptors and Effects of Adrenal Medullary Hormone Stimulation on Selected Organs and Tissues

Organ or Tissue	Receptors	Effects
Heart	$Beta_1$	Chronotropic action Inotropic action
Blood vessels	Alpha $Beta_2$	Vasoconstriction Vasodilation
Gastrointestinal tract	Alpha	Increased sphincter tone
	Beta	Decreased motility
Kidney	$Beta_2$	Increased renin release
Bronchioles	$Beta_2$	Relaxation; dilation
Bladder	Alpha $Beta_2$	Sphincter contractions Relaxation of detrusor muscle
Skin	Alpha	Increased sweating
Fat cells	Beta	Increased lipolysis
Liver	Alpha	Increased gluconeogenesis and glycogenolysis
Pancreas	Alpha	Decreased glucagon and insulin release
	Beta	Increased glucagon and insulin release
Eyes	Alpha	Dilation of pupils

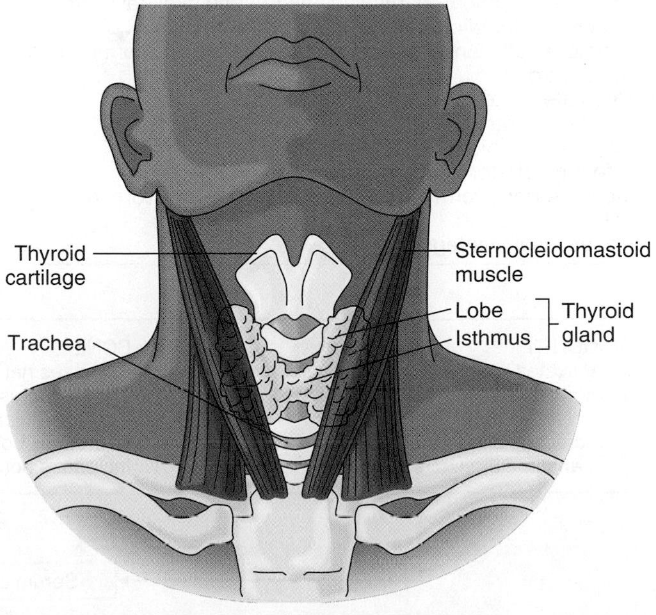

Figure 65-6 ■ Anatomic location of the thyroid gland.

Parafollicular cells produce and secrete **thyrocalcitonin** (calcitonin), which helps to regulate serum calcium levels.

Function

CONTROL OF METABOLISM

Both T_3 and T_4 increase metabolism, which causes an increase in oxygen use and heat production in all tissues. The two hormones differ in structure, but their functions are the same. Most circulating T_4 and T_3 is bound to plasma proteins. The proportion of bound hormone is in balance with the free hormone. The free hormone moves into the cell, where it binds to its receptor in the cell nucleus. Once in the cell, T_4 is converted to T_3, the most active thyroid hormone. The conversion of T_4 to T_3 is impaired by stress, starvation, dyes, beta blockers, amiodarone, corticosteroids, and propylthiouracil (PTU). Cold temperatures increase the conversion. Table 65-7 lists thyroid hormone functions.

The secretion of the thyroid hormones T_3 and T_4 is controlled by the hypothalamic-pituitary-thyroid gland axis, or feedback mechanism. The hypothalamus secretes thyrotropin-releasing hormone (TRH). TRH triggers the anterior pituitary gland to secrete thyroid-stimulating hormone (TSH), which then stimulates the thyroid gland to make and release thyroid hormones. If thyroid hormone levels are high, TSH release is inhibited; if low, TSH release is increased. This is an example of a negative feedback system. Cold and stress are two factors that cause the hypothalamus to secrete TRH, which then stimulates the anterior pituitary to secrete TSH.

Thyroid hormone production involves a series of steps. Dietary intake of protein and iodine is needed to produce thyroid hormones. Iodine is absorbed from the intestinal tract as iodide. The thyroid gland withdraws iodide from the blood and concentrates it. After iodide is in the thyroid, it enters into a series of reactions to form T_4 and T_3. These hormones bind to thyroglobulin and are stored in the follicular cells of the thyroid gland. With stimulation, T_4 and T_3 break off from thyroglobulin and are released into the blood. They enter many cells, bind to the nucleus, and turn on genes important in metabolism. Thus the presence of T_4 and T_3 directly regulate basal metabolic rate (BMR).

TABLE 65-7 Functions of Thyroid Hormones

- Fetal development, particularly neural and skeletal systems
- Control metabolic rate of all cells
- Promote sufficient pituitary secretion of growth hormone and gonadotropins
- Regulate protein, carbohydrate, and fat metabolism
- Exert chronotropic and inotropic cardiac effects
- Increase red blood cell production
- Affect respiratory rate and drive
- Increase bone formation and decrease bone resorption of calcium
- Act as insulin antagonists

CALCIUM AND PHOSPHOROUS BALANCE

Calcitonin (also called thyrocalcitonin, or TCT) is another hormone produced in the thyroid gland. Calcitonin lowers serum calcium and serum phosphorous levels by reducing bone resorption (breakdown). It works in opposition to parathyroid hormone (PTH).

The serum calcium level determines calcitonin secretion. Low serum calcium levels suppress the release of calcitonin; elevated serum calcium levels increase its secretion. Other factors that increase calcitonin release are pregnancy, a high-calcium diet, and an increased secretion of gastrin.

Parathyroid Glands

Structure

The parathyroid glands consist of four small glands located close to, embedded in, or attached to the back surface of the thyroid gland (see Figure 65-1). The chief cells of the parathyroid glands produce and secrete PTH.

Function

Parathyroid hormone regulates calcium and phosphorous metabolism by acting on bone, kidney, and the intestinal tract (Figure 65-7). Bone is the main storage site of calcium. PTH increases bone resorption, thus increasing serum calcium. In the kidneys, PTH activates vitamin D, which then increases the absorption of calcium and phosphate from the intestines. In the kidney tubules, PTH allows calcium to be reabsorbed and put back into the blood.

Serum calcium level is the major controlling factor of PTH secretion. PTH secretion decreases when serum calcium levels are high, and it increases when serum calcium levels are low. Serum phosphorous levels also affect PTH secretion, most likely because of the effect on serum calcium levels. PTH and calcitonin work together to maintain a normal level of ionic calcium in the blood and extracellular fluid.

Pancreas

Structure

The pancreas lies behind the stomach and has endocrine and exocrine functions. The islets of Langerhans areas perform the endocrine functions of the pancreas (Figure 65-8). About one million islet cells are found throughout the pancreas.

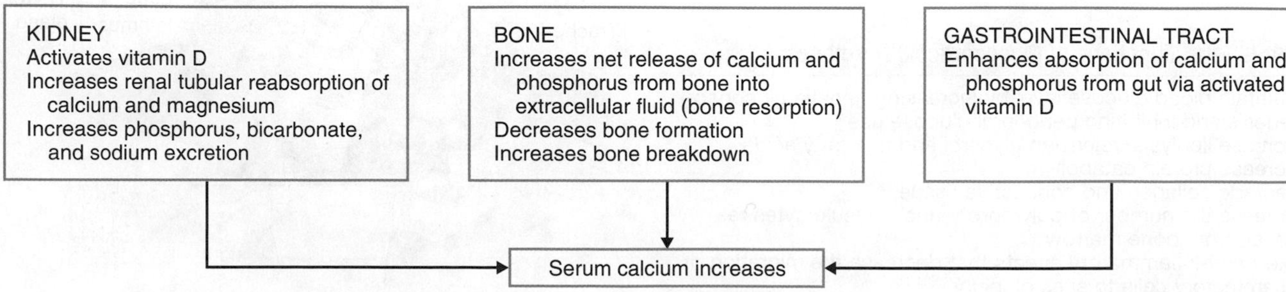

Figure 65-7 ■ Effects of parathyroid hormone on target organs.

The islets have three distinct cell types: alpha cells, which secrete glucagon; beta cells, which secrete insulin; and delta cells, which secrete somatostatin. Glucagon and insulin affect carbohydrate, protein, and fat metabolism. Somatostatin, which is secreted not only in the pancreas but also in the intestinal tract and the brain, inhibits the release of glucagon and insulin from the pancreas. It also inhibits the release of gastrin, secretin, and other gastrointestinal (GI) peptides.

Function

The exocrine function of the pancreas involves the secretion of digestive enzymes through ducts that empty into the duodenum (see Chapter 56). The main endocrine function of the pancreas is to regulate blood glucose (sugar).

Glucagon is a hormone that increases blood glucose levels. It is triggered by decreased blood glucose levels and increased blood amino acid levels. Together with epinephrine, growth hormone (GH), and cortisol, glucagon maintains blood glucose levels. In the liver (the main target organ of glucagon), it causes **glycogenolysis** (the conversion of glycogen to glucose). Glucagon also enhances amino acid transport from muscle and promotes **gluconeogenesis** (the conversion of amino acids to glucose). In fat metabolism, glucagon enhances **lipolysis** (fat breakdown) and ketone formation.

Insulin, an **anabolic** hormone (one that stimulates growth), promotes the movement and storage of carbohydrate (CHO), protein, and fat (Table 65-8). Insulin lowers blood glucose levels by enhancing glucose movement across cell membranes in many tissues. Basal levels of insulin are secreted continuously to control metabolism. Insulin secretion rises in response to an increase in blood glucose levels. CHO is the major stimulus for insulin secretion; amino acids trigger a lower-level response. More information on insulin is presented in Chapter 68.

Endocrine Changes Associated with Aging

The effects of aging on the endocrine system vary widely. The three endocrine tissues most commonly observed to have reduced function with aging include the gonads, the thyroid gland, and the endocrine pancreas. It is difficult to distinguish normal from abnormal endocrine activity because of the following other age-related variables:

- Acute and chronic illnesses
- Alterations in diet, activity, and lean body mass-fat ratio
- Disturbances in sleep patterns
- Decreased metabolic clearance rate of hormones
- Increased use of multiple drugs that may affect hormone function

It is important to consider these factors when assessing the older adult with endocrine dysfunction.

Encourage the older adult client to participate in regular screening examinations, including fasting and postprandial blood glucose checks, calcium level determinations, and thyroid function testing. Chart 65-1 lists the endocrine changes that occur in the older adult.

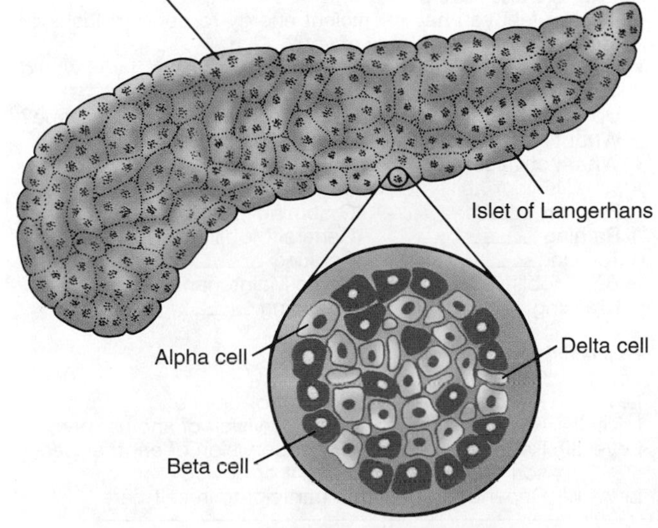

Figure 65-8 ■ The islets of Langerhans of the pancreas.

ASSESSMENT TECHNIQUES

History

Use a systems approach to obtain the history of clients with a suspected endocrine problem. This approach can be difficult because of the variety and combination of clinical manifestations. Identify the client's response to actual or perceived changes, and discuss the potential diagnostic and treatment plan. Chart 65-2 presents some assessment questions based on Gordon's Functional Health Patterns. Although endocrine problems can disturb any health pattern, the patterns most commonly affected are Nutritional-Metabolic, Activity, Elimination, Sleep-Rest, and Sexuality-Reproductive. These data are combined with physical, psychosocial, and laboratory findings for a complete assessment of endocrine function.

DEMOGRAPHIC DATA

The age and gender of the client provide baseline assessment data. Certain disorders are more common in older than in younger clients, such as diabetes mellitus, loss of ovarian function, and decreased thyroid function.

Manifestations of endocrine disorders can be gender related, such as the sexual effects of hyperpituitarism and hypopituitarism (see Chapter 66).

FAMILY HISTORY AND GENETIC RISK

Ask the client about any family history of obesity, growth or development difficulties, diabetes mellitus, infertility, or

TABLE 65-8 Anabolic Effects of Insulin

Effects on Liver
- Promotes glycogen synthesis and storage
- Inhibits glycogenolysis, gluconeogenesis, and ketogenesis
- Increases triglyceride synthesis

Effects on Muscle
- Promotes protein synthesis
- Increases amino acid transport
- Promotes glycogenesis

Effects on Fat
- Increases fatty acid synthesis
- Promotes triglyceride storage
- Decreases lipolysis

CHART 65-1

NURSING FOCUS on the OLDER ADULT

Changes in the Endocrine System Related to Aging

Physiologic Change	Nursing Interventions	Rationales
Decreased antidiuretic hormone (ADH)	Assess for diluted urine and polyuria.	Ongoing assessment helps to detect early signs of complications.
	Monitor fluid intake and output. Encourage fluid intake unless contraindicated.	A sufficient fluid intake may help prevent dehydration.
Decreased ovarian function	Teach the client the signs and symptoms of estrogen deficiency.	The client's ability to cope with changes may be enhanced with knowledge.
	Promote exercise and calcium intake.	Sufficient exercise and calcium intake delay bone loss and prevent osteoporosis.
Decreased glucose tolerance	Identify at-risk clients by obtaining a family history of diabetes mellitus and obesity. Assess for greater-than-ideal body weight or body mass index, little physical exercise, frequent yeast infections, polydipsia, polyuria.	Identification of at-risk clients helps in early detection of complications and conditions such as diabetes.
	Teach the client the signs and symptoms of hyperglycemia.	Knowledge helps to improve the client's ability to recognize hyperglycemia.
Decreased peripheral metabolism	Assess for signs and symptoms of hypothyroidism, especially constipation, lethargy, dry skin, and mental deterioration.	Ongoing assessment helps to differentiate hypothyroidism from the clinical features of aging.

CHART 65-2

Endocrine Assessment

USING GORDON'S FUNCTIONAL HEALTH PATTERNS

Nutritional-Metabolic Pattern
- What is your typical daily food intake? Describe a day's meals, snacks, and vitamins.
- How much salt do you typically add to your food? Do you use salt substitutes?
- How is your appetite?
- Do you have any difficulty chewing or swallowing?
- What is your typical daily fluid intake? What types of fluids (water, juices, soft drinks, coffee, tea)? How much?
- Have you had any recent change in your weight? Weight gain? Weight loss? How much?
- Have you noticed a change in the tightness of your rings or shoes? Tighter? Looser?
- Have you noticed any change in thirst?

Elimination Pattern
- What is your usual bowel elimination pattern? Frequency? Character? Discomfort? Laxatives?
- What is your usual urinary elimination pattern? Frequency? Amount? Color? Odor? Control?
- Have you noticed a change in the amount of urine?
- Do you have any problem with excessive perspiration?
- Do you have any other type of drainage?

Sleep-Rest Pattern
- Do you have any difficulty falling asleep when you go to bed?
- Is there a change in the number of hours you sleep per night?
- Do you take any medication to help you sleep?
- About how many times do you awaken during the night?
- Do you have any difficulty getting back to sleep?
- Are you bothered by nightmares or vivid dreams?
- Do you have difficulty awakening in the morning?
- Do you feel generally rested and ready for daily activities after sleep?
- Do you take scheduled naps or rest periods during the day?
- Do you find yourself falling asleep at work or at home while reading or watching television?
- Have you noticed any difficulty in your ability to concentrate?

Sexuality-Reproductive Pattern
- Are you sexually active?
- Are you satisfied with your level of sexual activity?
- Do you participate in sex as often as you would like?
- Do you participate in sex as often as your partner would like?
- Have you noticed a change in your interest in having sex over the past year?

Female:
- At what age did menstruation start?
- How regular are your periods?
- Do you have any pain, cramping, or clotting during your periods?
- Have you ever been pregnant? What was the outcome of the pregnancy(ies)?
- Do you use contraceptives? What type? Have you had any problems with your chosen method of contraception?

Activity-Exercise Pattern
- Do you feel you have sufficient energy to perform tasks or routines that are required of you?
- Do you feel you have sufficient energy to do what you would like to do?
- Do you exercise? How often? For how long each time? What type(s) of exercise do you perform?
- What activities do you perform in your spare time?
- What is your ability to perform the following tasks?

Feeding _____	Grooming _____
Bathing _____	General Mobility _____
Toileting _____	Cooking _____
Bed Mobility _____	Home Maintenance _____
Dressing _____	Shopping _____

Functional Levels Code

Level 0: Full self-care
Level I: Requires use of equipment or device
Level II: Requires assistance or supervision of another person
Level III: Requires assistance or supervision of another person and use of equipment or device
Level IV: Dependent; does not participate in self-care

Based on Gordon, M. (2002). *Manual of nursing diagnosis* (10th ed.). St. Louis: Mosby.

thyroid disorders. These problems may have an autosomal dominant, recessive, or cluster pattern of inheritance.

PERSONAL HISTORY

Assess the client for a history of endocrine dysfunction, manifestations that could indicate an endocrine disorder, and hospitalizations. Ask asked about past and current drugs, such as hydrocortisone, levothyroxine, oral contraceptives, and antihypertensive agents.

DIET HISTORY

Nutritional changes or GI tract disturbances may reflect many different endocrine problems. Ask about a history of nausea, vomiting, and abdominal pain. An increase or decrease in food or fluid intake may also indicate specific disorders. For example, diabetes insipidus triggers excessive thirst, and adrenal hypofunction triggers salt craving. Hunger and thirst may also be increased in diabetes mellitus. Rapid changes in weight without diet changes can signal the onset of a number of endocrine disorders, including diabetes mellitus and thyroid problems.

SOCIOECONOMIC STATUS

Because the client's socioeconomic status is a sensitive issue, explore with the client whether his or her resources are adequate for a healthy diet, needed drugs, and consistent health care follow-up. It may be appropriate to involve social service and home care agencies at an early stage.

CURRENT HEALTH PROBLEMS

Focus on the client's reason for seeking health care, asking questions such as the following:

- Did the symptoms occur gradually, or was the onset sudden?
- Has the client been treated for this problem in the past?
- How have the current symptoms affected the activities of daily living (ADLs)?

Such questions provide clues to specific endocrine disorders. Also explore changes in energy levels, elimination patterns, sexual and reproductive functions, and physical features.

Energy Levels

Changes in energy levels occur with many endocrine problems, especially thyroid problems (see Chapter 67) and adrenal problems (see Chapter 66). Ask the client about any change in ability to perform ADLs and assess the client's current energy level. For instance, has the client been sleeping longer, or does he or she have fatigue or generalized weakness?

Elimination

Elimination is also affected by the endocrine system. Identify the client's past pattern of elimination to determine deviations from the normal routine. Ask about the amount and frequency of urination. Does he or she urinate frequently in large amounts? Does the client wake during the night to urinate **(nocturia),** or is pain present with urination **(dysuria)?** Information about the frequency of bowel movements and their consistency and color may provide clues to problems in fluid balance or metabolic rate (i.e., thyroid function).

Sex and Reproduction

Sexual and reproductive functions are greatly affected by endocrine disturbances. Ask women about any changes in the menstrual cycle, such as increased flow, duration, and frequency of menses; pain or excessive cramping; or a recent change in the regularity of menses. Ask men whether they have experienced impotence. Question both men and women about a change in libido or any fertility problems.

Physical Appearance

Discuss any changes that the client perceives in physical features. Overt changes are identified during the physical assessment, but clients may be able to describe some of the more subtle changes. Ask the client about changes in the following:

- Hair texture and distribution
- Facial contours and eye protrusion
- Voice quality
- Body proportions
- Secondary sexual characteristics

For example, you might ask a man whether he is shaving less often or a woman if she has noticed an increase in facial hair. These changes may be associated with pituitary, thyroid, parathyroid, or adrenal dysfunction.

Critical Thinking Challenge

The client is a 44-year-old woman who tells you that she feels fatigued, although she goes to bed early. She says that she awakens frequently and has a hard time getting back to sleep. Some of the physical changes she has noticed over the past 6 months include a thinning of her pubic hair and a weight gain of about 15 lbs. Her periods have become less predictable and vary in amount of flow from scant to heavy. A home pregnancy test indicates that she is not pregnant.

1. Which endocrine glands or tissues should be assessed for causing the problems she has noticed?
2. What questions could you ask to try and quantify her sense of fatigue?
3. Are there any questions you should ask about the information she has already provided?

evolve For suggested answer guidelines, go to http://evolve.elsevier.com/Iggy/.

Physical Assessment

INSPECTION

An endocrine problem can change physical features because of its effect on growth and development, regulation of sex hormone levels, fluid and electrolyte balance, and the body's use of nutrients. Different clinical findings can occur with multiple endocrine disorders or with nonendocrine problems.

Use a head-to-toe approach to inspect the client. Observe the client's general appearance, and assess height, weight, fat distribution, and muscle mass in relation to age. It is important to remember that heredity and age rather than a health problem may be responsible for some physical features (e.g., short stature).

When examining the head, focus on abnormalities of facial structure, features, and expression, such as the following:

- Prominent forehead or jaw
- Round or puffy face

- Dull or flat expression
- Exophthalmos (protruding eyeballs and retracted upper lids)

Check the lower half of the neck for a visible enlargement of the thyroid gland. Normally the thyroid tissue cannot be observed. The isthmus may be noticeable when the client swallows. Jugular vein distention may be seen on inspection of the neck and can indicate fluid overload (see Chapter 15).

Skin changes may reflect a specific endocrine dysfunction. Observe skin color, and look for areas of pigment loss (hypopigmentation) or hyperpigmentation. Fungal skin infections, slow wound healing, bruising, and petechiae are often seen in clients with adrenal hyperfunction. Skin infections, foot ulcers, and slow wound healing are common among clients with diabetes mellitus. In secondary hypofunction of the adrenal glands, the skin over the finger joints, elbows, and knees, as well as any scar tissue, may show increased pigmentation due to increased levels of ACTH and melanocyte-stimulating hormone.

Vitiligo (patchy areas of pigment loss with increased pigmentation at the edges) is seen with primary hypofunction of the adrenal glands and is due to autoimmune destruction of melanocytes in the skin. Areas of pigment loss most often occur on the face, neck, and extremities. Mucous membranes may have large areas of uneven pigmentation. Document the location, color, distribution, and size of skin color changes and lesions.

Inspect the client's fingernails for malformation, thickness, or brittleness, all of which may suggest thyroid gland problems. Examine the extremities and the base of the spine for edema, which suggests a fluid and electrolyte imbalance.

Inspection of the trunk can show signs of specific endocrine dysfunction. Check for any abnormalities in chest size and symmetry. Truncal obesity, supraclavicular fat pads, and a "buffalo hump" may indicate adrenocortical excess. Hormonal imbalance may also change secondary sexual characteristics. Inspect the breasts of both men and women for size, symmetry, pigmentation, and discharge. **Striae** (reddish purple "stretch marks") on the breasts or abdomen are often seen with adrenocortical excess.

Assess the client's hair distribution for indications of endocrine gland dysfunction. Changes can include **hirsutism** (excessive growth of body hair, especially on the face, chest, and the linea alba of the abdomen of women), excessive hair loss, or changes in hair texture.

Examination of the genitalia may reveal a dysfunction in hormone secretion. Observe the size of the scrotum and penis or of the labia and clitoris in relation to standards for the client's age. The distribution and quantity of pubic hair are often affected in hypogonadism.

PALPATION

The thyroid gland and the testes can be examined by palpation. Chapters 76 and 79 discuss examination of the testes. The thyroid gland is palpated for size, symmetry, general shape, and the presence of nodules or other irregularities.

Palpate the thyroid gland by standing either behind or in front of the client (Figure 65-9); the posterior approach may be easier. Asking the client to swallow sips of water during the examination helps the clinician palpate the thyroid gland.

Ask the client to sit and to lower the chin. Using the posterior approach, place the thumbs of both your hands on the back of the client's neck, with the fingers curved around to the front of the neck on either side of the trachea. Ask the client to swallow, and then locate the isthmus of the thyroid as you feel it rising. Identify the anterior surface of the thyroid lobe. To examine the right lobe, proceed in the following way:

- Turn the client's head to the right
- Displace the thyroid cartilage to the right with the fingers of your left hand
- Palpate the right lobe with your right hand

Reverse this procedure to examine the left lobe.

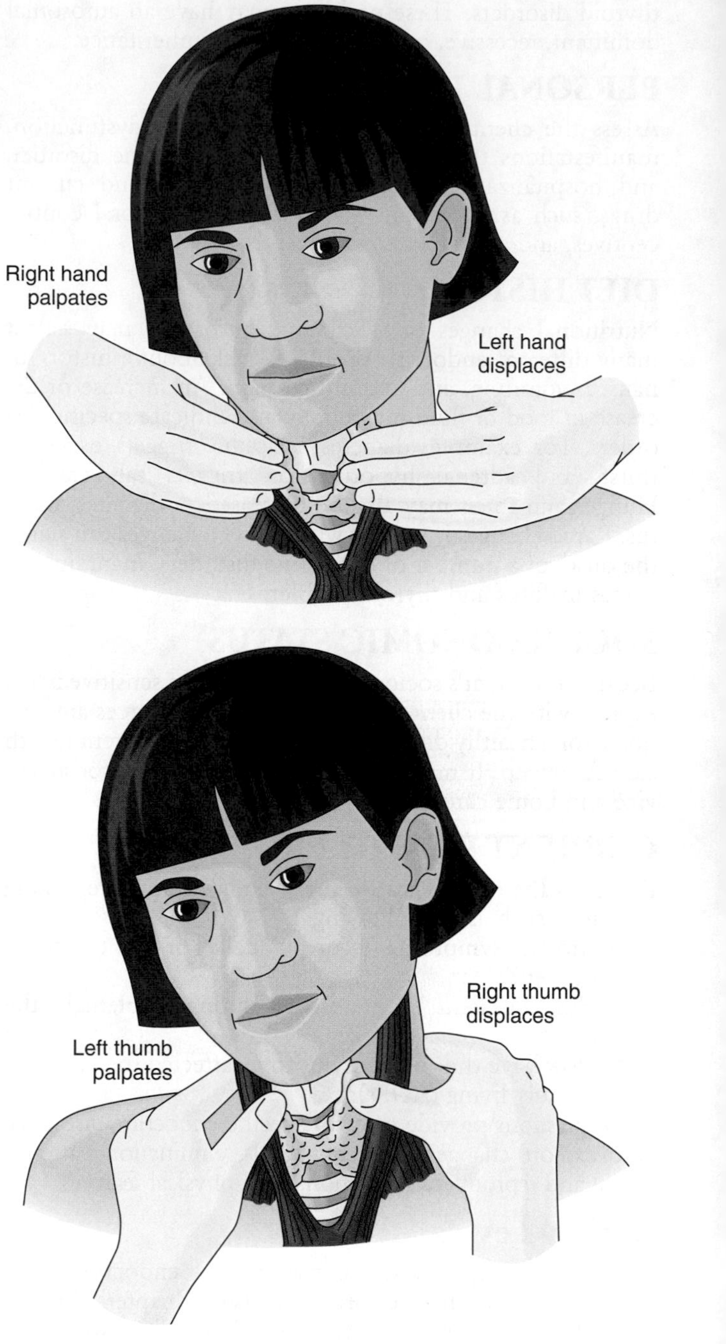

Figure 65-9 ■ Palpation of the thyroid gland.

AUSCULTATION

Auscultate the client's chest to establish baseline vital signs and to assess cardiac rate and rhythm. Some endocrine problems induce dysrhythmias. Many endocrine disturbances can cause dehydration and volume depletion. Therefore document any difference in the client's blood pressure and pulse in the lying, standing, or sitting positions (orthostatic vital signs).

If an enlarged thyroid gland is palpated, auscultate the area of enlargement for bruits. Hypertrophy of the thyroid gland causes an increase in vascular flow, which may result in bruits.

Psychosocial Assessment

Information obtained from the history and physical examination may help to identify psychosocial problems. Assess the client's coping skills, support systems, and health-related beliefs.

A number of endocrine disorders affect the client's perception of self. For example, body features can change significantly in disorders of the pituitary, adrenal, and thyroid glands. Infertility, impotence, and other changes in sexual function may result from endocrine dysfunction. Ask about any difficulty in coping with such changes.

Clients with endocrine problems may require lifelong drugs and follow-up care. Assess the client's readiness to learn and his or her ability to carry out specific self-management skills. Clients may also face financial difficulties resulting from a prolonged medical regimen or loss of employment. A referral to social service agencies may be needed.

Diagnostic Assessment

LABORATORY TESTS

For the client with possible endocrine dysfunction, laboratory tests are an essential part of the diagnostic process. The specialized testing for specific disorders is described in Chapters 66 to 68. Best practices for the collection of specimens for general endocrine testing are listed in Chart 65-3.

Stimulation/Suppression Tests

Measurement of specific hormone levels does not always distinguish between the normal and the abnormal. The wide normal range for some hormones makes it necessary to trigger responses by stimulation or suppression tests.

For the client who might have underactivity of an endocrine gland, a stimulus may be provided to determine whether the gland is capable of normal hormone production. This method is called *stimulation testing.* Measured amounts of selected hormones are given to stimulate the target gland to maximal production. Hormone levels are then measured and compared with expected normal values. Failure of the hormone level to rise with stimulation indicates hypofunction.

Suppression tests are used when hormone levels are high or in the upper range of normal. Failure of suppression of hormone production during testing indicates hyperfunction. (See the specific tests in Chapters 66 and 67.)

Assays

An assay measures the level of a specific hormone in blood or other body fluid. Some assays are indirect, such as the radioimmunoassay. In this test, radioactively labeled amounts of hormone (antigen) compete with unlabeled hormones from the plasma or serum for antibody binding sites. Various techniques measure the amount of unbound and bound hormone. The unbound hormone is the active hormone.

CHART 65-3

BEST PRACTICE for Endocrine Testing

- Explain the procedure to the client.
- Emphasize the importance of taking a medication prescribed for the test on *time.* Tell the client to set an alarm if the medication is to be taken during the night.
- Instruct the client to begin the urine collection (whether for 2, 4, 8, 12, or 24 hours) by emptying his or her bladder. Tell the client *not* to save the urine specimen that begins the collection. The timing for the urine collection begins after this specimen. To end the collection, the client empties his or her bladder at the end of the timed period and adds that urine to the collection.
- Make sure that the preservative has been added to the collection container at the beginning of the collection, if necessary. Tell the client of its presence in the container.
- Check your laboratory's method of handling hormone test samples. Blood samples drawn for certain hormones (e.g., catecholamines) must be placed on ice and taken to the laboratory immediately.
- If you are drawing blood samples from a line, clear the intravenous (IV) line thoroughly. Do not use a double- or triple-lumen line to obtain samples; contamination or dilution from another port is possible.

Other hormone assay methods include immunometric assays, chromatographic assays, and mass spectrometry. An immunometric assay uses a large antibody with a component that "captures" the hormone and a second component that creates a signal when the antibody binds to the hormone (antigen). Chromatographic assays separate molecules in the serum by size, light absorption, and other properties. Each hormone has very specific properties that allow it to separate from other blood substances and form a unique bandwidth. Mass spectrometry methods also allow individual hormones to separate from other serum molecules based on the amount (mass) and charge of individual components. On a graph these separate hormones each show as a unique "spike" pattern. Many different hormone concentrations can be analyzed at the same time by this method.

Urine Tests

Hormone levels and the metabolites of specific hormones in the urine are often measured to determine endocrine function. Because many of the endocrine hormones are secreted in a pulsatile fashion, measurement of a specific hormone in a 24-hour urine collection better reflects the overall function of certain glands, such as the adrenal gland. Teach the client how to collect a 24-hour urine sample (see also Chart 65-3).

Certain hormones require additives in the container at the beginning of the collection. Instruct the client not to discard the preservative from the container and to use caution when handling it because some solutions are caustic. Remind the client that this collection is timed for *exactly* 24 hours. Instruct the client to avoid taking any unnecessary drugs during endocrine testing because some drugs can interfere with the laboratory assays.

Tests for Glucose

Tests for functions of the islet cells of the pancreas are indirect; they measure the *result* of pancreatic islet cell function. Blood glucose values and the oral glucose tolerance test help to diagnose diabetes mellitus. The glycosylated hemoglobin (HbA_{1C}) value reveals the *average* blood glucose level over a period of 2 to 3 months. Its primary use is in assessing overall control of glucose level in diabetes mellitus. (See Chapter 68 for a full discussion of diabetes mellitus.)

RADIOGRAPHIC EXAMINATIONS

Anterior, posterior, and lateral skull x-rays may be used to visualize the sella turcica. Erosion of the sella turcica indicates invasion of the wall from an abnormal growth.

Magnetic resonance imaging (MRI) with contrast is the most sensitive method of imaging the pituitary gland, although computed tomography (CT) scans can also be used to evaluate it. The thyroid, parathyroid glands, ovaries, and testes are evaluated by ultrasound. In addition, CT scans are used to evaluate the adrenal glands, ovaries, and pancreas.

OTHER DIAGNOSTIC TESTS

Needle biopsy is a relatively safe and quick outpatient procedure used to indicate the composition of thyroid nodules. It is used to determine whether surgical intervention is needed.

Critical Thinking Challenge

The 44-year-old client with fatigue, menstrual changes, weight gain, and loss of pubic hair is scheduled to have blood drawn for follicle-stimulating hormone (FSH) levels, thyroid hormone levels, and blood glucose levels; an ultrasound of the ovaries; a 24-hour urine collection for estradiol beta-17 levels, and a CT scan of the head. In addition, she is to return for a glucose tolerance test. She is very anxious about the tests and the results.

1. How should you prepare her physically for each test?
2. What special instructions should you provide for the 24-hour urine test?
3. The client is very concerned about pain and modesty. What reassurances can you provide for the level of pain expected?
4. Is the client's modesty at risk with any of these procedures? If so, how? What precautions can be taken to reduce exposure?

evolve For suggested answer guidelines, go to http://evolve.elsevier.com/Iggy/.

GET READY for the NCLEX Examination!

KEY POINTS

Safe Effective Care Environment

- Use good handwashing technique and precautions to reduce the spread of infection to any client who is taking exogenous corticosteroids or who has a problem that increases corticosteroid production.

Health Promotion and Maintenance

- Teach all clients that abusing hormones or steroids can have an adverse effect on endocrine function.

Psychosocial Integrity

- Explain all diagnostic procedures, restrictions, and follow-up care to the client scheduled for tests.
- Allow the client to express fears or concerns about a change in appearance or a reduction in fertility.
- Ask family members about changes in the client's personality or behavior.

Physiological Integrity

- Ask the client about other family members with endocrine disorders because some endocrine problems have a genetic component.
- Ask the client what prescribed and over-the-counter drugs are taken on a regular basis because some drugs can alter endocrine function (see Table 65-4).

ADDITIONAL STUDY RESOURCES

Go to your Student CD-ROM for Review Questions for the NCLEX Examination.

evolve Go to http://evolve.elsevier.com/Iggy/ for Integrated Management of Care Questions for the NCLEX Examination.

SELECTED BIBLIOGRAPHY

Berne, R., et al. (2004). *Physiology* (5th ed.). St. Louis: Mosby.

Ebersole, P., Hess, P., & Luggen, A. (2004). *Toward healthy aging: Human needs and nursing response* (6th ed.). St. Louis: Mosby.

Gordon, M. (2002). *Manual of nursing diagnosis* (10th ed.). St. Louis: Mosby.

Holcomb, S. (2003). Detecting thyroid disease, part 1. *Nursing 2003, 33*(8), 32cc1-32cc4.

Holcomb, S. (2003). Detecting thyroid disease, part 2. *Nursing 2003, 33*(9), 32cc1-32cc4.

Jarvis, C. (2004). *Physical examination and health assessment* (4th ed.). Philadelphia: W.B. Saunders.

Klee, G. (2003). Laboratory techniques for recognition of endocrine disorders. In P.R. Larsen, et al. (Eds.). *Williams' textbook of endocrinology* (10th ed., pp. 65-79). Philadelphia: W.B. Saunders.

Lamberts, S. (2003). Endocrinology and aging. In P.R. Larsen, et al. (Eds.). *Williams' textbook of endocrinology* (10th ed., pp. 1287-1301). Philadelphia: W.B. Saunders.

Larsen, P.R., et al. (Eds.). (2003). *Williams' textbook of endocrinology* (10th ed., pp. 65-79). Philadelphia: W.B. Saunders.

Melmed, S., & Kleinberg, D. (2003). Anterior pituitary. In P.R. Larsen, et al. (Eds.). *Williams textbook of endocrinology* (10th ed., pp. 177-279). Philadelphia: W.B. Saunders.

Pagana, K., & Pagana, T. (2002). *Mosby's manual of diagnostic and laboratory tests* (2nd ed.). St. Louis: Mosby.

Robinson, A., & Verbalis, J. (2003). Posterior pituitary gland. In P.R. Larsen, et al. (Eds.). *Williams' textbook of endocrinology* (10th ed., pp. 281-329). Philadelphia: W.B. Saunders.

CHAPTER

66

Interventions for Clients with Pituitary and Adrenal Gland Problems

M. LINDA WORKMAN

LEARNING OUTCOMES

After studying this chapter, you should be able to:

1. Compare the common clinical manifestations associated with pituitary hypofunction and pituitary hyperfunction.
2. Interpret clinical changes and laboratory data to determine the effectiveness of therapy for pituitary hypofunction.
3. Identify the teaching priorities for the client taking hormone replacement therapy for pituitary hypofunction.
4. Prioritize nursing care for the client immediately after a transsphenoidal hypophysectomy.
5. Interpret clinical changes and laboratory data to determine the effectiveness of therapy for pituitary hyperfunction.
6. Compare the problems associated with oversecretion and undersecretion of antidiuretic hormone on blood and on urine volumes and blood and urine osmolarities.
7. Describe the mechanisms of action, side effects, and nursing implications for pharmacologic management of diabetes insipidus.
8. Interpret clinical changes and laboratory data to determine the effectiveness of interventions for diabetes insipidus.
9. Develop a community-based teaching plan for the client with diabetes insipidus.
10. Interpret clinical changes and laboratory data to determine the effectiveness of interventions for SIADH.
11. Develop a community-based teaching plan for the client with SIADH.
12. Compare the clinical manifestations of Cushing's syndrome and Addison's disease.
13. Interpret clinical changes and laboratory data to determine the effectiveness of interventions for Cushing's syndrome.
14. Develop a community-based teaching plan for the client with Cushing's syndrome or disease.
15. Describe the mechanisms of action, side effects, and nursing implications for pharmacologic management of adrenal insufficiency.
16. Interpret clinical changes and laboratory data to determine the effectiveness of therapy for adrenal insufficiency.
17. Develop a community-based teaching plan for the client with adrenal insufficiency.
18. Prioritize nursing interventions for the client experiencing acute adrenal insufficiency.

Go to your Student CD-ROM for Review Questions for the NCLEX Examination keyed to these Learning Outcomes.

Pituitary and adrenal gland problems can be caused by, or can cause, oversecretion or undersecretion of one or more hormones. At times, the correct amount of hormone may be produced but cannot be used because of receptor site failure.

Hormones secreted from the anterior pituitary gland regulate growth, metabolism, and sexual development. These functions are affected when the pituitary gland secretes too much or too little of one or more hormones. The posterior pituitary gland secretes **vasopressin** (antidiuretic hormone [ADH]).

Posterior pituitary problems result in fluid and electrolyte imbalance. The adrenal gland produces and secretes hormones that influence homeostasis and are life sustaining. The effects of these endocrine problems occur throughout the body and may induce psychological, as well as physical, changes. Nursing care for the client with pituitary or adrenal gland disorders includes assessment, client education, evaluation of client response to therapy, and providing support.

A complete history and physical examination are performed to detect specific clinical findings. The client also often undergoes many diagnostic tests and relies on the nurse for specific instructions and explanations. Surgical intervention may be indicated. The client often needs lifelong hormone replacement therapy. Physical and emotional support is critical.

Disorders of the Pituitary Gland

DISORDERS OF THE ANTERIOR PITUITARY GLAND

The anterior pituitary gland **(adenohypophysis)** controls growth, metabolic activity, and sexual development through the actions of the following hormones:

- Growth hormone (GH; somatotropin)
- Prolactin (PRL)
- Thyrotropin (thyroid-stimulating hormone [TSH])
- Corticotropin (adrenocorticotropic hormone [ACTH])
- Follicle-stimulating hormone (FSH)
- Luteinizing hormone (LH)
- Melanocyte-stimulating hormone (MSH)

Disorders of hormones secreted by the anterior pituitary gland can result from problems arising within the anterior pituitary gland itself **(primary pituitary dysfunction)** or from problems in the hypothalamus that change anterior pituitary function **(secondary pituitary dysfunction)**. In either case, one or more hormones may be undersecreted **(pituitary hypofunction)** or oversecreted **(pituitary hyperfunction)**.

Hypopituitarism

PATHOPHYSIOLOGY

A person with hypopituitarism has a deficiency of one or more anterior pituitary hormones, resulting in metabolic problems and sexual dysfunction. Decreased production of *all* of the anterior pituitary hormones is an extremely rare condition known as **panhypopituitarism**.

More commonly, there is a marked decrease in the secretion of one hormone and a lesser decrease in the other hormones. Deficiencies of adrenocorticotropic hormone (ACTH) and thyroid-stimulating hormone (TSH) are the *most* life threatening because they result in a corresponding decrease in the secretion of vital hormones from the adrenal and thyroid glands. Adrenal gland hypofunction is discussed on pp. 1470 to 1473; hypothyroidism is discussed in Chapter 67.

Deficiency of the **gonadotropins** (luteinizing hormone [LH] and follicle-stimulating hormone [FSH]—hormones that stimulate the ovaries and testes to produce sex hormones) changes sexual function in both men and women. In men, gonadotropin deficiency results in testicular failure, with decreased testosterone production from the Leydig cells and decreased or absent spermatogenesis. Decreased testosterone levels in men cause sterility. In women, gonadotropin deficiency results in ovarian failure, amenorrhea, and infertility.

TABLE 66-1 Causes of Hypopituitarism

Causes of Primary Hypopituitarism
- Pituitary tumor (adenomas, granulomas, meningiomas)
- Partial or total surgical hypophysectomy
- Radiation of the brain
- Infarction following systemic shock
- Metastatic cancer
- Trauma

Causes of Secondary Hypopituitarism
- Infection
- Trauma
- Brain tumor

Growth hormone (GH) deficiency changes tissue growth patterns indirectly. GH itself has little effect on tissues and cells. Rather, the presence of GH stimulates the liver to produce substances known as somatomedins. These somatomedins, especially somatomedin C (insulin-like growth factor-1 [IGF-1]), then enhance growth activities in cells and tissues. Somatomedin C is responsible for bone and cartilage growth and maintenance.

GH deficiency may be a result of decreased GH production, failure of the liver to produce somatomedins, or a failure of the cells or tissues to respond to the somatomedins. GH deficiency in children leads to short stature and other manifestations of growth retardation. GH deficiency in adults does not affect height but does increase the rate of bone destructive activity, leading to thinner, more fragile bones **(osteoporosis).**

The cause of hypopituitarism varies. Benign or malignant pituitary tumors can compress and destroy pituitary tissue. Pituitary function can be impaired by severe malnutrition or rapid loss of body fat, such as in people with **anorexia nervosa** (a disorder in which people see themselves as overweight and eat so little that starvation results). Shock or severe hypotension reduces blood flow to the pituitary gland, leading to hypoxia and infarction. Other causes of hypopituitarism are listed in Table 66-1. Idiopathic hypopituitarism is an isolated hormone deficiency with an unknown cause.

Postpartum hemorrhage is the most common cause of pituitary infarction, which results in decreased hormone secretion. This clinical problem is known as Sheehan's syndrome. The pituitary gland normally enlarges during pregnancy, and when hypotension results from hemorrhage, ischemia and necrosis of the gland occur. Usually this condition develops immediately after delivery, although some cases have occurred several years later.

◆COLLABORATIVE MANAGEMENT

◆Assessment

Changes in physical appearance and target organ function occur with deficiencies of specific pituitary hormones (Chart 66-1). Gonadotropin (LH and FSH) deficiency results in the

CHART 66-1

KEY FEATURES of Pituitary Hypofunction

Deficient Hormone	Clinical Manifestations
Anterior Pituitary Hormones	
Growth hormone (GH)	Decreased bone density Pathologic fractures Decreased muscle strength Increased serum cholesterol levels
Gonadotropins (luteinizing hormone [LH], follicle-stimulating hormone [FSH])	Women: ▪ Amenorrhea ▪ Anovulation ▪ Low circulating estrogen levels ▪ Breast atrophy ▪ Loss of bone density ▪ Decreased axillary and pubic hair ▪ Decreased libido ▪ Fine facial wrinkles Men: ▪ Decreased facial hair ▪ Decreased ejaculate volume ▪ Reduced muscle mass ▪ Loss of bone density ▪ Decreased body hair ▪ Decreased libido ▪ Impotence ▪ Fine facial wrinkles
Thyrotropin	Decreased circulating TSH levels
Thyroid-stimulating hormone [TSH]	Decreased circulating thyroid hormone levels Weight gain Intolerance to cold Scalp alopecia Hirsutism Menstrual abnormalities Decreased libido Slowed cognition Lethargy
Adrenocorticotropic hormone (ACTH)	Decreased serum cortisol levels Pale, sallow complexion Malaise and lethargy Anorexia Postural hypotension Headache Hypoglycemia Hyponatremia Decreased axillary and pubic hair (women)
Posterior Pituitary Hormones	
Vasopressin (antidiuretic hormone [ADH])	Diabetes insipidus ▪ Greatly increased urine output ▪ Low urine specific gravity (<1.005) ▪ Hypovolemia Hypotension Dehydration ▪ Increased plasma osmolarity ▪ Increased thirst ▪ Output does not decrease when fluid intake decreases

Data from Melmed, S., & Kleinberg, D. (2003). Anterior pituitary. In P.R. Larsen, et al. (Eds.). *Williams textbook of endocrinology* (10th ed., pp. 281-329). Philadelphia: W. B. Saunders, and from Robinson, A., & Verbalis, J. (2003). Posterior pituitary gland. In P.R. Larsen, et al. (Eds.). *Williams textbook of endocrinology* (10th ed., pp. 177-279). Philadelphia: W. B. Saunders.

loss of or change in secondary sex characteristics in men and women. While assessing the male client, look for facial and body hair loss. Ask about episodes of impotence and decreased libido (sex drive). Women may report **amenorrhea** (absence of menstrual periods), **dyspareunia** (painful intercourse), **infertility** (difficulty becoming pregnant), and decreased libido. While examining the female client, check for dry skin, breast atrophy, and a decreased amount or absence of axillary and pubic hair.

Neurologic manifestations of hypopituitarism due to tumor growth often first occur as changes in vision. Assess the client's visual acuity, especially peripheral vision, for changes or loss. Temporal headaches are a common finding. Other manifestations may include **diplopia** (double vision) and ocular muscle paralysis, limiting eye movement.

Laboratory findings vary widely with hypopituitarism. Some pituitary hormone levels may be measured directly. Often, however, the *effects* of the hormones, rather than their actual levels, are assessed. Basal levels of triiodothyronine (T_3) and thyroxine (T_4) from the thyroid, as well as testosterone and estradiol from the gonads, are measured easily. If levels of one or all of these hormones are low or in the low-normal range, further evaluation is necessary. Levels of pituitary gonadotropins (LH and FSH) and TSH are sufficient if function of the target organ is apparent. Function of LH and FSH is assessed by observing for the presence of secondary sexual characteristics; function of TSH is assessed by measuring circulating levels of thyroid hormones. ACTH levels may be normal or low, and prolactin (PRL) levels are low to high.

Some tests for pituitary function involve injecting agents that are known to stimulate secretion of specific pituitary hormones and then measuring the response. Such tests are called **stimulation tests**. For example, insulin injection in people with normal pituitary function causes an increased release of GH and ACTH. The stimulation test for either GH or ACTH assessment involves injecting the client with regular insulin (0.05 to 1 units/kg of body weight) and checking the circulating levels of GH and ACTH. The stimulation test for TSH involves injecting thyrotropin-releasing hormone (TRH) and measuring the blood levels of thyroid hormones. The stimulation test for LH and FSH involves giving gonadotropin-releasing hormone (GnRH). In people with no pituitary problems, this injection results in a peak release of LH and FSH within 15 to 45 minutes after the injection. Stimulation testing for PRL is the same as for TSH.

Pituitary problems may cause changes in the sella turcica (the bony nest where the pituitary gland rests) that can be seen with skull x-rays. Changes may include enlargement, erosion, and calcifications as a result of pituitary tumors. Computed tomography (CT) and magnetic resonance imaging (MRI) can more distinctly define bone or soft-tissue lesions. An angiogram may be used to rule out the presence of an aneurysm or congenital vascular malformations before any surgical intervention.

Interventions

Management of the adult with hypopituitarism focuses on replacement of deficient hormones. Older clients or those with a chronic disease often require a lower amount of hormone replacement. Men who have gonadotropin deficiency receive sex steroid replacement therapy with **androgens** (testosterone). The most effective route of androgen replacement is intramuscular (IM), although use of transdermal testosterone patches is increasing. Instruct the client in self-administration. Therapy begins with high-dose testosterone and is continued until **virilization** (presence of male secondary sex characteristics) is achieved. Maximal effects of treatment include increases in penis size, libido, muscle mass, bone size, and bone strength. Chest, facial, pubic, and axillary hair growth also increases, and the voice deepens. Clients usually report improved self-esteem and body image after therapy is initiated. The dose may then be decreased, but therapy continues throughout life.

Androgen therapy is avoided in men with prostate cancer. Side effects of testosterone therapy include **gynecomastia** (the development of breast tissue in men), acne, baldness, and prostate enlargement.

Achieving fertility in these clients is difficult and requires additional parenteral testosterone therapy and injections of human chorionic gonadotropin (hCG). Teach the client about the course of additional therapy and provide emotional support because the outcome of fertility treatment is uncertain.

Women who have gonadotropin deficiency receive hormone replacement with a combination of estrogen and progesterone. The risk for hypertension or thrombosis (formation of blood clots in deep veins) is increased with estrogen therapy, especially among women who smoke. Emphasize measures to reduce risk and the need for regular health visits. For women who wish to become pregnant, clomiphene citrate (Clomid) may be given to induce ovulation. Gonadotropin-releasing hormone (GnRH) and human chorionic gonadotropin (hCG) are used to stimulate ovulation when therapy with clomiphene citrate fails.

Adult clients with GH deficiency may be treated with injections of GH, although this treatment is rare.

Hyperpituitarism

PATHOPHYSIOLOGY

Hyperpituitarism is hormone oversecretion that occurs with pituitary tumors or hyperplasia. Tumors occur most often in the anterior pituitary cells that produce growth hormone (GH), prolactin (PRL), and adrenocorticotropic hormone (ACTH). Overproduction of PRL also may occur in response to tumors that overproduce GH and ACTH. Hypersecretion of ACTH may occur with increased secretion of melanocyte-stimulating hormone (MSH).

The most common cause of hyperpituitarism is a pituitary adenoma, a benign tumor. Adenomas are classified by size, invasiveness, and the hormone secreted. An invasive pituitary adenoma involves a portion or all of the sella turcica. When the sella turcica is not involved, the adenoma is "enclosed."

As an adenoma gets larger and compresses brain tissue, neurologic symptoms, as well as endocrine symptoms, may occur. Such symptoms may include visual changes, headache, and increased intracranial pressure.

PRL-secreting tumors are the most common type of pituitary adenoma. Excessive PRL inhibits the secretion of gonadotropins and sex hormones in men and women, resulting in galactorrhea (breast milk production), amenorrhea, and infertility.

Overproduction of GH results in **gigantism** (Figure 66-1) or **acromegaly** (Figure 66-2). The onset of the disease may be gradual with slow progression, and changes may remain unnoticed for years before diagnosis of the disorder. Early detection and treatment are essential to prevent irreversible changes in the soft tissues, such as those of the face, hands, feet, and skin. These changes are, to a certain extent, reversible after treatment, but skeletal changes are permanent.

In the client with gigantism, the onset of GH hypersecretion occurs *before* puberty, which causes rapid proportional growth in the length of all bones. In the client with acromegaly, excessive GH secretion occurs *after* puberty and produces increased skeletal thickness, hypertrophy of the skin, and enlargement of many visceral organs, such as the liver and heart.

Bone thinning and bone cell overgrowth occur slowly. Degeneration of joint cartilage and hypertrophy of ligaments, vocal cords, and eustachian tubes are common. Nerve entrapment occurs because of tissue overgrowth and myelin loss in peripheral nerves. Because GH is an insulin **antagonist** (blocks the action of insulin), **hyperglycemia** (elevated blood glucose levels) is also common.

Excess ACTH overstimulates the adrenal cortex. The result is excessive production of glucocorticoids, mineralocorticoids, and androgens, which leads to the development of Cushing's disease (see Hypercortisolism [Cushing's Syndrome], p. 1474).

Etiology and Genetic Risk

Most cases of hyperpituitarism result from hormone-secreting adenomas arising from one pituitary cell type. Hyperpituitarism can also be caused by hypothalamic problems in which excessive amounts of releasing hormones are produced and then overstimulate the normal pituitary gland.

> **Genetic Considerations**
>
> Adenomas can develop in clients without a family history or as part of a syndrome known as multiple endocrine neoplasia (MEN). This familial disorder, inherited as an autosomal dominant trait, may include parathyroid and pancreatic tumors.

Incidence/Prevalence

Hyperpituitarism is a rare disorder. The most common tumors are prolactinomas, followed by GH-producing adenomas. Tumors secreting gonadotropin or thyroid-stimulating hormone (TSH) are the least common. About 70% of all pituitary tumors secrete one or more hormones.

◆COLLABORATIVE MANAGEMENT

PHARM e REVIEW

◆Assessment

HISTORY

The manifestations of hyperpituitarism vary, depending on which hormone is produced in excess. Obtain data about the client's age, gender, and family history. Ask the client about any change in hat, glove, ring, or shoe size. Fatigue and lethargy are common. The client with high GH levels may have backache and **arthralgias** (joint pain) from bone changes. Ask specifically about headaches and changes in vision.

The client with hypersecretion of PRL often reports difficulties in sexual functioning. Ask women about menstrual changes (e.g., amenorrhea, irregular menses, and difficulty in becoming pregnant) and about decreased libido or dyspareunia (painful intercourse). Men may report decreased libido and impotence.

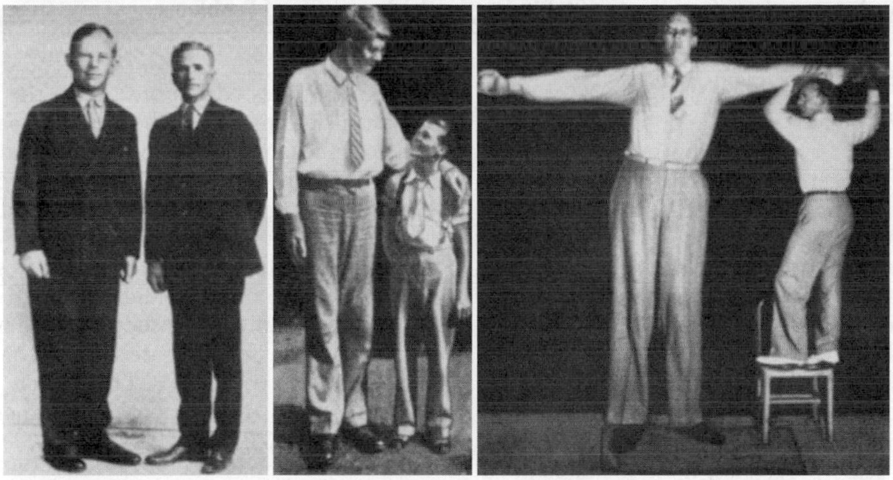

Figure 66-1 ■ The clinical features of growth hormone excess. Robert Wadlow, the "Alton giant," weighed 9 pounds at birth but grew to 30 pounds by the time he was 6 months old. By his first birthday, he had reached 62 pounds. At the time of his death at age 22 from cellulitis of the feet, he was 8 feet 11 inches tall and weighed 475 pounds.

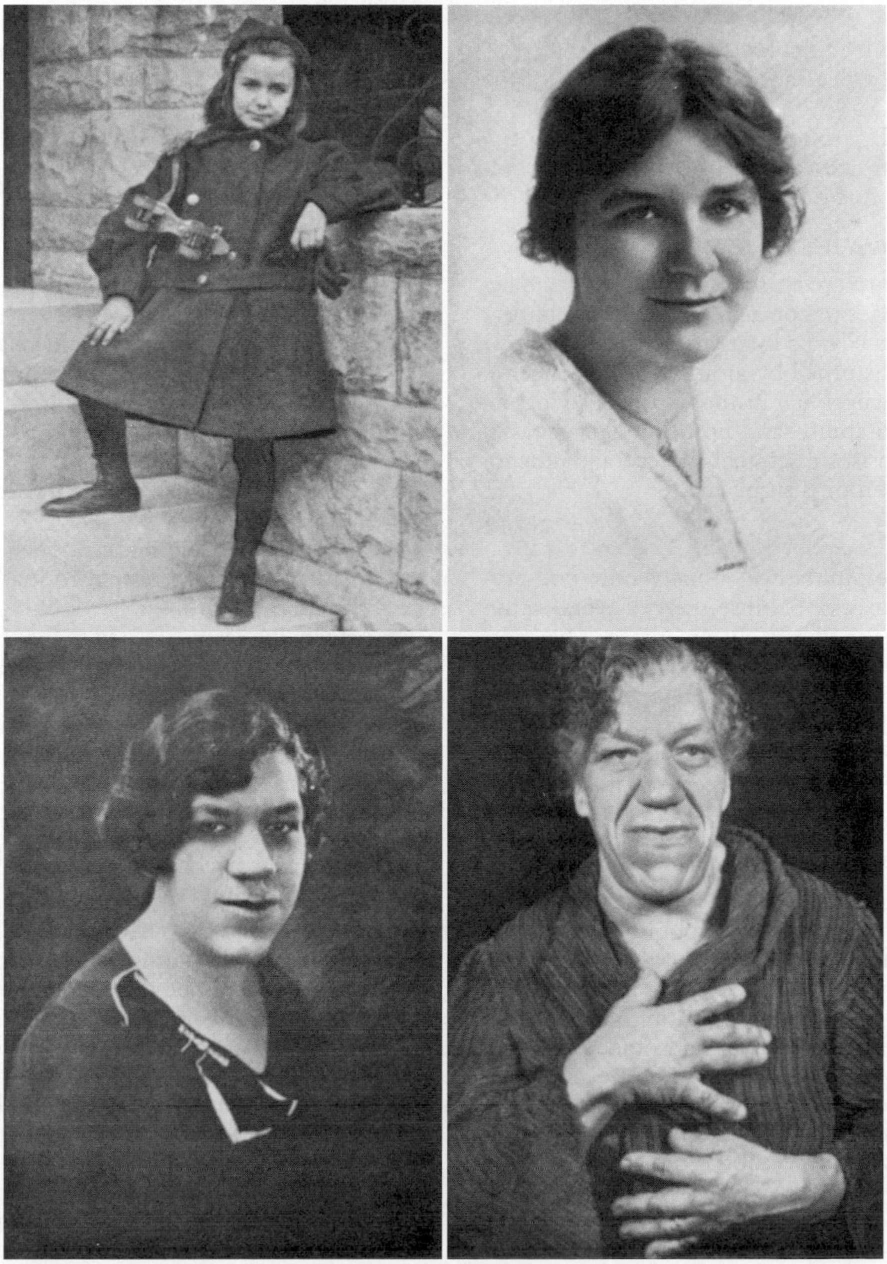

Figure 66-2 ■ The progression of acromegaly.

PHYSICAL ASSESSMENT/CLINICAL MANIFESTATIONS

Some changes in appearance and target organ function occur with excesses of specific anterior pituitary hormones (Chart 66-2). Initial manifestations of GH hypersecretion are changes in the facial features, including increases in lip and nose sizes and a prominent brow ridge; and increases in head, hand, and foot sizes. **Prognathism**, a projection of the jaw beyond the facial features, becomes marked. Assess the client for difficulty in chewing and for dentures that no longer fit. Arthritic changes causing joint pain and decreased mobility may also be noted. Fingers and toes may be thick with an arrowhead shape at the tips. At onset, acromegaly causes increased metabolism and strength. As the disease progresses, these manifestations are replaced with lethargy and weakness.

Assess the client's vision for any changes related to compression of the optic nerves. The client may also have increased perspiration and oil secretion on the skin. Other prominent features include the following:

- Organomegaly (cardiac or hepatic)
- Hypertension
- Dysphagia caused by an enlarged tongue
- Deepening of the voice caused by hypertrophy of the larynx

Hypersecretion of PRL is often observed, along with hypogonadism and galactorrhea. Galactorrhea may be present in either gender but occurs more often in women.

PSYCHOSOCIAL ASSESSMENT

The client with hyperpituitarism often seeks health care because of dramatic changes in appearance. Assess the impact of these changes on the client's interpersonal relationships.

In clients who are disturbed by an inability to conceive, identify symptoms of emotional distress, such as crying, reports of depression, irritability, and hostility. They may express fear of the diagnosis, subsequent surgery, and prognosis, especially when a tumor is suspected.

LABORATORY ASSESSMENT

In a person with hyperpituitarism, usually only one hormone is produced in excess, because the cell types within the pituitary gland are so discretely organized. The most common hormones produced in excess are PRL, ACTH, and GH. Tumors producing TSH, luteinizing hormone (LH), or follicle-stimulating hormone (FSH) are rare. Elevated levels of any of these hormones warrant evaluation. Elevations of LH and FSH, however, are normal in the postmenopausal woman.

RADIOGRAPHIC ASSESSMENT

Radiographic assessment of the client with hyperpituitarism is identical to that for a client with hypopituitarism. Skull x-rays are used to identify abnormalities of the sella turcica. Computed tomography (CT) and magnetic resonance imaging (MRI) can define soft-tissue lesions, and angiography can rule out an aneurysm or vascular malformations.

OTHER DIAGNOSTIC ASSESSMENTS

Rather than just measuring the blood level of a specific hormone, some tests measure how well the endocrine gland responds to stimulation changes. Suppression tests help diagnose hyperpituitarism. These tests involve giving agents that induce a suppressed response from the pituitary gland, and they can determine whether the normal negative feedback control mechanisms for hormonal regulation are intact. For example, high blood glucose levels suppress the release of GH. In a suppression test, 100 g of oral glucose or 0.5 g/kg of body weight is given intravenously (IV). GH levels are measured serially for up to 120 minutes. GH levels that do not fall below 5 ng/mL indicate a positive (abnormal) result.

Another example of a suppression test is the giving of IV cortisol in the form of dexamethasone (Decadron). This drug should suppress ACTH. When ACTH production continues in the presence of dexamethasone, the client may have pituitary Cushing's disease.

◆Analysis

COMMON NURSING DIAGNOSES AND COLLABORATIVE PROBLEMS

The following are priority nursing diagnoses for clients with hyperpituitarism with excesses of prolactin (PRL) and growth hormone (GH):

1. Disturbed Body Image related to illness or illness treatment
2. Sexual Dysfunction related to disease (related to loss of libido, infertility, impotence)

ADDITIONAL NURSING DIAGNOSES AND COLLABORATIVE PROBLEMS

In addition to the common nursing diagnoses, clients with excessive prolactin or growth hormone also may have one or more of the following:

- Acute Pain and Chronic Pain related to compression of tissues by tumor (e.g., discomfort, headache), backache, or arthralgia secondary to the effects of excessive GH levels or to dyspareunia secondary to excessive PRL levels
- Fear related to a perceived threat of death from an intracranial tumor
- Anxiety related to a threat of or change in health status
- Ineffective Coping related to inadequate level of perception of control
- Activity Intolerance related to the effects of excessive GH levels (e.g., pain or discomfort, lethargy, and weakness)
- Disturbed Sensory Perception (Visual) related to altered sensory reception, transmission, or integration
- Deficient Knowledge (diagnosis and treatment regimen) related to unfamiliarity with information resources

◆Planning and Implementation

DISTURBED BODY IMAGE

NOC **PLANNING: EXPECTED OUTCOMES.** The client with hyperpituitarism is expected to have a sense of congruence between body reality, body ideal, and body presentation. Indicators include that the client consistently or often demonstrates the following behaviors:

- Adjustment to changes in body function
- Willingness to use strategies to enhance appearance
- Willingness to touch affected body part
- A positive internal picture of self

INTERVENTIONS. The goals of therapy for the client who has hyperpituitarism are to return hormone levels to

CHART 66-2

KEY FEATURES of Pituitary Hyperfunction

Excess Hormone	Clinical Manifestations
Anterior Pituitary Hormones	
Prolactin (PRL)	Hypogonadism (loss of secondary sexual characteristics) Decreased gonadotropin levels Galactorrhea Increased body fat Increased serum prolactin levels
Growth hormone (GH)	Acromegaly ▪ Thickened, oily skin (facial) ▪ Thickened lips ▪ Folding of the scalp skin ▪ Deepening of the voice ▪ Enlarged hands and feet ▪ Increasing head size ▪ Protrusion of the lower jaw ▪ Joint enlargement and pain (knees, hips, and shoulders) ▪ Kyphosis and backache ▪ "Barrel chest" ▪ Excessive sweating (especially of the hands, feet, head, and face) ▪ Coarse facial features ▪ Tufting of the fingertips ▪ Hyperglycemia ▪ Airway narrowing, sleep apnea ▪ Enlarged heart, lungs, and liver
Adrenocorticotropic hormone (ACTH)	Cushing's disease (pituitary) ▪ Elevated plasma cortisol levels ▪ Weight gain ▪ Truncal obesity ▪ "Moon face" ▪ Extremity muscle wasting ▪ Loss of bone density ▪ Hypertension ▪ Hyperglycemia ▪ Purple striae ▪ Acne ▪ Thin, easily damaged skin ▪ Hyperpigmentation
Thyrotropin (thyroid-stimulating hormone [TSH])	Elevated plasma TSH levels Elevated plasma thyroid hormone levels Weight loss Tachycardia Heat intolerance Increased gastrointestinal (GI) motility Fine tremors
Gonadotropins (luteinizing hormone [LH], follicle-stimulating hormone [FSH])	Men: ▪ Elevated LH and FSH levels ▪ Hypogonadism or hypergonadism Women: ▪ Normal LH and FSH levels (The most common clinical manifestations in men and women are related to the physical presence of a tumor rather than to excessive hormone secretion.)
Posterior Pituitary Hormones	
Vasopressin (antidiuretic hormone [ADH])	Syndrome of inappropriate antidiuretic hormone (SIADH) ▪ Decreased urine output ▪ Increased urine osmolarity ▪ Increased plasma volume ▪ Decreased plasma osmolarity ▪ Weight gain ▪ Hyponatremia ▪ Nonpitting edema ▪ Central nervous system (CNS) changes (confusion, seizures)

Data from Melmed, S., & Kleinberg, D. (2003). Anterior pituitary. In P.R. Larsen, et al. (Eds.). *Williams textbook of endocrinology* (10th ed., pp. 281-329). Philadelphia: W. B. Saunders, and from Robinson, A., & Verbalis, J. (2003). Posterior pituitary gland. In P.R. Larsen, et al. (Eds.). *Williams textbook of endocrinology* (10th ed., pp. 177-279). Philadelphia: W. B. Saunders.

normal or near normal, reduce or eliminate headache and visual disturbances, prevent complications, and reverse as many of the body changes as possible.

NONSURGICAL MANAGEMENT. Encourage the client to express concerns and fears about his or her altered physical appearance. Help the client identify personal strengths and positive characteristics, reinforcing each client's uniqueness and importance.

Galactorrhea, gynecomastia, and reduced sexual functioning can disturb body image and personal identity. Reassure the client that treatment may reverse some of these problems. Encourage the client to discuss his or her feelings.

Drug Therapy. Drug therapy may be used alone or in combination with surgery and/or radiation. The most common drugs used are dopamine agonists, especially bromocriptine mesylate (Parlodel) and cabergoline (Dostinex). These drugs stimulate dopamine receptors in the brain and inhibit the release of many pituitary hormones, most specifically GH and PRL. In most cases, small tumors decrease until the pituitary gland is of normal size. Large pituitary tumors usually decrease to some extent. In clients with acromegaly, bromocriptine reduces GH levels and decreases tumor size, especially when GH levels remain high after surgery or before the full effect of radiation therapy has occurred.

Side effects of bromocriptine include **orthostatic** (postural) hypotension, gastric irritation, nausea, headaches, abdominal cramps, and constipation. Give bromocriptine with a meal or a snack to reduce some of these side effects. Treatment starts with a low dose and is gradually increased until the desired level (usually 7.5 mg/day) is reached. *If pregnancy occurs, the drug is stopped immediately.*

Other agents used for acromegaly are the somatostatin analogues, especially octreotide (Sandostatin), and a growth hormone receptor blocker, pegvisomant (Somavert). Octreotide inhibits GH release through negative feedback. Pegvisomant blocks growth hormone (GH) receptor activity and production of insulin-like growth factor (IGF). Although these therapies are effective, a disadvantage is that they must be given as an injection on a daily or weekly schedule. A major side effect is gallbladder disease. Pegvisomant may cause an increase in tumor size.

Radiation Therapy. Radiation therapy is not useful in the immediate management of acute hyperpituitarism. These therapy regimens take a long time to complete, and several years may pass before a therapeutic effect can be seen. Side effects of radiation therapy include hypopituitarism, optic nerve damage, reduced coordinated eye movement, and visual field defects. Use of the gamma knife procedure is increasing the accuracy of radiation therapy.

SURGICAL MANAGEMENT. Surgical removal of the pituitary gland and tumor **(hypophysectomy)** is the most common treatment for hyperpituitarism.

Preoperative Care. Explain that hypophysectomy decreases hormone levels, relieves headaches, and may reverse changes in sexual functioning. Body changes, organ enlargement, and visual changes are not usually reversible. Explain that because nasal packing is present for 2 to 3 days after surgery, it will be necessary to breathe through the mouth, and a "mustache" dressing ("drip" pad) will be placed under the nose. Instruct the client not to brush teeth, cough, sneeze, blow the nose, or bend forward after surgery. These activities can open the muscle graft, increase intracranial pressure, and delay healing of the incision. Nasal and oral mucous membrane swab specimens for bacterial culture and sensitivity are obtained before surgery because the surgery can move organisms from these areas into the blood and cause systemic infection.

Operative Procedures. A transsphenoidal approach to the pituitary gland is most commonly used (Figure 66-3). Transsphenoidal hypophysectomy is microscopic surgery performed with the client under general anesthesia and in a semi-sitting position. The surgeon makes an incision just above the upper lip and reaches the pituitary gland through the sphenoid sinus. After the gland is removed, a muscle graft is taken, often from the thigh, to support the area and prevent leakage of cerebrospinal fluid (CSF). Nasal packing is inserted after the incision is closed. A mustache dressing is then applied. If the tumor cannot be reached by this approach, a craniotomy may be indicated (see Chapter 48).

Postoperative Care. Monitor the client's neurologic response and document any changes in vision, mental status, altered level of consciousness, or decreased strength of the extremities. Observe the client for complications (e.g., transient diabetes insipidus).

In a client with diabetes insipidus, urine specific gravity is low and urine output is excessive. Monitor the intake of IV fluid, urge fluid intake in response to thirst, and give vasopressin as indicated. A Foley catheter may be inserted for accurate measuring of urine output, and daily weights are taken.

Teach the client to report any postnasal drip, which might indicate leakage of CSF. Keep the head of the bed elevated after surgery. Assess nasal drainage for quantity, quality, and the presence of glucose (which indicates that the fluid is CSF). A light yellow color at the edge of the clear drainage on the dressing is called the "halo sign" and indicates CSF. If the client has persistent, severe headaches, CSF fluid may have leaked into the sinus area. Most CSF leaks resolve with bedrest. If the CSF leak persists, the physician may perform a spinal tap to reduce CSF pressure. Surgical intervention is rarely necessary.

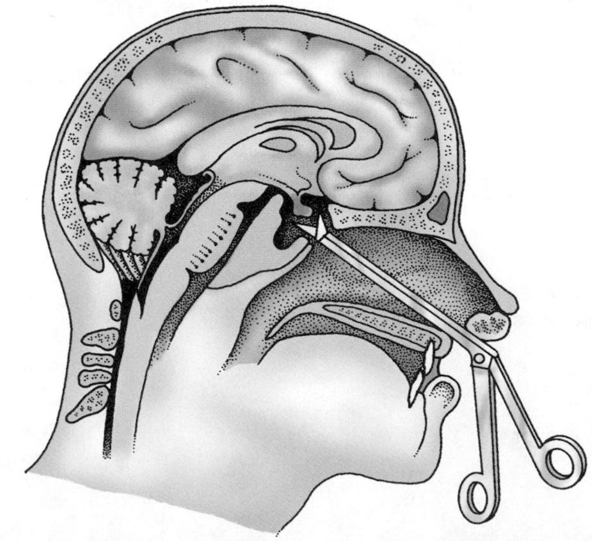

Figure 66-3 ■ The transsphenoidal surgical approach to the pituitary gland. Selective adenomectomy leaves normal pituitary tissue undisturbed.

Teach the client to avoid coughing early after surgery because it increases pressure in the incision area and may lead to a CSF leak. Remind the client to perform deep breathing exercises hourly while awake to prevent pulmonary problems. Clients may also have mouth dryness from mouth breathing. Perform frequent oral rinses and apply petroleum jelly to dry lips.

Infection can occur after surgery. Specifically assess for manifestations of meningitis, such as headache, fever, and nuchal (neck) rigidity. The surgeon may prescribe antibiotics, analgesics, and antipyretics.

If the entire pituitary gland has been removed, thyroid hormones and glucocorticoids must be replaced. Best practices for care after surgery are listed in Chart 66-3.

SEXUAL DYSFUNCTION

NOC **PLANNING: EXPECTED OUTCOMES.** The client with hyperpituitarism is expected to achieve a personally desired level of sexual expression and performance. Indicators include client consistently or often demonstrating the following:

- Expresses sexual interest
- Attains sexual arousal
- Adapts sexual techniques as needed

INTERVENTIONS. Identify the specific problems that the client is experiencing. Encourage the client to discuss any effect that sexual dysfunction has had on his or her sexual partner. Drug therapy with bromocriptine can decrease prolactin (PRL) levels in clients with PRL-secreting tumors. After PRL levels are decreased, gonadotropin function often returns to normal. Clients may have sexual dysfunction from gonadotropin deficiency and need hormone replacement (discussed earlier under Interventions [Hypopituitarism], p. 1459).

Community-Based Care

HOME CARE MANAGEMENT

Clients who have advanced acromegaly may have arthritic changes. Assess the degree of mobility impairment and identify appropriate adaptations, such as the use of ambulatory aids (cane or walker) and the accessibility of bathroom facilities.

After treatment, the client with hyperpituitarism needs daily self-management regimens and frequent checkups. The client may also need to develop strategies to reduce stress. Perform a focused assessment during the first several home visits to a client who has undergone a hypophysectomy (Chart 66-4). Review drug regimens and manifestations of infection and cerebral edema with the family.

HEALTH TEACHING

After a transsphenoidal hypophysectomy, advise the client to avoid activities that might interfere with healing. Bending over from the waist to pick up objects or tie shoes must be avoided because this position increases intracranial pressure (ICP). Teach the client to bend the knees and then lower the body to pick up fallen objects. ICP also increases when the client strains to have a bowel movement. Suggest techniques to prevent constipation, such as eating high-fiber foods, drinking plenty of fluids, and using stool softeners or laxatives. Activities that increase ICP should be avoided for up to 2 months after surgery.

The client must avoid toothbrushing for about 2 weeks after surgery until the incision has healed. Frequent mouth care (every 4 to 6 hours) with mouthwash and daily flossing provides adequate oral hygiene. Numbness in the area of

CHART 66-3

BEST PRACTICE for
The Client After Hypophysectomy

- Monitor the client's neurologic status hourly for the first 24 hours, then every 4 hours.
- Monitor fluid balance, especially for output greater than intake, because transient diabetes insipidus can occur.
- Encourage the client to maintain pulmonary hygiene through deep breathing exercises.
- Instruct the client *not* to cough, blow the nose, or sneeze.
- Instruct the client to use dental floss and oral mouth rinses because brushing the teeth is not permitted until the incision heals sufficiently.
- Instruct the client to avoid bending at the waist for any reason, because this position increases intracranial pressure.
- Monitor the nasal drip pad for the type and amount of drainage. The presence of the halo sign may indicate a CSF leak.
- Monitor bowel movements to prevent constipation and subsequent "straining."
- Teach the client self-administration of the prescribed hormones.

CSF, Cerebrospinal fluid.

CHART 66-4

HOME CARE ASSESSMENT of
The Client Who Has Undergone Transsphenoidal Hypophysectomy for Hyperpituitarism

Assess cardiovascular status:
- Vital signs, including apical pulse, pulse pressure, presence or absence of orthostatic hypotension, and the quality/rhythm of peripheral pulses.

Assess cognition and mental status:
- Level of consciousness
- Orientation to time, place, and person
- Accurate reading of a seven-word sentence containing no words longer than three syllables

Assess condition of operative site:
- Observe nasal area for drainage.
  - If present, note color, clarity, and odor.
  - Test clear drainage for the presence of glucose.

Assess neuromuscular status:
- Reactivity of patellar and biceps reflexes
- Oral temperature
- Handgrip strength
- Steadiness of gait
- Visual fields
- Distant and near visual acuity
- Pupillary responses to light

Assess renal system:
- Observe urine specimen for color, odor, cloudiness, and amount.

Ask about:
- Headaches or visual disturbances
- Ease of bowel movements
- 24-hour fluid intake and output
- 24-hour diet recall
- 24-hour activity recall
- Over-the-counter and prescribed medications taken

Assess client's understanding of illness and adherence with treatment:
- Signs and symptoms to report to health care provider
- Medication plan (correct timing and dose)

the incision and a decreased sense of smell are expected after surgery and usually last 3 to 4 months. Advise the client to use a mirror to check the gums for bleeding, because reduced sensation increases the risk for injury.

After a hypophysectomy, hormone replacement with vasopressin may be needed to maintain fluid balance (see later discussion under Interventions [Diabetes Insipidus], p. 1467). If the anterior portion of the pituitary gland is removed, instruct the client in cortisol, thyroid, and gonadal hormone replacement. Teach the client to report the return of any symptoms of hyperpituitarism immediately to the primary health care provider.

HEALTH CARE RESOURCES

The client with decreased mobility related to acromegaly or who has had recent surgery may require a home care aide or nurse to help maintain activities of daily living (ADLs). The client with hyperpituitarism must have hormone levels monitored at regular intervals to detect tumor recurrence. Regularly scheduled follow-up with the health care team is essential.

◆Evaluation: Outcomes

Evaluate the care of the client with hyperpituitarism on the basis of the identified nursing diagnoses and collaborative problems. The expected outcomes include that the client will:

- Experience an improvement in body image
- Achieve a personal desired level of sexual functioning

Specific indicators for these outcomes are listed for each nursing diagnosis under the Planning and Implementation section (see earlier).

DISORDERS OF THE POSTERIOR PITUITARY GLAND

Disorders of the posterior pituitary gland **(neurohypophysis)** are related to a deficiency or excess of the hormone vasopressin (antidiuretic hormone [ADH]). Diabetes insipidus occurs with ADH deficiency, and the syndrome of inappropriate antidiuretic hormone (SIADH) occurs with ADH excess.

Diabetes Insipidus

PATHOPHYSIOLOGY

Diabetes insipidus (DI) is a water metabolism problem caused by an ADH deficiency (either a decrease in ADH synthesis or an inability of the kidneys to respond to ADH). ADH deficiency results in the excretion of large volumes of dilute urine. Without ADH, distal kidney tubules and collecting ducts remain impermeable to water. Water is excreted as urine rather than being absorbed in these areas, which leads to **polyuria** (excessive water loss through urination) and dehydration.

Dehydration caused by this massive diuresis increases plasma osmolarity, which stimulates the osmoreceptors to relay a sensation of thirst to the cerebral cortex. Thirst promotes increased fluid intake and aids in maintaining water homeostasis. If the thirst mechanism is poor or absent, or if the person is unable to obtain water, dehydration becomes more severe.

ADH deficiency is classified as nephrogenic, drug-related, primary, or secondary, depending on whether the problem is caused by insufficient production of ADH or an inability of the kidney to respond to the presence of ADH.

Nephrogenic diabetes insipidus is an inherited disorder. The renal tubules do not respond to the actions of ADH, which results in poor water reabsorption by the kidney. The actual amount of hormone produced is not deficient.

Primary diabetes insipidus is caused by a defect in the hypothalamus or pituitary gland, resulting in a lack of ADH production or release. Secondary diabetes insipidus can result from tumors within or adjacent to the hypothalamus or pituitary gland, head trauma, infectious processes, surgical procedures (hypophysectomy), or metastatic tumors, usually from the lung or the breast. Less often, it is caused by brain hemorrhage, brain disease, or cerebral aneurysm, which reduce ADH production.

Drug-related diabetes insipidus is caused by lithium carbonate (Eskalith, Lithobid, Carbolith✱) and demeclocycline (Declomycin). These drugs can interfere with the response of the kidneys to ADH.

◆COLLABORATIVE MANAGEMENT

◆Assessment

Most manifestations of DI are related to dehydration (Chart 66-5). The key manifestations are an increase in the frequency of urination and excessive thirst. Ask about a history of any known etiologic factors, such as recent surgery, head trauma, or drug use (e.g., lithium). Although increased fluid

CHART 66-5

KEY FEATURES of Diabetes Insipidus

Cardiovascular Manifestations
- Hypotension
- Decreased pulse pressure
- Tachycardia
- Peripheral pulses weak, easily obliterated
- Hemoconcentration
  - Increased hemoglobin
  - Increased hematocrit
  - Increased BUN

Renal/Urinary Manifestations
- Increased urine output
  - Dilute, low specific gravity
  - Hypo-osmolar

Integumentary Manifestations
- Poor turgor
- Dry mucous membranes

Neurologic Manifestations
- Increased sensation of thirst
  - Irritability*
  - Decreased cognition*
  - Hyperthermia*
  - Lethargy to coma*
  - Ataxia*

BUN, Blood urea nitrogen.
*Occurs when access to water is limited and rapid dehydration results.

intake prevents serious dehydration and volume depletion, the client who is deprived of fluids or who cannot increase oral fluid intake may develop shock from fluid loss. Manifestations of dehydration, such as poor skin turgor and dry or cracked mucous membranes or skin, may be present in varying degrees. (See Chapter 15 for further discussion of dehydration.)

Water loss produces changes in blood and urine tests. The initial step in diagnosis is to measure a 24-hour fluid intake and output. The amount of the client's food and fluid is not restricted during this measurement. Urine output must be more than 4 L during this period for diabetes insipidus to be diagnosed. The amount of urine excreted in 24 hours may vary from 4 to 30 L/day. Urine is dilute with a low specific gravity (less than 1.005) and low osmolarity (50 to 200 mOsm/kg). Dehydration and hypertonic saline tests are also used for diagnosis of the disorder (Table 66-2).

Common Nursing Diagnoses and Collaborative Problems

Nursing diagnoses and collaborative problems that may apply to clients with diabetes insipidus include the following:

- Deficient Fluid Volume related to excessive fluid loss or inadequate fluid intake
- Decreased Cardiac Output related to decreased plasma volume
- Impaired Oral Mucous Membrane related to inadequate oral secretions
- Potential for Dysrhythmias

Interventions

Medical management is aimed at controlling manifestations with drug therapy (Chart 66-6). If only a partial deficit of ADH is present, effective control can be achieved with oral chlorpropamide (Diabinese, Novo-Propamide✱). This drug increases the action of existing ADH and possibly has a stimulating effect on the production of ADH in the hypothalamus.

When ADH deficiency is severe, ADH is replaced in amounts sufficient to maintain water balance. Desmopressin acetate (DDAVP) is a synthetic form of vasopressin given intranasally in a metered spray and is the drug of choice. Chart 66-7 lists some NIC interventions for nasal drugs. The frequency of dosing varies with client responses. Each metered spray delivers 10 mcg, and the client with mild DI may need only one to two doses in 24 hours. For the client with more severe DI, one to two metered doses two to three times daily may be needed. Lypressin (Diapid) is a short-acting form of the drug and is given by nasal spray or subcutaneously when an immediate response is needed. Injections last only 3 to 6 hours. During severe dehydration, ADH may be given IV or IM. Ulceration of the mucous membranes, allergy, a sensation of chest tightness, and pulmonary inhalation of the spray may occur with use of the intranasal preparations. If side effects occur, or if the client has an upper respiratory infection, subcutaneous vasopressin is used.

Nursing management is aimed at the early detection of dehydration and maintaining adequate hydration. Interventions include accurately measuring fluid intake and output, checking urine specific gravity, and recording the client's weight daily.

Urge the client to drink fluids in an amount equal to urine output. If fluids are given IV, ensure the patency of the access catheter and accurately monitor the amount infused hourly.

The client with permanent DI requires lifelong vasopressin therapy. Assess the client's ability to follow instructions and participate in health care. Teach the client that polyuria and polydipsia are signals for the need for another dose. *Teach all clients taking vasopressin to weigh themselves daily to identify weight gain.* Emphasize the importance of using the same scale and weighing at the same time of day while wearing a similar amount of clothing. If weight gain occurs, instruct the client to notify the health care provider. Clients with DI should wear a medical alert bracelet identifying the disorder and the drugs.

TABLE 66-2 Care of the Client Undergoing Special Tests for Diabetes Insipidus

Nursing Interventions	Rationales
Dehydration Test	
Obtain baseline vital signs; then check them hourly.	Assessment permits detection of changes, especially postural hypotension and tachycardia.
Deprive the client of fluid. Observe the client for adherence to fluid restriction.	Fluid restriction must be maintained for test results to be of diagnostic importance.
Measure urine output, specific gravity, and osmolarity hourly.	Urine testing results determine whether testing can proceed.
Weigh the client hourly.	Testing can proceed if urine osmolarity stabilizes for three samples and 3% weight loss is noted.
Give 5 units of aqueous vasopressin (subcutaneously), as prescribed. Continue hourly urine measurements.	Vasopressin triggers—and ongoing assessment detects—changes in urine specific gravity and osmolarity. Specific gravity and osmolarity decrease with primary and secondary diabetes insipidus. No response is seen with nephrogenic diabetes insipidus.
Hypertonic Saline Test (to Stimulate Release of ADH)	
Administer a normal water load to the client, followed by infusion of hypertonic saline. Measure urine output hourly.	The procedure detects ADH release. A sudden decrease in urine output is a sign of ADH release.

ADH, Antidiuretic hormone.

CHART 66-6

DRUG THERAPY for Diabetes Insipidus

Drug	Usual Dosage	Nursing Interventions	Rationales
Lypressin (Diapid)	4-8 sprays (5-10 pressor units) (nasal spray) in divided doses	Monitor for upper respiratory tract infections or allergy.	The effectiveness of nasal sprays is affected by upper respiratory tract infections.
Desmopressin (DDAVP)	0.1-0.4 mL in single or divided dose (nasal spray)	Teach the client the proper method of administration.	Some clients may have difficulty with measuring and inhaling.
Aqueous vasopressin [1](Pitressin)	5-20 units in divided doses (SC, IM, or nasal spray)	Instruct the client to sit upright when spraying.	An upright position promotes effective absorption in the nasal mucosa.
		Instruct the client to hold his or her breath when using nasal spray.	Holding one's breath prevents nasal spray from entering the lungs and potentially causing pneumonia.
		Monitor the client's intake and output.	Intake and output measurement helps to guide dosage regulation.
		Have the client space fluid intake during waking hours.	Extra fluid intake at night can cause nocturia.
		Monitor the client frequently (every 3-4 hr) for a recurrence of symptoms.	Monitoring detects the need for additional doses of these short-acting medications.
		Monitor the client's weight.	Water retention can be detected by weight gain.
[2]Chlorpropamide (Diabinese, Novo-Propamide♣)	125-250 mg PO every other day *Older adults:* 100-125 mg PO every other day	Monitor the client for signs and symptoms of hypoglycemia.	Hypoglycemia is a potentially severe side effect.
Indomethacin (Indocin, Indameth♣)	25-50 mg PO three times daily	Teach client to observe for bruising and for bleeding gums.	Disrupts platelet activity.
		Drug should be discontinued before surgery or dental work.	Excessive bleeding could result.

[1]***Med Error Alert!*** *Do not confuse with Pitocin, an oxytocic hormone used to induce labor.*

[2]***Med Error Alert!*** *Do not confuse with chlorpromazine, an antiemetic, or with chlorothiazide, a diuretic.*

SC, Subcutaneous; *SIADH,* syndrome of inappropriate antidiuretic hormone.

Critical Thinking Challenge

The client is your neighbor, a 34-year-old man who is being treated for gastroesophageal reflux disease with omeprazole (Prilosec) daily for this problem. He also has bipolar disorder for which he takes lithium. During the fall pollen season, he uses over-the-counter Benadryl and also takes ibuprofen occasionally for muscle and joint aches. He tells you that he thinks he may have diabetes mellitus or prostate problems like his father because he has to get up at least five times per night to urinate. In addition, he tells you that he is constantly thirsty and drinks a lot of water and coffee.

1. How are diabetes mellitus and diabetes insipidus similar and how are they different?
2. Which of this client's drugs could contribute to manifestations of diabetes insipidus?
3. Is his father's history of diabetes mellitus or prostate problems important in this client's health consideration?

evolve For suggested answer guidelines, go to http://evolve.elsevier.com/Iggy/.

CHART 66-7

NIC INTERVENTION ACTIVITIES for The Client with Diabetes Insipidus

Medication Administration: Nasal: *Preparing and giving medications via nasal passages*

- Instruct client to blow nose gently prior to administration of nasal medication, unless contraindicated.
- Instruct client to remain upright and to not tilt head backward when nasal spray is administered.
- Insert nozzle into nostril and squeeze bottle quickly and firmly when nasal spray is administered.
- Instruct client not to blow nose for several minutes after administration.
- Monitor client to determine response to medication.

NIC intervention activities selected from Dochterman, J.M., & Bulechek, G.M. (Eds.). (2004). *Nursing interventions classification (NIC)* (4th ed.). St. Louis: Mosby.

Syndrome of Inappropriate Antidiuretic Hormone

PATHOPHYSIOLOGY

The **syndrome of inappropriate antidiuretic hormone (SIADH)** occurs when vasopressin (antidiuretic hormone [ADH]) is secreted even when plasma osmolarity is low or normal. A decrease in plasma osmolarity normally inhibits ADH production and secretion. SIADH is also known as the Schwartz-Bartter syndrome. SIADH is also discussed in Chapter 28 as a complication of cancer and cancer therapy. SIADH occurs with many pathologic conditions and specific drugs. Table 66-3 lists common causes of SIADH.

In SIADH, the feedback mechanisms that regulate ADH do not function properly. ADH continues to be released even when plasma is hyposmolar. Water is *retained,* which results in dilutional **hyponatremia** (a decreased serum sodium level) and expansion of the extracellular fluid volume. The increase in plasma volume causes an increase in the glomerular filtration rate and inhibits the release of renin and aldosterone. The combined effect is an increased sodium loss in urine, leading to greater hyponatremia.

TABLE 66-3 Conditions Causing the Syndrome of Inappropriate Antidiuretic Hormone

Malignancies	CNS Disorders
■ Small cell carcinoma of the lung	■ Trauma
■ Pancreatic, duodenal, and GU carcinomas	■ Infection
■ Thymoma	■ Tumors (primary or metastatic)
■ Hodgkin's lymphoma	■ Strokes
■ Non-Hodgkin's lymphoma	■ Porphyria
	■ Systemic lupus erythematosus
Pulmonary Disorders	**Drugs**
■ Viral and bacterial pneumonia	■ Exogenous ADH
■ Lung abscesses	■ Chlorpropamide
■ Active tuberculosis	■ Vincristine
■ Pneumothorax	■ Cyclophosphamide
■ Chronic lung diseases	■ Carbamazepine
■ Mycoses	■ Opioids
■ Positive-pressure ventilation	■ Tricyclic antidepressants
	■ General anesthetics

ADH, Antidiuretic hormone; *CNS,* central nervous system; *GU,* Genitourinary.

COLLABORATIVE MANAGEMENT

Assessment

HISTORY

Ask the client about his or her medical history, which may reveal conditions that occur with the development of SIADH. Information about the following conditions should be obtained:

- Recent head trauma
- Cerebrovascular disease
- Tuberculosis or other pulmonary disease
- Cancer
- All past and current drug use

PHYSICAL ASSESSMENT/CLINICAL MANIFESTATIONS

The early manifestations of SIADH are related to water retention. Gastrointestinal (GI) disturbances, such as loss of appetite, nausea, and vomiting, may occur first. Weigh the client and document any recent weight gain. In clients with SIADH, free water (not salt) is retained and dependent edema is not usually present, even though water is retained.

Water retention, hyponatremia, and fluid shifts affect central nervous system function, especially when the serum sodium level drops below 115 mEq/L. The client may have lethargy, headaches, hostility, disorientation, and a change in level of consciousness. Manifestations can progress from lethargy and headaches to decreased responsiveness, seizures, and coma. Assess deep tendon reflexes, which are often decreased.

Vital sign changes include tachycardia (caused by the increased fluid volume) and hypothermia (caused by central nervous system disturbance). Chapter 16 presents other findings that occur with hyponatremia.

DIAGNOSTIC ASSESSMENT

Water retention changes both plasma and urine osmolarity. Urine volume decreases and urine osmolarity increases. Plasma volume increases and plasma osmolarity decreases. Elevated urine sodium levels and specific gravity reflect increased urine concentration. Serum sodium levels are decreased, often as low as 110 mEq/L, because of fluid retention and sodium loss.

Radioimmunoassay of ADH can diagnose SIADH when ADH levels are inappropriately elevated when plasma osmolarity is normal or decreased.

Interventions

Interventions to treat SIADH focus on restricting fluid intake, promoting the excretion of water, replacing lost sodium, interfering with the action of ADH, and preventing injury.

Fluid Restriction. Fluid restriction is essential because fluid intake further dilutes the plasma sodium levels. In some cases, fluid intake may be kept as low as 500 to 600 mL/24 hr. Dilute tube feedings with a solution other than plain water, and use saline to irrigate GI tubes. Mix drugs to be given by GI tube with saline.

Measure intake, output, and daily weights to assess the degree of fluid restriction needed. A weight gain of 2 pounds or more per day or a gradual increase over several days is cause for concern. A 1-kg weight increase is equal to a 1000-mL fluid retention (1 kg = 1 L). The client is uncomfortable during fluid restriction. Keep mucous membranes moist by offering frequent oral rinsing (remind the client not to swallow the rinses).

Drug Therapy. Diuretics may be used to treat SIADH, particularly if heart failure results from fluid overload. Be aware of the diuretic effects on sodium loss. Sodium loss can be potentiated, further contributing to the problems caused by SIADH.

Hypertonic saline (i.e., 3% sodium chloride [3% NaCl]) is often used to treat SIADH. Give IV saline cautiously because it may add to existing fluid overload and promote heart failure. If the client needs routine IV fluids, a saline solution rather than a water solution is prescribed.

Drugs such as lithium carbonate (Eskalith, Lithobid, Carbolith✱) and demeclocycline (Declomycin) may help treat SIADH. Lithium is seldom used because of its toxicity; demeclocycline is used more commonly.

Providing a Safe Environment. Observe for and document changes in the client's neurologic status. Assess for subtle changes, such as muscle twitching, before they progress to seizures or coma. Check orientation to time, place, and person every 2 hours because disorientation or confusion may be present. Reduce environmental noise and lighting to prevent overstimulation.

Flow sheets with continuing information about the level of consciousness, motor and sensory neurologic assessments, and laboratory data are helpful in detecting neurologic trends. The frequency of neurologic checks depends on the client's status. For the client with SIADH who is hyponatremic but alert, awake, and oriented, neurologic checks every 4 hours are sufficient. For the client who has had a change in level of consciousness, perform neurologic checks at least every hour. Inspect the environment every shift, making sure that basic safety measures, such as siderails being securely in place, are observed.

Disorders of the Adrenal Gland

ADRENAL GLAND HYPOFUNCTION

PATHOPHYSIOLOGY

Production of adrenocortical steroids may decrease as a result of inadequate secretion of adrenocorticotropic hormone (ACTH), dysfunction of the hypothalamic-pituitary control mechanism, and dysfunction of adrenal gland tissue. Manifestations may develop gradually or occur quickly with stress. In acute adrenocortical insufficiency **(adrenal crisis)**, life-threatening manifestations may appear without warning.

Loss of the adrenal medulla, which produces **catecholamines** (dopamine, norepinephrine, and epinephrine), does not upset the maintenance of homeostasis. This is because catecholamines are also released from other areas in the sympathetic nervous system.

However, insufficiency of adrenocortical steroids causes problems through the loss of aldosterone and cortisol action. Impaired secretion of cortisol results in decreased **gluconeogenesis** (making glucose from proteins) along with depletion of liver and muscle glycogen, leading to **hypoglycemia** (low blood glucose levels). The glomerular filtration rate and gastric acid production decrease, leading to reduced urea nitrogen excretion, causing anorexia and weight loss.

Reduced aldosterone secretion causes potassium, sodium, and water imbalances. Potassium excretion is decreased, causing hyperkalemia. Sodium and water excretion is increased, causing hyponatremia and hypovolemia. Potassium retention also promotes reabsorption of hydrogen ions, which can lead to acidosis.

Low adrenal androgen levels decrease the body, axillary, and pubic hair, especially in women, because the adrenals produce most of the androgens in females. The severity of symptoms is related to the degree of hormone deficiency.

Acute adrenal insufficiency, or **Addisonian crisis**, is a life-threatening event in which the need for cortisol and aldosterone is greater than the available supply. Often, acute insufficiency occurs in response to a stressful event (e.g., surgery, trauma, or severe infection), especially when the adrenal hormone output is already reduced. The problems of acute adrenal insufficiency are almost the same as that of chronic insufficiency. In clients with acute adrenal crisis related to bilateral adrenal hemorrhage, however, sodium and potassium levels may be normal because the time between the event and the presentation may be too short for a change in electrolyte composition to occur. Unless intervention is initiated promptly, however, sodium levels fall and potassium levels rise rapidly. More severe hypotension results from the blood volume depletion that occurs with the loss of aldosterone. Best practices for emergency care of clients with acute adrenal insufficiency are listed in Chart 66-8.

CHART 66-8

BEST PRACTICE for Emergency Care of the Client with Acute Adrenal Insufficiency

EMERGENCY CARE

Hormone Replacement
- Start rapid infusion of normal saline or dextrose 5% in normal saline.
- Initial dose of hydrocortisone sodium succinate (Solu-Cortef) is 100 to 300 mg or dexamethasone 4 to 12 mg as an IV bolus.
- Infuse additional 100 mg of hydrocortisone sodium succinate by continuous IV drip over the next 8 hours.
- Give hydrocortisone 50 mg IM concomitantly every 12 hours.
- Initiate an H_2 histamine blocker (e.g., ranitidine) IV for ulcer prevention.

Hyperkalemia Management
- Administer insulin (20 to 50 units) with dextrose (20 to 50 mg) in normal saline to shift potassium into cells.
- Administer potassium binding and excreting resin (e.g., Kayexalate).
- Give loop or thiazide diuretics.
- Avoid potassium-sparing diuretics.
- Initiate potassium restriction.
- Monitor intake and output.
- Monitor heart rate, rhythm, and ECG for manifestations of hyperkalemia (slow heart rate, block, tall peaked T-waves, fibrillation, asystole).

Hypoglycemia Management
- Administer IV glucose.
- Administer glucagon, as needed.
- Maintain IV access.
- Monitor blood glucose level hourly.

ECG, Electrocardiogram.

Adrenal insufficiency is classified as primary or secondary. Causes of primary and secondary adrenal insufficiency are listed in Table 66-4. One of the most common causes of secondary adrenal insufficiency is the sudden cessation of long-term, high-dose glucocorticoid therapy. This therapy suppresses production of glucocorticoids through negative feedback by causing atrophy of the adrenal cortex. Glucocorticoid drugs must be withdrawn gradually to allow for pituitary production of ACTH and activation of adrenal cells to produce cortisol.

◆COLLABORATIVE MANAGEMENT

◆Assessment

HISTORY

While taking a history from the client with possible adrenal insufficiency, ask questions about manifestations and factors that cause adrenal hypofunction. Ask about any change in activity level, because lethargy, fatigue, and muscle weak-

TABLE 66-4 Causes of Primary and Secondary Adrenal Insufficiency

Primary Causes	Secondary Causes
▪ Idiopathic (autoimmune) disease*	▪ Pituitary tumors
▪ Tuberculosis	▪ Postpartum pituitary necrosis (Sheehan's syndrome)
▪ Metastatic cancer	▪ Hypophysectomy
▪ Fungal lesions	▪ High-dose pituitary radiation
▪ AIDS	▪ High-dose whole-brain radiation
▪ Hemorrhage	
▪ Gram-negative sepsis (Waterhouse-Friderichsen syndrome)	
▪ Adrenalectomy	
▪ Abdominal radiation therapy	
▪ Drugs (mitotane) and toxins	

*Most common cause.

CHART 66-9

KEY FEATURES of Adrenal Insufficiency

Neuromuscular Manifestations
- Muscle weakness
- Fatigue
- Joint/muscle pain

Gastrointestinal Manifestations
- Anorexia
- Nausea, vomiting
- Abdominal pain
- Bowel changes (constipation/diarrhea)
- Weight loss
- Salt craving

Integumentary Manifestations
- Vitiligo
- Hyperpigmentation

Cardiovascular Manifestations
- Anemia
- Hypotension
- Hyponatremia
- Hyperkalemia
- Hypercalcemia

ness are often present. Include questions about salt intake because salt craving often occurs with hypofunction.

Gastrointestinal (GI) problems, such as anorexia, nausea, vomiting, diarrhea, and abdominal pain, often occur. Ask about weight loss during the past months. Women may have menstrual changes related to weight loss, and men may report impotence.

Ask whether the client has had radiation to the abdomen or head. Document medical problems (e.g., tuberculosis or previous intracranial surgery) and all past and current drugs, especially steroids, anticoagulants, opioids, or cytotoxic drugs.

PHYSICAL ASSESSMENT/CLINICAL MANIFESTATIONS

The manifestations of adrenal insufficiency vary, and the severity is related to the degree of hormone deficiency (Chart 66-9). In clients with primary insufficiency, plasma ACTH and melanocyte-stimulating hormone (MSH) levels are elevated because of the loss of the adrenal-hypothalamic-pituitary feedback system. Elevated MSH levels result in areas of increased pigmentation (Figure 66-4). In primary autoimmune disease, areas of decreased pigmentation may occur because of destruction of pigment-producing cells in the skin (melanocytes). Body hair may also be decreased. In secondary disease, there is no change in skin pigmentation.

Assess for manifestations of hypoglycemia (e.g., sweating, headaches, tachycardia, and tremors) and volume depletion (postural hypotension and dehydration). **Hyperkalemia** (elevated blood levels of potassium) can cause dysrhythmias with an irregular heart rate and result in cardiac arrest.

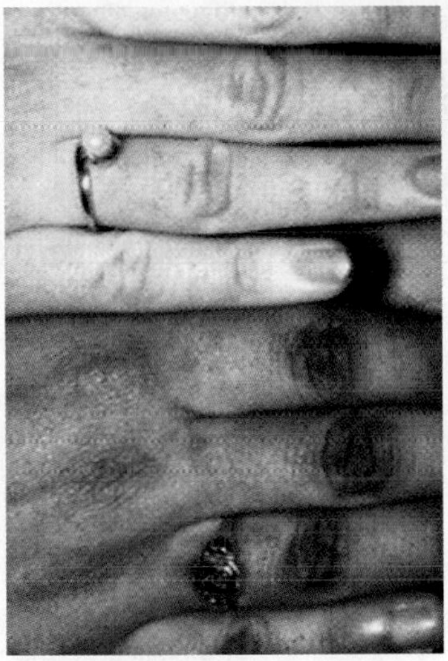

Figure 66-4 ▪ The increased pigmentation seen in primary adrenocortical insufficiency.

PSYCHOSOCIAL ASSESSMENT

Depending on the degree of imbalance, clients may appear lethargic, depressed, confused, and even psychotic. Observe the client and check his or her orientation to person, place, and time. Families may report that the client has a decreased energy level, experiences wide mood swings, and is forgetful.

DIAGNOSTIC ASSESSMENT

Laboratory findings include low serum cortisol, low fasting blood glucose, low sodium, elevated potassium, and increased serum blood urea nitrogen (BUN) levels (Chart 66-10). In primary disease, the eosinophil count and ACTH level are elevated. Plasma cortisol levels do not rise during stimulation tests.

Urinary 17-hydroxycorticosteroids are the glucocorticoid metabolites, and 17-ketosteroid levels reflect the adrenal androgen metabolites. Both levels are in the low or low-normal range in adrenal hypofunction. Table 66-5 lists drugs that can interfere with test results.

Skull x-rays, computed tomography (CT), magnetic resonance imaging (MRI), and arteriography may help determine the cause of pituitary problems leading to adrenal insufficiency.

Noninvasive procedures of the adrenal gland, such as CT scans without dye, may show atrophy of the gland. CT scans may help determine adrenal hypofunction.

An ACTH stimulation test is the most definitive test for adrenal insufficiency. A rapid ACTH stimulation test may be performed on an outpatient basis. ACTH 0.25 to 1 mg is given IV, and plasma cortisol levels are obtained at 30-minute and 1-hour intervals. In primary insufficiency, the cortisol response is absent or markedly decreased; in secondary insufficiency, it is increased.

A longer ACTH stimulation test uses a continuous infusion of 50 units of ACTH in saline for 24 hours or an 8-hour infusion daily for 4 to 5 days, with simultaneously collected 24-hour urine samples. Levels of urinary 17-hydroxycorticosteroids and urinary free cortisol are also measured. In primary adrenal insufficiency, the response is low or absent; in

CHART 66-10

LABORATORY PROFILE
Adrenal Gland Assessment

		Significance of Abnormal Findings	
Test	**Normal Range for Adults**	**Hypofunction of the Adrenal Gland**	**Hyperfunction of the Adrenal Gland**
Sodium	136-145 mEq/L	Decreased	Increased
Potassium	3.5-5.0 mEq/L	Increased	Decreased
Glucose	70-115 mg/dL *Older adults:* slightly increased	Normal to decreased	Normal to increased
Calcium	9-10.5 mg/dL (total) 4.5-5.6 mg/dL (ionized) *Older adults*: slightly decreased	Increased	Decreased
Bicarbonate	21-28 mEq/L	Increased	Decreased
BUN	10-20 mg/dL *Older adults:* may be slightly higher	Increased	Normal
Cortisol	6 AM to 8 AM 5-23 mcg/dL or 138-635 SI units (nmol/L) 4 PM to 6 PM 3-16 mcg/dL or 83-359 SI units (nmol/L)	Decreased	Increased

BUN, Blood urea nitrogen; *SI*, System Internationale.

TABLE 66-5 Drugs That Interfere with Tests for Urinary 17-Hydroxycorticosteroids and Urinary 17-Ketosteroids

- Acetaminophen
- Acetazolamide
- Acetylsalicylic acid
- Amphetamines
- Ascorbic acid
- Barbiturates
- Calcium gluconate
- Carbon disulfide
- Chloral hydrate
- Chlordiazepoxide
- Chlormerodrin
- Chlorothiazide
- Chlorpromazine
- Chlorthalidone
- Colchicine
- Corticotropin
- Cortisone
- Dexamethasone
- Diazepam
- Digitoxin
- Digoxin
- Diphenhydramine
- Diphenylhydantoin
- Erythromycin
- Estrogens
- Fructose
- Glutethimide
- Hydralazine
- Iodides
- Medroxyprogesterone
- Meperidine
- Meprobamate
- Metyrapone
- Mitotane
- Morphine
- Nalidixic acid
- Oral contraceptives
- Paraldehyde
- Penicillin
- Pentazocine
- Perphenazine
- Phenobarbital
- Phenothiazines
- Phenylbutazone
- Promazine
- Propoxyphene
- Quinidine
- Quinine
- Reserpine
- Secobarbital
- Spironolactone
- Testosterone
- Vitamin K

secondary insufficiency, the value for 17-hydroxycorticosteroids fails to rise above 20 mg per total volume.

Common Nursing Diagnoses and Collaborative Problems

Nursing diagnoses that may apply to clients with adrenal gland hypofunction include the following:

- Decreased Cardiac Output related to decreased vascular volume and hyperkalemia
- Risk for Injury related to hypoglycemia
- Fatigue related to disease state

Interventions

Nursing interventions aim to promote fluid balance and monitor for fluid deficit (Chart 66-11). Weigh the client daily and record intake and output. Assess vital signs every 1 to 4 hours, depending on the client's condition and the presence of dysrhythmias or postural hypotension. Monitor laboratory values to identify hemoconcentration (e.g., increased hematocrit or BUN). Chapter 15 discusses fluid volume deficit in detail.

Cortisol and aldosterone deficiencies are corrected by replacement therapy. Hydrocortisone corrects glucocorticoid deficiency (Chart 66-12). Therapy replacement regimens vary. Generally, divided doses are given, with two thirds given in the morning and one third in the late afternoon to mimic the normal release of this hormone. Although most clients do well on this regimen, some may not tolerate the dosage or may need more.

An additional mineralocorticoid hormone, such as fludrocortisone (Florinef), may be needed to maintain electrolyte balance (especially sodium and potassium). Dosage adjustment may be needed, especially in hot weather, when more sodium is lost because of excessive perspiration. *Salt restriction or diuretic therapy should not be started without considering whether it might lead to an adrenal crisis.*

Critical Thinking Challenge

The client is a 60-year-old woman who was taking 80 mg of oral prednisone daily for 10 weeks because of a severe pulmonary problem. Her pulmonary problem has resolved and she tapered down her prednisone dose by 10 mg daily for 8 days. It has now been 10 days since her last dose. She is brought to the emergency department by her family who say that she is too weak to walk, has poor memory, and seems confused. They tell you about her prednisone therapy. On admission, her

CHART 66-11

NIC INTERVENTION ACTIVITIES for
The Client with Adrenal Insufficiency

Electrolyte Management: Hyperkalemia: *Promotion of potassium balance and prevention of complications resulting from serum potassium levels higher than desired*

- Administer electrolyte-binding and electrolyte-excreting resins (e.g., Kayexalate) as prescribed, if appropriate.
- Monitor lab values for changes in oxygenation or acid-base balance, as appropriate.
- Administer prescribed medications to shift potassium into the cell (e.g., 50% dextrose and insulin, sodium bicarbonate, calcium chloride, and calcium gluconate), as appropriate.
- Avoid potassium-sparing medications (e.g., spironolactone [Aldactone] and triamterene [Dyrenium]), as appropriate.
- Maintain potassium restrictions.
- Administer prescribed diuretics, as appropriate.
- Monitor fluid status, including intake and output, as appropriate.
- Monitor potassium levels after diuresis.
- Monitor cardiac manifestations of hyperkalemia (e.g., decreased cardiac output, heart blocks, peaked T waves, fibrillation, or asystole).
- Respond to cardiac arrest.

Hypoglycemia Management: *Preventing and treating low blood glucose levels*

- Determine recognition of hypoglycemia signs and symptoms.
- Monitor blood glucose levels, as indicated.
- Monitor for signs and symptoms of hypoglycemia (e.g., shakiness, tremor, sweating, nervousness, anxiety, irritability, impatience, tachycardia, palpitations, chills, clamminess, light-headedness, pallor, hunger, nausea, headache, tiredness, drowsiness, weakness, warmth, dizziness, faintness, blurred vision, nightmares, crying out in sleep, paresthesias, difficulty concentrating, difficulty speaking, incoordination, behavior change, confusion, coma, seizure).
- Provide simple carbohydrate, as indicated.
- Administer glucagon, as indicated.
- Maintain IV access, as appropriate.
- Instruct client and significant others on signs and symptoms, risk factors, and treatment of hypoglycemia.
- Instruct client to have simple carbohydrate available at all times.
- Instruct client to obtain and carry/wear appropriate emergency identification.

NIC intervention activities selected from Dochterman, J.M., & Bulechek, G.M. (Eds.). (2004). *Nursing interventions classification (NIC)* (4th ed.). St. Louis: Mosby.

CHART 66-12

DRUG THERAPY for
Hypofunction of the Adrenal Gland

Drug	Usual Dosage	Nursing Interventions	Rationales
Cortisone	25-50 mg PO either once daily in AM or daily in divided doses	Instruct the client to take the drug with meals or a snack.	Gastrointestinal irritation can occur.
Hydrocortisone (Cortef, Hycort✱)	20-50 mg PO either once daily in AM or daily in divided doses	Instruct the client to report the following signs or symptoms of excessive drug therapy: ▪ Rapid weight gain ▪ Round face ▪ Fluid retention	Cushing's syndrome, which indicates a need for dosage adjustment, can occur.
! Prednisone (Winpred✱)	5-10 mg PO either once daily in AM or daily in divided doses		
Fludrocortisone (Florinef)	0.05-0.2 mg PO daily	Instruct the client to report illness, such as: ▪ Severe diarrhea ▪ Vomiting ▪ Fever	Other conditions may indicate a need for dosage change. The usual daily dosage may not be adequate during periods of illness or severe stress.
		Monitor the client's blood pressure.	Hypertension is a potential side effect.
		Instruct the client to report weight gain or edema.	Sodium-related fluid retention is possible.

*! **Med Error Alert!** Drug name is similar to prednisolone, another corticosteroid that is 4 to 5 times more potent than prednisone.*

vital signs are T 97; P 58, thready, with some "dropped" beats; R 14 and shallow; BP 92/50.

1. Should this client be seen in the emergency department or should she be told to make an appointment with either her primary care physician or her pulmonologist?
2. What other assessment data should you obtain?
3. What is the probable cause of this client's manifestations?
4. Should this client be started on oxygen? Why or why not?
5. Should an IV line be started on this client? If so, what fluid should you use?

evolve For suggested answer guidelines, go to http://evolve.elsevier.com/Iggy/.

ADRENAL GLAND HYPERFUNCTION

The adrenal gland may oversecrete just one hormone or all adrenal hormones. Hypersecretion by the adrenal cortex results in hypercortisolism (e.g., **Cushing's disease** or **Cushing's syndrome**), **hyperaldosteronism** (excessive mineralocorticoid production), or excessive androgen production.

Hyperstimulation of the adrenal medulla caused by a tumor **(pheochromocytoma)** results in excessive secretion of catecholamines, of which 80% is epinephrine and the remainder is norepinephrine.

Hypercortisolism (Cushing's Disease)

PATHOPHYSIOLOGY

Cushing's disease exaggerates the normal actions of glucocorticoids, causing widespread problems. Excessive stimulation of adrenocorticotropic hormone (ACTH) of either pituitary or ectopic origin causes adrenocortical hyperplasia, which disrupts normal hormone secretion rhythms. The client's endocrine tissues are less responsive to releasing hormones, especially prolactin (PRL), thyrotropin, and gonadotropin. Many clients also have abnormal sleep patterns. These changes are due to excessive amounts of glucocorticoids.

The client with Cushing's disease has problems in nitrogen, carbohydrate, and mineral metabolism. An increase in total body fat results from slow turnover of plasma fatty acids. This fat is redistributed to produce the typical body pattern of truncal obesity, "buffalo hump," and "moon face" (Figure 66-5). Increases in the breakdown of tissue protein and an increase in urine nitrogen excretion also occur, resulting in decreased muscle mass, thin skin, and bone density loss.

High levels of corticosteroids kill lymphocytes and shrink organs containing lymphocytes, such as the liver, the spleen, and the lymph nodes. Eosinophils and macrophages are reduced. Although the number of neutrophils may be increased, the reduction of cytokines makes these cells less active. Thus protection of the inflammatory and immune responses is reduced.

In most cases, increased androgen production causes acne, **hirsutism** (increased hair growth), and occasionally clitoral hypertrophy. Increased androgen production can also interrupt the normal hormone feedback mechanism for the ovary, decreasing the ovary's production of estrogens and progesterone. **Oligomenorrhea** (scant or infrequent menses) occurs as a result.

Cushing's disease or syndrome is a group of clinical problems caused by an excess of cortisol, secreted by the adrenal cortex (**endogenous** [Cushing's disease) or given for another clinical disorder (**exogenous** or **iatrogenic** [Cushing's syndrome]). Table 66-6 lists causes of cortisol excess. Women are more likely than men to develop Cushing's disease. Clients of either gender are at equal risk for Cushing's syndrome as a result of chronic use of exogenous corticosteroids.

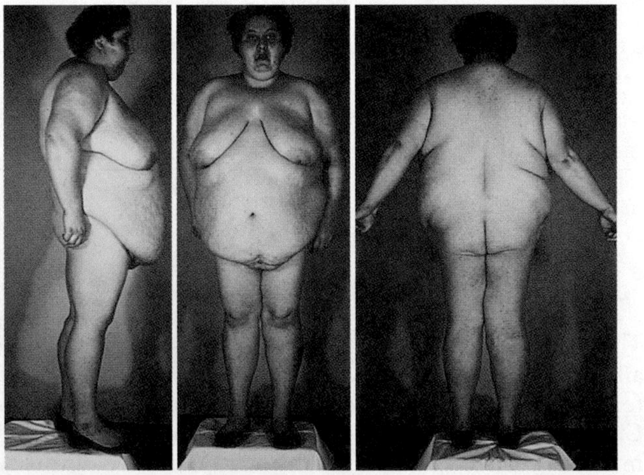

Figure 66-5 ■ The typical appearance of a client with Cushing's disease or syndrome. Note truncal obesity, moon face, buffalo hump, thinner arms and legs, and abdominal striae. (From Jarvis, C. [2000]. Physical examination and health assessment [3rd ed.]. Philadelphia: W. B. Saunders, p. 210. Reprinted with permission.)

COLLABORATIVE MANAGEMENT

Assessment

HISTORY

The client with hypercortisolism has many changes because of the widespread effect of excessive cortisol levels. Ask about changes in activity or sleep patterns, fatigue, and muscle weakness. Ask about bone pain or a history of fractures because osteoporosis is common in hypercortisolism. Ask about a history of frequent infections and easy bruising, which suggest hypercortisolism. Women may report a cessation of menses. Gastrointestinal (GI) problems include ulcer formation from increased hydrochloric acid secretion and decreased production of protective gastric mucous.

Check the client's medical history. Steroid or alcohol abuse can induce the manifestations of Cushing's syndrome.

PHYSICAL ASSESSMENT/CLINICAL MANIFESTATIONS

The client with hypercortisolism has specific physical changes (see Figure 66-5 and Chart 66-13). Observe the client's general appearance. Changes in fat distribution may result in fat pads on the neck, back, and shoulders ("buffalo hump"); an enlarged trunk with thin arms and legs; and a round face ("moon face"). Other changes include muscle wasting and weakness.

Inspect for skin changes resulting from increased blood vessel fragility, such as bruises, thin or translucent skin, and wounds that have not healed. Reddish purple **striae** ("stretch marks") are often present on the abdomen, thighs, and upper arms because of the degradative effect of cortisol on collagen.

Excessive cortisol secretion may result in acne and a fine coating of hair over the face and body. In women, look for the presence of hirsutism, clitoral hypertrophy, and male pattern balding related to androgen excess.

Elevated blood glucose levels are common. Hypertension may occur from water and sodium retention.

TABLE 66-6 Conditions Causing Increased Cortisol Secretion

Endogenous Secretion (Cushing's Disease)
- Bilateral adrenal hyperplasia*
- Pituitary adenoma increasing the production of ACTH (pituitary Cushing's disease)
- Malignancies: carcinomas of the lung, gastrointestinal tract, pancreas
- Adrenal adenomas or carcinomas

Exogenous Administration (Cushing's Syndrome)
- Therapeutic use of ACTH or glucocorticoids—most commonly for treatment of:
  - Asthma
  - Autoimmune disorders
  - Organ transplantation
  - Cancer chemotherapy
  - Allergic responses
  - Chronic fibrosis

ACTH, Adrenocorticotropic hormone.
*Most common cause.

The client with chronic hypercortisolism is immunosuppressed. The excess cortisol reduces the number of circulating lymphocytes, inhibits maturation of macrophages, reduces antibody synthesis, and inhibits production of cytokines and inflammatory chemicals (e.g., histamine). Not only are these clients at greater risk for infection, they may not have the expected inflammatory manifestations (fever, purulent exudate, redness in the affected area) when an infection is present.

PSYCHOSOCIAL ASSESSMENT

Hypercortisolism can result in emotional lability. Ask about mood swings, irritability, confusion, or depression. The client may have neurotic or psychotic behavior as a result of high blood cortisol levels.

DIAGNOSTIC ASSESSMENT

Plasma cortisol levels are high in clients with hypercortisolism. Blood for cortisol assays is obtained at the same time of day because levels vary throughout the day. Further diagnostic testing is performed to confirm the diagnosis of hypercortisolism, because an increase in cortisol levels is also seen in acute illness and trauma. Plasma ACTH levels vary, depending on the cause of hypercortisolism. In ectopic (ACTH-producing) syndromes, ACTH levels are elevated. In primary Cushing's disease or when Cushing's syndrome results from chronic steroid use, ACTH levels are very low. Additional laboratory findings include the following:

- Increased blood glucose level
- Decreased lymphocyte count
- Increased sodium level
- Decreased serum calcium level
- Decreased serum potassium level

Urine is tested to measure levels of free cortisol and the metabolites of cortisol and androgens (17-hydroxycorticosteroids and 17-ketosteroids). Instruct the client to save *all* urine for 24 hours. In Cushing's disease, levels of urine cortisol, 17-ketosteroids, and 17-hydroxycorticosteroids are all elevated, as are urine calcium, potassium, and glucose levels.

X-rays, computed tomography (CT) scans, magnetic resonance imaging (MRI), and arteriography may identify lesions of the adrenal or pituitary glands, lung, GI tract, or pancreas.

The *overnight dexamethasone suppression test* is an initial screening test for Cushing's disease. Instruct the client not to take drugs, especially phenytoin (Dilantin) or phenobarbital, for at least 2 days before the test. Normally, plasma cortisol levels are lower than 5 mg/dL. Higher levels indicate that further testing is needed.

For the *3-day, low-dose* dexamethasone suppression test, the client must take no drugs for at least 2 days before the test (if possible) and have no stressful procedures (e.g., barium enema, myelogram, or an intense physical therapy session) performed during the test. Table 66-5 lists drugs that interfere with testing. A baseline 24-hour urine sample is collected on day 1. Dexamethasone 0.5 mg is given every 6 hours on days 2 and 3, during which time 24-hour urine collections are taken. The 24-hour urine collections are tested for 17-ketosteroids, 17-hydroxycorticosteroids, creatinine, and urine cortisol. Normally, urinary 17-hydroxycorticosteroid excretion and cortisol levels are suppressed by dexamethasone, and Cushing's disease is ruled out. If these levels are not suppressed, a higher-dose dexamethasone test is performed.

The *high-dose* (8-mg) dexamethasone suppression test distinguishes between bilateral adrenocortical hyperplasia (e.g., Cushing's disease) and an adrenocortical neoplasm as the cause of hypercortisolism. This test can be performed as an overnight test or a 2-day test and uses higher doses of dexamethasone. In the overnight test, the client with Cushing's disease has a reduced plasma cortisol level that is less than 50% of baseline. This test is more reliable than the 2-day high-dose test.

CHART 66-13

KEY FEATURES of Hypercortisolism (Cushing's Disease/Syndrome)

General Appearance
- Fat redistribution
  - Moon face
  - Buffalo hump
  - Truncal obesity
- Weight gain

Cardiovascular Manifestations
- Hypertension
- Increased risk for thromboembolic events
- Frequent dependent edema
- Capillary fragility
  - Bruising
  - Petechiae

Musculoskeletal Manifestations
- Muscle atrophy (most apparent in extremities)
- Osteoporosis (bone density loss)
  - Pathologic fractures
  - Decreased height with vertebral collapse
  - Aseptic necrosis of the femur head
  - Slow or poor healing of bone fractures

Skin Manifestations
- Thinning skin ("paper-like" appearance, especially on the back of the hands)
- Striae
- Increased pigmentation (with ectopic or pituitary production of ACTH)

Immune System Manifestations
- Increased risk for infection
- Decreased immune function
  - Decreased circulating lymphocytes
  - Decreased production of immunoglobulins (antibodies)
- Decreased inflammatory responses
  - Decreased eosinophil count
  - Slight increase in neutrophil count but activity is reduced
- Decreased production of proinflammatory cytokines, histamine, and prostaglandins
- Manifestations of infection/inflammation may be masked

Common Nursing Diagnoses and Collaborative Problems

Nursing diagnoses that may apply to clients with Cushing's disease or Cushing's syndrome include the following:

- Disturbed Body Image related to illness
- Fatigue related to sleep deprivation
- Excess Fluid Volume related to excess water and sodium reabsorption
- Risk for Infection related to immunosuppression and inadequate primary defenses

- Risk for Injury related to poor wound healing and bone density loss
- Deficient Knowledge (Illness and Treatment) related to lack of interest in learning and unfamiliarity with information resources
- Imbalanced Nutrition: More Than Body Requirements related to excess intake in relation to metabolic need as a result of appetite stimulation by cortisol

◆Interventions

Goals of treatment for hypercortisolism are the reduction of plasma cortisol levels, removal of tumors, prevention of complications, and restoration of normal or acceptable body appearance.

NONSURGICAL MANAGEMENT. Weigh the client daily and monitor intake and output to assess hydration status. Fluid intake restriction is sometimes needed to maintain fluid balance.

Drug Therapy. Most clients with endogenous hypercortisolism undergo surgery. Drugs that interfere with adrenocorticotropic hormone (ACTH) production or adrenal hormone synthesis, however, may be used for temporary relief. Mitotane (Lysodren) is an adrenal cytotoxic agent used for inoperable adrenal tumors. Aminoglutethimide (Elipten, Cytadren) and metyrapone (Metopirone) use different pathways to decrease cortisol production. For clients with hypercortisolism from increased ACTH production, cyproheptadine (Periactin) may be used because it interferes with ACTH production. Assess the client for therapy effectiveness and side effects or toxicity.

Radiation Therapy. Radiation may be used to treat hypercortisolism caused by pituitary adenomas. However, radiation is not always effective and often destroys normal tissue. Observe for any changes in the client's neurologic status, such as headache, elevated blood pressure or pulse, disorientation, or changes in pupil size or reaction. The client may have skin dryness, redness, flushing, or alopecia at the radiation site. Review these possible side effects with the client. Chapter 48 discusses radiation therapy to the head.

SURGICAL MANAGEMENT. The surgical treatment of adrenocortical hypersecretion depends on the cause of the disease. When adrenal hyperfunction is due to increased pituitary secretion of ACTH, removal of a pituitary adenoma may be attempted. In many instances, a total **hypophysectomy** (surgical removal of the pituitary gland) is needed. Hypophysectomy is performed via the transsphenoidal or transfrontal craniotomy route. (See earlier discussion of hypophysectomy on pp. 1464-1465; see also Chapter 48 for nursing care of clients undergoing a craniotomy.) If hypercortisolism is caused by adrenal tumors, a partial or complete **adrenalectomy** (removal of the adrenal gland) may be needed.

Preoperative Care. Electrolyte imbalances are corrected before surgery. Continue to monitor blood potassium, sodium, and chloride levels. Dysrhythmias from potassium imbalance may occur, and cardiac monitoring is needed. Hyperglycemia is controlled before surgery, and blood glucose levels are monitored.

The client with hypercortisolism is at risk for complications such as infections and fractures. Prevent infection with handwashing and aseptic technique. Decrease the risk for falls by raising bed siderails and encouraging the client to ask for assistance when getting out of bed. A high-calorie, high-protein diet is prescribed before surgery.

Glucocorticoid preparations are given before surgery. The client continues to receive glucocorticoids during surgery to prevent adrenal crisis because the removal of the tumor results in a sudden drop in cortisol levels. Before surgery, discuss the care needs for after surgery and the need for long-term drug therapy.

Operative Procedures. A unilateral adrenalectomy is performed when one gland is involved. A bilateral adrenalectomy is needed when ectopic ACTH-producing tumors cannot be treated by other means or when both adrenal glands are diseased.

Surgery can be abdominal or through the lateral flank. Abdominal surgery causes a higher degree of illness and risk. The flank approach is preferred because the abdominal cavity is not entered and complications are reduced. A laparoscopic adrenalectomy may reduce complications after surgery.

Postoperative Care. After an adrenalectomy, the client is usually sent to a critical care unit. Immediately after surgery, assess the client every 15 minutes for shock (e.g., hypotension, a rapid, weak pulse, and a decreasing urine output) due to possible insufficient glucocorticoid replacement. Monitor ongoing vital signs and other hemodynamic variables (central venous pressure, pulmonary wedge pressure), intake and output, daily weights, and serum electrolyte levels.

After a bilateral adrenalectomy, clients require lifelong glucocorticoid replacement, starting immediately after surgery. In unilateral adrenalectomy, glucocorticoid replacement continues until the remaining adrenal gland increases hormone production. This therapy may be needed for up to 2 years after surgery.

Preventing Complications. The client who has hypercortisolism is at risk for injury from skin breakdown, bone fractures, and gastrointestinal (GI) bleeding. Prevention of such injuries is a major nursing care focus.

Skin Breakdown. Assess the client's skin for reddened areas, excoriation, breakdown, and edema. If mobility is decreased, turn the client every 2 hours and pad bony prominences.

Instruct the client to avoid activities that can result in skin trauma. To reduce tissue injury, teach the client to use a soft toothbrush and an electric shaver. Instruct clients to keep the skin clean and to dry it thoroughly after washing. Excessive dryness can be prevented by using a moisturizing lotion.

Adhesive tape often causes skin breakdown. Use tape sparingly and use caution when removing it. After venipuncture or arterial puncture, the client may have increased bleeding because of blood vessel fragility. Exert pressure over the site for longer than normal to prevent bleeding and bruising.

Pathologic Fractures. Hypercortisolism causes bone density loss and osteoporosis. Teach the client about safety issues and dietary needs. The client is at risk for fractures as a result of minor falls or bumps. When helping the client to move in bed, use a lift sheet instead of grasping him or her. Instruct the client to call for help when ambulating. Review the use of ambulatory aids (walkers or canes), if needed. Keep rooms free of extraneous objects that might cause a fall.

Consult with a dietitian to counsel the client about diet therapy. A high-calorie diet is prescribed that includes items from all of the major food groups and increased amounts of calcium and vitamin D. Generous amounts of milk, cheese, yogurt, and green leafy and root vegetables add calcium. Advise the client to avoid caffeine and alcohol, which increase the risk for GI ulcers and may promote bone density loss.

Gastrointestinal Bleeding. Interventions aim to reduce gastric irritation, usually through drug therapy. Drug therapy involves agents that protect the GI mucosa and those that decrease the secretion of hydrochloric acid.

AGENTS PROTECTING THE GASTROINTESTINAL MUCOSA. Antacids buffer stomach acids and protect the GI mucosa. Teach the client that these drugs should be taken on a regular schedule, rather than on an as-needed basis.

AGENTS INHIBITING THE SECRETION OF HYDROCHLORIC ACID. Some agents block the H_2-receptor site in the gastric mucosa. When histamine binds to this receptor site, a series of actions occur that release hydrochloric acid. Drugs that block the H_2-receptor site include cimetidine (Tagamet, Peptol✱, Novo-Cimetine✱), ranitidine (Zantac, Apo-Ranitidine✱), famotidine (Pepcid), and nizatidine (Axid). Omeprazole (Losec✱, Prilosec) and esomeprazole (Nexium) inhibit the gastric proton pump and prevent the formation of hydrochloric acid.

PREVENTION OF IRRITATION. Encourage the client to reduce or eliminate habits that contribute to gastric irritation, such as consuming alcohol or caffeine, smoking, and fasting. Discuss other prescribed and over-the-counter drugs that the client may be taking. Nonsteroidal anti-inflammatory drugs (NSAIDs) and drugs that contain aspirin or other salicylates can cause gastritis and intensify GI bleeding.

CLIENT EDUCATION. Lifelong hormone replacement is needed after bilateral adrenalectomy. Teach the client and family about adherence with the drug regimen and its side effects (Chart 66-14). Wearing a medical alert bracelet is essential.

Hyperaldosteronism

PATHOPHYSIOLOGY

In clients with hyperaldosteronism, increased secretion of aldosterone results in mineralocorticoid excess. Primary hyperaldosteronism (Conn's syndrome) results from excessive secretion of aldosterone from one or both adrenal glands. Most often, this is caused by an adrenal adenoma. In a person with secondary hyperaldosteronism, the excessive secretion of aldosterone is caused by high levels of angiotensin II that are stimulated by high plasma renin levels. Causes of high renin levels include renal hypoxemia and the use of thiazide diuretics.

Increased aldosterone levels affect the renal tubules and cause sodium retention with potassium and hydrogen ion excretion. Hypernatremia, hypokalemia, and metabolic alkalosis result. Sodium retention increases blood volume, which raises blood pressure and suppresses renin production. The elevated blood pressure may cause strokes and renal damage. Peripheral edema rarely occurs because of the "renal escape mechanism," in which the kidney decreases sodium reabsorption. However, no compensatory mechanism exists to stop or reverse potassium loss. (See Chapter 16 for discussion of electrolyte imbalances.)

CHART 66-14

CLIENT EDUCATION GUIDE
Cortisol Replacement Therapy

- Take your medication in divided doses, the first dose in the morning and the second dose between 4 and 6 PM.
- Take your medication with meals or snacks.
- Weigh yourself daily.
- Increase your dosage as directed for increased physical stress or severe emotional stress, including surgery, dental work, influenza, fever, pregnancy, and family problems.
- Never skip a dose of medication. If you have persistent vomiting or severe diarrhea and cannot take your medication by mouth for 24 to 36 hours, call your physician. If you cannot reach your physician, go to the nearest emergency department. You may need an injection to take the place of your usual oral medication.
- Always wear your medical alert bracelet or necklace.
- Make regular visits for health care follow-up.
- Learn how to give yourself an intramuscular injection of hydrocortisone.

COLLABORATIVE MANAGEMENT

Assessment

Problems from hypokalemia and elevated blood pressure are the most common issues of the client with hyperaldosteronism. The client may have headache, fatigue, muscle weakness, **nocturia** (excessive urination at night), and loss of stamina. **Polydipsia** (excessive fluid intake) and **polyuria** (excessive urine output) occur less frequently. **Paresthesias** (sensations of numbness and tingling) may occur if potassium depletion is severe. The client may have visual changes related to hypertension.

The diagnosis of hyperaldosteronism is made on the basis of laboratory studies, x-rays, and imaging with CT or MRI. Serum potassium levels are decreased, and sodium levels are elevated. Plasma renin levels are low; aldosterone levels are high. Increased hydrogen ion loss leads to metabolic alkalemia (elevated blood pH). Urine has a low specific gravity and high aldosterone levels.

Interventions

Surgery is the most common treatment for early stage hyperaldosteronism. One or both adrenal glands may be removed. Surgery is not performed, however, until the client's potassium levels are normal. Drugs used to increase potassium levels include spironolactone (Aldactone, Novospiroton✱, Sincomen✱), a potassium-sparing diuretic and aldosterone antagonist. Potassium supplements may be prescribed to increase potassium levels before surgery. The client may also benefit from a low-sodium diet before surgery, but sodium restriction is not needed after surgery because aldosterone levels should return to normal.

The client who has undergone a unilateral adrenalectomy may need temporary glucocorticoid replacement. Replacement is lifelong if both adrenal glands are removed. Glucocorticoids are given before surgery to prevent adrenal crisis. The client receiving long-term replacement therapy should wear a medical alert bracelet. (See the discussion of adrenalectomy under Hypercortisolism [Cushing's syndrome], p. 1476, for more discussion of care after surgery and client education.)

When surgery cannot be performed, spironolactone therapy is continued to control hypokalemia and hypertension. *Because spironolactone is a potassium-sparing diuretic, hyperkalemia can occur in clients who have impaired renal function or excessive potassium intake.* Advise the client to avoid potassium supplements and foods rich in potassium (see Chart 16-6). Hyponatremia can occur with spironolactone therapy and the client may need increased dietary sodium. Instruct the client to report symptoms of hyponatremia, such as dryness of the mouth, thirst, lethargy, or drowsiness. Teach clients to report any additional side effects of spironolactone therapy, including gynecomastia, diarrhea, drowsiness, headache, rash, **urticaria** (hives), confusion, erectile dysfunction, hirsutism, and amenorrhea.

Pheochromocytoma

PATHOPHYSIOLOGY

Pheochromocytoma is a catecholamine-producing tumor that arises in chromaffin cells. These tumors usually occur as a single lesion in the right adrenal gland, although they can be bilateral or in the abdomen. Pheochromocytomas are most often benign, but about 10% are malignant. The tumors produce and store catecholamines.

Pheochromocytomas release epinephrine and norepinephrine (NE). Excessive epinephrine and NE stimulate alpha receptors and beta receptors and can have wide-ranging adverse effects mimicking the action of the sympathetic division of the autonomic nervous system.

The cause is unknown but some pheochromocytomas occur with inherited disorders such as neurofibromatosis and multiple endocrine neoplasia (MEN) syndromes. These tumors are rare and occur slightly more often in women. They can occur at any age but appear most commonly in clients between 40 and 60 years of age.

COLLABORATIVE MANAGEMENT

Assessment

The client often has intermittent episodes of hypertension or attacks that vary in length from a few minutes to several hours. During these episodes, the client has severe headaches, palpitations, profuse diaphoresis, flushing, apprehension, or a sense of impending doom. Pain in the chest or abdomen, with nausea and vomiting, can also occur. Increased abdominal pressure, urination, and vigorous abdominal palpation, can provoke a hypertensive crisis. Drugs, such as tricyclic antidepressants, droperidol, glucagon, metoclopramide, phenothiazines, and naloxone can induce a hypertensive crisis in the client with pheochromocytoma. Foods or beverages high in tyramine (e.g., aged cheese, red wine) also induce hypertension. The client may also report heat intolerance, weight loss, and tremors.

Diagnostic tests include 24-hour urine collections for vanillylmandelic acid (VMA) (a product of catecholamine metabolism), metanephrine, and catecholamines, all of which are elevated in the presence of a pheochromocytoma. Best practices for VMA testing are listed in Chart 66-15. Plasma catecholamine levels are elevated after the client has rested for at least 30 minutes. The clonidine suppression test is used in the diagnosis of a pheochromocytoma when the catecholamine levels are not consistent. When oral clonidine hydrochloride (Catapres, Dixarit✱) is given to a person who does not have a pheochromocytoma, the clonidine suppresses catecholamine release and reduces the serum catecholamine levels. This response is not seen in the client who has a pheochromocytoma.

CHART 66-15

BEST PRACTICE for Vanillylmandelic Acid Testing

- Describe the test to the client and explain that his or her participation is needed for accurate test results.
- Instruct the client on the special vanillylmandelic acid (VMA)–restricted diet that starts 2 or 3 days before the 24-hour urine collection.
- Restricted foods include those containing caffeine (coffee, tea, cola, and chocolate or cocoa), certain fruits (citrus fruits and bananas), vanilla-containing foods, and licorice. Check your laboratory for a more inclusive food list.
- Confer with the physician about which medications should not be given during the 3- or 4-day test. Medications usually withheld include aspirin and antihypertensive agents.
- Be aware that strenuous physical activity, stress, and starvation can increase VMA levels; monitor, intervene, and teach the client as appropriate.
- Instruct the client about how to collect an accurate 24-hour urine sample: the collection is started with an empty bladder, and then all urine formed over the next 24 hours is collected in one container. At the end of the 24-hour period, the client voids and adds that urine to the collection.
- Obtain a urine collection container with preservative from the laboratory. Check with the laboratory about keeping the collection on ice.
- When the collection is complete, send the urine to the laboratory promptly.
- Help the client understand the test results; normal VMA excretion in 24 hours is 2 to 7 mg, or 10 to 35 μmol.

Catecholamine stimulation tests, such as with glucagon, can help diagnose a pheochromocytoma; however, the danger of uncontrolled hypertension and effects on the heart limit the usefulness of this type of testing.

MRI or CT scans can precisely locate tumors in the adrenal gland. After diagnosis, computed tomography (CT) scans of the chest and abdomen may be used to locate any other tumors.

Interventions

Surgery is the main treatment for a pheochromocytoma. One or both adrenal glands are removed (depending on whether the tumor is bilateral). After surgery, focus on promoting adequate tissue perfusion, nutritional needs, and comfort measures.

Hypertension is the hallmark of the disease. Monitor the blood pressure regularly and place the cuff consistently on the same arm, with the client in lying and standing positions. Identify stressors that may lead to a hypertensive crisis and attempt to reduce them. Instruct the client not to smoke, drink caffeine-containing beverages, or change position suddenly. *Do not palpate the abdomen because this action could cause a sudden release of catecholamines and severe hypertension.* Provide a diet rich in calories, vitamins, and minerals.

The client often benefits from hydration before surgery because decreased blood volume increases the risk for hypotension during and after surgery. Assess the client's hydration status and report manifestations of dehydration or fluid overload.

Provide a calm, restful environment for the client who has a severe headache. Instruct the client to limit activity. A private, darkened room helps promote rest. If the client is sleeping, avoid interruptions if possible.

The client's blood pressure is stabilized with alpha-adrenergic blocking agents before surgery because of the increased risk for severe hypertension during surgery. Anesthetic agents and touching of the tumor during surgery can cause a catecholamine release. Short-acting alpha-adrenergic blockers are given by IV bolus or drip for a hypertensive crisis. Phenoxybenzamine (Dibenzyline) produces long-acting alpha-adrenergic blockade and is often used for management of hypertension before surgery. It is also used for management of the client who is not a candidate for surgery.

The drug dosages are adjusted for 2 to 3 weeks before surgery until blood pressure is controlled and hypertensive attacks do not occur. The blood volume expands, and blood pressure in the supine position returns to normal.

Beta-adrenergic blocking agents are avoided in clients with a pheochromocytoma until after alpha-adrenergic blockade is in effect, because these drugs may cause a rebound rise in blood pressure. After alpha-adrenergic blockade, low doses of propranolol (Inderal, Detensol✱) or labetalol (Trandate) may be used to treat tachycardia and dysrhythmias. Other drugs used for blood pressure control before surgery include calcium channel blockers, such as nicardipine (Cardene) and agents that suppress catecholamine synthesis such as metyrosine (Demser).

Nursing care after surgery is similar to that for the client who has undergone an adrenalectomy (see Hypercortisolism [Cushing's Syndrome], p. 1474). Closely monitor the client for hypotension (from the sudden decrease in catecholamine levels) and for hypovolemia. Hemorrhage and shock are possible, and plasma expanders or fluids may be needed. Monitor vital signs, as well as fluid intake and output. If opioids are given, check for their effect on blood pressure.

Tumors may be inoperable because of the client's other medical conditions. Treatment then is medical, with alpha-adrenergic and beta-adrenergic blocking agents, because the tumors do not respond well to chemotherapy or radiation therapy. For clients who are medically managed, self-measurement of blood pressure with home monitoring equipment is essential.

GET READY for the NCLEX Examination!

KEY POINTS

Safe Effective Care Environment

- Handle all clients with bone density loss carefully, using lift sheets whenever possible.
- Teach the client and family about the clinical manifestations of infection and when to seek medical advice.
- Use good handwashing techniques before providing any care to a client who is immunocompromised from hypercortisolism.

Health Promotion and Maintenance

- Teach all people about the hazards of using any unprescribed hormonal or steroid agents.

Psychosocial Integrity

- Allow the client the opportunity to express fear or anxiety regarding a change in health status.
- Explain all diagnostic procedures, restrictions, and follow-up care to the client scheduled for tests.
- Allow clients who experience a change in physical appearance to mourn this change.

Physiological Integrity

- Ensure that hormone replacement drugs are given as close to the prescribed times as possible.
- Use bleeding precautions for clients who have hypercortisolism.
- Teach clients who have permanent endocrine hypofunction the proper techniques and timing of hormone replacement therapy.
- During the immediate period after a transsphenoidal hypophysectomy, teach the client to avoid activities that increase intracranial pressure (e.g., bending at the waist, straining to have a bowel movement, coughing).
- Measure intake and output accurately on clients who have either diabetes insipidus or syndrome of inappropriate antidiuretic hormone (SIADH).
- Teach clients with diabetes insipidus the proper way to self-administer vasopressin nasal spray.
- Teach the client with diabetes insipidus the manifestations of dehydration.
- Instruct the client with adrenal insufficiency to wear a medical alert bracelet and to carry simple carbohydrates with them at all times.
- Do not palpate the abdomen of a client who has a pheochromocytoma.

ADDITIONAL STUDY RESOURCES

Go to your Student CD-ROM for Review Questions for the NCLEX Examination.

evolve Go to http://evolve.elsevier.com/Iggy/ for Integrated Management of Care Questions for the NCLEX Examination.

SELECTED BIBLIOGRAPHY

Ackley, B., & Ladwig, G. (2002). *Nursing diagnosis handbook: A guide to planning care* (5th ed.). St. Louis: Mosby.

Carson, P. (2000). Emergency: Adrenal crisis. *American Journal of Nursing, 100*(7), 49-50.

Castiglione, V. (2000). Emergency: Hyperkalemia. *American Journal of Nursing, 100*(1), 55-56.

Daub, K. (2002). Pheochromocytoma, up close and personal. *Nursing2002, 32*(3), 32hn1-32hn4.

Dluhy, R., Lawrence, J., & Williams, G. (2003). Endocrine hypertension. In P.R. Larsen, et al. (Eds.), *Williams textbook of endocrinology* (10th ed., pp. 551-585). Philadelphia: W. B. Saunders.

Dochterman, J., & Bulechek, G. (Eds.). (2004). *Nursing interventions classification (NIC)* (4th ed.). St. Louis: Mosby.

Ebersole, P., Hess, P., & Luggen, A. (2004). *Toward healthy aging: Human needs and nursing response* (6th ed.). St. Louis: Mosby.

Facts and Comparisons. (2004). *Drug facts and comparisons* (58th ed.). St. Louis: Author.

Goldberg, M. (2000). The diagnostic challenge–Hyperaldosteronism caused by bilateral adrenal hyperplasia. *Emergency Medicine, 32*(3), 55-56.

Holcomb, S. (2002). Stopping the cascade of diabetes insipidus. *Nursing2002, 32*(3), 32cc1-32cc6.

Kearney, K. (2000). Emergency: Adrenal crisis. *American Journal of Nursing, 100*(7), 49-50.

Langfeldt, L., & Cooley, M. (2003). Syndrome of inappropriate antidiuretic hormone secretion in malignancy: Review and implications for nursing management. *Clinical Journal of Oncology Nursing, 7*(4), 425-430.

Larsen, P.R., et al. (Eds.). *Williams textbook of endocrinology* (10th ed.). Philadelphia: W. B. Saunders.

LoBuono, C. (2001). Managing geriatric endocrine disorders. *Patient Care for the Nurse Practitioner, 4*(11), 26-36.

McCance, K., & Huether, S. (2002). *Pathophysiology: The biologic basis for disease in adults and children* (4th ed.). St. Louis: Mosby.

McConnell, E. (2002). Myths and facts about Addison's disease. *Nursing2002, 32*(8), 79.

Melmed, S., & Kleinberg, D. (2003). Anterior pituitary. In P.R. Larsen, et al. (Eds.), *Williams textbook of endocrinology* (10th ed., pp. 177-279). Philadelphia: W. B. Saunders.

Moorhead, S., Johnson, M., & Maas, M. (Eds.). (2004). *Nursing outcomes classification (NOC)* (3rd ed.). St. Louis: Mosby.

Mosso, L., et al. (2003). Primary hyperaldosteronism and hypertensive disease. *Hypertension, 42*(1), 161-165.

Nayback, A. (2000). Hyponatremia as a consequence of acute adrenal insufficiency and hypothyroidism. *Journal of Emergency Nursing, 26*(2), 130-133.

Pagana, K., & Pagana, T. (2002). *Mosby's manual of diagnostic and laboratory tests* (2nd ed.). St. Louis: Mosby.

Reincke, M. (2000). Subclinical Cushing's syndrome. *Endocrinology and Metabolism Clinics of North America, 29*(1), 43-56.

Robinson, A., & Verbalis, J. (2003). Posterior pituitary gland. In P.R. Larsen, et al. (Eds.), *Williams textbook of endocrinology* (10th ed., pp. 281-329). Philadelphia: W. B. Saunders.

Sachse, D. (2001). Acromegaly. *American Journal of Nursing, 101*(11), 69-74.

Stewart, P. (2003). The adrenal cortex. In P.R. Larsen, et al. (Eds.), *Williams textbook of endocrinology* (10th ed., pp. 491-551). Philadelphia: W. B. Saunders.

CHAPTER 67

Interventions for Clients with Problems of the Thyroid and Parathyroid Glands

M. LINDA WORKMAN

LEARNING OUTCOMES

After studying this chapter, you should be able to:

1. Compare the common clinical manifestations of hyperthyroidism with those of hypothyroidism.
2. Explain the pathophysiology of Graves' disease.
3. Describe the mechanisms of action, side effects, and nursing implications for pharmacologic management of hyperthyroidism.
4. Interpret clinical changes and laboratory data to determine the effectiveness of interventions for hyperthyroidism.
5. Prioritize nursing care for the client during the first 24 hours after a total thyroidectomy.
6. Explain the pathophysiology of Hashimoto's thyroiditis.
7. Identify teaching priorities for the client taking thyroid hormone replacement therapy.
8. Interpret clinical changes and laboratory data to determine the effectiveness of interventions for hypothyroidism.
9. Compare the clinical manifestations of hyperparathyroidism with those of hypoparathyroidism.
10. Prioritize nursing care for the client during the first 24 hours after a parathyroidectomy.
11. Interpret clinical changes and laboratory data to determine the effectiveness of interventions for parathyroid problems.

Go to your Student CD-ROM for Review Questions for the NCLEX Examination keyed to these Learning Outcomes.

Hormones from the thyroid and parathyroid glands affect overall metabolism, electrolyte balance, and excitable membrane activity. Therefore problems of either thyroid or parathyroid function usually have widespread effects and manifestations. With mild disturbances, the problems are subtle. With more severe disturbances, the problems may be life threatening.

THYROID DISORDERS

Hyperthyroidism

PATHOPHYSIOLOGY

Excessive thyroid hormone secretion leads to **hyperthyroidism.** The manifestations of hyperthyroidism are called **thyrotoxicosis.** Thyroid hormones affect metabolism in all body organs. Increased thyroid function produces many different manifestations. Hyperthyroidism can be temporary or permanent, depending on the cause.

In hyperthyroidism the normal feedback control over thyroid hormone secretion fails. Because thyroid hormones stimulate most body systems, excessive thyroid hormones produce hypermetabolism and increased sympathetic nervous system activity. Many of the manifestations are caused by the body's response to the demands of hypermetabolism (Chart 67-1).

Thyroid hormones directly stimulate the heart. The resulting increased heart rate and stroke volume cause increased cardiac output and blood flow.

Elevated thyroid hormone levels affect protein, lipid, and carbohydrate metabolism. Protein **synthesis** (buildup) and **degradation** (breakdown) are increased. Breakdown ex-

CHART 67-1

KEY FEATURES of Hyperthyroidism

Skin Manifestations
- Diaphoresis (excessive sweating)
- Fine, soft, silky hair (body)
- Smooth, warm, moist skin
- Thinning of scalp hair

Pulmonary Manifestations
- Shortness of breath with or without exertion
- Rapid, shallow respirations
- Decreased vital capacity

Cardiovascular Manifestations
- Palpitations
- Chest pain
- Increased systolic blood pressure
- Widened pulse pressure
- Tachycardia
- Dysrhythmias

Gastrointestinal Manifestations
- Weight loss
- Increased appetite
- Increased stools
- Hypoproteinemia

Musculoskeletal Manifestations
- Muscle weakness
- Muscle wasting

Neurologic Manifestations
- Blurred or double vision
- Eye fatigue
- Corneal ulcers or infections
- Increased tears
- Injected (red) conjunctiva
- Photophobia
- Eyelid retraction, eyelid lag*
- Globe lag*
- Hyperactive deep tendon reflexes
- Tremors
- Insomnia

Metabolic Manifestations
- Increased basal metabolic rate
- Heat intolerance
- Low-grade fever
- Fatigue

Psychological/Emotional Manifestations
- Decreased attention span
- Restlessness
- Irritability
- Emotional lability
- Manic behavior

Reproductive Manifestations
- Amenorrhea
- Decreased menstrual flow
- Increased libido

Other Manifestations
- Goiter
- Wide-eyed (startled) appearance*
- Decreased total white blood cell count
- Enlarged spleen

*Present in Graves' disease only.

TABLE 67-1 Causes of Hyperthyroidism

Cause	Mechanism
Graves' disease (toxic diffuse goiter)	Autoimmune in nature. Antibodies (TSH-Ab) bind to TSH receptors and keep them activated, increasing the size of the gland and increasing the production of thyroid hormones.
Toxic multinodular goiter	Multiple thyroid nodules, resulting in thyroid hyperfunction.
Thyroid adenoma	Uncontrolled secretion of T_3 and T_4 from benign thyroid tumor.
Pituitary hyperthyroidism	Pituitary adenoma resulting in excessive TSH secretion.
Thyroiditis (radiation-induced)	T_3 and T_4 secretion increased before destruction of gland. Hyperthyroid state usually transient.
T_3 thyrotoxicosis	Increase in thyroid secretion of T_3. Cause unknown.
Factitious hyperthyroidism	Ingestion of excessive amounts of thyroid hormone.
Jod-Basedow phenomenon (iodine induced)	Administration of iodine to an individual with endemic goiter, resulting in excessive production of thyroid hormone.
Thyroid carcinoma	Uncommon, usually occurs with large follicular carcinomas.
Tumors elsewhere in the body	Secrete TSH or thyroid hormones (T_3 and T_4) mimicking hyperthyroid activity.

T_3, Triiodothyronine; *T_4*, thyroxine; *TSH*, thyroid-stimulating hormone.

ceeds buildup, causing a net loss of protein known as a **negative nitrogen balance.** Glucose tolerance is decreased, and the client has **hyperglycemia** (elevated blood glucose levels). Fat metabolism is increased, and body fat decreases. Although the client has an increased appetite, food intake does not meet energy demands, and the client loses weight. With prolonged hyperthyroidism, the client has chronic nutritional deficiency.

Thyroid hormones are produced in response to the stimulation hormones secreted by the hypothalamus and anterior pituitary glands. Thus oversecretion of thyroid hormones changes the secretion of hormones from the hypothalamus and anterior pituitary gland. In addition, thyroid hormones have some influence over sex hormone production in both men and women. Women have menstrual problems and decreased fertility. Both men and women with hyperthyroidism have an increased libido (sexual urge or interest).

Etiology and Genetic Risk

Hyperthyroidism has many causes (Table 67-1), the most common cause of which is **Graves' disease,** also called toxic diffuse goiter. The client with Graves' disease usually has hyperthyroidism, a **goiter** (enlargement of the thyroid gland), **exophthalmos** (abnormal protrusion of the eyes), and **pretibial myxedema** (dry, waxy swelling of the front surfaces of the lower legs). *Not all clients with a goiter have hyperthyroidism.*

Graves' disease is an autoimmune disorder in which antibodies are made and attach to the thyroid stimulating hormone (TSH) receptor sites on the thyroid tissue. When these antibodies, known as thyroid-stimulating immunoglobulins (TSIs), bind to the thyroid gland, the gland increases in size and overproduces thyroid hormones.

Genetic Considerations

Although no specific gene or gene mutation has been identified as a cause of Graves' disease, its high incidence among family members suggests a genetic component for risk. The pattern of inheritance appears to be familial clustering and may involve mutations in different genes. The risk for Graves' disease is increased in people who have other autoimmune disorders such as type 1 diabetes mellitus and pernicious anemia.

Hyperthyroidism caused by multiple thyroid nodules is termed **toxic multinodular goiter.** The nodules may be enlarged thyroid tissues or adenomas. These clients usually have had a goiter for years. The overproduction of thyroid hormones is usually milder than that seen in Graves' disease, and the client does not have exophthalmos or pretibial edema.

Hyperthyroidism also can be caused by excessive use of thyroid replacement hormones. This type of problem is called **exogenous hyperthyroidism.**

A condition called thyroid storm or thyroid crisis can occur when hyperthyroidism is untreated or poorly controlled or when the client is severely stressed. This condition is an extreme state of hyperthyroidism in which all manifestations are more severe and life threatening.

Incidence/Prevalence

Hyperthyroidism is a common endocrine disorder. Graves' disease can occur at any age but is diagnosed most often in women between 20 and 40 years of age. Toxic multinodular goiter usually occurs after the age of 50 and affects women four times as often as men.

COLLABORATIVE MANAGEMENT

Assessment

HISTORY

The client may have noticed many changes and problems because hyperthyroidism affects all body systems. Record age, gender, and usual weight. The client may report a recent weight loss, an increased appetite, and an increase in the number of bowel movements per day.

A hallmark of hyperthyroidism is heat intolerance. The client may have **diaphoresis** (increased sweating) even when environmental temperatures are comfortable for others. He or she often wears lighter clothing in cold weather. The client may also report palpitations or chest pain as a result of the cardiovascular effects. Ask about changes in breathing patterns because dyspnea (with or without exertion) is common.

Visual changes may be the earliest problem the client notices, especially ophthalmopathy with Graves' disease (Figure 67-1). Ask the client about changes in vision, such as blurring or double vision and tiring of the eyes.

Ask whether the client has noticed a change in energy level or in the ability to perform activities of daily living (ADLs). Fatigue, weakness, and insomnia are common.

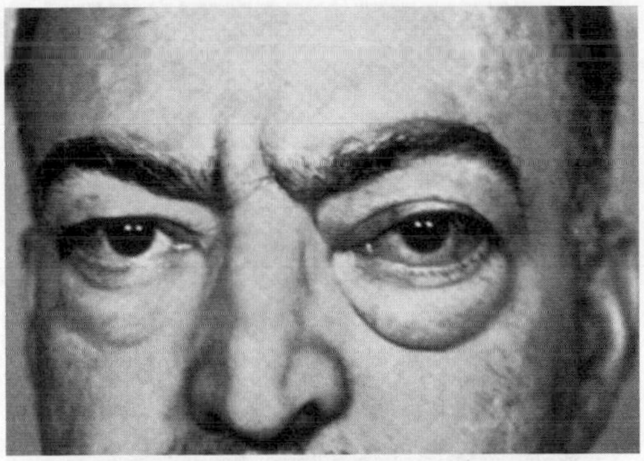

Figure 67-1 ■ Ophthalmopathy. The client has proptosis.

Family and friends may report that the client has become irritable or depressed.

Ask women about changes in menses because amenorrhea or a decreased menstrual flow is common. Initially both men and women may have an increase in libido.

Explore the client's medical history. Previous thyroid surgery or radiation therapy to the neck is important because some people remain hyperthyroid after surgery or are resistant to radiation therapy. Ask about past and current drugs, especially the use of thyroid hormone replacement or antithyroid drugs.

PHYSICAL ASSESSMENT/CLINICAL MANIFESTATIONS

Observe the client's general appearance. Two types of **ophthalmopathy** (abnormal eye appearance or function) are common with hyperthyroidism: eyelid retraction (eyelid lag) and globe (eyeball) lag. In eyelid lag, which occurs in all forms of thyrotoxicosis, the upper eyelid fails to descend when the client gazes slowly downward. In globe lag, the upper eyelid pulls back faster than the eyeball when the client gazes upward. During assessment ask the client to look down and then up, and document the response.

Infiltrative ophthalmopathy, which leads to exophthalmos, is common in clients with Graves' disease (Figure 67-2). The wide-eyed or "startled" look is due to edema in the extraocular muscles and increased fatty tissue behind the eye, which pushes the eyeball forward. Pressure on the optic nerve may impair vision. Swelling and shortening of the muscles may cause problems with focusing. If the eyelid fails to close completely and the eye is unprotected, the eye may become overdry and develop corneal ulcers or infection. Observe the client's eyes for excessive tearing and a bloodshot appearance, and ask about sensitivity to light **(photophobia).**

Observe the size and symmetry of the thyroid gland. Palpate the thyroid gland to assess the presence of a mass or general enlargement. In goiter, a generalized thyroid enlargement, the thyroid gland may increase to four times its normal size (Figure 67-3). Goiters are classified by size (Table 67-2). Bruits (turbulence from increased blood flow) may be heard with a stethoscope. (See Chapter 65 for a discussion of thyroid palpation and auscultation.)

The cardiac problems of hyperthyroidism include increased systolic blood pressure, tachycardia, and other dysrhythmias. Usually the diastolic pressure is decreased, causing a widened pulse pressure.

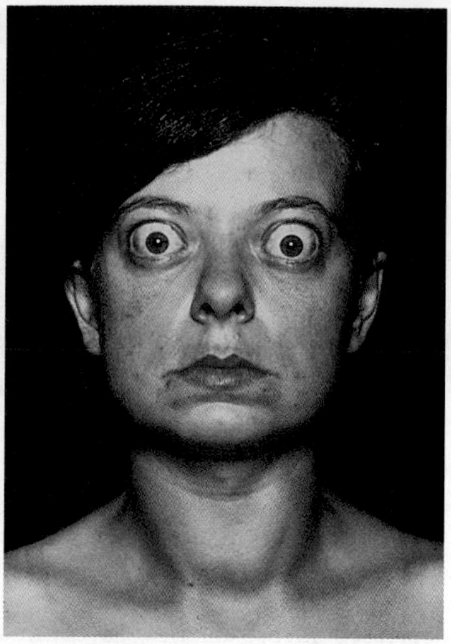

Figure 67-2 ■ Exophthalmos.

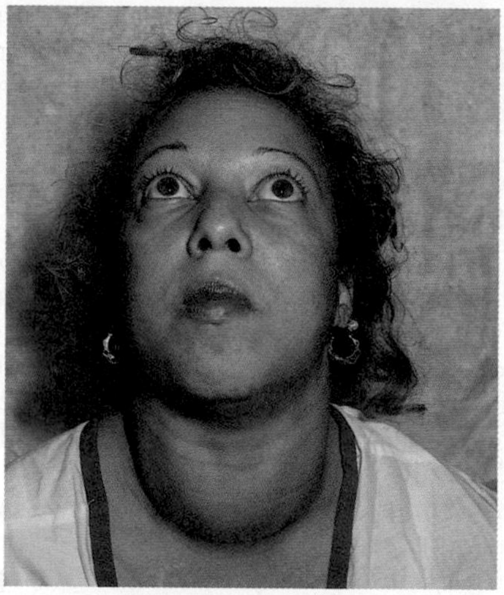

Figure 67-3 ■ Goiter.

Inspect the client's hair and skin. Fine, soft, silky hair and smooth, moist skin are common with hyperthyroidism. The client may have muscle weakness, hyperactive deep tendon reflexes, or tremors. Observe gross motor movements for tremors, especially of the hands. Reflexes may be hyperactive. The client may appear extremely restless, irritable, and fatigued.

PSYCHOSOCIAL ASSESSMENT

The client with hyperthyroidism often has wide mood swings, irritability, decreased attention span, and manic behavior. Mild to severe hyperactivity often leads to fatigue because of the inability to sleep well. Ask the client whether he or she has been crying or laughing inappropriately or has had difficulty concentrating. Family members often report these changes in mental or emotional status.

LABORATORY ASSESSMENT

Testing for hyperthyroidism includes measurement of the following blood values: triiodothyronine (T_3), thyroxine (T_4), T_3 resin uptake (T_3RU), and thyroid-stimulating hormone (TSH). Antibodies to TSH (TSH-RAb) are measured to determine the presence of Graves' disease. Laboratory changes in hyperthyroidism are listed in Chart 67-2.

TABLE 67-2 Goiter Classification

Goiter Grade	Description
0	No palpable or visible goiter.
1	Mass is not visible with neck in the normal position. Goiter can be palpated and moves up when the client swallows.
2	Mass is visible as swelling when the neck is in the normal position. Goiter is easily palpated and is usually asymmetric.

OTHER DIAGNOSTIC ASSESSMENTS

THYROID SCAN. The thyroid scan evaluates the position, size, and functioning of the thyroid gland. Radioactive iodine (RAI [^{123}I]) is given by mouth, and the uptake of iodine by the thyroid gland (RAIU) is measured. The half-life of ^{123}I is short, and radiation precautions are not needed. Pregnancy, however, should be ruled out before the scan is performed.

Normally the thyroid has an uptake of 5% to 35% of the given dose when measured at 24 hours. RAIU is increased in clients with hyperthyroidism.

Assess whether the client has undergone procedures or has taken drugs that might affect the results of the scan. Procedures that use iodine-containing dye (e.g., renography) should not be performed for at least 4 weeks before a thyroid scan is done. Any drug that contains iodine should be discontinued for 1 week before the scan.

ULTRASONOGRAPHY. Ultrasonography of the thyroid gland can determine its size and the composition of any masses or nodules. This procedure takes about 30 minutes to perform. Reassure the client that it is painless.

ELECTROCARDIOGRAPHY. An electrocardiogram (ECG) usually shows tachycardia. Other ECG changes with hyperthyroidism include atrial fibrillation and changes in P and T waveforms.

Common Nursing Diagnoses and Collaborative Problems

Nursing diagnoses and collaborative problems that may apply to the client with hyperthyroidism include the following:

- Imbalanced Nutrition: Less Than Body Requirements related to inadequate intake in relation to metabolic needs
- Hyperthermia related to increased metabolic rate
- Fatigue related to sleep deprivation
- Potential for Hypertension and Cardiac Failure

Critical Thinking Challenge

One of the nurses on your med-surg unit is having a difficult time getting along with her co-workers. She has become very critical of others and very defensive when anyone suggests that her performance is less than perfect. Recently she was passed over for the assistant director position. You have noticed that she

CHART 67-2

LABORATORY PROFILE
Thyroid Function

Test	Normal Range for Adults	Significance of Abnormal Findings	
		Hyperthyroidism	Hypothyroidism
Serum T_3	70-205 ng/dL, or 1.2-3.4 SI units	Increased	Decreased
Serum T_4	4-12 mcg/dL, or 51-154 SI units	Increased	Decreased
Free T_4 index	0.8-2.4 ng/dL, or 10-31 SI units	Increased	Decreased
T_3 resin uptake	24%-34% (varies with different laboratories)	Increased	Decreased
TRH stimulation test	Doubling of baseline TSH 30 min after IV injection of 500 mcg TRH (women have greater response)	Little or no TSH response	Delayed or poor TSH response in secondary hypothyroidism (pituitary failure) Elevated two or more times the normal in primary hypothyroidism (thyroid gland failure)
Thyroid suppression test	N/A	Fails to suppress RAIU or T_4 levels	No change in RAIU or T_4 levels
TSH stimulation test (thyroid stimulation test)	>10% in RAIU or >1.5 mcg/dL	N/A (test differentiates primary from secondary hypothyroidism)	No response in primary hypothyroidism Normal response in secondary hypothyroidism
Thyroid antibodies (antithyroglobulan antibody)	Titer <1:100	High titer of antithyroglobulin antibodies	Increased titers
Thyrotropin receptor antibodies (TSH-RAb)	Titer <130% of basal activity	High titers indicate Graves' disease	No response
TSH	2-10 μU/mL or 2-10 SI units	Low in Graves' disease High in secondary or tertiary hyperthyroidism	High in primary disease Low in secondary or tertiary disease

N/A, Not applicable; *RAIU*, radioactive iodine uptake; *SI*, Système Internationale; T_3, triiodothyronine; T_4, thyroxine; *TRH*, thyrotropin-releasing hormone; *TSH*, thyroid-stimulating hormone.

has lost weight and is about 10 lbs underweight for her height. Her eyes seem to bulge a little. When you ask her if she is feeling okay, she tells you that she thinks she is losing her mind, that she is having a hard time getting to sleep at night, and that she seems to overreact to everything. She bursts into tears and says, "Nobody likes me. I don't even like myself anymore." You escort her down to employee health. Her vital signs there are as follows: T 99.4; P 102, slightly irregular; R 32; BP 130/68.

1. What questions about her health should you ask?
2. What additional questions should you ask related to her weight?
3. What diagnostic tests do you anticipate will be requested?
4. Is drug abuse a possible cause of her manifestations of hyperthyroidism?

evolve For suggested answer guidelines, go to http://evolve.elsevier.com/Iggy/.

Interventions

Because Graves' disease is the most common form of hyperthyroidism, the interventions discussed in the following sections include those specific for the problems that occur with Graves' disease. The goals of management are to decrease the effect of thyroid hormone on cardiac function and to reduce thyroid hormone secretion.

NONSURGICAL MANAGEMENT. Monitor the client's apical pulse, BP, and temperature at least every 4 hours. Instruct the client to report immediately any palpitations, dyspnea, vertigo, or chest pain.

Encourage the client to rest. Keep the environment as quiet as possible. Use frequent bed linen changes, sponge baths, and a cool environment to decrease discomfort caused by diaphoresis and heat intolerance.

Drug Therapy. The most commonly used antithyroid drugs are the thioamides, including propylthiouracil (PTU), methimazole (Tapazole), and carbimazole (Neo-Mercazole✱), which block thyroid hormone production (Chart 67-3). The response to these drugs is delayed because the client may have large amounts of stored thyroid hormones that continue to be released. Other drugs are needed to control the cardiac manifestations until hormone production and release are reduced.

Iodine preparations decrease blood flow through the thyroid gland. This action reduces the production and release of thyroid hormone. Improvement usually occurs within 2 weeks, but weeks may be needed before metabolism returns to normal. This treatment can result in hypothyroidism, and the client must be closely monitored for the need for drug regimen changes.

Lithium carbonate also inhibits thyroid hormone release. However, its use is limited because of side effects such as depression, diabetes insipidus, tremors, nausea, and vomiting. Lithium may be used for a client who cannot tolerate other antithyroid drugs.

Beta-adrenergic blocking drugs, such as propranolol (Inderal, Detensol✱), relieve diaphoresis, anxiety, tachycardia, and palpitations.

CHART 67-3

DRUG THERAPY for Hyperthyroidism

Drug	Usual Dosage	Nursing Interventions	Rationales
Propylthiouracil (PTU, Propyl-Thyracil*)	100-150 mg PO three times daily	Give at 8-hr intervals around the clock.	Spreading out dosage helps maintain suppression of hormone.
Methimazole (Tapazole)	5-15 mg PO three times daily	Monitor vital signs. Weigh the client weekly. Observe for sore throat, fever, headache, and skin eruptions.	Changes in vital signs or weight and appearance or other signs and symptoms may indicate adverse reactions, which may necessitate discontinuation of drug use.
Carbimazole (Neo-Mercazole*)	10-15 mg twice daily	Instruct the client to avoid crowds and sick people.	Drug reduces immune and inflammatory responses.
Iodine products Strong iodine (Lugol's) solution Saturated solution of potassium iodide (SSKI) Potassium iodide tablets, solution, and syrup	Dosage varies, depending on the type of iodine prescribed, the manufacturer, and the form supplied (tablet, solution, or syrup)	Give in fruit juice or water. Observe for fever, rash, metallic taste, sore mouth, severe GI distress, and burning mouth and throat. Instruct the client to take tablets after meals.	Giving in fruit juice or water improves taste. Signs of iodism may necessitate discontinuation drug use. Taking after meals enhances absorption.
Lithium carbonate (Lithobid, Carbolith* Lithizine*)	Individualized 900-1200 mg PO daily in divided doses	Observe for signs of hypothyroidism. Instruct the client to drink 10-12 glassfuls of fluid per day. Instruct the client to maintain normal sodium intake.	Signs of hypothyroidism may indicate drug-induced thyroid enlargement. Extra fluid intake helps to prevent dehydration. Reduced sodium intake can cause retention of the drug.
Dexamethasone (Decadron)	2 mg q6h	Instruct client to avoid crowds and sick people.	Drug reduces immune and inflammatory responses.
Propranolol (Inderal, Detensol*) ***Med Error Alert!** Do not confuse Inderal with Toradol, an anti-inflammatory agent.*	20-80 mg four times daily in divided doses	Weigh the client daily. Measure intake and output. Instruct the client to take the drug with food. Instruct the client to avoid smoking. Monitor the client's pulse.	Increased weight and decreased output may indicate congestive heart failure. Taking the drug with food enhances absorption. The drug's effect is reduced by smoking. Tachycardia is a sign of hyperthyroidism.

GI, Gastrointestinal.

Radioactive Iodine Therapy. *Radioactive iodine (RAI) therapy is not used in pregnant women because ^{131}I crosses the placenta and can damage the fetal thyroid gland.* The client with hyperthyroidism may receive RAI in the form of oral ^{131}I. The dosage depends on the thyroid gland's size and sensitivity to radiation. The thyroid gland picks up the RAI, and some of the cells that produce thyroid hormone are destroyed by the local radiation. Because the thyroid gland stores thyroid hormones to some degree, the client may not have complete symptom relief until 6 to 8 weeks after RAI therapy. Additional drug therapy for hyperthyroidism is still needed during the first few weeks after RAI treatment.

RAI therapy is performed on an outpatient basis. One dose may be sufficient, although some clients need a second or third dose. The radiation dose is low enough that radiation precautions are not needed. Reassure the client that the radioactivity is quickly eliminated. The degree of thyroid destruction is variable. Some clients become hypothyroid as a result of treatment. This problem may occur within a few weeks, or it may take several years to develop. The client then needs lifelong thyroid hormone replacement. All clients who have undergone RAI therapy should be monitored regularly for changes in thyroid function.

SURGICAL MANAGEMENT. Antithyroid drugs and RAI therapy are now the most common treatments for clients with hyperthyroidism. Surgery to remove all or part of the thyroid gland may be needed for clients who have a large goiter causing tracheal or esophageal compression or who do not have a good response to antithyroid drugs. Removal of all **(total thyroidectomy)** or part **(subtotal thyroidectomy)** of the thyroid tissue decreases the production of thyroid hormones. After a total thyroidectomy, clients must take lifelong thyroid hormone replacement.

Preoperative Care. If possible the client is treated with drug therapy first and returns to near-normal thyroid function **(euthyroid)** before thyroid surgery. The euthyroid state is achieved with antithyroid drugs that decrease the secretion of thyroid hormones. Iodine preparations are used to decrease thyroid size and vascularity, thereby reducing the risk for hemorrhage and the potential for thyroid storm during surgery.

Hypertension, dysrhythmias, and tachycardia must be controlled before surgery. The client with hyperthyroidism is often not at an optimal weight and may need to follow a high-protein, high-carbohydrate diet for days or weeks before surgery.

Instruct the client to perform coughing and deep-breathing exercises. Teach the client how to support the neck when coughing or moving. Placing both hands behind the neck when moving reduces the strain on the suture line. Explain that hoarseness may be present for a few days as a result of endotracheal tube placement during surgery.

Clients often fear thyroid surgery, perhaps because the incision is on the neck. Reassure the client by calmly explaining the surgery and the care after surgery. Answer any questions the client and family have.

Operative Procedures. A thyroidectomy is performed with the client under general anesthesia. The client's neck is extended, and the surgeon makes a "collar" incision just above the clavicle. The parathyroid glands and recurrent laryngeal nerves are avoided to reduce the risk for complications and injury.

With a subtotal thyroidectomy, the remaining thyroid tissues are sutured to the trachea. With a total thyroidectomy, the parathyroid glands are left with an intact blood supply, but the entire thyroid gland is removed.

Postoperative Care. Monitor vital signs every 15 minutes until the client is stable and then every 30 minutes. Increase or decrease the monitoring of vital signs based on changes in the client's condition.

Assess the client's level of discomfort. Use sandbags or pillows to support the head and neck. Place the client, while he or she is awake, in a semi-Fowler's position. When positioning the client, decrease tension on the suture line by avoiding neck extension. Give prescribed pain medications as needed.

Humidifying the air promotes easier respiration and thins respiratory secretions. Assist the client to cough and deep-breathe every 30 minutes to 1 hour. Suction oral and tracheal secretions when necessary.

Thyroid surgery can cause hemorrhage, respiratory distress, parathyroid gland injury (resulting in **hypocalcemia** [low serum calcium levels] and **tetany** [hyperexcitability of nerves and muscles]), damage to the laryngeal nerves, and thyroid storm. Remain alert to the potential for complications and identify manifestations early.

Hemorrhage. Hemorrhage is most likely to occur during the first 24 hours after surgery. Inspect the neck dressing and behind the client's neck for blood. A drain may be present and have a moderate amount of serosanguineous drainage. Hemorrhage may also be seen as bleeding at the incision site or as respiratory distress caused by tracheal compression.

Respiratory Distress. Respiratory distress can result from swelling or tetany. Laryngeal **stridor** (harsh, high-pitched respiratory sounds) is heard in acute respiratory obstruction. Keep emergency tracheostomy equipment in the client's room. Check that oxygen and suctioning equipment are nearby and in working order. In some instances, nurses are instructed to remove clips or sutures when medical assistance is not immediately available and swelling at the surgical site is obstructing the airway.

Hypocalcemia and Tetany. The parathyroid glands can be damaged or their blood supply impaired during thyroid surgery. Hypocalcemia and tetany result when parathyroid hormone (PTH) levels decrease. Ask the client about any tingling around the mouth or of the toes and fingers. Assess for muscle twitching as signs of calcium deficiency. Calcium gluconate or calcium chloride for intravenous (IV) use must be available in an emergency situation. (For information on the later signs of hypocalcemia, see Postoperative Care [Hyperparathyroidism], p. 1495, and Assessment [Hypoparathyroidism], p. 1495. The care of clients with hypocalcemia is discussed in Chapter 16.)

CHART 67-4

BEST PRACTICE for
Emergency Care of the Client During Thyroid Storm

EMERGENCY CARE

- Maintain a patent airway and adequate ventilation.
- Give antithyroid drugs as prescribed: propylthiouracil (PTU, Propyl-Thyracil*), 300 to 900 mg daily; methimazole (Tapazole), up to 60 mg daily.
- Administer sodium iodide solution, 2 g IV daily as prescribed.
- Give propranolol (Inderal, Detensol*), 1 to 3 mg IV as prescribed. Give slowly over 3 minutes; the client should be connected to a cardiac monitor, and a central venous pressure catheter should be in place.
- Give glucocorticoids as prescribed: hydrocortisone, 100 to 500 mg IV daily; prednisone, 4 to 60 mg IV daily; or IM dexamethasone 2 mg every 6 hours.
- Monitor continually for cardiac dysrhythmias.
- Monitor vital signs every 30 minutes.
- Provide comfort measures, including a cooling blanket.
- Give nonsalicylate antipyretics as prescribed.
- Correct dehydration with normal saline infusions.
- Give aspirin or other antipyretic.
- Apply cooling blanket or ice packs to reduce fever.

Laryngeal Nerve Damage. Hoarseness and a weak voice may occur if the laryngeal nerve is injured during surgery. Assess the client's voice at 2-hour intervals, and document any changes. Reassure the client that hoarseness is usually temporary.

Thyroid Storm. **Thyroid storm** or **thyroid crisis** is a life-threatening event that occurs in clients with uncontrolled hyperthyroidism and is usually caused by Graves' disease. Manifestations of crisis develop quickly. Thyroid storm is often triggered by stressors such as trauma, infection, diabetic ketoacidosis, and pregnancy. Other conditions that can lead to thyroid storm include vigorous palpation of the goiter, exposure to iodine, and radioactive iodine (RAI) therapy. Although thyroid storm after surgery is rare because clients receive antithyroid drugs, beta blockers, and iodides before thyroid surgery, it can still occur.

The manifestations of thyroid storm are caused by excessive thyroid hormone release, which dramatically increases metabolic rate. *Key manifestations include fever, tachycardia, and systolic hypertension.* The client may have gastrointestinal problems such as abdominal pain, nausea, vomiting, and diarrhea. Often the client with thyroid storm is very anxious and has tremors. As the crisis progresses, he or she may become restless, confused, psychotic, and may have seizures, leading to coma. *Even with treatment, thyroid storm has a mortality rate of 25%.*

Emergency measures to prevent death vary with the intensity and type of specific symptoms. After the cause has been identified, interventions focus on maintaining airway patency, providing adequate ventilation, reducing fever, and stabilizing the hemodynamic status. Chart 67-4 outlines the best practices for emergency management of thyroid storm.

INFILTRATIVE OPHTHALMOPATHY. Treatment for hyperthyroidism does not correct the eye and vision problems of Graves' disease. Treatment of infiltrative ophthalmopathy is symptomatic. Instruct the client with mild symptoms to elevate the head of the bed at night and to use artificial tears. If **photophobia** (sensitivity to light) is present, dark glasses or eye patches are often helpful. For the client who cannot close the eyelids completely, recommend gently taping the lids closed with nonallergenic tape. These actions prevent irritation and injury. If pressure behind the eye continues and forces the eye forward, blood supply to the eye can be compromised, leading to ischemia and blindness.

In severe cases short-term steroid therapy is prescribed to reduce swelling and halt the infiltrative process. Prednisone (Deltasone, Winpred✱) is given in high doses (often 120 mg daily) at first and then is tapered down according to the client's response. Explain the need to reduce the prednisone gradually, and review its side effects with the client.

Diuretics may be prescribed to decrease edema around the eye. Surgical intervention (orbital decompression) may be needed if loss of sight or damage to the eyeball is possible.

HEALTH TEACHING. Review with the client the manifestations of hyperthyroidism and instruct him or her to report an increase or recurrence of symptoms. Teach the client about the manifestations of hypothyroidism (discussed in the next section) and the need for thyroid hormone replacement. Reinforce the need for regular follow-up because hypothyroidism can occur several years after radioactive iodine therapy.

If the client has had surgery, the surgeon usually removes the sutures on the third or fourth postoperative day. Instruct the client to inspect the incision area and to report redness, tenderness, drainage, or swelling the health care provider.

The discharged client may continue to have mood changes as a result of hyperthyroidism. Explain the reason for mood swings to the client and family and reassure them that it will decrease with continued treatment.

Critical Thinking Challenge

The nurse with manifestations of hyperthyroidism is diagnosed as having Graves' disease. She has an iodine allergy and undergoes a partial thyroidectomy. You are caring for her about 12 hours after surgery. She puts on her call light, and when you come into the room she is sweating and anxious. She tells you that she feels "jittery" and that her heart is racing. She also tells you that she feels like she has a lump in her throat.

1. What should you do first?
2. What is the most likely cause of her current manifestations?

evolve For suggested answer guidelines, go to http://evolve.elsevier.com/Iggy/.

Hypothyroidism

PATHOPHYSIOLOGY

The manifestations of hypothyroidism (Chart 67-5) are the result of decreased metabolism from low levels of thyroid hormones. Hypothyroidism can occur anytime throughout the life span.

Thyroid cells may fail to produce sufficient levels of thyroid hormones (THs) for several reasons. Sometimes the cells themselves are damaged and no longer function normally. Other times the thyroid cells are functional, but the person does not ingest enough of the substances needed to make

CHART 67-5

KEY FEATURES of Hypothyroidism

Skin Manifestations
- Cool, pale or yellowish, dry, coarse, scaly skin
- Thick, brittle nails
- Dry, coarse, brittle hair
- Decreased hair growth, with loss of eyebrow hair
- Poor wound healing

Pulmonary Manifestations
- Hypoventilation
- Pleural effusion
- Dyspnea

Cardiovascular Manifestations
- Bradycardia
- Dysrhythmias
- Enlarged heart
- Decreased activity tolerance
- Hypotension

Metabolic Manifestations
- Decreased basal metabolic rate
- Decreased body temperature
- Cold intolerance

Musculoskeletal Manifestations
- Muscle aches and pains
- Delayed contraction and relaxation of muscles

Neurologic Manifestations
- Slowing of intellectual functions
  - Slowness or slurring of speech
  - Impaired memory
  - Inattentiveness
- Lethargy or somnolence
- Confusion
- Hearing loss
- Paresthesia (numbness and tingling) of the extremities
- Decreased tendon reflexes

Psychological/Emotional Manifestations
- Apathy
- Depression
- Paranoia
- Withdrawal

Gastrointestinal Manifestations
- Anorexia
- Weight gain
- Constipation
- Abdominal distention

Reproductive Manifestations

Women
- Changes in menses (amenorrhea or prolonged menstrual periods)
- Anovulation
- Decreased libido

Men
- Decreased libido
- Impotence

Other Manifestations
- Periorbital edema
- Facial puffiness
- Nonpitting edema of the hands and feet
- Hoarseness
- Goiter (enlarged thyroid gland)
- Thick tongue
- Increased sensitivity to opioids and tranquilizers
- Weakness, fatigue
- Decreased urine output
- Anemia
- Easy bruising
- Iron deficiency
- Folate deficiency
- Vitamin B_{12} deficiency

thyroid hormones, especially iodide and tyrosine. When the production of thyroid hormones is too low or absent, the blood levels of TH are very low and the client has a decreased metabolic rate. This lowered metabolism causes the hypothalamus and anterior pituitary gland to make stimulatory hormones, especially thyroid-stimulating hormone (TSH), as compensation. The TSH binds to thyroid cells and causes the thyroid gland to enlarge, forming a goiter.

Most tissues and organs are affected by the low metabolic rate caused by hypothyroidism. Cellular energy is decreased, and metabolites build up. The metabolites are compounds of proteins and sugars called glycosaminoglycans. These compounds build up inside cells, which increases the mucous and water, forms cellular edema, and changes organ texture. The edema is mucinous (called **myxedema**) rather than edema caused by water alone (Figure 67-4). This edema changes the client's appearance. Nonpitting edema forms everywhere, especially around the eyes, in the hands and feet, and between the shoulder blades. The tongue thickens and edema forms in the larynx, making the voice husky. General physiologic function is decreased.

Myxedema coma is a rare, serious complication of untreated or poorly treated hypothyroidism. The decreased metabolism causes the heart muscle to become flabby and the chamber size to increase. The result is decreased cardiac output and decreased perfusion to the brain and other vital organs. The decreased perfusion makes the already slowed cellular metabolism worse, resulting in tissue and organ failure. *The mortality rate for myxedema coma is extremely high, and this condition is considered a life-threatening emergency.* Myxedema coma can be caused by a variety of events or conditions (Table 67-3).

Etiology

Most cases of hypothyroidism in the United States occur as a result of thyroid surgery and radioactive iodine (RAI) treatment of hyperthyroidism. Worldwide, hypothyroidism is common in areas where the soil and water have little natural iodide, causing endemic goiter. (This problem was common in the Midwest region of the United States before iodide was added to table salt and before saltwater fish was widely available.) Hypothyroidism is also caused by a variety of other conditions (Table 67-4).

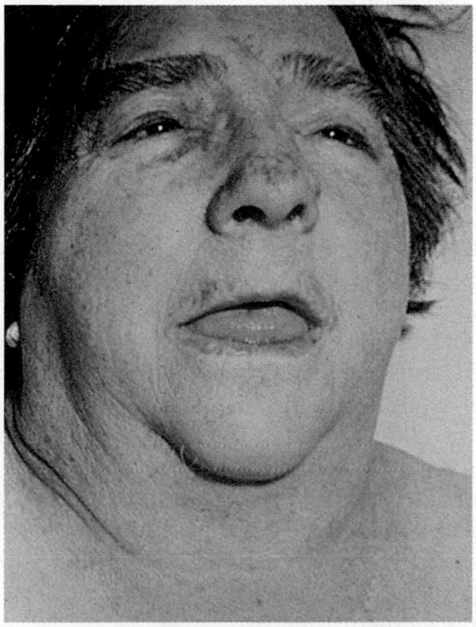

Figure 67-4 ■ Myxedema.

Incidence/Prevalence

Hypothyroidism occurs most often in women between 30 and 60 years of age. Women are affected 7 to 10 times more often than men (McCance & Huether, 2002). An association exists between the development of hypothyroidism and diabetes mellitus.

◆COLLABORATIVE MANAGEMENT

PHARM REVIEW

◆Assessment

HISTORY

A decrease in thyroid hormones produces many manifestations related to decreased metabolism. The client often reports an increase in time spent sleeping, sometimes up to 14 to 16 hours daily. Generalized weakness, anorexia, muscle aches, and paresthesias may also be present. Constipation is common. The client often has cold intolerance. Ask whether more blankets at night or sweaters and extra clothing in warm weather have been needed.

Both men and women with hypothyroidism may report a decrease in libido. Women may have had difficulty becoming pregnant or have changes in menses (heavy, prolonged bleeding or amenorrhea). Men can have problems with impotence and infertility.

TABLE 67-3 Conditions or Events Precipitating Myxedema Coma

■ Acute illness	■ Rapid withdrawal of thyroid medications
■ Anesthesia	■ Untreated hypothyroidism
■ Surgery	■ Inadequately treated hypothyroidism
■ Hypothermia	
■ Chemotherapy	
■ Sedatives/opioids	

TABLE 67-4 Causes of Hypothyroidism

Primary Causes

Decreased Thyroid Tissue
- Surgical removal of the thyroid
- Radiation-induced thyroid destruction
- Autoimmune thyroid destruction
- Congenital thyroid agenesis
- Congenital thyroid hypoplasia
- Congenital thyroid dysgenesis
- Cancer (thyroidal or metastatic)

Decreased Synthesis of Thyroid Hormone
- Endemic iodine deficiency
- Excessive exposure to iodine
- Medications
  - Lithium
  - Phenylbutazone
  - Propylthiouracil
  - Sodium or potassium perchlorate
  - Aminoglutethimide

Secondary Causes

Inadequate Production of Thyroid-Stimulating Hormone
- Pituitary tumors, trauma, infections, or infarcts
- Congenital pituitary defects
- Hypothalamic tumors, trauma, infections, or infarcts

Ask the client about current or previous use of drugs, such as lithium, aminoglutethimide, sodium or potassium perchlorate, thiocyanates, or cobalt. All these drugs can impair thyroid hormone production.

PHYSICAL ASSESSMENT/CLINICAL MANIFESTATIONS

Observe the client's overall appearance. Figure 67-4 shows the typical appearance of an adult with hypothyroidism. Common changes include coarse features, edema around the eyes and face, a blank expression, and a thick tongue. The client's overall muscle movement is slow.

PSYCHOSOCIAL ASSESSMENT

Hypothyroidism causes many problems in psychosocial functioning. Depression is the most common reason for seeking medical attention. Family members often bring the client for the initial evaluation. The client may be too lethargic, apathetic, or drowsy to recognize changes in his or her condition. Families may report that the client is withdrawn. Assess the client's attention span and memory, both of which can be impaired by hypothyroidism.

LABORATORY ASSESSMENT

Laboratory findings for hypothyroidism are the opposite of those for hyperthyroidism. Triiodothyronine (T_3) and thyroxine (T_4) serum levels are decreased. TSH levels are high in primary hypothyroidism but can be decreased or near-normal in clients with secondary hypothyroidism (see Chart 67-2).

> **Critical Thinking Challenge**
>
> The client is a 78-year-old woman. She has resided in a nursing home for the past 3 years because a stroke paralyzed her left side and she is unable to care for herself. She does talk, although her speech is slow and sometimes she uses the wrong word to describe something. For several weeks you have noted that her speech is becoming less understandable and that she is sleeping more. Today the nursing assistant tells you that the client's heart rate is 34 beats/min and her temperature is 96.2°F. She also tells you that the client had trouble opening her eyes and swallowing.
>
> 1. What should you do first?
> 2. Should oxygen be applied? Why or why not?
> 3. What indications do you have that the changes in her health status are not related to her stroke?

evolve For suggested answer guidelines, go to http://evolve.elsevier.com/Iggy/.

Analysis

COMMON NURSING DIAGNOSES AND COLLABORATIVE PROBLEMS

The following are priority nursing diagnoses for clients with hypothyroidism:

1. Decreased Cardiac Output related to altered heart rate and rhythm as a result of decreased myocardial metabolism
2. Ineffective Breathing Pattern related to decreased energy, obesity, and fatigue
3. Disturbed Thought Processes related to impaired brain metabolism and edema

The major collaborative problem is the Potential for Myxedema Coma.

ADDITIONAL NURSING DIAGNOSES AND COLLABORATIVE PROBLEMS

In addition to the common nursing diagnoses and collaborative problems, clients with hypothyroidism may have one or more of the following:

- Imbalanced Nutrition: More Than Body Requirements related to excessive intake in relation to metabolic need
- Hypothermia related to decreased metabolic rate
- Constipation related to decreased motility of the gastrointestinal tract
- Disturbed Body Image related to illness
- Deficient Knowledge of condition, diagnosis, and treatment related to cognitive limitation

Additional collaborative problems for clients with hypothyroidism are Potential for Paralytic Ileus and Potential for Cardiomyopathy.

Planning and Implementation

DECREASED CARDIAC OUTPUT

NOC **PLANNING: EXPECTED OUTCOMES.** The client with hypothyroidism is expected to have cardiovascular function that is either not compromised or mildly compromised. Indicators include that the client:

- Maintains heart rate above 60 beats/min
- Maintains blood pressure within normal limits for his or her age and general health
- Has no dysrhythmias, peripheral edema, or neck vein distension

INTERVENTIONS. NIC interventions for the client with hypothyroidism are listed in Chart 67-6. The client with hypothyroidism can have decreased blood pressure, bradycardia, and dysrhythmias. Monitor blood pressure, heart rate, and rhythm, and observe closely for signs of shock, such as hypotension, decreasing urine output, and changes in mental status.

If hypothyroidism has been chronic, the client may have cardiovascular disease. *Instruct the client to report episodes of chest pain or discomfort immediately.*

The client with hypothyroidism requires lifelong thyroid hormone replacement. Synthetic hormone preparations are usually prescribed; the most common is levothyroxine sodium (Synthroid, T_4, Eltroxin✱). Therapy is started with low doses and gradually increased over a period of weeks. *The client with more severe symptoms of hypothyroidism is started on the lowest dose of thyroid hormone replacement.* This caution is especially important when the client has known cardiac problems. Starting at too high a dose or increasing the dose too rapidly can cause severe hypertension, heart failure, and myocardial infarction.

Assess the client for chest pain and dyspnea during initiation of therapy. The final dosage is determined by blood levels of TSH and the client's physical responses. The dosage and time required for symptom relief vary with each client. Monitor for and teach the client about the manifestations of hyperthyroidism (see Chart 67-1), which can occur with replacement therapy.

CHART 67-6

NIC **INTERVENTION ACTIVITIES for**
The Client with Hypothyroidism

Respiratory Monitoring: *Collection and analysis of client data to ensure airway patency and adequate gas exchange*
- Monitor rate, rhythm, depth, and effort of respirations.
- Note chest movement, watching for symmetry, use of accessory muscles, and supraclavicular and intercostal muscle refractions.
- Monitor breathing patterns for bradypnea.
- Monitor for diaphragmatic muscle fatigue (paradoxical motion).
- Note changes in Sao_2 and Svo_2, end tidal CO_2 and ABG values, as appropriate.
- Monitor client's ability to cough effectively.
- Monitor for dyspnea and events that decrease and worsen it.

Shock Prevention: *Detecting and treating a client at risk for impending shock.*
- Monitor temperature and respiratory status.
- Monitor circulatory status: BP, skin color, skin temperature, heart sounds, heart rate and rhythm, presence and quality of peripheral pulses, and capillary refill.
- Monitor for signs of inadequate tissue oxygenation.
- Monitor for apprehension, increased anxiety, and changes in mental status.
- Monitor intake and output.
- Administer oxygen and/or mechanical ventilation, as appropriate.
- Administer antiarrhythmic agents, as appropriate.

Hypothermia Treatment: *Rewarming and surveillance of a client whose core body temperature is below 35° C.*
- Monitor client's temperature, using a low-recording thermometer if necessary.
- Place on a cardiac monitor, as appropriate.
- Cover with warmed blankets, as appropriate.
- Administer heated oxygen, as appropriate.
- Monitor vital signs, as appropriate.
- Monitor skin color and temperature.
- Monitor intake and output.
- Avoid giving IM or subcutaneous medications during the hypothermic state.
- Give client warm oral fluids, if alert and able to swallow.
- Teach client to consume a caloric intake sufficient to maintain a normal body temperature.
- Emphasize the importance of wearing warm, protective clothing when going into a cold environment.

Sao_2, Arterial oxygen saturation; Svo_2, venous oxygen saturation.

INEFFECTIVE BREATHING PATTERN

PLANNING: EXPECTED OUTCOMES. The client with hypothyroidism is expected to have respiratory function be not compromised or only mildly compromised. Indicators include the following:
- Maintenance of Spo_2 of at least 88%
- Absence of cyanosis
- Maintenance of cognitive orientation

INTERVENTIONS. Observe and record the rate and depth of respirations. Auscultate the lungs for any problems, such as a decrease in breath sounds. If hypothyroidism is severe, the client may have such severe respiratory distress that ventilatory support is required. Severe respiratory distress often occurs with myxedema coma.

Sedating a client with hypothyroidism can make respiratory difficulties worse and is avoided, if possible. When sedation is needed, the dosage is reduced because hypothyroidism increases sensitivity to these drugs. Assess the client receiving sedation for respiratory adequacy.

CHART 67-7

BEST PRACTICE for
Emergency Care of the Client During Myxedema Coma

EMERGENCY CARE
- Maintain a patent airway.
- Replace fluids with IV normal or hypertonic saline.
- Give levothyroxine sodium IV as prescribed.
- Give glucose IV as prescribed.
- Give corticosteroids as prescribed.
- Check the client's temperature hourly.
- Monitor blood pressure hourly.
- Cover the client with warm blankets.
- Monitor for changes in mental status.
- Turn every 2 hours.
- Institute aspiration precautions.

DISTURBED THOUGHT PROCESSES

PLANNING: EXPECTED OUTCOMES. The client with hypothyroidism is expected to have thought processes not compromised or only mildly compromised with correction of the hypothyroidism. Indicators include that the client:
- Demonstrates immediate memory
- Communicates clearly and appropriately for age and ability
- Is attentive during conversations

INTERVENTIONS. Observe for and record the presence and severity of lethargy, drowsiness, memory deficit, poor attention span, and difficulty communicating. These problems should decrease with thyroid hormone treatment, and mental awareness usually returns to normal levels within 2 weeks. Orient the client to person, place, and time, and explain all procedures slowly and carefully. Provide a safe environment.

Family members may have difficulty coping with the client's behavior. Encourage them to accept the mood changes and mental slowness as manifestations of the disease. Remind the family that these problems should improve with therapy.

MYXEDEMA COMA

Any client with hypothyroidism who has any other health problem or who is newly diagnosed is at risk for myxedema coma. Factors leading to myxedema coma are listed in Table 67-3. Problems that often occur with this condition include the following:
- Coma
- Respiratory failure
- Hypotension
- Hyponatremia
- Hypothermia
- Hypoglycemia

Untreated myxedema coma leads to shock, organ damage, and death. Assess the client with hypothyroidism every shift for changes that indicate increasing severity, especially changes in mental status.

Treatment is instituted quickly according to the client's manifestations and without waiting for laboratory confirmation. Best practices for emergency care of the client with myxedema coma are listed in Chart 67-7.

CHART 67-8

NURSING FOCUS on the OLDER ADULT
Thyroid Problems

Teach the client the following facts about changes in the thyroid gland related to aging:

- The thyroid gland decreases in size with increasing age.
- Thyroid hormone secretion decreases with age, but the hormone level remains stable because cellular clearance of the hormone also decreases with age.
- The basal metabolic rate decreases with age, usually as a result of decreased activity. This decrease changes the body composition from predominantly muscular to predominantly fatty.
- Older clients require lower doses of replacement thyroid hormone. Too large a dose may adversely affect the heart muscle.

CONSIDERATIONS FOR OLDER ADULTS

Metabolic rate and production of thyroid hormone both decrease with advancing age (Chart 67-8), particularly among people older than 80 years of age. Until recently, however, data regarding normal levels of T_3 and T_4 were established only for adults between the ages of 20 and 30 years. By such criteria, older people with T_3 and T_4 levels 15% to 20% below "normal levels" (established for a younger population) were considered to have hypothyroidism and therapy with thyroid hormone was initiated. In fact many of these clients were not truly hypothyroid, and therapy caused pseudohyperthyroidism, stressing many tissues and organs. Daily thyroid hormone therapy decreases the activity of the anterior pituitary gland and the thyroid gland, creating actual hypothyroidism. Health care providers need to assess more than just laboratory data to determine hypothyroidism in the older adult.

Community-Based Care

Hypothyroidism is usually a chronic condition. Clients with hypothyroidism are managed on an outpatient basis and may reside anywhere. Clients in acute care settings, subacute care settings, and rehabilitation centers may have long-standing hypothyroidism in addition to other acute or chronic health problems. Ensure that whoever is responsible for overseeing the client's daily care is aware of the condition and understands its treatment.

HOME CARE MANAGEMENT

The client with hypothyroidism does not usually require changes in the home unless cognition has decreased to the point that he or she poses a danger to himself or herself. Activity intolerance and fatigue may necessitate one-floor living for a short time. If manifestations have not improved before discharge, discuss the need for extra heat or clothing because of cold intolerance. The client who has a decreased attention span may need help with the drug regimen. Discuss this issue with the family and client, and develop a plan for drug therapy. One person should be clearly designated as responsible for drug preparation and delivery so that doses are neither missed nor duplicated.

HEALTH TEACHING

The most important educational need for the client with hypothyroidism is about hormone replacement therapy and its side effects. Emphasize the need for lifelong drugs, and review the manifestations of both hyperthyroidism and hypothyroidism. Instruct the client to wear a medical alert bracelet. Teach the client and family when to seek medical interventions for dosage adjustment. Instruct the client not to take any over-the-counter (OTC) drugs because thyroid hormone preparations interact with many other drugs. Older clients may need additional information about the effects of aging on the thyroid gland (see Chart 67-8).

Advise the client to eat a well-balanced diet with adequate fiber and fluid intake to prevent constipation. Caution clients that use of fiber supplements may interfere with the absorption of thyroid hormone. Remind the client about the importance of adequate rest. Encourage family members to voice their concerns to the health care provider.

Assist the family in understanding that the time required for resolution of hypothyroidism varies. During this time the client may continue to have mental dullness or slowness. Teach the family to orient the client often and to explain everything clearly and simply.

CHART 67-9

HOME CARE ASSESSMENT of
The Client with Thyroid Dysfunction

Assess cardiovascular status.
- Vital signs, including apical pulse, pulse pressure, presence or absence of orthostatic hypotension, and the quality and rhythm of peripheral pulses
- Presence or absence of peripheral edema
- Weight gain or loss

Assess cognition and mental status.
- Level of consciousness
- Orientation to time, place, and person
- Accurately reading a seven-word sentence containing no words greater than three syllables
- Can the client count backward from 100 by threes?

Assess condition of skin and mucous membranes.
- Moistness of skin, most reliable on chest and back
- Skin temperature and color

Assess neuromuscular status.
- Reactivity of patellar and biceps reflexes
- Oral temperature
- Handgrip strength
- Steadiness of gait
- Presence or absence of fine tremors in the hand

Ask about the following:
- Sleep in the past 24 hours
- Client warm enough or too warm indoors
- 24-hour diet recall
- 24-hour activity recall
- Over-the-counter and prescribed medications taken
- Last bowel movement

Assess client's understanding of illness and adherence with treatment.
- Manifestations to report to health care provider
- Medication plan (correct timing and dose)

HEALTH CARE RESOURCES

Immediately after returning home, the client may need a support person to stay and provide more attention than could be given by a visiting nurse or home care aide. Contact with the health care team is needed for follow-up and identification of potential problems. The client taking thyroid drugs may have manifestations of hypothyroidism if the dosage is inadequate or manifestations of hyperthyroidism if the dose is too high. Perform a focused assessment at every home visit to the client under treatment for thyroid dysfunction (Chart 67-9).

Evaluation: Outcomes

Evaluate the care of the client with hypothyroidism on the basis of the identified nursing diagnoses and collaborative problems. The expected outcome is that the client will:

- Maintain normal cardiovascular function
- Maintain adequate respiratory function
- Experience improvement in thought processes

Specific indicators for these outcomes are listed for each nursing diagnosis and collaborative problem under the Planning and Implementation section (see earlier).

Thyroiditis

PATHOPHYSIOLOGY

Thyroiditis is an inflammation of the thyroid gland. There are three types: acute, subacute, and chronic. Chronic thyroiditis (Hashimoto's disease) is the most common type.

Acute thyroiditis is caused by bacterial invasion of the thyroid gland. Manifestations include pain, neck tenderness, malaise, fever, and **dysphagia** (difficulty swallowing). It usually resolves with antibiotic therapy.

Subacute or granulomatous thyroiditis results from a viral infection of the thyroid gland after a cold or other upper respiratory infection. Manifestations include fever, chills, dysphagia, and muscle and joint pain. Pain can radiate to the ears and the jaw. The thyroid gland feels hard and enlarged on palpation. Thyroid function can remain normal, although hyperthyroidism or hypothyroidism may develop.

Chronic thyroiditis (Hashimoto's disease) is a type of hypothyroidism that affects women more often than men, most often clients in their 30s to 50s. Hashimoto's disease is an autoimmune disorder. The thyroid becomes invaded with antithyroid antibodies and lymphocytes, causing thyroid tissue destruction. When large amounts of the gland are destroyed, serum thyroid hormone levels are low and secretion of thyroid-stimulating hormone (TSH) is increased.

COLLABORATIVE MANAGEMENT

The manifestations of Hashimoto's disease are dysphagia and painless enlargement of the gland. Diagnosis is based on circulating antithyroid antibodies and needle biopsy of the thyroid gland. Serum thyroid hormone levels, TSH levels, and radioactive iodine uptake (RAIU) vary with disease stage.

The client is given thyroid hormone to prevent hypothyroidism and to suppress TSH secretion, which decreases the size of the thyroid gland. Surgery (subtotal thyroidectomy) is needed if the goiter does not respond to thyroid hormone, is disfiguring, or compresses other structures.

Nursing interventions focus on promoting comfort and teaching the client about hypothyroidism, drugs, and surgery (see Surgical Management [Hyperthyroidism], pp. 1486 to 1487.)

Thyroid Cancer

PATHOPHYSIOLOGY

The four distinct types of thyroid cancer are papillary, follicular, medullary, and anaplastic. The initial manifestation of thyroid cancer is a single, painless lump or nodule in the thyroid gland. Additional manifestations depend on the presence and location of **metastasis** (spread of cancer cells).

Papillary carcinoma, the most common type of thyroid cancer, occurs most often in younger women. It is a slow-growing tumor that can be present for years before spreading to nearby lymph nodes. When the tumor is confined to the thyroid gland, the chance for cure is good with a partial or total thyroidectomy.

Follicular carcinomas are about 25% of all thyroid cancers. They occur most often in older clients. The cancer invades blood vessels and spreads to bone and lung tissue. It can adhere to the trachea, neck muscles, great vessels, and skin, resulting in **dyspnea** (difficulty breathing) and **dysphagia** (difficulty swallowing). When the tumor involves the recurrent laryngeal nerves, the client may have a hoarse voice. The prognosis is fair when metastasis is minimal at diagnosis.

Medullary carcinoma accounts for 5% to 10% of all thyroid cancers and is most common in clients older than 50 years of age. This tumor often occurs as part of multiple endocrine neoplasia (MEN) type II, a familial endocrine disorder. The tumor usually secretes calcitonin, adrenocorticotropic hormone (ACTH), prostaglandins, and serotonin.

Anaplastic carcinoma is a rapid-growing, aggressive tumor that directly invades nearby structures. Manifestations include stridor (harsh, high-pitched respiratory sounds), hoarseness, and dysphagia. The prognosis is poor.

COLLABORATIVE MANAGEMENT

Surgery is the treatment of choice for papillary, follicular, and medullary carcinomas. A total thyroidectomy is usually performed with a nodal neck dissection if regional lymph nodes are involved. The physician prescribes suppressive doses of thyroid hormone for 3 months after surgery. A radioactive iodine uptake (RAIU) study is performed after drugs are withdrawn. If there is RAI uptake, the client is treated with **ablative** (enough to destroy the tissue) amounts of RAI. If thyroid cancer does not respond to RAI, a course of chemotherapy is initiated.

PARATHYROID DISORDERS

Hyperparathyroidism

PATHOPHYSIOLOGY

The parathyroid glands maintain calcium and phosphate balance (Figure 67-5). Serum calcium level is normally maintained within a narrow range; phosphate levels vary more widely. Increased levels of parathyroid hormone (PTH) act directly on the kidney, causing increased kidney reabsorption of calcium and increased phosphate excretion. These processes cause **hypercalcemia** (excessive calcium) and **hypophosphatemia** (inadequate phosphate) in the client with hyperparathyroidism.

In bone, excessive PTH levels increase bone resorption (bone loss of calcium) by decreasing **osteoblastic** (bone production) activity and increasing **osteoclastic** (bone destruction) activity. This process releases calcium and phosphate into the blood and reduces bone density. With chronic calcium excess, as in long-standing hypercalcemia, calcium is deposited in soft tissues.

Although the exact triggering mechanisms are unknown, primary hyperparathyroidism results when one or more parathyroid glands do not respond to the normal feedback of serum calcium. The most common cause is a

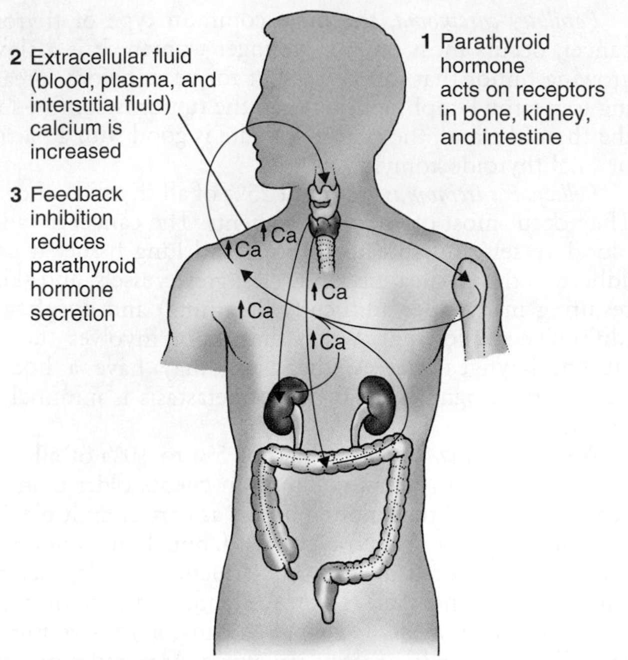

Figure 67-5 ■ The physiologic actions of parathyroid hormone.

TABLE 67-5 Causes of Parathyroid Dysfunction

Causes of Hyperparathyroidism
- Parathyroid adenoma
- Parathyroid carcinoma
- Congenital hyperplasia
- Neck trauma or radiation
- Vitamin D deficiency
- Chronic renal failure with hypocalcemia
- Parathyroid hormone-secreting carcinomas of the lung, kidney, or gastrointestinal tract

Causes of Hypoparathyroidism
- Surgical or radiation-induced thyroid ablation
- Parathyroidectomy
- Congenital dysgenesis
- Idiopathic (autoimmune) hypoparathyroidism
- Hypomagnesemia

benign tumor in one parathyroid gland. Table 67-5 lists other causes of hyperparathyroidism.

COLLABORATIVE MANAGEMENT

Assessment

Ask the client about any bone fractures, recent weight loss, arthritis, or psychological distress. Determine whether the client has received radiation treatment to the head or neck. The client with long-standing disease may have a waxy pallor of the skin and bone deformities in the extremities and back.

Manifestations of hyperparathyroidism may be related either to the effects of excessive PTH or to the effects of the accompanying hypercalcemia.

High levels of PTH cause **renal calculi** (kidney stones) and deposits of calcium in the soft tissue of the kidney. Bone lesions are due to an increased rate of bone destruction and may result in pathologic fractures, bone cysts, and osteoporosis.

Gastrointestinal manifestations (e.g., anorexia, nausea, vomiting, epigastric pain, constipation, weight loss) are common, particularly when serum calcium levels are high. Elevated serum gastrin levels are caused by hypercalcemia and lead to peptic ulcer disease. Fatigue and lethargy may be present and become more severe as the serum calcium levels increase. When serum calcium levels are greater than 12 mg/dL, the client may have psychosis with mental confusion, which leads to coma and death if left untreated. (See Chapter 16 for more information about hypercalcemia.)

Serum PTH, calcium, and phosphate levels and urine cyclic adenosine monophosphate (cAMP) are the most commonly used laboratory tests to detect hyperparathyroidism (Chart 67-10). X-rays may show kidney stones, calcium deposits, and bone lesions, such as cysts or fractures. Loss of bone density occurs in the client with chronic hyperparathyroidism. Other diagnostic tests include arteriography, computed tomography (CT), venous catheterization of the thyroid veins with sampling of the blood for PTH levels, and ultrasonography. Explain the procedures and care for the client undergoing diagnostic tests.

Interventions

NONSURGICAL MANAGEMENT

Diuretic and Fluid Therapy. The most common therapy for reducing serum calcium levels in clients who are not candidates for surgery is hydration and furosemide (Lasix, Uritol✱), a diuretic that increases kidney excretion of calcium. IV saline in large volumes also promotes renal calcium excretion.

Monitor cardiac function and intake and output every 2 to 4 hours during hydration therapy. Continuous cardiac monitoring may be needed. Closely monitor serum calcium levels, and immediately report any precipitous drop to the physician. Sudden drops in calcium levels may cause tingling and numbness in the muscles.

Drug Therapy. When hydration and furosemide cannot reduce hypercalcemia, or if it is necessary to discontinue IV fluids, other drugs can help to reduce the manifestations of hyperparathyroidism, especially those related to hypercalcemia.

Phosphates. Oral phosphates inhibit bone resorption and interfere with calcium absorption. IV phosphates are used only when serum calcium levels must be lowered rapidly.

Calcitonin. Calcitonin decreases the release of skeletal calcium and increases the kidney excretion of calcium. Calcitonin is not effective when used alone because of its short duration of action. Its therapeutic effects are greatly enhanced if given along with glucocorticoids.

Calcium Chelators. Some drugs lower calcium levels by binding (chelating) calcium, which reduces the levels of free calcium. Mithramycin, a cytotoxic agent, is the most effective and potent calcium chelator used to lower serum calcium levels. In most clients a single IV dose of 10 to 15 mg/kg of body weight by slow infusion can lower serum calcium levels within 48 hours. However, the toxic effects limit its use to two or three doses. Thrombocytopenia (decreased circulating platelets and an increased tendency to bleed) and kidney and liver toxicity can result after only one dose. Liver function studies, blood urea nitrogen and creatinine, complete blood count (CBC), and serum calcium levels are closely monitored

CHART 67-10

LABORATORY PROFILE
Parathyroid Function

Test	Normal Range for Adults	Significance of Abnormal Findings: Hyperthyroidism	Significance of Abnormal Findings: Hypothyroidism
Serum calcium	Total: 9.0-10.5 mg/dL or 2.25-2.75 SI units Ionized (active): 4.64-5.28 mg/dL or 1.16-1.32 SI units	Increased in primary hyperparathyroidism	Decreased
Serum phosphate	3.0-4.5 mg/dL or 0.97-1.45 SI units *Older adults:* May be slightly lower	Decreased	Increased
Serum parathyroid hormone	C-terminal 50-330 pg/mL	Increased	Decreased

SI, Système Internationale.

in the client receiving mithramycin. Another calcium chelator is penicillamine (Cuprimine, Pendramine).

SURGICAL MANAGEMENT. Surgical management of hyperparathyroidism involves a parathyroidectomy.

Preoperative Care. Before surgery the client is stabilized and calcium levels are decreased to near normal. If mithramycin has been used to lower serum calcium levels, studies to determine bleeding and clotting times are needed, as is a CBC to determine bone marrow function.

Advise the client that coughing and deep-breathing exercises should be performed after surgery and that talking may be painful for the first day or two. Teach about neck support by having the client place both hands behind the neck to assist in elevating the head.

Operative Procedures. Using general anesthesia and with the client's neck hyperextended, the surgeon makes a transverse incision in the lower neck. All four parathyroid glands are examined for enlargement. If only one gland on a side is enlarged, a frozen section is done on both glands. If a tumor is present on one side but the other side is normal, the surgeon removes the tumor and leaves the remaining gland intact.

Postoperative Care. Observe the client for respiratory distress, which may occur from compression of the trachea by hemorrhage or swelling of neck tissues. Ensure that emergency equipment, including suction, oxygen, and tracheostomy equipment, is at the bedside. If severe swelling occurs, the surgeon may need to remove clips from the incision to preserve the airway. Monitor vital signs, identify any change in status, and check the neck dressing for abnormal amounts of drainage or bleeding. A small amount (1 to 5 mL) of drainage is normal.

The remaining glands, which may have atrophied as a result of PTH overproduction, require several days to several weeks to return to normal function. A hypocalcemic crisis can occur during this critical period. Check serum calcium levels immediately after surgery and every 4 hours thereafter until calcium levels stabilize. Monitor for manifestations of hypocalcemia, such as tingling and twitching in the extremities and face. Check for Trousseau's and Chvostek's signs, either of which signal potential tetany (see Chapter 16).

Damage to the recurrent laryngeal nerve can occur. Assess the client for changes in voice patterns and hoarseness.

When hyperparathyroidism is due to **hyperplasia** (tissue overgrowth), three glands plus half of the fourth gland are usually removed. If all four glands are removed, a small portion of a gland may be implanted in the forearm, where it produces PTH and maintains calcium homeostasis. If all these maneuvers fail, the client will need lifelong treatment with calcium and vitamin D because the resulting hypoparathyroidism is permanent.

Hypoparathyroidism

PATHOPHYSIOLOGY

Hypoparathyroidism is a rare endocrine disorder in which parathyroid function is decreased. Problems are directly related to a lack of parathyroid hormone (PTH) secretion or to decreased effectiveness of PTH on target tissue. Whether the problem is a lack of PTH secretion or an ineffectiveness of PTH on tissues, the result is the same: hypocalcemia.

Iatrogenic hypoparathyroidism, the most common form, is caused by the removal of all parathyroid tissue during total thyroidectomy or by deliberate surgical removal of the parathyroid glands.

Idiopathic hypoparathyroidism can occur spontaneously. The exact cause is unknown, but an autoimmune basis is suspected in many clients. Hypoparathyroidism may occur with other autoimmune disorders such as adrenal insufficiency, hypothyroidism, diabetes mellitus, pernicious anemia, and vitiligo.

Hypomagnesemia (decreased serum magnesium levels) may also cause hypoparathyroidism. Hypomagnesemia is seen in alcoholics and in clients with malabsorption syndromes, chronic renal disease, and malnutrition. It causes impairment of PTH secretion and may interfere with the effects of PTH on the bones and kidneys.

◆COLLABORATIVE MANAGEMENT

◆Assessment

Ask about any head or neck surgery or radiation therapy because these treatments may cause hypoparathyroidism. Assess whether the client has any manifestations of hypoparathyroidism, which may range from mild tingling and numbness to tetany. Tingling and numbness around the mouth or in the hands and feet reflect mild to moderate hypocalcemia. Severe muscle cramps, carpopedal spasms, and seizures (with no loss of consciousness or incontinence) reflect a more severe hypocalcemia. The client or caregiver may notice mental changes ranging from irritability to psychosis.

The physical assessment may show excessive or inappropriate muscle contractions that cause finger, hand, and elbow flexion; this can signal an impending attack of tetany. Check for Chvostek's sign and Trousseau's sign; positive responses indicate potential tetany. Bands or pits may encircle the crowns of the teeth, which indicates a loss of calcium from the teeth and causes enamel loss.

Diagnostic tests for hypoparathyroidism include electroencephalography (EEG), blood tests, and computed tomography (CT). EEG changes revert to normal with correction of hypocalcemia. Serum calcium, phosphate, magnesium, vitamin D, and urine cyclic adenosine monophosphate (cAMP) levels may be used in the diagnostic workup for hypoparathyroidism (see Chart 67-10). The CT scan can show brain calcifications, which indicate chronic hypocalcemia.

◆Interventions

Management of hypoparathyroidism focuses on correcting hypocalcemia, vitamin D deficiency, and hypomagnesemia. For clients with acute and severe hypocalcemia, IV calcium is given as a 10% solution of calcium chloride or calcium gluconate over 10 to 15 minutes. Acute vitamin D deficiency is treated with calcitriol (Rocaltrol), 0.5 to 2 mg daily. Acute hypomagnesemia is corrected with 50% magnesium sulfate in 2-mL doses (up to 4 g daily) either intramuscularly or intravenously (IV). Long-term oral therapy for hypocalcemia involves the intake of calcium, 0.5 to 2 g daily, in divided doses.

Long-term therapy for vitamin D deficiency is 50,000 to 400,000 units of ergocalciferol daily. The dosage is adjusted to keep the client's calcium level in the low-normal range (slightly hypocalcemic), enough to prevent symptoms of hypocalcemia. It must also be low enough to prevent increased urine calcium levels, which can lead to stone formation.

Nursing management includes teaching about the drug regimen and interventions to reduce anxiety. Instruct the client to eat foods high in calcium but low in phosphorus. Milk, yogurt, and processed cheeses are avoided because of their high phosphorus content. *Stress that therapy for hypocalcemia is lifelong.* Advise the client to wear a medical alert bracelet. With adherence to the prescribed drug and diet regimen, the calcium level usually remains high enough to prevent a hypocalcemic crisis.

GET READY for the NCLEX Examination!

KEY POINTS

Safe Effective Care Environment

- Use a gait belt when assisting a client with muscle weakness to walk.
- Collaborate with the dietitian to teach clients about diets that are restricted in calcium or phosphate.
- Use a lift sheet to move or reposition a client with hypocalcemia.
- Keep the environment of a client at risk for thyroid storm cool, dark, and quiet.
- Keep emergency suctioning and tracheostomy equipment in the room of a client who has had thyroid or parathyroid surgery.

Health Promotion and Maintenance

- Teach all clients to take drugs as prescribed, especially diuretics, antihypertensives, and cardiac drugs.
- Include the person who prepares the client's meals when teaching about dietary electrolyte restrictions.

Psychosocial Integrity

- Be accepting of client behavior.
- Help clients and family members understand that changes in cognition and behavior are usually temporary.
- Allow the client who has a permanent change in appearance (such as exophthalmia) to mourn about the change.
- Assess clients who have a sudden change in cognition for electrolyte imbalances.
- Determine the client's food preferences and dislikes when planning an electrolyte-restricted diet.

Physiological Integrity

- Monitor the hydration status of clients who have hypercalcemia.
- Teach clients that hormone replacement therapy for hypothyroidism is lifelong.
- Teach clients to use clinical manifestations, such as the number of bowel movements per day and the ability to sleep, as indicators of therapy effectiveness and when the dose of thyroid hormone replacement may need to be adjusted.
- Assess the bowel sounds; deep tendon reflexes; heart rate, rhythm and quality; and hand grasps to evaluate the client's responses to therapy for an electrolyte imbalance.

ADDITIONAL STUDY RESOURCES

Go to your Student CD-ROM for Review Questions for the NCLEX Examination.

evolve Go to http://evolve.elsevier.com/Iggy/ for Integrated Management of Care Questions for the NCLEX Examination.

SELECTED BIBLIOGRAPHY

Abbas, A., & Lichtman, A. (2003). *Cellular and molecular immunology* (5th ed.). Philadelphia: W.B. Saunders.

Ackley, B., & Ladwig, G. (2002). *Nursing diagnosis handbook: A guide to planning care* (5th ed.). St. Louis: Mosby.

American Cancer Society. (2005). *Cancer facts and figures 2005.* Report No. 00-300M-No. 5008.05. Atlanta: Author.

Dahlen, R. (2002). Managing patients with acute thyrotoxicosis. *Critical Care Nurse, 22*(1), 62-69.

Davies, T., & Larsen, P.R. (2003). Thyrotoxicosis. In P.R. Larsen, et al. (Eds.). *Williams' textbook of endocrinology* (10th ed., pp. 374-422). Philadelphia: W.B. Saunders.

Dochterman, J., & Bulechek, G. (Eds.). (2004). *Nursing interventions classification (NIC)* (4th ed.). St. Louis: Mosby.

Ebersole, P., Hess, P., & Luggen, A. (2004). *Toward healthy aging: Human needs and nursing response* (6th ed.). St. Louis: Mosby.

Elliott, B. (2000). Diagnosing and treating hypothyroidism. *The Nurse Practitioner, 25*(3), 92-105.

Facts and Comparisons. (2004). *Drug facts and comparisons* (58th ed.). St. Louis: Author.
Germano, T. (2001). The parathyroid gland and calcium-related emergencies. *Topics in Emergency Medicine, 23*(4), 51-56.
Holcomb, S. (2003). Detecting thyroid disease, part 1. *Nursing 2003, 33*(8), 32cc1-32cc4.
Holcomb, S. (2003). Detecting thyroid disease, part 2. *Nursing 2003, 33*(9), 32cc1-32cc4.
Husein, M., et al. (2002). Predicting calcium status post thyroidectomy with early calcium levels. *Otolaryngology-Head and Neck Surgery, 127*(4), 289-293.
Klee, G. (2003). Laboratory techniques for recognition of endocrine disorders. In P.R. Larsen, et al. (Eds.). *Williams' textbook of endocrinology* (10th ed., pp. 65-79) Philadelphia: W.B. Saunders.
Klein, I., & Ojamaa, K. (2001). Thyroid hormone and the cardiovascular system. *New England Journal of Medicine, 344*(7), 501-509.
Kumrow, D., & Dahlen, R. (2002). Thyroidectomy: Understanding the potential for complications. *MEDSURG Nursing, 11*(5), 228-235.
Kuritzky, L. (2001). Hypothyroidism. *The American Journal for Nurse Practitioners, 5*(5), 26-39.
Larsen, P.R., & Davies, T. (2003). Hypothyroidism and thyroiditis. In P.R. Larsen, H.M., et al. (Eds.). *Williams' textbook of endocrinology* (10th ed., pp. 423-455). Philadelphia: W.B. Saunders.
Larsen, P.R., et al. (2003). Thyroid physiology and diagnostic evaluation of patients with thyroid disorders. In P.R. Larsen, et al. (Eds.). *Williams' textbook of endocrinology* (10th ed., pp. 331-373). Philadelphia: W.B. Saunders.
Larsen, P.R., et al. (Eds.). (2003). *Williams' textbook of endocrinology* (10th ed.). Philadelphia: W.B. Saunders.
Li, T-M. (2002). Hypothyroidism in elderly people. *Geriatric Nursing, 23*(2), 88-93.
Malchiodi, L. (2002). Emergency: Thyroid storm. *American Journal of Nursing, 102*(5), 33-35.
McCance, K., & Huether, S. (2002). *Pathophysiology: The biologic basis for disease in adults and children* (4th ed.). St. Louis: Mosby.
Mead, M. (2000). Thyroid function tests. *Practice Nurse, 19*(6), 283.
Michalek, A., Mahoney, M., & Calebaugh, D. (2000). Hypothyroidism and diabetes mellitus in an American Indian population. *Journal of Family Practice, 49*(7), 638-640.
Moorhead, S., Johnson, M., & Maas, M. (Eds.). (2004). *Nursing outcomes classification (NOC)* (3rd ed.). St. Louis: Mosby.
Nussbaum, R., McInnes, R., & Willard, H. (2001). *Thompson & Thompson: Genetics in medicine* (6th ed.). Philadelphia: W.B. Saunders.
Pagana, K., & Pagana, T. (2002). *Mosby's manual of diagnostic and laboratory tests* (2nd ed.). St. Louis: Mosby.
Schlumberger, M.-J., Filetti, S., & Hay, I. (2003). Nontoxic goiter and thyroid neoplasia, In P.R. Larsen, et al. (Eds.). *Williams' textbook of endocrinology* (10th ed., pp. 457-490). Philadelphia: W.B. Saunders.
Schori-Ahmed, D. (2003). Thyroid disease: Defenses gone awry. *RN, 66*(6), 38-43.
Waltman, P., Brewer, J., & Lobert, S. (2004). Thyroid storm during pregnancy: A medical emergency. *Critical Care Nurse, 24*(2), 74-79.

CHAPTER

68 Interventions for Clients with Diabetes Mellitus

M. ELAINE MCLEOD

LEARNING OUTCOMES

After studying this chapter, you should be able to:

1. Compare the age of onset, clinical manifestations, and pathologic mechanisms of type 1 and type 2 diabetes mellitus.
2. Identify clients at risk for type 2 diabetes mellitus.
3. Explain the effects of insulin on carbohydrate, protein, and fat metabolism.
4. Evaluate laboratory data to determine whether the client is using the prescribed dietary, medication, and exercise interventions for diabetes.
5. Explain the effect of aerobic exercise on blood glucose levels.
6. Describe the significance of ketone bodies in the urine of a diabetic client.
7. Discuss the dietary requirements of clients taking Humalog insulin before meals.
8. Identify eating habits and patterns that place the diabetic client at increased risk for hypoglycemia and hyperglycemia.
9. Compare the mechanisms of action of the sulfonylureas, meglitinide analogs, biguanides, alpha glucosidase inhibitors, and thiazolidinediones as antidiabetic agents.
10. Explain the effect of hypertension on the development of diabetic nephropathy and diabetic retinopathy.
11. Identify clients at risk for hypoglycemia.
12. Prioritize nursing interventions for the client with mild to moderate hypoglycemia and moderate to severe hypoglycemia.
13. Identify clients at risk for diabetic ketoacidosis (DKA).
14. Prioritize nursing interventions for clients with DKA.
15. Identify clients at risk for hyperglycemic-hyperosmolar nonketotic syndrome (HHNS).
16. Prioritize nursing interventions for clients with HHNS.
17. Use laboratory data and clinical manifestations to determine the effectiveness of the interventions for DKA and HHNS.
18. Describe the steps required for subcutaneous insulin administration.
19. Describe the correct technique to use when mixing different types of insulin in the same syringe.
20. Compare the clinical manifestations of hyperglycemia and hypoglycemia.
21. Perform foot assessment and foot care for the client with diabetes.

Go to your Student CD-ROM for Review Questions for the NCLEX Examination keyed to these Learning Outcomes.

Diabetes mellitus is a common chronic disease requiring lifelong behavioral and lifestyle changes. It is best managed with a team approach to empower the client to successfully manage the disease. As part of the team, the nurse plans, organizes, and coordinates care among the various health disciplines involved; provides care and education; and promotes the client's health and well-being.

Diabetes is a major public health problem worldwide. Its complications cause many devastating health problems. The financial cost of diabetes is discussed in the Resource Management box on p. 1499. In the United States, diabetes is the leading cause of new cases of blindness, end-stage renal disease requiring dialysis or transplantation, and foot or leg amputations. Many people with diabetes are undiagnosed. Many who are diagnosed have unacceptably high blood glucose levels.

RESOURCE MANAGEMENT

DIABETES MELLITUS

Cost of Care

- Although people diagnosed with diabetes comprise 4% of the U.S. population, almost $1 out of every $5 spent on health care is for a person with diabetes.
- The annual cost of diabetes in medical expenses and lost workdays increased from $98 billion in 1997 to $132 billion in 2002.
- The per capita annual costs of health care for people with diabetes rose from $10,000 in 1997 to $13,242 in 2002—an increase of more than 3%. Health care costs for clients without diabetes amounted to $2560 in 2002.
- In 2002, the direct cost of diabetes was estimated to be $91.8 billion—19% of total personal health care costs.
- In 2002, about $40.3 billion dollars was spent for inpatient hospital care, $13.8 billion for nursing home care, and $10 billion for office visits.
- In 2002, indirect costs of diabetes was estimated to be $39.8 billion.
- In 2002, diabetes accounted for a loss of nearly 88 million disability days.
- In 2002, 176,000 cases of permanent disability were caused by diabetes at a cost of $7.5 billion.

Implications for Nursing

If costs related to diabetes are to be reduced, attention must be directed to the prevention and treatment of chronic complications of diabetes. Therapies are available to reduce the incidence of blindness, medications are available to reduce the incidence of kidney and coronary artery disease, and regular sensory evaluation of the feet can reduce the incidence of amputation. The challenge for the nurse is to assist the diabetic client in achieving and maintaining meticulous blood glucose control so that long-term complications are prevented.

Data from American Diabetes Association. (2003). Reviews: Economic costs of diabetes in the U.S. in 2002. *Diabetes Care, 26*(3), 917-932, and from American Association of Diabetes Educators. Diabetes facts and statistics. Available at http://www.aadenet.org/GeneralDiabetesInfo/GovStats.html.

Studies confirm that **glycemic** (blood glucose) control reduces complications of diabetes. Treatment of hypertension and **hyperlipidemia** (high blood fat levels) is essential to prevent complications of diabetes.

The nurse's challenge is to help the client with diabetes achieve and maintain lifestyle changes that prevent long-term complications by keeping blood glucose levels as close to normal as possible. New insulins, oral antidiabetic drugs, and tools are available to help clients achieve normal glucose levels.

PATHOPHYSIOLOGY

Classification of Diabetes

For all types of diabetes mellitus, the main feature is chronic **hyperglycemia** (high blood glucose level) resulting from problems with insulin secretion, insulin action, or both. The disease is classified by the underlying problem causing a lack of insulin and the severity of the insulin deficiency. Table 68-1 outlines the types of diabetes.

The Endocrine Pancreas

The endocrine portion of the pancreas has about 1 million small glands, the islets of Langerhans, scattered through the gland. The islet cells are only a small portion of the gland. Most of the gland has digestive functions. Two types of islet cells are important to glucose control. Alpha cells produce glucagon; beta cells produce insulin. **Glucagon** is a major "counterregulatory" hormone that has actions opposite those of insulin. It causes the release of glucose from cell storage sites whenever blood glucose levels are low. Insulin allows body cells to use and store carbohydrate, fat, and protein.

TABLE 68-1 Classification of Diabetes Mellitus

Type 1 Diabetes

- Primary beta cell destruction leading to absolute insulin deficiency
  - Autoimmune process
  - Idiopathic

Type 2 Diabetes

- Ranges from insulin resistance with an insulin deficiency to secretory deficit with insulin resistance

Other Specific Types (Conditions Resulting in Hyperglycemia)

- Genetic defects of beta cell function
- Genetic defects in insulin action
- Diseases of the exocrine pancreas: pancreatitis, trauma, neoplasia, cystic fibrosis, hemochromatosis
- Endocrinopathies: acromegaly, Cushing's disease glucagonoma, pheochromocytoma, hyperthyroidism, aldosteronoma
- Drug- or chemical-induced conditions (from use of pentamidine, nicotinic acid, glucocorticoids, thyroid hormone, diazoxide, beta-adrenergic agonists, thiazides, Dilantin, interferon-alpha, other drugs)
- Infections: congenital rubella, cytomegalovirus
- Uncommon forms of immune-related diabetes
- Other genetic syndromes associated with diabetes: Down syndrome, Klinefelter syndrome, Turner's syndrome, Huntington disease, and others

Gestational Diabetes Mellitus (GDM)

- Carbohydrate intolerance with onset or first recognized during pregnancy
- Children of mothers with GDM are at greater risk for neonatal mortality, congenital malformation, and macrosomia (large body size).
- Children of mothers with GDM have an increased risk of obesity and impaired glucose tolerance in late adolescence and young adulthood.
- Clients with GDM are at high risk for developing diabetes after pregnancy.
- Diagnosis is based on the results of a 100-g oral glucose tolerance test during pregnancy.

Data from American Diabetes Association. (2003). Committee report: Report of the Expert Committee on the Diagnosis and Classification of Diabetes Mellitus. *Diabetes Care, 26*(Suppl. 1), 5-20, and American Diabetes Association. (2000). Position statement: Gestational diabetes mellitus. *Diabetes Care, 26*(Suppl. 1), 103-105.

Insulin Physiology

Insulin is a protein made up of 51 amino acids in two peptide chains: an alpha chain and a beta chain. Preproinsulin is produced initially. This protein is a precursor molecule. It is inactive and must be made smaller before becoming the active hormone insulin. Preproinsulin is cut by enzymes to **proinsulin** (a precursor that includes the alpha and beta chains of the insulin molecule) and an additional fragment, the C-peptide chain. Proinsulin is converted in the beta cells into equal amounts of insulin and C-peptide (Figure 68-1). C-peptide levels are used to measure the rate that beta cells secrete insulin.

Insulin allows glucose in the blood to move into cells to make energy. Thus, insulin is like a key to open cell membranes to glucose. Insulin starts by binding to insulin receptors on the cell membranes. The liver is the first major organ

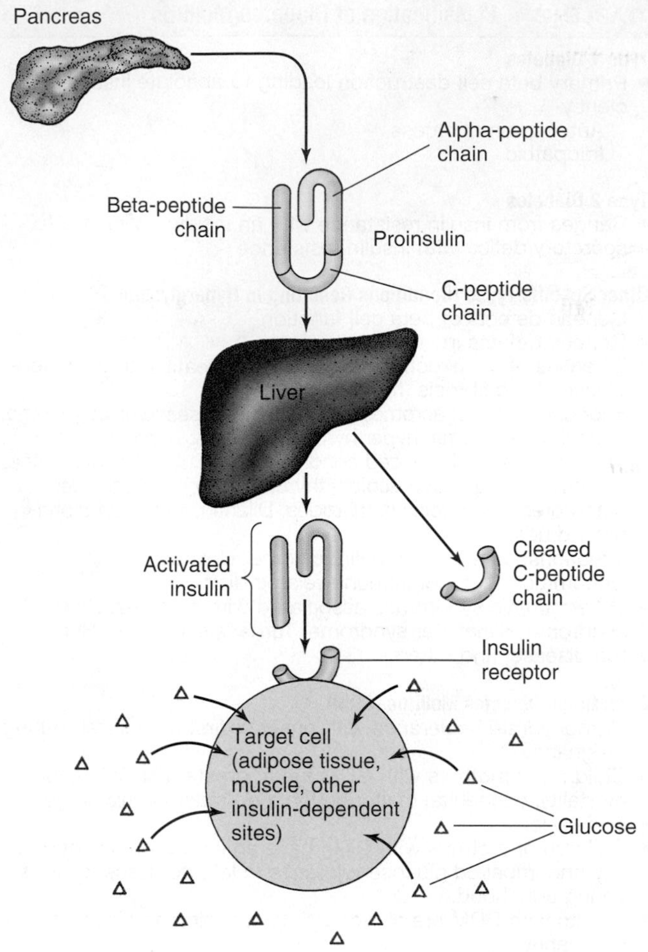

Figure 68-1 ■ Proinsulin, secreted by and stored in the beta cells of the islets of Langerhans in the pancreas, is transformed by the liver into activated insulin. Insulin attaches to receptors on target cells, where it promotes glucose transport into the cells through the cell membranes.

to be reached by insulin in the blood. In the liver, insulin promotes the production and storage of glycogen **(glycogenesis)** at the same time that it inhibits glycogen breakdown into glucose **(glycogenolysis)**. Insulin increases protein and lipid (fat) synthesis. Insulin inhibits tissue breakdown by inhibiting liver glycogenolysis, **ketogenesis** (conversion of fats to acids), and **gluconeogenesis** (conversion of proteins to glucose). In muscle, insulin promotes protein and glycogen synthesis. In fat cells, insulin promotes triglyceride storage. Overall, insulin keeps blood glucose levels from becoming too high and helps keep blood lipid levels in the normal range.

The pancreas secretes about 40 to 50 units of insulin daily directly into liver circulation in a two-step manner. Insulin is secreted at low levels during fasting **(basal insulin secretion)** and at increased levels after eating **(prandial)**. An early burst of insulin secretion occurs within 10 minutes of eating. This is followed by an increasing insulin release that lasts as long as hyperglycemia is present.

Glucose Homeostasis

Glucose is the main fuel for central nervous system (CNS) cells. Because the brain cannot produce or store much glucose, it needs a continuous supply from circulation. Fatty

TABLE 68-2 Physiologic Response to Insufficient Insulin

- Decreased glycogenesis (conversion of glucose to glycogen)
- Increased glycogenolysis (conversion of glycogen to glucose)
- Increased gluconeogenesis (formation of glucose from non-carbohydrate sources, such as amino acids and lactate)
- Increased lipolysis (breakdown of triglycerides to glycerol and free fatty acids)
- Increased ketogenesis (formation of ketones from free fatty acids)
- Proteolysis (breakdown of protein with amino acid release in muscles)

acids can be used as fuel when glucose is not available. The circulating fuels of glucose and free fatty acids are stored inside cells as glycogen in the liver and muscles and as triglyceride in fat cells. Fat, in the form of triglyceride, is the most efficient means of storing energy. Fat has 9 calories of stored energy per gram. Protein and carbohydrate have only 4 calories per gram. Although protein can be used as fuel during starvation, it is not used for fuel under normal conditions.

The combined actions of insulin and counterregulatory hormones (discussed in the next section) keep blood glucose levels in the range of 68 to 105 mg/dL (3.6 to 5.8 mmol/L) to support brain functions. When glucose levels fall, insulin secretion stops and glucagon is released. Glucagon causes the release of glucose from the liver. Liver glucose is made through **glycogenolysis** (breakdown of glycogen to glucose) and **gluconeogenesis.** When liver glucose is unavailable, **lipolysis** (breakdown of fat) and **proteolysis** (breakdown of amino acids) provide fuel for energy.

Counterregulatory hormones increase blood glucose by actions opposite those of insulin when more energy is needed. Glucagon is the main counterregulatory hormone. Other hormones that increase blood glucose levels are epinephrine, norepinephrine, growth hormone, and cortisol.

Absence of Insulin

Insulin is needed to move glucose into most body tissues. The lack of insulin in diabetes, from either a lack of production or a problem with insulin use at its cell receptor, prevents some cells from using glucose for energy. Without insulin, the body enters a serious state of breaking down body fat and protein. Levels of counterregulatory hormones increase in an attempt to make glucose from other sources. Table 68-2 outlines the body's response to insufficient insulin.

Without insulin, glucose builds up in the blood, causing **hyperglycemia** (high blood glucose levels). Hyperglycemia causes fluid and electrolyte imbalances, leading to the classic symptoms of diabetes: polyuria, polydipsia, and polyphagia.

Polyuria (frequent and excessive urination) results from an osmotic diuresis caused by excess glucose in the urine. As a result of diuresis, sodium, chloride, and potassium are excreted in the urine, and water loss is severe. Dehydration results and **polydipsia** (excessive thirst) occurs. Because the cells receive no glucose, cell starvation triggers **polyphagia** (excessive eating). Despite eating vast amounts of food, the person remains in starvation until insulin is available to move glucose into the cells.

With insulin deficiency, fats break down, releasing free fatty acids. Conversion of fatty acids to **ketone bodies** (small acids) provides a backup energy source. Because ketone bodies, or "ketones," are abnormal breakdown products of fatty acids, they may accumulate in the blood when insulin is not available. This accumulation causes metabolic acidosis.

The dehydration that occurs with diabetes leads to **hemoconcentration** (increased blood concentration), **hypovolemia** (decreased blood volume), **hyperviscosity** (thick, concentrated blood), **hypoperfusion** (decreased circulation) of tissues, and poor tissue oxygenation **(hypoxia)**. Hypoxic cells do not metabolize glucose efficiently, the Krebs cycle is blocked, and lactic acid increases, causing more acidosis. Restoring tissue perfusion and oxygenation by giving insulin halts lactic acid production.

The excess acids caused by absence of insulin increase hydrogen ion (H^+) and carbon dioxide (CO_2) levels in the blood. These products trigger the respiratory control areas of the brain to increase the rate and depth of respiration in an attempt to excrete more carbon dioxide and acid. This type of breathing is known as **Kussmaul respiration**. Acetone is exhaled, giving the breath a "fruity" odor. When the lungs can no longer offset acidosis, the pH drops. Arterial blood gas studies show a metabolic acidosis (decreased pH with decreased arterial bicarbonate [HCO_3^-] levels) and compensatory respiratory alkalosis (decreased partial pressure of arterial carbon dioxide [$Paco_2$]) (see Chapter 19).

Insulin lack causes potassium depletion. Because of the increased fluid loss with hyperglycemia, excessive potassium is excreted in the urine, leading to low serum potassium levels. However, high serum potassium levels may occur in acidosis because of the shift of potassium from inside the cells to the blood and other extracellular fluids. Serum potassium levels in diabetes, then, may be low **(hypokalemia)**, high **(hyperkalemia)**, or normal, depending on hydration, the severity of acidosis, and the client's response to treatment. Chapters 18 and 19 discuss acid-base balance and acidosis in more detail.

Acute Complications of Diabetes

Three glucose-related emergencies can occur in clients with diabetes: diabetic ketoacidosis (DKA) caused by lack of insulin and ketosis; hyperglycemic-hyperosmolar-nonketotic syndrome (HHNS) caused by insulin deficiency and profound dehydration; and hypoglycemia from too much insulin or too little glucose. All three problems require emergency treatment and can be fatal if treatment is delayed or incorrect. These problems and their interventions are described later.

Chronic Complications of Diabetes

Diabetes mellitus can lead to health problems and early death because of changes in large blood vessels **(macrovascular)** and small blood vessels **(microvascular)** in tissues and organs. Complications result from poor tissue circulation and cell death. Macrovascular complications, including coronary heart disease, cerebrovascular disease, and peripheral vascular disease, lead to increased early death among those with diabetes. Microvascular complications of blood vessel structure and function lead to **nephropathy** (kidney dysfunction), **neuropathy** (nerve dysfunction), and **retinopathy** (vision problems). Three theories have been used to explain these diabetic vascular complications:

- Chronic hyperglycemia causes irreversible structural changes resulting in basement membrane thickening and organ damage.
- Glucose toxicity directly or indirectly affects functional cell integrity.
- Chronic ischemia in microcirculatory branches causes connective tissue hypoxia and microischemia.

Chronic high blood glucose levels are the main cause of microvascular complications and allow premature development of macrovascular complications (Bell, 2002). Macrovascular complications in people with type 2 diabetes seem more related to hypertension, a sedentary lifestyle, high blood lipid levels, and smoking than to hyperglycemia. Obesity is also important for people with type 2 diabetes. About 80% of clients with type 2 diabetes are obese, and cardiovascular events account for most of their deaths.

The National Diabetes Data Group of the National Institutes of Health estimates that type 2 diabetes starts 9 to 12 years before the disorder is diagnosed. During this time of no treatment, complications develop. Up to 21% of clients have retinopathy at the time of diagnosis (American Diabetes Association [ADA], 2003e). Many older diabetic clients have no classic signs of high blood glucose levels, and the diagnosis is made when the person seeks treatment for another illness or for complications of diabetes.

The Diabetes Control and Complications Trial (DCCT), a study involving 29 medical centers and more than 1400 people with type 1 diabetes, showed that hyperglycemia is a critical factor for long-term diabetic complications. Intensive therapy with blood glucose levels as close to normal as possible delays the onset and progression of retinopathy, nephropathy, and neuropathy. Additional studies show that intensive therapy with lowered blood glucose levels reduced the onset of retinopathy, nephropathy, and neuropathy in clients with type 2 diabetes. A strong relationship exists between risks for microvascular complications and blood glucose levels. For every percentage point decrease in HbA1c, a 35% reduction in the risk for kidney and eye complications has been shown (ADA, 2003j).

MACROVASCULAR COMPLICATIONS

CARDIOVASCULAR DISEASE. Cardiovascular disease (CVD) is the most common complication of diabetes mellitus. Diabetic clients have a two to three times greater risk for CVD compared to nondiabetic clients. This excess risk occurs in both type 1 and type 2 diabetes, affects women more than men, and is influenced by ethnicity. More than 50% of clients with diabetes have some degree of CVD at the time of diagnosis. Complications of atherosclerosis cause about 80% of deaths in clients with diabetes and 75% of hospitalizations for diabetic complications (Spanheimer, 2001).

Myocardial infarction (MI) is the leading cause of death among clients with diabetes. They tend to have extensive coronary artery disease, cardiomyopathy, and abnormal blood clotting. Left ventricular dysfunction with heart failure and fatal dysrhythmias are common in diabetic clients after MI. Heart failure occurs in up to 50% of diabetic clients after MI (Tang & Young, 2001).

Diabetes is a major cardiovascular risk factor. Furthermore, clients with type 2 diabetes are more likely to have the risk factors of obesity, hypertension, dyslipidemia (excessive blood levels of cholesterol and other fats), and a sedentary lifestyle–a combination of factors known as "metabolic syndrome" (see later discussion). Renal disease, indicated by albumin in the urine, increases the risk for coronary heart disease and mortality from MI (Watkins, 2003).

Cardiovascular disease rates can be reduced through management of hyperglycemia, hypertension, and hyperlipidemia. The American Diabetes Association (ADA) recommends that blood pressure be maintained below 130/80 mm Hg and that low-density lipoprotein (LDL) cholesterol be kept below 100 mg/dL [<2.60 mmol/L] (ADA, 2003r). The American Heart Association recommends replacing saturated fat with monounsaturated fat (Safeer & Cornell, 2000).

CEREBROVASCULAR DISEASE. Diabetes damages cerebrovascular arterial circulation and is a risk factor for stroke. Hypertension, hyperlipidemia, nephropathy, peripheral vascular disease, and alcohol and tobacco abuse, along with diabetes, further increase the risk for stroke (Ingall, 2000).

Diabetes affects stroke outcomes as well. Elevated blood glucose levels at the time of the stroke may lead to greater brain injury and higher mortality (Beckman et al., 2002).

MICROVASCULAR COMPLICATIONS

EYE AND VISION COMPLICATIONS. Legal blindness (a corrected visual acuity of 20/200 or less) is 25 times more common in people with diabetes. In the United States, diabetic retinopathy is the most frequent cause of new blindness among adults 20 to 74 years of age. Retinopathy is strongly related to the duration of diabetes. After 20 years of diabetes, nearly all clients with type 1 diabetes and 78% of those with type 2 diabetes have some degree of retinopathy (Skyler, 2001).

The cause and progression of diabetic retinopathy are related to problems that block retinal blood vessels and cause them to leak, leading to retinal hypoxia. **Nonproliferative diabetic retinopathy (NPDR)** (Figure 68-2) causes structural problems in retinal vessels, but growth of new blood vessels is not stimulated. There are areas of poor retinal circulation, edema, hard fatty deposits in the eye, and retinal hemorrhages. **Microaneurysms** (small capillary wall dilations in retinal vessels) form throughout the eye. They leak fluid and blood into the retina, causing retinal edema and hard exudates. Other retinal problems include retinal hemorrhages, nerve fiber atrophy from hypoxia, and venous beading. **Venous beading** is the abnormal appearance of retinal veins in which areas of swelling and constriction along a segment of vein resemble links of sausage. Venous beading occurs in areas of retinal ischemia and is a predictor of proliferative diabetic retinopathy (PDR). NPDR develops slowly and rarely causes blindness. Clients with severe NPDR have a 45% chance of developing proliferative diabetic retinopathy (Franz, 2001).

Proliferative diabetic retinopathy (PDR) is the growth of new retinal blood vessels **(neovascularization).** When retinal circulation is poor and hypoxia develops, retinal cells secrete a "growth factor" that stimulates formation of new blood vessels in the eye. These new vessels are thin, fragile, and bleed easily. They lead to eye hemorrhage and more vision loss (Figure 68-3). Fibrous tissue bands, developing along with new blood vessels, cause retinal detachment and permanent vision loss. Chapter 50 discusses treatment of retinal problems.

Retinopathy is linked to fasting blood glucose levels above 129 mg/dL. Hyperglycemia and hypertension increase the rate of retinopathy development in clients with type 1 diabetes. Intensive diabetes management to obtain **near-euglycemic** (near-normal blood glucose) levels prevents or delays diabetic retinopathy (ADA, 2003e).

Vision loss also occurs from macular degeneration, corneal scarring, and changes in lens shape or clarity. Hyperglycemia may cause blurred vision, even with eyeglasses. Hypoglycemia may cause double vision. Cataracts occur at a younger age and progress faster among people with diabetes. Open-angle glaucoma also is more common in clients with diabetes. The management of cataracts and glaucoma are the same as for nondiabetic clients (see Chapter 50).

CONSIDERATIONS FOR OLDER ADULTS

The older client with diabetic retinopathy also has visual changes from aging. As a result, the older diabetic client's ability to perform self-care may be more seriously affected than that of a younger person with diabetes (see Chapter 50). The ability to discriminate among blues, greens, and violets decreases with normal aging. This problem makes performing visual blood glucose monitoring more difficult.

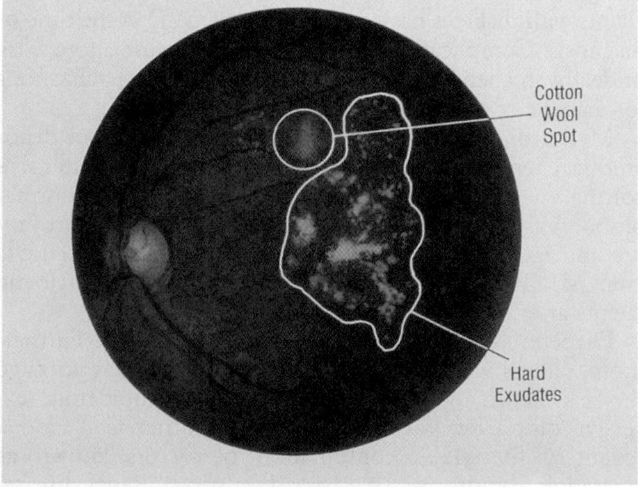

Figure 68-2 ■ Select ophthalmic changes seen in nonproliferative diabetic retinopathy (NPDR).

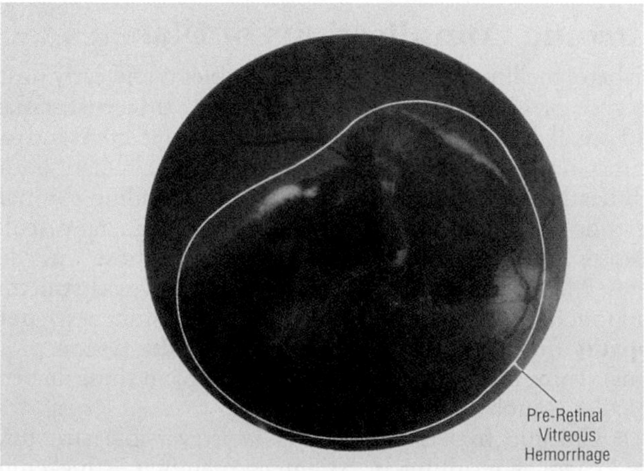

Figure 68-3 ■ Ophthalmic hemorrhage that is possible with proliferative diabetic retinopathy.

DIABETIC NEUROPATHY. **Neuropathy** is a progressive deterioration of nerves that results in loss of nerve function. It is a common complication of diabetes and often involves all parts of the body. Damage to sensory nerve fibers results in either pain or loss of sensation. Damage to motor nerve fibers results in muscle weakness. Damage to nerve fibers in the autonomic nervous system results in widespread loss of many functions.

Diabetic neuropathy can be focal or diffuse, each with different causes, rates of progression, and treatments. The most common neuropathies in diabetes are diffuse. They involve widespread nerve function loss, have a slow onset, affect both sides of the body, involve motor and sensory nerves, progress slowly, and are permanent. Diffuse neuropathies include autonomic nerve dysfunction. Late complications include foot ulcers and deformities.

Focal neuropathies affect a single nerve or nerve group. They usually are caused by an acute ischemic event (ischemic neuropathy) or by the physical trapping of a nerve (entrapment neuropathy). Both types lead to nerve damage or nerve death. Ischemic neuropathies occur when the blood supply to a nerve or group of nerves is disrupted. The symptoms begin suddenly, affect only one side of the body or body area, and are self-limiting in duration. Recovery time varies. Entrapment neuropathies stem from compression of a nerve in a body compartment or between tissues. Symptoms begin gradually and can occur anywhere. They may be bilateral, having a waxing and waning course without spontaneous recovery. An example of focal entrapment neuropathy is carpal tunnel syndrome.

Hyperglycemia leads to neuropathy through blood vessel changes that cause nerve hypoxia. Both the axon and its myelin sheath are damaged by reduced blood flow, resulting in blocked nerve impulse transmission. Excessive glucose is converted to sorbitol, which accumulates in nerves. The increased sorbitol also impairs motor nerve conduction. Common diabetic neuropathies are listed in Table 68-3. Autonomic nervous system neuropathy leads to problems in cardiovascular, gastrointestinal (GI), and urinary function. Keeping blood glucose levels in the normal range delays the onset and reduces the severity of diabetic neuropathies.

The cardiovascular problems of **orthostatic** (postural) hypotension and **syncope** (brief loss of consciousness) increase the risk for falls. In addition, the neuropathy can mask the pain of MI. Common GI symptoms from diabetic neuropathy are **dysphagia** (difficulty swallowing), heartburn, nausea and vomiting, and bowel elimination problems. Diarrhea caused by diabetes is chronic, may be severe, and often occurs at night. Constipation, the most common GI symptom, is intermittent and may alternate with bouts of diarrhea. **Gastroparesis** (delay in gastric emptying) is a cause of hypoglycemia. Loss of nerve input to the bladder results in incomplete emptying, which leads to urinary infection and kidney problems.

DIABETIC NEPHROPATHY. **Nephropathy** is pathologic change in the kidney that reduces kidney function and leads to renal failure. Diabetes mellitus is the leading cause of end-stage renal disease (ESRD) and renal failure in the United States. Diabetic nephropathy affects 20% to 30% of those with type 1 diabetes 20 years after onset. Although less than 20% of clients with type 2 diabetes have nephropathy, about 60% of the clients with ESRD have type 2 diabetes (Skyler, 2001). Native Americans/American Indians, Hispanics (especially Mexican Americans), and African Americans have much

TABLE 68-3 Features of Diabetic Neuropathy

	Complication	Manifestation
Diffuse Neuropathies		
Distal symmetric polyneuropathy	Sensory alterations	Paresthesias: burning/tingling sensations, starting in toes and moving up legs Dysesthesias: burning, stinging, or stabbing pain Anesthesia: loss of sensation
	Motor alterations in intrinsic muscles of foot	Foot deformities: high arch, claw toes, hammertoes; shift of weight bearing to metatarsal heads and tips of toes
Autonomic neuropathy	Anhidrosis	Drying, cracking of skin
	Gastroparesis	Delayed gastric emptying, constipation, nausea, anorexia
	Diabetic diarrhea	Diarrhea and bowel incontinence
	Neurogenic bladder	Atonic bladder, urinary retention
	Impotence	Erectile dysfunction
	Loss of cardiac reflexes	Orthostatic hypotension, resting tachycardia
	Defective counterregulation	Loss of warning signs of hypoglycemia
Focal Neuropathies		
Focal ischemia	Thoracolumbar radiculopathy with sensory and reflex loss	Pain radiating across back, side, and front of chest or abdomen
	Cranial nerve palsies, third and sixth nerves	Sudden diplopia or ptosis; eye pain
	Amyotrophy	Pain; asymmetric weakness; wasting of iliopsoas, quadriceps, and adductor muscles
Entrapment neuropathies	Median nerve	Carpal tunnel syndrome
	Popliteal nerve/knee	Footdrop
	Posterior tibial nerve at tarsal tunnel	Tarsal tunnel syndrome: sensory impairment in sole of foot; weakness of intrinsic muscles of foot; burning pain and paresthesias at ankle and plantar surface

TABLE 68-4 Differentiation of Type 1 and Type 2 Diabetes

Features	Type 1	Type 2
Former names	Juvenile-onset diabetes Ketosis-prone diabetes Insulin-dependent diabetes mellitus (IDDM)	Maturity-onset diabetes Ketosis-resistant diabetes Non–insulin-dependent diabetes mellitus (NIDDM)
Age at onset	Usually under 30 yr of age, occurs at any age	Peaks in 50s; may occur earlier
Symptoms	Abrupt onset, thirst, weight loss	Frequently none; thirst, fatigue, visual blurring, vascular or neural complications
Etiology	Viral infection	Not known
Pathology	Pancreatic beta cell destruction	Insulin resistance Dysfunctional pancreatic beta cell
Antigen patterns	HLA-DR4, HLA-DR3	None
Antibodies	ICAs present at diagnosis	None
Endogenous insulin and C-peptide	None	Low, normal, or high
Inheritance	Recessive	Dominant, multifactorial
Nutritional status	Usually nonobese	60% to 80% obese
Insulin	All dependent on insulin	Required for 20% to 30%
Sulfonylurea therapy	None	Effective for most clients
Medical nutrition therapy	Mandatory	Mandatory

ICAs, Islet cell antibodies.

higher risks for developing ESRD than non-Hispanic whites. Keeping blood glucose levels in the normal range can delay the onset of nephropathy and, in some cases, may prevent it.

Risk factors for diabetic nephropathy include a 10- to 15-year history of diabetes, diabetic retinopathy, poor blood glucose control, uncontrolled hypertension, and genetic predisposition (Sweny, 2002). In addition, clients with diabetes who also produce excess collagen (such as people who form keloid scars) are at greater risk for developing diabetic nephropathy.

The earliest clinical sign of nephropathy is **microalbuminuria** (very small amounts of albumin in the urine). Annual testing for microalbuminuria is recommended for clients who have had type 1 diabetes for at least 5 years and in all clients with type 2 diabetes (ADA, 2003r).

Chronic high blood glucose levels cause hypertension in kidney blood vessels and excess kidney perfusion. The increased pressure damages the kidney in many ways. The blood vessels become more leaky, especially in the glomerulus. This leakiness allows filtration of larger particles (including albumin and other proteins), which then form deposits in the kidney tissue and blood vessels. Deposits narrow the vessels, decreasing kidney oxygenation and leading to kidney cell hypoxia and cell death. These processes worsen over time. Blood vessels in the glomerulus become scarred and unable to filter urine from the blood, leading to renal failure.

Renal damage is also related to increased mean arterial blood pressure in diabetic clients with cardiovascular disease. Both systolic and diastolic hypertension greatly speed the progression of diabetic nephropathy.

MALE ERECTILE DYSFUNCTION. Erectile dysfunction (ED) is the inability to achieve or maintain a penile erection sufficient for satisfactory sexual performance. ED occurs at a higher rate and an earlier age among men with diabetes as compared with the general population. About half of diabetic men have ED. This occurs 10 to 15 years earlier than in the general population (Paty & Hirsch, 2000). In diabetes, ED is related to poor blood glucose control, obesity, hypertension, heavy cigarette smoking, and the presence of other chronic microvascular and macrovascular complications.

ED may be caused by neuropathy, vascular disease, psychological factors, or endocrine disorders. Autonomic neuropathy or vascular changes are responsible for persistent ED in diabetes. Chapter 79 discusses erectile function problems in depth.

Etiology and Genetic Risk

TYPE 1 DIABETES

Type 1 diabetes is an autoimmune disorder in which beta cells are destroyed in a genetically susceptible person (Table 68-4). The immune system fails to recognize normal body cells as "self" and takes destructive actions against them. In type 1 diabetes, immune system cells and cell products attack and destroy insulin-secreting cells in the islets. Although the exact cause of a person's immune system being attacked by normal body cells is not known, people with certain tissue types are more likely to develop autoimmune diseases, including type 1 diabetes. Specifically, people who have the tissue types HLA-DR3 or HLA-DR4 are at an increased risk for type 1 diabetes. Certain viral infections, such as mumps, congenital rubella, and coxsackievirus infection, appear to trigger autoimmune destruction of pancreatic beta cells.

Indicators or markers of immune damage to insulin-producing cells (a key feature of type 1 diabetes) are the presence of blood antibodies directed against the beta cells themselves or against substances made by beta cells. Most clients with type 1 diabetes have islet cell antibodies (ICAs), insulin autoantibodies (IAAs), autoantibodies to glutamic acid decarboxylase (GAD), or autoantibodies to tyrosine phosphates. Circulating ICA and IAA may be present before manifestations of type 1 diabetes develop.

Genetic Considerations

Risk for type 1 diabetes is determined by inheritance of the HLA-DR3 and HLA-DR4 genes. However, although inheritance of these genes increases the risk, most people with these genes do not develop type 1 diabetes. Development of the disease is an interactive effect of genetic predisposition and exposure to certain environmental factors. The risk for type 1 diabetes in the general population ranges from 1 in 400 to 1 in 1000. The risk greatly increases for those who have at least one parent with diabetes (from 1 in 20 to 1 in 50) (Franz, 2001). It is unclear why some genetically susceptible people develop diabetes and others do not.

TYPE 2 DIABETES AND METABOLIC SYNDROME

Type 2 diabetes is a progressive disorder in which the pancreas makes less insulin over time. Clients with type 2 diabetes have a reduced ability of most cells to respond to insulin **(insulin resistance)**, poor control of liver glucose output, and decreased beta-cell function, eventually leading to beta-cell failure. Most people with type 2 diabetes are obese adults. With the increased rate of obesity occurring in younger people, the age of onset for type 2 diabetes is also decreasing. The specific causes of type 2 diabetes are not known. Both insulin resistance and beta-cell failure have many genetic and nongenetic causes. Heredity plays a major role in the development of type 2 diabetes. Offspring of clients with type 2 diabetes have a 15% chance of developing the disease and a 30% risk of having impaired glucose tolerance. Specific gene defects have been identified in certain groups with high incidence rates of type 2 diabetes. Pima Indians have a 50% prevalence of type 2 diabetes (Franz, 2001).

Metabolic syndrome, also called **syndrome X,** is a group of disorders with insulin resistance as a main feature. Other features of the syndrome include obesity (particularly with excessive fat tissue around the waist and abdomen, giving the person a round, "apple-like" shape), low levels of physical activity, hypertension, and high blood levels of cholesterol. The syndrome is not a single disease but is a collection of related health problems thought to represent a gene-environment interaction. A genetic predisposition to type 2 diabetes increases the risk for the other metabolic syndrome health problems when compounded by obesity and a sedentary lifestyle. Any one of these health problems increases the rate of atherosclerosis and the risk for stroke, coronary heart disease, and early death. Together with metabolic syndrome, these health problems greatly increase the risk for potentially lethal cardiovascular complications. Although metabolic syndrome does not respond readily to drug therapy for any one of the health problems, lifestyle changes (e.g., getting regular aerobic exercise, achieving an ideal body weight) can reduce the insulin resistance and diabetic manifestations, reduce the high blood levels of cholesterol, and lower blood pressure.

Incidence/Prevalence

Diabetes mellitus is the seventh leading cause of death in the United States, where it affects 17 million people, or 6.2% of the population. In the United States, the incidence of diabetes is rising–up 49% from 1990 to 2000, with projections indicating a 165% increase by the year 2050. An additional 5.9 million people are unaware they have the disease (Lachuk et al., 2002).

About 90% of diabetic persons have type 2 diabetes. Diagnosed diabetes is most common among middle-aged and older adults, affecting about 6% of people 45 to 64 years of age and 11% of those over 65 years of age. About 10% of clients diagnosed with diabetes are older than 70 years of age. After 40 years of age, new-onset diabetes is usually type 2. The prevalence of diabetes is similar for men and women. Although type 2 diabetes is a disease of middle-aged and older adults, recent surveys show an increase of the disorder in childhood and adolescence as a result of obesity (El-Kebbi et al., 2003).

Because the prevalence of obesity is rising in the United States, diabetes will become even more common. Body mass index (BMI) is one of the strongest indicators of diabetes. Among clients diagnosed with diabetes, 68% have a BMI of at least 27 kg/m^2, and 46% have a BMI of at least 30 kg/m^2. Risk for diabetes increases dramatically as the degree of overweight increases.

HEALTH PROMOTION/ILLNESS PREVENTION

The fact that diabetes is a common disorder and causes many preventable but devastating complications makes the disease a major public health problem. The U.S. government has identified control of diabetes and its complications as a major focus for health promotion activities (see the Meeting Healthy People 2010 box on p. 1506).

No interventions are successful in preventing type 1 diabetes. Health promotion for clients with type 1 diabetes focuses on controlling hyperglycemia to reduce its long-term complications.

Type 2 diabetes can be prevented or delayed by weight loss and increased physical activity. Strategies to reduce the cardiovascular risk factors of tobacco use, hypertension, and high blood lipid levels also reduce the incidence of type 2 diabetes and its long-term complications. Drug therapy is not recommended for routine use to prevent diabetes (ADA, 2003t).

CULTURAL CONSIDERATIONS

Diabetes is a significant health problem for African Americans, Native Americans/American Indians, and Mexican Americans. The prevalence rates for this disease are 1.6 and 1.9 times higher, respectively, than the rate for white individuals. The increase in obesity and sedentary lifestyles in the U.S. population is the probable cause of this growing problem (El-Kebbi, 2003). The American Diabetes Association (ADA) has identified individuals who should be tested for diabetes in Table 68-5.

Racial and ethnic differences affect clinical outcomes for diabetic clients. The prevalence of hypertension in diabetic clients is at least twice the rate of nondiabetic clients, with non-Hispanic whites and African Americans having the highest prevalence. Microvascular complications of the eyes, nerves, and kidneys are more common in African Americans and Native Americans/American Indians with diabetes than in non-Hispanic whites with diabetes (Harris, 2001).

Meeting HEALTHY PEOPLE 2010 Objectives

DIABETES MELLITUS

Objective 18.4: Reduce the diabetes death rates (diabetes as the underlying cause) to no more than 12.0 per 100,000 persons.

- Encourage all people to have a yearly screening physical examination that includes blood testing for diabetes.
- Inform all clients who have a sedentary lifestyle and who are overweight about the risk factors for and complications of diabetes.
- Assist diabetic clients who smoke to reduce or quit smoking.
- Instruct clients with diabetes mellitus to achieve and maintain body weight within 5 pounds of identified ideal weight for age and body size.
- Provide one-to-one educational sessions, group education sessions, and printed and videotape information on diabetes treatment and care to clients diagnosed with diabetes.
- Educate clients about the specific medications prescribed to manage their disease.
- Demonstrate the use of the diet strategy individually planned for the client with diabetes.
- Encourage all clients with diabetes to participate in an individualized education program at least 3 days per week.
- Assist those clients with diabetes who also have hypertension to understand the importance of adhering to the prescribed drug therapies for both health problems.
- Instruct clients with diabetes to obtain annual vaccinations against influenza.
- Teach clients with diabetes to maintain adequate hydration, especially when any other illness is present.
- Participate in mass screenings to identify people with undiagnosed type 2 diabetes among the general population.
- Develop culturally sensitive and literacy-appropriate education materials targeted to high-risk minority populations.

Objective 18.9: Reduce the frequency of foot ulcers in persons with diabetes.

- Include foot assessment whenever caring for a client with diabetes.
- Include sensory testing of the feet for all people with diabetes.
- Instruct the client with diabetes about proper foot care.
- Teach the client with diabetes the importance of always wearing protective footwear whenever the client is out of bed.
- Show the client the proper type of footwear to prevent foot injury.
- Find resources for those diabetic clients who are unable to afford properly fitting shoes.
- Teach the client how to monitor the circulatory status of his or her feet.
- Encourage the client to see a podiatrist twice a year.
- Refer the client with foot lesions to a wound management specialist.
- Encourage the client with diabetes who smokes to reduce or quit smoking.

Objective 18.23 Increase to 52% the proportion of persons with diabetes who have received formal diabetes education.

- Evaluate the diabetes education materials and programs currently in place at your institution for currency, literacy, cultural sensitivity, and adequacy.
- Identify resources within your agency and community for diabetes education and support.
- Meet with the diabetes educator at your agency and establish means for collaboration and referral.
- If a diabetes educator is not available at your agency, work with existing personnel to enhance diabetes knowledge and awareness.
- Assist in policy-making decisions within your agency to develop a formalized teaching plan for all clients with diabetes, regardless of whether the clients are newly diagnosed or have had diabetes for a long time.
- Develop and offer diabetes education programs within your community in a variety of settings.

Critical Thinking Challenge

You are caring for a 31-year-old man who has had type 1 diabetes for 8 years. He runs 5 miles three times per week, is about 10 pounds overweight, and is relatively healthy. His blood pressure is 138/88 and his urine is negative for microalbumin. He is newly married and works as an editor for a local newspaper. He worries about whether or not he should have children and whether they will have diabetes. His 58-year-old mother had a myocardial infarction 2 years ago. The client is concerned that he is doomed to an early death by heart attack or renal failure and that he may end up having a foot or leg amputated.

1. Explain the genetic influence for type 1 diabetes.
2. Is this client's family history of MI important? Why or why not?
3. How could this client reduce his risk for or delay complications?

evolve For suggested answer guidelines, go to http://evolve.elsevier.com/Iggy/.

COLLABORATIVE MANAGEMENT

PHARM e REVIEW

Assessment

HISTORY

Ask questions about risk factors and symptoms related to diabetes. The client's age is important because type 2 diabetes is more common in older people, especially among African Americans and Mexican Americans. Ask women how large their children were at birth because many women who develop type 2 diabetes had gestational diabetes or were glucose intolerant during pregnancy. These women often have given birth to infants weighing 9 pounds or more.

Assessing weight and weight change is important because excess weight and obesity are risk factors for type 2 diabetes. The client with type 1 diabetes often has weight loss with increased appetite during the weeks before diagnosis. For both types of diabetes, clients usually have fatigue, polyuria, and

TABLE 68-5 Major Risk Factors for Type 2 Diabetes

Testing for diabetes should be considered in individuals 45 years of age and older, particularly in those with a BMI greater than 25 kg/m^2. If normal, it should be repeated at 3-year intervals.

Testing should be considered at a younger age or be carried out more frequently in individuals who are overweight (BMI $>$25 kg/m^2) and have additional risk factors:

- Have a first-degree relative with diabetes
- Are habitually physically inactive
- Are members of a high-risk ethnic population (e.g., African American, Hispanic American, Native American/American Indian, Asian American, or Pacific Islander).
- Deliver a baby weighing more than 9 pounds or have been diagnosed with GDM
- Are hypertensive ($>$140/90 mm Hg)
- Have a high-density lipoprotein cholesterol (HDL) level less than 35 mg/dL (0.90 mmol/L) and/or a triglyceride level greater than 250 mg/dL (2.82 mmol/L)
- Have polycystic ovary syndrome
- Have IFG or IGT on previous testing
- Have a history of vascular disease

Data from American Diabetes Association. (2003). Committee report: Report of the Expert Committee on the Diagnosis and Classification of Diabetes Mellitus. *Diabetes Care 26*(Suppl. 1), 5-20.

BMI, Body mass index, *IFG,* impaired fasting glucose; *IGT,* impaired glucose tolerance.

polydipsia. Ask clients about recent major or minor infections. In particular, ask women about frequent vaginal yeast infections. Ask all clients whether they have noticed that small skin injuries become infected more easily or take longer to heal.

Explore the family history for parents and siblings with diabetes. If the client has one or more relatives with diabetes, it is important to determine whether these relatives use insulin or control their disease with diet, exercise, or oral antidiabetic drugs.

LABORATORY ASSESSMENT

BLOOD TESTS. Blood glucose values are used to diagnose diabetes. The nurse, the client, or a family member monitors the ongoing status of the disease by performing capillary blood glucose testing using a blood glucose meter. The physician and the nurse assess the overall result of treatment through review of glycosylated hemoglobin (hemoglobin A1c [HbA1c]) and fructosamine levels.

Instructions for blood glucose testing are listed in Chart 68-1. The American Diabetes Association (ADA) defines normal blood glucose values in Chart 68-2. ADA criteria for diagnosing adult diabetes mellitus are listed in Table 68-6.

FASTING BLOOD GLUCOSE TEST. Fasting blood glucose test results are most accurate when the blood is obtained by venipuncture. The client should fast for at least 8 hours (water is permitted). Draw the blood before insulin or oral antidiabetic agents have been taken. Diabetes is diagnosed when two separate test results exceed 126 mg/dL (7 mmol/L) (ADA, 2003a).

ORAL GLUCOSE TOLERANCE TEST. The oral glucose tolerance test (OGTT) is the most sensitive test for diagnosing diabetes, although it is not routinely used except in gestational diabetes. The test is inconvenient to clients, costly, and time consuming compared with the fasting blood glucose measure. Before the test, review instructions from Chart 68-1 with the client. Carbohydrate restriction or bedrest before the test alters glucose tolerance. The client drinks a beverage containing a glucose load of 75 g, and blood samples are collected at 30-minute intervals for 2 hours. A diagnosis of diabetes is made if the blood glucose is greater than 200 mg/dL (11.1 mmol/L) at 120 minutes.

GLYCOSYLATED HEMOGLOBIN ASSAYS. Blood glucose permanently attaches to hemoglobin. The higher the blood glucose level is over time, the more glycosylated hemoglobin becomes. Thus glycosylated hemoglobin

CHART 68-1

CLIENT EDUCATION GUIDE
Blood Glucose Testing

Fasting Plasma Blood Glucose
- Do not eat any food or drink any liquid for at least 8 hours.

Oral Glucose Tolerance Test
- Eat a balanced diet with carbohydrate intake of at least 150 g for a minimum of 3 days while maintaining normal physical activity.
- Carbohydrate restriction, bedrest, acute illness, and certain drugs interfere with the test. Phenytoin (Dilantin), anovulatory drugs, diuretics, nicotinic acid, and glucocorticoids adversely affect results.
- The test is performed in the morning after a 10- to 12-hour fast.
- A fasting blood sample is obtained.
- You will be asked to drink 300 mL (75 g) of a flavored beverage within 5 minutes of the fasting blood sample.
- Blood samples are drawn at 30-minute intervals for 2 hours.
- During the test, you will remain at rest and not be able to smoke or drink liquids.
- Report any signs suggesting hypoglycemia, such as weakness, dizziness, nervousness, and confusion.

TABLE 68-6 Criteria for the Diagnosis of Type 2 Diabetes

Symptoms of diabetes plus casual blood glucose concentration greater than 200 mg/dL (11.1 mmol/L). *Casual* is defined as any time of day without regard to time since last meal. The classic symptoms of diabetes include polyuria, polydipsia, and unexplained weight loss.

Or

Fasting plasma glucose greater than 126 mg/dL (7.0 mmol/L). *Fasting* is defined as no caloric intake for at least 8 hr.

Or

2-hr plasma glucose greater than 200 mg/dL during an oral glucose tolerance test. The test should be performed using a glucose load containing the equivalent of 75 g glucose dissolved in water.

NOTE: Each test must be confirmed, on a subsequent day, under similar circumstances.

Data from American Diabetes Association. (2003). Committee report: Report of the Expert Committee on the Diagnosis and Classification of Diabetes Mellitus. *Diabetes Care, 26*(Suppl. 1), 5-20.

CHART 68-2

LABORATORY PROFILE
Blood Glucose Values

Test	Normal Range for Adults	Significance of Abnormal Results
Fasting blood glucose test	<110 mg/dL (6.1 mmol/L) *Older adults:* Levels rise 1 mg/dL per decade of age.	Levels >110 mg/dL (6.1 mmol/L) but <126 mg/dL (7.0 mmol/L) indicate impaired fasting glucose (IFG). Levels >126 mg/dL (7.0 mmol/L) obtained on at least two occasions are diagnostic of diabetes, even in older adults.
Glucose tolerance test (2-hr postload result)	<140 mg/dL (7.8 mmol/L)	Levels >140 mg/dL (7.8 mmol/L) and <200 mg/dL (11.1 mmol/L) indicate impaired glucose tolerance (IGT). Levels >200 mg/dL (11.1 mmol/L) indicate provisional diagnosis of diabetes.
Glycosylated hemoglobin (hemoglobin A_{1c} [HbA_{1c}]) test	4%-6%	Levels >8% indicate poor diabetic control and need for adherence to regimen or changes in therapy.

Data from American Diabetes Association. (2003). Committee report: Report of the Expert Committee on the Diagnosis and Classification of Diabetes Mellitus. *Diabetes Care, 26*(Suppl. 1), 5-20, and the American Diabetes Association. (2003). Position statement: Tests of glycemia in diabetes. *Diabetes Care, 26*(Suppl. 1), 106-108.

(HbA1c) is a good indicator of the average blood glucose levels. Measurement of HbA1c shows the average blood glucose level during the previous 120 days–the life span of red blood cells. HbA1c testing is used to assess long-term glycemic control, as well as to predict the risk for complications. Unlike the fasting blood glucose test, HbA1c test results are not altered by eating habits the day before the test. HbA1c testing is performed at diagnosis and at specific intervals to evaluate the treatment plan. Hemolysis, blood loss, and pregnancy all increase red blood cell turnover and reduce HbA1c levels. Triglycerides and bilirubin interfere with the assay, leading to overestimation of HbA1c levels in clients with hypertriglyceridemia. HbA1c testing is recommended at least twice yearly in clients who are meeting treatment goals and have stable blood glucose control. Quarterly assessment is recommended for clients whose therapy has changed or who are not meeting glycemic goals (ADA, 2003r).

GLYCOSYLATED SERUM PROTEINS AND ALBUMIN. Serum proteins and albumin become increasingly glycosylated with elevated blood glucose levels in the same way that hemoglobin does. However, because proteins and albumin turn over in 14 days, compared with 120 days for red blood cells, an assay of glycosylated serum proteins can indicate blood glucose control over a shorter period. These measures are useful when tight control of blood glucose levels is needed (e.g., pregnancy) or for follow-up of treatment changes. Available tests are called GSA (glycosylated serum albumin), GSP (glycosylated serum protein), and fructosamine.

URINE TESTS

URINE TESTING FOR KETONES. Ketones are a waste product of fat metabolism. Their presence in urine may indicate impending ketoacidosis. The ADA recommends testing urine for ketones during acute illness or stress, when blood glucose levels consistently exceed 300 mg/dL (16.7 mmol/L), during pregnancy, or when any symptoms of ketoacidosis are present (ADA, 2003s). Ketone testing is recommended for diabetic clients following a weight loss program.

URINE TESTING FOR RENAL FUNCTION. The presence of urine protein without renal symptoms may indicate microvascular changes in the kidney. Urine albumin excretion rates of 20 to 200 g/min (30 to 300 mg/hr) indicate microalbuminuria. Even minor elevations of albumin excretion are linked to increased mortality.

Once clinical proteinuria has been detected, kidney function (e.g., glomerular filtration rate) is assessed by creatinine clearance tests (see Chapter 72). In clients with nephropathy, a rise in serum creatinine levels is related to both poor blood glucose control and hypertension.

URINE TESTING FOR GLUCOSE. Blood glucose may be measured indirectly by urine testing for glucose, although this method is less precise than blood testing. Fluid intake, urine concentration, time since last voiding, and certain drugs affect the results.

OTHER DIAGNOSTIC ASSESSMENTS

Although not commonly used, other tests can help determine whether a client has type 1 or type 2 diabetes. Type 1 diabetes is an autoimmune disease with the presence of autoantibodies to proteins. Measuring levels of islet cell antibodies (ICAs) is an indicator of type 1 diabetes. Measurement of C-peptide levels indicates beta secretory function of the pancreas. C-peptide levels correlate well with insulin levels and are used to diagnose type 1 diabetes.

◆Analysis

COMMON NURSING DIAGNOSES AND COLLABORATIVE PROBLEMS

The following are priority nursing diagnoses for clients with diabetes:

1. Risk for Injury related to hyperglycemia
2. Risk for Delayed Surgical Recovery related to endocrine and vascular effects of diabetes
3. Risk for Injury related to sensory alterations (diabetic neuropathy)
4. Chronic Pain related to peripheral nerve dysfunction (diabetic neuropathy)
5. Risk for Injury related to disturbed sensory perception: visual (diabetic retinopathy)
6. Ineffective Tissue Perfusion (Renal) related to impaired transport of oxygen across capillary membranes

The following are primary collaborative problems:

1. Potential for Hypoglycemia
2. Potential for Diabetic Ketoacidosis
3. Potential for Hyperglycemic-Hyperosmolar Nonketotic Syndrome and Coma

ADDITIONAL NURSING DIAGNOSES AND COLLABORATIVE PROBLEMS

In addition to the common nursing diagnoses and collaborative problems, clients with diabetes may have one or more of the following:

- Imbalanced Nutrition: More Than Body Requirements related to an imbalance of food intake and physical activity, lack of knowledge, and ineffective coping skills
- Risk for Deficient Fluid Volume related to fluid shifts, failure of regulatory mechanisms, hyperglycemic diuresis, polyuria, vomiting, diarrhea, decreased oral intake, and dehydration
- Impaired Oral Mucous Membrane related to microvascular circulatory changes and uncontrolled blood glucose levels
- Deficient Knowledge about diabetes management related to a lack of familiarity with information resources about disease, diet, exercise, drugs, weight control, and foot care
- Impaired Urinary Elimination and Urinary Retention (with Overflow Incontinence) related to diabetic neuropathy
- Constipation related to diabetic neuropathy
- Diarrhea related to diabetic neuropathy
- Risk for Impaired Skin Integrity related to decreased circulation, increased blood glucose levels, decreased mobility, and decreased sensation
- Risk for Infection related to increased blood glucose levels, decreased tissue perfusion, inadequate primary defenses, and the effects of chronic disease
- Risk for Infection related to wounds, urinary tract infection, intravenous (IV) access site, or oral mucous membranes
- Risk for Ineffective Sexuality Patterns (Male) related to autonomic neuropathy, decreased circulation, or psychological problems
- Risk for Ineffective Sexuality Patterns (Female) related to the stressors of diabetes
- Sexual Dysfunction related to impotence, impaired lubrication, painful intercourse with the changes in neu-

rologic control of the genitalia, the effects of actual or perceived limitations imposed by the disease or therapy, and altered self-concept

- Situational Low Self-Esteem related to an inability to deal with the self-care demands of the diabetic regimen
- Anxiety related to diagnosis of diabetes, potential complications of diabetes, and self-care regimens
- Fear related to diagnosis of diabetes, potential complications of diabetes, and self-care regimens
- Ineffective Coping and Compromised Family Coping related to a chronic disease, a complex self-care regimen, and decreased social support
- Powerlessness related to the complications of diabetes (blindness, amputations, renal failure, and neuropathy)
- Social Isolation related to visual impairment or blindness
- Noncompliance with self-care related to the complexity and duration of the prescribed regimen
- Ineffective Health Maintenance related to insufficient knowledge of diet restriction, weight control, weight maintenance, benefits and risks of exercise, self-monitoring of blood glucose, medications, sick-day care, foot care, hypoglycemia, and available resources

Planning and Implementation

The management of diabetes mellitus is complicated and involves considerable client cooperation and education. The Concept Map on p. 1510 highlights care issues for the client with type 2 diabetes mellitus.

RISK FOR INJURY RELATED TO HYPERGLYCEMIA

NOC **PLANNING: EXPECTED OUTCOMES.** The client with diabetes is expected to manage diabetes mellitus and prevent disease progression by maintaining blood glucose levels in the expected range. Indicators are that the client consistently demonstrates the following behaviors:

- Performs treatment regimen as prescribed
- Follows recommended diet
- Demonstrates correct procedure for blood glucose testing
- Monitors blood glucose
- Treats symptoms of hyperglycemia
- Seeks health care if blood glucose levels fluctuate outside of recommended parameters
- Follows recommended activity level
- Uses drugs as prescribed
- Maintains optimum weight

INTERVENTIONS

NONSURGICAL MANAGEMENT. Nonsurgical management of diabetes mellitus involves dietary interventions, blood glucose monitoring, a planned exercise program, and in some instances, medications to lower blood glucose levels. The nurse, together with the client, physician, dietitian, pharmacist, and in some cases, physical therapist, plans, organizes, and delivers care.

The American Diabetes Association (ADA) has proposed the following treatment goals for glycosylated hemoglobin (HbA1c) and blood glucose levels (ADA, 2003r):

- HbA1c levels should be maintained at 7% or below.
- The majority of premeal **(preprandial)** blood glucose levels should be 80 to 120 mg/dL (4.4 to 6.7 mmol/L).
- Blood glucose values at bedtime should be between 100 and 140 mg/dL (5.6 to 7.8 mmol/L).

Drug Therapy. Antidiabetic drugs are indicated when a client with type 2 diabetes does not have blood glucose control with diet changes, regular exercise, and stress management. See Table 68-7 for the cost of diabetes medications.

Oral Therapy. Oral agents are prescribed after dietary control has proven insufficient or if the client is highly symptomatic.

Sulfonylurea Agents. Sulfonylurea agents are used only for clients with some remaining pancreatic beta-cell function. These drugs stimulate insulin secretion (which reduces liver glucose output and increases cell uptake of glucose) and enhance the number or sensitivity of cell receptor sites for interaction with insulin. These drugs differ in strength, overall effects, metabolism, and risk for complications (Chart 68-3).

Hypoglycemia is the most serious complication of sulfonylurea therapy. Hypoglycemic episodes are more likely to occur with chlorpropamide (Diabinese, Novo-Propamide✱) because of its long duration of action. Underweight older clients with cardiovascular, liver, or kidney impairment are more susceptible to hypoglycemia.

Other less common side effects include leukopenia, thrombocytopenia, hemolytic anemia, allergic skin reactions, and gastrointestinal (GI) effects (nausea, epigastric fullness, heartburn). In addition, many drugs can potentiate or interfere with sulfonylureas (Table 68-8 on p. 1516).

Meglitinide Analogs. Repaglinide (Prandin) has actions and adverse effects similar to those of sulfonylureas. The drug is taken before meals and has a rapid onset with a limited duration of action. Adverse effects include hypoglycemia, GI disturbances, upper respiratory tract infection, arthralgia or back pain, and headache.

Nateglinide (Starlix) lowers blood glucose by triggering insulin secretion via interaction with the adenosine triphosphate (ATP)-sensitive potassium channel on pancreatic beta cells. The drug is rapidly absorbed and stimulates insulin secretion within 20 minutes of ingestion. It is taken just before meals to control mealtime hyperglycemia and improves overall glycemic control in clients with type 2 diabetes. The major adverse effect is hypoglycemia. Clients who skip meals should also skip their scheduled dose of Starlix to reduce the risk for hypoglycemia.

Biguanides. Metformin (Glucophage) lowers glucose by decreasing liver glucose release and decreasing cellular insulin resistance. It does not stimulate insulin release. When given alone, it does not cause hypoglycemia. It should not be given to anyone with renal disease and elevated blood creatinine levels. It should be withheld for 48 hours before and after using contrast material and surgical procedures requiring anesthesia (Slagle, 2002).

Metformin can cause lactic acidosis in diabetic clients with renal insufficiency and should not be used in conditions that decrease drug clearance, such as renal insufficiency, liver disease, alcoholism, severe congestive heart failure, or in clients older than 80 years of age (Bell, 2002). The symptoms of lactic acidosis are often nonspecific. Teach the client to report symptoms of fatigue, unusual muscle pain, difficulty breathing, unusual or unexpected stomach discomfort, dizziness, light-headedness, or irregular heartbeats

Text continued on p. 1516.

CONCEPT MAP Diabetes Mellitus—Type 2

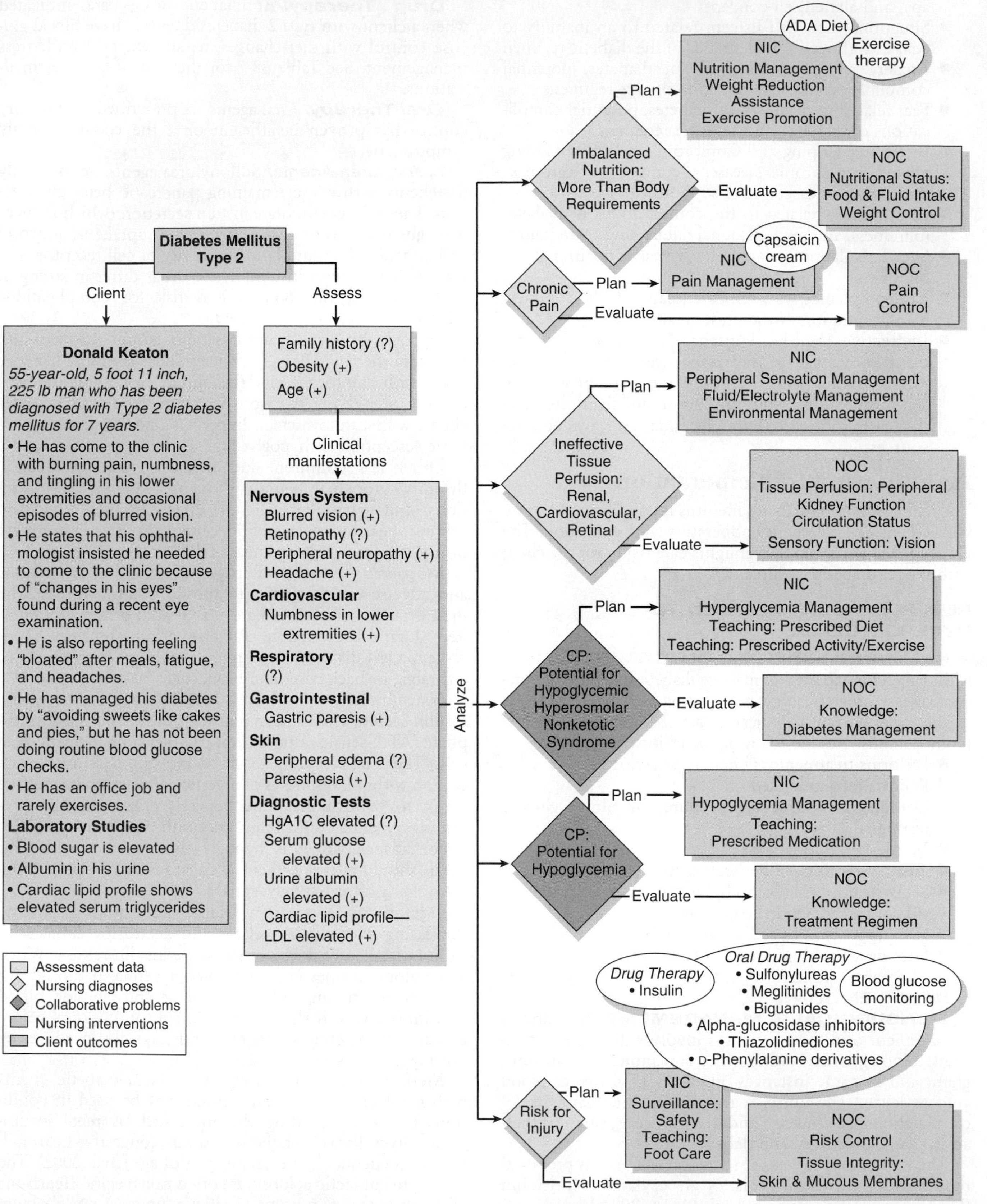

Concept Map by Elaine Bishop Kennedy, EdD, RN

TABLE 68-7 Cost of Diabetes Medications

Medications	Specific Product	Size	Price*
Humulin insulins	Humulin R	100 units/mL, 10-mL vial	$26.56
	Humulin N	100 units/mL, 10-mL vial	$26.56
	Humulin L	100 units/mL, 10-mL vial	$26.56
	Humulin U	100 units/mL, 10-mL vial	$26.56
	Humulin R U-500	500 units/mL, 20 mL vial	$191.09
	Humulin N Pen	100 units/mL, 3 mL, #5	$78.54
	Humulin 70/30 pen	70 units - 30 units/mL, 3 mL, #5	$78.54
Humalog insulin	Insulin lispro	100 units/mL, 10-mL vial	$50.09
	Humalog pen	100 units/mL, 3 mL cartridge, #5	$100.80
Novolin insulins (Novo Nordisk)	Novolin R	100 units/mL, 10-mL vial	$25.30
	Novolin N	100 units/mL, 10-mL vial	$25.30
	Novolin L	100 units/mL, 10-mL vial	$26.65
	70/30	70 units - 30 units/mL, 10-mL vial	$25.30
NovoLog insulin	Insulin aspart	100 units/mL, 10-mL vial	$50.09
Combination insulins	Humulin 50/50	50 units - 50 units/mL, 10-mL vial	$26.56
	Humulin 70/30	70 units - 30 units/mL, 10-mL vial	$26.56
	Novolin 70/30	70 units - 30 units/mL, 10-mL vial	$50.09
	Humalog mix 75/25	75 units - 25 units/mL, 10-mL vial	$50.09
Lantus	Insulin glargine	100 units/mL, 10-mL vial	$46.99
Iletin insulins	Iletin II Regular pork	100 units/mL, 10-mL vial	$47.98
	Iletin II NPH pork	100 units/mL, 10-mL vial	$47.98
	Iletin II Lente pork	100 units/mL, 10-mL vial	$47.98
Oral agents	Chlorpropamide	100 mg, # 100	$18.37
		250 mg, # 100	$38.85
	Glipizide	5 mg, # 100	$6.99
		10 mg, # 100	$9.44
	Glyburide	1.5 mg, # 100	$25.50
		3 mg, # 100	$32.02
	Glimepiride	1 mg, # 100	$28.62
		4 mg, # 100	$87.47
	Metformin	500 mg, # 100	$70.35
	Repaglinide	0.5 mg, # 100	$92.96
		2 mg, # 100	$92.96
	Acarbose	100 mg, # 100	$74.22
	Pioglitazone	15 mg, # 90	$276.89
		30 mg, # 90	$426.71
	Rosiglitazone	4 mg, # 100	$256.09
		8 mg, # 100	$473.84

Data from *2002 Drug Topics Red Book.* (2002). Montvale, NJ: Medical Economics Company.
*Average wholesale price.

CHART 68-3

DRUG THERAPY for Diabetes Mellitus: Oral Blood Glucose Lowering Agents

Drug	Dosage and Duration	Nursing Interventions	Rationales
First-Generation Sulfonylurea Agents			
Acetohexamide (Dymelor, Dimelor✱)	*Usual:* 0.25-1.5 g daily *Maximum:* 1.5 g daily *Duration:* 12-24 hr	Instruct client in measures to prevent and treat hypoglycemia.	Older, debilitated, or malnourished clients are more susceptible to hypoglycemia with acetohexamide.
		Caution clients to avoid drinking alcohol when taking acetohexamide.	Disulfiram-like reaction may occur when alcohol is consumed with acetohexamide. Symptoms include flushing of face, pulsating headache, sweating, confusion, and slurred speech. Severe reaction can cause sudden death.
Chlorpropamide (Diabinese, Novo-Propamide✱)	*Usual*: 100-500 mg q24h (take with breakfast) *Maximum*: 500 mg daily *Duration*: 24-60 hr	Instruct client in measures to prevent and treat hypoglycemia.	Chlorpropamide is associated with a high incidence of hypoglycemia. Blood glucose lowering effects can persist for long after drug is discontinued.
		Monitor weight and intake and output patterns.	Chlorpropamide may potentiate antidiuretic hormone secretion and result in the syndrome of inappropriate antidiuretic hormone secretion (SIADH).
		Caution clients to avoid drinking alcohol when taking chlorpropamide.	Alcohol, even in small amounts, can cause a disulfiram-like reaction.

Continued

CHART 68-3

DRUG THERAPY for
Diabetes Mellitus: Oral Blood Glucose Lowering Agents—*cont'd*

Drug	Dosage and Duration	Nursing Interventions	Rationales
Tolazamide (Tolinase)	*Usual:* 100-500 mg q24h (take with meals) *Maximum*: 2000 mg daily *Duration*: 12-24 hr	Administer with meals.	Taking with meals helps to avoid gastrointestinal upset.
		Caution clients to avoid drinking alcohol when taking tolazamide.	Alcohol, even in small amounts, can cause a disulfiram-like reaction.
Tolbutamide (Orinase, Mobenol✱)	*Usual:* 750-1500 mg/12-24hr *Maximum*: 3000 mg daily *Duration*: 6-10 hr	Administer 30 min before meals.	Taking 30 min before meals gives the best reduction in postmeal hyperglycemia.
		Instruct client in measures to prevent and treat hypoglycemia.	Symptoms of a hypoglycemic reaction in an older client receiving a beta blocker may be masked. Teach family to observe for subtle signs of hypoglycemia.
		Caution clients to avoid drinking alcohol when taking tolbutamide.	Alcohol, even in small amounts, can cause a disulfiram-like reaction.
Second-Generation Sulfonylurea Agents			
Glipizide		Administer 30 min before meals.	Absorption of glipizide is delayed by food.
(Glucotrol)	*Usual:* 2.5-5 mg q12-24h (30 min before meals) *Maximum:* 40 mg daily *Duration:* 12-24 hr	Instruct client in measures to prevent and treat hypoglycemia.	Hypoglycemia is more likely to occur with insufficient caloric intake.
(Glucotrol XL)	*Usual:* 5-20 mg daily *Maximum:* 40 mg daily *Duration:* 24 hr	Instruct clients taking Glucotrol XL that tablets must be swallowed whole and never crushed or chewed.	Glucotrol XL is designed to be slowly absorbed from the gastrointestinal tract. Crushing or chewing the tablet alters absorption of the drug.
Glyburide		Administer with first main meal.	Administration with food helps reduce gastrointestinal side effects.
(DiaBeta Micronase✱)	*Usual:* 1.25-20 mg daily with meals (single or divided doses) *Maximum:* 20 mg daily *Duration:* 24 hr	Instruct client in measures to prevent and treat hypoglycemia.	Hypoglycemia is more likely to occur with insufficient caloric intake.
(Glynase PresTabs)	*Usual:* 0.75-12 mg daily (divide doses >6 mg) *Maximum:* 12 mg daily *Duration:* 24 hr		
Glimepiride (Amaryl)	*Usual:* 1-4 mg once daily *Maximum:* 8 mg daily *Duration:* 24 hr	Administer with first main meal. Instruct client in measures to prevent and treat hypoglycemia.	Debilitated or malnourished clients and clients with impaired renal or hepatic function are more sensitive to blood glucose–lowering effects of glimepiride.
Meglitinide Analogs			
Repaglinide (Prandin)	*Usual:* 0.5-4 mg daily *Maximum:* 16 mg daily *Duration:* Less than 4 hr	Administer 30 min before meals.	Taking drug 30 min before meals gives the best reduction in postmeal hyperglycemia.
		Instruct client to omit medication when skipping a meal. Instruct client to add a dose if an extra meal is eaten.	Drug reduces the risk of hypoglycemia. Duration of action of repaglinide is 4 hr. A dose of medication needs to be available for each meal eaten.
		Instruct client in measures to prevent and treat hypoglycemia.	Older, debilitated, or malnourished clients are more susceptible to hypoglycemia with repaglinide.
		Store at 15°-30° C (59°-86° F) in a tightly closed container and protect from moisture and heat.	Proper storage prevents deterioration of the drug.
Nateglinide (Starlix)	*Usual:* 60-120 mg before meals *Maximum:* Optimal dose not determined *Duration:* 4 hr	Administer 1-30 min before meals.	Stimulates rapid secretion of insulin to reduce increases in blood glucose levels that occur soon after eating.
		Instruct client to omit medication when skipping a meal. Instruct client to add a dose if an extra meal is eaten.	Drug reduces the risk of hypoglycemia. Duration of action of nateglinide is 4 hr. A dose of medication needs to be available for each meal eaten.

CHART 68-3

DRUG THERAPY for Diabetes Mellitus: Oral Blood Glucose Lowering Agents—*cont'd*

Drug	Dosage and Duration	Nursing Interventions	Rationales
Biguanides			
Metformin		Administer with food.	Slow titration adjustment and administration with food reduces gastrointestinal side effects.
(Glucophage)	*Starting dose:* 500 mg twice daily or 850 mg once daily with meals. *Maintenance dose:* Individualized *Maximum:* 2550 mg daily in divided doses	Monitor renal function.	Renal impairment increases the risk of lactic acidosis. Metformin is contraindicated in renal disease (serum creatinine >1.5 mg/dL in males, >1.4 mg/dL in females).
		Withhold metformin for 48 hr before use of iodinated contrast materials used in certain radiographic studies.	Iodinated contrast materials can alter renal function and increase the risk for lactic acidosis. Metformin therapy is restarted when renal function has returned to normal.
		Monitor cardiopulmonary status throughout therapy.	Conditions associated with hypoxia increase the risk for lactic acidosis.
(Glucophage XR [extended release])	*Starting dose:* 500 mg daily with largest meal *Maintenance dose:* Individualized *Maximum:* 2000 mg daily	Instruct the client taking metformin to report symptoms of lactic acidosis: malaise, unusual muscle pain, respiratory distress, increasing somnolence, and abdominal distress.	Onset of lactic acidosis is subtle and accompanied by nonspecific symptoms.
		Instruct clients taking metformin to report any illness that causes severe vomiting, diarrhea, or fever.	Precipitating events for lactic acidosis include hypoxemia, dehydration, and sepsis.
		Instruct clients taking Glucophage XL that tablets must be swallowed whole and never crushed or chewed.	Glucophage XL is designed to be slowly absorbed from the gastrointestinal tract. Crushing or chewing the tablet alters absorption of the drug.
Alpha-Glucosidase Inhibitors			
Acarbose (Precose)	*Usual:* 50-100 mg three times daily *Maximum:* 100 mg three times daily *Duration:* 2-4 hr	Instruct client to take with the first bite of each of the three main meals.	Acarbose must be taken at the beginning of a meal to be fully effective.
		Monitor renal function.	Drug may accumulate in clients with renal dysfunction; drug not recommended for clients with serum creatinine >2 mg/dL.
		Monitor for abdominal pain, diarrhea, and flatulence.	Gastrointestinal side effects are very common. Symptoms can be reduced by slow titration adjustment of dose.
		Monitor liver function tests. Emphasize need to report symptoms of unexplained nausea, vomiting, abdominal pain, fatigue, anorexia, or dark urine.	Acarbose is associated with an elevation in serum transaminase levels.
		Instruct clients receiving acarbose and other hypoglycemic medications to treat hypoglycemia with glucose tablets, glucose gel, or low-fat milk.	Acarbose does not cause hypoglycemia when given alone. Hypoglycemia caused by other agents should be treated with oral dextrose. Sucrose (table sugar or candy bars) will not reverse symptoms of hypoglycemia due to the actions of acarbose.
		Instruct client to store the medication according to manufacturer's directions.	Remove from foil wrapper immediately before administration to prevent deterioration of acarbose.
Miglitol (Glyset)	*Usual:* 50 mg three times daily *Maximum:* 100 mg three times daily *Duration:* 2-4 hr	Instruct client to take with the first bite of each main meal.	Miglitol must be taken at the beginning of a meal to be fully effective.
		Monitor renal function.	Drug may accumulate in clients with renal dysfunction; drug is not recommended for clients with serum creatinine >2 mg/dL.
		Monitor for abdominal pain, diarrhea, and flatulence.	Gastrointestinal side effects are very common. Symptoms can be reduced by slow adjustment of dose.

Continued

CHART 68-3

DRUG THERAPY for
Diabetes Mellitus: Oral Blood Glucose Lowering Agents—*cont'd*

Drug	Dosage and Duration	Nursing Interventions	Rationales
Miglitol (Glyset)—*cont'd*		Monitor liver function tests. Emphasize need to report symptoms of unexplained nausea, vomiting, abdominal pain, fatigue, anorexia, or dark urine.	Miglitol is associated with an elevation in serum transaminase levels.
		Instruct clients receiving miglitol and other hypoglycemic medications to treat hypoglycemia with glucose tablets, glucose gel or low-fat milk. Treat hypoglycemia symptoms with dextrose.	Miglitol does not cause hypoglycemia when given alone. Hypoglycemia caused by other agents should be treated with oral dextrose. Sucrose (table sugar or candy bars) will not reverse symptoms of hypoglycemia due to the actions of miglitol.
Thiazolidinediones			
Pioglitazone (Actos)	*Starting dose:* 500 mg daily with largest meal *Usual:* 15 to 30 mg daily with or without food *Maximum*: 45 mg daily	Emphasize need for liver function tests as recommended. Emphasize need to report symptoms of unexplained nausea, vomiting, abdominal pain, fatigue, anorexia, or dark urine.	Rare cases of liver failure have occurred with pioglitazone. Liver function tests are measured at the start of therapy and at regular times thereafter.
		Advise women of childbearing age to use adequate contraception.	Administration of pioglitazone with certain oral contraceptives may reduce the plasma concentration of the oral contraceptive.
		Monitor weight and assess for edema.	Major side effects are fluid retention, weight gain, and congestive heart failure.
Rosiglitazone (Avandia)	*Usual:* 4 mg daily with or without food *Maximum:* 8 mg daily	Emphasize need for liver function tests as recommended. Emphasize need to report symptoms of unexplained nausea, vomiting, abdominal pain, fatigue, anorexia, or dark urine.	Rare cases of liver failure have occurred with rosiglitazone. Liver function tests are measured at the start of therapy and at regular times thereafter.
		Advise women of childbearing age to use adequate contraception.	Administration of rosiglitazone with certain oral contraceptives may reduce the plasma concentration of the oral contraceptive.
		Monitor weight and assess for edema.	Major side effects are fluid retention, weight gain, and congestive heart failure.
Fixed Combinations			
Glucovance (Glyburide and metformin) 1.25 mg/250 mg 2.5 mg/500 mg 5 mg/500 mg	*Initial therapy*: 1.25 mg/250 mg once or twice daily with meals *Maintenance*: Individualized *Maximum*: 20 mg glyburide and 2000 mg metformin daily *Previously treated clients*: 2.5 mg/500 mg or 5 mg/500 mg twice daily with meals. *Maintenance*: Individualized *Maximum*: 20 mg glyburide and 2000 mg metformin daily	Give in divided doses with meals.	Slow adjustment and administration with food minimizes hypoglycemia and gastrointestinal effects.
		Instruct client in measures to prevent and treat hypoglycemia.	Hypoglycemia can occur in clients with insufficient oral intake, excess exercise, or alcohol intake, or those who are older and debilitated.
		Monitor renal and hepatic function.	Renal or hepatic impairment increases blood levels of both drugs and increases the risk of hypoglycemia and lactic acidosis. Metformin is contraindicated in renal disease (serum creatinine >1.5 mg/dL in males, >1.4 mg/dL in females).

CHART 68-3

DRUG THERAPY for
Diabetes Mellitus: Oral Blood Glucose Lowering Agents—*cont'd*

Drug	Dosage and Duration	Nursing Interventions	Rationales
Avandamet (Rosiglitazone and metformin) 1 mg/500 mg 2 mg/500 mg 4 mg/500 mg	*Previously on metformin alone*: add 4 mg daily to current regimen *Previously on rosiglitazone alone*: add metformin 1000 mg to current regimen *Maximum*: 8 mg rosiglitazone and 2000 mg metformin daily	Give in divided doses with meals.	Slow adjustment and administration with food minimizes hypoglycemia and gastrointestinal effects.
		Monitor renal and hepatic function.	Rare cases of liver failure have occurred with rosiglitazone. Liver function tests are measured at the start of therapy and at regular times thereafter. Metformin is contraindicated in renal disease (serum creatinine >1.5 mg/dL in males, >1.4 mg/dL in females).
		Monitor weight and assess for edema.	Major side effects are fluid retention, weight gain, and congestive heart failure.
		Monitor cardiopulmonary status throughout therapy. Instruct the client taking metformin to report symptoms of lactic acidosis: malaise, unusual muscle pain, respiratory distress, increasing somnolence, and abdominal distress.	Conditions associated with hypoxia increase the risk for lactic acidosis. Onset of lactic acidosis is subtle and accompanied by nonspecific symptoms.
		Instruct clients taking metformin to report any illness that causes severe vomiting, diarrhea, or fever.	Precipitating events for lactic acidosis include hypoxemia, dehydration, and sepsis.
		Instruct client in measures to prevent and treat hypoglycemia.	Older, debilitated, or malnourished clients are more susceptible to hypoglycemia.
		Advise women of childbearing age to use adequate contraception.	Administration of rosiglitazone with certain oral contraceptives may reduce the plasma concentration of the oral contraceptive.
Metaglip (Glipizide and metformin) 2.5 mg/250 mg 2.5 mg/500 mg 5 mg/500 mg	*Initial therapy*: 2.5 mg/250 mg once or twice daily with meals. *Maintenance*: Individualized *Maximum*: 20 mg glipizide and 2000 mg metformin daily *Previously treated clients*: 2.5 mg/500 mg or 5 mg/500 mg twice daily with meals *Maintenance*: Individualized *Maximum*: 20 mg glipizide and 2000 mg metformin daily	Give in divided doses with meals.	Slow adjustment and administration with food minimizes hypoglycemia and gastrointestinal effects.
		Instruct client in measures to prevent and treat hypoglycemia.	Hypoglycemia can occur in clients with insufficient oral intake, excess exercise, or alcohol intake, or in those who are older and debilitated.
		Monitor renal and hepatic function.	Renal or hepatic impairment increases blood levels of both drugs and increases the risk of hypoglycemia and lactic acidosis. Metformin is contraindicated in renal disease (serum creatinine >1.5 mg/dL in males, >1.4 mg/dL in females).

TABLE 68-8 Drug Interactions with Sulfonylurea Agents

Potentiate Hypoglycemia	Worsen Hyperglycemia
Allopurinol (Zyloprim)	Amphetamines
Ammonium chloride	Asparaginase (Elspar)
Androgens (testosterone [Testoderm])	Bumetanide (Bumex)
Angiotensin-converting agents (captopril [Capoten], enalapril [Vasotec])	Calcium channel blockers (diltiazem, nifedipine)
Anticoagulants, oral (warfarin)	Cholestyramine (Questran)
Antifungal azoles, systemic (fluconazole [Diflucan], miconazole [Monistat])	Chlorthalidone (Hygroton)
Barbiturates	Clonidine (Catapres)
Beta-adrenergic blocking agents (atenolol, propranolol)	Corticosteroids (prednisone)
Bromocriptine	Corticotropin (adrenocorticotropin hormone)
Calcium channel blockers (verapamil)	Danazol (Danocrine)
Clofibrate (Atromid-S)	Diazoxide, parenteral (Hyperstat)
Disopyramide (Norpace)	Dextrothyroxine (Choloxin)
Ethanol	Diuretics, thiazide (hydrochlorothiazide)
Fenfluramine (Pondimin)	Estrogen (Estrace, Premarin)
Fluoroquinolone anti-infectives (ciprofloxacin)	Estrogen-progesterone-containing oral contraceptives (Brevicon, Depo-Provera, Estrostep)
Guanethidine (Ismelin)	Furosemide (Lasix)
Histamine H_2 antagonists (cimetidine [Tagamet], ranitidine [Zantac])	Gemfibrozil (Lopid)
Monoamine oxidase (MAO) inhibitors (phenelzine [Nardil])	Glucagon
Methyldopa (Aldomet)	Isoniazid (INH)
NSAIDs (indomethacin [Indocin], ibuprofen [Advil])	Lithium (Lithobid)
Octreotide (Sandostatin)	Morphine (morphine sulfate)
Probenecid (Benemid, Probalan)	Nicotinic acid (Nicolar)
Pyridoxine (vitamin B_6)	Pentamidine (pentamidine isethionate)
Quinidine (quinidine gluconate)	Phenothiazines (prochlorperazine [Compazine], trifluoperazine [Stelazine])
Quinine (quinine sulfate)	Phenytoin (Dilantin)
Sulfinpyrazone (Anturane)	Rifampin (Rifadin)
Sulfonamides (trimethoprim/sulfamethoxazole [Bactrim], sulfisoxazole [Gantrisin])	Salicylates (large doses)
Tetracycline	Thyroid hormones (liothyronine [Cytomel], levothyroxine [Levothroid, Synthroid])

to the primary care provider. Instruct clients to take metformin with meals to reduce GI effects. Caution against excessive alcohol intake because alcohol increases the risk for lactic acidosis.

Alpha-Glucosidase Inhibitors. Alpha-glucosidase inhibitors reduce hyperglycemia after meals by slowing intestinal digestion and absorption of carbohydrate. These agents inhibit enzymes in the intestinal tract, delaying carbohydrate digestion. The prolonged digestion time reduces the rate of glucose absorption and lowers blood glucose levels. Total glucose absorption is unchanged, and there is no weight loss or gain. The most common side effects are flatulence, diarrhea, and abdominal discomfort. There are two drugs in this class. Acarbose (Precose) is well tolerated when started at a low dose (25 mg once daily to three times daily with meals) and increased slowly. At higher doses, poor carbohydrate absorption can occur. Miglitol (Glyset) should be taken three times daily with the first bite of each main meal.

Alpha-glucosidase inhibitors do not cause hypoglycemia unless given with sulfonylureas or insulin. Because alpha-glucosidase inhibitors delay carbohydrate absorption and interfere with the conversion of complex sugars to glucose, many of the standard products used to treat hypoglycemia result in a delayed blood glucose response (see Chart 68-14). Alpha-glucosidase inhibitors do not inhibit absorption of glucose or lactose. Instruct clients to use oral glucose tablets, glucose gel, or low-fat milk to treat hypoglycemia. Severe hypoglycemia may require glucose infusion or glucagon injection.

Thiazolidinedione Antidiabetic Agents. Thiazolidinediones enhance insulin action, thus promoting glucose utilization in peripheral tissues. They are known as "insulin sensitizers" and include rosiglitazone (Avandia) and pioglitazone (Actos). These drugs improve sensitivity to insulin in muscle and fat tissue and inhibit gluconeogenesis. They can be used with a sulfonylurea or insulin to improve blood glucose control because their mechanisms of action are different. Clients taking these drugs should have periodic liver function studies performed because of the potential liver damage.

All drugs in this class have effects on serum lipid levels. Other side effects of these drugs include infection, headache, peripheral edema, and pain. They can reduce the effectiveness of oral contraceptives. About 15% of clients taking these drugs gain weight. Ensure that these clients receive instructions about following a low-sodium diet.

Combination Agents. Some oral agents combine drugs with different mechanisms of action. Glucovance, for example, combines glyburide with metformin. Combining drugs with different mechanisms of action may be highly effective in maintaining desired blood glucose control. Some clients may need a combination of oral agents and insulin to control blood glucose levels.

Drug Administration. Drugs are started at the lowest effective dose and increased every 1 to 2 weeks until the client reaches acceptable blood glucose control or the maximum dosage. If the maximal dosage does not control blood glucose levels, a different oral agent is used. Insulin therapy is indicated when blood glucose cannot be controlled after the use of two or three different oral agents.

Antidiabetic drugs are not a substitute for dietary modification and exercise. Teach the client about the need for continuing dietary restrictions and regular exercise while taking antidiabetic drugs. To avoid adverse drug interactions, teach the client to consult with the primary care provider or pharmacist before using any over-the-counter drugs.

Drug Selection. The choice of oral antidiabetic drug is based on cost, the client's ability to manage multiple drug doses, and the client's age and response to the drugs. Sulfonylureas are less expensive than other oral antidiabetic agents, can be taken once daily, and have few side effects. Metformin (Glucophage) can have more GI side effects than sulfonylureas. Acarbose must be taken before each meal.

Beta-cell function in type 2 diabetes often declines over time, reducing the effectiveness of some oral antidiabetic drugs. The treatment regimen for the client with type 2 diabetes may eventually require insulin therapy either alone or with oral agents.

Insulin Therapy. Insulin therapy is needed for type 1 diabetes and is used frequently for type 2 diabetes. The safety of insulin therapy in older clients may be affected by reduced vision, mobility and coordination problems, and decreased memory. There are many types of insulin and regimens, all aimed at achieving normal blood glucose levels.

TABLE 68-9 Insulin Preparations

Type	Source
Insulin Analog	
■ Humalog (Lilly)	DNA technology
■ Insulin aspart (Novo Nordisk)	DNA technology
■ Insulin glulisine (Aventis)	DNA technology
Short-Acting Insulin	
Insulin injection (regular crystalline insulin):	
■ Iletin II R (Lilly)	Pork (purified)
Insulin human injection (regular human insulin):	
■ Humulin R (Lilly)	DNA technology
■ Novolin R (Novo Nordisk)	DNA technology
■ Velosulin BR (Novo Nordisk)	Semisynthetic
■ Velosulin BR (Novo Nordisk)	DNA technology
Concentrated Insulin	
Insulin injection (regular crystalline insulin):	
■ Iletin II U-500 (Lilly)	Pork (purified)
Intermediate-Acting Insulin	
Isophane insulin suspension (NPH insulin):	
■ Iletin II (Lilly)	Pork (purified)
■ Humulin N (Lilly)	DNA technology
■ Novolin N (Novo Nordisk)	DNA technology
Insulin zinc suspension (Lente insulin):	
■ Iletin II (Lilly)	Pork (purified)
■ Humulin L (Lilly)	DNA technology
■ Novolin L (Novo Nordisk)	DNA technology
Fixed-Combination Insulin	
■ Humulin 50/50 (Lilly)	DNA technology
■ Humulin 70/30 (Lilly)	DNA technology
■ Novolin 70/30 (Novo Nordisk)	DNA technology
■ Humalog Mix 75/25	DNA technology
Long-Acting Insulin	
■ Humulin U (Lilly)	DNA technology
■ Insulin glargine (Aventis)	DNA technology

Types of Insulin. Insulin is obtained from animal sources (beef or pork pancreas), combined animal sources and semisynthetic human insulin, and synthetic human insulin (made through recombinant DNA technology). There are differences in strength and onset of action between human and animal-source insulins. Thus, dose and timing need adjustment when a client changes from one type of insulin to another. Human insulin has a more rapid onset of action, a shorter peak action, and a shorter duration of action than animal-source insulin. Human insulin is preferred for pregnant women or women considering pregnancy, clients with allergies or resistance to animal-source insulins, clients beginning insulin therapy, and clients who use insulin intermittently (ADA, 2003k).

Rapid-, short-, intermediate-, and long-acting forms of insulin can be injected separately and some can be mixed in the same syringe. Insulin is available in 100 units/mL (U-100) and 500 units/mL (U-500). U-500 is used only in rare cases of insulin resistance. U-500 and all analogs are the only insulins that need a prescription.

Teach the client that the insulin types, the injection technique, the site of injection, and the individual response can all affect the absorption, onset, degree, and duration of insulin activity. Reinforce that changing insulins may affect blood glucose control and should be done only under careful supervision (ADA, 2003k). Table 68-9 reviews the types and sources of insulin preparations, and Table 68-10 outlines the time activity of subcutaneous human insulin.

Insulin Regimens. Insulin regimens try to duplicate the normal release pattern of insulin from the pancreas. The pancreas produces a constant (basal) amount of insulin that balances liver glucose production with glucose use and maintains normal blood glucose levels between meals. The pancreas also produces additional (prandial) insulin, stimulated by food, that prevents blood glucose elevations after meals. The insulin dose required for blood glucose control varies among clients. A usual starting dose is between 0.5 and 1 unit/kg of body weight per day. For multiple-dose regimens or continuous subcutaneous insulin infusion (CSII), basal insulin makes up about 40% to 50% of the total daily dosage, with the remainder divided into premeal doses of regular insulin. Dosage adjustments are based on the results of blood glucose monitoring. Because the rate of absorption is slowed by increasing the dosage, adjustments in dosage should be made no more than every 3 to 4 days.

Basal insulin coverage can be provided by NPH insulin. Humulin U Ultralente insulin provides a lower basal rate and may be used instead of NPH insulin for a client with frequent hypoglycemic episodes. Insulin glargine (Lantus), a long-acting insulin analog, is available for once-daily injection for basal insulin coverage. The client determines the effect of long-acting insulin by monitoring fasting blood glucose values. Insulin protocols (regimens or programs) are shown in Figure 68-4.

SINGLE DAILY INJECTION PROTOCOL. Many clients inject insulin only once daily. This protocol may include only intermediate-acting insulin or combined short- and intermediate-acting insulin. A single dose of intermediate-acting insulin may not match the blood insulin level with food intake. When fasting glucose levels are elevated, a multiple-injection protocol should be considered.

TWO-DOSE PROTOCOL. Combinations of short- and intermediate-acting insulin are injected twice daily. Two thirds of the daily dose is given before breakfast and one third before the evening meal. At first, intermediate-acting and regular insulin are usually given in a 2:1 ratio, and the evening (or bedtime) dose is given in a 1:1 ratio. Changes in these ratios are based on results of blood glucose monitoring.

THREE-DOSE PROTOCOL. A combination of short- and intermediate-acting insulin is given before breakfast, short-acting insulin is given before the evening meal, and intermediate-acting insulin is given at bedtime. Giving intermediate-acting insulin at bedtime lowers fasting and after-breakfast blood glucose levels. This schedule avoids nighttime hypoglycemia but may not provide enough coverage for the noon meal (Franz, 2001).

FOUR-DOSE PROTOCOL. Giving short-acting insulin 30 minutes before meals allows the greatest amount of insulin to be present during the time of greatest insulin need. Basal insulin is provided by twice-daily injection of intermediate-acting insulin or a once daily injection of long-acting insulin. Injection of premeal short-acting insulin based on anticipated carbohydrate intake allows some clients with diabetes to have more flexibility in meal timing and size. Insulin lispro should be given within 15 minutes of eating a meal; action usually peaks in 30 to 90 minutes. Because this dura-

TABLE 68-10 Time Activity of Subcutaneous Human Insulin

Preparation	Brand	Onset (hr)	Peak (hr)	Duration (hr)
Rapid Acting				
Insulin aspart injection	NovoLog	0.25	1-3	3-5
Insulin lispro injection	Humalog	0.25	0.5-1.5	3-4
Insulin glulisine injection	Apidra	0.3	0.5-1.5	5
Short Acting				
Regular human insulin injection	Humulin R Novolin R	0.5 0.5	2-4 2.5-5	6-8 8
Buffered regular human insulin injection	Velosulin BR	0.5	1-3	8
Intermediate Acting				
Human insulin isophane suspension	NPH	1.5	4-12	24
Human insulin zinc suspension	Lente	2.5	7-15	22
Long Acting				
Human insulin extended zinc suspension	Ultralente	4-6	8-20	28
Insulin glargine injection	Lantus	2-4	None	24
Combination Insulin				
70% Insulin aspart protamine suspension/30% insulin aspart injection	NovoLog Mix 70/30	0.25	1-4	24
75% Insulin lispro protamine suspension/25% insulin lispro injection	Humalog Mix 75/25	0.25	1-2	24
70% Human insulin isophane suspension (NPH)/30% human insulin injection (regular)	Humulin 70/30 Novolin 70/30	0.5 0.5	2-12 2-12	24 24
50% Human insulin isophane suspension (NPH)/50% human insulin injection (regular)	Humulin 50/50	0.5	3-5	24

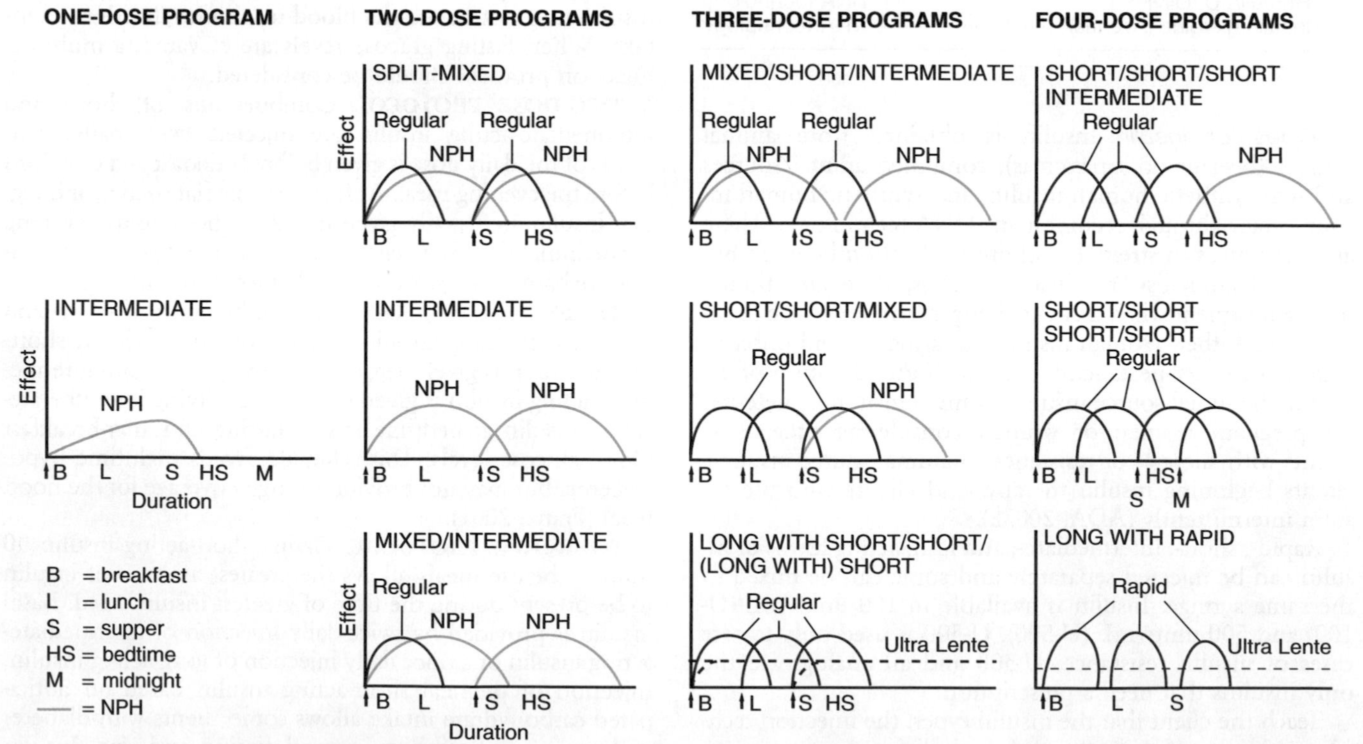

Figure 68-4 ■ Insulin regimens. One injection a day of short-acting or intermediate-acting insulin may be enough to control blood glucose levels. However, split doses (two, three, or four injections of the daily dose) or split mixed doses (a mixture of short-acting and longer acting insulins) may give better control.

tion of action is short, the client taking insulin lispro also needs longer-acting insulin for basal insulin requirements.

COMBINATION THERAPY. A combination of oral agents and intermediate-acting insulin is given to clients with type 2 diabetes who do not have blood glucose control with oral agents alone. Obese clients with higher fasting C-peptide levels are still making some insulin and may be more likely to respond to combination therapy than to single therapy.

INTENSIFIED THERAPY REGIMENS. Intensified regimens are a basal dose of intermediate-acting or long-acting insulin and a bolus dose of short-acting or rapid-acting insulin designed to bring the next blood glucose value into the target range. The client's blood glucose patterns determine insulin dosage. Frequency of blood glucose monitoring is based on the timed action of short- and intermediate-acting insulins and may occur as often as eight times daily. Blood glucose testing 1 to 2 hours after meals and within 10 minutes before the next meal helps determine the adequacy of the bolus dose. The client determines the effects of basal insulin by monitoring pre-evening meal and fasting blood glucose values. Blood glucose values at 3 AM detect nighttime hypoglycemia and indicate adequacy of both short- and intermediate-acting insulin doses.

Clients on intensified insulin regimens need extensive education to achieve target blood glucose values. They need to know how to adjust insulin doses and understand nutrition therapy to maintain dietary flexibility and target blood glucose values. Clients must also be able to perform accurate blood glucose monitoring so that therapy decisions can be based on accurate data.

Pharmacokinetics of Insulin. The action of insulin to move glucose into the cells after insulin injection depends on physical factors and injection techniques.

INJECTION SITE. Figure 68-5 shows common insulin injection sites. The site of injection affects the speed of insulin absorption. Absorption is fastest in the abdomen, followed by the deltoid, thigh, and buttocks. Rotating injection sites prevents lipohypertrophy (increased fat deposits in the skin) or lipoatrophy (loss of fatty tissue, leaving an uneven appearance). Rotation *within* one anatomic site is preferred to rotation from one site to another to prevent day-to-day changes in absorption. The abdomen (except for a 2-inch radius around the navel) is the preferred site because it provides the most rapid insulin absorption.

ABSORPTION RATE. Insulin properties affect its absorption. The longer the duration of action, the more unpredictable is absorption. Ultralente has less consistent absorption than shorter-acting insulins. The larger the dose of insulin, the more prolonged the absorption. Factors that increase blood flow from the injection site, such as local application of heat, massage of the area, and exercise of the injected area, increase insulin absorption. Scarred sites often become favorite injection sites because they are less sensitive to pain. Areas of lipohypertrophy usually slow the rate of insulin absorption (ADA, 2003k).

INJECTION DEPTH. Injections are made into the subcutaneous tissue. Most clients lightly grasp a fold of skin and inject at a 90-degree angle. Aspiration for blood is not necessary. A thin person may need to pinch the skin and inject at a 45-degree angle to avoid intramuscular (IM) injection. IM injection has a faster absorption and is not recommended for routine insulin use (ADA, 2003k). Assess the older client's ability to inject insulin and arrange for assistance when self-care is no longer possible.

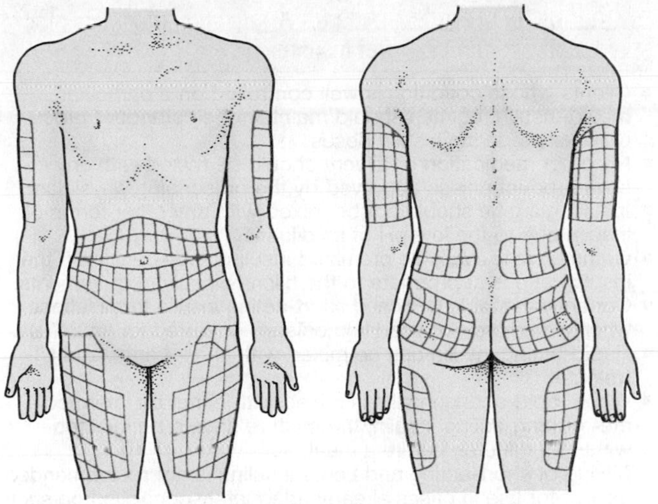

Figure 68-5 ■ Common insulin injection sites.

TIME OF INJECTION. Injecting regular insulin 30 minutes before meals provides a greater amount of plasma free insulin at mealtime. Eating within a few minutes after (or before) injecting short-acting insulin reduces the ability of insulin to prevent rapid rises in blood glucose after meals and may increase the risk for delayed hypoglycemia (Kissin & Katzeff, 2002). Humalog (insulin lispro), NovoLog (insulin aspart), and insulin glulisine (Apidra) should be given 5 to 15 minutes before a meal.

MIXING INSULINS. Caution clients that mixing different types of insulin can change the timing of peak action. Mixtures of short- and intermediate-acting insulins produce a more normal blood glucose response in some clients than does a single dose. The response to mixed insulin may differ from the response to the same insulins given separately.

When rapid-acting (Humalog or NovoLog) or short-acting (regular) insulin is mixed with a longer-acting insulin, draw the shorter-acting dose into the syringe first. This procedure prevents contamination of the shorter-acting insulin vial with the longer-acting insulin. Short-acting and NPH insulins may be used immediately when mixed, or they may be stored (ADA, 2003k). *Insulin glargine (Lantus) must not be diluted or mixed with any other insulin or solution.* Mixing clouds the solution and makes the onset of action and peak effect time less predictable. Follow American Diabetes Association (ADA) guidelines for mixing insulins (Table 68-11).

Complications of Insulin Therapy. Hypoglycemia from insulin excess has many causes. Its effects and treatment are discussed later under Potential for Hypoglycemia, p. 1539.

Lipoatrophy is a loss of fat tissue in areas of repeated injection that results from an immune reaction to impurities in beef or pork insulin. Treatment consists of injection of human insulin at the edge of the atrophied area. **Lipohypertrophy** is an increased swelling of fat that occurs at the site of repeated insulin injections. The overlying skin has decreased sensitivity, and the area can become large and unsightly. Treatment consists of rotating the injection site among different body areas (White & Hirsch, 2000). Instruct

TABLE 68-11 American Diabetes Association Guidelines for the Mixing of Insulins

- Clients whose condition is well controlled on a particular mixed-insulin regimen should maintain their standard procedure for preparing insulin doses.
- No other medication or diluent should be mixed with any insulin product unless approved by the prescribing physician.
- Insulin glargine should not be mixed with any other forms of insulin due to the low pH of its diluent.
- Commercially available premixed insulins may be used if the insulin ratio is appropriate to the client's insulin requirements.
- Currently available NPH and short-acting insulin formulations when mixed may be used immediately or stored for future use.
- Rapid-acting insulin can be mixed with NPH, Lente, and Ultralente.
- When rapid-acting insulin is mixed with either an intermediate- or long-acting insulin, the mixture should be injected within 15 minutes before a meal.
- Mixing of short-acting and Lente insulins is not recommended except for use in cases already adequately controlled on such a mixture. If short-acting and Lente mixtures are to be used, the client should standardize the interval between mixing and injection.
- Phosphate-buffered insulins (e.g., NPH) should not be mixed with Lente insulins.
- Insulin formulations may change; therefore, the manufacturer should be consulted when their recommendations appear to conflict with the American Diabetes Association guidelines.

Data from American Diabetes Association. (2003). Position statement: Insulin administration. *Diabetes Care 26*(Suppl. 1), 121-124.

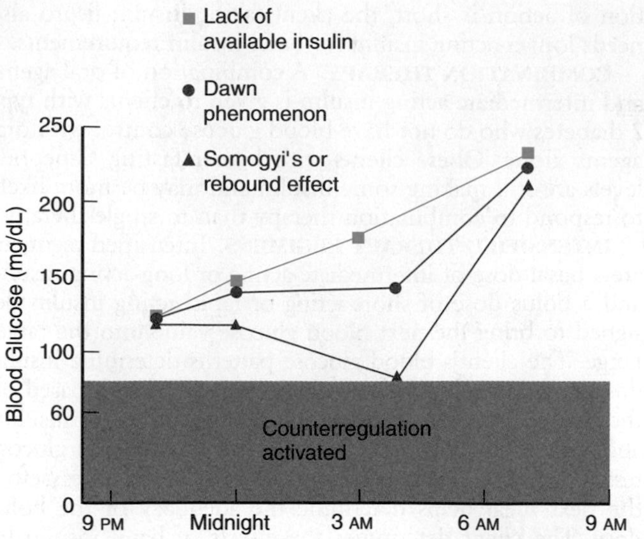

Figure 68-6 ■ Three blood glucose phenomena in diabetic clients.

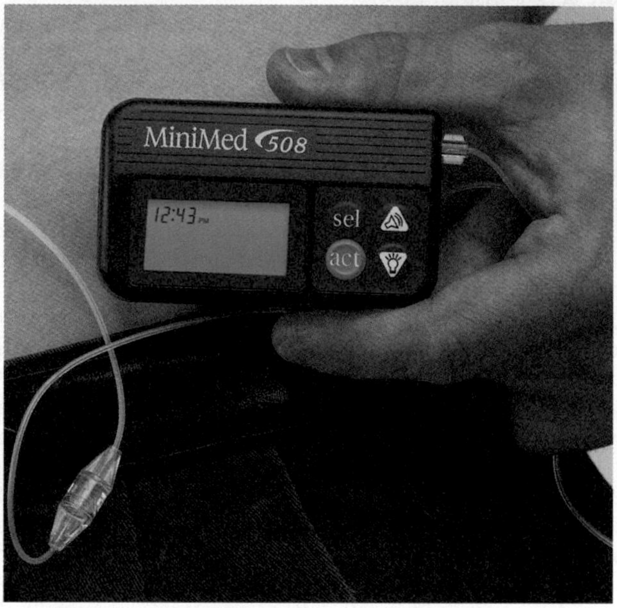

Figure 68-7 ■ External insulin pump. (Courtesy Medtronic MiniMed, Inc., Northridge, CA.)

clients who take insulin to rotate injection sites to prevent lipohypertrophy.

Two conditions of fasting hyperglycemia can occur (Figure 68-6). **Dawn phenomenon** results from a nighttime release of growth hormone that causes blood glucose elevations at about 5 to 6 AM. Dawn phenomenon is treated by providing more insulin for the overnight period (e.g., giving the evening dose of intermediate-acting insulin at 10 PM). **Somagyi's phenomenon** is morning hyperglycemia from the effective counterregulatory response to nighttime hypoglycemia. Somagyi's phenomenon is treated by ensuring adequate dietary intake at bedtime and evaluating the insulin dose and exercise programs to prevent conditions that lead to hypoglycemia. Both phenomena are diagnosed by blood glucose monitoring during the night. Help identify these problems and educate the client and family about management.

Alternative Methods of Insulin Administration. Many methods of insulin delivery are available in addition to traditional intermittent subcutaneous injections.

CONTINUOUS SUBCUTANEOUS INFUSION OF INSULIN. Continuous subcutaneous infusion of a basal dose of insulin (CSII) with increases in insulin at mealtimes is more effective in controlling blood glucose levels than a multiple-injection schedule. CSII allows for flexibility in meal timing, because if a meal is skipped, the mealtime dose of insulin is not given. CSII is given by an externally worn pump containing a syringe and reservoir with rapid- or short-acting insulin and is connected to the client by an infusion set. Teach the client to adjust the amount of insulin received based on data from blood glucose monitoring. Both Humalog (lispro) and NovoLog (insulin aspart) are appropriate for insulin infusion pumps (Figure 68-7).

Skin infections occur when the infusion site is not cleaned or the needle is not changed every 3 days. When the client is receiving rapid-acting insulin and has normal blood glucose levels, stopping the infusion quickly results in hyperglycemia. CSII may lead to more frequent and more severe ketoacidosis than other methods of insulin delivery. Ketoacidosis is related to inexperience in using the pump, infection, accidental cessation of insulin infusion, infusion set obstruction, or mechanical pump problems. Buffered insulin may be used to prevent precipitation of insulin crystals in the catheter. Stress the importance of regular testing for ketones.

Clients using CSII need intensive education. Because of the risk for hypoglycemia or hyperglycemia, the client must perform all the following functions to ensure accurate insulin delivery. Teach the client to operate the pump, adjust the settings, and respond appropriately to alarms. Removing

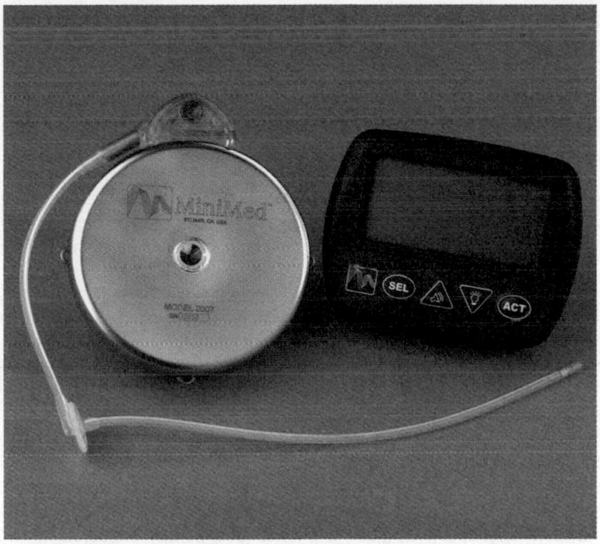

Figure 68-8 ■ Internal insulin pump. (Courtesy Medtronic MiniMed, Inc., Northridge, CA.)

the pump for any length of time can result in hyperglycemia. Provide supplemental insulin schedules for times when the pump is not operational. CSII is more costly than traditional insulin injections, and not all costs are covered by insurance.

IMPLANTED INSULIN PUMPS. Pumps are implanted in the peritoneal cavity, where insulin is absorbed by local blood vessels in a manner similar to that of natural insulin release (Figure 68-8). The pump is surgically implanted in a subcutaneous pocket in the lower abdomen. The pump reservoir is refilled with U-400 insulin every 1 or 2 months. Complications of implanted insulin pumps (IIPs) are catheter blockage, inflammation in the subcutaneous pocket, and mechanical pump failure. Because mechanical problems with the pump, catheter, and insulin delivery remain, the implantable pump is not widely available.

INJECTION DEVICES. In addition to traditional insulin syringes, injection devices include a needleless system and a pen-type injector. With a needleless device, the needle is replaced by an ultrathin liquid stream of insulin forced through the skin under high pressure. Insulin given by jet injection is absorbed at a faster rate, with a resulting shorter duration of action. Cost is a primary drawback to this system (Clarke, 2002).

Pen-type injectors hold small, lightweight, prefilled insulin cartridges. The injectors are easy to carry and make intensive therapy with multiple injections easier. These devices allow greater accuracy than traditional insulin syringes, especially when measuring doses smaller than 5 units (Robertson, Glazer, & Campbell, 2000). Discuss how to maintain the insulin cartridges at an appropriate temperature when using this device away from home. Be cautious when recommending pen-type injectors for visually or neurologically impaired clients. These devices are not meant for independent use by visually impaired people (Fleming, 2000).

NEW TECHNOLOGY. Inhaled insulin is currently under development. The insulin is contained in a pellet that is vaporized in an inhaler or delivered as a dry powder inhaled through a mouthpiece. These systems deliver insulin with a particle size of less than 5 micrometers in diameter able to reach deep lung tissues with a slow, deep inhalation by means of a handheld nebulizer. These particles quickly dissolve in the alveoli and pass into circulation. Systems are being developed to deliver both rapid-acting and long-acting insulins. Pulmonary insulin delivery appears to be safe and effective (White & Campbell, 2001).

Transdermal (through the skin) patch delivery of insulin is being tested. This method is predictable but slower than delivery by injection (Robertson, Glazer, & Campbell, 2000).

Client Education: Prescribed Medication. Provide specific instructions about insulin therapy. Chart 68-4 lists NIC activities for self-medication.

STORAGE. Refrigerate insulin not in use to maintain potency, prevent exposure to sunlight, and inhibit bacterial growth. Insulin in use may be kept at room temperature for up to 28 days to limit irritation at the injection site, which cold insulin may cause.

To prevent loss of drug potency, teach the client to avoid exposing insulin to temperatures below 36° F (2.2° C) or above 86° F (30° C) or to excessive shaking. Insulin lispro (Humalog) and insulin glargine (Lantus) should be stored in a refrigerator (2° to 8° C [36° to 46° F]). Neither type of insulin should be allowed to freeze. If refrigeration is not possible, the vial or cartridge of insulin lispro can be left unrefrigerated for up to 28 days, as long as it is kept as cool as possible (not above 86° F [30° C]) and away from direct heat and light. Discard any unused insulin after 28 days.

Instruct the client to always have a spare bottle of each type of insulin used. A slight loss in potency may occur after the bottle has been in use for more than 30 days even when the expiration date has not passed. When refrigerated, prefilled syringes are stable up to 30 days. If possible, store syringes in the upright position, needle pointing upward, so that insulin particles do not clog it. Teach clients to roll predrawn syringes between their hands before using. The effect of premixing insulins on blood glucose control is assessed by examining blood glucose levels.

DOSE PREPARATION. The person giving the insulin inspects the insulin before each use for changes (e.g., clumping, frosting, precipitation, or change in clarity or color) that may signal loss in potency. Rapid-, short-acting, and glargine insulins should be clear, and all other types of insulin should be uniformly cloudy after gently rolling the vial between the hands. If potency is questionable, another vial of the same type of insulin should be used.

SYRINGES. Standard insulin administration involves injection with syringes marked in insulin units. Insulin syringes are available in 1-mL (100-U), $\frac{1}{2}$ mL (50-U), and $\frac{3}{10}$ mL (30-U) sizes. The unit scale on the barrel of the syringe differs with the syringe size and manufacturer. Insulin syringe needle gauges are measured in 28 gauge, 29 gauge, and 30 gauge and in lengths of $\frac{1}{2}$ inch and $\frac{5}{16}$ inch. Short needles are not used for obese clients because of variability of insulin absorption. To ensure accurate insulin measurement, instruct the client to always buy the same type of syringes. Charts 68-5 and 68-6 review instructions for drawing up a single insulin injection and for mixing regular and NPH insulin in the same syringe.

Manufacturers of disposable syringes and pen needles recommend that needles be used only once. Reuse of an insulin

CHART 68-4

NIC INTERVENTION ACTIVITIES for The Diabetic Client with Hyperglycemia

Hyperglycemia Management: *Preventing and treating above normal blood glucose levels*

- Monitor blood glucose levels, as indicated.
- Monitor for signs and symptoms of hyperglycemia: polyuria, polydipsia, polyphagia, weakness, lethargy, malaise, blurring of vision, or headache.
- Monitor urine ketones, as indicated.
- Monitor ABG, electrolyte, and betahydroxybutyrate levels, as available.
- Monitor orthostatic blood pressure and pulse, as indicated.
- Administer insulin, as prescribed.
- Encourage oral fluid intake.
- Monitor fluid status (including intake and output), as appropriate.
- Maintain IV access, as appropriate.
- Administer IV fluids, as needed.
- Administer potassium, as prescribed.
- Consult physician if signs and symptoms of hyperglycemia persist or worsen.
- Identify possible causes of hyperglycemia.
- Anticipate situations in which insulin requirements will increase (e.g., intercurrent illness).
- Restrict exercise when blood glucose levels are >250 mg/dL, especially if urine ketones are present.
- Instruct client and significant others on prevention, recognition, and management of hyperglycemia.
- Encourage self-monitoring of blood glucose levels.
- Instruct on urine ketone testing, as appropriate.
- Instruct client and significant others on diabetes management during illness, including use of insulin and/or oral agents, monitoring fluid intake, carbohydrate replacement, and when to seek health professional assistance, as appropriate.
- Provide assistance in adjusting regimen to prevent and treat hyperglycemia (e.g., increasing insulin or oral agent), as indicated.

Teaching: Prescribed Medication: *Preparing a client to safely take prescribed medications and monitor for their effects*

- Instruct the client to recognize distinctive characteristics of the medication(s), as appropriate.
- Inform the client of both the generic and brand names of each medication.
- Instruct the client on the purpose and action of each medication.
- Instruct the client on the dosage, route, and duration of each medication.
- Instruct the client on the proper administration/application of each medication.
- Evaluate the client's ability to self-administer medications.
- Instruct the client to perform needed procedures before taking a medication (e.g., check pulse, glucose), as appropriate.
- Inform the client what to do if a dose of medication is missed.
- Inform the client of consequences of not taking or abruptly discontinuing medication(s), as appropriate.
- Instruct the client on which criteria to use when deciding to alter the medication dosage/schedule, as appropriate.
- Instruct the client on possible adverse effects of each medication.
- Instruct the client how to relieve and/or prevent certain side effects, as appropriate.
- Instruct the client on appropriate actions to take if side effects occur.
- Instruct the client on the signs and symptoms of overdosage/underdosage.
- Inform the client of possible drug-food interactions, as appropriate.
- Instruct the client how to properly store the medication(s).
- Instruct the client on the proper care of devices used for administration.
- Instruct the client on proper disposal of needles and syringes at home, as appropriate, and where to dispose of the sharps container in his or her community.
- Provide the client with written information about the action, purpose, side effects, and so on, of medication.
- Assist the client to develop a written medication schedule.
- Instruct the client to carry documentation of his or her prescribed medication regimen.
- Instruct the client how to fill his or her prescription(s), as appropriate.
- Inform the client of possible changes in appearance and/or dosage when filling generic medication prescription(s).
- Warn the client of the risks associated with taking expired medication.
- Determine the client's ability to obtain required medications.
- Provide information on medication reimbursement, as appropriate.
- Provide information on cost savings programs/organizations to obtain medications and devices, as appropriate.
- Provide information on medication alert devices and how to obtain them.
- Reinforce information provided by other health care team members, as appropriate.
- Include the family/significant others, as appropriate.

Teaching: Prescribed Diet: *Preparing a client to correctly follow a prescribed diet*

- Appraise the client's current level of knowledge about prescribed diet.
- Determine the client's/significant other's feelings/attitude toward prescribed diet and expected degree of dietary compliance.
- Instruct the client on the proper name of the prescribed diet.
- Explain the purpose of the diet.
- Instruct the client about how to keep a food diary, as appropriate.
- Instruct the client on allowed and prohibited foods.
- Inform the client of possible drug-food interactions, as appropriate.
- Assist the client to accommodate food preferences into the prescribed diet.
- Assist the client in substituting ingredients to conform favorite recipes to the prescribed diet.
- Instruct the client about how to read labels and select appropriate foods.
- Observe the client's selection of foods appropriate to prescribed diet.
- Instruct the client about how to plan appropriate meals.
- Provide written meal plans, as appropriate.
- Reinforce information provided by other health care team members, as appropriate.
- Refer client to dietitian/nutritionist, as appropriate.
- Include the family/significant others, as appropriate.

NIC intervention activities selected from Dochterman, J.M., & Bulechek, G.M. (Eds.). (2004). *Nursing interventions classification (NIC)* (4th ed.). St. Louis: Mosby.

ABG, Arterial blood gas.

CHART 68-5

CLIENT EDUCATION GUIDE

Subcutaneous Insulin Administration

- Wash your hands.
- Inspect the bottle for the type of insulin and the expiration date.
- Gently roll the bottle of intermediate-acting insulin in the palms of your hands to mix the insulin.
- Clean the rubber stopper with an alcohol swab.
- Remove the needle cover and pull back the plunger to draw air into the syringe. The amount of air should be equal to the insulin dose. Push the needle through the rubber stopper and inject the air into the insulin bottle.
- Turn the bottle upside down and draw the insulin dose into the syringe.
- Remove air bubbles in the syringe by tapping on the syringe or injecting air back into the bottle. Redraw the correct amount.
- Make certain the tip of the plunger is on the line for your dose of insulin. Magnifiers are available to assist in measuring accurate doses of insulin.
- Remove the needle from the bottle. Recap the needle if the insulin is not to be given immediately.
- Select a site within your injection area that has not been used in the past month.
- Clean your skin with an alcohol swab. Lightly grasp an area of skin and insert the needle at a 90-degree angle.
- Push the plunger all the way down. This will push the insulin into your body. Release the pinched skin.
- Pull the needle straight out quickly. Do not rub the place where you gave the shot.
- Dispose of the syringe and needle without recapping in a puncture-proof container.

Data from American Diabetes Association. (2003). Position statement: Insulin administration. *Diabetes Care, 26*(Suppl. 1), 121-124.

CHART 68-6

CLIENT EDUCATION GUIDE

How to Mix a Prescribed Dose of 10 Units of Regular Insulin and 20 Units of NPH Insulin

- Wash your hands.
- Inspect the bottle for the type of insulin and the expiration date.
- Gently roll the bottle of intermediate insulin in the palms of your hands to mix the insulin.
- Clean the rubber stopper with an alcohol swab.
- Inject 20 units of air into the NPH insulin bottle. The amount of air should be equal to the dose of insulin needed. Always inject air into the intermediate-acting insulin first. Withdraw the syringe.
- Inject 10 units of air into the regular insulin bottle. The amount of air is equal to the dose of insulin desired.
- Withdraw 10 units of regular insulin. Be sure that the syringe is free of air bubbles. Always withdraw the shorter-acting insulin first.
- Withdraw 20 units of NPH insulin with the same syringe, being careful not to inject any short-acting insulin into the bottle. (A total of 30 units should be in the syringe.)

Data from American Diabetes Association. (2003). Position statement: Insulin administration. *Diabetes Care, 26*(Suppl. 1), 121-124.

syringe and needle can compromise insulin sterility. Most insulins contain products that inhibit growth of bacteria commonly found on the skin. Some clients, however, have an increased risk of infection with syringe or needle reuse. A far more important reason to not reuse needles has arisen with the advent of new, smaller (30 and 31 gauge) needles. Even with one injection, the needle tip can become bent to form a hook, which can lacerate tissue or break off to leave needle fragments

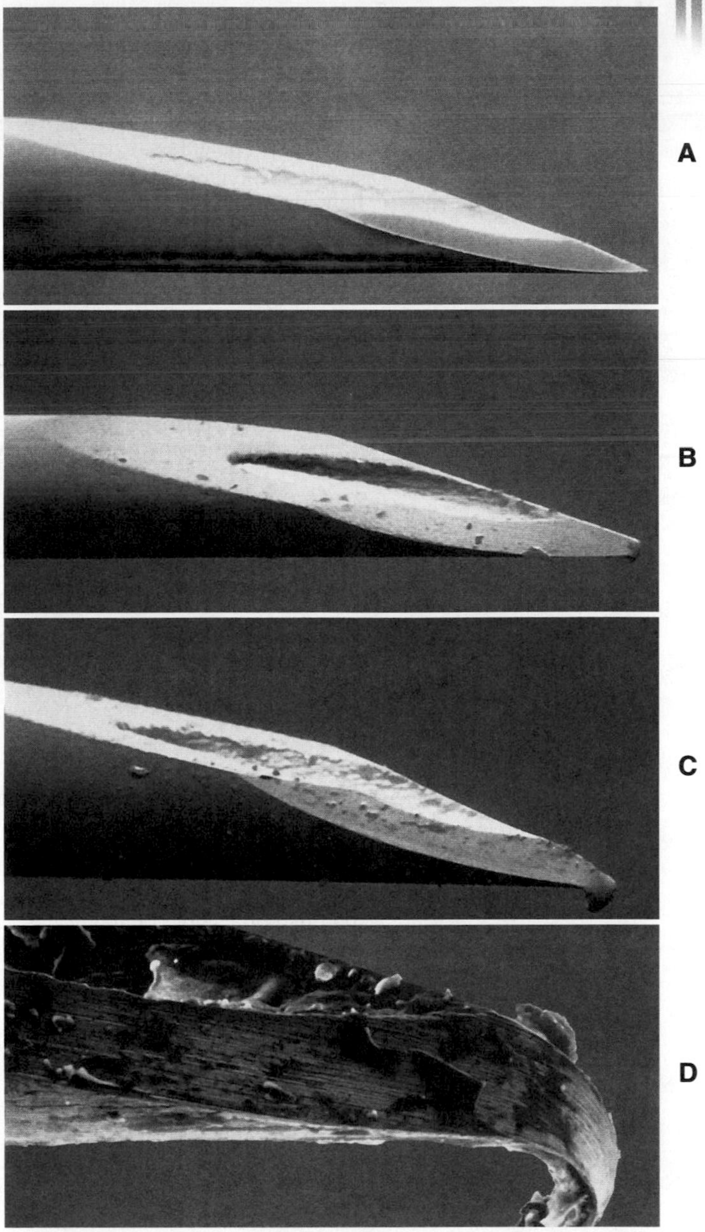

Figure 68-9 ■ Reuse of insulin needle. **A,** A new needle. **B,** A needle that has been used once. **C,** A needle that has been used twice. **D,** A needle that has been used six times. (Courtesy of BD Medical, Franklin Lakes, NJ.)

in the skin (Figure 68-9). Instruct the client to discard the syringe and needle after one use. The Environmental Protection Agency recommends that needles, syringes, lancets, and other sharp objects be placed in a hard-plastic or metal container with a screw-on lid or a tightly secured lid that is clearly marked "Not for Recycling" and discarded with other household trash (http://www.epa.gov/epaoswer/other/medical).

Client Education: Blood Glucose Monitoring. Self-monitoring of blood glucose levels (SMBG) provides information that allows the client to adjust therapy. Teach the client to use the prescribed formulas to (1) self-adjust diet, exercise, or pharmacologic therapy; (2) identify and properly treat hyperglycemia and hypoglycemia; and (3) improve decision making and problem solving. See Table 68-12 for costs of glucose monitors and strips.

TABLE 68-12 Blood Glucose Monitors

Meter	Features	Cost	Test strips (50)	Test Strips (100)
Bayer Diagnostics				
Ascensia ELITE	20 test memory with dates and times Easy to use meter with no buttons; turns on by inserting test strip Approved for multiple site testing	System: $39.95* (Rebate: $35.00)*	$36.99* (foil wrapped strips)	$64.99* (foil wrapped strips)
Ascensia DEX 2	Disk-based monitor eliminates need to handle strips 100-test memory with dates, times, and four daily averages Approved for multiple site testing Data management software available	System: $64.95* (Rebate: $55.00)	$37.99* (5 cartridges of 10 test strips)	$67.99* (10 cartridges of 10 tests each)
Ascensia ELITE XL	120-test memory with dates, times, and 14-day average Easy to use meter with no buttons; turns on by inserting test strip Approved for multiple site testing Advanced data management capability	System: $49.95* (Rebate: $45.00)*	$36.99* (foil wrapped strips)	$64.99* (foil wrapped strips)
Lifescan				
One Touch Ultra	150-test memory and plasma values; 14- and 30-day averaging Approved for multiple site testing Advanced data management capability	System: $59.95* (Rebate: $30.00)*	$39.49*	$71.44*
Medisense				
Precision QID	125-test memory Data management software available	System: $49.95* (Rebate: $20.00)	$39.44*	$70.99*
Precision Xtra	450-test memory Measures both blood glucose and ketone levels Advanced data management capability	System: $64.95* (Rebate: $20.00)*	$39.44* 8 ketone test strips: $27.95	$70.99*
Sof-Tact	A one-button automatic testing system: brings blood to skin surface, pricks the skin, draws the sample, and transfers it to the test strip with the push of a single button Stores up to 450 results with date and time Approved for multiple site testing Data management software available	Unit price: $195.99*	$39.44*	
Roche Diagnostics				
Accu-Chek Active	200-test memory with 7- and 14-day averaging of data Approved for multiple site testing Data management software available	Care Kit: $17.95*	$25.95*	
Accu-Chek Compact	Easy to use meter for clients with limited dexterity Clients insert a drum containing 17 test strips into the meter. It has a 100-test memory and reports highest, lowest, and average values Approved for multiple site testing Data management software available	System: $64.95* (Rebate $25.00)*	$ 39.99* (3 drums of 17 tests each)	$75.99* (6 drums of 17 tests each)
Accu-Chek Advantage	Easy to use meter, even for young children 100-test memory that stores the date and time for each test Data management software available	Meter: $49.99* (Rebate $25.00)*	Comfort Curve & Advantage strips $39.88*	Comfort Curve & Advantage strips $71.99*
Accu-Chek Complete	1000-test memory with date and time for each test Advanced data management capability	System: $97.95* (Rebate $25.00)	Comfort Curve & Advantage strips $39.88*	Comfort Curve & Advantage strips $71.99*
Accu-Chek Voicemate	Clear voice prompt to guide the visually impaired step-by-step through the blood glucose testing process using the Accu-Chek Advantage meter Insulin vial identification system for Lilly insulin Prescription required with visual impairment of 20/200 or greater for insurance reimbursement	System: $495.00*	Comfort curve strips $39.88*	Comfort Curve strips $71.99*

Pricing data for meters and strips from http://www.diabeticpromotions.com* and http://www.diabeticsupplies.com.

TABLE 68-12 Blood Glucose Monitors—*cont'd*

Meter	Features	Cost	Test strips (50)	Test Strips (100)
Therasense				
FreeStyle	250-test memory Approved for multiple site testing Data management software available	System: $64.95* (Rebate: $40.00)*	$38.99*	$68.95*
FreeStyle Tracker	2500-test memory Comprehensive data management system that combines a blood glucose meter, diabetes manager, and personal digital assistant (PDA) in one device Approved for alternate site testing	System: $299.00* (Rebate $75.00)*	Uses FreeStyle testing strips	

Pricing data for meters and strips from http://www.diabeticpromotions.com* and http://www.diabeticsupplies.com.

The American Diabetes Association (ADA) recommends SMBG for clients taking insulin or oral therapy. Assessment of blood glucose levels is very important for the following clients:

- Any diabetic client trying to keep glucose levels in the near-normal range
- Pregnant clients
- Clients with a tendency to develop severe ketosis or hypoglycemia
- Clients with hypoglycemic unawareness
- Clients undergoing intensive treatment programs, especially those using portable infusion devices, or taking multiple daily insulin injections

The principles of most self-monitoring systems are the same. The finger is pricked and a drop of blood is made to flow over a reagent pad on a testing strip. Meters measure blood glucose by using color reflectance or sensor technology. With reflectance meters, the glucose in a drop of blood reacts with an enzyme in the strip, changing the color of the strip. The meter reads the color of the strip and gives a number for the blood glucose value. Meters that use sensor technology measure small electrical currents produced by the interaction between the glucose in the blood and the chemicals on the strip (Peragallo-Dittko, 2002b). Clients can also perform visual blood glucose monitoring by comparing the color on a test strip with a color key on the vial.

There is some variation between glucose level in whole blood by SMBG systems and that measured by a clinical laboratory. The ADA has set the performance goal to be a total error of no more than 5% at glucose levels between 30 and 400 mg/dL (1.6 and 22.2 mmol/L) (Sacks et al., 2002). The accuracy of SMBG systems decreases at hypoglycemic and hyperglycemic levels. The overall performance of SMBG systems depends on the accuracy of the specific blood glucose meter, operator proficiency, and test strip quality. Results are influenced by the amount of blood on the strip; the meter's calibration to the strip currently in use; environmental conditions of altitude, temperature, and moisture; and client-specific conditions of hematocrit level, triglyceride level, and presence of hypotension.

Most meters indicate blood glucose results as a number, but some have voice readouts, memories that can be displayed, or graphic displays. A client's vision problems, including color blindness, determine the method of SMBG selected. Some models have large, bold display screens and simple, user-friendly procedures.

Teach the client to follow Centers for Disease Control and Prevention (CDC) guidelines for infection control during SMBG. The chances of becoming infected from blood glucose monitoring processes are reduced by handwashing before monitoring and by not reusing lancets. Instruct clients not to share their blood glucose monitoring equipment. Hepatitis B virus can survive in a dried state for at least 1 week. Infection can be spread by the lancet holder even when the lancet itself has been changed. Small particles of blood can stick to the device and infect multiple users. Regular cleaning of the meter is critical for infection control. Health care staff who perform blood glucose testing and family members who help with testing should wear gloves (American Association of Diabetes Educators, 2003b).

INTERPRETATION OF RESULTS. Accuracy of blood glucose measurements is reduced by errors in technique or by equipment failure. Data obtained from SMBG are evaluated with other measures of blood glucose levels (e.g., glycosylated hemoglobin, or hemoglobin A1c [HbA1c], values) or periodic laboratory blood glucose tests. Even when SMBG is performed correctly, the results are affected by hematocrit values (anemia falsely elevates glucose values; polycythemia falsely depresses them) and may be unreliable in the hypoglycemic or severe hyperglycemic ranges. Accuracy of the meter itself is also an issue. Even when highly trained personnel tested meters under optimal conditions, wide variation exists in accuracy and precision among capillary blood glucose monitoring devices. Laboratory glucose determinations are more accurate than SMBG.

FREQUENCY OF TESTING. The frequency of testing varies with the complexity of the drug schedules and the goals of therapy. Clients with unstable blood glucose levels, as well as those using intensive treatment regimens, require frequent monitoring. Clients using simple treatment regimens designed to prevent symptomatic hyperglycemia or clients with type 2 diabetes using oral agents need less frequent testing.

BLOOD GLUCOSE THERAPY GOALS. Work with the client to reach set goals for therapy. Target blood glucose levels are set individually for each client. The American Diabetes Association (ADA) recommends that clients with type 1 diabetes aim for hemoglobin A1c (HbA1c) values less than 7%, premeal glucose levels of 90 to 130 mg/dL (5.0 to 7.2 mmol/L), and postmeal glucose levels less than 180 mg/dL (10.0 mmol/L) (ADA, 2003r).

ACCURACY OF SELF-MONITORING OF BLOOD GLUCOSE LEVELS. All meters are reasonably accurate when the manufacturer's directions are followed. Results are technique dependent regardless of whether test strips are read visually or with a meter. Help the client select a meter based on cost of the meter and strips, ease of use, availability of repair and servicing, and ability to see color. Provide training, explain and demonstrate procedures, assess visual acuity, and check the client's ability to perform the procedure through a return demonstration. Assess color discrimination for those who do not use a blood glucose meter.

Common errors in SMBG involve failure to obtain a sufficient blood drop, poor storage of test strips, and not changing the code number on the meter to match the strip bottle code. Continued retraining of clients performing SMBG helps ensure accurate results because performance accuracy deteriorates over time.

ALTERNATE SITE TESTING. Blood samples for SMBG are usually obtained by pricking the fingertip, where blood glucose levels closely match arterial blood glucose levels. Some meters test blood glucose levels in the forearm, upper arm, abdomen, thigh, and calf. However, blood glucose levels from these alternate sites are not the same as those from the fingertip. Comparison studies indicate that these sites can vary by as much as 100 mg/dL from the fingertip. This variance is from circulation differences at times when blood glucose values are changing rapidly. Teach clients that there is a lag time for blood glucose levels between the fingertip and other sites when blood glucose levels are changing rapidly and that the fingertip reading is the only safe choice at those times.

Clients with a history of hypoglycemic unawareness should not test at alternative sites (Peragallo-Dittko, 2002). Alternative site testing is safe before a meal and 2 hours after a meal. Instruct the client to use only fingertip testing in the following situations:

- When hypoglycemic
- When risk for hypoglycemia is greater (at time of peak activity of basal insulin, or within 2 hours after injecting rapid-acting insulin)
- After exercise
- During an illness
- When blood glucose levels are changing rapidly (e.g., within 2 hours after a meal)
- Before driving

CONSIDERATIONS FOR OLDER ADULTS

Visual interpretation of blood glucose values is affected by normal age-related changes in color perception. The ability to discriminate shades of blue, violet, and green become less accurate, making performance of visual blood glucose monitoring more difficult. Also, older clients need more light to see things clearly. Placing a high-intensity light on the object or surface is more effective than increasing light for the entire room.

New Technology. Current methods of measuring blood glucose are not sufficiently adequate for adjusting insulin doses for clients receiving intense insulin therapy. Continuous blood glucose monitoring with an implanted sensor could allow more adequate insulin delivery and earlier detection of hypoglycemia (Gerritsen, 2000).

The GlucoWatch (Cygnus) sends a tiny electrical current through the skin to measure glucose from interstitial fluid just beneath the skin. It analyzes glucose every 20 minutes for up to 12 hours and appears best suited for detecting unsuspected hypoglycemia. The GlucoWatch is meant to supplement, not replace, finger stick tests. Insulin should only be given after confirming the results of the GlucoWatch with a finger stick test (Table 68-13).

The Continuous Glucose Monitoring System (Medtronic MiniMed) is a subcutaneous glucose sensor connected to an externally worn monitor. Blood glucose values, obtained every 5 minutes for up to 72 hours, are downloaded into computer for analysis. The data show blood glucose changes over the day, allowing more accurate adjustments in intensive insulin therapy.

Systems for obtaining blood without finger sticks are being developed. The Professional Lancette gets a drop of blood by vaporizing a pinpoint of skin on the finger with a laser beam.

Diet Therapy. Effective self-management of diabetes requires that the meal plan, education, and counseling programs be individualized for each client. A registered dietitian should be a member of the treatment team. The nurse, dietitian, client, and family work together on all aspects of the meal plan, which must be realistic and as flexible as possible.

Goals of Diet Therapy. Diet therapy focuses on the following goals:

- Keeping blood glucose and glycosylated hemoglobin levels as near normal as possible
- Having optimal serum lipid levels: low-density lipoprotein (LDL) cholesterol below 100 mg/dL (2.60 mmol/L), high-density lipoprotein (HDL) cholesterol above 40 mg/dL, and triglyceride levels below 150 mg/dL (1.7 mmol/L) (ADA, 2003l)
- Having a blood pressure consistently less than 130/80 mm Hg (ADA, 2003r)
- Ensuring adequate calories for achieving reasonable weight for adults, meeting increased metabolic needs during pregnancy and lactation, or promoting recovery from illness
- Preventing and treating the acute complications of hypoglycemic drugs, short-term illness, and exercise-related problems

TABLE 68-13 Cost of Blood Glucose Monitoring Products

Product	Cost	Cost of Supplies	Comments
Lasette	$495.00	Disposable cartridge: $12.90 for a two-pack system ($0.13 per test)	Cartridge is good for 120 uses. Battery is rechargeable, with 50 uses per charge.
GlucoWatch	$872.00	Auto sensor: $9.38	Auto sensor must be changed every 12 hr. Watch should last 2-3 yr.

Data from the following:
Lasette: Cell Robotics International (http://www.cellrobotics.com; http://www.diabeteswebsite.com; 800-846-0590); GlucoWatch: Automatic glucose biography (http://www.glucoewatch.com; 866-GLWATCH).

- Preventing and treating complications of diabetes (renal disease, neuropathy, and cardiovascular disease)
- Improving overall health through healthy food choices and physical activity
- Facilitating changes in eating habits that reduce insulin resistance and improve metabolic status
- Meeting the nutritional and psychosocial needs of older individuals
- Providing self-management education for clients treated with insulin or sulfonylureas for treatment and prevention of hypoglycemia, acute illness, and exercise related blood glucose problems
- For clients at risk for diabetes, encouraging food choices that facilitate moderate weight loss or at least prevent weight gain (ADA, 2003r)

Principles of Nutrition in Diabetes. The dietitian develops a meal plan based on the client's usual food intake. Day-to-day consistency in the timing and amount of food eaten helps control blood glucose. Clients receiving insulin therapy need to eat at consistent times that are coordinated with the timed action of insulin. Teach clients using intense insulin therapy to adjust premeal insulin to allow for timing and quantity changes in their meal plan (ADA, 2003f).

Protein. The usual protein intake (15% to 20% of total daily calories) is appropriate for diabetic clients with normal kidney function. In clients with microalbuminuria, reduction of protein to 10% of calories (0.8 g/kg) may slow progression of kidney failure (ADA, 2003f).

Fat and Carbohydrate. The amount of calories from fat and carbohydrates is based on individual goals. Of the remaining 80% to 90% of calories, less than 10% should be from saturated fat and up to 10% should be from polyunsaturated fat. Foods high in trans-fatty acids are avoided or severely limited. The remaining 60% to 70% of calories are from monounsaturated fat and carbohydrates (ADA, 2003f).

Further fat restrictions for clients with diabetes are determined by a dietitian based on specific lipid abnormalities. Adults with diabetes should be tested annually for lipid abnormalities. These tests include fasting serum cholesterol, triglyceride, high-density lipoprotein (HDL) cholesterol, and calculated LDL cholesterol levels (ADA, 2003l).

The percentage of calories obtained from carbohydrates is determined for each client. Various starches have different blood glucose responses. Emphasis is placed on the total amount of carbohydrate consumed each day rather than the source of the carbohydrate. Little scientific evidence supports the assumption that sugars are more rapidly absorbed than starches and cause blood glucose values to increase more rapidly.

Fiber. High-fiber diets improve carbohydrate metabolism and lower cholesterol levels. Teach the client to select foods with moderate to high amounts of dietary fiber (e.g., legumes, lentils, roots, leafy green vegetables, all types of whole-grain cereals, and fruits). Intake of 20 to 35 g of dietary fiber per day is ideal.

Teach the client that adding high-fiber foods to the diet gradually can reduce abdominal cramping, loose stools, and flatulence. An increase in fluid intake should accompany increased fiber intake. The nurse and the client should pay careful attention to blood glucose levels because hypoglycemia can result when dietary fiber intake increases significantly.

Nonnutritive Sweeteners. The use of products to enhance the taste of food while not disturbing blood glucose control is desirable. The FDA has approved four nonnutritive sweeteners for use: saccharin, aspartame, acesulfame K, and sucralose.

Fat Replacers. Fat replacers in foods create good-tasting, lower-fat foods but may increase carbohydrate content. Teach clients how to incorporate fat replacers into their meal plan. Guidelines regarding the use of fat replacers are as follows (ADA, 2001b):

- Fat replacer should be less than 20 calories or less than 5 g of carbohydrate per serving if it is a "free food."
- Limit fat replacer to three servings per day.
- From 6 to 10 g of carbohydrate per serving is one half of a carbohydrate choice.
- From 11 to 20 g of carbohydrate per serving is one carbohydrate choice.

Alcohol. Blood glucose levels are not affected by *moderate* use of alcohol when diabetes is well controlled. Teach clients using insulin that two alcoholic beverages for men and one for women can be ingested with, and in addition to, the usual meal plan. (One alcoholic beverage equals 12 ounces of beer, 5 ounces of wine, or 1.5 ounces of distilled spirits.) Because of the potential for alcohol-induced hypoglycemia, instruct the client to ingest alcohol only with or shortly after meals. Alcohol raises plasma triglycerides; thus, reducing or abstaining from alcohol is important for clients with hyperlipidemia. One alcoholic beverage is substituted for two fat exchanges when calculating caloric intake (ADA, 2003f).

Food Labeling. Nutrient and ingredient information help clients make good food and portion choices. For clients with diabetes, foods containing sucrose or other sugars are not restricted. These foods are used sparingly and substituted for other carbohydrates in the individual meal plan. Teach the client to use the food label to determine carbohydrate content.

Client Education: Prescribed Diet. No one meal plan is right for all clients with diabetes. Each client's nutrition recommendations are based on blood glucose monitoring results, total blood lipid levels, and glycosylated hemoglobin. These tests help to determine whether current meal and exercise patterns need adjustment or whether present habits need reinforcement. A specific dietary prescription is developed for each client.

Support and reinforce nutrition information provided by the dietitian. The diabetic client needs to understand how to make adjustments in food intake during illness, planned exercise, and social occasions (such as restaurant meals) where the usual time of eating is delayed. The client may be unable to follow the prescribed diet because of an inability to see, read, or understand printed materials. Share dietary information with the person who prepares the meals. The dietitian sees each client at least yearly to identify changes in lifestyle and make appropriate diet therapy changes. Some clients, such as those with weight control problems or low incomes, may need more frequent evaluation and counseling.

Meal-Planning Strategies. Many meal-planning approaches are available. Each approach emphasizes different aspects of nutrition.

EXCHANGE SYSTEM. The exchange system is based on three food groups: carbohydrates, meat and meat substitutes, and fat. The exchange list for meal planning assumes

TABLE 68-14 Exchange System of Medical Nutrition Therapy

Food Content	Carbohydrate (g)	Protein (g)	Fat (g)	Calories	Example
Carbohydrate					
Breads/grains	15	3	1 or less	80	1 slice bread ½ bagel ½ hamburger bun ½ cup corn ½ cup mashed potato
Fruit	15	0	0	60	1 small apple ½ medium banana ½ grapefruit
Milk					
Skim	12	8	0-3	90	1 cup skim milk (½%-1%)
Low-fat	12	8	5	120	1 cup 2% milk
Whole	12	8	5	150	1 cup whole milk
Other carbohydrates	15	Varies	Varies	Varies	Brownie, unfrosted (2-inch square) Fruit juice bar 1 tablespoon jelly, regular
Vegetables	5	2	0	25	Carrots, green beans, spinach, ½ cup cooked, 1 cup raw 1 large tomato
Meat or Meat Substitute					
Very lean	0	7	0-1	35	1 oz chicken (white meat, skinless), 1 oz fat-free cheese (1 g fat or less)
Lean	0	7	3	55	1 oz lean beef (trimmed rump roast), dark meat chicken (skinless), or salmon; ¼ cup cottage cheese (4.5% fat)
Medium-fat	0	7	5	75	1 oz ground beef, pork cutlet, lamb, or dark meat chicken with skin
High-fat	0	7	8	100	1 oz pork sausage, 1 tablespoon peanut butter, 1 oz American cheese
Fat	0	0	5	45	1 teaspoon butter or margarine, 1 strip bacon

that foods with similar nutrient content affect blood glucose levels similarly. Diets based on the exchange system produce predictable blood glucose responses. The client's prescription identifies how many items from each food group are to be eaten at a meal or snack. Table 68-14 provides an example of the exchange system of diet therapy.

CARBOHYDRATE COUNTING. Carbohydrate (CHO) counting is a simple approach to meal planning that uses label information of the nutritional content of packaged food items. Because fat and protein have little effect on postmeal blood glucose levels, CHO counting focuses on the nutrient that has the greatest impact on these levels. CHO counting uses total grams of carbohydrate, regardless of the food source. The dietitian determines the number of grams of carbohydrate to be eaten at each meal and snack and helps the client to make appropriate food choices. CHO counting is effective in achieving overall blood glucose control when carbohydrate intake is consistent from day to day.

Clients using intensive insulin or pump therapies can use CHO counting to determine insulin coverage. After the amount of insulin needed to cover the usual meal is determined, insulin may be added or subtracted for changes in carbohydrate intake. An initial formula of 1 unit of rapid-acting insulin for each 15 g of carbohydrate provides flexibility to meal plans. The client determines the grams of carbohydrate in a specific meal or snack by label reading or weighing and measuring of each item. The total grams of carbohydrate are used to calculate the bolus dose of insulin based on their individual insulin to carbohydrate ratio. See Table 68-15 for an example of carbohydrate counting.

SPECIAL CONSIDERATIONS FOR TYPE 1 DIABETES. A meal plan based on the client's usual food intake is developed, and insulin therapy is integrated into the usual eating and exercises patterns. To match the effects of insulin, the daily caloric intake is spread among three main meals and any between-meal or bedtime snacks. Blood glucose monitoring before and within 1 to 2 hours after meals determines whether the insulin/carbohydrate ratio is correct. For clients who are on fixed insulin regimens and do not adjust premeal insulin dosages, consistency of carbohydrate intake at each meal is important. Clients using intensified insulin therapy with multiple daily injections of insulin or an insulin pump have more flexibility in the choice and timing of meals and snacks. The need for between-meal or bedtime snacks is based on the peak action time of insulin and the need to prevent hypoglycemia. Additional carbohydrate may be needed before unplanned exercise to prevent exercise-related hypoglycemia.

Besides maintaining blood glucose levels within a target range, a second goal for clients with type 1 diabetes is to avoid gaining weight. Hyperinsulinemia (chronic high blood insulin levels) can occur with intensive treatment

TABLE 68-15 Carbohydrate Counting

	Food Source	Grams of Carbohydrates	Total	Insulin Dose* (1:15 ratio)
Breakfast	2 slices honey grain bread	32		
	¼ cup egg substitute	0		
	½ cup orange juice	15		
	1 Tablespoon lower-fat margarine	0	47	3
Lunch	2 oz tuna, canned in water	0		
	1 hamburger bun	30		
	Fat-free Pringles (#15)	15		
	1 Tablespoon reduced-fat mayonnaise	0		
	1 tomato and 1 lettuce slice	0		
	1 medium dill pickle	0		
	Sugar-free pudding made with fat-free milk	15	60	4
Supper	3 oz chicken breast, grilled	0		
	1 small (3 oz) baked potato	15		
	1 cup steamed broccoli	10		
	1 French roll	25		
	1 Tablespoon lower-fat margarine	0		
	2 Tablespoons reduced-fat sour cream	0		
	½ cup canned pineapple (in own juice)	15	65	4

*Insulin dosage has been rounded off to the nearest whole unit. Tenths of units of insulin can only be given with an insulin pump.

schedules and may result in weight gain. These clients may need to treat hyperglycemia by restricting calories rather than increasing insulin. Weight gain can be minimized by following the prescribed meal plan, getting regular exercise, and avoiding overtreatment of hypoglycemia.

SPECIAL CONSIDERATIONS FOR TYPE 2 DIABETES. Many clients with type 2 diabetes are overweight and insulin resistant. Diet therapy stresses lifestyle changes that reduce calories eaten and increase calories expended through physical activity. Many clients with diabetes also have abnormal blood fat levels (metabolic syndrome) and hypertension, making reductions of saturated fat, cholesterol, and sodium desirable. A moderate caloric restriction (250 to 500 calories less than average daily intake) and an increase in physical activity improves diabetic control and weight control. Decreases of more than 10% of body weight can result in significant improvement in glycosylated hemoglobin (hemoglobin A1c) (King & Wofford, 2000). Decreasing intake of cholesterol-raising fatty acids helps reduce the risk of cardiovascular disease.

When clients with type 2 diabetes need treatment with insulin, consistency in timing and carbohydrate content of meals is important. Division of the total daily calories into three meals or into smaller meals and snacks is based on individual preference.

CONSIDERATIONS FOR OLDER ADULTS

Older clients are at increased risk for malnutrition, hypoglycemia, and especially dehydration, a factor in the development of the hyperglycemic hyperosmolar nonketotic (HHNS) syndrome. Many factors contribute to malnutrition. Older clients who prepare their own food or have tooth loss or poorly fitting dentures may not eat enough food. Neuropathy with gastric retention or diarrhea compounds poor food intake. Impaired cognition and depression may disrupt self-care. Older clients may have a marginal food supply because of inadequate income, may have poor understanding of meal planning goals, or may live alone and have reduced incentive to prepare or eat proper meals. They may eat in restaurants or live in situations in which they have little control over meal preparation. Regular visits by home health nurses can assist older clients in following a diabetic meal plan.

A realistic approach to diet therapy is essential for the older diabetic client. Changing the eating habits of 60 to 70 years is very difficult. The nurse, dietitian, and client assess the client's usual eating patterns. Teach the older client taking antidiabetic drugs about the importance of eating meals and snacks at the same time every day, eating the same amount of food from day to day, and eating all food allowed on the diet.

Exercise Therapy. Regular exercise is an essential part of a diabetic treatment plan. Exercise has beneficial effects on carbohydrate metabolism and insulin sensitivity. It also improves the client's sense of well-being and reduces the risk for atherosclerosis (ADA, 2003n). Motivation to start an exercise program, especially among people who are sedentary, can be difficult. A large study indicated that gender differences rather than racial or ethnic differences were a better predictor of exercise success. (See the Evidence-Based Practice for Nursing Box on p. 1530.)

In the person without diabetes, glucose use during exercise is matched by glucose production by the liver; thus exercise does not induce hyperglycemia or hypoglycemia. The client with type 1 diabetes is unable to make these hormonal changes. Without an adequate insulin supply, cells are unable to use glucose. Low insulin levels trigger release of glucagon and epinephrine to increase hepatic glucose production, further raising blood glucose levels. In the absence of insulin, free fatty acids become the source of energy. Exercise in the client with uncontrolled diabetes results in further hyperglycemia and the formation of ketone bodies. Diabetic clients may have prolonged elevated blood glucose levels after vigorous exercise.

Exercise in the person with diabetes can cause hypoglycemia because of increased muscle glucose uptake and inhibited glucose release from the liver. Hypoglycemia can occur during exercise and for up to 24 hours after exercise. Replacement of muscle and liver glycogen stores, along with

EVIDENCE-BASED PRACTICE for Nursing

Do exercise practices among people with diabetes vary with ethnicity?

Wood, F. (2002). Ethnic differences in exercise among adults with diabetes. *Western Journal of Nursing Research, 24*(5), 502-515.

Exercise has been identified as an important strategy to reduce complications among adults who have diabetes. Previous studies of exercise patterns among adult Americans are largely confined to white men. This study sought to identify exercise patterns among men and women with diabetes from racially and ethnically diverse backgrounds. The study examined data previously collected by the National Health and Nutrition Examination Survey (NHANES) III Household Adult Data Files from 1988 through 1994. Sixteen questions from the original survey provided information about diabetes, gender, ethnicity/race, and exercise. Data obtained as responses to these 16 survey items were reanalyzed to compare exercise patterns among adults with diabetes from diverse ethnic backgrounds: African American, Hispanic American, and European American. Survey and interview data from 1614 adults with diabetes were examined. Fifty-nine percent (953) of the subjects were women, 41% (661) of the subjects were men. About half were over 56 years of age. Twenty-seven percent (448) were African American and 29% (505) were Hispanic American. This secondary analysis revealed that about one third of subjects did not engage in any form of regular exercise or physical activity. Rates and types of exercise were not statistically different among the three different ethnic/racial groups. Overall, men of all ethnicities were more physically active than women. Walking and gardening were the two most widely practiced forms of exercise or physical activity.

Level of Evidence: 3—Well-designed trial without randomization.

Critique. This secondary analysis used data collected from a large, cross-sectional sample that originally oversampled nonwhite individuals and people older than 60 years of age. The findings of this secondary analysis support the findings of other studies indicating little or no performance of regular physical activity in individuals older than 60 years of age.

Implications for Nursing. The benefits of mild to moderate exercise for clients with diabetes are well-documented. This study indicates that many people with diabetes of all ethnicities do not participate in any form of exercise. What is not known is why some individuals do not exercise. Providing information to clients with diabetes that exercise is beneficial is not sufficient. Nurses must assess each client's level of physical activity and determine what factors prevent the person from participating in regular physical exercise as well as what factors enhance participation in regular exercise. In this way, nurses can help individualize an exercise program for each client with the potential to increase overall participation in regular physical activity.

increased insulin sensitivity following exercise, causes insulin requirements to drop.

Benefits of Exercise. Regular, moderate-intensity exercise helps regulate blood glucose levels and lowers insulin requirements for clients with type 1 diabetes. It also improves control by increasing insulin sensitivity, enhancing cell uptake of glucose, and promoting weight loss.

Regular exercise decreases risk factors for cardiovascular disease. For clients with type 1 diabetes, exercise decreases most blood lipid levels and increases high-density lipoproteins (HDLs). Exercise decreases blood pressure and improves cardiovascular function. Regular vigorous physical activity prevents or delays type 2 diabetes by reducing body weight, insulin resistance, and glucose intolerance.

Risks Related to Exercise. Assess the diabetic client for risk for injury related to exercise. Prolonged hypoglycemia or hyperglycemia can occur, particularly after sustained high-intensity exercise.

Several complications of diabetes can be made worse by exercise. The client with proliferative retinopathy is advised to avoid the Valsalva maneuver (breath-holding while bearing down) and activities that increase blood pressure. Heavy lifting, rapid head motion, or jarring activities can cause eye hemorrhage or retinal detachment. Exercise may increase proteinuria in clients with diabetic nephropathy. The risk for foot and joint injury rises for clients with peripheral neuropathy. Autonomic neuropathy can cause orthostatic hypotension after exercise.

Screening Before Starting an Exercise Program. Advise a diabetic client to have a complete physical examination before starting an exercise program. Regular physical activity increases the risk for musculoskeletal injury and life-threatening cardiovascular events. The ability of the heart to respond to increasing levels of exercise on a treadmill, as well as the presence of other risk factors, forms the basis of the exercise prescription. For clients who are unable to perform vigorous exercise, the heart's ability to tolerate exercise is tested with cardiac stressor drugs (e.g., coronary vasodilators, dipyridamole thallium scans). The client needs to be carefully evaluated for vascular complications that may be worsened by exercise (ADA, 2003n).

Guidelines for Exercise. The client checks blood glucose levels before exercise. When levels exceed 250 mg/dL (13.8 mmol/L), the client tests the urine for ketones. The absence of urine ketones indicates that enough insulin is available for glucose transport and use, and that exercise should be effective in lowering blood glucose levels. When urine ketones are present, the client should **not** exercise. Ketones indicate that current insulin levels are not adequate and that exercise would elevate blood glucose levels.

Low-intensity aerobic exercise for longer durations is most effective in achieving desired health effects for clients with diabetes. These exercises require slow, submaximal effort, continue for more than 12 to 15 minutes, and moderately elevate the heart rate (above 50% of maximal rate). Such activities include walking briskly, running, jogging, stationary or regular bicycling, swimming, dancing, rowing, and cross-country skiing. These activities improve cardiac output.

For clients with type 1 diabetes, the aerobic exercise should last for 20 to 40 minutes and be performed 4 to 7 days per week. A 5- to 10-minute warm-up period with stretching and low-intensity exercise before exercise and a 5- to 10-minute cool-down period after exercise reduce the risk for dysrhythmias. Daily exercise increases total energy expenditure, helps weight loss, and improves blood glucose control.

Client Education: Exercise Promotion. Chart 68-7 lists NIC intervention activities for exercise. Instruct the client to wear shoes with good traction and cushioning and to examine the feet daily and after exercise. Discourage exercise in extreme heat or cold or during periods of poor blood glucose control. Advise the client to stay hydrated, especially during and after exercise in a warm environment.

Teach clients not to exercise within 1 hour of insulin injection or at the peak time of insulin action. Exercise can increase absorption of insulin from the injection site, increasing blood insulin levels. The risk for hypoglycemia increases when insulin is injected into an area that is exercised.

CHART 68-7

NIC INTERVENTION ACTIVITIES for The Diabetic Client Needing to Increase Physical Activity

Exercise Promotion: *Facilitation of regular physical activity to maintain or advance to a higher level of fitness and health*

- Appraise individual's health beliefs about physical exercise.
- Encourage verbalization of feelings about exercise or need for exercise.
- Include family/caregivers in planning and maintaining the exercise program.
- Inform individual about health beliefs and physiologic effects of exercise.
- Instruct individual about appropriate type of exercise for level of health, in collaboration with physician and/or exercise physiologist.
- Instruct individual about desired frequency, duration, and intensity of the exercise program.
- Instruct individual about conditions warranting cessation of or alteration in the exercise program.
- Instruct individual on proper warm-up and cool-down exercises.
- Instruct the individual in techniques to avoid injury while exercising.
- Assist individual to develop an appropriate exercise program to meet needs.
- Assist individual to set short-term and long-term goals for the exercise program.
- Assist individual to schedule regular periods for the exercise program into weekly routine.
- Monitor individual's response to exercise program.
- Provide positive feedback for individual's efforts.

Vital Signs Monitoring: *Collection and analysis of cardiovascular, respiratory, and body temperature data to determine and prevent complications*

- Monitor blood pressure, pulse, temperature, and respiratory status, as appropriate.
- Monitor for and report signs and symptoms of hypothermia and hyperthermia.
- Monitor presence and quality of pulses.
- Monitor cardiac rhythm and rate.
- Monitor respiratory rate and rhythm (e.g., depth and symmetry).
- Monitor for abnormal respiratory patterns (e.g., Cheyne-Stokes, Kussmaul, Biot, apneustic, ataxic, and excessive sighing).
- Monitor skin color, temperature, and moistness.
- Identify possible causes of changes in vital signs.

NIC intervention activities selected from Dochterman, J.M., & Bulechek, G.M. (Eds.). (2004). *Nursing interventions classification (NIC)* (4th ed.). St. Louis: Mosby. No part of this work is to be altered without prior written permission from the Publisher.

Make sure clients engaging in exercise know the risk for hypoglycemia, and teach preventive measures. Clients taking oral drugs or insulin should monitor blood glucose levels to determine the effects of exercise. Teach the client that snacks containing rapidly absorbable carbohydrate may be eaten before and during exercise to maintain blood glucose levels within normal ranges. Extra carbohydrate may be needed for up to 24 hours after exercise to prevent hypoglycemia. The amount of additional carbohydrate is directed by the results of blood glucose monitoring. Instruct the client to decrease insulin dosage before planned exercise as directed.

Clients with type 1 diabetes should perform vigorous exercise only if blood glucose levels are 80 to 250 mg/dL (4.4 to 13.8 mmol/L) and no ketones are present in the urine. Advise the non-obese client who is taking insulin to have a carbohydrate-containing snack before exercise if at least 1 hour has elapsed since the last food was eaten or if high-intensity exercise is planned. There is no need for additional carbohydrate intake when the blood glucose level exceeds 100 mg/dL (5.6 mmol/L) before exercise and the planned activity is of low intensity and short duration. When vigorous activity of long duration is planned, the client should eat an additional 15 to 30 g of carbohydrate for every 30 to 60 minutes of exercise. Snacks such as fruit, fruit juice, bread products, and whole milk are effective in preventing hypoglycemia. Instruct the client to carry a simple sugar (hard candy) to eat if symptoms of hypoglycemia occur. Also instruct the client to carry identifying information about having diabetes.

CONSIDERATIONS FOR OLDER ADULTS

With age, the ability of the heart and lungs to deliver oxygen to tissues and organs declines. These changes may result more from a decline in muscle mass than to changes in cardiac output. Aerobic activities are important in maintaining muscle mass. Healthy older clients are able to maintain cardiac output by increasing stroke volume during exercise.

In the absence of retinopathy-related restrictions, strength (resistance) training for major muscles of the legs, arms, stomach, and trunk, performed two or three times weekly helps preserve muscle mass and minimizes general functional decline (Flood & Constance, 2002).

SURGICAL MANAGEMENT. Surgical interventions for diabetes mellitus include transplantation of all or part of the pancreas. Successful pancreas and islet cell transplantations are the only therapies that achieve blood glucose control by providing normal insulin secretion that responds to feedback regulation (Robertson et al., 2000). Clients' quality of life is improved when they no longer have to take insulin injections and are free of diabetic dietary restrictions.

Whole-Pancreas Transplantation. Improved surgical techniques and newer immunosuppressive therapies have improved pancreatic transplantation outcomes. The 1-year survival rate is above 90%, with more than 80% of clients remaining free of insulin injection and diet restrictions after 1 year (Cattral et al., 2000). The degree of tissue-type matching affects the results.

Pancreatic transplantation is performed in one of three ways: transplant of the pancreas alone (PTA), transplant of the pancreas after successful kidney transplant (PAK), and simultaneous pancreas and kidney transplant (SPK). The ideal procedure for diabetic clients with uremia is SPK. These clients are generally poor surgical candidates because of complications from the diabetes. The problems of diabetes must be severe enough to balance the toxicity of immunosuppressive drugs. Pancreatic transplant is only partially successful in reversing the long-term complications of diabetes (ADA, 2003m).

Operative Procedures. Most pancreatic transplants are from cadaver donors using a total pancreas still attached to the exit of the pancreatic duct. The pancreas is placed in the pelvis and the pancreatic duct outlet is attached to the urinary bladder. Endocrine hormones from the pancreas drain into systemic circulation and exocrine hormones drain into the urinary bladder (systemic venous-bladder). Pancreatic transplant is successful when the client no longer needs insulin therapy and all blood measures of glucose are normal.

Chronic loss of pancreatic secretions can cause dehydration and electrolyte imbalance, and drainage of exocrine hormones into the urinary bladder causes irritation. Some techniques allow drainage of endocrine hormones into the portal venous system and intestinal drainage of exocrine secretions (portal venous-enteric).

Rejection Management. A combination of drugs and antibodies are used to reverse rejection. (See Chapter 23 for a listing of agents used to prevent or treat transplant rejection.) Clients undergoing immunosuppressive therapy first receive drugs to prevent viral, bacterial, and fungal infection because of the risk for opportunistic infections.

In nearly 90% of rejections, kidney problems occur before pancreatic problems. An increase in serum creatinine indicates rejection of both the transplanted kidney and the pancreas. In clients with bladder drainage of pancreatic hormones, a decrease in the urine amylase level by 25% is an indication to treat rejection. High blood glucose levels are a later marker of rejection and usually indicate irreversible graft failure.

Long-Term Effects. Long-term immunosuppressive therapy increases the risk for infection, cancer, and atherosclerosis. The transplanted pancreas does not duplicate all the functions of a normal pancreas. When insulin drains into systemic rather than portal circulation, circulating insulin levels rise (hyperinsulinemia) and increase the risk for hypertension and macrovascular disease.

Complications. Complications are common in clients taking long-term immunosuppressive therapy. Pancreatic transplant complications include venous thrombosis, rejection, and infection. Monitor laboratory values, fluid and electrolyte status, physical manifestations, and changes in vital signs to identify possible complications. Early removal of IV and intra-arterial lines, use of sterile technique with dressing changes and catheter irrigations, strict handwashing by health care personnel, and good pulmonary hygiene all help prevent infection.

Pancreatic blood vessel thrombosis occurs in about 30% of clients after transplantation. Observe for and report any sudden drop in urine amylase levels, rapid increases in blood glucose, gross **hematuria** (bloody urine), and tenderness or pain in the graft area (iliac fossa).

Assess the client for manifestations of rejection. In acute rejection, decreased kidney function is indicated by increased serum creatinine, decreased urine output, hypertension, increased weight, graft tenderness, and fever. Proteinuria is often the first indicator of chronic graft rejection. Check for increased blood amylase, lipase, or glucose; decreased urine amylase; graft tenderness; hyperglycemia; and fever. It is especially important to assess for signs of infection and start appropriate treatment. Fever can signal both infection and rejection.

Monitor for side effects of the immunosuppressive drugs. Cyclosporine (Neoral) is toxic to the kidney. Signs of toxicity are elevated creatinine and decreased urine output. Monitor white blood cell counts daily, because azathioprine (Imuran) can suppress bone marrow function. Prednisone has many side effects, including elevated blood glucose levels. Common side effects of tacrolimus (Prograf) are hypertension, kidney toxicity, neurotoxicity, gastrointestinal (GI) toxicity, and glucose intolerance.

The client's quality of life improves as a result of freedom from the need for insulin, a less restricted lifestyle, and a return to a normal diet. You must stress, however, the potential need for insulin injections to treat hyperglycemia caused by immunosuppressive drugs.

Islet Cell Transplantation. Islet cell transplantation eliminates the need for insulin and provides protection from the complications of diabetes. Wider use of this procedure is hindered by the limited supply of beta cells available for transplantation and by problems caused by antirejection drugs. Islet cells from tissue-typed (HLA-matched) cadaver pancreas glands are injected into the portal vein. The new cells lodge in the liver and begin to function, secreting insulin and maintaining near perfect blood glucose control. Successful transplantation has occurred in a small number of clients, and this therapy is currently experimental (ADA, 2003m).

RISK FOR DELAYED SURGICAL RECOVERY

NOC **PLANNING: EXPECTED OUTCOMES.** The client with diabetes undergoing a surgical procedure is expected to recover completely without complications. Indicators include the following:

- Wound healing
- Absence of infection
- Maintenance of blood glucose levels within expected range
- Discharge readiness

INTERVENTIONS. Surgery is a physical and emotional stressor, and the diabetic client has a higher than average risk for complications. Acute stress increases the blood glucose levels. Counterregulatory hormones suppress insulin action, increasing the risk for ketoacidosis and metabolic acidosis. Fasting worsens ketoacidosis. Diuresis from hyperglycemia can cause severe dehydration and electrolyte loss.

Coronary artery disease, diabetic nephropathy, and autonomic neuropathy further increase the risk for surgical complications. Diabetic nephropathy complicates fluid management. Cardiac dysrhythmias may result from the combined effect of anesthesia and autonomic neuropathy. Autonomic neuropathy may cause paralytic ileus and urinary retention after surgery.

Blood glucose must be controlled to prevent hypoglycemia, diabetic ketoacidosis (DKA), and hyperglycemic-hyperosmolar nonketotic syndrome (HNNS). Blood glucose control is needed to reduce infection and promote wound healing. For best healing, the blood glucose level should be less than 200 mg/dL (11.1 mmol/L) (Franz, 2001).

Preoperative Care. Chlorpropamide (Diabinese) is stopped for at least 36 hours before surgery. Metformin (Glucophage) is stopped 48 hours before surgery and restarted only after renal function is normal. All other oral drugs are stopped the day of surgery. Insulin is adjusted based on blood glucose levels before surgery. IV access is used to maintain hydration, monitor blood glucose results, and allow insulin delivery.

Surgery for clients with type 1 diabetes is performed early in the day to cause the least disruption in blood glucose control. When surgery is performed later in the day, IV insulin is used to stabilize blood glucose levels. Withholding insulin can cause hyperglycemia, ketosis, and electrolyte problems. Monitor blood glucose often during the perioperative period to determine the need for additional insulin.

Plan ahead for pain control after surgery. Pain, a stressor, triggers the release of counterregulatory hormones, increasing blood glucose levels and insulin needs. Opioid analgesics slow gastrointestinal (GI) motility and alter blood glucose levels. The older client who receives opioids is more at risk for confusion, paralytic ileus, hypoventilation, and hypotension. Compared with IM opioids, patient-controlled analgesia (PCA) systems cause fewer respiratory complications and less confusion. (See Chapter 7 for pain interventions and Chapter 20 for general preoperative care.)

Intraoperative Care. The frequency of blood glucose assessment depends in part on the type of anesthetic agent used. Epidural anesthesia has little effect on glucose metabolism. During general anesthesia, glucose levels increase early and remain elevated through surgery. Surgery lasting 3 to 5 hours or longer leads to greater hyperglycemia, with these clients needing supplemental short-acting insulin.

The goal is to keep the glucose level between 140 and 200 mg/dL during surgery to prevent hypoglycemia. Levels below 200 mg/dL reduce the risk for wound infection. IV delivery of short-acting insulin in 5% to 10% glucose is recommended for all insulin-treated clients, as well as in clients with poorly controlled type 2 diabetes who are receiving general anesthesia. Larger than normal insulin doses may be needed during surgery because stress releases glucagon and epinephrine. Insulin/glucose infusion rates are based on hourly capillary glucose tests.

NIC intervention activities for vital sign monitoring are listed in Chart 68-7. Monitor the client's temperature; it may be lowered deliberately in some surgical procedures and inadvertently in others. Low operating room temperatures and large incisions also lower body temperature. Hypothermia decreases metabolic needs, depresses heart rate and contractility, causes vasoconstriction, and impairs insulin release, resulting in high blood glucose levels. Monitor arterial blood gas values for acidosis.

Postoperative Care. Continue glucose and insulin infusions, as prescribed, until the client is stable and can tolerate oral feedings. Supplemental short-acting insulin may be needed to control blood glucose levels until the client's usual drug regimen is restarted. Short-term insulin therapy may be needed after surgery for the client who usually uses oral agents alone. For the client receiving insulin therapy, the usual dosage may change until the stress of surgery subsides. To prevent insulin allergy, use only human insulin for short-term therapy.

Monitoring. Clients with autonomic neuropathy or vascular disease need close monitoring to avoid hypotension or respiratory arrest. Clients who take beta blockers for hypertension need close monitoring for hypoglycemia because these drugs mask hypoglycemia. Clients with **azotemia** (increased nitrogen waste products in the blood) may have problems with fluid management. Check central venous pressure or pulmonary artery pressure as needed.

Hyperkalemia (high blood potassium level) is common in clients with mild to moderate kidney failure and can lead to an acute cardiac dysrhythmia. In other clients, **hypokalemia** (low blood potassium level) may occur and be made worse by insulin and glucose given during surgery. Watch the client's cardiac rhythm and serum potassium values.

CARDIOVASCULAR MONITORING. Serial electrocardiograms (ECGs) are recommended for older diabetic clients, those with long-standing type 1 diabetes, and those with heart disease. Diabetic clients are at higher risk for myocardial infarction (MI) after surgery with a higher mortality rate. Changes in ECG or in potassium level may indicate a silent MI.

RENAL MONITORING. Monitoring fluid balance helps detect acute kidney failure. Diagnosis of renal impairment may require the use of x-ray studies using dyes, which may be nephrotoxic. Treatment of infections may require the use of nephrotoxic antibiotics. Ensure adequate hydration when these drugs are used. Watch for impending renal failure by assessing fluid and electrolyte status.

Nutritional Care. Using total parenteral nutrition (TPN) in diabetic clients can cause severe metabolic changes. Monitor blood glucose often to determine the need for supplemental short-acting insulin. After the insulin dose is stabilized, it can be added to the TPN solution and the frequency of capillary blood glucose monitoring decreased.

Returning to a normal meal plan as soon as possible after surgery promotes healing and metabolic balance. When oral foods are tolerated, make sure the client takes at least 150 to 200 g of carbohydrate daily to prevent hypoglycemia.

RISK FOR INJURY RELATED TO SENSORY ALTERATIONS

NOC **PLANNING: EXPECTED OUTCOMES.** The client with diabetes is expected to identify factors that increase the risk for injury, practice proper foot care, and maintain intact skin on the feet. Indicators include that the client consistently demonstrates the following behaviors:

- Following preventive foot care practices
- Cleansing and inspecting the feet daily
- Wearing properly fitting shoes
- Avoiding walking in bare feet
- Trimming toenails properly
- Reporting non-healing breaks in the skin of the feet to the health care provider

INTERVENTIONS. Clients with diabetes need intensive teaching about foot care. Foot injury is the most common complication of diabetes leading to hospitalization. Diabetes is the leading cause of amputation worldwide. The overall risk for amputation is 15 times greater in diabetic clients than in nondiabetic clients. For clients with a previous amputation, the risk for amputation in the second leg is 10 to 20 times greater than among the general population. The 5-year mortality rate after leg or foot amputation ranges from 39% to 68%. Factors related to an increased risk for amputation include duration of diabetes, poor glucose control, and low levels of high-density lipoprotein (HDL) cholesterol.

Sensory neuropathy, ischemia, and infection are the leading causes of foot disease among clients with diabetes. Peripheral sensory neuropathy occurs in 60% to 90% of diabetic foot ulcers (Inlow, Orsted, & Sibbald, 2000). Loss of pain, pressure, and temperature sensation in the foot increases the risk for injury and ulceration. Impaired blood flow to the foot limits wound healing.

Claw toe deformity is common in diabetic neuropathy (Inlow, Orsted, & Sibbald, 2000). Toes are hyperextended, which increases pressure on the metatarsal heads ("ball" of the foot), resulting in ulceration. Thinning or shifting of the fat pad under the metatarsal heads decreases cushioning and increases areas of pressure. These changes predispose the client to callus formation, ulceration, and infection. Figure 68-10 shows hallux valgus (turning of the great toe), and Figure 68-11 shows a hammertoe.

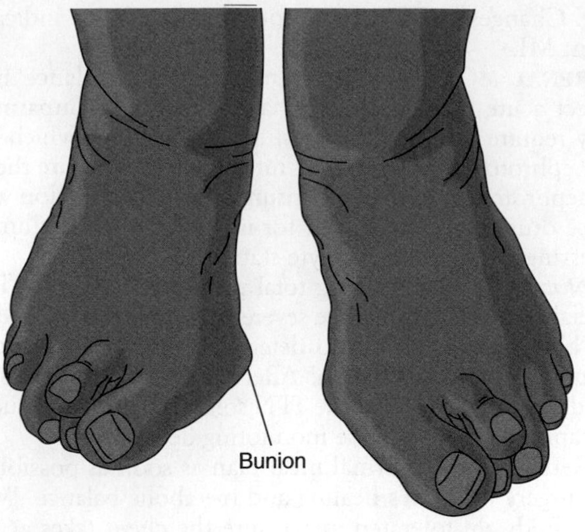

Figure 68-10 ■ The appearance of hallux valgus with a bunion.

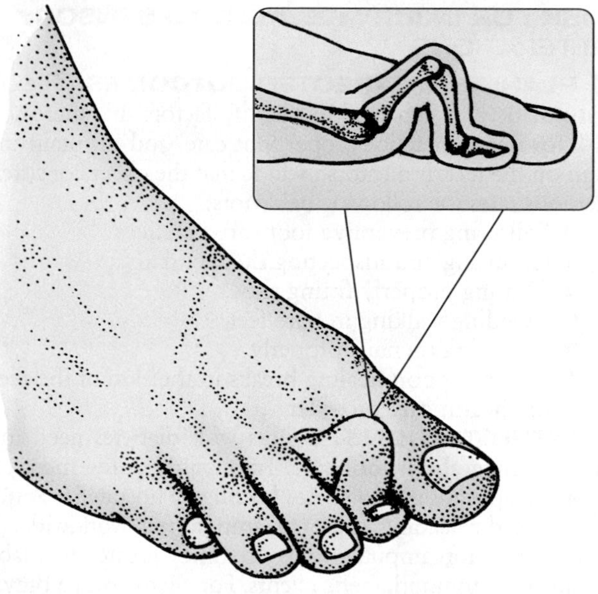

Figure 68-11 ■ Hammertoe of the second metatarsophalangeal (MTP) joint.

The Charcot foot is a type of diabetic foot deformity. The foot is warm, swollen, and painful. Walking collapses the arch, shortens the foot, and gives the foot a "rocker bottom" shape.

Sensory neuropathy may cause tingling or burning, but more often it produces numbness and reduced sensation. Neuropathy causes loss of normal sweating and skin temperature regulation, resulting in dry, thinning skin. Skin cracks and fissures increase the risk for infection.

Without sensation, the client does not notice physical, thermal, or chemical injuries to the foot and does not treat them. Foot injuries can be caused by walking barefoot, wearing ill-fitting shoes, sustaining thermal injuries from hot water (e.g., water bottles, heating pads, baths), or receiving caustic burns from over-the-counter corn treatments. Because the blood supply to the diabetic foot is poor, these injuries sometimes lead to amputation.

Ulcers result from continued pressure. Plantar ulcers (on the sole, usually the ball) are from standing or walking. Ulcers on the top or sides of the foot usually are from shoes. The increased pressure causes calluses. Ulcers usually form over or around the great toe, under the metatarsal heads, and on the tops of claw toes.

Broken skin increases the risk for infection. Skin tends to break in areas of pressure. Infection is common in diabetic foot ulcers and, once present, is difficult to treat. Infection also impairs glucose control, leading to higher blood glucose levels and reduced immune defense mechanisms. Decreased immune function further increases the risk for infection.

Prevention of High Risk Conditions. Neuropathy of the feet and legs can be delayed by keeping blood glucose levels as near normal as possible. Poor blood glucose control increases the risk for neuropathy and amputation. Intensive therapy reduces the risk for peripheral sensory neuropathy by 60%. Encourage smoking cessation to reduce the risk for vascular complications.

The risk for ulcers or amputation increases with duration of diabetes. Other risk factors are male gender; poor glucose control; and cardiovascular, retinal, or renal complications. Foot-related risks include poor gait and stepping mechanics, peripheral neuropathy, increased pressure (callus, erythema, hemorrhage under a callus, limited joint mobility, foot deformities, or severe nail pathology), peripheral vascular disease, and a history of ulcers or amputation (ADA, 2003p).

NIC **Peripheral Sensation Management.** The feet should be evaluated closely at least annually (ADA, 2003p). Chart 68-8 lists NIC intervention activities for peripheral sensation management and foot care, and Table 68-16 lists foot risk categories. The Evidence-Based Practice for Nursing box on p. 1536 supports the need for continued education on foot care practices.

Complete a full foot assessment as outlined in Chart 68-9. Sensory examination with Semmes-Weinstein monofilaments is the most practical measure of the risk for foot ulcers. The nylon monofilament is mounted on a holder standardized to exert a 10-g force. There is no agreement on the exact number of sites to test. A person who cannot feel the 10-g pressure at any point is at increased risk for ulcers. Perform the examination in the following way:

- Provide a quiet and relaxed setting. Ask the client to close his or her eyes during the test.
- Test the monofilament on the client's cheek so he or she knows what to expect.
- Test the sites noted in Figure 68-12.
- Apply the monofilament at a right angle to the skin surface.
- Apply enough force to bend the filament using a smooth, not jabbing motion (Figure 68-13).
- The approach, contact, and removal of the filament at each site should take 1 to 2 seconds.
- Apply the filament along the perimeter and **not** on an ulcer site, callus, scar, or necrotic tissue. Do not slide the filament across the skin or make repeated contact at the test site.
- Randomize the sequence of applying the filament throughout the examination. Have the client identify where the filament touched (*Feet Can Last a Lifetime*, 2001).

Footwear. All clients with any degree of peripheral neuropathy need to wear protective shoes. They must be fitted by an experienced shoe fitter, such as a certified podiatrist. The shoe should be ½ to ⅝ inch longer than the

CHART 68-8

NIC **INTERVENTION ACTIVITIES for**
The Diabetic Client with Reduced Sensation in the Lower Extremities

Peripheral Sensation Management: *Prevention or minimization of injury or discomfort in the client with altered sensation.*
- Monitor sharp/dull and/or hot/cold discrimination.
- Monitor for paresthesia: numbness, tingling, hyperesthesia, and hypoesthesia.
- Encourage client to use the unaffected body part to determine temperature of food, liquids, bathwater, and so on.
- Instruct client or family to monitor position of body parts while the client is bathing, sitting, lying, or changing position.
- Instruct client or family to examine skin daily for alteration in skin integrity.
- Monitor fit of bracing devices, prostheses, shoes, and clothing.
- Instruct client or family to use thermometer to test water temperature.
- Encourage use of gloves or other protective clothing over affected body part when body part is in contact with objects that—because of their thermal, textural, or other characteristics—may be potentially hazardous.
- Avoid or carefully monitor use of heat or cold, such as heating pads, hot water bottles, and ice packs.
- Encourage client to wear well-fitting, low-heeled, soft shoes.
- Check shoes, pockets, and clothing for wrinkles or foreign objects.
- Instruct client to use timed intervals, rather than presence of discomfort, as a signal to alter position.
- Protect body parts from extreme temperature changes.
- Discuss or identify causes of abnormal sensation or sensation changes.
- Instruct client to visually monitor position of body parts, if proprioception is impaired.

Foot Care: *Cleansing and inspecting the feet for the purposes of relaxation, cleanliness, and healthy skin*
- Inspect skin for irritation, cracking, lesions, corns, calluses, deformities, or edema.
- Inspect client's shoes for proper fit.
- Dry carefully between toes.
- Apply lotion.
- Clean nails.
- Apply moisture-absorbing powder, as indicated.
- Discuss with client usual foot care routine.
- Instruct client/family on the importance of foot care.
- Offer positive feedback about self-care foot activities.
- Monitor client's gait and weight distribution on feet.
- Monitor cleanliness and general condition of shoes and stockings.
- Instruct client to inspect inside of shoes for rough areas.
- Monitor hydration level of feet.
- Monitor for arterial insufficiency in lower legs.
- Monitor legs and feet for edema.
- Instruct client to monitor temperature of feet using the back of the hand.
- Instruct client in the importance of inspection, especially when sensation is diminished.
- Cut normal-thickness toenails when soft, using a toenail clipper and using the curve of the toe as a guide.
- Refer to podiatrist for trimming of thickened nails, as appropriate.

NIC intervention activities selected from Dochterman, J.M., & Bulechek, G.M. (Eds.). (2004). *Nursing interventions classification (NIC)* (4th ed.). St. Louis: Mosby. No part of this work is to be altered without prior written permission from the Publisher.

TABLE 68-16 Foot Risk Categories

Risk Categories	Management Categories
Risk Category 0 ■ Has disease that leads to insensitivity ■ Has protective sensation ■ Has not had a plantar ulcer	***Management Category 0*** ■ Examine feet at each visit, at least four times per year ■ Foot clinic once a year ■ Client education
Risk Category 1 ■ Does not have protective sensation ■ Has not had a plantar ulcer ■ Does not have a foot deformity	***Management Category 1*** ■ Examine feet at each visit, at least four times per year ■ Foot clinic visit every 6 months ■ Soft insoles ■ Client education
Risk Category 2 ■ Does not have protective sensation ■ Has not had a plantar ulcer ■ Does have a foot deformity	***Management Category 2*** ■ Examine feet at each visit, at least 4 times per year ■ Foot clinic visit every 3-4 months ■ Custom-molded insoles ■ Prescription footwear ■ Client education
Risk Category 3 ■ Does not have protective sensation ■ Has history of plantar ulcer	***Management Category 3*** ■ Examine feet at each visit, at least four times per year ■ Foot clinic visit every 1 to 2 months ■ Custom-molded insoles ■ Prescription footwear ■ Client education

From Gillis W. Long Hansen's Disease Center Rehabilitation Branch. (1992). *Foot screening: Care of the foot in diabetes: The Carville approach.* Carville, LA: Department of Health and Human Services.

longest toe. Heels should be less than 2 inches high. Shoes that are too tight damage tissue when worn for 4 hours or longer. Teach the client to change shoes by midday and again in the evening. Socks or stockings need to fit properly and be appropriate for the planned activity. Stockings should feel soft and have no thick seams, creases, or holes. They should pad the foot and absorb excess moisture. Teach clients to avoid tight stockings or those that have constricting bands. Clients with toe deformities should buy custom shoes with high, wide toe boxes and extra depth. Clients with severely deformed feet, such as Charcot feet, need specially molded shoes. All new shoes need a long break-in period with frequent inspection for irritation or blistering.

Foot Care. Teach clients about preventive foot care and the need for examination of the feet and legs at each visit to a health care provider. Identify clients with high-risk foot conditions and teach them about foot care. Explain problems caused by loss of protective sensation, the importance of monitoring the feet daily, proper care of the feet (including nail and skin care), and how to select appropriate footwear. Advise clients with neuropathy to break in new shoes slowly to reduce blisters (ADA, 2003p).

Teach clients to inspect their feet daily. Assess the client's ability to inspect all areas of the foot and to perform foot care. Teach family members how to inspect and care for client's feet if the client cannot (ADA, 2003p). Chart 68-10 lists foot care instructions.

Wound Care. The standards of care for diabetic ulcers are a moist wound environment, debridement of necrotic tissue, and elimination of pressure (off-loading).

EVIDENCE-BASED PRACTICE for Nursing

Rural-dwelling diabetics are at risk for foot ulcers

Neil, J.A. (2002). Assessing foot care knowledge in a rural population with diabetes. *Ostomy/Wound Management, 48*(1), 50-56.

This study follows a group of rural-dwelling individuals with diabetes who received education in foot care and foot wear management at some time during their illness. All of the participants had "diminished protective sensation" on Semmes-Weinstein monofilament testing. The purpose of the study was to evaluate foot care practices among rural persons with diabetes mellitus and diminished protective sensation. The study sample included 61 persons (average 46 years of age). At the time of the study, 24% to 39% of the participants had a foot ulcer. The participants were divided into two groups, those with ulcers, and those without foot ulcers. Subjects were interviewed to determine their foot cares practices. Foot care behaviors were determined by use of the Siriraj Foot-Care instrument, a previously validated tool on client knowledge of foot care.

Improper foot care practices were evident in a group of diabetic clients who already had foot ulcers as well as in those who were at high risk for developing ulcers. Reasons given for not performing foot care by subjects in the study were that they were unable to reach their feet or that they could not see their feet. Diabetic retinopathy and obesity were common in the study group. No statistical differences were found between the two groups on daily examination of their feet for reddened areas, blisters, corns, calluses, or open areas, for daily foot cleansing with warm water, or for nail cutting practices. Statistically significant differences were found in answers to questions about going barefoot. Those without ulcers were more likely to go barefoot inside the house. Poor foot care practices such as not adequately washing their feet, using knives or razor blades to trim nails, and going barefoot inside and outside the house were noted for both groups.

Level of Evidence: 6—Uncontrolled descriptive study.

Critique. The methods used were appropriate for this descriptive study.

Implications for Nursing. Nurses need to teach all clients with diabetes about appropriate foot care practices, especially for those clients identified at being at high risk for foot injury. The American Diabetes Association estimates that 50% of amputations are preventable. This study supports the work of others that indicates the need for frequent education for prevention of foot ulcers in people with diabetes mellitus.

Wound Environment. Dressings reduce or prevent infection, allow debridement, reduce wound pain, and stimulate granulation tissue. Many commercial products are available. Antiseptics such as povidone iodine, hydrogen peroxide, and chlorhexidine interfere with wound healing. Dressings that keep the wound moist are essential.

Debridement. Debridement removes dead tissues that support bacterial growth. It is accomplished with surgery, topical debriding agents, and dressings. Mechanical debridement, although helpful, can delay wound healing by removing newly formed tissue (Ayello, Cuddigan, & Kerstein, 2002).

Elimination of Pressure. Eliminating pressure on an infected area is essential to wound healing. Teach clients with foot ulcers to not wear a shoe on the foot while the ulcer is healing. Clients with poor sensation keep walking on an ulcer because it does not hurt. This results in pressure necrosis that delays healing and increases ulcer size. Pressure is reduced by specialized orthotic devices, custom-molded shoes inserts, or shoe adjustments that redistribute weight.

The best way to avoid weight-bearing is with a contact cast (Levin, 2002). Casting material is molded to the foot and leg so pressure is spread along the entire surface of contact, thereby reducing vertical force. The almost complete elimination of motion of the total-contact cast reduces plantar shear forces. The cast is removed 24 to 48 hours after application and weekly thereafter until the ulcer is healed. *Teach the client that foot ulcers will recur unless weight is permanently redistributed.*

Growth Factors. Growth factors applied to wounds increase the rate of healing by stimulating new tissue and enhancing cell growth. This treatment has helped heal foot ulcers present for many months or even years. Because it is costly and based on having other aspects of diabetes controlled, growth factor therapy is usually performed in specialized treatment centers.

CHART 68-9

FOCUSED ASSESSMENT of The Diabetic Foot

Assess the client for risk of diabetic foot problems:
- History of previous ulcer
- History of previous amputation

Assess the foot for abnormal skin and nail conditions:
- Dry, cracked, fissured skin
- Ulcers
- Toenails: thickened, long nails; ingrown nails
- Tinea pedis; onychomycosis (mycotic nails)

Assess the foot for status of circulation:
- Symptoms of claudication
- Presence or absence of dorsalis pedis or posterior tibial pulse
- Prolonged capillary filling time (greater than 25 seconds)
- Presence or absence of hair growth on the top of the foot

Assess the foot for evidence of deformity:
- Calluses, corns
- Prominent metatarsal heads (metatarsal head is easily felt under the skin)
- Toe contractures: clawed toes, hammertoes
- Hallux valgus or bunions
- Charcot foot ("rocker bottom")

Assess the foot for loss of strength:
- Limited ankle joint range of motion
- Limited motion of great toe

Assess the foot for loss of protective sensation:
- Numbness, burning, tingling
- Semmes-Weinstein monofilament testing at 10 points on each foot

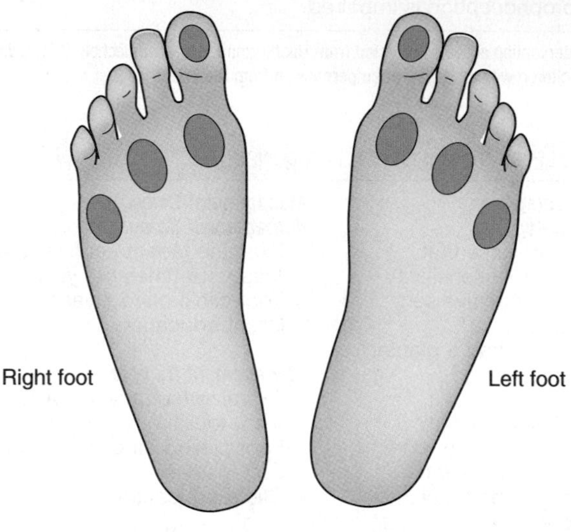

Figure 68-12 ■ Placement sites of monofilaments for testing of protective sensation.

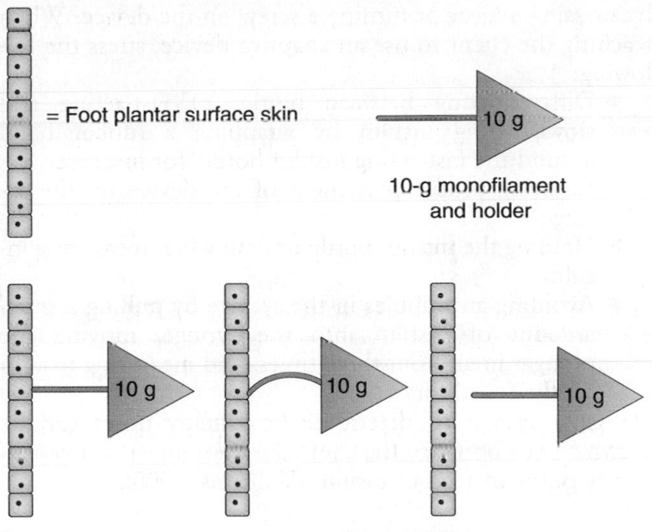

Figure 68-13 ■ Correct technique for sensation testing with 10-g monofilament. **A,** Apply monofilament to designated areas of the foot sole (intact skin, see Figure 68-12). **B,** Apply pressure to the filament until either the client states he or she can feel the pressure or until the filament bends (see p. 1534). **C,** Quickly remove the filament without sliding the filament or touching other areas of the foot.

CHRONIC PAIN

NOC **PLANNING: EXPECTED OUTCOMES.** The client with neuropathic pain is expected to experience relief of pain. Indicators include the following consistent behaviors:

- Using preventive measures
- Using available resources to increase comfort
- Reporting pain controlled.

INTERVENTIONS. NIC intervention activities to manage pain are listed in Chart 68-11. Maintaining normal blood glucose levels prevents neuropathy and relieves symptoms of acute nerve dysfunction. Anticonvulsants and antidepressants are often used to treat the pain of neuropathy. Drugs such as gabapentin (Neurontin) can reduce pain and improve quality of life (Bowker & Pfeifer, 2001). Tricyclic antidepressants, particularly amitriptyline hydrochloride (Elavil, Levate✱) and nortriptyline (Pamelor), also are used for neuropathic pain. Smaller doses are needed for analgesia than for antidepressant effects.

The burning of neuropathy may respond to capsaicin cream 0.075% (Axsain✱, Zostrix-HP). This drug reduces amounts of substance P, which is involved in pain transmission (see Chapter 7). Teach the client how to apply it four times daily for several weeks. Neuropathic pain may worsen for several days after therapy is started before improving.

RISK FOR INJURY RELATED TO DISTURBED SENSORY PERCEPTION: VISUAL

PLANNING: EXPECTED OUTCOMES. The client with diabetes is expected to be free of injury related to decreased visual acuity and to maintain current level of vision. Indicators include the following:

- No further reduction of visual fields
- No double vision

INTERVENTIONS.

Blood Glucose Control. Poor blood glucose control, proteinuria, diastolic hypertension, and long duration of diabetes are risk factors for diabetic retinopathy and vision loss. Surgical intervention for retinal hemorrhage or new retinal blood vessel growth can reduce vision loss.

Only about 10% of all visually impaired clients are totally blind. The rest have reduced vision. Besides regular eye examinations to evaluate retinopathy, urge the diabetic client with impaired vision to have an optometrist or ophthalmologist assess the remaining vision and prescribe appropriate eyewear. A functional vision assessment, performed by a low-vision technician, rehabilitation teacher, or diabetes educator, determines the client's use of lighting, contrast, nonoptical and low-vision devices, and large-print options. Included in this assessment is whether the client uses central or peripheral vision. Clients with macular edema have loss of central vision. This process causes difficulty seeing details, reading printed materials, preparing insulin syringes for injection, and self-monitoring blood glucose levels (SMBG).

Environmental Management. Not all visually impaired clients need special devices. Adjustments in lighting, contrast, color, distance, type size of printed materials, and eye movement often improve visual abilities. Instruct the client to supplement overhead fluorescent lighting with an incandescent lamp directed toward the workspace. Placing dark equipment against a white or yellow background (or vice versa) provides contrast to enhance vision. Coding objects such as vials of insulin with bright colors or with felt tipped markers help identify the correct bottle. Bringing the blood glucose lancet or insulin syringe close to the eye

CHART 68-10

CLIENT EDUCATION GUIDE
Foot Care Instructions

- Inspect your feet daily, especially the area between the toes.
- Wash your feet daily with lukewarm water and soap. Dry thoroughly.
- Apply moisturizing cream to your feet after bathing. Do not apply to the area between your toes.
- Change into clean cotton socks every day.
- Do not wear the same pair of shoes 2 days in a row, and wear only leather shoes.
- Check your shoes for foreign objects (nails, pebbles) before putting them on. Check inside the shoes for cracks or tears in the lining.
- Purchase shoes that have plenty of room for your toes. Buy shoes later in the day, when feet are normally larger. Break in new shoes gradually.
- Wear socks to keep your feet warm.
- Trim your nails straight across with a nail clipper. Smooth the nails with an emery board.
- See your physician or nurse immediately if you have blisters, sores, or infections. Protect area with a dry, sterile dressing. Do not use adhesive tape to secure dressing.
- Do not treat blisters, sores, or infections with home remedies.
- Do not smoke.
- Do not step into the bathtub without checking the temperature of the water with your wrist. Optimal temperature is 95° F (29.4° to 35° C).
- Do not use very hot or cold water. Never use hot water bottles, heating pads, or portable heaters to warm your feet.
- Do not treat corns, blisters, bunions, calluses, or ingrown toenails yourself.
- Do not go barefooted.
- Do not wear sandals with open toes or straps between the toes.
- Do not cross your legs or wear garters or tight stockings that constrict blood flow.
- Do not soak your feet.

CHART 68-11

NIC INTERVENTION ACTIVITIES for The Diabetic Client Experiencing Pain

Analgesic Administration: *Use of pharmacologic agents to reduce or eliminate pain*
- Determine pain location, characteristics, quality, and severity before medicating client.
- Check medical order for drug, dose, and frequency of analgesic prescribed.
- Attend to comfort needs and other activities that assist in relaxation to facilitate response to analgesia.
- Set positive expectations regarding the effectiveness of analgesics to optimize client response.
- Document response to analgesic and any untoward effects.
- Teach about the use of analgesics, strategies to decrease side effects, and expectations for involvement in decisions about pain relief.

Teaching: Individual: *Planning, implementation, and evaluation of a teaching program designed to address a client's particular needs*
- Establish rapport.
- Determine the client's learning needs.
- Appraise the client's current level of knowledge and understanding of content.
- Appraise the client's educational level.
- Appraise the client's cognitive, psychomotor, and affective abilities/disabilities.
- Determine the client's ability to learn specific information (i.e., developmental level, physiologic status, orientation, pain, fatigue, unfulfilled basic needs, emotional state, and adaptation to illness).
- Set mutual, realistic learning goals with the client.
- Identify learning objectives necessary to reach goals.
- Determine the sequence for presenting the information.
- Appraise the client's learning style.
- Select appropriate teaching method/strategies.
- Select appropriate educational materials.
- Tailor the content to the client's cognitive, psychomotor, and/or affective abilities/disabilities.
- Adjust instruction to facilitate learning, as appropriate.
- Provide an environment conducive to learning.
- Instruct the client, when appropriate.
- Evaluate the client's achievement of the stated objectives.
- Reinforce behavior, as appropriate.
- Correct information misinterpretations, as appropriate.
- Provide time for the client to ask questions and discuss concerns.
- Select new teaching methods/strategies, if previous ones were ineffective.
- Refer the client to other specialists/agencies to meet the learning objectives, as appropriate.
- Document the content presented, the written materials provided, and the client's understanding of the information or client behaviors that indicate learning on the permanent medical record.
- Include the family/significant others, as appropriate.

makes it easier to see. Suggest large type or bold print to ease reading. Teach the client to use peripheral vision.

Certain devices can help the client self-administer insulin independently. Some syringes may have a magnifier attached to the syringe. Other devices include preset dose gauges (which measure the space between the end of the syringe barrel and the plunger) to help the client draw up the correct amount of insulin by feeling this distance. Variable dose gauges draw insulin in variable and mixed doses of 1-, 2-, and 10-unit increments. The client sets the desired dose by pressing a lever or turning a screw on the device. When teaching the client to use an adaptive device, stress the following:
- Differentiating between bottles of fast-acting and slower-acting insulin by wrapping a rubber band around the fast-acting insulin bottle, for instance
- Ensuring proper placement of the device on the syringe
- Holding the insulin bottle upright when measuring insulin
- Avoiding air bubbles in the syringe by pulling a small amount of insulin into the syringe, moving the plunger in and out three times, and measuring insulin on the fourth draw

Design a system to determine how many doses can be drawn from a bottle so the client does not inject air from an empty bottle instead of insulin (Williams, 2000).

Critical Thinking Challenge

The client has had type 2 diabetes for many years and now needs insulin for glucose control. He has severe vision impairment. His wife has normal vision, but does not want "to stick him with needles," either for glucose testing or giving insulin. He would like to be as independent as possible in his two-dose protocol. He also has arthritis in his dominant shoulder (right side) and cannot reach around behind him.

1. What role can the wife have in blood glucose monitoring and insulin delivery?
2. What procedures could this client perform safely by himself?
3. Should the wife be taught insulin injection techniques? Why or why not?

evolve For suggested answer guidelines, go to http://evolve.elsevier.com/Iggy/.

INEFFECTIVE TISSUE PERFUSION: RENAL

NOC **PLANNING: EXPECTED OUTCOMES.** The client with diabetes is expected to maintain a normal urine elimination pattern. Indicators include the following:
- Urine protein levels within normal limits
- 24-hour intake and output balance
- Blood urea nitrogen (BUN) and serum creatinine within the normal ranges
- Serum electrolytes within the normal ranges

INTERVENTIONS

Prevention. Tight control of blood glucose levels may slow renal disease in clients with type 1 diabetes. Control of hypertension also slows diabetic nephropathy and the complications of hypertensive nephropathy (ADA, 2003r).

Stress the need for yearly evaluation of kidney function according to American Diabetes Association (ADA) Standards of Care. Screening is performed by three methods: (1) random, spot urine collection to measure the albumin-creatinine ratio, (2) 24-hour urine collection to measure creatinine clearance, and (3) timed urine collection (e.g., 4 hours or overnight) (ADA, 2003r). Timed urine collections are not reliable in clients with neuropathy and incomplete bladder emptying. Random urine albumin/creatinine testing is recommended as the standard measurement of proteinuria in clients with diabetes (Loon, 2003). Explain the implications of the test and help the client collect the specimen if necessary.

Aggressive control of blood glucose and hypertension in diabetic clients without microalbuminuria can avoid nephropathy. Once microalbuminuria develops, treatment is aimed at controlling blood pressure and blood glucose, restricting dietary protein, avoiding nephrotoxic agents, promptly treating urinary tract infections (UTIs), and preventing dehydration.

Control of blood pressure and blood glucose levels requires the client's effort. Prescribed drugs must be taken according to schedules, and dietary restriction must be maintained. Teach diabetic clients about the roles of blood pressure and blood glucose levels in renal disease. Help the client maintain normal blood glucose levels and blood pressure levels below 130/80 mm Hg (ADA, 2003d). Stress the need for yearly screening for microalbuminuria.

Any UTI can lead to kidney infection and further reduce renal function. Explain the manifestations of UTI. Urge the client to take antibiotics exactly as prescribed, completing the course of treatment. Reinforce the need for follow-up urine cultures to reduce the risk of renal damage. Avoid indwelling urinary catheters when possible.

Drugs can affect renal function either through toxic effects on the kidney or by an acute but reversible reduction in function. The most common nephrotoxic drugs are antifungal agents (amphotericin B); aminoglycoside antibiotics such as amikacin (Amikin), streptomycin, kanamycin (Kantrex), gentamicin (Garamycin), and tobramycin (Tobrex); and nonsteroidal anti-inflammatory drugs such as ibuprofen (Advil) or naproxen (Aleve). Radiocontrast dyes can also affect renal function (Singri, Ahya, & Levin, 2003). To prevent accidental ingestion of nephrotoxic drugs, caution the client to check with a health care provider before taking over-the-counter or prescription drugs.

Diet Therapy. Clients with nephropathy should restrict dietary protein to 0.8 g/kg of body weight per day. Once the glomerular filtration rate (GFR) starts falling, further reducing protein to 0.6 g/kg may slow the decline in renal function (ADA, 2003d). Because lifelong dietary restrictions are difficult, provide ongoing teaching to encourage adherence.

NIC **Fluid/Electrolyte Management.** Fluid and electrolyte management can prevent more loss of renal function. NIC intervention activities for fluid and electrolyte management are listed in Chart 68-12. Avoiding dehydration is important for renal perfusion and function. Any illness that leads to dehydration or hypotension is treated with isotonic saline for volume replacement (Singri, Ahya, & Levin, 2003). Assess fluid balance, and use measures to prevent dehydration. The most common cause of dehydration in clients with diabetes is overuse of diuretics. Teach clients to report edema or symptoms of orthostatic hypotension and provide ongoing education to promote dietary goals.

Dialysis for clients with diabetes and renal failure is the same as for clients without diabetes (see Chapter 75). The dosage of insulin needs to be adjusted when dialysis starts.

POTENTIAL FOR HYPOGLYCEMIA

Central nervous system (CNS) function depends on a continuous supply of glucose in the blood. The brain cannot make glucose and stores only a few minutes' supply as glycogen. This needed supply is not maintained when blood glucose levels fall below critical levels.

The first defense against falling blood glucose levels in the nondiabetic client is decreased insulin secretion, decreased glucose use, and increased glucose production. Normally, insulin secretion decreases when blood glucose levels drop to about 83 mg/dL (4.5 mmol/L). Counterregulatory hormones are activated at about 68 mg/dL (3.8 mmol/L), a level well above the threshold for symptoms of hypoglycemia. The main counterregulatory hormone is glucagon; epinephrine also becomes important in diabetic clients who are deficient in glucagon. Both glucagon and epinephrine raise blood glucose levels by stimulating liver glycogenolysis and gluconeogenesis. Epinephrine also limits insulin secretion.

Type 1 diabetes disrupts the body's response to hypoglycemia, a change that occurs within 1 to 5 years of diagnosis. Regulation of circulating insulin levels is lost because the insulin comes from an injection rather than from the pancreas. As blood glucose levels fall, insulin levels do not decrease. Over time, the pancreas loses its ability to secrete glucagon in response to hypoglycemia. After a few more years of type 1 diabetes, the response of epinephrine to falling blood glucose levels is also reduced. It does respond, but it takes a lower blood glucose level to become active. These problems dramatically increase the risk for severe hypoglycemia.

A second problem with long-standing type 1 diabetes is *hypoglycemic unawareness*. Clients no longer have the warning symptoms of impending hypoglycemia that should prompt them to take preventive action. Hypoglycemic unawareness occurs in about 25% of diabetic clients and about 50% of all clients who have had type 1 diabetes for 30 years or longer.

Symptoms of hypoglycemia are neuroglycopenic or neurologic. Neuroglycopenic symptoms occur when brain glucose gradually declines to a low level. Neurologic symptoms result from autonomic nervous activity triggered by a rapid decline in blood glucose (Table 68-17).

The blood glucose level at which symptoms of hypoglycemia occur varies among clients. Many have symptoms when blood glucose levels are well above 50 mg/dL (2.8 mmol/L), especially if the level dropped rapidly or they are used to chronic hyperglycemia. Thus, clinical criteria are used to categorize hypoglycemic severity rather than blood glucose levels. In mild hypoglycemia, the client remains alert and able to treat symptoms. In severe hypoglycemia, neurologic function is so impaired that the client needs another person's help.

PLANNING: EXPECTED OUTCOMES. The diabetic client is expected to have decreased episodes of hypoglycemia and remain oriented to person, place, and time, as indicated by a Glasgow Coma Scale score above 7.

INTERVENTIONS. Because symptoms of hypoglycemia commonly occur at levels above 50 mg/dL, a blood glucose level below 70 mg/dL requires an assessment (Franz, 2001) (Table 68-18; see Table 68-17).

NIC **Hypoglycemia Management.** NIC intervention activities for hypoglycemia appear in Chart 68-13. Monitor blood glucose levels before giving antidiabetic drugs, before meals, before bedtime, and when the client is symptomatic. All clients who take insulin or other antidiabetic drugs are at risk for hypoglycemia, especially if they are older, have liver or kidney impairment, or are taking drugs that enhance the effects of antidiabetic drugs. Proper client selection, drug dosage, and instructions are important factors in avoiding severe hypoglycemia. Hypoglycemia may be difficult to rec-

CHART 68-12

NIC INTERVENTION ACTIVITIES for The Diabetic Client Experiencing Fluid and Electrolyte and Acid-Base Imbalances

Fluid/Electrolyte Management: *Regulation and prevention of complications from altered fluid and/or electrolyte levels*

- Monitor for abnormal serum electrolyte levels, as available.
- Obtain laboratory specimens for monitoring of altered fluid or electrolyte levels (e.g., hematocrit, BUN, protein, sodium, and potassium levels), as appropriate.
- Weigh client daily and monitor trends.
- Promote oral intake (e.g., provide oral fluids that are the client's preference, place in easy reach, provide a straw, and provide fresh water), as appropriate.
- Set an appropriate intravenous infusion (or blood transfusion) flow rate.
- Monitor laboratory results relevant to fluid balance (e.g., hematocrit, BUN, albumin, total protein, serum osmolarity, and urine specific gravity levels).
- Monitor hemodynamic status, including CVP, MAP, PAP, and PCWP levels, if available.
- Keep an accurate record of intake and output.
- Monitor for signs and symptoms of fluid retention.
- Monitor vital signs, as appropriate.
- Maintain intravenous solution containing electrolyte(s) at a constant flow rate, as appropriate.
- Monitor client's response to prescribed electrolyte therapy.
- Monitor for manifestations of electrolyte imbalance.
- Assess client's buccal membranes, sclera, and skin for indications of altered fluid and electrolyte balance (e.g., dryness, cyanosis, and jaundice).
- Consult physician if signs and symptoms of fluid and/or electrolyte imbalance persist or worsen.
- Administer prescribed supplemental electrolytes, as appropriate.
- Monitor for fluid loss (e.g., bleeding, vomiting, diarrhea, perspiration, and tachypnea).

Acid-Base Management: Metabolic Acidosis: *Promotion of acid-base balance and prevention of complications resulting from serum HCO_3 levels lower than desired.*

- Obtain ordered specimens for laboratory analysis of acid-base balance (e.g., ABG, urine, and serum levels), as appropriate.
- Monitor ABG levels for decreasing pH level, as appropriate.
- Maintain patent IV access.
- Monitor intake and output.
- Monitor determinants of tissue oxygen delivery (e.g., Pao_2, Sao_2, and hemoglobin levels and cardiac output) if available.
- Monitor for electrolyte imbalances associated with metabolic acidosis (e.g., hyponatremia, hyperkalemia or hypokalemia, hypocalcemia, hypophosphatemia, and hypomagnesemia), as appropriate.
- Monitor for decreasing bicarbonate from excessive nonvolatile acids (e.g., renal failure, diabetic ketoacidosis, tissue hypoxia, and starvation), as appropriate.
- Administer prescribed alkaline medications (e.g., sodium bicarbonate), as appropriate, based on ABG results.
- Prevent complications from excessive $NaHCO_3$ administration (e.g., metabolic alkalosis, hypernatremia, volume overload, decreased oxygen delivery, decreased cardiac contractility, and enhanced lactic acid production).
- Administer fluids as prescribed.
- Administer insulin and fluid hydration (isotonic and hypotonic) for diabetic ketoacidosis, causing metabolic acidosis, as appropriate.
- Institute seizure precautions.
- Monitor for CNS manifestations of metabolic acidosis (e.g., headache, drowsiness, decreased mentation, seizures, and coma), as appropriate.
- Monitor for cardiopulmonary manifestations of metabolic acidosis (e.g., hypotension, hypoxia, arrhythmias, and Kussmaul respiration), as appropriate.
- Monitor for GI manifestations of metabolic acidosis (e.g., anorexia, nausea, and vomiting), as appropriate.
- Provide comfort measures to deal with the GI effects of metabolic acidosis.
- Instruct the client and/or family on actions instituted to treat the metabolic acidosis.

NIC intervention activities selected from Dochterman, J.M., & Bulechek, G.M. (Eds.). (2004). *Nursing interventions classification (NIC)* (4th ed.). St. Louis: Mosby. No part of this work is to be altered without prior written permission from the Publisher.

ABG, Arterial blood gas; *BUN*, blood urea nitrogen; *CNS*, central nervous system; *CVP*, central venous pressure; *GI*, gastrointestinal; *MAP*, mean arterial pressure; *$NaHCO_3$*, sodium bicarbonate; *Pao_2*, partial pressure of arterial oxygen; *PAP*, pulmonary artery pressure; *PCWP*, pulmonary capillary wedge pressure; Sao_2, arterial oxygen saturation.

ognize in older clients and those who take beta-blocking drugs.

Diet Therapy. When the client is hypoglycemic, start carbohydrate replacement per physician prescription or standing protocols. If the client can swallow, give a liquid form of carbohydrate, although any source of carbohydrate can be used to treat hypoglycemia. Specific recommendations appear in Chart 68-14. The blood glucose level determines the form and amount of glucose used. Fluid is absorbed much more quickly from the gastrointestinal (GI) tract than solids. Concentrated sweet fluids, such as juice with sugar added or a soft drink, may slow absorption. Commercially available products provide predictable glucose absorption.

Drug Therapy. Glucagon given subcutaneously or IM and 50% dextrose given IV is the therapy for diabetic clients who cannot swallow. Glucagon converts liver glycogen to glucose but is not effective in severely starved clients. Take care to prevent aspiration in clients receiving glucagon, because it often causes vomiting. Give 50% dextrose carefully to avoid extravasation. The effects of glucagon and dextrose are temporary. After the client responds, give a simple sugar followed by a small snack or meal. IV glucose is used to maintain mild

TABLE 68-17 Symptoms of Hypoglycemia

Neuroglycopenic Symptoms	Neurogenic Symptoms
▪ Warmth	▪ Adrenergic
▪ Weakness	Shaky/tremulous
▪ Fatigue	Heart pounding
▪ Difficulty thinking	Nervous/anxious
▪ Confusion	▪ Cholinergic
▪ Behavior changes	Sweaty
▪ Emotional lability	Hungry
▪ Seizures	Tingling
▪ Loss of consciousness	
▪ Brain damage	
▪ Death	

TABLE 68-18 Differentiation of Hypoglycemia and Hyperglycemia

Feature	Hypoglycemia	Hyperglycemia
Skin	Cool, clammy	Hot, dry*
Dehydration	Absent	Present
Perspiration	Profuse*	Absent
Respirations	No particular or consistent change	Rapid, deep*; Kussmaul type; acetone odor ("fruity" odor) to breath
Mental status	Anxious, nervous,* irritable, mental confusion,* seizures, coma	Varies from alert to stuporous, obtunded, or frank coma
Symptoms	Weakness,* double vision, blurred vision, hunger, tachycardia, palpitations	No specific symptoms for DKA Acidosis; hypercapnia; abdominal cramps, nausea and vomiting Dehydration: decreased neck vein filling, orthostatic hypotension, tachycardia, poor skin turgor
Glucose	50 mg/dL (2.8 mmol/L)	>250 mg/dL (13.8 mmol/L)
Ketones	Negative	Positive

DKA, Diabetic ketoacidosis.
*Classic symptoms.

CHART 68-13

NIC INTERVENTION ACTIVITIES for The Diabetic Client Experiencing or at Risk for Hypoglycemia

Hypoglycemia Management: *Preventing and treating low blood glucose levels*

- Identify client at risk for hypoglycemia.
- Monitor blood glucose levels, as indicated.
- Monitor for signs and symptoms of hypoglycemia (e.g., shakiness, tremor, sweating, nervousness, anxiety, irritability, impatience, tachycardia, palpitations, chills, clamminess, light-headedness, pallor, hunger, nausea, headache, tiredness, drowsiness, weakness, warmth, dizziness, faintness, blurred vision, nightmares, crying out in sleep, paresthesias, difficulty concentrating, difficulty speaking, incoordination, behavior change, confusion, coma, seizure).
- Provide simple carbohydrate, as indicated.
- Provide complex carbohydrate and protein, as indicated.
- Administer glucagon, as indicated.
- Contact emergency medical services, as necessary.
- Administer intravenous glucose, as indicated.
- Maintain patent airway, as necessary.
- Maintain IV access, as appropriate.
- Protect from injury, as necessary.
- Review events prior to hypoglycemia to determine probable cause.
- Provide feedback regarding appropriateness of self-care management of hypoglycemia.
- Instruct client and significant others on signs and symptoms, risk factors, and treatment of hypoglycemia.
- Instruct client to have simple carbohydrates available at all times.
- Instruct client to obtain and carry/wear appropriate emergency identification.
- Instruct significant others on the use and administration of glucagon, as appropriate.
- Instruct on interaction of diet, insulin/oral agents, and exercise.
- Provide assistance in making self-care decisions to prevent hypoglycemia (e.g., reducing insulin/oral agents and/or increasing food intake for exercise).
- Encourage self-monitoring of blood glucose levels.
- Encourage ongoing telephone contact with diabetes care team for consultation regarding adjustments in treatment regimen.

NIC intervention activities selected from Dochterman, J.M., & Bulechek, G.M.(Eds.). (2004). *Nursing interventions classification (NIC)* (4th ed.). St. Louis: Mosby.

CHART 68-14

CLIENT EDUCATION GUIDE Treatment of Hypoglycemia at Home

For *mild* hypoglycemia (hungry, irritable, shaky, weak, headache, fully conscious; blood glucose usually less than 60 mg/dL [3.4 mmol/L]):

- Treat the symptoms of hypoglycemia with 10 to 15 g of carbohydrate. You may use one of the following:
  - Glucose tablets or glucose gel (dosage is printed on the package)
  - ½ cup of fruit juice
  - ½ cup of regular (nondiet) soft drink
  - 8 ounces of skim milk
  - 6 to 10 hard candies
  - 4 cubes of sugar
  - 4 teaspoons of sugar
  - 6 saltines
  - 3 graham crackers
  - 1 tablespoon of honey or syrup
- Retest blood glucose in 15 minutes.
- Repeat this treatment if symptoms do not resolve.
- Eat a small snack of carbohydrate and protein if your next meal is more than an hour away.

For *moderate* hypoglycemia (cold, clammy skin; pale; rapid pulse; rapid, shallow respirations; marked change in mood; drowsiness; blood glucose usually less than 40 mg/dL [2.2 mmol/L]):

- Treat the symptoms of hypoglycemia with 15 to 30 g of rapidly absorbed carbohydrate.
- Take additional food, such as low-fat milk or cheese, after 10 to 15 minutes.

For *severe* hypoglycemia (unable to swallow; unconsciousness or convulsions; blood glucose usually less than 20 mg/dL [1.0 mmol/L]):

Treatment administered by family members:

- Administer 1 mg of glucagon as intramuscular or subcutaneous injection.
- Administer a second dose in 10 minutes if the person remains unconscious.
- Notify a primary care provider immediately, and follow instructions.
- If still unconscious, transport the person to the emergency department.
- Give a small meal when the person wakes up and is no longer nauseated.

hyperglycemia. Diazoxide (Proglycem), an antidote to sulfonylurea-induced hypoglycemia, or octreotide (Sandostatin), which inhibits sulfonylurea-induced insulin release, may be needed if blood glucose levels cannot be maintained by infusion alone (Herbel & Boyle, 2000).

Evaluate response by monitoring blood glucose levels for several hours. Symptoms may persist for an hour or more after treatment. A target blood glucose level is 70 to 110 mg/dL (3.9 to 6.2 mmol/L).

Prevention Strategies. Teach the client how to prevent future episodes of hypoglycemia. Four common causes of hypoglycemia are (1) excess insulin, (2) deficient intake or absorption of food, (3) exercise, and (4) alcohol intake.

Insulin Excess. Even when insulin is injected correctly, variable absorption can cause hypoglycemia. Excess insulin also can be caused by lowered insulin resistance, which occurs with termination of pregnancy or resolution of an infection. Increased insulin sensitivity can occur with weight loss or exercise programs. Differences in insulin formulation can result in hypoglycemia. Instruct the client not to change insulin brands or change from animal-source to human insulin without medical supervision.

Deficient Food Intake. Inadequate or incorrectly timed meals can result in hypoglycemia. Changes in gastric absorption sometimes cause hypoglycemia in clients with delayed gastric emptying. This problem is more common in clients with diabetes of long duration, is more severe with solid than with liquid meals, and is made worse by illness or poor glucose control. Instruct the client about the importance of regularity in timing and quantity of food eaten.

Exercise. Blood glucose levels usually fall during exercise in a client with type 1 diabetes. Prolonged exercise increases cellular glucose uptake for several hours after exercise. Teach the client about blood glucose monitoring and carbohydrate consumption during exercise.

Alcohol. The main cause of alcohol-induced hypoglycemia is inhibited liver glucose production. Alcohol is more likely to cause hypoglycemia when fasting is prolonged and glycogen stores are depleted before drinking begins. Alcohol interferes with the counterregulatory response to insulin-induced hypoglycemia and impairs glycogen breakdown, making exercise-induced hypoglycemia more severe. Teach clients to ingest alcohol only with or shortly after eating a meal with enough carbohydrate to prevent hypoglycemia (ADA, 2003f). Caution clients to avoid excess alcohol at bedtime to prevent nighttime hypoglycemia.

Client Education. The cause of hypoglycemia may be subtle. At the onset of menses, a fall in hormone levels decreases insulin needs and contributes to hypoglycemia. When clients switch to a new bottle of insulin, hypoglycemia may occur because the fresh insulin has greater potency. Some clients have hypoglycemia when they change injection sites. Drugs such as propranolol (Inderal, Detensol✱) or other beta blockers mask warning signs and thus predispose clients to severe hypoglycemia. Some episodes of hypoglycemia occur without an obvious cause, and many are due to the erratic absorption of insulin, a problem for even the most careful client.

Help each diabetic client develop a personal treatment plan for hypoglycemia. Routinely taking 10 to 15 g of carbohydrate results in overtreatment of hypoglycemia in some clients and undertreatment in others. The exact glucose rise from a set amount of carbohydrate varies. Using the estimate that each 5 g of carbohydrate raises blood glucose about 20 mg/dL, a personal treatment plan can be developed. For example, the client may be directed to take the following (Farkas-Hirsch, 2000):

- 20 to 30 g of carbohydrate if the blood glucose level is 50 mg/dL (2.8 mmol/L) or less
- 10 to 15 g of carbohydrate if the blood glucose level is 51 to 70 mg/dL (2.9 to 3.9 mmol/L)

Use blood glucose monitoring results to revise or reinforce this plan.

Instruct the client to wear a medical alert bracelet and help the client obtain one. This bracelet is helpful if the client becomes hypoglycemic and is unable to provide self-care.

Teach the client and family about the manifestations of hypoglycemia. Emphasize that delaying a meal for more than 30 minutes raises the risk for hypoglycemia when using some insulin regimens. Instruct the client to keep a carbohydrate source nearby at all times.

Hypoglycemia is a major risk for clients receiving intensive insulin protocols who engage in exercise programs. Explain that nightmares or headaches on days after prolonged or severe exercise occur with hypoglycemia.

Establishing Treatment Plans. Blood glucose monitoring directs hypoglycemia treatment. Treatment continues until blood glucose levels reach and stay in the target range. Once blood glucose control is regained, the specific cause of each hypoglycemic episode must be determined and measures taken to prevent recurrence.

CONSIDERATIONS FOR OLDER ADULTS

Older clients who take antidiabetic drugs are at increased risk for hypoglycemia. Age-related changes in liver and kidney function slow metabolism of these drugs, predisposing the client to prolonged and recurrent hypoglycemia. Older clients may have a delayed release of epinephrine in response to falling blood glucose levels and are less likely to notice and act on hypoglycemic symptoms. Physical symptoms such as confusion may make the older client unable to correct hypoglycemia.

Instruct the older diabetic client and family to monitor blood glucose values when symptoms such as unsteadiness, lightheadedness, poor concentration, trembling, or sweating occur. Assess eating patterns to make sure the client is eating sufficient foods at appropriate times. Encourage a client with a poor appetite to eat a small snack at bedtime to prevent hypoglycemia during the night.

When possible, an antidiabetic drug with low hypoglycemia potential is selected for older clients. The highest risk for severe or fatal hypoglycemia is among older adults taking glyburide (Dailey, 2002). Drug regimens that require meals to be eaten on time only increase the risk for hypoglycemia.

POTENTIAL FOR DIABETIC KETOACIDOSIS

Metabolic problems of diabetic ketoacidosis (DKA) are caused by a total or partial lack of insulin combined with the action of counterregulatory hormones (Figure 68-14). Laboratory diagnosis of DKA is shown in Table 68-19. DKA occurs in 2% to 5% of clients with type 1 diabetes and most often starts from infection. *Death occurs in 1% to 10% of these cases even with appropriate treatment.* Mortality is highest for older clients who also have infection, stroke, myocardial infarction, vascular thrombosis, intestinal obstruction, or pneumonia.

Polyuria, polydipsia, and polyphagia start before DKA. Central nervous system (CNS) depression changes consciousness from lethargy to coma. The client is dehydrated with severe fluid loss. Kussmaul respiration, abdominal pain, nausea, and vomiting occur. Initial serum sodium levels may be low or normal. Initial potassium levels depend on how long DKA lasts before treatment. After therapy starts, serum potassium levels drop quickly.

TABLE 68-19 Differences Between Diabetic Ketoacidosis and Hyperglycemic-Hyperosmolar Nonketotic Syndrome

	Diabetic Ketoacidosis (DKA)	Hyperglycemic-Hyperosmolar Nonketotic Syndrome (HHNS)
Onset	Sudden	Gradual
Precipitating factors	Infection Other stressors Inadequate insulin dose	Infection Other stressors Poor fluid intake
Manifestations	Ketosis: Kussmaul respiration, "fruity" breath, nausea, abdominal pain Dehydration or electrolyte loss: polyuria, polydipsia, weight loss, dry skin, sunken eyes, soft eyeballs, lethargy, coma	Altered central nervous system function with neurologic symptoms Dehydration or electrolyte loss: same as for DKA
Laboratory Findings		
Serum glucose	>300 mg/dL (16.7 mmol/L)	>800 mg/dL (44.5 mmol/L)
Osmolarity	Variable	>350 mOsm/L
Serum ketones	Positive at 1:2 dilutions	Negative
Serum pH	<7.35	>7.4
Serum HCO_3	<15 mEq/L	>20 mEq/L
Serum Na	Low, normal, or high	Normal or low
Serum K	Normal; elevated with acidosis, low following dehydration	Normal or low
BUN	>20 mg/dL; elevated because of dehydration	Elevated
Creatinine	>1.5 mg/dL; elevated because of dehydration	Elevated
Urine ketones	Positive	Negative

BUN, Blood urea nitrogen; *HCO_3*, bicarbonate.

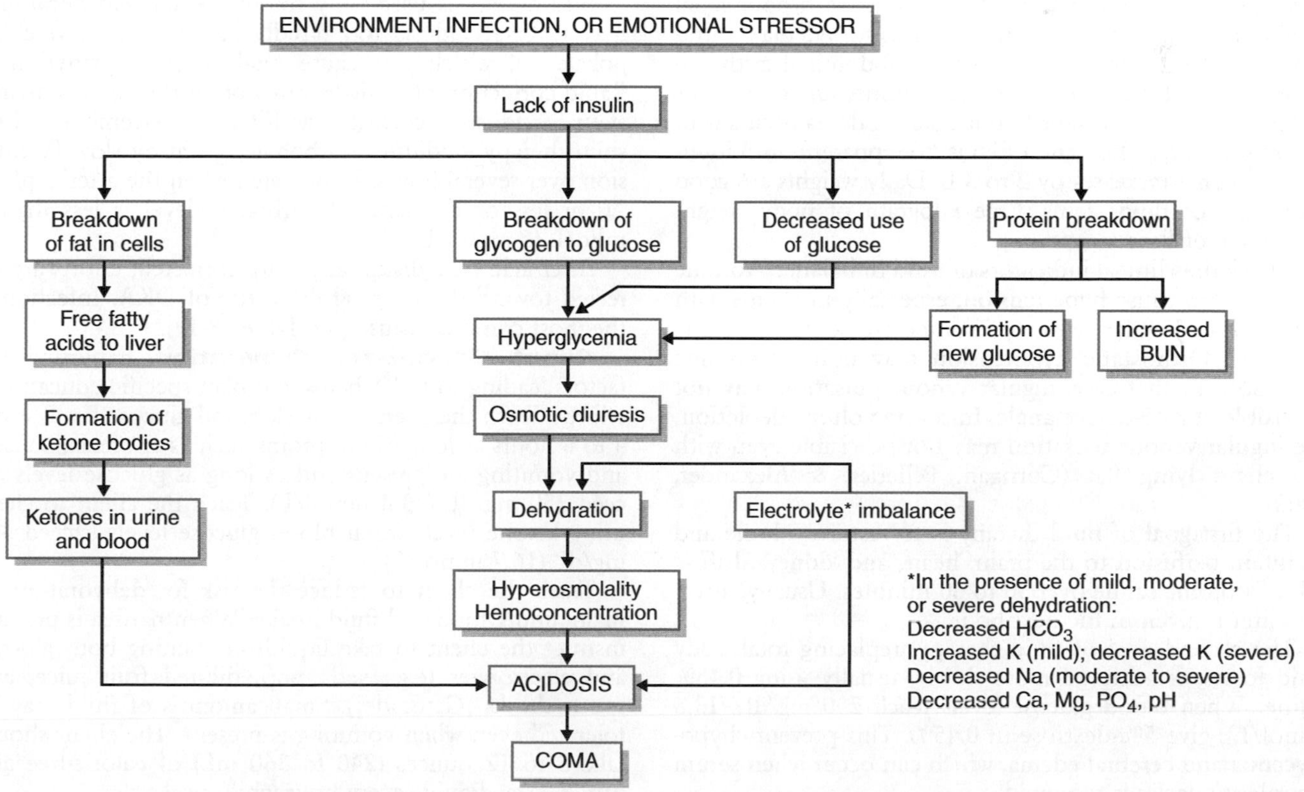

Figure 68-14 ■ The pathophysiologic mechanism of diabetic ketoacidosis.

NOC **PLANNING: EXPECTED OUTCOMES.** The client is expected to have few episodes of hyperglycemia and avoid diabetic ketoacidosis. Indicators include that the client consistently demonstrates the following behaviors:

- Maintains blood glucose levels within the target range
- Adjusts insulin doses to match eating patterns and blood glucose levels during illness
- Describes correct procedure for urine ketone testing
- Describes when to seek help from health care professional

INTERVENTIONS

Hyperglycemic Management. Monitor for manifestations of DKA (see Table 68-19 and Figure 68-14). *First assess the airway, level of consciousness, hydration status, electrolytes, and blood glucose level.* Early in treatment, check the client's blood pressure, pulse, and respirations every 15 minutes until stable. Record urine output, temperature, and mental status every hour. When a central venous catheter is present, assess central venous pressure every 30 minutes or as prescribed. After treatment starts and these values are stable, monitor and record vital signs every 4 hours. Use blood glucose values to assess therapy and determine when to switch from saline to dextrose-containing solutions.

Fluid and Electrolyte Management. *Closely assess the client's fluid status.* The kidneys are less able to respond to changes in pH or fluid and electrolyte balance, to concentrate urine, or to regulate blood osmolarity. The risk for kidney failure rises with age. Impaired bicarbonate reabsorption and acid excretion in poorly functioning renal tubules can lead to acidosis. Cardiovascular disease can cause fluid retention. The dehydrated client's lips and mouth may be dry, and the tongue furrowed. Temperature may be elevated. Age-related skin changes, such as loss of elasticity and dryness, make skin turgor an unreliable sign of dehydration in the older client. In clients with poor renal function and excess fluid volume, assess for edema around the eyes and in the limbs, increasing abdominal girth, increasing blood pressure and pulse volume, jugular venous distention, and orthostatic hypotension. Edema occurs with excess interstitial fluid and often is not apparent until interstitial volume increases by 2 to 3 L. Daily weights are good indicators of fluid status. One kilogram of body weight equals 1 L of fluid.

Check the clinical indicators of fluid imbalance. Volume overload can cause hypertension, especially in clients with renal failure. Jugular venous pressure increases with volume overload. Orthostatic hypotension may indicate volume depletion. In that case, jugular venous pulsation may not be visible at a 45-degree angle. In severe volume depletion, the jugular venous pulsation may not be visible even with the client lying flat (Corrigan, Pelletier, & Alexander, 2000).

The first goal of fluid therapy is to restore volume and maintain perfusion to the brain, heart, and kidneys. Infuse 1 L of isotonic saline over 30 to 60 minutes. Usually, a second liter is given in the next hour.

The second goal of fluid therapy, replacing total body fluid losses, is achieved more slowly, usually using 0.45% saline. When blood glucose levels reach 250 mg/dL (13.8 mmol/L), give 5% dextrose in 0.45%. This prevents hypoglycemia and cerebral edema, which can occur when serum osmolarity declines too rapidly.

During the first 24 hours of treatment, the client needs enough fluids to replace the actual volume deficit and ongoing losses. This may be as much as 6 to 10 L. Watch for signs of congestive heart failure and pulmonary edema. Central venous pressure may be monitored for older clients and those with myocardial disease.

Drug Therapy. The goal of insulin therapy is to lower serum glucose by about 75 to 150 mg/dL/hr. The best way to accomplish this goal is controversial. "Low-dose" insulin therapy results in less hypokalemia and hypoglycemia than a "high-dose" regimen. Although both IM and IV routes are used, continuous IV delivery of regular insulin is recommended because other routes have more erratic absorption. A steady-state level of insulin can be reached in 25 to 30 minutes. Effective blood insulin levels are reached quickly when an IV bolus dose is given at the start of the infusion. Usually, regular insulin is given in an initial IV bolus dose of 0.1 unit/kg, followed by an IV drip of 0.1 unit/kg/hr. Continuous insulin infusion is used because of the 4-minute half-life of IV insulin. Subcutaneous insulin is started when the client can take oral fluids and ketosis has stopped. Assess therapy effectiveness by hourly blood glucose measurements.

Acidosis Management. Regardless of the initial potassium value, there is a large total-body potassium deficit. With insulin therapy, serum potassium levels fall rapidly as potassium shifts into the cells. *Watch for signs of hypokalemia, including fatigue, malaise, confusion, muscle weakness, shallow respirations, abdominal distention or paralytic ileus, hypotension, and weak pulse.* An electrocardiogram (ECG) shows cardiac conduction changes related to potassium. Hypokalemia is a significant cause of death in the treatment of DKA. *Before giving IV potassium, make sure the client produces at least 30 mL/hr of urine.*

Bicarbonate is used only for severe acidosis because it may reverse acidosis too rapidly and lead to severe hypokalemia, which can cause fatal cardiac dysrhythmias. Rapid correction of acidosis can worsen the client's mental status. Acidosis is corrected with fluid replacement and insulin therapy. Sodium bicarbonate, given by slow IV infusion over several hours, is indicated when the arterial pH is 7.0 or less or the serum bicarbonate level is less than 5 mEq/L (5 mmol/L).

After acid-base disturbances are corrected, efforts are directed toward determining the cause of DKA. Infection is the most common cause (see Table 68-19).

Client Education: Prevention. Exploring the factors leading to DKA helps you plan specific educational efforts. Teach the client to check blood glucose levels every 4 to 6 hours as long as symptoms such as anorexia, nausea, and vomiting are present and as long as glucose levels exceed 250 mg/dL (13.8 mmol/L). Teach the client to check urine ketone levels when blood glucose levels exceed 300 mg/dL (16.7 mmol/L).

Teach the client to reduce the risk for dehydration by maintaining food and fluid intake. When nausea is present, instruct the client to take liquids containing both glucose and electrolytes (e.g., soda pop, diluted fruit juice, and sports drinks [Gatorade]). Small amounts of fluid may be tolerated even when vomiting is present. The client should take 8 to 12 ounces (240 to 360 mL) of calorie-free and caffeine-free liquids every hour while awake.

Liquids containing carbohydrate can be taken if the diabetic client cannot eat solid food. Ingesting at least 150 g of carbohydrate daily reduces the risk for starvation ketosis. After consulting a primary care provider, urge the client to take additional rapid-acting (lispro) or short-acting (regular) insulin based on blood glucose levels.

CHART 68-15

CLIENT EDUCATION GUIDE
Sick Day Rules

- Notify your health care provider that you are ill.
- Monitor your blood glucose at least every 4 hours.
- Test your urine for ketones when your blood glucose level is greater than 240 mg/dL (13.8 mmol/L).
- Continue to take insulin or oral antidiabetic agents.
- To prevent dehydration, drink 8 to 12 ounces of sugar free liquids every hour that you are awake.
- Continue to eat meals at regular times.
- If unable to tolerate solid food because of nausea, consume more easily tolerated foods or liquids equal to the carbohydrate content of your usual meal.
- Call your primary care provider for any of the following danger signals:
  - Persistent nausea and vomiting
  - Moderate or large ketones
  - Blood glucose elevation after two supplemental doses of insulin
  - High (101.5° F [38.6° C]) temperature or increasing fever; fever for more than 24 hours
- Treat symptoms (e.g., diarrhea, nausea, vomiting, and fever) as directed by your primary care provider.
- Get plenty of rest.

Instruct the client to consult the primary care provider when the following problems occur:

- Blood glucose exceeds 250 mg/dL (13.8 mmol/L).
- Ketonuria lasts for more than 24 hours.
- The client cannot take food or fluids.
- Illness lasts more than 1 to 2 days.

Also instruct the client or family to detect hyperglycemia by performing SMBG whenever the client is ill. Illness can result in dehydration with DKA, hyperglycemic-hyperosmolar nonketotic syndrome, or both. The sooner the client seeks treatment, the less severe the metabolic alteration. The client should understand not to omit insulin therapy during illness. Chart 68-15 reviews guidelines for the ill client.

POTENTIAL FOR HYPERGLYCEMIC-HYPEROSMOLAR NONKETOTIC SYNDROME AND COMA

Hyperglycemic-hyperosmolar nonketotic syndrome (HHNS) is a hyperosmolar (increased blood osmolarity) state caused by hyperglycemia. The processes of HHNS are outlined in Figure 68-15. Although both HHNS and diabetic ketoacidosis (DKA) are caused by hyperglycemia, HHNS is different from DKA because of the absence of ketosis and the much higher blood glucose levels and blood osmolarity. Blood glucose levels may exceed 800 mg/dL (44.5 mmol/L) and blood osmolarity may exceed 350 mOsm/L. Other biochemical problems with HHNS also are more severe than those with DKA. Table 68-19 lists the differences between DKA and HHNS.

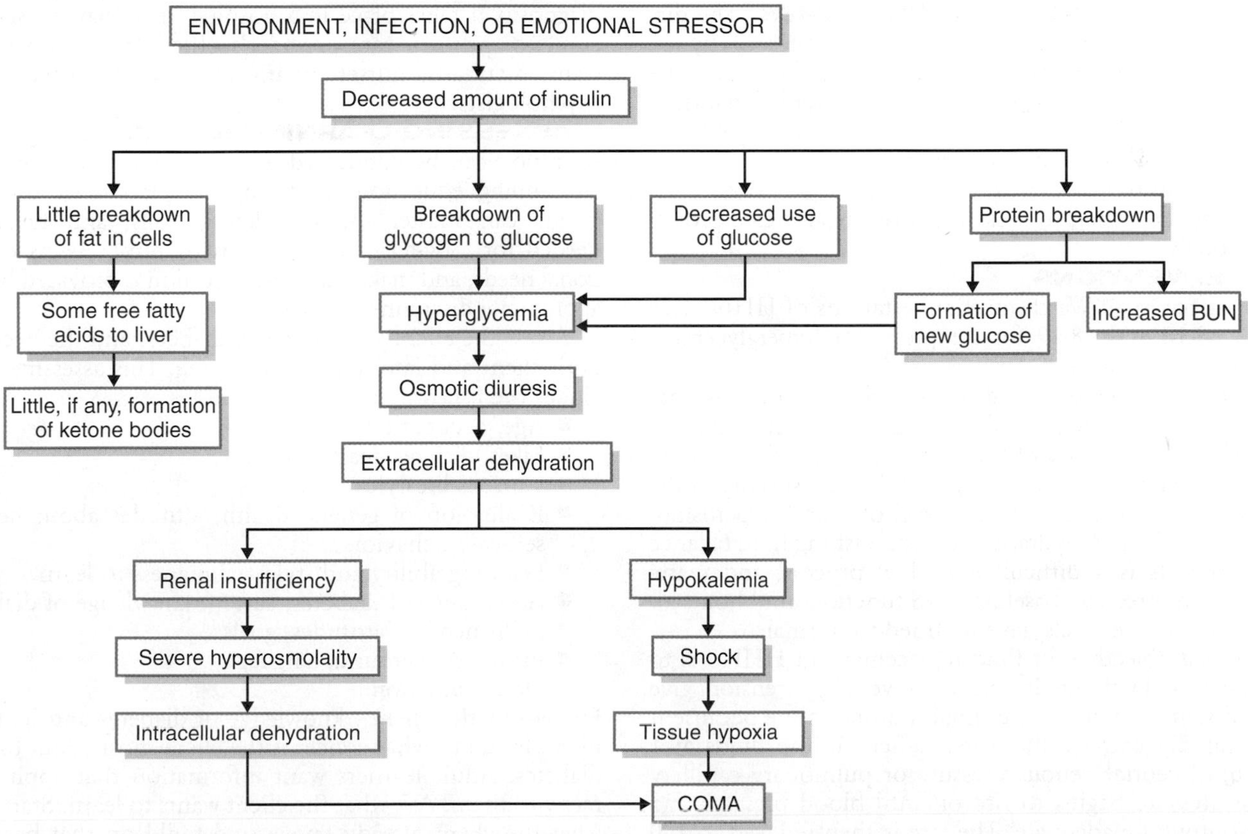

Figure 68-15 ■ The pathophysiologic mechanism of hyperglycemic-hyperosmolar nonketotic syndrome.

CONSIDERATIONS FOR OLDER ADULTS

HHNS occurs most often in older clients with type 2 diabetes mellitus, many of whom did not know that they had diabetes. Mortality rates in older clients are as high as 40% to 70%. The onset of HHNS is slow and may not be recognized. The older client often seeks medical attention later and is sicker than the younger client. HHNS does not occur in adequately hydrated people. Older diabetic clients are at greater risk for dehydration and HHNS because of age-related changes in thirst perception and poor urine-concentrating abilities.

Myocardial infarction, sepsis, pancreatitis, and stroke, and some drugs (glucocorticoids, diuretics, phenytoin [Dilantin], propranolol [Inderal], and calcium channel blockers) also may cause HHNS. Central nervous system (CNS) changes range from confusion to complete coma. Unlike DKA, clients with HHNS may have seizures, myoclonic jerking, and reversible paralysis.

The development of HHNS rather than DKA is related to residual insulin secretion. In HHNS, the client secretes just enough insulin to prevent ketosis but not enough to prevent hyperglycemia. The hyperglycemia of HHNS is more severe than that of DKA, greatly increasing the blood osmolarity and causing profound diuresis. Severe dehydration and electrolyte loss occur, and the client may lose 15% to 25% of body fluid. When dehydration is severe, glucose is not filtered into the urine, causing even greater hyperglycemia and hyperosmolarity. Impairment of the thirst center in the brain occurs, making it impossible for the client to drink enough fluid to prevent dehydration.

NOC **PLANNING: EXPECTED OUTCOMES.** The diabetic client is expected to have few episodes of hyperglycemia and avoid HHNS. Indicators include that the client consistently demonstrates the following behaviors:

- Maintains blood glucose levels within the target range
- Uses antidiabetic drugs appropriately
- Remains well hydrated
- Describes when to seek help from health care professionals

INTERVENTIONS

Monitoring. Watch for manifestations of HHNS (see Tables 68-18 and 68-19 for symptoms of hyperglycemia). Continually assess fluid status.

Fluid Therapy. The goal of therapy is to rehydrate the client and restore normal blood glucose levels within 36 to 72 hours. The choice of fluid replacement and the rate of infusion are critical in managing HHNS. The severity of the CNS problems is related to the level of blood hyperosmolarity and cellular dehydration. Re-establishing fluid balance in brain cells is a difficult and slow process, and many clients do not recover baseline CNS function until hours after blood glucose levels have returned to normal.

The *first* objective for fluid replacement in HHNS is to increase blood volume. In shock or severe hypotension, give normal saline. Otherwise, use half-normal saline because it more rapidly corrects the water deficit. Infuse fluids at 1 L/hr until central venous pressure or pulmonary capillary wedge pressure begins to rise or until blood pressure and urine output are adequate. The rate is then reduced to 100 to 200 mL/hr. Half of the estimated water deficit is replaced in the first 12 hours, and the rest is given during the next 36 hours. Body weight, urine output, kidney function, and the presence or absence of pulmonary congestion and jugular venous distention determine the rate of fluid infusion. In clients with congestive heart failure, renal insufficiency, or acute kidney failure, monitor central venous pressure. *Assess the client hourly for signs of cerebral edema; abrupt changes in mental status, abnormal neurologic signs, and coma. Immediately report changes in the level of consciousness; changes in pupil size, shape, or reaction; or seizures.* Lack of improvement in level of consciousness may indicate inadequate rates of fluid replacement or reduction in plasma osmolarity. Regression after initial improvement may indicate a too rapid reduction in plasma osmolarity. A slow but steady improvement in CNS function is the best evidence that fluid management is satisfactory.

Continuing Therapy. IV insulin given at 10 units/hr is often needed to reduce blood glucose levels. Although fluid replacement reduces hyperglycemia, it cannot alone return blood glucose levels to normal. A reduction of blood glucose by 10% per hour is a reasonable goal (Delaney et al., 2000). Potassium loss occurs in HHNS, although not to the degree it does in DKA. Because of the initial low urine output **(oliguria)** or absent urine output **(anuria)**, potassium replacement may not be needed at the start of therapy. Client education and interventions to minimize dehydration are similar to those for ketoacidosis.

Community-Based Care

HEALTH TEACHING

Education about blood glucose control begins at the time of diagnosis. It takes place in a hospital or outpatient setting, clinic, or primary care provider's office. It involves physicians, dietitians, nurses, pharmacists, social workers, and psychologists.

ASSESSING LEARNING NEEDS. Although some education can be conducted in groups, most is one-to-one. Continuing education needs to take place over time, so clients can master the knowledge, skills, and flexibility needed for long-term blood glucose control. Assess educational needs, and make sure that education is provided by the appropriate disciplines.

Assess the client's awareness of diabetes and the needs of both client and family before teaching. This assessment includes the following:

- Age, occupation
- Likes, dislikes, fears
- Current lifestyle
- Evaluation of general health, attitudes about health, self-care behaviors
- Learning ability and style, willingness to learn
- Acceptance of diabetes, current knowledge of diabetes
- Skills needed, attitudes, goals
- Ethnic background, language
- Home situation

First assess the client's knowledge of diabetes and its treatment. Find out what concerns the client most about having diabetes. Adult learners want information that applies directly to them. Ask what the client wants to learn. Start with what the client already knows and build on that base. To capture interest and motivate clients for learning, present material relevant to their first questions. Because they will be managing their own care after discharge, clients tend to focus on issues most important to them. Treatment measures that need to start soon after diagnosis may be of more interest to the client than long-term control.

The client's physical condition dictates the timing of teaching. When blood glucose levels are fluctuating, the client does not have the energy to learn complex information. Explaining that well-controlled blood glucose levels improve the sense of well-being can help the client accept the therapy plan. Use an informal teaching program until the client feels able to attend a formal class. Teach and observe the client's technique for injections and blood glucose monitoring.

Each client learns in an individual way. A successful diabetic education program combines several teaching methods. Some clients learn better when they read pamphlets. Others learn better when they watch videotapes. Learning improves when the equipment is handled, techniques are practiced, success is rewarded, and errors are corrected immediately.

ASSESSING PHYSICAL, COGNITIVE, AND EMOTIONAL LIMITATIONS. Assess the client's education and reading level to determine what level of information to present. Assess the client's ability to read printed information, insulin labels, and markings on syringes and equipment. Many clients with type 2 diabetes have **presbyopia** (age-related far-sightedness) and other visual difficulties made worse by blurred vision caused by fluctuating blood glucose levels. The client must be able to understand the printed material. Even highly educated clients do not want to read complicated information when they are sick. Much of the printed material from drug companies is printed at the sixth- or seventh-grade level. The International Diabetes Center prepares printed diabetic education material at the second- and third-grade levels. Develop creative teaching strategies for the client who cannot read.

Assess the client's ability to conceptualize. Adjusting insulin dosage based on blood glucose monitoring is a difficult concept and may not be appropriate for clients who cannot understand it. Managing drugs, exercise, and diet requires complex interpretation and behavior.

Assess manual dexterity for any physical limitations that may alter the teaching plan. A hand injury, tremors, or severe arthritis may require a change in insulin preparation.

Information is best learned when the client is ready. Clients with newly diagnosed diabetes are facing a life crisis. Some are motivated to learn information and are willing to change lifelong behaviors. Others may grieve the loss of their previous lifestyle and use denial as a means of coping. In this instance, the client may not be able to learn needed information right away.

EXPLAINING SURVIVAL SKILLS. The initial phase of diabetic education involves basic survival skills. The physical changes of diabetes and the relationship of diet, drugs, and exercise to overall control are important.

A dietitian provides the initial diet instruction. The client needs to understand what to eat, how much to eat, and when to eat. Stress the importance of eating on time and the dangers of skipping meals. The client must know how to maintain food intake during illness. Reinforce dietary instruction, answer questions, and refer questions to the dietitian or physician as indicated.

After being taught, the client should be able to identify the drugs needed to control blood glucose levels. If insulin is needed, the client must be able to prepare and give the dose accurately using sterile technique. The client must also be able to state when insulin is to be injected, where insulin is injected, and how insulin is stored. Stress the dangers of skipping doses. Carefully review drug interactions, especially with older clients taking oral antidiabetic drugs.

The client should be able to state a plan for regular physical activity. The client must be able to describe the relationship between exercise and blood glucose control and identify situations when activity should not be performed. Provide guidelines for additional carbohydrate intake to prevent hypoglycemia from excessive exercise.

The diabetic client also must be able to state the plan for monitoring blood glucose. The person doing the monitoring must be able to do the procedure accurately and understand the results. Explain when blood glucose should be monitored, acceptable ranges, and actions to take when results are out of these ranges. If the client cannot perform SMBG due to illness, ensure that a resource (e.g., home care agency, health clinic, or primary care provider's office) will be available to do the monitoring.

The most important part of diabetes education is to ensure that the client understands the significance, symptoms, causes, and treatment of hypoglycemia. The client must be able to state the causes of hypoglycemia and the activities needed to prevent it. He or she must be able to describe appropriate carbohydrates to have available and the need to notify the physician of hypoglycemic episodes.

The client also must understand the significance of hyperglycemia and its relationship to illness. The client must describe actions to take during illness and when to communicate with the primary care provider.

Most of this information is best retained when the client is ready to learn. Education is a challenge because clients tend to be hospitalized for shorter periods. All diabetic education may be provided in an outpatient setting, where contact with the client is limited. Important information must be squeezed into the time available. Many clients do not progress in self-management beyond the survival level because of psychological barriers.

COUNSELING. The major goal of in-depth counseling is to help the client become self-sufficient in diabetes management. Educational sessions with client and family are needed to individualize the diabetes regimen for their needs and abilities. Education is often provided by a team of a physician, nurse educator, dietitian, social worker, pharmacist, psychologist, and other health care professionals as needed. Education may occur in various outpatient settings.

Besides knowledge gained at the survival level, the client should be able to discuss the action of insulin in the body and the effects of insulin deficiency. The client should also be able to explain the effects of diet, drugs, and activity on blood glucose. He or she should be able to relate maintaining normal blood glucose levels to preventing complications. This includes relating changes in glucose level to the possible need for a change in insulin dosage.

The client must be able to describe the meal plan and explain the adjustments needed to meet diabetic diet requirements. He or she should state how food intake should be altered when eating out or increasing exercise. *The client must be able to list specific foods to be eaten to prevent and treat hypoglycemia, as well as adjustments to make when ill.*

The client must be able to prepare and give insulin accurately. He or she should be able to discuss the onset, peak, and duration of the insulin used. In reviewing insulin administration, stress the importance of injection site selection and rotation. Review adjustments in insulin based on SMBG results (when permitted by the physician) and explain that follow-up SMBG results are needed to evaluate the effects of additional insulin. The client should know how to protect insulin when traveling. For clients at risk for severe hypoglycemia, teach a family member to inject glucagon. If the client takes an oral diabetic drug, ask him or her to identify the drug and describe its prescribed schedule. The client must identify over-the-counter drugs with the potential to cause adverse interactions and the need to inform all care providers of the drug regimen.

Within health status–imposed physical limitations, the client should be able to perform desired physical activities. The client must state blood glucose levels that are safe for exercise, the frequency of SMBG during exercise, food required before exercise, and what food to have available during exercise. He or she should be aware of the risk for injury during exercise and explain the importance of protective footwear.

The goals of in-depth education are to help the diabetic client solve problems of blood glucose fluctuation through the use of SMBG. The client should be able to identify practices, such as travel (Chart 68-16), that cause blood glucose to fluctuate and to treat these problems with supplemental insulin, changes in activity, or changes in diet. Ask the client to demonstrate urine ketone testing and to describe when urine ketones should be measured.

The client must be able to describe a plan for periodic evaluation of blood glucose control by the primary care provider, as well as periodic dental and eye examinations. He or she must be able to perform foot care, wear properly fitting shoes, and describe hazards related to foot care. The client must be able to describe ways to reduce specific risk factors, such as cigarette smoking and hypertension.

The client must state that diabetes is a lifelong disease that requires lifestyle changes, describe the changes being made, and indicate those that need to be made. He or she should be able to identify stress-producing situations and discuss ways to reduce stress.

PSYCHOSOCIAL PREPARATION

The diagnosis of diabetes may represent a loss of control. All but a few clients lose flexibility. Life becomes ordered and routines must be followed. Certain events surrounding diabetes are predictable. Taking an insulin injection and not eating for several hours causes hypoglycemia. Poorly controlled diabetes leads to complications and premature death. Tight control of blood glucose levels prevents complications.

The stress of diabetes is in addition to the demands of normal daily life. The client must be able to integrate the demands of diabetes into daily and recreational schedules while keeping blood glucose stable.

You can assist in healthy psychological adaptation to diabetes by providing successful educational experiences. Mastery of blood glucose monitoring helps the client feel that he or she has control over the disease. Knowing the effects of extra activities, extra food, or extra insulin is helpful in learning to adjust the regimen.

Feeling a sense of control over the condition does much to promote a positive attitude about diabetes. Success in injecting insulin provides concrete evidence that he or she can mas-

CHART 68-16

CLIENT EDUCATION GUIDE
Travel Tips for Diabetic Clients

Before traveling visit your primary care provider and diabetes educator.
- See your physician to make certain you do not have any other health problems.
- Obtain a letter from your physician (typed on office letterhead) that indicates you have diabetes and lists the medications you are taking.
- Obtain any needed immunizations or inoculations.
- Obtain prescriptions from your physician for your medications, including glucagon if you take insulin, and prescriptions for motion sickness, nausea and vomiting, and traveler's diarrhea.
- Develop a plan for changing strengths of insulin if you are traveling to a country that does not carry the type of insulin you use. Learn how to use a U-100 syringe to draw up U-40 insulin.
- Develop a plan for meal and medication adjustment across time zones. Eastbound travel will shorten the day, requiring a reduction in the amount of medication needed. Westbound travel may add an extra meal to the day and require additional medication.
- Obtain a list of foods from your diabetes educator that you can substitute for food served in restaurants or airplanes.

If you are traveling by air, train, or boat, call ahead and request special meals for individuals with diabetes.
- Plan for delays in eating.
- Eat something every 4 hours.
- Drink a glass of water every 2 hours to prevent dehydration.
- Do not assume that special meals will be available; substitute items you cannot eat with foods you have in your travel kit.

Notify airline and hotel personnel that you have diabetes.
- Always wear medical alert identification and keep your medical alert card in your wallet.

While traveling:
- Check your blood glucose level frequently.
- Do not engage in activities when blood glucose levels are lower than 65 mg/dL.
- Stretch and walk around every 2 hours to help your circulation.
- Check your feet frequently for blisters and sores. You may be doing more walking than usual.
- Take extra shoes with you, and plan to change shoes often when walking more than normal.
- Protect your skin against exposure to the sun. Drug-induced photosensitivity can occur with some oral hypoglycemic agents.

Always have your travel kit with you; do not check your kit along with the rest of your luggage. Include these items in your travel kit:
- Insulin bottles in boxes with prescription labels
- Twice as much medication and twice as many supplies as you think you will need (Pack medications separately from checked luggage.)
- Insulin stored in an insulated carrying case that will maintain temperatures according to the manufacturer's directions
- The letter from your physician (typed on office letterhead) that indicates you have diabetes and lists the medications you are taking
- A supply of fast-acting sugar (such as glucose tablets or gel, hard candy, and sugar cubes), as well as longer-acting foods (such as cheese and crackers and peanut butter and crackers)
- A self-monitoring diary

CHART 68-17

FOCUSED ASSESSMENT of
The Insulin-Dependent Diabetic Client During a Home or Clinic Visit

Assess overall mental status, wakefulness, ability to converse.
Take vital signs and weight:
- Fever could indicate infection.
- Are blood pressure and weight within target range? Why or why not?

Question client regarding any change in visual acuity; check current visual acuity.
Inspect oral mucous membranes, gums, and teeth.
Question client about injection areas used; inspect areas being used; assess whether client is using areas and sites appropriately.
Inspect skin for intactness, wounds that have not healed, new sores, ulcers, bruises, or burns; assess any previously known wounds for infection, progression of healing.
Question client regarding foot care.
Assess lower extremities and feet for peripheral pulses, lack of or decreased sensation, abnormal sensations, breaks in skin integrity, condition of toes and nails.
Question client regarding color and consistency of stools and frequency of bowel movements; assess abdomen for bowel sounds.
Review client's home health diary:
- Is blood glucose within targeted range? Why or why not?
- Is glucose monitoring being recorded often enough?
- Is the client's food intake adequate and appropriate? Why or why not?
- Is exercise occurring regularly? Why or why not?

Assess client's ability to perform self-monitoring of blood glucose.
Assess client's procedures for obtaining and storing insulin and syringes, cleaning equipment, disposing of syringes and needles.
Assess client's insulin preparation and injection technique.

ter the disease. Teach by breaking a task into small, achievable units to ensure mastery; for example, a client may begin learning how to inject insulin by first obtaining an accurate dose.

Devote as much teaching time as possible to insulin injection and blood glucose monitoring. Clients with newly diagnosed diabetes are often fearful of giving themselves injections. After this technique has been mastered, clients become less anxious and are able to attend to other tasks.

HOME CARE MANAGEMENT

Clients with diabetes self-manage their disease. Each day the client decides what to eat, whether to exercise, and whether to take prescribed drugs. Maintaining blood glucose control depends on the accuracy of self-management skills. The main role of the health care professional is to provide support and education and to empower the client to make informed decisions. Self-management education allows clients to identify their problems and provides techniques to help them make decisions, take appropriate actions, and alter these actions as needed.

Provide information about resources. The client must know whom to contact in case of emergency. Older adults who live alone must have daily telephone contact with a friend or neighbor. The client may also need help shopping and preparing meals. He or she may have limited access to transportation and may not have sufficient supplies of food, particularly in bad weather. Because of the likelihood of visual problems in older clients, they may need assistance in preparing insulin syringes for injection or in monitoring blood glucose. Make referrals to home care or public health agencies as needed. Referral is especially important for older women who are insulin dependent. Chart 68-17 identifies areas for assessment during a home or clinic visit.

TABLE 68-20 Outcome Criteria for Diabetic Teaching

Before being discharged to home, the diabetic client or the significant other should be able to:
- Tell why insulin or an oral hypoglycemic agent is being prescribed.
- Name which insulin or oral hypoglycemic agent is being prescribed, and name the dosage and frequency of administration.
- Discuss the relationship between mealtime and the action of insulin or the oral hypoglycemic agent.
- Discuss plans to follow diabetic diet instructions.
- Prepare and administer insulin accurately.
- Test blood for glucose, or state plans for having blood glucose levels monitored.
- Test urine for ketones, and state when this test should be done.
- Verbalize how to store insulin.
- List symptoms that indicate a hypoglycemic reaction.
- Tell what carbohydrate sources are used to treat hypoglycemic reactions.
- Tell what symptoms indicate hyperglycemia.
- Tell what dietary changes are needed during illness.
- Verbalize when to call the physician or the nurse (frequent episodes of hypoglycemia, symptoms of hyperglycemia).
- Verbalize the procedures for proper foot care.

HEALTH CARE RESOURCES

A wide array of diabetic education material is available from drug companies. The American Diabetes Association (ADA) will refer a diabetic client to specific agencies or resources (phone 800-DIABETES [800-342-2383] in the United States; 800-BANTING [800-226-8464] in Canada). The American Association of Diabetes Educators can refer a diabetic client to a local certified diabetes educator (phone [800] TEAM-UP-4). Additional resources are listed in the bibliography.

Critical Thinking Challenge

A 68-year-old client has had type 2 diabetes for several years. She has come to the clinic for a 6-month evaluation. During the interview, she complains of burning and tingling sensations in her feet and tells you that her feet are always cold. She keeps her feet warm with a hot water bottle. Examination of her feet reveals the skin to be very dry with deep cracks and fissures. Her feet are cold to the touch with calluses over the metatarsal heads. Her toenails are long and thickened. She has a history of an ulcer on the plantar surface of her left foot, which developed after she stepped on a sharp object on her kitchen floor.

1. List four parameters you would assess to determine the client's risk for foot injury.
2. Discuss three elements of education that are especially important for this client.
3. What referrals would you make for this client?

evolve For suggested answer guidelines, go to http://evolve.elsevier.com/Iggy/.

Evaluation: Outcomes

Evaluate the care of the client with diabetes on the basis of the identified nursing diagnoses and collaborative problems. Outcome success for diabetic education is the ability of the client to maintain blood glucose levels within the normal range. General outcome criteria are listed on the next page and in Table 68-20. More specific outcomes are listed with each nursing diagnosis and collaborative problem. The expected outcomes include that the client will:

- Achieve blood glucose control
- Avoid acute and chronic complications of diabetes
- Have a satisfactory and complete postoperative recovery without complications
- Avoid injury
- Experience relief of pain
- Maintain optimal vision
- Maintain a urine elimination pattern in the expected range
- Have an optimal level of mental status functioning
- Have decreased episodes of hypoglycemia
- Have decreased episodes of hyperglycemia

Specific indicators for these outcomes are listed for each nursing diagnosis and collaborative problem under the Planning and Implementation section (see earlier).

GET READY for the NCLEX Examination!

KEY POINTS

Safe Effective Care Environment

- Use aseptic technique during all central line dressing changes or any invasive procedure.
- Use good handwashing techniques before providing any care to a client who has diabetes.
- Wash your hands before and after testing the client's blood glucose levels.

Health Promotion and Maintenance

- Encourage all people to maintain weight within an appropriate range.
- Encourage all people, including clients with diabetes, to participate regularly in exercise or physical activity appropriate to their health status.
- Teach the client and family about the clinical manifestations of infection and when to seek medical advice.
- Instruct clients with diabetes to wear a medical alert bracelet.
- Instruct clients not to share blood glucose monitoring equipment.
- Reinforce to all clients with diabetes that tight control over blood glucose levels reduces the risk for the vascular complications of diabetes.
- Remind the diabetic client to have yearly eye examinations by an ophthalmologist.
- Teach diabetic clients with peripheral neuropathy to use a bath thermometer to test water for bathing, to avoid walking barefoot, and to inspect their feet daily.
- Encourage all clients who smoke cigarettes to quit smoking.
- Help clients who want to stop smoking find an appropriate smoking cessation program.

Psychosocial Integrity

- Explore with the client what the diagnosis of diabetes means to him or her.
- Allow the client the opportunity to express fear or anxiety regarding the diagnosis of diabetes or the treatment regimen.
- Explain all procedures, restrictions, medications, and follow-up care to the client and family.
- Pace your education sessions to match the learning needs and style of the individual client.
- Use return demonstration strategies when teaching the client about medication regimen, insulin injection, blood glucose monitoring, and foot assessment.
- Refer clients newly diagnosed with diabetes to local resources and support groups.
- Assess clients' visual acuity and peripheral tactile sensation to determine needed adjustments in teaching self-medication and self-monitoring of blood glucose levels.

Physiological Integrity

- Teach the client about any drugs to be continued after discharge from the hospital.
- Instruct the client and family in the manifestations of complications and when to seek assistance.
- Instruct all clients with diabetes to avoid becoming dehydrated and to drink at least 3 L of water each day unless another medical condition requires fluid restriction.
- Instruct clients who are taking sulfonylurea antidiabetic agents, especially chlorpropamide, about an increased risk for hypoglycemic reactions.
- Teach clients who are taking metformin the clinical manifestations of lactic acidosis (fatigue, dizziness, difficulty breathing, stomach discomfort, irregular heartbeat).
- Warn the client not to take over-the-counter drugs with their oral antidiabetic drugs without consulting their primary care provider.
- When mixing different kinds of insulin together, draw the shorter-acting insulin into the syringe before drawing up the longer-acting insulin.
- Never dilute or mix insulin glargine with any other insulin or solution.
- Teach clients to rotate insulin injection areas within one site rather than to other sites, to prevent changes in absorption.
- Avoid injecting insulin within a 2-inch radius of the umbilicus.
- Avoid intramuscular insulin injection.
- Teach clients who experience Somagyi's phenomenon (early morning hyperglycemia) to ensure an adequate dietary intake at bedtime.
- Instruct the client to always carry a glucose source.
- Teach clients who exercise to test urine for ketone bodies if blood glucose levels are greater than 250 mg/dL before engaging in strenuous exercise.
- Instruct clients in foot care as outlined in Chart 68-10.

ADDITIONAL STUDY RESOURCES

Go to your Student CD-ROM for Review Questions for the NCLEX Examination.

evolve Go to http://evolve.elsevier.com/Iggy/ for Integrated Management of Care Questions for the NCLEX Examination.

SELECTED BIBLIOGRAPHY

Asterisk indicates a classic or definitive work on this subject.

2002Drug topics red book. (2002). Montvale, NJ: Medical Economics Company.

Ahern, J. (2001). Site rotation. *Diabetes Forecast, 54*(4), 66-68.

American Association of Diabetes Educators. (2003a). Diabetes–Facts and Statistics. Available at http://www.aadenet.org/GeneralDiabetesInfo/GovStats.html.

American Association of Diabetes Educators. (2003b). Position statement: Educating providers and persons with diabetes to prevent transmission of bloodborne infections and avoid injuries from sharps. Available at http://www.aadenet.org.
American Association of Diabetes Educators. (2003c). Position statement: Special considerations for the education and management of older adults with diabetes. *The Diabetes Educator, 29*(1), 93-96.
American Diabetes Association. (2001a). Consensus statement: Postprandial blood glucose. *Diabetes Care, 24*(4), 775-778.
American Diabetes Association. (2001b). Position statement: Role of fat replacers in diabetes medical nutrition therapy. *Diabetes Care, 24*(Suppl. 1), 104-105.
American Diabetes Association. (2003a). Committee report: Report of the Expert Committee on the Diagnosis and Classification of Diabetes. *Diabetes Care, 26*(Suppl. 1), 5-20.
American Diabetes Association. (2003b). Position statement: Aspirin therapy in diabetes. *Diabetes Care, 26*(Suppl. 1) 87-88.
American Diabetes Association. (2003c). Position statement: Continuous subcutaneous insulin infusion. *Diabetes Care, 26*(Suppl. 1), 125.
American Diabetes Association. (2003d). Position statement: Diabetic nephropathy. *Diabetes Care, 26*(Suppl. 1), 94-98.
American Diabetes Association. (2003e). Position statement: Diabetic retinopathy. *Diabetes Care, 26*(Suppl. 1), 99-102.
American Diabetes Association. (2003f). Position statement: Evidence-based nutrition principles and recommendations for the treatment and prevention of diabetes and related complications. *Diabetes Care, 26*(Suppl. 1), 51-61.
American Diabetes Association. (2003g). Position statement: Gestational diabetes mellitus. *Diabetes Care, 26*(Suppl. 1), 103-105.
American Diabetes Association. (2003h). Position statement: Hyperglycemic crisis in patients with diabetes mellitus. *Diabetes Care, 26*(Suppl. 1), 109-117.
American Diabetes Association. (2003i). Position statement: Implications of the Diabetes Control and Complications Trial. *Diabetes Care, 26*(Suppl. 1), 25-27.
American Diabetes Association. (2003j). Position statement: Implications of the United Kingdom Prospective Diabetes Study. *Diabetes Care, 26*(Suppl. 1), 28-32.
American Diabetes Association. (2003k). Position statement: Insulin administration. *Diabetes Care, 26*(Suppl. 1), 121-124.
American Diabetes Association. (2003l). Position statement: Management of dyslipidemia in adults with diabetes. *Diabetes Care, 26*(Suppl. 1), 83-86.
American Diabetes Association. (2003m). Position statement: Pancreas transplantation. *Diabetes Care, 26*(Suppl. 1), 120.
American Diabetes Association. (2003n). Position statement: Physical activity/exercise and diabetes mellitus. *Diabetes Care, 26*(Suppl. 1), 73-77.
American Diabetes Association. (2003o). Position statement: Prevention of type 1 diabetes mellitus. *Diabetes Care, 26*(Suppl. 1), 140.
American Diabetes Association. (2003p). Position statement: Preventive foot care in people with diabetes. *Diabetes Care, 26(*Suppl. 1), 78-79.
American Diabetes Association. (2003q). Position statement: Screening for type 2 diabetes. *Diabetes Care, 26*(Suppl. 1), 21-24.
American Diabetes Association. (2003r). Position statement: Standards of medical care for patients with diabetes mellitus. *Diabetes Care, 25*(Suppl. 1), 33-49.
American Diabetes Association. (2003s). Position statement: Tests of glycemia in diabetes. *Diabetes Care, 26*(Suppl. 1), 106-108.
American Diabetes Association. (2003t). Position statement: The prevention or delay of type 2 diabetes. *Diabetes Care, 26*(Suppl. 1), 62-69.
American Diabetes Association. (2003u). Position statement: Treatment of hypertension in adults with diabetes. *Diabetes Care, 26*(Suppl. 1), 80-86.
American Diabetes Association. (2003v). Reviews: Economic costs of diabetes in the U.S. in 2002. *Diabetes Care, 26*(3), 917-932.
American Dietetic Association. (2003). *Exchange lists for meal planning*. (2003). Chicago: Author.
Arauz-Pacheco, C., Parrott, M.A., & Raskin, P. (2002). The treatment of hypertension in adult patients with diabetes. *Diabetes Care, 25*(1), 134-147.
Ayello, E., Cuddigan, J., & Kerstein, M. (2002). Skip the knife: Debriding wounds without surgery. *Nursing2002, 32*(9), 58-63.
Bailes, B. (2002). Diabetes mellitus and its chronic complications. *AORN Journal, 76*(2), 265-282.
Barr, R.G., et al. (2002). Tests of glycemia for the diagnosis of type 2 diabetes mellitus. *Annals of Internal Medicine, 137*(4), 263-272.
Bartol, T. (2002). Putting a patient with diabetes in the driver's seat. *Nursing2002, 32*(2), 53-55.
Beckman, J.A., Creager, M.A., & Libby, P. (2002). Diabetes and atherosclerosis: Epidemiology, pathology and management. *Journal of the American Medical Association, 287*(19), 2570-2581.
Beebe, C., & O'Donnell, M. (2001). Educating patients with type 2 diabetes. *Nursing Clinics of North America, 36*(2), 375-386.
Begany, K. (2000). Over the counter drugs: What's safe to take? *Diabetes Self-Management. 17*(6), 46-52.
Bell, D.S.H. (2002). Chronic complications of diabetes. *Southern Medical Journal, 95*(1), 30-34.
Bergenstal, R., et al. (2000). Identifying variables associated with inaccurate self-monitoring of blood glucose: Proposed guidelines to improve accuracy. *The Diabetes Educator, 26*(6), 981-989.
Berkowitz, K. (2002). Lantus? or Lente? *American Journal of Nursing, 102*, 8, 55.
Bishop, M.L., & Duben-Engelkirk, J.L. (2000). *Clinical chemistry*. Philadelphia: Lippincott Williams & Wilkins.
Blonde, L. (2001). Optimizing therapy in type 2 diabetes. *Patient Care for the Nurse Practitioner, 4*(Suppl. Fall, 2001), 8-14.
Bode, B.W., Sabbah, H., & Davidson, P.C. (2001). What's ahead in glucose monitoring? *Postgraduate Medicine, 109*(4), 41-49.
Bodenheimer, T., et al. (2002). Patient self-management in chronic disease in primary care. *Journal of the American Medical Association, 288*(19), 2469-2475.
*Bowker, J.H., & Pfeifer, M.A. (2000). Levin and O'Neal's *the diabetic foot* (6th ed.). St. Louis: Mosby.
Buse, J.B., Sisca, T.S., & Menke, M. (Eds.). (2002). Diabetic ketoacidosis in the adult patient. Available at http://www.novonordisk.com.
Caballero, E., Habershaw, G.M., & Pinzur, M.S. (2000). Preventing amputation in patients with diabetes. *Patient Care for the Nurse Practitioner, 3*(9), 17-45.
Caffrey, R.M. (2003). Diabetes under control: Are all syringes created equal? *American Journal of Nursing, 103*(6), 46-49.
Cameron, B.L. (2002). Making diabetes management routine. *American Journal of Nursing, 102*(2), 26-33.
Canobbio, M.M. (2000). *Handbook of patient teaching*. St. Louis: Mosby.
Cattral, M.S., et al. (2000). Portal venous and enteric exocrine drainage versus venous and bladder exocrine drainage of pancreatic grafts. *Annals of Surgery, 232*(5), 688-695.
Chan, J.L., & Abrahamson, M.J. (2003). Pharmacologic management of type 2 diabetes mellitus: Rationale for rational use of insulin. *Mayo Clinic Proceedings, 78*(4), 459-468.
Chau, D., & Edelman, S. (2001). Clinical management of diabetes in the elderly. *Clinical Diabetes, 19*(4), 172-175.
Chu, N.V., & Edelman, S. (2001). Diabetes and erectile dysfunction. *Clinical Diabetes, 19*(1), 45-47.
Clark, W.L. (2000). Beta cell replacement and islet cell transplantation. *Diabetes Self-Management, 17*(1), 52-54.
Clarke, K. (2002). New insulin therapy: No needles needed. *Nursing2002, 32*(5), 49-51.
Colwell, J.A., et al. (2000). Strategies for managing diabetes. *Patient Care for the Nurse Practitioner, 3*(9), 2-16.

Conlon, P.C. (2001). A practical approach to type 2 diabetes. *Nursing Clinics of North America, 36*(2), 193-202.

Corrigan, A.M., Pelletier, G., & Alexander, M. (Eds.). (2000). *Core curriculum for intravenous nursing*. Philadelphia: J.B. Lippincott.

Creviston, T., & Quinn, L. (2001). Exercise and physical activity in the treatment of type 2 diabetes. *Nursing Clinics of North America, 36*(2), 243-272.

Crump, V. (2004). Hyperglycemic crisis: Regaining control. *RN, 67*(4), 23-28.

Cryer, P.E., & Childs, B.P. (2002). Negotiating the barrier of hypoglycemia in diabetes. *Diabetes Spectrum, 15*(1), 20-27.

Cunningham, M.A. (2001). Glucose monitoring in type 2 diabetes. *Nursing Clinics of North America, 36*(2), 361-374.

Dagogo-Jack, S., & Alberti, K.G. (2002). Management of diabetes mellitus in surgical patients. *Diabetes Spectrum, 15*(1), 44-48.

Dahmen, R., Haspels, B., Koomen, B., et al. (2001). Therapeutic footwear for the neuropathic foot. *Diabetes Care, 24*(4), 705-709.

Dailey, G. (2002). Hypoglycemia in elderly patients treated with oral agents. *Practical Diabetology, 21*(2), 7-14.

Daly, A., et al. (2003). Diabetes medical nutrition therapy: Practical tips to improve outcomes. *Journal of the American Academy of Nurse Practitioners, 15*(5), 206-211.

Deedwania, P.C. (2000). Hypertension and diabetes. *Archives of Internal Medicine, 160*(11), 1585-1594.

Delaney, M.F., Zisman, A., & Kettyle, W.M. (2000). Diabetic ketoacidosis and hyperglycemic hyperosmolar nonketotic syndrome. *Endocrinology and Metabolism Clinics of North America, 29*(4), 683-705.

Devlin, J.T. (2001). Exercise therapy in the management of diabetes. *Practical Diabetology, 20*(1), 38-44.

Diabetic foot disorders: A clinical practice guideline. (2000). Available at http://acfas.org/diabeticpg.html.

Dinsmoor, R.S. (2000a). High blood sugar after meals: Why it matters. *Diabetes Self-Management, 17*(4), 46-49.

Dinsmoor, R.S. (2000b). Insulin resistance at the root of type 2 diabetes. *Diabetes Self-Management, 17*(3), 38-41.

Donovan, D.S. (2001). Gaining control: A guide to aggressive management of monotherapy failure. *Consultations in Primary Care, 41*(13), 22-31.

Dowell, M., et al. (2004). Economic and clinical disparities in hospitalized patients with type 2 diabetes. *Journal of Nursing Scholarship, 36*(1), 66-72.

El-Kebbi, I.M., et al. (2003). Association of younger age with poor glycemic control and obesity in urban African Americans with type 2 diabetes. *Archives of Internal Medicine, 163*(1), 69-75.

Ellison, J.M., et al. (2001). Rapid changes in postprandial blood glucose produce concentration differences at finger, forearm, and thigh sampling sites. *Diabetes Care, 25(6*), 961-964.

Fain, J. (2002). Delivering insulin 'round the clock. *Nursing2002, 32(8*), 54-56.

Farkas-Hirsch, R. (2000). All about hypoglycemia. *Diabetes Self-Management, 17*(1), 21-27.

Feet can last a lifetime. (2001). Available at http://www.niddk.nih.gov.

Fleming, D. (2000). Mightier than the syringe. *American Journal of Nursing, 100*(11), 44-48.

Flood, L., & Constance, A. (2002). Diabetes & exercise safety. *American Journal of Nursing, 102*(6), 47-55.

*Franz, M. (Ed.). (2001). *A core curriculum for diabetes educators*. Chicago: American Association of Diabetes Educators.

Fritschi, C. (2001). Preventive care of the diabetic foot. *Nursing Clinics of North America, 36*(2), 303-320.

Funnell, M.M., & Barlage, D.L. (2000). Oral diabetes drugs. *Nursing2000, 30*(11), 34-39.

Funnell, M.M., & Barlage, D.L. (2004). Managing diabetes with "Agent Oral." *Nursing2004, 34*(3), 36-43.

Gavin, J.R. (2001). The pathophysiology of type 2 diabetes. *Patient Care for the Nurse Practitioner, 4*(Suppl. Fall, 2001) 4-7.

Gehling, E. (2000). Injecting insulin 101. *Diabetes Self-Management, 17*(5), 7-15.

Gerritsen, M. (2000). Problems associated with subcutaneously implanted glucose sensors. *Diabetes Care, 22*(2), 143-145.

Gonsalves, M.Y. Coordinating care for patients with type 2 diabetes. *Patient Care for the Nurse Practitioner*, 3(9), 15-36.

Green, M.F., Zarrintaj, A., & Green, B.T. (2002). Diabetic foot: Evaluation and management. *Southern Medical Journal, 95*(1), 95-101.

Gregg, E.W., et al. (2002). Is diabetes associated with cognitive impairment and cognitive decline among older women? *Archives of Internal Medicine, 160*(2), 174-180.

Harris, M.I. (2001). Racial and ethnic differences in health care access and health outcomes for adults with type 2 diabetes. *Diabetes Care, 24*(3), 454-459.

Herbel, G., & Boyle, P. (2000). Hypoglycemia: Pathophysiology and treatment. *Endocrinology and Metabolism Clinics of North America, 29*(4), 725-743.

Hunt, D. (2002). Using evidence in practice: Foot care in diabetes. *Endocrinology and Metabolism Clinics of North America, 31*(3), 603-611.

Ingall, T.J. (2000). Preventing ischemic stroke: Current approaches to primary and secondary prevention. *Postgraduate Medicine, 107*(6), 34-50.

Inlow, S., Orsted, H., & Sibbald, R.G. (2000). Best practices for the prevention, diagnosis and treatment of diabetic foot ulcers. *Ostomy Wound Management, 46*(11), 55-67.

Insulin delivery systems for the management of diabetes. (2002). Available at http://www.novonordisk.com.

Insulin: New products, new strategies. (2002). Available at http://www.novonordisk.com.

Jacober, S., & Sowers, J.R. (2001). Management of diabetes in patients undergoing surgery. *Practical Diabetology, 201*(42), 7-14.

Jungheim, K., & Koschinsky, T. (2002). Glucose monitoring at the arm. *Diabetes Care, 25*(6), 956-960.

Kim, R.P., Edelman, S.V., & Kim, D.K. (2001). Musculoskeletal complications of diabetes mellitus. *Clinical Diabetes, 19*(3), 132-135.

King, D.S., & Wofford, M.R. (2000). Obesity and new-onset diabetes mellitus. Available at http://www.drugtopics.com.

Kissin, A., & Katzeff, H. L. (2002). New insulin therapies for the management of diabetes mellitus. *Practical Diabetology, 21*(1), 14-20.

Kulkarni, K. (2003). Managing type 2 diabetes. Available at http://www.clinicianreviews.com.

Lachuk, L., McGee, K.H., & Voris, J.C. (2002). Current guidelines for managing diabetes mellitus. *Federal Practitioner, 20*(11), 54 61.

Laffel, L. (2000). Sick-day management in type 1 diabetes. *Endocrinology and Metabolism Clinics of North America, 29*(4), 707-723.

Lenhard, M.J., & Reeves, G.D. (2001). Continuous subcutaneous insulin infusion. *Archives of Internal Medicine, 161*(19), 2293-2300.

Levetan, C.S., & Magee, M.F. (2000). Hospital management of diabetes. *Endocrinology and Metabolism Clinics of North America, 29*(4), 745-770.

Levin, M. (2002). Management of the diabetic foot: Preventing amputation. *Southern Medical Journal, 95*(1), 10-20.

Loon, N.R. (2003). Diabetic kidney disease: Preventing dialysis and transplantation. *Clinical Diabetes, 21*(2), 55-62.

Lorig, K. (2001). *Patient education: A practical approach* (3rd ed.). London: Sage Publications.

Lower, J. (2002). Facing neuro assessment fearlessly. *Nursing2002, 32*(2), 58-64.

McCloskey, J.C., & Bulechek, G.M. (Eds.). (2000). *Nursing interventions classification (NIC)* (3rd ed.). St. Louis: Mosby.

McCormick, J.L., & Deeg, M.A. (2000). Pharmacologic treatment of dyslipidemia. *American Journal of Nursing, 100*(2), 55-60.

Meece, J., & Campbell, R.K. (2002). Insulin lispro update. *The Diabetes Educator. 28*(2), 269-277.

Mokdad, A.H., et al. (2000). Diabetes trends in the U. S.: 1990-1998. *Diabetes Care, 23*(9), 1278-1283.
Mudaliar, S., & Edelman, S.V. (2001). Insulin therapy in type 2 diabetes. *Endocrinology and Metabolism Clinics of North America, 30*(4), 935 982.
Nath, C., & Ponte, C.D. (2000). Lessons learned about insulin therapy. *Nursing 2000, 30*(11), 40-45.
National Task Force on the Prevention and Treatment of Obesity. (2000). Overweight, obesity and health risk. *Archives of Internal Medicine, 160*(7), 898-904.
Neil, J.A. (2002). Assessing foot care knowledge in a rural population with diabetes. *Ostomy/Wound Management, 48*(1), 50-56.
Nurse Practitioner's Prescribing Reference. (2003). New York: Prescribing Reference, Inc.
Paty, B.W., & Hirsch, I. (2000). Erectile dysfunction in diabetes. *Practical Diabetology, 19*(2), 16-23.
Peragallo-Dittko, V. (2002a). Alternate site testing. *Practical Diabetology, 21*(4), 48-49.
Peragallo-Dittko, V. (2002b). Blood glucose monitoring update. *Diabetes Self-Management, 19*(1), 46-52.
Peragallo-Dittko, V. (2000c). How accurate is your meter? *Diabetes Self-Management, 17*(5), 78-85.
Plodkowski, R.A., & Edelman, S. (2001). Pre-surgical evaluation of diabetic patients. *Clinical Diabetes, 19*(1), 92-95.
Quinn, L. (2001a). Diabetes emergencies in patients with type 2 diabetes. *Nursing Clinics of North America, 36*(2), 341-360.
Quinn, L. (2001b). Type 2 diabetes: Epidemiology, pathophysiology, and diagnosis. *Nursing Clinics of North America, 36*(2), 175-192.
Quinn, L. (2002a). Pharmacologic treatment of the critically ill patient with diabetes. *Critical Care Clinics of North America, 14*(1), 87-98.
Quinn, L. (2002b). Pharmacologic management of the patient with diabetes. *Nursing Clinics of North America, 36*(2), 217-242.
Rao, S.H. (2001). Treating to target: A rational approach based on pathophysiology. *Consultations in Primary Care, 41*(13), 14-21.
Reasner, C.A. (2002). Aggressive control of type 2 diabetes using oral agents. Available at http://www.cliniciansCME.com.
Rezabek, K.M. (2001). Medical nutrition therapy in type 2 diabetes. *Nursing Clinics of North America, 36*(2), 203-216.
Robertson, K.E., Glazer, N.B., & Campbell, R.K. (2000). The latest development in insulin injection devices. *The Diabetes Educator, 26*(1), 135-152.
Robertson, R.P., et al. (2000). Pancreas and islet transplantation for patients with diabetes. *Diabetes Care, 23*(1), 112-116.
Sacks, D.B., et al. (2002). Guidelines and recommendations for laboratory analysis in the diagnosis and management of diabetes mellitus. *Clinical Chemistry, 48*(3), 436-472.
Safeer, R.S., & Cornell, M.O. (2000). The emerging role of HDL cholesterol. *Postgraduate Medicine, 108*(7), 87-98.
Saleh, M., & Grunberger, G. (2001). Hypoglycemia: An excuse for poor glycemic control? *Clinical Diabetes, 19*(4), 161-167.
Sammer, C. (2001). How should you respond to hypoglycemia? *Nursing2001, 31*(7), 48-50.
Seley, J. (2003).Giving the fingers a rest: Alternative site testing eases blood glucose monitoring. *American Journal of Nursing, 103*(3), 73-77.
Seley, J.J. (2001). The role of insulin in type 2 diabetes. *Patient Care for the Nurse Practitioner*, 4(Suppl. Fall, 2001), 15-20.
Singri, N., Ahya, S., & Levin, M.L. (2003). Acute renal failure. *Journal of the American Medical Association, 289*(6), 747-751.
Skelly, A. (2002). Elderly patients with diabetes. *American Journal of Nursing, 102*(2), 15-16.
Skyler, J. (2001). Microvascular complications: Retinopathy and nephropathy. *Endocrinology and Metabolism Clinics of North America, 29*(4), 833-856.
Slagle, M. (2002). Medication update: Diabetes mellitus. *Southern Medical Journal, 95*(1), 50-55.
Spanheimer, R.G. (2001). Cardiovascular risk in diabetes. *Postgraduate Medicine, 109*(4), 26-36.
Stevens, R.B., Matsumoto, S., & Marsh, C.L. (2001). Is islet cell transplantation a realistic therapy for treatment of type 1 diabetes in the near future? *Clinical Diabetes, 19*(1), 51-60.
Strock, E. (2001). Strategies for patient care and education. *Consultations in Primary Care, 41*(13), 6-13.
Sweny, S. (2002). Toward a better understanding of diabetic nephropathy. *The Diabetes Educator, 28*(1), 72-75.
Tang, W.H.W., & Young, J.B. (2001). Cardiomyopathy and heart failure in diabetes. *Endocrinology and Metabolism Clinics of North America, 29*(4), 1031-1046.
Tkacs, N.C. (2002). Hypoglycemia unawareness. *American Journal of Nursing, 102*(2), 34-41.
Tripp-Reimer, T., et al. (2001). Cultural barriers to care: Inverting the problem. *Diabetes Spectrum, 14*(1), 13-22.
Umpierrez, G.E., Murphy, B.E., & Kitabchi, A.E. (2002). Diabetic ketoacidosis and hyperglycemic hyperosmolar syndrome. *Diabetes Spectrum, 15*(1), 28-36.
U.S. Environmental Protection Agency. (2005). Medical waste. Retrieved February 3, 2005 from http://www.epa.gov/epaoswer/other/medical.
Valentine, V. (2000). When diabetes affects the stomach. *Diabetes Self-Management, 17*(4), 52-56.
Valentine, V. (2002). Using a laser to make a point. *Nursing2002, 32*(110), 56-57.
Valk, G.D., Kriegsman, D.M.W., & Assendelft, W.J.J. (2002). Patient education for preventing food ulceration: A systematic review. *Endocrinology and Metabolism Clinics of North America, 31*(3), 634-658.
van Bijsterveld, O.O. (Ed.). (2000). *Diabetic retinopathy*. London: Martin Dunitz Ltd.
Vijan, S., & Hayward, R.A. (2003). Treatment of hypertension in type 2 diabetes mellitus: Blood pressure goals, choice of agents, and setting priorities in diabetes care. *Annals of Internal Medicine, 138*(7), 593-602.
Vinik, A.I., et al. (2003). Diabetic autonomic neuropathy. *Diabetes Care, 26*(5), 1553-1579.
Watkins, P.J. (2003). Cardiovascular disease, hypertension, and lipids. *British Medical Journal, 326*(7394), 874-976.
White, J.R., & Campbell, R.K. (2000). Dangerous and common drug interactions in patients with diabetes mellitus. *Endocrinology and Metabolism Clinics of North America, 29*(4), 789-803.
White, J.A., & Hirsh, I.R. (2000). Nonhypoglycemic drug reactions of agents used to treat diabetes. *Endocrinology and Metabolism Clinics of North America, 29*(4), 803-811.
White, J.R., & Campbell, R.K. (2001). Inhaled insulin: An overview. *Clinical Diabetes, 19*(1), 13-16.
Williams, A.S. (2000). Helpful odds and ends. *Diabetes Self-Management, 17*(2), 22-27.
Wilson, B.A., Shannon, M.T., & Stang, C.L. (2002). *Nurse's drug guide.* Upper Saddle River, N J: Prentice Hall.
Wilson, P.W.F. (2001). Diabetes mellitus and coronary artery disease. *Endocrinology and Metabolism Clinics of North America, 29*(4), 857-881.
Wood, F. (2002). Ethnic differences in exercise among adults with diabetes. *Western Journal of Nursing, 24*(5), 502-515.

INTERNET REFERENCES

U.S. Department of Health and Human Services, Bureau of Primary Health Care: The LEAP Program: http://www.bphc.hsra.gov/leap
Centers for Disease Control and Prevention: http://www.cdc.gov/health/diabetes.htm

Cell Robotics International:
http://www.cellrobotics.com/perslasette.html
Diabeteswebsite.com:
http://www.diabeteswebsite.com
U.S. Environmental Protection Agency:
http://www.epa.gov/epaoswer/other/medical/dispose1.pdf
GlucoWatch: Automatic Glucose Biographer:
http://www.glucowatch.com
National Institutes of Diabetes and Digestive and Kidney Diseases:
http://www.niddk.nih.gov
Diabetes Prevention Program:
http://www.gwu.edu/dpp/index.htmlvdoc
Discount Diabetic Supplies:
http://www.diabeticpromotions.com
Diabetic Supplies.com:
http://www.diabeticsupplies.com

UNIT **FIFTEEN**

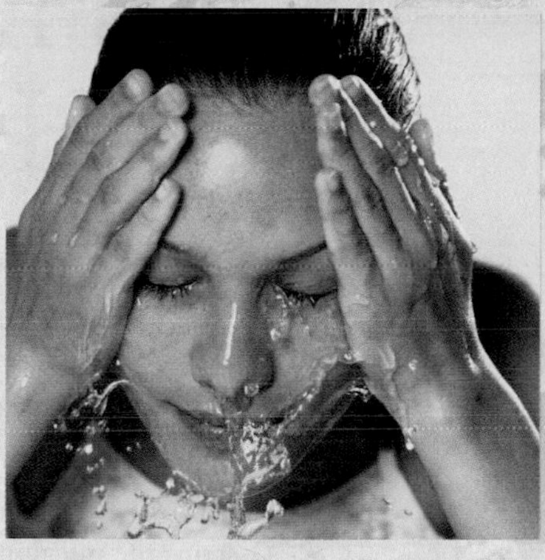

PROBLEMS of PROTECTION

Management of Clients with Problems of the Skin, Hair, and Nails

CHAPTER 69

Assessment of the Skin, Hair, and Nails

JANICE CUZZELL • M. LINDA WORKMAN

LEARNING OUTCOMES

After studying this chapter, you should be able to:

1. Compare the structures and function of the dermis with those of the epidermis.
2. Describe the integumentary changes associated with aging.
3. Use proper terminology to describe different skin lesions.
4. Describe techniques to assess skin changes in clients with dark skin.
5. Distinguish between normal variations and abnormal skin manifestations with regard to skin color, texture, warmth, and moisture.
6. Explain the role of melanocytes in determining skin color.
7. Describe the ABCD method of assessing skin lesions for cancer.
8. Prioritize the educational needs for the client undergoing an excisional biopsy for a skin lesion.

Go to your Student CD-ROM for Review Questions for the NCLEX Examination keyed to these Learning Outcomes.

The integumentary system is composed of the skin, hair, and nails. This system is the first line of defense in protecting the inner organs from the external environment. The skin is the largest organ of the body, and it plays a major role in homeostasis. Not only is it a barrier to organisms, but it also helps to regulate body temperature and maintains fluid and electrolyte balance. Changes in the skin can communicate information about a person's health and well-being.

Emotional stress, systemic disease, and skin injury or disease can alter the function, appearance, and texture of the skin. Therefore examine the skin for important clues about the client's health. Because the skin has many sensory receptors, the client can report subjective skin sensations that might indicate specific health problems. The sensory function of the skin allows the use of touch as a therapeutic intervention to provide comfort, relieve pain, and communicate caring.

ANATOMY AND PHYSIOLOGY REVIEW

Structure of the Skin

As shown in Figure 69-1, the skin has three layers: fat, dermis, and epidermis. Each layer has unique properties that contribute to the skin's ability to maintain its complex functions.

SUBCUTANEOUS FAT (ADIPOSE TISSUE)

The innermost layer of the skin, which lies over muscle and bone, is the site for fat formation and storage. Fat cells serve as an energy reserve in the event extra calories are needed to power the body. These cells also act as heat insulators for the body. They absorb shock and protect against injury by padding internal structures. Fat distribution varies with body area, age, and gender. Many blood vessels go through the fatty layer and extend into the dermal layer, forming capillary networks that supply nutrients and remove wastes.

DERMIS (CORIUM)

Above the fat layer lies the **dermis,** a layer of connective tissue that contains no cells. The dermis is composed of collagen and elastic fibers that are interwoven to give the skin both flexibility and strength.

Collagen, the main component of dermal tissue, is a protein formed by dermal cells called fibroblasts. Collagen production increases in areas of tissue injury and helps to form scar tissue. Fibroblasts also produce **ground substance,** a lubricant composed of protein and sugar groups that surrounds the dermal cells and fibers and contributes to the skin's normal suppleness and turgor.

The elasticity of the skin depends on both the amount and quality of the elastic fibers, which are scattered among the collagen fibers. The major component of the elastic fiber is **elastin.**

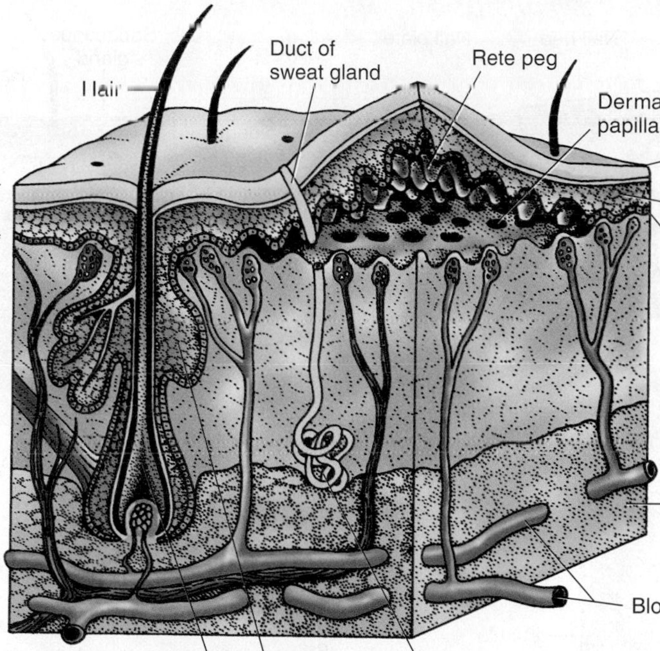

Figure 69-1 ■ Anatomy of the skin.

The dermis houses a network of capillaries and lymph vessels in which the exchange of oxygen and heat occurs. The dermis is also rich in sensory nerves that transmit the sensations of touch, pressure, temperature, pain, and itch.

EPIDERMIS

The outermost skin layer, the **epidermis,** is anchored to the dermis by fingerlike projections of dermal tissue **(dermal papillae).** The fingers of epidermal tissue that project into the dermis are called **rete pegs.** The epidermis is less than 1 mm thick, but it is the protective barrier between the body and the environment.

The epidermis does not have a separate blood supply. It receives its nutrients by diffusion from the many blood vessels in the dermal layer through a porous basement membrane at the dermal-epidermal junction. Attached to the basement membrane are the keratinocytes. The basal cells (those keratinocytes capable of cell division and located closest to the basement membrane) continuously divide to form new cells. Older keratinocytes are pushed upward to form the stratified layers of the epithelium **(malpighian layers).** As keratinocytes move toward the surface, they flatten and eventually die. The outermost skin layer, the **stratum corneum** (horny layer), is composed of these dead cells. **Keratin,** the protein produced by keratinocytes, makes the horny layer waterproof. A keratinocyte takes about 28 to 45 days to move from the basement membrane to the skin surface, where it is shed (exfoliated).

Vitamin D is activated in the epidermis by ultraviolet (UV) light. It is then distributed by the blood to other body areas.

Melanocytes are pigment-producing cells found at the level of the basement membrane in a ratio of about one melanocyte for every 10 keratinocytes. These cells give color to the skin and account for the racial differences in skin tone. Darker skin tones are not caused by increased numbers of melanocytes; rather, the size of the pigment granules (melanin) contained in each cell determines the color. Freckles, birthmarks, and age spots are caused by patches of melanin within the skin. UV light stimulates the production of melanin, which protects against the harmful effects of sun exposure. Melanin production increases locally in response to endocrine changes or inflammation. Specialized cells called Langerhans cells also are present in the epidermis. If the skin is damaged, these cells engulf any foreign substances (antigens) that invade the body. These cells then alert the immune system to the presence of the antigen.

Structure of the Skin Appendages

HAIR

Hair, a remnant of the thick protective pelt worn by most mammals, is mainly a cosmetic feature for modern humans. Hair growth varies with race, gender, age, and genetic predisposition. Individual hairs can differ in both structure and rate of growth, depending on body location.

Hair follicles are located in the dermal layer of the skin but are actually extensions of the epidermal layer (see Figure 69-1). Within each hair follicle, a round column of keratin forms the hair shaft. Hair keratin contains more sulfur than do skin cells, which toughens the hair shaft as it forms. Hair color is genetically determined by a person's rate of melanin production.

Hair growth occurs in cycles; a growth phase (anagen) is followed by a resting phase (telogen). Local and systemic stressors can alter the growth cycle and result in temporary hair loss. Permanent baldness, such as male pattern baldness, is genetic in origin and is seldom influenced by personal or environmental factors.

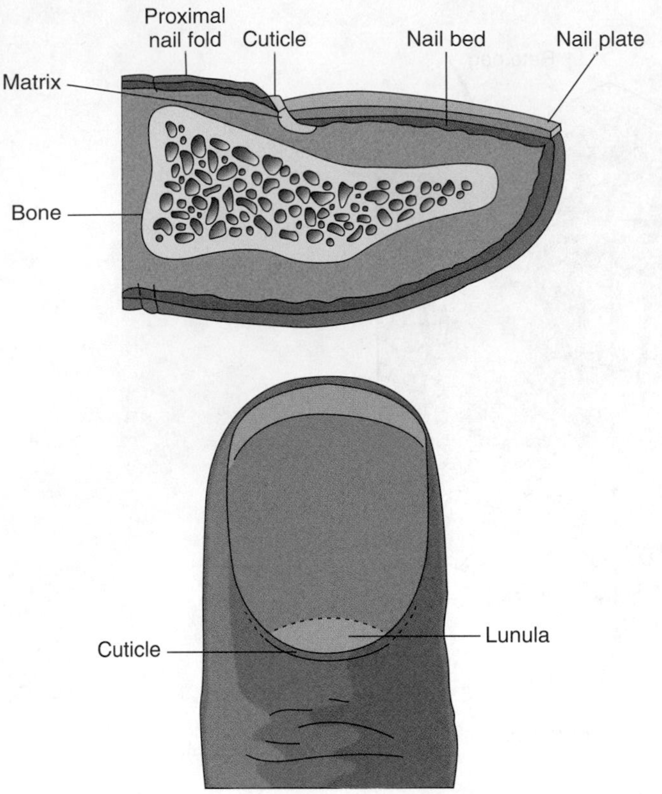

Figure 69-2 ■ Anatomy of the nail.

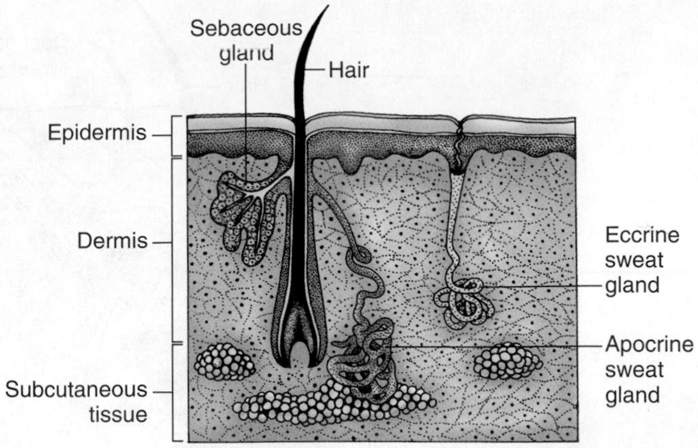

Figure 69-3 ■ Anatomy of the hair follicle and sebaceous and sweat glands.

NAILS

Well-groomed fingernails and toenails have cosmetic value and serve as useful tools with which to scrape and grasp. Like hair follicles, the nails are extensions of the keratin-producing epidermal layers of the skin.

The white crescent-shaped portion of the nail at the lower end of the nail plate **(lunula)** reflects the underlying nail matrix, where nail keratin is formed and nail growth begins (Figure 69-2). Unlike hair growth, which is cyclic, nail growth is a continuous but slow process. Total replacement of a fingernail requires 3 to 4 months. Total replacement of a toenail may take up to 12 months.

The **cuticle,** a layer of keratin at the nail fold, attaches the nail plate to the soft tissue of the nail fold. The nail body is translucent, and the pinkish hue reflects a rich blood supply beneath the nail surface. Nail growth and appearance are often altered during systemic disease or serious illness.

GLANDS

SEBACEOUS GLANDS. The sebaceous glands are distributed over the entire skin surface, except for the palms of the hand and soles of the feet. Most sebaceous glands are directly connected to the hair follicles (Figure 69-3). The sebaceous glands of the eyelids, nipple areolae, and genitalia are freestanding.

Sebaceous glands produce **sebum,** a mildly bacteriostatic, fat-containing substance. Sebum lubricates the skin and reduces water loss from the skin surface.

SWEAT GLANDS. The skin has two types of sweat glands: eccrine and apocrine. Eccrine sweat glands arise from the epithelial cells. They are found over the entire skin surface and are not associated with the hair follicle. The odorless, colorless, isotonic secretions of the eccrine glands are an important factor in the regulation of body temperature. Stimulation of sweat from these glands and the resultant water evaporation can cause the body to lose as much as 10 to 12 L of fluid in a single day.

Apocrine sweat glands are in direct contact with the hair follicle. They are found mostly in the axillae, perineal, nipple areolae, and periumbilicus body areas. The interaction of skin bacteria with the secretions of the apocrine glands causes the distinctive body odor.

Functions of the Skin

The skin is a complex organ responsible for the regulation of many body functions throughout the life span (Table 69-1). In addition to the skin's protective and regulatory functions, its location on the outside of the body makes it an important way to communicate a client's state of health and body image.

Skin Changes Associated with Aging

The process of aging begins at birth. As changes in physiology progress with aging, the skin also undergoes age-related changes in both structure and function (Chart 69-1). Figures 69-4 through 69-15 show some common age-related skin changes.

Individual differences exist in how quickly and to what degree the skin ages. Although genetic background, hormonal changes, and systemic disease may change the appearance of the skin over time, chronic sun exposure is the single most important factor leading to degeneration of the skin components (Figure 69-16).

ASSESSMENT TECHNIQUES

History

Before examining the skin, take an accurate history from the client so that actual and potential skin problems can be readily identified. Chart 69-2 lists the best practices for obtaining a history from a client with a skin problem. Begin by gathering information about skin changes and current skin care practices.

TABLE 69-1 Functions of the Skin

Epidermis	Dermis	Subcutaneous Tissue
Protection		
Keratin provides protection from injury by corrosive materials Inhibits proliferation of microorganisms because of dry external surface Mechanical strength through intercellular bonds	Provides fibroblasts for wound healing. Provides mechanical strength. ▪ Collagen fibers ▪ Elastic fibers ▪ Ground substance	Mechanical shock absorber. Energy reserve.
Homeostasis (Water Balance)		
Low permeability to water and electrolytes prevents systemic dehydration and electrolyte loss	Lymphatic and vascular tissues respond to inflammation, injury, and infection.	
Temperature Regulation		
Eccrine sweat glands allow dissipation of heat through evaporation of sweat secreted onto the skin surface	Cutaneous vasculature, through dilation or construction, promotes or inhibits heat conduction from the skin surface.	Fat cells act as insulators and assist in retention of body heat.
Sensory Organ		
Transmits a variety of sensations through the neuroreceptor system	Encloses an extensive network of nerve endings for relaying sensations to the brain.	Contains large pressure receptors.
Vitamin Synthesis		
7-Dehydrocholesterol is present in large concentrations in malpighian cells; photoconversion to vitamin D takes place	No function.	No function.
Psychosocial		
Body image alterations occur with many epidermal diseases, such as generalized psoriasis	Body image alterations occur with many dermal diseases, such as scleroderma.	Body image alterations may result from increases, decreases, and redistribution of body fat stores.

CHART 69-1

NURSING FOCUS on the OLDER ADULT

Changes in the Integumentary System Related to Aging

Physical Changes	Clinical Findings	Changes in Functional Ability
Epidermis		
Decreased thickness in epidermal layer	Increased skin transparency and fragility	
Decreased epidermal mitotic activity	Delayed wound healing	Decreased cell replacement
Decreased epidermal mitotic homeostasis	Skin hyperplasia, such as hyperkeratoses and skin cancers (especially in sun-exposed areas)	
Increased epidermal permeability	Increased susceptibility to irritant reactions	Decreased barrier function
Decreased number of Langerhans cells	Decreased cutaneous inflammatory response	Decreased injury response
Decreased number of active melanocytes	Increased sensitivity to sun exposure	
Hyperplasia of melanocytes at the dermal-epidermal junction (especially in sun-exposed areas)	Mottled hyperpigmentation and hypopigmentation (e.g., liver spots, age spots)	
Decreased vitamin D production	Increased susceptibility to osteomalacia	Decreased vitamin D production
Flattening of the dermal-epidermal junction	Increased susceptibility to shearing forces, with resultant blisters, purpura, skin tears, and pressure-related skin problems	
Dermis		
Decreased dermal blood flow	Increased susceptibility to dry skin (xerosis)	Decreased chemical clearance
Decreased vasomotor responsiveness	Increased thermoregulatory alterations (predisposition to heat stroke and hypothermia)	Decreased vascular responsiveness
Decreased dermal thickness	Paper-thin, transparent skin with an increased susceptibility to trauma	Decreased injury response
Degeneration of elastic fibers	Decreased tone and elasticity (wrinkles)	Body image alterations
Benign proliferation of capillaries	Cherry hemangiomas	
Abnormal nerve endings	Alterations in sensory perception	Decreased sensory perception

Continued

CHART 69-1

NURSING FOCUS on the OLDER ADULT

Changes in the Integumentary System Related to Aging—*cont'd*

Physical Changes	Clinical Findings	Changes in Functional Ability
Subcutaneous Layer		
Redistribution of adipose tissue	"Bags," cellulite, double chin, abdominal apron	Body-image alterations
Thinning of subcutaneous fat layer	Increased susceptibility to hypothermia Decreased resistance to mechanical injury (especially pressure necrosis)	Decreased thermoregulation Decreased injury response
Hair		
Decreased number of hair follicles and rate of growth	Increased hair thinning	Decreased cell replacement
Decreased number of active melanocytes in follicle	Gradual loss of hair color (graying)	Body image alterations
Nails		
Decreased rate of growth	Increased susceptibility to fungal infections	Decreased cell replacement
Decreased blood flow beneath the nail bed	Longitudinal nail ridges	
Glands		
Decreased sebum production despite sebaceous gland hyperplasia	Increased size of pores (especially on nose); large comedones in malar region	Decreased sebum production
Decreased eccrine and apocrine gland activity	Increased susceptibility to dry skin Decreased perspiration, leading to decreased cooling effect Decreased need for antiperspirants	 Decreased sweat production Decreased thermoregulation

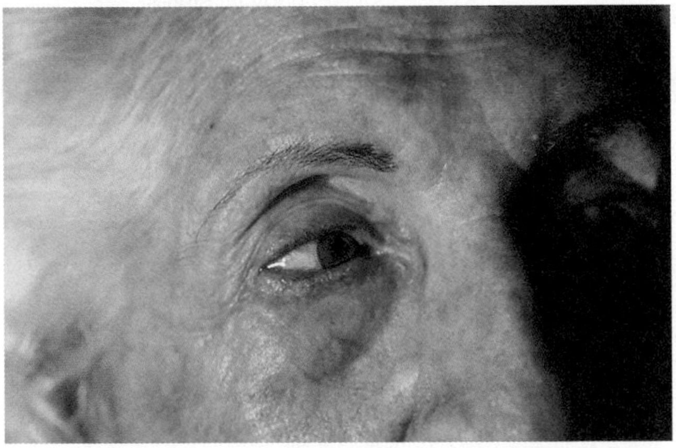

Figure 69-4 ■ Eyelid eversion.

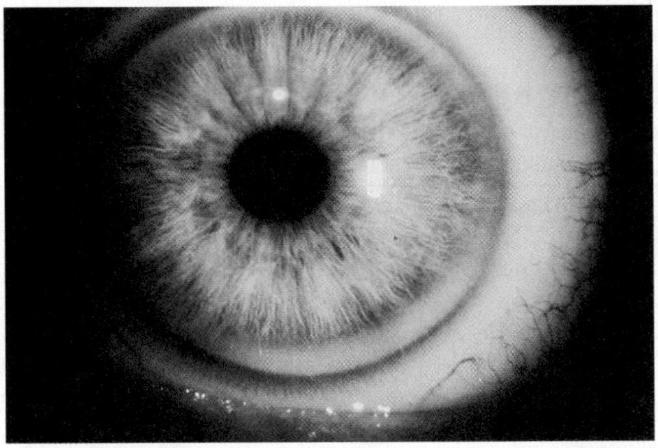

Figure 69-6 ■ Arcus senilis of the iris.

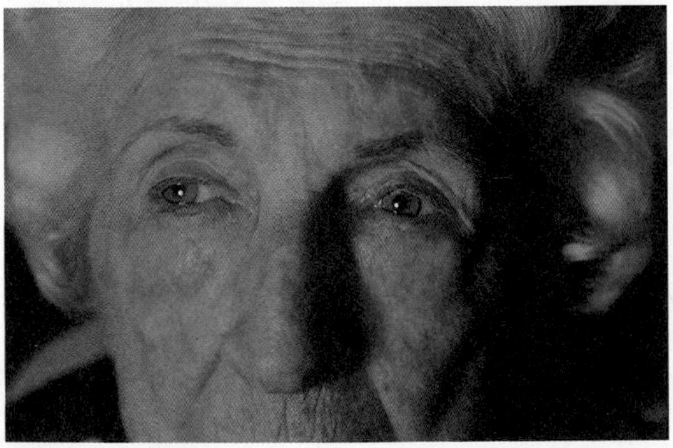

Figure 69-5 ■ Deepening of the orbit.

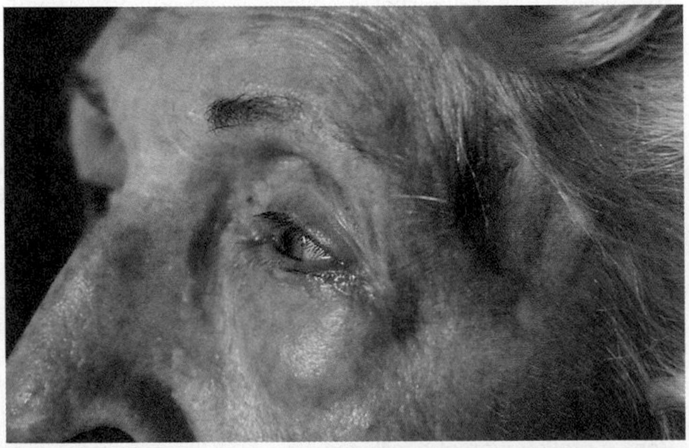

Figure 69-7 ■ Changes in the body contour: "bags" under the eyes.

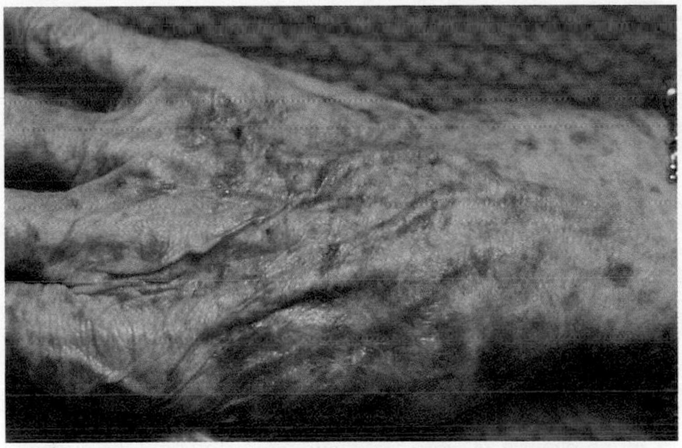

Figure 69-8 ■ Paper-thin, transparent skin.

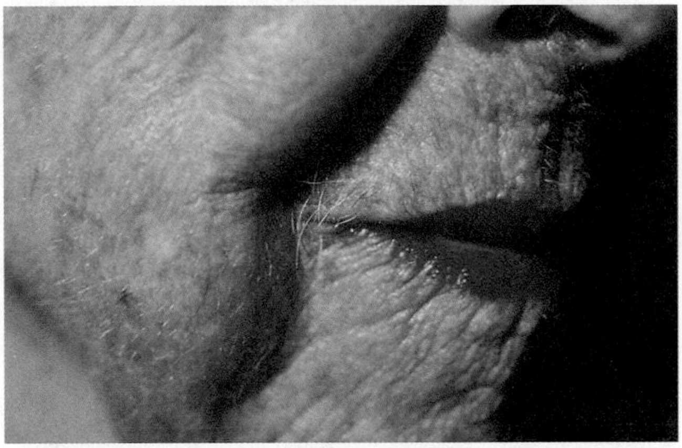

Figure 69-9 ■ Wrinkles.

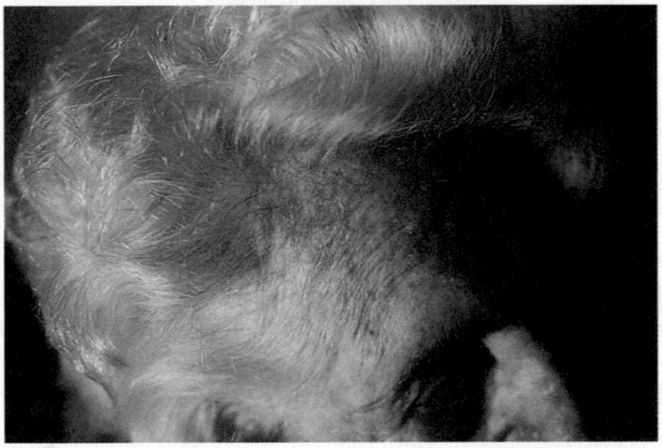

Figure 69-10 ■ Graying and thinning of the hair.

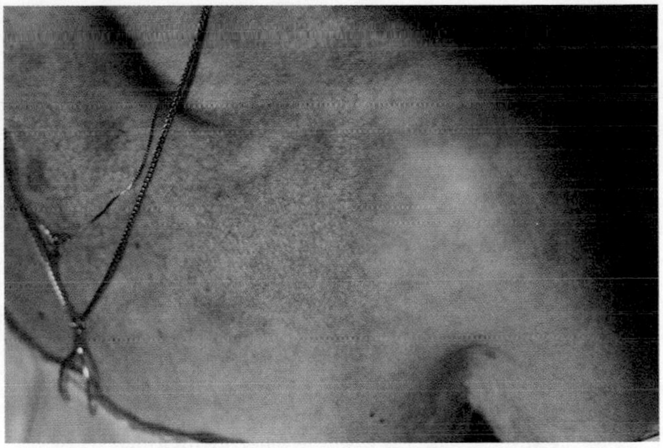

Figure 69-11 ■ Xerosis (dry skin).

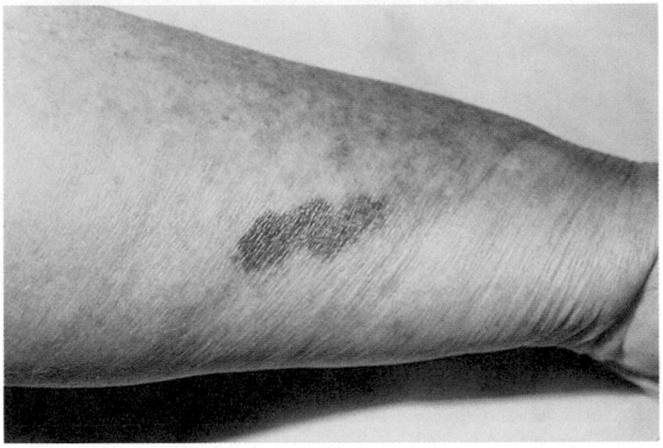

Figure 69-12 ■ Actinic purpura.

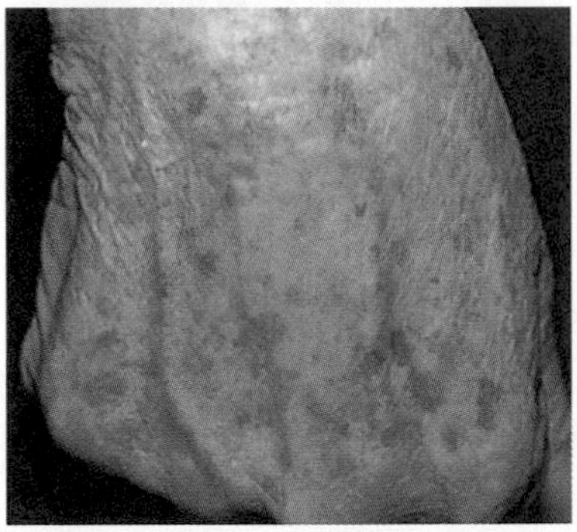

Figure 69-13 ■ Actinic lentigo (liver spots).

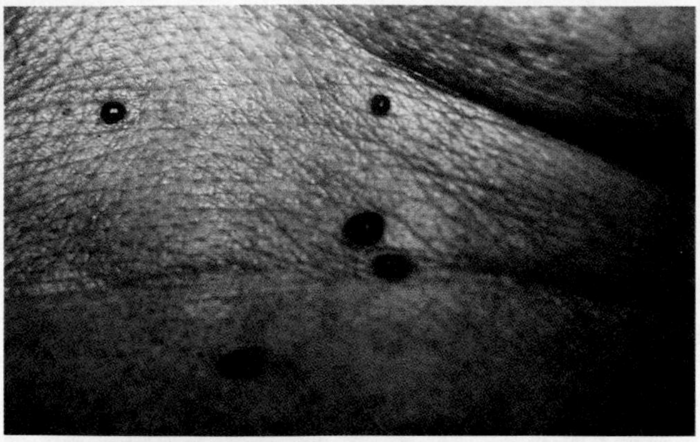

Figure 69-14 ■ Senile (cherry) angiomas.

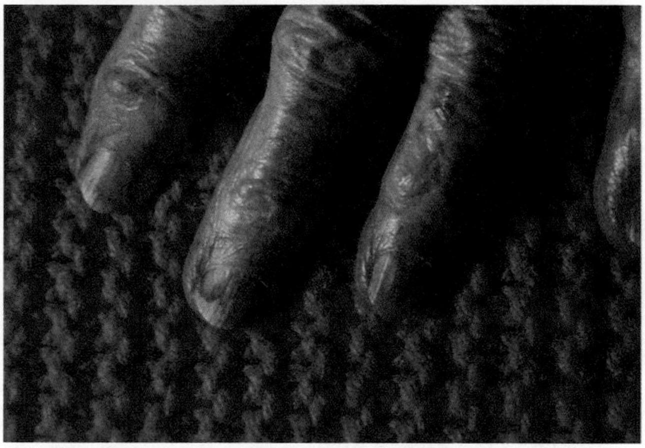

Figure 69-15 ■ Nail changes: longitudinal ridges and thickening.

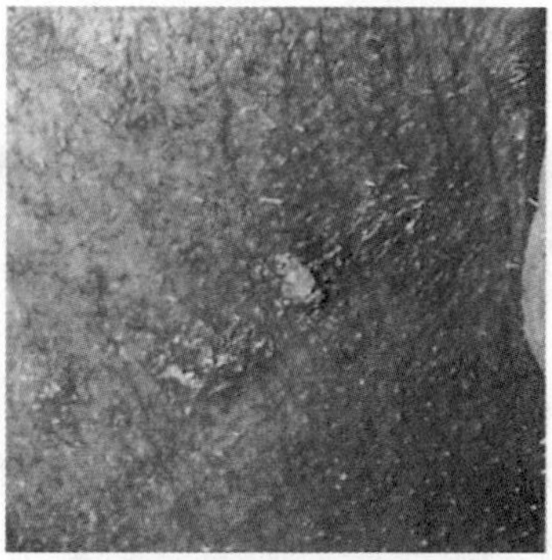

Figure 69-16 ■ Actinic (solar) keratosis.

CHART 69-2

BEST PRACTICE for

Obtaining an Accurate Nursing History of the Client with a Skin Problem

Medical-Surgical History

- Does the client have any current or previous medical problems?
- Has the client undergone any recent or previous surgical procedures?

Family History

- Is there any family tendency toward chronic skin problems?
- Do any members of the immediate family have recent skin complaints?

Medication History

- Is the client allergic to any systemic or topical medication? If so, have the client describe the reaction.
- What prescription drugs has the client taken recently? When was the drug started? What is the dose or frequency of administration? When was the last dose taken?
- What over-the-counter drugs has the client taken recently? When was the drug started? What is the dose or frequency of administration? When was the last dose taken?

Social History

- What is the client's occupation?
- What recreational activities does the client enjoy?
- Has the client traveled recently?
- What is the client's nutritional status?

Current Health Problem

- When did the client first notice the skin problem?
- Where on the body did the problem begin?
- Has the problem gotten better or worse?
- Has a similar skin condition ever occurred before? If so, have the client describe the typical course and how it was treated.
- Is the problem associated with any of the following: itching, burning, stinging, numbness, pain, fever, nausea and vomiting, diarrhea, sore throat, cold, stiff neck, new foods, new soaps or cosmetics, new clothing or bed linens, or stressful situations?
- Does anything seem to make the problem worse (e.g., sun exposure, medications, heat or cold, and menses)?
- Does anything seem to make the problem better?

DEMOGRAPHIC DATA

Obtain demographic data from clients with actual or potential skin disorders. Age is important because many changes in the integumentary system are normal manifestations of the aging process.

Race and nationality can also be important. Some variations in the appearance of skin are normal among clients of specific races and ethnicities but are abnormal for clients of other races or ethnicities.

Information regarding the client's occupation and hobbies can provide clues to chronic skin exposure to chemicals, irritants, abrasive substances, and other environmental factors that can contribute to skin problems.

FAMILY HISTORY AND GENETIC RISK

Many skin disorders have a familial predisposition or can be inherited. Therefore explore any family tendency toward chronic skin problems. Ask about all immediate family members' current health status to identify a communicable disease that has been transferred between family members.

PERSONAL HISTORY

Take the client's medical history, including previous or current illnesses and surgical procedures. This information helps to determine whether skin changes are a manifestation of an underlying systemic disorder.

MEDICATION HISTORY

Skin reactions to systemic drugs are common. Ask the client about any recent use of prescription and over-the-counter (OTC) drugs (e.g., laxatives, antacids, and cold remedies). Determine when each drug was started, the dose and frequency of the drug, and the time the last dose was taken. A drug history also helps identify skin changes that result from the treatment of other health problems, such as the changes that occur with long-term steroid or anticoagulant therapy.

DIET HISTORY

Document the client's weight, height, body build, and food preferences. Poor nutrition, especially protein deficiencies, vitamin deficiencies, and obesity, can increase the client's risk for skin lesions and delay wound healing. Fat-free diets and chronic alcoholism can lead to vitamin deficiencies and related skin changes. Some skin diseases, such as chronic urticaria and acne, may be worsened by certain foods or food additives.

SOCIOECONOMIC STATUS

Ask the client about his or her social and economic background to identify environmental factors that might contribute to skin disease. Recent travel may be a source of skin infections or unusual lesions.

If the client is well tanned, ask about the amount of time spent in the sun and tanning booths and whether he or she has any skin problems from sun exposure.

Skin problems related to poor hygiene are common. Ask about living conditions, bathing practices, and the availability of running water.

CURRENT HEALTH PROBLEMS

If a skin problem is identified, obtain more information about the specific problem, such as the following:

- When did the client first notice the rash or skin change?
- Where on the body did the rash begin?
- Has the problem improved or become worse?

If a similar problem has occurred before, ask the client to describe the course of the skin lesion and how it was treated. Try to link the problem with specific symptoms, such as itching, burning, numbness, pain, fever, sore throat, stiff neck, or nausea and vomiting. Ask the client to identify anything that seems to make the problem better or worse.

Skin Assessment

INSPECTION

Skin changes may be related to specific skin diseases and may also reflect an underlying systemic disorder. By using skin assessment skills, you are in a unique position to identify clues about a client's state of health.

A thorough assessment of the skin is best performed with the client partially or completely undressed. Incorporate skin examination for actual or potential impairments into the routine part of daily care while bathing or assisting the client.

Inspect the client's skin surfaces in a well-lighted room; natural or bright fluorescent lighting enhances the visibility of subtle skin changes. Although no special equipment is needed, use a penlight for close inspection of lesions and to illuminate the mouth.

Assess each skin surface systematically, including the scalp, hair, nails, and mucous membranes. Give particular attention to the skin-fold areas. The moist, warm environment of skin folds can harbor organisms, such as yeast or bacteria. Observe and document the following features:

- Obvious changes in color and vascularity
- Presence or absence of moisture
- Edema
- Skin lesions
- Skin integrity

Check the cleanliness of the various body areas to determine whether the client's self-care activities need to be evaluated.

Color

Skin color is affected by a number of factors, including blood flow, oxygenation, body temperature, and pigment production. In addition to these factors, the wide variation in natural skin tones may require different techniques for clients who have darker skin. (See Cultural Considerations, p. 1571, for suggestions for assessing clients with darker skin.)

Describe changes in skin color by their appearance (Table 69-2). Document changes in color, and describe whether the changes are generalized or localized. Color changes can be seen most easily in the areas of least pigmentation, such as the oral mucosa, sclera, nail beds, and the palms and soles. Inspect these areas to help confirm more subtle color changes of general body areas.

Lesions

Skin disease is clinically described in terms of primary and secondary lesions (Figure 69-17). **Primary lesions** are an initial reaction to a problem that alters one of the structural components of the skin. **Secondary lesions** are changes in the appearance of the primary lesion. These changes occur with progression of an underlying disease or in response to a topical or systemic therapeutic intervention.

For example, acute dermatitis often occurs as primary vesicles with associated **pruritus** (itching). Secondary lesions in the form of crusts occur as the client scratches, the vesicles are opened, and the exudate dries. With chronic dermatitis, the skin often becomes **lichenified** (thickened) because of the client's continual rubbing of the area to relieve itching.

Describe lesions in terms of their color, size, location, and configuration. Document whether the lesions occur as isolated changes or are grouped and form a distinct pattern. Table 69-3 defines terms commonly used to describe lesions.

Assess each lesion for the following ABCD features that are associated with skin cancer:

A Asymmetry of shape
B Border irregularity
C Color variation within one lesion
D Diameter greater than 5 mm

A client who has a lesion with one or more of the ABCD features should be evaluated by a dermatologist or surgeon.

In describing the location of lesions, determine whether they are generalized or localized. If the lesions are localized, identify the specific body areas involved. This information is important because some diseases have a specific pattern of skin lesions. Involvement of only the sun-exposed areas of the body is important information when a possible cause is being considered. Rashes limited to the skin fold areas (e.g., on the axillae, beneath the breasts, in the groin) may reflect problems related to friction, heat, and excessive moisture.

TABLE 69-2 Common Alterations in Skin Color

Alteration	Underlying Cause	Location	Significance
White (pallor)	Decreased hemoglobin level Decreased blood flow to the skin (vasoconstriction)	Conjunctivae Mucous membranes Nail beds Palms and soles Lips	Anemia Shock or blood loss Chronic vascular compromise Sudden emotional upset Edema
	Genetically determined defect of the melanocyte (decreased pigmentation)	Generalized	Albinism
	Acquired patchy loss of pigmentation	Localized	Vitiligo, tinea versicolor
Yellow-orange	Increased total serum bilirubin level (jaundice)	Generalized Mucous membranes Sclera	Increased hemolysis of red blood cells Liver disorders
	Increased serum carotene level (carotenemia)	Perioral Palms and soles Ears and nose Absent in sclera and mucous membranes	Increased ingestion of carotene-containing foods (carrots) Pregnancy Thyroid deficiency Diabetes
	Increased urochrome level	Generalized Absent in sclera and mucous membranes	Chronic renal failure (uremia)
Red (erythema)	Increased blood flow to the skin (vasodilation)	Generalized	Generalized inflammation (e.g., erythroderma)
		Localized (to area of involvement)	Localized inflammation (e.g., sunburn, cellulitis, trauma, and rashes)
		Face, cheeks, nose, upper chest Area of exposure	Fever, increased alcohol intake Exposure to cold
Blue	Increase in deoxygenated blood (cyanosis)	Nail beds Mucous membranes Generalized	Cardiopulmonary disease Methemoglobinemia
	Bleeding from vessels into tissue: ▪ Petechiae (1-3 mm) ▪ Ecchymosis (>3 mm)	 Localized Localized	 Thrombocytopenia Increased blood vessel fragility
Reddish blue	Increased overall amount of hemoglobin Decreased peripheral circulation	Generalized Distal extremities, nose	Polycythemia vera Inadequate tissue perfusion
Brown	Increased melanin production	Localized (to area of involvement) Pressure points, areolae, palmar creases, and genitalia Face, areolae, vulva, and linea nigra	Chronic inflammation Exposure to sunlight Addison's disease Pregnancy; oral contraceptives (melasma)
	Café au lait spots (tan-brown patches) ▪ <6 spots ▪ >6 spots	 Localized Generalized	 Nonpathogenic Possible neurofibromatosis
	Melanin and hemosiderin deposits (bronze or grayish tan color)	Distal lower extremities Exposed areas or generalized	Chronic venous stasis Hemochromatosis

Edema

The presence of edema causes the skin to appear shiny, **taut** (tightly stretched), and paler than uninvolved skin. During skin inspection, document the location, distribution, and color of any areas of edema.

Skin elasticity is also affected by edema. Using moderate pressure, place the tip of the index finger against edematous tissue to determine the degree of indentation, or pitting (see Chapters 14 and 15).

Moisture

Examine skin for moisture content, noting the thickness and consistency of secretions. Normally, increased moisture in the form of sweat occurs with increased activity or elevated environmental temperatures. Dampness of skin fold areas is common because of decreased air circulation where the skin surfaces touch. Excess moisture can cause eventual skin breakdown in bedridden and debilitated clients.

Overly dry skin can be caused by factors such as a dry environment, poor skin lubrication, inadequate fluid intake, and the normal processes of aging. Dry skin usually has scaling of the stratum corneum. Dry skin may be especially marked in areas of limited circulation, such as the feet and lower legs. Dry skin becomes a problem for most adults during the winter months, when the air contains less moisture, and in the hospital environment, where humidity is often poorly controlled.

Vascular Markings

Vascular changes are classified as normal or abnormal, depending on the cause. Normal vascular markings include birthmarks, cherry angiomas (see Figure 69-14), spider angiomas, and venous stars (Table 69-4). Bleeding into the tissue is abnormal and results in purpuric lesions: petechiae and ecchymosis.

Petechiae are small, reddish purple lesions (<0.5 mm in di-

PRIMARY LESIONS

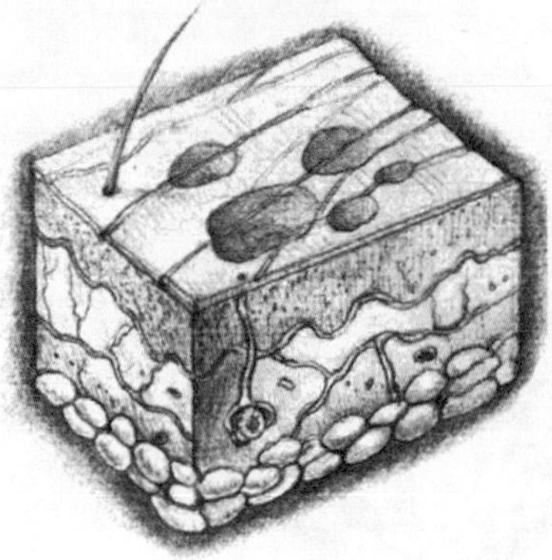

Macules (such as *freckles, flat moles, or rubella*) are flat lesions of less than 1 cm in diameter. Their color is different from that of the surrounding skin—most often white, red, or brown.

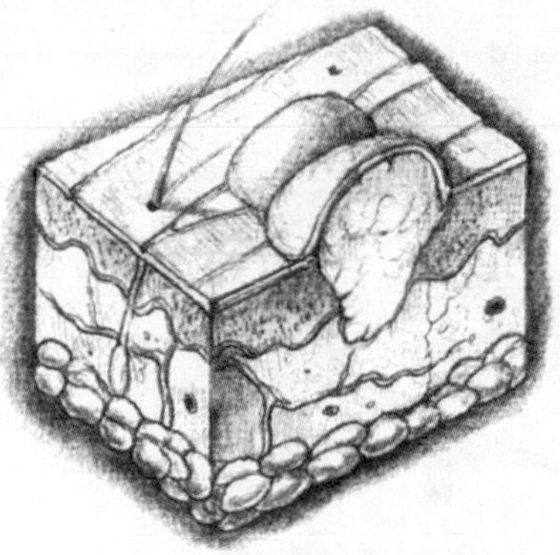

Nodules (such as *lipomas*) are elevated, marble-like lesions more than 1 cm wide and deep.

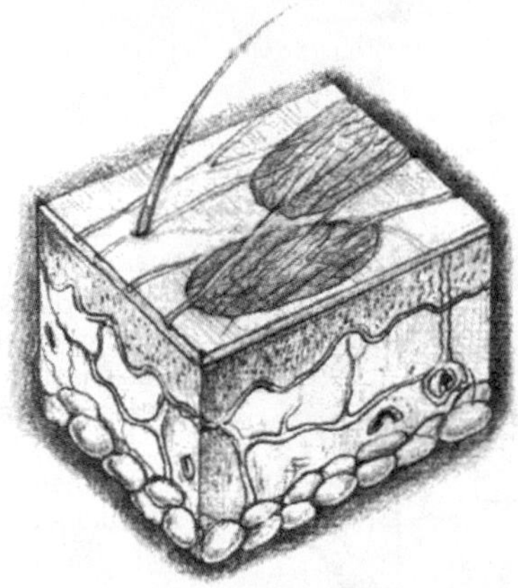

Patches (such as *vitiligo or café au lait spots*) are macules that are larger than 1 cm in diameter. They may or may not have some surface changes—either slight scale or fine wrinkles.

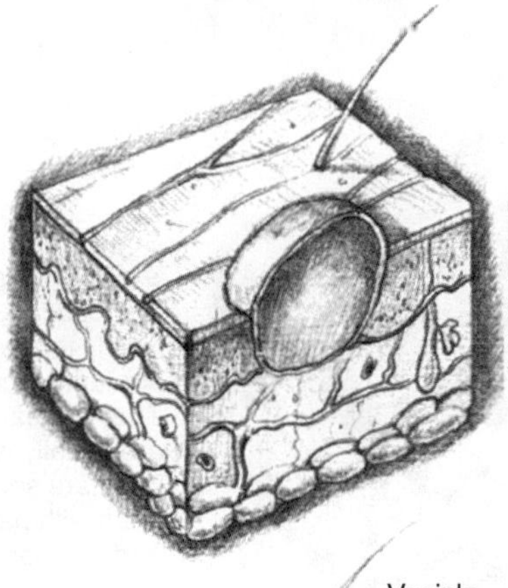

Cysts (such as *sebaceous cysts*) are nodules filled with either liquid or semisolid material that can be expressed.

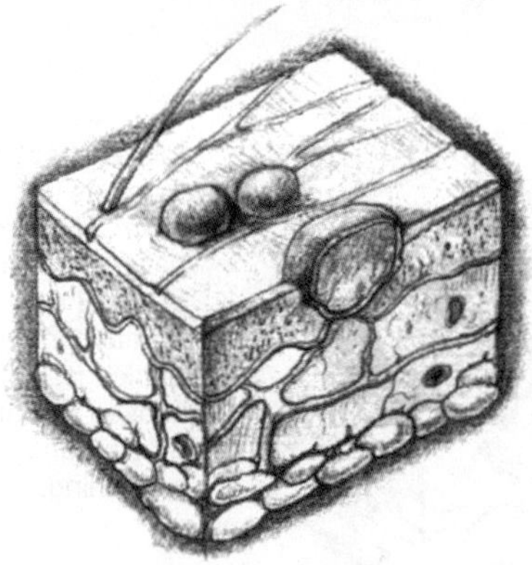

Papules (such as *warts* or *elevated moles*) are small, firm, elevated lesions less than 1 cm in diameter.

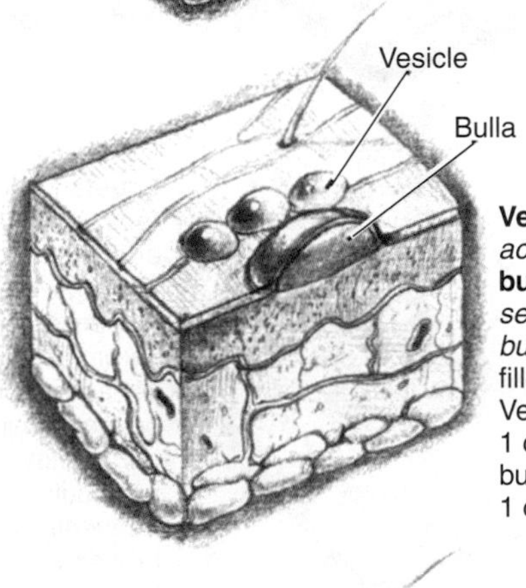

Vesicles (such as in *acute dermatitis*) and **bullae** (such as *second-degree burns*) are blisters filled with clear fluid. Vesicles are less than 1 cm in diameter, and bullae are more than 1 cm in diameter.

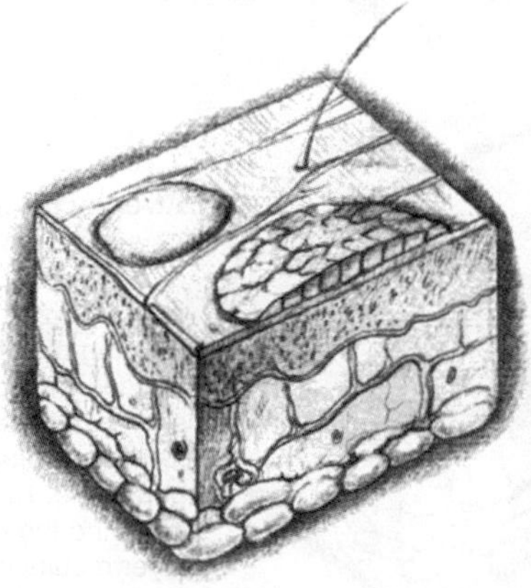

Plaques (such as in *psoriasis* or *seborrheic keratosis*) are elevated, plateau-like patches more than 1 cm in diameter that do not extend into the lower skin layers.

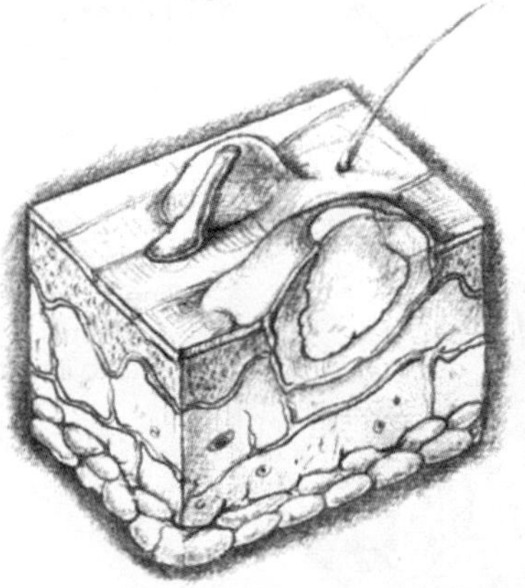

Pustules (such as in *acne* and *acute impetigo*) are vesicles filled with cloudy or purulent fluid.

Figure 69-17 ■ Classification of skin lesions.

Continued

PRIMARY LESIONS—cont'd

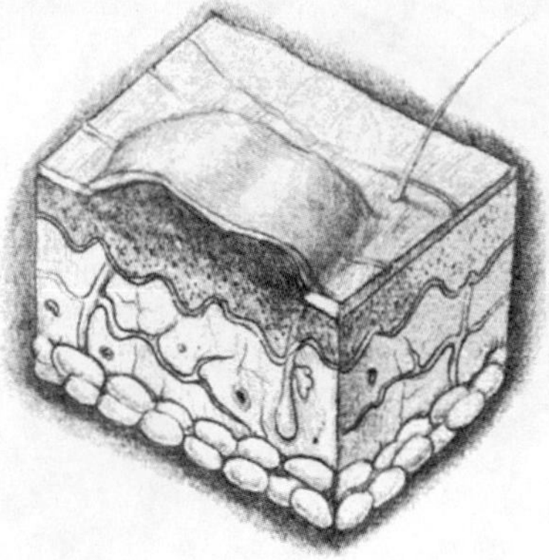

Wheals (such as *urticaria* and *insect bites*) are elevated, irregularly shaped, transient areas of dermal edema.

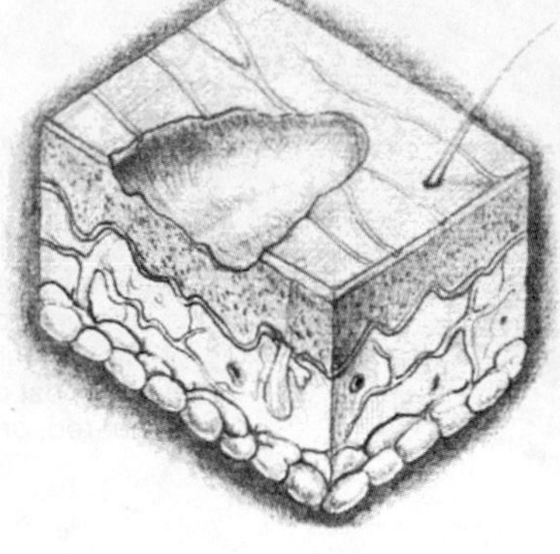

Erosions (such as in *varicella*) are wider than fissures but involve only the epidermis. They are often associated with vesicles, bullae, or pustules.

SECONDARY LESIONS

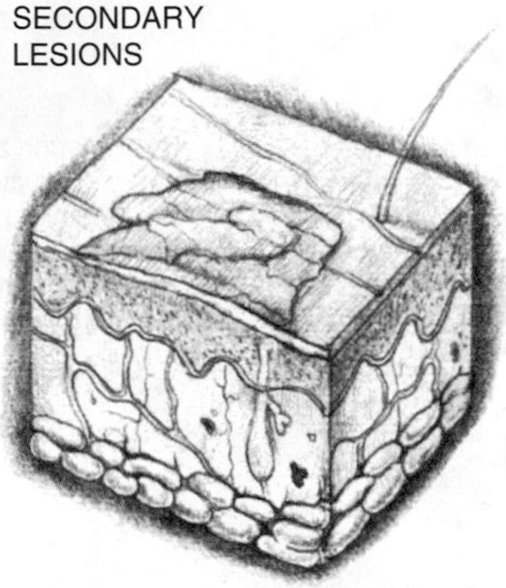

Scales (such as in *exfoliative dermatitis* and *psoriasis*) are visibly thickened stratum corneum. They appear dry and are usually whitish. They are seen most often with papules and plaques.

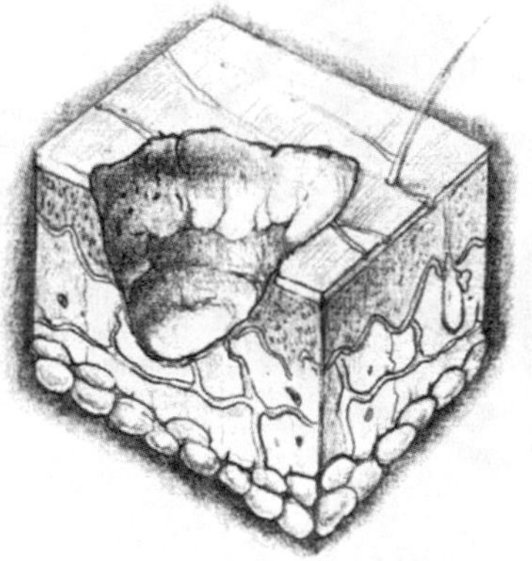

Ulcers (such as *stage 3 pressure sores*) are deep erosions that extend beneath the epidermis and involve the dermis and sometimes the subcutaneous fat.

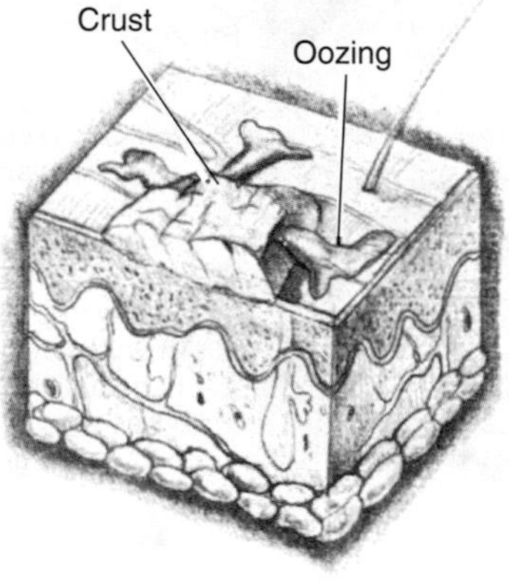

Crusts and oozing (such as in *eczema* and *late-stage impetigo*) are composed of dried serum or pus on the surface of the skin, beneath which liquid debris may accumulate. Crusts frequently result from broken vesicles, bullae, or pustules.

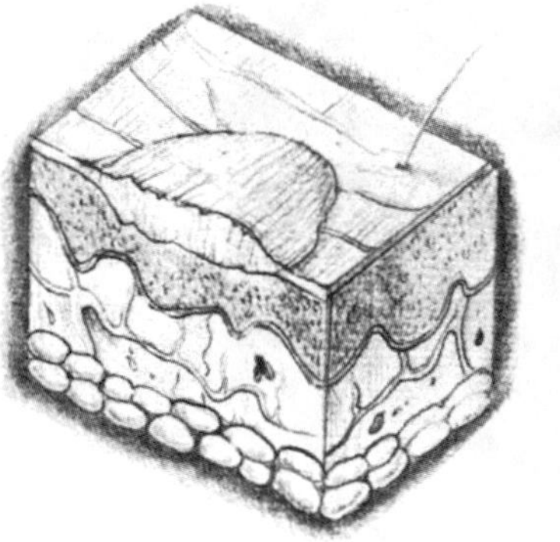

Lichenifications (such as in *chronic dermatitis*) are palpably thickened areas of epidermis with accentuated skin markings. They are caused by chronic rubbing and scratching.

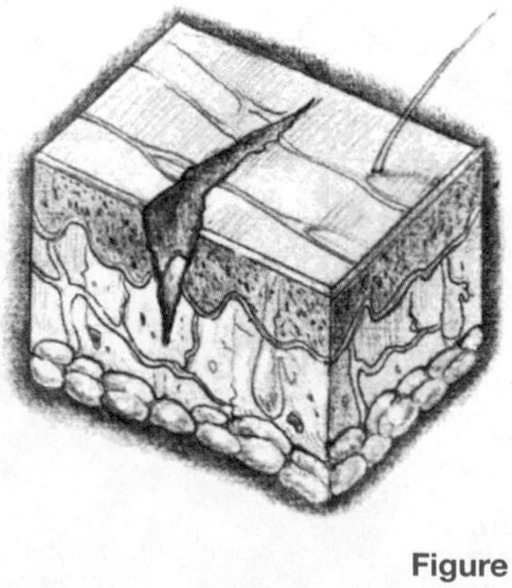

Fissures (such as in *athlete's foot*) are linear cracks in the epidermis, which often extend into the dermis.

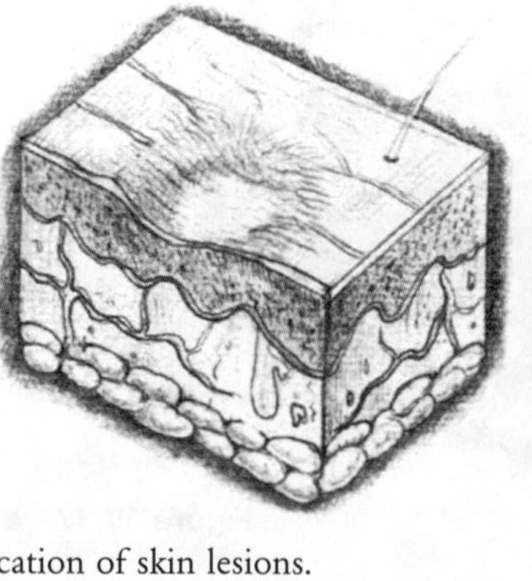

Atrophy (such as *striae* [stretch marks] and *aged skin*) is characterized by thinning of the skin surface with loss of skin markings. The skin is translucent and paper-like. Atrophy involving the dermal layer results in skin depression.

Figure 69-17, cont'd ■ Classification of skin lesions.

ameter) that do not fade or blanch when pressure is applied (Figure 69-18). They often indicate increased capillary fragility. Petechiae of the lower extremities often occur with stasis dermatitis, a condition commonly seen in clients with a history of chronic venous insufficiency.

Ecchymoses (bruises) are larger areas of hemorrhage that range in size from several millimeters to many centimeters. In older adults, bruising is common after minor trauma to the skin, especially on sun-exposed areas of the body. Certain drugs and low platelet counts lead to easy or excessive bruising. Anticoagulants and decreased numbers of platelets disrupt clotting action, resulting in ecchymosis.

Integrity

Thoroughly examine areas with actual breaks in skin integrity. For example, skin tears are a common finding in older people as a result of a flattening of the dermal-epidermal junction with aging. The thin, fragile skin is easily damaged by friction or shearing forces, especially if bruising is already present. Look for skin tears in the following areas:

- In areas where constricting clothing rubs against the skin
- On the upper extremities, where the skin is grasped when assisting a client to ambulate or change position
- In areas where adhesive tapes or dressings have been applied and removed

Check for the presence of multiple abrasions or early pressure-related skin changes. These problems may signal previously unrecognized impairments in physical mobility or changes in sensory perception.

Describe breaks in skin integrity by their location, size, color, and distribution as well as by the presence of drainage or any signs of infection. The evaluation of partial-thickness and full-thickness wounds, including objective criteria that describe progress toward healing, is discussed in Chapter 70.

Cleanliness

Evaluate the cleanliness of the skin to gain information about self-care needs. Inspect the hair, nails, and skin closely for excessive soiling and offensive odor. Depending on a client's degree of self-care deficit, hard-to-reach areas (e.g., perirectal and inguinal skin folds, axillae, feet) may be less clean than other skin surface areas.

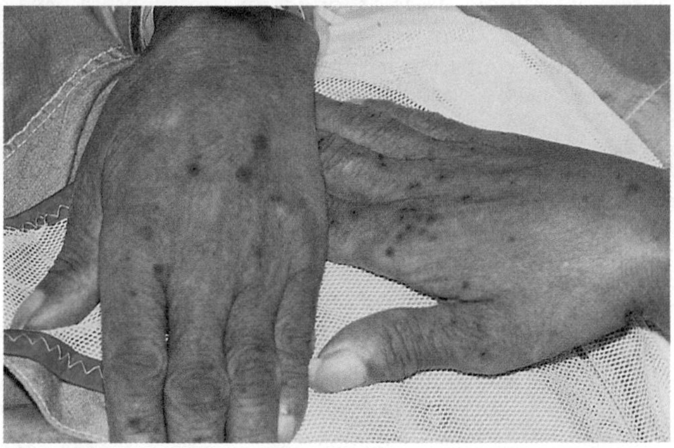

Figure 69-18 ■ Petechiae.

TABLE 69-3 Terms Commonly Used to Describe Skin Lesion Configurations

annular Ringlike with raised borders around flat, clear centers of normal skin
circinate Circular
circumscribed Well-defined with sharp borders
clustered Several lesions grouped together
coalesced Lesions that merge with one another and appear confluent
diffuse Widespread, involving most of the body with intervening areas of normal skin; generalized
linear Occurring in a straight line
serpiginous With wavy borders, resembling a snake
universal All areas of the body involved, with no areas of normal-appearing skin

TABLE 69-4 Common Vascular Skin Lesions

Lesion	Clinical Findings	Location	Significance
Cherry angioma (senile angioma)	Bright to dusky red, dome-shaped papule 2-5 mm in diameter Adjacent lesions may vary in size and color Partial blanching on palpation	Chest and back	Normal skin change with aging
Spider angioma	Bright red, starlike lesion varying in size from small to 2 cm Center of "star" is sometimes raised and may pulsate when palpated	Face, neck, and upper trunk	Associated with liver disease, pregnancy (change in estrogen level), and vitamin B deficiency May be normal finding
Telangiectasia	Reddish blue linear or star-like lesion caused by enlargement of the superficial blood vessels	Face and trunk	Associated with sun exposure and prolonged alcohol intake May be seen in systemic scleroderma and after continued use of potent topical steroids
Venous star	Spider-like blue marking varying in size from small to several inches May have a "cascading" appearance Does not blanch with pressure	Legs (near veins) and anterior chest Face, scalp, and groin	Associated with increased pressure in superficial veins (varicose veins)
Port-wine stain	Large, dark-red to purple area of discoloration Does not blanch with pressure	Any body location Very common on the face and the back of the neck	Congenital abnormality If on the face, may be associated with neurologic disorders and ocular abnormalities

PALPATION

Skin inspection alone can be misleading. Use palpation to gather additional information about skin lesions, moisture, temperature, texture, and turgor (Table 69-5).

Palpation confirms the size of the lesions and determines whether they are flat or slightly raised. The consistency of larger lesions can vary from soft and pliable to firm and solid. Subtle changes, such as the difference between a fine **macular** (flat) rash and a **papular** (raised) rash, may best be determined by palpating with your eyes closed. Ask the client whether he or she has pain or tenderness during palpation of the skin.

In areas of excess dryness, rub your finger against the skin surface to determine the degree of flaking or scaling. Both generalized and localized changes in skin temperature can be detected by placing the back of a hand on the skin surface. Before assessing for changes in skin temperature, make certain to have warm hands. Cold hands interfere with accurate assessment and are uncomfortable for the client.

Palpate skin surfaces to assess texture, which differs according to body region and exposure to environmental irritants. For example, areas of long-term sun exposure have a rougher texture than that of protected skin surfaces. The client whose occupation requires repeated exposure to harsh soaps or chemicals may show skin changes related to this exposure. Increased skin thickness from scarring, lichenification, or edema usually decreases elasticity.

Turgor indicates the amount of skin elasticity. Skin turgor can be altered by a number of factors, including water content and aging. Gently pinch the client's skin between your thumb and forefinger and then release. If skin turgor is normal, the skin immediately returns to its original state when released. Poor skin turgor is evidenced by "tenting" of the skin, with a gradual return to the original state (see Chapter 14). Normal loss of elasticity with aging makes the assessment of skin turgor difficult in an older client. Assess skin turgor of an older client on the forehead or chest.

Hair Assessment

During the skin assessment, inspect and palpate the hair for cleanliness, distribution, quantity, and quality. Hair is normally found in an even distribution over most of the body surfaces, with the hair on the scalp, in the pubic region, and in the axillary folds thicker and coarser than hair on the trunk, arms, and legs. Although color and growth patterns vary widely, sudden or marked changes in hair characteristics may reflect an underlying disease process.

TABLE 69-5 Common Clinical Findings in Skin Palpation

Clinical Findings	Cause	Location	Examples of Predisposing Conditions
Edema			
Localized	Inflammatory response	Area of injury or involvement	Trauma
Dependent or pitting	Fluid and electrolyte imbalance Venous and cardiac insufficiency	Ambulatory: dorsum of foot and medial ankle Bedridden: buttocks, sacrum, and lower back	Congestive heart failure Renal disease Hepatic cirrhosis Venous thrombosis or stasis
Nonpitting	Endocrine imbalance	Generalized, but more easily seen over the tibia	Hypothyroidism (myxedema)
Moisture			
Increased	Autonomic nervous system stimulation	Face, axillae, skin folds, palms, and soles	Fever, anxiety, activity Hyperthyroidism
Decreased	Dehydration Endocrine imbalance	Buccal mucous membranes with progressive involvement of other skin surfaces	Fluid loss Postmenopausal status Hypothyroidism Normal aging
Temperature			
Increased	Increased blood flow to the skin	Generalized Localized	Fever, hypermetabolic states Inflammation
Decreased	Decreased blood flow to the skin	Generalized Localized	Impending shock, sepsis, anxiety Hypothyroidism Interference with vascular flow
Turgor			
Decreased	Decreased elasticity of the dermis (tenting when pinched)	Abdomen, forehead, or radial aspect of the wrist	Severe dehydration Sudden, severe weight loss Normal aging
Texture			
Roughness or thickness	Irritation, friction	Pressure points (e.g., soles, palms, elbows)	Calluses Chronic eczema Atopic skin diseases
	Sun damage Excessive collagen production	Areas of sun exposure Localized or generalized	Normal aging Scleroderma Keloids
Softness or smoothness	Endocrine disturbances	Generalized	Hyperthyroidism

As with skin changes, check any abnormal findings by obtaining an in-depth history of the circumstances surrounding any change.

How well the hair is groomed, including the cleanliness of areas of thicker hair growth, can confirm information already gathered about a client's social history and health care needs. If the client has intense itching or scratches continually, examine the scalp and pubis for lice and **nits** (lice eggs). Inspect the scalp for scaling, redness, lesions, excoriation, crusting, and tenderness.

Dandruff, an accumulation of patchy or diffuse white or gray scales that appear on the surface of the scalp, is common. Dandruff is mainly a cosmetic problem, but a very oily scalp can induce inflammatory changes with redness and itching. Severe inflammatory dandruff can extend to the eyebrows and the skin of the face and neck. *If severe dandruff is not treated, hair loss can occur.*

Although gradual hair loss occurs with aging, sudden asymmetric or patchy hair loss at any age is of concern. Assess the scalp for distribution and thickness of the hair, and document variations.

Hirsutism is excessive growth of body hair or hair growth in abnormal body areas. Increased hair growth across the face and chest in women is a sign of hirsutism. Hirsutism is one manifestation of hormonal imbalance. If hirsutism is present, look for changes in fat distribution and capillary fragility, which can occur in Cushing's disease, and for clitoral enlargement and deepening of the voice, which may indicate ovarian dysfunction.

Nail Assessment

Dystrophic (abnormal) nails may occur with a serious systemic illness or local skin disease involving the epidermal keratinocytes. Evaluate the fingernails and toenails for color, shape, thickness, texture, and the presence of lesions.

Many variations in color, texture, and grooming of the nails are influenced by factors unrelated to disease, such as occupation. When assessing the older adult, observe for minor variations associated with the aging process (see Figure 69-15), such as a gradual thickening of the nail plate, the presence of longitudinal ridges, or a yellowish gray discoloration.

Color

The color of the nail plate depends on many factors, including nail thickness and transparency, amount of red blood cells, arterial blood flow, and pigment deposits (Table 69-6). Figure 69-19 shows normal variations in nail color. Changes in color can be caused by external factors, such as the chemical damage that occurs with some occupations and in the long-term use of nail polish.

During examination, the client's fingers and toes should be free of any surface pressure that might interfere with local blood flow or alter the appearance of the digits. To differentiate between color changes attributable to the underlying vascular supply and those resulting from pigment deposition, blanch the nail bed to see whether a color change occurs with pressure. Do this by gently squeezing the end of the finger or toe, exerting downward pressure on the nail bed, and then releasing the pressure. Color caused by vascular alterations changes as pressure is applied and returns to the original state when pressure is released. Color caused by pigment deposition remains unchanged.

Shape

Nail shape may indicate early or late changes specific to systemic disease. For example, fingernail clubbing occurs with impaired gas exchange.

Evaluate the nail shape by examining the curve of the nail plate and surrounding soft tissue from all angles. Palpate the fingertips to define areas of sponginess, tenderness, or edema. Table 69-7 describes common variations in nail shape.

TABLE 69-6 Common Alterations in Nail Color

Alteration	Clinical Findings	Significance
White	Horizontal white banding or areas of opacity Generalized pallor of nail beds	Chronic hepatic or renal disease (hypoalbuminemia) Shock Anemia Early arteriosclerotic changes (toenails) Myocardial infarction
Yellow-brown	Diffuse yellow to brown discoloration	Jaundice Peripheral lymphedema Bacterial or fungal infections of the nail Psoriasis Diabetes Cardiac failure Staining from tobacco, nail polish, or dyes Long-term tetracycline therapy Normal aging (yellow-gray color)
	Vertical brown banding extending from the proximal nail fold distally	Normal finding in dark-skinned clients Nevus or melanoma of nail matrix in light-skinned clients
Red	Thin, dark-red vertical lines 1-3 mm long (splinter hemorrhages)	Bacterial endocarditis Trichinosis Trauma to the nail bed Normal finding in some clients
	Red discoloration of the lunula	Cardiac insufficiency
	Dark-red nail beds	Polycythemia vera
Blue	Diffuse blue discoloration that blanches with pressure	Respiratory failure Methemoglobinuria Venous stasis disease (toenails)

A 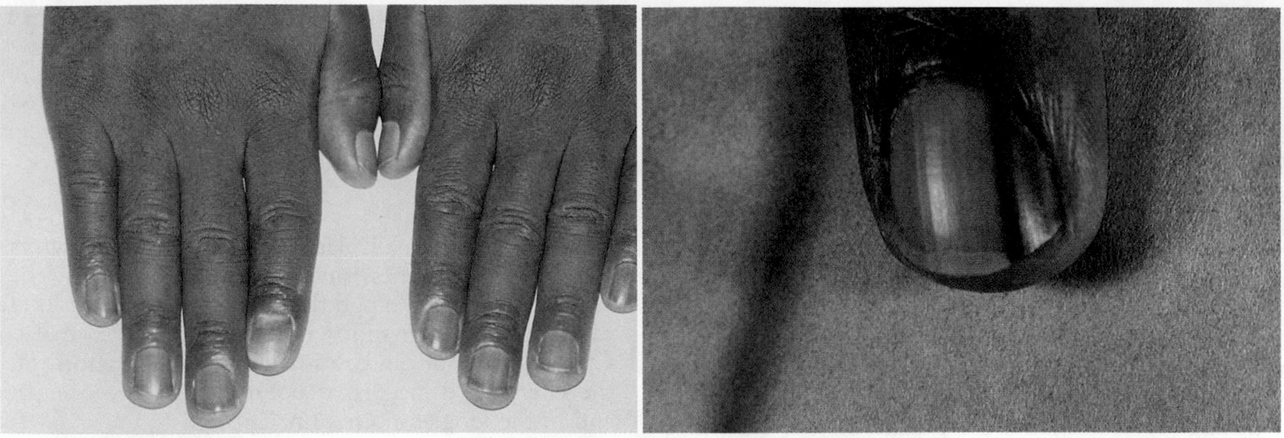 B

Figure 69-19 ■ **A,** Diffuse nail pigmentation. **B,** Linear nail pigmentation.

TABLE 69-7 Common Variations in Nail Shape

Nail Shape	Clinical Findings		Significance
Normal	Angle of 160 degrees between the nail plate and the proximal nail fold ■ Nail surface slightly convex ■ Nail base firm when palpated	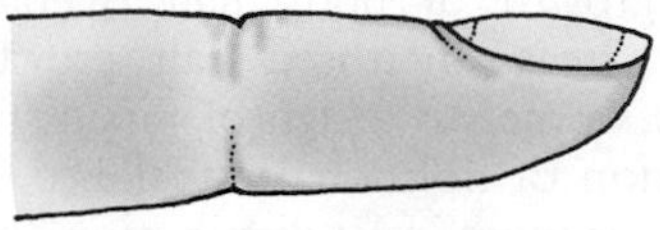	Normal finding
Clubbing Early clubbing	Straightening of angle between the nail plate and the proximal nail fold to 180 degrees ■ Nail base spongy when palpated	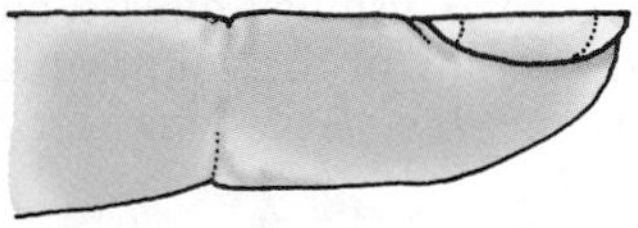	Hypoxia Lung cancer
Late clubbing	Angle between the nail plate and the proximal nail fold exceeds 180 degrees ■ Nail base visibly edematous and spongy when palpated ■ Enlargement of the soft tissue of the fingertips gives a "drumstick" appearance when viewed from above	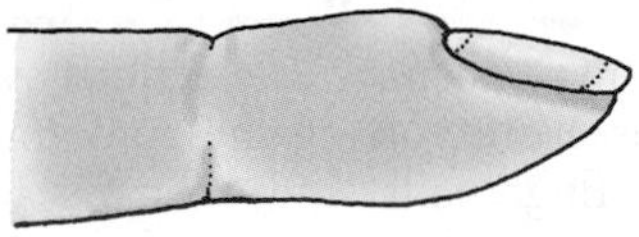	Prolonged hypoxia Emphysema Chronic obstructive pulmonary disease Advanced lung cancer
Spoon nails (koilonychia) Early koilonychia	Flattening of the nail plate with an increased smoothness of the nail surface	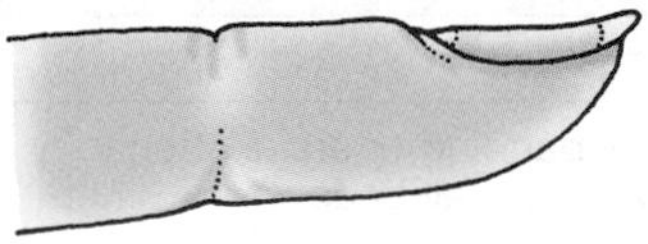	Iron deficiency (with or without anemia) Poorly controlled diabetes >15 yr in duration
Late koilonychia	Concave curvature of the nail plate		Local injury Psoriasis Chemical irritants Developmental abnormality
Beau's grooves	1-mm wide horizontal depressions in the nail plates caused by growth arrest (involves all nails)	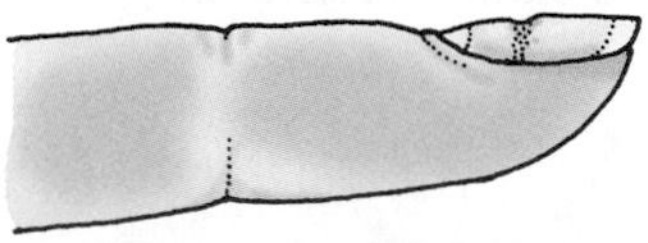	Acute, severe illness Prolonged febrile state Isolated periods of severe malnutrition
Pitting	Small, multiple pits in the nail plate ■ May be associated with plate thickening and onycholysis ■ Most often involves the fingernails (several or all)	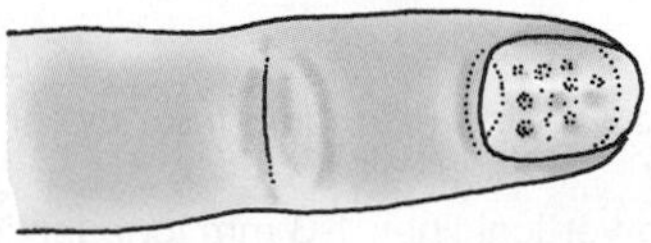	Psoriasis Alopecia areata

Thickness

The nail plate can thicken as a result of trauma, chronic dermatologic disease, or decreased arterial blood flow. In older clients, look for a "heaped-up" appearance of the toenails, which may occur with fungal infection (onychomycosis).

Consistency

Nail consistency is described as hard, soft, or brittle. Nail plates may become hard, with increased thickening. A warm-water soak or lubrication with petroleum jelly is required to soften the nail plates before they can be trimmed.

Soft nail plates, which are thin and bend easily with pressure, are associated with malnutrition, chronic arthritis, myxedema, and peripheral neuritis.

Brittle nails can split, as in the client with onychomycosis or advanced psoriasis. Splitting of the nail plate is also caused by repeated exposure to water and detergents, which damage the plate over time.

Lesions

Separation of the nail plate from the nail bed (onycholysis) creates an air pocket beneath the nail plate. The pocket first appears as a grayish white opacity. The color may change as dirt and keratin collect in the pocket, and the area begins to have a bad odor. Onycholysis is common with fungal infections and after trauma. Separation of the nail plate may also occur with psoriasis or as a result of prolonged contact with chemicals.

Inspect the soft-tissue folds around the nail plate for redness, heat, swelling, and tenderness. Inflammation of the skin around the nail **(acute paronychia)** usually occurs with a torn cuticle or an ingrown toenail. If acute paronychia occurs in an immunocompromised client, an opportunistic infection caused by the *Staphylococcus* organism is probable.

Chronic paronychia is more common and is an inflammation that persists for months. People at risk for chronic paronychia are men and women with frequent exposure to water, such as homemakers, bartenders, and laundry workers.

CULTURAL CONSIDERATIONS

Pallor, erythema, cyanosis, and other color changes reflective of the physical state are less visible in clients with naturally dark skin tones. Although physiologic processes are the same for both light-skinned and dark-skinned clients, the amount of skin pigmentation greatly alters how the skin appears in response to physiologic alterations. Consequently assessment skills to detect the more subtle color changes are needed. Become familiar with the normal appearance of a dark-skinned client's mucous membranes, nail beds, and skin tone so that variations from normal can be identified. Chart 69-3 lists specific assessment techniques for skin manifestations of health in people with dark skin.

Skin Assessment Techniques for Clients with Dark Skin

ASSESSMENT OF PALLOR IN DARK-SKINNED CLIENTS

To detect generalized pallor, inspect the mucous membranes for an ash-gray color. If the lips and the nail beds are not heavily pigmented, they appear paler than normal for that client. Use good lighting to assess for the absence of the underlying red tones that normally give heavily pigmented skin a healthy glow. With generalized decreased blood flow to the skin, brown skin appears yellow-brown, and very dark brown skin is ash gray.

ASSESSMENT OF CYANOSIS IN DARK-SKINNED CLIENTS

If impaired gas exchange is suspected, examine the lips, tongue, nail beds, conjunctivae, and palms and soles at regular intervals for subtle color changes. In a client with cyanosis, the lips and tongue are gray, and the palms, soles, conjunctivae, and nail beds have a bluish tinge. To support these findings, assess for other obvious manifestations of hypoxia, including tachycardia, hypotension, changes in respiratory rate or rhythm, decreased breath sounds, changes in level of consciousness, and any increase in the amount or viscosity of secretions.

CHART 69-3

BEST PRACTICE for Assessing Changes in Dark Skin

Cyanosis
- Examine lips and tongue for gray color.
- Examine nail beds, palms, and soles, for blue tinge.
- Examine conjunctiva for pallor.

Inflammation
- Compare affected area with nonaffected area for increased warmth.
- Examine the skin of the affected area to determine whether it is shiny, taut, or pits with pressure.
- Compare the skin color of affected area to the same area on the opposite side of the body.
- Palpate the affected area and compare it with unaffected area to determine whether there is a difference in texture (affected area may feel hard or "woody").

Jaundice
- Check for yellow tinge to oral mucous membranes, especially the hard palate.
- Examine the sclera nearest to the iris rather than the corners of the eye.

Bleeding
- Compare the affected area with the same area on the unaffected body side for swelling or skin darkening.
- If the client has thrombocytopenia, petechiae may be present on the oral mucosa or conjunctiva.

ASSESSMENT OF INFLAMMATION IN DARK-SKINNED CLIENTS

Use the back of your hand to palpate areas of suspected inflammation for the increased warmth that occurs when blood flow to the skin increases. With the fingertips, palpate for hardened areas deep in the tissue, which may give the skin a "woody" feeling. Inflamed skin is tender and edematous. If edema is extensive, the skin is taut and shiny.

Areas of the body where inflammation (e.g., inflammatory rash or cellulitis) has recently resolved appear darker than the normal skin tone. This change is due to stimulation of the melanocytes during the inflammatory process and to the increased pigment production that continues after inflammation subsides. More extensive injury to the skin with destruction of melanocytes (e.g., deep ulcer, full-thickness burn) may heal with color changes that are lighter than the normal skin tone. Unlike acute changes, chronic inflammatory changes seldom produce tenderness on palpation. If scar tissue is present, the skin may feel less supple, especially over the joints. If chronic inflammatory changes are suspected, ask the client about a history of skin problems in that area of the body.

ASSESSMENT OF JAUNDICE IN DARK-SKINNED CLIENTS

Jaundice in a client with dark skin is best assessed by inspecting the oral mucosa, especially the hard palate, for yellow discoloration. Inspection of the conjunctivae and adjacent sclera may be misleading because normal deposits of fat produce a yellowish hue that is visible in contrast to the dark skin around the eyes. Examine the sclera closest to the cornea for a more accurate determination of jaundice. The palms and soles of dark-skinned clients may appear yellow if they are callused; a callus should not be mistaken for jaundice.

ASSESSMENT OF SKIN BLEEDING IN DARK-SKINNED CLIENTS

Purpuric lesions may not be visible in areas of deep pigmentation. Areas of ecchymosis appear darker than normal skin; they may be tender and easily palpable, depending on whether hematoma is present. In most cases, the client relates a history of trauma to the area that confirms the assessment. Petechiae are rarely visible in dark skin and may be seen only in the oral mucosa and conjunctiva.

Psychosocial Assessment

Skin changes, especially when more visible skin surfaces (e.g., face, hair, hands) are involved, often affect a person's body image. Assess the client's body language for clues indicating a disturbance in self-concept. For example, the avoidance of eye contact or the use of garments to cover the affected areas communicates concern about physical appearance. Clients with chronic skin diseases often relate a history of social isolation related to a fear of rejection by others or a belief that the skin problem is contagious.

Skin changes linked to poor hygiene are common in clients from low socioeconomic backgrounds. Assess the client's overall appearance for excessive soiling, matted hair, body odor, or other self-care deficits. Confirm unsanitary living conditions by obtaining a social history. Clients may relate similar skin problems among family members, friends, and sexual contacts.

If skin problems related to poor hygiene are identified in older clients, also evaluate any physical limitations that might contribute to poor health maintenance. For example, visual or mobility problems can make it difficult for clients to see or reach skin surfaces to clean them.

Critical Thinking Challenge

The client is a 73-year-old Hispanic woman who has hypertension and some degree of heart failure. Her lower legs are swollen and have reddish purple patches with a few small open areas. When you ask her how long these areas have been present, she tells you that they started in the wintertime and are very itchy. On closer inspection, you can see scratches around the open areas. She tells you she has been putting alcohol on the open areas to prevent infection.

1. What additional health history information should you obtain?
2. What further assessment of the skin problem should you perform?
3. Should she continue to use the alcohol? Why? Why not?

evolve For suggested answer guidelines, go to http://evolve.elsevier.com/Iggy/.

Diagnostic Assessment

LABORATORY TESTS

When a fungal, bacterial, or viral pathogen is suspected as the cause of certain skin changes, confirmation by microscopic examination is necessary.

Cultures for Fungal Infections

When superficial fungal **(dermatophyte)** infections are suspected, gently scrape scales from the skin lesions into a clean container and send to the laboratory for culture. Collect fingernail clippings and hair in a similar manner. Unfortunately waiting for culture results can delay treatment of a superficial fungal infection. For this reason the specimen is also treated with a potassium hydroxide (KOH) preparation and examined microscopically. Fungal infections show branched hyphae when viewed under a microscope after treatment with KOH. A positive KOH test often eliminates the need for a culture.

For deeper fungal infections, a piece of tissue is obtained for culture. The physician obtains the specimen by punch biopsy (see Skin Biopsy below). When a specimen is needed for cell analysis and special fungal stains, either two specimens are obtained or one biopsy tissue specimen is bisected before being sent to the laboratory.

Cultures for Bacterial Infections

Specimens for bacterial culture are obtained from intact primary lesions (bullae, vesicles, or pustules), if possible. Express material from the lesion, collect it with a cotton-tipped applicator, and place the material in a bacterial culture medium. For intact lesions, **unroofing** (lifting or puncturing of the outer surface) may be needed using a sterile small-gauge needle before the material can be easily expressed. If crusts are present, remove the crusts and swab the underlying exudate.

A biopsy of deep bacterial infections may be required to obtain a specimen for culture. If bacterial cellulitis is suspected, nonbacteriostatic saline can be injected deep into the tissue and aspirated; the aspirant is sent for culture.

Cultures for Viral Infections

Viral cultures are indicated if a herpes virus infection is suspected. A cotton-tipped applicator is used to obtain vesicle fluid from intact lesions. Unlike bacterial and fungal specimens, which can remain at room temperature until being transported to the laboratory, viral culture tubes are placed on ice immediately after the specimen is obtained and are transported to the laboratory as soon as possible.

OTHER DIAGNOSTIC TESTS

Skin Biopsy

A small piece of skin tissue is obtained for pathologic study to establish an accurate diagnosis or assess the effectiveness of an intervention. Before preparing the client, check with the physician to determine the number, location, and type of skin biopsies to be performed.

TYPES OF BIOPSIES

Depending on the size, depth, and location of the skin changes, the physician may perform a punch biopsy, shave biopsy, or scalpel excision (excisional biopsy).

PUNCH BIOPSY. The punch biopsy is the most common technique. A small circular cutting instrument, or punch, ranging in diameter from 2 to 6 mm is used. After the site is injected with a local anesthetic, a small plug of tissue is cut to the depth of the subcutaneous fat and removed with forceps and scissors. The site may be closed with one or two sutures if it is on the face or leg. Some physicians allow the biopsy site to heal without suturing.

SHAVE BIOPSY. A shave biopsy removes only the portion of the skin elevated above the surrounding tissue when injected with a local anesthetic. A scalpel or razor blade is moved parallel to the skin surface to remove the tissue specimen. Shave biopsies are usually indicated for superficial or raised lesions. Suturing is not necessary.

EXCISIONAL BIOPSY. In rare instances, larger or deeper specimens are obtained by excision with a scalpel. Deep incisions are made and then sutured after the specimen is removed. Unlike punch and shave biopsies, excisional biopsies involve more discomfort for the client while the site is healing.

CLIENT PREPARATION. Explain to the client what to expect. Emphasize that a biopsy is a minor procedure with few, if any, complications. If a punch or shave biopsy is planned, reassure the client that scarring is minimal because of the small size of the tissue removed. If an excisional biopsy is planned, tell the client that a scar similar to that of a healed surgical incision will result.

PROCEDURE. Establish a sterile field and assemble all needed supplies and instruments. Local anesthesia is provided by local infiltration using a small-gauge needle (no. 25) to reduce discomfort during injection. Although preparation of the biopsy site differs according to the physician's preference, the skin is simply wiped with alcohol in most cases.

The most uncomfortable time for the client is during the injection of a local anesthetic agent, which produces a burning or stinging sensation. Reassure the client that the discomfort will subside as the anesthetic takes effect. Talking the client through the procedure with a quiet voice, in combination with a gentle touch, has a calming effect.

After removal tissue specimens for routine pathologic study are placed directly in 10% formalin for fixation. Specimens for culture are placed in sterile saline solution. Bleeding of the biopsy site may be controlled by applying a topical hemostatic agent. If topical treatment does not stop the bleeding, suturing is considered.

FOLLOW-UP CARE. After bleeding is under control and any sutures have been placed, the site is covered with an adhesive bandage or a dry gauze dressing. Instruct the client to keep the dressing dry and in place for a minimum of 8 hours. Teach the client to clean the site daily after the dressing is removed. Tap water or saline can be used to remove any dried blood or crusts. An antibiotic ointment may be prescribed to reduce the risk for infection. The biopsy site may be left open unless a covering is preferred for cosmetic reasons or because the site is an area often soiled. Instruct the client to report any redness or excessive drainage. Sutures are usually removed 7 to 10 days after biopsy.

Wood's Light Examination

A handheld, long-wave length ultraviolet (black) light or Wood's light is sometimes used during physical examination. Exposure of some skin infections with this light produces a specific color, such as blue-green or red, that can be used to identify the infection. Hypopigmented skin is more prominent when it is viewed under black light, which makes evaluation of pigment changes in fair-skinned clients easier.

Wood's light examination of the skin is always carried out in a darkened room. Reassure the client that no discomfort occurs with a Wood's light examination.

Diascopy

Diascopy is a noninvasive and painless technique that eliminates erythema caused by increased blood flow to the skin, thereby easing the inspection of skin lesions. A glass slide or lens is pressed down over the area to be examined, blanching the skin and revealing the shape of the lesions.

Skin Testing

If a client's rash might be an allergic contact dermatitis, patch testing may identify the allergen. The technique for skin testing for allergy is described in Chapter 26.

Critical Thinking Challenge

The client is an 84-year-old white woman who has several slightly raised, bright red lesions on her upper back. They are smaller than 2 mm and are in a line with about 1 inch between the lesions. She tells you these lesions have been there for about 10 years and she is afraid that they might be skin cancer.

1. What additional questions should you ask this client about these lesions?
2. What additional physical assessment data should you obtain regarding these lesions?
3. Should these lesions be examined by a surgeon or dermatologist? Why or why not?

evolve For suggested answer guidelines, go to http://evolve.elsevier.com/Iggy/.

GET READY for the NCLEX Examination!

KEY POINTS

Safe Effective Care Environment

- Assist all clients with limited mobility to change positions at least every 2 hours while awake.
- Wash your hands before and after touching any skin lesions.
- Use standard precautions when providing care to a client who has any areas of nonintact skin.

Health Promotion and Maintenance

- Encourage all clients to reduce sun exposure and exposure to ultraviolet (UV) light.
- Teach clients how to examine all skin areas on a monthly basis for new lesions and changes to existing lesions. The client should keep a record or "body map" of skin lesions.
- Encourage all clients to bathe, shampoo the hair, and keep fingernails clean and trimmed on a regular basis.
- Teach all clients the ABCD method of evaluating a lesion for melanoma.

Psychosocial Integrity

- Allow the client the opportunity to express feelings about a change in body image that results from changes in the skin, hair, or nails.
- Explain all procedures, restrictions, medications, and follow-up care to the client and family.
- Check the cognitive function of any client whose hygiene of the skin, hair, and nails appears inadequate.
- Offer alternative therapies for reducing skin discomfort or itching, such as massage, music therapy, and guided imagery.

Physiological Integrity

- Document any known specific allergies that have skin manifestations.
- Keep skin-fold areas on clients clean and dry.
- Position clients who are confined to bed in a way that promotes air circulation to skin-fold areas.
- Ask any client who has started taking a newly prescribed or over-the-counter drug whether he or she has noticed any skin changes that occurred since starting the medication.

ADDITIONAL STUDY RESOURCES

Go to your Student CD-ROM for Review Questions for the NCLEX Examination.

evolve Go to http://evolve.elsevier.com/Iggy/ for Integrated Management of Care Questions for the NCLEX Examination.

SELECTED BIBLIOGRAPHY

Asterisk indicates a classic or definitive work on this subject.

American Cancer Society. (2005). *Cancer facts and figures 2005.* Report No. 00-300M-No. 5008.05. Atlanta: Author.

Carter, K., Dufour, L., & Ballard, C. (2004). Identifying secondary skin lesions. *Nursing 2004, 34*(1), 68.

Cole, J., & Gray-Miceli, D. (2002). The necessary elements of a dermatologic history and physical evaluation. *Dermatology Nursing, 14*(6), 377-383.

*Gaskin, F.C. (1986). Detection of cyanosis in the person with dark skin. *Journal of the National Black Nurses Association, 1*(1), 52-60.

Guyton, A., & Hall, J. (2000). *Textbook of medical physiology* (10th ed.). Philadelphia: W.B. Saunders.

Harris, J. (2000). A plan to promote the prevention and early detection of melanoma. *Dermatology Nursing, 12*(5), 329-333.

Jarvis, C. (2004). *Physical examination and health assessment* (4th ed.). Philadelphia: W.B. Saunders.

Lookingbill, D.P., & Marks, J.G., Jr. (2000). *Principles of dermatology* (3rd ed.). Philadelphia: W.B. Saunders.

Nussbaum, R., McInnes, R., & Willard, H. (2001). *Thompson & Thompson: Genetics in medicine* (6th ed.). Philadelphia: W.B. Saunders.

Pagana, K., & Pagana, T. (2002). *Mosby's manual of diagnostic and laboratory tests* (2nd ed.). St. Louis: Mosby.

Zulkowski, K. (2003). Protecting your patient's aging skin. *Nursing 2003, 33*(1), 84.

CHAPTER 70

Interventions for Clients with Skin Problems

JANICE CUZZELL • M. LINDA WORKMAN

LEARNING OUTCOMES

After studying this chapter, you should be able to:

1. Prioritize nursing care for a client with dry skin.
2. Compare wound healing by first, second, and third intention.
3. Identify clients at risk for pressure ulcer development.
4. Plan an individualized strategy for pressure ulcer prevention for a specific client at increased risk.
5. Differentiate the clinical manifestations for stage I through stage IV pressure ulcers.
6. Prioritize the nursing interventions for a client with a stage III pressure ulcer.
7. Evaluate the effectiveness of interventions for pressure ulcer management.
8. Compare the clinical manifestations and modes of transmission for bacterial, viral, and fungal skin infections.
9. Prioritize nursing care and educational needs for clients who have parasitic skin infections.
10. Describe the mechanisms of action, side effects, and nursing implications for pharmacologic management of psoriasis.
11. Explain the rationale for ultraviolet therapy for psoriasis.
12. Develop a community-based teaching plan for the client with psoriasis.
13. Identify interventions for prevention of skin cancer.
14. Describe the clinical manifestations of melanoma.

Go to your Student CD-ROM for Review Questions for the NCLEX Examination keyed to these Learning Outcomes.

Skin problems are common, and often the cause is not known. In addition to direct skin functions, the skin reflects other body conditions. Thus skin problems may truly arise in the skin, or they may be a symptom of a systemic disease or injury. Drugs and other interventions for any health problem can trigger a skin response or reaction. Skin problems can interfere with the medical or surgical treatment of other conditions. Age-related skin changes and problems arising from immobility, chronic disease, debility, and change in immune function place the older client at an increased risk for skin damage.

MINOR SKIN IRRITATIONS

Dryness

PATHOPHYSIOLOGY

Dry skin **(xerosis)** is a common problem, especially in older clients. It is seen as a fine flaking of the **stratum corneum** (outermost skin layer), and it is usually worse on the lower legs. Generalized **pruritus** (itching) often occurs with dry skin. In clients with chronic skin conditions, unrelieved itching causes the client to scratch and rub the skin in an attempt to relieve the intense itching. These actions may result in secondary skin lesions, excoriations, **lichenification** (thickening), and infection.

Xerosis is worse in dry climates. Central heating and air-conditioning reduce the humidity in the air and increase skin dryness. Wind, cold, and sunlight also worsen the problem. Frequent bathing with harsh soap and hot water further dries the skin, especially if moisturizers are not applied after bathing.

COLLABORATIVE MANAGEMENT

Nursing interventions aim to rehydrate the skin and relieve itching. Bathing with moisturizing soaps, oils, and lotions may reduce dryness. Using soap only in soiled or skin-fold areas can also reduce dryness. A 20-minute soak in a warm bath, followed by application of an emollient cream or lotion, can rehydrate the skin and reduce itching. If the client cannot take a tub bath, wrap the trunk and extremities in warm, moist towels covered by plastic sheeting and additional blankets to prevent chilling. Always apply skin creams or lotions to slightly damp skin within 2 to 3 minutes after bathing.

Contrary to popular belief, the cream or lotion is *not* what makes the skin soft and supple. Water is the agent that softens the outer skin layers. Lubricating creams and lotions seal in the moisture provided by water, promoting suppleness and preventing flaking. Some skin lotions are **hydrophilic** (water seeking) and actually draw moisture from the skin, making the dryness worse if they are not applied directly to damp skin.

Teach clients and family members how to maintain healthy skin. Chart 70-1 lists practical ways to avoid drying the skin.

Pruritus

PATHOPHYSIOLOGY

Pruritus, or itching, is a distressing symptom that may or may not occur with skin disease. Pruritus is caused by stimulation of itch-specific nerve fibers at the dermal-epidermal junction. Physical or chemical agents either act directly on these nerve fibers or activate chemical mediators, such as histamine, which then act on the itch receptors.

Itching is a subjective symptom similar to pain. Thus the sensation varies among clients in location and severity. Regardless of the underlying cause, clients usually report that itching is worse at night. Other conditions that make itching worse include poor skin hydration, increased skin temperature, perspiration, and emotional stress.

CHART 70-1

CLIENT EDUCATION GUIDE

Prevention of Dry Skin

- Use a room humidifier during the winter months or whenever the furnace is in use.
- Take a complete bath or shower only every other day (wash face, axillae, perineum, and any soiled areas with soap daily).
- Use tepid water.
- Use a superfatted, nonalkaline soap instead of deodorant soap.
- Rinse the soap thoroughly from your skin.
- If you like bath oil, add the oil to the water at the end of the bath.
- Pat rather than rub skin surfaces dry.
- Avoid clothing that continuously rubs the skin, such as tight belts, nylon stockings, or pantyhose.
- Maintain a daily fluid intake of 3000 mL unless contraindicated for another medical condition.
- Do not apply rubbing alcohol, astringents, or other drying agents to the skin.
- Avoid caffeine and alcohol ingestion.

COLLABORATIVE MANAGEMENT

Clients usually try to relieve itching by scratching or rubbing the skin, a response that further stimulates the itch receptors and causes a pattern referred to as the **"itch-scratch-itch" cycle.** When the skin lesions are present with itching, relief can usually be obtained by treatment of the underlying skin disorder with topical or systemic medications. Systemic diseases, such as liver and venous disorders, can also cause itching without skin lesions.

Plan care to promote comfort and prevent disruption of skin integrity that can result from vigorous scratching. Because dry skin worsens itching, emphasize proper bathing and skin lubrication techniques (see Chart 70-1). Encourage clients to keep the fingernails trimmed short, with rough edges filed, to reduce skin damage. Tell clients that wearing mittens or splints at night can help to prevent inadvertent scratching during sleep.

A cool sleeping environment along with a larger dose of sedating antihistamines at bedtime (when the side effect of drowsiness is welcome) may provide an uninterrupted night's sleep. Therapeutic baths **(balneotherapy)** with colloidal oatmeal preparations or tar extracts may give temporary relief (Table 70-1).

If antihistamines are prescribed, closely monitor the client's response to therapy so that the dosage can be adjusted as needed. The anti-inflammatory properties of topical steroid preparations are increased if the drug is applied to slightly damp skin.

TABLE 70-1 Uses of Therapeutic Baths

Agents	Disease	Purpose
Antibacterial Baths		
Potassium permanganate (1:32,000; 1:64,000)	Infected eczema Pemphigus Multiple infected ulcerations	To lower skin bacterial load
Colloidal Baths		
Starch and baking soda (1 c. each per tub) Aveeno colloidal oatmeal (1 c. per tub) Aveeno oilated colloidal oatmeal	Atopic eczema Psoriasis Chickenpox	To relieve itching To soothe To lubricate
Emollient Baths*		
Bath oils; Alpha Keri Lubath Mineral oil	Any dry skin condition	To clean and hydrate the skin
Tar Baths*		
Bath oils with tar: Balnetar, Zetar, Polytar Coal tar concentrate (liquor carbonis, detergents)	Scaly dermatosis Psoriasis Eczema	To loosen scale To relieve itching To potentiate ultraviolet A or ultraviolet B light therapy

Modified from Rosen, T., Lanning, M.B., & Hill, M.J. (1983). *The nurse's atlas of dermatology.* Boston: Little, Brown & Co. Copyright 1983 by Theodore Rosen and Marilyn B. Lanning.

* For emollient and tar baths, add 3 to 6 capfuls of therapeutic agent per standard bathtub.

Sunburn

PATHOPHYSIOLOGY

Sunburn is a first-degree or superficial burn and a very common skin injury. Excessive exposure to ultraviolet (UV) light injures the dermis and dilates the capillaries, leading to redness, tenderness, edema, and occasional blister formation. When large areas of the body are sunburned, systemic symptoms, such as headache, nausea, and fever, are produced.

◆COLLABORATIVE MANAGEMENT

Redness **(erythema)** and pain begin within a few hours after sunburn has occurred and increase in intensity for 1 to 2 days before subsiding. Treatment is directed toward comfort and includes cool baths and soothing lotions, such as bland lubricants or refrigerated moisturizing lotions. Antibiotic ointments are used only if blistering of the skin causes infection. If pain is severe, topical corticosteroids may decrease the inflammation temporarily.

Urticaria

PATHOPHYSIOLOGY

Urticaria (hives) is the presence of white or red edematous papules or plaques of various sizes. Urticaria is usually caused by exposure to a specific substance (different for different people), which releases histamine in the dermal tissue, causing blood vessel dilation and leakage of plasma protein to form lesions or wheals. Unfortunately the exact cause of urticaria is rarely identified. The following factors are thought to cause urticaria: drugs, foods, infections, autoimmune diseases, malignancies, physical stimuli, and psychogenic responses.

◆COLLABORATIVE MANAGEMENT

Treatment is aimed at removal of the triggering substance and relief of symptoms. Because the skin reaction is caused by histamine release, antihistamines are helpful. Instruct the client to avoid overexertion, alcohol consumption, and warm environments, which contribute to blood vessel dilation and make the symptoms worse.

TRAUMA

PATHOPHYSIOLOGY

Skin trauma can vary from an aseptic surgical incision to a grossly infected, draining pressure ulcer with deep-tissue destruction. Injury to the skin starts a series of actions to repair the skin and re-establish this protective barrier.

Phases of Wound Healing

Wound healing occurs in three phases: the inflammatory, or "lag," phase; the fibroblastic, or connective tissue repair phase; and the maturation, or remodeling, phase. Table 70-2 lists the key events of normal wound healing. The length of each phase depends on the type of injury and whether the wound is healing by first, second, or third intention (Figure 70-1).

A wound without tissue loss, such as a clean laceration or a surgical incision, can be closed with sutures or staples. The wound edges are brought together with the skin layers lined up in correct anatomic position **(approximated)** and held in place until healing is complete. Because the wound can be easily closed and dead space eliminated, healing by **first intention** shortens the phases of tissue repair. Inflammation resolves quickly, and connective tissue repair is minimal, resulting in a thin scar.

Deeper tissue injuries or wounds with tissue loss, such as a chronic pressure ulcer or venous stasis ulcer, result in a cavity-like defect that requires gradual filling in of the dead space with connective tissue. This healing occurs by **second intention** and prolongs the repair process.

Wounds with a high risk for infection, such as surgical incisions that enter a nonsterile body cavity or traumatic wounds that occur under unclean conditions, may be intentionally left open for several days. After debris and exudate have been removed and inflammation has subsided, the wound is closed by first intention. This type of healing involves delayed primary closure **(third intention)** and results in a scar similar to that found in wounds that heal by first intention. As shown in Table 70-3, healing can be impaired by a number of factors.

Mechanisms of Wound Healing

When injury occurs, the body restores skin integrity through three processes: re-epithelialization, granulation, and wound contraction. The extent to which these processes contribute to tissue repair depends on the depth of injury and the extent of tissue loss.

PARTIAL-THICKNESS WOUNDS

Partial-thickness (superficial) wounds involve damage to the epidermis and upper layers of the dermis. These wound heal

TABLE 70-2 Normal Wound Healing

Inflammatory Phase
- Begins at the time of injury or cell death and lasts 3-5 days.
- Immediate responses are vasoconstriction and clot formation.
- After 10 minutes, vasodilation with increased capillary permeability and leakage of plasma (and plasma proteins) into the surrounding tissue.
- Migration of white blood cells (especially macrophages) into the wound.
- Clinical manifestations of local edema, pain, erythema, and warmth.

Fibroblastic Phase
- Begins about the fourth day after injury and lasts 2 to 4 weeks.
- Fibrin strands form a scaffold or framework.
- Mitotic fibroblast cells migrate into the wound, attach to the framework, divide, and stimulate the secretion of collagen.
- Collagen, together with ground substance, builds tough and inflexible scar tissue.
- Capillaries in areas surrounding the wound form "buds" that grow into new blood vessels.
- Capillary buds and collagen deposits form the "granulation" tissue in the wound, and the wound contracts.
- Epithelial cells grow over the granulation tissue bed.

Maturation Phase
- Begins as early as 3 weeks after injury and may continue for a year.
- Collagen is reorganized to provide greater tensile strength.
- Scar tissue gradually becomes thinner and paler in color.
- The mature scar is firm and inelastic when palpated.

The Process of Wound Healing

▶ Healing by First Intention

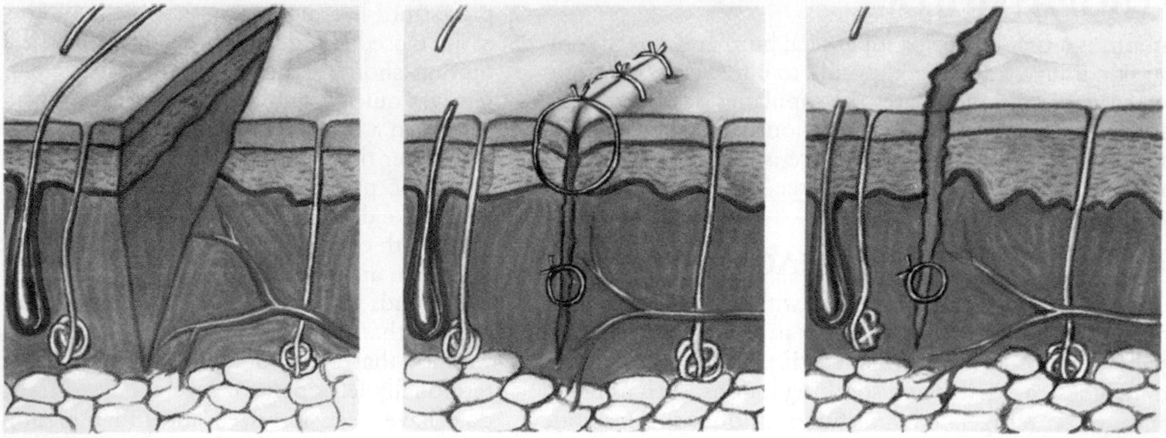

Clean incision | Early suture | "Hairline" scar

An aseptically made wound with minimal tissue destruction and minimal tissue reaction begins to heal as the edges are approximated by close sutures or staples. No open areas or dead spaces are left to serve as potential sites of infection.

▶ Healing by Second Intention (Granulation) and Contraction

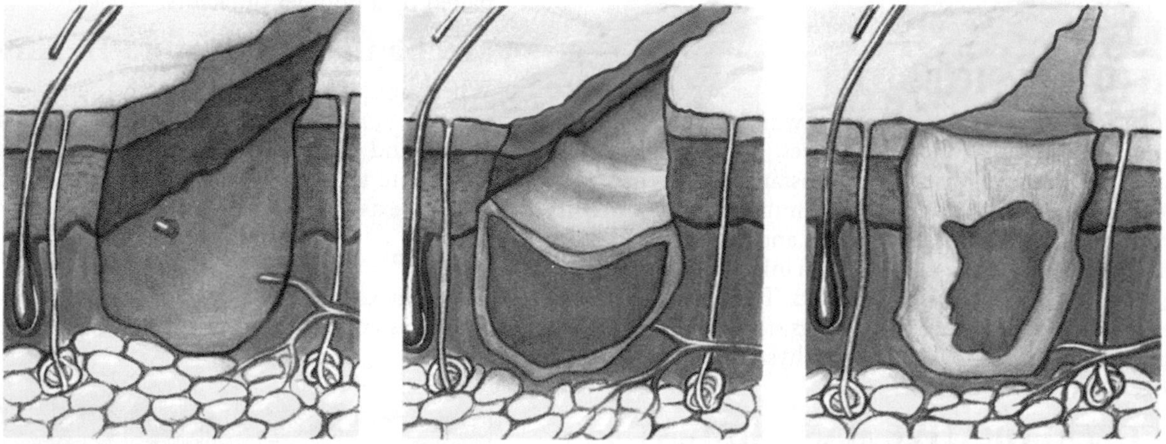

Gaping, irregular wound | Granulation and contraction | Growth of epithelium over scar

An infected or chronic wound or one with tissue damage so extensive that the edges cannot be smoothly approximated is usually left open and allowed to heal from the inside out. The nurse periodically cleans and assesses the wound for healthy tissue production. Scar tissue is extensive, and healing is prolonged.

▶ Healing by Third Intention (Delayed Closure)

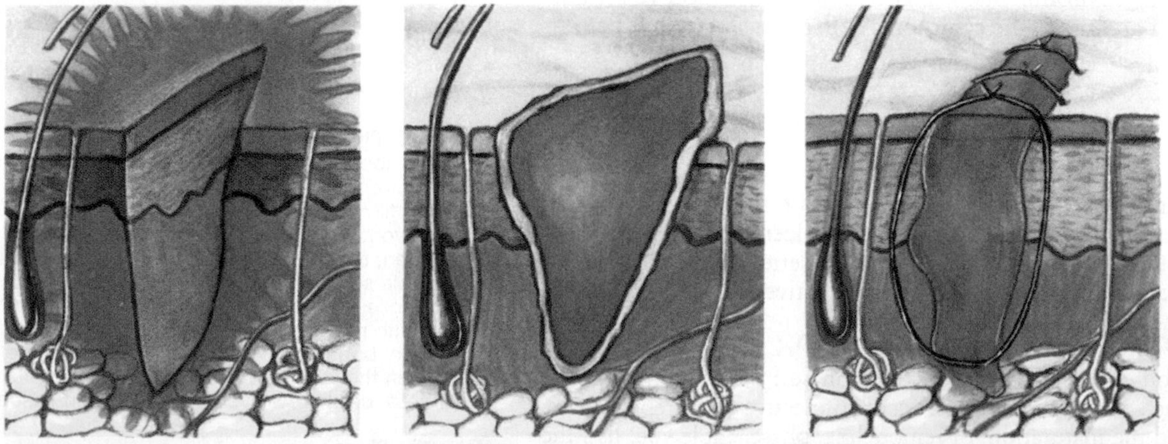

Infected wound | Granulation | Closure with wide scar

A potentially infected surgical wound may be left open for several days. If no clinical signs of infection occur, the wound is then closed surgically.

Figure 70-1 ■ The process of wound healing.

TABLE 70-3 Causes of Impaired Wound Healing

Cause	Mechanism
Altered Inflammatory Response	
Local	
Arteriosclerosis Diabetes Vasculitis Thrombosis Venous insufficiency Lymphedema Pharmacologic vasoconstriction Irradiated tissue Crush injuries Primary closure under tension	Reduced local tissue circulation, resulting in ischemia, impaired leukocytic response to wounding, and increased probability of wound infection
Systemic	
Leukemia Prolonged administration of high-dose anti-inflammatory drugs ▪ Corticosteroids ▪ Aspirin	Systemic inhibition of leukocytic response, resulting in impaired host resistance to infection
Impaired Cellular Proliferation	
Local	
Wound infection Foreign body Necrotic tissue Repeated injury or irritation Movement of wound (e.g., across a joint) Wound desiccation or maceration	Prolonged inflammatory response, which can result in low tissue oxygen tension and further tissue destruction
Systemic	
Aging Chronic stress Nutritional deficiencies ▪ Calories ▪ Protein ▪ Vitamins ▪ Minerals ▪ Water Impaired oxygenation ▪ Pulmonary insufficiency ▪ Heat failure ▪ Hypovolemia Cirrhosis Uremia Prolonged hypothermia Coagulation disorders Cytotoxic drugs	Impaired cellular proliferation and collagen synthesis Decreased wound contraction

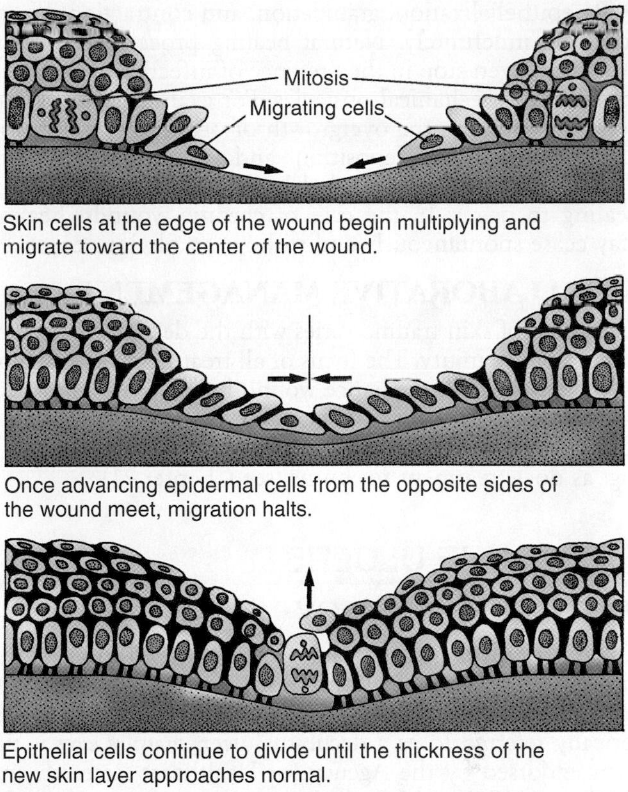

Figure 70-2 ■ Re-epithelialization. (Modified from Swaim, S.F. [1980]. *Surgery of traumatized skin.* Philadelphia: W.B. Saunders.)

by **re-epithelialization,** the production of new skin cells by undamaged epidermal cells in the basal layer of the dermis and lining the epidermal appendages (Figure 70-2). Skin injury is followed immediately by local inflammation. The inflammatory response causes the formation of a fibrin clot and the release of chemical messengers (growth factors) that stimulate epidermal cell division (mitosis). New skin cells move into "cell-free" spaces on the wound surface, where the fibrin clot acts as a frame or scaffold to guide cell movement. Regrowth across the open area **(resurfacing)** is only one cell layer thick at first. As healing continues, the cell layer thickens and stratifies to resemble normal skin. A healed wound re-establishes the barrier properties of the skin with keratin production.

In a healthy client, healing of a partial-thickness wound by re-epithelialization takes about 5 to 7 days. This process occurs most rapidly in tissue that is hydrated, oxygenated, and has few organisms present.

FULL-THICKNESS WOUNDS

In deep partial-thickness and full-thickness wounds, damage extends into the lower layers of the dermis and underlying subcutaneous tissue. As a result most, if not all, the epithelial cells at the base of the wound have been destroyed and cannot replicate. Removal of the damaged tissue results in a defect that must be filled with scar tissue **(granulation)** for healing to occur. During the proliferative phase of healing, new blood vessels form at the base of the wound and fibroblastic cells begin moving into the wound space. Fibroblasts deposit new collagen to replace the damaged tissue.

Some of these fibroblasts take on the features of smooth-muscle cells and begin to pull the wound edges inward along the path of least resistance **(contraction)** (see Figure 70-1). This causes the wound to decrease in size at a uniform rate of about 0.6 to 0.75 mm/day. Complete closure of a wound by contraction depends on the mobility of the surrounding skin as tension is applied to it. If tension in the surrounding skin exceeds the counter force of wound contraction, healing will be delayed until undamaged epidermal cells at the wound edges are able to bridge the defect. Unlike re-epithelialization in partial-thickness wounds, which results in the return of a near-normal epithelial barrier, the bridging of epithelial cells across a large area of granulation tissue results in an unstable barrier. A venous leg ulcer is one example of a skin defect that heals poorly by contraction. Re-epithelialization of these chronic wounds often results in a thin epidermal barrier that is easily reinjured.

Re-epithelialization, granulation, and contraction do not continue indefinitely. Natural healing processes can slow down and even stop in the presence of infection, unrelieved pressure, or mechanical obstacles. For example, dead tissue not only supports the overgrowth of organisms, but it also obstructs collagen deposition and wound contraction. Therefore thorough wound debridement is necessary for healing to occur. In the case of chronic wounds, healing may cease spontaneously and without an obvious cause.

COLLABORATIVE MANAGEMENT

Treatment of skin trauma varies with the depth and circumstances of the injury. The focus of all treatment for any type of skin trauma is to enhance wound healing, prevent infection, and restore function to the area. Management for pressure ulcers presents interventions common to wound healing, as does treatment for burns (see Chapter 71).

PRESSURE ULCERS

PATHOPHYSIOLOGY

A **pressure ulcer** is tissue damage caused when the skin and underlying soft tissue are compressed between a bony prominence and an external surface for an extended period. Historically referred to as a decubitus ulcer, *pressure ulcer* is the term endorsed by the Agency for Healthcare Research and Quality (AHRQ). Although they commonly occur over the sacrum, hips, and ankles, pressure ulcers can occur on any body surface. For example, nasal cannula tubing that is too tight can cause pressure ulcers behind the ear or in the nares.

Tissue compression from pressure restricts blood flow to the skin, resulting in tissue anoxia and cell death. These ulcers commonly occur in people with limited mobility because they are unable to change their position to relieve pressure. Sensory impairment is also a contributing factor. Clients who are unable to feel or communicate the pain that occurs with unrelieved pressure are more likely to develop pressure ulcers. Once formed, these chronic wounds are slow to heal, resulting in increased morbidity and health care costs.

In addition to pressure, other factors may predispose a client to pressure ulcers. Friction and shear are mechanical forces that impair skin integrity and set the stage for skin breakdown. Excessive skin moisture, such as urinary incontinence, increases the risk for skin damage when mechanical forces are applied. Nutritional status is also a concern. Protein malnutrition not only makes normal tissue more prone to breakdown, but it also delays healing.

Mechanical Forces

PRESSURE

Pressure occurs as a result of gravity. Dependent tissues in contact with a fixed surface experience varying degrees of pressure. Pressure is determined by the amount of weight exerted at the point of contact, the distribution of weight at the point of contact, and the density of the contacting surface. Excessive or prolonged pressure can compress blood vessels at the point of contact, leading to ischemia, inflammation, and tissue necrosis. Pressure occurs when the client is positioned on a hard surface that does not diffuse the weight or when he or she remains in the same position too long.

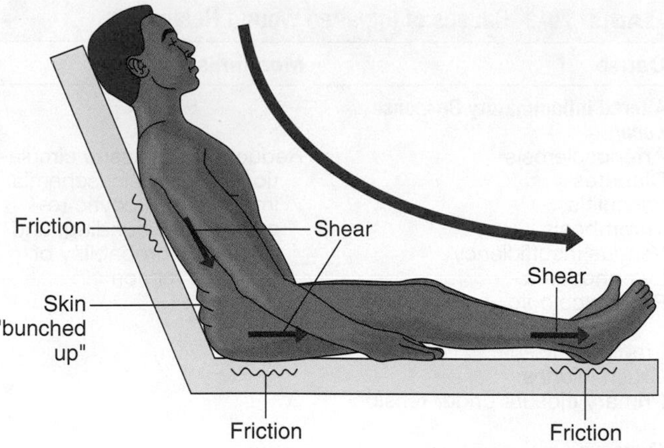

Figure 70-3 ■ Shearing forces pulling skin layers away from deeper tissue. The skin is "bunched up" against the back of the mattress while the rest of the bone and muscle in the area press downward on the lower part of the mattress. Blood vessels become kinked, obstructing circulation and leading to tissue death.

FRICTION

Friction occurs when surfaces rub the skin and irritate or directly pull off epithelial tissue. Such forces are generated when the client is dragged or pulled across bed linen.

SHEAR

Shear or shearing forces are generated when the skin itself is stationary and the tissues below the skin (such as fat and muscle) shift or move (Figure 70-3). The movement of the deeper tissue layers reduces the blood supply to the skin, leading to skin hypoxia, anoxia, ischemia, inflammation, and necrosis.

Gravity plays a role in the development of shearing forces. A shear injury usually occurs when a client is in bed in a semisitting position and gradually slides downward. Often the skin over the sacrum does not slide down at the same pace as the deeper tissues; thus the skin is mechanically "sheared," causing blood vessels to stretch and leading to soft-tissue ischemia, although no break in external skin integrity is observed.

> **CONSIDERATIONS FOR OLDER ADULTS**
>
> Older adults are at particular risk for pressure ulcers because of the presence of age-related skin changes. Progressive flattening of the dermal-epidermal junction predisposes older people to skin tears from mechanical shearing forces, such as the removal of adhesive tape and friction from tightly applied restraints. In addition, skin moisture and irritation from incontinence and friction over bony prominences can lead to partial-thickness skin destruction and early pressure ulcer formation. *If pressure is unrelieved, tissue destruction progresses to full-thickness injury.*

Incidence/Prevalence

Pressure ulcer development is a problem found among clients in the acute care setting, long-term care facility, and home care setting. Although client care has improved in many ways and new products are available for prevention and treatment, 3% to 14% of hospitalized clients still experience pressure ulcer formation.

CHART 70-2

NIC **INTERVENTION ACTIVITIES for**
The Client at Risk for or with Pressure Ulcers

Pressure Ulcer Prevention: *Prevention of pressure ulcers for a client at high risk for developing them*
- Use an established risk assessment tool to monitor client's risk factors (e.g., Braden scale).
- Document skin status on admission and daily.
- Monitor any reddened areas closely.
- Remove excessive moisture on the skin resulting from perspiration, wound drainage, and fecal or urinary incontinence.
- Apply protective barriers, such as creams or moisture-absorbing pads, to remove excess moisture, as appropriate.
- Turn every 1 to 2 hours, as appropriate.
- Turn with care (e.g., avoid shearing) to prevent injury to fragile skin.
- Post a turning schedule at the bedside, as appropriate.
- Inspect skin over bony prominences and other pressure points when repositioning at least daily.
- Avoid massaging over bony prominences.
- Position with pillows to elevate pressure points off the bed.
- Keep bed linens clean, dry, and wrinkle free.
- Utilize specialty beds and mattresses, as appropriate.
- Use devices on the bed (e.g., sheepskin) that protect the individual.
- Moisturize dry, unbroken skin.
- Avoid hot water and use mild soap when bathing.
- Apply elbow and heel protectors, as appropriate.
- Facilitate small shifts of body weight frequently.
- Ensure adequate dietary intake, especially protein, vitamins B and C, iron, and calories, using supplements, as appropriate.
- Instruct family member/caregiver about signs of skin breakdown, as appropriate.

Pressure Ulcer Care: *Facilitation of healing in pressure ulcers*
- Describe characteristics of the ulcer at regular intervals, including size (L × W × D), stage (I-IV), location, exudate, granulation or necrotic tissue, and epithelialization.
- Monitor color, temperature, edema, moisture, and appearance of surrounding skin.
- Keep the ulcer moist to aid in healing.
- Cleanse the skin around the ulcer with mild soap and water.
- Debride ulcer, as needed.
- Cleanse the ulcer with the appropriate nontoxic solution, working in a circular motion from the center.
- Note characteristics of any drainage.
- Apply dressings, as appropriate.
- Monitor for signs and symptoms of infection in the wound.
- Position every 1 to 2 hours to avoid prolonged pressure.
- Use specialty beds and mattresses, as appropriate.
- Ensure adequate dietary intake.
- Monitor nutritional status.
- Teach individual or family member(s) wound care procedures.
- Initiate consultation services of the enterostomal therapy nurse, as needed.

Pressure Management: *Minimizing pressure to body parts*
- Place client on an appropriate therapeutic mattress/bed.
- Place client on a polyurethane foam pad, as appropriate.
- Refrain from applying pressure to the affected body part.
- Elevate injured extremity.
- Turn the immobilized client at least every 2 hours, according to a specific schedule.
- Facilitate small shifts of body weight.
- Monitor skin for areas of redness and breakdown.
- Use an established risk assessment tool to monitor client's risk factors (e.g., Braden scale).
- Monitor the client's nutritional status.
- Monitor for sources of pressure and friction.

NIC intervention activities selected from Dochterman, J.M., & Bulechek, G.M. (2004). *Nursing interventions classification (NIC)* (4th ed.). St. Louis: Mosby.

HEALTH PROMOTION/ILLNESS PREVENTION

Pressure ulcers can be prevented if the risk is recognized and intervention begins early (Charts 70-2 and 70-3). Key health care team members for pressure ulcer prevention and management are the enterostomal therapist (ET), the certified wound specialist, and the registered dietitian (RD).

A pressure ulcer prevention program consists of two steps: (1) identification of high-risk clients and (2) implementation of aggressive intervention for prevention with the use of pressure relief or reduction devices. Many facilities do not recognize the value of preventing pressure ulcers through appropriate consultation, the use of pressure relief and pressure reduction products, and ensuring adequate nutrition. The costs of such prevention strategies is more than justified by the savings seen in comparison with the costs of interventions for care when actual ulceration is present (see the Resource Management box on p. 1582).

Risk identification and prevention measures must include education of the client and the caregiver. Documentation of risk assessment, prevention measures implemented, and education of all individuals involved in the care of the client at risk for pressure ulcer formation are key to the plan's success. Periodic reassessment of risk and continuing evaluation of the implemented plan are necessary as client conditions change.

Identification of High-Risk Clients

All clients admitted to a health care facility or home care agency should be assessed for pressure ulcer risk, as recommended by the AHRQ. The use of a risk assessment tool increases the chances of identifying those clients at greater risk for skin breakdown. The two risk assessment tools recommended by the AHRQ guidelines are the Norton Scale and the Braden Scale (Figure 70-4). Other factors to consider when determining the risk category for pressure ulcer formation are mental status, activity/mobility, nutritional status, and incontinence.

MENTAL STATUS/DECREASED SENSORY PERCEPTION

The client's mental status determines whether he or she is a partner in the prevention of pressure. When the client understands that turning and shifting of weight prevent tissue damage, the risk for pressure ulcers decreases. When he or she has a mental status problem because of stroke, head injury, organic brain disease, Alzheimer's disease, or other problem with cognition, the risk for pressure ulcer formation increases.

ACTIVITY/MOBILITY

The level of the client's independent mobility is a direct factor in the risk for pressure ulcer formation. Clients who

CHART 70-3

BEST PRACTICE for
Preventing Pressure Ulcers

Positioning
- Pad contact surfaces with foam, silicon gel, or air pads.
- Do not keep the head of the bed elevated above 30 degrees.
- Use a lift sheet to move client in the bed. Avoid dragging or sliding the client.
- When positioning a client on his or her side, do not position directly on the trochanter.
- Reposition an immobile client every 2 hours while in bed and every 1 hour while sitting in a chair.
- Do not place a rubber ring or doughnut under the client's sacral area.
- When moving an immobile client from a bed to another surface use a designated slide board well lubricated with talc.
- Place pillows or foam wedges between two bony surfaces.
- Keep the client's skin directly off plastic surfaces.
- Keep the client's heels off the bed surface.

Nutrition
- Ensure a fluid intake between 2000 and 3000 mL/day.
- Help the client maintain an adequate intake of protein and calories.

Skin Care
- Use moisturizers daily on dry skin, and apply when skin is damp.
- Keep moisture from prolonged contact with skin.
  - Dry areas where two skin surfaces touch, such as the axilla and under the breasts.
  - Place absorbent pads under areas where perspiration collects.
  - Use moisture barriers on skin areas where wound drainage or incontinence occurs.
- Do not massage bony prominences.
- Humidify the room.

Skin Cleaning
- Clean the skin as soon as possible after soiling occurs and at routine intervals.
- Use a mild, heavily fatted soap.
- Use tepid rather than hot water.
- While cleaning, use the minimal scrubbing force necessary to remove soil.
- Gently pat rather than rub the skin dry.

have unimpaired mobility and can respond to physical sensation changes are at low risk for pressure ulcer formation. Any client, regardless of age, who requires assistance with turning and positioning or who is less aware of physical sensation changes is at high risk for pressure ulcer formation. A client who is confined to bed or a chair is at higher risk than a client who requires assistance with ambulation.

NUTRITIONAL STATUS

Nutritional status is a critical risk factor for pressure ulcer development. Intact skin and wound healing are dependent on a positive nitrogen balance and adequate serum protein levels. The client in a negative nitrogen balance not only heals more slowly but also is at greater risk for tissue destruction. In addition, draining wounds are a route of protein loss.

Adequate nutrition is critical in the prevention of pressure ulcer formation. A dietitian or nutrition specialist should be a part of the pressure reduction team or program.

Nutritional status assessment includes laboratory studies; evaluation of weight and weight change; ability of the client to consume an adequate diet; and the need for vitamin, mineral, or protein supplementation. Nutrition is inadequate when the client's serum albumin level is lower than 3.5 mg/dL or the lymphocyte count is less than 1800/mm^3. Other indicators of inadequate nutrition include a weight loss of 15% of total body weight or greater.

A positive nitrogen balance requires an intake of 30 to 35 calories per kilogram of body weight daily with a protein intake of 1.25 to 1.5 g/kg/day. Up to 2 g/kg/day of protein may be needed when nutritional deficits are severe or protein loss is ongoing. Vitamin supplementation is based on the client's nutritional status.

RESOURCE MANAGEMENT

PRESSURE ULCER PREVENTION

Cost of Care
- Medicare reimbursement for medically complex residents of long-term care decreased from an average of $408 to $231 per day, beginning in 1997.
- Most residents with complex wounds and stage III or IV pressure ulcers fall into the category of medically complex.
- Pressure relief/reduction devices and appropriate dressing materials cost more than the available reimbursement.
- Many long-term care facilities made product choices based on cost alone.
- Use of pressure relief/reduction devices for prevention of pressure ulcers was limited.
- The number and severity of pressure ulcers among residents of long-term care facilities increased during this budget reduction period.

Implications for Nursing
An ounce of prevention may be worth tons rather than pounds of cure. Although on the surface, pressure relief/reduction devices, high protein diets, and appropriate dressing materials appear expensive, the actual cost in nursing hours, equipment, devices, and consumable supplies when caring for a client with even one pressure ulcer is far greater. Legislation signed in 1999 allows prevention costs as well as care costs to be justly reimbursed. Nurses need to consider pressure ulcer prevention in care setting as a number one priority of care.

Data from Motta, G. (2000). Reimbursement relief. *Continuing Care, 19*(4), 14-16.

INCONTINENCE

Incontinence results in prolonged contact of the skin with such substances as urea, bacteria, yeast, and enzymes carried in urine and feces. These substances are irritants and lead to skin breakdown. Excessive moisture macerates intact skin, increasing the risk for breakdown. Daily inspection of the skin for any areas of redness or skin breakdown is a major part of pressure ulcer prevention. Maintenance of clean, intact skin also assists in the prevention process. The skin should be washed with a pH-balanced soap to maintain the normal acid level. Creams or lotions are used to lubricate and moisturize the skin. Barrier ointment protection is needed whenever incontinence is present. Absorbent pads or garments must be changed quickly with each incontinence episode to avoid prolonged skin contact with urine or feces. *Reddened areas are never massaged because this action can damage capillary beds and increase tissue necrosis.*

Pressure-Relieving Techniques

The cornerstone in the prevention (and treatment) of pressure ulcers is adequate pressure relief. A factor in pressure re-

Client's name ______	Evaluator's name ______			Date of assessment		
Sensory perception Ability to respond meaningfully to pressure-related discomfort	**1. Completely limited** Unresponsive to painful stimuli (does not moan, flinch, or grasp) because of diminished level of consciousness or sedation OR limited ability to feel pain over most of body surface	**2. Very limited** Responds only to painful stimuli; cannot communicate discomfort except by moaning or restlessness OR has a sensory impairment that limits the ability to feel pain or discomfort over half of the body	**3. Slightly limited** Responds to verbal commands but cannot always communicate discomfort or need to be turned OR has some sensory impairment that limits ability to feel pain or discomfort in one or two extremities	**4. No impairment** Responds to verbal commands; has no sensory deficit that would limit ability to feel or voice pain or discomfort		
Moisture Degree to which skin is exposed to moisture	**1. Constantly moist** Skin is kept moist almost constantly by perspiration, urine; dampness is detected every time the client is moved or turned	**2. Very Moist** Skin is often but not always moist; linen must be changed at least once a shift	**3. Occasionally moist** Skin is occasionally moist, requiring an extra linen change approximately once a day	**4. Rarely moist** Skin is usually dry; linen requires changing only at routine intervals		
Activity Degree of physical activity	**1. Bedfast** Confined to bed	**2. Chairfast** Ability to walk severely limited or nonexistent; cannot bear own weight and must be assisted into chair or wheelchair	**3. Walks occasionally** Walks occasionally during the day but for very short distances, with or without assistance; spends the majority of each shift in bed or chair	**4. Walks frequently** Walks outside the room at least twice a day and inside the room at least once every 2 hours during waking hours		
Mobility Ability to change or control body position	**1. Completely immobile** Does not make even slight changes in body or extremity position without assistance	**2. Very limited** Makes occasional slight changes in body or extremity position but unable to make frequent or significant changes independently	**3. Slightly limited** Makes frequent though slight changes in body or extremity position independently	**4. No limitations** Makes major and frequent changes in position without assistance		
Nutrition Usual food intake pattern	**1. Very poor** Never eats a complete meal; rarely eats more than a third of any food offered; eats two servings or less of protein (meat or dairy products) per day; takes fluids poorly; does not take a liquid dietary supplement OR is NPO or maintained on clear liquids or IV for more than 5 days	**2. Probably inadequate** Rarely eats a complete meal and generally eats only about half of any food offered; protein intake includes only three servings of meat or dairy products per day; occasionally will take a dietary supplement OR receives less than optimal amount of liquid diet or tube feeding	**3. Adequate** Eats over half of most meals; eats a total of four servings of protein (meat, dairy products) each day; occasionally will refuse a meal, but will usually take a supplement if offered OR is receiving tube feeding or total parenteral nutrition, which probably meets most nutritional needs	**4. Excellent** Eats most of every meal; never refuses a meal; usually eats a total of four or more servings of meat and dairy products; occasionally eats between meals; does not require supplementation		
Friction and shear	**1. Problem** Requires moderate to maximum assistance in moving; complete lifting without sliding against sheets is impossible; frequently slides down in bed or chair, requiring frequent repositioning with maximum assistance; spasticity, contractures, or agitation leads to almost constant friction	**2. Potential problem** Moves feebly or requires minimum assistance during a move; skin probably slides to some extent against sheets, chair, restraints, or other devices; maintains relatively good position in chair or bed most of the time but occasionally slides down	**3. No apparent problem** Moves in bed and in chair independently and has sufficient muscle strength to lift up completely during move; maintains good position in bed or chair at all times			
Scoring system: 15-16 = mild risk, 12-14 = moderate risk, <11 = severe risk				Total score		

Figure 70-4 ■ The Braden Scale for predicting pressure ulcer risk. IV, Intravenous; NPO, nothing by mouth. (From Barbara Braden and Nancy Bergstrom. Copyright 1988. Reprinted with permission.)

lief is the **capillary closing pressure,** which is the amount of pressure needed to occlude skin capillary blood flow, in the area at risk. The normal capillary closing pressure ranges from 12 to 32 mm Hg. Any device used must provide pressure relief below the capillary closing pressure to prevent tissue ischemia. *Most devices have a standardized guaranteed pressure relief reading; however, these readings do not ensure that capillary blood flow for any given client is adequate. You must observe skin color, integrity, and temperature to determine capillary flow adequacy.*

Devices are classified according to whether they relieve pressure or merely reduce pressure. In addition, devices are further classified as dynamic or static. Dynamic systems alternate inflation and deflation of the device through the use of electricity. Static devices made of gel, water, foam, or air are in a constant state of inflation that distributes the client pressure load over a larger area and reduce the pressure any one area experiences.

Pressure relief/reduction products come in many forms, such as specialty beds, mattress replacements, overlays, and assistive devices. Choosing the correct product is important in the success of the prevention plan. The product selected is reevaluated daily for effectiveness in reducing pressure, comfort, and elimination of "bottoming out," wherein the client's bony prominences sink into the mattress or cushion, causing him or her to have pressure even with the product in place.

PRESSURE-RELIEF DEVICES

Pressure-relief devices consistently reduce pressure below capillary closing pressure. These devices are recommended for clients who need the following:

- Prevention of skin breakdown because they cannot turn
- Prevention of extension of skin breakdown that has already occurred
- Promotion of healing for breakdown present on several turning surfaces

PRESSURE-REDUCTION DEVICES

Pressure-reduction devices lower pressure below that of a standard hospital mattress or chair surface but do not reduce pressure consistently below the capillary closing pressure. Such devices must be used along with a turning schedule.

POSITIONING

A good plan for positioning is the 30-degree rule. This plan ensures that the client is positioned and propped so that whatever part of the body is elevated is tilted back at least 30 degrees to the mattress rather than resting directly on a dependent bony prominence. This rule applies to side-lying as well as head-of-bed elevation positions. The client who must be elevated to a full 90 degrees because of respiratory difficulties should be tilted forward even more than 90 degrees, with pillows behind the back to keep pressure off of the sacral/coccyx area.

The client at risk for pressure ulcers in bed is also at risk while sitting. Carefully assess for proper wheelchair or regular chair cushioning. Consult with physical therapists and rehabilitation specialists for selection of these products.

Even with an appropriate mattress or cushion, the client must change or be helped to change positions periodically. Many facilities require turning and positioning every 2 hours. *However, pressure can occur in less time, and the actual turning or repositioning schedule for each client must be individualized.*

Use pillows and other positioning/padding devices to keep heels pressure-free at all times for high-risk clients. Assess heel positioning frequently to ensure that pressure is not redistributed to another high-risk area, such as the sides of the feet. Assess even more frequently when devices that hide the feet, such as boots, are used, especially if the client has a peripheral vascular problem.

COLLABORATIVE MANAGEMENT

The Concept Map on p. 1585 addresses some of the assessment and nursing care issues for clients who have or who are at risk for developing pressure ulcers.

Assessment

HISTORY

When taking a history from the client with a pressure ulcer, identify the underlying cause of skin loss as well as factors that may impair healing. Ask about the specific circumstances of the skin loss. In general, clients with chronic pressure ulcerations usually have a history of delayed healing or recurrence of the ulcer after healing has occurred. Because pressure-related skin loss is common among severely debilitated clients, determine whether a client has any of the following contributing factors:

- Prolonged bedrest
- Immobility
- Incontinence
- Inadequate nutrition or hydration
- Altered mental status (decreased sensory perception)

PHYSICAL ASSESSMENT/CLINICAL MANIFESTATIONS

Inspect the entire body, including the back of the head, for areas of skin injury or pressure. Give special attention to bony prominences (such as the heels, sacrum, elbows, trochanter, posterior and anterior iliac spines) and areas that are vulnerable to excessive moisture. In addition, assess the client's general appearance for issues related to skin health. Such issues include body weight and the proportion of weight to height because obese persons as well as thin persons are at increased risk for pressure ulcer formation. Check overall cleanliness of the skin, hair, and nails. Determine whether any loss of mobility or range of joint motion has occurred.

WOUND ASSESSMENT

The appearance of pressure ulcers changes with the depth of the injury. Chart 70-4 lists the features of the four stages of pressure ulceration, and Figures 70-5 to 70-8 show examples.

Assess wounds for location, size, color, extent of tissue involvement, cell types in the wound base and margins, exudate, condition of surrounding tissue, and the presence of foreign bodies. Document this initial assessment to serve as a starting point for determining the intervention plan and its effectiveness. How often a wound is assessed is determined by the written policies and procedures at the facility or agency. Weekly documented assessment is the standard in many facilities. *However, also assess the wound at each dress-*

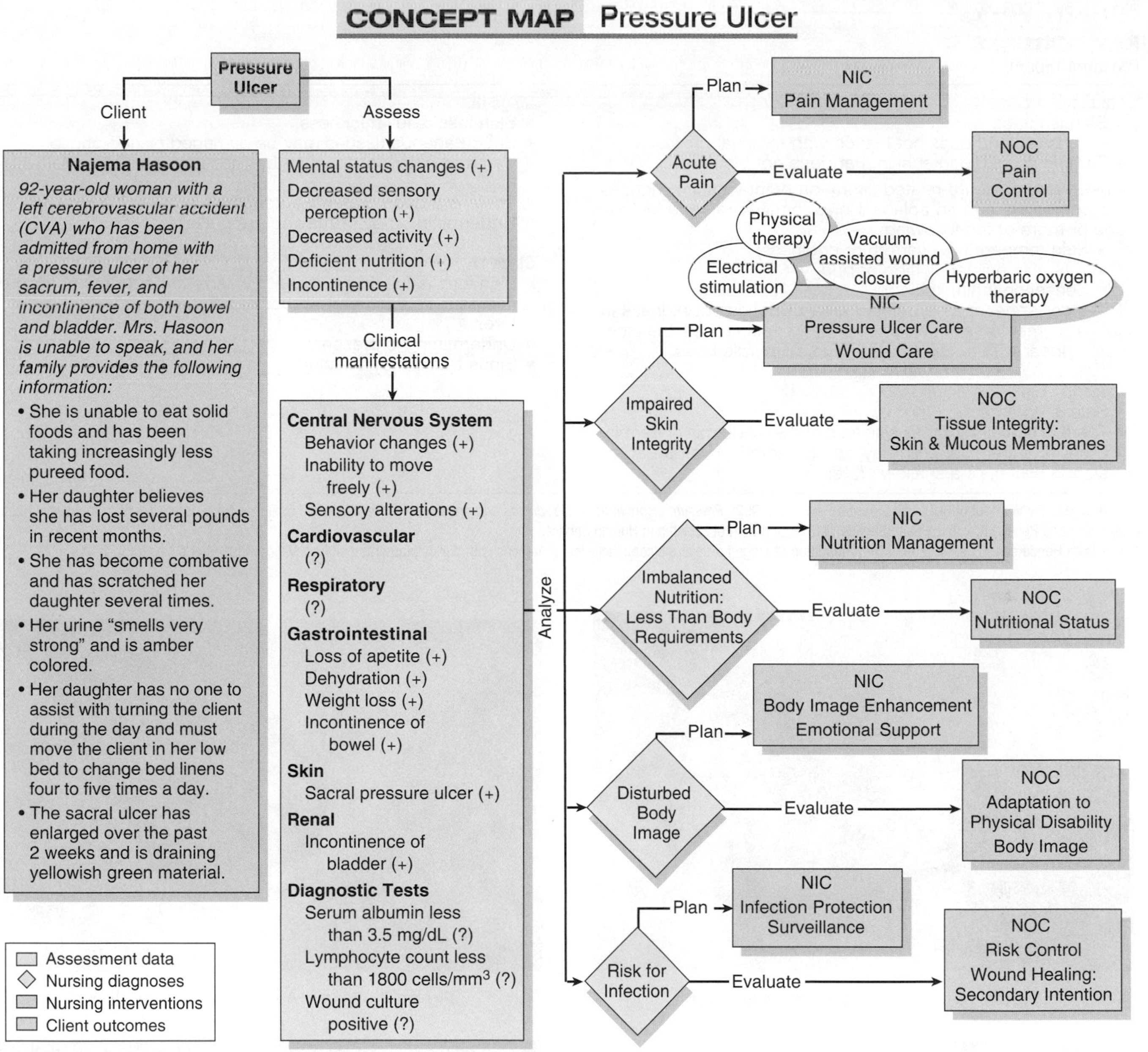

Concept Map by Elaine Bishop Kennedy, EdD, RN

ing change, comparing the existing wound features with those documented previously to determine the current state of healing or deterioration.

Record the location and size of the wound first. Wounds are sized by length, width, and depth using millimeters or centimeters. In standardizing wound size for documentation and communication purposes, assess the wound as a clock face with 12 o'clock in the direction of the client's head and 6 o'clock in the direction of the client's feet. Always measure the length from 12 o'clock to 6 o'clock and the width between 9 o'clock and 3 o'clock. Measure depth as the distance from the deepest portion of the wound base to the skin level. When all caregivers use this format, measurement is accurate and wound progress can be determined.

Inspect the wound margins for **cellulitis** (inflammation of the skin cells) extending beyond the area of injury. Progressive tissue destruction, seen as an increase in the size or depth of the ulcer and increased wound drainage, usually indicates an impairment in the client's ability to resist infection if proper measures have been taken to relieve pressure.

Inspect the wound for the presence or absence of necrotic tissue. Because of the depth of tissue destruction, a full-thickness pressure ulcer is often covered by a layer of black, gray, or brown nonviable, denatured collagen called wound **eschar.**

In the early stages of wound healing, the eschar is dry, leathery, and firmly attached to the wound surface. As the inflammatory phase of wound healing begins and removal of wound debris progresses, the eschar starts to lift and separate from the tissue beneath. This nonliving eschar is a good breeding ground for bacteria normally found on the skin surface as well as those introduced by other means. As bacteria increase, they release enzymes, which softens necrotic tissue. This tissue becomes softer and more yellow.

CHART 70-4

KEY FEATURES of Pressure Ulcers

Stage I
- Skin is intact.
- Area is red and does not blanch with external pressure.
- For clients with darker skin that does not blanch:*

Observable pressure-related alteration of intact skin; changes are compared with an adjacent or opposite area and include one or more of the following:
- Skin temperature (warmth or coolness)
- Tissue consistency (firm or boggy)
- Sensation (pain, itching)

The ulcer appears as a defined area of persistent redness in lightly pigmented skin, whereas in darker skin tones, the ulcer may appear with persistent red, blue, or purple hues.

Stage II
- Skin is not intact.
- There is partial-thickness skin loss of the epidermis or dermis.
- Ulcer is superficial and may be characterized as an abrasion, a blister, or a shallow crater.

Stage III
- Skin loss is full thickness.
- Subcutaneous tissues may be damaged or necrotic.
- Damage extends down to but not through the underlying fascia.
- There is a deep crater-like appearance or eschar present.
- Undermining may or may not be present.

Stage IV
- Skin loss is full thickness with extensive destruction, tissue necrosis, or damage to muscle, bone, or supporting structures.
- Undermining is present.
- Sinus tracts may develop.

Data from U.S. Department of Health and Human Services. (1992). *Pressure ulcers in adults: Prediction and prevention.* Clinical Practice Guideline No. 3. Rockville, MD: Agency for Health Care Policy and Research, Public Health Service, U.S. Department of Health and Human Services.

* Data from Henderson, C., et al. (1997). Draft definition of stage I pressure ulcers: Inclusion of persons with darkly pigmented skin. *Advances in Wound Care, 10*(5), 16-19.

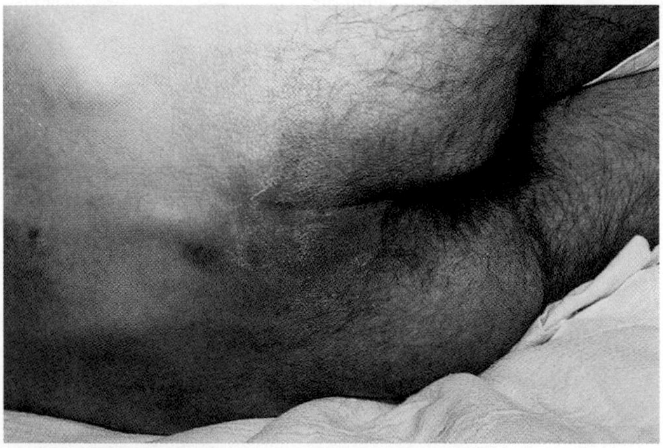

Figure 70-5 ■ A stage I pressure ulcer.

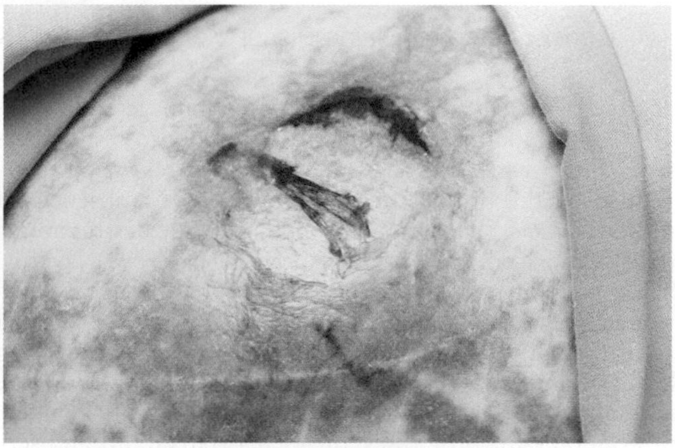

Figure 70-6 ■ A stage II pressure ulcer.

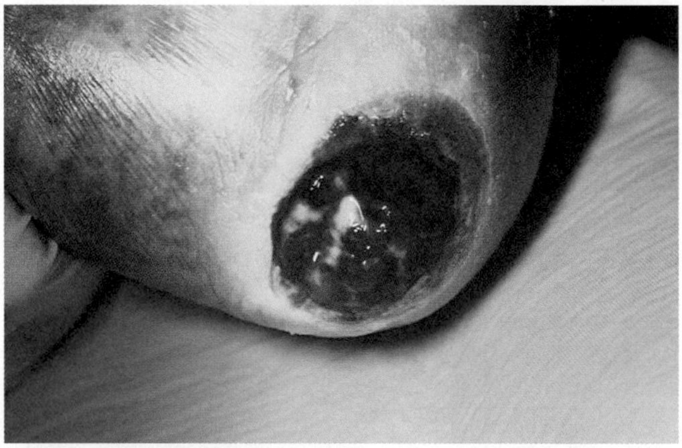

Figure 70-7 ■ A stage III pressure ulcer.

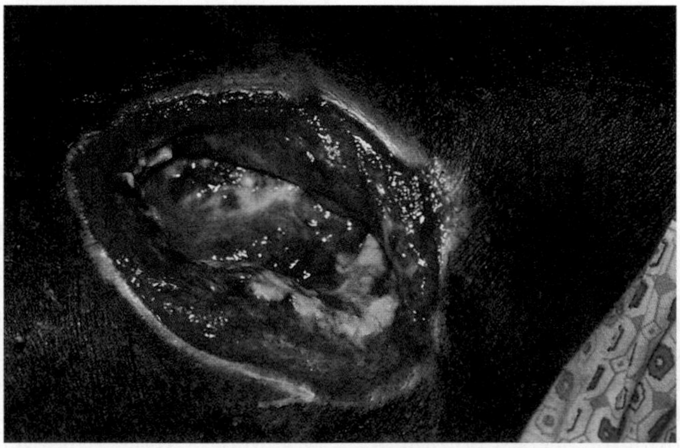

Figure 70-8 ■ A stage IV pressure ulcer.

TABLE 70-4 Types of Wound Exudate

Characteristics	Significance
Serosanguineous Exudate	
Blood-tinged amber fluid consisting of serum and red blood cells	Normal for first 48 hr after injury Sudden increase in amount precedes wound dehiscence in wounds closed by first intention
Purulent Exudate	
Creamy yellow pus	Colonization with *Staphylococcus*
Greenish blue pus causing staining of dressings and accompanied by a "fruity" odor	Colonization with *Pseudomona*
Beige pus with a "fishy" odor	Colonization with *Proteus*
Brownish pus with a "fecal" odor	Colonization with aerobic coliform and *Bacteroides* (usually occurs after intestinal surgery)

In the presence of bacterial colonization, wound exudate increases substantially; the color and odor of wound exudate indicate the major organism present. The features of wound exudate are listed in Table 70-4.

Beneath the separating dead tissue, granulation tissue appears. Early granulation is pale pink, progressing to a beefy red color as it grows and fills the wound. A wound with poor local arterial blood supply appears dry with pale, immature granulation tissue present. Venous obstruction causes an excessively moist ulcer surface with a deep red color (reflective of the deoxygenated blood beneath the ulcer surface).

Palpate the wound to determine the texture of the granulations. Healthy granulations have a slightly spongy texture. Pressure ulcers may involve more extensive tissue destruction than is first seen on inspection. Separation of the skin layers at the wound margins from the underlying granulation tissue is known as **undermining.** Inspect undermined areas for gradual filling with healthy granulations and for wound-healing progress. Palpate the bony prominences for deep hardening of the surrounding soft tissue, which often suggests tissue ischemia well beneath the surface of the skin.

After ischemia has occurred, continued pressure over the area of injury allows progression of tissue destruction from the deep tissue layers toward the surface. This "hidden" wound may first have a small opening in the skin with purulent drainage. If you observe such an opening, use a cotton-tipped applicator to probe gently for a much larger pocket of necrotic tissue beneath the opening.

PSYCHOSOCIAL ASSESSMENT

The client with pressure ulcers may have an altered body image. Ineffective coping patterns emerge as the client and family or significant others strive to adhere to changes in lifestyle that are needed for healing. In addition, chronic, slow-healing ulcers are often painful and costly to treat.

Assess the client's and family's knowledge of the treatment goals at each stage of the healing process as well as adherence to the prescribed treatment regimen. Also assess the client's skills in cleaning the wound and applying a dressing. Poor adherence to pressure ulcer care procedures may reflect an inability to accept the diagnosis or to cope with the pain, cost, or potential scarring associated with prolonged healing. Depending on the client's activity level and the location of the ulcer, assistance of a family member or home care nurse may be needed to care for the pressure ulcer at home.

Explore with the client specific changes in activities of daily living (ADLs) that are needed to relieve pressure and promote healing. Promote increased activity whenever possible to enhance circulation to the affected tissue. Bedrest with elevation of the legs may be needed for healing when ulcers occur on the lower legs, especially for the client with poor venous blood flow and lower-leg edema. When the client is bedridden, frequent repositioning to relieve pressure (every 2 hours in bed, every 1 hour in a chair) can be labor intensive. In the home environment, repositioning, incontinence management, and dressing changes are often needed around the clock, disrupting family routines and contributing to stress.

LABORATORY ASSESSMENT

A wound that is exposed is always *contaminated* but is not always *infected.* **Contamination** is the presence of organisms without any clinical manifestation of infection. The normal immune defenses of the body keep the number of bacteria to a minimum and prevent infection. **Wound infection** is contamination with pathogenic organisms to the degree that growth and spread cannot be controlled by the body's immune defenses. Wounds that are inflamed, indurated, red, have an odor, and have moderate to heavy exudate should be cultured to identify the causative organism and determine its sensitivity to antibiotics. The presence of pus as exudate alone does not indicate an infection because pus formation occurs when necrotic tissue debrides and liquefies.

If wounds are extensive, if the client is severely immunocompromised, or if local blood supply to the wound is impaired, bacterial growth may exceed the body's ability to defend against invasion into deeper tissue layers. The result is deep wound infection and eventually bacteremia and **sepsis** (systemic infection).

Swab cultures are helpful only in identifying the types of bacteria present on the ulcer surface and may be misleading when trying to identify or quantify bacteria in deeper tissues. Tests such as quantitative wound biopsies allow the numbers of bacteria to be analyzed. Unfortunately these tests are time consuming, costly, and unavailable in many laboratories. Therefore clinical indicators of infection (cellulitis, progressive increase in ulcer size or depth, changes in the quantity and quality of exudate) and systemic signs of bacteremia are important criteria in the diagnosis and treatment of an infection.

OTHER DIAGNOSTIC ASSESSMENTS

Additional laboratory studies are performed on the basis of the suspected cause of the wound. For pressure ulcers to show progress toward healing, the factors contributing to delayed healing must be diagnosed and treated. For example, noninvasive and invasive arterial blood flow studies are indicated if arterial occlusion is suspected in delayed healing of a pressure ulcer on the heel or ankle. Blood tests to establish specific nutritional deficiencies are helpful in treating the debilitated, malnourished client with a pressure ulcer.

Critical Thinking Challenge

The client is a 72-year-old woman who has had type 2 diabetes for 20 years. She is a widow who lives alone and is being admitted for bacterial pneumonia. She also has mild to moderate heart failure controlled with furosemide (Lasix, Furoside*) and an ACE inhibitor. She weighs 180 lbs and is 5 feet 1 inch tall.

1. What risk factors does this client have for pressure ulcer development? How do these factors increase her risk?
2. What additional assessment data should you obtain?
3. Given her diagnosis, in what position do you expect to place her? Does this position increase or decrease her risk for pressure ulcer formation? If so, where is/are the ulcer(s) likely to develop?

evolve For suggested answer guidelines, go to http://evolve.elsevier.com/Iggy/.

Analysis

COMMON NURSING DIAGNOSES AND COLLABORATIVE PROBLEMS

The most common nursing diagnosis for clients with pressure ulcers is Impaired Skin Integrity related to vascular insufficiency and trauma. The most common collaborative problem is Risk for Infection and Wound Extension.

ADDITIONAL NURSING DIAGNOSES AND COLLABORATIVE PROBLEMS

In addition to the common nursing diagnoses and collaborative problems, clients with pressure ulcers may have one or more of the following:

- Acute Pain or Chronic Pain related to skin trauma, wound infection, and wound treatment
- Disturbed Body Image related to altered appearance
- Ineffective Coping related to the chronicity of the ulcer, alteration in body image, and changes in lifestyle required to promote healing
- Imbalanced Nutrition: Less Than Body Requirements related to inability to ingest food due to biologic, psychological, or economic factors
- Ineffective Tissue Perfusion (Peripheral) related to mechanical reduction of venous or arterial blood flow
- Deficient Knowledge (treatment) related to cognitive limitation or unfamiliarity with information resources

Planning and Implementation

IMPAIRED SKIN INTEGRITY

NOC **PLANNING: EXPECTED OUTCOMES.** The client with a pressure ulcer is expected to experience complete wound healing and not experience the formation of new pressure ulcers. Indicators include the following:

- Presence of granulation, re-epithelialization, and scar tissue formation
- Decreased wound size
- Absence of new pressure ulcers

INTERVENTIONS. Wound care techniques for pressure ulcers vary according to each client's needs and the physician's preferences. Surgery with aggressive removal of necrotic tissue may be indicated for some clients, whereas a nonsurgical approach to ulcer debridement is preferred for an older client who has adequate defenses but is too ill or debilitated for surgery.

TABLE 70-5 Common Dressing Techniques for Wound Debridement

Technique	Mechanism of Action
Wet-to-dry saline-moistened gauze	Dry, necrotic debris is softened by the saline, allowing it to become more effectively entrapped in the interstices as the gauze dries and shrinks. Dressing may also entrap healing tissue.
Wet-to-damp saline-moistened gauze	As with the wet-to-dry technique, necrotic debris is mechanically removed but with less trauma to healing tissue.
Continuous wet gauze	The wound surface is continually bathed with a wetting agent of choice, promoting dilution of viscous exudate and softening of dry eschar.
Topical enzyme preparations	Proteolytic action on thick, adherent eschar causes breakdown of denatured protein and more rapid separation of necrotic tissue.
Moisture-retentive dressing	Spontaneous separation of necrotic tissue is promoted by autolysis.

NONSURGICAL MANAGEMENT. The NIC interventions for pressure ulcer prevention and management are listed in Chart 70-2. Nonsurgical intervention of pressure ulcers is often left to the discretion of the nurse, who collaborates with the physician to select a method of wound dressing on the basis of the identified goal of wound management.

Dressings. A properly designed dressing can speed healing by removing unwanted debris from the ulcer surface, protecting exposed healthy tissues, and creating a barrier between the body and the environment until the ulcer is closed. For a client with a draining, necrotic ulcer, the dressing must also remove excessive exudate and loose debris without damaging epithelial cells or newly formed granulation tissue. If necrosis is extensive and the eschar is thick, dead tissue must be surgically or chemically removed before further debridement with dressings will be effective. Depending on the dressing material used, dressings help to remove debris either through mechanical entrapment and detachment of dead tissue or by creating an environment that promotes self-digestion of dead tissues by the bacterial enzymes (autolysis) (Table 70-5).

After all the dead tissue has been removed, protection of any exposed vital structures, such as tendon, bone, and newly formed collagen, is critical to pressure ulcer care. The ideal environment for healing is a clean, *slightly* moist ulcer surface with minimal bacterial colonization. Heavy moisture from an excessively draining ulcer or a dressing that is too wet interferes with healing by promoting the growth of organisms and causing maceration of healthy tissue. Likewise, if a clean ulcer surface is exposed to air or if highly absorbent dressing materials are used for prolonged periods, the drying effect can dehydrate surface cells, form scabs, or convert the wound to a deeper injury.

Assess the ulcer for necrotic tissue and the quantity of exudate. Select a dressing material with properties that promote an optimal environment for healing (Table 70-6). For example, a material that does not stick to the wound surface and does not remove fragile epithelial cells when it is

TABLE 70-6 Commonly Used Dressing Materials

	Alginates	Biologic Dressings	Cotton Gauze Dressing	Foams	Hydrocolloidal Wafers	Hydrogel Dressing	Transparent Films
Indications	Absorption Protection	Debridement after eschar removal* Protection Test before skin grafts (pigskin and cadaver skin) Burns Dormant, nonhealing wounds that do not respond to other topical therapies	***Continuous Dry*** Absorption Protection (nonadherent contact layer) ***Continuous Wet*** Delivery of topical agent Debridement (autolysis) Protection ***Wet to Damp*** Atraumatic mechanical debridement ***Wet to Dry*** Aggressive mechanical debridement	Absorption Protection	Debridement* Absorption Protection	Debridement* Absorption Protection	Debridement* Protection (partial-thickness lesions) Secondary (cover) dressing
Advantages	Highly absorbent Biodegradable Easy application Nonadhesive Can be used as packing for deep wounds Can be used for infected wounds	Most "natural" wound covering Reduces pain Conforms to uneven wound surfaces Acts as a catalyst for healing Alternative to autograft	Readily available Good mechanical debridement *if used properly* Effective delivery of topical agents	Absorbent Insulates wound Easy application Nonadhesive (most products) Conforms to uneven wound surfaces	Absorbent Excludes bacteria Waterproof Reduces pain Easy application Easy to store	Absorbent Nonadhesive Reduce pain Conducive to use with topical agents Conforms to uneven wound surfaces Amorphous form can be used as a filler Easy to store	Wound visualization Good adhesion Waterproof Reduces pain Cost-effective Easy to store
Disadvantages	Requires secondary dressing to secure Can cause desiccation of tissue if drainage is minimal	Requires secondary dressing to secure Very expensive Skin substitutes require skill to apply	Delayed healing if used improperly Pain on removal Requires frequent dressing changes	Poor barrier function Requires secondary dressing to secure	Nontransparent Softening and loss of shape with pressure, heat, and friction Odor with dressing removal Expensive Requires use of "fillers" for deep, draining lesions	Poor barrier function Only partial wound visualization Requires secondary dressing to secure Can promote growth of *Pseudomonas* and other microorganisms	Difficult to apply properly Nonabsorbent Adhesive to normal and healing tissue Limited to superficial lesions
Dressing changes	When dressing is saturated (q3-5 days) or more frequently	Topical growth factors: Daily skin substitutes: Varies (similar to grafts)	Necrotic base: q4-6h Clean base: q12-24h	When dressing is saturated or more frequently	Necrotic base: q24h Clean base: on leakage of exudate	Necrotic base: q6-8h Clean base: q24h	Necrotic base: q24h Clean base: on leakage of exudate

*Use with caution in clients with leukopenia or vascular disease.

changed is the dressing of choice for protecting new tissue. Depending on the amount of drainage, select either a hydrophobic or a hydrophilic material:

- A **hydrophobic** (nonabsorbent, waterproof) material is useful when the wound is relatively free of drainage and the purpose is to protect the ulcer from external contamination.
- A **hydrophilic** (absorbent) material draws excessive drainage away from the ulcer surface, preventing maceration.

A variety of synthetic materials with hydrophilic and hydrophobic properties is available. Unlike cotton gauze dressings, these may be left intact for extended periods. Biologic and synthetic skin substitutes are available that can also prevent tissue dehydration and promote healing (see Chapter 71). However, the use of these products for chronic wounds is often cost prohibitive.

The frequency of dressing changes depends on the amount of necrotic material or exudate. Dry gauze dressings are changed when "strike through" occurs or when the outer layer of the dressing first becomes saturated with exudate. Gauze dressings used for debridement, such as those placed on a wound wet, allowed to dry, and then removed, are changed often enough to take off any loose debris or exudate, usually every 4 to 6 hours. Synthetic dressings are changed when exudate causes the adhesive seal to break and leakage to occur.

Before reapplying any dressing, gently clean the ulcer surface with saline or a nontoxic wound cleanser as prescribed. If an antibacterial cleanser is prescribed, dilute the agent to reduce tissue toxicity and then rinse and dry the surface thoroughly before applying the dressing.

Physical Therapy. The use of daily whirlpool treatments along with dressing changes for debridement can help remove dead tissue. The ulcerated area is immersed in warm tap water that contains an antibacterial cleansing agent. Continuous agitation of the water loosens the debris and washes away exudate and particulate matter. During treatment, clean the ulcer surface with a gauze pad. After treatment the therapist or certified wound specialist often uses instruments to trim away any obvious bits of dead tissue that are still loosely attached to the ulcer surface.

Drug Therapy. Clean, healthy granulation tissue has a blood supply and is capable of providing white blood cells and antibodies to the ulcer surface to combat infection. If extensive necrosis is present or if local tissue defenses are impaired, topical antibacterial agents are often needed to control bacterial growth. (Chapter 71 details the advantages and uses of topical antimicrobial agents.) In the absence of infection, antibiotics are avoided because of the danger of the development of resistant strains of bacteria.

Diet Therapy. Successful healing of pressure ulcers depends on adequate nutritional stores of calories, protein, vitamins, minerals, and water (Zulkowski & Albrecht, 2003). Nutritional deficiencies are common among older adults and chronically ill clients. Such deficiencies increase the risk for skin breakdown and delayed healing of wounds that are already present. Severe protein deficiency inhibits all stages of the healing process and impairs host defenses against bacterial invasion.

To promote healing, encourage the client to eat a well-balanced diet, emphasizing foods containing nutrients vital to cell growth and collagen synthesis (Table 70-7). If the client cannot eat sufficient amounts of food, nasogastric feedings and hyperalimentation via a central venous catheter may be needed to increase protein and caloric intake. Vitamin and mineral supplements are also indicated.

New Technologies. For chronic ulcers that remain open for months, new technologies have had some success. These include electrical stimulation, vacuum-assisted wound closure, and hyperbaric oxygen therapy.

Electrical Stimulation. Applying a low-voltage current to a wound area can increase blood vessel growth and promote granulation (Kloth, 2002). This treatment is usually performed by a certified wound care specialist. A single electrode can be applied directly to a wound through a sterile dressing, or multiple electrodes can be applied around a wound. When multiple electrodes are used, the positive and negative poles are arranged to allow the current to move through the wound area. Voltage intensities ranging from 50 to 150 are delivered in "pulses" that may cause the client to feel a "tingling" sensation. Usually electrical stimulation is performed for one hour each day five to seven times per week. This form of treatment is not used with clients who have a pacemaker or who have a wound over the heart.

Vacuum-Assisted Wound Closure. Vacuum-assisted wound closure has been used successfully to reduce or even close chronic ulcers by enhancing the formation of granulation tissue (Patel, Kinsey, Koperski-Moen, & Bungum, 2000). This technique requires that a suction tube be covered by a special sponge and sealed in place for 48 hours. During that time, continuous low-level negative pressure is applied through the suction tube. Duration of the treatment is determined by the wound's response.

Hyperbaric Oxygen Therapy. Hyperbaric oxygen (HBO) therapy is the administration of oxygen under high pressure, raising the tissue oxygen concentration (Leifer, 2001). This type of therapy is costly and usually reserved for life- or limb-threatening wounds such as burns, necrotizing soft tissue infections, brown recluse spider bites, osteomyelitis, and diabetic ulcers. The client is enclosed in a large chamber and exposed to 100% oxygen at pressures greater than normal atmospheric (sea level) pressure. Systemic oxygen enhances the ability of white blood cells to kill bacteria and reduce swelling. Treatment usually lasts from 60 to 90 minutes. Topical oxygen delivery devices are also available. These devices are applied directly over an open wound to promote local tissue oxygenation. Studies supporting the benefits of topical oxygen are limited, and more research in this area is needed.

SURGICAL MANAGEMENT. Surgical management of a pressure ulcer includes removal of necrotic tissue and skin grafting to close wounds that cannot heal by epithelialization and contraction.

Preoperative Care. Preoperative care is focused on preparing the ulcer to accept a skin graft. Monitor potential donor sites, taking care to maintain the integrity of the donor skin and to avoid minor injuries that may result in infection and graft loss.

Operative Procedures. The operative procedures used for surgical management of pressure ulcers include debridement and grafting. One or both of these procedures may be done.

Debridement, or sharp excision of thick, adherent wound eschar using a scalpel or scissors, may be performed

TABLE 70-7 Foods That Promote Wound Healing

Food	Function
Protein Sources	
Meat Fish Poultry Milk Cheese Eggs Soybeans Legumes Nuts Nutritional supplements	Maintenance and healing of body tissues Antibody production Energy
Carbohydrate Sources	
Whole grains (preferable to enriched because of higher nutritional and fiber content) Enriched grain and cereal products Fruit Juices Vegetables (especially starchy ones: corn, peas, potatoes) Milk Desserts and sweets	Energy Sparing of protein (if diet does not contain sufficient nonprotein calories, protein from body tissues will be broken down to supply energy) Wound healing
Sources of Vitamin C	
Berries Broccoli Brussels sprouts Cabbage Citrus fruits and juices Green peppers Kale Melons Spinach and dark green vegetables Tomatoes Vitamin C-enriched juices	Collagen synthesis Immunity
Zinc Sources	
Same as protein sources Beef Organ meat Shellfish Salmon Poultry Cheese Whole grains Dried beans	Tissue repair (zinc-deficient diet causes poor wound healing, decreased ability to taste, and poor appetite) Protein synthesis
Iron Sources*	
Liver Meat Baked beans Dried fruits Legumes Eggs Dark-green leafy vegetables Blackstrap molasses Whole-grain breads and cereals	Cellular respiration Hemoglobin synthesis
Sources of Vitamin B_{12}	
Liver Organ meats Muscle meats Fish Eggs Shellfish Milk Yogurt Cheese	Protein synthesis
Sources of Vitamin B_6	
Meats Liver Some vegetables (including potatoes) Wheat germ Wheat bran Whole-grain cereals and breads Fish Brewer's yeast Dried beans	Amino acid metabolism
Folate Sources	
Liver Yeast Leafy vegetables Dried beans Green vegetables Nuts Fresh oranges Whole-wheat cereals and breads	Protein synthesis
Water Sources	
Water Milk Juices Gelatin Tomatoes Citrus fruit Melons Vegetables Berries Broths Soups Tea Coffee Carbonated beverages	Maintain condition of the skin (dehydration can lead to tissue breakdown, poor appetite, and constipation)

From Ross, R., & Noe, J. (1983). *Chronic problem wounds.* Boston: Little, Brown & Co.
* Iron cooking utensils add iron to the diet.

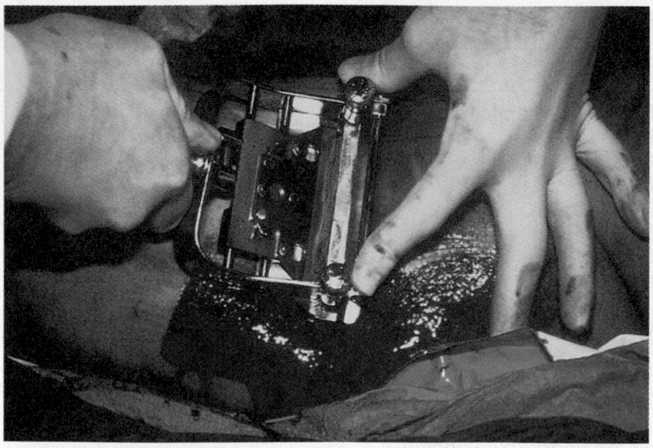

Figure 70-9 ■ Removal of a partial-thickness (split-thickness) skin graft.

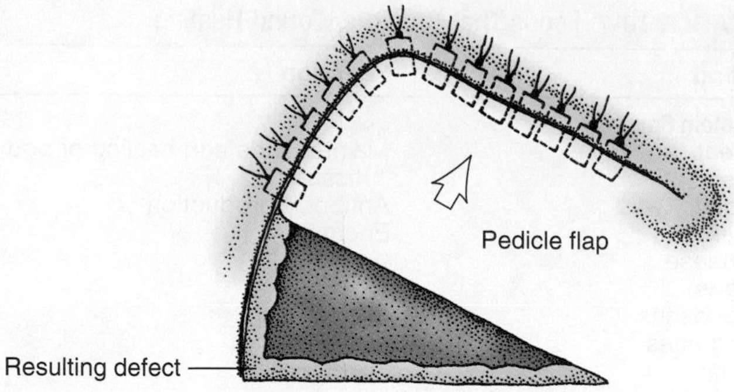

Figure 70-10 ■ A full-thickness pedicle flap of skin is separated and rotated to cover the wound. Blood vessels are left intact. The resultant defect is either primarily closed or covered with skin grafts. The flap is held in place with staples or sutures.

to hasten the removal of the dead tissue, a potential source of infection. Surgical debridement is indicated for severely immunosuppressed clients or those with large, full-thickness ulcers because of the extensive time required for spontaneous separation of eschar. The longer open wounds exist, the greater the risk for systemic sepsis or prolonged hospitalization. Depending on the size and depth of the ulcer and the projected blood loss, debridement can be performed at the bedside, in the treatment room, or in an operating room.

Grafting is used for wound closure when full-thickness ulcers are unable to close and when natural healing would result in loss of joint function, an unacceptable cosmetic appearance, or a high potential for wound recurrence. Successful skin grafting requires a clean and granulating or freshly excised ulcer bed. Partial-thickness (split-thickness) or full-thickness strips of skin are removed from the donor area (Figure 70-9), transferred to the ulcer, and sutured or stapled in place. Full-thickness free grafts and myocutaneous flaps are used to cover deep, massive ulcers or ulcers in which vital structures, such as bone or tendon, are exposed.

Unlike free grafts, a pedicle flap is a full-thickness flap of skin that is raised and rotated to cover the defect, with one edge of the flap still attached to the site of origin to provide a blood supply (Figure 70-10). Because all skin layers are removed, full-thickness donor sites are closed surgically or covered with additional split-thickness skin grafts. Partial-thickness donor sites heal spontaneously if infection is avoided.

Postoperative Care. Postoperative graft sites are immobilized with bulky cotton pressure dressings for 3 to 5 days to allow vascularization, or "take," of the newly grafted skin. Do not disturb the dressing, and encourage elevation and complete rest of the grafted area. Any activity that might cause movement of the dressing against the body and separation of the graft from the wound is prohibited.

After dressings are removed, monitor the graft for indications of failure to vascularize, nonadherence to the wound, or graft necrosis. If a pedicle flap has been used to cover the wound, inspect the edges of the flap at least every 4 hours for changes in color. A pale flap with delayed capillary filling when blanched may have inadequate arterial perfusion. A dusky color or sharp line of color change suggests inadequate venous or lymphatic drainage. Other techniques to monitor trends of blood flow in the graft, depending on the graft's location, include pulse oximetry, Doppler ultrasonography, and transcutaneous oxygen determination.

Postoperative care of donor sites aims to protect the area from injury and infection until healing can occur and to promote comfort. A pressure dressing is usually placed over the donor area to promote hemostasis. After 24 to 48 hours, this outer dressing is removed, revealing a single wound contact layer of fine-mesh gauze or synthetic mesh material.

If the donor site is treated with dry exposure, promote air circulation to the wound by positioning the client to avoid pressure on the site and using an overbed cradle to tent the sheets. In the rare instance when heat lamps are prescribed, place the 60- to 100-watt bulb at least 2 feet from the wound to prevent thermal injury to the skin. After the dressing has dried and formed a "scab," keep the wound dry and undisturbed until healing is evident (at 10 to 14 days). As the donor site heals, the gauze and dried blood lift away from the new epithelium beneath. Trimming the separating gauze close to the skin surface reduces the chance of the client's catching the loose end of the dressing on an object and removing the still adherent gauze before healing is complete. Today most surgeons prefer to dress donor sites with moisture-retentive dressings, such as synthetic transparent films, instead of the traditional dry exposure method of treatment (see Table 70-6).

Because exposed donor sites are initially more painful than graft sites, give pain medication as prescribed and provide other comfort measures as needed. Reposition the client during the immediate period after surgery to promote comfort only if movement of the graft site can be avoided. Offer back rubs to help relieve muscle spasms that occur with reduced mobility. Pay attention to relieving pressure over unaffected bony prominences that may lead to additional ulcers.

Graft and donor sites on posterior body surfaces present a particular problem. For the graft or flap to become fully vascularized or for the donor sites to dry, the client must be immobilized in a side-lying or prone position for 7 to 10 days.

An alternative to this positioning is the use of special low-pressure or air-fluidized beds, which not only reduce ischemia of the graft or flap while the client is supine but also help prevent breakdown of intact skin. A major limitation to the use

TABLE 70-8 Monitoring the Wound

Variable	Frequency of Assessment	Rationale
Wounds Without Tissue Loss		
Examples		
Surgical incisions and clean lacerations closed primarily by sutures or staples		
Observations (Using First Postoperative Dressing Change as Baseline)		
Check for the presence or absence of increased: ■ Localized tenderness ■ Swelling of the incision line ■ Erythema of the incision line >1 cm on each side of wound ■ Localized heat	At least every 24 hr until sutures or staples are removed	To detect cellulitis (bacterial infections)*
Check for the presence or absence of: ■ Purulent drainage from any portion of the incision site ■ Localized fluctuance (from fluid accumulation) and tenderness beneath a *portion* of the wound when palpated	At least every 24 hr until sutures or staples are removed	To detect abscess formation related to presence of foreign body (suture material) or deeper would infection*
Check for the presence or absence of approximation (sealing) of wound edges with or without serosanguineous drainage	At least every 24 hr until sutures or staples are removed	To detect potential for wound dehiscence
Wounds with Tissue Loss		
Examples		
Partial- or full-thickness skin loss caused by pressure necrosis, vascular disease, trauma, etc., and allowed to heal by secondary intention		
Observations		
Wound Size		
Measure wound size at greatest length and width using a metric ruler or, for asymmetric ulcers, by tracing the wound onto a piece of plastic film or sheeting (plastic template). Compare all subsequent measurements against the initial measurement.	At least every week	To detect increase in wound size and depth secondary to infectious process
Ulcer Base		
Check for the presence or absence of: ■ Necrotic tissue (loose or adherent) ■ Presence or absence of foul odor from wound when dressing is changed Note the frequency of dressing changes or dressing reinforcements owing to drainage.	At least every 24 hr	To detect the need for debridement or the response to treatment (necrotic tissue) and to detect local wound infection (frequent dressing changes and foul odor)
Wound Margins		
Check for the presence or absence of: ■ Erythema and swelling extending outward >1 cm from wound margins ■ Increased tenderness at wound margins	At least every 24 hr or at each dressing change	To detect wound infection*
Systemic Response		
Check for the presence or absence of elevated body temperature, WBCs, or positive blood culture	As needed	To detect bacteremia

WBCs, White blood cells.
*The wounds of clients who are severely immunosuppressed or those wounds with compromised blood supply may not exhibit a typical inflammatory response to local wound infection.

of these beds is cost, which is usually outweighed by the potential for decreased morbidity and length of hospital stay.

RISK FOR INFECTION AND WOUND EXTENSION

NOC **PLANNING: EXPECTED OUTCOMES.** The client with a pressure ulcer is expected to remain free of wound infection or systemic sepsis. Indicators include that the client will have mild or no:

- White blood cell elevation
- Wound site culture colonization
- Purulent drainage
- Increase in wound size or depth

INTERVENTIONS. Closely monitor the ulcer's progress so that timely treatment with topical and systemic antibiotics can be started if ulcer deterioration occurs. Steps are taken to reduce introduction of pathogenic organisms to the ulcer through direct contact.

Monitoring Ulcer Progress. Monitoring the ulcer's appearance using objective criteria allows evaluation of the response to treatment and early recognition of infection. If an ulcer shows no progress toward healing within 3 weeks, the treatment plan should be re-evaluated. Table 70-8 outlines objectives of monitoring wounds with and without tissue loss. Clients who are at highest risk for infection are those who are older, have white blood cell disorders, are receiving steroid therapy, or have wounds with a compromised blood supply.

Prevention of Infection and Wound Extension. Complications of infection and wound extension are avoided by monitoring of the ulcer's progress and by prevention of new ulcer formation. Report the following signs to the physician:

- Sudden deterioration of the ulcer as evidenced by an increase in the size or depth of the lesion
- Changes in the color or texture of the granulation tissue
- Changes in the quantity, color, or odor of exudate

Also check for the classic signs of wound infection: increased redness, edema, purulent and malodorous drainage, and tenderness of the wound margins. These manifestations may occur with or without clinical signs of bacteremia, such as fever, an elevated white blood cell count, and positive blood cultures. Use appropriate interventions to prevent the formation of new pressure ulcers and to prevent early-stage ulcers from progressing to deeper wounds (Chart 70-3; see also Chart 70-2).

Maintaining a Safe Environment. Because of the variety of organisms in the hospital environment, keeping an ulcer totally free of bacteria is impossible. Optimal ulcer management is based on maintaining acceptably low levels of organisms through meticulous wound care and reducing contamination with pathogenic organisms. All personnel must use standard precautions to prevent direct contact with ulcer secretions and cross-contamination among clients. All personnel must practice thorough handwashing before and after dressing changes and properly dispose of soiled dressings and linens.

Community-Based Care

Clients with pressure ulcers may be in acute care, subacute care, long-term care, or home care settings. If pressure ulcer therapy requires hospitalization, most clients with pressure ulcers are discharged before complete wound closure is achieved. Discharge may be to the home setting or to a long-term care facility, depending on the degree of debilitation and other client factors.

HOME CARE MANAGEMENT

Care of the ulcer in the client's home is similar to care in the hospital. Most dressing supplies and pressure-relief devices can be easily obtained at the local pharmacy or medical supply store. If debridement of the ulcer is still needed, a handheld shower device or forceful irrigation of the wound with a 35-mL syringe and 19-gauge angiocatheter can be substituted for whirlpool therapy.

Clients with chronic pressure ulcers are often depressed about their debilitated state, which may affect their adherence to wound care measures. Many clients cannot change their own dressings because of distress over an altered body image or the pain of dressing removal. Others are dependent on family members or support personnel because of limited physical mobility or inability to reach the wound.

For some clients, drastic changes in daily activities are needed to promote healing. Clients with pressure ulcers on the legs may need frequent rest periods with leg elevation to avoid or reduce edema. Immobile clients with pressure ulcers require around-the-clock repositioning as often as every 2 to 4 hours to prevent further breakdown, which takes its toll on family members or caregivers. Explain the rationale for activity changes to the client and family and explore alternative ways of coping with these changes.

HEALTH TEACHING

Before the client is discharged, the client or person who will be performing the wound care should demonstrate facility in removing the dressing, cleaning the wound, and applying the dressing. When choosing a dressing to be used at home, consider the client's or caregiver's ability to apply the dressing properly. If the client's finances are limited, also address the cost of the dressing material. Some dressings may be easier to apply and less expensive than other materials. At times, the more expensive dressing materials that require less frequent changing may be preferred. Explain the manifestations of wound infection.

Encourage the client to eat a balanced diet with frequent high-protein snacks. Discuss diet preferences with the client, and suggest foods that promote wound healing (see Table 70-7). The health care provider may prescribe vitamin and mineral supplements if there are dietary deficiencies.

If the client is incontinent, emphasize the need to keep the skin clean and dry. If bowel and bladder training is not possible, discuss the use of absorbent underpads, briefs, and topical moisture barrier creams and ointments as a method to reduce skin exposure to urine and feces.

HEALTH CARE RESOURCES

A home care nurse may be needed to follow wound progress after the client is discharged. The hospital nurse provides details of ulcer size and appearance and any special wound care needs to the nurse in the home, who can then accurately judge changes in ulcer appearance. Chart 70-5 is guideline for a focused assessment of the client with pressure ulcers.

To reduce waste and to help decrease the overall cost of treatment, emphasize proper use of dressing materials. Clean tap water and nonsterile supplies are acceptable for treatment of chronic wounds in the home and are less costly than sterile products. Nonsterile dressing materials can often be purchased in bulk from a local medical supply store at reduced cost. However, items reused in the home can become contaminated with pathogens and pose a risk to some clients. (See the Evidence-Based Practice for Nursing box on p. 1595.) Stress the importance of proper cleaning of reused items and of handwashing when before touching any supplies.

The client with activity restrictions may need daily assistance from a home care aide. Consultation with a physical therapist may be appropriate to help the client and family or significant others continue rehabilitation efforts in the home.

Critical Thinking Challenge

Despite preventive care, the diabetic client with pneumonia developed a stage II pressure ulcer on her left heel. She is being discharged to home today. She has stated that she will keep her foot in the "down" position to relieve pressure on the heel.

1. Is keeping the foot in the down position a good strategy? Why or why not?

CHART 70-5

HOME CARE ASSESSMENT of
The Client at Risk for Pressure Ulcers

Assess cardiovascular status:
- Presence or absence of peripheral edema
- Hand-vein filling in the dependent position
- Neck-vein filling in the recumbent and sitting positions
- Weight gain or loss

Assess cognition and mental status:
- Level of consciousness
- Orientation to time, place, and person
- Can the client accurately read a seven-word sentence containing no words greater than three syllables?

Assess condition of skin:
- Assess general skin cleanliness.
- Observe all skin areas, paying particular attention to bony prominences and those areas in greatest contact with the bed and other firm surfaces.
- Measure and record any areas of redness or loss of integrity.
- If possible, photograph areas of concern.
- Note the presence or absence of skin tenting over the sternum or the forehead.
- Note the moistness of skin and mucous membranes.
- If wounds are present, remove dressings (noting condition of dressings), cleanse the wound, and compare with previous notations of wound condition.
  - Presence, amount, and nature of exudate
  - Use a ruler to measure wound diameter and depth
  - Amount (%) and type of necrotic tissue
  - Presence of granulation/epithelium
  - Presence or absence of cellulitis
  - Presence or absence of odor

Take the client's temperature.

Assess the client's understanding of illness and compliance with treatment:
- Manifestations to report to health care provider
- Mediation plan (correct timing and dose)
- Ambulation or positioning schedule
- Dressing changes/skin care
- Diet modifications (24-hour diet recall)

Assess the client's nutritional status:
- Change in muscle mass
- Lackluster nails, sparse hair
- Recent weight loss of more than 10% of usual weight
- Impaired oral intake
- Difficulty swallowing
- Generalized edema

2. What care techniques will you teach this client to help heal this ulcer? (You may want to review diabetic foot care in Chapter 68.)

evolve For suggested answer guidelines, go to http://evolve.elsevier.com/Iggy/.

Evaluation: Outcomes

Evaluate the care of the client with a pressure ulcer on the basis of the identified nursing diagnoses and collaborative problems. The expected outcomes include that the client will:
- Experience wound healing by secondary intention as evidenced by granulation, epithelialization, and resolution of wound size
- Develop skin thickness in expected range at ulcer area
- Remain infection free

Specific indicators for these outcomes are listed for each nursing diagnosis and collaborative problem under the Planning and Implementation section (see earlier).

EVIDENCE-BASED PRACTICE for Nursing

Reuse of supplies increases contamination risk

Zwanziger, P., & Roper, S. (2002). Bacterial counts and types found on wound care supplies used in the home setting. *Journal of Wound, Ostomy, and Continence Nursing. 29*(2), 83-87.

The purpose of this prospective, descriptive study was to determine the length of time needed for wound care supplies left in the home setting to become contaminated. Homes of 17 clients with wounds were selected as study sites. The level of home cleanliness varied from filthy to clean. Forty-seven wound care supplies used by home care nurses, caregivers and clients were cultured before placement in the homes and recultured after 7 days in the home setting. New supplies were then cultured, placed in the homes, and recultured after 14 days. The supplies included scissors, plastic wound-measuring guides, plastic cleanser nozzles, forceps, normal saline irrigant, and gauze sponges, squares and strips. Caregivers and clients were instructed in the proper use and cleaning methods for the supplies.

Data collection occurred at 7 and 14 days. Data collectors used sterile gloves and appropriate containers to transport the study items to the laboratory for culture. Handling of the items for culture and culture techniques were within recommended guidelines to prevent accidental contamination.

Seventy-five percent of items had some degree of contamination after being in the home. Items left in the home for 14 days had greater numbers of bacterial colonies and more varieties of bacteria than did those left in the home for only seven days. Multiple use items, such as scissors and wound measuring devices, harbored some of the more virulent pathogens commonly associated with wound infection.

Level of Evidence: 6—Descriptive study.

Critique. The study was appropriately designed for the research questions. Although the use of the supplies and cleanliness of the homes varied, this condition is consistent with the reality of home care.

Implications for Nursing. Many protocols stress that clean technique rather than sterile technique can be used for wound care and dressing changes in the home because the home environment tends to harbor fewer pathogenic organisms than do acute care environments. However, such protocols may erroneously lead nurses, clients, and caregivers to believe that wound infections are not likely in the home setting. Reusing supplies and equipment for wound care requires appropriate cleaning to prevent serious wound infections. Nurses must ensure that caregivers and clients understand how microorganisms are transmitted from one object to another and how to properly use/clean/dispose of these items. Appropriate cleaning and storage of wound care supplies is critical to the objective of wound closure and infection prevention.

COMMON INFECTIONS

PATHOPHYSIOLOGY

Bacterial Infections

Bacterial skin lesions usually start at the hair follicle, where bacteria easily collect and grow in the warm, moist environment. **Folliculitis** is a superficial infection involving only the upper portion of the follicle and is usually caused by *Staphylococcus* (Figure 70-11). **Furuncles** (boils) are also caused by *Staphylococcus*, but the infection is much deeper in the follicle (Figure 70-12). **Cellulitis** is a generalized infection with either *Staphylococcus* or *Streptococcus* and involves the deeper connective tissue.

Minor skin trauma usually occurs before the appearance of folliculitis and furuncles and may or may not contribute

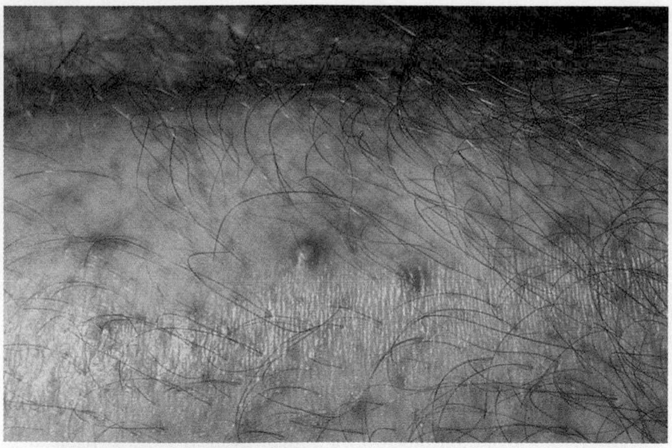

Figure 70-11 ■ Folliculitis.

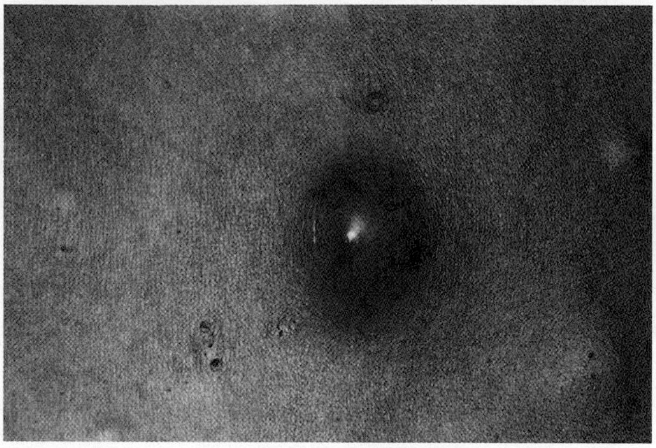

Figure 70-12 ■ A furuncle.

to the development of cellulitis. Clients may spread the infection to other parts of their bodies by scratching or rubbing the skin with fingernails that have organisms under them. Furuncles are more likely to occur in areas of heat and moisture, such as in the hair-bearing skin-fold areas. Cellulitis can occur as a result of secondary bacterial infection of an open wound, or it may be unrelated to skin trauma.

Viral Infections

HERPES SIMPLEX VIRUS

Herpes simplex virus (HSV) infection is the most common viral infection of adult skin. HSV infections are of two types. Type 1 (HSV 1) infections cause the classic recurring cold sore. The severity of the disease increases with age and is worse when the client is immunosuppressed. Genital herpes, caused by type 2 infection (HSV-2), is also recurrent (see Chapter 80).

After the first infection, the virus remains in the body in a dormant state in the nerve ganglia, and the client has no symptoms. Reactivation stimulates the virus to travel the pathway of sensory nerves to the skin, where lesions reappear. In healthy people, recurrence of HSV infection is triggered by physical or psychological stressors, such as sunburn, trauma, fever, menses, and fatigue. The virus can also be spread by direct contact between an actively infected person and a susceptible host. *Autoinoculation,* or transfer of either viral type from one part of the body to another, is also possible.

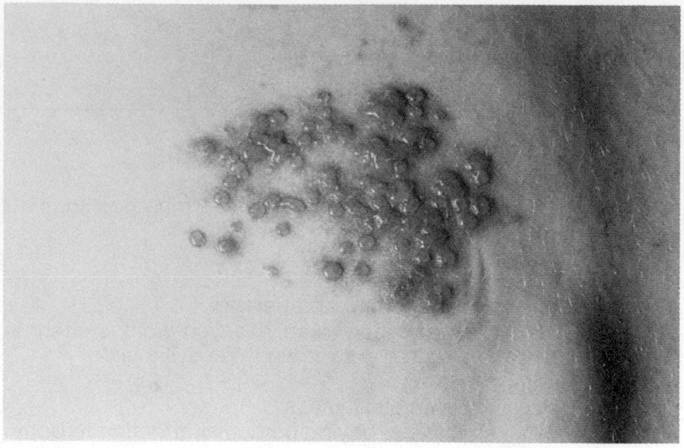

Figure 70-13 ■ Herpes simplex.

The time span between episodes and the severity of each attack varies. Outbreaks of oral herpes simplex usually last 3 to 10 days. The client sheds virus and is contagious for the first 3 to 5 days. The client may have tingling or burning of the lip before any lesion is evident.

The most common clinical picture of HSV 1 infection is isolated or grouped vesicles on a red base (Figure 70-13). The infection can occur anywhere on the skin and may be spread by respiratory droplets or by direct contact with an active lesion or virus-containing fluid (such as saliva).

Herpetic whitlow is a form of herpes simplex infection occurring on the fingertips of medical personnel who have come in contact with viral secretions. This form of herpes can easily be spread to clients. Immunosuppressed clients are at increased risk for severe and persistent eruptions that can lead to life-threatening complications.

HERPES ZOSTER

Herpes zoster (shingles) is caused by reactivation of the dormant varicella-zoster virus in clients who have previously had chickenpox. The dormant virus resides in the dorsal root ganglia of the sensory cranial and spinal nerves. The lesions of herpes zoster infections are similar to those of herpes simplex, but they have a different distribution pattern (Figure 70-14). Multiple lesions occur in a segmental distribution on the skin area innervated by the infected nerve. Herpes zoster eruptions usually occur after several days of discomfort, which may vary from minor irritation and itching to severe, deep pain. The eruption usually lasts several weeks. **Postherpetic neuralgia,** pain persisting after the lesions have resolved, is a common complication in older clients.

Herpes zoster is a disease of immunosuppression, occurring most often and with greater severity in older people or in anyone who is immunosuppressed for any reason. The disorder can be accompanied by fever and malaise, often progressing to visceral involvement. Herpes zoster is contagious to people who have not previously had chickenpox.

Complications include full-thickness skin necrosis, Bell's palsy, or eye infection, and scarring if the virus is introduced into the eye.

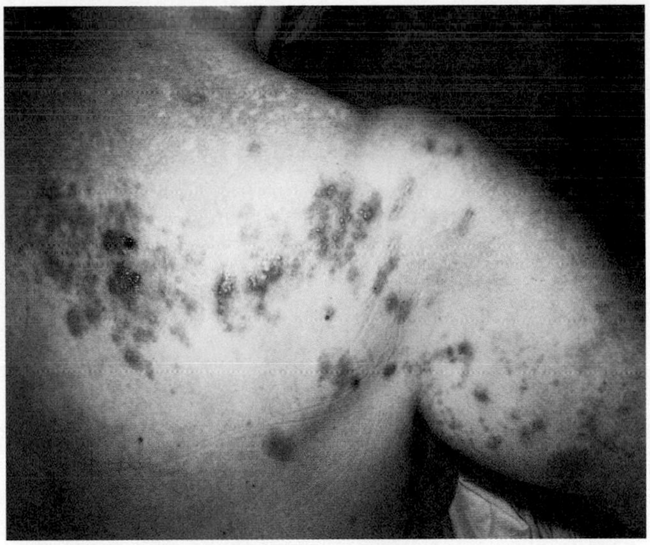

Figure 70-14 ■ Herpes zoster.

TABLE 70-9 Tinea Infections

Infection	Location
Tinea pedis	Feet (athlete's foot)
Tinea manus	Hands
Tinea cruris	Groin (jock itch)
Tinea corporis	Smooth skin surfaces (ringworm)
Tinea capitis	Scalp
Tinea barbae	Beard

Fungal Infections

Superficial fungal (dermatophyte) infections can differ in lesion appearance, anatomic location, and species of the infecting organism. The term *tinea* is used to describe dermatophytoses. Table 70-9 lists the anatomic locations of the various categories of infection.

Depending on the species, dermatophytes live mainly in the soil, on animals, and on humans. Superficial infection can start only if conditions are right for inoculation and maintenance of the organism in the outer layers of the skin.

Dermatophyte infections occur when the infecting organism comes in contact with impaired skin in a susceptible host. Most infections are spread by direct contact with infected humans or animals. Certain types of infections, such as tinea capitis and tinea corporis, can be transmitted by means of inanimate objects. For example, tinea capitis can be spread by the sharing of contaminated combs, brushes, hats, pillowcases, and similar objects from people with poor personal hygiene.

◆COLLABORATIVE MANAGEMENT

◆Assessment

HISTORY

The manifestations of the skin infection provide direction for questions and collection of data to confirm a suspected diagnosis. To differentiate among the possible causes of the lesions, concentrate on risk factors for each type of infection. If the location and appearance of lesions suggest a bacterial infection, explore any recent history of skin trauma as well as past or current staphylococcal or streptococcal infections. Ask whether fever and malaise are also present.

Lesions appearing on the lips, in the mouth, or in the genital region are more likely to be a possible viral infection. Ask about the following:

- A history of similar lesions in the same location
- Signs of burning, tingling, or pain
- Recent stress factors that may have precipitated the outbreak
- Recent contact with an infected person

Information that the same type of lesions has occurred before is important in helping to differentiate viral from bacterial lesions. If herpes zoster is suspected, ask whether the client has had chickenpox in the past and about a history of shingles.

The type of information you should ask a client with probable dermatophyte infection depends on the location of the lesions. If tinea corporis or tinea capitis is present, assess the social and environmental factors that may have contributed to infection, such as direct contact with an infected person, poor personal hygiene practices, or frequent contact with animals. If tinea cruris and tinea pedis are suspected, ask the client about the type and frequency of athletic activities.

PHYSICAL ASSESSMENT/CLINICAL MANIFESTATIONS

Because most skin infections are contagious, take precautions to prevent the spread of infection when performing a physical assessment. Chart 70-6 lists the manifestations of common skin infections.

LABORATORY ASSESSMENT

When pustules are present in bacterial infections, the infecting organism is confirmed by swab culture of the purulent material. Blood cultures may be helpful, especially if the client is showing clinical signs of bacteremia.

Viral infections are confirmed by *Tzanck's smear* and viral culture. Tzanck's smear is a cytologic examination in which cells from the base of a lesion are examined under a microscope. The presence of multinucleated giant cells confirms a viral infection, although the exact virus is not identified.

Fungal infections are confirmed by a potassium hydroxide (KOH) test. Scales from the lesions are scraped, prepared with KOH, and examined under a microscope. The presence of fungal hyphae confirms the diagnosis. In addition to a KOH test, a fungal culture may be needed. Occasionally a skin biopsy is performed to obtain organisms for identification.

◆Interventions

Most skin infections heal well with nonsurgical management. Surgery may be required when an infectious agent is present in deep tissue layers.

NONSURGICAL MANAGEMENT. Nursing interventions focus on meticulous skin care and prevention of infection spread. In some instances, drug therapy is needed.

Skin Care. Instruct clients with bacterial infections to bathe daily with an antibacterial soap. Instruct the client to remove any pustules or crusts gently so that topical drugs can be more easily absorbed. Teach the client to apply warm

CHART 70-6

KEY FEATURES of
Common Skin Infections

Clinical Manifestations	Distribution
Bacterial Infections	
Folliculitis	
Isolated erythematous pustules occur singly or in groups; hairs grow from centers of many of the lesions. Occasional papules are present. There is little or no associated discomfort. There is no residual scarring.	Areas of hair-bearing skin, especially buttocks, thighs, beard area, and scalp
Furuncle	
Small, tender erythematous nodules become pus filled and more tender over time. Lesions may be single or multiple and also recurrent. Regional lymphadenopathy is sometimes present; fever is rare. Occasional scarring results.	Areas of hair-bearing skin, especially buttocks, thighs, abdomen, posterior neck regions, and axillae
Cellulitis	
Localized area of inflammation may enlarge rapidly if not treated. Redness, warmth, edema, tenderness, and pain are present. On rare occasions, blisters are present. Cellulitis is often accompanied by lymphadenopathy and fever.	Lower legs, areas of persistent lymphedema, and areas of skin trauma (leg ulcer, puncture wound, and others)
Viral Infections	
Herpes Simplex	
Grouped vesicles are present on an erythematous base. Vesicles evolve to pustules, which rupture, weep, and crust. Older lesions may appear as punched-out, shallow erosions with well-defined borders. Lesions are associated with itching, stinging, or pain. Secondary bacterial infection with necrosis is possible in immunocompromised clients.	Type 1 classically on the face and type 2 on the genitalia, but either may develop in any area where inoculation has occurred; recurrent infections occur repeatedly in the same skin area
Herpes Zoster	
Lesions are similar in appearance to herpes simplex and also progress with weeping and crusting. Grouped lesions present unilaterally along a segment or skin following the pathway of a spinal or cranial nerve (dermatomal distribution). Eruption is preceded by deep pain and itching. Postherpetic neuralgia is common in older adults. Secondary infection with necrosis is possible in immunocompromised clients.	Anterior or posterior trunk following involved dermatome; face, sometimes involving trigeminal nerve and eye
Fungal Infections	
Dermatophytosis	
Annular or serpiginous patches are present with elevated borders, scaling, and central clearing. Itching is common. Lesions may be single or multiple.	Anywhere on the body
Candidiasis	
Erythematous macular eruption occurs with isolated pustules or papules at the border (satellite lesions). Candidiasis is associated with burning and itching. Oral lesions (thrush) appear as creamy white plaques on an inflamed mucous membrane. Cracks or fissures at the corners of the mouth may be present.	Skin-fold areas: perineal and perianal region, axillae, beneath breasts, and between the fingers; under wet or occlusive dressings Lesions possibly present on the oral or vaginal mucous membranes

compresses twice a day to furuncles or areas of cellulitis to increase comfort.

Applying astringent compresses, such as Burow's solution, to viral lesions for 20 minutes three times a day promotes crust formation and healing. Compresses also relieve the irritation and pain associated with herpetic infection. Instruct the client to avoid constricting garments that might rub the lesions and increase irritation.

Most superficial skin infections resolve more quickly if the involved skin is allowed to dry between treatments. Excessive moisture, especially if occluded by dressings, clothing, or bedding, promotes growth of organisms. If the client is bedridden, position him or her for optimal air circulation to the area and avoid occlusive dressings or garments.

Isolation Precautions. Take precautions to reduce the spread of pathogenic organisms to other people. For most superficial bacterial infections, proper handwashing prevents cross-contamination. However, when hospitalized clients are colonized with *Staphylococcus* that is resistant to antibiotic therapy, strict adherence to isolation procedures is necessary.

Of the dermatophyte infections, tinea capitis, tinea corporis, and tinea pedis are most easily transmitted to others. Instruct clients to avoid sharing personal items, such as hairbrushes, articles of clothing, or footwear. Repeated infections transmitted by dogs or cats may mean that clients might have to get rid of a family pet to control infections.

Drug Therapy. Commonly used topical drugs for the treatment of bacterial, viral, and fungal skin infections are listed in Chart 70-7.

Mild bacterial infections of the skin usually resolve with topical antibacterial treatment. Clients with extensive infections, especially if fever or lymphadenopathy is present, require systemic antibiotic therapy.

Acyclovir (Zovirax) or penciclovir (Denavir) is used for the treatment of viral infections. Topical treatment decreases the numbers of active virus on the skin surface and reduces pain in primary herpetic infections and localized lesions in immunocompromised clients. Topical treatment is of little benefit in recurrent infection. Intravenous (IV) administration is limited to severe primary infections and immunosuppressed clients with symptoms of systemic infection.

Topical antifungal agents are used for clients with dermatophyte and yeast infections. An imidazole cream is applied to the infected skin at least twice a day until the lesions have cleared. To prevent recurrence, therapy is usually continued for 1 to 2 weeks after clearing. In some instances, antifungal powders may also help to suppress fungal growth. For widespread or resistant fungal infections, systemic antifungal agents, such as ketoconazole (Nizoral), are given.

SURGICAL MANAGEMENT. Surgery is not usually performed for a superficial skin infection, except for incision and drainage of furuncles. In severely immunocompromised clients, superficial lesions can progress to full-thickness wounds requiring surgical excision.

CUTANEOUS ANTHRAX

PATHOPHYSIOLOGY

Cutaneous anthrax is an infection caused by the spores of the bacterium *Bacillus anthracis.* The infection can be confined to the skin, or it may be systemic. At first a raised vesicle appears on an exposed body area such as the head or arms. The lesion may itch and often resembles an insect bite. Within a few days, the center of the vesicle becomes hemorrhagic and sinks inward. An area of necrosis and ulceration begins. Usually this process is painless. The tissue around the wound swells and can become quite edematous. With necrosis an eschar forms. The two features that distinguish anthrax lesions from insect bites or other skin lesions are the fact that it is painless and that eschar forms regardless of treatment. Clients may have only one lesion, or there may be multiple lesions, usually in the same body area.

Some clients develop glandular symptoms with cutaneous anthrax. The entire area becomes edematous and tender. Fever and chills may be present, as may enlarged lymph nodes.

COLLABORATIVE MANAGEMENT

Diagnosis is made based on the appearance of the lesions, a culture that is positive for the organism, or the presence of anthrax antibodies in the client's blood. Cultures are most easily obtained in the vesicle stage. Once the eschar is formed, a biopsy may be needed for culture. Blood cultures should be obtained from clients who have a fever.

Oral antibiotics for 60 days are indicated for clients who have no edema, systemic symptoms, and the lesions are not located on the head or neck. The antibiotics of choice are ciprofloxacin (Cipro) or doxycycline (Doryx, Vibramycin). For clients who have a fever, have lesions on the head or neck, are pregnant, or have extensive edema, antibiotics are given intravenously and then followed by an oral course of 60 days.

PARASITIC DISORDERS

Parasitic skin disorders occur most often in clients with poor hygiene and substandard living conditions. Any client who shows obvious signs of a self-care deficit should be examined for these contagious parasitic infections.

Pediculosis

PATHOPHYSIOLOGY

Pediculosis is an infestation by human lice: *pediculosis capitis* (head lice), *pediculosis corporis* (body lice), and *pediculosis pubis* (pubic, or crab, lice). Human lice are oval and 2 to 4 mm long. The female louse lays hundreds of eggs, called *nits,* which are deposited at the hair shaft base in hair-bearing areas.

COLLABORATIVE MANAGEMENT

The most common symptom of pediculosis is itching **(pruritus).** Excoriation from scratching may or may not be present. In addition to causing discomfort, these parasites can also be carriers of disease such as typhus and recurrent fever.

Assessment

Pediculosis capitis occurs more commonly in women than in men, especially on the sides and back of the scalp. Itching, the result of biting of the scalp by the parasites, is intense. A secondary infection may also be present from scratching.

Because the louse is difficult to see, examine the scalp for visible white flecks, the nits of the female louse. Matting and crusting of the scalp along with a foul odor indicates a probable secondary infection.

Pediculosis corporis is caused by lice that live and lay eggs in the seams of clothing. The parasites also cause itching. The only visible sign of infestation may be excoriations on the trunk, abdomen, or extremities.

Pediculosis pubis causes intense itching of the vulvar or perirectal region. Pubic lice, which are more compact and crablike in appearance than body lice, can be contracted from infested bed linens or during sexual intercourse with an infected person. Although lice are usually found in the genital region, it can also infest the axillae, the eyelashes, and the chest.

Interventions

The treatment of pediculosis is chemical killing of the parasites with agents such as lindane (Bio-Well, Kwell, Kwellada)

CHART 70-7

DRUG THERAPY for Skin Disorders

Drug	Usual Dosage	Nursing Interventions	Rationales
Antibacterial Drugs			
Ointments			
Neomycin sulfate Combination antibiotics (Neosporin, Bacitracin, Polysporin, Mycitracin) Gentamicin (Garamycin) Chloramphenicol (Chloromycetin) Povidone-iodine (Betadine) Bactroban	Apply a thin layer to the affected area three times daily. Dressing is optional.	Gently clean affected areas with saline, half-strength peroxide, or tap water before applying ointments. Avoid rubbing ointment into skin. Apply with downward strokes in direction of hair growth. Assess for worsening of problem in spite of topical therapy. Discontinue use if rash appears.	Atraumatic cleaning promotes healing by preventing further injury to skin cells. Cleaning helps to remove exudate, crusts, and residual medication and increases the effectiveness of therapy. Ointments can irritate hair follicles and lead to folliculitis. Client may become allergic to active ingredients, the ointment base, or added preservatives.
Creams			
Silver sulfadiazine (Silvadene, SSD, Flamazine ✱)	Apply in layer about 1⁄16-inch thick to affected areas three times daily and PRN. Dressing is optional.	Assess for allergy to sulfa drugs. Gently clean affected areas with saline, half-strength hydrogen peroxide, or tap water before reapplying. If affected areas are left open without dressings, reapply cream PRN between cleanings to maintain a layer of cream at all times. Monitor white blood cell count for drop to $<5000/mm^3$.	Use should be avoided in clients with a suspected or known sulfa allergy. Cleaning removes crusts, exudate, and caked-on medication while promoting percutaneous absorption of drug. Cream base melts with an increase in body or room temperature and is easily rubbed off with movement if left uncovered. Use of silver sulfadiazine over large skin surface areas has been associated with a transient leukopenia (cause unknown).
Antifungal Drugs			
Ointments and Creams			
Clotrimazole (Lotrimin, Mycelex, Canesten ✱) Nystatin (Mycolog II, Mycostatin, Nilstat) Ciclopirox olamine (Loprox) Miconazole nitrate (Monistat-Derm 2%) Econazole (Spectazole, Ecostatin ✱) Tolnaftate (Tinactin) Haloprogin (Halotex ✱) Undecylenic acid (Desenex) Ketoconazole (Nizoral)	Apply a thin layer to the affected area three times daily.	Teach the importance of thoroughly drying the skin before applying medication. Position bedridden clients for maximal air circulation to involved areas. Emphasize wearing nonconstricting cotton garments to absorb perspiration.	Moist environment promotes the growth of fungal organisms. Increasing air circulation to the affected areas promotes drying. Cream base is easily removed with perspiration, decreasing the effectiveness of therapy.
Powders			
Nystatin (Mycostatin) Tolnaftate (Zeasorb-AF 1%)	Apply a thin dusting of powder to the affected area three times daily.	Teach the client to thoroughly dry skin before applying powder.	In addition to discouraging the growth of fungal organisms, a dry skin surface minimizes caking of powder in skin fold areas.
Oral Preparations			
Nystatin (Mycostatin oral suspension, Nilstat oral suspension)	Rinse the mouth four times daily with 4-6 mL (400,000-600,000 units) and swallow.	Teach the client to coat the entire oral cavity with drug and hold the suspension in the mouth for several minutes before swallowing.	Effectiveness of drug is dependent on good contact of drug with mucous membrane surfaces.
Clotrimazole (Mycelex troche)	Take 1 troche five times daily.	Teach the client to let troche dissolve slowly in the mouth.	

CHART 70-7

DRUG THERAPY for Skin Disorders—*cont'd*

Drug	Usual Dosage	Nursing Interventions	Rationales
Anti-Inflammatory Drugs **Potent Fluorinated Steroid Preparations** Clobetasol propionate (Temovate 0.05%) Triamcinolone acetonide (Aristocort 0.5%, Kenalog 0.5%, Triaderm✱ 0.5%) Amcinonide (Cyclocort 0.1%)	Apply a small amount to affected areas no more than 4 times in 24 hr.	Teach the client to use the least amount of drug possible to cover the treatment site and to use the drug *only* under the direction of a physician.	Overuse of topical steroid preparations can cause serious side effects, including skin thinning (atrophy), superficial dilated blood vessels (telangiectasia), acne-like eruptions, and adrenal suppression. The incidence of side effects increases proportionately with the potency of the steroid and is most common with prolonged widespread use of the high-potency preparations.
Betamethasone dipropionate (Diprosone 0.05%, Betaderm✱ 0.5%) Diflorasone diacetate (Maxiflor 0.05%, Florone 0.05%) Halcinonide (Halog 0.025%) Fluocinonide (Lidex 0.05%, Topsyn gel✱ 0.05%, Lidemol✱ 0.05%, Topsyn✱ 0.05%) Fluocinolone acetonide (Synalar-HP 0.2%, Fluoderm✱ 0.2%) Desoximetasone (Topicort 0.25%) Betamethasone benzoate (Uticort 0.025%, Novobetamet✱ 0.025%)		Never apply highly potent steroid preparations to the face, genital area, or skin fold areas.	Absorption of topical steroids is much higher in these areas, and the associated side effects are more severe.
Medium-Potency Fluorinated Steroid Preparations Triamcinolone acetonide (Kenalog 0.025%, 0.1%; Aristocort 0.025%, 0.1%) Flurandrenolide (Cordran 0.5%, 0.025%) Fluocinolone acetonide (Fluonid 0.025%, Synalar 0.025%) Desoximetasone (Topicort LP 0.05%) Betamethasone valerate (Valisone 0.1%)		Teach the client to hydrate the skin before applying a topical steroid.	Skin hydration increases percutaneous absorption and maximizes the effectiveness of topical treatment.
Low-Potency Nonfluorinated Steroid Preparations Hydrocortisone 0.5%, 1.0%, 2.5% Desonide (Tridesilon) Hydrocortisone valerate (Westcort)		Teach the client to hydrate the skin before applying a topical steroid.	Skin hydration increases percutaneous absorption and maximizes the effectiveness of topical treatment.
Antiviral Drugs **Ointments** Acyclovir (Zovirax)	Apply to affected areas six times daily.	Teach the client to use topical acyclovir only under the direction of a physician for primary infections.	Topical acyclovir has no proven clinical benefit in the prevention or treatment of recurrent infections.
		Emphasize precautionary measures to prevent transmission of infection while the lesion is present.	There is no evidence that topical treatment prevents transmission of infection.

or topical malathion (Ovide, Prioderm). In the case of pediculosis capitis, areas where the client's head has rested (such as on pillows or chair backs) are also treated. Clothing and bed linens should be washed in hot water or dry-cleaned. The use of a fine-toothed comb can help remove nits from an infested scalp but alone does not cure the infection. In all cases of louse infestation, social contacts are treated when possible.

Scabies

PATHOPHYSIOLOGY

Scabies is a contagious skin disease caused by mite infestations. Scabies infections are transmitted by close and prolonged contact with an infested companion or infested bedding. Infestation is common among clients with poor hygiene or crowded living conditions. The scabies mite is carried by pets and is found among schoolchildren and institutionalized older clients.

COLLABORATIVE MANAGEMENT

Scabies is manifested by curved or linear ridges in the skin. The itching is more intense than with pediculosis, and clients often report that the itching becomes unbearable at night.

The visible white skin ridges are formed by burrowing of the mite into the outer skin layers. Closely examine the skin between the fingers and on the palms and inner aspects of the wrists, where these ridges are most common. A hypersensitivity reaction to the mite results in excoriated erythematous papules, pustules, and crusted lesions on the elbows, nipples, lower abdomen, buttocks, thighs, and in the axillary folds. Male clients can also have excoriated papules on the penis.

Infestation is confirmed by taking a scraping of a lesion and examining it under the microscope for mites and eggs. Close contacts also should be examined for possible infestation.

Treatment involves the use of scabicides, such as lindane (Kwell, Kwellada) or topical sulfur preparations. Laundering of clothes and personal items is sufficient to eliminate the mites.

COMMON INFLAMMATIONS

PATHOPHYSIOLOGY

The inflammatory skin conditions have a variety of nonspecific manifestations, including severe itching, lesions with indistinct borders, and different distribution patterns. The cause of the eruption may or may not be identifiable. Inflammatory rashes can evolve from acute to chronic conditions.

Most inflammatory rashes are related to allergic immune responses. The responses may be triggered by external skin exposure to allergens or by exposure of the internal environment to allergens and irritants. The result is tissue destruction or skin changes induced by antibodies or cellular mediators of the immune system. (A more detailed description of these immune mechanisms is presented in Chapter 23.)

The specific cause of inflammatory rashes is not always known. When this is the case, the catch-all diagnosis of nonspecific eczematous dermatitis, or *eczema,* is often used.

Contact dermatitis is an acute or chronic rash caused by either direct contact with an irritant substance, resulting in toxic injury to the skin, or by contact with an allergen, resulting in a cell-mediated immune reaction.

Atopic dermatitis is a chronic rash that occurs with respiratory allergies and atopic skin disease. The mechanism is unknown, but atopic dermatitis is made worse by factors that include dry or irritated skin, food allergies, chemicals, or stress. (Atopic reactions are described in Chapter 26.)

COLLABORATIVE MANAGEMENT

Assessment

Because all the inflammatory skin eruptions appear similar, data collected from the client are needed to identify the cause. Inflammatory skin problems differ from eczematous dermatitis in the chronicity of the disease, the distribution of lesions, and associated symptoms. Chart 70-8 lists the manifestations of many types of inflammatory skin conditions. Diagnosis is based on historical and clinical data.

Interventions

If the cause of the rash is identified, avoidance therapy is used to reverse the reaction and clear the rash. Even when the cause is unclear, certain irritants may cause the rash to worsen and increase discomfort. Additional interventions promote comfort through suppression of the inflammatory response.

Steroids. Topical, intralesional, or systemic steroids are prescribed to suppress inflammation. The vehicle used to deliver a topical steroid depends on the body area involved. Because a side effect of oral corticosteroids is adrenal suppression, clients receiving long-term therapy must taper their drug dosages rather than come to an abrupt halt.

Corticosteroids never cure. During active disease, these drugs reduce manifestations and relieve associated discomfort. Moisten dressings with warm tap water and place over topical steroids for short periods to increase absorption.

Oil-Based Products. Avoid applying oil-based ointments and pastes to the sweaty skin fold areas because maceration and blocking of pores may result in folliculitis. Instead, water-soluble creams are the vehicle of choice for these areas. Lotions and gels prevent matting of the hair and are more appropriate for hairy areas, such as the scalp. Stiff pastes are used to apply therapy to localized areas because this vehicle clings to the skin where it is applied and resists spreading to uninvolved skin.

Creams are used when the client has acute dermatitis with oozing and weeping. Chronic dermatitis responds more favorably to oil-based ointments that seal in moisture and help combat dryness and scaling.

Antihistamines. Antihistamines provide some relief of itching but may not keep the client totally symptom free. The sedative effects of antihistamines can be reduced if the client takes most of the daily dose near bedtime.

Compresses and Baths. Cool, moist compresses and lukewarm baths with bath additives have a soothing effect, decrease inflammation, and help to debride crusts and

CHART 70-8

KEY FEATURES of
Common Inflammatory Skin Conditions

Clinical Manifestations	Distribution
Nonspecific Eczematous Dermatitis	
Evolution of lesions from vesicles to weeping papules and plaques. Lichenification occurs in chronic disease. Oozing, crusting, fissuring, excoriation, or scaling may be present. Itching is common.	Anywhere on the body; localized eczema commonly involves the hands or feet
Contact Dermatitis	
Localized eczematous eruption with well-defined, geometric margins that are consistent with contact by an irritant or allergen. Usually seen in the acute form, but may become chronic if exposure is repeated. Allergy to plants (e.g., poison ivy or oak) classically occurs as linear streaks of vesicles or papules.	Cosmetic/perfume allergy: head and neck Hair product allergy: scalp Shoe/rubber allergy: dorsum of feet Nickel allergy: earlobes Mouthwash/toothpaste allergy: perioral region Airborne contact allergy (e.g., paint and ragweed): generalized
Atopic Dermatitis	
Hallmark in adults is lichenification with scaling and excoriation. Extremely itchy. Face involvement is seen as dry skin with mild to moderate erythema, perioral pallor, and skin folds beneath the eyes (Dennie-Morgan lines). Associated with linear markings on the palms.	Face, neck, upper chest, and antecubital and popliteal fossae
Drug Eruption	
Bright red erythematous macules and papules are found. Skin blisters in extreme cases. Lesions tend to be confluent in large areas. Moderately itchy. Fever is rare. Dehydration and hypothermia can occur with extensive involvement. Condition clears only after offending medication has been discontinued.	Generalized Involvement begins on trunk, proceeds distally (legs are the last to be involved)

scales. Colloidal oatmeal preparations, tar extracts, cornstarch, or oils are often added to baths to relieve itching (see Table 70-1).

PSORIASIS

PATHOPHYSIOLOGY

Psoriasis is a lifelong disorder that has exacerbations and remissions. Even though psoriasis cannot be cured, clients can usually achieve control of symptoms with proper treatment.

Psoriasis is a scaling disorder with underlying dermal inflammation. The problem involves an abnormality in the growth of epidermal cells in the outer skin layers. Normally cells at the basement membrane of the epidermis take about 27 days to reach the outermost layer, where they are shed. In a person with psoriasis, the rate of cell division is speeded up so that cells are shed every 4 to 5 days.

Etiology and Genetic Risk

Although the antigens responsible for psoriasis have yet to be identified, psoriasis appears to be an autoimmune reaction resulting from over stimulation of the immune system. Langerhans cells in the skin respond to the unknown antigen, leading to T-lymphocyte activation. These cells target the keratinocytes, causing increased cell division and plaque formation.

A genetic predisposition has been recognized in some cases; however, often there is no family history of the disease. Many environmental factors lead to outbreaks and influence the severity of clinical symptoms, but these vary from person to person. Triggering factors may be local or systemic. A psoriatic lesion may appear after skin trauma (Koebner's phenomenon in which a previously injured area is more susceptible to development of cancer or chronic skin problems), such as surgery, sunburn, or excoriation.

Clients with psoriasis seem to improve in warmer climates, where there is more exposure to sunlight. Systemic factors that can aggravate the disease include infections (severe streptococcal throat infection, *Candida* infection, upper respiratory tract infection), hormonal changes (during puberty and menopause), psychological stress, drugs (lithium, beta-blocking agents, indomethacin, antimalarials), obesity, and the presence of other diseases.

Some clients with psoriasis also develop a debilitating arthritis. Psoriatic arthritis may be mild or can lead to severe joint changes similar to those seen in rheumatoid arthritis. The association of arthritis with psoriasis strongly suggests that psoriasis is really a systemic connective tissue disorder rather than a simple skin disease. See Chapter 24 for more discussion of connective tissue disorders.

COLLABORATIVE MANAGEMENT

Assessment

HISTORY

In addition to collecting routine epidemiologic data, ask the client about any family history of psoriasis, including the age at onset, a description of the disease progression, and the pattern of recurrences. Ask the client to describe the current flare-up of psoriasis, including whether the onset was gradual or sudden, where the lesions first appeared, whether there have been any changes in severity over time, and whether fever and itching are present. Explore possible precipitating factors, including recent skin trauma, upper respiratory tract infection, recent surgeries, menopause status, past and current use of drugs, and recent stress. Ask about previous interventions and the effectiveness of each in reducing symptoms.

PHYSICAL ASSESSMENT/CLINICAL MANIFESTATIONS

The appearance of psoriasis and its course vary among clients. Typically during flare-ups of the disease, lesions thicken and extend to involve new areas of the body. As psoriasis responds to treatment, lesions become thinner with less scaling.

PSORIASIS VULGARIS. Psoriasis vulgaris is the most common type of psoriasis and presents as thick reddened papules or plaques covered by silvery white scales (Figure 70-15). Borders between the lesions and normal skin are sharply defined. Patches are less red and more moist in skin fold areas because of sweat-induced maceration. Lesions are usually present in the same areas on both sides of the body. The more common sites are the scalp, elbows, trunk, knees, sacrum, and outside surfaces of the limbs. The facial skin is rarely affected. The client may have only a few isolated lesions, or the entire skin surface may be affected.

EXFOLIATIVE PSORIASIS. Exfoliative psoriasis (erythrodermic psoriasis) is an explosively eruptive and inflammatory form of the disease with generalized erythema and scaling that do not form obvious lesions. Examine for signs of dehydration and hypothermia or hyperthermia related to this severe inflammatory reaction. The increased blood vessel dilation and blood flow to the skin can reduce fluid volume through evaporative water loss from the skin surface.

A

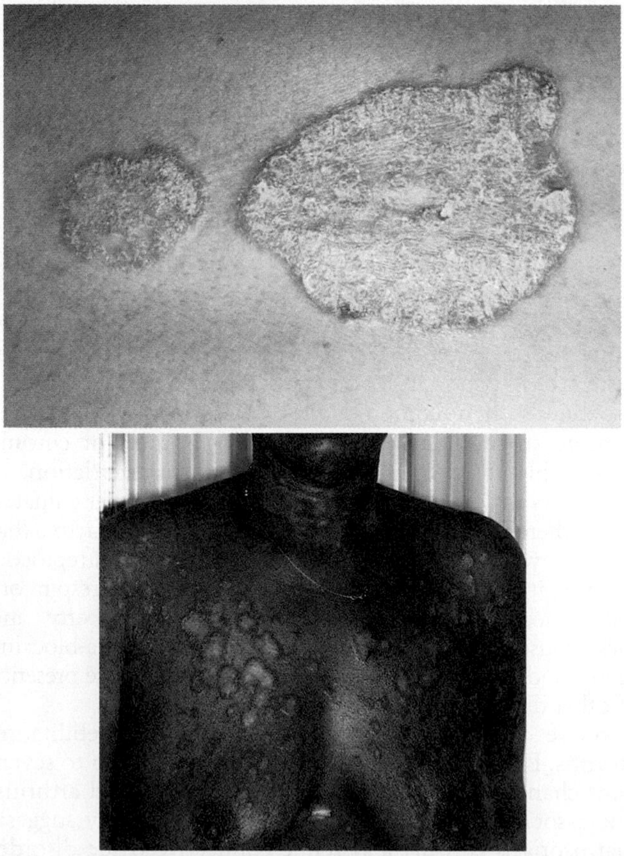

B

Figure 70-15 ■ **A,** Psoriasis vulgaris in a light-skinned client. **B,** Psoriasis vulgaris in a dark-skinned client.

Common Nursing Diagnoses and Collaborative Problems

Nursing diagnoses that may apply to the client with psoriasis include the following:

- Disturbed Body Image related to altered appearance
- Ineffective Coping related to the chronicity of the disease and alteration in body image
- Deficient Knowledge (Treatment) related to lack of exposure or unfamiliarity of information resources
- Chronic Low Self-Esteem related to alteration in body image
- Social Isolation related to alteration in physical appearance.

Interventions

The different approaches to therapy are based on the extent of disease, the client's distress, the physician's preference, and the response of the psoriasis to treatment. Clients must understand that no cure for psoriasis exists yet. Therapy is aimed at reducing cell proliferation and the inflammation.

Topical Therapy. The topical agents used to treat psoriasis are topical steroids, topical tar and anthralin preparations, and ultraviolet (UV) light.

Topical Steroids. Corticosteroids have anti-inflammatory actions. When they are applied to psoriatic lesions, they suppress cell division. The effectiveness of a topical steroid depends on its potency and ability to be absorbed into the skin. The more potent agents are used to treat clients with psoriasis.

A simple way to enhance the skin penetration of these drugs is to apply the steroid directly to the skin. Follow this step with warm, moist dressings and an occlusive outer wrap of plastic (film, gloves, booties, or similar garments). When large surface areas are involved, limit occlusive therapy to 12 hours per day because of the increased risk of local and systemic side effects.

Tar Preparations. When a tar preparation is applied to the skin, it suppresses cell division and reduces inflammation. Coal tar derived preparations are available as solutions, ointments, lotions, gels, and shampoos. The use of coal tar ointments is usually limited to inpatient care and specialized outpatient treatment clinics because these ointments are messy, cause staining, and have an unpleasant odor.

Topical therapy with anthralin (Anthraforte✱, Drithocreme, Lasan), a hydrocarbon similar in action to tar, also relieves chronic psoriasis. These drugs can be used alone or in combination with coal tar baths and UV light.

Apply high-potency anthralin, suspended in a stiff paste, to each lesion for short periods (not exceeding 2 hours). Anthralin is a strong irritant and can cause chemical burns. During therapy observe for local tissue reaction and prevent this drug from coming into contact with uninvolved skin. Anthralin is not used to treat acute, spreading psoriasis because it tends to induce Koebner's phenomenon (see Skin Cancer, p. 1608).

Newer topical therapy with calcipotriene (Dovonex) as a cream, ointment, or lotion is effective for many clients with mild to moderate psoriasis. This drug is a synthetic form of vitamin D that regulates skin cell division. Tazarotene (Tazorac), a vitamin A derivative primarily used for acne, has been helpful for treatment of psoriasis in clients who have lesions on less than 20% of the body surface. This drug is teratogenic (can cause birth defects) even when used topically. In addition, methotrexate delivered as a topical agent can help control psoriasis. Other immunosuppressive agents are being tested for effectiveness in a topical form.

Ultraviolet Light Therapy. Ultraviolet (UV) radiation is a physical agent commonly used as a topical treatment in many skin conditions, including psoriasis. Ultraviolet B (UVB) light, which produces more energy, is responsible for the obvious biologic effects of the sun, such as burning. Ultraviolet A (UVA) light emits a lower level of energy, requiring longer exposure time before cellular destruction occurs. Although the sun is an inexpensive source of UV radiation, better availability and intensity control occur with the use of artificial light sources. These sources include lamps or cabinets containing UV tubes. *The use of commercial tanning beds is not recommended for the client with psoriasis.*

Ultraviolet therapy is limited by the potency and distance of the source from the skin as well as the exposure time. Potency and distance remain constant, and the time of exposure is gradually increased to achieve a mild suntan effect without burning or tenderness. The client's skin type, ranging from fair to darkly pigmented, affects his or her risk for burning and determines the exposure times. Because of the extremely high intensity of most artificial UVB light sources, treatments are measured in seconds of exposure; clients must wear eye protection during treatment.

Teach clients to inspect the skin carefully each day for signs of overexposure. If clients have tenderness on palpation and have clinical signs of severe erythema or blister formation, notify the physician before therapy is resumed.

Psoralen and UVA (PUVA) treatments are more common on an outpatient basis (Figure 70-16). Clients ingest psoralen, a photosensitizing agent, 2 hours before exposure to UVA light. Because UVA light produces less energy than UVB light, the onset of erythema and skin darkening may be delayed as long as 96 hours after exposure. Treatments are limited to two or three times a week and are not given on consecutive days. Exposure is gradually increased until tanning occurs. As with UVB exposure, dosages are adjusted according to the erythema reaction of normal skin as well as the response of psoriatic lesions.

Observe for generalized redness with edema and tenderness. If these symptoms are present, treatment must be interrupted until they subside. Because of the strong photosensitizing properties of psoralen, clients must wear dark glasses during treatment and for the remainder of the day.

Long-term side effects of both UVB and PUVA therapies include premature aging of the skin, actinic keratosis, and an increased risk for skin cancer.

Systemic Therapy. Some clients have severe psoriasis that is resistant to topical therapy. In these instances, systemic treatment with a cytotoxic agent, such as methotrexate (Folex, Mexate), is warranted. Because of the liver-damaging side effects of methotrexate, liver studies are recommended before therapy is started and at least yearly thereafter. Small doses are usually effective in clearing the lesions. This treatment of last resort is avoided for clients who have liver damage, bone marrow suppression, or impaired renal function.

Because psoriasis has an autoimmune basis, some systemic agents that induce immunosuppression are used when lesions do not respond to other therapies. Such agents include cyclosporine (Sandimmune) and azathioprine (Imuran). The many health risks associated with these therapies must be considered along with the potential benefits.

A better understanding of the role of the immune system in the cause of psoriasis has led to biologic therapies to treat moderate to severe disease. This treatment is most successful for clients with moderate to severe plaque disease who are candidates for systemic therapy or phototherapy. Biologic agents alter the acquired immune response, thus preventing over stimulation of keratinocytes. Although precautions vary with the specific mechanism of action, these drugs induce immunosuppression, and clients are at an increased risk for infection.

Approved biologic agents include alefacept (Amevive) and efalizumab (Raptiva). Alefacept is given by intramuscular

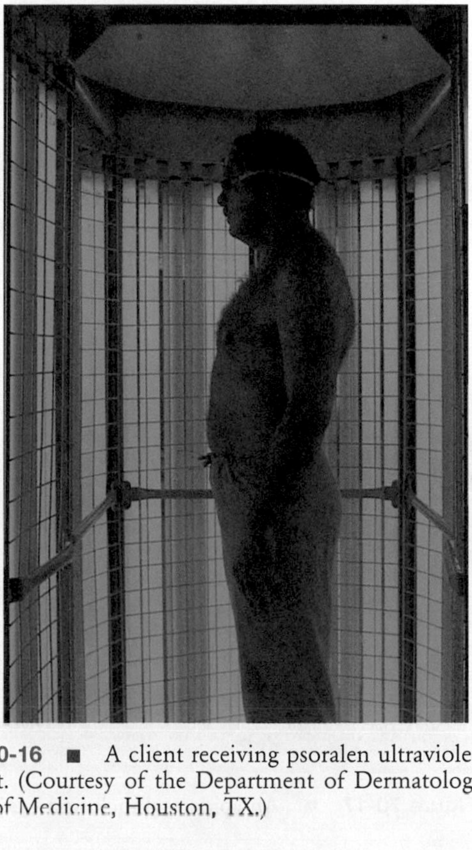

Figure 70-16 ■ A client receiving psoralen ultraviolet (PUVA) treatment. (Courtesy of the Department of Dermatology, Baylor College of Medicine, Houston, TX.)

(IM) injection weekly for 12 weeks. Efalizumab is given by subcutaneous injections once per week.

Emotional Support. Often clients' self-esteem suffers not only because of the presence of skin lesions but also because of the unpleasantness of some of the treatments. Tar not only looks dirty but also has a very unpleasant odor. Bed linens and pajamas become stained, further discouraging social interaction.

Encourage contact with other clients who have similar problems. Group discussions with family members or significant others can increase the socialization process.

The use of touch takes on an added significance for clients with psoriasis. For example, shake the client's hand during an introduction or place a hand on the client's shoulder when explaining a procedure. Do not wear gloves during these social interactions. Touch, more than any other gesture, communicates acceptance of the person and the skin problem.

BENIGN TUMORS

Cysts

PATHOPHYSIOLOGY

Cysts are firm flesh-colored nodules that contain liquid or semisolid material. Unlike cancerous growths, which are hard and firmly attached to underlying structures, a cyst moves and indents on palpation. Often there is a central pore through which the material can be expressed if the lesion is squeezed.

The most common cyst is an epidermal inclusion cyst. These growths are often asymptomatic and can be located anywhere, but they occur most often on the head and trunk (Figure 70-17). The most common cyst on the scalp is the sebaceous, or pilar, cyst.

COLLABORATIVE MANAGEMENT

If the client wants to have a cyst removed for appearance or any reason, surgical excision with primary closure is performed with a local anesthetic agent. The surgeon removes the entire cyst wall during excision to prevent recurrence.

A pilonidal cyst is a lesion of the sacral area that often has a sinus track extending into deeper tissue structures. As this cyst fills or becomes infected, it can become tender. An incision and drainage can be performed. Often the cyst is surgically removed and the area heals by second intention.

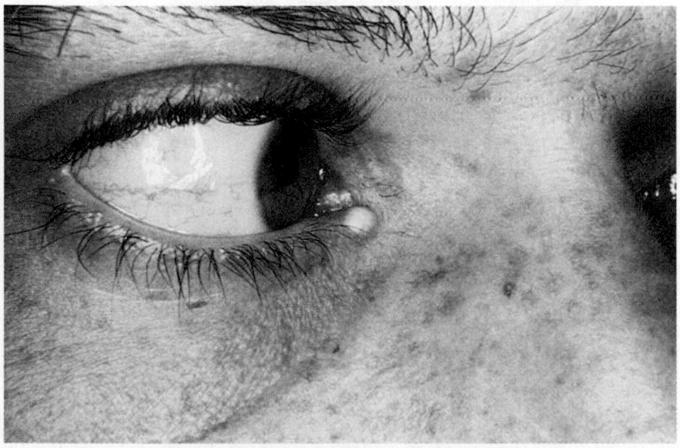

Figure 70-17 ■ An epidermal inclusion cyst.

Seborrheic Keratoses

PATHOPHYSIOLOGY

Seborrheic keratoses are a common problem of older people. These benign epidermal neoplasms are gradually acquired after middle age and are often mistaken for actinic keratoses or pigmented skin cancers. These growths may occur anywhere but are more commonly found on the face, neck, upper trunk, and arms.

COLLABORATIVE MANAGEMENT

On inspection, seborrheic keratoses appear as multiple "pasted-on" papules or plaques ranging in color from flesh tones to brown or black (Figure 70-18). The surface of the lesion has a rough, greasy, wartlike texture on palpation.

Seborrheic keratoses are removed only for cosmetic reasons or if a lesion becomes irritated from friction. Cryosurgery or curettage with or without a local anesthetic is performed.

Keloids

PATHOPHYSIOLOGY

A keloid is overgrowth of a scar with an excessive accumulation of collagen and ground substance. Keloids are more common in darker-skinned people and often arise at sites of surgical incisions, burns, and ear piercing (Figure 70-19).

COLLABORATIVE MANAGEMENT

On physical examination, a keloid is an elevated, protruding lesion that extends beyond the edges of the original injury. These lesions can be cosmetically disfiguring. Treatment is difficult and not always successful. Because surgical excision alone can result in an even larger scar, surgery is usually combined with another form of therapy, such as intralesional steroid injections or low-dose radiotherapy. Pressure dressings or elastic garments worn over the skin for 1 year after excision or steroid injection may also help to keep the lesion flat.

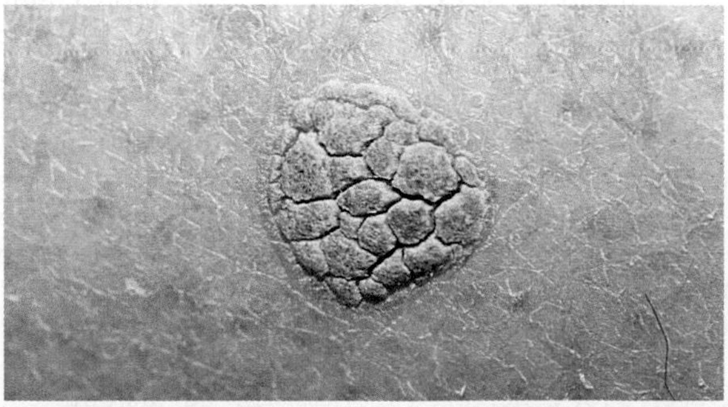

Figure 70-18 ■ Seborrheic keratosis. (From Lookingbill, D.P., & Marks, J.G. [2000]. Principles of dermatology [3rd ed.]. Philadelphia: W.B. Saunders.)

Nevi

PATHOPHYSIOLOGY

A **nevus,** or mole, is a benign growth of the pigment-forming cells. These lesions are classified according to their location within the layers of the skin.

COLLABORATIVE MANAGEMENT

Normal nevi have regular, well-defined borders and are uniform in color, ranging from light colors to dark brown (Figure 70-20). The lesion's surface may be rough or smooth. Because about 50% of malignant melanomas arise from moles, nevi with irregular or spreading borders and those with multiple colors should be considered highly suspicious. Other abnormal findings include sudden changes in the size of the lesion and complaints of itching or bleeding.

Unsightly nevi or those subject to repeated irritation or trauma can be removed. Biopsy of any suspicious lesions is performed to rule out malignancy.

Warts

PATHOPHYSIOLOGY

Warts, or **verrucae,** are small tumors caused by papillomavirus infection of the skin cells. They may occur singly or in groups and are classified according to their anatomic location.

Common warts are raised, flesh-colored papules with a rough surface (Figure 70-21). Although they may grow anywhere on the skin surface, they often occur on the hands and fingers.

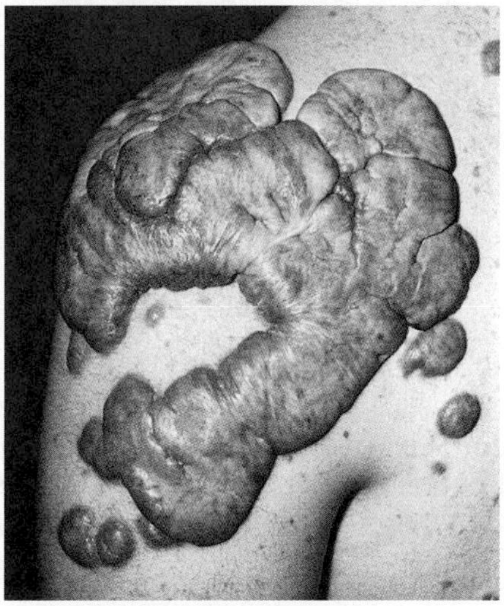

Figure 70-19 ■ A keloid.

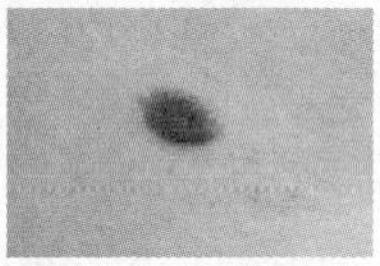

Figure 70-20 ■ A typical nevus (mole).

Flat warts range in size from 2 to 4 mm. They appear as slightly elevated reddish brown or flesh-colored papules with flat tops and minimal scale. These warts often multiply and affect the hands and the face.

An often painful wart occurring on the bottom of the foot is the plantar wart. Plantar warts have a thick callus that, when removed, reveals tiny black dots (thrombosed capillaries).

COLLABORATIVE MANAGEMENT

The treatment of warts is aimed at destroying the skin cells containing the virus, a process that can be destructive and painful. Treatment modalities include surgical excision, electrodesiccation and curettage, and cryosurgery. Cryosurgery is usually preferred because a local anesthetic is not required and scarring is less likely. Topical caustic agents, including salicylic acid and lactic acid, are also used. These agents are painted onto the surface of the lesion and result in destruction of the cells and peeling of the infected skin area.

Hemangiomas

Hemangiomas (angiomas) are blood vessel tumors and are common benign tumors. The appearance varies from lesions that appear shortly after birth and gradually regress to those that are present at birth and gradually expand with growth.

Nevus flammeus is a congenital hemangioma involving the capillaries. These lesions are usually found on the face and the upper body. They are well-demarcated macular patches ranging in color from pink to bluish purple. Although nevus flammeus may gradually fade during the first years of life, a form of this neoplasm, the port-wine stain, grows with the child and remains unchanged in adult life. Port-wine stains usually occur as solitary lesions that vary in size.

The problem of nevus flammeus is cosmetic. Depending on the size of the lesion, surgical excision with or without skin grafting may be indicated. Treatment with laser therapy is also an alternative to surgery. Noninvasive treatment consists of masking the lesion by covering it with an opaque makeup.

Cherry hemangiomas are often seen in older adults. These lesions are small, dome-shaped papules ranging in color from red to purple (see Figure 69-14). Treatment is not indicated except when the client is unhappy with his or her appearance.

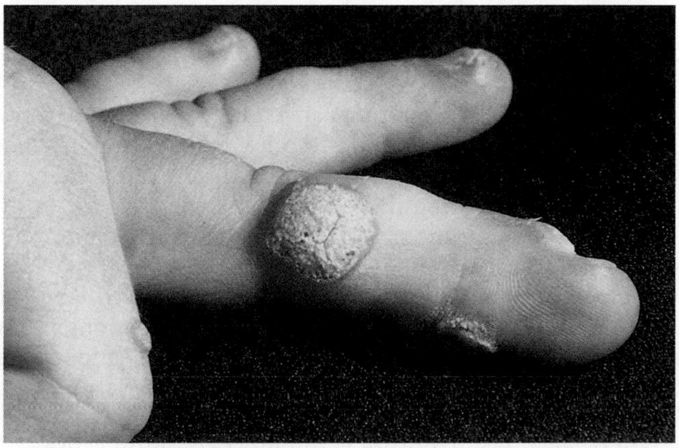

Figure 70-21 ■ A common wart.

TABLE 70-10 Common Skin Cancers

Clinical Manifestations	Distribution	Course
Actinic Keratosis (Premalignant)		
Small (1-10 mm) macule or papule with dry, rough, adherent yellow or brown scale Base may be erythematous Associated with yellow, wrinkled, weather-beaten skin Thick, indurated keratoses more likely to be malignant	Cheeks, temples, forehead, ears, neck, backs of hands, and forearms	May disappear spontaneously or reappear after treatment. Slow progression to squamous cell carcinoma is possible.
Squamous Cell Carcinoma		
Firm, nodular lesion topped with a crust or with a central area of ulceration Indurated margins Fixation to underlying tissue with deep invasion	Sun-exposed areas, especially head, neck, and lower lip Sites of chronic irritation or injury (e.g., scars, irradiated skin, burns, and leg ulcers)	Rapid invasion with metastasis via the lymphatics occurs in 10% of cases. Larger tumors are more prone to metastasis.
Basal Cell Carcinoma		
Pearly papule with a central crater and rolled, waxy borders Telangiectasias and pigment flecks visible on close inspection	Sun-exposed areas, especially head, neck, and central portion of face	Metastasis is rare. May cause local tissue destruction. 50% recurrence rate related to inadequate treatment.
Melanoma		
Irregularly shaped, pigmented papule or plaque Variegated colors, with red, white, and blue tones	Can occur anywhere on the body especially where nevi (moles) or birthmarks are evident Commonly found on upper back and lower legs Soles of feet and palms in dark-skinned individuals	Horizontal growth phase followed by vertical growth phase. Rapid invasion and metastasis with high morbidity and mortality.

SKIN CANCER

PATHOPHYSIOLOGY

Overexposure to sunlight is the major cause of skin cancer, although other factors are associated. Because sun damage is an age-related skin finding, screening for suspicious lesions is an important part of physical assessment of the older adult. The most common skin cancers are actinic or solar keratosis, squamous cell carcinoma, basal cell carcinoma, and melanoma. Table 70-10 lists common skin cancers.

Etiology and Genetic Risk

Actinic keratoses are premalignant lesions of the cells of the epidermis. These lesions are common in people with chronically sun-damaged skin (see Figure 69-16). Progression to squamous cell carcinoma may occur if lesions are untreated.

Squamous cell carcinomas are cancers of the epidermis. They can invade locally and are potentially metastatic. Lesions on the ear, lip, and external genitalia are more likely to invade and spread than those found elsewhere on the body (Figure 70-22). Chronic skin damage from repeated injury or irritation also predisposes to this malignancy.

Basal cell carcinomas arise from the basal cell layer of the epidermis (Figure 70-23). Early malignant lesions often go unnoticed, and although metastasis is rare, underlying tissue destruction can progress to include vital structures. Genetic predisposition and chronic irritation are risk factors; however, UV exposure is the most common cause.

Melanomas are pigmented cancers arising in the melanin-producing epidermal cells (Figure 70-24). Risk factors include genetic predisposition, excessive exposure to UV light, and the presence of one or more precursor lesions that resemble unusual moles. *This skin cancer is highly metastatic, and a person's survival depends on early diagnosis and treatment.*

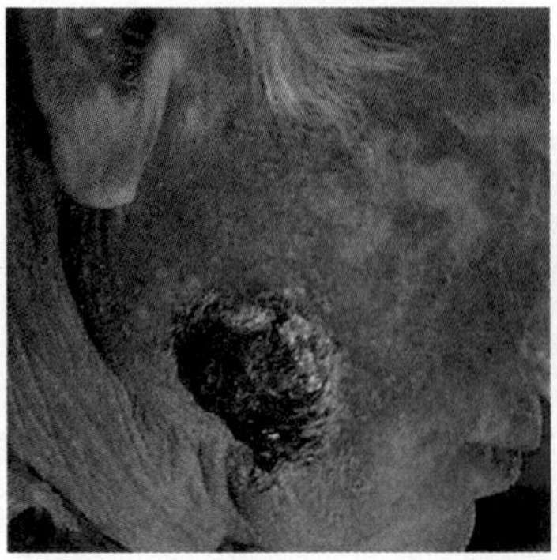

Figure 70-22 ■ Squamous cell carcinoma.

Lighter skin and less pigmentation are genetically inherited traits. Additionally, a genetic mutation that is inherited in an autosomal-dominant pattern has been found for some cases of familial melanoma. The mutation occurs in a suppressor gene resulting in loss of tumor suppressor function. Two such mutated genes are *PTCH* and *CDKN2* (Nussbaum, McInnes, & Willard, 2001).

Incidence/Prevalence

The incidence of skin cancer is highest among light-skinned races and individuals older than 60 years of age (American Cancer Society, 2005). The incidence is higher among indi-

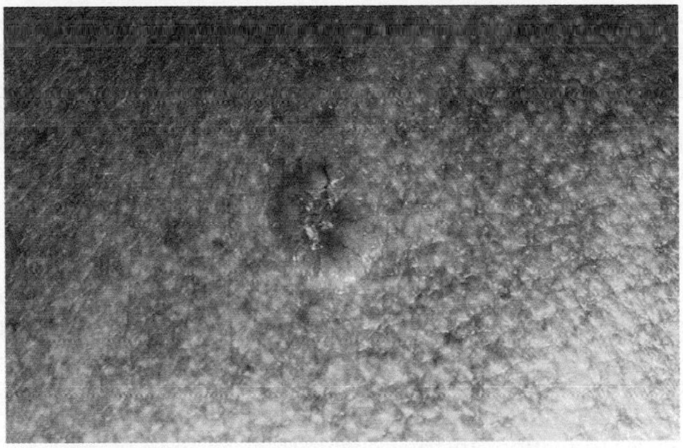

Figure 70-23 ■ Basal cell carcinoma.

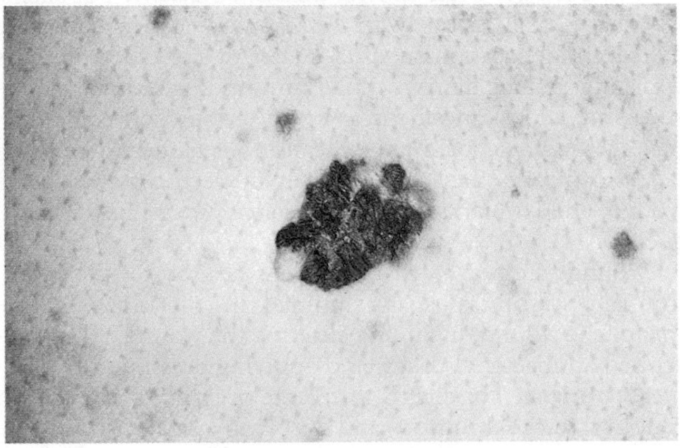

Figure 70-24 ■ Melanoma.

viduals who work outdoors and live at higher altitudes or lower latitudes. Occupational exposure to arsenic or other chemical carcinogens also increases risk. The incidence of melanoma has increased during the past 30 years, accounting for 2% of all cancers and 1% of all cancer deaths (American Cancer Society, 2005).

HEALTH PROMOTION/ILLNESS PREVENTION

The single most effective prevention strategy for skin cancer is avoiding or reducing skin exposure to sunlight. However, even when people understand the cause of skin cancer and the seriousness of the disease, preventive behaviors are not always practiced (see the Evidence-Based Practice for Nursing box above). Chart 70-9 lists methods of prevention that clients can use to reduce their risk for skin cancer.

◆COLLABORATIVE MANAGEMENT

◆Assessment

In addition to age and race, ask the client about any family history of skin cancer and any past surgery for removal of skin growths. Recent changes in the size, color, or sensation of any mole, birthmark, wart, or scar are also significant. Ask the client about which geographic regions he or she has lived in and where he or she currently resides. Obtain information about occupational and recreational activities in relation to sun exposure as well as any occupational history of exposure to chemical carcinogens (e.g., arsenic, coal tar, pitch, radioactive waste, radium). Ask whether any skin lesions are repeatedly irritated by the rubbing of clothes against them.

EVIDENCE BASED PRACTICE for Nursing

Good role modeling requires knowing your risk!

Grubbs, L., & Tabano, M. (2000). Use of sunscreen in health care professionals. *Cancer Nursing, 23*(1), 164-167.

The purpose of this descriptive study was to examine the relationship between perceived risk for skin cancer and use of sunscreen among a convenience sample of 98 health care professionals living in a high sun exposure area of the United States. The health care professionals group was comprised of registered nurses, pharmacists, psychologists, nurse practitioners, and physicians. The level of education in this group was high with 63% having postgraduate or professional degrees. Most of the participants were white women.

The study involved completion of a questionnaire that included demographic and skin cancer risk assessment questions. A total of 90 questionnaires were returned (92% response rate). The perceived risk for skin cancer among this group was 50% low perceived risk, 44% high perceived risk, and 6% neutral. The actual risk for skin cancer, based on family history, burn history, and skin type was 7% low risk, 48% average risk, and 45% high risk. Statistical analysis confirmed that subjects at high risk and those at low risk had an accurate perception of actual risk. The subjects at average risk overwhelmingly reported their perceived risk as low. There was no relationship between perceived risk and consistent use of sunscreen.

Level of Evidence: 6—Correlational descriptive study.

Critique. The study was appropriately designed as a descriptive pilot study. Subject homogeneity limits the generalizability of the study results beyond this group.

Nursing Implications. Nurses and other health care professionals are perceived by the general public as role models of healthy behaviors. With a preventable cancer, such as skin cancer, nurses can have the greatest impact by the encouragement of prevention practices. An inaccurate perception of personal risk and inconsistent use of protective or preventive practices reduce this positive impact.

CHART 70-9

CLIENT EDUCATION GUIDE
Prevention of Skin Cancer

- Avoid sun exposure between 11:00 AM and 3:00 PM.
- Use sunscreens with the appropriate skin protection factor for your skin type.
- Wear a hat, opaque clothing, and sunglasses when you are out in the sun.
- Examine your body monthly for possibly cancerous or precancerous lesions.
- Seek medical advice if you note any of the following:
  - A change in the color of a lesion, especially if it darkens or shows evidence of spreading
  - A change in the size of a lesion, especially rapid growth
  - A change in the shape of a lesion, such as a sharp border becoming irregular or a flat lesion becoming raised
  - Redness or swelling of the skin around a lesion
  - A change in sensation, especially itching or increased tenderness of a lesion
  - A change in the character of a lesion, such as oozing, crusting, bleeding, or scaling

Skin that has been injured previously is at greater risk for cancer development, an effect known as *Koebner's phenomenon*. Ask the client if he or she has ever experienced a severe skin injury that resulted in a scar. Examine all scarred skin areas for the presence of potentially cancerous lesions.

The skin cancers vary in their appearance and distribution. Although most skin cancers appear in sun-exposed areas of the body, inspect the entire skin surface. Systematically examine the skin for any unusual lesions, particularly moles, warts, birthmarks, and scars. Also examine hair-bearing areas of the body, such as the scalp and genitalia. Palpate lesions to determine surface texture. Document the location, size, color, and surface features of all lesions and any subjective reports of tenderness or itching. Use the ABCD method of evaluating all lesions for possible melanoma (see Chapter 69).

Table 70-10 lists facts about common skin cancers. Punch, shave, or excisional biopsy of suspicious lesions is necessary to determine whether a skin lesion is benign or malignant.

Interventions

Nonsurgical and surgical interventions are combined for the effective management of skin cancer. Treatment is determined by the size and severity of the malignancy, the location of the lesion, and the age and general health of the client.

NONSURGICAL MANAGEMENT

Drug Therapy. Topical chemotherapy with 5-fluorouracil cream is used for treatment of multiple actinic keratoses or for widespread superficial basal cell carcinoma that would require several surgical procedures to eradicate. Therapy is continued for several weeks, and the treated areas become increasingly tender and inflamed as the lesions crust, ooze, and erode. Prepare the client for an unsightly appearance during therapy, and reassure the client that the cosmetic result will be positive.

After treatment is discontinued, cool compresses and topical corticosteroid preparations help to decrease inflammation and promote comfort.

Systemic chemotherapeutic agents are used in the treatment of skin cancer, except when the prognosis is poor, as in advanced melanoma.

Drug therapy with interferon, a biological response modifier, is now an accepted treatment after surgery for melanomas that are at stage III or higher. The client is first started on high-dose (20,000,000 units/m^2) interferon infusions daily for 5 days per week for 4 weeks after the surgical wound is well healed. Maintenance doses of 10,000,000 units/m^2 are continued three times per week for 1 year. The maintenance doses are given subcutaneously, and the client must learn to self-inject the drug.

Radiation Therapy. Radiation therapy for skin cancer is limited to older clients with large, deeply invasive basal cell tumors and to those who are poor risks for surgery. Malignant melanoma is resistant to radiation therapy; however, radiation therapy may be helpful for clients with metastatic disease when used in combination with systemic corticosteroids.

Immunotherapy. An experimental treatment available at some centers for clients with melanoma that has spread to distant sites is a melanoma vaccine. This treatment takes advantage of distinctive cell surface proteins found on some melanomas that can act like antigens. Although this therapy is new and as yet unapproved, it shows promise for melanoma.

SURGICAL MANAGEMENT. Surgical intervention ranges from local removal of small lesions, with minimal discomfort and positive cosmetic results, to massive excision of large areas of the skin.

Cryosurgery. Cryosurgery involves the local application of liquid nitrogen (−200° C) to isolated lesions, causing cell death and tissue destruction. Local anesthesia is seldom needed because most clients have only minor discomfort during the procedure. Prepare clients for swelling and increased tenderness of the treated area when the skin thaws. Tissue freezing is followed in 1 or 2 days by hemorrhagic blister formation. Instruct clients to clean the sites with hydrogen peroxide to prevent infection. A topical antibiotic may also be prescribed.

Curettage and Electrodesiccation. For clients who have small lesions with well-defined borders, curettage and electrodesiccation are used to destroy the cancerous cells while minimizing damage to the surrounding uninvolved tissue. After a local anesthetic is given, the surgeon uses a dermal curette to scrape away the cancerous tissue. After curettage is complete, the surgeon places an electric probe on the wound, and remnants of the tumor are destroyed by thermal energy.

Wounds created by this treatment heal by second intention, and scarring is usually minimal. Instruct clients in caring for the wound, including cleaning the wound, using prescribed antibacterial drugs, and applying dressings.

Excision. For clients with large or poorly defined skin cancers, recurrent tumors, and deeply invasive cancers, wide excision is used to remove the cancer. If the size and location of the lesion permit, surgical excision with primary closure is the preferred method. If the tumor has already been removed several times or if radiation therapy has damaged the surrounding skin, healing by second intention is indicated. This procedure allows the wound to be monitored for cancer recurrence. Skin grafts and flaps are used to repair large defects if tissue destruction is deep.

A specialized form of excision, Mohs' surgery, is used to treat basal and squamous cell carcinomas. The cancerous tissue is sectioned horizontally in layers, and each layer is examined histologically to determine the presence of residual tumor cells. Although the procedure is long and tedious, cure rates are high and there is less removal of healthy tissue compared with other surgical methods.

PLASTIC OR RECONSTRUCTIVE SURGERY

PATHOPHYSIOLOGY

The aim of plastic or reconstructive surgery is to correct functional defects and alter physical appearance (processes that influence a person's self-image). Plastic surgery is usually an elective procedure. Such intervention is sought by clients who cannot perform activities of daily living (ADLs) as a result of an anatomic problem or by those who are unsatisfied with their body image. In the United States the decision to undergo plastic surgery is often a response to social and cultural norms about beauty. Clients become self-conscious about scars, facial lesions, disproportionate anatomic features, or changes in physical features associated with aging. For some clients, severe trauma or extensive surgery causes functional problems that warrant surgical correction. For example, breast reconstruction is commonly performed after a mastectomy. This surgery not only serves an aesthetic purpose for some clients but also replaces lost anatomy and negates the need for a prosthesis.

Clients may request plastic surgery as a remedy for the normal changes in appearance that occur with aging. Loss of skin elasticity and changes in fatty tissue distribution are progressive and especially noticeable around the eyes, near the cheeks, and on the neck. Fine facial wrinkles around the eyes and mouth are one of the first signs of aging. These changes are followed by gradual stretching and downward displacement of the soft tissue of the lower two thirds of the face. Similar changes are seen as skin wrinkling and looseness on the arms, chest, abdomen, buttocks, and thighs. These changes are also seen after dramatic weight loss. Appearance of skin lesions associated with chronic sun exposure may trouble the aging client.

COLLABORATIVE MANAGEMENT

Assessment

HISTORY

When taking a history from a client who elects to have plastic surgery, use a nonjudgmental approach, and be careful not to assume the reason for surgery on the basis of physical appearance. Often what might appear to be unsightly to you is of little concern to the client, who wishes to change something else. Observe for any nonverbal communication that might establish the emotional state of the person or reveal feelings of embarrassment or guilt. Encourage the client to describe the problem, including why it is bothersome and what he or she expects as a result of the change. Ask about his or her health history and recent medical problems, including obesity and trauma, to predict the amount of surgery needed to correct the defect and potential complications.

PHYSICAL ASSESSMENT/CLINICAL MANIFESTATIONS

The client seeking plastic surgery may have changes in appearance ranging from minor to significant deformity. Depending on the location of the problem, the client may need to undress before the examination. Ensure privacy because the client may be embarrassed by the problem.

Begin the physical assessment by closely examining the area of involvement to determine the extent of the deformity or problem. Have the client assume different normal sitting and standing postures to provide better visibility of nonfacial defects. Document asymmetry of anatomic features, wrinkling or skin redundancy, scars or disfiguring skin marks, and obvious skin lesions.

PSYCHOSOCIAL ASSESSMENT

Address the client's expectations of plastic surgery. Often people who seek plastic surgery have unrealistic expectations or are uncertain about what they actually want. For example, the client with minor deformities who is seeking perfection is sure to be disappointed. The client who wants an operation mainly to please the spouse or partner is also a poor candidate. His or her psychological outlook before surgery should be positive if results are to be therapeutic.

Interventions

SURGICAL MANAGEMENT. Depending on the planned intervention, surgery is performed either in the outpatient setting with the client under local anesthesia or in the hospital. Most clients scheduled for plastic surgery have had consultations with their surgeon to discuss the planned intervention, possible complications, and postoperative expectations. The indications and complications of common cosmetic procedures are listed in Table 70-11.

Many plastic surgeons use photography both as a visual aid when discussing clients' problems and as a means of documenting before and after surgical intervention. Pictures taken of clients are confidential. Showing clients pictures of other clients is done only after proper consent is obtained.

Preoperative Care. Because of the large amount of blood loss associated with skin (particularly facial) surgery, instruct the client to avoid aspirin and other nonsteroidal anti-inflammatories for several weeks before and after the procedure. Immediate preoperative care is focused on collection of any routine laboratory test data required before general anesthesia and preparation of the operative site. In most cases, the procedure for shaving and washing the skin is dictated by the physician's preference.

Clients undergoing facial surgery, specifically **rhytidectomy** (face-lift), are often asked to wash their hair several times with antibacterial soap to decrease bacterial flora near the incision site. Instruct clients to remove any makeup and to avoid using face creams before surgery. If a **rhinoplasty** (reconstruction of the nose) is scheduled, explain the need for nasal packing and review mouth-breathing techniques.

Operative Procedures. Reconstructive procedures vary depending on the location, purpose, and extent of reconstruction. Ironically, in performing plastic surgery, the surgeon must make a wound to correct existing skin deformities.

Postoperative Care. Care after surgery focuses on monitoring for complications (see Chapter 22). Pressure dressings may be applied at the time of surgery and left in place for several days to control hemorrhage and edema formation. Check dressings and any nasal packing for bright red bleeding, and monitor changes in vital signs and level of consciousness indicating active hemorrhage.

Repeated swallowing followed by belching after rhinoplasty is a sign of postnasal bleeding and must be reported immediately to the surgeon. The client who has had breast surgery may have drains in place after surgery. Monitor the amount and color of drainage. Place the client who has had any facial reconstruction in a semi-Fowler's position to reduce edema and promote comfort.

Use additional comfort measures, such as the application of ice packs or cold compresses, as prescribed. Support garments are used after breast augmentation surgery to reduce edema and tension on the suture line from the weight of the breast tissue.

Monitor for wound infection and progress toward healing. Of particular concern are any areas of skin necrosis or eschar formation near the operative site, a complication from excessive tension on the suture line as a result of edema and blood vessel obstruction. Table 70-8 lists wound monitoring criteria.

TABLE 70-11 Common Plastic Surgery Procedures

Description	Indications	Complications
Blepharoplasty		
Excision of bulging fat and redundant skin of the periorbital area with primary closure	Bags under the eyes	Hematoma Ectropion Corneal injury Visual loss (rare) Wound infection (rare)
Breast Augmentation (Augmentation Mammoplasty)		
Insertion of synthetic breast-shaped implants through a skin incision	Inadequate breast volume or contour	Hematoma or hemorrhage Wound infection (with gram-positive organisms) Phlebitis
Breast Reduction (Reduction Mammoplasty)		
Excision of excessive breast tissue and skin with primary closure	Hypertrophy of breast tissue caused by elevated hormone levels, endocrine abnormalities, or obesity Weight of large breasts can contribute to back pain	Hematoma or hemorrhage Nipple, areola, and skin flap necrosis Wound infection Fat necrosis Wound dehiscence
Dermabrasion		
Abrasive removal of the facial epidermis and portion of the dermis followed by healing by second intention	Moderate to severe acne scar Deep wrinkling Multiple actinic keratoses Hyperpigmentation (postinflammatory or after the use of estrogens)	Hypertrophic scarring Altered skin pigmentation Acne flare Wound infection (rare)
Rhinoplasty		
Removal of excessive cartilage and tissue from the nose with correction of septal defects if indicated	Disproportionate anatomy Post-traumatic nasal deformity Difficulty breathing through the nose	Hematoma or hemorrhage Ecchymosis and edema (temporary) Wound infection (with gram-positive organisms) Septal perforation Minor skin irritation
Rhytidectomy (Face Lift)		
Removal of excess skin and tissue from the face at the level of the hairline followed by primary closure	Excessive wrinkling or sagging of facial skin	Hematoma or hemorrhage Facial nerve damage (temporary or permanent) Wound infection Ecchymosis and edema (temporary) Skin necrosis Hair loss
Liposuction (Suction Lipectomy)		
Removal of subcutaneous fat from localized areas of accumulation such as the hips, abdomen, neck, and arms	Disproportionate distribution of adipose tissue	Hematoma Severe pain Infection Emboli Sagging of skin (if skin is not elastic enough to contract after fat removal)

Regardless of the planned procedure, inform the client to expect edema and discoloration of the operative site. Swelling and bruising alter the facial features and may not resolve for several weeks after surgery. Remind the client that the true results of surgery will not be visible until healing is complete, usually 6 months to a year or longer after surgery.

OTHER SKIN DISORDERS

Acne

PATHOPHYSIOLOGY

Acne is a red pustular eruption that affects the sebaceous glands of the skin. It is a common condition that, despite popular belief, is not confined to adolescents. Lesions result from increased sebum production, which is stimulated by androgenic hormones and obstruction of the sebaceous canal outlet. Debris collection promotes bacterial growth and rupture of the gland into the surrounding dermis with inflammation.

COLLABORATIVE MANAGEMENT

Acne is a progressive disorder that manifests as several types of skin lesions, including non-inflammatory **comedones** (blackheads and whiteheads), inflammatory papules, pustules, and cysts. These lesions are usually present only on the face and upper trunk (Figure 70-25).

Control of acne is possible, with spontaneous remission occurring over time. However, severe eruptions or chronic inflammation can lead to extensive scarring.

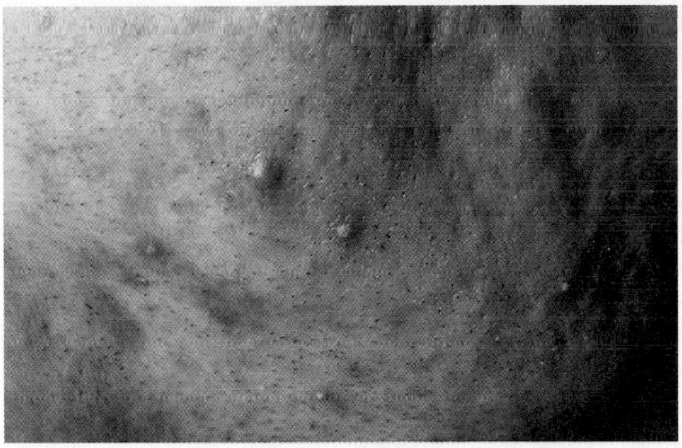

Figure 70-25 ■ Acne.

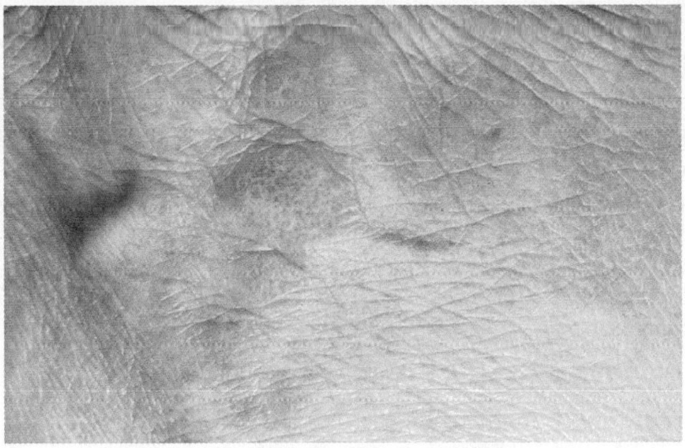

Figure 70-26 ■ Lichen planus.

For clients with superficial lesions, topical agents (retinoic acid, benzoyl peroxide, antibiotic solutions) are used. Systemic antibiotics are indicated for those with inflammatory disease. Clients with severe acne may have improvement after receiving isotretinoin (Accutane, Accutane Roche✱). Side effects include elevated liver function test results; dry, chapped skin; and depression in some clients. The most important concern, however, is the teratogenic effect of systemic retinoic acid. A pregnancy test is required before therapy, and strict birth control measures must be used during therapy.

Lichen Planus

PATHOPHYSIOLOGY

Lichen planus is a common skin disorder of purple, flat-topped papules that are itchy. Although viral infections and emotional stress may be possible causes, the actual etiology of lichen planus is not known. The course of the disease can be chronic, or it can resolve spontaneously.

COLLABORATIVE MANAGEMENT

Lesions of lichen planus are usually occur over the wrists and the inner surfaces of the forearms, but they may also be present on the lower legs, genitalia, and other body areas. Oral lesions may occur alone or with other skin changes. Unlike the skin lesions, oral lesions have a white lacelike appearance. These lesions usually occur on the oral mucosa and are often confused with thrush (Figure 70-26).

Treatment is determined by the symptoms. Topical steroids help to reduce inflammation, and antihistamines help to relieve itching. Systemic steroids may be prescribed when lesions are widespread, but long-term use is avoided because of the side effects.

Pemphigus Vulgaris

PATHOPHYSIOLOGY

Pemphigus vulgaris is a rare, chronic blistering disease with high morbidity and mortality. It is caused by an autoimmune disorder that occurs most often during middle and old age.

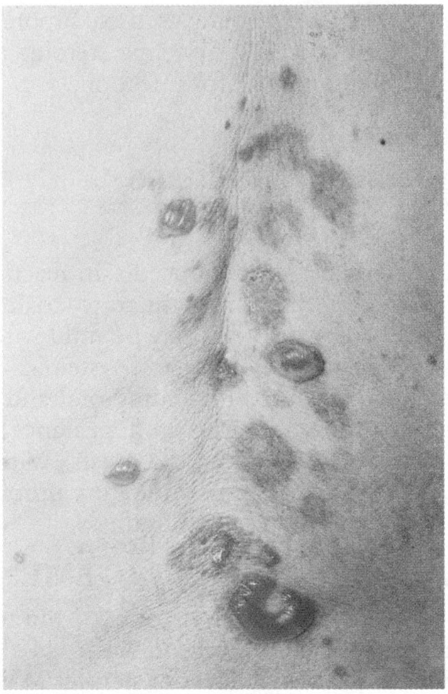

Figure 70-27 ■ Pemphigus vulgaris.

COLLABORATIVE MANAGEMENT

The acute lesions occur on normal-appearing skin or mucous membrane surfaces as fragile, flaccid bullae (Figure 70-27). Breaking the bullae leaves partial-thickness wounds that bleed, weep, and eventually form crusts.

Lesions can occur anywhere. The initial lesions usually occur on the oral mucosa, and later lesions form on the trunk. Spread of the disease is seen with the appearance of new lesions on the face and in skin-fold areas while older lesions are in the process of healing. Oral lesions are common and can make chewing and swallowing difficult.

Treatment of pemphigus vulgaris is aimed at suppressing the immune response that causes the blister formation. Systemic steroids and cytotoxic agents are used to bring about remission. Topical antibiotic creams or ointments are used to reduce bacterial infection of the unhealed lesions.

Toxic Epidermal Necrolysis

PATHOPHYSIOLOGY

Toxic epidermal necrolysis (TEN) is a rare acute drug reaction of the skin resulting in diffuse erythema and large blister formation. Mucous membranes are often involved, and systemic toxicity is evident. The most common causative drugs are sulfonamides, pyrazolones, barbiturates, and antibiotics. Removal of the drug is usually followed by gradual healing in 2 to 3 weeks, with widespread peeling of the epidermis.

COLLABORATIVE MANAGEMENT

The drug thought to be causing a toxic reaction is discontinued, and therapy is aimed at systemic support and prevention of secondary infection. Clients with TEN are often admitted to burn units, where fluid and electrolyte balance, caloric intake, and hypothermia can be closely monitored. Topical antibacterial agents are used to suppress bacterial growth until healing occurs. Systemic steroids are avoided because of the increased risk for infection.

Stevens-Johnson Syndrome

PATHOPHYSIOLOGY

This disorder is often a drug-induced skin reaction through an immunologic mechanism, similar to toxic epidermal necrolysis (TEN). The disorder may be mild with only skin involvement, or it may be severe and systemic. The skin lesions are widely distributed (including oral and respiratory mucous membranes) and varied in appearance. The client has a mix of vesicles, erosions, and crusts. With severe involvement, the client may have respiratory problems, excessive fluid loss, renal failure, and blindness.

COLLABORATIVE MANAGEMENT

Removal of the offending drug is critical. Mild forms of the disorder are usually self-limiting in 10 to 14 days. Severe manifestations require high doses of steroids to suppress the immune and inflammatory reactions. Supportive care may include fluid replacement, mechanical ventilation, and even renal replacement therapy.

Frostbite

PATHOPHYSIOLOGY

Cold injury of the skin depends on the intensity of the external temperature, the duration of exposure to cold temperatures, and the relative hypoxia of the tissues at the time of exposure. Cell death occurs as a result of poor tissue oxygenation owing to cold-induced blood vessel constriction. With continued exposure to the cold, vascular necrosis and gangrene result. Factors that increase the risk for cold injury are age, immobility, alcohol use, vascular disease, and psychiatric disorders.

COLLABORATIVE MANAGEMENT

Acute frostbite is treated in the hospital setting, with rapid and continuous rewarming of the tissue in a water bath (90° to 107° F [32° to 42° C]) for 15 to 20 minutes or until flushing of the skin occurs. Slow thawing or interrupted periods of warmth are avoided because this can increase cell damage. Thawing can cause considerable pain, and analgesics are needed.

After thawing, the wound is left exposed so that local tissue changes can be monitored. Blisters are left intact. With time, the degree of actual tissue destruction becomes evident as an eschar forms. After eschar has formed, local care of the wound is similar to that for skin trauma. Complications of cold injury include amputation, scarring, depigmentation, and thickened nail plates.

Leprosy

PATHOPHYSIOLOGY

Leprosy (Hansen's disease) is a chronic contagious, systemic mycobacterial infection of the peripheral nervous system with skin involvement. The clinical course of the disease is either progressive or self-limiting, depending on the immunologic status of the host. Hansen's disease is still found in the United States. Most cases are reported in Florida, Louisiana, Texas, New York, California, and Hawaii.

The exact mechanism of infection remains unknown. Studies suggest transmission via the airborne route, by insects, or through direct contact with skin lesions.

COLLABORATIVE MANAGEMENT

Manifestations of leprosy, including skin changes, are directly related to how resistant the client is to the mycobacteria:

- Localized (high-immunity) leprosy–one or two isolated, red, anesthetic, hairless plaques that are sometimes scaly
- Generalized (low-immunity) leprosy–widespread, faintly red macules, papules, nodules, and plaques
- Varying degrees of reduced skin sensation of the lesions are caused by peripheral nerve damage

Treatment is available on an outpatient basis. The aim is to control bacterial growth and reduce physical deformities. The drug of choice is dapsone (DDS; Avlosulfon), a sulfone with relatively few side effects that clients must take for life. In clients with sulfone-resistant disease, clofazimine (Lamprene) is indicated. This drug has a slow bactericidal effect on the organism that causes leprosy. Major side effects include skin discoloration (pink to brownish black) and abdominal discomfort.

NAIL DISORDERS

Ingrown Toenail

PATHOPHYSIOLOGY

Although seemingly a minor problem, an ingrown toenail **(unguis incarnatus)** can be troublesome. Pain and infection result when the edge of the nail plate grows into the soft pulp of the toe.

COLLABORATIVE MANAGEMENT

Management is aimed at controlling local infection while encouraging the nail edges to grow beyond the level of the pulp, where the nail plate can be trimmed. Teach clients to soak the foot in warm water (to which an antiseptic has been added) for 20 to 30 minutes. The softened nail plate then is gently lifted, and a small piece of gauze is inserted between the nail and the flesh on each side. This procedure is repeated twice daily until the nail has grown beyond the flesh so that it can be cut.

An ingrown toenail can be treated more aggressively with surgical removal of the nail plate. However, the pain of surgical removal can be severe, and recurrence is possible if the nail bed is not completely destroyed.

GET READY for the NCLEX Examination!

KEY POINTS

Safe Effective Care Environment

- Assist all clients with limited mobility to change positions at least every 2 hours while awake.
- Evaluate the pressure ulcer risk for all clients on admission and regularly thereafter.
- Be proactive in the use of pressure-relieving devices for any client who is identified to be at risk for pressure ulcer formation (i.e., requires prolonged bedrest, is an older adult, has some degree of immobility, is incontinent, has some degree of malnutrition, is dehydrated, has decreased sensory perception, or has an altered mental state).
- Wash your hands before and after touching any skin lesions.
- Use standard precautions when providing care to a client who has any areas of nonintact skin.
- Use a tongue depressor or gloved finger to remove topical medication from a jar or other type of open container.
- Do not reuse disposable supplies between clients.
- Use a lift sheet to move immobilized older clients rather than pulling or dragging them across bed linens.

Health Promotion and Maintenance

- Encourage all clients to reduce sun exposure and exposure to ultraviolet (UV) light.
- Teach clients how to examine all skin areas on a monthly basis for new lesions and changes to existing lesions. The client should keep a record or "body map" of skin lesions.
- Teach clients who have skin scarring from a previous skin injury to examine this area at least monthly for changes related to cancer development or chronic skin conditions (Koebner's phenomenon).
- Encourage all clients to bathe, shampoo the hair, and keep fingernails clean and trimmed on a regular basis.
- Teach all clients the ABCD method of evaluating a lesion for melanoma.
- Keep the skin of clients who are incontinent clean and dry.
- Ensure that female clients in their child-bearing years who are receiving isotretinoin therapy understand the teratogenic effects of this therapy and are using at least two forms of contraception during treatment.

Psychosocial Integrity

- Allow the client the opportunity to express feelings about a change in body image as a result of changes in the skin, hair, or nails.
- Explain all procedures, restrictions, medications, and follow-up care to the client and family.
- Touch the client who has skin problems to show acceptance.
- Ask the client who plans to have plastic surgery what he or she expects as a result of the surgery.

Physiological Integrity

- Keep skin-fold areas on clients clean and dry.
- Avoid applying oil-based ointments or pastes to skin fold areas.
- Ask any client who has started taking a newly prescribed drug whether he or she has noticed if any skin changes have occurred since starting the medication.
- Avoid rubbing any area of the skin that has been subjected to pressure.
- Encourage clients with itching to avoid scratching the skin.
- Teach clients to avoid using over-the-counter cortisone preparations on skin lesions until the cause has been identified.
- Teach clients who have a skin infection how to avoid spreading the infection to either other parts of their own bodies or to other people.
- Evaluate any open skin area on a client daily for size, depth, exudate, and presence of infection.

ADDITIONAL STUDY RESOURCES

Go to your Student CD-ROM for Review Questions for the NCLEX Examination.

evolve Go to http://evolve.elsevier.com/Iggy/ for Integrated Management of Care Questions for the NCLEX Examination.

SELECTED BIBLIOGRAPHY

Asterisk indicates a classic or definitive work on this subject.

Abbas, A., & Lichtman, A. (2003). *Cellular and molecular immunology* (5th ed.). Philadelphia: W.B. Saunders.

Ackley, B., & Ladwig, G. (2002). *Nursing diagnosis handbook: A guide to planning care* (5th ed.). St. Louis: Mosby.

American Academy of Dermatology. (2002). Actinic keratoses and skin cancer. *Dermatology Nursing, 14*(6), 397-399.

American Cancer Society. (2005). *Cancer facts and figures 2005.* Report No. 00-300M-No. 5008.05. Atlanta: Author.

Ayello, E. (2003). Predicting pressure ulcer sore risk. *Dermatology Nursing, 15*(1), 62, 65.

Ayello, E., Cuddigan, J., & Kerstein, M. (2002). Skip the knife: Debriding wounds without surgery. *Nursing 2002, 32*(9), 58-63.

Ayello, E., et al. (2004). Time heals all wounds. *Nursing 2004, 34*(4), 36-41.

Ayers, D.M. (2004). Melanoma. *Nursing 2004, 34*(4), 52-53.

Bamberg, R., Sullivan, P.K., & Conner-Kerr, T. (2002). Diagnosis of wound infections: Current culturing practices of U.S. wound care professionals. *Wounds, 14*(9), 314-327.

Baranoski, S. (2000). Skin tears: The enemy of frail skin. *Advances in Skin and Wound Care, 13*(3), 123-126.

Beitz, J. (2004). Anticoagulant-induced skin necrosis. *American Journal of Nursing, 104*(4), 31-32.

Bielan, B. (2000). What's your assessment? *Dermatology Nursing, 12*(5), 350-351.

Bruce, S. (2004). Radiation-induced xerostomia: How dry is your patient? *Clinical Journal of Oncology Nursing, 8*(1), 61-67.

Carter, K., Dufour, L., & Ballard, C. (2004). Identifying secondary skin lesions. *Nursing 2004, 34*(1), 68.

Clark, J. (2002). Wound repair and factors influencing healing. *Critical Care Nursing Quarterly, 25*(1), 1-12.

Cloote, H. (2000). Psoriasis. *Nursing Standard, 14*(45), 47-52.

Cole, J., & Gray-Miceli, D. (2002). The necessary elements of a dermatologic history and physical evaluation. *Dermatology Nursing, 14*(6), 377-383.

Cuzzell, J. (2002a). Wound assessment and evaluation of wound dressings - Confusion or choice? *Dermatology Nursing, 14*(3), 187-188, 191.

Cuzzell, J. (2002b). Wound assessment and evaluation: Wound documentation guidelines. *Dermatology Nursing, 14*(4), 265-266.

Cuzzell, J. (2002c). Wound healing: Translating theory into clinical practice. *Dermatology Nursing, 14*(4), 257-261.

Davidson, M. (2002). Sharpen your wound assessment skills. *Nursing 2002, 32*(10), 32hn1-32hn4.

DeBoer, S., & Zeglin, D. (2001). Necrotizing fasciitis. *American Journal of Nursing, 101*(4), 37-38.

Dochterman, J., & Bulechek, G. (eds). (2004). *Nursing interventions classification (NIC)* (4th ed.). St. Louis: Mosby.

Ebersole, P., Hess, P., & Luggen, A. (2004). *Toward healthy aging: Human needs and nursing response* (6th ed.). St. Louis: Mosby.

Facts and Comparisons. (2004). *Drug facts and comparisons* (58th ed.). St. Louis: Author.

Ferguson, M., et al. (2000). Pressure ulcer management: The importance of nutrition. *MEDSURG Nursing, 9*(4), 163-176.

Fink, A., & DeLuca, G. (2002). Necrotizing fasciitis: Pathophysiology and treatment. *Dermatology Nursing, 14*(5), 324-327.

Fishman, T. (2000). Wound assessment and evaluation. *Dermatology Nursing, 12*(3), 194-195.

Friedberg, E., Harrison, M., & Graham, I. (2002). Current home care expenditures for persons with leg ulcers. *Journal of Wound, Ostomy, and Continence Nursing, 29*(4), 186-192.

Gray, M., Ratliff, C., & Donovan, A. (2002). Tender mercies: Providing skin care for an incontinent patient. *Nursing 2002, 32*(7), 51-54.

Grubbs, L., & Tabano, M. (2000). Use of sunscreen in health care professionals. *Cancer Nursing, 23*(1), 164-167.

Hallett, C., Caress, A., & Luker, K. (2000). Wound care in the community setting: Clinical decision-making in context. *Journal of Advanced Nursing, 31*(4), 783-793.

Harris, J. (2000). A plan to promote the prevention and early detection of melanoma. *Dermatology Nursing, 12*(5), 329-333.

Harrison-Mackey, C., & Colquitt, E.C. (2001). The hidden culprit: Stevens-Johnson syndrome. *American Journal of Nursing, 101*(5), 24AA-24CC.

Hayes, J. (2003). Are you assessing for melanoma? *RN, 66*(2), 36-40.

Hess, C. (2000). Skin care basics. *Advances in Skin and Wound Care, 13*(3), 127-128.

Hilton, D., Williams, L., & Nesbitt, L. (2000). Systemic glucocortico-steroid therapy in dermatology. *Dermatology Nursing, 12*(4), 258-263.

Hockett, K. (2004). Stevens-Johnson syndrome and toxic epidermal necrolysis: Oncologic considerations. *Clinical Journal of Oncology Nursing, 8*(1), 27-30, 55.

Kaufman, M., & Pahl, D. (2003). Vacuum-assisted closure therapy: Wound care and nursing implications. *Dermatology Nursing, 15*(4), 317-325.

Kloth, L. (2002). How to use electrical stimulation for wound healing. *Nursing 2002, 32*(12), 17.

Lang, P. (2000). Dermatoses in African-Americans. *Dermatology Nursing, 12*(2), 87-98.

Lapka, D. (2000). Oncology today: Skin cancer. *RN, 63*(7), 32-39.

Leifer, G. (2001). Hyperbaric oxygen therapy. *American journal of Nursing, 101*(8), 26-34.

Leininger, S. (2002). The role of nutrition in wound healing. *Critical Care Nursing Quarterly, 25*(1), 13-21.

Levine, N. (2000). Exfoliative erythroderma: Skin biopsy is required to determine the cause of this pruritic eruption. *Geriatrics, 55*(8), 25.

Liao, D. (2003). Management of acne. *The Journal of Family Practice, 52*(1), 43-51.

Lindow, K., & Warren, C. (2001). Understanding rosacea. *American Journal of Nursing, 101*(10), 44-51.

Lookingbill, D.B., & Marks, J.G., Jr. (2000). *Principles of dermatology* (3rd ed.). Philadelphia: W.B. Saunders.

Markova, T. (2002). What is the most effective treatment for tinea pedis (athlete's foot)? *The Journal of Family Practice, 51*(1), 21.

McCance, K., & Huether, S. (2002). *Pathophysiology: The biologic basis for disease in adults and children* (4th ed.). St. Louis: Mosby.

McKay, S. (2000). Why we need to worry about warts. *RN, 63*(9), 68-72.

Moorhead, S., Johnson, M., & Maas, M. (Eds.). (2004). *Nursing outcomes classification (NOC)* (3rd ed.). St. Louis: Mosby.

Moss, R., Moss, C., & Broadway, D. (2000). Body contouring with ultrasound-assisted lipoplasty. *AORN Journal, 71*(2), 370-385.

Motta, G. (2000). Reimbursement relief. *Continuing Care, 19*(4), 14-16.

Novatnack, E., & Steven, S. (2002). HERPES: A bigger problem than you think. *RN, 65*(6), 31-38.

Nussbaum, R., McInnes, R., & Willard, H. (2001). *Thompson & Thompson: Genetics in medicine* (6th ed.). Philadelphia: W.B. Saunders.

Oprica, C., Emtestam, L., & Nord, C. (2002). Overview of treatments for acne. *Dermatology Nursing, 14*(4), 242-246.

Pagana, K., & Pagana, T. (2002). *Mosby's manual of diagnostic and laboratory tests* (2nd ed.). St. Louis: Mosby.

Palmissano, C., & Norman, R. (2000). Geriatric dermatology in chronic care and rehabilitation. *Dermatology Nursing, 12*(2), 116-123.

Patel, C., et al. (2000). Vacuum-assisted wound closure. *American Journal of Nursing, 100*(12), 45-48.

Peters, J. (2000). Toxic epidermal necrolysis. *Nursing Times, 96*(36), 43-44.

Pirrung, M. (2001). Management of toxic epidermal necrolysis. *Journal of Intravenous Nursing, 24*(2), 107-113.

Randolph, S. (2002). When candida turns deadly. *RN, 65*(3), 41-45.

Rapaport, M. (2000). Eyelid dermatitis. *Dermatology Nursing, 12*(5), 352-354.

Rayner, V. (2000). Cosmetic rehabilitation. *Dermatology Nursing, 12*(4), 267-271.

Rivera, E., Walsh, A., & Bradley, M. (2000). Using behavior modification to promote wound healing. *Home Healthcare Nurse, 18*(9), 579-586.

Roy, D., & Stotts, N. (2002). Targeting cellulitis. *Nursing 2002, 32*(12), 46-47.

Rudy, S., & Parham-Vetter, P. (2003). Percutaneous absorption of topically applied medication. *Dermatology Nursing, 15*(2), 145-152.

Schiech, L. (2002). Malignant cutaneous wounds. *Clinical Journal of Oncology Nursing, 6*(5), 305-312.

Scholl, D., & Langkamp-Henken, B. (2001). Nutrient recommendations for wound healing. *Journal of Intravenous Nursing, 24*(2), 124-132.

Sheppard, C., & Brenner, P. (2000). The effects of bathing and skin care practices on skin quality and satisfaction with an innovative product. *Journal of Gerontological Nursing, 25*(10), 36-45.

Sibbald, G., et al. (2000). Preparing the wound bed: Debridement, bacterial balance, and moisture balance. *Ostomy Wound Management, 46*(11), 14-35.

Stanley, W. (2003). Nailing a key assessment. *Nursing 2003, 33*(10), 50-51.

Stotts, N., & Hopf, H. (2003). The link between tissue oxygen and hydration in nursing home residents with pressure ulcers: Preliminary data. *Journal of Wound, Ostomy, and Continence Nursing, 30*, 184-190.

Thompson, J. (2003). Maximizing your pressure ulcer care. *RN, 66*(4), 16-24.

*U.S. Department of Health and Human Services. (1992a). *Pressure ulcers in adults: Prediction and prevention.* Clinical Practice Guideline No. 3. Rockville, MD: Agency for Health Care Policy and Research, Public Health Service, U.S. Department of Health and Human Services.

*U.S. Department of Health and Human Services. (1992b). *Preventing pressure ulcers: A patient's guide.* Clinical Practice Guideline No. 3. Rockville, MD: Agency for Health Care Policy and Research, Public Health Service, U.S. Department of Health and Human Services.

U.S. Preventive Services Task Force (2004). Counseling to prevent skin cancer: Recommendations and rationale. *American Journal of Nursing, 104*(4), 87-91.

Van Rijswijk, L. (2004). Wound wise: Moist dressings are better than dry ones. *American Journal of Nursing, 104*(2), 28-31.

Weiss, S., et al. (2003). Quality of life considerations in psoriasis treatment. *Dermatology Nursing, 15*(2), 120-127.

Wilson, J., & Clark, J. (2003). Obesity: Impediment to wound healing. *Critical Care Nursing Quarterly, 26*(2), 119-132.

Worley, C. (2004a). The wound healing process symphony: Part I. *Dermatology Nursing, 16*(1), 67, 72.

Worley, C. (2004b). The wound healing process symphony: Part II. *Dermatology Nursing, 16*(2), 179-180.

Young, M. (2003). Preparing dermatology nurses: Biologic therapies for psoriasis. *Dermatology Nursing, 15*(2), 413-423.

Zulkowski, K., & Albrecht, D. (2003). How nutrition and aging affect wound healing. *Nursing 2003, 33*(8), 70-71.

Zwanziger, P., & Roper, S. (2002). Bacterial counts and types found on wound care supplies used in the home setting. *Journal of Wound, Ostomy, and Continence Nursing, 29*(2), 83-87.

CHAPTER 71

Interventions for Clients with Burns

TAMMY L. COFFEE

LEARNING OUTCOMES

After studying this chapter, you should be able to:

1. Identify burn clients at risk for inhalation injury.
2. Compare the clinical manifestations of superficial, partial-thickness, and full-thickness burn injuries.
3. Explain the expected clinical manifestations of neural and hormonal compensation during the emergent phase of burn injury.
4. Calculate the total body surface area (TBSA) involved in a burn injury.
5. Identify clients at risk for problems of oxygenation.
6. Prioritize nursing care for the client during the emergent phase of burn injury.
7. Use laboratory data and clinical manifestations to determine the effectiveness of fluid resuscitation during the emergent phase of burn injury.
8. Use the Parkland formula to establish the correct rate and timing of fluid replacement.
9. Describe methods to prevent infection from autocontamination and cross-contamination in clients with burn injuries.
10. Prioritize nursing care for the client during the acute phase of burn injury.
11. Explain the alteration of nutritional needs for the burn client during the acute phase of burn injury.
12. Evaluate wound healing in the client during the acute phase of burn injury.
13. Compare pain management strategies for clients in the emergent and acute phases of burn injury.
14. Describe the characteristics of infected burn wounds.
15. Explain the positioning and range-of-motion interventions for the prevention of mobility problems in the client with burns.
16. Prioritize nursing care for the client during the rehabilitation phase of burn injury.
17. Discuss the potential psychosocial problems associated with burn injury.
18. Develop a community-based teaching plan for the client recovering from a burn injury.
19. Identify populations at risk for burn injury and discuss preventive measures.

Go to your Student CD-ROM for Review Questions for the NCLEX Examination keyed to these Learning Outcomes.

Clients who have burn injuries experience many physiologic, metabolic, and psychological changes. Burn injuries can range from a "sunburn" to complex injuries involving all layers of the skin. When the skin is injured, fluid loss and large inflammatory responses change the function of most body systems. The burn client needs comprehensive care for weeks to months in order to survive the injury, reduce complications, and return to his or her best possible functional status. A multidisciplinary team of health care providers is essential to ensure best care and client outcomes.

INTRODUCTION TO THE BURN PROBLEM

PATHOPHYSIOLOGY OF BURN INJURY

The tissue destruction caused by a burn injury leads to many local and systemic problems. Such problems include fluid and protein losses, sepsis, and changes in metabolic, endocrine, respiratory, cardiac, hematologic, and immune functioning. The extent of local and systemic problems is related to age, general health, extent of injury, depth of injury, and the specific body area injured. Even after healing, the burn injury results in late complications such as contracture formation and scarring. Therefore the prevention of infection and closure of the burn wound are vitally important. A lack of or delay in healing is a key factor for all systemic problems and causes much morbidity and mortality among clients who are burned.

Skin Changes Resulting from Burn Injury

ANATOMIC CHANGES

The skin is the largest organ of the body (see Chapter 69). Each of its two major layers, the epidermis and dermis, has several sublayers. The epidermis, the outer layer of skin, is a superficial layer of stratified epithelial cells about 0.15 mm thick (somewhat thinner in older adults). This layer can grow back after a burn injury because the epidermal cells surrounding sweat and oil glands and hair follicles extend into dermal tissue and regrow to heal partial-thickness wounds. Together, the sweat and oil glands and the hair follicles are the **dermal appendages.** The depth of the dermal appendages varies from one body area to another. The sweat and oil glands in the palm of the hand and the sole of the foot, for example, extend deep into the dermis. This allows for healing of fairly deep burns in these areas. The epidermis has no blood vessels. Nutrients to this layer are diffused from the second layer of skin, the dermis.

The basement membrane, a thin noncellular protein surface, separates the dermis from the epidermis. The dermis is sometimes called the "true skin" because it is not constantly shed and replaced. The dermis is thicker than the epidermis and ranges in thickness from 0.60 to 1.2 mm. The dermis is the thicker part of the skin and is made up of collagen, fibrous connective tissue, and elastic fibers. Within the dermis are the blood vessels, sensory nerves, hair follicles, lymph vessels, sebaceous glands, and sweat glands.

When burn injury occurs, the skin can regenerate as long as parts of the dermis are present. When the entire layer of dermis is burned, all epithelial cells and dermal appendages are destroyed, and the skin can no longer restore itself. The subcutaneous tissue, or superficial fascia, varies in thickness and lies below the dermis. With deep burns, the subcutaneous tissues may be damaged, leaving bones, tendons, and muscles exposed.

FUNCTIONAL CHANGES

The skin has many functions (see Table 69-1). The skin is a protective barrier against injury and microbial invasion from the environment. A burn injury breaks this barrier, greatly increasing the risk for infection.

The skin also helps maintain the delicate fluid and electrolyte balance essential for life. After a burn injury, massive fluid loss occurs through evaporation. Evaporate through burn-injured skin occurs four times as rapidly as from intact skin. The rate of evaporation is in proportion to the total body surface area (TBSA) burned and the depth of injury.

The skin is an excretory organ through sweating. Full-thickness burns destroy the sweat glands, reducing excretory ability.

The skin is the largest sensory organ of the body. Pain, pressure, temperature, and touch are sensed on the skin in normal daily activities, which allows a person to react to changes in the environment. All burn injuries are painful. With partial-thickness burns, nerve endings are exposed, increasing sensitivity and pain. With full-thickness burns, nerve endings are completely destroyed. At first these wounds are completely **anesthetic** (do not transmit sensation) when a sharp stimulus is applied. Despite this destruction, clients often have dull or pressure-type of pain in these areas.

Skin exposed to sunlight activates vitamin D. Partial-thickness burns reduce the activation of vitamin D. Activation of vitamin D is lost completely in full-thickness burns.

The skin helps determine physical identity. The skin's cosmetic quality is part of each person's unique appearance. With a change in appearance through a major burn, psychological problems may develop.

TEMPERATURE. The internal body temperature remains within a narrow range (about 84.2° to 109.4° F [29° to 43° C]) compared with the wide temperature changes in the external environment. Several processes normally adjust to wide differences in external temperature. Circulating blood both provides and dissipates heat efficiently. When heat is applied to the skin, the temperature of the immediate subdermal layer rises rapidly. As soon as the heat source is removed, compensatory processes quickly return the area to a normal temperature. If the heat source is not removed, or if it is applied at a rate that exceeds the skin's capacity to dissipate it, cells are destroyed.

The skin can tolerate temperatures up to 104° F (40° C) without injury. At temperatures of 158° F (71° C) and above, cell destruction is so rapid that even brief exposure damages the skin and subcutaneous levels. Figure 71-1 shows the relationship between temperature and exposure time for burn injury.

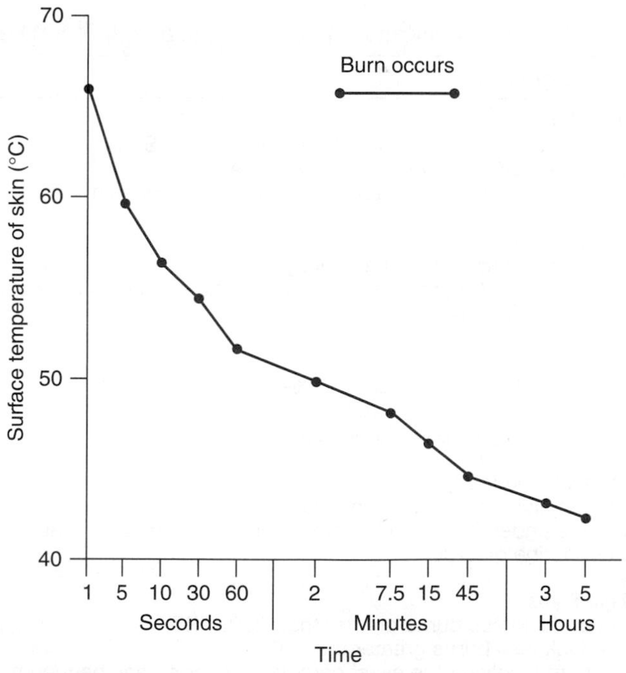

Figure 71-1 ■ Relationship between intensity of heat and the duration of exposure. Exposure for prolonged periods causes burns, even with milder temperatures. At more extreme temperatures, tissue damage results after only seconds. (Modified from Mortiz, A.R. [1947]. Studies of thermal injuries. II: The relative importance of time and surface temperature in causation of cutaneous burns. *American Journal of Pathology,* 23, 695.)

DEPTH OF BURN INJURY. The severity of a burn is determined by the extent of the body surface area involved and the depth of the burn. The degree of tissue damage is related to what agent caused the burn and to the temperature and duration of exposure to the heat source.

Differences in skin thickness in various parts of the body also affect burn depth. In areas where the skin is thin (e.g., eyelids, ears, nose, genitalia, tops of the hands and feet, fingers, and toes), a short exposure to high temperatures causes a deep burn injury. The skin is thinner in older adults, which predisposes them to increased burn severity, even at lower temperatures of shorter duration.

Burn wounds are classified as superficial-thickness wounds, partial-thickness wounds, full-thickness wounds, and deep full-thickness wounds. The partial-thickness wounds are further divided into superficial and deep subgroups. Table 71-1 lists the clinical differences of these burns.

The American Burn Association (ABA) describes burns as minor, moderate, or major depending on the depth, extent, and location of injury (Table 71-2). Figure 71-2 shows

TABLE 71-1 Classification of Burn Depth

Characteristic	Superficial	Partial-Thickness Superficial	Deep Partial-Thickness	Full-Thickness	Deep Full-Thickness
Color	Pink to red	Pink to red	Red to white	Black, brown, yellow, white, red	Black
Edema	Mild	Mild to moderate	Moderate	Severe	Absent
Pain	Yes	Yes	Yes	Yes and no	Absent
Blisters	No	Yes	Rare	No	No
Eschar	No	No	Yes, soft and dry	Yes, hard and inelastic	Yes, hard and inelastic
Healing time	3-5 days	~2 wk	2-6 wk	Weeks to months	Weeks to months
Grafts required	No	No	Can be used if healing is prolonged	Yes	Yes
Example	Sunburn, flash burns	Scalds, flames, brief contact with hot objects	Scalds; flames; prolonged contact with hot objects, tar, grease, chemicals	Scalds; flames; prolonged contact with hot objects, tar, grease chemicals, electricity	Flames, electricity, grease, tar, chemicals

TABLE 71-2 Classification of Burn Injury and Burn Center Referral Criteria

Characteristics	Comments
Minor Burns Deep partial-thickness burns less than 15% TBSA Full-thickness burns less than 2% TBSA No burns of eyes, ears, face, hands, feet, or perineum No electrical burns No inhalation injury No complicated concomitant injury Client is under 60 years and has no chronic cardiac, pulmonary, or endocrine disorder	Clients in this category should receive emergency care at the scene and be taken to a hospital emergency department. A special expertise hospital or designated burn center is not necessary.
Moderate Burns Deep partial-thickness burns 15%-25% TBSA Full-thickness burns 2%-10% TBSA No burns of eyes, ears, face, hands, feet, or perineum No electrical burns No inhalation injury No complicated concomitant injury Client is under 60 yr and has no chronic cardiac, pulmonary, or endocrine disorder	Clients in this category should receive emergency care at the scene and be transferred either to a special expertise hospital or to a designated burn center.
Major Burns Partial-thickness burns greater than 25% TBSA Full-thickness burns greater than 10% Any burn involving the eyes, ears, face, hands, feet, perineum Electrical injury Inhalation injury Client over 60 yr of age Burn complicated with other injuries (e.g., fractures) Client has cardiac, pulmonary, or other chronic metabolic disorders	Clients who meet *any one* of the criteria for a major burn should receive emergency care at the nearest emergency department and then be transferred to a designated burn center as soon as possible.

TBSA, Total body surface area.

the tissue layers involved with different depths of injury and describes the criteria for referral to a burn center.

SUPERFICIAL-THICKNESS WOUNDS. Of all burn types, superficial-thickness wounds have the least damage because the epidermis is the only part of the skin that is injured. The epithelial cells and basement membrane, needed for total regrowth, are present.

Superficial-thickness wounds are caused by prolonged exposure to low-intensity heat (e.g., sunburn) or short (flash) exposure to high-intensity heat. Redness with mild edema, pain, and increased sensitivity to heat occur as a result. Peeling of dead skin **(desquamation)** occurs for 2 to 3 days after the burn. The area heals rapidly in 3 to 5 days without a scar or other complication.

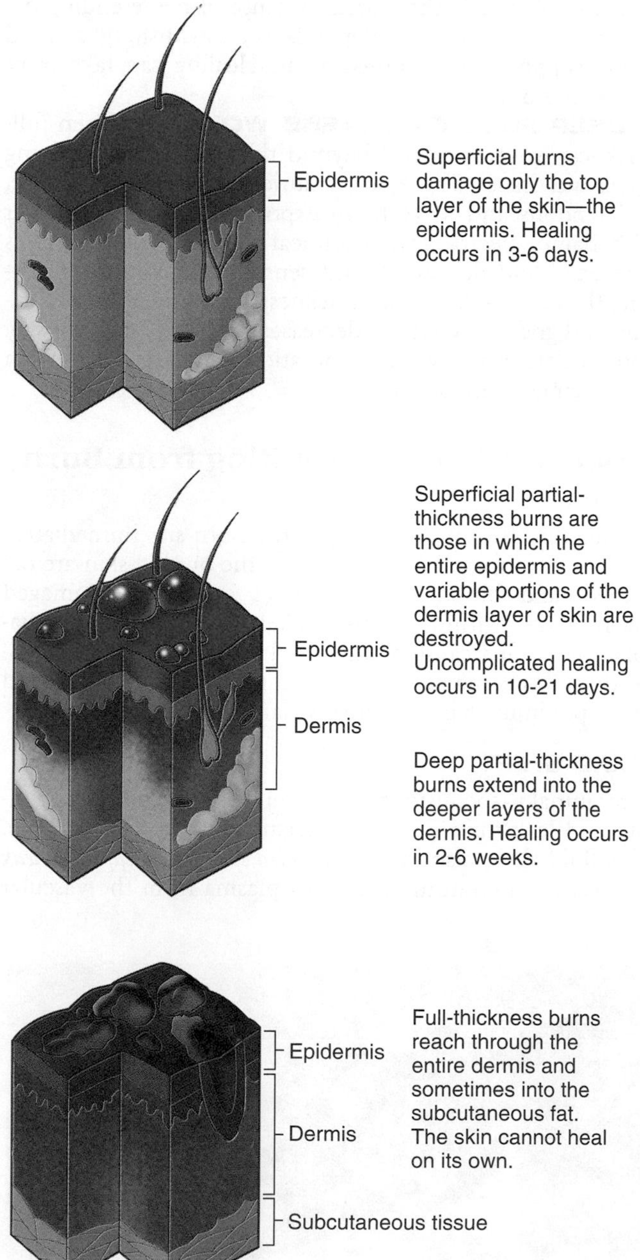

Figure 71-2 ■ The tissues involved in burns of various depths.

PARTIAL-THICKNESS WOUNDS. A partial-thickness wound involves the entire epidermis and varying depths of the dermis. Depending on the amount of dermal tissue damaged, partial-thickness wounds are further subdivided into superficial partial-thickness and deep partial-thickness injuries.

Superficial Partial-Thickness Wounds. Superficial partial-thickness wounds are caused by heat injury to the upper third of the dermis leaving a good blood supply. These wounds are red, moist, and **blanch** (whiten) when pressure is applied (Figure 71-3). The small vessels perfusing this area are injured, resulting in the leakage of large amounts of plasma, which in turn lifts off the heat-destroyed epidermis, causing blister formation. The blisters continue to increase in size after the burn as cell and protein breakdown occurs. When intact, the blister is a sterile environment, which can protect the wound from infection and water loss. Large or numerous blisters are opened to promote healing and prevent immunosuppression.

Superficial partial-thickness wounds increase pain sensation. Nerve endings are exposed, and any stimulation (touch or temperature change) causes intense pain. With standard care these burns heal in 10 to 21 days with no scar, but some minor pigment changes may occur.

Deep Partial-Thickness Wounds. Deep partial-thickness wounds extend deeper into the skin dermis, and fewer healthy cells remain. In these clients, blister formation does not usually occur because the dead tissue layer is so thick and sticks to underlying viable dermis that it does not readily lift off the surface. The wound surface is red and dry with white areas in deeper parts (dry because fewer

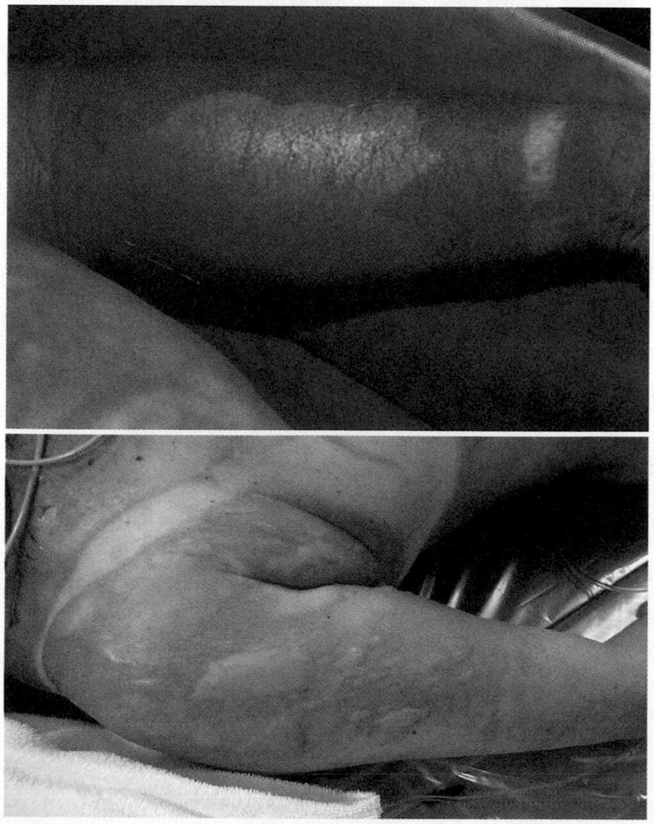

Figure 71-3 ■ The typical appearance of superficial partial-thickness burn injury.

blood vessels are patent). When pressure is applied to the burn, it may blanch slowly or not at all (Figure 71-4). Edema is moderate; pain is present to a lesser degree than with superficial burns because more of the nerve endings have been destroyed.

The blood supply to these areas is reduced by blood vessel constriction. Progression to deeper injury can occur from hypoxia and ischemia. Adequate hydration, nutrients, and oxygen are needed for regrowth of skin cells and prevention of conversion to deeper burns. Partial-thickness wounds can convert to full-thickness wounds when tissue damage increases with infection, hypoxia, or ischemia. Deep partial-thickness wounds generally heal in 3 to 6 weeks, but scar formation results. Surgical intervention with skin grafting can reduce healing time.

FULL-THICKNESS WOUNDS. A full-thickness wound occurs with destruction of the entire epidermis and dermis, leaving no residual epidermal cells to repopulate (Figure 71-5). This wound, therefore, does not re-epithelialize and whatever area of the wound is not closed by wound contraction (see Chapter 70) will require grafting.

The full-thickness injury has a hard, dry, leathery **eschar** (burn crust) that forms from coagulated particles of destroyed dermis. *The eschar is dead tissue; it must slough off or be removed from the burn wound before healing can occur.* The thick particles often stick to the subcutaneous layer by collagen fibers, which makes eschar removal difficult. Edema is pronounced under the eschar in a full-thickness wound. When the injury completely surrounds an extremity or the thorax **(circumferential),** blood flow and chest movement for breathing may be reduced by tight eschar. **Escharotomies** (incisions through the eschar) or **fasciotomies** (incisions through eschar and fascia) may be needed to relieve pressure and allow normal blood flow and breathing (see Surgical Management [Ineffective Tissue Perfusion], p. 1634).

A full-thickness burn wound may be waxy white, deep red, yellow, brown, or black. Thrombosed vessels may be visible beneath the surface of the burn because the dermal blood vessels are heat coagulated, causing the burned tissue to be without a blood supply **(avascular).** Sensation is reduced or absent in these areas because of nerve ending destruction. Healing time depends on establishing a good blood supply in the injured areas. Healing can take from weeks to months.

DEEP FULL-THICKNESS WOUNDS. Deep full-thickness wounds extend beyond the skin into underlying fascia and tissues. These deep injuries damage muscle, bone, and tendons and leave them exposed. These burns occur with flame, electrical, or chemical injuries. The wound is blackened and depressed, and sensation is completely absent (Figure 71-6). All full-thickness burns need early excision and grafting. Grafting decreases pain and length of stay and accelerates recovery. Amputation may be needed when an extremity is involved.

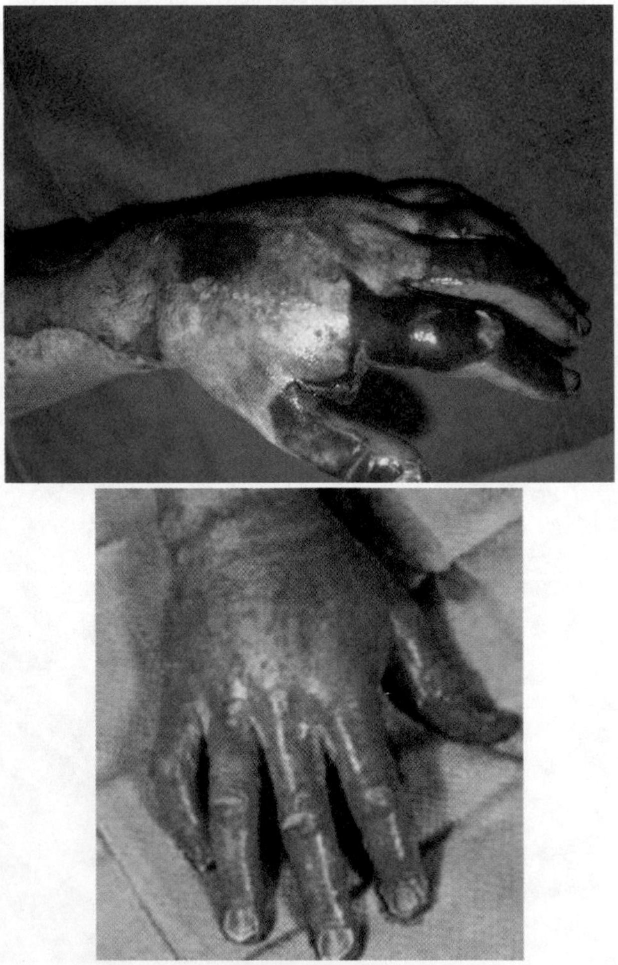

Figure 71-4 ■ The typical appearance of a deep partial-thickness burn injury.

Vascular Changes Resulting from Burn Injuries

Circulatory disruption occurs at the burn site immediately after a burn injury. Blood vessels to the burned skin are occluded, and blood flow decreases or ceases. Damaged macrophages within the tissues release chemicals (mediators) that at first cause blood vessel constriction. Blood vessel thrombosis may occur, causing necrosis, which can lead to deeper injuries in the already damaged areas.

FLUID SHIFT

After initial vasoconstriction, blood vessels near the burn dilate and leak fluid into the interstitial space (Figure 71-7). This fluid shift, also known as *third spacing* or *capillary leak syndrome,* is a continuous leak of plasma from the vascular

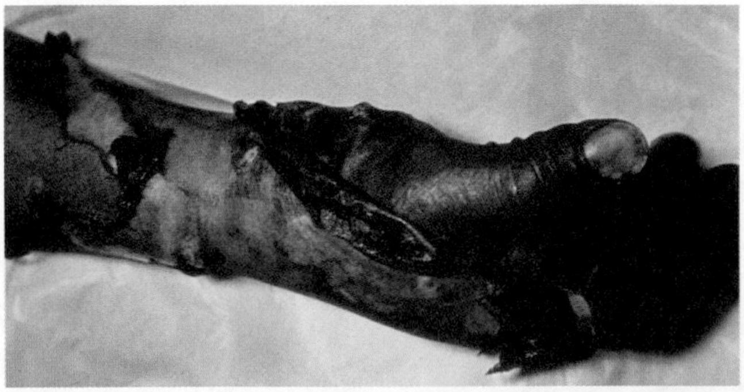

Figure 71-5 ■ The typical appearance of a full-thickness burn injury.

space into the interstitial space. The loss of plasma fluids and proteins decreases blood volume and blood pressure. Leakage of fluid and electrolytes from the vascular space continues, causing extensive edema, even in areas that were not injured. Fluid shift, with excessive weight gain, usually occurs in the first 12 hours after the burn and can continue for 24 to 36 hours.

The amount of fluid shifted depends on the extent and severity of injury. Capillary leak occurs in both burned and unburned area when tissue damage is extensive (i.e., greater than 20% to 30% total body surface area **[TBSA]**). Edema develops as plasma and electrolytes escape into the interstitial space. The proteins now in the interstitial space increase the movement of fluids out from the vascular space.

Profound imbalances of fluid, electrolytes, and acid-base occur as a result of the fluid shift and cell damage. These imbalances usually include hypovolemia, metabolic acidosis, **hyperkalemia** (elevated blood potassium levels), and **hyponatremia** (decreased blood sodium levels). Hyperkalemia occurs as a result of direct cell injury that releases large amounts of cellular potassium. Sodium is retained by the body as a result of the endocrine response to stress. Aldosterone secretion increases, leading to increased sodium reabsorption by the kidney. This sodium, however, quickly passes into the interstitial spaces of the burned area with the fluid shift; therefore despite the increased amount of sodium in the body, most of the sodium is trapped in the interstitial space, and a sodium deficit occurs in the blood. **Hemoconcentration** (elevated blood osmolarity, hematocrit, and hemoglobin) develops from vascular dehydration. Hemoconcentration increases blood viscosity, reducing flow through small vessels and increasing tissue hypoxia.

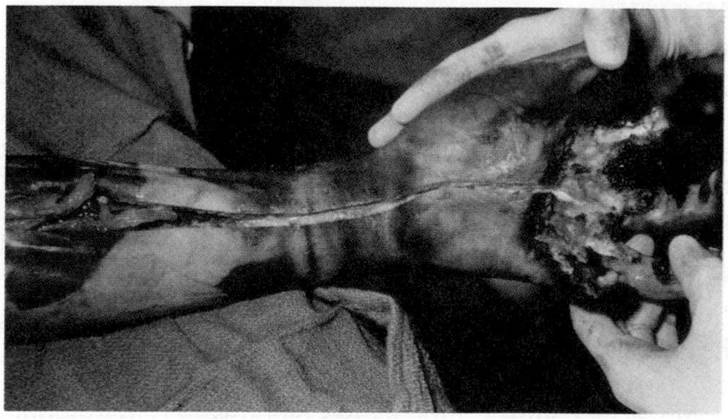

Figure 71-6 ■ The typical appearance of a deep full-thickness burn injury.

FLUID REMOBILIZATION

At about 24 hours after injury, the capillary leak stops and capillary integrity is restored. The diuretic stage begins at about 48 to 72 hours after the burn injury as capillary membrane integrity returns and edema fluid shifts from the interstitial spaces into the vascular space. Blood volume increases, leading to increased renal blood flow and diuresis unless renal damage has occurred. Body weight returns to normal over the next several days as edema subsides.

During this phase, **hyponatremia** (low blood sodium level) develops because of increased renal sodium excretion and the loss of sodium from wounds. **Hypokalemia** (low blood potassium level) results from potassium moving back into the cells and being excreted in urine output. Anemia often develops as a result of hemodilution, but it is generally not severe enough to require blood transfusions. Transfusions are needed if the client's hematocrit is less than 20% to 25% and the client has manifestations of hypoxia. Transfusions are given only when absolutely necessary. Protein continues to be lost from the wounds. Metabolic acidosis remains a possibility because of the loss of sodium bicarbonate in the urine and the increased fat metabolism secondary to decreased carbohydrate intake.

Cardiac Changes Resulting from Burn Injury

Heart rate increases and cardiac output decreases because of the initial fluid shifts and hypovolemia that occur after a burn injury. Cardiac output may remain low until 18 to 36 hours after the burn injury occurs. Cardiac output increases with fluid resuscitation and reaches normal levels before plasma volume is restored completely. Proper fluid resuscitation and support with adequate oxygenation prevent further complications.

Pulmonary Changes Resulting from Burn Injury

Direct injury to the lung from contact with flames rarely occurs. Rather, respiratory problems are caused by superheated air, steam, toxic fumes, or smoke. Such problems are a major

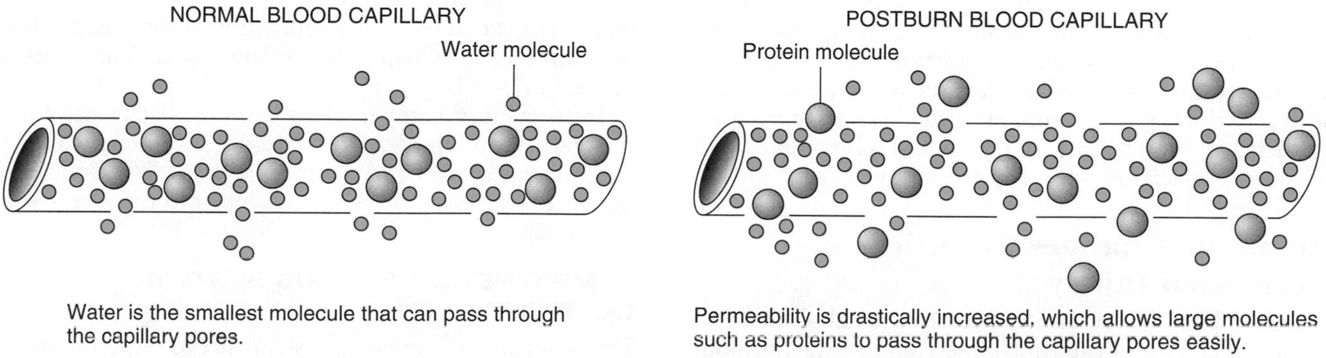

Figure 71-7 ■ The capillary response to burn injury (early phase). This response is also known as "capillary leak syndrome."

cause of death in clients with burns. Respiratory failure with burn injuries can result from airway edema during fluid resuscitation, pulmonary capillary leak, circumferential chest burns that restrict chest movement, and carbon monoxide poisoning.

Respiratory damage from an inhalation injury can occur in the upper and major airways and the lung tissue. The upper airway is affected when inhaled smoke or irritants cause edema and obstruct the trachea. Irritants coming in contact with the upper airway cause a reflex closure of the vocal cords. This protective reflex decreases the amount of smoke and toxic gases entering the lungs. Although air is a poor conductor of heat, some heat does reach the upper airway, causing an inflammatory response that leads to edema of the mouth and throat with the potential of airway obstruction.

More airway injury is caused by chemicals and toxic gases (rather than heat) that are produced during combustion. The ciliated membranes lining the trachea normally trap bacteria and foreign materials. Smoke and combustion products slow this activity, which allows foreign particles to enter the bronchi. The lining of the trachea and bronchi may slough 48 to 72 hours after injury, enter the airway, narrow the tracheal lumen, and obstruct the lower airways.

Lung tissue injuries result from toxic irritant damage to the alveoli and capillaries. Leaking capillaries cause alveolar edema. This edema can occur immediately or as late as 1 week after the injury. The fluid that diffuses into the lung tissue spaces contains proteins that form fibrinous membranes and lead to respiratory distress. Progressive pulmonary failure develops with acute pulmonary insufficiency and infection.

Gastrointestinal Changes Resulting from Burn Injury

The fluid shifts and decreased cardiac output that occur after injury divert blood flow to the brain, heart, and liver. As a result, other organs, including the gastrointestinal (GI) tract, have decreased perfusion. Gastric mucosal integrity and motility are impaired. The sympathetic nervous system stress response increases secretion, especially of epinephrine and norepinephrine, which inhibit GI motility and reduce the flow of blood to the area. Peristalsis decreases, and a paralytic ileus may develop. Secretions and gases collect in the intestines and stomach, causing abdominal distention.

Curling's ulcer (acute ulcerative gastroduodenal disease) may develop within 24 hours after a severe burn injury because of reduced GI blood flow and mucosal damage. The mucosal membrane normally acts as a barrier to the absorption of hydrogen ions secreted into the gastric lumen. With decreased gastric mucosal function, this barrier is disrupted and hydrogen ion production is increased. Ulcerations may develop as a result. However, this complication is now less common because of the use of H_2 histamine blockers, mucoprotectants, and early enteral nutrition.

Metabolic Changes Resulting from Burn Injury

A serious burn injury greatly increases metabolism by increasing secretion of catecholamines, antidiuretic hormone, aldosterone, and cortisol. With this hypermetabolism, the client's oxygen and calorie needs are high.

The catecholamines activate the stress response. The increased production (and loss) of heat breaks down protein and fat **(catabolism),** rapidly uses glucose and calories, and increases urine nitrogen loss. The heat and water lost from the burn also increase metabolic and catabolic rates, which increase calorie needs. Depending on the extent of injury, the client's calorie needs double or triple normal energy needs. These increased rates peak 4 to 12 days after the burn and can remain elevated for months until all wounds are closed.

The hypermetabolic condition also increases core body temperature. The client loses heat through the burned skin because the protective barrier is lost. Core body temperature increases as a response to the adjustment in the hypothalamus. Central body temperature control changes to adapt to the hypermetabolic state and a low-grade fever commonly develops. Essentially what occurs is a "resetting" of the body's normal temperature-control system.

Immunologic Changes Resulting from Burn Injury

Burn injury disrupts the protective barrier of the skin, increasing the risk for infection. The injury activates the inflammatory response and often suppresses immune function (see Chapter 23). Antibody-mediated immunity and cell-mediated immunity are both suppressed. Topical and systemic antibiotics, general anesthesia, blood transfusion, and the stress of surgery further reduce immune function.

Compensatory Responses to Burn Injury

Any tissue injury is a threat to homeostasis and is a stressor. Two compensatory responses have immediate benefit: the inflammatory response and the sympathetic nervous system stress response. Together these responses cause changes that result in many of the manifestations seen in the first 2 to 3 days after a burn injury.

INFLAMMATORY COMPENSATION

Inflammatory compensation can be helpful by triggering healing in the injured tissues. It also is responsible for some of the serious problems that occur with the fluid shift. Inflammatory compensation causes blood vessels to leak fluid into the interstitial space and white blood cells to release chemicals that trigger local tissue reactions. These responses cause the massive fluid shift, edema, and hypovolemia that are seen in the **emergent phase** (first 48 hours) after a burn injury. The extent of the inflammatory response depends on the burn severity. Chapter 23 explains the inflammatory responses in detail.

Inflammatory compensation is immediately helpful to the body when injury occurs. These actions are intended to function on a local and short-term basis. When these actions are widespread or persistent, they can cause severe tissue damage.

SYMPATHETIC NERVOUS SYSTEM COMPENSATION

The sympathetic nervous system stress response occurs when any physical or psychological stressors are present. Changes caused by sympathetic compensation are most ev-

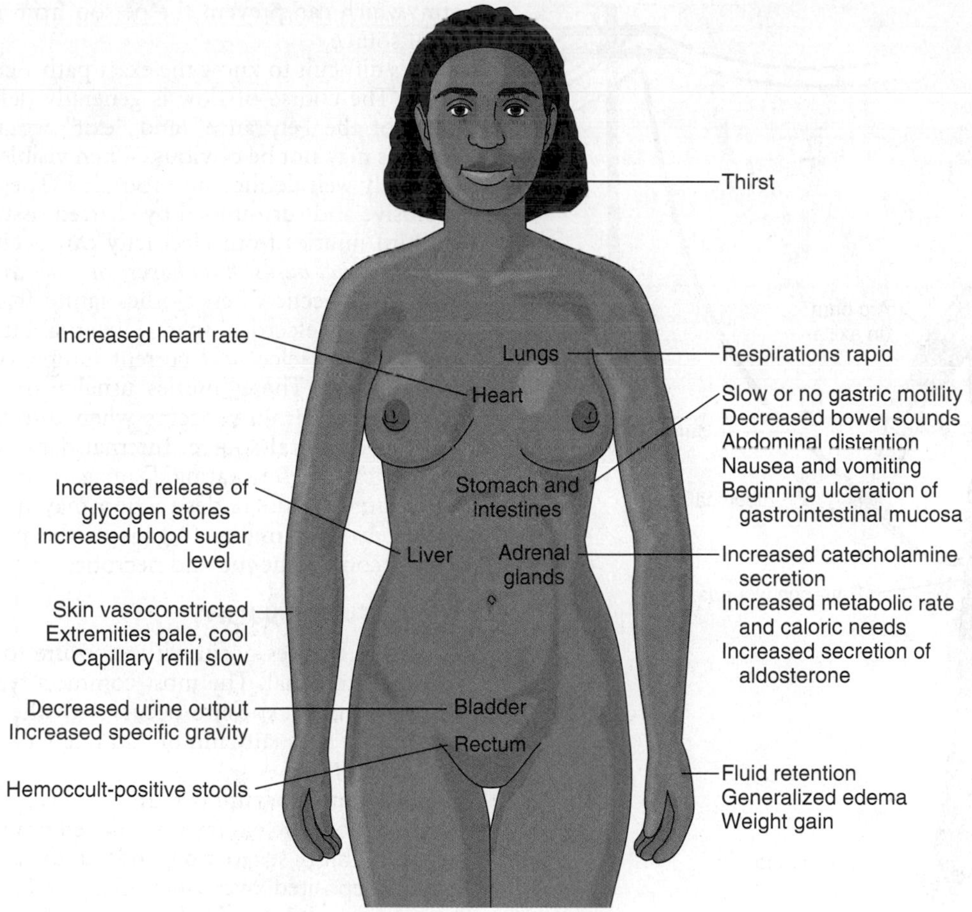

Figure 71-8 ■ The physiologic actions of the sympathetic nervous system compensatory responses to burn injury (early phase).

ident in the cardiovascular, respiratory, and gastrointestinal (GI) systems. Figure 71-8 shows the results of sympathetic nervous system stimulation.

Etiology of Burn Injury

Burn injuries are caused by dry heat (flame), moist heat (scald), contact with hot surfaces, chemicals, electricity, and ionizing radiation. The cause of the injury affects both the prognosis and the treatment.

DRY HEAT

Dry heat injuries are caused by open flame. The most common flame injuries occur in house fires and explosions. Ignited clothing from an open flame accounts for most of the injuries. Explosions usually result in flash burns because they produce a brief exposure to very high temperatures.

MOIST HEAT

Moist heat (scald) injuries are caused by contact with hot liquids or steam. Scald injuries are most common among older adults (Stone, Ahmed, & Evans, 2000). Hot liquid spills usually burn the upper, frontal surfaces of the body, whereas immersion scald injuries usually involve the lower body.

CONTACT BURNS

Hot metal, tar, and grease can cause full-thickness burns when they contact the skin. Hot metal injuries occur when a body part contacts a hot surface, such as a space heater or iron. They also can occur in industrial settings from molten metals. Tar and asphalt temperatures usually are greater than 400° F, and serious deep injuries occur within seconds when the skin is immersed in or splashed with the agent. Hot grease injuries from cooking are usually deep because of the temperature of the grease.

CHEMICAL INJURY

Chemical burns occur as a result of accidents in homes or industry. They can also be the result of a deliberate assault on an individual. Tissue injury occurs when chemicals come in direct contact with the skin and epithelial tissues or are ingested. The severity of the injury depends on the duration of contact, the concentration of the chemical, the amount of tissue exposed, and the action of the chemical.

Alkalis found in oven cleaners, fertilizers, drain cleaners, and heavy industrial cleaners damage the tissue by causing tissues to liquefy and proteins to denature. This allows for deeper spread of the chemical and more severe burns. Acids found in bathroom cleaners, rust removers, chemicals for swimming pools, and industrial drain cleaners damage tissue by coagulating cells and proteins, which tends to limit the depth of tissue damage. Organic compounds are found in many chemical disinfectants and in gasoline. Organic compounds cause damage due to their fat solvent action. Once absorbed they can produce toxic effects on the kidneys and liver.

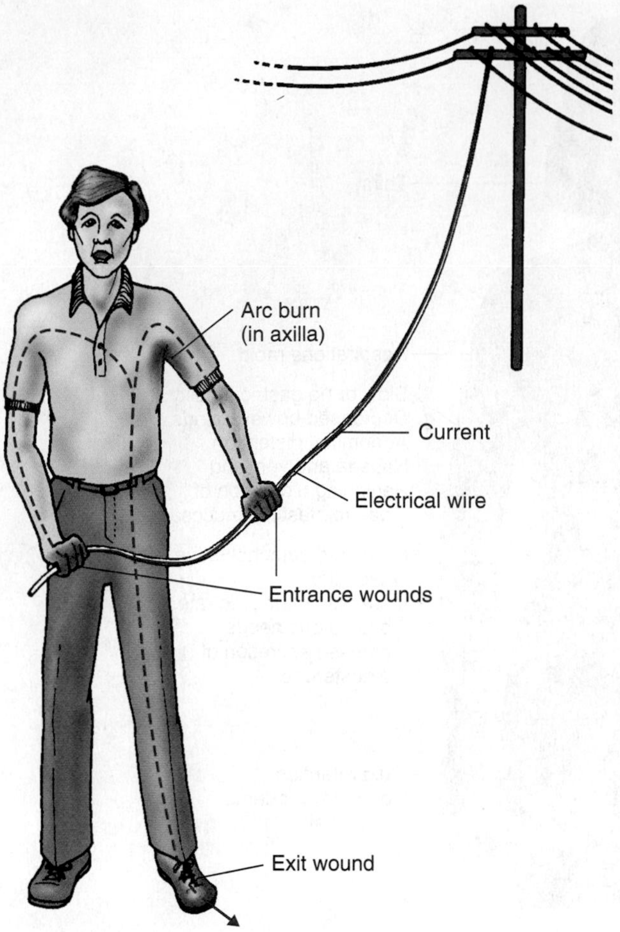

Figure 71-9 ■ The mechanism of electrical injury: Currents passing through the body follow the path of least resistance to the ground.

ELECTRICAL INJURY

An electrical injury is a burn occurring when an electrical current enters the body (Figure 71-9). Electrical injuries have been called the "grand masquerader" of burn injuries because small surface injuries may be associated with devastating internal injuries. Electrical injuries are divided into high and low voltage with high voltage being greater than 1000 volts. Tissue injury from electrical trauma results from electrical energy being converted to heat energy. The extent of injury depends on the type of current, the pathway of flow, the local tissue resistance, and the duration of contact. The skin is the most resistant organ; the greatest resistance is in the epidermis of the skin. At high voltages the difference in tissue resistance is clinically unimportant. Although various underlying tissues have different resistance to current flow, once skin resistance is overcome, the body acts as a conductor and current flows throughout the involved body part. Bone has a very high resistance because of its density. Current flows along the surface of the bone, and the heat generated damages adjacent muscle. As a result, deep muscle injury may be present even when superficial muscles appear normal or uninjured.

The longer the electricity is in contact with the body, the greater the damage. The duration of contact is increased by tetanic contractions of the strong flexor muscles in the forearm, which can prevent the person from releasing the electrical source.

It is difficult to know the exact path a current takes in the body. The course of flow is generally defined by the locations of the "entrance" and "exit" wounds. At first, the wounds may not be obvious. When visible, the entrance site is usually well defined and rounded. The exit site is usually explosive and surrounded by charred tissue.

Burn injuries from electricity can occur in one of three ways: *thermal burns, flash burns,* or *true electrical injury.* Thermal burns occur when clothes ignite from heat or flames produced by electrical sparks. External burn injuries can occur when the electrical current jumps, or "arcs," between two surfaces. These injuries usually are severe and deep. True electrical injury occurs when direct contact is made with an electrical source. Internal damage results, and the injuries can be devastating. Damage starts on the inside and goes out; deep-tissue destruction may not be apparent immediately after injury. Organs in the path of the current may become ischemic and necrotic.

RADIATION INJURY

Radiation injuries occur with exposure to large doses of radioactive material. The most common type of tissue injury from radiation exposure occurs with therapeutic radiation. This injury is usually minor and rarely causes extensive skin damage.

Radiation exposure is more serious in industrial settings where radioactive energy is produced or radioactive isotopes are used. Injury severity depends on the amount and type of energy deposited over time. Chapter 28 discusses the potential for tissue damage from alpha, beta, and gamma radiation. The severity of injury is determined by the type of radiation, distance from the source, duration of exposure, absorbed dose, and depth of penetration into the body.

Incidence/Prevalence of Burn Injury

The incidence of burn injuries in the United States has declined significantly in the past two decades. As of the early 1990s, the rate of reportable burn injuries in the United States had declined from 10 in 10,000 to 4.2 in 10,000.

An estimated 4500 fire and burn deaths occur each year. This total includes deaths from fires and motor vehicle or aircraft crashes, electricity, chemicals, hot liquids and substances, and any other sources of burn injury. Fire and burn deaths in the United States declined about 50% from 1971-1998. The death rate from burns has declined by 60%. Of the clients who seek medical attention, 45,000 are hospitalized each year. Half of the hospitalizations occur in the 125 specialized burn treatment centers. The average TBSA affected in burn victims admitted to a burn center is 14%. Fifty-four percent of burn center admissions are for burns affecting 10% or less TBSA, whereas 4% of admissions are for burns affecting greater than 60% TBSA.

Burns are the sixth leading cause of accidental death in the United States. Causes vary among different age-groups (Table 71-3). The highest risk is among those 75 years and older. Men are at slightly higher risk for fatal and nonfatal burn injuries.

Death from burn injuries decreases with appropriate intervention. Factors that increase the risk for death include age older than 60 years, a burn greater than 40% total body

TABLE 71-3 Percentage of Burn Injuries by Age in the United States

Age	Dry Heat (Flame)	Moist Heat (Scalds)	Contact	Chemical	Electrical	Ionizing Radiation
Birth-23 mo	10	72	15	1	2	<1
2-4 yr	34	54	8	1	3	<1
5-12 yr	70	23	4	1	2	<1
13-18 yr	69	20	5	2	4	<1
19-35 yr	56	26	10	4	4	<1
36-54 yr	44	33	13	4	6	<1
55 yr and older	73	21	4	1	1	<1

CHART 71-1

BEST PRACTICE for Emergency Management of Burns

EMERGENCY CARE

General Management for All Types of Burns
- Assess for airway patency.
- Administer oxygen as needed.
- Cover the client with a blanket.
- Keep the client on NPO status.
- Elevate the extremities if no fractures are obvious.
- Obtain vital signs.
- Initiate an IV line and begin fluid replacement.
- Administer tetanus toxoid for prophylaxis.
- Perform a head-to-toe assessment.

Specific Management

Flame Burns
- Smother the flames.
- Remove smoldering clothing and all metal objects.

Chemical Burns
- Brush off any dry chemicals present on the skin or clothing.
- Remove the client's clothing.
- Ascertain the type of chemical causing the burn.
- Do not attempt to neutralize the chemical unless it has been positively identified and the appropriate neutralizing agent is available.

Electrical Burns
- At the scene, separate the client from the electrical current.
- Smother any flames that are present.
- Initiate cardiopulmonary resuscitation.
- Obtain an electrocardiogram (ECG).

Radiation Burns
- Remove the client from the radiation source.
- If the client has been exposed to radiation from an unsealed source, remove the client's clothing (using tongs or lead protective gloves).
- If the client has radioactive particles on his or her skin, send the client to the nearest designated radiation decontamination center.
- Help the client to bathe or shower.

surface area (TBSA), and the presence of an inhalation injury. When a client has all three risk factors, the risk for mortality is 90%.

The successful treatment of burns can be attributed to many therapeutic advances including vigorous fluid resuscitation, early burn wound excision, improved critical care monitoring, early enteral nutrition, improved topical and systemic antibiotics, and the use of specialized burn centers.

EMERGENT PHASE OF BURN INJURY

OVERVIEW

Burns can be a devastating and dehumanizing injury. Events within the first hour after injury can make the difference between life and death for the client with a burn injury. Immediate care focuses on maintaining an open airway, ensuring adequate breathing and circulation, limiting the extent of injury, and maintaining the function of vital organs. Chart 71-1 outlines the emergency management of a burn injury.

The **emergent phase** is the first phase of a burn injury. It begins at the onset of injury and continues to about 48 hours. During this phase the injury is evaluated and the immediate problems of fluid loss, edema, and reduced blood flow are assessed. The goals of management during this period are to (1) secure the airway, (2) support circulation by fluid replacement, (3) keep the client comfortable with analgesics, (4) prevent infection through careful wound care, (5) maintain body temperature, and (6) provide emotional support.

◆COLLABORATIVE MANAGEMENT

◆Assessment

HISTORY

Knowledge of circumstances surrounding the burn injury is extremely valuable in the management of a burn victim. If possible, obtain information directly from the client. If this is not possible, ask significant others or witnesses. Ask questions that include the circumstances of the injury, the time and place of injury, and the source and cause of injury. Obtain a detailed description of how the burn occurred, and the events occurring from the time of injury until help arrived. Also obtain demographic data, health history (including pre-existing illness), drug use, any accompanying injuries, and pain information.

Demographic data include age, weight, and height. The rate of serious complications and death from burn injuries is increased among adults over 50 years of age. Chart 71-2 lists the age-related differences in the older adults' response to a burn injury. The client's preburn weight is used to calculate fluid rates, energy requirements, and drug doses. The preburn weight often is referred to as "dry weight," because it represents the client's weight before edema begins to form. Calculations based on a weight obtained after fluid replacement is started are not accurate because of water-induced weight gain. Height is important in determining body surface area **(BSA)**, which is used to calculate nutritional needs.

A health history, including any pre-existing illnesses, must be known for appropriate treatment to be given. Obtain information from the client specifically about his or her history of cardiac or renal impairment, chronic alcoholism, substance abuse, and diabetes mellitus; any of these problems

CHART 71-2

NURSING FOCUS on the OLDER ADULT

Age-Related Changes That Increase Mortality and Morbidity from Burns

- Older adults are at a higher risk for burn injury because of thinner skin, decreased mobility and reaction time, and visual and hearing impairment.
- The skin of an older adult person is thinner and more easily damaged than that of a younger person. Therefore burn injuries tend to be more extensive in older clients, even when exposure to causative agent is shorter.
- Healing time is slower in the older adult, which increases risk for infection and other complications.
- Cardiac impairment in the older client with burns limits the amount and type of fluids used in resuscitation. As a result, older clients are more likely to develop complications from hypovolemic shock and inadequate renal perfusion.
- The immune responses of the older client may be reduced, which increases the risk for infection and sepsis. In addition, the older adult may not have a fever when an infection is present.
- Decreased elasticity of the thoracic cage and decreased number and efficiency of alveoli make older adults more likely to develop hypoxia, hypoventilation, and atelectasis.
- Older adults are more likely to have pre-existing medical condition (e.g., diabetes mellitus, cardiovascular disorders, pulmonary or renal impairment, or immunosuppression) that may further compromise vital organ function or interfere with resuscitation and treatment.

influence fluid resuscitation. The physiologic stress seen with a burn can make a latent disease process develop symptoms or worsen an active process. Obtain a drug history that includes allergies, current drugs, and immunization status from the client or family. Determine the dose and time the last drug was taken. Ask whether or not the client smokes or drinks alcohol daily; these factors can influence treatment and physical responses.

Other injuries are unusual but may occur at the time of the burn. The most common causes of associated injuries are falls and motor vehicle accidents. Such injuries increase the client's risk for complications or death. Determine whether additional injuries such as fractures, chest injuries, and abdominal trauma are causing pain or discomfort.

PHYSICAL ASSESSMENT/CLINICAL MANIFESTATIONS

Physical assessment findings in the emergent phase vary greatly from findings later in the course of the injury. Use a systematic approach to ensure that no problem is missed. The systems assessed first are those that can have immediate, life-threatening changes in function.

RESPIRATORY ASSESSMENT. Clients with major burn injuries and those with inhalation injury are at risk for respiratory problems. Respiratory manifestations common with a burn injury are listed in Table 71-4.

DIRECT AIRWAY INJURY. Inhalation injuries are present in 20% to 50% of the clients admitted to burn centers. The degree of inhalation damage depends on the fire source, temperature, environment, and types of toxic gases generated. Ask about the source of the fire, duration of exposure, and history of being in an enclosed space. Assess the respiratory system by visually inspecting the mouth, nose, and pharynx. Burns of the lips, face, ears, neck, eyelids, eyebrows, and eyelashes are strong indicators that an inhalation injury may be present. Burns inside the mouth and singed nasal hairs indicate potentially serious injuries. Carbonaceous particles in the nose, mouth, and sputum along with edema of the nasal septum indicate smoke inhalation, as does a "smoky" smell to the client's breath.

TABLE 71-4 Factors Determining Inhalation Injury or Airway Obstruction

- Individuals who were injured in a closed space
- Clients with extensive burns or with burns of the face
- Intra-oral charcoal, especially on teeth and gums
- Clients who were unconscious at the time of injury
- Clients with singed hairs, nasal hairs, eyelids, or eyelashes
- Clients who are coughing up carbonaceous sputum
- Changes in voice such as hoarseness or brassy cough
- Use of accessory muscles or stridor
- Poor oxygenation or ventilation
- Edema, erythema, and ulceration of airway mucosa
- Wheezing, bronchospasm

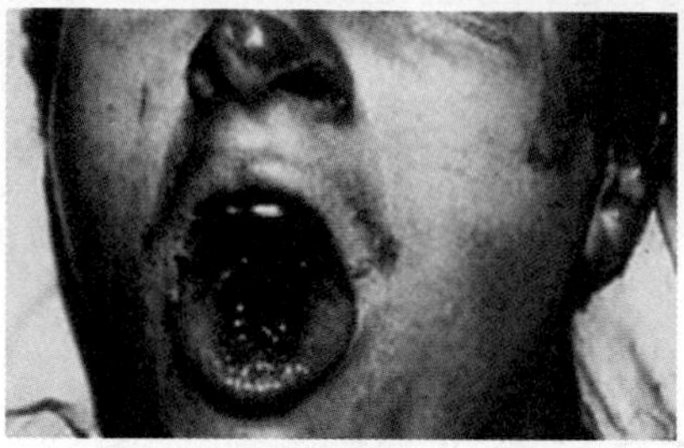

A change in respiratory pattern may indicate a pulmonary injury. The client may:

- Become progressively hoarse
- Develop a brassy cough
- Drool or have difficulty swallowing
- Produce expiratory sounds that include audible wheezes, crowing, and stridor

Upper airway edema and inhalation injury are most common in the trachea and mainstem bronchi. Auscultation of these areas may reveal wheezes, which are a sign of obstruction. Clients with severe inhalation injuries may have such rapid obstruction that within a short time they cannot force air through the narrowed airways. As a result, the wheezing sounds disappear. *This finding indicates impending airway obstruction and demands immediate intubation.* Many clients are intubated when an inhalation injury is suspected rather than waiting until obstruction makes endotracheal or nasotracheal intubation difficult or impossible.

CARBON MONOXIDE POISONING. Carbon monoxide is one of the leading causes of death associated with fires. It is a colorless, odorless, tasteless gas released as oxygen is being consumed in the process of combustion. Inhalation injury is a risk for carbon monoxide poisoning.

Carbon monoxide is rapidly transported across the alveolar membrane and preferentially binds to hemoglobin in place of oxygen to form carboxyhemoglobin (COHb). In addition, CO causes the oxyhemoglobin dissociation curve to shift to the left, thereby impairing oxygen unloading at the tissue level. This shift results in a substantial reduction in oxygen delivery, given that 98% of the oxygen supplied to the tissues comes bound to hemoglobin. Even though the oxygen-carrying capacity of the hemoglobin is reduced,

TABLE 71-5 Physiologic Effects of Carbon Monoxide Poisoning

Carbon Monoxide Level	Physiologic Effects
1%-10% (normal)	Increased threshold to visual stimuli Increased blood flow to vital organs
11%-20% (mild poisoning)	Headache Decreased cerebral function Decreased visual acuity Slight breathlessness
21%-40% (moderate poisoning)	Headache Tinnitus Nausea Drowsiness Vertigo Altered mental state Confusion Stupor Irritability Decreased blood pressure, increased and irregular heart rate Depressed ST segment on ECG and dysrhythmias Pale to reddish purple skin
41%-60% (severe poisoning)	Coma Convulsions Cardiopulmonary instability
61%-80% (fatal poisoning)	Death

ECG, Electrocardiogram.

the partial pressure of arterial oxygen (PaO_2) is normal. The vasodilating action of carbon monoxide causes the "cherry red" color in these clients. Clinical manifestations vary with the concentration of COHb. Table 71-5 lists the effects of carbon monoxide poisoning.

THERMAL (HEAT) INJURY. Except for rare events such as steam inhalation, aspiration of scalding liquid or explosion occurring while a client is breathing very high concentrations of oxygen or flammable gases under pressure, thermal burns to the respiratory tract are limited to the upper airway above the glottis (nasopharynx, oropharynx, and larynx). The respiratory tract's heat exchange capability is so efficient that most damage occurs above the true vocal cords. Heat damage of the pharynx is often severe enough to produce upper airway obstruction, which can occur any time during resuscitation. In the unresuscitated client, supraglottic edema may be delayed in onset until fluid resuscitation is well underway. Early intervention with intubation may be preferred.

Inhaled steam can injure the lower respiratory tract because water holds heat better than does dry air. The respiratory tract down to the major bronchioles can be damaged by steam. Ulcerations, redness, and edema of the mouth and epiglottis are the first manifestations, with rapid edema formation progressing to upper airway obstruction. Stridor, hoarseness, and shortness of breath result.

SMOKE POISONING. Smoke poisoning, or chemical injury from the inhalation of combustion by-products, is the most common type of inhalation injury. Toxic by-products, especially hydrogen cyanide, are produced when plastics or home furnishings are burned. Cyanide binds to the cytochrome system, thereby inhibiting cell metabolism and adenosine triphosphate (ATP) production. This problem disrupts cell function.

PULMONARY FLUID OVERLOAD. Pulmonary edema can result even when the lung tissues have not been damaged directly. Other damaged tissues release such large amounts of histamine and other inflammatory mediators causing capillary leak that even lung capillaries leak fluid into the pulmonary tissue spaces.

Circulatory overload from fluid resuscitation may cause left-sided heart failure. This problem creates such high hydrostatic pressure within pulmonary blood vessels that even more fluid is lost from the pulmonary vascular space into the tissue spaces. Excess lung tissue fluid makes gas exchange difficult. The client is short of breath and has dyspnea in the supine position. Crackles are heard on auscultation.

EXTERNAL FACTORS. In addition to pulmonary problems, clients with burn injuries may have breathing problems as a result of external factors. The most common external factor affecting breathing is tight eschar from deep circumferential chest burns. The eschar either restricts chest movement or compresses structures in the neck and throat to such an extent that ventilation is impaired. Inspect the client's chest for ease of respiration, amount of chest movement, rate of breathing, and effort required to breathe. Use pulse oximetry to assess breathing effectiveness in maintaining blood oxygen levels.

CARDIOVASCULAR ASSESSMENT. Changes in the cardiovascular system begin immediately after the burn injury and include shock from various causes. *Shock is a common cause of death in the emergent phase in clients with serious injuries.* See Chapter 40 for discussion of all types of shock.

At first, cardiac manifestations reflect hypovolemia and decreased cardiac output. Monitor the degree of edema and assess cardiac status by measuring central and peripheral pulses, blood pressure, capillary refill, and pulse oximetry. Noninvasive blood pressure readings are inaccurate in clients with large burns involving the upper extremities. Thus invasive monitoring may be needed for blood pressure measurement. At first, the client has tachycardia, decreased blood pressure, and decreased peripheral pulses. Peripheral capillary refill is slow or absent as tissue blood flow decreases. With fluid resuscitation, peripheral edema increases, as does the client's body weight.

Electrocardiographic (ECG) changes indicate electrical damage to the heart. These changes are most common with electrical burn injuries or with stress that induces a myocardial infarction. Obtain baseline ECG tracings at the time of admission to the hospital or burn center.

RENAL/URINARY ASSESSMENT. Changes in renal function with burn injury are related to decreased renal blood flow and to the presence of cellular debris. During the fluid shift of the emergent period, blood flow to the kidney may not be adequate for glomerular filtration. As a result, urine output is greatly decreased compared with intravenous (IV) fluid intake. The urine is highly concentrated and has a high specific gravity.

Other substances may be present in the blood that flows through the kidney. Destroyed red blood cells release hemoglobin and potassium. When muscle damage occurs from a major burn or electrical injury, a large oxygen-carrying protein called **myoglobin** is released from damaged muscle and

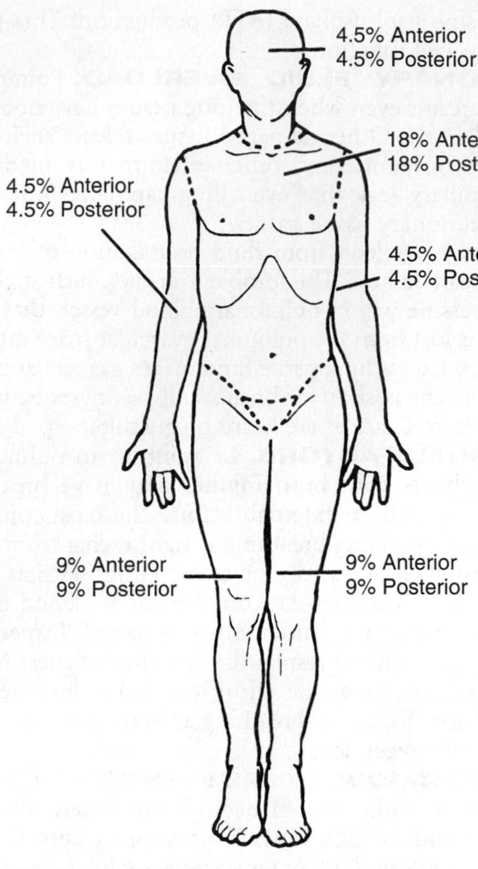

Figure 71-10 ■ The rule of nines for estimating burn percentage.

circulates to the kidney. Most damaged cells release proteins that form uric acid. All of these large molecules in the blood may precipitate in the kidney tubular system. This precipitation blocks kidney blood and urine flow and may cause renal failure.

Assess renal function by accurately measuring urine output and comparing this value with fluid intake. Urine output is decreased during the first 24 hours of the emergent phase. Fluid resuscitation is provided at the rate needed to maintain adult urine output at 30 to 50 mL or 0.5 mL/kg/hr. Assess response to fluid resuscitation by measuring urine specific gravity, blood urea nitrogen (BUN), serum creatinine, and serum sodium levels in addition to urine output. Examine the urine for color, odor, and the presence of particles or foam.

SKIN ASSESSMENT. Assess the skin to determine the size and depth of burn injury. The size of the injury is first estimated in comparison to the total body surface area (TBSA). For example, a burn that involves 40% of the TBSA is a 40% burn. The size of the injury is important not only for diagnosis and prognosis but also for calculating drug doses, fluid replacement volumes, and caloric needs.

Inspect the skin to identify injured areas and changes in color and appearance. Except with electrical burns, this initial size assessment usually can be made accurately with specific assessment tools and charts.

The most rapid method for calculating the size of a burn injury in adult clients whose weights are in normal proportion to their heights is the *rule of nines* (Figure 71-10). With this method, the body is divided into areas that are multiples of 9%. Although the rule of nines is useful at the site of injury and in emergency departments, overestimation of the TBSA involved can easily occur.

The Lund-Browder and Berkow methods are more accurate for evaluating the size of the injury (Figure 71-11). These methods take into account changes in body surface area from birth through adulthood.

Because specific treatments are related to the depth of the burn injury, initial assessment of the skin includes estimations of burn depth. Criteria for depth of injury are based on appearance and associated characteristics (see Depth of Burn Injury, p. 1620).

GASTROINTESTINAL ASSESSMENT. Although the gastrointestinal (GI) tract usually is not directly injured (except in those with chemical burns), changes in GI function are expected in all burn clients. The decreased blood flow and sympathetic stimulation during the emergent phase causes reduced GI motility and paralytic ileus. Auscultate the abdomen to assess bowel sounds. Bowel sounds are commonly reduced or absent in a client with severe burns. Other manifestations include nausea, vomiting, and abdominal distention. Clients with burns of 25% TBSA or who are intubated generally require a nasogastric (NG) tube inserted to prevent aspiration and remove gastric secretions. Assess the tube for placement and patency after insertion. Because of the potential for ulcer formation in the GI tract, you must examine the stool and vomitus for the presence of gross blood or other material indicative of partially digested blood. Tests for the presence of occult blood are performed.

LABORATORY ASSESSMENT

Changes in laboratory test values are found in different phases of postburn recovery and reflect tissue damage or compensatory responses. However, other changes in specific laboratory findings may suggest complications.

During the emergent phase and before the start of fluid resuscitation, venous blood analysis reflects the fluid shift and direct tissue damage. Baseline laboratory test values and early postburn variations are listed in Chart 71-3.

Changes in the total white blood cell (WBC) count and differential count reflect immune function and inflammatory responses to the burn injury. The burn client's total WBC count, especially the neutrophil percentage, first rises and then drops rapidly, with a "left shift" (see Chapter 23) as the immune system becomes unable to sustain its defenses. If sepsis occurs, the total WBC count may be as low as 2000 cells/mm^3.

Other laboratory tests that provide useful information about the burn client's status include urine electrolyte assays, urine cultures, liver enzyme studies, and clotting studies. Drug and alcohol screens are obtained if drug or alcohol intoxication is suspected.

CULTURAL CONSIDERATIONS

For African-American clients, a sickle cell preparation may be appropriate if sickle status is unknown. Trauma often triggers a sickle cell crisis in clients who have the disease and in those who carry the trait.

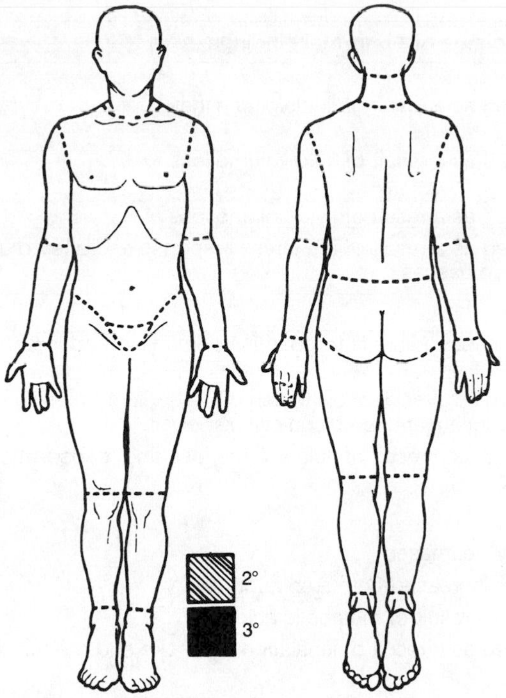

Date: ______________________

Height: ____________ Weight: ____________

2° ________ + 3° ________ = ________%

Percent surface area burned
(Berkow formula)

AREA	0-1 YEAR	1-4 YEARS	5-9 YEARS	10-14 YEARS	15 YEARS	ADULT	2°	3°
Head	19	17	13	11	9	7		
Neck	2	2	2	2	2	2		
Ant. Trunk	13	13	13	13	13	13		
Post.Trunk	13	13	13	13	13	13		
R. Buttock	2½	2½	2½	2½	2½	2½		
L. Buttock	2½	2½	2½	2½	2½	2½		
Genitalia	1	1	1	1	1	1		
R. U. Arm	4	4	4	4	4	4		
L. U. Arm	4	4	4	4	4	4		
R. L. Arm	3	3	3	3	3	3		
L. L. Arm	3	3	3	3	3	3		
R. Hand	2½	2½	2½	2½	2½	2½		
L. Hand	2½	2½	2½	2½	2½	2½		
R. Thigh	5½	6½	8	8½	9	9½		
L. Thigh	5½	6½	8	8½	9	9½		
R. Leg	5	5	5½	6	6½	7		
L. Leg	5	5	5½	6	6½	7		
R. Foot	3½	3½	3½	3½	3½	3½		
L. Foot	3½	3½	3½	3½	3½	3½		
TOTAL								

Figure 71-11 ■ Estimation of the extent of burn injury by the Berkow method. *Ant.,* Anterior; *Post.,* posterior; *R.,* right; *L.,* left; *R.U.,* right upper; *L.U.,* left upper; *R.L.,* right lower; *L.L.,* left lower.

CHART 71-3

LABORATORY PROFILE
Burn Assessment During the Emergent Period

Test	Normal Range for Adults	Significance of Abnormal Findings
Serum Studies		
Hemoglobin	12-16 g/dL (women) 14-18 g/dL (men)	Elevated as a result of fluid volume loss
Hematocrit	37%-47% (women) 42%-52% (men)	Elevated as a result of fluid volume loss
Urea nitrogen	10-20 mg/dL	Elevated as a result of fluid volume loss
Glucose	70-105 mg/dL	Elevated as a result of the stress response and altered uptake across injured tissues
Electrolytes		
Sodium	136-145 mEq/L (mmol/L)	Decreased; sodium is trapped in edema fluid and lost through plasma leakage
Potassium	3.5-5.0 mEq/L (mmol/L)	Elevated as a result of disruption of the sodium-potassium pump, tissue destruction, and red blood cell hemolysis
Chloride	98-106 mEq/L (mmol/L)	Elevated as a result of fluid volume loss and reabsorption of chloride in urine
Arterial Blood Gas Studies		
Pao_2	80-100 mm Hg	Slightly decreased
$Paco_2$	35-45 mm Hg	Slightly increased from respiratory injury
pH	7.35-7.45	Low as a result of metabolic acidosis
Carboxyhemoglobin	0%-10%	Elevated as a result of inhalation of smoke and carbon monoxide
Other		
Total protein	6.4-8.3 g/dL	Low; protein exudate is lost through the wound
Albumin	3.5-5.0 g/dL	Low; protein is lost through the wound and through vascular membranes because of increased permeability

Pao_2, Partial pressure of arterial oxygen; *$Paco_2$*, partial pressure of arterial carbon dioxide.

RADIOGRAPHIC ASSESSMENT

Standard x-rays and scans do not provide direct assessment data about the burn wound. These assessments are not performed unless other trauma is suspected.

OTHER DIAGNOSTIC ASSESSMENTS

In addition to routine laboratory tests, specific studies of involved organs are performed. For example, when burn injuries involve the eye, an ophthalmic evaluation detects corneal damage (see Chapters 49 and 50 for specific eye and vision evaluation procedures).

Specific diagnostic studies are performed when deep organ trauma is suspected. Such studies include IV renograms, computed tomography (CT), ultrasonography, bronchoscopy, and magnetic resonance imaging (MRI).

Critical Thinking Challenge

The client is a 57-year-old woman admitted directly to the burn center after being rescued from a house fire. She apparently was reading in bed and fell asleep while smoking. Following rescue from the burning house, she was given oxygen, 12 L/min through nasal prongs. She has partial-thickness burns on her face and anterior neck. Full-thickness circumferential burns are present on the upper trunk and both upper limbs. Estimated TBSA burn is 41%. The client is disoriented and complaining of shortness of breath as well as pain in the face and neck area. Further assessment reveals a hoarse, productive cough of carbonaceous sputum and carbon deposits on the tongue and throughout the oral pharynx. The client has a 20-gauge IV line in the left hand.

1. Is this client at risk for an inhalation injury? Why or why not?
2. What initial consideration must be given in moving the client from the stretcher to the bed?
3. Once the client is found to have an adequate airway and level of consciousness, what is your next priority?

evolve For suggested answer guidelines, go to http://evolve.elsevier.com/Iggy/.

◆Analysis

A burned client has dramatic changes not only in the directly damaged tissues but also in many other body systems. During the course of the illness, most burn clients experience all of the common and many of the additional nursing diagnoses listed in the following sections.

COMMON NURSING DIAGNOSES AND COLLABORATIVE PROBLEMS

The following are priority nursing diagnoses for clients with burn injuries in the emergent phase who have sustained a burn injury greater than 25% of the total body surface area (TBSA):

1. Decreased Cardiac Output related to altered stroke volume from an increase in capillary permeability
2. Deficient Fluid Volume related to active fluid volume loss, electrolyte imbalance, and inadequate fluid resuscitation

3. Ineffective Tissue Perfusion (Cerebral, Cardiopulmonary, Renal, Gastrointestinal, and Peripheral) related to hypovolemia from extravascular fluid shifts, decreased cardiac output, constriction of eschar, and edema
4. Ineffective Breathing Pattern related to respiratory distress from upper airway edema, pulmonary edema, airway obstruction, or pneumonia
5. Acute Pain and Chronic Pain related to biologic injury, damaged or exposed nerve endings, debridement, dressing changes, invasive procedures, and donor sites

The following are primary collaborative problems:

1. Potential for Pulmonary Edema
2. Potential for Acute Respiratory Distress Syndrome (ARDS)

ADDITIONAL NURSING DIAGNOSES AND COLLABORATIVE PROBLEMS

In addition to the common nursing diagnoses and collaborative problems, clients with burn injuries in the emergent phase may have one or more of the following:

- Excess Fluid Volume related to massive IV fluid administration
- Risk for Ineffective Thermoregulation related to trauma, hypermetabolism, and a loss of the protective barrier
- Disturbed Sensory Perception (Visual, Auditory, and Tactile) related to periorbital edema or ulcerations, hospital environment, noise, infections, and dressings
- Anxiety related to threat of death, initial burn trauma, situational crisis, painful procedures, unfamiliar environment, separation from significant others, and loss of control
- Fear related to pain, knowledge deficit, therapeutic procedures, hospitalization, separation, and social re-entry

Planning and Implementation

DECREASED CARDIAC OUTPUT; DEFICIENT FLUID VOLUME; INEFFECTIVE TISSUE PERFUSION

NOC **PLANNING: EXPECTED OUTCOMES.** With appropriate intervention, the client is expected to have cardiac output restored to normal. Indicators include that the client should:

- Have normal or only mildly compromised blood pressure and heart rate
- Have normal or only mildly compromised peripheral pulses
- Have normal or only mildly compromised oxygen saturation, partial pressure of arterial oxygen (PaO_2), partial pressure of arterial carbon dioxide ($PaCO_2$), and arterial pH

INTERVENTIONS. Interventions are aimed at increasing blood fluid volume, supporting compensatory mechanisms, and preventing complications. Chart 71-4 lists some NIC intervention activities for the burn client with decreased cardiac output, deficient fluid volume, and ineffective tissue perfusion. Nonsurgical management is often sufficient for achieving these aims. Surgical management is required most often for full-thickness burns.

NONSURGICAL MANAGEMENT. Fluid volume and tissue blood flow are restored through IV fluid therapy, plasma exchange therapy, and drug therapy.

CHART 71-4

NIC INTERVENTION ACTIVITIES for The Burn Client with Decreased Cardiac Output, Deficient Fluid Volume, and Ineffective Tissue Perfusion

Fluid Monitoring: *Collection and analysis of client data to regulate fluid balance*

- Monitor serum and urine electrolyte values, as appropriate.
- Monitor blood pressure, heart rate, and respiratory status.
- Monitor orthostatic blood pressure and change in cardiac rhythm, as appropriate.
- Monitor weight.
- Keep an accurate record of intake and output.
- Note presence or absence of vertigo on rising.
- Monitor color, quantity, and specific gravity of urine.

Fluid Resuscitation: *Administering prescribed intravenous fluids rapidly*

- Obtain and maintain a large-bore IV.
- Administer IV fluids, as prescribed.
- Monitor hemodynamic response.
- Monitor oxygen status.
- Monitor for fluid overload.
- Monitor output of various body fluids (e.g., urine and nasogastric drainage, and chest tube drainage)
- Monitor BUN, creatinine, total protein, and albumin levels.
- Monitor for pulmonary edema and third spacing.

Fluid Management: *Promotion of fluid balance and prevention of complications resulting from abnormal or undesired fluid levels*

- Administer IV therapy, as prescribed.
- Give fluids, as appropriate.
- Distribute the fluid intake over 24 hours, as appropriate.

NIC intervention activities selected from Dochterman, J.M., & Bulechek, G.M. (Eds.). (2004). *Nursing interventions classification (NIC)* (4th ed.). St. Louis: Mosby. No part of this work is to be altered without prior written permission from the Publisher.
BUN, blood urea nitrogen.

IV Fluid Therapy. Infusion of IV fluids is needed to maintain sufficient blood volume for normal cardiac output, mean arterial pressure, and tissue oxygenation. Clients with burns involving 15% to 20% of the TBSA require IV fluid resuscitation. Many formulas for calculating fluid requirements exist. Table 71-6 lists the formulas commonly used for the therapy of adult clients. Although the types and amounts of electrolytes, crystalloids, and colloids vary, the purpose of all of these formulas is to prevent shock by maintaining adequate circulating blood fluid volume. The optimal formula and infusion schedules remain controversial.

Resuscitation for a severe burn requires large fluid loads in a short time to maintain blood flow to vital organs. The Parkland formula recommends that half of the calculated fluid volume for 24 hours be given in the first 8 hours after injury. The other half is given over the next 16 hours for a total of 24 hours. Fluid boluses are avoided because they increase capillary pressure and worsen edema. In the second 24-hour period after a burn injury, the volume and content of the IV fluids are based on the client's specific fluid volume and electrolyte imbalances and his or her response to treatment.

Fluid replacement formulas are calculated from the time of injury and not from the time of arrival at the hospital. For example, if a burn injury occurred at 8 AM but the client was not admitted to the hospital until 10 AM, the first 8-hour period would be completed at 4 PM, or 8 hours after the injury. Thus if resuscitation was delayed by 2 hours until admission

TABLE 71-6 Common Fluid Resuscitation Formulas for the First 24 Hours After a Burn Injury

	Formula	Solution	Rate of Administration
Modified Brooke	0.5 mL/kg/% TBSA burn 1.5 mL/kg/% TBSA burn	Protenate or 5% albumin in isotonic saline Lactated Ringer's without dextrose	½ given in first 8 hr ½ given in next 16 hr
Parkland (Baxter)	4 mL/kg/% TBSA burn for 24-hr period	Crystalloid only (lactated Ringer's)	½ given in first 8 hr ½ given in next 16 hr
Monafo		Crystalloid (hypertonic saline: sodium = 250 mEq/L)	Adjust to maintain urine output of 30 mL/hr
Modified Parkland	4 mL/kg/% TBSA burn + 15 mL/m² of TBSA	Crystalloid only (lactated Ringer's)	½ given in first 8 hr ½ given in next 16 hr
Winski	2 mL/kg/% burn + maintenance fluid	Crystalloid only (lactated Ringer's)	½ given in first 8 hr ½ given in next 16 hr

to the hospital, calculated fluids would need to be given over the next 6-hour period rather than an 8-hour period. All burn resuscitation formulas are used as *guides.* The client's response to therapy determines exact fluid requirements. No single formula has been found to provide superior results over another.

The management of extensive burns may require placement of a large-bore central venous catheter so that massive fluid loads can be given. Peripheral lines are less useful because they become dislodged or fluid flow is cut off when massive peripheral edema compresses the IV catheter.

Plasma Exchange Therapy. Shock may persist in the postburn period despite adequate fluid resuscitation. The cause of this persistent shock is unknown, but toxic serum factors have been suggested. Plasma exchange therapy is used in some burn centers for clients with massive burns who fail to respond from burn shock with fluid resuscitation.

The plasma exchange process either removes the client's plasma and replaces it with fresh frozen plasma **(plasmapheresis)** or removes the client's blood and replaces it with whole blood **(exchange transfusion).** Plasma exchange can decrease the amount of required fluid and increase urine output, thus helping those clients who do not respond to conventional fluid therapy.

Monitoring. Monitor client responses to determine the adequacy of fluid resuscitation for hydration and adequate blood perfusion of the brain, heart, and kidneys. Urine output is the most common and most sensitive noninvasive assessment parameter for cardiac output and tissue perfusion (see Chapters 15 and 40). Regardless of the total amount of fluid calculated as needed to meet the fluid requirements of the client, the amount of fluid given depends on how much IV fluid per hour is needed to maintain the hourly urine output at 0.5 mL/kg (about 30 mL/hr). Adjustment of the IV fluid rate on the basis of urine output plus serum electrolyte values is known as the **titration** of fluid. *In clients with burns larger than 35% TBSA, the use of urine output and vital signs to guide resuscitation may be insufficient. Invasive monitoring of cardiac and pulmonary function is necessary to ensure optimal fluid resuscitation.*

Burn clients often develop severe hypovolemic shock and need invasive cardiac monitoring. Vital parameters such as central venous pressure, pulmonary artery pressures, and cardiac output are obtained on a frequent to continuous basis.

Monitor the electrocardiographic (ECG) activity of clients who have sustained large burns. Nonburn-related dysrhythmias, such as atrial fibrillation, are often present in older clients.

Drug Therapy. A common mistake in treatment is giving diuretics to increase urine output rather than changing the amount and rate of fluid administration. *Diuretics do not increase cardiac output; they actually decrease circulating volume and cardiac output by pulling fluid from the circulating blood volume to enhance diuresis.* This effect reduces blood flow to other vital organs (especially the heart, lungs, and brain) and greatly increases the risk for severe hypovolemic shock. Therefore diuretics are not generally used to improve urine output for burn clients. An exception is the client with a burn injury caused by electrical energy. Muscle and deep tissue damage release large protein molecules (myoglobin), which precipitate in and obstruct the renal tubules. Although the diuretic mannitol (Osmitrol) is often used in this situation, it should always be given after adequate urine output has been established.

In older clients or those with cardiac disease, a complicating factor in reduced cardiac output may be heart failure or myocardial infarction. Drugs that increase cardiac output, such as dopamine (Intropin), or that strengthen the force of myocardial contraction, such as digoxin (Lanoxin), may be used along with fluid therapy.

SURGICAL MANAGEMENT. The surgical procedure for the treatment of inadequate tissue perfusion is *escharotomy.* An incision through the burn eschar relieves pressure caused by the constricting force of circumferential burns on the extremity or chest and improves circulation. If the pressure is not relieved, arterial compression can occur with a loss of blood flow to the extremity leading to ischemia and possible necrosis. Incisions are made along sides of the extremity and extend into the subcutaneous tissue (Figures 71-6 and 71-12). This procedure relieves the tourniquet effect of the eschar. If tissue pressure remains elevated after escharotomy, a *fasciotomy* (a deeper incision extending through the fascia) may be needed.

Escharotomies and fasciotomies are often performed at the bedside. No anesthesia is needed for escharotomy because nerve endings have been destroyed by the burn injury, but sedation and analgesia are given to reduce anxiety. Assure the client that he or she will be made as comfortable as possible during the procedure. Remove the dressings and thoroughly cleanse the areas to be incised. After the procedure, apply topical antimicrobial agents and dressings to the

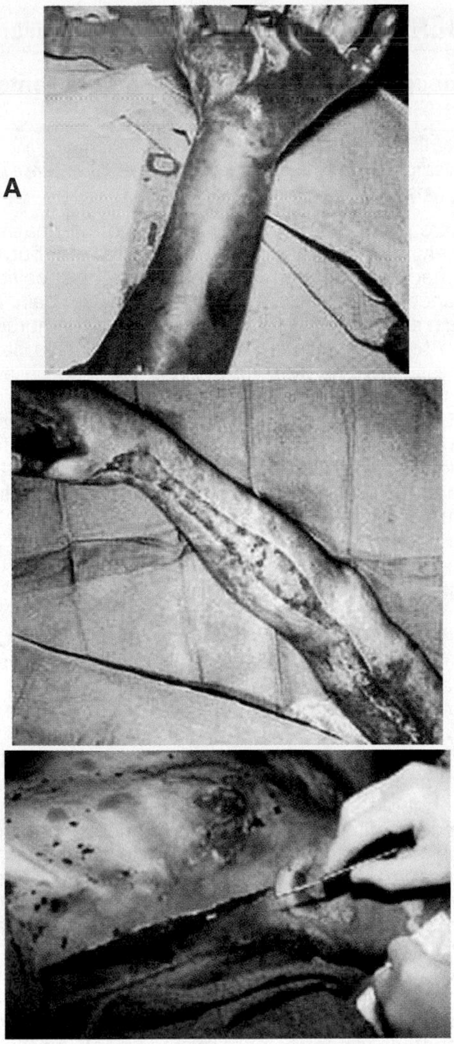

Figure 71-12 ■ Escharotomy to release circumferential burn eschar and improve circulation to a distal extremity or to improve ventilation. **A,** Tight circumferential eschar restricting swelling as edema forms in the tissue beneath the eschar. Edema compresses blood vessels, which inhibits blood flow to the distal extremity. **B,** An escharotomy incision allows outward swelling of edematous tissues. Restricted blood flow through the vessels to the distal extremity is relieved. **C,** An anterior axillary incision is made bilaterally to relieve respiratory distress.

area. Carefully monitor escharotomy sites for bleeding. Fasciotomies generally require large doses of narcotics or anesthesia for pain management.

INEFFECTIVE BREATHING PATTERN

NOC **PLANNING: EXPECTED OUTCOMES.** With proper intervention, the client is expected to maintain a patent airway and have an effective breathing pattern. Indicators include that the client should have either mildly compromised or not compromised oxygen saturation, PaO_2, $PaCO_2$, and arterial pH.

INTERVENTIONS. Interventions are aimed at supporting normal pulmonary function and preventing pulmonary problems. Specific plans for pulmonary management depend on the cause of the breathing problem and the status of the respiratory tract.

NONSURGICAL MANAGEMENT. Interventions include airway maintenance, promotion of ventilation, monitoring gas exchange, oxygen therapy, drug therapy, positioning, and deep breathing.

Airway Maintenance. Maintenance of the airway begins at the burn scene in an unconscious client and may involve only a chin lift or a head tilt maneuver. Upper airway edema becomes pronounced 8 to 12 hours after the beginning of fluid resuscitation. These clients often require nasal or oral intubation if crowing, stridor, or dyspnea is present.

A bronchoscopy is performed to examine the vocal cords and airways of clients at risk for obstruction. Clients with severe smoke inhalation or poisoning may require a bronchoscopy on admission and routinely thereafter for examination of the respiratory tract, deep suctioning of the lungs, and removal of sloughing necrotic tissue. Assess the endotracheal tube hourly to ensure patency and location in intubated clients.

Other causes of airway obstruction are excessive secretions and sloughed tissue from damaged lungs. Suction as indicated based on clinical assessment or clinician order. Vigorous endotracheal or nasotracheal tube suctioning is performed after chest physiotherapy and aerosol treatments. Clients report that deep endotracheal suctioning is extremely painful. Therefore suctioning the endotracheal tube often requires increased analgesia or sedation.

Promotion of Ventilation. Respiration depends on skeletal muscle movement of the chest for ventilation. Chest movement can be restricted by tight dressings that cover the neck, chest, and abdomen. Observe the client for ease of respiratory movements and loosen tight dressings as needed to assist with ventilation.

Monitoring Gas Exchange. Monitor the effectiveness of gas exchange by using laboratory tests (e.g., arterial blood gas, carboxyhemoglobin levels) and by assessing for cyanosis, disorientation, and increased pulse rate. Other data to monitor in critically ill clients include chest x-ray, pulmonary artery catheters, and central venous pressure measurement.

The possibility of cyanide poisoning is considered in clients involved in house fires. An elevated plasma lactate level is a useful indicator of cyanide toxicity in clients who do not have severe burns.

Oxygen Therapy. Management of impaired breathing patterns includes giving humidified oxygen by face mask, cannula, or hood. Arterial oxygenation less than 60 (PaO_2 <60 mm Hg) is an indication for intubation and mechanical ventilation. Keep emergency airway equipment at or near the client's bedside. This equipment must include oxygen, masks, cannulas, manual resuscitation bags, laryngoscope, endotracheal tubes, and equipment for tracheostomy. Chapter 35 addresses specific nursing actions for clients during mechanical ventilation.

Drug Therapy. When pneumonia or other pulmonary infections impair breathing, antibiotics are prescribed. Drug selection is based on known culture and sensitivity reports or on the specific microflora common to that burn unit. Impaired breathing from cardiac failure and increased pulmonary pressures may be treated with drugs that improve cardiac output and enhance urine output.

When a client's activity during mechanical ventilation severely compromises respiratory mechanics, it may be necessary to use a paralytic drug, such as atracurium (Tracrium) or vecuronium (Norcuron). This situation is often referred to as "bucking" the ventilator. Paralytic agents remove all breathing control from the client, making mechanical ventilation easier. *These drugs do not prevent the client from seeing and hearing or from experiencing fear, pain, and loss of control. Any client receiving neuromuscular blockade drugs must also receive agents for sedation, analgesia, and antianxiety unless clinically contraindicated.* Extreme care must be taken to ensure that all alarms are operative and that clients are checked frequently, because the client cannot call for help if he or she becomes extubated.

Positioning and Deep Breathing. To improve breathing patterns and oxygenation, turn the client frequently and assist him or her out of bed to a chair as much as possible. Teach the client to use coughing and deep breathing exercises. Encourage the client to use incentive spirometry every 2 hours while awake. Chest physiotherapy may be helpful to mobilize lung secretions, depending on the client's clinical condition and the clinician's prescription.

SURGICAL MANAGEMENT. A tracheostomy may be needed when long-term intubation is expected. A tracheostomy increases the risk for infection in burn clients even more than in nonburned clients. Emergency tracheostomies are performed when an airway becomes occluded and oral or nasal intubation cannot be achieved.

Other surgical procedures for improving the burn client's breathing pattern include inserting chest tubes and performing an escharotomy. Chest tubes are used to re-expand the lung when a pneumothorax or hemothorax has occurred (see Chapters 33 and 35). Tight eschar on the neck, chest, or abdomen can restrict respiratory movement. Escharotomies (described on p. 1634) can relieve this restriction and permit greater respiratory movement.

ACUTE PAIN; CHRONIC PAIN

The pain with burn injuries is both chronic and acute. Many factors contribute to burn pain and may be altered to reduce pain perception. Pain from the actual injury is worse when painful procedures are performed. Many nursing procedures needed by burn clients increase pain. Accurate assessment of the client's pain before and during procedures is an essential part of pain management. Visual analog scales and pain assessment scales that use color or faces have been used successfully to assess pain in the client with burns (see the Evidence-Based Practice for Nursing box at right).

NOC **PLANNING: EXPECTED OUTCOMES.** The pain level of a client with a burn injury is expected to be alleviated or reduced. Indicators include that the client should rarely demonstrate the following behaviors:

- Report pain
- Moan and cry
- Make facial expressions of pain
- Lose his or her appetite

INTERVENTIONS. The plan for pain management is tailored to the client's tolerance for pain, coping mechanisms, and physical status.

NONSURGICAL MANAGEMENT. Interventions for the client having pain include drug therapy, complementary therapy measures, and environmental manipulation.

Drug Therapy. Opioid and non-opioid analgesics, such as morphine sulfate, hydromorphone (Dilaudid), and fentanyl, are given often. However, these drugs rarely offer more than moderate relief during acutely painful procedures, and they depress respiratory function and reduce intestinal motility.

During the emergent postburn phase, the IV route is used for giving opioid drugs because of problems with absorption from the muscle and stomach. When these drugs are given by the intramuscular or subcutaneous route, they remain in the spaces and do not relieve pain. In addition, when edema is present, cumulative doses are rapidly absorbed when the fluid shift is resolving. This delayed absorption can result in lethal blood levels of analgesics.

Anesthetic agents, such as ketamine (Ketalar), pentobarbital sodium (Nembutal, Novopentobarb✱), and nitrous oxide, also reduce pain. Use strict protocols when giving these agents to prevent serious complications.

EVIDENCE-BASED PRACTICE for Nursing

Pain management—Are we meeting our clients' goals?

Carrougher, G.J., et al. (2003). Comparison of patient satisfaction and self-reports of pain in adult burn-injured patients. *Journal of Burn Care and Rehabilitation, 24*(1), 1-8.

Health care providers place a great deal of emphasis on pain assessment and management in hospitalized burn clients. Current medical practices include the use of specific opioids and adjunctive treatment to obtain effective pain management. Pain assessment tools have provided the nurse with information to guide treatment effectiveness. This study took pain assessment one step further and focused on evaluating whether the treatments used to prevent and treat burn-related pain met the client's analgesic goals. Background, procedural pain, and treatment goals were assessed in 84 clients.

In addition to obtaining pain scores, twice-weekly client self-reports of worst and average procedural pain, background pain, treatment goals, and overall satisfaction with pain management plans were assessed. Data were also collected regarding type and amount of analgesia and nonpharmacologic adjunct therapy.

Sixty-seven of the participants were male and 17 were female. A total of 351 assessments were performed on these 84 clients. The mean age was 36.9, 85% white, mean TBSA 13.3%, and average length of hospital stay was 18 days. Eighty percent of the burns were a result of a scald or flame injury.

The results of this study indicated that client satisfaction with pain management is highest in those who experience the least amount of burn care pain. The opposite result was found in treatment satisfaction being the highest in those whose pain experiences most closely matched treatment analgesics goals. Reasons stated for this outcome may be related to the high pain scores reported during procedures. When the average pain scores were analyzed, the researchers were more successful in meeting the clients' goals.

Level of Evidence: 3—Well-designed trial without randomization (cohort study).

Critique. The authors of this study have brought to our attention another aspect of pain management. As they stated, pain assessment is more than just asking for a number. No data were provided regarding the percentage of partial- or full-thickness burn of the wound. The study could have been strengthened by correlating the size of burn and degree of satisfaction with pain management. There is a need for further studies of this type.

Implications for Nursing. Managing pain related to burn injuries continues to be a challenge for health care professionals. To achieve effective pain management, the nurse must not only accurately assess the level of pain but also obtain client self-reports and evaluate the individualized treatment goals with the pain regimen.

Complementary and Alternative Therapy. Complementary and alternative therapy measures include relaxation techniques, meditative breathing, guided imagery, music therapy, massage, and healing or therapeutic touch. Hypnosis and autohypnosis can be used by lucid, cooperative clients under the direction of trained therapists. Therapeutic touch, acupuncture, and acupressure are used to a limited extent for burn clients; the results are variable. Nontraditional and complementary therapy types of pain intervention are detailed in Chapter 7.

Environmental Change. You can increase the client's comfort by providing a quiet environment, using nonpainful tactile stimulation, and increasing the client's control. Sleep deprivation increases the client's discomfort. Increasing sleep or rest time in a quiet environment helps reduce the adverse effects of sleep deprivation, replenishes catecholamine stores, helps prevent critical care unit psychosis, and restores the diurnal effects of endorphins. Health care providers need to ensure that most procedures are performed during the client's waking hours.

Tactile stimulation can reduce pain. Help the client change positions every 2 hours to reduce pressure on any specific area, improve circulation to painful areas, and ease pain. Massage nonburn areas to reduce pain transmission and stimulate endorphin release. Apply heat and maintain warm room temperatures to prevent shivering.

To reduce anxiety and increase feelings of confidence and independence, encourage the client to participate in pain control measures. For example, make a contract with the client that specifies how long a painful procedure will last. This helps clients deal with the pain for that particular period. Patient-controlled analgesia (PCA) also reduces pain in burned clients. Important issues and techniques for the best use of PCA include the following: give an initial bolus of 5 to 10 mg of morphine (or equivalent drug), increasing the PCA dose as needed to achieve pain relief, and plan for a change in dosing regimens at night (e.g., giving a bolus dose at bedtime).

SURGICAL MANAGEMENT. Early surgical excision of the burn wound is used in many burn centers (see Surgical Excision, p. 1642). Early excision under anesthesia reduces the pain from daily debridement at the bedside or during hydrotherapy.

POTENTIAL FOR PULMONARY EDEMA

PLANNING: EXPECTED OUTCOMES. With intervention, the client with a burn injury is expected to be free of pulmonary edema.

INTERVENTIONS. Pulmonary edema can arise from lung injury or from fluid resuscitation and myocardial overload. Even a young healthy person can become fluid overloaded. These clients usually receive digoxin or other drugs to improve left ventricular function and prevent or treat pulmonary edema. Diuretics, a mainstay of therapy for pulmonary edema from other causes, may or may not be used in the emergent phase depending on the client's blood volume and renal function.

POTENTIAL FOR ACUTE RESPIRATORY DISTRESS SYNDROME

PLANNING: EXPECTED OUTCOMES. The client with a burn injury is expected to:

- Not experience acute respiratory distress
- Have arterial blood gases (ABGs) within normal limits
- Maintain normal lung compliance

INTERVENTIONS. Clients who develop acute respiratory distress syndrome (ARDS) as a result of burn injury require thorough assessments and interventions. The interventions are aimed at increasing lung compliance and improving Pa_{O_2} (partial pressure of arterial oxygen) levels.

In collaboration with the physician and respiratory therapist, give positive end-expiratory pressure (PEEP) to augment the decreased lung volume by providing a continuous positive pressure in the airways and alveoli. This procedure enhances the diffusion of oxygen across the alveolar-capillary membrane. PEEP can be combined with intermittent mandatory volume (IMV) to enhance its effectiveness.

Assess and document the client's response so that needed ventilator changes can be made. Document and report any signs of respiratory distress or change in respiratory patterns. Monitor pulse oximetry and arterial blood gas (ABG) levels to assess changes in respiratory status.

Neuromuscular blocking agents (atracurium) can be used in clients receiving mechanical ventilation to reduce oxygen consumption (see the discussion of specific nursing care under Drug Therapy [Ineffective Breathing Pattern], p. 1635).

Critical Thinking Challenge

The client who sustained a 41% TBSA burn (36% full-thickness) injury described earlier is started on fluid resuscitation. You notice that her urine is becoming darker and has a high specific gravity.

1. Do you expect that this client needs more fluid for resuscitation as a person who has only a partial-thickness burn? Why or why not?
2. What should be your first action upon viewing the change in the character of this client's urine?
3. What additional drugs or adjustments in resuscitation should you expect to be prescribed?

evolve For suggested answer guidelines, go to http://evolve.elsevier.com/Iggy/.

ACUTE PHASE OF BURN INJURY

OVERVIEW

The acute phase of burn injury begins about 36 to 48 hours after injury and lasts until wound closure is complete. During this phase, a multidisciplinary approach to care is needed. Care is directed toward continued assessment and maintenance of the cardiovascular and respiratory systems, as well as toward gastrointestinal and nutritional status, burn wound care, pain control, and psychosocial interventions.

◆COLLABORATIVE MANAGEMENT

PHARM REVIEW

◆Assessment

PHYSICAL ASSESSMENT/CLINICAL MANIFESTATIONS

CARDIOPULMONARY ASSESSMENT. In the acute phase of burn injury, the cardiovascular and respiratory systems are assessed for maintaining these systems and treating or preventing potential complications. At this time, the client may develop pneumonia that can result in respiratory failure requiring mechanical ventilation. Although cardiovascular problems should be resolved, the client is at risk for infection and sepsis, which affect cardiovascular function. The interventions used in the emergent phase also may be needed for these new problems.

NEUROENDOCRINE ASSESSMENT. The increased metabolic demands placed on the body after a severe burn injury can severely deplete nutritional stores. Weigh the client daily without dressings or splints and compare it to his or her preburn weight. A 2% loss of body weight indicates a mild deficit. A 10% or greater weight loss is important and requires the evaluation and modification of calorie intake. For very accurate calorie requirements, indirect calorimetry may be used. This method determines kilocalories of energy expenditure by measuring oxygen consumption (V_{O_2}) and carbon dioxide production (V_{CO_2}). Measurements are taken while the client is at rest and preferably at least 30 minutes after the most recent dressing changes or other stressful procedures. Indirect calorimetry often is performed shortly after admission and at least once each week until the wounds are closed.

TABLE 71-7 Local and Systemic Signs of Infection

Local Signs
- Conversion of a partial-thickness injury to a full-thickness injury
- Ulceration of healthy skin at the burn site
- Erythematous, nodular lesions in uninvolved skin and vesicular lesions in healed skin
- Edema of healthy skin surrounding the burn wound
- Excessive burn wound drainage
- Pale, boggy, dry, or crusted granulation tissue
- Sloughing of grafts
- Wound breakdown after closure
- Odor

Systemic Signs
- Altered level of consciousness
- Changes in vital signs (tachycardia, tachypnea, temperature instability, hypotension)
- Increased fluid requirements for maintenance of a normal urine output
- Hemodynamic instability
- Oliguria
- Gastrointestinal dysfunction (diarrhea, vomiting, abdominal distention, paralytic ileus)
- Hyperglycemia
- Thrombocytopenia
- Change in total white blood cell count (above normal or below normal)
- Metabolic acidosis
- Hypoxemia

IMMUNE ASSESSMENT. The client with a burn injury is at risk for infection as a result of open wounds and reduced immune function. Burn wound sepsis is a serious complication of burn injury, and infection is the leading cause of death during the acute phase of recovery. Continually assess the client for signs of local and systemic infections (Table 71-7), including changes in wound appearance, changes in neurologic and GI function, and subtle changes in vital signs. Monitor for the manifestations of gram-positive, gram-negative, and fungal infections (Table 71-8). Enforce meticulous handwashing by all health care personnel. Use aseptic technique in caring for wounds and during invasive monitoring to prevent infections.

MUSCULOSKELETAL ASSESSMENT. Clients with a burn injury are at risk for musculoskeletal problems as a result of other injuries, immobility, healing processes, and treatment. The musculoskeletal status is first evaluated on admission to the hospital or burn center and throughout the acute phase of injury. Assess active and passive range of motion for all joints, including the neck. Give special attention to joints within the burn area. Ranges and limitations are documented for future reference.

◆Analysis

During the acute phase of the burn injury, the client with a burn injury has resolution of some earlier problems, may have initial problems that extend into the acute phase, and may develop new problems.

COMMON NURSING DIAGNOSES AND COLLABORATIVE PROBLEMS

The following are priority nursing diagnoses for clients with burn injuries greater than 25% TBSA in the acute phase of recovery:

1. Impaired Skin Integrity related to burn wound, graft site, or donor site, and physical immobilization
2. Risk for Infection related to inadequate primary defenses (wounds), the presence of multiple invasive catheters, reduced immune function, and malnutrition
3. Imbalanced Nutrition: Less Than Body Requirements related to increased metabolic rate; reduced calorie intake; and increased urinary nitrogen losses
4. Impaired Physical Mobility related to open burn wounds, pain, and scars and contractures
5. Disturbed Body Image related to trauma, changes in physical appearance and lifestyle, as well as alterations in sensory and motor function

TABLE 71-8 Signs and Symptoms of Sepsis Caused by Different Organisms

Sign/Symptom	Gram-Positive	Gram-Negative	Fungal
Onset	Insidious, 2-6 days	Rapid, 12-36 hr	Delayed
Sensorium	Severe disorientation and lethargy	Mild disorientation	Mild disorientation
Ileus	Severe	Severe	Mild
Diarrhea	Rare	Severe	Occasional
Temperature	Hyperpyrexia	Hypothermia	Hyperpyrexia
Hypotension	Late	Early	Late
White blood cell count	Neutrophilia	Neutropenia	Neutrophilia
Platelets	Normal	Low	Low

The primary collaborative problem is Wound Care Management.

ADDITIONAL NURSING DIAGNOSES AND COLLABORATIVE PROBLEMS

In addition to the common nursing diagnoses and collaborative problems, clients with burn injuries in the acute phase may have one or more of the following:

- Anticipatory Grieving related to loss of significant others, loss of possessions, physical disfigurement, and changes in body image
- Disabled Family Coping related to loss of home, family, or significant others; crises resulting from burn injury; disturbances in normal functions; role changes; and prolonged hospitalization and rehabilitation
- Ineffective Coping related to situational crises, disfigurement, separation, and sensory overload
- Self-Care Deficits (Feeding, Bathing/Hygiene, Dressing/Grooming, Toileting) related to pain; contractures; and loss of function in the hands, extremities, and other body parts
- Sexual Dysfunction related to trauma; perineal, genital, and breast burns; immobility, fatigue, and depression; and disturbance in body image
- Disturbed Sleep Pattern related to pain, treatment regimen, and environmental noise
- Social Isolation related to the altered state of wellness, protective isolation treatment regimen, and alterations in physical appearance
- Deficient Knowledge (treatment regimen and healing process) related to unfamiliarity of information resources and cognitive limitation
- Potential for Pneumonia
- Potential for Septicemia

Planning and Implementation

IMPAIRED SKIN INTEGRITY; WOUND CARE MANAGEMENT

NOC **PLANNING: EXPECTED OUTCOMES.** With appropriate intervention, the client with a burn injury is expected to have no further loss of skin integrity and to have skin integrity restored. Indicators include that the client:

- Has presence of granulation, re-epithelialization, and scar tissue formation
- Has decreased wound size
- Has no new wounds

INTERVENTIONS. Interventions aim to preserve the integrity of nonburned skin, enhance wound healing of burned skin, and prevent complications.

NONSURGICAL MANAGEMENT. Nonsurgical burn wound management involves removing exudates and necrotic tissue, cleaning the area, stimulating granulation and revascularization, and applying dressings. Restoring skin, whether by natural healing or grafting, starts with the removal of eschar and other cellular debris from the burn wound. This removal is called **debridement.** Nonsurgical treatment allows debris removal through mechanical and enzymatic actions that separate eschar over time. The goal is to have the wound prepare itself for grafting and wound closure by a natural process.

Mechanical Debridement. Burn wounds are debrided and cleaned one to two times each day during **hydrotherapy** (the application of water for treatment). Nurses, unlicensed nursing personnel, and physical therapists perform hydrotherapy daily to debride and examine the wounds. Hydrotherapy can be performed by immersing the client in a tub, showering the client on a specially designed shower table, or washing only small areas of the wound at the bedside. Showering enhances wound inspection and allows water temperature to be kept constant.

Nurses and skilled technicians use forceps and scissors to remove loose, nonviable tissue during hydrotherapy. The care of intact blisters is controversial. At most burn units, small blisters are left alone because they serve as a protective barrier that promotes wound healing. Because the protein-filled fluid within blisters can cause some reduced immune function, many units open larger blisters. Washcloths or gauze sponges are used to debride soft "cheesy" eschar. During hydrotherapy, wash burn areas thoroughly and gently with mild soap or detergent and water. Then rinse these areas with room temperature water.

Enzymatic Debridement. Enzymatic debridement can occur naturally by autolysis or artificially by the application of exogenous agents. **Autolysis** is the disintegration of tissue by the action of the client's own cellular enzymes. This process is seldom used in North America for larger burns because it is slow and results in a prolonged hospital stay.

Topical enzyme agents, such as collagenase (Santyl), are used for rapid wound debridement. When these agents are applied directly to the burn wound in a once-a-day dressing change, the enzymes digest collagen in necrotic tissues. They require a moist environment within a specific pH range for activation. Polysporin powder is often used with this topical agent to prevent infection.

Dressing the Burn Wound. After burn wounds are cleaned and debrided, topical antibiotics are reapplied to prevent infection (see Risk for Infection, p. 1643). Some type of dressing is then applied to the burn wound. Burn dressings include standard wound dressings, biologic dressings, and synthetic dressings and artificial skin. (Table 71-9 describes the features of many types of dressings.)

Standard Wound Dressings. Standard wound dressings are multiple layers of gauze applied over the topical agents on the burn wound. The number of gauze layers depends on the following:

- Depth of the injury
- Amount of drainage expected
- Area injured
- Client's mobility
- Frequency of dressing changes

The gauze layers are held in place with roller-type gauze bandages applied in a distal to proximal direction or with circular net fabrics. Cover gauze dressings on the client's arms and legs with elastic wraps, especially if the client is ambulatory. Dressings are generally changed and reapplied every 8 to 24 hours after thoroughly cleaning the areas.

Biologic Dressings. Biologic wound dressings are often used for temporary wound coverage and closure. Biologic dressings are skin or membranes obtained from human tissue donors (homograft or allograft) or animals (heterograft or xenograft). When applied over open wounds, a biologic dressing rapidly adheres and promotes healing or prepares the wound for permanent skin graft coverage.

TABLE 71-9 Advantages and Disadvantages of Dressings and Dressing Systems for Burns

Product	Description	Action	Advantages	Disadvantages	Interventions
Acticoat	Prepackaged in sheets	Silver-coated antimicrobial Broad-spectrum coverage	Painless Change dressing every 3 days Effective against antibiotic-resistant *Pseudomonas*, vancomycin-resistant *Enterococcus* (VRE), methicillin-resistant *Staphylococcus aureus*, and fungi May be used in sulfa-allergic clients Provides moist (nonmacerating) wound coverage	Expensive May cause transient discoloration of tissue Known sensitivity to silver Not compatible with oil-based products	Must be moistened with sterile water before application. Dressings must be wetted down every 8 hours with sterile water. Use on partial-thickness wounds, grafts or donor sites. Do not combine with any other topical anti-microbial. Not compatible with magnetic resonance imaging procedures. Should not come into contact with electrodes or conductive gels during electronic measurements.
Accuzyme	Water insoluble Derived from fruit of papaya melon tree (Papain)	Enzymatic debrider Breaks down nonviable tissue	Harmless to viable tissue Once-a-day dressing	Painful Infection	Apply directly to wound. Cover with normal saline gauze. Use on deep-partial thickness wounds. Discontinue use when wound is free of eschar.
Xeroform	Petroleum-based gauze impregnated with 3% bismuth tribromophenate	Contains no antimicrobial action Encourages migration of epithelial cells	Acts as barrier dressing Prevents wound desiccation Prevents loss of body fluid Inexpensive	Allows bacterial growth due to minimal antibacterial properties	Use daily dressings. Use on clean partial-thickness burns or donor sites. Only place a single layer. Monitor for signs of infection.
Scarlet Red	Vaseline-impregnated gauze containing red dye	Encourages spread of epithelial cells at faster rate than Xeroform	Use on clean partial-thickness wounds or donor site Inexpensive	Promotes bacterial growth if infection is present No antimicrobials	Change daily or every other day. Apply single layer. Red dye permanently stains clothes, furniture, and the like. Dye on skin is not permanent. Monitor for signs of infection.
Mepitel	Pliable nonadherent dressing Fine mesh netting coated with silicone	Mild antimicrobial properties Provides protective barrier dressing to allow for epithelial growth	Pores allow for drainage of exudates Does not adhere to wound May use on grafts	Sensitivity/allergy reactions Provides no antimicrobial effect	May leave in place for 5 days when used with grafts. May apply topical solutions over Mepitel.

Biobrane	Biosynthetic skin substitute (nylon and Silastic membrane combined with collagen derivative)	Promotes epithelialization Physiologic barrier Allows water vapor to escape Adherence due to wound binding to collagen then by tissue growth into nylon fabric	One time application Visualization of wound progression through Biobrane Decreased pain medication required	Expensive Infection or wound conversion prohibits adherence Recommended application time within 6 hours of injury No antimicrobials	Use on clean partial-thickness wounds, donor sites, grafts. May not reapply once removed. Must apply dull side down. Monitor for infection and adherence. Once Biobrane is adherent, may change dressing every other day. Keep in place until wound is healed.
Transcyte	Human fibroblast-derived temporary skin substitute Contains human dermal matrix, growth factors, essential structural proteins Consists of polymer membrane and newborn human fibroblast cells cultured under aseptic conditions in vitro on nylon mesh	Provides physiologic barrier Accelerates re-epithelialization Provides tissue matrix	One time application Visualization of wound through Transcyte Decrease pain medication Apply within 24 hours of burn injury	Expensive Infection of wound conversion prohibits adherence No antimicrobials Use only on clean partial-thickness wounds	Monitor adherence to wound. Monitor for infection. Maintained frozen, must use within 2 hours after thawing.
Pigskin (xenograft, heterograft)	Biologic skin substitute Skin harvested from pigs, cryopreserved for long-term storage	Provides biologic covering of clean wounds	Decreases pain Prevents water, electrolyte, and protein losses Used on wounds as bridge to skin grafting	Infection No antimicrobials	Monitor for infection. Monitor for wound adherence. Remove dressing daily for inspection; replace if purulent drainage or nonadherent.
Homograft (allograft)	Skin harvested from human	Provides biologic covering of clean wounds	Decreases pain Prevents wound drying Promotes healing Remains adherent until rejection occurs or is surgically removed	Disease transmission Hypersensitivity reaction	Client eventually rejects skin. Monitor for infection and adherence. Use on newly excised wounds.
Alloderm	Cadaver skin in which the epidermis is removed and allogenic cells are removed.	Provides dermal base to excised wounds Thin graft placed over Alloderm	Requires thinner autograft to be harvested Used in extensive burns with limited donor tissue		Managed identical to skin grafts.
Integra	Biosynthetic dermal regeneration template	Dermal template for the formation of a neodermis within 14-21 days Consists of bovine collagen dermal layer and silicone epidermis	Used in extensive burns with limited donor tissue Potentially less scarring Requires thinner autografts to be harvested	Expensive Requires two-stage surgical procedure 14-21 days apart	Monitor for infection. Limit motion and friction. Monitor for adherence.

TABLE 71-10 Biologic Dressings

Uses
- Debridement of untidy wounds after separation of eschar
- Promotion of re-epithelialization of deep partial-thickness wounds
- Temporary coverage after excision of the burn wound
- Protection of granulation tissue between autografts
- Test graft before autografting

Advantages
- Early adherence to the wound
- Reduction of evaporative heat loss
- Reduction of evaporate water loss
- Prevention of desiccation of granulation tissue
- Reduction of exudate protein losses
- Reduction of pain
- Assistance in wound debridement
- Enhancement of healing with partial-thickness injuries
- Protection of exposed neovascular tissue
- Inhibition of bacterial proliferation

Disadvantages
- Early lysis resulting in bacterial proliferation
- Expensive
- Rejection responses
- Possible burn wound sepsis if applied over eschar
- Not readily available
- Storage (some may require refrigeration or freezing)
- Possible transmission of diseases, such as hepatitis

Biologic materials are used in healing partial-thickness and granulating full-thickness wounds that are clean and free of eschar. Table 71-10 outlines the advantages and disadvantages of biologic dressings. The type of biologic dressing selected depends on the type of wound to be covered and the availability of the material.

Homograft. A **homograft** or **allograft** is human skin obtained from a cadaver and provided through a skin bank. It is fresh or frozen; frozen skin is thawed in a warm bath of sterile normal saline before application. Disadvantages to the use of homografts are the high costs ($750 to $1000 per square foot) and the risk of transmitting a bloodborne infection.

Heterograft. A **heterograft** or **xenograft** is skin obtained from another species. Pigskin is the most common heterograft and is compatible with human skin. Pigskin is assessed daily for adherence and need for replacement.

Amniotic Membrane. Amniotic membrane is another form of biologic dressing used on burn wounds. Its large size, low cost, and availability have helped with its success. In full-thickness injuries, the amniotic membrane adheres to the wound. With partial-thickness areas, the amniotic membrane is effective as a dressing until epithelial cell regrowth occurs. The membrane requires frequent changes because it does not develop a blood supply and it disintegrates in about 48 hours.

Cultured Skin. Cultured skin can be grown from a small specimen of epidermal cells from an unburned portion of the client's body. The cells are grown in a laboratory to produce cell sheets that can be grafted on the client to generate a permanent skin surface. The length of time for culturing and growing the skin is prolonged, and the cell sheets are not durable. Take care when applying these sheets to ensure adherence and prevent sloughing. This process is very costly.

Artificial Skin. Artificial skin is an alternative approach to closure of the burn wound. This substance has two layers, a Silastic epidermis and a porous dermis made from bovine hide collagen and shark cartilage.

After the artificial skin is applied to a clean, excised wound surface, fibroblasts move into the collagen part of the artificial skin and create a structure similar to normal dermis. The artificial dermis slowly dissolves and is replaced with normal blood vessels and connective tissue (*neodermis*). The neodermis supports a standard autograft placed over it when the Silastic layer is removed.

Biosynthetic Wound Dressings. Biosynthetic wound dressings are a combination of biosynthetic and synthetic materials. Biobrane is commonly used and effective in the treatment of clean superficial partial-thickness burns such as scalds, as a covering for meshed autografts, and as donor site dressings.

Biobrane is made up of a nylon fabric that is partially embedded into a silicone film. Collagen is incorporated into both the silicone and nylon components. The nylon fabric comes into contact with the wound surface and forms an adherent bond until epithelialization has occurred. The porous silicone film allows exudates to pass through.

Synthetic Dressings. Synthetic dressings are made of solid silicone and plastic membranes (e.g., polyvinyl chloride and polyurethane). They may be substituted for standard or biologic dressings. Synthetic dressings are applied directly to the surface of a clean or surgically prepared wound and remain in place until they fall off or are removed. Because many of these dressings are transparent or translucent, the wound can be inspected without removing the dressing. Pain is reduced at the site because these agents also prevent contact of the wound with air. These dressings also are used to cover donor sites where skin was obtained for autografting.

Transparent film appears to be the best dressing for the care of donor site wounds. This dressing type promotes faster healing with low infection rates, minimal pain, and reduced cost (Rakel et al., 1998).

Another strategy to manage donor site pain is the topical application of lidocaine to donor harvest sites. The resulting analgesic effects reduce opioid requirements, lower pain scores, and do not cause systemic effects when used for small areas (less than 15% TBSA) (Jellish et al., 1999).

SURGICAL MANAGEMENT. Surgical management of burn wounds focuses on excision and wound covering. Surgical excision is performed early in the postburn period. Grafting may be performed throughout the acute phase as burn wounds are made ready and donor sites are available. Early grafting reduces the time clients are at risk for infection and sepsis.

Wound covering through autografting involves taking skin from an area of the client's intact, healthy skin and transplanting it to an excised burn wound.

Surgical Excision. Surgical excision is the most common treatment for full-thickness and deep partial-thickness wounds. The client is taken to the operating room within the first 5 days after injury and again as needed until all wounds are closed permanently.

The burn wound is excised by either a tangential or a fascial excision technique. In the tangential technique, the surgeon excises very thin layers of the necrotic burn surface until bleeding tissue is encountered. Bleeding indicates that a bed of healthy dermis or subcutaneous fat has been reached.

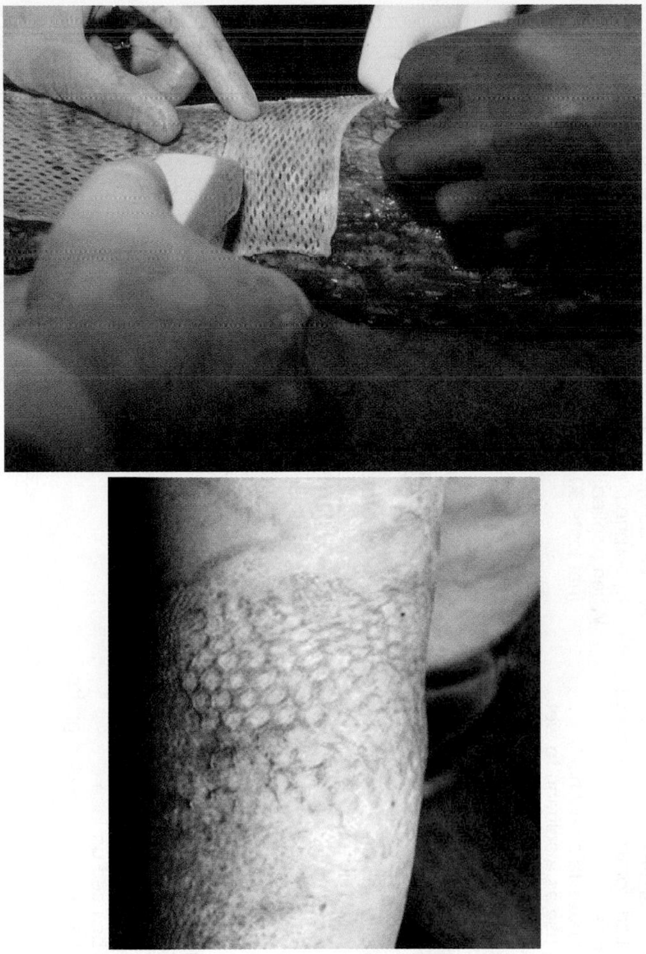

Figure 71-13 ■ The typical appearance of meshed autografts. **A,** Appearance during application of meshed autograft. **B,** Appearance of meshed autograft after healing.

In the fascial technique, the surgeon excises the burn wound to the level of superficial fascia. Fascial excision usually is reserved for very deep and extensive burns. Blood loss is minimal, and grafting is usually successful.

Wound Covering. Permanent skin coverage for large full-thickness injuries is achieved by applying an autograft. Skin for an autograft is taken from the client's own body. The surgeon removes a piece of skin from a remote unburned area of the body and transplants it to cover the burn wound. Skin grafts are generally of split thickness (0.015 inch) and a partial-thickness injury is formed at the site of surgical removal (the donor site). Grafts are placed either on a clean granulated bed or over a surgically excised area of burn (see also Chapter 70).

The availability of donor sites for larger burns is small. Clients with larger burns may have only 5% to 20% of healthy skin surface available to cover the 80% to 95% burned area. Coverage is accomplished in the following ways:

- Successive reharvesting of the available donor site. Time is allowed between harvests for healing.
- Meshing the split-thickness skin grafts (Figure 71-13) to allow a small graft to cover a larger area. Healing time is slower for a meshed graft because the skin must fill in open meshed areas (interstices) as well as attach to the granulation bed.

RISK FOR INFECTION

Burn wound infection occurs through **autocontamination,** in which the client's own normal flora overgrows and penetrates the internal environment; and **cross-contamination,** in which organisms from elsewhere are transferred to the client.

NOC **PLANNING: EXPECTED OUTCOMES.** The client is expected to remain free from infection by cross-contamination and not develop septicemia. Indicators include that the client will exhibit only mild instances or none of the following manifestations:

- Foul-smelling discharge
- Fever
- Blood culture colonization
- Wound site colonization
- White blood cell count elevation

INTERVENTIONS. Interventions aim to prevent infection and remove infected tissue.

NONSURGICAL MANAGEMENT. Nonsurgical management consists of minimizing exposure of the burn client to exogenous organisms, reducing the risk for autocontamination, and recognizing the manifestations of infection early. Drug therapy, isolation therapy, and environmental manipulation are strategies for preventing and managing infection.

Drug Therapy for Infection Prevention. Burn wound conditions promote the growth of *Clostridium tetani* and all burn clients are at risk for this dangerous infection. Tetanus toxoid, 0.5 mL given IM, enhances acquired immunity to *C. tetani.* This agent is a routinely given when the client is admitted to the hospital. Tetanus immune globulin (human) (Hyper-Tet) injection is recommended when the client's history of tetanus immunization is not known.

The use of topical antimicrobial drugs is an important intervention for infection prevention in burn wounds. The goal of this therapy is to reduce bacterial growth into the wound and prevent systemic sepsis.

Topical antibiotics are applied by either the *open* or the *closed* technique. With the open technique, use either aseptic or clean methods to apply the drug directly to the burn wound without further dressing the wound. Clean the wound every 8 to 24 hours and apply fresh antimicrobial drugs. With the more common closed technique, dress the burn wound after applying the topical drugs.

Two of the more commonly used drugs are silver sulfadiazine (Silvadene, Flamazine✱) and mafenide acetate (Sulfamylon). Topical antimicrobial drugs are not applied to freshly grafted areas because they may inhibit cell growth. Chart 71-5 lists the features of various topical antimicrobial drugs.

Drug Therapy for Treatment of Infection. Systemic antibiotics are used when burn clients have symptoms of an actual infection, including septicemia. Broad-spectrum antibiotics are given until the results of blood cultures and sensitivity status are available. At that time, more specific antibiotics, including the aminoglycosides such as amikacin (Amikin) or gentamicin (Garamycin, Alcomicin✱) and cephalosporins such as cephalothin (Keflin) or ceftriaxone (Rocephin), are used. Because of increased metabolism,

CHART 71-5

DRUG THERAPY for Burns

Agent	Description	Action	Advantages	Disadvantages	Interventions
Silver sulfadiazine (Silvadene, Thermazene)	Nontoxic salt of silver sulfadiazine in water-based cream	Binds to bacterial cell membranes and interferes with DNA synthesis	Does not cause hypochloremia, hyponatremia, electrolyte imbalance, or kidney disease Painless Wide-spectrum antimicrobial action against gram-positive and gram-negative organisms Long shelf life Delays eschar separation to a lesser degree than do many other topical drugs	Absorbed into eschar less than other drugs May cause rash, pruritus, burning, and leukopenia Not consistently effective for burns covering 60% of the body Not effective against *Pseudomonas*	Watch for signs of infection, such as soupiness of wound area. Watch for allergic reaction causing a drop in white blood cell count. Do not use if reaction to sulfonamide has occurred. Use on deep-partial or full-thickness wounds.
Collagenase (Santyl) with Polysporin powder	Topical enzymatic debriding agent with 250 collagenase units/g of white petroleum	Digests collagen in necrotic tissue	Painless Daily dressing changes No side effects Quick debridement action Easy to apply Not harmful to healthy tissue Specific only to nonviable tissue	Expensive	Apply once a day. Painless. Use on deep-partial wound with eschar. Monitor wounds for infection. May be used with barrier dressing such as Xeroform.
Mafenide acetate (Sulfamylon)	Soft, white, non-staining water-based cream Available in solution	Bacteriostatic action against many gram-positive and gram-negative organisms	Effective against *Pseudomonas* Long shelf life Excellent for treating electrical burns Penetrates thick eschar May use as a solution to wet down grafts or wounds	May lead to infection May cause metabolic acidosis, hyperpnea, and rash When applied, may cause pain that lasts 30-40 minutes	Premedicate for pain before application. Monitor blood gas and serum electrolyte levels. Monitor for infection.
Nitrofurazone (Furacin)	Cream, solution, or water-soluble ointment, or foam	Wide-spectrum anti-bacterial	Effective against *Staphylococcus aureus* and some antibiotic-resistant organisms Causes neither pain nor maceration	May cause contact dermatitis (rare) Messy to apply in cream form May cause renal problems if used in extensive burns	Observe carefully for signs of allergic reaction and evidence of superinfection.
Gentamicin sulfate (Garamycin, Gentamar)	Available as a cream or solution for topical use	Antibiotic action against organisms resistant to other drugs	Effective against *Pseudomonas* Does not cause pain	May have ototoxic and nephrotoxic effects May result in resistance by certain organisms	Use with caution in clients with decrease renal function. Monitor serum and urine creatinine clearance before and during treatment.
Polymyxin B-bacitracin	Topical cream	Wide-spectrum antimicrobial	Painless Effective against many gram-positive and gram-negative organisms Can be used on face Can be placed on healed grafts to lubricate	May cause urticaria, burning, and inflammation Does not penetrate eschar	Apply q2-8h to keep areas moist.

burn clients generally require a larger than normal dose of these drugs to maintain therapeutic blood levels. If aminoglycosides are used, serial peak and trough blood levels are monitored to determine the efficacy of treatment and evaluate potential ear and kidney toxicity.

Isolation Therapy. Some burn care philosophy believes that isolation therapy effectively reduces cross-contamination. However, methods of isolation are varied and controversial. Some burn centers practice virtually no isolation, whereas others use near-total sterile conditions. All isolation methods emphasize proper and consistent handwashing as the most effective technique for preventing infection transmission.

Environmental Management. All health care personnel wear gloves during all contact with open wounds. The use of sterile versus clean gloves for routine wound care varies by agency and is a matter of debate. Regardless of sterility, change gloves when handling wounds on different areas of the body and between handling old and new dressings.

The equipment on burn units is not shared among clients. Disposable items (e.g., pillows, syringes, and dishes) are used as much as possible. Assign to each client any equipment used in daily routine care (e.g., thermometers, blood pressure cuffs, and stethoscopes). Daily cleaning of the equipment and general housekeeping are essential for infection control. All equipment must be cleaned after use on one client and before use on another. Because *Pseudomonas* has been shown to sequester in plants, the presence of plants and flowers is prohibited. Some burn units do not permit clients to eat raw foods (such as salads, fruit, and pepper) to reduce exposure to organisms. Rugs and upholstered articles are difficult to clean and may harbor organisms; their use is also restricted.

Visitors are restricted when the client is immunosuppressed. Ill people, small children, and other clients should not come into direct contact with the burn client. Some burn units recommend that all visitors wear protective clothing (gowns, gloves, masks, and shoe and hair covers) in the room of the burn client, but no data support the effectiveness of this approach.

Secondary Prevention/Early Detection. Carefully monitor the burn wounds at each dressing change. Examine the wounds for the following signs of infection:

- Pervasive odor
- Color changes–focal, dark red, brown discoloration in the eschar
- Change in texture
- Purulent drainage
- Exudate
- Sloughing grafts
- Redness at the wound edges extending to nonburned skin

Laboratory cultures and biopsies are recommended. Quantitative biopsies of the eschar and granulation tissue are performed routinely and as needed to monitor the proliferation of organisms and are considered the gold standard for wound monitoring.

SURGICAL MANAGEMENT. Infected burn wounds with colony counts of or approaching 10^5 colonies per gram of tissue are life threatening, even with antibiotic therapy. Surgical excision of the burn wound may be necessary.

IMBALANCED NUTRITION: LESS THAN BODY REQUIREMENTS

NOC **PLANNING: EXPECTED OUTCOMES.** The client is expected to maintain adequate nutrient intake for meeting the body's calorie needs. Indicators include that the client should have mild or no deviations from the normal ranges of the following:

- Weight/height ratio
- Food intake
- Hematocrit and hemoglobin
- Serum albumin
- Blood glucose

INTERVENTIONS. Interventions aim to calculate the client's calorie needs and provide an adequate daily source of calories and nutrients that the client can ingest and metabolize.

Diet therapy begins with calculating the client's current daily calorie needs. Several formulas and charts are used for this calculation. Nutritional requirements for a client with a large burn area can exceed 5000 kcal/day. In addition to a high-calorie intake, the burn client requires a diet high in protein for wound healing. Collaborate with the dietitian and the client to plan additions to standard nutritional patterns.

Oral diet therapy may be delayed for several days after the injury until the GI tract is motile. Nasoduodenal tube feedings are often started soon after admission. Beginning enteral feedings early helps to decrease weight loss, gut atrophy, bacterial translocation, and sepsis. These feedings often are started within 4 hours of beginning fluid resuscitation. This type of supplement prevents nutritional deficits in severely burned clients.

Encourage clients who can eat solid foods to ingest as many calories as possible. Take the client's preferences into consideration for diet planning and food selection. Encourage clients to request food whenever they feel they can eat, not just according to the hospital's standard meal schedule. Offer frequent high-calorie, high-protein supplemental feedings. Keep an accurate calorie count for foods and beverages that are actually ingested by the client.

Clients who cannot swallow but who have adequate gastric motility may meet calorie and nutrition needs through enteral tube feedings (see Chapter 64). Parenteral nutrition may be given IV when the GI tract is not functional or when the client's nutritional needs cannot be met by oral and enteral feeding. This method is used as a last resort because it is invasive and can lead to infectious and metabolic complications.

IMPAIRED PHYSICAL MOBILITY

NOC **PLANNING: EXPECTED OUTCOMES.** The client with a burn injury is expected to regain and maintain an optimal ability to move purposefully. Indicators include that the client should be mildly compromised or not compromised in the following actions:

- Muscle movement
- Joint movement
- Walking
- Body positioning performance

INTERVENTIONS. Interventions aim to maintain the client's preburn range of joint motion and prevent contracture formation.

CHART 71-6

BEST PRACTICE for
Positioning to Prevent Contractures

Affected Body Part	Position of Function	Intervention
Head and neck	Hyperextension	No pillow. Place a towel roll under the client's neck or shoulder. Neck splint.
Posterior neck	Flexion	Have client turn the head from side to side.
Upper chest and chest	Shoulder retraction	Place client in supine position. Place a folded towel under the spine, between the scapulae.
Lateral trunk	Flexion to uninvolved side	Place the client supine with arm on the affected side up over the head.
Anterior shoulder	Abduction and external rotation	Maintain the upper arm at 90 degrees of abduction from the lateral aspect of the trunk.
Posterior shoulder	Slight flexion and interior rotation	Keep the arm slightly behind the midline.
Axilla	Abduction with 10-15 degree forward flexion and external rotation	Support the abducted arm with suspension from IV pole or bedside table. Axilla splint
Elbow	Extension and supination	Keep the joint in the extended position.
Wrist	30-45 degrees of extension	Use a splint.
Fingers		
MP joints	70-90 degrees of flexion	Use a splint.
PIP and DIP joints	Extended	Use a splint.
Ankle	90 degrees of dorsiflexion	Use a padded footboard or splint with heels free of pressure.
Legs	15-20 degrees of abduction	Place small pillow between legs.
Hip	Extension and neutral rotation	Supine with lower extremity extended. Trochanter roll. Foam wedge along lateral aspect of thigh.

NONSURGICAL MANAGEMENT. Nonsurgical management includes positioning, range-of-motion exercises, ambulation, and pressure dressings.

Positioning. Positioning is critical for clients with burn injuries because the position of comfort for the client is often one of joint flexion, which predisposes him or her to contracture development. Maintain the client in a neutral body position with minimal flexion. Best practice for the prevention of contractures is listed in Chart 71-6. Splints and other conforming devices may assist in maintaining position. These devices are used most often on the joints of the hands, elbows, knees, neck, and axillae.

Range-of-Motion Exercises. Range-of-motion exercises are performed actively at least three times a day. If the client cannot move a joint actively, perform passive range-of-motion exercises. Give burned hands special attention. Encourage the client to perform active range-of-motion exercises for the hand, thumb, and fingers every hour while he or she is awake.

Ambulation. Ambulation is started as soon as possible after the fluid shifts have resolved. Clients with a variety of attached equipment (IV catheters, nasogastric tubes, electrocardiographic leads, extensive dressings) can ambulate with preparation and assistance. Ambulation is performed two or three times a day and progresses in length each time. Ambulation inhibits the loss of bone density, strengthens muscles, stimulates immune function, promotes ventilation, and prevents many complications.

Pressure Dressings. After the graft heals, pressure dressings are applied to help prevent contractures and tight hypertrophic scars, which can inhibit mobility. These dressings also inhibit venous stasis and edema formation in areas with decreased lymphatic outflow. Pressure dressings may be elastic wraps or specially designed, custom-fitted, elasticized clothing that provide continuous pressure over the burned area. Figure 71-14 shows such garments. For best effectiveness, pressure garments must be worn at least 23 hours a day, every day, until the scar tissue is mature (12 to 24 months). Pressure garments cause some personal discomfort with itchiness and increased warmth. Reinforce to the client that wearing pressure garments is very beneficial in maintaining mobility and reducing scarring.

SURGICAL MANAGEMENT. Surgical management restores mobility rather than prevents immobility. Surgical release of contractures is most commonly performed in the neck, axilla, elbow flexion areas, and hand. Specific surgical procedures to improve movement vary for each client.

Nursing responsibilities after surgery include interventions to prevent contractures from reforming as well as the care of new grafts and suture lines. Constantly reinforce the need for the client to adhere to exercise and splinting regimens to prevent the recurrence of joint immobility.

DISTURBED BODY IMAGE

NOC **PLANNING: EXPECTED OUTCOMES.** Following intervention, the client with a burn injury is expected to have a positive perception of his or her own appearance and body functions. Indicators include that the client should consistently demonstrate the following behaviors:

- Willingness to touch the affected body part
- Adjustment to changes in body function
- Willingness to use strategies to enhance appearance and function

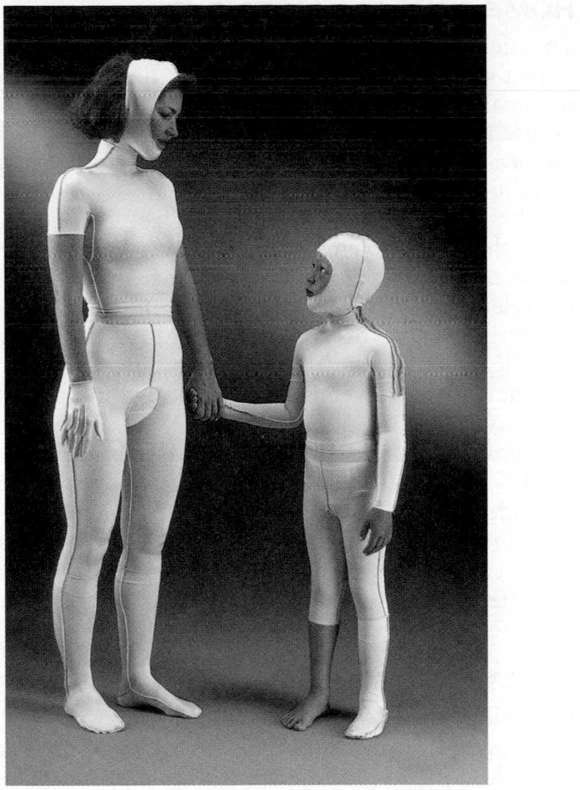

Figure 71-14 ■ Models wearing pressure garments. (Courtesy of Beiersdorf-Jobst, Inc., Charlotte, NC.)

- Successful progression through the grieving process
- Use of support systems

INTERVENTIONS. Nonsurgical and surgical interventions can assist clients who have body image disturbances as a result of burn injury.

NONSURGICAL MANAGEMENT. Understanding the stages of grief is helpful for the client, family, and health professionals. Assess which stage of grief the client is currently experiencing and help interpret his or her behaviors. The client often is unaware of or is confused by his or her feelings. Reassure the client that feelings of grief, loss, anxiety, anger, fear, and guilt are normal. The client may be grieving the loss of body parts, appearance, role identity, and social identity. Collaborate with other health care team members (e.g., psychologist, psychiatrist, social worker, or clergy or religious leader) in addressing these problems.

Accept the physical and psychological characteristics of the client. Present clients and families with realistic expected outcomes for the client's functional capacity and physical appearance. Provide information sessions and counseling for the family to help identify effective patterns of support. Facilitate client's use of these systems and the development of new support systems. Make referrals to support groups. To identify the effectiveness of such assistance and possible gaps in support, evaluate support resources throughout the course of illness.

Engaging in decision making and independent activities fosters feelings of self-worth, which are closely linked to body image. To this end, plan and encourage the client's active participation in self-care activities. Assist family members to understand that it is more beneficial for the client to perform these activities than to have them performed by someone else. Encourage families to include the client in family decision making to the same degree that he or she participated in this process before the injury.

SURGICAL MANAGEMENT. Reconstructive and cosmetic surgery can be performed for many years after the burn injury. Restoring function and improving appearance through surgical techniques often increase the client's feelings of self-worth and promote a positive body image. Many clients have unrealistic expectations of reconstructive surgery and envision an appearance identical or equal in quality to the preburn state. Teach the client and family about expected cosmetic outcomes.

Critical Thinking Challenge

The 57-year-old who sustained a 41% TBSA flame burn was grafted with split-thickness meshed grafts to her bilateral upper limbs and hands taken from her thighs. When performing the initial postoperative dressing, you note that the graft has a dusky appearance and that the edges of the graft are beginning to curl. The margins of the wound are firm and red with some purulent drainage. You also note a greenish blue color in the burned area next to the graft.

1. What is your first action?
2. Should range-of-motion exercises be performed to the upper extremities at this time? Why or why not?
3. What is the best position for the upper extremities and hands to prevent contractures?
4. What additional assessment data should you obtain about the graft and the surrounding burn wound?

evolve For suggested answer guidelines, go to http://evolve.elsevier.com/Iggy/.

REHABILITATIVE PHASE OF BURN INJURY

OVERVIEW

Although rehabilitation efforts are started from the time of admission, the technical rehabilitative phase begins with wound closure and ends when the client returns to the highest possible level of functioning. The emphasis during this phase is the psychosocial adjustment of the client, the prevention of scars and contractures, and the resumption of preburn activity, including resuming work, family, and social roles. This phase may take years or even a lifetime as clients adjust to permanent limitations that may not be apparent until long after the initial injury.

COLLABORATIVE MANAGEMENT

Although attention is placed first on the physical interventions for the burn injury, psychological care is equally important. Provide psychosocial support to the client and family throughout hospitalization but more extensively in the rehabilitative phase.

Information from the client and family aids in the assessment and diagnosis of psychological problems and allows treatment to be instituted. Explore the client's feelings about the burn injury. It is extremely difficult for clients to concentrate on the many tasks before them when obstacles such as guilt and grief are in the forefront.

TABLE 71-11 Needs to Address Before Discharge of the Client with Burns

- Early client assessment
- Financial assessment
- Evaluation of family resources
- Weekly discharge planning meeting
- Psychological referral
- Client and family teaching (home care)
- Designation of principal learners (specific family members or significant others who will help with care)
- Development of teaching plan
- Training for wound care
- Rehabilitation referral
- Home assessment (on-site visit)
- Medical equipment
- Public health nursing referral
- Evaluation of community resources
- Visit to referral agency
- Re-entry programs for school or work environment
- Nursing home placement
- Environmental interventions
- Auditory testing
- Speech therapy
- Prosthetic rehabilitation

Ask the client or family member whether there is a history of psychological problems. Assess and document the type of coping mechanisms the client has used successfully during times of stress to assist with a future plan of care. Also assess the client's family unit and the family members' history of interaction. Identify cultural and ethnic factors and take these into consideration when planning psychosocial interventions.

Throughout the hospitalization the client progresses through a variety of stages and exhibits many feelings, including denial, regression, and anger. Assess the client's feelings during each stage so appropriate plans of care can be developed and carried out.

Community-Based Care

Discharge planning for the client with a burn injury begins at the time of admission to the hospital or burn center. In most burn centers, the multidisciplinary team meets regularly to plan for discharge. In helping the client reach mutually established discharge goals, the team evaluates the progress of each discipline. Table 71-11 lists common discharge needs of the client with burns.

PSYCHOSOCIAL PREPARATION

During the recovery period and for some time after discharge from the hospital, clients with severe burn injuries are likely to have psychological problems that require intervention. Such problems include posttraumatic stress disorder, sexual dysfunction, and severe depression. Assistance is coordinated with the client, family, and health care team. Psychosocial assistance is best provided by a professional counselor with experience in helping burn clients.

One specific area to address with the client is the reaction of others to the sight of healing wounds and disfiguring scars. Clients with facial burns are especially subjected to stares and other reactions from the general public. Visits from friends and short public appearances before discharge may help the client begin adjusting to this problem. Community reintegration programs can assist the psychosocial and physical recovery of the client with serious burns.

HOME CARE MANAGEMENT

The client with severe burns is discharged from the acute care setting when life-threatening complications are resolved and minimal wound areas remain open. During the first weeks at home, the client usually needs at least daily wound care, physical therapy, nutritional support, symptom management, and drug therapy.

Although the client usually views going home in a positive light, the problems of physical care and the psychological stresses from changes in appearance, role, function, and lifestyle may overwhelm the client and family. Successful discharge depends on extensive planning and preparation of the client, family, and home environment through education and the involvement of appropriate support agencies and services.

Preparation for discharge includes assessment of the family and home care situation from physical and social perspectives. Consider the needs of the client when evaluating the home for cleanliness; access to bathing facilities, electricity, and running water; stairways; number of occupants; temperature control; and safety. If the burn injuries occurred in a house fire, a new residence may need to be established.

HEALTH TEACHING

Education about burn care and living with the consequences of burn injuries begins when the client is admitted to the hospital or burn center. A weekly plan for client education is outlined; the goal is progression toward independence for the client and family. Critical for this goal is teaching clients and family members to perform such care tasks as dressing changes. Allow clients and family members to first observe dressing changes, then to assist in performing the changes, and finally to change the dressings independently under your supervision.

Before discharge, all people who will be involved in the client's home care participate in discharge planning and teaching sessions. In addition to details about dressing changes, explain the following:

- Signs and symptoms of infection
- Drug regimens
- Proper use of prosthetic and positioning devices
- Correct application and care of pressure garments
- Comfort measures to reduce pruritus
- Dates for follow-up appointments

HEALTH CARE RESOURCES

The health care team evaluates the family in terms of capacity and willingness to assist in providing care to the client after discharge. A visiting nurse or case manager referral can assist the family with care problems arising at home. In addition, the visiting nurse can help the family determine what special equipment, supplies, or services will be needed. The frequency of home visits depends on the client's condition and the ability of family members to function as care providers. *It is imperative that the visiting nurse have extensive experience in providing burn care.* The home care nurse may need a brief visit to the client while in the hospital and observation of burn wound care.

The home care of a client after a serious burn often involves daily physical therapy and rehabilitation sessions at special centers. Address and resolve transportation problems before the client is discharged. In some instances, the burn center has arrangements for transportation. Some community volunteer agencies provide transportation by private car.

When rehabilitation is prolonged, the client may be discharged to a rehabilitation facility. Consult with the rehabilitation team and provide copies of the care and teaching plans used with the client.

Critical Thinking Challenge

The 57-year-old client who sustained a flame injury and received skin grafting is being prepared for discharge. You notice that your client's appetite has decreased, she refuses to participate in her occupational therapy, and she complains of fatigue despite staying in her bed all day. Your assessment reveals that she is depressed.

1. Are these symptoms the client is experiencing part of the complex systemic response to burn injuries? Why or why not?
2. What resources or referrals would be most appropriate for this client at this time?
3. What other needs should be addressed before discharge?

evolve For suggested answer guidelines, go to http://evolve.elsevier.com/Iggy/.

◆Evaluation: Outcomes

Evaluate the care of the client with a burn injury on the basis of the identified nursing diagnoses and collaborative problems. The expected outcomes include that the client should:

- Have cardiac output restored to normal
- Maintain adequate oxygenation and circulation to all vital organs
- Maintain a patent airway
- Have an effective breathing pattern
- Have pain alleviated or reduced
- Experience no further loss of skin integrity
- Have skin integrity restored without complications
- Remain free from infection by cross-contamination
- Not experience septicemia
- Maintain an adequate nutrient intake for meeting the body's calorie needs
- Regain and maintain an optimal ability to move purposefully
- Have a positive perception of his or her own appearance and body functions

Specific indicators for these outcomes are listed for each nursing diagnosis and collaborative problem under the Planning and Implementation section (see earlier).

GET READY for the NCLEX Examination!

KEY POINTS

Safe Effective Care Environment

- Use strict aseptic technique when caring for clients who have open burn wounds.
- Check ventilator alarms hourly for clients who are receiving paralytic drugs during mechanical ventilation.

Health Promotion and Maintenance

- Encourage all people to have and maintain home smoke detectors.
- Warn clients who smoke about not smoking in bed or when taking any substance that induces sedation (drugs or alcohol).
- Instruct clients who have reduced sensation in hands or feet to use a bath thermometer to check water temperature before bathing.
- Teach clients to avoid exposing the burned skin areas to the sun or to temperature extremes.

Psychosocial Integrity

- Allow clients time to grieve over a change in body image.
- Reassure clients that pain will be managed effectively.
- Explain all procedures to the client.
- Give analgesics, sedatives, and antianxiety drugs to clients receiving paralytic drugs during mechanical ventilation.
- Encourage the client to actively participate in pain control measures.
- Encourage the client to look at and touch burned areas.

Physiological Integrity

- Assess the burn client's airway and adequacy of breathing before assessing any other body system.
- Keep an endotracheal kit or tracheostomy kit at the bedside of any client with facial burns, burns inside the mouth, singed nasal hairs, or a "smoky" smell to the breath.
- Notify the physician immediately if the client with an inhalation injury becomes more dyspneic or audible wheezes disappear.
- Give half of the fluid volume calculated for the first 24 hours after burn injury in the first 8 hours postburn.
- Give prescribed opioid analgesics by the IV route during the emergent phase of burn recovery.
- Position clients to prevent contractures and promote joint function.
- Assist clients to ambulate several times each day as soon as the fluid shifts have resolved.
- Encourage clients to use the prescribed splints and pressure garments to prevent joint immobility.

ADDITIONAL STUDY RESOURCES

Go to your Student CD-ROM for Review Questions for the NCLEX Examination.

evolve Go to http://evolve.elsevier.com/Iggy/ for Integrated Management of Care Questions for the NCLEX Examination.

SELECTED BIBLIOGRAPHY

Asterisk indicates a classic or definitive work on this subject.

Ackley, B., & Ladwig, G. (2002). *Nursing diagnosis handbook: A guide to planning care* (5th ed.). St. Louis: Mosby.

American Burn Association. (2002). U.S. trauma and burn statistics. Available at http://www.ameriburn.org.

Badger, J. (2001). Burns: The psychological aspects. *American Journal of Nursing, 101*(11), 38-44.

Carrougher, G., et al. (2003). Comparison of patient satisfaction and self-reports of pain in adult burn-injured patients. *Journal of Burn Care and Rehabilitation, 24*(1), 1-8.

*Covington, D., Wainwright, D., & Parks, D. (1996). Prognostic indicators in the elderly patient with burns. *Journal of Burn Care and Rehabilitation, 17*(3), 222-230.

Demling, R., & DeSanti, L. (2002). The rate of re-epithelialization across meshed skin grafts is increased with exposure to silver. *Burns, 28*(3), 264-266.

DiLuigi, K. (2001). Hydrofluoric acid burns. *American Journal of Nursing 101*(6), 24AAA-24DDD.

Dochterman, J., & Bulechek, G. (Eds). (2004). *Nursing interventions classification (NIC)* (4th Ed.). St. Louis: Mosby.

Ebersole, P., Hess, P., & Luggen, A. (2004). *Toward healthy aging: Human needs and nursing response* (6th ed.). St. Louis: Mosby.

Facts and Comparisons. (2004). *Drug facts and comparisons* (58th ed.). St. Louis: Author.

*Flynn, M. (1999). Identifying and treating inhalation injuries in fire victims. *DCCN: Dimensions of Critical Care Nursing, 18*(4), 18-23.

Gosain, A., & Gamelli, R. (2005). The role of the gastrointestinal tract in burn sepsis. *Journal of Burn Care and Rehabilitation, 26*(1), 85-91.

*Hansbrough, J., et al. (1995). Wound healing in partial-thickness burn wounds treated with collagenase ointment versus silver sulfadiazine cream. *Journal of Burn Care and Rehabilitation, 16*(3), 241-247.

Helvig, E. (2002). Managing thermal injuries within WOCN practice. *Journal of Wound Ostomy, and Continence Nursing, 29*(2), 76-82.

Hunt, J., et al. (2000). Occupation-related burn injuries. *Journal of Burn Care: Rehabilitator 21*(4), 327-332.

Iraniha, S., et al. (2000). Determination of burn depth with noncontact ultrasonography. *Journal of Burn Care and Rehabilitation, 21*(4), 333-338.

*Jellish, W.S., et al. (1999). Effect of topical local anesthetic application to skin harvest sites for pain management in burn patients undergoing skin-grafting procedures. *Annals of Surgery, 229*(1), 115-120.

Kagan, R., & Smith, S. (2000). Evaluation and treatment of thermal injuries. *Dermatology Nursing, 12*(5), 334-335, 338-344, 347-350.

Koschel, M.J. (2002). Where there's smoke, there may be cyanide. *American Journal of Nursing, 102*(8), 39-42.

Kraft, P. (2000). The osmotic shift. *Journal of Intravenous Nursing, 23*(4), 220-224.

*Kravitz, M., et al. (1989). A randomized trial of plasma exchange in the treatment of burn shock. *Journal of Burn Care and Rehabilitation, 10*(1), 17-26.

Lawrence, J., & Fauerbach, J. (2003). Personality, coping, chronic stress, social support and PTSD symptoms among adult burn survivors: A path analysis. *Journal of Burn Care and Rehabilitation, 24*(1), 63-72.

*Mayes, T., Gottschlich, M., & Warden, G. (1997). Clinical nutrition protocols for continuous quality improvements in the outcomes of patients with burns. *Journal of Burn Care and Rehabilitation, 18*(4), 365-368.

McCance, K., & Huether, S. (2002). Pathophysiology: The biologic basis for disease in adults and children (4th ed.). St. Louis: Mosby.

McGwin, G., et al. (2003). Long-term trends in mortality according to age among adult burn patients. *Journal of Burn Care and Rehabilitation, 24*(1), 21-25.

Milner, S., Mottar, R., & Smith, C. (2001). The burn wheel: An innovative method for calculating the need for fluid resuscitation in burned patients. *American Journal of Nursing, 101*(11), 35-37.

Moorhead, S., Johnson, M., & Maas, M. (Eds.). (2004). *Nursing outcomes classification (NOC)* (3rd ed.). St. Louis: Mosby.

*Moritz, A.R. (1947). Studies of thermal injuries: II. The relative importance of time and surface temperature in the causation of cutaneous burns. *American Journal of Pathology, 23,* 695.

Nanchalhal, J., Dover, R., & Otto, W. (2002). Allogeneic skin substitutes applied to burns patients. *Burns, 28*(3), 254-257.

*Nguyen, T.T., et al. (1996). Current treatment of severely burned patients. *Annals of Surgery, 223*(1), 14-25.

Pagana, K., & Pagana, T. (2002). *Mosby's manual of diagnostic and laboratory tests* (2nd ed.). St. Louis: Mosby.

*Rakel, B., et al. (1998). Split-thickness skin graft donor site care: A quantitative synthesis of the research. *Applied Nursing Research, 11*(4), 174-182.

Scholl, D., & Langkamp-Henken, B. (2001). Nutrient recommendations for wound healing. *Journal of Intravenous Nursing, 24*(2), 124-132.

Sheridan, R. (2000). Evaluating and managing burn wounds. *Dermatology Nursing, 12*(1), 17-28.

Sibbald, G., et al. (2000). Preparing the woundbed: Debridement, bacterial balance, and moisture balance. *Ostomy Wound Management, 46*(4), 14-35.

Stone, M., Ahmed, J., & Evans, J. (2000). The continuing risk of domestic hot water scalds to the elderly. *Burns, 26*(4), 347-350.

Wiebelhaus, P., & Hansen, S. (2001). What you should know about managing burn emergencies. *Nursing2001, 31*(1), 36-41.

*Winfrey, M., Cochran, M., & Hegarty, M. (1999). A new technology in burn therapy: Integra artificial skin. *Dimensions of Critical Care Nursing, 18*(1), 14-20.

UNIT **SIXTEEN**

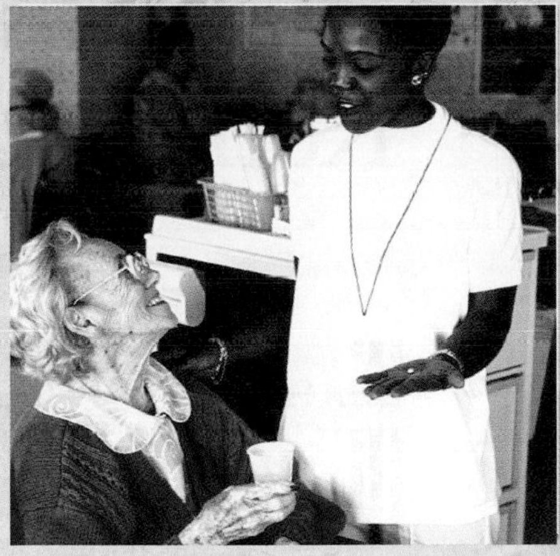

PROBLEMS of EXCRETION

Management of Clients with Problems of the Renal/Urinary System

CHAPTER

72 Assessment of the Renal/Urinary System

CHRIS WINKELMAN

LEARNING OUTCOMES

After studying this chapter, you should be able to:

1. Compare and contrast kidney function with functions of the ureters, bladder, and urethra.
2. Describe the roles of the afferent and efferent arterioles in glomerular filtration.
3. Explain the influence of antidiuretic hormone and aldosterone on urine formation and composition.
4. Describe age-related changes in the renal/urinary system.
5. Use laboratory data to distinguish between dehydration and renal impairment.
6. Describe how to obtain a sterile urine specimen from a client with a Foley catheter.
7. Identify teaching priorities for a client who needs to obtain a 24-hour urine specimen.
8. Identify teaching priorities for a client who needs to obtain a "clean-catch" urine specimen.
9. Describe the correct techniques to use in physically assessing the renal system.
10. Prioritize nursing care for the client during the first 24 hours following intravenous (IV) urography.

Go to your Student CD-ROM for Review Questions for the NCLEX Examination keyed to these Learning Outcomes.

Kidneys help maintain health in several ways. Their primary role is to maintain body fluid volume and composition and to filter waste products for elimination. The kidneys also help regulate blood pressure, participate in acid-base balance, produce erythropoietin for red blood cell (RBC) synthesis, and metabolize vitamin D to an active form.

The renal system includes the kidneys and the entire urinary tract. The ureters, bladder, and urethra are the drainage route for the excretion of urine. Structural or functional problems in the kidney or urinary tract usually alter fluid, electrolyte, and acid-base balance.

Assessment of the client at risk for or with actual problems of the renal system begins with a history and physical assessment. Understanding the anatomy, physiology, and diagnostic tests of the renal system helps you in problem-solving about renal function in the clinical setting. It also assists you in teaching the client about the purpose of tests or procedures and in physically and emotionally preparing the client for assessment.

ANATOMY AND PHYSIOLOGY REVIEW

Kidneys

Structure

GROSS ANATOMY

Normally, two kidneys are located behind the peritoneum, not really in the abdominal cavity, one on either side of the spine (Figure 72-1). The adult kidney is 4 to 5 inches (11 to 13 cm) long, 2 to 3 inches (5 to 7 cm) wide, and about 1 inch (2.5 to 3 cm) thick. It weighs about 8 ounces (250 g). The left kidney is slightly longer and narrower than the right kidney. Kidney size is can be determined via ultrasound. Larger-than-usual kidneys may indicate renal obstruction or polycystic disease, whereas smaller-than-usual kidneys may indicate chronic renal disease.

Several layers of tissue surround the kidney, providing protection and support. On the outer surface of the kidney is a layer of fibrous tissue called the **renal capsule** (Figure 72-2). This capsule covers most of the kidney except the **hilum,** the area in which the renal artery and nerve plexus enter and the renal vein and ureter exit. The renal capsule is surrounded by layers of fat and connective tissue (Gerota's fascia).

Lying beneath the renal capsule are the two layers of functional kidney tissue, the cortex and the medulla. The **renal cortex,** or outer tissue layer, is covered by the renal capsule. The **medulla,** or medullary tissue, lies below the cortex in the shape of many fans. Each "fan" is called a **pyramid,** and there are 12 to 18 pyramids per kidney. The **renal columns** (columns of Bertin) are cortical tissue that dip down into the interior of the kidney and separate the pyramids.

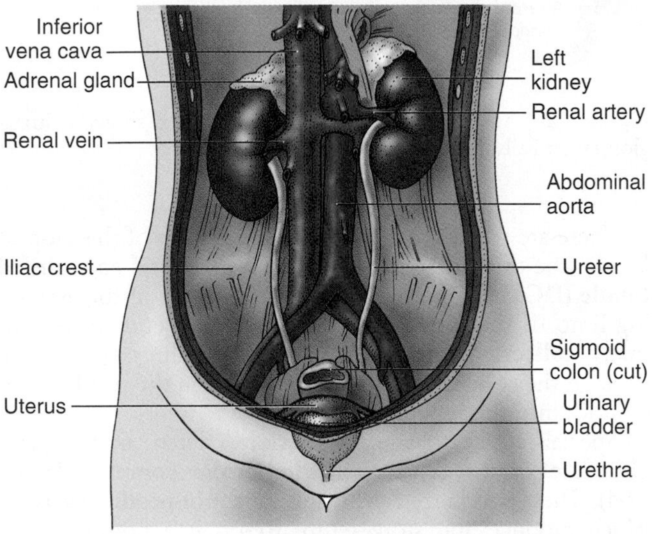

Figure 72-1 ■ Anatomic location of organs of the renal/urinary system.

The tip, or end, of each pyramid is called a **papilla.** The papillae drain urine into the collecting system. A cuplike structure called a **calyx** collects the urine at the end of each papilla. The calices join together to form the **renal pelvis,** which narrows to become the ureter.

The kidneys receive 20% to 25% of the total cardiac output. Renal blood flow per minute varies from about 600 to 1300 mL/min. The blood supply to each kidney comes from the **renal artery,** which branches from the abdominal aorta (Table 72-1). The renal artery divides into progressively smaller arteries, supplying all areas of the renal tissue **(parenchyma)** and the nephrons. The smallest arteries, the afferent arterioles, feed the nephrons directly to form urine.

Venous blood from the kidneys starts with the capillaries surrounding each nephron. These capillaries drain into progressively larger veins, with blood eventually returned to the inferior vena cava through the renal vein.

MICROSCOPIC ANATOMY

The **nephron** is the "working" unit of the kidney, and it is here that urine is actually formed from blood. There are

TABLE 72-1 The Sequence of Renal Blood Flow from the Renal Artery to the Renal Vein

1. Renal artery
2. Interlobar artery
3. Arcuate artery
4. Interlobular artery
5. Afferent arteriole
6. Glomerulus
7. Efferent arteriole
8. Peritubular capillaries or vasa recta
9. Stellate vein
10. Interlobular vein
11. Arcuate vein
12. Interlobar vein
13. Renal vein

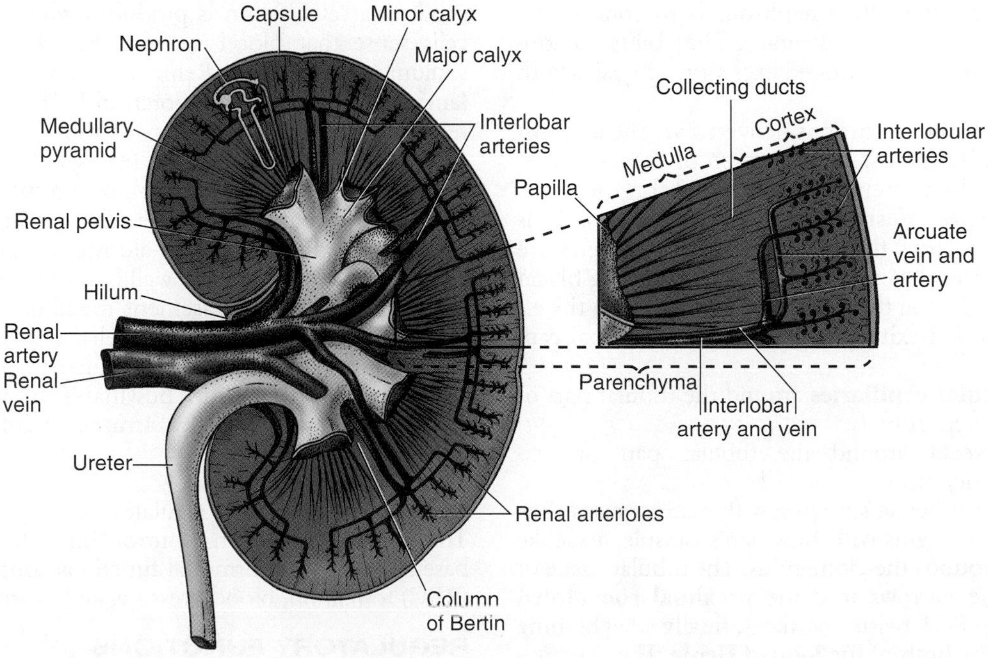

Figure 72-2 ■ Bisection of the kidney showing the major structures of the kidney.

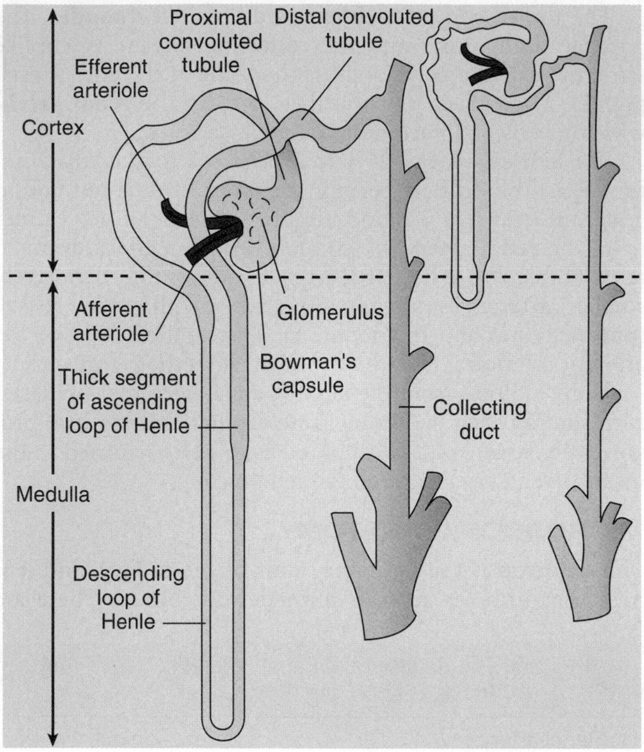

Figure 72-3 ■ Anatomy of the nephron, the functional unit of the kidney. Note that the particular nephron labeled here is a juxtamedullary nephron.

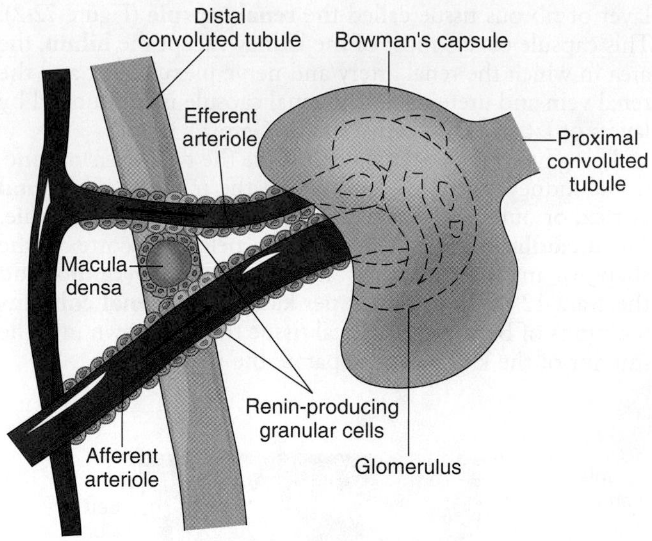

Figure 72-4 ■ The juxtaglomerular complex showing juxtaglomerular cells and the macula densa.

about 1 million nephrons per kidney, and each nephron separately makes urine from blood.

There are two types of nephrons: cortical nephrons and juxtamedullary nephrons. The cortical nephrons are short, with all parts located in the renal cortex. The juxtamedullary nephrons (about 20% of all nephrons) are longer, and their tubes and blood vessels dip deeply into the medulla. The purpose of the juxtamedullary nephrons is to concentrate urine during times of low fluid intake. The ability to concentrate urine allows for continued excretion of wastes with less fluid loss.

Blood supply to the nephron is delivered via the **afferent arteriole,** the smallest, most distal portion of the renal arterial system. From the afferent arteriole, blood flows into the **glomerulus,** a series of specialized capillary loops. It is through these capillaries that water and small particles are filtered from the blood to make urine. The remaining blood leaves the glomerulus via the **efferent arteriole.** From the efferent arteriole, blood exits into one of two additional capillary systems:

- The **peritubular capillaries** around the tubular part of the cortical nephrons
- The **vasa recta** around the tubular part of juxtamedullary nephrons

Each nephron is a tubelike structure with distinct parts (Figure 72-3). The tube begins with Bowman's capsule, a saclike structure that surrounds the glomerulus. The tubular tissue of Bowman's capsule narrows into the **proximal convoluted tubule (PCT).** The PCT twists and turns, finally straightening into the descending limb of the **loop of Henle.** The descending loop of Henle dips in the direction of the medulla but forms a hairpin loop and comes back up into the cortex.

There are two segments of ascending limb of the loop of Henle: the thin and thick segments. The **distal convoluted tubule (DCT)** forms from the thick segment of the ascending limb of the loop of Henle. The DCT ends in one of many **collecting ducts** located in the kidney tissue. The urine in the collecting ducts passes through the papillae and empties into the renal pelvis.

Special cells in the afferent arteriole, efferent arteriole, and DCT are known as the **juxtaglomerular complex** (Figure 72-4). These specialized cells are the **renin-producing cells,** which produce and store renin. **Renin** is a hormone that helps to regulate blood flow, glomerular filtration rate (GFR), and blood pressure. Renin is secreted when sensing cells in the DCT (called the **macula densa**) sense changes in blood volume and pressure. The macula densa lies next to the renin-producing cells. Renin is produced when the macula densa cells sense that blood volume, blood pressure, or blood sodium levels are low. Renin then converts renin substrate (angiotensinogen) into angiotensin I. This leads to a series of reactions that cause secretion of the hormone **aldosterone** (Figure 72-5). Aldosterone increases kidney reabsorption of sodium and water, restoring blood pressure, blood volume, and blood sodium levels. (See Chapter 14 for more discussion of the renin-angiotensin-aldosterone pathway).

The glomerular capillary wall has three layers (Figure 72-6): the endothelium, the basement membrane, and the epithelium. The endothelial and epithelial cells lining these capillaries are separated by pores that filter water and small particles from the blood into Bowman's capsule. This fluid is called the **filtrate** (also **ultrafiltrate**), or early urine.

Function

The kidneys have both regulatory and hormonal functions. The regulatory functions control fluid, electrolyte, and acid-base balance. The hormonal functions control red blood cell (RBC) formation, blood pressure, and vitamin D activation.

REGULATORY FUNCTIONS

The kidney processes that maintain fluid, electrolyte, and acid-base balance are glomerular filtration, tubular reab-

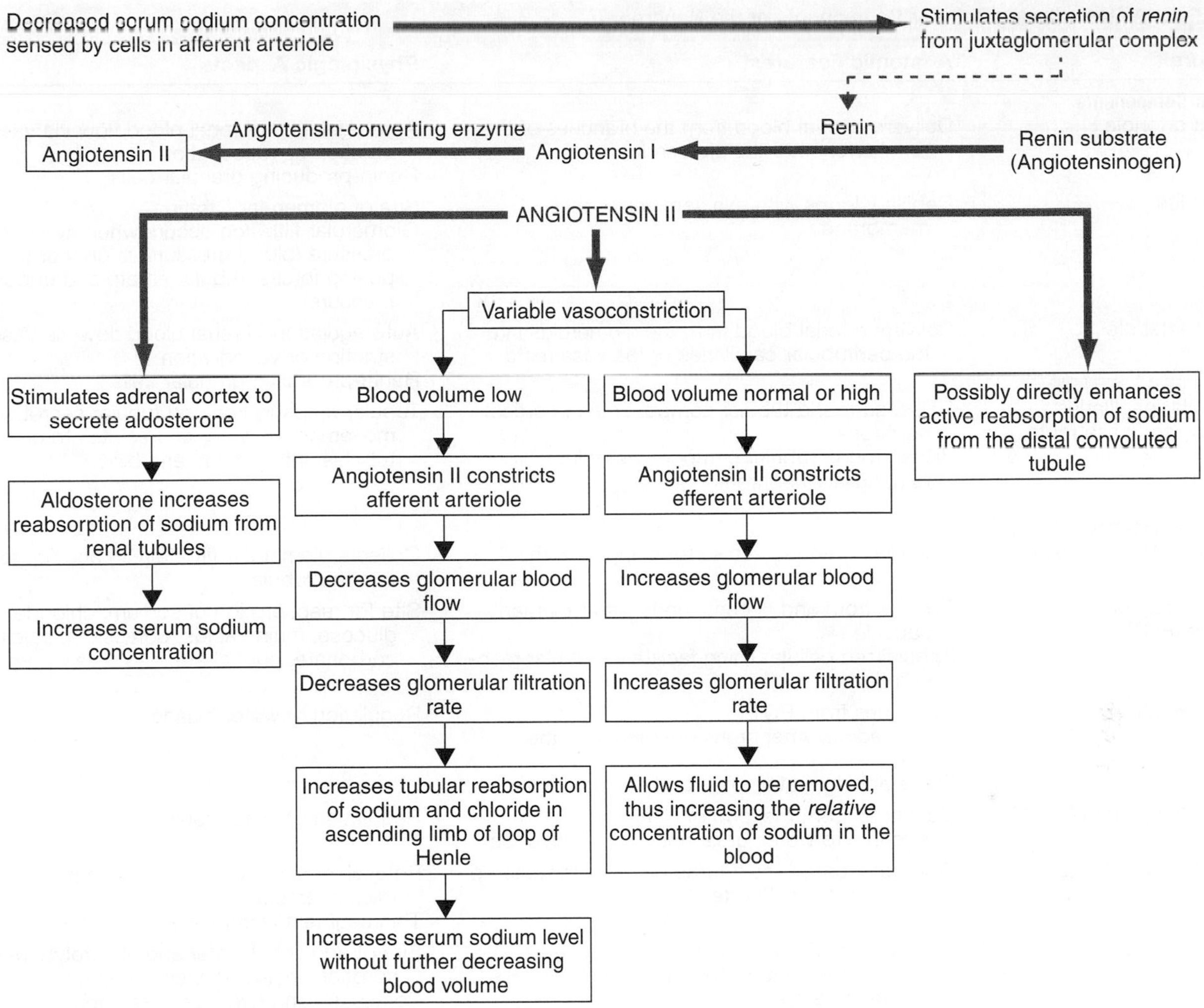

Figure 72-5 ■ The role of aldosterone, renin substrate (angiotensinogen), angiotensin I, and angiotensin II in the renal regulation of water and sodium.

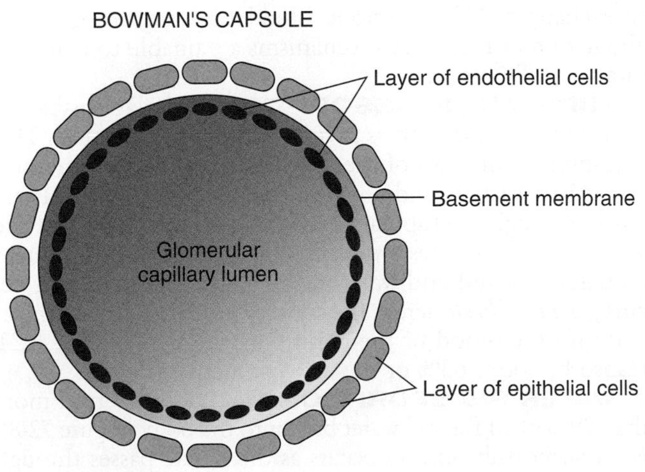

Figure 72-6 ■ Glomerular capillary wall.

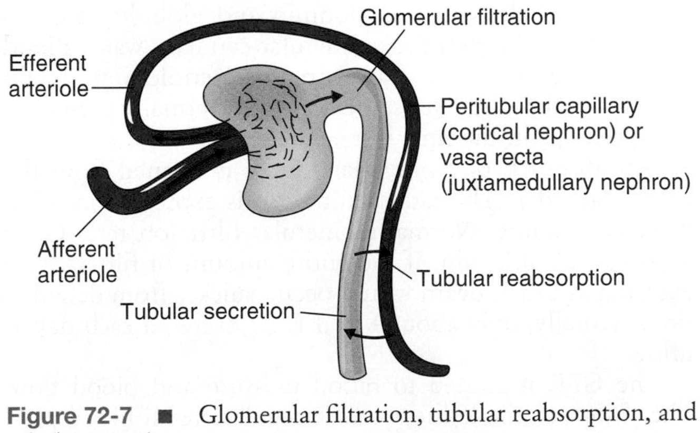

Figure 72-7 ■ Glomerular filtration, tubular reabsorption, and tubular secretion.

sorption, and tubular secretion (Figure 72-7). These processes use filtration, diffusion, active transport, and osmosis. (See Chapter 14 for a review of these actions.) Table 72-2 lists the functions of nephron tubules and blood vessels.

GLOMERULAR FILTRATION. Glomerular filtration is the first process in urine formation. As blood passes from the afferent arteriole into the glomerulus, water, electrolytes, and other small particles (e.g., creatinine, urea nitrogen, and glucose) are filtered across the glomerular membrane into the Bowman's capsule to form *glomerular* filtrate. As the filtrate enters the proximal convoluted tubule (PCT), it is called *tubular* filtrate.

TABLE 72-2 Vascular and Tubular Components of the Nephron

Structure	Anatomic Features	Physiologic Aspects
Vascular Components		
Afferent arteriole	Delivers arterial blood from the branches of the renal artery into the glomerulus	Autoregulation of renal blood flow via vasoconstriction or vasodilation Renin-producing granular cells
Glomerulus	Capillary loops with thin semipermeable membrane	Site of glomerular filtration Glomerular filtration occurs when hydrostatic pressure (blood pressure) is greater than opposing forces (tubular filtrate and oncotic pressure)
Efferent arteriole	Delivers arterial blood from the glomerulus into the peritubular capillaries or the vasa recta	Autoregulation of renal blood flow via vasoconstriction or vasodilation Renin-producing granular cells
Peritubular capillaries (PTCs) and vasa recta (VR)	PTCs: surround tubular components of cortical nephrons VR: surround tubular components of juxtamedullary nephrons	Tubular reabsorption and tubular secretion allow movement of water and solutes to or from the tubules, interstitium, and blood
Tubular Components		
Bowman's capsule (BC)	Thin membranous sac surrounding ⅞ of the glomerulus	Collects glomerular filtrate (GF) and funnels GF into the tubule
Proximal convoluted tubule (PCT)	Evolves from and is continuous with Bowman's capsule Specialized cellular lining facilitates tubular reabsorption	Site for reabsorption of sodium, chloride, water, glucose, amino acids, potassium, calcium, bicarbonate, phosphate, and urea
Loop of Henle	Continues from PCT Juxtamedullary nephrons dip deep into the medulla Permeable to water, urea, and sodium chloride	Regulation of water balance
Descending limb (DL)	Continues from the loop of Henle Permeable to water, urea, and sodium chloride	Regulation of water balance
Ascending limb (AL)	Emerges from DL as it turns and is redirected up toward the renal cortex	Potassium and magnesium reabsorption in the thick segment Thin segment is impermeable to water
Distal convoluted tubule (DCT)	Evolves from AL and twists so the macula densa cells lie adjacent to the juxtaglomerular cells of afferent arteriole	Site of additional water and electrolyte reabsorption, including bicarbonate Potassium and hydrogen secretion
Collecting ducts	Collects formed urine from several tubules and delivers it into the renal pelvis	Receptor sites for antidiuretic hormone regulation of water balance

Large particles, such as albumin and globulin, are too large to filter through the glomerular capillary walls. Blood cells also are too large to pass from the arterioles into the filtrate. Therefore these substances are not normally present in the filtrate or in the final urine.

About 180 L of glomerular filtrate is formed from the blood each day. The rate of filtration is expressed in milliliters per minute. Normal glomerular filtration rate (GFR) averages 125 mL/min. If the entire amount of filtrate were excreted as urine, death would occur quickly from dehydration. Actually, only about 1 to 3 L are excreted each day as urine.

The GFR is related to blood pressure and blood flow. The ability of the kidneys to self-regulate renal blood pressure and renal blood flow keeps GFR constant. GFR is controlled by selectively constricting and dilating the afferent and efferent arterioles. When the afferent arteriole is constricted or the efferent arteriole is dilated, pressure in the glomerular capillaries falls and filtration decreases. When the afferent arteriole is dilated or the efferent arteriole is constricted, pressure in the glomerular capillaries rises and filtration increases. Through this process the kidney can maintain a constant GFR, even when systemic blood pressure changes. When systolic blood pressure drops below about 70 mm Hg, these mechanisms are unable to compensate and GFR stops.

TUBULAR REABSORPTION. Tubular reabsorption is the second process involved in urine formation. This reabsorption of most of the filtrate keeps normal urine output at 1 to 3 L/day and prevents dehydration. As the filtrate passes through the tubular parts of the nephron, most of the water and electrolytes are reabsorbed. Reabsorption returns particles **(solutes)** and water to the blood. Reabsorption occurs *from the filtrate* across the tubular lumen of the nephron and into the blood of the peritubular capillaries. The PCT reabsorbs about 65% of the total glomerular filtrate.

WATER REABSORPTION. The tubules return more than 99% of all filtered water back into the body (Figure 72-8). Most water reabsorption occurs as the filtrate passes through the PCT. Water reabsorption continues as the filtrate flows down the descending loop of Henle. The thin and thick segments of the ascending loop of Henle is *not* permeable to water and water reabsorption does not occur here.

The distal convoluted tubule (DCT) can be permeable to water, and some water reabsorption can occur as the filtrate continues to flow through the tubule. The membrane of the

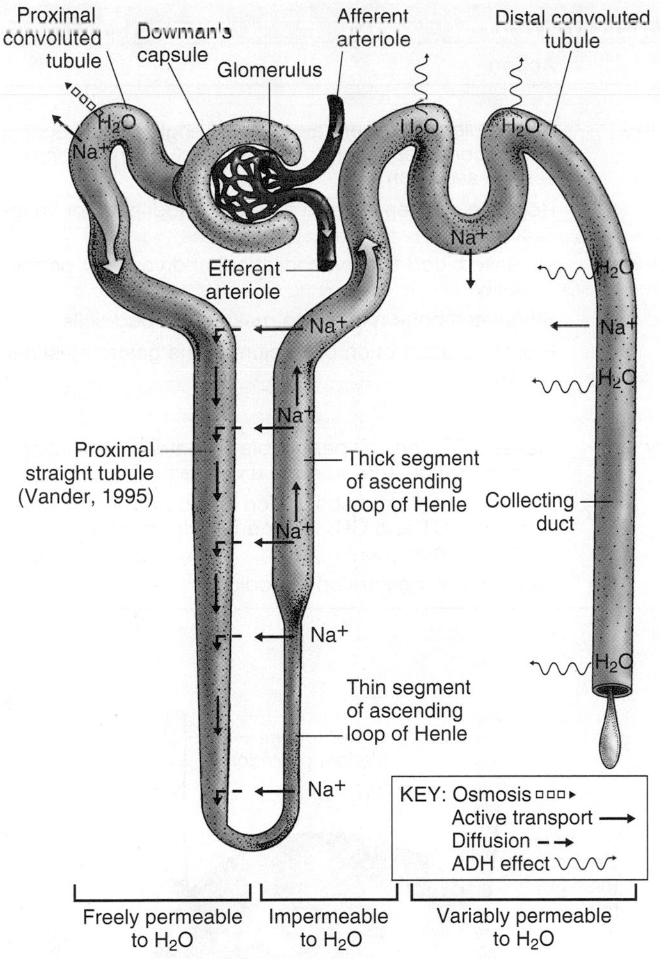

Figure 72-8 ■ Sodium and water reabsorption by the tubules of a cortical nephron.

DCT may be made more permeable to water through the action of the hormones **antidiuretic hormone (ADH)** and aldosterone. ADH increases membrane permeability to water and enhances water reabsorption. Aldosterone promotes the reabsorption of sodium in the DCT; water reabsorption occurs as a result of the movement of sodium (where sodium goes, water follows).

The ability of the kidneys to vary the volume or concentration of urine helps regulate total water balance regardless of water intake. In this way, the healthy kidney can prevent dehydration when fluid intake is low and prevent circulatory overload when fluid intake is excessive.

SOLUTE REABSORPTION. Some particles in the tubular filtrate are *returned to the blood.* This process is called **tubular reabsorption** and is selective. About 50% of all urea in the early urine is reabsorbed. On the other hand, no creatinine is reabsorbed.

Most sodium, chloride, and water reabsorption occurs in the PCT. The collecting ducts are the other site of sodium, chloride, and water reabsorption. Here reabsorption is caused by aldosterone. Potassium is also mostly reabsorbed in the PCT, with an additional 20% to 40% reabsorbed in the thick segment of the ascending loop of Henle.

Bicarbonate, calcium, and phosphate are mostly reabsorbed in the PCT. Bicarbonate reabsorption helps neutralize acids and maintain a normal blood pH. Blood levels of calcitonin and parathyroid hormone (PTH) (see Chapters 16 and 67) control calcium reabsorption and excretion.

The kidney reabsorbs some of the glucose filtered from the blood. However, there is a limit to how much glucose the kidney can reabsorb. This limit is called the **renal threshold** for glucose reabsorption or the **transport maximum** for glucose reabsorption. The usual renal threshold for glucose is about 220 mg/dL. This means that at a blood glucose level of 220 mg/dL or less, all glucose is reabsorbed and returned to the blood, with no glucose present in final urine. When blood glucose levels are greater than 220 mg/dL, some glucose stays in the filtrate and is present in the urine. Normally, almost all glucose and any filtered amino acids or proteins are reabsorbed and are not present in the urine.

TUBULAR SECRETION. Tubular secretion is the third process involved in urine formation. Like glomerular filtration, it allows substances to move *from the blood* into the early urine. During tubular secretion, substances move from the peritubular capillaries, across capillary membranes, and into the cells that line the tubules. From the cells, these substances are moved into the urine and are excreted from the body. Potassium (K^+) and hydrogen ions (H^+) are some of the substances moved in this way to maintain homeostasis of electrolytes and pH.

HORMONAL FUNCTIONS

The kidneys produce renin, prostaglandins, bradykinin, erythropoietin, and activated vitamin D (Table 72-3). Other kidney products, such as the kinins, change renal blood flow and capillary permeability. The kidneys also help break down and excrete insulin.

RENIN. As discussed earlier under Microscopic Anatomy (p. 1653), renin assists in blood pressure control. Renin is formed and released when there is a decrease in blood flow, volume, or pressure through the renal arterioles or when too little sodium is present in renal blood. These conditions are detected through the receptors of the juxtaglomerular complex.

Renin release causes the production of *angiotensin II* through a series of steps (see Figure 72-5). Angiotensin II increases systemic blood pressure through powerful blood vessel constricting effects and stimulates the release of aldosterone from the adrenal cortex. Aldosterone increases the reabsorption of sodium in the distal tubule of the nephron. Therefore more water is reabsorbed and blood pressure is increased because of increases in blood volume. When renal blood flow is reduced, this renin-angiotensin-aldosterone system of blood pressure control regulates pressures in the nephron as well as systemic blood pressure (see also Chapter 14).

PROSTAGLANDINS. Prostaglandins are produced in many tissues, including the kidney. Specific prostaglandins produced in the kidney are prostaglandin E_2 (PGE_2) and prostacyclin (PGI_2). These substances help regulate glomerular filtration, kidney vascular resistance, and renin production. PGE_2 acts on the distal tubule and collecting duct to increase sodium and water excretion.

BRADYKININ. The presence of angiotensin II, prostaglandins, and ADH stimulates the release of bradykinin in the kidney. **Bradykinin** dilates the afferent arteriole and increases capillary membrane permeability to some solutes. These actions maintain kidney blood flow and reabsorption even when other conditions cause systemic blood vessel constriction.

TABLE 72-3 Renal Hormone Production and Hormones Influencing Renal Function

	Site	Action
Renal Hormone Production		
Renin	Renin-producing granular cells	Raises blood pressure as result of angiotensin (local vasoconstriction) and aldosterone (volume expansion) secretion
Prostaglandins	Renal tissues	Regulate intrarenal blood flow by vasodilation or vasoconstriction
Bradykinins	Juxtaglomerular cells of the arterioles	Increase blood flow (vasodilation) and vascular permeability
Erythropoietin	Renal parenchyma	Stimulates bone marrow to make red blood cells
Activated vitamin D	Renal parenchyma	Promotes absorption of calcium in the gastrointestinal tract
Hormones Influencing Renal Function		
Antidiuretic hormone (ADH, vasopressin)	Released from posterior pituitary	Makes DCT and CD permeable to water to maximize reabsorption and produce a concentrated urine
Aldosterone	Released from adrenal cortex	Promotes sodium reabsorption and potassium secretion in DCT and CD; water and chloride follow sodium movement
Natriuretic hormones	Cardiac atria, brain	Cause tubular secretion of sodium

DCT, Distal convoluted tubule; *CD*, collecting ducts.

ERYTHROPOIETIN. **Erythropoietin** is produced and released in response to decreased oxygen tension in the renal blood supply. Erythropoietin triggers red blood cell (RBC) production in the bone marrow. When kidney tissue is nonfunctional, erythropoietin production decreases and the person becomes anemic.

VITAMIN D ACTIVATION. A series of steps are needed for vitamin D, a hormone, to become active. Some of these steps take place in the skin when it is exposed to ultraviolet light and then more processing occurs in the liver. From there, vitamin D is converted to its active form (1,25-dihydroxy-cholecalciferol) in the kidney. Activated vitamin D is needed to absorb calcium in the intestinal tract and to regulate calcium balance.

Ureters

Structure

Each kidney has a single ureter, a hollow tube that connects the renal pelvis with the urinary bladder. The ureter is about ½ inch (1.25 cm) in diameter and about 12 to 18 inches (30 to 45 cm) in length.

The diameter of the ureter narrows in three areas:

- In the upper third of the ureter, at the point at which the renal pelvis becomes the ureter, is a narrowing known as the **ureteropelvic junction (UPJ).**
- The ureter also narrows as it bends toward the abdominal wall (aortoiliac bend).
- Each ureter narrows at the point it enters the bladder; this point is called the **ureterovesical junction (UVJ).**

The ureter tunnels through bladder tissue for a short distance and then opens into the bladder at the **trigone** (Figure 72-9).

The ureter has three layers: an inner lining of mucous membrane (urothelium), a middle layer of smooth muscle fibers, and an outer layer of fibrous tissue. The outer layer of the ureter contains the blood supply. The middle layer of muscle fibers is controlled by several nerve pathways from the lower spinal cord.

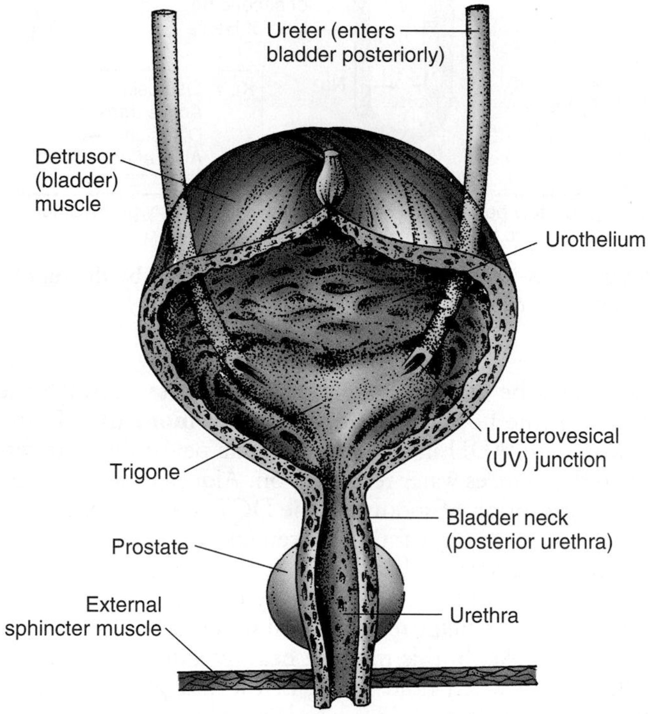

Figure 72-9 ■ Gross anatomy of the urinary bladder.

Function

Contractions of the smooth muscle in the ureter move urine from the renal pelvis of the kidney to the bladder. Stretch receptors in the renal pelvis regulate this movement. For example, a large volume of urine in the renal pelvis triggers the stretch receptors, which respond by increasing ureteral contractions and peristalsis.

Urinary Bladder

Structure

The urinary bladder is a muscular sac. The upper surface lies next to the peritoneal cavity. In men, the bladder is in front of the rectum. In women, the bladder is in front of the vagina. The bladder lies directly behind the pubic bone.

The bladder is composed of the **body** (the rounded sac portion) and the **bladder neck** (posterior urethra), which connects to the bladder body. The bladder has three linings, an inner lining of epithelial cells **(urothelium),** middle layers of smooth muscle **(detrusor muscle),** and an outer lining. The **trigone** is an area on the posterior wall between the points of ureteral entry (ureterovesical junctions [UVJs]) and the urethra.

The **internal urethral sphincter** is the smooth detrusor muscle of the bladder neck and elastic tissue. The **external urethral sphincter** is skeletal muscle that surrounds the urethra.

In men, the external sphincter surrounds the urethra at the base of the prostate gland. In women, the external sphincter is at the base of the bladder. The pudendal nerve from the spinal cord controls the external sphincter.

Function

The bladder is a temporary urine storage site. The bladder also provides continence and enables voiding. The secretions of the bladder lining resist bacteria.

Continence is the ability to voluntarily control bladder emptying. Bladder continence occurs during bladder filling through the combination of detrusor muscle relaxation, internal sphincter muscle tone, and external sphincter contraction. As the bladder fills with urine, stretch sensations are transmitted to spinal sacral nerves S2 and S3.

MAINTAINING CONTINENCE

Continence is maintained by the interaction of the nerves that control the muscles of the bladder, bladder neck, urethra, and pelvic floor, as well as by factors that close the urethra. During bladder filling, the sympathetic nervous system fibers prevent detrusor muscle contraction. These control centers are located in the cerebral cortex, the brainstem, and the sacral part of the spinal cord. For urethral closure to be adequate for continence, the mucosal surfaces must be in contact and must be adhesive. Contact depends on the presence and proper function of the involved nerves and muscles. Adhesion depends on the adequate secretion of mucus-like substances.

MICTURITION

Micturition (voiding) is a reflex of autonomic control that triggers contraction of the detrusor muscle at the same time as relaxation of the external sphincter and the muscles of the pelvic floor. With detrusor muscle contraction, the UVJ of the ureter closes, and the normally round bladder assumes the shape of a funnel. Voiding is a voluntary act as the result of a learned response and is controlled by the cerebral cortex and the brainstem. Contraction of the external sphincter inhibits the micturition reflex and prevents voiding.

Urethra

Structure

The urethra is a narrow tube lined with mucous membranes and epithelial cells. The **urethral meatus,** or opening, is the end point of the urethra. In men, the urethra is about 6 to 8 inches (15 to 20 cm) long, with the meatus located at the tip of the penis. The male urethra has three sections:

- The prostatic urethra, which extends from the bladder to the prostate gland
- The membranous urethra, which extends to the wall of the pelvic floor
- The cavernous urethra, which is external and extends through the length of the penis

In women, the urethra is about 1 to 1.5 inches (2.5 to 3.75 cm) long and exits the bladder through the pelvic floor. The meatus lies slightly below the clitoris and directly in front of the vagina and rectum.

Function

The urethra is a tube for eliminating urine from the body. The passing of urine normally removes bacteria from the urethra.

Renal/Urinary System Changes Associated with Aging

RENAL CHANGES

Structural and functional changes occur in the kidney as a result of the aging process. These changes often have clinical significance. The kidney loses cortical tissue and gets smaller by 80 years of age. This cortical loss is caused by reduced renal blood flow. The medulla is not affected by aging, and the juxtamedullary nephron functions are preserved. However, the glomerular and tubular basement membranes thicken, reducing filtrating ability. Both the number of glomeruli and their surface areas decrease with aging. Tubule length also decreases.

Kidney function also changes with aging (Chart 72-1). Blood flow to the kidney decreases by about 10% per decade as blood vessels thicken. Glomerular filtration rate (GFR) decreases with age, especially after 45 years of age. By age 65, the GFR is about 65 mL/min (half the rate in a young adult). This decline is more rapid in clients with diabetes or hypertension.

Tubular changes with aging decrease the ability to concentrate urine, resulting in **nocturnal polyuria** (increased urination at night). The excretion and regulation of sodium, acids, and bicarbonate remain effective but are less efficient. Along with an age-related impairment in the thirst mechanism, these changes increase the risk for dehydration and **hypernatremia** (increased blood sodium levels) in the older adult (Brenner, 2000). Hormonal changes include a decrease in renin secretion, aldosterone levels, and activation of vitamin D.

CULTURAL CONSIDERATIONS

African Americans have more rapid age-related decreases in GFR than do white individuals (Brenner, 2000). The renal excretion of sodium is less effective in hypertensive African Americans who have high sodium intake, and the kidneys have about 20% less blood flow as a result of anatomic changes in small renal ves-

Continued

CHART 72-1

NURSING FOCUS on the OLDER ADULT
Changes in the Renal/Urinary System Related to Aging

Physiologic Change	Nursing Interventions	Rationales
Decreased glomerular filtration rate (GFR)	Monitor hydration status.	With aging, the ability of the kidneys to regulate water balance is decreased.
	Ensure adequate fluid intake.	The kidneys are less able to conserve water when necessary.
	Administer potentially nephrotoxic agents or drugs carefully.	Dehydration results in decreased renal blood flow and increases the nephrotoxic potential of many agents. Acute or chronic renal failure may result.
Nocturia	Ensure adequate nighttime lighting and a hazard-free environment.	Nocturia may occur from decreased renal concentrating ability associated with aging.
	Ensure the availability of a toilet, bedpan, or urinal.	The desire to maintain continence prompts individuals to seek the bathroom. Falls and injuries are common among older clients seeking bathroom facilities.
	Discourage excessive fluid intake for 2-4 hr before the client retires for the evening.	Excessive fluid intake at nighttime may increase nocturia.
	Evaluate medications and timing.	Some drugs increase urine output.
Decreased bladder capacity	Encourage the client to use the toilet, bedpan, or urinal at least q2h. Respond as soon as possible to the client's indication of the need to void.	By emptying the bladder on a regular basis, urinary incontinence from overflow may be avoided.
Weakened urinary sphincter muscles and shortened urethra in women	Respond as soon as possible to the client's indication of the need to void.	A quick response may alleviate episodes of urinary stress incontinence.
	Provide thorough perineal care after each voiding.	The shortened urethra increases the potential for bladder infections. Good perineal hygiene may prevent skin irritations and urinary tract infection (UTI).
Tendency to retain urine	Observe the client for urinary retention (e.g., bladder distention) or urinary tract infection (e.g., dysuria, foul odor, confusion).	Urinary stasis may result in a UTI. UTIs may become bloodstream infections, resulting in septicemia or septic shock.
	Provide privacy, assistance, and voiding stimulants such as warm water over the perineum as needed.	Nursing interventions can help to initiate voiding.
	Evaluate medications for possible contribution to retention.	Anticholinergic drugs promote urinary retention.

sels and intrarenal responses to renin (Price et al., 2001; Shulman & Hall, 1991). Thus African American clients are at greater risk for renal failure than are white clients. Yearly health examinations should include urinalysis and checking for the presence of microalbuminuria.

URINARY CHANGES

Changes in the detrusor muscle elasticity lead to decreased bladder capacity and reduced ability to retain urine. The urge to void may cause immediate bladder emptying because the urinary sphincters lose muscle tone and often become weaker with age. In women, weakened muscles shorten the urethra and promote incontinence. In men, an enlarged prostate gland makes starting the urine stream difficult and may cause urinary retention.

ASSESSMENT TECHNIQUES

History

One way to assess renal and urologic function is to use Gordon's Functional Health Patterns (Gordon, 2002). The patterns most related to the renal system are Nutritional/Metabolic and Elimination (Chart 72-2).

FAMILY HISTORY AND GENETIC RISK

The family history of the client with a suspected kidney or urologic problem is important because some disorders have a familial inheritance pattern. Ask the client whether his or her siblings, parents, parents' siblings, or grandparents have had renal problems. Past terms used for kidney disease include Bright's disease, nephritis, and nephrosis. Clients may use these terms to describe kidney disease as it was known by their parents or grandparents years ago. Adult polycystic kidney disease can occur in clients of either gender.

DEMOGRAPHIC DATA AND PERSONAL HISTORY

Age, gender, race, and ethnicity are important to assess in the client with any renal or urinary problem. A sudden onset of hypertension in clients older than 50 years of age suggests possible kidney disease. Clinical changes with adult polycystic kidney disease typically occur in clients in their

CHART 72-2

Renal/Urinary Assessment
USING GORDON'S FUNCTIONAL HEALTH PATTERNS

Nutritional/Metabolic Pattern
- What is your typical daily food intake? Describe a day's meals, snacks, and vitamins.
- How much salt do you typically add to your food? Do you use salt substitutes?
- How is your appetite?
- Have you experienced any nausea or vomiting?
- What is your typical daily fluid intake?
- What types of fluids do you drink (water, juices, soft drinks, coffee, tea)?
- How much fluid do you drink each day?
- Have you had any recent change in your weight? Weight gain? Weight loss? How much?
- Have you noticed a change in the tightness of your rings or shoes? Tighter? Looser?
- Have you noticed any skin changes lately? More dry? Less dry? Itchy?

Elimination Pattern
- What is your usual bowel elimination pattern? Frequency? Character? Discomfort? Laxatives?
- What is your usual urinary elimination pattern? Frequency? Amount? Color? Odor? Control?
- Have you noticed a change in the amount of urine?
- Do you have any problem with excessive perspiration?
- Do you have any other type of drainage?

Based on Gordon, M. (2002). *Manual of nursing diagnosis* (10th ed.). St. Louis: Mosby.

40s or 50s. In men older than 50 years of age, altered urine patterns accompany prostate disease.

Anatomic gender differences make some disorders worse or more common. For example, men rarely have urinary tract infections unless there are abnormalities, such as ureteral reflux or prostatic enlargement. Women have a shorter urethra and more commonly develop **cystitis** (bladder infection) because bacteria pass more readily into the bladder.

Ask the client about any previous renal or urologic problems, including tumors, infections, stones, or urologic surgery. A history of any chronic health problems, such as diabetes mellitus or hypertension, increases the risk for development of renal disease.

Identify all of the client's prescription drugs. Ask the client about the duration of drug use and whether there have been any recent changes in prescribed drugs. Drugs for diabetes mellitus, hypertension, cardiac disorders, hormonal disorders, cancer, arthritis, and psychiatric disorders are potential causes of renal dysfunction. Antibiotics, such as gentamicin (Garamycin, Cidomycin✱), may also cause sudden renal dysfunction.

Explore the use of over-the-counter (OTC) drugs or agents, including vitamin and mineral supplements and replacements, laxatives, analgesics, and nonsteroidal anti-inflammatory drugs (NSAIDs). Many of these drugs affect renal function. The long-term use of NSAIDs can seriously reduce renal function.

Ask the client about chemical exposures at the work place or with hobbies. Exposure to hydrocarbons (e.g., gasoline, oil), heavy metals (mercury, lead), and some gases (e.g., chlorine, toluene) can impair kidney function.

Specifically ask the client whether he or she has ever been told about the presence of protein or albumin in the urine. The question "Have you ever been told that your blood pressure is high?" may prompt a different response than "Do you have high blood pressure?" Ask women about health problems during pregnancy (e.g., proteinuria, high blood pressure, gestational diabetes, and urinary tract infections). Obtain information about the following:

- Chemical or environmental toxin exposure in occupational or other settings
- Recent travel to geographic regions that pose infectious disease risks
- Recent physical injuries
- Trauma
- Sexual contacts
- A history of altered patterns of urinary elimination

DIET HISTORY

Ask the client with known or suspected renal or urologic disorders about his or her usual diet and any recent changes in the diet. Note any excessive intake or omission of certain food categories. Ask about food and fluid intake. If the client has followed a diet for weight reduction, the details of the diet plan are important. A high-protein intake can result in temporary renal problems. Clients at risk for **calculi** (stone) formation who ingest large amounts of calcium-containing foods or have a poor fluid intake may form new stones.

Ask about any change in appetite or in the ability to discriminate tastes. These symptoms can occur with the accumulation of nitrogenous waste products from renal failure. Changes in thirst or fluid intake may also cause changes in urine output. Endocrine disorders may also cause changes in thirst, fluid intake, and urine output (see Chapter 65).

SOCIOECONOMIC STATUS

The client's socioeconomic status may influence health care practices. People with limited income or no health insurance often ignore physical problems or delay seeking health care because they lack the funds to pay for tests or treatment. They may also have difficulty following medical advice, having prescriptions filled, and keeping follow-up appointments.

Educational level may affect health-seeking practices and the client's understanding of a disease or its symptoms. Recurring urinary tract infections often result from inadequate or incomplete treatment, including lack of follow-up to ensure eradication. The lack of money to pay for antibiotics or nutritious foods may inhibit or delay recovery.

The client's health beliefs affect the approach to health and illness. Cultural background or religious affiliation may influence the belief system.

The language used by clients may be different from that used by the health care professional. Anatomic or medical terms may have no meaning for the client (Table 72-4). When obtaining a history, listen to and explore the terms used by the client. By using the client's own terms, you may help him or her to provide a more complete description of the problem. This technique may increase the amount of information obtained and decrease the client's discomfort when discussing bodily functions.

CURRENT HEALTH PROBLEM

The effects of renal failure result in changes in all body systems. Therefore document all of the client's current health problems. Encourage the client to describe all

TABLE 72-4 Commonly Used Renal and Urinary Terms

anuria Total urine output of less than 100 mL in 24 hours
azotemia Increased blood urea nitrogen and serum creatinine levels suggestive of renal impairment but without outward symptoms of renal failure
dysuria Discomfort or pain associated with micturition
frequency Feeling the need to void often, usually voiding small amounts of urine each time; may void every hour or even more frequently than hourly
hesitancy Difficulty in initiating the flow of urine, even when the bladder has sufficient urine to initiate a void and the sensation of the need to void is present
micturition The act of voiding
nocturia Awakening prematurely from sleep because of the need to empty the bladder
oliguria Decreased urine output; total urine output between 100 and 400 mL in 24 hours
polyuria Increased urine output; total urine output usually greater than 2000 mL in 24 hours
uremia Full-blown manifestations of renal failure; sometimes referred to as the uremic syndrome, especially if the cause of the renal failure is unknown
urgency A sudden onset of the feeling of the need to void immediately; may result in incontinence if the client is unable to locate or get to toileting facilities quickly

health concerns, because some renal disorders cause systemic problems or problems in other body systems. Recent upper respiratory problems, generalized muscle and joint pain, or gastrointestinal (GI) problems may be related to problems of kidney function.

Assess the kidney and urologic system specifically. Ask the client about any changes in the appearance (color, odor, clarity) of the urine, pattern of urination, ability to initiate or control voiding, and other unusual symptoms. Urine that is reddish, dark brown or black, greenish, or otherwise different from the usual yellowish, straw color usually prompts the client to seek health care assistance. Urine typically has a mild but distinct odor of ammonia. An increase in the intensity of color, a change in odor quality, or a decrease in urine clarity may suggest infection.

Ask the client about changes in urination patterns, such as **nocturia** (urination at night), frequency, or an increase or decrease in the amount of urine. The normal urine output for adults is 1 mL/kg/hr, or about 1500 to 2000 mL/day. The client usually does not know the exact amount of urine produced; a bladder diary may provide useful data. Also ask the following:

- If the client has difficulty initiating urine flow
- If a burning sensation or other discomfort occurs with urination
- If the force of the urine stream is decreased (in men)

Ask about any loss of urinary continence, especially when coughing, sneezing, or laughing. Clients may also report a persistent dribbling of urine.

The onset of pain in the flank, in the lower abdomen or pelvic region, or in the perineal area is often of great concern and usually prompts the client to seek assistance. Ask about the onset, intensity, and duration of the pain, its location, and its association with any activity or event.

Pain associated with renal or ureteral irritation is often severe and spasmodic. Pain that radiates into the perineal area, groin, scrotum, or labia is described as **renal colic.** Renal colic pain occurs with distention or spasm of the ureter, such as in an obstruction or the passing of a stone. Renal colic pain may be intermittent or continuous and may be accompanied by pallor, diaphoresis, and hypotension. These general symptoms occur because of the location of the nerve tracts near or in the kidneys and ureters.

Because the kidneys are close to the GI organs and the nerve pathways are similar, GI manifestations may be part of the presenting history. These **renointestinal reflexes** often complicate the description of the renal problem.

Uremia results from the accumulation of nitrogenous waste products in the blood, a result of renal failure. Manifestations include anorexia, nausea and vomiting, muscle cramps, **pruritus** (itching), fatigue, and lethargy.

Physical Assessment

The physical assessment of the client with a known or suspected renal or urologic disorder includes general appearance, a general review of body systems, and specific structure and functions of the renal/urinary systems.

Assess the general appearance of the client and check for a yellowish skin color and the presence of any rashes, bruising, or other discoloration. The skin and tissues may show edema, which with renal disorders may be detected in the **pedal** (foot), **pretibial** (shin), sacral tissues, and around the eyes. Auscultate the lungs to determine whether fluid is present. Weigh the client and take his or her blood pressure as a baseline for later comparisons.

Assess the client's level of consciousness and level of alertness, recording any deficits in concentration, thought processes, or memory. Family members may report subtle changes. Such cognitive changes may be the result of accumulated waste products when renal disease is present.

ASSESSMENT OF THE KIDNEYS, URETERS, AND BLADDER

Assess the kidneys, ureters, and bladder during an abdominal assessment. Auscultate before percussion and palpation because these activities can enhance bowel sounds and obscure abdominal vascular sounds.

Inspection

Inspect the abdomen and the flank regions with the client in both the supine and the sitting position. Observe the client for asymmetry (e.g., swelling) or discoloration (e.g., bruising or redness) in the flank region, especially in the area of the **costovertebral angle (CVA).** The CVA is located between the lower portion of the twelfth rib and the vertebral column.

Auscultation

Listen for a bruit over each renal artery on the midclavicular line. A **bruit** is an audible swishing sound produced when the volume of blood or the diameter of the blood vessel changes. A bruit often occurs with blood flow through a narrowed vessel, as in renal artery stenosis.

Palpation

Renal palpation can help locate masses and areas of tenderness in or around the kidney. Lightly palpate the abdomen in all quadrants. Ask about areas of tenderness or discom-

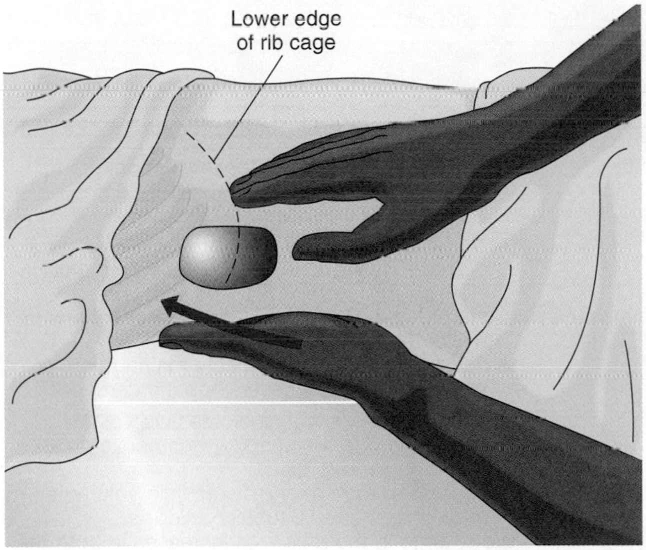

Figure 72-10 ■ Advanced technique for palpation of the kidney.

fort and examine nontender areas first. The outline of the bladder may be seen as high as the umbilicus in clients with severe bladder distention. Special training and practice under the guidance of a qualified practitioner are necessary; therefore appropriate education is essential before attempting the procedure. If tumor or aneurysm is suspected, palpation may harm the client.

Because the kidneys are located deep and posterior, palpation is easier in thin clients who have little abdominal musculature. For palpation of the right kidney, the client assumes a supine position while you place one hand under the right flank and the other hand over the abdomen below the lower right part of the rib cage. Use the lower hand to raise the flank, and the upper hand to depress the abdomen as the client takes a deep breath (Figure 72-10). The left kidney is deeper and rarely palpable. A transplanted kidney is readily palpable in either the lower right or left abdominal quadrant. The kidney should feel smooth, firm, and nontender.

Percussion

A distended bladder sounds dull when percussed. After gently palpating to determine the outline of the distended bladder, begin percussion on the lower abdomen and continue in the direction of the umbilicus until dull sounds are no longer produced.

If the client identifies flank pain or tenderness, percuss the nontender flank first. Have the client assume a sitting, side-lying, or supine position, and then form one of your hands into a clenched fist. Place your other hand flat over the CVA of the client. Then quickly deliver a firm thump to your hand over the CVA area. Costovertebral tenderness often occurs with kidney infection or inflammation. Clients with inflammation or infection in the kidney or adjacent structures may describe their pain as severe or as a constant, dull ache.

ASSESSMENT OF THE URETHRA

Using a good light source and wearing gloves, inspect the urethra by examining the meatus and surrounding tissues. Record any unusual discharge such as blood, mucus, or purulent drainage. Inspect the skin and mucous membranes of surrounding tissues, documenting the presence of lesions, rashes, or other abnormalities of the penis or scrotum or of the labia or vaginal opening. Urethral irritation is suspected when the client reports discomfort with urination.

Psychosocial Assessment

Concerns about the urologic system may evoke fear, anger, embarrassment, anxiety, guilt, or sadness in the client. Childhood learning often includes privacy with regard to urination habits. Urologic disorders may bring up forgotten memories of difficult toilet training and bedwetting or of childhood experiences of exploring one's body. The client may ignore symptoms or delay seeking health care because of emotional responses or cultural taboos about the urogenital area.

Critical Thinking Challenge

The client is a 67-year-old woman who has a change in mental status: she is lethargic and, when roused, not clearly able to state the correct place or time. Her daughter, with whom the client lives because of limited mobility due to rheumatoid arthritis, states that her mom was able to take care of herself and was quite alert 3 days ago. Since then she had a 2-day episode of "stomach flu" and this morning was not able to get out of bed, becoming increasingly confused. She has not voided for 24 hours. This woman is about 5 feet tall and weighs 95 pounds. The admitting diagnosis indicates that this woman is dehydrated, leading to decreased cerebral perfusion and mental status changes.

1. What personal or demographic data should you obtain?
2. How would you proceed in gathering physical assessment data?
3. Given this client's health problems, what drugs might she be taking that could affect kidney function or her hydration status?

evolve For suggested answer guidelines, go to http://evolve.elsevier.com/Iggy/.

Diagnostic Assessment

LABORATORY TESTS

Blood Tests

SERUM CREATININE

Serum creatinine is an end product of muscle and protein metabolism. Creatinine is filtered by the kidneys and excreted in the urine. Because muscle mass and metabolism are usually constant, the serum creatinine level is a good indicator of kidney function. Normal serum creatinine levels vary with age, gender, and body muscle mass. The normal serum creatinine level is slightly higher in men than in women (Chart 72-3). In general, men have a larger muscle mass than do women, but there are exceptions. Muscle mass and the amount of creatinine produced decrease with age. Because of decreased rates of creatinine clearance, however, the serum creatinine level remains relatively constant in older adults unless renal disease is present.

No common pathologic condition other than renal disease increases the serum creatinine level. The serum creatinine level does not increase until at least 50% of the renal function is lost, and therefore *any* elevation of serum creatinine values is important.

CHART 72-3

LABORATORY PROFILE
Renal Function Blood Studies

Test	Normal Range for Adults	Significance of Abnormal Findings
Serum creatinine	*Males:* 0.6-1.2 mg/dL (53-106 mmol/L) *Females:* 0.5-1.1 mg/dL (44-97 mmol/L) *Older adults:* may be decreased	An *increased level* indicates renal impairment. A *decreased level* may be caused by a decreased muscle mass.
Blood urea nitrogen (BUN)	10-20 mg/dL (3.6-7.1 mmol/L) *Older adults:* 60-90 yr: 8-23 mg/dL (2.9-8.2 mmol/L) Over 90 yr: 10-31 mg/dL (3.6-11.1 mmol/L)	An *increased level* may indicate hepatic or renal disease, dehydration or decreased renal perfusion, a high-protein diet, infection, stress, steroid use, GI bleeding, or other situations in which there is blood in body tissues. A *decreased level* may indicate malnutrition, fluid volume excess, or severe hepatic damage.
BUN/creatinine ratio	Mass ratio: 12:1 to 20:1 Mole ratio: 48.5:1 to 80.8:1	An *increased ratio* may indicate fluid volume deficit, obstructive uropathy, catabolic state, or a high-protein diet. A *decreased ratio* may indicate fluid volume excess or acute renal tubular acidosis. *No change* in the ratio with increases in both the BUN and creatinine levels indicates renal impairment.

Data from Pagana, K.D., & Pagana, T.J. (2002). *Mosby's manual of diagnostic and laboratory tests* (2nd ed.). St. Louis: Mosby.
GI, Gastrointestinal.

BLOOD UREA NITROGEN

Blood urea nitrogen (BUN) measures the renal excretion of urea nitrogen, a by-product of protein metabolism in the liver. Urea nitrogen is mostly produced from liver metabolism of food sources of protein. The kidneys filter urea nitrogen from the blood and excrete the nitrogenous waste in urine. BUN levels indicate the extent of renal clearance of this nitrogenous waste product.

Other factors influence the BUN level, and an elevation does not always mean renal disease is present (see Chart 72-3). For example, rapid cell destruction from infection or steroid therapy may elevate BUN level. In addition, blood is a protein. Blood in the tissues rather than in the blood vessels is reabsorbed as if it were a general protein. Thus reabsorbed blood protein is processed by the liver and increases BUN levels. This means that injured tissues can result in increased BUN levels even when kidney function is normal.

The liver must function properly to produce urea nitrogen. When liver and kidney dysfunction are both present, urea nitrogen levels are actually decreased because the liver failure limits urea production. The BUN level is not always elevated with kidney disease and is not the best indicator of kidney function. However, an elevated BUN level is highly *suggestive* of kidney dysfunction.

RATIO OF BLOOD UREA NITROGEN TO SERUM CREATININE

The BUN/creatinine ratio can help determine whether nonrenal factors, such as dehydration or poor renal perfusion, are causing the elevated BUN level rather than kidney damage. When blood volume is deficient (dehydration) or blood pressure is low, the BUN level rises more rapidly than the serum creatinine level. As a result, the ratio of BUN to creatinine is *increased.*

When both the BUN and serum creatinine levels increase at the same rate, the BUN/creatinine ratio remains normal. However, the elevated serum creatinine and BUN levels suggest renal dysfunction that is not related to dehydration or poor perfusion.

Urine Tests

URINALYSIS

Urinalysis is a part of any complete physical examination but is particularly useful for clients with suspected kidney or urologic disorders (Chart 72-4). Ideally, the urine specimen is collected at the morning's first voiding. Specimens obtained at other times may not be adequately concentrated. The specimen may be collected by several techniques (Table 72-5).

COLOR, ODOR, AND TURBIDITY. Urine color comes from urochrome pigment. Color variations may result from increased levels of urochrome or other pigments, changes in the concentration or dilution of the urine, and the presence of drug metabolites in the urine. Urine smells faintly like ammonia and is normally clear without **turbidity** (cloudiness) or haziness.

SPECIFIC GRAVITY. The specific gravity of urine is density of urine compared to water. Density is related to the number of particles in a specific volume of urine. The specific gravity of urine ranges from 1.000 (the specific gravity of water) to greater than 1.035. In kidney disease, changes in specific gravity do not reflect systemic fluid volume. For example, dilute urine with a low specific gravity may occur in a dehydrated client who has a lack of nephron receptors for antidiuretic hormone (ADH).

An *increase* in specific gravity occurs with dehydration, decreased kidney perfusion, or the presence of ADH. (ADH production is normally increased with stress, surgery, anesthetic agents, and certain drugs such as morphine and oral antidiabetic agents.) In these situations the normal kidney response is to reabsorb water and decrease urine output. As a result, the urine produced is more concentrated.

A *decrease* in specific gravity occurs with increased fluid intake, diuretic administration, and diabetes insipidus. In

CHART 72-4

LABORATORY PROFILE
Urinalysis

Test	Normal Range for Adults	Significance of Abnormal Findings
Color	Pale yellow	*Dark amber* indicates concentrated urine. *Very pale yellow* indicates dilute urine. *Dark red or brown* indicates blood in the urine; brown also may indicate increased urinary bilirubin level, red may also indicate the presence of myoglobin. *Other color changes* may result from diet or medications.
Odor	Specific aromatic odor, similar to ammonia	*Foul smell* indicates possible infection, dehydration, or ingestion of certain foods or drugs.
Turbidity	Clear	*Cloudy urine* indicates infection, sediment, or high levels of urinary protein.
Specific gravity	Usually 1.005-1.030; possible range 1.000-1.030 (after 12-hr fluid restriction, >1.025) *Older adult*: Decreased because of decreased concentrating ability	*Increased* in decreased renal perfusion, inappropriate antidiuretic hormone secretion, or congestive heart failure. *Decreased* in chronic renal insufficiency, diabetes insipidus, malignant hypertension, diuretic administration, and lithium toxicity.
pH	Average: 6; possible range: 4.6-8	*Changes* are caused by diet, the administration of medications, infection, freshness of the specimen, acid-base imbalance, and altered renal function.
Glucose	<0.5 g/day (<2.78 mmol/L)	*Presence* reflects hyperglycemia or a decrease in the renal threshold for glucose.
Ketones	None	*Presence* reflects incomplete metabolism of fatty acids, as in diabetic ketoacidosis, prolonged fasting, anorexia nervosa.
Protein	0.8 mg/dL	*Increased amounts* may indicate stress, infection, recent strenuous exercise, or glomerular disorders.
Bilirubin (urobilinogen)	None	*Presence* suggests hepatic or biliary disease or obstruction.
Red blood cells (RBCs)	0-2 per high-power field	*Increased* amounts are normal with indwelling or intermittent catheterization or menses but may reflect tumor, stones, trauma, glomerular disorders, cystitis, or bleeding disorders.
White blood cells (WBCs)	*Males:* 0-3 per high-power field *Females:* 0-5 per high-power field	*Increased* amounts may indicate an infectious or inflammatory process anywhere in the renal/urinary tract, renal transplant rejection, fever, or exercise.
Casts	A few or none, composed of RBC or WBC, protein or tubular cell casts	*Increased amounts* indicate the presence of bacteria or protein, which is seen in severe renal disease and could also indicate urinary calculi.
Crystals	None	*Presence* of normal or abnormal crystals may indicate that the specimen has been allowed to stand.
Bacteria	<1000 colonies/mL	*Increased amounts* indicate the need for urine culture to determine the presence of urinary tract infection.
Parasites	None	*Presence* of *Trichomonas vaginalis* indicates infection, usually of the urethra, prostate, or vagina.
Leukoesterase	None	*Presence* suggests urinary tract infection
Nitrites	None	*Presence* suggests bacteria, usually *Escherichia coli.*

these situations, the normal kidney response is to excrete more water; thus urine output is increased. In kidney disease, the specific gravity decreases because the damaged kidneys reabsorb less water. The specific gravity does not vary with changes in plasma osmolarity (e.g., it becomes fixed).

pH. A pH value less than 7 is acidic, and a value greater than 7 is alkaline. Many factors influence urine acidity or alkalinity. A diet high in certain fruits and vegetables results in a more alkaline urine, whereas a high-protein diet produces a more acidic urine. The presence of *Escherichia coli* in the urine also results in an acidic urine.

Urine specimens become more alkaline when left standing unrefrigerated for more than 1 hour, if bacteria are present, or if a specimen is left uncovered. Alkaline urine increases cell breakdown; thus the presence of red blood cells may be missed on analysis. Ensure that urine specimens are covered and delivered to the laboratory promptly or refrigerated. During acidosis or alkalosis, the kidneys, along with blood buffers and the lungs, normally respond to keep serum pH normal. Chapters 18 and 19 discuss acid-base balance and imbalance.

GLUCOSE. Glucose is filtered by the glomerulus and is reabsorbed in the proximal tubule of the nephron. When the blood glucose level rises above 220 mg/dL, the renal threshold for reabsorption is exceeded, and some glucose is present in the urine. Changes in the renal threshold for glucose occur in many clients, such as those with infection or those with long-standing diabetes mellitus. It is possible that their serum glucose level may be high (e.g., greater than 400 mg/dL), and glucose may still not be present in the urine.

KETONE BODIES. Ketone bodies are by-products of the incomplete metabolism of fatty acids. Three types of

TABLE 72-5 Collection of Urine Specimens

Nursing Interventions	Rationales
Voided Urine	
Collect the first specimen voided in the morning.	Urine is more concentrated in the early morning.
Send the specimen to the laboratory as soon as possible.	After urine is collected, cellular breakdown results in more alkaline urine.
Refrigerate the specimen if a delay is unavoidable.	Refrigeration delays the alkalinization of urine. Bacteria are more likely to multiply in an alkaline environment.
Clean-Catch Specimen	
Explain the purpose of the procedure to the client.	Correct technique is needed to obtain a valid specimen.
Instruct the client to self-clean before voiding.	Surface cleaning is necessary to remove secretions or bacteria from the urethral meatus.
Instruct the female client to separate the labia and use the sponges and solution provided to wipe with three strokes over the urethra. The first two wiping strokes are over each side of the urethra; the third wiping stroke is centered over the urethra (from front to back).	
Instruct the male client to retract the foreskin of the penis and to similarly clean the urethra, using three wiping strokes with the sponge and solution provided (from the head of the penis downward).	
Instruct the client to initiate voiding after cleaning. The client then stops and resumes voiding into the container. Only 1 ounce (30 mL) is needed; the remainder of the urine may be discarded into the commode.	A midstream collection further removes secretions and bacteria because urine flushes the distal portion of the internal urethra. An improperly collected specimen may result in inappropriate or incomplete treatment.
Ensure that the client understands the procedure. Assist the client as needed.	The client's understanding and the nurse's assistance ensure proper collection.
Catheterized Specimen	
For non-indwelling (straight) catheters:	The one-time passage of a urinary catheter may be necessary to obtain an uncontaminated specimen for analysis or to measure the volume of residual urine.
Avoid routine use. Follow the facility's procedures for catheterization technique.	These procedures minimize bacterial entry.
For indwelling catheters:	Collection of urine from an indwelling catheter or tubing is performed when clients have catheters for continence or long-term urinary drainage.
Apply a clamp to the drainage tubing, distal to the injection port.	Clamping allows urine to collect in the tubing at the location where the specimen is obtained.
Clean the injection port cap of the catheter drainage tubing with an appropriate antiseptic. Povidone-iodine solution or alcohol is acceptable.	Surface contamination is prevented by following the cleaning procedures.
Insert a sterile 5-mL syringe into the port and aspirate the quantity of urine required.	A minimum of 5 mL is needed for culture and sensitivity (C&S) testing.
Inject the urine sample into a sterile specimen container.	A sterile container is used for C&S specimens.
Remove the clamp to resume drainage.	
Properly dispose of the syringe.	
24-Hour Urine Collection	
Instruct the client thoroughly.	A 24-hr collection of urine is necessary to quantify or calculate the rate of clearance of a particular substance.
Provide written materials to assist in instruction. Place signs appropriately. Inform all personnel or family caregivers of test in progress.	Instructional materials for clients, signs, and so on remind clients and staff to ensure that the total collection is completed.
Check laboratory or procedure manual on proper technique for maintaining the collection (e.g., on ice, in a refrigerator, or with a preservative).	Proper technique prevents breakdown of elements to be measured.
On initiation of the collection, ask the client to void, discard the urine, and note the time. If a Foley catheter is in use, empty the tubing and drainage bag at the start time and discard the urine. Collect all urine of the next 24 hr. Twenty-four hours after initiation, ask the client to empty the bladder and add that urine to the container.	Proper techniques ensure that *all* urine formed within the 24-hr period is collected.
Do not remove urine from the collection container for other specimens.	Urine in the container is not considered a "fresh" specimen and may be mixed with preservative.

ketone bodies are acetone, acetoacetic acid, and beta-hydroxybutyric acid. Normally there are no ketones in urine. Ketone bodies are produced when fat is used instead of glucose for cellular energy. Ketones present in the blood are partially excreted in the urine.

PROTEIN. Protein, such as albumin, is not normally present in the urine. Levels greater than 300 mg/24 hr, or 200 mcg/min, are abnormal. Protein molecules are too large to pass through intact glomerular membranes. When glomerular membrane permeability is increased, protein molecules pass through and are excreted in the urine. Increased membrane permeability is caused by infection, inflammation, or immunologic problems. Some systemic problems cause production of abnormal proteins, such as globulin. These proteins are not detected by routine urinalysis, and require electrophoresis or other tests for detection.

A random finding of proteinuria followed by a series of negative (normal) findings does not imply renal disease. If infection is the cause of the **proteinuria** (protein in the urine), urinalyses after elimination of the infection should be negative for protein. Persistent proteinuria needs further investigation.

Microalbuminuria is the presence of albumin in the urine that is not measurable by a urine dipstick or usual urinalysis procedures. Specialized assays are used to quickly analyze a freshly voided urine specimen for microscopic levels of albumin. The normal microalbumin levels in a freshly voided specimen should range between 2.0 and 20 mg/mmol for men and between 2.8 and 28 mg/mmol for women. Higher levels indicate microalbuminuria and could mean the presence of very early kidney disease, especially in clients with diabetes mellitus. In 24-hour urine specimens, levels of 30 to 300 mg/24 hr, or 20 to 200 mcg/min, indicate microalbuminuria.

LEUKOESTERASE. Leukoesterase is an enzyme found in some white blood cells, especially neutrophils. When the number of these cells increases in the urine or they are lysed, the urine will contain measurable amounts of leukoesterase. The presence of leukoesterase and nitrites in the urine is a sensitive screen for assessing urinary tract infections. A normal reading is no leukoesterase in the urine. A positive test (+ sign) indicates increasing leukocytes in the urine.

NITRITES. Urine does not usually contain nitrites. Many types of bacteria, when present in the urine, convert nitrates (normally found in urine) into nitrites. A positive finding is associated with urinary tract infection.

SEDIMENT. Urine sediment is precipitated particles in the urine. These particles include cells, casts, crystals, and bacteria.

CELLS. Normally, urine contains few, if any, cells. Types of cells abnormally present in the urine include tubular cells (from the tubule of the nephron), epithelial cells (from the lining of the urinary tract), red blood cells (RBCs), and white blood cells (WBCs).

CASTS. Casts are structures formed around other particles. There may be casts of cells, bacteria, or protein. When cells, bacteria, or proteins are present in the urine, minerals and gelatinous materials clump around them and form a cast. Casts are described by the type of particle they have surrounded (e.g., RBC cast, WBC cast, tubular epithelial cast) or the stage of cast breakdown. Casts are described as "granular" (coarse or fine) and "waxy."

CRYSTALS. Urine crystals come from various mineral salts. These minerals may be a result of diet, drugs, or disease. Common salt crystals are formed from calcium, oxalate, urea, phosphate, magnesium, or other substances. Some drugs, such as the sulfates, can also form crystals.

BACTERIA. Bacteria in a urine sample multiply quickly, so the specimen must be analyzed promptly. Normally urine is sterile, but is easily contaminated by perineal bacteria during collection.

URINE FOR CULTURE AND SENSITIVITY

Urine is analyzed for the number and types of organisms present. Manifestations of infection and unexplained bacteria in a urine specimen are indications for urine culture and sensitivity testing. Bacteria from urine are placed in a medium with different antibiotics to determine which drugs are effective in killing or stopping the growth of the bacteria **(sensitivity)**. In this way we can know which antibiotics are effective in killing the organisms (organisms are "sensitive") and which are not effective (organisms are "resistant"). A clean-catch or catheter-derived specimen is best for culture and sensitivity testing.

COMPOSITE URINE COLLECTIONS

Some urine collections are made for a specified number of hours (e.g., 24 hours) for more quantitative analysis of one or more substances. These collections are often used to measure urine levels of creatinine or urea nitrogen, sodium, chloride, calcium, catecholamines, or other components (Chart 72-5). For a composite urine specimen, *all* urine within the designated time frame must be collected (see Table 72-5). If other voided or catheterized specimens must be obtained while the collection is in progress, measure and record the amount collected but not added to the timed collection.

The urine collection may need to be refrigerated or stored on ice to prevent changes in the urine during the collection time. Follow the procedure from the laboratory for urine storage. The urine collection must be free from fecal contamination. Menstrual blood and toilet tissue also contaminate the specimen and can invalidate the results.

The collection of urine for a 24-hour period is often more difficult than it seems. With hospitalized clients, the cooperation of staff personnel, the client, family members, and visitors is essential. Placing signs in the bathroom, instructing the client and family, and emphasizing the need to save the urine are helpful.

CREATININE CLEARANCE

Creatinine clearance is a calculated measure of glomerular filtration rate. It is the best indication of overall kidney function. The amount of creatinine cleared from the blood (e.g., filtered into the urine) is measured in the total volume of urine excreted in a defined period. A urine specimen for a creatinine clearance test is usually collected for 24 hours, but it can be collected for shorter periods (e.g., 8 or 12 hours). The calculation compares the urine creatinine level with the blood creatinine level, and therefore a blood specimen or creatinine must also be collected.

The laboratory or care provider calculates the creatinine clearance. The client's age, gender, height, weight, diet, and activity level influence the expected amount of creatinine to be excreted. Thus these factors are considered when interpreting creatinine clearance test results.

The following formula is used to calculate creatinine clearance:

$$\text{Creatinine clearance} = U \times V/P \times T$$

where U is creatinine in urine (mg/dL), V is volume of urine (mL/24 hr), P is creatinine in plasma or blood (mg/dL), and T is time (minutes).

The rate of creatinine clearance is expressed as milliliters per minute per square meter of body surface area. The range

CHART 72-5

LABORATORY PROFILE
24-Hour Urine Collections

Component	Normal Range for Adults	Significance of Abnormal Findings
Creatinine	0.8-2 g/24 hr *Males:* 1-2 g/24 hr or 14-26 mg/kg/24 hr (124-230 μmol/kg/24 hr or 7.1-17.7 mmol/24 hr) *Females:* 0.6-1.8 g/24 hr or 11-20 mg/kg/24 hr (97-177 μmol/kg/24 hr or 5.3-15.9 mmol/24 hr) *Older adults:* 10 mg/kg/24 hr (88.4 μmol/kg/24 hr) at 90 yr	*Decreased amounts* indicate a deterioration in renal function caused by renal disease, shock, hypovolemia, or any condition affecting muscle. *Increased amounts* occur with infections, exercise, diabetes mellitus, and meat meals.
Urea nitrogen	12-20 g/24 hr (0.43-0.71 mmol/24 hr)	*Decreased amounts* occur when renal damage or liver disease is present. *Increased amounts* commonly result from a high-protein diet, dehydration, trauma, or sepsis.
Sodium	40-220 mEq/24 hr (40-220 mmol/24 hr)	*Decreased amounts* are seen in hemorrhage, shock, hyperaldosteronism, and prerenal acute renal failure. *Increased amounts* are common with diuretic therapy, excessive salt intake, hypokalemia, and acute tubular necrosis.
Chloride	110-250 mEq/24 hr (110-250 mmol/24 hr) *Older adults:* 95-195 mEq/24 hr (95-195 mmol/24 hr)	*Decreased amounts* are seen in certain renal diseases, malabsorption syndrome, pyloric obstruction, prolonged nasogastric tube drainage, diarrhea, diaphoresis, heart failure, and emphysema. *Increased amounts* are seen with hypokalemia, adrenal insufficiency, and massive diuresis.
Calcium	100-400 mg/24 hr (2.50-7.50 mmol/kg/24 hr)	*Decreased amounts* are often associated with hypocalcemia, hypoparathyroidism, nephrosis, and nephritis. *Increased amounts* are commonly seen with calcium renal stones, hyperparathyroidism, sarcoidosis, certain cancers, immobilization, and hypercalcemia.
Total catecholamines*	<100 mcg/24 hr (<591 mmol/24 hr)	*Increased amounts* occur with pheochromocytoma, neuroblastomas, stress, or strenuous exercise.
Protein	1-14 mg/dL (10-140 mg/L) or 50-80 mg/24 hr at rest	*Increased amounts* indicate glomerular disease, nephrotic syndrome, diabetic nephropathy, urinary tract malignancies, and irritations.

*Epinephrine and norepinephrine only; dopamine is not measured.

for normal creatinine clearance is 90 to 139 mL/min for adult males and 80 to 125 mL/min for females.

Creatinine clearance values are used to determine the client's current kidney function. Decreases in the creatinine clearance rate may require reducing drug doses and often signifies the need to further explore the cause of kidney deterioration.

URINE ELECTROLYTES

Urine samples can be analyzed for electrolyte levels (e.g., sodium and chloride). Normally the amount of sodium excreted in the urine is nearly equal to that consumed. Urine sodium levels of less than 10 mEq/L indicate that the tubules are able to conserve (reabsorb) sodium.

OSMOLARITY

Osmolarity measures the concentration of particles in solution. The particles in urine contributing to osmolarity include electrolytes, glucose, urea, and creatinine.

BLOOD/PLASMA OSMOLARITY. The kidneys excrete or reabsorb water to keep blood osmolarity in the range of 285 to 295 mOsm/L. Osmolarity is slightly higher in older adults (285 to 301 mOsm/L). When blood osmolarity is decreased, the release of antidiuretic hormone (ADH) is inhibited. Without ADH, the distal tubule and collecting ducts are *not* permeable to water. As a result, water is *excreted,* not reabsorbed, and blood osmolarity increases. When blood osmolarity increases, ADH is released. ADH increases the permeability of the distal tubule to water. Then water is reabsorbed, and blood osmolarity decreases.

URINE OSMOLARITY. Urine osmolarity can vary from 50 to 1400 mOsm/L, depending on the client's hydration status and kidney function. With average fluid intake, the range for urine osmolarity is 300 to 900 mOsm/L. Electrolytes, acids, and other wastes of normal metabolism are continually produced. These particles are the solute load that must be excreted in the urine on a regular basis. This is referred to as *obligatory solute excretion.* If the client loses excessive fluids, the renal response is to save water while excreting wastes by excreting small amounts of highly concentrated urine. Diet, drugs, and activity can change urine osmolarity. Thus urine with an increased osmolarity is concentrated urine with less water and more solutes. Urine with a decreased osmolarity is dilute urine with more water and fewer solutes.

Bedside Sonography/Bladder Scanners

The use of portable ultrasound scanners in the hospital and rehabilitation setting by nurses is a noninvasive method of estimating bladder volume. Bladder scanners are used to screen clients for postvoid residual volumes and to determine the need for intermittent catheterization based on the amount of urine in the bladder rather than the time between catheterizations. The scan does not require client preparation beyond an explanation of what to expect. There is no discomfort associated with the scan.

PROCEDURE. Explain the rationale for the procedure and share information about sensations commonly experienced during the procedure. For example, "This test will measure the amount of urine in your bladder. I will place a gel pad just above your pubic area, then place the probe that is a little bigger and heavier than a stethoscope on the gel."

Before scanning, select the male or female icon on the bladder scanner. Using the female icon allows the scanner software to subtract the volume of the uterus from any measurement. Use the male icon on all men and any woman who has undergone a hysterectomy.

Place an ultrasound gel pad right above the symphysis pubis (pubic bone) or moisten the round dome of the scan head area with 5 mL of conducting gel to improve ultrasound conduction. Use conducting gel on the scanner head for obese clients and those with heavy body hair in the area to be scanned. Place the probe midline over the abdomen about 1.5 inches (4 cm) above the pubic bone. Aim the scan head so the ultrasound is projected toward the expected location of the bladder, typically toward the client's coccyx. Press and release the scan button; the scan is complete with the sound of a beep and a volume is displayed. Two readings are recommended for best accuracy. An aiming icon on the portable bladder scanner indicates whether the bladder image is centered on the crosshairs of the scan head. If the crosshairs on the aiming icon are not centered on the bladder, the measured volume may not be accurate.

Critical Thinking Challenge

The 67-year-old client described earlier has the following vital signs and laboratory data: T 98.4; P 112, thready, slightly irregular; R 30 and shallow; BP 98/50; oxygen saturation 95%; serum potassium 2.9 mEq/L; serum sodium 151 mEq/L; hematocrit 47%.

1. Which of these data support a diagnosis of dehydration?
2. What alterations in BUN, and creatinine do you anticipate?
3. What findings in a urinalysis would suggest a urinary tract infection?

evolve For suggested answer guidelines, go to http://evolve.elsevier.com/Iggy/.

RADIOGRAPHIC EXAMINATIONS

Radiographic and other procedures are used to diagnose abnormalities within the urinary system (Table 72-6). Explain the procedures thoroughly to the client, prepare the client, and provide follow-up care.

Kidney, Ureter, and Bladder X-rays

An x-ray of the kidneys, ureters, and bladder (KUB) is a plain film of the abdomen obtained without any specific client preparation. The KUB study shows gross anatomic features and obvious stones, strictures, calcifications, or obstructions in the urinary tract. This test identifies the shape, size, and relationship of the organs to other parts of the urinary tract. Other tests are needed to diagnose functional or structural problems.

There is no discomfort or risk from this procedure. Tell the client that the x-ray will be taken while the client is in a supine position. No specific follow-up care is needed.

Intravenous Urography

Other names for IV urography include excretory urography and (the older term) IV pyelography (IVP).

CLIENT PREPARATION. Before urography, assess the client (Chart 72-6), perform bowel preparation, and teach the client. Report allergy information to the physician. Contrast reactions can be minor (nausea and vomiting, urticaria, itching, sneezing), moderate (nephrotoxic effects, congestive heart failure, pulmonary edema), or severe (bronchospasm, anaphylaxis). If the diagnostic test must be performed in a client with a minor allergy to the contrast dye, drugs such as a steroid (prednisone or methylprednisolone), and an antihistamine (diphenhydramine hydrochloride [Benadryl, Allerdryl✱]) are prescribed before the procedure to reduce an allergic response. Explain the rationale for the procedure to the client.

Some preparations may be needed to ensure that urinary structures are not obscured by bowel contents. Some radiologists recommend a light evening meal or clear liquids, then fasting (NPO status) from midnight on the night before the procedure. Others recommend increased fluid intake to prevent dehydration up until the time of the procedure. Because some clients may vomit as a reaction to the IV contrast, some physicians prefer the client to remain on NPO status for a few hours before the procedure. Hydration with IV fluids may be prescribed.

A bowel preparation is prescribed to remove fecal contents, fluid, and air from the gut, any of which could obscure part of the outline of the kidneys, ureters, and bladder. Bowel preparation procedures vary but usually include the use of laxatives the day before the procedure. Enemas also may be prescribed but their use is controversial because some air and fluid can be retained.

CONSIDERATIONS FOR OLDER ADULTS

Bowel preparation procedures increase the risk for dehydration, especially in older adult clients. To help prevent dehydration, contact the testing department and ask that urograms be scheduled early in the day for older clients.

The contrast dye is potentially nephrotoxic. The risk for *contrast-induced renal failure* is greatest in clients who are older or dehydrated, who have some renal insufficiency (e.g., serum creatinine levels greater than 1.5 mg/dL), or who are also taking other nephrotoxic drugs. These clients need additional IV fluids before the procedure to maintain hydration and decrease the nephrotoxic risk. Acetylcysteine (an antioxidant) or fenoldopam (a dopamine-1 agonist) may be used to prevent contrast-induced nephrotoxic effects in radiologic procedures. Diuretics may be given immediately after the dye is injected to enhance dye excretion.

Instruct the client in the preparation procedures for the urogram and explain the procedure so that he or she knows what to expect (Chart 72-7). Intervene on behalf of the client to ensure that questions are answered *before* the procedure.

PROCEDURE. A radiopaque dye is injected intravenously with the client in a supine position. As blood (with

TABLE 72-6 Common Radiologic and Special Diagnostic Tests for Clients with Disorders of the Renal/Urinary System

Test	Purpose	Comments
Radiography of kidneys, ureters, and bladder (KUB) (plain film of abdomen)	To screen for the presence of two kidneys To measure kidney size To detect gross obstruction	
Excretory urography	To measure kidney size To detect obstruction To assess parenchymal mass	Radiopaque contrast media may cause an allergic (hypersensitivity) reaction in iodine-sensitive clients. Contrast agent is also hypertonic and increases the risk of acute renal failure in adults with serum creatinine levels greater than 1.5 mg/dL, diabetes mellitus, multiple myeloma, or dehydration. Nephrotoxic complications can be prevented by parenteral fluid administration, the use of mannitol, and daily monitoring of serum creatinine levels.
Nephrotomography	To assess various planes of kidney tissue for cysts, tumors, or calculi	Same as for excretory urogram.
Computed tomography (CT)	To measure kidney size To evaluate contour to assess for masses or obstruction	Contrast medium may provoke acute renal failure. See comments with excretory urography for high-risk clients and preventive measures related to contrast. May be performed without contrast medium and still obtain adequate visualization.
Cystography and cystoscopy	To identify abnormalities of the bladder wall and urethral and ureteral occlusions To treat small obstructions or lesions via fulguration, lithotripsy, or removal with a stone basket	Instrumentation of the urinary tract increases the risk of infection. Monitor for infection for 48-72 hr after the procedure.
Voiding cystourethrography (VCUG)	To outline bladder's contour and detect urinary reflux from vesicourethral junctions	The risk of infection is similar to that in cystography because urinary catheterization is necessary. Monitor for postprocedure infection.
Renal arteriography	To identify vascular abnormalities within each kidney and adjacent aorta	Contrast medium may provoke acute renal failure. See comments with excretory urography for high-risk clients and preventive measures related to contrast. Essential for diagnosis and treatment of some vascular abnormalities, such as renal artery stenosis. Monitor for bleeding after the procedure.
Ultrasonography (US)	To identify the size of the kidneys or obstruction in the kidneys or the lower urinary tract May detect tumors or cysts	Ultrasonography entails minimal risk to the client. Ultrasonography is a good alternative to excretory urography.
MAG3 study 99m	To assess renal function, structural abnormalities, renal failure, obstruction, and renal calculi	Radioactive material (technetium Tc mertiatide) is used for this test.
Intravenous pyelography (fluoroscopy)	To assess renal function, identify anomalies To image renal/urinary calculi (size, location, radiodensity) To screen for renal injury after trauma	Contraindicated during pregnancy (ionizing radiation is a risk to the fetus). Contrast dye can cause renal dysfunction. Colonic cleaning improves quality of image.
Magnetic resonance imaging (MRI)	Staging of cancers, similar to CT	Client must be able to lie still (motion can interfere with imaging).
Renal scan	Evaluation of renal blood flow Estimation of renal glomerular filtration rate Provides functional information without exposing the client to iodinated contrast dye	ACE inhibitors should be held for 48 hours before the test. ACE inhibitors may be given during the test, placing the client at risk for episodes of hypotension. Ensure adequate hydration for best results.

ACE, Angiotensin converting enzyme.

CHART 72-6

BEST PRACTICE for
Assessing the Client About to Undergo a Diagnostic Test or Interventional Procedure Using Contrast Media

Before the procedure:
- Ask the client if he or she has ever had a reaction to contrast media. (Such a client has the highest risk for having another reaction.)
- Ask the client about a history of asthma. (Clients with asthma have been shown to be at greater risk for contrast reactions than the general public; when reactions do occur, they are more likely to be severe.)
- Ask the client about known hay fever or food or medication allergies, especially to seafood, eggs, milk, or chocolate. (Contrast reactions have been reported to be as high as 15% in these clients.)
- Ask the clients to describe any specific allergic reactions (e.g., hives, facial edema, difficulty breathing, bronchospasm).
- Assess for a history of renal insufficiency and for conditions that have been implicated in increasing the chance of developing renal failure after contrast media (e.g., diabetic nephropathy, class IV heart failure, dehydration, concomitant use of potentially nephrotoxic medications such as the aminoglycosides or NSAIDs, and cirrhosis).
- Ask the client if he or she is taking metformin (Glucophage). (Metformin must be discontinued at least 48 hours before any study using contrast media because the life-threatening complication of lactic acidosis, although rare, could occur.)
- Assess hydration status by checking blood pressure, heart and respiratory rates, mucous membranes, skin turgor, and urine concentration.
- Ask the client when he or she last ate or drank anything.

From Cohan, R.H., & Ellis, J.H. (1997). Iodinated contrast material in uroradiology. Choice of agent and management of complications. *Urologic Clinics of North America, 24*(3), 471-491.
NSAIDs, Nonsteroidal anti-inflammatory drugs.

CHART 72-7

CLIENT EDUCATION GUIDE
Excretory Urogram

- The urogram outlines your urinary tract and helps determine any problems there.
- Notify your nurse or physician if you have had any reactions (allergic or otherwise) to any food or drugs, especially shellfish (shrimp, scallops, crab, lobster, and so on) or iodine, or to x-ray "dyes" such as contrast media; if you have a history of asthma; or if you are taking metformin (Glucophage) or Glucovance.
- The day before the test, follow the instructions about changes in your diet and fluid intake to be sure that as much information as possible is gained from the test.
- After you start the bowel preparation, you may need to be close to toileting facilities. The preparation medications usually work quickly.
- You will be lying on an x-ray table with the x-ray machine above you for most of the procedure.
- A pressure band, similar to a large blood pressure cuff, may be placed around your stomach or abdomen to help obtain better x-rays.
- If you do not already have an IV access site, one will be started to give you the contrast agent.
- After the contrast is injected, you may feel a sense of warmth or heat as it travels throughout your body. You also may have a taste in your mouth that is sometimes described as metallic. These sensations last only a few seconds or minutes.
- When the pressure band is inflated, you may feel some tightness around your abdomen. The sensation is similar to the feeling on your arm when you have your blood pressure taken.
- A series of x-rays will be taken. You may be asked to empty your bladder and return to the table for more films. You also may be asked to have a standing film taken.
- After the test is completed, you are usually able to resume your normal activities and diet.
- You will not notice any change in the color or characteristics of your urine.
- Please do not hesitate to ask your nurse, physician, or x-ray technologist any question, no matter how slight the question may seem to you. It is important that you have as much understanding as possible.

the dye) rapidly circulates into the kidney blood vessels and is filtered by the glomeruli, the dye is excreted in the urine. A series of x-rays are taken at various times after injection. Nephrotomograms may be taken at the same time as the urogram. Tomograms take images of different planes of tissue and show any abnormalities present at varying depths. The technologist then asks the client to empty the bladder and return for a few more x-rays. An outline of the kidneys, ureters, and bladder result as urine containing the dye is excreted.

The urogram provides information about the following:
- The number, size, shape, and location of the kidneys
- The adequacy of filling and the rate of excretion of contrast medium
- The number, size, location, appearance, and patency of the calices, pelves, and ureters
- The size, location, and nature of the urinary bladder

FOLLOW-UP CARE. After the urogram, monitor the client for altered renal function and other effects from the dye. Ensure adequate hydration by urging the client to take oral fluid or by giving IV fluids. Hydration reduces the risk for renal damage. Monitor blood creatinine levels to assess ongoing renal function.

Computed Tomography

CLIENT PREPARATION. Inform the client that a computed tomography (CT) scan provides three-dimensional information about the kidneys, ureters, bladder, and surrounding tissues. A CT scan is usually performed after other diagnostic procedures and can provide information about tumors, cysts, abscesses, other masses, obstruction, and certain blood vessel abnormalities.

Some hospitals require clients having abdominal CT scans to be NPO for some period before the scan. For the scan using contrast, extra hydration may be needed before the test, especially if the client has reduced renal function. Ask about allergy to dyes and intervene as with IV urography.

PROCEDURE. The CT scan is performed in a special room, usually in the radiology department. An IV injection of radiopaque dye may be given before starting the imaging procedures. Dye use may be eliminated in clients at risk for contrast media-induced acute renal failure, but the images produced are less distinct.

FOLLOW-UP CARE. No special follow-up care is needed unless dye was used. In that case, the follow-up care is the same as for IV urography.

Cystography and Cystourethrography

CLIENT PREPARATION. Explain the procedure to the client. A urinary catheter is temporarily needed to instill contrast dye. The dye is needed to enhance x-ray visibility of the lower urinary tract.

PROCEDURE. In both cystography and cystourethrography, dye is instilled into the bladder via a urethral catheter. After bladder filling, x-rays are taken from the front, back, and side positions. For the voiding cystourethrogram (VCUG), the client is requested to void, and x-rays are taken during the voiding. A VCUG is obtained to determine whether a vesicoureteral reflux is present. The cystogram is often used in cases of trauma when urethral or bladder injury is suspected.

FOLLOW-UP CARE. Monitor for the development of infection as a result of catheter placement. In this test, the dye is not nephrotoxic because it does not enter the bloodstream. Encourage fluid intake to dilute the urine and reduce the burning sensation from catheter irritation after removal. Also monitor for changes in urine output because pelvic or urethral trauma may be present.

OTHER RENAL DIAGNOSTIC TESTS

Renal Arteriography (Angiography)

Indications for this test include suspected causes of decreased renal function such as renovascular hypertension, other vessel abnormalities, and bleeding from trauma.

CLIENT PREPARATION. Inform the client that this procedure is used to assess the arterial blood supply of the kidneys. A bowel preparation may be needed before the test if a barium study has been performed recently. A light evening meal is given, and the client is on NPO status until after the procedure. An IV may be placed before the procedure and fluids may be given to ensure adequate hydration because dye is used in this study.

Review the procedure with the client, answer questions, and review the drug regimen and blood study results as indicated. For example, review the medication record for drugs affecting blood clotting, such as heparin, Lovenox, warfarin (Coumadin, Warfilone✱), or aspirin. The client needs to sign an informed consent statement.

PROCEDURE. The injection of a radiopaque dye into the renal arteries requires entry into an artery, usually the femoral artery in the groin. After the client is sedated and the skin is prepared and draped, the radiologist injects a local anesthetic. An arterial puncture is then performed and the angiographic catheter is inserted.

Using fluoroscopy, the radiologist guides the catheter into the abdominal aorta and the renal artery. When the tip of the catheter is positioned at each renal artery, dye is injected and x-rays are taken. The speed of distribution of the dye and any areas of blood vessel narrowing are recorded. Arterial blockage is found when the dye fails to circulate within the kidney. **Extravasation** (infiltration) of dye into surrounding tissue indicates vessel rupture, which could be present after trauma.

FOLLOW-UP CARE. Bleeding from the catheter insertion site is the most common delayed complication of renal arteriography. Monitor the insertion site for bleeding or swelling. If the site bleeds or if a hematoma forms, hold manual, non-occlusive pressure on the entry site and notify the radiology department for an evaluation.

Monitor vital signs as per the physician's prescription or according to the agency's policy, usually every 15 minutes for 1 hour, then every 30 minutes for 2 hours, then every hour for 4 hours, and then every 4 hours. Check the temperature and color of the extremities and distal pulses. A sudden absence of pulses in the catheterized vessel may reflect hematoma formation or embolization.

The period of absolute bedrest (to prevent bleeding) after arteriography varies. Usually bedrest is maintained for 4 to 6 hours. Instruct the client about the importance of keeping the leg in a straight position for those 4 to 6 hours. A restraint may be used on the leg with the client's consent. Encourage ankle flexing and weight shifting to prevent deep vein thrombosis. If there is no evidence of bleeding after 4 to 6 hours, the client may be permitted to stand to void or may use a bedside commode.

Serum creatinine is measured for several days after the arteriogram to determine whether the test has affected kidney function. For some clients with renal insufficiency, the dye may cause an episode of acute renal failure severe enough to require short-term dialysis. Because the test is used to determine the need for interventions to restore kidney blood flow and preserve kidney function, many clients accept the risk of short-term dialysis to prevent the need for permanent dialysis. Urge clients to drink fluids after the procedure to enhance dye excretion.

Renal Biopsy

CLIENT PREPARATION. Explain that a kidney biopsy can help to determine a cause of for unexplained renal problems and to direct or change therapy. Most renal biopsies are performed **percutaneously** (through the skin and other tissues) using ultrasound or CT guidance. The client signs an informed consent. Clients are NPO for 4 to 6 hours before the procedure.

Because of the risk for postprocedure bleeding, coagulation studies such as platelet count, activated partial thromboplastin time (aPTT), prothrombin time (PT), and bleeding time are performed before surgery. A blood transfusion may be needed to correct anemia before biopsy. Hypertension and uremia increase the risk for bleeding and antihypertensive drugs or dialysis may be ordered before a biopsy.

PROCEDURE. In a percutaneous biopsy, the nephrologist or radiologist obtains tissue samples without an incision. Clients receive sedation and are monitored throughout the procedure. The client is placed in the prone position on the procedure table. The entry site is selected after taking preliminary images. The area is prepped and sterilely draped. A local anesthetic is injected and the physician then inserts the biopsy device into the tissues toward the kidney. Needle depth and placement is confirmed by ultrasound or CT. While the client holds his or her breath, the needle is advanced into the renal cortex. Samples are then taken with a spring-loaded coring biopsy needle and sent for pathologic analysis.

FOLLOW-UP CARE. After a percutaneous biopsy, the major risk is bleeding from the biopsy site. For 24 hours after the biopsy, monitor the dressing site, vital signs, urine output, hemoglobin level, and hematocrit. Even if the dressing is dry and there is no hematoma, the client could be bleeding from the site. An internal bleed is not readily visible but is suspected with flank pain, decreasing blood pressure, decreasing urine output, or other signs of hypovolemia or shock.

The client follows a plan of strict bedrest, lying in a supine position with a back roll for additional support for 2 to 6 hours after the biopsy. The head of the bed may be elevated, and the client may resume oral intake of food and fluids. After bedrest, the client may have limited bathroom privileges if there is no evidence of bleeding.

Monitor for hematuria, the most common complication of renal biopsy. Hematuria occurs microscopically in most clients, but 5% to 9% have gross hematuria. This problem usually resolves without treatment in 48 to 72 hours after the biopsy but can persist for 2 to 3 weeks. In rare cases, transfusions and surgery are required. There should be no obvious blood clots in the urine.

The client may have some local discomfort after the percutaneous renal biopsy. If aching originates at the biopsy site and begins to radiate to the flank and around the front of the abdomen, bleeding may have started or a perinephric hematoma is forming. This pattern of discomfort with bleeding occurs because blood in the tissues around the kidney increases pressure on local nerve tracts.

If bleeding occurs, IV fluid, packed red blood cells, or both may be needed to prevent shock. In general, a small amount of bleeding creates enough pressure to compress bleeding sites; this is called a "tamponade effect." If tamponade does not occur and bleeding is extensive, surgery for hemostasis or even nephrectomy may be needed. A hematoma in, on, or around the kidney may become infected, requiring treatment with antibiotics and surgical drainage.

If no bleeding occurs, the client can resume general activities after 24 hours. Instruct him or her to avoid lifting heavy objects, exercising, or performing other strenuous activities for 1 to 2 weeks after the biopsy procedure. Driving may also be restricted. Refer to Chapter 22 for general postoperative care for the client undergoing an open renal biopsy.

Renography (Kidney Scan)

CLIENT PREPARATION. Explain that a kidney scan is performed to provide general information about renal blood flow. A small amount of radioactive material, a radionuclide, is used. Reassure the client that there is no danger from the small amount of radioactive material present in the agent.

PROCEDURE. For a kidney scan, the radionuclide is injected intravenously. After injection, the radionuclide is absorbed into kidney tissue and gives off low-level radioactive emissions (scintillations). The amount of emission is measured by a scintillation counter. A special camera records the emissions and produces an image. At the same time, the rate and location of the emissions are recorded by computer, and information about renal blood flow, or glomerular filtration, is provided.

In some cases, captopril (Capoten), an antihypertensive drug, is given at the start of the procedure to change blood flow in the kidney. This procedure is a "captopril renal scan." The drug can cause severe hypotension during and after the procedure.

FOLLOW-UP CARE. If the client is able, urination into a commode is acceptable without risk from the small amount of radioactive material excreted. If the client is incontinent, change the bed linens promptly and wear gloves to maintain standard precautions. If captopril was used during the procedure, assess the client's blood pressure frequently. Caution the client to avoid rapid position changes and about the risk for falling as a result of orthostatic (positional) hypotension.

Ultrasonography

CLIENT PREPARATION. Inform the client that ultrasonography does not cause discomfort and is without risk. This test usually requires a full bladder. Ask the client to drink water, if needed, to help fill the bladder. This test applies sound waves to structures of different densities to produce images of the kidneys, ureters, and bladder and surrounding tissues. Ultrasonography allows assessment of kidney size, cortical thickness, and status of the calices. The test can identify obstruction in the urinary tract, tumors, cysts, and other masses without the use of nephrotoxic contrast material (dye).

PROCEDURE. The client undergoing renal ultrasound is usually placed in the prone position. Sonographic gel is applied to the skin over the back and flank areas to enhance sound wave conduction. A transducer in contact with and moving across the skin delivers sound waves and measures the echoes. Images of the internal structures are produced.

FOLLOW-UP CARE. Skin care to remove the gel is all that is needed after ultrasonography.

OTHER URINARY TRACT DIAGNOSTIC TESTS

Cystoscopy and Cystourethroscopy

CLIENT PREPARATION. Cystoscopy and cystourethroscopy are operative procedures and require completion of a preoperative checklist and a signed informed consent statement. The physician provides a complete description of and reasons for the procedure and the nurse reinforces this information. Cystoscopy may be performed for diagnosis or treatment. This test is used to examine for bladder trauma (cystoscopy) or urethral trauma (cystourethroscopy) and to identify causes of urinary tract obstruction. Cystoscopy may be used to remove bladder tumors or an enlarged prostate gland.

Cystoscopy may be performed under general or local anesthesia with sedation. The client's age, general health, and the expected duration of the procedure are considered in the decision about anesthesia. A light evening meal may be eaten. Usually the client is NPO after midnight on the night before the cystoscopy. A bowel preparation with laxatives or enemas is performed the evening before the procedure.

PROCEDURE. The cystoscopy is performed in a designated cystoscopic examination room. If the procedure is performed in a surgical suite under general anesthesia, the usual surgical support personnel are present (see Chapter 21). This procedure is often performed in clinics, ambulatory surgery or short-procedure units, or a urologist's office.

Assist the client onto a table and, after sedation, place him or her in the lithotomy position. After the anesthesia is given and the area cleansed and draped, the urologist inserts a cystoscope through the urethra into the urinary bladder. This exam commonly includes the use of both the cystoscope and the urethroscope.

FOLLOW-UP CARE. After cystoscopic examination with general anesthesia, the client is returned to a postanesthesia care unit (PACU) or area. If local anesthesia and sedation were used, the client may be returned directly to the hospital room. Clients undergoing cystoscopic examinations as outpatients are transferred to an area for monitoring before discharge to home. Monitor the client for airway patency and breathing, changes in vital signs (including temperature), and changes in urine output. Also observe for the complications of bleeding and infection.

A catheter may or may not be present after cystoscopy. The client without a catheter has urinary frequency due to irritation from the procedure. The urine may be pink tinged, but gross bleeding is not expected. Bleeding or the presence of clots may obstruct the catheter and decrease urine output. Monitor urine output and notify the physician of obvious blood clots or a decreased or absent urine output. Irrigate the Foley catheter with sterile saline, if prescribed. Notify the physician if the client has a fever (with or without chills) or an elevated white blood cell (WBC) count, which suggests infection. Encourage the client to take oral fluids to promote adequate urine output (which helps prevent clotting) and to reduce the burning sensation on urination.

Retrograde Procedures

Retrograde means going against the normal flow of urine. A retrograde examination of the ureters and pelves (pyelogram), the bladder (cystogram), and the urethra (urethrogram) involves instilling dye into the lower urinary tract. Because the dye is instilled directly to obtain an outline of the structures desired, the dye does not enter the bloodstream. Therefore the client is not at risk for dye-induced acute renal failure or a systemic allergic response.

CLIENT PREPARATION. The client is prepared for retrograde procedures (retrograde pyelography, retrograde cystography, and retrograde urethrography) in the same way as for cystoscopy.

PROCEDURE. Retrograde x-rays are obtained during the cystoscopy. After placement of the cystoscope by the urologist, catheters are placed into each ureter, and contrast dye is instilled into each ureter and renal pelvis. The catheters are removed by the urologist, and x-rays are taken by the radiology technician to outline these structures as the dye is excreted. The procedure identifies obstruction or structural abnormalities.

For clients undergoing retrograde cystoscopy or urethrography, contrast dye is instilled similarly into the bladder or urethra. Cystography and urethrography identify structural problems, such as fistulas, diverticula, and tumors.

FOLLOW-UP CARE. After retrograde procedures, monitor the client for infection caused by placing instruments in the urinary tract. Because these procedures are performed during cystoscopic examination, follow-up care is the same as that for cystoscopy.

Urodynamic Studies

Urodynamic studies examine the processes of voiding and include the following:

- Tests of bladder capacity, pressure, and tone
- Studies of urethral pressure and urine flow
- Tests of perineal voluntary muscle function

These tests are often used along with voiding urographic or cystoscopic procedures to evaluate problems with urine flow.

CYSTOMETROGRAPHY

The purpose of a cystometrogram (CMG) is to determine how well the bladder wall (detrusor) muscle functions and how sensitive it is to stretching as the bladder fills. This test provides information about bladder capacity, bladder pressure, and voiding reflexes.

CLIENT PREPARATION. Explain the procedure and inform the client that a urinary catheter may be needed temporarily during the procedure.

PROCEDURE. Ask the client to void normally. Record the amount, rate of flow, and time of voiding. Insert a urinary catheter to measure the residual urine volume. The cystometer is attached to the catheter, and fluid is instilled via the catheter into the bladder. The point at which the client first notes a feeling of the urge to void and the point at which the client notes a strong urge to void are recorded. Bladder capacity and bladder pressure readings are recorded graphically. The client is asked to void when the bladder instillation is complete (about 500 mL). The residual urine after voiding is recorded, and the catheter is removed. Electromyography of the perineal muscles may be performed during the cystometric examination.

FOLLOW-UP CARE. As with any procedure that involves inserting instruments into the urinary tract, monitor for infection. Record the client's temperature, the character of the urine, and the amount of urine output.

URETHRAL PRESSURE PROFILE

A urethral pressure profile (also called a urethral pressure profilometry [UPP]) can provide information about the nature of urinary incontinence or urinary retention.

CLIENT PREPARATION. Explain the procedure and inform the client that a urinary catheter may be needed temporarily during the procedure.

PROCEDURE. A special catheter with pressure-sensing capabilities is inserted into the bladder. Variations in the pressure of the smooth muscle of the urethra are recorded as the catheter is slowly withdrawn.

FOLLOW-UP CARE. As with any study involving inserting instruments into the urinary tract, monitor the client for manifestations of infection.

ELECTROMYOGRAPHY

Electromyography (EMG) of the perineal muscles tests the strength of the muscles used in voiding. This information may help to identify methods of improving continence.

CLIENT PREPARATION. Inform the client that some temporary discomfort may accompany placement of the electrodes. Any discomfort is usually mild and of short duration.

PROCEDURE. In EMG of the perineal muscles, electrodes are placed in either the rectum or the urethra to measure muscle contraction and relaxation.

FOLLOW-UP CARE. After the completion of EMG, administer analgesics as prescribed to promote the client's comfort. Any discomfort is usually mild and of short duration.

URINE STREAM TEST

A urine stream test is used to evaluate pelvic muscle strength and the effectiveness of pelvic muscles in stopping the flow of urine. It is useful in assessing urinary incontinence.

CLIENT PREPARATION. Explain the procedure and reassure the client that efforts will be made to ensure privacy.

PROCEDURE. The client is asked to begin urinating. Three to five seconds after urination begins, the examiner gives the client a signal to stop urine flow. The length of time required to stop the flow of urine is recorded.

FOLLOW-UP CARE. Cleaning the perineal area, as after any voiding, is all that is necessary after the urine stream test.

Critical Thinking Challenge

The client, a 62-year-old man with type 2 diabetes and benign prostatic hyperplasia (BPH), is scheduled to have an IV urogram. He asks you whether he should take his oral antidiabetic drugs in the morning before the procedure. He also asks if the procedure will be painful and if he can attend a baseball game the evening after the procedure.

1. Should this client take his usual antidiabetic medication before the procedure? Why or why not?
2. What will you tell this client about activity restrictions?
3. How will you reassure this client about pain management during and after the procedure?
4. What effect can the BPH have on this procedure?

evolve For suggested answer guidelines, go to http://evolve.elsevier.com/Iggy/.

GET READY for the NCLEX Examination!

KEY POINTS

Safe Effective Care Environment

- Use sterile technique when inserting a catheter or any other instrument into the urinary system.
- Use contact precautions with any client who has drainage from the genitourinary tract.

Health Promotion and Maintenance

- Teach clients the proper way to clean the perineal area after voiding, having a bowel movement, or after sexual intercourse.
- Encourage all clients to maintain an adequate fluid intake (minimum of 3 L/day unless another condition requires fluid restriction.
- Teach clients who come into contact with chemicals in their workplaces or for leisure time activities, to avoid direct skin or mucous membrane contact with these chemicals.

Psychosocial Integrity

- Pace your interview to match the learning needs and style of the individual client.
- Allow the client the opportunity to express fear or anxiety regarding tests of the renal and urinary tract or about a potential change in renal function.
- Assess the client's level of comfort in discussion issues related to elimination and the urogenital area.
- Explain all diagnostic procedures, restrictions, and follow-up care to the client scheduled for tests.
- Provide as much privacy as possible for clients undergoing examination or testing of the renal/urinary tract.
- Use language and terminology that the client can understand during discussions of renal/urinary assessment.

Physiological Integrity

- Ask the client about renal problems in any other members of the family because some problems have a genetic component.
- Ask the client whether or not any nephrotoxic medications have ever been used.
- Ask the client if he or she has ever had an allergic reaction to radiopaque contrast dye, shellfish, or iodine.
- Assess urine output closely after any procedure in which contrast dye is used intravenously.
- Assess the client for bleeding or manifestations of infection after any invasive test of renal/urinary function.

ADDITIONAL STUDY RESOURCES

Go to your Student CD-ROM for Review Questions for the NCLEX Examination.

evolve Go to http://evolve.elsevier.com/Iggy/ for Integrated Management of Care Questions for the NCLEX Examination.

SELECTED BIBLIOGRAPHY

Asterisk indicates a classic or definitive work on this subject.

Aranout, M. (2001). Molecular genetics and the pathogenesis of autosomal dominant polycystic kidney disease. *Annual Review of Medicine, 52,* 93-123.

Beck, L.H. (2000). The aging kidney. Defending a delicate balance of fluid and electrolytes. *Geriatrics, 55*(4), 31-32.

Brenner, B.M. (Eds.). (2000). *Brenner & Rector's the kidney* (6th ed.). Philadelphia: W.B. Saunders.

*Driver, D.S. (1996). Renal assessment: Back to basics. *American Nephrology Nurses' Association Journal, 23*(4), 361-368.

*Duthrie, E.H., & Katz, P.R. (1998). *Practice of geriatrics* (3rd ed.). Philadelphia: W.B. Saunders.

Ebersole, P., Hess, P., & Luggen, A. (2004). *Toward healthy aging: Human needs and nursing response* (6th ed.). St. Louis: Mosby.

Gordon, M. (2002). *Manual of nursing diagnosis* (10th ed.). St. Louis: Mosby.

Guyton, A.C., & Hall, J.E. (2000). *Textbook of medical physiology* (10th ed.). Philadelphia: W.B. Saunders.

Jarvis, C. (2004). *Physical examination and health assessment* (4th ed.). Philadelphia: W.B. Saunders.

Lancaster, L.E. (Ed.). (2001). *Core curriculum for nephrology nursing* (4th ed.). Pitman, NJ: A.J. Janetti.

Little, C. (2000). Renovascular hypertension. *American Journal of Nursing, 100*(2), 46-51.

Kee, J.L. (2002). *Laboratory and diagnostic tests with nursing implications.* Upper Saddle River, NJ: Prentice-Hall.

Maddox, T.G. (2002). Adverse reactions to contrast material: recognition, prevention, and treatment. *American Family Physician, 66*(7), 1229-1231.

Manjunath, G., Sarnak, M.J., Levey, A.S. (2001). Estimating the glomerular filtration rate: Dos and don'ts for assessing kidney function. *Postgraduate Medicine, 110* (6), 55-62.

O'Farrell, B., et al. (2001). Evaluation of portable bladder ultrasound: Accuracy and effect on nursing practice in an acute care neuroscience unit. *Journal of Neuroscience Nursing, 33*(6), 310-319.

Price, D.A., et al. (2001). Renal perfusion and function in healthy African Americans. *Kidney International, 59*(3), 1037-1043.

Schaeffer, A.J. (2002). Infections and inflammations of the genitourinary tract. In P.C. Walsh, et al. (Eds.). *Campbell's urology.* Philadelphia: W.B. Saunders.

Shinopulos, N. (2000). Bedside urodynamic studies: Simple testing for urinary incontinence. *The Nurse Practitioner, 25*(6), 19-20, 22, 25-26, 28, 33-34, 37.

*Shulman, N.B., & Hall, W.D. (1991). Renal vascular disease in African-Americans and other racial minorities. *Circulation, 83*(4), 1477-1479.

Thompsom, E.J., & King, S.L. (2003). Acetylcysteine and fenoldopam: Promising new approaches for preventing effects of contrast nephrotoxicity. *Critical Care Nurse, 23*(3), 39-46.

U.S. Renal Data Systems. (2002). *USRDS 2002 annual data report.* Bethesda, MD: The National Institutes of Health, National Institute of Diabetes and Digestive and Kidney Diseases.

Vander, A.J,. & Navar, L.G. (2003) *Renal physiology* (6th ed.). New York, McGraw-Hill.

Walsh, P.C., Retik, A.B., & Vaughn, E. D. (Eds.). (2002). *Campbell's urology* (8th ed.). Philadelphia, W.B. Saunders

*Yucha, C., & Keen, M. (1996). Renal regulation of extracellular fluid volume and osmolality. *American Nephrology Nurses' Association Journal, 23*(5), 487-497.

CHAPTER 73

Interventions for Clients with Urinary Problems

CHRIS WINKELMAN

LEARNING OUTCOMES

After studying this chapter, you should be able to:

1. Describe the clinical manifestations of cystitis.
2. Develop a community-based teaching plan for a person at risk for cystitis.
3. Describe nursing interventions to prevent urinary tract infections among hospitalized clients.
4. Compare the pathophysiology and manifestations of stress incontinence, urge incontinence, overflow incontinence, mixed incontinence, and functional incontinence.
5. Describe the mechanisms of action, side effects, and nursing implications for the management of a urinary tract infection with sulfonamide and fluoroquinolone antibiotics.
6. Describe the techniques used to assess pelvic floor strength in the client who is experiencing some incontinence.
7. Explain the proper application of exercises to strengthen pelvic floor muscles.
8. Explain the drug therapy for different types of incontinence.
9. Develop a community-based teaching plan for the client who must perform intermittent self-catheterization for incontinence.
10. Prioritize nursing care for the client with renal colic.
11. Describe the manifestations of urinary obstruction.
12. Describe the common clinical manifestations of bladder cancer.
13. Develop a community-based teaching plan for continuing care of clients who have a urinary diversion for bladder cancer.

Go to your Student CD-ROM for Review Questions for the NCLEX Examination keyed to these Learning Outcomes.

Urinary problems affect the storage or elimination of urine. Both acute and chronic urinary problems are common and costly. More than 20 million people in the United States are treated annually for urinary tract infections, cystitis, kidney and ureter stones, or urinary incontinence (U.S. Renal Data Systems, 2002). Although life-threatening complications are rare with urinary problems, clients may have significant functional, physical, and psychosocial changes that reduce quality of life. Nursing interventions are directed toward prevention, detection, and management of urologic disorders.

INFECTIOUS DISORDERS

Infections of the urinary tract and kidneys are common, especially among women. Manifestations of urinary tract infection (UTI) account for more than 6.5 million health care visits annually in the United States, and 1.5 million hospital discharges involve a diagnosis of UTI (National Kidney and Urologic Diseases Information Clearinghouse, 2004). In the hospital, UTIs are the most prevalent nosocomial infection (Foxman, 2002). Total direct and indirect costs for adult urinary tract infections are estimated at $1.6 billion each year.

Urinary tract infections are described by their location in the tract. Acute infections in the lower urinary tract include urethritis (urethra), cystitis (bladder), and prostatitis (prostate gland). Acute **pyelonephritis** is an upper urinary tract (kidney) infection. The site of infection is important to know because site, along with the specific type of bacteria present, determines treatment. Several risk factors are associated with occurrence of UTIs (Table 73-1).

Cystitis

PATHOPHYSIOLOGY

Cystitis is an inflammation of the bladder. It can be caused by infection from bacteria, viruses, fungi, or parasites. Infectious cystitis is the most common of the UTIs. Noninfectious cystitis is caused by irritation from chemicals or

TABLE 73-1 Factors Contributing to Urinary Tract Infections

Factor	Mechanism	Interventions
Obstruction	Incomplete bladder emptying creates a continuous pool of urine where bacteria can grow, prevents flushing out of bacteria, and allows bacteria to ascend more easily to higher structures.	Relieve or bypass the obstruction to promote complete bladder emptying.
	Bacteria have a greater chance of multiplying the longer they remain in residual urine.	Increase liquids to dilute urine and encourage more frequent voiding.
	Overdistention of the bladder damages the mucosa and allows bacteria to invade the bladder wall.	Use intermittent catheterization to keep the bladder from becoming distended.
Stones (calculi)	Large stones can cause obstruction to urine flow.	Remove stones and/or treat the underlying condition that causes the stones to form.
	The rough surface of a stone irritates mucosal surfaces and creates a spot where bacteria can establish and grow.	
	Bacteria can live within stones and cause reinfection.	
Vesicoureteral reflux	Bacteria-laden urine is forced backward from the bladder up into the ureters and kidneys, where pyelonephritis can develop.	The affected ureters may be able to be surgically reimplanted in the bladder to eliminate the reflux.
	Reflux of sterile urine can cause renal scarring, which may promote renal dysfunction.	
Diabetes mellitus	Excess glucose in urine provides a rich medium for bacterial growth.	Maintain good glucose control in clients with diabetes.
	Peripheral neuropathy affects bladder innervation and leads to a flaccid bladder and incomplete bladder emptying.	
Characteristics of urine	Alkalotic urine promotes bacterial growth.	Acidify urine by taking vitamin C tablets, not citrus fruits. Such fruits make the urine alkaline.
	Concentrated urine promotes bacterial growth.	Increase urine dilution by increasing fluid intake.
Gender	Female clients are susceptible to periurethral colonization with coliform bacteria.	Explain the importance of perineal hygiene (wiping front to back) to prevent large amounts of coliform bacteria from remaining in the perineal area.
	Bladder displacement during pregnancy predisposes women to cystitis and the development of pyelonephritis.	Routine monitoring of pregnant women for UTIs prevents complications.
	A diaphragm or pessary that is too large can cause an obstruction to urine flow or trauma to the urethra.	Be sure diaphragms and pessaries are properly fitted.
Age	Obstruction may be caused by incomplete bladder emptying as a result of an enlarged prostate in men and cystocele and prolapse in women.	Do not rush older clients during toileting; provide regular and private toileting times to promote complete bladder emptying.
	Neuromuscular conditions that cause incomplete bladder emptying, such as Parkinson's disease and strokes, affect older adults more frequently.	Straight catheter for residual and Credé maneuver to promote more complete emptying.
	The use of anticholinergic medications in older adults contributes to delayed bladder emptying.	Monitor and report this medication side effect.
	Fecal incontinence contributes to poor perineal hygiene.	Promptly clean clients after episodes of incontinence.
	Hypoestrogenism in older women adversely affects the cells of the vagina and urethra, making them more susceptible to infections.	Give vaginal estrogen cream as directed to improve the health of the client's vaginal and urethral cells.
Sexual activity	Irritation of the perineum and urethra during intercourse can promote migration of bacteria from the perineal area to the urinary tract in some women.	Empty the bladder before and after intercourse. Drink 8 oz of fluid (especially water) after intercourse.
	Spermicides can alter vaginal pH, increasing potential numbers of pathogens.	Consider alternate method of birth control if experiencing repeated UTIs.
	Inadequate vaginal lubrication may exacerbate potential urethral irritation.	Use an artificial vaginal lubricant.
	Bacteria may be introduced into the man's urethra during anal intercourse or during vaginal intercourse with a woman who has a bacterial vaginitis.	Use a condom.

radiation. **Interstitial cystitis** is an inflammatory process of unknown etiology.

Infectious agents, most commonly bacteria, move up the urinary tract from the external urethra to the bladder. Less common, spread of infection through the blood and lymph fluid can occur. Once bacteria enter the urinary tract, several factors influence the outcome (Table 73-2).

Asymptomatic bacteriuria is common in older adults and is a benign condition. No studies have demonstrated a relationship between asymptomatic bacteriuria and progression

TABLE 73-2 Important Factors Influencing the Outcome of Urinary Tract Infection

Facilitating Aspects	Protective Aspects
Anatomy	
Females: Short length of the urethra and its proximity to the vagina and rectum facilitate colonization of coliform bacteria. *Males:* With age, the prostate enlarges and may obstruct the normal flow of urine, producing stasis.	*Males:* Long length of the urethra and its distance from the rectum provide protection from colonization with coliform bacteria.
Physiology	
Females: Pregnancy predisposes a woman to ureteral reflux and subsequent pyelonephritis; with age the decline in estrogen facilitates colonization of *Escherichia. coli.* *Males:* With age, prostatic secretions lose their antibacterial characteristics and predispose to bacterial proliferation in the urine.	*Females:* Well-estrogenized mucosa in the urethra and trigone may inhibit bacterial colonization. *Males:* Normal prostatic secretions inhibit bacterial growth. *Both males and females:* Mucin is produced by urothelial cells lining the bladder—this helps to maintain mucosal integrity and prevent cellular damage; mucin may also prevent bacteria from adhering to urothelial cells.
Trauma	
Females: Vaginal penetration with sexual intercourse may traumatize the urethra and bladder base, leading to postcoital (or honeymoon) cystitis; a vaginal diaphragm that is too large can place pressure on the urethra, causing trauma; vaginal childbirth can cause permanent damage to the urethra. *Males:* Sexually transmitted diseases may cause urethral strictures that obstruct the flow of urine and predispose to urinary stasis. *Both males and females:* Urethral instrumentation (such as catheterization) may disturb the urothelial surface and predispose to adherence of bacteria that would ordinarily not be pathogenic.	*Females:* Adequate lubrication, either natural or artificial, with intercourse may prevent any trauma.
Infectious Agent	
Some organisms are better able to adhere to host cells and secrete substances that induce inflammation.	A small inoculum (number of microorganisms) introduced into the body) is more easily flushed away by the flow of urine.

to acute infection or renal insufficiency in clients without other pathologic problems.

Etiology and Genetic Risk

UTIs, like other infections, are the result of interactions between a pathogen and the host. A high bacterial virulence is necessary to overcome usual strong host resistance. However, a compromised host is more likely to be infected with a pathogen that has a low virulence. Genetically, invading bacteria with special adhesions are more likely to cause ascending urinary tract infections (UTIs). Host genetic factors such as blood group secretor status and ability to generate bladder surface biofilms may influence the risk for UTI (Moore, Day, & Albers; 2002).

The most common organisms in infectious cystitis are from the intestinal tract. About 90% of UTIs are caused by *Escherichia coli.* Less common organisms include *Staphylococcus saprophyticus, Klebsiella pneumoniae,* and organisms from the *Proteus* and *Enterobacter* species (Moore, Day, & Albers, 2002).

In most cases, organisms first grow in the perineal area, then move into the urethra as a result of irritation, trauma, or catheterization of the urinary tract, and finally ascend to the bladder. Catheters are the most common predisposing factor for UTIs in the hospital setting. Within 48 hours of catheter insertion, bacterial colonization begins. About 50% of clients with indwelling catheters become infected within 1 week of catheter insertion.

The etiology of catheter-related infections varies between genders. Bacteria from a women's perineal area are more likely to ascend to the bladder by moving along the catheter. In men, bacteria tend to gain access to the bladder from inside the lumen of the catheter (Warren et al, 1999). Any break in the closed urinary drainage system allows bacteria to migrate through the urinary tract. Best practices to reduce the risk of catheter contamination are listed in Chart 73-1.

Organisms other than bacteria can cause cystitis. Fungal infections, such as those caused by *Candida,* can occur during long-term antibiotic therapy, because antibiotics change normal flora. Clients who are severely immunocompromised, are receiving corticosteroids or other immunosuppressive agents, or have diabetes mellitus or acquired immunodeficiency syndrome (AIDS) are at higher risk for fungal UTIs.

Viral and parasitic infections are rare and usually are transferred to the urinary tract from an infection at another site. For example, *Trichomonas,* a parasite found in the vagina, can also be found in the urine. Treatment of the vaginal infection (see Chapter 78) also resolves the UTI.

Noninfectious cystitis may result from chemical exposure, such as to drugs (e.g., cyclophosphamide [Cytoxan, Procytox✱]), from radiation therapy, and from immunologic responses, as with systemic lupus erythematosus (SLE).

Interstitial cystitis is a rare, chronic inflammation of the entire lower urinary tract (bladder, urethra, and adjacent pelvic muscles) that is not a result of infection. The condition affects women more often than men (in a 10:1 ratio), and the diagnosis is difficult to make. Manifestations are similar to those of infectious cystitis with more intense urgency and bladder pain. Results from urinalysis and urine

CHART 73-1

BEST PRACTICE for Minimizing Catheter-Related Infection

- Avoid long-term use (>3 days) during active illness or perioperatively.
- Use aseptic routine when handling catheter devices; manipulation can promote an environment favorable to pathogens.
- Use strict sterile technique to insert the catheter (in the hospital setting); a break in technique can introduce pathogens into the urinary tract.
- Ensure that catheter tubing connections are sealed securely; disconnections can introduce pathogens into the urinary tract.
- Keep urine collection bags below the level of the bladder at all times; elevating the collection bag above the bladder causes reflux of pathogens from the bag into the urinary tract.
- Secure the catheter to the client's thigh (female) or lower abdomen (male); catheter movement can cause urethral friction and irritation.
- Perform daily catheter care by washing the perineum and proximal portion of the catheter with soap and water, drying gently (removes pathogens and reduces pathogenic population).
- Consider the use of silver-iodide coated catheters for clients requiring indwelling catheters for more than 3 to 5 days. This coating reduces bacterial colonization along the catheter.
- *Application of antiseptic solutions or antibiotic ointments to the perineal area of catheterized clients has not been demonstrated to have any beneficial effect.*

culture are negative for infection (Gray, Albo, & Huffstutler, 2002).

Although cystitis is not life threatening, infectious cystitis can lead to life-threatening complications, including pyelonephritis and sepsis. The risk for kidney tissue damage and subsequent kidney failure as a result of bacteria ascending from the bladder to the kidney is controversial. Severe kidney damage is a rare complication unless the client also has other predisposing factors, such as anatomic abnormalities, pregnancy, obstruction, reflux, calculi, or diabetes mellitus.

The spread of the infection from the urinary tract to the bloodstream is termed **urosepsis**. Sepsis from any source is a systemic infection that can lead to overwhelming organ failure, shock, and death. The most common cause of sepsis in the hospitalized client is a UTI (Warren et al., 1999). Sepsis has a high mortality and prolongs hospital stays (see Chapter 40).

Incidence/Prevalence

The incidence of UTI is second only to that of upper respiratory infections in primary care. Clients who have **frequency** (an urge to urinate frequently in small amounts), **dysuria** (pain or burning with urination), and **urgency** (the feeling that urination will occur immediately) account for more than 5 million health care visits annually. About 50% of these clients will have a confirmed UTI (National Kidney and Urologic Diseases Information Clearinghouse, 2004).

CONSIDERATIONS FOR OLDER ADULTS

The prevalence of UTIs varies with age and gender. Women of any age are more commonly affected with UTIs than men. In men 65 to 73 years old, the incidence of UTI is 3%; after 73 years of age, however, the incidence is 20%. In women, the prevalence of UTIs increases from 20% among all women to 50% in those older than 80 years of age. Skin and mucous membrane changes from a lack of estrogen appear to account for much of the increased risk in older women. Prostate disease increases risk for UTIs in men.

COLLABORATIVE MANAGEMENT

Assessment

PHYSICAL ASSESSMENT/CLINICAL MANIFESTATIONS

Frequency, urgency, and dysuria are the common clinical manifestations of a urinary tract infection (UTI), but other manifestations may be present (Chart 73-2). Urine may be cloudy, foul smelling, or blood tinged. Risk factors for UTI are included in the assessment (see Table 73-1).

Before performing the physical assessment, ask the client to void so that the urine can be examined and the bladder emptied before palpation. Assess vital signs to help rule out sepsis. Inspect the lower abdomen and palpate the urinary bladder. Distention after voiding indicates incomplete bladder emptying.

Using standard precautions (see Chapter 29), record any skin lesions around the urethral meatus and vaginal opening. To help differentiate between a vaginal and a urinary tract infection, note whether there is any vaginal discharge (i.e., vaginal discharge and irritation are more indicative of vaginal infection). Women often report burning with urination when normal, acidic urine touches labial tissues that are inflamed or ulcerated by vaginal infections or sexually transmitted diseases (STDs). Maintain privacy with drapes during the examination.

The prostate is palpated by rectal examination for size, change in shape or consistency, and tenderness. The physician or advanced practice nurse performs the rectal prostate assessment.

LABORATORY ASSESSMENT

Laboratory assessment for a UTI is a urinalysis with testing for leukocyte esterase and nitrate. The combination of a positive leukocyte esterase and nitrate is 85% to 90% sensitive and 95% specific in the diagnosis of a UTI (Bass, Jarvis, and Mitchell, 2003). Although more time-consuming and expensive, a urinalysis can include a microscopic count of bacteria, white blood cells (WBCs), and red blood cells (RBCs). The presence of 100,000 colonies/mL or the presence of WBCs (**pyuria**) with RBCs (**hematuria**) indicate infection.

A urinalysis is performed on a clean-catch midstream specimen. If the client cannot produce a clean-catch specimen, you may need to obtain the specimen with a small-caliber (6 Fr) catheter. For a routine urinalysis, 10 mL of urine is required; smaller quantities are sufficient for culture.

A urine culture confirms the type of organism and the number of colonies. Urine culture is expensive and takes 48 hours to obtain results. It is indicated when the UTI is complicated, does not respond to usual therapy, or if the diagnosis is uncertain. A UTI is confirmed when there are more than 10^5 colony-forming units in the urine from any client. In clients who have UTI manifestations, as few as 10^3 colony-forming units may be diagnostic. Multiple types of organisms in low colony counts indicate a contaminated specimen.

CHART 73-2

KEY FEATURES of Urinary Tract Infection

Common Clinical Manifestations
- Frequency
- Urgency
- Dysuria
- Hesitancy or difficulty in initiating urine stream
- Low back pain
- Nocturia
- Incontinence
- Hematuria
- Pyuria
- Bacteriuria
- Retention
- Suprapubic tenderness or fullness
- Feeling of incomplete bladder emptying

Rare Clinical Manifestations
- Fever
- Chills
- Nausea
- Vomiting
- Malaise
- Flank pain

Atypical Clinical Manifestations That May Occur in the Older Adult
- The only symptom may be something as vague as increasing mental confusion or frequent, unexplained falls.
- A sudden onset of incontinence or a worsening of incontinence may be the only symptom of an early UTI.
- Fever, tachycardia, tachypnea, and hypotension, even without any urinary symptoms, may be signs of urosepsis.
- Loss of appetite, nocturia, and dysuria are common symptoms.

UTI, Urinary tract infection.

Sensitivity testing follows culture results when complicating factors are present, such as stones or recurrent infection, or when the client is older.

Occasionally the serum WBC count may be elevated, with the differential WBC count showing a "left shift" (see Chapter 23). This shift indicates that the number of immature WBCs is increasing in response to the infection. As a result, the number of bands, or immature WBCs, is elevated. Left shift most often occurs with urosepsis and rarely occurs with uncomplicated cystitis.

OTHER DIAGNOSTIC ASSESSMENTS

The diagnosis of cystitis is based on the history, physical examination, and laboratory data. If urinary retention and obstruction of urine outflow are suspected, urography, abdominal sonography, or computed tomography (CT) may be needed to locate the site of obstruction or the presence of calculi. Voiding cystourethrography (see Chapter 72) is needed when vesicoureteral reflux is suspected.

Cystoscopy (see Chapter 72) may be performed when the client has recurrent UTIs (more than three or four a year). The urine is sterilized with antibiotic therapy before the procedure to reduce the risk for sepsis. Cystoscopy identifies abnormalities that increase the risk for cystitis. Such abnormalities include bladder calculi, bladder diverticula, urethral strictures, foreign bodies (such as sutures from previous surgery), and **trabeculation** (an abnormal thickening of the bladder wall caused by urinary retention and obstruction). Retrograde pyelography, along with the cystoscopic examination, shows outlines and images of the drainage tract. Areas of obstruction or malformation and the presence of reflux are then identified early.

Cystoscopy is needed to accurately diagnose interstitial cystitis. A urinalysis usually shows WBCs and RBCs but no bacteria. Common findings in interstitial cystitis are a small-capacity bladder, the presence of **Hunner's ulcers** (a type of bladder lesion), and small hemorrhages after bladder distention.

◆Common Nursing Diagnoses and Collaborative Problems

Nursing diagnoses and collaborative problems that may apply to clients with cystitis include the following:
- Acute Pain related to bladder spasms
- Deficient Knowledge (risk factors for cystitis and drug regimen) related to information misinterpretation or unfamiliarity with information resources
- Urge Urinary Incontinence related to irritation of bladder stretch receptors causing spasm (e.g., bladder infection)
- Risk for Impaired Skin Integrity related to moisture from incontinence
- Risk for Sepsis

◆Interventions

NONSURGICAL MANAGEMENT

Drug Therapy. Drugs used to treat bacteriuria and promote client comfort include urinary antiseptics or antibiotics, analgesics, and antispasmodics. Cure of a UTI is dependent on the antibiotic levels achieved in the urine (Chart 73-3). Antifungal agents are prescribed for fungal infections. Amphotericin B is most often given in daily bladder instillations, and ketoconazole (Nizoral) is usually given orally. Antispasmodic drugs decrease bladder spasm and promote complete bladder emptying.

Antibiotic therapy is used for bacterial UTIs (see Chart 73-3). Guidelines indicate that a 3-day course of trimethoprim/sulfamethoxazole or fosfomycin is effective in treating an uncomplicated, community-acquired UTI in women (Bass, Jarvis, & Mitchell, 2003). Single-dose therapy with long-acting fluoroquinolones is under investigation. The shorter courses increase adherence and reduce cost. Longer antibiotic treatment (7 to 21 days) is required for hospitalized clients, those with complicating factors, such as indwelling catheters or calculi, and those with diabetes or immunosuppression.

Long-term antibiotic therapy is recommended for chronic, recurring infections caused by structural abnormalities or calculi. Trimethoprim 100 mg daily may be used for long-term management of the older client with frequent UTIs. For women who have recurrent UTIs after intercourse, one low-dose tablet of trimethoprim (TMP) (Proloprim, Trimpex) or TMP/sulfamethoxazole (half- or single-strength Bactrim, Cotrim, Septra) or nitrofurantoin (Macrodantin, Nephronex✱, Novofuran✱) after intercourse is often recommended (McLaughlin & Carson, 2004). Estrogen used as an intravaginal cream may prevent recurrent UTIs in the postmenopausal woman; the benefits of systemic estrogen replacement therapy in preventing UTIs may not outweigh the risks of hormone replacement therapy for most clients (Maloney, 2002).

CHART 73-3

DRUG THERAPY for Urinary Tract Infection

Drug	Usual Dosage	Nursing Interventions	Rationales
Antimicrobials			
Quinolones		Avoid use in pregnancy and in those under 18 yr.	Drug can interfere with cartilage formation in weight-bearing joints.
Ciprofloxacin (Cipro)	250 mg PO twice daily for 3 days with uncomplicated cystitis, for 7 days with complicated cystitis, and for 10-14 days with uncomplicated pyelonephritis	Avoid taking with aluminum- or magnesium-containing antacids. Give 1 hr before or 2 hr after food or drink. Avoid caffeinated beverages, and use with caution in clients receiving theophylline.	Food, calcium, and antacids interfere with drug adsorption. Quinolones prolong the half-life of caffeine and theophylline.
[1]Lomefloxacin (Maxaquin)	400 mg PO daily for 3 days for uncomplicated cystitis, for 7 days for complicated cystitis, and for 10-14 days for uncomplicated pyelonephritis	As above. Avoid the sun.	As above. Drug causes photosensitivity.
[2]Levofloxacin (Levaquin)	250 mg PO daily for 3 days for uncomplicated cystitis, for 7 days for complicated cystitis, and for 10-14 days for uncomplicated pyelonephritis	As above. Avoid the sun.	As above. Drug causes photosensitivity.
Norfloxacin (Noroxin)	400 mg PO twice daily for 3 days for uncomplicated cystitis, for 7 days for complicated cystitis, and for 10-14 days for uncomplicated pyelonephritis	As above.	As above.
Ofloxacin (Floxin)	200 mg PO twice daily for 3 days for uncomplicated cystitis, for 7 days for complicated cystitis, and for 10-14 days for uncomplicated pyelonephritis	As above.	As above.
[3]Sparfloxacin (Zagam)	400 mg PO for 1 day, then 200 mg daily for 2 days for uncomplicated cystitis, for 7 days for complicated cystitis, and for 10-14 days for uncomplicated pyelonephritis	As above.	As above.

[1]***Med Error Alert!*** *Do not confuse with Maxidex, a glucocorticoid, or Maxalt, an antimigraine agent.*

[2]***Med Error Alert!*** *Do not confuse with levothyroxine, a synthetic thyroid hormone.*

[3]***Med Error Alert!*** *Do not confuse with Zantac, an H_2 histamine blocker.*

CHART 73-3

DRUG THERAPY for Urinary Tract Infection—*cont'd*

Drug	Usual Dosage	Nursing Interventions	Rationales
Antimicrobials—*cont'd*			
Penicillins		Inquire about penicillin allergy.	
Amoxicillin (Amoxil)	500 mg PO twice daily for 3 days	Give with food.	Food reduces GI upset.
Amoxicillin/ clavulanate (Augmentin, Clavulin ✱)	500 mg/125 mg PO twice daily for 3 days	Give with food.	Food reduces GI upset.
Cephalosporins		Inquire about allergy to cephalosporin or penicillin.	There is a 1% to 20% cross-reactivity between penicillin and cephalosporins.
Cefadroxil (Duricef)	1000 mg PO daily for 3 days for uncomplicated cystitis, or 1000 mg twice daily for 10 days for complicated cystitis		
[4]Cefixime (Suprax)	400 mg PO daily for 3 days for uncomplicated cystitis, for 7 days for complicated cystitis, and for 10-14 days for uncomplicated pyelonephritis		
Fosfomycin (Monurol)	3 g PO (1 packet) as a single dose	Avoid use of GI drugs during dosing.	Drug is less effective if given with drugs that increase GI motility.
Sulfonamide			
Trimethoprim/ sulfamethoxazole (Bactrim, Septra, Sulfatrim Roubac ✱)	1 double-strength tablet (DS or 160/800 mg) for 3 or 10 days for uncomplicated cystitis, or single-strength PO (80/400 mg) after coitus for prophylaxis	Provide adequate fluid intake. Avoid ascorbic acid and ammonium chloride that acidify urine.	Sulfa can crystallize in acidic or concentrated urine.
		Use with caution in clients with asthma, G6PD deficiency, or multiple allergies.	Sulfa allergies are relatively common; monitor client for potential reaction.
Urinary Antiseptic			
Nitrofurantoin (Macrobid Macrodantin, Nephronex ✱, Novofuran ✱)	*Macrobid:* 100 mg PO twice daily for 7 days *Macrodantin:* 100 mg PO four times daily for 7 days	Give with food or milk.	Food or milk decreases GI upset.
		Monitor for flulike symptoms in older clients and in those with pulmonary disease.	Rare case of interstitial pneumonitis can occur in susceptible clients.
Analgesic			
Phenazopyridine (Pyridium, Urogesic, [5]Phenazo ✱)	100-200 mg PO three times daily for 2-3 days	Give with food.	Food helps reduce GI upset.
		Advise client that urine will become red or orange.	Urine discoloration is normal.
		Help the client to understand the difference between a urinary analgesic and antibiotic.	A complete dosing schedule is not necessary.
Antispasmodic			
Hyoscyamine (Anaspaz, Cystospaz-M, others)	0.125-0.5 PO three times daily and at bedtime	Assess for safety, constipation, and urinary retention.	Anticholinergics cause drowsiness, blurred vision, dry mouth, constipation, and urinary retention.

[4]***Med Error Alert!*** *Do not confuse with Surfak, a stool softener.*

[5]***Med Error Alert!*** *Do not confuse with pyridostigmine, an anticholinesterase.*

GI, Gastrointestinal; *G6PD*, glucose-6-phosphate dehydrogenase deficiency.

NIC **Urinary Elimination Management.** The goal is to maintain an optimal urinary elimination pattern. Nursing interventions for the management of cystitis are listed in Chart 73-4.

> **WOMEN'S HEALTH CONSIDERATIONS**
>
> Pregnant women with a bacterial UTI require vigorous intervention because of the tendency of simple cystitis to lead to acute pyelonephritis during pregnancy. Pyelonephritis in pregnancy can cause preterm labor and adversely affect the fetus.

Diet Therapy. The diet should include all food groups and include increased calories for the increased metabolism caused by infection. Urge clients to drink at least 2 to 3 L of fluid each day unless another condition requires fluid restriction. There is no evidence that additional fluid intake alters the course of a UTI (Gray, Albo, & Hufstutler, 2002). Although a critical review of the literature suggests that there is not enough evidence to routinely ingest cranberry products to prevent UTIs, one study suggests that 50 mL of concentrated cranberry juice consumed daily decreases bacterial adherence to the urinary tract, decreasing the incidence of UTIs in some clients. Cranberry juice must be consumed for 3 to 4 weeks to be effective (Jepson, Mihaljevic, & Craig, 2002; Kontiokari et al., 2001).

Other Pain Relief Measures. A warm sitz bath taken two or three times a day for 20 minutes may provide comfort and some relief of local symptoms. If burning with urination is severe or urinary retention occurs, instruct the client to sit in the sitz bath and urinate into the warm water.

SURGICAL MANAGEMENT. Surgery for cystitis treats the conditions that predispose to recurrent UTIs (e.g., removal of obstructions and repair of vesicoureteral reflux). Procedures may include cystoscopy (see Chapter 72) to identify and remove calculi or obstructions.

Community-Based Care

Assess the client's level of understanding of the problem. The client's knowledge about factors contributing to the development of cystitis is the basis on which further teaching interventions are planned.

CHART 73-4

NIC INTERVENTION ACTIVITIES for The Client with a Urinary Tract Infection

Urinary Elimination Management: *Maintenance of an optimum urinary elimination pattern*

- Monitor urinary elimination, including frequency, consistency, odor, volume, and color, as appropriate.
- Teach client signs and symptoms of urinary tract infection.
- Obtain midstream voided specimen for urinalysis, as appropriate.
- Refer to physician if signs and symptoms of urinary tract infection occur.
- Instruct client to respond immediately to urge to void, as appropriate.
- Teach client to drink eight ounces of liquid with meals, between meals, and in early evening.
- Assist client with development of toileting routine, as appropriate.

NIC intervention activities selected from Dochterman, J.M., & Bulechek, G.M. (Eds.). (2004). *Nursing interventions classifications (NIC)* (4th ed.). St. Louis: Mosby.

Teach the client how to take prescribed drugs. Emphasize the need for correct spacing of doses throughout the day and the need to complete all of the prescribed drugs. If the drug will change the color of the urine, as it does with phenazopyridine (Pyridium, Urogesic, Phenazo✱), inform the client to expect this occurrence. Offer techniques for remembering the drug schedule, such as the use of a daily calendar or the association of drugs with usual activities (e.g., mealtimes).

Clients may associate symptoms of discomfort with sexual activities and have feelings of guilt and embarrassment. Frank and sensitive discussions with a woman who experiences frequent recurrences of UTI after sexual intercourse can help her find techniques to handle the problem (see Table 73-1). Explore with the woman the factors that contribute to her infections, such as diaphragm use and her general resistance to infection. Remind the client that vigorous cleaning of the perineum with harsh soaps and vaginal douching may irritate the perineal tissues and increase the risk for UTI. At the client's request, discuss the problem with the client and her partner to help them find ways of maintaining their intimate relationship. Chart 73-5 lists actions for preventing UTIs.

> ***Critical Thinking Challenge***
>
> The client is a 22-year-old woman who comes to the clinic saying that she has to "pee" all the time and that it burns. She did not complete high school and currently works as a waitress at a truck stop. Her symptoms started 5 days ago and she says that she is so busy at work that she couldn't get off work to come to the clinic sooner. She uses street language to describe her symptoms and body areas. She also tells you that she is sexually active and uses a diaphragm for birth control. She is afraid that she may give this infection to her partner.

CHART 73-5

CLIENT EDUCATION GUIDE
Preventing a Urinary Tract Infection

- Drink 1 to 3 L of fluid every day.
- Drink 300 mL of cranberry juice daily.
- Be sure to get enough sleep, rest, and nutrition daily.
- [For women] Clean your perineum (the area between your legs) from front to back.
- [For women] Avoid irritating substances, such as bubble bath, nylon underwear, and scented toilet tissue. Wear loose-fitting cotton underwear.
- [For women] Empty your bladder before and after intercourse.
- If you experience burning when you urinate, if you have to urinate frequently, or if you find it difficult to begin urinating, notify your physician or other health care provider right away, especially if you have a chronic medical condition (such as diabetes) or are pregnant.
- Empty your bladder as soon as you feel the urge to urinate.
- Empty your bladder regularly (e.g., every 4 hours), even if you do not feel the urge to urinate.
- You may try the following home therapies:
  - Cranberry juice (pure) 50 mL daily.
  - Apple cider vinegar, 2 tablespoons three times daily in juice.
  - Vitamin C 500 mg daily to acidify the urine.
- To prevent recurrent infection:
  - Take your medication as directed even after the symptoms go away.
  - Schedule a follow-up appointment for 10 to 14 days after you finish taking your medication. At your follow-up visit, another urine sample may be taken for analysis or culture.

1. Should you use medical terminology during your assessment with this client? Why or why not?
2. What factors may have contributed to this client's infection?
3. What other assessment data should you obtain and why?
4. What is the risk that the client's infection could be passed on to her sexual partner?
5. What interventions will you teach her for comfort and treatment of this infection?
6. What interventions will you teach her for prevention of future episodes of cystitis?

evolve For suggested answer guidelines, go to http://evolve.elsevier.com/Iggy/.

Urethritis

PATHOPHYSIOLOGY

Urethritis is an inflammation of the urethra that causes symptoms similar to urinary tract infection (UTI). In men, manifestations of urethritis are burning or difficulty with urination and a discharge from the urethral meatus. The most common cause of urethritis in men is sexually transmitted diseases (STDs). These include gonorrhea or nonspecific urethritis caused by *Ureaplasma* (a gram-negative bacterium), *Chlamydia* (a sexually transmitted gram-negative bacterium), or *Trichomonas vaginalis* (a protozoan found in both the male and female genital tract).

In women, urethritis causes manifestations similar to those of bacterial cystitis. Urethritis is known by several other terms: *pyuria-dysuria syndrome, frequency-dysuria syndrome, trigonitis syndrome,* and *urethral syndrome.* Urethritis is most common in postmenopausal women and is probably caused by tissue changes related to low estrogen levels.

◆COLLABORATIVE MANAGEMENT

◆Assessment

Ask the client about a history of STD, painful or difficult urination, discharge from the penis or vagina, and discomfort in the lower abdomen. Urinalysis may show **pyuria** (white blood cells [WBCs]) without a large number of bacteria; however, results of urethral culture may indicate an STD. In women, the diagnosis may be made by exclusion when urinalysis and urethral culture are negative for bacteria and symptoms persist. In such cases, pelvic examination may reveal tissue changes from low estrogen levels in the vagina. Urethroscopy may show low estrogen changes with inflammation of urethral tissues.

◆Interventions

STDs are treated with antibiotic therapy. More information on STDs can be found in Chapter 80.

Postmenopausal women often have improvement in their urethral symptoms with the use of estrogen vaginal cream. Estrogen cream applied locally to the vagina increases the amount of estrogen in the urethra as well, and irritating symptoms are reduced.

NONINFECTIOUS DISORDERS

Urethral Strictures

PATHOPHYSIOLOGY

Urethral strictures are narrowed areas of the urethra. These problems may be caused by complications of an STD (usually gonorrhea) and from trauma during catheterization, urologic procedures, or childbirth. Strictures occur more often in men than in women. They may be a factor in other urologic problems, such as recurrent UTIs, urinary incontinence, and urinary retention.

◆COLLABORATIVE MANAGEMENT

The most common symptom of urethral stricture is obstruction of urine flow. Strictures rarely cause pain. Because urine stasis can result when flow is obstructed, the client with a stricture is at risk for developing a UTI and may have overflow incontinence. **Overflow incontinence** is the involuntary loss of urine when the bladder is overdistended. Assess the client for these two problems.

A urethral stricture is treated surgically. Dilation of the urethra (using a local anesthetic) is only a temporary measure, not a curative one. The best chance of long-term cure is with **urethroplasty,** surgical removal of the affected area with or without grafting to create a larger opening. The recurrence rate after surgery is still high, and most clients need repeated procedures.

Urinary Incontinence

PATHOPHYSIOLOGY

Continence (control over the time and place of urination) is unique to humans and some domestic animals. Continence is a learned behavior whereby a person can suppress the urge to urinate until a socially appropriate location is available (e.g., a toilet). Efficient bladder emptying (i.e., coordination between bladder contraction and urethral relaxation) is needed for continence.

Incontinence is an involuntary loss of urine severe enough to cause social or hygienic problems. Incontinence is *not* a normal consequence of aging or childbirth. Incontinence is stigmatizing and an underreported health problem. Many people suffer in silence, are socially isolated, and may be unaware that treatment is available. In addition, costs associated with incontinence are enormous for individuals and institutions.

Continence occurs when pressure in the urethra is greater than pressure in the bladder. For normal voiding to occur, the urethra must relax and the bladder must contract with enough pressure and duration to empty completely. Voiding should occur in a smooth and coordinated manner under a person's conscious control. Incontinence has several possible causes and can be either temporary or chronic (Table 73-3). Temporary causes usually do not involve a disorder of the urinary tract. The most common forms of urinary incontinence in adults are stress incontinence, urge incontinence, overflow incontinence, functional incontinence, and a mixed form.

Stress Incontinence

Stress incontinence is the most common type of incontinence. It is characterized by the loss of small amounts of urine during coughing, sneezing, jogging, or lifting. In the continent person, the urethra can be relaxed and tightened under conscious control because skeletal muscles of the pelvic floor surround it. When a person feels the urge to urinate, the conscious contraction of the urethra can override a bladder contraction if the urethral contraction is strong enough.

TABLE 73-3 Types of Urinary Incontinence

Type	Definition/Description	Cause	Clinical Manifestations
Stress incontinence	The involuntary loss of urine during activities that increase abdominal and detrusor pressure. Clients cannot tighten the urethra sufficiently to overcome the increased detrusor pressure; leakage of urine results.	Weakening of bladder neck supports; associated with childbirth. Intrinsic sphincter deficiency caused by such congenital conditions as epispadias (abnormal location of the urethra on the dorsum of the penis) or myelomeningocele. Acquired anatomic damage to the urethral sphincter (from repeated incontinence surgeries, prostatectomy, radiation therapy, and trauma).	Urine loss with physical exertion, cough, sneeze, or exercise. Usually only small amounts of urine are lost with each exertion. Normal voiding habits (≤8 times per day, 2 or fewer times per night). Postvoid residual usually ≤50 mL. Pelvic examination shows hypermobility of the urethra or bladder neck with Valsalva maneuvers.
Urge incontinence	The involuntary loss of urine associated with a strong desire to urinate. Clients cannot suppress the signal from the bladder muscle to the brain that it is time to urinate.	Unknown.	An abrupt and strong urge to void. May have loss of large amounts of urine with each occurrence.
Detrusor hyperreflexia (reflex incontinence)	The abnormal detrusor contractions result from neurologic abnormalities.	Central nervous system (CNS) lesions from stroke, multiple sclerosis, and parasacral spinal cord lesions. Local irritating factors such as caffeine, medications, or bladder tumor.	Postvoid residual <50 mL.
Overflow incontinence	The involuntary loss of urine associated with overdistention of the bladder when the bladder's capacity has reached its maximum. The urethra is obstructed, so it fails to relax sufficiently to allow urine to flow, resulting in incomplete bladder emptying or complete urinary retention, causing overflow incontinence.	Diabetic neuropathy; side effects of medication; after radical pelvic surgery or spinal cord damage; outlet obstruction. Causes external to the mechanism of the urethra: an enlarged prostate (male clients) and large genital prolapse (female clients). When the cause is intrinsic to the urethra, abnormal contraction of the skeletal muscle occurs, causing obstruction. This condition, called *detrusor dyssynergia*, is seen in clients with spinal cord injuries and multiple sclerosis.	Bladder distention, often up to the level of the umbilicus. Constant dribbling of urine.
Mixed incontinence	A combination of stress, urge, and overflow incontinence.	As with each separate disorder.	As with each separate disorder.
Functional incontinence	Leakage of urine caused by factors other than disease of the lower urinary tract.		Quantity and timing of urine leakage vary; patterns are difficult to discern.
Transient causes	Transient causes improve with treatment of the underlying condition.	Loss of cognitive functioning. Loss of awareness that urination is to occur in a socially acceptable place.	Altered mental state, as in delirium, confusion, depression, dementia, sepsis, mental illness, or severe psychological stress.
		Abnormal openings in the urinary tract, such as a fistula or diverticulum.	Urinary drainage noted from areas other than the urinary meatus.
		Medications, such as sedatives, hypnotics, diuretics, anticholinergics, decongestants, antihypertensives, and calcium channel blockers.	Some medications cause altered mental state; others cause increased urine production.
		Diabetes insipidus or psychogenic polydipsia.	Increased urine output.
		Inability to get to toileting facilities.	Restraints, restricted mobility.
		Direct bladder pressure or urethral obstruction.	Constipation or fecal impaction.
Permanent causes	Permanent causes are organic but may be improved with treatment.	Cognitive impairment. Traumatic or surgical effects. Those factors contributing to stress incontinence, urge incontinence, and overflow incontinence. Structural or functional defects of the bladder or the sphincters. Injuries or diseases of the spinal cord, brainstem, or cerebral cortex (neurogenic bladder). Congenital defects, including exstrophy of the bladder (bladder turned "inside out") and spina bifida.	Clinical manifestations depend on the cause.

Clients who have *stress incontinence* cannot tighten the urethra enough to overcome the increased detrusor pressure. Stress incontinence is common after childbirth, when the pelvic muscles are stretched and weakened. The weakened pelvic floor allows mobility and displacement of the urethra during exertion. If the pelvic muscles are not strengthened, this condition continues. Low estrogen levels after menopause also contribute to stress incontinence. Vaginal, urethral, and pelvic floor muscles become thin and weak without estrogen.

Urge Incontinence

Bladder contractions are perceived as an urge to urinate. When the bladder is full, contraction of the smooth muscle fibers of the bladder detrusor muscle normally signals the brain that it is time to urinate. Continent persons override that signal and relax the detrusor muscle for the time it takes to locate a toilet. Those who suffer from urge incontinence cannot suppress the signal and leak large amounts of urine associated with a sudden, strong urge to void. Urge incontinence is also known as an "overactive bladder" or an unstable bladder. Overactivity may have no known cause or be the result of abnormal detrusor contractions related to other problems. Such problems include stroke, Parkinson's disease, multiple sclerosis, and spinal tumors or disease; UTI; benign prostatic enlargement; bladder irritability from concentrated urine or artificial sweeteners, caffeine, alcohol, and citric intake; use of diuretics and other drugs; nicotine; and atrophic vaginitis (Rigsby, 2003).

Mixed Incontinence

Many clients with urinary incontinence fall into the mixed category. Often urine loss is related to both stress and urge incontinence. The manifestations have aspects of more than one subtype. This category is more common in older women.

Overflow Incontinence

When the detrusor muscle fails to contract, the bladder becomes overdistended. Overflow incontinence (also known as "reflex incontinence") occurs when the bladder has reached its absolute maximal capacity and some urine must leak out to prevent bladder rupture. Causes for the underactive (acontractile) bladder may or may not be determined.

The urethra can be obstructed so that it fails to relax enough to allow urine flow. Incomplete bladder emptying or urinary retention due to urethral obstruction results in overflow incontinence.

Functional Incontinence

Factors other than the abnormal function of the bladder and urethra result in functional incontinence. A common factor is the loss of cognitive function in clients affected by dementia. To maintain continence, a person must be aware that urination needs to occur in a socially acceptable place; clients with dementia may not have that awareness.

Etiology and Genetic Risk

Incontinence may have temporary or permanent causes. Evaluation of the incontinent client means considering all possible causes, beginning with those that are temporary and correctable. Surgical and traumatic causes of urinary incontinence are related to procedures or surgery in the lower pelvic structures, areas that contain complex nerve pathways. Radical urologic, prostatic, and gynecologic procedures for treatment of pelvic cancers may result in urinary incontinence. Injury to segments S2 to S4 of the spinal cord may cause incontinence from impairment of normal nerve pathways.

Inappropriate bladder contraction may result from disorders of the brain and nervous system or from bladder irritation due to chronic infection, stones, chemotherapy, or radiation therapy. Failure of bladder contraction occurs with the autonomic neuropathy of diabetes mellitus and syphilis.

CONSIDERATIONS FOR OLDER ADULTS

Many factors contribute to urinary incontinence in older adults (Chart 73-6). An older person may have decreased mobility from disease, neurologic dysfunction, or musculoskeletal degeneration. In the hospital or extended care setting, mobility is limited when the older client is restrained or placed on bedrest. Vision and hearing impairments may also prevent the client from locating a call bell to notify the nurse or assistive personnel of the need to void. Assess for these factors and minimize them to prevent urinary incontinence.

Incidence/Prevalence

Incontinence is a major health problem that affects more than 13 million people of all ages in the United States (AHCPR, 1996); about 85% are women. It is most common in older adults, including 15% to 30% of community-dwelling older people and at least one half of all nursing home residents (AHCPR, 1996).

CHART 73-6

NURSING FOCUS on the OLDER ADULT
Factors Contributing to Urinary Incontinence*

Medications
- Central nervous system depressants, such as opioid analgesics, decrease the client's level of consciousness and the urge to void, and they contribute to constipation.
- Diuretics cause frequent voiding, often of large amounts of urine.
- Multiple medications can contribute to changes in mental status or mobility, and they can irritate the bladder.

Disease
- Cerebrovascular accidents and other neurologic disorders decrease mobility, sensation, or cognition.
- Arthritis decreases mobility and causes pain.
- Parkinson's disease causes muscle rigidity and an inability to initiate movement.

Depression
- Depression decreases the energy necessary to maintain continence.
- Decreased self-esteem and feelings of self-worth decrease the importance to the client of maintaining continence.

Inadequate Resources
- Clients who have glasses or use a cane, walker, or slippers may be afraid to ambulate.
- Products that help clients manage incontinence are often costly.
- No one may be available to assist the client to the bathroom or help with incontinence products.

*These factors are in addition to the physiologic changes of aging given in Chapter 5.

In adult clients under 65 years of age, urinary incontinence occurs twice as often in women as in men. Incontinence in women of this age may occur after one or more pregnancies. Men in this age group rarely experience incontinence unless they have prostate disease or a spinal cord injury.

◆COLLABORATIVE MANAGEMENT

◆Assessment

HISTORY

Effective screening includes asking clients to respond "always," "sometimes," or "never" to the following questions (Castina, Boyington, & Dougherty, 2002):

- Do you ever leak urine or water when you don't want to?
- Do you ever leak urine or water when you cough, laugh, or exercise?
- Do you ever leak urine or water on the way to the bathroom?
- Do you ever use pads, tissue, or cloth in your underwear to catch urine?

If any answer is always or sometimes, proceed with a focused assessment (AHCPR, 1996; Bates, 2002) (Chart 73-7). Incontinence may be underreported because health care professionals do not ask clients about urine loss. Do not assume that clients will volunteer the information without specifically being asked.

CHART 73-7

FOCUSED ASSESSMENT of The Client with Urinary Incontinence

Note the presence of risk factors for urinary incontinence:
- Age
- If female, menopausal status
- Neurologic disease
  - Parkinson's disease
  - Dementia
  - Multiple sclerosis
  - Stroke
  - Spinal injury
- Diabetes mellitus
- Childbirth
- Urologic procedures
- Medications
- Bowel patterns
- Stress/anxiety level

Detail the symptoms of urinary incontinence:
- Leakage
- Frequency
- Urgency
- Nocturia
- Sensation of full bladder before leakage

Obtain a 24-hour intake and output record:
- Time and amount of oral intake and continent voidings
- Time and estimated amount of incontinent leakages
- Activity around the time of leakage

Assess client's:
- Mobility
- Self-care ability
- Cognitive ability
- Communication patterns

Assess the environment for barriers to toileting:
- Privacy
- Restrictive clothing
- Access to toilet

Data from Mather, K. (2002). Nursing assistants' perceptions of their ability to provide continence care. *Geriatric Nursing, 23*(2), 76-81; and Agency for Health Care Policy and Research. (1996). *Urinary incontinence in adults: Acute and chronic management. Clinical practice guideline.* AHCPR Publication No. 96-0682. Rockville, MD: Agency for Health Care Policy and Research, Public Health Service, U.S. Department of Health and Human Services; http://www.ahcpr.gov/clinic/uhistory.html (Clinical Practice Guidelines Online: Urinary Incontinence Guideline: Real World Examples of Use).

PHYSICAL ASSESSMENT/CLINICAL MANIFESTATIONS

Assess the abdomen to estimate bladder fullness, to rule out palpable hard stool, and to evaluate bowel sounds. With a physician's order, determine the amount of postvoid residual urine by portable ultrasound or catheterizing the client immediately after voiding. Urinary incontinence is confirmed by evaluating the force and character of the urine stream during voiding by the client. Asking the client to cough while wearing a perineal pad is useful in evaluating stress incontinence; a wet pad with forceful coughing may indicate stress incontinence. A cystometrogram (see Chapter 72) is used for diagnosis in most cases (Walsh et al., 2002).

For women, inspect the external genitalia to determine whether there is apparent urethral or uterine prolapse, **cystocele** (herniation of the bladder into the vagina), or rectocele. These conditions occur with pelvic floor muscle weakness. An advanced practice nurse puts on an examination glove and inserts two fingers into the vagina to assess the strength of these muscles. Strength is described as weak, adequate, or strong on the basis of the amount of pressure felt by the nurse as the client tightens her vaginal muscles. Describe and document the color, consistency, and odor of any secretions from the genitourinary orifices. The urine stream interruption test (see Chapter 72) is another method of determining pelvic muscle strength. For men, inspect the urethral meatus for any discharge.

A digital rectal examination is performed on both male and female clients. This examination provides information about the integrity of the nerve supply to the bladder. The examiner determines whether there is tactile sensation in the anorectal area by observing whether the rectal sphincter is relaxed or contracted on digital insertion. Because nerve supply to the bladder is similar to nerve supply to the rectum, the presence of tactile sensation and a rectal sphincter that contracts suggest that the nerve supply to the bladder is intact. A fecal impaction may be discovered during rectal examination. The health care provider assesses for prostate enlargement in men.

LABORATORY ASSESSMENT

A urinalysis is useful to rule out infection. This test is the first step in the assessment of incontinent clients of any age. The presence of red blood cells (RBCs), white blood cells (WBCs), leukocyte esterase, or nitrites is an indication for culturing the urine. Any infection is treated before further assessment of incontinence.

RADIOGRAPHIC ASSESSMENT

Radiographic assessment is rarely needed unless surgery is being considered. Urography is the most useful for locating the kidneys and ureters. A voiding cystourethrogram (VCUG) may be performed to assess the size, shape, support, and function of the bladder. Problems identified by this test include obstruction (especially prostate obstruction in men), or postvoid residual (PVR). Assessment of PVR also can be made with a portable ultrasonographic bladder scanner.

OTHER DIAGNOSTIC ASSESSMENTS

Clients who have unusual symptoms, medical complications, or a history of failed incontinence surgery may need urodynamic studies to determine the cause of their incontinence. Such studies are not standardized procedures and may consist of any combination of the following tests:

- Cystourethroscopy to examine the inside of the bladder and urethra directly
- Cystometrogram (CMG) to measure the pressure inside the bladder as it fills
- Urethral pressure profilometry (UPP) to measure the pressure in the urethra in relation to the bladder pressure during various activities
- Uroflowmetry to measure rate and degree of bladder emptying

Testing may take several hours and more than one visit (see Chapter 72).

Electromyography (EMG) of the pelvic muscles may be a part of the urodynamic studies. A perineometer is a tampon-shaped instrument inserted into the vagina to measure the strength of pelvic muscle contractions. The graph shows the amplitude of muscle contraction to the client as a method of biofeedback.

> **Critical Thinking Challenge**
>
> The client is a 78-year-old woman who is being admitted to an assisted living environment. When you ask her what she needs help with and what she can do independently, she confides in you that she has trouble getting to the bathroom in time and has frequent "accidents." She states, "It seems my bladder is smaller than ever. When I have to go, I really have to go right then." She wears paper towels in her underwear to catch the urine before she wets her clothes. She says that she expected this to happen because her mother and sisters all had bladder problems when they got old. She also says "That's what happens when you have nine pound babies." She says she tries to drink very little so that she will remain dry.
>
> 1. What other questions should you ask?
> 2. What type or types of incontinence is she most likely to have from the information she has provided thus far?
> 3. Is this problem likely to be genetic? Why or why not?
> 4. Which nursing diagnoses would be priority for this client?

evolve For suggested answer guidelines, go to http://evolve.elsevier.com/Iggy/.

Analysis

COMMON NURSING DIAGNOSES AND COLLABORATIVE PROBLEMS

The following are priority nursing diagnoses for clients with urinary incontinence:

1. Stress Urinary Incontinence related to weak pelvic muscles and structural supports
2. Urge Urinary Incontinence related to decreased bladder capacity, bladder spasms, diet, and neurologic impairment
3. Reflex Urinary Incontinence related to neurologic impairment
4. Functional Urinary Incontinence related to impaired cognition or neuromuscular limitations
5. Mixed or Total Urinary Incontinence related to many causes

ADDITIONAL NURSING DIAGNOSES AND COLLABORATIVE PROBLEMS

In addition to the common nursing diagnoses, clients with urinary incontinence may have one or more of the following:

- Social Isolation related to altered state of wellness or fear of embarrassment
- Risk for Impaired Skin Integrity related to excessive moisture from urinary excretions
- Disturbed Body Image related to odor, need to alter clothing selections, or need to wear protective briefs or supplies
- Risk for Infection related to increased environmental exposure to pathogens from retained or refluxing urine

Planning and Implementation

Several interventions are useful for each type of incontinence. Collaborative management uses these interventions, as well as medication, surgical repair, and diet therapy (Newman & Palmer, 2003).

STRESS URINARY INCONTINENCE

NOC **PLANNING: EXPECTED OUTCOMES.** With appropriate therapy, the client with urinary incontinence is expected to develop urinary continence. Indicators include that the client rarely or never demonstrates the following actions:

- Urine leakage between voidings
- Urine leakage with increased abdominal pressure (e.g., sneezing, laughing, lifting)

INTERVENTIONS. Initial interventions for clients with stress incontinence include keeping a diary, behavioral interventions, and drugs. Surgery also may be an option if other interventions are not effective. Explain the purpose of a detailed diary in which the client records times of urine leakage, activities, and foods eaten. The diary is then used by the health care practitioner to plan and evaluate interventions. Collection devices, absorbent pads, and undergarments may be used during the sometimes lengthy process of assessment and treatment and by those clients who elect not to pursue further interventions.

NONSURGICAL MANAGEMENT. Drug therapy and behavioral interventions (primarily diet and exercise) for stress incontinence require the client's active participation for success; however, these efforts have had significant proven success (see the Evidence-Based Practice for Nursing box on p. 1690). Providing ongoing encouragement, clarification, and support is extremely valuable for maximizing the effects of all interventions.

Exercise Therapy. Pelvic floor (Kegel) exercises for women with stress incontinence strengthen the muscles of the pelvic floor (circumvaginal muscles). These muscles become strengthened, as any other skeletal muscle does, by frequent, systematic, and repeated contractions.

The most important step in teaching pelvic muscle exercises is to help the client become aware of which muscle to exercise. During the pelvic examination in women and the rectal examination in men or women, instruct the client to tighten the pelvic muscles around your fingers. Then provide feedback about the strength of the contraction. Biofeedback devices, such as electromyography (EMG) or perineometers (see earlier discussion under Other Diagnostic Assessments), measure the strength of contraction. Retention of a vaginal weight is also evidence that the client

EVIDENCE-BASED PRACTICE for Nursing

Low tech is effective when reinforced by nurses

Goode, P., et al. (2003). Effect of behavioral training with or without pelvic floor electrical stimulation on stress incontinence in women. *Journal of the American Medical Association, 290*(3), 345-352.

The purpose of this prospective randomized controlled clinical trial was to determine whether pelvic floor electrical stimulation (PFES) could increase the efficacy of behavioral training for continence improvement among community-dwelling women with stress incontinence. The sample consisted of 200 women between 40 and 78 years of age with stress incontinence or mixed incontinence in which stress incontinence was dominant. Incontinence was confirmed with clinical evaluation and urodynamic studies. The subjects were randomly assigned to one of three treatment groups. One group received 8 weeks of behavioral training for pelvic floor exercises, including four visits from a nurse practitioner. A second group received the same 8-week behavioral training and additionally used PFES. The third group did not receive nurse-guided behavioral training or PFES; these subjects used a self-administered behavior training booklet for performing pelvic floor exercises. All subjects used bladder diaries throughout the study period to document episodes of incontinence. Evaluation of change in incontinence was determined by data in the bladder diaries and changes in urodynamic study results.

Of the 200 subjects who began the study, 155 completed the study. The group using the self-administered program had the highest attrition rate (37.3%) and the group receiving behavioral training plus PFES had the lowest attrition rate (11.9%). A significant reduction in incontinence was found across all groups (52.5% to 71.9%). Although greatest reduction was seen in the group receiving behavioral training plus PFES, it was not significantly different from the group receiving only the behavioral training. The investigators concluded that pelvic floor exercises are effective in improving pelvic muscle tone and reducing stress incontinence. They also concluded that having nurses teach, reinforce, and monitor behavior activities is a key factor in improving adherence to the behavioral intervention.

Level of Evidence: 2—Properly designed randomized controlled trial of appropriate size.

Critique. The study was well designed and used multiple objective measures as well as subjective measures to determine outcome. A major strength is the number of subjects. The study could have been strengthened by having a fourth group of subjects with stress incontinence who did not receive an intervention during the 8 weeks, but did receive four visits by a nurse.

Implications for Nursing. Stress incontinence is a common and costly problem for middle-aged and older women. Consistently and correctly performing pelvic floor exercises can reduce the severity of stress incontinence for many women; however, improvement is not immediate and requires adherence to the regimen. Nurses can provide the encouragement and recognition of positive advances to help women continue this therapeutic regimen. Nurses should ask about the presence of stress incontinence in all female clients older than 40 years of age and instruct clients in the correct techniques for progressive pelvic floor exercise.

has identified the proper muscle. The ability to start and stop the urine stream or stop the passage of flatus is evidence that the client has correctly identified the pelvic muscles.

Instructions for pelvic muscle exercises are given in Chart 73-8. Although improvement may take several months, most clients notice a positive change after 6 weeks. Teach clients to continue the exercises to maintain the improvement.

Diet Therapy. A diet plan for weight reduction is helpful for obese clients because stress incontinence is made worse by increased abdominal pressure from obesity. Instruct the client to avoid alcohol, nicotine, artificial sweeteners, citrus, and caffeine (bladder irritants). Refer the client to the dietitian as needed.

Drug Therapy. Because bladder pressure is greater than urethral resistance in clients with stress incontinence, drugs may be used to improve urethral resistance (Chart 73-9).

Estrogen is used to treat postmenopausal women with stress incontinence, although its exact mechanism of action is unknown. Estrogen may increase the blood flow and tone of the circumvaginal and periurethral muscles, thus improving the client's ability to contract those muscles during times of increased intra-abdominal stress.

Vaginal Cone Therapy. Vaginal cones are a set of five small, cone-shaped weights. They are of equal size but of varying weights and are used with pelvic muscle exercise. The woman inserts the lightest cone, labeled 1, into her vagina (Figure 73-1), with the string to the outside, for a 1-minute test period. If she can hold the first cone in place without its slipping out while she walks around, she proceeds to the second cone, labeled 2, and repeats the procedure. The client begins her treatment with the heaviest cone she can comfortably hold in her vagina for the 1-minute test period. Treatment periods are 15 minutes twice a day. When the client can comfortably hold the cone in her vagina for the 15-minute period, she progresses to the next heaviest weight. Treatment is completed with the cone labeled 5.

Weighted vaginal cones are helpful in strengthening the pelvic muscles and decreasing stress incontinence but may not help pelvic prolapse. Vaginal cones are available without prescription.

CHART 73-8

CLIENT EDUCATION GUIDE
Pelvic Muscle Exercises

- The pelvic muscles are composed of a sling of muscles that support your bladder, urethra, and vagina. Like any other muscles in your body, you can make your pelvic muscles stronger by alternately contracting (tightening) and relaxing them in regular exercise periods. By strengthening these muscles, you will be able to stop your urine flow more effectively.
- *To identify your pelvic muscles*, sit on the toilet with your feet flat on the floor about 12 inches apart. Begin to urinate, then try to stop the urine flow. Do not strain down, lift your bottom off the seat, or squeeze your legs together. When you start and stop your urine stream, you are using your pelvic muscles.
- *To perform pelvic muscle exercises*, tighten your pelvic muscles for a slow count of 10, then relax for a slow count of 10. Do this exercise 15 times while you are lying down, sitting up, and standing (a total of 45 exercises). Repeat, this time rapidly contracting and relaxing the pelvic muscles 10 times. This should take no more than 10 to 12 minutes for all three positions, or 3 to 4 minutes for each set of 15 exercises.
- Begin with 45 exercises a day in three sets of 15 exercises each. You will notice faster improvement if you can do this twice a day, or a total of 20 minutes each day. Remember to exercise in all three positions so your muscles learn to squeeze effectively despite your position. At first, it is helpful to have a designated time and place to do these exercises because you will have to concentrate to do them correctly. After you have been doing them for several weeks, you will notice improvement in your control of urine; however, many people report that improvement may take as long as 3 months.

CHART 73-9

DRUG THERAPY for Urinary Incontinence

Drug	Usual Dosage	Nursing Interventions	Rationales
Estrogen (Premarin, C.E.S.*)	0.3-1.25 mg PO daily 1-2 g every other day per vagina	Report any unusual vaginal bleeding or calf pain.	Estrogen use can increase the risk of endometrial cancer and thrombophlebitis.
Anticholinergics/antispasmodics Propantheline (Pro-Banthine, Propanthel*) Oxybutynin (Ditropan) (Ditropan XL) Dicyclomine hydrochloride (Bentyl, Di-Spaz, Bentylol*, Formulex*, Lomine*)	7.5-30 mg PO three to four times daily 2.5-5 mg PO three to four times daily 5-15 mg PO daily 10-20 mg PO three times daily	Check the client's intraocular pressure before starting the regimen. Offer fluids and hard candy to moisten the mouth. Give the drug between meals. Increase fluids and fiber in the client's diet.	Anticholinergics can increase intraocular pressure and are contraindicated in the presence of narrow-angle glaucoma. Anticholinergics cause extreme dryness of the mouth. Food interferes with absorption of the drug. Anticholinergics decreases GI motility and can cause constipation.
Tolterodine [1](Detrol) (Detrol LA)	2 mg PO twice daily 4 mg PO daily	Warn the client to check that daily urine output is equal to intake.	Drug can cause urinary retention.
Tricyclic antidepressants Imipramine (Tofranil, Novo-Pramine*)	25-100 mg PO daily	Administer the full dose at bedtime if possible and warn clients that dizziness may occur on arising in the morning.	Tricyclics have a high potential to cause postural hypotension.
Desipramine (Norpramin) Nortriptyline [2](Pamelor)	10-25 mg PO three times daily 10-25 mg PO three times daily	Warn clients about other anticholinergic and alpha-adrenergic side effects.	Tricyclics have a combination of anticholinergic and alpha-adrenergic effects.

[1]*Med Error Alert!* *Do not confuse with Detensol, a beta blocker.*

[2]*Med Error Alert!* *Do not confuse Pamelor with pamidronate, a drug used to prevent osteoporosis.*

A

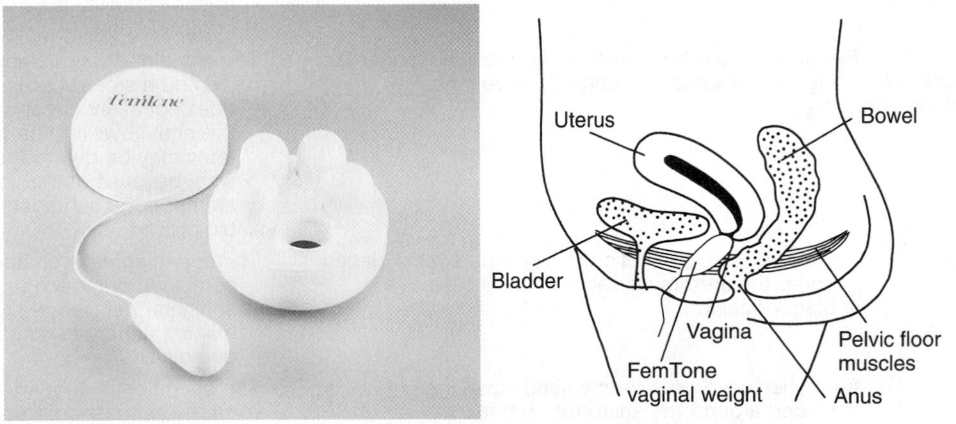

B

Figure 73-1 ■ **A,** FemTone vaginal weights, or cones. The number on the top of each cone represents increasing weight up to the heaviest cone, a 5. **B,** Diagram showing the correct positioning of a vaginal weight, or cone, in place. (**A** courtesy of ConvaTec, A Bristol-Meyers Squibb Company, a Division of E.R. Squibb & Sons, Inc., Princeton, NJ; **B** from ConvaTec. [1996]. FemTone vaginal weights: A training aid for pelvic floor exercises [brochure]. Princeton, NJ: Author.)

Other Therapy. Other interventions for stress incontinence include behavior modification, psychotherapy, and electrical stimulation devices to strengthen urethral contractions. Many intravaginal and intrarectal electrical stimulation devices have been used with varying degrees of success. More research is needed to determine the ideal level of stimulation and methods of reducing discomfort before electrical stimulation becomes a standard treatment for incontinence.

The Reliance insert is like a tiny tampon that the client inserts into the urethra. After insertion, the client inflates a tiny balloon, which rests at the bladder neck and prevents the flow of urine. To void, the client pulls a string to deflate the balloon and removes the device. The applicator is reusable, although the tampon part is disposed of after each void.

SURGICAL MANAGEMENT. Stress incontinence may be corrected by vaginal, abdominal, or retropubic surgeries. Success rates vary between 50% and 90% for most procedures, but these rates are difficult to evaluate because of the varying definitions of cure. Cure also may vary between short-term and long-term (over 5 years) results. Complications can be significant, with rates ranging from less than 2% for collagen or Siloxane injection to 50% for bladder neck suspension.

Preoperative Care. Teach the client about the procedure and clarify events surrounding the surgery. Extensive urodynamic testing (see Chapter 72) is often performed before surgery, and the need for such thorough assessment should be explained to the client.

Operative Procedures. The surgical procedures used for women include repositioning the urethra and bladder, changing the structure of the involved tissues, or inserting artificial devices to improve function (Table 73-4).

Postoperative Care. After surgery, assess for and intervene to prevent or detect complications. For prevention of movement or traction on the bladder neck, secure the urethral catheter with tape or a tube holder. If a suprapubic catheter is used instead of a urethral catheter, monitor the dressing for urine leakage and other drainage. Catheters are usually in place until the client can urinate easily and has postvoid residual urine of less than 50 mL. (See Chapters 20 and 22 for a discussion of general care before and after surgery.)

URGE URINARY INCONTINENCE

NOC **PLANNING: EXPECTED OUTCOMES.** The client with urinary incontinence is expected to use techniques to prevent or manage urge incontinence. Indicators include that the client often or consistently demonstrates the following behaviors:

- Responds to urge in a timely manner
- Gets to toilet between urge and passage of urine
- Avoids substances that stimulate the bladder (e.g., caffeine and alcohol)

INTERVENTIONS. Interventions for clients with urge incontinence or overactive bladder include behavioral

TABLE 73-4 Surgical Procedures for Stress Incontinence

Procedure	Purpose	Nursing Considerations
Anterior vaginal repair (colporrhaphy)	Elevates the urethral position and repairs any cystocele.	Because the operation is performed by vaginal incision, it is often done in conjunction with a vaginal hysterectomy. Recovery is usually rapid, and a urethral catheter is in place for 24-48 hr.
Retropubic suspension (Marshall-Marchetti-Krantz or Burch colposuspension)	Elevates the urethral position and provides longer-lasting results.	The operation requires a low abdominal incision and a urethral or suprapubic catheter for several days postoperatively. Recovery takes longer, and urinary retention and detrusor instability are the most frequent complications.
Needle bladder neck suspension (Pereyra or Stamey procedure)	Elevates the urethral position and provides longer-lasting results without a long operative time.	The combined vaginal approach with a needle and a small suprapubic skin incision does not allow direct vision of the operative site; however, the high complication rates may be due to the selection of clients who, because of their medical condition, are not good candidates for longer retropubic procedures.
Pubovaginal sling procedures	A sling made of synthetic or fascial material is placed under the urethrovesical junction to elevate the bladder neck.	The operation uses an abdominal, vaginal, or combined approach to treat intrinsic sphincter deficiencies. Temporary or permanent urinary retention is common postoperatively.
Artificial sphincters	A mechanical device to open and close the urethra is placed around the anatomic urethra.	The operation is done more frequently in men. The most common complications include mechanical failure of the device, erosion of tissue, and infection.
Periurethral injection of collagen or Siloxane	Implantation of small amounts of an inert substance through several small injections provides support around the bladder neck.	The procedure can be done in an ambulatory care setting and can be repeated as often as necessary. Certain compounds may migrate after injection; an allergy test to bovine collagen must be performed before implantation.

Data from Schultz, J.A., & Drutz, H.P. (1999). The surgical management of recurrent urinary stress incontinence. *Current Opinions in Obstetrics and Gynecology, 11*(5), 489-494; and Lighter, D.J., & Itano, N.M. (1999). Treatment options for women with stress urinary incontinence. *Mayo Clinic Proceedings, 74*(11), 1149-1156.

interventions and drugs (Newman & Giovannini, 2002). Surgery is not the recommended treatment of this condition. Collection devices and absorbent pads and undergarments may be used.

Drug Therapy. Because the hypertonic bladder contracts involuntarily in clients with urge incontinence, drugs that relax the smooth muscle and increase the bladder's capacity are prescribed (see Chart 73-9).

The most effective drugs are anticholinergics, such as propantheline (Pro-Banthine, Propanthel✽), and anticholinergics with smooth muscle relaxant properties, such as oxybutynin (Ditropan and Ditropan XL), tolterodine (Detrol and Detrol LA), and dicyclomine hydrochloride (Bentyl, Formulex✽, Spasmoban✽, Viscerol✽). This class of drugs has serious side effects and is used in conjunction with behavioral interventions. These drugs inhibit the nerve fibers that stimulate bladder contraction. Tricyclic antidepressants with anticholinergic and alpha-adrenergic agonist activity, such as imipramine (Tofranil, Novopramine✽), have been used successfully. The effectiveness of other drugs, such as flavoxate (Urispas) and the antihistamines, nonsteroidal anti-inflammatory agents, beta-adrenergic agonists, and calcium channel blockers, have yet to be determined.

Diet Therapy. Instruct the client to avoid foods that have a direct bladder-stimulating or diuretic effect, such as caffeine and alcohol. Spacing fluids at regular intervals throughout the day (e.g., 120 mL every hour or 240 mL every 2 hours) and limiting fluids after the dinner hour (e.g., only 120 mL at bedtime) help avoid fluid overload on the bladder and allow urine to accumulate at a steady pace.

Behavioral Interventions. Behavioral interventions for urge incontinence include bladder training, habit training, exercise therapy, and electrical stimulation.

NIC interventions for urinary bladder training and urinary habit training are listed in Chart 73-10. It can be difficult for clients to use these interventions because they involve a significant amount of client participation. Provide ongoing encouragement, clarification, and support to maxi-

CHART 73-10

NIC **INTERVENTION ACTIVITIES for**
The Client with Urinary Incontinence

Urinary Bladder Training: *Improving bladder function for those with urge incontinence by increasing the bladder's ability to hold urine and the client's ability to suppress urination*

- Determine ability to recognize urge to void.
- Keep a continence specification record for 3 days to establish voiding pattern.
- Establish interval of initial toileting schedule, based on voiding pattern.
- Establish beginning and ending time for toileting schedule, if not for 24 hours.
- Establish interval for toileting of not less than 1 hour and preferably not less than 2 hours.
- Toilet client or remind client to void at prescribed intervals.
- Provide privacy for toileting.
- Use power of suggestion (e.g., running water or flushing toilet) to assist client to void.
- Avoid leaving client on toilet for more than 5 minutes.
- Reduce toileting interval by one half hour if there are more than three incontinence episodes in 24 hours.
- Increase toileting interval by 1 hour if client has no incontinence episodes for 3 days until optimal 4-hour interval is achieved.
- Teach the client to consciously hold urine until the scheduled toileting time.
- Discuss daily record of continence with client to provide reinforcement.

Urinary Habit Training: *Establishing a predictable pattern of bladder emptying to prevent incontinence for persons with limited cognitive ability who have urge, stress, or functional incontinence.*

- Keep a continence specification record for 3 days to establish voiding pattern.
- Establish interval of initial toileting schedule, based on voiding pattern and usual routine (e.g., eating, rising, and retiring).
- Establish beginning and ending time for the toileting schedule, if not for 24 hours.
- Establish interval for toileting of preferably not less than 2 hours.
- Assist client to toilet and prompt to void at prescribed intervals.
- Provide privacy for toileting.
- Use power of suggestion (e.g., running water or flushing toilet) to assist client to void.
- Avoid leaving the client on toilet for more than 5 minutes.
- Reduce toileting interval by one half hour if there are more than two incontinence episodes in 24 hours.
- Maintain toileting interval if there are two or fewer incontinence episodes in 24 hours.
- Increase the toileting interval by one half hour if client has no incontinence episodes in 48 hours until optimal 4-hour interval is achieved.
- Discuss daily record of continence with staff to provide reinforcement and encourage compliance with toileting schedule.
- Maintain scheduled toileting to assist in establishing and maintaining voiding habit.
- Give positive feedback or positive reinforcement (e.g., 5 minutes of social conversation) to client when he/she voids at scheduled toileting times, and make no comment when client is incontinent.

Urinary Catheterization: *Intermittent: Regular periodic use of a catheter to empty the bladder*

- Teach client/family purpose, supplies, method, and rationale of intermittent catheterization.
- Teach client/family clean intermittent catheterization technique.
- Provide quiet private room for the procedure.
- Demonstrate procedure and have a return demonstration, as appropriate.
- Determine catheterization schedule based on comprehensive urinary assessment.
- Adjust frequency of catheterization to maintain output of 300 cc or less.
- Maintain client on prophylactic antibacterial therapy for 2 to 3 weeks at initiation of intermittent catheterization, as appropriate.
- Complete a urinalysis about every 2 weeks to 1 month.
- Establish a catheterization schedule based on individual needs.
- Maintain a detailed record of catheterization schedule, fluid intake, and output.
- Teach client/family signs and symptoms of urinary tract infection.
- Monitor color, odor, and clarity of urine.

NIC intervention activities selected from Dochterman, J.M., & Bulechek, G.M. (Eds.). (2004). *Nursing interventions classification (NIC)* (4th ed.). St. Louis: Mosby.

mize the effects of all interventions. Behavioral interventions are often combined with drug therapy for maximal effect.

Bladder Training. Bladder training is an education program for the client that begins with a thorough explanation of the problem of urge incontinence. Instead of the bladder being in control of the client, the client learns to control the bladder. For the program to succeed, he or she must be alert, aware, and able to resist the urge to urinate.

Start a schedule for voiding, beginning with the longest interval that is comfortable for the client, even if the interval is only 30 minutes. Instruct the client to void every 30 minutes and to ignore any urge to urinate between the mandated intervals. Once the client is comfortable with the initial schedule, increase the interval by 15 to 30 minutes. Instruct the client to follow the new schedule until success is again achieved. As the interval increases, the bladder gradually tolerates more volume. Teach the client relaxation and distraction techniques to maximize success in the retraining. Provide positive reinforcement for maintaining the prescribed schedule.

Habit Training. Habit training (scheduled toileting) is a type of bladder training that is successful in reducing incontinence in cognitively impaired clients. To use habit training, caregivers assist the client in voiding at specific times (e.g., every 2 hours on the even hours). The goal is to get the client to the toilet before incontinence occurs. There is no effort to increase bladder capacity by gradually lengthening the voiding intervals.

Prompted voiding, a supplement to habit training, attempts to increase the client's awareness of the need to void and to prompt him or her to ask for toileting assistance. Habit training otherwise relies completely on a time schedule.

Exercise Therapy. Pelvic muscle exercises for urge incontinence have been helpful and are taught in the same way as for stress incontinence (see Chart 73-8). Improved urethral resistance helps the client overcome abnormal detrusor contractions long enough to get to the toilet.

Electrical Stimulation. Many different intravaginal and intrarectal electrical stimulation devices are available to treat both urge and stress incontinence.

REFLEX URINARY INCONTINENCE

NOC **PLANNING: EXPECTED OUTCOMES.** With appropriate intervention, the client with urinary incontinence is expected to achieve continence. Indicators include that the client often or consistently demonstrates the following behaviors:

- Recognizes the urge to void
- Maintains a predictable pattern of voiding
- Responds to urge in a timely manner
- Empties bladder completely
- Keeps urine volume in the bladder within normal limits to prevent bladder overdistention

INTERVENTIONS. Interventions for the client with reflex (overflow) incontinence caused by obstruction of the bladder outlet may include surgery to relieve the obstruction. The most common surgical procedures are prostate removal (see Chapter 79) and repair of genital prolapse (see Chapter 78). For overflow incontinence related to detrusor muscle weakness, the most effective method of treatment is intermittent catheterization. Behavioral interventions such as bladder compression and intermittent self-catheterization are the primary management techniques for urinary retention with overflow incontinence.

Drug Therapy. Drugs are prescribed for short-term management of urinary retention, often after surgery. They are not used in long-term management of overflow incontinence caused by a hypotonic bladder. The most commonly used drug is bethanechol chloride (Urecholine), an agent that increases bladder pressure.

Behavioral Interventions. The most common behavioral interventions are bladder compression and intermittent self-catheterization.

Bladder Compression. Techniques that promote bladder emptying include the Credé method, the Valsalva maneuver, double-voiding, and splinting.

In the Credé method, instruct the client in external compression of the urinary bladder or parasympathetic stimulation via tugging at pubic hair or massaging the genital area. These techniques manually assist the bladder in emptying. In the Valsalva maneuver, breathing techniques increase intrathoracic and intra-abdominal pressure. This increased pressure is then directed toward the bladder during exhalation. With the technique of double-voiding, the client empties the bladder and then, within a few minutes, attempts a second bladder emptying.

For women who have a large cystocele (prolapse of the bladder into the vagina), a technique called *splinting* both compresses the bladder and moves it into a better position. The woman inserts her fingers into her vagina, gently pushes the cystocele back into the vagina, and begins to urinate.

Intermittent Self-Catheterization. NIC interventions for intermittent urinary catheterization are listed in Chart 73-10. Teach intermittent self-catheterization to clients with long-term problems of incomplete bladder emptying. Self-catheterization is effective and can be learned fairly easily. The following points are important in teaching this technique:

- Proper handwashing and cleaning of the catheter reduce the frequency of infection.
- A small lumen and good lubrication of the catheter prevent urethral trauma.
- A regular schedule for bladder emptying prevents bladder overdistention and mucosal trauma.

Clients must be able to understand instructions and have the manual dexterity to manipulate the catheter. Caregivers or family members in the home can also be taught to perform straight catheterization using a clean (rather than sterile) technique with good outcomes.

FUNCTIONAL URINARY INCONTINENCE

NOC **PLANNING: EXPECTED OUTCOMES.** The client with functional urinary incontinence is expected to remain dry. Indicators include that the client often or consistently demonstrates the following behaviors:

- Uses urine containment or collection measures to ensure dryness
- Manages clothing independently

INTERVENTIONS. Causes of functional (or chronic intractable) incontinence vary greatly; some are reversible, and others are not. The focus of intervention is treatment of reversible causes. When incontinence is not reversible, urinary habit training (see Habit Training, p. 1694) is used to establish a predictable pattern of bladder emptying to prevent incontinence. A final strategy focuses on containment of the urine and protection of the client's skin. Nonsurgical interventions include applied devices, containment, and catheterization.

Applied Devices. Applied devices include intravaginal pessaries for women and penile clamps for men. The intravaginal pessary supports the uterus and vagina and helps maintain the correct position of the bladder. (See Chapter 78 for further discussion of pessaries.) The penile clamp is applied externally to compress the urethra and prevent leakage of urine.

The dangers of pessaries and penile clamps include damage to the tissues and infection from constant pressure in sensitive areas. Both devices require either that the client have manual dexterity or that a caregiver applies and removes the device. Instruct the client or caregivers in the use of these devices. Male clients may use an external collecting device, such as a condom catheter. Design of an effective external collecting device for women has not been as successful.

Containment. Absorbent pads and briefs are designed to collect urine and keep the client's skin and clothing dry. Many types and sizes of pads are available:

- Shields or liners inserted inside a panty
- Undergarments consisting of full-sized pads with waist straps
- Plastic-lined protective underpants with or without elastic legs
- Combination pad and pant systems
- Absorbent bed pads

A major concern with the use of protective pads is the risk that skin breakdown will occur. Materials and costs vary. Some are reusable; others are disposable. The disposal of these products raises ecologic concerns. Avoid use of the word "diaper" when discussing these adult protective pants, however, because of the usual association of diapers with babies.

Urinary Catheterization. Catheterization for control of incontinence may be intermittent or involve an indwelling catheter. Intermittent catheterization is preferred to an indwelling catheter because of the reduced risk for infection. Indwelling urinary catheters should be used temporarily and only when all other interventions have been unsuccessful. A long-term indwelling urinary catheter is appropriate for clients with skin breakdown who need a dry environment for healing, clients who are terminally ill and need comfort, and clients who are critically ill and require careful measurement of urine output.

MIXED OR TOTAL URINARY INCONTINENCE

Mixed or total urinary incontinence is a combination of two or more types of involuntary urine loss syndromes. For example, stress incontinence and urge incontinence often occur together in perimenopausal and postmenopausal women. For the client with mixed or total incontinence, combinations of assessment techniques (as discussed under each syndrome) are used. Interventions are similarly combined to promote continence. The problems and interventions for mixed incontinence are the same as they are for each specific type of incontinence separately. After identifying the specific types of incontinence experienced by the client with mixed incontinence, apply the appropriate nursing diagnoses, collaborative problems, interventions, and expected outcomes discussed earlier with each incontinence type.

> *Critical Thinking Challenge*
>
> Your older client in assistive living (previously described) is diagnosed with mixed stress and urge incontinence. Her environment has no barriers to toileting. She has been prescribed to take tolterodine (Detrol) for her urge incontinence. Additionally, she is to use vaginal cones for improving her pelvic floor muscles for the stress incontinence. She tells you she isn't sure she should be touching herself "down there."
>
> 1. What should you teach her about the effects and side effects of her newly prescribed drug?
> 2. How could she strengthen her pelvic floor muscles without touching herself?
> 3. How can you help evaluate this client's response to exercise and the prescribed drug to improve continence?

evolve For suggested answer guidelines, go to http://evolve.elsevier.com/Iggy/.

Community-Based Care

Community-based care for the client with urinary incontinence considers his or her personal, physical, emotional, and social resources. Important personal resources for self-care include mobility, vision, and manual dexterity. When planning care, consider who will be the primary caregiver and what factors may influence the effectiveness of the plan.

HOME CARE MANAGEMENT

Assess the home environment for barriers that impede access to the toileting facilities. Eliminate hazards that might slow walking or contribute to injury. These hazards might include small area rugs (throw rugs), tables or chairs with legs that extend into the walking area, slippery waxed or polished floors, and inadequate lighting.

If the client must climb stairs to reach a bathroom, handrails should be installed and stairs should be kept free of obstacles. Toilet seat extenders may help provide the right level of seating so that maximal abdominal pressure may be applied to encourage voiding. Portable commodes may be obtained for homes in which ambulatory access to toilets is impractical or impossible. Physical and occupational therapists are valuable resources for assisting with home care management.

HEALTH TEACHING

Teach the client and family about the cause of the specific type of incontinence and discuss available treatment options for its management. The teaching plan addresses the prescribed drugs (purpose, dosage, method and route of administration, and expected and potential side effects). Instruct the client and family about the importance of weight reduction and dietary modification to help control urinary incontinence.

When external devices or protective pads are needed, describe the possible options, discuss the advantages and disadvantages of each, and help the client make a selection that considers lifestyle and resources. For clients who will use intermittent catheterization or those with artificial urinary sphincters, demonstrate the correct technique to the client or caregiver. Evaluate return demonstrations for correct technique. Chart 73-11 also addresses teaching.

PSYCHOSOCIAL PREPARATION

The embarrassment of incontinence can be devastating to a client's self-esteem, body image, and interpersonal relationships. The unpredictability of incontinence creates anxiety. Clients are often embarrassed to seek help, and even when resources are identified, they may need assistance to feel

CHART 73-11

CLIENT EDUCATION GUIDE
Urinary Incontinence

- Maintain a normal body weight to reduce the pressure on your bladder.
- Do not try to control your incontinence by limiting your fluid intake. Adequate fluid intake is necessary for kidney function and health maintenance.
- If you have a catheter in your bladder, follow the instructions given to you about maintaining the sterile drainage system.
- If you are discharged with a suprapubic catheter in your bladder, inspect the entry site for the tube daily, clean the skin around the opening gently with warm soap and water, and place a sterile gauze dressing on the skin around the tube. Report any redness, swelling, drainage, or fever to your physician.
- Do not put anything into your vagina, such as tampons, medications, hygiene products, or exercise weights, until you check with your physician at your 6-week checkup after surgery.
- Do not have sexual intercourse until after your 6-week postoperative checkup.
- Do not lift or carry anything heavier than 5 lb or participate in any strenuous exercise until your physician gives you postoperative clearance. In some cases, this could be as long as 3 months.
- Avoid exercises, such as running, jogging, step or dance aerobic classes, rowing, cross-country ski or stair-climber machines, and mountain biking. Brisk walking without any additional hand, leg, or body weights is allowed. Swimming is allowed after all drains and catheters have been removed and your incision is completely healed.
- If Kegel exercises are recommended, ask your nurse for specific instructions.

comfortable in using the resources. Even buying supplies at a local store can be a threat to their privacy.

Accept and acknowledge the personal concerns of the client and caregiver. Never minimize the concerns or make them seem trivial. Help the client learn methods of controlling or managing the fear or anxiety. As the client learns the specifics of the plan that will allow control of urinary incontinence, the confidence to resume social interactions should return.

HEALTH CARE RESOURCES

Referral to home care agencies for help with personal care and to continence clinics that specialize in evaluation and treatment may be helpful. In many continence clinics, nurses collaborate with physicians and other health care professionals to evaluate and manage clients. The treatment plan is specific for each client; supplies and products are custom selected.

Clients may benefit from education and from the support of others who experience similar concerns. The National Association for Continence (NAFC) (http://www.nafc.org), Access to Continence Care and Treatment (http://www.wellweb.com/INCONT/acct/contents.htm), and the Wound, Ostomy, and Continence Nurses (http://www.wocn.org) publish newsletters and educational materials written with simple, easy-to-understand explanations. The American Foundation for Urologic Disease (http://www.afud.com) provides information on several areas of bladder dysfunction. The Agency for Healthcare Research and Quality (AHRQ) has also published a caregiver guide (AHCPR Publication No. 96-0683) for the public that is available on the Internet or by calling (800) 358-9295. Local hospitals, in collaboration with the NAFC, may conduct local support groups.

Evaluation: Outcomes

Evaluate the care of the client with urinary incontinence on the basis of the identified nursing diagnoses. The expected outcomes are that the client will:

- Describe the type of urinary incontinence experienced
- Demonstrate knowledge of proper use of medications and correct procedures for self-catheterization, use of the artificial sphincter, or care of an indwelling urinary catheter
- Demonstrate effective use of the selected exercise or bladder training program
- Select and use incontinence devices and products
- Have a reduction in the number of incontinence episodes

Specific indicators for these outcomes are listed for each nursing diagnosis under the Planning and Implementation section (see earlier).

Urolithiasis

PATHOPHYSIOLOGY

Urolithiasis is the presence of calculi (stones) in the urinary tract. Stones are often asymptomatic until they pass into the lower urinary tract, where they can cause excruciating pain. **Nephrolithiasis** is the formation of stones in the kidney. Formation of stones in the ureter is **ureterolithiasis.**

Urologic stones are caused by many metabolic disorders. However, the exact mechanism of stone formation is not entirely understood. Everyone excretes crystals in the urine at some time, but fewer than 10% of people form stones. About 75% of stones contain calcium as one part of the stone complex, which may be calcium oxalate or calcium phosphate. Struvite (15%), uric acid (8%), and cystine (3%) make up the less common stones.

Formation of stones seems to involve three conditions:

- Slow urine flow, resulting in supersaturation of the urine with the particular element (such as calcium) that first becomes crystallized and later becomes the stone
- Damage to the lining of the urinary tract (i.e., from crystals)
- Decreased inhibitor substances in the urine that would otherwise prevent supersaturation and crystal aggregation

High urine acidity (as with uric acid and cystine stones) or alkalinity (as with calcium phosphate and struvite stones) as well as drugs (as with triamterene, indinavir, and acetazolamide) contribute to stone formation.

One example of a metabolic problem causing stone formation begins when excessive amounts of calcium are absorbed through the intestinal tract (the most common cause of hypercalciuria). As blood circulates through the kidneys, the excess calcium is filtered into the urine, causing supersaturation of calcium in the urine. If fluid intake is inadequate, such as when a client is dehydrated, supersaturation is more likely to occur, and the risk for calcium combining with another compound to form a larger molecule increases. Calcium complexes often serve as a center for other deposits, and eventually a stone forms.

TABLE 73-5 Metabolic Defects That Commonly Cause Calculi

Metabolic Deficit	Etiology
Hypercalcemia	
Primary	Absorptive: increased intestinal calcium absorption Renal: decreased renal tubular excretion of calcium
Secondary	Resorptive: hyperparathyroidism, vitamin D intoxication, renal tubular acidosis, prolonged immobilization
Hyperoxaluria	
Primary	Genetic: autosomal recessive trait resulting in high oxalate production
Secondary	Dietary: excess oxalate from foods such as spinach, rhubarb, Swiss chard, cocoa, beets, wheat germ, pecans, peanuts, okra, chocolate, and lime peel
Hyperuricemia	
Primary	Gout is an inherited disorder of purine metabolism (20% of clients with gout have uric acid calculi)
Secondary	Increased production or decreased clearance of purine from myeloproliferative disorders, thiazide diuretics, carcinoma
Struvite	Made of magnesium ammonium phosphate and carbonate apatite; formed by urea splitting by bacteria, most commonly, *Proteus mirabilis;* needs an alkaline urine to form
Cystinuria	Autosomal recessive defect of amino acid metabolism that precipitates insoluble cystine crystals in the urine

Stones that form in the kidney and then pass into the ureter often lodge in the ureteropelvic angle, the aortoiliac bend, or the ureterovesical angle. When the stone occludes the ureter and blocks the flow of urine, the ureter dilates. Enlargement of the ureter is called **hydroureter**.

The pain associated with ureteral spasm is excruciating and may cause the client to go into shock from stimulation of nearby sympathetic nerves. In addition, **hematuria** (bloody urine) may result from damage to the urothelial lining. If the obstruction is not removed, urinary stasis can cause infection and impair kidney function on the side of the blockage. As the blockage persists, **hydronephrosis** (enlargement of the kidney caused by blockage of urine lower in the tract and filling of the kidney with urine) and permanent kidney damage may develop.

Etiology and Genetic Risk

The cause of urolithiasis is unknown. At least 90% of clients who form stones have a metabolic risk factor. Table 73-5 lists some metabolic defects that commonly cause stone formation.

A diet high in calcium is not believed to cause stones unless a metabolic defect or renal tubular defect already exists. Data suggest that a normal-calcium diet that is relatively low in animal protein, salt, or both may be effective in preventing stone formation. A low calcium diet does not prevent stone formation (Borghi et al., 2002). Urinary stasis, urinary retention, immobilization, and dehydration all contribute to a stone-forming environment. Except for the use of the thiazides for calcium oxalate stones, diuretics can cause volume depletion and thus may promote the formation of stones.

Genetic Considerations

More than 30 genetic variations are associated with the formation of renal stones (Danpure, 2000). Single gene disorders are rare. More commonly, nephrolithiasis is a complex disease, with genetic variation in intestinal calcium absorption, renal calcium transport, or renal phosphate transport all associated with stone formation (Frick & Bushinsky, 2003).

Incidence/Prevalence

The incidence of stone disease is high and varies with geographic location, race, and family history. About 12% of adults will have at least one episode of renal stone disease. The incidence is higher in men; however, struvite stones are twice as common in women. Recurrence rates vary depending on the type of treatment. The recurrence rate of untreated calcium oxalate stones is 35% to 50% in 5 to 10 years. A higher recurrence of stones occurs in clients with a family history of stone disease and in those who had their first occurrence by age 25 years.

CULTURAL CONSIDERATIONS

The incidence of stone disease is most common in the southeastern United States, Japan, and Western Europe. Calcium stone disease is more common in men than in women and tends to occur in young adults or during early middle adulthood. Kidney stone disease occurs more often in younger adults than older adults and more commonly among white individuals. For clients in these higher-risk groups, nursing care should include teaching family members, as well as clients, about the manifestations of a stone and interventions to reduce stone formation.

COLLABORATIVE MANAGEMENT

Assessment

HISTORY

Ask the client about a personal or family history of urologic stones. Obtain a diet history, including fluid intake patterns. If the client has a history of stone formation, ask about past treatment, whether chemical analysis of the stone was performed, and what preventive measures are followed.

PHYSICAL ASSESSMENT/CLINICAL MANIFESTATIONS

The major manifestation of stones is severe pain, commonly called **renal colic.** Flank pain suggests that the stone is in the kidney or upper ureter. Flank pain that radiates abdominally or into the scrotum and testes or the vulva suggests that stones are in the ureters or bladder. Pain is most intense when the stone is moving or when the ureter is obstructed.

Renal colic begins suddenly and is often described as "unbearable." Nausea, vomiting, pallor, and diaphoresis often accompany the pain. A large stationary stone in the kidney (staghorn calculus), however, rarely causes much pain because it is not moving. Frequency and dysuria occur when a stone reaches the bladder. **Oliguria** (scant urine output) or **anuria** (absence of urine output) suggests obstruction, possibly at the bladder neck or urethra. *Urinary tract obstruction is an emergency and must be treated immediately to preserve kidney function.*

Examine the client to detect bladder distention. The client may appear pale, ashen, and diaphoretic, and suffer from excruciating pain. Vital signs may be moderately elevated with pain; body temperature and pulse are elevated with infection. Blood pressure may decrease if the severe pain causes shock.

LABORATORY ASSESSMENT

Urinalysis is performed in clients with suspected calculi. Hematuria is a common finding; blood may make the urine appear smoky or rusty. RBCs are usually caused by stone-induced direct trauma on the lining of the ureter, bladder, or urethra. WBCs and bacteria may be present as a result of urinary stasis. Increased turbidity and odor are manifestations of infection that may accompany urolithiasis Microscopic examination of the urine may identify crystals from which stones could form. Urinary pH is measured to determine acidity or alkalinity.

The serum WBC count is elevated with infection. Increases in the serum calcium, serum phosphate, or serum uric acid levels indicate excess minerals are present and may contribute to stone formation.

RADIOGRAPHIC ASSESSMENT

Stones are easily seen on x-rays of the kidneys, ureters, and bladder (KUB) (Figure 73-2), or on intravenous (IV) pyelograms, computed tomography (CT) scans, or magnetic resonance imaging (MRI) scans. Noncontrast helical CT has the highest sensitivity for the identification of urinary tract stones (Portis & Sudaram, 2001). These procedures confirm the presence and location of the stones.

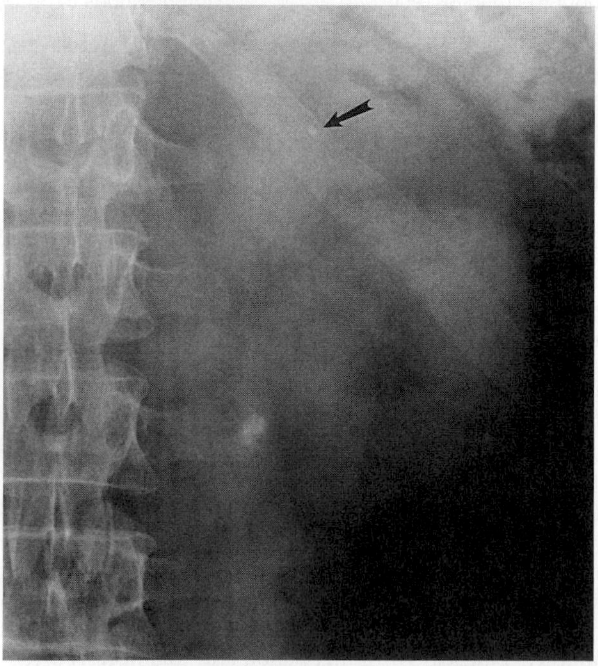

Figure 73-2 ■ Urinary stones on x-ray of the kidneys, ureters, and bladder (KUB). (From Pollack, H.M. [2000]. Clinical urography [2nd ed.] Philadelphia: W.B. Saunders.)

IV pyelography is useful for identifying whether urinary tract obstruction is present. However, because of the risk of acute renal failure induced by contrast dye, other diagnostic tests may be chosen for high-risk clients (older adults and clients with diabetes mellitus, multiple myeloma, or elevated serum creatinine levels). CT or MRI is needed to identify cystine or uric acid stones, neither of which can be seen on x-ray.

OTHER DIAGNOSTIC ASSESSMENTS

Renal ultrasonography creates images from sound waves. Structures of varying density are imaged. Solid structures, such as stones, are extremely dense; therefore the images of stones are clear. Small stones are harder to identify and locate.

Common Nursing Diagnoses and Collaborative Problems

Nursing diagnoses that may apply to clients with urolithiasis include the following:

- Acute Pain related to presence of stone in the urinary tract
- Deficient Knowledge (risk factors for stone formation) related to information misinterpretation and unfamiliarity with information resources
- Fear related to potential recurrence of the stone
- Risk for Infection related to trauma of the ureter, bladder, or urethra lining
- Risk for Injury (renal) related to obstruction

Interventions

Nursing interventions focus on pain management and prevention of infection and urinary obstruction. Most clients can expel the stone without invasive procedures. The most important factors regarding whether a stone will pass on its own are its composition, size, and location. The larger the stone and the higher up in the urinary tract it is, the less likely it is to be passed. Other interventions may be needed when the client does not pass the stone spontaneously (Portis & Sudaram, 2001) (Figure 73-3).

PAIN RELIEF MEASURES

Nonsurgical and surgical approaches are used to assist the client with a kidney stone in achieving an acceptable degree of pain relief.

NONSURGICAL MANAGEMENT. Nonsurgical measures to relieve pain include strategies to enhance stone passing as well as direct pain management.

Drug Therapy. Pain is usually most severe in the first 24 to 36 hours. Opioid analgesics are often needed to control the severe pain caused by stones in the urinary tract. Opioid agents, such as morphine sulfate (Statex✱), are often given IV to ensure prompt and adequate absorption. Nonsteroidal anti-inflammatory drugs (NSAIDs) such as ketorolac (Toradol) in the acute phase may be quite effective. The antiplatelet effects of NSAIDs are a contraindication to the use of extracorporeal shock wave lithotripsy.

Control of pain is more effective when drugs are given at regularly scheduled intervals or via a constant delivery system (e.g., skin patch) instead of as needed (PRN). Spasmolytic drugs, such as oxybutynin chloride (Ditropan) and propantheline bromide (Pro-Banthine, Propanthel✱), are important for the relief and control of pain (see Chart 73-9). Give the drugs and assess the response by asking the client to rate the discomfort on a rating scale.

Complementary and Alternative Therapy. Relaxation techniques, such as hypnosis and imagery, therapeutic or healing touch, and acupuncture, can relieve pain. Clients often have difficulty finding a comfortable position in which to relax. Thus assisting the client with positioning can often aid in relaxation. Breathing techniques, such as those used in childbirth, can also help clients relax.

Other Management Techniques. Avoiding overhydration and underhydration in the acute phase helps make the spontaneous passage of a stone less painful. Strain the urine to monitor for stone passage. Send any stone passed to the laboratory for analysis because preventive therapy is based on stone composition.

Lithotripsy. Lithotripsy, also known as extracorporeal shock wave lithotripsy (ESWL), is the use of sound, laser, or dry shock wave energies to break the stone into small fragments. The client receives conscious sedation and lies on a flat table with the lithotriptor aimed at the stone, which is located by fluoroscopy. A local anesthetic cream is applied to the skin site over the stone 45 minutes before the procedure. During the procedure, cardiac rhythm is monitored by electrocardiography (ECG), and the shock waves are delivered in synchrony with the R wave. About 500 to 1500 shock waves are applied in 30 to 45 minutes. Continuous ECG monitoring for dysrhythmia and fluoroscopic observation for stone destruction are maintained.

After lithotripsy, strain the urine to monitor the passage of stone fragments. Some bruising may occur on the flank of the affected side after extracorporeal shock wave lithotripsy (ESWL). Occasionally a stent is placed in the ureter before ESWL to ease passage of the stone fragments. Cystine stones are often resistant to ESWL.

SURGICAL MANAGEMENT. Minimally invasive surgical and open surgical procedures are indicated if urinary obstruction occurs or if the stone is too large to be passed spontaneously.

Minimally Invasive Surgical Procedures. Minimally invasive surgical (MIS) procedures include stenting, retrograde ureteroscopy, and percutaneous ureterolithotomy and nephrolithotomy.

Stenting. A **stent** is a small tube that is placed in the ureter by ureteroscopy. The stent dilates the ureter and enlarges the passageway for the stone or stone fragments. This procedure prevents the passing stone from coming in contact with the ureteral mucosa, thereby reducing pain. A Foley catheter may be placed to facilitate passage of the stone through the urethra.

Retrograde Ureteroscopy. Retrograde ureteroscopy is an endoscopic procedure. The ureteroscope is passed through the urethra and bladder into the ureter. Once the stone is seen, it is removed using grasping baskets, forceps, or loops. Lithotripsy also can be performed through the ureteroscope. A Foley catheter may be placed to facilitate passage of the stone fragments through the urethra.

Percutaneous Ureterolithotomy and Nephrolithotomy. The client lies prone or laterally and receives local or general anesthesia. The physician identifies the ideal entry point with fluoroscopy and then passes a needle into the collecting system of the kidney. Once a tract has been made in the kidney, other equipment, such as an **intracorporeal** (inside the body) ultrasonic or laser lithotriptor, can be used to break up and remove the stone. An endoscope with a special attachment to grasp and extract the stone can be used. Often a nephrostomy tube is left in place at first to prevent the stone fragments from passing through the normal urinary tract.

Provide routine nephrostomy tube care and monitor the client for complications after the procedure. Complications include bleeding at the site or through the tube, pneumothorax, and infection.

Open Surgical Procedures. When other stone removal attempts have failed, or when risk of a lasting injury

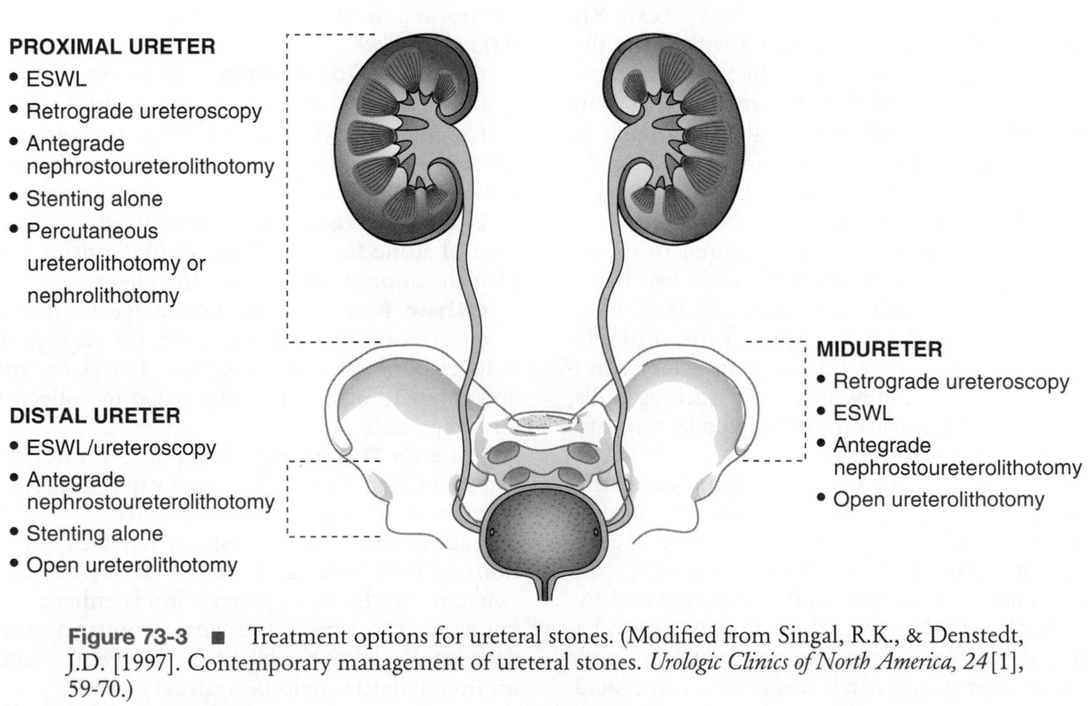

Figure 73-3 ■ Treatment options for ureteral stones. (Modified from Singal, R.K., & Denstedt, J.D. [1997]. Contemporary management of ureteral stones. *Urologic Clinics of North America, 24*[1], 59-70.)

to the ureter or kidney is possible, an open ureterolithotomy (into the ureter), pyelolithotomy (into the kidney pelvis), or nephrolithotomy (into the kidney) procedure may be indicated. These procedures are used for a large or impacted stone.

Preoperative Care. Prepare the client for the selected procedure by explaining how, when, and where the procedure will be performed. Describe what the client can expect to see, hear, and feel before and after the procedure. The client is given nothing by mouth and also receives preoperative bowel preparation. (See Chapter 20 for routine care before surgery.)

Operative Procedures. The retroperitoneal area is entered through a large flank incision, as for nephrectomy (see Chapter 74), pyelolithotomy, or nephrolithotomy, and through a lower abdominal incision for ureterolithotomy. The urinary tract is entered surgically and the stone is removed. Before closure, tubes and drains may be placed (e.g., nephrostomy tube, ureteral stent, Penrose or other wound drainage device, and Foley catheter).

Postoperative Care. Follow routine procedures for assessment of the client who has received anesthesia. (See Chapter 22 for routine care after surgery.) Monitor the amount of bleeding from incisions and in the urine. Maintain adequate fluid intake. Strain the urine to monitor the passage of stone fragments. Teach the client how to prevent future stones through dietary changes.

PREVENTION OF INFECTION

Control of infections before invasive and noninvasive procedures is critical for the prevention of urosepsis. Interventions include giving appropriate antibiotics, either to eliminate an existing infection or to prevent new infections, and the maintenance of adequate nutrition and fluid intake. Because infection always occurs with struvite stone formation, the health care team plans for long-term infection prevention.

Drug Therapy. Broad-spectrum antibiotics, such as the aminoglycosides (e.g., gentamicin [Garamycin]) and cephalosporins (e.g., cephalexin [Keflex, Novo-Lexin✱]), are first prescribed for infections occurring with stone disease. The broad coverage is effective against gram-negative organisms. After the results of the culture and sensitivity (C&S) studies are obtained, more specific antibiotics may be prescribed. C&S studies are often done 48 hours after the start of antibiotic therapy and again 48 hours after completion of the prescribed course of therapy.

Blood levels of antibiotics may be measured to ensure that adequate levels have been reached. If the desired blood level of these antibiotics is exceeded, toxic effects and kidney damage may result. If the blood level of the antibiotic is not adequate, organisms may not be completely eliminated. Clinical evidence of a new infection (such as chills, fever, or altered mental status) warrants the collection of a urine sample for repeated C&S tests.

For the client with struvite stones, periodic and long-term monitoring of the urine for infection are needed. Urine cultures are checked monthly for 3 months, then quarterly for 1 year. Drugs that prevent bacteria from splitting urea, such as acetohydroxamic acid (Lithostat) and hydroxyurea (Hydrea), are often prescribed on a long-term basis for clients with struvite stones. Serum creatinine levels are monitored in clients receiving acetohydroxamic acid. This drug is stopped if creatinine levels are above 2 mg/dL. Review interventions aimed at preventing urinary tract infection (UTI) (see Interventions [Cystitis], p. 1681).

Diet Therapy. The client's diet ideally includes adequate calorie intake with a balance of all food groups. Encourage a fluid intake of 2 to 3 L/day unless another condition requires fluid restriction.

PREVENTION OF OBSTRUCTION

Measures to prevent urinary obstruction by stones include a high intake of fluids (3 L/day or more) and careful measures of intake and output. A liberal but not excessive fluid intake helps prevent dehydration, promotes the flow of urine, and decreases the chance of crystals forming a stone. Interventions also depend on the type of stone. Drugs, diet modification, and fluid intake are the major strategies available.

Drug Therapy. Drug selection to prevent obstruction depends on what is promoting the formation of stones and the type of stone formed. Teach the client the reason for the drug and assess for side effects or adverse drug reactions.

Calcium-Containing Stones. Drugs to treat hypercalciuria (high levels of calcium in the urine) include thiazide diuretics (e.g., chlorothiazide [Diuril] or hydrochlorothiazide [HydroDIURIL, Urozide✱]), orthophosphate, and sodium cellulose phosphate. Thiazide diuretics promote calcium resorption from the renal tubules back into the body, thereby reducing urine calcium loads. Orthophosphates alter calcium-phosphorus metabolism, resulting in decreased urine saturation of calcium oxalate. Sodium cellulose phosphate reduces intestinal absorption of calcium.

Oxalate-Containing Stones. For clients with hyperoxaluria (high levels of oxalic acid in the urine), allopurinol (Zyloprim) and vitamin B_6 (pyridoxine) are used.

Uric Acid–Containing Stones. For clients with chronic gout, allopurinol helps prevent the formation of urate (uric acid) stones. To alkalinize the urine, drugs such as potassium citrate, 50% sodium citrate, and sodium bicarbonate are used. The desired urine pH is 6 to 6.5. Because the normal urine pH averages 5 to 6, the desired values are termed *alkaline*.

Cystine-Containing Stones. For clients with cystinuria (high levels of cystine in the urine), both alpha-mercaptopropionylglycine (AMPG) and captopril (Capoten) lower urine cystine levels. They are used when hydration and urine alkalinization have not been successful.

Diet Therapy. Diet modification depends on the type of stone formed (Table 73-6). Consult the dietitian to plan the appropriate diet for the client.

Other Measures. Encourage the client to walk as often as possible. Walking promotes passage of stones and reduces bone calcium resorption. Check the urine pH daily and strain all urine with filter paper to collect passed stones and fragments.

Health Teaching. Key points for health teaching are listed in Chart 73-12. The client often has great anxiety and fear that a stone and its pain may recur. In addition to anxiety about the pain, the risk for repeated surgical interventions or permanent and serious kidney damage is of major concern. Psychosocial preparation is enhanced when clients know what to expect and what actions to take if problems develop. Reassure the client that preventive and health promotion activities help prevent recurrence.

TABLE 73-6 Dietary Treatment for Renal Stones

Stone Type	Dietary Interventions	Rationales
Calcium oxalate	Avoid oxalate sources, such as spinach, black tea, and rhubarb (see also Table 73-5).	Reduction of urinary oxalate content may help prevent these stones from forming. Urinary pH is not a factor.
	Decrease sodium intake.	High sodium intake reduces renal tubular calcium reabsorption.
Calcium phosphate	Limit intake of foods high in animal protein to 5-7 servings per week and never more than 2 per day.	Reduction of protein intake reduces acidic urine and prevents calcium precipitation.
	Some clients may benefit from a reduced calcium intake (milk, other dairy products).	Reduction of urine calcium concentration may prevent calcium precipitation and crystallization.
	Decrease sodium intake.	High sodium intake reduces renal tubular calcium reabsorption.
Struvite (magnesium ammonium phosphate)	Limit high-phosphate foods, such as dairy products, red, and organ meats, and whole grains.	Reduction of urinary phosphate content may help prevent these stones from forming.
Uric acid (urate)	Decrease intake of purine sources, such as organ meats, poultry, fish, gravies, red wines, and sardines.	Reduction of urinary purine content may help prevent these stones from forming.
Cystine	Limit animal protein intake (as above).	Reduces urinary uric acid.
	Encourage oral fluid intake (500 mL every 4 hours while awake and 750 mL at night).	Increased fluid helps dilute the urine and prevents the cystine crystals from forming.

CHART 73-12

CLIENT EDUCATION GUIDE
Urinary Calculi

- Finish your entire prescription of antibiotics to ensure that you will not get a urinary tract infection.
- You may resume your usual daily activities.
- Remember to balance regular exercise with sleep and rest.
- You may return to work 2 days to 6 weeks after surgery, depending on the type of intervention, your personal tolerance, and your physician's directives.
- Depending on the type of stone you had, your diet may be restricted to prevent further stone formation.
- Remember to drink at least 3 L of fluid a day to dilute potential stone-forming crystals, prevent dehydration, and promote urine flow.
- Monitor urine pH as directed (possibly up to three times per day).
- Expect bruising after lithotripsy. The bruising may be quite extensive and may take several weeks to resolve.
- Your urine may be bloody for several days after surgery.
- Pain in the region of the kidneys or bladder may signal the beginning of an infection or the formation of another stone. Report any pain, fever, chills, or difficulty with urination immediately to your physician or nurse.
- Keep follow-up appointments to check on infection, have repeat cultures done, and so forth.

Urothelial Cancer

PATHOPHYSIOLOGY

Urothelial cancers are malignant tumors of the urothelium, the lining of transitional cells in the kidney, renal pelvis, ureters, urinary bladder, and urethra. Most urothelial cancers occur in the bladder. Consequently, the term *bladder cancer* is often used to describe this condition.

In the United States, about 73% of urinary tract cancers are transitional cell carcinomas of the bladder (American Cancer Society [ACS], 2005). The second most common site of urinary tract cancer is the kidney and renal pelvis (27%). Urothelial cancers are usually low grade, have multiple points of origin (**multifocal**), and are recurrent. Once the cancer spreads beyond the transitional cell layer, they are highly invasive and metastatic. Because of the multifocal and recurrent nature of this cancer, clients may have recurrence up to 10 years after being cancer free.

Table 73-7 shows the staging of bladder cancer. Tumors confined to the mucosa are treated by simple excision, whereas carcinoma in situ (CIS), or stage T_{is}, is treated with excision plus **intravesical** (inside the bladder) chemotherapy. Cancer that has spread beyond CIS is treated with more extensive surgery, often a radical **cystectomy** (removal of the bladder and surrounding tissue) with urinary diversion. Chemotherapy and radiation therapy are used in addition to surgery. If untreated, the tumor invades surrounding tissues, spreads to distant sites (liver, lung, and bone), and ultimately leads to death.

Exposure to toxins, especially chemicals used in the hairdressing, rubber, paint, electric cable, and textile industries, increases the risk for bladder cancer. The greatest risk factor for bladder cancer is tobacco use. Other risks include *Schistosoma haematobium* (a parasite) infection, excessive use of drugs containing phenacetin, and long-term use of cyclophosphamide (Cytoxan, Procytox✱).

About 54,300 new cases of bladder cancer are diagnosed each year in the United States and about 12,400 deaths occur each year from the disease (ACS, 2005). This cancer is rare in adults younger than age 40, and is most common after 60 years of age.

◆COLLABORATIVE MANAGEMENT

◆Assessment

PHYSICAL ASSESSMENT/CLINICAL MANIFESTATIONS

Ask about the client's perception of his or her general health. Document the gender and age of the client. Ask about active and passive exposure to cigarette smoke. To detect exposure to harmful environmental agents, ask the client to describe his or her occupation in detail. Also ask

TABLE 73-7 Staging of Bladder Cancer

Primary Tumor (T)	
T_x	Primary tumor cannot be assessed
T_0	No evidence of primary tumor
T_{is}	Carcinoma in situ: "flat tumor"
T_1	Tumor invades submucosa (subepithelial connective tissue)
T_2	Tumor invades superficial muscle (inner half)
T_3	Tumor invades deep muscle or perivesical fat
T_{3a}	Tumor invades deep muscle (outer half)
T_{3b}	Tumor invades perivesical fat
T_4	Tumor invades any of the following: prostate, uterus, vagina, pelvic wall, abdominal wall
T_{4a}	Tumor invades prostate, uterus, vagina
T_{4b}	Tumor invades pelvic or abdominal wall
Lymph Node (N)	
N_x	Regional lymph nodes cannot be assessed
N_0	No regional lymph node metastasis
N_1	Metastasis in a single lymph node, 2 cm or less in greatest dimension
N_2	Metastasis in a single lymph node, more than 2 cm but not more than 5 cm in greatest dimension, or multiple lymph nodes, none more than 5 cm in greatest dimension, pelvic only
Distant Metastasis (M)	
M_x	Presence of distant metastasis cannot be assessed
M_0	No distant metastasis
M_1	Distant metastasis or nodes positive above aortic bifurcation

Modified from American Joint Committee on Cancer. (1992). In O.H. Beahrs (Ed.), *Manual for staging of cancer* (4th ed.). Philadelphia: Lippincott-Raven; and Bennett, J.C., & Plum, F. (Eds.). (2002). *Cecil textbook of medicine* (22nd ed.). Philadelphia: W.B. Saunders.

the client to describe any change in the color, frequency, or amount of urine and any abdominal discomfort.

Observe the overall appearance of the client, especially skin color and general nutritional status. Inspect, percuss, and palpate the abdomen for asymmetry, tenderness, and bladder distention.

Examine the urine for color and clarity. Hematuria is the major sign occurring with bladder cancer. It may be gross or microscopic and is usually painless and intermittent. Dysuria, frequency, and urgency are common when infection or obstruction is also present.

PSYCHOSOCIAL ASSESSMENT

Assess the client's emotions, including his or her response to a tentative diagnosis of bladder cancer, and note anxiety, fear, sadness, anger, or guilt. Early manifestations are painless, and many clients ignore hematuria because it is intermittent. Clients also may be reluctant to seek treatment because they suspect a sexually transmitted disease (STD). Consequently, they may have guilt or anger about their own delays in seeking medical attention.

Assess the client's methods of coping and the degree of support from family members. Social support may provide motivation and improve coping during convalescence.

DIAGNOSTIC ASSESSMENT

The only significant finding on a routine urinalysis is gross or microscopic hematuria. Cytologic testing on voided urine specimens is not usually helpful. Bladder-wash specimens and bladder biopsies are the most specific tests for cancer.

Cystoscopy with retrograde pyelography is usually performed to evaluate painless hematuria. A biopsy of a visible bladder tumor can be performed during cystoscopy. This is essential for staging and is usually performed in a day-surgery unit before admission to the hospital for treatment. IV pyelography may be used in the presence of hematuria. Excretory urography is useful in identifying obstructions, especially at the ureterovesical junction. Computed tomography (CT) scans show tumor invasion of surrounding tissues. Ultrasonography shows masses but is less valuable for tumor staging. Magnetic resonance imaging (MRI) may help to assess deep, invasive tumors.

◆Common Nursing Diagnoses and Collaborative Problems

Nursing diagnoses that may apply to clients with bladder cancer include the following:

- Fear or Anxiety related to potential diagnosis of a malignant disease
- Disturbed Body Image related to surgery-induced changes in urinary habits, or changes in appearance from chemotherapy
- Risk for Infection related to invasive procedures or side effects of systemic chemotherapy
- Risk for Impaired Skin Integrity related to surgical incision or urinary diversion
- Risk for Social Isolation related to altered physical appearance, embarrassment, or odors

◆Interventions

Therapy for the client with bladder cancer usually begins with surgical removal of the tumors for diagnosis and staging of disease. For tumors extending beyond the mucosa, surgery is followed by intravesical chemotherapy or immunotherapy. High-grade or recurrent tumors are treated with more radical surgery plus intravesical chemotherapy, radiotherapy, or both. Systemic chemotherapy is reserved for clients with distant metastases. (See Chapter 28 for general care of the client receiving chemotherapy or radiation therapy.)

NONSURGICAL MANAGEMENT. Prophylactic immunotherapy with intravesical instillation of bacille Calmette-Guérin (BCG), a compound used to vaccinate against tuberculosis in some countries, is used to prevent tumor recurrence of superficial cancers (stage T_1 or lower). This procedure is more effective than single-agent chemotherapy.

Multiagent chemotherapy is successful in prolonging life after distant metastasis has occurred but rarely results in a cure. Radiation therapy is also useful in prolonging life.

SURGICAL MANAGEMENT. The type of surgery for bladder cancer depends on the type and stage of the cancer and the client's general health. Complete bladder removal (cystectomy) with additional removal of surrounding muscle and tissue offers the best chance of a cure for large, invasive bladder cancers. Four alternatives are used after cystectomy: ileal conduit, continent pouch, bladder reconstruction also known as neobladder, and ureterosigmoidostomy (Oosterlinck et al., 2002).

Preoperative Care. Specific client education depends on the type and extent of the planned surgical procedure. Coordinate education before surgery with the surgeon

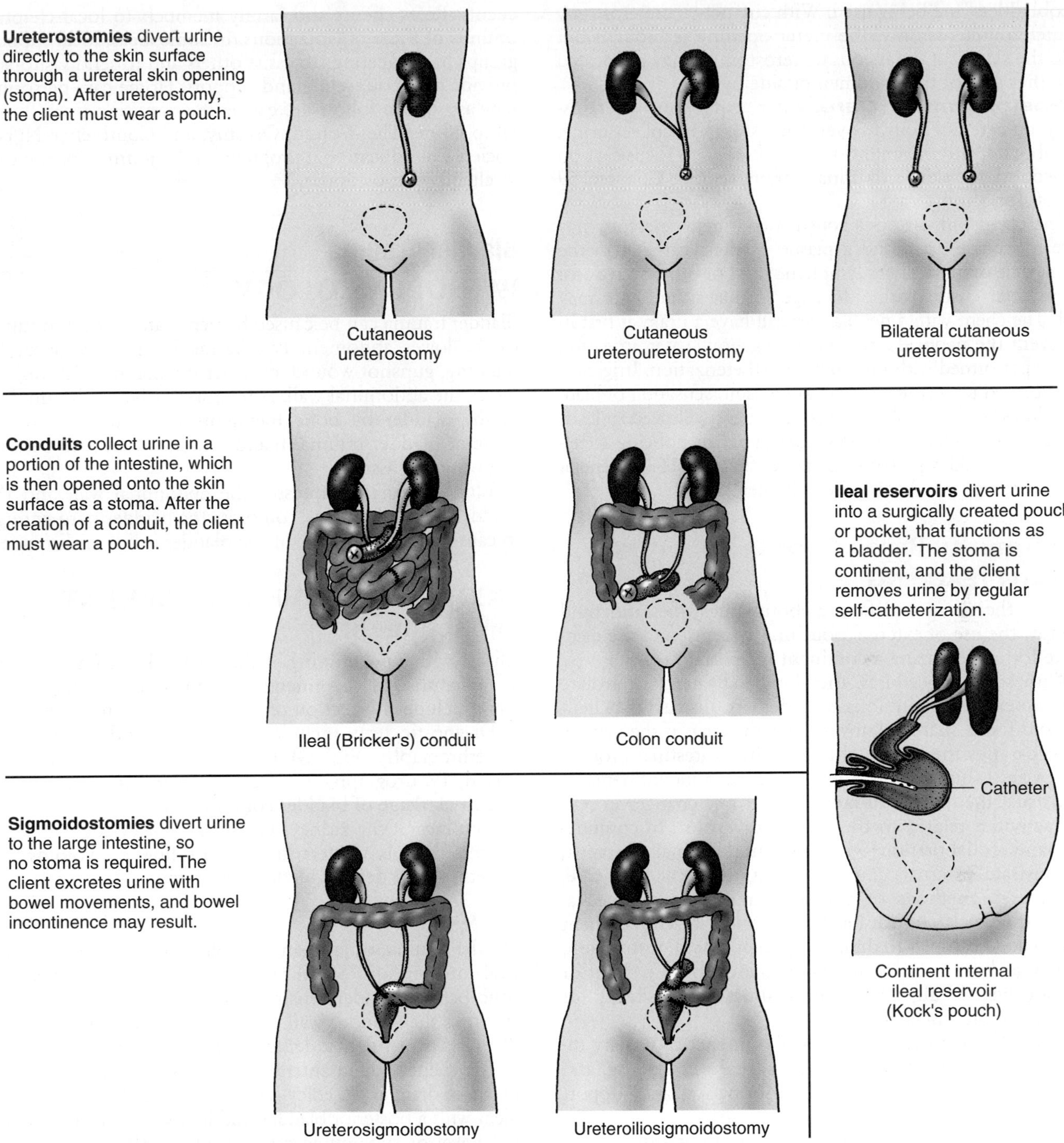

Figure 73-4 ■ Urinary diversion procedures used in the treatment of bladder cancer.

and enterostomal therapist. Discuss the type of planned urinary diversion and the selection of a site for the stoma. The goal is for the client to have a positive attitude about body image and a positive self-image. Use educational counseling to ensure understanding about self-care practices, methods of pouching, control of urine drainage, and management of odor.

The site selected for the stoma should be visible and avoid folds of skin, bones, and scar tissue. When possible, the client's waistline or belt area is avoided. Prepare the client for the number and type of drains that will be present after surgery. General care before surgery is discussed in Chapter 20.

Operative Procedures. Transurethral resection of the bladder tumor (TURBT) or partial cystectomy is performed for small, early, superficial tumors. In a partial (segmental) cystectomy, a portion of the bladder is removed. This procedure is used when there is only a single isolated bladder tumor.

When the entire bladder must be removed (complete **cystectomy**), the ureters are diverted into a collecting reservoir. Techniques for urinary diversion are shown in Figure 73-4. With an ileal conduit, the ureters are surgically placed in the ileum, and urine is collected in a pouch on the skin around the stoma. More often, continent reservoirs or "neobladders" are being used. With cutaneous ureterostomy or ureteroureterostomy, the ureter opening is brought out onto the skin. The cutaneous ureterostomies may be located on either side of the abdomen or side by side.

Postoperative Care. After cutaneous ureterostomy, an external pouch covers the ostomy to collect urine. Collaborate with the enterostomal therapist to focus care on the wound, the skin, and urinary drainage. (See Chapters 59 and 60 for ostomy care.)

The client with a Kock's pouch, a continent reservoir, may have a Penrose drain and a plastic Medena catheter in the stoma. The drain removes lymphatic fluid or other secretions; the catheter ensures urine drainage so that suture lines may heal. The client with a neobladder will have a drain at first in the event the neobladder requires irrigation. Later, irrigation can be performed with intermittent catheterization. Irrigation is performed to ensure patency. There is no sensation of bladder fullness with a neobladder, so the client will need to learn new cues to void, such as prescribed times or noticing a feeling of neobladder pressure (Beitz & Zuzelo, 2003). General care after surgery is discussed in Chapter 22.

Community-Based Care

HEALTH TEACHING

Educate the client and family about drugs, diet and fluid therapy, the use of external pouching systems, and the technique for catheterizing a continent reservoir.

With some procedures, the client may need electrolyte replacement to prevent long-term deficits. Instruct the client to avoid foods that are known to produce gas if the urinary diversion uses the intestinal tract. When intestinal production of gas is limited, flatus will not induce incontinence.

Instruct the client and family about any changes in self-care activities related to the urinary diversion. In conjunction and collaboration with the enterostomal therapist, demonstrate external pouch application, local skin care, pouch care, methods of adhesion, and drainage mechanisms. If a Kock's pouch has been created, teach the client how to use a catheter to drain the pouch. For all instruction, observe at least one return demonstration by the client or the caregiver. Ideally, the client assumes responsibility for self-care before discharge.

Assist the client to prepare for the impact of urinary diversion on self-image, body image, sexual functioning, and self-esteem. Counseling provides information and support to reduce feelings of powerlessness.

Through discussions with the client about usual social situations, help the client gain control over new toileting practices. Men with a urinary diversion into the sigmoid colon need to learn the habit of sitting to urinate. For clients of either gender, promote confidence in social situations by encouraging frequent emptying of urinary collection devices before traveling or attending social functions. Resumption of sexual activity is a major concern for many clients, regardless of age. Address this topic openly and with sensitivity. Cystectomy causes impotence in men, but treatment is available (see Chapter 79).

HEALTH CARE RESOURCES

The United Ostomy Association and the American Cancer Society have educational materials that may be useful to clients. Refer clients and family members to local chapters or units of these organizations. In some areas, local support groups have meetings to assist others and to send visitors to provide peer counseling and support. Home care personnel may assist with follow-up, easing the transition from hospital to home. The Wound, Ostomy, and Continence Nurses Society has educational programs and a journal for the care of clients with ostomies.

Bladder Trauma

PATHOPHYSIOLOGY

Bladder trauma can be caused by penetrating or blunt injury to the lower abdomen. Penetrating injury may occur by stabbing, gunshot wound, or other trauma in which objects pierce the abdominal wall. A fractured pelvis with puncture of the bladder by bone fragments is the most common cause of bladder trauma. Bladder trauma may also be a result of sexual assault.

Blunt trauma compresses the abdominal wall and the bladder. A seat belt may compress the bladder hard enough to cause injury, especially if the bladder is full or distended.

COLLABORATIVE MANAGEMENT

Assessment

Clients with a penetrating bladder wound often have anuria or hematuria. In the emergency department, initial assessment includes inspection of the urinary meatus for blood.

Diagnostic tests include cystography and voiding cystourethrography (VCUG). If renal or ureteral trauma is suspected, IV urography is scheduled before cystography so that any leakage of bladder contrast medium does not mask the outlines of the kidneys or ureters. The cystogram shows whether there is a defect in bladder filling; the voiding cystourethrogram defines bladder emptying.

Interventions

Bladder trauma, other than a simple contusion, requires surgical intervention. Stabilization of any fractures usually is done before bladder repair. Surgical interventions include repairing the bladder wall and peritoneal membrane. Usually, repairs of the bladder are closure procedures.

The client with an anterior bladder wall injury usually has a Penrose drain and a Foley catheter in place after surgery. The client with a posterior bladder wall injury has a Penrose drain and Foley or suprapubic catheter after surgery. In some instances, vaginal or rectal fistulas may also require repair.

Psychosocial support is critical for clients who have sustained traumatic injuries. Refer the client to counseling resources to assist in dealing with psychosocial issues.

GET READY for the NCLEX Examination!

KEY POINTS

Safe Effective Care Environment

- Use sterile technique when inserting a catheter or any other instrument into the urinary system.

- Use contact precautions with any client who has drainage from the genitourinary tract.

Health Promotion and Maintenance

- Teach clients the proper way to clean the perineal area after voiding, having a bowel movement, or after sexual intercourse.
- Encourage all clients to maintain an adequate fluid intake (minimum of 2 L daily unless another condition requires fluid restriction).
- Instruct women who have stress incontinence the proper way to perform pelvic floor strengthening exercises.
- Teach clients who come into contact with chemicals in their workplaces or with leisure time activities to avoid direct skin or mucous membrane contact with these chemicals.

Psychosocial Integrity

- Pace your interview to match the learning needs and style of the individual client.
- Allow the client the opportunity to express fear or anxiety regarding a potential cancer diagnosis.
- Use a nonjudgmental approach in caring for clients with urinary incontinence.
- Avoid referring to protective pads or pants as "diapers."
- Recognize the need for the client undergoing cystectomy and urinary diversion to grieve about the body image change.
- Assess the client's level of comfort in discussing issues related to elimination and the urogenital area.
- During renal/urinary assessment, use language and terminology that is comfortable for the client.
- Refer clients to community resources and support groups.

Physiological Integrity

- Identify hospitalized clients at risk for urosepsis.
- Report immediately any condition that obstructs urine flow.
- Instruct clients with UTI to complete all prescribed antibiotic therapy even when symptoms of infection are absent.
- Avoid maintaining indwelling catheters long term in hospitalized clients.
- Teach clients the expected side effects and any adverse reactions to prescribed drugs.
- Assess the client's manual dexterity and cognitive awareness before teaching a regimen of intermittent self-catheterization.

ADDITIONAL STUDY RESOURCES

Go to your Student CD-ROM for Review Questions for the NCLEX Examination.

evolve Go to http://evolve.elsevier.com/Iggy/ for Integrated Management of Care Questions for the NCLEX Examination.

SELECTED BIBLIOGRAPHY

Asterisk indicates a classic or definitive work on this subject.

*Agency for Health Care Policy and Research. (1996). (Reviewed 2001). *Urinary incontinence in adults: Acute and chronic management. Clinical practice guideline.* AHCPR Publication No. 96-0682. Rockville, MD: Agency for Health Care Policy and Research, Public Health Service, U.S. Department of Health and Human Services.

American Cancer Society. (2005). *Cancer facts and figures–2005.* Report No. 01-300M-No. 5008.05. Atlanta: Author.

Barkin, J. (2003). Interstitial cystitis: The great imposter! Epidemiology, etiology, diagnosis, and management. *Journal of Sexual and Reproductive Medicine, 3*(2), 57-64.

Bass, P.F., Jarvis, J.W., & Mitchell, C.K. (2003). Urinary tract infections. *Primary Care: Clinics in Office Practice, 30*(1), 1-16.

Bates, F. (2002). Assessment of the female patient with urinary incontinence. *Urologic Nursing, 22*(5) 305-314.

Beisel, B., Hale, W., & Graves, R., (2002). Does postcoital voiding prevent urinary tract infections in young women? *The Journal of Family Practice, 51*(11), 977.

Beitz, J., & Zuzelo, P. (2003). The lived experience of having a neobladder. *Western Journal of Nursing Research, 25*(3), 294-316.

Borghi, L., et al. (2002). Comparison of two diets for the prevention of recurrent stones in idiopathic hypercalciuria. *The New England Journal of Medicine, 346*(2), 77-84.

Castina, S., Boyington, A., & Dougherty, M. (2002). Urinary incontinence. *American Journal of Nursing 102*(8), 85-87.

Choe, J. (2002). Interstitial cystitis: Pelvic pain from the bladder. *The Clinical Advisor, 5(11/12)*, 118-127.

Cohen, M., & Rothmann, M. (2001). Gemcitabine and cisplatin for advanced metastatic bladder cancer. *Journal of Clinical Oncology, 19*(4), 1229-1231.

Danpure, C.J. (2000). Genetic disorders and urolithiasis. *Urologic Clinics of North America, 27*(2), 1-16.

Diering, C., & Palmer, M. (2001). Professional information about urinary incontinence on the World Wide Web: Is it timely? Is it accurate? *Journal of Wound, Ostomy, and Continence Nursing, 28*(1), 55-62.

Dochterman, J., & Bulechek, G. (Eds.). (2004). *Nursing interventions classification (NIC)* (4th ed.). St. Louis: Mosby.

Foxman, B. (2002). Epidemiology of urinary tract infections: incidence, morbidity, and economic costs. *American Journal of Medicine, 113*(Suppl. 1A), 5S-13S.

Frick, K.K., & Bushinsky, D.A. (2003). Molecular mechanisms of primary hypercalciuria. *Journal of the American Society of Nephrology, 14*(4), 222-224.

Goode, P., et al. (2003). Effect of behavioral training with or without pelvic floor electrical stimulation on stress incontinence in women. *Journal of the American Medical Association, 290*(3), 345-352.

Gray, M. (2000a). Urinary retention management in the acute care setting, Part 1. *American Journal of Nursing, 100*(7), 40-48.

Gray, M. (2000b). Urinary retention management in the acute care setting, Part 2. *American Journal of Nursing, 100*(8), 36-44.

Gray, M. (2004). Stress incontinence in women. *Journal of the American Academy of Nurse Practitioners, 16*(5), 188-197.

Gray, M. (2003). Gender, race, and culture in research on UI. *American Journal of Nursing, 103*(Suppl. 3), 20-25.

Gray, M., & Krissovich, M. (2003). Does fluid intake influence the risk for urinary incontinence, urinary tract infection, and bladder cancer? *Journal of Wound, Ostomy, and Continence Nursing, 30*, 126-131.

Gray, M., Albo, M., & Huffstutler, S. (2002). Interstitial cystitis: A guide to recognition, evaluation, and management for nurse practitioners. *Journal of Wound Care, Ostomy, and Continence Nursing, 29*(2), 93-102.

Hay-Smith, E.J.C., et al. (2003). Pelvic floor training for urinary incontinence in women. *Cochrane Database of Systemic Reviews* (*www.gateway2.ovid.com*). Accessed June, 2003. Last updated January, 2003.

Hess, B. (2002). Nutritional aspects of Stone disease. *Endocrinology and Metabolism Clinics, 31*(4), 1-11.

Hruska, K. (2001). Renal calculi. In J.C. Bennett & F. Plum (Eds.), *Cecil textbook of medicine* (22nd ed.). Philadelphia: W.B. Saunders.

Ingelfinger, J. (2002). Diet and kidney stones. *The New England Journal of Medicine, 346*(2), 74-76.

Jepson, R.G., Mihaljevic, L., & Craig, J. (2002). Cranberries for preventing urinary tract infections. Cochrane Renal Group. *Cochrane Database of Systematic Reviews*. Accessed June, 2003.

Johnson, S. (2000). From incontinence to confidence. *American Journal of Nursing, 100*(2), 69-76.

Johnson, V. (2001). Effects of a submaximal exercise protocol to recondition the pelvic floor musculature. *Nursing Research, 50*(1), 33-41.

Kiel, R., & Nashelsky, M. (2003). Does cranberry juice prevent or treat urinary tract infection? *The Journal of Family Practice, 52*(2), 154-155.

Kincade, J., Peckous, B., & Busby-Whitehead, J. (2001). A pilot study to determine predictors of behavioral treatment completion for urinary incontinence. *Urologic Nursing, 21*(1), 39-44.

Kontiokari, T., et al. (2001). Randomised trial of cranberry-ligonberry juice and *Lactobacillus* GG drink for the prevention of urinary tract infection in women. *British Medical Journal, 332,* 1571-1573.

Lehmann, S., & Dietz, C. (2002). Double-J stents: They're not trouble free. *RN, 65*(1), 54-60.

Lekan-Rutledge, D., & Colling, J. (2003). Urinary incontinence in the frail elderly. *American Journal of Nursing, 103*(3 Suppl.), 36-46.

Lopez, R., Smith, P., & Thering, A. (2002). What are the indications for urodynamic testing in older adults with incontinence? *The Journal of Family Practice, 51*(12), 1077.

Lyons, S., & Specht, J. (2000). Prompted voiding protocol for individuals with urinary incontinence. *Journal of Gerontological Nursing, 20*(6), 5-13.

Maloney, C. (2002). Estrogen and recurrent UTI in postmenopausal women. *American Journal of Nursing, 102*(8), 44-53.

Maloney, C., & Cafiero, M. (2001). Non-invasive evaluation and treatment of bladder control problems in the primary care setting. *The American Journal for Nurse Practitioners, 5*(5), 42, 45-46, 49-50, 53-54.

Mather, K., & Bakas, T. (2002). Nursing assistants' perceptions of their ability to provide continence care. *Geriatric Nursing, 23*(2), 76-81.

McCance, K., & Huether, S. (2002). Pathophysiology: The biologic basis for disease in adults and children (4th ed.). St. Louis: Mosby.

McLaughlin, S.P., & Carson, C.C. (2004). Urinary tract infections in women. *Medical Clinics of North America, 88*(2), 417-429.

Miller, C. (2002). Anticholinergics: The good and the bad. *Geriatric Nursing, 23*(5), 286-287.

Miller, C. (2002). Recently approved and forthcoming drugs for elders. *Geriatric Nursing, 23*(1), 51-52.

Moore, K., Day, R., & Albers, M. (2002). Pathogenesis of urinary tract infections: A review. *Journal of Clinical Nursing, 11*(5), 568-574.

Moorhead, S., Johnson, M., & Maas, M. (Eds.). (2004). *Nursing outcomes classification (NOC)* (3rd ed.). St. Louis: Mosby.

Mueller, C., & Cain, H. (2002). Comprehensive management of urinary incontinence through quality improvement efforts. *Geriatric Nursing, 23*(2), 82-87.

National Kidney and Urologic Diseases Information Clearinghouse. (2004). *Kidney and urologic diseases statistics for the United States.* NIH Pub. No. 04-3895. Bethesda, MD. National Institutes of Health. Available at http://kidney.niddk.nih.gov/kudiseases/pubs/kustats/index.htm.

Newman, D. (2003). Stress urinary incontinence in women. *American Journal of Nursing, 103*(8), 46-55.

Newman, D., & Giovannini, D. (2002). Overactive bladder: A nursing perspective. *American Journal of Nursing, 102*(6), 36-46.

Newman, D.K., & Palmer, M.H. (2003). State of the science on urinary incontinence. *American Journal of Nursing, 103*(March Suppl.), 3-56.

Oosterlinck, W., et al. (2002). Guidelines on bladder cancer. *European Urology, 41*, 105-112.

Portis, A.J., & Sudaram, C.P. (2001). Diagnosis and management of kidney stones. *American Family Physician, 63*(7), 1329-1338.

*Resnick, M.I. (Ed.). (1997). Urolithiasis. *Urologic Clinics of North America, 24*(1), entire issue.

Rigsby, D. (2003). The overactive bladder. *Nursing Standard, 17*(39), 45-54.

Saint, S. (2000). Clinical and economic consequences of nosocomial catheter-related bacteriuria. *American Journal of Infection Control, 28*, 68-75.

Sampselle, C. (2003). Behavioral interventions in young and middle-age women. *American Journal of Nursing, 103*(Suppl. 3), 9-19.

Sampselle, C. (2003). Teaching women to use a voiding diary. *American Journal of Nursing, 103*(11), 62-64.

U.S. Renal Data Systems. (2002). *USRDS 2002 annual data report.* Bethesda, MD: The National Institutes of Health, National Institute of Diabetes and Digestive and Kidney Diseases.

Vaughn, D., & Malkowicz, S. (2001). Recent advances in bladder cancer chemotherapy. *Cancer Investigation, 19*(1), 77-85.

Walsh, P.C., et al. (2002). *Campbell's urology* (8th ed.). Philadelphia: W.B. Saunders.

*Warren, J.W., et al. (1999). Guidelines for antimicrobial treatment of uncomplicated acute bacterial cystitis and acute pyelonephritis in women. *Clinics in Infectious Disease, 29*(4), 745-758.

Wyman, J. (2003). Treatment of urinary incontinence in men and older women. *American Journal of Nursing, 103*(Suppl. 3), 26-35.

*Young-McCaughan, S. (1999). Invasive bladder cancer. In C. Miaskowski & P. Buchsel (Eds.), *Oncology nursing: Assessment and clinical care* (pp. 1055-1087). St. Louis: Mosby.

CHAPTER 74

Interventions for Clients with Renal Disorders

CHRIS WINKELMAN

LEARNING OUTCOMES

After studying this chapter, you should be able to:

1. Prioritize nursing care for the client with polycystic kidney disease.
2. Describe the clinical manifestations of hydronephrosis.
3. Identify clients at risk for pyelonephritis.
4. Describe the mechanisms of action, side effects, and nursing implications for drug therapy for pyelonephritis.
5. Use laboratory data and clinical manifestations to determine the effectiveness of therapy for pyelonephritis.
6. Compare the pathophysiology and clinical manifestations of acute glomerular nephritis and nephrotic syndrome.
7. Explain the relationship between hypertension and renal disease.
8. Prioritize nursing care for the client during the first 24 hours after a nephrectomy.
9. Explain how diabetic nephropathy can affect glucose metabolism and control in the client with diabetes mellitus.
10. Develop a community-based teaching plan for the client who has had a nephrectomy for renal cell carcinoma.
11. Describe strategies to prevent renal trauma.

Go to your Student CD-ROM for Review Questions for the NCLEX Examination keyed to these Learning Outcomes.

Renal disorders reduce the ability of the kidney to filter wastes and to balance fluid, electrolytes, acids, and bases. The kidneys work together with many other organ systems; thus renal disorders affect systemic health and can lead to life-threatening outcomes. Renal disorders are classified as congenital, obstructive, infectious, glomerular, and degenerative. Renal tumors and renal trauma are also described in this chapter. Renal failure is discussed in Chapter 75.

CONGENITAL DISORDERS

Polycystic Kidney Disease

PATHOPHYSIOLOGY

Polycystic kidney disease (PKD) is an inherited disorder in which fluid-filled cysts develop in the nephrons. In the dominant form, only a few nephrons have cysts until the person reaches his or her 30s. In the recessive form of the disease, nearly 100% of nephrons have cysts from birth. Cysts develop anywhere in the nephron as a result of kidney cell division, altered secretion, and abnormal cell matrix biology (Calvet & Grantham, 2001; Igarashi & Somlo, 2002).

Over time, small cysts become much larger (up to a few centimeters in diameter) and more widely distributed. The growing cysts damage the glomerular and tubular membranes. As the cysts fill with fluid and enlarge, the nephron functions become less effective.

The kidney tissue is eventually replaced by nonfunctioning cysts, which look like clusters of grapes (Figure 74-1). The kidneys are grossly enlarged; each cystic kidney may enlarge to two or three times its normal size, becoming as large as a football. Other abdominal organs are displaced, and the client has discomfort or pain. The fluid-filled cysts are also at increased risk for infection, rupture, and bleeding.

Most clients with PKD have high blood pressure. The cause of hypertension is thought to be related to renal ischemia from the enlarging cysts. As the vessels are compressed and renal blood flow decreases, the renin-angiotensin system is activated, raising blood pressure. Control of hypertension

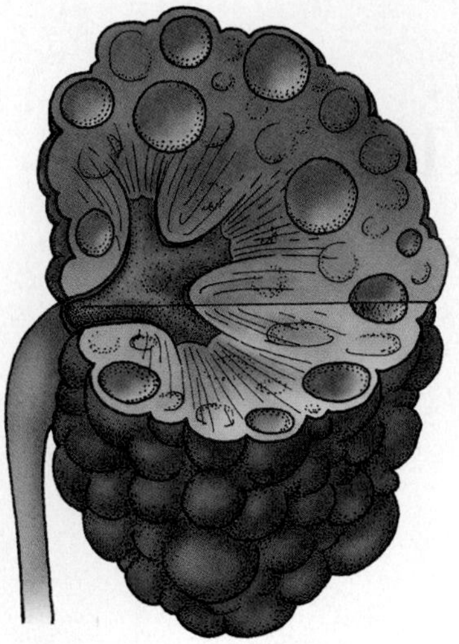

Figure 74-1 ■ Polycystic kidney.

is a top priority because proper treatment can disrupt the process that leads to renal ischemia.

Cysts may also occur in other tissues, such as the liver, blood vessels of the brain, and cardiac blood vessels. Cysts may reduce liver function or result in bleeding into the brain from ruptured intracranial vascular cysts *(berry aneurysms)*, causing sudden death. For reasons as yet unknown, kidney stones occur in 8% to 36% of the clients with PKD. Heart valve abnormalities (e.g., mitral valve prolapse), left ventricular hypertrophy, and colonic diverticula also are common in clients with PKD.

Etiology and Genetic Risk

PKD has several inherited forms. It can be inherited as either an autosomal dominant trait or, less commonly, as an autosomal recessive trait. People who inherit the recessive form of PKD usually die in early childhood. The 5% to 10% incidence of PKD in clients with no family history occurs as a result of a spontaneous gene mutation.

Genetic Considerations

The autosomal dominant form of PKD (ADPKD) is the most common form of polycystic disease. Children of parents who have the autosomal dominant form of PKD have a 50% chance of inheriting the gene that causes the disease. Manifestations of ADPKD can vary for age of onset, manifestations, and illness severity, even within one family. However, ADPKD is fully penetrant, meaning that nearly 100% of people who inherit a PKD gene will develop renal cysts by age 30 (Igarashi & Somlo, 2002). Half of these people develop renal failure by age 50 years. ADPKD-1 is the most common and most severe form of the autosomal dominant disease. ADPKD-2 has a slower rate of cyst formation so that symptoms occur later in life and there is delayed progression to renal failure and other complications. The gene products of ADPKD-1 and ADPKD-2 are both polycystins, cell membrane proteins important to ion transport (Arnaout, 2001; Online Mendelian Inheritance in Man, 2004).

Autosomal recessive PKD is rare, caused by a different gene mutation than the dominant form. To inherit a recessive gene, both parents must carry a copy of the mutated allele and both mutated alleles must be inherited. Thus each child has a 1 in 4 chance of inheriting autosomal recessive polycystic disease (ARPKD).

At present, there is no way to prevent PKD, although early detection and management of hypertension may slow the progression of renal impairment. Genetic counseling and evaluation may be useful for adults who have one parent or both parents with PKD.

CHART 74-1

KEY FEATURES of Polycystic Kidney Disease

- Abdominal or flank pain
- Hypertension
- Nocturia
- Increased abdominal girth
- Constipation
- Bloody or cloudy urine
- Kidney stones

Incidence/Prevalence

Polycystic kidney disease (PKD) is a common disorder, affecting 250,000 to 500,000 people in the United States. PKD is more common in white individuals than in people of other races. Men and women have an equal chance of inheriting the disease because the gene responsible for PKD is not located on the sex chromosomes (Polycystic Kidney Disease Foundation, 2004).

COLLABORATIVE MANAGEMENT

Assessment

HISTORY

Explore the family history of a client with suspected or actual PKD and ask whether either parent was known to have PKD or whether there is any family history of kidney disease. The age at which signs and symptoms developed in the parent and any related complications are important to obtain. Ask the client about constipation, abdominal discomfort, a change in urine color or frequency, high blood pressure, headaches, and a family history of sudden death from a stroke.

PHYSICAL ASSESSMENT/CLINICAL MANIFESTATIONS

Chart 74-1 lists key features of PKD. Pain is often the first manifestation. Inspect the abdomen. A distended abdomen is common as the cystic kidneys swell and push the abdominal contents forward. Polycystic kidneys are easily palpated because of their increased size. Proceed with *gentle* abdominal palpation because the cystic kidneys and nearby tissues may be tender, and palpation is uncomfortable.

The client also may have flank pain as a dull ache or as sharp and intermittent discomfort. Dull, aching pain is caused by increased kidney size with distention or from infection within the cyst. Sharp, intermittent pain occurs when a cyst ruptures or a stone is present. When a cyst ruptures, the client may have bright red or cola-colored urine. Infection is suspected if the urine is cloudy or foul smelling or if there is **dysuria** (pain on urination).

Nocturia (the need to urinate excessively at night) is an early manifestation and occurs because of decreased urine concentrating ability. As renal function further declines, the client has increasing hypertension, edema, and uremic problems such as anorexia, nausea, vomiting, pruritus, and fatigue (see Chapter 75). Because berry aneurysms often occur in clients with PKD, a severe headache with or without neurologic or vision changes deserves particular attention.

PSYCHOSOCIAL ASSESSMENT

As an inherited disorder, PKD may cause complex psychosocial responses. The client often has seen the effects and problems of the disease in close family members. He or she may have had a parent who died or close relatives who required dialysis or transplantation. While obtaining the family history, listen carefully for spoken and unspoken feelings of anger, resentment, futility, sadness, or anxiety; such feelings may need further exploration. The focus of the feelings may be one or both parents or the process of diagnosis and treatment. Feelings of guilt and concern for the client's children may also complicate the issue.

DIAGNOSTIC ASSESSMENT

Urinalysis shows **proteinuria** (protein in the urine) once the glomeruli are involved. **Hematuria** (blood in the urine) may be gross or microscopic. Bacteria in the urine indicate infection, usually in the cysts. Obtain a urine sample for culture and sensitivity testing when there is clinical or laboratory evidence of infection. As kidney function deteriorates, serum creatinine and blood urea nitrogen (BUN) levels rise. With decreasing kidney function, creatinine clearance decreases. Changes in renal handling of sodium may cause either sodium losses or sodium retention.

Diagnostic studies include renal sonography, computed tomography (CT), and magnetic resonance imaging (MRI). Small cysts are detected by sonography, CT, or MRI. Renal sonography provides diagnostic evidence of PKD, with minimal risk cases.

◆Common Nursing Diagnoses and Collaborative Problems

Nursing diagnoses and collaborative problems that may apply to clients with polycystic kidney disease (PKD) include the following:

- Acute Pain related to cyst rupture or stone formation
- Chronic Pain related to enlarging kidneys compressing abdominal contents
- Constipation related to compression of intestinal tract
- Risk for Infection related to the presence of cysts and decreased renal blood flow
- Potential for Hypertension
- Potential for Stone Formation
- Potential for Renal Failure

◆Interventions

Chart 74-2 lists NIC interventions for clients with renal disorders. (See Chapter 73 for information on urinary infections and stone formation. See Chapter 75 for care of the client with renal failure.)

Acute and Chronic Pain. Comfort strategies include drug therapy and complementary approaches. A combination may be most effective. Nonsteroidal anti-inflammatory drugs (NSAIDs) are used cautiously because of their tendency to reduce renal blood flow. Aspirin-containing compounds are avoided to reduce the risk for bleeding.

If cyst infection causes discomfort, lipid-soluble antibiotics such as trimethoprim/sulfamethoxazole (Bactrim, Septra, Trimpex) or ciprofloxacin (Cipro), are prescribed. These drugs penetrate the cyst wall. Monitor the serum creatinine levels because antibiotic therapy can be nephrotoxic. Apply dry heat to the abdomen or flank to promote comfort when renal cysts are infected. When pain is severe or debilitating, cysts can be reduced by percutaneous needle aspiration and drainage.

Teach the client methods of enhancing relaxation and promoting comfort via deep breathing, guided imagery, or other strategies. The overall goal is client self-management. (See Chapter 7 for pain management.)

Constipation. Teach the client how to prevent constipation (see Bowel Management in Chart 74-2). Include teaching about maintaining adequate fluid intake, increasing dietary fiber when fluid intake is more than 2500 mL/24 hr, and the need for regular exercise. Explain that pressure on the large intestine may further impede peristalsis as the polycystic kidneys increase in size. The client should know that these recommendations for bowel management might change, particularly if renal failure also develops. Advise the client about the use of stool softeners and bulk agents, including the careful use of laxatives, to prevent chronic constipation.

Hypertension and Renal Failure. Blood pressure control is necessary to reduce cardiovascular complications and slow the progression of renal dysfunction. Nursing interventions include education to promote self-management and understanding (see Medication Management in Chart 74-2 and Chapter 39 for information on hypertension). When renal impairment results in decreased urine concentration with nocturia and low urine specific gravity, urge the client to drink at least 2 L of fluid per day to prevent dehydration, which further reduces renal function. Restricting sodium intake may help control blood pressure.

Drug therapy for blood pressure control includes antihypertensive agents and diuretics. Antihypertensive agents include angiotensin-converting enzyme (ACE) inhibitors, calcium channel blockers, beta blockers, and vasodilators (see Chart 39-2). ACE inhibitors may help control the cell proliferation aspects of PKD and reduce microalbuminuria. If PKD progresses to chronic renal failure or end-stage renal disease, treatment approaches are similar to those in Chapter 75.

Teach the client, family, or significant other how to measure and record blood pressure. Help the client establish a schedule for self-administering drugs, monitoring daily weights, and keeping blood pressure records (Chart 74-3). Explain the potential side effects of the drugs. Make available written materials, such as drug teaching cards and booklets.

A low-sodium diet is often prescribed to control the hypertension that usually accompanies PKD. However, some clients may have salt wasting and should not follow a sodium-restricted diet. As the disease progresses, the client's protein intake may need to be limited to slow the development of renal failure. Assist the client, family, or significant other in understanding the diet plan and clarify its rationale. Work closely with the dietitian to foster the client's understanding. You may also refer the client for nutritional counseling.

CHART 74-2

NIC **INTERVENTION ACTIVITIES for**
The Client with Renal Problems

Pain Management: *Alleviation of pain or a reduction in pain to a level of comfort that is acceptable to the client*
- Observe for nonverbal cues of discomfort, especially in those unable to communicate effectively.
- Ensure that client receives attentive analgesic care.
- Consider cultural influences on pain response.
- Utilize a developmentally appropriate assessment method that allows for monitoring of change in pain and that will assist in identifying actual and potential precipitating factors (e.g., flow sheet, daily diary).
- Control environmental factors that may influence the client's response to discomfort (e.g., room temperature, lighting, noise).
- Consider type and source of pain when selecting pain relief strategy.
- Provide the person optimal pain relief with prescribed analgesics.
- Implement the use of patient-controlled analgesia (PCA), if appropriate.
- Use pain control measures before pain becomes severe.
- Evaluate the effectiveness of the pain control measures used through ongoing assessment of the pain experience.
- Institute and modify pain control measures on the basis of the client's response.

Bowel Management: *Establishment and maintenance of a regular pattern of bowel elimination*
- Note pre-existent bowel problems, bowel routine, and use of laxatives.
- Teach client about specific foods that assist in promoting bowel regularity.
- Initiate a bowel training program, as appropriate.
- Instruct client on foods high in fiber, as appropriate.
- Evaluate medication profile for gastrointestinal side effects.

Medication Management: *Facilitation of safe and effective use of prescription and over-the-counter drugs*
- Monitor client for the therapeutic effect of the medication.
- Monitor for signs and symptoms of drug toxicity.
- Monitor for adverse effects of the drug.
- Develop strategies with the client to enhance compliance with prescribed medication regimen.
- Teach the client and/or family members the expected action and side effects of the medication.
- Instruct client when to seek medical attention.

Energy Management: *Regulating energy use to treat or prevent fatigue and optimize function*
- Determine client's physical limitations.
- Determine client's/significant other's perceptions of causes of fatigue.
- Encourage verbalization of feelings about limitations.
- Determine what and how much activity is required to build endurance.
- Monitor nutritional intake to ensure adequate energy resources.
- Monitor client for evidence of excess physical and emotional fatigue.
- Monitor cardiorespiratory response to activity (e.g., tachycardia, other dysrhythmias, dyspnea, diaphoresis, pallor, hemodynamic pressures, and respiratory rate).
- Monitor location and nature of discomfort or pain during movement/activity.
- Promote bed rest/activity limitation (e.g., increase number of rest periods).
- Encourage alternate rest and activity periods.
- Provide calming diversionary activities to promote relaxation.
- Plan activities for periods when the client has the most energy.
- Encourage physical activity (e.g., ambulation or performance of activities of daily living, consistent with client's energy resources).

Fluid Monitoring: *Collection and analysis of client data to regulate fluid balance*
- Monitor weight.
- Monitor intake and output.
- Monitor serum and urine electrolyte values, as appropriate.
- Monitor serum albumin and total protein levels.
- Monitor serum and urine osmolality levels.
- Keep an accurate record of intake and output.
- Monitor for distended neck veins, crackles in the lungs, peripheral edema, and weight gain.
- Restrict and allocate fluid intake, as appropriate.
- Administer pharmacologic agents to increase urinary output, as appropriate.
- Administer dialysis, as appropriate, noting client response.

Urinary Retention Care: *Assistance in relieving bladder distention*
- Provide privacy for elimination.
- Provide Credé maneuver, as necessary.
- Use double-voiding technique.
- Insert urinary catheter, as appropriate.
- Monitor degree of bladder distention by palpation and percussion.
- Catheterize for residual, as appropriate.
- Implement intermittent catheterization, as appropriate.

Infection Protection: *Prevention and early detection of infection in a client at risk*
- Monitor for systemic and localized signs and symptoms of infection.
- Maintain asepsis for client at risk.
- Inspect condition of any surgical incision/wound.
- Instruct client to take antibiotics as prescribed.
- Obtain cultures, as needed.

NIC intervention activities selected from: Dochterman, J.,M., & Bulechek, G.M. (Eds.). (2004). *Nursing interventions classification (NIC)* (4th ed.). St. Louis: Mosby.

Health Care Resources

The Polycystic Kidney Research Foundation (http://www.pkdcure.org) and the National Kidney and Urologic Disease division and the National Institute of Health (http://www.niddk.nih.gov) conduct research and provide education about PKD. Many pamphlets are available; there is a fee for some materials. Chapters of the National Kidney Foundation (NKF) and the American Association of Kidney Patients (AAKP) also have resources for information and support.

OBSTRUCTIVE DISORDERS

Hydronephrosis, Hydroureter, and Urethral Stricture

PATHOPHYSIOLOGY

Hydronephrosis and hydroureter are problems of urine outflow obstruction. Urethral strictures also obstruct outflow. Prompt recognition and treatment are crucial to prevent permanent renal damage.

CHART 74-3

CLIENT EDUCATION GUIDE
Polycystic Kidney Disease

- Measure and record your blood pressure daily.
- Take your temperature if you suspect you have a fever.
- Weigh yourself every day at the same time of day and with the same amount of clothing; notify your physician or nurse if you have a sudden weight gain.
- Limit your intake of salt to help control your blood pressure.
- Notify your physician or nurse if your urine is foul smelling or if there is blood in your urine.
- Notify your physician or nurse if you have a headache that does not go away or if you have visual disturbances.
- Monitor bowel movements to prevent constipation.

In **hydronephrosis,** the kidney enlarges as urine collects in the pelvis and kidney tissue. Because the capacity of the renal pelvis is normally 5 to 8 mL, obstruction in the pelvis or at the ureteropelvic junction (UPJ) quickly distends the renal pelvis. Kidney pressure increases as the volume of urine increases. Over time, sometimes in only a matter of hours, the blood vessels and renal tubules can be damaged extensively (Figure 74-2).

In clients with **hydroureter** (enlargement of the ureter), the effects are similar but the obstruction is lower in the urinary tract. The ureter is most easily obstructed where the iliac vessels cross or where the ureters enter the bladder. Ureter dilation occurs above the obstruction and enlarges as urine collects (see Figure 74-2).

In clients with a **urethral stricture,** the obstruction is very low in the urinary tract, causing bladder distention before hydroureter and hydronephrosis. The problems and kidney damage are similar without prompt treatment.

Urinary obstruction causes damage when pressure builds up directly on tissue. Tubular filtrate pressure also increases in the nephron as drainage through the collecting system is impaired. With this added pressure, glomerular filtration decreases or ceases, and renal failure results. Nitrogenous waste products (urea, creatinine, and uric acid) and electrolytes (sodium, potassium, chloride, and phosphorus) are retained in the blood, and acid-base balance is impaired.

Causes of hydronephrosis or hydroureter include tumors, stones, trauma, congenital structural defects, and fibrosis. In clients with cancer, obstructed ureters may result from pelvic radiation or surgical intervention. Early treatment of the causes can prevent hydronephrosis and hydroureter and thus prevent permanent renal damage. The specific time needed to prevent permanent damage depends on the client's renal health. Permanent damage can occur in less than 48 hours in some clients and after several weeks in other clients.

COLLABORATIVE MANAGEMENT

Assessment

Obtain a history from the client, focusing on known renal or urologic disorders. A history of childhood urinary tract problems may indicate previously undiagnosed structural defects. Ask about the client's pattern of urination, especially amount, frequency, color, clarity, and odor. Ask the client about recent flank or abdominal pain. Chills, fever, and malaise may be present with a urinary tract infection (UTI).

Inspect each flank to identify asymmetry, which may occur with a renal mass, and *gently* palpate the client's abdomen to locate areas of tenderness. Palpate and percuss the bladder to detect distention. Gentle pressure on the abdomen may cause urine leakage, which reflects a full bladder and possible obstruction.

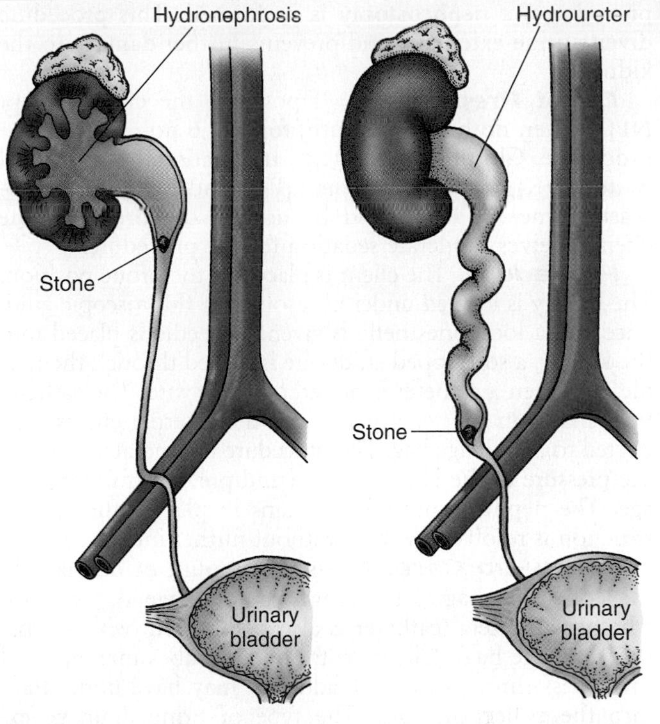

Figure 74-2 ■ Hydronephrosis is caused by obstruction in the upper part of the ureter; hydroureter is caused by obstruction in the lower part of the ureter.

Urinalysis may show bacteria or white blood cells if infection is present. When urinary tract obstruction is prolonged, microscopic examination may reveal tubular epithelial cells. Blood chemistries are normal unless decreased glomerular filtration has occurred. Blood creatinine and blood urea nitrogen (BUN) levels increase with a reduced glomerular filtration rate (GFR). Serum electrolyte levels may be altered with hyperkalemia, hyperphosphatemia, hypocalcemia, and metabolic acidosis (bicarbonate deficit).

Intravenous urography shows ureteral or renal pelvis dilation. Urinary outflow obstruction can be seen with sonography (renal echography) or computed tomography (CT).

Interventions

Urinary retention and potential for infection are the primary problems. (See Fluid Monitoring, Urinary Retention Care, and Infection Protection in Chart 74-2.) Failure to treat the cause of obstruction leads to infection and renal failure.

Urologic Interventions. If the stricture is caused by a stone, it can be located and retrieved using cystoscopic or retrograde pyelogram procedures. The urologist uses a cystoscope to guide a stone basket over the stone and removes it through the bladder. After stone removal, a plastic stent is usually left in the ureter for a few weeks to improve urine flow in the area irritated by the stone. The stent is later removed via another cystoscopic procedure.

Radiologic Intervention. When a stricture is causing hydronephrosis and cannot be corrected with urologic procedures, a **nephrostomy** is performed. This procedure diverts urine externally and prevents further damage to the kidney.

Client Preparation. If possible, the client is kept NPO (given nothing by mouth) for 4 to 6 hours before the procedure. Clotting studies (e.g., International Normalized Ratio [INR], prothrombin time [PT], and partial thromboplastic time [PTT]) should be normal or corrected. The client receives moderate sedation for the procedure.

Procedure. The client is placed in the prone position. The kidney is located under ultrasound or fluoroscopic guidance and a local anesthetic is given. A needle is placed into the kidney, a soft-tipped guidewire is placed through the needle, and then a catheter is placed over the wire. The catheter tip remains in the renal pelvis and the external end is connected to a drainage bag. The procedure immediately relieves the pressure in the kidney system and prevents further damage. The nephrostomy tube remains in place until the obstruction is resolved (with or without further intervention).

Follow-up Care. Assess the amount of drainage in the collection bag. The amount of drainage depends on whether a ureteral catheter is also being used (with a separate drainage bag). Clients with ureteral tubes may have all urine pass through to the bladder or may have urine drain into the collection bags. The type of urine drainage expected should be clearly communicated in the chart. If urine is expected to drain into the collection bag, assess the amount of drainage hourly for the first 24 hours. If the amount of drainage decreases and the client has back pain, the tube may be clogged or dislodged. Notify the physician immediately.

Monitor the nephrostomy site for leaking urine or blood. If either occurs, notify the physician immediately. Urine drainage may be red-tinged for the first 12 to 24 hours after the procedure and should gradually clear. Assess the client for manifestations of infection, including fever or a change in urine character.

INFECTIOUS DISORDERS

The urinary system normally excretes sterile urine. The unobstructed and complete passage of urine from the renal and urinary systems is critical in maintaining a sterile urinary tract. When any structural abnormality is present, the risk for damage as a result of infection is greatly increased. **Urinary tract infection (UTI)** is an infection in this normally sterile system. **Pyelonephritis** is a bacterial infection in the kidney and renal pelvis–the *upper* urinary tract. Infections in the *lower* urinary tract are described in Chapter 73.

Pyelonephritis

PATHOPHYSIOLOGY

Pyelonephritis is either the presence of active organisms in the kidney or the effects of kidney infections. **Acute pyelonephritis** is the active bacterial infection, whereas **chronic pyelonephritis** results from repeated or continued upper urinary tract infections or the effects of such infections. Chronic pyelonephritis often occurs with an anatomic urinary tract anomaly, obstruction or, most commonly, vesicoureteral urine reflux. The vesicoureteral junction is the point at which the ureter joins the bladder. **Reflux** is the reverse or upward flow of urine toward the renal pelvis and kidney.

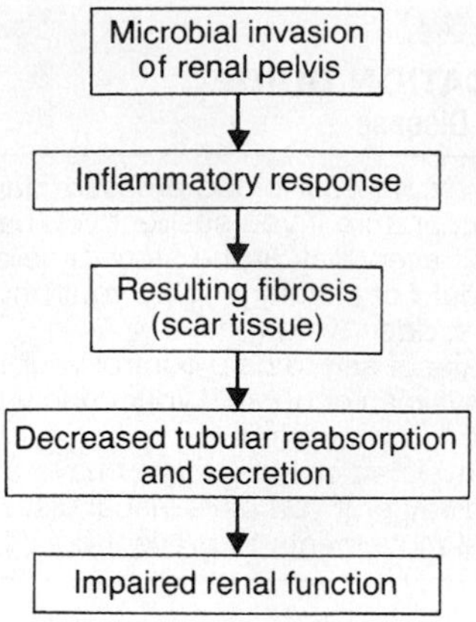

Figure 74-3 ■ Pathophysiology of chronic pyelonephritis.

In pyelonephritis, organisms ascend from the lower urinary tract into the renal pelvis. Descending infection transmitted by organisms in the blood may occur, but not often. Bacteria trigger the inflammatory response, and local edema results.

Acute pyelonephritis involves acute interstitial inflammation, tubular cell necrosis, and possible abscess formation. **Abscesses**, pockets of local infection, can occur in the capsule, cortex, or medulla. The infection is scattered within the kidney; healthy tissues can lie next to infected areas. Fibrosis and scar tissue develop from the inflammation. The calices thicken and scars develop in the interstitial tissue.

Reflux of infected urine from the bladder into the ureters and kidney is responsible for most cases of chronic pyelonephritis. Reflux within the kidney can occur when some papillae in the kidney do not close properly. Inflammation and fibrosis lead to deformity of the renal pelvis and calices. Repeated or continuous infections create additional scar tissue, changing blood vessel, glomerular, and tubular structure. As a result, filtration, reabsorption, and secretion are impaired, and renal function is reduced (Figure 74-3).

Etiology and Genetic Risk

Single episodes of *acute* pyelonephritis may result from the entry of bacteria associated with pregnancy, obstruction, or reflux. *Chronic* pyelonephritis is usually associated with structural deformities or obstruction with reflux. Reflux or obstruction leading to chronic pyelonephritis is often caused by stones or neurogenic impairment of voiding. Reflux is more common in children, who as adults have scarring with chronic pyelonephritis. Chronic pyelonephritis in adults who did not have reflux as a child usually occurs with spinal cord injury, bladder tumor, prostatic enlargement, or urinary tract stones.

Acute or chronic pyelonephritis occurs often in clients who have undergone manipulation of the urinary tract (e.g., placement of a urinary catheter), those with diabetes mellitus or chronic renal calculi, or those who overuse analgesics. In clients with diabetes mellitus, the development of bladder atony increases the risk for pyelonephritis. In clients with chronic stone disease, stones may retain organisms resulting in ongoing infection and renal scarring. Nonsteroidal anti-inflammatory drug (NSAID) use is associated with papillary necrosis and reflux.

The most common pyelonephritis-causing organism is *Escherichia coli. Enterococcus faecalis* is common in hospitalized clients. Both organisms are in the intestinal tract. Other organisms that cause pyelonephritis in hospitalized clients include *Proteus mirabilis, Klebsiella,* and *Pseudomonas aeruginosa*. When the infection is bloodborne, common infecting organisms include *Staphylococcus aureus* and the *Candida* and *Salmonella* species.

Other possible causes of kidney scarring leading to renal impairment include antibody reactions, cell-mediated immunity against the bacterial antigens, or autoimmune reactions.

Incidence/Prevalence

The exact incidence and prevalence of pyelonephritis are not known because this diagnosis is not separately reported from all urinary tract infections. Acute conditions of the kidneys or urinary tract, nephritic syndrome, urethral stricture, and cystitis account for more than 7 million new cases annually in community-dwelling Americans (NIDDK National Kidney and Urologic Diseases Information Clearinghouse, 2004). Women have more cases of pyelonephritis. After 65 years of age, rates for men increase greatly because of the increased incidence of prostatitis.

◆COLLABORATIVE MANAGEMENT

PHARM e REVIEW

◆Assessment

HISTORY

Ask the client about a history of urinary tract infections (UTIs), diabetes mellitus, stone disease, and other abnormalities of the genitourinary tract. Determine whether the UTIs occurred with pregnancy and ask the client about any previous episodes of pyelonephritis or similar symptoms. Recurrences are common and may lead to a decline of renal function.

PHYSICAL ASSESSMENT/CLINICAL MANIFESTATIONS

Ask the client about manifestations of acute pyelonephritis (Chart 74-4). Chronic pyelonephritis has a less dramatic presentation, with manifestations related to the infection or renal function. Ask the client to describe any vague or nonspecific urinary symptoms or abdominal discomfort. Inquire about any history of repeated, low-grade fevers. The client with chronic pyelonephritis often has asymptomatic bacteremia. Chart 74-5 outlines the renal effects of chronic pyelonephritis.

Inspect the flanks and gently palpate the costovertebral angle (CVA). Inspect both CVAs for enlargement, asymmetry, edema, or erythema, all of which can be manifestations of inflammation. If there is no tenderness to light palpation in either CVA, a specially trained nurse firmly percusses each area. Tenderness or discomfort may indicate infection or inflammation.

PSYCHOSOCIAL ASSESSMENT

The client with any problem in the genitourinary area may have feelings of anxiety, embarrassment, or guilt. Listen carefully for evidence of anxiety or specific fears, and prevent embarrassment during assessment. Feelings of guilt, often associated with sexual habits or practices, may be masked through delay in seeking treatment or through vague, nonspecific responses to specific or direct questions. Encourage clients to tell their own story in familiar, comfortable language.

CHART 74-4

KEY FEATURES of Acute Pyelonephritis

- Fever
- Chills
- Tachycardia and tachypnea
- Flank, back, or loin pain
- Tender costal vertebral angle (CVA)
- Abdominal, often colicky, discomfort
- Nausea and vomiting
- General malaise or fatigue
- Burning, urgency, or frequency of urination
- Nocturia

CHART 74-5

KEY FEATURES of Chronic Pyelonephritis

- Hypertension
- Inability to conserve sodium
- Decreased concentrating ability (nocturia)
- Tendency to develop hyperkalemia and acidosis

LABORATORY ASSESSMENT

Urinalysis shows a positive leukocyte esterase and nitrite dipstick test and the presence of white blood cells and bacteria. Occasional red blood cells, white blood cell casts, and proteinuria may be present. The urine is cultured to determine whether gram-positive or gram-negative organisms are causing the infection. The urine sample for culture and sensitivity testing, obtained by the clean-catch method, shows the bacterial species and susceptibility or resistance of the specific organism to various antibiotics. In clients with recurrent episodes of pyelonephritis or upper UTIs, more specific testing of bacterial antigens and antibodies may help determine whether the same organism is responsible for the recurrent infections.

Blood cultures are obtained for specific organisms. Other blood tests include the C-reactive protein and erythrocyte sedimentation rate.

RADIOGRAPHIC ASSESSMENT

An x-ray of the kidneys, ureters, and bladder (KUB) and intravenous (IV) pyelography are performed to determine the presence of stones or obstructions. A cystourethrogram is indicated for some clients. These procedures define urinary tract structures and identify any structural defects. Specific defects to be identified include foreign bodies, such as stones; obstruction to the outflow of urine, such as tumors, structural defects, or prostate enlargement; and urine reflux caused by incompetent ureterovesical valve closure. (See Chapter 72 for more information on radiographic assessment.)

OTHER DIAGNOSTIC ASSESSMENTS

Other diagnostic tests include examining antibody-coated bacteria in urine, certain enzymes (e.g., lactate dehydrogenase isoenzyme 5), and radionuclide scintillation (e.g., gallium scan). Examining urine for antibody-coated bacteria helps identify clients who may need long-term antibiotic therapy. High molecular-weight enzymes in urine, such as lactate dehydrogenase isoenzyme 5, are present with any renal tissue deterioration problem and give trend data. The gallium scan can identify active pyelonephritis or abscesses in or around the kidney.

Critical Thinking Challenge

The client is a 21-year-old female nursing student who has flank and CVA pain, dysuria, urgency, nocturia, and frequency. She tells you she started to feel unwell about 3 days ago but is much worse now. She says she has had cystitis about six times in the past year but has never been this sick with it. She says "I usually work as a nursing assistant at night but had to call off because I was so tired and nauseated." Her vital signs are P 114, BP 130/90, R 22, T 102. Her urine is cloudy, amber, and foul smelling, positive for both leukocyte esterase and nitrate, with white blood cells and gram-negative bacteria.

1. What additional assessment data should you obtain?
2. Which manifestations are specific to cystitis, which are specific to pyelonephritis, and which are common to both?
3. What risk factors for pyelonephritis are present for this client?

evolve For suggested answer guidelines, go to http://evolve.elsevier.com/Iggy/.

Analysis

COMMON NURSING DIAGNOSES AND COLLABORATIVE PROBLEMS

The primary common nursing diagnosis for the client with pyelonephritis is Acute Pain (Flank and Abdominal) related to inflammation and infection. A common collaborative problem is Potential for Renal Failure.

ADDITIONAL NURSING DIAGNOSES AND COLLABORATIVE PROBLEMS

In addition to the common nursing diagnoses and collaborative problems, clients with pyelonephritis may have one or more of the following:

- Infection or Risk for Infection related to inadequate primary defenses (urinary stasis) or instrumentation
- Deficient Knowledge regarding the medical diagnosis and therapy related to unfamiliarity with information resources
- Activity Intolerance related to fatigue, debilitation, and generalized weakness associated with the infection
- Fear of development of chronic renal failure related to an inability to control recurrent infections
- Hyperthermia related to increased metabolic rate from infection

An additional collaborative problem is Potential for Sepsis and Septic Shock.

Planning and Implementation

ACUTE PAIN

NOC **PLANNING: EXPECTED OUTCOMES.** With proper intervention, the client with pyelonephritis is expected to achieve an acceptable state of comfort. Indicators include that the client often or consistently demonstrates the following behaviors:

- Uses nonanalgesic relief measures
- Uses analgesics appropriately
- Reports pain controlled

INTERVENTIONS. Interventions may be nonsurgical or surgical. (See Pain Management in Chart 74-2.) The success of several noninvasive techniques that crush stones, such as lithotripsy and percutaneous ultrasonic pyelolithotomy (see Chapter 73), have decreased the need for surgery.

NONSURGICAL MANAGEMENT. Nonsurgical interventions include the use of drug therapy, diet and fluid therapy, and teaching to ensure the client's understanding of the treatment.

Drug Therapy. Antibiotics are prescribed to treat the infection. At first, the antibiotics are broad spectrum. After urine and blood culture and sensitivity results are known, more specific antibiotics may be prescribed. Urinary antiseptic drugs (e.g., nitrofurantoin [Macrodantin]) may also be prescribed to provide comfort. See Medication Management in Chart 74-2 for nursing intervention activities.

Diet Therapy. For healing to occur, the client's nutritional intake must include adequate calories and all food groups. Fluid intake is recommended at 2 to 3 L/day unless another condition requires fluid restriction.

SURGICAL MANAGEMENT. Surgical interventions can correct structural problems causing urine reflux or obstruction of urine outflow or to eradicate the source of infection.

Preoperative Care. Antibiotics are given, usually intravenously, to achieve adequate blood levels or sterile blood culture results. Teach the client the nature and purpose of the proposed surgery, the expected outcome, and how the client can participate.

Operative Procedures. The surgical procedures may be one of the following: **pyelolithotomy** (stone removal from the kidney), **nephrectomy** (removal of the kidney), ureteral diversion, or reimplantation of ureter to restore proper bladder drainage.

A pyelolithotomy is needed for removal of a large stone in the renal pelvis that blocks urine flow and causes infection. Nephrectomy is a last resort when all other measures to eradicate infection have failed. For clients with poor ureterovesical valve closure or dilated ureters, **ureteroplasty** (ureter repair or revision) or ureteral reimplantation (through another site in the bladder wall) preserves renal function and eliminates infections.

Postoperative Care. See Chapter 73 for nursing care after surgery for the client undergoing urologic surgery.

POTENTIAL FOR RENAL FAILURE

NOC **PLANNING: EXPECTED OUTCOMES.** The client under treatment for pyelonephritis is expected to conserve existing renal function for as long as possible and have a slow progression of renal failure once the process of renal failure begins. Indicators include that the client consistently demonstrates the following behaviors:

- Describes the role of antibiotics and self-administration of medications
- Explains and offers techniques to ensure adequate nutrition and hydration

- Describes the plan for post-treatment follow-up, including knowledge of recurrent symptoms
- Modifies prescribed regimen as directed by a health care professional

INTERVENTIONS. Specific antibiotics are prescribed to treat the infection. Stress the importance of completing the drug therapy as directed. Discuss with the client and family the importance of regular follow-up examinations and completing the recommended diagnostic tests.

Blood pressure control is needed to slow the progression of renal dysfunction. When renal impairment decreases concentrating ability, encourage the client to drink at least 2 L of fluid per day to prevent dehydration, which could further reduce renal function. When dietary protein is restricted, refer the client to the dietitian as needed. Other interventions related to the progression of chronic renal failure are covered in Chapter 75.

Community-Based Care

Pyelonephritis causes fear and anxiety in the client and family. The severity of the acute process and its potential to develop into a chronic process are frightening. The client and the family need reassurance that treatment and preventive measures can be accomplished.

HOME CARE MANAGEMENT

If no surgery is performed, the client may need assistance with self-care, nutrition, and drug management at home. If surgery is performed, the client may need help with incision care, self-care, and transportation for follow-up appointments.

HEALTH TEACHING

After assessing the client and family's understanding of pyelonephritis and its therapy, explain the following:

- Drug regimen (purpose, timing, frequency, duration, and possible side effects)
- The role of nutrition and adequate fluid intake
- The need for a balance between rest and activity, including any limitations after surgery
- The manifestations of disease recurrence
- The use of previously successful coping mechanisms

Advise the client to complete all prescribed antibiotic regimens and to report any side effects or unusual symptoms to the physician rather than stopping the drugs. Refer the client and family for nutritional counseling as needed, because many clients have special nutritional requirements, such as those caused by diabetes mellitus or pregnancy.

HEALTH CARE RESOURCES

The client may also briefly need a community health nurse to help with drug or nutrition therapy at home. Housekeeping services may be helpful while the client is regaining strength.

Evaluation: Outcomes

Evaluate the care of the client with pyelonephritis on the basis of the identified nursing diagnoses and collaborative problems. Expected outcomes may include that the client will:

- Report that pain is controlled
- Be knowledgeable about the disease, its treatment, and interventions to prevent or reduce disease progression

Specific indicators for these outcomes are listed for each nursing diagnosis and collaborative problem under the Planning and Implementation section (see earlier).

Critical Thinking Challenge

The client described earlier (p. 1714) is diagnosed with acute pyelonephritis. She is initially prescribed IV ciprofloxacin (Cipro) for pyelonephritis but was changed to gentamicin after a urine culture indicated that the infecting organism is *Lactobacillus*, an organism that is considered normal flora of the vagina and seldom the cause of major infections. After the client's manifestations have resolved, she undergoes cystography because of the frequency of cystitis episodes. The perineal examination and the cystography show that her urethral meatus is located abnormally close to her vagina and that she also has a mild degree of vesicoureteral reflux. She has no scarring of the kidney at this time and surgery is not planned.

1. Explain whether this client's acute pyelonephritis is an ascending or a descending infection.
2. How do the findings of the physical examination and the cystography relate as a cause of her acute pyelonephritis?
3. In addition to adherence to any chronic antiseptic or antibiotic therapy, what could you suggest as measures for this client to reduce her risk for future episodes of pyelonephritis and cystitis (you may need to review Chapter 73)?

evolve For suggested answer guidelines, go to http://evolve.elsevier.com/Iggy/.

Renal Abscess

PATHOPHYSIOLOGY

An **abscess** is a collection of fluid and cells caused by an inflammatory response to bacteria. It may occur within the kidney tissue (renal abscess), in Gerota's fascia (perinephric abscess), or in the flank. An abscess is suspected when manifestations are not relieved promptly by antibiotic therapy.

COLLABORATIVE MANAGEMENT

A renal or perirenal abscess is diagnosed via sonography or a computed tomography (CT) scan. Arteriography and radionuclide scintillation methods (e.g., gallium scan) also may be useful for diagnosis. Manifestations include fever, flank pain, and general malaise. Local flank edema and redness may be observed.

Drainage by surgical incision or needle aspiration is often necessary. Broad-spectrum antibiotics are also prescribed.

Renal Tuberculosis

PATHOPHYSIOLOGY

The urinary tract is the most common site of tuberculosis (TB) outside of the lungs. About 10% of new cases of TB occur outside the lungs (Tolkoff-Rubin, Cotran, & Rubin, 2000). TB of the kidney is sometimes called *granulomatous nephritis.* After TB invades the kidneys by the bloodborne route, an inflammatory response is triggered and forms scar tissue **(granuloma)** that replaces normal kidney tissue.

COLLABORATIVE MANAGEMENT

Clients may have urinary frequency, dysuria, hematuria and/or proteinuria, flank pain or renal colic with the pas-

TABLE 74-1 Primary Glomerular Diseases and Syndromes

- Acute glomerulonephritis
- Rapidly progressive glomerulonephritis (RPGN)
- Chronic glomerulonephritis
- Nephrotic syndrome
- Persisting urinary abnormalities with few or no symptoms

sage of clots or stones, pyuria, and hypertension. Skin test (e.g., purified protein derivative [PPD]) or chest x-ray evidence of tuberculosis (TB) may or may not be present.

Clients with current or previous pulmonary TB who show signs of unexplained fever, hematuria, and sterile pyuria are at high risk for renal TB. The diagnosis is made through a urine culture of three clean-catch, first-morning specimens. Other genitourinary sites for tuberculosis include the prostate, epididymis, ureters, testes, bladder, and seminal vesicles.

Antitubercular therapy with a 2-month course of rifampin, isoniazid, and pyrazinamide followed by 4 months of rifampin and isoniazid is the main therapy. Three to six more months of rifampin and isoniazid are recommended for men who have the organism in the prostate (Tolkoff-Rubin, Cotran, & Rubin, 2000).

Complications include renal failure, kidney stones, obstruction, and bacterial superinfection of the urinary tract. Surgical excision of diseased tissue may be needed to preserve renal function.

IMMUNOLOGIC RENAL DISORDERS

Glomerulonephritis (GN) is the third leading cause of end-stage renal disease (ESRD) (NIDDK, 2004). Both primary and secondary diseases or syndromes result in glomerular injury. Glomeruli are usually involved in primary disease (Table 74-1); the nonrenal effects of primary disease stem from the glomerular injury. Most primary diseases and syndromes have an immunologic component, and many have an underlying genetic basis. Secondary glomerular diseases are those situations in which glomerular involvement is part of another disease. For example, systemic diseases and infections can have renal effects and cause glomerular injury (Table 74-2). Conditions that cause secondary glomerular disease include systemic lupus erythematous and diabetic nephropathy.

Each primary or secondary disease or syndrome has a specific pathophysiology and clinical manifestations. Their *glomerular* effects are caused by injury to the glomeruli and result in proteinuria, hematuria, decreased glomerular filtration rate (GFR), edema, and hypertension. The extent and duration of renal injury, prognosis, and specific cause vary among these syndromes.

Immunologic changes injure the glomeruli, interstitium, or tubules, and the effects may be acute or chronic. Both antibody and cellular immune responses are involved. The resultant renal disorder can be systemic or localized to the kidneys.

Most forms of glomerulonephritis (GN) occur with a collection of immune complexes in the glomeruli (Figure 74-4). An immune complex is made up of antigens and antibodies. The antigen can be any normal kidney tissue, or it can be dissolved in a body fluid (e.g., blood). Bacteria and viruses are also antigens. Exposure to bacteria, viruses, drugs, or other toxins is believed to be the trigger for glomerular injury.

Antibody reaction with antigens can lead to immune complex formation and deposition in glomerular tissue. The

TABLE 74-2 Secondary Glomerular Diseases and Syndromes

- Systemic lupus erythematosus (SLE)
- Schönlein-Henoch purpura
- Goodpasture's syndrome
- Systemic necrotizing vasculitis
- Wegener's granulomatosis
- Periarteritis nodosa (also called polyarteritis nodosa)
- Amyloidosis
- Diabetic glomerulopathy
- HIV-associated nephropathy
- Alport's syndrome
- Multiple myeloma
- Viral hepatitis B
- Viral hepatitis C
- Cirrhosis
- Sickle-cell disease
- Nonstreptococcal postinfectious acute glomerulonephritis
- Infective endocarditis
- Hemolytic-uremic syndrome
- Thrombotic thrombocytopenic purpura

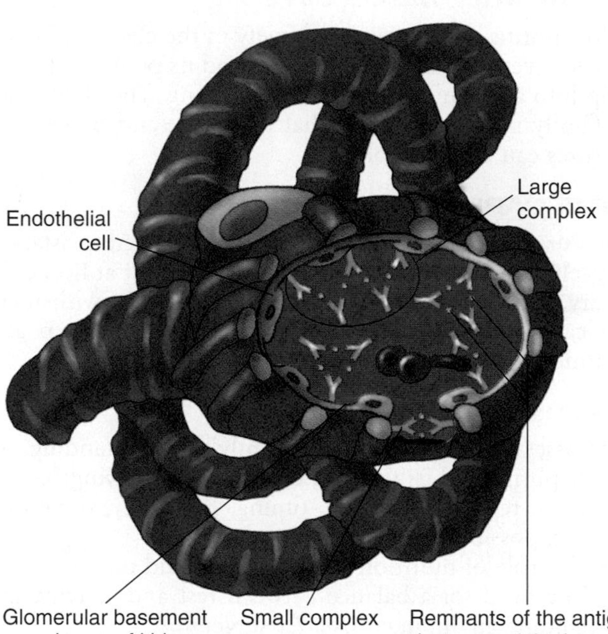

Figure 74-4 ■ An immune complex precipitating in the glomerulus of a client with glomerulonephritis.

immune complexes trigger many inflammatory mediators, such as complement, white blood cells, and blood clotting proteins, which also damage the renal tissue. Actions that cause tissue injury include damage to cell membranes, local edema, movement of white blood cells to the site of inflammation, and platelet activation.

Acute Glomerulonephritis

PATHOPHYSIOLOGY

An infection often occurs before the renal manifestations of acute glomerulonephritis (GN). The onset of symptoms is about 10 days from the time of infection. Usually, clients recover quickly and completely from acute GN. The term *acute nephritic syndrome* also describes this disorder.

Most causes of acute GN are infectious (Table 74-3) or are related to other systemic diseases (see Table 74-2). The

TABLE 74-3 Infectious Causes of Acute Glomerulonephritis

- Group A beta-hemolytic *Streptococcus*
- Staphylococcal or gram-negative bacteremia or sepsis
- Pneumococcal, *Mycoplasma*, or *Klebsiella* pneumonia
- Syphilis
- Visceral abscesses
- Infective endocarditis
- Hepatitis B
- Infectious mononucleosis
- Measles
- Mumps
- Rocky Mountain spotted fever
- Cytomegaloviral infection
- Histoplasmosis
- Toxoplasmosis
- Varicella
- *Chlamydia psittaci* infection
- Coxsackievirus infection
- Any bacterial, parasitic, fungal, or viral infection (potentially)

incidence of acute GN is unknown. GN after a systemic streptococcal infection is more common in men.

COLLABORATIVE MANAGEMENT

Assessment

HISTORY

Ask about recent infections, particularly of the skin or upper respiratory tract, and about recent travel or other activities with possible exposure to viruses, bacteria, fungi, or parasites. Recent illnesses, surgery, or other invasive procedures may suggest infections. Ask about any known systemic diseases, such as systemic lupus erythematosus (SLE), which could cause acute GN.

PHYSICAL ASSESSMENT/CLINICAL MANIFESTATIONS

Inspect the client's skin for lesions or recent incisions and the face, eyelids, hands, and other areas for edema (present in about 75% of the clients with acute GN). Assess for fluid overload and circulatory congestion (which may accompany the sodium and fluid retention occurring with acute GN). Ask about any difficulty in breathing, nocturnal or exertional dyspnea, or orthopnea. Assess for crackles in the lung fields, an S_3 heart sound (gallop rhythm), and neck vein distention.

Ask about changes in urination pattern and any change in urine color. Microscopic hematuria occurs up to 66% of the time, and clients often describe their urine as smoky, reddish-brown, rusty, or cola colored. Ask about dysuria or oliguria. Weigh the client to assess for fluid retention.

Take the client's blood pressure and compare it with the baseline blood pressure. Mild to moderate hypertension often occurs with acute GN due to sodium and fluid retention. The client may have fatigue, a lack of energy, anorexia, nausea, and/or vomiting if uremia from renal failure is present.

CONSIDERATIONS FOR OLDER ADULTS

The less common manifestations of acute GN are more likely to occur in older adults. Circulatory congestion often dominates the client's clinical picture. Acute GN is easily confused with congestive heart failure.

LABORATORY ASSESSMENT

Urinalysis shows red blood cells **(hematuria)** and protein (proteinuria). An early morning specimen of urine is preferred for urinalysis because the urine is most acidic and formed elements are more intact at that time. Microscopic examination often shows red blood cell casts as well as casts from other substances. The urine sediment assay is usually positive.

The glomerular filtration rate (GFR), measured by the 24-hour urine test for creatinine clearance, may be decreased to 50 mL/min. Blood urea nitrogen (BUN) levels are usually increased. The older client may have a greater decline in GFR.

A 24-hour urine collection for total protein assay is also obtained. The protein excretion rate for clients with acute GN may be increased from 500 mg to 3 g/24 hr in most clients. Serum albumin levels are decreased because of the protein lost in the urine and because of fluid retention causing dilution.

Specimens from the blood, skin, or throat are obtained for culture, if indicated. Other serologic tests include antistreptolysin-O titers, C3 complement levels, cryoglobulins (immunoglobulin G [IgG]), antinuclear antibodies (ANAs), and circulating immune complexes.

Antistreptolysin-O titers are increased after group A beta-hemolytic *Streptococcus* infections. Complement levels are decreased when the complement system is activated. Type III cryoglobulins may be found during acute illness. ANAs suggest an autoimmune response, and SLE is just one possibility. Circulating immune complexes containing IgG and C3 are often detected.

OTHER DIAGNOSTIC ASSESSMENTS

A renal biopsy provides a precise diagnosis of the pathologic condition, assists in determining the prognosis, and helps outline treatment (see Chapter 72). The specific tissue morphology is determined by light microscopy, immunofluorescent stains, and electron microscopy to identify cell type, the presence of immunoglobulins, or the type of tissue deposits.

Interventions

Interventions focus on treating the underlying infectious process, preventing complications, and providing appropriate client education.

Management of Infection. Treatment for acute GN with an infectious cause is an appropriate antibiotic. Penicillin, erythromycin, or azithromycin are prescribed for GN resulting from streptococcal infection. Check the client's known allergies before giving any drug. To prevent infection spread, antibiotics for persons in immediate close contact with the client may be prescribed. Stress personal hygiene and basic infection control principles (e.g., handwashing) to prevent spread of the organism.

Prevention of Complications. For clients with fluid overload, hypertension, and edema, diuretics and a sodium and water restriction are prescribed. Antihypertensive drugs may be needed to control hypertension (see Chart 39-3). The usual fluid allowance is equal to the 24-hour urine output plus 500 to 600 mL. Clients with oliguria usually have increased serum levels of potassium and blood urea nitrogen (BUN). Potassium and protein intake may be restricted to prevent hyperkalemia and uremia as a result of the elevated BUN.

Nausea, vomiting, or anorexia indicates that uremia is present. Dialysis is necessary if uremic symptoms or fluid volume excess cannot be controlled (see Chapter 75). **Plasmapheresis** (removal and filtering of the plasma to eliminate antibodies) also may be attempted (see Chapter 43).

To conserve the client's energy, assist him or her in maintaining a restful environment, balancing activity and rest, and coordinating needed therapeutic activities. Encourage the client to practice relaxation techniques and to participate in diversional activities to reduce emotional stress.

Client Education. Instruct the client and family members about the purpose and desired effects of prescribed drugs, the dosage and schedule, and potential adverse side effects. Ensure that the client and family understand dietary or fluid modifications, including methods of detecting fluid retention. Advise the client to weigh himself or herself and measure blood pressure daily at the same time each day. Instruct the client to notify the health care provider of any sudden increase in weight or blood pressure.

If short-term dialysis is required to control fluid volume excess or uremic symptoms, explain peritoneal or vascular access care and dialysis schedules and routines (also see Chapter 75).

Rapidly Progressive Glomerulonephritis

Rapidly progressive glomerulonephritis (RPGN), a type of acute nephritis, is also called *crescentic glomerulonephritis* because of the presence of crescent-shaped cells in the Bowman's capsule. RPGN develops over several weeks or months and causes a significant loss of renal function. Clients become quite ill quickly and have manifestations of renal failure (fluid volume excess, hypertension, oliguria, electrolyte imbalances, and uremic symptoms).

The client may have has previous infection or systemic disease, such as systemic lupus erythematosus (SLE). The renal deterioration often progresses to end-stage renal disease (ESRD).

Chronic Glomerulonephritis

PATHOPHYSIOLOGY

Chronic glomerulonephritis, or *chronic nephritic syndrome,* develops over 20 to 30 years or even longer. The exact onset of the disorder is rarely identified. In many instances the cause of the disease is not known because the kidneys are atrophied and tissue is not available for biopsy or diagnosis. Mild proteinuria and hematuria, hypertension, and occasional edema are often the only manifestations.

Although the exact cause is not known, changes in the renal tissue result from hypertension, infections and inflammation, or altered metabolism and poor blood flow to the kidneys. Kidney tissue atrophies, and the number of functional nephrons is greatly reduced. Biopsy in the late stages of atrophy may show glomerular changes, cell loss, protein and collagen deposits, and fibrosis of the kidney tissue. Microscopic examination shows deposits of immune complexes.

The loss of nephrons reduces glomerular filtration. Hypertension and renal arteriole sclerosis are often present. The glomerular damage allows proteins to enter the urine. Eventually, chronic glomerulonephritis always leads to renal failure (see Chapter 75).

COLLABORATIVE MANAGEMENT

Assessment

HISTORY

Ask the client about other health problems, including systemic diseases, renal or urologic disorders, infectious diseases (e.g., streptococcal infections), and recent exposures to infections. Ask about his or her overall health status and whether increasing fatigue and lethargy have been experienced.

Identify the client's pattern of voiding. Ask whether the frequency of voiding has increased or the quantity of urine has decreased. Ask about changes in urine color, odor, or clarity and whether dysuria or incontinence have occurred.

Assess the client's general comfort and ask whether any dyspnea at rest or with exertion has occurred because fluid overload can occur with decreased urine output. Ask about and observe for changes in mental functioning, such as irritability or an inability to read or to perform job-related functions or other processes requiring concentration. Changes in memory and the ability to concentrate occur as waste products collect in the blood.

PHYSICAL ASSESSMENT/CLINICAL MANIFESTATIONS

Assess for systemic circulatory overload. Auscultate lung fields for crackles, observe the respiratory rate and depth, and measure blood pressure and weight. Auscultate the heart for rate, rhythm, and the presence of an S_3 heart sound. Inspect the neck veins for venous engorgement and check for edema in the pedal, pretibial, and presacral tissues.

Assess for uremic symptoms, such as slurred speech, ataxia, tremors, or **asterixis** (flapping tremor of the fingers or the inability to maintain a fixed posture with the arms extended and wrists hyperextended). Inspect skin for a yellowish color, texture, bruises, rashes, or eruptions. Document areas of dryness and any excoriation from scratching.

DIAGNOSTIC ASSESSMENT

Urine output decreases but the urine appears normal unless a urinary tract infection (UTI) also is present. Urinalysis shows proteinuria, usually less than 2 g in a 24-hour collection. The specific gravity is fixed at a constant level of dilution (around 1.010). There may be red blood cells and casts in the urine.

The glomerular filtration rate (GFR), measured by creatinine clearance, is low. The serum creatinine level is elevated, usually greater than 6 mg/dL but may be as high as 30 mg/dL or more. Blood urea nitrogen (BUN) is increased, often as high as 100 to 200 mg/dL.

Decreased renal function causes abnormal serum electrolyte levels. Sodium retention is common, but dilution of the plasma from excess fluid can result in a falsely normal serum sodium level (135 to 145 mEq/L) or a dilutional hyponatremia (<135 mEq/L). When oliguria develops, potassium retention occurs causing hyperkalemia when levels exceed 5.4 mEq/L.

Hyperphosphatemia develops with serum levels greater than 4.7 mg/dL. Serum calcium levels are usually at the lower end of the normal range or are slightly below normal.

Acidosis develops from hydrogen ion retention and loss of bicarbonate. However, there may be a decrease in serum carbon dioxide (CO_2) levels as clients breathe more rapidly to compensate for the acidosis. If respiratory compensation is present, the pH of arterial blood is between 7.35 and 7.45. A pH of less than 7.35 means that the client's respiratory system is not completely compensating for the acidosis (see Chapter 19).

The kidneys are abnormally small on x-ray, IV urography, and when measured by sonography or computed tomography (CT).

A renal biopsy is important in the early stages of glomerulonephritis, when proteinuria or hematuria is first present. Tissue changes include a variety of cells infiltrating the glomerular tissue, deposition of immune complexes, and blood vessel sclerosis. In advanced disease, when the kidneys are small, renal biopsy is not usually performed.

Interventions

Interventions focus on slowing the progression of the disease and preventing complications. Treatment consists of diet changes, fluid intake sufficient to prevent reduced blood flow volume to the kidneys, and drug therapy to control the problems from uremia. Eventually, the client requires dialysis or transplantation to prevent death from the systemic effects of uremia. (Nursing care for the client with ESRD requiring dialysis or transplantation is discussed in Chapter 75.)

Nephrotic Syndrome

PATHOPHYSIOLOGY

Nephrotic syndrome (NS) is a condition of increased glomerular permeability that allows larger molecules to pass through the membrane into the urine and be removed from the blood. This process causes massive loss of protein into the urine, edema formation, and decreased plasma albumin levels. Many agents and disorders are possible causes of NS.

The most common cause of glomerular membrane changes is an immune or inflammatory processes. Defects in glomerular filtration can also occur as a result of genetic flaws resulting in defective proteins in the glomerular filtering system (Jalanko et al., 2001; Online Mendelian Inheritance in Man, 2004). Altered liver activity may occur with nephrotic syndrome, resulting in increased lipid production and hyperlipidemia.

COLLABORATIVE MANAGEMENT

The main feature of nephrotic syndrome (NS) is severe proteinuria (>3.5 g of protein in 24 hours). Clients also have hypoalbuminemia (serum albumin <3 g/dL), hyperlipidemia, lipiduria, edema, and hypertension (Chart 74-6). Renal vein thrombosis often occurs at the same time as NS, either as a cause of the problem or as an effect. NS may progress to ESRD, but progression can be prevented with treatment.

Treatment varies depending on what process is causing the disorder (identified by renal biopsy). Immunologic processes may improve with suppressive therapy using steroids and cytotoxic or immunosuppressive agents. Angiotensin-converting enzyme (ACE) inhibitors can decrease proteinuria, and cholesterol-lowering drugs can improve hyperlipidemia. Heparin may lower proteinuria and reduce renal insufficiency. Diet changes are often prescribed. If the glomerular filtration rate (GFR) is normal, dietary intake of complete proteins is needed. If the GFR is decreased, dietary protein intake must be decreased. Mild diuretics (Chart 74-7) and sodium restriction may be needed to control edema and hypertension. Assess the client's hydration status, as vascular dehydration is common. If the plasma volume is depleted, renal problems worsen. Acute renal failure may be avoided if good renal blood flow is maintained.

CHART 74-6

KEY FEATURES of Nephrotic Syndrome

- Massive proteinuria
- Hypoalbuminemia
- Edema
- Lipiduria
- Hyperlipidemia
- Increased coagulation
- Renal insufficiency

Immunologic Interstitial and Tubulointerstitial Disorders

Interstitial and tubulointerstitial disorders in the kidney are usually caused by immune alterations. These renal changes may be acute or chronic. The acute effects often occur with drugs such as penicillins, cephalosporins, sulfonamides, or nonsteroidal anti-inflammatory drugs (NSAIDs). Chronic interstitial nephritis has many causes, including analgesic use, complement activation, cyclosporin use, polycystic kidney disease, autoimmune disorders, multiple myeloma, sickle cell disease, obstructive disorders, and radiation nephritis. Drug-induced problems often occur with a rash or an elevated eosinophil count. Fever is common in interstitial nephritis of unknown cause. Progression to ESRD occurs unless the causative problem is identified and removed.

DEGENERATIVE DISORDERS

Degenerative disorders that change renal function often occur with a multisystem disorder. Many of these degenerative disorders result from changes in kidney blood vessels.

Nephrosclerosis

PATHOPHYSIOLOGY

Nephrosclerosis is a problem of thickening in the nephron blood vessels, resulting in narrowing of the vessel lumen. This change decreases renal blood flow and kidney tissue is chronically hypoxic. Ischemia and fibrosis develop over time.

Nephrosclerosis occurs with all types of hypertension, atherosclerosis, and diabetes mellitus. The more severe the hypertension, the greater the risk for severe kidney damage. Nephrosclerosis is rarely seen when blood pressure is consistently below 160/110 mm Hg. The changes caused by hypertension may be reversible or may progress to end-stage renal disease (ESRD) within months or years.

Hypertension is the second leading cause of ESRD. About 30% of clients requiring renal replacement therapy (e.g., dialysis or transplantation) have hypertension as the cause of their renal failure (NIDDK, 2004).

CHART 74-7

DRUG THERAPY for
Diuretics Used to Increase Urine Output

Drug	Usual Dosage	Indication	Nursing Interventions	Rationales
Osmotic Diuretics (act on glomerulus and renal tubular system)				
Mannitol (Osmitrol*), urea	50-100 g IV as a 5%-25% solution	Causes rapid diuresis (e.g., after contrast media infusion)	Measure fluid intake and output.	Severe dehydration is possible.
			Check vial for crystals. If crystals are present, warm vial between the hands.	Mannitol may crystallize while on the shelf. Crystals dissolve with body warmth.
			Administer through a filter.	This prevents remaining crystals from entering the body.
Thiazide and Thiazide-Like Diuretics (act on cortical diluting site of ascending limb of loop of Henle)				
Chlorothiazide (Diuril)	250 mg PO, IV once to four times daily	Hypertension	Observe for signs and symptoms of electrolyte imbalance.	Common complications include hypokalemia and hypercalcemia.
Hydrochlorothiazide (HydroDIURIL, Apo-Hydro*, Urozide*)	25-100 mg PO once or twice daily	Congestive heart failure (CHF) with edema	Monitor heart sounds for S_3, lung sounds for crackles, and other signs of CHF.	Ongoing monitoring detects complications and helps ensure prompt treatment.
Chlorthalidone (Hygroton, Uridon*)	25-100 mg PO daily	Edema, hypertension	Do not give with NSAIDs.	A decreased diuretic effect is seen with concomitant use of NSAIDs.
[1]Metolazone (Zaroxolyn)	5-20 mg PO daily	Edema, hypertension	Do not give with NSAIDs.	A decreased diuretic effect is seen with concomitant use of NSAIDs.
Loop Diuretics (act on ascending limb of loop of Henle)				
Furosemide (Lasix, Furoside*)	20-80 mg PO or IV once or twice daily; maximum daily dose 600 mg	Hypertension	Observe for orthostatic hypotension.	An early sign of rapid fluid volume depletion may be orthostatic hypotension.
Bumetanide [2](Bumex)	0.5-2 mg PO daily	CHF	Monitor for possible hyponatremia and hypokalemia.	These agents increase excretion of both sodium and potassium.
Potassium-Sparing Diuretics (act on distal convoluted tubule)				
Spironolactone [3](Aldactone, Novospiroton*)	25-200 mg PO once or twice daily	Primary aldosteronism	Observe for signs and symptoms of electrolyte imbalance.	Hyperkalemia with cardiac manifestations is a common complication.
Triamterene (Dyrenium)	25-100 mg once or twice daily; maximum daily dose 300 mg	Hypertension (with other drugs to decrease potassium loss)	Teach client to avoid unprotected sun exposure.	Photosensitivity reactions are possible.
Amiloride [4](Midamor*)	5-10 mg daily	Edema, hypertension	Give with food or milk.	Stomach upset is possible.

[1]*Med Error Alert!* *Do not confuse with metoprolol, a beta blocker.*

[2]*Med Error Alert!* *Do not confuse with Buprenex, an opioid analgesic.*

[3]*Med Error Alert!* *Do not confuse with Aldomet, an antihypertensive.*

[4]*Med Error Alert!* *Do not confuse with Midodrine, a drug used to treat orthostatic hypotension.*

NSAID, Nonsteroidal anti-inflammatory drug.

CULTURAL CONSIDERATIONS

Hypertension is more common in African Americans, and the risks of ESRD from hypertension are also greater for African Americans (Bakris et al., 2000; Sowers et al., 2002). Between 25 and 45 years of age, the ratio of African Americans to Caucasians at risk for ESRD from hypertension is nearly 20:1 (Richardson & Piepho, 2000). At any health care encounter with an African American client, blood pressure should always be assessed. If hypertension is present, treatment and client education can help reduce the risk for development of ESRD.

COLLABORATIVE MANAGEMENT

Treatment aims to control high blood pressure and preserve renal function. Although many antihypertensive drugs may lower blood pressure, the client's response is important in ensuring long-term adherence to the prescribed therapy. Factors promoting adherence include once-a-day dosing, low cost, and minimal side effects.

Lack of knowledge or misinformation about hypertension poses many challenges to health care providers working with clients who have hypertension. When renal disease occurs, adherence to therapy is even more important for preserving health.

Many drugs can control high blood pressure (see Chart 39-3), and more than one agent may be necessary. Angiotensin-converting enzyme (ACE) inhibitors are particularly useful in reducing hypertension and preserving renal function. Diuretics can maintain fluid and electrolyte balance in the presence of renal insufficiency. Hyperkalemia needs to be prevented when potassium-sparing diuretics, alone or in combination, are used to treat hypertensive clients with known renal disease.

Renovascular Disease

PATHOPHYSIOLOGY

Processes affecting the renal arteries may severely narrow the lumen and profoundly reduce blood flow to the kidney tissues. Uncorrected renovascular disease, such as renal artery stenosis, atherosclerosis, or thrombosis, causes ischemia and atrophy of renal tissue.

Clients with renovascular disease often have a sudden onset of hypertension, particularly in clients older than 50 years of age. Clients with high blood pressure but with no family history of hypertension also may potentially have renal artery stenosis (RAS). RAS from atherosclerosis or blood vessel hyperplasia is the main cause of renovascular disease. Other causes include thrombosis and renal aneurysms.

Atherosclerotic changes in the renal artery often occur with sclerosis in the aorta and other major vessels. Changes in the renal artery are often located where the renal artery and aorta meet. Fibrotic changes of the blood vessel wall occur throughout the length of the renal artery.

COLLABORATIVE MANAGEMENT

Assessment

Key features of renovascular disease are listed in Chart 74-8. Hypertension usually first occurs after 40 to 50 years of age, and often the client does not have a family history of hypertension. Diagnosis is made by magnetic resonance angiography (MRA), renal duplex ultrasonography, radionuclide imaging, renal arteriography, and renal vein renin levels. MRA provides an excellent image of the renal vasculature and kidney anatomy. Radionuclide imaging is a noninvasive way of evaluating renal blood flow and excretory function. Combining radionuclide imaging with ingestion of an angiotensin-converting enzyme (ACE) inhibitor such as captopril improves the accuracy of the test. A renal arteriogram makes the features of the renal blood vessels visible. The comparison of renal vein renin levels *may* reveal which kidney is producing more renin.

CHART 74-8

KEY FEATURES of
Renovascular Disease

- Significant, difficult-to-control blood pressure
- Elevated serum creatinine
- Decreased creatinine clearance

Interventions

Viewing the type of defect, extent of narrowing, and condition of the surrounding blood vessels is critical for treatment choice. The client's overall health and the size of the atrophied kidney also influence treatment decisions. Many clients with renovascular disease also have cardiovascular disease and both conditions require evaluation and treatment.

RAS may be treated by drugs to control high blood pressure and by procedures to restore the renal blood supply. Drugs may control high blood pressure but may not lead to long-term preservation of kidney function. In young and middle-aged adults, a lifetime of treatment with many drugs for high blood pressure may make treatment difficult and the outcomes uncertain.

Balloon angioplasty with or without stent placement to open renal vessels is less risky and requires less time for recovery than does renal artery bypass surgery (see Chapter 39). Renal artery bypass surgery is a major procedure and requires 2 or more months for recovery. A bypass may be performed for either one or both renal arteries.

Renal angioplasty with metal stent placement is one safe and effective method to permanently repair RAS. Following angioplasty, the client usually remains in ICU for 24 hours to monitor for sudden blood pressure fluctuations as the kidneys adjust to increased blood flow.

A synthetic blood vessel graft is inserted to redirect blood flow from the abdominal aorta into the renal artery, beyond the area of narrowing. A splenorenal bypass can also restore renal blood flow. The process is similar to other arterial bypass procedures (see Chapter 38).

Diabetic Nephropathy

PATHOPHYSIOLOGY

Diabetes mellitus is the leading cause of end-stage renal disease (ESRD) among white individuals in the United States. About 36% of clients requiring dialysis or renal transplantation have diabetes mellitus (NIDDK, 2004). The cost of preventing or reducing renal problems among clients with

RESOURCE MANAGEMENT

DIABETES AND RENAL DISEASE

Cost of Care

- A common complication of both type 1 and type 2 diabetes mellitus (DM) is nephropathy leading to end-stage renal disease.
- Diabetic clients are 5 times more likely to develop end-stage renal disease than others in their cohort.
- Abnormal renal function increased diabetes treatment costs by $1350 and advanced renal disease by $4000 per individual treated.
- Intensive therapy increases costs to maintain blood glucose values between 90 and 140 mg/dL in both type 1 and type 2 diabetes. This type of therapy significantly reduces complications and prolongs renal function.

Implications for Nursing

Although the cost of maintaining tight control is two to three times the costs of conventional therapy, economic modeling predicts that tight control could reduce end-stage renal disease from 24% to 7%. Thus the costs of maintaining tight control are offset by savings related to reduced need for diagnosis and treatment of DM-related renal disease.

Renal disease is an expensive diagnosis, not only in dollar costs, but also in social, psychological, and functional costs as clients undergo extensive diagnostic workup and work-limiting treatment. Preventing the renal complications of DM saves money; it also saves individuals from a heavy biopsychosocial burden.

Data from Nathan, D.M. (1993). Diabetes Control and Complications Trial Research Group: The effect of long-term intensified insulin treatment on development of microvascular complications of diabetes. *New England Journal of Medicine, 329*(14), 977-986; Palmer, A.J. (2001). Intensive glucose control is more costly than conventional treatment but also has more benefits for people with type-2 diabetes. *Evidence-Based Health Care, 5*(1), 17-18; and U.S. Renal Data Systems. (2002). *USRDS 2002 annual data report.* Bethesda, MD: The National Institutes of Health, National Institute of Diabetes and Digestive and Kidney Diseases.

diabetes is offset by the high cost of treating severe renal disease (see the Resource Management box above). Diabetic nephropathy occurs with either type 1 or type 2 diabetes mellitus. Severity of diabetic renal disease is related to the extent, duration, and effects of atherosclerosis, hypertension, and neuropathy, which promotes bladder atony, urinary stasis, and urinary tract infection.

COLLABORATIVE MANAGEMENT

Diabetic nephropathy is a *microvascular* complication of diabetes. Its first manifestation is persistent albuminuria (as shown by dipstick or a urinary albumin excretion rate above 0.3 g/dL), without evidence of other renal disease. Diabetic renal disease is progressive (Table 74-4).

Structural and functional changes occur in the kidneys of diabetic clients. Initially, kidney size is slightly increased and glomerular filtration rates (GFR) are higher than normal. Microlevels of albumin are first detected in the urine. Progressive renal damage occurs before dipstick procedures can detect protein in the urine. For most clients, proteinuria (albuminuria) indicates the need for a renal biopsy for further diagnosis. For the client with diabetes, observed microvascular changes in the retina correlate well with the renal microvascular changes. Examination of the retina showing capillary leakage, fibrosis, and the typical changes of diabetic retinopathy eliminates the need for a risky renal biopsy.

Proteinuria may be mild, moderate, or severe. Diabetic clients are always considered to be at risk for renal failure. If possible, nephrotoxic agents (e.g., radiopaque contrast media or aminoglycosides) and dehydration are avoided. Clients with worsening renal function may begin to have frequent hypoglycemic episodes and a reduced need for insulin or oral antidiabetic agents. Explain to the client that the kidneys metabolize and excrete insulin. When renal function is reduced, the insulin is available for a longer time and thus less of it is needed. Unfortunately, many clients believe this means their diabetes is improving. The result is a more rapid progression to ESRD. (See Chapter 68 for specific information on diabetic nephropathy.)

TABLE 74-4 The Stages of Progression of Type 1 Diabetic Renal Disease

- **Stage I, at the time diabetes is diagnosed.** Kidney size and glomerular filtration rate are increased. Blood sugar control can reverse the changes.
- **Stage II, 2 to 3 years after diagnosis.** Glomerular and tubular capillary basement membrane changes result in microscopic changes, with loss of filtration surface area and scar formation. Glomerular changes are referred to as glomerulosclerosis.
- **Stage III, 7 to 15 years after diagnosis.** Microalbuminuria is present. The glomerular filtration rate (GFR) may still be normal or may be increased.
- **Stage IV.** Albuminuria is detectable by dipstick. GFR is decreased. Blood pressure is increased, and retinopathy is present.
- **Stage V.** GFR decreases at an average rate of 10 mL/min/yr.

TUMORS

Cysts and Benign Tumors

PATHOPHYSIOLOGY

Benign urinary tract growths include cysts and tumors of the kidney tissue or urinary bladder. Because cancer can occur within cystic structures, a thorough evaluation is needed.

A simple renal cyst grows out of renal cortical tissue, rather than tubular tissues. The cyst fills with fluid and causes local tissue damage as it enlarges. Many cysts cause no symptoms and are discovered by accident during other procedures or on autopsy.

Cysts are a structural birth defect that occurs in fetal life. The incidence of renal cysts and benign tumors is unknown.

COLLABORATIVE MANAGEMENT

Diagnosis of a simple renal cyst is usually made by ultrasound. If hematuria or other suspicious manifestations are present, computed tomography (CT) may be needed to rule out other problems. CT can determine whether the cyst is filled with serous fluid, urine, or blood.

Once determined to be a simple cyst, the cyst may be drained by percutaneous aspiration if it becomes painful. Surgical exploration with the potential for total or subtotal nephrectomy is rarely needed.

Renal Cell Carcinoma

PATHOPHYSIOLOGY

Renal cell carcinoma is also known as *adenocarcinoma of the kidney*. As with other cancers, the healthy tissue of the kidney is damaged and replaced by cancer cells.

TABLE 74-5 Staging Renal Tumors

- **Stage I.** Tumors up to 2.5 cm are situated within the capsule of the kidney; the renal vein, perinephric fat, and adjacent lymph nodes have no tumor.
- **Stage II.** Tumors are larger than 2.5 cm and extend beyond the capsule but are within Gerota's fascia; the renal vein and lymph nodes are not involved.
- **Stage III.** Tumors extend into the renal vein, lymph nodes, or both.
- **Stage IV.** Tumors include invasion of adjacent organs beyond Gerota's fascia or metastasize to distant tissues.

Data from American Cancer Society. (2005). *Cancer facts and figures 2005.* Report No. 00-300M–No. 5008.05. Atlanta: Author.

Systemic effects occurring with this cancer type are called **paraneoplastic syndromes** and include anemia, erythrocytosis, hypercalcemia, liver dysfunction with elevated liver enzymes, hormonal effects, increased sedimentation rate, and hypertension.

Anemia and erythrocytosis may appear contradictory; however, most clients with this cancer have either anemia or erythrocytosis, not both at the same time. There is some blood loss from hematuria, but the small amount lost does not cause anemia. The cause of the anemia and the erythrocytosis is related to kidney cell production of erythropoietin. At times, the tumor cells produce large amounts of erythropoietin, causing erythrocytosis. Other times, the tumor cells destroy the erythropoietin-producing kidney cells and anemia results. Hypertension may result from increased blood levels of renin.

Parathyroid hormone produced by tumor cells can cause hypercalcemia. Other hormone changes include increased renin levels (causing hypertension) and increased human chorionic gonadotropin (hCG) levels, which decreases libido and changes secondary sex features. The cause of the increased sedimentation rate and changes in liver function studies is not known.

Renal cell carcinoma has four distinct histologic patterns. Genetic differences cause a predisposition to develop tumors of each of these histologic types. The most well known genetic familial syndrome that includes renal cancer is von Hippel-Lindau syndrome. These cancers are highly vascular and may occur with cancers of the pancreas, central nervous system, and adrenal glands.

Renal tumors are classified into four stages (Table 74-5). Complications include metastasis and urinary tract obstruction. Metastasis usually occurs to the adrenal gland, liver, lungs, long bones, or the other kidney. When the cancer surrounds a ureter, hydroureter and obstruction may result.

The exact cause of renal cell carcinoma is unknown, but the risk is slightly higher for people who use tobacco or are exposed to lead, phosphate, and cadmium.

Renal cancers account for about 28,800 new cases and 11,300 deaths annually in the United States. The 5-year survival rate is 60% in the United States. Renal cell carcinoma occurs most often in clients between 55 and 60 years of age (Kidney Cancer Association, 2005).

COLLABORATIVE MANAGEMENT

Assessment

HISTORY

Ask the client about age, known risk factors (e.g., smoking or chemical exposures), weight loss, changes in urine color, abdominal or flank discomfort, and fever. Also ask whether any other family member has ever been diagnosed with cancer of the kidney, bladder, ureter, prostate gland, uterus, or ovary.

PHYSICAL ASSESSMENT/CLINICAL MANIFESTATIONS

Only about 5% to 10% of clients with renal cell cancer have flank pain, gross hematuria, and a palpable renal mass. Ask about the nature of the flank or abdominal discomfort. Clients often describe the pain as dull and aching. The pain may be more intense if bleeding into the tumor or kidney occurs. Inspect the flank area, checking for asymmetry or an obvious bulge. You may be able to feel an abdominal mass through *gentle* palpation. A renal bruit may be heard on auscultation.

Hematuria is a *late* common sign. Blood in the urine may be visible as bright red flecks or clots, or the urine may appear smoky or cola colored. Without gross hematuria, microscopic examination may or may not reveal red cells.

Inspect the skin for pallor, darkening of the nipples and, in men, breast enlargement. Other findings may include muscle wasting, weakness, poor nutritional status, and weight loss. All tend to occur late in the disease.

DIAGNOSTIC ASSESSMENT

Urinalysis may show red blood cells. Hematologic studies reveal decreased hemoglobin and hematocrit values, hypercalcemia, increased erythrocyte sedimentation rate, and increased levels of adrenocorticotropic hormone, human chorionic gonadotropin (hCG), cortisol, renin, and parathyroid hormone.

Renal masses may be detected by surgical exploration, IV urogram with nephrograms, or sonography. The mass and surrounding tissues may be outlines by CT with contrast or by magnetic resonance imaging (MRI).

Interventions

Interventions focus on controlling the cancer and preventing metastasis.

NONSURGICAL MANAGEMENT. Radiofrequency ablation has shown some promise in treating renal cancer. Radiofrequency ablation is a minimally invasive procedure carried out during magnetic resonance imaging (MRI). MRI can monitor the results of tumor destruction immediately because MRI is sensitive to temperature changes. Radiofrequency ablation is still undergoing evaluation to determine its effectiveness and is not widely available (Bonn, 2002).

Chemotherapy has limited effectiveness against this cancer type. Use of biological response modifiers (BRMs) such as interleukin-2 (IL-2), interferon (INF), and tumor necrosis factor (TNF) have lengthened survival time (see Chapters 23 and 28).

SURGICAL MANAGEMENT. Renal cell carcinoma is usually treated surgically by **nephrectomy** (kidney removal). Renal cell tumors are highly vascular and blood loss during surgery is a major concern. Before surgery, the arteries supplying the kidney may be occluded (embolized) by radiation to reduce bleeding during nephrectomy.

Preoperative Care. Instruct the client about surgical routines (see Chapters 20, 21, and 22). Explain the probable site of incision and the presence of dressings, drains, or other equipment after surgery. Reassure the client about pain relief. Care before surgery may include giving blood and fluids intravenously to ensure hemodynamic stability.

Operative Procedures. The client is placed on his or her side with the kidney to be removed uppermost. Usually, the client's trunk area is flexed to increase exposure of the kidney area. Removal of the eleventh or twelfth rib is needed to provide better access to the kidney. The surgeon removes the entire kidney and all visible tumor, renal artery and vein, and fascia after tying off the ureter. The adrenal gland is left intact. A drain may be placed in the wound before closure.

When a *radical* nephrectomy is performed, the periaortic lymph nodes are also removed. The surgical approach may be transthoracic (as discussed in the previous paragraph), lumbar, or through the abdomen depending on the size and location of the tumor. Radiation therapy may follow a radical nephrectomy.

Postoperative Care. Refer to Chapter 22 for care of the client after surgery. Assessment of urologic and renal function is essential to determine function in the remaining kidney.

Monitoring. Assess the client for hemorrhage and adrenal insufficiency. Inspect the client's abdomen for distention from bleeding. Check the bed linens under the client, because bleeding may be present. Hemorrhage or adrenal insufficiency cause hypotension, decreased urine output, and an altered level of consciousness.

A decrease in blood pressure is an early sign of both hemorrhage and adrenal insufficiency. With hypotension, urine output also decreases immediately. Large water and sodium losses in the urine occur in clients with adrenal insufficiency. As a result, a large urine output is followed by hypotension and oliguria (<400 mL/24 hr or less than 25 mL/hr). IV replacement of fluids and packed red blood cells may be needed.

The second kidney is expected to provide adequate renal function. Assess urine output hourly for the first 24 hours after surgery (urine output of 30 to 50 mL/hr is acceptable). Output of less than 25 to 30 mL/hr suggests decreased renal blood flow. The hemoglobin level, hematocrit values, and white blood cell count may be measured every 6 to 12 hours for the first day or two after surgery.

Monitor the client's temperature, pulse rate, and respiratory rate at least every 4 hours. Accurately measure and record fluid intake and output. Weigh the client daily.

The client may be in a special care unit for 24 to 48 hours after surgery for monitoring of bleeding and/or adrenal insufficiency. A drain placed near the site of incision removes residual fluid. Because of the discomfort of deep breathing, the client is at risk for atelectasis. Fever, chills, thick sputum, or decreased breath sounds suggest pneumonia.

Pain Management. After surgery, opioid analgesics (e.g., hydromorphone [Dilaudid] and morphine sulfate [Statex✱]) are given parenterally. The incision was made through major muscle groups used with breathing and movement. Liberal use of analgesics is needed for 3 to 5 days to manage the pain after surgery. Oral agents may be tried when the client is permitted to eat and drink.

Prevention of Complications. Antibiotics may be prescribed during and after surgery to prevent infection. These drugs are usually given as single-dose prescriptions. The need for additional antibiotics is based on clinical and laboratory evidence of infection. Steroid replacements may be needed in clients who have adrenal insufficiency.

RENAL TRAUMA

PATHOPHYSIOLOGY

Trauma to one or both kidneys is always a concern in penetrating wounds or blunt injuries to the back, flank, or abdomen. Blunt trauma to the back, flank, or abdomen accounts for 85% of all renal injuries; most blunt renal injuries are not serious (Rakel & Bope, 2003). Injury to the kidney can be minor, major, or pedicle (Figure 74-5). Strategies to prevent trauma are reviewed in Chart 74-9.

Minor injuries include contusions, small lacerations, and tearing of the parenchyma and the calyx (forniceal disruption). With a contusion, one or both kidneys are bruised because of the major impact. Small blood vessels may be damaged, causing some hematuria. Small lacerations may result in small, local hematomas. A small hematoma also may occur at the site of forniceal disruption. Common causes include falls, contact sports, and blows to the back and torso.

Major injuries include lacerations to the cortex, medulla, or branches of the renal artery or vein. Deep tissue injuries may extend throughout the kidney and cause hematomas within or through the capsule. Injuries involving the cortex can cause tissue shattering. The capsule may remain intact or be ruptured.

A major injury most commonly follows penetrating abdominal, flank, or back wounds (such as is seen with gunshot wounds, knife wounds, or motor vehicle accidents). Bleeding is extensive, and surgical exploration is often needed. Because of the hemorrhage, decreased renal blood flow can produce short-term or long-term renin-induced hypertension.

Pedicle injuries are lacerations or breaks in the renal artery or renal vein. Hemorrhage is extensive and rapid, and death may occur unless diagnosis and intervention are prompt.

◆COLLABORATIVE MANAGEMENT

◆Assessment

Obtain a history of the client's usual health and the events involved in the trauma from the client, a witness, or emergency personnel. Critical information to know is a history of renal or urologic disease, surgical intervention, or health problems such as diabetes mellitus or hypertension.

Ureteral or renal pelvic injury often cause diffuse abdominal pain, local collections of urine, and infection. Ask the client about pain in the flank or abdominal pain. Is the pain dull? Sharp? Constant? Intermittent? Made worse by coughing?

Take the client's blood pressure, apical and peripheral pulses, respiratory rate, and temperature. Inspect both flanks for asymmetry or penetrating injuries of the lower thorax or back. Also inspect the abdomen for bruising or penetrating wounds. Percuss the abdomen for distention. Inspect the urethra for gross bleeding.

Urinalysis usually shows hemoglobin or red blood cells from renal blood vessel rupture. Microscopic examination may also show red blood cell casts, which suggest tubular damage. Hemoglobin and hematocrit values decrease with blood loss. If inflammation or infection is present, the white blood cell count is elevated.

Diagnostic procedures include IV urography and computed tomography (CT). CT scan shows the location of the in-

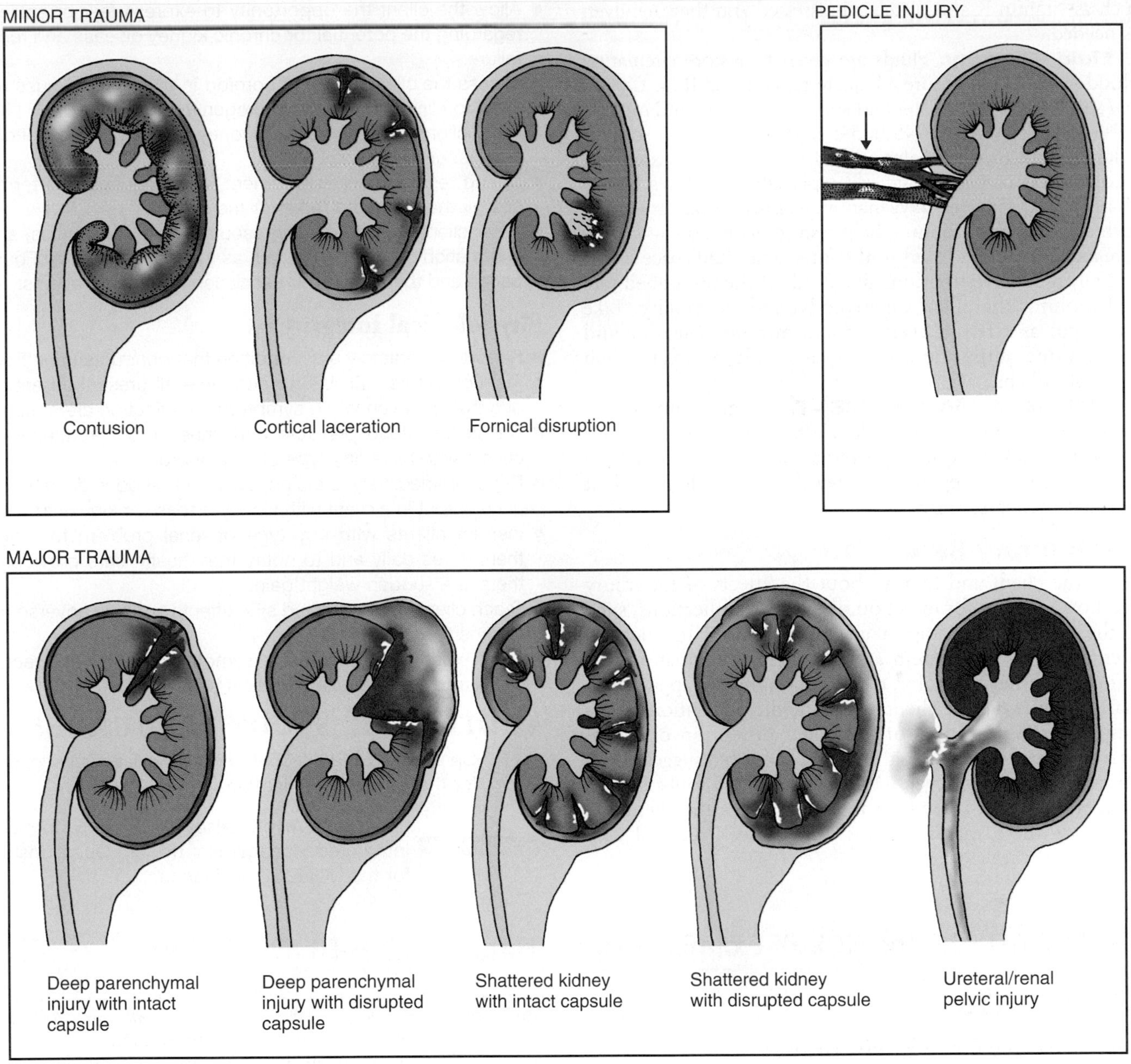

Figure 74-5 ■ Common types and locations of renal trauma.

CHART 74-9

CLIENT EDUCATION GUIDE
Preventing Renal and Genitourinary Trauma

- Wear a seat belt.
- Practice safe walking habits.
- Use caution when riding bicycles and motorcycles.
- Wear appropriate protective clothing when participating in contact sports.
- Avoid all contact sports and high-risk activities if you have only one kidney.

jury as well as blood vessel and tissue integrity. Hematomas within or through the renal capsule are seen with CT scan. A urogram reveals the integrity and patency of the collecting system. Renal sonography can be used instead if there is a need to avoid contrast dye, especially in clients with elevated serum creatinine levels.

◆Common Nursing Diagnoses and Collaborative Problems

Nursing diagnoses that may apply to clients with renal trauma include the following:

- Ineffective Tissue Perfusion (Renal) related to interruption of arterial flow
- Anxiety related to threat to health status
- Acute Pain related to physical injury
- Impaired Urinary Elimination related to renal damage and shock
- Risk for Infection related to altered immune function

◆Interventions

NONSURGICAL MANAGEMENT

Drug Therapy. Prescribed IV dopamine (Revimine✱, others) promotes renal perfusion. The need for clotting factors such as vitamin K and platelets is assessed and they are given as needed.

Fluid Therapy. Fluids are given to restore circulating blood volume and ensure adequate renal blood flow. *Crystalloid* solutions replace water and some electrolytes and include 0.9% sodium chloride (NSS), 5% dextrose in 0.45% sodium chloride, and Ringer's solution. When bleeding is extensive, whole blood or packed red cell replacement restores hemoglobin and promotes oxygenation. *Plasma volume expanders,* such as dextran or albumin, help restore plasma oncotic pressure and reduce fluid shift to the interstitial fluid space.

During fluid restoration, give fluids at the prescribed rate and monitor the client for hemodynamic instability. Take vital signs as often as every 5 to 15 minutes. Measure and record urine output hourly. Output should be greater than 25 to 30 mL/hr.

SURGICAL MANAGEMENT. Nephrectomy or partial nephrectomy may be needed. When major blood vessels are torn, the kidney may be removed, repaired, and then reimplanted. This repair of kidney tissue outside the client is called "bench surgery."

Community-Based Care

Teach the client and family about the effects of the injury and how to assess for infection or other complications, such as the onset of bleeding or urinary retention. Instruct the client to check the pattern and frequency of urination and to note whether the color, clarity, and amount appear normal. Also instruct the client to seek medical attention if anything appears abnormal or if bladder distention or inadequate bladder emptying occurs, which suggests an obstruction. Chills, fever, lethargy, or cloudy, foul-smelling urine indicate a urinary tract infection. Warn the client not to ignore these manifestations and to seek medical care promptly if they occur.

GET READY for the NCLEX Examination!

KEY POINTS

Safe Effective Care Environment

- Use sterile technique when inserting a catheter or any other instrument into the urinary system.
- Use contact precautions with any client who has drainage from the genitourinary tract.

Health Promotion and Maintenance

- Encourage all clients to maintain an adequate fluid intake (minimum of 3 L/day unless another condition requires fluid restriction).
- Encourage clients with diabetes to adhere to regimens for glucose control to prevent hypertension and renal disease.
- Teach clients who come into contact with nephrotoxic chemicals in their workplaces or for leisure time activities, to avoid direct skin or mucous membrane contact with these chemicals (you may need to review Chapter 72).

Psychosocial Integrity

- Pace your interview to match the learning needs and style of the individual client.
- Allow the client the opportunity to express fear or anxiety regarding the potential for chronic kidney disease and renal failure.
- Assess the client's level of comfort in discussing issues related to elimination and the urogenital area.
- Refer clients with polycystic kidney disease to a geneticist or a genetic counselor.
- During renal/urinary assessment, use language and terminology that is comfortable for the client.
- Refer clients to community resources, support groups, and information organizations such as the National Kidney Foundation and the American Association of Kidney Patients.

Physiological Integrity

- Report immediately any condition that obstructs urine flow.
- Instruct clients with UTI to complete all prescribed antibiotic therapy even when symptoms of infection are absent.
- Check the blood pressure and urine output frequently in clients who have any type of kidney problem.
- Report immediately to the physician, any sudden decrease of urine output in a client with kidney disease or kidney trauma.
- Instruct clients with any type of renal problem to weigh themselves daily and to notify their health care provider if there is a sudden weight gain.
- Teach clients the expected side effects and any adverse reactions to prescribed drugs.
- Teach clients the signs and symptoms of disease recurrence and when to seek medical help.

ADDITIONAL STUDY RESOURCES

Go to your Student CD-ROM for Review Questions for the NCLEX Examination.

evolve Go to http://evolve.elsevier.com/Iggy/ for Integrated Management of Care Questions for the NCLEX Examination.

SELECTED BIBLIOGRAPHY

Asterisk indicates a classic or definitive work on this subject.

American Cancer Society. (2005). *Cancer facts and figures 2005.* Report No. 00-300M-No. 5008.05. Atlanta: Author.

Appel, G.B., Radhakrishnan, J., & D'Agati, V. (2000). Secondary glomerular diseases. In B.M. Brenner & F.C. Rector (Eds.), *Brenner & Rector's the kidney* (5th ed., pp. 1350-1416). Philadelphia: W.B. Saunders.

Arnaout, M.A. (2001). Molecular genetics and pathogenesis of autosomal dominant polycystic kidney disease. *Annual Review of Medicine, 52,* 93-123.

Bakris, G., et al. (2000). Preserving renal function in adults with hypertension and diabetes: A consensus approach. National Kidney Foundation Hypertension and Diabetes Executive Committee Working Group. *American Journal of Kidney Disease, 36*(3), 646-661.

Bonn, D. (2002). Radiofrequency ablation: First-line treatment for renal cancer? *The Lancet Oncology, 3*(1), 3-4.

Calvet, J., & Grantham, J. (2001). The genetics and physiology of polycystic kidney disease. *Seminars in Nephrology, 21*(2), 107-123.

Dagher, P.C., et al. (2003). Newly developed techniques to study and diagnose acute renal failure. *Journal of the American Society of Nephrology, 14,* 2188-2198.

Dochterman, J., & Bulechek, G. (Eds). (2004). *Nursing interventions classification (NIC)* (4th ed.). St. Louis: Mosby.

Facts and Comparisons. (2004). *Drug facts and comparisons* (58th ed.). St. Louis: Author.

Falk, J., Jennett, J., & Nachman, S. (2000). Primary glomerular disease. In B.M. Brenner & S.A. Levine (Eds.), *Brenner & Rector's the kidney* (6th ed., pp. 1263-1349). Philadelphia: W.B. Saunders.

George, A.L., & Neilson, E.G. (2000). Genetics of kidney disease. *American Journal of Kidney Diseases, 35*(4), S160-S169.

Goolsby, M. (2002). National Kidney Foundation Guidelines for chronic kidney disease: Evaluation, classification, and stratification. *Journal of the American Academy of Nurse Practitioners, 14*(6), 238-242.

Igarashi, P., & Somlo, S. (2002). Genetics and pathogenesis of polycystic kidney disease. *Journal of the American Society of Nephrology, 13*(9), 2384-2398.

Jalanko, H., et al. (2001). Genetic kidney diseases disclose the pathogenesis of proteinuria. *Annals of Medicine, 33*(8), 526-533.

Kelly, C.J., & Neilson, E.G. (2000). Tubulointerstitial diseases. In B.M. Brenner & S.A. Levine (Eds.), *Brenner & Rector's the kidney* (6th ed., pp. 1506-1536). Philadelphia: W.B. Saunders.

Kidney Cancer Association. (2005). Available at http://www.curekidneycancer.org/.

Kikkawa, R., Koya, D., & Haneda, M. (2003). Progression of diabetic nephropathy. *American Journal of Kidney Diseases, 41*(3), 519-521.

Kneipp, S., & Himmelstein, S.B. (2000). Nephrotic syndrome secondary to amyloidosis. *The Nurse Practitioner, 25*(6), 78-93.

Lancaster, L.E. (Ed.). (2001). *Core curriculum for nephrology nursing* (4th ed.). Pitman, NJ: American Association of Nephrology Nurses.

Laragh, J.H., & Blumenfeld, J.D. (2000). Essential hypertension. In B.M. Brenner & S.A. Levine (Eds.), *Brenner & Rector's the kidney* (6th ed., pp. 1967-2006). Philadelphia: W.B. Saunders.

Laudicina, P.F. (2001). Diagnostic imaging of the genitourinary system. *Seminars in Radiologic Technology, 9*(2), 48-65.

Lehmann, S., & Dietz, C. (2002). Double J stents: They're not trouble-free. *RN, 65*(1), 54-60.

Lerman, L., & Textor, S.C. (2001). Pathophysiology of ischemic neuropathy. *Urologic Clinics of North America, 28* (4), 793-803.

Leung, D.A., et al. (2002). MR angiography of the renal arteries. *Radiology Clinics of North American, 40*(4), 847-865.

Little, C. (2000). Renovascular hypertension. *American Journal of Nursing, 100*(2), 46-51.

Maranchie, J.K., & Linehan, W.M. (2003). Genetic disorders and renal cell carcinoma. *Urologic Clinics of North America, 30*(1), 133-141.

McCance, K., & Huether, S. (2002). Pathophysiology: The biologic basis for disease in adults and children (4th ed.). St. Louis: Mosby.

Moorhead, S., Johnson, M., & Maas, M. (Eds.). (2004). *Nursing outcomes classification (NOC)* (3rd ed.). St. Louis: Mosby.

Munson, B.L. (2004). Myths and facts about polycystic kidney disease. *Nursing2004, 34*(3), 75.

*Nathan, D.M. (1993). Diabetes Control and Complications Trial Research Group: The effect of long-term intensified insulin treatment on development of microvascular complications of diabetes. *The New England Journal of Medicine, 329*(14), 977-986.

NIDDK National Kidney and Urologic Diseases Information Clearinghouse. (2004). *Kidney and urologic diseases statistics for the United States.* NIH Publication No. 04-3895. Bethesda, MD: National Institutes of Health. Available at http://kidney.niddk.nih.gov/kudiseases/pubs/kustats/index.htm.

Nussbaum, R., McInnes, R., & Willard, H. (2001). *Thompson & Thompson: Genetics in medicine* (6th ed.). Philadelphia: W.B. Saunders.

Olin, J.W. (2002). Atherosclerotic renal disease. *Cardiology Clinics, 20*(4), 547-562.

Online Mendelian Inheritance in Man. (2004). Retrieved November 17, 2004, from http://www.ncbi.nlm.nih.gov/Omim.

Palmieri, P.A. (2002). Obstructive nephropathy: Pathophysiology, diagnosis, and collaborative management. *Nephrology Nursing Journal, 29*(1), 15-21.

Polycystic Kidney Disease Foundation. (2004). Accessed November 2004 from http://www.pkdcure.org/home.html.

Rakel, R.E., & Bope, E.T. (2003). Conn's current therapy. Philadelphia: W.B. Saunders.

Richardson, A., & Piepho, R. (2000). Effect of race on hypertension and antihypertensive therapy. *International Journal of Clinical Pharmacology, 38*(2), 75-79.

Rodriguez-Itrube, B. (2000). Post-infectious glomerulonephritis. *American Journal of Kidney Disease, 35*(1), xlvi-xlviii.

Schmelzer, M., & Stam, M. (2000). A hidden menace: Hemolytic uremic syndrome. *American Journal of Nursing, 100*(11), 26-32.

Schwarz, A. (2001). New aspects of the treatment of nephrotic syndrome. *Journal of the American Society of Nephrology, 12*(Suppl. 17), 544-547.

*See, W.A., & Williams, R.D. (1992). Tumors of the kidney, ureter, and bladder. *Western Journal of Medicine, 156*(5), 523-534.

Sowers, J.R., et al. (2002). Hypertension-related disease in African-Americans. *Postgraduate Medicine, 112* (4) 24-33.

Steeg, C., Walsh, C., & Glickstein, J. (2001). Rheumatic fever: No cause for complacence. *Patient Care for the Nurse Practitioner, 4*(10), 15-16, 18, 23-24, 26.

Stegbauer, C. (2000). Nephrotic syndrome secondary to amyloidosis. *The Nurse Practitioner, 25*(6), 78, 81, 85-86, 88, 91-93.

Stuart, R., & Nigam, S. (2000). Developmental biology of the kidney. In B.M. Brenner & S.A. Levine (Eds.), *Brenner & Rector's the kidney* (6th ed., pp. 68-92). Philadelphia: W.B. Saunders.

Szromba, C., Theis, M.A., & Ossman, S.S. (2002). Advancing chronic kidney disease: New imperatives for recognitions and intervention. *Nephrology Nursing Journal, 29*(6), 547-561.

Tillou, A., et al. (2001). Renal vascular injuries. *Surgical Clinics of North America, 81*(6), 1417-1430.

Tolkoff-Rubin, N., Cotran, R., & Rubin, R. (2000). Urinary tract infection, pyelonephritis, and reflux nephropathy. In B.M. Brenner & S.A. Levine (Eds.), *Brenner & Rector's the kidney* (6th ed., pp. 1449-1508). Philadelphia: W.B. Saunders.

U.S. Renal Data Systems. (2003). *USRDS 2003 annual data report.* Bethesda, MD: The National Institutes of Health, National Institute of Diabetes and Digestive and Kidney Diseases.

Wright, J.T., et al. (2002). Effect of blood pressure lowering and antihypertensive drug class on progression of hypertensive kidney disease: Results from the AASK trial. *Journal of the American Medical Association, 288*(19), 2421-2431.

CHAPTER 75

Interventions for Clients with Acute and Chronic Renal Failure

LINDA A. LaCHARITY

LEARNING OUTCOMES

After studying this chapter, you should be able to:

1. Compare the pathophysiology and causes of acute renal failure (ARF) with those of chronic renal failure (CRF).
2. Identify clients at risk for development of ARF.
3. Identify clients at risk for development of CRF.
4. Use laboratory data and clinical assessment to determine the effectiveness of therapy for renal failure.
5. Discuss interventions to prevent ARF.
6. Prioritize nursing care for the client with ARF.
7. Describe the mechanisms of action, side effects, and nursing implications for pharmacologic management of renal failure.
8. Compare the clinical manifestations of stage I, stage II, and stage III CRF.
9. Discuss the mechanisms of peritoneal dialysis (PD) and hemodialysis (HD) as renal replacement therapies.
10. Prioritize nursing care for the client with end-stage renal disease.
11. Prioritize teaching needs for the client using continuous ambulatory PD.
12. Develop a community-based teaching plan for the client with a permanent vascular access for long-term HD.
13. Compare the dietary modifications needed for the client undergoing HD with those for the client undergoing PD.
14. Plan prevention strategies for the complications of PD.
15. Discuss the criteria for kidney donation.
16. Prioritize nursing care for the client during the first 24 hours after kidney transplantation.
17. Develop a community-based teaching plan for the client who has received a kidney transplant.

Go to your Student CD-ROM for Review Questions for the NCLEX Examination keyed to these Learning Outcomes.

Acute renal failure (ARF) and chronic renal failure (CRF) have become increasingly more common in the United States, resulting in considerable morbidity and mortality. ARF is responsible for 7% of all hospital admissions and for 2% to 5% of clients admitted to medical-surgical hospital units. The prevalence of end-stage renal disease (ESRD) has more than doubled in the last decade (U.S. Renal Data Systems, 2002). Renal failure has many causes. Complications related to poorly controlled diabetes are the most common cause (43.4%), followed by hypertension (25.5%) and glomerulonephritis (8.4%).

Kidney functions include excretion of waste, water and salt balance, acid-base balance, and hormone secretion. When renal function declines gradually, as occurs most often with CRF, 90% to 95% of the nephrons must be destroyed before renal failure is obvious. The client may have many years of decreased renal reserve and chronic renal insufficiency before the uremia of end-stage renal failure develops. During this time of decreased renal reserve and chronic renal insufficiency, the client is at increased risk for acute renal failure because of the reduced functioning of remaining nephrons.

When renal decline is sudden, the work capacity of functioning nephrons is exceeded more quickly, and renal failure may develop with the loss of only 50% of functioning nephrons. Acute renal failure and chronic renal failure are

TABLE 75-1 Characteristics of Acute and Chronic Renal Failure

Characteristic	Acute Renal Failure	Chronic Renal Failure
Onset	Sudden (hours to days)	Gradual (months to years)
Percentage of nephron involvement	≈50%	90%-95%
Duration	2-4 wk; less than 3 mo	Permanent
Prognosis	Good for return of renal function with supportive care, high mortality in some situations	Fatal without a renal replacement therapy, such as dialysis or transplantation

compared in Table 75-1. Acute renal failure affects *many* body systems; chronic renal failure affects *every* body system. Renal failure problems are related to the effects of the following:

- Fluid-volume excess
- Electrolyte and acid-base abnormalities
- Accumulated nitrogenous wastes
- Hormonal inadequacies

When renal function decreases to the point that the kidneys can no longer meet the body's homeostatic demands, renal replacement therapy is needed to prevent death from potentially life-threatening consequences.

ACUTE RENAL FAILURE

PATHOPHYSIOLOGY

Acute renal failure (ARF) is a rapid decrease in renal function, leading to the collection of metabolic wastes in the body. ARF can result from conditions that cause inadequate kidney perfusion **(prerenal failure);** damage to the glomeruli, interstitial tissue, or tubules **(intrarenal/intrinsic renal failure);** or obstruction urine flow **(postrenal failure)** (Nally, 2002). ARF in clients with chronic renal insufficiency (CRI) may result in **end-stage renal disease (ESRD),** or it may resolve to nearly the pre-ARF level of renal function. Many factors contribute to renal insults in ARF, but the acute syndrome may be reversible, especially with prompt intervention.

The pathologic process of ARF is related to the cause of the sudden decrease in kidney function and to the affected kidney sites(s). Reduced blood flow **(hypoperfusion),** toxins, tubular ischemia, infections, and obstruction have different effects on the renal system. Any of these processes can reduce glomerular filtration rate (GFR), disrupt tubular cell membranes, and obstruct urine flow in the renal tubules.

With shock or other problems causing an acute reduction in renal blood flow (hypoperfusion), the kidney compensates with autoregulatory responses (e.g., renal blood vessel constriction, activation of renin-angiotensin-aldosterone pathway, and release of antidiuretic hormone [ADH]). These responses increase blood volume and improve renal perfusion. However, these same responses reduce urine volume, resulting in **oliguria** (urine output less than 400 mL/day). Tubular cell injury is more likely to occur from the increasing ischemia related to hypoperfusion. Toxins can cause blood vessel constriction in the kidney, leading to reduced renal blood flow and renal ischemia.

Kidney tissue inflammation caused by infection, drugs, or cancer result in immune-mediated changes in renal tissue. With extensive tubular damage, tubular cells slough and combine with other formed elements (e.g., red blood cell [RBC] casts), which then obstruct the tubular lumen and prevent urine outflow. Obstruction anywhere within the urinary tract may result in full or partial obstruction to the formation and outflow of urine.

When pressure in the renal tubules (intrarenal pressure) exceeds glomerular hydrostatic pressure, glomerular filtration stops. This problem allows nitrogenous wastes to collect in the blood, increasing the blood urea nitrogen (BUN) and serum creatinine levels. When the BUN rises faster than the serum creatinine level, the cause is usually related to protein breakdown or volume depletion. When both the BUN and the creatinine levels rise and the ratio between the two remains constant, renal failure is present.

Types of Acute Renal Failure

Several syndromes describe the types of ARF. These include prerenal azotemia, intrarenal (intrinsic) ARF, and postrenal azotemia. Table 75-2 lists the causes and problems of ARF.

Prerenal azotemia can be reversed by correcting blood volume, increasing blood pressure, and improving cardiac output. Prolonged, untreated hypoperfusion can lead to severe ischemic injury and intrarenal failure.

The term *intrarenal ARF* is often shortened to just *ARF* in the clinical setting. Other terms include **acute tubular necrosis (ATN)** and **lower nephron nephrosis.** Infections (bacteria, viral, fungal), drugs (especially aminoglycoside antibiotics and nonsteroidal anti-inflammatory drugs [NSAIDs]), and invading tumors (e.g., lymphomas or leukemias) can cause acute interstitial nephritis. Other causes of intrarenal ARF include inflammation of the glomeruli **(glomerulonephritis)** or of the small vessels of the kidneys **(vasculitis),** or an obstruction of renal blood flow.

Postrenal azotemia develops from obstruction to the outflow of formed urine anywhere within the renal or urinary tract.

Phases of Acute Renal Failure

When a client's renal function declines, the phases of ARF begin (Table 75-3). Some clients have a *nonoliguric* form of ARF in which urine output remains near normal. The phases of this form of ARF are similar to those listed in Table 75-3 except for the references to urine output. The treatment of these clients is less complicated because renal replacement therapy is rarely needed. Interventions to restore circulating volume, improve cardiac output, or increase blood pressure may prevent progression of the phases when hypoperfusion is present.

Etiology

Many types of renal insults can reduce renal function. Severe hypotension from shock or dehydration reduces renal blood flow and can lead to prerenal ARF. Cardiac disease or

TABLE 75-2 Causes of the Three Types of Acute Renal Failure

Pathologic Change	Causes
Prerenal	
Decreased blood flow to the kidneys leading to ischemia in the nephrons; prolonged hypoperfusion can lead to tubular necrosis and ARF	Conditions that cause decreased cardiac output Shock HF Pulmonary embolism Anaphylaxis Pericardial tamponade Sepsis
Intrarenal (Intrinsic)	
Actual tissue damage to the kidney caused by inflammatory or immunologic processes or from prolonged hypoperfusion	Acute interstitial nephritis Exposure to nephrotoxins Acute glomerulonephritis Vasculitis Hepatorenal syndrome ATN Renal artery or vein stenosis/thrombosis
Postrenal	
Obstruction of the urine collecting system anywhere from the calyces to the urethral meatus Obstruction of the bladder must be bilateral to cause postrenal failure unless only one kidney is functional	Urethral or bladder cancer Renal, ureteral, or bladder stones Atony of bladder Prostatic hyperplasia or cancer Cervical cancer Urethral stricture

ARF, Acute renal failure; *ATN*, acute tubular necrosis; *HF*, heart failure.

TABLE 75-3 The Phases of Oliguric Acute Renal Failure

Phase	Description	Characteristics	Duration
Onset phase	Begins with the precipitating event and continues until oliguria develops.	The gradual accumulation of nitrogenous wastes, such as serum creatinine and BUN, may be noted.	Can last hours to several days.
Oliguric phase	Characterized by a urine output to 100-400 mL/24 hr that does not respond to fluid challenges or diuretics.	Laboratory data include increasing serum creatinine and BUN levels, hyperkalemia, bicarbonate deficit (metabolic acidosis), hyperphosphatemia, hypocalcemia, and hypermagnesemia. Sodium retention occurs, but this is masked by the dilutional effects of water retention. Urinary indices are typically low and fixed; regulation of water balance by the kidneys is impaired, so urine specific gravity and urine osmolarity do not vary as plasma osmolarity changes.	Typically lasts 8-15 days but can last for several weeks, especially in older clients or those having pre-existing renal insufficiency.
Diuretic phase (high-output phase)	Often has a prompt onset, with urine flow increasing rapidly over a period of several days. The diuresis can result in an output of up to 10 L/day of dilute urine.	Electrolyte losses typically precede clearance of nitrogenous wastes. Later in the diuretic phase, the BUN level starts to fall and continues to fall until the level reaches normal limits or reaches a plateau. Normal renal tubular function is reestablished during this phase.	Usually occurs 2-6 wk after the onset of oliguric acute renal failure and continues until the BUN level ceases to rise.
Recovery phase (convalescent phase)	In this phase, the client begins to return to normal levels of activity.	The client functions at a lower energy level and has less stamina than before the illness. Residual renal insufficiency may be noted through regular monitoring of renal function. Renal function may never return to preillness levels, but renal function sufficient for a long and healthy life is likely.	Renal function may continue to improve for up to 12 mo after oliguric acute renal failure began. The client is particularly vulnerable to additional renal injury during this time.

BUN, Blood urea nitrogen.

heart failure also can reduce renal blood flow. The client may be oliguric or even **anuric** (less than 100 mL/24 hr) if the dehydration or renal blood flow reduction is severe. The following other conditions can lead to ARF:

- Nephrotoxic agents (antibiotics, NSAIDs) (Table 75-4)
- Disseminated intravascular coagulation (DIC)
- Obstruction by thrombosis or stenosis
- Uric acid crystals or other obstructing precipitates
- Acute hemolytic transfusion reactions
- Complications of infection (e.g., endotoxins or sepsis)
- Acute glomerulonephritis
- Vasculitis
- Severe hypertension
- Hepatorenal syndrome of cirrhosis

Incidence/Prevalence

Acute renal failure affects 15% to 20% of all critically ill clients and has a 50% to 80% mortality rate (U.S. Renal Data Systems, 2002). Eighty percent of ARF episodes are due to acute tubular necrosis (ATN) and worsening of chronic renal insufficiency (CRI). Volume depletion leading to prerenal azotemia is the most common cause of ARF and is reversible in most cases with prompt intervention.

For clients who survive the precipitating event, the chance for return of renal function is good. However, complications during the course of AFR can greatly increase mortality. Bloodstream infections from contamination through intravenous (IV) lines are the most often common complications that lead to death. However, the highest mortality occurs with trauma (70%) and surgery. ARF caused by nephrotoxic substances has the lowest rates (10% to 26%) of recovery. The prognosis for ARF caused by obstruction or glomerulonephritis is much better.

TABLE 75-4 Some Potentially Nephrotoxic Substances

Drugs ***Antibiotics/Anti-infectives*** ▪ Amphotericin B ▪ Colistimethate ▪ Methicillin ▪ Polymyxin B ▪ Rifampin ▪ Sulfonamides ▪ Tetracycline hydrochloride ▪ Vancomycin ***Aminoglycoside Antibiotics*** ▪ Gentamicin ▪ Kanamycin ▪ Neomycin ▪ Netilmicin sulfate ▪ Tobramycin ***Antineoplastics*** ▪ Cisplatin ▪ Cyclophosphamide ▪ Methotrexate ***Nonsteroidal Anti-inflammatory Drugs (NSAIDs)*** ▪ Celecoxib ▪ Flurbiprofen ▪ Ibuprofen ▪ Indomethacin ▪ Ketorolac ▪ Meclofenamate ▪ Meloxicam ▪ Nabumentone ▪ Naproxen ▪ Oxaprozin ▪ Rofecoxib ▪ Tolmetin	***Other Drugs*** ▪ Acetaminophen ▪ Captopril ▪ Cyclosporine ▪ Fluorinate anesthetics ▪ D-Penicillamine ▪ Phenazopyridine hydrochloride ▪ Quinine **Other Substances** ***Organic Solvents*** ▪ Carbon tetrachloride ▪ Ethylene glycol ***Nondrug Chemical Agents*** ▪ Radiographic contrast dye ▪ Pesticides ▪ Fungicides ▪ Myoglobin (from breakdown of skeletal muscle) ***Heavy Metals and Ions*** ▪ Arsenic ▪ Bismuth ▪ Copper sulfate ▪ Gold salts ▪ Lead ▪ Mercuric chloride

HEALTH PROMOTION/ILLNESS PREVENTION

Keep in mind that severe blood volume depletion can lead to renal failure even in people who have no known kidney problems. Encourage all clients to maintain an adequate fluid intake to avoid dehydration. This is especially important for athletes or any person who engages in strenuous exercise and sweats heavily.

Nurses have an essential role in the prevention of acute renal failure (ARF) in hospitalized clients. Always be on the lookout for signs of impending renal impairment through careful physical assessment and closely monitoring laboratory values. Early recognition and correction of problems causing reduced renal blood flow usually restore renal function before tissue damage can occur. Evaluate the client's fluid status. Accurately measure intake and output, and check body weight to identify trends in fluid balance. Assess for manifestations of blood volume depletion, such as decreased urine output, postural hypotension, and tachycardia. Prompt fluid replacement in the prerenal stage can prevent renal tissue damage and renal failure.

Also monitor laboratory values for any changes that reflect poor renal function. Decreased urine specific gravity indicates a loss of urine-concentrating ability and is the earliest sign of renal tubular damage. Other laboratory values that are helpful in monitoring renal function include serum creatinine, urine and serum electrolytes, and blood urea nitrogen (BUN).

Be aware of nephrotoxic substances that the client may ingest or be exposed to (see Table 75-4). Question any prescription for potentially nephrotoxic drugs, and validate the dose before the client receives the drug. Antibiotics are common drugs that have nephrotoxic side effects. NSAIDs can cause or increase the risk for ARF. Combining two or more nephrotoxic drugs dramatically increases the risk for ARF. If a client must receive a potentially nephrotoxic drug, monitor laboratory values, including BUN, creatinine, and drug peak and trough levels, closely for indications of renal dysfunction.

◆COLLABORATIVE MANAGEMENT

◆Assessment

HISTORY

The accurate diagnosis of ARF, including its type and its cause, depends on a detailed history of potential causes of ARF. Ask the client about exposure to nephrotoxins, recent surgery or trauma, transfusions, or other factors that might lead to reduced renal blood flow. Obtain a drug history, especially treatment with antibiotics, angiotensin-converting enzyme (ACE) inhibitors, and NSAIDs. Ask the client whether he or she has recently had an x-ray requiring injection of a contrast dye. These dyes can cause ARF, especially in older clients with reduced renal reserve. ARF must be differentiated from chronic renal insufficiency (CRI). Ask the client about diseases that impair renal function, such as diabetes mellitus, systemic lupus erythematosus, other connective tissue diseases, and chronic hypertension.

To identify possible acute glomerulonephritis, ask about acute illnesses such as influenza, colds, gastroenteritis, and sore throats. Ask the client whether urine color has become darker or appears smoky.

Reversible prerenal azotemia may occur after any episode of acute hypotension, hemorrhage or shock, burns, heart failure, or any problem in which the blood volume is depleted. Extensive bowel preparations and being allowed nothing by mouth (NPO) before surgery along with fluid loss during surgery can cause prerenal azotemia in some clients.

Postrenal renal failure is identified by focusing on urinary obstructive problems. Ask the client about any difficulty in starting the urine stream, changes in the amount or appearance of the urine, narrowing of the urine stream, nocturia, urgency, or symptoms of renal stones. Also ask about any cancer history that may cause urinary obstruction.

PHYSICAL ASSESSMENT/CLINICAL MANIFESTATIONS

The manifestations of ARF are related to the collection of nitrogenous wastes **(azotemia)** as well as to as the underlying cause (Chart 75-1). Manifestations of *prerenal* azotemia are hypotension, tachycardia, decreased urine output, decreased cardiac output, decreased central venous pressure (CVP), and lethargy. The appearance of a client with prerenal azotemia is similar to that of a client with heart failure or dehydration, depending on the cause of the poor renal blood flow.

Intrarenal (intrinsic) ARF usually occurs with damage to the glomeruli, interstitial tissue, or tubules. Manifestations are decreased urine output **(oliguria)** or absence of urine **(anuria)**, edema, hypertension, tachycardia, shortness of breath, distended neck veins, elevated central venous pressure, weight gain, respiratory crackles, anorexia, nausea, vomiting, and lethargy or varying levels of consciousness. Manifestations of electrolyte imbalances, such as electrocardiographic (ECG) changes, may also be present.

In clients with *postrenal* failure, monitor for oliguria or intermittent anuria, symptoms of uremia, and lethargy. Report changes in the urine stream or difficulty starting urination.

LABORATORY ASSESSMENT

The many changes in laboratory values in the client with ARF are similar to those occurring in chronic renal failure (CRF) (Chart 75-2; see also Laboratory Assessment [Chronic Renal Failure], p. 1745). Expect to see rising BUN, creatinine, and abnormal blood electrolytes values. Table 75-5 shows electrolyte values common to renal failure. Clients with ARF, however, do *not* have the anemia associated with CRF unless there is hemorrhagic blood loss. However, uremic hemolysis can develop and may be the cause of anemia in the early phase of ARF.

In the early phases of ARF, urine tests may provide diagnostic information. Urine sodium levels are often less than 10 to 20 mEq/L in clients with prerenal azotemia. The urine is often concentrated, with a specific gravity greater than 1.020. The presence of urine sediment (red blood cells [RBCs], RBC casts, tubular cells), myoglobin, or hemoglobin; a urine sodium level lower than 40 mEq/L; and a specific gravity of 1.010 indicate intrarenal failure. In postrenal failure, urine sodium levels may be normal to 40 mEq/L, with a specific gravity of 1.000 to 1.010.

CHART 75-1

KEY FEATURES of
Acute Renal Failure

Prerenal Azotemia
- Hypotension
- Tachycardia
- Decreased cardiac output
- Decreased central venous pressure
- Decreased urine output
- Lethargy

Intrarenal (Intrinsic) ARF and Postrenal Azotemia
- Renal manifestations
  - Oliguria or anuria
  - Increased urine specific gravity
- Cardiac manifestations
  - Hypertension
  - Tachycardia
  - Jugular venous distention
  - Increased central venous pressure
  - ECG changes: tall T waves
- Respiratory manifestations
  - Shortness of breath
  - Orthopnea
  - Rales or crackles
  - Pulmonary edema
  - Friction rub
- Gastrointestinal manifestations
  - Anorexia
  - Nausea
  - Vomiting
  - Flank pain
- Neurologic manifestations
  - Lethargy
  - Headache
  - Tremors
  - Confusion
- General manifestations
  - Generalized edema
  - Weight gain

ARF, Acute renal failure; *ECG,* electrocardiogram.

RADIOGRAPHIC ASSESSMENT

X-rays help to determine the cause of ARF. A flat-plate x-ray of the abdomen is used to determine the size of the kidneys. Enlarged kidneys, possibly due to obstruction, may result from hydronephrosis. This x-ray may show stones obstructing the renal pelvis, ureters, or bladder.

Renal ultrasonography is a noninvasive procedure using high-energy sound waves. It is useful in the diagnosis of urinary tract obstruction. Dilation of the renal calyces and collecting ducts, as well as stones, can be detected.

Computed tomography (CT) scans without contrast dye can identify obstruction or tumors. Contrast dyes are usually avoided to prevent further renal damage. Ultrasonography is preferred to renography to determine kidney size and the patency of the ureters. A nuclear medicine study called *MAG3* may be used to determine the nature of the renal failure, GFR, or tubular function and its severity. A renal scan can determine whether blood flow to the kidneys is sufficient.

Aortorenal angiography may be used to examine renal blood vessels and blood flow. The procedure involves the

CHART 75-2

LABORATORY PROFILE
Renal Failure

Test	Normal Range for Adults	Values in Renal Failure	Comments
Test to Evaluate Removal of Nitrogenous Wastes			
Serum creatinine	*Male:* 0.6-1.2 mg/dL *Female:* 0.5-7 mg/dL *Older adults:* Decreased	**In Chronic Renal Failure** May increase by 0.5-1.0 mg/dL every 1-2 yr May be as high as 15-30 mg/dL *before* symptoms of CRF are present **In Acute Renal Failure** Gradual increase of 1-2 mg/dL every 24-48 hr May increase 1-6 mg/dL in 1 wk or less	Consistently elevated levels indicate decreased renal function. Serum creatinine levels are used to evaluate the effectiveness of dialysis treatments.
Blood urea nitrogen	10-20 mg/dL *Older adults:* May be slightly increased	**In Chronic Renal Failure** May reach 180-200 mg/dL *before* symptoms develop **In Acute Renal Failure** Often increases by 10-20 mg/dL at same pace as serum creatinine level May reach 80-100 mg/dL within 1 wk	Increases depend on protein intake and other factors (see text). Rate of increase is controlled by limiting protein intake. This intervention is believed to decrease the rate of onset of systemic symptoms, such as anorexia, nausea, and vomiting. Elevations have multiple causes, including diminished renal function excessive protein intake, sepsis GI bleeding, dehydration, and tissue catabolism.
Electrolyte Studies			
Serum sodium	136-145 mEq/L; 136-145 mmol/L (SI units)	Normal or decreased	Clients with renal failure retain sodium. With associated water retention, serum sodium levels seem normal. With excessive water retention, serum sodium levels seem decreased owing to hemodilution. Assess the client for evidence of fluid volume excess: edema, weight increase, or elevation of diastolic blood pressure. Limit fluid intake as directed. Avoid excessive sodium intake Monitor for signs of hypernatremia dry skin, excessive thirst, dry mucous membranes, elevated body temperature, and flushed skin. Client may need diuretics or dialysis.
Serum potassium	3.5-5.0 mmol/L (SI units)	Increased	Advise the client to avoid salt substitutes and to limit potassium-containing foods. Monitor for rapidly increasing serum potassium levels in ARF. ECG changes occur with serum potassium levels ≥6.5. Monitor for signs of hyperkalemia: dizziness, weakness, cardiac irregularities, muscle cramps, diarrhea, and nausea. May require administration of sodium polystyrene sulfonate (Kayexalate) or other treatment.
Serum phosphorus (phosphate)	3.0-4.5 mg/dL, 0.97-1.45 mmol/L (SI units) *Older adults:* May be slightly decreased	Increased	Short-term increases have potential to cause rapid decrease in serum calcium level and cardiac rhythm disturbances. Long-term increases demineralize bones of calcium and enhance fracture potential. Phosphate-binding medications help control hyperphosphatemia and prevent calcium depletion from the bones.

ARF, Acute renal failure; *ECG*, electrocardiogram; *CRF*, chronic renal failure; *GI*, gastrointestinal; *GFR*, glomerular filtration rate *RBCs*, red blood cells; *SI*, Système Internationale; *WBCs*, white blood cells.

Continued

CHART 75-2

LABORATORY PROFILE
Renal Failure—*cont'd*

Test	Normal Range for Adults	Values in Renal Failure	Comments
Serum calcium	Total calcium: 9.0-10.5 mg/dL; 2.25-2.75 mmol/L (SI units) Ionized calcium: 4.5-5.6 mg/dL, 1.05-1.3 mmol/L (SI units) *Older adults:* Slightly decreased	Decreased	Decreases in ARF may necessitate replacement. Decreases in CRF may only be slight and may or may not necessitate replacement. As the serum phosphate level increases, the serum calcium level decreases. Chronic calcium deficiency leads to renal osteodystrophy. Control of phosphate excess is usually essential before calcium replacement is initiated. Monitor for manifestations of hypocalcemia: abdominal cramps, hyperactive reflexes, tingling fingertips, and spasms in feet and wrists (see also Chapter 16).
Serum magnesium	1.3-2.1 mEq/L; 0.65-1.05 mmol/L (SI units)	Increased	Advise the client to avoid compounds containing magnesium (e.g., laxatives).
Serum carbon dioxide combining power (bicarbonate)	23-30 mEq/L (venous); 23-30 mmol/L (SI units)	Decreased	Replace bicarbonate. Monitor respiratory rate and depth. Monitor for decreased orientation.
Arterial blood pH	7.35-7.45	Decreased (in metabolic acidosis) or normal	The respiratory system attempts to compensate by hyperventilation (increased rate and depth of respiration). Values are within the normal range if blood buffers and lungs can compensate. Monitor breathing rate and depth. Monitor level of consciousness.
Arterial blood bicarbonate (HCO_3^-)	21-28 mEq/L	Decreased	Provide replacement PO, IV, or by hemodialysis or peritoneal dialysis.
Arterial blood $Paco_2$	35-45 mm Hg	Decreased	Monitor for respiratory fatigue (the client breathes more rapidly and deeply to "blow off" carbon dioxide).
Other Blood Studies			
Hemoglobin	*Female:* 12-16 g/dL, 7.4-9.9 mmol/L (SI units) *Male:* 14-18 g/dL, 8.7-11.2 mmol/L (SI units) *Older adults:* Slightly decreased	Decreased	Decreased levels indicate anemia. Monitor for pallor, weakness, lethargy, dizziness, possible shortness of breath, and activity intolerance.
Hematocrit	*Female:* 37%-47% *Male:* 42%-52% *Older adults:* May be slightly decreased	Decreased to 20%	Same as for hemoglobin. With erythropoietin therapy, may be able to obtain levels as high as 36%.
Urinalysis*			
Specific gravity	Usually 1.010-1.025 Possible range: 1.005-1.030	Usually decreased and fixed	Reflects inability of the tubules to produce a concentrated or diluted urine in response to changes in plasma osmolarity. Monitor for fluid volume deficit or excess.
pH	Average: 5.5-6 Possible range: 4.6-8	May be fixed; pH does not change with dietary changes	Collect a freshly voided specimen for testing
Glucose	None or $<$15 mg/dL Usually detectable in urine of nondiabetic clients when blood level is 160-180 mg/dL	Increased	The renal threshold is often increased; therefore the blood glucose level may be $>$160-180 mg/dL before glucose is detectable in the urine. Monitor *blood* glucose levels.

ARF, Acute renal failure; *ECG*, electrocardiogram; *CRF*, chronic renal failure; *GI*, gastrointestinal; *GFR*, glomerular filtration rate *RBCs*, red blood cells; *SI*, Système Internationale; *WBCs*, white blood cells.

*Urine may become cloudy with heavy sediment. Urine output and appearance vary, depending on remaining renal function.

CHART 75-2

LABORATORY PROFILE

Renal Failure—*cont'd*

Test	Normal Range for Adults	Values in Renal Failure	Comments
Urinalysis*—*cont'd*			
Protein	0-8 mg/dL	Increased when there is glomerular damage or disease	Increases may be an incidental and benign finding. Transient increases occur with extreme exercise, fever, stress, or infection. Persistent proteinuria requires 24-hr collection for determination of total quantity excreted. Persistent proteinuria may indicate a serious renal problem. Instruct the client about the need for follow-up. Instruct the client in the correct procedure for collection of 24-hr specimen (see Chapter 72).
Occult blood	No RBCs or occasionally 2 or 3 RBCs per high-power field No hemoglobin	More than 2 or 3 RBCs per high-power field Detectable hemoglobin	Hemoglobin is detectable when hemolysis of RBCs has occurred. Intact RBCs are detectable only with microscopic examination. Collect a freshly voided specimen for testing.
WBCs	0-5 per high-power field	Increased in urinary tract infection	Often indicates need for urine culture.
Bacteria	Fewer than 1000 colonies/mL	Increased in the presence of infection, with or without an increase in WBCs	Obtain urine culture.
Casts	None or a few; composed of RBCs, WBCs, protein, or tubular cell casts such as hyaline	Casts present	Casts may be a benign occurrence or may signify that some renal injury or disease is present. Collect a freshly voided specimen for direct microscopic examination.
Creatinine clearance	*Male:* 107-139 mL/min *Female:* 87-107 mL/min *Older adults:* Progressively decreased with advancing age	Decreased	Change reflects decreases in GFR. Creatinine clearance is determined from a 24-hr urine collection and a serum creatinine value.

ARF, Acute renal failure; *ECG*, electrocardiogram; *CRF*, chronic renal failure; *GI*, gastrointestinal; *GFR*, glomerular filtration rate *RBCs*, red blood cells; *SI*, Système Internationale; *WBCs*, white blood cells.

*Urine may become cloudy with heavy sediment. Urine output and appearance vary, depending on remaining renal function.

TABLE 75-5 Effects of Renal Failure on Electrolyte Balance

Electrolyte	Effects of Renal Failure	Problems	Treatments
Potassium	Retained with oliguria (increased)	Hyperkalemia Cardiac dysrhythmias Asystole	Kayexalate, PO or rectal Regular IV insulin with 5% to 50% dextrose IV calcium gluconate Dialysis
Sodium	Retained (increased)	Dilutional hyponatremia Fluid volume excess Hypertension Heart failure Pulmonary edema	Diuretics until no longer responsive Dialysis Fluid restriction Sodium restriction
Phosphate	Retained (increased)	Hyperphosphatemia Metastatic calcium phosphate deposits Renal bone disease	Phosphate-binding agents Limit phosphorus intake Vitamin D analogues
Calcium	Decreased gastrointestinal absorption Binds to phosphate (decreased)	Bone demineralization Pathologic fractures	Replace vitamin D Calcium supplements
Hydrogen	Retained (increased)	Binds with bicarbonate for excretion through respiratory compensation	Dialysis Bicarbonate supplements
Bicarbonate	Depleted (decreased)	Used for blood buffering to prevent metabolic acidemia	Dialysis Bicarbonate supplements
Magnesium	Retained (decreased)	Potential for hypermagnesemia	Avoid magnesium-containing antacids and laxatives

risk of using contrast dye but can reveal any occlusion of major renal vessels by thrombus, embolus, or stenosis. Cystoscopy or retrograde pyelography may be needed to identify obstructions of the lower urinary tract.

OTHER DIAGNOSTIC ASSESSMENTS

Renal biopsy is performed if the cause of ARF is uncertain, an immunologic disease is suspected, or the reversibility of the renal failure needs to be determined after ARF has persisted for an extended period. Prepare the client before the test, and provide follow-up care. You must be aware of all test results and understand how they might affect the treatment regimen. (See Chapter 72 for a detailed discussion of renal diagnostic tests.)

◆Common Nursing Diagnoses and Collaborative Problems

Nursing diagnoses and collaborative problems that may apply to clients with acute renal failure include the following:

- Excess Fluid Volume related to compromised regulatory mechanisms (inability of the kidneys to maintain body fluid balance)
- Potential for Pulmonary Edema
- Potential for Electrolyte Imbalances

◆Interventions

The client with ARF may move from the oliguric phase (in which fluid and electrolytes are retained) to the diuretic phase. If the client moves to the diuretic phase, hypovolemia and electrolyte *loss* are the main problems. The client in the diuretic phase of ARF needs a plan of care that focuses on fluid and electrolyte *replacement* and monitoring.

These examples of output variation reflect the continually changing nature of ARF and the need for the plan of care to be constantly updated to reflect the stages of the disease process. Drug therapy, diet therapy, and renal replacement therapy (peritoneal dialysis [PD], hemodialysis [HD], or hemofiltration) are commonly used to manage ARF.

Drug Therapy. Clients with ARF receive many drugs. As kidney function changes, drug dosages are modified. You must be knowledgeable about the site of drug metabolism and especially careful when giving drugs. Constantly monitor for possible side effects and interactions of the drugs that the client with ARF is receiving (Chart 75-3; see also Drug Therapy [Chronic Renal Failure], p. 1748). Diuretics may be used to increase urine output.

In clients with prerenal azotemia, fluid challenges and diuretics are often used to promote renal blood flow. In clients without manifestations of fluid volume excess, 500 to 1000 mL of normal saline may be infused over a 1-hour period. In prerenal azotemia, the client responds to the fluid challenge by producing urine soon after the initial bolus. Diuretics such as furosemide (Lasix) also may be prescribed along with a fluid bolus. If oliguric renal failure is diagnosed, the fluid challenges and diuretics are discontinued. Low-dose (1 to 3 mcg/kg) dopamine may be given in a continuous infusion to enhance renal blood flow and to increase blood pressure (Chart 75-4). These clients often require central venous pressure (CVP) monitoring or measurement of pulmonary arterial pressure by means of a pulmonary artery catheter for an exact evaluation of their hemodynamic status. They also require constant nursing supervision for assessment of the response to fluid and drug therapy. Carefully monitor for signs of possible fluid overload.

Calcium channel blockers may be used to treat ARF resulting from nephrotoxic acute tubular necrosis (ATN). These drugs prevent the influx of calcium into the kidney cells, maintain kidney cell integrity, and improve the glomerular filtration rate (GFR) by improving renal blood flow.

Diet Therapy. Clients who have ARF often have a high rate of protein breakdown. The exact cause for this state is not well understood. Increases in metabolism and protein breakdown may be related to the stress of a critical illness, causing an increase in blood levels of catecholamines, cortisol, and glucagon. The rate of protein breakdown correlates with the severity of uremia and azotemia. This hypercatabolic state causes the breakdown of muscle for protein, which leads to an increase in azotemia and an even more elevated blood urea nitrogen (BUN) level.

If the client with ARF has an adequate dietary intake (see Imbalanced Nutrition: Less Than Body Requirements [Chronic Renal Failure], p. 1746), nutritional support may not be needed. Consultation with a dietitian, who will calculate the client's caloric needs, may be prescribed. Work with the dietitian to provide a diet with specified amounts of protein, sodium, and fluids. For the client who does not require dialysis, 0.6 g/kg of body weight or 40 g/day of protein is usually prescribed. For clients who do require dialysis, the protein level needed will range from 1 to 1.5 g/kg. The amount of dietary sodium ranges from 60 to 90 mEq. If hyperkalemia is present, dietary potassium is restricted to 60 to 70 mEq. The amount of fluid permitted is generally calculated to equal the urine volume plus 500 mL. Continually assess oral intake to make certain that caloric intake is adequate.

Many clients with ARF are too ill or have too poor an appetite to eat enough food. For these clients, some form of nutritional support (e.g., total parenteral nutrition [TPN] or hyperalimentation) is needed. The goals of nutritional support in ARF are to provide sufficient nutrients to maintain or improve nutritional status, to preserve lean body mass, to restore or maintain fluid balance, and to preserve renal function.

If TPN is used, the solutions are mixed to meet the client's specific needs. Because kidney function is unstable in ARF, constantly monitor the serum electrolyte concentrations and indicate when the hyperalimentation solution needs to be changed. IV fat emulsion (Intralipid) infusions can provide a nonprotein source of calories. In uremic clients, fat emulsions are used in place of glucose to avoid the problems of excessive sugars.

Dialysis Therapies. If necessary, hemodialysis (HD) and peritoneal dialysis (PD) may be implemented for clients with ARF. The following are indications for dialysis in ARF:

- Uremia
- Persistent hyperkalemia
- Uncompensated metabolic acidosis
- Fluid volume excess unresponsive to diuretics
- Uremic pericarditis
- Uremic encephalopathy

Immediate vascular access for HD in clients with ARF is made by placement of a dual- or triple-lumen catheter specific for HD. When HD is expected to be used for several

CHART 75-3

DRUG THERAPY for Renal Failure

Drug	Usual Dosages	Indications	Nursing Interventions	Rationales
Cardioglycosides				
Digoxin (Lanoxin, Novodigoxin✱)	0.125-0.25 mg PO or IV daily or every other day *Older adults:* 0.0625-0.125 PO or IV daily or every other day	Decreased stroke volume Decreased strength of cardiac contractions	Monitor for signs of digoxin toxicity and hypokalemia. Monitor for bradycardia (pulse $<$50-60 beats/min). Monitor serum drug levels.	Digoxin remains in the body longer when renal function is impaired. Bradycardia is a sign of digoxin toxicity. A toxic digoxin level is $>$2.5 ng/mL.
Vitamins and Minerals				
Folic acid (vitamin B_9, Folvite, Novofolacid✱)	0.1 mg PO, SC, or IM daily	Dietary supplement	Usually given after dialysis.	Water-soluble vitamins are removed during dialysis.
Ferrous sulfate (Feosol, Novoferrosulfa✱)	325 mg PO three or four times daily	Anemia	Monitor for constipation. Note any change in the stools, which normally become blackish green.	Constipation is a common and uncomfortable side effect associated with oral iron supplements. The color is caused by the presence of unabsorbed iron and is harmless.
Biological Response Modifiers				
Erythropoietin alpha (Epogen, Procrit)	50-100 units/kg IV or SC 3 times/wk	Anemia associated with CRF	Monitor hematocrit twice weekly until maintenance dose is achieved. Monitor blood pressure.	The dose is based on response as measured by hematocrit changes. Rapid rise in hematocrit can cause hypertension.
Phosphate Binders				
Aluminum hydroxide gel (Amphojel, AlternaGEL, Alu-Cap, Nephrox) Aluminum carbonate gel (Basaljel)	500 mg–2 g PO twice to four times daily as tablets, capsules, or oral suspension	Phosphate binder Prevention of renal osteodystrophy	Monitor for constipation, which occurs frequently. Monitor for signs of hypophosphatemia. Monitor serum aluminum levels.	Constipation is a frequent side effect of many drugs that bind phosphorus. These drugs can prevent intestinal absorption of phosphorus to the extent that the client develops hypophosphatemia. Aluminum toxicity may cause bone disease and dementia.
Sevelamer hydrochloride (Renagel)	Serum phosphorus 6.0-7.5 mg/dL: 2 capsules three times daily Serum phosphorus 7.6-8.9 mg/dL: 3 capsules three times daily Serum phosphorus $>$9.0 mg/dL: 4 capsules three times daily	Hyperphosphatemia	Give with meals. Tell client to swallow capsule whole; do not chew. Monitor serum phosphorus levels.	Drug binds with phosphorus in food, preventing absorption. Drug expands when capsule is broken. Drug can cause hypophosphatemia.
Calcium carbonate (Tums, OsCal, CalciChew)	1-3 tablets PO daily (in divided doses three or four times daily)	Dietary supplement Phosphate binder	Give only when serum phosphate levels are normal. Monitor for hypercalcemia, constipation, and soft-tissue calcifications. Give after meals.	Calcium supplements may cause a *decrease* in serum phosphate levels because these two minerals exist in blood in a balanced, *reciprocal* relationship. Giving binders after meals enhances binding capacity.
Stool Softeners and Laxatives				
Docusate sodium (Colace) Bisacodyl (Dulcolax, Bisco-Lax, Laxit✱)	100-300 mg daily 5-10 mg PO or PR daily or every other day	Prevention of constipation caused by limited fluid intake, iron supplements, and phosphate binders	Observe for abdominal cramps and diarrhea. Monitor bowel movements.	These gastrointestinal effects indicate drug overdose. Monitoring bowel movements is a way of determining medication effectiveness.

Med Error Alert! *Watch dose; it is very low (0.125-0.25 mg).*

SC, Subcutaneous.

CHART 75-4

BEST PRACTICE for
Administering Renal-Dose Dopamine

- Take an accurate weight because the dose is prescribed according to the client's weight.
- Know the hospital's policy regarding who is responsible for calculating the rate of infusion (i.e., physician, pharmacist, or nurse). Renal-dose dopamine is 1 to 5 mcg per kilogram of body weight per minute but is converted to mL/min for an IV infusion.
- Before hanging the dopamine infusion, double-check the amount of dopamine added to the solution, the total volume of solution (usually 250 mL), and the calculation milliliters per minute.
- Do not hang the dopamine infusion until all questions about the calculation are clarified.
- If dopamine is to be infused into a peripheral vein, be sure that the line is intact and secured.
- Once the infusion is started, check the client's blood pressure and pulse according to hospital policy or at least every 2 hours.
- Notify the physician of changes in vital signs per policy.
- Monitor the IV site hourly for infiltration.
- If infiltration occurs, stop the infusion but do not discontinue the IV catheter. Prepare for phentolamine (Regitine, Rogitine*) administration through the IV catheter and subcutaneously into the infiltrated tissue.

weeks, the catheter is usually placed in the subclavian or internal jugular vein. If only one or two HD treatments are needed, as for removal of drugs or toxins, a femoral site may be selected. Longer use of the femoral site is discouraged because the client's mobility is restricted and complications, such as hematomas and infection, are common. Repeatedly accessing the femoral site increases the risk for hematoma formation and makes repeated use of the vein impossible.

The subclavian vein is preferred over the femoral site because the catheter can be left in place between dialysis treatments. However, the longer the catheter is left in this place, the greater the chance for infection. The subclavian dialysis catheter (Figure 75-1) is inserted at the bedside. A physician or nurse practitioner performs the sterile procedure, and then the catheter is covered with a sterile dressing. Catheter placement is checked by chest x-ray before its use.

If hemodialysis is needed for more than a few days, a long-term dialysis catheter may be used. Most of these catheters are placed in the radiology department using a tunneling technique. The client receives moderate sedation. Under sonographic or fluoroscopic guidance, the physician makes a small incision where the internal jugular vein passes behind the clavicle. A 6- to 8-cm subcutaneous tunnel is created out from the side of the incision. A long-term hemodialysis catheter is inserted through the tunnel and into the jugular vein. Keeping a segment of the catheter within the subcutaneous tissues before entering the jugular vein reduces the risk for infection.

Hemodialysis catheters have two lumens, one for outflow and one for inflow. As a result, the outflow of blood for dialysis is separated from the dialyzed blood returned through the inflow lumen. A triple-lumen catheter for HD is available. The third lumen is an access for drawing venous blood or giving drugs and fluid without interruption of dialysis.

Peritoneal dialysis (PD) may also be used in the treatment of ARF, although some clients, such as those being

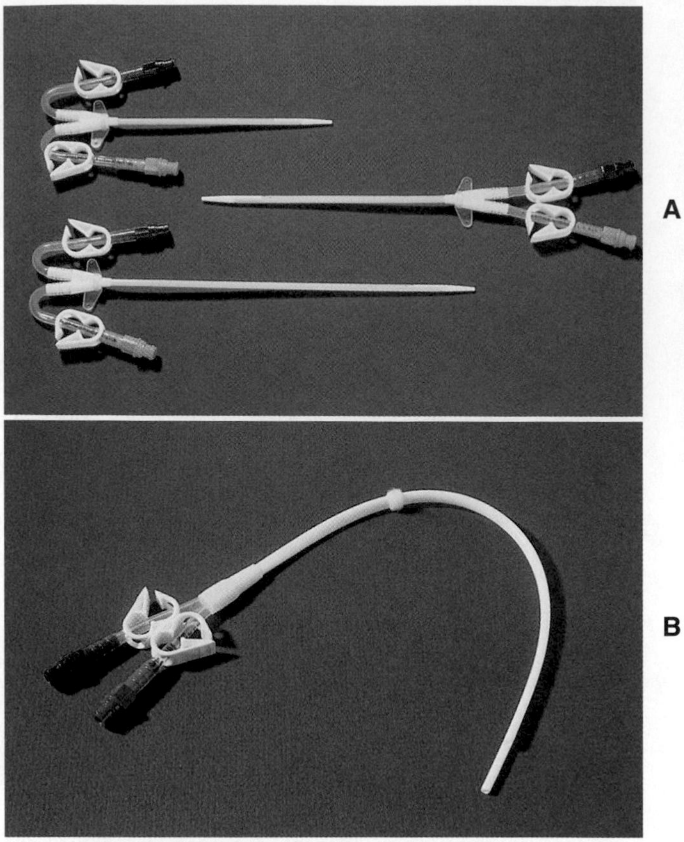

Figure 75-1 ■ Subclavian dialysis catheters. These catheters are radiopaque tubes that can be used for hemodialysis access. The Y-shape tubing allows arterial outflow and venous return through a single catheter. **A,** Mahurkar catheters, made of polyurethane and used for short-term access. **B,** A PermCath catheter, which is made of silicone and used for long-term access. (Courtesy of Kendall Company, Bothell, WA.)

mechanically ventilated, may not be able to tolerate the accompanying abdominal distention. PD uses the peritoneum as the dialyzing membrane. The dialysate is infused through a catheter implanted in the peritoneum. A complete discussion of PD is provided later in this chapter under Chronic Renal Failure, pp. 1757 to 1759).

Continuous Renal Replacement Therapy. Continuous renal replacement therapies (CRRTs) are the standard treatment for ARF. Renal replacement therapies in the form of hemofiltration are often better tolerated than HD for critically ill clients because this method avoids rapid shifts of fluids and electrolytes.

Continuous arteriovenous hemofiltration (CAVH) and continuous arteriovenous hemodialysis and filtration (CAVHD) are additional renal replacement therapies for clients with ARF. These procedures are similar to HD, but indications for their use are more specific.

CAVH is indicated for clients who have fluid volume overload, are resistant to diuretics, and are hemodynamically unstable. The use of CAVH requires placement of both arterial and venous catheters, and a mean arterial pressure of at least 60 mm Hg. CAVH continuously removes large amounts of plasma water, wastes, and electrolytes. Electrolytes are replaced through prescribed amounts of IV electrolyte solutions. A major disadvantage of arteriovenous (AV) filtration is the risk for bleeding caused by anticoagulants used to prevent membrane clotting.

A double-lumen dialysis catheter inserted into a large vein (subclavian, jugular) is the access for CAVHD. CAVHD uses a **dialysate** (a solution composed of water, glucose, sodium chloride, potassium, magnesium, calcium, and bicarbonate) delivery system to remove waste products in addition to plasma water in clients with limited cardiac output, those with severe hypotension, or those who do not respond to diuretic therapy. These clients cannot tolerate standard HD, and PD would be inadequate for the fluid removal required.

Continuous venovenous hemofiltration (CVVH) is often the treatment of choice for critically ill clients. CVVH uses only a double-lumen venous catheter for access and is powered by a pump, making the rate of filtration more reliable than methods using mean arterial pressure. The pump increases the risk for an air embolus, but most pumps have alarms that detect air. These systems also require the use of anticoagulants, but at lower doses than needed for AV systems. These procedures are used in critical care units, and clients require continuous nursing care.

Posthospital Care. The care for a client with ARF after discharge from the hospital varies widely, depending on the status of the disease when the client is discharged. The course of ARF varies, with recovery lasting up to several months. If the renal failure is resolving, follow-up care may be provided by a nephrologist or by the family physician in consultation with the nephrologist. However, ARF may result in permanent renal damage and the need for chronic dialysis or even transplantation. In these cases, follow-up care is similar to that needed for clients with chronic renal failure (see Community-Based Care, p. 1763).

If the ARF is beginning to resolve, the follow-up care may involve many services. Frequent medical visits are necessary, as are scheduled laboratory blood and urine tests to monitor renal function. A dietary consult is needed to modify the client's diet according to the degree of renal function and ongoing nutritional requirements. Teach clients continuing dialysis after discharge to limit foods high in potassium and sodium and to observe protein restrictions. Also teach about any needed fluid intake limitation.

Some clients may need temporary dialysis until their kidneys can eliminate fluid and waste products. The dialysis started while the client was an inpatient can be continued at an outpatient dialysis center. Teaching about the type of dialysis, how to care for vascular access sites, dietary restrictions, fluid restrictions, and prevention of complications is ongoing throughout the recovery phase. Depending on their level of independence and family support, some clients may also need home care nursing or social work assistance.

Critical Thinking Challenge

The client is a 32-year-old woman who was struck by a car while jogging on a country road during the afternoon of a very hot day. When she arrives at the emergency department by ambulance 3 hours after the accident, she is able to talk, does not have an IV, and is in extreme pain. She tells you that she had been jogging for an hour when she was hit. Her husband tells you that she is in great health and works full-time as an aerobics instructor. She is 5 feet 1 inch tall and weighs 110 lb. Her only drugs include oral contraceptives, a multivitamin, and 800 mg daily of ibuprofen. She has a compound fracture of her left femur and considerable bruising on left hip and pelvis. Her vital signs are T 99.4, P 116 and thready, R 30, and BP 90/58.

1. For what type(s) of acute renal failure is she at risk? Why?
2. Do any of her usual drugs increase her risk for ARF? Which one(s) and why?
3. Is there any specific assessment data you could obtain without a prescription to evaluate her risk for acute renal failure?

The physician prescribes the following interventions:

- IV placement with an 18-gauge cannula, NS at 200 mL/hr
- Hematocrit and hemoglobin levels
- Morphine sulfate 2 mg IV push
- Foley catheter placement
- Type and crossmatch for 4 units of packed red blood cells
- X-rays of the left hip and leg and KUB

4. In what order (and why) should you perform these interventions?

evolve For suggested answer guidelines, go to http://evolve.elsevier.com/Iggy/.

CHART 75-5

KEY FEATURES of Uremia

Metallic taste in the mouth	Fatigue and lethargy
Anorexia	Hiccups
Nausea	Edema
Vomiting	Dyspnea
Muscle cramps	Muscle cramps
Itching	Paresthesias

CHRONIC RENAL FAILURE

PATHOPHYSIOLOGY

Unlike ARF, chronic renal failure (CRF) is a progressive, irreversible kidney injury. Kidney function does not recover. When kidney function is too poor to sustain life, CRF is termed *end-stage renal disease* (ESRD). Terms used with renal failure include **azotemia** (collection of nitrogenous wastes in the blood), **uremia** (azotemia with clinical symptoms [Chart 75-5]), and **uremic syndrome** (the systemic clinical and laboratory manifestations of ESRD). ARF and CRF are compared in Table 75-1.

Stages of Chronic Renal Failure

The kidneys fail in an organized fashion. Progression toward ESRD usually starts with a gradual decrease in renal function of 30% to 50% (Table 75-6). At first, there is a *diminished renal reserve.* A 24-hour urine specimen for monitoring creatinine clearance is used to detect that renal reserve is less than normal. In this stage, reduced renal function occurs without accumulation of metabolic wastes in the blood because the unaffected nephrons overwork to compensate for the diseased nephrons. Renal damage increases systemic blood pressure, which also increases glomerular pressure and the pressure in remaining unaffected nephrons. Eventually the unaffected nephrons may be damaged by this long-term increased pressure, causing the progressive renal

TABLE 75-6 Progression Toward Chronic Renal Failure

Stage I: Diminished Renal Reserve
- Renal function is reduced, but no accumulation of metabolic wastes occurs.
- The healthier kidney compensates for the diseased kidney.
- Ability to concentrate urine is decreased, resulting in nocturia and polyuria.
- A 24-hour urine collection for creatinine clearance is necessary to detect that renal reserve is less than normal.

Stage II: Renal Insufficiency
- Metabolic wastes begin to accumulate in the blood because the unaffected nephrons can no longer compensate.
- Responsiveness to diuretics is decreased, resulting in oliguria and edema.
- The degree of insufficiency is determined by the decreasing GFR and is classified as mild, moderate, or severe.
- Treatment is medical.

Stage III: End-Stage Renal Disease
- Excessive amounts of metabolic wastes such as urea and creatinine accumulate in the blood.
- The kidneys are unable to maintain homeostasis.
- Treatment is by dialysis or other renal replacement therapy.

GFR, Glomerular filtration rate.

damage of CRF. Although no manifestations of renal failure are usually present at this stage, if the client is stressed with infection, fluid overload, or dehydration, renal function at this stage can appear reduced.

In the next stage, *renal insufficiency,* metabolic wastes begin to collect in the blood because not enough healthy nephrons remain to compensate completely for the nonfunctioning nephrons. Levels of blood urea nitrogen (BUN), serum creatinine, uric acid, and phosphorus are elevated in proportion to the amount of nephrons lost. Careful management of fluid volume, blood pressure, electrolytes, dietary intake, and drug therapy slows, but does not halt, the progression of renal failure.

Over time most clients progress to ESRD. Excessive amounts of urea and creatinine build up in the blood, and the kidneys cannot maintain homeostasis. Severe fluid, electrolyte, and acid-base imbalances occur. Without renal replacement therapy, fatal complications are likely.

Kidney Changes

Renal failure causes many problems, including decreased glomerular filtration rate (GFR), abnormal urine production, poor water excretion, electrolyte imbalances, and metabolic abnormalities. Because the healthy nephrons hypertrophy and work harder, the kidneys can maintain an effective GFR until 70% to 80% of renal function is lost. Homeostasis is maintained until late in the course of renal failure. When fewer than 20% of the nephrons are functional, the GFR is decreased despite hypertrophy of the remaining nephrons. This problem occurs because the hypertrophied nephrons can maintain waste excretion only by decreasing water reabsorption. Thus, at this stage of renal failure, **hyposthenuria** (the loss of urine concentrating ability) and **polyuria** (increased urine output) occur. Both hyposthenuria and polyuria are early signs of CRF and, if the problem is untreated at this stage, can cause severe dehydration.

As the disease progresses, the ability to produce dilute urine is reduced, resulting in urine with a fixed osmolarity **(isosthenuria).** As renal function continues to decline, the BUN increases and urine output decreases. When renal function declines to this level, the client is at risk for fluid overload.

Metabolic Changes

UREA AND CREATININE

Renal failure disrupts urea and creatinine excretion. Creatinine is derived from creatine and phosphocreatine, which are present in skeletal muscle. The normal rate of creatinine excretion depends on muscle mass, physical activity, and diet. Without major changes in diet or physical activity, the serum creatinine level remains constant. Creatinine is partially excreted by the renal tubules, and a decrease in renal function leads to a buildup of serum creatinine. Urea is a product of protein metabolism and is excreted by the kidneys. The BUN level normally varies directly with protein intake.

The method for assessing the GFR is to measure the creatinine clearance. As renal function and GFR decline, creatinine clearance decreases and blood creatinine levels rise (see Chapter 72).

SODIUM

Changes in sodium excretion are common. Early in CRF, the client is at risk for hyponatremia (sodium depletion) because reduced numbers of functional nephrons are present to reabsorb sodium; thus sodium is lost in the urine. The polyuria often seen in early renal failure also causes sodium depletion.

In the later stages of renal failure, kidney excretion of sodium is reduced as urine production decreases. Then sodium retention and hypernatremia can occur with only modest increases in dietary sodium intake. This problem leads to severe fluid and electrolyte imbalances (see Chapters 15 and 16). Sodium retention causes hypertension and edema.

Even with sodium retention, the serum sodium level may appear normal because plasma water is retained at the same time. If fluid retention occurs at a greater rate than sodium retention, the serum sodium level is falsely low (hyponatremia) because of dilution (see Table 75-5).

POTASSIUM

The kidney is responsible for potassium excretion. Any increase in potassium load during the later stages of renal disease can lead to **hyperkalemia** (excessive potassium retention). Normal serum potassium levels of 3.5 to 5 mEq/L are maintained until the 24-hour urine output falls below 500 mL. Hyperkalemia then develops quickly, and serum potassium levels may reach 7 to 8 mEq/L or greater. Severe electrocardiographic (ECG) changes result from this elevation, and fatal dysrhythmias can occur. Other factors contribute to hyperkalemia in renal failure, including the ingestion of potassium in drugs, failure to restrict potassium in the diet, tissue breakdown, blood transfusions, and bleeding or hemorrhage. (See Chapter 16 for discussion of hyperkalemia.)

ACID-BASE BALANCE

In the early stage of renal failure, blood pH changes little because the remaining healthy nephrons increase their rate of acid excretion. As more nephrons are lost, acid excretion is reduced and metabolic acidosis results (see Chapter 19).

Many factors lead to metabolic acidosis in renal failure. First the kidneys are unable to excrete excessive hydrogen ions (acids). Normally, tubular cells move hydrogen ions into the urine for excretion, but ammonium and bicarbonate are needed for this movement to occur. In clients with renal failure, ammonium production is decreased and reabsorption of bicarbonate does not occur. This process leads to a buildup of hydrogen ions and reduced levels of bicarbonate (base deficit). In the presence of hyperkalemia, renal ammonium production and excretion are further inhibited.

As renal failure advances and acid retention increases, respiratory compensation is needed to keep blood pH normal. The respiratory system compensates for the decreased blood pH levels by increasing the rate and depth of breathing to excrete carbon dioxide through the lungs. This breathing pattern, called **Kussmaul respiration,** increases with worsening renal failure. Although hydrogen ions (acids) can leave the body this way, when too much carbon dioxide is "blown off," respiratory alkalosis results. Serum bicarbonate measures the extent of metabolic acidosis (bicarbonate deficit). Clients with CRF usually need alkali replacement to counteract acidosis.

CALCIUM AND PHOSPHORUS

A complex, balanced reciprocal relationship between calcium and phosphate is influenced by vitamin D (see Chapter 16). The kidney produces a hormone needed to activate vitamin D, which then enhances intestinal absorption of calcium.

In renal failure, phosphate retention and a deficiency of active vitamin D disrupt the calcium and phosphate balance. Normally, excessive dietary phosphate is excreted by the kidneys in the urine. Parathyroid hormone (PTH) controls the amount of phosphate in the blood by causing tubular excretion of phosphate when there is an excess. An early effect of CRF is reduced phosphate excretion (Figure 75-2). As plasma phosphate levels increase **(hyperphosphatemia),** calcium levels decrease **(hypocalcemia).** Chronic hypocalcemia causes chronic stimulation of the parathyroid glands. Under the influence of additional PTH, calcium is released from storage areas in bones **(bone resorption),** which results in bone demineralization and bone density loss. The additional calcium is needed to compensate, or balance, the excess plasma phosphate level. The problem of hypocalcemia is compounded because decreased renal function also causes decreased production of active vitamin D. Thus less calcium is absorbed through the intestinal tract in the absence of sufficient vitamin D.

The problems in bone metabolism and structure caused by renal failure-induced hypocalcemia and hyperphosphatemia are called **renal osteodystrophy.** Bone mineral loss from hyperparathyroidism causes bone pain, spinal sclerosis, fractures, bone density loss, osteomalacia, and tooth calcium loss.

Metastatic calcifications, crystals formed from excessive calcium phosphate, may precipitate in various parts of the body. When the plasma level of the calcium-phosphate product (serum calcium level multiplied by the serum phosphate level) exceeds 70 mg/dL, the crystals may lodge in the kidneys, heart, lungs, major blood vessels, joints, eyes (causing

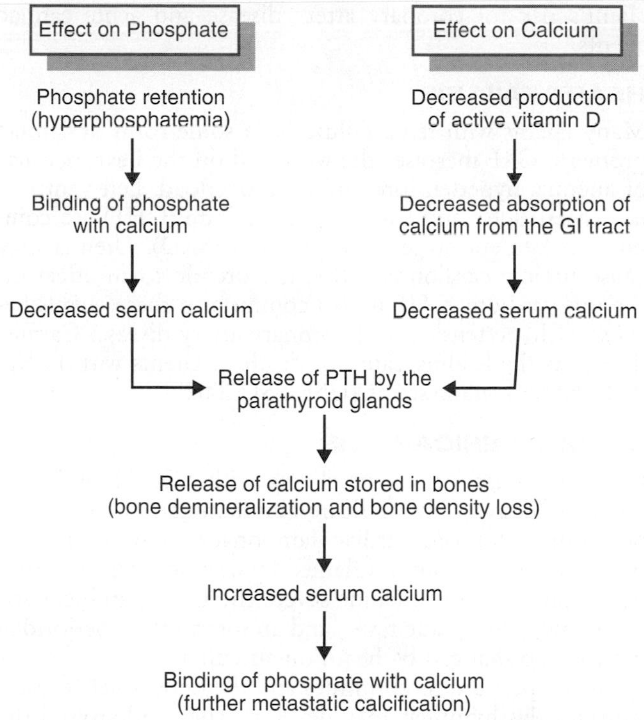

Figure 75-2 ■ The effects of renal failure on phosphate and calcium balance.

conjunctivitis), and brain. Uremic pruritus also results from calcium-phosphate imbalances and excess PTH production.

Cardiac Changes

HYPERTENSION

Most clients with CRF have hypertension. Hypertension may be either the cause or the result of CRF. In clients who have nonrenal causes of hypertension, the increased blood pressure damages the delicate capillaries in the glomerulus, and eventually renal failure results.

Renal failure itself elevates blood pressure by causing fluid and sodium overload and the malfunction of the renin-angiotensin-aldosterone system. The retention of sodium and water causes circulatory overload, which elevates blood pressure. The kidneys respond to a decrease in renal blood flow or to low serum sodium levels by trying to improve the renal blood flow. The release of renin stimulates the production of angiotensin and aldosterone. Angiotensin causes blood vessel constriction and increases blood pressure. Aldosterone, a hormone released by the adrenal glands, stimulates kidney tubules to reabsorb sodium and water. This action expands plasma volume and raises blood pressure. The damaged kidneys do not recognize the increase in blood pressure and continue to produce renin. The result is severe hypertension that is difficult to treat and worsens renal function. Many clients with CRF also have cardiomyopathy and left ventricular hypertrophy from the prolonged hypertension.

HYPERLIPIDEMIA

Chronic renal failure (CRF) changes fat metabolism, resulting in increased triglyceride, total cholesterol, and low-density lipoprotein (LDL) levels. These changes increase the client's risk for coronary artery disease and acute cardiac events.

HEART FAILURE

Many clients with renal failure have some form of cardiac problem. CRF increases the workload on the heart because of anemia, hypertension, and fluid overload. Left ventricular hypertrophy and chronic heart failure (CHF) are common in late end-stage renal disease (ESRD). Uremia may cause uremic cardiomyopathy, the uremic toxin effect on the myocardium. CHF is also common in these clients because of hypertension and coronary artery disease. Cardiac disease is the leading cause of death in clients with ESRD (U.S. Renal Data Systems [USRDS], 2002).

UREMIC PERICARDITIS

Pericarditis also occurs in clients with CRF. If it is not treated effectively, this pericardial inflammation can lead to pericardial effusion, cardiac tamponade, and death. The pericardial sac becomes inflamed by uremic toxins or infection. Manifestations include severe chest pain, an increased pulse rate, a low-grade fever, and an intermittent pericardial friction rub that can be heard on auscultation.

As the pericarditis continues and the pericardial effusion worsens, dysrhythmias may develop. The fluid around the heart makes heart tones softer and harder to hear. Blood pressure decreases, and the client may have shortness of breath. If left untreated, pericardial effusion causes cardiac tamponade, an emergency in which pulse pressure decreases and bradycardia or asystole results. Treatment of pericardial tamponade requires removal of pericardial fluid by placement of a needle, catheter, or drainage tube into the pericardium.

Hematologic Changes

Anemia is a common problem in clients with CRF, and it worsens the CRF manifestations. The causes of anemia include a decreased erythropoietin level that decreases red blood cell (RBC) production, decreased RBC survival time resulting from uremia, iron and folic acid deficiencies, and increased bleeding as a result of uremia-induced impaired platelet function.

Gastrointestinal Changes

Uremia affects the entire gastrointestinal (GI) system. The normal flora of the mouth changes with uremia. The mouth contains the enzyme urease, which breaks down urea into ammonia. The ammonia generated from this reaction causes uremic halitosis and may also cause uremic **stomatitis** (mouth inflammation).

Anorexia, nausea, vomiting, and hiccups are common in clients with uremia. The specific cause of these problems is unknown but may be related to high BUN and creatinine levels as well as acidosis.

Peptic ulcer disease is also common in clients with uremia; however, the exact cause is unclear. Uremic colitis with profound watery diarrhea or constipation may also be present in clients with uremia. Ulcerations may occur in the stomach or small or large intestine, causing erosion of blood vessels. The blood loss caused by these erosions may result in melena or, in more serious cases, hemorrhagic shock from severe GI bleeding.

TABLE 75-7 Selected Causes of Chronic Renal Failure

Morphologic	Etiologic
Glomerular Disease ▪ Glomerulonephritis ▪ Basement membrane disease ▪ Goodpasture's syndrome ▪ Intercapillary glomerulosclerosis	***Infection*** ▪ Pyelonephritis ▪ Tuberculosis
Tubular Disease ▪ Chronic hypercalcemia ▪ Chronic potassium depletion ▪ Fanconi's syndrome ▪ Heavy metal (lead) poisoning	***Systemic Vascular Disease*** ▪ Intrarenal renovascular hypertension ▪ Extrarenal renovascular hypertension
Vascular Disease of the Kidney ▪ Ischemic disease of the kidney ▪ Bilateral renal artery stenosis ▪ Nephrosclerosis ▪ Hyperparathyroidism	***Metabolic Renal Disease*** ▪ Amyloidosis ▪ Gout (hyperuricemic nephropathy) ▪ Diabetic nephropathy ▪ Milk-alkali syndrome ▪ Sarcoidosis
Urinary Tract Disease ▪ Obstructive uropathy	***Connective Tissue Disease*** ▪ Progressive systemic sclerosis ▪ Systemic lupus erythematosus ▪ Polyarteritis
Inherited or Genetic Conditions ▪ Hypoplastic kidneys ▪ Medullary cystic disease ▪ Polycystic kidney disease	

NOTE: List is not all inclusive.

Etiology and Genetic Risk

The causes of CRF are complex (Table 75-7). More than 100 different disease processes can result in progressive loss of renal function (see also Chapter 74). Three main causes of ESRD include diabetes mellitus (43.4%), hypertension (25.5%), and glomerulonephritis (8.4%) (USRDS, 2002). African American clients are four times more likely to develop ESRD and seven times more likely to have hypertensive ESRD.

Although not a common cause of CRF, a variety of genetic disorders can affect renal function. Polycystic kidney disease (PKD) (see Chapter 74) is a hereditary renal disorder in adults that leads to CRF. PKD has both an autosomal-dominant and an autosomal-recessive pattern of inheritance.

Incidence/Prevalence

The number of clients with CRF is increasing. The 2002 U.S. Renal Data Systems annual report stated that more than 375,000 people in the United States are receiving treatment for ESRD. In 2002 the reported incidence of renal disease (new clients per year requiring renal replacement therapy) was close to 100,000. More than 75,000 deaths related to ESRD occurred in 2002. ESRD occurs more often in men than in women (USRDS, 2002). The greatest increase in ESRD is in clients 65 years of age and older. Chart 75-6 addresses the prevention of renal and urinary problems. In 2002 more than 275,000 people were estimated to be receiving renal replacement therapy in the United States (USRDS, 2002).

HEALTH PROMOTION/ILLNESS PREVENTION

The health-promotion activities to prevent or delay the onset of chronic renal failure (CRF) focus on controlling the diseases that lead to its development, such as diabetes mel-

CHART 75-6

CLIENT EDUCATION GUIDE
Prevention of Renal and Urinary Problems

- Be alert to the general appearance of your urine. Note any changes in its color, clarity, or odor.
- Changes in the frequency or volume of urine passage occur with changes in fluid intake. More frequent, or infrequent, voiding not associated with changes in fluid intake may signal potential problems.
- Any discomfort or distress with the passage of urine is not normal. Pain, burning, urgency, aching, or difficulty with initiating urine flow or complete bladder emptying is of some concern.
- The kidneys need 1 to 2 quarts of fluid a day to flush out your body wastes. Water is the ideal flushing agent.
- Reduce your intake of soda pop soft drinks.
- Changes in kidney function are often silent for many years. Periodically ask your health care provider to measure your kidney function with a blood test (serum creatinine) and a urinalysis.
- If you have a history or renal disease, diabetes mellitus, hypertension (high blood pressure), or a family history of kidney disease, you should know your serum creatinine level and your 24-hour creatinine clearance. At least one checkup per year that includes laboratory blood and urine testing of kidney function is recommended.
- If you are identified as having decreased kidney function, ask about whether any prescribed medication, diet, diagnostic test, or therapeutic procedure will present a risk to your current kidney function. Check out all nonprescription medications with your physician or pharmacist before using them.

litus and hypertension. Identifying clients who have these disorders at an early stage is critical to CRF prevention. Client education to promote adherence to drug and diet regimens and engaging in regular physical activity are key in preventing the blood vessel changes that lead to kidney damage. Teach clients with diabetes to keep their blood glucose levels within the prescribed range. Teach clients with hypertension that drug therapy is not a cure and must be continued. Encourage clients with diabetes or hypertension to have yearly testing for microalbuminuria.

Teach everyone treated for an infection anywhere in the renal/urinary system to take all antibiotics as prescribed. Encourage everyone to drink at least 3 L of water daily unless a health problem requires fluid restriction. Caution people who use over-the-counter nonsteroidal anti-inflammatory drugs (NSAIDs) to avoid abusing these drugs because they reduce renal perfusion and their long-term use reduces kidney function.

◆COLLABORATIVE MANAGEMENT

◆Assessment

HISTORY

When taking a history from a client with suspected chronic renal failure (CRF), focus on the manifestations of CRF. Document the client's age and gender. Obtain accurate weight and height measurements, and ask about usual weight and recent weight gain or loss. Weight gain may indicate fluid retention caused by poorly functioning kidneys. Weight loss may be the result of anorexia from uremic syndrome.

Obtain a complete history of known renal or urologic disorders, long-term health problems, drug use, and current health problems. Ask the client about any existing renal disease or family history of renal disease that might indicate a hereditary disorder. A history of kidney infection or stones may imply past kidney damage. Explore the possibility of long-term health problems because illnesses such as hypertension, diabetes, systemic lupus erythematosus, arthritis, cancer, and tuberculosis can cause decreased renal function.

Document the use of prescription and over-the-counter drugs because many drugs are nephrotoxic and can cause renal damage.

Examine the client's nutritional habits and discuss any present GI problems. A change in the taste of foods often occurs with CRF. Clients may report that sweet foods are not as appealing or that meats have a metallic taste. Ask about the presence of nausea, vomiting, anorexia, hiccups, diarrhea, or constipation. These manifestations may be the result of excess wastes that the body cannot excrete because of renal malfunction.

Ask the client about his or her energy level and any recent injuries or bleeding. Explore changes in the client's daily routine as a possible *result* of fatigue. Weakness, drowsiness, and shortness of breath suggest impending pulmonary edema or neurologic degeneration. Ask about bruising or bleeding, which can be caused by hematologic changes from uremia.

Discuss the client's urine elimination in detail, including frequency of urination, appearance of the urine, and any difficulty starting or controlling urination. These data can help to identify existing urologic disorders that may influence the preservation of existing renal function.

PHYSICAL ASSESSMENT/CLINICAL MANIFESTATIONS

Chronic renal failure (CRF) causes changes in many body systems (Chart 75-7). Most manifestations are related to changes in fluid volume, electrolyte and acid-base imbalances, and buildup of nitrogenous wastes.

NEUROLOGIC MANIFESTATIONS. Neurologic manifestations of CRF and uremic syndrome are numerous (see Chart 75-7) and vary widely. Observe for problems ranging from lethargy to seizures or coma, which indicate uremic encephalopathy. Assess for sensory changes that appear in a glove and stocking pattern over the hands and feet. Check for weakness in the upper or lower extremities (e.g., uremic neuropathy).

If untreated, uremic encephalopathy progresses to seizures and coma. Dialysis is used to treat CRF when neurologic problems result. The manifestations of uremic encephalopathy resolve with dialysis. However, improvement in neuropathy is limited if the neuropathy is severe and motor function is impaired.

CARDIOVASCULAR MANIFESTATIONS. The manifestations of CRF and uremia cause fluid volume excess, hypertension, heart failure (HF), uremic pericarditis, and potassium-induced dysrhythmias. Assess for signs of reduced sodium and water excretion. Circulatory fluid overload, if untreated, leads to HF, pulmonary edema, peripheral edema, and hypertension.

Assess heart rate and rhythm, listening for extra beats (particularly an S_3), irregular patterns, or a pericardial friction rub. Unless a hemodialysis (HD) vascular access has been created, measure blood pressure in each arm. Assess the jugular veins

CHART 75-7

KEY FEATURES of Chronic Renal Failure

Neurologic Manifestations
- Lethargy and daytime drowsiness
- Inability to concentrate or decreased attention span
- Seizures
- Coma
- Slurred speech
- Asterixis
- Tremors, twitching, or jerky movements
- Myoclonus
- Ataxia (alteration in gait)
- Paresthesias

Cardiovascular Manifestations
- Cardiomyopathy
- Hypertension
- Peripheral edema
- Heart failure
- Uremic pericarditis
- Pericardial effusion
- Pericardial friction rub
- Cardiac tamponade

Respiratory Manifestations
- Uremic halitosis
- Tachypnea
- Deep sighing, yawning
- Kussmaul respirations
- Uremic pneumonitis
- Shortness of breath
- Pulmonary edema
- Pleural effusion
- Depressed cough reflex
- Crackles

Hematologic Manifestations
- Anemia
- Abnormal bleeding and bruising

Gastrointestinal Manifestations
- Anorexia
- Nausea
- Vomiting
- Metallic taste in the mouth
- Changes in taste acuity and sensation
- Uremic colitis (diarrhea)
- Constipation
- Uremic gastritis (possible GI bleeding)
- Uremic fetor
- Stomatitis
- Diarrhea

Urinary Manifestations
- Polyuria, nocturia (early)
- Oliguria, anuria (later)
- Proteinuria
- Hematuria
- Diluted, strawlike appearance

Integumentary Manifestations
- Decreased skin turgor
- Yellow-gray pallor
- Dry skin
- Pruritus
- Ecchymosis
- Purpura
- Soft-tissue calcifications
- Uremic frost (late, premorbid)

Musculoskeletal Manifestations
- Muscle weakness and cramping
- Bone pain
- Pathologic fractures
- Renal osteodystrophy

Reproductive Manifestations
- Decreased fertility
- Infrequent or absent menses
- Decreased libido
- Impotence

GI, Gastrointestinal.

for distention, and assess for pedal, pretibial, presacral, and periorbital edema. Shortness of breath with exertion and nocturnal dyspnea suggest fluid volume excess.

RESPIRATORY MANIFESTATIONS. Respiratory manifestations of CRF vary widely (e.g., breath that smells like urine [*uremic fetor* or uremic halitosis], deep sighing, yawning, shortness of breath). Observe the rhythm, rate, and depth of breathing. **Tachypnea** (increased rate of breathing) and **hyperpnea** (increased depth of breathing) occur with worsening metabolic acidosis.

With severe metabolic acidosis, you may see extreme hyperventilation (Kussmaul respirations). A few clients have hilar pneumonitis, or *uremic lung.* In these clients, assess for thick sputum, minimal coughing, tachypnea, and fever. A pleural friction rub may be heard with a stethoscope. Clients often have pleuritic pain with breathing. Auscultate the lungs for crackles, which indicate fluid volume overload.

HEMATOLOGIC MANIFESTATIONS. Hematologic problems include anemia and abnormal bleeding. Check for indicators of anemia (e.g., fatigue, pallor, lethargy, weakness, shortness of breath, dizziness). Check for abnormal bleeding by observing for bruising, petechiae, purpura, mucous membrane bleeding in the nose or gums, abnormal vaginal bleeding, or intestinal bleeding (black, tarry stools **[melena]**).

GASTROINTESTINAL MANIFESTATIONS. Assess for foul breath and mouth ulceration or inflammation. Document any abdominal pain, cramping, or vomiting. Test all stools for occult blood.

URINARY MANIFESTATIONS. The urinary findings in renal failure reflect the kidneys' decreasing function. At first changes occur in the amount, frequency, and appearance of the urine. Proteinuria or hematuria also may be present.

The amount and composition of the urine change as renal function decreases. With the onset of end-stage renal disease (ESRD), the urine may be more dilute and clearer as tubular reabsorption is reduced. The actual urine output in a client with CRF varies with the amount of remaining renal function. The client with ESRD usually has oliguria, but some clients remain able to produce 1 L or more per 24 hours. Daily urine volume usually changes again after dialysis is started.

SKIN MANIFESTATIONS. In clients with uremia, urochrome pigment is deposited in the skin, causing a yellowish coloration. Some African Americans report a darkening of the skin. The anemia of CRF causes a sallowness, which appears as a faded suntan on lighter-skinned clients.

Skin oils and turgor are decreased in clients with uremia. A distressing problem of uremia is severe **pruritus** (itching). **Uremic frost,** a layer of urea crystals from evaporated sweat, may appear on the face, eyebrows, axilla, and groin in clients with advanced uremic syndrome. Assess for bruises **(ecchymoses),** purple patches **(purpura),** and rashes.

PSYCHOSOCIAL ASSESSMENT

Chronic renal failure and its treatment disrupt many aspects of a client's life. You are in a unique position to evaluate the client with newly diagnosed renal failure and to assist with adjustments.

Psychosocial assessment and support are part of the nurse's role from the time that CRF is first diagnosed. Ask about the client's understanding of the diagnosis and what the treatment regimen means to him or her (e.g., diet, drugs, dialysis). Assess for anxiety and for the coping styles used by the client or family members. Psychosocial issues affected by CRF include family relations, social activity, work patterns, body image, and sexual activity. The chronicity of

ESRD, the variety of treatment options, and the uncertainties about the course of the disease and its treatment require ongoing psychosocial assessment.

LABORATORY ASSESSMENT

Chronic renal failure causes extreme changes in many laboratory values (see Chart 75-2). Monitor the following blood values: creatinine, blood urea nitrogen (BUN), sodium, potassium, calcium, phosphate, bicarbonate, hemoglobin, and hematocrit.

Initially a urinalysis is performed, and a 24-hour urine specimen for creatinine and urea clearance is obtained. In the early stages of CRF, urinalysis may show excessive protein, glucose, red blood cells (RBCs), white blood cells (WBCs), and decreased or fixed specific gravity. Urine osmolarity is usually decreased. A 24-hour creatinine clearance is calculated after blood and urine creatinine levels are collected and quantified. These data, along with weight and height, are used to calculate renal creatinine clearance. As renal failure progresses, the urine output decreases dramatically.

Changes in renal function are monitored by measurements of the serum creatinine and BUN levels. Serum creatinine levels may increase gradually over a period of years, reaching levels of 15 to 30 mg/dL or more, depending on the client's muscle mass. BUN levels are directly related to dietary protein intake. Without protein restriction, BUN levels may rise 10 to 20 times the value of the serum creatinine level. With dietary protein restriction, BUN levels are elevated but less than those of nonprotein-restricted clients. Fluid balance also affects BUN. Chapter 72 describes the significance of BUN and creatinine levels as well as creatinine clearance.

RADIOGRAPHIC ASSESSMENT

Few x-ray finding are abnormal with CRF. Bone x-rays of the hand can show renal osteodystrophy. With long-term ESRD, the kidneys are atrophic and may be 8 to 9 cm or smaller. This small size results from renal atrophy and fibrosis. If ESRD progresses suddenly, a renal ultrasound or computed tomography (CT) scan without contrast media may be used to rule out an obstruction. (See Chapter 72 for a complete description of renal diagnostic tests.)

Critical Thinking Challenge

The client is a 77-year-old woman admitted to your unit with suspected CRF. She has had type 2 diabetes for 25 years and is also being treated for hypertension. She admits that when her money is low, she stops buying the blood pressure drugs because she feels that if she has to choose between the two, it is more important to continue her antidiabetic drugs. She says she has noticed that her heartbeat is irregular, her rings and shoes are tight, and that she has gained 8 pounds over the last 10 days.

1. What other assessment data should you obtain?
2. What risk factors for the development of CRF are noted in her past medical history? Provide a rationale for your choices.
3. What cardiac and respiratory manifestations might you find on physical examination of this client?

evolve For suggested answer guidelines, go to http://evolve.elsevier.com/Iggy/.

Analysis

The client with CRF has usually had a progressive reduction of renal function and is often hospitalized for adjustment of the treatment plan. The focus of care is to manage symptoms and prevent complications.

COMMON NURSING DIAGNOSES AND COLLABORATIVE PROBLEMS

The following are priority nursing diagnoses for clients with CRF:

1. Imbalanced Nutrition: Less Than Body Requirements related to inability to ingest, digest food, or absorb nutrients as a result of physiologic factors
2. Excess Fluid Volume related to compromised regulatory mechanisms (inability of the kidneys to maintain body fluid balance)
3. Decreased Cardiac Output related to altered stroke volume (reduced) as a result of dysrhythmias and mechanical malfunction (increased preload [excess volume] and increased afterload [increased peripheral vascular resistance])
4. Risk for Infection related to inadequate primary defenses (broken skin), chronic disease, or malnutrition
5. Risk for Injury related to internal biochemical risk factors associated with renal failure (increased susceptibility to bleeding, falls, and fractures)
6. Fatigue related to disease states, altered metabolic energy production, and anemia
7. Anxiety related to threat to or change in health status, economic status, relationships, role function, systems, or self-concept; situational crisis; threat of death; lack of knowledge (diagnostic tests, disease process, treatment); loss of control; or disrupted family life

The primary collaborative problem is Potential for Pulmonary Edema.

ADDITIONAL NURSING DIAGNOSES AND COLLABORATIVE PROBLEMS

In addition to the common nursing diagnoses and collaborative problems, clients with CRF may have one or more of the following:

- Diarrhea related to chemical or electrolyte imbalances or side effects of drugs
- Impaired Oral Mucous Membrane related to limited fluid intake, malnutrition, and elevated levels of uremic toxins
- Impaired Skin Integrity related to altered chemical balance and uremic toxins
- Social Isolation related to altered state of wellness or alterations in physical appearance
- Interrupted Family Processes related to situational crisis, reduced income, unemployment, or effects of chronic illness
- Sexual Dysfunction related to altered body function, disease process, effects of drugs, depression, or disturbance in body image
- Disturbed Thought Processes related to irritation, central nervous system (CNS) depression, side effects of drugs, sleep deprivation, or clinical depression
- Deficient Knowledge (disease process, care regimen, and follow-up care) related to lack of informational resources and magnitude of the care issues
- Potential for Sepsis
- Potential for Malnutrition
- Potential for Electrolyte Imbalances
- Potential for Metabolic Acidosis

CONCEPT MAP End-Stage Renal Disease

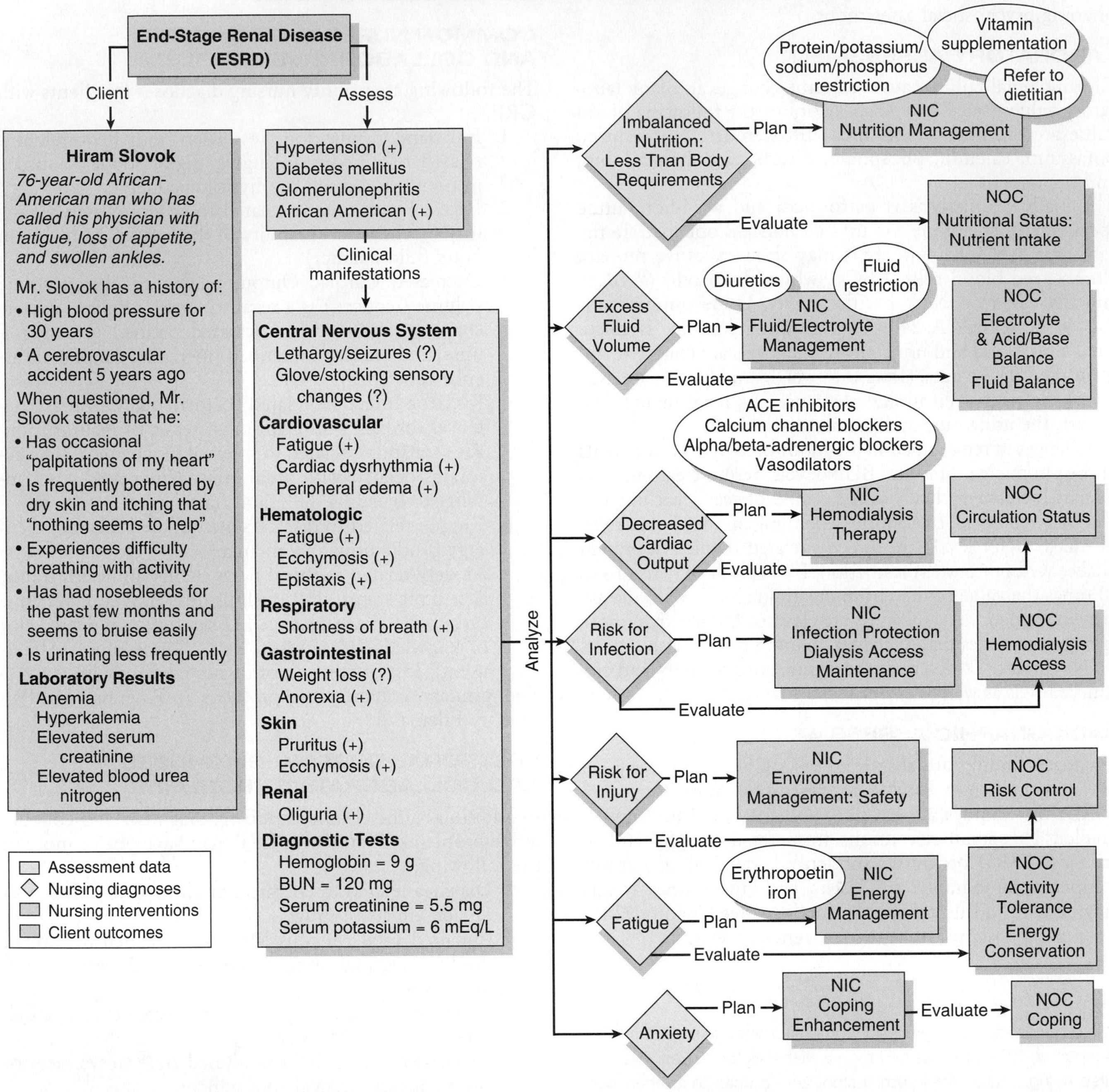

Concept Map by Elaine Bishop Kennedy, EdD, RN

Planning and Implementation

The Concept Map above addresses care issues related to clients who have end-stage renal disease (ESRD).

IMBALANCED NUTRITION: LESS THAN BODY REQUIREMENTS

NOC **PLANNING: EXPECTED OUTCOMES.** The client with CRF is expected to attain and maintain adequate nutrition. Indicators include that the client should have mild or no deviation from the normal ranges for the following parameters:

- Food intake
- Weight-height ratio
- Muscle tone
- Laboratory values (serum albumin, hematocrit, hemoglobin)

INTERVENTIONS. The nutritional needs and diet restrictions for the client with CRF vary according to the degree of remaining renal function and the type of renal replacement therapy used (Table 75-8).

Nutrition Therapy. The purpose of nutrition therapy is to provide the food and fluids needed to support the metabolism for a client who is at high risk for becoming malnourished. Clients starting hemodialysis (HD) have an increase in catabolism and a decrease in intake that results

TABLE 75-8 Dietary Restrictions for the Client with Renal Failure

Dietary Component	With Chronic Uremia	With Hemodialysis	With Peritoneal Dialysis
Protein	0.55-0.60 g/kg/day	1.0-1.5 g/kg/day	1.2-1.5 g/kg/day
Fluid	Depends on urine output, but may be as high as 1500-3000 mL/day	500-700 mL/day plus amount of urine output	Restriction based on fluid weight gain and blood
Potassium	60-70 mEq/day	70 mEq/day	Usually no restriction
Sodium	1-3 g/day	2-4 g/day	Restriction based on fluid weight gain and blood pressure
Phosphorus	700 mg/day	700 mg/day	800 mg/day

in a loss of lean body mass. NIC nutrition interventions are listed in Chart 75-8.

The client is referred to a registered dietitian for dietary teaching and planning. In collaboration with the dietitian, teach the client about diet changes that are needed as a result of CRF. Such changes include control of protein intake; fluid intake limitation; restriction of potassium, sodium, and phosphorus intake; taking vitamin and mineral supplements; and eating enough calories to meet metabolic demand.

If adequate calories are not supplied, the body will use muscle protein for energy, which leads to a negative nitrogen balance and malnutrition. The dietitian assists in determining the number of calories and types of nutrients required to meet body needs.

Protein Restriction. Early protein restriction prevents some of the symptoms of CRF and may preserve kidney function. Protein is restricted on the basis of the degree of renal impairment and the severity of the symptoms. Accumulation of waste products from protein metabolism is the primary cause of uremia. Although lower protein levels are recommended, protein-calorie malnutrition must be avoided in clients receiving HD. At least 1.5 g of protein per kilogram of body weight per day may be needed for weight gain and improved nutritional status in clients receiving maintenance HD.

The glomerular filtration rate (GFR) is used as an indicator of renal function and as a guide to safe levels of protein intake. A client with a severely reduced GFR who is *not* undergoing dialysis is usually permitted 0.55 to 0.60 g of protein per kilogram of body weight (e.g., 40 g of protein daily for a 150-pound [70-kg] adult). If proteinuria is present, protein is added to the diet in amounts equal to that lost in the urine. Protein requirements are calculated based on actual body weight (corrected for edema), not ideal body weight.

The client receiving dialysis needs more protein because some protein is lost through dialysis. While receiving HD, protein requirements are individually tailored according to the client's post-dialysis, or "dry" weight. Generally HD clients are allowed about 1 to 1.5 g of protein/kg/day. Peritoneal dialysis (PD) clients are allowed 1.2 to 1.5 g of protein/kg/day because protein is lost with each exchange. The protein should be of high biologic value, such as milk, meat, or eggs. If protein intake is inadequate, a negative nitrogen balance develops and causes muscle wasting. BUN and albumin levels are used to monitor the adequacy of protein intake. Decreased serum albumin levels indicate inadequate protein intake. Excessive protein intake increases BUN levels in clients with CRF.

CHART 75-8

NIC INTERVENTION ACTIVITIES for The Client with Chronic Renal Failure

Nutrition Therapy: *Administration of food and fluids to support metabolic processes of a client who is malnourished or at high risk for becoming malnourished*

- Complete a nutritional assessment, as appropriate.
- Determine—in collaboration with dietitian, as appropriate—the number of calories and type of nutrients needed to meet nutritional requirements.
- Refer to diet teaching and planning, as needed.
- Instruct client and family about prescribed diet.
- Provide needed nourishment within limits of prescribed diet.
- Give client and family written examples of prescribed diet.
- Monitor food/fluid ingested and calculate daily caloric intake, as appropriate.
- Offer herbs and spices as an alternative to salt.
- Monitor lab values, as appropriate.

Fluid Management: *Promotion of fluid balance and prevention of complications resulting from abnormal or undesired fluid levels*

- Maintain accurate intake and output record.
- Monitor hydration status (e.g., moist mucous membranes, adequacy of pulses, and orthostatic blood pressure), as appropriate.
- Monitor for indications of fluid overload/retention (e.g., crackles, elevated CVP or pulmonary capillary wedge pressure, edema, neck vein distention, and ascites), as appropriate.
- Weigh client daily and monitor trends.
- Monitor laboratory results relevant to fluid retention (e.g., increased specific gravity, increased BUN, decreased hematocrit, and increased urine osmolality levels).
- Monitor client's weight change before and after dialysis, if appropriate.
- Assess location and extent of edema, if present.
- Administer prescribed diuretics, as appropriate.
- Distribute the fluid intake over 24 hours, as appropriate.
- Consult physician if signs and symptoms of fluid volume excess persist or worsen.

NIC intervention activities selected from Dochterman, J.M., & Bulechek, G.M. (Eds.) (2004). *Nursing interventions classification (NIC)* (4th ed.). St. Louis: Mosby. No part of this work is to be altered without prior written permission from the Publisher.
CVP, Central venous pressure; *BUN*, blood urea nitrogen.

Sodium Restriction. Monitor fluid and sodium intake. In clients with little or no urine output, fluid and sodium retention causes edema, hypertension, and heart failure (HF). Most clients with CRF retain sodium; a few cannot conserve sodium.

Estimate the client's fluid and sodium retention status by monitoring body weight and blood pressure. In uremic clients not receiving dialysis, sodium is limited to 1 to 3 g daily, and fluid intake depends on urine output. In oliguric clients receiving dialysis, the sodium restriction is 2 to 4 g daily, and fluid intake is limited to 500 to 700 mL plus the amount of any urine output. Instruct the client not to add salt at the table or during cooking. Foods high in sodium (e.g., processed foods, fast foods, potato chips, pretzels, pickles, ham, bacon, and sausage) are permitted in moderation. Herbs and spices can be used in place of salt to enhance food flavor.

Potassium Restriction. Monitor potassium intake because hyperkalemia can cause dangerous cardiac dysrhythmias. Monitor the ECG for tall, peaked T waves caused by hyperkalemia. Document serum potassium levels. Instruct the client with advanced CRF to limit potassium intake to 60 to 70 mEq/day. Teach the client to read labels of seasoning agents carefully for sodium and potassium content. Instruct clients to avoid salt substitutes composed of potassium chloride. Clients receiving PD or who are producing urine may not need potassium restriction.

Phosphorus Restriction. Control of phosphate levels is started early in CRF to avoid osteodystrophy. Monitor serum phosphate levels. Dietary phosphorus restrictions and drugs to assist with phosphate control may be prescribed. Phosphate binders must be taken at mealtime. Most clients with CRF already restrict their protein intake, and because high-protein foods are also high in phosphorus, their phosphorus consumption is also reduced. Chapter 14 lists foods high in potassium, sodium, and phosphorus.

Vitamin Supplementation. Most clients with CRF need daily vitamin and mineral supplements. Low-protein diets are also low in vitamins, and water-soluble vitamins are removed from the blood during dialysis. Anemia also is a problem in clients with CRF because of the limited iron content of low-protein diets and decreased kidney production of erythropoietin. Thus supplemental iron is needed. Calcium and vitamin D supplements may be needed, depending on the client's serum calcium levels and bone status.

Individualizing the Diet for Peritoneal Dialysis. Clients undergoing PD require a slightly different diet from those undergoing HD. Because protein is lost with the dialysate in PD, replacing lost protein is needed. Often 1.2 to 1.5 g of protein per kilogram of body weight per day is recommended. Clients may have anorexia and have difficulty eating enough protein. High-calorie enteral supplements may also be needed. Sodium restriction varies with fluid weight gain and blood pressure. Usually dietary potassium does not need to be restricted because the dialysate is potassium free. The potassium restriction, if any, is determined by the serum potassium level.

Collaborate with the dietitian to assess each client's nutritional needs. Teach the client and evaluate his or her understanding of and adherence with dietary regimens. Give written examples of the prescribed diet to the client and family to promote adherence. Help clients adapt the diet to their budget, ethnic background, and food preferences to maximize caloric intake within the diet's restrictions.

EXCESS FLUID VOLUME

NOC **PLANNING: EXPECTED OUTCOMES.** The client with CRF is expected to achieve and maintain an acceptable fluid balance. Indicators include that the following parameters are only mildly compromised or not compromised:

- Blood pressure
- Stable body weight
- Central venous pressure
- Serum electrolytes

INTERVENTIONS. Management of the client with CRF includes drug therapy, diet therapy, fluid restriction, and dialysis. Diet therapy is discussed under Imbalanced Nutrition, p. 1746, and dialysis is discussed under Renal Replacement Therapies, p. 1751).

The purpose of fluid management is to promote fluid balance and prevention of complications of fluid overload (see Chart 75-8). Monitor the client's intake and output and hydration status. Assess for manifestations of fluid volume excess (e.g., crackles in the bases of the lungs, edema, and distended neck veins).

Drug Therapy. Diuretics are prescribed for clients with renal insufficiency for treatment of fluid retention or to help control blood pressure. The diuresis produced from these drugs helps to reduce fluid overload in clients who still have some urine output. Diuretics are seldom used in clients with ESRD after dialysis has been initiated because, as kidney function is reduced, these drugs can have harmful side effects on the remaining kidney cells and on the hearing structures.

Assess fluid status by obtaining daily weights and reviewing the client's intake and output. Daily weight gain in these clients indicates fluid retention rather than true body weight gain. Estimate the amount of fluid retained: 1 kg of weight equals about 1 L of fluid retained. Weigh the client daily at the same time each day, on the same scale, with the client wearing the same amount of clothing, and after the client has voided (if the client is not anuric). Monitor weight for changes before and after dialysis.

Fluid Restriction. The amount of fluid restriction prescribed is discussed under Sodium Restriction, p. 1747. Consider all forms of fluid intake, including oral, IV, and fluid or drugs given through gastric tubes, when calculating fluid intake. Assist the client in spreading oral fluid intake over a 24-hour period. Monitor the client's response to fluid restriction, and notify the health care provider if manifestations of fluid excess persist or worsen.

DECREASED CARDIAC OUTPUT

NOC **PLANNING: EXPECTED OUTCOMES.** The client with CRF is expected to attain and maintain adequate cardiac output. Indicators include that the following parameters are either only mildly compromised or not compromised:

- Systolic and diastolic blood pressures
- Ejection fraction
- Peripheral pulses
- Cognitive status

INTERVENTIONS. Many clients with long-standing hypertension have renal insufficiency, and some progress to CRF and ESRD. Therefore control of hypertension is essential in preserving renal function. To control hypertension, the physician may prescribe calcium channel blockers, angiotensin-converting enzyme (ACE) inhibitors, alpha-adrenergic and beta-adrenergic blockers, and vasodilators. ACE inhibitors appear to be the most effective drugs to slow the progression of renal failure (Levine, 1997). More information on the specific drugs for hypertension can be found in Chapter 39. Indications vary depending on the client, and these drugs are used carefully to avoid hyperkalemia and hypotension. Many combinations and doses may be tried until blood pressure control is adequate and side effects are minimized. Calcium channel blockers seem to improve the GFR and renal blood flow.

Instruct the client and family to measure blood pressure. Evaluate the client's ability to measure and record blood pressure accurately using the client's own equipment. Periodically recheck measurement accuracy. The client and family must understand the relationship of blood pressure control and regulation to diet and drug therapy. Also instruct the client to weigh himself or herself daily and to bring records of blood pressure measurements and weights for discussion with the physician, nurse, or dietitian.

Assesses the client on an ongoing basis for manifestations of decreased cardiac output, heart failure, and dysrhythmias. These topics are discussed in Chapters 36 through 38.

RISK FOR INFECTION

NOC **PLANNING: EXPECTED OUTCOMES.** The client with CRF is expected to remain free of infection. Indicators include that the client will have only mild or absent:

- Fever
- Lymphadenopathy
- Urine culture colonization
- Wound site (dialysis access site) culture colonization
- White blood count elevation

INTERVENTIONS. Provide meticulous care to any areas where skin integrity has been broken (incisions, site of drains, puncture sites, cracked or excoriated skin, pressure sores), and provide preventive skin care to intact areas. For clients undergoing dialysis, inspect the vascular access site or PD catheter insertion site every shift for redness, swelling, pain, and drainage. Monitor vital signs for any manifestation of infection (e.g., fever, tachycardia).

RISK FOR INJURY

NOC **PLANNING: EXPECTED OUTCOMES.** The client with CRF is expected to remain free of injury. Indicators include that the client should not have any of the following problems:

- Fall or experience injury from a fall
- Pathologic fractures
- Bleeding
- Toxic effects of prescribed drugs

INTERVENTIONS. Managing drug therapy in clients with CRF is a complex clinical problem. Many over-the-counter drugs contain ingredients that alter renal function. Therefore it is important to obtain a detailed drug history. You must be aware of the use of each drug, its side effects, and its site of metabolism. Monitor the client closely for drug-related complications, and ensure that dosages are adjusted as needed.

Certain drugs must be avoided, and the dosages of others must be adjusted according to the degree of remaining renal function. As the client's renal function decreases, repeated dosage adjustments are necessary. Assess for side effects and signs of drug toxicity, and notify the physician as appropriate.

Many drugs are routinely given to clients with renal failure (see Chart 75-3). You must understand the rationale for these drugs and the indicated nursing interventions. Many clients have cardiac disease and may require cardiac drugs such as digoxin. Clients with renal failure are particularly at risk for digoxin toxicity because the drug is excreted by the kidneys. When caring for clients with CRF who are receiving digoxin, monitor for signs of toxicity, such as nausea, vomiting, anorexia, visual disturbances, restlessness, headache, fatigue, confusion, cardiac irregularities (particularly **bradycardia** [pulse rate less than 50 to 60 beats/min] and **tachycardia** [pulse rate greater than 100 beats/min]). Monitor the serum drug levels to be certain they are in the therapeutic range (0.8-2 ng/mL). Also closely monitor the serum potassium levels of any client receiving digoxin.

Drugs to control an excessively high phosphate level include phosphate-binding compounds. Calcium acetate, calcium carbonate, and aluminum hydroxide are used as phosphate-binding agents in clients with renal failure. These drugs help prevent renal osteodystrophy and related injuries. Stress the importance of these agents and all prescribed drugs.

Hypercalcemia (excessively high serum calcium levels) is a possible complication for clients taking calcium-containing compounds to control phosphate excess. **Hypophosphatemia** (low serum phosphorus levels) is also a complication of phosphate binding, especially in clients who are not eating adequately but who are continuing to take phosphate-binding drugs. In clients taking aluminum-based phosphate binders for prolonged periods, aluminum deposits may cause bone disease or permanent neurologic problems. Monitor the client for muscle weakness, anorexia, malaise, tremors, or bone pain.

Teach clients with renal disease to avoid antacids containing magnesium. Clients with renal failure cannot excrete magnesium and thus should avoid additional intake.

In addition to the drugs used to treat renal failure, the use of certain other drugs requires special attention. These drugs include antibiotics, opioids, antihypertensives, diuretics, insulin, and heparin.

Many antibiotics are safe for clients with CRF, but those excreted by the kidney require dose adjustment. To prevent complications of bloodstream infections from mouth bacteria, prophylactic antibiotic treatment is given to clients with CRF before any dental procedures. The antibiotic used varies with the client's needs and the physician's preference.

Give opioid analgesics cautiously in clients with renal failure because the effects often last much longer than in people with healthy kidneys. Clients with uremia are more sensitive to the respiratory depressant effects of these drugs. Because opioids are broken down by the liver and not the kidneys, the dosages are often the same regardless of the level of renal function. Monitor the client closely after opioids are given, and evaluate the client's reaction to determine whether adjustments are needed.

As CRF progresses, the client with diabetes often must have insulin or oral antidiabetic drug dosages reduced because the failing kidneys do not excrete or metabolize these drugs well. Thus the drugs are effective longer, increasing the risk for hypoglycemia. Monitor the client's blood glucose levels at least four times per day to determine whether a dosage change is needed. Urine glucose measurements are less accurate when CRF is present.

Poor platelet function and capillary fragility in renal failure make anticoagulant therapy risky. Monitor clients receiving heparin, warfarin, or other anticoagulants every shift for bleeding.

FATIGUE

NOC **PLANNING: EXPECTED OUTCOMES.** The client with chronic renal failure (CRF) is expected to conserve energy by balancing activity and rest. Indicators include that the following parameters are either only mildly compromised or not compromised:

- Performance of self-care
- Interest in surroundings
- Concentration

INTERVENTIONS. Some causes of fatigue in the client with CRF include vitamin deficiency, anemia, and buildup of urea. All clients are given some type of vitamin and mineral supplement because of diet restrictions and vitamin losses from dialysis. Avoid giving the client these vitamin supplements before hemodialysis (HD) treatment because they will be dialyzed out of the body and the client will receive no benefit.

The anemic client with CRF is treated with erythropoietin (Epogen, Procrit). The goal of this therapy is to maintain a hematocrit of 30% to 35%. Erythropoietin therapy is effective in triggering bone marrow production of red blood cells if the client has adequate iron stores. Iron supplements may be needed if clients are iron deficient. Many clients who receive erythropoietin report improved appetite and sexual function along with decreased fatigue. The increased cell production from this therapy may induce hypertension in some clients. The improved appetite challenges clients in their attempts to maintain protein, potassium, and fluid restrictions and requires additional education.

ANXIETY

NOC **PLANNING: EXPECTED OUTCOMES.** The client with CRF is expected to reduce feelings of apprehension and tension. Indicators include that the client often or consistently demonstrates the following behaviors:

- Seeking information to reduce anxiety
- Using effective coping strategies
- Reporting an absence of physical manifestations of anxiety

INTERVENTIONS. A team of health care professionals, including nurses, collaborates to provide support and counseling for the client and family, often over many years of treatment. The nurse has the most contact with the client with CRF when the client is hospitalized or undergoing in-center dialysis treatments. Perform an ongoing assessment of the client's anxiety level to determine the level of nursing intervention required. Observe the client's behavior for cues indicating anxiety (e.g., anxious facial expressions or gestures and an increased pulse rate). Evaluate the support systems, such as the involvement of family and friends with the client's care.

Unfamiliar settings and lack of knowledge about treatments and tests can increase the client's anxiety level. Explain all procedures, tests, and treatments. Identify the client's knowledge deficits about normal renal function and renal failure. Provide instruction appropriate to the client's needs and ability to understand.

Provide continuity of care, whenever possible, to establish a consistent nurse-client relationship to decrease anxiety and promote discussions of client and family concerns. As you develop the nurse-client relationship, encourage the client to discuss current problems or concerns.

Encourage the client to ask questions and discuss fears about the diagnosis of renal failure. An open atmosphere that allows for discussion can decrease anxiety level. Facilitate discussions with family members about the prognosis and the potential impact on the client's lifestyle.

POTENTIAL FOR PULMONARY EDEMA

PLANNING: EXPECTED OUTCOMES. The client with CRF is expected to remain free of pulmonary edema by maintaining optimal fluid balance.

INTERVENTIONS. In the client with CRF, pulmonary edema can result from either left-sided heart failure or from vascular injury. In left-sided heart failure, the heart is unable to eject blood adequately from the left ventricle, leading to an increased pressure in the left atrium and in the pulmonary blood vessels. The increased pressure causes fluid to cross the capillaries into the pulmonary tissue, forming edema. Pulmonary edema can also occur from injury to the pulmonary blood vessels as a result of uremia. This condition causes inflammation and capillary leak. Fluid then leaks into the lung tissue and the alveoli.

Assess the client for early signs of pulmonary edema, such as restlessness, heightened anxiety, tachycardia, dyspnea, and crackles that begin at the base of the lungs. As pulmonary edema worsens, the level of fluid in the lungs rises. Auscultation reveals increased crackles, decreased air exchange. The client may have frothy, blood-tinged sputum. As cardiac and pulmonary function decrease further, the client becomes diaphoretic and cyanotic.

The client with pulmonary edema is admitted to the intensive care unit for aggressive treatment and continuous cardiac monitoring. Place the client in a high Fowler's position, and give oxygen to enhance lung expansion and improve gas exchange. Drug therapy with renal failure and pulmonary edema is difficult because of potential adverse drug effects on the kidneys. Treatment of pulmonary edema involves giving loop diuretics, such as furosemide (Lasix), IV. Renal impairment increases the risk for ototoxicity with the use of furosemide; thus IV doses are given cautiously. Diuresis usually begins within 5 minutes of giving IV furosemide. Measure urine output every 15 to 30 minutes during the acute episode and every hour thereafter until the client is stabilized. Monitor vital signs and assess breath sounds at least every 2 hours to evaluate the client's response to this treatment.

Intravenous morphine sulfate (1 to 2 mg) is often prescribed to reduce myocardial oxygen demand by triggering blood vessel dilation and to provide sedation. Dosage adjustments are needed to achieve the desired response and avoid respiratory depression. Monitor the client's respiratory rate and blood pressure hourly during this therapy. Other vasodilators, such as nitroglycerin, also may be given as a continuous infusion to reduce pulmonary vascular pressure. Monitor vital signs at least hourly because this drug combination may cause severe hypotension.

Monitor serum electrolyte levels daily, and report abnormalities to the physician so that imbalances can be corrected quickly. Monitor electrocardiography at least every 2 hours to identify potential dysrhythmias. Monitor oxygen saturation levels by pulse oximetry and arterial blood gas values. Adjust the oxygen delivery system to maintain adequate oxygen saturation levels. Monitor the client for worsening of the condition, manifested as increasing pulmonary edema and hypoxemia. The client may require temporary intubation and mechanical ventilation to prevent death.

Clients with CRF who have existing cardiac problems, hypertension, or chronic fluid retention are at increased risk for developing pulmonary edema. Such clients are less likely to respond quickly to treatment and are more likely to develop adverse effects from drug therapy. Ultrafiltration may be used with these clients to reduce fluid volume.

Renal Replacement Therapies

Renal replacement therapy is needed when the physiologic changes of chronic renal failure (CRF) are potentially life threatening or pose continuing discomfort to the client. When the client can no longer be managed with conservative therapies, such as diet, drugs, and fluid restriction, dialysis is indicated. Transplantation may be discussed at any time.

HEMODIALYSIS

Hemodialysis (HD) is one of several renal replacement therapies used for the treatment of renal failure (Table 75-9). Dialysis removes excess fluids and waste products and restores chemical and electrolyte balance. HD involves passing the client's blood through an artificial semipermeable membrane to perform the filtering and excretion functions of the kidney.

Client Selection. Any client may be considered for HD therapy. Starting this therapy depends on client symptoms, not on the creatinine clearance. Dialysis is started immediately for clients who have the following: fluid overload that does not respond to diuretics, pericarditis, uncontrolled hypertension, neurologic problems, and development of bleeding diathesis. More commonly, dialysis is started when clients have uremic manifestations, such as nausea and vomiting, decreased attention span, decreased cognition, worsening anemia, and pruritus.

TABLE 75-9 A Comparison of Hemodialysis and Peritoneal Dialysis as Renal Replacement Treatment Options

Hemodialysis	Peritoneal Dialysis
Advantages	
More efficient clearance	Easy access
Short time needed for treatment	Few hemodynamic complications
Complications	
Disequilibrium syndrome	Protein loss
Muscle cramps	Peritonitis
Hemorrhage	Hyperglycemia
Air embolus	Respiratory distress
Hemodynamic changes (hypotension, cardiac dysrhythmias, and anemia)	Bowel perforation
Contraindications	
Hemodynamic instability	Extensive peritoneal adhesions
	Peritoneal fibrosis
	Recent abdominal surgery
Access	
Vascular access route	Intra-abdominal catheter
Procedure	
Complex	Simple
Specially trained registered nurses required	Training less complex than for hemodialysis
Nursing Implications	
Vascular access care	Abdominal catheter care
Restrict diet	More flexible diet

Many clients survive for years with HD therapy and others may only live a few months. How long the client survives using HD therapy depends on the client's age, the cause of renal failure, and the presence of other diseases, such as coronary artery disease, hypertension, or diabetes. The following are general client selection criteria:

- Presence of irreversible renal failure when other therapies are unacceptable or ineffective
- Absence of illnesses that would seriously complicate HD
- Expectation of rehabilitation
- The client's acceptance of the regimen

Dialysis Settings. Clients with CRF may receive HD treatments in many settings, depending on specific needs. Regardless of the setting for therapy, the client needs ongoing nursing support to maintain this complex and lifesaving treatment.

Clients may be dialyzed in an acute care (hospital-based) center if they have recently started treatment or have complicated conditions that require close supervision. Stable clients not requiring intense supervision may be dialyzed in a community or free-standing HD center. Selected clients may participate in complete or partial self-care in an outpatient center or with in-home HD.

In-home HD is the least disruptive form of therapy and allows for adaptation of the regimen to the client's lifestyle. Unfortunately many clients cannot participate in in-home dialysis because they lack an appropriate partner to assist with the therapy and manage the dialysis machine. Some clients and partners find the responsibilities of in-home dialysis to be too stressful. In addition, a water treatment system must be installed in the home to provide a safe, clean water supply for the dialysis process.

Procedure. Dialysis works using the passive transfer of toxins by diffusion. **Diffusion** is the movement of molecules from an area of higher concentration to an area of lower concentration. The rate of diffusion during dialysis occurs more rapidly when the membrane pores are large, there is a large surface area of membrane, the temperature of the solutions is higher, and there is a greater difference in the solute concentrations. Molecules that are too large, such as RBCs and most plasma proteins, cannot pass through the membrane.

When HD is started, blood and **dialysate** (dialyzing solution) flow in opposite directions across an enclosed semipermeable membrane. The dialysate contains a balanced mix of electrolytes and water that closely resembles human plasma. On the other side of the membrane is the client's blood, which contains metabolic waste products, excess water, and excess electrolytes. During HD, the waste products move from the blood into the dialysate because of the difference in their concentrations **(diffusion).** Excess water is also removed from the blood into the dialysate **(osmosis).** Electrolytes can move in either direction, as needed, and take some fluid with them. Potassium and sodium typically move out of the plasma into the dialysate. Bicarbonate and calcium generally move from the dialysate into the plasma. This circulating process continues for a preset length of time, restoring water, electrolyte, and acid-base balance and removing wastes. Water volume may be removed from the plasma by applying positive or negative pressure to the system.

The HD system includes a dialyzer, dialysate, vascular access routes, and an HD machine. The artificial kidney, or **dialyzer** (Figure 75-3), has four parts: a blood compartment, a dialysate compartment, a semipermeable membrane, and an enclosed structure to support the membrane.

Dialysate is made from clear water and chemicals and is free of any waste products or drugs. Bacteria and other organisms are too large to pass through the membrane; therefore dialysate does not need to be sterile. The water used in dialysate must meet specific standards and usually requires special treatment before mixing the dialysate. The dialysate composition may be altered according to the client's needs for treatment of electrolyte imbalances. During HD, the dialysate is warmed to 100° F (37.8° C) to increase the rate of diffusion and to prevent hypothermia.

The HD machine has alarm systems to monitor for potential problems, including the following:

- Changes in dialysate temperature
- Air in the blood tubing
- A blood leak in the dialysate compartment
- Changes in the pressure within the blood and the dialysate compartments
- Changes in composition of the blood or dialysate

If any of these problems are detected, an alarm sounds to protect the client from life-threatening complications.

All models of HD machines function in a manner similar to that shown in Figure 75-4. Figure 75-5 shows one type of HD machine. Figure 75-6 shows a client receiving HD. The number and length of each treatment depend on the amount of wastes and fluid to be removed, the clearance capacity of the dialyzer, and the blood flow rate to and from the machine. Most clients require about 12 hours per week of total dialysis time. This time is usually divided into three 4-hour treatments. For clients with some ongoing urine production, two 5- to 6-hour treatments a week may be adequate. If the client gains large amounts of fluid weight, a longer treatment time may be needed to remove the fluid without hypotension or severe side effects.

Anticoagulation. To prevent blood clots from forming within the dialyzer or the blood tubing, anticoagulation is needed during HD treatments. Heparin is the most commonly used drug to prevent clots from forming when blood comes in contact with foreign surfaces. Client response to heparin varies, and the dose is adjusted on the basis of each client's need. Clients receiving erythropoietin may require additional heparin.

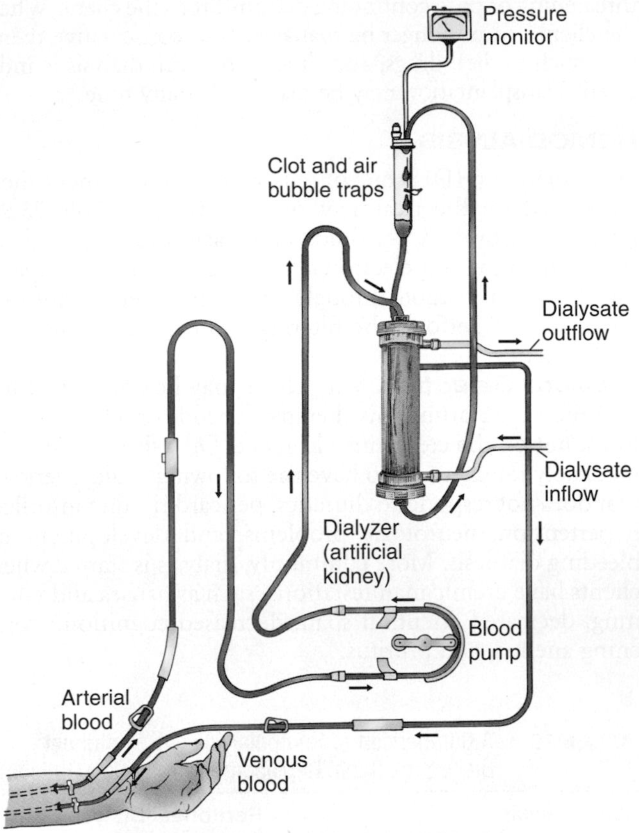

Figure 75-4 ■ A hemodialysis circuit.

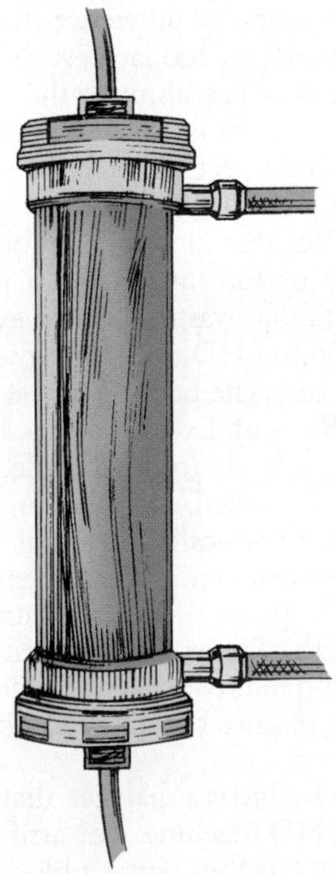

Figure 75-3 ■ Artificial kidney (dialyzer) used in hemodialysis.

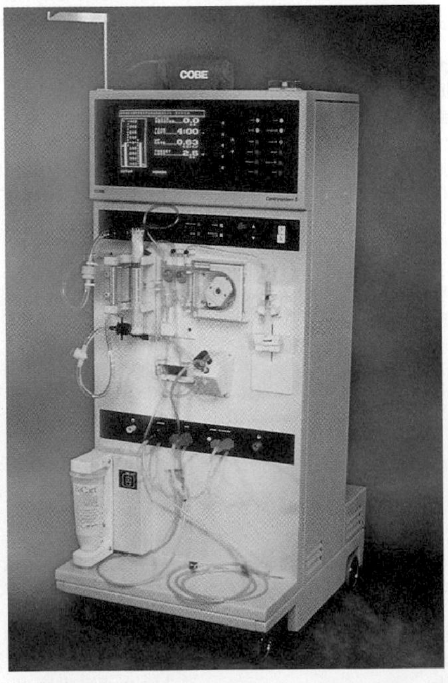

Figure 75-5 ■ Hemodialysis machine. (Courtesy of GAMBRO Healthcare, Stockholm, Sweden.)

Heparin remains active in the body for 4 to 6 hours after dialysis, making the client at risk for hemorrhage during and immediately after HD treatments. Invasive procedures must be avoided during that time. Monitor the client closely for any signs of bleeding or hemorrhage. Clotting tendencies can be monitored during HD with a bedside machine (e.g., the Homochron), by whole-blood clotting times (Lee-White clotting test), or by activated partial thromboplastin times (aPTT) during and after HD. Protamine sulfate is an antidote to heparin and should be available in the dialysis setting.

Vascular Access. Vascular access is required for hemodialysis (Table 75-10). The procedure requires the easy availability of a large amount of blood flow: at least 250 to 300 mL/min, usually for a period of 3 to 4 hours. Normal venous cannulation does not provide this rate of blood flow.

Long-Term Vascular Access. An internal access is used for most clients having long-term HD (see Table 75-10). The two common choices are an internal arteriovenous (AV) fistula or an AV graft (Figure 75-7). *AV fistulas* are formed by connecting **(anastomosis)** an artery to a vein. The most commonly used vessels are the radial or brachial artery and the cephalic vein of the nondominant arm. Fistulas increase venous blood flow to 250 to 400 mL/min, the amount needed for effective dialysis.

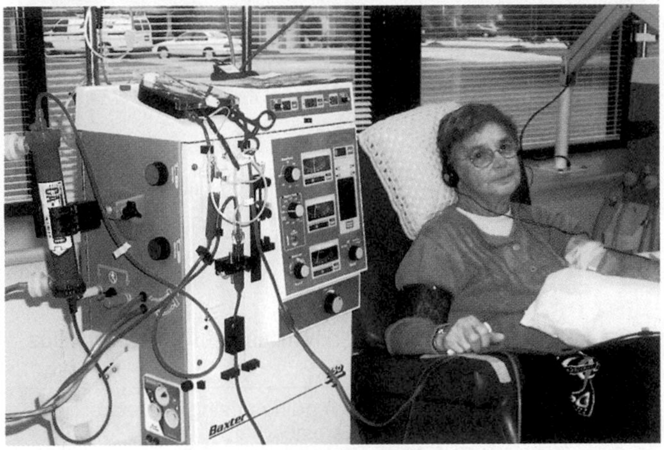

Figure 75-6 ■ Client receiving hemodialysis.

Time is needed after anastomosis for the AV fistula to develop. As the AV fistula "matures," the increased pressure of the arterial blood flow into the vein causes the vessel walls to thicken. This thickening increases their strength and suitability for repeated cannulation. Clients differ in the amount of time needed for the fistula to mature. Some fistulas may not be ready for use for as long as 4 months after the surgery, and a temporary vascular access (AV shunt or HD catheter) is used during this time.

To access a fistula, cannulate it by inserting two needles, one toward the venous blood flow and one toward the arterial blood flow. This procedure allows the HD machine to draw the blood out through the arterial needle and return it through the venous needle.

Arteriovenous grafts are used when the AV fistula does not develop or when complications limit its use. The polytetrafluoroethylene (PTFE) graft is a synthetic material (Gore-Tex). This type of graft is commonly used in older clients undergoing HD. Figure 75-8 shows a client's AF graft.

PRECAUTIONS. Some precautions are needed to ensure the functioning of an internal AV fistula or AV graft. First assess for adequate circulation in the fistula or graft as well as in the distal portion of the extremity. Then check for a bruit or a thrill by auscultation or palpation over the access site. *Repeated compression can result in the loss of the vascular access; therefore avoid taking the blood pressure or performing venipunctures in the arm with the vascular access.* The AV fistula or graft is *not* used for delivery of IV fluids. Chart 75-9 lists best practices for care of the client with an HD access.

COMPLICATIONS. Complications can occur regardless of the type of access. The most common problems are

TABLE 75-10 Types of Vascular Access for Hemodialysis

Access Type	Description	Location	Initial Use
Permanent			
AV fistula	An internal anastomosis of an artery to a vein	Forearm	2-4 mo or longer
AV graft	Synthetic vessel tubing tunneled beneath the skin, connecting an artery and a vein	Forearm Upper arm Inner thigh	1-2 wk
Dual-lumen hemodialysis catheter	An extended-use catheter, surgically tunneled under the skin with a barrier cuff	Subclavian vein	Immediately postoperatively and after x-ray confirmation of placement
Temporary			
Hemodialysis catheter (dual- or triple-lumen)	A specially designed catheter with two or three lumens Two lumens are for blood outflow and inflow for hemodialysis; a third lumen allows venous access without accessing dialysis lumens	Subclavian, internal jugular, or femoral vein	Immediately after insertion and x-ray confirmation of placement
AV shunt (relatively uncommon)	An external loop of Silastic tubing connecting an artery and a vein Each section of tubing is sutured into a vessel and brought through a skin stab wound	Forearm	Immediately after insertion
Subcutaneous device	An internal device with two metallic access ports and two catheters inserted into large central veins	Subclavian	Immediately after insertion

AV, Arteriovenous.

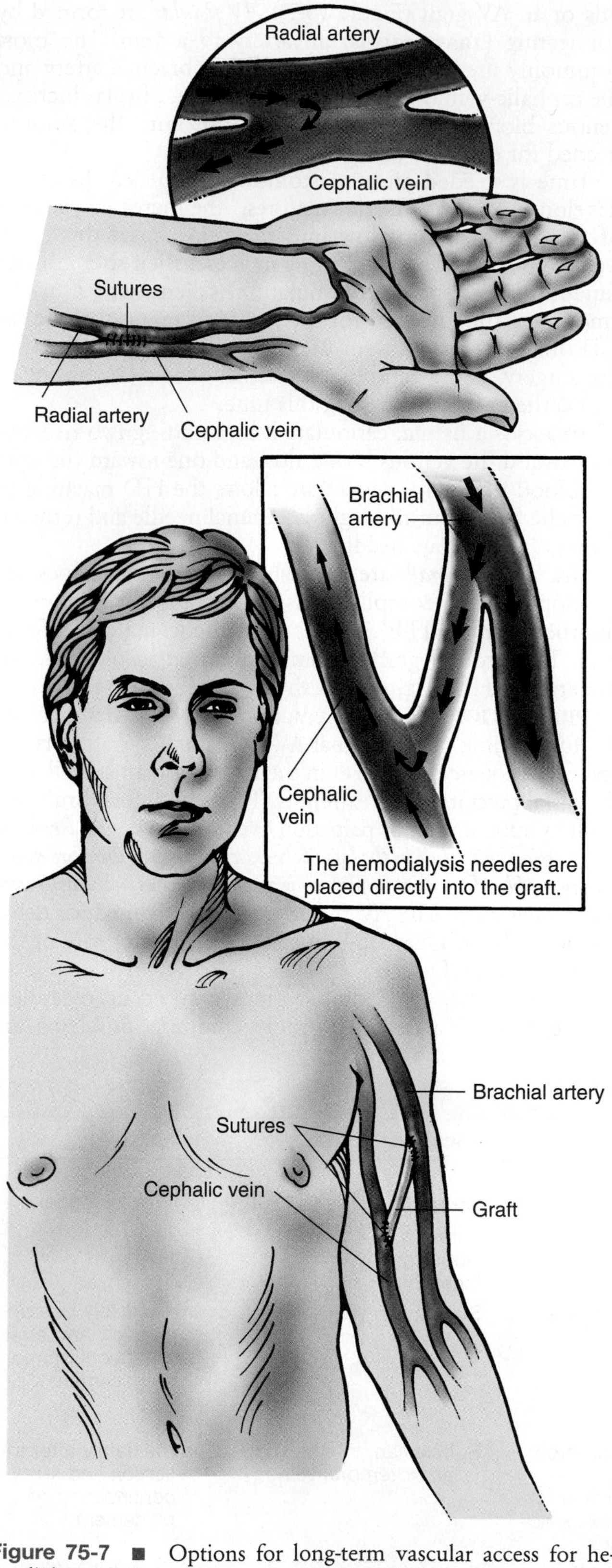

Figure 75-7 ■ Options for long-term vascular access for hemodialysis. **A,** A surgically created venous fistula. The increased pressure from the artery forces blood into the vein. This process causes the vein to dilate enough for fistula needles to be placed for hemodialysis. When the vein dilates in this manner, the fistula is said to be "developed." **B,** A surgically placed straight vascular graft in the upper arm. The graft creates a shunt between arterial and venous blood.

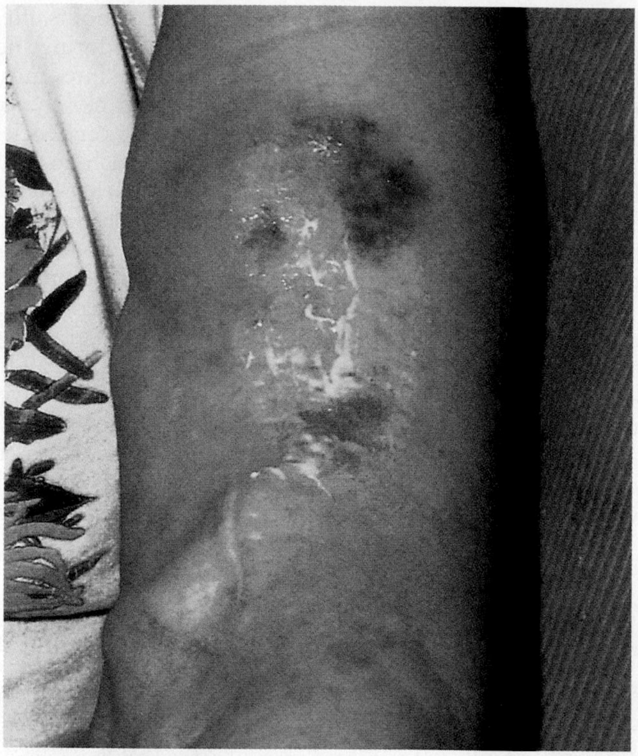

Figure 75-8 ■ Hemodialysis access.

CHART 75-9

BEST PRACTICE for
Caring for the Client with an Arteriovenous Fistula, Arteriovenous Graft, or Arteriovenous Shunt

- Do not take blood pressure readings using the extremity in which the vascular access is placed.
- Do not perform venipunctures or start an IV line in the extremity in which the vascular access is placed.
- Palpate for thrills and auscultate for bruits every 4 hours while the client is awake.
- Assess the client's distal pulses and circulation.
- Elevate the affected extremity postoperatively.
- Encourage routine range-of-motion exercises.
- Check for bleeding at needle insertion sites or shunt tubing insertion sites. (Keep small clamps handy on the dressing of the AV shunt.)
- Assess for manifestations of infection at needle sites and shunt tubing insertion sites.
- Instruct the client not to carry heavy objects or anything that compresses the extremity in which the vascular access if placed.
- Instruct the client against sleeping with his or her body weight on top of the extremity in which the vascular access is placed.

AV, Arteriovenous.

thrombosis or stenosis, infection, aneurysm formation, ischemia, and heart failure.

Thrombosis, or clotting of the AV access, is the most frequent complication. Some clients are at greater risk for clotting than others and may be given anticoagulants. Interventional radiology can treat failing grafts. Most grafts fail because of high-pressure arterial flow entering the venous system. The muscle layers of the veins react to this increased pressure by thickening. The venous thickening reduces or oc-

TABLE 75-11 Nursing Interventions for Prevention of Complications in Hemodialysis Vascular Access

Access Type	Bleeding	Infection	Clotting
AV fistula or AV graft	Apply pressure to the needle puncture sites.	Ensure adequate site cleaning before cannulation	Avoid constrictive devices. Rotate needle insertion sites with each hemodialysis treatment. Assess for thrill and bruit.
AV shunt	Keep clamps available.	Perform exit site care 3 times/wk.	Avoid constrictive devices. Assess for thrill and bruit.
Hemodialysis catheters (temporary and permanent)	Monitor the access site.	Use aseptic technique. Change the dressing 3 times/wk.	Place a heparin or heparin/saline dwell solution after hemodialysis treatment. Not used between treatments.

AV, Arteriovenous.

cludes blood flow. Radiologists inject a thrombolytic drug (such as urokinase or tPA) to dissolve the clot. The clot usually dissolves within minutes, and often a stricture is revealed at the point where the graft and the vein connect. The stricture can be treated by balloon angioplasty (Table 75-11).

Most infections of the vascular access are caused by *Staphylococcus aureus* introduced during cannulation. Use sterile technique during cannulation to prevent infection (see Table 75-11).

Aneurysms can form in the fistula and are caused by repeated needle punctures at the same site. Large aneurysms may cause loss of the fistula's function and require surgical repair.

Ischemia occurs in a few clients with vascular access when the fistula decreases arterial blood flow to areas distal to the fistula. Ischemic symptoms *("steal syndrome")* vary from cold or numb fingers to gangrene. If the collateral circulation is inadequate, the fistula may need to be tied off and a new one created in another area to preserve extremity circulation.

The shunting of blood directly from the arterial system to the venous system, through the fistula, can cause heart failure in clients with a limited cardiac reserve (see Chapter 38). This complication is rare, but if it does occur, the fistula may need to be revised to reduce arterial blood flow.

Temporary Vascular Access. An older type of vascular access is the external *arteriovenous (AV) shunt* (Figure 75-9; see also Table 75-10). This shunt is created by surgical placement of one end of a piece of silicone rubber (Silastic) tubing into an artery and the other end into a nearby vein. Part of the tubing is left external to provide a readily available vascular access. Few clients still have this type of access.

Temporary vascular access with special catheters has replaced the use of the AV shunt for most clients requiring immediate HD. A catheter designed for HD may be inserted into the subclavian, internal jugular, or femoral vein. The lumens of these devices are much smaller than the permanent accesses, and more time (4 to 8 hours) is required to complete each dialysis session.

Subcutaneous devices may also be surgically inserted to provide temporary access for HD. Implanted beneath the skin, these devices are composed of two small metallic ports with attached catheters that are inserted into large central veins (Figure 75-10). The ports of subcutaneous devices have internal mechanisms, which open when needles are inserted and close when needles are removed. Blood from one port flows from the body to the HD machine and returns to the body via the other port. These devices may be ideal for clients awaiting permanent access placement or kidney transplantation.

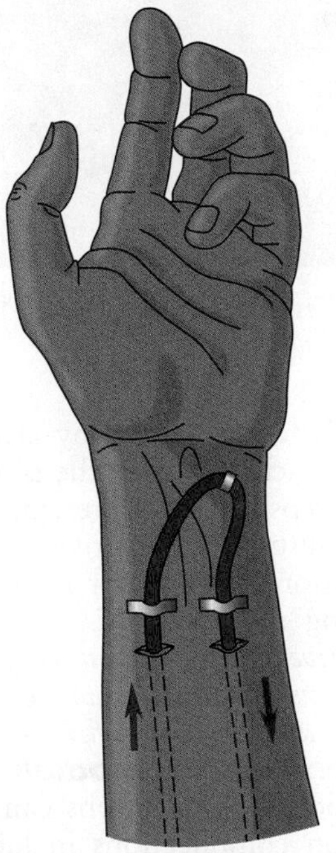

Figure 75-9 ■ An arteriovenous shunt in the forearm. One part of the shunt cannula is placed in an artery; the other part in a vein. The ends of the shunt cannula are joined when dialysis is not in progress.

Hemodialysis Nursing Care. Many client drugs are dialyzable (i.e., can be partially removed from the blood during dialysis). Vasoactive drugs can cause hypotension during HD and may also be held until after treatment. Consult with the physician to assess the client's drug regimen and determine which drugs should be held until after HD treatment. Table 75-12 lists common dialyzable and vasoactive drugs that should be given after HD.

Post-Dialysis Care. Closely monitor the client immediately and for several hours after dialysis for any side effects from the treatment. Common complications include hypotension, headache, nausea, malaise, vomiting, dizziness, and muscle cramps.

Obtain vital signs and weight for comparison with predialysis measurements. Blood pressure and weight are expected to be reduced as a result of fluid removal. Hypotension may require rehydration with IV fluids, such as normal

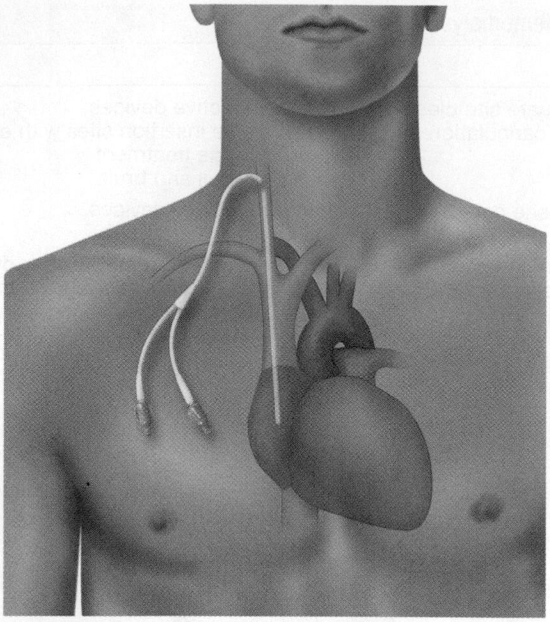

Figure 75-10 ■ Temporary subcutaneous hemodialysis access.

saline. The client's temperature may also be elevated because the dialysis machine warms the blood slightly. If the client has a fever, sepsis may be present, and a blood sample is needed for culture and sensitivity.

The heparinization required for hemodialysis (HD) increases the clotting time and thus the risk for excessive bleeding. *All invasive procedures must therefore be avoided for 4 to 6 hours after dialysis. Continually monitor the client for hemorrhage during dialysis and for 1 hour after dialysis* (Chart 75-10).

Complications of Hemodialysis. Many fluid-related and infectious complications can occur from HD. The most common complications include disequilibrium syndrome and viral infections.

Dialysis disequilibrium syndrome may develop during HD or after HD has been completed. The cause is thought to be due to the rapid decrease in fluid volume and blood urea nitrogen (BUN) levels during HD. The change in urea levels can cause cerebral edema and increased intracranial pressure. Neurologic complications can result (e.g., headache, nausea, vomiting, restlessness, decreased level of consciousness, seizures, coma, or death). Early recognition of the syndrome and treatment with anticonvulsants and barbiturates may prevent a life-threatening situation. Dialysis disequilibrium syndrome may be prevented by starting HD for short periods with low blood flows so that rapid changes in plasma composition are avoided.

Infectious diseases transmitted by blood transfusion are a serious complication of long-term HD. Two of the most serious blood-transmitted infections are hepatitis and human immunodeficiency virus (HIV).

Hepatitis infection (B and C) in clients with chronic renal failure (CRF) has decreased because the use of erythropoietin has reduced the need for blood transfusions to maintain red blood cell counts. Hepatitis is a problem because of the blood access and the risk for contamination during HD. The viruses can be transmitted through the use of contaminated needles or instruments, by entry of contaminated blood through open wounds in the skin or mucous membranes, or through transfusions with contaminated blood. Monitor all clients receiving HD for manifestations of hepatitis (see Chapter 62).

HIV is a blood-borne and body fluid–borne virus that poses some risk for clients undergoing HD. Fortunately the risks for HIV transmission are reduced by the consistent practice of standard precautions (blood and body fluids), routine screening of donated blood for HIV, and decreased

TABLE 75-12 Dialyzable and Vasoactive Drugs

Dialyzable Drugs	Vasoactive Drugs
Aminoglycosides	***Antidysrhythmics***
Amikacin	Flecainide
Gentamycin	Lidocaine
Tobramycin	Procainamide
	Quinidine
Antiviral Agents	
Acyclovir	***Antihypertensives***
Ganciclovir	Atenolol
	Captopril
Penicillins	Diltiazem
Amoxicillin	Enalapril
Ampicillin	Lisinopril
Cloxacillin	Methyldopa
Dicloxacillin	Nifedipine
Mezlocillin	Propranolol
Penicillin G	Verapamil
Ticarcillin	
	Narcotics
Anticonvulsants	Codeine
Ethosuximide	Morphine
Gabapentin	
Phenobarbital	***Sedatives***
	Midazolam
Cephalosporins	Phenobarbital
Cefaclor	Propofol
Cefazolin	
Cefoxitin	***Vasodilators***
Ceftizoxime	Hydralazine
Ceftriaxone	Nitroglycerin
Cefuroxime	Nitroprusside
Antituberculosis	
Ethambutol	
Isoniazid	
Miscellaneous	
Aztreonam	
Cimetidine	
Vitamins	

CHART 75-10

BEST PRACTICE for
Caring for the Client Undergoing Hemodialysis

- Weigh the client before and after dialysis.
- Know the client's dry weight.
- Discuss with the physician whether any of the client's medications should be withheld until after dialysis.
- Be aware of events that occurred during the dialysis treatment.
- Measure blood pressure, pulse rate, respirations, and temperature.
- Assess for symptoms of orthostatic hypotension.
- Assess the vascular access site.
- Observe for bleeding.
- Assess the client's level of consciousness and assess for headache, nausea, and vomiting.

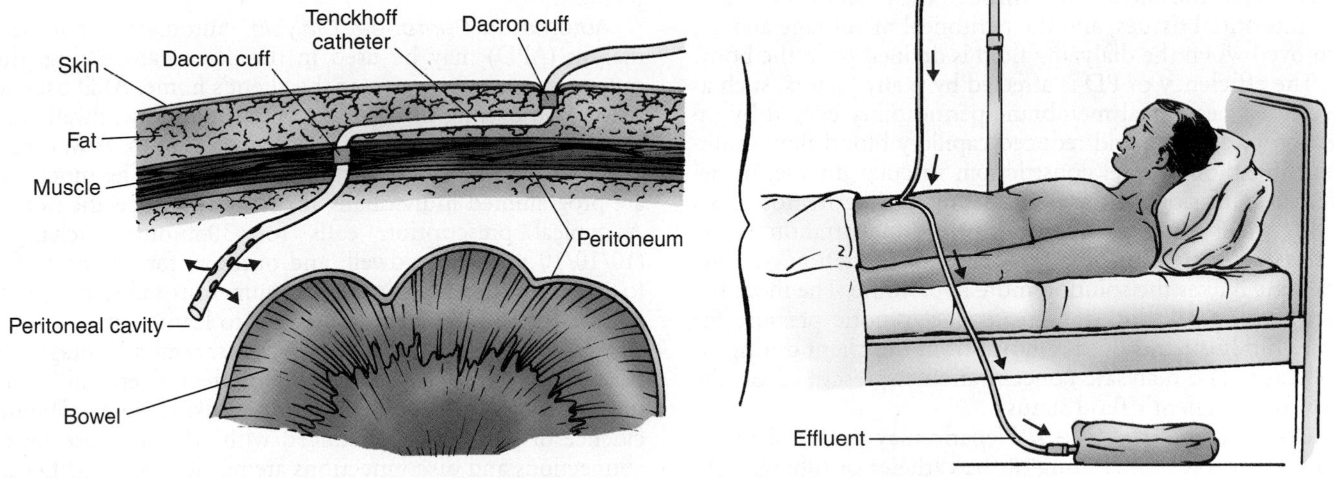

Figure 75-11 ■ Manual peritoneal dialysis via an implanted abdominal catheter (Tenckhoff catheter).

need for blood transfusions for clients with end-stage renal disease (ESRD). Despite this progress, however, some clients have already been infected with the HIV virus. Clients who have been undergoing HD or received frequent transfusions during the early to mid-1980s are at risk for acquired immunodeficiency syndrome (AIDS) (see also Chapter 25).

CONSIDERATIONS FOR OLDER ADULTS

The occurrence of ESRD is greater in clients 65 to 74 years of age. In the past decade the incidence of ESRD in individuals aged 45 to 65 has increased by 5.3% and in those 75 years of age and older by 9.5% (USRSD, 2002). Clients over age 65 who are receiving HD are more at risk for dialysis-induced hypotension. These clients require more frequent monitoring during and after dialysis.

Critical Thinking Challenge

Your client (described earlier on p. 1745) has been diagnosed as having ESRD. The health care provider has prescribed dietary teaching and outpatient HD three times per week. She asks whether she can eventually have a kidney transplant.

1. What instructions should you provide regarding the dietary and fluid needs for this client?
2. How will you explain to the client and her family that HD, rather than transplantation, is the best choice of renal replacement therapy for her?
3. What changes, if any, will need to be made in her therapy for diabetes and hypertension?
4. What complications should you monitor the client for during and immediately following dialysis?

evolve For suggested answer guidelines, go to http://evolve.elsevier.com/Iggy/.

PERITONEAL DIALYSIS

Peritoneal dialysis (PD) occurs in the peritoneal cavity. PD is slower than hemodialysis (HD), however, and more time is needed to achieve the same effect.

Client Selection. Most clients with chronic renal failure (CRF) can select either HD or PD. For clients who are hemodynamically unstable and for those who cannot tolerate anticoagulation, PD is less hazardous than HD. For some clients, vascular access problems may eliminate HD as an option. At times a client may use PD until a new arteriovenous (AV) fistula matures. PD is also often the treatment of choice for older adults because it offers more flexibility if the client's status changes frequently.

Peritoneal dialysis cannot be performed if peritoneal adhesions are present or if extensive intra-abdominal surgery has been performed. In these cases the surface area of the peritoneal membrane is not sufficient for adequate dialysis exchange. Peritoneal membrane fibrosis may occur after repeated infections, which decreases membrane permeability.

Procedure. A siliconized rubber (Silastic) catheter is surgically placed into the abdominal cavity for infusion of dialysate (Figure 75-11). Usually 1 to 2 L of dialysate is infused by gravity *(fill)* into the peritoneal space over a 10- to 20-minute period, according to the client's tolerance. The fluid *dwells* in the cavity for a specified time prescribed by the physician. The fluid then flows out of the body *(drains)* by gravity into a drainage bag. The peritoneal outflow contains the dialysate and the excess water, electrolytes, and nitrogenous waste products. The dialyzing fluid is called peritoneal *effluent* on outflow. The three phases of the process (infusion, or "fill"; dwell; and outflow, or drain) make up one PD exchange. The number and frequency of PD exchanges are prescribed by the physician, depending on the client's manifestations and laboratory data.

Process. Peritoneal dialysis occurs through diffusion and osmosis across the semipermeable peritoneal membrane and capillaries. The peritoneal membrane is large and porous. It allows solutes and water to move from an area of higher concentration in the blood to an area of lower concentration in the dialyzing fluid (diffusion).

The peritoneal cavity is rich in capillaries and is a ready access to the blood supply. The fluid and waste products dialyzed from the client move through the blood vessel walls, the interstitial tissues, and the peritoneal membrane and are removed when the dialyzing fluid is drained from the body.

The efficiency of PD is affected by many factors, such as decreased peritoneal membrane permeability caused by infection or scarring and reduced capillary blood flow resulting from blood vessel constriction, vascular disease, or decreased perfusion of the peritoneum. Unlike hemodialysis (HD), water removal depends on the concentration of the dialysate. Increasing the glucose concentration of the dialysate makes the solution more hypertonic. The more hypertonic the solution, the greater the osmotic pressure for water filtration and fluid removal from the client during an exchange. The dialysate concentration is prescribed on the basis of the client's fluid status.

Dialysate Additives. Heparin may be added to the dialysate to prevent clotting of the catheter or tubing. Usually intraperitoneal (IP) heparin is needed only after new catheter placement or if peritonitis occurs. IP heparin is not absorbed systemically and does not affect blood clotting.

Other agents that may be given in the dialysate include potassium and antibiotics. Commercially prepared dialysate does not contain potassium. Some clients need potassium added to the dialysate so that hypokalemia does not occur. Antibiotics may be given by the IP route when peritonitis is present or suspected. Potassium and antibiotics are not mixed in the same dialysate bag because interactions may reduce the antibiotic effect.

Types of Peritoneal Dialysis. Many types of PD are available, including continuous ambulatory PD, multiple-bag continuous ambulatory PD, automated PD, intermittent PD, and continuous-cycle PD. The type selected depends on the client's ability and lifestyle.

Continuous Ambulatory Peritoneal Dialysis. In continuous ambulatory peritoneal dialysis (CAPD), the client performs self-dialysis by infusing four 2-L exchanges of dialysate into the peritoneal cavity, where the dialysate remains for 4 to 8 hours, 7 days a week. During the dwell period, the client can use a continuous connect system or a disconnect system.

With the continuous *connect* system (straight transfer set), the dialysate bag is attached to the catheter by 48-inch tubing. The empty bag and tubing are folded and worn beneath the clothing until they are used for outflow. After draining, the client removes the bag and connects a new bag to repeat the process.

With the *disconnect system* (Y-transfer set), the client removes the connecting tubing and empty dialysate bag after inflow and attaches a cap to the PD catheter. The disconnect system eliminates the need to wear the tubing and bag but requires opening the system two extra times with each exchange. The extra opening of the system increases the risk for infection.

With CAPD treatment, no machine is necessary and no partner is required. However, it is best for a partner also trained in CAPD to be available as a support for the client if illness occurs. Devices to assist in the safe, aseptic connection of the tubing spike with the dialysate bag are available. These devices are useful for clients with impaired vision, limited manual dexterity, or decreased hand and arm strength. CAPD allows constant removal of fluid and wastes and more nearly resembles renal function than does HD. Some clients even perform their own exchanges while hospitalized.

Automated Peritoneal Dialysis. Automated peritoneal dialysis (APD) may be used in the acute care setting, the outpatient dialysis center, or the client's home. APD uses an automated cycling machine for dialysate inflow, dwell, and outflow according to preset times and volumes. A warming chamber for dialysate is part of the machine. The functions are programmed individually for the client's specific needs. A typical prescription calls for 30-minute exchanges (10/10/10 for inflow, dwell, and outflow) for a period of 8 to 10 hours. The machines have numerous safety monitors and alarms and are relatively simple to learn to use.

Automated peritoneal dialysis has several advantages. It permits in-home dialysis while the client sleeps, allowing him or her to be dialysis free during waking hours. The incidence of peritonitis is reduced with APD because fewer connections and disconnections are needed. Also, APD can be used to administer larger volumes of dialysis solution for clients who need higher clearances.

Intermittent Peritoneal Dialysis. Intermittent peritoneal dialysis (IPD) combines osmotic pressure gradients with true dialysis. The client usually requires exchanges of 2 L of dialysate at 30- to 60-minute intervals, allowing 15 to 20 minutes of drain time. For most clients, 30 to 40 exchanges of 2 L three times weekly are needed. IPD treatments can be automated or manual.

Continuous-Cycle Peritoneal Dialysis. Continuous-cycle peritoneal dialysis (CCPD) uses an automated cycling machine. Exchanges occur at night while the client sleeps. The final exchange of the night is left to dwell through the day and is drained the next evening as the process is repeated. CCPD offers the advantage of 24-hour dialysis, as in CAPD, but the sterile catheter system is violated less often.

Complications. Complications are possible with PD, but many can be prevented with careful nursing care.

Peritonitis. Peritonitis is the major complication of PD. The most common cause of peritonitis is connection site contamination. To prevent peritonitis, use meticulous sterile technique when caring for the PD catheter and when hooking up or clamping off dialysate bags (Chart 75-11).

Manifestations of peritonitis include cloudy dialysate outflow (effluent), fever, abdominal tenderness, abdominal pain, general malaise, nausea, and vomiting. Cloudy or opaque effluent is the earliest sign of peritonitis. Examine all effluent for color and clarity to detect peritonitis early. When peritonitis is suspected, send a specimen of the dialysate outflow for culture and sensitivity study, Gram stain, and cell count to identify the infecting organism.

Pain. Pain during the inflow of dialysate is common when clients are first started on PD therapy. Usually this pain no longer occurs after a week or two of PD. Cold dialysate increases discomfort. Thus you should warm the dialysate bags before instillation by using a heating pad to wrap the bag or by using the warming chamber of the auto-

CHART 75-11

BEST PRACTICE for
Caring for the Client with a Peritoneal Dialysis Catheter

- Mask yourself and your client. Wash your hands.
- Put on sterile gloves. Remove the old dressing. Remove the contaminated gloves.
- Assess the area for signs of infection, such as swelling, redness, or discharge around the catheter site.
- Use aseptic technique:
  Open the sterile field on a flat surface, and place two precut 4 × 4 inch gauze pads on the field.
  Place three cotton swabs soaked in povidone-iodine on the field. Put on sterile gloves.
- Use cotton swabs to clean around the catheter site. Use a circular motion starting from the insertion site and moving away toward the abdomen. Repeat with all three swabs.
- Apply precut gauze pads over the catheter site. Tape only the edges of the gauze pads.

mated cycling machine. *Microwave ovens are not recommended for the warming of dialysate.*

Exit Site and Tunnel Infections. The exit site from a PD catheter should be clean, dry, and without pain or inflammation. Exit site infections (ESIs) can occur with any type of PD catheter. These infections are difficult to treat and can become chronic. Exit site and tunnel infections can lead to peritonitis, catheter failure, and hospitalization. Dialysate leakage and pulling or twisting of the catheter predispose the client to ESIs. A Gram stain and culture should be performed when exit sites have purulent drainage.

Tunnel infections occur in the path of the catheter from the skin to the cuff. Manifestations include redness, tenderness, and pain. ESIs are treated with antimicrobials. Deep cuff infections usually require catheter removal.

Poor Dialysate Flow. Constipation is the main cause of inflow or outflow problems. To prevent constipation, the physician prescribes a bowel preparation before placing the PD catheter. An enema before starting PD may also prevent flow problems. A high-fiber diet and stool softeners are often needed for prevention of constipation. Other causes of flow difficulty include kinked or clamped connection tubing, the client's position, fibrin clot formation, and PD catheter displacement.

Ensure that the drainage bag is lower than the client's abdomen to enhance gravity drainage. Inspect the connection tubing and PD system for kinking or twisting, and ensure that clamps are open. If inflow or outflow drainage is still inadequate, reposition the client to stimulate inflow or outflow. Turning the client to the other side or making sure that he or she is in good body alignment may help. Having the client in a supine low-Fowler's position reduces intra-abdominal pressure. Increased intra-abdominal pressure from sitting or standing, or from coughing, contributes to leakage at the PD catheter site.

Fibrin clot formation may occur after PD catheter placement or with the onset of peritonitis. Milking the tubing may dislodge the fibrin clot and improve flow. An x-ray is needed to identify PD catheter placement. If displacement has occurred, the physician repositions the PD catheter.

Dialysate Leakage. Dialysate leakage is seen as clear fluid coming from the catheter exit site. When dialysis is first started, small volumes of dialysate are used. It may take clients 1 to 2 weeks to tolerate a full 2-L exchange without leakage around the catheter site. Leakage occurs more often in obese or diabetic clients, older adults, and those on long-term steroid therapy. During periods of catheter leak, clients may require hemodialysis (HD) support.

Other Complications. When PD is first started, the outflow may be bloody or blood tinged. This condition normally clears within a week or two. After PD is well-established, the effluent should be clear and light yellow. Observe for and document any change in the color of the outflow. Brown-colored effluent is associated with a bowel perforation. If the outflow is the same color as urine and has the same glucose concentration, a possible bladder perforation should be investigated. Cloudy or opaque effluent indicates infection.

Nursing Care During Peritoneal Dialysis. In the hospital setting, PD is routinely initiated and monitored by the nurse. Before the treatment, evaluate baseline vital signs, including blood pressure, apical and radial pulse rates, temperature, quality of respirations, and breath sounds. Weigh the client, always on the same scale, before the procedure and at least every 24 hours while receiving treatment. Baseline laboratory tests, such as electrolyte and glucose levels, are obtained before starting PD and are repeated at least daily during the PD treatment.

Continually monitor the client during PD. Take and record vital signs every 15 to 30 minutes. Assess the client for signs of respiratory distress, pain, or discomfort. Check the dressing around the catheter exit site every 30 minutes for wetness during the procedure. Monitor the prescribed dwell time and initiate outflow. Assess blood glucose levels in clients who absorb glucose.

Observe the outflow pattern (outflow should be a continuous stream after the clamp is completely open). Accurately record the total amount of outflow after each exchange. Maintain accurate inflow and outflow records when hourly PD exchanges are performed. When outflow is less than inflow, the difference is retained by the client during dialysis and is counted as intake. Weigh the client daily to monitor fluid status.

RENAL TRANSPLANTATION

Dialysis and transplantation are life-sustaining *treatments* for end-stage renal disease (ESRD). Renal transplantation is not considered a "cure." Each client, in consultation with a nephrologist, determines which type of therapy is best suited to that client's physical condition and lifestyle. As of August 2003, 10,485 kidney transplants had been performed in that year. Currently more than 82,000 people are awaiting renal transplantation in the United States (United Network for Organ Sharing [UNOS], 2003).

Candidate Selection Criteria. Candidates for transplantation must be free of medical problems that might increase the risks from the procedure. The usual age range for transplantation is 2 to 70 years of age. Clients older than 70 years of age are considered for transplantation on an individual basis because complications are more common in the older adult.

A thorough assessment of the client is performed before the client is considered for transplantation. Clients who have advanced, uncorrectable cardiac disease are excluded from transplantation because these problems are made worse by the procedure. Other conditions that preclude transplantation include metastatic cancer, chronic infection, and severe psychosocial problems such as chemical dependency (Bartucci, 1999). Long-standing pulmonary disease increases the risk for complications and death from respiratory infections. Clients with diseases of the gastrointestinal system may require treatment before consideration for transplantation. Such problems as peptic ulcer and diverticulosis are made worse by the large doses of steroids used after transplantation.

The urinary system is completely evaluated to ensure normal urine flow. Many clients with ESRD have not used their lower urinary tract for years, and ureteral or bladder problems may require surgical correction before renal transplantation.

Clients with a recent history of cancer are treated with dialysis because of the shortage of donor organs and the limited life expectancy of these clients. In addition, the drugs used after transplantation increase the risk for cancer recurrence. If more than 2 to 5 years have passed since eradication of the cancer, the client can be considered for a transplant.

Diabetes mellitus and other endocrine problems cause even greater risks. These clients can have a renal transplant, but they require intense observation and management to limit complications. Other complicating conditions are considered on an individual basis, depending on the client's current health status. Renal transplantation can be considered for many of those with ESRD and is the optimal therapy for many people. Most people who have undergone this procedure are satisfied with their quality of life for years after the transplant (see the Evidence-Based Practice for Nursing box at right).

Donors. Kidney donors may be living donors (related or unrelated to the client), non–heart-beating donors (NHBDs), and cadaveric donors. The available kidneys are matched on the basis of tissue type similarity between the donor and the recipient. Living donors are most often blood relatives, but unrelated donors have been used. NHBDs are persons declared dead by cardiopulmonary criteria. Kidneys from NHBDs are harvested immediately after death in cases where clients have previously given consent for organ donation. If immediate removal must be delayed, in situ preservation is performed with infusion of a cool preservation solution inserted into the abdominal aorta after death is declared and until surgery can be performed. Cadaveric donors are usually individuals who suffered irreversible brain injury, most often as a result of trauma. These donors are maintained with mechanical ventilation and must have sufficient renal perfusion for the kidneys to remain viable (Bartucci, 1999).

The size of the kidney is seldom a problem in adults. Pediatric cadaveric kidneys hypertrophy to meet adult needs within a few months.

Organs from living *related* donors (LRDs) have the highest rates of renal graft survival (90%). Donors are usually at least 18 years old and are seldom older than 65 years of age. Physical criteria for donors include the following:

- Absence of systemic disease and infection
- No history of cancer
- No hypertension or renal disease
- Adequate renal function as determined by diagnostic studies

EVIDENCE-BASED PRACTICE for Nursing

Life satisfaction after kidney transplant influenced by other health problems

Siegal, B., Halbert, R., & McGuire, M. (2002). Life satisfaction among kidney transplant recipients: Demographic and biological factors. *Progress in Transplantation, 12*(4), 293-298.

The Transplant Learning Center (TLC), an organization dedicated to providing education and support to recipients of solid organ transplants, found that no current quality-of-life instrument was specific enough to include dimensions of concern to transplant recipients. This group developed the Life Satisfaction Index (LSI), which attempted to capture the issues considered by transplant recipients to most affect their level of life satisfaction. The investigators used a descriptive correlational study to determine which specific factors influenced the perception of life satisfaction among solid organ transplant recipients. This study reports the findings specifically for recipients of kidney transplants.

This instrument was mailed to the 9000 solid organ transplant recipients who had joined the TLC program. Analyses were performed on the questionnaires returned over a 2-year period by the 3676 kidney transplant recipients who participated in the initial survey round. Internal consistency of the total LSI is reported as having a Cronbach's alpha of 0.85 with a range on the individual items from 0.82 to 0.88. In addition to demographic data questions, the LSI included 8 questions related to life satisfaction, 11 questions related to comorbid health conditions, 11 questions related to adverse effects of the post-transplant regimen, and 6 questions related to adherence to post-transplant drug regimens.

Highest life satisfaction scores correlated with an age over 64 years, male gender, higher mean income and education, and being married. Lowest life satisfaction scores correlated with medical comorbidities, particularly emotional/psychological problems and eye/vision problems. Subjects who reported more frequent failure to adhere to the prescribed post-transplant drug regimen also had lower life satisfaction scores.

Level of Evidence: 6—Uncontrolled correlational, descriptive study.

Critique. The strengths of this study include the large sample size and the high level of internal consistency of the instrument. However, the sample is biased in several ways. First, only transplant recipients who were enrolled in the TLC were contacted for participation in the study. Of these, data were collected only on those subjects who returned their questionnaires, which may represent only those kidney transplant recipients who had higher levels of life satisfaction. This study relied solely on self-reports. The study could have been strengthened by having subjects also complete other established instruments to measure life satisfaction or quality of life and to compare the results with those obtained on the LSI.

Implications for Nursing. Life satisfaction for recipients of kidney transplants resembles that of other individuals in that it is multidimensional. Nurses need to help clients with end-stage renal disease who are planning for kidney transplantation to understand that the transplant will solve only renal-related issues. Other pre-existing health, psychological, financial, or personal issues will remain after the transplant and will continue to have some influence on the client's quality of life.

In addition, LRDs must express a clear understanding of the surgery and a willingness to give up a kidney. Some transplant centers require a psychiatric evaluation to assess the donor's motivation.

Because of advances in immunosuppressant therapy and medical management, the United Network of Organ Sharing (UNOS) reports 1-year renal transplant graft survival to be 90% for all centers in the United States (UNOS, 2003).

Preoperative Care. Many issues related to client health and the actual transplant procedure must be addressed before surgery. The Clinical Pathway on the Evolve website highlights care needs for the client undergoing renal transplantation.

Immunologic Studies. The major barrier to transplantation success after a suitable donor kidney is available is the body's ability to reject "foreign" tissue. This immunologic process can attack the transplanted kidney and destroy it. For immunologic problems to be overcome, in-depth tissue typing is performed on all candidates. These studies include simple blood typing and human leukocyte antigen (HLA) studies as well as other tests. The HLAs are the main immunologic feature used to match transplant recipients with compatible donors. The more similar the antigens of the donor are to those of the recipient, the more likely it is that the transplant will be successful and rejection will be avoided (see Chapter 23).

Surgical Team. The specialized surgical team includes circulating and scrub nurses, clinical nurse specialists, transplant surgeons, anesthesiologists, and nephrologists. Preoperative nursing responsibilities include the following:

- Teaching about the procedure and postoperative care
- In-depth client assessment
- Coordination of diagnostic tests
- Development and implementation of treatment plans

The client usually requires dialysis within 24 hours of the surgery. In addition, the recipient often receives a blood transfusion before surgery. Usually blood from the kidney donor is transfused into the recipient. This procedure increases graft survival of organs from LRDs.

Operative Procedures. The donor nephrectomy procedure varies depending on whether the donor is an NHBD, cadaveric donor, or living donor. The NHBD or cadaveric donor nephrectomy is a sterile autopsy in the operating room. All arterial and venous vessels and a long piece of ureter are preserved. After removal, the kidneys are preserved until time for implantation into the recipient. The technique for kidney removal from living donors is a delicate procedure that lasts 3 to 4 hours. A flank incision is used, and care is taken to avoid scarring. Donors usually have more pain after surgery than do recipients. They also need nursing care and support for the psychological adjustment to loss of a body part.

The transplantation surgery usually takes 4 to 5 hours. The transplanted kidney is usually placed in the right anterior iliac fossa (Figure 75-12) instead of the usual anatomic position. This placement allows easier connection of the ureter and the renal artery and vein. It also allows for kidney assessment by palpation. The recipient's own nonfunctioning kidneys are not usually removed unless chronic infection is present in one or both kidneys. After surgery, the client is taken to the postanesthesia unit and then, when stable, to a designated unit in the transplant center or to a critical care unit.

Postoperative Care. Care of the recipient after surgery requires that nurses be knowledgeable about the expected clinical findings and potential complications. Nursing care includes ongoing physical assessment with an emphasis on evaluation of renal function. The transplant recipient requires close attention because the immunosuppressive drug therapy used to prevent tissue rejection impairs healing and increases the risk for infection.

Urologic management is essential to graft success. These clients always have a large indwelling (Foley) catheter for accurate measurements of urine output and decompression of the bladder. Decompression prevents stretch on suture and ureter attachment sites on the bladder.

Assess urine output at least hourly during the first 48 hours. An abrupt decrease in urine output may indicate complications such as rejection, acute tubular necrosis (ATN), thrombosis, or obstruction. Examine the urine color. The urine is pink and bloody right after surgery and gradually returns to normal over several days to several weeks, depending on renal function. Obtain daily urine specimens for urinalysis, glucose measurement, the presence of acetone, specific gravity measurement, and culture (if needed).

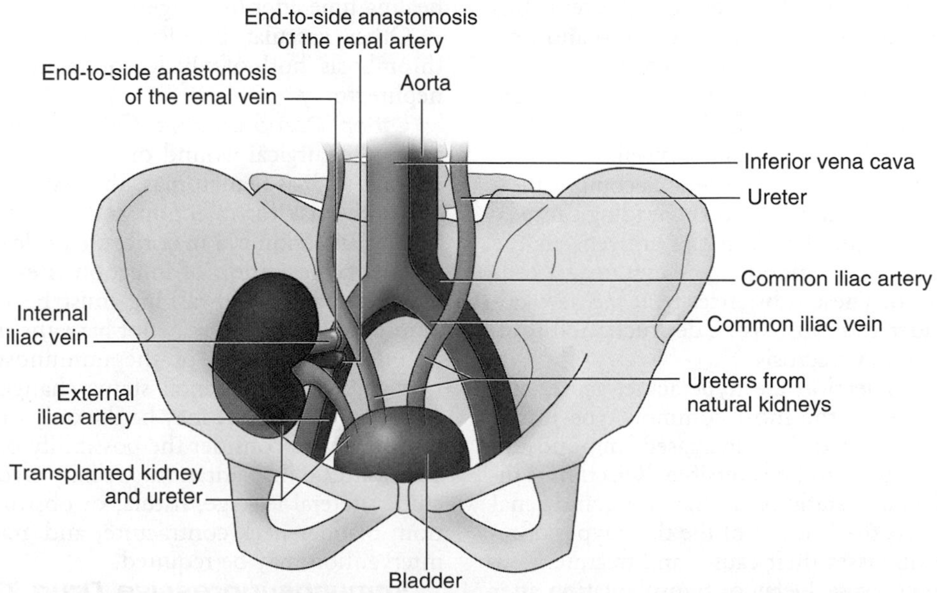

Figure 75-12 ■ Placement of a transplanted kidney in the right iliac fossa.

TABLE 75-13 A Comparison of Hyperacute, Acute, and Chronic Post-Transplant Rejection

Hyperacute Rejection	Acute Rejection	Chronic Rejection
Onset		
Within 48 hr after surgery	1 wk to 2 yr postoperatively (most common in first 2 wk)	Occurs gradually during a period of months to years
Clinical Manifestations		
Increased temperature Increased blood pressure Pain at transplant site	Oliguria or anuria Temperature over 100° F (37.8° C) Increased blood pressure Enlarged, tender kidney Lethargy Elevated serum creatinine, BUN, potassium levels Fluid retention	Gradual increase in BUN and serum creatinine levels Fluid retention Changes in serum electrolyte levels Fatigue
Treatment		
Immediate removal of the transplanted kidney	Increased doses of immunosuppressive drugs	Conservative management until dialysis is required

BUN, Blood urea nitrogen.

Occasionally a continuous bladder irrigation is prescribed to decrease the formation of blood clots, which could increase pressure in the bladder and endanger the graft. Perform routine catheter care, according to your agency's policy, to reduce catheter contamination. The catheter is removed as soon as possible to avoid infection, usually 3 to 7 days after surgery. After surgery the function of the transplanted kidney (renal graft) can result in either oliguria or diuresis. Oliguria may occur as a result of ischemia and ATN, rejection, or other complications. To increase urine output, the physician may prescribe diuretics and osmotic agents, such as mannitol. Closely monitor the client's fluid status because fluid overload can cause hypertension, heart failure, and pulmonary edema. Evaluate the client's fluid status by taking daily weights, measuring blood pressure every 2 to 4 hours, and accurately measuring intake and output.

Instead of oliguria, the client may have diuresis, especially with a kidney from a living related donor (LRD). Carefully monitor intake and output, and observe for electrolyte imbalances, such as hypokalemia and hyponatremia. Excessive diuresis may cause hypotension. Prevent this problem because hypotension reduces blood flow and oxygen to the new kidney, threatening graft survival.

Complications. Many potential complications are possible after renal transplantation. Early detection and intervention improve the chances of graft survival.

Rejection. The most common and serious complication of transplantation is rejection, which is the leading cause of graft loss. A reaction occurs between the antigens in the transplanted kidney and the antibodies and cytotoxic T-cells in the recipient's blood. These substances treat the new kidney as a foreign invader and cause tissue destruction, thrombosis, and eventual kidney necrosis.

The three types of rejection are hyperacute, acute, and chronic. Acute rejection is the most common type in the transplant client. It is treated with increased immunosuppressive therapy and often can be reversible. Rejection is diagnosed by clinical manifestations, a renal scan, and renal biopsy. Table 75-13 lists the features of the three types of rejection. Chapter 23 discusses their causes and treatment.

Acute Tubular Necrosis. Delay of transplantation after kidneys have been harvested can result in ischemic damage to the kidney and the client having acute tubular necrosis (ATN) after surgery. These clients may need dialysis until adequate urine output returns and the blood urea nitrogen (BUN) and creatinine levels normalize. ATN is often difficult to distinguish from acute rejection, and clients need to undergo weekly biopsies to assess the need for further immunosuppression if rejection is occurring.

Thrombosis. Thrombosis of the major renal blood vessels may occur during the first 2 to 3 days after transplantation. A sudden decrease in urine output may signal impaired perfusion resulting from thrombosis. Ultrasound examination of the kidney may reveal decreased or absent blood supply. Emergency surgery is required to prevent ischemic damage or graft loss.

Renal Artery Stenosis. Stenosis of the renal artery may result in hypertension. Other manifestations include a bruit over the artery anastomosis site and decreased renal function. A renal scan can quantify the blood flow to the kidney. The involved artery may be repaired surgically or by balloon angioplasty in the radiology department. The decision to perform a balloon repair is determined by the amount of healing time after the surgery.

Other vascular problems include vascular leakage or thrombosis, both of which require an emergency transplant nephrectomy.

Other Complications. Other complications may involve the surgical wound or urinary tract. Wound complications, such as hematomas, abscesses, and lymphoceles, increase the risk for infection and exert pressure on the new kidney. Infection is a major cause of death in the transplant recipient. Prevention of infection is essential. Strict aseptic technique and handwashing must be rigorously enforced. Transplant recipients may not have the usual manifestations of infection because of the immunosuppressive therapy. Low-grade fevers, mental status changes, and vague complaints of discomfort may be the only manifestations before sepsis. Always consider the possibility of infection with any client after transplantation. Urinary tract complications include ureteral leakage, fistula, or obstruction; stone formation; bladder neck contracture; and graft rupture. Surgical intervention may be required.

Immunosuppressive Drug Therapy. The success of renal transplantation depends on changing the client's immunologic response so that the new kidney is not rejected as a foreign organ. Immunosuppressive drugs protect the transplanted organ. These drugs include corticosteroids, anti-lymphocyte preparations, monoclonal antibodies, and cyclosporine (Cyclosporin A). Chapter 23 discusses the mechanisms of action for these agents and the associated client responses. Clients taking these drugs are at an increased risk for death by viral, fungal, bacterial, or protozoal infection.

Community-Based Care

HOME CARE MANAGEMENT

Because of the complex nature of CRF, its progressive course, and many treatment modalities, a case manager is helpful in the planning, coordination, and evaluation of care. As the renal disease progresses, the client is seen by a physician or nurse practitioner regularly and may be hospitalized often. Together with the dietitian and social worker, evaluate the home environment and determine equipment needs before discharge. Once the client is discharged, home care nurses direct care and monitor progress. Chart 75-12 provides a focused assessment guide for the client after transplantation.

Provide health teaching about the diet in renal disease and the progression of renal disease. As CRF approaches end-stage renal disease (ESRD), one of the following courses of treatment is chosen: hemodialysis (HD), peritoneal dialysis (PD), or transplantation. For each form of treatment, the client must learn about the procedures and consider his or her personal lifestyle, support systems, and methods of coping. Decision making about treatment type, or even whether to pursue treatment, is difficult for clients and families. Provide information and emotional support to assist clients with these decisions.

Teach clients who select hemodialysis (HD) about the dialysis machine and vascular access care. If in-home HD is selected, preparations are needed for installation of the appropriate equipment, including a water treatment system. Regardless of whether the treatment occurs at home or in a center, provide ongoing physical assessment and health teaching to promote independence at home.

The client receiving PD needs extensive training in the procedure. The client also needs assistance in obtaining equipment and the many supplies needed. Home care nurses assess clients, monitor vital signs, assess adherence with drug and diet regimens, and monitor for manifestations of peritonitis.

The nurse plays a vital role in the long-term care of the client with a renal transplant. This client is usually discharged 3 to 4 weeks after surgery. Stress that adherence to the prescribed immunosuppressive drug therapy is essential for the survival of the kidney. Facilitate acceptance and understanding of this regimen as a part of daily life. Carefully monitor for signs of graft rejection and for complications, such as infection.

HEALTH TEACHING

Instruct clients and family members in all aspects of diet therapy, drug therapy, and complications. Teach clients and family members to report complications, such as fluid overload and infection. When a client requires a more advanced form of therapy, such as dialysis or transplantation, focus teaching on the chosen therapeutic intervention.

CHART 75-12

FOCUSED ASSESSMENT of
The Client with Chronic Renal Failure

Assess cardiovascular and respiratory status, including the following:
- Vital signs, with special attention to blood pressure
- Presence of S_3 or pericardial friction rub
- Presence of chest pain
- Presence of edema (periorbital, pretibial, sacral)
- Jugular vein distention
- Presence of dyspnea
- Presence of crackles, beginning at the bases and extending upward

Assess nutritional status, including the following:
- Weight gain or loss
- Presence of anorexia, nausea, or vomiting

Assess renal status, including the following:
- Amount, frequency, and appearance of urine (in non-anuric clients)
- Presence of bone pain
- Presence of hyperglycemia secondary to diabetes

Assess hematologic status, including the following:
- Presence of petechiae, purpura, ecchymoses
- Presence of fatigue or shortness of breath

Assess gastrointestinal status, including the following:
- Presence of stomatitis
- Presence of melena

Assess integumentary status, including the following:
- Skin integrity
- Presence of pruritus
- Presence of skin discoloration

Assess neurologic status, including the following:
- Changes in mental status
- Presence of seizure activity
- Presence of sensory changes
- Presence of lower extremity weakness

Assess laboratory data, including the following:
- BUN
- Serum creatinine
- Creatinine clearance
- CBC
- Electrolytes

Assess psychosocial status, including the following:
- Presence of anxiety
- Presence of maladaptive behavior

BUN, Blood urea nitrogen; *CBC*, complete blood count.

Hemodialysis (HD) is the most complex form of therapy for the client and family to understand. Even if clients receive HD in a dialysis center instead of at home, they are expected to have some knowledge of the HD machine. The client or a family member must be taught to care for the vascular access and to report signs of infection and stenosis. The client who plans to have in-home HD will need a partner. Both the client and the partner must be taught the entire process of HD and must be able to perform it independently before the client is discharged.

Peritoneal dialysis (PD) involves extensive health teaching. This instruction can be given to the client alone or to the client and a family member if the client cannot perform the procedure. Emphasize sterile technique because peritonitis is the most common complication of PD. Instruct clients to report any manifestation of peritonitis, especially cloudy effluent and abdominal pain. If peritonitis develops, teach clients how to give themselves antibiotics by the intraperitoneal (IP) route. Stress the importance of completing the antibiotic regimen. Remind clients that repeated episodes of peritonitis can reduce the effectiveness of PD, which may require the transfer to HD.

The client receiving a renal transplant also needs extensive health teaching. Provide instruction about drug regimens, home monitoring, immunosuppression, manifestations of rejection, infection, and prescribed changes in the diet and activity level.

PSYCHOSOCIAL PREPARATION

Provide psychological support for the client and family. Help the client adjust to the diagnosis of renal failure and eventually accept the treatment regimens.

Many clients view dialysis as a cure instead of a required lifelong treatment. For many clients, the reduction of uremic symptoms in the first weeks after starting dialysis treatment creates a sense of euphoria and well-being (the "honeymoon" period). They feel better physically, and their mood may be happy and hopeful. At this time they tend to overlook the discomfort and inconvenience of dialysis. Use this time to begin health care teaching. Stress that although the uremic symptoms are reduced, the client will not return completely to the previous state of well-being.

Many clients become discouraged during the first year of treatment. This mood state may last a few months to a year or longer. The difficulties of incorporating dialysis into daily life are staggering, and clients may become depressed as problems occur. They may struggle with the idea of having to be permanently dependent on a disruptive therapy. Clients may feel helpless and dependent. Some people retreat into complete or partial denial of the disease and the need for treatment. They may deny the need for dialysis or may not adhere to drug therapy and diet restrictions. Monitor any behaviors that may contribute to nonadherence, and suggest psychiatric referrals. Help the client and family to focus on the positive aspects of the treatments. Continue health care education with clients as active participants and decision makers.

Most clients with CRF eventually enter a phase of acceptance or resignation. The idea of a chronic illness may be devastating for some people, and each person reacts differently. To make this long-term adaptation, the client must adjust to continuous change. Specific concerns depend on the client's health and particular treatment method.

After clients have accepted or become resigned to the chronic aspect of their disease, they usually attempt to return to their previous activities. Resuming the previous level of activity, however, may not be possible. Help clients to set realistic goals that allow them to lead active, productive lives.

HEALTH CARE RESOURCES

Professionals from various disciplines are resources for the client with renal failure. Home care nurses monitor the client's status and evaluate maintenance of the prescribed treatment regimen (HD or PD). A client with advanced renal failure may need a home care aide to help perform activities of daily living. Social services are often involved because of the complex process of applying for financial aid to pay for the required medical care. A physical therapist may be beneficial in helping to improve the client's functional health. A dietitian can assist the client and family members in understanding the special dietary needs. A psychiatric evaluation may be needed if depressive symptoms are present. Clergy and pastoral care specialists offer spiritual support.

Clients with CRF are routinely followed by a physician, usually a nephrologist. Organizations such as the National Kidney Foundation (NKF), the American Kidney Fund, and the National Association of Patients on Hemodialysis and Transplantation (NAPHT) may be helpful to clients and families.

◆Evaluation: Outcomes

Evaluate the care of the client with chronic renal failure (CRF) on the basis of the identified nursing diagnoses and collaborative problems. The expected outcomes are that the client should:

- Achieve and maintain appropriate fluid volume
- Maintain an adequate nutritional status
- Use effective coping strategies
- Report an absence of physical manifestations of anxiety

Specific indicators for these outcomes are listed for each nursing diagnosis and collaborative problem under the Planning and Implementation section (see earlier).

GET READY for the NCLEX Examination!

KEY POINTS

Safe Effective Care Environment

- Use sterile technique when cannulating a vascular access or connecting peritoneal dialysis tubing.
- Handle clients with chronic renal failure gently to prevent fractures.
- Assess all clients at risk for dehydration or hypovolemia for adequacy of renal perfusion.

Health Promotion and Maintenance

- Encourage clients with renal failure to follow fluid and dietary restrictions regarding sodium, potassium, and protein.
- Instruct clients on immunosuppressive therapy to avoid crowds and people who are ill.
- Teach clients on immunosuppressive therapy to assess themselves daily for fever, general malaise, and nausea or vomiting.

Psychosocial Integrity

- Pace your interview to match the learning needs and style of the individual client.
- Allow the client the opportunity to express fear or anxiety regarding the risk for death and the disruption of lifestyle as a result of treatment for renal failure.
- During renal/urinary assessment use language and terminology that are comfortable for the client.
- Assess the client for depression and nonacceptance of his or her diagnosis or treatment plan.
- Refer clients to community resources and support groups.

Physiological Integrity

- Report immediately any condition that obstructs urine flow.
- Teach clients the expected side effects and any adverse reactions to prescribed drugs.
- Collaborate with the dietitian to teach clients about needed fluid, sodium, potassium, or dietary protein restriction.

- Teach clients in the early stages of renal failure the manifestations of dehydration.
- Teach clients in the later stages of chronic renal failure the manifestations of fluid overload and hyperkalemia.
- Avoid taking blood pressure measurements or drawing blood from an arm with a vascular access (AV fistula or graft).
- Do not use an AV fistula or graft site for IV fluid administration.
- Avoid all invasive procedures within 4 to 6 hours after the client has undergone hemodialysis.
- Use meticulous sterile technique when caring for the peritoneal dialysis catheter and when hooking up or clamping off dialysate bags.
- Teach clients using peritoneal dialysis the manifestations of peritonitis.

ADDITIONAL STUDY RESOURCES

Go to your Student CD-ROM for Review Questions for the NCLEX Examination.

evolve Go to http://evolve.elsevier.com/Iggy/ for Integrated Management of Care Questions for the NCLEX Examination.

SELECTED BIBLIOGRAPHY

Asterisk indicates a classic or definitive work on this subject.

Abbas, A., & Lichtman, A. (2003). *Cellular and molecular immunology* (5th ed). Philadelphia: W.B. Saunders.

Ackley, B., & Ladwig, G. (2002). *Nursing diagnosis handbook: A guide to planning care* (5th ed). St. Louis: Mosby.

American Association of Kidney Patients. (2003). Understanding your hemodialysis access options. Available at http://kidney.niddk.nih.gov/kudiseases/pubs/vascularaccess/index.htm.

*Baer, C. (1998). Care of the critically ill chronic renal failure patient: Crisis, challenges and choices. *Critical Care Nursing Clinics of North America, 10*(4), 433-448.

Baker, J., & Thomas, A. (2001). Progressive renal insufficiency program planning: A technique for evaluation and improvement. *Nephrology Nursing Journal, 28*(1), 13-18.

Barone, C., Martin-Watson, A., & Barone, G. (2004). The postoperative care of the adult renal transplant recipient. *MEDSURG Nursing, 13*(5), 296-302.

*Bartucci, M.R. (1999). Kidney transplantation: State of the art. *AACN Clinical Issues: Advanced Practice in Acute and Critical Care, 10*(2), 153-163.

Behrens, J. (2001). Assessing anemia secondary to hemolysis in hemodialysis patients. *Nephrology Nursing Journal, 28*(2), 253-258.

Blanchet, P., et al. (2000). Urinary complications after kidney transplantation can be reduced. *Transplant Proceedings, 32*, 2769.

Burrows-Hudson, S. (2005). Chronic kidney disease: An overview. *American Journal of Nursing, 105*(2), 40-49.

Campbell, D. (2003). How acute renal failure puts the brakes on kidney function. *Nursing 2003, 33*(1), 59-64.

Cannon, J. (2004). Recognizing chronic renal failure. *Nursing 2004, 34*(1), 50-53.

Coburn, S., & Mitchell, S. (2002). Acute renal failure. *American Journal of Nursing, 102*(4), 6-12.

Dochterman, J., & Bulechek, G. (Eds.). (2004). *Nursing interventions classification (NIC)* (4th ed). St. Louis: Mosby.

Drummond, D. (2000). Caring for your patient with a permanent hemodialysis access. *Nursing 2000, 30*(3), 41-46.

Ebersole, P., Hess, P., & Luggen, A. (2004). *Toward healthy aging: Human needs and nursing response* (6th ed). St. Louis: Mosby.

Facts and Comparisons. (2004). *Drug facts and comparisons* (58th ed). St. Louis: Author.

*Giuliano, K., & Sims, T.W. (1999). Transplant issues: Infections and immunosuppressant drugs. *Dimensions of Critical Care Nursing, 18*(2), 16-19.

Hagren, B., et al. (2001). The haemodialysis machine as a lifeline: Experiences of suffering from end-stage renal disease. *Journal of Advanced Nursing, 34*(2), 196-202.

Hayes, D. (2000). Caring for your patient with a permanent renal dialysis access. *Nursing 2000, 30*(3), 41-46.

Kaplow, R., & Barry, R. (2002). Continuous renal replacement therapies. *American Journal of Nursing, 102*(11), 26-34.

Kearney, K. (2000). Dialysis disequilibrium syndrome. *American Journal of Nursing, 100*(2), 53-54.

Kellum, J. (2000). An evaluation of pharmacological strategies for the prevention and treatment of acute renal failure. *Drugs, 59*(1), 79-91.

King, B. (2000). Meds and the dialysis patient. *RN, 63*(7), 54-59.

Kuhlmann, M.K., Schmidt, F., & Kohler, H. (1999). High protein/energy vs. standard protein: Energy nutritional regimen in the treatment of malnourished hemodialysis patients. *Mineral and Electrolyte Metabolism, 25*(4-6), 306-310.

*Levine, D.Z. (1997). *Caring for the renal patient* (3rd ed.). Philadelphia: W.B. Saunders.

Manns, B., Doig, C., Lee, H., Dean, S., Tonelli, M., Johnson, D., & Donalson, C. (2003). Cost of acute renal failure requiring dialysis in the intensive care unit: Clinical and resource implications of renal recovery. *Critical Care Medicine, 31*(2), 449-455.

Martins, L., et al. (2000). Renal osteodystrophy: Histologic evaluation after renal transplantation. *Transplantation Proceedings, 32*, 2599-2601.

McCance, K., & Huether, S. (2002). *Pathophysiology: The biologic basis for disease in adults and children* (4th ed). St. Louis: Mosby.

Medline Plus (2003). Acute renal failure, chronic renal failure. Available at http://www.nlm.nih.gov/medlineplus/ency/encyclopedia_R.htm.

*Mehrotra, R., & Nolph, K.D. (1999). Low protein diets are not needed in chronic renal failure. *Mineral and Electrolyte Metabolism, 25*(4-6), 311-316.

Merck Manual B Home Edition (2003). Kidney failure. Available at http://www.merck.com/mrkshared/mmanual_home/sec11/123.jsp

Moorhead, S., Johnson, M., & Maas, M. (Eds.). (2004). *Nursing outcomes classification (NOC)* (3rd ed.). St. Louis: Mosby.

Nally, J. (2002). Acute renal failure in hospitalized patients. *Cleveland Clinic Journal of Medicine, 60*(7), 569-574.

National Kidney and Urologic Diseases Information Clearinghouse (2003). Treatment methods for kidney failure: Hemodialysis, Peritoneal Dialysis, Kidney Transplantation. Available at http://kidney.niddk.nih.gov/kudiseases/pubs/.

Nussbaum, R., McInnes, R., & Willard, H. (2001). *Thompson & Thompson: Genetics in medicine* (6th ed). Philadelphia: W.B. Saunders.

Pagana, K., & Pagana, T. (2002). *Mosby's manual of diagnostic and laboratory tests* (2nd ed.). St. Louis: Mosby.

Polkinghorne, K., & Kerr, P. (2002). Predicting vascular access failures: A collective review. *Nephrology 2002*(7), 170-176.

Ray, T. (2000). Chronic and acute renal failure: Primary care issues. *ADVANCE for Nurse Practitioners, 8*(8), 69-72.

Ro, Y., et al. (2002). The effects of aromatherapy on pruritus in patients undergoing hemodialysis. *Dermatology Nursing, 14*(4), 231-234, 237-239.

Sehgal, A.R. (2000). Outcomes of renal replacement therapy among blacks and women. *American Journal of Kidney Diseases, 35*(4 Suppl 1), S148-S152.

Siegal, B., Halbert, R., & McGuire, M. (2002). Life satisfaction among kidney transplant recipients: Demographic and biological factors. *Progress in Transplantation, 12*(4), 293-298.

Sofer, D. (2003). Chronic kidney disease: The emerging epidemic. *American Journal of Nursing, 103*(12), 23.

*Stark, J. (1998). Acute renal failure: Focus on advances in acute tubular necrosis. *Critical Care Nursing Clinics of North America, 10*(2), 159-170.

Tanyi, R. (2002). Sexual unattractiveness: A patient's story. *MEDSURG Nursing, 11*(2), 95-99.

Tran, M., & Rutecki, G. (2000). Renal disease: Tips on prevention and early recognition. *Consultant, 40*(2), 222-229.

United Network for Organ Sharing online. (2003). Available at http://www.unos.org.

U.S. Renal Data Systems. (2002). *USRDS 2002 annual data report.* Bethesda, MD: National Institutes of Health, National Institute of Diabetes and Digestive and Kidney Diseases.

UNIT **SEVENTEEN**

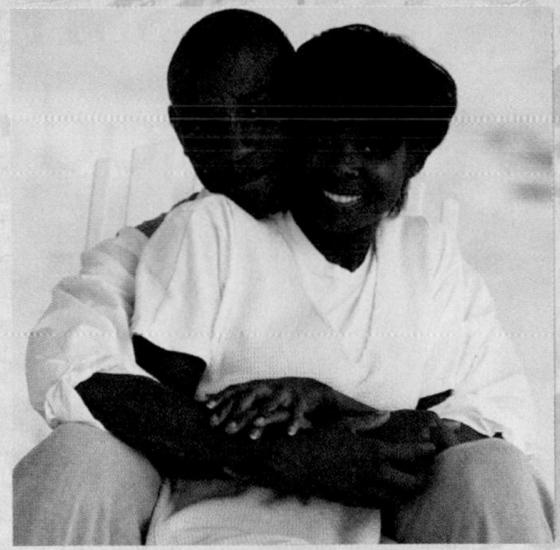

PROBLEMS of REPRODUCTION

Management of Clients with Problems of the Reproductive System

CHAPTER

76 Assessment of the Reproductive System

DEITRA LEONARD LOWDERMILK

LEARNING OUTCOMES

After studying this chapter, you should be able to:

1. Review the anatomy and physiology of the male and female reproductive systems.
2. Discuss the components of a health history for reproductive health problems using Gordon's Functional Health Patterns.
3. Explain the procedures for physical assessment of the male and female reproductive systems.
4. Describe the client preparation for common reproductive diagnostic tests.
5. Interpret common reproductive laboratory diagnostic test findings.
6. Develop a teaching plan for a client undergoing one of the endoscopic studies for reproductive health problems.
7. Explain the importance of selected reproductive screening tests in promoting and maintaining health (e.g., Pap test).

Go to your Student CD-ROM for Review Questions for the NCLEX Examination keyed to these Learning Outcomes.

The nurse is often the first health care professional to assess the client with a reproductive system disorder. Basic assessment of the male and female reproductive systems should be part of every complete physical examination. The nurse should be comfortable with his or her sexuality and be nonjudgmental about differences in sexual practices.

This chapter describes basic reproductive system assessment. Chapters 77, 78, and 79 provide additional assessment data. The student is also referred to a fundamentals or basic nursing text for a review of human sexuality.

ANATOMY AND PHYSIOLOGY REVIEW

Structure and Function of the Female Reproductive System

Females begin to develop secondary sex characteristics at a wide range of ages. The average age for a girl to begin puberty is 11 years of age. Delayed puberty may be caused by the following:

- A familial history of late growth
- A low percentage of body fat
- Problems of the pituitary gland, ovaries, or hypothalamus
- Congenital structural abnormalities

EXTERNAL GENITALIA

The external female genitalia, or **vulva,** extends from the mons pubis to the anal opening. The **mons pubis** is a fat pad that covers the symphysis pubis and protects it during **coitus** (sexual intercourse). The mons becomes prominent and covered with hair during puberty.

The **labia majora** are two vertical folds of adipose tissue that extend posteriorly from the mons pubis to the perineum. The size of the labia majora varies depending on the amount of fatty tissue present. The skin over the labia majora is usually darker than the surrounding skin and is highly vascular. The labia become prominent during puberty and develop hair on the outer surfaces. The labia majora protect inner vulval structures and enhance sexual arousal.

The labia majora surround two thinner, vertical folds of reddish epithelium called the **labia minora.** The labia minora are highly vascular and have a rich nerve supply. Emotional or physical stimulation produces marked swelling and sensitivity. Numerous sebaceous glands in the labia minora lubricate the entrance to the vagina. The **clitoris** is a small, cylindric organ that is composed of erectile tissue with a high concentration of sensory nerve endings. During sexual arousal, the clitoris becomes larger and increases sexual sensation.

The **vestibule** is a longitudinal area between the labia minora, the clitoris, and the vagina that contains Bartholin's

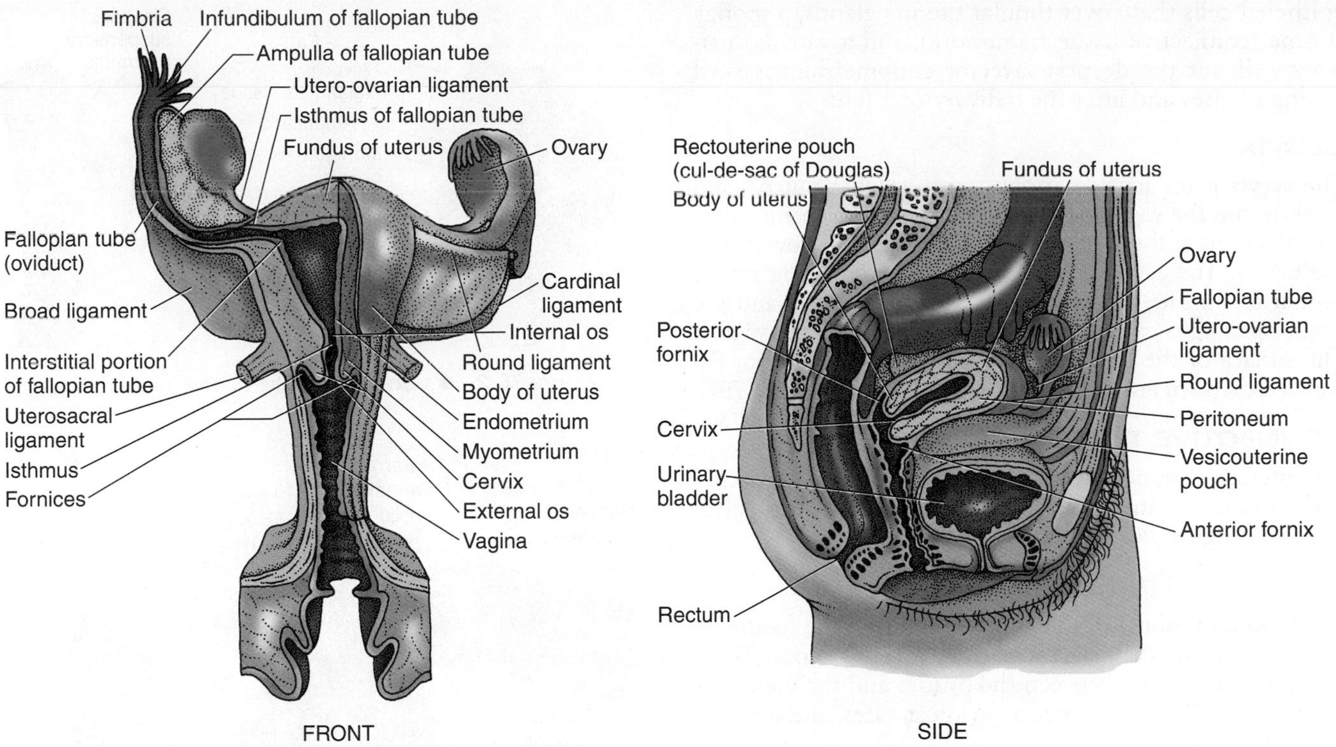

Figure 76-1 ■ Internal female genitalia.

glands and the openings of the urethra, Skene's glands (paraurethral glands), and vagina. The two Bartholin's glands, located deeply toward the back on both sides of the vaginal opening, secrete lubrication fluid during sexual excitement. Their ductal openings are usually not visible.

The area between the vaginal opening and the anus is the **perineum.** The skin of the perineum covers the muscles, fascia, and ligaments that support the pelvic structures.

INTERNAL GENITALIA

The internal female genitalia are shown in Figure 76-1.

Vagina

The **vagina** is a collapsible hollow tube that extends from the vestibule to the uterus. In addition to being the channel for the passage of the menstrual flow, the vagina allows reception of the penis during intercourse and passage of the fetus during a vaginal birth. Mucous membrane and many blood vessels line the thin, muscular walls of the vagina. This tissue lies in folds **(rugae)** during the reproductive years and is very stretchable. Reduced estrogen levels, occurring during postpartum periods, lactation, and menopause, cause the vaginal wall to become dry, thinner, and smoother.

The amounts of glycogen and lubricating fluid secreted by the vaginal cells are influenced by ovarian hormones. Döderlein's bacilli, the normal vaginal flora, interact with the secretions to produce lactic acid and maintain an acidic pH (4 to 5) in the vagina. This acidity reduces the susceptibility of the vagina to infection.

At the upper end of the vagina, the uterine cervix projects into a cup-shaped vault of thin vaginal tissue. The recessed pockets around the cervix (the fornices) permit palpation of the internal pelvic organs. The posterior area provides access into the peritoneal cavity (through the cul-de-sac of Douglas) for diagnostic or surgical purposes.

Uterus

The **uterus** is a thick-walled, muscular organ attached to the upper end of the vagina. This inverted pear-shaped organ is located within the true pelvis, between the bladder and the rectum. The uterus is composed of the corpus (body) and the cervix. The uterus responds to hormonal stimulation and prepares to receive, nurture and, finally, expel the products of conception.

The size of the uterus depends on the woman's developmental stage and obstetric history. In women who have never been pregnant, the average uterine dimensions are $3\frac{1}{2}$ inches × 2 inches × 1 inch (7.5 cm × 5 cm × 2.5 cm).

CORPUS

The upper segment of the uterine body, between the insertion sites of the fallopian tubes, is referred to as the fundus. Although the uterus is a hollow organ, its walls are in such close proximity in the nonpregnant state that its cavity is merely a slit. The uterine walls are composed of three layers: the perimetrium, the myometrium, and the endometrium.

The **perimetrium** is the outer layer that separates the uterus from the abdominal cavity. The **myometrium** is the thick, middle, muscular layer of the body of the uterus. Contraction of these muscle fibers can expel the products of conception and can constrict the blood vessels to control bleeding after childbirth.

The inner mucosal layer of the uterine body is the **endometrium**. The monthly cyclic effects of estrogen and progesterone change the thickness of this tissue (from 0.5 to 5 mm). The endometrium consists of a single layer of epithelial cells that cover tubular uterine glands, a spongy stroma (connective tissue framework), and a vascular network. All but the deepest layer of endometrium is shed during menses and after the delivery of a fetus.

CERVIX

The **cervix** is the lower, narrowed portion of the uterus and extends into the vagina. It is the passage site for sperm to enter the uterus and the passage site for menstrual flow to exit the uterus. The cervix is about 1 inch (2.5 cm) long with a central canal. The upper opening is the internal os and the lower opening is external os, which projects into the vagina. The surface of the cervix and the canal are the sites for Papanicolaou (Pap) testing. (See the later discussion on p. 1781.)

CONNECTIVE TISSUE SUPPORT

The uterus is supported by the broad, round, uterosacral, and cardinal ligaments and by the muscles of the pelvic floor (see Figure 76-1).

Fallopian Tubes

The **fallopian tubes** (uterine tubes) insert into the fundus of the uterus and extend laterally close to the ovaries. These tubes provide a duct between the ovaries and the uterus for the passage of ova and sperm. In most cases, the ovum is fertilized in these tubes.

Each tube is about $3\frac{1}{8}$ to $5\frac{1}{2}$ inches (8 to 14 cm) long and is covered by one of the peritoneal folds of the broad ligament. The tubes are lined with ciliated and secretory cells, which help move the ovum to the uterus.

The uterine tubes have four anatomic sections (see Figure 76-1). The interstitial portion is closest to the uterus, the isthmus and the ampulla are the middle segments, and the infundibulum is the most distal portion. The fimbriated ends of the infundibulum extend almost to each ovary and facilitate the capture of a released ovum during ovulation.

Ovaries

The **ovaries** are a pair of almond-shaped organs located near the lateral walls of the upper pelvic cavity. After menopause, they become smaller. These small organs develop and release ova. **Ovulation** is the cyclic maturation of a dominant follicle (the graafian follicle) and the subsequent release of the ovum. The ovaries also produce the sex steroid hormones (estrogen, progesterone, androgen, and relaxin). Adequate amounts of these steroidal sex hormones are needed for normal female growth and development and for the maintenance of a pregnancy.

BREASTS

The female **breasts** are a pair of mammary glands that develop in response to secretions from the hypothalamus, pituitary gland, and ovaries. The breasts are an accessory of the reproductive system meant to nourish the infant after birth. They also are an organ for sexual arousal in the mature adult.

The breasts are located between the second and sixth ribs, between the edge of the sternum and the midaxillary line. About two thirds of the breast lies over the greater pectoral muscle.

The structure of a mature female breast is shown in Figure 76-2. The nipple rises from the center of the pigmented

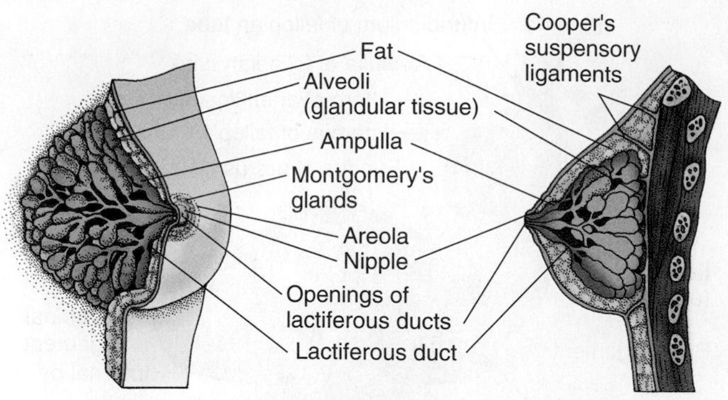

Figure 76-2 ■ Structure of the mature female breast.

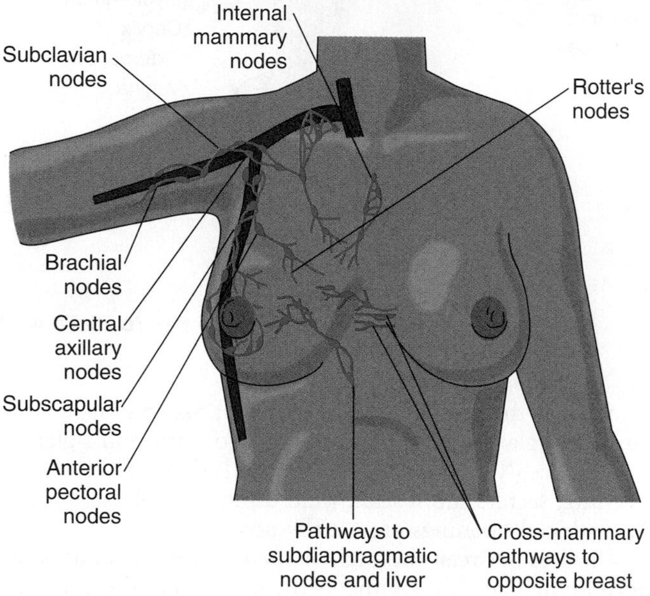

Figure 76-3 ■ Lymphatic drainage of the female breast.

areola, which is usually located slightly lateral to the midline of each breast. Montgomery's glands are small, round sebaceous glands that appear as elevations on the areola. These glands are thought to secrete a fatty substance that protects the nipple during breastfeeding.

Breast tissue is composed of a network of glandular and ductal tissue, fibrous tissue, and fat. The proportion of each component of breast tissue depends on genetic factors, nutrition, age, and obstetric history. The breast is supported by Cooper's suspensory ligaments that are attached to underlying muscles. The breasts have abundant blood supply and lymph flow. Lymph drains from an extensive network toward the axilla (Figure 76-3).

Animation: Lymphatic Drainage

The breasts may not develop symmetrically during puberty but are usually symmetric in size and contour by adulthood. It is not unusual for the breast on the woman's dominant side (on the basis of right-handedness or left-handedness) to appear larger because of the more developed pectoral muscle base.

In many women, the breasts become slightly larger and tender during the premenstrual period. The tissue may also feel nodular at this time. Increasing levels of estrogen and progesterone 3 to 4 days before menses affect the breasts by

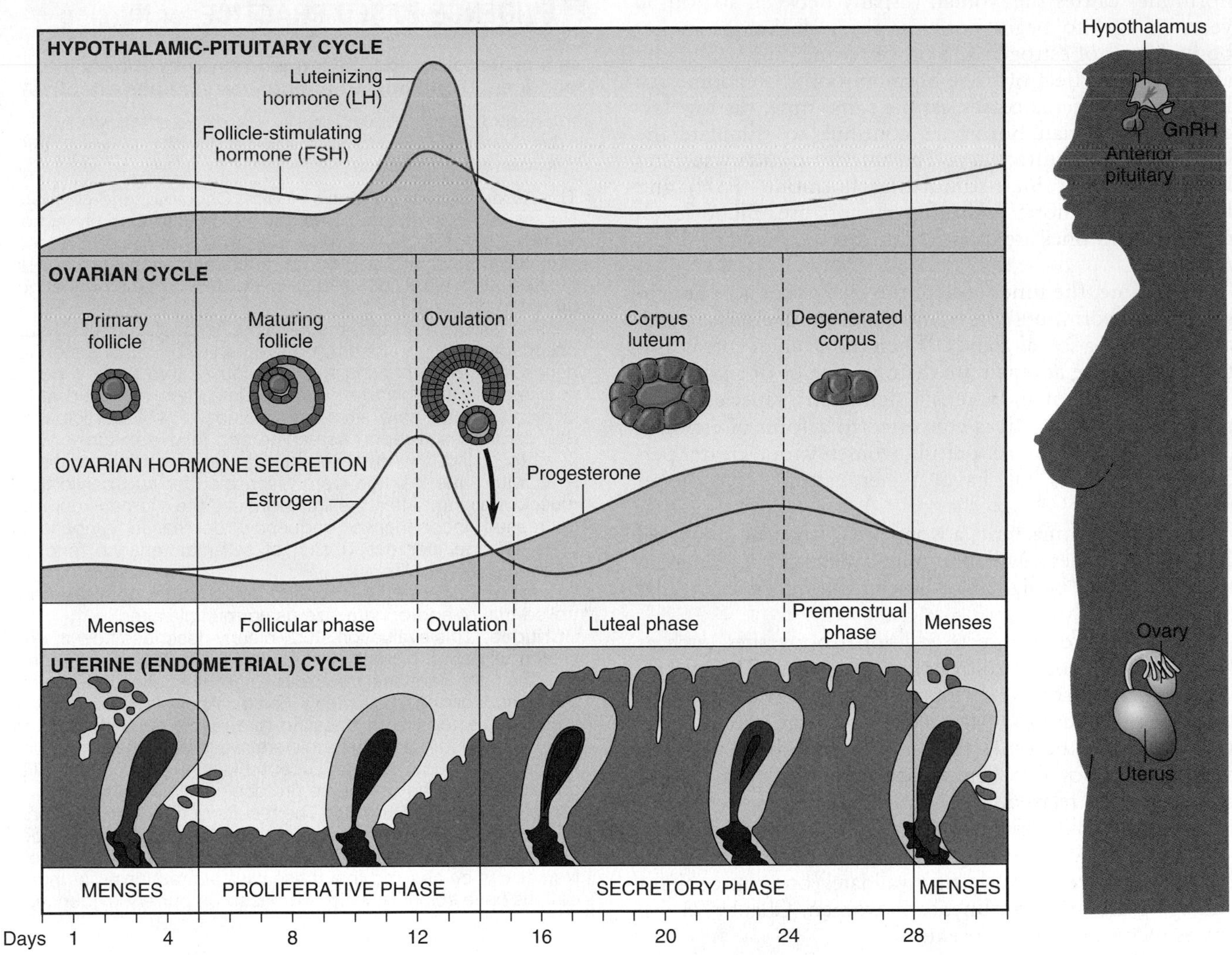

Figure 76-4 ■ Interrelationships of the events of the menstrual cycle. *GnRH,* Gonadotropin-releasing hormone.

increasing blood flow, inducing the growth of the ducts and alveoli, and promoting water retention.

MENSTRUATION AND MENOPAUSE

Normal Menstrual Cycle

Animation: Menstrual Cycle

Menstruation is the cyclic shedding of the endometrial lining of the uterus. The term **menarche** refers to the female's first menstruation and is one sign of puberty. Most girls begin to menstruate between 10 and 16 years of age.

The occurrence of cyclic menstruation and reproduction depends on maturation of the hypothalamic-pituitary-ovarian-uterine axis. Normally this cycle is not achieved for the first 1 to 2 years after menarche. The first menstrual cycles are typically anovulatory and irregular.

The menstrual cycle is under a feedback control system of three interrelated cycles: the hypothalamic-pituitary cycle, the ovarian cycle, and the uterine (or endometrial) cycle. The relationship of these cycles is illustrated in Figure 76-4.

The idealized menstrual cycle is 28 days, but variation is normal. The first day of the menstrual cycle is the first day of monthly menstrual bleeding. The menstrual flow is referred to as the **menses.** Ovulation occurs about 14 days before the beginning of the next menstrual cycle. Regular menstrual cycles indicate normal sex hormone production and the occurrence of ovulation. Variations in the length of the menstrual cycle occur in response to variations in hormone levels and surges.

Menopause and the Climacteric

NATURAL MENOPAUSE

Menopause is the biologic end of reproductive ability, but the term applies to only the last menstrual period. The actual date of menopause cannot be determined until at least 1 year has passed without menses. The phase of a woman's life from the initial decline in the amount of estrogen produced by the ovaries to the end of symptoms is called the **climacteric**. The lay term for this phase is "the change of life." Menopause is only one sign of the climacteric.

The follicles in the ovary atrophy continuously during a woman's life. The progressive decline in the number of follicles that can produce estrogen in response to pituitary hormones causes the woman (usually between 40 and 50 years of age) to begin noticing physical changes in her body. Levels of estrogen and progesterone diminish gradually until the effect of these hormones on the endometrial lining of the uterus ceases. At the same time, the low levels of the ovarian hormones continue to stimulate the hypothalamic-pituitary axis. The anterior pituitary secretes high levels of follicle-stimulating hormone (FSH) and luteinizing hormone (LH) after menopause. Blood levels of these hormones are used to confirm the presence of climacteric.

For a time, the inner core of the ovary produces **androgens** (male hormones). In women, most androgens are produced by the adrenal glands. When the ovarian core ceases to function, the adrenals are the only source of androgens. The production of androgens is significant, especially after menopause, because it is converted to a form of estrogen (estrone) in body fat. As a result, women with a greater percentage of body fat have higher estrone levels after menopause.

During the climacteric, a woman has irregular menstrual and ovarian cycles. Ovulation often fails to occur. The menstrual flow may be lighter or heavier during these irregular cycles.

Reduced estrogen affects additional body sites, such as bone density and cardiovascular function. The uterus, cervix, ovaries, labia, and clitoris shrink in size. The low estrogen levels cause the vagina to narrow and shorten. The vaginal mucosa becomes thin and dry, which makes intercourse uncomfortable. The muscular support to the pelvis becomes more relaxed. The loss of tone also reduces bladder support, which results in urinary incontinence for many women. The accompanying Evidence-Based Practice box at right summarizes a study that validates one protocol for managing urinary incontinence in women. Chapter 73 discusses incontinence in more detail.

Bone density is a concern after estrogen production decreases. Estrogen is needed by bone tissue for calcium uptake. It also increases the metabolism of vitamin D, which is needed for the absorption of calcium from the intestines. Bone density decreases in clients with decreased calcium uptake. The reduction in the amount of bone mass is called **osteoporosis** (see Chapter 54). Thus women are more at risk for bone fractures after menopause.

One of the most common symptoms that occurs during the climacteric is the hot flash, which is caused by vasomotor instability. The cause is not clear, but it is thought that surges of FSH and LH cause vasodilation and increased heat production (Fogel, 2004). In addition to physical changes during the climacteric, the woman may also experience emotional changes (including mood changes) and fatigue.

ARTIFICIAL MENOPAUSE

Menopause may occur for reasons other than the natural changes of the climacteric. Artificial menopause is the abrupt end of menstruation by some artificial means, such as an oophorectomy (surgical removal of the ovaries) or radiation to the ovaries. A premenopausal woman who experiences artificial menopause may need estrogen and progesterone therapy; however, the risks and benefits of such therapy need to be understood before making a decision (ACOG, 2003).

EVIDENCE-BASED PRACTICE for Nursing

Is a protocol for identifying women with urinary incontinence and implementing interventions effective?

Sampselle, C., et al. (2000). Continence for women: A test of AWHONN's Evidence-based protocol in clinical practice. *Journal of Obstetric, Gynecologic, and Neonatal Nursing, 29*(1), 18-26.

The Association of Women's Health, Obstetric, and Neonatal Nurses (AWHONN) sponsored a research utilization project on urinary incontinence. In phase I, an evidence-based protocol was developed and a plan for implementation was set. In phase II, data were collected, and evaluation of the project occurred in phase III.

This study reported the effectiveness of the evidence-based protocol for identifying women with urinary incontinence and for improving their outcomes through the pelvic floor muscle and bladder training. Data were collected at 21 women's health care sites and included 1474 participants. Standardized self-report screening and follow-up forms were used to collect the data. Women (57%) who reported problems with urine leakage were given bladder and pelvic floor muscle training. After the intervention, the women reported decreased incontinence frequency, decreased amount of urine leakage, decreased cost of self-maintenance, and increased quality of life.

Level of Evidence: 2—Properly designed randomized controlled trial of appropriate size using multiple sites.

Critique. This evaluation study clearly describes how the research utilization project investigated the research questions, how the data were analyzed, and what the implications are for clinicians working in women's health. Analysis included only those cases for whom baseline (pretreatment) and 4-month follow-up (posttreatment) data were available. The sample was fairly diverse, supporting an acceptable level of generalizability and supporting the use of the protocol in clinical practice.

Implications for Nursing. The results of this AWHONN project support widespread application of the screening and behavioral interventions for urinary incontinence in women. Nurses can be assured that these clinical practice recommendations have scientific rationale based on current evidence.

Structure and Function of the Male Reproductive System

EXTERNAL GENITALIA

The external male genitalia undergo many changes during puberty. The first visible sign of puberty is enlargement of the scrotum and testes, which typically occurs between 11 and 13½ years of age.

These changes occur in response to an increase in testosterone production at puberty. The release of gonadotropin-releasing hormone (GnRH) from the hypothalamus stimulates the anterior pituitary to secrete LH (luteinizing hormone) and FSH (follicle-stimulating hormone). As the levels of these hormones increase, the amount of testosterone greatly increases. Other signs of puberty that occur as a result of the presence of testosterone are the growth of axillary hair, lengthening and thickening of the vocal cords, increased sebaceous gland activity, and a general increase in muscle mass and body size.

Testosterone production is relatively constant in the adult male. Only a slight and gradual reduction of testosterone production occurs in the older adult male. Lower testosterone levels decrease muscle mass, reduce skin elasticity, and induce postural changes and changes in sexual performance.

Penis

The **penis** is an organ for urination and intercourse. It consists of the body or shaft and the glans penis (the distal end of the penis). The body is made up of three circular layers or columns of erectile tissue. Engorgement of these highly vascular, erectile columns with blood during sexual excitement causes the penis to expand and elongate and become firm and erect. The glans is the smooth end of the penis and contains the slitlike opening of the urethral meatus. The urethra is the pathway for the exit of both urine and semen.

The penis is covered by thin skin that is loosely attached to the underlying fascia. This loose skin allows the penis to enlarge during erections. The skin is darker than that of the rest of the body, and hair is present only at the base. A continuation of penile skin covers the glans and folds back on itself to form the prepuce (foreskin). Surgical removal of the foreskin (**circumcision**) for religious or cultural reasons is a common procedure in the United States.

The penis is richly innervated through branches of the sympathetic and parasympathetic nervous systems and by nerves of cerebral origin. Penile erection is under the control of the autonomic nervous system. Erection can also be induced by local reflex mechanisms (tactile stimulation) and by psychogenic mechanisms (auditory, visual, tactile, or imaginative stimulation). Sympathetic fibers control the rhythmic muscle contractions that lead to the ejaculation of semen.

Scrotum

The **scrotum** is a thin-walled, fibromuscular pouch that is behind the penis and suspended below the pubic bone. This pouch protects the testes, epididymis, and vas deferens in a space that is slightly cooler than inside the abdominal cavity. Normal sperm production and maturation **(spermatogenesis)** requires a controlled temperature. The slightly lower temperature, about 6° F (2° C) less than body temperature, is optimal for sperm production and viability.

The scrotal skin is darkly pigmented and contains sweat glands, sebaceous glands, and few hair follicles. The skin is arranged in horizontal folds called **rugae.** The rugae are more apparent when the scrotum is retracted toward the body. The scrotum contracts with cold, exercise, tactile stimulation, and sexual excitement.

INTERNAL GENITALIA

The internal male genitalia are shown in Figure 76-5.

Testes and Spermatic Cord

The testes are a pair of oval organs that produce sperm and testosterone. Each testis is suspended in the scrotum by the spermatic cord, which provides vascular, lymphatic, and nerve supply to the testis. The cord also covers the epididymis and a portion of the vas deferens. The cord and testes are surrounded by fascia and the cremaster muscle. Sympathetic nerve fibers are located on the arteries in the cord, and sympathetic and parasympathetic fibers are on the vas deferens. When the testes are traumatized, these autonomic nerve fibers transmit excruciating pain and a sensation of nausea.

EPIDIDYMIS

The **epididymis** is the first portion of a ductal system that transports sperm from the testes to the urethra. It is a site of sperm maturation. The epididymis is comma shaped, lies to one side of each testis, and is divided into a head, body, and tail. The tail merges into the vas deferens and is a storage site for maturing sperm.

VAS DEFERENS

The **vas deferens**, or ductus deferens, is a firm, muscular tube that continues from the tail of each epididymis. The

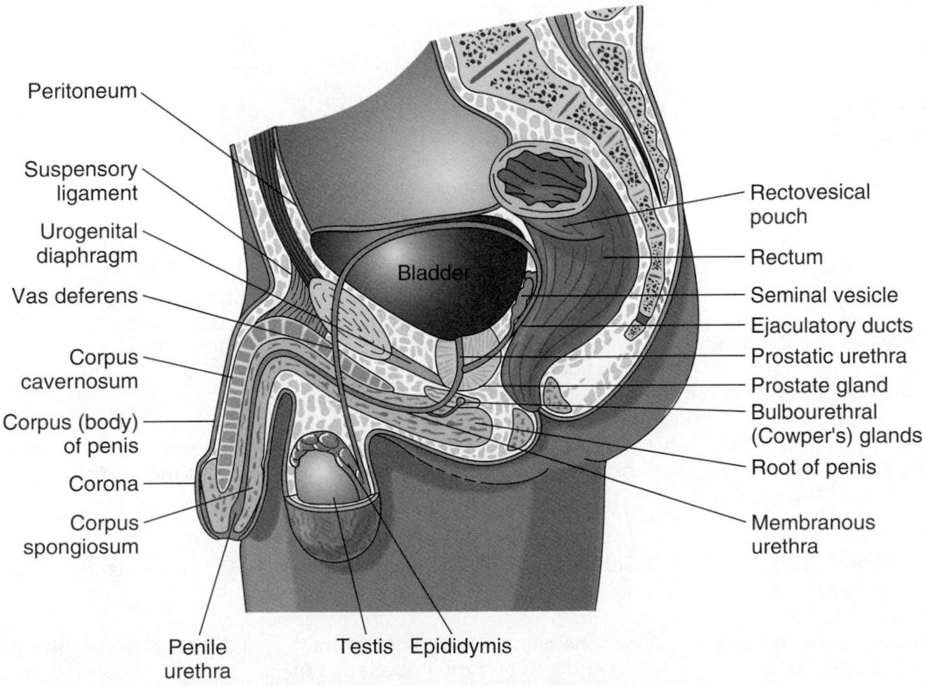

Figure 76-5 ■ Internal male genitalia.

end of each vas deferens is a reservoir for sperm and tubular fluids. They merge with ducts from the seminal vesicle to form the ejaculatory ducts at the base of the prostate gland. Sperm from the vas deferens and secretions from the seminal vesicles are transported through the ejaculatory duct to mix with prostatic fluids in the prostatic urethra.

Seminal Vesicles and Ejaculatory Ducts

The seminal vesicles are paired glands that secrete most of the volume of the ejaculate. Each vesicle ends in a small duct that joins with the end of the vas deferens to form an ejaculatory duct. The two ejaculatory ducts descend through the prostate gland and empty into the prostatic urethra.

Prostate Gland

The **prostate gland** is a large accessory gland of the male reproductive system. It is a chestnut-shaped, glandular, and fibromuscular organ. It secretes a milky alkaline fluid that adds bulk to the semen, enhances sperm motility, and neutralizes acidic vaginal secretions.

During **emission**, the first stage of the male orgasm, the prostate gland secretes its fluid at the same time as the vas deferens. The average pH of the combined secretions of semen is about 7.5, whereas secretions from the vagina normally have a pH of 3.5 to 4. Sperm need a surrounding fluid pH of 6 to 6.5 before they become optimally motile.

The prostate gland is located between the neck of the bladder and the urogenital diaphragm. It is separated from the anterior wall of the rectum by a thin fascial sheath. The prostate gland can be palpated through the rectum and should not project more than 3/8 inch (1 cm) into the rectal lumen.

As men age, the prostate gland becomes clinically significant. The gland is small at birth, but during puberty it rapidly enlarges to its normal adult size. By 40 years of age, about 10% of men have an enlarged prostate (benign prostatic hyperplasia), which can cause problems such as overflow incontinence and nocturia (Jarvis, 2004). Prostate function depends on adequate levels of testosterone. As men age, testosterone production decreases.

Inguinal Area

The inguinal area (groin) is located between the superior iliac spine and the symphysis pubis and is the junction of the lower abdominal wall and thigh. The area is a common site for a **hernia**, which is a loop of bowel that protrudes through a weak spot in the muscles (Jarvis, 2004).

Reproductive Changes Associated with Aging

Age affects the function of both the male and the female reproductive systems. After puberty, hormones produced by the gonads (testis and ovary) affect many body systems. Many changes in the reproductive system occur in older adults (Chart 76-1).

ASSESSMENT TECHNIQUES

History

DEMOGRAPHIC DATA

Use data about the client's age, gender, and culture to assess the risk for certain diseases and in evaluating the reproductive system. The age at which secondary sexual characteristics developed in the client are compared with the typical ranges for males or females (see the Cultural Considerations box on p. 1775).

CHART 76-1

NURSING FOCUS on the OLDER ADULT
Changes in the Reproductive System Related to Aging

Physiologic Change	Nursing Interventions	Rationales
Women		
Graying and thinning of the pubic hair Decreased size of the labia majora and clitoris	Discuss changes with the client (applies to all structures for both women and men).	Education helps prevent problems with body image (applies to all structures for both women and men).
Drying, smoothing, and thinning of the vaginal walls	Provide information about vaginal estrogen therapy and water-soluble lubricants.	Education enables the client to make informed decisions about the treatment of vaginal dryness, which can cause painful intercourse.
Decreased size of the uterus Atrophy of the endometrium Decreased size and marked convolution of the ovaries Loss of tone and elasticity of the pelvic ligaments and connective tissue	Provide information about Kegel exercises to strengthen pelvic muscles. Urinary incontinence can be a major problem.	Strengthening exercises may prevent or reduce pelvic relaxation and urinary incontinence.
Increased flabbiness and fibrosity of the breasts, which hang lower on the chest wall; decreased erection of the nipples	Teach or reinforce the importance of breast self-examination (BSE).	BSE may detect lumps or other changes that may indicate the presence of cancer.
Men		
Graying and thinning of the pubic hair Increased pendulousness (drooping) of the scrotum and loss of rugae	Teach or reinforce the importance of testicular self-examination (TSE).	TSE may detect changes that may indicate cancer.
Prostate enlargement, with an increased likelihood of urethral obstruction	Teach the client the signs of urethral obstruction and the importance of prostate cancer screening.	Education helps the client detect enlargement or obstruction, which may indicate the presence of cancer.

CULTURAL CONSIDERATIONS

Cultural beliefs and practices influence lifestyle and sexual practices. These beliefs and expectations account for differences in acceptable gender-related identity. A person's attitude and behavior about the meaning and use of genitals begin in early childhood and are modeled on the behavior of significant adults. Religious preferences may parallel those of a specific culture and strongly affect sexual activity. A person's religious beliefs often influence specific sexual practices, the acceptable number of partners, contraceptive use, and the decision to terminate a pregnancy, end fertility, or remove barriers to infertility (D'Avanzo & Geissler, 2003).

FAMILY HISTORY AND GENETIC RISK

The family history, including that of the parents, grandparents, siblings, and spouse, helps determine the client's risk for conditions that affect reproductive functioning. A delayed or early development of secondary sex characteristics may be a familial pattern.

The current age and health status of family members are of interest. The cause of and age at death of specific family members may also be important. Evidence of medical diseases or reproductive problems in family members (e.g., diabetes, endometriosis, complications of pregnancy, and reproductive cancer) allows better interpretation of the client's presenting symptoms. For example, daughters of women who were given diethylstilbestrol (DES) to control bleeding during pregnancy are at increased risk for infertility and reproductive tract cancer.

Recent advances in genetics determined the hereditary component of many diseases including those of the reproductive system. For example, about 10 % of all cancers have a hereditary component, but only a small percent of breast cancers are hereditary. Specific BRCA 1 and BRCA 2 gene mutations do increase the overall risk for breast or ovarian cancer (DiSaia & Creasman, 2002; Zawacki & Phillips, 2002). Men with first-degree relatives (e.g., father, brother) with prostate cancer are at greater risk for the disease than men in the general population. Testicular cancer can also be familial (O'Rourke, 2001).

PERSONAL HISTORY

Assess the client's health habits, such as diet, sleep, and exercise patterns. Low levels of body fat may be related to ovarian dysfunction. Assess the client's alcohol, tobacco, and drug use because **libido** (sex drive), sperm production, and **potency** (the ability to have and sustain an erection) can be affected by such substances (Raines, 2004).

The client's personal medical history provides data about his or her general health. Certain childhood illnesses can have an effect on the reproductive system. Women need to be screened for sufficient rubella titers and should be treated, if necessary, to prevent possible **teratogenic** effects (development of birth defects) on their unborn children if they get rubella during the first trimester of pregnancy. Mumps or smallpox in men after puberty may cause **orchitis** (painful inflammation and swelling of the testes) and occasionally leads to testicular atrophy and sterility.

Assess for any major adult illnesses or chronic illnesses that may severely affect reproductive function. Endocrine disorders may affect the hypothalamic-pituitary-gonadal function of men or women. Almost any disease that disturbs a woman's metabolism or nutrition can depress ovarian function and cause **amenorrhea** (absence of menses). Failure of ovulation is associated with a greater risk for endometrial cancer. Clients with diabetes mellitus may experience physiologic changes such as vaginal dryness or impotence. Chronic disorders of the nervous system, respiratory system, or cardiovascular system can alter the sexual response. Some drugs, especially antihypertensives, opioids, antidepressants, and histamine antagonists, may impair fertility (Raines, 2004).

Reproductive system dysfunction can also result from irradiation, prolonged use of corticosteroids, external estrogen or testosterone use, and chemotherapy drugs. In addition, past severe infections can alter a person's reproductive ability. For example, pelvic inflammatory disease or a ruptured appendix followed by peritonitis can cause strictures or adhesions in the fallopian tubes and pelvic scarring. **Salpingitis** (tubal infection) is usually caused by chlamydial infection and often results in female infertility. Infections or prolonged fever in males may damage sperm production or cause obstruction of the seminal tract, which leads to infertility. Explore the client's history of illnesses, surgeries, serious injuries, current medications, and allergies. Each of these can affect reproductive structure or function.

GENITOREPRODUCTIVE HISTORY

Obtain genitoreproductive history for both men and women. Chart 76-2 describes assessment data using Gordon's Functional Health Patterns.

Female Client

Ask the female client about her menses, including age of menarche, cycle frequency and duration, amount of flow, spotting between periods, **dysmenorrhea** (painful menstrual periods), and premenstrual symptoms. If the client is of menopausal age, determine the date of her last menstrual period, the presence of climacteric symptoms, and any drugs or alternative therapies used for these symptoms. Ask all women about the presence of vaginal discharge, a history and treatment of sexually transmitted diseases, the date and the result of the most recent Papanicolaou (Pap) test, breast self-examination practices, and vulvar self-examination practices (National Women's Health Resource Center, 2001).

Obtain an obstetric history. Women who have never had children have higher rates of ovarian, endometrial, and breast cancer than do women who have had children. If the woman has ever been pregnant, ask about the outcome of the pregnancies. Collect information about the following: the date and mode of deliveries or termination of the pregnancy; complications during pregnancy, labor, and delivery; birth weight and gestational age of the infants; and the health of the infants at birth and at present.

Data about sexual activity is important to obtain as part of the history. Heterosexual activity should not be assumed. Homosexual (gay) and bisexual issues are most often not assessed by the nurse or discussed by the client. Explore information about sexual practices in a nonjudgmental manner.

An early age at first intercourse and multiple sex partners are associated with an increased risk for cervical cancer. Ask about satisfaction with sexual response, any pain or bleeding with sexual intercourse, and contraceptive use. Religious

CHART 76-2

Reproductive Assessment
USING GORDON'S FUNCTIONAL HEALTH PATTERNS

Health Perception/Health Management Pattern
- Has anyone in your family had cancer of the breast or reproductive organs? Who and what type of cancer?
- If you engage in sexual activities, do you practice "safer" sex?
- What do you do to keep healthy—regular health checkups, self-examination (breast, genital [vulvar, testicular]), healthy diet, exercise, use of medications or alternative therapies?

Sexuality-Reproductive Pattern
- *Male and Female:* Are you sexually active? Do you find your sexual relationship satisfying? Have there been any changes in your relationship? Are you having any problems in your sexual relationship?
- Do you use contraceptives? If so, do you have any problems with the method of contraception?
- Have you had any sexually transmitted diseases? If yes, when and what type did you have?
- *Female:* When did you first start menstruating? When was your last menstrual period? Do you have any menstrual problems?
- Have you ever been pregnant? If so, how many times and what were the outcomes?
- Have you had any symptoms of menopause?
- *Male:* Do you have any problems with getting and maintaining an erection, or do you have difficulty with ejaculation?
- Have you ever had a hernia or pain in the groin?

Self-Perception/Self-Concept Pattern
- How would you describe yourself? Do you feel good or not so good about yourself?
- Have you experienced changes in your body appearance or function? If so, are these problematic for you? Have you felt anxious, fearful, or depressed about these changes?

Based on Gordon, M. (2002). *Manual of nursing diagnosis* (10th ed.). St. Louis: Mosby.

TABLE 76-1 Abuse Screening Questions*

1. Are you with a spouse or partner who threatens or physically hurts you?
2. In the past year has anyone hurt, slugged, kicked, or otherwise hurt you?
3. Has your spouse or partner forced you to have sexual activity that made you uncomfortable?
4. Are you afraid of your spouse or partner?

*Never ask questions with partner present.

Source: American College of Obstetricians and Gynecologists. (2002). *Screening tools for domestic violence.* ACOG Violence Against Women Homepage. Retrieved June 13, 2003, from http://www.acog.org.

beliefs or type of sex (oral, anal, and vaginal) may dictate the contraceptive practices. Assessment for intimate partner abuse may be included at this point of the interview or at another point during the interview for all women. Table 76-1 lists suggested questions that you should ask regarding potential abuse.

Male Client

Ask the male client about testicular changes and self-examination practices, problems with urination, discharge from the penis, rectal problems, history and treatment of sexually transmitted diseases, and symptoms related to hernias.

Ask about sexual functioning. Reproductive history and contraceptive use, current problems or changes in sexual response, any difficulty with erection, ejaculation, or infertility, and the use of drugs or treatments direct the physical assessment. The type of sex practiced also allows attention to be focused on the body area involved.

DIET HISTORY

A diet history is often critical for the correct interpretation of reproductive system problems. For example, fatigue and low libido may occur with poor diet and anemia. Obesity raises the risk for uterine cancer. High-fat diets may increase the risk for cancer of the breast, ovary, and prostate gland (ACS, 2005). Ask the client to recall his or her dietary intake for a recent 24-hour period to assess diet quality.

Compare the client's height, weight, and body mass index with the dietary recall. The client may be hesitant to divulge practices such as bingeing, purging, anorexic behaviors, or excessive exercise; however, these practices may affect the reproductive system. A certain level of body fat and weight is necessary for the onset of menses and the maintenance of regular menstrual cycles. Decreased body fat results in insufficient estrogen levels for the maintenance of normal ovulatory cycles.

Women have special dietary needs. The diet of women who use oral contraceptives should have increased sources of folic acid and vitamins B_6, B_{12}, and C. Heavy menstrual bleeding, particularly in women who have intrauterine devices, may require oral iron supplements. Teach all women about their body's need for calcium. Although adequate calcium intake throughout life is optimal, it is especially important during and after menopause. The bone density loss at this time because of reduced estrogen levels predisposes perimenopausal women to osteoporosis and fractures (see Chapter 54).

SOCIOECONOMIC STATUS

The social history of the client provides insight into the whole person, including stressors, job history, education, and support systems. Ask about smoking and the use of alcohol and drugs. All of these factors can influence reproductive system health.

Stressors

Stress is associated with menstrual and ovulatory problems and infertility. Ask the client about leisure time activities that pose a high risk of injury to the reproductive system. For example, men who lounge for long periods in hot tubs or saunas may experience decreased sperm production. Women who exercise vigorously have lower levels of body fat and more menstrual problems (Sabatini, 2001).

Occupation

The client's work may directly affect the reproductive system. Occupational exposure to potential teratogenic substances (agents capable of producing birth defects in offspring) results in a higher incidence of abnormal sperm and low sperm counts in men or miscarriages in women. People who work around certain chemicals, radiation, and heavy metals are at risk. Trauma and exposure to extremely high temperatures in the workplace are potential causes of male infertility. Exposure to some industrial agents, such as cadmium, may be related to the development of cancers of the reproductive system.

Education

Assess the educational level of the client to individualize health teaching. Lay language for body parts and functions is commonly used when discussing the reproductive system (e.g., the term "womb" for uterus). Be familiar with such terms and be comfortable in their use. Clients may try to evoke a particular response in you by using certain words, or they may know no other terms to express the problem. Responding with shock or disdain displays a judgmental attitude that hinders successful data gathering. Use these teaching opportunities to provide more appropriate terminology.

Support Systems

The client's general satisfaction with life and the support systems available can directly relate to the current health problem. Questions that elicit information about daily routines often give insight into the client's perception of the quality of life and outlook for the future.

CURRENT HEALTH PROBLEMS

If a client seeks medical attention for a problem related to the reproductive system, ask additional questions to explore the chief complaint. Most problems concern pain, bleeding, discharge, masses, and reproductive functioning (Chart 76-3).

Pain

Pain related to reproductive system disorders may be confused with that associated with gastrointestinal or urinary tract problems. Ask the client to describe the nature of the pain, including its type, intensity, timing and location, duration, and relationship to menstrual, sexual, urinary, or gastrointestinal function. Assess the factors that **exacerbate** (worsen) the pain or give relief.

Bleeding

Heavy bleeding or a lack of bleeding may concern the client. Consider the possibility of pregnancy in any sexually active woman with amenorrhea. Any postmenopausal bleeding needs to be evaluated. Ask the client to describe the amount and character of abnormal vaginal or penile bleeding. Assess whether the bleeding occurs in relation to the menstrual cycle or menopause, intercourse, trauma, or strenuous exercise. Ask about any associated symptoms, such as pain, cramping or abdominal fullness, a change in bowel habits, urinary difficulties, and weight changes. Many factors can cause bleeding, and sites other than the genital tract need to be considered.

Discharge

Discharge from either the male or female reproductive tract can cause severe irritation of the surrounding tissues, itching, pain, embarrassment, and anxiety. Ask about the amount, color, consistency, odor, and chronicity of the discharge. Drugs (e.g., antibiotics) and clothing (e.g., tight jeans and synthetic underwear fabric) may cause or worsen genital discharge. Many types of discharge are caused by sexually transmitted diseases (see Chapter 80). The body location of these infections depends on the client's sexual practices. Ask the client about lesions, bleeding, itching, and pain related to the genitals and orifices used during sexual activity. Ask about the presence of symptoms in the sexual partner.

Masses

Any reported masses in the breasts, testes, or inguinal area need to be evaluated. Some masses change in character or size, and the client can often relate these changes to menstrual cycles, heavy lifting, straining, or trauma. Ask about associated symptoms such as tenderness, heaviness, pain, dimpling, and tender lymph nodes.

CHART 76-3

BEST PRACTICE for
Client Complaints Related to the Reproductive System

Complaint	Nursing Assessment
Pain	Type and intensity of pain Location and duration of pain Factors that relieve or worsen pain Relationship to menstrual, sexual, urinary, or gastrointestinal function Medications
Bleeding	Presence or absence of bleeding Character and amount of bleeding Relationship of bleeding to events or other factors (e.g., menstrual cycle) Onset and duration of bleeding Presence of associated symptoms, such as pain
Discharge	Amount and character of discharge Presence of genital lesions, bleeding, itching, or pain Presence of symptoms or discharge in sexual partner
Masses	Location and characteristics of mass Presence of associated symptoms, such as pain Relationship to menstrual cycle

Critical Thinking Challenge

Client 1—A 20-year-old woman who runs cross-country for her college has come to the clinic complaining of amenorrhea. She is sexually active but not using any birth control method on a regular basis.

Client 2—A 55-year-old man has come to the clinic complaining that he has trouble urinating and when he is done he still has the urge. He discloses that he drinks beer daily and eats a diet high in fat. He has engaged in unprotected sexual intercourse recently.

For each of these clients:

1. What other data about the present health status, past health history, or family history are needed to explore these complaints?
2. What is your rationale for asking for these data?
3. What other physical assessment data should you obtain?
4. How should you address this client's need for protection against unwanted pregnancy or sexually transmitted disease?

evolve For suggested answer guidelines, go to http://evolve.elsevier.com/Iggy/.

Physical Assessment

ASSESSMENT OF THE FEMALE REPRODUCTIVE SYSTEM

Examination of the breasts, axillae, and lymph nodes precedes that of the anterior thorax in a complete physical examination. Inspection of the female genitalia and the pelvic examination are usually performed at the end of the physical examination. The client is often more apprehensive about these portions of the examination than about any other segment. Pain or lack of privacy during previous pelvic or breast examinations may prevent the client from relaxing.

Show the client the equipment to be used, along with three-dimensional models, to demonstrate the assessment procedures. Teach the client relaxation and breathing techniques to enhance the client's sense of control. Inform the client about what is going to be done and what she may feel as the examination proceeds to allow her to incorporate learned coping mechanisms more successfully than if she were not expecting any discomfort. If the client displays signs of pain or exceptional concern during the procedures, the examination should stop and adjustments made in the assessment plan or techniques. For example, clients who have been sexually abused may become upset during pelvic examinations (Zdanuk, 2004). The presence of a support person or having the examination performed by an examiner who is the same gender as the client may be of benefit to the client during the examination.

A pelvic examination is indicated to assess the presence or amount of the following:

- Menstrual irregularities
- Unexplained abdominal pain
- Vaginal discharge or infection
- Appropriateness of a desired contraceptive
- Rape trauma
- Physical changes in the vagina, cervix, uterus, and adnexa
- Infertility

The woman should not douche for at least 24 hours before the pelvic examination, because doing so may prevent an accurate evaluation of smears, cultures, and cytologic data.

Before the pelvic and breast examinations, ask the client to empty her bladder and undress completely. Drape the woman adequately to protect modesty throughout the examination. If she is not wearing a gown, a small towel can be placed over the breasts under the larger drape. Remove drapes only over the region being examined and replace them when that area has been examined. Drapes that prevent eye contact between the examiner and the client dehumanize the client and prevent successful assessment of comfort during the examination. Mirrors can be used to facilitate teaching if the client so desires. The examination is performed in a room with adequate lighting for body inspection, a comfortable temperature, and the assurance of privacy.

Breast Examination

The physical examination of the reproductive system often includes the breasts (see Chapter 77).

Abdominal Examination

After the breast examination, the examiner generally completes the thoracic and cardiovascular examinations and then inspects, auscultates, and palpates the abdomen. The client's arms should be at her sides or over her chest to allow better relaxation of the abdominal muscles. During the gynecologic examination, the examiner palpates for symptomatic and asymptomatic abdominopelvic masses. A mass can be of reproductive, intestinal, or urinary tract origin. Careful history taking combined with the physical examination can usually determine the origin of a mass. Gynecologic masses, such as ovarian and adnexal masses, can be further differentiated from lesions on the body of the uterus during the bimanual portion of the pelvic examination.

CHART 76-4

CLIENT EDUCATION GUIDE
Vulvar Self-Examination

- Perform a vulvar self-examination monthly between menstrual periods if you are older than 18 years of age or if you are sexually active.
- Sit in a well-lighted area on a soft surface (bed or carpeted floor).
- Use a handheld mirror to see your external genitalia.
- Examine the area around the vaginal opening from the mons pubis to the perianal area.
- Feel and visually inspect the area.
- Report to your health care provider new nodes, warts, growths of any type, ulcers, sores, blisters, change in skin color, painful areas, areas of itching or inflammation, or any change in vaginal discharge.

Examination of the External Genitalia

◄ Video Clip: External Genitalia

After the abdominal examination, prepare the client for the inspection of the external genitalia and the pelvic examination. Assist the woman into the lithotomy position and ask her to place her arms at her sides or over her chest. The client's buttocks extend slightly beyond the edge of the table, and her thighs are abducted. All equipment for the vaginal and speculum examination and cytologic studies is prepared. The examiner wears gloves to protect against possible disease and potential cross-contamination from other clients. The client is informed that the genitalia will be touched and separated.

The initial inspection and palpation of the external genitalia provide an assessment of age-appropriate development. Hair color and distribution over the symphysis pubis and vulva suggest the woman's age and hormonal functioning. The pubic hair is inspected for the presence of lice or scabies. The skin and mucosa of the vulva are inspected in a systematic pattern from anterior to posterior for signs of inflammation, infestation, swelling, lesions, and discharge.

The paraurethral glands (Skene's glands) are barely visible on either side of the urethral meatus. If infection is suspected, the urethra should be gently "milked" by inserting the index finger into the vagina and gently pressing the finger pad against the anterior vaginal wall as the finger is being withdrawn. This procedure usually produces no pain or discharge unless there is inflammation or infection. The openings of the ducts from the Bartholin's glands cannot be seen. The area just outside the lower vaginal orifice is palpated carefully to assess for inflammation, tenderness, or swelling. Any discharge from these ducts is cultured, because these structures are often involved in gonorrheal infections.

The examination of the external female genitalia is an excellent time for teaching about **vulvar self-examination (VSE).** The incidence of precancerous conditions and infectious diseases of the vulva is increasing, especially in young women (DiSaia & Creasman, 2002). VSE can easily be taught and can lead to early diagnosis of vulvar conditions (Chart 76-4).

Perineal support and the strength of the vaginal walls are assessed by asking the woman to squeeze the vaginal open-

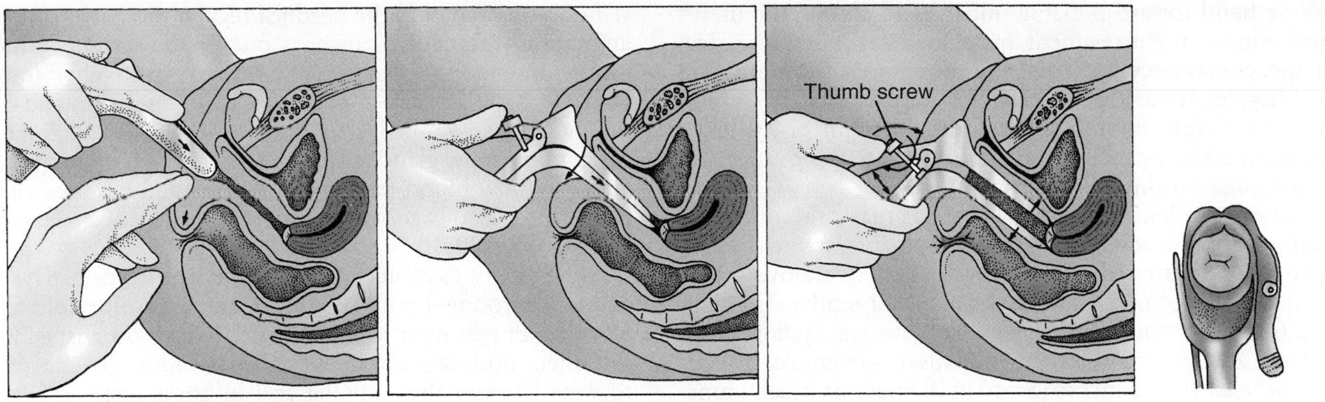

1. With the speculum blades positioned vertically, the nurse presses down on the perineal body just inside the vagina as the speculum is inserted.

2. The nurse removes the fingers from the vagina while continuing to insert the closed blades of the speculum to their full length and rotating them into a horizontal position.

3. The nurse opens the blades and maneuvers the speculum for optimal visualization of the cervix, then tightens the thumb screw to lock the blades in place.

View of the cervix through the speculum

Figure 76-6 ■ Internal examination of the cervix.

ing closed after the examiner has inserted two fingers. The client is then asked to strain downward while the examiner assesses for urinary incontinence or any bulging of the anterior or posterior vaginal walls that would indicate a cystocele or rectocele, respectively.

Pelvic Examination

Video Clip: Speculum Examination

▶ EXAMINATION WITH A SPECULUM

After the correct speculum size is selected, the speculum may be warmed and lubricated with warm water. Lubricant should not be used if cytologic studies are to be collected because it interferes with specimen analysis. Tell the woman when the speculum is going to be inserted. The examiner's fingers can ease insertion of the speculum by pressing down on the perineal body just inside of the vaginal orifice (Figure 76-6, step 1). The woman can also be asked to breathe slowly and to bear down. The closed speculum is inserted in an oblique position, with the pressure exerted toward the posterior vaginal wall. The examiner removes his or her fingers and then rotates the closed blades of the speculum to a horizontal position while inserting the speculum to its full length (see Figure 76-6, step 2). The blades are opened, and the speculum is maneuvered to enable visualization of the cervix. The blades are locked in place by tightening the thumbscrew of the speculum (see Figure 76-6, step 3).

Video Clip: Bimanual Examination

The cervix is inspected for color, shape, and dilation of the os and for erosions, nodules, masses, discharge, and bleeding.

Herpes simplex, syphilis, and carcinomas can produce characteristic lesions on the cervix. Specimens are obtained from the cervix, endocervix, and vaginal pool for cytologic studies (see Microscopic Studies, p. 1784). After completion of the cervical examination, the thumbscrew of the speculum is loosened to close the blades and the speculum is rotated slowly to a vertical position as it is withdrawn. The vaginal tissue is inspected for lesions or inflammation during withdrawal.

▶ BIMANUAL EXAMINATION

After withdrawing the speculum, proceed with the bimanual examination. Use a new glove and lubricant, stand and insert one or two fingers of one hand into the client's vagina (Figure 76-7). Palpate the posterior vaginal wall and check for masses or tenderness. The cervix and fornix around the cervix are identified. Place the opposite hand on the client's abdomen–between her umbilicus and symphysis pubis–and press downward. Lift the cervix and uterus with the

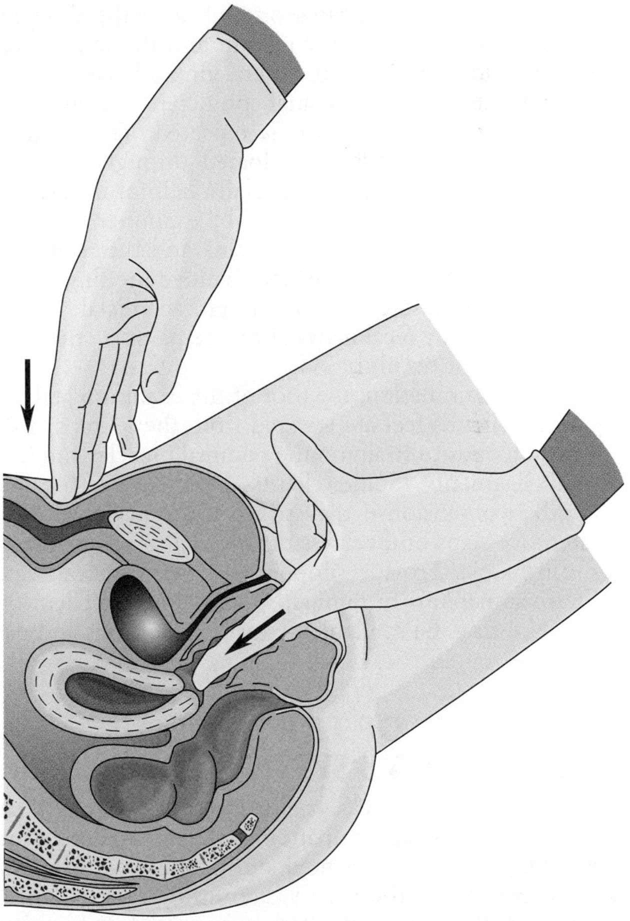

Figure 76-7 ■ Technique of bimanual pelvic examination.

pelvic hand toward the abdominal hand to trap the uterus and adnexa for assessment by palpation. Assess the size, shape, consistency, location, and mobility of the uterus and for any tenderness or masses. To palpate each ovary and tube, press the abdominal hand into the right or left lower quadrant. The fingers in the fornix palpate the ovaries and adnexa against the opposite hand.

Obesity or tense abdominal muscles may prevent the examiner from locating the ovaries. If palpable, the ovaries are 3 cm long, 2 cm wide, and 1 cm thick; they are ovoid, feel firm and smooth, and may feel somewhat tender. The uterine tubes are not usually palpable. Ovarian cysts may be painful and recurrent in premenopausal women. An ovarian cyst smaller than 2 inches (5 cm) in diameter is usually functional and responds to hormonal influence. Cysts larger than 2 inches in diameter are possible neoplasms. The ovaries are normally atrophied and not palpable 3 to 5 years after menopause; therefore any palpable structure in this area of postmenopausal women suggests cancer.

RECTOVAGINAL EXAMINATION

The rectovaginal and rectal examination is the last part of the pelvic examination. Change and lubricate the glove and place the middle finger in the rectum and the index finger in the vagina. Insertion of the rectal finger is easier if the client strains and relaxes the anal sphincter. The procedure for the bimanual examination is repeated. The posterior vaginal and uterine walls are palpated through the rectal mucosa. This examination is especially helpful in assessing a retroflexed or retroverted uterus. The examiner can assess the tissue structure between the vagina and the rectum by palpating between the two fingers. Remove the finger from the vagina and fold into the palm. Rotate the rectal finger as it is withdrawn; any fecal material that remains on the glove may be tested for occult blood.

After the examination, the foot of the examining table is raised. The client's feet are lowered from the stirrups at the same time to reduce strain on the perineal muscles and lumbosacral ligaments. Some clients experience orthostatic (postural) hypotension if they sit up too quickly. Evaluate the client for signs of dizziness before letting her get off the examining table. Provide supplies, such as perineal wipes and perineal napkins or minipads, and allow the client privacy for dressing. Be available to answer questions and provide support.

ASSESSMENT OF THE MALE REPRODUCTIVE SYSTEM

Unless a male client seeks health care for a genital tract problem, inspection and palpation of the male genitalia and rectum may not be performed during physical examinations, depending on the health care setting and the age of the client. Male clients are often embarrassed and anxious when the reproductive system is assessed. This concern may be worse when the examiner is a woman. The client may be concerned about discomfort, the developmental stage of his genitalia, or the likelihood of an erection during the examination. If the client does have an erection, the examiner should assure him that this is a normal response to a tactile stimulus and should continue the examination.

The examination of the male genitalia is a good opportunity to teach the client about contraceptives, testicular self-examination, and the need for regular prostate gland examinations. Testicular cancer is one of the most common cancers in young men and can be treated effectively if found early. Prostate cancer is common in older men, and the prognosis is favorable if diagnosed early. Annual digital rectal and prostate gland examinations and prostate-specific antigen (PSA) blood tests are recommended for men older than 50 years of age with a life expectancy of at least 10 years (ACS, 2005).

Wear gloves to protect against possible infection. The examination room should be private and a comfortable temperature. Proper light sources are needed for the inspection. The client undresses completely but should be given a gown to wear because the genitalia and buttocks need to be exposed. As with examinations of other body systems, explain each step of the assessment procedure before performing it. The client needs to be reassured that the examiner will stop and change the assessment plan or technique if the client perceives pain during the examination. Relaxation techniques and support during the examination can increase the tolerance of minimal discomfort.

Video Clips: Inspection (Standing) ◀

Examination of the External Genitalia

The client may be in a lying or a standing position for inspection and palpation of the external genitalia. Sit on a chair in front of the client. A general observation is made of the secondary sex characteristics. Note the age appropriateness of the developmental stage, including the distribution pattern of the pubic hair, the descent and size of the testes, and the size of the scrotum and penis. Inspect the pubic hair for the presence of lice or scabies.

Inspect the skin of the penis for intactness; the dorsal vein should be apparent. Note any lesions or ulcers on the penis, and scrape a specimen for cytologic study if needed. If the client has not been circumcised, he is asked to retract the foreskin. This should be accomplished easily unless the client has **phimosis** (a tight foreskin that cannot be retracted). Inspect the glans penis for possible inflammation, fungal infection, syphilitic chancres, and carcinomas. **Smegma,** a white, cheesy secretion from the sebaceous glands in the glans, may accumulate under the foreskin. This secretion is not present in the circumcised male.

The glans is also inspected for placement of the urinary meatus. Positions other than at the distal end of the glans are abnormal. By compressing the glans between the thumb and index finger, the meatus is separated and any discharge present can be determined. Urethral discharge is not normal, and a specimen should be obtained for culture. The foreskin is replaced if it has been retracted. The body of the penis is palpated between the thumb and first two fingers; note tenderness, hard areas under the skin, and signs of inflammation.

Inspection of the scrotum and inguinal areas is best accomplished by having the client hold the penis up and to the side. Document the shape and contour of the scrotum. Normally, the left side of the scrotum is lower than the right because the left testicle has a longer spermatic cord. Both the anterior and posterior surfaces of the scrotum are inspected for lesions, nodules, rashes, pain, and edema. Swelling of the scrotum may indicate a hydrocele (collection of serous fluid in the scrotal sac), infection, or torsion (twisting) of the spermatic cord.

Palpation of the scrotum, testes, epididymis, and spermatic cords is best accomplished in a warm environment so the scrotum hangs low and relaxed. Hold the scrotum gently between the thumb and two fingers and compare the contents of each side of the scrotal pouch. Locate and examine each testis for size, shape, symmetry, tenderness, nodules, and consistency.

The normal testis has smooth borders, is somewhat sensitive to light palpation, and feels rubbery. The epididymis can be palpated on the posterior surface of the testis. It is examined for size, shape, and tenderness. In clients with infection of the epididymis, its outline cannot be distinguished. Palpate the spermatic cord along its length between the epididymis and the superficial inguinal ring; nodules and swelling are noted and further evaluated. Varicose veins of the spermatic cord (varicocele) feel like a "bag of worms" above the testis.

Any swollen area of the scrotum should be transilluminated. The examining room is darkened for this procedure, and the beam from the penlight is directed through the scrotal swelling from the posterior surface of the scrotum. The light transmits a red glow if the swelling contains serous fluid. Blood and solid tissue do not transmit the light.

Stroke the inner thigh with a blunt instrument (e.g., the handle of the reflex hammer) to elicit the **cremasteric reflex**. If this reflex is intact, the testicle and scrotum rise on the stroked side.

Video Clip: Inguinal Hernia Evaluation

Examination for Inguinal Hernia

To palpate for inguinal hernias, the client stands in front of the examiner. Use the right index finger to examine the client's right side and the left index finger to examine the left side. To provide sufficient mobility of the examining finger, place a fingertip low on the scrotal pouch and direct the loose skin of the pouch toward the inguinal canal. The slitlike opening of the external inguinal ring is located by following the direction of the spermatic cord. If possible, gently press the finger into the canal, ask the client to cough or bear down, and be alert for a tapping or pushing sensation against the finger–a sign that a hernia may be present.

Examination of the Rectum and Prostate

The final assessment of the male reproductive system is an examination of the rectum and the prostate gland. This examination can be performed with the client in a knee-chest position, in a lithotomy position, in a left lateral with knees flexed position, or standing and leaning over the examining table with the feet turned inward to relax the buttocks.

Proper lighting is necessary to visualize the anus and surrounding tissue. Note and record any lesions, ulcerations, masses, or fissures.

To assess the prostate gland, press the pad of a well-lubricated, gloved index finger against the anus. As the sphincter relaxes, slowly insert the finger in the direction of the umbilicus and rotate it to palpate the anterior rectal wall. The posterior surface of the prostate gland is felt extending less than $^3/_8$ inch (1 cm) into the rectum. Inform the client that he may feel an urge to urinate as the prostate is being examined but that he will not do so. Note the size of the lateral prostate lobes and their contour and consistency. The prostate should feel firm (the consistency has been equated to that of a pencil eraser), smooth, and slightly mobile. It should be nontender across its diameter.

Extend the finger further to attempt to palpate the seminal vesicles, which are palpable only if they are inflamed. If any discharge is secreted from the penis during palpation of the prostate gland and seminal vesicles, obtain specimens for culture and microscopic examination. Remove the examining finger, and test any fecal material for occult blood.

Psychosocial Assessment

The psychosocial assessment may suggest some contributory factors to the client's illness. During the social history, ask about the client's sources of support, strengths, and likely reactions to illness or dysfunction.

A client's personal history or beliefs may negatively influence his or her ability to enjoy a satisfactory sexual life. These factors may include the following:

- Sexual trauma or abuse inflicted during childhood or adulthood
- Punishment or reproach for masturbation
- Psychological trauma
- Cultural influences, such as the idea of female passivity during intercourse
- Concerns about sexual partners or sexual lifestyle
- Use of alcohol or street drugs

Fears may affect the client's satisfaction with sexuality or body image. He or she may also be concerned about the potential or actual reaction of family members to reproductive health problems (see Chart 76-2).

Diagnostic Assessment

LABORATORY TESTS

Papanicolaou Test

The **Papanicolaou test,** or **Pap smear,** is a cytologic study that is effective in detecting precancerous and cancerous cells from the cervix (Adams, 2002). Health care providers vary in their recommendations for the frequency of routine Pap tests. The American Cancer Society (ACS) advises all women to begin having an annual Pap test within 3 years of becoming sexually active or by 21 years of age. Annual screening is recommended to 30 years of age (with the conventional Pap test or every 2 years if a liquid-based test is used. After three or more consecutive negative test results, Pap tests may be performed less frequently until 65 to 70 years of age. Women who have had no abnormal tests for 10 years may choose to discontinue getting tested (ACS, 2005; U.S. Preventive Services Task Force, 2003). Women who have had a hysterectomy may need less frequent screening or may not need screening at all (DiSaia & Creasman, 2002; Saraiya et al., 2001). However, many clinicians continue to suggest that the test be performed annually during routine physical examinations.

Cytologic examinations can also detect viral, fungal, and parasitic disorders. Examination of cells from the vaginal walls can evaluate the function of steroid hormones.

CLIENT PREPARATION. The Pap test should be scheduled between the client's menstrual periods so that the menstrual flow does not interfere with the test interpretation. The woman should not douche, use vaginal medications or deodorants, or have sexual intercourse for at least 24 hours before the test.

Assist the woman into the lithotomy position. Relaxation techniques, including concentrating on breathing patterns or a visual focal point, may help the apprehensive

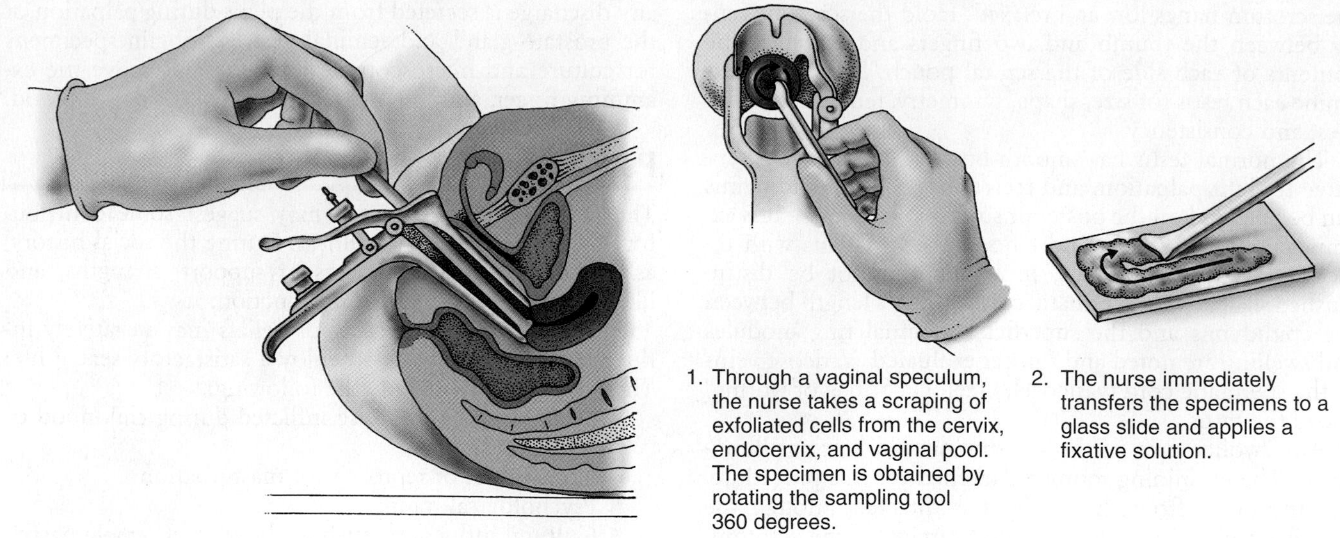

Figure 76-8 ■ Procedure for obtaining a cervical smear (Pap test).

client. All steps of the examination are explained to the client before they are performed.

PROCEDURE. A speculum is inserted into the vagina. Usually, the cervix is visualized and then scraped with one of the various sampling tools available, such as a cytology brush, cotton-tipped applicator, endocervical aspirator, or wooden or plastic spatula. The use of brushes improves the quality of cells obtained for analysis (Jarvis, 2004).

One sample is taken from the endocervical canal and a second from the ectocervical and squamocolumnar junction (Figure 76-8). Both specimens are immediately transferred to glass slides and are either sprayed with or immersed in a fixative solution. If the smear dries on the slide before the fixative is applied, the diagnosis will be inaccurate. The slides are sent to a laboratory for interpretation (Huff, 2000).

The liquid-based test (e.g., ThinPrep Pap Test) is an improved method of sample preservation. After the sample is obtained, the cells are rinsed into a vial filled with a preserving solution. The vial is sent to the laboratory, where an automated instrument separates the cells from blood and mucus. The thinner layer of cells can then be better visualized under a microscope, which improves the accuracy of the test (Biscotti et al., 2002).

FOLLOW-UP CARE. Provide the client with a perineal pad, if needed, to protect her clothes from any bleeding from the cervix. The test results may be shared with the client in person, by telephone, or by letter. If a woman's smear has atypical cells, she is urged to have follow-up testing.

DNA Human Papillomavirus (HPV)

Testing with the HC2 High-Risk HPV DNA test can identify 13 high-risk types of HPV associated with the development of cervical cancer. This test can be done at the same time as the Pap test for women older than 30 years of age as well as for a woman of any age who has had an abnormal Pap test result (U.S. Food and Drug Administration, 2003). It does not take the place of the Pap test because it tests for the viruses that can cause cell changes in the cervix that, if not treated, could lead to cancer. Cells are collected from the cervix and sent to a laboratory for analysis. Women who have normal Pap test results and no HPV infection are at very low risk for developing cervical cancer; conversely women with an abnormal Pap result and a positive HPV test are at higher risk if not treated.

Critical Thinking Challenge

Three women, a 21-year-old African-American student, a 35-year-old Hispanic prostitute, and a 65-year-old white widow, need teaching about the importance of screening for cervical cancer.

1. How would you present the screening recommendations for each of these women that would demonstrate age and cultural appropriateness as well as the latest screening guidelines?

evolve For suggested answer guidelines, go to http://evolve.elsevier.com/Iggy/.

Blood Studies

PITUITARY GONADOTROPIN

Determinations of the quantitative levels of follicle-stimulating hormone (FSH), luteinizing hormone (LH), and prolactin are helpful in the diagnosis of male and female reproductive tract disorders. No dietary restrictions are necessary before the test. Chart 76-5 gives the normal values and the significance of abnormal findings.

STEROID HORMONES

The radioimmunoassay technique can detect estrogen, progesterone, and testosterone levels in men and women.

SEROLOGIC TESTS

Serologic studies detect antigen-antibody reactions that occur in response to foreign organisms. This form of diagnostic testing is beneficial only after an infection has become well established. Serologic testing can be used in the evaluation of exposure to organisms causing syphilis, rubella, and herpes simplex virus type 2 (HSV2). Results may be read as nonreactive, weakly reactive, or reactive. A single titer is not

CHART 76-5

LABORATORY PROFILE
Reproductive Assessment

Test	Normal Range for Adults	Significance of Abnormal Findings
Serum Studies		
Follicle-stimulating hormone (FSH) (Follitropin)	*Men:* 1.42-15.4 IU/mL *Women:* follicular phase, 1.37-9.9 IU/mL; midcycle, 6.17-17.2 IU/mL; luteal phase, 1.09-9.2 IU/mL; postmenopause, 19.3-100.6 IU/mL	Decreased levels indicate possible infertility, anorexia nervosa, neoplasm. Elevations indicate possible Turner's syndrome.
Luteinizing hormone (LH) (Lutropin)	*Men:* 1.24-7.8 IU/mL *Women:* follicular phase, 1.68-15 IU/mL, midcycle, 21.9-56.6 IU/mL; luteal phase, 0.61-16.3 IU/mL; postmenopause, 14.2-52.3 IU/mL	Decreased levels indicate possible infertility, anovulation. Elevations indicate possible ovarian failure, Turner's syndrome.
Prolactin	*Men:* 0-20 ng/mL *Women:* 0-20 ng/mL *Pregnant women:* 20-400 ng/mL	Elevations indicate possible galactorrhea (breast discharge), pituitary tumor, disease of hypothalamus or pituitary gland, hypothyroidism.
Estradiol	*Men:* 10-50 pg/mL *Women:* follicular phase, 20-350 pg/mL; midcycle, 150-750 pg/mL; luteal phase, 30-450 pg/mL; postmenopause, ≤20 pg/mL	Elevations of estradiol, total estrogens, and estriol in men indicate possible gynecomastia, decreased body hair, increased fat deposits, feminization.
Estriol	*Men and nonpregnant women:* <2.0 ng/dL	Decreased levels or estradiol, total estrogens, and estriol in women indicate possible amenorrhea, climacteric, impending abortion, hypothalamic disorders.
Progesterone	*Men:* 10-50 ng/dL *Women:* follicular phase, <50 ng/dL; luteal phase, 300-2500 ng/dL	Decreased levels in women indicate possible inadequate luteal phase, amenorrhea. Elevations in women indicate possible ovarian luteal cysts.
Testosterone	*Men:* 3-10 ng/dL or 10-35 mmol/L *Women:* <1 ng/dL or <3.5 mmol/L	Decreased levels in men indicate possible hypogonadism, Klinefelter syndrome, hypopituitarism, orchidectomy. Elevations in women indicate possible adrenal neoplasm, polycystic ovaries, ovarian tumors.
Urine Studies		
Total estrogens	*Men:* 4-25 mcg/24 hr *Women*: 4-60 mcg/24 hr	Elevations indicate possible testicular tumors, adrenal tumors, ovarian tumors, pregnancy. Decreased levels indicate possible ovarian dysfunction, intrauterine death, menopause.
Pregnanediol	*Men:* 0-1.9 mg/24 hr *Women:* follicular phase, <2.6 mg/24 hr; luteal phase, 2.6-10.6 mg/24 hr	Elevations indicate possible luteal ovarian cysts, ovarian neoplasms, adrenal disorders. Decreased levels indicate possible amenorrhea.
17-Ketosteroids	*Men (20-50 yr):* 6-20 mg/24 hr *Women (20-50 yr):* 6-17 mg/24 hr Values decrease with age	Elevations indicate possible Cushing's syndrome, increased androgen or cortisol production, severe stress. Decreased levels indicate possible Addison's disease, hypopituitarism.

Data from Pagana, K.D., & Pagana, T.J. (2002). *Mosby's manual of diagnostic and laboratory tests* (2nd ed.). St. Louis: Mosby.
1 ng, 1 nanogram or 1 billionth of a gram; *1 pg,* 1 picogram or 1 trillionth of a gram; *mcg,* 1 microgram or 1 millionth of a gram.

as revealing as serial titers, which can detect the rise in antibody reactions as the body continues to fight the infection.

SYPHILIS DETECTION

The VDRL (Venereal Disease Research Laboratory) test, serologic test for syphilis (STS), and the rapid plasma reagin test (RPR) are used to detect, confirm, and monitor cases of syphilis. These tests are recommended for all pregnant women and persons at high risk for syphilis (Centers for Disease Control and Prevention [CDC], 2002). These antigen tests are used to screen for the presence of nonspecific reagin antibodies that appear and increase in titer after infection. They are not totally specific or sensitive for syphilis, but they are economical and highly diagnostic. Some acute and chronic conditions that cause false-positive results are the following:

- Tuberculosis
- Infectious mononucleosis
- Recent smallpox vaccination
- Rheumatoid arthritis
- Systemic lupus erythematosus
- Subacute bacterial endocarditis

- Hepatitis
- Recent ingestion of alcohol

Test results vary with the stage of syphilis. The serologic test result is usually positive about 2 weeks after the client has become infected. If the primary syphilis is treated, the serologic titers almost always return to nonreactive levels within 4 months.

If the VDRL or RPR test is positive, the diagnosis must be confirmed by a more specific test for *Treponema pallidum,* such as the fluorescent treponemal antibody absorption test (FTA-ABS). This expensive and time-consuming test is positive 4 to 6 weeks after infection. Most positive test results for *Treponema pallidum* remain positive for the rest of the person's life.

PROSTATE-SPECIFIC ANTIGEN

The prostate-specific antigen (PSA) test is used to screen for prostate cancer and to monitor the disease after treatment. PSA levels of less than 4 ng/mL are normal; elevated PSA levels are associated with prostate cancer. If combined with a digital rectal examination, almost 90% of all prostate cancers can be detected (Pagana & Pagana, 2002).

The client should not ejaculate at least 24 hours before the test to avoid a false-positive result. For the same reason, draw the blood for the PSA test before doing the digital rectal examination (Haese & Partin, 2001).

Urinalysis for Steroid Hormones

The health care provider may order 24-hour urine samples for levels of total estrogens and pregnanediol (a urinary byproduct of progesterone) to detect ovulation.

Microscopic Studies

WET PREPARATION (WET SMEARS)

Secretions can be obtained from the vaginal pool at the beginning of a speculum examination. Specimens can also be obtained from the vaginal walls, labia, or vulva during the examination. The specimens are placed on glass slides and are treated with a wet preparation such as saline and potassium hydroxide (KOH). The slides are examined under a microscope to confirm or rule out the presence of a pathogen. Table 76-2 lists common types of wet preparations used to diagnose selected vaginal problems.

TABLE 76-2 Wet Preparations Used for the Diagnosis of Common Vaginal Problems

Wet Preparation	Problems
Normal saline	Cervicitis Trichomoniasis Bacterial vaginosis Atrophic vaginitis
Potassium hydroxide (KOH)	Candidiasis *(Candida albicans, Monilia)* Bacterial vaginosis
Gram stain	Mucopurulent cervicitis

CULTURES

Cultures identify pathogenic organisms and are used to determine the correct antibiotic therapy. The examiner obtains specimens for culture analysis from any discharge or orifice of the male or female reproductive system. Routine bacteriologic cultures and antibiotic sensitivity studies are performed when a nonspecific bacterial infection is suspected.

The culture to detect *Neisseria gonorrhoeae* is one of the most important in evaluating the reproductive system. This culture is the only means of confirming a diagnosis of gonorrhea in asymptomatic women. Cervical cultures can be taken after the Pap specimen is obtained. Specimens from men can be taken directly from any penile discharge. Additional specimens from men or women can also be obtained from the urethra, rectum, and throat. The swab is then placed in a culture tube and sent to the laboratory for incubation and analysis.

Cultures to detect *Chlamydia trachomatis* use antigen detection methods. Tissue cultures are the most accurate but take several days for results and are expensive. Less expensive and more widely available are a direct immunofluorescent test and an enzyme-linked immunosorbent assay (ELISA) (Pagana & Pagana, 2002). Nucleic acid amplification tests can be used to detect *N. gonorrhoeae and C. trachomatis* in first-voided urine specimens or in specimens collected from the cervix (CDC, 2002). Cultures are taken from the cervix in women and from the urethra in men.

RADIOGRAPHIC EXAMINATIONS

General X-rays

A kidney, ureter, and bladder (KUB) x-ray of the abdomen shows these structures and is used in the assessment of disorders of either the male or female reproductive system. Pelvic masses, calcified tumors or fibroids, dermoid cysts, and metastatic bone changes may be evident. Urologic studies may enhance the film by the use of contrast media. No specific preparation is needed.

Bone scans, intravenous (IV) pyelograms, barium enema studies, and chest x-rays are also included in the workup of the client with suspected metastatic cancer. They help determine the extent of the cancer spread and obstruction or displacement of the organs. These tests are discussed elsewhere in this text.

Computed Tomography

Computed tomography (CT) scans for reproductive system disorders involve the abdomen and the pelvis. They can detect and evaluate masses and lymphatic enlargement from metastasis. This scan can differentiate solid tissue masses from cystic or hemorrhagic structures.

Hysterosalpingography

A **hysterosalpingogram** is an x-ray of the cervix, uterus, and fallopian tubes and is performed after the injection of a contrast medium. This test is used in infertility workups to evaluate tubal anatomy and patency and uterine problems such as fibroids, tumors, and fistulas. The study should not be attempted for at least 6 weeks after abortion, delivery, or dilation and curettage. Other contraindications include reproductive tract infection or uterine bleeding.

CLIENT PREPARATION. The examination is scheduled in a radiology department 2 to 5 days after the end of the client's normal menses. The scheduling is important to prevent the accidental flushing of a fertilized ovum from the fallopian tube or the exposure of a fetus to radiation.

The client is usually instructed to take a laxative the evening before the test, followed by an enema or rectal suppository on the morning of the examination. These procedures reduce the distortion of the x-rays by gas shadows.

On the day of the examination, confirm the date of the client's last menstrual period and record it in the medical record. Ask about allergies to iodine dye or shellfish. The client signs a consent form for the procedure. Because discomfort is anticipated during the examination, premedication with analgesics or nonsteroidal anti-inflammatory drugs may be prescribed. Inform the client that she may experience some nausea and vomiting, abdominal cramping, or faintness. Provide support and assistance with relaxation techniques.

PROCEDURE. The client is placed in the lithotomy position. A speculum is inserted, and the cervix is visualized. Dye is injected through the cervix to fill and highlight the interior of the cervix, uterus, and fallopian tubes. If the fallopian tubes are patent, the contrast material spills into the peritoneal cavity. Usually, only two or three films are obtained to show the path and distribution of the contrast medium.

FOLLOW-UP CARE. The client may experience pelvic pain after the study and should receive analgesic drugs accordingly. She may also have referred pain to the shoulder because of irritation of the phrenic nerve. Provide a perineal pad after the test to prevent the soiling of clothes as the dye drains from the cervix. Instruct the woman to contact her health care provider if bloody discharge continues for 4 days or longer and to report any signs of infection, such as lower quadrant pain, fever, malodorous discharge, or tachycardia.

Mammography

Mammography is an x-ray of the soft tissue of the breast. Mammograms assess differences in the density of breast tissue. They are especially helpful in evaluating poorly defined masses, multiple masses or nodules, nipple changes or discharge, skin changes, and pain. Mammography can detect many cancers that are not palpable by physical examination; however, some actual cancers may not appear on mammography or may appear as benign.

In young women's breasts there is little difference in the density between normal glandular tissue and malignant tumors, which makes the mammogram less useful for evaluation of breast masses in these women. For this reason, annual screening mammograms are not recommended for women younger than 40 years of age (ACS, 2005). In older women, the amount of fatty tissue is higher and the fatty tissue appears lighter than neoplasms. Cancer and cysts may have the same density. Cysts usually have smooth borders, and cancers often have starburst-shaped margins.

CLIENT PREPARATION. No dietary restrictions are necessary before the mammogram. Remind the client not to use creams, powders, or deodorant on the breasts or underarm areas before the study, because these products can show on the x-ray and confound the interpretation. If there is any possibility that the client is pregnant, the test should be rescheduled. Explain the purpose of the examination and its anticipated discomforts. Provide a cover gown and adequate privacy for the client to undress above the waist. The client also needs support and may need time to express her concerns about the mammogram and the presence of any lumps. Because this is a time when the client is anxious about the health of her breasts, it is a good opportunity to teach or reinforce the importance of breast self-examination.

PROCEDURE. The technician positions the client next to the x-ray machine with one breast exposed. A film plate and the platform of the machine are placed on opposite sides of the breast to be examined. The technician includes as much breast tissue as possible between the plates. The woman may experience some temporary discomfort when the breast is compressed during the positioning and the test. The test takes about 15 minutes, but the client is usually asked to wait until the films are developed in case a view needs to be repeated. A screening mammogram uses two low-dose x-ray views of each breast: a view from the side and a view from above.

FOLLOW-UP CARE. If the results are not communicated at the time of the mammogram, the woman should know when to expect the report. Assess her knowledge of breast self-examination and give instructions if needed.

OTHER DIAGNOSTIC TESTS

Ultrasonography

Ultrasonography is a technique that is routinely used to assess problems such as uterine fibroids, ovarian cysts, and pelvic masses. It can be used to locate intrauterine devices and to monitor the progress of tumor regression after medical treatment. Ultrasonography is also useful in differentiating solid tumors from cysts in breast examinations. In men, ultrasound can test for varicoceles, scrotal abnormalities, and problems of the ejaculatory ducts and seminal vesicles and the vas deferens (Pagana & Pagana, 2002; Zahalsky & Nagler, 2001).

No specific preparations are needed for this study. Women should have a full bladder to enable visualization of the uterus and to make the location of other structures more distinct with abdominal ultrasonography. A full bladder is not needed for breast, scrotal, transvaginal or transrectal scans.

For an abdominal, breast, or scrotal scan, the technician exposes the area and applies oil or gel to the area to be scanned. These substances provide better transmission of sound waves from the transducer through the client's skin. The transducer is moved in a linear pattern across the area being tested to outline and define soft-tissue masses and to differentiate tumor type, ascites, and encapsulated fluid.

For a transvaginal or transrectal scan, the transducer is covered with a condom or vinyl glove onto which transmission gel has been placed. The transducer is then inserted.

The client may want to watch the oscilloscope screen and can be helped by a brief explanation of the landmarks and structures visualized. There is no special follow-up care for the client after this procedure except to provide wipes to remove the gel.

Magnetic Resonance Imaging

Magnetic resonance imaging (MRI) uses a magnetic field and radiofrequency energy to scan for pelvic tumors. This scan distinguishes between normal and malignant tissues. MRIs are also being investigated for use in the diagnosis of breast cancer (Stenchever et al., 2001). Because of the expense, MRIs are not yet recommended for general screening.

Endoscopic Studies

COLPOSCOPY

The colposcope allows three-dimensional magnification and intense illumination of epithelium with suspected disease.

Colposcopy is suited for inspection of the cervical epithelium, vagina, and vulvar epithelium. This procedure can locate the exact site of precancerous and malignant lesions for biopsy.

CLIENT PREPARATION. The woman is placed in the lithotomy position and provided the same support as for a pelvic examination. The client should not douche or use vaginal preparations for 24 to 48 hours before the test. This nearly painless procedure is better tolerated if it is explained in advance and if the instrument is shown to the client.

Colposcopy provides accurate site selection for tissue biopsy; therefore the client should also be prepared for a biopsy. Materials for cytologic studies and biopsy should be readily available.

PROCEDURE. The physician locates the cervix, or vaginal site, through a speculum examination. Lubricants other than water should not be used. Cells in the area may be stained or left unstained to enhance visibility. The physician cleans and moistens the cervix with normal saline. This increases the visibility of vascular patterns and the junction between the columnar epithelium and the squamous epithelium. Acetic acid, 3%, is applied to the cervix to draw moisture from the tissue and to accentuate important features. The physician then uses a colposcope or colpomicroscope to inspect the area in question. A biopsy specimen may also be taken if abnormal cells are seen (see discussion on cervical biopsy on p. 1787).

FOLLOW-UP CARE. After the procedure, assist the woman as you would for a pelvic examination and provide supplies to clean the perineum. Also give her a perineal pad to absorb any dye or discharge. If a biopsy specimen is taken, additional follow-up care is needed.

LAPAROSCOPY

Laparoscopy is a direct examination of the pelvic cavity through an endoscope. This procedure can rule out an ectopic pregnancy, evaluate ovarian disorders and pelvic masses, and aid in the diagnosis of infertility and unexplained pelvic pain. Laparoscopy is also used during surgical procedures such as the following:

- Tubal sterilization
- Ovarian biopsy
- Cyst or graafian follicle aspiration (to retrieve ova for in vitro fertilization)
- Lysis of adhesions around the fallopian tubes
- Retrieval of "lost" intrauterine devices

A laparoscopy is used instead of a laparotomy for minor surgical procedures because it requires only a small incision, involves less discomfort, and hospitalization is not needed.

CLIENT PREPARATION. The physician explains the procedure, risks (complications associated with the use of general anesthesia, postoperative shoulder pain, and the rare occurrence of infection or electrical burns), and anticipated discomforts and obtains the client's consent. The procedure can be performed with either a regional or general anesthetic. Clients should expect mild discomfort from the incision site and may experience referred shoulder pain from phrenic nerve irritation (Raines, 2004).

PROCEDURE. The client is anesthetized and placed in the lithotomy position. A urinary catheter is inserted to drain the bladder. The operating table is placed in a slight Trendelenburg position to cause the intestines to fall away from the pelvis. The cervix is held with a cannula to allow movement of the uterus during laparoscopy (Figure 76-9). The surgeon inserts a needle below the umbilicus to infuse carbon dioxide into the pelvic cavity, which distends the abdomen and permits better visualization of the organs. The surgeon inserts a trocar and a cannula into the incision. After the trocar and cannula are in place in the abdominal cavity, the surgeon removes the trocar and inserts the laparoscope. The surgeon can then visualize the pelvic cavity and reproductive organs. Further instrumentation is possible through a second small incision. The laparoscope is removed at the end of the procedure, and the abdomen is deflated. The small incision is closed with absorbable sutures and dressed with an adhesive bandage.

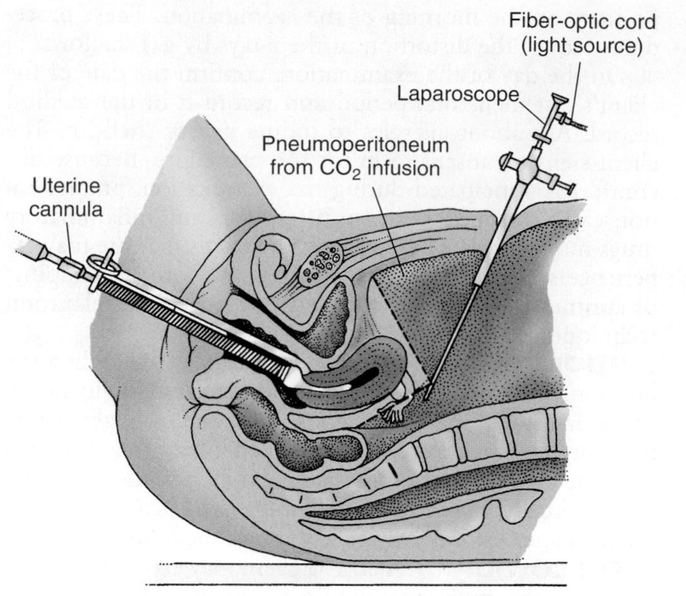

Figure 76-9 ■ Laparoscopy.

FOLLOW-UP CARE. Care after surgery is similar to that for other clients after general anesthesia. The client is usually discharged on the day of the surgery. Discomfort from the incision is usually alleviated by oral analgesics. The greatest discomfort is due to referred shoulder pain caused by residual gas in the peritoneal cavity. Most of these sensations disappear within 48 hours. Instruct the client to change the small adhesive bandage as needed and to observe the incision for signs of infection or hematoma. Remind the client to avoid strenuous activity for the first week after the procedure.

HYSTEROSCOPY

Hysteroscopy is an endoscopic examination done to visualize the interior of the uterus and the cervical canal. The hysteroscope includes a fiberoptic camera. Aqueous carbon dioxide is the medium used to distend the uterus. Hysteroscopy can be used for the removal of intrauterine devices and as a complement to other diagnostic tests for infertility and unexplained bleeding (Stenchever et al., 2001).

CLIENT PREPARATION. The surgeon informs the client of all aspects of the procedure and obtains consent. The preparation is the same as for a pelvic examination. The procedure is best performed 5 days after menses have ceased to reduce the possibility of pregnancy. The client is placed in the lithotomy position and is usually anesthetized with a pericervical or other regional block.

PROCEDURE. After the client is anesthetized, the cervix is dilated. The physician inserts the hysteroscope through the cervix. Because a medium distends the uterus, cells can be pushed through the fallopian tubes and into the pelvic cavity. Therefore hysteroscopy is contraindicated in clients with suspected cervical or endometrial cancer, in clients with infection of the reproductive tract, and in pregnant clients.

FOLLOW-UP CARE. Care is the same as that after a pelvic examination. Analgesics may be prescribed if the client has cramping or shoulder pain.

Biopsy Studies

CERVICAL BIOPSY

In a cervical biopsy, cervical tissue is removed for cytologic study. A biopsy is indicated in a client with an identifiable cervical lesion, regardless of the cytologic findings. The physician usually performs a biopsy in conjunction with colposcopy as a follow-up to a suspicious Pap test finding. The procedure may be performed in a clinic or office setting.

Several techniques can be used for a cervical biopsy. If a lesion is clearly visible, an endocervical curettage can be performed as an outpatient procedure and with little or no anesthetic. **Conization** (removal of a cone-shaped sample of tissue) and loop electrosurgical excision procedures (LEEP) are usually not done unless the cervical biopsy findings are positive or the results of the colposcopy are unsatisfactory (Lowdermilk, 2004). Conization can be done as a cold-knife procedure, a laser excision, or an electrosurgical incision.

CLIENT PREPARATION. The biopsy is usually scheduled when the client is in the early proliferative phase of the menstrual cycle, when the cervix is least vascular. The procedure is explained to the client. Because a biopsy evaluates potentially malignant cells, most women are anxious and need time to discuss their feelings and fears. The use of relaxation techniques may assist comfort. The client is assisted into the lithotomy position and prepared in the same way as for a pelvic examination. Further preparation depends on the type of procedure to be performed.

PROCEDURE. The physician may anesthetize the client according to the needs of the chosen procedure. The physician visualizes the cervix and obtains the tissue sample. All specimens are immediately placed into a formalin solution.

FOLLOW-UP CARE. The type of anesthetic used for the procedure determines the type of immediate care needed after the procedure. Discharge instructions are listed in Chart 76-6.

CHART 76-6

CLIENT EDUCATION GUIDE
The Client Recovering from Cervical Biopsy

- Do not lift any heavy objects until the site is healed (about 2 weeks).
- Rest for 24 hours after the procedure.
- Report any excessive bleeding (more than that of a normal menstrual period) to your health care provider.
- Report signs of infection (fever, increased pain, foul smelling drainage) to your health care provider.
- Do not douche, use tampons, or have vaginal intercourse until the site is healed (about 2 weeks).
- Keep the perineum clean and dry by using antiseptic solution rinses (as directed by your health care provider) and changing pads frequently.

ENDOMETRIAL BIOPSY AND ASPIRATION

Both endometrial biopsy and aspiration are used to obtain cells directly from the lining of the uterus to assess for cancer of the endometrium. Biopsy also helps assess menstrual disturbances (especially heavy bleeding) and infertility (corpus luteum dysfunction).

When menstrual disturbances are being evaluated, the biopsy is generally done in the immediate premenstrual period to provide an index of progesterone influence and ovulation. A biopsy performed in the second half of the menstrual cycle (about days 21 and 22) evaluates corpus luteum function and the presence or absence of a persistent secretory endometrium. Postmenopausal women may undergo biopsies at any time.

CLIENT PREPARATION. Menstrual data are obtained from the client and are included on the specimen slip for the pathologist. The client is given the same preparation as for a pelvic examination. Advise the woman that she may experience some cramping when the cervix is dilated. Analgesia before the procedure and relaxation and breathing techniques during the procedure are often of value.

PROCEDURE. An endometrial biopsy is often performed as an office procedure with or without anesthesia. After the uterus is sounded (measured) and the cervix dilated, the physician inserts the curette or intrauterine cannula into the uterus. A portion of the endometrium is withdrawn using either the cuplike end of the curette or with suction equipment. The client usually has moderate cramping. The specimens are placed in a formalin solution and sent for histologic examination.

FOLLOW-UP CARE. Allow the client to rest on the examining table until the cramping has subsided. Provide a perineal pad and a wipe to clean the perineum. Tell the client that spotting may be present for 1 to 2 days, but any signs of infection or excessive bleeding should be reported to the physician. Instruct the client to refrain from intercourse or douching until all discharge has ceased. Results of the biopsy are usually available within 72 hours.

BREAST BIOPSY AND ASPIRATION

An incisional biopsy is the surgical removal of tissue from a breast mass. An excisional biopsy removes the mass itself for histologic (cellular) evaluation. Aspiration biopsy is the removal of fluid or tissue from the breast mass through a large-bore needle. Figure 76-10 shows these three types of breast biopsy.

Any breast mass needs to be evaluated for the possibility of cancer. Fibrocystic lesions, fibroadenomas, and intraductal papillomas can be differentiated by biopsy. Any discharge from the breasts is examined histologically.

CLIENT PREPARATION. The instructions to the client depend on the type of biopsy and the type of anesthesia. Tell the woman to expect pulling or probing sensations during the procedure.

PROCEDURE. Aspiration biopsy is often performed in an outpatient setting without an anesthetic. The mass is located by palpation of the breast. The surgeon then directs the needle into the lump and aspirates the contents into the

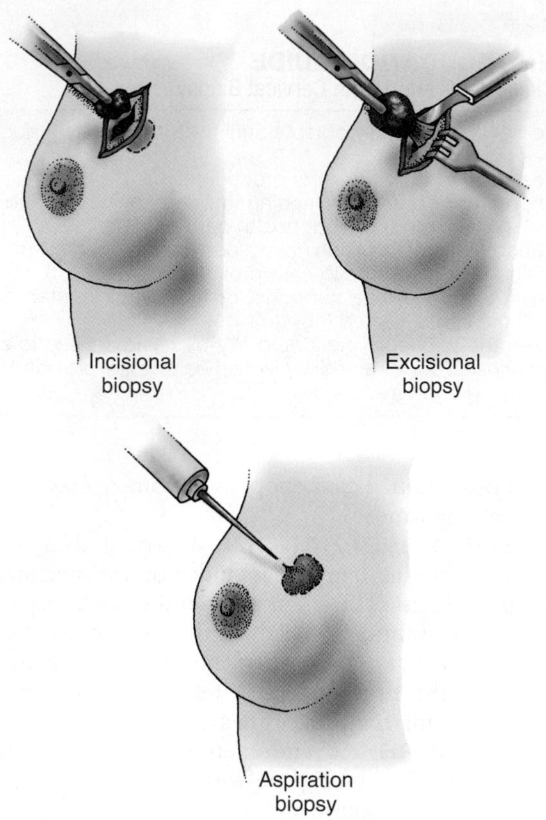

Figure 76-10 ■ Breast biopsy techniques.

syringe. The contents are placed on a slide for Pap evaluation. Fluid from benign cysts may appear clear to dark green-brown; bloody fluid suggests cancer. If no fluid is aspirated, the mass is examined by incisional biopsy.

Biopsies are often performed as same-day procedures with local or general anesthesia. The specimen undergoes histologic evaluation. If cancer is found, the tissue is sent to the laboratory for estrogen receptor analysis.

FOLLOW-UP CARE. Discomfort after surgery is usually mild and is controlled with analgesics or the use of a heating pad. Teach the client how to assess the incision for bleeding and edema. Tell her to wear a properly supportive bra continuously for 1 week after surgery. Instruct the client to avoid cold temperatures to prevent nipple contractions that can cause stress the incision. Numbness around the biopsy site may last 2 to 3 months. Assess the client's knowledge of breast self-examination and provide instructions if needed. If cancer is identified, provide emotional support as well as information about follow-up treatment alternatives.

NEEDLE BIOPSY OF THE PROSTATE

When prostate cancer is suspected, the physician performs a needle aspiration biopsy of the prostate gland for histologic study. This procedure is often performed at the same time as cystoscopy, with the client under anesthesia. The physician can perform needle biopsies without anesthesia or with the client under local anesthesia.

CLIENT PREPARATION. Preparation for the procedure depends on the technique used to puncture the gland. Explain about the expected discomforts. Teach the client about breathing and relaxation techniques for use during the examination. Because the purpose of this procedure is to evaluate prostate cells for cancer, the man needs support and time to discuss his fears. Preparation for a transrectal biopsy involves the use of cleansing enemas. Prophylactic antibiotics are given to reduce the risk for bacterial contamination of the blood or prostate tissue. Local anesthesia is used for transperineal biopsy.

PROCEDURE. The client is placed in the same position as for a rectal examination. After injecting a local anesthetic for the transperineal biopsy, the physician places a finger in the rectum to help guide the needle to the prostate. For the transrectal biopsy, the physician places the needle against the examining finger and then inserts it into the rectum to the prostate. From this site, the needle is advanced through the rectal mucosa and into the prostate gland. The aspiration may be repeated several times to obtain a satisfactory specimen.

FOLLOW-UP CARE. Sepsis is a life-threatening complication of transrectal biopsy. Report any manifestations of infection (e.g., fever, or low back pain) or sepsis immediately. Prophylactic antibiotics are usually prescribed.

Semen Analysis

A complete semen analysis may be done as a test of male infertility. The client collects a semen specimen usually by ejaculation into a clean specimen container. Abstinence from ejaculation for 2 to 5 days before the collection is recommended. The specimen should be examined in a laboratory within 2 hours after it is collected. It should not be exposed to excessive heat or cold. Accepted values for characteristics of semen are listed in Chart 76-7.

CHART 76-7

LABORATORY PROFILE
Semen Analysis

Selected Parameter	Normal Ranges*
Liquefaction	Complete within 10 to 30 minutes
Semen volume	2 mL or greater
Semen pH	7.2 to 8.0
Total sperm count	>40 million/mL
Sperm density	20 to 200 million/mL
% Normal morphology	30% or greater
Sperm motility (forward moving)	50% or greater

*Based on World Health Organization. (1992). *Laboratory manual for the examination of human semen and sperm-cervical mucus interaction.* Cambridge, UK: WHO. Values vary according to source used as a reference.

GET READY for the NCLEX Examination!

KEY POINTS

Safe Effective Care Environment

- Ask all women about intimate partner abuse at any health visit.
- Encourage all pregnant women and women at high risk for syphilis to be screened for this sexually transmitted disease.

- Ask any woman scheduled for a hysterosalpingography about allergy to iodine dye or shellfish because she may have an allergic reaction to the radiopaque dye used during the procedure.
- Use standard precautions for all examinations of the external and internal genitalia for both males and female clients.
- Use sterile technique when collecting specimens for laboratory testing.

Health Promotion and Maintenance

- Encourage all women to follow recommended Pap screening guidelines for early detection of precancerous and cancerous cells from the cervix.
- Teach women about pelvic floor muscle exercises to reduce or prevent pelvic relaxation and urinary incontinence.
- Assess cultural issues when identifying risks for certain reproductive problems as well as when evaluating health promotion practices.
- Assess/teach all women for breast and vulvar self-examination practices because these practices can lead to early identification of cancer and other conditions.
- Assess/teach all men about performing testicular self-examinations.
- Ask all clients about the use of safer sex practices because sexually transmitted diseases can increase the risk for some cancers and infertility, as well as unplanned pregnancy.

Psychosocial Integrity

- Allow the client the opportunity to express fear or anxiety regarding tests of the reproductive system or about a potential change in sexual or reproductive function.
- Assess the client's level of comfort in discussing issues related to reproduction and sexuality.
- Explain all diagnostic procedures, restrictions, and follow-up care to the client scheduled for tests.
- Provide as much privacy as possible for clients undergoing examination or testing of the reproductive system.
- Use language and terminology that the client can understand and that the client is comfortable with during discussions of the reproductive system.
- Encourage clients to express feelings of anxiety or discomfort related to genital examinations.
- Offer to teach relaxation techniques to use during examinations.

Physiological Integrity

- Always consider the possibility of pregnancy in a sexually active woman who has amenorrhea.
- Urge clients with pain, bleeding, discharge, masses, or changes in reproductive function to seek health care advice.
- Teach clients who have undergone invasive testing of the reproductive tract about the manifestations of infection (e.g., fever, increased pain, foul-smelling drainage).
- Instruct women to report manifestations of infection to their health care provider after hysterosalpingography and biopsies of the breast, cervix, and endometrium.
- Instruct men to report manifestations of infection to their health care provider after a transrectal biopsy of the prostate.

ADDITIONAL STUDY RESOURCES

Go to your Student CD-ROM for Review Questions for the NCLEX Examination.

evolve Go to http://evolve.elsevier.com/Iggy/ for Integrated Management of Care Questions for the NCLEX Examination.

SELECTED BIBLIOGRAPHY

Asterisk indicates a classic or definitive work on this subject.

Ackley, B., & Ladwig, G. (2002). *Nursing diagnosis handbook: A guide to planning care* (5th ed.). St. Louis: Mosby.

Adams, K. (2002). Confronting cervical cancer: Screening is the key to stopping this killer. *AWHONN Lifelines*, *6*(3), 216-222.

American Cancer Society. (2005). *Cancer facts and figures 2005*. Report No. 00-300M-No. 5008.05. Atlanta: Author.

American College of Obstetrics and Gynecology. (2002). Screening tools for domestic violence. *AGOG Violence against women homepage*. Retrieved June 16, 2003, from http://www.acog.org.

American College of Obstetrics and Gynecology. (2003). Questions and answers on hormone replacement therapy. Retrieved June 17, 2003, from http://www.acog.org.

Biscotti, C., et al. (2002). Thin-layer Pap test vs. conventional Pap smear. Analysis of 400 split samples. *Reproductive Medicine*, *47*(1), 9-13.

Boyer, L., et al. (2001). Hispanic women's perceptions regarding cervical cancer screening. *Journal of Obstetric, Gynecologic, and Neonatal Nursing, 30*(2), 240-245.

Centers for Disease Control and Prevention (CDC). (2002). Sexually transmitted diseases treatment guidelines. *Morbidity & Mortality Weekly Report, 51*(RR-6), 1-80.

D'Avanzo, C., & Geissler, E. (2003). *Cultural health assessment* (3rd ed.). St. Louis: Mosby.

DiSaia, P., & Creasman, W. (2002). *Clinical gynecologic oncology* (6th ed.). St. Louis: Mosby.

Ebersole, P., Hess, P., & Luggen, A. (2004). *Toward healthy aging: Human needs and nursing response* (6th ed.). St. Louis: Mosby.

Fogel, C. (2004). Reproductive system concerns. In D. Lowdermilk & S. Perry (Eds.), *Maternity and women's health care* (8th ed., pp. 155-184). St. Louis: Mosby.

Gordon, M. (2002). *Manual of nursing diagnosis* (10th ed.). St. Louis: Mosby.

Haese, A., & Partin, A. (2001). New serum tests for the diagnosis of prostate cancer. *Drugs Today*, *37*(9), 607-616.

Halcon, L., et al. (2002). Pap test results among low-income youth: Prevalence of dysplasia and practice implications. *Journal of Obstetric, Gynecologic, and Neonatal Nursing, 31*(3), 294-304.

Huff, B. (2000). Screening for cervical cancer: It's time to check your technique. *AWHONN Lifelines 4*(3), 53-55.

Jarvis, C. (2004). *Physical examination and health assessment* (4th ed.). Philadelphia: W.B. Saunders.

Lowdermilk, D. (2004). Structural disorders and neoplasms of the reproductive system. In D. Lowdermilk & S. Perry (Eds.), *Maternity and women's health care* (8th ed., pp. 289-326). St. Louis: Mosby.

National Women's Health Resource Center. (2001). Screening tests and women's health. *National Women's Health Report, 23*(6), 1-7.

Nussbaum, R., McInnes, R., & Willard, H. (2001). *Thompson & Thompson: Genetics in medicine* (6th ed.). Philadelphia: W.B. Saunders.

O'Rourke, M. (2001). Genitourinary cancer. In S. Otto (Ed.), *Oncology nursing* (4th ed.). St. Louis: Mosby.

Pagana, K., & Pagana, T. (2002). *Mosby's manual of diagnostic and laboratory tests* (2nd ed.). St. Louis: Mosby.

Raines, C. (2004). Infertility. In D. Lowdermilk & S. Perry (Eds.), *Maternity and women's health care* (8th ed., pp. 246-266). St. Louis: Mosby.

Sabatini, S. (2001). The female athlete triad. *American Journal of the Medical Sciences, 322*(4), 193-195.

Sampselle, C., et al. (2000). Continence for women: A test of AWHONN's evidence-based protocol in clinical practice. *Journal of Obstetric, Gynecologic, and Neonatal Nursing, 29*(1), 18-26.

Saraiya, M., et al. (2001). Self-reported Papanicolaou smears and hysterectomies among women in the United States. *Obstetrics and Gynecology, 98*(2), 269-278.

Stenchever, M., et al. (2001). *Comprehensive gynecology* (4th ed.). St. Louis: Mosby.

U.S. Food and Drug Administration. (2003). FDA approves expanded use of HPV test. *FDA News.* Retrieved June 18, 2003, from http://www.fda.gov.

U.S. Preventive Services Task Force. (2003). *Screening for cervical cancer.* AHRQ Publication 03515A. Rockville, MD: Agency for Healthcare and Quality.

*World Health Organization. (1992). *Laboratory manual for the examination of human semen and sperm-cervical mucus interaction.* Cambridge, UK: WHO.

Zahalsky, M., & Nagler, H. (2001). Ultrasound and infertility: Diagnostic and therapeutic uses. *Current Urology Report, 2*(6), 437-447.

Zawacki, K., & Phillips, M. (2002). Cancer genetics and women's health. *Journal of Obstetric, Gynecologic, and Neonatal Nursing, 31*(2), 208-216.

Zdanuk, J. (2004). Assessment and health promotion. In D. Lowdermilk & S. Perry (Eds.), *Maternity and women's health care* (8th ed., pp. 91-130). St. Louis: Mosby.

CHAPTER 77

Interventions for Clients with Breast Disorders

ANGELA SAMMARCO

LEARNING OUTCOMES

After studying this chapter, you should be able to:

1. Compare assessment findings associated with benign breast lesions with those of malignant breast lesions.
2. Describe the three-pronged approach to early detection of breast masses: mammography, clinical breast examination (CBE), and breast self-examination (BSE).
3. Teach a client how to do BSE.
4. Explain the options available to a woman at high genetic risk for breast cancer.
5. Analyze assessment data to determine priority nursing diagnoses and collaborative problems for a woman with breast cancer.
6. Develop a plan of care for a client with breast cancer.
7. Discuss the psychosocial aspects related to having breast cancer and undergoing surgery for breast cancer.
8. Formulate a community-based teaching plan for clients undergoing surgery for breast cancer.
9. Explain what options are available to a client considering breast reconstruction.

Go to your Student CD-ROM for Review Questions for the NCLEX Examination keyed to these Learning Outcomes.

After skin cancer, breast cancer is the most commonly diagnosed cancer in women in the Western world, with more than 211,300 new cases identified annually and more than 40,200 deaths attributed to the cancer in the United States alone (American Cancer Society, 2005). Although breast disorders affect both men and women, women are most often affected. The most common manifestation associated with a breast disorder is a palpable mass. The discovery of a mass in a woman's breast, whether the discovery is by the woman herself, her partner, or a health care provider, is a frightening experience. Even if the woman is aware that 90% of all breast lumps are benign, she may fear that the lump is cancerous. This fearful reaction stays with the woman through the period of diagnosis, decision making, and treatment. Regardless of the severity of the diagnosis, you must incorporate the physiologic and emotional factors involved to provide effective nursing care.

BENIGN BREAST DISORDERS

Most breast lumps are benign. Because the incidence of breast disease is related to age, breast disorders are described in an age-related order (Table 77-1).

Fibroadenoma

Fibroadenomas are the most common cause of breast masses during adolescence, although they may occur into the 30s. A fibroadenoma is a solid, slowly enlarging, benign mass of connective tissue that is unattached to the surrounding breast tissue and is typically discovered by the client herself. Although the immediate fear is that of breast cancer, only 0.9% of these masses are malignant. The mass is usually round, firm, easily movable, nontender, and clearly delineated from the surrounding tissue.

TABLE 77-1 Typical Presentation of Benign Breast Disorders

Breast Disorder	Description	Incidence
Fibroadenoma	Most common benign lesion; solid mass of connective tissue that is unattached to the surrounding tissue	During teenage years into the 30s
Fibrocystic breast disease (FBD)	*First stage:* Characterized by premenstrual bilateral fullness and tenderness *Second stage:* Presence of bilateral, multicentric nodules *Third stage:* Presence of microscopic and macroscopic cysts	Late teens and 20s
Ductal ectasia	Hard, irregular mass or masses with nipple discharge, enlarged axillary nodes, redness, and edema; difficult to distinguish from cancer	Women approaching menopause
Intraductal ectasia	Mass in duct that results in nipple discharge; mass is usually not palpable	Women 40 to 55 yr of age

Data from National Cancer Institute.

Fibroadenomas are usually located in the upper outer quadrant of the breast. Enlargement is more likely in pregnancy. The health care provider may order a breast ultrasound examination or may perform a needle aspiration to establish whether the lump is cystic or solid. If the lesion is solid, outpatient excision using local anesthesia is the treatment of choice.

Fibrocystic Breast Disease

PATHOPHYSIOLOGY

Fibrocystic changes, or physiologic nodularity of the breast, often referred to as **fibrocystic breast disease (FBD),** are the most common breast problem of women between 20 and 30 years of age. Over the life span, about 90% of women have fibrocystic changes. These changes are thought to be caused by an imbalance in the normal estrogen to progesterone ratio. This imbalance results in an excess of estrogen exposure and a reduction of progesterone exposure (McCance & Huether, 2002). Fibrocystic changes may proceed through several clinical stages or may present in only one form.

The first stage commonly occurs between the late teens and early 20s. Premenstrual fullness and tenderness in both breasts are present, especially in the outer upper quadrant. Symptoms usually resolve after menstruation and then recur before the next menstrual period in a cyclic fashion.

The second stage usually occurs in the late 20s and throughout the 30s. Multiple nodular areas can be felt in both breasts. These areas feel like small marbles and occur with the fullness and soreness.

The third stage generally occurs between 35 and 55 years of age. Microscopic or macroscopic cysts appear suddenly and are associated with pain, tenderness, or burning. They are usually three-dimensional, smooth, mobile, and well delineated. Although the cysts may recede somewhat before menstruation, they do not disappear completely. Mammography is generally indicated, and fine-needle aspiration may be performed. Older clients receiving hormone replacement therapy may develop painful fluid-filled cysts. Biopsy is indicated in the following situations:

- No fluid is aspirated.
- The mammogram shows suspicious findings.
- A mass remains palpable after aspiration.
- The cytology of the aspirated fluid reveals malignant cells.

Symptoms often resolve after menopause in the absence of estrogen supplementation.

◆COLLABORATIVE MANAGEMENT

Management of FBD is generally symptomatic. Hormonal manipulation is the main focus of drug therapy. Oral contraceptives can suppress oversecretion of estrogen, and progestins may be used to correct luteal insufficiency. Danazol (Danocrine, Cyclomen✱) suppresses ovarian function and estrogen stimulation of breast tissue. However, because hormonal therapy with danazol does not cure FBD, and because its side effects are undesirable, it is generally used only in clients with recurrent and severe fibrocystic disease.

Drug therapy may also include the use of vitamins C, E, and B complex. Diuretics may be prescribed to decrease premenstrual breast engorgement. Clients are counseled to avoid the use of caffeine; however, the role of caffeine in FBD is controversial.

Encourage the client to continue prescribed drug therapy and monitor the effectiveness of these interventions. Suggest supportive measures, such as the use of mild analgesics or limiting salt intake before menses, to help decrease swelling. The client may want to wear (both day and night) a well-padded, supportive bra to decrease tension on ligaments. Local application of ice or heat may provide temporary relief of pain. Promote the practice of BSE and teach the procedure when necessary.

Ductal Ectasia

Ductal ectasia is a benign breast problem that is usually seen in women approaching menopause. The disease is caused by dilation and thickening of the collecting ducts in the subareolar area. These ducts become distended and filled with cellular debris, which activates an inflammatory response. Two manifestations result from these changes:

- A mass develops that feels hard, has irregular borders, and may be tender.
- A greenish brown nipple discharge, enlarged axillary nodes, and redness and edema over the site of the mass are noted.

These masses are often difficult to distinguish from breast cancer. Because the risk for breast cancer is increased among women in the menopause age-group, accurate diagnosis is vital. A microscopic examination of the nipple discharge is performed to detect any atypical or malignant cells, and the affected area is excised. Nursing care is directed at reducing the anxiety associated with the threat of breast cancer and at supporting the woman through the diagnostic and treatment procedures.

Intraductal Papilloma

Intraductal papilloma occurs most often in women 40 to 55 years of age. A benign process in the epithelial lining of the duct forms a **papilloma** (pedunculated outgrowth of tissue). As the papilloma grows, trauma and erosion within the duct result in a bloody or serous nipple discharge. A mass is rarely palpable.

Diagnosis is aimed first at ruling out breast cancer. Microscopic examination of the nipple discharge and surgical excision of the mass and ductal area are usually indicated.

Issues of Large-Breasted Women

Although Western society emphasizes large breasts as positive attributes, women with excessive breast tissue do have some difficulties and discomfort. For instance, because fashion is directed at the small-breasted figure, a woman with large breasts may have difficulty finding clothes that fit well and in which she feels attractive. The breast size may be out of proportion to the rest of the body, which adds to the problem of finding clothes that fit. Larger bras are expensive and may need to be specially ordered. The client may have large dents in the shoulders from bra straps. In addition, many large-breasted women develop fungal infections under the breasts, especially in hot weather, because it is difficult to keep this area dry and exposed to air.

Backaches from the added weight are also common. The only alternative for this condition, if well-fitting bras do not help and obesity is not part of the problem, may be breast reduction surgery. The surgeon removes excess breast tissue, and then repositions the nipple and remaining skin flaps to produce an optimal cosmetic effect. This operation is a major surgical procedure and is termed a *reduction mammoplasty*.

The decision to undergo the procedure is usually made after years of living with the discomfort of excessive breast size. Become involved in the decision-making stage by listening to the client verbalize her feelings and provide information as appropriate. The nursing diagnoses and goals after surgery are similar to those for the woman undergoing reconstructive surgery (see Breast Reconstruction, p. 1815).

Issues of Smaller-Breasted Women

Many women choose to have breast augmentation surgery to enhance the size, shape, or symmetry of their breasts. Whereas most surgeries involve the implantation of saline-filled or silicon prostheses, some are constructed from the women's own tissue in much the same way as for reconstruction after mastectomy. Cosmetic or "plastic surgery" for breast augmentation is discussed in Chapter 70.

One issue for clients who have breast augmentation surgery is that of breast cancer surveillance. Breast self-examination (BSE) and clinical breast examination (CBE) are easily performed after prostheses are placed for breast augmentation. The prosthesis is placed behind the woman's normal breast tissue, actually pushing it forward. Mammography, however, may be somewhat more uncomfortable for the woman who has a prosthesis. The anatomic breast must be pulled more forward, slightly away from the implant, during mammography. There are no data to support the possibility that breast augmentation changes the woman's risk for breast cancer.

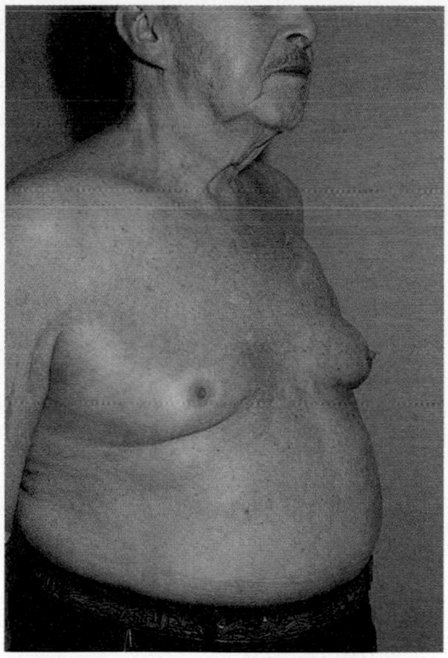

Figure 77-1 ■ Gynecomastia. (From Schwartz, M.H. [1998]. *Textbook of physical diagnosis: History and examination* [3rd ed.]. Philadelphia: W.B. Saunders.)

Gynecomastia

Gynecomastia literally means "female breasts" and is a symptom rather than a disease. It is usually a benign condition of breast enlargement in *men* (Figure 77-1). However, gynecomastia can be a result of a primary cancer such as lung cancer. The enlargement is usually bilateral, but enlargement is asymmetric in about 10% of cases. The condition is caused by abnormal growth of the glandular tissue, including the mammary ducts and ductal stroma. In many instances, it is difficult to distinguish gynecomastia from breast enlargement related to excess adipose tissue. Causes of gynecomastia include the following:

- Drugs
- Aging
- Obesity
- Underlying disease causing estrogen excess, such as malnutrition, liver disease, or hyperthyroidism
- Androgen-deficiency states, such as age, chronic renal failure, or alcoholism

Although gynecomastia is not common, men with abnormal breast findings, especially a breast mass, are carefully evaluated for breast cancer.

BREAST CANCER

PATHOPHYSIOLOGY

Breast cancer is the most commonly diagnosed invasive cancer in women and is second only to lung cancer as a cause of cancer deaths. The goal of early diagnosis is to reduce mortality by identifying women at risk for breast cancer and predicting the prognosis and response to different therapies. Because of the high incidence of the disease, almost every woman has had a close personal association with another woman with the disease. Thus most women have strong reactions to the threat of breast cancer. These reactions greatly influence a woman's health habits, including breast self-

TABLE 77-2 Types of Invasive Breast Cancer

Breast Cancer Type	Percent of Breast Cancers	Specific Features
Ductal carcinoma	~80%	Shows as a characteristic "spicule" pattern and calcifications on mammography
Lobular carcinoma	10%	More likely to affect both breasts and to have multiple sites within each breast Forms a palpable lump but does not always show on mammography
Medullary carcinoma	1%-5%	Occurs more frequently in younger women, especially those who are BRCA1 or BRCA2 positive
Colloid (mucinous) carcinoma	1%-6%	Occurs more frequently in older women Soft and slow-growing, may be hard to distinguish from cysts or benign breast disease on palpation or mammography Good prognosis
Inflammatory carcinoma	>1%	Rapidly growing, often with metastasis present at diagnosis First manifestations are breast skin edema and redness

Data from Cotran, R., Kumar, V., & Collons, T. (1999). *Robbins pathologic basis of disease* (6th ed.). Philadelphia: W.B. Saunders.

examination (BSE) and her readiness to seek care when a suspicious area is discovered.

Until prevention becomes a viable option, early detection is the key to effective treatment and survival. The 5-year relative survival rate is lower for women who are diagnosed with a more advanced stage of breast cancer. The 5-year survival rate for women with localized breast cancer is 97%, whereas the rate drops to 79% when the breast cancer has spread to the regional lymph nodes. Survival drops to only 23% when the breast cancer is metastatic (spread to distant sites) (American Cancer Society, 2005).

Types of Breast Cancer

There are many types of breast cancer (Table 77-2), but the most common, accounting for more than 80% of cases, is **infiltrating ductal carcinoma.** As the name implies, the disease originates in the mammary ducts and grows in the epithelial cells lining these ducts. The rate of cancer growth varies and partially depends on hormonal influences. It takes an estimated 5 to 9 years for a cancer cell to divide enough to form a palpable lesion.

As long as the cancer remains within the duct, it is noninvasive. The cancer is classified as **invasive** when it penetrates the tissue surrounding the duct. Most breast cancers arise from the intermediate ducts and are invasive. Once invasive, the cancer grows into the tissue around it in an irregular pattern; for this reason, once the lesion is palpable, it is felt as an irregular, poorly defined mass.

As the tumor continues to grow, **fibrosis** (replacement of normal cells with connective tissue and collagen) develops around the cancer. This fibrosis may cause shortening of Cooper's ligaments and the resulting typical skin dimpling that is seen with more advanced disease (Figure 77-2).

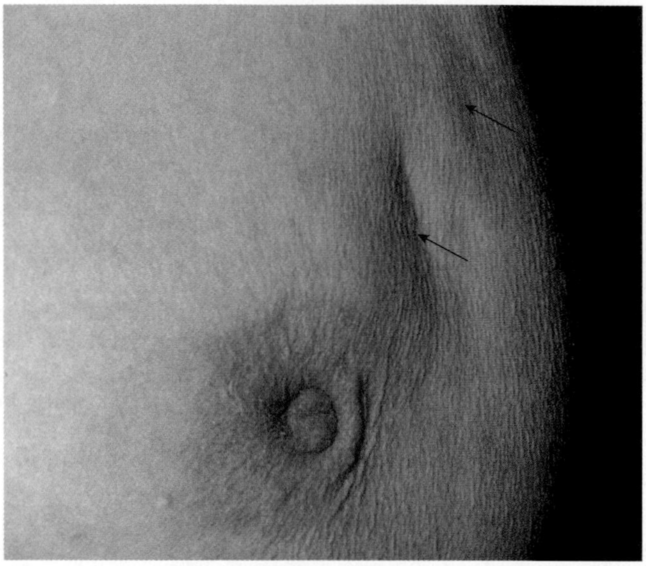

Figure 77-2 ■ Skin dimpling on a breast as a result of fibrosis or breast cancer. (Arrows indicate dimples.) (From Evans, A.J. et al. [1998]. *Atlas of breast disease management:* 50 illustrative cases. Philadelphia: W.B. Saunders.)

Complications of Breast Cancer

The tumor also invades the lymphatic channels, blocking skin drainage and causing skin edema and an "orange peel" appearance of the skin **(peau d'orange)** as shown in Figure 77-3. Invasion of the lymphatic channels carries cancer cells to the lymphatic nodes, including those in the axillary region. For this reason, pathologic examination of the axillary nodes is imperative for staging the disease. The cancer eventually replaces the skin itself, and ulceration of the overlying skin occurs. Metastasis results from seeding of the cancer cells into the blood and lymph systems, which permits spread of these cells to distant sites. The most common sites of metastatic disease from breast cancer are bone, lungs, brain, and liver.

The course of metastatic breast cancer is related to the site affected and to the function impaired. The processes involved in cancer development are described in Chapter 27.

Breast Cancer in Men

About 1% of all cases of breast cancer occur in men. The average age of onset is 60 years. Most cases of breast cancer in men occur in those with a genetic mutation in either the BRCA1 or the BRCA2 gene. (See later discussion of genetic risk.)

Men usually present with a hard, nonpainful, and subareolar mass. Gynecomastia may be present. Occasionally the man may have nipple discharge, retraction, erosion, or ulceration. Although nipple discharge is not a common manifestation, about 75% of the men who present with nipple discharge are diagnosed with breast carcinoma. Breast cancer in men is staged in the same manner as in women. Breast cancer in men is often a widely spread disease because it is usually detected

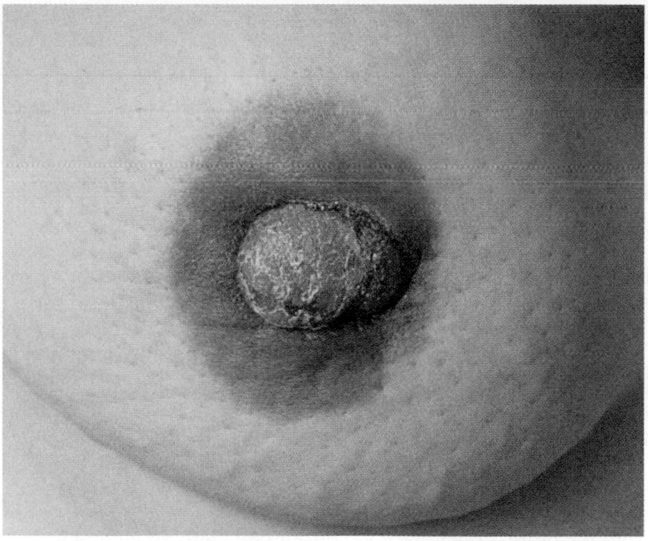

Figure 77-3 ■ Breast edema giving the skin an "orange peel" (peau d'orange) appearance. (From Mansel, R. [1995]. *Color atlas of breast diseases.* London: Mosby.)

at a later stage than in women. This fact gives men lower survival rates than women. Treatment of breast cancer in men is the same as in women at a similar stage of disease.

Etiology and Genetic Risk

There is no single known etiologic agent for breast cancer. Breast cancer can be attributed to multiple factors. Being an older woman is the primary risk factor, although some women are at higher risk than others. As age increases, so does risk. More than 85% of cases are diagnosed in clients older than 45 years of age. At 25 years of age, the overall risk for breast cancer is about 1 in 20,000. By 75 years of age, this risk increases to 1 in 11.

Women with a family history of breast cancer, particularly a history of a first-degree relative (mother, sister, or daughter) with premenopausal breast cancer, have a threefold risk increase. This risk is further increased if the relative either had breast cancer in both breasts or was diagnosed before 40 years of age (American Cancer Society, 2005). Family history includes multiple relatives with breast cancer, early age at diagnosis, and in some families, ovarian cancer.

Genetic Considerations

Inherited mutations in several genes are related to hereditary breast cancer. The most common genes tested for an inherited susceptibility for breast cancer are BRCA1 and BRCA2. Women who have specific mutations in either one of these genes are at a 40% to 89% risk for developing breast cancer. However, only about 5% of all breast cancers are hereditary. These mutations are more common among women with an Ashkenazi Jewish ethnicity.

Breast cancer is usually a **sporadic** (not having an identifiable genetic pattern of inheritance) rather than an inherited or a familial disorder. Many personal and environmental interactions are related to its development. Known risk factors that increase risk include exposure to high-dose ionizing radiation to the thorax (especially before 20 years of age), early menarche (before 12 years of age), and late menopause (after 50 years of age). A history of previous breast cancer, **nulliparity** (no pregnancies), and first birth after 30 years of age appear to heighten risk. Table 77-3 lists known risk factors for breast cancer development.

Other less well-explained risk factors include a diet high in animal fats, alcohol consumption, and long-term estrogen replacement therapy (McPherson, Steel, & Dixon, 2000). Studies have shown a small increase in the risk for breast cancer in postmenopausal women receiving hormone replacement therapy (HRT) after 5 or more years of use. Obesity may be a factor associated with the development of breast cancer in postmenopausal women.

Incidence/Prevalence

Each year, breast cancer is diagnosed in more than 200,000 women and 1300 men in the United States. Of these, more than 40,000 women and 400 men die of the disease. Although these numbers are staggering, there is a trend toward earlier diagnosis. Breast cancer incidence rates have continued to climb since 1980 with a slowing of the rate of increase occurring in the 1990s (American Cancer Society, 2005). Breast cancer accounts for 1 in 4 cancers in women. It occurs most commonly in older adults, and its prevalence increases with age. One of every eight American women will develop breast cancer in her lifetime.

CULTURAL CONSIDERATIONS

Although the incidence of breast cancer is lower in African Americans than in white individuals, death rates are higher for African-American women at every stage of the disease. The 5-year survival rate for African Americans is 62% compared with 79% for white individuals. Research suggests that poverty, less education, and inadequate access to screening are related to higher cancer morbidity and mortality rates in African Americans (American Cancer Society, 2003a).

Like the African-American female population, Latino and Hispanic women have a lower incidence of breast cancer than white women but a higher death rate. The differences in survival rates reflect the stage at which the cancer is diagnosed. Breast cancer is the most common cancer in immigrant Asian and Pacific Island women; the incidence and death rates are higher for Hawaiian women than for all other ethnic groups (Shinagawa, 2000).

Better access to screening techniques for minority women could help decrease these health disparities. Nursing research is needed in the area of the development and testing of culturally sensitive and appropriate breast cancer screening and treatment information.

HEALTH PROMOTION/ILLNESS PREVENTION

Early detection by screening for breast masses involves a three-pronged approach: mammography, breast self-examination (BSE), and clinical breast examination (CBE).

Mammography

The American Cancer Society (ACS) has established guidelines for breast cancer screening. The ACS recommends a baseline screening mammogram (x-ray of the breast) at 40 years of age and yearly screening for women beginning at age 40 (American Cancer Society, 2003b) (Table 77-4).

TABLE 77-3 Risk Factors for Breast Cancer

Factor	Degree of Risk	Comments
Female gender	Increased	Ninety-nine percent of all breast cancers occur in women.
History of a previous breast cancer	Increased	The risk of developing a cancer in the opposite breast is 5 times greater than for the average population at risk.
Age >40 yr	Increased	Incidence increases with age and peaks in the sixth decade.
Menstrual history Early menstruation or late menopause, or both	Increased	The risk for breast cancer rises as the interval between menarche and menopause increases. Women who undergo bilateral oophorectomy before age 35 have only 40% of the risk for breast cancer than do women who undergo natural menopause.
Reproductive history Nulliparity First child born after age 30	Increased	Childless women have an increased risk, as do women who bear their first child near or after age 30.
Family history Mother or sister or both	Increased	Risk increases 3 or more times if the mother or a sister has had breast cancer and is further increased if the relative was younger than 40 years of age or if the cancer was bilateral, or if the relative also developed ovarian cancer.
Diet	Controversial	Animal data and descriptive epidemiology of breast cancer incidence suggest an association of dietary factors, specifically a high-fat diet, with an increased risk for breast cancer. The association is stronger if the client is also obese.
Alcohol	Unknown	A suggested small increase in risk with moderate alcohol consumption has been reported, although limitations in methodology have been cited and results require confirmation.
Obesity	Controversial	Weight, obesity (especially increased abdominal fat), increased body mass, insulin resistance, and hyperglycemia have been reported to be associated with an increased risk for breast cancer.
Ionizing radiation	Increased	Women who received frequent low-level radiation exposure to the thorax had an increased risk, especially if the exposure occurred during periods of rapid breast formation.
Benign breast disease	None	Fibrocystic breast disease is not associated with breast cancer. However, biopsy-proven atypical hyperplasia is associated with an increased risk.
Oral contraceptives	None	There is no evidence that suggests a causal relationship between oral contraceptives and the incidence of and survival from breast cancer. Small studies have indicated a possible protective effect of oral contraceptives.
Exogenous (external) hormones	Controversial	Several studies report no link with replacement hormones and breast cancer, and those that do appear to identify only subsets of clients at risk: those who have taken replacement estrogens for more than 5 yr and those who have taken large cumulative doses.

Modified from McPherson, C.M., et al. (2000). ABC of breast disease: Breast cancer-epidemiology, risk factors, and genetics. *British Medical Journal 321*(9), 624-628.

TABLE 77-4 American Cancer Society Breast Cancer Screening Guidelines for Asymptomatic Women*

Age	Screening Activity
20 to 39 yr	Breast self-examination (BSE), monthly Clinical breast examination (CBE), every 3 years
40 yr and older	BSE monthly CBE annually Screening mammography (two views of each breast), annually

*Asymptomatic women who are identified to be at higher risk need to have an individualized screening plan that may differ from these guidelines.

Information from American Cancer Society. (2003). *Cancer prevention and early detection. Facts and figures-2003.* Report No. 8600.03. Atlanta: Author.

Barriers to mammography compliance may include fear of radiation, fear of results, concern about pain, and lack of education (Rawl et al., 2000; Strzelczyk & Dignan, 2002). Awareness of barriers to mammography adherence as well as how factors such as ethnicity and age interact with these barriers can assist in the development of interventions that help increase adherence to mammogram guidelines (Rawl et al., 2000).

Breast Self-Examination

Breast self-examination (BSE) is an inexpensive means for detecting breast cancer that has been encouraged by health care providers for decades. The goal of screening for breast cancer is *early detection because BSE does not prevent breast cancer.* Detection of breast cancer before axillary node invasion increases the chance of survival. BSE, used in conjunction with mammography and CBE, is effective in detecting early breast cancer and reducing mortality rates. BSE *alone* as a screening technique has not been of equal value. The American Cancer Society recommends monthly BSE as a screening option for all women beginning in their 20s. Most women have heard of BSE, but many do not practice it regularly or correctly.

Whether the client seeks health care because she has found a breast lump, because she needs a routine physical examination, or because she has an unrelated health problem, BSE should be taught. Do not assume that women who practice BSE do so competently and regularly. Women who are taught BSE on an individual or group basis practice BSE more often, more proficiently, and more confidently than do women who learn the technique from pamphlets.

PREPARATION FOR TEACHING BREAST SELF-EXAMINATION

Before teaching BSE, assess the psychological factors influencing the client's motivation to practice BSE. Lack of knowledge about the technique and the benefits of early detection, uneasiness about self-assessment, and lack of confidence in self-assessment may be reasons why women fail to perform BSE regularly. Stress that treatment for breast cancer is more successful when the disease is detected earlier. It is also important for the client to develop confidence in her ability to detect breast changes. A yearly breast examination by a health care provider cannot substitute for BSE.

Emphasize the advantages of early detection and help the client review risk factors to determine her risk for developing breast cancer. Ask the client whether she has ever had a breast problem in the past. Women must believe that there are benefits to practicing BSE and that the barriers to practicing it are minimal. Addressing these issues will increase the client's knowledge and practice of BSE.

Discussing the client's fears, beliefs, and concerns about breast disease and BSE with her is an important step. Discuss the proper timing for BSE. Instruct premenopausal women to examine their breasts 1 week after the menstrual period. At this time, hormonal influence on breast tissue is minimal, so that fluid retention and tenderness are reduced. Instruct women whose breast tissue is no longer influenced by hormonal fluctuations, such as after a total hysterectomy or menopause, to pick a day each month to do BSE, such as the first day of the month.

TEACHING BREAST SELF-EXAMINATION

Ensure that the setting in which you demonstrate BSE is private and comfortable. Ask the woman to undress from the waist up and provide a gown and sheet. Before teaching the technique of breast palpation, assess the client's technique by asking her to demonstrate her own method. If the woman is unsure or has not performed BSE before, slowly lead her through the examination while explaining the rationale for the technique and answering questions. It is also helpful to point out different findings at this time, especially those that the client might perceive as abnormal. For example, nodular breast tissue may normally feel lumpy, which may be interpreted as widespread cancer in the unknowledgeable woman. Placing the client's hand directly on the involved area and showing her precisely what is normal for her can build self-confidence.

Indicate the inframammary ridge, the area of the breast where the skin folds under the breast. This thickened area may be perceived as a lump instead of a normal finding. In thin or small-breasted women, the ribs may be mistaken for masses. Demonstrate how to follow the rib to the sternum to be sure that what she is feeling is bone and not breast tissue. Teach the client to stand in front of a mirror to inspect the breast for abnormalities. She should raise her arms above her head and press her hands on her hips to emphasize any changes in the shape of the breasts. The breasts are examined in a lying position and while bathing or showering.

Additionally, demonstrate the proper amount of pressure needed to palpate the breast tissue and the correct position of the hands. The finger pads, which are more sensitive than the fingertips, are used when palpating the breasts. Teach the client to press firmly enough to detect the underlying tissue, but not to compress the tissue on the ribs, because this may falsely feel like a mass.

Use teaching models of normal and abnormal breasts when teaching BSE. Demonstrate the correct technique of examining the breasts with the arm overhead while lying down instead of having the arm by her side. Showing the difference in the two techniques, especially in large-breasted women, reveals the advantage of using the correct method, which spreads the tissue over the chest wall for more effective palpation (Figure 77-4).

Clinical Breast Examination

Clinical breast examination (CBE) is typically performed by advanced practice nurses and physicians. However, nurses in general practice who are skilled in the technique can perform this examination. The examination can be done before, after, or during the teaching session. It is recommended that the CBE be part of a periodic health examination, at least every 3 years for women in their 20s and 30s, and annually for asymptomatic women at least 40 years of age (American Cancer Society, 2003b). The same guidelines of providing a private and comfortable setting, maintaining dignity, and allowing time for discussion apply.

Video Clip: Inspection (Sitting) ◀

Taking a breast history is vital. Results may be recorded on a breast evaluation form, which is a part of the client's record (Figure 77-5). This record helps establish the relative risk for breast disease and the need for follow-up diagnostic tests, such as mammograms, and teaching.

The physical assessment begins with inspection. The woman undresses from the waist up and first sits or stands with her hands by her sides. The examiner inspects the breasts for symmetry and size, contour, skin changes (color, texture, and venous patterns), nipple changes, and lesions.

One breast may be larger than the other, and inverted nipples are common. Ask the client whether these findings are normal for her. Any change in symmetry may indicate a problem. The contour should be even, and the skin should have a smooth texture. Venous patterns may be visible but should be similar bilaterally. The nipples and areola should be equal or nearly equal in size and should be a similar color. The nipples may be wrinkled or smooth, and Montgomery's tubercles on the areola are normal. Supernumerary nipples (extra nipples), although rare, are also normal and may appear anywhere on the chest. If present, they should be examined in the same manner as the normal nipples.

If a mass is palpated, note its position by visualizing the breast as a clock face (with 12 o'clock being toward the client's head) and noting the "area of the clock" where the mass is located. If it is necessary to move the arms away from the body, the woman should rest her arm on the examiner's to prevent flexion of the underlying muscles. While the arms are by the side and relaxed, the axillae can be palpated. Palpate the axilla and the area above and below the clavicle for enlarged lymph nodes. The woman is then asked to raise her arms over her head, which exposes the sides and underneath portions of the breast for inspection. Finally, she is asked to place her hands on her hips and press, thus flexing the pectoral muscles. This action accentuates skin dimpling, retractions, or masses.

Video Clips: Inspection (Supine) ◀

The remainder of the examination is done with the client lying supine. Place a pillow or rolled sheet under the client's

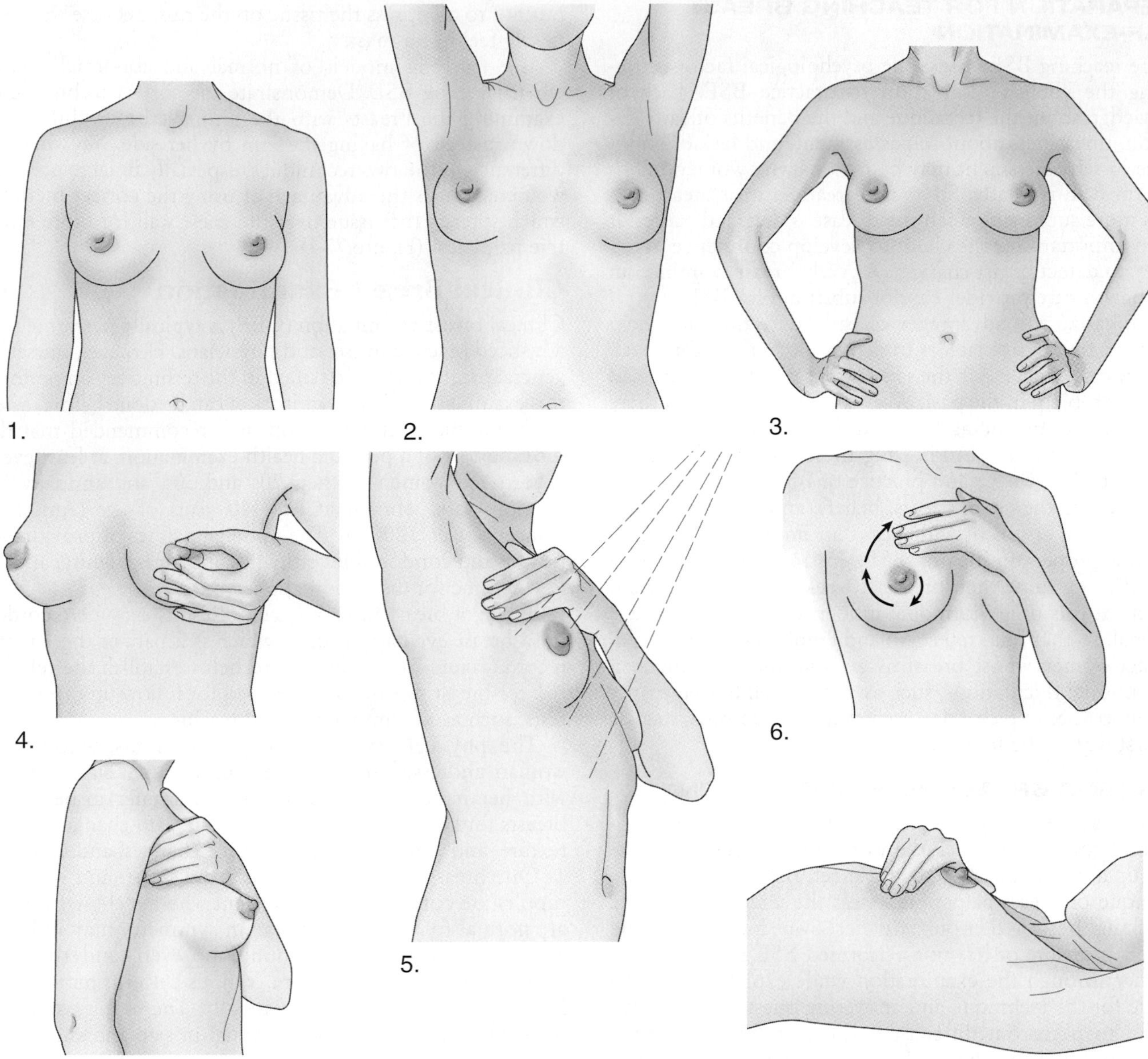

Figure 77-4 ■ A woman performing breast self-examination (BSE). From…

shoulder, and the arm on that side is raised above the head. Each breast is palpated separately while the other breast remains covered. If the woman has identified a problem in one breast, the other, "normal" breast is examined first to establish a baseline for comparison.

Palpate in a vertical pattern, in a horizontal pattern, or in concentric circles, covering every inch of the breast tissue, including the tail of Spence, which extends from the upper outer quadrant of the breast into the axilla. The supraclavicular lymph nodes are palpated for the presence of enlarged nodes by hooking the fingers over the clavicle.

Finally, the nipple is gently compressed to detect the presence of a discharge. If a discharge is produced, note the "area of the clock" where the breast was compressed when the discharge was released. If there is a history of discharge, the client may be able to express the discharge more successfully than the examiner can and should be asked to do so.

CONSIDERATIONS FOR OLDER ADULTS

As women age, the breast tissue becomes flattened and elongated and is suspended loosely from the chest wall. On palpation, the breast tissue of the older woman has a finer, more granular feel than the lobular feel in a younger woman. The inframammary ridge may be more prominent as a result of atrophy of the breast tissue. Breast examination in older clients may be easier because of tissue atrophy and relaxation of the suspensory ligaments (Cooper's ligaments).

Discovery of a suspicious lesion or discharge during the examination requires consultation or referral to a health care provider who specializes in caring for breast disorders. Follow-up usually involves mammography and possibly ultrasound. If there is a dominant mass or high genetic risk, the woman should be referred for biopsy even if the mammogram is negative.

CLIENT'S NAME ______________________ Gender ________ Race ____________ Age ______

Weight ____________ Ideal Weight ____________ Marital Status ______________________

HISTORY	Yes	No	Comments
Family history of breast cancer			
Personal history of breast cancer			
Previous mammograms			
Previous biopsy (findings)			
Nipple discharge			
Hormone use (specify)			
BSE Practice			
High-fat diet			
ETOH/smoking			
Current medications (list)			

Age at menses ____________ Age at menopause ____________

COMMENTS

____

PHYSICAL FINDINGS

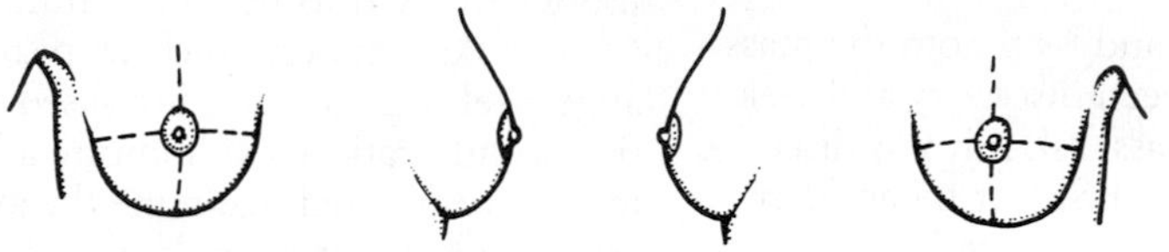

Mammogram Report ______________________________

Biopsy/Cytology Results ______________________________

BSE Return Demonstration ______________________________

Plan ______________________________

CLIENT EDUCATION ______________________________

Figure 77-5 ■ A breast evaluation form.

Cancer Surveillance

Cancer surveillance is a prevention option preferred by most *high-risk* women. Cancer surveillance is also referred to as "secondary prevention" and is used to detect cancer early in the initial stages. For breast cancer surveillance in high-risk women, the same combination of breast self-examination (BSE), clinical breast examination (CBE), and mammography are recommended as in the asymptomatic population. The difference for high-risk women is in the timing of examinations and starting age of mammography. The recommendations include monthly BSE beginning by 20 years of age, CBE every 6 to 12 months beginning at 25 to 35 years of age, and annual mammography beginning at 25 to 35 years of age (Sakorafas, 2003).

Prophylactic Mastectomy

Prophylactic (preventive) **mastectomy** (surgical breast removal) is another option for reducing the risk of breast cancer. It remains a highly controversial practice. Even though a woman may elect to undergo a prophylactic mastectomy, there is a small risk that breast cancer will develop in residual breast glandular tissue, because no mastectomy reliably removes all mammary tissue. Therefore when prophylactic mastectomy is selected by the client, careful and regular long-term follow-up is indicated (Sakorafas, 2003).

Chemoprevention

Another management option for women at high risk for breast cancer is chemoprevention with the use of selective estrogen receptor modifiers (SERMs), such as tamoxifen citrate (Nolvadex, Tamofen✱, Tamone✱). This strategy has been found to significantly reduce the incidence of breast cancer in women at high risk for breast cancer (Sakorafas, 2003). Other drugs in this class include raloxifene (Evista), toremifene (Fareston), droloxifene, and idoxifene (Sakorafas, 2003; Workman, 2002).

◆COLLABORATIVE MANAGEMENT

PHARM e REVIEW

◆Assessment

HISTORY

Often, the history is taken after a mass has been discovered but before definitive diagnosis has been made. For some clients, the history may be obtained at the time the woman is seen for treatment of an identified cancer. The interview should focus on three major areas: risk factors, the breast mass, and health maintenance practices.

RISK FACTORS. Record age, gender, marital status, weight, and height. Marital status and identification of the client's primary support person provide information about those to be included in the woman's care, teaching, and support. Ask specific information on personal and family histories of breast cancer. In addition to increasing the woman's own risk, these factors also affect any sisters' or daughters' risk and should be incorporated into later counseling.

Ask the following information about the client's gynecologic and obstetric history:

- Age at menarche
- Age at menopause
- Symptoms of menopause
- Age at first child's birth
- Number of children

Prolonged hormonal stimulation (e.g., early menses or late menopause) increases a woman's risk, as do birth of the first child after 30 years of age and nulliparity.

HISTORY OF THE BREAST MASS. This information reveals not only the course of the disease but also data related to health care seeking practices and health-promoting behaviors.

Ask the client about how, when, and by whom the mass was discovered and the interval between discovery and seeking care. If the woman found the mass, ask if it was discovered through breast self-examination (BSE) or by accident? The answer to this question highlights the need for discussion and teaching about BSE regardless of whether the mass proves to be malignant. If there was a delay between discovery and seeing the health care provider, ask what caused the delay. These questions are linked to the psychosocial assessment but also reveal the length of time that the tumor has been present. Ask the client what procedures have been performed to diagnose the problem. Also, ask the client if she has noticed any other changes in her body within the past year. This information can help determine whether there has been obvious cancer spread. Ask especially about the presence of joint or bone pain.

HEALTH MAINTENANCE PRACTICES. In addition to asking the client about the knowledge, practice, and regularity of BSE, take a mammographic history. The existence of previous mammograms allows the health care provider to compare current mammograms with past ones to facilitate diagnosis.

A brief diet history, in which the client is asked to recall a typical day's menu and alcoholic intake per week, reveals the usual intake of fat and alcohol. A high alcohol and fat intake *may* increase the risk of breast cancer.

Ask the client what types of prescribed and over-the-counter drugs she uses, specifically, hormonal supplements, such as estrogen. Estrogen can be taken orally, intravaginally, or via a transdermal patch. Document the type and form of hormones (birth control pills or patches, supplements) and length of use. Use of estrogen creams intravaginally is common among postmenopausal women and also is a source of estrogen.

Critical Thinking Challenge

A middle-aged woman is hospitalized for a bowel resection for colon cancer. Before discharge, she tells you that she is very concerned about her risk for breast cancer. The disease was diagnosed in her sister 2 years ago. She tells you that she thinks because she already has colon cancer, that her risk is increased for breast cancer.

1. How should you respond to her at this time?
2. What questions should you ask her about her family history, including her sister's breast cancer?
3. What questions should you ask her to help assess her risk for breast cancer?
4. What options does she have for health promotion and disease prevention?

evolve For suggested answer guidelines, go to http://evolve.elsevier.com/Iggy/.

PHYSICAL ASSESSMENT/CLINICAL MANIFESTATIONS

The approach to physical assessment is discussed earlier under Breast Self-Examination (p. 1796) and under Clinical Breast Examination (p. 1797). Check for and document specific information about the breast mass (Chart 77-1). Describe the mass in terms of location (using the "face of the clock" method), shape, size, consistency, and whether it is mobile or fixed to the surrounding tissues.

Any skin change, such as peau d'orange (dimpling, orange peel appearance), increased vascularity, nipple retraction, or ulceration, can indicate advanced disease and needs to be documented. Examine the axillary and supraclavicular areas thoroughly by palpating deeply for enlarged lymph nodes and documenting their presence and location in the client's record. The presence of pain or soreness in the affected breast is evaluated. After gathering this information, draw a diagram on the chart (see Figure 77-5) that will be helpful for others involved in the client's care.

PSYCHOSOCIAL ASSESSMENT

The client with potential or diagnosed breast cancer faces three major issues: (1) the fear of cancer, (2) threats to body image, sexuality, intimate relationships, and survival, and (3) decisional conflict related to treatment options.

The woman needs information about how advanced the disease is, the likelihood of cure, treatment options and side effects, how treatment will affect her life and self-image, how her family or partner will be affected, and home self-care. A woman's previous experience with cancer, and especially with other women with breast cancer, influences her reactions to the disease. Ask the client whether she has known anyone with breast cancer and what types of experiences she has had with breast disease and cancer in

CHART 77-1

BEST PRACTICE for
Assessing a Breast Mass

- Identify the location of the mass by using the "face of the clock" method.
- Describe the shape, size, and consistency of the mass.
- Assess whether the mass is fixed or movable.
- Note any skin changes around the mass, such as dimpling *(peau d'orange),* increased vascularity, nipple retraction, and ulceration.
- Assess the adjacent lymph nodes, both axillary and supraclavicular nodes.
- Ask the client if she experiences pain or soreness in the area around the mass.

general. Explore the woman's feelings about the disease because her choices of treatment, her recovery, and her ability to learn are influenced by these emotions. Assess the client's and family's knowledge of breast cancer, the stage of the disease, and treatment options. The client's level of education is a significant influencing factor in her treatment choices for stage I breast cancer. Her perception of her situation is often influenced by outdated information. Perhaps she knew someone who had a Halsted radical mastectomy more than 30 years ago and thus associates breast surgery with the chest deformity and lymphedema experienced by that woman. Dispel myths or misconceptions by providing current information.

Also assess the client for problems related to sexuality. Three critical areas of distress–psychological, physiologic, and relational–contribute to the psychosexual morbidity of these clients. Ask about her frequency of, and satisfaction with, sexual relations with her partner. The client should reflect on the relationship with the partner and be asked whether and how the breast cancer has changed the intimate relations with, sexual function of, or types of touch by the partner.

Evaluate the need for additional resources at this time. Will extra psychological counseling be needed? Are there financial concerns that need to be discussed with social services? Will the client's partner, family, or friends support her throughout this period? How much support and teaching do they need? When does the client expect to hear about her pathology results, and whom would she like to have with her when she hears the results? Answers to these types of questions provide guidelines in establishing expected outcomes and in planning nursing care.

LABORATORY ASSESSMENT

The diagnosis of breast cancer relies on pathologic examination of tissue from the breast mass. After the presence of cancer is established, laboratory tests, including pathologic study of the lymph nodes, help detect possible metastases. Elevated liver enzyme levels indicate possible liver metastases, and increased serum calcium and alkaline phosphatase levels suggest bone metastases.

RADIOGRAPHIC ASSESSMENT

Mammography is a sensitive screening tool for breast cancer. However, it must be combined with BSE for optimal early detection and with clinical breast examination (CBE) for full interpretation of the findings. These three methods together are effective in detecting breast cancer as early as possible. The uniqueness of mammography results from its ability to reveal preclinical lesions (masses too small to be palpated manually). Client preparation and the procedure for mammography are discussed in Chapter 76.

Other radiographic procedures may be used before surgery to rule out metastases. A chest x-ray to screen for lung metastases is routine. Bone, liver, and brain scans and computed tomography (CT) scans of the chest and abdomen can reveal distant metastases.

OTHER DIAGNOSTIC ASSESSMENTS

Ultrasonography of the breast is an additional diagnostic tool used to clarify findings on mammography. If the mammogram reveals a lesion, ultrasonography is helpful in differentiating a fluid-filled cyst from a solid mass.

Pathologic examination of the breast tissue, or breast biopsy, is the key to diagnosis of breast cancer. Breast tissue is obtained by one of several types of biopsies (see Chapter 76).

Several other tests are useful for establishing the stage of disease and prognosis after the diagnosis is made. These tests include a pathologic examination of the lymph nodes on the affected side. Other prognostic factors include the following (Rosenzweig, Rust, & Hoss, 2000):

- Presence or absence of estrogen receptors (ER) or progesterone receptors (PR)
- S-phase index, or growth rate (done by flow cytometry to determine the S-phase fraction, also known as mitotic index)
- DNA ploidy (the amount of DNA in a tumor cell compared with the amount in a normal cell to determine whether the number of chromosomes in the cancer cells is normal **(euploid)** or abnormal **(aneuploid)**
- Histologic or nuclear grade
- HER2/neu gene expression

Estrogen and progesterone receptors are cytoplasmic proteins present in breast cancer cells that bind to estrogen and progesterone. In some cancers, when estrogen or progesterone binds to these receptors, the growth rate of the cell increases. Cancer cells that contain estrogen receptors (ER positive) or progesterone receptors (PR positive) have a better prognosis and usually respond to hormonal therapy. More postmenopausal women than premenopausal women are ER positive.

DNA ploidy and calculation of the number of cells in S phase by flow cytometry can reveal the growth rate of cells. Tumors with a high growth rate index and altered DNA content have a worse prognosis (Rosenzweig, Rust, & Hoss, 2000).

Tumor cells are also examined for specialization or differentiation. Because well-differentiated tumors tend to be less aggressive than poorly differentiated ones, a woman with a well-differentiated breast cancer has a better prognosis than the woman with a poorly differentiated tumor. Figure 77-6 illustrates the four stages of breast cancer.

Genetic Considerations

Breast cancer cells also are analyzed for the presence of excessive numbers of the HER2/neu receptor on or in the cancer cells. This receptor is related to the growth potential of the cancer cell. When breast cancer cells have excessive numbers of these receptors (overexpress the HER2/neu gene), they grow more rapidly and are relatively resistant to standard therapies. However, there is a targeted therapy, trastuzumab (Herceptin), that blocks these receptors and slows or stops the breast cancer cell growth. It is only effective for women whose breast cancer cells overexpress the HER2/neu gene.

Analysis

COMMON NURSING DIAGNOSES AND COLLABORATIVE PROBLEMS

A common nursing diagnosis for clients with breast cancer is Anxiety related to the diagnosis of cancer. A common collaborative problem is Potential for Metastasis.

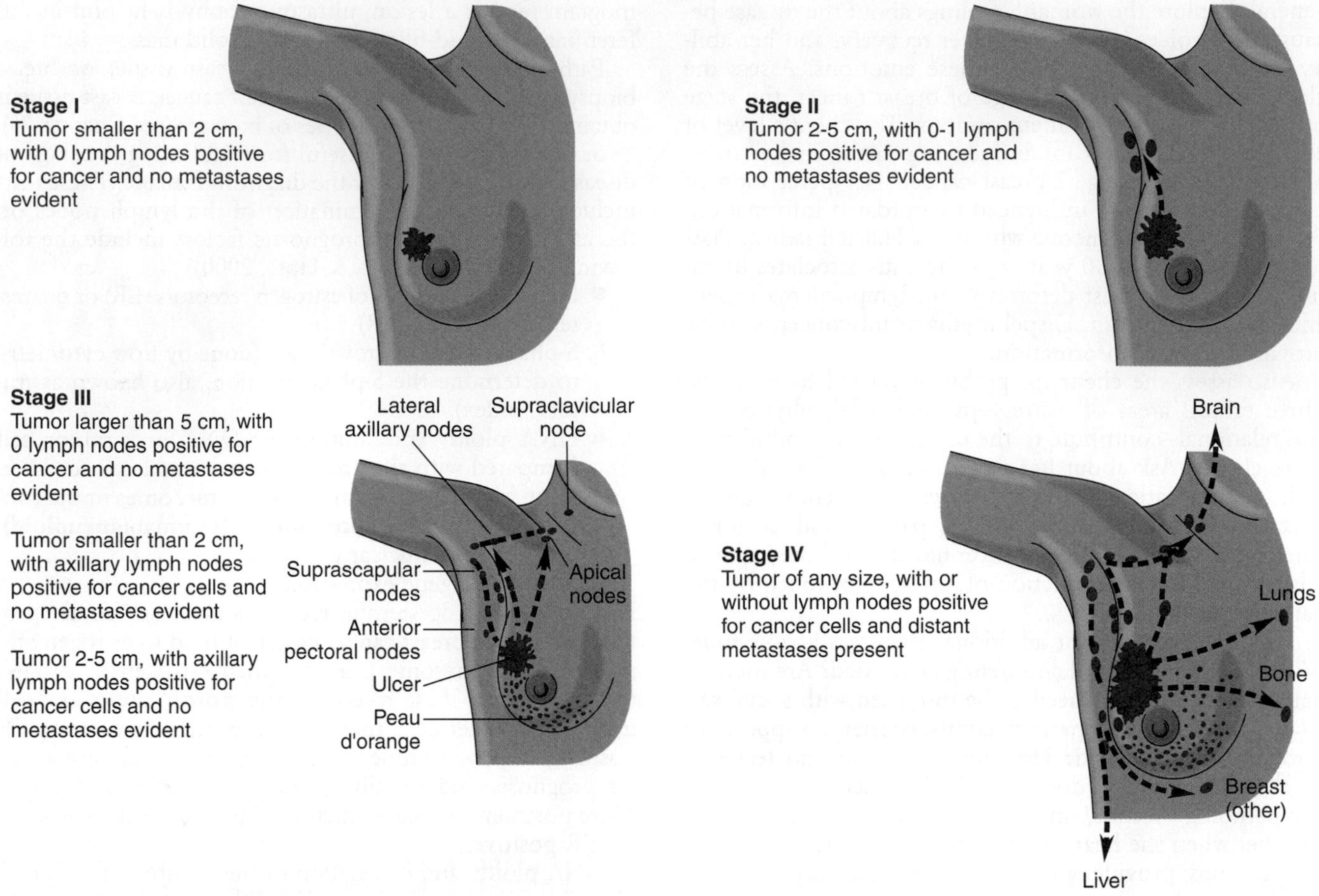

Figure 77-6 ■ Staging of breast cancer.

ADDITIONAL NURSING DIAGNOSES AND COLLABORATIVE PROBLEMS

In addition to the common nursing diagnoses and collaborative problems, clients with breast cancer (particularly advanced breast cancer) may have one or more of the following:

- Anticipatory Grieving related to loss and possible or impending death
- Acute Pain related to tumor compression on nerve endings
- Disturbed Sleep Pattern related to pain and anxiety
- Disturbed Body Image related to illness treatment, surgery, or loss of a body part
- Sexual Dysfunction related to surgery, disease process, or altered body structure

Planning and Implementation

ANXIETY

NOC **PLANNING: EXPECTED OUTCOMES.** The client with breast cancer is expected to reduce anxiety to acceptable levels. Indicators include that the client often or consistently demonstrates the following behaviors:

- Seeks information to reduce anxiety
- Uses effective coping strategies
- Uses relaxation techniques to reduce anxiety
- Maintains social relationships
- Maintains adequate sleep

INTERVENTIONS. The woman with breast cancer is usually admitted to the health care facility with a definitive diagnosis established through an outpatient biopsy of the mass. The practice of admitting a woman with a suspicious lesion and using general anesthesia for a biopsy, frozen section, and possible mastectomy has largely been abandoned. Women who have an interval between the biopsy and treatment, during which they actively participate in the choice of treatment, cope more effectively after surgery, no matter which treatment is chosen.

The anxiety for the woman with breast cancer begins the moment the lump is discovered. The level of anxiety may be related to past experiences and personal associations with the disease. Many women have an intuitive feeling about a cancer diagnosis even before it is established. The likelihood that the lesion is or is not cancer is irrelevant to the level of fear. Assess the client's perceptions of her own situation and personal level of anxiety. Allow the client to ventilate these feelings even if a diagnosis has not been established (Chart 77-2).

If the mass has been diagnosed as cancer, many women feel a partial sense of relief to be dealing with a known entity. A feeling of shock or disbelief may predominate. It is difficult to accept a diagnosis of cancer when one feels basically well. Clients and their families or significant others deal in individual ways with the mix of feelings, which include shock, disbelief, and grief. Some may want to read and discuss any available information. Others may want to

CHART 77-2

NIC **INTERVENTION ACTIVITIES for The Client with Breast Cancer**

Anxiety Reduction: *Minimizing apprehension, dread, foreboding, or uneasiness related to an unidentified source of anticipated danger*

- Listen attentively.
- Use a calm, reassuring approach.
- Provide factual information concerning diagnosis, treatment, and prognosis.
- Encourage verbalization of feelings, perceptions, and fears.
- Identify when level of anxiety changes.
- Support the use of appropriate defense mechanisms.
- Determine client's decision-making ability.

know as little as possible and resent attempts at teaching. Although one woman may want to talk at length about her concerns, another may want to be alone. Flexibility is the key to nursing care. Adjust your approach to care as the client's emotional state changes. An integral part of the plan to meet these emotional needs is the use of outside resources. Most health care providers view such groups as the American Cancer Society's Reach to Recovery as a source of support after surgery, but these groups can be suggested in the preoperative phase.

Health care providers working with clients who have breast cancer may know other clients willing to make a preoperative visit. These resource people may be chosen on the basis of the client's concerns. The woman who is worried in particular about the side effects of radiation therapy may benefit more from talking to someone who has undergone radiation than from talking to the nurse about secondhand experiences.

In addition to Reach to Recovery, formal and informal community support groups, such as ENCORE (Encouragement, Normalcy, Counseling, Opportunity, Reaching Out, and Energies Revived), may be available. These groups can be reached through the health care provider, the local hospital, visiting nurse associations, or by word of mouth.

POTENTIAL FOR METASTASIS

NOC **PLANNING: EXPECTED OUTCOMES.** The client with breast cancer is expected to remain free of metastases or recurrence of disease.

INTERVENTIONS. There are many surgical and nonsurgical options for breast cancer treatment. Because of the various options, the woman with breast cancer often faces difficult decisions.

Although most women with metastatic breast cancer eventually succumb to the disease, chemotherapy, hormonal therapy, radiotherapy, and limited surgery are all helpful for palliative care, improvement in quality of life, and prolongation of life. Once cancer is diagnosed, the extent and location of metastases determine the overall therapeutic strategy. Treatment is tailored specifically to each client, taking into account other health problems and the client's ability to tolerate a particular therapy. Most importantly, the woman's specific goals and the particular outcome she seeks from therapy are thoroughly discussed.

NONSURGICAL MANAGEMENT. For clients with late-stage breast cancer, nonsurgical treatment may be the only alternative. If the disease is in a late stage, such as stage IV, with the presence of confirmed metastasis, or if the client cannot withstand a major surgical procedure, the tumor may be removed with a local anesthetic. Follow-up treatment may include hormonal therapy, chemotherapy, and sometimes radiation. If the tumor is attached to the skin or the underlying muscle, resection may be impossible. Follow-up therapy involves radiation, usually in conjunction with chemotherapy. Chapter 28 describes the nursing care associated with chemotherapy and radiation.

For women with breast cancer at a stage for which surgery is the main treatment, follow-up with adjuvant radiation, chemotherapy, hormone therapy, or targeted therapy is commonly prescribed. These therapy options are discussed under adjuvant therapy on p. 1817.

SURGICAL MANAGEMENT. The most common types of breast surgery are illustrated in Figure 77-7. Although controversy exists concerning the best treatment for breast cancer, experts agree that the mass itself should be removed to reduce the risk for local recurrence. Removal of the axillary lymph nodes for staging purposes may also be recommended. Axillary lymph node dissection (ALND) is usually performed for clients with palpable axillary lymph nodes. It is unclear whether clients with nonpalpable nodes should also have ALND because these nodes could have micrometastasis, which, if not removed or treated, could result in recurrence. However, the long-term effects of ALND are significant. Thus women who have stage I breast cancer have not always had an ALND.

The technique of sentinel lymph node biopsy (SLNB) is a promising method of identifying clients with axillary involvement who do not have palpable nodes but who may have microscopic disease in one or more nodes (Zack, 2001). In this method, the one or two sentinel lymph nodes, which receive all of the lymphatic drainage from an anatomic region are identified through a lymph node mapping procedure. Mapping involves injecting the area immediately around a tumor with a blue dye and/or radioactive colloid 1 to 8 hours before the lymph node biopsy. The main lymph channels for the tumor area carry the marker dye or radioactivity to the first nodes. The nodes that take up the dye (or give off a certain level of radiation picked up by a handheld counter) are removed and examined for the presence of cancer cells. It is believed that if cancer cells have traveled through the lymph channels, the cells would have lodged in the sentinel nodes. Travel beyond these nodes to higher level nodes would have occurred as a secondary event. Therefore the absence of cancer cells in the sentinel nodes is an indicator that no other nodes in the regional basin should be involved. This method has been helpful in limiting axillary dissections only to those with positive nodes (Zack, 2001).

Preoperative Care. Care of the woman facing surgery for breast cancer focuses on psychological preparation and preoperative teaching. The issues related to anxiety and lack of knowledge are primary. Direct efforts toward educating the client include the husband or partner who may be experiencing similar stress and confusion.

Review the type of procedure planned. Use open-ended questions (e.g., "What type of surgery are you having? Can

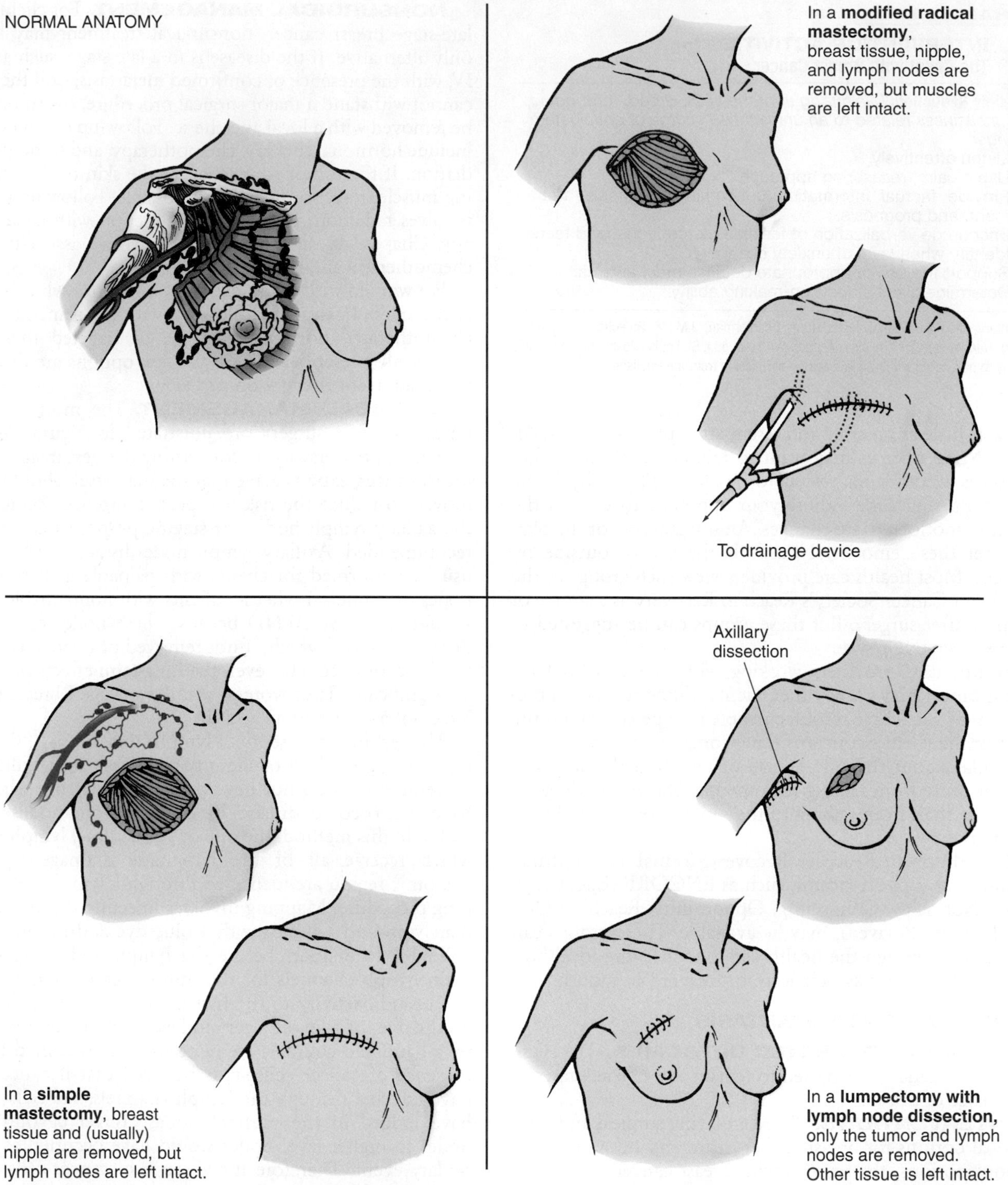

Figure 77-7 ■ Surgical management of breast cancer.

you explain what will happen?") to assess the client's level of knowledge. The client should be knowledgeable about the type of procedure. Provide postoperative information, including the following:

- The need for a drainage tube
- The location of the incision
- Mobility restrictions
- The length of the hospital stay (if any)
- The possibility of adjuvant therapy
- Basic before and after surgery information needed by any surgical client (see Chapters 20 and 22)

Because of short hospital stays or same-day surgery procedures, supplement teaching with written materials for the client and family to take home as references. This information should include who to call in case there are any complications. Address body image issues before surgery to correct misconceptions about appearance after surgery and help the client begin adjusting to changes after surgery. If available, clients and their caregivers may attend classes before surgery in an ambulatory care setting, such as a surgical clinic, to promote successful early discharge from the hospital. These programs, which may provide emotional support, information, and opportunities for discussion related to sexuality, body image, preoperative instructions, and care after surgery enhance the care of the short-stay mastectomy client.

Operative Procedures. During breast-conserving surgery, the surgeon removes the bulk of the tumor. Typically, radiation therapy follows to eradicate residual tumor cells. Radiation therapy plays a critical role in the therapeutic regimen and is effective treatment for nearly all sites where breast cancer can metastasize. The most common site for metastasis is to bone tissue.

The following types of breast-conserving surgery are used as primary treatment for stage I and stage II breast cancer:

- Lumpectomy, also known as tylectomy or local excision, is gross resection of the tumor.
- Partial mastectomy, which includes wide excision, quadrantectomy, or segmental mastectomy, is removal of the portion of the breast that contains the tumor.

Breast-conserving procedures are usually performed in same-day surgical settings. The breast-conserving results in 5- and 10-year survival and local recurrence rates are no worse than those of the modified radical mastectomy. The cosmetic results have been good to excellent, and other long-term problems are comparable to those of more radical procedures. For many women, the psychological benefits of avoiding breast removal are significant and lead them to choose this option.

The modified radical mastectomy does *not* conserve the breast; the affected breast is completely removed. This procedure differs from the older Halsted radical mastectomy in that the surgeon leaves the pectoral muscles and nerves intact. Thus the breast tissue and skin and the axillary nodes are removed, and the underlying muscles are left in place. The typical incision is a 5- to 6-inch-long elliptic incision from the midchest to the axilla (see Figure 77-7). If reconstruction is to follow the procedure, the plastic surgeon may recommend a different location for the incision. When reconstruction is to be performed at the same time as the mastectomy, less invasive techniques, such as incising a 1.5-inch flap of skin around the nipple (excising the same amount of breast tissue as with conventional mastectomy), may be performed. Skin flaps or implants may be used to create a breast mound at the time of the original procedure.

The use of carbon dioxide laser procedures in place of cutting and cauterizing for mastectomies is an option that is becoming more available. Advantages of laser procedures include less blood loss and faster recovery.

Postoperative Care. Care after surgery in the hospital and at home for the woman undergoing a modified radical mastectomy or breast-conserving surgery is provided in the Plan of Care on pp. 1806 to 1815. Before the woman returns from surgery, place a sign over the client's bed to warn nurses and other personnel to avoid using the affected arm for taking blood pressure measurements, giving injections, or drawing blood. The woman returns from the postanesthesia care unit (PACU) as soon as vital signs return to baseline levels and if no complications have occurred. On the client's return, the focus is on maintaining physiologic stability and comfort. Assess vital signs on a schedule of decreasing frequency, such as every 30 minutes for two times, every hour for two times, and then every 4 hours. During these checks, assess the dressing for bleeding.

Care of Drainage Tubes. During a modified radical mastectomy, the surgeon places one or two drainage tubes, usually Jackson-Pratt drains, under the skin flaps and attaches the tubes to a small collection chamber. Gentle suction is exerted, and fluid that would accumulate under the flaps and delay healing is collected. Various drains are available, but all allow the drainage to be seen and measured. When taking vital signs, monitor the drain for the amount and color of drainage. Add this information to the intake and output record. Clients undergoing a lumpectomy may also have drainage tubes (usually Jackson-Pratt drains) placed if the lump is large or if axillary node dissection is performed.

Observe the wound for signs of swelling and infection throughout the client's recovery. Drainage tubes are removed by the surgeon when drainage is less than 25 mL in 24 hours. With short hospital stays, drainage tubes are usually removed about 1 week after hospital discharge, when the client returns for her first postoperative office visit. Inform the client that tube removal may be painful although these tubes lie just under the skin.

Comfort Measures. Assess the client's position to ensure that the drainage tubes or collection device are not pulled or kinked. The client should sit with the head of the bed up at least 30 degrees, with the affected arm (the arm on the same side as the axillary dissection) elevated on a pillow, while awake. Keeping the affected arm elevated promotes lymphatic fluid return after removal of axillary lymph nodes and channels. Provide other basic comfort measures, such as repositioning and analgesics, as prescribed, on a regular basis until pain ceases.

Mobility and Diet. The hospital stay after a modified radical mastectomy is short, often same-day or just overnight, and recovery is usually not complicated. Because some managed care companies will not authorize an overnight stay in the hospital following a mastectomy, several states have enacted legislation mandating inpatient benefits. The client who chooses an early discharge should have a home care visit within 24 hours of the discharge.

Ambulation and a regular diet are resumed by the day after surgery. While the client is in an upright position, the arm on the affected side may need to be supported at first. Gradually, the arm should be allowed to hang straight by the side while the client is walking. Instruct the client to avoid the hunched-back position with the arm flexed because of the risk for elbow contracture. Beginning exercises that do not stress the incision can usually be started on the first day after surgery. These exercises include squeezing the affected hand around a soft, round object (a ball or rolled washcloth) and flexion/extension of the elbow. The progression to more strenuous exercises depends on the subsequent procedures planned (such as reconstruction) and the surgeon's prescription.

As soon as the woman is fully ambulatory, eating well, and surgical pain is under control, she is discharged to

Text continued on p. 1815.

PLAN of CARE — MEDICAL DIAGNOSIS: MASTECTOMY (WITH CHEMOTHERAPY/RADIATION)

NURSING DIAGNOSIS NO. 1 ■ Anxiety

	Expected Outcomes	Nursing Interventions	Rationales
RELATED FACTORS		NIC **Anxiety Reduction**	
Situational/maturational crises Threat of death Threat to self, self-concept Threat to or change in:	Denies fatigue Denies weakness No verbal report or observation of alteration in sleep patterns	D Use a calm, reassuring approach.	The client may perceive fast-paced questioning and procedures as tension and worry from health care team members.
Role status Health status Interaction patterns Role function	No verbal report or observation of alteration in appetite No verbal report or observation of irritability	D Stay with the client.	The presence of a health care team member may serve to promote safety and reduce fear.
Environment Economic status	No verbal report or observation of self-focusing behavior	Create an atmosphere to facilitate trust.	A calm, reassuring, and truthful approach facilitates trust.
		Control stimuli, as appropriate, for the client's needs.	Noise, fast-paced activity, and bright lights serve to increase tension.
		Support the use of appropriate defense mechanisms.	Appropriate coping strategies help the client to feel more in control and less powerless.
		Administer medications to reduce anxiety, as appropriate.	Hypnotics/sedatives will promote rest and relaxation, which enhances coping abilities. Anxiolytics will decrease the client's perception of anxiety.
		Provide factual information concerning diagnosis, treatment, and prognosis.	In addition to establishing trust, accurate information will help the client marshal the appropriate coping strategies and the ability to make reasonable decisions.
		Other Interventions	
		Acknowledge the client's successes with anxiety management.	Positive reinforcement encourages the client to continue with anxiety management.
		Continuing Care Considerations	
		Monitor the client's verbal and nonverbal behaviors for anxiety.	The client may be unaware of his or her anxiety level in a subacute setting.
		Assist the client to set realistic expectations and plans for anxiety management.	Establishing a plan and setting realistic goals will help the client to feel more control over circumstances.

NURSING DIAGNOSIS NO. 2 ■ Anticipatory Grieving

	Expected Outcomes	Nursing Interventions	Rationales
RELATED FACTORS		NIC **Grief Work Facilitation**	
Future change in body shape Loss of a body part Possible reduction of life span	No verbal report or observation of alteration in sleep patterns	Identify the loss.	The client's perception of loss may be different from the circumstances.
DEFINING CHARACTERISTICS	No verbal report or observation of alteration in activity level	Assist the client to identify personal coping strategies.	The client may need to have his or her strengths reinforced.
Potential loss of significant object (e.g., people, possessions, job, status, home, ideals, parts and processes of the body)	No verbal report of alteration in libido Able to express the significance of potential loss	Encourage the client to express his or her feelings about the loss.	The client may need to repeatedly express his or her feelings about the loss to diminish the burden of anguish.
Verbal expression of distress at loss Sleep patterns: Change in Activity patterns: Changes in	No verbal report or observation of alteration in communication pattern No verbal report or observation of anger	Communicate acceptance of discussing loss.	Nurses facilitate the expression of grief by giving the client permission to express herself or himself. The nurse's manner and words show that these expressions of grief are acceptable and expected.

D Indicates tasks that can be delegated to unlicensed assistive nursing personnel at the discretion of the nurse.

PLAN of CARE MEDICAL DIAGNOSIS: MASTECTOMY (WITH CHEMOTHERAPY/RADIATION)—*cont'd*

NURSING DIAGNOSIS NO. 2 ■ Anticipatory Grieving—*cont'd*

Expected Outcomes	Nursing Interventions	Rationales
	Encourage identification of the client's greatest fears concerning the loss.	Helping the client to identify his or her fears permits the client and family to implement strategies to control the feared event.
	Assist the client in identifying needed lifestyle modifications.	The client may need assistance with services ranging from prosthetic devices to mobility equipment. A realistic appraisal of needs will save the client effort, time, and money in the adjustment period.
	Instruct the client regarding phases of the grieving process, as appropriate.	Clients need to know that grieving is an uneven process that may take months or years to complete. Many are surprised to find that one day is tranquil and the next is stormy.
	NIC **Active Listening**	
	D Display an awareness of and sensitivity to emotions.	Active listening techniques such as clarification and rephrasing help the client to trust that his or her feelings are being conveyed.
	Focus completely on the interaction by suppressing prejudice, bias, assumptions, preoccupying personal concerns, and other distractions.	The client should receive the nurse's complete attention and impartial ear. Listening without advising helps the client to sort through feelings and beliefs.
	Listen for unexpressed messages and feelings, as well as the content, of the conversation.	Nonverbal cues are often the greatest indicator of the client's meaning.
	Avoid barriers to active listening.	Minimizing feelings, offering easy solutions, interrupting, talking about self, and premature closure indicate to the client that his or her feelings and thoughts are unimportant.
	Other Interventions	
	Refer the client to community resources (e.g., hospice care, Reach to Recovery), as appropriate.	The client and family may find support and additional resources for coping with loss through community agencies.
	Continuing Care Considerations	
	Assess the family's adjustments to the changes the client has made in response to the loss.	Clients may become withdrawn, angry, restless, or demanding as they attempt to cope with their changed circumstances.
	Assure the caregiver and family that assistance is readily available.	Caregivers may feel overwhelmed with the care regimen and with the amount of work required to assist the grieving person. Clear and simple directions for seeking assistance will help the caregiver maintain a sense of control.

Continued

PLAN of CARE MEDICAL DIAGNOSIS: MASTECTOMY (WITH CHEMOTHERAPY/RADIATION)—*cont'd*

NURSING DIAGNOSIS NO. 3 ■ Acute Pain

	Expected Outcomes	Nursing Interventions	Rationales
RELATED FACTORS Injury agents (biologic, chemical, physical, psychological) **DEFINING CHARACTERISTICS** Verbal or coded report of pain Protective gestures Facial mask Self-focus	Denies experiencing pain greater than 5 on a 0 to 10 pain scale No verbal report or observation of guarding or protective gestures No verbal report or observation of alteration in sleep patterns No verbal report or observation of self-focusing behavior No verbal report or observation of facial mask of pain No verbal report or observation of alteration in activity level	NIC **Pain Management** Perform a comprehensive pain assessment that includes location, characteristics, onset/duration, frequency, quality, intensity or severity of pain, and precipitating factors.	A plan for pain management must be based on the client's unique responses to pain.
		Observe for nonverbal cues of discomfort, especially in clients who are unable to communicate effectively.	Nonverbal cues provide support for the existence of pain.
		Evaluate past experiences with pain to include the individual or family history of chronic pain or resulting disability, if appropriate.	Past experiences with pain may affect the perception of and response to pain.
		Reduce or eliminate factors that precipitate or increase the pain experience.	Preventing a pain experience is preferred to trying to control or eliminate pain.
		Select and implement a variety of measures to facilitate pain relief, as appropriate.	Pharmacologic, nonpharmacologic, and interpersonal strategies may provide pain relief depending on the client's unique responses to the therapeutic interventions.
		Use pain control measures before pain becomes severe.	Medicating the client in a timely manner prevents pain from reaching acutely unpleasant levels.
		Provide information about the pain, such as causes, how long it will last, and anticipated discomforts from procedures.	The client is better able to monitor his or her own discomfort and to intervene appropriately when informed.
		NIC **Analgesic Administration** D Monitor the client's vital signs before and after administering opioid analgesics with the first-time dose or if unusual signs are noted.	Opioid analgesics may depress respirations or cause other adverse effects.
		Choose the IV route rather than the IM route for frequent pain medication injections, when possible.	The IV route avoids tissue trauma and unpredictable absorption of medication.
		Administer analgesics around-the-clock.	Administration around-the-clock prevents peaks and troughs of analgesia, especially with severe pain.
		Institute safety precautions for those receiving opioid analgesics, as appropriate.	Opioid analgesics may impair the client's judgment and/or coordination.
		Evaluate the effectiveness of the analgesic at regular frequent intervals after each administration, but especially after the initial dose; in addition, observe for any manifestations of untoward effects.	Frequent evaluation of analgesic effectiveness permits the nurse to adjust the dose and timing interval to the client's need and provides an early warning of adverse responses.

D Indicates tasks that can be delegated to unlicensed assistive nursing personnel at the discretion of the nurse.

PLAN of CARE MEDICAL DIAGNOSIS: MASTECTOMY (WITH CHEMOTHERAPY/RADIATION)—*cont'd*

NURSING DIAGNOSIS NO. 3 ■ Acute Pain—*cont'd*

Expected Outcomes	Nursing Interventions	Rationales
	Document the client's response to the analgesic and any untoward effects.	Documentation provides the health care team with the information needed to accurately evaluate the client's response to the analgesic regimen.
	Implement actions to decrease the untoward effects of analgesics.	Actions taken to prevent the predictable but unwanted effects of narcotic analgesics (e.g., constipation) increase client comfort.
	Collaborate with the physician if drug, dose, route of administration, or interval changes are indicated, making specific recommendations based on equianalgesic principles.	The nurse working with the client is often in the best position to observe the client's response to the analgesic regimen.
	Instruct the client to request PRN pain medication before the pain becomes severe.	Pain may be managed with lower doses of analgesics and fewer untoward effects if PRN drugs are administered before pain becomes severe.
	Inform the client that drowsiness sometimes occurs during the first 2 to 3 days of opioid administration and then subsides.	Drowsiness poses a hazard to the client, making accidents more likely to occur.
	Correct the misconceptions/myths that the client or family members may hold regarding analgesics, particularly opioids.	A client's misconceptions may prevent him or her from using opioid analgesics.
	Teach about the use of analgesics, strategies to decrease side effects, and expectations for involvement in decisions about pain relief.	Information about analgesics and the expectation for involvement increase the client's sense of control over his or her pain.
	NIC **Patient-Controlled Analgesia (PCA) Administration**	
	Validate that the client can use a PCA device.	To use a PCA, the client must be able to communicate, comprehend explanations, and follow directions.
	Assist the client or family member to administer an appropriate bolus loading dose of analgesic.	The initial or bolus loading dose helps to establish baseline pain relief.
	Consult with the client, family members, and physician to adjust the lockout interval, basal rate, and demand dosage.	The client's response to the analgesic will determine the PCA settings.
	Document the client's pain, amount and frequency of drug dosing, and response to pain treatment on a pain flow sheet.	Information on the pain flow sheet will assist the health care team to adjust the analgesic regimen to the client's needs.

Continued

PLAN of CARE MEDICAL DIAGNOSIS: MASTECTOMY (WITH CHEMOTHERAPY/RADIATION)—*cont'd*

NURSING DIAGNOSIS NO. 3 ■ Acute Pain—*cont'd*

	Expected Outcomes	Nursing Interventions	Rationales
		Teach the client and family to monitor pain intensity, quality, and duration.	This information will help the client and family determine when to administer a bolus dose of analgesic, if appropriate, or when to request an increase in basal rate of the analgesic.
		Teach the client and family to monitor respiratory rate and blood pressure.	This information will help the health care team adjust analgesic doses to the client's responses and will decrease untoward effects.
		NIC **Environmental Management: Comfort**	
		Determine sources of discomfort, such as damp dressings, positioning of tubing, constrictive dressings, wrinkled bed linens, and environmental irritants.	Control of environmental discomforts may decrease the need for pharmacologic intervention.
		D Prevent unnecessary interruptions and allow for rest periods.	Rest may improve the client's pain tolerance.
		Facilitate hygiene measures to keep the client comfortable.	Hygiene measures may improve the client's overall sense of well-being.
		Other Interventions	
		Refer the client to the Pain Advisory Committee.	The Pain Advisory Committee is a multidisciplinary committee with wide expertise in pain relief interventions.
		Continuing Care Considerations	
		Refer the client to an advanced practice nurse pain specialist, social worker, home care nurse, and/or psychologist, as appropriate.	Health care team members are able to provide continuing support for the client facing chronic pain.

NURSING DIAGNOSIS NO. 4 ■ Disturbed Body Image

	Expected Outcomes	Nursing Interventions	Rationales
RELATED FACTORS Psychosocial Biophysical Illness Surgery Illness treatment **DEFINING CHARACTERISTICS** Verbal report of feelings that reflect an altered view of one's body in appearance, structure, or function Nonverbal response to actual or perceived change in body structure and/or function Behavior: Avoidance of monitoring or acknowledgment of one's body Missing body part Hiding or overexposing body part (intentional or unintentional)	Views, monitors, and acknowledges body Social involvement remains at pre-illness baseline Acknowledges changes in body that reflect a realistic appraisal of altered appearance or function Acknowledges loss of significant objects Does not verbalize self-negating statements Denies alteration in relationship with significant other	NIC **Body Image Enhancement** Use anticipatory guidance. Assist the client to discuss changes caused by illness or surgery, as appropriate. Help the client determine the extent of actual changes in the body or its level of functioning. Assist the client to separate physical appearance from feelings of personal worth, as appropriate.	Anticipatory guidance prepares the client for predictable changes in body image. The client who experiences changes caused by illness or surgery may be reluctant to verbalize his or her feelings. The client may be unable to realistically determine the extent of actual changes in the body or its level of functioning because of grieving for the changes. The client's feeling of personal worth may be strongly tied to physical appearance so that negative changes in appearance trigger feelings of low self-worth.

D Indicates tasks that can be delegated to unlicensed assistive nursing personnel at the discretion of the nurse.

PLAN of CARE MEDICAL DIAGNOSIS: MASTECTOMY (WITH CHEMOTHERAPY/RADIATION)—*cont'd*

NURSING DIAGNOSIS NO. 4 ■ Disturbed Body Image—*cont'd*

	Expected Outcomes	Nursing Interventions	Rationales
DEFINING CHARACTERISTICS—cont'd Actual change in structure and/or function Preoccupation with change or loss Verbal report: Negative feelings about body (e.g., feelings of helplessness, hopelessness, or powerlessness) Change in social involvement		Assist the client to discuss stressors affecting body image.	Stressors affecting body image may be due to congenital condition, injury, disease, or surgery.
		Identify the influence of the client's culture, religion, race, gender, and age on body image.	Culture, religion, race, gender, and age influence the client's perception of positive or negative body image.
		D Monitor whether the client can look at the changed body part.	The client's inability to look at the changed body part may indicate that he or she has strong negative feelings about the change.
		Determine the client's and family's perceptions of the alteration in body image versus reality.	The client's and family's perceptions of the alteration in body image may vary significantly from the reality of the change.
		Determine if a change in body image has contributed to increased social isolation.	A client who experiences a negative change in body image may withdraw from social contact.
		Assist the client in identifying the parts of his or her body that have positive perceptions associated with them.	The client may need assistance in identifying a positive body image if he or she is focused solely on a negative change.
		Identify means of reducing the impact of any disfigurement.	The use of clothing, wigs, or cosmetics may reduce the impact of any disfigurement.
		Assist the client to identify actions that will enhance appearance.	Assisting the client to enhance his or her appearance will improve self-concept.
		Other Interventions	
		Assess the client's readiness to accept a change in body functioning.	Cues that the client is ready to begin dealing with body changes include questions about how to manage an aspect of his or her care or how to adapt familiar activities to the changed capability.
		Provide an atmosphere of caring and acceptance.	A client with traumatic changes in body parts or functioning may be especially sensitive to cues that indicate an aversive reaction.
		Continuing Care Considerations	
		Refer the client to restorative specialists, as appropriate.	Restorative specialists have expertise in body enhancement and techniques to maximize appearance to improve self-concept.
		Refer the client to a support group of others who have experienced the same loss.	The client may receive useful information and support from others who are experiencing the same circumstances.

Continued

PLAN of CARE MEDICAL DIAGNOSIS: MASTECTOMY (WITH CHEMOTHERAPY/RADIATION)—*cont'd*

NURSING DIAGNOSIS NO. 5 ■ Disturbed Sleep Pattern

	Expected Outcomes	Nursing Interventions	Rationales
RELATED FACTORS Ruminative thoughts before sleep Depression **DEFINING CHARACTERISTICS** Sleep onset greater than 30 minutes Early-morning insomnia Awakening earlier or later than desired Verbal: Complaints of not feeling well rested Decreased ability to function	Denies difficulty falling asleep Verbally reports feeling well rested No verbal report or observation of early-morning insomnia No verbal report or observation of sleep onset greater than 30 minutes Denies waking earlier or later than desired	NIC **Sleep Enhancement** Approximate the client's regular sleep/wake cycle in planning care.	Care activities should not interfere with the client's preferred sleep cycle.
		Determine the effects of the client's medications on the sleep pattern.	Medications may interfere with sleep patterns by causing insomnia or by increasing the sleep cycle.
		Monitor the client's sleep pattern and note circumstances that interrupt sleep.	Physical difficulties (e.g., sleep apnea, obstructed airway, pain/discomfort, and urinary frequency) and/or psychological difficulties (e.g., fear or anxiety) may interrupt the client's normal sleep cycle.
		D Adjust light, noise, temperature, mattress, and bed.	Adjustments to the environment may promote sleep.
		Assist the client to eliminate stressful situations before bedtime.	Stressful situations increase anxiety, heart rate, respiratory rate, and mental activity, which interfere with the transition to sleep.
		Instruct the client how to perform autogenic muscle relaxation.	Autogenic muscle relaxation may facilitate sleep.
		Adjust the medication administration schedule.	Administer medications during the client's awake cycle to support his or her sleep/wake cycle.
		Regulate environmental stimuli to maintain normal day-night cycles.	Providing quiet for sleep cycles and light and activity for awake cycles helps the client to maintain physiologic balance.
		Other Interventions Discourage the use of alcohol.	Alcohol speeds the onset of sleep but disrupts rapid eye movement (REM) sleep.
		Suggest the use of L-tryptophan or an increased consumption of milk, cheese, and meats, as appropriate.	L-tryptophan may help the client sleep.
		D Offer the client a position change and a backrub at bedtime.	A backrub and repositioning increase the client's physical comfort and may help him or her achieve restful sleep.
		Continuing Care Considerations Adjust the height of the head of the bed, as necessary.	Clients who are troubled with esophageal reflux may need the head of their bed elevated to prevent reflux, which may interfere with sleep.
		Teach the client to void before going to sleep.	Voiding at bedtime may prevent awakening during the sleep cycle to void.

D Indicates tasks that can be delegated to unlicensed assistive nursing personnel at the discretion of the nurse.

PLAN of CARE MEDICAL DIAGNOSIS: MASTECTOMY (WITH CHEMOTHERAPY/RADIATION)—*cont'd*

NURSING DIAGNOSIS NO. 6 ■ Sexual Dysfunction

	Expected Outcomes	Nursing Interventions	Rationales
RELATED FACTORS Vulnerability Altered body structure (e.g., drugs, surgery, disease processes, trauma, radiation) Threat to self-concept Misinformation or lack of knowledge **DEFINING CHARACTERISTICS** Altered relationship with significant other Altered sense of achieving sexual satisfaction Actual or perceived limitations imposed by disease and/or therapy Altered sense of achieving perceived sex role	No verbal report or observation of change in libido Denies alteration in relationship with significant other Verbal report of ability to achieve desired satisfaction	NIC **Sexual Counseling** Establish a therapeutic relationship based on trust and respect.	Discussions of sexuality and sexual functioning are often hampered by cultural proscriptions, which indicate that these areas are private and are not to be discussed.
		Preface questions about sexuality with a statement that tells the client that many people experience sexual difficulties.	Clients may be reluctant to discuss sexual function. Helping clients to understand that the nurse is aware that others have experienced difficulties makes them less likely to feel abnormal.
		Discuss the effect of the illness/health situation and/or medication on sexuality.	The client should be questioned about the specific effects of the illness and/or medication so an appropriate plan of care can be developed.
		Encourage the client to verbalize fears and ask questions.	Information about what the client knows, fears, and has questions about form the basis for health teaching and referrals.
		Help the client to express grief and anger about alterations in body functioning/appearance. Avoid displaying aversion to an altered body part.	Encouraging the client to acknowledge alterations in body parts or appearance starts the grieving process. Calm acceptance of the client's altered appearance provides assurance that others do not regard him or her as mutilated.
		In collaboration with other health care team members, introduce the client to positive role models who have successfully conquered a similar problem, as appropriate.	Introductions to others who have faced similar problems may be supportive and reassuring.
		Collaborate with other health care team members to provide services, as necessary.	Other health care team members, such as sex therapists, may offer the client additional strategies for managing the sexual disturbance.
		Other Interventions Use humor carefully.	Humor may help to relieve uneasiness or anxiety without causing the client a loss of self-respect.
		Include the client's significant other in counseling (with permission from the client).	Sexual dysfunction impacts both partners engaged in intimacy.
		Continuing Care Considerations Refer the client to appropriate health care professionals, as necessary.	Sexual dysfunction may be an ongoing problem related to health matters. The client and significant other may need ongoing support from health care team members.

Continued

PLAN of CARE MEDICAL DIAGNOSIS: MASTECTOMY (WITH CHEMOTHERAPY/RADIATION)—*cont'd*

NURSING DIAGNOSIS NO. 7 ■ Ineffective Protection

RELATED FACTORS
- Leukopenia
- Thrombocytopenia
- Anemias
- Inadequate nutrition
- Drug therapies (e.g., antineoplastics, corticosteroids)
- Surgery
- Radiation

DEFINING CHARACTERISTICS
- Impaired healing
- Diaphoresis
- Fatigue
- Cough
- Appetite: Loss of

Expected Outcomes
- Denies fatigue
- Denies weakness
- No verbal report or observation of alteration in sleep patterns
- No verbal report or observation of restlessness
- Has skin that remains intact with no bruising or rashes
- No verbal report or observation of delayed healing
- No verbal report or observation of alteration in appetite

Nursing Interventions	Rationales
NIC **Infection Protection**	
D Monitor for systemic and localized manifestations of infection.	Elevated temperature, pulse, respirations, and fever indicate systemic infection, whereas redness, heat, swelling, and pain indicate a local infection.
Monitor absolute granulocyte count, white blood cell (WBC) count, and differential results.	Elevations in these laboratory tests demonstrate the body's response to infection.
Inspect the condition of any surgical incision/wound.	A surgical incision may be slightly reddened and swollen from tissue damage but remains free of purulent drainage, excess swelling, or excess local pain (which indicate infection).
D Provide appropriate skin care to edematous areas.	Edematous skin is particularly susceptible to injury, and edematous tissue may encourage the growth of pathogenic agents.
D Maintain asepsis for the client at risk.	Asepsis minimizes the client's exposure to pathogenic agents and thus minimizes the incidence of infection.
D Promote sufficient nutritional intake.	Adequate nutrition is essential for immune system cell formation and for the repair of damaged body tissues to provide protection against external pathogens.
D Encourage rest.	Mending tissues require energy. A fatigued client is stressed and requires greater expenditure of energy to accomplish tasks.
Numerous visitors should be limited and visits from individuals with known infections should be discouraged.	Visitors may provide a needed diversion, but too many visitors may result in fatigue and unwanted exposure to pathogens.
Report positive cultures to infection control personnel.	Early intervention to treat infection improves the client's response to therapy.
Teach the client and family about the manifestations of infection and when to report them to the health care provider.	Early intervention to treat infection prevents untoward complications from the infection and its therapy.
NIC **Infection Control**	
Promote safe food preservation and preparation.	Clients who are immunosuppressed may be susceptible to pathogens from foods that are improperly prepared or stored.
Administer antibiotic therapy, as appropriate.	Antibiotic therapy should assist the body to destroy pathogens.
NIC **Surveillance: Safety**	
Monitor the client for alterations in physical or cognitive function.	Changes in physical or cognitive function may lead to unsafe behavior.

D Indicates tasks that can be delegated to unlicensed assistive nursing personnel at the discretion of the nurse.

PLAN of CARE MEDICAL DIAGNOSIS: MASTECTOMY (WITH CHEMOTHERAPY/RADIATION)—*cont'd*

NURSING DIAGNOSIS NO. 7 ■ Ineffective Protection—*cont'd*

Expected Outcomes	Nursing Interventions	Rationales
	NIC **Surveillance: Safety—*cont'd***	
	Communicate information about the client's risk to other nursing staff.	Caregivers in the environment are better able to prevent injury when high-risk clients are identified and monitored continuously.
	Other Interventions	
	Avoid overexertion, stress, temperature extremes, and people with upper respiratory tract infection.	Stressors exacerbate fatigue.
	Continuing Care Considerations	
	Consider the use of complementary and alternative therapies.	Complementary and alternative therapies may be used to cope with chronic disease and disability, especially if chronic pain is a problem.

CHART 77-3

CLIENT EDUCATION GUIDE
Postmastectomy Exercises

Hand Wall Climbing
- Face the wall, and put the palms of your hands flat against the wall at shoulder level.
- Flex your fingers so that your hands slowly "walk" up the wall.
- Stop when your arms are fully extended.
- Slowly "walk" your hands back down the wall until they return to shoulder level.

Pulley Exercise
- Drape a 6-foot-long rope over a shower curtain rod or over the top of a door. If you use a door for this exercise, have someone put a nail or hook at the top of the door so that the rope does not slip off.
- Grab the ends of the rope, one in each hand, and extend your arms out to your sides until they are straight.
- Keeping your arms straight, pull down with your left arm to raise your right arm as high as you can.
- Pull down with your right arm to raise your left arm as high as you can.

Rope Turning
- Tie a rope to the knob of a closed door.
- Hold the other end of the rope and step back from the door until your arm is almost straight out in front of you.
- Swing the rope in a circle. Start with small circles and gradually increase to larger circles as you become more flexible.

home. Common instructions for exercises after mastectomy are listed in Chart 77-3.

Breast Reconstruction. Breast reconstruction after mastectomy is common, with few complications. Clients now consult with the reconstructive surgeon and have definite ideas regarding the type of reconstruction, timing of the procedure, and technique desired. Many women want breast reconstruction immediately after mastectomy using their own tissue (autogenous reconstruction). Breast reconstruction at the time of mastectomy, both autogenous and prosthetic, appears to lessen the psychological strain associated with undergoing a mastectomy.

The surgeon should offer the option of breast reconstruction before surgery is performed. If the client does not choose immediate reconstructive surgery, a temporary prosthesis is given to the client. Some surgeons allow women to use a temporary prosthesis in the immediate postoperative period as a part of the postoperative dressing. If this is the case, the client returns from surgery with a surgical bra and temporary sterile prosthesis in place. The nurse or social worker can refer the client to the American Cancer Society's Reach to Recovery program. In this program, a volunteer who has had breast cancer surgery visits the client at home, offering information on breast forms, clothing, coping with breast cancer, and possible reconstructive options. For this intervention to be as helpful as possible, the volunteer should be about the same age as the client and have experienced the same surgical procedure.

Evaluate the client's level of satisfaction with her prosthesis several weeks after surgery. Assess the client's attitude by asking about future plans for restoring appearance. Although reconstruction is not appropriate for some clients and others may not be interested in it, the surgeon should discuss the indications and contraindications, advantages and disadvantages, and typical recovery. If immediate reconstruction is chosen, the surgeon should be aware of this before so that the surgeon's plans can be coordinated with those of the plastic surgeon.

Several procedures are available for restoring the appearance of the breast (Table 77-5). Reconstruction may begin during the original operative procedure or later in one to several stages. The following are some of the more common techniques (Resnick & Belcher, 2002):

- Use of a flap of skin and muscle from the abdomen, back, or hip to create a breast mound

TABLE 77-5 Examples of Breast Reconstruction Procedures

Procedure	Description	Procedure	Description
Implantation	An implant matching the size of the other breast is placed under the muscle on the operative side to create a breast mound. 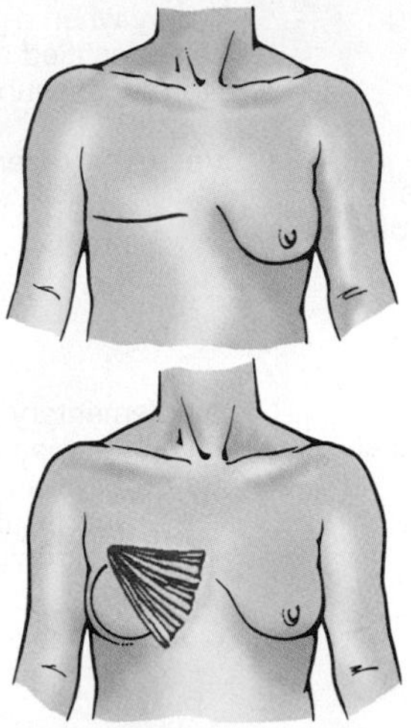	Myocutaneous flaps	A flap of skin, fat, and muscle is transferred from the donor site to the operative area. The flap contains an appropriate amount of fat to match the other breast and is similar in appearance to breast tissue. A blood supply is established by reanastomosis of vessels from the operative area to those with the flap when possible. A new nipple may be created with tissue from areas such as the labia or upper, inner thigh. Nipples can also be created by tattooing. Latissimus dorsi musculocutaneous flap 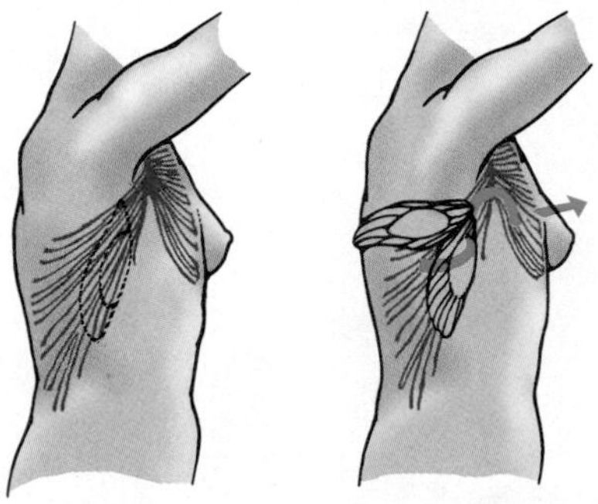
Tissue expansion	A tissue expander is placed under the muscle and gradually expanded with saline to stretch the overlying skin and create a pocket. After several weeks, the tissue expander is exchanged for an implant. 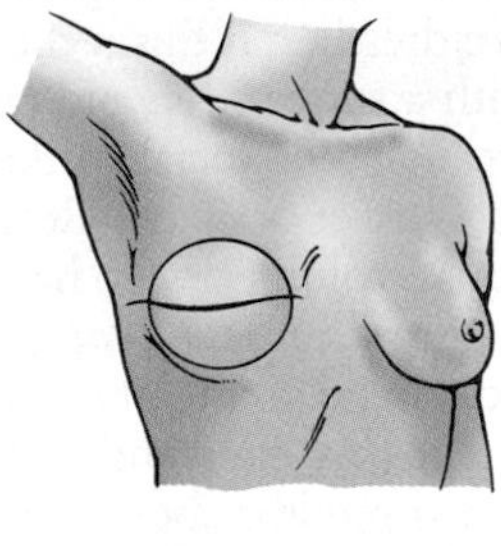		Abdominal myocutaneous flap 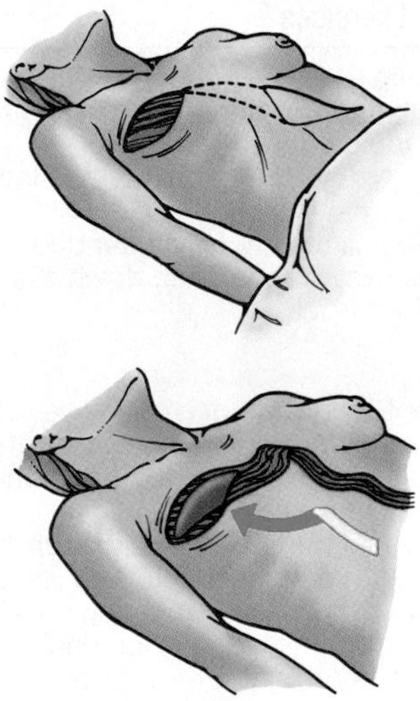

- Placement of a saline- or gel-filled prosthesis
- Use of progressive tissue expanders to slowly create a pocket under the mastectomy site for placement of a permanent implant.

Reconstruction of the nipple-areola complex is the last stage in the reconstruction of the breast. If necessary, a new nipple may be created with other body tissue, such as from the labia or inner thigh.

After concerns about the safety and effectiveness of silicone gel implants were voiced in the early 1990s, the Food and Drug Administration (FDA) restricted the use of silicone gel implants to women in FDA-approved safety studies. The studies were open to women seeking implants after breast cancer surgery or traumatic injury (McSpedon, 2002). Although no conclusive evidence indicates that silicone gel implants put women at risk for connective tissue diseases, some research findings suggest that ruptured silicone gel implants may lead to the development of fibromyalgia (Brown, 2001; Janowsky, 2000). Further research in this area is needed to support these findings.

The transverse rectus abdominis myocutaneous (TRAM) flap, a commonly used method of reconstruction, provides women with naturally appearing breasts without the risks associated with the silicone gel implant. This procedure has become the first choice for breast reconstruction and can be combined with tissue expanders and implants to obtain symmetry (Moran et al., 2000). Nursing care of the woman who has undergone breast reconstruction is outlined in Chart 77-4.

CHART 77-4

BEST PRACTICE for
Postoperative Care of the Client After Breast Reconstruction

- Assess the incision and flap for signs of infection (excessive redness, drainage, odor) during dressing changes.
- Assess the incision and flap for signs of poor tissue perfusion (duskiness, decreased capillary refill) during dressing changes.
- Avoid pressure on the flap and suture lines by positioning the client on her nonoperative side and avoiding tight clothing.
- Monitor and measure drainage in collection devices, such as Jackson-Pratt drains.
- Teach the client to return to her usual activity level gradually and to avoid heavy lifting.
- Remind the client to avoid sleeping in the prone position.
- Teach the client to avoid participation in contact sports or other activities that could cause trauma to the chest.
- Teach the client to minimize pressure on the breast during sexual activity.
- Remind the client to refrain from driving until advised by the physician.
- Remind the client to ask at the 6-week postoperative visit when full activity can be resumed.
- Reassure the client that optimal appearance may not occur for 3 to 6 months postoperatively.
- If implants have been inserted, teach the proper method of breast massage to enhance expansion and prevent capsule formation (consult with the physician).
- Review the breast self-examination procedure and the need to continue this practice monthly.
- Remind the client that mammograms should be scheduled at least yearly for the rest of her life.

Adjuvant Therapy. The decision to follow the original surgical procedure with chemotherapy, radiation, hormonal, or targeted therapy is based on the following:

- The stage of the disease
- The client's age and menopausal status
- Client preferences
- Pathologic examination
- Hormone receptor status
- Presence of a known genetic predisposition

The purpose of adjuvant therapy is to decrease the risk of recurrence for the client who has no evidence of but is at risk for metastasis or to prolong survival after metastasis occurs. Adjuvant therapy for stage I and stage II (early-stage) breast cancer consists of breast-conserving surgery with radiotherapy after surgery or of modified radical mastectomy.

Radiation Therapy. The purpose of radiation therapy is to kill breast cancer cells that may remain near the site of the original tumor. This therapy can be delivered to the whole breast by external beam given daily for 6 to 7 weeks. Skin changes are a major side effect during this therapy (see Chapter 28). An alternative approach is partial breast brachytherapy. In this procedure, small catheters are threaded through the breast in the tumor bed. Then, twice each day for 5 days, radioactive seeds are place in the catheters for a specified exposure period (usually 5 to 10 minutes). The total dose of radiation to the breast is the same for both procedures.

Chemotherapy. Chemotherapy is usually **adjuvant** therapy (in addition to surgery) for breast cancer. Its purpose is to kill breast cancer cells that may have left the original tumor and moved to more distant sites. Usually, it is used for stage II or higher breast cancer although determination of when it is needed is controversial. Chemotherapy is unpleasant, expensive, and can have dangerous short-term and long-term side effects. Therefore the risks and the benefits of its use must be examined for each client. Although chemotherapeutic regimens differ among treatment centers, multiple-agent combinations are used. Most combinations include paclitaxel (Taxol) and doxorubicin (Adriamycin). The length of treatment may also vary. Some protocols involve giving chemotherapy before surgery; more commonly, it is given after surgery.

Although some side effects are specific to a given drug, chemotherapy is systemic treatment and affects many tissues. Common side effects include nausea and vomiting, hair loss (**alopecia**), and an increased risk for infection because of bone marrow suppression. Chapter 28 discusses issues and interventions for clients receiving systemic chemotherapy.

Hormonal Therapy. Women who have estrogen receptor (ER)-positive tumors may be given estrogen receptor blocking agents such tamoxifen (Nolvadex, Tamofen✱), toremifene (Fareston), raloxifene (Evista), droloxifene, and idoxifene, or agents that reduce the circulating levels of estrogen, such as inhibitors of estrogen synthesis and aromatase inhibitors. When hormonal therapy is appropriate, the response rate is 50% to 60%. Tamoxifen therapy has a higher risk for endometrial cancers for women who still have a uterus. For these women, other estrogen receptor blockers that are more specific to the ER receptors in the breast are used.

Drugs that inhibit estrogen synthesis include leuprolide (Lupron) and goserelin (Zoladex). These drugs suppress the hypothalamus from making luteinizing hormone-releasing hormone (LH-RH). Under the influence of LH-RH, the ovaries are stimulated to produce estrogen. When LH-RH is inhibited, the ovary does not produce estrogen.

A small but significant source of estrogen is that made in the adrenal gland, kidney, and a few other organs through the action of the enzyme aromatase. The drugs anastrozole (Arimidex), letrozole (Femara), exemestane (Aromasin), and fulvestrant (Faslodex) all reduce circulating levels of estrogen by blocking the activity of aromatase. These drugs have eliminated the need for an adrenalectomy or pituitary gland removal to control the estrogen influence on breast cancer cells.

Stem Cell Transplantation. Autologous and allogeneic stem cell transplantation are options for clients with a high risk for recurrence or who have advanced disease. **Autologous** bone marrow transplantation (taken from the client's bone marrow), peripheral blood stem cell transplantation (taken from the client's circulating blood), or **allogeneic** bone marrow transplantation (taken from a healthy donor's bone marrow or peripheral blood) are performed as a means of rescue therapy following very high doses of chemotherapy. A discussion of the care of the client undergoing bone marrow or stem cell transplantation is given in Chapter 43.

Targeted Therapy. For clients whose breast cancer cells overexpress the HER2/neu gene product and have large numbers of HER2 receptors, targeted therapy with trastuzumab (Herceptin) is effective in slowing cancer cell growth. Although not many tumors are HER2/neu-positive, the development of targeted therapy for breast cancer is an important step in improving the outcome for this disease. Common side effects of Herceptin when used alone include headaches, skin rashes, diarrhea, and flu-like symptoms of fever, chills, and muscle aches.

Critical Thinking Challenge

You are an RN assigned to a group of clients with an LPN and patient care technician (PCT) on your team. A client in your group has just returned from the PACU following a left modified radical mastectomy. She has a pressure dressing over the surgical site (which is dry and intact) and two drains. When performing her postoperative assessment, you note that her vital signs are stable, and she states that her pain is under control. The client's life partner and daughter are with her in the room.

1. What is this client's priority for care at this time?
2. What position should you place the client in and why?
3. What part of the client's postoperative assessment, if any, would you assign to the LPN? Explain your rationale?
4. What nursing tasks or activities, if any, would you delegate to the PCT? Explain your rationale.
5. What roles do the life partner and daughter have in planning continuing care for this client?

evolve For suggested answer guidelines, go to http://evolve.elsevier.com/Iggy/.

Community-Based Care

HOME CARE MANAGEMENT

Home care preparation should be initiated when the decision to have surgical therapy is made. Referral to a case manager can ensure that the educational needs of the client are met early in the perioperative period. The preadmission testing center or the surgeon could make referrals. Preoperative teaching and arrangements for home care management and referrals (Reach to Recovery, social services, home care) can be initiated before hospitalization. Planning ahead for the client's discharge needs facilitates discharge.

The client who has undergone breast surgery can be discharged to the home setting unless other physical disabilities exist. Some are discharged a day after surgery with Jackson-Pratt or other types of drains in place. Many clients are discharged to home on the same day that surgery is performed. These clients need assistance at home with drain care, dressings, and activities of daily living because of pain and impaired range of motion of the affected arm. Summaries of discharge instructions are given in Charts 77-5 and 77-6.

It is not necessary to modify the home for the client after breast surgery. Activities involving stretching or reaching for heavy objects should be avoided temporarily. This restriction can be discussed with a family member or significant other who can perform these tasks or place the objects within easy reach of the client.

HEALTH TEACHING

The teaching plan for the client after surgery includes the following:

- Measures to optimize a positive body image
- Information to enhance interpersonal relationships and roles
- Exercises to regain full range of motion
- Measures to prevent infection of the incision
- Measures to avoid injury, infection, and swelling of the affected arm
- Care of the incision and drainage device

Explain incisional care to the client and family. The client may wear a light dressing to prevent irritation. Explain that no lotions or ointments should be used on the area and that the use of deodorant under the affected arm should be delayed until healing is complete. Although swelling and redness of the scar itself are normal for the first few weeks, swelling, redness, increased heat, and tenderness of the surrounding area indicate infection and should be reported to the surgeon. If a lymph node dissection was performed, instruct the client to elevate the affected arm on a pillow for at least 30 minutes a day for the first 6 months. The client should have someone bring a loose-fitting, nonwired bra or camisole for her to try before discharge with a soft cotton-filled or polyester fiber-filled form supplied by the hospital or by Reach to Recovery. The client wears this form until the incision is completely healed and the health care provider approves the fitting of a more sophisticated prosthesis, usually 6 to 8 weeks after discharge. Encourage the client to dress in loose-fitting street clothes at home, not pajamas, to further enhance a positive self-image.

Teach the client to continue performing the exercises that began in the hospital. Active range-of-motion exercises should begin 1 week after surgery or when sutures and drains

CHART 77-5

CLIENT EDUCATION GUIDE
Recovery from Breast Cancer Surgery

- There may be a dry gauze dressing over the incision when you leave the hospital. You may change this dressing if it becomes soiled.
- A small, dry dressing will be around the site where a drain is placed. Often there is some leakage of fluid around the drain. Check the gauze dressing for drainage, and change it if it becomes soiled. Some leakage is normal, but if the dressing becomes soaked more than once a day, call your health care provider.
- Your nurse has shown you how to empty the reservoir from your drain and how to measure the volume of drainage. You should empty the drain twice a day and record the measurements.
- Drains are generally removed when drainage is less than 25 mL in 24 hours.
- Drains are often removed at the same time as the stitches or staples, generally 7 to 10 days after surgery.
- You may take sponge baths or tub baths, making certain that the area of the drain and incision stays dry. You may shower after the stitches, staples, and drains are removed.
- You can begin using your arm for normal activities, such as eating or combing your hair. Exercises involving the wrist, hand, and elbow, such as flexing your fingers, circular wrist motions, and touching your hand to your shoulder, are very good. You can usually resume more strenuous exercises after the drains have been removed.
- You can expect some discomfort or mild pain after surgery, but within 4 to 5 days most women have no need for pain medication or require medication only at bedtime.
- Numbness in the area of the surgery and along the inner side of the arm from the armpit to the elbow occurs in virtually all women. It is the injury to the nerves that causes sensation to the skin in those areas. Women have described sensations of heaviness, pain, tingling, burning, and "pins and needles." These sensations change over the months and usually resolve by 1 year.
- Pamphlets on exercises, hand and arm care, and general facts about breast cancer are available from your nurse or volunteer visitor. The American Cancer Society has volunteers who have had surgery similar to yours and are available to visit you.

Modified from Thomas, S., & Greifzu, S. (2000). Breast cancer. *RN, 63,* 40-47.

CHART 77-6

HOME CARE ASSESSMENT of
Clients Recovering from Breast Cancer Surgery

Assess cardiovascular, respiratory, and urinary status:
- Vital signs
- Lung sounds
- Urine output patterns

Assess for pain and effectiveness of analgesics.
Assess dressing and incision site:
- Excess drainage
- Manifestations of infection
- Wound healing
- Intact staples

Assess drain and site:
- Drainage around drain site and in drain
- Color and amount of drainage
- Manifestations of infection

Review client's recordings of drainage.
Evaluate client's ability to care for and empty drain.
Assess status of affected extremity:
- Range of motion
- Ability to perform exercise regimen
- Lymphedema

Assess nutritional status:
- Food and fluid intake
- Presence of nausea and vomiting
- Bowel sounds

Assess functional ability:
- Activities of daily living
- Mobility and ambulation

Assess home environment:
- Safety
- Structural barriers

Assess client's compliance and knowledge of illness and treatment plan:
- Follow-up appointment with surgeon
- Manifestations to report to health care provider
- Hand and arm care guidelines
- Referral to Reach to Recovery

Assess client and caregiver coping skills:
- Determine if client has looked at incision site.
- Assess client's reaction to incision site.

are removed. Emphasize that reaching and stretching exercises should continue only to the point of pain or pulling, never beyond that. ENCORE, a YWCA program, is appropriate for women as early as 3 weeks after surgery and includes exercise to music, exercise in water, and psychological support. Before discharge, the surgeon may prescribe precautions or limitations specific to plans for future procedures, such as reconstruction.

Provide information needed to help the client avoid infection and subsequent lymphedema of the affected arm after the mastectomy. Teach the client to avoid having blood pressure measurements taken on, having injections in, or having blood drawn from the arm on the side of the mastectomy. Instruct the client to wear a mitt when using the oven, wear gloves when gardening, and treat cuts and scrapes appropriately. If lymphedema occurs, the arm should be elevated when possible and special attention paid to the aforementioned warnings. In addition, if lymphedema occurs, it can be managed with the use of an arm sleeve (similar to a Ted or Jobst stocking) or a sequential compression device. Management of lymphedema is directed toward measures that promote drainage of the affected arm; however, prevention is the best cure.

CONSIDERATIONS FOR OLDER ADULTS

With the projected increase in the older adult population, especially women, during the next half-century, breast cancer will be an even greater health concern. Older breast cancer survivors require more time for assessment and follow-up care. They require careful assessment for differentiation of symptoms that may be treatment related, associated with development of chronic diseases, or physical decline from aging. Older breast cancer survivors should be provided with thorough information and encouraged to participate in treatment decision making. They should be assisted to identify their sources of support and encouraged to expand their support networks with supportive friends and relatives. Age-specific support groups enable older survivors to broaden their support networks by introducing them to other survivors, which provides an opportunity for information sharing and the formation of new friendships.

PSYCHOSOCIAL PREPARATION

Concerns about appearance after surgery are common and are often a threat to the client's self-concept as a woman. Before breast surgery, the woman and her partner can benefit from an explanation of the expected postoperative appearance. After a modified radical mastectomy, the chest wall is fairly smooth and has a horizontal incision from the axilla to the midchest area. After breast-conserving surgery, scars vary according to the amount of breast tissue removed. Scars may be red and raised at first, but these features lessen in the first few months. After surgery, encourage the woman to look at her incision before she goes home and offer to be present when she does so.

Much of one's body image is a reflection of how others respond. Therefore the response of the client's family or partner to the surgery is crucial in determining the effect on self-concept. These people may also need the support of the nurse. They may have concerns about their ability to accept the changes and need to discuss these feelings with an objective listener. They may also need help with communicating their feelings, both negative and positive, with their loved one. Involving them in teaching may also help reinforce learning and increase retention.

Discuss sexual concerns before discharge. Sexual intercourse can be resumed whenever the client is comfortable. Clients may prefer to lay a pillow over the surgical site or wear a bra or camisole to prevent contact with the surgical site during intercourse. The client may be embarrassed to broach the topic. Be sensitive to possible concerns and approach the subject first.

For women of childbearing age (about 25% of breast cancer clients), issues related to childbearing may be a concern. Chemotherapy and radiation are considered serious teratogenic (birth defect–causing) agents, and sexually active clients receiving chemotherapy or radiotherapy should be advised to use birth control during therapy. The method and length of birth control is discussed with the health care provider.

For older women, issues such as fear and uncertainty about treatment outcomes, reduced functional status, concurrent chronic diseases, disease recurrence, future well-being and independence, and reduced social resources may be encountered (Sammarco, 2003). Be aware of the specific con-

EVIDENCE-BASED PRACTICE for Nursing

What is the quality of life of breast cancer survivors of different psychosocial stages and places in life?

Sammarco, A. (2003). The quality of life of older breast cancer survivors. *Cancer Nursing. 26*(6), 431-438.

This study investigated the relationship between perceived social support, uncertainty, and quality of life among older breast cancer survivors. A sample of 103 breast cancer survivors older than 50 years of age completed questionnaires that measured their perceived social support, uncertainty, and quality of life. The study results showed that as age increased, the women perceive less support and more uncertainty in their lives, which could adversely affect their quality of life.

Level of Evidence: 5—Well-conducted case control study (qualitative of sufficient size).

Critique. The results of this study cannot be generalized to the population of older breast cancer survivors due to use of a convenience sample. However, the study results underscore the importance of social support in reducing illness uncertainty and improving the quality of life of older breast cancer survivors.

Implications for Nursing. The study findings provide useful information that can assist nurses in increasing their awareness regarding the interplay of the developmental stage and place in life of older breast cancer survivors with quality of life. The current health care environment is one of attenuating resources and narrow margins of opportunity for contact with breast cancer clients. Nurses are constantly challenged to meet the supportive needs of older breast cancer survivors and contribute to improved quality of life outcomes. It should be recognized that the quality of life needs of older breast cancer survivors differ considerably from those of younger survivors and require interventions that are tailored to the specific psychosocial life-stage of the individual.

cerns of the older clients and plan interventions accordingly (see the Evidence-Based Practice for Nursing box above).

HEALTH CARE RESOURCES

Resources available to the client after discharge include personal support and community programs. After discharge, the spouse or partner may need help in planning support for home responsibilities. For example, a partner who may be assuming additional duties at home and work may feel stressed. Exploring temporary relief resources for child care, cleaning, or cooking may be helpful until the woman regains her previous energy level. Discussing the need for ongoing emotional support is also beneficial to both the client and her partner. Leaving the hospital and appearing normal do not end the anxiety and fear. Identifying a support person with whom the client or couple can explore these feelings and discussing the need to ventilate feelings enhance personal and family recovery.

As mentioned, Reach to Recovery and ENCORE are two community resources for women with breast cancer. Reach to Recovery provides a volunteer who visits the client in the hospital or at home. She brings a personal message of hope, informational materials on breast cancer recovery, and a soft, temporary breast form. Some communities offer additional resources such as support groups and exercise classes.

◆Evaluation: Outcomes

Evaluate the care of the client with breast cancer on the basis of the identified nursing diagnoses and collaborative problems. The expected outcomes include that the client will:

- Be able to cope with the diagnosis
- Remain free of metastasis

Specific indicators for these outcomes are listed for each nursing diagnosis and collaborative problem under the Planning and Implementation section (see earlier).

GET READY for the NCLEX Examination!

KEY POINTS

Safe Effective Care Environment

- In collaboration with the health care team, assess the physiologic stability and comfort level of clients who have undergone surgical intervention for breast cancer.
- After breast cancer surgery, assess vital signs, dressings, drainage collection tubes, and amount of drainage in collection container.
- Clients who have had lymph node dissection in addition to breast surgery must be placed on arm precautions to prevent lymphedema. The arm of the surgical side cannot be used for blood pressures, blood drawing, or injections. A sign to that effect must be placed over the client's bed and the health care team notified.
- Use standard precautions when managing the drains of a client after mastectomy.

Health Promotion and Maintenance

- Identify clients at higher risk for breast cancer, especially women with family history of breast cancer, those who have had early menarche, late menopause, first pregnancy after 30 years of age, or those who are nullipara.
- Teach women how to perform breast self-examination (BSE) as a means of early detection of breast cancer.
- Encourage women to have screening mammography according to recommended guidelines. Baseline screening should begin at 40 years of age and continue yearly. In high-risk women, screening should be started between 25 and 35 years of age.
- Encourage women to have clinical breast examination (CBE) according to recommended guidelines.

Psychosocial Integrity

- Assess women's reactions to the diagnosis of breast cancer and the affect of breast cancer treatment on their body image and sexuality.
- Identify resources that facilitate their grief work and coping skills.
- Allow the client opportunities to express feelings of grief, fear, and anxiety.
- Teach client ways to minimize surgical area deformity and enhance body image, such as use of a breast prosthesis or the option of breast reconstruction.
- Address the reactions of family and significant others to the diagnosis of breast cancer; provide support and education.
- For clients with advanced metastatic breast cancer, provide end-of-life care, including referral to hospice care.

Physiological Integrity

- Assess the return of arm and shoulder mobility after breast surgery and axillary dissection.
- Assess for the presence of lymphedema and assist client to perform therapeutic measures to reduce lymphedema in the affected arm.

- Teach the client measures to prevent lymphedema after axillary node dissection.
- Observe for and report other complications of breast cancer surgery or breast reconstruction, especially infection and inadequate vascular perfusion.
- For clients with advanced breast cancer, evaluate the client's ability to perform activities of daily living (ADLs); refer or consult with social worker if home care is needed.
- For clients with advanced metastatic breast cancer, manage chronic pain with drug therapy as prescribed and nonpharmacologic measures, such as relaxation, aromatherapy, and imagery.
- After an axillary lymph node dissection, elevate the affected arm on a pillow.
- Encourage ambulation, a regular diet, and mild arm exercises to maintain mobility and enhance recovery.
- Use strict aseptic technique in dressing changes and care of drainage apparatus.

ADDITIONAL STUDY RESOURCES

Go to your Student CD-ROM for Review Questions for the NCLEX Examination.

evolve Go to http://evolve.elsevier.com/Iggy/ for Integrated Management of Care Questions for the NCLEX Examination.

SELECTED BIBLIOGRAPHY

Asterisk indicates a classic or definitive work on this subject.

American Cancer Society. (2003a). *Cancer facts and figures for African Americans-2003.* Report No. 8614.03. Atlanta: Author.

American Cancer Society. (2003b). *Cancer prevention and early detection. Facts and figures-2003.* Report No. 8600.03. Atlanta: Author.

American Cancer Society. (2005). *Cancer facts and figures–2005.* Report No. 00-300M-No. 5008.05. Atlanta: Author.

*Ashing-Giwa, K., et al. (1999). Quality of life of African-American and white long term breast carcinoma survivors. *Cancer, 85*(2), 418-426.

Austin, L., et al. (2002). Breast and cervical cancer screening in Hispanic women: A literature review using the health belief model. *Women's Health Issues, 12*(3), 122-128.

Baltzell, K., Eder, S., & Wrensch, M. (2005). Breast carcinogenesis: Can the examination of ductal fluid enhance our understanding? *Oncology Nursing Forum, 32*(1), 33-39.

Baquet, C., & Commiskey, P. (2000). Socioeconomic factors and breast carcinoma in multicultural women. *Cancer, 88*(5), 1256-1264.

Baron, R., et al. (2002). Eighteen sensations after breast cancer surgery: A comparison of sentinel lymph node biopsy and axillary lymph node dissection. *Oncology Nursing Forum, 29*(4), 651-659.

Barroso, J., et al. (2000). Comparison between African-American and white women in their beliefs about breast cancer and their health locus of control. *Cancer Nursing, 23*(4), 268-276.

Berry, J. (2001). Breast pain: All that hurts is not cancer. *The American Journal for Nurse Practitioners, 5*(4), 9-18.

Boehmke, M. (2004). Measurement of symptom distress in women with early-stage breast cancer. *Cancer Nursing, 27*(2), 144-152.

Bragg Leight, S., et al. (2000). The effect of structured training on breast self-examination search behaviors as measured using biomedical instrumentation. *Nursing Research, 49*(5), 283-289.

Brown, S., et al. (2001). Silicone gel breast implant rupture, extracapsular silicone, and health status in a population of women. *Journal of Rheumatology, 28*(5), 996-1003.

Campbell, J. (2002). Breast cancer race, ethnicity, and survival: A literature review. *Breast Cancer Research and Treatment, 74,* 187-192.

Coleman, E., et al. (2003). Developing and testing lay literature about breast cancer screening for African-American women. *Clinical Journal of Oncology Nursing, 7*(1), 66-70.

Conto, S., & Myers, J. (2002). Risk factors and health promotion in families of patients with breast cancer. *Clinical Journal of Oncology Nursing, 6*(2), 83-87.

Dell, D. (2003). Control of pain after breast reconstruction procedure. *Clinical Journal of Oncology Nursing, 7*(3), 335-336, 338.

DuVal, S. (2004). Inflammatory breast disease. *RN, 67*(2), 43-44.

Facione, N.C., et al. (2000). Perceived risk and help-seeking behavior for breast cancer: A Chinese-American perspective. *Cancer Nursing, 23*(4), 258-267.

Garmon-Bibb, S. (2001). The relationship between access and stage at diagnosis of breast cancer in African American and Caucasian women. *Oncology Nursing Forum, 28*(4), 711-719.

Gaston-Johansson, F., et al. (2000). The effectiveness of the comprehensive coping strategy on clinical outcomes in breast cancer autologous bone marrow transplantation. *Cancer Nursing, 23*(4), 277-285.

Greifzu, S. (2004). Breast cancer. *RN, 67*(2), 36-42.

Hancock, C. (2003). Fulvestrant antiestrogen for treatment of breast cancer. *Clinical Journal of Oncology Nursing, 7*(2), 201-202.

*Hartmann, L., et al. (1999a). Clinical options for women at high risk for breast cancer. *Surgical Clinics of North America, 79*(5), 1189-1204.

*Hartmann, L., et al. (1999b). Efficacy of bilateral prophylactic mastectomy in women with a family history of breast cancer. *New England Journal of Medicine, 340*(2), 77-84.

Hilton, B.A., et al. (2000). Men's perspectives on individual and family coping with their wives' breast cancer and chemotherapy. *Western Journal of Nursing Research, 22*(4), 438-459.

Horden, A. (2000). Intimacy and sexuality for the woman with breast cancer. *Cancer Nursing, 23*(3), 230-236.

Hunter, C. (2000). Epidemiology, stage at diagnosis, and tumor biology of breast carcinoma in multiracial and multiethnic populations. *Cancer, 88*(5), 1193-1202.

Hutson, S. (2003). Attitudes and psychological impact of genetic testing, genetic counseling, and breast cancer risk assessment among women at increased risk. *Oncology Nursing Forum, 30*(2), 241-246.

Janowsky, E., et al. (2000). Meta-analysis of the relation between silicone breast implants and the risk of connective tissue diseases. *New England Journal of Medicine, 342*(11), 781-790.

Kang, D. (2002). Oxidative stress, DNA damage, and breast cancer. *AACN Clinical Issues, 13*(4), 540-549.

Kimmick, G., & Balducci, L. (2000). Breast cancer and aging. *Hematology/Oncology Clinics of North America, 14*(1) 213-234.

Lengacher, C., et al. (2002). Frequency of use of complementary and alternative medicine in women with breast cancer. *Oncology Nursing Forum, 29*(10), 1445-1452.

MacDonald, D. (2002). Women's decisions regarding management of breast cancer risk. *MEDSURG Nursing, 11*(4), 183-186.

Mahon, S., & Casey, M. (2003). Patient education for women being fitted for breast prostheses. *Clinical Journal of Oncology Nursing, 7*(2), 194-199.

McCance, K., & Huether, S. (2002). *Pathophysiology: The biologic basis for disease in adults and children* (4th ed.). St. Louis: Mosby.

McPherson, K., Steel, C.M., & Dixon, J.M. (2000). ABC of breast diseases: Breast cancer–epidemiology, risk factors, and genetics. *British Medical Journal 321*(9), 624-628.

McSpedon, C. (2002). Silicone safety. *American Journal of Nursing, 102*(4), 31.

Moore, S. (2002). Cutaneous metastatic breast cancer. *Clinical Journal of Oncology Nursing, 6*(5), 255-260.

Moran, S.L., et al. (2000). TRAM flap breast reconstruction with expanders and implants. *AORN Journal, 71*(2), 354-362.

Nissen, M., Swenson, K., & Kind, E. (2002). Quality of life after postmastectomy breast reconstruction. *Oncology Nursing Forum, 29*(3), 547-553.

Nogueira, S.M., & Appling, S.E. (2000). Breast cancer: Genetics, risks, and strategies. *Nursing Clinics of North America, 35*(3), 663-669.

*Northouse, L., et al. (1999). The quality of life of African-American women with breast cancer. *Research in Nursing and Health, 22,* 449-460.

Partin, M., & Slater, J. (2003). Promoting repeat mammography use: Insights from a systematic needs assessment. *Health Education & Behavior, 30*(1), 97-112.

Rawl, S., et al. (2000). The impact of age and race on mammography practices. *Health Care for Women International, 21,* 583-595.

Resnick B., & Belcher, A. (2002). Breast reconstruction: Options, answers, and support for patients making a difficult personal decision. *American Journal of Nursing, 102*(4), 26-33.

Ridner, S. (2002). Breast cancer lymphedema: Pathophysiology and risk reduction guidelines. *Oncology Nursing Forum, 29*(9), 1285-1294.

Rosenzweig, M., Rust, D., & Hoss, J. (2000). Prognostic information in breast cancer care: Helping patients utilize important information. *Clinical Journal of Oncology Nursing, 4*(6), 271-278.

Sakorafas, G. (2002). Women at high risk for breast cancer: Preventive strategies. *The Mount Sinai Journal of Medicine, 69*(4), 264-266.

Sakorafas, G. (2003). The management of women at high risk for the development of breast cancer: Risk estimation and prevention. *Cancer Treatment Reviews, 29,* 79-89.

Sammarco, A. (2001a). Perceived social support, uncertainty, and quality of life of younger breast cancer survivors. *Cancer Nursing, 24*(3), 212-219.

Sammarco, A. (2001b). Psychosocial stages and quality of life of women with breast cancer. *Cancer Nursing, 24*(4), 272-277.

Sammarco, A. (2003). The quality of life of older breast cancer survivors. *Cancer Nursing, 26*(6), 431-438.

Sandau, K. (2002). Free TRAM flap breast reconstruction. *American Journal of Nursing, 102*(4), 36-43.

Shinagawa, S. (2000). The excess burden of breast carcinoma in minority and medically underserved communities. *Cancer, 88*(5), 1217-1223.

Shuster, T., et al. (2000). Multidisciplinary care for patients with breast cancer. *Surgical Clinics of North America, 80*(2), 505-533.

Strzelczyk, J., & Dignan, M. (2002). Disparities in adherence to recommended follow-up on screening mammography: Interaction of sociodemographic factors. *Ethnicity & Disease, 12,* 77-86.

Templeman, C., & Hertweck, S. (2000). Breast disorders in the pediatric and adolescent patient. *Obstetric and Gynecology Clinics, 27*(1), 19-31.

Thomas, S., & Greifzu, S. (2000). Breast cancer. *RN, 63*(4), 40-48.

Versea, L., & Rosenzweig, M. (2003). Hormonal therapy for breast cancer: Focus on fulvestrant. *Clinical Journal of Oncology Nursing, 7*(3), 307-312.

Workman, M.L. (2002). Breast cancer: New strategies to beat an old enemy. *Nursing2002, 32*(10), 58-63.

Yu, M., Seetoo, A., & Qu, M. (2002). Challenges of identifying Asian women for breast cancer screening. *Oncology Nursing Forum, 29*(3), 585-587.

Zack, E. (2001). Sentinel lymph node biopsy in breast cancer: Scientific rationale and patient care. *Oncology Nursing Forum, 28*(6), 2001.

CHAPTER 78

Interventions for Clients with Gynecologic Problems

KAREN NOVAK

LEARNING OUTCOMES

After studying this chapter, you should be able to:

1. Compare the pathophysiology, manifestations, and treatments of common menstrual cycle disorders.
2. Discuss common assessment findings associated with menopause.
3. Describe the mechanisms of action, side effects, and nursing implications for pharmacologic management of endometriosis.
4. Develop a teaching plan for a client with a vagina inflammation or infection.
5. Prioritize care after surgery for the client undergoing an anterior and/or posterior repair.
6. Analyze assessment data for clients with leiomyomas to determine nursing diagnoses and collaborative problems.
7. Formulate a plan of care for a client undergoing a hysterectomy.
8. Identify the risk factors for gynecologic cancers.
9. Discuss the psychosocial issues associated with gynecologic cancers.
10. Explain the purpose of radiation and chemotherapy for clients with gynecologic cancers.
11. Develop a community-based plan of care for clients with gynecologic cancers.

Go to your Student CD-ROM for Review Questions for the NCLEX Examination keyed to these Learning Outcomes.

The most common reasons for seeking gynecologic care are pain, vaginal discharge, and bleeding. Nurses can play an important role in assessing gynecologic disorders by being knowledgeable about disease manifestations, being sensitive to the client's problems, and encouraging discussion about menstrual or other reproductive problems. Teaching women about their bodies, helping them to recognize when professional help should be sought, and teaching them how to make informed decisions about treatments are major goals for nurses working with female clients in any setting. Nurses also need to assess the effects of gynecologic problems on sexual health.

MENSTRUAL CYCLE DISORDERS

Primary Dysmenorrhea

PATHOPHYSIOLOGY

Dysmenorrhea, or painful menstrual flow, is one of the most common gynecologic problems, occurring most often in women in their teens and early 20s. More than 50% of all women report some degree of dysmenorrhea, but only a small percentage are unable to function. Primary dysmenorrhea alone does not involve pelvic pathologic changes, whereas secondary dysmenorrhea usually begins with an underlying disease condition such as anovulatory cycles or endometriosis. Pelvic congestion (larger ovarian and uterine vein diameters) is a syndrome of secondary dysmenorrhea.

Primary dysmenorrhea usually occurs after ovulation is established. Dysmenorrhea is painful uterine cramping with spasmodic lower abdominal pain that begins with the onset of menstrual flow and lasts 12 to 48 hours. The pain often radiates to the lower back and thighs. Nausea and vomiting, fatigue, and nervousness may occur with the pain. Less common manifestations include headache, syncope, diarrhea, bloating, and breast tenderness.

The cause of primary dysmenorrhea is thought to be increased production and release of uterine prostaglandins. Prostaglandins are produced by the endometrium during the luteal phase of the menstrual cycle, and the levels peak at the onset of menses. Excessive prostaglandin levels stimulate the myometrium and cause severe spasms, which constrict uterine blood flow, resulting in ischemia and pain. Other causes for primary dysmenorrhea are **adenomyosis** (increased vascular supply to the uterus), adhesions, salpingo-oophoritis, ovarian remnant syndrome, tumors or cysts of the reproductive organs, endometriosis, and myomas (fibroids).

COLLABORATIVE MANAGEMENT

Assessment

A thorough history of the client includes the following:

- Age at **menarche** (onset of menstruation)
- Characteristics of menstruation
- Obstetric history
- Contraceptive history
- Type of pain
- Previous therapy
- The need for contraception

Ask the client whether she has any conditions suggestive of pelvic problems. To plan care, also assess emotional factors, such as each woman's response to dysmenorrhea, her attitudes about menstruation, and the extent to which she believes that dysmenorrhea disrupts her life.

Interventions

Interventions for primary dysmenorrhea include prevention, education, support, and therapeutic measures that are tailored to each woman's needs.

Drug Therapy. Prostaglandin synthetase inhibitors (nonsteroidal anti-inflammatory drugs [NSAIDs]), such as ibuprofen (Motrin, Apo-Ibuprofen*) and naproxen sodium (Anaprox, Naprosyn), are currently recommended for pain relief. In addition, numerous over-the-counter ibuprofen products, such as Advil and Nuprin, provide pain relief for many clients with primary dysmenorrhea. Aspirin is a mild prostaglandin synthetase inhibitor and may relieve mild dysmenorrhea. All these drugs can cause gastrointestinal (GI) distress and should therefore be taken with meals or milk. Bextra, a cyclooxygenase-2 (COX-2) inhibitor, also inhibits the release of prostaglandins and aids in some pain relief caused by dysmenorrhea (Anderson, Knobmen, & Troutman, 2002). Bextra does not inhibit platelet aggregation, as seen with aspirin or NSAIDS. However, drugs similar to Bextra have been found to increase the risk for acute cardiac problems.

Before treatment, the client's contraception needs are assessed. When contraception is not needed, prostaglandin synthetase inhibitors are the treatment of choice because they are needed only when manifestations are present. If contraception is a consideration, ovulation suppression with oral contraceptives is the treatment of choice.

Complementary and Alternative Therapies. Complementary therapies that may alleviate or prevent pain include acupressure, aerobic exercise, swimming, yoga or other meditation, application of heat or cold, massage, biofeedback, and relaxation techniques. Dietary measures for the prevention of pain may include increasing the intake of vitamin B_6, calcium, magnesium, and protein and reducing the intake of sodium to reduce fluid retention.

Premenstrual Syndrome

PATHOPHYSIOLOGY

Many women experience problems that recur regularly in the luteal phase of each menstrual cycle. These problems are termed **premenstrual syndrome (PMS).** About 5% of menstruating women have severe premenstrual symptoms, and many more have moderate symptoms. Neuroendocrine mechanisms appear to influence PMS. Serotonin is a neurotransmitter that is present in the central nervous system and affects mood. A noted change in serotonin synthesis during a woman's luteal phase of the menstrual cycle increases the symptoms of PMS. Fortunately most affected women can be helped.

Premenstrual syndrome is a collection of symptoms that are cyclic in nature. These symptoms are followed by relief with menses and a symptom-free phase. PMS affects women of all races, socioeconomic levels, and educational levels. It is more prevalent in women 30 to 40 years of age. The severity increases with aging until menopause. Women are at greater risk for PMS after pregnancy, childbirth, and tubal ligation; during the perimenopausal years; and during major life stresses.

Currently there is no agreement on a single set of diagnostic criteria for PMS. Three elements are found in defining PMS: symptoms, severity level, and timing. Many women report six or more manifestations across emotional, physical, and cognitive categories.

Emotional symptoms include irritability, easily precipitated crying spells, low self-esteem, anxiety, and depression. Physical manifestations include breast tenderness, bloating, fluid retention, increased appetite and food cravings, insomnia, fatigue, hot flushes, headaches, and musculoskeletal discomfort. Cognitive problems include short-term memory problems, difficulty concentrating, and unclear thinking.

COLLABORATIVE MANAGEMENT

Assessment

There is no objective means of diagnosing PMS, although some patterns have been identified. Determining the timing of the symptoms is as critical as noting the type of symptoms. The most effective assessment tool is a menstrual chart. Instruct the client to keep a chart for at least three consecutive cycles, showing the length of the menstrual cycle, the duration of bleeding, and the occurrence of symptoms. If the woman has PMS, the symptoms recur during the luteal phase (from ovulation to menstruation), which is followed by a symptom-free period (at least 7 days).

When taking a menstrual history, assess to what extent the woman believes her activities of daily living (ADLs) are disrupted by the symptoms. Often reassurance that the symptoms are legitimate and that other women share these problems can help the client learn more about PMS. Manifestations vary greatly among women and affect many body systems (Chart 78-1).

Interventions

Management of PMS focuses on eliminating the uncomfortable symptoms. The syndrome is highly individualized; however, one of the most important interventions is education. Each woman needs information about her body, especially the menstrual cycle, so that she can begin to understand the physiologic basis of PMS.

Women may need to express their feelings and discuss their experiences with PMS. Self-help groups and support groups are helpful resources. These groups also encourage significant others to participate because PMS usually affects not only the woman but also her family and friends. For ex-

CHART 78-1

KEY FEATURES of
Premenstrual Syndrome

Dermatologic Manifestations
- Acne
- Urticaria
- Herpes

Respiratory Manifestations
- Sinusitis
- Asthma
- Rhinitis
- Colds

Urologic Manifestations
- Oliguria
- Cystitis
- Enuresis
- Urethritis

Ophthalmologic Manifestations
- Conjunctivitis
- Styes
- Glaucoma

Neurologic Manifestations
- Headaches
- Migraine
- Syncope
- Vertigo
- Numbness of hands and feet
- Epilepsy (if susceptible)

Metabolic Manifestations
- Edema
- Breast tenderness

Emotional or Psychological Manifestations
- Depression
- Irritability
- Tension
- Panic attacks
- Change in libido
- Mood swings
- Anxiety

Behavioral Manifestations
- Lowered work performance
- Food cravings
- Alcohol and drug overindulgence
- Confusion
- Sleeplessness
- Lack of coordination
- Suicide
- Lethargy
- Child abuse
- Assaultive behavior

Other Manifestations
- Allergies
- Hypoglycemia
- Joint pain
- Backache
- Palpitations
- Water retention

ample, increased family conflict, communication problems with family and friends, and decreased family cohesion occur. Other coping strategies for the woman with PMS may include spiritual support, especially participating in religious services and seeking advice from spiritual leaders. Chart 78-2 lists NIC interventions for PMS.

Diet Therapy. Diet and nutrition are useful in managing PMS. If hypoglycemia (low blood glucose) occurs, instruct the woman to eat six small meals a day and to limit her intake of sugar, red meat, alcohol, coffee, tea, and chocolate.

Eliminating caffeine may help reduce irritability. Salt and sodium intake should be limited if edema occurs. Calcium, magnesium, and vitamins A, B_6, and C have also been used for relief of PMS.

Drug Therapy. Drug therapy remains controversial, but some drugs may be been effective. Mild potassium-sparing diuretics taken for 10 days before menstruation can provide relief for some women. Women may need to decrease their intake of potassium-containing foods if they are receiving this therapy.

Progesterone may relieve physical and psychological symptoms. Natural progesterone is preferable to synthetic progesterone, even though the drug must be specially made by a pharmacist at the time prescribed. The daily dosage is 50 to 100 mg IM from ovulation to menstruation. Long-term side effects are unknown.

Bromocriptine mesylate (Parlodel) 2.5 mg two or three times daily with meals during the luteal phase can relieve breast symptoms. The side effects (light-headedness and

CHART 78-2

NIC **INTERVENTION ACTIVITIES for**
The Client with Gynecologic Problems

Premenstrual Syndrome (PMS) Management: *Alleviation/attenuation of physical and/or behavioral symptoms occurring during the luteal phase of the menstrual cycle*
- Instruct individual in the prospective identification of the major premenstrual symptoms (e.g., bloating, cramping, irritability), use of a prospective calendar checklist or symptom log, and recording of timing and severity of each symptom.
- Review symptom log/checklist.
- Collaborate with individual to identify most problematic symptoms.
- Discuss the complexity of management and need for stepwise approach to alleviate individual symptoms.
- Collaborate with the individual to select and institute stepwise approach to eliminating symptoms.
- Provide information about symptom-specific self-care measures (e.g., exercise and calcium supplementation).
- Monitor changes in symptoms.
- Encourage individual to participate in PMS support group if available.

Hormone Replacement Therapy: *Facilitation of safe and effective use of hormone replacement therapy*
- Determine reason for choosing hormone replacement therapy.
- Review alternatives to hormone replacement therapy.
- Monitor client for therapeutic effect.
- Monitor for adverse effects.
- Review information regarding beneficial and adverse effects of the different hormonal components (e.g., estrogen, progesterone, androgen).
- Review information regarding interaction effects of adjunct therapies (e.g., calcium and vitamin D supplementation, exercise, thiazide use).
- Review information regarding the different methods of administration (e.g., oral continuous combined, oral sequential, dermal, vaginal).
- Facilitate the decision to continue/discontinue.
- Recommend clients make short-term annual decisions about continuation.

NIC intervention activities selected from Dochterman, J.M., & Bulechek, G.M. (Eds.) (2004). *Nursing interventions classification (NIC)* (4th ed.). St. Louis: Mosby. No part of this work is to be altered without prior written permission from the Publisher.

hypotension) may not be well tolerated. Other drugs for PMS that have been used include birth control pills, gonadotropin-releasing hormone (GnRH) agonists, antidepressants, and prostaglandin inhibitors, such as nonsteroidal anti-inflammatory drugs (NSAIDs).

Sarafem is an antidepressant agent that belongs to the selective serotonin reuptake inhibitors (SSRI) class of drugs. It is approved for use in women with PMS during the luteal phase of a menstrual cycle. The precise action of Sarafem is not fully understood, but it is believed that the most important effect is the enhancement of the action of serotonin that results from the highly specific serotonin reuptake blockades at the neuronal membrane (Anderson et al, 2002).

Amenorrhea

PATHOPHYSIOLOGY

Amenorrhea (the absence of menstrual periods) can be either primary (menstruation that has failed to occur by age 16 years) or secondary (menstruation that has started but has since stopped and has not recurred for at least 3 months). Primary amenorrhea often occurs with anomalies

TABLE 78-1 Common Causes of Amenorrhea

Primary
- Congenital anomalies
- Hypothalamic and pituitary disorders, such as delayed puberty
- Systemic disease
  - Thyroid and adrenal dysfunction
  - Diabetes mellitus
  - Extreme malnutrition
- Ovarian disease
- Malformations of the reproductive tract

Secondary
- Pregnancy
- Menopause
- Lactation
- Cervical stenosis
- Polycystic ovary disease
- Pituitary tumor or insufficiency
- Psychogenic stress
- Excessive physical activities
- Medications
  - Antihypertensive agents
  - Birth control pills
  - Phenothiazines
- Nutritional disorders
  - Obesity
  - Anorexia nervosa
  - Sudden weight loss
- Ovarian disease, failure, or destruction

of the reproductive tract, and the prognosis for fertility is poor. Secondary amenorrhea is usually a functional disorder, and the prognosis for fertility is better. Amenorrhea can cause a woman much distress and concern.

Menstruation is a complex process that relies on the interplay of the hypothalamic, pituitary, ovarian, endometrial functions, and anatomy. Dysfunction related to any of these five factors may cause amenorrhea (Table 78-1). Primary amenorrhea is relatively uncommon and is associated with congenital factors or factors caused by ovarian, pituitary, or hypothalamic disease. Pregnancy, **lactation** (breastfeeding), and menopause are the most common causes of secondary amenorrhea.

COLLABORATIVE MANAGEMENT

Assessment

Assess both the menstrual history and the obstetric history. Ask about possible sexual activity and symptoms of pregnancy. A medical history may identify a systemic disease as a cause of amenorrhea. Ask about current eating habits and any history of dieting because both obesity and starvation (e.g., anorexia nervosa) can contribute to amenorrhea. Strenuous exercise associated with competitive athletics, such as long-distance running, can cause stress or a reduction in body fat, resulting in amenorrhea. Assess for manifestations of hormone deficiencies, such as those associated with menopause (hot flushes and vaginal dryness). Ask about the use of drugs (e.g., oral contraceptives, phenothiazines, antihypertensives) and about recent stressors. Check for **galactorrhea** (watery or milky breast secretions in nonbreastfeeding or women who have not been pregnant and **hirsutism** (unusual hair growth in women), both of which are related to polycystic ovary disease and subsequent amenorrhea.

TABLE 78-2 Common Causes of Postmenopausal Bleeding

Benign	Malignant
Atrophic vaginitis	Endometrial cancer
Cervical polyps	Cervical cancer
Endometrial hyperplasia	Ovarian cancer
Uterine fibroids	Vaginal cancer
Cervical erosion	Tubal cancer
Estrogen therapy	

Interventions

Explain amenorrhea in easily understandable terms, and answer questions about tests and treatments. Provide counseling and emotional support. Amenorrhea may be a threat to a woman's self-concept; she usually needs to ventilate her feelings about sexuality or fertility.

Interventions for specific causes of amenorrhea are based on each woman's needs. Medical and surgical management of amenorrhea is directed at the underlying causes. Treatment includes hormone replacement, ovulation stimulation, and periodic progesterone withdrawal.

Postmenopausal Bleeding

PATHOPHYSIOLOGY

Postmenopausal bleeding (vaginal bleeding occurring after a 12-month cessation of menses after the onset of menopause) is a manifestation rather than a disease. Bleeding is considered serious and should be evaluated. Gynecologic cancer occurs in 20% to 40% of women who have postmenopausal bleeding.

Postmenopausal bleeding can be caused by many benign and malignant conditions (Table 78-2). The three most common causes are atrophic vaginitis, cervical polyps, and endometrial hyperplasia.

In a client with **atrophic vaginitis,** the vaginal mucosa is thin and dry and easily traumatized by sexual intercourse and infection, causing spotting. Cervical polyps are usually soft, red, oval tissue masses that appear within the cervical canal. They may bleed spontaneously or after intercourse.

The most serious cause of postmenopausal bleeding is **endometrial hyperplasia** (tissue overgrowth), a precursor of endometrial cancer. Bleeding is caused by declining ovarian function that leads to prolonged estrogen stimulation, producing the hyperplasia that eventually breaks down and bleeds. Estrogen stimulation can also be caused by estrogen replacement therapy (ERT).

Because many women who report postmenopausal bleeding need medical or surgical interventions, assessment is the major focus. Assess the menstrual history and family history initially, including the following:

- The client's age at menopause
- The frequency and amount of bleeding
- Previous bleeding episodes
- Use of drugs (especially estrogen-only [unopposed estrogen] replacement therapy [ERT])
- Gastrointestinal (GI) or genitourinary symptoms

Also identify women who are at high risk for endometrial cancer (e.g., women who are obese, hypertensive, or diabetic or who have never had children).

CHART 78-3

CLIENT EDUCATION GUIDE
Estrogen Replacement Therapy

For All Types of Estrogen Replacement Therapy
- Call your health care provider if you have pain in your calves or groin, if you suddenly become short of breath, if you have abnormal vaginal bleeding, if you feel a lump in your breast, if you have a severe headache, or if you feel weak or numb in your arms or legs.
- Use sunscreen if you are in the sun for a prolonged period.
- Keep appointments for checkups.
- If your health care provider has prescribed progesterone to decrease your risk of endometrial cancer, take it as prescribed.

For Oral Therapy
- Take 1 pill daily for the first 25 days each month.
- If you feel nauseated or have intestinal upset, take your medication with food.

For Transdermal or Subdermal Administration
- Rotate the sites for the patches or injections to avoid skin irritation.
- Change the patches twice a week or according to your prescribed schedule.

For Vaginal Therapy
- Use an applicator to insert the suppository or cream daily as prescribed.
- You may need to wear a minipad to protect your clothing from soiling or staining by the drug.

Urine and stool specimens can be collected and tested for blood to differentiate other sources of bleeding. Blood specimens may be drawn for hemoglobin or hematocrit levels because clients are often anemic from excessive bleeding. Prepare the woman for physical and pelvic examinations, including obtaining a specimen for a Papanicolaou (Pap) test, or smear, to evaluate the cause of bleeding.

COLLABORATIVE MANAGEMENT

Nursing interventions focus on providing information and support for diagnostic and treatment procedures directed at the specific causes of bleeding. An endometrial biopsy can evaluate the presence of malignancy. A diagnostic dilation and curettage (D&C) procedure can be used to determine malignancy (see Dysfunctional Uterine Bleeding, p. 1828). Atypical hyperplasia is often treated with a hysterectomy (see Uterine Leiomyomas, p. 1838). Cancer is usually treated with a combination of surgery, radiation therapy, and chemotherapy (see Endometrial [Uterine] Cancer, p. 1842).

The medical treatment of a woman receiving unopposed estrogen therapy may include the monthly administration of progesterone daily for the last 10 days of the estrogen therapy (days 16 to 25) or a once-per-month IM progesterone injection. This treatment can reduce the abnormal endometrial growth and is suggested for the prevention of endometrial and breast cancer.

Atrophic vaginitis is managed by the use of estrogen via the vaginal, oral, transdermal, or subdermal route. Teach the client about ERT (Chart 78-2 and Chart 78-3). Inform women who use vaginal estrogen cream that it can cause systemic effects. Women who take estrogen may be at risk for gallbladder disease, hypertension, breast cancer, endometrial cancer, and coronary artery disease.

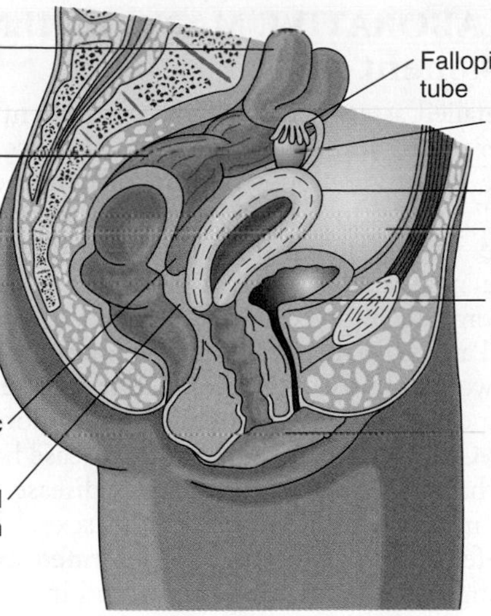

Figure 78-1 ■ Common sites of endometriosis.

Over-the-counter use of Replens vaginal lubricant can often ease the symptoms of vaginal dryness and irritation that occur with atrophic vaginitis. A water-based lubricant, such as Astroglide, used during intercourse helps reduce vaginal discomfort during intercourse.

Endometriosis

PATHOPHYSIOLOGY

Endometriosis is usually a benign problem of endometrial tissue implantation outside the uterine cavity. The tissue typically appears on the ovaries and the cul-de-sac and less commonly on other pelvic organs and structures (Figure 78-1). A "chocolate" cyst is an area of endometriosis inside an ovary.

Endometrial tissue located outside the uterus responds to hormonal stimulation similarly to the response of the intrauterine endometrium and goes through the same cyclic changes. Bleeding occurs at the site of implantation, and the blood is trapped in the tissues. Scarring and adhesions result from blood reabsorption. Endometriosis progresses slowly. It regresses during pregnancy and at menopause. Rarely does endometriosis become a malignant disease.

The cause of endometriosis is unknown, but possible causes include transportation and formation. Transportation involves implantation and vascular or lymphatic dissemination. With implantation, endometrial tissue flows back through the fallopian tubes during menstruation and then implants on pelvic structures. With vascular or lymphatic dissemination, endometrial tissues are transported through the vascular and lymphatic system to foreign locations. This possible cause explains implantation in areas outside the pelvis, such as the lungs and the kidneys. It is also possible that endometrial tissue develops outside the uterus as a birth defect.

The disorder is most often found in women during their reproductive years (i.e., their late 20s to 30s). Only about 1% to 2% of women have endometriosis, although the incidence among infertile women is about 15% to 25% (DeCherney & Nathan, 2003). It is also common in women who have not been pregnant and in those whose mothers had endometriosis.

◆COLLABORATIVE MANAGEMENT

◆Assessment

Make a detailed assessment, including the client's menstrual history, her sexual history, and the characteristics of bleeding. Pain is the most common symptom of endometriosis. The pain usually peaks just before the menstrual flow and is thought to be stimulated from estrogen and progesterone during the menstrual cycle. The endometrial implants enlarge, undergo secretory changes, and bleed (DeCherney et al., 2003). Pain is usually located in the lower abdomen, causing many women to feel a sense of rectal pressure. The degree of pain is not related to the extent of the endometriosis but to the site. Often women with minimal disease have more severe pain than do women with extensive disease. Other manifestations include **dyspareunia** (painful sexual intercourse), painful defecation, low backache, **hypermenorrhea** (excessive, prolonged, or frequent bleeding), and infertility.

A pelvic examination may reveal pelvic tenderness, nodular uterosacral ligaments, and fixed or limited movement of the uterus. Psychosocial assessment may reveal anxiety because of uncertainty about the diagnosis. The woman may also have concerns about her self-concept if she is infertile and wants to become pregnant.

Diagnostic studies include blood tests (erythrocyte sedimentation rate [ESR] and white blood cell [WBC] count) to rule out pelvic inflammatory disease (PID). Ultrasonography is used to differentiate pelvic masses that might be mistaken for endometriosis. Laparoscopy is the key diagnostic procedure for pelvic endometriosis. Examination of tissue specimens obtained during laparoscopy confirms the diagnosis.

Critical Thinking Challenge

The client is a 26-year-old nurse who has been having progressively more pain before and during menstruation. She has missed work and family events because of pain and other discomforts. She tells you that she took oral contraceptives (OC) for the first two years of her marriage and was pain-free at that time. She has been off OC for 2 years because she and her husband are trying to get pregnant. One of the residents has told her that her problem might be pelvic inflammatory disease (PID) and this comment upset her considerably because she says she has never had sex with anyone but her husband and had these symptoms throughout her teenage years before she became sexually active. She asks whether tampon use could have caused her problems.

1. What is the relationship between PID and endometriosis?
2. Could tampon use have caused endometriosis? Give a rationale for your answer.
3. Is a diagnosis of endometriosis likely to interfere with pregnancy? Why or Why not?
4. What information and emotional support can you give this client?

evolve For suggested answer guidelines, go to http://evolve.elsevier.com/Iggy/.

◆Interventions

Hormonal and surgical management may be used, depending on the symptoms, the extent of disease, and the client's desire for childbearing. Nursing management is aimed at the following:

- Reducing pain
- Restoring sexual function that was impaired by dyspareunia (painful sexual intercourse)
- Alleviating anxiety related to the manifestations of the disease and the uncertainty of the diagnosis
- Educating the client about the disease and its treatment
- Alleviating fear related to the possibility of laparoscopy or surgery
- Preventing self-esteem disturbance related to infertility

Several organizations, such as the Endometriosis Society and RESOLVE (an organization for infertile couples), offer information on endometriosis that is helpful in planning care.

NONSURGICAL MANAGEMENT

Drug Therapy. Nonsurgical management involves the use of mild analgesics or nonsteroidal anti-inflammatory drugs (NSAIDs) for pain relief. Hormonal therapies may relieve pain by suppressing ovulation. The hormonal therapies produce pseudopregnancy, pseudomenopause, or medical oophorectomy.

Pseudopregnancy is induced with oral contraceptives or progesterone. Usually a 6-month course of a low-dose estrogen oral contraceptive is prescribed, followed by cyclic oral contraceptive use or therapy with progesterone alone.

Other hormonal treatment causes ovarian suppression, or pseudomenopause, by the use of danazol (Danocrine, Cyclomen✱), an antigonadotropin drug. This approach is the current choice of many health care providers, but it is expensive ($120 to $180 per month) and may cause undesirable side effects, including acne, hirsutism (abnormal hair growth in unwanted areas), weight gain, decreased breast size, hot flushes, and cardiovascular disease. It is suggested that danazol use should not exceed 8 months (DeCherney et al., 2003).

Gonadotropin-releasing hormone (GnRH) agonists can be used to produce a reversible medical oophorectomy. The drug can be given by IM or subcutaneous injection or by nasal spray. Side effects include hot flushes, vaginal dryness, insomnia, and elevated liver enzymes. A decrease in bone density occurs within 6 months of using a GnRH agonist; thus suggested length of therapy is 6 to 8 months (DeCherney et al, 2003).

Complementary and Alternative Therapies. Strategies to relieve pain include the application of a heating pad to the abdomen or sacrum, relaxation techniques, yoga, and biofeedback. These approaches may decrease muscle tissue hypoxia and hypertonicity and relieve ischemia by increasing blood flow to the affected areas.

SURGICAL MANAGEMENT. Surgical management of endometriosis for a woman who wants to remain fertile is conservative and involves the removal of endometrial implants and adhesions. The surgeon may use a laser to treat endometriosis by vaporizing adhesions and endometrial implants. If the client does not wish to have children, the uterus and ovaries may be removed.

Dysfunctional Uterine Bleeding

PATHOPHYSIOLOGY

Dysfunctional uterine bleeding (DUB) is a nonspecific term to describe bleeding that is excessive or abnormal in amount or frequency without predisposing anatomic or systemic conditions. DUB occurs most often at either end of the span of a woman's reproductive years–when ovulation is becoming established or when it is becoming irregular at menopause.

Normally the menstrual cycle is a series of complex hormonal events related to balanced hypothalamic, pituitary, ovarian, and uterine functions. **Menses,** the sloughing of the endometrial lining, is an expected result. DUB occurs when there is a breakdown of these functions, causing hormonal imbalance.

The mechanism of DUB is unknown, but it may be linked to endometrial or myometrial dysfunction. Excessive fibrinolytic activity in the endometrium and changes in prostaglandin production in the uterus may also cause DUB.

Generally DUB occurs in the absence of ovulation caused by ovarian dysfunction. Estrogen stimulation of the endometrium is prolonged, and the endometrium grows past its hormonal support, causing bleeding and desquamation (shedding of uterine lining).

Anovulatory DUB during the reproductive years is associated with the following:

- Endocrine disturbances
- Polycystic ovary disease
- Stress
- Extreme weight changes
- Long-term drug use (e.g., anticholinergics, morphine, or oral contraceptives)
- Anatomic abnormalities

Ovulatory causes of DUB are uncommon and are related to a dysfunctional corpus luteum, irregular maturation, and shedding of the endometrium.

◆COLLABORATIVE MANAGEMENT

◆Assessment

When interviewing a woman with DUB, take a complete menstrual history. Ask about illnesses, changes in weight or diet, exercise, drug ingestion, and whether she has pain.

Observe for symptoms of anemia or systemic disease, such as the following:

- Renal or hepatic disease
- Obesity
- Undernutrition
- Abnormal hair growth related to hormonal dysfunction
- Evidence of abdominal pain or masses

An examination that includes inspection of the external genitalia and a bimanual pelvic and rectal examination is essential to identify lesions or tenderness. A physician or an advanced practice nurse performs the internal pelvic examination.

Pelvic ultrasonography and transvaginal ultrasound use may reveal polyps or lesions and measure an excessively thick endometrium. Hysteroscopy is a valuable tool for the diagnosis of anatomic lesions that affect the endometrial cavity (DeCherney et al., 2003). In addition, the surgeon usually does an endometrial biopsy by suction aspiration or dilation and curettage (D&C). These are important procedures for women over 40 years of age, who are at greater risk for endometrial cancer.

◆Interventions

NONSURGICAL MANAGEMENT. Nonsurgical management is usually the treatment of choice, although surgery may be needed to treat DUB. Most women can be treated successfully with hormonal manipulation. For those with anovulatory DUB, the health care provider may prescribe medroxyprogesterone acetate (Depo-Provera) or combination oral contraceptives. If the client takes oral contraceptives, she should take one pill daily for 21 or 28 days, beginning on the first day of the menstrual cycle. Medroxyprogesterone is taken on days 16 to 25 of each month. Monthly withdrawal bleeding is expected with both therapies. Usually the use of progestin therapy will control the abnormality once uterine pathology is ruled out (DeCherney et al., 2003).

Women with ovulatory DUB may be treated with progestins during the luteal phase or with oral contraceptives, prostaglandin inhibitors, or danazol. In cases of young women, anovulatory bleeding may occur with excessive endometrial buildup, a delay in diagnosis, or heavy blood loss. Low-dose oral contraceptives (combined progestin-estrogen) are useful. The contraceptive pills are taken in the following regimen: one pill twice daily for 5 to 7 days. Warn the client that cessation of blood flow will happen in 12 to 24 hours. They should also anticipate heavy bleeding and cramping 2 to 4 days after stopping therapy. If this therapy is successful, a low-dose combination oral contraceptive (one pill daily) is started on the fifth day of flow. This sequence is repeated for several 3-week treatments, allowing 1 week for withdrawal bleeding.

Estrogen therapy is indicated when bleeding is heavy and acute. Conjugated estrogens (25 mg) are given intravenously (IV) every 4 hours until bleeding stops or for 12 hours. When bleeding is less, low doses of oral estrogen are given to the client for 7 to 10 days (DeCherney et al., 2003). Explain the desired effects and the side effects of these drugs, and evaluate the woman's knowledge of the effects, dosage, and schedule.

SURGICAL MANAGEMENT. Surgical management includes D&C, laser or balloon endometrial ablation, and hysterectomy. A D&C is used to treat an acute episode of bleeding, but the problem often returns. Laser or balloon endometrial ablation is a safe alternative for women who do not respond to medical management or who do not need a hysterectomy. A hysterectomy is usually performed only after other treatments have failed. Table 78-3 compares the care of clients undergoing a D&C or endometrial ablation. Hysterectomy is discussed later under Operative Procedures (see Uterine Leiomyomas), p. 1838. If the woman has undergone a D&C or laser ablation, instruct her about care after surgery (Chart 78-4).

Menopause

PATHOPHYSIOLOGY

Menopause is a normal biologic event marked for most women by the end of menstrual periods (6 to 12 months of amenorrhea). It signifies the depletion of estradiol, a hormone produced by the ovaries. Although the meaning of menopause is the last menstrual period, it is more clinically relevant to look at the months or years surrounding this event.

During the past decade there has been an explosion of interest among health care providers about all aspects of menopause: endocrinologic, metabolic, pathologic, sociocultural, and psychological. Of particular interest is the role

TABLE 78-3 Nursing Care of Clients Undergoing Surgery for Dysfunctional Uterine Bleeding

	Dilation and Curettage (D&C)	Endometrial Ablation
Usual site	Outpatient	Outpatient.
Anesthesia	Local, regional, general	Regional, general.
Procedure	The cervical os is dilated; the endometrium is scraped.	The laser fiber is passed into the uterus through a hysteroscope; the endometrium is destroyed by laser energy, and tissues are removed by irrigating the uterine cavity with saline.
Preoperative care	Assess the client's knowledge of the procedure. The client is NPO after midnight. Teach postoperative expectations.	Same as for D&C. The client may be given danazol or GnRH agonist for 1 mo before surgery to decrease endometrial thickness. Counsel the client about the likelihood of sterility as a result of uterine scarring.
Postoperative care	Monitor vital signs every 15 min until client is stable. Assess the need for pain relief. Assess for vaginal bleeding. Expect discharge when the client is stable.	Same as for D&C. Same as for D&C. Assess for spotting and vaginal drainage. Same as for D&C.

GnRH, Gonadotropin-releasing hormone; *NPO*, nothing by mouth.

CHART 78-4

CLIENT EDUCATION GUIDE

Endometrial Ablation and Dilation and Curettage

Endometrial Ablation

- Spotting and vaginal drainage are normal for several days after the procedure.
- If you have abdominal cramping, take mild analgesics, such acetaminophen (Tylenol, Atasol✱), or prostaglandin inhibitors, such as ibuprofen (Motrin).
- You can return to your normal activities within 2 or 3 days.
- You will probably be sterile because of uterine scarring.

Dilation and Curettage

- Take your temperature once a day for the next 2 days. If your oral temperature is more than 100° F (38° C), call the clinic or your doctor.
- Avoid sexual intercourse, tub baths, and the use of tampons for 2 weeks to allow healing and prevent infection.
- Slight bleeding is normal. However, if bleeding is as heavy as during your normal menstrual period or if bleeding lasts longer than 2 weeks, call the clinic or health care provider.
- You can use a heating pad or hot water bottle to relieve abdominal cramping if it occurs.
- You can take mild analgesics, such as acetaminophen, for pain.

of hormone replacement therapy (HRT) in the management of symptoms.

Much interest in menopause is directed at the health problems common to postmenopausal women that may be affected by hormonal change. Such problems include osteoporosis, coronary heart disease, and breast and endometrial cancer.

Women experience menopause as individuals, and care should be taken not to make generalizations. Women become menopausal in a variety of ways, including by surgery when the uterus and ovaries are removed and by medical treatment for cancer. Natural menopause is experienced across a wide age range, from as early as the 30s or 40s or as late as the 60s. The average age at which women have their last menstrual period is between 50 and 52 years. All women under 40 who have early menopause, regardless of cause, are at higher risk for osteoporosis and related fractures. It is thought that these clients also may be at higher risk for cardiovascular disease.

Several factors may affect the timing of menopause. These include the following:

- Autoimmune disease
- Chromosomal abnormalities
- Genetic influence
- Early **menarche** (beginning of menses)
- Hysterectomy
- Smoking
- Cancer treatment (chemotherapy or radiation)

COLLABORATIVE MANAGEMENT

Assessment

Menopause transition, or **perimenopause,** are those changes in spontaneous ovarian function that precede the last menstrual period and occur gradually. Common features of the transition are a change in the woman's usual menstrual periods and the beginning of vasomotor symptoms, such as hot flushes and night sweats. These symptoms may disturb the woman's usual sleep pattern. Vaginal dryness and mood changes may also occur. Urogenital atrophy, decreased libido, decrease in cognitive function, and back pain are also symptoms associated with menopause (DeCherney et al., 2003). Ask the client about these changes, and reassure her that they are normal during perimenopause. In addition to manifestations, laboratory tests can support the presence of menopause (Table 78-4).

The most common early change in the bleeding pattern is a shortening of the time between menstrual periods, which may be accompanied by an increase in menstrual flow. As the transition evolves, about 70% of women find that their periods become lighter and farther apart until they finally stop.

Some women simply stop menstruating without further change. The remaining women experience heavier bleeding, which can be either regularly timed or unpredictable. In addition, abnormal bleeding in this age-group can be caused

TABLE 78-4 Laboratory Studies That Confirm Menopause

Test	Normal Range	Menopausal Range
Estradiol (serum)	20-750 pg/mL	<20 pg/mL
FSH	1.09-17.2 IU/mL	19.3-100.6 IU/mL
LH	0.61-56.6 IU/mL	14.2-52.3 IU/mL

FSH, Follicle stimulating hormone; *LH,* luteinizing hormone; *pg,* picograms.

by endometrial cancer, endometrial polyps, or uterine fibroid tumors.

Most women pass through the menopause transition and into the postmenopause phase with minimal symptoms and never seek treatment for menopause-related problems. About 20% of women, however, seek care for one or more symptoms related to menopause.

Interventions

Hormone replacement therapy (HRT), a combination of estrogen and progestin (progesterone), is a common medical intervention for menopause. Estrogen given alone can cause gynecologic cancers and thromboembolic conditions, such as deep vein thrombosis. Finding the right estrogen-progestin combination takes time. HRT has recently been discovered not to provide cardiac protective effects, thus changing the risk to benefit ratio of this therapy. Each woman, together with her health care provider, needs to base the decision whether or not to use HRT on the severity of symptoms and personal risk factors for other health problems.

Estrogen is available as oral, transdermal, intravaginal, and IM preparations. Because the oral estrogens have similar effects on symptoms and health risks, the choice of preparation for most women can be based on cost and individual side effect experience. Transdermal estrogen offers a useful alternative route of administration for women who prefer not to take pills; who cannot tolerate oral therapy because of gastrointestinal (GI) side effects; or who have abnormalities in liver-function tests. Side effects of estrogen occur and persist in about 10% of women.

The most common side effects are bloating, nausea, and breast tenderness. These problems often resolve after a few months of estrogen use. Chart 78-2 lists some NIC interventions for the client choosing HRT.

INFLAMMATIONS AND INFECTIONS

Vaginal discharge and itching are two common problems of female clients. Women may need information about the normal vaginal physiology, causes of symptoms, and methods of treatment. The nurse must be well informed about these topics to provide comprehensive care to clients with vaginal infections.

Vaginal infections are sometimes considered sexually transmitted diseases (STDs) because their causative organisms may be transmitted to sexual partners. However, many infections can develop without sexual contact, and sexual partners do not always become infected. True STDs, such as gonorrhea, syphilis, chlamydial infection, and herpes simplex virus infection, are discussed in Chapter 80. Acquired immunodeficiency syndrome (AIDS) is covered in Chapter 25.

CHART 78-5

BEST PRACTICE for
Care of the Client with Simple Vaginitis

In taking a client history, ask about the following:
- Onset of symptoms
- Characteristics of the discharge, especially the color and odor
- Associated symptoms such as itching and dysuria
- Types of contraceptives used
- Recent use of antibiotics
- Client's sexual activity
- Any history of vaginal infection
- Client's hygiene practices: douching and using tampons

In performing a physical examination, do the following:
- Palpate the abdomen for tenderness or pain.
- Inspect the external genitalia for erythema, edema, excoriation, odor, and discharge.
- If you are qualified, perform a speculum examination to visualize the vagina and cervix, and note the source of any discharge or inflammation.

If you are qualified, perform the following laboratory tests as ordered: a saline or potassium hydroxide wet smear and a Nitrazine paper test of vaginal pH.

Simple Vaginitis

PATHOPHYSIOLOGY

Vaginitis can develop whenever there is a disturbance of the balance of hormones and bacterial interaction in the vagina as a result of one or more of the following:
- Menopause
- STDs *(Trichomonas vaginalis)*
- Fungal (yeast) infections *(Candida albicans)*
- Changes in the normal flora
- Alkaline pH
- Insertion of foreign bodies, such as tampons and condoms
- Chemical irritations, such as from douches or sprays
- Drugs, especially antibiotics
- Health problems, such as diabetes

Vaginitis is an inflammation of the lower genital tract. Its occurrence is rising in frequency. Women who are sexually active are at greater risk for vaginitis (DeCherney et al., 2003). Assess for vaginitis by asking questions about the symptoms, assisting with a pelvic examination, and obtaining vaginal smears for laboratory testing (Chart 78-5). Use a nonjudgmental approach, and provide reassurance during the assessment because the client may be embarrassed or afraid to discuss her symptoms.

COLLABORATIVE MANAGEMENT

Interventions for vaginitis depend on the causes and the specific vaginal infection (Table 78-5). Proper health habits can be beneficial to treatment. Instruct the client to get enough rest and sleep, observe good dietary habits, get regular exercise, and use good personal hygiene. Popular, but not scientifically tested, hygiene practices to prevent vaginitis include the following:
- Perineal cleaning (wiping front to back) after urinating or defecating
- Wearing cotton underwear
- Avoiding strong douches and feminine hygiene sprays
- Avoiding tight-fitting pants

TABLE 78-5 Common Vaginal Infections

	Assessment		
Sexual Transmission	**Physical Findings**	**Laboratory Findings**	**Drug Therapy**
***Candida albicans* Infection**			
Unlikely	Odorless, white, curdlike discharge Patches on vaginal walls and cervix Inflamed vaginal walls and cervix Itching	Hyphae and spores visible on potassium hydroxide wet slide Vaginal pH 4.5 or less	Miconazole nitrate (Monistat), clotrimazole (Gyne-Lotrimin), or nystatin (Mycostatin) vaginal creams or suppositories for 7 days Terconazole (Terazol) cream or suppositories for 7 days or double strength for 3 days Tioconazole (Vagistat) single-dose vaginal application
***Trichomonas vaginalis* Infection**			
Yes	None or fishy Itching Strawberry spot on vaginal surface and cervix	Flagellated, pear-shaped protozoa on saline wet slide Vaginal pH 6-7	Oral metronidazole (Flagyl), single 2-g dose for client and sexual partners
Bacterial Vaginosis/*Gardnerella vaginalis* Infection			
Yes	Gray-white or green discharge Fishy odor Itching Normal vaginal mucosa 10%-40% asymptomatic	"Clue" cells or examination of saline wet slide Positive "whiff" test finding Vaginal pH 5-6	Oral metronidazole 500 mg four times daily for 7 days or ampicillin or tetracycline Clindamycin 450 mg four times daily for 7 days
Cervicitis			
Yes	Mucopurulent discharge from endocervix Pelvic pain, postcoital and intermenstrual bleeding The cervix may be inflamed and bleed when touched	Need to rule out herpes, gonorrhea, and chlamydial infection Vaginal pH 4.5 or less	Depends on diagnosis
Atrophic Vaginitis			
No	Pale, thin, dry mucosa Itching No odor Scant white, yellow, gray, or green discharge Dyspareunia, postcoital bleeding	Parabasal cells Leukocyte predominance Vaginal pH 6	Topical conjugated estrogen cream ½ to 1 application at night for 7 nights, then twice weekly

CHART 78-6

CLIENT EDUCATION GUIDE
Vaginal Infections

- Your risk for getting vaginal infections increases if you have sex with more than one person.
- When you have a vaginal infection, do not have sexual intercourse, or at least make sure that your partner wears a condom.
- Sexual partners may need to be treated for infection.
- The only way to identify what infection you have is to be examined by a health care provider and to get the results of laboratory tests.
- Take your medicine as prescribed, not just until your symptoms go away.

Estrogen creams are used intravaginally if no infection is present or after antibiotic therapy has been successful. Assess whether or not the client finds using an estrogen vaginal cream acceptable. If the client has a personal history of breast or uterine cancer, she may not want to use an estrogen vaginal product because some of the drug is absorbed systemically. An estradiol ring, which is changed every 90 days, is an acceptable delivery route for many women because of its long duration. Vagifem one tablet inserted intravaginally daily for 2 weeks, then 2 times per week for at least 3 to 6 months, is another treatment option (DeCherney et al., 2003).

If antibiotics are prescribed, eating yogurt or taking *Lactobacillus* culture (Lactinex) tablets may help restore the natural flora of the vagina. Teach the client about preventive measures and infection transmission (Chart 78-6).

Vulvitis

PATHOPHYSIOLOGY

Vulvitis is an inflammatory condition of the vulva that is associated with symptoms of pruritus (itching) and a burning sensation. The vulvar skin is sensitive to hormonal, metabolic, and allergic influences. Symptoms can be caused by systemic conditions, direct contact with irritants, and extension of infection from the vagina.

The most common skin disease affecting the vulva is contact dermatitis, which can be caused by an irritant, such as feminine hygiene sprays, fabric dyes, soaps and deter-

CHART 78-7

BEST PRACTICE for
Prevention of Vulvitis

- Wear cotton underwear.
- Avoid wearing tight clothing, such as pantyhose or tight jeans, because they can cause chafing. You can also get hot and sweaty, which can cause an infection.
- Always wipe front to back after having a bowel movement or urinating.
- Do not douche or use feminine hygiene sprays.
- If your sexual partner has an infection of the sex organs, do not have intercourse with him or her until he or she has been treated.
- You are more likely to get an infection if you are pregnant, have diabetes, take oral contraceptive drugs, or are menopausal.
- Practice vulvar self-examination monthly (see Chapter 76).

gents, or allergens. Primary infections that affect the vulva include herpes genitalis and condylomata acuminata (venereal warts) (see Chapter 80). Secondary infections of the vulva are caused by organisms responsible for the many numerous types of vaginitis, including candidiasis. Pediculosis pubis (crab lice) and scabies (itch mite) are common parasitic infestations of the skin of the vulva. Other causes of vulvitis include the following:

- Atrophic vaginitis
- Vulvar kraurosis (postmenopausal disorder causing dryness and atrophy)
- Vulvar leukoplakia (postmenopausal atrophy and thickening of vulvar tissues)
- Cancer
- Urinary incontinence

COLLABORATIVE MANAGEMENT

Assessment usually identifies symptoms of itching and burning sensation. **Erythema** (redness), edema, and superficial skin ulcers also may be present. Some women may have an itch-scratch-itch cycle, in which the itching leads to scratching, which causes excoriation that then must heal. As healing takes place, itching occurs again, which leads to further scratching. If the cycle is not interrupted, the condition may become chronic, causing the vulvar skin to become white and thickened (leathery). This skin is dry and scaly and cracks easily, increasing the woman's risk for infection.

Treatment of clients with vulvitis depends on the cause. Nursing interventions to relieve itching include applying wet compresses, sitz baths for 30 minutes several times a day, and applying the prescribed topical drugs, such as hydrocortisone and fluorinated corticosteroids (betamethasone valerate [Valisone, Betaderm✱] or fluocinolone acetonide [Synalar, Fluoderm]).

The health care provider prescribes oral antibiotics if infection is the underlying cause. Encourage the removal of any irritant or allergen, such as by changing detergents. Treatment of pediculosis and scabies is instituted if needed and includes applying lindane (1% gamma benzene hexachloride [Kwell, Kwellada✱]) lotion, shampoo, or cream to the affected area as directed; cleaning affected clothes, bedding, and towels; and disinfecting the home environment (lice cannot live for more than 24 hours away from the body).

If the vulvitis is chronic or severe, laser therapy (see pp. 1846 to 1847) or a "skinning" vulvectomy (see p. 1851) may be performed. Preventive measures that may be helpful for vulvitis are listed in Chart 78-7.

Toxic Shock Syndrome

PATHOPHYSIOLOGY

Toxic shock syndrome (TSS) was first recognized in 1980, when it was found to be related to menstruation and tampon use. Other conditions associated with TSS include surgical wound infection, nonsurgical focal infections, postpartum conditions, and nonmenstrual vaginal conditions. Use of the diaphragm, cervical cap, and vaginal contraceptive sponge also has been linked to TSS.

The pathophysiology of TSS is not clearly understood. Certain strains of *Staphylococcus aureus* produce a toxin that leads to the symptoms of TSS. The actual mechanism of *S. aureus* absorption in TSS is unknown. The vagina may be highly susceptible to the toxin released by *S. aureus.*

In menstrually related TSS, the risk appears to be associated with tampon use. Risk for TSS increased with the degree of absorbency of the tampon. The following are possible explanations:

- Toxins readily cross the vaginal mucosa.
- Highly absorbent tampons reduce vaginal moisture, causing fissures in the vaginal walls; they also rub the vaginal walls and cause ulceration, allowing movement of the toxins.
- Prolonged or continued tampon use can cause chronic vaginal ulcerations through which *S. aureus* is absorbed.
- Plastic tampon inserters can cause ulceration through which toxins are transported.
- Toxin producing *S. aureus* has a growth requirement for magnesium (some tampons contain magnesium).

COLLABORATIVE MANAGEMENT

Influenza-like symptoms for the first 24 hours are common. The abrupt onset of a high fever along with a headache, sore throat, vomiting, diarrhea, generalized rash, and hypotension is often present. The most common manifestations are skin changes (initially a rash resembling a severe sunburn that changes to a macular erythema similar to a drug-related rash). Because not all women have all these manifestations, the criteria established by the Centers for Disease Control and Prevention (CDC) are used to verify cases of TSS (Chart 78-8).

Management focuses on client education and prevention. Instruct the client on the prevention of TSS related to the use of tampons, vaginal sponges, and diaphragms (Chart 78-9).

Treatment when the infection is present includes fluid replacement because dehydration and electrolyte imbalance result from vomiting and diarrhea. Antibiotics, most often penicillin, are the mainstay of treatment. Other antibiotics are needed if the penicillin-resistant strain of *S. aureus* is the cause of TSS. Vancomycin is the drug of choice to treat *S. aureus* TSS if the client is allergic to penicillin (DeCherney et al., 2003). Other measures may include transfusions to reverse low platelet counts, corticosteroids to treat skin changes, and drugs to treat hypotension.

PELVIC STRUCTURE SUPPORT PROBLEMS

Uterine Prolapse

PATHOPHYSIOLOGY

The stages of **uterine prolapse** are described by the degree of descent of the uterus (Figure 78-2). Uterine prolapse can be caused by congenital defects, persistent high levels of intra-abdominal pressure related to heavy physical labor or exertion, or any other event that weakens the pelvic supports.

CHART 78-8

KEY FEATURES of
Toxic Shock Syndrome

- Fever (temperature >102° F [38.9° C]
- Diffuse rash resembling sunburn
- Peeling of skin—primarily the soles of the feet and the palms of the hands—1 to 2 wk after onset of the illness.
- Hypotension (systolic blood pressure <90 mm Hg or orthostatic syncope)
- Involvement of three or more of the following:
  - Gastrointestinal system: vomiting, diarrhea at the onset of the syndrome
  - Musculoskeletal system: severe aching or a serum creatinine phosphatase level twice the normal level
  - Respiratory system: acute respiratory distress syndrome (ARDS)
  - Renal/urinary system: decreased urine output, pyuria
  - Cardiovascular system: decreased left ventricular contractility; ischemic changes shown on the electrocardiogram
  - Liver: total bilirubin, aspartate aminotransferase (serum glutamic-oxaloacetic transaminase), and alanine aminotransferase (serum glutamic-pyruvic transaminase) levels elevated; jaundice; disseminated intravascular coagulation (DIC)
  - Hematologic system: platelet levels below normal
  - Central nervous system: disorientation, altered consciousness in the absence of fever or hypertension
  - Mucous membranes: hyperemia of the vaginal walls, the throat, or the conjunctiva of the eye
- Negative results for the following: Rocky Mountain spotted fever, measles, scarlet fever, and throat, blood, and cerebrospinal fluid cultures
- Positive culture for *Staphylococcus aureus* from blood, urine, or stool

CONSIDERATIONS FOR OLDER ADULTS

Prolapse is often a complication of childbirth injuries and repetitive stresses occurring many years later, but it also occurs in older adults who have never had children. The pelvic floor that supports the uterus is weakened by aging.

COLLABORATIVE MANAGEMENT

Assessment findings include the client's sensation of feeling as if "something is in my vagina," **dyspareunia** (painful sexual intercourse), backache, a feeling of heaviness or pressure in the

CHART 78-9

CLIENT EDUCATION GUIDE
Prevention of Toxic Shock Syndrome

Tampon Use
- Wash your hands before inserting a tampon.
- Do not use a tampon if it is dirty.
- Insert the tampon carefully to avoid injuring the delicate tissue in your vagina.
- Change your tampon every 3 to 6 hours.
- Do not use superabsorbent tampons.
- Use sanitary napkins at night.
- Call your health care provider if you suddenly experience a high temperature, vomiting, or diarrhea.
- Do not use tampons at all if you have had toxic shock syndrome.
- Not using tampons almost guarantees that you will not get toxic shock syndrome.

Vaginal Sponge Use
- Wash your hands before inserting a vaginal sponge.
- Use only clean water to wet the sponge.
- Do not use the sponge if it is dirty.
- Do not use the sponge for more than 30 hours at a time.
- Call your health care provider if you have two or more symptoms of toxic shock syndrome.

Diaphragm Use
- Wash your hands and the diaphragm before insertion.
- Remove the diaphragm within 24 hours after intercourse.
- Do not use the diaphragm during your menstrual period.
- After you take out the diaphragm, wash it with mild soap, rinse it, and dry it. Coating the diaphragm with a small amount of cornstarch will absorb any excess water and prevent damage to the latex rubber. Store it in a clean, dry place.

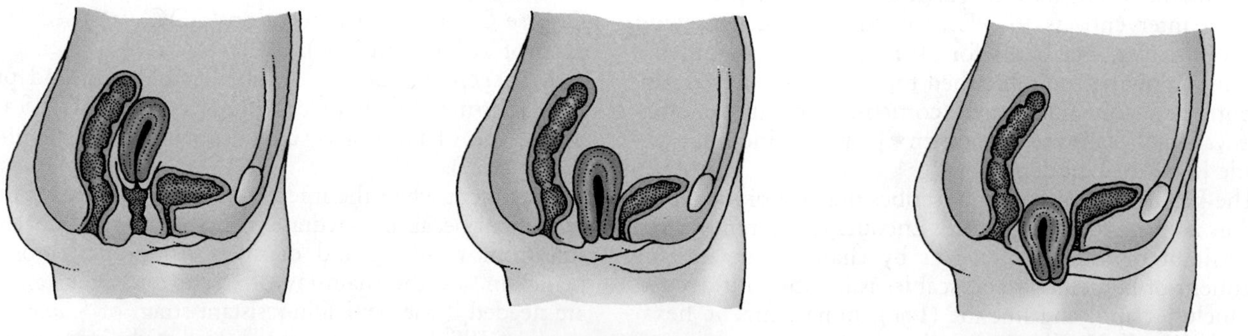

In **grade I uterine prolapse**, the uterus bulges into the vagina, but the cervix does not protrude through the entrance to the vagina.

In **grade II uterine prolapse**, the uterus bulges farther into the vagina, and the cervix protrudes through the entrance to the vagina.

In **grade III uterine prolapse**, the body of the uterus and the cervix protrude through the entrance to the vagina. The vagina is turned inside out.

Figure 78-2 ■ Types of uterine prolapse.

pelvis, and bowel or bladder problems (if cystocele or rectocele is also present). A pelvic examination may reveal a protrusion of the cervix when the woman is asked to bear down.

Interventions are based on the degree of prolapse. Conservative treatment, such as the use of pessaries, is preferred over surgical treatment when possible. Chart 78-10 lists NIC interventions for pessary use. Vaginal hysterectomy with repair is the usual surgical procedure (see Operative Procedures [Uterine Leiomyomas], p. 1839). Before surgical intervention, ask the woman about her desire for future childbearing (surgery may be delayed) and her desire for sexual intercourse. Surgery usually shortens and narrows the vagina, possibly causing painful intercourse.

Whenever the uterus is displaced, other structures, such as the bladder, rectum, and small intestine, are affected and can protrude through the vaginal walls.

CHART 78-10

NIC INTERVENTION ACTIVITIES for The Client with Weak Pelvic Floor Muscles

Pessary Management: *Placement and monitoring of a vaginal device for treating stress urinary incontinence, uterine retroversion, genital prolapse, or incompetent cervix*
- Determine ability to perform self-care of pessary.
- Discuss maintenance regimen and cleaning procedures with client prior to fitting pessary (e.g., fit is trial and error; frequent follow-up visits are required).
- Review manufacturer's directions regarding specific type of pessary.
- Instruct on method for pessary removal, as appropriate.
- Instruct on contraindications for intercourse or douching based on pessary type.
- Instruct to report discomfort; dysuria; changes in color, consistency, or frequency of vaginal discharge.
- Determine therapeutic response to pessary use.

Pelvic Muscle Exercise: *Strengthening and training the levator ani and urogenital muscles through voluntary, repetitive contraction to decrease stress, urge, or mixed types of urinary incontinence*
- Determine ability to recognize the urge to void.
- Instruct female individual to locate the levator ani and urogenital muscles by placing her finger in the vagina and squeezing.
- Instruct individual to tighten, then relax, the ring of muscle around urethra and anus, as if trying to prevent urination or bowel movement.
- Instruct individual to perform muscle tightening exercises, working up to 300 contractions each day, holding the contraction for 10 seconds each and resting at least 10 seconds between each contraction, per agency protocol.
- Inform individual that it takes 6 to 12 weeks for exercises to be effective.
- Teach individual to monitor response to exercise by attempting to stop urine flow no more often than once a week.
- Provide written instructions describing the intervention and the recommended number of repetitions.

NIC intervention activities selected from Dochterman, J.M., & Bulechek, G.M. (Eds.) (2004). *Nursing interventions classification (NIC)* (4th ed.). St. Louis: Mosby.

Cystocele

PATHOPHYSIOLOGY

A **cystocele** is a protrusion of the bladder through the vaginal wall (Figure 78-3). It is due to weakened pelvic structures. This protrusion can be caused by obesity, advanced age, childbearing, or genetic predisposition. The development of a cystocele occurs more often in the postmenopausal years, when estrogen loss also weakens tissue supports and can cause relaxation of the supports.

COLLABORATIVE MANAGEMENT

Assessment findings may include the following:
- Difficulty in emptying the bladder
- Urinary frequency and urgency
- Urinary tract infection
- Stress urinary incontinence (loss of urine during activities that increase intra-abdominal pressure, such as laughing, coughing, sneezing, or lifting heavy objects)

A pelvic examination reveals a large bulge of the anterior vaginal wall when the woman is asked to bear down. Diagnostic tests include cystography (to show the presence of bladder herniation), measurement of residual urine by catheterization or bladder ultrasound, and urine culture and sensitivity testing. Radiographic imaging of the urinary tract and a voiding cystourethrography are useful in determining the degree of cystocele. Radiographic imaging of the urinary tract includes an intravenous urogram (IVU) to define urinary anatomy. A voiding cystourethrography (VCUG) is done to determine the following: the degree of the cystocele

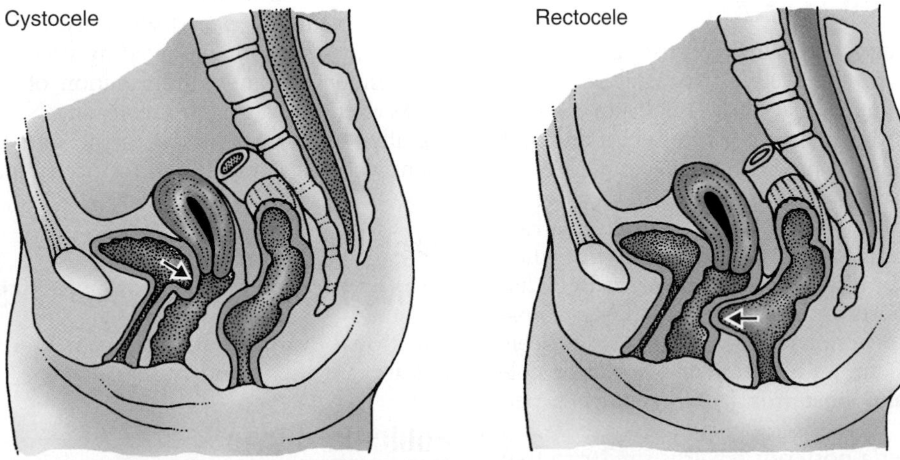

Figure 78-3 ■ In cystocele, the urinary bladder is displaced downward, causing bulging of the anterior vaginal wall. In rectocele, the rectum is displaced, causing bulging of the posterior vaginal wall.

in the standing position, the amount of a postvoid residual, and urethral abnormalities. A cystometrogram measures bladder storage. Uroflowmetry evaluates characteristics of the woman's voiding pattern. Failure to empty the bladder because of poor bladder contraction can be identified during this test (DeCherney et al., 2003).

If the client has only mild symptoms, management is conservative. The health care provider may recommend a pessary to support the bladder in some clients. Estrogen therapy may be prescribed for the postmenopausal woman to prevent atrophy and weakening of vaginal walls. Kegel exercises may help strengthen perineal muscles (see Chart 78-10). Teach the woman Kegel exercises, telling her to tighten and relax the perineal muscles; the woman presses the buttocks together and holds the position for at least 5 seconds. Instruct the client to repeat the exercise often throughout the day. An alternative exercise is to try to stop the flow of urine after urination has started and then hold the position for a few seconds before letting the urine flow again.

Surgery may be recommended for severe symptoms. An **anterior colporrhaphy** (anterior repair) tightens the pelvic muscles for better bladder support. A vaginal surgical approach is used. Nursing care of a woman undergoing an anterior repair is similar to that for a woman undergoing a vaginal hysterectomy (see Operative Procedures [Uterine Leiomyomas], p. 1839).

After surgery, instruct the client to limit her activities, not lift anything heavier than 5 pounds, avoid strenuous exercises, and avoid sexual intercourse for 6 weeks. Tell the woman to notify her health care provider if she has signs of infection, such as fever, persistent pain, or purulent, foul-smelling discharge. Encourage the client to keep her follow-up appointment after surgery.

Rectocele

PATHOPHYSIOLOGY

A **rectocele** is a protrusion of the rectum through a weakened vaginal wall (see Figure 78-3). This problem usually results from the pressure of an infant's head during a difficult delivery, a traumatic forceps delivery, or a congenital defect of the supporting tissues. Symptoms do not typically appear until the woman is older than 35 years of age.

COLLABORATIVE MANAGEMENT

The woman usually relates symptoms of constipation, hemorrhoids, fecal impaction, and feelings of rectal or vaginal fullness. A pelvic examination may show a bulge of the posterior vaginal wall when the woman is asked to bear down. A rectal examination reveals the presence of a rectocele. A barium enema study also confirms the presence of a rectocele.

Management focuses on promoting bowel elimination. The health care provider usually prescribes a high-fiber diet, stool softeners, and laxatives. The surgical procedure that strengthens pelvic supports and reduces the bulging is **posterior colporrhaphy** (posterior repair). If both a cystocele and a rectocele are present, an **anterior and posterior colporrhaphy (anterior and posterior [A&P] repair)** is performed.

The nursing care after a posterior repair is similar to that after any rectal surgery. After surgery a low-residue (low-fiber) diet is prescribed to prevent bowel movements and allow time for the incision to heal. Instruct the client not to strain when she does have a bowel movement so that she does not put pressure on the suture line. Bowel movements are often painful, and the client may need pain medication before having a bowel movement. Sitz baths may relieve discomfort. Instructions for the client undergoing a posterior repair are similar to those for undergoing an anterior repair.

Fistulas

PATHOPHYSIOLOGY

Fistulas are abnormal openings between two adjacent organs or structures. Vaginal fistulas can occur between the vagina and the urethra (urethrovaginal), the vagina and the bladder (vesicovaginal), or the vagina and the rectum (rectovaginal). Trauma is the main cause of fistulas, although they can result from complications of surgery, vaginal-delivery complications, malignancy, or radiation therapy for cancer.

COLLABORATIVE MANAGEMENT

Symptoms depend on the location of the fistula. A fistula may result in any of the following problems:

- Leakage of urine, flatus, or feces into the vagina
- Irritation or excoriation of the vulva and vaginal tissues
- An unpleasant odor (fecal or urine) in the vagina
- A feeling of wetness or dribbling in the vagina

Women who have fistulas may be embarrassed to seek help until symptoms are severe. The client may withdraw from social activities or from relationships with significant others as the symptoms become more difficult to manage.

Management depends on the fistula's location. Surgery is not recommended if infection or inflammation is present. Surgery may not be successful. Nursing care focuses on assisting the woman with the frequent and time-consuming perineal hygiene, including sitz baths; perineal cleaning with mild, unscented soap and water; and low-pressure douching with commercial deodorizing solutions or homemade solutions (1 teaspoon [5 mL] of nonchlorine household bleach to 1 quart [about 1 L] of water). The woman may need to wear sanitary napkins or disposable undergarments (such as Depends) if there is leakage of urine or feces. Other interventions may include the application of A and D ointment to excoriated tissues.

If the fistula is repaired surgically, nursing care focuses on preventing infection and avoiding stress on the repaired area (low-residue diet and administration of stool softeners for 2 weeks after rectovaginal fistula repair). Nursing care and teaching after surgery are similar to the care and teaching of the client who has a cystocele or rectocele repair (see text at left).

BENIGN NEOPLASMS

FUNCTIONAL OVARIAN CYSTS

Functional ovarian cysts can occur in a woman of any age but are rare after menopause.

Follicular Cysts

Follicular cysts usually occur in young, menstruating women. These cysts are not malignant and do not grow without hormonal influences. A cyst can develop when a mature follicle fails to rupture or an immature follicle fails to reabsorb follicular fluid during the second half of the menstrual cycle. The cyst is usually small (2.4 to 3.2 inches [6 to 8 cm]) and may be asymptomatic unless it ruptures. Rupture of a follicular cyst or **torsion** (twisting) may cause acute, severe pelvic pain. The pain usually resolves after several days of bedrest and use of mild analgesics. If the cyst does not rupture, it usually disappears within two or three menstrual cycles without intervention. If the cyst does not shrink, the health care provider may prescribe oral contraceptives for one or two menstrual cycles to depress ovulation. When the cyst is managed conservatively, follow-up care is necessary to confirm that it has disappeared.

If the cyst is larger than 6 to 8 cm, a neoplasm may be suspected, and evaluation by ultrasonography or laparoscopy is needed. Larger cysts often occur with menstrual irregularities.

Surgery is recommended only after menopause or when cysts are larger than 3.2 inches (7 cm). A **cystectomy** (removal of the cyst) is performed instead of an **oophorectomy** (removal of the ovary).

Corpus Luteum Cysts

Corpus luteum cysts occur after ovulation and often occur with increased secretion of progesterone. The cysts are usually small, averaging 1.5 inches (4 cm). They are purplish red as a result of hemorrhage within the corpus luteum. These cysts occur with a delay in the onset of menses and irregular or prolonged flow. They may occur with low abdominal or pelvic pain that is usually described as dull or aching. If the cyst ruptures, intraperitoneal hemorrhage can occur.

Corpus luteum cysts may disappear in one or two menstrual cycles or with suppression of ovulation. The treatment is the same as that for follicular cysts.

Theca-Lutein Cysts

Theca-lutein cysts are uncommon and often occur with a hydatidiform molar pregnancy. Theca-lutein cysts develop as a result of prolonged stimulation of the ovaries by excessive amounts of human chorionic gonadotropin (hCG).

These cysts regress spontaneously within 3 months with the removal of the molar pregnancy or the source of excessive hCG. Usually no other treatment is necessary.

Polycystic Ovary

Polycystic ovary, or Stein-Leventhal syndrome, results when high levels of luteinizing hormone (LH) overstimulate the ovaries, which produces multiple cysts on one or both ovaries. High levels of estrogen are produced by these cysts and are unopposed by postovulatory progesterone. Endometrial **hyperplasia** (tissue overgrowth) or even carcinoma may result.

A typical client is obese, is **hirsute** (hairy), has irregular menses, and may be infertile because of lack of ovulation. Treatment depends on which disorder is of greatest concern to the woman. The best treatment is the use of oral contraceptives because they inhibit LH production. The health care provider may advise a woman who is older than 35 years of age and no longer desires childbearing to undergo a **bilateral salpingo-oophorectomy (BSO)** (removal of both tubes and ovaries) and **hysterectomy** (removal of the uterus and cervix). Women who desire fertility can be treated with drugs such as clomiphene citrate (Clomid) to stimulate ovulation.

OTHER BENIGN OVARIAN CYSTS AND TUMORS

Dermoid Cysts

Dermoid cysts are common germ cell tumors and are usually benign. These cysts more commonly occur in childhood, although they can develop in a female of any age.

Dermoid cysts may contain hair, skin, teeth, and other calcifications. They are usually asymptomatic unless they grow large and put pressure on other organs, such as the bladder and the bowel. The cysts develop on both ovaries in some cases. They are often attached to the ovary by a **pedicle** (stalk).

Management of dermoid cysts is surgical removal (cystectomy). If the cysts are not removed, they usually continue to grow and rupture, causing hemorrhage and infection.

Ovarian Fibromas

Fibromas are the most common benign, solid ovarian neoplasms. These pearly white tumors of connective tissue origin rarely become malignant. Fibromas can range in size from a small nodule to a mass weighing more than 50 pounds (22.7 kg). The average size is 2.4 inches (6 cm) in diameter, slightly smaller than a tennis ball. Most affect only one ovary. On examination, they feel firm, have a slightly irregular contour, and are mobile. Larger fibromas may cause ascites and feelings of pelvic pressure or abdominal enlargement. Unless rupture or torsion occurs, the fibroma is usually asymptomatic. Fibromas often occur postmenopausally.

Solid ovarian neoplasms are surgically removed. The surgeon may perform an oophorectomy for borderline tumors (when there is a question of possible cancer). Nursing care of a woman undergoing an oophorectomy is similar to that for a woman undergoing a tubal ligation. When both ovaries are removed, artificial menopause occurs in a premenopausal women. The woman then often develops decreased vaginal lubrication, hot flashes, and atrophy of the vaginal epithelium. These symptoms may be treated with estrogen replacement therapy (ERT) (see Chart 78-3).

Epithelial Ovarian Tumors

Epithelial ovarian tumors, serous and mucinous cystadenomas, occur in women between the ages of 30 and 50 years. Serous cystadenomas usually affect both ovaries and are more likely to become malignant than mucinous cystadenomas. Both tumors can be irregular and smooth, but mucinous cystadenomas tend to grow large, some to more than 100 pounds (45 kg).

Management of cystadenomas is **unilateral salpingo-oophorectomy** (surgical removal of a fallopian tube and ovary) because it is often impossible to tell whether the tumor is benign or malignant. Small cysts may be removed by cystectomy, but the larger ones are difficult to resect from the ovary.

Uterine Leiomyomas

PATHOPHYSIOLOGY

Leiomyomas, also called myomas and fibroids, are benign, slow-growing solid tumors of the uterus. They are the most commonly occurring pelvic tumors.

Leiomyomas develop from the uterine myometrium. As they grow, fibroids stay attached to the myometrium by means of a pedicle. Leiomyomas are classified according to their position in the layers of the uterus. The most common types of leiomyomas are intramural, submucosal, and subserosal (Figure 78-4).

Intramural leiomyomas are contained in the uterine wall within the myometrium. Submucosal leiomyomas protrude into the cavity of the uterus. Subserosal leiomyomas protrude through the outer surface of the uterine wall. Subserosal leiomyomas may grow laterally and extend to the broad ligament.

Although most fibroids develop within the uterine wall, about 5% may appear in the cervix. Rarely, a fibroid breaks off the pedicle and attaches to other tissues (parasitic fibroid).

Etiology

The cause of leiomyomas is not precisely known. Leiomyomas usually result from excessive local growth of smooth muscle cells. The stimulus for growth may be physical or mechanical and may operate at points of maximal stress within the myometrial layer of the uterine wall. Because there are multiple points of stress caused by the contractions of the uterine muscle, multiple fibroids develop. The growth of leiomyomas may be related to estrogen stimulation; fibroids often enlarge during pregnancy and diminish in size after menopause.

Incidence/Prevalence

Leiomyomas occur in about 20% to 30% of women older than age 30. The rationale for why leiomyomas develop in some women and not in others is not known.

COLLABORATIVE MANAGEMENT

PHARM REVIEW

Assessment

HISTORY

Many women with uterine leiomyomas are asymptomatic, but abnormal bleeding is common. Because African American women and premenopausal women are at greatest risk for leiomyomas, any abnormal bleeding should be discussed. Menstrual bleeding may be increased **(menorrhagia);** the bleeding may occur between menstrual periods **(metrorrhagia),** or it may be continuous.

PHYSICAL ASSESSMENT/CLINICAL MANIFESTATIONS

Women with fibroids do not usually have pain, although acute pain may occur with twisting of the fibroid on its stalk. A woman may report a feeling of pelvic pressure, constipation, or urinary frequency or retention. These symptoms result when an enlarged fibroid presses on other organs. The client may notice that her abdomen has increased in size with or without noticeable weight gain. Painful sexual intercourse and infertility may also occur with leiomyomas.

Abdominal, vaginal, and rectal examinations usually establish the presence of a uterine enlargement that may indicate a leiomyoma. Other diagnostic procedures are needed to differentiate benign tumors from malignant ones.

PSYCHOSOCIAL ASSESSMENT

A woman who is symptomatic may fear that she has a malignancy. She may be anxious about abnormal bleeding or her failure to conceive. She may also be concerned if surgery is recommended. Assess the woman's feelings and concerns about her symptoms and fears of the unknown. If surgery is recommended, explore the significance of the loss of the uterus for the woman.

LABORATORY ASSESSMENT

A complete blood count identifies iron deficiency anemia (related to bleeding). A pregnancy test is done to determine

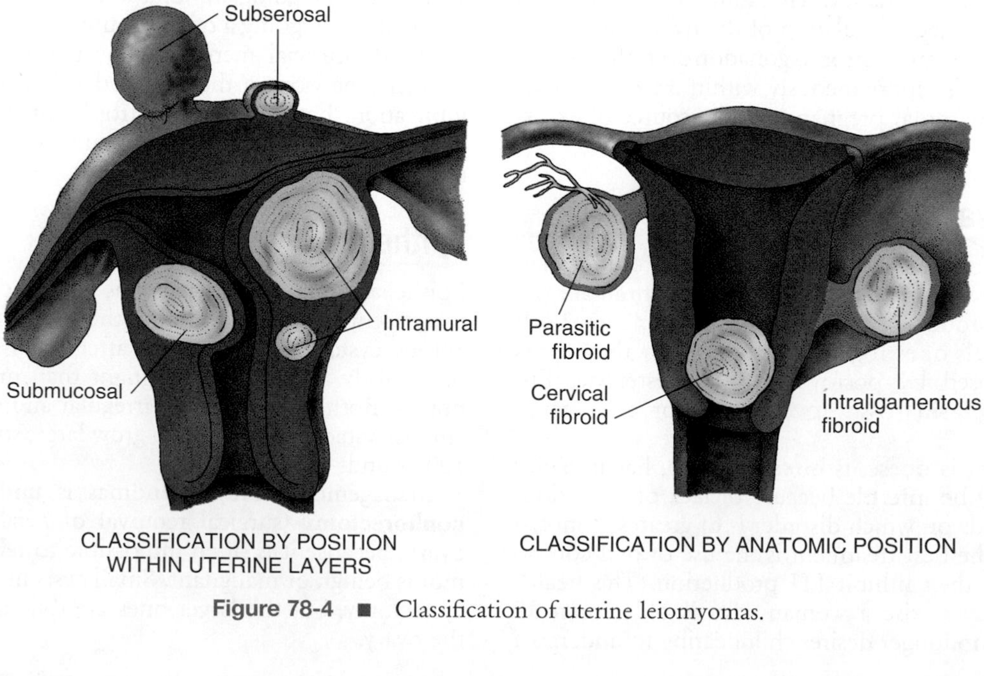

Figure 78-4 ■ Classification of uterine leiomyomas.

whether pregnancy is the cause of the uterine enlargement. An endometrial biopsy may be performed to determine whether the lesion is malignant.

RADIOGRAPHIC ASSESSMENT

Computed tomography (CT) may be of some value. However, CT scans do not differentiate between benign and malignant myomas. Magnetic resonance imaging (MRI) can differentiate between benign and malignant lesions.

OTHER DIAGNOSTIC ASSESSMENTS

Ultrasonography may help differentiate causes of pelvic masses, such as ovarian masses and pregnancy. Culdoscopy or laparoscopy may help differentiate a uterine fibroid from an ovarian mass. These tests are described in Chapter 76.

Analysis

COMMON NURSING DIAGNOSES AND COLLABORATIVE PROBLEMS

The most common collaborative problem for clients with leiomyomas is Potential for Hemorrhage.

ADDITIONAL NURSING DIAGNOSES AND COLLABORATIVE PROBLEMS

In addition to the common collaborative problems, clients with leiomyomas may have one or more of the following:

- Anxiety and Fear related to a threat to or change in health status (uncertain diagnosis; potential surgical treatment)
- Acute Pain related to physical pressure from tumors
- Anticipatory Grieving or Dysfunctional Grieving related to perceived or actual loss of the uterus or reproductive function
- Sexual Dysfunction related to altered body structure and dyspareunia
- Ineffective Coping related to uncertainty or depression as a response to treatment

Planning and Implementation

POTENTIAL FOR HEMORRHAGE

NOC **PLANNING: EXPECTED OUTCOMES.** The client with leiomyomas is expected to be free of bleeding complications. Indicators include that the client should have only mild or no deviations of the following parameters:

- Vaginal bleeding
- Anxiety
- Decreased hematocrit (Hct)
- Decreased hemoglobin (Hgb)

INTERVENTIONS. Observation of the leiomyomas over time, myomectomy, and hysterectomy are the methods of management. The choice depends on the size and symptoms of the fibroids and the woman's desire for future childbearing.

NONSURGICAL MANAGEMENT. If the client has few symptoms or desires childbearing, the health care provider typically suggests observation and examination every 4 to 6 months. If the woman is menopausal, the fibroids usually shrink, and surgery may not be necessary. However, a client who is receiving estrogen replacement therapy (ERT) for menopausal symptoms should know that the fibroids may continue to grow because of the estrogen stimulation.

A new alternative to surgery is radiologic management by uterine artery embolization (UFE). This treatment for leiomyomas is to embolize (occlude) the blood flow to the tumors using a percutaneous catheter approach. Under moderate sedation, the radiologist places a tiny catheter in both uterine arteries and injects embolic particles into the tumor's blood supply. This 1- to 2-hour procedure is usually effective in shrinking tumors, thereby reducing pain and bleeding.

SURGICAL MANAGEMENT. If the woman desires childbearing, the surgeon may perform a **myomectomy** (the removal of leiomyomas with preservation of the uterus) regardless of the size, number, or location of the fibroids. A laser may be used to remove the tumors. Myomectomy is usually performed in the proliferative phase of the menstrual cycle to minimize blood loss and to avoid the possibility of interrupting an unsuspected pregnancy. A small percentage of leiomyomas that are removed recur. Nursing care is similar to that of a woman undergoing a hysterectomy, as described below under Operative Procedures.

Preoperative Care. Teaching by the physician begins in his or her office. Preoperative teaching is usually done on an individual basis. Explain procedures that routinely take place before surgery, including laboratory tests and expected drugs, such as prophylactic antibiotics. Teach about the need for turning, coughing, deep breathing exercises; incentive spirometry; early ambulation; and the need for pain relief (see Chapter 20).

Psychological assessment is essential. First explore the significance of the loss of the uterus for the client. She may feel a great loss if she wishes to retain her childbearing ability, relates her uterus to her self-image and femininity, or believes that her sexual function is related to her uterus. A woman may have misconceptions about the effects of hysterectomy (e.g., associating it with masculinization and weight gain). Identify any misconceptions, and provide correct information. Assess the client's support system. The client may fear rejection by her sexual partner. Urge inclusion of the partner in all teaching sessions unless this practice is not culturally acceptable.

Operative Procedures. A **total abdominal hysterectomy (TAH)** is usually performed for leiomyomas larger than the size of a 12-week pregnancy. The uterus and cervix are removed through a horizontal incision (traditional approach) or via laparoscopic surgery, which requires a very small umbilical incision.

A uterus that has smaller fibroids may be removed via a **total vaginal hysterectomy (TVH)**. The surgeon removes the uterus and cervix through the vagina without an external surgical incision. In both vaginal and abdominal hysterectomies, the surgeon removes the uterus from the five supporting ligaments, which are then attached to the vaginal cuff so that normal depth of the vagina is maintained (Table 78-6).

In selected cases (e.g., submucous fibroids, menorrhagia), minimally invasive uterine surgery may be performed, such as a **transcervical endometrial resection (TCER).** A hysteroscope is inserted into the uterus, and the endometrium is destroyed using a diathermy resectoscope (similar to the scope used with prostate surgery) or with radioablation. Po-

TABLE 78-6 Common Gynecologic Surgeries

Total Hysterectomy
All the uterus, including the cervix, is removed. The procedure may be vaginal, abdominal, or laparoscopic.

Subtotal Hysterectomy
All the uterus, except the cervix, is removed. This procedure is rarely performed.

Bilateral Salpingo-Oophorectomy
Fallopian tubes and ovaries are removed.

Panhysterectomy
Total abdominal hysterectomy and bilateral salpingo-oophorectomy. The uterus, ovaries, and fallopian tubes are removed abdominally.

Radical Hysterectomy
All the uterus is removed abdominally. The lymph nodes, the upper third of the vagina, and the surrounding tissues (parametrium) are also removed.

CHART 78-11

FOCUSED ASSESSMENT of
The Client After Total Abdominal Hysterectomy

Assess cardiovascular, respiratory, renal, and gastrointestinal status, including the following:
- Vital signs
- Heart, lung, and bowel sounds
- Urine output
- Temperature and color of the skin
- Red blood cell, hemoglobin, and hematocrit levels
- Activity tolerance
- Dressing and drains for color and amount of drainage
- Peripads for vaginal bleeding and clots
- Fluid intake (IVs until bowel sounds return and client is tolerating oral intake)
- Signs of thrombophlebitis

Teach the client to use the following interventions to prevent postoperative complications:
- Cough and deep breathing exercises
- Incentive spirometry
- Sequential compression devices
- Ambulation
- Avoidance of heavy lifting or strenuous activity

Assess the home care teaching needs of the client related to the illness and surgery, including:
- Physiologic effects of the surgery
- Signs or symptoms to report
- Side or toxic effects of medications
- Activity limitations related to driving and use of stairs
- Follow-up care
- Postoperative restrictions related to sexual activity, use of tampons, and bathing
- Care of wound and/or drains

Assess the client's coping skills and reaction to the diagnosis and surgical procedure.

tential complications of hysteroscopic surgery include the following:
- Fluid overload (fluid used to distend the uterine cavity can be absorbed)
- Embolism
- Hemorrhage
- Perforation of the uterus, bowel, or bladder and ureter injury
- Persistent increased menstrual bleeding
- Incomplete suppression of menstruation

TABLE 78-7 Common Postoperative Complications of Traditional Abdominal and Vaginal Hysterectomies

Traditional Abdominal Hysterectomy
- Intestinal obstruction (paralytic ileus)
- Thromboembolism
- Atelectasis
- Pneumonia
- Wound dehiscence (especially in obese clients)
- Urinary retention

Vaginal Hysterectomy
- Hemorrhage
- Urinary tract complications, especially infection or retention
- Wound infection
- Urinary retention

There is a small risk of subsequent pregnancy and the possibility of cancer developing in the scar. Hysterectomy is the procedure of choice for women who have other problems, especially those with cancer or symptomatic uterovaginal prolapse.

Postoperative Care. Care of the woman who has undergone a TAH is similar to that of any client who has undergone abdominal surgery (see Chapter 22). For clients who have undergone a TAH, assess the following (Chart 78-11):
- Vaginal bleeding (there should be less than one saturated perineal pad in 4 hours)
- Abdominal bleeding at the incision site (a small amount is normal)
- Intactness of the incision
- Urine output per Foley catheter for 24 hours or less for a traditional surgical approach
- Pain

Specific interventions for a vaginal hysterectomy include the following:
- Assessment of vaginal bleeding (there should be less than one saturated pad in 4 hours)
- Foley catheter care
- Perineal care (sitz baths or ice packs)

The surgeon usually removes the abdominal sutures or clips at the first postoperative visit, whereas vaginal sutures are usually absorbed. Monitor for complications associated with hysterectomies (Table 78-7).

CONSIDERATIONS FOR OLDER ADULTS

Older women are at greater risk for all complications, particularly pulmonary embolism. Obese women are more at risk for thromboembolism. These clients need more frequent monitoring after surgery. Psychological complications can occur with both abdominal and vaginal procedures. Depression is the most frequent reaction reported. Other reactions are perceived loss of femininity and decreased libido. Loss of femininity may be the problem if a woman was interested in her appearance before surgery but afterward has no interest, even when she is feeling better. Decreased sexual desire is often temporary, if it occurs, and is usually related to discomfort.

Community-Based Care

The client with uterine leiomyomas is managed on an ambulatory care basis unless surgery is performed. After discharge, the client usually returns to her home.

HOME CARE MANAGEMENT

Planning for home care management begins at the time of admission. The woman is usually discharged to the home setting 1 to 2 days after a traditional TAH, depending on the age and health of the client. TVH, laparoscopic surgery, or TCER may be performed as same-day surgery in an ambulatory setting. The client who has undergone a hysterectomy usually needs to limit stair climbing for several weeks. If the client lives in a two-story house with a bathroom only on one level, advise the client to rent a bedside commode. If the client lives alone and is not permitted to drive for 2 to 6 weeks, she will need to make arrangements for transportation to follow-up visits.

HEALTH TEACHING

Teach the client who has undergone an abdominal hysterectomy about the expected physical changes, any activity restrictions, diet, sexual activity, any needed wound care, complications, and the need for follow-up care. Chart 78-12 lists education issues to stress for the client after surgery.

PSYCHOSOCIAL PREPARATION

Women who have undergone a hysterectomy need information about possible emotional reactions. Generally, women adjust well to surgery if they have completed childbearing, work, have interests outside the home, have no misconceptions about the effects of hysterectomy, and have support from the family, especially their sexual partner.

Reactions may be different after vaginal and abdominal procedures because women who have undergone a vaginal hysterectomy have no external focus (no obvious change in body image) for their feelings. Psychological reactions can occur months to years after surgery. Women identified as being at high risk for psychological problems may need long-term follow-up care or referral. Women may need to be counseled about signs of depression. Intermittent sadness is normal, but continued feelings of low self-esteem or loss of interest or pleasure in usual activities and pastimes is not normal and should be evaluated. Providing written materials and discussing the positive aspects of the client's life can help to decrease adverse psychological reactions.

HEALTH CARE RESOURCES

Usually no special home equipment is needed for a woman who has undergone a hysterectomy. A home care nurse may be needed to assess and monitor the older client's progress after surgery if other conditions (e.g., uncontrolled diabetes) are present. Financial assistance may be needed, and referral to the hospital's department of social services or case management department may be indicated if the woman has no insurance coverage. Provide a referral for psychological or sexual counseling if potential problems are identified before discharge.

◆Evaluation: Outcomes

Evaluate the care of the client who has undergone surgery for leiomyomas on the basis of the identified nursing diagnoses and collaborative problems. The expected outcomes include that the client should:

- Be free of hemorrhage
- Recover from surgery without complications

Specific indicators for these outcomes are listed for each collaborative problem under the Planning and Implementation section (see earlier).

CHART 78-12

CLIENT EDUCATION GUIDE
Care After a Total Abdominal Hysterectomy

Expected Physical Changes
- You will no longer have a period, although you may have some vaginal discharge for a few days after you go home.
- It will not be possible for you to become pregnant, and birth control methods are no longer needed.
- If your ovaries were removed, you may have some menopause symptoms such as hot flushes, night sweats, and vaginal dryness.
- It is normal to tire more easily and require more sleep and rest during the first few weeks after surgery (this may last for 2 to 3 months).

Activity
- Limit stair climbing to less than five times per day.
- Take showers rather than tub baths.
- Do not lift anything heavier than 5 lbs.
- Walk indoors for the first week. Then gradually increase walking as exercise but stop before you become fatigued.
- Avoid the sitting position for any extended period. When you sit, do not cross your legs at the knees.
- Avoid jogging, aerobic exercise, participating in sports, or any strenuous activity for 6 weeks.
- Do not drive for at least 4 weeks or until your surgeon has told you it is alright.

Diet
- Eat a well-balanced diet with extra protein and vitamin C to help heal your tissues.
- Drink at least 3 quarts of fluid, especially water, each day unless you have another health problem (like heart failure or kidney disease) that requires fluid restriction.
- If gas is a problem, avoid foods and beverages that increase gas.

Sexual Activity
- Do not engage in sexual intercourse for 4 to 6 weeks, as prescribed by your surgeon.
- If you had a vaginal "repair" as part of your surgery, the first time you have intercourse you may have some tenderness or pain because the vaginal walls are tighter. Careful intercourse and the use of water-based lubricants can help reduce this discomfort. This discomfort usually goes away with time and stretching of the vagina.

Follow-up Care
- If antibiotics are prescribed, take them as directed until all the drugs are gone.
- Make and keep your follow-up appointment(s) with your surgeon.

Complications
- Take your temperature twice each day for the first 2 weeks after surgery.
- Check your incision daily for signs of infection (increasing redness, open areas, drainage that is thick or foul-smelling, incision pain).

Report Any of the Following to Your Surgeon
- Increased vaginal drainage or change in drainage (more bloody, thicker, foul-smelling)
- Temperature over 100° F
- Pain, tenderness, redness, or swelling in your calves
- Pain or burning on urination

Bartholin Cyst

PATHOPHYSIOLOGY

Bartholin cyst is a common disorder of the vulva. The cysts result from obstruction of the duct of the Bartholin gland. The secretory function of the gland continues, and the fluid fills the obstructed duct. The main causes of the obstruction are infection, thickened mucus near the ductal opening, or trauma, such as lacerations or episiotomy.

COLLABORATIVE MANAGEMENT

Assessment

The client may be asymptomatic if the cyst is small. Often the client has dyspareunia, inadequate genital lubrication, or a mass in the perineal area. A large cyst usually causes constant local pain and may cause difficulty walking or sitting. Physical examination of the vulva reveals a swelling immediately beneath the skin in the posterior portion of the vulva. The cyst may appear brown or bloody, depending on its contents. Usually a cyst is present only on one side and ranges from 3/8 to 4 inches (1 to 10 cm) in size.

If the cyst is draining, fluid is sent to the laboratory for culture (for gonorrhea and aerobic and anaerobic organisms) and sensitivity testing. If the woman is older than 40 years of age, a specimen of the cyst should be sent for pathologic examination to determine whether the lesion is benign or malignant.

Interventions

If the woman is asymptomatic, no intervention is needed. If symptoms are present, simple incision and drainage (I&D) may provide temporary relief; however, cysts tend to recur when the opening of the duct reobstructs. Usually the surgeon establishes a permanent opening for drainage. Marsupialization (formation of a pouch that is a new duct opening) is performed using local, regional, or general anesthesia. Discomfort after surgery may be relieved with analgesics and sitz baths. Prophylactic antibiotics may be prescribed.

Often Bartholin cysts are infected and abscesses form when bacteria, such as *Escherichia coli* or *Staphylococcus aureus,* result in infection that closes the duct. An abscess usually ruptures spontaneously within 72 hours of formation. Interventions for the woman with an abscess include analgesics and application of moist heat (sitz baths or hot wet packs) to the vulva. Antibiotics are prescribed to treat the infection. I&D of the abscess may provide temporary relief.

The Bartholin glands may be totally excised in older women when cancer is suspected or if infections with abscess formation recur. Care after surgery includes the following:

- Application of ice packs or sitz baths several times a day for comfort and promotion of healing
- Analgesics for pain
- Prophylactic antibiotics
- Assessment of the incision for signs of healing or infection

Cervical Polyps

Cervical polyps are **pedunculated** (on stalks) tumors that arise from the mucosa and extend to the opening of the cervical os. Polyps result from a hyperplastic condition of the endocervical epithelium. They may also be due to inflammation or from an abnormal local response to hormonal stimulation or localized vascular congestion of the cervical blood vessels (DeCherney et al., 2003). Polyps are the most common benign growth of the cervix. They occur most often women older than 40 years of age who have had several children.

A woman may be asymptomatic, have premenstrual or postmenstrual bleeding, or have bleeding after coitus. A speculum examination may reveal small single or multiple polyps. They are bright red, are soft and fragile, and may bleed when touched.

Polyp removal is a simple office procedure. The base of the polyp is grasped with a clamp, and the polyp is twisted off and sent to the pathology laboratory for evaluation. Cautery usually stops any bleeding at the site of removal. After the procedure, instruct the client to avoid tampon use, douches, and sexual intercourse for a week or until healing has taken place.

MALIGNANT NEOPLASMS

Endometrial (Uterine) Cancer

PATHOPHYSIOLOGY

Endometrial cancer (cancer of the uterus) is a reproductive cancer; adenocarcinoma is the most common type (American Cancer Society, 2005). It arises from the glandular part of the endometrium and may be preceded by endometrial overgrowth. These cancers are divided into three grades based on tumor growth and the degree of differentiation (normal cell appearance). Grade 1 cancers are identified by endometrial glands that are well differentiated, whereas grade 3 tumors have a solid growth pattern and are poorly differentiated (DeVita et al., 2001). The initial growth of the cancer is within the uterine cavity, followed by extension into the myometrium and the cervix. Spread outside the uterus occurs as follows:

- Through lymphatic spread to the ovaries and parametrial, pelvic, inguinal, and para-aortic lymph nodes
- By blood, to the lungs, liver, or bone
- By transtubal or intra-abdominal spread to the peritoneal cavity

This type of cancer is asymptomatic in its early development and has a good prognosis in 80% to 90% of cases.

Etiology and Genetic Risk

Personal risk factors for endometrial cancer are listed in Table 78-8. The use of menopausal estrogen replacement therapy (ERT) and long-term tamoxifen therapy also appear to increase the risk for endometrial cancer. Although most cases of endometrial cancer do not have a genetic predisposition, it is more common in families who have gene mutations for hereditary nonpolyposis colon cancer (HNPCC).

Incidence/Prevalence

More than 40,100 new cases of endometrial cancer occur annually in the United States (American Cancer Society, 2005). Thus about 1 of every 100 women in the United States has endometrial cancer. The average age at diagnosis is 60 years.

CONSIDERATIONS FOR OLDER ADULTS

Endometrial cancer is a slow-growing tumor mainly occurring in postmenopausal women. The average age at onset is 61 years. The incidence declines after the age of 70 years. It is important to teach older women that any instance of postmenopausal bleeding should be evaluated by a health care provider.

TABLE 78-8 Risk Factors for Endometrial Cancer and Cervical Cancer

Endometrial Cancer	Cervical Cancer
Age 50 to 70 yr	African American
Family history of endometrial cancer or HNPCC	Native American/American Indian
Diabetes mellitus	Multiparity
Hypertension	<18 yr of age at first intercourse
Obesity	<18 yr of age at first pregnancy
Uterine polyps	Multiple sex partners
Late menopause	Smoking
Nulliparity	Infection with herpes simplex virus (HSV)
Smoking	Infection with human papilloma virus (HPV)
	Infection with cytomegalovirus (CMV)
	HIV/AIDS
	Lower socioeconomic status
	Sexual partner had a previous partner who developed cervical cancer
	Intrauterine exposure to diethylstilbestrol (DES)

HNPCC, Hereditary nonpolyposis colon cancer.

COLLABORATIVE MANAGEMENT

Assessment

The main symptom of endometrial cancer is postmenopausal bleeding. Some women also have a watery, bloody vaginal discharge, low back or abdominal pain, and low pelvic pain (caused by pressure of the enlarged uterus). A pelvic examination may reveal the presence of a palpable uterine mass or uterine polyp. The uterus is enlarged if the cancer is advanced.

DIAGNOSTIC ASSESSMENT

Basic diagnostic tests to determine the client's overall status and the presence of metastasis include the following:

- CA-125 tumor marker to rule out ovarian involvement
- Chest x-ray
- Intravenous pyelography (IVP), or excretory urography, to assess renal function and to assess for renal metastasis
- Barium enema study to assess for intestinal metastasis
- Computed tomography (CT) of the pelvis to identify the spread of the tumor
- Liver and bone scans to assess for distant metastasis

Dilation and curettage (D&C [scraping individual sections of the uterus]) and endometrial biopsy are the definitive diagnostic procedures for endometrial cancer. Other tests that may be useful include proctosigmoidoscopy, ultrasonography, and endoscopic examination of the uterus.

PSYCHOSOCIAL ASSESSMENT

Before a diagnosis is made, the client may deny that the symptoms are related to cancer. During the diagnostic phase, the woman may express fears and concerns about having cancer. After the diagnosis is confirmed, she may express disbelief, anger, depression, anxiety, or withdrawal behaviors.

Interventions

Nonsurgical interventions (radiation therapy and chemotherapy) and surgery may be used alone or in combination, depending on the stage of the cancer.

NONSURGICAL MANAGEMENT. Radiation therapy and chemotherapy are the two major nonsurgical methods used to treat endometrial cancer.

Radiation Therapy. The oncologist prescribes radiation therapy (external and internal) if the stage of cancer is hard to determine and if surgery is planned for stage II and III cancers. Radiation therapy may be used before or after surgery and can be delivered either by external beam **(teletherapy)** or with an internal source **(brachytherapy)**.

An older method was to deliver radiation therapy to the client for 6 weeks before surgery to shrink the tumor and possibly inhibit recurrence. Although this method is still used, it is not the standard of care.

Intracavitary Radiation. If intracavitary radiation therapy (IRT [brachytherapy]) is selected, the radiologist places an applicator within the woman's uterus through the vagina while she is anesthetized. After the correct position of the applicator is confirmed by x-ray, the client is taken to the hospital room and a radiologist places a radioactive isotope in the applicator, which remains for 1 to 3 days. The goal of intracavity radiation is to prevent vaginal recurrence.

Before the procedure, instruct the client about activities she will need to perform (e.g., deep breathing and leg exercises) and restrictions during the time the radiation source is in place. While the radioactive implant is in place, the client is strictly isolated, usually in a private room, because radiation is emitted and can affect other people. The amount of time needed for the therapy depends on the amount of radiation emitted from the source. The radiologist calculates the time need for a specific dose of radiation. Usually this time ranges from 35 to 60 hours.

Inform the client that she is restricted to bedrest on her back with the head of the bed flat or slightly elevated. Movement in bed is restricted to prevent dislodgment of the radioactive source. Assess the skin for breakdown over bony pressure points during the activity restriction period.

A Foley catheter is inserted into the bladder before the implant to prevent dislodgment of the implant, which can be caused by a full bladder or attempts to void. Encourage fluid intake to prevent urine stasis and infection. A low-residue diet is prescribed (to prevent bowel movements that might dislodge the implant). The health care provider usually prescribes the following:

- Antiemetics
- Broad-spectrum antibiotics (to prevent bladder infections)
- Tranquilizers (to help the client relax)
- Analgesics
- Heparin or Lovenox (to prevent thromboembolism)
- Antidiarrheal medications (to prevent bowel movements)

Practice radiation precautions while the implant is in place. Organize care so that minimal time is spent close to the radiation source. Chart 78-13 lists the best practices for care of the client with sealed implant radiation sources.

External Radiation. External radiation therapy may be used to treat any stage of endometrial cancer in combination with surgery. Depending on the extent of the tumor, external radiation is given on an ambulatory care basis for 4 to 6 weeks. Tissue around the tumor and pelvic wall nodes also are irradiated. Specific instructions for the woman undergoing external radiation for endometrial cancer include monitoring for signs of skin breakdown, especially in the perineal area; no sunbathing; and not removing the markings outlining the treatment site. Inform the client that cystitis, diarrhea, and

CHART 78-13

BEST PRACTICE for
Care of the Client with Sealed Implants of Radioactive Sources

- Assign the client to a private room with a private bath.
- Place a "Caution: Radioactive Material" sign on the door of the client's room.
- Wear a dosimeter film badge at all times while caring for clients with radioactive implants. The badge offers no protection but measures an individual's exposure to radiation. Each badge should be used by only one individual.
- Wear a lead shielding apron; always face the radiation source (do not turn your back toward the source).
- Stay as far away from the radiation source as possible.
- Pregnant nurses, or those who are trying to become pregnant, should not care for these clients; do not allow pregnant women or children younger than 16 years of age to visit.
- Limit each visitor to one-half hour per day. Be sure visitors are at least 6 feet from the source.
- Never touch the radioactive source with bare hands. In the rare instance that it is dislodged, use a long-handled forceps to retrieve it. Deposit the radioactive source in the lead container kept in the client's room.
- Save all dressings and bed linens until after the radioactive source is removed. After the source is removed, dispose of dressings and linens in the usual manner. Other equipment can be removed from the room at any time.

anorexia are common during the weeks of therapy (see also Chapter 28).

Chemotherapy. Chemotherapy is an adjuvant treatment used when the risk for distant spread exceeds 20%. Usually combinations of three agents are given for chemotherapy. Although the combination can vary, the three most common agents recommended as chemotherapy for endometrial cancer are doxorubicin, cisplatin, and paclitaxel. Chapter 28 lists specific information about these agents and nursing care needs for clients during treatment. Chemotherapy is used as palliative treatment in advanced and recurrent disease.

Other Drug Therapy. Hormone therapy can be used for stage I and II cancers that are estrogen dependent and for palliative treatment of stage IV cancer. The hormones commonly prescribed are medroxyprogesterone acetate (Depo-Provera) and megestrol acetate (Megace). Tamoxifen citrate (Nolvadex✱, Tamofen✱), an anti-estrogen, is also used. The progestational agents do not cause acute side effects, but nausea and vomiting and hot flushes are associated with tamoxifen.

SURGICAL MANAGEMENT. Surgical management is the standard for tumors that are stage IC and higher if the client's general health permits. The gynecology oncologist usually performs a total abdominal hysterectomy (TAH) (removal of the uterus and cervix) and bilateral salpingo-oophorectomy (removal of both tubes and ovaries) for stage I tumors without cervical involvement. A radical hysterectomy (see Table 78-6) with bilateral pelvic lymph node dissection is performed for stage II cancer. Nursing care for a radical hysterectomy is the same as that for a TAH except that the woman's hospitalization is usually longer and her convalescence may be extended.

Critical Thinking Challenge

You are the charge nurse of a small medical-surgical nursing unit. Three of your clients are undergoing radiation therapy with a sealed radiation source. One client, a woman in her 70s, has just been admitted from the radiology department, where a position-fixing device was placed to hold a sealed radiation source. Within the next hour, she will be receiving radiation therapy with a sealed source for the next 50 hours. She has a number of medications prescribed for her heart failure (which is why she is having radiation therapy rather than surgery). She had a hip replacement last year. All together, you have 22 clients in your care. Your personnel include one LPN who is pregnant, two unlicensed assistive personnel, and another RN. This nurse is assigned to care for both of the other clients receiving brachytherapy.

1. Which person should you assign to care for this 70-year-old client? Provide a rationale for your choice.
2. What precautions will you institute to prevent skin breakdown?
3. Your unit does not have a lead-lined room. What type of room arrangements should you make to reduce radiation exposure to other clients, visitors, and staff?

evolve For suggested answer guidelines, go to http://evolve.elsevier.com/Iggy/.

Community-Based Care

HOME CARE MANAGEMENT

The client with endometrial cancer is managed at home unless surgery is indicated. After surgery, the client is usually discharged to her home. Home care after surgery for endometrial cancer is the same as that after a hysterectomy (see Operative Procedures [Uterine Leiomyomas], p. 1839). Clients who are receiving chemotherapy or external radiation therapy are usually treated on an ambulatory care basis. Help the client and her family plan daily activities around trips to the clinic or the health care provider's office. If the tumor recurs and cure is not likely, the client and her family need to think about hospice care and whether the client can be cared for in the home.

HEALTH TEACHING

For the woman who has undergone a hysterectomy for endometrial cancer, the teaching plan is the same as that for the woman who has undergone a hysterectomy for uterine leiomyomas (see Postoperative Care [Uterine Leiomyomas], p. 1840). Side effects to report to the health care provider include vaginal or rectal bleeding, foul-smelling discharge, abdominal pain or distention, and hematuria.

The high dose of radiation causes sterility, and vaginal shrinkage can occur. Vaginal dilators can be used with water-soluble lubricants for 10 minutes each day until sexual activity resumes (in 10 days to 6 weeks). Reassure the woman that she is not radioactive and that her partner will not "catch" cancer by engaging in sexual intercourse. A normal diet can be resumed.

Review all prescribed drugs, including the dosage and schedule, effects, and side effects. Emphasize the importance of keeping appointments for follow-up care.

PSYCHOSOCIAL PREPARATION

Clients need to discuss their concerns about the presence of cancer and the potential for recurrence. Provide emotional support and create an atmosphere that encourages the woman to ask questions or express her fears and concerns.

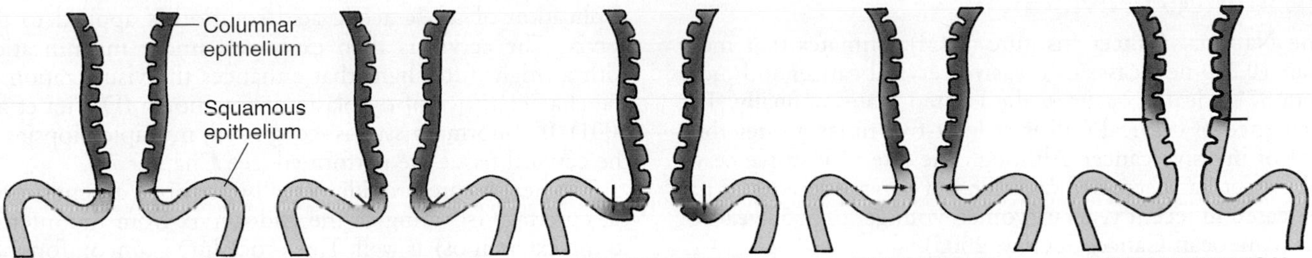

Figure 78-5 ■ The location of the translocation zones at various stages of adult development.

Include family members or significant others in discussions when possible.

Reactions to radiation therapy vary. Some clients may feel radioactive or "unclean" after treatments and may exhibit withdrawal behaviors. Correct such misconceptions.

Clients who have chemotherapy may be upset if **alopecia** (hair loss) occurs. Warn the client of this possibility before treatment starts. Wigs, scarves, or turbans can be worn until regrowth occurs.

Often clients experience emotional crises because of the physical effects of cancer treatments. Radical hysterectomy may be seen as mutilating, and both radiation and chemotherapy have side effects that change the client's appearance. A client may have a grief reaction to this perceived change in body image. The feelings of loss depend on the visibility of the loss, the function of the loss, and the amount of emotional investment. Help the client adapt to the body changes. One way to do this is to encourage self-care as soon as the client's condition is stable. Use a calm, accepting attitude.

Death can occur with or without treatment. Clients and their families or significant others have concerns about recurrence. All want to pass the 5-year survival mark without a recurrence. If there is a recurrence, the client may be hostile and may have manifestations of a grief reaction. Encourage clients to ventilate their feelings. Response to loss and grieving are discussed in Chapter 9.

HEALTH CARE RESOURCES

In the United States, local American Cancer Society chapters provide written materials about endometrial cancer as well as information about local support groups. If the client is in the terminal stages of cancer, hospice care may be appropriate (see Chapter 9). If nursing care is needed at home, the hospital nurse or case manager refers the client and her family to a community health or home care agency. A referral to a social services agency may be needed if the client is unable to meet the financial demands of treatment and long-term follow-up.

Cervical Cancer

PATHOPHYSIOLOGY

Cervical cancer is a common reproductive cancer among women in the United States. This disorder is a progression from totally normal cervical cells to premalignant changes in appearance of cervical cells (dysplasia), to changes in function and, ultimately, transformation to cancer.

TABLE 78-9 Clinical Staging of Cervical Cancer*

Stage	Characteristics
I	Carcinoma is strictly confined to cervix (extension to corpus should be disregarded).
II	Carcinoma extends beyond cervix but has not extended to pelvic wall; it involves vagina, but not as far as lower third.
III	Carcinoma has extended to pelvic wall; on rectal examination, there is no cancer-free space between tumor and pelvic wall; tumor involves lower third of vagina; all cases with hydronephrosis or nonfunctioning kidney should be included unless they are known to be due to another cause.
IV	Carcinoma has extended beyond true pelvis or has clinically involved mucosa of bladder or rectum

*An a, b, or c designation at any stage indicates specific degree or depth of spread within that stage.

Premalignant changes are described on a continuum from dysplasia (the earliest premalignant change) to carcinoma in situ (CIS) (the most advanced premalignant change).

Once cervical cancer has developed, it is described as preinvasive or invasive. Preinvasive cancer is limited to the cervix; invasive cancer is in the cervix and other pelvic structures. Preinvasive lesions usually begin in the area called the *transformation zone* (Figure 78-5). This area includes the squamocolumnar junction, which is located near the external cervical os, where changes in the squamous and columnar (glandular) epithelium normally occur. Preinvasive cancers are also termed *cervical intraepithelial neoplasia (CIN)* and classified according to severity:

- CIN I: mild
- CIN II: moderate
- CIN III: severe to carcinoma in situ

Most cervical cancer (90%) arises from the squamous cells, and only 5% arise from the mucous secreting cells (adenocarcinoma). Squamous cell cancers spread by direct extension to the vaginal mucosa, lower uterine segment, parametrium, pelvic wall, bladder, and bowel. Metastasis is usually confined to the pelvis, but distant spread can occur through lymphatic spread and the circulation to the liver, lungs, or bones. Table 78-9 shows the staging of cervical cancer.

Etiology

The exact cause of squamous cell cervical cancer is unknown, but many factors appear to be involved. Table 78-8 lists risk factors for cervical cancer.

Incidence/Prevalence

The National Cancer Institute (NCI) estimates that more than 10,370 new cases of invasive cervical cancer and more than 3710 deaths occur in the United States annually. The incidence of cervical CIS is at least five times greater than that of invasive cancer. Although the rate of invasive cervical cancer has decreased over the last several decades, it has increased in recent years in women younger than 50 years of age (American Cancer Society, 2005).

Cervical intraepithelial neoplasia (CIN) occurs mainly in young women; the peak incidence of dysplasia occurs in clients in their mid-20s. CIS occurs in women about 30 years old, and invasive cancer occurs most commonly in the late 40s.

Invasive cervical cancer is the third most common cause of death related to reproductive cancers (American Cancer Society, 2005). Death rates for cervical cancer have dropped 50% in the past two decades because of mass screening of premalignant and early stage cancer through Pap tests.

◆COLLABORATIVE MANAGEMENT

◆Assessment

PHYSICAL ASSESSMENT/CLINICAL MANIFESTATIONS

The client who has preinvasive cancer is often asymptomatic. The classic symptom of invasive cancer is painless vaginal bleeding. The bleeding may start as spotting between menstrual periods or after coitus or douching. As the cancer grows, bleeding increases in frequency, duration, and amount and may become continuous.

The client may also have a watery, blood-tinged vaginal discharge that becomes dark and foul-smelling as the disease progresses. Leg pain (along the sciatic nerve) or swelling of one leg may be a late symptom or may indicate recurrent disease. Flank pain may be a late symptom of hydronephrosis, indicating advanced disease or recurrence. Other signs of recurrence or metastasis include unexplained weight loss, pelvic pain (caused by pressure of the tumor on the bladder or the bowel), **dysuria** (painful urination), **hematuria** (bloody urine), rectal bleeding, chest pain, and coughing. A physical examination may not reveal any abnormalities in early preinvasive cervical cancer; the internal pelvic examination may identify late-stage disease.

DIAGNOSTIC ASSESSMENT

Diagnostic assessment for cervical cancer begins with a Pap smear. If the results are abnormal, the smear is repeated before further studies are done. If abnormal tissue is detected on a subsequent Pap test, further testing is done, depending on the type of abnormality present (squamous atypia, inflammatory atypia, or minor atypia). These atypical cells are categorized more definitely, regardless of whether dysplasia is present, by the Bethesda System (TBS) for the specific type of follow-up needed. If invasive cervical cancer is diagnosed, laboratory tests such as those described earlier for the investigation of endometrial cancer are performed (see Assessment [Endometrial Cancer], p. 1843).

The health care provider may perform a colposcopic examination to view the transformation zone, where dysplasia, cervical intraepithelial neoplasia (CIN), and carcinoma in situ (CIS) often arise. Colposcopy is a procedure in which application of a 3% acetic acid solution is applied to the cervix. The cervix is then examined under magnification with a bright filter light that enhances the visualization of the characteristics of dysplasia or carcinoma (DeVita et al., 2001). If abnormal tissue is recognized, multiple biopsies of the cervical tissue are performed (see Chapter 76).

The health care provider usually performs an endocervical curettage (scraping of the endocervix from the internal to the external os) as well. This procedure is uncomfortable, and you may need to encourage the client to use relaxation or breathing exercises to cope with the cramping and pain. Inform the client that a small amount of bleeding is expected for up to 2 weeks after the biopsies.

◆Interventions

Care of the client with cervical cancer is similar to that for endometrial cancer. Interventions discussed here are those that differ from those for the client with endometrial cancer.

NONSURGICAL MANAGEMENT. Nonsurgical interventions for cervical cancer depend on the stage of disease. Early management techniques include local ablation therapies of electrosurgical excision, laser therapy, or cryosurgery. Radiation therapy or chemotherapy is usually used along with surgery for later-stage disease. Factors that influence the choice of localized treatment versus surgical intervention include client health, tumor size, stage, cancer cell type, degree of lymph node involvement, risk factors for surgical complications, and client preference.

Loop Electrosurgical Excision Procedure. The loop electrosurgical excision procedure (LEEP) is rapidly becoming the nonsurgical management of choice for intraepithelial lesions. This procedure is short (10 to 30 minutes) and is performed in a physician's office or in a clinic setting with a local anesthetic injected into the cervix. A thin loop-wire electrode that transmits a painless electrical current is used to cut away or "peel off" affected tissue. Unlike laser or cryotherapy, in which tissue is destroyed, LEEP results in a specimen that can be examined by a pathologist to ensure the lesion was completely removed.

Little discomfort is associated with this procedure. Spotting after the procedure is common. Instruct clients to adhere for 3 weeks to the restrictions listed in Chart 78-14.

Laser Therapy. Laser therapy is an office procedure used for CIN. A laser beam is directed to the abnormal tissues, where energy from the beam is absorbed by the fluid in the tissues, causing them to vaporize. A small amount of bleeding occurs with the procedure, and the client may have a slight vaginal discharge. Healing occurs in 6 to 12 weeks.

CHART 78-14

CLIENT EDUCATION GUIDE
Care After Local Cervical Ablation Therapy

- Refrain from sexual intercourse.
- Do not use tampons.
- Do not douche.
- Take showers rather than tub baths.
- Avoid lifting heavy objects.
- Report any heavy vaginal bleeding, foul-smelling drainage, or fever.

The usual time period for these restrictions is 3 weeks. Your health care provider may prescribe a different (longer or shorter) time frame for you.

A disadvantage of this procedure is that no specimen is available for study.

Cryotherapy. Cryotherapy is another common treatment for CIN. A probe is placed against the cervix to cause freezing of the tissues and subsequent necrosis. The procedure is painless, although some clients have slight cramping after the procedure. The client has a heavy watery discharge for several weeks after the procedure. Instruct her to follow the restrictions in Chart 78-14.

Radiation Therapy. Radiation therapy is reserved for invasive cervical cancer. For cancer that has extended beyond the cervix but not to the pelvic wall, radiation therapy is as effective as a radical hysterectomy. Intracavitary and external radiation therapies are used in combination, depending on the extent and location of the lesion. Intracavitary implants are usually used after the client has completed 5 to 6 weeks of external pelvic radiation in combination with chemotherapy. The procedure is similar to that described for endometrial cancer. Nursing care related to radiation therapy is presented in the earlier discussion of endometrial cancer (see p. 1843 and Chapter 28).

Chemotherapy. Cervical cancer generally responds poorly to chemotherapy. These agents are usually reserved for locally advanced carcinomas, unresectable recurrent tumors, or widely metastatic disease (DeVita et al., 2001). Agents shown to be somewhat effective for cervical cancer include paclitaxel, carboplatin, ifosfamide, hydroxyurea, fluorouracil, and irinotecan. See Chapter 28 for more information about these drugs.

SURGICAL MANAGEMENT. The surgical procedure for cervical cancer depends on the extent of the disease and whether the client wants to have children. Clinical staging is performed before surgery to establish the extent of the disease. Small tumors that are only microinvasive are managed conservatively with excisional conization or hysterectomy. Early stage invasive cancers are managed with radical surgery and radiation. Locally advanced cancers are managed with radiation.

Conization. Conization is used to treat clients with microinvasive cervical cancer, especially when preservation of fertility is desired. This procedure is done when the lesion cannot be visualized by colposcopic examination. A cone-shaped area of cervix is removed surgically and sent to the laboratory to determine the extent of the cancer. Potential complications from this procedure include hemorrhage, uterine perforation, incompetent cervix, cervical canal narrowing, and preterm labor for future pregnancies. Long-term follow-up care is needed because new lesions can develop.

Hysterectomy. A simple hysterectomy may be performed as treatment of microinvasive cancer if the client does not desire childbearing. A vaginal approach is commonly used. A radical hysterectomy and bilateral pelvic lymph node dissection are as effective as radiation is for treating cancer that has extended beyond the cervix but not to the pelvic wall. Care for clients undergoing hysterectomy is found under Operative Procedures (Uterine Leiomyomas), p. 1839.

Pelvic Exenteration. One of the most radical surgical procedures is **pelvic exenteration.** It is performed for recurrent cancers if there is no evidence of tumor outside the pelvis and no lymph node involvement.

Preoperative Care. Assess the client scheduled for a pelvic exenteration for anxiety, concerns about the impact on sexual function, and the ability to adjust to her altered body image. Involve family members or partners in discussions about postoperative expectations. Physical preparation includes selection of stoma sites, extensive bowel preparation, and extensive radiographic and laboratory tests to assess for spread of cancer outside the pelvis. Teach the client about the following:

- Recovery after surgery in a critical care unit
- Pain management
- Presence of numerous intravenous (IV) and arterial catheters
- Nasogastric suction
- Colostomy and/or urinary diversion (e.g., ileal conduit, Kock ileal urinary pouch)

Operative Procedures. The three types of exenteration are anterior, posterior, and total (Figure 78-6). Anterior exenteration is the removal of the uterus, cervix, ovaries, fal-

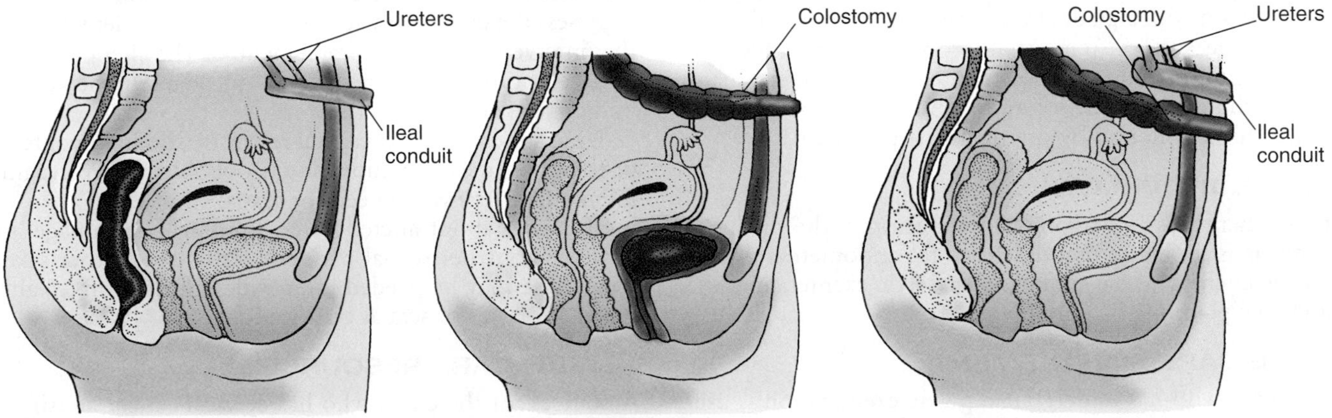

Anterior exenteration is removal of all pelvic organs except the descending colon, rectum, and anal canal. Urine can be diverted into an ileal conduit or urinary Kock pouch.

Posterior exenteration is removal of all pelvic organs except the bladder. A colostomy is created for the passage of feces.

Total exenteration is removal of all pelvic organs with creation of an ileal conduit or urinary Kock pouch and a colostomy.

Figure 78-6 ■ Pelvic exenteration.

lopian tubes, vagina, bladder, urethra, and pelvic lymph nodes. Posterior exenteration is the removal of the uterus, cervix, ovaries, fallopian tubes, descending colon, rectum, and anal canal. Total exenteration is a combination of anterior and posterior procedures. When the bladder is removed, urine is diverted through a urinary diversion (e.g., ileal conduit or Kock ileal urinary pouch). When the colon, rectum, and anal canal are removed, a colostomy is created for passage of feces. The stomas are located on the abdomen, the colostomy on the left and the ileal conduit on the right.

Postoperative Care. After surgery, the client often is admitted to a critical care unit for the first 1 to 2 days because of the high risk for complications resulting from this massive surgery. Assess for the following:

- Hemorrhage and shock
- Pulmonary complications such as atelectasis and pneumonia
- Fluid and electrolyte imbalances such as metabolic acidosis or alkalosis and dehydration
- Renal or urinary complications
- Pain

Assist the client with deep breathing and coughing hourly. Monitor urine output and specific gravity, parenteral nutrition, and provide colostomy and urinary diversion care.

Once the client's condition is stable, she returns to the medical-surgical unit when normal postoperative interventions are continued. During the recovery period, assess for the following:

- Late cardiovascular complications such as deep vein thrombosis and pulmonary emboli
- Gastrointestinal (GI) complications, such as paralytic ileus
- Wound infections
- Wound dehiscence or evisceration
- Pain

Prophylactic heparin or low-molecular weight heparin (enoxaparin [Lovenox]) may be prescribed. Maintain the use of anti-embolism stockings or sequential compression devices (SCDs) for the prevention of thrombosis. Auscultate the lungs at least twice per shift. Assess the abdomen for the presence of bowel sounds and the wound for indications of healing or infection. Give antibiotics as prescribed, and manage pain with a gradual withdrawal of opioid analgesics.

After the surgeon removes the operative dressings, perineal irrigations may be implemented. Irrigation is usually done with normal saline solution applied with an Asepto syringe. This is followed by drying of the perineum.

Community-Based Care

If the client has undergone a hysterectomy, the discharge planning is similar to that described for endometrial cancer. For the client who has undergone a pelvic exenteration, the discharge planning is more involved.

HOME CARE MANAGEMENT

The client who has undergone a pelvic exenteration is usually in the hospital for at least 1 week after surgery. She may be discharged to a skilled nursing facility or subacute unit for continued recovery and care or may be discharged directly to home. When the client returns home, she needs assistance. She is not able to engage in strenuous activities associated with most household work for up to 6 months. The family may need to consider outside help if there is no one in the family who can assume household responsibilities.

No special equipment is needed in the home, although a foam mattress or other special pressure-relieving device may be placed on the bed to prevent skin breakdown and to increase comfort. Colostomy and ureterostomy pouches and equipment for changing the pouches can be purchased in local pharmacies.

HEALTH TEACHING

Collaborate with the wound and ostomy care nurse to teach the woman who has undergone a pelvic exenteration how to manage new functions with equipment (colostomy and urinary diversion). Teach the client or family how to provide wound care and other aspects of self-care. The perineal opening may drain mucus for several months to a year. The client can wear sanitary napkins if they are beltless (so as not to interfere with the stomas). The client may need help in adjusting her diet to maintain high nutritional requirements for healing while selecting foods that are tolerated. Teach the client about the effects, dosages, and side effects of all prescribed drugs.

Sexual function is different after exenteration (even if an artificial vagina is constructed), and the couple may need counseling about alternatives to intercourse. Even with vaginal reconstruction, the use of vaginal dilators is necessary to achieve desired sexual function.

Physical activities are limited during convalescence. Until walking is permitted, encourage range-of-motion exercises. Follow-up care is important. Counsel the client about keeping all follow-up appointments. Provide information about late complications (e.g., infection, bowel obstruction) so that the client can seek medical care promptly.

PSYCHOSOCIAL PREPARATION

Usually by 3 to 5 days after surgery, the client begins expressing grief about her body changes. At first she may deny changes by refusing to look at the wound or stoma sites. Later she may become depressed or withdrawn or even angry or hostile. She may then move to reality testing by asking questions about her care, watching the nurses do wound care, and becoming actively involved in self-care.

Assess the client daily for manifestations of depression so that interventions can be implemented. The client needs intense emotional support if she is to adapt to her altered body image and functions.

Unless the client has vaginal reconstruction after anterior or total pelvic exenteration, she is not able to have vaginal intercourse. Assess the need for sexual counseling by listening for cues about altered perceptions of body image and anxiety about her sexual partner's response. Further sexual counseling may be needed to provide information on alternative methods of sexual gratification.

HEALTH CARE RESOURCES

Resources for the client who has cervical cancer are similar to those for the client with endometrial cancer. However, the client who has undergone a pelvic exenteration will need much assistance for several months. Help her arrange for transportation and home care. A home care nurse can assist with dressing changes, ostomy care, and perform assessments for several weeks after discharge to home. Assistance

TABLE 78-10 Risk Factors for Ovarian Cancer and Vulvar Cancer

Ovarian Cancer	Vulvar Cancer
Age over 40 years	Age over 40 years
Family history	Cervical cancer
Diabetes mellitus	Diabetes mellitus
Nulliparity	Hypertension
>30 years of age at first pregnancy	Obesity
Breast cancer	Infection with human papilloma virus (types 16, 18)
Colorectal cancer	Cervical cancer
Infertility	Smoking
BRCA1 or BRCA2 gene mutations	

with self-care, meal preparation, and home maintenance are usually needed.

Ovarian Cancer

PATHOPHYSIOLOGY

Etiology and Genetic Risk

Of all ovarian cancers, more than 90% are epithelial tumors; the most common type is serous adenocarcinoma. These tumors grow rapidly, spread quickly, and are often bilateral. In addition to metastasizing by direct extension into nearby organs and through blood and lymph circulation to distant sites, ovarian cancer also spreads through the abdomen by seeding free-floating cancer cells. This type of spread usually occurs with ascites.

The cause of ovarian cancer is not precisely known. Table 78-10 lists known and suspected risk factors for ovarian cancer.

Genetic Considerations

About 10% of ovarian cancer cases are related to known gene mutations. Hereditary breast-ovarian cancer syndrome (HBOC) is associated with specific mutations of the *BRCA1* gene locus that are inherited in an autosomal dominant pattern. Testing to determine gene carrier status for *BRCA1* mutations is available for clients with a family predisposition to breast or ovarian cancer. Hereditary ovarian cancer also may be a part of the hereditary nonpolyposis colorectal cancer syndrome (HNPCC). See Chapter 11 for more information about hereditary ovarian cancer.

Incidence/Prevalence

Ovarian cancer is the leading cause of death from female reproductive cancers. About 23,300 new cases are diagnosed each year, and 13,900 deaths occur each year (American Cancer Society, 2005). Survival rates continue to be low because ovarian cancer is not often detected in its early stages. The incidence increases in women older than 50 years of age and peaks at 60 to 64 years of age.

◆COLLABORATIVE MANAGEMENT

◆Assessment

Clients with ovarian cancer may complain of abdominal pain or swelling or have vague symptoms of abdominal discomfort, such as dyspepsia, indigestion, gas and distention, and other mild GI disturbances. The client may have a history of ovarian imbalance, such as evidenced by premenstrual tension, heavy menstrual flow or dysfunctional bleeding, or infertility.

TABLE 78-11 Clinical Staging of Ovarian Cancer*

Stage	Characteristics
I	Growth is limited to ovaries.
II	Growth involves one or both ovaries with pelvic extension.
III	Tumor involves one or both ovaries with peritoneal implants outside the pelvis or positive retroperitoneal or inguinal nodes; superficial liver metastasis but with histologically proven malignant extension to small bowel or omentum.
IV	Growth involving one or both ovaries with distant metastases; if pleural effusion is present, there must be positive cytologic findings to allot a case to stage IV; parenchymal liver metastasis equals stage IV.

*An a, b, or c designation at any stage indicates specific degree or depth of spread within that stage.

The only sign may be an abdominal mass, which may be noticed only after it reaches a size of 6 inches (15 cm). Most pelvic examinations do not identify abnormalities. However, an enlarged ovary found after menopause should be evaluated as though it were malignant.

The client with ovarian cancer has concerns similar to those described for the client with endometrial cancer. Because the cancer is often diagnosed in an advanced stage, fears of death and dying are common and may be more of a concern than the proposed treatments.

Cytologic examination has limited application because a Pap smear is abnormal in only 20% to 30% of clients with ovarian cancer, even in advanced cases. Diagnosis depends on surgical exploration. Usually a complete laboratory workup is done before exploratory surgery, including a complete blood count, urinalysis, and liver studies if ascites occurs.

The level of ovarian antibody designated as CA-125 may be elevated if ovarian cancer is present. This test may be useful in monitoring a client's progress after treatment, but it may not be as useful for diagnostic purposes. The CA-125 tumor marker is often elevated by benign conditions, such as endometriosis, fibroids, pelvic inflammatory disease (PID), liver disease, heart failure, and diverticulitis (DeVita et al., 2001).

Ultrasonography, intravenous pyelography (IVP), computed tomography (CT), and radiography are used in detecting ovarian tumors. In addition, a barium enema study and an upper GI radiographic series can be performed to rule out tumor in the adjacent structures.

Exploratory laparotomy is performed to diagnose and stage ovarian tumors. Ovarian cancer is staged when it is removed (Table 78-11).

Critical Thinking Challenge

The client is a 34-year-old woman who has been diagnosed with ovarian cancer. She is a twin, and her sister was diagnosed with breast cancer 1 year ago. Her mother died from

Continued

ovarian cancer at 40 years of age. The client has one child. Her other health problems include pregnancy-induced hypertension and rheumatoid arthritis. She had cryotherapy for cervical dysplasia when she was 25 years old. Her history and physical examination revealed the following problems or manifestations: migraine headaches, 10-lb weight gain in the past 6 months, seasonal pollen allergies, GERD, irregular menses, and intermittent constipation.

1. What risk factors, if any, does she have for ovarian cancer?
2. Which of her previous or current health problems or manifestations may contribute to or be a result of ovarian cancer?
3. She is scheduled for a hysterectomy and an oophorectomy and surgical staging procedure.
4. What preoperative teaching will you emphasize?
5. How will you approach the issue of fertility with this client?

evolve For suggested answer guidelines, go to http://evolve.elsevier.com/Iggy/.

Interventions

Nursing care of the client with ovarian cancer is similar to that of the client with endometrial or cervical cancer. The options for treatment depend on the extent of the cancer and include chemotherapy, immunotherapy, radiation therapy (external or intraperitoneal), and surgery.

NONSURGICAL MANAGEMENT. After surgery, chemotherapy and radiation therapy are the two most common nonsurgical options for ovarian cancer.

Chemotherapy. The oncologist usually prescribes chemotherapy after surgery for all stages of ovarian cancer. Cisplatin, carboplatin, and paclitaxel (Taxol) are the most common agents used for treating ovarian cancer. Chemotherapy is usually given every 3 to 4 weeks for six cycles on an inpatient or an ambulatory basis.

Radiation Therapy. External radiation therapy is used after surgery if tumors have invaded other pelvic or abdominal organs. It may be given with chemotherapy or alone (see Chapter 28).

SURGICAL MANAGEMENT. Total abdominal hysterectomy and bilateral salpingo-oophorectomy are the surgical procedures for all stages of ovarian cancer. Surgery confirms disease, allows for surgical staging, and can debulk or remove the tumor. When cancer has spread to other abdominal organs or lymph nodes, they can be resected during the surgery. Some clients with advanced disease may undergo neoadjuvant chemotherapy before tumor debulking surgery.

Ovarian cancer is staged during surgery (see Table 78-11). The client usually has a vertical incision instead of a horizontal incision. This incision improves the surgeon's ability to assess disease in the upper abdomen. If disease is present on the omentum, it is removed. The upper abdomen evaluation continues with inspection of the diaphragm, liver serosa, and parenchyma. Peritoneal washings; frozen sections of the pelvic mass; and biopsies of the pelvic organs, diaphragm, and lymph nodes are sent to pathology during the surgery.

After surgery, nursing care of the client is similar to that of the client undergoing a hysterectomy for uterine leiomyomas. The vertical incision is assessed in the same fashion as a horizontal abdominal incision.

A "second-look" procedure (laparoscopy or laparotomy) is performed, usually after 1 year of chemotherapy, to confirm the absence or presence of tumor and to remove any new or residual tumor if it was too large to be removed at the first operation. Nursing care is similar to that of the client after any major abdominal surgery.

The client who is faced with the diagnosis of advanced ovarian cancer may be concerned about dying. Encourage her to ventilate her feelings about her diagnosis. Provide realistic assurance as well as accurate information about treatments. Providing continuity of care, with at least one regular caregiver, may be helpful. Encourage the client to use her support system, including family members, friends, and a spiritual leader, such as a rabbi or other clergy member. A visit from another woman who has survived a similar disease may decrease fears.

If there is recurrence, the client may deny symptoms at first or express feelings of anger and grief. The family is often fearful of the outcome (see the Evidence-Based Practice for Nursing box above). Provide encouragement and support during this difficult time, and help the client and her family work through their grief and prepare for death.

EVIDENCE-BASED PRACTICE for Nursing

What impact does ovarian cancer have on women and their families?

Howel, D, Fitch, M.I., & Deane, K.A. (2003). Impact of ovarian cancer perceived by women. *Cancer Nursing, 26*(1):1-9.

This study was conducted to increase health care professionals' understanding of the following: about the impact of ovarian cancer on day-to-day living, the major challenges women and their families face in dealing with ovarian cancer, and the availability of support systems for clients and their families. The researchers in this study interviewed 18 women diagnosed with ovarian cancer. The participants were asked to describe their experiences in living with this disease. The participant's ages ranged from 35 to 73 years. The diagnosis of ovarian cancer occurred as recently as 5 months to 12 years before the interview. More than half of the women were married and had children, had higher education levels, and were unemployed because of their age or disability.

Level of Evidence: 6—Uncontrolled case series, qualitative study.

Critique. The investigators used accepted techniques for qualitative study to ensure data collection to saturation and validated the results with the participants.

Implications for Nursing. Nurses are often the first line of support for clients with cancer, and these clients rely on nurses for help. It is critical, therefore, that nurses understand the concept of family-centered care. This study reveals the need for sensitivity in dealing with: life changes, financial support, disability, coping skills, anxiety or depression, and access to palliative care programs. Further nursing research focusing on the impact of living with the uncertainty of death and ovarian cancer in the clients and their families, particularly children, is needed.

Vulvar Cancer

PATHOPHYSIOLOGY

Etiology

Most vulvar cancers (90%) are squamous cell carcinomas. The remaining 10% are adenocarcinomas, sarcomas, and Paget's disease. Most vulvar cancers do not have premalignant changes in the epithelium.

Vulvar cancer is slow growing, stays localized for a long time, and metastasizes late. The first change is usually vulvar atypia or mild dysplasia (vulvar intraepithelial neoplasia [VIN] I), followed by moderate dysplasia (VIN II) and then severe dysplasia or carcinoma in situ (VIN III) until the lesion becomes invasive. Vulvar cancer can spread directly to the urethra, the vagina, or the anus and through the lymphatic system to the inguinal, femoral, and deep iliac pelvic nodes.

The cause of vulvar cancer is unknown, although a strong relationship exists between vulvar cancer and herpes simplex type II, human papillomavirus, and capsid antigen. Other risk factors for vulvar cancer are listed in Table 78-10. Guidelines for the early detection and prevention of vulvar cancer include performing monthly vulvar self-examination, having an annual pelvic examination, and practicing "safer sex."

Incidence/Prevalence

About 4000 new cases are diagnosed each year, and 800 deaths result from this disease annually (American Cancer Society, 2005). Vulvar cancer occurs most commonly in women 50 to 70 years of age. More than 50% of the cases of vulvar cancer occur in women older than 60 years of age.

COLLABORATIVE MANAGEMENT

Assessment

Women with vulvar lesions often report irritation or itching in their perineal area. Sometimes they describe a "sore that will not heal." Bleeding is a late symptom. Women usually try to treat themselves before seeking medical help. Often a lesion has been present for months or even years. Embarrassment may be one reason why older women delay seeking medical care.

Pelvic examinations usually show multifocal lesions, most often on the labia. The lesions may be whitish or reddish, and the vulvar skin may be excoriated as a result of irritation.

The client may be anxious or fearful about the diagnosis of cancer. She may have fears that her partner will reject her because of the diagnosis, or she may worry about disfigurement related to surgery. Assess the client's past experiences in coping with stressful situations and whether she has the psychological resources to cope with the current crisis.

A Pap smear and colposcopic examination of the vulva (see Assessment [Cervical Cancer], p. 1846) may aid in diagnosis. A toluidine blue test may be used to identify abnormal cells for biopsy. The solution is applied to the vulva and allowed to dry. Then a 1% acetic acid solution is applied. Biopsy of the areas that remain blue is performed. The test chemical stains nuclei in the superficial epithelium, where cells do not normally contain nuclei. An abnormal finding does not diagnose cancer because ulcerations also stain.

A biopsy of the lesion is needed for diagnosis. This is easily accomplished with a Keyes dermal punch (a device that removes a disk of tissue). Depending on the site of the lesion, one or more biopsy specimens may be taken. Excisional biopsies are preferred for smaller lesions.

Prognosis is related to lesion size, contour, mitotic activity, and whether cancer is present in the lymph nodes. Lesions larger than 5 cm in diameter with infiltrating margins and extensive necrosis are the most likely to recur after surgical resection. Clients with seven or more positive lymph nodes have a poorer prognosis (DeVita et al., 2001).

Interventions

Surgery is the major treatment aimed at curing vulvar cancer. Radiation therapy may be used for advanced cancer or for palliation.

NONSURGICAL MANAGEMENT

Laser Therapy. If a woman has premalignant vulvar lesions, laser therapy may be used (see p. 1846). The treatment is usually done on an outpatient basis; local, regional, or general anesthesia is used. Healing occurs over a period of several weeks, usually without scarring.

Radiation Therapy. External radiation therapy to the deep pelvic nodes may be used after surgery (see earlier discussion of endometrial cancer [p. 1843] and Chapter 28). Radiation treatments cause ulceration and dermatitis, which can be uncomfortable for the woman.

SURGICAL MANAGEMENT. The surgeon performs a vulvectomy to remove the cancerous vulvar lesions.

Preoperative Care. The surgeon provides a complete explanation of the extent of the surgical procedure to be performed. Reinforce the information provided by the surgeon. Photographs of a healed vulvectomy or reconstructed vulva may help reassure the client about the expected cosmetic outcome. Specific care before a vulvectomy may include an abdominal or perineal shave, an enema, douching, and insertion of an indwelling catheter into the bladder.

Operative Procedures. Several surgical procedures are used for the treatment of vulvar cancer. A local wide excision may be used to remove the abnormal area (for carcinoma in situ [CIS]). A simple **vulvectomy** (removal of the vulva, the labia majora, the labia minora, and possibly the clitoris) may also be performed for CIS, but this disfiguring surgery is used less often today. Instead, a **skinning vulvectomy**—the removal of superficial vulvar skin (without removal of the clitoris) and replacement of removed skin with split-thickness grafts—is performed (Figure 78-7). Sexual function is less affected, and the appearance of the vulva is less changed.

For invasive cancer, a modified radical or **radical vulvectomy** (removal of the entire vulva skin, labia, clitoris, subcutaneous tissues, and possibly inguinal and femoral node dissection), may be performed, depending on node involvement (see Figure 78-7). Tumors that involve the anus, rectum, rectovaginal septum, or urethra usually require a pelvic exenteration with radical vulvectomy and bilateral groin dissection.

Postoperative Care. After surgery, multiple suction drains (Hemovac or Jackson-Pratt drains) are present in the inguinal or vulvar areas for wound drainage for 7 to 10 days. A pressure-reducing mattress may be placed on the bed to prevent pressure ulcers and increase comfort. A bed cradle may be used to keep linens off the incision site. The client usually wears antiembolism stockings or sequential compression devices to prevent thromboembolism and leg edema.

Providing Wound Care. The major focus of nursing care is wound healing. Change the dressings over the incision frequently because of the amount of wound drainage and the risk for infection. Wound complications, such as infection and dehiscence, often occur after vulvectomies, and the healing process may take up to 6 months. Meticulous

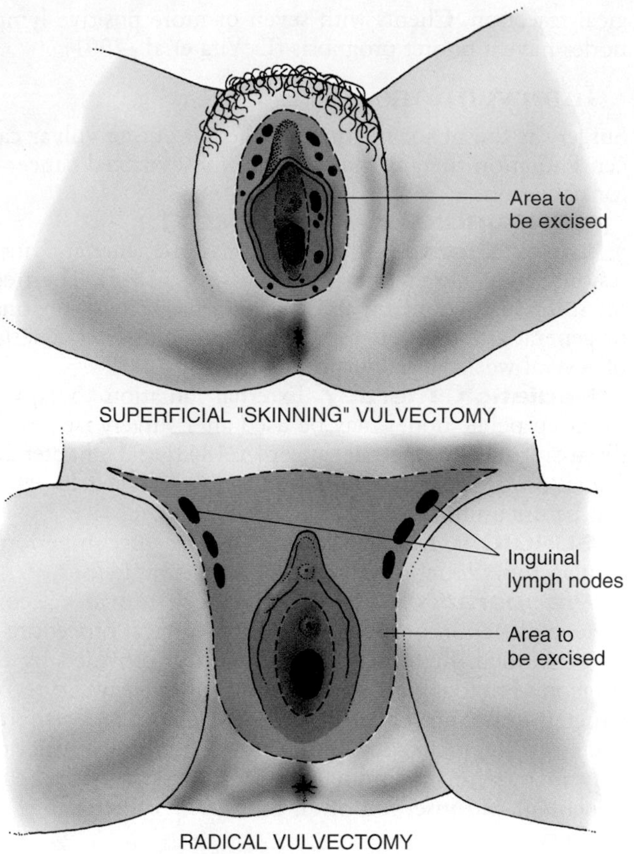

Figure 78-7 ■ Vulvectomy.

wound care is needed and may involve debridement. Rinse the area with a normal saline solution, using a bulb syringe or a water pick (on low pressure). Then dry the wound using a heat lamp or air-dry it with a hair dryer (using warm air). Wound care is usually done three or four times a day.

Depending on the client's hygiene and home situation, she may use a sitz bath, tub, or whirlpool bath once or twice a day for wound care. Teach the client that the tub should be meticulously cleaned each time before she uses it. A half cup of salt may be added to the water. If the client does not have access to a tub or whirlpool, a squeeze bottle or squirt gun can be filled with warm water or a saline solution and poured or squirted over the wound area.

Instruct the client to include foods rich in vitamin C, iron, and protein to promote wound healing.

Promoting Urinary and Bowel Elimination. The Foley catheter remains in the bladder for 7 to 10 days to prevent ureteral stenosis and incontinence. After the catheter is removed, the urine stream may be deflected down the leg as a result of edema or even may be uncontrolled. Having the client stand while voiding may decrease the incidence of these annoying problems. Antiperistaltic drugs are usually given for 7 to 10 days to prevent defecation and decrease the risk for wound infection. Then stool softeners may be given to prevent straining and decrease discomfort related to bowel movements. Perineal care or sitz baths after voidings or bowel movements may prevent contamination of the incision site.

Managing Pain. Discomfort after surgery is usually controlled with opioid analgesics during the first couple of days after surgery. Medicating for pain before wound care may help the client to relax and tolerate the procedure with less distress.

Addressing Sexuality. Provide complete explanations of the changes that occur as a result of surgery. If a radical vulvectomy is performed, the clitoris is removed and loss of orgasm usually occurs. Dyspareunia may result from any of the surgical procedures. Vaginal dilators may be useful to stretch the remaining vaginal tissues. Discomfort can also be reduced during sexual intercourse by having the couple use water-soluble lubricants or a side-lying position. The couple may need counseling about alternatives to vaginal intercourse. Encourage the client to express feelings of grief related to her loss of normal sexual function.

A vulvectomy can be devastating to a client's self-concept. She often has a grief reaction related to the loss of the vulva and subsequent disfigurement. She may fear rejection from her sexual partner and may be reluctant to make herself vulnerable by getting involved in any relationship. Fears of recurrence or metastasis may be present. Encourage the client to vent her feelings and concerns about her perceived or actual losses and body changes. Urge family members or significant others to share their feelings and concerns with the woman. A visit by a woman who has successfully recovered from similar surgery could be beneficial.

Vaginal Cancer

PATHOPHYSIOLOGY

Invasive vaginal cancer is rare, accounting for less than 2% of all gynecologic cancers. Usually vaginal cancer is an extension of cervical, endometrial, or vulvar cancers. Most vaginal cancers are squamous cell carcinomas that develop in the upper one third of the vagina. They occur most often in women older than 50 years of age; 90% of cases develop after menopause. Adenocarcinoma of the vagina is found in women between the ages of 14 and 30 years and is associated with intrauterine exposure to diethylstilbestrol (DES) as a result of maternal ingestion during pregnancy.

The cause of vaginal cancer is unknown. Risk factors include repeated pregnancies; vaginal trauma; sexually transmitted diseases (STDs), especially syphilis and herpes simplex virus type 2 and papillomavirus infections; and prior radiation.

The spread of vaginal cancer depends on the location of the tumor. Upper vaginal lesions spread in the same manner as cervical cancer, whereas lower lesions spread similarly to vulvar cancer. Because of the rich lymphatic drainage in the vaginal area, metastasis can occur early.

◆COLLABORATIVE MANAGEMENT

◆Assessment

Premalignant lesions (vaginal intraepithelial neoplasia) are often asymptomatic, and an abnormal Pap smear may be the only indication. Late symptoms include pain, foul-smelling vaginal discharge, painless vaginal bleeding, pruritus, and urinary symptoms from the pressure of the lesion on the bladder.

A pelvic examination may reveal a lesion. Premalignant changes are diagnosed through colposcopic examination and biopsy.

Survival rates are better when tumors are smaller and no lymph nodes are involved.

Interventions

NONSURGICAL MANAGEMENT. Noninvasive malignancy and early stage vaginal cancers may be treated nonsurgically with a variety of techniques. Laser therapy (see p. 1846) may be used. The health care provider stains the abnormal tissues with an iodine solution to identify the area for treatment. A vaginal discharge may be present for several days after treatment, and healing normally takes a few weeks. Close follow-up is necessary and includes a Pap smear and colposcopic examination every 4 months for 1 year and then every 6 to 12 months.

Topical chemotherapy with local application of 5-fluorouracil (5-FU) cream to the vagina daily for 1 week is another treatment option. This drug is irritating to the skin, and often zinc oxide ointment application is recommended to protect the vulvar area. The treatment is repeated in 3 to 4 weeks, and follow-up is the same as that for laser therapy.

Radiation therapy can be used for all stages of vaginal cancer. Intracavitary radiation therapy (IRT, brachytherapy) is usually used alone for the treatment of cancer limited to the vaginal wall, and external radiation therapy is combined with IRT for cancer that extends beyond the vaginal wall. Complications of radiation therapy include vaginal stenosis, adhesions, and discharge. Women need to use vaginal dilators after treatment, and assessment for sexual dysfunction is suggested.

SURGICAL MANAGEMENT. A local wide excision may be performed for localized lesions. A partial or total **vaginectomy** (removal of part or all the vagina) is performed for invasive disease. Vaginectomy affects sexual function. Without surgical reconstruction, vaginal intercourse is impossible. The client and her sexual partner need counseling about alternative activities for achieving sexual satisfaction. A radical hysterectomy or pelvic exenteration may also be performed, depending on the extent of the cancer.

Fallopian Tube Cancer

PATHOPHYSIOLOGY

Fallopian tube cancer is the rarest of gynecologic cancers, with an incidence of less than 1%. It occurs in women older than 50 years of age; 80% to 90% of cases are metastases from ovarian and endometrial cancers.

The cause of squamous cell fallopian tube cancer is unknown. Adenocarcinoma of the fallopian tube may result from pelvic inflammatory disease (PID) and chronic salpingitis. Nulliparity and infertility (inability to conceive) have also been cited as risk factors.

Most fallopian tube carcinomas are serous adenocarcinomas. The spread of this disease is very similar to that of epithelial ovarian cancer. The initial lesion is confined to the lumen of the tube. From there it invades the serosa and spreads intraperitoneally to the bowel, omentum, and peritoneum. Lymphatic spread is to the para-aortic and retroperitoneal lymph nodes.

COLLABORATIVE MANAGEMENT

Clients who have fallopian tube cancer often have only a few manifestations. The most common manifestations are postmenopausal bleeding, increasing abdominal pain, watery vaginal discharge, and leukorrhea. Later manifestations include lower abdominal pain or distention and feelings of pressure.

Diagnosis is rare before surgery. Pap smears are abnormal in only 10% of cases. A mass may be felt on examination in late stages. Vaginal ultrasonography, computed tomography (CT), or laparoscopy may be used to confirm a mass.

Treatment of cancer limited to the fallopian tube is a total abdominal hysterectomy and bilateral salpingo-oophorectomy with **omentectomy** (removal of the connective tissues covering these organs). Care of the client with fallopian tube cancer is similar to that described for cancer of the ovary (see Interventions [Ovarian Cancer], p. 1850). Chemotherapy may be used before surgery in later stages or for recurrence. The lesions respond to alkylating agents (see Chapter 28). External radiation therapy has been used after surgery for late-stage tumors.

GET READY for the NCLEX Examination!

KEY POINTS

Safe Effective Care Environment

- Use clean technique when emptying wound drains following pelvic exenteration surgery.
- Have clients report any manifestations of infection when caring for a urinary catheter in the home.
- Teach clients not to do any heavy lifting (>15 pounds) after a hysterectomy or cervical ablative procedures.
- Do not allow pregnant women or children under 18 years of age to enter the room where radioactive implants are in use.

Health Promotion and Maintenance

- Teach women at risk for ovarian or endometrial cancer to follow the American Cancer Society's screening guidelines.
- Teach all women to have regular Pap tests based on their risk factors.
- Teach women to practice safer sex to prevent infections of the reproductive organs.
- Teach women who use tampons to wash their hands before inserting the tampon, not to leave the tampon in place for more than 6 hours, and to use sanitary napkins (rather than tampons) at night.
- Urge women who have an increased genetic risk for endometrial or ovarian cancer to see their gynecological health care provider annually.

Psychosocial Integrity

- Use language and terminology the client is comfortable with when discussing reproductive issues, sexuality, and gynecologic problems.
- Reassure women who suffer from premenstrual syndrome (PMS) that their manifestations have a physiologic basis.
- Explain all tests, procedures, and treatments, especially if they cause discomfort during or after the procedures.
- Assess the client's anxiety before any gynecologic surgery.
- Encourage women who are having procedures that may interfere with fertility to express feelings of fear or grief.
- Encourage women with chronic or serious health problems to consider using support groups or counseling.

Physiological Integrity

- Help clients to be informed enough to make appropriate decisions about whether or not to use hormone replacement therapy during or after menopause.
- Urge any women who experiences postmenopausal vaginal bleeding to consult with her gynecologic health care provider as soon as possible.
- Teach clients taking danazol for endometriosis about the side effects of the drug (hirsutism, weight gain, decreased breast size, acne).
- Monitor all clients who have pelvic surgery for the presence of deep vein thrombosis after surgery.
- Instruct clients prescribed to use pessaries the proper way to use and care for the device.
- Teach clients about specific restrictions after local cervical ablation therapy (see Chart 78-14).
- When caring for a client who has a radioactive implant, wear your dosimeter and lead apron whenever you are in the room, always face the radiation source, and do not spend more than 30 minutes per day in the room.
- Teach the client who is going home after a hysterectomy how to monitor herself for infection or other complications.
- Instruct clients receiving external beam radiation to the abdomen to gently wash the area; not to apply creams or lotions (unless prescribed by the radiologist); not to wash off marking; to avoid exposing the area to sunlight or temperature extremes; and to wear soft, nonirritating clothing.

ADDITIONAL STUDY RESOURCES

Go to your Student CD-ROM for Review Questions for the NCLEX Examination.

evolve Go to http://evolve.elsevier.com/Iggy/ for Integrated Management of Care Questions for the NCLEX Examination.

SELECTED BIBLIOGRAPHY

Asterisk indicates a classic or definitive work on this subject.

Ackley, B., & Ladwig, G. (2002). *Nursing diagnosis handbook: A guide to planning care* (5th ed.). St. Louis: Mosby.

Ahlberg, K., et al. (2004). Fatigue, psychological distress, coping, and quality of life in patients with uterine cancer. *Journal of Advanced Nursing, 45*(2), 205-213.

Ahmedin, J., et al. (2003). Cancer statistics 2003. *CA: A Cancer Journal for Clinicians, 53*(1), 5-26.

Almadrones, L., et al. (2004). Psychometric evaluation of two scales assessing functional status and peripheral neuropathy associated with chemotherapy for ovarian cancer: A gynecological oncology study group study. *Oncology Nursing Forum, 31*(3), 615-623.

American Cancer Society. (2005). *Cancer facts and figures 2005.* Report No. 00-300M-No. 5008.05. Atlanta: Author.

Anderson, P.O., Knobmen, J.E., & Troutman, W.G. (2002). Handbook of clinical drug data, 10th ed. New York: McGraw-Hill Medical Publishing Division.

Baily, D., et al. (2004). Uncertainty intervention for watchful waiting in prostate cancer. *Cancer Nursing, 27*(5), 339-346.

*Barrett, R.J., et al. (1995). Endometrial cancer: Stage at diagnosis and associated factors in black and white patients. *American Journal of Obstetrics and Gynecology, 173*(2), 414-422.

*Barrow, C. (1999). Balloon endometrial ablation as a safe alternative to hysterectomy. *AORN Journal, 70*(1), 80, 83-86, 89-90.

Barton, D., & Loprinzi, C. (2004). Making sense of the evidence regarding nonhormonal treatment for hot flashes. *Clinical Journal of Oncology Nursing, 8*(1), 39-42.

Barton, D., et al. (2004). Libido as part of sexuality in female cancer survivors. *Oncology Nursing Forum, 31*(3), 599-607.

Bond, S. (2003). New guidelines for Pap screening and management of results. *Journal of Midwifery & Women's Health, 49*(1), 57-59.

Choma, K.K. (2003). ASC-US HPV testing. *American Journal of Nursing, 103*(2), 42-51.

Christman, N., Oakley, M., & Cronin, S. (2001). Developing and using preparatory information for women undergoing radiation therapy for cervical or uterine cancer. *Oncology Nursing Forum, 28*(1), 93-98.

DeCherney, A.H., & Nathan, L. (2003). *Current obstetric & gynecologic diagnosis & treatment.* New York: McGraw-Hill Medical Publishing Division.

Denny, E. (2004). Women's experience of endometriosis. *Journal of Advanced Nursing, 46*(6), 641-648.

DeVita, V.T., Hellman, S., & Rosenberg, S.A. (2001). *Cancer: principles and practice of oncology, 6th ed.,* Philadelphia: Lippincott, Williams, & Wilkins.

Dochterman, J., & Bulechek, G. (eds). (2004). *Nursing interventions classification (NIC)* (4th ed.). St. Louis: Mosby.

Donovan. H., & Ward, S. (2005). Representations of fatigue in women receiving chemotherapy for gynecologic cancers. *Oncology Nursing Forum, 32*(1), 113-116.

Ebersole, P., Hess, P., & Luggen, A. (2004). *Toward healthy aging: Human needs and nursing response* (6th ed.). St. Louis: Mosby.

Ekwall, W., Ternestedt, B., & Sorbe, B. (2003). Important aspects of health care for women with gynecologic cancer. *Oncology Nursing Forum, 30*(2), 313-319.

Facts and Comparisons. (2004). *Drug facts and comparisons* (58th ed.). St. Louis: Author.

Fey, M., & Beal, M. (2004). Role of human papilloma virus testing in cervical cancer prevention. *Journal of Midwifery & Women's Health, 49*(1), 4-13.

Hackley, B., & Rousseau, M. (2004). Managing menopausal symptoms after the women's health initiative. *Journal of Midwifery & Women's Health, 49*(2), 87-95.

Howel, D., Fitch, M.I., & Deane, K.A. (2003). Impact of ovarian cancer perceived by women. *Cancer Nursing, 26*(1):1-9.

Iannacchione, M.A. (2004). The vagina dialogues: Do you douche? *American journal of Nursing, 104*(1), 40-45.

Janicek, M.F., & Averette, H.E. (2001). Cervical cancer: Prevention, diagnosis, and therapeutics. *CA: Cancer Journal for Clinicians, 51,* 92-114.

*Johnson, S. (1998). Menopause and hormone replacement therapy. *Medical Clinics of North America, 82*(2), 297-320.

*Kim, K., et al. (1999). Cervical cancer screening knowledge and practices among Korean-American women. *Cancer Nursing, 22*(4), 297-302.

Koldjeski, D., et al. (2004). Health seeking related to ovarian cancer. *Cancer Nursing, 27*(5), 370-378.

Lee, C., (2000a). Gynecologic Cancers: Part I Risk factors. *Clinical Journal of Oncology Nursing, 4*(2), 67-71.

Lee, C., (2000b). Gynecologic Cancers: Part II Risk assessment and screening. *Clinical Journal of Oncology Nursing, 4*(2), 73-77.

*Lessick, M., Wickham, R., & Rehwaldt, M. (1997). Breast and ovarian cancer: Genetic update and implications for nursing. *MEDSURG Nursing, 6*(6), 341-349.

Likes, W., & Itano, J. (2003). Human papillomavirus and cervical cancer: Not just a sexually transmitted disease. *Clinical journal of Oncology Nursing, 7*(3), 271-276.

Lockwood-Rayerman, S. (2004). Characteristics of participation in cervical cancer screening. *Cancer Nursing, 27*(5), 353-363.

Loitmen, J. (2002). Transdermal fentanyl in ovarian cancer. *Journal of Pain and Symptom Management, 23*(1), 5-6.

*Lowdermilk, D.L. (1995). Reproductive surgery. In C.I. Fogel & N.F. Woods (Eds.), *Women's health care* (pp. 629-650). Springhouse, PA: Springhouse.

Lyndaker, C., & Hulton, L. (2004). The influence of age on symptoms of perimenopause. *Journal of Gynecologic and Neonatal Nursing, 33*(3), 340-347.

McCance, K.L., & Huether, S.E. (2002). *Pathophysiology: The biological basis for disease in adults and children* (4th ed.). St. Louis: Mosby.

Mick, J.A., Hughes, M., & Cohen, M. (2004). Using the BETTER model to assess sexuality. *Clinical Journal of Oncology Nursing, 8*(1), 84-86.

Moore-Higgs, G.J., et al. (2000). *Women and cancer: A gynecologic oncology nursing perspective*, 2nd ed., Boston: Jones & Bartlett.

Moorhead, S., Johnson, M., & Maas, M. (Eds.). (2004). *Nursing outcomes classification (NOC)* (3rd ed.). St. Louis: Mosby.

O'Rourke, J., & Mahon, S. (2003). A comprehensive look at the early detection of ovarian cancer. *Clinical Journal of Oncology Nursing, 7*(1), 41-47.

*Pearl, M.L., et al. (1999). Transcutaneous electrical nerve stimulation as an adjunct for controlling chemotherapy-induced nausea and vomiting in gynecologic oncology. *Cancer Nursing, 22*(4), 307-311.

*Rose, P.G. (1996). Endometrial carcinoma. *New England Journal of Medicine, 335*(9), 640-649.

Ryan, M., et al. (2003). The experience of lower limb lymphedema for women after treatment for gynecologic cancer. *Oncology Nursing Forum, 30*(3), 417-423.

Shinn, S. (2004). Taking a stand against cervical cancer. *Nursing 2004, 34*(5), 36-41.

Smith, L. (2004). Shedding light on photodynamic therapy. *Nursing 2004, 34*(5), 32hn1-32hn2.

*Spies, J.B., et al. (1999). Initial results from uterine fibroid embolization for symptomatic leiomyomata. *Journal of Vascular and Interventional Radiology, 10*(9), 1149-1157.

Stekler, J., & Elmore, J. (2002). Cervical cancer screening: Who, when, why? *The Clinical Advisor, (October 2002),* 107-114.

Swenson, M., et al. (2003). Quality of life among ovarian germ cell cancer survivors: A narrative analysis. *Oncology Nursing Forum, 30*(3), E56-E62.

*Taylor, L.K., et al. (1998). The effect of music in the postanesthesia care unit on pain levels in women who have had abdominal hysterectomies. *Journal of Perianesthesia Nursing, 13*(2), 88-94.

Tiffen, J., & Novak, K. (2004). Ovarian cancer. *Clinical Journal of Oncology Nursing, 8*(1), 80-82.

Wade, J., et al. (2000). Hysterectomy: What do women need and want to know? *Journal of Obstetric, Gynecologic, and Neonatal Nursing, 29*(1), 33-42.

Yarbro, C.H., et al. (2000). *Cancer nursing: principles & practice,* 5th ed., Boston: Jones & Bartlett.

Zimmerman, V. (2002). BRCA gene mutations and cancer. *American Journal of Nursing, 102*(8), 28-36.

CHAPTER

79 Interventions for Male Clients with Reproductive Problems

LINDA J. CAPUTI

LEARNING OUTCOMES

After studying this chapter, you should be able to:

1. Describe common physical assessment findings for the client with benign prostatic hyperplasia (BPH).
2. Describe the mechanisms of action, side effects, and nursing implications for pharmacologic management of BPH.
3. Discuss options for surgical management of the client with BPH.
4. Develop a postoperative plan of care for a client undergoing a transurethral resection of the prostate (TURP).
5. Identify the procedures for prostate cancer screening.
6. Explain the role of hormonal therapy in treating prostate cancer.
7. Develop a community-based plan of care for a client with prostate cancer.
8. Describe the options for treating erectile dysfunction.
9. Describe the mechanisms of action, side effects, and nursing implications for pharmacologic management of erectile dysfunction.
10. Discuss cultural considerations related to male reproductive problems.
11. Analyze assessment data to determine priority nursing diagnoses and collaborative problems for a man with testicular cancer.
12. Develop a plan of care for a client with testicular cancer.
13. Formulate a community-based teaching plan for continuing care of clients with testicular cancer.
14. Compare hydrocele, spermatocele, and varicocele.
15. Compare the four types of prostatitis.
16. Discuss issues related to sexuality and body image for a man experiencing male reproductive health problems.

Go to your Student CD-ROM for Review Questions for the NCLEX Examination keyed to these Learning Outcomes.

Apply knowledge of the anatomy and physiology of male reproductive functions when instructing clients about the impact of a disease process or treatment on their reproductive ability. Include the client and his spouse, sexual partner, or significant other in the decision-making process and work with members of the interdisciplinary team in providing collaborative care.

BENIGN PROSTATIC HYPERPLASIA

PATHOPHYSIOLOGY

In a young adult male, the prostatic capsule is thin and attached to the underlying tissue. With aging, the glandular units in the prostate undergo tissue **hyperplasia** (an increase in the number of cells), resulting in prostatic **hypertrophy**

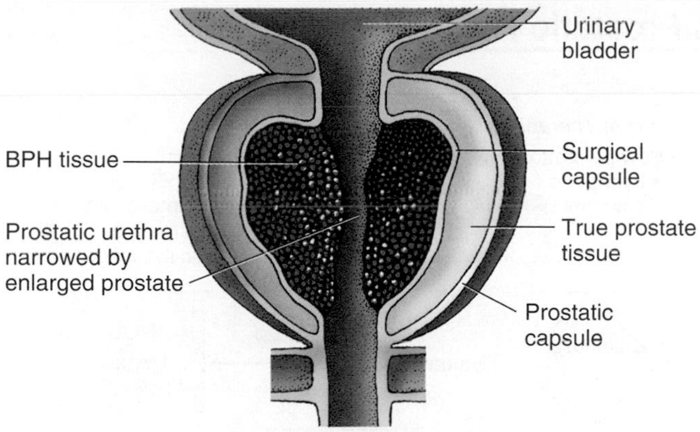

Figure 79-1 ■ Benign prostatic hyperplasia (BPH) grows inward, causing narrowing of the urethra.

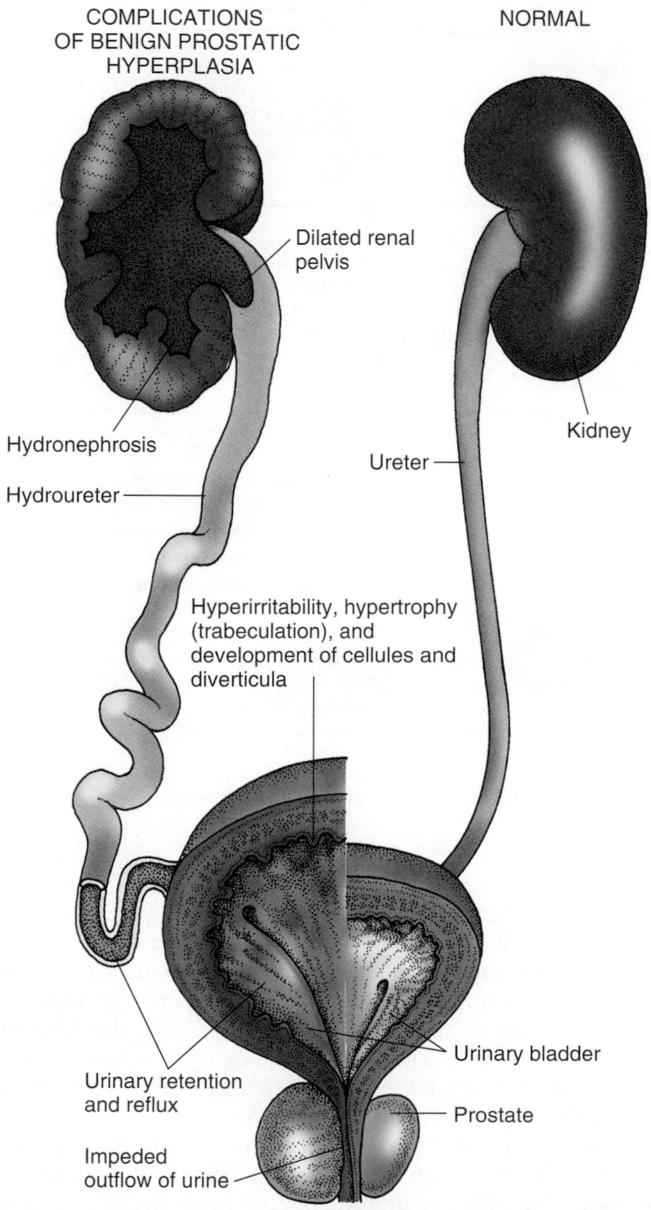

Figure 79-2 ■ Potential complications of benign prostatic hyperplasia. The right side of the illustration shows a normal male urologic system. The left side shows potential complications.

(enlargement). Although benign prostatic hypertrophy is the more common term used to describe this problem, **benign prostatic hyperplasia (BPH)** is the correct term for the pathologic process.

When the prostate gland enlarges, it extends upward, into the bladder, and inward, narrowing the prostatic urethral channel. This obstructs urine outflow by encroaching on the bladder opening (Figure 79-1). In response to this outlet resistance, the bladder is affected in several ways (Figure 79-2). It may become hyperirritable, which causes urgency and frequency. As the bladder tries to compensate for its increased workload, muscles in the bladder wall hypertrophy and may develop cellules and diverticula. If allowed to continue, this obstruction of urine flow can cause a gradual dilation of the ureters **(hydroureter)** and kidneys **(hydronephrosis).** The enlarged prostate may also obstruct the bladder neck or the prostatic urethra, causing urinary retention or incomplete bladder emptying. **Overflow urinary incontinence** is common; the urine "leaks" around the enlarged prostate, causing dribbling. Urinary stasis can result in urinary tract infections.

Etiology

The exact cause of BPH is unknown. Because BPH development is almost universal in older men, several theories have been examined (Marks, 2003).

- The effect of chronic inflammation of the prostate gland
- The role of general metabolic and nutritional factors (diet)
- The possible contribution of atherosclerosis

Although demographic data (such as race) and social factors (such as socioeconomic status and heredity) have been examined as predictors for the BPH development, it appears to result from a systemic hormonal alteration. Support for this theory is based on the fact that aging is the major contributing factor and that another factor is the presence of testicular androgen. BPH does not occur in men who were castrated before puberty (testicular androgen is absent). Men with BPH have a regression of this problem if the testes are surgically removed.

Incidence/Prevalence

CONSIDERATIONS FOR OLDER ADULTS

The incidence of BPH consistently increases with age. Thus BPH is a disease of men older than 40 years of age, and the incidence increases with each decade of life. By 50 years of age, at least 50% of all men have some degree of BPH, although not all are symptomatic (Ebersole, Hess, & Luggen, 2004).

◆COLLABORATIVE MANAGEMENT

The Concept Map on p. 1858 discusses nursing assessment and care issues related to management of the client with BPH.

◆Assessment

HISTORY

Pay particular attention to the client's report of his urinary pattern. Commonly the client reports frequency, **nocturia** (voiding at night), and other symptoms of bladder neck obstruction. Together these problems are known as **lower urinary tract symptoms (LUTS).** The symptoms of LUTS include hes-

CONCEPT MAP Benign Prostatic Hyperplasia

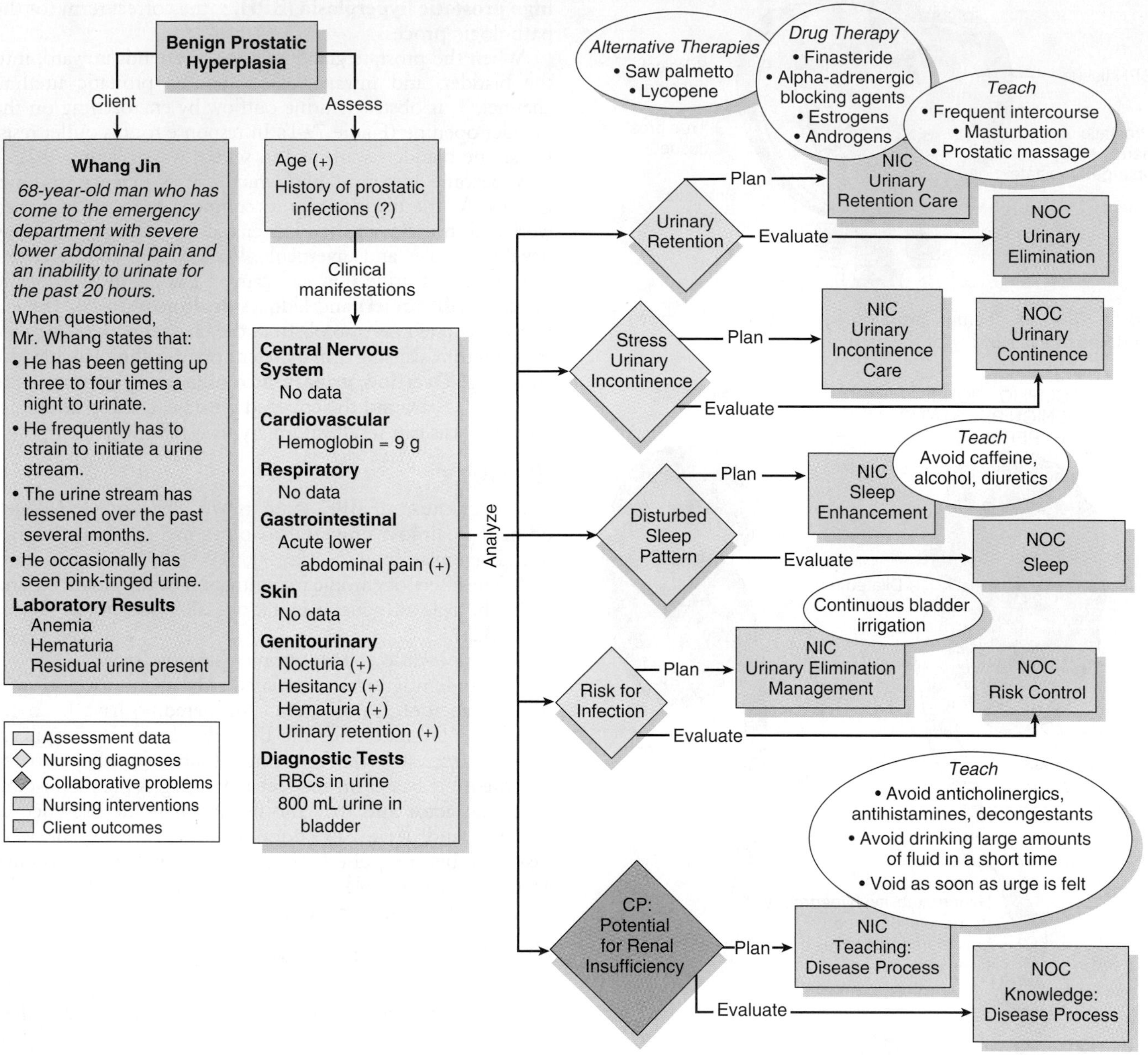

Concept Map by Elaine Bishop Kennedy, EdD, RN

itancy, intermittency, reduced force and size of the urinary stream, a sensation of incomplete bladder emptying, and postvoid dribbling. If frequency and nocturia are not accompanied by symptoms of restricted flow, the possibility of a nonobstructive etiology, such as infection, is considered.

Ask whether the client has experienced any **hematuria** (blood in the urine) when starting the urine stream or at the end of urination. BPH is a common cause of hematuria in men older than 60 years of age.

PHYSICAL ASSESSMENT/CLINICAL MANIFESTATIONS

Instruct the client to void before the physical assessment. Inspect, palpate, and percuss the abdomen for a distended bladder. Normally the bladder must contain 150 mL of urine to be outlined during palpation and percussion. A bladder with a larger amount of urine may be visible on inspection. An enlarged bladder may be palpated as a mass in the lower abdomen. If the client has a sense of urgency when pressure is applied to the bladder area, the bladder may be distended. The bladder of an obese client is best identified through percussion or bedside bladder scanner rather than by inspection or palpation.

Prepare the client for examination of the prostate gland. Tell him that he may feel the urge to urinate as the prostate is palpated. Because the prostate is close to the rectal wall, it is easily examined by **digital rectal examination (DRE).** Help the client to bend over the examination table or assume a side-lying fetal position. The health care provider examines the prostate for size and consistency. Benign prostatic hyper-

Animation: Rectal Examination

CHART 79-1

KEY FEATURES of
Benign Prostatic Hyperplasia

- Urinary frequency
- Nocturia
- Urinary hesitancy, particularly on initiation of voiding
- Hematuria
- Diminished force of the urinary stream
- Postvoid dribbling (overflow incontinence)
- Bladder distention
- Possible evidence of renal insufficiency, including edema, pallor, and pruritus
- A uniform, elastic, nontender palpable prostate

plasia (BPH) usually presents as a uniform, elastic, nontender enlargement, whereas cancer of the prostate gland usually presents as a stony-hard nodule (Chart 79-1). Advise the client that after the prostate gland is palpated, it may be massaged to obtain a fluid sample for examination to rule out **prostatitis** (inflammation of the prostate).

LABORATORY ASSESSMENT

A urinalysis may be performed to detect any urine problems, and a culture may be obtained for evidence of urinary tract infection. Urinalysis includes glucose, protein, occult blood, and pH levels. If infection is present, the specimen may contain white blood cells (WBCs) or red blood cells (RBCs).

Blood studies that may be performed at the initial evaluation, depending on the client's condition and third-party payer, include the following:

- A complete blood count (CBC) to evaluate any evidence of infection (elevated WBCs) or anemia (decreased RBCs)
- Blood urea nitrogen (BUN) and serum creatinine levels to evaluate renal function (both are elevated with renal disease)
- A prostate-specific antigen (PSA) and a serum acid phosphatase measurement if prostate cancer is suspected (PSA is elevated with prostate cancer) (see Physical Examination and Prostate Cancer Screening, p. 1865)

If prostatic fluid is expressed during the examination, send the fluid to the laboratory for microscopic examination and cultures.

RADIOGRAPHIC ASSESSMENT

Radiologic studies that may be conducted in the workup of the client with suspected BPH include x-rays of the kidneys, ureters, and bladder (KUB) and intravenous (IV) urography to assess the entire urinary/renal system. The KUB outlines the structure of the urinary tract in the abdomen. Urography is useful in studying both the structure and function of the urinary tract.

OTHER DIAGNOSTIC ASSESSMENTS

Urodynamic studies are important in the diagnosis and evaluation of clients with bladder neck obstruction. Urodynamic flow studies include flow rate analysis **(flowmetry)** and assessment of residual urine. Flow rate analysis is simply a way of assessing the activity of the bladder and the outlet during the emptying phase of micturition.

During a cystourethroscopic examination, the physician uses a cystoscope to view the interior of the bladder, the bladder neck, and the urethra. This examination is used to study the presence and effect of bladder neck obstruction. The procedure is usually done in an ambulatory care setting. See Chapter 72 for a detailed description of cystoscopy.

Residual urine may be determined by bladder scan immediately after the client voids. As an alternative, because the client always voids before cystourethroscopy, residual urine may be measured at that time.

Common Nursing Diagnoses and Collaborative Problems

Nursing diagnoses and collaborative problems that may apply to clients with benign prostatic hyperplasia include the following:

- Urinary Retention related to blockage from enlarged prostate gland
- Urinary Incontinence related to overdistension of the bladder
- Disturbed Sleep Pattern related to urinary urgency, nocturia
- Risk for Infection related to inadequate primary defenses (stasis of urine)
- Potential for Renal Insufficiency

Interventions

Traditionally, the only effective treatment for the relief of the symptoms caused by BPH has been surgical. However, drug therapy is now becoming a popular option. Chart 79-2 lists NIC interventions for clients with BPH.

NONSURGICAL MANAGEMENT. In some cases where clients are not yet bothered by the symptoms of BPH, "watchful waiting" may be appropriate. In watchful waiting, the client is examined every year to determine whether the BPH is causing urinary difficulties and getting worse. Medical management of BPH includes drug therapy and other measures to reduce obstruction.

Drug Therapy. The health care provider may prescribe finasteride (Proscar) to shrink the prostate gland and improve urine flow. Finasteride lowers the level of **dihydrotestosterone (DHT),** a major cause of prostate growth. In some men, decreasing the DHT levels can shrink the enlarged prostate. The client may need to take the drug for as long as 6 months before improvement is noticed. The major side effects of the drug are erectile dysfunction (ED) and decreased libido, although these effects are not common.

The presence of alpha-adrenergic receptors in the prostatic smooth muscle makes it respond to alpha-blocking agents, such as terazosin (Hytrin), doxazosin (Cardura), and tamsulosin (Flomax). When alpha-blocking agents are given, the prostate gland constricts, thereby reducing urethral pressure and improving urine flow. A variety of hormonal agents, including estrogens and androgens, alone or in combination, also have been used less successfully to alter BPH and its effects on voiding.

Complementary and Alternative Therapies. Some herbs and natural products that have been used to manage BPH include saw palmetto extract (a natural herb) and lycopene (a botanical found in tomatoes). Many men with early to moderate BPH believe these agents have relieved their symptoms and prefer this treatment over prescription drugs or surgery. Clinical trials for both agents are now under way.

CHART 79-2

NIC **INTERVENTION ACTIVITIES for The Client with Benign Prostatic Hyperplasia**

Urinary Retention Care: *Assistance in relieving bladder distension*
- Perform a comprehensive urinary assessment focusing on incontinence (e.g., urinary output, urinary voiding pattern, cognitive function, and preexisting urinary problems).
- Monitor use of nonprescription agents with anticholinergic or alpha-agonist properties.
- Provide privacy for elimination.
- Use the power of suggestion by running water or flushing the toilet.
- Provide enough time for bladder emptying (10 minutes).
- Provide Credé maneuver, as necessary.
- Insert urinary catheter, as appropriate.
- Monitor intake and output.
- Monitor degree of bladder distension by palpation and percussion.
- Catheterize for residual, as appropriate.
- Implement intermittent catheterization, as appropriate.

Bladder Irrigation: *Instillation of a solution into the bladder to provide cleansing or medication*
- Determine whether the irrigation will be continuous or intermittent.
- Observe universal precautions.
- Explain the procedure to the client.
- Set up sterile irrigating supplies, maintaining sterile technique per agency protocol.
- Cleanse site of entry or end of Y-connector with alcohol wipe.
- Instill irrigating fluid, per agency protocol.
- Monitor and maintain correct flow rate, as necessary.
- Record amount of fluid used, characteristics of fluid, amount returned, and client responsiveness, according to agency protocol.

NIC intervention activities selected from Dochterman, J.M., & Bulechek, G.M. (Eds.) (2004). *Nursing interventions classification (NIC)* (4th ed.). St. Louis: Mosby.

Other Measures. Other nonsurgical measures that reduce obstructive symptoms include those that cause the release of prostatic fluid, such as prostatic massage, frequent sexual intercourse, and masturbation. These measures are helpful for the client whose obstructive symptoms result from an enlarged prostate with a large amount of retained prostatic fluid. Instruct the client to avoid drinking large amounts of fluid in a short time; to avoid alcohol, diuretics, and caffeine; and to void as soon as the urge is felt. These measures are aimed at preventing overdistention of the bladder, which may result in loss of detrusor muscle tone. Teach clients to avoid any drugs that can cause urinary retention, especially anticholinergics, antihistamines, and decongestants. Emphasize the importance of telling the health care provider about the diagnosis of BPH so that these drugs are not prescribed.

SURGICAL MANAGEMENT. Because most older men have some degree of BPH, the mere presence of the condition does not mean that the client requires surgical intervention. Some or all of the following criteria are typically present when surgical intervention is necessary:
- Acute urinary retention
- Chronic urinary tract infections secondary to residual urine in the bladder
- Hematuria
- Hydronephrosis
- Bladder neck obstruction symptoms that bother the client, such as urinary frequency and nocturia

The goals of surgical intervention are to relieve the symptoms of bladder neck obstruction and to improve quality of life. Accomplishment of these goals allows the client to void at normal intervals while retaining adequate urinary control and normal sexual functioning.

Preoperative Care. When planning surgical interventions, the client's general physical condition, the size of the prostate gland, and the client's preferences are considered.

CONSIDERATIONS FOR OLDER ADULTS

The client is evaluated for any other diseases that are common in older persons, such as cardiovascular disease, chronic pulmonary disease, diabetes mellitus, or renal disease. If the client has renal disease, an indwelling catheter may be inserted. Closely monitor the client's intake, output, and serum electrolyte and creatinine levels until renal status has improved. In some cases, the client may have another medical condition that makes surgery too risky. In such cases, bladder neck obstruction may be relieved by permanent indwelling urinary drainage. The client is also assessed for the presence of urinary tract infection. Any infection is treated before surgery.

The client may have many fears and misconceptions about prostatic surgery, such as believing that automatic loss of sexual functioning or permanent incontinence will occur. Assess the client's anxiety, correct any misconceptions about the surgery, and provide accurate information to him and his family or significant others. Regardless of the type of surgery to be performed, provide information about anesthesia (see Chapter 21). The client may have other medical problems that increase the risk for complications of general anesthesia and may be advised to have regional anesthesia. Epidural or spinal anesthesia may be used for any of the procedures and are the most common types of anesthesia used for a transurethral resection of the prostate. Because the client is awake, it is easier to assess for hyponatremia, fluid overload, and water intoxication.

It is important to include the topic of urinary catheters in the teaching plan before surgery. After prostatic surgery, all clients have an indwelling urethral catheter for at least a day. Be sure that the client knows that he will feel the urge to void while the catheter is in place. Tell the client that he may also have continuous bladder irrigation (CBI) and traction on the catheter, but this may not be known until the client returns from the postanesthesia care unit (PACU). Also explain before surgery that it is normal for the urine to be blood-tinged after surgery. Small blood clots and tissue debris may pass while the catheter is in place and immediately after it is removed.

Operative Procedures. Several surgical procedures are possible for removing the enlarged portion of the prostate gland (Figure 79-3). In all approaches, the surgeon removes the hyperplastic tissue and leaves the prostatic capsule.

In the last few years, a variety of less invasive surgical procedures for BPH have emerged. These procedures are recommended as alternatives to drug therapy or when drug therapy fails. These procedures are generally recommended for clients in the early stages of the disease. Such procedures include the following:
- Transurethral thermotherapy (uses microwave thermotherapy)
- Transurethral needle ablation B, also known as TUNA procedure (uses low level radio frequency energy)

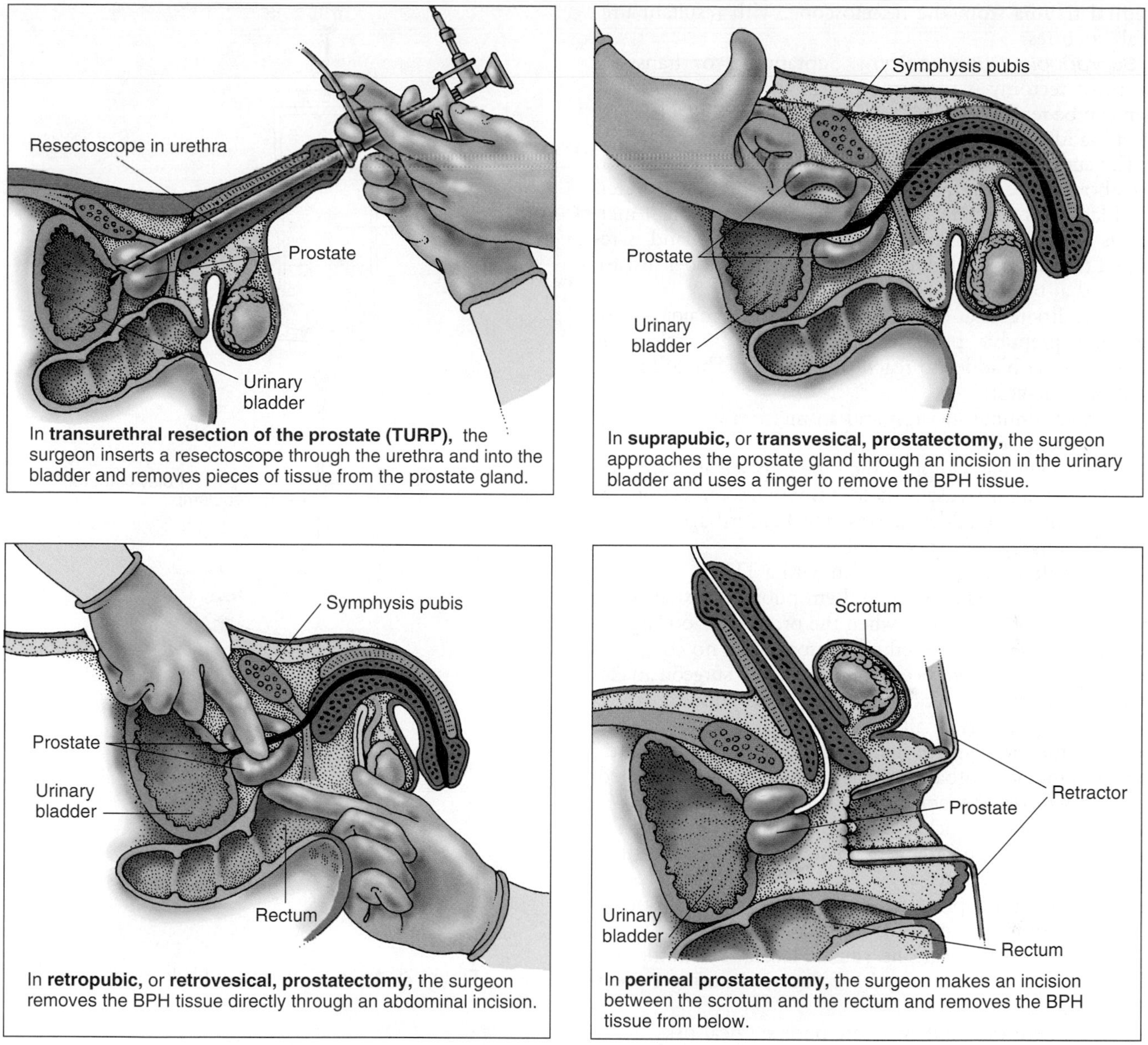

In **transurethral resection of the prostate (TURP),** the surgeon inserts a resectoscope through the urethra and into the bladder and removes pieces of tissue from the prostate gland.

In **suprapubic,** or **transvesical, prostatectomy,** the surgeon approaches the prostate gland through an incision in the urinary bladder and uses a finger to remove the BPH tissue.

In **retropubic,** or **retrovesical, prostatectomy,** the surgeon removes the BPH tissue directly through an abdominal incision.

In **perineal prostatectomy,** the surgeon makes an incision between the scrotum and the rectum and removes the BPH tissue from below.

Figure 79-3 ■ Prostatectomy procedures. *BPH,* Benign prostatic hyperplasia.

- Visual laser ablation (uses laser energy)
- Electrovaporization (uses electrocautery) of the prostate.

The advantages of these minimally invasive procedures are that there is less bleeding after surgery and the client can be discharged from the hospital within 24 hours with a retention catheter. Teach the client to monitor for catheter patency, hematuria, and infection after surgery. Also tell clients and their caregivers that delayed hematuria and urinary retention may occur days to weeks after the electrovaporization procedure.

Transurethral Resection of the Prostate. The traditional **transurethral resection of the prostate (TURP)** is a "closed" surgical procedure and is still commonly performed. The prostate may also be removed using an "open" procedure because of the need for a surgical incision. The choice of procedure depends on the following:

- The size of the prostate gland
- The location of the enlargement
- Whether surgery on the bladder is also needed
- The client's age and physical condition

To perform the TURP procedure, the surgeon inserts a resectoscope (an instrument similar to a cystoscope, but with a cutting and cauterizing loop) through the urethra. The enlarged portion of the prostate gland is then resected in small pieces (prostate chips).

This procedure is used when the area of major enlargement is in the medial lobe of the prostate that directly surrounds the urethra and when the amount of tissue to be removed is relatively small. A TURP is safer for the client who is at high risk for open surgery because a surgical incision is not used. Hospitalization and convalescence are shorter than with any other type of **prostatectomy** (prostate removal).

The disadvantage of a TURP is that because only small pieces of the gland are removed, remaining prostate tissue may continue to grow and cause urinary obstruction, requiring additional TURPs. There is also the possibility of urethral trauma from the resectoscope, with resultant urethral strictures.

Suprapubic Prostatectomy. Suprapubic, or transvesical, prostatectomy is performed when the prostate is larger than can be removed transurethrally and if the client has any other bladder problems that can be treated at the same time.

The surgeon makes a low horizontal abdominal incision just above the symphysis pubis and exposes the bladder. The bladder is then distended with fluid, and a small incision is made in the bladder wall. The prostate gland is removed through the bladder cavity, and any bladder disease is treated at this time.

The ability to treat bladder problems is the major advantage of suprapubic prostatectomy because an incision is made into the bladder to reach the prostate. The following are disadvantages:

- An abdominal incision and an incision into the bladder are necessary.
- The client has a suprapubic tube in place after surgery.
- There is an increased risk for urinary tract infection, incontinence, bladder spasms, and hemorrhage.
- The surgery is more painful.
- Convalescence is longer than with a TURP.

Retropubic Prostatectomy. Retropubic, or extravesical, prostatectomy is performed when the prostate is too large to be resected via the transurethral approach but no coexisting bladder problems have been identified. The surgeon makes an abdominal incision above the symphysis pubis to expose the prostate gland. A small incision is made in the prostate capsule, and the gland is removed. This procedure differs from suprapubic approach in that the bladder is not entered.

Perineal Prostatectomy. Perineal prostatectomy is mainly performed to achieve the following:

- Removal of an enlarged prostate gland that is filled with calculi (stones)
- Treatment of prostatic abscesses that have not responded to conservative treatment
- Repair of complications, such as lacerations in the prostatic capsule, that may have occurred during a previous surgery
- Treatment of clients who are poor surgical risks

The client is placed in an exaggerated lithotomy position, and the knees are positioned on the chest. The surgeon makes a U-shaped incision between the scrotum and the rectum. The prostatic capsule is then opened and the tissue removed. This procedure provides direct access to the prostate gland.

The major disadvantage of this procedure is the loss of sexual potency resulting from damage to the pudendal nerve. Clients with peripheral vascular disease or chronic pulmonary problems cannot tolerate the exaggerated lithotomy position and are not candidates for this procedure. Other disadvantages include a greater risk for infection, the possibility of damage to the rectum and anal sphincter, and the possibility of urinary incontinence. Thus this approach is not commonly used.

Postoperative Care. The care after surgery for the client who has undergone prostatic surgery is similar regardless of the type of procedure done and the type of anesthesia used (see Chapter 22). However, be aware of several differences because they affect nursing care.

Nursing Care After a Transurethral Resection Prostatectomy. After a TURP, the surgeon inserts a three-way urinary catheter with a 30- to 45-mL retention balloon through the urethra into the bladder (Figure 79-4). The catheter is pulled down into the prostatic fossa to help prevent bleeding. Traction is often applied on the catheter by pulling it taut and taping it to the client's abdomen or thigh.

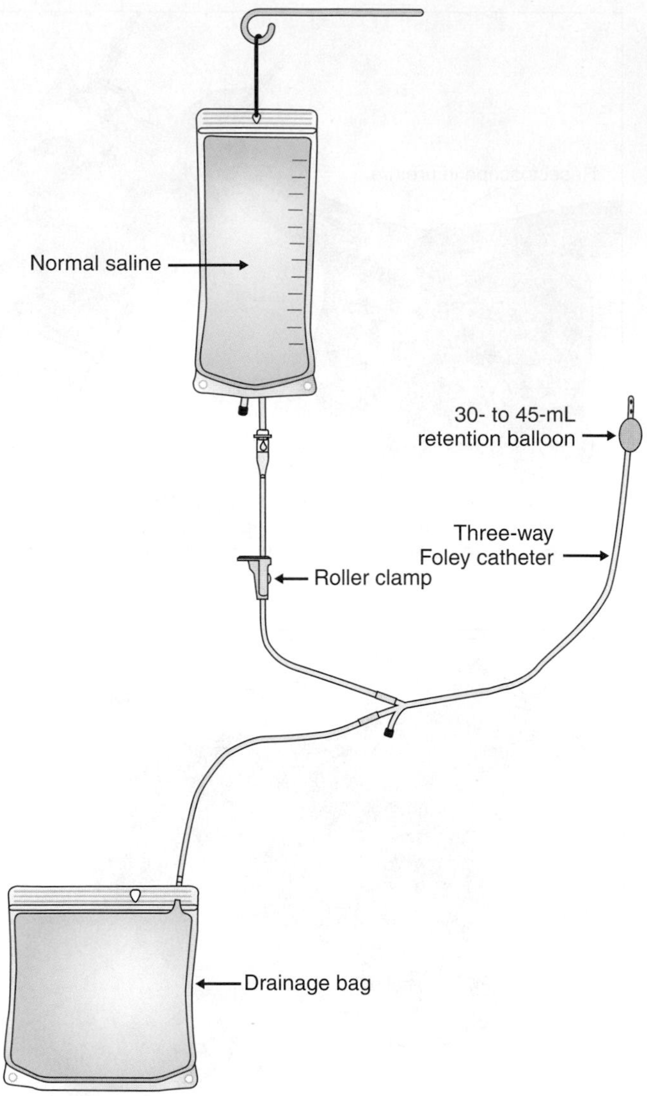

Figure 79-4 ■ Continuous bladder irrigation.

CATHETER CARE AND CONTINUOUS BLADDER IRRIGATION. Chart 79-2 lists intervention activities for the client after prostate surgery. If the catheter is taped to the client's thigh, instruct him to keep his leg straight. The surgeon determines when the traction should be removed; usually it is removed on the first day after surgery.

Explain that because of the retention catheter's large diameter and the pressure of the retention balloon on the internal sphincter of the bladder, the client will feel the urge to void continuously. This is a normal sensation, not a surgical complication. Advise the client not to try to void around the catheter, which causes the bladder muscles to contract and may result in painful bladder spasms. Reassure him that an antispasmodic drug can be given to keep him comfortable.

CONSIDERATIONS FOR OLDER ADULTS

When caring for older men who may become confused after surgery, reorient them frequently and remind them not to pull on the catheter. If the client is restless or "picks" at tubes, provide a familiar object, such as a family picture, for him to hold for distraction and a feeling of security. The client should not be restrained unless all other alternatives have failed.

Continuous bladder irrigation (CBI) with normal saline or other solution, as prescribed, helps to keep the catheter free of obstruction and facilitates detection of obstruction or other complications. Adjust the irrigation fluid rate to maintain a colorless or light pink drainage return. (For the nursing care of the client undergoing CBI, see Chart 79-3.) The continuous irrigation is usually discontinued 24 hours after a TURP. The retention catheter is usually removed when CBI is discontinued.

POSTCATHETERIZATION CARE. When the urinary catheter is removed, the client may experience some burning on urination as well as some urinary frequency, dribbling, and leakage. Reassure the client that these symptoms are normal and will subside. The client may also pass small clots and tissue debris for several days after the TURP. Instruct him to increase fluid intake to at least 2000 to 2500 mL daily, which helps to decrease the dysuria and keep the urine clear. An older client who has renal disease or who is at risk for heart failure may not be able to tolerate this much fluid. By the time of discharge (usually 2 days after surgery), he should be voiding 150 to 200 mL of clear yellow urine every 3 to 4 hours. By discharge, pain is minimal and analgesics may not be required.

COMPLICATIONS OF TRANSURETHRAL RESECTION OF THE PROSTATE. Clients who undergo a TURP or open prostatectomy are at risk for bleeding or hemorrhage after surgery. Bleeding is most common within the first 24 hours. Bladder spasms or movement may trigger fresh bleeding from previously controlled vessels. This bleeding may be arterial or venous, but venous bleeding is more common.

Monitor the client's urine output every 2 hours and vital signs every 4 hours. If the bleeding is arterial, the urinary drainage is bright red or ketchup-like with numerous clots. If arterial bleeding occurs, notify the surgeon immediately and increase the CBI rate or intermittently irrigate the catheter with normal saline solution. The surgeon may prescribe aminocaproic acid (Amicar) to control bleeding. Keep in mind that if the drug does not work, surgical intervention may be needed to clear the bladder of clots and to stop the bleeding.

If the bleeding is venous, the urine output is burgundy, with or without any change in vital signs. Inform the surgeon of any manifestations of bleeding. The surgeon may apply traction on the catheter for a few hours, which may control venous bleeding. Assess the success of this procedure in stopping the bleeding. Be aware that the traction on the catheter is quite uncomfortable and increases the risk for bladder spasms. Analgesics or antispasmodics, such as dicyclomine hydrochloride (Bentyl, Antispas, Formulex✱, Lomine✱), oxybutynin (Ditropan), or belladonna and opium (B&O) suppositories, are usually prescribed to decrease painful bladder spasms.

Closely monitor the client's hemoglobin (Hgb) and hematocrit (Hct) levels for anemia as a result of blood loss. Some clients may require blood transfusions to return the Hgb and Hct values to baseline levels.

CHART 79-3

BEST PRACTICE for
Care of the Client After Prostate Surgery

- Monitor the client closely for signs of infection. Older clients undergoing prostate surgery often also have underlying chronic diseases (such as cardiovascular disease, chronic lung disease, or diabetes) and multiple invasive lines that predispose them to infections.
- Help the client out of the bed to the chair as soon as permitted to prevent complications of immobility. Older clients may need assistance because of underlying changes in the musculoskeletal system, such as decreased range of motion and stiffness in joints. These clients are at *high risk* for falls.
- Encourage the client to turn, cough, and deep breathe and to use the incentive spirometer every 2 hours to prevent atelectasis and pneumonia. Older adults are at risk for pneumonia because of the decreases in lung elasticity and vital capacity associated with aging.
- Assess the client's pain every 2 to 3 hours, and give pain medication as needed.
- Provide a safe environment for the client. Anticipate a temporary change in mental status for the older client in the immediate postoperative period as a result of anesthetics and unfamiliar surroundings. Reorient the client frequently. Keep IV lines and catheter tubes secure.
- Use normal saline solution for the bladder irrigant unless otherwise prescribed. Normal saline solution is isotonic.
- Adjust the rate of the irrigation solution to the physician's specifications. The physician may prescribe a solution rate that keeps the output clear and free of clots.
- Monitor the color, consistency, and amount of urine output.
- Check the drainage tubing frequently for external obstructions (such as kinks) and internal obstructions (such as blood clots and decreased output).
- Assess the client for reports of bladder spasms, which may indicate obstruction.
- If the urinary catheter is obstructed, turn off the continuous bladder irrigation (CBI), and irrigate the catheter with 30 to 50 mL of normal saline solution using a large piston syringe.
- Notify the physician immediately if the obstruction does not resolve by hand irrigation or if the urinary return becomes "ketchupy."

Nursing Care After Suprapubic Prostatectomy. If the client has undergone a suprapubic prostatectomy, a suprapubic catheter, in addition to a urethral catheter, will be in place. Each catheter is connected to a separate closed drainage system and drains the bladder via gravity. Be aware that catheter traction is not effective for the client who has bleeding after a suprapubic prostatectomy. This client needs brisk CBI via the catheter. If the CBI does not control the bleeding, the client needs surgical intervention.

If the client has a suprapubic catheter in place, the urethral catheter is generally removed on the second day after surgery. After the retention catheter is removed, clamp the suprapubic catheter and instruct the client to attempt to void. After the client has urinated, check the residual urine in the bladder by unclamping the suprapubic tube. The client may be discharged from the hospital with a suprapubic catheter in place. When the client consistently empties his bladder and the residual urine in the bladder is 75 mL or less, the suprapubic catheter is then removed. An antimicrobial ointment may be applied daily to the site, depending on hospital's policy or the physician's preference.

The client with a suprapubic catheter in place is at increased risk for bladder spasms. Observe the incision dressing at least twice per shift, and change it frequently because the dressing becomes saturated with urine until the incision heals. If the suprapubic drain is not connected to gravity drainage, enclose the drain with an ostomy bag to measure the output accurately and to prevent any skin problems or breakdown.

Nursing Care After Retropubic Prostatectomy. After a retropubic prostatectomy, the urinary sphincter muscles are seldom damaged, the bladder is not entered, and no urinary drainage should be seen on the abdominal dressing. Notify the surgeon of any urinary or purulent drainage, fever, or increased pain because these symptoms indicate a serious complication such as a deep wound infection or pelvic abscess.

Nursing Care After Perineal Prostatectomy. After the perineal approach to prostatectomy, the client has an incision dressing and may or may not have an incision drain. Rectal thermometers and rectal tubes or enemas are not used because they may cause trauma or bleeding.

Community-Based Care

The client with benign prostatic hyperplasia (BPH) is typically managed at home. Clients who have surgery are also discharged to their home.

HOME CARE MANAGEMENT

Unless there is a complication of surgery, such as a wound infection or an unusual problem with voiding, the client does not have a dressing or indwelling catheter at the time of discharge. In some cases, the suprapubic tube may remain in place for several weeks after discharge.

HEALTH TEACHING

After any type of prostatectomy, some clients, especially those who have undergone a transurethral resection of the prostate (TURP), may have temporary loss of control of urination or a dribbling of the urine. Reassure the client that these symptoms are almost always temporary and will resolve. Assist the client and his family in devising ways to keep his clothing dry until sphincter control returns. Instruct him to contract and relax his sphincter frequently to re-establish urinary control (Kegel exercises). External urinary (condom or Texas) catheters are not used except in extreme cases because they may give the client a false sense of security and delay his urinary control.

Provide specific instructions for each client on the basis of the type of surgical procedure performed and any interventions he may need in the future. Discharge instructions for a client undergoing surgery of the prostate gland are listed in Chart 79-4.

CHART 79-4

CLIENT EDUCATION GUIDE

Care After a Transurethral Resection of the Prostate

- Drink 12 to 14 glasses of water each day, preferably before 8 PM, *unless otherwise contraindicated.*
- Use alcohol, caffeinated beverages, and spicy foods in moderation to avoid overstimulation of your bladder.
- If your urine becomes bloody, rest quietly and increase your fluid intake. If the bleeding does not subside shortly, contact your doctor.
- Avoid strenuous activities, such as driving and working, during the first 2 to 3 weeks after surgery.
- Schedule a follow-up appointment with your doctor after you leave the hospital.

The client who undergoes prostatic surgery usually needs emotional support. The client who undergoes a perineal prostatectomy is at risk for permanent sexual dysfunction. Inform the client of the options, such as a penile prosthesis, that are available to treat erectile dysfunction (ED) (see Interventions [Erectile Dysfunction], p. 1871).

Other surgical procedures for prostate removal should not cause physiologic ED. However, some clients may have functional ED for a short time after surgery during the recovery phase.

Critical Thinking Challenge

You are starting a new shift and are caring for a man who returned from the PACU 3 hours ago after a TURP. He received epidural anesthesia for this surgery. He is receiving continuous bladder irrigation with normal saline. The flow sheet at the bedside indicates that a 1500-mL bag of normal saline was hung 1 hour ago. The bag is now empty, and there is only 200 mL of fluid in the drainage bag of the three-way catheter.

1. What assessment data should you obtain?
2. What action should you take as soon as possible?
3. Should the next bag of irrigation solution be started now? Why or Why not?
4. Which staff member should be assigned to care for this client during the rest of the shift: registered nurse, LPN, nursing assistant? Provide a rationale for your choice.

evolve For suggested answer guidelines, go to http://evolve.elsevier.com/Iggy/.

PROSTATE CANCER

PATHOPHYSIOLOGY

Prostate cancer is the most common invasive cancer among American men. It follows lung cancer as the second leading cause of cancer deaths in this group (American Cancer Society, 2005a).

Of all cancers of the prostate, 95% are adenocarcinomas. These cancers arise from the epithelial cells of the prostate and are usually located in the posterior lobe or outer portion of the gland (Figure 79-5). The remaining types of prostatic neoplasms are classified as *nonepithelial* carcinomas and include ductal carcinomas, transitional cell carcinomas, squamous cell carcinomas, and sarcomas.

Of all malignancies, prostate cancer is one of the slowest growing, and it metastasizes in a predictable pattern. Common sites of metastasis are the nearby lymph nodes; bone marrow; and the bones of the pelvis, sacrum, and lumbar spine.

Spread to the visceral organs occurs late in the course of the disease. Common organ sites of metastasis for prostate cancer are the lungs, liver, adrenals, and kidneys.

Tumor grade is an important factor in the management of prostate cancer. Grading is the pathologist's interpretation of the aggressiveness of the cancer. Usually the Gleason grading system is used. Normal prostate tissue cells are given a score of 1 (best), and abnormal cells are given a score of up to 5 (worst). The scores of the two most common cell types found in the specimen are added to give the tumor a grade between 2 and 10.

Etiology and Genetic Risk

Although the cause of prostate cancer remains unclear, several factors influence its development. First, an intact hypothalamic-pituitary-testicular pathway must be present. Men who have been castrated before puberty are at little risk for prostate cancer. Second, the advancing age of the client increases his risk of prostate cancer.

Other contributing factors include a family history of prostate cancer, heavy metal exposure, and a history of vasectomy or sexually transmitted disease (STD). Several viruses, including cytomegalovirus and herpesvirus type 2, are present more commonly in prostate cancer cells than in normal cells.

Genetic Considerations

Most prostate cancers are sporadic in nature, meaning that no clear pattern of inheritance emerges. However, some genetic influences for prostate cancer have been discovered. The risk for prostate cancer is greater among men who have a first-degree relative (father, brother, or son) with prostate cancer. Inherited forms of prostate cancer are suspected, and some are known. People who have specific *BRCA-2* gene mutations have an increased risk for breast cancer and an increased risk for prostate cancer among male carriers. For individuals who have these gene mutations, prostate cancer develops at an earlier age and usually has a more aggressive profile. Other gene mutations are being studied in the hope of developing a test to more accurately assess risk for prostate cancer development.

Incidence/Prevalence

Prostate cancer is the sixth most common cancer worldwide. It is mainly a cancer of older men and occurs rarely before age 39 years. The rate increases after age 40 to as many as one in six between the ages of 60 and 79 (American Cancer Society, 2005a). Recent increases in incidence rates in the United States are related to earlier diagnosis through an increase in mass screenings with prostate specific antigen (PSA) levels and digital rectal examinations (DRE). The actual incidence in the United States has stabilized. The American Cancer Society estimates that 232,090 new cases of prostate cancer will be diagnosed in 2005 and that 30,350 deaths will result from the disease. Prostate cancer has a higher incidence in less affluent countries and a low incidence in Asian countries.

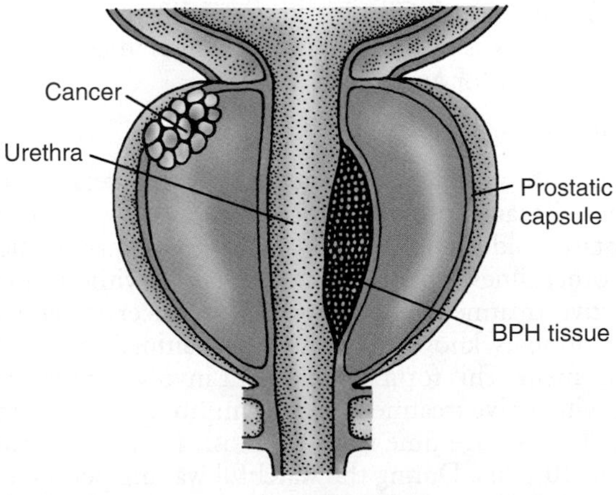

Figure 79-5 ■ The prostate gland with cancer and benign prostatic hyperplasia (BPH). Note that cancer normally arises in the periphery of the gland, whereas BPH occurs in the center of the gland.

CONSIDERATIONS FOR OLDER ADULTS

The incidence of prostate cancer increases with age. More than 75% of all prostate cancers are diagnosed in men over 65 years of age (American Cancer Society, 2005a). Include questions about prostate problems whenever you are assessing the health of an older adult male.

CULTURAL CONSIDERATIONS

African-American men tend to be affected at an earlier age and have more advanced disease at diagnosis. The American Cancer Society estimates that 27,000 African-American men will be diagnosed with prostate cancer in 2005 and that 5300 will die of the disease. Lack of cancer awareness may be one cause of increased mortality rates. Reduced access to primary care and screening is another factor. New guidelines for prostate cancer screening recommend that African-American men begin screening by age 45 years (ACS, 2005a; ACS, 2005b).

◆COLLABORATIVE MANAGEMENT

◆Assessment

HISTORY

As with any cancer, accurate staging is needed for treatment planning and for monitoring the course of the disease. As in BPH, the first symptoms that the client may experience are related to bladder neck obstruction, such as difficulty in initiating urination, recurrent bladder infections, and urinary retention. Gross, painless hematuria is the most common presenting manifestation.

A client may be undergoing treatment for BPH and is discovered to have prostate cancer. Bone pain is a symptom of a more advanced stage of prostate cancer. The client who has symptoms of urinary obstruction (urinary hesitancy, back pain) and bone pain is likely to have metastatic disease at diagnosis.

PHYSICAL EXAMINATION AND PROSTATE CANCER SCREENING

The most effective screening procedures for prostate cancer are the **digital rectal examination (DRE)** and the PSA test. Chart 79-5 lists the American Cancer Society's prostate cancer screening guideline. Beginning at age 50 years, all men should have an annual DRE and PSA test. Men at higher risk for prostate cancer, including African Americans or men who have a first-degree relative with prostate cancer, should start screening at 45 years of age.

DIGITAL RECTAL EXAMINATION. On rectal examination, a prostate that is found to be stony hard and with palpable irregularities or indurations is suspected to be malignant.

PROSTATE-SPECIFIC ANTIGEN. **Prostate-specific antigen (PSA)** is a glycoprotein produced solely by the prostate. The normal blood level of PSA is less than 4 ng/mL.

CHART 79-5

CLIENT EDUCATION GUIDE
American Cancer Society Prostate Screening and Detection Guidelines (2005)

- An annual digital rectal examination (DRE) and prostate-specific antigen (PSA) test should be offered to the following clients:
  - Men beginning at age 50 years
  - Men who have a life expectancy of at least 10 years
  - Younger men who are at high risk (at least by age 45 years)
- Men at high risk include those with a strong familial predisposition (e.g., two or more first-degree relatives with prostate cancer) and African-American men.
- DRE should be performed by health care professionals skilled in recognizing subtle prostate abnormalities.
- DRE is less effective than PSA in detecting prostate cancer. An abnormal PSA test result is a value above 4.0 ng/mL.

PSA levels are higher in clients with increased prostatic tissue as a result of BPH, prostatic infarction, prostatitis, and prostate cancer. The levels associated with prostate cancer are usually much higher than those occurring with other prostate tissue enlargement.

Prostate-specific antigen blood levels should never be used as a screening test without a digital rectal examination (DRE) of the prostate. *The PSA serum level does not replace the DRE but is to be used in conjunction with it.* Because other prostate problems also increase the PSA level, it is not specifically diagnostic for cancer. In addition, about 25% of clients with prostate cancer have PSA levels less than 4 ng/mL.

The PSA is not elevated in healthy men or in men with cancer in other organs. However, the normal PSA level is slightly higher in older adults and in African Americans. An elevated PSA level should decrease a few days after a prostatectomy. An increase in the PSA level several weeks after surgery usually indicates that the disease has recurred.

OTHER DIAGNOSTIC ASSESSMENTS

After screening by DRE and PSA, some clients undergo a transrectal ultrasound study of the prostate. The urologist inserts a small probe into the rectum and obtains an ultrasonogram of the prostate. A specimen for biopsy may also be obtained with the rectal probe.

BIOPSY

When the diagnosis of prostatic cancer is suspected, a biopsy is necessary for confirmation. Prostatic ultrasonography may be performed to isolate the area of the prostate for biopsy. One of several procedures may be used to obtain the biopsy specimen. The most common procedure is the needle-core or aspiration biopsy.

After a transrectal ultrasound with biopsy, instruct the client about possible complications, including hematuria with clots, signs of infection, and perineal pain. Instruct the client to report fever, chills, bloody urine, and any difficulty voiding. Usually antibiotics are prescribed. Stress to the client the importance of completing the entire course. Advise the client to avoid strenuous physical activity and drink plenty of fluids, especially in the first 24 hours after the procedure.

After the diagnosis of prostate cancer is made, the client undergoes radiographic and blood studies to ascertain the extent of the disease. Common tests include computed tomography (CT) of the pelvis and abdomen and magnetic resonance imaging (MRI) to assess the status of the pelvic and para-aortic lymph nodes. A bone scan is performed to detect metastatic disease. An enlarged liver or abnormal liver function study results indicate possible liver metastases.

Clients with advanced prostate cancer may have elevated levels of serum acid phosphatase. About 90% of clients with bone metastasis have elevated serum alkaline phosphatase levels.

Critical Thinking Challenge

The client is a 70-year-old man who tells you he has had the following symptoms for a year: hesitancy, nocturia, hematuria, reduced size of the urinary stream, pain in the lower back and legs, and dribbling after voiding. He has never had a DRE or a PSA test. He tells you he is worried about possibly having prostate cancer for two reasons; one is that his father died of prostate cancer at age 75, and the other is that he had gonorrhea when he was 22 years old.

1. Which of this client's manifestations are more specific to prostate cancer, and which are common to prostate cancer and BPH?
2. Is this client's history of gonorrhea important to his current health problem? Why or why not?
3. Does the fact that this client's father died of prostate cancer increase the client's risk for it? Why or why not?

evolve For suggested answer guidelines, go to http://evolve.elsevier.com/Iggy/.

Common Nursing Diagnoses and Collaborative Problems

Nursing diagnoses and collaborative problems that may apply to clients with prostate cancer include the following:

- Anxiety related to a threat to or change in health status and treatment options
- Acute Pain or Chronic Pain related to effects of metastasis, bone pain, and spinal cord compression
- Impaired Urinary Elimination related to sensory motor impairment, blockage, or trauma
- Risk for Sexual Dysfunction related to altered body structure or function (secondary to disease process and treatment)
- Dysfunctional Grieving or Anticipatory Grieving related to loss of a body part or changes in body function
- Potential for Metastasis

Interventions

Clients with prostate cancer are faced with several treatment options. Because prostate cancer is slow growing with late metastasis, older adult clients who are asymptomatic and have other illness may choose observation without immediate active treatment, especially if the cancer is early stage. This option is known as "watchful waiting," or expectant management. This form of treatment involves initial surveillance with active treatment if the symptoms become bothersome. The average time from diagnosis to start of treatment is up to 10 years. During the watchful waiting period, clients are monitored at regular intervals through DRE and PSA testing. Factors that are considered in choosing watchful waiting include potential side effects of treatment (e.g., urinary incontinence, erectile dysfunction, bowel dysfunction), estimated life expectancy, and the risk for increased morbidity and mortality from not seeking active treatment.

Clients who have stage 0 cancer of the prostate who choose watchful waiting require only close follow-up by their health care provider. If obstruction occurs, repeated needle biopsies or transurethral resection of the prostate (TURPs) should be part of the screening.

Active treatment options for the client with prostate cancer include surgery, radiation therapy, and drug therapy. Management is based on the extent of the disease and the client's physical condition. The client may undergo surgery for a biopsy, staging and removal of the tumor, or palliation to control the spread of disease or relieve distressing symptoms. As with watchful waiting, the health care provider and client must weigh the benefits of treatment against potential adverse effects such as incontinence and erectile dysfunction (ED).

SURGICAL MANAGEMENT. Because as many as 30% of localized prostate cancers are resistant to radiation, surgery is the standard treatment. Usually a radical prostatectomy is performed. The surgical approaches for prostatectomy are similar to those for BPH (see Surgical Management [Benign Prostatic Hyperplasia], p. 1860). However, the surgery is much more extensive.

Preoperative Care. The surgeon advises clients who are undergoing radical perineal prostatectomy that they may have erectile dysfunction (ED) after the surgery. This consequence is directly related to any damage done to the pudendal nerve (which is needed for erection and orgasm) during the surgery. Another consequence of this surgery is the possibility of urinary incontinence. To help reduce the severity of incontinence, teach the client how to perform **Kegel exercises** (exercises that strengthen the pubococcygeus muscle) before surgery. These exercises are continued after surgery.

For the client undergoing a radical prostatectomy, the preoperative procedure includes bowel cleansing using a cathartic such as GoLYTELY. The client is usually permitted to have a clear liquid diet the day before surgery, with nothing by mouth after midnight. Drugs for other pre-existing conditions may be taken the morning of surgery with only sips of water. Provide psychosocial and spiritual supportive measures as needed.

Operative Procedures. The radical prostatectomy can be performed via a retropubic, perineal, or suprapubic approach. The surgeon removes the entire prostate gland along with the prostatic capsule, the cuff at the bladder neck, the seminal vesicles, and the regional lymph nodes. The remaining urethra is anastomosed to the bladder neck. The removal of tissue at the bladder neck allows the seminal fluid to travel upward into the bladder rather than down the urethral tract, resulting in retrograde ejaculations. The client is sterile.

Often the pudendal nerves are damaged or severed during a radical prostatectomy. The surgeon may perform a "nerve-sparing" prostatectomy in the following cases:

- There is no evidence of disease in adjacent lymph nodes.
- Serum acid phosphatase levels are not elevated.
- There is no evidence of cancer beyond the prostate gland.

As the name of the procedure implies, the surgeon keeps the nerves responsible for penile erection intact. After surgery, the client may experience temporary ED, but normal function usually returns in 3 to 12 months.

CHART 79-6

BEST PRACTICE for
Care of the Client After a Radical Prostatectomy

- Encourage the client to use patient-controlled analgesia (PCA) as needed. The PCA device may be used through the second postoperative day.
- Keep the client on bedrest on the day of surgery. Help the client to get out of bed and ambulate for a short distance by the first postoperative day.
- Maintain the sequential compression device until the client begins to ambulate. Apply antiembolic stockings until discharge.
- Monitor the client for deep vein thrombosis and pulmonary embolus.
- Keep an accurate record of intake and output, including Jackson-Pratt or other drainage device drainage.
- Keep the urinary meatus clean using soap and water.
- Avoid rectal procedures or treatments.
- Teach the client how to care for the urinary catheter because he will be discharged with the catheter in place.
- Teach the client how to use a leg bag.
- Emphasize the importance of not straining during bowel movement. Advise the client to avoid suppositories or enemas.
- Remind the client about the importance of follow-up appointments with the physician to monitor progress.

Postoperative Care. Care of the client after radical prostatectomy is listed in Chart 79-6. Activities include all the typical care for a client undergoing major surgery. These issues include maintaining hydration with IV therapy, caring for wound drains, preventing emboli, and preventing pulmonary complications (see Chapter 22).

Drug therapy after surgery includes antibiotics to prevent infection and analgesics for pain. Pain is managed with opioids given IV with patient-controlled analgesia (PCA), a common method of delivery. A laxative and stool softener may be given to prevent possible constipation from the drugs.

The client has an indwelling urinary catheter to straight drainage. An antispasmodic may be prescribed to decrease bladder spasm induced by the indwelling urinary catheter. Belladonna and opium suppositories are avoided because rectal manipulation may injure the surgical site. Kegel exercises, taught before surgery, should be performed consistently throughout the day.

The client may have a nasogastric tube (NGT) to low intermittent suction because of the extensive surgery. The NGT is usually discontinued on the second day after surgery. The client is then permitted clear liquids. Solid foods are introduced as tolerated when bowel sounds return.

Ambulation begins early, usually by the second day after surgery. Provide assistance in ambulating the client at least twice a day. Scrotal or penile swelling may occur from the disruption in pelvic lymph flow. If this occurs, elevate the scrotum and penis and apply ice to the area intermittently (20 minutes on and 20 minutes off) for the first 24 to 48 hours.

Complications. Common potential long-term complications of radical prostatectomy are urinary incontinence and erectile dysfunction.

Urinary Incontinence. Incontinence is possible because the internal and external sphincters of the bladder lie close to the prostate gland and are often damaged during the surgery.

EVIDENCE-BASED PRACTICE for Nursing

Clients and society are not prepared for male incontinence

Palmer, M.H., et al. (2003). Incontinence after prostatectomy: Coping with incontinence after prostate cancer surgery. *Oncology Nursing Forum, 30*(2), 229-238.

The purpose of this survey study was to describe the nature of postprostatectomy urinary incontinence, determine how men manage postsurgery urinary incontinence, identify men's perceptions of adequacy of preoperative counseling, and identify men's expectations regarding the probability of postsurgery incontinence. Subjects were a convenience sample of 154 men postprostatectomy who belonged to the support group, "US TOO." Subjects self-selected to complete a questionnaire with both forced-choice items and open-ended questions.

Of the 154 subjects responding to the survey, 105 indicated that incontinence was or remained a significant problem with social, economic, and emotional effects. Subjects indicated that problems away from home, such as the availability of continence pads or garments, appropriate disposal sites, and the expectation of other men that continence is expected, were of greatest concern. Additionally, this study found that the incidence of persistent incontinence after prostate cancer surgery was greater than reported in the medical literature and that most men were not well-prepared to deal with the problem.

Level of Evidence: 6—Uncontrolled, descriptive study.

Critique. The use of a convenience sample and the self-selection may have biased study results toward the relatively high incidence of persistent incontinence. However, this study was valuable because it uncovered areas of need for male clients with any degree of incontinence.

Implications for Nursing. The study found that it is extremely important for nurses to give these clients information on more than one occasion. Preoperative information should be reinforced with additional follow-up information, emotional support, and practical assistance with management strategies for urinary incontinence. Nurses should promote the continued use of Kegel exercises to improve urine control. Because use of these exercises appeared to decline over time, continued teaching and reinforcement of the need to perform these exercises are important. Nurses can also be helpful by providing information on what types of continence care supplies are available and at what economic costs. Developing a "tip" sheet for how to manage incontinence away from home would also be useful.

Kegel perineal exercises have been shown to reduce the severity of urinary incontinence after radical prostatectomy (see the Evidence-Based Practice for Nursing box above).

Teach the client perineal exercises to help facilitate the return of urinary continence after surgery or after removal of the retention catheter. To perform the exercises, the client contracts and relaxes the perineal and gluteal muscles in several ways. For one of the exercises, teach the client to do the following:

1. Tighten the perineal muscles for 3 to 5 seconds as if to prevent voiding and then relax.
2. Bear down as if having a bowel movement.
3. Relax and repeat the exercise.

Show the client how to inhale through pursed lips while tightening the perineal muscles and how to exhale when he relaxes. To regain urinary control, teach the client to practice holding an object, such as a pencil, in the fold between the buttock and the thigh. He may also sit on the toilet with the knees apart while voiding and start and stop the stream several times.

Other interventions for incontinence that may be helpful after radical prostatectomy include biofeedback retraining and the surgical placement of an artificial urinary sphincter

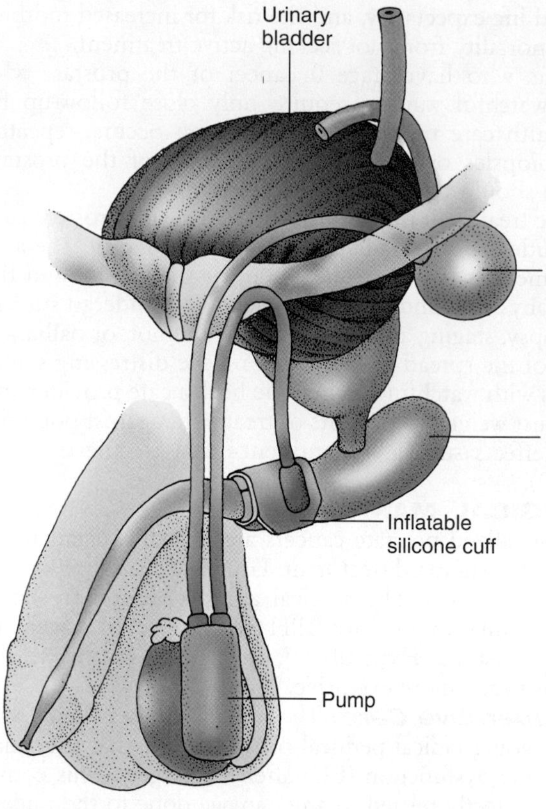

Figure 79-6 ■ An artificial urinary sphincter is a fluid-filled system with a silicone cuff that surrounds the urethra and functions as a urinary sphincter. A pump is placed in the scrotum, and a fluid reservoir is placed in the abdomen. When the pump is squeezed, fluid leaves the urethral cuff and flows into the reservoir, allowing the client to empty his bladder.

(Figure 79-6). Artificial sphincters have been more successful in men than in women, possibly because of the difference in urethral length. After sphincter implantation, instruct the client to report fever, pain on inflation of the device, edema or cellulitis in the genitalia (manifestations of infection), or recurrence of incontinence (indicating a possible mechanical malfunction of the device).

Erectile Dysfunction. Difficulty having or maintaining and erection is possible after radical prostatectomy because of damage to the pudendal nerves. Interventions for erectile dysfunction are presented on pp. 1870 to 1871.

Cryosurgical Ablation. **Cryoablation** is a minimally invasive procedure that can be an alternative to radical prostatectomy. This surgery is reserved for clients for whom the cancer is known to be confined to the prostate gland. During surgery, the client is placed in the lithotomy position, and a transrectal ultrasound probe is placed in the rectum. The probe helps to determine the size of the prostate and the subsequent number of small cryoprobes that are positioned around the prostate gland. Liquid nitrogen freezes the gland and results in prostate cell death. The dead cells are then absorbed gradually by the body.

The advantages of this procedure are minimal blood loss, minimal pain, decreased risk for urinary incontinence, and a short hospital stay. Most clients are able to return to their usual activity level in about 1 week after surgery. The procedure can be repeated if necessary.

CHART 79-7

DRUG THERAPY for Prostate Cancer: Hormone Therapy

Drug	Usual Dosage	Nursing Interventions
Leuprolide acetate (Lupron)	7.5 mg IM q mo	Use at least a 22-gauge needle. Mix the solution well; it is a milky suspension. Observe for side effects, including "hot flashes" and sweating. Be aware that the client's symptoms may temporarily worsen, caused by a temporary testosterone increase.
Flutamide (Eulexin, Euflex✱)	750 mg PO in 3 daily divided doses	Teach the client that side effects include "hot flashes," loss of libido, and impotence. Diarrhea and nausea with vomiting are less common.
Goserelin acetate (Zoladex)	3.6 mg SC every 28 days	The prefilled syringe cannot be aspirated. If a blood vessel is damaged, blood will enter the syringe. Teach the client that side effects include "hot flashes," sexual dysfunction, and decreased erections.

SC, Subcutaneous.

Bilateral Orchiectomy. **Bilateral orchiectomy** (removal of both testes) is palliative surgery and is not intended to cure the prostate cancer. The intent of the surgery is to arrest cancer spread by removing testosterone. This procedure is described later in this chapter under Testicular Cancer, p. 1874.

NONSURGICAL MANAGEMENT. Nonsurgical management is usually an adjunct to surgery but may be done as an alternative intervention. Modalities include radiation therapy, hormonal therapy, chemotherapy, and targeted therapy.

Radiation Therapy. External beam radiation therapy is used in the treatment of prostate cancer for the following purposes:

- As an alternative curative treatment to surgery for locally contained tumors
- As an adjunct to radical prostatectomy when surgical margins or regional lymph nodes show cancer cells after surgery
- For palliation of the client's symptoms

Palliative radiation therapy relieves pain caused by bone metastases and relieves ureteral or bladder neck obstruction.

Radiation therapy also can be performed by implanting low-dose radiation seeds directly into and around the prostate gland. This treatment includes ultrasonically guided iodine-125 or pallidium-103 interstitial brachytherapy (radiation therapy) or radioactive seed implantation. These procedures are done on an ambulatory care basis and are the most cost-effective treatment for early stage prostate cancer. Reassure the client that the dose of radiation is low and that he will not pose a hazard to himself or others. These treatments are well tolerated and have minimal complications.

Drug Therapy. Drug therapy may consist of either hormonal therapy or chemotherapy. A vaccine to locate and destroy prostate cancer cells is also being investigated (Marks, 2003).

Hormonal Therapy. Because prostate cancer is hormone dependent, clients with extensive tumors or those with metastatic disease are usually managed by androgen deprivation. Manipulating the hormonal environment in the client may be accomplished in two ways:

- The testosterone influence can be removed by a bilateral orchiectomy.
- Estrogens or gonadotropin-releasing hormone (GnRH) agonist analogs can be given (Chart 79-7).

Estrogens such as diethylstilbestrol (DES) inhibit the release of luteinizing hormone (LH) from the pituitary gland. Clients with significant cardiovascular disease may not be candidates for estrogen therapy because of the side effects of estrogens, such as sodium and water retention and thromboembolic episodes. Other hormonal drugs, such as megestrol (Megace) and medroxyprogesterone (Depo-Provera), are sometimes used if first-line hormonal treatments lose their effectiveness.

Leuprolide acetate (Lupron), a GnRH agonist analogue (which suppresses LH release by the pituitary) reduces serum testosterone levels without any of the estrogenic side effects of DES. Flutamide (Eulexin, Euflex✱), an oral androgen-blocking agent, inhibits tumor progression by blocking the uptake of testicular and adrenal androgens at the prostate tumor site.

Goserelin acetate (Zoladex), a potent GnRH agonist analogue, may be prescribed for palliation of advanced prostatic carcinoma. This drug is an alternative treatment when orchiectomy or estrogen administration is not acceptable or not indicated for the client.

Chemotherapy. Systemic cytotoxic chemotherapy has not proved effective as the main treatment of prostate cancer. It is used for the client who fails to respond to hormonal manipulation. Agents approved for this use are a combination of docetaxel (Taxotere) and prednisone. Estramustine (Emcyt) is another drug that combines an estrogen with the chemotherapy drug mechlorethamine. Although these therapies prolong survival, they do not cure the disease. Clinical trials are testing the effectiveness of thalidomide (Celgene), a drug that inhibits blood vessel formation, on prostate cancer. (See Chapter 28 for a discussion of chemotherapy.)

Targeted Therapy. A promising area of treatment for prostate cancer is targeted therapy. These therapies take advantage of one or more differences in a cancer cell that is either not present or only slightly present in normal cells. Agents used as targeted therapies are either antibodies that "target" a cellular element of the cancer cell or "antisense" drugs that work at the gene level. Some agents being tested as targeted therapy for prostate cancer are targeted to the

CHART 79-8

CLIENT EDUCATION GUIDE
Catheter Care at Home

- Once a day gently wash the first 6 inches of the catheter starting at the penis and washing outward with mild soap and water.
- Rinse and dry the catheter well.
- If you have not been circumcised, push the foreskin back to the clean the catheter site; when finished, push the foreskin forward.
- Change the drainage bag at least once a week.
  - Hold the catheter with one hand and the tubing with the other hand and twist in opposite directions to disconnect.
  - Place the end of the catheter in a clean container to catch leakage of urine.
  - Remove the rubber cap from the tubing of the leg bag or clean drainage bag.
  - Clean the end of the new tubing with alcohol swabs.
  - Insert the end of the new tubing into the catheter and twist to connect securely.
- Clean the drainage bag just removed by pouring a solution of one part vinegar to two parts water through the tubing and bag. Rinse well with water and allow the bag to dry.

epidermal growth factor receptor. Another targeting drug in clinical trials for prostate cancer is bortezomib (Velcade), a proteosome inhibitor.

Community-Based Care

Nursing management of the client with prostate cancer always includes his spouse or sexual partner. Clients with prostate cancer may require nursing interventions in a wide variety of settings: at the hospital, the radiation therapy department, the oncologist's office, or home and at any stage of the disease process. The following interventions focus on the needs of clients who have undergone radical prostatectomy for prostate cancer.

HOME CARE MANAGEMENT

Discharge planning and health teaching start early, even before surgery. A client can better plan home care management when he knows what to expect. A case manager working with the client throughout treatment is helpful in coordinating the efforts of the physician, surgical unit nursing staff, and home care nurse. The client then has one person with whom he can feel connected and can rely on for information and referral. The case manager provides continuity.

HEALTH TEACHING

An important area of teaching for the client going home after radical prostatectomy is catheter care. An indwelling urinary catheter may be in place for up to 3 weeks. Teach the client how to care for the catheter, use a leg bag, and identify manifestations of infection and other complications. See Chart 79-8 for information on teaching clients about catheter care in the home.

Walking short distances is encouraged, but lifting is restricted to no more than 15 pounds for up to 6 weeks. Clients need to maintain an upright position and not walk bent or flexed. Vigorous exercise such as running or jumping should be avoided for at least 12 weeks and then gradually introduced.

Instruct the client not to strain to defecate. A stool softener may be prescribed to reduce the need for straining. If an opioid is prescribed for pain management, encourage the client to drink plenty of water to prevent constipation.

Instruct the client to shower rather than soak in a bathtub for the first 2 to 3 weeks. Teach him how to inspect the incision site daily for signs of infection. Follow-up appointments are scheduled in 1 week for removal of the staples and in 2 to 3 weeks for removal of the urinary catheter. PSA blood tests are taken 6 weeks after surgery and then every 4 to 6 months to monitor progress.

HEALTH CARE RESOURCES

Refer the client and family to agencies or support groups such as the American Cancer Society's Man to Man program to help cope with prostate cancer. This program provides one-on-one education, personal visits, educational presentations, and the opportunity to engage in open and candid discussions. Another prostate cancer support group is "US TOO," sponsored by the American Foundation for Urologic Disease. This group provides education and support with national and international chapters.

ERECTILE DYSFUNCTION

PATHOPHYSIOLOGY

Erectile dysfunction (ED), previously known as impotence, is the inability to achieve or maintain an erection for sexual intercourse. It affects about 10 to 20 million men in the United States. During the last decade, there has been a major change in the management of men with ED as a result of increased understanding of the physiology of erectile function and the development of new, effective therapies. There are two classes of ED: organic and functional.

Organic Erectile Dysfunction

Organic ED is a gradual deterioration of function. The man first notices diminishing firmness and a decrease in frequency of erections. Causes include the following:

- Inflammation of the prostate, urethra, or seminal vesicles
- Surgical procedures such as prostatectomy
- Pelvic fractures
- Lumbosacral injuries
- Vascular disease, including hypertension
- Chronic neurologic conditions, such as Parkinson disease or multiple sclerosis
- Endocrine disorders, such as diabetes mellitus or thyroid disorders
- Smoking and alcohol consumption
- Drugs
- Poor overall health that prevents sexual intercourse

Functional Erectile Dysfunction

If the client has episodes of ED, it usually has a functional (psychological) cause. Men with functional ED have normal nocturnal (nighttime) and morning erections. Onset is usually sudden and preceded by a period of high stress.

COLLABORATIVE MANAGEMENT

Assessment

For a man to have an erection, he must have normal innervation and a normal **libido** (sex drive). Therefore a medical, social, and sexual history along with a complete physical examination is needed. The first step is to determine whether there is an organic cause. Diagnostic testing is done to rule out possible organic causes.

If test results are negative, the evaluation then focuses on the specific causes that may have been indicated in the client's medical history. For example, hormone testing is used for clients who have a poor libido, small testicles, or sparse beard growth. Serum levels of testosterone and gonadotropins are also measured.

Duplex Doppler ultrasonography is another test to evaluate ED. It provides information about arterial and venous blood flow to the penis. It can also be used to determine the best treatment for ED. A nocturnal penile tumescence test that measures nighttime erections is done in a sleep laboratory. Usually an erection is expected with each rapid eye movement (REM) episode. This study can determine whether ED is caused by an organic or functional problem. If the man has nocturnal erections, the ED is functional. Sexual counseling is needed in this case, and the client is referred to a certified sexual therapist.

◆Interventions

Current methods of treatment include oral drug therapy, vacuum devices, intracorporal injections, intraurethral applications, and prostheses.

Drug Therapy. Drugs used to manage erectile dysfunction work by causing relaxation of the smooth muscles in the corpora cavernosa so blood flow to the penis is increased. The veins exiting the corpora are compressed, limiting outward blood flow, resulting in penile **tumescence** (swelling). Clients are instructed to take the pill 1 hour before sexual intercourse. For some drugs, such as sildenafil (Viagra) and vardenafil (Levitra), sexual stimulation is needed within a half hour to 1 hour to promote the erection. With other drugs, such as tadalafil (Cialis), erection can be stimulated over a longer period. Because the erection occurs more naturally compared with other treatment options, most men and their partners prefer this option.

Instruct clients to abstain from alcohol before sexual intercourse because it may impair the ability to have an erection. Common side effects of these drugs include headaches, facial flushing, and diarrhea. If more than one pill a day is being taken, leg and back cramps, nausea, and vomiting also may occur. Men who take nitrates should not take these drugs because the vasodilation effects can cause a profound hypotension and reduce blood flow to vital organs.

Vacuum Devices. The basic design of a vacuum device is a cylinder that fits over the penis and sits firmly against the body. Using a pump, a vacuum is created to draw blood into the penis to maintain an erection. A rubber ring (tension band) is placed around the base of the penis to maintain the erection, and the cylinder is removed.

The advantage of this procedure is that the device is easy and safe to use. The disadvantage is its clumsiness and lack of spontaneity. In addition, the man may experience pain from the rubber ring or from pumping the device too quickly. The ring should be removed after an hour, or tissue damage may occur.

Intracorporal Injections. Injecting the penis with vasoconstrictive drugs can make the penis erect. The most common agents used for this purpose today are papaverine, phentolamine (Regitine), and alprostadil. These drugs may be used alone but are most often given in combination. The drug is injected into the side of the penis using a 27- or 30-gauge needle. Adverse effects include priapism (prolonged erection), penile scarring, fibrosis, bleeding, bruising at the injection site, pain, infection, and vasovagal responses.

Intraurethral Applications. Prostaglandin E (alprostadil [Muse]) is a self-administered suppository that is placed in the urethra with an applicator. The drug is absorbed into the corpora, which causes an erection in about 10 minutes; erections last 30 to 60 minutes. Advantages include the simplicity of the procedure and noninvasiveness. Disadvantages are a decrease in spontaneity, syncope, and burning of the urethra after the application. Rubbing the penis between the client's hands helps relief the discomfort.

Prostheses. Penile implants are used when other modalities fail. Devices include semirigid, malleable, or hydraulic inflatable and multicomponent or one-piece instruments. The three-piece inflatable device is the most commonly implanted prosthesis. A reservoir is placed in the scrotum. Tubes carry the fluid into the inflatable pieces that are placed in the penis. To inflate the prosthesis, the man squeezes the pump located in the scrotum. To deflate the prosthesis, a release button is activated. Advantages include the man's ability to control his erections. The major disadvantages include device failure and infection.

The device is implanted as an ambulatory surgical procedure. Instruct the client to observe the surgical site for bleeding and infection.

CHART 79-9

CLIENT EDUCATION GUIDE
Testicular Self-Examination

- Examine your testicles monthly immediately after a bath or a shower, when your scrotal skin is relaxed.
- Examine each testicle by gently rolling it between your thumbs and fingers. Testicular tumors tend to appear deep in the center of the testicle.
- Look and feel for any lumps; smooth, rounded masses; or any change in the size, shape, or consistency of the testes.
- Report any lump or swelling to your doctor as soon as possible.

TESTICULAR CANCER

PATHOPHYSIOLOGY

Testicular cancer is not common. It represents fewer than 2% of all cancers in men. However, testicular cancer is the most common malignancy in men 15 to 35 years of age (American Cancer Society, 2005a). It strikes young men at a productive time of life and thus has significant economic, social, and psychological impact on the client and his family or partner. Although testicular cancer occurs more often in younger men, middle-aged and older men also may be affected. With early detection by testicular self-examination (TSE) (Chart 79-9) and treatment with combination chemotherapy, testicular cancer can be cured.

Primary testicular cancers fall into two major groups:

- Germ cell tumors arising from the sperm-producing cells (account for 95% of testicular cancers).

TABLE 79-1 Classification of Testicular Tumors

Germ Cell Germinal Tumors	Non–Germ Cell (Nongerminal) Tumors
■ Seminoma	■ Interstitial cell tumor
■ Nonseminoma	■ Androblastoma
Embryonal carcinoma	
Teratoma	
Choriocarcinoma	

- Non–germ cell tumors arising from the stroma, interstitial, or Leydig cells that produce testosterone (account for 2% to 4% of testicular cancers).

Germ Cell Tumors

Testicular germ cell tumors are classified into two broad categories: seminomas and nonseminomas (Table 79-1).

SEMINOMAS

The most common type of testicular tumor is seminoma. Clients with pure seminomatous tumors have the most favorable prognoses because the tumors are usually localized and metastasize late. Seminomas often are diagnosed when they are still confined to the testicles and retroperitoneal lymph nodes. These cancers respond extremely well to radiation therapy. Clients with early stage seminomas have a 5-year survival rate of about a 95% with surgery (orchiectomy) and radiation therapy (American Cancer Society, 2005a).

NONSEMINOMAS

Nonseminomatous germ cell tumors include three types: embryonal carcinoma, teratoma, and choriocarcinoma. These tumors are not as sensitive to treatment with radiation therapy. They are treated with surgery or chemotherapy, depending on the extent of the disease at diagnosis.

Embryonal carcinomas tend to spread earlier than seminomas, usually to the nearby lymph nodes. This tumor may also spread to more distant body sites such as the lung or the liver. Teratomas rarely occur and are usually malignant in adults. Choriocarcinoma is a highly malignant cancer that spreads rapidly throughout the body. Usually metastasis is present at diagnosis.

Non–Germ Cell Tumors

Non–germ cell tumors are classified as either *interstitial cell tumors* or *androblastomas* (testicular adenomas). Most of these tumors do not metastasize. Interstitial cell tumors arise from the Leydig cells, which secrete testosterone into the bloodstream. These tumors secrete an excessive amount of androgenic hormones, which cause young boys with such tumors to undergo early puberty. Androblastomas sometimes secrete estrogen, which accounts for the feminization and **gynecomastia** (breast enlargement) occasionally seen in these clients.

Etiology and Genetic Risk

The cause of testicular cancer is unknown. The risk for testicular tumors is reported to be higher in males who have an undescended testis **(cryptorchidism).** In males with cryptorchidism, the testicular cancer usually develops in the undescended testis (80%), and there is a 25% chance of cancer developing in the normally descended testis. Seminoma is the most common type of testicular cancer associated with cryptorchidism. The undescended testis undergoes gradual involution and degeneration over time, which may contribute to tumor development. It is not known why the normally descended testis is at risk for cancer. Brothers and close male relatives of clients with testicular cancer have a slightly greater risk for testicular cancer than the general population, suggesting a genetic influence.

Although a history of trauma or infection is common in clients with testicular cancer, neither is a cause of testicular cancer. Testicular trauma or infection can make changes in the shape, size, or texture of the testes more difficult to determine. The client with testicular trauma or infection should be examined by a health care provider after the acute episode subsides to rule out the presence of a tumor.

Testicular cancer is rarely bilateral. Other cancers, however, such as leukemia, lymphoma, plasmacytoma, and metastatic carcinomas may invade the testes. A client with bilateral testicular tumors is more likely to have metastatic disease to the testes than bilateral primary testicular tumors.

Incidence/Prevalence

In the United States it is estimated that 8010 new cases of testicular cancer will be diagnosed each year, and an estimated 390 males will die of the disease. This cancer is the most common solid tumor diagnosed in men between the ages of 15 and 40 years. Testicular cancer can occur during infancy and middle age (after age 50); however, the peak incidence is between the ages of 18 and 40 years (American Cancer Society, 2005a).

◆COLLABORATIVE MANAGEMENT

PHARM e REVIEW

◆Assessment

HISTORY

When taking a history from a client with a suspected testicular tumor, consider the risk factors. It is important to collect data about age and race because the disease occurs most often in young white males. Be alert to other risk factors, including a history or presence of an undescended testis and a family history of testicular cancer.

Ask the client whether he has noticed a discomfort such as heaviness or aching in the lower abdomen or the scrotum. Determine how long any manifestations have been present.

Assess the client's family situation. Is the client sexually active? Does he have children? Does he want children in the future? Depending on the treatment plan chosen, would he be interested in sperm storage in a sperm bank?

If the client has one healthy testis, he can function sexually and may not have any reproductive dysfunction. If the client undergoes a retroperitoneal lymph node dissection or chemotherapy, he may become sterile because of treatment effects on the sperm-producing cells or surgical trauma to the sympathetic nervous system, resulting in retrograde ejaculations.

PHYSICAL ASSESSMENT/CLINICAL MANIFESTATIONS

The testes, lymph nodes, and abdomen are thoroughly examined. Palpate the testes for lumps or swelling (Chart 79-10), the most common manifestations of testicular cancer. The presence of any lymph node swelling, abdominal masses, or gynecomastia often indicates metastatic disease.

CHART 79-10

FOCUSED ASSESSMENT of
A Male Client with a Testicular Lump

Obtain a medical history from the client:
- When was the lump discovered?
- Are there any other symptoms (sensation of heaviness, dragging in testicle, pain, discharge from penis)?
- Is there a history of cryptorchidism?

Assess the genital system. Always wear gloves during the examination of the male genitalia.
- Inspect and palpate the scrotal contents. Have the client perform a Valsalva maneuver, and palpate for a varicocele.
- Any lump or enlargement that does not transilluminate should be suspected as malignant.

Palpate for any enlarged lymph nodes. Most common lymphadenopathy is in the inguinal or supraclavicular regions.
Assess the abdomen for a possible mass or hepatomegaly.

PSYCHOSOCIAL ASSESSMENT

Because testicular cancer and its treatment often lead to sexual difficulties, pay close attention to the psychosocial outcomes of the disease. Sexuality is an issue for men of any age, but it may be even more of an issue for younger men. Even if the cancer is detected at an early stage and the client is cured after orchiectomy, he may be afraid that he will be sexually handicapped. Even if the client's disease is arrested with surgery, radiation, or chemotherapy, he may think of himself as less than a whole man. These fears can disrupt the psychosocial and sexual development of the young male and can threaten the identity of adult males. The client may be afraid that he will be unable to perform sexually, will no longer be sexually attractive or desirable, and will face rejection. Feelings of sexual inadequacy may be denied, repressed, or displaced, causing increased stress on the man's personal and work relationships.

Perform a psychosocial assessment with these clients because problems may arise anytime. Referrals are made to other resources as appropriate.

LABORATORY ASSESSMENT

An important diagnostic indicator for testicular cancer is the presence of certain "marker proteins" (tumor markers). These are proteins that normally were produced during embryonic development and their presence in adults is abnormal. Benign testicular tumors do not elevate the levels of any of these marker proteins.

Common tumor markers for testicular cancer are alpha-fetoprotein (AFP) and the beta subunit of human chorionic gonadotropin (hCG). About 90% of clients with embryonal carcinoma, teratoma, or choriocarcinoma have elevated blood levels of AFP, hCG, or both. Clients with a pure seminoma do not have an elevated AFP level, and only 10% have a slightly elevated hCG level. This level resolves after orchiectomy.

If a client has a diagnosis of seminoma and also has an elevated AFP level, the tumor specimen must be re-examined for evidence of a component of nonseminomatous cancer. This step is necessary because the treatments differ for seminomatous and nonseminomatous tumors.

The AFP and hCG blood levels are also used to evaluate responses to therapy for testicular cancer and to document the presence of residual or recurrent disease. With effective treatment, the levels of abnormal markers fall. The persistence of elevated levels of markers after orchiectomy is evidence that the client has metastatic disease, even if x-rays and scans do not show a tumor presence. The reappearance of the tumor markers indicates recurrence of the cancer. Therefore marker levels must be monitored regularly during the follow-up of clients treated for testicular cancer.

OTHER DIAGNOSTIC ASSESSMENTS

When a client has a change in testis size, shape, or texture, ultrasonography can determine whether the mass is solid or fluid filled. It also can help differentiate benign masses from malignant ones.

After the diagnosis of testicular cancer, the client should have a computed tomography (CT) scan of the abdomen and the chest, or chest tomograms, to identify small metastatic lesions.

Magnetic resonance imaging (MRI) is used to detect enlarged lymph nodes and abnormal nodules in certain organs that may indicate metastasis from the testicles. Chest x-rays and bone scans may also be performed if metastasis is suspected.

Clients with a pure seminoma may undergo bipedal lymphangiography as part of the staging workup to assess for retroperitoneal lymph node involvement. Lymphangiograms are also helpful in determining the extent of radiation therapy fields.

◆Analysis

COMMON NURSING DIAGNOSES AND COLLABORATIVE PROBLEMS

A common nursing diagnosis in clients with testicular cancer is Risk for Sexual Dysfunction related to altered body structure and function from disease or treatment. A common collaborative problem is Potential for Metastasis.

ADDITIONAL NURSING DIAGNOSES AND COLLABORATIVE PROBLEMS

In addition to the common nursing diagnoses and collaborative problems, clients with testicular cancer may have one or more of the following:
- Dysfunctional Grieving or Anticipatory Grieving related to loss of a body part or changes in body function
- Disturbed Body Image related to the diagnosis of cancer and its treatment
- Acute Pain or Chronic Pain related to tumor compression or effects of metastasis
- Anxiety related to threat to health status from the diagnosis of cancer

◆Planning and Implementation

RISK FOR SEXUAL DYSFUNCTION

NOC **PLANNING: EXPECTED OUTCOMES.** The client with testicular cancer is expected to maintain an acceptable level of sexual function. Indicators include that the client often or consistently demonstrates the following behaviors:
- Attains sexual arousal
- Adapts sexual technique as needed
- Expresses comfort with sexual expression
- Expresses comfort with his body

INTERVENTIONS. At diagnosis the incidence of **oligospermia** (low sperm count) and **azoospermia** (absence of living sperm) is increased in clients with testicular cancer. This problem is thought to be related to higher testicular temperatures created by cancer cell metabolism. The client may not discover that he has reduced sperm numbers count until he has a sperm count performed before surgery.

Health teaching about reproduction, fertility, and sexuality is started in the pretreatment phase. Normal reproductive function is reviewed as well as the possible effects of cancer and its treatment on reproductive function. Explore with the client various reproductive options (e.g., sperm banks and artificial insemination) (Chart 79-11). The sperm bank facility provides comprehensive information on semen collection, storage of semen, the storage contract, costs, and the insemination process.

When preparing the client for the collection and storage of sperm, assume the role of client advocate and keep in mind the effect of the cancer diagnosis on the client. The psychological benefit of having stored sperm may be important for the client and may influence his response to treatment. Knowing that the potential for being a father still exists may help the client cope with other assaults to his masculinity, such as alopecia or erectile dysfunction (ED).

The client should arrange for semen storage as soon as possible after diagnosis. Sperm collection should be completed *before* he begins radiation therapy or chemotherapy or undergoes a radical lymph node dissection. After radiation therapy or chemotherapy has been started, the client is at increased risk for producing mutagenic sperm, which may not be viable or may result in fetal abnormalities.

The recommended number of samples to optimize the chances of later fertilization is three to six ejaculates, collected 2 to 4 days apart. The process of sperm collection can delay treatment for as long as 1 month, especially if the client is still recovering from surgery and multiple procedures or tests.

The client's diagnosis and his physical condition may not allow treatment to be postponed, thus making sperm storage an unfeasible reproductive option. Also, some clients may have personal or religious beliefs that do not allow sperm storage. For clients who are not candidates for sperm storage in a sperm bank and for those who choose not to bank, discuss other reproductive options such as donor insemination, adoption, or not fathering children.

POTENTIAL FOR METASTASIS

NOC **PLANNING: EXPECTED OUTCOMES.** The client with testicular cancer is expected not to experience disease metastasis or recurrence.

CHART 79-11

CLIENT EDUCATION GUIDE
Sperm Banking

- You may want to investigate sperm storage in a sperm bank as a way to preserve your sperm for future use.
- No one knows how long sperm can be stored successfully, but pregnancies have resulted from sperm stored for longer than 10 years.
- Check with the sperm bank to see how much it charges to process and store your sperm and to see whether you must pay when the service is provided.
- Investigate whether your health insurance company will reimburse you for sperm collection and storage.

INTERVENTIONS. Surgery is the main treatment for testicular cancer. It is often combined with nonsurgical management to prevent metastatic disease (or to alleviate symptoms of metastasis) and to bring about tumor regression.

SURGICAL MANAGEMENT. The surgeon performs a unilateral orchiectomy for diagnosis and for surgical management. Every effort is made to remove the cancerous testis as an intact organ to prevent releasing cancer cells into the surgical site.

Clients with testicular cancer may also undergo a radical retroperitoneal lymph node dissection. With this procedure, the disease can be staged accurately and the tumor volume **debulked** (reduced in size) so that other therapies are more effective.

Preoperative Care. Like most clients with cancer, the client with testicular cancer is usually apprehensive. Offer support and reinforce the teaching provided by the surgeon. Anticipate the client's postoperative needs and plan interventions before surgery. Inform the client and his family or partner about what to expect after surgery. The surgical incision for a retroperitoneal lymph node dissection is extensive. Depending on the extent of the dissection and the need for surgical exploration, the surgeon might make not only a midline incision but also a transthoracic incision or a combination of the two incisions (thoracoabdominal).

Inform the client and family that radical retroperitoneal lymph node dissections are long operations, lasting 6 to 12 hours. Tell the client that he may be cared for in a critical care unit after surgery for close observation.

Operative Procedures. To perform a radical retroperitoneal lymph node dissection, the surgeon removes the retroperitoneal nodes in the iliac and lumbar regions. Because the blood supply and the lymphatic vessels of the testes and kidneys are directly related, an extensive midline incision from the xiphoid process to the pubis is necessary. The lymph nodes around the kidney along with the nodes near the aorta and both kidneys are removed. Node removal also includes those in the inguinal area on the affected side. During the lymph node removal, the sympathetic ganglia around the lower lumbar lymphatics are dissected. Removal of the sympathetic ganglia eliminates peristalsis in the vas deferens and contractions of the seminal vesicles. This disruption results in sterility because the client's ejaculate no longer contains sperm. However, having a normal erection and experiencing orgasm usually are not affected.

A gel-filled silicone prosthesis can usually be surgically implanted into the scrotum at the time of the orchiectomy or later if the client desires. Reassure the client that this procedure does not impair fertility or sexual function; the client cosmetically appears to have two testes.

Postoperative Care. Because of the length of the surgery, manipulation of the abdominal and retroperitoneal viscera, and the loss of a major part of the lymphatic fluid, nodes, and channels, observe and assess the client for any of the complications of major abdominal surgery (see Chapter 22). Intervene for any of the following expected problems:

- Pain from surgical incisions
- Immobility related to prolonged maintenance of surgical positioning and pain after surgery
- Injuries related to any invasive catheters or tubes

The client is usually hospitalized for 3 to 4 days after a radical retroperitoneal lymph node dissection. During this time explain care after discharge.

NONSURGICAL MANAGEMENT. Chemotherapy and radiation therapy are indicated for clients at high risk for metastatic disease or those with metastatic disease.

Chemotherapy. Combination chemotherapy may be used as adjuvant therapy for nonseminomatous testicular tumors or as primary treatment when there is evidence of metastatic disease. Combination chemotherapy is effective in treating nonseminomatous testicular cancer, particularly if cisplatin (Platinol) is used. This agent is a part of any successful chemotherapy regimen for treating testicular cancer.

The following are other drugs commonly used in combination with cisplatin:

- Bleomycin sulfate (Blenoxane) (most common)
- Etoposide (VP-16, VePesid) (most common)
- Vinblastine sulfate (Velban, Velbe✱)
- Dactinomycin (Cosmegen)
- Cyclophosphamide (Cytoxan, Procytox✱)
- Doxorubicin (Adriamycin)

The specific combination of drugs and the frequency, cycling, and duration of treatment vary from client to client, depending on the extent of the disease and the protocol being followed. For many clients, the acute side effects are severe enough that the client is admitted to the hospital for chemotherapy. Chapter 28 discusses the nursing care issues for the client receiving chemotherapy.

Radiation Therapy. After **orchiectomy** (removal of one or both testes), external beam radiation therapy is the treatment of choice for clients with a pure seminoma. This type of testicular cancer is highly radiosensitive. Before radiation therapy, a staging lymphangiogram is used to determine the treatment fields. An advantage of using radiation therapy instead of radical lymph node dissection is that reproductive function is preserved because surgical dissection of the nerves is avoided.

For the client undergoing radiation therapy to the retroperitoneal lymph nodes, the remaining testis is shielded with a lead cup to preserve reproductive function. Even with these precautions, the client may have a temporary decreased sperm count as a result of radiation scatter. Normally the sperm count returns to the pretreatment level within 24 to 30 months after the radiation treatment is completed. If metastases develop outside the lymphatic system, the client may still be cured with radiation therapy if the area of involvement is limited. If lymphatic involvement is extensive, or if the visceral organs are involved, combination chemotherapy is used.

Stem Cell Transplantation. Studies are being conducted to explore whether high-dose chemotherapy with stem cell transplantation may be valuable in treating men with advanced germ cell cancer. In this procedure, the client's blood-forming stem cells are removed from the blood and preserved by freezing while the client receives high-dose chemotherapy. Once the chemotherapy is completed, the stem cells are returned to the client. This procedure helps to prevent the infection and anemia that occur with chemotherapy.

Community-Based Care

After an orchiectomy, the client is typically hospitalized for 1 to 2 days. This period may need to be extended if he must undergo additional surgery or chemotherapy. Because it may not be known until after the orchiectomy whether the client has cancer, what type of testicular cancer he has, or whether he needs additional surgery or treatment with radiation therapy or chemotherapy, specific discharge planning may need to be deferred until after surgery.

HOME CARE MANAGEMENT

After an orchiectomy, unless the client has a wound complication, he is discharged without a dressing on the inguinal incision. He may want to wear a dressing to prevent clothing from rubbing on the sutures and causing irritation. Tell the client that the sutures will be removed in the physician's office 7 to 10 days after surgery.

HEALTH TEACHING

For the client who has undergone testicular surgery, emphasize the importance of scheduling a follow-up visit with the surgeon to examine the incision for healing and complications. Instruct the client to notify the surgeon if any of the following symptoms occur: chills, fever, increasing tenderness or pain around the incision, drainage, or dehiscence of the incision.

These manifestations may indicate infection for which antibiotics are needed. Instruct the client that he will be able to resume most of his usual activities within 1 week after discharge, except for lifting heavy objects (objects weighing 15 pounds [9.1 kg]) or stair climbing. Remind him to ask his surgeon when strenuous activities may be resumed.

Inform the client that he may make arrangements with his surgeon to have a silicone prosthesis inserted into the scrotum if a prosthesis was not inserted during the orchiectomy.

Explain the importance of performing monthly testicular self-examination (TSE) on the remaining testis and scheduling follow-up examinations with the physician. The client who has had testicular cancer should schedule tests for urinary and serum levels of tumor markers and computed tomography (CT) or magnetic resonance imaging (MRI) studies as part of his routine follow-up for at least 3 years.

Depending on the pathologic findings and the stage of the cancer, the client may need further treatment. This information may not be known at the time of discharge. If it is known that the client needs further surgery, he and his family need information about the future surgery. If it is known that he must undergo radiation therapy or chemotherapy, he needs education about a radiation therapy and chemotherapy regimen.

The client who has testicular cancer may need emotional support. If permanent sterility occurs and sperm storage has not been feasible, the man may need counseling about other reproductive options.

HEALTH CARE RESOURCES

The client may be referred to agencies or support groups, such as the American Fertility Society or RESOLVE (an organization for infertile couples).

Evaluation: Outcomes

Evaluate the care of the client who has been treated for testicular cancer on the basis of the identified nursing diagnoses and collaborative problems. The expected outcomes include that the client will:

- Not experience a recurrence of cancer or metastases
- Have an acceptable level of sexual function

Specific indicators for these outcomes are listed for each nursing diagnosis and collaborative problem under the Planning and Implementation section (see earlier).

Critical Thinking Challenge

The client is a 28-year-old man who is 4 days postoperative from a radical retroperitoneal lymph node dissection and orchiectomy for testicular cancer. His cancer is stage III, and he is scheduled to start chemotherapy in about 1 month. He is engaged to be married. Whenever you are providing care, he makes sexual jokes and talks about having sex with you. When you suggest he might be more comfortable with an older nurse or a male nurse, he becomes very upset and apologizes. However, his behavior is the same the next time you enter his room.

1. Should you tell him you do not appreciate this kind of talk? Why or Why not?
2. What concerns might be driving his behavior?
3. Should you tell his fiancée about his behavior? Why or Why not?

evolve For suggested answer guidelines, go to http://evolve.elsevier.com/Iggy/.

OTHER COMMON PROBLEMS AFFECTING THE TESTES AND ADJACENT STRUCTURES

Problems that develop inside the scrotum usually occur as a mass or as scrotal edema. Some problems produce pain, but others do not. Figure 79-7 shows some of the most common conditions found in the male, including hydrocele, spermatocele, varicocele, and scrotal torsion.

Hydrocele

PATHOPHYSIOLOGY

A hydrocele is a cystic mass, usually filled with straw-colored fluid that forms around the testis (see Figure 79-7). It results from impaired lymphatic drainage of the scrotum, causing a swelling of the tissue surrounding the testes. Unless the swelling becomes large and uncomfortable or begins to impair blood flow to the testis, no treatment is necessary. Hydroceles are usually painless. It is important that the cause of the hydrocele is investigated to rule out a serious condition. The cause may be determined by examination and ultrasound. A small hydrocele may go untreated with no further problems. However, a hydrocele may become very large, which makes clothing uncomfortable and may be cosmetically unacceptable.

◆COLLABORATIVE MANAGEMENT

A hydrocele may be drained via a needle and syringe, or it may be removed surgically. To correct a hydrocele surgically, an incision is made in the scrotum and the hydrocele is removed. The client may or may not have a drain at the incision site. Usually the surgery is performed on an outpatient basis. If the client requires hospitalization, it is for only 1 or 2 days. The recurrence rate for hydrocele is about 1% to 2%.

Instruct the client that if an incision drain is present, some serosanguineous drainage may be present for the first 24 to 48 hours after surgery. Explain the importance of wearing a scrotal support. The scrotal support keeps the scrotal dressing in place and keeps the scrotum elevated, which helps to prevent edema.

The degree of pain experienced after this surgery varies. Assess and observe the client for pain every 2 to 3 hours immediately after surgery. Moderate incision pain is expected for the first 24 hours after surgery and should markedly decrease within 1 or 2 days. If the client's pain does not resolve within this time, be alert to the possible development of wound complications, such as infection or bleeding.

Instruct the client to schedule a follow-up visit with the surgeon to have the wound evaluated for healing. Stress the importance of continuing to wear a scrotal support to promote drainage and comfort. The scrotum can remain swollen from residual inflammation and edema for as long

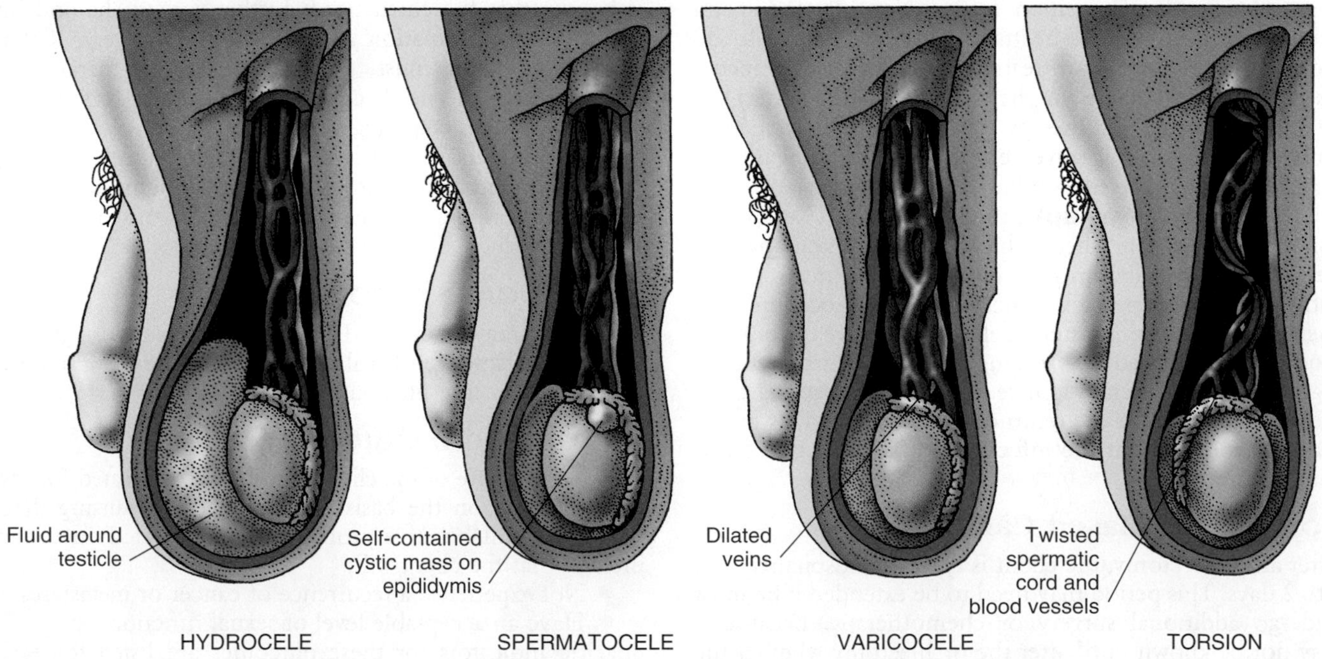

Figure 79-7 ■ Common problems affecting the testes and adjacent structures.

as several weeks. Instruct the client to stay off his feet for 3 to 5 days and to limit physical activity for a week. Reassure him that this swelling is normal and eventually subsides.

Spermatocele

PATHOPHYSIOLOGY

A spermatocele is a sperm-containing cyst that develops on the epididymis alongside the testicle (see Figure 79-7). Trauma, infection, congenital abnormalities, or often for no identifiable reason results in the widening of a portion of the epididymis creating a small cavity where sperm collects.

COLLABORATIVE MANAGEMENT

Normally spermatoceles are small and asymptomatic, and no interventions are needed. If the spermatocele becomes large enough to cause discomfort, a spermatocelectomy is performed. In this simple procedure, the spermatocele is excised through a small scrotal incision. Routinely no incision drain is used because drainage and swelling are minimal. About 5% of clients have recurrence.

Varicocele

PATHOPHYSIOLOGY

A varicocele is a cluster of dilated veins behind and above the testis (see Figure 79-7). Varicosity of the testicles may result from the increased fluid secondary to damaged or incompetent valves in the testicular veins. The diagnosis is made by scrotal palpation, particularly when the client performs a Valsalva maneuver, creating additional pressure in the varicose veins. The scrotum feels "wormlike" when palpated. If the varicocele is very small and cannot be palpated, thermography, which detects pockets of heat, or a Doppler, which magnifies the sound of the blood flowing through the veins, is used.

Varicoceles can be either unilateral or bilateral, but most are unilateral. They occur most often on the left side of the scrotum. In many cases, varicoceles are asymptomatic, and no treatment is required. In a few men varicoceles are painful and must be removed surgically.

Varicoceles can also cause infertility. It is thought that they increase scrotal temperature from the venous stasis near the testis, altering spermatogenesis. Surgical correction of a varicocele may resolve the infertility.

COLLABORATIVE MANAGEMENT

A **varicocelectomy** (surgical removal of the varicocele) is usually performed through an inguinal incision, in which the spermatic veins are ligated in the cord. It can also be performed through an incision near the superior iliac spine, in which the spermatic veins are ligated in the retroperitoneal space. A varicocelectomy may be done on an ambulatory care basis, or the client may be hospitalized overnight.

Before surgery explain to the client that persistent venous congestion of the scrotum is common after this type of surgery because of the changed circulation in the area. To promote drainage of the scrotum, place a rolled towel under the scrotum while the client is in bed. Ice may be applied to the scrotum if needed. Any intervention that facilitates drainage and decreases swelling from the area promotes relief. Instruct the client about the importance of wearing a scrotal support while ambulating. Usually the client can resume normal activities, including sexual activities, within a week.

At discharge, instruct the client to make a follow-up appointment with the surgeon to have the sutures removed. Remind him to notify the surgeon of any increasing discomfort at the incision site or in the scrotum, which might indicate an infection. Increasing scrotal discomfort can mean that the circulation to the testis has been impaired. Testicular atrophy, a rare complication of a varicocelectomy, may occur if the blood supply to the testis becomes insufficient.

Scrotal Torsion

PATHOPHYSIOLOGY

Because of the mobility of the scrotum, scrotal injuries are relatively rare. Torsion of the testes involves the twisting of the spermatic cord and occurs most often during puberty (see Figure 79-7). Torsion may occur after strenuous exercise or trauma, although for many cases no specific causative event is identified. Because the testes are sensitive to any decrease in blood flow, torsion of the testis is a surgical emergency.

The client experiences pain, which does not subside with scrotal elevation. In addition to pain, he usually has nausea and vomiting. Other manifestations include blood in the semen, lower abdominal pain, a lump in the testicle, and red and swollen testicle(s). Diagnosis is made by history and physical examination. Because manifestations of testicular torsion are similar to epididymitis, a color Doppler sonography may be used to identify the absence of blood flow through the twisted testicle. A urinalysis or culture may be used to rule out a bacterial infection.

COLLABORATIVE MANAGEMENT

In addition to caring for the client's physical needs, be attuned to his psychosexual needs. Of primary concern to the client with an injury to his external genitalia are his masculinity and sexuality. An awareness of crisis intervention techniques and knowledge about sexuality are helpful when assisting the client to adjust to an injury in the genital area.

Surgical intervention may be required to untwist the torsion. Evaluation of the condition of the testicles can be made at that time, including looking for signs of necrosis. Any dead tissue may have to be removed, or one or both of the testicles may be excised. If the testicles are found to be healthy, they may be sutured to the scrotal wall to prevent recurrence of the torsion.

At discharge, instruct the client to maintain ice to the scrotum for at least 72 hours, and elevate the scrotum to minimize edema. Instruct him to avoid lifting heavy objects for 4 to 6 weeks, limit stair climbing, and suspend strenuous physical activity for 1 month. Remind the client to wear a scrotal support for at least 3 weeks.

Cryptorchidism

PATHOPHYSIOLOGY

Before birth the testicles develop in the abdominal cavity and descend into the scrotum. Cryptorchidism results when the testicles fail to descent and is mainly a pediatric problem.

Three percent of full-term male infants and 20% of premature infants have an undescended testis. In 80% of cases, the undescended testis descends spontaneously during the infant's first year. When the testicles reside in the scrotum, sperm production and fertility are enhanced and testicular cancer can be detected. Undescended testicles often result in infertility and are at an increased risk of cancer.

COLLABORATIVE MANAGEMENT

If the testicles do not spontaneously descend, medical or surgical intervention may be needed. Medically, hormonal injections of β-hCG, luteinizing hormone-releasing hormone, or testosterone may be used to promote descent of the testicles into the scrotum. If the testicles do not descend, surgery, an **orchidopexy** (surgical placement of the testicle into the scrotum) may be performed to prevent irreversible damage, causing infertility, and to allow examination of the testicles for tumors. If left untreated until adulthood, an orchidopexy may be performed for cosmetic and psychosexual reasons as well. In a small percent of clients, no testicles are found at surgery. This is known as a "vanished" or absent testis.

During an orchidopexy, an inguinal incision is made and the spermatic cord is released from the surrounding fascia to obtain maximal length. The surgeon then creates a pouch and places the testis between the skin and the dartos muscle of the scrotum. The testis is sutured to the dartos muscle, and the inguinal incision and the scrotal incision (if there is one) are then closed, and a dressing is applied. If there is an incision in the scrotum, it is also covered with a dressing and the client is instructed to wear a scrotal support. The site should be checked for bleeding and infection. The client should rest for 2 to 3 days and avoid strenuous activity for at least a month.

Cancer of the Penis

PATHOPHYSIOLOGY

Cancer of the penis represents fewer than 1% of all malignancies in men in the United States. The overall 5-year survival rate is 50%. Most penile cancers (95%) are epidermoid (squamous) carcinomas developing from the squamous cells. These tumors tend to grow slowly and can develop anywhere on the penis but most commonly occur on the foreskin or the glans. When the cancer is confined to the skin of the penis it is called carcinoma in situ (CIS). Other types of penile cancers include melanomas, basal cell cancer, and sarcomas.

Circumcision (the surgical removal of the prepuce from the penis) in infancy almost eliminates the possibility of penile cancer in that chronic irritation and inflammation of the glans penis predispose uncircumcised men to penile cancer. Because of the ongoing controversy about neonatal circumcision, teach men and new mothers of boys that strict personal hygiene is an important preventive measure against penile cancer.

COLLABORATIVE MANAGEMENT

Assessment

Penile cancer usually occurs as a painless, wartlike growth or ulcer on the glans under the **prepuce** (foreskin) and may be mistaken for a venereal wart. A penile carcinoma may also appear as a reddened lesion with plaque.

Interventions

Small lesions involving only the skin may be controlled by excisional biopsy. When the lesion is not curable by excisional biopsy or radiation therapy, a **penectomy** (partial or total removal of the penis) may be required.

Partial Penectomy. When the lesion is limited to the glans, a partial penectomy is performed. The distal portion of the corpus cavernosum and the corpus spongiosum is amputated. The urethra is anastomosed to the skin, and a dressing is applied. A retention catheter is in place for 3 to 5 days after surgery until the edema surrounding the urethra subsides. Assess the dressing for drainage, which should be minimal. Check the urinary catheter for patency every 4 hours for the first 24 hours.

Total Penectomy. A total penectomy is required when the lesion has penetrated the shaft of the penis or when the tumor has recurred after a partial penectomy or radiation therapy. An incision is made from the pubic bone, which encircles the penis and extends into the perineum. The bases of both corpora cavernosa are exposed and excised, and the penis is amputated. An incision drain is placed in the wound before it is sutured. Clients who undergo a total penectomy also have a perineal urethrotomy (anastomosis of the urethra to the skin in the perineum) for urinary drainage.

After a total penectomy, observe the incision dressing every 2 to 4 hours during the first 24 to 48 hours. A moderate amount of serosanguineous drainage from the incision drains is expected.

Be aware that regardless of how accepting the client may appear before surgery, he may experience severe emotional problems after surgery. After a partial penectomy, the client must adjust to considerable changes in body image and sexuality. Encourage him to verbalize his feelings about the loss of his penis. After a total penectomy, the client can no longer have penile-vaginal or penile-anal intercourse and cannot urinate in a standing position. It is difficult for most clients to accept the possibility that they might die because of a lesion on the penis, especially because they rarely experience any systemic cancer symptoms and are otherwise healthy. Help the client to realize that removal of his penis may save his life. Be aware of the possibility of suicide attempts because the client's penis may be more important to him than his life. The nurse may be the one to detect the need for professional psychological assistance for the client or his partner. Early interventions can make a tremendous difference in the client's or partner's well-being.

Phimosis and Paraphimosis

PATHOPHYSIOLOGY

In a man with phimosis, the prepuce is constricted so that it cannot be retracted over the glans. The prepuce remains down, around the tip of the penis. Instruct uncircumcised men about the importance of cleaning the prepuce.

In paraphimosis the prepuce has not been returned to its normal position after being retracted and forms a constricting band around the glans. This constricts lymph drainage, causing the penis to swell. Blood flow becomes impeded, and tissue death can occur. This problem is an emergency requiring immediate treatment. Uncircumcised males are at risk. Causes include infection, not returning the foreskin to the original position after urethral catheterization, poor hygiene, vigorous sexual intercourse, and penile piercing.

COLLABORATIVE MANAGEMENT

Phimosis is corrected by **circumcision** (surgical removal of the prepuce or foreskin). This procedure also may be performed for other medical reasons or for aesthetic reasons.

Circumcision in the adult male is usually performed in a same-day surgical setting. If the client has a dressing, instruct him to soak in a warm bath that evening to allow the dressing to loosen. If the dressing falls off before the next day, caution the client not to replace it. Explain that the sutures will be absorbed and need not be removed. No residual or side effects result from this surgery, and the client should be able to resume normal activities within 1 week. Sexual intercourse may be resumed after 1 to 2 weeks.

The client may be discharged with a prescription for a barbiturate sleeping medication to be taken for several nights after surgery. Emphasize that these drugs suppress the rapid-eye-movement (REM) phase of sleep so that normal nocturnal erections do not occur. This prevents tension on the sutures by an erection. Nonbarbiturate sleeping medications do not inhibit the nocturnal erection pattern. Explain the relationship between barbiturate sleeping medications and nocturnal erections because the client may not adhere with the instructions to take the drug, especially if he is not having any difficulty sleeping.

Advise the client to notify his physician if he has any wound complications, such as swelling at the incision area or drainage, and to schedule a postoperative office visit.

Priapism

PATHOPHYSIOLOGY

Priapism is an uncontrolled, long-maintained erection without sexual desire, which causes the penis to become large, hard, and painful. Priapism affects the two corpora cavernosa; the corpus spongiosum and glans penis are not affected.

Priapism can occur from neural, vascular, or pharmacologic causes, including the following:

- Thrombosis of the veins of the corpora cavernosa (usually resulting from trauma)
- Leukemia
- Sickle cell disease
- Diabetes mellitus
- Malignancies

Sickle cell disease causes priapism through the collection of erythrocytes within the corporal bodies. Leukemia may cause priapism because the increased number of white blood cells (WBCs) permits persistent engorgement of the corporal bodies. Cancer may also infiltrate the corporal bodies, causing persistent engorgement. Priapism can also result from an abnormal neurogenic reflex, psychotropic drugs, antidepressants, antihypertensive drugs, and drugs used to treat erectile dysfunction. Other risk factors include recreational drugs (cocaine, ecstasy, marijuana), overdose of injectable drugs for erectile dysfunction, and prolonged sexual activity.

COLLABORATIVE MANAGEMENT

Priapism is a urologic emergency because the circulation to the penis may be compromised and the client may not be able to void with an erect penis. The goal of intervention is to improve the venous drainage of the corpora cavernosa. Conservative measures involve prostatic massage, sedation, and bedrest.

Meperidine (Demerol) is usually given immediately because of its hypotensive effect. Warm enemas may be given to cause venous dilation and thus increase the outflow of the trapped blood. Urinary or suprapubic catheterization is required if the client cannot void.

If conservative therapy is unsuccessful, treatment may proceed to aspiration of the corpora cavernosa with a large-bore needle or surgical intervention. The priapism should be resolved within the first 24 to 30 hours to prevent penile ischemia, gangrene, fibrosis, and erectile dysfunction. If a cause of priapism is identified, treatment is directed toward that underlying cause.

When caring for the client with priapism, be sensitive to his emotional needs. The client may be uncomfortable and in crisis but at the same time embarrassed by his erection and loss of control. Reassure the client that it is understood that he is not in control of his erection, and provide him with privacy.

Prostatitis

PATHOPHYSIOLOGY

Prostatitis is an inflammation of the prostate gland. The four types of prostatitis are acute bacterial (ABP), chronic bacterial (CBP), nonbacterial (NBP)/chronic pelvic pain syndrome (CPPS), and asymptomatic inflammatory prostatitis. Duration of symptoms, presence or absence of WBCs in the urine, and urinary culture results determine the classification.

Bacterial Prostatitis

Bacterial prostatitis often occurs with urethritis or an infection of the lower urinary tract. Organisms may reach the prostate via the bloodstream or the urethra. The most common organisms are *Escherichia coli, Enterobacter, Proteus,* and group D streptococci. Acute bacterial prostatitis may be manifested by fever, chills, **dysuria** (painful urination), urethral discharge, and a boggy, tender prostate. Gentle palpation of the prostate usually results in a urethral discharge, which has WBCs in the prostatic secretions.

Chronic bacterial prostatitis generally occurs in older men and has a less dramatic presentation than acute bacterial prostatitis and without the systemic manifestations. The client reports experiencing hesitancy, urgency, dysuria, difficulty initiating and terminating the flow of urine, and decreased strength and volume of urine. Additionally, there may be discomfort in the perineum, scrotum, and penis.

Nonbacterial/Chronic Pelvic Pain Syndrome

A bacterial prostatitis can occur after a viral illness or may be associated with sexually transmitted diseases (STDs), especially in young males. Although an infection may be the cause, bacteria is not found on urinalysis and culture. Other causes may be autoimmune disorders, neuromuscular etiologies, allergy-mediated reactions, and psychosexual problems. In many instances, an exact cause of the perineal discomfort cannot be found. The client reports mild urgency and dysuria. Rectal, perineal, and ejaculatory pain may be present. Decreased libido may also be present.

Prostatodynia (pelvic floor pain) is a related condition in which manifestations of prostatitis are present, but there is no inflammation of the prostate and the urine culture is negative. Additionally, the client has low back pain with unilateral testicular pain, narrowed force of the urinary stream, and post-void dribbling.

COLLABORATIVE MANAGEMENT

The client with chronic prostatitis usually reports backache, perineal pain, mild dysuria, and urinary frequency. Hematuria may be present. The prostate may feel irregularly enlarged, firm, and slightly tender when palpated. Segmented specimens are obtained. This is referred to as the *Stamey-Meares Method.* Four specimens are taken. Comparison of the number of WBCs in the specimens and the presence of bacteria assists in making a diagnosis. The first specimen is the first 10 mL of urine obtained by voiding, which is used to diagnose urethritis. The second is 50 mL of midstream urine used to diagnose cystitis. For the third specimen, prostatic secretions are collected following prostate massage and the urethra milked to express any prostatic secretions (expressed prostatic secretions, EPS). The fourth specimen is then collected by a post-massage bladder voiding into a sterile container. The third and fourth specimens may show WBCs, but no bacterial growth if nonbacterial prostatitis is present. The third and fourth specimens will contain greater bacterial growth than the first or second specimens in bacterial prostatitis. Prostatodynia is present in the absence of bacteria in the sequential cultures, along with normal expressed prostatic secretions.

Complications of prostatitis are **epididymitis** (inflammation of the epididymis) and **cystitis** (inflammation of the bladder). A rare complication is a prostatic abscess. The client with either acute or chronic bacterial prostatitis is likely to develop urinary tract infections. Sexual functioning may be reduced because of discomfort.

Early diagnosis and treatment of prostatitis with antimicrobials, 160 mg/800 mg of trimethoprim/sulfamethoxazole (Bactrim DS) every 12 hours or carbenicillin indanyl sodium (Geocillin, Geopen Oral), or fluoroquinolones (ciprofloxacin [Cipro]) can help to prevent an abscess. After culture results are obtained, other antibiotics may be required. Treatment may last from 4 weeks to many months because there is poor penetration of antibiotics into prostatic tissue. Acute bacterial prostatitis may require hospitalization with aggressive IV antibiotics.

Emphasize the importance of comfort measures, such as sitz baths, donut-shaped cushions, and nonsteroidal anti-inflammatory drugs. Stool softeners are prescribed to prevent straining and rectal irritation of the prostate during a bowel movement. Instruct clients to avoid alcohol, coffee, tea, and spicy foods that irritate symptoms. Over-the-counter cold preparations containing decongestants or antihistamines may result in urinary retention.

Teach the client with chronic prostatitis about the long-term nature of the problem. Because prostatitis can cause other urinary tract infections, explain the importance of increasing fluid intake and long-term antibiotic therapy. It is important to teach the client to take the prescribed antibiotics on schedule. Because trimethoprim (Bactrim, Septra) diffuses into the prostatic fluid, it is the antibiotic of choice. Instruct the client about activities that drain the prostate (sexual intercourse, masturbation, prostatic massage), which may help in the management of chronic prostatitis. Inform the client that prostatitis is not infectious or contagious.

Epididymitis

PATHOPHYSIOLOGY

Epididymitis is an inflammation of the epididymis. This inflammation may be a result of an infection or noninfectious source, such as trauma. Bacterial infection is the most common cause of epididymitis. The infection may spread from other structures such as the prostate, bladder, or urethra. It can be a complication of an STD, such as gonorrhea or chlamydia. Although not common, epididymitis can also be a complication of long-term use of an indwelling urinary catheter, prostatic surgery, or a cystoscopic examination.

Organisms such as *Staphylococcus* and *E. coli* commonly cause epididymitis. In men younger than 35 years of age, the major causative organism in epididymitis is *Chlamydia trachomatis,* which is transmitted sexually (see Chapter 80). The infective organism passes upward through the urethra and the ejaculatory duct and then along the vas deferens to the epididymis.

The client with epididymitis usually reports pain along the inguinal canal and along the vas deferens, followed by pain and swelling in the scrotum and the groin. If epididymitis is untreated, the epididymis becomes swollen and painful and fever may be present. Pyuria and bacteriuria may develop, with resultant chills and fever. An abscess may form, requiring an **orchiectomy** (removal of one or both testes).

COLLABORATIVE MANAGEMENT

Instruct the client with epididymitis to remain in bed with his scrotum elevated on a towel to prevent traction on the spermatic cord, to facilitate venous drainage, and to relieve pain. A scrotal support should be worn when the client is ambulating. A smear or culture of the urine or prostate secretions may be obtained to identify the causative organism. Antibiotics appropriate to the specific organism can then be prescribed. These antibiotics are taken until all acute manifestations are gone. If the epididymitis is chlamydial or gonorrheal in origin, the client's sexual partners are also treated with antibiotics. Nonsteroidal anti-inflammatory drugs such as ibuprofen or naproxen (Naprosyn) may be used to decrease inflammation and promote comfort.

The client may find other comfort measures effective, such as applying cold compresses or ice to the scrotum intermittently and taking sitz baths. Advise him to avoid lifting, straining, or sexual activity until the infection is under control (which may take as long as 4 weeks).

In clients with epididymitis, there must always be the suspicion of a testicular tumor, especially if the condition does not resolve in a week or two. Ultrasound study is often done to rule out an abscess or tumor. Clients with recurrent or chronic painful conditions may require an **epididymectomy** (excision of the epididymis from the testicle).

Orchitis

PATHOPHYSIOLOGY

Orchitis is an acute testicular inflammation resulting from trauma or infection. The infection may be caused by the direct spread of bacteria through the urethra or by an infection elsewhere in the body, such as pneumonia, tuberculosis, gonorrhea, syphilis, or mumps. Usually both the testes and the epididymis are involved (epididymo-orchitis). Risk factors for orchitis include recurrent urinary tract infections, recurrent STDs, congenital abnormalities of the urogenital tract, instrumentation, and chronic indwelling urethral urinary catheter.

Orchitis may be unilateral or bilateral. If the orchitis is bilateral, the client is at increased risk for sterility because of the testicular atrophy and fibrosis that occur during healing.

The manifestations of orchitis are the same as those of epididymitis and include scrotal pain, edema, reports of heavy feelings in the involved testicle(s), dysuria, pain on ejaculation, blood in the semen, and discharge from the penis. In addition, the client may experience nausea and vomiting and pain radiating to the inguinal canal.

COLLABORATIVE MANAGEMENT

The treatment of orchitis is the same as for epididymitis and includes the following:

- Bedrest with scrotal elevation
- Application of ice
- Administration of analgesics and antibiotics

Mumps orchitis, which occurs in about 20% of males who have mumps after puberty, is usually bilateral and develops 4 to 6 days after the parotitis. Any adult male who has not had mumps and is exposed to or contracts mumps is usually given gamma globulin. Although gamma globulin does not prevent mumps, the clinical course of the disease is likely to be less severe, with fewer complications. However, the outcome is unpredictable, and sterility still may result. Childhood vaccination against mumps is an important preventive measure.

GET READY for the NCLEX Examination!

KEY POINTS

Safe Effective Care Environment

- Use sterile technique when empty wound drains following prostatectomy.
- Provide assistance when ambulating clients immediately after prostate surgery.
- Monitor the client's oxygen saturation status when on PCA following prostate surgery.
- Use the information listed in Chart 79-8 to teach clients urinary catheter care.
- Have clients report signs of infection when caring for a urinary catheter in the home.
- Teach clients about no heaving lifting (>15 pounds) following prostate surgery.

Health Promotion and Maintenance

- Teach men at risk for prostate cancer to follow the American Cancer Society's screening guidelines.
- Teach men to report any lower urinary tract symptoms that may be indicative of BPH.
- Teach men how to perform testicular self-examination.
- Teach men to practice safer sex to prevent infections of the reproductive organs.

Psychosocial Integrity

- Because most clients with testicular cancer are young adults, assess their reaction to the possible loss of reproductive ability.
- Because of the high incidence of erectile dysfunction following radical prostatectomy, assess the client's adjustment to these changes in body function.
- Assess the client's anxiety preceding prostate surgery, and allow him to express feelings of fear or grief.
- Teach clients with prostate cancer about American Cancer Society's Man to Man program and the American Foundation for Urologic Disease's US TOO program to help men and their partners cope with prostate cancer.

Physiological Integrity

- Observe for and report complications following radical prostatectomy.
- Observe for and report bloody urine with clots following TURP.
- Maintain traction on the urinary catheter following a TURP.
- Teach clients about drug therapies used to treat BPH.
- Teach clients to avoid any drugs that can cause urinary retention, especially anticholinergics, antihistamines, and decongestants if BPH is present.
- Following discharge after prostate or testicular surgery, instruct the client to notify the physician if any of the following symptoms occurs before the scheduled appointment: chills, fever, increasing tenderness or pain around the incision, drainage, or dehiscence of the incision.
- Teach the client the importance of taking the prescribed barbiturate sleeping medication for several nights postoperatively following penile surgery. Emphasize that barbiturate sleeping medications suppress the REM phase of sleep so that normal nocturnal erections do not occur.

ADDITIONAL STUDY RESOURCES

Go to your Student CD-ROM for Review Questions for the NCLEX Examination.

evolve Go to http://evolve.elsevier.com/Iggy/ for Integrated Management of Care Questions for the NCLEX Examination.

SELECTED BIBLIOGRAPHY

Asterisk indicates a classic or definitive work on this subject.

Abel, L., et al. (2003). Treatment outcomes and quality-of-life issues for patients treated with prostate brachytherapy. *Clinical Journal of Oncology Nursing, 7*(1), 48-54.

Ackley, B., & Ladwig, G. (2002). *Nursing diagnosis handbook: A guide to planning care* (5th ed). St. Louis: Mosby.

American Cancer Society. (2003). *Cancer prevention and early detection. Facts & figures–2003.* Report No. 8600.03. Atlanta: Author.

American Cancer Society. (2005a). *Cancer facts and figures 2005.* Report No. 00-300M-No. 5008.05. Atlanta: Author.

American Cancer Society. (2005b). *Cancer facts and figures for African Americans–2005-2006.* Report No. 8614.05. Atlanta: Author.

Baily, D., et al. (2004). Uncertainty intervention for watchful waiting in prostate cancer. *Cancer Nursing, 27*(5), 339-346.

Balmer, L., & Greco, K. (2004). Prostate cancer recurrence fear: The prostate-specific antigen bounce. *Clinical Journal of Oncology Nursing, 8*(4), 361-366.

Carlson, S. (2004). Prostate disease. *RN, 67*(9), 54-59.

Coleman, E., Hutchins, L., & Goodwin, J. (2004). An overview of cancer in the older adult. *MEDSURG Nursing, 13*(2), 75-80, 109.

Dest, V. (2002). Nursing care for radiation treatment. In M. Wallace & L. Powell (Eds.). *Prostate cancer: Nursing assessment, management, and care* (pp. 89-109). New York: Springer.

Dochterman, J., & Bulechek, G. (Eds.). (2004). *Nursing interventions classification (NIC)* (4th ed). St. Louis: Mosby.

Dorey, G. (2002). Clinical outcome measures for erectile dysfunction: Literature review. *British Journal of Nursing, 11*(1), 54-64.

Ebersole, P., Hess, P., & Luggen, A. (2004). *Toward healthy aging: Human needs and nursing response* (6th ed). St. Louis: Mosby.

Facts and Comparisons. (2004). *Drug facts and comparisons* (58th ed). St. Louis: Author.

Flack, J. (2002). The effect of doxazosin on sexual function in patients with benign prostatic hyperplasia, hypertension, or both. *International Journal of Clinical Practice, 56*(7), 527-530.

Forristal, H. (2002). Benign prostatic hyperplasia and prostate cancer. *Practice Nurse, 24*(9), 37-38, 41, 43.

Galbraith. M.E., Ramirez, J.M., & Pedro, L.W. (2001). Quality of life, health outcomes, and identity for patients with prostate cancer in five different treatment groups. *Oncology Nursing Forum, 28*(3), 551-560.

Hedestig, O., Sandman, P., & Widmark, A. (2003), Living with untreated localized prostate cancer. *Cancer Nursing, 26*(1), 55-60.

Held-Warmkessel, J. (2000). *Contemporary issues in prostate cancer: A nursing perspective.* Subury, MA: Jones & Bartlett.

Held-Warmkessel, J. (2002). What your patient needs to know about prostate cancer. *Nursing 2002, 32*(12), 36-42.

*Jackson, J., et al. (1996). Biofeedback: A noninvasive treatment for incontinence after radical prostatectomy. *Urology Nursing, 16*(2), 50-54.

Kirby, R., Brawer, M., & Denis, L. (2003). *Fast facts: prostate cancer* (4th ed.). Oxford: Health Press.

*Klingman, L. (1999). Assessing the male genitalia. *American Journal of Nursing, 99*(7), 47-50.

Leak, B., et al. (2002). Relevant patient and tumor considerations for early prostate cancer treatment. *Seminars in Urologic Oncology, 20*(1), 39-44.

Lee, E.H. (2002). Assessment, screening and diagnosis of prostate cancer. In M. Wallace & L. Powell (Eds.). *Prostate cancer: Nursing assessment, management, and care* (pp. 33-45). New York: Springer Publishing.

Lewis, J., Rosen, R., & Goldstein, I. (2005). Patient education guide: Erectile dysfunction. *Nursing 2005, 35*(2), 64.

Maliski, S., Clerkin, B., & Litwin, M. (2004). Describing a nurse case manager intervention to empower low-income men with prostate cancer. *Oncology Nursing Forum, 31*(1), 57-64.

Marks, L.S., et al. (2000). Effects of a saw palmetto herbal blend in men with symptomatic benign prostatic hyperplasia. *Journal of Urology, 163*(5), 1451-1456.

Marks, S. (2003). *Prostate and cancer* (3rd ed.). Cambridge, MA: Perseus Publishing.

Marschke, P. (2002). Nursing care for radical prostatectomy. In M. Wallace & L. Powell (Eds.). *Prostate cancer: Nursing assessment, management, and care* (pp. 77-88). New York: Springer.

McCance, K., & Huether, S. (2002). *Pathophysiology: The biologic basis for disease in adults and children* (4th ed). St. Louis: Mosby.

Moorhead, S., Johnson, M., & Maas, M. (Eds.). (2004). *Nursing outcomes classification (NOC)* (3rd ed). St. Louis: Mosby.

Nussbaum, R., McInnes, R., & Willard, H. (2001). *Thompson & Thompson: Genetics in medicine* (6th ed). Philadelphia: W.B. Saunders.

O'Rourke, M. I. (2003). Ketoconazole in the treatment of prostate cancer. *Clinical Journal of Oncology Nursing, 7*(2), 235-236.

Palmer, M.H., et al. (2003). Incontinence after prostatectomy: Coping with incontinence after prostate cancer surgery. *Oncology Nursing Forum, 30*(2), 229-238.

Pickett, M., et al. (2000). Prostate cancer elder alert: Living with treatment choices and outcomes. *Journal of Gerontological Nursing, 26*(2), 22-34.

Russell, I. (2002). Overcoming erectile dysfunction. *Practice Nursing, 13*(9), 415-416, 418.

Scura, K.W., Budin, W., & Garting, E. (2004). Telephone social support and education for adaptation to prostate cancer: A pilot study. *Oncology Nursing Forum, 31*(2), 335-338.

Stevenson, T., & McNeill, J. (2004). Surgical management of testicular cancer. *Clinical Journal of Oncology Nursing, 8*(4), 355-360.

Stipetich, R.L., et al. (2002). Nursing assessment of sexual function following permanent prostate brachytherapy for patients with early-stage prostate cancer. *Clinical Journal of Oncology Nursing, 6*(6), 271-274.

Wallace, M., & Powell, L. (2002). *Prostate cancer: Nursing assessment, management, and care.* New York: Springer Publishing.

Wallace, M. (2003). Uncertainty and quality of life of older men who undergo watchful waiting for prostate cancer. *Oncology Nursing Forum, 30*(2) 303-309.

Wallner K. (2000). Prostate cancer: A non-surgical perspective. Seattle, WA: SmartMedicine.

Weinrich, S.P., et al. (2000). Barriers to prostate screening. *Cancer Nursing, 23,* 117-121.

Weinrich, S.P., et al. (2002). Interest in genetic prostate cancer susceptibility testing among African American men. *Cancer Nursing, 25*(1), 28-34.

CHAPTER 80

Interventions for Clients with Sexually Transmitted Diseases

SHIRLEY E. VAN ZANDT

LEARNING OUTCOMES

After studying this chapter, you should be able to:

1. Explain how sexually transmitted diseases (STDs) can be prevented.
2. Compare the stages of syphilis.
3. Prioritize nursing care for the client with syphilis at each stage.
4. Identify the role of drug therapy in managing clients with genital herpes (GH).
5. Discuss the psychosocial effects of having an STD.
6. Develop a community-based teaching plan for clients diagnosed with gonorrhea.
7. Describe the assessment findings that are typical in clients with *Chlamydia trachomatis* infection.
8. Analyze assessment data to determine common nursing diagnoses for women with pelvic inflammatory disease (PID).
9. Formulate a collaborative plan of care for a client with PID.
10. Describe the mechanisms of action, side effects, and nursing implications for drug therapy of PID.
11. Develop a community-based teaching plan for clients with PID.
12. Evaluate care for a client with PID.
13. Identify common causes of vaginal infections.

Go to your Student CD-ROM for Review Questions for the NCLEX Examination keyed to these Learning Outcomes.

Sexually transmitted diseases (STDs)* are caused by infectious organisms that have been passed from one person to another through intimate contact, usually oral, or vaginal intercourse. Some organisms that cause these diseases are transmitted only through sexual contact. Other organisms are transmitted by parenteral exposure to infected blood, fecal-oral transmission, intrauterine transmission to the fetus, and perinatal transmission from mother to neonate (Table 80-1).

With improved diagnostic techniques, increased knowledge about organisms that can be sexually transmitted, and changes in sexual attitudes and practices, the number of cases of STDs continues to increase. Sexual issues are often controversial, and nurses must respect the choices that clients make. Providing confidentiality is essential for clients to receive correct information, make informed decisions, and obtain appropriate care (see the Legal/Ethical Issues box on p. 1884).

*NOTE: This text uses the term *sexually transmitted diseases (STDs)* to be consistent with the language used by the Centers for Disease Control and Prevention (CDC).

The prevalence of STDs is a major health concern worldwide. External factors, such as increasing population, cultural factors (e.g., later marriage, earlier first intercourse), political and economic policies, as well as international travel and migration, affect the prevalence of STDs in any given geographic area. The prevalence is also affected by changing human physiology patterns such as earlier menarche. Sexual attitudes and behaviors and access to care play a major role in the risk of acquiring an STD. STDs also cause complications that can contribute to severe physical and emotional suffering, including infertility, ectopic pregnancy, cancer, and death. Some of the most common complications caused by sexually transmitted organisms are listed in Table 80-2.

Chlamydia, gonorrhea, syphilis, and AIDS (acquired immunodeficiency syndrome) are reportable to local health authorities in every state (Centers for Disease Control and Prevention [CDC], 2002a). Other STDs, such as genital herpes (GH), HIV infection, and chancroid, may or may not be reported, depending on local legal requirements. Rigorous reporting and a follow-up effort by local public health

TABLE 80-1 Sexually Transmitted Diseases

- Human immunodeficiency virus infection
- Chancroid
- Syphilis
- Lymphogranuloma venereum
- Genital herpes simplex virus infection
- Genital warts
- Gonococcal infection
- Chlamydial infection
- Nongonococcal urethritis
- Mucopurulent cervicitis
- Epididymitis
- Pelvic inflammatory disease
- Sexually transmitted enteritis
- Sexually transmitted proctitis
- Trichomoniasis
- Candidal infection
- Bacterial vaginosis
- Viral hepatitis
- Cytomegalovirus infection
- Ectoparasitic infection
  - Pediculosis pubis
  - Scabies

From Centers for Disease Control and Prevention. (1998). 1998 Guidelines for treatment of sexually transmitted diseases. *Morbidity and Mortality Weekly Report, 47*(No. RR-1), 1-103.

LEGAL/ETHICAL ISSUES

SEXUAL DECISION MAKING AND CONFIDENTIALITY FOR CLIENTS WITH SEXUALLY TRANSMITTED DISEASES

Sexual issues are surrounded with much controversy in the United States. Personal values, cultural mores, and public health standards often collide as clients make decisions about their sexual health. Americans hold strongly to the principle of autonomy. Autonomy in sexual decision making (e.g., about whether to be sexually active, how to choose sexual partners, and the type of sexual behavior that is appropriate) is held as a high value. The standard of confidentiality protects this principle of autonomy in some clinical situations and under some state laws.

As nurses aim to respect this principle of autonomy about sexual decision making and confidentiality, they are challenged by the public health concerns of protecting the health of the entire community versus the autonomy of each person to make his or her own decisions. Increasing rates of chlamydial infection, especially in the teenage population, with the costly risk of infertility complications, make the idea of autonomy in sexual decision making more problematic. Clients who refuse to discuss their sexually transmitted disease with their partners, or partners who choose not to get tested or treated also pose challenges to our respect for autonomy in light of the overwhelming public health concerns. Nurses feel the conflict between their commitment to confidentiality (autonomy) and their commitment to promotion of the public's health (beneficence).

departments and health care professionals is one intervention for decreasing the incidence of STDs.

Nurses in a variety of community settings are responsible for identifying clients at risk for STDs, caring for clients with diagnosed STDs, and preventing further cases through education and case finding. Nurses in secondary and tertiary care settings, such as hospitals, also have a responsibility to recognize clients who are at risk for or who have STDs.

The Centers for Disease Control and Prevention (CDC) updates its guidelines for treatment of STDs. The 2002 guidelines provide information, treatment standards, and counseling advice to help decrease the spread of STDs (CDC, 2002a).

TABLE 80-2 Complications Caused by Sexually Transmitted Organisms

Complication	Causative Organisms
Salpingitis, infertility, and ectopic pregnancy	*Neisseria gonorrhoeae* *Chlamydia trachomatis* *Mycoplasma hominis* *Ureaplasma urealyticum*
Reproductive loss (abortion/miscarriage)	*N. gonorrhoeae* *C. trachomatis* Herpes simplex virus *M. hominis* *U. urealyticum* *Treponema pallidum*
Puerperal infection	*N. gonorrhoeae* *C. trachomatis*
Perinatal infection	Hepatitis B virus Human immunodeficiency virus Human papillomavirus *N. gonorrhoeae* *C. trachomatis* Herpes simplex virus *T. pallidum* Cytomegalovirus Group B streptococcus
Cancer of genital area	*C. trachomatis* Herpes simplex virus Human papillomavirus
Male urethritis	*M. hominis* Herpes simplex virus *N. gonorrhoeae* *C. trachomatis* *U. urealyticum*
Vulvovaginitis	Herpes simplex virus *Trichomonas vaginalis* Bacteria causing vaginosis *Candida albicans*
Cervicitis	*N. gonorrhoeae* *C. trachomatis* Herpes simplex virus
Proctitis	*N. gonorrhoeae* *C. trachomatis* Herpes simplex virus *Campylobacter jejuni* *Shigella* species *Entamoeba histolytica*
Hepatitis	*T. pallidum* Hepatitis A, B, and C virus
Dermatitis	*Sarcoptes scabiei* *Phthirus pubis*
Genital ulceration or warts	*C. trachomatis* Herpes simplex virus Human papillomavirus *T. pallidum* *Haemophilus ducreyi* *Calymmatobacterium granulomatis*

WOMEN'S HEALTH CONSIDERATIONS

Women, because of the extensive and heavily vascular mucous membranes of the vagina, are more easily infected with STDs than are men and are at greater risk for health problems caused by STDs. Young women who are sexually active have unprotected sexual intercourse more often than do older women and are at greatest risk because of the following:

- Lack of knowledge about the risk of disease
- Their belief that they are not vulnerable to disease

- Their mistaken belief that oral contraceptives; contraceptive patches, sponges, and foams; and intrauterine devices protect them from STDs as well as from pregnancy
- Alcohol consumption, which promotes risky sexual behavior

Postmenopausal women also may be at high risk for STDs because many perceive that pregnancy is no longer a risk and, thus do not use barrier protection. Mucosal tears from vaginal atrophy in postmenopausal women may also place them at greater risk.

Women have more asymptomatic infections that may delay diagnosis and treatment. This delay increases the likelihood of more serious problems, including irreversible damage to reproductive organs and systemic illness. Embarrassment, denial, or fear about STDs may further delay treatment, increasing the potential for serious complications.

ACQUIRED IMMUNODEFICIENCY SYNDROME

Acquired immunodeficiency syndrome (AIDS), a disease caused by infection with the human immunodeficiency virus (HIV), causes immunosuppression and affects the body's ability to fight disease. HIV is transmitted through infected body fluids (e.g., semen, vaginal secretions, blood and blood products, breast milk) infected with HIV. Adults at high risk include the following:

- People who engage in anal sexual activity
- People who share needles
- People who have unprotected sexual intercourse with multiple partners
- People who have unprotected sexual intercourse with partners infected with HIV
- People who have hemophilia or other clotting disorders
- People who used untested blood and blood products before 1985
- Health care workers
- Sexual partners of anyone at risk for HIV (of both sexes)

Men and women with HIV disease are at greater risk for acquiring other STDs (Williams, 2003). HIV affects the immune system and can be transmitted in ways other than by sexual contact; it is discussed in detail in Chapter 25.

INFECTIONS ASSOCIATED WITH ULCERS

Syphilis

PATHOPHYSIOLOGY

Etiology

Syphilis is a complex sexually transmitted disease (STD) that can become systemic and cause serious complications and even death. The causative organism of syphilis is *Treponema pallidum,* a spirochete with a slender, spiral shape that resembles a corkscrew. Nonpathogenic *Treponema* species are found in the mouth, intestinal tract, and genital areas of people and animals. Although the organism can be seen only with a darkfield microscope, several serologic tests may be used to screen for the presence of syphilis antigen or antibody. *T. pallidum* is damaged by dry air or any known disinfectant. The organisms die within hours at temperatures of 105.8° to 107.6° F (41° to 42° C) and are not airborne. The infection is usually transmitted by sexual contact, but transmission can occur through close body contact and kissing.

Meeting HEALTHY PEOPLE 2010 Objectives

SEXUALLY TRANSMITTED DISEASES

Objective 25.3: Eliminate sustained domestic transmission of primary and secondary syphilis.

Objective 25.6: Reduce the proportion of females who have ever required treatment for pelvic inflammatory disease.

- Teach sexually active clients of all ages to use protection during sexual intercourse.
- Teach clients how and when to use condoms.
- Educate clients and partners about the medical complications of STDs and pelvic inflammatory disease (PID).
- Target nonwhite groups for education and screening because these groups have the highest incidence of STDs and PID.
- Target clients who are substance abusers for education and screening because they have a high incidence of STDs and PID.
- Participate in health fairs and surveillance programs to screen at-risk groups.
- Develop culturally appropriate education materials.
- Ensure that education materials are written or presented at no greater than a fourth grade literacy level.

Incidence/Prevalence

Before penicillin was available in the 1940s, syphilis affected nearly 25% of the U.S. population. Cases of primary and secondary syphilis peaked in 1948 and then declined sharply until 1958. From that time until 1990 there was a slow rise in the rates of syphilis despite successful treatment. In 1990, the number of cases increased significantly to a post-World War II peak of more than 50,000. Because of strong public health efforts between 1990 and 2000, there was a 90% decrease in cases to an all-time low in 2000, followed by an increase in 2002 and 2003 (CDC, 2004). Areas of the southern United States and men who have sex with men have the highest rates of new syphilis cases. African Americans have a 16 times greater rate of acquiring syphilis than white individuals; however, this rate is much lower than it was in previous years (CDC, 2004). One of the Healthy People 2010 objectives is to eliminate syphilis in the United States (see the Meeting Healthy People 2010 Objectives box above).

Syphilis progresses through stages: primary, secondary, latency, and tertiary.

Primary Syphilis

The appearance of an ulcer, called a **chancre,** is the first sign of syphilis. The chancre develops at the site of entry (inoculation) of the organism from 10 to 90 days after exposure (3 weeks is average). Chancres may be found on any area of the skin or mucous membranes but occur most often on the genitalia, lips, nipples, and hands and in the oral cavity, anus, and rectum.

During this highly infectious stage, the chancre begins as a small papule. Within 3 to 7 days, it breaks down into its typical appearance: a painless, indurated, smooth weeping lesion. Regional lymph nodes enlarge, feel firm, and are not painful. Without treatment, the chancre usually disappears

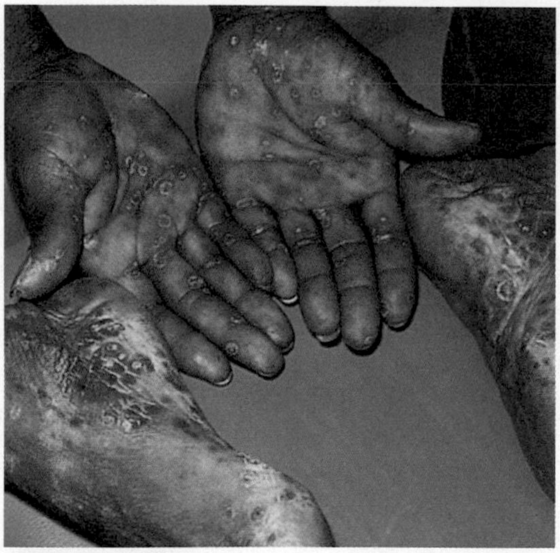

Figure 80-1 ■ Palmar and plantar secondary syphilis. (From Morse, S., et al. [2003]. *Atlas of sexually transmitted diseases and AIDS* [3rd ed.]. Edinburgh: Mosby.)

within 6 weeks. However, the organism spreads throughout the body, and the client is still infectious.

Secondary Syphilis

Secondary syphilis develops 6 weeks to 6 months after the onset of primary syphilis. Secondary syphilis is a systemic disease because the spirochetes circulate throughout the bloodstream. Manifestations include malaise, low-grade fever, headache, muscular aches and pains, and sometimes a sore throat.

These symptoms are often mistaken for those of influenza. A generalized rash develops, which involves the palms and soles of the feet. Although the rash has no typical appearance, it tends to evolve from papules to squamous papules to pustules. Other skin lesions include psoriasis-like rashes (Figure 80-1), wartlike lesions (condyloma lata), and mucous patches. The lesions are highly contagious and should not be touched without gloves. The rash subsides without treatment in 4 to 12 weeks.

Early and Late Latent Syphilis

After the second stage of syphilis, there is a period of latency. *Early* latent syphilis occurs during the first year after infection, and infectious lesions can recur. *Late* latent syphilis is a disease of more than 1 year's duration after infection. This stage is not infectious except to the fetus of a pregnant woman. Clients with latent syphilis may or may not have reactive serologic test findings.

Tertiary Syphilis

Tertiary, or late, syphilis occurs after a highly variable period, from 4 to 20 years. This stage develops in untreated cases and can mimic almost any pathologic condition because any organ system can be affected. The following are manifestations of late syphilis:

- Benign lesions (gummas) of the skin, mucous membranes, and bones
- Cardiovascular syphilis, usually in the form of aortic valvular disease and aortic aneurysms
- Neurosyphilis, causing central nervous system problems (e.g., meningitis, hearing loss, generalized paresis)

HEALTH PROMOTION/ILLNESS PREVENTION

The most important aspect for prevention of most sexually transmitted diseases (STDs), including syphilis, is education. All people, regardless of age, gender, ethnicity, or sexual orientation, are susceptible to STDs. STDs are largely preventable through education that includes safer sex practices. *Do not assume that a person is not sexually active because of his or her age, profession, or religion.* Discuss prevention methods frankly with all clients who are sexually active. Safer sex practices are those that reduce the risk of nonintact skin or mucous membranes coming in contact with infected body fluids and blood. Such practices include using the following:

- A latex condom for genital and anal intercourse
- A condom or latex barrier (dental dam) over the genitals or anus during oral-genital or oral-anal sexual contact
- Latex gloves for finger or hand contact with the vagina or rectum

Abstinence and decreasing the number of sexual partners also decrease the risk for acquiring an STD. Chapter 25 describes specific sexual acts that carry the greatest risk for STDs.

◆COLLABORATIVE MANAGEMENT

◆Assessment

Assessment of the client who has manifestations of syphilis begins with a history to gather information about any lesions or rash. The history should include a risk assessment and sexual history and whether previous testing or treatment for syphilis or other STDs has ever been done (Chart 80-1). Ask about allergic reactions to drugs, especially penicillin. A woman may present with inguinal lymph node enlargement, the location that drains the area of the vagina and cervix. She may state a history of sexual contact with a male partner who had an ulcer that she noticed during the encounter. Men usually discover the chancre on the penis or scrotum.

Conduct a physical examination, including inspection and palpation, to identify manifestations of syphilis. Wear gloves while palpating any lesions because of the highly contagious treponemes that are present. Women frequently have the chancre on areas that are not easily visible to them, such as the vagina or cervix. Observe for and document rashes of any type because of the variable presentation of secondary syphilis.

After the physical examination, the health care provider obtains a specimen of the chancre for examination under a darkfield microscope. Diagnosis of primary or secondary syphilis is confirmed if *T. pallidum,* the characteristic spirochete, is present. If the first slide is negative for *T. pallidum,* the procedure should be repeated in 3 days because many conditions can cause a false-negative result.

Blood tests are also used to diagnose syphilis. The usual screening test is the Venereal Disease Research Laboratory (VDRL) serum test. This test is based on an antibody-antigen reaction that determines both the presence and the amount of antibodies produced by the body in response to an infection by *T. pallidum.* The VDRL test becomes reactive 2 to 6 weeks after infection. VDRL titers are also used to monitor

CHART 80-1

FOCUSED ASSESSMENT of
The Client with a Sexually Transmitted Disease

Assess history of present illness:
- Chief complaint
- Symptoms by quality and quantity, precipitating and palliative factors
- Any treatments taken (self-prescribed or over-the-counter products)

Assess past medical history:
- Major health problems—including any history of STDs/PID
- Surgeries—obstetric and gynecologic, circumcision

Assess current health status:
- Menstrual history for irregularities
- Sexual history
  - Type and frequency of sexual activity
  - Number of sexual contacts
  - Sexual orientation
- Contraceptive history
- Medications
- Allergies
- Lifestyle risks—drugs, alcohol, tobacco

Assess preventive health care practices:
- Pap smears
- Regular STD screening
- Use of barrier contraceptives to prevent STDs and pregnancy

Assess physical examination findings:
- Vital signs
- Oropharyngeal findings
- Abdominal findings
- Genital or pelvic findings
- Anorectal findings

Assess laboratory data:
- Urinalysis
- Hematology
- Cervical, urethral, oral, rectal specimens
- Lesion samples for microbiology and virology
- Pregnancy testing

PID, Pelvic inflammatory disease; *STDs*, sexually transmitted diseases.

treatment effectiveness. The antibodies are not specific to *T. pallidum,* and false-positive reactions often occur from such conditions as drug addiction, cancer, hepatitis, some viral diseases, and systemic lupus erythematosus (SLE).

If a positive VDRL result is obtained, the health care provider orders a more specific test, such as the *fluorescent treponemal antibody absorption (FTA-ABS)* test or the *microhemagglutination assay for T. palladium* (MHA-TP), to confirm the infection. These tests are more sensitive for all stages of syphilis, although false-positive results may still occur.

Interventions

Drug Therapy. Antibiotics are the main therapy for the client with syphilis. The drug therapy of choice is benzathine penicillin G, given intramuscularly as a single 2.4 million unit dose. Allergic reactions to the antibiotic can occur. Therefore it is important to monitor for allergic manifestations (e.g., rash, edema, shortness of breath, chest tightness, anxiety). Penicillin desensitization is recommended for penicillin-allergic clients. The client who has never had penicillin previously should have a skin test before receiving a penicillin injection. Keep all clients at the health care agency for at least 30 minutes after they have received injections of antibiotics, so that manifestations of an allergic reaction can be detected and treated. If an allergic reaction does occur, treatment can begin immediately. The most severe reaction is anaphylaxis. All health care professionals working in clinics or offices where injections of penicillin are given must be familiar with the symptoms and treatment of anaphylaxis (see Chapter 26).

The **Jarisch-Herxheimer reaction** may also follow antibiotic therapy for syphilis. This reaction is caused by the rapid release of products from the disruption of the cells of the organism. Onset occurs within 2 hours after therapy, with a peak at 4 to 8 hours. Symptoms include generalized aches, pain at the injection site, vasodilation and hypotension, and a rise in temperature. These symptoms do not always occur and often are benign. This reaction may be treated symptomatically with analgesics and antipyretics.

TABLE 80-3 Selected Nursing Diagnoses for Clients with Sexually Transmitted Diseases

- Risk for Injury related to the disease process
- Ineffective Coping related to high degree of threat, fear, guilt, or anger
- Noncompliance (treatment and/or partner follow-up) related to cost, significant other, access and convenience of care, cultural influences
- Sexual Dysfunction related to disease process, fear of transmission
- Impaired Skin Integrity related to the presence of genital ulcers, warts, or rash
- Ineffective Health Maintenance related to lack of resources and information about the mode of transmission, disease process, or need for treatment
- Impaired Social Interaction related to self-concept disturbance or social stigma
- Acute Pain related to the physical agent (infection process)
- Anxiety related to threat to health status (possible infertility) as a result of having an STD
- Chronic Low Self-Esteem/Situational Low Self-Esteem related to disturbed body image as a result of having an STD

Nursing Management. Nursing interventions are based on data gained during the history and physical assessment. Nursing diagnoses for clients with syphilis, as well as other STDs, are listed in Table 80-3.

Reinforce the information provided to the client about the cause of infection (sexual transmission); treatment, including side effects, possible complications of untreated or incompletely treated disease; and the need for follow-up care. All sexual partners must be adequately treated as soon as possible. Discuss with the client the importance of partner notification and treatment, including the risk for reinfection if the partner goes untreated. Inform the client that the disease must be reported to the local health authority and that all information will be held in strict confidence. Encourage the client to provide accurate information for this follow-up to ensure that all at-risk partners are treated appropriately. Provide a setting that offers privacy and encourages open discussion.

Urge the client to adhere to the treatment regimen, which includes follow-up visits. Also urge sexual abstinence until the treatment is completed.

The emotional responses to syphilis vary and may include feelings of fear, depression, guilt, and anxiety. Clients may experience guilt if they have infected others or anger if they have been infected by a partner. If further psychosocial interventions are needed, encourage the client to discuss these feelings or refer him or her to other resources such as psychotherapy groups, self-help support groups, or STD clinics.

Genital Herpes

PATHOPHYSIOLOGY

Etiology

Genital herpes (GH) is an acute, recurring, incurable viral disease. Two serotypes of herpes simplex virus (HSV) affect the genitalia: type 1 (HSV-1) and type 2 (HSV-2). Most nongenital lesions, such as cold sores, are caused by HSV-1; HSV-2 causes most of the genital lesions. However, this distinction is academic because the transmission, symptoms, diagnosis, and treatment are nearly identical for the two types. Either type can produce oral or genital lesions through oral-genital contact with an infected person.

The incubation period is 2 to 20 days, with the average period being 1 week. Many people are asymptomatic during the primary infection. When symptoms do occur, they may be severe during the first infection and may require hospitalization.

Itching or a tingling sensation may be felt in the skin 1 to 2 days before an outbreak. These sensations are followed by the appearance of **vesicles** (blisters) in a typical cluster (see Figure 70-13) on the penis, scrotum, vulva, perineum, vagina, cervix, or perianal region. The blisters rupture spontaneously in a day or two and leave painful erosions. These lesions can become extensive, and other symptoms, such as headaches, fever, general malaise, and swelling of inguinal lymph nodes, may be present. Urination may be painful, and clients with urinary retention may need to be catheterized. Lesions resolve within 2 to 6 weeks.

After the lesions heal, the virus remains in a dormant state in the nerve ganglia (specifically, in the sacral ganglia). Periodically, the virus may activate, and symptoms recur. These recurrences may be triggered by many factors, including stress, fever, sunburn, poor nutrition, menses, and sexual activity.

Recurrences are not caused by reinfection. Recurrent episodes are usually less severe and of shorter duration than the primary infection. Some clients have no symptoms at all during recurrence or viral reactivation. *However, there is viral shedding, and the client is infectious.* Long-term complications of GH include the risk of neonatal transmission and an increased risk for acquiring HIV infections. The risk for neonatal transmission is greater in a pregnant woman who has a primary infection than in one who has a recurrence.

Incidence/Prevalence

On the basis of serologic studies, not symptoms, 50 million persons in the United States may have HSV-2 (CDC, 2002a). HSV-2 is believed to cause 70% to 95% of the primary episodes of GH and recurs more often than HSV-1. Most people infected with GH have not been diagnosed (CDC, 2002a). About 19% of the U.S. population between the ages of 14 and 49 years are thought to be infected (McQuillan, 2000). Most people infected with HSV have not received a diagnosis because they have mild symptoms and shed virus intermittently.

COLLABORATIVE MANAGEMENT

Assessment

The diagnosis of GH is usually based on the client's history and physical examination and is confirmed through a viral culture (see Chart 80-1). Cultures are most accurate if specimens are obtained within 48 hours of the first outbreak of the blisters. Fluid from inside the blister should be obtained to ensure a correct diagnosis. GH is often diagnosed without cultures if the presenting manifestations are classic.

CHART 80-2

BEST PRACTICE for
Care of the Client with Genital Herpes

- Administer oral analgesics as prescribed.
- Apply local anesthetic sprays or ointments as prescribed
- Apply ice packs or warm compresses to the client's lesions.
- Administer sitz baths three or four times a day.
- Encourage an increase in fluid intake.
- Encourage frequent urination.
- Pour water over the client's genitalia while the client is voiding, or encourage voiding while the client is sitting in a tub of water or standing in a shower.
- Catheterize the client as necessary.
- Encourage genital hygiene, and encourage keeping the skin clean and dry.
- Wash hands thoroughly after contact with lesions, and launder towels that have had direct contact with lesions.
- Wear gloves when applying ointments.
- Advise the client to avoid sexual activity when lesions are present.
- Advise the client to use latex or polyurethane condoms during all sexual exposures.
- Instruct the client in the use, side effects, and risks versus benefits of antiviral agents.

Interventions

Treatment of HSV-infected clients is usually symptomatic. The goals of management are to decrease the discomfort from painful ulcerations, to promote healing without secondary infection, to decrease viral shedding, and to prevent infection transmission (Chart 80-2).

Drug Therapy. Antiviral drugs are used to treat GH. *The drugs do not cure the infection* but do decrease the severity, promote healing, and decrease the frequency of recurrent outbreaks. Drug therapy is recommended for most people with an initial outbreak. Topical therapy is not as effective as oral therapy. Acyclovir (Zovirax, Avirax✱), famciclovir (Famvir), or valacyclovir (Valtrex) may be used. The main differences in these drugs are cost and frequency of use. Dosage and length of treatment differ for primary outbreaks (lasting 7 to 10 days) and recurrent outbreaks (lasting 5 days) (Chart 80-3). Mild recurrent episodes do not show a reasonable benefit from antiviral treatment, and the cost may outweigh the benefit. Therapy for severe recurrent outbreaks may be beneficial if it is started within 1 day of the appearance of lesions or during the period of itching or tingling before lesions appear.

Clients who have frequent recurrences (more than six in a year) may benefit from daily suppressive treatment with antivirals. Suppression may reduce recurrences by 70% to 80% in clients with frequent outbreaks. However, suppression only reduces but does not prevent viral shedding even when symptoms are not present (CDC, 2002a). Clients receiving continuous therapy should stop after 1 year for reassessment of recurrences.

The cost of care for clients with GH is enormous, making it a major public health problem with a large economic burden. Annual direct medical costs in the United States are estimated at $207 million. Of that amount, health care provider visits accounted for 36%, and drug therapy accounted for 64% (Tao et al., 2000).

CHART 80-3

DRUG THERAPY for
Genital Herpes: First Clinical Episode of Genital Herpes

Drug	Dosage	Nursing Interventions	Rationales
Acyclovir (Zovirax, Avirax✱)	400 mg PO three times daily for 7 to 10 days	Instruct client that nausea and vomiting may occur when taking the drug.	The client is prepared for possible side effect.
	Or 200 mg PO five times daily for 7 to 10 days	Same as above.	Same as above.
Famciclovir (Famvir)	*Or* 250 mg PO three times daily for 7 to 10 days	Instruct client that the drug is most effective if started within the first 48 hours of symptoms.	Efficacy has not been established for the first dose started more than 72 hours after the onset of symptoms.
Valacyclovir (Valtrex)	*Or* 1 g PO twice daily for 7 to 10 days	Observe for side effects, including gastrointestinal disturbances, headaches, and dizziness.	The client is prepared for possible side effects.

Nursing Management. Nursing management includes client counseling and education about the infection, the potential for recurrent episodes, the correct use and possible side effects of antiviral therapy, viral shedding even when clients are symptom free, and sexual transmission. Discussion about sexual activity is extremely important. Remind clients to abstain from sexual activity while lesions are present. Urge condom use during all sexual exposures because of the increased risk for HSV transmission, because viral shedding can occur even when lesions are not present. Teach the client about how and when to use condoms (Chart 80-4).

Assess the client's psychological responses to the diagnosis of genital herpes. Many clients are initially shocked and need reassurance that they can manage the disease. Infected clients have reported feelings of disbelief, uncleanness, isolation, and loneliness. They have also reported anger at their partners for transmitting the infection or fear of rejection by partners because they have the infection. Help clients cope with the diagnosis by being sensitive and supportive during assessments and interventions. Encourage social support and refer clients to support groups such as HELP (local support groups of the National Herpes Resource Center). Symptomatic care may include oral analgesics, topical anesthetics, sitz baths, and increased oral fluid intake.

Health Promotion. Emphasize the risk of fetal infection to all clients, both male and female. Women and men who have genital herpes need to inform the maternity care provider of their history during future pregnancies.

CHART 80-4

CLIENT EDUCATION GUIDE
Use of Condoms

- Use latex or polyurethane condoms rather than natural membrane condoms.
- Use a condom with every sexual encounter (including oral, vaginal, and anal).
- Female condoms (Reality)—polyurethane sheaths in the vagina—are effective in preventing transmission of viruses, including HIV.
- Condoms infrequently (2 per 100) break during sexual intercourse, unless used incorrectly.
- Keep condoms (especially latex) in a cool, dry place, out of direct sunlight.
- Do not use condoms that are in damaged packages or that are brittle or discolored.
- Always handle a condom with care to avoid damaging it with fingernails, teeth, or other sharp objects.
- Put condoms on before any genital contact. Hold the condom by the tip and unroll it on the penis. Leave a space at the tip to collect semen.
- If you use a lubricant with condoms, make sure that the lubricant is water based and washes away with water. Oil-based products may damage latex condoms.
- Use of spermicide (nonoxynol-9) with condoms, either lubricated condoms or vaginal application, has *not* been proved to be more or less effective against STDs than use without spermicide. *Spermicide-coated condoms have been associated with* Escherichia coli *urinary tract infections in women. Nonoxynol-9 may increase risk for transmission of HIV during vaginal intercourse and anal intercourse. Its use is discouraged for anal intercourse.*
- If a condom breaks, replace it immediately.
- After ejaculation, withdraw the erect penis carefully, holding the condom at the base of the penis to prevent the condom from slipping off.
- Never use a condom more than once.

Modified from Centers for Disease Control and Prevention. (2002). Sexually transmitted diseases treatment guidelines. *Mortality and Morbidity Weekly Report, 517*(RR-6), 1-80.

Critical Thinking Challenge

The client is a 50-year-old woman who is a lawyer. She has been a widow for 10 years and her children are grown. She has come to the GYN clinic because she has painful blisters on her perineum and vulva. She says that although she has some burning with urination, she doesn't think she has a bladder infection because the urine doesn't smell and she does not have frequency. She also tells you that she has a lump in her right groin and just feels fatigued. She asks if all these problems could mean she is entering menopause. Her last Pap smear, GYN examination, and mammogram were performed 18 months ago.

When you inspect her genital region, you see many clustered vesicles and some eroded and crusted lesions.

1. What additional information should you obtain?
2. What infectious process is most likely?
3. How will you prepare her for the diagnostic tests?
4. Why does she have burning on urination?

evolve For suggested answer guidelines, go to http://evolve.elsevier.com/Iggy/.

Lymphogranuloma Venereum

PATHOPHYSIOLOGY

Etiology

Lymphogranuloma venereum (LGV) is the result of genital infection with one of three serotypes of *Chlamydia trachomatis,* which is spread systemically until it localizes in the genital or rectal lymph nodes. The incubation period is 3 to 30 days. The primary lesion, at the point of entry, is transient, painless, and often not noticed by the client. The lesion usually appears on the penis in men and on the vaginal wall in women. However, sores may also be located in the mouth and rectum. Five times as many men are diagnosed with this disease as are women.

Lesions vary in form from herpes-like blisters (vesicles), to ulcers, papules, or pustules. Within 1 to 2 weeks after the primary lesion appears, secondary signs of infection appear. Lymphadenopathy (primarily inguinal and femoral) is present, more commonly in men than in women. Swelling from the enlarged lymph nodes occurs on both sides of the inguinal ligament and forms the characteristic "groove sign" of LGV. This sign is only present in about 10% to 15% of clients (Schacter & Stephens, 2003). Women and men who have had anal sex may have inflamed perianal or perirectal tissues (CDC, 2002a). Other manifestations may include headache, malaise, arthralgia, and anorexia. Most clients seek care at this point.

Lymphadenopathy can recede or develop into an abscess or firm bubo. The bubo may become more **fluctuant** (softer and fluid filled). When the bubo ruptures, healing occurs slowly. Sinus tracts, formed as a result of the infection, drain thick, viscous pus for several weeks, leaving behind deep scars.

Complications of the infection include fistulas, rectal strictures, chronic enlarged lymph nodes, and proctitis. Systemic involvement can cause carditis, arthritis, and pneumonia.

Incidence/Prevalence

LGV is common in areas of South America, Asia, Africa, and the Caribbean. It is far less common in more affluent countries. The actual incidence is not known because LGV is difficult to distinguish from other lesion-producing infections. Because it is more common in other areas of the world, ask clients about recent travel to endemic areas by themselves or by their partners.

◆COLLABORATIVE MANAGEMENT

The diagnosis of LGV is usually made on physical examination and serologic testing. The serologic test, an antibody complement fixation test (LGV-CF), is considered positive if the titer is higher than 1:64. Detection of *Chlamydia trachomatis* in material aspirated from a bubo, rather than from an open lesion, is most diagnostic for LGV. Detection of the organism can be made with the use of a test kit using gene amplification methods, although this type of test is relatively new for LGV (Mabey & Peeling, 2002). Regular cultures from the enlarged lymph nodes or bubo can be used to isolate organism but this method is not very sensitive (Schacter & Stephens, 2003).

The health care provider prescribes doxycycline (Monodox, Doxy-Caps, Doxycin✱) 100 mg orally twice daily or an erythromycin-based drug 500 mg orally four times daily for 21 days. Antibiotic treatment cures the infection and prevents further tissue damage. Infected lymph nodes may be aspirated by needle or incised and drained to prevent ulcer formation. Surgical intervention may be needed for late complications, such as perianal or perirectal strictures and fistulas. Nursing management and client education is similar to that for syphilis.

Sexual partners should be tested for cervical or urethral chlamydial infection. They should be treated if they had sexual contact with the client during the 30 days before the client's onset of symptoms.

Chancroid

PATHOPHYSIOLOGY

Etiology

Chancroid lesions are painful genital ulcerations caused by infection with *Haemophilus ducreyi,* a gram-negative bacteria. Chancroid ulcers are soft, genital lesions. These lesions and inguinal lymphadenopathy without systemic illness are the usual presentation. The infection develops as a result of sexual exposure or self-contamination from a lesion elsewhere on the body. The incubation period for chancroid varies from 3 to 10 days. A tender papule appears at the site of inoculation. This lesion rapidly breaks down to form an irregularly shaped, deep ulcer that has a purulent discharge and bleeds easily.

Complications include inguinal adenitis, balanitis, phimosis, and urethral fistulas. Chancroids differ from chancres caused by syphilis in that chancroids are soft and painful. Transmission of the disease is through contact with the ulcer or with the discharge from the infected local lymph glands during sexual activity.

Incidence/Prevalence

Although chancroid has a worldwide distribution, it is most common in less affluent tropical and subtropical countries, such as Africa, the West Indies, and Asia. It also can be found in parts of the United States. In 2000, 99 U.S. cases were reported (Ballard & Morse, 2003).

Chancroid is a cofactor for HIV transmission, leading to high rates of HIV infection of those with chancroid. About 10% of clients with chancroid acquired in the United States are co-infected with syphilis and herpes simplex virus (HSV). The rate of co-infection appears higher for those clients who acquired the disease outside the United States (CDC, 2002a). This co-infection appears to be the result of the open genital lesions. Uncircumcised men may be at greater risk for infection than circumcised men, and men are more frequently infected than women.

◆COLLABORATIVE MANAGEMENT

The health care provider obtains cultures from the ulcers to isolate the *Haemophilus ducreyi* organism. Gram staining of the exudate from the ulcer can be difficult because of multiple microbial contamination, but the gram-negative rods may be seen. Usually the diagnosis is based on the presence of ulcerative genital lesions, lymphadenopathy, and the absence of systemic symptoms. Syphilis and herpes are excluded by appropriate testing.

Management for chancroid consists of azithromycin (Zithromax) 1 g orally in a single dose, ceftriaxone (Rocephin) 250 mg intramuscularly in a single dose, ciprofloxacin (Cipro) 500 mg orally twice daily for 3 days, or erythromycin

(E-Mycin, Apo-Erythro✱) 500 mg orally four times daily for 7 days. These antibiotics cure the infection, resolve the symptoms, and prevent transmission. Clients should be observed periodically by a health care provider until ulcers heal, usually in 7 days.

Client education is similar to that for syphilis. Sexual contacts must be located and treated whether or not they are symptomatic if they have had sexual contact with the client in the 10 days before the client's onset of symptoms. The nurse's responsibility in management of the client with chancroid is similar to that for other STDs.

Granuloma Inguinale

PATHOPHYSIOLOGY

The causative organism of granuloma inguinale, or donovanosis, is *Calymmatobacterium granulomatis.* A nodule appears at the site of inoculation after 1 to 12 weeks. This lesion ulcerates, and others are formed. They are painless and grow together, becoming a spreading ulcer on the genitalia. Left untreated, these lesions can be mutilating. Inguinal lymphadenopathy does not occur, thus the name of this disease may be inappropriate. The ulcerated lesions are very vascular and bleed easily on contact. As open areas, the ulcerated lesions can become infected with bacteria or other STDs.

Granuloma inguinale is common in some less affluent countries, especially those that are tropical. Highest areas of prevalence are India, Papua, New Guinea, the Caribbean, South America, Vietnam, northern and central Australia, and southern Africa. Even in these endemic areas, granuloma inguinale makes up only about 10% of ulcerative genital lesions (Bowden, 2003).

◆COLLABORATIVE MANAGEMENT

Biopsy and cytologic smears from the ulcers are the only conclusive methods for diagnosis. Definitive diagnosis depends on finding characteristic Donovan bodies in these samples. This can be difficult, and often treatment is started before results of these tests are available.

Granuloma inguinale is treated with doxycycline 100 mg orally twice daily or trimethoprim/sulfamethoxazole double strength (Bactrim D.S., Septra D.S.) twice daily for a minimum of 3 weeks. Treatment needs to continue until all the lesions are completely healed. Relapse can occur within 6 to 18 months, even after successful initial treatment.

Nursing management of the client with granuloma inguinale is similar to that for other STDs. Obtain a thorough history that includes sexual contacts, travel abroad, and contact with partners who may have traveled to or are from endemic areas (see Chart 80-1). Asking about genital lesions that may have disappeared or changed provides information to help accurately diagnose the infection.

Explain cultures, biopsies, or other diagnostic tests that will be done to make a correct diagnosis. Provide comfort measures and emotional support, because some procedures may be invasive or painful. Teach the client about the diagnosis, the risk for complications if the disease is left untreated or incompletely treated, and the antibiotics prescribed.

Encourage the client to provide the names of sexual contacts for follow-up and treatment. Concerns about coping with the disease may arise. Encourage the client to verbalize concerns and/or refer him or her for further counseling. Because these infections are relatively rare, the client may have the added discomfort and inconvenience of being evaluated by specialists to get a correct diagnosis, which may contribute to his or her anxiety.

Persons having sexual contact with the client within 60 days of the onset of symptoms or those displaying any signs or symptoms should be treated. Despite this recommendation, benefit of treatment when no symptoms are present is not known (CDC, 2002a).

Critical Thinking Challenge

The client described on p. 1889 is diagnosed with genital herpes; HSV-2 is cultured from the blisters. She is shocked when she is told the diagnosis and says "How can this have happened? I haven't even had intercourse." When you ask about her intimate relationships, she says that, until recently, she had not had any sexual contact since her husband died 10 years ago. She has been intimate for the past month with a 60-year-old co-worker, but they have not had vaginal intercourse because he has erectile dysfunction. She does tell you that he has orally stimulated her and has rubbed his genitals against her to bring her to orgasm. She says she didn't think this type of sexual activity carried any risk for pregnancy or disease.

1. What should you tell her about the risks associated with the type of sexual activity she described?
2. Is the partner a likely source for the infection? Why or why not?
3. She says she doesn't want to tell him about the problem. Is this a reportable disease? How should you respond to this statement?
4. What measures should you suggest to reduce her physical discomfort?

evolve For suggested answer guidelines, go to http://evolve.elsevier.com/Iggy/.

INFECTIONS OF THE EPITHELIAL STRUCTURES

Condylomata Acuminata

PATHOPHYSIOLOGY

Etiology

Condylomata acuminata (also known as genital *warts*) are caused by certain types of human papillomavirus (HPV), mainly types 6 and 11. These types rarely result in invasive cancer of the genital tract. However, HPV types 16, 18, 31, 33, and 35 (of the nearly 70 different HPV genotypes) are found on the skin of the genitalia and increase the risk for genital cancers, especially cervical cancer. Infection with several HPV types can occur at the same time. Sites commonly affected include the urinary meatus, labia, vagina, cervix, penis, scrotum, anus, and perineal area. Pregnancy may increase the growth rate of the lesions. The incubation period is usually 2 to 3 months.

The genital warts are initially single, small papillary growths that may grow into large cauliflower-like masses (Figure 80-2). Bleeding may occur if the wart is disrupted. Warts may regress spontaneously without treatment.

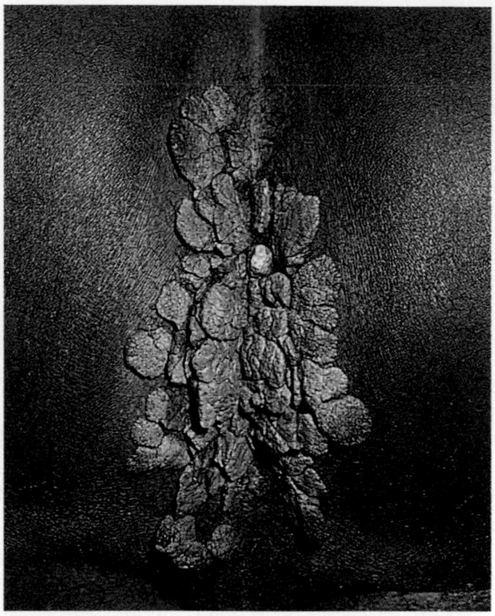

Figure 80-2 ■ Perianal condyloma acuminata. (From Morse, S., et al. [2003]. Atlas of sexually transmitted diseases and AIDS [3rd ed.]. Edinburgh: Mosby.)

Incidence/Prevalence

Genital warts are the most common sexually transmitted viral disease and are often seen with other infections. About 5.5 million people in the United States become infected with HPV each year. Possibly 75% of the reproductive age population is infected. An estimated 20 million people currently have HPV infections that can be transmitted to others (CDC, 2001).

COLLABORATIVE MANAGEMENT

Assessment

The diagnosis of condylomata acuminata is made by examination of the lesions, which appear wartlike. A Pap smear is obtained to assess for cervical dysplasia and is useful in the isolation and diagnosis of HPV from the cervix. HPV can also be detected in genital swab specimens using DNA probes. To rule out the presence of other infections, a VDRL test and cultures for chlamydial and gonorrhea infections are obtained. If a wartlike lesion bleeds easily, appears infected, is atypical or persistent, a specimen for biopsy is obtained to rule out other pathologic problems. Colposcopy with biopsies should be performed for any lesions on the cervix (see Chapter 78).

Interventions

The goals of management are to remove the warts, treat the symptoms, and prevent development of atypical or dysplastic cells to cancer. No current therapy eradicates HPV; therefore recurrences after treatment are likely. It is not known whether removal of visible warts, thus decreasing viral presence, decreases the risk for disease transmission (CDC, 2002a).

Treatment Options. The treatment options for external warts are client applied or provider applied. Clients may apply podofilox 0.5% solution or gel twice daily for 3 days with no treatment for the next 4 days. This regimen should be repeated for four cycles. Another option is imiquimod 5% cream applied topically at bedtime three times a week for up to 16 weeks.

Cryotherapy, podophyllin, and trichloroacetic acid (TCA) are provider-applied treatments. **Cryotherapy** (freezing), usually with liquid nitrogen, can be used every 1 to 2 weeks until lesions are resolved. Podophyllin resin 10% to 25% in a compound of tincture of benzoin can be applied weekly but needs to be washed off 1 to 4 hours after application. Trichloroacetic acid (80% to 90%) can be applied weekly. Extensive warts have been treated with the carbon dioxide laser, intralesional interferon injections, and surgical removal.

For effective management of condylomata acuminata, sexual partners must also be evaluated and treated (if warts are present). Teach clients to avoid intimate sexual contact until external lesions are healed.

Nursing Management. Nursing management focuses on client education about the mode of transmission, incubation period, treatment, and complications, especially the association with cervical cancer. Reinforce instructions about local care of the lesions or patient-applied treatment. Inform clients that after treatment with cryotherapy, podophyllin, or TCA, they may experience discomfort, bleeding or discharge from the site, or sloughing of parts of warts. Instructs the client to keep the area clean (shower or bath) and dry, and to be alert for any signs or symptoms of infection or side effects of the treatment.

Condoms are recommended to help reduce transmission (see Chart 80-4). Inform clients that recurrence is likely and that repeated treatments may be needed. Urge women who have had condylomata acuminata to have an annual Pap smear. As with other STDs, provide emotional support and refer for counseling as needed.

Gonorrhea

PATHOPHYSIOLOGY

Etiology

Gonorrhea, a sexually transmitted bacterial infection occurs in both men and women. Infants can be infected during childbirth. The causative organism is *Neisseria gonorrhoeae,* a gram-negative intracellular diplococcus. *N. gonorrhoeae* is transmitted by direct sexual contact with mucosal surfaces (vaginal intercourse, orogenital contact, or anogenital contact). Although the organism has been found on inanimate surfaces where it has been artificially inoculated, there is no evidence that transmission occurs naturally in this manner.

The first symptoms of gonorrhea may appear 3 to 10 days after sexual contact with an infected person. The infection can be asymptomatic in both men and women, but women have asymptomatic, or "silent," infections more often than do men. If symptoms are present, men usually notice dysuria and a penile discharge that can be either profuse yellowish green fluid or scant clear fluid. The urethra is most commonly affected, but infection can extend to the prostate, the seminal vesicles, and the epididymis. Men seek curative treatment sooner, usually because they have symptoms, and thereby avoid some of the serious complications.

Women may report a change in vaginal discharge (yellow, green, profuse, odorous), urinary frequency, or dysuria. The

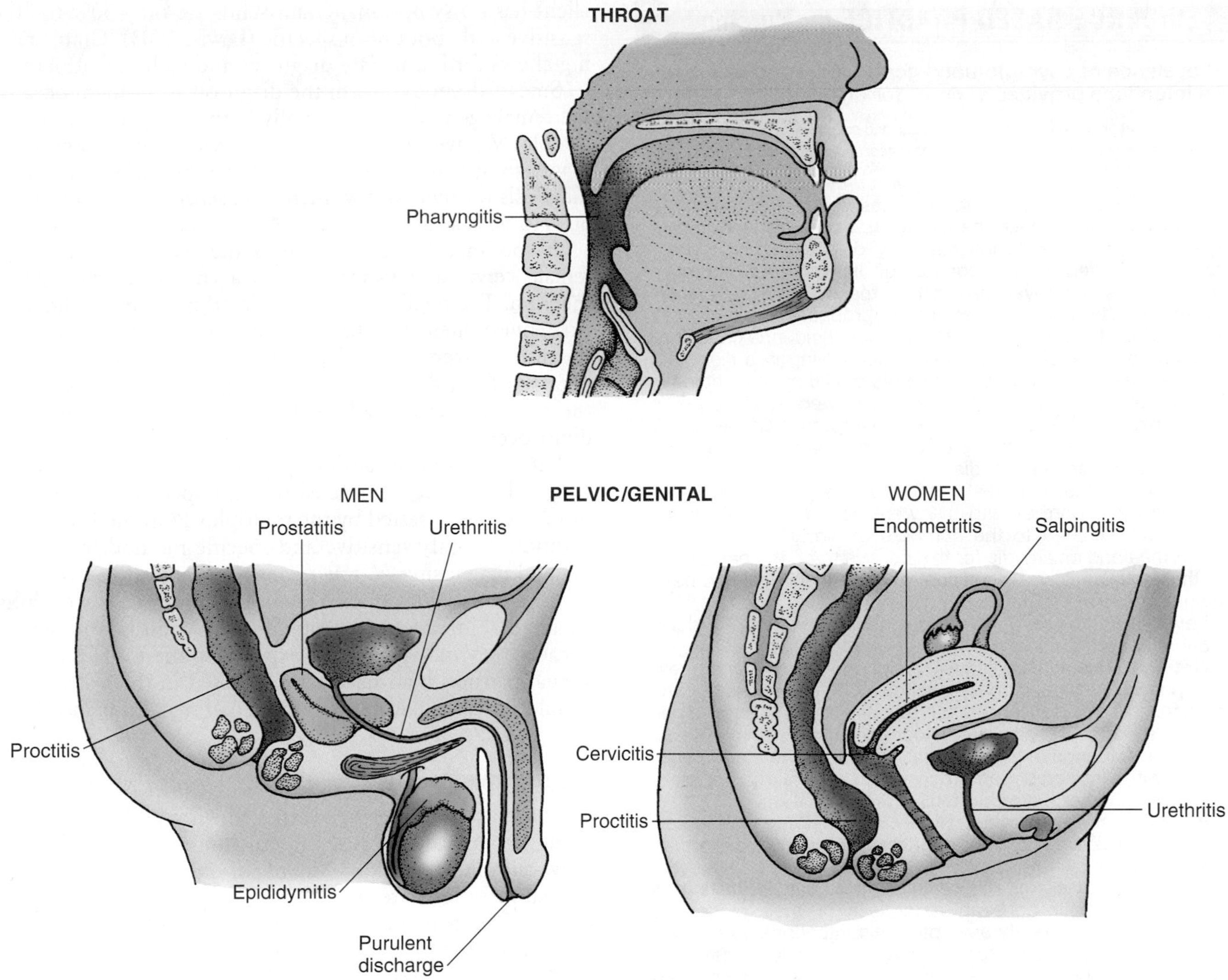

Figure 80-3 ■ Areas of involvement of gonorrhea in men and women.

cervix and urethra are the most common sites of infection. Gonorrhea can be present without symptoms in the cervix and can be transmitted or progress without warning. Ascending spread of the organism can cause pelvic infection **(pelvic inflammatory disease [PID]), endometritis** (endometrial infection), **salpingitis** (fallopian tube infection), and pelvic peritonitis. Infections with or without symptoms can lead to PID and tubal scarring. Rare complications of gonorrhea in adults include arthritis, meningitis, hepatitis, and disseminated infection.

Anal manifestations may include anal itching and irritation, rectal bleeding or diarrhea, and painful defecation. Oral manifestations, related to throat infection, are seldom noted but may include a sore throat, ulcerated lips, tender gingivae, and blisters in the throat. Figure 80-3 shows common sites of gonococcal infections.

Clients without symptoms may be found to have positive cultures for gonorrhea when they have a routine physical examination, are admitted to a hospital, or during preoperative testing. Others may seek screening and care because the sexual partner has been diagnosed with the infection. Universal screening of all sexually active men and women for gonorrhea may be a useful public health tool to avoid spread of asymptomatic infection (see the Evidence-Based Practice for Nursing box on p. 1894).

Incidence/Prevalence

Gonorrhea is the most reported communicable disease in the United States and may be on the rise. An estimated 650,000 new infections occur each year (CDC, 2001). The incidence is highest in 15- to 19-year-old women and 20- to 24-year-old men (CDC, 2002a). Fluoroquinolone-resistant *N. gonorrhoeae* has increased from 0.1% of cases in 1998 to 0.7% of cases in 2001; however, there are regional differences (CDC, 2002a).

COLLABORATIVE MANAGEMENT

Assessment

A complete history includes reviewing possible symptoms of gonorrhea, taking a sexual history that includes sexual orientation and sites of intercourse, and assessing for allergies to antibiotics (see Chart 80-1). Using a nonjudgmental approach helps elicit more complete information. This approach may

EVIDENCE-BASED PRACTICE for Nursing

Prevalence of asymptomatic gonococcal and chlamydial infections provides support for universal screening

Turner, C., et al. (2002). Untreated gonococcal and chlamydial infections in a probability sample of adults. *Journal of the American Medical Association, 287*(6), 726-733.

Untreated sexually transmitted diseases such as gonorrhea and chlamydia increase the risk for transmission and for sequelae such as pelvic inflammatory disease, ectopic pregnancy, and infertility. The concept of universal asymptomatic screening is controversial but has the potential to identify asymptomatic individuals so that appropriate treatment can occur. This study sought to establish the incidence of asymptomatic, and therefore untreated, adults living in a high STD rate census tract. A purposive sample of 728 adults ranging in age from 18 to 35 years were interviewed about specific health habits, STD risks, and current symptoms. Of these, 579 people without symptoms provided urine samples for testing for gonorrhea and chlamydia.

Based on the urine tests, 5.3% of this population tested positive for gonorrhea and 3% were positive for chlamydia. When extrapolated to the numbers of individuals who had gonorrhea and chlamydia for this census tract, the prevalence of these diseases was significantly higher than what had been actually reported to the health department.

Level of Evidence: 3—Well-designed trial without randomization (cohort study).

Critique. This study was well designed to answer the question posed. The ligand chain reaction (LCR) urine assay for the presence of these diseases has a sensitivity of 90% to 94%, which is not as sensitive as endocervical or urethral swabs; thus the incidence of asymptomatic adults in the study population with untreated gonorrhea or chlamydia may actually have been higher than reported.

Implications for Nursing. Nurses who provide care in settings where STD testing is not offered or routinely performed may consider offering noninvasive gonorrhea and chlamydia urine testing to clients. Universal testing, that is, testing all clients (with their consent) regardless of their presenting symptoms, may identify asymptomatic infections. Admission screening in acute care settings also could include these additional tests. Applying these testing recommendations could help reduce the incidence of STDs by identifying infected individuals and starting appropriate therapy. Nurses can use these findings to emphasize to clients, during educational sessions, the possibility of asymptomatic infection and the consequences of delayed treatment.

decrease the client's anxiety and fear about having a sexually transmitted disease (STD).

Physical assessment includes inspection for discharge from the urethra, cervix, and rectum. Palpation of the lower abdomen may reveal tenderness. Fever may be present, especially if an ascending or systemic infection has occurred. Gonorrheal infections that have become systemic may develop quickly. Manifestations of disseminated gonococcal infection (DGI) include fever, chills, skin lesions on distal extremities, and joint pain, with or without swelling, heat, or redness.

Definitive diagnosis involves laboratory testing. Identification of gonorrhea in men can be made with smears of the discharge that has been swabbed onto a glass slide, dried, and Gram stained. The presence of gram-negative diplococci is diagnostic for gonococcal urethritis. Gram stains of urethral discharge, if the client has symptoms, are 90% to 95% sensitive and about 97% specific for gonorrhea. If the client has no symptoms, Gram stains are only 50% to 70% sensitive and about 86% specific (Lewis, 2003). Gram staining allows for immediate diagnosis and earlier treatment.

Smears do not confirm the diagnosis in women, because the female genital tract normally harbors organisms that resemble *N. gonorrhoeae.* Cultures provide a more definitive diagnosis and are the most reliable method of confirming a diagnosis for men and women. The sensitivity of cultures is 80% to 98% and greater than 99% specific (Lewis, 2003).

A specimen is obtained from the male urethra or the female cervix and swabbed onto a chocolate agar culture medium. The medium must be placed in a carbon dioxide–rich environment for the organism to grow. Depending on the history given by the client, culture specimens may also be obtained from the throat and rectum. After 24 to 48 hours, the culture is examined for the presence of gram-negative diplococci.

Direct fluorescent antibody tests, collected on a swab as with cultures, are very sensitive and specific. First-voided urine specimens tested by the multiplex PCR method are an additional highly sensitive and specific method for screening and diagnosing *N. gonorrhoeae.*

All clients with gonorrhea should be tested for syphilis, chlamydial infection, hepatitis B and C, and HIV infection because they may have been exposed to these STDs as well. Sexual partners who have been exposed in the last 30 days should be examined, and specimens for culture should be obtained.

◆Interventions

Uncomplicated gonorrhea is treated with antibiotics. Treatment has changed because of penicillin-resistant strains and now quinolone-resistant strains of *N. gonorrhoeae.* Chlamydial infections are frequently found in clients with gonorrhea. Clients treated for gonorrhea should also be treated with drugs that eradicate *Chlamydia.*

Drug Therapy. Drug therapy recommended by the Centers for Disease Control and Prevention (CDC) is ceftriaxone (Rocephin) 125 mg intramuscularly, ciprofloxacin (Cipro) 500 mg orally, *or* ofloxacin (Floxin) 400 mg orally, *each* in a single dose *plus* azithromycin (Zithromax) 1 g orally in a single dose *or* doxycycline (Monodox, Doxy-Caps, Doxycin✱) 100 mg orally twice daily for 1 week if *Chlamydia* has not been ruled out. These combinations seem to be effective for all mucosal gonorrheal infections; treatment failure is rare.

The quinolones (ciprofloxacin, ofloxacin) are not recommended in areas with reported high quinolone resistance (e.g., Hawaii, California, Asia, and the Pacific rim) (CDC, 2002b). The only nonquinolone antibiotic choice for clients in these areas is intramuscular ceftriaxone (Rocephin).

Sexual partners must be treated as well. A test of cure is not required, but the client is advised to return for a follow-up examination if symptoms persist after treatment. Reinfection is often the cause of these symptoms and indicates a need for more education of the client and sexual partner.

The use of single-dose treatment, especially among younger individuals at high risk, is recommended. Directly observed therapy (DOT) in the health care setting appears to improve adherence (Feroli & Burstein, 2003).

Treatment of DGI includes intravenous (IV) or intramuscular ceftriaxone 1 g every 24 hours. If symptoms resolve within 24 to 48 hours, the client may be discharged to home to continue oral antibiotic therapy for at least 1 week.

Meningitis and endocarditis occur rarely. Hospitalization for clients with these problems is recommended for the initial treatment. Treatment is with IV antibiotic therapy, usually ceftriaxone 1 to 2 g every 12 hours. If meningitis or endocarditis is present, therapy is continued for 10 to 14 days for meningitis and at least 4 weeks for endocarditis. Infectious disease specialists are consulted for management of these infections.

Nursing Management. Nursing interventions focus on teaching the client about transmission and treatment of gonorrhea. Clients must understand why medications should be taken for the prescribed time for maximal effectiveness. Discuss the possibility of reinfection, including the risk for pelvic inflammatory disease (PID), and resultant problems such as ectopic pregnancy, infertility, and chronic pelvic pain. Instruct clients to avoid sexual activity until the antibiotic therapy is completed and they no longer have symptoms. Urge men and women to use condoms, especially if abstinence is not possible. Explain that gonorrhea is a reportable disease. All sexual contacts need to be examined and treated for both gonorrhea and chlamydial infection.

When a diagnosis of gonorrhea is made, clients may have feelings of fear or guilt. They may be concerned that they have contracted other STDs or see the disease as a punishment for promiscuity or "unnatural" sex acts. They may believe that acquiring gonorrhea (or any STD) is a risk that they must take to pursue their desired lifestyle. Such feelings can impair relationships with sexual partners. Encourage clients to express their feelings during assessments and teaching sessions. Assuring privacy for client teaching and maintaining confidentiality of medical records are important nursing interventions in meeting the client's psychosocial needs.

Chlamydial Infection

PATHOPHYSIOLOGY

Etiology

C. trachomatis is an intracellular bacterium and the causative agent of genital chlamydial infections. It invades the epithelial tissues in the reproductive tract and causes manifestations similar to those of gonorrheal infections. The incubation period ranges from 1 to 3 weeks, but the pathogen may be present in the genital tract for months without producing symptoms. The average duration of infection before diagnosis is about 1 year in women and 5 months in men because of its frequent asymptomatic status.

In men, the main symptom is urethritis, occurring with dysuria, frequent urination, and a mucoid discharge that is more watery and less copious than a gonorrheal discharge. Some men have the discharge only in the morning on arising. Complications include epididymitis, prostatitis, infertility, and Reiter's syndrome, a type of connective tissue disease (see Chapter 24).

In contrast, many women may have no symptoms. Women with symptoms have a mucopurulent cervicitis with a change in vaginal discharge, easily induced cervical bleeding, urinary frequency, and abdominal discomfort or pain. The vaginal discharge typically becomes yellow and more opaque (Sellors et al., 2000). Complications of infection with *C. trachomatis* include salpingitis, PID, ectopic pregnancy, and infertility.

Incidence/Prevalence

Chlamydia trachomatis is the most common sexually transmitted disease in the United States. The disease is now reportable to local health departments in all states. In 2003, 877,478 cases were reported, an increase of more than 24% over 2000 (CDC, 2004). Four times more women than men are reported to have chlamydia, which in part reflects more screening of women than men. Up to 70% of women and 25% of men screened for chlamydia are asymptomatic (Schacter & Stephens, 2003). In men, about 10% to 20% of the cases of nongonococcal urethritis are caused by *C. trachomatis*. In women, 20% to 40% of those infected with *C. trachomatis* develop pelvic inflammatory disease (PID), discussed on p. 1896. Transmission to the newborn can occur during vaginal delivery, causing neonatal eye infections and pneumonia.

◆COLLABORATIVE MANAGEMENT

◆Assessment

Obtain a complete history, including medical, menstrual, and sexual history from the client (see Chart 80-1). Ask about the following:

- Presence of symptoms
- Any history of sexually transmitted diseases (STDs)
- Whether sexual partners have had symptoms or a history of STDs

Many women with chlamydial infections are asymptomatic. The client's history may reveal only risk factors associated with *C. trachomatis*. These factors include age younger than 20 years, being unmarried, nulliparity, having a higher number of sexual partners or a new sexual partner, use of a nonbarrier method of birth control (hormonal, intrauterine device [IUD]), and concurrent gonorrhea. As with all interviews concerning sexual behavior, use a nonjudgmental approach and provide privacy and confidentiality.

Diagnosis of chlamydial infections is made by sampling cells from the endocervix, the urethra, or both. Because chlamydiae can only reproduce inside cells, host cells that harbor the organism (or parts of it) are required in the sample. Gram staining of urethral or cervical samples can help exclude gonorrhea. The presence of polymorphonuclear leukocytes and the absence of gram-negative intracellular diplococci (suggestive of gonorrhea) points to a chlamydial infection. Absolute diagnosis of chlamydial infection is made with a tissue culture. Culture for *Chlamydia*, which detects 70% to 80% of cervical infections with *C. trachomatis*, has been the "gold standard." Special transport medium is required.

Gene amplification tests or DNA amplification tests (ligand chain reaction [LCR] and polymerase chain reaction [PCR]), are very sensitive and specific methods of detecting the presence of chlamydia on endocervical samples, urethral swabs, and urine (Lewis, 2003). The enzyme-linked immunoassay (ELISA) and direct fluorescent antibody (DFA) tests are less sensitive.

Screening asymptomatic women and men who may have risk factors for having chlamydial infections is strongly encouraged. The use of urine testing has been found to increase acceptability of testing and has resulted in increased identification of asymptomatic individuals (Turner et al., 2002).

Interventions

The treatment of choice for chlamydial infections is azithromycin (Zithromax) 1 g in a single dose or doxycycline (Monodox, Doxy-Caps, Doxycin✱) 100 mg twice daily for 7 days. The one-dose course, although more expensive, is preferred because of the ease in completing the treatment. Giving the drug while the client is in the health care facility helps ensure adherence. Sexual partners should be tested and treated if possible. Individuals with positive test results for chlamydia must be reported to the Health Department.

Client education is an important nursing intervention. Explain the following:

- The mode of disease transmission
- The incubation period
- Manifestations, including the possibility of asymptomatic infections
- Treatment of infection with antibiotics
- The need for abstinence from sexual intercourse until the client and partner(s) have completed treatment (7 days from the start of treatment, including a single-dose regimen)
- No test of cure is required, but all women should be re-screened 3 to 4 months after treatment because of the high risk for PID if reinfection occurs.
- The need to return for evaluation if symptoms recur or new symptoms develop (most recurrences are actually reinfections from a new or untreated partner)
- Possible complications of untreated or inadequately treated infection, such as PID, ectopic pregnancy, or infertility

OTHER GYNECOLOGIC CONDITIONS

Pelvic Inflammatory Disease

PATHOPHYSIOLOGY

Etiology

Pelvic inflammatory disease (PID) is a complex infectious process in which organisms from the lower genital tract migrate from the endocervix upward through the uterine cavity into the fallopian tubes. The spread of infection to other organs and tissues of the upper genital tract occurs from direct contact with mucosal surfaces or through the fimbriated ends of the tubes to the ovaries, parametrium, and peritoneal cavity (Figure 80-4). This may involve one or more pelvic structures, including the uterus, fallopian tubes, and adjacent pelvic structures. The most common site is the fallopian tube. Resultant infections include the following:

- Endometritis (infection of the endometrial cavity)
- Salpingitis (inflammation of the fallopian tubes)
- Oophoritis (ovarian infection)
- Parametritis (infection of the parametrium)
- Peritonitis (infection of the peritoneal cavity)
- Tubal or tubo-ovarian abscess

Many different pathogens are linked to PID. Sexually transmitted organisms are most often responsible for PID, especially *Chlamydia trachomatis* and *Neisseria gonorrhoeae.* Organisms that are part of the vaginal flora can also cause PID.

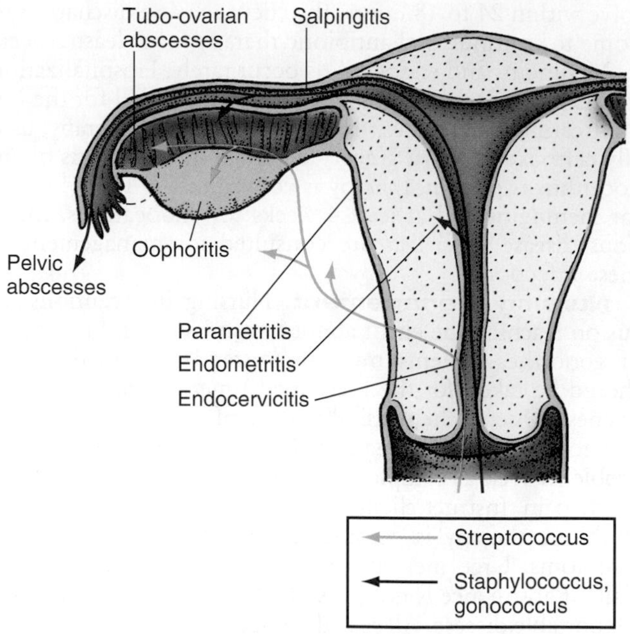

Figure 80-4 ■ The spread of pelvic inflammatory disease.

Chlamydia is the most common causative agent of PID in the United States and Europe. In addition, *Gardnerella vaginalis, Haemophilus influenzae, Staphylococcus, Streptococcus, Escherichia coli,* and other aerobic and anaerobic organisms have been identified in clients with PID. There is increasing evidence that the anaerobes involved in bacterial vaginosis may have a role in the development of PID (CDC, 2002a).

The infectious organisms invade the pelvis from an infection ascending from the vagina or cervix. Infections are spread during sexual intercourse, during childbirth (including the postpartum period), and after abortion. Rarely do infections result from transperitoneal spread from a ruptured appendix or intra-abdominal abscess. Sepsis and death can occur, especially if treatment is delayed or inadequate (Dulin & Akers, 2003).

Many practitioners use the terms *PID* and *salpingitis* synonymously for acute infections. PID is one of the leading causes of infertility and is related to the increase in the number of ectopic pregnancies reported in the United States. It is an acute syndrome resulting in tenderness in the tubes and ovaries (adnexa) and low, dull abdominal pain. However, many women experience only mild discomfort or menstrual irregularity; others experience no symptoms at all, so-called "silent" or "subclinical" PID. Diagnosis and treatment of PID in these women is challenging. Irreversible scarring or stricture, causing sterility, may occur before PID is diagnosed.

Incidence/Prevalence

The incidence of PID is on the rise. Accurate rates are unavailable because PID is not a reportable disease. Many of the same factors that place women at risk for STDs also place them at risk for PID. Risk factors for sexually active women include the following:

- Age younger than 20 years
- Multiple sexual partners
- Intrauterine device (IUD) in place
- Use of vaginal douches

- Smoking
- Chlamydial or gonococcal infection; bacterial vaginosis
- A history of sexually transmitted diseases (STDs)
- A history of PID

COLLABORATIVE MANAGEMENT

Assessment

HISTORY

Obtain a complete medical, family, menstrual, obstetric, and sexual history, including a history of previous episodes of pelvic inflammatory disease (PID) or other sexually transmitted diseases (see Chart 80-1). Assess for contraceptive use (especially the intrauterine device), a history of reproductive surgery, and other risk factors previously identified. The possibility of sexual abuse should be raised.

One of the most frequent symptoms of PID is lower abdominal pain. Other symptoms include menstrual irregularities or abnormal vaginal bleeding, dysuria, an increase or change in vaginal discharge, dyspareunia, malaise, fever, and chills.

PHYSICAL ASSESSMENT/CLINICAL MANIFESTATIONS

Observe whether the client has discomfort with movement. Often the client has a hunched-over gait that she uses to protect her abdomen. She may find it difficult to independently get on the examination table or stretcher. She may be fatigued and diaphoretic and have a fever.

Assess for lower abdominal tenderness, possibly with rigidity or rebound tenderness. A pelvic examination by the health care provider may reveal yellow or green cervical discharge and a reddened or **friable** cervix (a cervix that bleeds easily). On bimanual examination, uterine or cervical tenderness with motion and tender adnexa (tubes and ovaries) are often present. If the client is using an IUD for contraception, the device should be removed at the time of the examination if possible. Ectopic pregnancy and appendicitis must be ruled out as other potential causes of the pain.

PSYCHOSOCIAL ASSESSMENT

The woman who has symptoms of PID is usually anxious and fearful of the examination and unknown diagnosis. She may need much reassurance and support during the physical examination because her abdomen may be very tender and she may wish to avoid further pain. Explain what is taking place to help promote cooperation during the examination.

Because PID is often associated with an STD, the woman may feel embarrassed or uncomfortable discussing her symptoms or history. Use a nonjudgmental approach and encourage the client to express her feelings and concerns. The client's ability to follow through with the treatment plan (taking antibiotics, resting, returning for follow-up evaluation in 48 hours) is essential in deciding whether ambulatory care treatment is appropriate.

LABORATORY ASSESSMENT

The health care provider obtains cultures of the cervix, urethra, and rectum to determine the presence of *N. gonorrhoeae* or *C. trachomatis.* The white blood cell (WBC) count and erythrocyte sedimentation rate (ESR) may be elevated but are not specific for PID. Gram stains of endocervical secretions may show the presence of *N. gonorrhoeae.* A sensitive test that detects human chorionic gonadotropin in urine or blood should be performed to determine whether the client is pregnant. Microscopic examination of vaginal discharge should be done to evaluate for infection. The presence of more than 10 WBCs per high-power field in vaginal discharge correlates with infection. Bacterial vaginosis can be found by observing the diagnostic "clue" cells with microscopic examination of vaginal discharge.

OTHER DIAGNOSTIC ASSESSMENTS

Abdominal ultrasonography may be used to determine the presence of appendicitis and tubo-ovarian abscesses that need to be ruled out when the diagnosis of PID is made. Transvaginal ultrasound and magnetic resonance imaging (MRI) are used in some cases to detect tubal wall thickening, fluid-filled tubes, and free pelvic fluid or a tubo-ovarian abscess, all associated with PID.

Laparoscopy, although expensive, invasive, and requiring anesthesia, is the most definitive test. It provides an immediate, accurate diagnosis through direct inspection of the tubes and ovaries. Endometrial biopsy also has been used to increase the accuracy of the diagnosis.

Because of great variations in client signs and symptoms, the diagnosis of acute PID is difficult because women may have subtle symptoms not typical of PID. Delay in diagnosis and treatment may add to the sequelae of PID in the upper genital tract. Laparoscopy may not be feasible, so that PID is diagnosed on the basis of clinical signs and symptoms (Gaitan, 2002). The Centers for Disease Control and Prevention (CDC) have set minimum criteria for the diagnosis of PID, but there are no laboratory or physical examination techniques that alone are both sensitive and specific for the diagnosis of acute PID. The CDC recommends treatment with antibiotics if all of the minimum criteria have been met and no other causes of illness are found (Table 80-4).

Critical Thinking Challenge

The client is a 28-year-old Hispanic woman admitted to your medical-surgical unit for multiple fractures, lacerations, and abrasions sustained in a car accident. She drove the car into a tree after she found out that her boyfriend had been having sex with other women. On her second day after admission, she tells you that she is having a lot of lower abdominal pain and some yellowish vaginal discharge. She is receiving morphine sulfate IV by PCA to manage her pain from her trauma.

1. What specific questions should you ask her about her current and previous health?
2. What risk factors does she have for PID?
3. What additional assessment data should you obtain?
4. How will you approach the topic of the possibility of a sexually transmitted disease or problem?

evolve For suggested answer guidelines, go to http://evolve.elsevier.com/Iggy/.

Analysis

COMMON NURSING DIAGNOSES AND COLLABORATIVE PROBLEMS

The primary collaborative problem for clients with pelvic inflammatory disease (PID) is Infection related to invasion

TABLE 80-4 Diagnostic Criteria for Pelvic Inflammatory Disease

Minimum Criteria for Initiating Empiric Treatment for Pelvic Inflammatory Disease
- Uterine/adnexal tenderness *or*
- Cervical motion tenderness (chandelier sign)

Additional Criteria to Increase the Specificity of the Diagnosis of PID
- Oral temperature >101° F (>38.3° C)
- Abnormal cervical or vaginal mucopurulent discharge
- Presence of white blood cells on saline microscopy of vaginal secretions
- Elevated erythrocyte sedimentation rate
- Elevated C-reactive protein
- Laboratory documentation of cervical infection with *Neisseria gonorrhoeae* or *Chlamydia trachomatis*

Definitive Criteria for Diagnosing PID, Warranted in Selected Cases
- Histopathologic evidence of endometritis on endometrial biopsy
- Transvaginal sonography or other imaging techniques showing thickened fluid-filled tubes with or without free pelvic fluid or tubo-ovarian complex
- Laparoscopic abnormalities consistent with PID

Modified from Centers for Disease Control and Prevention. (2002). Sexually transmitted diseases treatment guideline. *Morbidity and Mortality Weekly Report, 51*(No. RR-6), 1-80.
PID, Pelvic inflammatory disease.

CHART 80-5

NIC INTERVENTION ACTIVITIES for The Client with Pelvic Inflammatory Disease

Infection Control: *Minimizing the acquisition and transmission of infectious agents*
- Encourage rest.
- Encourage fluid intake, as appropriate.
- Administer antibiotic therapy, as appropriate. *Or*
- Instruct client to take antibiotics, as prescribed.
- Promote appropriate nutritional intake.
- Teach client and family about signs and symptoms of infection and when to report them to the health care provider.
- Teach client and family members how to avoid infections.

Anxiety Reduction: *Minimizing apprehension, dread, foreboding, or uneasiness related to an unidentified source of anticipated danger*
- Create an atmosphere to facilitate trust.
- Listen attentively.
- Encourage verbalization of feelings, perceptions, and fears.
- Provide factual information concerning diagnosis, treatment, and prognosis.
- Instruct client in use of relaxation techniques.

NIC intervention activities selected from Dochterman, J.M., & Bulechek, G.M. (Eds.). (2004). *Nursing interventions classification (NIC)* (4th ed.). St. Louis: Mosby. No part of this work is to be altered without prior written permission from the Publisher.

of pelvic organs by pathogens. The following are common nursing diagnoses for clients with PID:

1. Acute Pain related to injuring agents (biologic) and the effects of the infectious process
2. Anxiety related to threat to health status and possible infertility as a result of infection

ADDITIONAL NURSING DIAGNOSES AND COLLABORATIVE PROBLEMS

In addition to the common nursing diagnoses and collaborative problems, clients with PID may have one or more of the following:

- Ineffective Health Maintenance related to knowledge deficit about risks, prevention, symptoms, treatment, and effects of PID
- Chronic Pain related to chronic presence of organisms that stimulate recurrent PID episodes
- Sexual Dysfunction related to altered body function from the effects of the infectious process
- Situational Low Self-Esteem/Chronic Low Self-Esteem related to disturbed body image or feeling guilty for having PID (associated with sexual transmission)

Planning and Implementation

INFECTION

NOC **PLANNING: EXPECTED OUTCOMES.** The client with PID is expected to have her infection resolved. Indicators include that the client should have mild or none of the following associated symptoms:

- Pain and tenderness of the pelvis
- Fever
- Discharge (vaginal)
- Culture colonization

INTERVENTIONS. Infection control is accomplished with the use antibiotics, self-care measures, and surgical intervention (rarely) (Chart 80-5).

Infection Control. Uncomplicated PID is usually treated on an ambulatory care basis. The CDC recommends hospitalization for PID if the client:

- Has appendicitis, ectopic pregnancy, or other surgical emergency that has not been excluded
- Is pregnant
- Does not respond to oral antibiotic therapy
- Is unable to follow or tolerate an outpatient regimen
- Has severe illness, nausea and vomiting, or high fever
- Has a tubo-ovarian abscess

There are no recommendations about whether HIV-infected women should be hospitalized. Your assessment of the ability of high-risk women to manage their care at home is an essential part of the plan of care. Their clinical condition and availability of support at home are considerations for care at home. If the infection has not responded to treatment, the client may need to be hospitalized for IV antibiotic therapy and further evaluation.

Drug Therapy. Drug therapy options for PID include oral and parenteral antibiotics (Chart 80-6). Treatment lasts for 14 days. All clients should be re-evaluated 48 to 72 hours after antibiotic therapy is started. If the infection has not responded to treatment, the client is hospitalized for IV antibiotic therapy and further evaluation. Inpatient therapy involves a combination of several IV antibiotics until the client shows signs of improvement (e.g., decreased pelvic tenderness for at least 24 hours). Then oral antibiotics are continued until the course of treatment has lasted 14 days.

Encourage clients treated as outpatients to rest, abstain from sexual intercourse, and check their temperature twice a day. These clients need to be seen by the health care provider 48 to 72 hours from starting the antibiotics and then 1 and 2 weeks from the time of the initial diagnosis.

In a small number of clients, the pain and tenderness may not be relieved by antibiotic therapy. The surgeon may perform a laparotomy to remove an abscess through a subumbilical incision that is several inches long to provide better access

CHART 80-6

DRUG THERAPY for Acute Pelvic Inflammatory Disease

Drug	Dosage	Nursing Interventions	Rationales
Parenteral Treatment (Inpatient)			
Regimen A			
Cefotetan (Cefotan)	2 g IV q12h, which can be changed to oral therapy after 24 hr of clinical improvement	Assess the client for rash, itching, and hypotension.	Assessment detects adverse reactions.
Or			
Cefoxitin (Mefoxin)	2 g IV q6h, which can be changed to oral therapy after 24 hr of clinical improvement	Assess the client for rash, itching, and hypotension.	Assessment detects adverse reactions.
		Observe the IV site for signs of redness, heat, and tenderness.	Phlebitis can be detected.
Plus			
[1]Doxycycline (Monodox, Doxy-Caps, Doxycin✱)	100 mg IV or PO q12h for 14 days (PO is preferred because of the pain associated with infusion)	Assess the client for rash, nausea, and diarrhea.	Assessment detects drug side effects.
		Encourage fluid intake.	Fluid intake decreases esophageal irritation.
		Instruct the client about possible photosensitivity and the need for sun protection.	This precaution prevents sunburn by limiting the client's exposure to the sun.
		Instruct the client that it is beneficial to take the drug with food.	Food decreases gastrointestinal upset.
Regimen B			
Clindamycin (Cleocin)	900 mg IV q8h	Observe the client for rash and urticaria.	Adverse reactions are detected.
		Observe the client for hypotension, dyspnea, and restlessness.	Anaphylactic reaction is detected.
		Observe the client for diarrhea.	This precaution avoids pseudomembranous colitis.
		Observe the IV site for redness, heat, and tenderness.	Phlebitis can be detected.
Plus			
Gentamicin (Garamycin IV)	2 mg/kg once IV or IM followed by 1.5 mg/kg q8h IV or IM until there have been signs of clinical improvement for 24 hr	Encourage oral intake of fluids.	Fluid intake prevents irritation to renal tubules.
		Observe the IV site for redness, heat, and tenderness.	Phlebitis can be detected.
		Measure fluid intake and output.	Oliguria or anuria can be detected.
		Observe the client for hearing loss, fever, or decreased renal function.	Ototoxicity, nephrotoxicity, and fever are known side effects.
		Draw serum for peak and trough levels.	Serum levels can vary, and drug has low threshold for toxic level.
Then			
Doxycycline (Monodox, Doxy-Caps, Doxycin✱)	100 mg PO twice daily to complete a total of 14 days of treatment	See above for doxycycline.	See above for doxycycline.
Or			
Clindamycin (Cleocin)	450 mg PO four times daily to complete a total of 14 days of treatment	Give with 8 oz of water.	Water decreases esophageal irritation.
		See above for clindamycin.	See above for clindamycin.
Oral Treatment (Outpatient)			
Regimen A			
Ofloxacin (Floxin)	400 mg PO twice daily for 14 days	Monitor the serum level if the client is taking theophylline.	This drug raises the serum level of theophylline.
		Do not administer this drug to clients younger than 18 yr of age.	The safety of this drug has not been established in clients younger than 18 yr of age.
		Administer or instruct the client to take this drug on an empty stomach.	Food decreases drug absorption.

[1]***Med Error Alert!*** *Do not confuse with doxepin, an antidepressant.*

Modified from Centers for Disease Control and Prevention. (1998). Guidelines for treatment of sexually transmitted disease. *Morbidity and Mortality Weekly Report, 47*(RR-1), 1-103.

Continued

CHART 80-6

DRUG THERAPY for
Acute Pelvic Inflammatory Disease—*cont'd*

Drug	Dosage	Nursing Interventions	Rationales
Oral Treatment (Outpatient)—*cont'd*			
Regimen A—*cont'd*			
Or			
Levofloxacin (Levaquin)	500 mg PO daily for 14 days	Do not give to pregnant women.	This drug disrupts fetal bone growth.
With or without			
Metronidazole (Flagyl, Novonidazol✱)	500 mg PO twice daily for 14 days	Monitor the serum level if the client is taking lithium. Avoid alcohol within 24 hr of use.	This drug raises the serum level of lithium. Alcohol causes disulfiram-like effect.
Regimen B			
Ceftriaxone (Rocephin)	250 mg IM one time only	Give deep IM injection in the outer upper quadrant of the gluteus maximus. Watch for fever, chills, and nausea. Tell the client that the injection may be painful.	Local irritation is avoided, and drug absorption is increased. Allergic reactions can be detected. The client is prepared for discomfort related to the inflammatory reaction.
Or			
Cefoxitin (Mefoxin)	2 g IM one time only	Give deep IM injection in the outer upper quadrant of the gluteus maximus. Watch for fever, chills, and nausea. Tell the client that the injection may be painful.	Local irritation is avoided, and drug absorption is increased. Allergic reactions can be detected. The client is prepared for discomfort related to the inflammatory reaction.
Plus			
[2]Probenecid (Benemid, Benuryl✱)	1 g PO one time only concurrently	Give with food. Encourage fluid intake (10 glasses per day).	Taking the medication with food avoids gastrointestinal upset. Fluid intake prevents formation of kidney stones.
Or			
Other parenteral third-generation cephalosporin (e.g., ceftizoxime or cefotaxime)			
Plus			
Doxycycline (for all of the above regimens)	100 mg PO twice daily for 14 days	See previous page for doxycycline.	See previous page for doxycycline.

[2]***Med Error Alert!***
Do not confuse with Procanbid, a drug used for cardiac dysrhythmias.

Modified from Centers for Disease Control and Prevention. (1998). Guidelines for treatment of sexually transmitted disease. *Morbidity and Mortality Weekly Report, 47*(RR-1), 1-103.

to the fallopian tubes. Before surgery, provide information about hospital routines and procedures. General preoperative care is described in Chapter 20. After surgery, the care of the woman with PID is similar to that of any client after abdominal surgery. One difference is that the client with PID may have a wound drain in place for drainage of abscess fluid that may not have been completely removed during surgery. Observe, measure, and record wound drainage every 4 to 8 hours as ordered.

ACUTE PAIN

NOC **PLANNING: EXPECTED OUTCOMES.** The client with PID is expected to have reduced pain and increased comfort. Indicators include that the client should rarely demonstrate the following behaviors:

- Reports of pain
- Moaning and crying
- Facial expressions of pain
- Loss of appetite

INTERVENTIONS. Pain management of PID begins with treatment of the infection. Antibiotic treatment relieves pain by decreasing the inflammation caused by infection. If the client is ill enough to be hospitalized, parenteral antibiotics are usually given. See the earlier section on drug therapy for PID.

Other pain relief measures include taking analgesics, using sitz baths, and applying heat to the lower abdomen or back. Bedrest in a semi-Fowler's position promotes gravity drainage and consolidation of the infection that may relieve pain.

ANXIETY

NOC **PLANNING: EXPECTED OUTCOMES.** The client with PID is expected to take actions to reduce anxiety about infertility. Indicators include that the client should often or consistently demonstrate the following behaviors:

- Use of effective coping patterns strategies
- Controlled anxiety response
- Use of available social support
- Seeking of professional help, as appropriate

INTERVENTIONS. Infertility is the most common complication of PID and affects at least 15% to 25% of women who have had one or more episodes of PID. Nursing interventions are aimed at understanding the client's perspective of the diagnosis and future complications.

If the client has anxiety, provide an atmosphere in which she feels comfortable expressing her feelings and asking questions. Give accurate information about the diagnosis, treatment, and prognosis. Providing information about the advantages of early diagnosis and treatment (which limit damage to one area of the pelvis) and the advances in treatments for infertility may reassure the client. Help the client assess the emotional support available from family members or significant others. Relaxation techniques may be useful to decrease the anxiety (see Chart 80-5).

Community-Based Care

The client with pelvic inflammatory disease (PID) needs to have regular follow-up with her health care provider to assess for complications and ensure that the infection has resolved. The ongoing role of the nurse is to assess for any continued risk for contracting PID again, signs of persistent or recurrent infection, and education to prevent exposure to and infection with all STDs (e.g., decrease the number of partners, consistent condom use). Establish an atmosphere of trust that encourages the client to return frequently, if needed, for education or reassurance.

HOME CARE MANAGEMENT

Parenteral antibiotic therapy may be given at home, but usually the health care provider changes the treatment regimen to oral antibiotics before hospital discharge (see Planning and Implementation, p. 1898).

HEALTH TEACHING

Client teaching focuses on providing information about PID, identifying recurrences (persistent pain, dysmenorrhea, low backache, fever), and urging early treatment to prevent complications. Review information for oral antibiotic therapy (Chart 80-7).

Counsel the client to contact her sexual partner(s) for examination and treatment. The partner is usually treated for gonorrhea and chlamydial infection. Remind the client about follow-up care and counsel her about the complications that can occur after an episode of PID, including increased risk for recurrence of PID, increased risk for ectopic pregnancy, increased risk for infertility, and chronic pelvic pain.

CHART 80-7

CLIENT EDUCATION GUIDE

Oral Antibiotic Therapy for Sexually Transmitted Diseases

- Take your medicine for the number of times a day it is prescribed and until it is completed.
- Your sexual partner must be tested and may need to be treated.
- Be sure to return for your follow-up appointment after completing your antibiotic treatment.
- Call if you have any questions or concerns.
- Do not have sex until after you complete your antibiotic therapy. If your partner is being treated, you can go back to having sex together 48 hours after he or she starts taking antibiotics if you use a condom.
- Drink at least 8 to 10 glasses of fluid a day while taking your antibiotics.
- Do not take antacids containing calcium, magnesium, or aluminum, such as Tums, Maalox, or Mylanta, with your antibiotics. They may decrease the effectiveness of the antibiotic.
- Take your antibiotics on an empty stomach unless your health care provider instructs you to take them with food.

Discuss contraception and the client's need or desire for it. This discussion includes methods that may decrease the risk for future episodes of PID, such as the use of barrier methods. Help the client understand lifestyle factors that heighten the risk for recurrent episodes of PID, including sexual intercourse with multiple partners and vaginal douching.

Psychosocial concerns may require teaching and counseling. A client who has PID may exhibit a variety of feelings (guilt, disgust, anger) about having a condition that may have been transmitted to her sexually. These feelings may affect her relationship with significant others and future sexual relationships. She may also have concerns about future fertility if PID has caused damage or scarring of the fallopian tubes and other reproductive organs. Provide nonjudgmental emotional support and allow time for the client to express her feelings.

HEALTH CARE RESOURCES

If infertility is a result of PID, the client may need referral to a clinic specializing in infertility treatment and counseling. The client can also contact support groups for infertile couples, which exist in many local communities.

The costs of antibiotics for care of clients with PID and other STDs may be a concern for those who are uninsured or underinsured. The case manager, social worker, or ambulatory care nurse seeks community resources for free or discounted medications for clients with financial limitations.

◆ Evaluation: Outcomes

Evaluate the care of the client with PID on the basis of the identified nursing diagnoses and collaborative problems. The expected outcomes include that the client should:

- Show evidence that the infection has resolved
- Report or demonstrate that pain is relieved or reduced and that she feels more comfortable
- Take action to manage anxiety about future infertility

Specific indicators for these outcomes are listed for each nursing diagnosis and collaborative problem under the Planning and Implementation section (see earlier).

SEXUALLY TRANSMITTED VAGINAL INFECTIONS

Vaginal infection associated with sexual activity may produce vaginal discharge or vulvar irritation. The following are common causes of vaginal infection:

- *Trichomonas vaginalis*
- *Candida,* primarily *C. albicans*
- Bacteria that produce bacterial vaginosis, including *Gardnerella vaginalis* and anaerobes

These infections can be spread by sexual contact. Men can also acquire these infections but are not always symptomatic. Several studies have shown that *T. vaginalis* is common in men, especially those who have other STDs, such as *Chlamydia trachomatis* (Bachmann et al., 2000; Joyner et al., 2000). However, because most of these infections are seen more commonly in women, assessments and interventions are discussed with other causes of vaginitis in Chapter 78.

Trichomoniasis and candida infections are limited to the vagina. They can be very irritating and bothersome but do not cause any long-term sequelae. The partner must also be treated for trichomoniasis if the infection is to be resolved. Candidiasis does not usually require partner treatment, but if the male partner is symptomatic (irritation of the genital skin), then treatment is indicated. It is important to remember that candida is a normal flora on the skin and can easily be translocated to the vagina. Although it can be transmitted sexually, candidiasis occurs among women who are not sexually active. Additionally, antibiotics that change the normal flora of the vagina (especially tetracyclines) contribute to candidiasis.

Bacterial vaginosis (BV) has been implicated in upper genital tract infections. Women undergoing surgery of the upper genital tract should be evaluated and treated if BV is found. There also is evidence that BV in pregnancy can lead to preterm labor and premature delivery. These findings are controversial, but evaluation for BV during pregnancy has been suggested (Carey et al., 2000; Hay, Ugwumadu, & Manvonda, 2001).

HEPATITIS A, B, AND C

In the United States, 12% to 26% of new cases of hepatitis A are reported to be acquired through household or sexual contact. Up to 55% of the new cases of hepatitis B (HBV) are transmitted sexually. Sexual transmission of hepatitis C (HCV) is inefficient, although about 5% of new cases is thought to be transmitted this way. Of those infected as adults, 2% to 6% of those with HBV and 75% to 85% of those with HCV develop chronic hepatitis, which can lead to cirrhosis and primary liver cancer. An estimated 0.5% of the total U.S. population have chronic HBV and 1.3% have chronic HCV (National Institutes of Health, 2002; Weinbaum, Lyerla, & Margolis, 2003). Hepatitis is discussed further in Chapter 62.

Prevention of sexually transmitted diseases (STDs) should include educating clients about the risks of contracting hepatitis A, B, and C. Currently, vaccines against HAV and HBV are available. Use of these vaccines have the potential to limit the spread of these diseases by sexual transmission. The CDC recommends that anyone who is treated for STDs, men who have sex with men, and injection drug users should be offered hepatitis vaccination (CDC, 2002a).

GET READY for the NCLEX Examination!

KEY POINTS

Safe Effective Care Environment

- Use standard precautions for all clients regardless of age, gender, race or ethnicity, sexual orientation, education level, and profession.
- Ask all women about intimate partner abuse at any health visit.
- Use gloves when examining the genitalia of any client.

Health Promotion and Maintenance

- Encourage all clients who are sexually active to use condoms and other precautions during sexual intimacy.
- Urge sexually active women to go for routine health maintenance visits and screenings.

Psychosocial Integrity

- Treat all clients, regardless of diagnosis, with dignity.
- Do not assume that any visitor or family member knows the client's diagnosis.
- Pace your interview to match the learning needs and style of the individual client.
- Provide as much privacy as possible for clients undergoing examination or testing for STDs.
- Use language and terminology that the client can understand and that the client is comfortable with during discussions of the reproductive system.
- Allow the client the opportunity to express fear or anxiety regarding a change in health status.
- Refer clients newly diagnosed with an STD to local resources and support groups.
- Encourage all clients who have an STD to inform their sexual partner(s) of their health status.

Physiological Integrity

- Encourage clients to adhere to their anti-infective drug regimen.
- Teach clients the expected side effects and possible adverse reactions to prescribed drugs.
- Urge clients to refrain from sexual activity while being treated for an STD.
- Teach female clients who have PID the clinical manifestations of ectopic pregnancy.

ADDITIONAL STUDY RESOURCES

Go to your Student CD-ROM for Review Questions for the NCLEX Examination.

evolve Go to http://evolve.elsevier.com/Iggy/ for Integrated Management of Care Questions for the NCLEX Examination.

SELECTED BIBLIOGRAPHY

Asterisk indicates a classic or definitive work on this subject.

Akande, V. (2002). Tubal pelvic damage: Prediction and prognosis. *Human Fertility, 5*(Suppl.), S15-S20.

Apoola, A., & Radcliffe, K. (2004). Antiviral treatment of genital herpes. *International Journal of SDT & AIDS, 15*(7), 429-433.

Bachmann, L.H., et al. (2000). Risk and prevalence of treatable sexually transmitted diseases at a Birmingham substance abuse treatment facility. *American Journal of Public Health, 90*(10), 1615-1618.

Ballard, R., & Morse, S. (2003). Chancroid. In S.A. Morse, et al. (Eds.). *Atlas of sexually transmitted diseases and AIDS* (3rd ed.). Edinburgh: Mosby.

Bartlett, J. (2002). *2002 Pocket book of infectious disease therapy.* Philadelphia: Lippincott Williams & Wilkins.

Blake, D., et al. (2003). Improving participation in chlamydia screening programs. *Archives of Adolescent Medicine, 157*, 523-529.

Bowden, F. (2003). Donovanosis. In S.A. Morse, et al. (Eds.). *Atlas of sexually transmitted diseases and AIDS* (3rd ed.). Edinburgh: Mosby.

Carey, J., et al. (2000). Metronidazole to prevent preterm delivery in pregnant women with asymptomatic bacterial vaginosis. *New England Journal of Medicine, 342*, 534-540.

Carpenito-Loyet, L. (2004). *Nursing diagnoses: Application to clinical practice* (10th ed.). Philadelphia: Lippincott Williams & Wilkins.

Centers for Disease Control and Prevention. (2001). Tracking the hidden epidemics: Trends in STDs in the United States 2000. Available at www.cdc.gov/nchstp/dstd/Stats_Trends/Trends2000.pdf.

Centers for Disease Control and Prevention. (2002a). Sexually transmitted diseases treatment guidelines 2002. *Morbidity and Mortality Weekly Report, 51*(RR-6), 1-80.

Centers for Disease Control and Prevention. (2002b). Increases in fluoroquinolone-resistant *Neisseria gonorrhoeae*–Hawaii and California, 2001. *Morbidity and Mortality Weekly Report, 51*, 1041-1044.

Centers for Disease Control and Prevention. (2002c). Notice to readers: Discontinuation of cefixime tablets–United States. *Morbidity and Mortality Weekly Report, 51*(46), 1052.

Centers for Disease Control and Prevention. (2004). Sexually transmitted disease surveillance, 2003. Atlanta, GA: U.S. Department of Health and Human Services, November 2004. Available at http://www.cdc.gov/std/stats/toc2003.htm.

Champion, J., et al. (2004). Abused women and the risk for pelvic inflammatory disease. *Western Journal of Nursing Research, 26*(2), 176-191.

Cothran, M., & White, J. (2002). Adolescent behavior and sexually transmitted diseases: The dilemma of human papillomavirus. *Health Care for Women International, 23*, 306-319.

Davidson, M. (2004). Sexually transmitted infections: Screening and counseling. *Clinician Reviews, 14*(6), 55-62.

Dochterman, J., & Bulechek, G. (Eds.). (2004). *Nursing interventions classification (NIC)* (4th ed.). St. Louis: Mosby.

Dulin, J., & Akers, M.C. (2003). Pelvic inflammatory disease and sepsis. *Critical Care Nursing Clinics of North America, 15*(1), 63-70.

Ebersole, P., Hess, P., & Luggen, A. (2004). *Toward healthy aging: Human needs and nursing response* (6th ed.). St. Louis: Mosby

Facts and Comparisons. (2004). *Drug facts and comparisons* (58th ed.). St. Louis: Author.

Feroli, K., & Burstein, G. (2003). Adolescent sexually transmitted diseases. *Maternal Child Nursing, 28*(2), 113-118.

Gaitan, H., et al. (2002). Accuracy of five different diagnostic techniques in mild-to-moderate pelvic inflammatory disease. *Infectious Diseases in Obstetrics and Gynecology, 10*, 171-180.

*Hauth, J., et al. (1995). Reduced incidence of preterm delivery with metronidazole and erythromycin in women with bacterial vaginosis. *New England Journal of Medicine, 333*, 1732-1736.

Hay, P., Ugwumadu, A., & Manvonda, J. (2001). Oral clindamycin prevents spontaneous preterm birth and mid trimester miscarriage in pregnant women with bacterial vaginosis. *International Journal of Sexually Transmitted Diseases and AIDS, 12*(Suppl 2), 70-71.

*Hiller, S., et al. (1995). Association between bacterial vaginosis and preterm delivery of a low birth-weight infant. *New England Journal of Medicine, 333*(26), 1737-1742.

Honey, E., et al. (2002). Cost effectiveness of screening for *Chlamydia trachomatis*: A review of published studies. *Sexually Transmitted Infections, 78*, 406-412.

Joyner, J.L., et al. (2000). Comparative prevalence of infection with *Trichomonas vaginalis* among men attending a sexually transmitted disease clinic. *Sexually Transmitted Diseases, 27*(4), 236-240.

Lewis, J. (2003). Selection and evaluation of diagnostic tests. In S.A. Morse, et al. (Eds.). *Atlas of sexually transmitted diseases and AIDS* (3rd ed.). Edinburgh: Mosby.

Mabey, D., & Peeling, R. (2002). Lymphogranuloma venereum. *Sexually Transmitted Infections, 78*, 90-92.

Maw, R. (2004) Critical appraisal of commonly used treatment for genital warts. *International Journal of STD & AIDS, 15*(6), 357-364.

McQuillan, G. (2000). Implications of a national survey for STDs: Results from NHANES Survey. Presentation at 2000 Infectious Disease Society of America Conference. September 7-10, 2000, New Orleans.

Mehta, S., et al. (2003). Generalizability of STD screening in urban emergency departments: Comparison of results from inner city and urban sites in Baltimore, Maryland. *Sexually Transmitted Diseases, 30*(2), 143-148.

Moens, V., Baruch, G., & Fearon, P. (2003). Opportunistic screening for chlamydia at a community-based contraceptive service for young people. *British Medical Journal, 326*, 1252-1255.

Morse, S.A., et al. (2003). *Atlas of sexually transmitted diseases and AIDS* (3rd ed.). Edinburgh: Mosby.

National Institutes of Health (2002). Management of hepatitis C: 2002, Consensus Development Conference Statement, June 10-12, 2002. Available at http://consensus.nih.gov/cons/116/hepatitis_c_consensus.pdf.

Nsuami, M., et al. (2003). Screening for sexually transmitted diseases during sports examination of high school adolescents. *Journal of Adolescent Health, 32*, 336-339.

Pagana, K., & Pagana, T. (2002). *Mosby's manual of diagnostic and laboratory tests* (2nd ed.). St. Louis: Mosby.

Rein, D., et al. (2000). Direct medical cost of pelvic inflammatory disease and its sequelae: Decreasing but still substantial. *Obstetrics and Gynecology, 95*(3), 397-402.

Rein, M. (2001). Sexually transmitted disease. In G. Mandell. *Essential atlas of infectious diseases* (2nd ed., pp. 153-174). Philadelphia: Current Medicine.

Robinson, K. (2002). Sexually transmitted diseases. In K. McCance & S. Huether (Eds.), *Pathophysiology: The biologic basis for disease in adults and children* (4th ed., pp. 781-811). St. Louis: Mosby.

Roddy, R., et al. (2002). Effect of nonoxynol-9 gel on urogenital gonorrhea and chlamydia infections. *Journal of the American Medical Association, 287*(9), 1117-1122.

Schacter, J., & Stephens, R. (2003). Infections caused by *Chlamydia trachomatis*. In S.A. Morse, et al. (Eds.). *Atlas of sexually transmitted diseases and AIDS* (3rd ed.). Edinburgh: Mosby.

Scharbo-Dehaan, M., & Anderson, D. (2003). The CDC 2002 guidelines for the treatment of sexually transmitted diseases: Implications for women's health care. *Journal of Midwifery and Women's Health, 48*(2), 96-104.

Schillinger, J., et al. (2003). Patient-delivered partner treatment with azithromycin to prevent repeated *Chlamydia trachomatis* infection among women: A randomized, controlled trial. *Sexually Transmitted Diseases, 30*(1), 49-56.

Sellors, J.W., et al. (2000). A new visual indicator of chlamydial cervicitis? *Sexually Transmitted Infections, 76*(1), 46-48.

Skidmore-Roth, L. (2003). *Mosby's nursing drug reference.* St. Louis: Mosby.

Tao, G., et al. (2000). Medical care expenditures for genital herpes in the United States. *Sexually Transmitted Diseases, 27*(1), 32-38.

Turner, C., et al. (2002). Untreated gonococcal and chlamydial infections in a probability sample of adults. *Journal of the American Medical Association, 287*(6), 726-733.

Weinbaum, C., Lyerla, R., & Margolis, H. (2003). Prevention and control of infections with hepatitis viruses in correctional settings. *Morbidity and Mortality Weekly Report, 52*(RR-1), 1-33.

Williams, A. (2003). Gynecologic care for women with HIV infections. *Journal of Obstetric, Gynecologic, and Neonatal Nursing, 32*, 87-93.

Workman, M.L. (2003). The cellular basis of bacterial infection. *Critical Care Clinics of North America, 15*(1), 1-11.

APPENDIX

Abbreviations

AAA	abdominal aortic aneurysm
AACN	American Association of Critical Care Nurses
AAKP	American Association of Kidney Patients
ABC	airway, breathing, and circulation
ABG	arterial blood gas
ABI	ankle-brachial index
ABPM	ambulatory blood pressure monitoring
ABVD	Adriamycin, bleomycin, vinblastine, dacarbazine
AC	assist-control; alternating current
ACE	angiotensin-converting enzyme
ACh	acetylcholine
AChRAb	acetylcholine receptor antibody
ACL	anterior cruciate ligament
ACLS	advanced cardiac life support
ACS	acute compartment syndrome; American Cancer Society
ACTH	adrenocorticotropic hormone
AD	autosomal dominant
ADC	AIDS dementia complex
ADH	antidiuretic hormone
ADLs	activities of daily living
ADP	adenosine diphosphate
ADPKD	autosomal dominant polycystic kidney disease
AED	automatic external defibrillation
aFP	alpha-fetoprotein
AGC	absolute granulocyte count
AGN	acute glomerulonephritis
AGR	abdominal-gluteal ratio
AHA	American Heart Association
AHRQ	Agency for Healthcare Research and Quality
AIDS	acquired immunodeficiency syndrome
AIVR	accelerated idioventricular rhythm
AJCC	American Joint Committee on Cancer
AKA	above-knee amputation
AL	ascending limb
ALA	American Lung Association
ALG	antilymphocyte globulin
ALL	acute lymphocytic leukemia
ALP	alkaline phosphatase
ALS	amyotrophic lateral sclerosis
AMI	antibody-mediated immunity
AML	acute myelocytic leukemia
AMSN	Academy of Medical-Surgical Nurses
ANA	American Nurses' Association; antinuclear antibody
ANC	absolute neutrophil count
ANOVA	analysis of variance
ANP	atrial natriuretic peptide
ANS	autonomic nervous system
AORN	Association of periOperative Room Nurses
AP	anteroposterior
APSAC	anisoylated plasminogen streptokinase activator complex
APSGN	acute poststreptococcal glomerulonephritis
aPTT	activated partial thromboplastin time
AR	autosomal recessive
ara-A	adenine arabinoside
ARDS	acute respiratory distress syndrome
ARF	acute renal failure
ASA	acetylsalicylic acid
ASPEN	American Society of Parenteral and Enteral Nutrition
AST	aspartate aminotransferase
ATG	antithymocyte globulin
ATN	acute tubular necrosis
ATP	adenosine triphosphate
ATPase	adenosine triphosphatase
AV	atrioventricular, arteriovenous
AVM	arteriovenous malformation
AVN	avascular necrosis
AZA	azathioprine
BBIAT	Baird Body Image Assessment Tool
BC	Bowman's capsule
BCG	bacille Calmette-Guérin
BCNU	carmustine
BCS	Body Cathexis Scale
BE	barium enema
BGMS	blood glucose monitoring strip
BKA	below-knee amputation
BMI	body mass index
BMT	bone marrow transplantation
BP	blood pressure
BPEG	British Pacing and Electrophysiology Group
BPH	benign prostatic hyperplasia (hypertrophy)
BRM	biologic response modifier
BSE	breast self-examination
BSI	body substance isolation
BSO	bilateral salpingo-oophorectomy
BUN	blood urea nitrogen
c	cup(s)
C&S	culture and sensitivity
CABG	coronary artery bypass graft
CAD	computer-assisted design; coronary artery disease
CAH	chronic active hepatitis
CAL	chronic airflow limitation
CALLA	common acute lymphoblastic leukemia antigen
CAM	complementary and alternative medicine
cAMP	cyclic adenosine monophosphate
CAPD	continuous ambulatory peritoneal dialysis
CAVH	continuous arteriovenous hemofiltration
CAVHD	continuous arteriovenous hemofiltration and dialysis

CBC complete blood count
CBD common bile duct
CBE charting by exception
CBI continuous bladder irrigation
CCA circumflex coronary artery
CCP critical closing pressure
CCPD continuous-cycle peritoneal dialysis
CD Cotrel-Dubousset; collecting duct
CD4 cluster of differentiation 4
CDC Centers for Disease Control and Prevention; chenodeoxycholic acid
CEA carcinoembryonic antigen
CFU colony-forming unit
CGN chronic glomerulonephritis
CHF congestive heart failure
CIC Certified in Infection Control
CIN cervical intraepithelial neoplasia
CIS carcinoma in situ
CK creatine kinase
CLE centrilobular emphysema
CLL chronic lymphocytic leukemia
cm centimeter(s)
CMG cystometrogram
CMI cell-mediated immunity
CML chronic myelocytic leukemia
CMS circulation, movement, sensation
CMV cisplatin, methotrexate, vinblastine; cytomegalovirus
CNS central nervous system
CO cardiac output
COHb carboxyhemoglobin
COLD chronic obstructive lung disease
COPD chronic obstructive pulmonary disease
COPES Family Crisis-Oriented Personal Evaluation Scale
CPAP continuous positive airway pressure
CPB cardiopulmonary bypass
CPK creatine phosphokinase
CPM continuous passive motion
CPN chronic pyelonephritis
CPO certified prosthetist-orthotist
CPP cerebral perfusion pressure
CPR cardiopulmonary resuscitation
cps cycles per second
CQI continuous quality improvement
CREST calcinosis, Raynaud's phenomenon, esophageal dysfunction, sclerodactyly, telangiectasia
CRF chronic renal failure
CRH corticotropin-releasing hormone
CRI chronic renal insufficiency
CRNA certified registered nurse anesthetist
CS crush syndrome
CSA cyclosporine A
CSF cerebrospinal fluid
CST certified surgical technologist
CT computed tomography
CTD connective tissue disease
CTS carpal tunnel syndrome
CVA cerebrovascular accident (stroke); costovertebral angle
CVC central venous catheter
CVP central venous pressure
D&C dilation and curettage
DARE Drug Awareness Resistance Education
dB decibel(s)
DCCT Diabetes Control and Complications Trial
DCM dilated cardiomyopathy
DCT distal convoluted tubule
DDAVP desmopressin acetate
ddI dideoxyinosine (didanosine)
DDS dapsone
DES diethylstilbestrol
DHE dihydroergotamine
DHHS U.S. Department of Health and Human Services
DHT dihydrotestosterone
DI diabetes insipidus
DIC disseminated intravascular coagulation
DIP distal interphalangeal joint
DJD degenerative joint disease
dL deciliter(s)
DL descending limb
DLCO diffusion capacity for carbon monoxide
DLE discoid lupus erythematosus
DNA deoxyribonucleic acid
DNP dinitrophenol
DNR do not resuscitate
DOE dyspnea on exertion
DP dopamine
DPOA durable power of attorney
DRE digital rectal examination
DRG diagnosis-related group
DS double-strength
DSA digital subtraction angiography
DTIC dacarbazine
DTR deep tendon reflex
DUB dysfunctional uterine bleeding
DVT deep vein thrombosis
EAT Eating Attitudes Test
EBL estimated blood loss
EBV Epstein-Barr virus
ECCC Emergency Cardiac Care Committee
ECCE extracapsular cataract extraction
ECF extracellular fluid
ECG electrocardiogram
EDI Eating Disorder Inventory
EGD esophagogastroduodenoscopy
EHDP etidronate disodium
EIA enzyme immunoassay
ELISA enzyme-linked immunosorbent assay
EMD electromechanical dissociation
EMG electromyography
EMS emergency medical services
EMT emergency medical technician
ENCORE encouragement, normalcy, counseling, opportunity, reaching out, revived energies
ENG electronystagmography
ENT ear, nose, and throat
EOM extraocular movement
EPO erythropoietin
EPS electrophysiologic study
ER estrogen receptor
ERCP endoscopic retrograde cholangiopancreatography

ERS	endoscopic retrograde sphincterotomy
ERT	estrogen replacement therapy
ESR	erythrocyte sedimentation rate
ESRD	end-stage renal disease
ET	enterostomal therapist; endotracheal tube
ETDR	early treatment diabetic retinopathy
ETT	exercise tolerance test
EVS	early vitrectomy study
FACT	fruits, animals, colors, and towns
FAM	fluorouracil, Adriamycin, and mitomycin C
FANA	fluorescent antinuclear antibody
FAST	fluoroallergosorbent test
FBD	fibrocystic breast disease
FBSS	failed back surgery syndrome
FDA	U.S. Food and Drug Administration
FEF	forced expiratory flow
FES	fat embolism syndrome
FEV	forced expiratory volume
FEV_1	forced expiratory volume in 1 second
FEV_1/FVC	ratio of expiratory volume in 1 second to forced vital capacity
FFP	fresh frozen plasma
FIM	Functional Independence Measure
$F\textsc{io}_2$	fraction of inspired oxygen
FNB	Food and Nutrition Board
FNCR	family nursing chart review
FOBT	fecal occult blood test
FR	flutter rate
Fr	French
FRC	functional residual capacity
FS	full-strength
FSBS	fingerstick blood sugar
FSH	follicle-stimulating hormone
Ft	foot (feet)
FTA-ABS	fluorescent treponemal antibody absorption test
5-FU	5-fluorouracil
FUDR	floxuridine
FVC	forced vital capacity
FWB	full weight-bearing
g	gram(s)
g/day	gram(s) per day
G6PD	glucose-6-phosphate dehydrogenase
GABA	gamma-aminobutyric acid
GAS	general adaptation syndrome
GB	gallbladder
GBS	Guillain-Barré syndrome
GCS	Glasgow Coma Scale
GCSF	granulocyte colony-stimulating factor
GDM	gestational diabetes mellitus
GE	gastroenteritis
GF	glomerular filtrate
GFR	glomerular filtration rate
GH	growth hormone
GH-IH	growth hormone–inhibiting hormone
GH-RH	growth hormone–releasing hormone
GI	gastrointestinal
GM-CSF	granulocyte-macrophage colony-stimulating factor
Gn-RH	gonadotropin-releasing hormone
GSW	gunshot wound
GVHD	graft-versus-host disease
Gy	gray(s)
h	hour(s)
HAT	hearing assessment test
Hb	hemoglobin
HBIG	hepatitis B immunoglobulin
HBO	hyperbaric oxygen
HBV	hepatitis B virus
hCG	human chorionic gonadotropin
HCM	hypertrophic cardiomyopathy
Hct	hematocrit
HCV	hepatitis C virus
HD	hemodialysis
HDL	high-density lipoprotein
HDV	hepatitis delta virus
HEPA	high-efficiency particulate air
HEV	hepatitis E virus
Hgb	hemoglobin
HIDA	hepatobiliary iminodiacetic acid analogue (radionuclide labeled with technetium-99m)
HIP	Help for Incontinent Persons
HITT	heparin-induced thrombocytopenia/thrombosis
HLA	human leukocyte antigen
HMO	health maintenance organization
HPA	hypothalamic-pituitary-adrenal
HPV	human papillomavirus
hr	hour
HR	heart rate
HSV	herpes simplex virus
5-HT	5-hydroxytryptamine (serotonin)
HTLV	human T-cell lymphotropic virus
Hz	hertz
I&D	incision and drainage
IABP	intra-aortic balloon pumping
IBS	irritable bowel syndrome
IBW	ideal body weight
ICD	implantable cardioverter-defibrillator
ICF	intracellular fluid
ICHD	Intersociety Commission for Heart Disease
ICP	intracranial pressure
ICS	intercostal space
ICU	intensive care unit
IEC	Institutional Ethics Committee
IF	interstitial fluid
Ig	immunoglobulin
IHSS	idiopathic hypertrophic subaortic stenosis
IL	interleukin
IL-2	interleukin-2
IL-3	interleukin-3
IL-4	interleukin-4
IL-5	interleukin-5
IL-8	interleukin-8
IM	intramedullary rod; intramuscular
IMF	intermaxillary fixation
IMV	intermittent mandatory ventilation
INF	interferon
INR	international normalized ratio
IOL	intraocular lens
IOP	intraocular pressure
IP	intraperitoneal
IPD	intermittent peritoneal dialysis
IPG	impedance plethysmography

IRT intracavitary radiation therapy
IS incentive spirometer
ITH idiosyncratic toxic hepatitis
ITP idiopathic thrombocytopenic purpura
IU international unit(s)
IU/L international unit(s) per liter
IUD intrauterine device
IV intravenous
IVC inferior vena cava
IVP intravenous pyelography
JCAHO Joint Commission on the Accreditation of Healthcare Organizations
JGC juxtaglomerular cell
JVD jugular venous distention
JVP jugular venous pressure
KCS keratoconjunctivitis sicca
kg kilogram(s)
kJ kilojoule(s)
KS Kaposi's sarcoma
KUB kidneys, ureters, and bladder
KW Keith-Wagner classification
LAC long arm cast
LAD left anterior descending
LAK lymphokine-activated killer (cell)
LAP leukocyte alkaline phosphatase
LAS localized adaptation syndrome
LATS long-acting thyroid stimulator
LBP low back pain
LCA left coronary artery
LDH lactate dehydrogenase
LDL low-density lipoprotein
LE lupus erythematosus; lower extremity
LES lower esophageal sphincter
LGV lymphogranuloma venereum
LH luteinizing hormone
LL left lateral
LLC long leg cast
LLQ left lower quadrant
LMN lower motor neuron
LOA leave of absence
LOC level of consciousness
LORS Level of Rehabilitation Scale
LP lumbar puncture; light perception
LPS lipopolysaccharide
LR lactated Ringer's (solution)
LRD living related donor
LTC long-term care
LUQ left upper quadrant
LVD left ventricular dysfunction
LVEDP left ventricular end-diastolic pressure
M-CSF monocyte-macrophage colony-stimulating factor
mA milliampere(s)
MAC *Mycobacterium avium* complex
MAO monoamine oxidase
MAP mean arterial pressure
MAST military antishock trousers
MAT multifocal atrial tachycardia
MB-CAPD multiple-bag continuous ambulatory peritoneal dialysis
MCA middle cerebral artery
mcg microgram(s)
MCH mean corpuscular hemoglobin
MCHC mean corpuscular hemoglobin concentration
MCL modified chest lead
MCP metacarpophalangeal
MCV mean corpuscular volume
MD muscular dystrophy
MDF myocardial depressant factor
MDI metered-dose inhaler
MEN multiple endocrine neoplasia
mEq milliequivalent(s)
mEq/L milliequivalent(s) per liter
MFH malignant fibrous histiocytoma
mg milligram(s)
MG myasthenia gravis
mg/dL milligram(s) per deciliter
MH malignant hyperthermia
MHAUS Malignant Hyperthermia Association of the United States
MHC major histocompatibility complex
MI myocardial infarction
MICU medical intensive care unit
MIH melanocyte-inhibiting hormone
min minute(s)
mL milliliter(s)
mL/kg milliliter(s) per kilogram
mm millimeter(s)
mm Hg millimeter(s) of mercury
mmol millimole(s)
mmol/L millimoles per liter
MMPI Minnesota Multiphasic Personality Inventory
MMSE Mini-Mental State Examination
MMV maximum mandatory ventilation
MODY maturity-onset diabetes of the young
MOPP mechlorethamine, Oncovin, procarbazine, prednisone
mOsm milliosmole(s)
mOsm/L milliosmole(s) per liter
MRB manual resuscitation bag
MRC Medical Research Council
MRI magnetic resonance imaging
MS multiple sclerosis; morphine sulfate
msec millisecond(s)
MSH melanocyte-stimulating hormone
MTP metatarsophalangeal
mU milliunit(s)
mU/mL milliunit(s) per milliliter
MUGA multigated angiography
mV millivolt(s)
MVA motor vehicle accident
MVAC methotrexate, vinblastine, Adriamycin, cisplatin
NANDA North American Nursing Diagnosis Association
NAON National Association of Orthopaedic Nurses
NAPHT National Association of Patients on Hemodialysis and Transplantation
NASPE North American Society for Pacing and Electrophysiology
NCI National Cancer Institute
NE norepinephrine
ng nanogram(s)
NG nasogastric

NHANES	National Health and Nutrition Examination Survey
NHIF	National Head Injury Foundation
NIC	Nursing Interventions Classification
NK	natural killer (cell)
NKF	National Kidney Foundation
NLN	National League for Nursing
NRC/NAS	National Research Council/National Academy of Sciences
NS	nephrotic syndrome; normal saline
NSAID	nonsteroidal anti-inflammatory drug
NSNA	National Student Nurse Association
NSR	normal sinus rhythm
NTP	noninvasive temporary pacing
NWB	non–weight-bearing
NYHA	New York Heart Association
OA	osteoarthritis
OBS	organic brain syndrome
OCG	oral cholecystogram
OFP	optimal functioning plan
OI	osteogenesis imperfecta
OR	operating room
ORIF	open reduction, internal fixation
ORT	oral rehydration therapy; operating room technician
OSHA	U.S. Occupational Safety and Health Administration
OT	occupational therapist
OTC	over-the-counter
oz	ounce(s)
PA	posteroanterior; physician's assistant
PAB	prealbumin
PAC	premature atrial complex
$Paco_2$	partial pressure of arterial carbon dioxide
PACU	postanesthesia care unit
Pao_2	partial pressure of arterial oxygen
Pap	Papanicolaou (test, smear)
PAP	pulmonary artery pressure
PASG	pneumatic antishock garment
PAT	paroxysmal atrial tachycardia
PAWP	pulmonary artery wedge pressure
PCA	patient-controlled analgesia; patient care assistant
PCAC	Patient Care Advisory Committee
PCM	protein-calorie malnutrition
PCN	penicillin
PCP	*Pneumocystis carinii* pneumonia
PCR	polymerase chain reaction
PCT	proximal convoluted tubule
PD	peritoneal dialysis
PE	pulmonary embolism; pharyngoesophageal
PEA	pulseless electrical activity
PEEP	positive end-expiratory pressure
PERRLA	pupils equal, round, and reactive to light and accommodation
PES	problem, etiology, symptoms
PES-EO-IO	problem, etiology, signs and symptoms; expected outcome, interventions, outcome
PET	positron emission tomography
PFT	pulmonary function test
PGE_2	prostaglandin E_2
PGI_2	prostaglandin I_2 (prostacyclin)
pH	the negative logarithm of the hydrogen ion concentration
PHP	plasma hydrostatic pressure
PHS	Public Health Service
PICC	peripherally inserted central catheter
PID	pelvic inflammatory disease
PIE	plan, interventions, evaluation
PIH	prolactin-inhibiting hormone
PIP	proximal interphalangeal; peak inspiratory pressure
PJC	premature junctional complex
PJT	premature junctional tachycardia
PKD	polycystic kidney disease
PLE	panlobular emphysema
PLP	phantom limb pain
PMI	point of maximal impact
PMN	polymorphonuclear cell
PMR	progressive muscle relaxation; polymyalgia rheumatica
PMS	premenstrual syndrome
PMT	premenstrual tension
PND	paroxysmal nocturnal dyspnea
PNS	parasympathetic nervous system; peripheral nervous system
PO	*per os* (by mouth)
POAG	primary open-angle glaucoma
POC	point-of-care
POR	problem-oriented record
PPD	purified protein derivative
ppm	parts per million
PPM	pulses per minute
PPN	partial parenteral nutrition
PPS	post-polio sequelae (syndrome)
PRL	prolactin
PRN	*pro re nata* (as needed)
PSA	prostate-specific antigen
PSE	portal systemic encephalopathy
PSS	progressive systemic sclerosis
PSV	pressure support ventilation
PSVT	paroxysmal supraventricular tachycardia
PT	physical therapy; physical therapist; prothrombin time
PTA	percutaneous transluminal angioplasty; peritonsillar abscess
PTC	peritubular capillary
PTCA	percutaneous transluminal coronary angioplasty
PTFE	polytetrafluoroethylene
PTH	parathyroid hormone (parathormone)
PTT	partial thromboplastin time
PUD	peptic ulcer disease
PULSES	physical condition, upper limb function, lower limb function, sensory components, excretory function, support factors
PUVA	psoralen and ultraviolet A
PV	polycythemia vera
PVC	premature ventricular contraction
PVD	peripheral vascular disease
PVR	postvoiding residual
PVS	persistent vegetative state
PWB	partial weight-bearing
q	*quaque* (every)

QOL	quality of life
QOLY	quality of life year(s)
RA	rheumatoid arthritis
rad	radiation absorbed dose
RAI	radioactive iodine
RAIU	radioactive iodine uptake
RAS	reticular activating system
RBC	red blood cell
RCA	right coronary artery
RDA	recommended daily allowance; recommended dietary allowance
REM	rapid eye movement
RFUT	radiofibrinogen uptake test
RIA	radioimmunoassay
RIND	reversible ischemic neurologic deficit
RL	right lateral
RLQ	right lower quadrant
RNA	ribonucleic acid
RNI	recommended nutrient intake
ROM	range of motion
RPGN	rapidly progressive glomerulonephritis
RSD	reflex sympathetic dystrophy
RTA	renal tubular acidosis
RUQ	right upper quadrant
RV	residual volume
SA	sinoatrial
SAC	short arm cast
SAECG	signal-averaged electrocardiography
SAM	smoking-attributable mortality
SaO_2	saturation of arterial oxygen
SBE	subacute bacterial endocarditis
SBFT	small bowel follow-through
SCD	sequential compression device
SCI	spinal cord injury
SCID	severe combined immunodeficiency
SCS	Self-Cathexis Scale
SDA	same-day admission
SDAT	senile dementia Alzheimer's type
SDS	same-day surgery
SEAPort	side-entry access port
sec	second(s)
SEP	somatosensory evoked potential
SF6	sulfahexafluoride
SFA	superficial femoral artery
SGOT	serum glutamic-oxaloacetic transaminase
SI	Système International d'Unites
SIADH	syndrome of inappropriate antidiuretic hormone
SIMV	synchronized intermittent mandatory ventilation
SLC	short leg cast
SLE	systemic lupus erythematosus
SLP	speech-language pathologist
SLR	straight-leg raise; sex-linked recessive
SMI	sustained minimal inspiration; self-management inventory
SMR	submucous resection
SMX	sulfamethoxazole
SNF	skilled nursing facility
SNS	sympathetic nervous system
SOAP	subjective data, objective data, analysis, plan
SOAPIER	subjective data, objective data, analysis, plan, interventions, evaluation, revision of plan
SP	suprapubic
SPD	supply processing and distribution
SPECT	single photon emission computed tomography
SPEP	serum protein electrophoresis
SPF	suntan photoprotection factor
SSKI	saturated solution of potassium iodide
STA	superficial temporal artery
STD	sexually transmitted disease
STS	serologic test for syphilis
STSG	split-thickness skin graft
SV	stroke volume
SVC	superior vena cava
T&A	tonsillectomy and adenoidectomy
t-PA	tissue plasminogen activator
T_3	triiodothyronine
T_3RU	triiodothyronine resin uptake
T_4	thyroxine
TAF	tumor angiogenesis factor
TAH	total abdominal hysterectomy
TB	tuberculosis
TBI	total body irradiation
TBSA	total body surface area
tbsp	tablespoon(s)
TCDB	turn, cough, and deep breathe
TCT	thyrocalcitonin
TDT	terminal deoxynucleotidyl transferase
TED	thromboembolic device
TEE	transesophageal echocardiography
TEF	tracheoesophageal fistula
TEN	toxic epidermal necrolysis
TENS	transcutaneous electrical nerve stimulation
THA	tetrahydroaminoacridine
THP	tissue hydrostatic pressure
THR	total hip replacement
TIA	transient ischemic attack
TIBC	total iron-binding capacity
TJR	total joint replacement
TKR	total knee replacement
TLC	total lung capacity; total lymphocyte count
TLS	tumor lysis syndrome
TLSO	thoracic lumbar sacral orthosis (thoracolumbosacral orthosis)
TMJ	temporomandibular joint
TMP	trimethoprim
TNF	tumor necrosis factor
TNM	tumor, node, metastasis
TOP	tissue osmotic pressure
TOPS	Take Off Pounds Sensibly
TPI	treponemal immobilization (test)
TPN	total parenteral nutrition
TQM	total quality management
TRH	thyrotropin-releasing hormone
TSE	testicular self-examination
TSH	thyroid-stimulating hormone
TSI	thyroid-stimulating immunoglobulin
TSM	transparent semipermeable membrane
tsp	teaspoon(s)
TSS	toxic shock syndrome
TTD	transtelephonic defibrillation/monitoring
TTO	transtracheal oxygen

TTP	thrombotic thrombocytopenic purpura
TURBT	transurethral resection of bladder tumor
TURP	transurethral resection of the prostate
TVH	total vaginal hysterectomy
UGI	upper gastrointestinal
UMN	upper motor neuron
UPJ	ureteropelvic junction
UPP	urethral pressure profilometry
US	ultrasonography
USDA	United States Department of Agriculture
UTI	urinary tract infection
UV	ultraviolet
UVA	ultraviolet A
UVB	ultraviolet B
UVJ	ureterovesical junction
$\dot{V}/\dot{Q}$	ventilation-perfusion
VAD	venous access device
VADS	Visual Analog Dyspnea Scale
VAS	visual analog scale
VC	vital capacity
VCUG	voiding cystourethrogram
VDRL	Venereal Disease Research Laboratory (test)
VEP	visual evoked potential
VF	ventricular fibrillation
VLS	vascular leak syndrome
VMA	vanillylmandelic acid
VO_2	oxygen consumption
VOD	veno-occlusive disease
VPB	ventricular premature beat
VR	vasa recta
VSE	vulvar self-examination
VT	ventricular tachycardia
V_T	tidal volume
VZV	varicella-zoster virus
WAIS	Wechsler Adult Intelligence Scale
WBC	white blood cell
WHO	World Health Organization
WHR	waist-to-hip ratio

Index

b indicates boxed material, *c* indicates charts, *f* indicates illustrations, and *t* indicates tables.

E

G

H

I

O

Q

T

U

Communication Quick Reference for Spanish-Speaking Clients–cont'd

OBTAINING BLOOD FROM A FINGER STICK

I need to take a few drops of blood from your finger.	Necesito sacarle unas gotas de sangre de uno de sus dedos.	*Neh-seh-SEE-toh sah-KAHR-leh OO-nahs GOH-tahs deh SAHN-greh deh OO-noh deh soos DEH-dohs.*

OBTAINING A URINE SAMPLE

We also need a urine sample.	También necesitamos una muestra de la orina.	*Tahm-BYEHN neh-seh-see-TAH-mohs OO-nah MWEHS-trah deh lah oh-REE-nah.*
It has to be from the middle of the stream.	Tiene que ser de la mitad del chorro.	*TYEH-neh keh sehr deh lah mee-TAHD dehl CHOH-rroh.*
Put the urine in this cup.	Ponga la orina en este vaso.	*POHN-gah lah oh-REE-nah ehn EHS-teh VAH-soh.*

OBTAINING A STOOL SPECIMEN

I need a sample of your stool.	Necesito una muestra de su excremento.	*Neh-seh-SEE-toh OO-nah MWEHS-trah deh soo ehks-kreh-MEN-toh.*
Please put a small amount in this cup.	Por favor ponga un poco en este vaso.	*Pohr fa-VOHR POHN-gah oon POH-koh ehn EHS-teh VAH-soh.*

OBTAINING A SPUTUM SPECIMEN

I need a sample of your sputum.	Necesito una muestra de su esputo.	*Neh-seh-SEE-toh OO-nah MWEHS-trah deh soo ehs-POO-toh.*
Please spit in this cup.	Por favor, escupa en este vaso.	*Pohr fah-VOHR, ehs-KOO-pah ehn EHS-teh VAH-soh.*

ORDERS

You need . . .	Necesita . . .	*Neh-seh-see-TAH . . .*
a bandage.	un vendaje.	*oon behn-DAH-heh.*
a blood transfusion.	una transfusión de sangre.	*OO-nah trahns-foo-SEE-ohn deh SAHN-greh.*
a cast.	una armadura de yeso.	*OO-nah ahr-mah-DOO-rah deh YEH-soh.*
gauze.	la gasa.	*lah GAH-sah.*
intensive care.	el cuidado intensivo.	*ehl kwee-DAH-doh een-tehn-SEE-boh.*
intravenous fluids.	los líquidos intravenosos.	*lohs LEE-kee-dohs een-trah-beh-NOH-sohs.*
an operation.	una operación.	*OO-nah oh-peh-rah-see-OHN.*
physical therapy.	la terapia física.	*lah teh-RAH-pee-ah FEE-see-kah.*
a shot.	una inyección.	*OO-nah een-yehk-see-OHN.*
x-rays.	los rayos equis.	*lohs RAH-yohs EH-kees.*
We're going to . . .	Vamos a . . .	*VAH-mohs ah . . .*
change the bandage.	cambiarle el vendaje.	*kahm-bee-AHR-leh ehl behn-DAH-heh.*
give you a bath.	darle un baño.	*DAHR-leh oon BAH-nyoh.*
take out the I.V.	sacarle el tubo intravenoso.	*sah-KAHR-leh ehl TOO-boh een-trah-beh-NOH-soh.*

DESCRIPTION OF TUBES

The tube in your . . .	El tubo en su . . .	*Ehl TOO-boh ehn soo . . .*
arm is for I.V. fluids.	brazo está para los líquidos intravenosos.	*BRAH-soh ehs-TAH PAH-rah LEE-kee-dohs een-trah-beh-NOH-sohs.*
bladder is for urinating.	vejiga es para orinar.	*beh-HEE-gah ehs PAH-rah oh-ree-NAHR.*
stomach is for the food.	estómago es para la comida.	*ehs-TOH-mah-goh ehs PAH-rah lah koh-MEE-dah.*
throat is for breathing.	garganta es para respirar.	*gahr-GAHN-tah ehs PAH-rah rehs-pee-RAHR.*

Communication Quick Reference for Spanish-Speaking Clients

THE BODY • EL CUERPO (ehl KWEHR-poh)

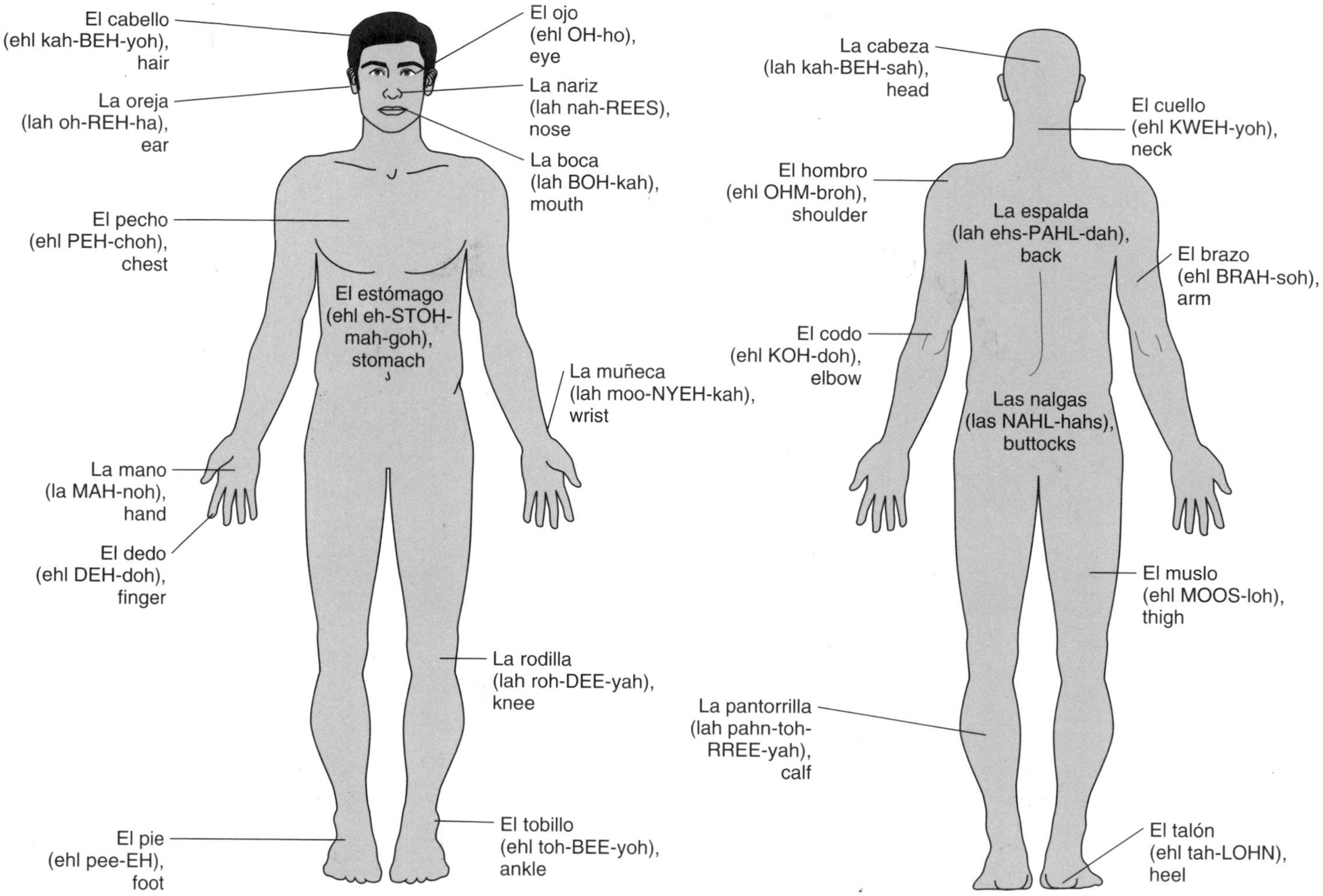

COMMON INSTRUCTIONS TO BE USED WITH THE BODY PARTS

Move the, Mueva *(mooh-EH-bah)*
Touch the, Toque *(TOH-keh)*
Point to the, Señale *(seh-NYAH-leh)*

MORE PARTS OF THE BODY

Armpit, la axila *(lah ahk-SEE-lah)*
Breasts, los senos *(lohs SEH-nohs)*
Collarbone, la clavícula *(lah klah-BEE-koo-lah)*
Diaphragm, el diafragma *(ehl dee-ah-FRAH-mah)*
Forearm, el antebrazo *(ehl ahn-teh-BRAH-soh)*
Groin, la ingle *(lah EEN-gleh)*
Hip, la cadera *(lah kah-DEH-rah)*
Kneecap, la rótula *(lah ROH-too-lah)*
Nail, la uña *(lah OON-yah)*
Pelvis, la pelvis *(lah PEHL-beece)*
Rectum, el recto *(ehl REHK-toh)*
Rib, la costilla *(lah koh-STEE-yah)*
Spine, el espinazo *(ehl ehs-pee-NAH-soh)*
Throat, la garganta *(lah gahr-GAHN-tah)*
Tongue, le lengua *(lah LEHN-gwah)*

ORGANS

Appendix, el apéndice *(ehl ah-PEHN-dee-seh)*
Bladder, la vejiga *(lah beh-HEE-gah)*
Brain, el cerebro *(ehl seh-REH-broh)*
Colon, el colon *(ehl KOH-lohn)*
Esophagus, el esófago *(ehl eh-SOH-fah-goh)*
Gallbladder, la vesícula biliar *(lah beh-SEE-koo-lah bee-lee-AHR)*
Genitals, los genitales *(lohs heh-nee-TAH-lehs)*
Heart, el corazón *(ehl koh-rah-SOHN)*
Kidney, el riñón *(ehl ree-NYOHN)*
Large intestine, el intestino grueso *(ehl een-tehs-TEE-noh groo-EH-so)*
Liver, el hígado *(ehl EE-gah-doh)*
Lungs, los pulmones *(lohs pool-MOH-nehs)*
Pancreas, el páncreas *(ehl PAHN-kreh-ahs)*
Small intestine, el intestino delgado *(ehl een-tehs-TEE-noh dehl-GAH-doh)*
Spleen, el bazo *(ehl BAH-soh)*
Thyroid gland, la tiroides *(lah tee-ROH-ee-dehs)*
Tonsils, las amígdalas *(lahs ah-MEEG-dah-lahs)*
Uterus, el útero *(ehl OO-teh-roh)*